evolve

ELSEVIER

YOU'VE JUST PURCHASED MORE THAN A TEXTBOOK!

Evolve Student Resources for *Maternal Child Nursing Care in Canada, Second Edition,* include the following:

- Answer Key – Textbook Critical Thinking Case Studies
- Audio Glossary
- Case Studies
- Key Points
- Nursing Care Plans
- Nursing Processes
- Nursing Skills
- Review Questions for Exam Preparation

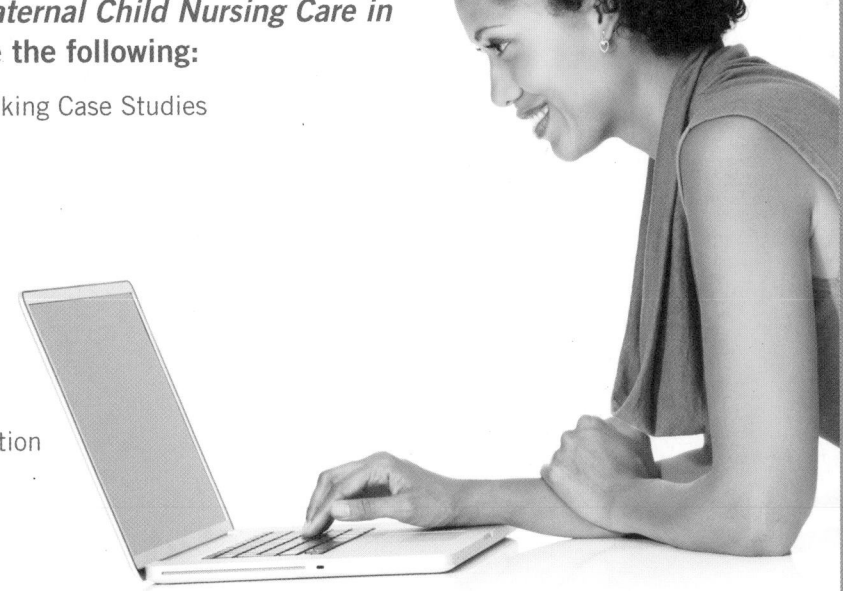

Activate the complete learning experience that comes with each textbook purchase by registering at

http://evolve.elsevier.com/Canada/Perry/maternal

REGISTER TODAY!

Maternal Child Nursing Care in Canada

SECOND EDITION

Maternal Child Nursing Care in Canada

Shannon E. Perry, RN, PhD, FAAN
Professor Emerita, School of Nursing
San Francisco State University
San Francisco, California

Marilyn J. Hockenberry, PhD, RN-CS, PNP, FAAN
Bessie Baker Distinguished Professor of Nursing
Professor of Pediatrics
Chair, Duke Institutional Review Board
Duke University
Durham, North Carolina

Deitra Leonard Lowdermilk, RNC, PhD, FAAN
Clinical Professor Emerita, School of Nursing
University of North Carolina at Chapel Hill
Chapel Hill, North Carolina

David Wilson, MS, RN,C (NIC)
Staff, PALS Coordinator
Children's Hospital at Saint Francis
Tulsa, Oklahoma

Lisa Keenan-Lindsay, RN, MN, LCCE, PNC(C)
Professor, School of Health Sciences
Seneca College of Applied Arts and Technology
Toronto, Ontario

Cheryl A. Sams, RN, BScN, MSN
Professor Emerita, School of Health Sciences
Seneca College of Applied Arts and Technology
Toronto, Ontario

ELSEVIER

ELSEVIER

Notices

Knowledge and best practice in this field are constantly changing. As new research and experience broaden our understanding, changes in research methods, professional practices, or medical treatment may become necessary.

Practitioners and researchers must always rely on their own experience and knowledge in evaluating and using any information, methods, compounds, or experiments described herein. In using such information or methods, they should be mindful of their own safety and the safety of others, including parties for whom they have a professional responsibility.

With respect to any drug or pharmaceutical products identified, readers are advised to check the most current information provided (i) on procedures featured or (ii) by the manufacturer of each product to be administered, to verify the recommended dose or formula, the method and duration of administration, and contraindications. It is the responsibility of practitioners, relying on their own experience and knowledge of their patients, to make diagnoses, to determine dosages and the best treatment for each individual patient, and to take all appropriate safety precautions.

To the fullest extent of the law, neither the Publisher nor the authors, contributors, or editors, assume any liability for any injury and/or damage to persons or property as a matter of products liability, negligence or otherwise, or from any use or operation of any methods, products, instructions, or ideas contained in the material herein.

The Publisher

Library and Archives Canada Cataloguing in Publication

Perry, Shannon E., author
Maternal child nursing care in Canada / Shannon E. Perry, Marilyn J. Hockenberry, Deitra Leonard Lowdermilk, David Wilson, Lisa Keenan-Lindsay, Cheryl Sams. – Second edition.

ISBN 978-1-77172-036-6 (hardback)

1. Maternity nursing–Textbooks. 2. Pediatric nursing–Textbooks. I. Title.

RG951.P477 2016 618.92′00231 C2016-902229-3

Vice President, Publishing: Ann Millar
Content Strategist (Acquisitions): Roberta A. Spinosa-Millman
Content Development Specialist: Sandy Matos
Publishing Services Manager: Jeffrey Patterson
Book Production Specialist: Carol O'Connell
Copy Editor: Jerrolyn Hurlbutt
Proofreader: Wendy Thomas
Cover Image: Mother and Child, artist Kellie Marian Hill
Book Designer: Ashley Miner
Typesetting and Assembly: Toppan Best-set Premedia Limited

Elsevier Canada
555 Richmond Street West, Suite 1100, Toronto, ON, Canada M5V 3B1
Phone: 1-866-896-3331
Fax: 1-855-215-5738

1 2 3 4 5 20 19 18 17 16

Ebook ISBN: 978-1-77172-067-0

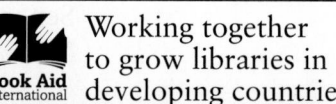

CONTENTS

PART 2

Perinatal Nursing

UNIT 2 INTRODUCTION TO PERINATAL NURSING

UNIT 3 WOMEN'S HEALTH

UNIT 5 CHILDBIRTH

UNIT 6 POSTPARTUM PERIOD

UNIT 7 NEWBORN

PART 3

Pediatric Nursing

UNIT 8 CHILDREN, THEIR FAMILIES, AND THE NURSE

UNIT 10 HEALTH PROMOTION AND SPECIAL HEALTH PROBLEMS

UNIT 11 SPECIAL NEEDS, ILLNESS, AND HOSPITALIZATION

UNIT 12 HEALTH PROBLEMS OF CHILDREN

APPENDICES

ABOUT THE AUTHORS

Shannon E. Perry is Professor Emerita, School of Nursing, San Francisco State University. She received her diploma in nursing from St. Joseph Hospital School of Nursing, Bloomington, Illinois; a Baccalaureate in Nursing from Marquette University; an MSN from the University of Colorado Medical Center; and a PhD in Educational Psychology with a specialty in Child Development from Arizona State University. She completed a 2-year postdoctoral fellowship in perinatal nursing at the University of California, San Francisco, as a Robert Wood Johnson Clinical Nurse Scholar.

Dr. Perry has had clinical experience as a staff nurse, head nurse, and supervisor in surgical nursing, obstetrics, pediatrics, gynecology, and neonatal nursing. She has served as expert witness and legal consultant. She has taught in schools of nursing in several states and was Interim Director and Director of the School of Nursing and Director of the Child and Adolescent Development Baccalaureate Program at San Francisco State University. She was Marquette University College of Nursing Alumna of the Year in 1999 and the University of Colorado School of Nursing Distinguished Alumna of the Year in 2000. She received the San Francisco State University Alumni Association Emeritus Faculty Award in 2005 and the Excellence in Education Award from the Beta Upsilon chapter of Sigma Theta Tau International in 2012.

She is a Fellow in the American Academy of Nursing and a member of the STTI Foundation Fellows Committee and the STTI International Services Task Force.

Dr. Perry's experience in international nursing includes teaching international nursing courses in the United Kingdom, Ireland, Italy, Thailand, Ghana, and China and participating in health missions in Ghana, Kenya, and Honduras. For her "exemplary contributions to nursing, public service, and selfless commitment and passion in shaping the future of international health," she received the President's Award from the Global Caring Nurses Foundation, Inc., in 2008. In January 2012, she and 47 other women climbed Mt. Kilimanjaro, the highest mountain in Africa, to raise awareness of human trafficking and to raise funds to support projects to combat human trafficking.

Marilyn J. Hockenberry is the Bessie Baker Distinguished Professor of Nursing and Professor of Pediatrics at Duke University. She serves as a Chair for the Duke Institutional Review Board and is Co-Chair of the Oncology Nursing Center of Excellence within the Duke Translational Nursing Institute. For over 18 years she served as the Director of the Pediatric Nurse Practitioner Program in the Texas Children's Cancer Center. Her research focuses on symptom management and treatment-related adverse effects experienced by children who have cancer. Dr. Hockenberry's current NIH-funded research studies are evaluating the treatment-related symptoms and neurocognitive deficits of leukemia treatment. She has authored over 80 articles and has served as the senior editor on the Wong nursing textbooks for many years.

Dr. Hockenberry completed her prenursing education at Mt. Vernon Nazarene College and received her Bachelors of Science from Capital University. She received her Masters of Science from Texas Woman's University and her Doctorate of Philosophy with distinction from the Medical College of Georgia. She is a Fellow of the American Academy of Nursing.

Deitra Leonard Lowdermilk is Clinical Professor Emerita, School of Nursing, University of North Carolina at Chapel Hill. She received her BSN from East Carolina University and her MEd and PhD in Education from the University of North Carolina at Chapel Hill. She is certified in In-Patient Obstetrics by the National Certification Corporation, and she is a Fellow in the American Academy of Nursing. In addition to being a nurse educator for over 34 years, Dr. Lowdermilk has clinical experience as a public health nurse and as a staff nurse in labour and birth, postpartum, and newborn units, and she has worked in gynecological surgery and cancer care units.

Dr. Lowdermilk has been recognized for her expertise in nursing education. She has repeatedly been selected as Classroom and Clinical Teacher of the Year by graduating seniors. She was a recipient of the Educator of the Year Award from both the District IV Association of Women's Health, Obstetric and Neonatal Nurses (AWHONN) and the North Carolina Nurses Association. She also received the 2005 AWHONN Excellence in Education Award.

She is active in AWHONN, having served as Chair of the North Carolina Section of AWHONN, and has served as chair and member of various committees in AWHONN at the national, district, state, and local levels. She has served as guest editor for the *Journal of Obstetric, Gynecologic, and Neonatal Nursing* and served on editorial boards for other publications.

Dr. Lowdermilk's most significant contribution to nursing has been to promote excellence in nursing practice and education in women's health through integration of knowledge into practice. In 2005 she received the first Distinguished Alumni Award from East Carolina University School of Nursing for her exemplary contributions to the nursing profession in the area of maternal-child care and the community. In 2011 she was inducted into the Hall of Fame for the College of Nursing at East Carolina University.

We remember **David Wilson**, who passed away March 7, 2015, after a long battle with cancer. A co-author of the Perry *Maternal Child Care* textbook, David was known as an expert clinical nurse and nurse educator. His last clinical position was at St. Francis Health Services in Tulsa, Oklahoma, where he worked in the Children's Day Hospital as the coordinator for Pediatric Advanced Life Support (PALS). He was known as an outstanding educator and supporter of nursing students; his attention to clinical excellence was evident in all his work. Those who contributed to the books and had the opportunity to work with David realize the important role he played as a leader in nursing education for students and faculty. David led by example in promoting and achieving excellence in clinical nursing practice.

Those who knew David well will miss his humour, loyalty to friends and colleagues, and never-ending support. He is missed greatly by those who worked closely with him on many Elsevier textbooks over the years. Most importantly, we miss his friendship; he was always there to support and to encourage. We have lost an amazing nurse who worked effortlessly over the years to improve the care of children and families in need. David will not be forgotten.

Lisa J. Keenan-Lindsay graduated from the University of Toronto for both her BScN and MN degrees. She worked in the area of pediatrics for the first several years of her career, mainly working in the pediatric intensive care unit at the Hospital for Sick Children. She has worked in the maternal-newborn area for over 25 years, holding a variety of positions, including staff nurse in labour and birth, and educator for a maternal-newborn department. Currently Lisa is a professor of nursing at Seneca College in the York University Collaborative BScN program. She has been involved in all aspects of nursing education, including curriculum development and incorporation of simulation into the curriculum.

Lisa has been an active board member of the Canadian Association of Perinatal and Women's Health Nurses (CAPWHN) since its inception and before that was a Section Leader for AWHONN-Canada. She was President of CAPWHN in 2014. Lisa has previously been involved with the Society of Obstetricians and Gynaecologists of Canada (SOGC) as an RN member for the Maternal-Fetal Medicine Committee for many years and co-authored many SOGC Clinical Practice Guidelines. Lisa has also been a Lamaze certified childbirth educator for many years and continues to practice in this role in her community. She is passionate about normalizing birth and works tirelessly at spreading the word in this endeavour.

Cheryl A. Sams is a graduate of Ryerson University (BScN) and D'Youville College (MSN). She has worked at the Hospital for Sick Children in Toronto since she graduated from nursing school. She has held many positions there, including staff nurse, clinical educator, manager, director, and clinical nurse specialist. Cheryl has held many teaching positions at Ryerson University in the Post RN Program and the Nurse Practitioner Program. She has also taught at the University of Toronto in the BScN program. Cheryl taught at Seneca College in the York University Collaborative BScN program until her recent retirement.

As an author, Cheryl enjoys contributing to the nursing body of literature. She has contributed chapters to the Canadian publication of Lewis et al.'s *Medical-Surgical Nursing* and Potter and Perry's *Fundamentals of Nursing*. She was one of the editors for *Mosby's Comprehensive Review for the Canadian RN Exam.*

CONTRIBUTORS

Janet Andrews, RN, BScN, MN
Trillium Health Partners
Mississauga, Ontario

Debbie Aylward, BScN, MScN
Perinatal Consultant
Champlain Maternal Newborn Regional Program
Ottawa, Ontario

Melanie Basso, RN, MSN, PNC(C)
Senior Practice Leader-Perinatal
BC Women's Hospital and Health Centre
Vancouver, British Columbia

Katherine Bertoni, BScN, MN, NP-F, CDE
Assistant Teaching Professor
Faculty of Human and Social Development, School of Nursing
University of Victoria
Victoria, British Columbia

Karen Breen-Reid, RN, BScN, MN
Manager, Nursing & Interprofessional Education
Collaborative for Professional Practice
The Hospital for Sick Children;
Adjunct Lecturer, Lawrence S. Bloomberg Faculty of Nursing
University of Toronto
Toronto, Ontario

Judy Buchan, RN, BScN, MN, PMP
Acting Manager, Family Health
Health Services
Peel Public Health
Mississauga, Ontario

Nancy Caprara, RN, BScN, MN
Professor, School of Health Science
Seneca College
Toronto, Ontario

Cheryl Dika, RN, MN, NP
Director, Nurse Practitioner Program
College of Nursing
Faculty of Health Sciences
University of Manitoba
Winnipeg, Manitoba

Kerry Lynn Durnford, MN, RN
Nursing Faculty
School of Health and Human Services
Aurora College
Yellowknife, Northwest Territories

Helen Edwards, RN, BA, MN
Director, Clinical Informatics and Technology Assisted Programs
The Hospital for Sick Children
Adjunct Lecturer, Lawrence S. Bloomberg Faculty of Nursing
University of Toronto
Toronto, Ontario

K. Ileen Gladding, RN, MN, PNC(C)
Clinical Educator, Birthing Services
Trillium Health Partners
Mississauga, Ontario

Denise Harrison, RN, PhD
Associate Professor and Chair in Nursing Care of Children, Youth and Families
University of Ottawa and Children's Hospital of Eastern Ontario (CHEO)
Ottawa, Ontario

Anne Hogarth, RN, BScN
Professor and Clinical Student Advisor
School of Health Sciences
Seneca College
King City, Ontario

France Morin, BScN, MScN
Perinatal Consultant
Champlain Maternal Newborn Regional Program
Ottawa, Ontario

Pat O'Flaherty, MEd, MN
Neonatal Nurse Practitioner
Champlain Maternal Newborn Regional Program
Ottawa, Ontario

Shelly Petruskavich, MN, BScN
Manager, Professional Practice Nursing
Trillium Health Partners
Mississauga, Ontario

Lauren Rivard, RN, BScN, MSc
Perinatal Consultant
Champlain Maternal Newborn Regional Program
Kingston, Ontario

Nancy Watts, RN, MN
Clinical Nurse Specialist
Perinatal
Mount Sinai Hospital
Toronto, Ontario

F. Maureen White, RN, MN
Assistant Professor
School of Nursing
Dalhousie University
Halifax, Nova Scotia

PEDIATRIC SECTION EDITOR

Andrea Logan, RN, MN, NP-Paediatrics
Assistant Clinical Services Manager of Paediatrics and NICU
William Osler Health System
Brampton, Ontario;
Registered Nurse, Emergency Department
The Hospital for Sick Children
Toronto, Ontario

PEDIATRIC ASSISTANT SECTION EDITOR

Martha Cope RN, BA, MScN(c)
Professor and Clinical Instructor
Health, Wellness and Sciences
Georgian College
Barrie, Ontario;
Registered Nurse, Surgical Inpatient Unit
Royal Victoria Regional Health Centre
Barrie, Ontario
Research Assistant
York University Institute for Health Research
Toronto, Ontario

REVIEWERS

Jacquie Bouchard, RN, BScN
Curriculum Developer
Practical Nurse Instructor
Northern Lakes College, Smoky River Campus
Slave Lake, Alberta

Jaime Charlebois, BScN, MScN
Professor and Clinical Instructor
Health, Wellness, and Sciences
Georgian College
Barrie, Ontario;
RN & OB Simulation Lead
Labour and Delivery, North York General
Toronto, Ontario

Sai Choon Choo
Faculty Member (Retired)
Douglas College
New Westminster, British Columbia

Dr. Shelley L. Cobbett, RN BN GnT MN EdD
Adjunct Assistant Professor
Dalhousie University School of Nursing—Yarmouth Site
Yarmouth, Nova Scotia

Marianne Cochrane, RN, MHSc(N)
Professor and Year 4 Coordinator, Collaborative BScN Program
University of Ontario Institute of Technology/Durham College
Oshawa, Ontario

Tracey Fallak, BScN, MN
Course Leader, Nursing
Red River College
Winnipeg, Manitoba

Mary Ann Fegan RN, MN
Associate Professor, Teaching Stream
Undergraduate Clinical Education Coordinator
Lawrence S. Bloomberg Faculty of Nursing
University of Toronto
Toronto, Ontario

Alison Fyfe-Carlson, RN, BN, MA-Ed
Course Leader, Nursing
Red River College
Winnipeg, Manitoba

Laurie Gedcke-Kerr, RN, BNSc, MSc
Lecturer, School of Nursing
Queen's University
Kingston, Ontario

Corinne Hart, RN, BScN, MHSc, PhD
Associate Professor
Daphne Cockwell School of Nursing
Ryerson University
Toronto, Ontario

Amy Klepetar, RN, BA, BScN, MSPH
Assistant Professor
School of Nursing
University of Northern British Columbia
Terrace, British Columbia

Krista Lussier RN, BScN, MSN
Chairperson, BScN Program
Senior Lecturer
Thompson Rivers University
Kamloops, British Columbia

Carla Shapiro, RN, MN
Senior Instructor
Faculty of Health Sciences
College of Nursing
University of Manitoba
Winnipeg, Manitoba

Kimberley Widger, RN, PhD CHPCN(C)
Assistant Professor
Lawrence S. Bloomberg Faculty of Nursing
University of Toronto
Toronto, Ontario
Nursing Research Associate
Paediatric Advanced Care Team (PACT)
The Hospital for Sick Children
Toronto, Ontario

SECTION REVIEWERS (CHAPTER 34: PAIN ASSESSMENT AND MANAGEMENT)

Franklin F. Gorospe IV, RN, BScN, MN
Daphne Cockwell School of Nursing
Ryerson University
Toronto, Ontario
Perioperative Services
University Health Network – Toronto General Hospital
Toronto, Ontario

Jacqueline Hanley, RN, MN
Clinical Nurse Specialist
Acute Pain Service
Department of Anaesthesia and Pain Medicine
The Hospital for Sick Children
Toronto, Ontario

PREFACE

This second edition of *Maternal Child Nursing Care in Canada* combines essential perinatal and pediatric nursing information into one text. The text focuses on the care of women during their reproductive years and the care of children from birth through adolescence. The first section of the text focuses on important issues related to perinatal and pediatric nursing in Canada, including an overview of family and culture, as well as community nursing care. The second section discusses the promotion of wellness and the care for women experiencing common health concerns throughout the lifespan and care of the child-bearing woman. The health care of children and child development in the context of the family is the focus for the third section. The text provides a family-centred care approach that recognizes the importance of collaboration with families when providing care. This second edition of *Maternal Child Nursing Care in Canada* is designed to address the changing needs of Canadian women during their child-bearing years and those of children during their developing years.

Maternal Child Nursing Care in Canada was developed to provide students with the knowledge and skills they need to become competent critical thinkers and to attain the sensitivity needed to become caring nurses. This second edition reflects the Canadian health care system, the importance of family-centred care, and the cultural diversity throughout the country. It includes the most accurate, current, and clinically relevant information available.

APPROACH

Professional nursing practice continues to evolve and adapt to society's changing health priorities. The rapidly changing health care delivery system offers new opportunities for nurses to alter the practice of perinatal and pediatric nursing and to improve the way in which care is given. Increasingly, nursing care must be artfully constructed using research to inform the care provided. It is incumbent on nurses to use the most up-to-date and scientifically supported information on which to base their care. To assist nurses in providing this type of care, Research Focus boxes with implications for practice are included throughout the text.

Consumers of perinatal and pediatric care vary in age, ethnicity, culture, language, social status, marital status, and sexual orientation. They seek care from a variety of health care providers in numerous health care settings, including the home. To meet the needs of these consumers, clinical education must offer students a variety of health care experiences in settings that include hospitals and birth centres, homes, clinics, private physicians' offices, shelters for the homeless or for women and children who require protection, and other community-based settings.

The focus in the chapters is on nursing care along with collaboration with other health care disciplines, as this combination provides the most comprehensive care possible to women and children. Included on the Evolve site for this edition are the Nursing Process boxes and the Nursing Care Plans. The Nursing Process boxes include assessments, nursing diagnoses, expected outcomes, nursing care implementation, and evaluation of nursing care, and the Nursing Care Plans reinforce the problem-solving approach to patient care. Throughout the discussion of assessment and care, warning signs and emergency situations are also highlighted, to alert the nurse to signs of potential problems.

Patient education is an essential component of nursing care of women and children. The chapters on women's health promotion and screening (Chapters 5 through 8) emphasize teaching for self-care to promote wellness and encourage preventive care. Chapter 23, on transition to parenthood, focuses on teaching to new families and infants. Special boxes highlight community care throughout the text. Family-Centred Teaching boxes incorporate family considerations important to care of women and children. Issues concerning grandparents, siblings, and various family constellations are also addressed. In the pediatric chapters (Part 3), these boxes focus on the special learning needs of families caring for their child. Legal Tips are integrated throughout the maternity section to emphasize these issues as they relate to the care of women and infants.

This second edition features a contemporary design with logical, easy-to-follow headings and an attractive four-colour design that highlights important content and increases visual appeal. Hundreds of colour photographs and drawings throughout the text, many of them new, illustrate important concepts and techniques to further enhance comprehension. To help students learn essential information quickly and efficiently, we have included numerous features that prioritize, condense, simplify, and emphasize important aspects of nursing care. In addition, students are encouraged to apply critical thinking in real-life scenarios presented in the Critical Thinking Case Studies.

NEW TO THIS EDITION

- Part 1 (Chapters 1 to 3) introduces the reader to issues surrounding maternal child nursing in Canada; Part 2 (Chapters 4 to 29) focuses on perinatal nursing; and Part 3 (Chapters 30 to 54) concentrates on pediatric nursing.
- Increased coverage is provided on health care in the LGBTQ community and in the Indigenous community.
- Discussion of perinatal mental health has been added in the chapters on pregnancy, and there is more content related to pediatric mental health throughout the Pediatric section.
- New and updated references, sources, and guidelines are provided, including:
  - Society of Obstetrician and Gynaecologists of Canada (SOGC) guidelines
  - Canadian Association of Perinatal and Women's Health Nurses (CAPWHN)

  - Sexually transmitted infection (STI) guidelines
  - Canadian Paediatric Society (CPS) standards
  - Canadian Association of Midwives (CAM)
  - Public Health Agency of Canada (PHAC)
  - Registered Nurses' Association of Ontario (RNAO)
  - Perinatal Services BC
  - American College of Obstetricians and Gynecologists (ACOG)
  - Centers for Disease Control and Prevention (CDC)
  - World Health Organization (WHO)
- There is increased emphasis on health promotion in the Perinatal and Pediatric sections of the text.
- Enhanced detail on anatomy and physiology is provided in the Pediatric section.

SPECIAL FEATURES

- **Objectives** focus students' attention on the important content to be mastered.
- **Atraumatic Care** boxes emphasize the importance of providing competent care while minimizing undue physical and psychological distress for the child and family.
- **Community Focus** boxes emphasize community issues, provide resources and guidance, and illustrate nursing care in a variety of settings.
- **Critical Thinking Case Studies** present students with real-life situations and encourage students to make appropriate clinical judgements. Answer guidelines are provided on the book's Evolve site.
- **Cultural Awareness** boxes describe beliefs and practices about pregnancy, childbirth, parenting, women's health concerns, and caring for sick children.
- **Emergency** boxes alert students to the signs and symptoms of various emergency situations and provide interventions for immediate implementation.
- **Family-Centred Teaching** boxes highlight the needs of families that should be addressed when family-centred care is provided.
- **Guidelines** boxes provide students with examples of various approaches to implementing care.
- **Home Care** boxes emphasize patient and family self-care and provide information to help students transfer learning from the hospital to the home setting.
- **Medication Guide** boxes include key information about medications used in maternity and newborn care, including their indications, adverse effects, and nursing considerations.
- **Patient Teaching** boxes assist students to help patients and families become involved in their own care with optimal outcomes.
- **Research Focus** boxes are incorporated throughout the book. Findings that confirm effective practices or that identify practices with unknown, ineffective, or harmful effects are located within the narrative.
- **Legal Tips** are integrated throughout Part 1 to provide students with relevant information to deal with important legal areas in the context of perinatal nursing.
- **Medication Alerts** provides important information regarding the safety of medications, including interactions with other medications and important nursing considerations.
- **Nursing Alerts** call the reader's attention to critical information that could lead to deteriorating or emergency situations.
- **Safety Alerts** call the reader's attention to potentially dangerous situations that should be addressed by the nurse.
- **Key Points**, located at the end of each chapter, help the reader summarize major points, make connections, and synthesize information. The Key Points are also available in a downloadable format and can be found on this book's Evolve site. 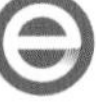
- **Additional Resources**, including websites and contact information for organizations and educational resources available for the topics discussed, are listed throughout.
- A highly detailed, cross-referenced **index** allows readers to quickly access needed information.

SUPPLEMENTAL RESOURCES

A comprehensive ancillary package is available to students and instructors using *Maternal Child Nursing Care in Canada*. The following supplemental resources have been thoroughly revised for this edition and can significantly assist in the teaching and learning of perinatal and pediatric nursing in classroom and clinical settings.

Evolve Website

Located at http://evolve.elsevier.com/Canada/Perry/maternal, the Evolve website for this book includes the following elements.

For Students

- More than 500 Review Questions for Exam Preparation
- Answers to Critical Thinking Case Studies from the book
- Key Points
- Nursing Care Plans
- Nursing Processes
- Nursing Skills
- Audio Glossary
- Case Studies

Throughout the text the authors have indicated areas where there is important information on the Evolve website. Look for these features. These assets include the following:

- **Nursing Care Plans** provide commonly encountered situations and disorders. Nursing diagnoses are included, as are rationales for nursing interventions that might not be immediately evident to students.
- **Nursing Processes** help students to easily identify information on some major diseases and conditions.
- **Nursing Skills** teach students how to implement concepts presented in the textbook and use them in real-life

situations. This will enhance student knowledge and give students a better understanding of concepts they learn while reading the textbook.

For Instructors

- **NEW** *TEACH for Nurses* Lesson Plans that focus on the most important content from each chapter and provide innovative strategies for student engagement and learning. These new Lesson Plans include strategies for integrating nursing curriculum standards, links to all relevant student and instructor resources, and an original instructor-only Case Study in most chapters.
- ExamView® Test Bank that features more than 1500 examination-format test questions (including alternate-item questions) with text page references, rationales, and answers. The robust ExamView® testing application, provided at no cost to faculty, allows instructors to create new tests; edit, add, and delete test questions; sort questions by category, cognitive level, and nursing process step; and administer and grade tests online, with automated scoring and gradebook functionality.
- PowerPoint® Lecture Slides consisting of more than 2100 customizable text slides for instructors to use in lectures
- An Image Collection with over 500 full-colour images from the book for instructors to use in lectures
- Access to all student resources listed above

Simulation Learning System (SLS)

The Simulation Learning System (SLS) is an online toolkit that helps instructors and facilitators effectively incorporate medium- to high-fidelity simulation into their nursing curriculum. Detailed patient scenarios promote and enhance the clinical decision-making skills of students at all levels. The SLS provides detailed instructions for preparation and implementation of the simulation experience, debriefing questions that encourage critical thinking, and learning resources to reinforce student comprehension. Each scenario in the SLS complements the textbook content and helps bridge the gap between lectures and clinical practice. The SLS provides the perfect environment for students to practice what they are learning in the text for a true-to-life, hands-on learning experience.

Virtual Clinical Excursions: Virtual Hospital and Workbook Companion

A virtual hospital and workbook package has been developed as a virtual clinical experience to expand student opportunities for critical thinking. This package guides the student through a computer-generated virtual clinical environment and helps the user apply textbook content to virtual patients in that environment. Case studies are presented that allow students to use this textbook as a reference to assess, diagnose, plan, implement, and evaluate "real" patients using clinical scenarios. The state-of-the-art technologies reflected on this virtual hospital and workbook package demonstrate cutting-edge learning opportunities for students and facilitate knowledge retention of the information found in the textbook. The clinical simulations and workbook represent the next generation of research-based learning tools that promote critical thinking and meaningful learning.

Elsevier eBooks

This exciting program is available to faculty who adopt a number of Elsevier texts, including *Maternal Child Nursing Care in Canada*. Elsevier eBooks is an integrated electronic study centre consisting of a collection of textbooks made available online. It is carefully designed to "extend" the textbook for an easier and more efficient teaching and learning experience. It includes study aids such as highlighting, e-note taking, and cut-and-paste capabilities. Even more importantly, it allows students and instructors to do a comprehensive search within the specific text or across a number of titles. Please check with your Elsevier Canada sales representative for more information.

ICONS AT A GLANCE

- ATRAUMATIC CARE
- COMMUNITY FOCUS
- CRITICAL THINKING CASE STUDY
- CULTURAL AWARENESS
- EMERGENCY
- FAMILY-CENTRED TEACHING
- GUIDELINES
- HOME CARE
- MEDICATION ALERT
- MEDICATION GUIDE
- NURSING ALERT
- PATIENT TEACHING
- RESEARCH FOCUS
- SAFETY ALERT

WE WELCOME YOUR FEEDBACK

We always welcome comments from instructors and students who use this book so that we may continue to make improvements and be responsive to your needs in future editions. Please send any comments you may have for us to the attention of the publisher, at a.millar@elsevier.com.

ACKNOWLEDGMENTS

I would like to offer thanks to the many perinatal contributors who worked diligently to provide this text with an updated and uniquely Canadian perspective as well as to the perinatal nurses across the country who continue to provide high-quality family-centred care to women and their families. I would also like to extend a very special thank you to my husband, John Lindsay, and to my three children, Katie (who makes me proud that she is also a perinatal nurse), Emily, and Jack, for their inspiration and encouragement.
Lisa Keenan-Lindsay

I would like to thank the many pediatric experts who have not only contributed to the "peds" part of this text but also made major contributions to the field of pediatric nursing in Canada. You make a difference every day to children and their families. I would also like to thank my husband, Stuart Sams, and my family for cheering me on.
Cheryl Sams

A special thank you goes to Sandy Matos, Jerri Hurlbutt, Carol O'Connell, Ann Millar, Roberta A. Spinosa-Millman, and the rest of the group at Elsevier for all of their exceptional support and encouragement throughout the development of this book. We also would like to thank all our chapter contributors, reviewers, and section editors whose advice, expertise, insight, and dedication greatly assisted us in completing this edition. We appreciate all your time and guidance.
Lisa and Cheryl

PART 1

Maternal Child Nursing

UNIT 1

Introduction to Maternal Child Nursing

CHAPTER

1

Contemporary Perinatal and Pediatric Nursing in Canada

Lisa Keenan-Lindsay

evolve WEBSITE

Visit the Evolve website for additional resources related to the content in this chapter such as Case Studies, Critical Thinking Case Study Answers, Nursing Care Plans, Nursing Processes, Nursing Skills, and Review Questions for Exam Preparation at: *http://evolve.elsevier.com/Canada/Perry/maternal/*

OBJECTIVES

On completion of this chapter the reader will be able to:

- Describe the scope of perinatal and pediatric nursing in Canada today.
- Examine the historical context of health care in Canada.
- Consider how the social determinants of health influence the health of women and children, and explore approaches needed to address health inequities.
- Describe the impact of residential schools on the health of Indigenous people.
- Describe how the Millennium Development Goals (MDGs) have worked to improve the health of people worldwide.
- Consider the role of research in perinatal and pediatric nursing.
- Explore ethical issues in contemporary perinatal and pediatric nursing.

The focus of the first part of this book is to provide an overview of perinatal and pediatric nursing in Canada from a national and global perspective. The role of social, cultural, and family influence on health promotion will also be discussed, as will the role of nurses in the community. Part 2 focuses on the care of child-bearing women and families, or perinatal nursing, as well as women's health promotion. Part 3, which begins with Chapter 30, addresses the issues and trends related to the health care of children.

PERINATAL AND PEDIATRIC NURSING

Nurses care for child-bearing women, children, and families in many settings, including the hospital, the home, and a variety of ambulatory and community settings. Nurses also work collaboratively with other health and social care providers, such as physicians, midwives, nutritionists, doulas, and social workers, to name a few. *Perinatal nurses* are those nurses who work collaboratively with women and families from the preconception period throughout the child-bearing year. Pediatric nurses care for children from birth up to age 18 years. Nurses caring for children also provide care for the family. Nursing may be provided in many settings, including inner-city, urban, or rural communities. The location of the care may have implications for the services that are offered, as remote and rural communities may not have all services necessary to provide comprehensive care (see discussion below). Most nurses working in hospitals provide acute care, while nurses working in a community setting may provide care that focuses on health promotion, although rehabilitative and palliative care are also provided in the community.

Nurses caring for women and children can help make the health care system more responsive to the needs of the patients in their care. Nurses have developed strategies to improve the well-being of women and their newborns as well as children, and have led efforts to develop and implement clinical practice guidelines that draw on current evidence or research. Through professional associations, nurses can have a voice in setting standards and influencing health policy by actively participating in the education of the public and that of local, provincial, and federal legislators.

THE HISTORY AND CONTEXT OF HEALTH CARE IN CANADA

Health services in Canada are organized provincially, and Medicare, Canada's government-funded health insurance program, provides universal medical and hospital services for all Canadians. New immigrants to Canada may wait 90 days for government health coverage, depending on which province or territory they will be living in. There is a program, the Interim Federal Health Program, that provides temporary health coverage for certain groups of refugees before they are covered under provincial or territorial health insurance plans. The principles of the Canada Health Act include public administration, comprehensive "medically necessary" care, universality, portability, and accessibility. Home care, extended care, pharmaceuticals, and dental care are not currently covered under Medicare provisions. Thus, to some extent, the Medicare program shapes the health services offered to Canadians. In an effort to control health care costs, interest has grown in restructuring health services and developing community-based programs and preventive health services.

Since the Lalonde Report was released in 1974, Canada has been a global leader in health promotion. In 1986, Canada hosted the first international conference on health promotion, which resulted in the Ottawa Charter. Three challenges for Canadians were identified: reducing health inequities, increasing prevention, and enhancing people's capacities to live with chronic disease and disability. The Charter also acknowledged the need for intersectoral collaboration, or looking beyond health, to include other sectors (e.g., income security, employment, education, housing, and transportation) (Public Health Agency of Canada [PHAC], 1986). In the late 1990s, interest expanded to creating evidence-informed programs that address all factors that impact health. With the HIV/AIDS epidemic, increasing rates of tuberculosis and other infectious diseases, the threat of bioterrorism, and the severe acute respiratory syndrome (SARS) epidemic, Canadians were reminded of the importance of immunizations and public health measures. In 2004, the federal government created the Public Health Agency of Canada (PHAC). While the PHAC initially focused on population health and health promotion, the emergence of avian influenza shifted the focus toward planning for a pandemic along with health promotion.

The delivery of health care within each community, province, and territory contains unique elements as each level of government tries to balance human resources, funding, and liability concerns with regulatory, educational, political, and demographic issues. Inequities in access to good-quality care have developed particularly in rural, remote, inner-city, and Indigenous communities compared with access to such care in other Canadian communities.

CONTEMPORARY ISSUES AND TRENDS

Social Determinants of Health

The emphasis in health care has shifted from treatment of illnesses to health promotion and prevention. In order to promote good health, the many complex influences on health need to be investigated and understood. To this end, the federal government has outlined the social *determinants of health* (Table 1-1). These determinants provide a blueprint for health care policies and help direct population health research with the goal of improving health for its citizens (PHAC, 2011). The determinants of health outline many factors that impact the health of Canadians (Fig. 1-1). The Canadian Nurses Association (CNA) position statement of the social determinants of health state that nurses in all domains of practice can address social inequities by:

- recognizing the significance of the social determinants of health at an individual and collective level and including them in assessments, diagnoses, outcomes planning, implementation, and evaluations;
- providing sensitive, empowering care at the individual, family, and community level to those experiencing inequities;
- engaging with health and social organizations in policy analysis and advocacy to promote health equity and for change in inequitable health and social policies, legislation, and regulations;
- advocating for publicly funded, not-for-profit health care services that are available to all; and
- supporting environmental preservation and restoration (Canadian Nurses Association [CNA], 2013).

Many health inequities also result from a lack of access to the social determinants of health, which creates conditions of vulnerability (Table 1-1), with poverty having the most significant influence on maternal child health (Pauly, MacKinnon, & Varcoe, 2009). The social determinants of health are conditions that can support or challenge health.

Socioeconomic Status

There is strong and growing evidence that higher social and economic status is associated with better health. In fact, these two factors seem to be the most important determinants of health (PHAC, 2011). The term *poverty* implies both visible and invisible impoverishment. It is a condition in which families live without adequate resources (Denburg & Daneman, 2010). *Visible poverty* refers to lack of money or material resources, which includes insufficient clothing, poor sanitation, and deteriorating housing. *Invisible poverty* refers to social and cultural deprivation, such as limited employment opportunities, inferior educational opportunities, lack of or inferior medical services and health care facilities, and an absence of public services. The sum of all aspects of a low-income family's living situation contributes to and compounds health problems; this includes crowded living conditions and poor sanitation, which facilitate transfer of disease (e.g., tuberculosis). Lack of funds or inaccessibility of health services can inhibit treatment for any but severe illness or injury. Sometimes health care is inadequate because of lack of information. Individuals may not have information regarding causes, treatment, outcome of the illness, or preventive measures.

Although Canada has no official definition of poverty, it is typically measured using the Low Income Cut-Offs

TABLE 1-1 SOCIAL DETERMINANTS OF HEALTH

HEALTH DETERMINANTS	DESCRIPTION
1. Income and social status	Greatest influence on health status and behaviours and use of health care services. Lower-income Canadians have poorer health, with more chronic illness and earlier death, than that of higher-income Canadians, regardless of age, gender, culture, race, or residence. Only 46% of Canadians with the least income rate their health as very good or excellent, compared with 73% for those in the highest income group.
2. Social support networks	Social contacts and support networks are linked with better health by providing emotional support, caregiving, and improved management of adversity.
3. Education and literacy	Higher education improves a person's state of health. Education increases opportunities for earning higher incomes and improves problem-solving capacity and access to health information.
4. Employment/working conditions	Unemployment or employment that is stressful or unsafe is linked to poorer health. Income, social contacts, and emotional health are all affected by the workplace.
5. Social environments	The community, region, province or territory, and country provide resource sharing and social networks that create safety nets and improve overall health for community members.
6. Physical environments	Environmental contaminants in the air, soil, water, and food can cause poor health, such as respiratory conditions or other serious illnesses. Environments in the built community can affect health in many ways, such as through poor air quality and unsafe building codes.
7. Personal health practices and coping skills	There are measures that individuals can carry out themselves to promote their own health and manage challenges. Self-sufficiency and making healthy choices will optimize their level of health.
8. Healthy child development	What happens to a child during the growing years will have an impact on the child's long-term health and may lead to the development of chronic illness—e.g., low–birth-weight infants have almost twice the incidence of lifelong diseases.
9. Biology and genetic endowment	Genetics play an important role in individuals' health status. Genetic predisposition to certain conditions, as well as environmental interrelationships, puts certain individuals at risk for specific diseases.
10. Health services	Availability of health services has a direct impact on individuals', families', groups', and communities' ability to prevent disease and adequately treat secondary conditions. There are still inequities in accessibility to these essential services—e.g., urban populations with increased access to health services have better morbidity and mortality rates than those of rural populations with less access to health care.
11. Gender	*Gender* refers to differences in biologics, roles in society, personalities, attitudes, values, and socioeconomic position. These differences have a direct bearing on health. There are also gender-specific predispositions toward certain disease states and treatments programs.
12. Culture	Health risks related to cultural and ethnic backgrounds can affect an individual and the family. A person's culture may influence his or her health choices. For example, access to health care may be difficult for new immigrants who do not know the language or how to enter and manoeuvre the health care system. It is essential that culturally appropriate care be available to everyone.

Adapted from Public Health Agency of Canada [2010]. *What makes Canadians healthy or unhealthy?* Retrieved from http://www.phac-aspc.gc.ca/ph-sp/determinants/index-eng.php

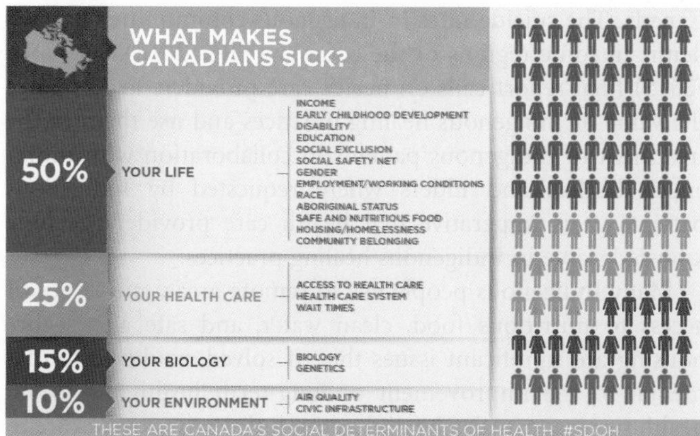

FIGURE 1-1 An infographic that shows the importance of the social determinants of health on health and wellness. (Source: Canadian Medical Association. Retrieved from http://healthcaretransformation.ca/infographic-social-determinants-of-health/)

(LICO)—before and after tax, the Low Income Measures (LIM)—before and after tax, and the Market Basket Measures (MBM) (Statistics Canada, 2013a). The LICO is meant to express the income level at which a family faces constraints because it has to spend a higher percentage of its income on basic resources—for example, shelter, clothes, food—than the average similar-size family. In 2011, Statistics Canada reported that 8.8% of Canadians had low incomes; this number is down from 15.2 in 1996 (Statistics Canada, 2013b). Poverty rates among Indigenous Canadians are significantly higher than for the rest of the population. Half of the status Indigenous children in Canada live in poverty, a figure that increases to two-thirds in Saskatchewan and Manitoba (MacDonald & Wilson, 2013).

Immigrants and Refugees

Of particular concern in Canada are immigrant and refugee women. It is difficult to assess the vulnerability of newcomers, as each situation is different and the specific events related to immigration become the determinants of health. The main issues faced by immigrant and refugee women are isolation from society, differing cultural values and beliefs, and the inability of large numbers of immigrant and refugee women to speak English or French. All of these factors will influence a woman's access to health care (see Chapter 2 for further discussion of culture).

Homelessness

Homeless individuals are those who lack resources and community ties necessary to provide for their own adequate shelter. It is estimated that there are at least 200,000 homeless people in Canada in a given year, living either in shelters or on the streets. Most nights, shelters accommodate at least 30,000 people. Although single men are the highest portion of homeless people in Canada, families with children living in poverty; street youth; Indigenous persons with mental illness; and new immigrants are disproportionately reflected in the homeless population (Gaetz et al., 2013).

There are a variety of causes of homelessness in Canada, including a lack of affordable housing, low income, job lay-offs, the gap between incomes and affordability of resources, mental illness, substance use, intimate partner conflict and violence, unexpected family crises, and inadequate discharge coordination between mental health services, justice facilities, and the social services system.

Culture

Another factor that affects the delivery and quality of health care is the fact that the Canadian population is diverse in terms of **culture**, **ethnicity**, race, and age. In 2011, 20.6% of people living in Canada were born outside the country (Statistics Canada, 2013c). Chinese, South Asians, and Blacks make up 61% of visible minorities. Statistics Canada predicts that by 2031, between 29 and 32% of Canadians will identify themselves as belonging to a visible minority and as many as 3 out of 5 people living in Toronto and Vancouver will identify as visible minorities (Statistics Canada, 2010).

Significant disparity exists in health outcomes among people of various racial and ethnic groups in Canada. People also have different health needs, practices, and health service preferences related to their ethnic or cultural backgrounds. They may have dietary preferences and health practices that are not understood by caregivers. To meet the health care needs of a culturally diverse society, nurses must provide culturally safe and responsive care (see Chapter 2).

Indigenous People

In Canada, the Constitution recognizes three groups of Indigenous people: First Nations (made up of more than 615 bands across the country), Métis (European–First Nation ancestry), and Inuit (Arctic-situated Indigenous peoples). In 2016, the term *Aboriginal* has been replaced with Indigenous people because the term Aboriginal does not recognize the inherent rights or Treaty rights of the various groups. Indigenous families living in poverty consistently have poorer health outcomes. Living in remote locations and lack of access to some of the social determinants of health account for some of these health inequities. Another reason is the historical context of Indigenous children being sent to residential schools.

Up until the 1990s the Canadian government, in partnership with a number of Christian churches, operated a residential school system for Indigenous children. The government-funded, usually church-run schools and residences were set up to assimilate Indigenous people into the Canadian mainstream by eliminating parental and community involvement in the intellectual, cultural, and spiritual development of Indigenous children in their communities. More than 150,000 Indigenous children were placed in these residential schools. The Truth and Reconciliation Commission (TRC) has worked to reveal the history and ongoing legacy of church-run residential schools in a manner that fully documents the harms perpetrated against Indigenous peoples, as well as leading the way to respect through reconciliation (TRC, 2012).

In these schools, children were often forbidden to speak their own language or engage in their own cultural and spiritual practices. Many children were abused either physically or sexually. Generations of children were traumatized by the experience. There was a lack of parental and family involvement in the upbringing of their own children, which also denied those same children the ability to develop parenting skills because they lacked effective role models. This has had an effect on generations of families as the impact of parenting difficulties has carried forward. In the TRC report, survivors described what happened after they left the schools: they no longer felt connected to their parents or their families; some said they felt ashamed of themselves, their parents, and their culture; some children found it difficult to forgive their parents for sending them to residential school. Parents also reported the difficulties of having their children away from home and the difficulties that occurred when they returned home (TRC, 2012).

The TRC highlighted that Indigenous people need specialized health supports available near where they live. This need is especially acute in the northern and more isolated regions of Canada. The suicide rates in Indigenous communities are epidemic in some regions of the country (TRC, 2012). The TRC (2015) final report calls on health care providers to recognize the value of Indigenous healing practices and use them in the treatment of Indigenous patients in collaboration with Indigenous healers and Elders where requested by Indigenous patients. It is imperative that health care providers become knowledgeable in Indigenous healing practices.

Many Indigenous people live in remote areas, and issues of access to nutritious food, clean water, and safe and secure housing are significant issues that, if solved, could be fundamental to the improvement of long-term health. Access to health services can also be difficult; solutions to provide care to remote communities need to be developed.

In 2011, the number of Indigenous people in Canada, which includes First Nations, Métis, and Inuit, was 1,400,685, which represents 4.3% of the Canadian population (Statistics Canada, 2014). Importantly for maternal child care provision between 2006 and 2011, the Indigenous population increased by 20%, compared with 5.2% for the non-Indigenous population.

Although the populations in many Canadian towns and cities are aging, in some Indigenous communities more than 46% of the residents are under 25 years of age. In 2011, Indigenous children aged 14 and under made up 28.0% of the total Indigenous population and 7.0% of all children in Canada (Statistics Canada, 2014).

Lesbian/Gay/Bisexual/Transsexual/Queer (LGBTQ) Health

LGBTQ people have many of the same health concerns as anyone else, but cultural differences and the impact of homophobia, biphobia, and transphobia and systemic discrimination mean that these health needs may be experienced quite differently (Rainbow Health Ontario [RHO], 2014). Due in part to negative past experiences, many LGBTQ people may delay or avoid seeking health care or choose to withhold personal information from health care providers.

In general, LGBTQ people end up receiving less quality health care than the population as a whole (RHO, 2014). LGBTQ people also have some unique health concerns and may be at increased risk for certain health issues, including mental health, substance use, smoking, cancer, and diet, weight, and body image concerns (RHO, 2014). Most health care providers are not trained in these LGBTQ health needs and may not be sensitive to the particular health risks or knowledgeable about how to work with LGBTQ people.

Nurses and other health care providers must provide care that is not seen to be heteronormative and that is inclusive of people of all sexualities. In providing care, questions need to be asked in a manner that does not make assumptions about sexuality or gender. Adding a "transgender" option to check boxes on patient visit records can help to better capture information about transgender patients and could be a sign of acceptance to that person (American College of Obstetricians and Gynecologists [ACOG], 2011). Nurses caring for pediatric patients must also be conscious of LGBTQ issues. Children and adolescents may have questions about their own sexuality and gender, and if a nurse develops a therapeutic relationship with the child, the child may feel comfortable enough to ask questions and seek appropriate resources. Throughout this text an attempt has been made to integrate LGBTQ issues into the respective sections. Although a comprehensive discussion is beyond the scope of the text, additional resources are also included when available. Throughout the text the term *patient* may be used instead of *woman* to ensure inclusivity of all people.

Integrative Healing

Integrative healing encompasses complementary and alternative therapies that are sometimes used in combination with conventional Western modalities of treatment. Many popular alternative healing modalities offer human-centred care based on philosophies that honour the individual's beliefs, values, and desires. The focus of these modalities is on the whole person, not just on a disease complex. Many patients often find that integrative modalities are more consistent with their own belief systems and allow for more autonomy in health care decisions. It is important that nurses understand the beliefs of patients to ensure that health care needs are met.

High-Technology Care

Advances in scientific knowledge have contributed to a health care system that emphasizes high-technology care. For example, maternity care has extended to preconception counselling, more scientific techniques to monitor the mother and fetus, more definitive tests for hypoxia and acidosis, and neonatal intensive care units, which have enhanced the life of premature children. Enhanced technology has also increased the life expectancy of many children with chronic diseases. Internet-based information is available to the public that enhances interactions among health care providers, families, and community providers. Point-of-care testing is available. Personal data assistants are used to enhance comprehensive care; the medical record is increasingly in electronic form.

Health information technology is also having a profound impact on the ways in which health services are delivered. **Telehealth** is an umbrella term for the use of communication technologies and electronic information to provide or support health care when the participants are separated by distance. It permits specialists, including nurses, to provide health care and consultation to those needing care. While this technology can increase access to health services for people living in geographically isolated communities, nurses must use caution and evaluate the effects of such emerging technologies. Another Web-based resource is Healthlink, which provides people with medically approved information on many health topics, medications, and tips for promoting healthy lifestyles in several provinces (see Additional Resources).

Social Media

Social media uses Internet-based technologies to allow users to create their own content and participate in dialogue. The most common social media platforms are Facebook, Twitter, and LinkedIn (Duffy, 2011). In addition to their own personal use of these technologies, nurses can connect with nurses with similar interests, share insights about patient care, and advocate for patients (Saver, 2010). However, there are pitfalls for nurses using this technology. Patient privacy and confidentiality can be violated, and institutions and colleagues can be cast in an unfavourable light, with negative consequences for those posting the information. Nursing students have been expelled from school and nurses have been fired or reprimanded by their College of Nursing for injudicious posts. To help make nurses aware of their responsibilities when using social media, the International Nurse Regulator Collaborative (INRC) published the 6 P's for social media use (Box 1-1). The paper details issues of confidentiality and privacy, possible consequences of inappropriate use of social media, common myths and misunderstandings of social media, and tips on how to avoid related problems.

Health Literacy

Health literacy involves a spectrum of abilities, ranging from reading an appointment slip to interpreting medication instructions. These skills must be assessed routinely to recognize a

BOX 1-1 6 P'S OF SOCIAL MEDIA USE

Professional—Act professionally at all times.
Positive—Keep posts positive.
Patient/Person-free—Keep posts patient or person free.
Protect yourself—Protect your professionalism, your reputation and yourself.
Privacy—Keep your personal and professional life separate; respect privacy of others.
Pause before you post—Consider implications; avoid posting in haste or anger.

Source: International Nurse Regulator Collaborative (2014). Position Statement: Social media use: Common expectations for nurses. Retrieved from http://www.cno.org/Global/docs/prac/INCR%20Social%20Media%20Use%20Common%20Expectations%20for%20Nurses.pdf

problem and accommodate patients with limited literacy skills. In Canada, health literacy is defined as "the ability to access, comprehend, evaluate and communicate information as a way to promote, maintain and improve health in a variety of settings across the life-course" (PHAC, 2014). Figures show that 60% of adults and 88% of older adults in Canada are not health literate. People who are not health literate have difficulty using the everyday health information that is routinely available in health care facilities, grocery stores, retail outlets, schools, through the media, and in their communities (PHAC, 2014).

As a result of the increasingly multicultural Canadian population, there is an urgent need to address health literacy as a component of culturally and linguistically competent care. Canadians with the lowest health-literacy skills were found to be more than two-and-a-half times as likely to be in fair or poor health as those with the highest skill levels (Canadian Council on Learning, 2008). Individuals and groups for whom English is a second language often lack the skills necessary to seek medical care and navigate the health care system. Health care providers can contribute to health literacy by speaking slowly and using simple, common words; avoiding jargon; and assessing whether the patient understands the discussion. The skillful use of an interpreter or telephone interpretation service can help promote understanding and **informed consent** (see Chapter 2).

SPECIALIZATION AND EVIDENCE-INFORMED NURSING PRACTICE

The increasing complexity of care required by women, their newborns, and children has contributed to the growth of specialized knowledge and skills needed by nurses working in the areas of maternal child nursing. This specialized knowledge is gained through experience, advanced degrees, and certification programs.

Advanced practice nurses, such as clinical nurse specialists, provide care for women and children with complex health challenges. Nurse practitioners may provide primary care throughout the life of a woman or child. Lactation consultants, many of whom are nurses, provide services in the hospital, on an outpatient basis, or in the woman's home. Maternal child nurses work collaboratively with public health nurses and an increasing array of health care providers. An example is working with registered midwives who may provide primary care during pregnancy and the early postpartum period. Public health nurses may also work with teachers in schools to provide quality education experiences for children who may have a chronic illness that impacts their ability to attend school.

Evidence-Informed or Research-Based Practice

Evidence-informed practice (EIP) is the collection, interpretation, and integration of valid, important, and applicable patient-reported, nurse-observed, and research-derived information. Evidence-informed nursing practice combines knowledge with clinical experience and intuition. It provides a rational approach to decision making that facilitates best practice. Although not all practice can be evidence-informed, nurses must use the best available information to guide their interactions and interventions.

Practising nurses should contribute to research because they are the individuals observing human responses to health and illness. The current emphasis on measurable outcomes to determine the efficacy of interventions (often in relation to the cost) demands that nurses know whether clinical interventions result in positive outcomes for their patients. This demand has influenced the current trend toward EIP, which involves questioning why something is effective and whether a better approach exists. The concept of EIP also involves analyzing published clinical research and translating it into the everyday practice of nursing. When nurses base their clinical practice on science and research and document their clinical outcomes, they are better able to validate their contributions to health, wellness, and cure—not only to their patients and institutions but also to the nursing profession. Evaluation is essential to the nursing process, and research is one of the best ways to accomplish this.

Research plays a vital role in establishing maternity, women's health, and child health science. It can validate that nursing care makes a difference. For example, although prenatal care is associated with healthier infants, no one knows exactly which interventions produce this outcome. In the past, medical researchers rarely included women in their studies; thus more research in this area is crucial. Many possible areas of research exist in maternity and women and children's health care. The clinician can identify problems in the health and health care of women and children. Through research nurses can make a difference for these patients. Nurses should promote research funding and conduct research on maternal child, pediatric, and women's health, especially concerning the effectiveness of nursing strategies for these patients (see Research Focus box).

Standards of Practice and Legal Issues in Delivery of Care

Nursing standards of practice reflect current knowledge, represent levels of practice agreed on by leaders in the specialty, and can be used for clinical benchmarking. In perinatal and women's health nursing, there are several organizations that publish standards of practice and education for perinatal nurses. These

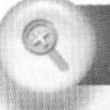

RESEARCH FOCUS

Searching for and Evaluating the Evidence

Throughout this text you will see Research Focus boxes. These boxes provide examples of how a nurse might conduct an inquiry into an identified practice question. Curiosity, access to a virtual or real library, and research critique skills are needed for the nurse to be confident that his or her practice is informed by a sound foundation of evidence.

Nurses construct their practice informed by research from many different sources. Categorizing evidence by "levels" is being replaced with embracing multiple ways of knowing that includes personal knowledge. Experienced nurses have practice knowledge that they need to share with other nurses through publication. Indigenous ways of knowing are increasingly being recognized, and patients are being acknowledged as experts in their own health care experiences (MacKinnon, 2006). Qualitative research has added to our understanding of a patient's experience with the health care system, whether during illness or wellness care.

In systematic reviews of quantitative research, such as those in the Cochrane Database, the research team uses a methodology to identify all studies relevant to a particular question. If the data are similar enough, they can be pooled into a meta-analysis. If the evidence is strong, some analyses will form the basis for recommendations for practice and guide further inquiry. Meta-synthesis of some forms of qualitative research has been developed, and the Cochrane review published the first systematic review of qualitative research in 2013. Recommendations for best practice stand on the shoulders of the systematic analysts, who in turn stand on the many shoulders of primary researchers.

Provided the professional organization is well respected and the process is rigorous, clinical practice guidelines and consensus statements reflect the current state of knowledge. Nurses need to also develop an inquiring mind and questioning attitude toward all forms of current evidence. In this way, the knowledge base required for maternal and child nursing will continue to grow and develop.

include the Canadian Association of Perinatal and Women's Health Nurses (CAPWHN) and the Association of Women's Health, Obstetric, and Neonatal Nurses (AWHONN), which publish standards of practice and education for perinatal nurses; and the National Association of Neonatal Nurses (NANN), which publishes standards of practice for neonatal nurses. The Canadian Nurses Association (CNA) Certification program also has competencies developed for perinatal, community, and pediatric critical care nurses.

In addition to these more formalized standards, agencies have their own policy and procedure books that outline standards to be followed in that setting. In legal terms the **standard of care** is that level of practice that a reasonably prudent nurse would provide in the same or similar circumstances.

LEGAL TIP *STANDARD OF CARE*

When there is uncertainty about how to perform a procedure, the nurse should consult the agency procedure book and follow the guidelines printed therein. These guidelines are the standard of care for that agency.

Patient Safety and Risk Management

Medical errors are a leading cause of death in the hospital or at home. According to the Canadian Adverse Events Study (Baker Study), the most quoted study in Canada regarding medical errors, 7.5% of hospitalized patients had an adverse event and of these, 16% died as a result (Baker et al., 2004). The cost of adverse events is staggering; a preliminary estimate of the economic burden of adverse events in Canada in 2009–2010 was $1.1 billion, including $397 million for preventable adverse events (Canadian Patient Safety Institute [CPSI], 2010). The actual numbers of adverse events is difficult to determine as there is a culture of silence surrounding patient errors. The Canadian Patient Safety Institute (CPSI) was developed as an integrated strategy for improving patient safety in Canadian health care (Box 1-2). The CPSI facilitates collaboration among governments and care providers to enhance patient safety and provides a number of useful resources, including the Canadian disclosure guidelines, an incident analysis framework, and the safety competencies framework. Achieving a culture of patient safety requires open, honest, and effective communication between health care providers and their patients. Patients are entitled to information about themselves and about their medical condition or illness, including the risks inherent in health care delivery (CPSI, 2011).

BOX 1-2 GOALS OF THE CANADIAN PATIENT SAFETY INSTITUTE (CPSI)

The CPSI four goals to improve patient safety:

- The CPSI will provide leadership on the establishment of a National Integrated Patient Safety Strategy.
- The CPSI will inspire and sustain patient safety knowledge within the system and, through innovation, enable transformational change.
- The CPSI will build and influence patient safety capability (knowledge and skills) at organizational and system levels.
- The CPSI will engage all audiences across the health system in the national patient safety agenda.

Source: The Canadian Patient Safety Institute. Retrieved from http://www.patientsafetyinstitute.ca/English/About/PatientSafetyForwardWith4/Pages/default.aspx

To decrease risk of errors in the administration of medications, the Institute of Safe Medication Practices (ISMP) developed a list of abbreviations, acronyms, and symbols *not* to use (Table 1-2).

Teamwork and Communication

Situation-Background-Assessment-Recommendation

The **situation-background-assessment-recommendation** (SBAR) technique gives a specific framework for communication among health care providers. SBAR is an easy-to-remember, useful, concrete mechanism for communicating important information that requires a clinician's immediate attention (Trentham et al., 2010) (Table 1-3). Failure to communicate is one of the major reasons for errors in health care. The SBAR technique has the potential to serve as a means to reduce errors.

TABLE 1-2 THE INSTITUTE OF SAFE MEDICATION PRACTICES CANADA (ISMP) "DO NOT USE" LIST

DO NOT USE	POTENTIAL PROBLEM	USE INSTEAD
U (unit)	Mistaken for "0" (zero), the number "4" (four), or "cc"	Use "unit"
IU (International Unit)	Mistaken for IV (intravenous) or the number 10 (ten)	Use "International Unit"
Abbreviations for drug names	Misinterpreted because of similar abbreviations for multiple drugs; e.g., MS, MSO_4 (morphine sulphate), $MgSO_4$ (magnesium sulphate) may be confused for one another	Write drug names in full
QD (daily), QOD (every other day)	Mistaken for one another, or as in "qid." The Q has also been misinterpreted as "2" (two).	Use "daily" or "every other day"
OD (daily)	Mistaken for "right eye" (OD = oculus dexter)	Use "daily"
OS, OD, OU (left eye, right eye, both eyes)	May be confused with one another	Use "left eye", "right eye", or "both eyes"
D/C (discharge)	Interpreted as "discontinue whatever medication follow"	Use "discharge"
µg (microgram)	Mistaken for mg (milligrams) resulting in one thousand-fold overdose	Use "mcg"
cc (cubic centimetre)	Mistaken for U (units) when poorly written	Use "mL" or "millilitres"
Trailing zero (X.0 mg)	Decimal point is overlooked, resulting in 10-fold dose error	Never use a zero by itself after a decimal point. Write "X mg"
Lack of leading zero (.X mg)	Decimal point is overlooked, resulting in 10-fold dose error	Write "0.X mg"
ADDITIONAL ABBREVIATIONS, ACRONYMS, AND SYMBOLS		
> (greater than)	Misinterpreted as the number "7" (seven) or the letter "L"; confused for one another	Use "greater than"
< (less than)		Use "less than"
@	Mistaken for the number "2" (two)	Write "at"

From Institute for Safe Medication Practices Canada (2006). *"Do Not Use" list*, https://www.ismp-canada.org/download/ISMPCanadaListOfDangerousAbbreviations.pdf. Reprinted with permission from ISMP Canada.

TABLE 1-3 SAMPLE SBAR REPORT TO PHYSICIAN ABOUT A CRITICAL SITUATION

S **Situation**
I am calling about Mary Smith.
I have just assessed her and she saturated a peripad in the last hour. Her blood pressure is 112/62, pulse 86, and respirations 18.
I think she is bleeding excessively.

B **Background**
Mrs. Smith is 12 hours postpartum after giving birth vaginally to a 4500 gm term infant after an uncomplicated pregnancy. She had a rapid labour, just over 4 hours, and had no analgesia. She plans to bottle-feed this baby. She had an IV with 10 units of oxytocin, but it was completed and discontinued about 2 hours ago.
This is her sixth birth. All were uncomplicated, and she had an uneventful recovery from them.

A **Assessment**
Her **fundus** becomes firm after massage but relaxes again. She has voided, and her bladder feels empty. I think she might have retained placenta and she needs to be examined.

R **Recommendation**
I would like you to come and examine her immediately.
Do you want her IV restarted?
Do you want her to have an Hb and HCT?

Hb, hemoglobin; *HCT*, hematocrit; *IV*, intravenous infusion; *SBAR*, situation-background-assessment-recommendation.

GLOBAL HEALTH

As the world becomes a smaller place because of travel and communication technologies, nurses and other health care providers are gaining a global perspective and participating in activities to improve the health and health care of people worldwide. Nurses participate in medical outreach; provide obstetrical, surgical, ophthalmological, orthopedic, or other services; attend international meetings; conduct research; and provide international consultation (Fig. 1-2). International student and faculty exchanges occur. More articles about health and health care in various countries are appearing in nursing journals.

Millennium Development Goals: A Global Challenge

The Millennium Development Goals (MDGs) were eight goals to be achieved by 2015 that responded to the world's main development challenges (Box 1-3). The MDGs are drawn from the actions and targets contained in the Millennium Declaration that was adopted by 189 nations and signed by 147 heads of state and governments during the United Nations Millennium Summit in September 2000 (http://www.un.org/millenniumgoals/). These goals were an ambitious pledge to uphold the principles of human dignity, equality, and equity and free the world from extreme poverty. Much work has been done on the MDGs, and they have made a profound difference in the lives of many people across the world (United Nations [UN], 2015). According to the United Nations (2015), global

BOX 1-3 THE UNITED NATIONS MILLENNIUM DEVELOPMENT GOALS

Goal 1—Eradicate extreme poverty and hunger
Goal 2—Achieve universal primary education
Goal 3—Promote gender equality and empower women
Goal 4—Reduce child mortality
Goal 5—Improve maternal health
Goal 6—Combat HIV/AIDS*, malaria, and other diseases
Goal 7—Ensure environmental sustainability
Goal 8—Develop a global partnership for development

**AIDS*, acquired immunodeficiency syndrome; *HIV*, human immunodeficiency virus.
From *Millennium Development Goals: 2011 Progress Chart*, by Statistics Division, Department of Economic and Social Affairs, United Nations, © 2011 United Nations. Reprinted with the permission of the United Nations.

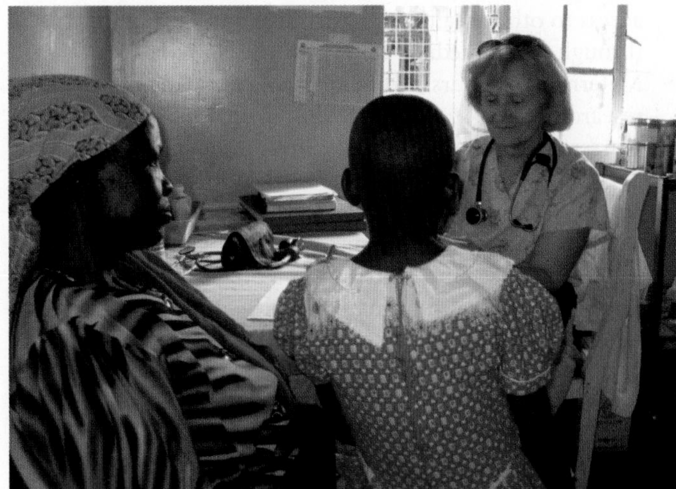

FIGURE 1-2 Nurse interviewing a young girl accompanied by her mother in a clinic in rural Kenya. (Courtesy of Shannon Perry.)

poverty has been halved; 90% of children in developing regions now enjoy primary education, and disparities between boys and girls in enrollment have narrowed; there are decreased rates of malaria and tuberculosis; the likelihood of a child dying before age 5 has been nearly cut in half over the last two decades; the number of people who do not have access to good water sources has been halved. Despite the significant gains that have been made for many of the MDG targets worldwide, the progress has been uneven across regions and countries, leaving significant gaps (UN, 2015). The post-2015 agenda goal is to build on the success and momentum of the MDGs; new global goals will break fresh ground to address inequalities, economic growth, decent jobs, cities and human settlements, industrialization, energy, climate change, sustainable consumption and production, and peace and justice (UN, 2015).

In 2010, with the signature of the Muskoka Accord, the Canadian government promised to assist developing countries in addressing health inequities that affect mothers and infants (Government of Canada, 2014). With its additional $1.1-billion commitment to maternal, newborn, and child health, Canada's total commitment to reducing child mortality (MDG 4) and improving maternal health (MDG 5) was $2.85 billion from 2010 to 2015 (Government of Canada, 2015).

Increasingly, Canadian nurses are working internationally in global health settings. This role is supported by the CNA (2011), which believes that nurses have the right and the responsibility to contribute to the advancement of global health and equity.

ETHICAL ISSUES IN MATERNAL CHILD NURSING

Ethical concerns and debates have multiplied with the increased use of technology and scientific advances. Nurses may face ethical issues regarding patient care, such as the use of life-saving measures for very low birth weight (VLBW) newborns or the terminally ill child's right to refuse treatment. They may struggle with questions involving truthfulness, balancing their rights and responsibilities in caring for children with AIDS, whistle-blowing, or allocating resources.

Ethical dilemmas arise when competing moral considerations underlie various alternatives. Parents, nurses, physicians, and other health care team members may reach different but morally defensible decisions by assigning different weight to the competing moral values. These competing moral values may include *autonomy*, the patient's right to be self-governing; *nonmaleficence*, the obligation to minimize or prevent harm; *beneficence*, the obligation to promote the patient's well-being; and *justice*, the concept of fairness. Nurses are important role models for demonstrating how to create an environment of mutual respect and understanding for patients and their families. Respect for the individuals they care for is the affirmation that other persons matter in the same way as the nurses themselves.

Nurses must prepare themselves systematically for collaborative ethical decision making. This can be accomplished through taking formal coursework and continuing education, reading contemporary literature, and working to establish an environment conducive to ethical discourse. Moreover, nurses need to be educated in the mechanisms for dispute resolution, case review by **ethics** committees, procedural safeguards, Canadian legislation, and case law.

The nurse can also use the professional code of ethics for guidance and as a means for professional self-regulation. The *Code of Ethics for Registered Nurses*, by the CNA, provides the framework and core responsibilities for nursing practice. The *Code of Ethics* focuses on the nurse's accountability and responsibility to the patient (CNA, 2008) and emphasizes the nursing role as an independent professional, one that upholds its own legal liability (see Additional Resources).

Ethical Guidelines for Nursing Research

Research with women and children may create ethical dilemmas for the nurse. For example, participating in research may cause additional stress for a woman concerned about outcomes of genetic testing or for one who is waiting for an invasive procedure. Obtaining amniotic fluid samples or performing cordocentesis poses risks to the fetus (see Chapter 13). Research on children must be conducted in ways that ensure informed consent of parents and for children, when possible (see Chapter 44, Consent for health research in children). Nurses must protect the rights of human participants in all research; women and children are already vulnerable, so they need to be reassured that their rights are being protected. For example, nurses may need to collect data on or care for patients who are participating in clinical trials. The nurse should ensure that the participants are fully informed and aware of their rights as participants. The nurse may be involved in determining whether the benefits of research outweigh the risks to the mother and her fetus or to children and needs to ensure that all research conducted has been approved by the appropriate research ethics board.

KEY POINTS

- Perinatal nursing focuses on caring for women and their families throughout the child-bearing year, and pediatric nurses care for children from birth to 18 years of age.
- Nurses can play an active role in shaping health policy and health systems to be responsive to the needs of Canadian women and children.
- The social determinants of health have an impact on the health of all people.
- Of the determinants of health, poverty remains the most important factor resulting in conditions of vulnerability such as homelessness.
- Women and children living in rural, remote, and Indigenous communities and in poverty in inner cities experience significant health challenges.
- Nurses must provide comprehensive, respectful care to all people, and knowledge about different cultural and diversity issues will assist in providing this care.
- Indigenous patients have unique health care issues that require health care providers to understand the historical context and impact of the social determinants of health.
- LGBTQ patients require health care providers that understand their specific health care needs.
- Integrative healing combines modern technology with ancient healing practices and encompasses the whole body, mind, and spirit.
- Technology has had a tremendous influence on health care through use of high-technology care modalities as well as access to other health care providers and to patients through social media.
- Maternal child nursing practice is increasingly informed by research.
- Nurses must ensure that safe care is provided to women and children by following safe medication practices and communicating with other members of the health care team in a manner that ensures clear understanding.
- At a global level, the Millennium Development Goals have improved the health of many people worldwide, although much work still needs to be done to reduce poverty, promote gender equality, and improve maternal and child health.
- Ethical concerns have multiplied with the increasing use of technology and scientific advances.

evolve WEBSITE

Visit the Evolve website for additional resources related to the content in this chapter such as Case Studies, Critical Thinking Case Study Answers, Nursing Care Plans, Nursing Processes, Nursing Skills, and Review Questions for Exam Preparation at: http://evolve.elsevier.com/Canada/Perry/maternal/

REFERENCES

American College of Obstetricians and Gynecologists, Committee on Healthcare for Underserved Women. (2011). Healthcare for transgendered individuals. Committee Opinion No. 512. *Obstetrics and Gynecology, 118*, 1454–1458. Retrieved from <http://www.acog.org/Resources-And-Publications/Committee-Opinions/Committee-on-Health-Care-for-Underserved-Women/Health-Care-for-Transgender-Individuals>.

Baker, G. R., Norton, P. G., Flintoft, V., et al. (2004). The Canadian adverse events study: The incidence of adverse events among hospital patients in Canada. *Canadian Medical Association Journal, 170*(11), 1678–1686.

Canadian Council on Learning. (2008). *Health literacy in Canada: A healthy understanding*. Ottawa: Author. Retrieved from <https://www.bth.se/hal/halsoteknik.nsf/bilagor/HealthLiteracyReportFeb2008E_pdf/$file/HealthLiteracyReportFeb2008E.pdf>.

Canadian Nurses Association. (2008). *Code of ethics for registered nurses*. Ottawa: Author. Retrieved from <http://www.cna-aiic.ca/~/media/cna/files/en/codeofethics.pdf>.

Canadian Nurses Association. (2011). *Position Statement: Global health partnerships*. Ottawa: Author. Retrieved March 5, 2015, from <http://www.cna-aiic.ca/~/media/cna/page-content/pdf-en/ps115_global_health_partnerships_2011_e.pdf?la=en>.

Canadian Nurses Association. (2013). *Position Statement: Social determinants of health*. Ottawa: Author. Retrieved from <http://www.cna-aiic.ca/~/media/cna/files/en/ps124_social_determinants_of_health_e.pdf?la=en>.

Canadian Patient Safety Institute. (2010). *The economics of patient safety in acute care: Technical report*. Ottawa: Author. Retrieved from <http://www.patientsafetyinstitute.ca/en/toolsResources/Research/commissionedResearch/EconomicsofPatientSafety/Documents/Economics%20of%20

Patient%20Safety%20-%20Acute%20Care%20-%20Final%20Report .pdf>.

Canadian Patient Safety Institute. (2011). *Canadian disclosure guidelines: Being open and honest with patients and families*. Edmonton, AB: Canadian Patient Safety Institute.

Denburg, A., & Daneman, D. (2010). The link between social inequality and child health outcomes. *Healthcare Quarterly, 14*, 21–31.

Duffy, M. (2011). Facebook, Twitter, and LinkedIn, Oh My! *American Journal of Nursing, 111*(4), 56–59.

Gaetz, S., Donaldson, J., Richter, T., & Gulliver, T. (2013). *The state of homelessness in Canada 2013*. Toronto: Canadian Homelessness Research Network Press. Retrieved from <http://www.wellesleyinstitute.com/wp-content/uploads/2013/06/SOHC2103.pdf>.

Government of Canada. (2014). *The Muskoka initiative: Background*. Retrieved from <http://mnch.international.gc.ca/en/topics/leadership-muskoka_background.html>.

Government of Canada. (2015). *Millennium development goals*. Ottawa: Author. Retrieved from <http://www.international.gc.ca/development-developpement/priorities-priorites/mdg-omd.aspx?lang=eng>.

MacDonald, D., & Wilson, D. (2013). *Poverty or prosperity: Indigenous children in Canada*. Ottawa: Canadian Centre for Policy Alternatives. Retrieved from: <https://www.policyalternatives.ca/sites/default/files/uploads/publications/National%20Office/2013/06/Poverty_or_Prosperity_Indigenous_Children.pdf>.

MacKinnon, K. (2006). Living with the threat of preterm labour: Women's work of keeping the baby in. *Journal of Obstetrical Gynecologic and Neonatal Nursing, 35*(6), 700–708.

Pauly, B., MacKinnon, K., & Varcoe, C. (2009). Revisiting "Who gets care?": Health equity as an arena for nursing action. *Advances in Nursing Science, 32*(2), 118–127.

Public Health Agency of Canada. (1986). *Ottawa charter for health promotion*. Ottawa: Author. Retrieved from <http://www.phac-aspc.gc.ca/ph-sp/docs/charter-chartre/pdf/charter.pdf>.

Public Health Agency of Canada. (2011). *What determines health?* Ottawa: Author. Retrieved from <http://www.phac-aspc.gc.ca/ph-sp/determinants/index-eng.php>.

Public Health Agency of Canada. (2014). *Health literacy*. Ottawa: Author. Retrieved from <http://www.phac-aspc.gc.ca/cd-mc/hl-ls/index-eng.php>.

Rainbow Health Ontario. (2014). *About LGBTQ health*. Retrieved from <http://www.rainbowhealthontario.ca/about-lgbtq-health/>.

Saver, C. (2010). *Social responsibility: Social media opportunities and pitfalls*. Retrieved from <https://news.nurse.com/2010/08/09/social-responsibility-social-media-opportunities-and-pitfalls/>.

Statistics Canada. (2010). *The ethnocultural diversity of the Canadian population*. Catalogue no. 89-638-X no. 2010004. Ottawa: Author. Retrieved from <http://www.statcan.gc.ca/pub/91-551-x/2010001/hl-fs-eng.htm>.

Statistics Canada. (2013a). *Low income lines: 2011-2012*. Ottawa: Author. Retrieved from <http://www.statcan.gc.ca/pub/75f0002m/75f0002m2013002-eng.htm>.

Statistics Canada. (2013b). *The daily*. Ottawa: Author. Retrieved from <http://www.statcan.gc.ca/daily-quotidien/130627/dq130627-eng.pdf>.

Statistics Canada. (2013c). *Projections of the diversity of the Canadian population, 2006–2031*. Ottawa: Author. Retrieved from <http://www.statcan.gc.ca/pub/91-551-x/91-551-x2010001-eng.htm>.

Statistics Canada. (2014). *Aboriginal peoples in Canada: First Nations people, Métis, and Inuit*. Ottawa: Author. Retrieved from <http://www12.statcan.gc.ca/nhs-enm/2011/as-sa/99-011-x/99-011-x2011001-eng.cfm>.

Trentham, B., Andreoli, A., Boaro, N., et al. (2010). *SBAR: A shared structure for effective team communication. An implementation toolkit* (2nd ed.). Toronto: Toronto Rehabilitation Institute. Retrieved from <http://www.uhn.ca/TorontoRehab/Education/SBAR/Documents/SBAR_Toolkit.pdf>.

Truth and Reconciliation Commission of Canada. (2012). *Truth and Reconciliation Commission of Canada: Interim report*. Retrieved from <http://www.myrobust.com/websites/trcinstitution/File/Interim%20report%20English%20electronic.pdf>.

Truth and Reconciliation Commission of Canada. (2015). *Truth and Reconciliation Commission of Canada: Calls to Action*. Retrieved from <http://www.trc.ca/websites/trcinstitution/File/2015/Findings/Calls_to_Action_English2.pdf>.

United Nations. (2015). *The millennium development goals report: 2015*. New York: Author. Retrieved from <http://www.un.org/millenniumgoals/2015_MDG_Report/pdf/MDG%202015%20rev%20%28July%201%29.pdf>.

ADDITIONAL RESOURCES

Alberta Health Services Healthlink. <http://www.albertahealthservices.ca/default.aspx>

Association of Ontario Midwives: Tip Sheet for Providing Care to Trans Men and All "Trans Masculine Spectrum" Clients. <http://www.rainbowhealthontario.ca/wp-content/uploads/woocommerce_uploads/2014/08/Midwives%20-%20Tip%20sheet%20for%20working%20with%20trans%20clients.pdf>.

Canadian Nurses Association certification process. <https://nurseone.ca/certification>

Canadian Nurses Association. Code of Ethics for Registered Nurses. <https://www.cna-aiic.ca/en/on-the-issues/best-nursing/nursing-ethics>

Healthlink BC. <http://www.healthlinkbc.ca/>

Poverty Trends Highlights 2013. <http://www.cpj.ca/files/docs/Poverty-Trends-Highlights-2013.pdf>

Public Health Agency of Canada Determinants of Health. <http://www.phac-aspc.gc.ca/ph-sp/determinants/index-eng.php#determinants>

Rainbow Health Ontario Resource Database—Reliable, up-to-date health resources to LGBTQ communities, service providers, and others with an interest in LGBTQ health. <http://www.rainbowhealthontario.ca/resource-search/>

Truth and Reconciliation Commission Canada. <http://www.trc.ca/websites/trcinstitution/index.php?p=3>

United Nations—Millennium Development Goals and Beyond 2015. <http://www.un.org/millenniumgoals/>

Upstream—Addresses the social determinants of health in order to build a healthier society. <http://www.thinkupstream.net/>

CHAPTER

2

The Family and Culture

Lisa Keenan-Lindsay

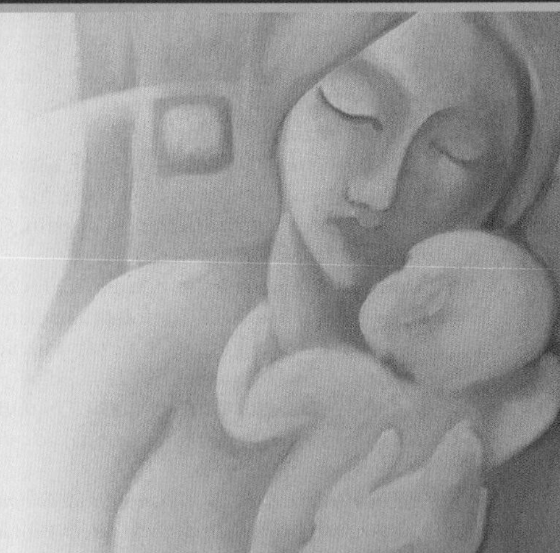

evolve WEBSITE

***Visit the Evolve website for additional resources related to the content in this chapter such as Case Studies, Critical Thinking Case Study Answers, Nursing Care Plans, Nursing Processes, Nursing Skills, and Review Questions for Exam Preparation at:** http://evolve.elsevier.com/Canada/Perry/maternal/*

OBJECTIVES

On completion of this chapter the reader will be able to:

- Describe the variety of family forms encountered by nurses in Canada today.
- Use the collaborative family-centred health framework to identify factors influencing family health.
- Explore and describe theories developed as guides to family nursing in Canada.
- Describe how different lenses contribute to our understanding of family health promotion.
- Explore and discuss how culture, broadly defined, influences the experiences of individuals and their families.
- Define culture, cultural safety, ethnocentrism, and cultural relativism.
- Describe the subcultural influences of socioeconomic status, poverty, religion, and schools on health.
- Describe what is meant by cultural competence and cultural respect and reflect on how this will influence nursing practice.
- Explore ways to provide culturally responsive nursing care.

THE FAMILY IN CULTURAL AND COMMUNITY CONTEXT

The family plays an important role in defining the work of perinatal and pediatric nurses. Despite modern stresses and strains, the family still forms a social network that acts as a potent support system for its members. Family care-seeking behaviour and relationships with providers are influenced by culturally related health beliefs and values. Ultimately, all of these factors have the power to affect maternal and child health outcomes. The current emphasis in working with families is on wellness and on empowerment of families to achieve control over their lives. Family-centred care treats the family as the unit of care delivery. Because the Canadian population has become increasingly diverse in terms of culture, ethnicity, and socioeconomic status, it is essential that nurses become culturally competent in order to provide the most appropriate care possible.

The Family in Society

The social context for the family can be viewed in relation to social and demographic trends that define the population as a whole. Each family sets up boundaries between itself and society. People are conscious of the difference between "family members" and "outsiders," or people without kinship status. Some families isolate themselves from the outside community; others have a wide community network that they can turn to in times of stress. Although boundaries exist for every family, family members set up channels through which they interact with society.

Defining Family

The family has traditionally been viewed as the primary unit of socialization—the basic structural unit within a community. The family plays a pivotal role in health care and is often the primary target of health care delivery for many nurses. As one of society's most important institutions, the family represents a primary social group that influences and is influenced by other people and institutions. A variety of family configurations exist.

The term **family** has been defined in many different ways according to the individual's own frame of reference, value judgement, or discipline. There is no universal definition of family; a family is what an individual considers it to be. Biologists describe the family as fulfilling the biological function of perpetuation of the species. Psychologists emphasize interpersonal aspects of family and its responsibility for personality development. Economists view the family as a productive unit providing for material needs. In sociology, the family is depicted as a social unit interacting with the larger society, creating contexts within which cultural values and identity are formed. Others define family in terms of the relationships of the persons who make up the family units. Some of the common types of family relationships are *consanguineous* (blood relationships), *affinal* (marital relationships), and *family of origin* (family unit a person is born into).

Earlier definitions of family emphasized that family members were related by legal ties or genetic relationships and lived in the same household with specific roles. Later definitions have been broadened to reflect structural and functional changes. A family can be defined as an institution in which individuals, related through biology or enduring commitments and representing similar or different generations and genders, participate in roles involving mutual socialization, nurturance, and emotional commitment.

Family Organization and Structure

Individuals define their own family and support system by choosing who is included and who is excluded. The definition of family may include one person or many different people (see Table 2-1). This may include parents, siblings, grandparents, partners, aunts and uncles, or friends.

The **nuclear family** has long represented the traditional North American family in which male and female partners and their children live as an independent unit sharing roles, responsibilities, and economic resources (Fig. 2-1). In contemporary society, this family structure actually represents a relatively small number of families, and that number is steadily decreasing. *Married-parent families* (biological or adoptive parents) make up 67% of Canadian families and this number has been steadily decreasing. *Common-law families* are those in which children live with two unmarried biological parents or two adoptive parents. The number of common-law families is steadily increasing; in 2011 the percentage of these families was 16.7% (Statistics Canada, 2014).

Multigenerational or extended families, consisting of grandparents, children, and grandchildren living in the same household, are becoming increasingly common (Fig. 2-2). In 2011, 45% of children under 14 lived with a grandparent in their home (Statistics Canada, 2014). This may create stress, as children must care for their parents as well as their own children. In other instances, the grandparents support the children and grandchildren or are sole caregivers for the grandchildren. For some groups such as Indigenous peoples, the family network is an important resource for promoting health and healing.

TABLE 2-1 DEFINITIONS OF FAMILY

TYPE OF FAMILY	DESCRIPTION
Nuclear	Male and female parent with children
Married-parent families	Biological or adoptive parents
Common-law families	Unmarried biological or adoptive parents
Multigenerational or extended family	Grandparents, children, and grandchildren living in same house
Married-blended families	Unrelated family members join to make a new household as result of death/divorce and remarriage
Lone-parent families	Unmarried biological or adoptive parent who may or may not be living with other adults. May be planned or unplanned
Same-sex parent families	May be married or common-law

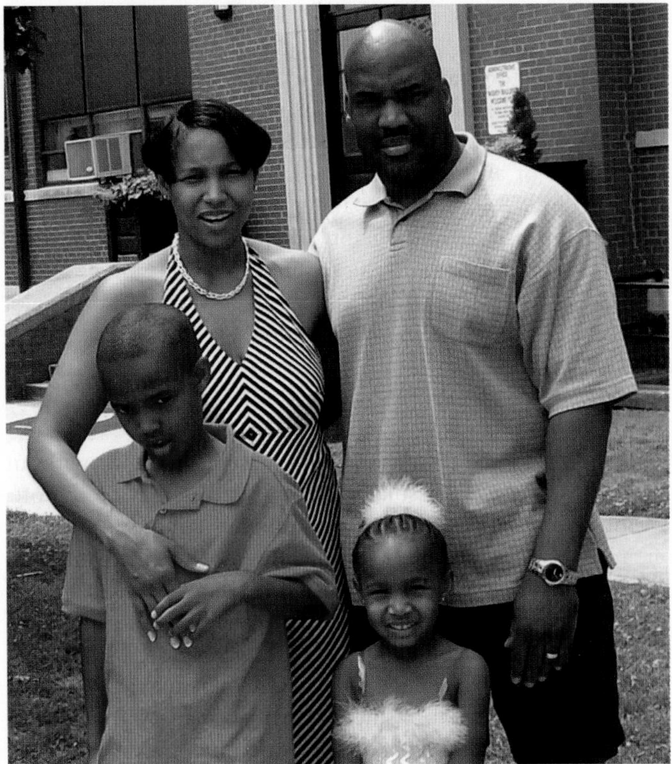

FIGURE 2-1 Nuclear family. (Courtesy Makeba Felton.)

Married-blended families, those formed as a result of divorce and remarriage, consist of unrelated family members (stepparents, stepchildren, and stepsiblings) who join to create a new household. These family groups frequently involve a biological or adoptive parent whose spouse may or may not have adopted the child.

Lone-parent families comprise an unmarried biological or adoptive parent who may or may not be living with other adults. The lone-parent family may result from the loss of a spouse by death, divorce, separation, or desertion; from either

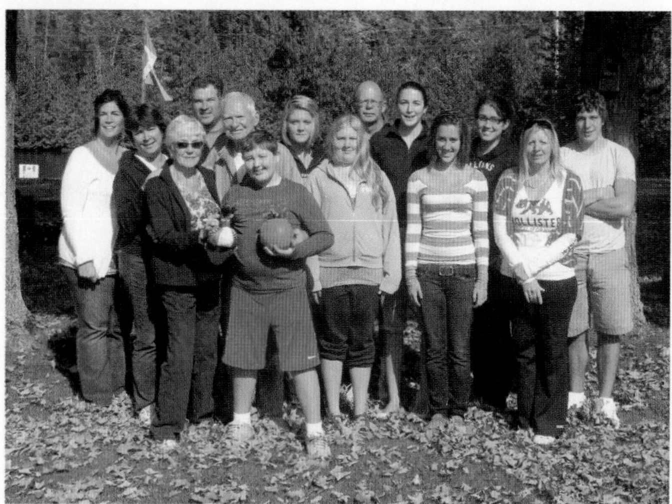

FIGURE 2-2 Extended (multigenerational) family. (Courtesy Lisa Keenan-Lindsay.)

an unplanned or planned pregnancy; or from the adoption of a child by an unmarried woman or man. This family structure has become common, with Statistics Canada (2014) reporting that 16.3% of all census families in 2011 were a lone-parent family. About 8 in 10 lone-parent families were female lone-parent families, accounting for 12.8% of all census families, while male lone-parent families represented 3.5% of all census families. This gender difference is significant because female-headed lone-parent families are more likely to have lower incomes and to experience poverty than male lone-parent families, which in turn can affect the health status of family members.

Same-sex couple families may live together with or without children. Children in lesbian and gay families may be the offspring of previous heterosexual unions, conceived by one member of a lesbian couple through therapeutic insemination, or adopted. Overall, same-sex couples accounted for 0.8% of all couples in Canada in 2011; this number has tripled since 2006. In 2011, same-sex couples in Canada were more likely to be male (54.5%) than female (45.5%), whether married or living in a common-law relationship (Statistics Canada, 2014). Transgendered couples also form families and often become parents, either through the use of fertility drugs, adoption, or transmen discontinuing the hormones they are taking so they can become pregnant themselves.

Family Dynamics

Ideally, the family uses its resources to provide a safe, intimate, and nurturing environment that supports the biopsychosocial development of family members. The family provides for the nurturing and socialization of children. Children form their earliest and closest relationships with their parents or parenting persons; these affiliations continue throughout a lifetime. Parent–child relationships may influence self-worth and the ability to form later relationships. The family also influences the child's perceptions of the outside world. The family provides the growing child with an identity that has both a past and a sense of the future. Cultural beliefs, values, and rituals are passed from one generation to the next through the family.

Over time, the family develops protocols for problem-solving, particularly those regarding important decisions such as having a baby or buying a house. The criteria used in making decisions are based on family values and attitudes about the appropriateness of the behaviour and the moral, social, political, and economic events of society. The power to make critical decisions is given to a family member through tradition or negotiation. All families have strengths and the potential for growth. It is important for the nurse to identify those strengths and potential in order to facilitate the growth of the family (Black & Lobo, 2008).

FAMILY NURSING

Family plays a pivotal role in health care, representing the primary target of health care delivery for perinatal and pediatric nurses. In treating the family with respect and dignity, health care providers listen to and honour perspectives and choices of the family. They share information with families in ways that are positive, useful, timely, complete, and accurate. The family is supported in participating in the care and decision making at the level of their choice.

Because so many variables affect ways of relating, the nurse must be aware that family members may interact and communicate with each other in ways that are distinct from those of the nurse's own family of origin. Families may hold some beliefs about health that are different from those of the nurse. Their beliefs can conflict with principles of health care management predominant in the Western health care system. Nurses must learn to incorporate these beliefs into the care that is provided.

Theories as Guides to Understanding and Working With Families

A **family theory** can be used to describe families and how the family unit responds to events both within and outside the family. Each family theory makes certain assumptions about the family and has inherent strengths and limitations. Most nurses use a combination of theories in their work with families. A brief synopsis of several theories useful in working with families is included in Table 2-2. Application of these concepts can guide assessment and interventions for the family and can be used when providing care in many perinatal and pediatric situations.

Family Assessment

When selecting a family assessment framework it is important to assess the focus of nursing care. An appropriate model for a perinatal nurse is one that is health promoting rather than an illness-care model. The family can be assisted in fostering a healthy pregnancy, childbirth, and integration of the newborn into the family. Women experiencing perinatal health challenges or conditions of vulnerability (e.g., poverty) or families with ill children have additional needs that the nurse may need to address while also promoting the health of the family.

TABLE 2-2 THEORIES AND MODELS RELEVANT TO FAMILY NURSING PRACTICE

THEORY	SYNOPSIS OF THEORY
Family Systems Theory (Wright & Leahy, 2013)	The family is viewed as a unit, and interactions among family members are studied rather than studying individuals. A family system is part of a larger suprasystem and is composed of many subsystems. The family as a whole is greater than the sum of its individual members. A change in one family member affects all family members. The family is able to create a balance between change and stability. Family members' behaviours are best understood from a view of circular rather than linear causality.
Family Life Cycle (Developmental) Theory (Carter & McGoldrick, 1999)	Families move through stages. The family life cycle is the context in which to examine the identity and development of the individual. Relationships among family members go through transitions. Although families have roles and functions, a family's main value is in relationships that are irreplaceable. The family involves different structures and cultures organized in various ways. Developmental stresses may disrupt the life cycle process.
Family Stress Theory (Boss, 2002)	This theory is concerned with ways families react to stressful events. Family stress can be studied within the internal and external contexts in which the family is living. The internal context involves elements that a family can change or control, such as family structure, psychological defences, and philosophical values and beliefs. The external context consists of the time and place in which a particular family finds itself and over which the family has no control, such as the culture of the larger society, the time in history, the economic state of society, the maturity of the individuals involved, the success of the family in coping with stressors, and genetic inheritance.
McGill Model of Nursing (Allen, 1997)	This model of situation-responsive nursing has a strength-based focus in clinical practice with families rather than a deficit approach. Identification of family strengths and resources, provision of feedback about strengths, and assistance given to the family to develop and elicit strengths and use resources are key interventions. The McGill model is particularly relevant for working with child-bearing families, as pregnancy can be considered a "teachable moment" for promoting the health of the entire family.
The Collaborative Partnership Approach (Gottlieb & Feeley, 2006)	This model builds on the McGill model of nursing and more fully develops a collaborative partnership approach to family nursing. A collaborative partnership is defined as "the pursuit of person-centred goals through a dynamic process that requires the active participation and agreement of all partners." Features of a collaborative partnership include mutual identification of an agreement on goals; sharing expertise and power; being respectful, accepting, and nonjudgemental; being open to learning together and learning to live with ambiguity; and being reflective and self-aware.

The Calgary Family Assessment Model

A family assessment tool such as the Calgary Family Assessment Model (CFAM) (Box 2-1) can be used as a guide for assessing aspects of the family. Such an assessment is based on "the nurse's personal and professional life experiences, beliefs, and relationships with those being interviewed" (Wright & Leahy, 2013) and is not "the truth" about the family but, rather, one perspective at one point in time.

The CFAM consists of three major categories: structural, developmental, and functional. There are several subcategories within each category. The three assessment categories and the many subcategories can be conceptualized as a branching diagram (Fig. 2-3). These categories and subcategories can be used to guide the assessment that will provide data to help the nurse better understand the family and formulate a plan of care. The nurse asks questions of family members about themselves to gain understanding of the structure, development, and function of the family at this point in time. Not all questions within the subcategories should be asked at the first interview, and some questions may not be appropriate for all families. Although individuals are the ones interviewed, the focus of the assessment is on interaction of individuals within the family.

Graphic Representations of Families

A *family genogram*, which is a family-tree format depicting relationships of family members over at least three generations (Fig. 2-4), provides valuable information about a family and can be placed in the nursing care plan for easy access by care providers. An *ecomap*, a graphic portrayal of social relationships of the individual and family, may also help the nurse understand the social environment of the family and identify support systems available to them (Fig. 2-5). Software is available to generate genograms and ecomaps (http://www.interpersonaluniverse.net).

Family Nursing as Relational Inquiry

Relational nursing challenges nursing practices based on structured assessment frameworks and proposes that nurses need to be "in relation" with patients and family members, taking cues from the family and collaboratively identifying capacity and adversity patterns and building knowledge together for health promotion (Doane & Varcoe, 2015). It recognizes that families are socially located in historical, cultural, and environmental contexts and that these factors have a significant impact on family members' experiences of health and child-bearing. Relational nursing moves beyond a health service provision approach toward one that recognizes the determinants of health and is more congruent with health promotion (Box 2-2).

This approach is understood as a process of inquiry, and it is this structure or process that forms the framework for thoughtful, interpretive, critical, and spiritual inquiry. Nurses learn together with the family members about what matters most to them, about family strengths and health challenges, and about how to work toward better health for the family.

BOX 2-1 CALGARY FAMILY ASSESSMENT MODEL

There are three major categories of the Calgary Family Assessment Model (CFAM)—structural, developmental, and functional. Each category has several subcategories. In this box, only the major categories are included. A few sample questions are included.

Structural Assessment

- Determine the members of the family, relationship among family members, and context of family.
- Genograms and ecomaps (see Figs. 2-4, 2-5) are useful in outlining the internal and external structures of a family.

Sample Questions

- Who are the members of your family?
- Has anyone moved in or out lately?
- Are there any family members who don't live with you?
- What impact did your parents' ideas have on your own ideas of masculinity and femininity?
- How many times have you moved in the past 5 years?

Developmental Assessment

- Describe the developmental life cycle for each family.

Sample Questions

- Which of your parents is most accepting of your career plans?
- What percentage of your time do you spend taking care of your children?
- What percentage of your time do you spend taking care of your marriage?
- When you think back, what do you most enjoy about your life?
- What do you regret about your life?
- Have you made plans for your care as your health declines?

Functional Assessment

- Evaluate the way in which individuals behave in relation to each other in instrumental and expressive aspects. (Instrumental aspects are activities of daily living; expressive aspects include communication, problem-solving, roles, etc.)

Sample Questions

- Who in your family shows the most distress when your father is drinking?
- To whom do most of you go when you need someone to talk to?
- Which one of the family is best at ensuring that your grandmother takes her medicine?

Data from Wright, L. M., & Leahy, M. (2013). *Nurses and families: A guide to family assessment and intervention* (6th ed.). Philadelphia: FA Davis.

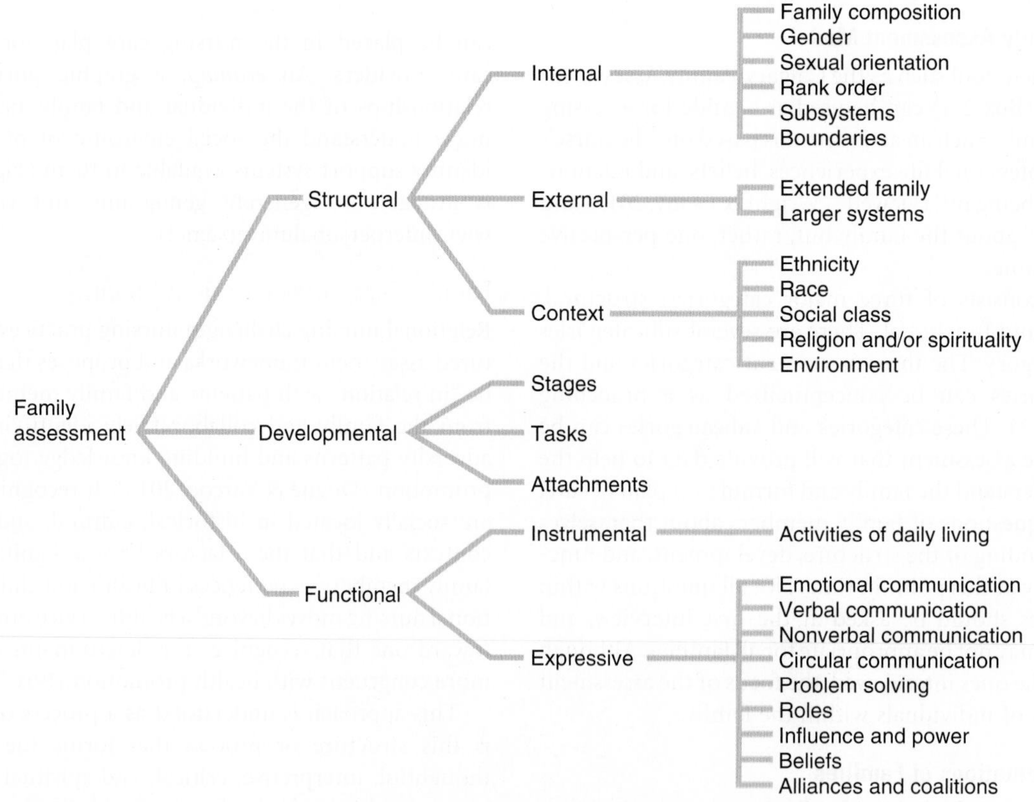

FIGURE 2-3 Branching diagram of Calgary Family Assessment Model (CFAM). (From Leahy, M. & Lorraine, W. [2013]. *Nurses and families: A guide to family assessment and intervention* [6th ed.]. Philadelphia: FA Davis, with permission.)

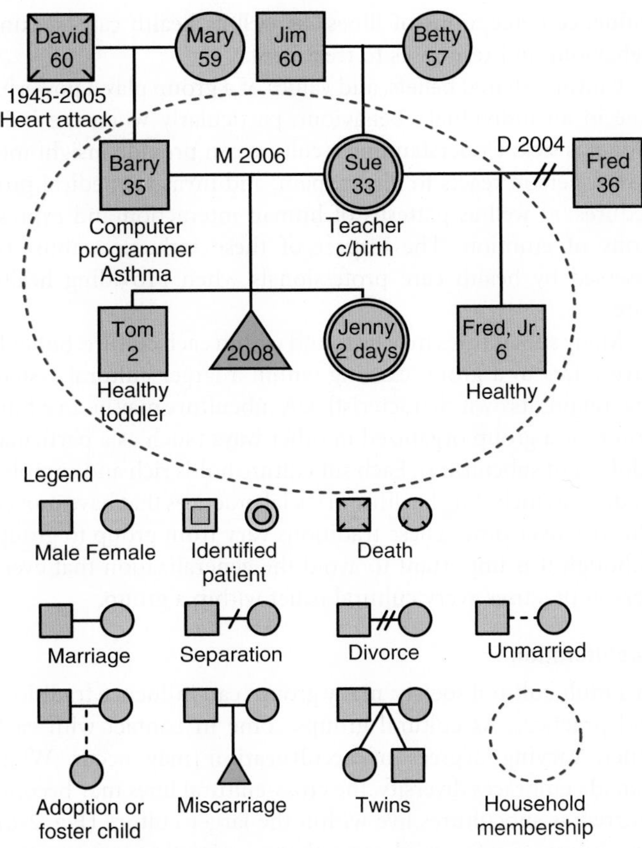

FIGURE 2-4 Example of a family genogram.

> **BOX 2-2 RELATIONAL NURSING PRACTICE: ASSESSING AND INTERVENING PROCESSES**
>
> 1. Entering into relation: Getting "in sync" with a family
> 2. Being in collaborative relation: Working together to assess and intervene
> 3. Inquiring into family health and healing experiences: What is meaningful and significant to the family?
> 4. Following the lead of families: Beginning from an unknowing stance, for example, one of curiosity and acceptance of diversity
> 5. Listening to and for: Listening by using the four lenses or perspectives described above
> 6. Self-observation: Reflecting on how you are "in relation" with this particular family right now
> 7. Letting be and change: Creating the opportunity for the family to discover their own patterns, capacities, challenges, and contextual constraints as a foundation for change
> 8. Collaborative knowledge development: Drawing on both family and nursing knowledge
> 9. Pattern recognition: Identifying underlying patterns of experience that influence health and well-being and possibilities for change
> 10. Naming and supporting capacity: Building upon family strengths
> 11. Emancipatory action: Naming health inequities and working together to address structural inequalities (social justice lens)

Adapted from Doane, G., & Varcoe, C. (2005). *Family nursing as relational inquiry*. Philadelphia: Lippincott, Williams & Wilkins.

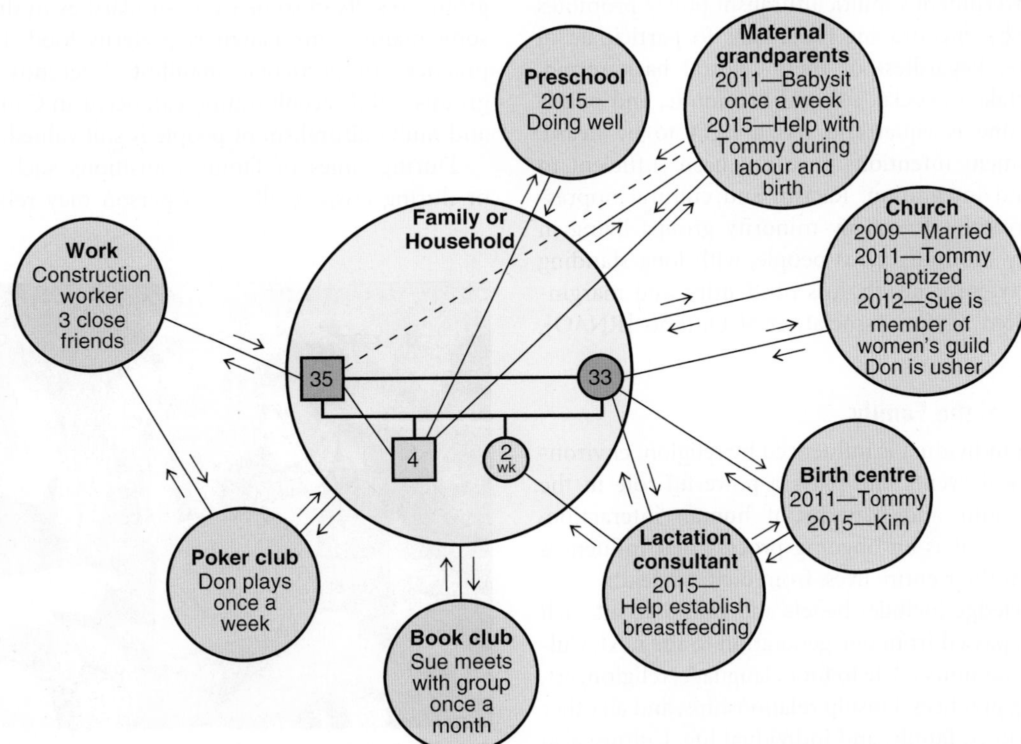

FIGURE 2-5 Example of an ecomap. An ecomap describes social relationships and depicts available supports.

This approach also considers the family from four lenses or perspectives: (1) a phenomenological lens, (2) a sociopolitical lens, (3) a spiritual lens, and (4) a socioenvironmental health promotion perspective. The phenomenological lens cues the nurse to learn more about the family members' experiences of health and illness. How does the family view illness? What do they do to enhance wellness? What is meaningful and significant to the family? The sociopolitical lens attends to power and gender, class, ethnic, racial, and professional relationships. The spiritual lens reminds us that health (e.g., child-bearing or child-rearing) has particular personal, cultural, and religious meanings and significance. A socioenvironmental perspective on health promotion is an understanding of health and health promotion that focuses on the family in their environmental context. It reminds nurses that nursing assessment and intervention are primarily about supporting individuals' and family choices and the capacity to live healthy, meaningful lives within their particular personal, physical or material, and social context.

CULTURAL FACTORS RELATED TO HEALTH

Multiculturalism in Canada

In 1971, Canada adopted multiculturalism as an official policy that confirmed the following:

- The value and dignity of all Canadians, regardless of their racial or ethnic origins, their language, or their religious affiliations
- The rights of Indigenous peoples
- The status of Canada's two official languages: French and English

The Canadian government's multiculturalism policy promotes multiculturalism by encouraging Canadians to participate in all aspects of life. Regardless of their cultural background, everyone can partake in social, cultural, economic, and political affairs. Everyone is equal and has a right to be heard. However, government intentions have not been sufficient to achieve equity and integration. Racism and cultural oppression have been realities for many minority groups living in Canada, especially the Indigenous people, with long-standing impacts of poverty, poor health, loss of identity, and marginalization (Registered Nurses Association of Ontario [RNAO], 2007).

Cultural Context of the Family

The culture of an individual is influenced by religion, environment, and historical events and plays a powerful role in the individual's behaviour and patterns of human interaction. Culture is not static; it is an ongoing process that influences people throughout their entire lives, from birth to death.

Cultural knowledge includes beliefs and values about each facet of life and is passed from one generation to the next. Cultural beliefs and traditions relate to food, language, religion, art, health and healing practices, kinship relationships, and all other aspects of community, family, and individual life. Culture also has been shown to have a direct effect on health behaviours. Values, attitudes, and beliefs that are culturally acquired may influence perceptions of illness as well as health care–seeking behaviour and responses to treatment.

Culture, shared beliefs, and values of a group play a powerful role in an individual's behaviour, particularly when the individual is sick. Understanding a culture can provide insight into how a person reacts to illness, pain, and invasive medical procedures, as well as patterns of human interaction and expressions of emotion. The impact of these influences must be assessed by health care professionals when providing health care.

Many subcultures may be found within each culture. Subculture refers to a group existing within a larger cultural system that retains its own characteristics. A subculture may be an ethnic group or a group organized in other ways (such as a particular adolescent subculture). Each subculture holds rich and complex traditions, including health and social practices that have proven effective over time. These traditions vary from group to group, although it is important to avoid the generalization that every person practises every cultural belief within a group.

Acculturation

In a multicultural society, many groups can influence traditions and practices. As cultural groups come in contact with each other, varying degrees of acculturation may occur. While Canada embraces diversity, the cross-cultural lines may become blurred as subcultures live within the larger culture (Fig. 2-6). Acculturation refers to changes that occur within one group or among several groups when people from different cultures come in contact with one another. People may retain some of their own culture while adopting some of the cultural practices of the dominant society. This familiarization among cultural groups results in some overt similarities in dress, lifestyle, and some mannerisms. Language patterns, food choices, and health practices in particular manifest differently among cultural groups. While acculturation can occur in Canada, the diversity and multiculturalism of people is still valued.

During times of family transitions such as child-bearing or during crisis or illness, a person may rely on old cultural

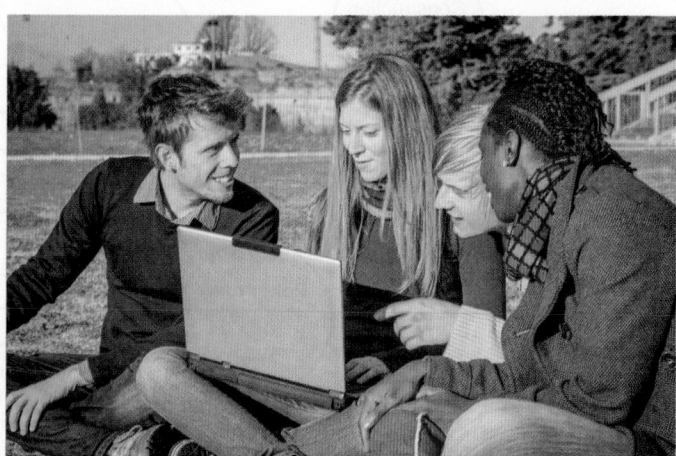

FIGURE 2-6 Teenagers from different cultural backgrounds interact within the larger culture. (From William Perugini/Shutterstock.com.)

patterns even after becoming acculturated in many ways. This is consistent with family developmental theory, which states that during times of stress, people revert to practices and behaviours that are most comfortable and familiar.

Providing Culturally Competent Nursing Care

The Canadian Nurses Association (CNA) (2010) has defined cultural competence in nursing as "the application of knowledge, skills, attitudes or personal attributes required by nurses to maximize respectful relationships with diverse populations of clients and co-workers." Values that underpin the provision of culturally competent care include respect, valuing difference, inclusivity, equity, and a commitment to providing culturally safe nursing care (RNAO, 2007). The CNA (2010) defines cultural safety as "both a process and an outcome whose goal is to promote greater [health] equity."

Nursing care is delivered in multiple cultural contexts. These contexts include the cultures of the family, the nurse, and the health care system, as well as the larger culture of the society in which health care is delivered. If any of these cultural groups is excluded from the nurse's assessment and consideration, nursing care may fail to achieve its goals and may be culturally insensitive or unsafe.

In addition to issues of preserving and promoting human dignity, the development of cultural competence is of equal importance in terms of health outcomes. Nurses who relate effectively with families are better able to promote health and address conditions of vulnerability.

As our society becomes more culturally diverse, it is essential that nurses become culturally competent. Nurses must examine their own beliefs so that they have a better appreciation and understanding of the beliefs of their patients. Understanding the concepts of ethnocentrism and cultural relativism may help nurses care for families in a multicultural society.

Ethnocentrism is the view that one's own way of doing things is best while all other ways are unnatural and inferior (Giger, 2013). *Ethnic stereotyping* or labelling stems from ethnocentric views of people. Ethnocentrism implies that all other groups are inferior and that their ways are not in the best interests of the group. It is a common attitude among a dominant ethnic group and strongly influences the ability of one person to objectively evaluate the beliefs and behaviours of others. This inherent viewpoint of individuals tends to bias their interpretation and understanding of the behaviour of others. The culturally competent nurse should be empathetic and aware of his or her own views and that they may differ from another's, based on culture or ethnicity. The nurse should be willing to ask questions that will provide a better understanding of individual or family views, when appropriate.

Cultural relativism is the opposite of ethnocentrism. It refers to learning about and applying the standards of another's culture to activities within that culture. The nurse recognizes that people from different cultural backgrounds may comprehend the same objects and situations differently. In other words, culture determines viewpoint.

Cultural relativism does not require nurses to accept the beliefs and values of another culture. Instead, nurses recognize that the behaviour of others may be based on a system of logic different from their own. Cultural relativism affirms the uniqueness and value of every culture.

To provide culturally competent care, the nurse must assess the beliefs, values, and practices of individuals and their families. Individuals and their families can be asked about their expectations so that nurses can learn collaboratively with the particular person and family. It is also important for nurses to understand and value diversity and avoid stereotyping the individuals and families they care for. Nurses should also consider all aspects of culture, including communication, space, time orientation, and family roles, when working with families.

Cultural competence is an ongoing, interactive process. It has been described as a set of congruent behaviours, attitudes, and policies that come together to enable a system, organization, or professionals to work effectively in cross-cultural situations. More recently it has been defined as cultural awareness that includes curiosity, perceptiveness, respect, and a desire to connect with the patient and family in order to determine the most appropriate goals and the interventions most likely to achieve those goals (Srivastava, 2007). Six elements of fostering cultural competence are as follows (CNA, 2010):

- Working on changing one's world view by examining one's own values and behaviours and striving to reject racism and institutions that support it
- Becoming familiar with core cultural issues by recognizing these issues and exploring them with individuals
- Becoming knowledgeable about the cultural groups one works with while learning about each individual's unique history
- Becoming familiar with core cultural issues related to health and illness and communicating in a way that encourages individuals to explain what an illness means to them
- Developing a relationship of trust with individuals and creating a welcoming atmosphere in the health care setting
- Negotiating for mutually acceptable and understandable interventions of care

! NURSING ALERT

Cultural knowledge helps nurses better understand the behaviour of individuals and families. This knowledge helps to ensure that nurses are not making assumptions about patients' behaviour in a clinical context. By performing a cultural assessment, the nurse can elicit the patient's and family's understanding of their illness and individualize the patient's care plan.

To begin to understand and work effectively with families in a multicultural community, nurses need to recognize the barriers to transcultural communication and work toward removing those barriers. Nurses, too, are a product of their own cultural background. They need to recognize that they are part of the "nursing culture." Nurses function within the framework of a professional culture with its own values and traditions and, as such, become socialized into their professional culture in their educational program and later in their work environments and professional associations.

Developing cultural competence means that the health professional becomes aware of one's own cultural attributes and biases, and their impact on others. Frequently, nurses and other health care workers are not aware of their own cultural values and how those values influence their thoughts and actions. Understanding one's own worldview and that of the "other" avoids stereotyping and the misapplication of scientific knowledge (RNAO, 2007). Self-awareness is the first step in achieving cultural competence. Evidence has shown that attitudes, whether one is conscious of them or not, have a direct and significant impact on the people around them. Through self reflection, health care providers are able to acknowledge their own cultural beliefs and values, which will aid them in achieving cultural competence in practice (RNAO, 2007). Recognizing that a behaviour may be characteristic of a culture places nurses at an advantage in their relationships with families. When nurses respect a family's cultural differences, they are better able to determine whether the behaviour is distinctive to the individual or a characteristic of the culture. It is important to understand that it is difficult to truly know everything about other cultures; nonetheless, nurses should be sensitive and learn how to respect others within all cultures.

Cultural standards and values, family structure and function, and experience with health care may influence a family's feelings and attitudes toward health, their children, and health care delivery systems. It is often difficult for nurses to be nonjudgemental and objective in working with families whose behaviours and attitudes differ from or conflict with their own. Nurses need to understand how their own cultural background influences the way in which they deliver care, and they need to be responsible and accountable for incorporating culturally competent care into their practice, regardless of domain (CNA, 2010). Relying on one's own values and experiences for guidance can result in frustration and disappointment. It is one thing to know what is needed to deal with a health problem; it is often quite another to implement a fruitful course of action within the cultural and socioeconomic framework of a particular family.

CRITICAL THINKING CASE STUDY

Culturally Competent Care in the Emergency Department

Arisha, a 37-year-old woman, accompanied by her 16-year-old son, Mahesh, is admitted to the emergency department (ED) with profuse vaginal bleeding. Arisha's primary language is Hindi, and she speaks very little English; Mahesh is fluent in Hindi and English. No health care providers present in the ED speak Hindi. The nurse assigned to care for Arisha must obtain a health history and perform an assessment. She wants to provide culturally competent care for Arisha.

QUESTIONS

1. Evidence—Is there sufficient evidence to determine what culturally competent nursing care consists of?
2. Assumptions—What assumptions can be made about culturally competent care and the role language plays in providing that care?
   a. How the nurse, who speaks no Hindi, might effectively communicate with Arisha
   b. How the nurse can obtain a health history with questions about vaginal bleeding, sexual activity, and pregnancy if Mahesh is the only person available who speaks Hindi
   c. How the nurse can provide culturally competent teaching
   d. What teaching materials and resources are appropriate; what questions are appropriate to gain information about sexual activity and the possibility of pregnancy
3. What implications and priorities for nursing care can be drawn at this time?
4. Does the evidence objectively support your conclusion?

Communication

Communication sometimes creates a challenging obstacle for nurses working with individuals from diverse cultural groups. Communication is not merely the exchange of words. Instead, it involves (1) understanding the individual's language, including subtle variations in meaning and distinctive dialects; (2) appreciation of individual differences in interpersonal style; and (3) accurate interpretation of the volume of speech, as well as the meanings of touch and gestures. For example, members of some cultural groups tend to speak more loudly, with great emotion, and with vigorous and animated gestures when they are excited; this is true whether their excitement is related to positive or negative events or emotions. Therefore, it is important for the nurse to avoid rushing to judgement regarding an individual's intent when the individual is speaking, especially in a language not understood by the nurse. In these situations it is critical that the nurse avoid instantaneous responses that may well be based on an incorrect interpretation of the person's gestures and meaning. Instead, the nurse should withhold an interpretation of what has been communicated until it is possible to clarify the person's intent. The nurse needs to enlist the assistance of a person who can help verify with the person the true intent and meaning of the communication (see Critical Thinking Case Study).

Use of interpreters. Inconsistencies between the language of family members and that of providers presents a significant barrier to effective health care. Because of the diversity of cultures and languages within the Canadian population, health care agencies are increasingly seeking the services of interpreters (of oral communication from one language to another) or translators (of written words from one language to another) to bridge these gaps and fulfill their obligation to provide linguistically appropriate health care.

Finding the best possible interpreter in these circumstances is critically important. A number of personal attributes and qualifications contribute to an interpreter's potential to be effective. Ideally, interpreters should have the same native language and be of the same religion or have the same country of origin as the patient. Interpreters should have specific health-related language skills and experience and help bridge the language and cultural barriers between the individual and the health care provider. The person interpreting should be mature enough to be trusted with private information. It is not appropriate to use a child or another family member to interpret health care information. However, because the nature of nursing care is not always predictable and because nursing care provided in a home or community setting does not always allow expert, experienced, or mature adult interpreters, ideal interpretive services are sometimes impossible to find when they are needed. In crisis or emergency situations or when family members are experiencing extreme stress or emotional upset, it may be necessary to use family members as interpreters. If this situation occurs, the nurse must ensure that the person is in agreement and comfortable with using the available interpreter to assist. Another alternative that has become more available in many settings is to access professional interpreters over the telephone when someone is not available in person. Most health care institutions have lists of staff members who may be available to interpret when required, although professional interpreters are the ideal.

When using an interpreter, the nurse needs to respect the family by creating an atmosphere of respect and privacy (see Box 2-3). Questions should be addressed to the person and not to the interpreter. Even though an interpreter will of necessity be exposed to sensitive and privileged information about the family, the nurse should take care to ensure that confidentiality is maintained. A quiet location free from interruptions is the ideal place for interpretive services to take place. In addition, culturally and linguistically appropriate educational materials that are easy to read, with appropriate text and graphics, should be available to assist the individual and family in understanding health care information. When using interpretive services, the nurse demonstrates respect for the person and helps maintain a sense of dignity by taking care to do all of the following:

- Respect the person's wishes
- Involve the person in the decisions about who will be the most appropriate person to interpret under the circumstances
- Provide as much privacy as possible

Personal Space

Cultural traditions define the appropriate personal space for various social interactions. Although the need for personal space varies from person to person and with the situation, the

BOX 2-3 WORKING WITH AN INTERPRETER

Step 1: Before the Interview

A. Outline your statements and questions. List the key pieces of information you want or need to know.

Step 2: Meeting with the Interpreter

A. Introduce yourself to the interpreter and converse informally. This is the time to find out how well he or she speaks English. No matter how proficient or what age the interpreter is, be respectful. Some ways to show respect are to acknowledge that you can learn from the interpreter or learn one word or phrase from the interpreter.

B. Emphasize that you would like to encourage the person to ask questions if they have any concerns and to feel comfortable doing so, as some cultures consider asking questions to be inappropriate.

C. Make sure that the interpreter is comfortable with the technical terms you need to use. If not, take some time to explain them.

Step 3: During the Interview

A. Ask your questions and explain your statements (see Step 1) directly to the person and maintain eye contact.

B. Make sure that the interpreter understands which parts of the interview are most important. You usually have limited time with the interpreter, and you want to have adequate time at the end for patient questions.

C. Try to get a "feel" for how much is "getting through." No matter what the language is, if in relating information to the person the interpreter uses far fewer or far more words than you do, "something else" is going on.

D. Stop every now and then and ask the interpreter, "How is it going?" You may not get a totally accurate answer, but you will have emphasized to the interpreter your strong desire to focus on the task at hand. If there are language problems, (1) speak slowly, (2) use gestures (e.g., fingers to count or point to body parts), and (3) use pictures.

E. Ask the interpreter to elicit questions. This may be difficult, but it is worth the effort.

F. Identify cultural issues that may conflict with your requests or instructions.

G. Use the interpreter to give insight into possibilities for solutions.

Step 4: After the Interview

A. Speak to the interpreter and try to get an idea of what went well and what could be improved related to the interpretation service. This will help you to be more effective with this or another interpreter.

B. Make notes on what you learned for your future reference or to help a colleague.

Remember:

Your interview is a *collaboration* between you and the interpreter. Listen as well as speak.

Notes

1. Be sensitive to cultural and situational differences (e.g., an interview with someone from an urban city will likely be different from an interview with someone from a transitional refugee camp).
2. Younger females telling older males what to do may be a problem for both a female nurse and a female interpreter. This is not the time to pioneer new gender relations. Be aware that in some cultures it is difficult for a woman to talk about some topics with a husband or a father present.

Courtesy Elizabeth Whalley, PhD, San Francisco State University.

actual physical dimensions of comfort zones differ from culture to culture. Actions such as touching, placing the person in proximity to others, taking away personal possessions, and making decisions for the individual can decrease personal security and heighten anxiety. Conversely, respecting the need for distance allows the person to maintain control over personal space and support personal autonomy, thereby increasing a sense of security. Nurses must touch patients, but they frequently do so without any awareness of the emotional distress they may be causing individuals. It is important to ask permission before touching any person.

Time Orientation

Time orientation is a fundamental way in which culture affects health behaviours. People in various cultural groups may be relatively more oriented to past, present, or future. Those who focus on the past strive to maintain tradition or the status quo and have little motivation for formulating future goals. In contrast, individuals who focus primarily on the present neither plan for the future nor consider the experiences of the past. These individuals do not necessarily adhere to strict schedules and are often described as "living for the moment" or "marching to the beat of their own drummer." Individuals oriented toward the future maintain a focus on achieving long-term goals.

The time orientation of the family may affect nursing care. For example, talking to a family about bringing the infant to the clinic for follow-up examinations (events in the future) may be difficult for the family that is focused on the present concerns of day-to-day survival. Because a family with a future-oriented sense of time plans far in advance and thinks about the long-term consequences of present actions, they may be more likely to return as scheduled for follow-up visits. Despite the differences in time orientation, each family may be equally concerned for the well-being of its newborn.

Family Roles

Family roles involve the expectations and behaviours associated with a member's position in the family (e.g., mother, father, grandparent). Social class and cultural norms also affect these roles, with distinct expectations for men and women clearly determined by social norms. For example, culture may influence whether a man actively participates in pregnancy and childbirth, yet maternity care practitioners working in the Western health care system expect fathers to be involved. This can create a significant conflict between the nurse and the role expectations of some very traditional families, who usually view the birthing experience as a female affair. Family roles may also dictate who in the family makes the major decisions regarding health care, for example which family member decides treatment options for a sick child. It is important to know this information, as it may dictate who is given information first. The way that health care practitioners facilitate such a family's care may mould the family's experience and perception of the Western health care system.

KEY POINTS

- Because there is no agreement about the definition of family, a family is what an individual considers it to be.
- Contemporary Canadian society recognizes, accepts, and values diverse family forms.
- The family is a social network that acts as an important support system for its members.
- Family theories provide nurses with useful guidelines for working with child-bearing families.
- Poverty and environmental factors, family resources and support systems, health challenges and responses to stress, and cultural and religious beliefs and practices are important factors influencing the health of the whole family.
- Culture is the pattern of assumptions, beliefs, and practices encompassing other products of human work and thoughts specific to members of an intergenerational group, community, or population.
- The beliefs and values of a culture are embedded in its economic, religious, kinship, and political structures and are reproduced through health and social practices.
- To provide quality care to perinatal and pediatric patients, nurses should be aware of the cultural beliefs, values, and practices important to particular families.
- The practice of cultural competence is continual and an important concept in nursing. Nurses can facilitate this process by recognizing cultural differences, integrating cultural knowledge, being aware of their own beliefs and practices, and acting in a respectful manner.
- No cultural group is homogenous; every racial and ethnic group contains great diversity.
- Nurses need to listen to the stories that individuals and family members tell them about their culture, their health care experiences, their resources, and their needs.
- Because verbal and nonverbal communication are important cultural considerations, nurses need to acknowledge and respect their patients' practices for productive interaction to occur.

evolve WEBSITE

Visit the Evolve website for additional resources related to the content in this chapter such as Case Studies, Critical Thinking Case Study Answers, Nursing Care Plans, Nursing Processes, Nursing Skills, and Review Questions for Exam Preparation at: http://evolve.elsevier.com/Canada/Perry/maternal/

REFERENCES

Allen, M. (1997). Comparative theories of the expanded role in nursing and implications for nursing practice: A working paper. *Nursing Papers, 9*(2), 38–45.

Black, K., & Lobo, M. (2008). A conceptual review of family resilience factors. *Journal of Family Nursing, 14*(1), 33–55. doi:10.1177/1074840707312237.

Boss, P. (2002). *Family stress management* (2nd ed.). Thousand Oaks, CA: Sage.

Canadian Nurses Association. (2010). *Position statement: Promoting cultural competence in nursing.* Ottawa: Author. Retrieved from <http://www.cna-aiic.ca/~/media/cna/page-content/pdf-en/ps114_cultural_competence_2010_e.pdf?la=en>.

Carter, B., & McGoldrick, M. (1999). *The expanded family life cycle: Individual, family, and social perspectives* (3rd ed.). Boston: Allyn & Bacon.

Doane, G., & Varcoe, C. (2015). *How to nurse: Relational inquiry with individuals and families in changing health and health care contexts.* Philadelphia: Lippincott, Williams & Wilkins.

Giger, J. N. (2013). *Transcultural nursing: Assessment and intervention* (6th ed.). St Louis: Mosby.

Gottlieb, L., & Feeley, N. (2006). *The collaborative partnership approach to care—A delicate balance.* Toronto: Mosby Elsevier.

Registered Nurses Association of Ontario (RNAO). (2007). *Embracing cultural diversity in health care: Developing cultural competence.* Toronto: Author. Retrieved from <http://rnao.ca/bpg/guidelines/embracing-cultural-diversity-health-care-developing-cultural-competence>.

Srivastava, R. (2007). *The healthcare professional's guide to clinical cultural competence.* Toronto: Elsevier Canada.

Statistics Canada. (2014). *Portrait of families and living arrangements in Canada.* Ottawa: Author. Retrieved from <http://www12.statcan.ca/census-recensement/2011/as-sa/98-312-x/98-312-x2011001-eng.cfm>.

Wright, L. M., & Leahey, M. (2013). *Nurses and families: A guide to family assessment and intervention* (6th ed.). Philadelphia: FA Davis.

ADDITIONAL RESOURCES

Aboriginal Nurses Association of Canada, Canadian Association of Schools of Nursing & Canadian Nurses Association: Cultural Competence and Cultural Safety in Nursing Education: A framework for First Nations, Inuit and Metis Nursing. <http://casn.ca/wp-content/uploads/2014/12/FINALReviewofLiterature.pdf>

Best Start—Many resources appropriate for use with different cultures. <http://www.beststart.org/>

Canadian Nurses Association. <http://www.cna-aiic.ca/en>

Family Nursing Resources. <http://www.familynursingresources.com/>

Indigenous Cultural Competency Training Program. <http://www.sanyas.ca/>

CHAPTER

3

Community Care

Judy Buchan, with contributions from Shannon E. Perry

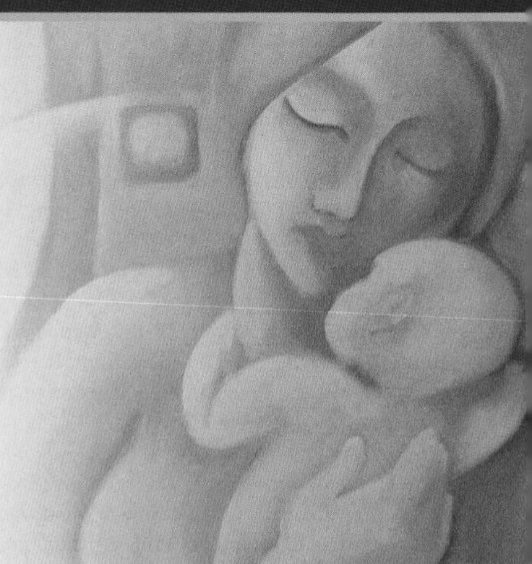

evolve WEBSITE

Visit the Evolve website for additional resources related to the content in this chapter such as Case Studies, Critical Thinking Case Study Answers, Nursing Care Plans, Nursing Processes, Nursing Skills, and Review Questions for Exam Preparation at: *http://evolve.elsevier.com/Canada/Perry/maternal/*

OBJECTIVES

On completion of this chapter the reader will be able to:

- Compare community-based home visiting programs and community health (population or aggregate-focused) care.
- List indicators of community health status and their relevance to maternal child health.
- Identify the various roles and functions that nurses have in the community.
- Describe three levels of preventive care and the differences between them.
- Discuss selected aspects of the epidemiological process.
- Explain the purpose of an economic evaluation.
- Discuss the components of the community nursing process.
- Describe data sources and methods for obtaining information about community health status.
- Identify key components of the community assessment process.
- Identify predisposing factors and characteristics of vulnerable populations within the context of the social determinants of health.
- Explore telephone contact centres and use of social media applications for nursing care options in maternal child nursing in Canada.
- Describe the nurse's role in maternal child home visiting.
- Describe the core competencies for community health nurses.
- List the potential advantages and disadvantages of home visits.
- Describe how home care fits within the continuum of care.
- Discuss safety and infection control principles as they apply to the care of patients in their homes.

Health care in Canada has evolved rapidly in recent years, with notable shifts in both the nature of health priorities and the ways in which health care is delivered to individuals, families, and populations. Today, greater emphasis is placed on health promotion and disease prevention than on the curative focus of past decades. This is in part a response to the skyrocketing costs of medical care and the realization that Canada's current health care system is unsustainable.

At a national level, the Public Health Agency of Canada's (PHAC) primary goal is to strengthen Canada's capacity to protect and improve the health of Canadians (Public Health Agency of Canada [PHAC], 2011a). This is done by promoting health; preventing and controlling chronic diseases, injuries, and infectious diseases; preparing and responding to public health emergencies; and strengthening public health capacity, through greater understanding of determinants of health and common factors that maintain health or lead to disease and injury. The Government of Canada has recognized the importance of health promotion by creating programs that address child health, healthy pregnancy and infancy, healthy living, injury prevention, mental health, family violence, obesity, physical activity, population health, rural health, and older adult health (PHAC, 2008). To carry out these programs, capacity building is required. This involves the implementation of health promotion initiatives to sustain positive health outcomes through active engagement of individuals, groups, organizations, and communities in all phases of planned change to increase their skills, knowledge, and willingness to take action to influence their own health outcomes in the future (Canadian Community Health Nursing [CCHN], 2008).

Another way to reduce the overall cost to the Canadian health care system is to reduce the length of hospital stay. By minimizing inpatient length of stay, inpatient nursing care has been transferred to home-based and community nursing care. There are many different roles that nurses have in the community, ranging from primary prevention, health promotion and protection, health education, surveillance, screening and immunization clinics to disaster management and emergency preparedness. Home health care nurses tend to provide specific nursing care in the home or at a clinic; such care will be discussed later in the chapter. Public health and community health nurses have a broader role and bring a unique set of knowledge and skills needed to plan, implement, and evaluate public health interventions.

The terms public health nurse and community health nurse are used in many different ways across the various jurisdictions in Canada. In some places, the term community health nurse means the same as, or is used instead of, the term public health nurse (Canadian Public Health Association [CPHA], 2010). In other areas, community health nurse is an overarching term that refers to the complete range of nurses working in the community, of which public health nurses are one group (CPHA, 2010).

Throughout this chapter, *community health nurse* refers to nurses who provide public health nursing in the community. *Home health care nurse* refers to nurses who provide care in a patient's home.

ROLES AND FUNCTIONS OF COMMUNITY HEALTH NURSES

Historically, the role of the community health nurse originates from the insights and wisdom of Florence Nightingale. Now recognized as a pioneer in epidemiology, disease prevention, and public health science, Nightingale used this knowledge to develop an educational training program for nurses for entering the profession. She was also a leader in the advancement of public health science through her work on sanitation, surveillance, and social reform (Savage & Kub, 2009). To understand the role of the nurse in public health, it is critical to examine the role of nurses who have the title of community health nurse and to look at the types of activities they engage in to promote the health of populations. Community nurses are equipped with knowledge of disease and wellness that is based on both their education and experience and includes an understanding of the clinical implications of public health interventions as well as the etiology and natural history of disease. Community health nursing practice is grounded in a holistic approach and considers the health of individuals, families, communities, and the population as a whole. The roles and functions of the community health nurse continue to evolve. In the future, many more nurses will be working in community settings (Underwood et al., 2009).

Community health nursing is a synthesis of nursing theory and public health science. The foundation for community health nursing includes a range of models and theories, such as population health promotion, illness and injury prevention, community participation, and community development (CPHA, 2010). Community health nurses work in the community to partner with people where they live, work, learn, meet, and play, in order to promote health. As nurses work in the community with families and individuals, the goal is to promote health, build individual and community capacity toward that goal, connect with and care for patients, facilitate access and equity, and demonstrate professional responsibility and accountability (Community Health Nurses of Canada [CHNC], 2009).

In community-based health care settings, both the aggregate (group of people who have shared characteristics) and the population become the focus of interventions. Health care providers are required to collaborate in order to determine health priorities for communities and develop successful plans of care to be delivered in a health clinic, community health centre, or a patient's home. Community-based health care, including public health services, is often under-resourced and is challenged to meet the demands of growing populations. Thus it is sometimes difficult to fully compensate for the gaps in health care service that currently exist.

Core Competencies

The PHAC (2011b) developed core competencies for all public health care professionals, which outlined the 36 competencies deemed essential to all disciplines practising in public health. To support the core competencies outlined by the PHAC, the Community Health Nurses Canada (CHNC) has developed discipline-specific practice competencies for community health nursing. There are two sets of competencies set out by the CHNC: one set for community health nurses (CHNC, 2009) and one for home health nurses (CHNC, 2010). Together, these competencies identify the required knowledge, abilities, attributes, and judgement for community health nursing practice within Canada. In 2010, the Canadian Public Health Association (CPHA) in collaboration with the CHNC and PHAC clarified and described the role and functions of community health nurses in Canada with the release of *Public Health/Community Health Nursing in Canada: Roles and Activities*, fourth edition (CPHA, 2010). Whereas previous editions had described public health/community health nursing roles as relating to communities, families, and individuals across the lifespan, the fourth edition has shifted in focus to populations and the broad determinants of health (CPHA, 2010).

Community health nurses can also become certified through the Canadian Nurses Association (CNA). This certification credential, part of a respected national certification program, is an important indicator to patients, employers, the public, and professional licensing bodies that the certified nurse is qualified, competent, and current in community health nursing.

NURSING ALERT

Nurses are required to work interprofessionally, speaking a common language laid out in the PHAC core competencies, as their work crosses many disciplines. This includes being able to understand terms used by demographers, epidemiologists, physicians, health promoters, researchers, and economists.

Public Health Decision Making

The use of research evidence plays an important role in public health decision making. The process of evidence-informed decision-making guides decision making by using the best research evidence available. However, research evidence is only one part of a larger picture. Decision makers must interpret and apply the research evidence in the context of four other sources of evidence (Fig. 3-1).

Public health expertise signifies the expertise that the public health practitioner contributes to the overall decision-making process. All the factors need to be weighed and balanced to make the most appropriate decision. When considering a policy or program change, it is important for the practitioner to understand the magnitude of the health issue in the local setting and how important this health issue is in comparison to others issues. This can help to ensure that those issues affecting the overall health status of the population receive priority over those which have a more limited impact on the public good (community health issues, local context). Community and political preferences and actions in Fig. 3-1 refers to the need to understand the political climate at the municipal, provincial, and federal level; it is important to know the community's views on an issue. Public health resources include budget, staff, and technological infrastructure. Decision makers must determine whether or not there are sufficient resources, both in terms of personnel and technology and in terms of funding, to successfully implement a program or policy. Finally, research evidence empowers the public health practitioner with an understanding of what the best available research says about an issue. All of these considerations help to bring evidence into practice, but they can only work as part of a comprehensive process and not independently of one another.

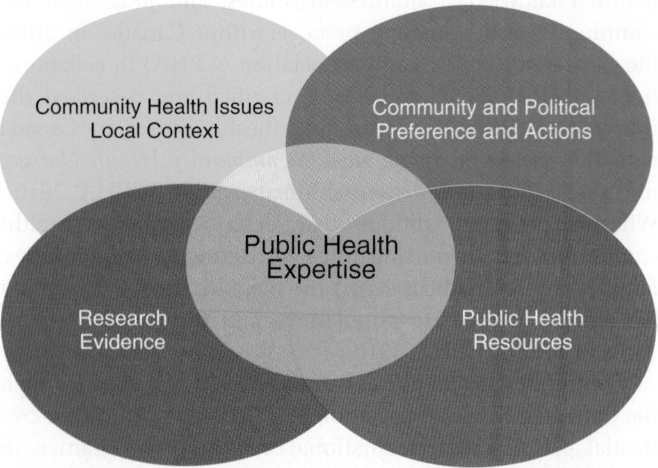

FIGURE 3-1 A model for evidence-informed decision making in public health. (Source: NCCMT National Collaborating Centres of Methods and Tools. http://www.nccmt.ca/eiph/index-eng.html.)

Community Health Promotion

Best practices in community-based health initiatives involve a thorough understanding of a community's health needs and priorities, the environmental context, power relationships, and available resources as well as participation of community leaders. A community-based framework helps to bring together multiple perspectives and diverse community resources to address a specific health priority. The emphasis on community-based health promotion has grown in recent years with the recognition that many health issues require the collaborative efforts of a diverse community network to achieve public health goals.

Economics

A basic understanding of the economics of health care enables the nurse to participate in decision making about the cost and benefits of health programs. Economists theorize that individuals and societies view health as a basic utility, that is, something that is perceived as valuable. Other basic utilities include food, shelter, and clothing. People may be willing to trade resources, such as money and time, for a program or intervention that will improve their health. Economists measure the amount of resources that individuals and communities are willing to pay for good health. Economic evaluation provides objective information to establish a program's value to the community.

Demography

Demography is the study of population characteristics. Demographic characteristics include age, gender, race and ethnicity, socioeconomic status, and education. Individuals, families, and communities may have demographic characteristics that affect their health risks (McFarlane & Gilroy, 2015). *Risk* is an increased probability of developing a disease, injury, or illness. Age is one of the most important risk factors for disease prevention and certain health conditions. For example, infants are more likely to die as a result of congenital malformations; children and adolescents, as a result of accidents; and middle-age adults, as a result of cancer (Statistics Canada, 2014). Gender also plays an important role. Males are at greater risk than females of having hemophilia A and B. Race and ethnicity have long been associated with increased risk for disease and disability, but it is now thought that, aside from genetic predisposition, there is a complicated relationship between minority status and socioeconomic status that increases the risk for disease and disability (PHAC, 2011c). Low socioeconomic status, an important determinant of health, predisposes children to a variety of problems. Poor children are more likely to be obese and to have untreated dental problems. They are more likely to be treated in emergency departments because they do not have a regular health care provider (PHAC, 2011c).

Epidemiology

Epidemiology is the science of population health applied to the detection of morbidity and mortality in a population. Through the epidemiological process, the distribution and causes of disease or injury across a population are identified (McFarlane & Gilroy, 2015). Epidemiology serves as an important component in developing health programs. For example, the Community Action Program for Children incorporated an epidemiological process to develop programs that promote the healthy development of young children from birth to 6 years (PHAC, 2015a). Health care professionals in community, provincial, and national organizations use the epidemiological process to guide the development of programs that will have the greatest impact on children's health.

Distribution of disease, injury, or illness. Morbidity rates are used to measure disease and injury and, along with birth and mortality rates, present an objective picture of a community's health status. There are two types of morbidity rates: incidence and prevalence. *Incidence* measures the occurrence of new events in a population during a period of time. *Prevalence* measures existing events in a population during a period of time. For example, the incidence of type 1 diabetes in a community is estimated by counting the new cases of type 1 diabetes in a population and dividing that figure by the size of the population at risk. The prevalence of type 1 diabetes is estimated by counting the existing cases of type 1 diabetes in a population and dividing that figure by the size of the population at risk. Both incidence and prevalence are usually given as rates per 1000, 10,000, or 100,000 population, depending on their frequency. Box 3-1 presents frequently used mortality and morbidity rates.

Epidemiological triangle. Three factors form the epidemiological triangle, and their interrelationship alters the risk of acquiring a disease or condition. These factors are *agent, host,* and *environment* (Fig. 3-2).

An agent is responsible for causing a disease. The agent may be an infectious agent, such as Mycobacterium tuberculosis; a chemical agent, such as lead in paint; or a physical agent, such as fire. Host factors are those that are specific to an individual or group. These may be genetic factors, which cannot be controlled, or they may be lifestyle factors, such as food selections or exercise patterns. Environmental factors provide a setting for the host and include the climatic conditions in which the host lives and factors related to the home, neighbourhood, and school.

Levels of Preventive Care

Population-based care may involve disease-prevention activities focused on specific needs that are identified through the community assessment process. These levels of prevention provide a framework for nursing interventions.

Primary prevention. *Primary prevention* involves health-promotion and disease-prevention activities to decrease the occurrence of illness and enhance general health and quality of life. Primary prevention precedes disease or dysfunction and encourages individuals to achieve the optimal level of health possible. Examples of primary prevention include health education and counselling about healthy lifestyle behaviours, including those related to nutrition and exercise. Other examples include well-child care clinics, immunization programs, water fluoridation, safety programs (bike helmets, car seats, seat belts,

BOX 3-1 FREQUENTLY USED MORTALITY AND MORBIDITY RATES

Crude Birth Rate

$$\frac{\text{Number of births in a population}}{\text{Total population}} \text{ within a time period} \times 1000$$

Crude Death Rate

$$\frac{\text{Number of deaths in a population}}{\text{Total population}} \text{ within a time period} \times 1000$$

Cause-Specific Death Rate

$$\frac{\text{Number of deaths in a population due to a certain disease}}{\text{Total population}} \text{ within a time period} \times 1000$$

Age-Specific Death Rate

$$\frac{\text{Number of deaths in a population in a certain age group}}{\text{Total population in that age group}} \text{ within a time period} \times 1000$$

Incidence of Disease

$$\frac{\text{Number of new events in a population}}{\text{Total at-risk population}} \text{ within a time period} \times 1000$$

Prevalence of Disease

$$\frac{\text{Number of existing events in a population}}{\text{Total at-risk population}} \text{ within a time period} \times 1000$$

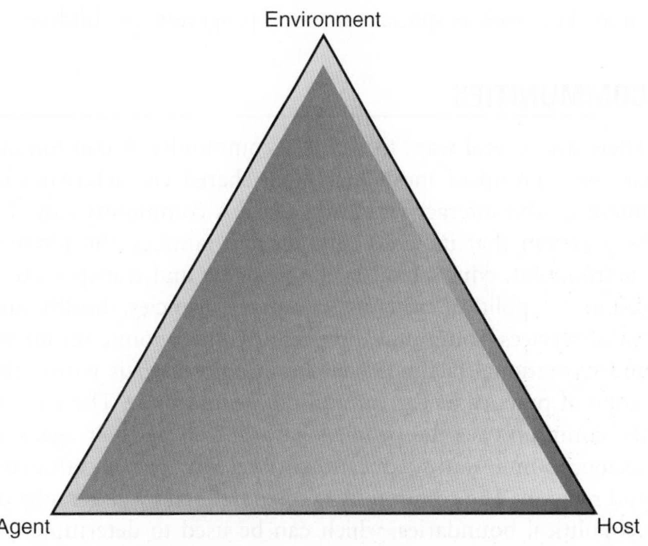

FIGURE 3-2 The epidemiological triangle.

child-proof containers), nutrition programs, environmental efforts (clean air programs), sanitation measures (chlorinated water, garbage removal, sewage treatment), and community parenting classes. Educational programs that teach healthy sexuality behaviours that reduce risk or that convey the dangers of smoking and drug use are also examples of primary prevention.

Secondary prevention. *Secondary prevention* is aimed at early detection of a disease and prompts treatment to either cure the disease or slow its progression and prevent subsequent disability. Screening programs to detect disease while persons are asymptomatic are the most frequent forms of secondary prevention. Examples of this level of prevention are community blood pressure and cholesterol screenings that identify persons at high risk for heart attack and stroke and facilitate early treatment. Another example is a Pap (Papanicolaou) test, which is used to screen women to detect premalignant and malignant cells on the cervix opening. If this condition is treated early, cervical cancer can be successfully prevented or cured. The goal of secondary prevention is to shorten disease duration and severity, thus enabling an individual to return to normal function as quickly as possible. However, screening is not appropriate for every condition. Although screening may bring benefits, a certain amount of risk is associated with any intervention. It is essential to determine the evidence for a proposed screening program before beginning it so that the benefits of screening exceed the risks and cost. It is also important to ensure there are adequate resources available to support and treat those with positive screening results.

Tertiary prevention. *Tertiary prevention* follows the occurrence of a disease or disability and is aimed at preventing disability through restoration of optimal functioning. Persons who have developed disease are provided with treatment and rehabilitation to prevent complications and further deterioration. Examples of tertiary prevention are early treatment and management of diabetes to reduce subsequent health problems, and rehabilitation of persons after a stroke. Other examples of tertiary interventions include rehabilitation and disease management programs for asthma, sickle cell disease, cancer, and anorexia as well as special education programs for children.

COMMUNITIES

There are several ways to define a community. A community can be a group of individuals with shared characteristics or interests who interact with each other. A community can also be a system that includes children and families, the physical environment, educational facilities, safety and transportation resources, political and governmental agencies, health and social services, communication resources, economic resources, and recreational facilities. The community itself is within the scope of practice of the community health nurse. The core of the community is the people, characterized by their age, sex, socioeconomic status, educational level, occupation, ethnicity, and religion. The community is often defined by geography or geopolitical boundaries, which can be used to determine the location of service delivery (Anderson & McFarlane, 2010). Community health initiatives are directed at either the general health of the community as a whole or specific populations within the community that have unique needs. In this context, populations can be described as groups of people who live in a community, for example, pregnant women or school-age children. Priority populations or subpopulations are more narrowly defined groups (e.g., unimmunized preschoolers, or obese middle school children) which are the focus of activities to improve the health status of individuals in the group. Common values often guide behaviours of populations and subpopulations in relation to health promotion and disease prevention (Williams, 2011).

A wide variety of strategies have been used to engage families and groups in health-promoting activities or community health programs. Some are more successful than others. Engaging participants in the planning process and empowering them to create internal solutions are considered key factors in developing effective interventions. Many communities have organized coalitions to address specific health-promotion agendas related to sharing information, educating community members, or advocating for health policies around maternal and child health issues. The benefits of partnership with faith-based organizations for community health improvement have been demonstrated in health-promotion efforts aimed at lifestyle choices, health education, and maternal child health outcomes.

Community Nursing Process

In community nursing, the nursing process shifts its focus from the individual patient and family to the community or target population (Box 3-2). The stages of the process (assessment, diagnosis, planning, implementation, and evaluation) are similar, whether the patient is one individual or a whole community.

Assessing the Community

A community health assessment is used to identify and measure the health status of the population of a given health authority or region (Community Health Assessment Network of Manitoba [CHANM], 2009). It is a complex but well-defined process through which the unique characteristics of the population, its assets, and needs are identified in order to facilitate collaborative action planning to improve community health status and quality of life (CHANM, 2009). The purpose of this process is

BOX 3-2 THE COMMUNITY NURSING PROCESS

Assessment and diagnosis—The nurse collects subjective and objective information about a community and develops a diagnosis based on community needs and problems.

Planning—The nurse develops community-centred goals to address the identified needs and problems.

Intervention—The nurse implements a program that enables community members to reach their goals.

Evaluation—The nurse conducts a systematic evaluation to determine that goals and program objectives were met by developing measureable outcomes.

to identify direct service and advocacy needs of the prioritized aggregate or group and to improve the health of the community. Engaging the community and key stakeholders in the process increases buy-in and ultimately leads to better outcomes for the proposed services.

During a community health assessment, data are collected, analyzed, and used to inform, educate, and mobilize communities; identify priorities; garner resources; and plan actions to improve the health of the public. Many models and frameworks of community assessment are available, but the actual process often depends on the extent and nature of the assessment to be performed, the time and resources available, and the way in which the information is intended to be used. For examples of community assessment tools, see the Additional Resources section at the end of the chapter.

The community-asset mapping approach provides an overview of community attributes and strengths that may facilitate long-term change and improved quality of life for community residents. Understanding community capacity involves looking at a community's ability to address social and health problems or to develop knowledge, systems, and resources that contribute to a community's health status. These approaches help to direct the health promotion process by identifying community priorities and areas of needed change. The community health nurse or home health nurse may assist with community capacity building by working with the community to develop skills in accessing resources, developing social networks, and learning from the experience of others (CPHA, 2010).

Data collection and sources of community health data. Data collection is often the most time-consuming phase of the community assessment process, but it provides an important understanding and description of the community. Measures of community health include health status data, access to care, level of provider services available, and other social and economic factors. Consideration of individual, interpersonal, community, organizational, and policy-level data and the interaction of these factors are important in providing a comprehensive framework for community health promotion. A community assessment model (Fig. 3-3) is often used to provide a comprehensive guide to data collection.

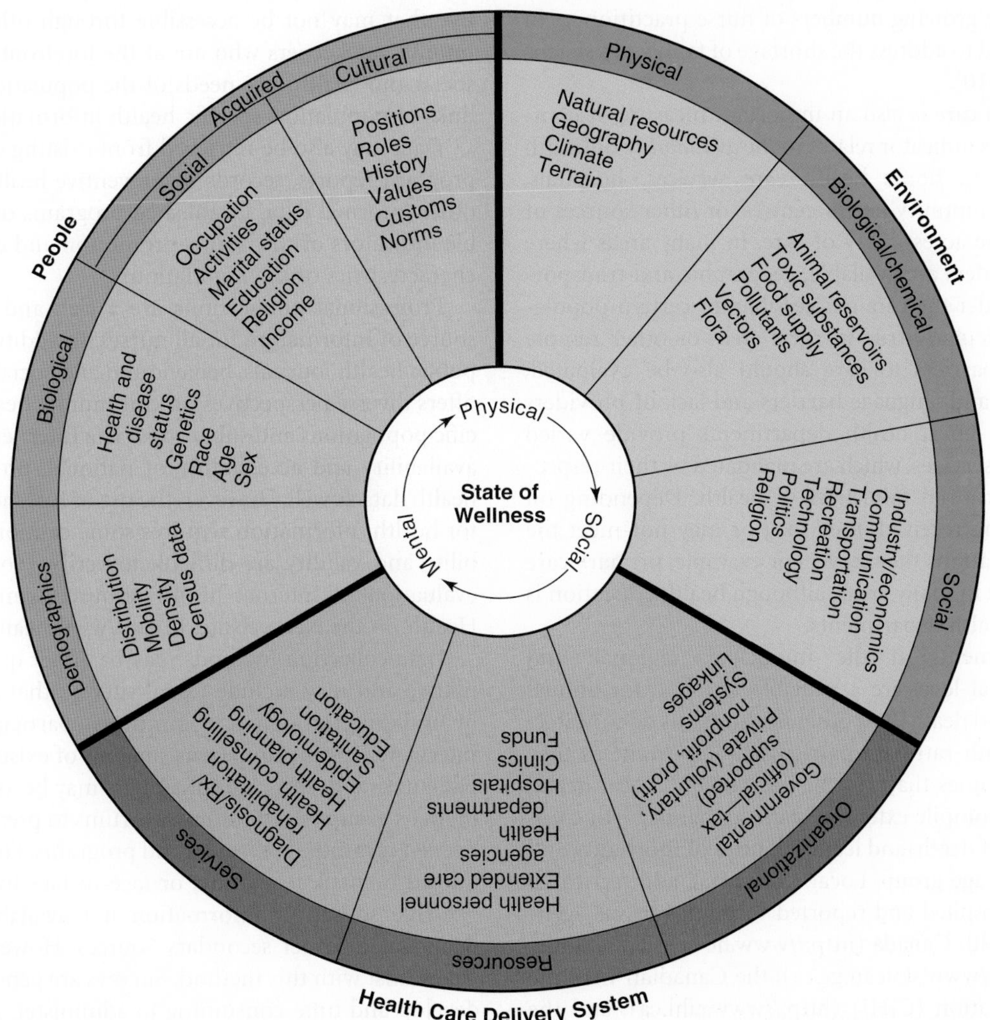

FIGURE 3-3 Community health assessment wheel. (From Clemen-Stone, S. [2002]. Community assessment and diagnosis. In Clemen-Stone, S., McGuire, S., & Eigsti, D. [Eds]. *Comprehensive community health nursing: Family, aggregate, and community practice* [6th ed.]. St. Louis: Mosby.)

Some important community indicators of maternal child health are as follows: maternal mortality, infant mortality, low birth weight (LBW), stillbirths, first-trimester prenatal care, enhanced 18-month well-baby visits, immunization rates, the Early Developmental Instrument, and rates for other screening tests. Nurses may use these indicators as a reflection of access, quality, and continuity of health care in a community. For women and children, access to a consistent source of health care is critical. Not having a regular medical doctor or nurse practitioner is associated with fewer health care visits with general practitioners and specialists who can play a role in screening and treating medical conditions early (Statistics Canada, 2010a). Over the past decade, the percentage of Canadians who report having a family doctor has declined slightly; remote areas in Canada report the lowest numbers of people with family doctors. In 2008, only 38% of residents of the Northwest Territories said that they had a family doctor, whereas in Nunavut, less than 15% reported having a regular physician (Statistics Canada, 2010). This is a significantly lower rate than that of the rest of the country, which ranges around 80%. When people do not have access to a primary health care provider they use walk-in clinics, hospital emergency departments, or community health centres. The growing numbers of nurse practitioners in Canada have helped to address the shortage of family physicians (DiCenso et al., 2010).

Access to health care is also an important measure of community health. This indicator relates to the *availability* of health department services, home health care services, hospitals, walk-in clinics, community health centres, or other sources of care and also to the accessibility of care. In many areas where facilities and providers are available, geographic and transportation barriers render the care inaccessible for certain populations. This is particularly true in rural areas or other remote locations. Other barriers to care should also be evaluated, including cultural and language barriers and lack of providers for specialty care. Local health departments provide varied levels and types of services, which are mandated by their respective provincial/territorial ministries of health. Depending on the level of funding received, they may or may not meet the needs of the populations they serve. For example, primary care services are limited in many areas, although health education is offered by most health departments.

Health departments at the municipal, regional, and provincial/territorial level are a valuable resource for annual reports of births and deaths and other health status data. Maternal and infant death rates are particularly important as they reflect health outcomes that may be preventable. Local health departments also compile extensive statistics about birth complications, causes of death, and leading causes of morbidity and mortality for each age group. Local, provincial, and territorial health data are compiled and reported through various agencies, including Health Canada (http://www.hc-sc.gc.ca), Statistics Canada (http://www.statcan.gc.ca), the Canadian Institute for Health Information (CIHI) (http://www.cihi.ca), and the Public Health Agency of Canada (PHAC) (http://www.phac-aspc.gc.ca). However, national data are only as accurate and reliable as the local data on which they are based; thus caution is needed in interpreting the data and applying them to specific population groups.

The Canadian government census provides data on population size, age ranges, sex, racial and ethnic distribution, socioeconomic status, educational level, employment, and housing characteristics. Summary data are available for most large metropolitan areas, arranged by postal code and census tract, which usually correspond to a neighbourhood comprising approximately 2000 to 8000 people. Assessment of individual census tracts within a community can help in identifying subpopulations or aggregates whose needs may differ from those of the larger community. For example, women at high risk for inadequate prenatal care according to age, race, and ethnic or cultural group may be readily identified, and outreach activities may be provided as appropriate.

Other sources of useful data are hospitals and voluntary health agencies. Community health resources include health care providers or administrators, government officials, religious leaders, and representatives of voluntary health agencies. Community or regional health councils exist in many areas, with oversight of specific health initiatives or programs for that region. These key informants often provide a unique perspective that may not be accessible through other sources. Community gatekeepers who are at the forefront of addressing the social and health care needs of the population are also critical links to population-specific health information.

Data may also be retrieved from existing community health program reports, records of preventive health screenings, and other informal data. Established programs often provide reliable indicators of the health-promotion and disease-prevention characteristics of the population.

Professional publications are a rich and readily accessible source of information for all nurses. In addition to nursing and public health journals, behavioural and social science literature offers diverse perspectives on community health status for specific populations and subgroups. The Internet has increased the availability and accessibility of national, provincial, and local health data as well. However, the use of Internet-based resources for health information requires some caution, since data reliability and validity are difficult to verify. (Some guidelines for evaluation of Internet health resources can be found at the Health on the Net website: https://www.healthonnet.org/).

Data collection methods may be either qualitative or quantitative and may include visual surveys that can be completed by walking through a community, participant observation, interviews, focus groups, and analysis of existing data. Potential patients and health care consumers may be asked to participate in focus groups or community forums to present their views on needed community services and programs. Formal surveys conducted by mail, telephone, or face-to-face interviews can be a valuable source of information not available from national databases or other secondary sources. However, several drawbacks exist with this method. Surveys are generally expensive to develop and time-consuming to administer. In addition to the cost of such surveys, poor response rates often preclude a sufficiently representative response on which to base nursing interventions.

A local walking survey is generally conducted by making a walk-through observation of the community (see Community Focus box), taking note of specific characteristics of the population, economic and social environment, transportation, health care services, safety, and other resources. This method allows the nurse to collect subjective data and may facilitate other aspects of the assessment. Participant observation is another useful assessment method, in which the nurse actively participates in the community to understand the community more fully and to validate observations.

COMMUNITY FOCUS

Community Walk-Through

As you observe the community, take note of the following:

Physical environment—Older neighbourhood or newer subdivision? Sidewalks, streets, and buildings in good or poor repair? Billboards and signs? What are they advertising? Are lawns kept up? Is there garbage in the streets? Parks or playgrounds? Parking lots? Empty lots? Industries? Air quality?

People in the area—Elderly, young, homeless, children, predominant ethnicity, language? Is the population homogeneous? What signs do you see of different cultural groups? Are people out and about in the community?

Stores and services available—Restaurants: chain, local, ethnic? Grocery stores: neighbourhood or chain? Department stores, gas stations, real estate or insurance offices, travel agencies, pawn shops, liquor stores, discount or thrift stores, convenience stores? Can people walk to shopping or do they need a car? Are there services for families with young children?

Social—Clubs, bars, fraternal organizations (e.g., Lion's Club, Canadian Legion), museums, community recreation centres?

Religious—Churches, synagogues, mosques? What denominations? Do you see evidence of their use other than on religious or holy days?

Health services—Drug stores, doctors' offices, clinics, dentists, mental health services, veterinarians, urgent care facilities, walk-in clinics, hospitals, shelters, nursing homes, home health agencies, public health services, local laboratory, traditional healers (e.g., herbalists, palmists)?

Transportation—Cars, bus, taxi, subway, light rail, sidewalks, bicycle paths, access for disabled persons?

Education—Schools, before-school and after-school programs, child care, libraries, bookstores? What is the reputation of the school?

Government—What is the governance structure? Is there a mayor? City council? Are meetings open to the public? Are there signs of political activity (e.g., posters, campaign signs)? Is there a local neighbourhood business community organization?

Safety—How safe is the community? What is the crime rate? What types of crimes are committed? Are police visible? Is there a fire station? Are people comfortable walking in their neighbourhood after dark?

Parks and Recreation Facilities—Are there local parks for toddlers and children? Are there recreational facilities for adults and children to participate in sports and recreation activities?

Evaluation of the community based on your observations—What is your impression of the community? Is the environment pleasing? Are services and transportation adequate? How difficult is it for residents to obtain needed services (i.e., how far do they have to travel)? Would you want to live in this community? Why or why not?

Finally, as part of the assessment process, nurses working in multiethnic and multicultural groups need an in-depth assessment of culturally based health behaviours.

Analysis and synthesis of data obtained during the assessment process help in generating a comprehensive picture of the community's health status, needs, and problem areas as well as its strengths and resources for addressing these concerns. The goals of this process are to assign priorities to community health needs and to develop a plan of action for correcting them. A comparison of community health data with provincial and national statistics may be useful in the identification of appropriate target populations and interventions to improve health outcomes.

Community Planning

After the assessment is completed, the community nurse can collaborate with team members to analyze the results of surveys and questionnaires and determine whether the needs described by community members can be met by existing community agencies. During the analysis, the community's demographic characteristics, morbidity rates, and mortality rates are compared with a standard. In time comparisons, the nurse contrasts the rates in the current year with the rates during an earlier period. In comparisons of place, the nurse contrasts the rates in the community with those of a standard population. Standard rates may come from another community or from city, province/territory, or national data. For example, the rate of tuberculosis in a group of preschool children in the community in 2016 could be compared with the rate of tuberculosis in preschool children in the province in 2016. A community health diagnosis or health issue is a reflection of health status, risk, or need. A community diagnosis is similar to that of an individual nursing diagnosis with a problem (need) and an etiology related to that problem (causative agent). An example of a community nursing diagnosis is childhood obesity related to poor socioeconomic environment.

The nurse can collaborate with community members to develop a plan that addresses the target population's needs and problems utilizing population health. To maximize the use of community resources, problems should first be prioritized on the basis of their severity, the community's identified needs, and the community nurse's ability to bring about change. The nurse or team works with community members to develop at least one goal for each problem. Goals are outcomes that give direction to interventions and provide a measure of the change the interventions produced. Community interventions frequently take the form of health programs for improving the target population's health status. Community health programs are based on the three levels of prevention: primary, secondary, and tertiary. For example, a goal for preventing bicycle injuries is "Within one year all students in the first grade will wear bicycle helmets." A nurse working within a group along with community members can then plan a program that includes health education about bicycle safety for students and their parents (primary prevention).

The planning group will consider the resources that are already available in the community and resources that will be needed for implementing a health program, including location, personnel, supplies, and equipment. Decisions are made about the program's timeline, the budget, and strategies to obtain funding. Program descriptions are found through professional contacts, online resources, and a review of the literature.

Community Intervention

During program implementation, the nurse or team and community members carry out the intervention. Whether the program is simple or complex, oversight is needed to ensure that everyone involved is communicating with one another, adhering to the plan's guidelines, keeping within the timeline, and documenting daily activities and expenses. The documentation will prove invaluable during the evaluation phase of the process.

Community Evaluation

Evaluation is used to identify whether the goals and program objectives were met. There are various models for measuring quality of health care. The most common framework used by health care organizations is the structure, process, and outcomes method described by Donabedian (1988). Donabedian conceptualized three quality-of-care dimensions: structure, process, and outcomes.

Structure—refers to the attributes of setting where the care is delivered. It is the context in which care is delivered that affects processes and outcomes—that is, the qualifications of personnel; the adequacy of buildings and offices, supplies, and equipment; and the target population's characteristics.

Process—whether or not good health care practices are followed.

Outcomes—the impact of the care on health status. Outcomes indicate the combined effects of structure and process—that is, whether program objectives and community goals were met.

To monitor outcomes is to monitor performances, which are conditional on structure and process. Only structure and process can be manipulated. Program evaluation should be ongoing so that an improvement in the way health care is delivered will affect the target population's health status.

VULNERABLE POPULATIONS WITHIN THE COMMUNITY

In Canada, maternal, infant, and childhood survival rates are among the best in the world. This is in part due to relatively high levels of education, economic and social well-being, and an effective universal health care system. However, it is important to recognize that Canada does have vulnerable populations who face significant disparities. There are many families in this country who do not have ideal outcomes and face considerable challenges and health risks. Rates of adverse pregnancy outcomes, including preterm birth and intrauterine growth restriction, generally rise with greater socioeconomic disadvantage. During pregnancy, women with low socioeconomic status are more likely to face stressful life events and chronic stressors and experience low gestational-weight gain. They are also less likely to initiate early prenatal care. All of these factors can translate into poor pregnancy outcomes. Poor fetal development is associated with many chronic diseases in later life (Marmot, 2010; Scientific Advisory Committee on Nutrition, 2011). This means that the impact of being disadvantaged can last a lifetime. Vulnerable women also face a higher risk of maternal death (United Nations Population Fund, 2012; Verstraeten et al., 2015). In terms of child well-being, Canada has room for improvement. It recently ranked in a middle position at 17 of 29 of the world's richest nations, based on UNICEF's Report Card 11 (UNICEF Office of Research, 2013).

The high burden of illness responsible for premature loss of life arises in large part from the conditions in which people are born, grow, live, work, and age (World Health Organization [WHO], 2008). These social determinants of health (see Table 1-1) have a significant effect on health outcomes and influence a wide range of diseases. Compared to people with higher income, people with lower income have a shorter life expectancy, a higher risk of exposure to poor living and working conditions, and higher mortality rates. A higher income leads to better health—not only because it leads to the ability to buy adequate food, housing, and other necessities but also because it leads to more choices and a feeling of control over one's life (Marmot, 2010).

There are many subpopulations living in Canada who experience significant health inequities. These include women with mental health issues, women working in the sex-trade industry, pregnant and parenting adolescents, and women whose newborn has been taken into custody by child protection services. The offspring of women belonging to these populations are also at increased risk for poor outcomes. Many of these poor outcomes are preventable through access to adequate nutrition, prenatal care, and use of preventive health practices; clearly, comprehensive, community-based care that is culturally relevant and accessible for all mothers, children, and families is needed. In the community, health care services range from individual care to group and community services and from primary prevention to tertiary care.

Women comprise 50.4% of the Canadian population (Statistics Canada, 2015). Generally, women in Canada report good health, except those in areas where vulnerable populations are concentrated. Women's health experiences differ within and between social groups. For example, immigrant women; Indigenous women; women in remote and rural areas; women with disabilities; women living with mental illness; women living in low-income situations; and lesbian, bisexual, queer, and transgendered women have differential access to health services and differing health care needs. Many women belonging to these vulnerable population groups struggle to find health care practitioners who are knowledgeable and respectful of their unique needs and who provide care that is culturally and socially sensitive.

Indigenous People

Among vulnerable populations are the Indigenous people, who face higher risks of adverse pregnancy and poor infant and child health outcomes. The increased infant death, preterm birth, and large-for-gestational-age rates among First Nations, Métis, and Inuit infants compared with those of non–First Nations infants are independent of neighbourhood socioeconomic status (Canadian Perinatal Surveillance System [CPSS], 2008; Smylie et al., 2010). These significant health issues are outcomes stemming from the legacy of colonization (Truth and Reconciliation Commission of Canada, 2015) (see Chapter 1, p. 6 for further discussion).

Immigrants and Refugees

Along with profound resilience and determination, refugees and immigrants have brought rich diversity to Canada in several important dimensions, including cultural heritage and customs, economic productivity, and enhanced national vitality. At the same time, multiple challenges accompany the dramatic influx of individuals and families from other countries.

Over the last decade there has been a steady increase in the number of immigrants moving to Canada. In 2006, 20.3% of all women living in Canada were born outside the country (Statistics Canada, 2012). Among recent immigrant women, the largest share came from the People's Republic of China (15%), followed by India (11%) and the Philippines (8%) (Chui, 2011). In 2015–2016 the Canadian government committed to welcoming 25,000 Syrian refugees, many of whom were women and children coming from difficult situations.

Canada's total female workforce has increased steadily, with the female labour force increasing 16.8% among the immigrant population and 7.4% among the Canadian-born (Statistics Canada, 2012). New immigrants often find themselves either underemployed or unemployed because of discrimination, complications around accreditation of foreign degrees, lack of available and affordable child care, and social isolation. Immigrant women's rate of participation in the labour force is considerably lower than that of immigrant men and Canadian-born women. Newly arrived immigrant women, those who had arrived up to 5 years prior to the 2006 Census, were more likely to be unemployed than those who had spent more time in Canada. However, among immigrant women aged 25 to 54, the challenge of finding work eased the longer they lived in Canada (Statistics Canada, 2012).

Refugee status imposes a particular type of vulnerability on affected individuals and groups. Of primary significance are the precipitating factors by which people are displaced suddenly or forced to leave their country of origin: persecution, civil unrest, or war. Families are forced from their homes to seek residence and employment elsewhere. Often these groups are extremely impoverished and face extreme physical and emotional stress when they arrive in Canada.

In general, refugees are more likely to live in poverty than are immigrants. Over time, health disparities that adversely affect health and well-being actually decline for the immigrant population as they become part of Canadian society. Many of the conditions or illnesses that immigrants and refugees acquire contribute to the persistence of disparities in their health outcomes.

Immigrants typically arrive in Canada with better health than that of the Canadian-born population. This is because immigrants are screened on medical and other health-related criteria before they are admitted to the country. However, over time, this "healthy immigrant effect" tends to diminish as their health status converges with that of the host population. Some medical problems may arise as immigrants age, as well as when they integrate and adopt behaviours that have negative health impacts. Other health problems may arise from the stress of immigration itself, which involves finding suitable employment and establishing a new social support network.

Adolescent Girls

While the adolescent population in Canada is generally considered healthy, this group of women is often vulnerable because of their high-risk behaviours. Adolescent girls, especially those from low-income or disrupted families, are more likely to engage in early sexual activity and other high-risk behaviours, with both immediate and long-term health consequences. The teenage pregnancy rate declined almost 41% in Canada from 1994 to 2006 (McKay, 2012). This is significantly lower than pregnancy rates in the United States and England (McKay, 2012). Although the Canadian teen pregnancy rate declined by 20.3% between the years 2001 and 2010, the national teen pregnancy rate increased from 2006 to 2010 by 1.1%. Despite the fact that this represents an upward trend in some provinces, it is likely that the relative stability of teen pregnancy rates since reaching a low in 2006 may represent a levelling off at the lower end of a range of teen pregnancy rate levels that might be expected in Canada and other Western countries (McKay, 2012). Young women who are feeling optimistic about their futures tend to delay child-bearing. Declining teen pregnancy rates for Canada in general are indicative of better sexual and reproductive health among young women. This decline in teen pregnancy can be attributed largely to more sexually active young people using reliable contraception such as condoms and birth control pills. The incidence of **sexually transmitted infections** (STIs), primarily chlamydia and gonorrhea, is on the rise in Canada, with the highest rates occurring in adolescents and young adult females (PHAC, 2015b) (see Chapter 6).

Adolescent health is another broad target area for community health promotion efforts, including health education and policy initiatives. Because adolescents often fail to perceive their own vulnerability, they need help navigating a complex environment and dealing with risk behaviours through preventive strategies that enhance decision making and increase protective factors.

Older Women

Women aged 65 and over constitute one of the fastest growing segments of the female population in Canada. The growth rate in the number of older adult women has been twice that for women under the age of 65 over the course of the past couple of decades. In addition, women now predominate in the ranks of Canadian older adults, in large part because the life expectancy of women has risen more rapidly than that of men during most of the last century.

While most older women report that their overall health is relatively good, almost all have a chronic health condition as diagnosed by a health care professional. Arthritis or rheumatism and high blood pressure are the most common chronic health problems reported by older women. However, there are preventive interventions that are effective in delaying or controlling age-related changes. Improving self-management activities such as diet and exercise are important health-promotion elements for this population.

The percentage of the female population accounted for by older adult women is expected to continue to rise during the next several decades. Canada had 4.8 million people aged 65 years and over on July 1, 2010 (Chui, 2011). Of this older adult population, 2.7 million, or 56%, were women, accounting for 16% of the total female population (Chui, 2011). By 2031, projections demonstrate that 9.6 million people will be aged 65 years and over, of whom 5.1 million will be women (53% of older adults and 24% of the total female population). The fact that women make up such a disproportionate share of the very oldest segments of the population has health implications. They tend to be the most vulnerable to serious health problems and the most likely to experience socioeconomic difficulties.

Homeless Women and Families

Homelessness among women is an increasing social and health issue in Canada. Women are at increased risk for hidden homelessness, living in overcrowded conditions, or having insufficient money for shelter (Gaetz et al., 2013). Family violence is a major cause of homelessness for women, a significant reason why they end up using homeless shelters. Homeless women comprise a population that is at high risk for chronic and infectious diseases and premature death. While both homeless women and men experience similar health problems, homeless women have distinct characteristics, vulnerabilities, and treatment needs. Homeless women may also be pregnant or have young children in their custody. Some of the health issues of particular significance to this group of women include access to birth control, prenatal care, breast and cervical cancer screening, and sexually transmitted infections (STIs). Homeless women are also disproportionately represented among those with mental health problems and substance use disorders. Poverty is the primary cause of homelessness. Low-income rates are more prevalent among certain subgroups of women. Indigenous and visible-minority women are nearly twice as likely as non–visible-minority women in Canada to have low incomes. Compared to two-parent families, lone mothers are almost five times more likely to have incomes that fall below the low-income cut-off (LICO) (Employment and Social Development Canada, 2011).

While homeless women are a heterogeneous group, they do share a number of similar features that may contribute to their overall poor health status. These include low income, unemployment, low levels of education, insufficient material resources, fear and mistrust of the health care system and of health care providers, and limited social support. Canada urgently needs to find new and innovative strategies that will address the barriers to health care that homeless women face both in cities and in more remote rural areas.

Children

Research conducted over the past two decades has emphasized the significance of the early years in the growth and development of children. The World Health Organization (WHO) identifies early child development (ECD) as a social determinant of health (SDH) and as the most important period of overall development throughout a person's lifespan; what children experience during the early years sets a critical foundation for their entire life course (Irwin, Siddiqi, & Hertzman, 2007). All facets of children's early development—those involving physical, social, emotional, and cognitive opportunities for growth—shape children's learning, school success, economic participation, social citizenry, and health. It is important to identify where children are most at risk for adversity and to intervene accordingly.

Of the 6,871,000 children living in Canada, 17% live in poverty (UNICEF, 2013). Canadian children are being raised in families that are squeezed financially and pressed for family time (UNICEF, 2013). These children living in poverty are more likely to be further disadvantaged, because poverty, in and of itself, is a significant risk factor. Most children fall into the middle socioeconomic gradient; this is where the greatest number of developmentally vulnerable children can be found (UNICEF, 2013). Indigenous children stand out as being disproportionately burdened in Canada. Recent statistics suggest that up to 40% of Canadian indigenous children are growing up in poverty, representing approximately 171,000 children (Gaetz et al., 2013). These children are growing up in deplorable conditions—some without running water, access to affordable nutritious food, housing, and a proper education.

Clearly, Canadian children are not doing as well as they could be. Canadian children ranked 17th out of 29 countries in a recent study of child well-being in rich countries (UNICEF, 2013). Of great concern is the high rate of obesity (27th of 29 countries), the high rate of bullying (21st of 29 countries), and the high rate of cannabis use—Canada ranked last. Canada's children also self-report that they have low life satisfaction; in fact, they are among the unhappiest in the industrialized world (UNICEF, 2013).

Implications for Nursing

Working in the community or in the home with the full spectrum of family organizational styles, vulnerable populations, and cultural groups may present challenges for the nurse. Whether nursing care is focused on women or children or on treatment and prevention of other health conditions in women and children, such as communicable diseases and STIs, nurses must exhibit a high degree of professionalism and competence. Cultural sensitivity, compassion, and a critical awareness of family strengths, dynamics, and social stressors that affect health-related decision making are critical components in developing an effective plan of care.

Successful health promotion among immigrant families depends on the resources, benefits, and policies that ensure their healthy development and successful social adjustment. Culturally competent health care and involvement of the immigrant community in health care programs are recommended strategies for improving the access to and effectiveness of health care for this population.

Nurses working with homeless women and families are challenged to locate these patients on a regular basis and to establish a therapeutic relationship with them. Health care providers may lack sufficient knowledge and sensitivity around the circumstances and special needs of this population and may inadvertently provide ineffective care. Many homeless women delay seeking health care or avoid it altogether because of having previous negative encounters with and lack of trust in health care providers.

Case management is recommended for coordinating the services and disciplines that may be involved in meeting the complex needs of these families. Whenever possible, general screening and preventive services must be provided when the family member seeks treatment, as this may be the only opportunity to provide health information and intervention. Building on existing coping strategies and strengths, the health care provider can help the patient to reconnect with a social support system. Nurses also have an important role in advocating for funding to support homeless health services and to improve access to preventive care for all homeless populations.

HOME CARE IN THE COMMUNITY

Within the current health care system, home care is an important component of health care delivery along the maternal and child continuum of care. The growing demand for home care is based on several factors:

- Shortened hospital stays
- Increase use of outpatient procedures and surgeries
- New technologies that facilitate home-based assessments and treatments
- Desire for the patient and family to be at home

Home care is the provision of technical, psychological, and other therapeutic support in the patient's home rather than in an institution. The scope of nursing care delivered in the home is necessarily limited to practices deemed safe and appropriate to be carried out in an environment that is physically separated from a health care institution and its resources. Nursing practice at home is consistent with provincial regulations that direct home care practice. The nurse demonstrates practice competence through formalized orientation and ongoing clinical education and performance evaluation in the respective home care agency.

Home health care can be viewed as an extension of in-hospital care. Essentially, the primary difference between health care in a hospital and home care is the absence of the continuous presence of professional health care providers in a patient's home. Generally, but not always, home health care entails intermittent care by a professional who visits the patient's home for a particular reason and/or provides care onsite for fewer than 4 hours at a time. The home health care agency maintains on-call professional staff to assist home care patients who have questions about their care and for emergencies, such as equipment failure. A wide range of professional health care services and products can be delivered or used in the home by means of technology and telecommunication. For example, telehealth and telemedicine make it possible for patients in the home to be interviewed and assessed by a specialist located hundreds of kilometres away.

Home care agencies are subject to regulation by governmental and professional organizations and provide interdisciplinary services including social work, nutrition, and occupational and physical therapy. Increasingly, their caseloads are made up of patients who require high-technology care, such as parenteral nutrition for women with hyperemesis or children requiring care of central lines for chemotherapy. Although the home health nurse develops the care plan, all care must be ordered by a physician or a nurse practitioner.

Patient Selection and Referral

The office or hospital-based nurse is often the key person in making effective referrals to home care. When considering a referral to home care, the following factors are evaluated:

- Health status of patient: Is the condition serious enough to warrant home care, and is it stable enough for intermittent observation to be sufficient?
- Availability of professionals to provide the needed services within the patient's community.
- Family resources, including psychosocial, social, and economic resources: Will the family be able to provide care between nursing visits? Are relationships supportive? Does the family have health benefits to support their care? Could a voluntary community agency provide needed care without payment?
- Cost-effectiveness: Is it more reasonable for the patient to receive these services at home or to go to a local outpatient facility to receive them?

Community referrals should not be limited to patients with physiological complications that require medical treatment. Patients at risk (e.g., young adolescents, families with a history of abuse, members of vulnerable population groups, developmentally disabled individuals) may need follow-up care at home. As we move more and more into an interdisciplinary health care society, it is crucial that nurses communicate with social workers to tap into valuable community resources that patients can use in their own communities after being discharged.

High-technology home care requires additional information to be collected from the chart and consultation with the referring physician and other members of the health care team before a home care referral is made. These additional data include the medical diagnosis, medical prognosis, prescribed therapies, medication history, drug-dosing information, potential ancillary supplies, type of infusion and access device, and the available systems of social support for the patient and family. The nursing assessment and therapy data provide baseline information for the home care nurse and other health care providers involved in the care plan.

Phone and Online Health Support

As health care continues to consist of frequent and brief contacts with health care providers during the perinatal and early child development periods, services that link patients to care have assumed greater importance. There are several different ways in which these linkages can be made. Most public health departments across the country offer telephone support lines or social media connections with families (Facebook, Twitter) to provide parents with support and education about pregnancy, breastfeeding, and parenting. Another Web-based resource is provincial websites that provide people with medically approved information on many health topics, medications, and tips for promoting health lifestyles, for example, HealthlinkBC.

Providers are using the Internet to communicate with patients who have an Internet service provider (ISP). Telephonic nursing care through services such as nurse advice lines and telephonic nursing assessments is a valuable means of managing health care problems and bridging the gaps between acute, outpatient, and home care services. Nursing care that occurs by telephone is interactive and responsive to immediate health care questions about particular health care needs. Telehealth is another option in which nurses guide callers through urgent health care situations, suggest treatment options, and provide health education.

Nursing Care

Home Visiting

The community health or home health nurse will review the home visiting referral, screening tool results, record of birth, available clinical data, demographic information, and any other relevant information and then set up the visit with the patient. During the telephone call to arrange a mutually convenient visiting time, the nurse will determine the goals of the visit. The nurse needs to review relevant policies and procedures, professional literature about any potential diagnosis, and community resources as part of the previsit preparation work (Box 3-3).

Before going on a home visit, the nurse will contact the patient or family in order to make necessary arrangements and obtain detailed instructions on the location of the home. In addition to establishing a convenient time to visit and the exact directions, through the initial contact by telephone the nurse is also setting the stage for the first home visit.

During this contact, the nurse should identify himself or herself by name, title, and agency. He or she can then begin to build rapport with the patient. The nurse will convey the purpose of the home visits, if necessary. The nurse should briefly explain what will occur during the visit and approximately how long the visit will last. The patient and family should be asked to restrain any pets that may be present during the visit.

First home visit. Making the first home visit can be stressful for both the nurse and the family. The home visiting nurse is faced with an unknown environment controlled by the patient and the family. The patient and the family can also experience feelings about the unknown, such as anxiety about the way the nurse will treat them or what the nurse will do during the visit. The challenge for the community health or home health nurse is to establish a nurse–patient relationship and provide the prescribed services within the time provided for the initial home visit. One of the most important tasks of the home health nurse is modelling health-related behaviours for the patient and others who are in the home during the visit.

During the first visit, after introductions have been made, the nurse will complete extensive assessment documentation with the patient. If the nurse needs to consult with the patient's physician, nurse practitioner, or other health care providers, a consent form will need to be signed by the patient. All patients have the right to participate actively in their plan of care. Explanation of these patient rights and responsibilities should begin the discussion about the nurse and patient roles during this initial visit.

Assessment. The primary goals of the assessment phase are to develop a trusting relationship and collect data by various methods to obtain a comprehensive patient profile. The major areas of the assessment are demographics, medical history, general health history, medication history, psychosocial assessment (Box 3-4), home and community environment, and physical assessment. It may not be feasible or appropriate to collect in-depth information about all areas of assessment during the first visit. However, in many instances the nurse may be limited to one visit and must obtain information pertinent to the current situation during that visit.

Establishing a trusting relationship begins with the previsit telephone call. An interview style that reflects sensitivity, conveys a nonjudgemental, accepting attitude, and shows respect for the patient's rights facilitates the development of that trusting relationship. A skillful interviewer avoids barriers to communication, such as false reassurance, advice-giving, excessive talking, and showing approval or disapproval. This nurse–patient relationship will continue to develop over the course of each home visit.

The nurse is a guest in the patient's home and should show respect for the patient's belongings. Some adaptation of the home visit schedule may need to be made if numerous distractions interrupt a visit, such as caring for the needs of small children. The nurse may ask to have the volume of the television reduced or suggest moving to another room where it is more quiet and private.

Plan of care and implementation. The nursing plan of care is developed in collaboration with the patient, based on the health care and learning needs of the individual. Home visiting nurses work from a standard care plan and make adjustments in order to meet the needs of each individual patient. The frequency of the skilled nursing visit may vary with the individual plan of care, and often a family visitor or lay home visitor will be recommended if additional support is suggested.

There are several areas of concern when caring for a patient in the home. In home care, the patient or family members may be responsible for administration of medications in the absence of the nurse. A careful medication history should be obtained to see if the patient is taking the medications correctly and understands their desired action and potential side effects. It is important that patients and caregivers have a clear understanding of medication regimens and are notified when medications change in any way. Even more important is ensuring that the patient and caregivers fully understand the information that they are provided by health care providers.

BOX 3-3 PROTOCOL FOR HOME VISITS

Previsit Interventions

1. Contact the family to arrange details for a home visit.
   a. Identify self, credentials, and role of the community health or home health nurse.
   b. Review the purpose of the home visit.
   c. Schedule a convenient time for the visit.
   d. Confirm address and route to the family home.
2. Review and clarify appropriate data.
   a. Review all available assessment data for the patient or family (i.e., referral forms, hospital discharge summaries, family-identified learning needs).
   b. Review records of any previous nursing contacts.
   c. Contact other professional caregivers as necessary to clarify data (e.g., physician, midwife, nurse, referring source).
3. Identify community resources and teaching materials that are appropriate to meet needs already identified.
4. Plan the visit and prepare any resources required for the visit.

In-Home Interventions: Establishing a Relationship

1. Reintroduce self and establish the purpose of the visit for the parents, child, and family; offer the family an opportunity to clarify their expectations of contact.
2. Spend a brief time socially interacting with the family to become acquainted and establish a trusting relationship.

In-Home Interventions: Working with a Family

1. Conduct a systematic assessment of the patient to determine physiological adjustment and any existing complications.
2. Throughout the visit, collect data to assess the emotional adjustment of individual patient and family members to illness or lifestyle changes.
3. Determine adequacy of the support system if appropriate.
   a. To what extent does someone help with cooking, cleaning, and other home management tasks?
   b. To what extent is help being provided in caring for the patient or other family members?
   c. Are support persons encouraging the patient to care for herself and get adequate rest?
4. Throughout the visit, observe the home environment for adequacy of resources (if appropriate):
   a. Space: privacy, safe play of children, sleeping
   b. Overall cleanliness and state of repair
   c. Number of steps the patient must climb
   d. Adequacy of cooking arrangements
   e. Adequacy of refrigeration and other food storage areas
   f. Adequacy of bathing, toilet, and laundry facilities
5. Throughout the visit, observe the home environment for overall state of repair and existence of safety hazards:
   a. Storage of medications, household cleaners, and other substances hazardous to children
   b. Presence of peeling paint on furniture, walls, or pipes
   c. Factors that contribute to falls, such as dim lighting, broken steps, scatter rugs
   d. Presence of vermin
   e. Use of crib or playpen that fails to meet safety guidelines
   f. Existence of emergency plan in case of fire; fire alarm or extinguisher
6. Provide care to the patient.
7. Provide teaching on the basis of previously identified needs.
8. Refer the family to appropriate community agencies or resources, such as telephone contact information lines and community support groups.
9. Ascertain that the patient and family know potential problems to watch for and whom to call if they occur.

In-Home Interventions: Ending the Visit

1. Summarize the activities and main points of the visit.
2. Clarify future expectations, including scheduling of the next visit.
3. Review the teaching plan and highlight important points.
4. Provide information about reaching the nurse or public health department if needed before the next scheduled visit.

Postvisit Interventions

1. Document the visit thoroughly, using the required agency forms.
2. Initiate the plan of care on which the next encounter with the patient or family will be based.
3. Communicate appropriately to other staff assigned to care for the family. This may include follow-up with other health care providers, if warranted.

It is also important that nurses are aware of how to use and educate patients and families on the use of all home care equipment such as infusion pumps and phototherapy lights. Nurses also have to be skilled at performing various procedures such as venipuncture and administration of intravenous medications or fluids. In addition to teaching about medications and equipment, nurses must be sure that patients and families know how to respond in emergency situations.

The provision of education during a home visit is a key component of the visit. Verbal explanations should be supplemented with clearly written instructions if the patient has difficulty remembering or if there is a language barrier. Many written resources are available in multiple languages to facilitate the transfer of information and knowledge.

Finally, as soon as home care has been provided, it is essential that the nurse document the assessment findings, care provided, recommendations for change, and any patient or family teaching done. Nursing documentation should reflect an objective description of the nursing assessment data collected at each visit and the associated outcomes. Once the home visiting outcomes are achieved or the patient is discharged from the program, documentation should include information about the patient's status at the time of discharge, progress toward attaining health care goals, and plans for any follow-up care. Appropriate care should be taken to complete the necessary home health care records accurately and in a timely manner and ensuring appropriate privacy rules are maintained. Documentation guidelines are agency specific but may include writing or dictating notes

BOX 3-4 PSYCHOSOCIAL ASSESSMENT

Language
Identify the primary language spoken in the home.
Assess whether there are any language barriers to receiving support.
Assess health literacy.

Community Resources and Access to Care
Identify primary and secondary means of transportation.
Identify community agencies that the family currently uses for health care and support.
Assess cultural and psychosocial barriers to receiving care.

Social Support
Determine the people living with the patient.
Identify who assists with household chores.
Identify who assists with child care and parenting activities.
Identify who the patient turns to with problems or during a crisis.
Social networks both formal and informal.

Interpersonal Relationship
Identify the way in which decisions are made in the family.
Identify the family's perception of the need for home visiting.
Identify roles of adults in caring for family members.

Caregiver
Identify the primary caregiver for the patient.
Identify other caregivers and their roles.
Assess the caregiver's knowledge of care required for the patient and the purpose of home visits.
Identify potential strain from the caregiver role.
Identify the level of satisfaction with the caregiver role.

Stress and Coping
Identify what the patient perceives as lifestyle changes and their impact on self and the family.
Identify the changes that the patient and family have made to adjust to the illness or life transition.

or using eDocumentation shortly after the visit. Many agencies have adopted a charting-by-exception policy which requires charting health findings that are exceptional according to professional and legal standards.

Safety issues for the home visiting nurse. Nurse safety and infection control are two important aspects specific to home care. The nurse should be fully aware of the home environment and the neighbourhood in which the home care will be provided. Unlike hospitals, in which the environment is more predictable and controlled, the patient's neighbourhood and home have the potential for uncertainty. Home visiting nurses should take necessary safety precautions and avoid dangerous situations.

Personal strategies recommended for nurses visiting families with a history of violence or substance use include (1) self-awareness, (2) environmental assessment, (3) using listening and observation skills with patients to be aware of behavioural changes that indicate aggression or lack of impulse control, (4) planning for dealing with aggressive behaviour (i.e., allowing personal space and taking a nonaggressive stance), (5) making visits in pairs, and (6) having access to a cell phone at all times.

Personal safety. The home care nurse must be aware of personal safety behaviours before going on a home visit. Dress should be casual but professional in appearance, with a first-name-only identification tag. Limited jewellery should be worn. Valuable personal items such as an expensive purse or coat should not be worn on a visit. Carrying an extra set of car keys in the nursing home care bag saves time and frustration if the nurse becomes locked out of the automobile. The same common-sense behaviours and precautions that guide a person's behaviour when alone in any setting should be followed by home visiting nurses.

The community health nurse should ensure that his or her employer knows the itinerary by keeping their electronic calendar up to date as per protocol. Many nurses carry agency-provided cell phones that allow the department to contact the nurse throughout the day in order to give information about patient updates or schedule changes. A cell phone is also useful for notifying patients when the nurse is delayed.

Home visiting nurses should park and lock their cars in a safe place that is visible from the street and the patient's home and away from hidden alleys. While driving to the patient's home, the nurse should assess the neighbourhood for safety, especially if it is unfamiliar. All valuable items should be stored out of sight before leaving the office. While walking to the patient's home, nurses should avoid groups of strangers hanging out in doorways or alleys and avoid entering into vacant buildings or entering a yard that has an unrestrained dog. The home or building should not be entered if the nurse has any safety concerns. All health departments have policies to follow for such situations.

Patient's home. Once inside the woman's home, the nurse may encounter unsafe situations, such as the presence of weapons, abusive behaviour, or health hazards. Each potentially hazardous situation must be dealt with according to agency policies and procedures. If abuse or neglect is reasonably suspected, the home care nurse should follow the department's and the province's regulations for reporting and documenting the situation. Nurses should maintain their own safety first and act accordingly throughout the visit.

Infection control. The importance of infection control does not diminish because nursing care is being provided in the patient's home. Patients are not likely to become infected because of their home environment, but the nurse may become exposed to an infectious disease.

Hand hygiene remains the single most important infection-control procedure, and the caregiver is in a position to educate the family about the importance of this practice in preventing disease. Hands should be washed before and after each patient contact; wearing gloves does not eliminate the necessity for hand hygiene. If running water or clean facilities are unavailable, hands can be cleaned with hand sanitizer. Although community health nurses do not usually provide hands-on care to the patient unless it is for breastfeeding support, home health nurses do. Specific nursing practice varies across the country from province to province.

KEY POINTS

- A *community* is defined as a locality-based entity composed of systems of societal institutions, informal groups, and aggregates that are interdependent and whose function is to meet a wide variety of collective needs.
- Caring for patients within a community requires a multidisciplinary approach.
- Community health nursing focuses on promoting and maintaining the health of individuals, families, and groups in the community setting.
- Economic evaluations provide objective information to establish a program's value to society.
- Individual families and communities may have demographic characteristics that affect their risk for disease or injury.
- Epidemiology is the science of population health applied to the detection of morbidity and mortality in a population.
- Community health programs are based on three levels of intervention: primary, secondary, and tertiary.
- A community needs assessment involves collection of subjective and objective information about the community.
- A community health diagnosis is a problem with a defined cause related to a community problem.
- Most changes aimed at improving community health involve partnerships between community residents, key stakeholders, and health care workers.
- Evaluation of effective community programs includes consideration of the structure, process, and outcomes related to the program.
- Methods of collecting data useful to the nurse working in the community include walking surveys, analysis of existing data, informant interviews, and participant observation.
- Vulnerable populations are groups that are at higher risk for developing physical, mental, or social health problems.
- Community health nurses must be aware of vulnerable populations within the community who may require additional care.
- Telephone contact centres, credible websites, and social media applications are low-cost health care services that facilitate continuous patient education, support, and health care decision making, even though health care is delivered in multiple sites.
- Nurses who provide care in the community incorporate knowledge from community health nursing, acute care nursing, family therapy, health promotion, and patient education.
- Home visiting nurses should incorporate personal safety and infection control practices in the nursing plan of care.

evolve WEBSITE

Visit the Evolve website for additional resources related to the content in this chapter such as Case Studies, Critical Thinking Case Study Answers, Nursing Care Plans, Nursing Processes, Nursing Skills, and Review Questions for Exam Preparation at: http://evolve.elsevier.com/Canada/Perry/maternal/

REFERENCES

Anderson, E. T., & McFarlane, J. (2010). Community assessment. Using a model for practice. In E. T. Anderson & J. McFarlane (Eds.), *Community as partner: Theory and practice in nursing* (7th ed.). Philadelphia: Lippincott Williams & Wilkins.

Canadian Community Health Nursing. (2008). *Canadian Community Health Nursing: Standards of practice*. Retrieved from <http://www.chnc.ca/documents/chn_standards_of_practice_mar08_english.pdf>.

Canadian Perinatal Surveillance System. (2008). *Canadian perinatal health report: 2008 edition*. Retrieved from <http://www.violapolomeno.com/cphr-rspc08-eng.pdf>.

Canadian Public Health Association (CPHA). (2010). *Public health/community health nursing practice in Canada: Roles and activities* (4th ed.). Retrieved from <http://www.cpha.ca/uploads/pubs/3-1bk04214.pdf>.

Chui, T. (2011). *Women in Canada: A gender-based statistical report*. Retrieved from <http://www.statcan.gc.ca/pub/89-503-x/2010001/article/11528-eng.pdf>.

Community Health Assessment Network of Manitoba. (2009). *Community health assessment guidelines*. Retrieved from <http://www.gov.mb.ca/health/rha/docs/chag.pdf>.

Community Health Nurses of Canada. (2009). *Public health nursing discipline specific competencies*, version 1.0. Retrieved from <http://www.chnc.ca/documents/competencies_june_2009_english.pdf>.

Community Health Nurses of Canada. (2010). *Home health nursing competencies*, version 1.0. Retrieved from <http://login.greatbignews.com/UserFiles/289/documents/HomeHealthNursingCompetenciesVersion1March2010.pdf>.

DiCenso, A., Bourgeault, I., Abelson, J., et al. (2010). Utilization of nurse practitioners to increase patient access to primary healthcare in Canada—Thinking outside the box. *Nursing Leadership, 23*, 239–259.

Donabedian, A. (1988). The quality of care: How can it be assessed? *JAMA: The Journal of the American Medical Association, 121*(11), 1145–1150. doi:10.1001/jama.1988.03410120089033.

Employment and Social Development Canada. (2011). *Indicators of well-being in Canada*. Retrieved from <http://www4.hrsdc.gc.ca/.3ndic.1t.4r@-eng.jsp?iid=23>.

Gaetz, S., Donaldson, J., Richter, T., & Gulliver, T. (2013). *The state of homelessness in Canada 2013*. Toronto: Canadian Homelessness Research Network Press.

Irwin, L., Siddiqi, A., & Hertzman, C. (2007). *Early child development: A powerful equalizer*. Final report for the WHO Commission on the Social Determinants of Health. Geneva: World Health Organization. Retrieved from <http://www.who.int/maternal_child_adolescent/documents/ecd_final_m30/en/>.

Marmot, M. (2010). *Marmot Review report: Fair society, healthy lives.* Retrieved from <http://www.local.gov.uk/health/-/journal_content/56/10180/3510094/ARTICLE>.

McFarlane, J., & Gilroy, H. (2015). Epidemiology, demography and community health. In E. T. Anderson & J. McFarlane (Eds.), *Community as partner: Theory and practice in nursing* (7th ed.). Philadelphia: Lippincott Williams & Wilkins.

McKay, A. (2012). Trends in Canadian national and provincial/territorial teen pregnancy rates: 2001–2010. *Canadian Journal of Human Sexuality, 21*(3–4), 160–175.

Public Health Agency of Canada. (2008). *Centre for health promotion.* Retrieved from <http://www.phac-aspc.gc.ca/chhd-sdsh/index-eng.php>.

Public Health Agency of Canada. (2011a). *Mandate.* Retrieved from <http://www.phac-aspc.gc.ca/about_apropos/what-eng.php>.

Public Health Agency of Canada. (2011b). *The community capacity building tool: A tool for planning, building and reflecting on community capacity in community-based health projects.* Retrieved from <http://www.phac-aspc.gc.ca/canada/regions/ab-nwt-tno/downloads-eng.php>.

Public Health Agency of Canada. (2011c). *What determines health?* Retrieved from <http://www.phac-aspc.gc.ca/ph-sp/determinants/index-eng.php>.

Public Health Agency of Canada. (2015a). *Community action program for children.* Retrieved from <http://www.phac-aspc.gc.ca/hp-ps/dca-dea/prog-ini/capc-pace/index-eng.php>.

Public Health Agency of Canada. (2015b). *Report on sexually transmitted infections in Canada: 2012.* Retrieved from <http://www.phac-aspc.gc.ca/sti-its-surv-epi/rep-rap-2012/sum-som-eng.php>.

Savage, C., & Kub, J. (2009). Public health and nursing: A natural partnership. *International Journal of Environmental Research and Public Health, 6*(11), 2843–2848.

Scientific Advisory Committee on Nutrition. (2011). *The influence of maternal, fetal and child nutrition on the development of chronic disease in later life.* Retrieved from <https://www.gov.uk/government/uploads/system/uploads/attachment_data/file/339325/SACN_Early_Life_Nutrition_Report.pdf>.

Smylie, J., Crengle, S., Freemantle, J., & Taualii, M. (2010). Indigenous birth outcomes in Australia, Canada, New Zealand and the United States—An overview. *Open Women's Health Journal, 4,* 7–17. doi:10.2174/1874291201004010007.

Statistics Canada. (2010). *Having a regular medical doctor 2008.* Ottawa: Author. Retrieved from <http://www.statcan.gc.ca/pub/82-625-x/2010001/article/11102-eng.htm>.

Statistics Canada. (2012). *Women in Canada at a glance statistical highlights.* Retrieved from <http://www.swc-cfc.gc.ca/rc-cr/stat/wic-fac-2012/sec11-eng.html>.

Statistics Canada. (2014). *The 10 leading causes of death, 2011.* Retrieved from <http://www.statcan.gc.ca/pub/82-625-x/2014001/article/11896-eng.htm>.

Statistics Canada. (2015). *Women in Canada: A gender-based statistical report* (7th ed.). Ottawa: Author (Cat No: 89-503-XWE). Retrieved from <http://www.statcan.gc.ca/bsolc/olc-cel/olc-cel?lang=eng&catno=89-503-X>.

Truth and Reconciliation Commission of Canada. (2015). *Truth and Reconciliation Commission of Canada: Calls to action.* Retrieved from <http://www.trc.ca/websites/trcinstitution/File/2015/Findings/Calls_to_Action_English2.pdf>.

Underwood, J. M., Mowat, D., Meagher-Stewart, D., et al. (2009). Building community and public health nursing capacity: A synthesis report of the National Community Health Nursing Study. *Canadian Journal of Public Health, 100*(5), 1–11.

UNICEF Office of Research. (2013). *Child well-being in rich countries: A comparative overview. Innocenti Report Card 11.* Florence: Author.

United Nations Population Fund. (2012). *Rich mother, poor mother: The social determinants of maternal death and disability.* Retrieved from <http://www.unfpa.org/sites/default/files/resource-pdf/EN-SRH%20fact%20sheet-Poormother.pdf>.

Verstraeten, B. S., Mijovic-Kondejewski, J., Takeda, J., et al. (2015). Canada's pregnancy-related mortality rates: Doing well but room for improvement. *Clinical and Investigative Medicine, 38*(1), E15–E22.

Williams, C. A. (2011). Populations-focused practice: The foundation of specialization in public health practice. In M. Stanhope & J. Lancaster (Eds.), *Community and public health nursing* (7th ed.). St. Louis: Mosby.

World Health Organization. (2008). *Commission on the Social Determinants of Health final report: Closing the gap in a generation. Health equity through action on the social determinants of health.* Geneva: Author. Retrieved from <http://whqlibdoc.who.int/publications/2008/9789241563703_eng.pdf>.

ADDITIONAL RESOURCES

Community Assessment Tools

Community Health Assessment Guidelines 2009. <http://www.gov.mb.ca/health/rha/docs/chag.pdf>

What Is a Community Health Assessment? <http://www.cdc.gov/stltpublichealth/cha/plan.html>

Community Health Organizations

Canadian Public Health Association (CPHA). <http://www.cpha.ca/en/default.aspx>

Community Health Nurses of Canada (CHNC). <http://www.chnc.ca/default.cfm>

HealthlinkBC. <http://www.healthlinkbc.ca/>

PART 2

Perinatal Nursing

UNIT 2

Introduction to Perinatal Nursing

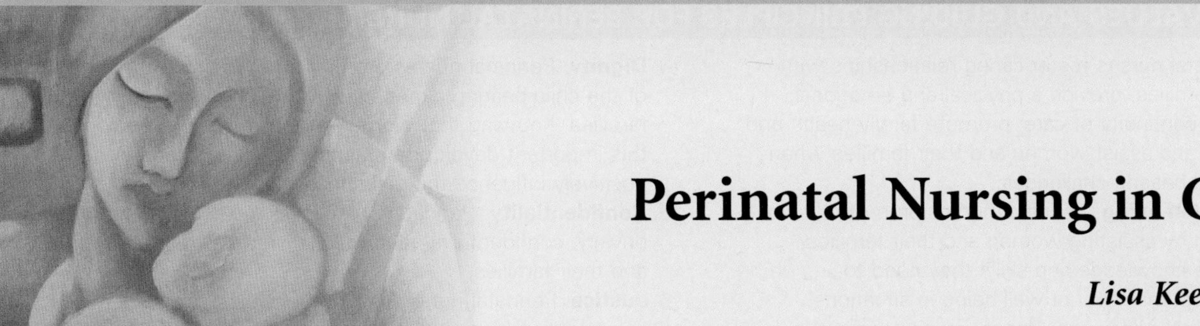

CHAPTER 4

Perinatal Nursing in Canada

Lisa Keenan-Lindsay

evolve WEBSITE

Visit the Evolve website for additional resources related to the content in this chapter such as Case Studies, Critical Thinking Case Study Answers, Nursing Care Plans, Nursing Processes, Nursing Skills, and Review Questions for Exam Preparation at: *http://evolve.elsevier.com/Canada/Perry/maternal/*

OBJECTIVES

On completion of this chapter the reader will be able to:

- Describe the scope of perinatal nursing in Canada today.
- Describe the history and context for perinatal care in Canada.
- Discuss guiding principles for working with child-bearing women and their families.
- Examine current trends in perinatal health and compare epidemiological data among groups and populations.
- Explore current issues affecting perinatal nursing practice and envision creative alternatives.
- Describe ethical issues facing perinatal nurses.

This chapter presents a general overview of Canadian issues and trends related to the health and health care of women, newborns, and families during the child-bearing year.

PERINATAL NURSING

Perinatal nursing is a recognized specialty in Canada. Perinatal nurses work collaboratively with child-bearing women and their families throughout the child-bearing year, from preconception through pregnancy and childbirth, and over the postpartum transition period. Perinatal nurses promote the physical, emotional, social, and spiritual well-being of the whole family and work to address health inequities that influence health outcomes (Box 4-1). Perinatal nurses care for child-bearing women and families in many settings, including the hospital, the home, and a variety of ambulatory and community settings. They also work collaboratively with other health and social care providers, such as physicians, midwives, nutritionists, doulas, and social workers, to name a few.

In Canada, perinatal nurses can be recognized for their expertise through the Canadian Nurses Association (CNA) certification program (see Additional Resources at the end of the chapter).

Nurses attempt to use evidence-informed practice to guide their interactions and interventions. The Society of Obstetricians and Gynaecologists of Canada (SOGC) has developed many clinical practice guidelines that are useful to perinatal nurses. Many regional health authorities have also developed guidelines that are available when providing care, for example, Perinatal Services BC and the Champlain Maternal Newborn Regional Program (see Additional Resources at the end of the chapter). Perinatal units can adapt these recommendations to their specific institutions, enabling nurses to become more informed about current evidence and provide more effective care for child-bearing families.

Perinatal Services in Canada

Maternal and newborn services have evolved from our colonial and Indigenous roots to the current system of regionalized perinatal and neonatal care. Box 4-2 provides an overview of the history over the past two centuries and shows the progress that has been made, although there is still room for improvement. Canada and the United States are unique internationally in that they have a very low percentage of well-woman care provided by midwives. Most perinatal care in Canada is provided by

BOX 4-1 VALUES AND GUIDING PRINCIPLES FOR PERINATAL NURSING IN CANADA

1. **Caring**: Perinatal nurses foster caring relationships with women and families, provide a physical and emotional presence and continuity of care, promote family health and development, and assist women and their families when they face child-bearing challenges.
2. **Health and Well-being**: Perinatal nurses promote health and well-being by assisting women and their families to develop the knowledge and skills they need to achieve their optimal level of well-being in situations of developmental transitions, illness, or injury or in the process of dying.
3. **Informed Decision Making**: Perinatal nurses have a holistic view of women and families and respect their capacity to set goals and make decisions. Women and families have the right to make informed choices that are congruent with their own beliefs and values.
4. **Dignity**: Perinatal nurses are privileged to share the intimacy of the child-bearing experience with women and their families. Knowing that women will have lasting memories of this important developmental process, nurses strive to positively influence the child-bearing experience.
5. **Confidentiality**: Perinatal nurses recognize the importance of privacy, confidentiality, and maintaining the trust of women and their families.
6. **Justice**: Perinatal nurses uphold principles of justice by safeguarding human rights, equity, and fairness as they work with child-bearing women, families, and newborns.
7. **Accountability**: Perinatal nurses act with integrity and in a manner consistent with their professional responsibilities and standards of practice.
8. **Quality Practice Environments**: Perinatal nurses advocate for safe, supportive, and respectful work environments.

Adapted from Association of Women's Health, Obstetric and Neonatal Nurses (AWHONN) (2009). *Standards for professional perinatal nursing practice and certification in Canada.* (2nd ed.). Washington, DC: Author. Retrieved from http://www.capwhn.ca

BOX 4-2 HISTORIC MILESTONES IN THE CARE OF MOTHERS AND INFANTS

1847—Ether used in Scotland for an internal podalic version (first reported use of obstetric anaesthesia)

1848—Soeurs de Misericorde (Montreal) provide maternity care for unwed mothers

1861—Ignaz Semmelweis writes *The Etiology, Concept, and Prophylaxis of Childbed Fever*

1892—A law is passed making it illegal to sell or advertise contraceptives in Canada

1897—Victoria Order of Nurses (VON) established to improve maternal and infant health and to train nurses

1908—Childbirth classes started and prenatal care provided by outpost and public health nurses working in cities, small towns, and rural communities

1911—First milk bank in the United States, established in Boston

1912—Medical Council of Canada formed and makes midwifery illegal in most locations

1916—Margaret Sanger establishes the first American birth control clinic, in Brooklyn, NY

1920—Midwifery legalized in the colony of Newfoundland

1923—First U.S. hospital centre for premature infant care, established in Chicago

1929—Modern tampon (with an applicator) invented and patented

1933—Sodium pentothal used as anaesthesia for childbirth; *Natural Childbirth* published by Grantly Dick-Read

1934—Dionne quintuplets born in Ontario and survive partly due to donated breast milk

1935—Sulphonamides introduced as cure for puerperal fever; Parents Information Bureau opened in Ontario to provide contraceptive information

1940—*Canadian Mother and Child* book first published and distributed free to Canadian mothers

1941—Penicillin used as treatment for infection

1944—Society of Obstetricians and Gynaecologists of Canada (SOGC) formed

1953—Apgar scoring system of neonatal assessment published by Virginia Apgar

1956—Oxygen determined to cause retrolental fibroplasia (now known as retinopathy of prematurity)

1957—Hospital Insurance and Diagnostic Services Act passed in Canada

1958—First fetal electrocardiogram from the maternal abdomen reported (first commercial electronic fetal monitor produced in the late 1960s); first clinical use of ultrasound to examine the fetus reported

1959—Agnes Higgins joins the Montreal Diet Dispensary and later develops an approach for improving nutrition for disadvantaged pregnant women (Higgins method); cytological studies demonstrate that Down syndrome is associated with a particular form of nondisjunction (trisomy 21); *Thank You, Dr. Lamaze* published by Marjorie Karmel

1960—American Society for Psychoprophylaxis in Obstetrics (ASPO/Lamaze) and the International Childbirth Education Association (ICEA) formed; birth control pill introduced for "menstrual regulation" since contraceptives could not be legally prescribed in Canada; condoms available behind the counter in most pharmacies

1962—Thalidomide found to cause birth defects

1963—Testing for PKU begun

1967—Rho(D) immune globulin produced for treatment of Rh incompatibility; Reva Rubin publishes article on maternal role attainment

1968—The *Medical Care Act* passed and provinces begin to implement health insurance plans; rubella vaccine available

1969—Nurses Association of the American College of Obstetricians and Gynecologists (NAACOG) founded in the United States; some Canadian nurses join this organization; contraception decriminalized in Canada; mammogram becomes available

1970s—Total of 20 human milk banks across Canada receive donated breast milk

BOX 4-2 HISTORIC MILESTONES IN THE CARE OF MOTHERS AND INFANTS—cont'd

1974—LaLonde Report recommends more attention to health promotion and disease prevention
1975—The Pregnant Patient's Bill of Rights published by ICEA
1976—First home pregnancy kits approved
1978—First test-tube baby born in Britain; outpost nursing program at Memorial University, Newfoundland, includes a 10-month nurse-midwifery program
1980—Canadian Obstetrical Gynaecological and Neonatal Nurses (COGNN) formed as a special interest group within NAACOG
1986—Ottawa Charter for Health Promotion recommends more attention to health determinants; midwifery education program in Povungnituk, Quebec, begins preparing Inuit midwives
1987—Safe Motherhood Initiative launched by the World Health Organization and other international agencies
1988—Abortion decriminalized in Canada; SOGC launches International Women's Health Program
1991—Canadian Paediatric Society recommends that a minimum of one person skilled in neonatal resuscitation be present at every birth
1993—Midwifery education program launched in Ontario; human embryos cloned in the United States; first Canadian statement on reducing the risk of Sudden Infant Death Syndrome (SIDS) released by Health Canada
1994—Midwifery legalized in Ontario; zidovudine guidelines published to reduce mother-to-fetus transmission of HIV; DNA sequences of BRCA1 and BRCA2 identified
1995—Canadian Perinatal Surveillance System (CPSS) launched
1998—Mandatory folic acid fortification of all breads and cereals sold in Canada
1998—COGNN becomes AWHONN Canada (Association of Women's Health, Obstetric and Neonatal Nurses Canada) and proposes to have perinatal nursing recognized as a specialty by the Canadian Nurses Association
1999—First emergency contraceptive pill for pregnancy prevention (Plan B) approved; midwifery legalized in Quebec with midwives practising in birth centres
2000—National guidelines for family-centred maternal and newborn care published; first Canadian Nurses Association Perinatal Nursing Certification exam; Canadian Association of Midwives (CAM) formed
2001—Joint Statement on Shaken Baby Syndrome released by Health Canada
2005—The Canadian Association of Neonatal Nurses (CANN) formed
2006—Human papillomavirus (HPV) vaccine first available
2008—Joint Policy Statement on Normal Birth released by SOGC; emergency contraception (Plan B) available over the counter in pharmacies
2009—*What Mothers Say: The Maternity Experiences Survey* published by the Public Health Agency of Canada, discussed Canadian women's experience of child-bearing
2010—One breast milk bank in Vancouver remains, although others are in development; midwifery recognized as a legal and regulated profession in many Canadian provinces and territories; SOGC releases policy statement "*Returning Birth to Aboriginal, Rural, and Remote Communities*"
2011—AWHONN Canada becomes the Canadian Association of Perinatal and Women's Health Nurses (CAPWHN)
2012—Breastfeeding Committee for Canada develops the Integrated Ten Steps Practice Outcome Indicators for Baby Friendly Initiative (BFI)
2013—Millennium Development Goals (MDG)—Canada commits to reducing child mortality (MDG 4) and improving maternal health (MDG 5) through major monetary contributions and recommitment beyond 2015
2015—78 hospitals/health centres have the Baby Friendly designation; four milk banks open in Canada with more under development

PKU, phenylketonuria; *SIDS*, sudden infant death syndrome.

physicians, with obstetricians providing increasing percentages of perinatal care. Most births in Canada take place in hospitals, some occur in birth centres; home births account for a very small proportion of births.

The delivery of maternity care within each community, province, and territory contains unique elements as each level of government tries to balance human resources, funding, and liability concerns with regulatory, educational, political, and demographic issues. Inequities in access to good-quality maternity care have developed particularly in rural, remote, inner-city, and Indigenous communities, compared with access to such care in other Canadian communities. Many of these health inequities result from conditions of vulnerability and lack of access to the social determinants of health (see Table 1-1 on p. 5).

Both the Canadian Perinatal Health Report (Canadian Perinatal Surveillance System [CPSS], 2008) and the Maternity Experiences Survey (Public Health Agency of Canada [PHAC], 2009) note that poor women (women living below the low income cut-off), Indigenous women, and young women with less education consistently have the poorest perinatal outcomes. Limited maternal education, young maternal age, poverty, and the lack of prenatal care appear to be associated with higher **infant mortality rates**. Poor nutrition, smoking and alcohol use, and overall poor maternal health or chronic conditions such as hypertension are also important contributors. To address the factors associated with infant mortality, there needs to be a shift from the current emphasis on highly technological medical interventions toward a focus on health promotion and preventive care for low-income families and women experiencing conditions of vulnerability.

Women and their families are also affected by geography and the availability of social resources and programs in their communities. For instance, rural, remote, and Indigenous communities may have well-developed social networks but have less access to specialized health services. Maternity services, an important part of primary health care services, are often more difficult to provide in rural and remote locations.

COLLABORATIVE WOMAN- AND FAMILY-CENTRED CARE

Collaborative woman- and family-centred maternity care is the overarching framework identified in the conceptual model for perinatal nursing in Canada (Association of Women's Health, Obstetric and Neonatal Nurses [AWHONN], 2009). This dynamic and complex process of providing safe, skilled, and individualized care is affected by women's beliefs and values, by the context for care, and by the availability of skilled maternity care providers.

Family-Centred Maternity and Newborn Care

Perinatal nurses made a significant contribution to the development of the guidelines, *Family-Centred Maternal and Newborn Care: National Guidelines* (PHAC, 2016), and continue to contribute to the updated version. This important document includes guiding principles and strategies for facilitating change to implement these evidence-informed guidelines (Box 4-3).

Collaborative woman- and family-centred maternity and newborn care is based on respect for pregnancy as a state of health and for childbirth as a normal physiological process. Among many cultures, birth is viewed as a completely normal process that can be managed with a minimum of involvement from health practitioners. The central objective of care for women, babies, and families is to maximize the probability of a healthy woman giving birth to a healthy baby. Health care providers share this aim and recognize each woman as an individual. For some women and families, however, the pregnancy may be unplanned or unwanted, and complications or adverse circumstances may occur. The birth itself may be complicated and the outcome unexpected. In these situations, collaborative woman- and family-centred care is even more important for supporting the family's unique needs.

Woman-Centred Care

Woman-centred care is grounded in the assumption that women know their own bodies and are experts in their own health (Box 4-4). Women are also frequently both organizers and providers of family caregiving. Woman-centred care also recognizes that women's child-bearing experiences vary, respects the many differences among women, and acknowledges that gender is an important determinant of health.

Caring for Families

Use of the collaborative woman- and family-centred framework for perinatal nursing (AWHONN, 2009) has brought greater understanding of how families need to be included in maternity care (see Box 4-1). Perinatal nurses' commitment to working in partnership with families can enhance the health and well-being of the whole family. Thus nurses must become competent in working collaboratively with families in a variety of contexts and settings. Relationships between women, their families, and health care providers are based on mutual respect and trust. Such mutual respect and collaborative partnerships will help women give birth safely with power and dignity in a way that promotes the health of the whole family. As well, it is crucial that the woman and her family respect and trust nurses and other health care providers who will be providing care for her during times of vulnerability and change or transition.

The core concepts of woman- and family-centred care include the need for respect and safety, involvement and participation, information sharing and collaboration, and active involvement in decision-making processes. When treating the woman and family with respect and dignity, health care providers listen to and honour their perspectives and choices. They share information with families in ways that are positive, useful, timely, complete, and accurate. The family is supported in participating in their care and decision making at the level of their choice. Collaboration with women and their families in the development, implementation, and evaluation of policy and programs, facility design, professional education, and delivery of care by all involved is essential for providing family-centred care.

BOX 4-3 GUIDING PRINCIPLES OF FAMILY-CENTRED MATERNITY AND NEWBORN CARE

1. A family-centred approach to maternal and newborn care is optimal
2. Pregnancy and birth are normal, healthy processes
3. Early parent–infant attachment is critical for newborn and child development and the growth of healthy families.
4. Family-centred maternal and newborn care applies to all care environments
5. Family-centred maternal and newborn care is informed by research evidence
6. Family-centred maternal and newborn care requires a holistic approach
7. Family-centred maternal and newborn care involves collaboration among care providers
8. Culturally appropriate care is important in a multicultural society
9. Indigenous peoples have distinctive needs during pregnancy and birth
10. Care as close to home as possible is ideal
11. Individualized maternal and newborn care is recommended
12. To make informed choices, women and their families require knowledge about their care
13. Women and their families play an integral role in decision making
14. Health care providers' attitudes and language have an impact on a family's experience of maternal and newborn care
15. Family-centred maternal and newborn care respects reproductive rights
16. Family-centred maternal and newborn care occurs within a system that requires ongoing evaluation
17. Best practices in family-centred maternal and newborn care from global settings may offer valuable options for Canadian consideration

Source: *Family-centered maternity and newborn care: National guidelines.* Public Health Agency of Canada, 2000. Adapted and reproduced with permission from the Minister of Health, 2016.

BOX 4-4 12 ELEMENTS OF THE FRAMEWORK FOR WOMAN-CENTRED HEALTH

Processes to Engage and Empower Women

1. Empowerment
2. Involvement and participation of women
3. Respect and safety
4. Collaborative work environments

Gender Differences That Affect Women's Health and Access to Health Care

5. Patterns or preferences in obtaining care
6. Forms of communication and interaction
7. Need for information
8. Decision-making processes

Support Structures and Approaches

9. Gender-inclusive approach to data
10. Gendered research and evaluation
11. Gender-sensitive training

Health Determinants and Systemic Inequalities

12. Intersecting oppressions and social justice concerns

Adapted from Cory, J. (March 2007). *Women-centred care: A curriculum for health care providers.* Vancouver: BC Women's Hospital and Health Centre. Retrieved from http://www.bcwomens.ca/NR/rdonlyres/FEDC2FC3-D01A-4F80-9D11-5A2FED19AEF4/59897/aaCurriculumforWomenCentredCareFinal2.pdf

Cultural Diversity and Child-bearing Families

Perinatal nurses may be working with families whose social class, sexual orientation, ethnicity, and cultural backgrounds differ from their own. Culturally congruent care can only occur when the individual's and family's cultural values, expressions, or patterns regarding care are known and used appropriately and in meaningful ways by health care providers.

Nurses need to ask women questions about their hopes and expectations regarding child-bearing, about their capacities, and about their needs for nursing assistance. Nurses can ask women about their place of birth (e.g., the country, rural or urban), about the length of time they have been in Canada, and about family and friends or their support network. Box 4-5 includes suggested questions to ask women when exploring their cultural expectations about child-bearing.

Valuing Diversity and Avoiding Stereotyping

Nurses working with child-bearing families should exercise sensitivity in working with every family, being careful to assess the ways in which they apply their own mixture of cultural traditions. Nurses need to reflect on their own beliefs, values, and practices (Box 4-6) to ensure they provide culturally competent care (see Chapter 2 for further discussion).

Pregnancy and childbirth within a biomedical perspective are viewed as processes with inherent risks that are most appropriately managed by using scientific knowledge and advanced technology. The medical perspective stands in direct contrast to the belief systems of many cultures. Among many women, birth is viewed as a completely normal process that can be managed with a minimum of involvement from health care practitioners. When encountering behaviour in women unfamiliar with the biomedical model or those who reject it, the nurse may become frustrated and impatient and may label the women's behaviour as inappropriate and believe that it conflicts with "good" health practices. If the Western health care system provides the nurse's only standard for judgement, the behaviour of the nurse is ethnocentric (see Chapter 2, p. 21).

BOX 4-5 QUESTIONS TO ASK TO EXPLORE CULTURAL EXPECTATIONS ABOUT CHILD-BEARING

1. What do you and your family believe that you should do to remain healthy during pregnancy?
2. What are the things you can or cannot do to improve your health and the health of your baby?
3. Tell me about any special dietary needs or foods that you cannot eat.
4. Tell me about any beliefs you have about pregnancy, birthing, and the postpartum period that would be important for me to know.
5. Tell me about any concerns or fears you or your family may have about hospitalization for childbirth.
6. Who do you want with you during your labour?
7. What actions are important for you and your family to take after the baby's birth?
8. Tell me about your expectations from the nurse(s) caring for you.
9. How will family members participate in your pregnancy, childbirth, and parenting?

BOX 4-6 PERSONAL REFLECTION FOR NURSES AND MATERNITY CARE PROVIDERS

Recognize the influence of your own ethnicity and culture and their effects on your life.
Recognize the diversity of needs and experiences of those you serve.
Obtain details based on personal information actually given by the woman or family members rather than making assumptions.
Use simple language when discussing procedures.
Explore what is acceptable and suited to the woman for her care.
Involve family members with the consent of the patient.
Work out a mutually acceptable schedule of caring for the woman or newborn.

Adapted from Best Start Resource Centre. (2009). *Giving birth in a new land: Strategies for service providers working with newcomers.* Toronto: Author. Retrieved from http://www.beststart.org/resources/rep_health/Newcomer_%20Guide_Final.pdf. Adapted with permission by the Best Start Resource Centre.

Cultural Practices and Nursing Interventions

In perinatal nursing, the nurse supports and nurtures beliefs that promote health, including those related to physical or emotional adaptation to child-bearing. However, if certain practices might be harmful, the nurse should carefully explore them with the woman and suggest modifications that promote family health.

Table 4-1 provides examples of some cultural beliefs and practices surrounding child-bearing. Rather than identifying particular cultural or ethnic groups, this table has been organized in a way that invites exploration of traditional beliefs and health practices and offers some strategies for nurses. These strategies aim to help nurses and other maternity care providers view these practices from a patient-centred perspective while taking into account Canadian practices and regulations.

In using Table 4-1 as a guide, nurses should exercise sensitivity in working with every family, being careful to assess the ways in which they adopt and adapt their own mixture of cultural traditions. Nurses are also reminded to reflect on the ways in which their own cultural practices (including the culture of nursing) may be interpreted by women and family members. Nurses may not agree with all cultural practices, but it is important to respect the woman's decisions. Perinatal nurses need to

TABLE 4-1 CULTURAL PRACTICES AND SUCCESSFUL STRATEGIES DURING CHILD-BEARING AND PARENTING

STAGE	STRATEGIES
Pregnancy	
• In some cultures, the announcement of the pregnancy may be done in a specific manner (e.g., by a father or by the parents of the woman).	• Find out from the woman what her wishes are around the announcement of the pregnancy and respect these wishes.
• Rituals may be performed to protect mother and child (e.g., reading from a sacred text, not going out at night, covering her head, wearing an amulet, giving to charity).	• Begin by asking each woman about beliefs and practices around health and acknowledge these without judging them.
• Parents may not have the social support they would have had in their home country.	• Highlight the benefits of building social support prior to the birth to reduce the risk of postpartum mood disorders and to facilitate breastfeeding. Show the woman specific ways of doing this through community, cultural, and religious groups, for example.
• In many cultures, women learn what they will need for pregnancy and childbirth through their mothers, sisters, and aunts.	• With the woman's permission, allow her partner, family, friends, and elders to accompany her to prenatal classes. • Respect the possibility that the partner may choose not to attend prenatal classes and that a family member will attend instead. • During the prenatal class, offer opportunities for participants to discuss their values and rituals related to pregnancy and birth as various topics come up. • Assist the participants in developing a birth and breastfeeding plan in class. • Clarify when the woman should come to the hospital and what she should bring. • Ensure that a supportive environment is created in the prenatal classes to help women build a social network.
• Language may be a barrier for some newcomers.	• If possible, use prenatal educators from linguistic communities similar to those of patients.
• Pregnancy information may be obtained from elders (e.g., mother, mother-in-law).	• Collaborate with elders, friends, and relatives to educate the woman about the benefits of consistent medical check-ups. • Provide culturally appropriate, medically sound information about pregnancy, childbirth, and infant care.
• Many prenatal tests and the concept of regular prenatal appointments may be unknown to the pregnant woman.	• Explain the importance of prenatal care. • Explain the relevance of tests and make sure they are understood.
• Women may have uncertainties regarding breastfeeding.	• Ask open-ended questions about the woman's beliefs, knowledge, and concerns about breastfeeding and make sure this information is in her files if it might have an impact on breastfeeding after the baby is born. • Give the woman information about where she can get help after the baby is born (breastfeeding clinic, lactation consultant, public health nurses, or breastfeeding peer mentor).
• The hospital may be a very unfamiliar setting to many newcomers. In many countries, home births are the norm.	• As with all expectant parents, a tour of the hospital is important to increase comfort levels. • Educate the woman about the birthing process and Canadian practices to avoid issues that may arise at the time of birth concerning medications, interventions, newborn care, etc. • Inform the woman about the possibility of using a midwife for a home birth or a doula as a birth assistant in the hospital.
• Some women may avoid certain foods in pregnancy.	• Discuss nutrition with the woman, focusing on promoting a healthy pregnancy. Ensure that her diet is not deficient.

TABLE 4-1 CULTURAL PRACTICES AND SUCCESSFUL STRATEGIES DURING CHILD-BEARING AND PARENTING—cont'd

STAGE	STRATEGIES
Labour and Birth	
• Some women may birth in silence and others may moan, groan, or scream.	• Respect cultural practices displayed by the woman during the birthing process. Ask her what she feels like doing.
• Women may squat or sit to assist in the birthing process.	• Encourage the woman to use the most comfortable position for her during the birthing process.
• Some women might avoid pain-relieving medications such as epidurals and spinal medication.	• Explain the procedures with diagrams and models. • Suggest nonintrusive alternatives (e.g., warm towel on the back). • Ensure that the woman provides informed consent.
Postpartum	
• There may be specific rituals performed to welcome the newborn.	• Accommodate the rituals, if possible, keeping in mind that these rituals may be particularly important for couples who are isolated from their extended families and removed from their culture.
• In many religions, the outcome of the birth (e.g., disability, Down syndrome, birth defect) is seen to be determined by God.	• These potential outcomes should be discussed during pregnancy. • Explain the short- and long-term consequences of the situation and the support options available. • Provide the family time to deal with the situation.
• In some cultures, female genital mutilation is a routine practice, involving the stitching of the inner layers of the labia minor or majora, the removal of the clitoris or other parts of the genitalia, or both.	• Educate yourself about the practice of female genital mutilation and the care required during childbirth.
• Women may refuse a Caesarean birth.	• During pregnancy, educate the woman and her partner about the need for the procedure and the consequences of refusal. • Ensure informed consent at birth.
• Women may prefer same-gender health care providers.	• Incorporate patient preferences in health-related decisions where possible and appropriate. • During pregnancy, let the woman know that it may not be possible to accommodate her preferences, depending on the staff on duty when she is admitted to the hospital.
• Women may expect nurses to do everything related to newborn care.	• During the prenatal stage, educate the woman about the roles and responsibilities of health care providers and other service providers in postpartum care. Encourage the involvement of family members in caregiving after the birth.
• The baby may sleep with the mother in bed.	• Educate the parents about safe sleeping guidelines.
• Personal hygiene practices may vary widely depending on the culture. Some women may not bathe or wash their hair or may bathe only once a week.	• Try to understand cultural hygiene practices and be understanding of a woman's preferences. • Explain the signs and symptoms of infection and the importance of contacting a health care provider if this occurs.

Adapted from Best Start Resource Centre. (2009). *Giving birth in a new land: Strategies for service providers working with newcomers.* Toronto: Author. Retrieved from http://www.beststart.org/resources/rep_health/Newcomer_%20Guide_Final.pdf. Adapted with permission by the Best Start Resource Centre.

listen to the stories that women and family members tell them about their culture, their child-bearing experiences, and their needs.

PERINATAL HEALTH INDICATORS: THE CANADIAN PERINATAL SURVEILLANCE SYSTEM

The Canadian Perinatal Surveillance System (CPSS) was developed in 1995 to monitor maternal and infant health across Canada. The CPSS collects data from a number of sources (for example, vital statistics and the Canadian Institute for Health Information [CIHI]), analyzes and interprets the data, and writes papers and reports to be used as the basis for health policy and action. The CPSS has identified more than 50 health indicators and ranked many of these indicators for importance on the basis of current research evidence and knowledge about the determinants of health and impact of health outcomes.

The CPSS plays an important role in monitoring the quality of epidemiological (population) data available to assist with health and social service planning. Through data collection it has been determined that not every province has the same birth registration practices. The CPSS has thus been working with some data collection agencies to improve the quality of the data collected so that provincial and international comparisons are more meaningful.

Nurses need to be aware that there are important differences in definitions for health indicators. An example is infant mortality rates, which have been identified as one of the best indicators of a nation's health status (CPSS, 2008). However, the infant mortality rate is a complex health indicator that is dependent on how "live births" are defined and registered and

BOX 4-7 COMMON PERINATAL HEALTH INDICATORS

Birth rate—Number of live births in 1 year per 1000 population
Fertility rate—Number of births per 1000 women between the ages of 15 and 44 (inclusive), calculated on a yearly basis
Infant mortality rate—Number of deaths of infants under 1 year of age per 1000 live births
Maternal mortality rate—Number of maternal deaths from births and complications of pregnancy, childbirth, and puerperium (the first 42 days after termination of the pregnancy) per 100,000 live births
Neonatal mortality rate—Number of deaths of infants under 28 days of age per 1000 live births
Perinatal mortality rate—Number of stillbirths and number of neonatal deaths per 1000 live births
Stillbirth—An infant who died in utero and at birth and demonstrates no signs of life, such as breathing, heartbeat, or voluntary muscle movements, with a birth weight of greater than 500 gm or gestational age of 20 weeks or more.

on how fetal and neonatal deaths are recorded. For example, Canada and the United States have adopted the World Health Organization (WHO) definition of live birth to include all products of conception that show signs of life at birth, without reference to birth weight or gestational age of the fetus. Many European countries have adopted different definitions; for example, in Sweden live births are considered to be at least 27 weeks' gestation and fetal deaths (stillbirths) are not recorded before 28 weeks' gestation. In Canada there has been a recent trend to include as "live births" more neonates born at less than 500 grams and 20 weeks' gestation, which may result in Canada and the United States comparing poorly with many European countries (CPSS, 2008). Box 4-7 defines maternal and infant health indicators commonly used for reporting in Canada.

The CPSS releases a new report every 2 years and focuses on perinatal health indicators that are deemed to be most important. The 2013 edition of the CPSS report includes 13 perinatal health indicators for which there is currently sufficient national data available. One of the success stories included in the report is the decreasing rate of neural tube defects (including spina bifida and anencephaly) since 1995 following the introduction of folic acid supplementation for child-bearing women.

Maternal Mortality

Worldwide, approximately 800 women die each day of problems related to pregnancy or childbirth. In Canada in 2010–11, the annual **maternal mortality rate** (number of maternal deaths per 100,000 live births) was 6.1 (PHAC, 2013). Although the overall number of maternal deaths is small, maternal mortality remains a significant problem because a high proportion of deaths are preventable, primarily through improving access to and use of prenatal care services.

The leading causes of maternal death attributable to pregnancy differ over the world. In general three major causes have persisted for the last 50 years: hypertensive disorders, infection, and hemorrhage. Unsafe abortion is an additional factor. Worldwide, strategies to reduce maternal mortality rates include improving access to skilled attendants at birth, providing post-abortion care, improving family planning services, and providing adolescents with better reproductive health services (Government of Canada, 2015). The leading causes of maternal mortality in Canada today are diseases of the circulatory system, gestational hypertension, hemorrhage, and other indirect causes (PHAC, 2013).

Maternal Morbidity

Although mortality is the traditional measure of maternal health and maternal health is often measured by neonatal outcomes, pregnancy complications are important to consider. In 2010–11, the rate of severe maternal morbidity in Canada was 15.4 per 1000 deliveries, although this statistic does not include Québec. The most common severe maternal morbidities included blood transfusion; postpartum hemorrhage and blood transfusion; hysterectomy; cardiac arrest or failure, myocardial infarction, or pulmonary edema; puerperal sepsis; uterine rupture during labour; and eclampsia (PHAC, 2013).

Maternal morbidity results in a high-risk pregnancy. The diagnosis of high risk imposes a **situational crisis** on the family. The combined efforts of medical and nursing personnel are required to care for these patients, who often need the expertise of physicians and nurses trained in both critical care obstetrics and intensive care medicine or nursing.

Trends in Fertility and Birth Rate

Fertility trends and birth rates reflect women's needs for health services. In recent years, more women living in Canada have delayed child-bearing until they are 35 years of age or older, and the rate of women conceiving over age 35 has steadily increased since 2001 (PHAC, 2013). Women who conceive at older ages are more likely to experience chronic illnesses, placental problems, and multiple pregnancy, and their fetuses are more likely to have chromosomal abnormalities (e.g., Down syndrome). However, older women also tend to be better educated, have higher income levels (less poverty), and seek early prenatal care.

The rate of live births to teenagers in Canada has been steadily decreasing, from 9.1% in 2001 to 7.7% in 2010 (PHAC, 2013). The decline in teen pregnancy may be attributed to the accessibility and use of reliable contraception such as condoms and birth control pills. Health problems associated with teen pregnancy include anemia and poor weight gain and twice the risk of delivering a preterm or low–birth weight baby (see Chapter 5). Teenage pregnancy can also influence the likelihood that women will not complete high school, which may result in underemployment and poverty. There are significant geographic variations in adolescent fertility rates for females ages 10 to 17, from the lowest in Quebec (1.6%) to the highest in Nunavut (29.4%), reflecting significant cultural differences and access to abortion services (PHAC, 2013).

Multiple Birth Rate

Multiple birth rates in Canada have increased from 2.8% in 2001 to 3.2% in 2010 of total births. Such pregnancies often occur in women who are of older maternal age at conception and are more likely to have used assisted reproductive technologies such as in vitro fertilization (IVF) (PHAC, 2013) (see Chapter 8). Multiple pregnancy can result in health problems for both women (anemia, pre-eclampsia, Caesarean birth) and their babies (preterm birth, low birth weight, perinatal death). There is growing evidence that decreasing the number of embryos may help decrease the poor health outcomes associated with higher-order (more than twins) multiple pregnancies.

Preterm Birth and Birth Weight

The proportion of preterm infants (born before 37 completed weeks' gestation) was 7.7% in 2010, although data from Ontario were not included in this analysis (PHAC, 2013). In industrialized nations, 60 to 80% of deaths of infants born without congenital anomalies are the result of preterm birth. Preterm birth is also associated with cerebral palsy and other long-term health problems. In 2010 there was significant regional variation in preterm birth rates, ranging from a low of 7.4% in Quebec and Saskatchewan to a high of 12.8% in Nunavut (PHAC, 2013).

Babies born both small (<10th percentile for sex-specific standardized birth weights) and large (>90th percentile) for gestational age experience significant health problems (see Chapter 28). Maternal cigarette smoking accounts for about 30 to 40% of small-for-gestational-age (SGA) babies born in industrialized countries, where malnutrition is not a predominant factor. Large-for-gestational-age (LGA) babies and their mothers are more likely to experience birth trauma (shoulder dystocia, nerve injuries, and postpartum hemorrhage). Maternal diabetes is an important risk factor. LGA babies are more common in Indigenous women (see Chapter 15).

Obesity

In Canada, 45% of women self-report that they are overweight or obese, and approximately 1 in 4 have a body mass index of greater than 30. The highest levels of obesity are found in Atlantic Canada, the Prairies, the Territories, and smaller cities in northern and southwestern Ontario (Navaneelan & Janz, 2014). There is a scarcity of data regarding the number of pregnant women who are obese, although rates are estimated to be between 11 and 20% (Davies et al., 2010). Obesity is accompanied by hypertension associated with pregnancy, diabetes, and decreased fertility, congenital anomalies, miscarriage, and fetal death. Obesity in pregnancy is also associated with increased Caesarean births, increased use of health care services, and longer hospital stays (Davies et al., 2010) (see further discussion in Chapter 15, p. 380).

Health Service Indicators

The CPSS also monitors a number of health service indicators, including, for example, rates of labour induction and Caesarean birth. The proportion of women delivering by Caesarean section has increased steadily, from 17.6% in 1995 to 28% in 2010–11 (PHAC, 2013). Most of this increase is due to a higher rate of primary (first-time) Caesarean births, although the vaginal birth after Caesarean (VBAC) rate also decreased over the same time period. There are some women who decide to have an elective Caesarean birth with no medical indications, although the number of Caesarean births done "by request" is fairly small and was found to be only 2% in British Columbia (Hanley, Janssen, & Greyson, 2010). These requests may be due to fear of pain or fear of being out of control, and sometimes counselling may help alleviate these fears. The overall trend is concerning, as evidence documents a higher risk of significant maternal morbidity (e.g., infection, thromboembolism, hysterectomy) for women who have a Caesarean birth.

THE CANADIAN MATERNITY EXPERIENCES SURVEY

The Canadian Maternity Experiences Survey was designed by the CPSS and included more than 300 questions asked of 6421 women from across Canada. The stratified sample was drawn from women who lived with an infant as identified in the 2006 Canadian census. Women were interviewed by telephone for 45 minutes when their baby was between 5 and 14 months of age. An attempt was made to include young; Indigenous; and immigrant women in the survey. The survey covered topics related to the experiences of pregnancy, childbirth, and the postpartum period and could be considered a snapshot in time and a rich source for the identification of concerns for further study. This report provides detailed information on many issues of concern for nurses (e.g., alcohol use, prenatal class attendance, social support, and stress). The report is available to download from the Public Health Agency of Canada website (see Additional Resources at the end of this chapter). At this time, there are no plans to repeat this survey.

CURRENT ISSUES AFFECTING PERINATAL NURSING PRACTICE

Promoting Healthy and Normal Birth

A guiding principle of the Family-Centred Maternity and Newborn Care national guidelines is that birth is a normal, healthy process (see Box 4-3). Women must be viewed holistically and in the context in which they live. Their physical, emotional, and social environment must be considered because these interdependent factors influence health and illness. Even the language that health care providers use to describe women and their concerns needs to be examined. For example, practitioners may describe women as having an "incompetent cervix," "failing to progress," or having an "arrest" of labour. They may describe a fetus as having intrauterine growth "retardation." They also may "allow" women a "trial" of labour. The use of these phrases implies failure or inadequacy on the part of the woman or fetus, and there is now more emphasis being placed on incorporating more positive language into the practitioner's vocabulary.

Vulnerable Populations in the Community

One of the primary factors compromising women's health is lack of access to acceptable-quality health care. The barriers to care may take many forms: living in a medically underserved area or an inability to obtain needed services, particularly basic services such as prenatal care. For example, some rural and remote areas have few physicians and midwives; women may have to travel hundreds of miles for this kind of care. Women often have lower incomes and less education than men and thus are considered at risk. Infant mortality is higher for infants of mothers without a high school education than for those of mothers with such education. See Chapter 3 (pp. 34–37) for further discussion of vulnerable populations.

Indigenous Women

Canada's history has influenced the health and the experience of pregnancy, childbirth, and parenting for Indigenous women (see Chapter 1, p. 6). One result of this history is that Indigenous women have an increased incidence of perinatal mood disorders (see Chapter 24). Having a healthy experience throughout pregnancy, childbirth, and parenting includes fostering positive mental and emotional health. Supporting individual resilience, creating supportive environments, and addressing the influence of the determinants of health are important considerations in promoting such an experience (British Columbia Reproductive Mental Health Program, 2011). Some Indigenous women face unique challenges in having healthy pregnancy, childbirth, and parenting experiences, often due to a lack of role models (e.g., mothers, aunts, sisters) around them who can support them and pass on important traditional practices. Supportive environments and relationships are especially important for Indigenous women as they become pregnant, go through childbirth, and become parents (British Columbia Reproductive Mental Health Program, 2011). Health care providers need to be aware of the impact of historical events on Indigenous women as well as their lack of access to some of the determinants of health, particularly their residing in remote locations, as perinatal morbidity and mortality are higher in Indigenous populations.

Immigrant and Refugee Women

Some immigrant and refugee women may also have higher rates of chronic disease, including diabetes and acquired immune deficiency syndrome (AIDS). Women with underlying health conditions are at especially high risk for poor obstetrical outcomes for themselves and their infants. They have high rates of preterm labour and gestational hypertension and often have intrauterine growth restriction, resulting in the birth of infants who are small for gestational age. Some immigrant and refugee women also have decreased access to social supports and may have a hard time navigating the health care system, often due to language difficulties, which can ultimately impact overall perinatal outcomes.

Homeless Women

Although little is known about pregnancy in this population, some women do become pregnant while homeless. Pregnancy is linked to a whole host of health issues for homeless women. The homeless woman is at risk for pregnancy complications because of a lack of prenatal care, poor nutrition, stress, and exposure to violence. Homeless women face multiple barriers to prenatal care, including lack of transportation, distance to travel for care, and not having a health care provider. The unsafe environment and high-risk lifestyles often result in adverse perinatal outcomes.

Perinatal Issues for LGBTQ Patients

Perinatal nurses must be aware of LGBTQ concerns when providing care (see Chapter 1, p. 7). Many lesbian, gay, and transsexual couples may become parents and deserve respectful care during the child-bearing experience as well as during health screening and wellness care. While this text cannot go into extensive detail, whenever possible, LGBTQ concerns are integrated throughout the chapters. The term *patient* may be used in situations where the person being cared for could be a woman or a man.

Community-Based Care

As health care costs continue to rise, Canada is faced with the challenge of providing safe and effective care that is innovative and cost-effective and meets the expectations of an increasingly more demanding and educated public. Some women who experience pregnancy complications are now cared for in the home by antepartum home care nurses. Portable fetal monitors and other forms of technology previously available only in the hospital are used. This change has affected the organizational structure of care, the costs of care, and the skills required to provide nursing care.

With the shorter length of hospital stay after birth, women and their babies are often discharged home before they are successfully breastfeeding, before they have mastered basic baby care activities, and without sufficient supports at home (Fig. 4-1). Public health departments and community agencies across the country must try to meet the needs of these new families. Changing demands on the community-based nurse have evolved out of these societal, economic, and health-related trends. Acuity of illness of home care patients is far greater than in the past, requiring the community nurse to become more adept in assessment, direct care, and health teaching. Assessment of the neonate requires knowledge of parameters for measuring the health of a newborn within the first days of life. Skill in assisting with breastfeeding is essential. Knowledge of an ever-widening array of diverse family traditions, beliefs, and expectations related to child-bearing has become even more critical for the nurse to effectively facilitate the transition involved when a family moves through the stages of incorporating a new member into their family (see Chapter 3 for further discussion of Community Health Nursing).

Enhancement of postpartum support services with the addition of homemakers, breastfeeding support services, and doulas may be needed to promote the health of Canadian families.

Perinatal nurses need to assess the resources that child-bearing women have to support them during the postpartum

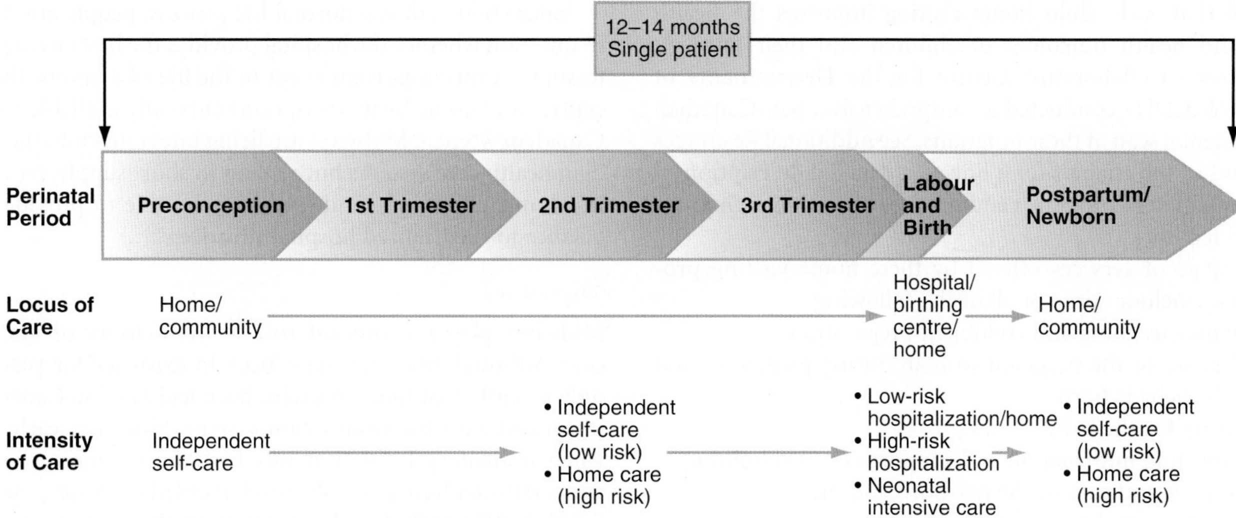

FIGURE 4-1 Perinatal continuum of care.

period at home. In many cultures, women are cared for by extended family members so that their primary responsibility is to breastfeed and recover from childbirth. In our independent North American culture, women may need to be encouraged to ask for help. At times, perinatal nurses may need to advocate for a delay of hospital discharge until the needed supports are put in place. Nursing care has become more community based, with nurses providing care for women and infants in homeless shelters and for adolescents in school-based clinics, and promoting health at community centres, churches, and shopping malls (see Community Focus box).

COMMUNITY FOCUS

Availability of Maternal Child Services in Your Community

To understand what services are available in your community, a good place to start is the Internet. Use the Internet to identify where the closest health department is located. Research what services are offered to child-bearing families.

- How many other agencies provide services for child-bearing families? Are they located in the area? What services do they offer?
- Are there registered nurses employed there? If not, what are the credentials of the people providing the services? Are there midwives and doulas also available?
- Is service provided in more than just English? If so, in what languages? Are interpreters available if needed?
- Do the agencies ever accept referrals for patients who cannot pay? Are there any bursaries or provisions made for families who cannot pay?
- Is there a maternal child home visiting program available in the community?

Based on the information you have gathered, are there adequate and appropriate services for pregnant women and their families in your area? If not, is there a postpartum care clinic where new mothers can access support for breastfeeding, hearing and dental screening, immunizations, well-baby care, and other related services?

Maternal Child Services in the Community

In Canada, community health and home health nurses provide most of the home visiting for child-bearing families. Early child home visiting programs have been delivered free of charge for many years in every province and territory in Canada by community health nurses. All programs are voluntary, and parents can decide whether they want to participate in the program. Referrals are received from many sources: perinatal nurses, obstetricians, family doctors, midwives, nurse practitioners, childbirth educators, and individual parents. Individual health departments may provide an array of other services for the child-bearing family. These may include childbirth education classes, breastfeeding clinics, mom and baby groups, postpartum mood disorder support services, and immunization clinics. Ideally, the community health nurse will begin to visit the family before the birth of the new baby to facilitate teaching about pregnancy, childbirth, and the transition to parenting. The nurse can assist families in preparation for childbirth and in arranging other community support services, if needed.

Across the country, home visiting programs vary, often because of the costs of providing services. Many home visiting programs may only offer telephone or clinic support in place of home visiting, whereas others only provide service after the birth of the baby. In this case, the community health nurse will call the patient after she is home from the hospital to answer any urgent questions she might have and to do an assessment of how the new mother and baby are doing. If the program has sufficient funding to visit all new mothers, the nurse will arrange a time to visit mom and baby. Otherwise, only those families assessed to be at high risk will be offered a home visit. Some programs offer additional visiting by lay home visitors (family visitors), who work with families on a more frequent basis to provide more in-depth teaching and support.

These programs have received renewed attention because of their impact on healthy child development outcomes. To identify the provincial/territorial similarities and differences in home visiting programs in Canada and to illuminate the evidence that early child home visiting improves the health equity and health outcomes of children and their families, the National Collaborating Centre for the Determinants of Health (NCCDH) conducted a comprehensive, pan-Canadian environmental scan of these programs. See Additional Resources at the end of the chapter for a link to a detailed description of the many different programs and services offered in each province and territory.

The range of services offered by these home visiting programs may include some or all of the following:

- Pregnancy teaching and childbirth preparation
- Taking care of the pregnant woman during pregnancy and after the baby is born
- Preparing for the baby
- Breastfeeding information and support and skill building
- Assessment and care of the newborn and mother
- Anticipatory guidance for parents
- Resources in the community
- Teaching how to transition to solid foods
- What to expect as the child grows to meet developmental outcomes
- How to keep children safe

Home visiting has many advantages for the new mother. She is able to stay at home and rest, and vulnerable newborns are not exposed to the weather or external sources of infection. She receives one-to-one supportive teaching and counselling free of charge and tailored specifically to her needs. The advantage for the nurse is that he or she can observe and interact with family members in their most natural and secure environment. Adequacy of resources and safety factors can be assessed. Teaching can be tailored to the actual home conditions, and other family members can be included. Some home visiting programs follow families until babies are 3 years of age.

While community-based care is ideal, the reality is that not all women have equal access to the services provided, either because not all communities are able to provide these services or because women within a community lack knowledge about available services or are unable to access them. For example, small northern communities may not have access to a health care provider who can provide all the services necessary due to location and cost. Indigenous health services are provided by the federal government rather than provincial health organizations and there may be differing priorities and funding formulas to provide these types of programs. There may also be difficulty in providing services in remote communities.

The Place of Birth and "High-Tech" Care

Advances in scientific knowledge and the identification of a large number of "high-risk" pregnancies have contributed to a health care system that emphasizes "high-tech" care. Maternity care has extended to include preconception counselling, more and better scientific techniques to monitor the mother and fetus, more definitive tests for genetic abnormalities and for identifying hypoxia and acidosis during labour, and neonatal intensive care units. Many women who labour in hospital settings are monitored electronically despite the lack of evidence that supports this practice.

Since childbirth is a normal life process, people are starting to question whether the hospital provides the best environment to support this important event in the life of a family. Birthing centres and home birth are options currently available to some Canadian women. Midwives are being integrated into the Canadian health care systems but remain in short supply. As experts in normal childbirth, midwives may be able to provide some balance to medicalized hospital practices.

Midwifery

Midwives play a significant role in the delivery of maternity care. Although midwives have been in existence for years, it is only recently that midwives have been legislated in Canada and integrated into the health care system. Since the early 1990s when midwifery legislation was first passed, most provinces and territories have gradually implemented midwifery-oriented health policy, including legalization of the profession, standardization of training, and the fees that are remunerated through their respective provincial insurance plans. In some provinces, for example, Ontario, women who do not have provincial health care may be able to access free midwifery care. Across Canada, less than 5% of births involve care by a midwife. Midwifery care may be provided differently across jurisdictions. Whereas many midwives are fully funded and work in independent practice, some provinces have developed programs that enhance interdisciplinary care in order to provide midwifery care to women who would not otherwise have access to it. An example is in Alberta, where the Rocky Mountain House midwives team up with the local Primary Care Network, providing care to women in three First Nations communities. They share calls with local physicians and provide breastfeeding support. In some jurisdictions where there are minimal numbers of midwives, a nurse will be the second care provider at the birth.

The Canadian Association of Midwives (CAM) is the national voice for midwifery in Canada. Midwives in Canada have their own regulations and education separate from nursing education. Integral to midwifery practice are the practices that support normal physiological birth and optimize women's childbirth experiences (Box 4-8).

Multidisciplinary Collaborative Maternity Care

A philosophy of respectful and collaborative work relationships between all different care providers underpins the framework for perinatal nursing in Canada. Nurses work with physicians, midwives, and doulas to provide appropriate care for families undergoing the childbirth experience. As contributors to the Multidisciplinary Collaborative Primary Maternity Care Project (MCP^2), which was funded in the context of a worsening shortage of maternity care providers, perinatal nurses helped to develop models and guidelines for multidisciplinary teams of professionals who work with child-bearing women and their families (MCP^2, 2006).

Breastfeeding in Canada

Breastfeeding is recognized internationally as the optimal method of infant feeding; 6 months of exclusive breastfeeding

BOX 4-8 COMPONENTS OF MIDWIFERY CARE MODEL

- Providing continuity of care to build trust and partnership with women
- Sharing information and offering choices, including the choice of birth place
- Actively supporting client decision making and autonomy
- Allowing adequate time for discussion of individual needs and concerns
- Preparing women for the realities of labour while anticipating a normal birth
- Creating a calm and intimate birth environment
- Providing a familiar presence and continuous support during active labour
- Using nonpharmacological methods to help women work with normal labour pain
- Encouraging free movement and instinctual behaviour in labour
- Encouraging fluid intake and nourishment as needed
- Encouraging spontaneous second-stage "pushing" in the woman's preferred position
- Supporting early labour at home, as appropriate
- Supporting birth at home or in a birthing centre, as appropriate

Adapted from Canadian Association of Midwives. (2010). *Midwifery care and normal birth.* Retrieved from http://www.canadianmidwives.org/DATA/DOCUMENT/CAM_ENG_Midwifery_Care_Normal_Birth_FINAL_Nov_2010.pdf

with continuation for up to 2 years or longer with complementary foods is currently recommended (Pound, Unger, & Canadian Pediatric Society [CPS], 2012/2015). While breastfeeding is well known to have benefits for newborns, there is also increasing evidence that breastmilk can improve the health of older children. Breastfeeding longer may have a protective effect against overweight and obesity in childhood and contributes to increased rates of immunity during the first and second years. Mothers who breastfeed their older infants and young children also report experiencing an increased sensitivity to and bonding with their child (Critch & CPS, Nutrition & Gastroenterology Committee, 2014). Breastfeeding initiation rates have been increasing steadily in Canada, with regional variation ranging from 57% in Newfoundland and Labrador to 96% in British Columbia and the Yukon. In 2012, 26% of Canadian women continued to breastfeed exclusively for 6 months or longer. While this rate increased from 17% in 2003, more work needs to be done to improve breastfeeding rates across the country (Statistics Canada, 2013). See Chapter 27 for further discussion on infant feeding.

Baby Friendly Initiative in Canada

The Breastfeeding Committee for Canada (BCC) identified the World Health Organization (WHO)/UNICEF Baby Friendly Initiative (BFI) as a primary strategy for the protection, promotion, and support of breastfeeding. The WHO/UNICEF guidelines for the BFI propose that each country identify a BFI national authority to facilitate the assessment and monitoring of the progress of BFI. The Breastfeeding Committee for Canada (BCC) is the national authority for the BFI in Canada.

The BFI protects, promotes, and supports breastfeeding through the Ten Steps to Successful Breastfeeding, developed by UNICEF and the WHO (see Box 27-2). As of 2015, just over 53 hospitals, birthing centres, and community health departments in Canada had received the Baby Friendly Designation (BCC, 2014; Government of Quebec, 2016) (see discussion in Chapter 27).

A Global Perspective

The fifth Millennium Development Goal (see Box 1-3 on p. 11) is to improve maternal health and reduce the maternal mortality rate by 75% between 1990 and 2015. As stated earlier, worldwide, approximately 800 women die each day of problems related to pregnancy or childbirth, with hemorrhage being the leading cause of death. There are great disparities in the maternal mortality rate between developing and developed countries. As well, nearly 3 million newborn babies die during the first month of life and a similar number are stillborn (WHO, 2014a). Most of the 3.2 million children living with human immunodeficiency virus (HIV) or AIDS acquired the infection through perinatal transmission and live in Sub-Saharan Africa. This difference illustrates the inequities that exist between industrialized and resource-poor parts of the world.

If women have access to appropriate health care in the event of a complication, the maternal mortality rate will decrease. The infant mortality rate could also be decreased using relatively simple interventions. Keeping the newborn warm, ensuring that the newborn is breathing, starting exclusive breastfeeding immediately, preventing malaria and tetanus, washing hands before touching the newborn, and enabling early recognition of illness and care seeking could have a large impact on reducing infant mortality rates (WHO, 2014a).

Another factor that can negatively affect maternal health is female genital mutilation, which is the removal of part or all of the female external genitalia for cultural or nontherapeutic reasons (WHO, 2014b). Worldwide, many women undergo such procedures. With the growing number of Canadian immigrants from Africa and other countries where female genital mutilation is practised, nurses will increasingly encounter women who have undergone the procedure. These women are significantly more likely to have adverse obstetrical outcomes. The United Nations, the International Council of Nurses, and other health professionals have spoken out against the procedures as harmful to women's health and a violation of human rights (see Chapter 5, p. 74, for further discussion).

Human trafficking is a $32-billion business that exists in North America and internationally (Dovydaitis, 2010). Health care professionals may interact with victims who are in captivity. If health care providers are appropriately trained, they may have opportunities to identify victims, intervene to help them obtain necessary health services, and provide information about ways to escape from their situation.

ETHICAL DECISION MAKING IN PERINATAL NURSING

Ethical concerns and debates have multiplied with the increased use of technology and with scientific advances. For example, with reproductive technology, pregnancy is now possible in women who thought they would never bear children, including some who are menopausal or postmenopausal. Should scarce resources be devoted to achieving pregnancies in older women? Is giving birth to a child at an older age worth the risks involved? Should older parents be encouraged to conceive a baby when they may not live to see the child reach adulthood? Should a woman who is HIV positive have access to assisted reproduction services? Who should pay for reproductive technologies, such as the use of induced ovulation and in vitro fertilization?

Questions about informed consent and allocation of resources must be addressed with innovations such as intrauterine fetal surgery, fetoscopy, therapeutic insemination, genetic engineering, stem cell research, surrogate child-bearing, surgery for **infertility**, "test-tube" babies, fetal research, and treatment of very preterm babies. For example, discussion is required when a 23-week gestation baby is born alive and decisions need to be made regarding what treatment will be provided based on the wants of the parents and the knowledge of health care providers. The introduction of long-acting contraceptives has created moral choices and policy dilemmas for health care providers and legislators (e.g., whether some women [substance users or women who are HIV positive] should be required to take the contraceptives). With the potential for great good that can come from fetal tissue transplantation, what research is ethical? What are the rights of the embryo? Should cloning of humans be permitted? Discussion and debate about these issues will continue for many years. Nurses and women, as well as scientists, physicians, lawyers, lawmakers, ethicists, and clergy, must be involved in the discussions.

ADDRESSING CURRENT CHALLENGES AND ENVISIONING THE FUTURE

Throughout this chapter the challenges currently faced by perinatal and women's health nurses have been discussed. In order to promote optimal health and growth and enhance child-bearing experiences for Canadian (and all) women and their families, these issues need to be addressed and goals established for the future (Box 4-9).

BOX 4-9 GOALS FOR PERINATAL NURSING: LOOKING AHEAD TO THE FUTURE

1. Recognize the importance of child-bearing for family health promotion and building collaborative relationships with women as family caregivers. Nurses will increasingly need to build upon strengths when working with women who experience child-bearing challenges due to conditions of vulnerability.
2. Decrease health service costs by expanding alternatives to highly technological hospital-based care, such as midwifery services, nurse practitioner–led health clinics, and alternative birth places, including birthing centres and women's homes
3. Expand multiprofessional teams, with nurses being more involved in helping women access appropriate health services (screening and referral services)
4. Recognize the contributions of traditional and integrative healers who support the belief systems and enhance health practices of child-bearing women and their families
5. Re-examine patient safety so that the important role nurses play in keeping patients safe, particularly in the hospital setting, is recognized
6. Promote normal birth within highly technological birth environments for women and newborns who require this level of care
7. Promote a culture of breastfeeding that also recognizes that breastfeeding may not be the right infant feeding option for all child-bearing women
8. Recognize perinatal nurses' knowledge and skills, and work to build respectful, collaborative interprofessional health care teams
9. Recognize the challenges experienced by both child-bearing women and maternity care providers who live and work in rural, remote, Indigenous and inner-city communities
10. Address health inequities by creating health policy and services that focus on the resources needed for health and access to health services
11. Utilize electronic technologies to provide enhanced continuing professional education and build communities of practice where knowledge exchange is supported

KEY POINTS

- Perinatal nursing focuses on women and their infants and families during the child-bearing cycle.
- Childbirth practices have changed to become more patient- and family-centred and include more alternatives in provider, birth place, and care.
- Collaborative woman- and family-centred maternal and newborn care is based on respect for pregnancy as a state of health and for childbirth as a normal physiological process.
- Perinatal nurses need to listen to the stories that women and family members tell about their culture, their child-bearing experiences, their resources, and their needs.
- Preterm birth, maternal obesity, and high Caesarean birth rates are current challenges in Canada.
- Women living in rural, remote, and Indigenous communities and in poverty in inner cities experience significant health challenges and have increased difficulty accessing appropriate care.

- Collaborative multidisciplinary maternity care based on mutual respect and trust is one strategy for addressing the critical shortages of maternity care providers.
- The Baby Friendly Initiative (BFI) is a primary strategy to improve breastfeeding rates and support across the country.
- Globally, women are still dying in childbirth, and infant mortality remains high.
- Ethical concerns have multiplied with increasing use of technology and scientific advances.
- Nurses caring for women can play an active role in shaping health care systems to be responsive to the needs of contemporary women.

evolve WEBSITE

Visit the Evolve website for additional resources related to the content in this chapter such as Case Studies, Critical Thinking Case Study Answers, Nursing Care Plans, Nursing Processes, Nursing Skills, and Review Questions for Exam Preparation at: *http://evolve.elsevier.com/Canada/Perry/maternal/*

REFERENCES

Association of Women's Health, Obstetric and Neonatal Nurses (AWHONN). (2009). *Standards for professional perinatal nursing practice and certification in Canada* (2nd ed.). Washington, DC: Author.

Breastfeeding Committee for Canada. (2014). *The baby friendly initiative in Canada: Status report 2014.* Retrieved from <http://breastfeedingcanada.ca/documents/BFI%20Status%20Report%202014%20with%20WHO%20Country%20report.pdf>.

British Columbia Reproductive Mental Health Program. (2011). *Celebrating the circle of life: Coming back to balance and harmony.* Retrieved from <http://www.perinatalservicesbc.ca/NR/rdonlyres/361F0C20-FDC5-499E-AC8D-D0F2A0494597/0/Circle_of_Life_FINAL_CompleteGuide_March2013.pdf>.

Canadian Perinatal Surveillance System. (2008). *Canadian perinatal health report: 2008 edition.* Retrieved from <http://www.phac-aspc.gc.ca/publicat/2008/cphr-rspc/pdf/overview-apercu-eng.pdf>.

Critch, J. N., & Canadian Paediatric Society, Nutrition and Gastroenterology Committee. (2014). Nutrition for healthy term infants, six to 24 months: An overview. *Paediatric & Child Health, 19*(10), 547–549. Retrieved from <http://www.cps.ca/en/documents/position/nutrition-healthy-term-infants-6-to-24-months>.

Davies, G. A., Maxwell, C., McLeod, L., et al. (2010). SOGC clinical practice guideline: Obesity in pregnancy. *Journal of Obstetrics and Gynaecology Canada, 32*(2), 165–173.

Dovydaitis, T. (2010). Human trafficking: The role of the health care provider. *Journal of Midwifery and Women's Health, 55*(5), 462–467.

Government of Canada. (2015). *Millennium development goals.* Ottawa: Author. Retrieved from <http://www.international.gc.ca/development-developpement/priorities-priorites/mdg-omd.aspx?lang=eng>.

Government of Quebec. (2016). *The baby initiative.* Retrieved from <http://www.msss.gouv.qc.ca/sujets/santepub/initiative-amis-des-bebes.php>.

Hanley, G. E., Janssen, P. A., & Greyson, D. (2010). Regional variation in the Cesarean delivery and assisted vaginal delivery rates. *Obstetrics & Gynecology, 115*(6), 1201–1208. doi:10.1097/AOG.0b013e3181dd918c.

Multidisciplinary Collaborative Primary Maternity Care Project (MCP^2). (2006). *Final report.* Retrieved from <http://www.sogc.org/wp-content/uploads/2013/09/repFinlHlthCA0606.pdf>.

Navaneelan, T., & Janz, T. (2014). Adjusting the scales: Obesity in the Canadian population after correcting for respondent bias. *Health at a Glance.* Statistics Canada Catalogue no. 82-624-X. Retrieved from <http://www.statcan.gc.ca/pub/82-624-x/2014001/article/11922-eng.htm>.

Pound, C. M., Unger, S. L., & Canadian Paediatric Society, Nutrition and Gastroenterology Committee. (2012). Reaffirmed in 2015. The Baby-Friendly Initiative: Protecting, promoting and supporting breastfeeding. *Paediatrics & Child Health, 17*(6), 317–321.

Public Health Agency of Canada. (2009). *What mothers say: The Canadian maternity experiences survey.* Ottawa: Author. Retrieved from <http://www.phac-aspc.gc.ca/rhs-ssg/survey-eng.php>.

Public Health Agency of Canada. (2013). *Perinatal health indicators for Canada 2013: A report of the Canadian Perinatal Surveillance System. Cat. No. HP7-1/2013E-PDF.* Ottawa: Author.

Public Health Agency of Canada. (2016). Pregnancy. In *Family-centred maternal and newborn care: National guidelines.* Ottawa: Author.

Statistics Canada. (2013). *Breastfeeding trends in Canada.* Ottawa: Author. Retrieved from <http://www.statcan.gc.ca/pub/82-624-x/2013001/article/11879-eng.htm>.

World Health Organization. (2014a). *Fact sheet: Children: Reducing mortality.* Geneva: Author. Retrieved from <http://www.who.int/mediacentre/factsheets/fs178/en/>.

World Health Organization. (2014b). *Fact sheet: Female genital mutilation.* Geneva: Author. Retrieved from <http://www.who.int/mediacentre/factsheets/fs241/en/>.

ADDITIONAL RESOURCES

Association of Ontario Midwives: Tip Sheet for Providing Care to Trans Men and All "Trans Masculine Spectrum" Clients. <http://www.rainbowhealthontario.ca/wp-content/uploads/woocommerce_uploads/2014/08/Midwives%20-%20Tip%20sheet%20for%20working%20with%20trans%20clients.pdf>.

Canadian Association of Perinatal and Women's Health Nurses (CAPWHN): <http://www.capwhn.ca>.

Canadian Nurses Association Certification: <http://nurseone.ca/certification/what-is-certification>.

Canadian Perinatal Surveillance System: <http://www.phac-aspc.gc.ca/rhs-ssg/index-eng.php>.

Canadian Perinatal Surveillance System: The Canadian Maternity Experiences Survey: <http://www.phac-aspc.gc.ca/rhs-ssg/survey-eng.php>.

Champlain Maternal Newborn Regional Program: <http://www.cmnrp.ca/en/cmnrp/Home_p2974.html>.

National Collaborating Centre for the Determinants of Health (NCCDH): <http://nccdh.ca/images/uploads/TK_KeyFactsGlossaryJune25_v61.pdf>.

Perinatal Services BC: <http://www.perinatalservicesbc.ca/>.

Public Safety Canada: Human Trafficking in Canada: <http://www.publicsafety.gc.ca/cnt/cntrng-crm/hmn-trffckng/index-eng.aspx>.

Society of Obstetricians and Gynaecologists of Canada: <http://www.sogc.org>.

UNIT 3

Women's Health

CHAPTER

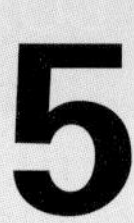

Health Promotion

Kerry Lynn Durnford

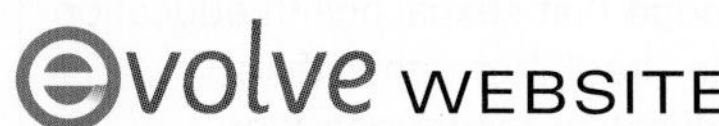

WEBSITE

***Visit the Evolve website for additional resources related to the content in this chapter such as Case Studies, Critical Thinking Case Study Answers, Nursing Care Plans, Nursing Processes, Nursing Skills, and Review Questions for Exam Preparation at:** http://evolve.elsevier.com/Canada/Perry/maternal/*

OBJECTIVES

On completion of this chapter the reader will be able to:

- Identify facilitators and barriers for women to access care in the health care system.
- Analyze the determinants of health that may affect a woman's decision to seek and follow through with health care.
- Describe the need for health promotion across the woman's lifespan.
- Analyze conditions and factors that increase health risks for women across the lifespan, including life stage, substance use, eating disorders, medical and health conditions, pregnancy, and intimate partner violence.
- Explain the cycle of violence and how an understanding of it can be used in assessment of and intervention for women who are victims of violence.
- Identify community resources to prevent violence against women.
- Outline health-screening schedules for women.
- Discuss how adult learning principles can be used in health-promotion education with women and families.

REASONS FOR ENTERING THE HEALTH CARE SYSTEM

Many women initially enter the health care system because of some reproductive system–related situation, such as pregnancy, irregular menses, a desire for **contraception**, or an episodic illness, for example, a vaginal **infection**. Once the woman is in the system, it is important that health care providers recognize the significance of health promotion and preventive health maintenance and offer these services across the lifespan. This chapter presents an overview of the nurse's role in encouraging health promotion and illness prevention in women. It includes a schedule of screening tests recommended for women at different stages of their lives. Barriers to seeking health care as well as an overview of conditions and circumstances that increase health risks for women across the lifespan are also included. Anticipatory guidance suggestions, such as nutrition and stress management, are included. Violence against women, particularly intimate partner violence (IPV) and battering of women, is discussed because it is often in the health care setting that the woman is able to acknowledge being in an abusive relationship.

Well-Woman Care Across the Lifespan

Maintaining optimal health is a goal for all women. Essential components of health maintenance are the identification of unrecognized problems and potential risks, and the education and health promotion needed to reduce them.

A holistic approach to women's health care goes beyond simple reproductive needs; it includes a woman's health needs throughout her lifetime, with attention to physical, mental or emotional, social, and spiritual health. Women's health is considered to be part of the primary health care delivery system, with assessment and screening focusing on a multisystem evaluation that emphasizes the maintenance and enhancement of wellness. Prevention of cardiovascular disease, promotion of mental health, and prevention of all forms of cancer, not just reproductive-related cancers, are all components of well-woman

BOX 5-1 TOP 10 LEADING CAUSES OF DEATH IN WOMEN IN CANADA

1. Malignant neoplasm (cancer)
2. Heart disease
3. Cerebrovascular disease (stroke)
4. Chronic lower respiratory disease
5. Accidents (unintentional injuries)
6. Alzheimer's disease
7. Diabetes mellitus
8. Influenza and pneumonia
9. Chronic liver disease and cirrhosis
10. Intentional self-harm (suicide)

Source: Statistics Canada. (2014). *The 10 leading causes of death, 2011*. Ottawa: Government of Canada. Retrieved from http://www.statcan.gc.ca/pub/82-625-x/2014001/article/11896-eng.htm

care. It is important to consider all aspects of women's health, particularly in light of the fact that the leading causes of death in women in Canada include more than just reproductive health–related conditions (Box 5-1).

Even when focusing on reproductive health, it is critical to take a holistic approach to the health of women. This is especially important for women in their child-bearing years because conditions that increase a woman's health risks are related not only to her well-being but also to the well-being of both mother and newborn in the event of a pregnancy. Prenatal care is an example of prevention that is practised after conception. However, prevention and health maintenance are also needed before conception because many of the mother's risks can be identified and modified then or perhaps even eliminated.

Health care needs vary with culture, religion, age, and personal differences. The changing responsibilities and roles of women, their socioeconomic status, and their personal lifestyles also contribute to differences in the health and behaviour of women. Employment outside the home, physical disability, lone parenthood, and sexual orientation also can affect women's ability to seek and receive health care in clinical settings. As women age, well-women's health care should continue to include a complete history, physical examination, age-appropriate screening, and health promotion.

Adolescents

As a female progresses through developmental ages and stages, she is faced with conditions that are age-related. All teens undergo progressive development of sex characteristics. They experience the developmental tasks of adolescence such as establishing identity and sexual orientation, separating from family, and establishing career goals. Some of these processes can produce great stress for the adolescent. Female teenagers who enter the health care system usually do so because of a problem, such as episodic illness or accidents or due to gynecological problems associated with menses (either bleeding irregularities or dysmenorrhea), vaginitis or leukorrhea, sexually transmitted infections (STIs), contraception, or pregnancy. The adolescent may also be at risk for use of street drugs, for eating disorders, and for stress, depression, and anxiety.

BOX 5-2 FRAMEWORK OF VALUES FOR SCHOOL-BASED SEXUAL HEALTH EDUCATION PROGRAM

Sexual health programming should:

- Focus on the self-worth, respect, and dignity of the individual
- Be provided in an age-appropriate, culturally sensitive manner that is respectful of individual sexual diversity, abilities, and choices
- Help individuals to become more sensitive and aware of the impact their behaviours and actions may have on others and society
- Not discriminate on the basis of age, race, ethnicity, gender identity, sexual orientation, socioeconomic background, physical/cognitive abilities, or religious background in terms of access to relevant, appropriate, accurate, and comprehensive information.

These statements acknowledge that sexual health education programs should not be "value -free" but rather that:

- Effective sexual health education recognizes that responsible individuals may choose a variety of paths to achieve sexual health
- Effective sexual health education supports informed decision making by providing individuals with the knowledge, personal insight, motivation, and behavioural skills that are consistent with each individual's personal values and choices.

Source: *Canadian guidelines on sexual health education*. Public Health Agency of Canada, Revised Edition: 2013. Adapted and reproduced with permission from the Minister of Health, 2016.

Most young women begin having sex in their mid- to late teens (Sexualityandu.ca, 2012). A sexually active teen who does not use contraception has a 90% chance of pregnancy within 1 year. Effective educational programs about sex and family life are imperative to control the rate of teen pregnancy and STIs. Most Canadian public schools have a sexual health and education component in their curriculum (Box 5-2).

Knowledge of and ability to apply growth and developmental concepts are critical for nurses in their work with adolescents. Involving adolescents in their care is important for establishing the nurse–patient relationship and for focusing on individual adolescents' strengths and resilience.

Teenage pregnancy. The rate of teenage pregnancy in Canada has decreased significantly. In 1995 the rate of teenage pregnancy was 28.2 per 1,000 and 15.8 per 1,000 in 2005 (McKay & Sex Information and Education Council of Canada, 2012). When teenage pregnancy does occur, it often introduces additional stress into an already challenging developmental period and there are greater risks than pregnancies for other women (Al-Sahab, Heifetz, Tamim, et al., 2012). The emotional level of teens who are less than 16 years of age can be characterized by impulsiveness and self-centred behaviour, and they often place primary importance on the beliefs and actions of their peers. In attempts to establish a personal and independent identity, many teens do not realize the consequences of their behaviour; their thinking processes do not include planning for the future.

From a public health perspective, the rate of teenage pregnancy is significant because teen pregnancy is more common among disadvantaged teenagers and may be a predictor of other social, educational, and employment barriers in later life (Ministry of Health and Long-Term Care [MHLTC], 2012). Al-Sahab et al. (2012) also found that the incidence of violence is higher for adolescent mothers (see discussion later).

Teenagers often lack the financial and social resources to support a pregnancy and may not have the maturity to avoid teratogens or to have prenatal care and instruction or follow-up care. Pregnant teens have a greater risk of developing health problems such as anemia, hypertension, eclampsia, and depressive disorders as well as of delivering newborns that are preterm or have low birth weight (MHLTC, 2012). Children of teen mothers may be at risk for abuse or neglect because of the teen's inadequate knowledge of child growth and development and of parenting. Implementation of specialized adolescent programs in schools, communities, and health care systems is demonstrating continued success in reducing the birth rate among teenagers.

Young and Middle Adulthood

Because women ages 20 to 40 years have a need for contraception, pelvic and breast screening, and pregnancy care, they may prefer to use their gynecological or obstetrical provider as their primary care provider. Women ages 20 to 40 may be "juggling" family, home, and career responsibilities, with resulting increases in stress-related conditions. Health maintenance includes not only pelvic and breast screening but also promotion of a healthy lifestyle (i.e., good nutrition, regular exercise, no smoking, moderate or no alcohol consumption, sufficient rest, stress reduction, and referral for medical conditions and other specific problems). Common conditions requiring well-woman care include urinary tract infections, menstrual variations, sexual and relationship issues, and pregnancy.

Parenthood after age 35. The woman older than 35 years does not have a different physical response to a pregnancy per se but rather has had health status changes as a result of time and the aging process. These changes may be responsible for age-related pregnancy conditions. Other chronic or debilitating diseases or conditions increase in severity with time, and these in turn may predispose these women to increased risks during pregnancy. Of significance to women in this age group is the risk for certain genetic anomalies (e.g., Down syndrome). The opportunity for genetic counselling should be available to all (see Chapter 9). Many women at this point in their lives are established in their careers and relationships and are preparing for a family. A thorough assessment of the woman and her fertility goals is important.

Late Reproductive Age

Women of later reproductive age often experience change and a reordering of personal priorities. In general, the goals of education, career, marriage, and family have been achieved; now the woman has more time and opportunity for new interests and activities. Divorce rates are high at this age, and children leaving home may produce an "empty nest syndrome," resulting in a potential increase in depression. Chronic diseases also become more apparent. Many women seek health care to discuss concerns with perimenopause (e.g., bleeding irregularities and vasomotor symptoms). Health maintenance screening continues to be of importance because some conditions such as breast disease or ovarian cancer occur more often during this stage.

APPROACHES TO CARE AT SPECIFIC STAGES OF A WOMAN'S LIFE

There are certain specific approaches to care of women at different stages of their lives. Several of these approaches are described in the next section.

Fertility Control and Infertility

Although information on unplanned pregnancies is not routinely collected, it is estimated that perhaps 40% of all pregnancies in Canada are unplanned. Education is key to encouraging women to make family planning choices based on preference and actual benefit-to-risk ratios. Health care providers can influence the woman's motivation and ability to use contraception correctly (see Chapter 8).

Women also enter the health care system because of their desire to become pregnant. Prevalence of infertility has increased in Canada, with estimates of 11.5 to 15.7% (Bushnik, Cook, Yuzper, et al., 2012). Many couples delay starting their families until they are in their 30s or 40s, which allows more time to be exposed to factors that affect fertility negatively (including age-related infertility for the woman). In addition, STIs, which can predispose to decreased fertility, are becoming more common, and many women and men are in workplaces and home settings where they may be exposed to reproductive environmental hazards.

Infertility can cause emotional pain for many couples. The inability to produce a child sometimes results in feelings of failure and places inordinate stress on the couple's relationship. Much time, money, and emotional investment may have been used for testing and treatment in efforts to build a family. A supportive health care team is important for the couple exploring fertility, struggling with fertility, or making choices for a life and career without children.

Steps toward prevention of infertility should be undertaken as part of ongoing routine health care. Such information is especially appropriate in preconception counselling. Primary care providers can undertake initial evaluation and provide counselling before couples are referred to specialists. For additional information about infertility, see Chapter 8.

Preconception Counselling and Care

Preconception health promotion provides women and their partners with information needed to make decisions about their reproductive future. This information can guide couples to identify and manage risk factors in their lives and in their environment. It can also be used to identify healthy behaviours that promote the well-being of the woman and her potential child.

BOX 5-3 COMPONENTS OF PRECONCEPTION CARE

Health Promotion: General Teaching
- Nutrition
- Healthy diet, including folic acid
- Optimal weight
- Exercise and rest
- Avoidance of use of substances (tobacco, alcohol, "recreational" drugs)
- Use of risk-reducing sex practices
- Attending to family and social needs

Risk Factor Assessment
- Chronic diseases
- Diabetes, heart disease, hypertension, asthma, thyroid disease, kidney disease, anemia, mental illness
- Infectious diseases
- HIV/AIDS, other sexually transmitted infections, vaccine-preventable diseases (e.g., rubella, hepatitis B, HPV)
- Reproductive history
- Contraception
- Pregnancies—unplanned pregnancy, pregnancy outcomes
- Infertility
- Genetic or inherited conditions (e.g., sickle cell anemia, Down syndrome, cystic fibrosis)
- Medications and medical treatment
- Prescription medications (especially those contraindicated in pregnancy), over-the-counter medication use, radiation exposure
- Personal behaviours and exposures
- Smoking, alcohol consumption, problematic drug use
- Overweight or underweight; eating disorders
- Spouse or partner and family situation, including intimate partner violence
- Availability of family or other support systems
- Readiness for pregnancy (e.g., age, life goals, stress)
- Environmental (home, workplace) conditions
- Safety hazards
- Toxic chemicals
- Radiation

Interventions
- Anticipatory guidance or teaching
- Treatment of medical conditions and results
- Medications
- Cessation or reduction in problematic substance use
- Immunizations (e.g., rubella, hepatitis)
- Nutrition, diet, weight management
- Exercise
- Referral for genetic counselling
- Referral to and use of:
  - Family planning services
  - Family and social services

AIDS, acquired immunodeficiency syndrome; *HIV*, human immunodeficiency virus. *HPV*, human papillomavirus.

Activities that promote health in mothers and babies must be initiated before the period of critical fetal organ development, which is between 17 and 56 days after fertilization. By the end of the eighth week after conception and certainly by the end of the first trimester, any major structural anomalies in the fetus are already present. Because many women do not realize that they are pregnant and do not seek prenatal care until well into the first trimester, the rapidly growing fetus may have already been exposed to many types of intrauterine environmental hazards during this most vulnerable developmental phase. These hazards include drugs, viruses, and chemicals. In many instances, counselling can aid in promoting behaviour modification before damage is done and in helping the woman make an informed decision about her willingness to accept potential hazards. Thus, preconception health care should occur well in advance of an actual pregnancy.

Preconception care is important for women who have had a problem with a previous pregnancy (e.g., miscarriage or preterm birth). Although causes are not always identifiable, in many cases problems can be identified and treated and do not recur in subsequent pregnancies. Preconception care is also important in order to minimize fetal malformations. For example, the children of women who have type 1 diabetes mellitus have significantly more congenital anomalies than do children of mothers without diabetes. The rate of malformation is greatly reduced when the insulin-dependent woman with diabetes has excellent blood glucose control when she becomes pregnant and maintains euglycemia (normal blood sugar) throughout the period of organ development in the fetus. The incidence of neural tube defects such as spina bifida and anencephaly is decreased significantly with the intake of folic acid. Health Canada (2013a) recommends a daily multivitamin of 400 mcg (0.4 mg) of folic acid at least 3 months prior to conception; higher doses may be required depending on risk factors. Women should consult their health care provider to collaborate on the safest and most appropriate dosage of folic acid.

The components of preconception care such as health promotion, risk assessment, and interventions are outlined in Box 5-3.

Pregnancy

A woman's entry into health care is often associated with pregnancy, for either confirmation of it or actual care. Early entry into prenatal care (i.e., within the first 12 weeks) enables identification of the woman at risk and initiation of measures to promote a healthy outcome. Early and consistent prenatal care improves outcomes for mothers and infants. Major goals of prenatal care, listed in Box 5-4, should be addressed during the first visit. More extensive discussion of pregnancy is found in Unit 4.

Menstrual Concerns

Irregularities or problems with the menstrual period are among the most common concerns of women and often cause them to seek help from a health care provider. Common menstrual disorders include amenorrhea, dysmenorrhea, premenstrual

BOX 5-4 MAJOR GOALS OF PRENATAL CARE

Establish a therapeutic relationship and collaborate with the mother to do the following:

- Define health status of mother and fetus.
- Determine the gestational age of the fetus and monitor fetal development.
- Identify the woman at risk for complications and minimize the risk whenever possible.
- Assess level of social support and history of previous loss.
- Assess learning needs related to pregnancy.
- Provide appropriate education and counselling.

syndrome, endometriosis, and menorrhagia or metrorrhagia. Simple explanation and counselling may handle the concern; however, history and examination must be completed, as well as laboratory or diagnostic tests, if indicated. Questions should never be considered inconsequential, and age-specific reading materials are recommended, especially for teenagers. See Chapter 7 for an in-depth discussion of menstrual concerns.

Perimenopause and Menopause

Perimenopause is the interval between regular cycles of ovulation occurring and menopause (permanent infertility). The body responds to this natural transition in a number of ways, most of which are caused by the decrease in estrogen. Most women seeking health care during the perimenopausal period do so because of irregular bleeding. Others are concerned about vasomotor symptoms (hot flashes and flushes). Although fertility is greatly reduced during this period, women are urged to maintain some method of birth control because pregnancies still can occur. All women need to receive factual information, have myths dispelled, and undergo a thorough examination. During menopause they should have periodic health screenings.

BARRIERS TO RECEIVING HEALTH CARE

The health of Canadians cannot be evaluated without consideration of the determinants of health (see Table 1-1 on p. 5). The Public Health Agency of Canada (PHAC) recognizes the following determinants of health: income and social status, social support networks, education and literacy, employment and working conditions, social environments, physical environments, personal health practices and coping skills, and healthy child development (Canadian Nurses Association [CNA], 2009; PHAC, 2010). Deficiencies in determinants of health and detrimental contextual factors may pose difficulties in accessing and receiving health care.

Financial Issues

Limited finances can be associated with lack of access to care, delay in seeking care, fewer illness prevention activities, and little accurate information about health and the health care system. Poverty is a significant health issue for Canadian women. It is estimated that more than 4.9 million Canadians live in poverty, including 21% of single mothers (Canada Without Poverty, 2016). In Canada, disparity among races and socioeconomic classes affects many facets of life, including health. Indigenous people in Canada are twice as likely as non-Indigenous people to live in a home in need of major repair, are 90 times more likely to have no piped water, and are 5 times more likely to have no bathroom facilities (Smylie, Fell, Ohlsson, et al., 2010). Infant mortality rates for Indigenous people in Canada have ranged from 1.7 to over 4 times national Canadian rates, and Indigenous children under the age of 6 are less likely to access health care than are non-Indigenous Canadian children (Smylie et al., 2010).

Socioeconomic status also affects birth outcomes. The rates of perinatal and maternal deaths, preterm births, and low-birth-weight babies are considerably higher in disadvantaged populations (Hogue & Silver, 2011). Single mothers with little to no employment skills are caught in the bind of insufficient income for child care, restricting their ability to search for and obtain more secure employment, and increasing their risks for health concerns. Social isolation, especially among immigrant women, prevents women from accessing the support they need during pregnancy (Reitmanova & Gustafson, 2008). Multiple roles for women in general produce overload, conflict, and stress, resulting in higher risks for psychological illness.

Cultural Issues

As our nation becomes more racially, ethnically, and culturally diverse, the health of minority groups has become a major issue. A variety of reasons are given to explain some of the differences in accessing care when financial barriers are adjusted. Some women experience racial discrimination or disrespectful, disillusioning, or discouraging encounters with community service providers such as social services and health care providers. Many women do not seek care from the health care system because of lack of trust (Yang, Matthews, & Hillemeier, 2011). A lack of cross-cultural communication also presents problems. Desired health outcomes are best achieved when the health care provider has knowledge of and understanding about the culture, language, values, priorities, and health beliefs of those in minority groups. Conversely, members of the group should understand the health goals to be achieved and the methods proposed to do so. Language differences can produce profound barriers between patients and providers. Even with an interpreter, misinformation can occur on both sides of the communication (see Chapter 2, p. 22).

Providers must consider culturally based differences that could affect the treatment of diverse groups of women, and the women themselves must share practices and beliefs that could influence their responses or their willingness to adhere to treatment. For example, women in some cultures value modesty to such an extent that they are reluctant to disrobe and as a result avoid physical examination unless it is absolutely necessary. Other women rely on their husbands to make major decisions, including those affecting the woman's health. Religious beliefs may dictate a plan of care, as with birth control measures or blood transfusions. Some cultural groups prefer traditional medicine, homeopathy, or prayer to Western medicine; others use a combination of some or all of these practices.

A history of residential school abuse in Canada has had a tremendous impact on the definition of health for Indigenous people (Allan & Smylie, 2015). Even in areas where health programs are well established, individuals may not access programs because of a legacy of mistrust of institutions. Recognition of how these factors may affect Indigenous people is essential in the establishment of culturally safe policy and programs. The Truth and Reconciliation Commission of Canada (2015) called for action by federal, provincial, and territorial governments to acknowledge and reduce disparities in the areas of education, child welfare, language, culture, health, and justice for Indigenous people in Canada (see Chapter 1 for further discussion).

Community collaboration is needed to ensure that health programs and policies are created in a culturally safe manner and that services will meet the needs of and be used by women and their families (see Chapter 2). It is not enough for health services to merely exist; they must be familiar and accessible to Canadians. This is especially important in the immigrant population, who may be struggling to navigate the Canadian health care system (Grewal, Bhagat, & Balneaves, 2008).

Gender Issues

Gender affects provider–patient communication and may influence access to health care in general. The most obvious gender consideration is that between men and women. Women tend to use primary care services more often than men and, some investigators believe, use them more effectively. The gender of the provider also plays a role. The concept of "gender concordance," in which the patient's gender matches the health care provider's gender, was found to be important for women seeking Pap tests (McAlearney, Oliveri, Post, et al., 2011). McAlearney et al. (2011) found that women were more comfortable having a Pap test performed by a female physician and having a female nurse present.

Sexual orientation may produce another barrier to adequate health care. Nurses need to understand the specific health care needs and issues related to sexual orientation (Brennan, Barnsteiner, de Leon Siantz, et al., 2012). Some women may not disclose their sexual orientation to health care providers because they feel they may be at risk for hostility, inadequate health care, or breach of confidentiality. In many health care settings heterosexuality is assumed, and the setting may be one in which the lesbian woman does not feel welcome (magazines, brochures, and the environment reflect heterosexual couples, or the health care provider shows discomfort interacting with the woman). This can result in a lack of medical care, as well as in health care providers giving incorrect advice or not providing appropriate screening for lesbian women. Not all gynecological cancers are related to sexual activity; women who have never had children may be more at risk for breast, ovarian, and endometrial cancer. Lesbian women's risk for heart disease, cancer of the lung, and colon cancer is not different from that of heterosexual women. To offset stereotypes, it is necessary for providers to develop an approach that does not assume that all patients are heterosexual. More content related to this issue needs to be included in nursing curricula and efforts are under way to do so.

IDENTIFICATION OF RISK FACTORS TO WOMEN'S HEALTH

In caring for women at all stages of life, it is important to understand the various and complex risk factors that can affect a woman's health. This section describes these risk factors.

Cultural and Genetic Factors

Differences exist among people from different socioeconomic levels and ethnic groups in terms of risk for illness and distribution of disease and death. Some diseases are more common among people of a specific ethnicity (e.g., sickle cell anemia in Blacks, Tay-Sachs disease in Ashkenazi Jews, adult lactase deficiency in Chinese, β-thalassemia in Mediterranean people, and cystic fibrosis in Northern Europeans). Cultural and religious influences can also increase health risks because the woman and her family may have life and societal values and a view of health and illness that dictate practices different from those expected in the Judeo-Christian Western model. Such practices may include food taboos or frequencies, methods of hygiene, effects of climate, care-seeking behaviours, willingness to undergo screening and diagnostic procedures, and value conflicts.

Substance Use

Use of illicit drugs and inappropriate use of prescription drugs continue to increase and are found in all age groups, races, and ethnic groups and at all socioeconomic levels. **Addiction** to substances is seen as a biopsychosocial disease, with several factors leading to risk. These include biogenetic predisposition, lack of resilience to stressful life experiences, and poor social support. Although women are less likely than men to abuse drugs, the rate of women who misuse drugs has risen significantly. Pregnant women who overuse substances have increased risk for development of their own health problems, and their offspring have increased risk for potential problems, including interference with optimal growth and development, and for physical dependence on the drug. Nurses must be aware of the potential impact of **substance use** and how to detect it, as many women who have addiction issues may not readily access health care or disclose about their addictions.

Cigarette Smoking

Tobacco use is the leading cause of preventable death and illness. Smoking is linked to cardiovascular disease, various types of cancers (especially lung and cervical), chronic lung disease, and negative pregnancy outcomes. Tobacco contains nicotine, which is an addictive substance that creates physical and psychological dependence. Smoking rates have declined overall in Canada in recent years: in 1999, 25% of Canadians smoked; the rate decreased to 16% in 2012 (Health Canada, 2013b). Smoking rates vary across Canada, with the highest rates existing in the three territories. Twenty-two percent of women age 20 to 34 smoke (Statistics Canada, 2015a). These

FAMILY-CENTRED TEACHING

Smoking Cessation

You are the nurse working in a family health team clinic; you observe that many of the young mothers with newborns seen in the clinic smoke cigarettes. One new mother said, "I know it's bad for me but I can't quit. At least I don't smoke around the baby." What advice could you provide for the young mothers about the effect of tobacco smoke on young infants, especially those under 6 months of age? Prepare a short presentation that can be shared with the young mothers about the effects of tobacco on an infant's long-term health. Discuss options and resources for smoking cessation that are available from local community agencies.

are the major child-bearing years, with significant consequences for pregnancy and the fetus. The Maternity Experience Survey found that 10.5% of women smoked cigarettes during their last 3 months of pregnancy (PHAC, 2009). Smoking in pregnancy is known to cause a decrease in placental perfusion and is one cause of low birth weight in infants. A Canadian national youth survey found that approximately 32% of adolescents in grades 7 to 12 had smoked menthol cigarettes, which may be incorrectly perceived as less harmful, thus encouraging nicotine dependence and a possible predictor of marijuana use and binge drinking (Azagba & Sharaf, 2014; Manske, Rynard, & Minaker, 2013). See Family-Centred Teaching box.

Cigarette smoking impairs fertility in both women and men, may reduce the age for menopause, and increases the risk for osteoporosis after menopause. Passive, or secondhand, smoke (environmental tobacco smoke) contains similar hazards and presents additional problems for the smoker and harm for the nonsmoker.

Caffeine

Caffeine is found in society's most popular drinks: coffee, tea, soft drinks, and energy drinks. It is a stimulant that can affect mood and interrupt body functions by producing anxiety and sleep interruptions. Heart arrhythmias may be made worse by caffeine, and there can be interactions with certain medications, such as lithium. Birth defects have not been related to caffeine consumption; however, high intake has been potentially related to a slight decrease in birth weight and may also increase the risk of miscarriage. Pregnant women should limit their consumption of caffeine to less than 300 mg/day, or a little more than two 240 mL (8-oz) cups (Health Canada, 2014; Motherisk, 2013). It is important for the nurse to educate the woman on the various sources of caffeine, as it is found in a variety of food and drink products.

Alcohol Consumption

The amount and frequency of alcohol consumption among young Canadian women is alarming: in 2012, 74% of Canadian women age 15 and older reported drinking alcohol; based on the amount of alcohol abused, 16% of those women are at risk for long-term complications and 10% at risk for acute illness (Canadian Centre on Substance Abuse, 2014a). Women who are problem drinkers are often depressed, have more motor vehicle injuries, and have a higher incidence of attempted suicide than do women in the general population. They are also at risk for alcohol-related liver damage. Early case finding and treatment are important for addressing alcoholism, for both the ill individual and family members.

Prenatal exposure to alcohol at high risk levels can have multiple, permanent cognitive and physical effects on the fetus (Senikas, Kluka, Wood, et al., 2010). Prenatal alcohol exposure has been found to increase the chance of birth defects significantly, with one study reporting a fourfold increase (O'Leary, Nassar, Kurinczuk, et al., 2011). Although fetal alcohol spectrum disorder (FASD) is a known consequence of prenatal alcohol intake, studies also indicate that other consequences include increased risk for miscarriage, stillbirth, preterm birth, and sudden infant death syndrome (SIDS). Clearly, alcohol consumption during pregnancy has wide-reaching effects (Bailey & Sokol, 2011).

FASD, which includes fetal alcohol syndrome (FAS), is the most serious complication. Children with FAS have facial abnormalities, including wide-set and narrow eyes, growth problems, and nervous system abnormalities. Low birth weight, intellectual disability, behavioural issues, and learning and physical problems are some of the symptoms of FASD (see Chapter 25). Recent research reveals that multivitamin supplement use during pregnancy may lessen the effects of prenatal alcohol exposure in the children of women who are unable or unwilling to curtail their alcohol use when pregnant (Avalos, Kaskutas, Block, et al., 2011). In addition, women may experience nutritional deficiencies, pancreatitis, alcoholic hepatitis, deficient milk ejection (let-down), and cirrhosis (Cunningham, Leveno, Bloom, et al., 2014).

Prescription Medication Use

Women are more likely than men to be prescribed mood-altering medications such as stimulants, sleeping pills, tranquilizers, and pain relievers (Poole & Dell, 2005). Such medications can bring relief from undesirable conditions such as insomnia, anxiety, depression, and pain. Because the medications have mind-altering capacity, misuse can produce psychological and physical dependency in the same manner as illicit drugs. Risk-to-benefit ratios should be considered when such medications are used for more than a very short period of time.

Depression and anxiety are the most common mental health problems in women (depression used to be considered the most common, but recently it has been noted that depression occurs comorbidly with anxiety). Many kinds of medications are used to treat depression and anxiety. All of these psychotherapeutic drugs can have some effect on the fetus and must be monitored very carefully in pregnant women.

Illicit Drug Use

Marijuana. Marijuana is a substance derived from the cannabis plant. It is usually rolled into a cigarette and smoked, but it also may be mixed into food and eaten. Marijuana produces distorted perceptions, difficulty with problem solving and with thinking and memory, altered state of awareness, relaxation, mild euphoria, and reduced inhibition (National Institute on Drug Abuse, 2015). In 2011, approximately one third of

Canadians age 15 and older reported using cannabis at least once in their lives, and 5.1% had ridden in a vehicle with someone who had used cannabis within 2 hours of driving (Canadian Centre on Substance Abuse, 2014a). In the pregnant woman, marijuana readily crosses the placenta and causes increased carbon monoxide levels in the mother's blood, which reduces the oxygen supply to the fetus. Research findings regarding the effects of marijuana demonstrate adverse outcomes on the fetus and infant (Hayatbakhsh, Flenady, Gibbons, et al., 2012).

Cocaine. Cocaine is a powerful central nervous system stimulant that is addictive because of the tremendous sense of euphoria it creates. It can be snorted, smoked, or injected. Crack, or rock cocaine, is a form of the drug that is exceedingly potent and even more highly addictive. (Some say that an individual is "hooked" after the first use or at least after two or three "hits.") After ingestion of cocaine, an intensely pleasurable high results that is followed by an uncomfortable low; this increases the urge to repeat the drug.

Predisposing factors and problems associated with cocaine use are polydrug use; poor nutrition; poverty; STIs; hepatitis B infection; dysfunctional family systems; employment difficulties; stress; anger; poor self-esteem; and previous or present physical, emotional, and sexual abuse. The clinical manifestations of cocaine use include tachycardia, pupillary dilation, and hypertension.

Cocaine affects all of the major body systems. Among other complications, it produces cardiovascular stress (including tachycardia and hypertension) that can lead to heart attack or stroke, liver disease, central nervous system stimulation that can cause seizures, and even perforation of the nasal septum. Needle-borne diseases such as hepatitis B and acquired immunodeficiency syndrome (AIDS) are common among cocaine users. If the user is pregnant, there is an increased incidence of miscarriage, preterm labour, small-for-gestational-age babies, abruption of placenta, and stillbirth. Anomalies have been reported (Canadian Centre on Substance Abuse, 2013).

One of the promising treatments for cocaine use in pregnancy is acupuncture. A component of traditional Chinese medicine, acupuncture is used to redirect energy flow (chi) within the body, reduce cravings, and enhance well-being. Acupuncture has been studied and shown to be effective in detoxification in people addicted to many different drugs (Schaub & Burt, 2013).

Opiates. The opiates include opium, heroin, meperidine, morphine, codeine, and methadone. Heroin is one of the most commonly used drugs of this class. It is usually taken by intravenous injection but can be smoked or "snorted." The signs and symptoms of heroin use are euphoria, relaxation, relief from pain, "nodding out" (apathy, detachment from reality, impaired judgement, and drowsiness), constricted pupils, nausea, constipation, slurred speech, and respiratory depression.

The incidence of heroin use among pregnant women is unknown because women with a dependency on heroin often use multiple drugs. Women who use opiates during pregnancy have a 6-times higher risk for problem outcomes (Keegan, Parva, Finnegan, et al., 2010). The recommended treatment is methadone maintenance, ideally done by stabilizing the treatment before as well as during pregnancy (Peles, Schreiber, Bloch, et al., 2012). This treatment must be closely monitored because, in pregnancy, methadone is metabolized more rapidly, leading to withdrawal symptoms in less than 24 hours in many women. Neonatal abstinence syndrome (NAS) is a serious concern for infants born to mothers who chronically use opioids (Canadian Centre on Substance Abuse, 2013) (see Chapter 29). Withdrawal symptoms can include fetal hyperactivity and, if severe, preterm labour or fetal death.

Methamphetamine. Methamphetamine is a relatively cheap and highly addictive stimulant. In 2012 there were an estimated 52,000 users in Canada, and at least 1% of high school students had used methamphetamine at least once in the previous year (Centre for Addiction and Mental Health [CAMH], 2012). Methamphetamine makes many users feel hypersexual and uninhibited, and this may lead to more sex and less protection from pregnancy.

The active metabolite of methamphetamine is amphetamine, a central nervous system stimulant known as both "speed" and "meth." The crystalline form, which is smoked, is known as "ice." Methamphetamine causes a person to experience an elevated mood state and pleasure as well as increased energy and creates addiction within a short period. It can lead to cardiac problems, including irregular heartbeat and hypertension and, over time, can create cognitive and mental as well as dental problems (Medline Plus, 2014). Most of the effects of amphetamines are similar to those of cocaine. Although fewer maternal and neonatal complications have been attributed to this class of substances than to cocaine, the rates of preterm births and intrauterine growth restriction with smaller head circumference are higher in methamphetamine-exposed pregnant women than in pregnant women who use other substances.

Other illicit drugs. A number of other street drugs pose risks to users. A few are derived from organic materials, but more and more are produced synthetically in laboratories. Sedatives such as "downers," "yellow jackets," or "red devils" are used to come off "highs." Hallucinogens alter perception and body function. PCP ("angel dust") and LSD produce vivid changes in sensation, often with agitation, euphoria, paranoia, and a tendency toward antisocial behaviour. Their use may lead to flashbacks, chronic psychosis, and violent behaviour. Hallucinogens taken during pregnancy may have negative neurobehavioural effects on the newborn.

Many prescription and nonprescription medications may also be transferred to the newborn via breast milk, and the potential impact must be discussed with breastfeeding women who use them.

Substance Use Cessation

All women at all ages will receive substantial and immediate benefits from stopping or decreasing their use of substances. However, this is not easy, and most people will attempt to stop several times before they accomplish their goal. Many are never able to do so.

New approaches are needed to increase cessation among smokers and to discourage smoking among young women,

BOX 5-5 REGISTERED NURSES' ASSOCIATION OF ONTARIO: INTEGRATING SMOKING CESSATION INTO DAILY NURSING PRACTICE

The most important outcome of this guideline is to motivate and support all health care providers to identify the tobacco use status of their clients and encourage providers to intervene with individuals who smoke, in a sensitive, nonjudgemental manner about the importance of cessation (RNAO, 2015). The RNAO has a four-step intervention for both minimal and intensive cessation that involves the 4A's: Ask, Advise, Assist, and Arrange. For more information visit http://tobaccofreernao.ca/en/4-s.

especially in adolescence and during pregnancy. Health care providers can have an impact on smoking behaviour and should attempt to motivate smokers to stop smoking. Raising questions about social consequences (e.g., stained teeth and foul-smelling breath and clothes) is sometimes effective with young people.

Those who wish to stop smoking can be referred to a smoking cessation program in which individualized methods can be implemented. At the very least, individuals should be guided to self-help materials available from Health Canada, the Canadian Lung Association, and the Canadian Cancer Society. Best practice guidelines regarding smoking cessation are also available from the Registered Nurses Association of Ontario (RNAO). See Additional Resources at the end of the chapter. The RNAO advocates the use of the 4 A's minimal smoking cessation intervention for all health care providers to use in their daily practice (see Box 5-5). There is good evidence that even brief advice from health professionals has a significant effect on smoking cessation rates; advice from a health care professional has been shown to decrease the proportion of people smoking by about 2% per year (RNAO, 2015).

Alcohol and other drugs exact a staggering toll on society, in terms of not only personal health but also their association with poverty and homelessness, family disorganization, violence, crime, motor vehicle injuries, reduced productivity, and economic costs. The use of alcohol and other drugs increases the risk of victimization and date rape and of acquiring HIV through shared needles or sexual contact. Alcohol and substance use are the leading preventable causes of birth defects.

While the legal drinking age varies among the provinces and territories (age 18 or 19), stronger regulation of advertising as well as health promotion and youth-designed programming, such as Students Against Drunk Driving (SADD), is having a positive impact. All primary care providers should screen for alcohol and other drug use, with an understanding of the obvious problem with relying on self-reporting of these behaviours. The use of over-the-counter medications by women should also be explored.

Counselling for women who appear to be drinking excessively or using drugs may include strategies to increase self-esteem and teaching of new coping skills to resist and maintain resistance to alcohol and substance use. Appropriate referrals should be made, with the health care provider arranging the contact and then following up to ensure that appointments are kept. General referral to sources of support should also be provided. Many organizations provide information and support for those who are chemically dependent and have local branches or contacts that are listed in the telephone book or online. Knowledge of harm reduction is important for the health care provider, to ensure that policies and programs exist that support reducing drug-related harm in the absence of abstention and are the first step in potential cessation of drug use (Canadian Harm Reduction Network, 2000).

Anticipatory guidance includes teaching about the health and safety risks of alcohol and mind-altering substances and discouraging drug experimentation among preteen and high school students. The use of drugs at an early age tends to predict greater involvement later.

Nutrition

Good nutrition is essential for optimal health. A well-balanced diet helps prevent illness and also is used to treat certain health problems. Conversely, poor eating habits, eating disorders, and obesity are linked to disease and debility. *Eating Well With Canada's Food Guide* (see Appendix A) provides a variety of educational tools for patients and health care providers to promote health and reduce risks for chronic diseases through diet and physical activity. The Heart and Stroke Foundation of Canada and EatRight Ontario also have a number of nutrition resources (see Additional Resources at the end of the chapter).

In addition to specific guidelines for healthy eating, environmental factors play an important role in nutrition. It is well known that social conditions and access to nutritious food are important contributors to women's health. Women who have access to healthy food have decreased obesity (Dubowitz, Ghosh-Dastidar, Eibner, et al., 2012).

Nutritional Deficiencies

Overt disease caused by a lack of certain nutrients is rarely seen in Canada. However, insufficient amounts or imbalances of nutrients do pose problems for individuals and families. Overweight or underweight status, malabsorption, listlessness, fatigue, frequent colds and other minor infections, constipation, dull hair and nails, and dental caries are examples of problems that could be related to poor nutrition and indicate the need for further nutritional assessment. Poor nutrition, especially that related to obesity and high fat and cholesterol intake, may lead to more serious conditions and contribute to heart disease, malignant neoplasms, cerebrovascular diseases, and diabetes—many of the leading causes of morbidity and mortality in Canada.

Other dietary extremes also produce risk. For example, insufficient amounts of calcium can lead to osteoporosis, too

TABLE 5-1 IDEAL BODY WEIGHT WITH BODY MASS INDEX AND RISK

	BMI RANGE	RISK OF DEVELOPING HEALTH PROBLEMS
Underweight	<18.5	Increased
Normal weight	18.5–24.9	Least
Overweight	25.0–29.9	Increased
Obese	>30.0	High

BMI, body mass index.
Adapted from Health Canada. (2011). *Canadian guidelines for body weight classification in adults.* Ottawa: Author. Retrieved from http://www.hc-sc.gc.ca/fn-an/nutrition/weights-poids/guide-ld-adult/qa-qr-pub-eng.php#a4

much sodium can aggravate hypertension, and megadoses of vitamins can cause adverse effects in several body systems. Fad weight-loss programs and yo-yo dieting (repeated and cyclical weight gain and weight loss) result in nutritional imbalances and, in some instances, medical problems. Such diets and programs are not appropriate for weight maintenance. Adolescent pregnancy produces special nutritional requirements, because the metabolic needs of pregnancy are superimposed on the teen's own needs for growth and maturation at a time when eating habits are not ideal.

Obesity

The number of women in Canada who report themselves to be obese rose from 14.5% in 2003 to 18.7% in 2014, and the rate of overweight women has been stable at 27.5% (Statistics Canada, 2015b) (Table 5-1). The likelihood of being overweight is greater among families living in low socioeconomic neighbourhoods, where the social environment is often less conducive to physical activity because of lack of safety and lack of available resources and opportunities.

There has been some controversy over whether the body mass index (BMI) remains an effective diagnostic tool of assessing for obesity, or if waist circumference offers more clinically relevant information. Both BMI and waist circumference (Box 5-6) appear to have their value in assessing the patient for risk of obesity, central obesity, and cardiovascular disease. Waist circumference provides an indicator of abdominal fat. Excess fat around the waist and upper body (also described as an "apple" body shape) is associated with greater health risk than fat located more in the hip and thigh area (described as a "pear" body shape) (Health Canada, 2011). BMI is defined as a measure of an adult's weight in relation to his or her height, specifically the adult's weight in kilograms divided by the square of his or her height in metres.

Overweight and obesity are known risk factors for premature death, diabetes, heart disease, stroke, hypertension, dyslipidemia, gallbladder disease, diverticular disease, constipation, osteoarthritis, gout, osteoporosis, respiratory dysfunction, sleep apnea, and some cancers (esophagus, uterine breast, colorectal, kidney, and endometrial) (National Cancer Institute, 2012). In addition, obesity is associated with high cholesterol, menstrual irregularities, hirsutism (excess body and facial hair), stress

BOX 5-6 WAIST CIRCUMFERENCE

Measure waist with clothing removed from abdomen. Place a measuring tape around waist, just above the hip bones.

Waist circumference = ___________ centimetres.

Assess health risk.

High Risk

A WC measurement of 88 cm or more for women is associated with an increased risk of developing health problems such as type 2 diabetes, coronary heart disease, and high blood pressure. As the cut-off points are approximate, a WC just below this measurement should also be taken seriously. The risk of developing health problems increases as WC measurement increases above the cut-off points.

WC, waist circumference.
Source: Health Canada (2011). *Canadian guidelines for body weight classification in adults.* Ottawa: Author. Retrieved from http://www.hc-sc.gc.ca/fn-an/nutrition/weights-poids/guide-ld-adult/qa-qr-pub-eng.php#a4.

incontinence, depression, complications of pregnancy, increased surgical risk, and shortened lifespan. Obese pregnant women are at risk for spontaneous **abortion**, hypertension, difficulties with fetal monitoring, and gestational diabetes as well as for intrapartum complications such as **macrosomia** and shoulder dystocia, Caesarean birth, and thromboembolism (Davies, Maxwell, MacLeod, et al., 2010) (see Chapter 15).

Eating Disorders

Anorexia nervosa and bulimia are two forms of eating disorders, although there are additional forms, such as subclinical eating disorders. Some women, especially adolescents, do not have symptoms that lend themselves to a diagnosis of anorexia nervosa or bulimia. These women are diagnosed as having a subclinical eating disorder, which is usually associated with disorders of mood and anxiety and requires accurate diagnosis and prompt treatment (Touchette, Henegar, Godart, et al., 2011). Recent research suggests that eating disorders are often associated with difficulties in intimate relationships, and interpersonal psychotherapy has been considered as an approach to treatment of women with eating disorders (Murphy, Straebler, Basden, et al., 2012).

It is important to assess for and treat women with eating disorders early because they are at increased risk for serious physical problems as well as diminished quality of life (Vallance, Latner, & Gleaves, 2011). Eating disorders during pregnancy are also associated with increased risk to the pregnant woman and her fetus (Pasternak, Weintraub, Shoham-Vardi, et al., 2012).

Anorexia nervosa. Some women have a distorted view of their bodies and, no matter what their weight, perceive themselves to be much too heavy. As a result, they undertake strict and severe diets and rigorous extreme exercise. This chronic eating disorder is known as **anorexia nervosa**. Women can carry this condition to the point of starvation, with resulting endocrine and metabolic abnormalities. If it is not corrected, significant complications of arrhythmias, amenorrhea, cardiomyopathy, and congestive heart failure occur and in the extreme

BOX 5-7 SCREENING FOR EATING DISORDERS: SCOFF QUESTIONS

Each question scores 1 point. A score of 2 or more indicates that the person may have anorexia nervosa or bulimia.

1. Do you make yourself **S**ick (i.e., induce vomiting) because you feel too full?
2. Do you worry about loss of **C**ontrol over the amount you eat?
3. Have you recently lost more than 6 kg in a 3-month period?
4. Do you think you are too **Fat** even if others think you are too thin?
5. Does **F**ood dominate your life?

Source: Morgan, J., Reid, F., & Lacey, J. (1999). The SCOFF questionnaire: Assessment of a new screening tool for eating disorders, *British Medical Journal, 319*(7223), 1467–1468.

can lead to death. The condition commonly begins during adolescence in young women who have some degree of personality disorder. They gradually lose weight over several months, have amenorrhea (see Chapter 7), and are abnormally concerned with body image. A coexisting depression usually accompanies anorexia.

There are no specific tests to diagnose anorexia nervosa. A medical history, physical examination, and screening tests help identify women at risk for eating disorders. Several tools are available to use in primary care settings. The SCOFF questionnaire, developed by Morgan, Reid, and Lacey (1999), is easy to administer and can help the nurse decide whether an eating disorder is likely and whether the woman needs further assessment and possibly psychiatric and medical intervention. More recently, Hautala, Junnila, Alin, et al. (2009) provided further evidence for the validity and usefulness of the SCOFF. See Box 5-7 for a description of the SCOFF.

Bulimia nervosa. **Bulimia** refers to secret, uncontrolled binge eating alternating with methods to prevent weight gain: self-induced vomiting, laxatives or diuretics, strict diets, fasting, and rigorous exercise. During a binge episode, large numbers of calories are consumed, usually consisting of sweets and "junk foods." Binges occur at least twice per week. Bulimia usually begins in early adulthood (ages 18 to 25) and is found primarily in females. Complications can include dehydration and electrolyte imbalance, gastrointestinal abnormalities, and cardiac arrhythmias. Bulimia is somewhat similar to anorexia in that it is an eating disorder and usually involves some degree of depression. Unlike those with anorexia, individuals with bulimia may feel shame or disgust about their disorder and tend to seek help earlier. The SCOFF screening assessment also can be used to assess patients with bulimia (see Box 5-7).

Lack of Exercise

Exercise contributes to good health by lowering risks for a variety of conditions that are influenced by obesity and a sedentary lifestyle. It is effective in the prevention of cardiovascular disease and in the management of chronic conditions such as hypertension, arthritis, diabetes, respiratory disorders, and osteoporosis (Fig. 5-1). Exercise also contributes to stress reduction and weight maintenance. Women report that engaging in regular exercise improves their body image and self-esteem and acts as a mood enhancer. Aerobic exercise produces cardiovascular involvement because increasing amounts of oxygen are delivered to working muscles. Anaerobic exercise such as weight training improves individual muscle mass without stress on the cardiovascular system. Because women are concerned about both cardiovascular and bone health, weight-bearing aerobic exercises such as walking, running, racket sports, and dancing are preferred. However, excessive or strenuous exercise can lead to **hormone** imbalances, resulting in amenorrhea and its consequences. Physical injury is also a potential risk.

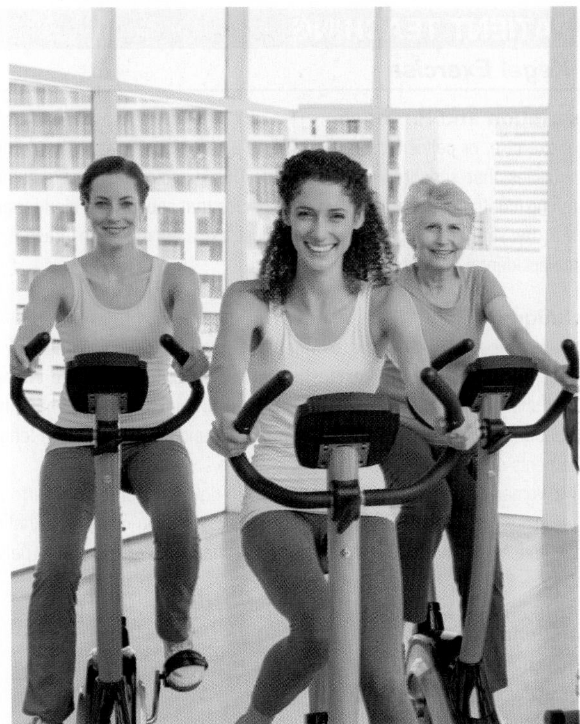

FIGURE 5-1 Exercise should be part of one's regular health routine. A cycle class is fun and provides moderate to vigorous exercise. (From wavebreakmedia/Shutterstock.com.)

One particular exercise that is important for women is *Kegel exercise*, or pelvic muscle exercise. These exercises are important for women to prevent urinary incontinence that can occur after childbirth and a variety of other conditions that may occur with age (Robert, Ross, et al., 2006). This exercise is used to strengthen the muscles that support the pelvic floor and should be practised regularly. Instructions for this exercise are in presented in the Patient Teaching box.

Physical activity and exercise counselling for persons of all ages should be available at schools, work sites, and primary care settings. Specific recommendations include 30 to 60 minutes of moderate activity most days of the week for adults and 60 to 90 minutes most days of the week for children and adolescents (Heart and Stroke Foundation, 2011). Few Canadians exercise this often, and physical inactivity increases with age, especially during adolescence and early adulthood. Even small increases in activity can be beneficial. During pregnancy, an ongoing

PATIENT TEACHING

Kegel Exercise

Description and Rationale

Kegel exercise, or pelvic muscle exercise, is a technique used to strengthen the muscles that support the pelvic floor. This exercise involves regularly tightening (contracting) and relaxing the muscles that support the bladder and urethra. By strengthening these pelvic muscles, a woman can prevent or reduce accidental urine loss.

Technique

The woman needs to learn how to target the muscles for training and how to contract them correctly. One suggestion for teaching is to have the woman pretend she is trying to stop the flow of urine in midstream or to have her think about how her vagina is able to contract around and move up the length of the penis during intercourse.

The woman should avoid straining or bearing-down motions while performing the exercise. She should be taught to avoid straining down by exhaling gently and keeping her mouth open each time she contracts her pelvic muscles.

Specific Instructions

- Each contraction should be as intense as possible without contracting the abdomen, thighs, or buttocks.
- Contractions should be held for at least 10 seconds. The woman may have to start with as little as 2 seconds per contraction until her muscles get stronger.
- She should rest for 10 seconds or more between contractions so that the muscles have time to recover and each contraction can be as strong as she can make it.
- She should feel the pulling up and over the three muscle layers so that the contraction reaches the highest level of her pelvis.
- Positive results can be achieved by performing the exercise for 15 minutes twice a day.
- The best position for learning how to do Kegel exercises is to lie supine with the knees bent. Another position to use is on the hands and knees. Once the woman learns the proper technique, she can perform the exercises in other positions such as standing or sitting.

Sources: Sampselle, C. M. (2000). Behavioural interventions for urinary incontinence in women: Evidence for practice. *Journal of Midwifery & Women's Health, 45*(2), 94–103; Sampselle, C. M., Burns, P. M., Dougherty, M. C., et al. (1997). Continence for women: Evidence-based practice. *Journal of Obstetric & Gynecologic Neonatal Nursing, 26*[4], 375–385; Robert, M., Ross, S., et al. (2006). SOGC Clinical practice guideline: Conservative management of urinary incontinence. *Journal of Obstetrics & Gynecology of Canada, 28*(12), 1113–1118.

BOX 5-8 STRESS SYMPTOMS

Physical

- Perspiration/sweaty hands
- Increased heart rate
- Trembling
- Nervous tics
- Dryness of throat and mouth
- Tiring easily
- Urinating frequently
- Sleeping problems
- Diarrhea, indigestion, vomiting
- Butterflies in stomach
- Headaches
- Premenstrual tension
- Pain in neck and lower back
- Loss of appetite or overeating
- Susceptibility to illness

Behavioural

- Stuttering and other speech difficulties
- Crying for no apparent reason
- Acting impulsively
- Startling easily
- Laughing in a high-pitched and nervous tone of voice
- Grinding teeth
- Increasing smoking
- Increasing use of drugs and alcohol
- Being accident prone

Psychological

- Feeling anxious
- Feeling scared
- Feeling irritable
- Feeling moody
- Having low self-esteem
- Being afraid of failure
- Being unable to concentrate
- Embarrassing easily
- Worrying about the future
- Being preoccupied with thoughts or tasks
- Forgetful

 It's your health: Mental health–coping with stress. Health Canada, 2007; Updated, January 2008. Adapted and reproduced with permission from the Minister of Health, 2016.

exercise regimen can be continued but should be decreased in intensity and duration.

Stress

Women are facing increasing levels of stress and, as a result, are prone to a variety of stress-induced illnesses. Stress often occurs because of conflict among multiple roles—for example, job and financial responsibilities can conflict with parenting and duties at home. To add to this burden, women are socialized to be caregivers, which is emotionally draining, creating additional stress. They also may find themselves in positions of minimal power that do not allow them to have control over their everyday environments. Some stress is normal and contributes to positive outcomes. Many women thrive in busy surroundings. However, excessive or high levels of ongoing stress trigger physical reactions such as rapid heart rate, elevated blood pressure, slowed digestion, release of additional neurotransmitters and hormones, muscle tenseness, and a weakened immune system. Consequently, constant stress can contribute to clinical illnesses such as exacerbations of arthritis or asthma, frequent colds or infections, gastrointestinal upsets, cardiovascular problems, and infertility. Box 5-8 lists symptoms that may be related to chronic or extreme stress. Psychological symptoms such as anxiety, irritability, eating disorders, depression, insomnia, and substance use have also been associated with stress.

Because it is neither possible nor desirable to avoid all stress, women must learn how to manage it. The nurse should assess each woman for signs of stress, using therapeutic communication skills to determine risk factors and the woman's ability to function. Women are twice as likely as men to suffer from depression, anxiety, or panic attacks. Nurses must be alert to the symptoms of serious mental disorders such as depression and anxiety and make referrals to counselling or other mental health practitioners when necessary. Women experiencing major life changes such as separation and divorce, bereavement, serious illness, and unemployment need special attention. A psychosocial assessment for stress and depression is recommended for pregnant women in each trimester (Kingston, Heaman, Fell, et al., 2012; PHAC, 2016). Thorough assessment allows for appropriate referrals and care planning.

Many centres offer support groups to help women prevent or manage stress. Social support and good coping skills can improve a woman's self-esteem and give her a sense of mastery. Anticipatory guidance for developmental or expected situational crises can help her plan strategies for dealing with potentially stressful events. Role-playing, relaxation techniques, biofeedback, meditation, desensitization, healing touch, imagery, assertiveness training, yoga, diet, exercise, and weight control are all techniques that nurses can include in their repertoire of helping skills.

Depression, Anxiety, and Other Mental Health Conditions

Women experience depression or anxiety frequently. In addition, depression is sometimes described as a co-traveller because it exists comorbidly with other physical conditions. Depression or anxiety create difficulties for quality of life and, at the extreme, create a risk for suicide. Recent research suggests that women with comorbid anxiety and depression are at greater risk for developing cardiac disease (Berecki-Gisolf, McKenzie, Dobson, et al., 2013). In addition to depression and anxiety, women experience other mental health disorders, such as bipolar disease.

Sleep Disorders

Many women suffer from sleep disorders, including difficulty initiating sleep or staying asleep and experiencing nonrestorative sleep (Zender & Olshansky, 2009). Restless leg syndrome may be a cause of sleep disorders or a comorbid condition. Sleep disorders are correlated with physical and mental health problems, including depression, pain, and fibromyalgia. Mong, Baker, Mahoney, et al. (2011) compiled a review of studies conducted on gender differences related to sleep which suggested that, while further research is needed, women experience insomnia significantly more than men. It is thus important that nurses talk with patients about their sleep patterns and discuss ways to improve sleep, such as avoiding alcohol before going to sleep and sleeping in a regular pattern.

Environmental and Workplace Hazards

A safe environment is a key determinant of health. Environmental hazards in the home, the workplace, and the community can contribute to poor health at all ages. Categories and examples of health-damaging hazards include the following: (1) pathogenic agents (viruses, bacteria, fungi, parasites); (2) natural and synthetic chemicals (natural toxins from animals, insects, and plants; consumer and industrial products such as pesticides and hydrocarbon gases; medical and diagnostic devices; tobacco; fuels; and drug and alcohol use); (3) radiation (radon, heat waves, sound waves); (4) food substances (added components that are not necessary for nutrition); and (5) physical objects (moving vehicles, machinery, weapons, water, and building materials). Canadians rate waste management, water quality, and air quality as the most important environmental issues facing their communities (Community Foundations of Canada, 2010).

Environmental hazards can affect fertility, fetal development, live birth, and the child's future mental and physical development. Children are at special risk for poisoning from lead found in paint and soil. The Canadian government has called for strict guidelines regarding the amount of lead in children's toys, a regulation that is nonexistent in the rest of the world. Everyone is at risk from air pollutants such as tobacco smoke, carbon monoxide, smog, suspended particles (dust, ash, and asbestos), and cleaning solvents; noise pollution; pesticides; chemical additives; and poor preparation of food. Workers also face safety and health risks caused by ergonomically poor work stations and stress. It is important that risk assessments continue to be in effect to identify and understand environmental problems in public health. Health Canada (2011) has published a helpful resource that summarizes the various risks posed in the environment to pregnant women and their fetuses. Motherisk is another excellent resource (see Additional Resources).

Safe drinking water is a basic determinant of health. A significant number of communities are placed under a boil water advisory each year in Canada. While some advisories are preventative of a possible risk, others are based on actual risk. Working with communities to advocate for safe drinking water, lobby for proper sanitation and consistently high quality controls, and educate the public about how to maintain health in the face of a boil water advisory is a key role of the community nurse.

Sexual Practices

Potential risks related to sexual activity include undesired pregnancy and STIs. The risks are particularly high for adolescents and young adults. Adolescents report many reasons for wanting to be sexually active: peer pressure, desire to love and be loved, experimentation, to enhance self-esteem, and to have fun. However, many teens do not have the decision-making or values-clarification skills needed to take this important step. They may also lack knowledge about contraception and STIs. Many do not believe that becoming pregnant or getting an STI will happen to them. An important role for the nurse is to ensure that youth have the correct information. SexualityandU is an excellent resource for more information for youth and is listed in the Additional Resources.

Although some STIs can be cured with antibiotics, many cause significant problems. Possible sequelae include **infertility**,

BOX 5-9 STI AND HIV PREVENTION

- Prevention of STIs and HIV is possible only if there is no oral, genital, or rectal exchange of body fluids or if a person is in a long-term, mutually monogamous relationship with an uninfected partner.
- Correct use of latex condoms, although greatly reducing risk, is not exclusively protective.
- Sexual partners should be selected with great care.
- Partners should be asked about history of STIs.
- Pre-exposure vaccination is one of the most effective methods for preventing transmission of some STIs (hepatitis A and hepatitis B, human papillomavirus).
- A new condom should be used for each act of sexual intercourse.
- Abstinence from sexual intercourse is encouraged for persons who are being treated for an STI or whose partners are being treated.
- Abstinence is also recommended if under the influence of drugs or alcohol.

STI, sexually transmitted infection; *HIV*, human immunodeficiency virus.
Adapted from SexualityandU: http://www.sexualityandu.ca

ectopic pregnancy, neonatal morbidity and mortality, genital cancers, AIDS, and even death. The incidence of some STIs is increasing rapidly and reaching epidemic proportions. Choice of contraception has an impact on the risk of contracting an STI. No method of contraception offers complete protection. (See Chapter 7 for a detailed discussion of STIs, and see Chapter 8 for a discussion of contraception.)

Prevention of STIs is predicated on the reduction of high-risk behaviours, through educating toward behavioural change. Behaviours that predispose to contracting an STI include having multiple sexual partners and carrying out unsafe sexual practices. Specific self-management measures to prevent STIs are listed in Box 5-9. The overuse of alcohol and drugs is also a high-risk behaviour, as it results in impaired judgement and thoughtless acts. Behavioural changes must come from within; therefore, the nurse must provide sufficient information for the individual or group to "buy into" the need for change. Education is a powerful tool in health promotion and prevention of STIs and pregnancy. However, it works best when delivered in a way that takes into account the language, culture, and lifestyle of the intended listener.

Medical Conditions

Most women of reproductive age are relatively healthy. Heart disease; lung, breast, colon, and other nongynecological cancers; chronic lung disease; and diabetes are all concerns for adult women because they are among the leading causes of death in women. Certain medical conditions present during pregnancy can have deleterious effects on both the woman and the fetus. Of particular concern are risks from all forms of diabetes, urinary tract disorders, thyroid disease, hypertensive disorders of pregnancy, cardiac disease, and seizure disorders. Effects on the fetus vary and include intrauterine growth restriction, macrosomia, anemia, prematurity, immaturity, and stillbirth. Effects on the woman also can be severe. These conditions are discussed in later chapters (see Chapter 15).

Gynecological Conditions

Women are at risk throughout their reproductive years for pelvic inflammatory disease, endometriosis, STIs and other vaginal infections, uterine fibroids, uterine deformities such as bicornuate uterus, ovarian cysts, interstitial cystitis, and urinary incontinence related to pelvic relaxation. These gynecological conditions may contribute negatively to pregnancy by causing infertility, miscarriage, preterm labour (see Chapter 7), and fetal and neonatal problems. Gynecological cancers also affect women's health, although risk factors depend on the type of cancer. The impact of developing a gynecological problem or cancer on women and their families is shaped by a number of factors, including the specific type of problem or cancer, the implications of the diagnosis for the woman and her family, and the timing of the occurrence in the woman's and family's lives.

Female Genital Mutilation

Female genital mutilation (FGM) is practised in more than 45 countries, most of which are in Africa. As individuals from these countries arrive in Canada, nurses will see patients who have had such procedures performed (see Cultural Awareness box).

Violence Against Women

Intimate partner violence (IPV), violence perpetrated by a spouse, partner, or someone with whom the person has had an ongoing intimate relationship, is the most common form of violence experienced by women worldwide, with a reported incidence of 1 out of every 6 women having been a victim of domestic violence. In Canada, IPV is a significant social problem that affects many women and men each year and costs millions of dollars in annual medical costs. It is estimated that approximately 1 in 3 Canadian women have experienced violence in their lives (Canadian Women's Foundation, 2011). Canadian Indigenous people are three times as likely to be victims of violence (Department of Justice Canada, 2015). Several factors present in Indigenous communities have been linked to this risk factor, including higher rates of unemployment, cohabitation, history of residential schools, alcohol use, and greater family size (Brownridge, 2008).

Although IPV is the preferred term, wife-battering, spouse abuse, and domestic or family violence are all terms that may be applied to a pattern of assaultive and coercive behaviours inflicted by a partner in a marriage or other significant, intimate relationship. It is also important to note that not all violence against women is caused by an intimate partner; non-IPV also occurs. Montero, Escriba, Ruiz-Perez, et al. (2011) studied both IPV and non-IPV, noting that violence in general has negative effects on women's health. They recommend that routine assessment of violence against women be included in primary care histories. Common elements of IPV are physical abuse; psychological or emotional abuse; sexual assault; isolation; and controlling all aspects of the victim's life, including money, shelter, time, and food.

CULTURAL AWARENESS

Female Genital Mutilation (FGM)

Defined by the World Health Organization (WHO), female genital mutilation (FGM) is "all procedures that involve partial or total removal of the external female genitalia, or other injury to the female genital organs for non-medical reasons" (WHO, 2012). This includes female circumcision and is an attempt to control women through controlling their sexuality. FGM is supposed to remove sexual desire so that the girl will not become sexually active until married (McGargill, 2009).

Female circumcision occurs in women of many different ethnic, cultural, and religious backgrounds. Although circumcision is usually performed during childhood, some communities circumcise infants or older females. The procedure involves the removal of a portion of the clitoris but may extend to the removal of the entire clitoris and labia minora. In addition, the labia majora, which are often stitched together over the urethral and vaginal openings, may be affected.

The extent of the circumcision site affects the seriousness of complications. Common complications include bleeding, pain, local scarring, keloid or cyst formation, and infection. Impaired drainage of urine and menstrual blood may lead to chronic pelvic infections, pelvic and back pain, and chronic urinary tract infections. On occasion the girl will die from complications. Some women may require surgery before vaginal examination, intercourse, or childbirth if the vaginal opening is obstructed. Caesarean birth may be necessary. The extent of the FGM site affects the seriousness of complications.

The practice of FGM is recognized internationally as a violation of human rights, and many countries have policies and legislation to ban it. The WHO is working to eliminate FGM, and most recently Nigeria banned it with the passing of the Violence Against Persons (Prohibition) Act (2015) (see Additional Resources). Canada and the U.S. federal government have criminalized the practice. "The practice also violates the rights to health, security and physical integrity of the person, the right to be free from torture and cruel, inhuman or degrading treatment, and the right to life when the procedure results in death" (WHO, 2012).

Nurses in Canada are providing care to a growing number of women who have emigrated from the Middle East, Asia, and Africa, where female circumcision is more common. Nurses must be sensitive to the unique needs of these patients, especially if these women have concerns about maintaining or restoring the intactness of the circumcision after childbirth.

Data from McGargill, P. (2009). Female genital mutilation. *On the Edge 15*(2 Summer). Retrieved from www.cinahl,com/cgi-bin/refsvc?jid=29638accno-2010331425; World Health Organization. (2012). *Female genital mutilation.* Retrieved from http:// www.who.int/mediacentre/factsheet/fs241/en/print.html

Battering is neither random nor constant; rather, it occurs in repeated cycles. Health care providers often refer to the "cycle of violence" (Fig. 5-2). A three-phase cycle includes a period of increasing tension leading to the battery. The battery consists of slaps, punches to the face and head, kicking, stomping, punching, choking, pushing, breaking of bones, burns from irons, and mutilations from knives and guns (see Box 5-10 for signs of IPV). The honeymoon phase is characterized by a period of calm and remorse in which the partner displays kind, loving behaviour and pleas for forgiveness. This honeymoon phase lasts until stress or other factors cause conflict and tension to mount again toward another episode of battering. Over time, the tension and battering phases last longer and the calm phase becomes shorter until there is no honeymoon phase (see Critical Thinking Case Study). Dating violence is also a growing concern among adolescents. A study among youth in a Canadian Atlantic province found that of 627 youth, ages 12 to 18, 62% of girls had experienced psychological violence, with many also experiencing physical abuse and sexual coercion (Sears & Byers, 2010). Knowledge of the potential for violence among youth in dating relationships is an important consideration for nurses when completing assessments with youth.

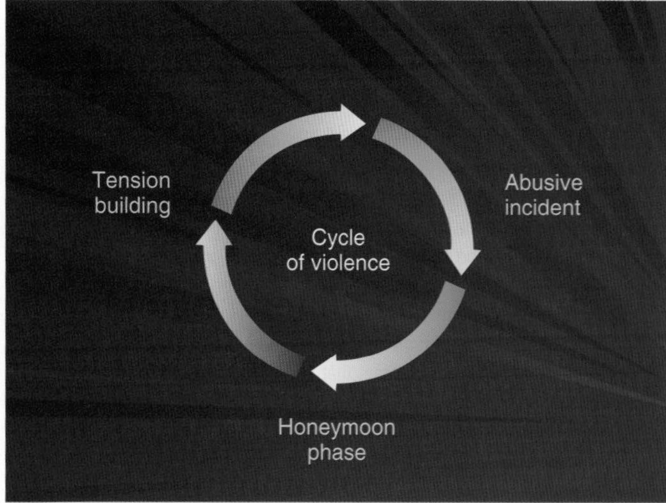

FIGURE 5-2 Cycle of violence.

BOX 5-10 SIGNS OF INTIMATE PARTNER VIOLENCE

- Overuse of health services
- Vague, nonspecific concerns
- Missed appointments
- Unexplainable injuries
- Untreated serious injuries
- Injuries not matching the description
- Intimate partner never leaving the patient's side
- Intimate partner insisting on telling the story of the injury

Source: Krieger, C. L. (2008). Intimate partner violence: A review for nurses. *Nursing & Women's Health, 12*(3), 224–234.

Cultural Considerations

Women of all races and of all ethnic, educational, religious, and socioeconomic backgrounds are affected by IPV. While all forms of abuse across the lifespan may be underreported, immigrant women may report IPV less than nonimmigrant women because of lack of social support, poor understanding of rights and the health care system, fear of deportation, and cultural beliefs from their home country. It is important that immigrant women to Canada know that they will not be deported if they leave their partner because of violence, even if the partner is their sponsor (Royal Canadian Mounted Police, 2012). Reporting rates may not reflect the magnitude of the problem, as many women do not disclose violence because of fear, embarrassment, or not having been asked by those from whom

CRITICAL THINKING CASE STUDY

Intimate Partner Violence

Annette is a 35-year-old married woman who comes to the clinic for complaints of abdominal pain and headaches. The nurse notices that Annette has bruises on her left cheek, forearms, and upper back. When the nurse asks about the cause of the bruises, Annette says that "she ran into a door." It is obvious to the nurse that the injuries could not have been caused by running into a door. What is the nurse's responsibility in this instance?

1. Evidence—Is there sufficient evidence to draw conclusions about the rights of Annette to privacy?
2. Assumptions—What assumptions can be made about the following risks for Annette of disclosing the fact that her injuries were caused by her husband?
   a. Annette's right to privacy
   b. Safety for Annette if she discloses domestic violence
   c. The nurse's responsibility to discuss domestic violence and offer a safety plan
   d. Determinants of health that may be a factor in this situation
3. What implications and priorities for nursing care can be drawn at this time?
4. Does the evidence objectively support your conclusion?

they seek help. Poor and uneducated women tend to be disproportionately represented because they are seen in emergency departments, they are financially more dependent, they have fewer resources and support systems, and they may have fewer problem-solving skills. Table 5-2 lists some myths and facts about abuse.

All women entering the health care system should be assessed for potential abuse. At least the following questions should be asked (Pellizzari, Mason, Grant, et al., 2005):

- "Have you been hit, kicked, punched, or otherwise hurt by someone within the past year?"
- "Do you feel safe in your current relationship?"
- "Have you ever been forced to have sex or engage in sexual activities against your will?"

These questions give a woman permission to disclose sensitive information.

A therapeutic relationship and skillful interviewing can help women disclose and describe their abuse (Box 5-11). Skillful use of language is important when talking with women. For example, the term *victim* connotes powerlessness and hopelessness; a more empowering term is *survivor*. Women who have

TABLE 5-2 MYTHS AND FACTS ABOUT INTIMATE PARTNER VIOLENCE

MYTHS	FACTS
Violence occurs in a small percentage of the population.	One third of all Canadian women have experienced violence in their life.
Being pregnant protects the woman from abuse.	From 4 to 8% of all women who are battered are battered during pregnancy. Battering frequently begins or escalates in frequency and intensity during pregnancy. Pregnancy may be the result of forced sex or of the man's control of contraception.
Violence occurs only in "problem" or lower-class families.	Intimate partner violence can occur in any family. Although lower-income families have a higher reported incidence of battering, it also occurs in middle- and upper-income families. Incidence is not accurately known because of the tendency of middle- and upper-income families to hide their battering.
Women like to be beaten and deliberately provoke the attack. They are masochistic.	Women are terrified of their assailants and go to great lengths to avoid a confrontation. In some cases, the woman may provoke her partner to release tension that, if left unchecked, might lead to a more severe beating and possible death.
Only men or women with psychological problems abuse women.	Many offenders are successful professionals. Research indicates that only a small number of abusers have psychological problems.
Only people who come from abusive families end up in abusive relationships.	Most women report that their partners were the first person to beat them.
Alcohol and drug use cause abuse.	Although alcohol may be involved in abusive incidents, it is not the cause. Many offenders use alcohol as an excuse for the violence and shift the blame to the alcohol.
Women would leave the relationship if the abuse were really that bad.	Women who stay in the relationship do so out of fear and financial dependence. Shelters have long waiting lists.
Abusers and survivors of violence cannot change.	Counselling may effectively help both the offenders and victims of violence.
Some women stay in abusive relationships because it is part of their culture.	Many women stay because of social isolation, language barriers, and poverty or for a sense of family responsibility. Many immigrant women may fear deportation.
Abuse does not happen in same-sex relationships.	Power dynamics can occur in any intimate relationship. Violence against a partner is a crime regardless of the gender.

Sources: British Columbia Ministry of Public Safety and Solicitor General. (2007). *Violence against women in relationships: Victim service worker handbook*. Retrieved from http://www.pssg.gov.bc.ca/victimservices/shareddocs/victim-service-worker-vawir.pdf; Canadian Women's Foundation. (n.d.). *The facts about violence against women*. Retrieved from http://www.canadianwomen.org/facts-about-violence; Canadian Women's Health Network. (2012). *Domestic violence in the LGBT community*. Retrieved from http://www.cwhn.ca/node/39623; Society of Obstetricians and Gynecologists of Canada. (2005). SOGC clinical practice guideline: Intimate partner violence consensus statement. *Journal of Obstetrics and Gynaecology Canada, 27*(4), 365–388.

BOX 5-11 WHAT NOT TO SAY TO A WOMAN WHO HAS BEEN SUBJECTED TO VIOLENCE AND WHAT YOU CAN SAY AND DO

What Not to Say

1. Do not ask "why." This question "re-victimizes" and blames the victim.
2. Do not talk negatively about the abuser to the victim. She may become defensive and stop talking.
3. Do not talk directly to the abuser about your suspicions of abuse. The abuser will assume the victim told you, and the victim risks retaliation.

What to Say

1. "I'm afraid for your safety (and the safety of your children)."
2. "I believe you."
3. "It is progressive and will only get worse."
4. "You deserve better than this. You deserve to be treated with respect."
5. "You are not alone."
6. "It is a crime."
7. "I'm here for you."

What to Do

1. Empower the woman.
2. Sit down with her.
3. Assure her of total privacy and confidentiality (but only if you can).
4. Use your best listening and relational practice skills.
5. Call 911 or call local police and report any incident of imminent danger.
6. Give the woman the telephone number and/or email address of the nearest women's shelter.
7. For further assistance, refer to a victim services division in the city or province if available.

BOX 5-12 SAFETY STRATEGIES

Survivors of intimate partner violence should try to maintain the following safety strategies:

- Always be aware of surroundings.
- Minimize time in kitchens, bathrooms, and closets when the abuser is near.
- Shop and bank at different places.
- Drive to work multiple ways.
- Get a protection order.
- Never lunch alone.
- Cancel joint credit cards and old bank accounts with the abuser.
- Provide a picture of the abuser to security at the workplace.
- Be escorted by workplace security to the car or transportation.
- When in danger, go to a place of safety and call 911 or local emergency response or police.
- Change locks on the house if the abuser has moved out.
- Get an unlisted telephone number.
- Block caller ID.

Source: Krieger, C. L. (2008). Intimate partner violence: A review for nurses. *Nursing & Women's Health, 12*[3], 224–234.

identified their abuse may appear passive, hostile, anxious, depressed, or hysterical because they may think they are at the mercy of their partner's temper or that the partner is "out of control." In addition, they may be embarrassed, afraid, angry, sad, and shocked. Many women are concerned about health care providers discovering their IPV (Catallo, Jack, Ciliska, et al., 2012). Demonstrating concern for women who are victims of violence, showing respect, exercising confidentiality, and conveying a nonjudegmental attitude are important attributes of health care providers to facilitate disclosure of violence (Catallo et al., 2012).

The most significant part of the intervention is to ensure that the woman has knowledge of the resources available to her and a plan of action should she stay with the violent partner. First, the nurse should provide services and telephone numbers of a hotline and of a women's shelter or other safe haven. The woman can be offered a telephone to call the shelter if this is an option she chooses. If she chooses to go back to the abuser, a safety plan includes necessities for a quick escape: a bag packed with personal items for an overnight stay (can be hidden or left with a neighbour), money or a chequebook, an extra set of car keys, and any legal documents for identification. Legal options such as those for restraining orders or arrest of the perpetrator also are important aspects of the safety plan (Box 5-12). A restraining order can be obtained 24 hours a day from the police department. Shelters also can be helpful with assistance in obtaining orders of protection. If the woman chooses not to act in the middle of a violent episode, she may use the hotline or shelter for some counselling when the threat of harm is no longer present. Of critical importance to addressing IPV on a wider scale is a coordinated approach to maintain the safety of women, good access to health care, and nonjudgemental treatment from health professionals (Cory & Dechief, 2007). Community involvement in developing a response to IPV is important to sustainable, safe, resilient communities (British Columbia Victim Services and Crime Prevention Division, 2010). Many victim services divisions have resources to help individuals, families, and communities, and nurses are in a prime position to engage in such community development work.

Violence During Pregnancy

In 2009, approximately 63,300 women reported experiencing IPV in the previous 5 years while they were pregnant (Sinha, 2013). Most women abused before pregnancy will be abused during pregnancy, and the incidence may escalate. Abuse also may happen for the first time during pregnancy. Pregnant adolescents are abused at higher rates than are adult women; thus they should be considered at high risk. Violence during pregnancy in teenagers constitutes a particularly difficult situation. Adolescents may be more trapped in the abusive relationship than adult women because of their inexperience. They may ignore the violence because the jealous and controlling behaviour is interpreted as love and devotion. Because pregnancy in young adolescent girls is frequently the result of sexual abuse, feelings about the pregnancy should be assessed.

During pregnancy the nurse should assess for abuse at each prenatal visit and on admission to labour. Violent episodes initiate or increase in pregnancy for a variety of reasons: (1) the biopsychosocial stresses of pregnancy may strain the relationship beyond the couple's ability to cope, and frustration is followed by violence; (2) the man may be jealous of the fetus, resenting the intrusion into the couple's relationship and the woman's displacement of attention; (3) the man may be angry at the unborn child or the woman; and (4) the beating may be the man's conscious or subconscious attempt to end the pregnancy. After birth, the mother may be so physically and emotionally drained that she may have difficulty bonding with her infant. She may be at risk for becoming an abusive mother whether or not she remains in the abusive relationship.

A pregnant woman is often accompanied by her husband to the prenatal appointment, especially if the woman does not speak English and the husband does. Unless an interpreter is available, it is difficult to interview the woman alone; in addition, asking questions about abuse through an interpreter is more difficult unless the interpreter is a woman and can communicate the nurse's sensitivity and concern accurately.

Prevention

Nurses can make a difference in stopping the violence and preventing further injury. Educating women that abuse is a violation of their rights and facilitating their access to protective and legal services is an important first step. Other helpful measures for nurses to take to discourage the risk of abusive relationships are promoting assertiveness and self-defence courses; suggesting support and self-help groups that encourage positive self-regard, confidence, and empowerment; and recommending educational and skills-development classes that will enhance independence and the ability to take care of oneself. Classes for English-language learners may be particularly helpful to immigrant women. Nurses can offer information on local classes.

Health Promotion and Illness Prevention

Over the last several decades women have made tremendous strides in education, careers, policy making, and overall participation in today's complex society. There have been costs for these advances, however; although women are living longer, they may not be living better. As a result, the health care system needs to include greater attention to the health consequences for women. Women also must be active participants in their own health promotion and illness prevention (see Community Focus box).

Nurses have a major opportunity and responsibility to help women understand risk factors and motivate them to adopt healthy lifestyles that prevent disease. Lifestyle factors that affect health—and over which the woman has some control—include diet; tobacco, alcohol, and substance use; exercise; sunlight exposure; stress management; and sexual practices. Other influences such as genetic and environmental factors may be beyond the woman's control, although some opportunities for prevention exist (e.g., through environmental legislative activism or genetic counselling services).

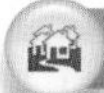

COMMUNITY FOCUS

Anticipatory Guidance for Health Promotion

Janie, a 30-year-old Cree woman who lives on reserve, comes to the clinic after attending a health fair in which she learned that her blood sugar is above normal, she is overweight, and her blood pressure is elevated. She informs the nurse that she doesn't want to end up like her grandmother, who had to have her toes amputated as a result of diabetes. Prepare a plan that uses community resources to meet Janie's needs to reduce her blood sugar and blood pressure and lose weight.

- Ascertain her opinion about her health status.
- Explore the determinants of health as they relate to Janie's health.
- Identify any need for counselling on nutrition, exercise, and stress management.
- Are physicians or nurse practitioners available in the community?
- What health education programs are available in the community?
- Working with Janie, develop an exercise program for her.
- What other community resources are available to her?

Knowledge alone is not enough to bring about healthy behaviours. The woman must be convinced that she has some control over her life and that healthy life habits, including periodic health examinations, are a sound investment. She must believe in the efficacy of prevention, early detection, and therapy and in her ability to perform self-management practices. Many people believe that they have little control over their health, or they become so immobilized by fear and anxiety in the face of life-threatening illnesses such as cancer that they delay seeking treatment. The nurse must explore the reality of each woman's perceptions about health behaviours and individualize teaching if it is to be effective.

Health Screening for Women Across the Lifespan

Periodic health screening includes history, physical examination, education, counselling, and selected diagnostic and laboratory tests. This regimen provides the basis for overall health promotion, prevention of illness, early diagnosis of problems, and referral for appropriate management. Such screening should be customized according to a woman's age and risk factors. In most instances it is completed in health care offices, clinics, or hospitals; however, portions of the screening are now being carried out at events such as community health fairs. An overview of health screening recommendations for women over 18 years of age is provided in Table 5-3. Consistent with information provided earlier in this chapter, it is important for the nurse to continually educate and counsel on diet, exercise, smoking cessation, alcohol moderation, help for substance use, and stress management.

Health Risk Prevention

Often simple safety factors are forgotten or perceived not to be important. Nonetheless, injuries continue to have a major impact on the health status of all age groups. Awareness of hazards and implementation of safety guidelines will reduce

TABLE 5-3 HEALTH SCREENING RECOMMENDATIONS FOR WOMEN AGE 18 YEARS AND OLDER

INTERVENTION	RECOMMENDATION
Physical Examination	
Blood pressure	All primary care visits, but at least every 2 years
Height and weight and BMI‡	At appropriate primary care visits, but at least every 2 years
Pelvic examination	Recommended to be done with Pap test unless symptomatic
Skin examination*	Yearly examinations or more frequently if risk factors; monthly self-examinations recommended of moles, birthmarks, healing skin
Oral cavity examination	Annually if history of mouth lesion or exposure to tobacco or excessive alcohol at least annually
Breast Examination	
Clinical examination‡	Not recommended in women who have no risk factors Annually after age 18 if high risk with history of premenopausal breast cancer in first-degree relative
Laboratory and Diagnostic Tests	
Blood cholesterol (fasting lipoprotein analysis)†	Screening at age 50 or postmenopausal Repeat yearly if have abnormal levels or risk factors for coronary artery disease; if low risk repeat every 3–5 years
Papanicolaou (Pap) test‡	<25 years of age: screening is not routinely recommended Every 3 years from ages 25 to 69 Over age of 70: may stop screening if have had 3 negative screens
Mammography‡	Ages 40 to 49: speak with health care provider about risk. Not routinely recommended Ages 50 to 69: every 2–3 years Ages 70 to 74: every 2–3 years Recommendations are different for women at higher risk for breast cancer
Colon cancer screening	Fecal occult blood test (FOBT) or fecal immunochemical test (FIT) every 2 years after age 50; more often if family history of colon cancer or polyps; screening colonoscopy at age 50 with schedule for this depending on what results show
Bone mineral density testing§	Over age 65 for everyone; earlier if risk factors (family history of osteoporosis, early menopause)
Risk Groups	
Fasting blood sugar or Hgb A_{1C}‡	Screen every 3–5 years
Hearing screen	Annually with exposure to excessive noise or when hearing loss is suspected
Sexually transmitted infection screen (e.g., gonorrhea, syphilis, herpes)	As needed if sexually active with multiple partners and engaging in risky sexual behaviours
Tuberculin skin test	Annually with exposure to persons with tuberculosis or in risk categories for close contact with the disease
Vision¶	Age 19 to 40: at least every 10 years Age 41 to 55: at least every 5 years Age 56 to 65: at least every 3 years Over age 65: at least every 2 years If high risk (e.g., diabetes, thyroid, lupus) Over age 40: at least every 3 years Over age 50: at least every 2 years Over age 60: at least once a year
Immunizations**	
Diphtheria, tetanus, acellular pertussis, and inactivated polio virus vaccine (DTaP-IPV)	Booster every 10 years after primary series (given as infant). Tdap vaccine once
Measles, mumps, rubella	Given once if no evidence of immunity (initial series given as infant)
Human papillomavirus (HPV)	Primary series of injections for ages 9 to 26. The recommended schedule is 3 doses at 0, 2, and 6 months, with a minimum interval of 1 month between the first 2 doses. May be given to women >26 if ongoing risk of exposure

Continued

TABLE 5-3 HEALTH SCREENING RECOMMENDATIONS FOR WOMEN AGE 18 YEARS AND OLDER—cont'd

INTERVENTION	RECOMMENDATION
Hepatitis A	Primary series of two injections for all who are in risk categories
Hepatitis B***	Three doses: the second dose should be administered at least 1 month after the first dose, and the third at least 2 months after the second dose. Provinces and territories differ as to when the first dose is given.
Influenza	Annually
Pneumococcal	1 dose after age 65; earlier if risk factors
Varicella (chickenpox)	Susceptible adults up to and including 49 years of age: 2 doses; if previously received 1 dose should receive a second dose
	Known seronegative adults 50 years of age and older: 2 doses; routine testing is not advised
Herpes zoster (shingles)	One dose at age 60 (can be given between 50 and 59 years of age)

‡Canadian Taskforce on Preventative Care. (2013). *CTFPHC Guidelines.* Retrieved from http://canadiantaskforce.ca/ctfphc-guidelines/overview/
†Anderson, T. J., Grégoire, J., Hegele, R. A., et al. (2012). Update of the Canadian Cardiovascular Society guidelines for the diagnosis and treatment of dyslipidemia for the prevention of cardiovascular disease in the adult. *Canadian Journal of Cardiology, 29,* 151–167.
§Papaioannou, A., Morin, S., Cheung, A. M., et al. (2010). 2010 clinical practice guidelines for the diagnosis and management of osteoporosis in Canada: Summary. *Canadian Medical Association Journal, 82*(17), 1864–1873. doi:10.1503/cmaj.100771.
¶Canadian Ophthalmological Society. *When should you see an ophthalmologist?* Retrieved from http://www.cos-sco.ca/vision-health-information/when-should-you-see-an-ophthalmologist/
*Canadian Cancer Society. (2015). *Prevention and screening.* Retrieved from www.cancer.ca
HealthLinkBC. (2014). *Skin cancer screening.* Retrieved from http://www.healthlinkbc.ca/healthtopics/content.asp?hwid=skc1179
**Immunization schedules vary among provinces and territories. See local public health agency for specific schedules.
***Some provinces and territories start the first hepatitis B injection after the newborn is 24 hours old, some at 2 months, and some not until age 13. Check individual provincial and territorial immunization schedules.

BOX 5-13 SAFETY GUIDELINES TO REDUCE RISK

- Wear seat belts at all times in a moving vehicle.
- Wear safety helmets when riding a motorcycle or bicycle.
- Follow driving rules of the road.
- Have working smoke alarms in place throughout the home and workplace; test them monthly.
- Avoid secondhand smoke.
- Reduce noise pollution or safeguard against hearing loss.
- Protect skin from ultraviolet light via sunscreen and clothing.
- Handle and store firearms appropriately.
- Practise water safety.

risks. The nurse should regularly reinforce practices that will protect the individual from injury (Box 5-13).

HEALTH TEACHING

Health education is the process of providing information, encouraging a learner to use the resources they have, and teaching health promotion strategies or how to manage an existing condition. Nurses must have the knowledge to provide effective teaching to different groups of people. There are many factors to consider when planning teaching, including the domains of learning, factors that can enhance or inhibit learning, adult learning principles, and effective teaching strategies that can be used.

Domains of Learning

Learning often occurs using one or a combination of the three domains of learning: cognitive (understanding), affective (attitudes), and psychomotor (motor skills) (Anderson & Krathwohl, 2001). When teaching patients, it is important to understand which domain is involved in order to plan the appropriate teaching strategy. See Box 5-14 for a discussion of teaching methods based on the domains of learning.

Cognitive Learning

Cognitive learning involves the acquiring of knowledge and development of intellectual skills, including the recall of specific facts. Bloom's taxonomy (knowledge, comprehension, application, analysis, synthesis, and evaluation) is frequently used to describe the increasing complexity of cognitive skills as learners move from beginner to more advanced in their knowledge of content. When considering which teaching strategies are appropriate to use for cognitive learning to occur see Box 5-14. An example of cognitive learning would be when teaching a patient about the different types of birth control methods that are available.

Affective Learning

Affective learning involves feelings, emotions, and values. Changing attitudes and values clarification are part of affective learning. This domain deals with attitudes, motivation, willingness to participate, valuing what is being learned, and ultimately incorporating values into a way of life. Discussing attitudes regarding the use of birth control is an example of incorporating affective learning in teaching.

Psychomotor Learning

The acquisition of a new motor skill involves psychomotor learning. This type of learning involves using physical movement. An example of this would be learning how to insert a diaphragm or how to put on a condom. Psychomotor skills are

BOX 5-14 APPROPRIATE TEACHING METHODS BASED ON DOMAINS OF LEARNING

Cognitive

Discussion (One-on-One or Group)

May involve nurse and one patient or nurse with several patients

Promotes active participation and focuses on topics of interest to patient

Facilitates peer support

Enhances application and analysis of new information

Storytelling

Can involve individual or group

Facilitates cultural relevance and safety

Enhances application of new information to a familiar context

Lecture

Is a more formal method of instruction because it is teacher controlled

Helps learner acquire new knowledge and gain comprehension

Question-and-Answer Session

Is designed specifically to address patient's concerns

Assists patient in applying knowledge

Role Play and Discovery

Encourages patient to actively apply knowledge in a controlled situation

Promotes synthesis of information and problem solving

Independent Projects (e.g., Computer-Assisted Instruction) and Field Experience

Assists patient to assume responsibility for learning at own pace

Promotes analysis, synthesis, and evaluation of new information and skills

Affective

Role Play

Encourages expression of values, feelings, and attitudes

Discussion (Group)

Enables patient to acquire support from other people in group

Encourages patient to learn from other people's experiences

Promotes responding, valuing, and organizing

Discussion (One-on-One)

Facilitates discussion of personal, sensitive topics of interest or concern

Psychomotor

Demonstration

Provides presentation of procedures or skills by nurse

Encourages patient to model nurse's behaviour

Allows nurse to control questioning during demonstration

Practice

Enables patient to perform skills by using equipment in a controlled setting

Allows repetition

Return Demonstrations

Enables patient to perform skill as nurse observes

Provides excellent source of feedback and reinforcement

Independent Projects and Games

Require teaching method that promotes adaptation and initiation of psychomotor learning

Enable learner to use new skills

Source: Potter, P. A., Perry, A. G., Ross-Kerr, J. C., et al. (Eds.). (2014). *Canadian fundamentals of nursing* (5th ed.). Toronto: Elsevier Canada.

often taught using demonstrations and return demonstrations (see Box 5-14).

Adult Learning

Malcolm Knowles (1970) identified adult learning as an approach to learning that is problem-based and collaborative. He focused on the equality between the learner and teacher. Knowles also identified six principles of adult learning:

1. Adults are internally motivated and self-directed—It is important to foster the internal motivation to learn and to facilitate learners' attitude toward being self-directed and responsible for their own learning. Adults resist learning when they feel it is being imposed on them.
2. Adults bring life experiences and knowledge to learning experiences—It is important to consider and build on learners' previous knowledge and experience; the ability to do this will enhance learning. Nurses should ask learners about their past experience and build on this information.
3. Adults are goal oriented—Learners will learn best when it is felt the information is important to them.
4. Adults are relevancy oriented—Adult learners like to know the relevance of what they are trying to achieve.
5. Adults are practical—it is important to ensure the learning applies to the specific situation.
6. Adult learners like to be respected—Nurses must convey respect and need to acknowledge the expertise and experience of the learner.

Learning Styles

Everyone processes information differently, therefore learners have different learning styles and preferences. Processing information involves seeing and hearing, reflecting and acting, reasoning logically and intuitively, and analyzing and visualizing (Hall & Edgecombe, 2014). Visual learners learn best by seeing what they are learning. Auditory learners want to hear the information, often in a lecture or through discussion. Kinesthetic learners want to be involved with the learning by doing hands-on practice. Nurses must first assess the learning style of the patient to ensure that the appropriate learning strategy is used. Assessing the type of environment the patient prefers to learn in is also necessary before providing teaching. Some people like to learn on their own and are very self-directed, whereas others like to learn in groups. Nurses also need to assess the preferred learning style of the learner and adapt strategies to meet the needs of the learner. When providing teaching in a group setting, it is often necessary to use several different teaching methods in order to ensure the needs of all the learners are met.

Teaching Methods

Nurses must consider the content being taught as well as how the patient learns best when deciding which method to use to provide the teaching. The nurse needs to assess the patient for their learning style and be prepared to modify the approach depending on how the patient responds. The most important factor when providing teaching is to provide an active learning environment; this is where the nurse and patient work together toward a common goal. See Patient Teaching box for strategies to use when providing patient teaching.

One-on-One Discussion

Many times nurses provide teaching in an individual session with a patient. Teaching one-on-one allows the learner to ask questions, and this should be encouraged. During the teaching session, the nurse can use pictures, written material, audiovisual aids, or models. The teaching aids that are used will depend on the learner's needs and how the person learns best.

Role Playing

Role playing is used to help a learner acquire new ideas and attitudes. The learner often takes the role of themselves or someone else in an unfamiliar situation and may practise a desired behaviour. An effective use for role playing is when a patient wants to feel more comfortable asking questions of a health care provider in an unfamiliar situation. The ability to practise the skill allows the learner to learn new skills and to feel more confident in situations when they are required.

Group Teaching

Teaching groups is often done through the use of lectures, although lecturing is not always the most effective method to enhance learning. Lectures can be very structured and limit interaction. A better way to provide teaching to groups is through discussion and practice (Hall & Edgecombe, 2014). People can learn well within group settings, especially if they are able to learn from other people's experiences. Nurses require practice and experience to feel comfortable facilitating group discussions rather than just lecturing.

Demonstration

Demonstration is an effective method to provide teaching regarding the acquisition of a psychomotor skill. Showing the learner how to do something can be effective, although a more effective method is to have the learner return the demonstration to ensure that learning is acquired. Teaching new parents how to do a baby bath or a teenager how to apply a condom are examples of skills that are effectively taught using demonstration.

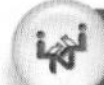

PATIENT TEACHING

Teaching Strategies

- Establish trust with the patient before beginning the teaching–learning session.
- Limit teaching objectives.
- Use simple terminology to enhance the patient's understanding.
- Schedule short teaching sessions at frequent intervals; minimize distractions during teaching sessions.
- Begin and end each teaching session with the most important information.
- Present information slowly, pacing to provide ample time for the patient to understand the material.
- Repeat important information.
- Provide many examples that have meaning to the patient; for example, relate new material to a previous life experience.
- Build on existing knowledge.
- Use visual cues and simple analogies when appropriate.
- Ask the patient for frequent feedback to determine whether the patient comprehends information.
- Demonstrate procedures such as measuring dosages; ask for return demonstrations (which provide opportunities to clarify instructions and time to review procedures).
- Provide teaching materials that reflect the reading level of the patient; use material written with short words and sentences, large type, and simple format (in general, information written on a Grade 5 reading level is recommended for adult learners).
- Provide teaching materials that reflect health literacy of the patient; use material that avoids jargon, acronyms, and unnecessary medical terminology and defines medical terms that are necessary.
- Model appropriate behaviour and use role playing to help the patient learn how to ask questions and ask for help effectively.
- Pace the delivery of material so that patients can progress at their own speed.
- Include family members or other caregivers in the education process.

Data from Bastable, S. (2008). *Nurse as educator: Principles of teaching and learning for nursing practice.* Sudbury, MA: Jones & Bartlett; Lowenstein, A. J., Foord-May, L., & Romano, J. C. (Eds.). (2009). *Teaching strategies for health education and health promotion: Working with patients, families and communities.* Sudbury, MA: Jones & Bartlett.

Factors That Influence Learning

Environment

An environment that is quiet with few distractions will enhance learning. The room should be well lit, well ventilated, and comfortable, as it is more difficult to learn in uncomfortable surroundings. It is important to determine whether the patient has pain or any other distractions, as these can affect learning. A new mother with a hungry, crying baby will find it difficult to concentrate on any teaching. The time of day may also have an impact on learning. People often learn better at different times of day. Nurses need to determine what is best for the patient when providing teaching.

Ability to Learn

The ability to learn depends on emotional, intellectual, and physical capabilities. If a patient's learning ability is impaired, the teaching may need to be postponed. For example, a patient who needs to learn to use a walker following hip surgery will not be able to learn this if the pain level is too high and the person has not been out of bed postoperatively. It is important not to assume that everyone has the same intellectual ability to learn. Furthermore, it is important not to make the assumption that all people are literate.

Health Literacy

In Canada, 42% of Canadian adults between the ages of 16 and 65 have low literacy skills, and 55% of working-age adults in Canada are estimated to have less than adequate health literacy skills (Canadian Literacy and Learning Network, 2016). Health literacy is closely related to literacy, but focuses specifically on health information demands. Health literacy requires the ability to solve problems, evaluate information, and know when to take action. Individuals and groups for whom English is a second language often lack the skills necessary to seek medical care and function adequately in the health care setting. Health literacy involves a spectrum of abilities, ranging from reading an appointment slip to interpreting medication instructions. Low health literacy may be an independent contributor to a disproportionate disease burden among disadvantaged populations. Nurses need to determine the level of reading ability before providing teaching and to ensure that written material is provided that meets the needs of the patient. The most commonly used measures of health literacy in clinical settings are the Rapid Assessment of Literacy in Medicine (REALM) test, which measures the ability to read health terms, and the Test of Functional Health Literacy in Adults (TOFHLA), which measures the ability to understand health information (Canadian Public Health Association, 2008). These tests offer approximations of reading skills but do not test health literacy.

Motivation to Learn

The motivation to learn can be influenced by many factors, including a learner's culture as well as the health beliefs of the learner. If a person does not have access to some of the determinants of health, it can be more difficult to teach preventive health strategies or ways to manage an existing illness. If someone does not see the value in quitting smoking, teaching on this topic is less likely be effective. Health teaching must be provided in a culturally competent manner and in a way that meets the needs of the patient.

Developmental level. The age and stage of development of a patient also can affect the ability to learn (see Box 5-15) as well as how the person learns best.

BOX 5-15 TEACHING METHODS BASED ON PATIENT'S DEVELOPMENTAL CAPACITY

Adolescent

Help the adolescent learn about feelings and need for self-expression.
Collaborate with the adolescent on teaching activities.
Let the adolescent make decisions about health and health promotion (safety, sex education, substance use).
Use problem solving to help the adolescent make choices.

Young or Middle-Age Adult

Encourage participation in the teaching plan by setting mutual goals.
Encourage independent learning.
Offer information so that the adult can understand effects of the health problem.

Older Adult

Teach when the patient is alert and rested.
Involve the adult in discussion or activity.
Focus on wellness and the person's strength.
Use approaches that enhance sensorially impaired patients' reception of stimuli.
Keep teaching sessions short.

Source: Potter, P. A., Perry, A. G., Ross-Kerr, J. C., et al. (Eds.). (2014). *Canadian fundamentals of nursing* (5th ed.). Toronto: Elsevier Canada.

KEY POINTS

- Many determinants of health, including culture and socioeconomic status, as well as personal circumstances, the uniqueness of the individual, and the stage of development, influence a person's recognition of need for care, the degree to which they will or will not access care, and the response to the health care system and therapy.
- Women have many reasons for accessing the health care system: well-woman care, fertility prevention, infertility, and pregnancy.
- Preconception counselling allows identification and possible remediation of potentially harmful personal and social conditions, medical and psychological conditions, environmental conditions, and barriers to care before pregnancy occurs.
- There are many risk factors related to women's health that must be considered when providing care, including, for example, nutrition, lack of exercise, stress, and substance use.
- Conditions that increase a woman's health risks also increase risks for her offspring.
- IPV against women is a major social and health care problem in Canada and includes physical, sexual, emotional, psychological, and economic abuse; it affects all races and all socioeconomic, educational, and religious groups.
- Periodic health screening provides the basis for overall health promotion, prevention of illness, early diagnosis of problems, and referral for management.

- Health promotion and prevention of illness can help women to actualize their health potential by increasing motivation, providing information, and suggesting how to access specific resources.
- Teaching should be timed to work with the patient's readiness and ability to learn.
- Teaching is most effective when it meets the needs of the learner.
- The use of different types of teaching methods can improve the learner's attentiveness and overall learning.

evolve EVOLVE WEBSITE

Visit the Evolve website for additional resources related to the content in this chapter such as Case Studies, Critical Thinking Case Study Answers, Nursing Care Plans, Nursing Processes, Nursing Skills, and Review Questions for Exam Preparation at: *http://evolve.elsevier.com/Canada/Perry/maternal/*

REFERENCES

Allan, B., & Smylie, J. (2015). *First Peoples, second class treatment: The role of racism in the health and well-being of Indigenous peoples in Canada.* Toronto: Wellesley Institute.

Al-Sahab, B., Heifetz, M., Tamim, H., et al. (2012). Prevalence and characteristics of teen motherhood in Canada. *Maternal Child Health Journal, 16*, 228–234. doi:10.1007/s10995-011-0750-8.

Anderson, L. W., & Krathwohl, D. R. (Eds.), (2001). *A taxonomy for learning, teaching and accessing: Revision of Bloom's taxonomy of educational objectives.* New York: Longman.

Avalos, L. A., Kaskutas, L., Block, G., et al. (2011). Does lack of multinutrient supplementation during early pregnancy increase vulnerability to alcohol-related preterm or small-for-gestational-age births? *Maternal Child Health Journal, 15*(8), 1324–1332.

Azagba, S., & Sharaf, M. F. (2014). Binge drinking and marijuana use among menthol and non-menthol adolescent smokers: Findings from the Youth Smoking Survey. *Addictive Behaviors, 39*, 740–743.

Bailey, B. A., & Sokol, R. J. (2011). Prenatal alcohol exposure and miscarriage, stillbirth, preterm delivery, and sudden infant death syndrome. *Alcohol Research & Health, 34*(1), 86–91.

Berecki-Gisolf, J., McKenzie, S. J., Dobson, A. J., et al. (2013). A history of co-morbid depression and anxiety predicts new onset of heart disease. *Journal of Behavioral Medicine, 36*(4), 347–353.

Brennan, A. M. W., Barnsteiner, J., de Leon Siantz, M. L., et al. (2012). Lesbian, gay, bisexual, transgendered, or intersexed content for nursing curricula. *Journal of Professional Nursing, 28*(2), 96–104.

British Columbia Victim Services and Crime Prevention Division. (2010, January). *Domestic violence response: A community framework for maximizing women's safety.* Retrieved from <http://www.pssg.gov.bc.ca/victimservices/shareddocs/pubs/domestic-violence-response.pdf>.

Brownridge, D. A. (2008). Understanding the elevated risk of partner violence against Aboriginal women: A comparison of two nationally representative surveys of Canada. *Journal of Family Violence, 23*, 353–367. doi:10.1007/s10896-008-9160-0.

Bushnik, T., Cook, J. L., Yuzpe, A., et al. (2012). Estimating prevalence of infertility in Canada. *Human Reproduction, 27*(3), 738–746.

Canada Without Poverty. (2016). *Just the facts.* Retrieved from <http://www.cwp-csp.ca/poverty/just-the-facts/>.

Canadian Centre on Substance Abuse. (2013). *Licit and illicit drug use during pregnancy: Maternal, neonatal and early childhood consequences.* Ottawa: Author.

Canadian Centre on Substance Abuse. (2014a). *Women and alcohol.* Retrieved from <http://www.ccsa.ca/Resource%20Library/CCSA-Women-and-Alcohol-Summary-2014-en.pdf>.

Canadian Centre on Substance Abuse. (2014b). *Cannabis use and risky behaviours and harms: A comparison of urban and rural populations in Canada.* Retrieved from <http://www.ccsa.ca/Resource%20Library/CCSA-Cannabis-use-Risky-behaviours-and-Harms-2014-en.pdf#search=risky%20behaviour>.

Canadian Harm Reduction Network. (2000). *Harm reduction: Policy and practice.* Retrieved from <http://www.canadianharmreduction.com/node/889>.

Canadian Literacy and Learning Network. (2016). *Literacy statistics.* Retrieved from <http://www.literacy.ca/literacy/literacy-sub/>.

Canadian Nurses Association. (2009). *Position statement: Determinants of health.* Ottawa: Author. Retrieved from <http://cna-aiic.ca/~/media/cna/page-content/pdf-en/ps_determinants_of_health_e.pdf>.

Canadian Public Health Association. (2008). *A vision for a health literate Canada: Report of the Expert Panel on Health Literacy.* Ottawa: Author. Retrieved from <http://www.cpha.ca/uploads/portals/h-l/report_e.pdf>.

Canadian Women's Foundation. (2011). *Report on violence against women, mental health and substance use.* Retrieved from <http://www.canadianwomen.org/sites/canadianwomen.org/files/PDF%20-%20VP%20Resources%20-%20BCSTH%20CWF%20Report_Final_2011_%20Mental%20Health_Substance%20use.pdf>.

Catallo, C., Jack, S. M., Cilska, D., & MacMillan, H. L. (2012). Minimizing the risk of intrusion: A grounded theory of intimate partner violence disclosure in emergency departments. *Journal of Advanced Nursing, 69*, 1366–1376. doi:10.1111/j.1365-2648.2012.06128.x.

Centre for Addiction and Mental Health. (2012). *Methamphetamines.* Retrieved from <http://www.camh.ca/en/hospital/health_information/a_z_mental_health_and_addiction_information/Methamphetamines/Pages/default.aspx>.

Community Foundations of Canada. (2010). *National public opinion survey: Local environment and sustainability.* Retrieved from <http://www.vitalsignscanada.ca/nr-2010-public-opinion-survey-e.html#envqual>.

Cory, J., & Dechief, L. (2007). *SHE framework: Safety and health enhancement for women experiencing abuse: A toolkit for health care providers and planners.* Retrieved from <http://endingviolence.org/files/uploads/SHE_Framework_F___122008_SEC1.pdf>.

Cunningham, F., Leveno, K., Bloom, S., et al. (2014). *Williams obstetrics* (24th ed.). New York: McGraw Hill.

Davies, G. A., Maxwell, C., MacLeod, L., et al.; Society of Obstetricians and Gynecologists of Canada. (2010). SOGC clinical practice guideline: Obesity in pregnancy. *Journal of Obstetrics and Gynaecology Canada, 32*(2), 165–173.

Department of Justice Canada. (2015). *Aboriginal victimization in Canada: A summary of the literature.* Retrieved from <http://www.justice.gc.ca/eng/rp-pr/cj-jp/victim/rd3-rr3/p3.html>.

Dubowitz, T., Ghosh-Dastidar, M., Eibner, C., et al. (2012). The women's health initiative: The food environment, neighborhood socioeconomic status, BMI, and blood pressure. *Obesity, 20*(4), 862–871.

Grewal, S. K., Bhagat, R., & Balneaves, L. G. (2008). Perinatal beliefs and practices of immigrant Punjabi women living in Canada. *Journal of Gynecologic and Neonatal Nursing, 37*, 290–300. doi:10.1111/j.1552-6909.2008.00234.x.

Hall, A. M., & Edgecombe, N. A. (2014). Patient education. In P. A. Potter, A. G. Perry, P. Stockert, et al. (Eds.), *Canadian fundamentals of nursing* (5th ed.). Toronto: Elsevier.

Hautala, L., Junnila, J., Alin, J., et al. (2009). Uncovering hidden eating disorders using the SCOFF questionnaire: Cross-sectional survey of adolescents and comparison with nurse assessments. *International Journal of Nursing Studies, 46*(11), 1439–1447.

Hayatbakhsh, M. R., Flenady, V. J., Gibbons, K. S., et al. (2012). Birth outcomes associated with cannabis use before and during pregnancy. *Pediatric Research, 71*(2), 215–219.

Health Canada. (2011). *Canadian guidelines for body weight classification in adults.* Ottawa: Author. Retrieved from <http://www.hc-sc.gc.ca/fn-an/nutrition/weights-poids/guide-ld-adult/qa-qr-pub-eng.php#a4>.

Health Canada. (2013a). *Prenatal nutrition guidelines for health professionals—folate contributes to healthy pregnancy.* Retrieved from <www.hc-sc.gc.ca/fn-an/pubs/nutrition/folate-eng.php>.

Health Canada. (2013b). *Canadian tobacco use monitoring survey 2012.* Ottawa: Author. Retrieved from <http://www.hc-sc.gc.ca/hc-ps/tobac-tabac/research-recherche/stat/ctums-esutc_2012-eng.php>.

Health Canada. (2014). *Caffeine and pregnancy.* Ottawa: Author. Retrieved from <http://www.phac-aspc.gc.ca/hp-gs/know-savoir/caffeine-eng.php>.

Heart and Stroke Foundation. (2011). *Basic principles of physical activity.* Retrieved from <http://www.heartandstroke.ab.ca/site/c.lqIRL1PJJtH/b.3651131/k.4EF0/Healthy_Living__Physical_Activity.htm>.

Hogue, C. J. R., & Silver, R. M. (2011). Racial and ethnic disparities in the United States—stillbirth rates: Trends, risk factors, and research needs. *Seminars in Perinatology, 35*(4), 221–233.

Keegan, J., Parva, M., Finnegan, M., et al. (2010). Addiction in pregnancy. *Journal of Addictive Diseases, 29,* 175–191.

Kingston, D., Heaman, M., Fell, D., et al. (2012). Factors associated with perceived stress and stressful life events in pregnant women: Findings from the Canadian maternity experiences survey. *Maternal Child Health Journal, 16,* 158–168. doi:10.1007/s10995-010-0732-2.

Knowles, M. S. (1970). *The modern practice of adult education. Andragogy versus pedagogy.* Englewood Cliffs, NJ: Prentice Hall/Cambridge.

Manske, S. R., Rynard, V., & Minaker, L. (2013). *Flavoured tobacco use among Canadian youth: Evidence from Canada's 2010/2011 youth smoking survey.* Waterloo: Propel Centre for Population Health Impact. Retrieved from <https://uwaterloo.ca/propel/sites/ca.propel/files/uploads/files/flavoured_tobacco_use_yss_20131007.pdf>.

McAlearney, A. S., Oliveri, J. M., Post, D. M., et al. (2011). Trust and distrust among Appalachian women regarding cervical cancer screening: A qualitative study. *Patient Education & Counseling, 86*(1), 120–126.

McKay, A., & Sex Information and Education Council of Canada. (2012). Trends in Canadian national and provincial/territorial teen pregnancy rates: 2001–2010. *Canadian Journal of Human Sexuality, 21*(3–4), 161–175.

Medline Plus. *Methamphetamine, 2014,* U.S. National Library of Medicine, National Institutes of Health. Retrieved from <www.nlm.nih.gov/medlineplus/methamphetamine.html>.

Ministry of Health and Long-Term Care. (2012). *Initial report on public health: Teen pregnancy.* Government of Ontario: Author. Retrieved from <http://www.health.gov.on.ca/en/public/publications/pubhealth/init_report/tp.html>.

Mong, J. A., Baker, F. C., Mahoney, M. M., et al. (2011). Sleep, rhythms, and the endocrine brain: Influence of sex and gonadal hormones. *Journal of Neuroscience, 31*(45), 16107–16116.

Montero, I., Escriba, V., Ruiz-Perez, I., et al. (2011). Interpersonal violence and women's psychological well-being. *Journal of Women's Health, 20*(2), 295–301.

Morgan, J., Reid, F., & Lacey, J. (1999). The SCOFF questionnaire: Assessment of a new screening tool for eating disorders. *British Medical Journal, 319*(7223), 1467–1468.

Motherisk. (2013, April). *Is caffeine consumption safe during pregnancy?* Retrieved from <http://www.motherisk.org/prof/updatesDetail.jsp?content_id=998>.

Murphy, R., Straebler, S., Basden, S., et al. (2012). Interpersonal psychotherapy for eating disorders. *Clinical Psychology & Psychotherapy, 19*(2), 150–158.

National Cancer Institute. (2012). *Obesity and cancer risk.* Retrieved from <http://www.cancer.gov/cancertopics/causes-prevention/risk/obesity/obesity-fact-sheet>.

National Institute on Drug Abuse. (2015). *Drug facts: Marijuana.* Retrieved from <www.drugabuse.gov/publications/drugfacts/marijuana>.

O'Leary, C., Nassar, N., Kurinczuk, J. J., et al. (2011). Prenatal alcohol exposure and risk of birth defects. *Obstetrical & Gynecological Survey, 66*(2), 88–90.

Pasternak, Y., Weintraub, A. Y., Shoham-Vardi, I., et al. (2012). Obstetric and perinatal outcomes in women with eating disorders. *Journal of Women's Health, 21*(1), 61–65.

Peles, E., Schreiber, S., Bloch, M., et al. (2012). Duration of methadone maintenance treatment during pregnancy and pregnancy outcome parameters in women with opiate addiction. *Journal of Addiction Medicine, 6*(1), 18–23.

Pellizzari, R., Mason, R., Grant, L., et al.; Society of Obstetricians and Gynaecologists of Canada. (2005). SOGC clinical practice guideline: Intimate partner violence consensus statement. *Journal of Obstetrics and Gynaecology Canada, 27*(4), 365–388.

Poole, N., Dell, C. A., & for Canadian Centre on Substance Abuse. (2005). *Girls, women and substance use.* Retrieved from <http://www.ccsa.ca/Resource%20Library/ccsa-011142-2005.pdf>.

Public Health Agency of Canada. (2009). *What mothers say: The Canadian maternity experiences survey.* Ottawa: Author.

Public Health Agency of Canada. (2010). *What determines health?* Retrieved from <http://www.phac-aspc.gc.ca/ph-sp/determinants/index-eng.php>.

Public Health Agency of Canada. (2016). Pregnancy. In *Family-centred maternity and newborn care: National guidelines.* Ottawa: Author.

Registered Nurses' Association of Ontario. (2015). *Engaging clients who use substances.* Toronto: Registered Nurses' Association of Ontario. Retrieved from <http://rnao.ca/sites/rnao-ca/files/Engaging_Clients_Who_Use_Substances_13_WEB.pdf>.

Reitmanova, S., & Gustafson, D. L. (2008). "They can't understand it": Maternity health and care needs of immigrant Muslim women in St. John's, Newfoundland. *Maternal Child Health Journal, 12,* 101–111. doi:10.1007/s10995-007-0213-4.

Robert, M., Ross, S., & Urogynaecology Committee. (2006). SOGC clinical practice guideline: Conservative management of urinary incontinence. *Journal of Obstetrics & Gynecology of Canada, 28*(12), 1113–1118.

Royal Canadian Mounted Police. (2012). *Intimate partner violence and abuse—it can be stopped.* Retrieved from <http://www.rcmp-grc.gc.ca/cp-pc/pdfs/int_par-rel_int-eng.pdf>.

Schaub, B. G., & Burt, M. M. (2013). Addiction and recovery counseling. In B. M. Dossey & L. Kegan (Eds.), *Holistic nursing: A handbook for practice* (6th ed., pp. 539–562). Burlington, MA: Jones & Bartlett.

Sears, H. A., & Byers, E. S. (2010). Adolescent girls' and boys' experiences of psychologically, physically, and sexually aggressive behaviors in their dating relationships: Co-occurrence and emotional reaction. *Journal of Aggression, Maltreatment and Trauma, 19,* 517–539.

Senikas, V., Kluka, S., Wood, R., et al.; Society of Obstetricians and Gynaecologists of Canada. (2010). SOGC clinical practice guideline: Alcohol use and pregnancy: Consensus clinical guidelines. *Journal of Obstetrics and Gynaecology Canada, 32*(8).

SexualityandU.ca. (2012). *Statistics on Canadian teen pregnancies.* Retrieved from <http://www.sexualityandu.ca/sexual-health/statistics1/statistics-on-canadian-teen-pregnancies>.

Sinha, M. (Ed.). (2013). *Measuring violence against women: Statistical trends (Component of Statistics Canada catalogue no. 85-002-X).* Ottawa: Minister of Industry. Retrieved from <http://www.statcan.gc.ca/pub/85-002-x/2013001/article/11766-eng.pdf>.

Smylie, J., Fell, D., Ohlsson, A., & The Joint Working Group on First Nations, Indian, Inuit, and Métis Infant Mortality of the Canadian Perinatal Surveillance System. (2010). Review of Aboriginal infant mortality rates in Canada: Striking and persistent Aboriginal/non-Aboriginal inequities. *Canadian Journal of Public Health, 101,* 143–148.

Statistics Canada. (2015a). *Smoking 2013*. Retrieved from <http://www.statcan.gc.ca/pub/82-625-x/2014001/article/14025-eng.htm>.

Statistics Canada. (2015b). *Overweight and obese adults (self-reported), 2014*. Retrieved from <http://www.statcan.gc.ca/pub/82-625-x/2015001/article/14185-eng.htm>.

Touchette, E., Henegar, A., Godart, N. T., et al. (2011). Subclinical eating disorders and their comorbidity with mood and anxiety disorders in adolescent girls. *Psychiatry Research, 185*(1), 185–192.

Truth and Reconciliation Commission of Canada. (2015). *Executive summary*. Retrieved from <http://www.trc.ca/websites/trcinstitution/File/2015/Honouring_the_Truth_Reconciling_for_the_Future_July_23_2015.pdf>.

Vallance, J. K., Latner, J. D., & Gleaves, D. H. (2011). The relationship between eating disorder psychopathology and health-related quality of life within a community sample. *Quality of Life Research, 20*(5), 675–682.

Yang, T. S., Matthews, S. A., & Hillemeier, M. M. (2011). Effect of health care system distrust on breast and cervical cancer screening in Philadelphia, Pennsylvania. *American Journal of Public Health, 101*(7), 1297–1305.

Zender, R., & Olshansky, E. (2009). Promoting wellness in women across the lifespan. *Nursing Clinics of North America, 44*(3), 281–291.

ADDITIONAL RESOURCES

Canadian Cancer Society: Smokers' Helpline: <http://www.smokershelpline.ca/>.

Canadian Centre on Substance Abuse: <http://www.ccsa.ca/Pages/default.aspx>.

EatRight Ontario—Access to nutrition and healthy eating information: <https://www.eatrightontario.ca/en/default.aspx>.

Family Health and Literacy: A Guide to Easy-to-Read Health Education Materials and Websites for Families: <http://healthliteracy.worlded.org/docs/family/fhl.pdf>.

Health Canada: Coping with Stress: <http://www.hc-sc.gc.ca/hl-vs/iyh-vsv/life-vie/stress-eng.php>.

Health Canada: Environmental and Workplace Health—Vulnerable Populations: <http://www.hc-sc.gc.ca/ewh-semt/contaminants/vulnerable/index-eng.php>.

Health Canada: Health Concerns—Quit Smoking: <http://www.hc-sc.gc.ca/hc-ps/tobac-tabac/quit-cesser/index-eng.php>.

Heart and Stroke Foundation of Canada—Risk factors and prevention: <http://www.heartandstroke.com/site/c.ikIQLcMWJtE/b.3483933/k.CD67/Stroke.htm>.

The Lung Association: Smoking and Tobacco: <http://www.lung.ca/quit>.

SexualityandU: <http://www.sexualityandu.ca>.

Motherisk—Research and counselling on reproductive risk or safety of drugs, chemicals and maternal disease in pregnancy: <http://motherisk.ca/>.

Nigeria: Violence Against Persons (Prohibition) Act (2015): <http://www.refworld.org/docid/556d5eb14.html>.

Registered Nurses' Association of Ontario. (2015, March). Engaging Clients Who Use Substances: <http://rnao.ca/bpg/guidelines/engaging-clients-who-use-substances>.

Registered Nurses' Association of Ontario Best Practice Guideline: Integrating Smoking Cessation Into Daily Nursing Practice: <http://www.rnao.ca/bpg/guidelines/integrating-smoking-cessation-daily-nursing-practice>.

Registered Nurses' Association of Ontario Best Practice Guideline: Women Abuse: Screening, Identification and Initial Response: <http://rnao.ca/sites/rnao-ca/files/Guideline__Supplement_PDF.pdf>.

Registered Nurses' Association of Ontario elearning series: Tobacco Free—A resource for health care professionals working with clients who use tobacco or other substance use disorders. <http://elearning.rnao.ca/>.

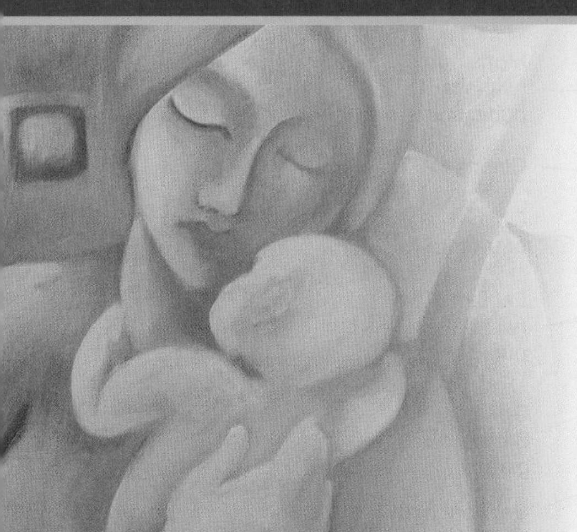

CHAPTER

6

Health Assessment

Lisa Keenan-Lindsay, with contributions from Ellen Olshansky

evolve WEBSITE

Visit the Evolve website for additional resources related to the content in this chapter such as Case Studies, Critical Thinking Case Study Answers, Nursing Care Plans, Nursing Processes, Nursing Skills, and Review Questions for Exam Preparation at: *http://evolve.elsevier.com/Canada/Perry/maternal/*

OBJECTIVES

On completion of this chapter the reader will be able to:

- Identify the structures and functions of the female reproductive system.
- Describe how to provide culturally competent care while completing a health assessment.
- Describe components of taking a woman's history and performing a physical examination.
- Identify how the history and physical examination can be adapted for women with special needs.
- Identify how to screen for intimate partner violence.
- Describe components of taking a woman's history and performing a physical examination.
- Identify the correct procedure for assisting with and collecting Papanicolaou test specimens.

The purpose of this chapter is to review female anatomy and physiology as well as gynecological health assessment.

FEMALE REPRODUCTIVE SYSTEM

The female reproductive system consists of external structures that are visible from the pubis to the perineum, and internal structures located in the pelvic cavity as well as the breasts. The external and internal female reproductive structures develop and mature in response to estrogen and progesterone. This process starts in fetal life and continues through **puberty** and the child-bearing years. Reproductive structures atrophy with age or in response to a decrease in ovarian hormone production. A complex nerve and blood supply supports the functions of these structures. The appearance of the external genitalia varies greatly among women. **Heredity**, age, race, and the number of children a woman has borne influence the size, shape, and colour of her external organs.

External Structures

The external genital organs, or *vulva*, include all structures visible externally from the pubis to the perineum. These include the mons pubis, labia majora, labia minora, clitoris, vestibular glands, vaginal vestibule, vaginal orifice, and urethral opening. The external genital organs are illustrated in Fig. 6-1.

The *mons pubis* is a fatty pad that lies over the anterior surface of the symphysis pubis. In the postpubertal female the mons is covered with coarse, curly hair. The *labia majora* are two rounded folds of fatty tissue covered with skin that extend downward and backward from the mons pubis. The *labia* are highly vascular structures that develop hair on the outer surfaces after puberty. They protect the inner vulvar structures. The *labia minora* are two flat, reddish folds of tissue visible when the labia majora are separated. There are no hair follicles on the labia minora, but many sebaceous follicles and a few sweat glands are present. The interior of the labia minora is composed of connective tissue and smooth muscle and is supplied with extremely sensitive nerve endings. Anteriorly the labia minora fuse to form the **prepuce** (the hoodlike covering of the clitoris) and the frenulum (the fold of tissue under the clitoris). The labia minora join to form a thin, flat tissue, called the *fourchette,* underneath the vaginal opening at midline. The *clitoris,* located underneath the prepuce, is a small structure composed of erectile tissue with numerous

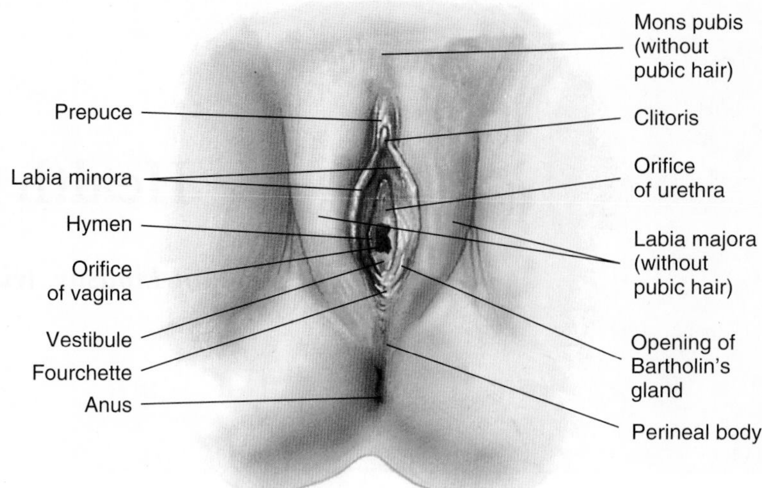

FIGURE 6-1 External female genitalia.

sensory nerve endings. During sexual arousal the clitoris increases in size.

The *vaginal vestibule* is an almond-shaped area enclosed by the labia minora that contains openings to the urethra, Skene glands, vagina, and Bartholin glands. The urethra is not a reproductive organ but is discussed here because of its location. It usually is found about 2.5 cm below the clitoris. Skene glands are located on each side of the urethra and produce mucus, which aids in lubrication of the vagina. The vaginal opening is in the lower portion of the vestibule and varies in shape and size. The *hymen*, a connective tissue membrane that surrounds the vaginal opening, can be perforated during strenuous exercise, insertion of tampons, masturbation, and vaginal intercourse. Bartholin glands lie under the constrictor muscles of the vagina and are located posteriorly on the sides of the vaginal opening, although the ductal openings usually are not visible. During sexual arousal, the glands secrete clear mucus to lubricate the vaginal introitus.

The area between the fourchette and the anus is the *perineum*, a skin-covered muscular area that covers the pelvic structures. The perineum forms the base of the perineal body, a wedge-shaped mass that serves as an anchor for the muscles, fascia, and ligaments of the pelvis. The muscles and ligaments form a sling that supports the pelvic organs.

Internal Structures

The internal structures include the vagina, uterus, uterine tubes, and ovaries.

The *vagina* is a fibromuscular, collapsible, tubular structure that lies between the bladder and rectum and extends from the vulva to the uterus. During the reproductive years, the mucosal lining is arranged in transverse folds called **rugae**. These rugae allow the vagina to expand during childbirth. Estrogen deprivation that occurs after childbirth, during lactation, and at **menopause** causes dryness and thinning of the vaginal walls and smoothing of the rugae. The vagina, particularly the lower segment, has few sensory nerve endings. Vaginal secretions are slightly acidic (pH 4 to 5), so vaginal susceptibility to **infections** is limited. The vagina serves as a passageway for menstrual flow, as a female organ of copulation, and as a part of the birth canal for childbirth. The uterine cervix projects into a blind vault at the upper end of the vagina. There are anterior, posterior, and lateral pockets called **fornices** (singular: fornix) that surround the cervix. The internal pelvic organs can be palpated through the thin walls of these fornices.

The *uterus* is a muscular organ shaped like an upside-down pear that sits midline in the pelvic cavity between the bladder and rectum and above the vagina. Four pairs of ligaments support the uterus: cardinal, uterosacral, round, and broad. Single anterior and posterior ligaments also support the uterus. The *cul-de-sac of Douglas* is a deep pouch, or recess, posterior to the cervix formed by the posterior ligament.

The uterus is divided into two major parts, an upper triangular portion called the *corpus* and a lower cylindrical portion called the *cervix* (Fig. 6-2). The **fundus** is the dome-shaped top of the uterus and is the site at which the uterine tubes (fallopian tubes) enter the uterus. The *isthmus*, or lower uterine segment, is a short, constricted portion that separates the corpus from the cervix.

The uterus serves for reception, implantation, retention, and nutrition of the fertilized ovum and later of the fetus during pregnancy and for expulsion of the fetus during childbirth. It is also responsible for cyclic menstruation.

The uterine wall is made up of three layers: the **endometrium**, the myometrium, and part of the peritoneum. The *endometrium* is a highly vascular lining made up of three layers, the outer two of which are shed during menstruation. The *myometrium* is made up of layers of smooth muscles that extend in three different directions (longitudinal, transverse, and oblique) (Fig. 6-3). Longitudinal fibres of the outer myometrial layer are found mostly in the fundus, and this arrangement assists in the expelling of the fetus during the birth process. The middle layer contains fibres from all three directions, which form a figure-eight pattern encircling large blood vessels. These fibres assist

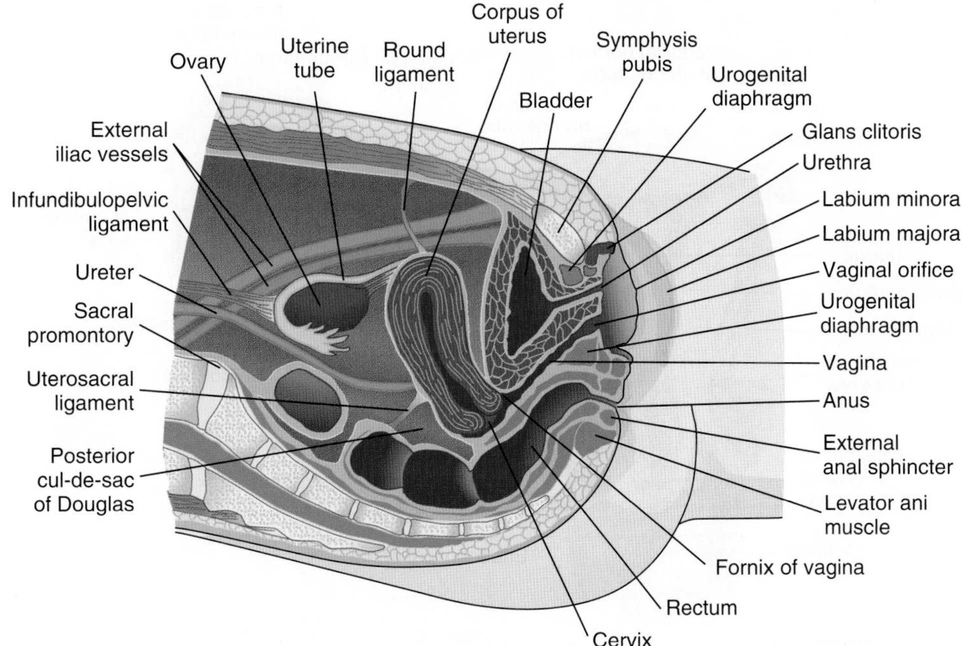

FIGURE 6-2 Midsagittal view of female pelvic organs.

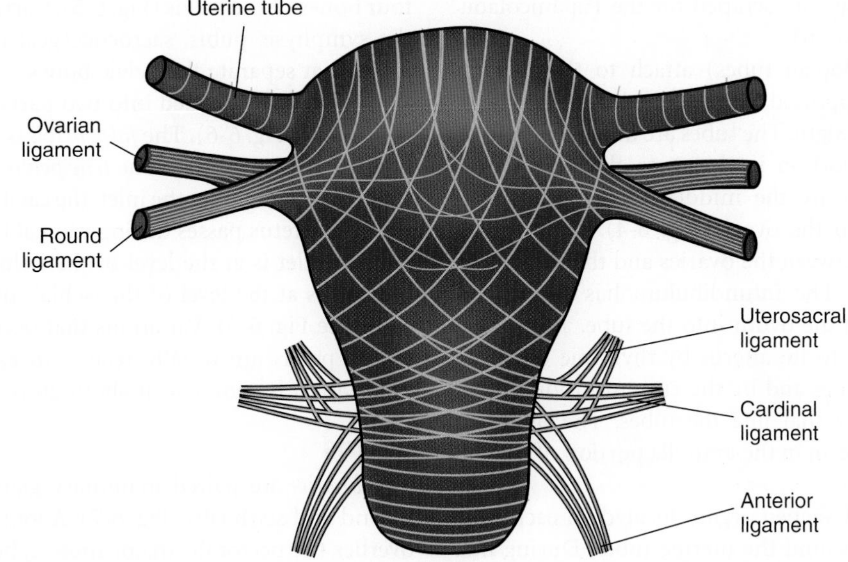

FIGURE 6-3 Schematic arrangement of directions of muscle fibres. Note that uterine muscle fibres are continuous with supportive ligaments of the uterus.

in ligating blood vessels after childbirth and controlling blood loss. Most of the circular fibres of the inner myometrial layer are around the site where the uterine tubes enter the uterus and around the internal cervical os (opening). These fibres help keep the cervix closed during pregnancy and prevent menstrual blood from flowing back into the uterine tubes during menstruation.

The cervix is made up of mostly fibrous connective tissues and elastic tissue, making it possible for the cervix to stretch during vaginal childbirth. The opening between the uterine cavity and the canal that connects the uterine cavity to the vagina (endocervical canal) is the *internal os.* The narrowed opening between the endocervix and the vagina is the *external os,* a small circular opening in women who have never been pregnant. The cervix feels firm (like the end of a nose) with a dimple in the centre that marks the external os.

The outer cervix is covered with a layer of squamous epithelium. The mucosa of the cervical canal is covered with columnar epithelium and contains numerous glands that secrete mucus in response to ovarian hormones. The squamo-columnar junction, where the two types of cells meet, is usually located just inside the cervical os. This junction also is called the

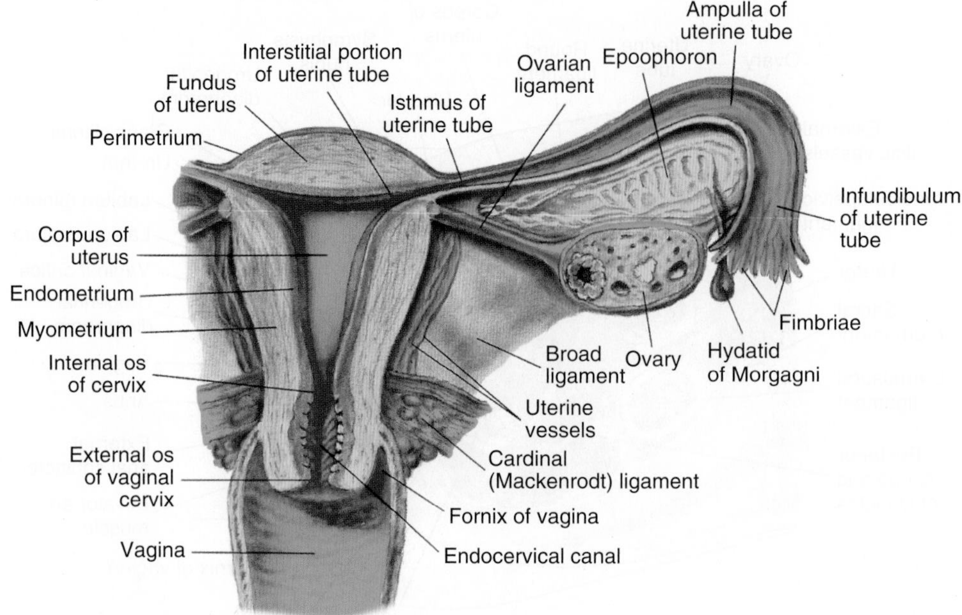

FIGURE 6-4 Cross section of uterus, fallopian tubes, ovaries, and upper vagina.

transformation zone and is the most common site for neoplastic changes. Cells from this site are scraped for the Papanicolaou (Pap) test (see later discussion).

The *uterine tubes* (fallopian tubes) attach to the uterine fundus. The tubes are supported by the broad ligaments and range from 8 to 14 cm in length. The tubes are divided into four sections: the interstitial portion is closest to the uterus; the isthmus and the ampulla are the middle portions; and the infundibulum is closest to the ovary (Fig. 6-4). The uterine tubes provide a passage between the ovaries and the uterus for movement of the ovum. The infundibulum has fimbriated (fringed) ends, which pull the ovum into the tube. The ovum is pushed along the tubes to the uterus by rhythmic contractions of muscles of the tubes and by the current produced by the movement of the cilia that line the tubes. The ovum is usually fertilized by the sperm in the ampulla portion of one of the tubes.

The *ovaries* are almond-shaped organs located on each side of the uterus below and behind the uterine tubes. During the reproductive years, they are approximately 3 cm long, 2 cm wide, and 1 cm thick; they diminish in size after menopause. Before menarche each ovary has a smooth surface; after menarche they are nodular because of repeated ruptures of follicles at ovulation. The two functions of the ovaries are ovulation and hormone production. **Ovulation** is the release of a mature ovum from the ovary at intervals (usually monthly). Estrogen, progesterone, and androgen are the hormones produced by the ovaries.

The Bony Pelvis

The bony pelvis serves three primary purposes: protection of the pelvic structures, accommodation of the growing fetus during pregnancy, and anchorage of the pelvic support structures. The two innominate (hip) bones (consisting of ilium, ischium, and pubis), the sacrum, and the coccyx make up the four bones of the pelvis (Fig. 6-5). Cartilage and ligaments form the symphysis pubis, sacrococcygeal joint, and two sacroiliac joints that separate the pelvic bones.

The pelvis is divided into two parts: the false pelvis and the true pelvis (Fig. 6-6). The *false pelvis* is the upper portion above the pelvic brim or inlet. The *true pelvis* is the lower curved bony canal, which includes the inlet, the cavity, and the outlet through which the fetus passes during vaginal birth. The upper portion of the outlet is at the level of the ischial spines, and the lower portion is at the level of the ischial tuberosities and the pubic arch (see Fig. 6-5). Variations that occur in the size and shape of the pelvis are usually related to age, race, and sex. Pelvic ossification is complete at about 20 years of age.

Breasts

The *breasts* are paired mammary glands located between the second and sixth ribs (Fig. 6-7). About two thirds of the breast overlies the pectoralis major muscle, between the sternum and midaxillary line, with an extension to the axilla referred to as the *tail of Spence*. The lower one third of the breast overlies the serratus anterior muscle. The breasts are attached to the muscles by connective tissue or fascia.

The breasts of the healthy, mature woman are approximately equal in size and shape but often are not absolutely symmetrical. The size and shape vary with the woman's age, heredity, and nutrition. However, the contour should be smooth with no retractions, dimpling, or masses. Estrogen stimulates growth of the breast by inducing fat deposition in the breasts, development of stromal tissue (i.e., increase in its amount and elasticity), and growth of the extensive ductile system. Estrogen also increases the vascularity of breast tissue.

Once ovulation begins in puberty, progesterone levels increase. The increase in progesterone causes maturation of

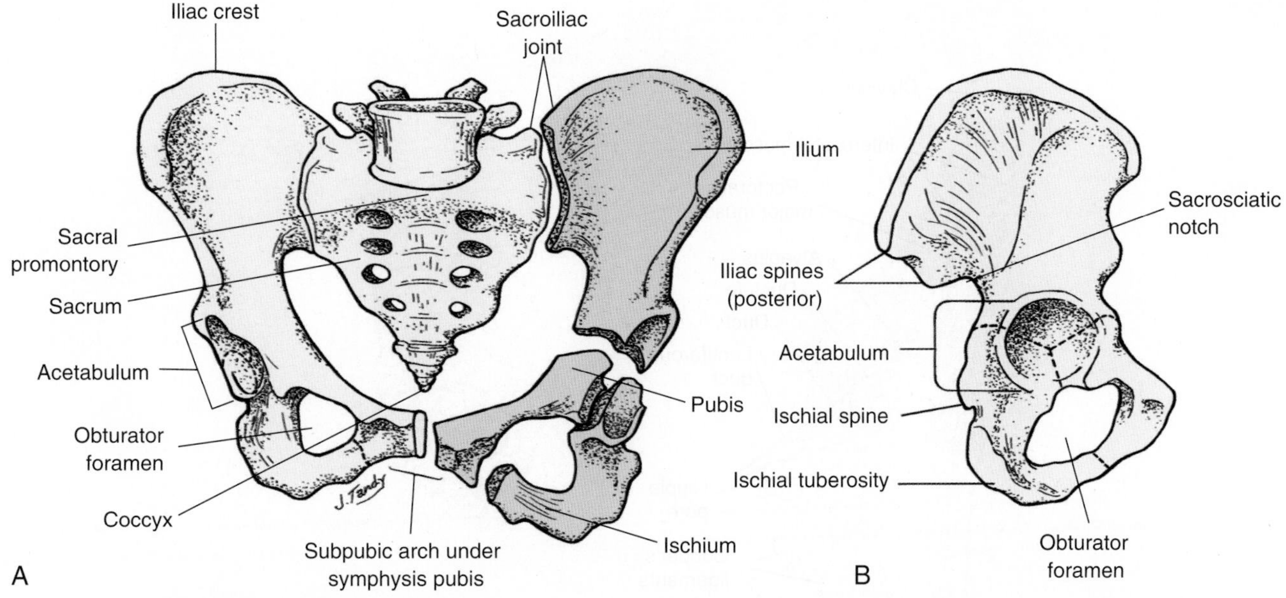

FIGURE 6-5 Adult female pelvis. **A:** Anterior view. **B:** External view of innominate bone (fused).

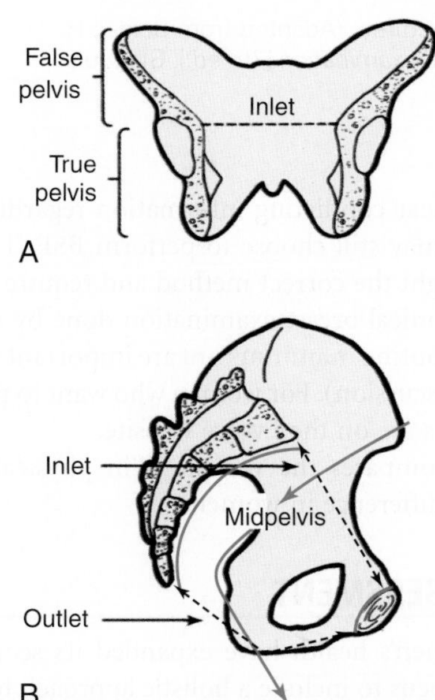

FIGURE 6-6 Female pelvis. **A:** The cavity of false pelvis is shallow. **B:** The cavity of true pelvis is an irregularly curved canal *(arrows)*.

mammary gland tissue, specifically the lobules and acinar structures. During adolescence fat deposition and growth of fibrous tissue contribute to the increase in the size of the glands. Full development of the breasts is not achieved until after the end of the first pregnancy or in the early period of lactation.

Each mammary gland is made of a number of lobes that are divided into lobules. *Lobules* are clusters of acini. An *acinus* is a saclike terminal part of a compound gland emptying through a narrow lumen or duct. The acini are lined with epithelial cells that secrete colostrum and milk. Just below the epithelium is the myoepithelium (*myo*, or muscle), which contracts to expel milk from the acini.

The ducts from the clusters of acini that form the lobules merge to form larger ducts draining the lobes. Ducts from the lobes converge in a single nipple (mammary papilla) surrounded by an areola. The anatomy of the ducts is similar for each breast but varies among women. Protective fatty tissue surrounds the glandular structures and ducts. *Cooper's ligaments,* or fibrous suspensory ligaments, separate and support the glandular structures and ducts. Cooper's ligaments provide support to the mammary glands while permitting their mobility on the chest wall (see Fig. 6-7). The round nipple is usually slightly elevated above the breast. On each breast the nipple projects slightly upward and laterally. It contains 4 to 20 openings from the milk ducts. The nipple is surrounded by fibromuscular tissue and covered by wrinkled skin (the *areola*). Except during pregnancy and lactation, there is usually no discharge from the nipple.

The nipple and surrounding areola are usually more deeply pigmented than the skin of the breast. The rough appearance of the areola is caused by sebaceous glands, Montgomery tubercles, directly beneath the skin. These glands secrete a fatty substance thought to lubricate the nipple. Smooth muscle fibres in the areola contract to stiffen the nipple to make it easier for the breastfeeding infant to grasp.

The vascular supply to the mammary gland is abundant. In the nonpregnant state, there is no obvious vascular pattern in the skin. The normal skin is smooth without tightness or shininess. The skin covering the breasts contains an extensive superficial lymphatic network that serves the entire chest wall and is continuous with the superficial lymphatic vessels of the neck and abdomen. The lymphatic vessels form a rich network in the deeper portions of the breasts. The primary deep lymphatic pathway drains laterally toward the axillae.

Besides their function of lactation, breasts function as organs for sexual arousal in the mature adult.

The breasts change in size and nodularity in response to cyclic ovarian changes throughout reproductive life. Increasing

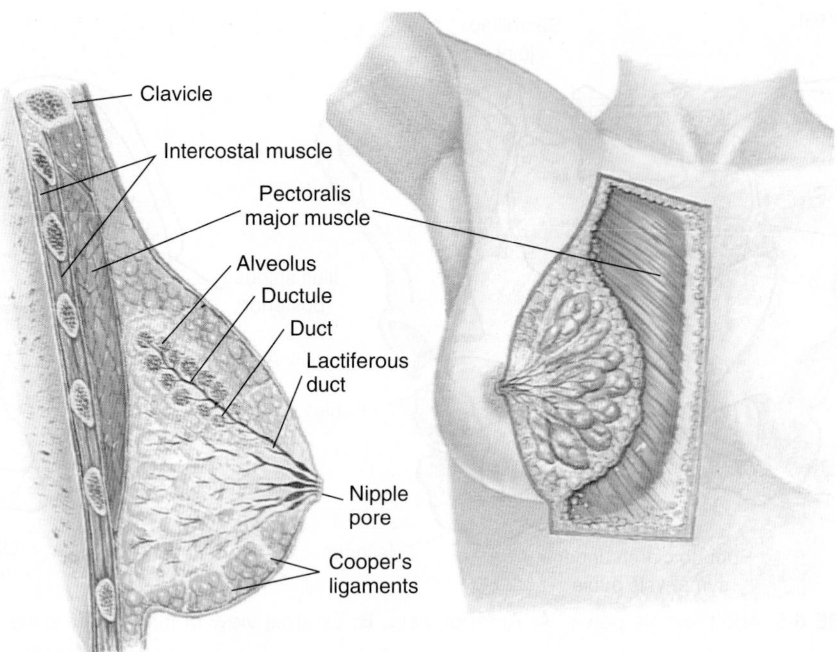

FIGURE 6-7 Anatomy of the breast, showing position and major structures. (Adapted from Seidel, H. M., Stewart, R. W., Ball, J. W., et al. [2011]. *Mosby's guide to physical examination* [7th ed.]. St. Louis: Mosby.)

levels of both estrogen and progesterone in the 3 to 4 days before menstruation increase the vascularity of the breasts, induce growth of the ducts and acini, and promote water retention. The epithelial cells lining the ducts proliferate in number, the ducts dilate, and the lobules distend. The acini become enlarged and secretory, and lipid (fat) is deposited within their epithelial cell lining. As a result, breast swelling, tenderness, and discomfort are common symptoms just before the onset of menstruation. After menstruation, cellular proliferation begins to regress, acini begin to decrease in size, and retained water is lost. After breasts have undergone changes numerous times in response to the ovarian cycle, the proliferation and involution (regression) are not uniform throughout the breast. In time, after repeated hormonal stimulation, small persistent areas of nodulations may develop. This normal physiological change must be remembered when breast tissue is examined. Nodules may develop just before and during menstruation, when the breast is most active. The physiological alterations in breast size and activity reach their minimum level about 5 to 7 days after menstruation stops. Breast self-examination (BSE) is best carried out during this phase of the menstrual cycle.

Routine monthly BSE, which is the systematic palpation of breasts to detect signs of breast cancer or other changes, is no longer recommended by the Society of Obstetricians and Gynaecologists of Canada (SOGC) (2006) and the Canadian Cancer Society (2014). Evidence-informed practice has changed because research has shown that BSE has not led to a decrease in mortality from breast cancer and has been linked to an increase in the number of unnecessary biopsies and other procedures. Women do need to know how their breasts feel and look and to watch for changes, but not on a regular schedule. Women may hear conflicting information regarding BSE, and some women may still choose to perform BSE. These women need to be taught the correct method and require information that a yearly clinical breast examination done by a health care provider and routine mammogram are important (see Chapter 7 for further discussion). For women who want to perform BSE, the instructions are on the Evolve website.

Table 6-1 compares the variations in physical assessment related to age difference in women.

HEALTH ASSESSMENT

Trends in women's health have expanded its scope beyond a reproductive focus to include a holistic approach to health care across the lifespan and place women's health within primary care. Women's health assessment and screening focus on a systems evaluation that begins with a careful history and physical examination. During assessment and evaluation, the woman's responsibility for self-management, health promotion, and enhancement of wellness is emphasized.

Often it is a nurse who takes the history, interprets test results, makes referrals, coordinates care, and directs attention to problems requiring medical intervention. Advanced practice nurses who specialize in women's health, such as nurse practitioners and clinical nurse specialists, order diagnostic tests and perform complete physical examinations, including gynecological examinations.

Interview

Contact with the woman usually begins with an interview, which is an integral part of the history. This interview should

TABLE 6-1 FEMALE REPRODUCTIVE PHYSICAL ASSESSMENT ACROSS THE LIFE CYCLE

	ADOLESCENT	ADULT	POSTMENOPAUSAL
Breasts	Tender when developing; buds appear; small, firm; one side may grow faster; areola diameter increases; nipples more erect	Grow to full shape in early adulthood; nipples and areola become darker	Become stringy, irregular, pendulous, and nodular; borders are less well delineated; may shrink and become flatter, elongated, and less elastic; ligaments weaken; nipples are positioned lower
Vagina	Vagina lengthens; epithelial layers thicken; secretions become acidic	Growth complete by age 20	Introitus constricts; vagina narrows, shortens, loses rugation; mucosa is pale, thin, and dry; walls may lose structural integrity
Uterus	Musculature and vasculature increase; lining thickens	Growth complete by age 20	Size decreases; endometrial lining thins
Ovaries	Increase in size and weight; menarche occurs between 8 and 16 years of age; ovulation occurs monthly	Growth complete by age 20	Size decreases to 1–2 cm; follicles disappear; surface convolutes; ovarian function ceases between 40 and 55 years of age
Labia majora	Become more prominent; hair develops	Growth complete by age 20	Labia become smaller and flatter; pubic hair becomes sparse and grey
Labia minora	Become more vascular	Growth complete by age 20	Become shinier and drier
Uterine tubes	Increase in size	Growth complete by age 20	Decrease in size

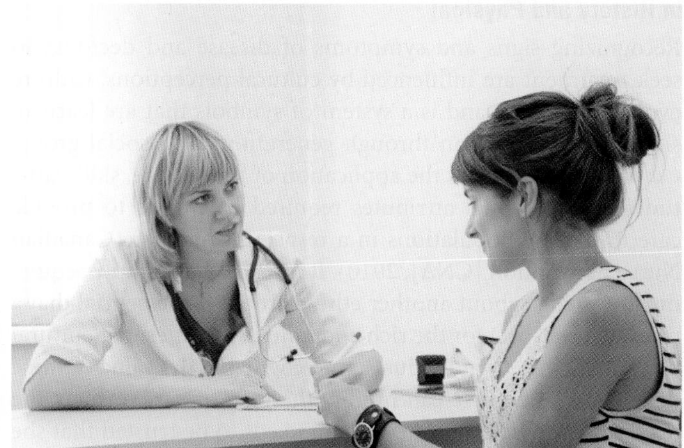

FIGURE 6-8 Nurse interviews patient as part of a routine history and physical examination. (© Can Stock Photo Inc./JackF.)

be conducted in a private, comfortable, and relaxed setting (Fig. 6-8). The nurse should be seated and make sure that the woman is comfortable. The woman should be addressed by her title and name (e.g., Mrs. Khan) and asked how she prefers to be addressed. Then the nurse can introduce herself or himself using name and title. It is important to phrase questions in a sensitive and nonjudgemental manner. Body language should match verbal communication. The nurse needs to be aware of a woman's vulnerability and assure her of strict confidentiality. For many women fear, anxiety, and modesty make the examination a dreaded and stressful experience. Women may feel that they do not have all the information a health professional has, may be misguided by myths, or be afraid that they will appear ignorant by asking questions about sexual or reproductive functioning. The woman needs to be assured that no question is irrelevant.

The history begins with an open-ended question, such as "What brings you into the office (or clinic or hospital) today?" and is furthered by other prompts, such as "Anything else?" and "Tell me about it." Additional ways of encouraging women to share information include the following:

Facilitation—Using a word or posture that communicates interest, such as leaning forward, making eye contact, or saying "Mm-hmmm" or "Go on"

Reflection—Repeating a word or phrase that the woman has used

Clarification—Asking the woman what is meant by a stated word or phrase

Empathic responses—Acknowledging the feelings of a woman through statements such as "That must have been frightening"

Confrontation—Identifying something about the woman's behaviour or feelings not expressed verbally or apparently inconsistent with her history

Interpretation—Putting into words what the nurse infers about the woman's feelings or about the meaning of her symptoms, events, or other matters

Nurses need to develop rapport and trust with their patients as they take a history; because communication within a caring context is core to nursing practice, nurses are well suited to taking a comprehensive patient history. Nurses should ask questions incrementally in order to build a comprehensive understanding. The nurse should ask about one item at a time and proceed from the general to the specific (Ball, Dains, Flynn, et al., 2014). The nurse should also share insights with the woman by eliciting her concerns or thoughts as well as offering clarification to her (Fawcet & Rhynas, 2012).

At a woman's first visit, she is often expected to fill out a form with biographical and historical data before meeting with the examiner. This form aids the health care provider in completing the history during the interview. Most forms include information within these categories:

- Biographical data
- Reason for seeking care
- Present health or history of present illness
- Past health

- Family history
- Screening for abuse
- Review of systems
- Functional assessment (activities of daily living)

Box 6-1 describes a complete health history based on the categories just mentioned.

Physical Examination

In preparation for the physical examination, the woman should be instructed on undressing and given a gown to wear during the examination. She is usually given the opportunity to undress privately. Objective data are recorded by system or location. A general statement of overall health status is a good way to start. Findings are described in detail.

- *General appearance:* age, sex, state of health, posture, height, weight, development, hygiene; affect, alertness, orientation, and communication skills
- *Vital signs:* temperature, pulse, respiration, blood pressure
- *Skin:* colour; integrity; texture; hydration; temperature; edema; excessive perspiration; unusual odour; presence and description of lesions; hair texture and distribution; nail configuration, colour, texture, and condition; presence of nail clubbing
- *Head:* size, shape, trauma, masses, scars, rashes, or scaling; facial symmetry; presence of edema or puffiness
- *Eyes:* pupil size, shape, reactivity; conjunctival injection, scleral icterus, fundal papilledema, hemorrhage, lids, extraocular movements, visual fields and acuity
- *Ears:* shape and symmetry, tenderness, discharge, external canal, and tympanic membranes; hearing—Weber test should be midline (loudness of sound equal in both ears) and Rinne test negative (no conductive or sensorineural hearing loss); should be able to hear whisper at 1 metre
- *Nose:* symmetry, tenderness, discharge, mucosa, turbinate inflammation, frontal or maxillary sinus tenderness; discrimination of odours
- *Mouth and throat:* hygiene; condition of teeth; dentures; appearance of lips, tongue, buccal and oral mucosa; erythema; edema; exudate; tonsillar enlargement; palate; uvula; gag reflex; ulcers
- *Neck:* mobility, masses, range of motion, trachea deviation, thyroid size, carotid bruits
- *Lymphatic:* cervical, intraclavicular, axillary, trochlear, or inguinal adenopathy; size, shape, tenderness, and consistency
- *Breasts:* skin changes, dimpling, symmetry, scars, tenderness, discharge, or masses; characteristics of nipples and areolae
- *Heart:* rate, rhythm, murmurs, rubs, gallops, clicks, heaves, or precordial movements
- *Peripheral vascular:* jugular vein distension, bruits, edema, swelling, vein distension, or tenderness of extremities
- *Lungs:* chest symmetry with respirations, wheezes, crackles, rhonchi, vocal fremitus, whispered pectoriloquy, percussion, and diaphragmatic excursion; breath sounds equal and clear bilaterally
- *Abdomen:* shape, scars, bowel sounds, consistency, tenderness, rebound, masses, guarding, organomegaly, liver span, percussion (tympany, shifting, dullness), costovertebral angle tenderness
- *Extremities:* edema, ulceration, tenderness, varicosities, erythema, tremor, abnormality
- *Genitourinary:* external genitalia, perineum, vaginal mucosa, cervix; inflammation, tenderness, discharge, bleeding, ulcers, nodules, or masses; internal vaginal support; bimanual and rectovaginal palpation of cervix, uterus, and adnexa
- *Rectal:* sphincter tone, masses, hemorrhoids, rectal wall contour, tenderness, stool for occult blood
- *Musculoskeletal:* posture, symmetry of muscle mass, muscle atrophy, weakness, appearance of joints, tenderness or crepitus, joint range of motion, instability, redness, swelling, spine deviation
- *Neurological:* mental status, orientation, memory, mood, speech clarity and comprehension, cranial nerves II to XII, sensation, strength, deep tendon and superficial reflexes, gait, balance, coordination with rapid alternating motions

Cultural Considerations and Communication Variations in History and Physical

Recognizing signs and symptoms of disease and deciding to seek treatment are influenced by cultural perceptions. Culture evolves over time and is a system of symbols that are learned, shared, and passed on through generations of a social group. *Cultural competence* is the application of knowledge, skills, attitudes, and personal attributes required by nurses to provide care to diverse populations in a respectful manner (Canadian Nurse Association [CNA], 2010). It is more than simply acquiring knowledge about another ethnic group. It is essential that a nurse have respect for the rich and unique qualities that cultural diversity brings to individuals. In recognizing the value of these differences, the nurse can modify the plan of care to meet the needs of each woman. The woman needs to be trusted that she is the expert on her life, culture, and experiences. If the nurse asks with respect and a genuine desire to learn, the woman will tell the nurse how to care for her. Modifications may be necessary in conducting the physical examination. In many cultures a woman examiner is preferred. In some cultures it may be considered inappropriate for the woman to disrobe completely for the physical examination.

Communication may be hindered by different beliefs, even when the nurse and woman speak the same language. Examples of communication variations are listed in the Cultural Awareness box.

Adolescents (Ages 13 to 19)

As a young woman matures, she should be asked the same questions that are included in any history. Particular attention should be paid to hints about risky behaviours, eating disorders, and depression. Sexual activity is addressed after rapport has been established. It is best to talk to a teen with the parent (or partner or friend) out of the room. The nurse should engage with the patient in a sensitive manner, using active listening and conveying a nonjudgemental manner.

Injury prevention should be a part of the counselling at routine health examinations, with special attention paid to use

BOX 6-1 HEALTH HISTORY AND REVIEW OF SYSTEMS

Identifying data: name, age, sex, marital status, occupation, and ethnicity

Reason for seeking care: a response to the question, "What problem or symptom brought you here today?" Is there more than one reason? Focus on the one she thinks is most important.

Present health: Current health status is described with attention to the following:

- *Use of safety measures:* seat belts, bicycle helmets, designated driver
- *Exercise and leisure activities:* regularity
- *Sleep patterns:* length and quality
- *Sexuality:* Is she sexually active? With men, women, or both? Risk-reducing sex practices?
- *Diet, including beverages:* 24-hour dietary recall
- *Nicotine, alcohol, illicit or recreational drug use:* type, amount, frequency, duration, and reactions
- *Environmental and chemical hazards:* home, school, work, and leisure setting; exposure to extreme heat or cold, noise, industrial toxins such as asbestos or lead, pesticides, radiation, cat feces, or cigarette smoke

History of present illness: a chronological narrative of the issue that includes a description of the following—location, quality or character, quantity or severity, timing (onset, duration, frequency), setting, factors that aggravate or relieve the issue, associated factors, and the woman's perception of the meaning of the symptom

Past health:

- *Infectious diseases:* e.g., measles, mumps, rubella, tuberculosis (TB), hepatitis, sexually transmitted infections (STIs)
- *Chronic disease and system disorders:* e.g., arthritis, cancer, diabetes, heart, lung, kidney, sickle cell anemia
- *Adult injuries, accidents*
- *Hospitalizations, operations, blood transfusions*
- *Obstetrical history*
- *Mental health concerns:* previous history of depression, anxiety, bipolar disorder; has this been treated?
- *Allergies:* medications, previous transfusion reactions, environmental allergies
- *Immunizations:* e.g., diphtheria, pertussis, tetanus, measles, mumps, rubella, influenza, hepatitis B, human papillomavirus (HPV), pneumococcal vaccine
- *Last date of screening tests:* e.g., Pap test, mammogram, cholesterol test, colonoscopy
- *Current medications:* name, dose, frequency, duration, reason for taking, and adherence to prescription regimen; home remedies, over-the-counter drugs, vitamin and mineral or herbal supplements used

Family history: information about the ages and health of family members. Check for history of diabetes, heart disease, or other chronic disorders.

Screen for abuse: Has she ever been hit, kicked, slapped, or forced to have sex against her wishes? Verbally or emotionally abused? History of childhood sexual abuse? If yes, has she received counselling or does she need a referral? (see Chapter 5, p. 74)

Review of systems: It is probable that all questions in each system will not be included every time a history is taken. The essential areas to be explored are listed in the following head-to-toe sequence. If a woman gives a positive response to a question about an essential area, more detailed questions should be asked.

- *General:* weight change, fatigue, weakness, fever, chills, or night sweats
- *Skin:* skin, hair, and nail changes; itching, bruising, bleeding, rashes, sores, lumps, or moles
- *Lymph nodes:* enlargement, inflammation, pain, or drainage
- *Head:* trauma, vertigo (dizziness), convulsive disorder, syncope (fainting); headache: location, frequency, pain type, nausea and vomiting, or visual symptoms present
- *Eyes:* glasses, contact lenses, blurriness, tearing, itching, photophobia, diplopia, inflammation, trauma, cataracts, glaucoma, or acute visual loss
- *Ears:* hearing loss, tinnitus (ringing), vertigo, discharge, pain, fullness, recurrent infections, or mastoiditis
- *Nose and sinuses:* trauma, rhinitis, nasal discharge, epistaxis, obstruction, sneezing, itching, allergy, or smelling impairment
- *Mouth, throat, and neck:* hoarseness, voice changes, soreness, ulcers, bleeding gums, goitre, swelling, or enlarged nodes
- *Breasts:* masses, pain, lumps, dimpling, nipple discharge, fibrocystic changes, or implants; breast examination practice
- *Respiratory:* shortness of breath, wheezing, cough, sputum, hemoptysis
- *Cardiovascular:* hypertension, rheumatic fever, murmurs, angina, palpitations, dyspnea, tachycardia, orthopnea, edema, chest pain, cough, cyanosis, cold extremities, ascites, phlebitis, or skin colour changes
- *Gastrointestinal:* appetite, nausea, vomiting, indigestion, dysphagia, abdominal pain, ulcers, bleeding with stools or black, tarry stools, diarrhea, constipation, bowel movement frequency, food intolerance, hemorrhoids, jaundice, or hepatitis
- *Genitourinary:* frequency, hesitancy, urgency, polyuria, dysuria, hematuria, nocturia, incontinence, stones, infection, or urethral discharge; menstrual history, dyspareunia, discharge, sores, or itching
- *Sexual health and sexual activity:* with men, women, or both; contraceptive use; sexually transmitted infections (STI)
- *Peripheral vascular:* coldness, numbness and tingling, leg edema, varicose veins, thromboses, or emboli
- *Endocrine:* heat and cold intolerance, dry skin, excessive sweating, polyuria, polydipsia, polyphagia, thyroid problems, diabetes, or secondary sex characteristic changes
- *Hematological:* anemia, easy bruising, bleeding, petechiae, purpura, or transfusions
- *Musculoskeletal:* muscle weakness, pain, joint stiffness, scoliosis, lordosis, kyphosis, range of motion, instability, redness, swelling, arthritis, or gout
- *Neurological:* loss of sensation, numbness, tingling, tremors, weakness, vertigo, paralysis, fainting, twitching, blackouts, seizures, convulsions, loss of consciousness or memory
- *Mental status:* moodiness, depression, anxiety, obsessions, delusions, illusions, or hallucinations
- *Functional assessment:* ability to care for self

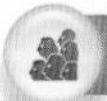

CULTURAL AWARENESS

Communication Variations

Conversational style and pacing—Silence may show respect or acknowledgement that the listener has heard. In cultures in which a direct "no" is considered rude, silence may mean no. Repetition or loudness may mean emphasis or anger.

Personal space—Cultural conceptions of personal space differ. For example, based on one's culture, someone may be perceived as being distant for backing off when approached or aggressive for standing too close.

Eye contact—Eye contact varies among cultures, from intense to fleeting. Consistent with the effort to refrain from invading personal space, avoiding direct eye contact may be a sign of respect.

Touch—The norms about how people should touch each other vary among cultures. In some cultures, physical contact with the same sex (embracing, walking hand in hand) is more appropriate than that with an unrelated person of the opposite sex.

Time orientation—In some cultures, involvement with people is more valued than being "on time." In other cultures, life is scheduled and paced according to clock time, which is valued over personal time.

Source: Mattson, S. (2000). Striving for cultural competence: Providing care for the changing face of the U.S. *AWHONN Lifelines, 4*(3), 48–52; Srivastava, R. (2006). *The healthcare professional's guide to clinical cultural competence.* St. Louis: Mosby.

of seat belts and helmets, recreational hazards, and sports involvement. The use of drugs and alcohol and the non-use of seat belts increase the risk of motor vehicle injuries, which account for the greatest proportion of accidental deaths in women. Information about contraceptives and sexually transmitted infection (STI) prevention may be needed for teens who are sexually active (see Chapter 7). Female athletes should have their weight assessed to ensure that they maintain an appropriate body mass index (BMI) (see Chapter 5).

To provide developmentally appropriate care, it is important to review the major tasks for women in this stage of life. Major tasks for teens include values assessment; education and work goal setting; formation of peer relationships that focus on love, commitment, and becoming comfortable with sexuality; and separation from parents. The teen is egocentric as she progresses rapidly through emotional and physical change. Her feelings of invulnerability may lead to misconceptions, such as the belief that unprotected sexual intercourse will not lead to pregnancy.

History and Physical Examination in Women With Disabilities

Women with emotional or physical disorders have special needs. Women who have vision, hearing, emotional, or physical disabilities should be respected and involved in the assessment and physical examination to the full extent of their capabilities. The nurse should communicate openly, directly, and with sensitivity. It is often helpful to learn about the disability directly from the woman, while maintaining eye contact. Family and significant others should be relied on only when absolutely necessary. The assessment and physical examination can be adapted to each woman's individual needs.

Communication with a woman who is hearing impaired can be accomplished without difficulty. Many women can read lips, write, or both. The interviewer who speaks and enunciates each word slowly and in full view may be easily understood. It is important that the interviewer not stand in front of a light source as this can make it more difficult for the woman to lip read. If a woman is not comfortable with lip reading, she may use an interpreter. In this case, it is important to continue to address the woman directly, avoiding the temptation to speak directly with the interpreter.

The visually impaired woman needs to be oriented toward the examination room and may have her guide dog with her. As with all patients, the visually impaired woman needs a full explanation of what the examination entails before proceeding. Before touching her, the nurse should explain, "Now I am going to take your blood pressure. I am going to place the cuff on your right arm." The woman can be asked if she would like to touch each of the items that will be used in the examination, to reduce her anxiety.

Women at Risk for Abuse

Nurses should screen all women who are entering the health care system for potential abuse. Abuse is a life-threatening public health problem that affects millions of women and their children. Prior to asking about abuse, all women should understand the reason for the questions being asked. A good way to present this is, "Because abuse happens to many women, we ask everyone about exposure to violence" (Rabin, Jennings, Campbell, et al., 2009). The risk for intimate partner violence (IPV) increases during pregnancy and after separation or divorce. Most women will not spontaneously provide information about family violence due to fear, guilt, and embarrassment; however, many women will often disclose if asked. Help for the woman may depend on the sensitivity with which the nurse screens for abuse, the discovery of abuse, and subsequent intervention. The nurse must be familiar with the laws governing abuse in the province in which she or he practises.

Pocket cards listing emergency numbers (abuse counselling, legal protection, and emergency shelter) may be obtained from local police departments, women's shelters, or emergency departments. It is helpful to have these on hand in the setting where screening is done. An abuse assessment screen (Fig. 6-9) can be used as part of the interview or written history. If a male partner is present, he should be encouraged to leave the room because the woman may not disclose experiences of abuse in his presence, or he may try to answer questions for her to protect himself. The same procedure applies for partners of lesbians or the adult children of older women.

Not all women will disclose abuse, but clues in the history and evidence of injuries on physical examination should elicit a high index of suspicion. The areas most commonly injured in women are the head, neck, chest, abdomen, breasts, and upper extremities. Burns and bruises in patterns resembling hands, belts, cords, or other weapons may be seen, as well as multiple traumatic injuries. Attention should be given to women who repeatedly seek treatment for somatic complaints such as

ABUSE ASSESSMENT SCREEN

1. Have you ever been emotionally or physically abused by your partner or someone important to you?

YES ☐ NO ☐

2. Within the last year, have you been hit, slapped, kicked, or otherwise physically hurt by someone?

YES ☐ NO ☐

If YES, by whom?________________

Number of times ________________

Mark the area of injury on body map.

3. Within the last year, has anyone forced you to have sexual activities?

YES ☐ NO ☐

If YES, who? ________________

Number of times ________________

4. Are you afraid of your partner or anyone you listed above?

YES ☐ NO ☐

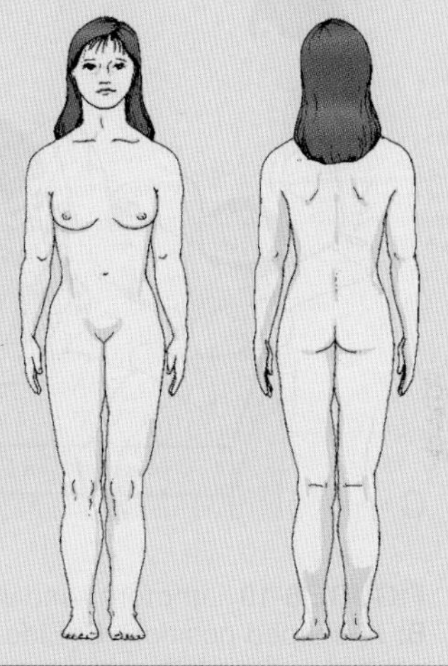

FIGURE 6-9 Screening for intimate partner violence. (Adapted from American College of Obstetrician and Gynecologists [2012]. *Are you being abused? Screening tool for domestic violence.* http://acog.org/About-ACOG/ACOG-Departments/Violence-Against-Women/Are-you-Being-Abused; Nursing Research Consortium on Violence and Abuse [1991].)

headaches; insomnia; choking sensations; hyperventilation; gastrointestinal symptoms; and pain in the chest, back, or pelvis. During pregnancy, the nurse should assess for injuries to the breasts, abdomen, and genitalia. See Chapter 5 for further discussion of IPV and the care provided to women.

Abusive relationships are often about power and control of the abuser over the woman (see Fig. 5-2). It is important to be aware of this when doing any physical examination, as any perception of power and control over the woman by a health care provider may exacerbate an abused woman's anxiety, discomfort, or fear. Women need to be shown respect and allowed control during the physical examination. All women should always be addressed using eye contact first, and they should always be asked for permission prior to any physical contact.

Transexuality

Although uncommon, there is an increasing number of individuals who transition from male to female or female to male. Health care providers need to provide respectful and sensitive care to transsexual men and women. A transsexual man who is in the process of transitioning may still have female reproductive organs and thus continues to need Pap tests, internal exams, and possibly breast examinations.

Transgender men with a cervix should be screened with Pap smears following the guidelines for all women. This examination may be emotionally difficult or painful for trans men. Several strategies may be employed to minimize the discomfort or trauma associated with this examination for some men.

Clinical breast examination as part of routine breast cancer screening is of questionable utility in trans women, but mammograms should be considered in trans women every 2 years if they are older than 50 years and on estrogen for more than 5 years. Initiation of screening may need to be considered at a younger age if additional risk factors are present (LGBT Health Program, 2015). See Additional Resources for further information on this topic.

Pelvic Examination

Many women fear the gynecological portion of the physical examination. The nurse can be instrumental in allaying these fears by providing information and assisting the woman to express her feelings to the examiner.

The woman should be assisted into the lithotomy position for the pelvic examination. If the woman is not comfortable in this position, then alternative positions may be used (Fig. 6-10). When she is in the lithotomy position, the woman's hips and

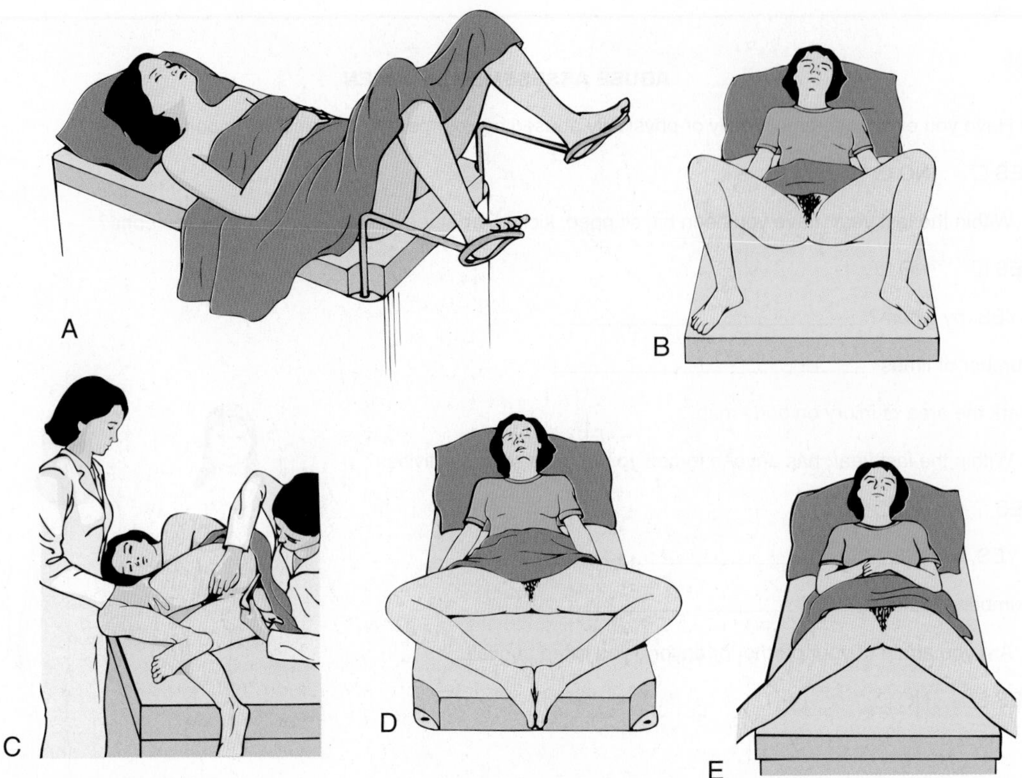

FIGURE 6-10 Lithotomy and variable positions for women who have a disability. **A:** Lithotomy position. **B:** M-shaped position. **C:** Side-lying position. **D:** Diamond-shaped position. **E:** V-shaped position.

knees are flexed, with buttocks at the edge of the table, and her feet are supported by heel or knee stirrups.

Many women and especially those with physical disabilities cannot comfortably lie in the lithotomy position for the pelvic examination. Several alternative positions may be used, including a lateral (side-lying) position, a V-shaped position, a diamond-shaped position, or an M-shaped position (see Fig. 6-10). The woman can be asked what has worked best for her previously. If she has never had a pelvic examination or has never had a comfortable pelvic examination, the nurse should proceed slowly by showing her a picture of various positions and asking her which one she prefers. The nurse's support and reassurance can help the woman to relax, which will make the examination go more smoothly.

Some women prefer to keep their shoes or socks on, especially if the stirrups are not padded. Women may express feelings of vulnerability and strangeness when in the lithotomy position. During the procedure, the nurse can assist the woman with relaxation techniques (see Box 6-2). Breathing techniques can be particularly helpful for the adolescent and for the woman whose introitus may be especially tight or for whom the experience is new or may provoke tension. Some women relax when they are encouraged to become involved with the examination by having a mirror placed so that they can view the area being examined. This type of participation helps with health teaching as well. Distraction is another technique that can be used effectively (e.g., placing interesting pictures on the ceiling over the head of the table).

Some women find it distressing to attempt to converse in the lithotomy position. Most women appreciate an explanation of the procedure as it unfolds, as well as coaching for the type of sensations they may expect. Generally, however, women prefer not to have to respond to questions until they are again upright and at eye level with the examiner. Being asked questions during the procedure, especially if they cannot see their questioner's eyes, may make some women tense.

A teenager's first speculum examination is the most important one because she will develop perceptions that will remain with her for future examinations. What the examination entails should be discussed with the teen while she is dressed. Models or illustrations can be used to show exactly what will happen. All of the necessary equipment should be assembled so that there are no interruptions. Pediatric specula that are 1 to 1.5 cm wide can be inserted with minimal discomfort. If the teen is sexually active, a small adult speculum may be used. See Critical Thinking Case Study.

External inspection. The examiner wears gloves and sits at the foot of the table for **inspection** of the external genitals and the speculum examination. In good lighting, external genitals are inspected for sexual maturity, including the clitoris, labia, and perineum, and for lesions indicative of STIs. After childbirth or other trauma there may be healed scars.

External palpation. Before touching the woman, the examiner should explain what is going to be done and what the woman should expect to feel (e.g., pressure). The examiner may touch the woman in a less sensitive area such as the inner thigh

BOX 6-2 PROCEDURE: ASSISTING WITH PELVIC EXAMINATION

1. Wash hands. Assemble the equipment (Fig. 6-11).
2. Ask the woman to empty her bladder before the examination (obtain clean-catch urine specimen as needed).
3. Assist with relaxation techniques. Have the woman place her hands on her chest at about the level of the diaphragm, breathe deeply and slowly (in through her nose and out through her O-shaped mouth), concentrate on the rhythm of breathing, and relax all body muscles with each exhalation.
4. Encourage the woman to become involved with the examination if she shows interest. For example, a mirror can be placed so that she can see the area being examined.
5. Assess for and treat signs of problems, such as supine hypotension.
6. Warm the speculum in warm water if a prewarmed one is not available.
7. Instruct the woman to bear down when the speculum is being inserted.
8. Apply gloves and assist the examiner with collection of specimens for cytological examination such as a Pap test. After handling specimens, remove gloves and wash hands.
9. Lubricate the examiner's fingers with water or water-soluble lubricant before bimanual examination.
10. Assist the woman to a sitting position upon completion of the examination.
11. Provide tissues to wipe lubricant from perineum.
12. Provide privacy for the woman while she is dressing.

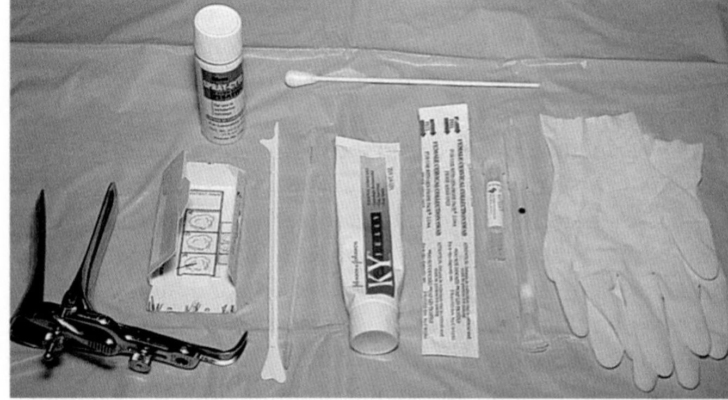

FIGURE 6-11 Equipment used for pelvic examination. (Courtesy Michael S. Clement.)

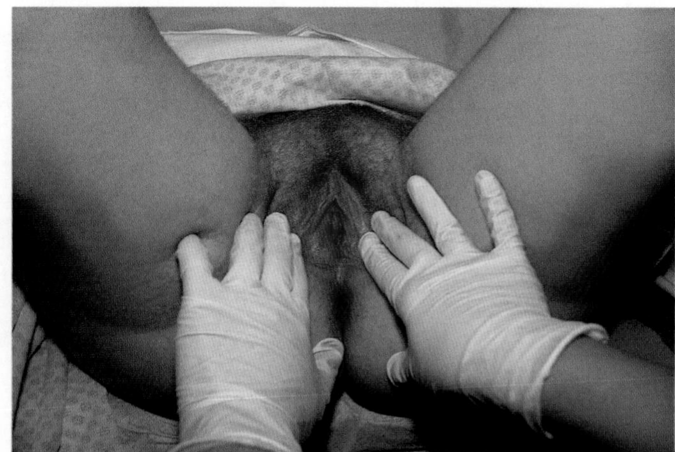

FIGURE 6-12 External examination. Separation of the labia. (From Wilson, S. F., & Giddens, J. F. [2013]. *Health assessment for nursing practice* [5th ed.]. St. Louis: Mosby.)

CRITICAL THINKING CASE STUDY

Caring for an Adolescent Having Her First Pelvic Examination

Nita, a 16-year-old adolescent, who has recently had sex for the first time with her boyfriend, comes to the clinic for information about birth control. Before prescribing any contraceptives, the nurse practitioner suggests that she perform a pelvic examination. Nita says she has never had one and has heard that they hurt and are "a terrible experience."

QUESTIONS

1. Evidence—Is there sufficient evidence to draw conclusions about the possibility of performing a pain-free pelvic examination on Nita?
2. Assumptions—What assumptions about the following factors can be made about performing a pelvic examination on an adolescent?
   a. Need for confidentiality; the need for a valid consent
   b. The nurse's usual assessment procedure
   c. Equipment needed for pelvic examination of a young girl or woman
   d. Necessary education about sexuality and prevention of sexually transmitted infections and pregnancy
3. What implications and priorities for nursing care can be drawn at this time?
4. Does the evidence objectively support your conclusion?

to alert her that the genital examination is beginning. This gesture may put the woman more at ease. The labia are spread apart to expose the structures in the vestibule: urinary meatus, Skene glands, vaginal orifice, and Bartholin glands (Fig. 6-12). To assess the Skene glands, the examiner inserts one finger into the vagina and "milks" the area of the urethra. Any exudate from the urethra or the Skene glands is cultured. Masses and erythema of either structure are assessed further. Ordinarily the openings to the Skene glands are not visible; prominent openings may be seen if the glands are infected (e.g., with gonorrhea). During the examination, the examiner needs to keep in mind the data from the review of systems, such as history of burning on urination.

The vaginal orifice is then examined. Hymenal tags are normal findings. With one finger still in the vagina, the examiner repositions the index finger near the posterior part of the orifice. With the thumb outside the posterior part of the labia majora, the examiner compresses the area of Bartholin glands located at the 8 o'clock and 4 o'clock positions and looks for swelling, discharge, and pain.

The support of the anterior and posterior vaginal wall is also assessed. The examiner spreads the labia with the index and middle fingers and then asks the woman to strain down. Any bulge from the anterior wall (urethrocele or cystocele) or posterior wall (rectocele) is noted and compared with the history, such as difficulty starting the stream of urine or with constipation.

The perineum (area between the vagina and anus) is assessed for scars from old lacerations or episiotomies, thinning, fistulas, masses, lesions, and inflammation. The anus is assessed for hemorrhoids, hemorrhoidal tags, and integrity of the anal sphincter. The anal area is also assessed for lesions, masses, abscesses, and tumours. If there is a history of STI, the examiner may want to obtain a culture specimen from the anal canal at this time. Throughout the genital examination, the examiner should note any odour, which may indicate infection or poor hygiene.

Internal examination. A vaginal speculum consists of two blades and a handle, and specula come in a variety of types and styles. A vaginal speculum is used to view the vaginal vault and cervix. The speculum is gently placed into the vagina and inserted to the back of the vaginal vault. The blades are opened to reveal the cervix and are locked into the open position. The cervix is inspected for position and appearance of the os: colour, lesions, bleeding, and discharge (Fig. 6-13, A to D). Cervical findings that are not within normal limits include ulcerations, masses, inflammation, and excessive protrusion into the vaginal vault. Anomalies such as a cockscomb (a protrusion over the cervix that looks like a rooster's comb), a hooded or collared cervix (seen in diethylstilbestrol daughters), or polyps should be noted.

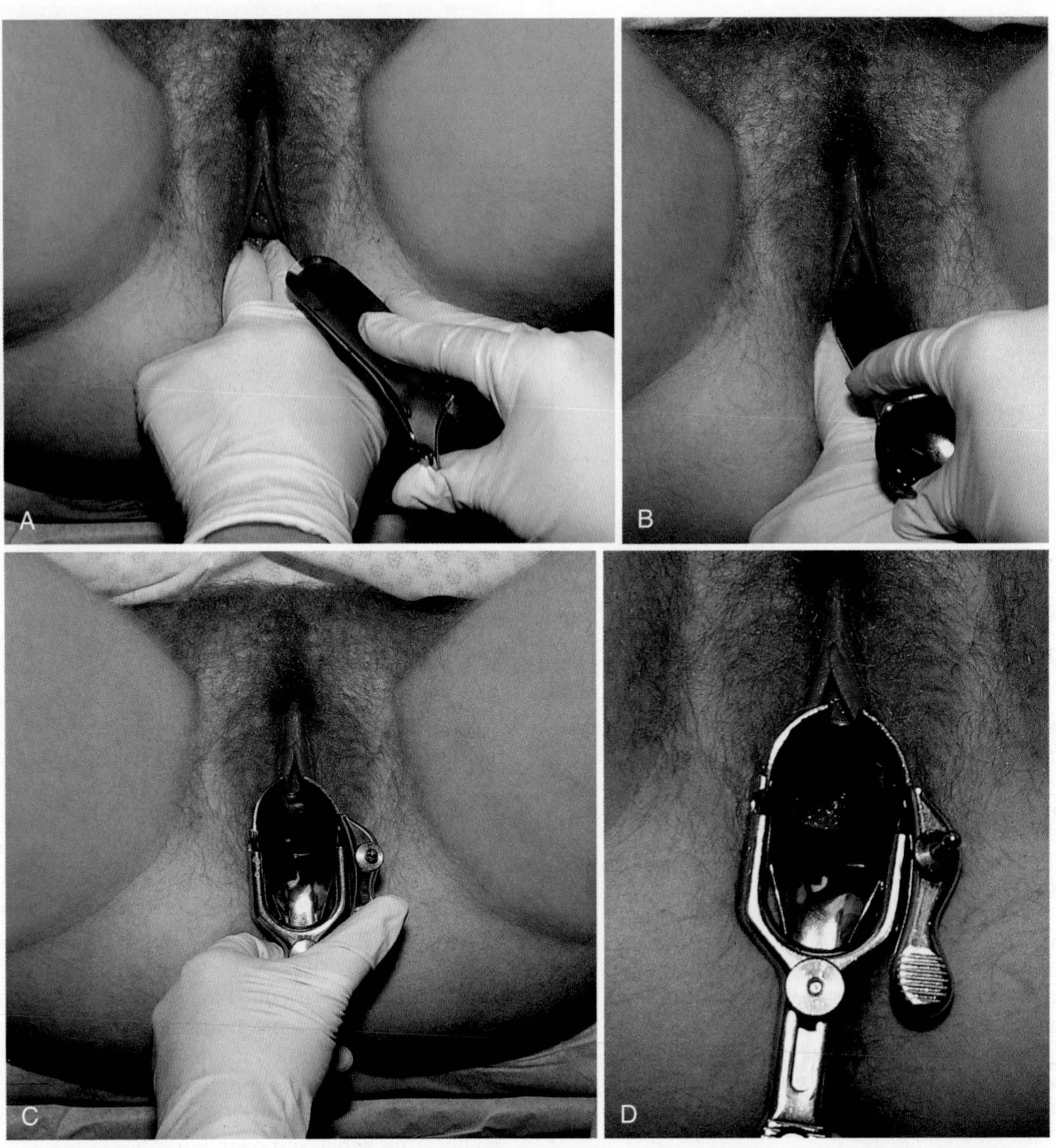

FIGURE 6-13 Insertion of speculum for vaginal examination. **A:** Opening of the introitus. **B:** Oblique insertion of the speculum. **C:** Final insertion of the speculum. **D:** Opening of the speculum blades. (From Wilson, S. F., & Giddens, J. F. [2013]. *Health assessment for nursing practice* [5th ed.]. St. Louis: Mosby.)

BOX 6-3 PROCEDURE: PAPANICOLAOU TEST

1. In preparation, make sure that the woman has not douched, used vaginal medications, or had sexual intercourse for at least 24 hours before the procedure. Reschedule the test if the woman is menstruating. Midcycle is the best time to test.
2. Explain to the woman the purpose of the test and what sensations she will feel as the specimen is obtained (e.g., pressure but not pain).
3. Assist the woman into a position that is most comfortable for her (usually lithotomy). A speculum is then inserted into the vagina.
4. The cytological specimen is obtained before any digital examination of the vagina is made or endocervical bacteriological specimens are taken. A cotton swab may be used to remove excess cervical discharge before the specimen is collected.
5. The specimen is obtained by using an endocervical sampling device (Cytobrush, Cervex-Brush, papette, or broom) (see Fig. 6-14). If the two-sample method of obtaining cells is used, the cytobrush is inserted into the canal and rotated 90 to 180 degrees, followed by a gentle smear of the entire transformation zone using a spatula. Broom devices are inserted and rotated 360 degrees 5 times. They obtain endocervical and ectocervical samples at the same time. If the patient has had a hysterectomy, the vaginal cuff is sampled. Areas that appear abnormal on visualization require colposcopy and biopsy. If using a one-slide technique, the spatula sample is smeared first. This is followed by applying the Cytobrush sample (rolling the brush in the opposite direction from which it was obtained), which is less subject to drying artifact; the slide is then sprayed with preservative within 5 seconds.
6. The ThinPrep Pap test is a liquid-based method of preserving cells that reduces blood, mucus, and inflammation. The Pap specimen is obtained in the manner described above except that the cervix is not swabbed before collection of the sample. The collection device (brush, spatula, or broom) is rinsed in a vial of preserving solution that is provided by the laboratory. The sealed vial with solution is sent off to the appropriate laboratory. A special processing device filters the contents, and a thin layer of cervical cells is deposited on a slide, which is then examined microscopically. The Papnet test is similar to the ThinPrep test. If cytology is abnormal, liquid-based methods allow follow-up testing for human papillomavirus (HPV) DNA with the same sample.
7. Label the slides or vial with the woman's name and site. Include on the form to accompany the slides the woman's name, age, last menstrual period, and parity and the reason for taking the cytological specimens.
8. Send specimens to the pathology laboratory promptly for staining, evaluation, and a written report, with special reference to abnormal elements, including cancer cells.
9. Advise the woman that repeat tests may be necessary if the specimen is not adequate.
10. Instruct the woman about routine checkups for cervical and vaginal cancer. It is recommended that Pap tests be initiated by age 25 and done every 3 years for women with no risk factors, although different provinces may have different guidelines. Women with abnormal Pap results need more frequent testing. Pap screening can be discontinued in a woman who is 70 years old and has had three negative smears in the past 10 years (Canadian Task Force on Preventative Health, 2013).
11. Record the examination date on the woman's record.

Source: Canadian Task Force on Preventative Health, 2013. Recommendations on screening for cervical cancer. *Canadian Medical Association Journal, 185*(1), 35–45. Retrieved from http://www.cmaj.ca/content/185/1/35.full

Collection of specimens. The collection of specimens for cytological examination is an important part of the gynecological examination. Infection can be diagnosed by examination of specimens collected during the pelvic examination. These infections include candidiasis, trichomoniasis, bacterial vaginosis, group B streptococcus, gonorrhea, chlamydia, and herpes simplex virus. Once the diagnoses have been made, treatment can be instituted (see discussion in Chapter 7).

Papanicolaou test. Carcinogenic conditions, whether potential or actual, can be determined by examination of cells from the cervix collected during the pelvic examination (i.e., a Pap test) (Box 6-3 and Fig. 6-14).

Vaginal wall examination. After the specimens are obtained, the vagina is viewed when the speculum is rotated. The speculum blades are unlocked and partially closed. As the speculum is withdrawn it is rotated; the vaginal walls are inspected for colour, lesions, rugae, fistulas, and bulging.

Bimanual palpation. The examiner stands for this part of the examination. A small amount of lubricant is placed on the first and second fingers of the gloved hand for the internal examination. To avoid tissue trauma and contamination, the thumb is abducted, and the ring and little fingers are flexed into the palm (Fig. 6-15).

The vagina is palpated for distensibility, lesions, and tenderness. The cervix is examined for position, shape, consistency, motility, and lesions. The fornix around the cervix is palpated.

The other hand is placed on the abdomen halfway between the umbilicus and symphysis pubis and exerts pressure downward toward the pelvic hand. Upward pressure from the pelvic hand traps reproductive structures for assessment by palpation. The uterus is assessed for position, size, shape, consistency, regularity, motility, masses, and tenderness.

With the abdominal hand moving to the right lower quadrant and the fingers of the pelvic hand in the right lateral fornix, the adnexa is assessed for position, size, tenderness, and masses. The examination is repeated on the woman's left side.

Just before the intravaginal fingers are withdrawn, the woman is asked to tighten her vagina around the fingers as much as she can. If the muscle response is weak, the woman is assessed for her knowledge about Kegel exercises.

Rectovaginal palpation. To prevent contamination of the rectum from organisms in the vagina, it is necessary to change

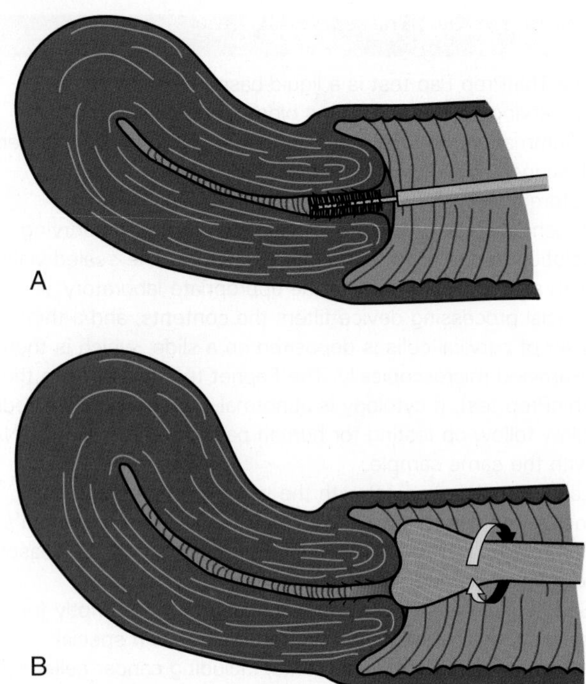

FIGURE 6-14 Pap test. **A:** Collecting cells from the endocervix using a cytobrush. **B:** Obtaining cells from the transformation zone using a wooden spatula. (From Lentz, G. M., Lobe, R. A., Gershenson, D. M., et al. [2012]. *Comprehensive gynecology* [6th ed.]. St. Louis: Mosby.)

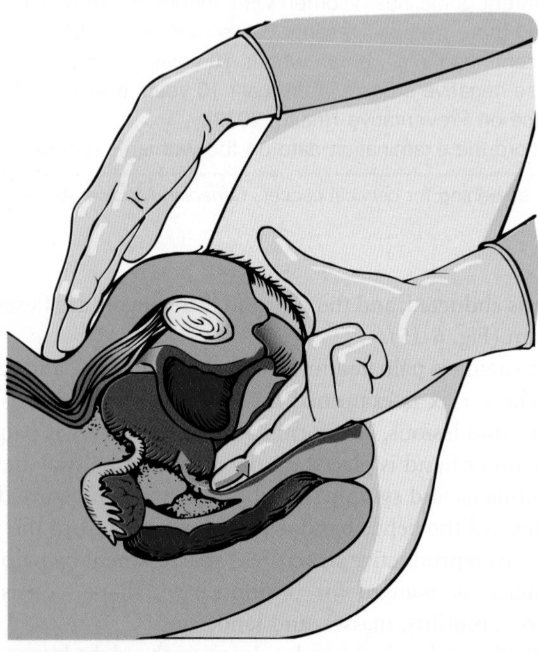

FIGURE 6-15 Bimanual palpation of the uterus. (From Seidel, H. M., Stewart, R. W., Ball, J. W., et al. [2011]. *Mosby's guide to physical examination* [7th ed., p. 566]. St. Louis: Mosby.)

gloves, add fresh lubricant, and then reinsert the index finger into the vagina and the middle finger into the rectum (Fig. 6-16). Insertion is facilitated if the woman strains down. The manoeuvres of the abdominovaginal examination are repeated. The rectovaginal examination enables assessment of the rectovaginal septum, the posterior surface of the uterus, and the

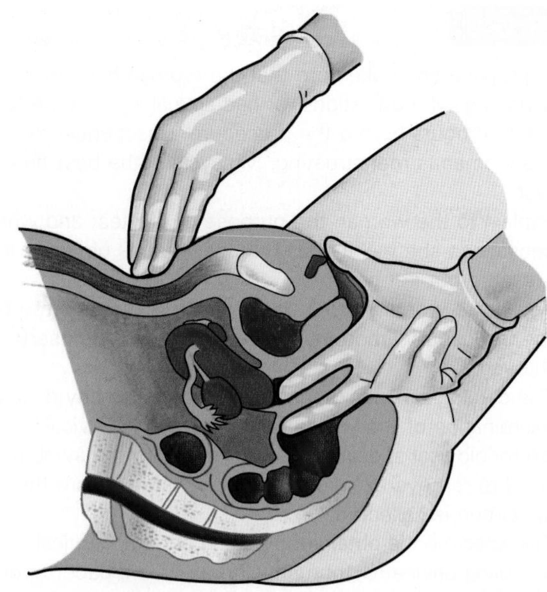

FIGURE 6-16 Rectovaginal examination. (From Seidel, H. M., Stewart, R. W., Ball, J. W., et al. [2011]. *Mosby's guide to physical examination* [7th ed., p. 568]. St. Louis: Mosby.)

region behind the cervix and the adnexa. The vaginal finger is removed and folded into the palm, leaving the middle finger free to rotate 360 degrees. The rectum is palpated for rectal tenderness and masses.

After the rectal examination is completed, the woman should be assisted into a sitting position, given tissues or wipes to cleanse herself, and given privacy to dress. The examiner returns after the woman is dressed, to discuss findings and the plan of care.

Pelvic examination during pregnancy. The pelvic examination during pregnancy is done in the same way as during a routine examination on a nonpregnant woman. Pelvic measurements are completed, and uterine size is estimated. A Pap test may be done initially and cytological specimens collected to test for gonorrhea, chlamydia, human papillomavirus, herpes simplex virus, and group B streptococcus.

While the pregnant woman is in lithotomy position, the nurse must watch for supine hypotension (decrease in blood pressure) caused by the weight of the uterus pressing on the vena cava and aorta. Symptoms of supine hypotension include pallor, dizziness, faintness, breathlessness, tachycardia, nausea, clammy skin, and sweating. The woman should be positioned on her side until symptoms resolve and vital signs stabilize. The vaginal examination can be done with the woman in lateral position.

Pelvic examination after hysterectomy. The pelvic examination after hysterectomy is done in much the same way as on a woman with a uterus. Vaginal screening using the Pap test is not recommended in women who have had a total hysterectomy with removal of the cervix for benign disease.

Vulvar self-examination. Approximately 15% of women who see a health care practitioner have some type of vulvar disease (Sexualityandu, 2012). The pelvic examination provides a good opportunity for the practitioner to emphasize the importance of regular *vulvar self-examination (VSE)* and to teach this procedure. VSE should be an integral part of preventive health care for all women who are sexually active or 18 years of age or older (Sexualityandu, 2012). VSE should be performed between menses, preferably monthly. Most lesions, including malignancy, condyloma acuminatum (wart-like growth), and Bartholin cysts, can be seen or palpated and are easily treated if diagnosed early.

It is important that women know what is normal so they can detect any changes. The VSE can be performed by the practitioner and woman together by using a mirror. A woman should be taught to perform the examination in a sitting position with adequate lighting, holding a mirror in one hand and using the other hand to expose the tissues surrounding the vaginal introitus. She then systematically examines the mons pubis, clitoris, urethra, labia majora, perineum, and perianal area and palpates the vulva, noting any changes in appearance or abnormalities, such as ulcers, lumps, warts, and changes in pigmentation.

Laboratory and Diagnostic Procedures

The following laboratory and diagnostic procedures are ordered at the discretion of the clinician, considering the patient and family history: hemoglobin, glycosalated hemoglobin ($HgbA_{1C}$), fasting blood glucose, total blood cholesterol, lipid profile, urinalysis, syphilis serology (Venereal Disease Research Laboratories [VDRL] or rapid plasma reagent [RPR]) and other screening tests for STIs, mammogram, tuberculosis skin testing, hearing, visual acuity, electrocardiogram, chest radiograph, pulmonary function, fecal occult blood, flexible sigmoidoscopy, and bone mineral density (dual energy X-ray absorptiometry [DEXA] scan). Results of these tests may be reported in person, by phone call, or by letter. Tests for HIV, hepatitis B, and drug screening may be offered with informed consent in high-risk populations. These test results are usually reported in person.

KEY POINTS

- The female's reproductive tract structures and breasts respond predictably to changing levels of sex steroids across her lifespan.
- The myometrium of the uterus is uniquely designed to expel the fetus and promote hemostasis after birth.
- Health promotion and illness prevention help women to actualize their health potential by increasing motivation, providing information, and suggesting how to access specific resources.
- Periodic health screening, including history, physical examination, and diagnostic and laboratory tests, provides the basis for overall health promotion, prevention of illness, early diagnosis of problems, and referral for management.
- Health screening needs to be performed in a way that is culturally sensitive.
- Routine screening mammography and annual breast examinations by skilled practitioners are recommended for early detection of breast cancer.

evolve WEBSITE

Visit the Evolve website for additional resources related to the content in this chapter such as Case Studies, Critical Thinking Case Study Answers, Nursing Care Plans, Nursing Processes, Nursing Skills, and Review Questions for Exam Preparation at: *http://evolve.elsevier.com/Canada/Perry/maternal/*

REFERENCES

Ball, J. W., Dains, J. A., Flynn, J. A., et al. (2014). *Mosby's guide to physical examination* (8th ed.). St. Louis: Mosby.

Canadian Cancer Society. (2014). *Breast cancer*. Screening for breast cancer. Retrieved from <http://www.cancer.ca/en/cancer-information/cancer-type/breast/screening/?region=on>.

Canadian Nurses Association. (2010). *Position statement: Promoting cultural competence in nursing*. Ottawa: Author. Retrieved from <http://www.cna-aiic.ca/~/media/cna/page-content/pdf-en/ps114_cultural_competence_2010_e.pdf?la=en>.

Canadian Task Force on Preventative Health. (2013). Recommendations on screening for cervical cancer. *Canadian Medical Association Journal, 185*(1), 35–45. Retrieved from <http://www.cmaj.ca/content/185/1/35.full>.

Fawcet, T., & Rhynas, S. (2012). Taking a patient history: The role of the nurse. *Nursing Standard, 26*(24), 41–46.

LGBT Health Program. (2015). *Guidelines and protocols for hormone therapy and primary health care for trans clients*. Toronto: Sherbourne Health Centre. Retrieved from <http://sherbourne.on.ca/wp-content/uploads/2014/02/Guidelines-and-Protocols-for-Comprehensive-Primary-Care-for-Trans-Clients-2015.pdf>.

Rabin, R. F., Jennings, J. M., Campbell, J. C., et al. (2009). Intimate partner violence screening tools: A systematic review. *American Journal of Preventative Medicine, 36*(5), 439–445.

Sexualityandu. (2012). *What are vulvar diseases?* Retrieved from <http://www.sexualityandu.ca/sexual-health/physical-problems/what-is-a-vulvar-disease>.

Society of Obstetricians and Gynaecologists of Canada. (2006). Breast self-examination. *Journal of Obstetrics and Gynaecology Canada, 28*(8), 728–730.

ADDITIONAL RESOURCES

Rainbow Health Ontario—LGBTQ health matters: <http//www.rainbowhealthontario.ca>

Rainbow Health Ontario—Tips for providing paps to trans men: <http://www.rainbowhealthontario.ca/wp-content/uploads/woocommerce_uploads/2014/09/Tips_Paps_TransMen.pdf>

CHAPTER

7

Reproductive Health

Lisa Keenan-Lindsay

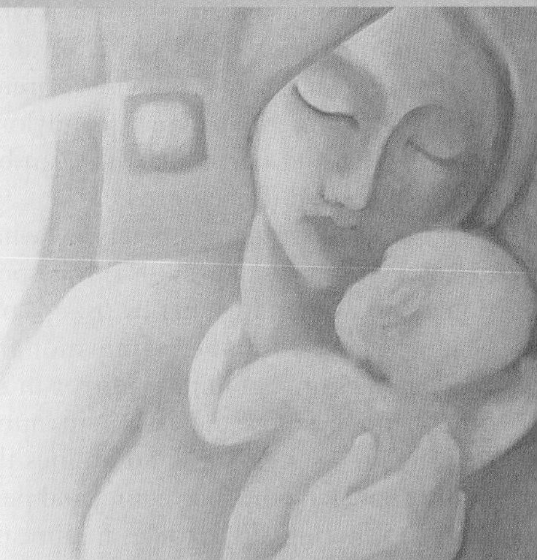

evolve WEBSITE

Visit the Evolve website for additional resources related to the content in this chapter such as Case Studies, Critical Thinking Case Study Answers, Nursing Care Plans, Nursing Processes, Nursing Skills, and Review Questions for Exam Preparation at: http://evolve.elsevier.com/Canada/Perry/maternal/

OBJECTIVES

On completion of this chapter the reader will be able to:

- Differentiate the menstrual cycle in relation to endometrial, hormonal, and ovarian responses.
- Differentiate among the signs and symptoms of common menstrual disorders.
- Develop a nursing care plan for the woman with primary dysmenorrhea.
- Outline patient teaching about premenstrual syndrome.
- Relate the pathophysiology of endometriosis to associated symptoms.
- Describe the etiology, significance, and management of abnormal uterine bleeding.
- Describe treatment for menopause symptoms.
- Describe prevention and treatment of sexually transmitted infections in women.
- Summarize the care of women with selected viral infections (i.e., human immunodeficiency virus and hepatitis B virus).
- Differentiate signs, symptoms, and management of selected vaginal infections.
- Discuss the pathophysiology and emotional effects of selected benign breast conditions and malignant neoplasms of the breasts that are found in women.

Health issues may occur at any point in a woman's life, especially during the reproductive years. Many factors, including anatomical abnormalities, physiological imbalances, and lifestyle, can affect the menstrual cycle. The average woman may have some concerns related to her menstrual and gynecological health at some point in her life and may experience bleeding, pain, discharge, or infections associated with her reproductive organs or functions. This chapter provides information on the menstrual cycle, common menstrual problems, sexually transmitted infections, and selected other infections that can affect reproductive functions. Benign breast conditions are also discussed. Breast cancer is addressed in this chapter because it is the most common reproductive cancer occurring in women.

MENSTRUATION

Menarche and Puberty

Young girls secrete small, rather constant amounts of estrogen, but a marked increase in secretion occurs between 8 and 11 years of age. The term **menarche** denotes first menstruation. **Puberty** is a broader term that denotes the entire transitional stage between childhood and sexual maturity. Increasing amounts and variations in gonadotropin and estrogen secretion develop into a cyclic pattern at least a year before menarche. In North America this occurs in most girls at about 13 years of age.

Initially, menstrual periods are irregular, unpredictable, painless, and anovulatory (no ovum is released from the ovary).

After 1 or more years, a hypothalamic–pituitary rhythm develops, and the ovary produces adequate cyclic estrogen to make a mature ovum. Ovulatory (ovum released from the ovary) periods tend to be regular, with estrogen dominating the first half of the cycle and progesterone dominating the second half of the cycle.

Although pregnancy can occur in exceptional cases of true precocious puberty, most pregnancies in young girls occur after the normally timed menarche. It is important that young adolescents of both sexes are informed that pregnancy can occur at any time after the onset of menses.

Menstrual Cycle

Menstruation is the periodic uterine bleeding that begins approximately 14 days after ovulation. It is controlled by a feedback system of three cycles: endometrial, hypothalamic–pituitary, and ovarian. The average length of a menstrual cycle is 28 days, but variations are normal. The first day of bleeding is designated as day 1 of the menstrual cycle, or menses (Fig. 7-1). The average duration of menstrual flow is 5 days (with a range of 3 to 6 days), and the average blood loss is 50 mL (with a range of 20 to 80 mL), but these vary greatly.

The menstrual blood clots within the uterus, but the clot usually liquefies before being discharged from the uterus. Uterine discharge includes mucus and epithelial cells in addition to blood.

The menstrual cycle is a complex interplay of events that occur simultaneously in the endometrium, the hypothalamus, the pituitary glands, and the ovaries. The menstrual cycle prepares the uterus for pregnancy. When pregnancy does not occur, menstruation follows. A woman's age, physical and emotional status, and environment influence the regularity of her menstrual cycles.

Endometrial Cycle

The four phases of the endometrial cycle are (1) the menstrual phase, (2) the proliferative phase, (3) the secretory phase, and (4) the ischemic phase (see Fig. 7-1). During the menstrual phase shedding of the functional two-thirds of the endometrium (the compact and spongy layers) is initiated by periodic vasoconstriction in the upper layers of the endometrium. The basal layer is always retained, and regeneration begins near the end of the cycle from cells derived from the remaining glandular remnants or stromal cells in this layer.

The proliferative phase is a period of rapid growth lasting from about the fifth day to the time of ovulation. The endometrial surface is completely restored in approximately 4 days, or slightly before bleeding ceases. From this point on, an 8-fold to 10-fold thickening occurs, with a levelling off of growth at ovulation. The proliferative phase depends on estrogen stimulation derived from ovarian follicles.

The secretory phase extends from the day of ovulation to about 3 days before the next menstrual period. After ovulation, larger amounts of progesterone are produced. An edematous, vascular, functional endometrium is now apparent. At the end of the secretory phase, the fully matured secretory endometrium reaches the thickness of heavy, soft velvet. It becomes luxuriant with blood and glandular secretions, a suitable protective and nutritive bed for a fertilized ovum.

Implantation of the fertilized ovum generally occurs about 7 to 10 days after ovulation. If fertilization and implantation do not occur, the corpus luteum, which secretes estrogen and progesterone, regresses. With the rapid decrease in progesterone and estrogen levels, the spiral arteries go into spasm. During the ischemic phase, the blood supply to the functional endometrium is blocked and necrosis develops. The functional layer separates from the basal layer, and menstrual bleeding begins, marking day 1 of the next cycle (see Fig. 7-1).

Hypothalamic–Pituitary Cycle

Toward the end of the normal menstrual cycle, blood levels of estrogen and progesterone decrease. Low blood levels of these ovarian hormones stimulate the hypothalamus to secrete gonadotropin-releasing hormone (GnRH). In turn, GnRH stimulates anterior pituitary secretion of follicle-stimulating hormone (FSH). FSH stimulates development of ovarian graafian follicles and their production of estrogen. Estrogen levels begin to decrease, and hypothalamic GnRH triggers the anterior pituitary to release luteinizing hormone (LH). A marked surge of LH and a smaller peak of estrogen (day 12) (see Fig. 7-1) precede the expulsion of the ovum from the graafian follicle by about 24 to 36 hours. LH peaks at about day 13 or 14 of a 28-day cycle. If fertilization and implantation of the ovum have not occurred by this time, regression of the corpus luteum follows. Levels of progesterone and estrogen decline, menstruation occurs, and the hypothalamus is once again stimulated to secrete GnRH. This process is called the *hypothalamic–pituitary cycle.*

Ovarian Cycle

The primitive graafian follicles contain immature oocytes (primordial ova). Before ovulation, from 1 to 30 follicles begin to mature in each ovary under the influence of FSH and estrogen. The preovulatory surge of LH affects a selected follicle. The oocyte matures, ovulation occurs, and the empty follicle begins its transformation into the corpus luteum. This follicular phase (preovulatory phase) (see Fig. 7-1) of the ovarian cycle varies in length from woman to woman. Almost all variations in ovarian cycle length are the result of variations in the length of the follicular phase. On rare occasions (i.e., 1 in 100 menstrual cycles) more than one follicle is selected, and more than one oocyte matures and undergoes ovulation.

After ovulation, estrogen levels drop. For 90% of women only a small amount of withdrawal bleeding occurs, and it goes unnoticed. In 10% of women there is sufficient bleeding for it to be visible, resulting in what is termed *midcycle bleeding.*

The luteal phase begins immediately after ovulation and ends with the start of menstruation. This postovulatory phase of the ovarian cycle usually requires 14 days (range 13 to 15 days). The corpus luteum reaches its peak of functional activity 8 days after ovulation, secreting the steroids estrogen and progesterone. Coincident with this time of peak luteal functioning, the fertilized ovum is implanted in the endometrium. If no implantation occurs, the corpus luteum regresses, and steroid levels drop. Two weeks after ovulation, if fertilization and

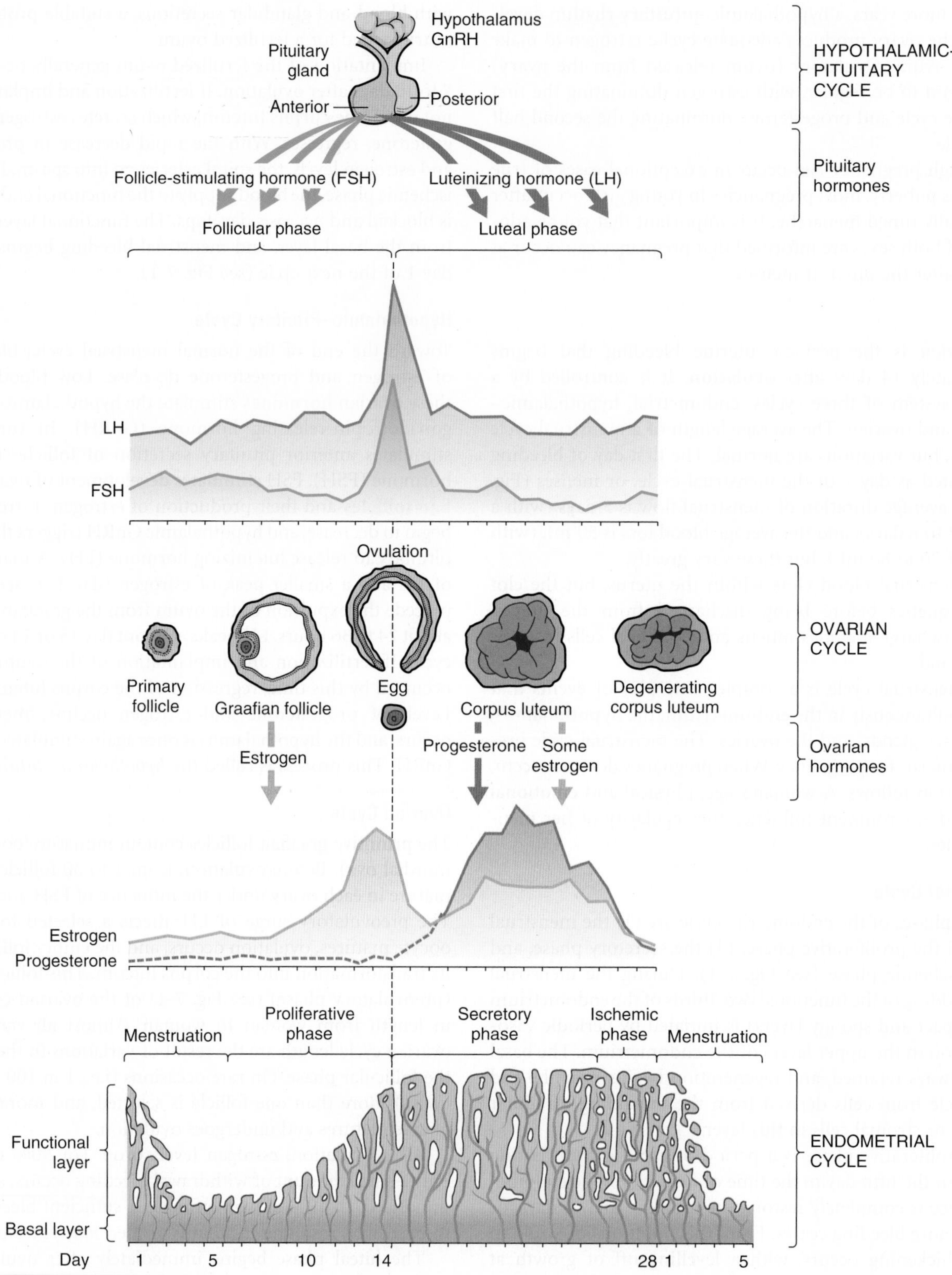

FIGURE 7-1 Menstrual cycle: hypothalamic–pituitary, ovarian, and endometrial. *GnRH*, gonadotropin-releasing hormone.

implantation do not occur, the functional layer of the uterine endometrium is shed through menstruation.

Other Cyclic Changes

When the hypothalamic–pituitary–ovarian axis functions properly, other tissues undergo predictable responses. Before ovulation, the woman's **basal body temperature** is often less than 37°C; after ovulation, with increasing progesterone levels, her basal body temperature rises. Changes in the cervix and cervical mucus follow a generally predictable pattern. Preovulatory and postovulatory mucus is viscous (thick) so that sperm penetration is discouraged. At the time of ovulation, cervical mucus is thin and clear. It looks, feels, and stretches like egg white. This stretchable quality is termed **spinnbarkeit**. Some women have localized lower abdominal pain, called **mittelschmerz** that coincides with ovulation. Some spotting may occur.

Prostaglandins

Prostaglandins (PGs) are oxygenated fatty acids classified as hormones. The different kinds of prostaglandins are distinguished by letters (PGE and PGF), numbers (PGE_2), and letters of the Greek alphabet ($PGF_{2\alpha}$).

PGs are produced in most organs of the body, including the uterus. Menstrual blood is a potent PG source. PGs are metabolized quickly by most tissues. They are biologically active in minute amounts in the cardiovascular, gastrointestinal, respiratory, urogenital, and nervous systems. They also exert a marked effect on metabolism, particularly on glycolysis. PGs play an important role in many physiological, pathological, and pharmacological reactions.

PGs affect smooth muscle contractility and modulation of hormonal activity. Indirect evidence indicates that PGs have an effect on ovulation, fertility, changes in the cervix and cervical mucus that affect receptivity to sperm, tubal and uterine motility, sloughing of endometrium (menstruation), onset of miscarriage and induced abortion, and onset of labour (term and preterm).

After exerting their biological actions, newly synthesized PGs are rapidly metabolized by tissues in such organs as the lungs, kidneys, and liver.

PGs may play a key role in ovulation. If PG levels do not rise along with the surge of LH, the ovum remains trapped within the graafian follicle. After ovulation PGs may influence production of estrogen and progesterone by the corpus luteum.

The introduction of PGs into the vagina or the uterine cavity (from ejaculated semen) increases the motility of uterine musculature, which may assist the transport of sperm through the uterus and into the oviduct.

PGs produced by the woman cause regression of the corpus luteum and regression and sloughing of the endometrium, resulting in menstruation. PGs increase myometrial response to oxytocic stimulation, enhance uterine contractions, and cause cervical dilation. They may be a factor in the initiation of labour, the maintenance of labour, or both. They may also be involved in dysmenorrhea (see discussion later in chapter) and preeclampsia and eclampsia (see Chapter 14).

MENSTRUAL CYCLE CONCERNS

Generally, a woman's menstrual frequency stabilizes at 28 days within 1 to 2 years after puberty, with a range of 26 to 34 days. Although no woman's cycle is exactly the same length every month, the typical month-to-month variation in an individual's cycle is usually plus or minus 2 days. However, greater but still normal variations are commonly noted.

Women typically have menstrual cycles for about 40 years. Once a cyclic, predictable pattern of monthly bleeding is established, women may worry about any deviation from that pattern or from what they have been told is normal for all menstruating women. A woman may be concerned about her ability to conceive and bear children or believe that she is not really a woman without monthly evidence. A sign such as amenorrhea or excess menstrual bleeding can be a source of severe distress and concern for a woman.

Amenorrhea

Amenorrhea, the absence of menstrual flow, is a clinical sign of a variety of conditions. Generally the following circumstances should be evaluated: (1) the absence of both menarche and secondary sexual characteristics by age 13 years; (2) the absence of menses by age 16.5 years, regardless of normal growth and development (primary amenorrhea); or (3) a 6-month cessation of menses after a period of menstruation (secondary amenorrhea) (Lobo, 2012a).

A moderately obese girl (20 to 30% above ideal weight) may have early-onset menstruation, whereas delay of onset is known to be related to malnutrition (starvation, such as that with anorexia). Girls who exercise strenuously before menarche can have delayed onset of menstruation until about age 18 (Lobo, 2012a).

Although amenorrhea is not a disease, it is often a sign of disease. It may occur from any defect or interruption in the hypothalamic–pituitary–ovarian–uterine axis (see Fig 7-1). It may also result from anatomical abnormalities, other endocrine disorders such as hypothyroidism or hyperthyroidism, chronic diseases such as type 1 diabetes, medications such as phenytoin (Dilantin), illicit drug use (opiates, marijuana, cocaine), eating disorders, strenuous exercise, emotional stress, and oral contraceptive use. Secondary amenorrhea is commonly the result of pregnancy.

Assessment of amenorrhea begins with a thorough history and physical examination. An important initial step is to be sure that the woman is not pregnant. Specific components of the assessment process depend on a patient's age—adolescent, young adult, or perimenopausal—and whether she has previously menstruated.

Hypogonadotropic Amenorrhea

Hypogonadotropic amenorrhea reflects a problem in the central hypothalamic–pituitary axis. In rare instances a pituitary lesion or genetic inability to produce FSH and LH is at fault.

Hypogonadotropic amenorrhea often results from hypothalamic suppression as a result of stress (in the home, school, or workplace) or a sudden and severe weight loss, eating disorders, strenuous exercise, or mental illness (Wambach & Alexander,

2012). Research on the interaction between nervous system or neurotransmitter functions and hormone regulation throughout the body has demonstrated a biological basis for the relation of stress to physiological processes. Women who are more than 20% underweight for height or who have had rapid weight loss and women with eating disorders such as anorexia nervosa may report amenorrhea. Amenorrhea is one of the classic signs of anorexia nervosa, and the interrelation of disordered eating, amenorrhea, and premature osteoporosis has been described as the *female athlete triad* (George, Leonard, & Hutchinson, 2011) (http://www.bodysense.ca/files/pdfs/BS-FemaleAthleteTriad-E.pdf). A loss of calcium from the bone, comparable to that seen in postmenopausal women, may occur with this type of amenorrhea.

Exercise-associated amenorrhea can occur in women undergoing vigorous physical and athletic training and is thought to be associated with many factors, including body composition (height, weight, and percentage of body fat); type, intensity, and frequency of exercise; nutritional status; and presence of emotional or physical stressors. Women who participate in sports emphasizing low body weight are at greatest risk, including the following:

- Sports in which performance is subjectively scored (e.g., dance, gymnastics)
- Endurance sports favouring participants with low body weight (e.g., distance running, cycling)
- Sports in which body contour–revealing clothing is worn (e.g., swimming, diving, volleyball)
- Sports with weight categories for participation (e.g., rowing, martial arts)
- Sports in which prepubertal body shape favours success (e.g., gymnastics, figure skating)

An important initial step, often overlooked, is to be sure that the woman is not pregnant. Once pregnancy has been ruled out by a β-human chorionic gonadotropin (hCG) pregnancy test, diagnostic tests may include FSH level, thyroid-stimulating hormone (TSH) and prolactin levels, radiographic or computed tomography (CT) scan of the sella turcica, and a progestational challenge (Lobo, 2012a).

Management. When amenorrhea is caused by hypothalamic disturbances, the nurse is an ideal health professional to assist women with this condition. Many of the causes are potentially reversible (e.g., stress, weight loss for nonorganic reasons). Counselling and education are primary interventions and appropriate nursing roles. When a stressor known to predispose a woman to hypothalamic amenorrhea is identified, initial management involves addressing the stressor. Together, the woman and nurse plan how the woman can decrease or discontinue medications known to affect menstruation, correct weight loss, deal more effectively with psychological stress, address emotional distress, and alter exercise routine.

The nurse can work with the woman to help her identify, cope with, and eliminate sources of stress in her life. Deep-breathing exercises and relaxation techniques are simple yet effective stress-reduction measures. Referral for biofeedback or massage therapy also may be useful. In some instances, referrals for psychotherapy may be indicated.

If a woman's exercise program is thought to contribute to her amenorrhea, several options exist for management. She may decide to decrease the intensity or duration of her training or to modify her diet to include the appropriate nutrition for her age. Accepting the former alternative may be difficult for a person who is committed to a strenuous exercise regimen. The woman and nurse may have several sessions before the woman elects to try exercise reduction. Many young female athletes may not understand the consequences of low bone density or osteoporosis; nurses can point out the connection between low bone density and stress fractures. The nurse and woman should also investigate other factors that may be contributing to the amenorrhea and develop plans for altering lifestyle and decreasing stress.

Although research on effectiveness is inconclusive, a daily calcium intake of 1200 to 1500 mg plus 400 to 800 International Units of vitamin D and 60 to 90 mg of potassium are recommended for women experiencing amenorrhea associated with the female athlete triad. Oral contraceptives have a positive effect on bone density in amenorrheic women but are usually not used in young women with amenorrhea associated with female athlete triad unless the woman is unable to come to terms with dietary and exercise recommendations or she continues to be amenorrheic even when following recommendations (Joy, 2012).

Dysmenorrhea

Dysmenorrhea, or pain during or shortly before menstruation, is one of the most common gynecological problems in women of all ages. Most adolescents have dysmenorrhea in the first 3 years after menarche. Young adult women ages 17 to 24 are most likely to report painful menses. Approximately 75% of women report some level of discomfort associated with menses, and approximately 15% report severe dysmenorrhea (Lentz, 2012); however, the amount of disruption in women's lives is difficult to determine. Menstrual problems, including dysmenorrhea, are relatively more common in women who smoke and are obese. Severe dysmenorrhea is also associated with early menarche, nulliparity, and stress (Lentz, 2012). Symptoms usually begin with menstruation, although some women have discomfort several hours before onset of flow. The range and severity of symptoms are different from woman to woman and from cycle to cycle in the same woman. Symptoms of dysmenorrhea may last several hours or several days.

Pain is usually located in the suprapubic area or lower abdomen. Women describe the pain as sharp, cramping, or gripping or as a steady dull ache. For some women pain radiates to the lower back or upper thighs. Traditionally dysmenorrhea is differentiated as primary or secondary.

Primary Dysmenorrhea

Primary dysmenorrhea is a condition associated with ovulatory cycles. Research has shown that primary dysmenorrhea has a biochemical basis and arises from the release of prostaglandins with menses. During the luteal phase and subsequent menstrual flow, prostaglandin F_2-alpha ($PGF_{2\alpha}$) is secreted. Excessive release of $PGF_{2\alpha}$ increases the amplitude and frequency of uterine contractions and causes vasospasm of the uterine arterioles, resulting in ischemia and cyclic lower abdominal cramps. Systemic responses to $PGF_{2\alpha}$ include backache, weakness, sweats, gastrointestinal symptoms (anorexia, nausea, vomiting, and diarrhea), and central nervous system symptoms (dizziness, syncope, headache, and poor concentration). Pain usually begins at the onset of menstruation and lasts 8 to 48 hours (Lentz, 2012).

Primary dysmenorrhea is not caused by underlying pathology. Rather, it is the occurrence of a physiological alteration in some women. Primary dysmenorrhea usually appears within 6 to 12 months after menarche when ovulation is established. Anovulatory bleeding, common in the first few months or years after menarche, is painless. Because both estrogen and progesterone are necessary for primary dysmenorrhea to occur, it is experienced only with ovulatory cycles. This problem is most common in women in their late teens and early 20s; the incidence declines with age. Psychogenic factors may influence symptoms, but symptoms are definitely related to ovulation and do not occur when ovulation is suppressed.

Management. Management of primary dysmenorrhea depends on the severity of the problem and an individual woman's response to various treatments. Women with symptoms of primary dysmenorrhea may not seek medical assistance and frequently do not make use of the prescription therapies that are available for a variety of reasons—including the belief that the pain is inevitable or lack of or limited accessibility to a health care provider. Education and support are important components of nursing care. Because menstruation is so closely linked to reproduction and sexuality, menstrual problems such as dysmenorrhea can have a negative influence on a woman's sense of sexuality and self-worth. Nurses can correct myths and misinformation about menstruation and dysmenorrhea by providing facts about what is normal.

Nurses can offer more than one alternative for alleviating menstrual discomfort and dysmenorrhea, which gives women options to try to decide which works best for them (see Critical Thinking Case Study).

Exercise helps relieve menstrual discomfort through increased vasodilation and subsequent decreased ischemia. It also releases endogenous opiates (specifically beta-endorphins), suppresses prostaglandins, and shunts blood flow away from the viscera, resulting in reduced pelvic congestion. One specific exercise that nurses can suggest is pelvic rocking (see Fig. 11-10).

In addition to maintaining good nutrition at all times, specific dietary changes may be helpful in decreasing some of the systemic symptoms associated with dysmenorrhea. Decreased salt and refined-sugar intake in the 7 to 10 days before expected menses may reduce fluid retention. Increasing water intake may serve as a natural diuretic. Including natural diuretics such as asparagus, cranberry juice, peaches, parsley, and watermelon in the diet may help reduce edema and related discomforts. A low-fat vegetarian diet may also help to minimize dysmenorrheal symptoms (Lentz, 2012).

Medications used to treat primary dysmenorrhea in women not desiring contraception include prostaglandin synthesis inhibitors, primarily nonsteroidal anti-inflammatory drugs

CRITICAL THINKING CASE STUDY

Management of Dysmenorrhea

Cheri, 16, has come to the adolescent health clinic for a checkup. She reports that she has "really bad cramps" for the first 2 days of her period. She has been taking Midol Menstrual Complete but says that it does not help "a lot." She wants to know if anything else can be done to relieve her pain. How should the nurse respond?

QUESTIONS

1. Evidence—Is evidence sufficient to draw conclusions about what advice the nurse should give?
2. Assumptions—Describe underlying assumptions about the following issues:
   a. Causes and symptoms of primary dysmenorrhea
   b. Self-help strategies (e.g., comfort measures, medications)
3. What implications and priorities for nursing care can be drawn at this time?
4. Does the evidence objectively support your conclusion?

(NSAIDs) (Lentz, 2012) (Table 7-1). NSAIDs are most effective if started several days before menses or at least by the onset of bleeding. All NSAIDs have potential gastrointestinal side effects, including nausea, vomiting, and indigestion. All women taking NSAIDs should be warned to report dark-coloured stools, which may be an indication of gastrointestinal bleeding. Approximately 80% of dysmenorrheic women obtain relief with prostaglandin inhibitors.

Over-the-counter (OTC) preparations indicated for primary dysmenorrhea contain the same active ingredients (e.g., ibuprofen or naproxen sodium) as those in prescription preparations. However, the labelled recommended dose may be subtherapeutic. Preparations containing acetaminophen are even less effective because acetaminophen does not have the antiprostaglandin properties of NSAIDs.

NURSING ALERT

If one NSAID is ineffective, often a different one may be effective. If the second drug is unsuccessful after a 6-month trial, combined oral contraceptive pills (OCPs) may be used. Women with a history of aspirin sensitivity or allergy should avoid all NSAIDs.

Oral contraceptive pills (OCPs) are a reasonable choice for women who may want to use contraception. The benefits of OCP use are attributed to decreased prostaglandin synthesis associated with an atrophic decidualized endometrium (Lentz, 2012). OCPs are effective in relieving symptoms of primary dysmenorrhea for approximately 90% of women. No single OCP has been shown to be superior to another for the relief of primary dysmenorrhea, including low-dose and extended-cycle OCPs (Lentz, 2012). OCPs are a particularly good choice for therapy because they combine contraception with a positive effect on dysmenorrhea, menstrual flow, and menstrual irregularities. Since OCPs have adverse effects, women may not wish to use them for dysmenorrhea. They may be contraindicated for some women. (See Chapter 8 for a complete discussion of

TABLE 7-1 MEDICATIONS USED TO TREAT DYSMENORRHEA

MEDICATION	RECOMMENED DOSAGE (ORAL)	COMMON ADVERSE EFFECTS	COMMENTS
Diclofenac (Voltaren)	50 mg tid or 100 mg initially, then 50 mg tid up to 150 mg/day	Nausea, diarrhea, constipation, abdominal distress, dyspepsia, heartburn, flatulence, dizziness, tinnitus, itching, rash	Enteric coated; immediate release
Ibuprofen (Motrin, Advil)	200–400 mg q4h up to max 1200 mg/day	See Diclofenac	If GI upset occurs, take with food, milk, or antacids; avoid alcoholic beverages; do not take with aspirin; stop taking and call care provider if rash occurs
Naproxen	500 mg initially, then 150 mg q 6–8 hr up to 1250 mg/day	See Diclofenac	See Ibuprofen
Mefenamic acid	500 mg initially, then 150 mg q 6 hr/day	See Diclofenac	Very potent and effective prostaglandin-synthesis inhibitor; antagonizes already formed prostaglandins; increased incidence of adverse GI effects
Aspirin	3.6–5.4 g/day in divided doses	See Ibuprofen	If GI upset occurs, take with food, milk; avoid alcoholic beverages
Acetaminophen	325–650 mg q4–6h; to maximum 4 g/day	Good GI tolerance Can cause liver damage with 3 or more alcoholic drinks/day	Does not have antiprostaglandin property of NSAIDs

Note: Risk with all NSAIDs is gastrointestinal ulceration, possible bleeding, and prolonged bleeding time. Incidence of adverse effects is dose related. Reported incidence, 3 to 9%. Do not give if patient has hemophilia or bleeding ulcers; do not give if patient has had an allergic or anaphylactic reaction to aspirin or another NSAID; do not give if patient is taking anticoagulant medication.
GI, gastrointestinal; *NSAID,* nonsteroidal anti-inflammatory drug.
(Source: Lentz, G. M. [2012]. Primary and secondary dysmenorrhea, premenstrual syndrome, and premenstrual dysphoric disorder: etiology, diagnosis, and management. In G. M. Lentz, R. A. Lobo, D. M. Gershenson, et al. [Eds.], *Comprehensive gynecology* [6th ed.]. Philadelphia: Mosby; Singh, S., et al., [2013] SOGC clinical practice guideline: Abnormal uterine bleeding in pre-menopausal women. *Journal of Obstetrics and Gynaecology Canada, 35*[5 eSuppl], S1–S28.)

OCPs.) Depot medroxyprogesterone acetate (DMPA) works by suppressing ovulation, which results in relief of dysmenorrhea symptoms. Levonorgestrel intrauterine system (Mirena) is an **intrauterine device (IUD)** that releases progestin inside the uterine cavity, causing a local effect on the endometrium, and can be considered for use with primary dysmenorrhea.

If dysmenorrhea is not relieved by one of the NSAIDs or OCPs, further investigation into the cause of the symptoms is necessary. Conditions associated with dysmenorrhea include Müllerian duct anomalies, **endometriosis**, and pelvic inflammatory disease (PID).

Complementary and alternative medicine (CAM) therapies have become increasingly popular. The use of heat (heating pad or hot bath) minimizes cramping by increasing vasodilation and muscle relaxation and minimizing uterine ischemia. Massaging the lower back can reduce pain by relaxing paravertebral muscles and increasing the pelvic blood supply. Soft, rhythmic rubbing of the abdomen (**effleurage**) is useful because it provides a distraction and an alternative focal point. Biofeedback, transcutaneous electrical nerve stimulation (TENS), progressive relaxation, hatha yoga, acupuncture, hypnosis, guided imagery, reiki, relaxation exercises, and meditation are also used to decrease menstrual discomfort, although evidence is inconclusive to determine their effectiveness (Dehlin & Schuiling, 2013; Lentz, 2012). Other CAM that may be useful in the treatment of primary dysmenorrhea include vitamin B_1, vitamin E, fish oil/vitamin B_{12} combination, magnesium, vitamin B_6, Toki-shakuyaku-san, and Neptune krill oil (Leyland, Casper, Laberge, et al., 2010). Herbal preparations, including Chinese herbal medicine, have long been used for management of menstrual problems, including dysmenorrhea (Table 7-2). However, it is essential that women understand that these therapies are not without potential toxicity and may cause drug interactions.

NURSING ALERT

Nurses must routinely ask women about the use of herbal and other alternative therapies and document their use. Nurses need to be aware of the potential for drug interactions with some herbal therapies.

Secondary Dysmenorrhea

Secondary dysmenorrhea is menstrual pain that develops later in life than primary dysmenorrhea, typically after age 25. It is associated with an underlying pelvic pathology such as adenomyosis, endometriosis, PID, endometrial polyps, or submucous or interstitial myomas (fibroids). Women with secondary dysmenorrhea often have other symptoms that may suggest the underlying cause. For example, heavy menstrual flow with dysmenorrhea suggests a diagnosis of leiomyomata, adenomyosis, or endometrial polyps. Pain associated with endometriosis often begins a few days before menses but can be present at ovulation and continue through the first days of menses or start after menstrual flow has begun. In contrast to primary

TABLE 7-2 HERBAL MEDICINALS TAKEN ORALLY FOR MENSTRUAL DISORDERS		
SYMPTOMS OR INDICATIONS	**HERBAL THERAPY***	**ACTION**
Menstrual cramping, dysmenorrhea	Black haw	Uterine antispasmodic
	Fennel	Uterotonic
	Catnip	Uterine antispasmodic
	Dong quai	Uterotonic; anti-inflammatory
	Ginger	Anti-inflammatory
	Motherwort	Uterotonic
	Wild yam	Uterine antispasmodic
	Valerian	Uterine antispasmodic
	Potentilla	Anti-inflammatory
Premenstrual discomfort, tension	Black cohosh root	Estrogen-like luteinizing hormone suppressant; binds to estrogen receptors
	Chamomile	Antispasmodic
Breast pain	Chaste tree fruit	Decreases prolactin levels
	Bugleweed	Antigonadotropic; decreases prolactin levels
Menorrhea, metrorrhagia	Lady's mantle	Uterotonic
	Raspberry	Uterotonic
	Shepherd's purse	Uterotonic

*Many women's herbs do not have rigorous scientific studies backing their use; most uses and properties of herbs have not been validated by Health Canada.
Data from Annie's Remedy: *Dysmenorrhea—Herbs for painful periods,* 2015, http://www.anniesremedy.com/chart_remedy_dysmenorrhea.php; National Center for Complementary and Alternative Medicine: *Herbs at a glance,* 2016, https://nccih.nih.gov/health/herbsataglance.htm.

dysmenorrhea, the pain of secondary dysmenorrhea is often characterized by dull, lower abdominal aching that radiates to the back or thighs. Often women experience feelings of bloating or pelvic fullness. In addition to a physical examination with a careful pelvic examination, diagnosis may be assisted by ultrasound examination, **dilation and curettage (D&C)**, endometrial biopsy, or laparoscopy.

Treatment is directed toward removal of the underlying pathology. Many of the measures described for pain relief of primary dysmenorrhea are also helpful for women with secondary dysmenorrhea. Surgical options may be used to decrease the pain in women when other medical alternatives have been refused or were unsuccessful, and hysterectomy can be considered when all other options have not worked and fertility is no longer a consideration (see the Nursing Process box on Evolve).

Premenstrual Syndrome

Approximately 30 to 80% of women experience mood or somatic symptoms (or both) that occur with their menstrual cycles (Lentz, 2012). Establishing a universal definition of **premenstrual syndrome (PMS)** is difficult, given that so many symptoms have been associated with the condition and at least two different syndromes have been recognized: PMS and **premenstrual dysphoric disorder (PMDD)**.

PMS is a complex, poorly understood condition that includes one or more of a large number (more than 150) of physical and psychological symptoms beginning in the luteal phase of the menstrual cycle. They occur to such a degree that lifestyle or work can be affected. Symptoms are then followed by a symptom-free period. PMS symptoms comprise distressing physical, mood, and behavioural experiences and can include fluid retention (abdominal bloating, pelvic fullness, edema of the lower extremities, breast tenderness, and weight gain); behavioural or emotional changes (depression, crying spells, irritability, panic attacks, and impaired ability to concentrate); premenstrual cravings (sweets, salt, increased appetite, and food binges); headache; fatigue; and backache.

All age groups are affected, with women in their 20s and 30s most frequently reporting symptoms. Ovarian function is necessary for the condition to occur. PMS does not occur before puberty, after menopause, or during pregnancy. The condition is not dependent on the presence of monthly menses; women who have had a hysterectomy without bilateral salpingo-oophorectomy (BSO) still can have cyclic symptoms.

A diagnosis of PMS is made when the following criteria are met (Taylor, Schuiling, & Sharp, 2013):

- Symptoms consistent with PMS occur in the luteal phase and resolve within a few days of menses onset.
- Symptom-free period occurs in the follicular phase.
- Symptoms are recurrent.
- Symptoms have a negative effect on some aspect of a woman's life.
- Other diagnoses that better explain the symptoms have been excluded.

PMDD is a more severe variant of PMS in which 3 to 8% of women have marked irritability, dysphoria, mood lability, anxiety, fatigue, appetite changes, and a sense of feeling overwhelmed (Lentz, 2012). The most common symptoms are those associated with mood disturbances.

For a diagnosis of PMDD, the following criteria must be met (American Psychiatric Association, 2013):

- Five or more affective and physical symptoms are present in the week before menses and absent in the follicular phase of the menstrual cycle.
- At least one of the symptoms is irritability, depressed mood, anxiety, or emotional lability.
- Symptoms interfere markedly with work or interpersonal relationships.
- Symptoms must be related to the menstrual cycle and are not caused by an exacerbation of another condition or disorder.

These criteria must be confirmed by prospective daily ratings for at least two menstrual cycles.

The etiology of PMS and PMDD is not clear, but there is general agreement that they are distinct psychiatric and medical syndromes rather than an exacerbation of an underlying psychiatric disorder. They do not occur if there is no ovarian function. A number of biological and neuroendocrine etiologies have been suggested; however, none have been substantiated conclusively as the causative factor. It is likely that biological, psychosocial, and sociocultural factors contribute to PMS and

PMDD (Lentz, 2012; Taylor et al., 2013). There are several risk factors for PMDD: personal history of a major mood disorder; family history of mood disorder; premenstrual depression; premenstrual mood changes; past history of sexual abuse; and past, present, or current domestic violence.

Management

There is little agreement on management of PMS. A careful, detailed history and daily log of symptoms and mood fluctuations spanning several cycles may give direction to a plan of management. Any changes that assist a woman with PMS to exert control over her life have a positive impact. For this reason, lifestyle changes are often effective in its treatment.

Education is an important component of the management of PMS. Nurses can advise women that self-help modalities often result in significant symptom improvement. Women have found a number of complementary and alternative therapies to be useful in managing the symptoms of PMS. Diet and exercise changes are a useful way to begin and provide symptom relief for some women. Nurses can suggest that patients not smoke and limit their consumption of refined sugar, salt, red meat, alcohol, and caffeinated beverages. Women can be encouraged to include whole grains, legumes, seeds, nuts, vegetables, fruits, and vegetable oils in their diet. Three small to moderate-size meals and three small snacks a day that are rich in complex carbohydrates and fibre have been reported to relieve symptoms (Lentz, 2012). Use of natural diuretics (see section on dysmenorrhea management earlier in this chapter) may help reduce fluid retention. Nutritional supplements may assist in symptom relief. Calcium (1200 mg/day), magnesium (300 to 400 mg/day), and vitamin B_6 have been shown to be moderately effective in relieving symptoms, to have few adverse effects, and to be safe. Daily supplements of evening primrose oil are reportedly useful in relieving breast symptoms with minimal side effects, but research reports are conflicting (Biggs & Demuth, 2011; Lentz, 2012). Other herbal therapies have long been used to treat PMS, although research on effectiveness and safety is not conclusive; specific suggestions are found in Table 7-2.

Regular exercise (aerobic exercise three to four times a week), especially in the luteal phase, is widely recommended for relief of PMS symptoms. A monthly program that varies in intensity and type of exercise according to PMS symptoms is best. Women who exercise regularly seem to have less premenstrual anxiety than do sedentary women. Researchers believe aerobic exercise increases β-endorphin levels to offset symptoms of depression and elevate mood. Yoga, acupuncture, hypnosis, light therapy, chiropractic therapy, and massage therapy have all been reported to have a beneficial effect on women with PMS, although further research is needed.

Nurses can explain the relation between cyclic estrogen fluctuation and changes in serotonin levels, that serotonin is one of the brain chemicals that assists in coping with normal life stresses, and the ways in which the different management strategies help maintain serotonin levels. Support groups or individual or couple counselling may be helpful. Stress-reduction techniques also may also assist with symptom management (Lentz, 2012). If these strategies do not provide significant symptom relief in 1 to 2 months, medication is often added. Many medications have been used in treatment of PMS, but no single medication alleviates all PMS symptoms. Medications often used in the treatment of PMS include diuretics, prostaglandin inhibitors (NSAIDs), progesterone, and OCPs. These have been used mainly for the physical symptoms. Studies of progesterone have not shown that it is an effective treatment (Ford, Lethaby, Roberts, et al., 2012). Serotonergic-activating agents, including the selective serotonin reuptake inhibitors (SSRIs) such as fluoxetine (Prozac), sertraline (Zoloft), and paroxetine (Paxil) are used as the first-line pharmacological therapy. Use of these medications during the luteal phase of the menstrual cycle results in a decrease in emotional premenstrual symptoms, especially depression (Biggs & Demuth, 2011; Lentz, 2012). Common adverse effects are headaches, sleep disturbances, dizziness, weight gain, dry mouth, and decreased libido.

Endometriosis

Endometriosis is characterized by the presence and growth of endometrial tissue outside of the uterus. The tissue may be implanted on the ovaries; anterior and posterior cul-de-sac; broad, uterosacral, and round ligaments; rectovaginal septum; sigmoid colon; appendix; pelvic peritoneum; cervix; and inguinal area (Fig. 7-2). Endometrial lesions have been found in the vagina and surgical scars, as well as on the vulva, perineum, and bladder. Lesions have also been found on sites far from the pelvic area, such as the thoracic cavity, gallbladder, and heart. A cystic lesion of endometriosis found in the ovary is sometimes described as a chocolate cyst because of the dark

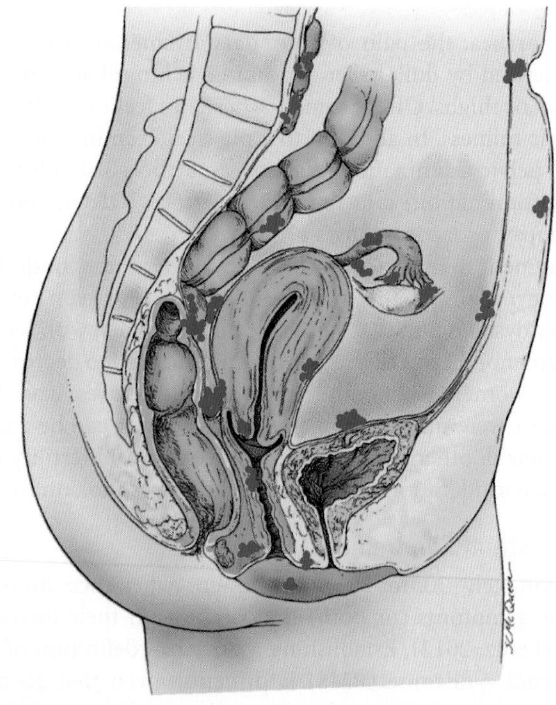

FIGURE 7-2 Common sites of endometriosis (*identified in blue*). (From Lentz, G. M., Lobo, D. M., Gershenson, D. M., et al. [2012]. *Comprehensive gynecology* [6th ed.]. Philadelphia: Mosby.)

colouring of the contents of the cyst caused by the presence of old blood.

Endometrial tissue responds to cyclic hormone stimulation in the same way that the uterine endometrium does but often out of phase with it. The endometrial tissue grows during the proliferative and secretory phases of the cycle. During or immediately after menstruation, the tissue bleeds, resulting in an inflammatory response with subsequent fibrosis and adhesions to adjacent organs.

The overall incidence of endometriosis is 5 to 10% in reproductive-age women, and 20 to 50% in women with persistent pelvic pain or infertility (Leyland et al., 2010). Although the condition usually develops in the third or fourth decade of life, endometriosis has been found in adolescents, with disabling pelvic pain or abnormal vaginal bleeding. Endometriosis may worsen with repeated cycles, or it may remain asymptomatic and undiagnosed, eventually disappearing after menopause. The condition appears equally in women of all cultures and it occurs across all socioeconomic levels. There appears to be a familial tendency to develop endometriosis; the condition is 3 to 10 times more prevalent in women who have a first-degree relative with endometriosis than in the general population (Leyland et al., 2010).

Several theories regarding the cause of endometriosis have been suggested. However, the etiology and pathology of this condition continue to be poorly understood. One of the most widely accepted theories is transplantation or retrograde menstruation. According to this theory, endometrial tissue is refluxed through the uterine tubes during menstruation into the peritoneal cavity, where it implants on the ovaries and other organs. Retrograde menstruation has been documented in a number of surgical studies and is estimated to occur in 90% of menstruating women. For most women, endometrial tissue outside the uterus is destroyed before it can implant or seed in the peritoneal cavity or elsewhere. Approaches to treatment have been improved on the basis of this theory of what causes endometriosis symptoms, but continued research is needed to better understand and manage the disorder (Leyland et al., 2010).

Symptoms ranging from nonexistent to incapacitating vary among women. The severity of symptoms can change over time and may not reflect the extent of the disease. Endometriosis may present as any of the following:

- Painful menstruation (dysmenorrhea)
- Painful intercourse (dyspareunia)
- Painful micturition (dysuria)
- Painful defecation (dyschezia)
- Lower back or abdominal discomfort
- Chronic pelvic pain (noncyclic abdominal and pelvic pain of at least 6 months' duration)

Less common symptoms include cyclic leg pain or sciatica, cyclic rectal bleeding or hematuria, and cyclic dyspnea (Leyland et al., 2010).

Impaired fertility may result from adhesions around the uterus that pull the uterus into a fixed, retroverted position. Adhesions around the uterine tubes may block the fimbriated ends or prevent the spontaneous movement that carries the ovum to the uterus.

Management

Treatment is based on the severity of symptoms and the goals of the woman. Women with endometriosis must be assessed for the level of pain they experience, their pain coping strategies, and the impact of the pain on their life. Women without pain who do not want to become pregnant need no treatment. In women with mild pain who may desire a future pregnancy, treatment may be limited to use of NSAIDs during menstruation (see earlier discussion of these medications).

Combined hormonal contraceptives, ideally administered continuously, should be considered as first-line agents. Continuous OCPs that have a low estrogen-to-progestin ratio are used to shrink endometrial tissue. Any low-dose OCPs can be used if taken for 15 weeks, followed by 1 week of withdrawal. This therapy is associated with minimal adverse effects and can be taken for extended periods (Leyland et al., 2010). Continuous combined hormone therapy (OCPs, estrogen/progestin patch, estrogen/progestin vaginal ring) for menstrual suppression and administration of NSAIDs are the usual treatment for adolescents under the age of 16 who have endometriosis. Limited data exist on the effectiveness of progestin-only medications for treating pain related to endometriosis (Brown, Kives, & Akhtar, 2012).

Suppression of endogenous estrogen production and subsequent endometrial lesion growth is one method of disease management and should be considered a second level of therapy. Two main classes of medications are used to suppress endogenous estrogen levels: GnRH agonists and androgen derivatives. GnRH agonist therapy (leuprolide [Lupron, Eligard], nafarelin [Synarel], and goserelin acetate [Zoladex]) acts by suppressing pituitary gonadotropin secretion. FSH and LH stimulation of the ovary declines markedly, and ovarian function decreases significantly. A medically induced menopause develops, resulting in anovulation and amenorrhea. Shrinkage of already established endometrial tissue, significant pain relief, and interruption in further lesion development follow. The hypoestrogenism results in hot flashes in almost all women. Trabecular bone loss is common, although most loss is reversible within 12 to 18 months after the medication is stopped (Leyland et al., 2010).

Leuprolide (3.75 mg intramuscular injection given once a month) and nafarelin (200 mg administered twice daily by nasal spray) and goserelin (3.6 mg every 28 days by subcutaneous implant) are effective and well tolerated. These medications reduce endometrial lesions and pelvic pain associated with endometriosis and have post-treatment pregnancy rates similar to that of danazol (Cyclomen) therapy (Leyland et al., 2010). Common adverse effects of these medications are those of natural menopause—hot flashes and vaginal dryness. Occasionally, women report headaches and muscle aches. Treatment is usually limited to 6 months to minimize bone loss. Although unlikely, it is possible for a woman to become pregnant while taking a GnRH agonist. Because the potential teratogenicity of this medication is unclear, women should use a barrier contraceptive during treatment.

Danazol, a mildly androgenic synthetic steroid, suppresses FSH and LH secretion, thus producing anovulation and hypogonadotropism. This results in decreased secretion of estrogen and progesterone and regression of endometrial tissue. Danazol can produce adverse effects severe enough to cause a woman to discontinue the medication. Adverse effects include masculinizing traits in the woman (weight gain, edema, decreased breast size, oily skin, hirsutism, and deepening of the voice), all of which often disappear when treatment is discontinued. Other adverse effects are amenorrhea, hot flashes, vaginal dryness, insomnia, and decreased libido. Migraine headaches, dizziness, fatigue, and depression are also reported. Danazol treatment has been reported to adversely affect lipids, with a decrease in high-density lipoprotein levels and an increase in low-density lipoprotein levels. Danazol should never be prescribed when pregnancy is suspected, and barrier contraception should be used with it because ovulation may not be suppressed. Danazol can produce pseudohermaphroditism in female fetuses. The medication is contraindicated in women with liver disease and should be used with caution in women with cardiac and renal disease. Danazol is less frequently used to treat endometriosis than other medical therapies (Leyland et al., 2010).

Surgical intervention is often needed for severe, acute, or incapacitating symptoms. Decisions regarding the extent and type of surgery are influenced by a woman's age, her desire for children, and location of the disease. For women who do not want to preserve their ability to have children, the only definite cure is total abdominal hysterectomy with bilateral salpingo-oophorectomy (TAH with BSO). In women who are in their child-bearing years and want children and in whom the disease does not prevent bearing children, reproductive capacity should be retained through careful removal by surgery or laser therapy (coagulation, vaporization, or resection) of all endometrial tissue possible, with retention of ovarian function (Leyland et al., 2010).

Regardless of the type of treatment (short of TAH with BSO), endometriosis recurs in approximately 40% of women. Thus, for many women, endometriosis is a chronic disease with conditions such as persistent pain or infertility. Counselling and education are critical components of nursing care for women with endometriosis. Women need an honest discussion of treatment options, with potential risks and benefits of each option reviewed. Because pelvic pain is a subjective, personal experience that can be frightening, support is important. Sexual dysfunction resulting from dyspareunia is common and may necessitate referral for counselling. Support groups for women with endometriosis may be found in some locations. The Infertility Awareness Association of Canada (see Additional Resources at end of chapter), an organization for infertile couples, may also be helpful. The nursing care discussed in the previous section on dysmenorrhea is appropriate for managing persistent pelvic pain and dysmenorrhea experienced by women with endometriosis (see Evolve resources for Nursing Care Plan for Woman with Endometriosis).

ABNORMAL UTERINE BLEEDING

Abnormal uterine bleeding (AUB) may be defined as any variation from the normal menstrual cycle and includes changes in regularity and frequency of menses, in duration of flow, or in amount of blood loss, as well as bleeding that is not related to menses. Abnormal uterine bleeding is a common condition affecting women of reproductive age that has significant social and economic impact due to loss of work time and possible decreased social interactions (Singh, Best, Dunn, et al., 2013). Box 7-1 lists possible causes of AUB. Inherited bleeding disorders may be an underlying cause of abnormal uterine bleeding, with von Willebrand's disease present in the majority of cases (Singh et al., 2013), and should be considered when other causes cannot be determined.

Management

The selection of a treatment for AUB will depend on the impact of the bleeding on the woman's overall health (Singh et al., 2013).

Acute Bleeding Episode

The most effective medical treatment of acute bleeding episodes of AUB is administration of high-dose estrogen and tranexamic acid. Surgery would only be done as a last resort because of the high morbidity associated with operating on patients with acute anemia and the resulting impaired healing, further bleeding, and infection. Surgical options in the acute setting include uterine curettage and hysteroscopic ablation, hysterectomy, and uterine artery embolization (Singh et al., 2013).

Once the acute phase has passed, the woman is maintained on an oral conjugated estrogen and progestin regimen for at least 3 months. Such long-term treatment will help prevent recurrence of the pattern of AUB and hemorrhage. If the woman wants contraception, she should continue to take OCPs. If the woman has no need for contraception, the treatment may be stopped to assess her bleeding pattern. If her menses do not resume, a progestin regimen 10 days before the expected date of her menstrual period may be prescribed. This is done to prevent persistent anovulation with chronic unopposed endogenous estrogen hyperstimulation of the endometrium, which can result in eventual atypical tissue changes (Singh et al., 2013).

Alterations in Cyclic Bleeding

Women often experience changes in amount, duration, interval, or regularity of menstrual cycle bleeding. Commonly, women worry about menstruation that is infrequent (**oligomenorrhea**), is scanty at normal intervals (**hypomenorrhea**), is excessive (**menorrhagia**), or occurs between periods (**metrorrhagia**).

Treatment depends on the cause and may include education and reassurance. For example, nurses should explain to women that OCPs can cause scanty menstrual flow and midcycle spotting. Progestin intramuscular injections and implants can also cause midcycle bleeding. A single episode of heavy bleeding may signal an early pregnancy loss such as a miscarriage or ectopic pregnancy. This type of bleeding is often thought to be a period that is heavier than usual, perhaps delayed, and is associated with abdominal pain or pelvic discomfort. When early pregnancy loss is suspected, hematocrit and pregnancy tests are indicated.

BOX 7-1 POSSIBLE CAUSES OF ABNORMAL UTERINE BLEEDING

Pregnancy-Related Conditions
Threatened or spontaneous miscarriage
Retained products of conception after elective abortion
Ectopic pregnancy
Placenta previa/placental abruption
Trophoblastic disease

Lower Reproductive Tract Infections
Cervicitis
Endometritis
Myometritis
Salpingitis

Benign Anatomical Abnormalities
Adenomyosis
Ovarian cyst
Leiomyomata
Polyps of the cervix or endometrium

Neoplasms
Endometrial hyperplasia
Cancer of the cervix and endometrium
Hormonally active tumours (rare)
Vaginal tumours (rare)

Malignant Lesions
Cervical squamous cell carcinoma
Endometrial adenocarcinoma
Estrogen-producing ovarian tumours
Testosterone-producing ovarian tumours
Leiomyosarcoma

Trauma
Genital injury (accidental, coital trauma, sexual abuse)
Foreign body
Lacerations

Systemic Conditions
Adrenal hyperplasia and Cushing's disease
Blood dyscrasias
Coagulopathies (e.g., von Willebrand's disease)
Hypothalamic suppression (from stress, weight loss, excessive exercise)
Polycystic ovary disease
Thyroid disease
Pituitary adenoma or hyperprolactinemia
Severe organ disease (renal or liver failure)

Iatrogenic Causes
Medications with estrogenic activity
Anticoagulants
Exogenous hormone use (oral contraceptives, menopausal hormone therapy)
Selective serotonin reuptake inhibitors
Tamoxifen
Intrauterine devices
Herbal preparation (e.g., ginseng)

Modified from Albers, J. R., Hull, S. K., & Wesley, R. M. (2004). Abnormal uterine bleeding. *American Family Physician, 69*, 1915–1926; 1931–1932; Singh, S., Best C., Dunn, S., et al. (2013). SOGC clinical practice guideline: Abnormal uterine bleeding in pre-menopausal women. *Journal of Obstetrics & Gynaecology Canada, 35*(5eSuppl), S1–S28.

Uterine **leiomyomas** (fibroids or myomas) are a common cause of menorrhagia. Fibroids are benign tumours of the smooth muscle of the uterus with an unknown cause. Fibroids occur in approximately one fourth of women of reproductive age; their incidence is higher in Black women (Katz, 2012). Other uterine growths ranging from endometrial polyps to adenocarcinoma and endometrial cancer are common causes of heavy menstrual bleeding and intermenstrual bleeding.

NURSING ALERT

If the woman considers the amount or duration of bleeding to be excessive, the problem should be investigated.

Treatment for menorrhagia depends on the cause of the bleeding. If the bleeding is related to contraceptive method (e.g., an intrauterine device [IUD]), provide factual information and reassurance and discuss other contraceptive options. Tranexamic acid (an antifibrolytic agent) has also been shown to be effective in reducing menstrual blood loss between 40 and 59% from baseline (Singh et al., 2013).

If there is no known cause for the bleeding and anatomical causes have been ruled out, therapy is aimed at reducing the amount of heavy bleeding. Current options for treatment include OCPs, NSAIDs, and other therapies: the levonorgestrel-releasing IUD, danazol, and antifibrinolytic agents (e.g., tranexamic acid) (Singh et al., 2013; Wilton, 2012).

If bleeding is related to the presence of fibroids, the degree of disability and discomfort associated with the fibroids and the woman's plans for child-bearing influence treatment decisions. Treatment options include medical and surgical management. Most fibroids can be monitored by frequent examinations to judge growth, if any, and correction of anemia if present. Warn women with metrorrhagia to avoid using aspirin because of its tendency to increase bleeding. Medical treatment is directed toward temporarily reducing symptoms, shrinking the myoma, and reducing its blood supply (Katz, 2012; Singh et al., 2013). This reduction is often accomplished with the use of a GnRH agonist. However, usually after cessation of this treatment, the myomas return to their pretreatment size (Singh et al., 2013). If the woman wishes to retain child-bearing potential, a myomectomy may be performed. Myomectomy, or removal of the tumours only by laparoscopic or hysteroscopic resection or laser surgery, is particularly difficult if multiple myomas must be removed. One in four women will have a hysterectomy performed within 20 years of having a myomectomy. If the woman does not want to preserve her child-bearing function or if she has severe symptoms (severe anemia, severe pain, considerable disruption of lifestyle), uterine artery embolization (UAE; procedure that blocks blood supply to fibroid) or hysterectomy (removal of uterus) may be performed. After UAE, 20 to 30% of women will undergo a hysterectomy within 5 years (Katz, 2012).

Nursing roles for the woman with abnormal uterine bleeding include informing patients of their options, counselling and education as indicated, and referring to the appropriate specialists and health care services.

PERIMENOPAUSE AND MENOPAUSE

The climacteric is a transitional phase during which ovarian function and hormone production decline. This phase spans the years from the onset of premenopausal ovarian decline to the postmenopausal time when symptoms stop. A natural part of aging, *menopause* is considered the point at which a woman has not had a menstrual period for 12 months. The average age for menopause to occur is 51.4 years, with an age range of 35 to 60 years. *Perimenopause* is the period of time prior to this when a woman experiences physical and emotional changes; this lasts an average of 5 years. During this time, ovarian function declines. Ova slowly diminish, and menstrual cycles may be anovulatory, resulting in irregular bleeding. The ovary stops producing estrogen, and eventually menses no longer occur. Any woman with postmenopausal bleeding always needs to be investigated for cancer.

Menopause symptoms may vary from mild to intense. The common symptoms that women report include vasomotor instability (hot flashes, night sweats), depression, anxiety, irritability, vaginal dryness, atrophic vaginitis, decreased libido, fatigue, aches and pains, and insomnia.

Some women will find that vasomotor symptoms decrease when they make lifestyle modifications, which include eating well, maintaining a healthy weight, regular exercise, reducing core body temperature (dressing in layers, use of a fan, and drinking cold fluids), smoking cessation, and limiting consumption of triggers (such as hot drinks and alcohol) (Reid, Abramson, Blake, et al., 2014). Stress management (relaxation, yoga, meditation) may also help with some psychological symptoms.

Hormonal replacement therapy (HRT) is used to decrease menopausal symptoms. Estrogen alone or combined with a progestin is the most effective therapy for the medical management of menopausal symptoms. There has been some increased risk of breast cancer, ovarian cancer, thromboembolism, and heart disease identified with estrogen/progesterone therapy, and estrogen-only therapy has been associated with an increased rate of strokes (Reid et al., 2014). Women for whom HRT is contraindicated or not desired may use nonhormonal therapies. These include certain antidepressant medications, gabapentin, clonidine, and bellergal, which may provide some relief from hot flashes. These medications have their own adverse effects (Reid et al., 2014).

The use of black cohosh and foods that contain phytoestrogens may improve mild menopausal symptoms, including hot flashes. Isoflavone (found in soy) and St. John's wort may also be used (Reid et al., 2014). Women should be asked about the use of any complementary therapies in order to decrease the risk of interactions with any medications. At present, the use of these therapies may be useful for some women, although research on the use of complementary and alternative therapy is limited, and women should be advised that alternative measures should be used with caution (Reid et al., 2014).

Every woman will go through the transition of menopause differently. Women need an understanding health care provider who can explain what is normal and provide support. An excellent resource for information for women is found at http://www.Menopauseandu.ca.

INFECTIONS

Infections of the reproductive tract can occur throughout a woman's life and are often the cause of significant reproductive morbidity, including ectopic pregnancy and tubal factor infertility. The direct economic costs of these infections can be substantial, and the indirect cost is equally overwhelming. Some consequences of maternal infection such as infertility last a lifetime. The emotional costs may include damaged relationships and lowered self-esteem.

Sexually Transmitted Infections

Sexually transmitted infections (STIs) comprise more than 25 infectious organisms that cause infections or infectious disease syndromes, transmitted primarily by close, intimate contact (Box 7-2). STIs continue to be a significant and increasing public health concern in Canada, with rates of the three nationally reportable bacterial STIs (chlamydia, gonorrhea, and syphilis) increasing, especially among women aged 15 to 24. The

BOX 7-2 SEXUALLY TRANSMITTED INFECTIONS

Bacteria
Chlamydia (Reportable to local health authority)
Gonorrhea (Reportable to local health authority)
Syphilis (Nationally reportable if infectious)
Chancroid
Lymphogranuloma venereum
Genital mycoplasmas

Viruses
Human immunodeficiency virus (Reportable to local health authority)
Herpes simplex virus, types 1 and 2
Cytomegalovirus
Viral hepatitis A and B
Human papillomavirus

Protozoa
Trichomoniasis

Parasites
Pediculosis (may or may not be sexually transmitted)
Scabies (may or may not be sexually transmitted)

COMMUNITY FOCUS

Sexually Transmitted Infections

While working in a clinic, interview a nurse about sexually transmitted infections commonly seen in the clinic.

- What are the most common infections seen in the clinic?
- Has the incidence of infections changed over the last 5 years? Which infections have increased and which have decreased in incidence during that time?
- Are adolescents seen in the clinic? Is there a special clinic for adolescents?
- How are patients diagnosed and treated for sexually transmitted infections?
- What patient teaching guidelines are available in the clinic? Are the guidelines available in languages other than English?

World Health Organization (WHO) has developed a global strategy for the prevention and control of STIs because of the health and economic burden of STIs (WHO, 2007) (see Community Focus box). The most common STIs in women are chlamydia, human papillomavirus (HPV), gonorrhea, herpes simplex virus (HSV) type 2, syphilis, and human immunodeficiency virus (HIV) infection. Neonatal effects of STIs are discussed in Chapter 28.

Prevention

Preventing infection (primary prevention) is the most effective way of reducing the adverse consequences of STIs for women and for society. Prompt diagnosis and treatment of current infections (secondary prevention) can prevent personal complications and transmission to others. Preventing the spread of STIs requires that women at risk for transmitting or acquiring infections change their behaviour related to sexual activity. A critical first step is for the nurse to include questions about a woman's sexual history, sexual risk behaviours, and drug-related risky behaviours as a part of the woman's assessment (Box 7-3). Effective techniques in providing prevention counselling include using open-ended questions; using understandable language; and reassuring the woman that treatment will be provided regardless of ability to pay, language spoken, or lifestyle (Public Health Agency of Canada [PHAC], 2013a). Prevention messages should include descriptions of specific actions to be taken to avoid acquiring or transmitting STIs (e.g., refraining from sexual activity if STI-related symptoms are present) and should be individualized for each woman, giving attention to her specific risk factors.

To be motivated to take preventive actions, a woman must believe that acquiring a disease will be serious for her and that she is at risk for infection. Most individuals tend to underestimate their personal risk of infection in a given situation. Thus, many women may not perceive themselves as being at risk for contracting an STI, and telling them that they should carry condoms may not be well received. Although levels of awareness of STIs are generally high, widespread misconceptions or specific gaps in knowledge also exist. Therefore, nurses have a responsibility to ensure that their patients have accurate, complete knowledge about transmission and symptoms of STIs and the behaviours that place them at risk for contracting an infection.

Primary preventive measures are individual activities aimed at avoiding infection. Risk-free options include complete abstinence from sexual activities that transmit semen, blood, or other body fluids or that allow for skin-to-skin contact (PHAC, 2013a). Involvement in a mutually monogamous relationship with an uninfected partner also eliminates risk of contracting STIs. When neither of these options is realistic for a woman, the nurse must focus on other, more feasible measures. It is important for nurses to be aware that some women do not have the ability or agency to take preventive action and may engage in high-risk behaviour because they have little choice or lack the confidence to do so. For these women, nurses need to provide individualized and respectful care.

Sexually transmitted infections/human immunodeficiency virus prevention strategies. An essential component of primary prevention is counselling the woman about sexual practices so that she can avoid acquiring or transmitting STIs. These practices include attaining knowledge of her partner, reducing her number of partners, practising low-risk sex, avoiding the exchange of body fluids, and vaccination.

Reducing the number of partners and avoiding partners who have had many previous sexual partners decreases a woman's chances of contracting an STI. Discussing each new partner's previous sexual history and exposure to STIs will augment other efforts to reduce risk; however, sexual partners are not always truthful about their sexual history.

Women should be taught low-risk sexual practices, as well as which sexual practices to avoid (see Box 5-9). Sexual fantasizing is safe, as are caressing, hugging, body rubbing, and massage. Mutual masturbation is low risk as long as there is no contact with a partner's semen or vaginal secretions. All sexual activities are safe when both partners are monogamous, trustworthy, and known (by testing) to be free of disease. Anal–genital intercourse, anal–oral contact, and anal–digital activity are high-risk sexual behaviours and should be avoided or done safely. Women need to be encouraged to think about the risk of STIs and to consider pre-sex testing before they become sexually active with a new partner so they can be proactive in preventing the risk of transmission. Women also need to discuss limiting alcohol or drug intake prior to sexual activity as these can impact decision-making and negotiation skills (PHAC, 2013a).

The physical barrier promoted for the prevention of sexual transmission of HIV and other STIs is the condom. The nurse should teach the woman to use a condom with every sexual encounter; to use latex or plastic male condoms rather than natural skin condoms for STI protection; to use a condom with a current expiration date; to use each one only once; and to handle it carefully in order to avoid damaging it with fingernails, teeth, or other sharp objects. Condoms should be stored away from high heat. Although it is not ideal, women may choose to carry condoms in wallets, shoes, or inside a bra. Women can be taught the differences among condoms: price ranges, sizes, and where they can be purchased. Explicit instructions for how to apply a male condom are included in Box 8-9.

BOX 7-3 FOCUSED RISK ASSESSMENT FOR SEXUALLY TRANSMITTED INFECTIONS

Information should be requested in a nonjudgemental manner, using language that is understandable.

Relationship

Do you have a regular sexual partner?
If yes, how long have you been with this person?
Do you have any concerns about your relationship?
If yes, what are they? (e.g., violence, abuse, coercion)

Sexual Risk Behaviour

When was your last sexual contact? Was that contact with your regular partner or with a different partner?
How many different sexual partners have you had in the past 2 months? In the past year? Are your partners men, women, or both?
Do you perform oral sex (i.e., Do you kiss your partner on the genitals or anus)?
Do you receive oral sex?
Do you have intercourse (i.e., Do you penetrate your partner in the vagina or anus [bum]? Or does your partner penetrate your vagina or anus [bum])?

Personal Risk Evaluation

Have any of your sexual encounters been with people from a country other than Canada? If yes, where and when?
How do you meet your sexual partners (when travelling, in a bathhouse, on the Internet)?
Do you use condoms? All the time, some of the time, never?
What influences your choice to use protection or not?
If you had to rate your risk for STI, would you say that you are no risk, low risk, medium risk, or high risk? Why?

STI History

Have you ever been tested for STI/HIV? If yes, what was your last screening date?
Have you ever had an STI in the past? If yes, what and when?

Current Concern

When was your last sexual contact of concern?
If symptomatic, how long have you had the symptoms you are experiencing?

Reproductive Health History

Do you and/or your partner use contraception? If yes, what? Any problems? If no, is there a reason?
Have you ever had any reproductive health problems? If yes, when? What?
Have you ever had an abnormal Pap test? If yes, when? Result, if known?
Have you ever been pregnant? If yes, how many times? What was the outcome (number of live births, abortions, miscarriages)?

Substance Use

Do you use alcohol? Drugs? If yes, frequency and type?
If you use injection drugs, have you ever shared equipment? If yes, what was your last sharing date?
Have you ever had sex while intoxicated? If yes, how often?
Have you had sex while under the influence of alcohol or other substances? What were the consequences?
Do you feel that you need help because of your substance use?
Do you have tattoos or piercings? If yes, were they done using sterile equipment (i.e., professionally)?

Psychosocial History

Have you ever

- traded sex for money, drugs, or shelter?
- paid for sex? If yes, what is the frequency, duration, and last event?
- been forced to have sex? If yes, when and by whom?
- been sexually abused?
- been physically or mentally abused? If yes, when and by whom?
- been physically or mentally abused? If yes, when and by whom?

Do you have a home? If no, where do you sleep?
Do you live with anyone?

HIV, human immunodeficiency virus; *STI*, sexually transmitted infection.

 Canadian guidelines on sexually transmitted infections. Public Health Agency of Canada, 2016. Adapted and reproduced with permission from the Minister of Health, 2016.

The female condom (a lubricated polyurethane sheath with a ring on each end that is inserted into the vagina) may be an effective mechanical barrier to viruses, including HIV. The consistent use of condoms for every act of sexual intimacy when there is the possibility of transmission of disease is ideal but not always possible in some situations. Women need to be encouraged to discuss concerns with their partner (Box 7-4).

Evidence has shown that vaginal spermicides do not protect against certain STIs (e.g., chlamydia, cervical gonorrhea) and that frequent use of spermicides containing nonoxynol-9 has been associated with genital lesions and may increase HIV transmission. Condoms lubricated with nonoxynol-9 are not recommended (PHAC, 2013a).

Vaccination is an effective method for the prevention of some STIs such as hepatitis B and HPV. Hepatitis B vaccine is recommended for women at high risk for STIs. A vaccine is available for HPV types 6, 11, 16, and 18 for girls and women 9 to 26 years of age (PHAC, 2014a) (see later discussion).

Women should be counselled to watch out for situations that make it hard to talk about and practise risk reduction. These situations include romantic times when condoms are not available and when alcohol or drugs make it difficult to make wise decisions.

Sexually Transmitted Bacterial Infections

Chlamydia

Chlamydia trachomatis is a reportable STI in Canada. Rates of chlamydia in Canada and elsewhere have been steadily increasing; between 1998 and 2007 the rate of chlamydia in females increased by 60% (PHAC, 2014b). In 2011 the reported rate

BOX 7-4 STRATEGIES TO ENHANCE A WOMAN'S NEGOTIATION AND COMMUNICATION SKILLS REGARDING CONDOM USE

- Suggest that the woman talk with her partner about condom use at a time not during sexual activity.
- Role play possible partner reactions with the woman and her alternative responses.
- For a woman who appears particularly uncomfortable, ask her to rehearse how she might approach the topic of condom use with her partner.
- Women may feel more comfortable and in control of the situation if they sort out their feelings and fears before talking with their partners. Reassure the woman that it is natural to be uncomfortable and that the hardest part is getting started.
- Suggest that the woman clarify for herself what she will and will not do sexually.
- Suggest that the woman begin the conversation by saying, "I need to talk with you about something that is important to both of us. It's hard for me, and I feel embarrassed, but I think we need to talk about ways to reduce risk when we have sex."
- The partner may need time to think about what he or she has heard.
- If the partner resists risk-reducing sexual behaviours, the woman may wish to reconsider the relationship.

among females (378.7 per 100,000) was almost twice as high as that among males (200.1 per 100,000). The highest rates of chlamydia were reported in those between the ages of 20 and 24 in both males and females (PHAC, 2014b). Risky behaviours, such as having sex with multiple partners and failure to use barrier methods of birth control, increase a woman's risk of chlamydial infection. Vulnerable populations (e.g., injection drug users, incarcerated individuals, sex trade workers, and street youth) are at increased risk for developing chlamydial infection (PHAC, 2013b). These infections are often silent and highly destructive. Their sequelae and complications can be very serious. In women, chlamydial infections are difficult to diagnose; the symptoms, if present, are nonspecific.

Acute salpingitis, or pelvic inflammatory disease, is the most serious complication of chlamydial infections. Past chlamydial infections are associated with an increased risk of ectopic pregnancy and tubal factor infertility. Furthermore, chlamydial infection of the cervix causes inflammation, resulting in microscopic cervical ulcerations that may increase risk of acquiring HIV infection. More than half of infants born to mothers with chlamydia will develop conjunctivitis or pneumonia after perinatal exposure to the mother's infected cervix. *C. trachomatis* is the most common infectious cause of ophthalmia neonatorum.

Screening and diagnosis. In addition to obtaining information about the presence of risk factors (see Box 7-3), the nurse should inquire about the presence of any symptoms. All pregnant women should have cervical cultures for chlamydia at the first prenatal visit. Screening late in the third trimester (36 weeks) may be carried out if the woman was positive previously or if she is younger than 25 years, has a new sex partner, or has multiple sex partners.

Although chlamydia infections are usually asymptomatic, some women may experience spotting or postcoital bleeding, mucoid or purulent cervical discharge, or **dysuria**. Bleeding results from inflammation and erosion of the cervical columnar epithelium.

Diagnosis of chlamydia is best done using nucleic acid amplification (NAAT), which is more sensitive and specific than culture, enzyme immunoassay (EIA), and direct fluorescent antibody assay (DFA). NAAT should be used whenever possible for urine, urethral, or cervical specimens. Results are highly dependent on the type of test available, specimen collection and transport, and laboratory expertise. Not all local laboratories will have the ability to provide all types of testing, so it is important to know what is available in the particular region (PHAC, 2013b).

Management. The Public Health Agency of Canada (PHAC) (2013b) recommendations for the treatment of chlamydial infections include doxycycline or azithromycin (Table 7-3). Azithromycin is often prescribed when adherence is a problem because only one dose is needed. Because chlamydia is often asymptomatic, the woman should be cautioned to take all medication prescribed. Women treated with recommended or alternative regimens do not need to be retested unless symptoms continue (PHAC, 2013b). All sexual partners who have had contact with the index case within 60 days before symptom onset must be tested and treated (PHAC, 2013b). Chlamydia is a reportable disease to the local health authority in all provinces and territories. Local public health authorities are able to help notify contacts.

Gonorrhea

Gonorrhea is probably the oldest communicable disease in Canada. Between 2002 and 2011, the overall rate of reported cases of gonorrhea increased by 40.8%. The reported rate, as in previous years, was higher among males than females (38.4 vs. 27.8 per 100,000 respectively) in 2011. Females between the ages of 15 and 24 and males between the ages of 20 and 24 accounted for the highest reported rates of gonorrhea (PHAC, 2014b). The incidence of medication-resistant cases of gonorrhea, in particular penicillinase-producing *Neisseria gonorrhoeae*, is increasing dramatically in North America.

Gonorrhea is caused by the aerobic, gram-negative diplococci *N. gonorrhoeae*. It is transmitted almost exclusively by sexual contact. The principal means of transmission is genital-to-genital contact during sexual activity; however, it is also spread by oral–genital and anal–genital contact. There is also evidence that infection may spread in females from vagina to rectum. Although the organism has been recovered from inanimate objects artificially inoculated with the bacteria, there is no evidence that natural transmission occurs this way.

Women are often asymptomatic; but, when they are symptomatic, they may have a greenish-yellow purulent endocervical discharge or may experience menstrual irregularities. Women may also have pain: chronic or acute severe pelvic or lower abdominal pain, or menses that last longer or are more painful than normal. Infrequently dysuria, vague abdominal pain, or low backache prompts a woman to seek care. Gonococcal rectal

TABLE 7-3 SEXUALLY TRANSMITTED INFECTIONS AND DRUG THERAPIES FOR WOMEN*

DISEASE	NONPREGNANT WOMEN (13–17 yr)	NONPREGNANT WOMEN (>18 yr)	PREGNANT/LACTATING WOMEN
Chlamydia	Doxycycline, 100 mg orally bid for 7 days *or* Azithromycin, 1 g orally once (if poor adherence is suspected)	Doxycycline, 100 mg orally bid for 7 days *or* Azithromycin, 1 g orally once (if poor adherence is suspected)	Amoxicillin, 500 mg orally tid for 7 days *or* Erythromycin 2 g/day orally in divided doses for 7 days *or* Erythromycin 1g/day orally in divided doses for 14 days *or* Azithromycin 1 g orally in a single dose, if poor adherence is expected **Doxycycline should not be used in pregnancy or while breastfeeding.**
Gonorrhea	Ceftriaxone, 250 mg IM once Plus zithromycin 1 g orally in a single dose *or* Cefixime 800 mg orally in a single dose Plus azithromycin 1 g orally in a single dose	Ceftriaxone, 250 mg IM once Plus zithromycin 1 g orally in a single dose *or* Cefixime 800 mg orally in a single dose Plus azithromycin 1 g orally in a single dose	Ceftriaxone, 250 mg IM once Zithromycin 1 g orally in a single dose
Syphilis	**Primary, secondary, early-latent disease:** Benzathine penicillin G, 2.4 million units IM once **Late-latent or unknown-duration disease:** Benzathine penicillin G, 7.2 million units total, administered as three doses, 2.4 million units each, at 1-week intervals **Penicillin allergy:** Doxycycline, 100 mg orally bid for 14 days *or* Tetracycline, 500 mg orally qid for 14 days	**Primary, secondary, early-latent disease:** Benzathine penicillin G, 2.4 million units IM once **Late-latent or unknown-duration disease:** Benzathine penicillin G, 7.2 million units total, administered as three doses, 2.4 million units each, at 1-week intervals **Penicillin allergy:** Doxycycline, 100 mg orally bid for 14 days *or* Tetracycline, 500 mg orally qid for 14 days	**Primary, secondary, early-latent disease:** Benzathine penicillin G, 2.4 million units IM for one to two doses **Late-latent or unknown-duration disease:** Benzathine penicillin G, 7.2 million units total, administered as three doses, 2.4 million units each, at 1-week intervals. No proven alternatives to penicillin in pregnancy. Pregnant women who have a history of allergy to penicillin should be desensitized and treated with penicillin.
Human papillomavirus	*For external genital warts:* **Patient-applied:** Podophyllotoxin/ Podofilox 0.5% solution to wart bid for 3 days followed by 4-day rest for ≤4 cycles *or* Imiquimod 3.75% cream, daily at hs for 8 weeks **Provider-applied:** Cryotherapy with liquid nitrogen or cryoprobe weekly up to 4 weeks *or* Podophyllin resin, 25% in tincture of benzoin compound weekly (wash off in 1–4 hr). Repeat up to 6 weeks *or* Trichloracetic acid (TCA) 50–90% solution in 70% alcohol weekly for 6–8 weeks	*For external genital warts:* **Patient-applied:** Podophyllotoxin/ Podofilox 0.5% solution to wart bid for 3 days followed by 4-day rest for ≤4 cycles *or* Imiquimod 3.75% cream, daily at hs for 8 weeks *or* Imiquimod, 5% cream, at hs 3 times a week for ≤16 weeks *or* Sinecatechins 10% ointment tid for ≤16 weeks **Provider-applied:** Cryotherapy with liquid nitrogen or cryoprobe *or* Podophyllin resin, 10–25% in tincture of benzoin compound weekly (wash off in 1–4 hr). Repeat weekly as necessary *or* TCA or Bichloroacetic acid (BCA) 80–90% weekly	*For external genital warts:* **Provider applied:** Cryotherapy with liquid nitrogen or cryoprobe *or* Trichloracetic acid (TCA) 50-90% solution in 70% alcohol weekly for 6–8 weeks. Imiquimod, podophyllin, podofilox/ podophyllotoxin, and sinecatechins should not be used in pregnancy or during lactation.

TABLE 7-3 **SEXUALLY TRANSMITTED INFECTIONS AND DRUG THERAPIES FOR WOMEN*—cont'd**

DISEASE	NONPREGNANT WOMEN (13–17 yr)	NONPREGNANT WOMEN (>18 yr)	PREGNANT/LACTATING WOMEN
Genital herpes simplex virus (HSV-1 or HSV-2)	**Primary infection:** Acyclovir, 200 mg orally 5 times a day for 5–10 days *or* Famciclovir, 250 mg orally tid for 5 days *or* Valacyclovir, 1 g orally bid for 10 days **Recurrent infection:** Valacyclovir, 500 mg orally bid or 1 g daily for 3 days *or* Famciclovir, 125 mg orally bid for 5 days *or* Ayclovir, 200 mg orally five times/day for 5 days **Suppression therapy:** *Take daily for 1 year:* Acyclovir, 200 mg orally three to five times/day *or* Famciclovir, 250 mg orally bid *or* Valacyclovir, 500 mg orally once a day (for patients with ≤ 9 recurrences/year) *or* Valacyclovir, 1 g orally once a day (if >9 recurrences/year)	**Primary infection:** Acyclovir, 200 mg orally 5 times a day for 5–10 days *or* Famciclovir, 250 mg orally tid for 5 days *or* Valacyclovir, 1 g orally bid for 10 days **Recurrent infection:** Valacyclovir, 500 mg orally bid or 1 g daily for 3 days *or* Famciclovir, 125 mg orally bid for 5 days *or* Ayclovir, 200 mg orally five times/day for 5 days **Suppression therapy:** *Take daily for 1 year:* Acyclovir, 200 mg orally three to five times/day *Or* Famciclovir, 250 mg orally bid *or* Valacyclovir, 500 mg orally once a day (for patients with ≤9 recurrences/year) *or* Valacyclovir, 1 g orally once a day (if >9 recurrences/year)	No increase in birth defects beyond the general population has been found with acyclovir use in pregnancy or while breastfeeding. Acyclovir, 400 mg orally tid for 7 days for first episode or severe recurrent infection; may be given IV if infection is severe **Suppression therapy:** 4 weeks before birth for women with recurrent infections can reduce the need for a Caesarean birth. Acyclovir 200 mg orally qid *or* Acyclovir 400 mg orally tid *or* Valacyclovir 500 mg orally bid

bid, Twice daily; *hs,* bedtime; *HSV,* herpes simplex virus; *IM,* intramuscularly; *IV,* intravenously; *qid,* four times daily; *tid,* three times daily.
*List is not inclusive of all drugs that may be used as alternatives.
Data from Public Health Agency of Canada. (2015). *Canadian guidelines on sexually transmitted infections.* Ottawa: Author. Retrieved from http://www.phac-aspc.gc.ca/std-mts/sti-its/cgsti-ldcits/index-eng.php#toc

infection may occur in women after anal intercourse; 10 to 30% of urogenital infections are accompanied by rectal infection. Individuals with rectal gonorrhea may be completely asymptomatic or, conversely, have severe symptoms with profuse purulent anal discharge, rectal pain, and blood in the stool. Rectal itching, fullness, pressure, and pain are also common symptoms, as is diarrhea. A diffuse vaginitis with vulvitis is the most common form of gonococcal infection in prepubertal girls. There may be few signs of infection; vaginal discharge, dysuria, and swollen, reddened labia may be present.

Gonococcal infections in pregnancy potentially affect both mother and infant. Women with cervical gonorrhea may develop salpingitis in the first trimester. Perinatal complications of gonococcal infection include postpartum endometritis or sepsis in the mother and ophthalmia neonatorum or systemic neonatal infection in the newborn (PHAC, 2013c). Amniotic infection syndrome—manifested by placental, fetal, and umbilical cord inflammation following premature rupture of the membranes—may result from gonorrheal infection during pregnancy.

Screening and diagnosis. Because gonococcal infections in women are often asymptomatic, the PHAC recommends screening all women at risk for gonorrhea (PHAC, 2014c). All pregnant women should be screened at the first prenatal visit, and infected women and those identified with risky behaviours rescreened at 36 weeks of gestation. Gonococcal infection cannot be diagnosed reliably by clinical signs and symptoms alone. Individuals may have "classic" symptoms, vague symptoms that may be attributed to a number of conditions, or no symptoms at all. Cultures should be obtained from the endocervix, the rectum, and, when indicated, the pharynx. Cultures are critical for improved public health monitoring of antimicrobial resistance patterns and trends (PHAC, 2014c). Depending on the clinical situation, consideration should be given for collection of samples using both culture and NAAT, especially in symptomatic patients. Because coinfection is common, any woman suspected of having gonorrhea should have a chlamydial culture and serological test for syphilis unless one has been done within the past 2 months.

Management. Management of gonorrhea is becoming more challenging as drug-resistant strains are increasing. The treatment of choice for uncomplicated urethral, endocervical, and rectal infections in pregnant and nonpregnant women is ceftriaxone given intramuscularly once. The PHAC also recommends concomitant treatment for chlamydia because coinfection is common (PHAC, 2014c) (see Table 7-3). All women with both gonorrhea and syphilis should also be treated for syphilis according to PHAC guidelines (see discussion of syphilis later in this chapter).

Gonorrhea is highly communicable. Recent (past 30 days) sexual partners must be notified and should be examined, cultured, and treated with appropriate regimens. Most treatment failures result from reinfection. The woman needs to be informed of this, as well as of the consequences of reinfection in terms of chronicity, complications, and potential infertility. Women should be counselled to use condoms. All women with gonorrhea should be offered confidential counselling and testing for HIV infection.

LEGAL TIP

Gonorrhea, chlamydia, infectious syphilis, and HIV are reportable communicable diseases in all provinces and territories. Health care providers are legally responsible for reporting all cases of these STIs to local public health authorities. Women should be informed that the case will be reported, told why it will be reported, and informed of the possibility of being contacted by a health department epidemiologist.

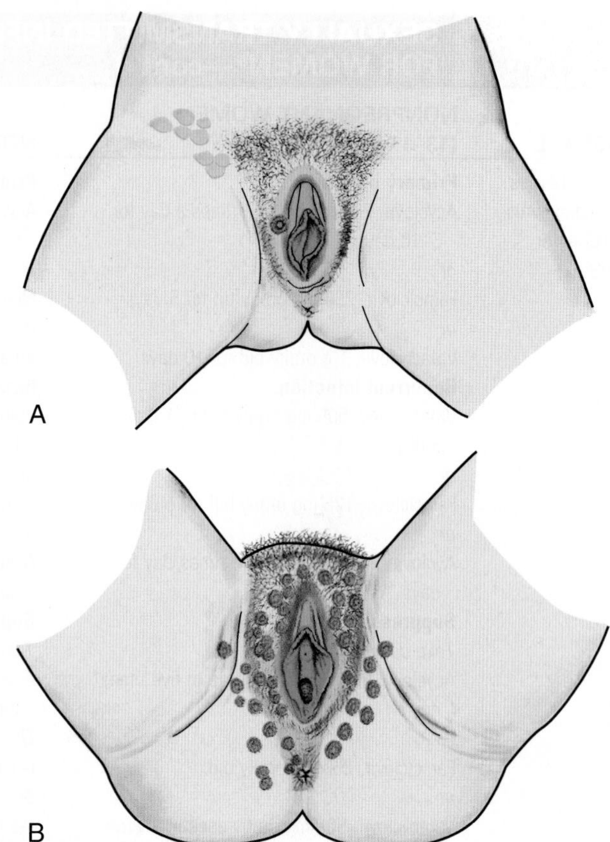

FIGURE 7-3 Syphilis. **A:** Primary stage: chancre with inguinal adenopathy. **B:** Secondary stage: condylomata lata.

Syphilis

Syphilis, one of the earliest described STIs, is caused by *Treponema pallidum*, a motile spirochete. Transmission is thought to occur by entry through microscopic abrasions in the subcutaneous tissue, which can happen during vaginal, anal, or oral sexual contact. The majority of infants with congenital syphilis are infected in utero, but they can also be infected by contact with an active genital lesion at the time of delivery. The risk of transmission in untreated women is 70 to 100% with primary or secondary syphilis, 40% with early latent syphilis, and 10% in late latent stages in pregnancy. About 40% of pregnancies in women with infectious syphilis result in fetal demise (PHAC, 2013e).

Infectious syphilis (primary, secondary and early latent stages) is the least common of the three nationally reportable bacterial STIs. The rate of infectious syphilis in Canada in 2008 was 4.2 per 100,000, an increase of 568% since 1999 (PHAC, 2014b). Much of the increase in cases was observed in men having sex with men (PHAC, 2014b). Syphilis is a complex disease that can lead to serious systemic disease and even death when untreated. Infection manifests itself in distinct stages with different symptoms and clinical manifestations. Primary syphilis is characterized by a primary lesion, the chancre, which appears 3 to 90 days after infection. This lesion often begins as a painless papule at the site of inoculation and then erodes to form a nontender, shallow, indurated, clean ulcer several millimetres to centimetres in size (Fig. 7-3A). Secondary syphilis occurs 2 to 6 months after the appearance of the chancre. It is characterized by a widespread, symmetrical, maculopapular rash on the palms and soles and generalized lymphadenopathy. The infected individual also may experience fever, headache, and malaise. Condylomata lata (broad, painless, pink-grey, wartlike infectious lesions) may develop on the vulva, perineum, or anus (Fig. 7-3B). If the woman remains untreated, she enters a latent phase that is asymptomatic for most individuals. Left untreated, about one third of these women will develop tertiary syphilis. Neurological, cardiovascular, musculoskeletal, or multiorgan system complications can develop in the third stage.

Screening and diagnosis. All women who are diagnosed with another STI or with HIV should be screened for syphilis. Universal screening of all pregnant women is important and remains the standard of care in most jurisdictions. The screening test should be repeated at 28 to 32 weeks and again during labour in women at high risk of acquiring syphilis (PHAC, 2013c). Diagnosis depends on microscopic examination of primary and secondary lesion tissue and serology during latency and late infection. A test for antibodies may not be reactive in the presence of active infection because it takes time for the body's immune system to develop antibodies to any antigens. Up to one third of people with early primary syphilis may have nonreactive serological tests. Two types of serological tests are used: nontreponemal and treponemal. Nontreponemal antibody tests such as VDRL (Venereal Disease Research Laboratories) and RPR (rapid plasma reagin) are used as screening tests. False-positive results are not unusual, particularly when conditions such as acute infection, autoimmune disorders, malignancy, pregnancy, and drug addiction exist, and after immunization or vaccination. The treponemal tests, fluorescent treponemal antibody absorbed and microhemagglutination assays for antibody to *T. pallidum*, are used to confirm positive results. Test results in patients with early primary or incubating syphilis may be negative. Seroconversion usually takes place 6 to 8 weeks after exposure; thus testing should be repeated in 1 to 2 months when a suggestive genital lesion exists.

Tests (e.g., wet preps and cultures) for concomitant STIs (e.g., chlamydia and gonorrhea) should be done and HIV testing offered, if indicated.

Management. Penicillin is the preferred medication for treating patients with all stages of syphilis, including pregnant women (see Table 7-3). Although doxycycline, tetracycline, and erythromycin are alternative treatments for penicillin-allergic patients, both tetracycline and doxycycline are contraindicated in pregnancy, and erythromycin is unlikely to cure a fetal infection. Therefore, if necessary, pregnant women should receive skin testing and be treated with penicillin or be desensitized (PHAC, 2013c).

! NURSING ALERT

Patients treated for syphilis may experience a Jarisch–Herxheimer reaction. This is an acute febrile reaction often accompanied by headache, myalgias, and arthralgias that develop within the first 24 hours of treatment. The reaction may be treated symptomatically with analgesics and antipyretics. If treatment precipitates this reaction in the second half of pregnancy, women are at risk for preterm labour and birth. They should be advised to contact their health care provider if they notice any change in fetal movement or have any contractions.

Monthly follow-up is important so that repeated treatment may be given, if needed. The nurse should emphasize the necessity of long-term serological testing even in the absence of symptoms. The woman should be advised to practise sexual abstinence until treatment is completed, all evidence of primary and secondary syphilis is gone, and serological evidence of a cure is demonstrated. Infectious syphilis is reportable in all provinces and territories to the PHAC. Noninfectious syphilis is reportable at the provincial/territorial level but not to the PHAC. All sexual or perinatal contacts must be notified and treated. Preventive measures should be discussed (PHAC, 2013e).

Pelvic Inflammatory Disease

Pelvic inflammatory disease (PID) is an infectious process that most commonly involves the uterine tubes, causing salpingitis; the uterus, causing endometritis; and, more rarely, the ovaries and peritoneal surfaces. Multiple organisms have been found to cause PID; most cases are associated with more than one organism. The pathogenic organisms can be categorized as sexually transmitted or endogenous (PHAC, 2013d). In the past, the most common causative agent was thought to be *N. gonorrhoeae*; however, *C. trachomatis* is now estimated to cause one half of all cases of PID. In addition to gonorrhea and chlamydia, a wide variety of anaerobic and aerobic bacteria cause PID.

Most PID results from the ascending spread of microorganisms from the vagina and endocervix to the upper genital tract. This spread most commonly happens at the end of or just after menses following reception of an infectious agent. During the menstrual period, several factors facilitate the development of an infection: the cervical os is slightly open, the cervical mucous barrier is absent, and menstrual blood is an excellent medium for growth. PID also may develop after a miscarriage or an induced **abortion**, pelvic surgery, or childbirth.

Risk factors for acquiring PID are those associated with the risk of contracting an STI, including young age, multiple partners, high rate of new partners, and a history of STIs. PID tends to recur and is a significant public health problem in Canada. There are approximately 100,000 cases of PID annually in Canada, although up to two thirds of cases go unrecognized, and underreporting is common (PHAC, 2013d).

Women who have had PID are at increased risk for ectopic pregnancy, infertility, and chronic pelvic pain. The incidence of long-term sequelae of PID is directly related to the number of episodes of PID. Other problems associated with PID include **dyspareunia**, *pyosalpinx* (pus in the uterine tubes), tubo-ovarian abscess, and pelvic adhesions.

The symptoms of PID vary, depending on whether the infection is acute, subacute, or chronic. However, pain is common to all clinical presentations. It may be dull, cramping, and intermittent (subacute) or severe, persistent, and incapacitating (acute). Women may also report one or more of the following: fever, chills, nausea and vomiting, increased vaginal discharge, symptoms of a urinary tract infection, and irregular bleeding. Abdominal pain is usually present and may include adnexal or cervical motion tenderness (PHAC, 2013d).

Screening and diagnosis. PID is difficult to diagnose because of the accompanying wide variety of symptoms. A complete abdominal and pelvic examination should be performed in any patient with lower abdominal pain. The PHAC recommends treatment for PID in all sexually active young women and others at risk for STIs if the following criteria are present and no other cause or causes of the illness are found: lower abdominal tenderness, bilateral adnexal tenderness, and cervical motion tenderness. Other criteria for diagnosing PID include an oral temperature of 38.3° C or above, abnormal cervical or vaginal discharge, elevated erythrocyte sedimentation rate, elevated C-reactive protein, and laboratory documentation of cervical infection with *N. gonorrhoeae* or *C. trachomatis* (PHAC, 2013d).

Management. The most important nursing intervention is prevention counselling (see earlier discussion). Early diagnosis and treatment are crucial in order to maintain fertility.

Although treatment regimens vary with the infecting organism, generally a broad-spectrum antibiotic is used (PHAC, 2013d). Treatment for PID may be intramuscular ceftriaxone plus oral doxycycline with or without metronidazole; or cefoxitin parenterally plus oral probenecid in a single dose concurrently once with doxycycline; or other parenteral third-generation cephalosporin (e.g., ceftizoxime or cefotaxime) with doxycycline. Regimens can be administered in inpatient or outpatient settings. PID can be difficult to treat if due to an antibiotic-resistant organism (specifically gonorrhea), and this needs to be determined. Also, the management of women with PID is considered inadequate unless their sexual partners are also clinically evaluated (PHAC, 2014d). All outpatients treated for PID should undergo evaluation 2 to 3 days after the initiation of treatment (PHAC, 2014d). When and if women with PID are hospitalized varies according to their particular circumstances. The PHAC recommends hospitalization for parenteral antibiotic treatment in the following situations (PHAC, 2013d):

- Surgical emergencies such as appendicitis cannot be excluded.
- The woman has a tubo-ovarian abscess.
- The woman is pregnant.
- The patient does not respond clinically to oral antimicrobial therapy.
- The patient is unable to follow or tolerate an outpatient oral regimen.
- The patient has severe illness, nausea and vomiting, or high fever.

The woman with acute PID should be on bed rest in a semi-Fowler's position. Comfort measures include analgesics for pain and all other nursing measures applicable to a patient confined to bed. Few pelvic examinations should be done during the acute phase of the disease. During the recovery phase, the woman should restrict her activity and make every effort to get adequate rest and a nutritionally sound diet. Follow-up laboratory work after treatment should include endocervical cultures for a test of cure.

Health education is central to effective management of PID. Nurses should explain the nature of the disease to affected women and encourage them to continue with all therapy and prevention recommendations, emphasizing the need to take all medication, even if symptoms disappear. Any potential problems (such as lack of money for prescriptions or lack of transportation to return for follow-up appointments) that would prevent a woman from completing a course of treatment should be identified, referrals made for assistance as needed, and the importance of follow-up visits stressed. Women should be counselled to refrain from sexual intercourse until their treatment is completed. Contraceptive counselling, including information on barrier methods such as condoms, the contraceptive sponge, and the diaphragm, should be provided.

The potential or actual loss of reproductive capabilities can be devastating and can adversely affect the woman's concept of herself. Part of the nurse's role is to help the woman adjust her self-concept to fit reality and to accept alterations in a way that promotes health. Because PID is so closely tied to sexuality, body image, and self-concept, the woman diagnosed with it will need supportive care. Her feelings should be discussed and her partner(s) included in the discussion, when appropriate.

Sexually Transmitted Viral Infections

Human Papillomavirus

Human papillomavirus (HPV) infection, also known as condylomatata acuminate, or genital warts, is the most common viral STI seen in ambulatory health care settings. It is estimated that 75% of the adult population will have at least one genital HPV infection over their lifetime, and prevalence among females is usually highest in those aged less than 25 years (PHAC, 2015).

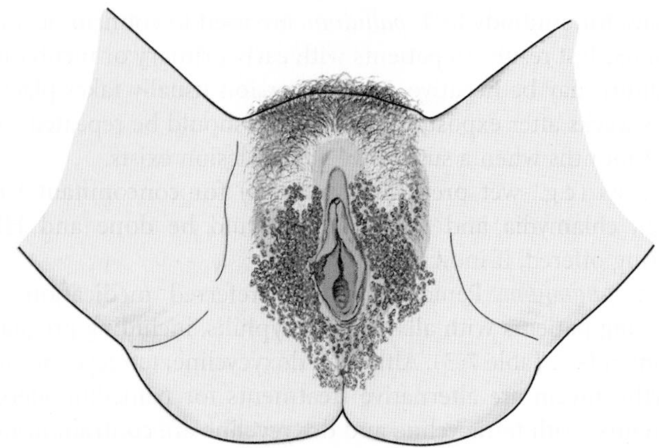

FIGURE 7-4 Human papillomavirus (HPV) infection. Genital warts or condylomata acuminata.

HPV prevalence in Canada appears to vary by subpopulation; recent data show that in females it ranged from 14 to 47% and was highest in those aged less than 20 years and living in low-income inner city settings and Indigenous communities (PHAC, 2015).

HPV, a double-stranded DNA virus, has more than 40 serotypes that can be transmitted sexually, 5 of which are known to cause genital wart formation and 8 of which are currently thought to have oncogenic (tumour-causing) potential (PHAC, 2015). HPV is the primary cause of cervical neoplasia (Canadian Cancer Society [CCS], 2014a).

In women, HPV lesions are most commonly seen in the posterior part of the introitus. Lesions also are found on the buttocks, vulva, vagina, anus, and cervix (Fig. 7-4). Typically the lesions are small (2 to 3 mm in diameter and 10 to 15 mm in height), soft, papillary swellings occurring singly or in clusters on the genital and anal–rectal region. Infections of long duration may appear as a cauliflower-like mass. In moist areas such as the vaginal introitus, the lesions may appear to have multiple fine, fingerlike projections. Vaginal lesions are often multiple. Flat-topped papules, 1 to 4 mm in diameter, are seen most often on the cervix. Often these lesions are visualized only under magnification. Warts are usually flesh coloured or slightly darker on White women, black on Black women, and brownish on Asian women. The lesions are usually painless, but they may be uncomfortable, particularly when very large, inflamed, or ulcerated. Chronic vaginal discharge, pruritus, or dyspareunia can occur.

During pregnancy, pre-existing HPV lesions may enlarge, a proliferation presumably resulting from the relative state of immunosuppression present during this period. Lesions may become so large during pregnancy that they affect urination, defecation, mobility, and fetal descent, although birth by Caesarean section is rarely necessary. Caesarean birth should be reserved for women with obstructions that do not allow the baby to pass through.

Screening and diagnosis. A woman with HPV lesions may have symptoms such as profuse, irritating vaginal discharge, itching, dyspareunia, or postcoital bleeding. She also may report "bumps" on her vulva or labia. History of a known exposure is important; however, because of the potentially long latency period and the possibility of subclinical infections in men, the lack of a history of known exposure cannot be used to exclude a diagnosis of HPV infection.

Physical inspection of the vulva, perineum, anus, vagina, and cervix is essential whenever HPV lesions are suspected or seen in one area. Because speculum examination of the vagina may block some lesions, it is important to rotate the speculum blades until all areas are visualized. When lesions are visible, the characteristic appearance previously described is considered diagnostic. However, in many instances cervical lesions are not visible, and some vaginal or vulvar lesions also may be unobservable to the naked eye. Because of the potential spread of vulvar or vaginal lesions to the anus, gloves should be changed between vaginal and rectal examinations.

Viral screening and typing for HPV is available but not standard practice. History, evaluation of signs and symptoms, Pap test, and physical examination are used in making a diagnosis. The HPV-DNA test can be used in women older than age 30 in combination with the Pap test to screen for types of HPV that are likely to cause cancer or in women with abnormal Pap test results (Canadian Cancer Society, 2014a; SOGC, 2007). The only definitive diagnostic test for the presence of HPV is histological evaluation of a biopsy specimen.

Management. Untreated warts may resolve on their own in young women since their immune systems may be strong enough to fight the HPV infection. Treatment of genital warts, if needed, is often difficult. No therapy has been shown to eradicate HPV. Therefore, the goal of treatment is removal of warts and symptom relief (PHAC, 2015). The patient often must make multiple office visits; frequently many different treatment modalities will be used.

Treatment of genital warts may be patient- (self) or clinician-applied and should be guided by preference of the woman; availability of resources; cost, size, shape, number, and site of lesions; convenience; potential adverse effects; and experience of the health care provider (PHAC, 2015). No one of the treatments is superior to all other treatments, and no one treatment is ideal for all warts (PHAC, 2015) (see Table 7-3). Imiquimod, polophyllin, and podofilox are common treatments but should not be used during pregnancy. Because the lesions can proliferate and become friable during pregnancy, many experts recommend their removal using cryotherapy or various surgical techniques (PHAC, 2015).

Women who have discomfort associated with genital warts may find that bathing with an oatmeal solution and drying the area with cool air from a hair dryer provides some relief. Keeping the area clean and dry also decreases the growth of the warts. Cotton underwear and loose-fitting clothes that decrease friction and irritation may lessen discomfort. Women should be advised to maintain a healthy lifestyle to aid the immune system and be counselled regarding diet, rest, stress reduction, and exercise.

Patient education is essential. Women must understand the virus, how it is transmitted, that no immunity is conferred with infection, and that reinfection is likely with repeated contact (PHAC, 2015). All sexually active women with multiple partners or a history of HPV should be encouraged to use latex condoms for intercourse to decrease acquisition or transmission of the infection.

Semiannual or annual health examinations are recommended to assess disease recurrence and to screen for cervical cancer. The provinces and territories have different cervical cancer screening guidelines for follow-up for women who have been treated for HPV infections and these should be referred to.

Women with HPV infection may radically alter their sexual practices both from fear of transmission to and from a partner and from genital discomfort associated with treatment, which may have a negative impact on their sexual relationships. Unless the partner accepts and understands the necessary precautions, it may be difficult for the woman to follow the treatment regimen. The nurse can offer to discuss feelings that the woman may have. When indicated, joint counselling can be suggested.

Prevention. The two most important preventive strategies are the use of condoms and prophylactic vaccination (PHAC, 2015). A vaccine against HPV was approved by Health Canada in 2006 and is recommended for females ages 9 to 26. Two vaccines, Cervarix and Gardasil, are available; other vaccines continue to be investigated. Cervarix prevents infection from HPV viruses 16 and 18, whereas Gardasil prevents infection from viruses 6, 11, 16, and 18. Both can be administered to girls and women ages 9 to 26 (PHAC, 2015). The HPV vaccine is highly effective and is given in three doses over a 7-month period (months 0, 2, and 6). All provinces and territories in Canada have implemented publicly funded HPV vaccine programs with the goal of reducing the risk of cervical cancer (PHAC, 2015). For provincial/territorial guidelines for immunizations see http://www.phac-aspc.gc.ca/im/is-vc-eng.php.

Herpes Simplex Virus

Unknown until the middle of the twentieth century, herpes simplex virus (HSV) infection is now widespread in Canada, especially in women. HSV infection results in painful, recurrent ulcers. It is caused by two different antigen subtypes of HSV: HSV type 1 (HSV-1) and HSV type 2 (HSV-2). HSV-2 is usually transmitted sexually and HSV-1, nonsexually. Although HSV-1 is more commonly associated with gingivostomatitis and oral labial ulcers (fever blisters) and HSV-2 with genital lesions, neither type is exclusively associated with the respective sites.

HSV infection is not a reportable disease in Canada, therefore the number of cases is unknown, although it is known that the incidence and prevalence of HSV-1 genital infection is increasing globally, with marked variation between countries (PHAC, 2013f). Recurrent HSV infections are much more common. Most persons infected with HSV-2 have not been diagnosed, and most infections are transmitted by persons unaware that they are infected. Genital herpes increases the risk of acquisition of HIV twofold (PHAC, 2013f).

An initial HSV genital infection is characterized by multiple painful lesions, fever, chills, malaise, and severe dysuria and may last 2 to 3 weeks. Women generally have a more severe clinical

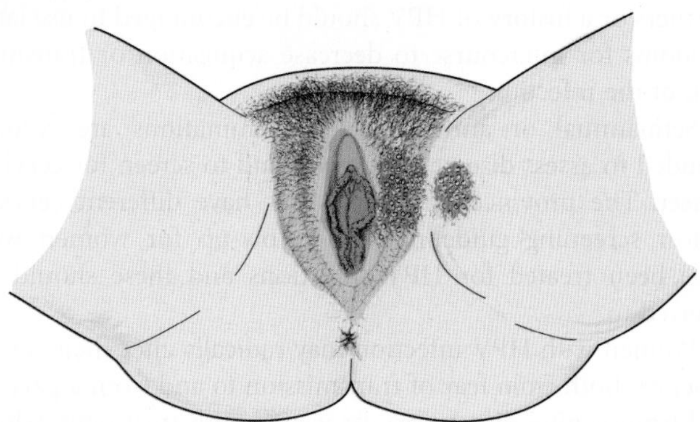

FIGURE 7-5 Herpes genitalis.

course than men do. Women with primary genital herpes have many lesions that progress from macules to papules; they then progress to form vesicles, pustules, and ulcers that crust and heal without scarring (Fig. 7-5). These ulcers are extremely tender, and primary infections may be bilateral. Women also may have itching, inguinal tenderness, and lymphadenopathy. Severe vulvar edema may develop, and women may have difficulty sitting. HSV cervicitis is common with initial HSV-2 infections. The cervix may appear normal or be friable, reddened, ulcerated, or necrotic. A heavy, watery-to-purulent vaginal discharge is common. Extragenital lesions may be present because of autoinoculation. Urinary retention and dysuria may occur secondary to autonomic involvement of the sacral nerve root.

Women with recurrent episodes of HSV infections commonly have only local symptoms that are usually less severe than those associated with the initial infection. Systemic symptoms are usually absent, although the characteristic prodromal genital tingling is common. Recurrent lesions are unilateral, are less severe, and usually last 9 to 11 days. Lesions begin as vesicles and progress rapidly to ulcers. Few women with recurrent disease have cervicitis.

During pregnancy maternal infection with HSV-2 can have adverse effects on both the mother and fetus. Viremia occurs during the primary infection, and congenital infection is possible although rare. The risk for neonatal infection is greatest when the maternal primary infection occurs in the third trimester. Primary infections during the first trimester have been associated with increased miscarriage rates (Money, Steben, et al., 2008).

Screening and diagnosis. Although a diagnosis of herpes infection may be suspected from the history and physical examination, it is confirmed by laboratory studies. A viral culture is obtained by swabbing exudate during the vesicular stage of the disease. A primary infection can be confirmed by demonstrating an absence of HSV antibody in an acute-phase blood sample and the presence of antibody in the convalescent sample (i.e., seroconversion). Most individuals seroconvert within 3 to 6 weeks; by 12 weeks, more than 70% will have seroconverted (PHAC, 2013f).

Management. Genital herpes is a chronic and recurring disease for which there is no known cure. Management is directed toward specific treatment during primary and recurrent infections, prevention, self-help measures, and psychological support.

Oral medications used for treating the first clinical HSV infection include acyclovir, famciclovir, and valacyclovir. These medications are considered for episodic or suppressive therapy for recurrent HSV. Intravenous acyclovir may be used for women with severe disease (PHAC, 2013f) (see Table 7-3). Acyclovir and valacyclovir may be used during pregnancy to reduce the symptoms of HSV and to suppress HSV close to the time of birth.

Cleaning lesions twice a day with saline helps prevent secondary infection. Bacterial infection must be treated with appropriate antibiotics. Measures that may increase comfort for women when lesions are active include warm sitz baths with baking soda; keeping lesions dry by using cool air from a hair dryer or by patting dry with a soft towel; wearing cotton underwear and loose clothing; using drying aids such as hydrogen peroxide, Burow solution, or oatmeal baths; and applying cool, wet, black tea bags to lesions. Women can also apply compresses with an infusion of cloves or peppermint oil and clove oil to lesions.

Oral analgesics such as aspirin or ibuprofen may be used to relieve pain and systemic symptoms associated with initial infections. Because the mucous membranes affected by herpes are extremely sensitive, any topical agents should be used with caution. Nonantiviral ointments, especially those containing cortisone, should be avoided. A thin layer of lidocaine ointment or an antiseptic spray may be applied to decrease discomfort, especially if walking is difficult.

Counselling and education are critical components of the nursing care of women with herpes infections. Information regarding the etiology, signs and symptoms, transmission, and treatment should be provided. The nurse should explain that each woman is unique in her response to herpes and emphasize the variability of symptoms. Women should be helped to understand when viral shedding and thus transmission to a partner are most likely. They should be counselled to refrain from sexual contact from the onset of prodrome until the complete healing of lesions.

Some authorities recommend consistent use of condoms for all persons with genital herpes. Condoms may not prevent transmission, particularly male-to-female transmission; however, this does not mean that the partners should avoid all intimacy. Women can be encouraged to maintain close contact with their partners while avoiding contact with lesions. Women should be taught how to look for herpetic lesions using a mirror and good light source and a wet cloth or finger covered with a finger cot to rub lightly over the labia. The nurse should ensure that women understand that when lesions are active, they should not share intimate articles (e.g., washcloths or wet towels) that come into contact with the lesions. Only plain soap and water are needed to clean hands that have come in contact with herpetic lesions; isolation is neither necessary nor appropriate.

Stress, menstruation, trauma, febrile illnesses, chronic illness, and ultraviolet light have all been found to trigger genital herpes. Women may wish to keep a diary to identify stressors that seem to be associated with recurrent herpes attacks so that they can then avoid these stressors when possible. The role of exercise in reducing stress can be discussed. Referral for stress-reduction therapy, yoga, or meditation classes may be indicated. Avoiding excessive heat, sun, and hot baths and using a lubricant during sexual intercourse to reduce friction may also be helpful. Women in their child-bearing years should be counselled about the risk of herpes infection during pregnancy. They should be instructed to use condoms if there is any risk of contracting an STI from a sexual partner. If they become pregnant while taking acyclovir, the risk of birth defects does not appear to be higher than that for the general population; however, continued use should be based on whether the benefits for the woman outweigh the possible risks to the fetus. Acyclovir does enter breast milk, but the amount of medication ingested during breastfeeding is very low and is usually not a health concern (Weiner & Buhimschi, 2009).

Because neonatal HSV infection is such a devastating disease, prevention is critical. Women should be questioned regarding the presence of HSV at the onset of labour. If visible lesions are not present when labour begins, vaginal birth is acceptable. Caesarean birth within 4 hours after labour begins or membranes rupture is recommended if visible lesions are present. Acyclovir oral therapy suppresses recurrent genital disease and asymptomatic shedding and thereby has been shown to reduce the need for Caesarean birth and should be offered to women at 36 weeks' gestation (see Table 7-3) (PHAC, 2013c). Infants who are born through an infected vagina should be observed carefully and cultured.

The emotional impact of contracting an incurable STI such as herpes can be considerable. The most common psychological patient concerns include the following:

- Fear of transmission
- Fear of being judged or rejected by her partner
- Loneliness, depression, and low self-esteem
- Anxiety concerning potential effect on child-bearing

Women need the opportunity to discuss their feelings and may need help in learning to live with the disease. A woman can be encouraged to think of herself as someone who is healthy and merely inconvenienced from time to time. Herpes can affect a woman's sexuality, her sexual practices, and her current and future relationships. She may need help in discussing her HSV status with her partner or with future partners.

Hepatitis

Five different viruses (hepatitis viruses A, B, C, D, and E) account for almost all cases of viral hepatitis in humans. While only hepatitis B is considered an STI, hepatitis A and C are discussed here. Hepatitis D and E viruses, common among users of intravenous drugs and recipients of multiple blood transfusions, are not included in this discussion.

Hepatitis A. Hepatitis A virus (HAV) infection is acquired primarily through a fecal–oral route by ingestion of contaminated food, particularly milk, shellfish, or polluted water, or person-to-person contact. People who are at risk for developing HAV include food workers who are exposed to contaminated food or water, injection drug users, household contacts of adopted children from countries with endemic HAV, incarcerated individuals, and household contacts of individuals with HAV (PHAC, 2014e). HAV infection is characterized by flu-like symptoms with malaise, fatigue, anorexia, nausea, pruritus, fever, and upper right quadrant pain. Serological testing to detect the immunoglobulin M (IgM) antibody is done to confirm acute infections. Because HAV infection is self-limited and does not result in chronic infection or chronic liver disease, treatment is usually supportive. Women who become dehydrated from nausea and vomiting or who have fulminating hepatitis A may need to be hospitalized. Medications that might cause liver damage or that are metabolized in the liver (e.g., acetaminophen, ethyl alcohol) should be used with caution. No specific diet or activity restrictions are necessary. Hepatitis A vaccine is effective in preventing most HAV infections and is recommended if travelling to areas with high levels of HAV. Hepatitis A vaccine should be considered for pregnant women in high risk situations when benefits outweigh risks (PHAC, 2014e).

Hepatitis B. Hepatitis B virus (HBV) infection is an STI and is the virus most threatening to the fetus and neonate. It is caused by a large DNA virus and is associated with three antigens and their antibodies: hepatitis B surface antigen (HBsAg), HBV antigen (HBeAg), HBV core antigen (HBcAg), antibody to HBsAg (anti-HBs), antibody to HBeAg (anti-HBe), and antibody to HBcAg (anti-HBc). HBsAg has been found in blood, saliva, sweat, tears, vaginal secretions, and semen. Screening for active or chronic disease or disease immunity is based on testing for these antigens and their antibodies.

Populations at greatest risk for HBV are listed in Box 7-5. Perinatal transmission most often occurs in infants of mothers who have acute hepatitis infection late in the third trimester or during the intrapartum or postpartum periods from exposure to HBsAg-positive vaginal secretions, blood, amniotic fluid, saliva, or breast milk. Although HBV can be transmitted via blood transfusion, the incidence of such infections has decreased significantly since the testing of blood for HBsAg became routine. The prevalence of HBV in Canada is estimated to be 0.5 to 1.0% with an increased rate in immigrants and Indigenous populations (PHAC, 2013g).

HBV infection is a disease of the liver and is often a silent infection. In the adult, its course can be fulminating and the outcome fatal. Symptoms of HBV infection are similar to those of hepatitis A: arthralgias, arthritis, lassitude, anorexia, nausea, vomiting, headache, fever, and mild abdominal pain. Later the woman may have clay-coloured stools, dark urine, increased abdominal pain, and jaundice. Between 5 and 10% of individuals with HBV have persistent HBsAg and become chronic hepatitis B carriers.

Screening and diagnosis. All women at high risk for contracting HBV should be screened on a regular basis. Since screening only individuals at high risk may not identify up to 50% of HBsAg-positive women, screening for the presence of HBsAg is recommended in all pregnant women at the first prenatal visit regardless of whether they have been tested previously; screening should be done on admission for labour and

BOX 7-5 HIGH-RISK GROUPS FOR HEPATITIS B

- Infants born to hepatitis B surface antigen (HBsAg)-positive mothers
- Injection drug users who share drug injection/preparation equipment
- Those with multiple sex partners
- Those born in or having sexual contact in areas of high endemicity
- Sexual and household contacts of an acute case or chronic carrier
- Health care workers and others with occupational blood exposure
- Those who are incarcerated or institutionalized
- Those infected with HIV or hepatitis C virus
- Those with a previous STI
- Staff and inmates of correctional facilities
- Travellers to HBV-endemic areas
- Children in childcare settings in which there is an HBV-infected child
- People who are HIV positive
- Sexual partners of any of those listed above

HBV, hepatitis B virus; *HBsAg*, hepatitis B surface antigen; *HIV*, human immunodeficiency virus.

birth for women at high risk for infection during pregnancy or if prenatal test results are not available (PHAC, 2013g).

The HBsAg screening test is usually performed, given that a rise in HBsAg occurs at the onset of clinical symptoms and usually indicates an active infection. If HBsAg persists in the blood, the woman is identified as a carrier. If the HBsAg test result is positive, further laboratory studies may be ordered: anti-HBe, anti-HBc, serum glutamic-oxaloacetic transaminase (SGOT), alkaline phosphatase, and liver panel.

Management. There is no specific treatment for hepatitis B. Recovery is usually spontaneous in 3 to 16 weeks. Pregnancies complicated by acute viral hepatitis are managed on an outpatient basis. Women should be advised to increase bed rest; eat a high-protein, low-fat diet; and increase their fluid intake. They should avoid alcohol and medications metabolized in the liver. Pregnant women with a definite exposure to HBV should be given hepatitis B immunoglobulin (HBIG) and begin the hepatitis B vaccine series within 14 days of the most recent contact to prevent infection (PHAC, 2013g). Vaccination during pregnancy is not thought to pose risks to the fetus.

Patient education includes explanation of the meaning of hepatitis B infection, including transmission, state of infectivity, and sequelae. The nurse should also explain the need for immunoprophylaxis for household members and sexual contacts. To decrease transmission of the virus, women with hepatitis B or who test positive for HBV should be advised to maintain a high level of personal hygiene (e.g., wash hands after using the toilet; carefully dispose of tampons, pads, and bandages in plastic bags; not share razor blades, toothbrushes, needles, or manicure implements; have her male partner use a condom if he is unvaccinated and without hepatitis; avoid sharing saliva through kissing or through sharing of silverware or dishes; and wipe up blood spills immediately with soap and water). Patients should inform all health care providers of their carrier state. Postpartum women should be reassured that breastfeeding is not contraindicated if the infant receives prophylaxis after birth and is currently on the immunization schedule.

Prevention. Primary prevention of HBV should be the focus for treatment. Primary prevention includes counselling and education regarding risk behaviours, harm reduction strategies (needle exchange programs), and hepatitis B vaccination (pre-exposure). All provinces and territories have either a universal school-based hepatitis B vaccination program aimed at children aged 9 to 13 or an infant vaccination program (PHAC, 2013g). Hepatitis B vaccine should also be offered to high-risk groups (see Box 7-5). The vaccine is given in a series of three (four if rapid protection is needed) doses over a 7-month period, with the first two doses given at least 1 month apart.

Secondary prevention is the administration of HBIG. This should be offered to affected individuals, including pregnant women who have percutaneous (needlestick) or mucosal exposure, up to 7 days after exposure and to sexual contacts within 14 days of exposure (ideally within 48 hours), followed by hepatitis B vaccine. For infants born to HBV-infected mothers, the first dose of hepatitis B vaccine should be administered within 12 hours of birth and HBIG given immediately after birth (efficacy decreases sharply after 48 hours) (PHAC, 2013g).

Hepatitis C. Hepatitis C (HCV) is an important cause of chronic liver disease and is becoming a major public health problem worldwide. In Canada it is estimated that approximately 242,500 individuals are infected with HCV (PHAC, 2014e). The most common risk factor is a history of intravenous drug use. Other risk factors include STIs such as hepatitis B and HIV, multiple sexual partners, tattoos and body piercing, and a history of blood transfusions. Hepatitis C is readily transmitted through exposure to blood.

Most patients with HCV are asymptomatic or have general flu-like symptoms similar to those of hepatitis A. HCV infection is confirmed by the presence of anti-C antibody during laboratory testing. Routine HCV testing is recommended for women who have ever injected drugs; women who received a blood transfusion before July 1992; children of HCV-positive women; health care, emergency, medical, and public safety workers; and women with chronic liver disease (Pinette, Cox, Heathcote, et al., 2009). Counselling and testing should be offered to pregnant women with known risk factors.

Interferon alfa-2b and ribavirin for 6 to 12 months are the main treatment for HCV infection, although the effectiveness of this treatment varies. New therapies called direct-acting antivirals act on the virus itself to eradicate it from the body, unlike interferon, which works by stimulating an immune response. In most situations, there is no need to use interferon, which is responsible for many adverse effects. The treatment duration is shorter (between 8 and 24 weeks) and effective with cure rates of over 90% (Canadian Liver Foundation, 2015). At the present time the medication is costly and not covered by many provincial or private insurance plans. Treatment for drug use is an important adjunct for many persons with HCV (Sherman, Shafran, Burak, et al., 2007).

Currently, there is no vaccine to prevent hepatitis C. Transmission of HCV through breastfeeding has not been reported, although women with cracked, bleeding nipples are advised to stop breastfeeding until the nipples heal.

Human Immunodeficiency Virus (HIV)

The number of people living with HIV (including acquired immunodeficiency syndrome [AIDS]) continues to rise, from an estimated 64,000 in 2008 to 75,500 in 2014 (Government of Canada, 2015). One reason for the increase in the number of people living with HIV is that new infections continue to increase at a greater number than HIV-related deaths, as new treatments have improved survival. An estimated 23% of cases of HIV are among women, and this number has increased since 2008. Although the incidence of HIV has decreased among the general population, the rate among Indigenous populations has been increasing (Government of Canada, 2015). Behaviours that place women at risk have been well documented; nonetheless, all women should be assessed for the possibility of HIV exposure.

Severe depression of the cellular immune system associated with HIV infection characterizes AIDS. The most commonly reported opportunistic diseases are *Pneumocystis carinii* pneumonia, *Candida* esophagitis, and wasting syndrome. Other viral infections such as HSV and cytomegalovirus infections seem to be more prevalent in women than in men. PID may be more severe in HIV-infected women, and rates of HPV and cervical dysplasia may be higher. The clinical course of HPV infection in women with HIV infection is accelerated and recurrence is more frequent.

Once HIV enters the body, seroconversion to HIV positivity usually occurs within 6 to 12 weeks. Although HIV seroconversion may be totally asymptomatic, it usually is accompanied by a viremic, influenza-like response. Symptoms include fever, headache, night sweats, malaise, generalized lymphadenopathy, myalgias, nausea, diarrhea, weight loss, sore throat, and rash.

Laboratory studies may reveal leukopenia, thrombocytopenia, anemia, and an elevated erythrocyte sedimentation rate. HIV has a strong affinity for surface-marker proteins on T lymphocytes. This affinity leads to significant T-cell destruction. Both clinical and epidemiological studies have shown that declining CD4 levels are strongly associated with increased incidence of AIDS-related diseases and death in many different groups of HIV-infected persons.

Transmission of the virus from mother to fetus can occur throughout the perinatal period. Exposure may occur to the fetus through the maternal circulation as early as the first trimester of pregnancy, to the infant during labour and birth by inoculation or ingestion of maternal blood and other infected fluids, or to the infant through breast milk (Bitnum, Brophy, Samson, et al., 2014).

Screening and diagnosis. Screening for HIV as well as teaching and counselling on risk factors, indications for being tested, and testing are major roles for nurses caring for women. A number of behaviours place women at risk for HIV infection, including intravenous drug use, high-risk sex practices, multiple sex partners, and a previous history of multiple STIs. HIV infection is usually diagnosed by using HIV-1 and HIV-2 antibody tests. Antibody testing is done first with a sensitive screening test such as the enzyme immunoassay. Reactive screening tests must be confirmed by an additional test such as the Western blot or an immunofluorescence assay. If a positive antibody test is confirmed by a supplemental test, it means that a woman is infected with HIV and is capable of infecting others. HIV antibodies are detectable in at least 95% of patients within 3 months after infection. Although a negative antibody test usually indicates that a person is not infected, antibody tests cannot exclude recent infection. Because the HIV antibody crosses the placenta, a definite diagnosis of HIV in children younger than 18 months is based on laboratory evidence of HIV in blood or tissues by culture, nucleic acid, or antigen detection (Bitnum et al., 2014).

An alternative method of rapid testing for HIV is available, which involves using a blood sample obtained by fingerstick or venipuncture, serum, or plasma or an oral fluid sample. The tests have accuracy rates of 98 to 99%. If the results are reactive, further testing is done. Health Canada requires that rapid test kits only be used in settings where pre- and post-test HIV counselling is available (PHAC, 2012).

Counselling for HIV testing. Counselling before and after HIV testing is standard nursing practice. It is a nurse's responsibility to assess a woman's understanding of the information that such a test would provide and to ensure that she thoroughly understands the emotional, legal, and medical implications of a positive or negative test before she is ready to take an HIV test. Given the strong social stigma attached to HIV infection, nurses must consider the issue of confidentiality and documentation before providing counselling and offering HIV testing to patients.

Unless rapid testing is done, there is generally a 1- to 3-week waiting period after testing for HIV; this can be a very anxious time for the woman. The nurse should inform her that this time period between blood drawing and test results is routine. Test results must always be communicated in person, and women should be told in advance that this is the procedure. Whenever possible, the person who provided the pretest counselling should also be the one to give the woman her test results.

The woman's reaction to a negative test should be explored by asking, "How do you feel?" Counselling sessions for women with an HIV-negative result are another opportunity to provide education. Emphasis can be placed on ways in which a woman can remain HIV-free. She should be reminded that if she has been exposed to HIV in the past 6 months she should be retested, and that she should have ongoing testing if she continues practising high-risk behaviours.

In post-test counselling of an HIV-positive woman, privacy with no interruptions is essential. Adequate time for the counselling sessions also should be provided. The nurse should make sure that the woman understands what a positive test means and review the reliability of the test results.

Risk-reduction practices should be re-emphasized. Referral for appropriate medical evaluation and follow-up should be made, and the need or desire for psychosocial or psychiatric referrals assessed. The public health unit needs to be notified regarding the positive status. Disclosure issues should be discussed with the woman, including the medico-legal requirement to disclose her HIV status to a potential sexual or drug-injecting partner. In general, persons with HIV infection should inform their primary health care provider and consider informing other health care providers (e.g., dentist). Disclosure in the workplace is usually not mandatory but should be individualized (e.g., where the person with HIV infection has direct patient-care responsibilities). The nurse should also discuss disclosing the diagnosis to friends or family; while not essential, it might be considered if there is potential for a positive outcome (e.g., positive family support).

The importance of early medical evaluation (to determine baseline health status) and the benefits of treatment and follow-up need to be stressed. If possible, the nurse should make a referral or appointment for the woman at the post-test counselling session.

Management. During the initial contact with an HIV-infected woman, the nurse should establish what the woman knows about HIV infection and determine whether she is being cared for by a medical practitioner or facility with expertise in caring for persons with HIV infections, including AIDS. Psychological referral also may be indicated. Resources such as counselling for financial assistance, legal advocacy, suicide prevention, and death and dying may be appropriate. Women who are drug users should be referred to a substance-use program. A major focus of counselling is prevention of transmission of HIV to partners.

Nurses counselling seropositive women wishing contraceptive information can recommend oral contraceptives and latex condoms, or tubal sterilization or vasectomy and latex condoms. Female condoms or abstinence should be suggested to women whose male partners refuse to use condoms.

No cure is available for HIV infections at this time. Rare and unusual diseases are characteristic of HIV infections. Opportunistic infections and concurrent diseases are managed vigorously with treatment specific to the infection or disease. Routine gynecological care for HIV-positive women should include a pelvic examination with thorough Pap screening every 6 months, twice and then at least annually depending on the results (PHAC, 2013h). In addition, HIV-positive women should be screened for syphilis, gonorrhea, chlamydia, and other vaginal infections and treated if infections are present. General prevention strategies are an important part of care (e.g., smoking cessation, sound nutrition) as is antiretroviral therapy. Discussion of the medical care of HIV-positive women or women with AIDS is beyond the scope of this chapter because of the rapidly changing recommendations. The reader is referred to the Centers for Disease and Prevention (CDC) (http://www.cdc.gov) and to Internet websites such as the Canadian Aids Treatment Information Exchange (http://www.catie.ca) for current information and recommendations. For care of the pregnant women with HIV see Chapter 15.

NURSING ALERT

Counselling associated with HIV testing has two components: pretest and post-test. During pretest counselling, a personalized risk assessment is conducted, the meaning of positive and negative test results is explained, informed consent for HIV testing is obtained, and the patient is helped to develop a realistic plan for reducing risk and preventing infection. Post-test counselling includes informing the patient of the test results, reviewing the meaning of the results, and reinforcing prevention messages. All pretest and post-test counselling should be documented.

Vaginal Infections

Vaginal discharge and itching of the vulva and vagina are among the most common reasons a woman seeks help from a health care provider. Women cite discomfort from vaginal discharge more than any other gynecological symptom. Women who have adequate endogenous or exogenous estrogen will have vaginal secretions. Vaginal discharge resulting from infection must be distinguished from normal secretions. Normal vaginal secretions (or leukorrhea) are clear to cloudy in appearance. The discharge may turn yellow after drying; is slightly slimy; is nonirritating; and has a mild, inoffensive odour. Normal vaginal secretions are acidic, with a pH range of 4 to 5. The amount of leukorrhea differs with phases of the menstrual cycle, with greater amounts occurring at ovulation and just before menses. Leukorrhea is also increased during pregnancy. Normal vaginal secretions contain lactobacilli and epithelial cells.

Vaginitis, or abnormal vaginal discharge, is an infection caused by a microorganism. The most common vaginal infections are bacterial vaginosis (BV), candidiasis, and trichomoniasis.

Vulvovaginitis (inflammation of the vulva and vagina) may be caused by vaginal infection; copious leukorrhea, which can cause maceration of tissues; and chemical irritants, allergens, and foreign bodies, which may produce inflammatory reactions.

Bacterial Vaginosis

BV, formerly called *nonspecific vaginitis*, *Haemophilus vaginitis*, or *Gardnerella*, is the most common type of vaginitis. The exact etiology of BV is unknown and it is not usually considered an STI. It is a syndrome in which normal hydrogen peroxide–producing lactobacilli are replaced with high concentrations of anaerobic bacteria (*Gardnerella* and *Mobiluncus*). With the proliferation of anaerobes, the level of vaginal amines is raised and the normal acidic pH of the vagina is altered. Epithelial cells slough, and numerous bacteria attach to their surfaces (clue cells). When the amines are volatilized, the characteristic odour of BV occurs.

Screening and diagnosis. A careful history may help distinguish BV from other vaginal infections if the woman is symptomatic. Most women with BV notice a characteristic "fishy odour" in the vaginal area, although not all note it. The odour may be noticed by the woman or her partner after heterosexual intercourse because semen releases the vaginal amines. When present, the BV discharge is usually profuse; thin; and white,

TABLE 7-4 WET SMEAR TESTS FOR VAGINAL INFECTIONS

INFECTION	TEST	POSITIVE FINDINGS
Trichomoniasis	Saline wet smear (vaginal secretions mixed with normal saline on a glass slide)	Presence of many white blood cell protozoa
Candidiasis	Potassium hydroxide (KOH) prep (vaginal secretions mixed with KOH on a glass slide)	Presence of hyphae and pseudohyphae (buds and branches of yeast cells)
Bacterial vaginosis	Normal saline smear	Presence of clue cells (vaginal epithelial cells coated with bacteria)
	Whiff test (vaginal secretions mixed with KOH)	Release of fishy odour

grey, or milky in appearance. Some women also may experience mild irritation or pruritus. Women with previous occurrence of similar symptoms, diagnosis, and treatment should be queried because women with BV often have been treated incorrectly due to misdiagnosis.

Microscopic examination of vaginal secretions is always done (Table 7-4). Both normal saline and 10% potassium hydroxide (KOH) smears should be made. The presence of clue cells confirmed by wet smear is highly diagnostic because the phenomenon is specific to BV (PHAC, 2013h). Vaginal secretions should be tested for pH and amine odour. Nitrazine paper is sensitive enough to detect a pH of 4.5 or greater. The fishy odour of BV will be released when KOH is added to vaginal secretions on the lip of the withdrawn speculum.

Management. Treatment of BV with oral metronidazole (Flagyl) is most effective (PHAC, 2013i), although vaginal preparations (e.g., metronidazole gel, clindamycin cream) are also used. Adverse effects of metronidazole are numerous and include a sharp, unpleasant metallic taste in the mouth; furry tongue; central nervous system reactions; and urinary tract disturbances. When oral metronidazole is taken, the patient is advised not to drink alcoholic beverages or she may experience severe adverse effects of abdominal distress, nausea, vomiting, and headache. Gastrointestinal symptoms are common whether alcohol is consumed or not. Treatment of sexual partners is not recommended because sexual transmission of BV has not been proven. BV during pregnancy is associated with premature rupture of the membranes, chorioamnionitis, preterm labour, preterm birth, and post-Caesarean delivery endometritis (PHAC, 2013i). Therefore, pregnant women should be treated to relieve vaginal symptoms and the signs of infection. Consideration should also be given to evaluation and treatment of asymptomatic women at high risk for preterm birth (PHAC, 2013i).

Candidiasis

Vulvovaginal candidiasis (VVC), or yeast infection, is the second most common type of vaginal infection in Canada. It is estimated that approximately 75% of women will have at least one episode of VVC in their lifetime (PHAC, 2013i). Although vaginal candidiasis infections are common in healthy women, those seen in women with HIV infection are often more severe and persistent. Genital candidiasis lesions may be painful, and coalescing ulcerations necessitate continuous, prophylactic therapy.

The most common organism is *Candida albicans.* It is estimated that 90% of yeast infections in women are caused by this organism. However, in the past 10 years the incidence of non–*C. albicans* infections has increased steadily. Women with chronic or recurrent infections often are infected with a higher percentage of non–*C. albicans* species than are women with their first infection or those who have few recurrences (PHAC, 2013i).

Numerous factors have been identified as predisposing a woman to yeast infections. These include antibiotic therapy, particularly broad-spectrum antibiotics such as ampicillin, tetracycline, cephalosporins, and metronidazole; diabetes, especially when uncontrolled; pregnancy; obesity; diets high in refined sugars or artificial sweeteners; use of corticosteroids and exogenous hormones; and immunosuppressed states. Clinical observations and research have suggested that tight-fitting clothing and underwear or pantyhose made of nonabsorbent materials create an environment in which a vaginal fungus can grow.

The most common symptom of yeast infection is vulvar and possibly vaginal pruritus. The itching may be mild or intense, may interfere with rest and activities, and may occur during or after intercourse. Some women report a feeling of dryness. Others may have painful urination as the urine flows over the vulva. The latter usually occurs in women who have excoriations resulting from scratching. Most often the discharge is thick, white, lumpy, and cottage cheese–like. The discharge may be found in patches on the vaginal walls, cervix, and labia. Commonly the vulva is red and swollen, as are the labial folds, vagina, and cervix. Although there is no odour characteristic of yeast infections, sometimes a yeasty or musty smell is noted.

Screening and diagnosis. In addition to noting the woman's symptoms, their onset, and their course, the history is a valuable screening tool for identifying predisposing risk factors. Physical examination should include a thorough inspection of the vulva and vagina. A speculum examination is always done. Commonly, saline and KOH wet smear and vaginal pH are obtained (see Table 7-4). Vaginal pH is normal (less than 4.5) with a yeast infection. The characteristic pseudohypha (bud or branching of a fungus) may be seen on a wet smear done with normal saline; however, they may be confused with other cells and artifacts.

Management. A number of antifungal preparations are available for the treatment of *C. albicans.* Fluconazole in a single dose can be prescribed, and other medications (e.g., miconazole [Monistat] and clotrimazole [Canesten]) are available as OTC agents. Fluconazole is contraindicated in pregnancy. The first time a woman suspects that she has a yeast infection she should see a health care provider for confirmation of the diagnosis and treatment recommendation. If she has another infection, she may wish to purchase an OTC preparation and self-treat. Treatments should begin to work in 2 to 3 days. If she elects to do

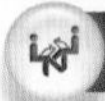

PATIENT TEACHING

Prevention of Genital Tract Infections in Women

- Practise genital hygiene.
- Choose underwear or hosiery with a cotton crotch.
- Avoid tight-fitting clothing (especially tight jeans).
- Select cloth car seat covers instead of vinyl.
- Limit the time spent in damp exercise clothes (especially swimsuits, leotards, and tights).
- Limit exposure to bath salts or bubble bath.
- Avoid coloured or scented toilet tissue.
- If sensitive, discontinue use of feminine hygiene deodorant sprays.
- Use condoms.
- Void before and after intercourse.
- Decrease dietary sugar.
- Drink yeast-active milk and eat yogurt (with lactobacilli).
- Do not douche.

this, she should always be counselled to seek care for numerous recurrent or chronic yeast infections. If vaginal discharge is extremely thick and copious, vaginal débridement with a cotton swab followed by application of vaginal medication may be effective.

Women who have extensive irritation, swelling, and discomfort of the labia and vulva may find sitz baths helpful in decreasing inflammation and increasing comfort. Adding colloidal oatmeal powder to the bath may also increase the woman's comfort. Not wearing underpants to bed may help decrease symptoms and prevent recurrences. Completion of the full course of treatment prescribed is essential to removing the pathogen. Medication should be continued even during menstruation. Women should be counselled not to use tampons during menses because the medication will be absorbed by the tampon. If possible, intercourse should be avoided during treatment; if this is not feasible, the woman's partner should use a condom to prevent introduction of more organisms. Suggested measures to prevent genital tract infections are in the Patient Teaching Box.

Trichomoniasis

Trichomonas vaginalis is almost always an STI and is also a common cause of vaginal infection (5 to 50% of all vaginitis) and discharge (Eckert & Lentz, 2012). Trichomoniasis is caused by *Trichomonas vaginalis*, an anaerobic, one-celled protozoan with characteristic flagella. Although trichomoniasis may be asymptomatic, commonly women have yellowish-to-greenish, frothy, mucopurulent, copious, and malodourous discharge. Inflammation of the vulva, vagina, or both may be present, and the woman may report irritation and pruritus. Dysuria and dyspareunia are often present. Typically the discharge worsens during and after menstruation. The cervix and vaginal walls demonstrate the characteristic "strawberry spots" or tiny petechiae in less than 10% of women, and the cervix may bleed on contact. In severe infections the vaginal walls, cervix, and, occasionally, the vulva may be acutely inflamed.

Screening and diagnosis. In addition to obtaining a history of current symptoms, a thorough sexual history should be taken. The nurse should note any history of similar symptoms in the past and treatment used. The nurse also needs to determine whether the woman's partner or partners were treated and if she has had subsequent relations with new partners.

A speculum examination is always done, even though it may be uncomfortable for the woman; relaxation techniques and breathing exercises may help the woman with the procedure. Any of the classic signs may or may not be seen on physical examination. The typical one-celled flagellate trichomonads are easily distinguished on a normal saline wet prep (Table 7-4). The pH of the discharge is greater than 5.0. Because trichomoniasis is an STI, once diagnosis is confirmed, appropriate laboratory studies for other STIs should be carried out.

Management. The recommended treatment is metronidazole (Flagyl), 2 g orally in a single dose or 500 mg orally bid for 7 days (PHAC, 2013i). The efficacy of the treatment will increase if the partner is also treated, even if symptoms are not present. If partners are not treated, the infection will likely recur. Women should be taught that they should not drink alcohol during and for 24 hours after therapy as there is a risk of a disulfuram (antabuse) reaction (PHAC, 2013i). Symptoms of this reaction include dizziness, headache, shortness of breath, palpitation, and nausea and vomiting.

Women with trichomoniasis need to understand the sexual transmission of this disease. Patients must know that the organism may be present without observable symptoms, perhaps for several months, and that determining when they became infected is impossible.

Effects of Sexually Transmitted Infections on Pregnancy and the Fetus

STIs in pregnancy are responsible for significant morbidity and mortality. Some consequences of maternal infection such as infertility and sterility last a lifetime. Congenitally acquired infection may affect a child's length and quality of life. Table 7-5 describes the effects of several common STIs on pregnancy and the fetus. It is difficult to predict these effects with certainty. Factors such as coinfection with other STIs and at what point in pregnancy the infection was treated can affect outcomes.

CONCERNS OF THE BREAST

Benign Problems

Fibrocystic Changes

Approximately 50% of women have a breast problem at some point in their adult lives. The most common benign breast problem is fibrocystic change (Katz & Dotters, 2012). Fibrocystic changes occur to varying degrees in breasts of healthy women. The etiological agent responsible for these changes has not been found. One theory is that estrogen excess and progesterone deficiency in the luteal phase of the menstrual cycle may cause changes in breast tissue.

Fibrocystic changes are characterized by lumpiness, with or without tenderness, in both breasts. Single simple cysts can also occur. Symptoms usually develop approximately a week before

TABLE 7-5 PREGNANCY AND FETAL EFFECTS OF COMMON SEXUALLY TRANSMITTED INFECTIONS

INFECTION	MATERNAL EFFECTS	FETAL EFFECTS
Chlamydia	Premature rupture of membranes* Preterm labour*	Low birth weight Conjunctivitis Pneumonia
Gonorrhea	Postpartum endometritis Postpartum sepsis	Ophthalmia neonatorum Systemic neonatal infection
Group B streptococci	Urinary tract infection Preterm labour Preterm labour rupture of membranes	Preterm birth Sepsis
Herpes simplex virus	Spontaneous abortion*	Congenital infection (rare) Neonatal infection Preterm birth* IUGR*
Human papillomavirus (HPV)	Excessive bleeding from lesions after birth	Recurrent respiratory papillomatosis (RRP) (rare)
Bacterial vaginosis	Premature rupture of membranes Preterm labour Postpartum endometritis	Preterm birth
Trichomoniasis	Premature rupture of the membranes Preterm labour	Low birth weight Preterm birth
Syphilis	Preterm labour	Preterm birth Stillbirth Congenital abnormalities Congenital infection

*Research is not convincing.
IUGR, intrauterine growth restriction.
Data from http://www.phac-aspc.gc.ca/std-mts/sti-its/cgsti-ldcits/section-6-4-eng.php

menstruation begins and subside approximately a week after menstruation ends. Symptoms include dull, heavy pain and a sense of fullness and tenderness often in the upper outer quadrants of the breasts. Physical examination may reveal excessive nodularity that many describe as feeling similar to a "plateful of peas" (Katz & Dotters, 2012). Larger cysts are often described as feeling like water-filled balloons. Women in their 20s report the most severe pain. Women in their 30s have premenstrual pain and tenderness; small multiple nodules are usually present. Women in their 40s usually do not report severe pain, but cysts are tender and often regress in size (Katz & Dotters, 2012).

Steps in the workup of a breast lump may begin with an ultrasound to determine whether it is fluid filled or solid. Fluid-filled cysts are aspirated, and the woman is monitored on a routine basis for the development of other cysts. If the lump is solid, a mammogram is obtained if the woman is older than age 50 years. A fine-needle aspiration (FNA) is performed, regardless of the woman's age, to determine the nature of the lump (Katz & Dotters, 2012).

Management depends on the severity of the symptoms. Women who have severe cyclic breast pain may find relief with eating dietary flaxseed (Chase, Wells, & Eley, 2011). Although research findings are contradictory, some practitioners advocate reducing consumption or eliminating methylxanthines (e.g., colas, coffee, tea, chocolate) and tobacco (Chase et al., 2011; Katz & Dotters, 2012).

Women may report decreased symptoms with such measures as eating a low-fat diet, decreasing sodium intake, or taking mild diuretics shortly before menses, but supporting evidence is lacking (Chase et al., 2011). Other pain-relief measures that include taking analgesics or NSAIDs, wearing a supportive bra, and applying heat or cold to the breasts are supported by research (Katz & Dotters, 2012).

Evening primrose oil and vitamin E supplements may be effective for some women, although more research is needed to support this claim (Chase et al., 2011). Oral contraceptives, danazol, bromocriptine, and tamoxifen have also been used with varying degrees of success (Katz & Dotters, 2012).

Fibroadenomas

The next most common benign neoplasm of the breast is a **fibroadenoma**. It is the single most common type of tumour seen in the adolescent population, although it can also occur in women in their 30s. Fibroadenomas are discrete, usually solitary lumps averaging 2.5 cm in diameter (Katz & Dotters, 2012). Occasionally the woman with a fibroadenoma experiences tenderness in the tumour during the menstrual cycle. Fibroadenomas do not increase in size in response to the menstrual cycle as cysts do. They increase in size during pregnancy and decrease in size as the woman ages. The cause of fibroadenomas is unknown.

Diagnosis is made by reviewing patient history and physical examination. Mammography, ultrasound, or magnetic resonance imaging (MRI) helps determine the type of lesion. FNA may be used to determine underlying pathological conditions. Surgical excision may be necessary if the lump is suspicious or if the symptoms are severe. Periodic observation of masses by professional physical examination or mammography may be all that is necessary for masses not needing surgical intervention (Katz & Dotters, 2012).

Lipomas

A *lipoma* is a tumour composed of fat that is soft and has discrete borders. The cause of lipoma is unknown. Lipomas are often found in women over 45 years of age, usually on the chest wall and breast. They are characterized as palpable soft masses that are mobile and nontender. Mammograms can be used to make a diagnosis; biopsy usually is not needed. Lipomas can be surgically excised if removal is desired.

Nipple Discharge

Nipple discharge is a common occurrence that affects many women. Although most nipple discharge is physiological, each

TABLE 7-6 COMPARISON OF COMMON MANIFESTATIONS OF BENIGN BREAST MASSES

FIBROCYSTIC CHANGES	FIBROADENOMA	LIPOMA	INTRADUCTAL PAPILLOMA	MAMMARY DUCT ECTASIA
Multiple lumps	Single lump	Single lump	Single or multiple	Mass behind nipple
Nodular	Well delineated	Well delineated	Not well delineated	Not well delineated
Palpable	Palpable	Palpable	Nonpalpable	Palpable
Movable	Movable	Movable	Nonmobile	Nonmobile
Round, smooth	Round, lobular	Round, lobular	Small, ball-like	Irregular
Firm or soft	Firm	Soft	Firm or soft	Firm
Tenderness influenced by menstrual cycle	Usually asymptomatic	Nontender	Usually nontender	Painful, burning, itching
Bilateral	Unilateral	Unilateral	Unilateral	Unilateral
May or may not have nipple discharge	No nipple discharge	No nipple discharge	Serous or bloody nipple discharge	Thick, sticky nipple discharge

woman who has this problem must be evaluated thoroughly, as a small percentage of women are found to have a serious endocrine disorder or malignancy. Most nipple discharge is elicited (i.e., discharge is a result of the breast being compressed or stimulated) and is usually not a concern unless the woman is postmenopausal or a mass is present in the breast (Lobo, 2012b).

Galactorrhea is another form of breast discharge not related to malignancy. Galactorrhea manifests as a bilaterally spontaneous, milky, sticky discharge. It is a normal finding in pregnancy. It can also occur as the result of elevated prolactin levels, caused by a thyroid disorder, pituitary tumour, or chest wall surgery or trauma. Obtaining a complete medication history on each woman is essential. Some tranquilizers (e.g., tricyclic antidepressants), narcotics, antihypertensive medications, and oral contraceptives can precipitate galactorrhea in some women (Lobo, 2012b). Diagnostic tests that may be indicated include a prolactin level, a microscopic analysis of the discharge, a thyroid profile, a pregnancy test, and a mammogram (Lobo, 2012b).

Mammary Duct Ectasia

Mammary duct ectasia is an inflammation of the ducts behind the nipple. It occurs most often in perimenopausal women and is characterized by a nipple discharge that is thick, sticky, and white, brown, green, or purple. The woman frequently experiences a burning pain, an itching, or a palpable mass behind the nipple.

The diagnostic workup includes a mammogram and aspiration and culture of fluid. Treatment is usually symptomatic; mild pain relievers, warm compresses applied to the breast, or wearing a supportive bra may provide relief. If a mass is present or an abscess occurs, treatment may include a local excision of the affected duct or ducts, provided that the woman has no future plans to breastfeed (Mayo Foundation for Medical Education and Research, 2012).

Intraductal Papilloma

Intraductal papilloma is a rare benign condition that develops within the terminal nipple ducts. The cause is unknown. It usually occurs in women between 30 and 50 years of age. The papilloma is usually too small to be palpated (less than 0.5 cm), and the characteristic sign is spontaneous unilateral nipple discharge that is serous, serosanguineous, or bloody. After eliminating the possibility of malignancy, the affected segments of the ducts and breasts are surgically excised (Katz & Dotters, 2012).

NURSING CARE

Assessment should include a careful history and physical examination. Table 7-6 compares common manifestations of benign breast masses. The history should focus on risk factors for breast diseases, events related to the breast mass, and health-maintenance practices. Risk factors for breast cancer are discussed later in this chapter. Information related to the breast mass should include how, when, and by whom the mass was discovered. The nurse should document the following patient information: pain, whether symptoms increase with menses, dietary habits, smoking habits, and the use of oral contraceptives. The woman's emotional status, including her stress level, fears, and concerns, and her ability to cope should also be assessed.

Physical examination may include assessment of the breasts for symmetry, masses (size, number, consistency, and mobility), and nipple discharge.

Nursing actions might include the following:

- Discuss the intervals for and facets of breast screening, including professional examination and mammography (see Table 7-6). Women with breast implants may need special views of the breast and precautions taken to avoid rupture of the implant during mammography.
- Provide written educational materials in the woman's primary language.
- Encourage expression of fears and concerns about treatment and prognosis.
- Provide specific information regarding the woman's condition and treatment, including dietary changes, drug therapy, comfort measures, stress management, and surgery.
- Describe pain-relieving strategies in detail and collaborate with the primary health care provider to ensure effective pain control.

- Encourage discussion of feelings about body image.
- Demonstrate correct breast self-examination technique if the woman wishes to practise it (see Chapter 6 and the Nursing Skills available on Evolve).

Cancer of the Breast

Mortality rates from breast cancer have declined since 1990. Nonetheless, 1 in 9 Canadian women will develop breast cancer in her lifetime, and 1 out of every 30 is expected to die from it (CCS, 2014b). The prognosis for and survival of the woman are improved with early detection. Therefore, women must be educated about risk factors, early detection, and screening.

Although the exact cause of breast cancer is still unknown, researchers have identified certain factors that increase a women's risk for developing a malignancy. These factors are listed in Box 7-6. The most important predictor of risk for breast cancer is age; a woman's risk increases as her age increases.

Much discussion has taken place about possible links between breast cancer and hormone therapy; several large research studies, including the Women's Health Initiative, have found that the risk of breast cancer increases when a woman is taking combined estrogen and progesterone but declines quickly once therapy is stopped. Researchers now believe that there is an increased risk in the development of breast cancer, but it is small and depends on the type of HRT that is used. For women taking estrogen-only HRT, this risk does not increase until after 7 years of use, and for those women taking combined HRT, this risk does not increase for 4 to 5 years (CCS, 2014b).

Although most breast cancers are not related to genetic factors, the identification of the *BRCA1* and *BRCA2* genes demonstrated the role of heredity and genetic mutations in this disease. Only approximately 5 to 10% of breast cancers are attributed to heredity. Women who have abnormalities in the *BRCA1* and *BRCA2* genes have up to an 80% chance of developing breast cancer (CCS, 2014b). Other genetic mutations that can cause breast cancer include mutations of the ataxia telangiectasia mutated (ATM) gene, the p53 tumour suppressor gene, the phosphatase and tensin homolog (PTEN) gene, and the checkpoint kinase 2 (CHEK2) gene (CCS, 2014b).

During breast cancer risk counselling, facts should be presented to women by their health care provider in a supportive, nondirective way, without personal opinions or preferences. Discussion should also include treatment options and prognosis of breast cancer, as well as risks and benefits of alternative methods of prevention and early diagnosis. A woman's recognition of having increased breast cancer risk can carry psychological consequences such as anxiety, guilt, depression, and reduced self-esteem. Enormous guilt may be experienced by high-risk women who pass specific genetic mutations on to their children. Psychological intervention may be offered to assist individuals in coping with these significant adverse sequelae.

BOX 7-6 RISK FACTORS FOR BREAST CANCER

Risks that are not modifiable:
- Age—risk increases with age
- Previous history of breast cancer
- Family history of breast cancer and other cancers, especially a mother or sister (particularly significant if premenopausal)
- Inherited genetic mutations in *BRCA1* and *BRCA2* genes
- Dense breasts
- Ashkenazi Jewish ancestry
- Rare genetic conditions
- Reproductive history
- Early menarche (before age 12)
- Late menopause (after age 55)
- Tall adult height
- Higher socioeconomic status

Lifestyle and modifiable risks:
- Nulliparity or first pregnancy after age 30
- Not breastfeeding
- Exposure to ionizing radiation
- Use of oral contraceptives
- Postmenopausal use of combined estrogen-progestin replacement therapy (HRT) for at least 5 years
- Obesity after menopause
- Alcohol consumption of more than one drink per day
- Sedentary lifestyle
- Vitamin D—low levels increase risk
- Smoking and secondhand smoke
- Night shift work

Source: Canadian Cancer Society. (2016). *Risk factors for breast cancer.* Retrieved from https://www.cancer.ca/en/cancer-information/cancer-type/breast/risks/?region=on

Ethical Considerations of Genetic Testing

Although knowing whether one is hereditarily predisposed to breast cancer may have benefits, the extent to which an individual can benefit from this information remains unclear. Confirming one's mutation status may provide a sense of control in life plans or it may create high levels of anxiety and distress. Genetic testing can alter decisions regarding family and intimate relationships, child-bearing, body image, and quality of life. Regardless of whether results are positive or negative for *BRCA1* and *BRCA2* mutations, the results can have a highly negative impact on women's lives. Women at increased risk for breast cancer need comprehensive information about the benefits and limitations of genetic testing to ensure that informed decisions about genetic testing can be made. Because decisions regarding genetic testing, genetic counselling, and breast cancer risk assessment are highly individualized, health care providers should be careful in making any generalizations about women at risk for breast cancer.

Prevention

Chemoprevention is the use of medications to reduce cancer risk. Tamoxifen and raloxifene both protect bone health but also have a role in blocking the effect of estrogen on breast tissue. Studies have shown that these two drugs can reduce the risk of breast cancer, although tamoxifen increases the risk of endometrial cancer. Women need information to weigh the risks and benefits of taking these medications. Surgical prophylaxis (bilateral mastectomy, oophorectomy) can reduce the risk of

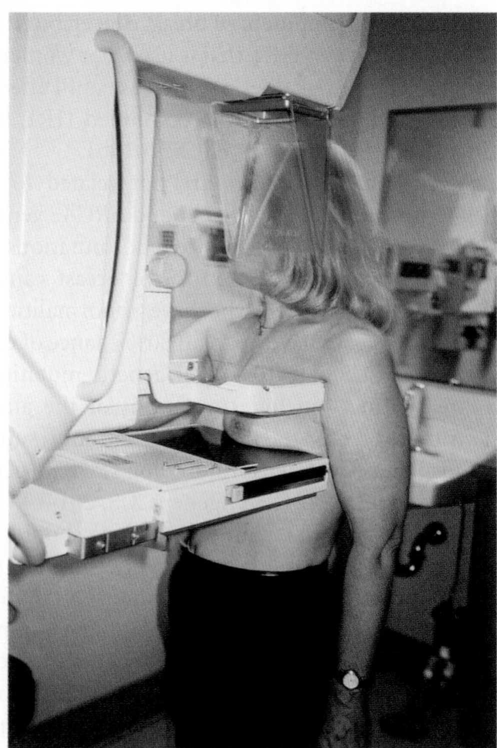

FIGURE 7-6 Mammography. (Courtesy Shannon Perry.)

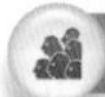

CULTURAL AWARENESS

Breast Screening Practices

Some women tend to have low breast screening rates. More than half of recent immigrants (less than 10 years) have not had a screening mammogram compared to 25% of Canadian-born women. Many factors play a role in influencing the screening practices of women, including unawareness of mammography screening, gender and modesty concerns unique to cultural beliefs, and fear resulting from a sense of vulnerability to breast cancer. Income, marital status, education, and language difficulties also contribute to rates of screening.

Interventions that encourage all women to participate in early breast cancer screen practices require women's input to improve our understanding of the barriers women have in getting screened; this would contribute to the design of community-driven interventions to enhance accessibility of breast cancer screening services. Existing research has suggested various strategies that place an emphasis on the need to develop tailored and culturally appropriate interventions for women to overcome knowledge and structural barriers, address misconceptions, and promote screening practices. Mobile breast cancer screening units may help women overcome obstacles to reaching optimal levels of health. Interventions that encourage women to participate in early breast cancer screening practices begin with the development of culturally sensitive community education programs designed to help women deal with barriers to reaching optimal levels of health.

Source: Mahamoud, A. (2014). *Breast cancer screening in racialized women: Implications for health equity.* Toronto: Wellesley Institute. Retrieved from http://www.wellesleyinstitute.com/publications/breast-cancer-screening-in-racialized-women/

breast cancer, but it should be considered only for people at very high risk (CCS, 2014b).

Screening and Diagnosis

Regular clinical examination by a qualified health care provider and screening mammography (x-ray filming of the breast) (Fig. 7-6) may aid in the early detection of breast cancers. A diagnostic mammogram is performed when a screening mammogram identifies something that needs further inspection or when the woman or examiner finds a breast symptom that is new. Women between the ages of 50 and 69 should have screening mammograms done every 2 years. Women aged 40 to 49 at high risk for developing breast cancer should consider mammograms earlier, in consultation with their health care provider. Women over 70 should discuss with their health care provider how often mammograms should be done.

More than half of all lumps are discovered in the upper outer quadrant of the breast. The woman may feel a lump or thickening of the breast. The lump may feel hard and fixed or soft and spongy. It may have well-defined or irregular borders. It may be fixed to the skin, thereby causing dimpling to occur. A bloody or clear unilateral nipple discharge may be present.

Early detection and diagnosis reduce the mortality rate because the cancer is found when it is smaller, lesions are more localized, and there tends to be a lower percentage of positive nodes.

Major obstacles to breast cancer screening include older age; knowledge, attitudinal, and behavioural barriers (e.g., fear, ignorance, lack of motivation); and organizational barriers (e.g., scheduling problems, lack of availability of mammography services, lack of physician referral). Strategies that may be helpful to health care providers in improving screening for breast cancer include related education and encouragement of older women; continuing education of providers; use of reminder systems in office practice; use of patient-directed literature; and interventions that reward, support, and prompt desired screening behaviours. All provinces and some territories have organized breast cancer screening programs for women 50 to 69 years of age. Women are automatically invited to take part in the breast screening program and are sent letters reminding them of next screening mammogram.

Cultural factors may influence a woman's decision to participate in breast cancer screening. Knowledge of these factors and use of culturally sensitive tailored messages and materials that appeal to the unique concerns, beliefs, and reading abilities of identified groups of women who do not participate in breast screening may assist the nurse in helping women overcome barriers to seeking care (see Cultural Awareness box).

When a suspicious finding on a mammogram is noted or when a lump is detected, diagnosis is confirmed by means of FNA, core needle biopsy, or surgical excision (Fig. 7-7).

Ultrasound may also be used to assess a specific area of abnormality found during a mammogram procedure (CCS, 2014b). Women need specific information regarding advantages and disadvantages of these procedures in making a decision about which one is most appropriate for them. Laboratory examination of breast tissue determines if cancer is present and, if so, the extent. Other tests performed to determine the spread

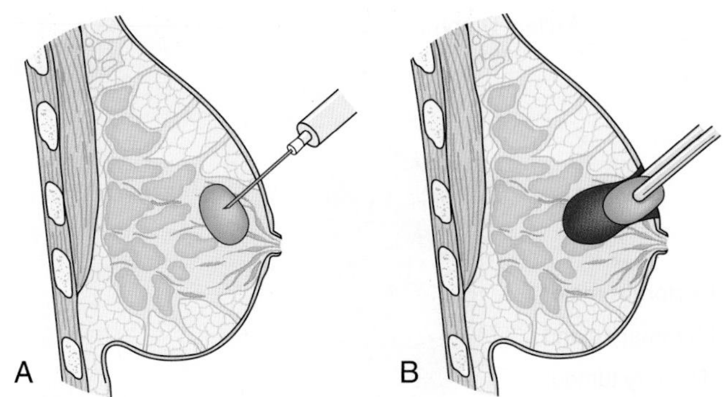

FIGURE 7-7 Diagnosis. **A**, Needle aspiration. **B**, Open biopsy. (Redrawn from National Women's Health Resource. [1995]. *National Women's Health Report, 13*[5], 3.)

of the cancer include chest x-ray film examination, bone scan, CT, MRI, and positron emission tomography (PET scan) (CCS, 2014b).

An important step in evaluating a breast cancer is to test for the presence of estrogen and progesterone receptors in the biopsied tissue. Cancer cells may contain one, both, or neither of these receptors. Breast cancers that contain estrogen receptors are often called *ER-positive* cancers, whereas those containing progesterone receptors are called *PR-positive* cancers. Women with hormone-positive tumours tend to respond better to treatment and have higher survival rates than the general population (Katz & Dotters, 2012).

An HER2 test also may be performed on the biopsied breast tissue. HER2 is a growth-promoting hormone; and in approximately 15% to 30% of breast cancers, excessive amounts of the hormone are present, causing the cancer to be more aggressive in spreading than other types of breast cancer (CCS, 2014b).

Breast Cancer During Pregnancy

Although breast cancer is the most common cancer diagnosed during pregnancy, it is rare. About 1 out of every 3000 pregnant women is diagnosed with breast cancer. Treatment decisions for breast cancer in pregnancy are based on the stage of breast cancer and the age of the fetus. Ending a pregnancy (therapeutic abortion) is not considered a necessary part of treatment because it does not improve a mother's prognosis or survival (CCS, 2014b).

Treatment for breast cancer during pregnancy often begins immediately and may include the following:

- Surgery to remove the lump or the affected breast. Surgery can be carried out at any stage in pregnancy.
- Chemotherapy—not given during the first 13 weeks of pregnancy as it may cause abnormalities in the baby
- Radiation—not usually offered as a treatment option until after the birth
- Tamoxifen—not recommended during pregnancy and will be delayed until after the birth (Royal College of Obstetricians and Gynecologists [RCOG], 2011)

Many women who are diagnosed with breast cancer during pregnancy are concerned that they can pass the breast cancer cells to their baby. There is no evidence that a fetus can get cancer from its mother while in the womb. There is also no evidence that a woman can pass cancer cells to her baby through breastfeeding. Women need correct information and discussion regarding how breast cancer treatment may affect fertility. The medical team should take into account any plans for future pregnancies and offer chemotherapy drugs that are less likely to affect fertility (CCS, 2014b).

BOX 7-7 DECISION-MAKING QUESTIONS TO ASK REGARDING BREAST CANCER TREATMENT

1. What kind of breast cancer is it (invasive or noninvasive)?
2. What stage is cancer (i.e., how extensive is the spread)?
3. Did the cancer test positive for hormone (estrogen) (may be slower growing)?
4. Which further tests are recommended?
5. What are the treatment options (pros and cons of each, including side effects)?
6. If surgery is recommended, what will the scar look like?
7. If a mastectomy is done, can breast reconstruction be done (at the time of surgery or later)?
8. How long will the woman be in the hospital? What kind of postoperative care will she need?
9. How long will treatment last if radiation or chemotherapy is recommended? What effects can the woman expect from these treatments?
10. What community resources are available for support?

Medical Management

Controversy continues regarding the best treatment for breast cancer. Nodal involvement, tumour size, receptor status, and aggressiveness are important variables for treatment selection. Medical management of breast cancer includes surgery, breast reconstruction, radiation therapy, adjuvant hormone therapy, biological targeted therapy, and chemotherapy. Many women face difficult decisions about the various treatment options. Box 7-7 lists questions that must be addressed in decision making. Treatment plans are designed to meet the unique needs of each person with cancer and are based on the following: stage of the breast cancer; if the woman has reached menopause; hormone receptor status of the cancer; HER2 status of the cancer; risk for recurrence (with early-stage breast cancer); the overall health of the woman; the woman's personal decision about certain treatments (CCS, 2014b).

Most health care providers recommend that the malignant mass and the axillary nodes, specifically the sentinel node, be removed for staging purposes (Katz & Dotters, 2012). The treatment can be conservative or more radical. Breast-conserving surgery such as a **lumpectomy** (Fig. 7-8, *A*) or partial mastectomy (e.g., quadrantectomy, wide excision) (Fig. 7-8, *B*) is the removal of the breast tumour and a small amount of surrounding tissue may be recommended. Sampling of axillary lymph nodes usually occurs through a separate incision at the time of these procedures, and the surgery is usually followed by radiation therapy to the remaining breast tissue (Katz & Dotters, 2012). These procedures are for the primary treatment of

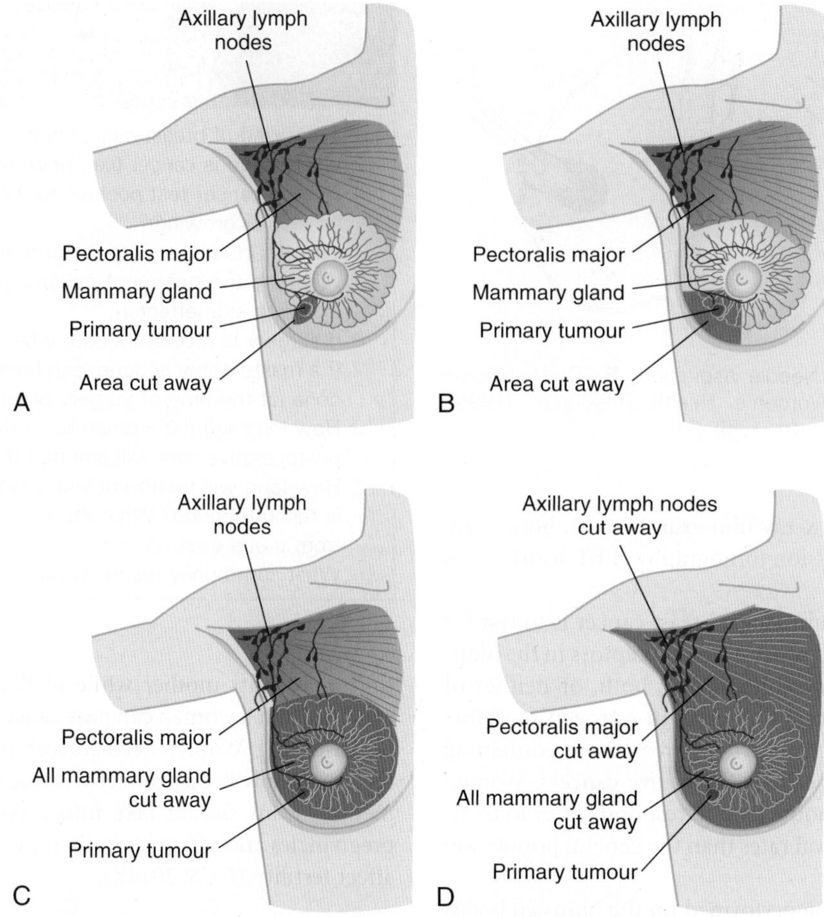

FIGURE 7-8 Surgical alternatives for breast cancer. **A:** Lumpectomy. **B:** Partial mastectomy (quadrantectomy, wide excision). **C:** Total (simple) mastectomy. **D:** Radical mastectomy.

women with early-stage (I or II) breast cancer. Lumpectomy offers survival equivalent to that with modified radical mastectomy. A total simple mastectomy (see Fig. 7-8, C) is the removal of the breast containing the tumour, whereas, a modified radical mastectomy is removal of the breast tissue, skin, and fascia of the pectoralis muscle and dissection of the axillary nodes. A radical mastectomy (see Fig. 7-8, D), although rarely performed, is removal of the breast and underlying pectoralis muscles and complete axillary node dissection. After surgery follow-up, treatment may include radiation, chemotherapy, or hormone therapy (Katz & Dotters, 2012). The decision to include follow-up therapy is based on the stage of disease, age and menopausal status of the woman, the woman's preference, and her hormone receptor status. Follow-up treatment is usually initiated to decrease the risk of recurrence in women who have no evidence of metastasis.

Radiation is usually recommended as follow-up therapy for women who have stage I or II cancer. Radiation can be external for 5 to 6 weeks or as short as 3 weeks. Internal radiation is in the form of needles, seeds, wires, or catheters filled with a radioactive substance that is inserted into the breast near the tumour.

Hormone therapy with tamoxifen, an estrogen agonist, is recommended for some women with breast cancer. In order to determine whether a woman is a candidate for hormone therapy, a receptor assay is performed. The cancer cells are examined for the presence of a receptor on the cell wall, which indicates that the woman is positive for that type of hormone receptor. If these receptors are present, the growth of the woman's breast cancer may be influenced by estrogen, progesterone, or both. It is unknown exactly how these hormones affect breast cancer growth. Some premenopausal women may undergo bilateral oophorectomy to decrease the supply of hormones available for tumour growth.

Tamoxifen is an oral anti-estrogen medication that mimics progesterone and estrogen. It attaches to the hormone receptors on cancer cells and prevents natural hormones from attaching to the receptors. When tamoxifen fits into the receptors, the cell is unable to grow. Adjuvant hormone therapy with tamoxifen is recommended for all postmenopausal women with breast cancer. Women treated with hormone therapy should receive therapy for at least 5 years (see Medication Guide [Tamoxifen]).

Aromatase inhibitors markedly suppress plasma estrogen levels in postmenopausal women by inhibiting or inactivating aromatase, the enzyme responsible for synthesizing estrogens from androgenic substrates. Aromatase inhibitors such as anastrozole, letrozole, and exemestane have been shown to be effective agents in hormone therapy for breast cancer. In early-stage breast cancer, adjuvant therapy with anastrozole appears to be superior to adjuvant therapy with tamoxifen in reducing recurrence in postmenopausal women (see Medication Guide

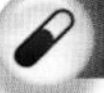

MEDICATION GUIDE

Tamoxifen (Nolvadex, Tamofen)

Action
Anti-estrogenic effects; attaches to hormone receptors on cancer cells and prevents natural hormones from attaching to the receptors

Indications
For treatment of advanced-stage or metastatic breast cancer; treatment of early-stage breast cancer after breast cancer surgery and radiation therapy; to reduce the incidence of breast cancer in women at high risk

Dosage
20 mg orally daily

Adverse Reactions
Common adverse effects include hot flashes, night sweats, nausea, vaginal bleeding or discharge, and mood swings. Hair loss is an uncommon effect. Serious adverse effects include deep vein thrombosis, increased risk of endometrial cancer, and stroke.

Nursing Considerations
The medication may be taken on an empty stomach or with food. Missed doses should be taken as soon as possible, but taking two doses at once is not recommended. A barrier or nonhormonal form of contraception is recommended in premenopausal women because tamoxifen may be harmful to the fetus if pregnancy should occur.

MEDICATION GUIDE

Anastrozole (Arimidex)

Action
An aromatase inhibitor; inhibits conversion of androgens to estrogen

Indication
For adjuvant treatment of early breast cancer in postmenopausal women who have received 5 years of tamoxifen therapy; first-line treatment of postmenopausal women with hormone receptor–positive or hormone receptor–unknown locally advanced or metastatic cancer; adjuvant treatment of postmenopausal women with hormone receptor–positive early breast cancer

Dosage and Route
1 mg once a day by mouth

Adverse Reactions
Common adverse effects include hot flashes, nausea, increased sweating, joint or muscle pain, fluid retention, vaginal dryness, constipation, dizziness, fatigue, headache; severe adverse effects include severe allergic reactions (e.g., rash, hives, difficulty breathing), vomiting, chest pain, severe bone pain, calf pain or tenderness

Nursing Considerations
The medication may be taken on an empty stomach or with food. The woman should use caution if driving or using machinery because this medication may cause drowsiness or dizziness. She should be advised that the medicine may decrease bone strength, increase her risk for fractures, and increase cholesterol.

[Anastrozole]). The aromatase inhibitors appear to be well tolerated, with a lower incidence of adverse effects than with tamoxifen (Saskatchewan Cancer Agency, 2012).

Chemotherapy is often given to premenopausal women who have positive nodes. Therapy for more advanced tumours usually includes surgery followed by chemotherapy, radiation, or both (Katz & Dotters, 2012). Chemotherapy with multiple drug combinations is used in the treatment of recurrent and advanced breast cancer, with positive results. Combination regimens and sequential single agents may be used. Some chemotherapeutic drugs provide additional treatment options for women with metastatic breast cancer.

Because chemotherapy drugs are designed to kill rapidly reproducing cells, normal body cells that rapidly reproduce (red and white blood cells, gastric mucosa, and hair) also can be affected during treatment. Thus chemotherapy can cause leukopenia, neutropenia, thrombocytopenia, anemia, gastrointestinal side effects (nausea, vomiting, anorexia, mucositis), and partial or full hair loss.

The goals of surgical breast reconstruction are achievement of symmetry and preservation of body image. Surgical reconstruction can be done immediately or at a later date. Immediate reconstruction at the time of mastectomy does not change survival rates or interfere with therapy or the treatment of recurrent disease.

The types of surgery for breast reconstruction include implants and flap procedures. Implants are made of silicone or saline or a combination of both and can be inserted at the same time as a mastectomy or later. They are placed underneath the chest muscle instead of on top of it, as in the case of breast augmentation. Silicone implants have been deemed safe and are options for women having breast reconstruction following mastectomy.

Flap procedures are done by plastic and reconstructive surgeons who specialize in microsurgery. During flap reconstruction a breast is created using tissue taken from other parts of the body, such as the abdomen, back, or buttocks, or thighs, which is then transplanted to the chest by reconnecting the blood vessels to new ones in the chest region.

After a woman has recovered from initial reconstructive surgery, she may choose to have nipple and areolar reconstruction. Nipple reconstruction is achieved by using an autologous skin graft to construct a nipple, either from tissue from the remaining nipple or from a donor site (Katz & Dotters, 2012).

NURSING CARE

Before surgery, women need to be assessed for psychological preparation and specific teaching needs. General preoperative teaching and care are given, including expectations regarding physical appearance, pain management, equipment to be used (e.g., intravenous therapy, drains), and emotional support. The emotional reaction to the diagnosis of cancer is always intense, and the many disruptions caused by the disease challenge the woman's and family's ability to cope. A visit from a woman who has had a similar experience may be beneficial both before and after surgery. The woman should be reminded that when she awakens after surgery, her arm on the affected side will feel tight.

Postoperative nursing care focuses on recovery. Special precautions must be observed to prevent or minimize lymphedema of the affected arm.

NURSING ALERT

Avoid taking blood pressure, giving injections, or taking blood from the arm on the affected side.

The affected arm is elevated with pillows above the level of the right atrium. Blood is not drawn from this arm, and it is not used for intravenous therapy. Early arm movement should be encouraged. Any increase in the circumference of that arm needs to be reported immediately.

Nursing care of the wound involves observation for signs of hemorrhage (dressing, drainage tubes, and Hemovac or Jackson-Pratt drainage reservoirs are emptied at least every 8 hours and more frequently as needed), shock, and infection. Dressings are reinforced as necessary. The woman is asked to turn (alternating between unaffected side and back), cough (while the nurse or the woman applies support to the chest), and deep-breathe every 2 hours. Breath sounds are auscultated every 4 hours. Active range-of-motion exercise of legs should be encouraged. Parenteral fluids need to be given until adequate oral intake is possible. Emotional support should be continued.

The woman is given self-management instructions and usually discharged to home after 24 hours or more, depending on the type of procedure done (see Home Care box). Lumpectomy is an outpatient procedure, and the patient usually returns home a few hours after surgery. A woman is discharged 24 to 48 hours after modified radical mastectomy. A referral for home nursing care can be made if the woman needs assistance caring for her incision. Through CancerConnection, a breast cancer survivor who has been trained in how to offer information can offer telephone support (see Community Focus box). The resources offered may include a list of sources for prostheses and lingerie. The woman should be encouraged to do arm exercises at least twice a day (see Patient Teaching box).

Exercise is increased as tolerated and stopped at the point of pain. Initially the woman will alternately clench and extend her fingers and then progress to wrist and elbow exercises, gradually abducting her arm and raising it to and over her head. She should be encouraged to exercise through assistance with her care—washing her face, brushing her teeth, and eating with her hand and arm on the affected side. Physiotherapy may be prescribed to improve strength and mobility of the affected arm.

Concerns about appearance after breast surgery may affect the woman's self-concept. Before surgery, the woman and her partner need to receive information about the woman's postoperative appearance. Some women may not want to view their surgical site, but it is important to give them the opportunity to do so and to provide emotional support at that time. Both the woman and her partner need to be able to discuss feelings and concerns about accepting the changes.

HOME CARE

After a Mastectomy

- Wash your hands well before and after touching the incision area or drains.
- Empty surgical drains twice a day and as needed, recording the date, time, drain site (if more than one drain is present), and amount of drainage in millilitres until your drains are removed. (Before discharge you may receive a graduated container for emptying drains and measuring drainage.)
- Avoid driving, lifting more than 5 kg, or reaching above your head until given permission by your surgeon.
- Take medications for pain as soon as pain begins.
- Perform arm exercises as directed.
- Call your physician if inflammation of the incision or swelling of the incision or the arm occurs.
- Avoid tight clothing, tight jewellery, and other causes of decreased circulation in the affected arm.
- Until drains are removed, wear loose-fitting underwear (camisole or half-slip) and clothes, pinning surgical drains inside clothing. (You will be taught how to do this safely.)
- After drains are removed and surgical sites are healing and still tender, wear a mastectomy bra or camisole with a cotton-filled, muslin temporary prosthesis. Temporary prostheses of this type are often available through the Canadian Cancer Society.
- Avoid depilatory creams; strong deodorants; and shaving of the affected chest area, axilla, and arm.
- Take sponge bath until drains are removed.
- Return to the surgeon's office for incision check, drain inspection, and possible drain removal as directed.
- Contact the Canadian Cancer Society for assistance in obtaining an external prosthesis and lingerie when dressings, drains, and staples are removed and the wound is healing and nontender.
- Contact your insurance company for information about coverage of the prosthesis and wig, if needed. Obtain prescriptions for a prosthesis and wig to submit with receipts of purchase for these items to the insurance company. If insurance does not pay for these items, contact the hospital or agency social worker or provincial Cancer Society for assistance.
- Encourage your mother, sisters, and daughters (if applicable) to have annual professional breast examinations and mammography (if appropriate).
- Keep follow-up visits for professional examination, a mammogram, and testing to detect recurrent breast cancer.
- Expect decreased sensation and tingling at incision sites and in the affected arm for weeks to months after surgery.
- Resume sexual activities as desired.

COMMUNITY FOCUS

Canadian Cancer Society

Check the Internet for the Canadian Cancer Society's website (http://www.cancer.ca) for their peer supports and services. Identify the services provided by the program and the requirements to become a volunteer. Visit the women's clinic in a local community health agency. Are materials about the different programs visible in the waiting areas? Talk to one of the nurses who work in the clinic (make an appointment for this conversation). What does the nurse know about CancerConnection? Does the nurse refer patients to this program? What is the nurse's evaluation of the program? Has the nurse met any of the volunteers? Do patients have positive things to say about the program?

PATIENT TEACHING

Exercises After Breast Surgery

It is important to talk to your doctor before starting any exercises. A physical or occupational therapist can help design an exercise program for you.

Exercises in Lying Position

These exercises should be performed on a bed or the floor while lying on your back with your knees and hips bent, feet flat.

Wand Exercise

This exercise helps increase the forward motion of the shoulders. You will need a broom handle, measuring stick, or other similar object to perform this exercise.

- Hold the wand in both hands with palms facing up.
- Lift the wand up over your head (as far as you can), using your unaffected arm to help lift the wand, until you feel a stretch in your affected arm.
- Hold for 5 seconds.
- Lower arms and repeat 5 to 7 times.

Elbow Winging

This exercise helps increase the mobility of the front of your chest and shoulder. It may take several weeks of regular exercise before your elbows will get close to the bed (or floor).

- Clasp your hands behind your neck with your elbows pointing toward the ceiling.
- Move your elbows apart and down toward the bed (or floor).
- Repeat 5 to 7 times.

Exercises in Sitting Position

Shoulder Blade Stretch

This exercise helps increase the mobility of the shoulder blades.

- Sit in a chair very close to a table with your back against the chair back.
- Place the unaffected arm on the table with your elbow bent and palm down. Do not move this arm during the exercise.
- Place the affected arm on the table, palm down with your elbow straight.
- Without moving your trunk, slide the affected arm toward the opposite side of the table. You should feel your shoulder blade move as you do this.
- Relax your arm and repeat 5 to 7 times.

Shoulder Blade Squeeze

This exercise also helps increase the mobility of the shoulder blade.

- Facing straight ahead, sit in a chair in front of a mirror without resting on the back of the chair.
- Arms should be at your sides with elbows bent.
- Squeeze shoulder blades together, bringing your elbows behind you. Keep your shoulders level as you do this exercise. Do not lift your shoulders up toward your ears.
- Return to the starting position and repeat 5 to 7 times.

Side Bending

This exercise helps increase the mobility of the trunk and body.

- Clasp your hands together in front of you and lift your arms slowly over your head, straightening your arms.
- When your arms are over your head, bend your trunk to the right while bending at the waist and keeping your arms overhead.
- Return to the starting position and bend to the left.
- Repeat 5 to 7 times.

Exercises in Standing Position

Chest Wall Stretch

This exercise helps stretch the chest wall.

- Stand facing a corner with your toes approximately 20 to 25 cm from the corner.
- Bend your elbows and place your forearms on the wall, one on each side of the corner. Your elbows should be as close to shoulder height as possible.
- Keep your arms and feet in position and move your chest toward the corner. You will feel a stretch across your chest and shoulders.
- Return to starting position and repeat 5 to 7 times.

Shoulder Stretch

This exercise helps increase the mobility in the shoulder.

- Stand facing the wall with your toes approximately 20 to 25 cm from the wall.
- Place your hands on the wall. Use your fingers to "climb the wall," reaching as high as you can until you feel a stretch.
- Return to starting position and repeat 5 to 7 times.

Source: American Cancer Society. (2010). *Exercises after breast surgery.* Retrieved from www.cancer.org/docroot/CRI/content/CRI_2_6x_Exercises_After_Breast_Surgery.asp?sitearea=CRI&viewmode=print&

Information about community resources and support groups such as CancerConnection may be beneficial. An invaluable resource is the Canadian Cancer Society, which provides via the Internet specific, up-to-date recommendations on breast cancer treatments.

Before discharge, considerable time should be spent counselling the woman and her family about the aspects of self-management. Printed instructions should be given to the woman and her family (see Nursing Care Plan: The Woman with Breast Cancer on the Evolve website).

KEY POINTS

- Normal feedback regulation of the menstrual cycle depends on an intact hypothalamic–pituitary–gonadal mechanism.
- The myometrium of the uterus is uniquely designed to expel the fetus and promote hemostasis after birth.
- Menstrual disorders may diminish the quality of life for affected women and their families.
- Primary dysmenorrhea is a condition associated with ovulatory cycles and is related to the release of prostaglandins with menses.

- PMS is a disorder with both physiological and psychological characteristics.
- Endometriosis is characterized by dysmenorrhea; infertility; and, less often, alterations in menstrual cycle bleeding and dyspareunia.
- Abnormal uterine bleeding has many causes; the treatment chosen is based on managing the cause of the bleeding.
- Menopause is a healthy transition that has different symptoms and may require different treatments.
- Key strategies for preventing STIs are the practice of and education in safer sex behaviours.
- STIs are responsible for substantial mortality and morbidity, personal suffering, and a heavy economic burden in Canada.
- HIV is transmitted through body fluids—primarily blood, semen, and vaginal secretions.
- HPV is the most common viral STI.
- Syphilis has re-emerged as a common STI.
- Rates of chlamydia are increasing and it is the most common cause of PID.
- The development of breast neoplasms, whether benign or malignant, can have a significant physical and emotional effect on the woman and her family.
- Approximately 50% of women experience a breast problem at some point in their adult lives; the risk of a Canadian woman developing breast cancer is 1 in 9.
- The primary therapy for most women with stage I or II breast cancer is breast-conserving surgery with axillary or sentinel lymph node sampling followed by radiation therapy.
- Tamoxifen is a common adjuvant therapy for breast cancers that are estrogen-receptor positive.

evolve WEBSITE

Visit the Evolve website for additional resources related to the content in this chapter such as Case Studies, Critical Thinking Case Study Answers, Nursing Care Plans, Nursing Processes, Nursing Skills, and Review Questions for Exam Preparation at: http://evolve.elsevier.com/Canada/Perry/maternal/

REFERENCES

American Psychiatric Association. (2013). *Diagnostic and statistical manual of mental disorders* (5th ed.). Washington, DC: Author.

Biggs, W. W., & Demuth, R. H. (2011). RH: Premenstrual syndrome and premenstrual dysphoric disorder. *American Family Physician, 84*(8), 918–924.

Bitnum, A., Brophy, J., Samson, L., et al. (2014). Prevention of vertical HIV transmission and management of the HIV-exposed infant in Canada in 2014. *Canadian Journal of Infectious Diseases and Medical Microbiology, 25*(2), 75–77.

Brown, J., Kives, S., & Akhtar, M. (2012). Progestagens and anti-progestagens for pain associated with endometriosis. *Cochrane Database of Systematic Reviews* (3). doi:10.1002/14651858.CD002122.pub2.

Canadian Cancer Society. (2014a). *Risk factors for cervical cancer*. Toronto: Author. Retrieved from <http://www.cancer.ca/en/cancer-information/cancer-type/cervical/risks/?region=on>.

Canadian Cancer Society. (2014b). *Breast cancer*. Toronto: Author. Retrieved from <http://www.cancer.ca/en/cancer-information/cancer-type/breast/breast-cancer/?region=on>

Canadian Liver Foundation. (2015). *Hepatitis C*. Retrieved from <http://liver.ca/liver-disease/types/viral_hepatitis/Hepatitis_C.aspx>.

Chase, C., Well, J., & Eley, S. (2011). Caffeine and breast pain: Revisiting the connection. *Nursing for Women's Health, 15*(4), 286–294.

Dehlin, L., & Schuiling, K. (2013). Chronic pelvic pain. In K. Schuiling & F. Likis (Eds.), *Women's gynecologic health*. Burlington, MA: Jones & Bartlett.

Eckert, L. O., & Lentz, G. M. (2012). Infections of the lower and upper genital tract: Vulva, vagina, cervix, toxic shock syndrome, endometritis, and salpingitis. In G. M. Lentz, R. A. Lobo, D. M. Gershenson, et al. (Eds.), *Comprehensive gynecology* (6th ed.). Philadelphia: Mosby.

Ford, O., Lethaby, A., Roberts, H., et al. (2012). Progesterone for premenstrual syndrome. *Cochrane Database Systematic Review*, (3), CD003415.

George, C. A., Leonard, J. P., & Hutchinson, M. R. (2011). The female athlete triad: A current concepts review. *South African Journal of Sports Medicine, 23*(2), 50–56.

Government of Canada. (2015). *Summary: Estimates of HIV incidence, prevalence and proportion undiagnosed in Canada, 2014*. Ottawa: Author. Retrieved from <http://healthycanadians.gc.ca/publications/diseases-conditions-maladies-affections/hiv-aids-estimates-2014-vih-sida-estimations/index-eng.php>.

Joy, E. (2012). Invited commentary: Is the pill the answer for patients with female athlete triad? *Current Sports Medicine, 11*(2), 54–55.

Katz, V. L. (2012). Benign gynecologic lesions. Vulva, vagina, cervix, uterus, oviduct, ovary, ultrasound imaging of pelvic structures. In G. M. Lentz, R. A. Lobo, D. M. Gershenson, et al. (Eds.), *Comprehensive gynecology* (6th ed.). Philadelphia: Mosby.

Katz, V. L., & Dotters, D. (2012). Breast disease: Diagnosis and treatment of benign and malignant disease. In G. M. Lentz, R. A. Lobo, D. M. Gershenson, et al. (Eds.), *Comprehensive gynecology* (6th ed.). Philadelphia: Mosby.

Lentz, G. M. (2012). Primary and secondary dysmenorrheal, premenstrual syndrome, and premenstrual dysphoric disorder. In G. M. Lentz, R. A. Lobo, D. M. Gershenson, et al. (Eds.), *Comprehensive gynecology* (6th ed.). Philadelphia: Mosby.

Leyland, N., Casper, R., Laberge, P., et al. (2010). SOGC clinical practice guideline: Endometriosis: Diagnosis and management. *Journal of Obstetrics and Gynaecology Canada, 32*(7) (Suppl 2), S1–S32.

Lobo, R. A. (2012a). Primary and secondary amenorrhea and precocious puberty. In G. M. Lentz, R. A. Lobo, D. M. Gershenson, et al. (Eds.), *Comprehensive gynecology* (6th ed.). Philadelphia: Mosby.

Lobo, R. A. (2012b). Hyperprolactinemia, galactorrhea, and pituitary adenomas: Etiology, differential diagnosis, natural history, management. In G. M. Lentz, R. A. Lobo, D. M. Gershenson, et al. (Eds.), *Comprehensive gynecology* (6th ed.). Philadelphia: Mosby.

Mayo Foundation for Medical Education and Research. (2012). *Mammary duct ectasia*. Retrieved from <www.mayoclinic.com/health/mammary-duct-ectasia/DS00751>.

Money, D., Steben, M., & Infectious Disease Committee. (2008). SOGC clinical practice guideline: Genital herpes: Gynaecological aspects. *Journal of Obstetrics and Gynaecology Canada, 30*(4), 347–353.

Pinette, G. D., Cox, J. J., Heathcote, J., et al. (2009). *Primary care management of chronic hepatitis C: Professional desk reference*. Retrieved from <http://www.catie.ca/sites/default/files/Primary-Care-Management-of-Chronic-Hepatitis-C-Professional-Desk-Reference.pdf>.

Public Health Agency of Canada. (2012). *Human immunodeficiency virus: HIV screening and testing guide*. Ottawa: Author. Retrieved from

<http://www.catie.ca/en/resources/human-immunodeficiency-virus-screening-and-testing-guide>.

Public Health Agency of Canada. (2013a). *Canadian guidelines on sexually transmitted infections. Primary care and sexually transmitted infections.* Ottawa: Author. Retrieved from <http://www.phac-aspc.gc.ca/std-mts/sti-its/cgsti-ldcits/section-2-eng.php#a4>.

Public Health Agency of Canada. (2013b). *Canadian guidelines on sexually transmitted infections. Management and treatment of specific infections: Chlamydia.* Ottawa: Author. Retrieved from <http://www.phac-aspc.gc.ca/std-mts/sti-its/cgsti-ldcits/section-5-2-eng.php>.

Public Health Agency of Canada. (2013c). *Canadian guidelines on sexually transmitted infections. Specific populations: Pregnancy.* Ottawa: Author. Retrieved from <http://www.phac-aspc.gc.ca/std-mts/sti-its/cgsti-ldcits/section-6-4-eng.php>.

Public Health Agency of Canada. (2013d). *Canadian guidelines on sexually transmitted infections. Management and treatment of specific infections: Pelvic inflammatory disease.* Ottawa: Author. Retrieved from: <http://www.phac-aspc.gc.ca/std-mts/sti-its/cgsti-ldcits/section-4-4-eng.php>.

Public Health Agency of Canada. (2013e). *Canadian guidelines on sexually transmitted infections. Syphilis.* Ottawa: Author. Retrieved from <http://www.phac-aspc.gc.ca/std-mts/sti-its/cgsti-ldcits/section-5-10-eng.php>.

Public Health Agency of Canada. (2013f). *Canadian guidelines on sexually transmitted infections. Management and treatment of specific syndromes: Genital herpes simplex virus (HSV) infections.* Ottawa: Author. Retrieved from <http://www.phac-aspc.gc.ca/std-mts/sti-its/cgsti-ldcits/section-5-4-eng.php>.

Public Health Agency of Canada. (2013g). *Canadian guidelines on sexually transmitted infections. Management and treatment of specific infections: Hepatitis B virus infections.* Ottawa: Author. Retrieved from <http://www.phac-aspc.gc.ca/std-mts/sti-its/cgsti-ldcits/section-5-7-eng.php>.

Public Health Agency of Canada. (2013h). *Canadian guidelines on sexually transmitted infections. Management and treatment of specific syndromes: Human immunodeficiency virus infections.* Ottawa: Author. Retrieved from <http://www.phac-aspc.gc.ca/std-mts/sti-its/cgsti-ldcits/section-5-8-eng.php>.

Public Health Agency of Canada. (2013i). *Canadian guidelines on sexually transmitted infections. Management and treatment of specific syndromes: Vaginal discharge (bacterial vaginosis, vulvovaginal candidiasis, trichomoniasis).* Ottawa: Author. Retrieved from <http://www.phac-aspc.gc.ca/std-mts/sti-its/cgsti-ldcits/section-4-8-eng.php>.

Public Health Agency of Canada. (2014a). *Canadian guidelines on sexually transmitted infections. Management and treatment of specific infections: Human papilloma virus.* Ottawa: Author. Retrieved from <http://www.phac-aspc.gc.ca/std-mts/sti-its/cgsti-ldcits/section-5-5-eng.php>.

Public Health Agency of Canada. (2014b). *Executive summary report on sexually transmitted infections in Canada: 2011.* Ottawa: Author. Retrieved from <http://www.phac-aspc.gc.ca/sti-its-surv-epi/rep-rap-2011/index-eng.php>.

Public Health Agency of Canada. (2014c). *Canadian guidelines on sexually transmitted infections. Management and treatment of specific infections: Gonococcal infections.* Ottawa: Author. Retrieved from <http://www.phac-aspc.gc.ca/std-mts/sti-its/cgsti-ldcits/section-5-6-eng.php>.

Public Health Agency of Canada. (2014d). *Canadian guidelines on sexually transmitted infections. Supplementary statement for recommendations related to the diagnosis, management, and follow-up of pelvic inflammatory disease: March 2014.* Ottawa: Author. Retrieved from <http://www.phac-aspc.gc.ca/std-mts/sti-its/cgsti-ldcits/pid-aip-eng.php>.

Public Health Agency of Canada. (2014e). *Hepatitis.* Ottawa: Author. Retrieved from <http://www.phac-aspc.gc.ca/hep/index-eng.php>.

Public Health Agency of Canada. (2015). *Canadian guidelines on sexually transmitted infections. Management and treatment of specific infections: Human papillomavirus (HPV) infections.* Ottawa: Author. Retrieved from <http://www.phac-aspc.gc.ca/std-mts/sti-its/cgsti-ldcits/section-5-5-eng.php>.

Reid, R., Abramson, B. L., Blake, J., et al. (2014). SOGC clinical practice guideline: Managing menopause. *Journal of Obstetrics and Gynaecology Canada, 36*(9 eSuppl A), S1–S80.

Royal College of Obstetricians and Gynecologists. (2011). *Pregnancy and breast cancer.* Green-top guideline No. 12. Retrieved from <https://www.rcog.org.uk/globalassets/documents/guidelines/gtg_12.pdf>.

Saskatchewan Cancer Agency. (2012). *Breast cancer treatment guidelines.* Retrieved from <http://www.saskcancer.ca/Breast%20CPGs%2005-12>.

Sherman, M., Shafran, S., Burak, K., et al. (2007). Management of chronic hepatitis C: Canadian consensus guidelines. *Canadian Journal of Gastroenterology, 21*(Suppl. C), 25C–34C.

Singh, S., Best, C., Dunn, S., et al. (2013). SOGC clinical practice guideline: Abnormal uterine bleeding in pre-menopausal women. *Journal of Obstetrics and Gynaecology Canada, 35*(5 eSuppl), S1–S28.

Society of Obstetricians and Gynaecologists of Canada. (2007). SOGC clinical practice guideline: Canadian consensus guideline on human papillomavirus. *Journal of Obstetrics and Gynaecology Canada, 29*(8), Supplement 3.

Taylor, D., Schuiling, K., & Sharp, B. (2013). Menstrual cycle pain and discomforts. In K. Schuiling & F. Likis (Eds.), *Women's gynecologic health* (2nd ed.). Burlington, MA: Jones & Bartlett.

Wambach, C. M., & Alexander, C. J. (2012). Menstrual disorders. In P. J. DiSaia, G. Chaudhuri, & L. C. Giudice et al. (Eds.), *Women's health review: A clinical update in obstetrics-gynecology.* Philadelphia: Saunders.

Weiner, C., & Buhimschi, C. (2009). *Drugs for pregnant and lactating women* (2nd ed.). Philadelphia: Saunders.

Wilton, J. M. (2012). Tranexamine acid: A new option for heavy menstrual bleeding. *Nursing for Women's Health, 16*(2), 146–150.

World Health Organization. (2007). *Global strategy for the prevention and control of sexually transmitted infections: 2006–2015: Breaking the chain of transmission.* Geneva: Author. Retrieved from <http://whqlibdoc.who.int/publications/2007/9789241563475_eng.pdf>.

ADDITIONAL RESOURCES

Bodysense: <http://www.bodysense.ca/>.

Breast Cancer Risk Assessment Tool: <http://www.cancer.gov/bcrisktool/>.

Canadian Cancer Society: <http://www.cancer.ca/.

Canadian Women's Health Network: <http://www.cwhn.ca/>.

Centers for Disease Control—2015 Sexually Transmitted Treatment Guidelines: <http://www.cdc.gov/std/tg2015/default.htm?s_CID=govd-std-057>.

Infertility Awareness Association of Canada: <http://www.iaac.ca/>.

Menopauseandu.ca: <http://www.Menopauseandu.ca>.

Provincial/Territorial STI Guidelines: <http://www.phac-aspc.gc.ca/std-mts/sti-its/pt-sti-its-eng.php>.

Public Health Agency of Canada: Canadian Guidelines on Sexually Transmitted Infections: <http://www.phac-aspc.gc.ca/std-mts/sti-its/index-eng.php>.

Sexualityandu.ca: <http://www.Sexualityandu.ca>.

Society of Obstetricians and Gynecologists of Canada—Managing Menopause: <http://sogc.org/wp-content/uploads/2014/09/gui311CPG1409Eabstract1.pdf>.

CHAPTER

8

Infertility, Contraception, and Abortion

Lisa Keenan-Lindsay, with contributions from Peggy Mancuso

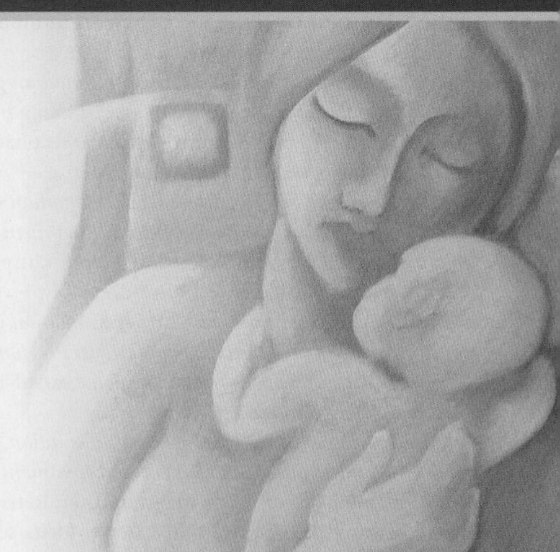

evolve WEBSITE

Visit the Evolve website for additional resources related to the content in this chapter such as Case Studies, Critical Thinking Case Study Answers, Nursing Care Plans, Nursing Processes, Nursing Skills, and Review Questions for Exam Preparation at: http://evolve.elsevier.com/Canada/Perry/maternal/

OBJECTIVES

On completion of this chapter the reader will be able to:

- List common causes of infertility.
- Discuss the psychological impact of infertility.
- Describe common diagnoses and treatments for infertility.
- Compare reproductive alternatives for couples experiencing infertility.
- State the advantages and disadvantages of the following methods of contraception: fertility awareness methods, barrier methods, hormonal methods, intrauterine devices, and sterilization.
- Explain common nursing interventions that facilitate contraceptive use.
- Describe the techniques used for medical and surgical interruption of pregnancy.
- Recognize ethical, legal, cultural, and religious considerations of infertility, contraception, and elective abortion.

INFERTILITY

Incidence

Infertility is a serious concern that affects the quality of life of 11.5 to 15.7% of reproductive-age couples (Bushnik, Cook, Yuzpe, et al., 2012). Commonly **infertility** is considered a diagnosis for couples who have not achieved pregnancy after 1 year of regular, unprotected intercourse when the woman is less than 35 years of age or after 6 months when the woman is older than 35 (Bushnik et al., 2012). *Fecundity* is the term used to describe the chance of achieving pregnancy and subsequent live birth within one menstrual cycle. Fecundity averages 20% in couples who are not experiencing reproductive problems.

The incidence of infertility has increased in Canada. A probable cause of infertility includes the trend toward delaying pregnancy until later in life, a time when fertility decreases naturally and the prevalence of diseases such as endometriosis and ovulatory dysfunction increases. Infertility increases with the age of the woman, with fertility rates in women ages 40 to 45 being 95% lower than that for women ages 20 to 24. It is unknown whether there has been an actual increase in male infertility or whether male infertility is more readily identified because of improvements in diagnosis.

For the couple experiencing infertility, diagnosis and treatment requires considerable physical, emotional, and financial investments over an extended period of time. Feelings connected with infertility are many and complex. The origins of some of these feelings are myths, superstitions, misinformation, or magical thinking about the causes of infertility. Other feelings of anxiety and helplessness arise from the need to undergo many tests and examinations, coping with expressed or unspoken expectations regarding pregnancy, and deciding when "enough is enough" (RESOLVE, 2015). Nurses who care for infertile couples should consider the following four goals:

- Provide the couple with accurate information about human reproduction, infertility treatments, and prognosis for pregnancy. Dispel any myths or inaccuracies from friends or the mass media that the couple may believe to be true.

- Help the couple and the health care team accurately identify and treat possible causes of infertility.
- Provide emotional support. The couple may benefit from anticipatory guidance, counselling, and support group meetings, either face-to-face or online. The Infertility Awareness Association of Canada (see Additional Resources as end of chapter) is an organization that provides support, advocacy, and education about infertility for those experiencing infertility as well as for health care providers.
- Guide and educate those who fail to conceive biologically as a couple about other forms of treatment, such as in vitro fertilization (IVF), donor eggs or semen, surrogate motherhood, and adoption. Support the couple in their decisions regarding their future family.

Nurses should also remember that among healthy women and men promotion of normal reproduction and prevention of infertility can be achieved if both partners maintain a normal body mass index (BMI) and avoid sexually transmitted infections (STIs) and exposures to substances or habits (such as smoking) that impair reproductive ability. As they make plans for their future family, adults should also know that, realistically, fertility decreases with age.

Factors Associated With Infertility

Although exact percentages vary somewhat with populations, approximately 80% of couples have an identifiable cause of infertility, with about 40% of these causes being related to factors in the female partner, 30% related to factors in the male partner, and 20% related to factors in both partners. About 10% or more couples will experience unexplained or idiopathic causes of infertility (Government of Canada, 2013). Nevertheless, the focus of infertility treatment has shifted from attempting to correct a specific pathology to recommending and initiating the treatment that is most effective in achieving pregnancy for this unique couple at this time in their reproductive lifespan. Assisted reproductive technologies (ARTs) have proven to be effective, even in couples who experience unexplained infertility.

Unassisted human conception requires a normally developed reproductive tract in both the male and female partners. For simplification, each live birth necessitates synchronization of the following:

- The male must deposit semen with sperm that has the capacity to fertilize an egg close to the cervix at the time of ovulation. The sperm must be able to ascend through the uterus and fallopian tubes (male factor).
- The cervix must be sufficiently open to allow semen to enter the uterus and provide a nurturing environment for sperm (cervical factor).
- The fallopian tubes must be able to capture the ovum, transport semen to the ovum, and transport the fertilized embryo to the uterus (tubal factor).
- Ovulation of a healthy oocyte must occur, ideally within the parameters of a regular, predictable menstrual cycle (ovarian factor).
- The uterus must be receptive to implantation of the embryo and capable of nourishing the growth and development of the fetus throughout the normal duration of pregnancy (uterine factor).

An alteration in one or more of these structures, functions, or processes results in some degree of impaired fertility. Boxes 8-1 and 8-2 list factors affecting female and male infertility. For conception to occur, both partners must have normal, intact hypothalamic–pituitary–gonadal hormonal axes that support the formation of sperm in the male and ova in the female. Sperm can remain viable within a woman's reproductive tract for at least 3 days and for as long as 5 days. The oocyte can only be successfully fertilized for 12 to 24 hours after ovulation (Cunningham, Leveno, Bloom, et al., 2014). The couple seeking pregnancy should be taught about the menstrual cycle and ways to detect ovulation (see discussion later in chapter). They should be counselled to have intercourse two to three times a week; or, if timed intercourse does not increase anxiety, they

BOX 8-1 FACTORS AFFECTING FEMALE FERTILITY

Ovarian Factors

- Developmental anomalies
- Anovulation—primary
  - Pituitary or hypothalamic hormone disorder
  - Adrenal gland disorders (rare)
  - Congenital adrenal hyperplasia (rare)
- Anovulation—secondary
  - Disruption of hypothalamic–pituitary–ovarian axis
  - Anorexia
  - Insufficient fat in athletic women
  - Increased prolactin levels
  - Thyroid disorders
  - Premature ovarian failure
  - Polycystic ovarian syndrome

Tubal/Peritoneal Factors

- Developmental anomalies of the tubes
- Reduced tubal motility
- Inflammation within the tube
- Tubal adhesions
- Disruption caused by tubal pregnancy
- Endometriosis

Uterine Factors

- Developmental anomalies of the uterus (see Fig. 8-1)
- Endometrial and myometrial tumours
- Asherman syndrome (uterine adhesions or scar tissue)

Vaginal–Cervical Factors

- Vaginal–cervical infections
- Cervical mucus inadequate
- Isoimmunization (development of sperm antibodies)

Other Factors

- Nutritional deficiencies
- Thyroid dysfunction
- Obesity
- Idiopathic conditions

BOX 8-2 FACTORS AFFECTING MALE FERTILITY

Hormonal Disorders
- Congenital disorders
- Tumours of the pituitary and hypothalamus
- Trauma to the pituitary or hypothalamus
- Hyperprolactinemia
- Excess of androgens, estrogen, cortisol
- Drugs and substance use (recreational and prescribed drugs)
- Chronic illnesses
- Nutritional deficiencies
- Obesity
- Endocrine disorders (e.g., diabetes)

Testicular Factors
- Congenital disorders
- Undescended testes
- Hypospadias
- Varicocele
- Viral infections (e.g., mumps)
- Sexually transmitted infections (gonorrhea, chlamydial infection)
- Obstructive lesions of the epididymis and vas deferens
- Environmental toxins
- Trauma
- Torsion
- Castration
- Systemic illnesses
- Changes in sperm from cigarette smoking or use of heroin, marijuana, amyl nitrate, butyl nitrate, ethyl chloride, or methaqualone
- Decrease in libido from use of heroin, methadone, selective serotonin reuptake inhibitors, or barbiturates
- Impotence from use of alcohol or antihypertensive medications
- Antisperm antibodies

Factors Associated With Sperm Transport
- Drugs
- Sexually transmitted infections of the epididymis
- Ejaculatory dysfunction
- Premature ejaculation

Idiopathic Male Infertility

BOX 8-3 RELIGIOUS CONSIDERATIONS CONCERNING INFERTILITY

The health care provider must be aware of civil laws and religious proscriptions about sexual activities. Conservative and reform Jewish couples accept most infertility treatment; however, the Orthodox Jewish husband and wife may face problems in infertility investigation and management because of religious laws governing marital relations. For example, according to Jewish law, the Orthodox couple may not engage in marital relations during menstruation or throughout the following seven "preparatory days." The wife then is immersed in a ritual bath *(Mikvah)* before relations can resume. Fertility problems can arise when the woman has a short cycle (i.e., a cycle of 24 days or fewer, when ovulation would occur on day 10 or earlier).

The Roman Catholic Church regards the embryo as a human being from the first moment of existence. Therefore, technical procedures such as in vitro fertilization (IVF), therapeutic donor insemination, and freezing embryos are not accepted or endorsed.

Other religious groups may have ethical concerns about infertility tests and treatments. For example, most Protestant denominations and Muslims support infertility management as long as IVF is done with the husband's sperm, there is no reduction of fertilized embryos after implantation, and insemination is done with the husband's sperm. These groups are less supportive of surrogacy and use of donor sperm and eggs. Christian Scientists do not permit surgical procedures or IVF but do permit insemination with husband and donor sperm.

Care providers should seek to understand the woman's religious views and how beliefs affect her perception of health care, especially in relation to infertility. Women may wish to seek infertility treatment but have questions about proposed diagnostic and therapeutic procedures because of religious proscriptions. These women should be encouraged to consult their minister, rabbi, priest, or other spiritual leader for advice.

Data from D'Avanzo, C. (2008). *Mosby's pocket guide to cultural health assessment* (4th ed.). St. Louis: Mosby.

should be encouraged to engage in intercourse the day before and the day of ovulation. Fertility decreases markedly 24 hours after ovulation.

NURSING CARE

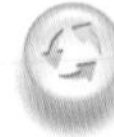

The nurse assists in the assessment and education of the infertile couple (see Nursing Process: Infertility, on Evolve). As part of the assessment process the nurse obtains information from the couple through interview and physical examination, regardless of whether this couple's situation is one of primary (never experienced pregnancy) or secondary (previous pregnancy) infertility. Religious, cultural, and ethnic data may place restrictions on use of available treatments. Box 8-3 describes some of the concerns related to religion that may affect the couple's choices regarding infertility treatment. The Cultural Awareness box notes cultural rituals and beliefs regarding fertility. In addition, the nurse will obtain and monitor results of diagnostic testing. Some of the information and data needed to investigate impaired fertility are of a sensitive, personal nature. The couple may experience feelings of invasion of privacy, and the nurse must exercise tact and express concern for their well-being throughout the interview. The tests and examinations associated with infertility diagnosis and treatment are occasionally painful and often intrusive. The couple's intimacy and feelings of romantic attachment are often frayed as they engage in this process. A high level of motivation is needed to endure the investigation and subsequent treatment. Because multiple factors involving both partners are common, the investigation of impaired fertility is conducted systematically and simultaneously for both male and female partners. Both partners must be interested in the solution to the problem. The medical investigation requires time (3 to 4 months) and considerable financial expense. Box 8-4 describes the status of insurance coverage for infertility treatment.

Assessment of Female Infertility

Evaluation for infertility should be offered to couples who have failed to become pregnant after 1 year of regular intercourse or after 6 months if the woman is over 35. Investigation of impaired fertility begins for the woman with a complete history and physical examination. A complete general physical examination should include height and weight and estimation of BMI. Both obesity and being underweight are associated with anovulation disorders. Signs and symptoms of androgen excess such as excess body hair or pigmentation changes should be noted. The general physical examination is followed by a specific assessment of the reproductive tract. A history of infection of the genitourinary system and any signs of infections, especially STIs that could impair tubal patency, should be assessed. Bimanual examination of internal organs may reveal lack of mobility of the uterus or abnormal contours of the uterus and adnexa. A woman may have an abnormal uterus and tubes (Fig. 8-1) as a result of congenital abnormalities during fetal development. These uterine abnormalities increase risk for early pregnancy loss.

Laboratory data, including routine urine and blood tests, are collected. The initial clinic visit serves as a preconceptual visit and as initial assessment of possible causes of infertility. The woman should be taking folic acid supplements, and all immunizations should be current to prepare for possible pregnancy.

Diagnostic testing. The basic infertility survey of the female involves evaluation of the cervix, uterus, tubes, and peritoneum; detection of **ovulation**; and hormone analysis. Timing and descriptions of common tests are presented in Table 8-1. Previous status regarding ovulation can be evaluated through menstrual history, serum hormone studies, and use of an ovulation predictor kit. If the woman is over age 35, the clinician may choose to assess "ovarian reserve" or how many potential ova remain within the ovaries. A common evaluation of ovarian reserve is measurement of follicle-stimulating hormone (FSH) levels on the third day of the menstrual cycle. The uterus and fallopian tubes can be visualized for abnormalities and tubal patency through hysterosalpingogram (x-ray film examination of the uterine cavity and tubes after instillation of radiopaque contrast material through the cervix). If the woman is at risk for endometriosis (implants of endometrial tissue outside of the uterus) or adhesions, diagnostic laparoscopy may be indicated. Test findings favourable to fertility are summarized in Box 8-5.

Assessment of Male Infertility

The systematic investigation of infertility in the male patient begins with a thorough history and physical examination. Assessment of the male patient proceeds in a manner similar to that of the female patient, starting with noninvasive tests.

Diagnostic testing and semen analysis. The basic test for male infertility is **semen analysis**. A complete semen analysis, study of the effects of cervical mucus on sperm forward motility and survival, and evaluation of the sperm's ability to penetrate an ovum provide basic information. Sperm counts vary from

BOX 8-4 INSURANCE COVERAGE FOR INFERTILITY

All provinces in Canada cover the cost of diagnostic testing and some medical and surgical treatment of infertility through provincial insurance plans. Presently, Ontario will pay for one IVF cycle with only one embryo to be transferred. Québec currently pays for one cycle for certain families although they must meet qualifying criteria. This is in contrast to the previously funded three cycles of IVF that were funded in Québec. The Canadian Fertility and Andrology Society strongly advocates for both regulation and public funding of in vitro fertilization across the country. Private insurance plans may pay for some aspects of treatment. Women need information about what they can expect from their private insurers and are encouraged to contact companies to obtain more complete information.

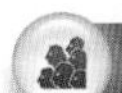

CULTURAL AWARENESS
Fertility and Infertility

Worldwide, cultures continue to use symbols and rites that celebrate fertility. One fertility rite that persists today is the custom of throwing rice at the bride and groom. Other fertility symbols and rites include passing out congratulatory cigars, candy, or pencils by a new father and baby showers held in anticipation of a child's birth.

In many cultures the responsibility for infertility is usually attributed to the woman. A woman's inability to conceive may be seen to be caused by previous sins, evil spirits, or personal inadequacies. In some cultures male virility remains in question until a man demonstrates his ability to reproduce by having at least one child (D'Avanzo, 2008).

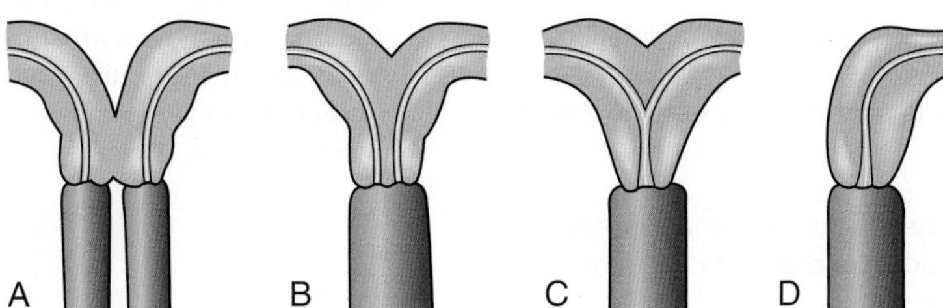

FIGURE 8-1 Abnormal uterus. **A:** Complete bicornuate uterus with vagina divided by a septum. **B:** Complete bicornuate uterus with normal vagina. **C:** Partial bicornuate uterus with normal vagina. **D:** Unicornuate uterus.

TABLE 8-1 GENERAL TESTS FOR IMPAIRED FERTILITY

TEST OR EXAMINATION	TIMING (MENSTRUAL CYCLE DAYS)	RATIONALE
Hysterosalpingogram (HSG) (uterine abnormalities, tubal patency)	7–10	Late follicular, early proliferative phase; will not disrupt a fertilized ovum; may open uterine tubes before time of ovulation
Chlamydia immunoglobulin G antibodies (tubal patency)	Variable	Negative antibody test may indicate tubal patency assessment (HSG); not needed in low-risk women
Hysterosalpingo-contrast sonography (uterine abnormalities, tubal patency)	7–10	Late follicular, early proliferative phase; will not disrupt a fertilized ovum; evaluates tubal patency, uterine cavity, and myometrium
Serum progesterone (ovulation)	7 days before expected menses	Midluteal-phase progesterone levels; check adequacy of corpus luteum progesterone production
Assessment of cervical mucus (ovulation)	Variable, ovulation	Cervical mucus should have low viscosity, high spinnbarkeit (ability to stretch) during ovulation
Basal body temperature (ovulation)	Chart entire cycle	Elevation occurs in response to progesterone; documents ovulation
Urinary ovulation predictor kit (ovulation)	Variable, ovulation	Detects timing of lutein hormone surge before ovulation
Semen analysis (male factor)	2–7 days after abstinence	Detects ability of sperm to fertilize egg
Sperm penetration assay (male factor)	After 2 days but ≤1 week of abstinence	Evaluation of ability of sperm to penetrate egg
Follicle-stimulating hormone (FSH) level (ovarian reserve)	Day 3	High FSH levels (>20) indicate that pregnancy will not occur with woman's own eggs; value <10 indicates adequate ovarian reserve
Clomiphene citrate challenge test (CCCT) (ovarian reserve)	Administer clomiphene 100 mg days 3 through 10	Assess FSH on days 3 and 10 in presence of clomiphene stimulation; high FSH levels (>20) indicate that pregnancy will not occur with woman's own eggs; FSH <15 suggestive of adequate ovarian reserve

BOX 8-5 SUMMARY OF FINDINGS FAVOURABLE TO FERTILITY

1. Follicular development, ovulation, and luteal development are supportive of pregnancy:
   a. Basal body temperature (presumptive evidence of ovulatory cycles) is biphasic, with temperature elevation that persists for 12 to 14 days before menstruation (see Fig. 8-9).
   b. Cervical mucus characteristics change appropriately during phases of the menstrual cycle (see discussion later in the chapter).
   c. Days 3 to 10 follicle-stimulating hormone (FSH) levels are low enough to verify presence of adequate ovarian follicles.
   d. Day 3 estradiol levels are low enough to verify presence of adequate ovarian follicles.
   e. Woman reports a history of regular, predictable menses with consistent premenstrual and menstrual symptoms.
2. The luteal phase is supportive of pregnancy:
   a. Levels of plasma progesterone are adequate to indicate ovulation.
   b. Luteal phase of menstrual cycle is of sufficient duration to support pregnancy.
3. Cervical factors are receptive to sperm during expected time of ovulation:
   a. Cervical os is open.
   b. Cervical mucus is clear, watery, abundant, and slippery and demonstrates good spinnbarkeit and arborization (fern pattern) at time of ovulation.
   c. Cervical examination reveals no lesions or infections.
4. The uterus and uterine tubes support pregnancy:
   a. Uterine and tubal patency are documented by (1) spillage of dye into the peritoneal cavity; and (2) outlines of uterine and tubal cavities of adequate size and shape, with no abnormalities.
   b. Laparoscopic examination verifies normal development of internal genitals and absence of adhesions, infections, endometriosis, and other lesions.
5. The male partner's reproductive structures are normal:
   a. There is no evidence of developmental anomalies of penis (e.g., hypospadius), testicular atrophy, or varicocele (varicose veins on the spermatic vein in the groin).
   b. There is no evidence of infection in the prostate, seminal vesicles, and urethra.
   c. Testes are more than 4 cm in largest diameter.
6. Semen is supportive of pregnancy:
   a. Sperm (number per millilitre) are adequate in ejaculate.
   b. Most sperm show normal morphology.
   c. Most sperm are motile, forward moving.
   d. No autoimmunity exists.
   e. Seminal fluid is normal.

BOX 8-6 SEMEN ANALYSIS

- Semen volume: 2–5 mL
- pH: 7.1–8.0
- Sperm concentration/density ≥20 million/mL
- Normal morphological features >5% (normal oval)
- Motility: At least 25% of the sperm exhibit sustainable rapid or slow progressive movement for at least 180 minutes
- Vitality: At least 50% of ejaculated sperm should be alive
- Liquefaction 20–30 minutes

NOTE: These values are not absolute but are only relative to final evaluation of the couple as a single reproductive unit. Values also differ according to source used as a reference.
Source: MyHealth.Alberta.ca. (2014). *Semen analysis.* Retrieved from https://myhealth.alberta.ca/health/Pages/conditions.aspx?hwid=hw5612#hw5641; World Health Organization (WHO). (2010). *Laboratory manual for the examination of human semen* (5th ed.). Geneva: Author.

day to day and depend on emotional and physical status and sexual activity. Therefore, a single analysis may be inconclusive. A minimum of two analyses must be performed several weeks apart to assess male fertility.

Semen is collected by ejaculation into a clean container or a plastic sheath that does not contain a spermicidal agent. The specimen is usually collected by masturbation following 2 to 5 days of abstinence from ejaculation. The semen is examined at the collection site or taken to the laboratory in a sealed container within 2 hours of ejaculation. Exposure to excessive heat or cold should be avoided. Commonly accepted values for semen characteristics are given in Box 8-6. If results are in the fertile range, no further sperm evaluation is necessary. If results are not within this range, the test is repeated. If subsequent results are still in the subfertile range, further evaluation is needed to identify the problem.

Hormone analyses are done for testosterone, gonadotropin, follicle-stimulating hormone (FSH), and luteinizing hormone (LH). The sperm penetration assay and other alternative tests can be used to evaluate the ability of sperm to penetrate an egg. Testicular biopsy may be warranted. Scrotal ultrasound is used to examine the testes for presence of varicoceles and to identify abnormalities in the scrotum and spermatic cord. Transrectal ultrasound is used to evaluate the ejaculatory ducts, seminal vesicles, and vas deferens.

Assessment of the Couple

Postcoital test. The postcoital test (PCT) is one method used to test for adequacy of coital technique, cervical mucus, sperm, and degree of sperm penetration through cervical mucus. The test is performed within several hours after ejaculation of semen into the vagina. A specimen of cervical mucus is obtained from the cervical os and examined under a microscope. The quality of mucus and the number of forward-moving sperm are noted. A PCT with good mucus and motile sperm is associated with fertility.

Intercourse is synchronized with the expected time of ovulation (as determined from evaluation of basal body temperature [BBT], cervical mucus changes, and usual length of menstrual cycle or use of LH detection kit to determine LH surge). Intercourse should occur only in the absence of vaginal infection. Couples may experience some difficulty abstaining from intercourse for 2 to 4 days before expected ovulation and then having intercourse with ejaculation on schedule. Sex on demand may strain the couple's relationship. A problem may arise if the expected day of ovulation occurs when facilities or the physician is unavailable (such as over a weekend or holiday).

Plan of Care and Implementation

Psychosocial Considerations

Infertility is recognized as a major life stressor that can affect self-esteem; relations with the spouse, family, and friends; and careers. Psychological responses to the diagnosis of infertility may tax a couple's capacity for giving and receiving physical and sexual closeness. The prescriptions and proscriptions for achieving conception may add tension to a couple's sexual functioning. Couples may report decreased desire for intercourse, orgasmic dysfunction, or midcycle erectile disorders. Treatment for infertility is complex and stressful, and 30% of couples quit treatment before becoming pregnant, because of the associated psychological distress (Boivin, Griffiths, & Venetis, 2011). Some women may feel that their stress levels will affect whether treatment is successful; however, Boivin et al. (2011) showed that emotional distress was unlikely to be a cause of infertility treatment failure. Couples need support and encouragement to express their concerns about infertility treatment.

In order to deal comfortably with a couple's sexuality, nurses must be comfortable with their own sexuality so that they can better help couples understand why the private act of lovemaking needs to be shared with health care professionals. Nurses need current factual knowledge about human sexual practices and must be accepting of the preferences and activities of others, without being judgemental. They must be skilled in interviewing and in therapeutic use of self, sensitive to the nonverbal cues of others, and knowledgeable about each couple's sociocultural and religious beliefs (see Critical Thinking Case Study).

The woman or couple facing infertility may exhibit behaviours of the grieving process that are associated with other types of loss. The loss of one's genetic continuity with the generations to come can lead to a loss of self-esteem, a sense of inadequacy as a woman or a man, a loss of control over one's destiny, and a reduced sense of self. Infertile individuals can perceive greater dissatisfaction with their marriages. Not all people will have all these reactions, nor can it be predicted how long any reaction will last for any one individual.

If the couple conceives, their concerns and problems with infertility may not be over. Many couples are overjoyed with the pregnancy; however, some are not. Some couples rearrange their lives, sense of self, and personal goals based on accepting their infertile state. The couple may think that those who worked with them to identify and treat impaired fertility expect them to be happy with the pregnancy. They may be shocked to find that they feel resentment because the pregnancy, once a cherished dream, now necessitates another change in goals,

CRITICAL THINKING CASE STUDY

Infertility

Diane is a 39-year-old accountant who has recently married for the first time. Charles is 41 and has two children from a previous marriage. Diane has a history of amenorrhea when she was in college and a member of the track team. Currently her menstrual periods are irregular. She wants to have a baby "before it's too late," and she and Charles have been having unprotected sex for almost a year. They have come to the fertility clinic today for an evaluation. Diane tells the nurse that she has heard a lot about the success of in vitro fertilization (IVF) and wants to know if she will be able to have it performed. How should the nurse respond to Diane's comments and questions?

QUESTIONS

1. Evidence—Is evidence sufficient to draw conclusions about what response the nurse should give?
2. Assumptions—Describe underlying assumptions about the following issues:
   a. Age and fertility
   b. Infertility as a major life stressor
   c. Success rates for IVF pregnancy and birth
   d. Causes of female infertility
   e. Costs of infertility treatment
3. What implications and priorities for nursing care can be drawn at this time?
4. Does the evidence objectively support your conclusion?

aspirations, and identities. The normal ambivalence toward pregnancy may be perceived as reneging on the original choice to become parents.

If the couple does not conceive, they should be assessed regarding their desire to be referred for help with adoption, donor eggs or semen, surrogacy, or other reproductive alternatives. The couple may choose to continue in a child-free state. The couple may find helpful a list of agencies, support groups, and other resources in their community, such as the Infertility Awareness Association of Canada and the Infertility Network (see Additional Resources at end of the chapter).

Nonmedical Treatments

Both men and women can benefit from healthy lifestyle changes that result in a BMI within the normal range; moderate daily exercise; and abstinence from alcohol, nicotine, and recreational drugs. For the woman with a BMI >27 and polycystic ovary syndrome, losing just 5 to 10% of body weight can restore ovulation within 6 months. Anovulatory women with a BMI <17 who have eating disorders or intense exercise regimens benefit from weight gain. Nevertheless, this population sometimes is reluctant to alter their behaviours, and counselling may be required.

Simple changes in lifestyle may be effective in the treatment of subfertile men. Only water-soluble lubricants should be used during intercourse because many commonly used lubricants contain **spermicides** or have spermicidal properties. High scrotal temperatures may be caused by daily hot tub baths or saunas that keep the testes at temperatures too high for efficient spermatogenesis. These conditions lead to only lessened fertility and should not be used as a means of contraception.

Most herbal remedies have not been proven clinically to promote fertility or to be safe in early pregnancy and should be taken by the woman only as prescribed by a health care provider who has expertise in herbology. Relaxation, osteopathy, stress management (e.g., aromatherapy, yoga), and nutritional and exercise counselling have been reported to increase pregnancy rates in some women. Herbs to avoid while trying to conceive include licorice root, yarrow, wormwood, ephedra, fennel, goldenseal, lavender, juniper, flaxseed, pennyroyal, passionflower, wild cherry, cascara, sage, thyme, and periwinkle. All supplements or herbs should be purchased from trusted sources to ensure that they do not contain contaminants.

Medical Therapy

One goal of infertility assessment and treatment is to determine which couples could respond to conventional therapies in a timely manner. Another goal is to refer couples who will need ARTs to conceive early in the process. In general, any fertility treatment is more likely to result in a live birth in women who are younger than age 35, with successful outcomes decreasing for women over age 40.

Pharmacological therapy for female infertility is often directed at treating ovulatory dysfunction by either stimulating or enhancing ovulation so more oocytes mature. These medications include (a) clomiphene citrate as initial therapy for many women with intermittent anovulation; (b) a combination of clomiphene and metformin for women with anovulation and insulin resistance; (c) human menopausal gonadotropin (HMG), FSH, and recombinant FSH (rFSH) to stimulate follicle formation in women who do not respond to clomiphene therapies; (d) human chorionic gonadotropin to induce ovulation when follicles are ripe; (e) gonadotropin-releasing hormone (GnRH) agonists at the beginning of a cycle to sequence HMG therapies; (f) progesterone to support the luteal phase of the cycle; and (g) bromocriptine for women who have excess prolactin.

Treatment of certain medical conditions can result in improved fertility. The woman who is hypothyroid benefits from thyroid hormone supplementation. Treatment of endometriosis could include trials of danazol, progesterone, continuous combined oral contraceptives, or GnRH agonists to suppress menstruation and shrink endometrial implants. This regimen would be followed by ovulation induction. Adrenal hyperplasia is treated with prednisone. Any infections present in the infertile couple should be treated with appropriate antimicrobial formulations.

Clomiphene citrate (with the possible addition of metformin) is often the initial pharmacological treatment of the infertile woman because it is inexpensive and the adverse effect profile is less than other medications that induce ovulation. There is an increased risk of giving birth to twins with clomiphene therapy.

The more powerful medications used to induce ovulation include GnRH agonists followed by gonadotropin therapy. These medications are extremely potent and require daily ovarian ultrasonography and monitoring of estradiol levels to prevent hyperstimulation of the ovaries. The incidence of multiple pregnancies with the use of these medications is greater than 25%. Combinations of these medications are used with ART to stimulate ovulation before harvesting eggs.

Drug therapy may be indicated for male infertility. Problems with the thyroid or adrenal glands are corrected with appropriate medications. Infections are identified and treated with antimicrobials. FSH, HMG, and clomiphene may be used to stimulate spermatogenesis in men with hypogonadism. Men who do not respond to these therapies are candidates for intracytoplasmic sperm injection (ICSI), which is a procedure that injects sperm directly into the egg as part of IVF. ICSI has enabled men with very low sperm counts to achieve biological reproduction.

The primary care provider is responsible for fully informing patients about the prescribed medications. The nurse must be ready to answer patients' questions and to confirm their understanding of the drug, its administration, potential adverse effects, and expected outcomes. Because information varies with each drug, the nurse must consult the medication package inserts, pharmacology references, the physician, and the pharmacist, as necessary. The nurse should also provide anticipatory guidance regarding the time needed for a medication trial before referral to a specialist in ART would be indicated if the couple wants to continue to attempt becoming pregnant.

Surgical therapies. A number of surgical procedures can be used for female infertility problems. Ovarian tumours must be excised. Whenever possible, functional ovarian tissue is left intact. Scar tissue adhesions caused by chronic infections may cover much or all of the ovary. These adhesions usually necessitate surgery to free and expose the ovary so that ovulation can occur.

Hysterosalpingography is useful for identification of tubal obstruction and for the release of blockage (Fig. 8-2). During laparoscopy, delicate adhesions may be divided and removed, and endometrial implants may be destroyed by electrocoagulation or laser (Fig. 8-3). Laparotomy and even microsurgery may be required for extensive repair of the damaged tube. Prognosis depends on the degree to which tubal patency and function can be restored. In general, laparoscopic surgery for tubal patency is most effective in younger women with distal tubal damage. Older women or those with significant proximal disease should be referred for ARTs that bypass the fallopian tube.

In women with uterine abnormalities, reconstructive surgery (e.g., the unification operation for **bicornuate uterus**) can improve the ability to conceive and carry the fetus to term. Surgical removal of tumours or fibroids involving the endometrium or muscular walls of the uterus could also improve the woman's chance of conceiving and maintaining the pregnancy to viability, depending on the location and size of the fibroid or tumour. Surgical treatment of uterine tumours or maldevelopment that results in successful pregnancy may require birth by Caesarean surgery near term gestation because the enlarging uterus can rupture as a result of weakness in the area of reconstructive surgery.

Chronic inflammation and infection can be eliminated by radial chemocautery (destruction of tissue with chemicals) or thermocautery (destruction of tissue with heat, usually electrical) of the cervix, cryosurgery (destruction of tissue by application of extreme cold, usually liquid nitrogen), or conization (excision of a cone-shaped piece of tissue from the endocervix). When the cervix has been deeply cauterized or frozen or when extensive conization has been performed, the cervix may produce less mucus. Therefore, the absence of a mucous bridge from the vagina to the uterus can make sperm migration difficult or impossible. Therapeutic intrauterine insemination may be necessary for the sperm to be carried directly through the internal os of the cervix.

Surgical procedures may also be used for problems causing male infertility. Surgical repair of varicocele has been relatively successful in increasing sperm count but not fertility rates. Microsurgery to reanastomose (restore tubal continuity) the sperm ducts after vasectomy can restore fertility.

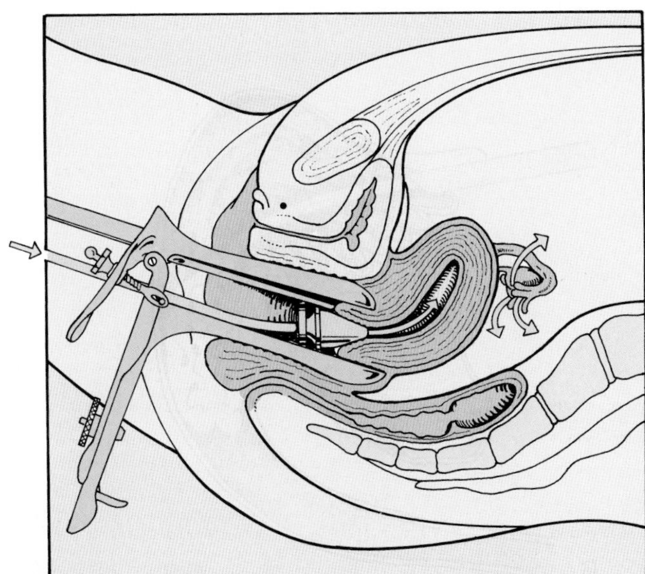

FIGURE 8-2 Hysterosalpingography. Note that the contrast medium flows through the intrauterine cannula and out through the uterine tubes.

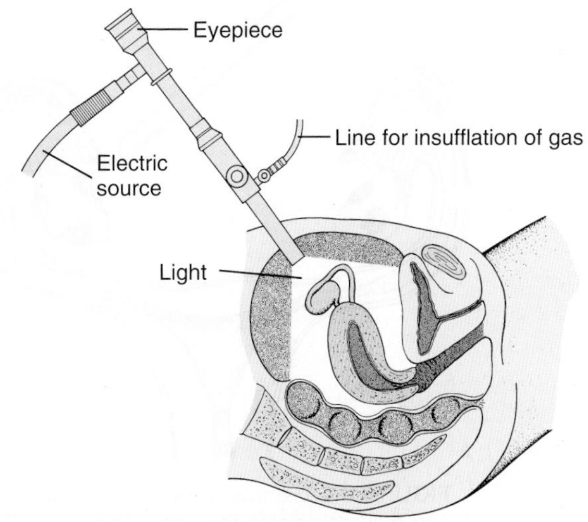

FIGURE 8-3 Laparoscopy.

Assisted Reproductive Technologies

Assisted reproductive technology (ART) is defined as fertility treatments in which both eggs and sperm are handled. In general these treatments involve removing the eggs from the woman, fertilizing the eggs in the laboratory, and returning the embryo or embryos to the woman or surrogate carrier. The Canadian Fertility and Andrology Society reported that in 2012 there were approximately 14,953 ART cycles with approximately 35% of these resulting in a pregnancy. Of these viable pregnancies, 82% were singletons, 17% were twins, and 1.1% were triplets or more. This represents a decrease in multiple pregnancy rate of 4 percentage points compared with 2011 (Canadian Fertility and Andrology Society, 2013). Although the use of ART is still relatively rare compared to the potential demand, its use has doubled over the past decade. Births conceived through ART comprise approximately 1% of all infants born in Canada every year.

Some of the ARTs for treatment of infertility include in vitro fertilization–embryo transfer (IVF-ET), gamete intrafallopian transfer (GIFT) (Fig. 8-4), zygote intrafallopian transfer (ZIFT), ovum transfer (oocyte donation), embryo adoption, embryo hosting and surrogate motherhood, therapeutic donor insemination (TDI), intracytoplasmic sperm injection (ICSI), assisted embryo hatching, and preimplantation genetic diagnosis (PGD). Table 8-2 describes these procedures and the possible indications for ARTs. Donor sperm and donor eggs can be used with ARTs. In addition, surrogates may carry the couple's biological child.

ARTs are associated with many ethical and legal issues (Box 8-7). The Assisted Human Reproduction Act sets legislation for all aspects of ART in Canada. The act prohibits human cloning and other unacceptable activities, while protecting the health and safety of people who use ART (Government of Canada, 2004). Nurses can provide relevant information to couples so that they have an accurate understanding of their chances for a successful pregnancy and live birth and can make an informed decision. Couples need to be counselled about the risks of multiple births to facilitate informed decision making regarding the number of embryos to transfer. The implications of having a multiple birth need to be explored, including the risk of preterm birth, possible admission to special care nurseries, and increased morbidity for multiples. Nurses also can provide anticipatory guidance about the moral and ethical dilemmas regarding the use of ARTs.

> **LEGAL TIP** ***CRYOPRESERVATION OF HUMAN EMBRYOS***
> Couples who have excess embryos frozen for later transfer must be fully informed before consenting to the procedure in order to make decisions about the disposal of embryos in the event of death, divorce, or the decision at a later time that the couple no longer wants the embryos.

Complications. Other than the established risks associated with laparoscopy and general anesthesia, few risks are associated with IVF-ET, GIFT, and ZIFT. The more common transvaginal needle aspiration requires only local or intravenous analgesia. Congenital anomalies occur no more frequently than among naturally conceived embryos, although the risk of pregnancy loss and chromosomal abnormality increases with maternal age. Multiple gestations are more likely and are associated with increased risks for both the mother and fetuses. Nevertheless, ectopic pregnancies do occur more often and pose significant maternal risk. There is no increase in maternal or perinatal complications with TDI and the same frequencies of anomalies (about 5%) and obstetric complications (between 5 and 10%) that accompany natural insemination (through sexual intercourse).

The percentage of multiple birth rates has decreased due to the work of a federal agency, Assisted Human Reproduction

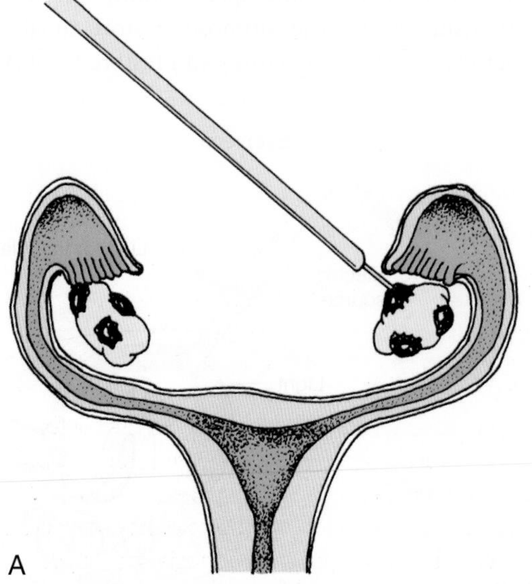

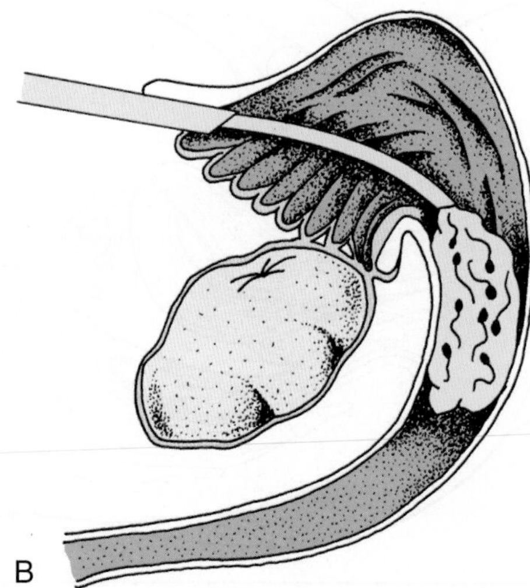

FIGURE 8-4 Gamete intrafallopian transfer (GIFT). **A:** Through laparoscopy a ripe follicle is located, and fluid containing the egg is removed. **B:** The sperm and egg are placed separately in the uterine tube, where fertilization occurs.

TABLE 8-2 ASSISTED REPRODUCTIVE TECHNOLOGIES

PROCEDURE	DEFINITION	INDICATIONS
In vitro fertilization–embryo transfer (IVF-ET)	A woman's eggs are collected from her ovaries, fertilized in the laboratory with sperm, and transferred to her uterus after normal embryo development has occurred.	Tubal disease or blockage; severe male infertility; endometriosis; unexplained infertility; cervical factor; immunological infertility
Gamete intrafallopian transfer (GIFT)	Oocytes are retrieved from the ovary, placed in a catheter with washed motile sperm, and immediately transferred into the fimbriated end of the uterine tube. Fertilization occurs in the uterine tube.	Same as for IVF-ET, except there must be normal tubal anatomy, patency, and absence of previous tubal disease in at least one uterine tube
IVF-ET and GIFT with donor sperm	This process is the same as that described for IVF-ET and GIFT except in cases where the man's fertility is severely compromised and donor sperm can be used; if donor sperm are used, the woman must have indications for IVF and GIFT.	Severe male infertility; azoospermia; indications for IVF-ET or GIFT
Zygote intrafallopian transfer (ZIFT)	This process is similar to IVF-ET; after IVF the ova are placed in one uterine tube during the zygote stage.	Same as for GIFT
Donor oocyte	Eggs are donated by an IVF procedure and the donated eggs are inseminated. The embryos are transferred into the recipient's uterus, which is hormonally prepared with estrogen–progesterone therapy.	Early menopause; surgical removal of ovaries; congenitally absent ovaries; autosomal or sex-linked disorders; lack of fertilization in repeated IVF attempts because of subtle oocyte abnormalities or defects in oocyte–spermatozoa interaction
Donor embryo (embryo adoption)	A donated embryo is transferred to the uterus of an infertile woman at the appropriate time (normal or induced) of the menstrual cycle.	Infertility not resolved by less aggressive forms of therapy; absence of ovaries; male partner is azoospermic or severely compromised
Gestational carrier (embryo host); surrogate mother	A couple undertakes an IVF cycle, and the embryo(s) is transferred to another woman's uterus (the carrier), who has contracted with the couple to carry the baby to term. The carrier has no genetic investment in the child. **Surrogate motherhood** is a process by which a woman is inseminated with semen from the infertile woman's partner and then carries the baby until birth.	Congenital absence or surgical removal of uterus; a reproductively impaired uterus, myomas, uterine adhesions, or other congenital abnormalities; a medical condition that might be life threatening during pregnancy, such as diabetes, immunological problems, or severe heart, kidney, or liver disease **It is illegal in Canada to pay someone to be a surrogate.**
Therapeutic donor insemination (TDI)	Donor sperm are used to inseminate the female partner.	Male partner is azoospermic or has a very low sperm count; couple has a genetic defect; male partner has antisperm antibodies; lesbian couple
Intracytoplasmic sperm injection	One sperm cell is selected to be injected directly into the egg to achieve fertilization. It is used with IVF.	Same as TDI
Assisted hatching	The zona pellucida is penetrated chemically or manually to create an opening for the dividing embryo to hatch and implant into the uterine wall.	Recurrent miscarriages; to improve implantation rate in women with previously unsuccessful IVF attempts; advanced age

Data from American Society for Reproductive Medicine. (2011). *Assisted reproductive technologies.* Retrieved from www.asrm.org; Government of Canada. (2004). *Assisted human reproduction act.* Ottawa: Minister of Justice. Retrieved from http://laws-lois.justice.gc.ca/eng/acts/A-13.4/

BOX 8-7 ISSUES TO BE ADDRESSED BY INFERTILE COUPLES BEFORE USING ASSISTED REPRODUCTIVE TECHNOLOGIES

- Risks of multiple gestation
- Possible need for multifetal reduction
- Possible need for donor oocytes, sperm, or embryos or for gestational carrier (surrogate mother)
- Whether or how to disclose facts of conception to offspring
- Freezing embryos for later use
- Possible risks of long-term effects of medications and treatment on women, children, and families
- Cost of treatment (emotional, monetary, and time)

Canada (AHRC). This agency was set up to oversee assisted reproduction and fertility treatments in Canada and has worked to increase the number of single embryo transfers over those of multiple embryos. Although AHRC closed in March 2013, the work of the agency has been taken over by Health Canada. With increased risk in multiple pregnancy for adverse maternal, obstetrical, and perinatal outcomes, couples need to be thoroughly counselled about the significant risks of multiple pregnancies associated with all assisted human reproductive treatments. The Society of Obstetricians and Gynaecologists of Canada (SOGC) recommends a policy of elective single embryo in couples with good prognosis for success (Okun, Sierra, Wilson, et al., 2014). To reduce the incidence of multiple pregnancy, health care policies that support public funding for assisted human reproduction, with regulations promoting best practice regarding elective single embryo transfer, should be strongly encouraged (Okun et al., 2014).

Preimplantation Genetic Diagnosis

Preimplantation genetic diagnosis (PGD) is a form of early genetic testing designed to eliminate embryos with serious genetic diseases before implantation through one of the ARTs and to avoid future termination of pregnancy for genetic reasons. Micromanipulation allows removal of a single cell from a multicellular embryo for genetic study (i.e., embryo biopsy) (Okun et al., 2014). Preimplantation screening for aneuploidy is associated with inconsistent findings for improving pregnancy outcomes. Patients need to know that currently there is no adequate information on the long-term effect of embryo single-cell biopsy (Okun et al., 2014). Couples must be counselled about their options and the implications of their choices when genetic analysis is considered.

LGBTQ Couples

Many LGBTQ couples may use ARTs in order to have biologically related children (LGBTQ Parenting Network, 2012). Couples need correct information in order to make informed choices. Health care providers need to provide sensitive and respectful care to couples and ensure that language, materials, and websites recognize and welcome LGBTQ clients (i.e., images depicting LGBTQ families, gender-neutral language, open-ended questions). It is beyond the scope of this text to discuss all options; readers are referred to the Additional Resources for excellent resources.

Adoption

Couples may choose to build their family by adopting children who are not genetically related. With increased availability of birth control and abortion and an increase in single mothers who choose to keep their babies, the availability of healthy newborn infants for adoption is extremely limited. Infants with diverse ethnic and racial heritages, infants with special needs, older children, and international adoptions are options that require careful consideration and sometimes significant time and financial investment (Fig. 8-5). Parents who adopt a child who has special needs or is from a different ethnic background face challenges that those who adopt a newborn may not. Often they must wait several years prior to adopting a child and this time can be challenging. Support groups can be an invaluable resource for these couples waiting for a child.

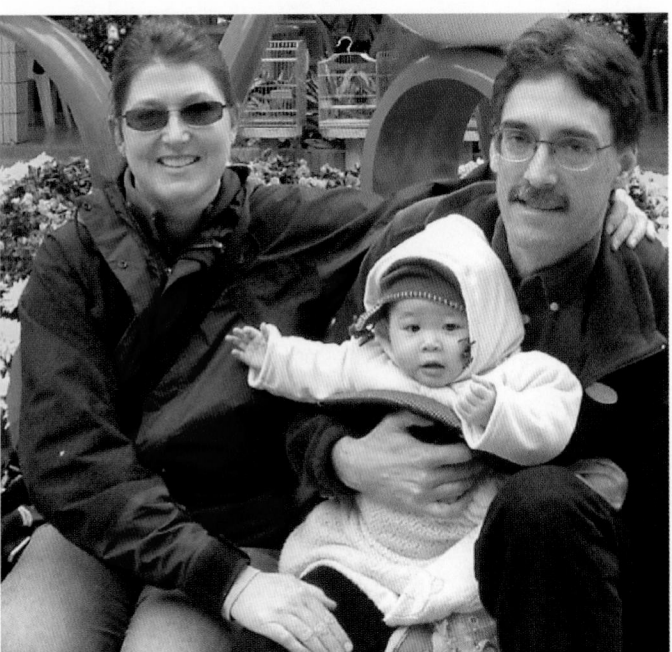

FIGURE 8-5 After two miscarriages, this couple chose international adoption. (Courtesy Shannon Perry.)

CONTRACEPTION

Contraception is the intentional prevention of pregnancy during sexual intercourse. *Birth control* is the device or practice used to decrease the risk of conceiving, or bearing, offspring. *Family planning* is the conscious decision regarding when to conceive or to avoid pregnancy throughout the reproductive years. The nurse can play a vital role in preventing unwanted pregnancy through counselling and education regarding family planning, contraception, and effective birth control. With the wide assortment of birth control options available, it is possible for a woman to use several different contraceptive methods at various stages throughout her fertile years. Nurses interact with the woman or couple to compare and contrast available options. Factors to consider include reliability, relative cost of the method, any protection from sexually transmitted infections (STIs), the individual's comfort level, and the partner's willingness to use a particular birth control method. Those who use contraception can still be at risk for pregnancy if their choice of contraceptive method results in one that is not used correctly. Providing adequate instruction about how to use a contraceptive method, when to use a backup method, and when to use emergency contraception (EC) can decrease the risk of unintended pregnancy.

NURSING CARE

A multidisciplinary approach may help a woman choose and correctly use an appropriate contraceptive method (see Nursing Process: Contraception, on Evolve). Nurses, midwives, nurse practitioners, and other advanced practice nurses and physicians have the knowledge and expertise to assist a woman in making decisions about contraception that will satisfy the woman's personal, social, cultural, and interpersonal needs.

Assessment for the couple desiring contraception involves assessment of the woman's reproductive history (menstrual, obstetrical, gynecological, contraceptive), physical examination, and sometimes current laboratory tests. The nurse must determine the woman's knowledge about reproduction, contraception, and STIs and possibly her sexual partner's commitment to any particular method. Fig. 8-6 illustrates contraceptive counselling. The nurse obtains information about the frequency of coitus, number of sexual partners (present and past), and any

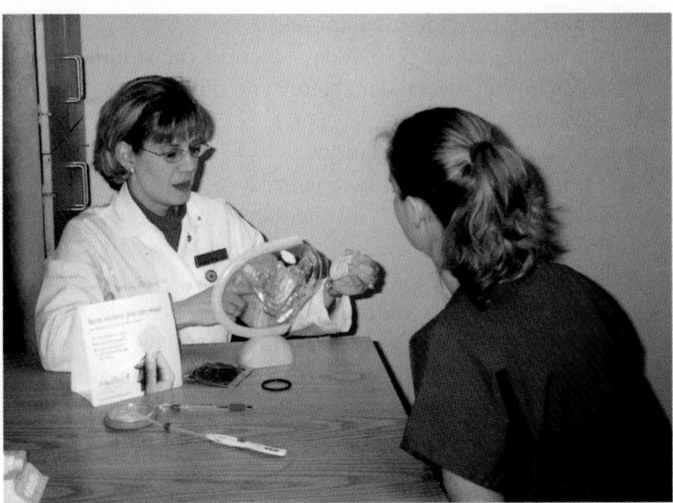

FIGURE 8-6 Nurse counselling woman about contraceptive methods. (Courtesy Dee Lowdermilk.)

BOX 8-8 FACTORS AFFECTING CONTRACEPTIVE METHOD EFFECTIVENESS

- Frequency of intercourse
- Motivation to prevent pregnancy
- Understanding of how to use the method
- Adherence to the method
- Consistent use of the method
- Provision of short-term or long-term protection
- Likelihood of pregnancy for the individual woman

objections that she or her partner might have about specific birth control methods. In addition, the nurse must determine a woman's willingness to touch her genitals. Religious and cultural factors may influence a woman or couple's choice regarding a particular contraceptive method. The woman/couple may believe in certain reproductive myths. Unbiased patient teaching is fundamental to initiating and maintaining any form of contraception. The nurse should counter myths with facts, clarify misinformation, and fill in gaps of knowledge. The ideal contraceptive should be safe, easily available, economical, acceptable, simple to use, and promptly reversible. Although no method may ever achieve all of these objectives, significant advances in the development of new contraceptive technologies have occurred over the past 30 years.

Contraceptive failure rate refers to the percentage of contraceptive users expected to have an unplanned pregnancy during the first year even when they use a method consistently and correctly. Contraceptive effectiveness varies from woman to woman and depends on both the properties of the method and the characteristics of the user (Box 8-8). Effectiveness of a method can be expressed as theoretical (i.e., how effective the method is with perfect use) and typical (i.e., how effective the method is with typical use). Failure rates decrease over time, either because a user gains experience with and uses a method more appropriately or because the less effective users stop using the method. Safety of a method may be affected by a woman's medical history (e.g., thromboembolic problems and contraceptive methods containing estrogen). Nevertheless, in most instances pregnancy would be more dangerous to the woman with medical problems than a particular contraceptive method. In addition, many contraceptive methods have health promotion effects. Barrier methods such as the male condom offer some protection from acquiring STIs, and oral contraceptives lower the incidence of ovarian and endometrial cancer.

Following assessment and analysis, the woman or couple determines possible contraceptive methods that are appropriate for their unique situation. Factors to consider when determining a contraceptive method are effectiveness, convenience, affordability, duration of action of method, reversibility of method, time of return to fertility, effects on uterine bleeding patterns, side effects, adverse events, health promotion effects of methods, effect of method on transmission of STIs, and medical contraindications for use.

The most effective reversible contraceptive methods at preventing pregnancy are the long–acting, reversible contraceptive (LARC) methods (e.g., contraceptive implants, intrauterine contraception). With these methods theoretical and typical pregnancy rates are the same because the method requires no user intervention after correct insertion. Effective methods include those that prevent pregnancy through exogenous hormones (estrogen or progestins) such as contraceptive injections, oral contraceptive pills, contraceptive patches, and vaginal rings. Each of these methods involves user interventions; thus typical-use pregnancy rates are higher than pregnancy rates with perfect use. The least effective contraceptive methods include the barrier methods and natural family planning. Examples include condoms, diaphragms, cervical caps, spermicides, withdrawal, and periodic abstinence during perceived ovulation. Effectiveness rates for these methods vary from user to user, depending on correct application of the method and consistency of use.

Expected outcomes related to contraceptive counselling are that the woman or couple will verbalize understanding about appropriate contraceptive methods, state that they are satisfied with the method chosen, use the method correctly and consistently, experience no adverse sequelae as a result of the chosen contraceptive method, and prevent unplanned pregnancy. The nurse assists with obtaining appropriate informed consent concerning contraception or sterilization, provides appropriate education to the couple, and documents the woman/couple's understanding of the contraceptive method chosen. Evaluation involves achievement of patient-centred outcomes when the couple engages in effective use of the chosen contraceptive device, experiences no adverse sequelae, and achieves pregnancy only when they desire to do so.

Methods of Contraception

The following discussion of contraceptive methods provides the nurse with information needed for patient teaching. After implementing the appropriate teaching for contraceptive use, the nurse supervises return demonstrations and practice to assess patient understanding (see Critical Thinking Case Study). The woman

CRITICAL THINKING CASE STUDY

Contraception for Adolescents

Marie is a 16-year-old Indigenous woman who comes to the nursing station on the reserve, seeking contraception. She has recently become sexually active and tells the nurse that she is concerned that her mother will find out. She also has many questions about the type of contraception to use. She seeks the nurse's advice to help in her decision making.

QUESTIONS

1. Evidence—Is there sufficient evidence to draw conclusions about what advice to give Marie? What is the age of consent?
2. Assumptions—What assumptions can be made about contraception for adolescents:
   a. Types of contraception
   b. Legal issues
   c. Implications of culture on choice
3. What implications and priorities for nursing care can be drawn at this time?
4. Does the evidence objectively support your conclusion?

or couple is given written instructions and telephone numbers or email contact information for questions. If the woman has difficulty understanding written instructions, she and her partner, if available, are offered graphic material, a telephone number to call as necessary, and an opportunity to return for further instruction. An excellent resource for information on all methods of contraception can be obtained from SexualityandU (see Additional Resources at the end of the chapter).

Coitus Interruptus

Coitus interruptus (withdrawal) involves the male partner withdrawing his penis from the woman's vagina before he ejaculates. Although coitus interruptus has been criticized as being an ineffective method of contraception, it is a good choice for couples who do not have another contraceptive method available. Effectiveness is similar to barrier methods and depends on the man's ability to withdraw his penis before ejaculation. The percentage of women who will experience an unintended pregnancy within the first year of typical use (failure rate) of withdrawal is about 19% (SexualityandU, 2012a). Coitus interruptus does not protect against STIs or human immunodeficiency virus (HIV) infection.

Natural Birth Control Methods

With natural birth control methods, women learn how to determine the beginning and the end of the fertile period of their menstrual cycle. Fertility awareness methods (FAMs) of contraception refer to a natural birth control method outside of a religious framework that supports the use of barrier methods (condom, diaphragm, and spermicide), emergency contraception, and abortion. Natural family planning (NFP) typically refers to natural birth control that is taught and practised within a religious framework, most commonly Catholic-centred organizations. It does not support the use of barrier methods, emergency contraception, or abortion. When women who want to use FAM/NFP are educated about the menstrual cycle, three phases are identified:

1. Infertile phase: before ovulation
2. Fertile phase: about 5 to 7 days around the middle of the cycle, including several days before and during ovulation and the day afterward
3. Infertile phase: after ovulation

The human ovum must be fertilized no later than 16 to 24 hours after ovulation. While motile sperm have been recovered from the uterus and the oviducts as long as 7 days after coitus, their ability to fertilize the ovum probably lasts no longer than 24 hours. Pregnancy is unlikely to occur if a couple abstains from intercourse for 4 days before and 3 or 4 days after ovulation (fertile period). Unprotected intercourse on the other days of the cycle (safe period) should not result in pregnancy. Nevertheless, the exact time of ovulation cannot be predicted accurately, and couples may find it difficult to abstain from sexual intercourse for several days before and after ovulation. Women with irregular menstrual periods have the greatest risk of failure with this form of contraception.

Although ovulation can be unpredictable in many women, teaching the woman about how she can directly observe her fertility patterns is an empowering tool. In addition, knowledge about the signs and symptoms of ovulation can be very helpful when the woman desires pregnancy. There are many categories of natural birth control methods. To prevent pregnancy, each one uses a combination of charts, records, calculations, tools, observations, and either abstinence (NFP) or barrier methods of birth control during the fertile period in the menstrual cycle. The charts and calculations associated with these methods can also be used to increase the likelihood of detecting the optimal timing of intercourse to achieve conception.

Advantages of these methods include low to no cost, absence of chemicals and hormones, and lack of alteration in the menstrual flow pattern. Disadvantages of FAM/NFP include adherence to strict record keeping, three to six cycles to learn, unintentional interference from external influences that may alter the woman's core body temperature and vaginal secretions, decreased effectiveness in women with irregular cycles (particularly adolescents who have not established regular ovulatory patterns), decreased spontaneity of coitus, and the necessity of attending possibly time-consuming training sessions by qualified instructors. The effectiveness of natural birth control methods depends on the users' ability to follow the plan. For the typical user, who may not follow all the rules, the effectiveness of FAM/NFP is 75 to 88%. With perfect use (user strictly follows rules to avoid pregnancy), the effectiveness is 95 to 98% (SexualityandU, 2012a). Natural birth control methods do not protect against STIs or HIV infection. FAM/NFP methods involve several techniques to identify high-risk, fertile days. The following discussion includes the most common techniques.

Rhythm (calendar) method. Practice of the calendar rhythm method is based on the number of days in each cycle, counting from the first day of the menstrual cycle. The fertile period is determined after accurately recording the length of menstrual cycles for 6 months. The beginning of the fertile period is estimated by subtracting 18 days from the length of the shortest cycle. The end of the fertile period is determined by subtracting 11 days from the length of the longest cycle. If the shortest cycle is 24 days and the longest is 30 days, application of the formula to calculate the fertile period is as follows:

Shortest cycle, 24 − 18 = day 6

Longest cycle, 30 − 11 = day 19

To avoid conception, the couple would abstain during the fertile period, days 6 through 19.

If the woman has very regular cycles of 28 days each, the formula indicates the fertile days to be as follows:

Shortest cycle, 28 − 18 = day 10

Longest cycle, 28 − 11 = day 17

To avoid conception, the couple would abstain days 10 through 17 because ovulation occurs on day 14 ± 2 days. A major drawback of the calendar method is that one is trying to predict future events with past data. The unpredictability of the menstrual cycle is also not taken into consideration. The calendar rhythm method alone is not recommended as a reliable method of birth control and is most useful as an adjunct to the basal body temperature (BBT) or cervical mucus method.

The standard days method (SDM) is essentially a modified form of the calendar rhythm method that has a "fixed" number of days of fertility for each cycle (i.e., days 8 to 19). A CycleBeads necklace (i.e., a colour-coded string of beads) can be purchased as a tool to track fertility (Fig. 8-7). Day 1 of the menstrual flow is counted as the first day to begin the counting. Women who use this device are taught to avoid unprotected intercourse on days 8 to 19 (white beads on CycleBeads necklace). Although this method is useful to women whose cycles are 26 to 32 days long, it is unreliable for those who have longer or shorter cycles (CycleBeads, 2016). Rhythm methods are the least effective natural birth control method and are not generally recommended (SexualityandU, 2012a).

Basal body temperature (BBT) method. The basal body temperature (BBT) is the lowest body temperature of a healthy person, taken immediately after waking and before getting out of bed. The BBT usually varies from 36.2° to 36.3°C during menses and for approximately 5 to 7 days afterward (Fig. 8-8).

About the time of ovulation, a slight drop in temperature (approximately 0.5°C) may occur in some women, but others may have no decrease at all. After ovulation, in concert with the increasing progesterone levels of the early luteal phase of the cycle, the BBT increases slightly (approximately 0.4° to 0.8°C). The temperature remains on an elevated plateau until 2 to 4 days before menstruation. Then BBT decreases to the low levels recorded during the previous cycle unless pregnancy has occurred. In pregnant women the temperature remains elevated. If ovulation fails to occur, the pattern of lower body temperature continues throughout the cycle.

To use this method, the fertile period is defined as the day of first temperature drop, or first elevation, through 3 consecutive days of elevated temperature. Abstinence begins the first day of menstrual bleeding and lasts through 3 consecutive days of sustained temperature rise (at least 0.2°C). The decrease and subsequent increase in temperature are referred to as the *thermal shift*. When the entire month's temperatures are recorded on a graph, the pattern described is more apparent. It is more difficult to perceive day-to-day variations without the entire picture (see Guidelines box). The thermometer used

GUIDELINES

Basal Body Temperature

- Discuss basal body temperature (BBT) with the woman.
- Show the woman a diagram depicting the phases of the menstrual cycle.
- Discuss the hormones in the woman's body that are responsible for her menstrual cycle and ovulation. Leave time for questions.
- Show the woman a sample BBT graph (see Fig. 8-8) and the biphasic line seen in ovulatory cycles.
- Show the woman the BBT thermometer and how it is calibrated.
- Provide a demonstration of how to take an oral temperature.
- Encourage the woman to demonstrate taking and reading the thermometer and graphing the temperature while the nurse watches.
- Encourage the woman to start a log to keep track of any other activity that might interfere with her true BBT.

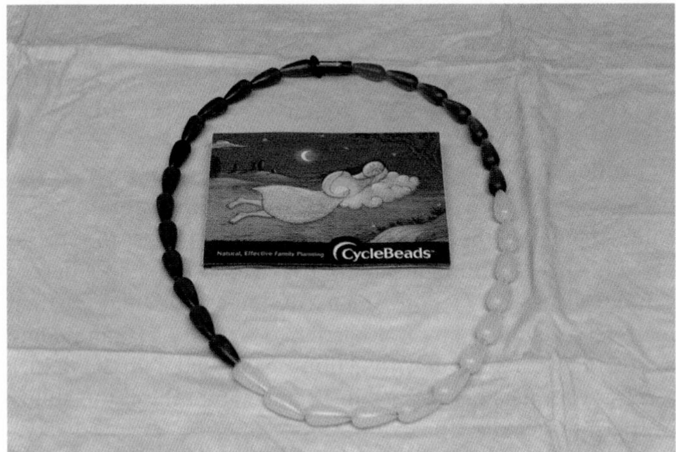

FIGURE 8-7 CycleBeads. Red bead marks the first day of the menstrual cycle. White beads mark days that are likely to be fertile days; therefore, unprotected intercourse should be avoided. Brown beads are days when pregnancy is unlikely and unprotected intercourse is permitted. (Courtesy Dee Lowdermilk.)

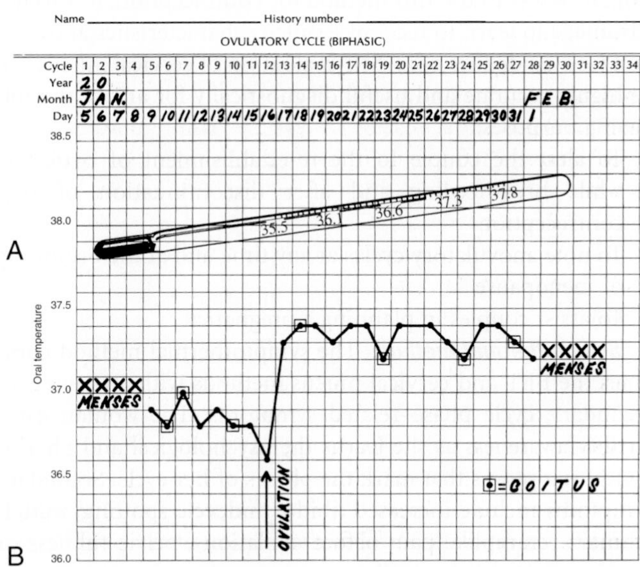

FIGURE 8-8 A: Special thermometer for recording basal body temperature, marked in tenths to enable the person to read more easily. **B:** Basal temperature record shows decrease and sharp increase at time of ovulation. Biphasic curve indicates ovulatory cycle.

must measure the temperature within one tenth of a degree. Infection, fatigue, less than 3 hours of sleep per night, awakening late, and anxiety may cause temperature fluctuations and alter the expected pattern. If a new BBT thermometer is purchased, this fact is noted on the chart because the readings may vary slightly. Jet lag, alcohol taken the evening before, or sleeping in a heated waterbed must also be noted on the chart because each affects the BBT. Therefore, the BBT alone is not a reliable method of predicting ovulation.

Cervical mucus ovulation-detection method. The cervical mucus ovulation-detection method (i.e., Billings method or Creighton model ovulation method) requires that the woman recognize and interpret the cyclic changes in the amount and consistency of cervical mucus that characterize her own unique pattern of changes at the time of ovulation. Cervical mucus changes before and during ovulation to facilitate and promote the viability and motility of sperm. Without adequate cervical mucus, coitus does not result in conception. This method requires that a woman check the quantity and character of mucus on the vulva or introitus with their fingers or with tissue paper each day for several months. This way she can learn how her cervical mucus responds to ovulation during her menstrual cycle. To ensure an accurate assessment of changes, the cervical mucus should be free from semen, contraceptive gels or foams, and blood or discharge from vaginal infections for at least one full cycle. Other factors that create difficulty in identifying mucus changes include douches and vaginal deodorants, being in the sexually aroused state (which thins the mucus), and taking medications such as antihistamines, which dry the mucus. Intercourse is considered safe without restriction beginning on the fourth day after the last day of wet, clear, slippery mucus, which would indicate that ovulation has occurred 2 to 3 days previously.

Some women find this method unacceptable if they are uncomfortable touching their genitals. Regardless of whether a woman wants to use this method for contraception, it is to her advantage to learn to recognize mucus characteristics at ovulation (see Guidelines box). Self-evaluation of cervical mucus can be highly accurate and useful diagnostically for any of the following purposes:

- To alert the couple to the re-establishment of ovulation while breastfeeding and after discontinuation of oral contraception
- To note anovulatory cycles at any time and at the beginning of menopause
- To assist couples in planning a pregnancy

Symptothermal method. The symptothermal method combines the BBT and cervical mucus methods with awareness of secondary, cycle phase–related symptoms. The woman gains fertility awareness as she learns the psychological and physiological symptoms that mark the phases of her cycle. Secondary symptoms include increased libido, midcycle spotting, mittelschmerz (cramplike pain before ovulation), pelvic fullness or tenderness, and vulvar fullness.

The woman is taught to palpate her cervix to assess for changes indicating ovulation: the cervical os dilates slightly, the cervix softens and rises in the vagina, and cervical mucus is copious and slippery. The woman notes days on which coitus, changes in routine, and illness have occurred (Fig. 8-9). Calendar calculations and cervical mucus changes are used to estimate the onset of the fertile period; changes in cervical mucus or the BBT are used to estimate its end.

If a woman's cycle does not follow a regular pattern, the use of natural birth control methods may be more difficult. In general, FAM/NFP methods are not recommended for women with the following difficulties: irregular cycles, inability to interpret the fertility signs correctly, or persistent infections that affect the signs of fertility (SexualityandU, 2012a).

Home predictor test kits for ovulation. All the methods previously discussed are indicative of ovulation but do not prove its occurrence or exact timing. The urine predictor test for ovulation is a major addition to the NFP/FAM methods to help women who want to plan the time of their pregnancies and for those who are trying to conceive. The urine predictor test for ovulation detects the sudden surge of LH that occurs approximately 12 to 24 hours before ovulation. Unlike BBT, the test is not affected by illness, emotional upset, or physical activity. For home use, a test kit contains sufficient material for several days' testing during each cycle. A positive response indicating an LH surge is noted by a colour change that is easy to read. Directions for use of urine predictor test kits vary with the manufacturer.

Breastfeeding: Lactational amenorrhea method. The lactational amenorrhea method (LAM) can be a highly effective, temporary method of birth control. It is more popular in underdeveloped countries and traditional societies where breastfeeding is used to prolong birth intervals.

When the infant suckles at the mother's breast, a surge of prolactin hormone is released, which inhibits estrogen production and suppresses ovulation and the return of menses. LAM works best if the mother is exclusively or almost exclusively breastfeeding, if the woman has not had a menstrual flow since giving birth, and if the infant is under 6 months of age. Effectiveness is enhanced by frequent feedings at intervals of less than 4 hours during the day and no more than 6 hours during the night, long duration of each feeding, and no bottle supplementation or limited supplementation by spoon or cup. The woman should be counselled that disruption of the breastfeeding pattern or supplementation can increase the risk of pregnancy and after 6 months, fertility could resume at any time. The typical failure rate is 2% (Kennedy & Trussell, 2011).

Nonhormonal Methods

Barrier contraceptives have gained in popularity not only as a contraceptive method but also as protection against the spread of STIs such as human papilloma virus (HPV) and herpes simplex virus (HSV). Some male condoms and female vaginal methods provide a physical barrier to several STIs, and some male condoms provide protection against HIV. **Spermicides** serve as chemical barriers against semen and inhibit the ability of sperm to fertilize the ovum.

The nurse should remember that any user of a barrier method of contraception must also be aware of emergency contraception options in case there is a failure of the method (see discussion later in chapter). An example of a barrier method failure would be if a condom broke during intercourse. In this instance emergency contraception would be indicated to prevent unplanned pregnancy.

Spermicides. Spermicides such as nonoxynol-9 (N-9) work by reducing the sperm's mobility; the chemicals attack the sperm flagella and body, thereby preventing the sperm from reaching the cervical os. N-9, the most commonly used spermicidal chemical in Canada, is a surfactant that destroys the sperm cell membrane; however, data now suggest that frequent use (more than two times a day) of N-9 or use as a lubricant during anal intercourse may increase the transmission of STIs and HIV and can cause lesions (SexualityandU, 2012b). Women with high-risk behaviours that increase their likelihood of contracting HIV and other STIs are advised to avoid the use of spermicidal products containing N-9, including lubricated condoms, diaphragms, and cervical caps to which N-9 is added.

Intravaginal spermicides are marketed and sold without prescriptions as aerosol foams, tablets, suppositories, creams, films, and gels (Fig. 8-10). Preloaded, single-dose applicators small enough to be carried in a small purse are available. Effectiveness of spermicides depends on consistent and accurate use. The spermicide should be inserted high into the vagina so that it makes contact with the cervix, not more than 1 hour before sexual intercourse. Spermicide must be reapplied for each additional act of intercourse, even if a barrier method is used. Studies have shown varying effectiveness rates for spermicidal use alone. Spermicide can also be used as a form of emergency contraception if inserted immediately after an accident with another contraceptive method. The failure rate for the use of spermicide is 31% for typical use and 18% for perfect use (SexualityandU, 2012b). Some female barrier methods (e.g., diaphragm, cervical caps) offer more effective protection against pregnancy with the addition of spermicides.

Male condoms. The male condom is a thin, stretchable sheath that covers the penis before genital, oral, or anal contact and is removed when the penis is withdrawn from the partner's orifice after ejaculation (Fig. 8-11, A). Condoms are made of latex rubber, which provides a barrier to sperm and STIs (including HIV); polyurethane (strong, thin plastic); or natural membranes (animal tissue). In addition to providing a physical barrier for sperm, nonspermicidal latex condoms also provide a barrier for STIs (particularly gonorrhea, chlamydia, and trichomonas) and HIV transmission. Condoms lubricated with N-9 are not recommended for preventing STIs or HIV and do not increase protection against pregnancy (Government of Canada, 2014). Latex condoms break down with oil-based lubricants (e.g., petroleum jelly and suntan oil) and should be used only with water-based or silicone lubricants. Because of the growing number of people with latex allergies, condom manufacturers have begun using polyurethane, which is thinner and stronger than latex.

! NURSING ALERT

All patients should be questioned about the potential for latex allergy. Latex condom use is contraindicated for patients with latex sensitivity.

Although polyurethane condoms are as effective for STI prevention as latex condoms, they are more likely to slip or lose contour than are latex condoms. Therefore, with perfect use latex condoms offer better protection against pregnancy. Polyurethane condoms do offer pregnancy protection equivalent to that of most barrier products. A small percentage of condoms are made from lamb cecum (natural skin). Natural skin condoms do not provide the same protection against STIs and HIV infection as that of latex condoms. Natural skin condoms contain small pores that could allow passage of viruses such as hepatitis B, HSV, and HIV and are not generally recommended.

A functional difference in condom shape is the presence or absence of a sperm reservoir tip. To enhance vaginal stimulation, some condoms are contoured and rippled or have ribbed or roughened surfaces. Thinner construction increases heat transmission and sensitivity; a variety of colours increases condom acceptability and attractiveness. A wet jelly or dry powder lubricates some condoms. Typical failure rate for the first year of use of the male condom is 15%. Effective condom use is a skill that must be taught. Box 8-9 summarizes advantages and disadvantages of male condoms.

! NURSING ALERT

It is a false assumption that everyone knows how to use condoms. To prevent unintended pregnancy and the spread of STIs, it is essential that condoms be used correctly. Proper instruction in use must be provided (Box 8-9). All types of condoms must be discarded after each single use. Condoms are available without prescription from a variety of sources, including vending machines.

Female condoms. The female condom is a vaginal sheath made of polyurethane and has flexible rings at both ends (see Fig. 8-11, A). The closed end of the pouch is inserted into the vagina and anchored around the cervix; the open ring covers the labia. A woman whose partner will not wear a male condom can use this as a protective mechanical barrier. Rewetting drops or oil- or water-based lubricants can be used to help decrease the distracting noise that is produced while penile thrusting occurs. The female condom is available in one size, is intended for single use only, and is sold over the counter. Disadvantages include difficulty for some women to insert them correctly and the cost per use. The female condom can also be inserted into the anus of both men and women for anal intercourse. When used this way, the inner ring of the condom is inserted into the rectum and the outside ring rests on the anus. Male condoms should not be used concurrently because the friction from both sheaths can increase the likelihood of either or both tearing. The typical failure rate is 21% (SexualityandU, 2012b).

Diaphragm. The contraceptive **diaphragm** is a shallow, dome-shaped, latex or silicone device with a flexible rim that covers the cervix (see Fig. 8-11, A). The diaphragm is a mechanical barrier to the meeting of sperm with the ovum. By holding spermicide in place against the cervix for the 6 hours it takes to destroy the sperm, the diaphragm also provides a chemical barrier to pregnancy. Diaphragms are available in a wide range

GUIDELINES

Cervical Mucus Characteristics

Setting the Stage

- Show charts of the menstrual cycle along with changes in the cervical mucus.
- Have the woman practise assessing mucus using raw egg white.
- Supply her with a basal body temperature (BBT) log and graph if she does not already have one (See Fig. 8-9).
- Explain that the assessment of cervical mucus characteristics is best when mucus is not mixed with semen, contraceptive jellies or foams, or discharge from infections.

Content Related to Cervical Mucus

- Explain to the woman (or couple) that a woman with a regular cycle will have the following sequence of events:
  - 3 to 7 days of menstruation
  - Several days where she does not feel or see mucus in her vagina or on her vulva
  - Several days of a "wet" or "slippery" sensation at her vulva or in the vagina where she sees or feels mucus. It is white or cream-coloured, thick to slightly stretchy, and breaks easily when stretched. Right before ovulation the mucus feels like a lubricant and can be stretched approximately 12 cm between the thumb and forefinger (similar to egg white); this is called *spinnbarkeit*. This characteristic indicates the period of maximum fertility. Sperm deposited in this type of mucus can survive until ovulation occurs.
- At ovulation it increases in amount and it becomes progressively more slippery, stretchy, and clear (like egg white) as ovulation approaches.
- After ovulation the mucus disappears from the vulva, and the vulva and vagina feel "drier."

Assessment Technique

- Stress that good hand hygiene is imperative to begin and end all self-assessment.
- Start observation from last day of menstrual flow.
- Assess cervical mucus several times a day for several cycles. Mucus can be obtained from vaginal introitus; there is no need to reach into the vagina to the cervix.
- Record findings on the same record on which her BBT is entered.

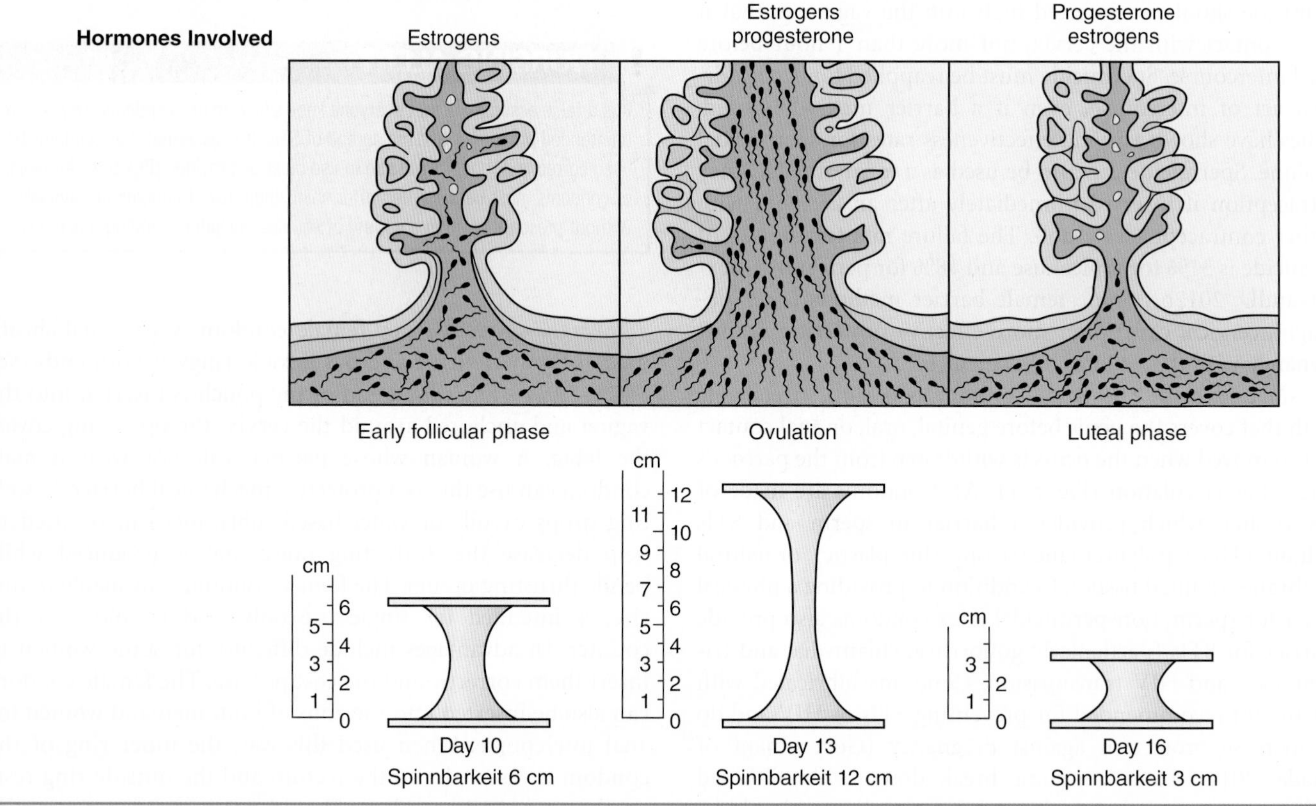

of diameters (50 to 95 mm) and differ in the inner construction of the circular rim. The types of rims are coil spring, arcing spring, and wide-seal rim. The diaphragm should be the largest size the woman can wear without being aware of its presence. It is 84 to 94% effective depending on how well the diaphragm is used (SexualityandU, 2012b).

Nursing considerations. The woman using a diaphragm needs an annual gynecological examination to assess the fit of the diaphragm. The device should be replaced every 2 years and may need to be refitted after a 20% weight loss or gain, birth, or second-trimester miscarriage and after any abdominal or pelvic surgery. Because various types of diaphragms are on the market, the nurse should use the package insert when teaching the woman how to use and care for the diaphragm (see Guidelines box).

Disadvantages of diaphragm use include the reluctance of some women to insert and remove the diaphragm. Although it

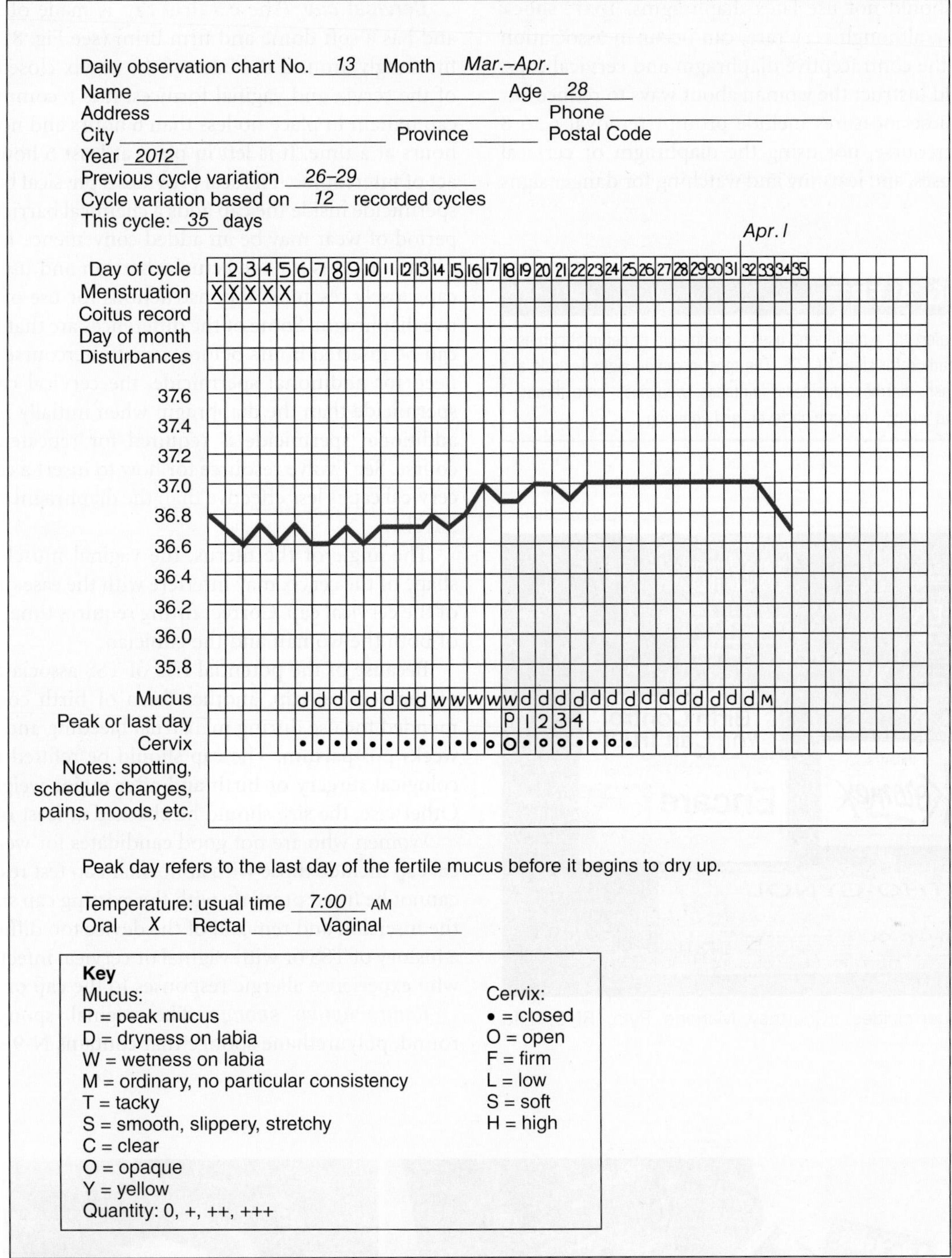

Daily observation chart No. 13 Month Mar.–Apr.
Name Age 28
Address Phone
City Province Postal Code
Year 2012
Previous cycle variation 26–29
Cycle variation based on 12 recorded cycles
This cycle: 35 days
Apr. I
Day of cycle 1 2 3 4 5 6 7 8 9 10 11 12 13 14 15 16 17 18 19 20 21 22 23 24 25 26 27 28 29 30 31 32 33 34 35
Menstruation X X X X X
Coitus record
Day of month
Disturbances
37.6
37.4
37.2
37.0
36.8
36.6
36.4
36.2
36.0
35.8
Mucus d d d d d d d d w w w w w d d d d d d d d d d d d d M
Peak or last day P 1 2 3 4
Cervix
Notes: spotting, schedule changes, pains, moods, etc.
Peak day refers to the last day of the fertile mucus before it begins to dry up.
Temperature: usual time 7:00 AM
Oral X Rectal Vaginal
Key
Mucus:
P = peak mucus
D = dryness on labia
W = wetness on labia
M = ordinary, no particular consistency
T = tacky
S = smooth, slippery, stretchy
C = clear
O = opaque
Y = yellow
Quantity: 0, +, ++, +++
Cervix:
• = closed
O = open
F = firm
L = low
S = soft
H = high

FIGURE 8-9 Example of completed symptothermal chart.

can be inserted up to 6 hours before intercourse, a cold diaphragm and a cold gel temporarily reduce vaginal response to sexual stimulation if insertion of the diaphragm occurs immediately before intercourse. Some women or couples object to the messiness of the spermicide. These annoyances of diaphragm use, along with failure to insert the device once foreplay has begun, are the most common reasons for failures of this method. Side effects may include irritation of tissues related to contact with spermicides.

The diaphragm is not a good option for women with poor vaginal muscle tone or recurrent urinary tract infections. For proper placement, the diaphragm must rest behind the pubic symphysis and completely cover the cervix. To decrease the chance of exerting urethral pressure, the woman should be reminded to empty her bladder before diaphragm insertion and immediately after intercourse.

Diaphragms are contraindicated for women with pelvic relaxation (uterine prolapse) or a large cystocele. Women with a latex allergy should not use latex diaphragms. Toxic shock syndrome (TSS), although very rare, can occur in association with the use of the contraceptive diaphragm and cervical caps. The nurse should instruct the woman about ways to reduce her risk for TSS. These measures include prompt removal 6 to 8 hours after intercourse, not using the diaphragm or cervical caps during menses, and learning and watching for danger signs of TSS.

> **NURSING ALERT**
>
> The nurse should alert the woman who uses a diaphragm or cervical cap as a contraceptive method for signs of TSS. The most common signs include a sunburn type of rash, diarrhea, dizziness, faintness, weakness, sore throat, aching muscles and joints, sudden high fever, and vomiting.

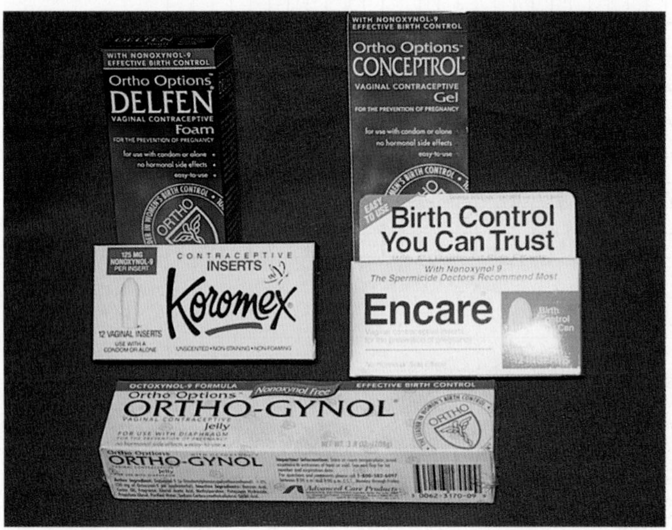

FIGURE 8-10 Spermicides. (Courtesy Marjorie Pyle, RNC, Life Circle.)

Cervical cap. The cervical cap is made of silicone rubber and has a soft dome and firm brim (see Fig. 8-11, A). The cap fits snugly around the base of the cervix close to the junction of the cervix and vaginal fornices. It is recommended that the cap remain in place no less than 6 hours and not more than 48 hours at a time. It is left in place at least 6 hours after the last act of intercourse. The seal provides a physical barrier to sperm; spermicide inside the cap adds a chemical barrier. The extended period of wear may be an added convenience for women.

Instructions for the actual insertion and use of the cervical cap closely resemble the instructions for use of the contraceptive diaphragm. Some of the differences are that the cervical cap can be inserted hours before sexual intercourse without a later need for additional spermicide, the cervical cap requires less spermicide than the diaphragm when initially inserted, and no additional spermicide is required for repeated acts of intercourse. See Evolve resource for how to insert a cervical cap. The cervical cap is less effective than the diaphragm (SexualityandU, 2012b).

The angle of the uterus, the vaginal muscle tone, and the shape of the cervix may interfere with the ease of fitting and use of the cervical cap. Correct fitting requires time, effort, and skill of both the woman and the clinician.

Because of the potential risk of TSS associated with the use of the cervical cap, another form of birth control is recommended for use during menstrual bleeding and up to at least 6 weeks postpartum. The cap should be refitted after any gynecological surgery or birth and after major weight loss or gain. Otherwise, the size should be checked at least once a year.

Women who are not good candidates for wearing the cervical cap include those with abnormal Pap test results, those who cannot be fitted properly with the existing cap sizes or who find the insertion and removal of the device too difficult, those with a history of TSS or with vaginal or cervical infections, and those who experience allergic responses to the cap or to spermicide.

Contraceptive sponge. The vaginal sponge is a small, round, polyurethane sponge that contains N-9 spermicide (see

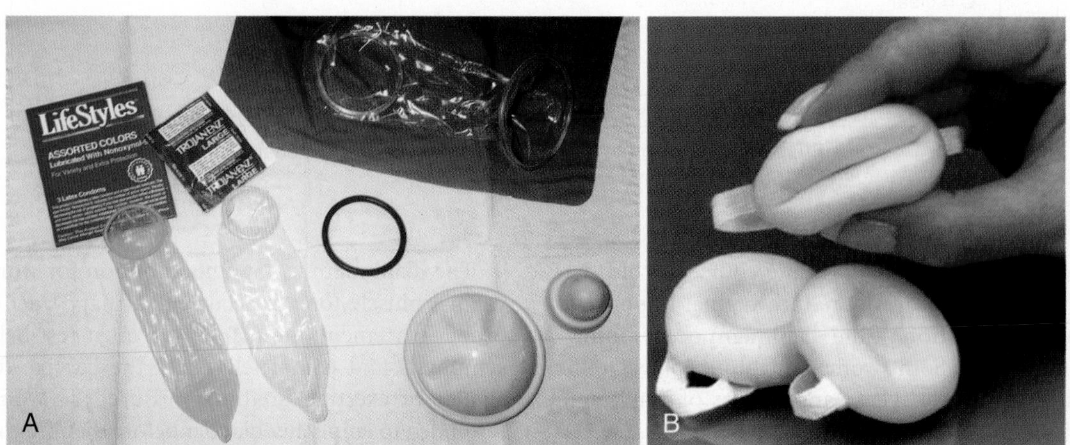

FIGURE 8-11 A: Mechanical barriers. Clockwise from top: female condom, cervical cap, diaphragm, types of male condoms, vaginal ring (hormonal) (centre). **B:** Contraceptive sponge. (**A,** Courtesy Donna Rowe, University of North Carolina Student Health. **B,** Courtesy Allendale Pharmaceuticals, Inc.)

BOX 8-9 MALE CONDOMS

Mechanism of Action

The sheath is applied over the erect penis before insertion or loss of pre-ejaculatory drops of semen. Used correctly, condoms prevent sperm from entering the cervix. Spermicide-coated condoms cause ejaculated sperm to be immobilized rapidly, thus increasing contraceptive effectiveness.

Failure Rate

- Typical users, 15%
- Correct and consistent users, 2%

Advantages

- Safe
- Inexpensive
- Latex and polyurethane condoms protect against sexually transmitted infections (STIs)
- No side effects
- Readily available
- Allows the male partner to assume some responsibility for birth control
- Premalignant changes in cervix can be prevented or ameliorated in women whose partners use condoms
- Method of male nonsurgical contraception

Disadvantages

- Must be available at time of intercourse
- May reduce sexual spontaneity and sensitivity for either partner
- Must be stored and handled properly
- Condoms occasionally may tear during intercourse.
- People with latex allergies cannot use latex condoms.
- The use of spermicide may cause irritation of the vaginal and rectal walls and increase the risks of contracting HIV.
- May interfere with the maintenance of an erection

STI Protection

If a condom is used throughout the act of intercourse and there is no unprotected contact with female genitals, a latex rubber condom, which is impermeable to viruses, can act as a protective measure against sexually transmitted infections.

Nursing Considerations

Teach the man or woman or both to do the following:

- Use a new condom (check expiration date) for each act of sexual intercourse or other acts between partners that involve contact with the penis.
- Place the condom after the penis is erect and before intimate contact.
- Place the condom on the head of the penis (A) and unroll it all the way to the base (B).
- Leave an empty space at the tip (A); remove any air remaining in the tip by gently pressing air out toward the base of the penis.

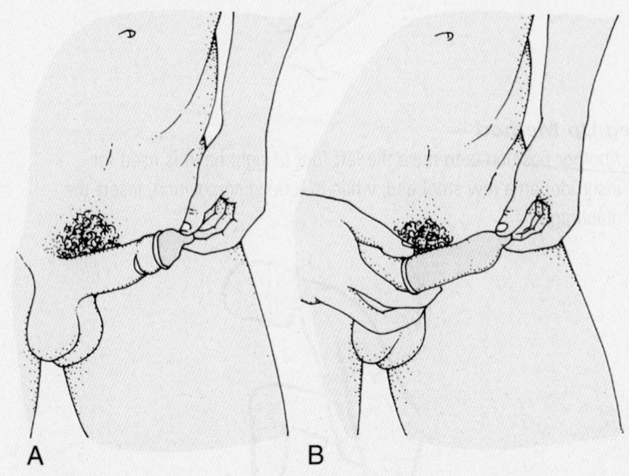

- If a lubricant is desired, use water-based products such as K-Y lubricating jelly. Do not use petroleum-based products because they can cause the condom to break.
- After ejaculation, carefully withdraw the still-erect penis from the vagina, holding onto the condom rim; remove and discard the condom.
- Store unused condoms in a cool, dry place.
- Do not use condoms that are sticky, brittle, or obviously damaged.

Source: SexualityandU. (2012). *Choosing a contraceptive that's right for u.* Retrieved from http://sexualityandu.ca/uploads/files/refContraceptiveComparativeChartFinalENG09.pdf

Fig. 8-11, B). It is designed to fit over the cervix (one size fits all). The side that is placed next to the cervix is concave for better fit. The opposite side has a woven polyester loop to be used for removal of the sponge.

The sponge must be moistened with water before it is inserted into the vagina to cover the cervix. It provides protection for up to 24 hours and for repeated instances of sexual intercourse. The sponge should be left in place for at least 6 hours after the last act of intercourse. Wearing it longer than 24 to 30 hours may put the woman at risk for TSS. The typical failure rate in the first year of use is 40% for parous women and 20% for nulliparous women.

Hormonal Methods

There are many different types of hormonal contraceptive formulations available in Canada. General classes are described in Table 8-3. Because of the wide variety of preparations available, the woman and nurse must read the package insert for information about specific products prescribed. Formulations include combined estrogen–progestin steroidal medications or progestational agents. The formulations are administered orally, transdermally, vaginally, or by injection.

Combined estrogen–progestin contraceptives

Oral contraceptives. The normal menstrual cycle is maintained by a feedback mechanism. FSH and LH are secreted in response to fluctuating levels of ovarian estrogen and progesterone. Regular ingestion of combined oral contraceptive pills (COCs) suppresses the action of the hypothalamus and anterior pituitary, leading to insufficient secretion of FSH and LH; therefore, follicles do not mature, and ovulation is inhibited.

Other contraceptive effects are induced by the combined steroids. Maturation of the endometrium is altered, making the

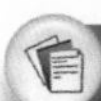

GUIDELINES

Use and Care of the Diaphragm

Positions for Insertion of Diaphragm

Squatting

- Squatting is the most commonly used position, and most women find it satisfactory.

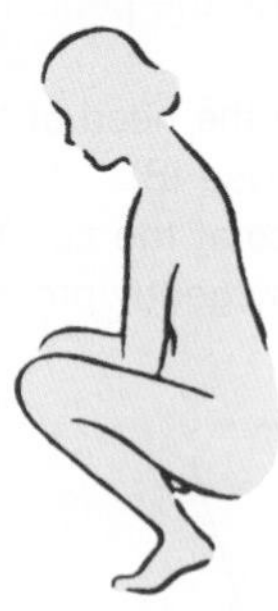

Leg-Up Method

- Another position is to raise the left foot (if right hand is used for insertion) on a low stool and, while in a bending position, insert the diaphragm.

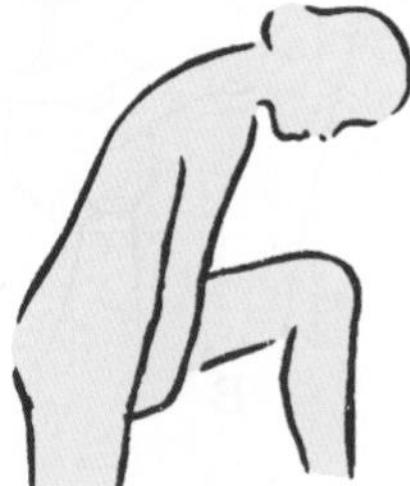

Chair Method

- Another practical method for diaphragm insertion is to sit far forward on the edge of a chair.

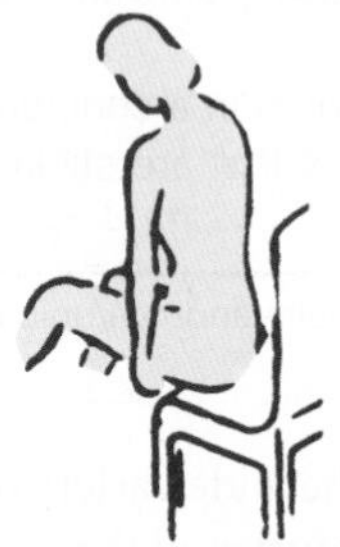

Reclining

- You may prefer to insert the diaphragm while in a semi-reclining position in bed.

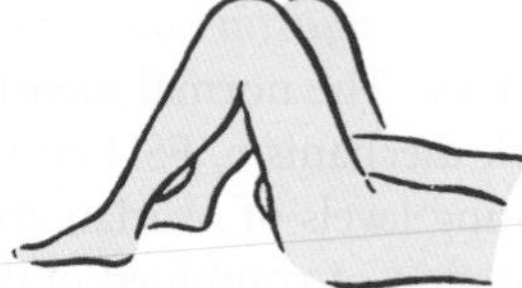

Inspection of Diaphragm

The diaphragm must be inspected carefully before each use. The best way to do this is to do the following:

- Hold the diaphragm up to a light source. Carefully stretch the diaphragm at the area of the rim, on all sides, to make sure that there are no holes. Remember, it is possible to puncture the diaphragm with sharp fingernails.
- Another way to check for pinholes is to carefully fill the diaphragm with water. If there is any problem, it will be seen immediately.
- If the diaphragm is puckered, especially near the rim, this could mean thin spots.
- The diaphragm should not be used if you see any of these; consult your health care provider.

Preparation of Diaphragm

- Rinse off cornstarch. The diaphragm must always be used with a spermicidal lubricant to be effective. Pregnancy cannot be prevented effectively by using the diaphragm alone.
- Always empty your bladder before inserting the diaphragm. Place about 10 mL (2 tsp) of contraceptive jelly or contraceptive cream on the side of the diaphragm that will rest against the cervix (or whichever way you have been instructed). Spread it around to coat the surface and the rim. This aids in insertion and offers a more complete seal. Many women also spread some jelly or cream on the other side of the diaphragm.

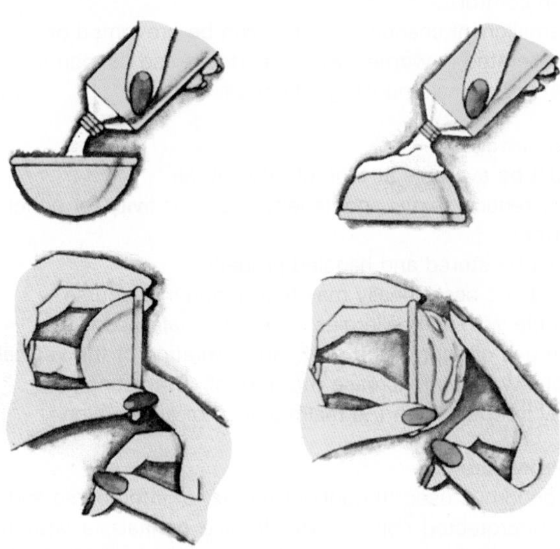

Insertion of Diaphragm

- The diaphragm can be inserted as long as 6 hours before intercourse. Hold the diaphragm between your thumb and fingers. The dome can either be up or down. Place your index finger on the outer rim of the compressed diaphragm.

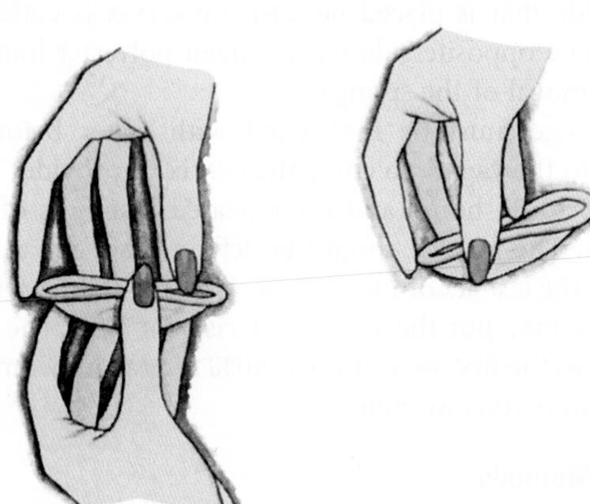

- Use the fingers of the other hand to spread the labia (lips of the vagina). This will assist in guiding the diaphragm into place.

GUIDELINES

Use and Care of the Diaphragm—cont'd

- Insert the diaphragm into the vagina. Direct it inward and downward as far as it will go to the space behind and below the cervix.

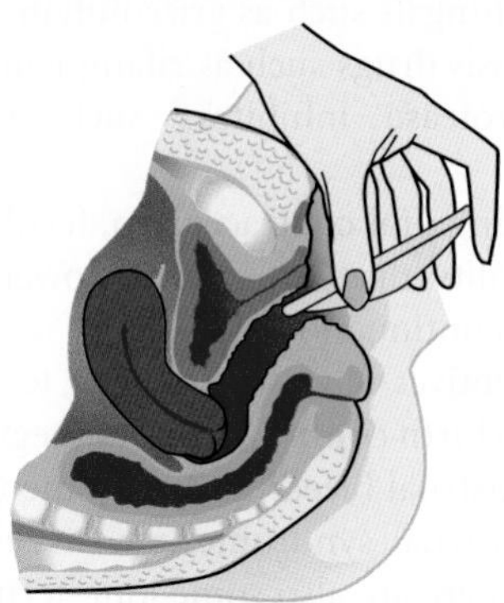

- Tuck the front of the rim of the diaphragm behind the pubic bone so that the rubber hugs the front wall of the vagina.

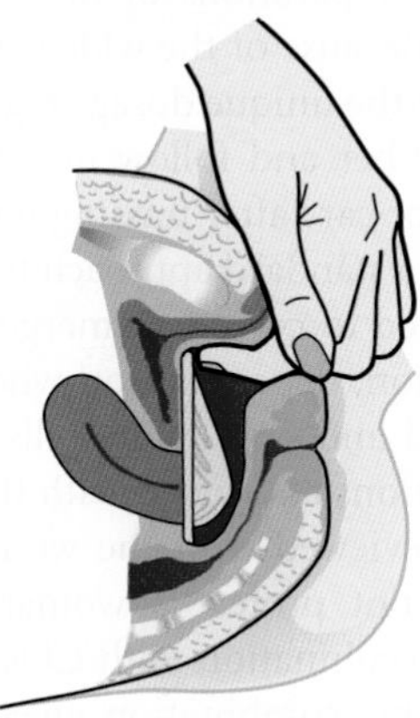

- Feel for the cervix through the diaphragm to be certain it is properly placed and securely covered by the rubber dome.

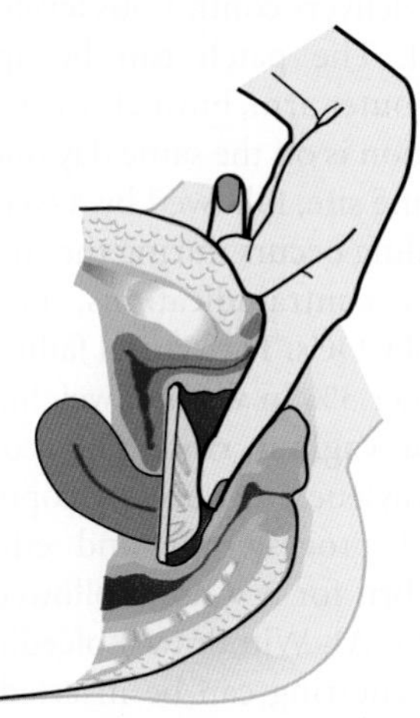

General Information

- Regardless of the time of the month, you must use your diaphragm every time intercourse takes place. The diaphragm must be left in place for at least 6 hours after the last intercourse. If you remove the diaphragm before the 6-hour period, your chance of becoming pregnant could be greatly increased. If you have repeated acts of intercourse, you must add more spermicide for each act of intercourse.

Removal of Diaphragm

- The only proper way to remove the diaphragm is to insert your forefinger up and over the top side of the diaphragm and slightly to the side.
- Next turn the palm of your hand downward and backward, hooking the forefinger firmly on top of the inside of the upper rim of the diaphragm, breaking the suction.
- Pull the diaphragm down and out. This avoids the possibility of tearing it with the fingernails. You should not remove the diaphragm by trying to catch the rim from below the dome.

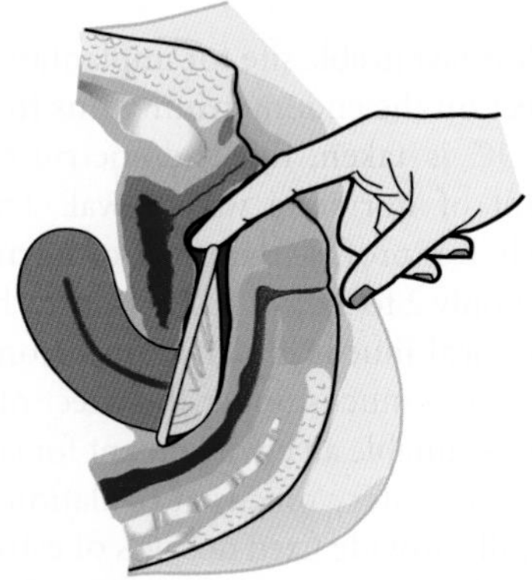

Care of Diaphragm

- When using a vaginal diaphragm, avoid using oil-based products such as body lubricants, mineral oil, baby oil, vaginal lubricants, or vaginitis preparations. These products can weaken the rubber.
- A little care means longer wear for your diaphragm. After each use, wash the diaphragm in warm water and mild soap. Do not use detergent soaps, cold-cream soaps, deodorant soaps, or soaps containing oil products because they can weaken the rubber.
- After washing, dry the diaphragm thoroughly. All water and moisture should be removed with a towel. Dust the diaphragm with cornstarch. Scented talc, body powder, baby powder, and the like should not be used because they can weaken the rubber.
- Place the diaphragm back in the plastic case for storage. Do not store it near a radiator or heat source or exposed to light for an extended period.

TABLE 8-3 HORMONAL CONTRACEPTION

COMPOSITION	ROUTE OF ADMINISTRATION	DURATION OF EFFECT
Combination estrogen and progestin (synthetic estrogens and progestins in varying doses and formulations)	Oral	24 hours; extended cycle—12 weeks
	Transdermal patch	7 days
	Vaginal ring insertion	3 weeks
Progestin only		
Norethindrone, norgestrel	Oral	24 hours
Medroxyprogesterone acetate	Intramuscular or subcutaneous injection	3 months
Levonorgestrel	Intrauterine system	5 years

uterine lining a less favourable site for implantation. COCs also have a direct effect on the endometrium; thus from 1 to 4 days after the last COC is taken, the endometrium sloughs and bleeds as a result of hormone withdrawal. The withdrawal bleeding is usually less profuse than that of normal menstruation and may last only 2 to 3 days. Some women have no bleeding at all. The cervical mucus remains thick from the effect of the progestin. Cervical mucus under the effect of progesterone does not provide as suitable an environment for sperm penetration as does the thin, watery mucus at ovulation.

Monophasic pills provide fixed dosages of estrogen and progestin. They alter the amount of progestin and sometimes the amount of estrogen within each cycle. These preparations reduce the total dosage of hormones in a single cycle without sacrificing contraceptive efficacy. To maintain adequate hormone levels for contraception and enhance compliance, COCs should be taken at the same time each day. Taken exactly as directed, COCs prevent ovulation, and pregnancy cannot occur. The overall effectiveness rate is almost 100%.

Because taking the pill does not relate directly to the sexual act, its acceptability may be increased. Improvement in sexual response may occur once the possibility of pregnancy is not an issue. For some women it is convenient to know when to expect the next menstrual flow.

Contraindications for COC use include a history of thromboembolic disorders, cerebrovascular or coronary artery disease, breast cancer, estrogen-dependent tumours, pregnancy, impaired liver function, liver tumour, lactation less than 6 weeks postpartum, smoking if older than 35 years of age, migraine with aura, surgery with prolonged immobilization or any surgery on the legs, hypertension (160/100), and diabetes mellitus (of more than 20 years' duration) with vascular disease. The risk of venous thromboembolism is rare although slightly increased over that of women who do not use COCs; women should undergo individualized risk assessments to determine who might benefit from another type of contraception (Reid et al., 2010).

The effectiveness of oral contraceptives is decreased when the following medications are taken simultaneously:

- Anticonvulsants such as barbiturates, oxycarbazepine, phenytoin, phenobarbital, carbamazepine, primidone, and topiramate
- Systemic antifungals such as griseofulvin
- Antituberculosis drugs such as rifampicin and rifabutin
- Anti-HIV protease inhibitors such as nelfinavir and amprenavir

After discontinuing oral contraception, fertility usually returns quickly, but fertility rates are slightly lower the first 3 to 12 months after discontinuation.

Oral contraceptives have been shown to have benefits that are not related to birth control, including regulation and reduction of both menstrual bleeding and dysmenorrhea, and treatment of premenstrual syndrome, menstrual migraines, acne, and hirsutism. There are also some long-term benefits, such as reduced rates of endometrial, ovarian, and colorectal cancer (Reid et al., 2010).

Many different preparations of oral hormonal contraceptives are available. Because of the wide variations, each woman must be clear about the unique dosage regimen for the preparation prescribed for her and follow directions on the package insert. Directions for care after missing one or two tablets vary. Fig. 8-12 illustrates a standard approach to missed pills. Women need to be instructed to consider emergency contraception or backup contraception, depending on when during the month the pills are missed and how many pills are missed. Signs of potential complications associated with the use of oral contraceptives must be reviewed with the woman (Box 8-10). Oral contraceptives do not protect a woman against STIs. Male condoms used in combination with COCs provide protection against STIs, and this combination gives excellent protection against unplanned pregnancy.

Transdermal contraceptive system. The **transdermal contraceptive patch** delivers continuous levels of progesterone and ethynyl estradiol. The patch can be applied to the lower abdomen, upper outer arm, buttock, or upper torso (except the breasts). Application is on the same day once a week for 3 weeks but not at the same site, followed by a week without the patch. Withdrawal bleeding occurs during the "no patch" week. Mechanisms of action, contraindications, and adverse effects are similar to those of COCs. The typical failure rate during the first year of use is under 3% in women weighing less than 90 kg.

Contraceptive vaginal ring. The **contraceptive vaginal ring** (made of ethylene vinyl acetate copolymer) delivers continuous levels of progesterone and ethynyl estradiol. One vaginal ring is worn for 3 weeks, followed by a week without the ring (Fig. 8-11, A). Withdrawal bleeding occurs during the "no ring" week. The ring can be inserted by the woman and does not have to be fitted. Some wearers may experience vaginal discomfort, usually related to increased vaginal discharge, but other wearers report that the ring alleviates symptoms of vaginitis. Mechanisms of action, contraindications, and adverse effects are similar to those of COCs. The typical failure rate of the vaginal contraceptive ring is reportedly under 2% during the first year of use.

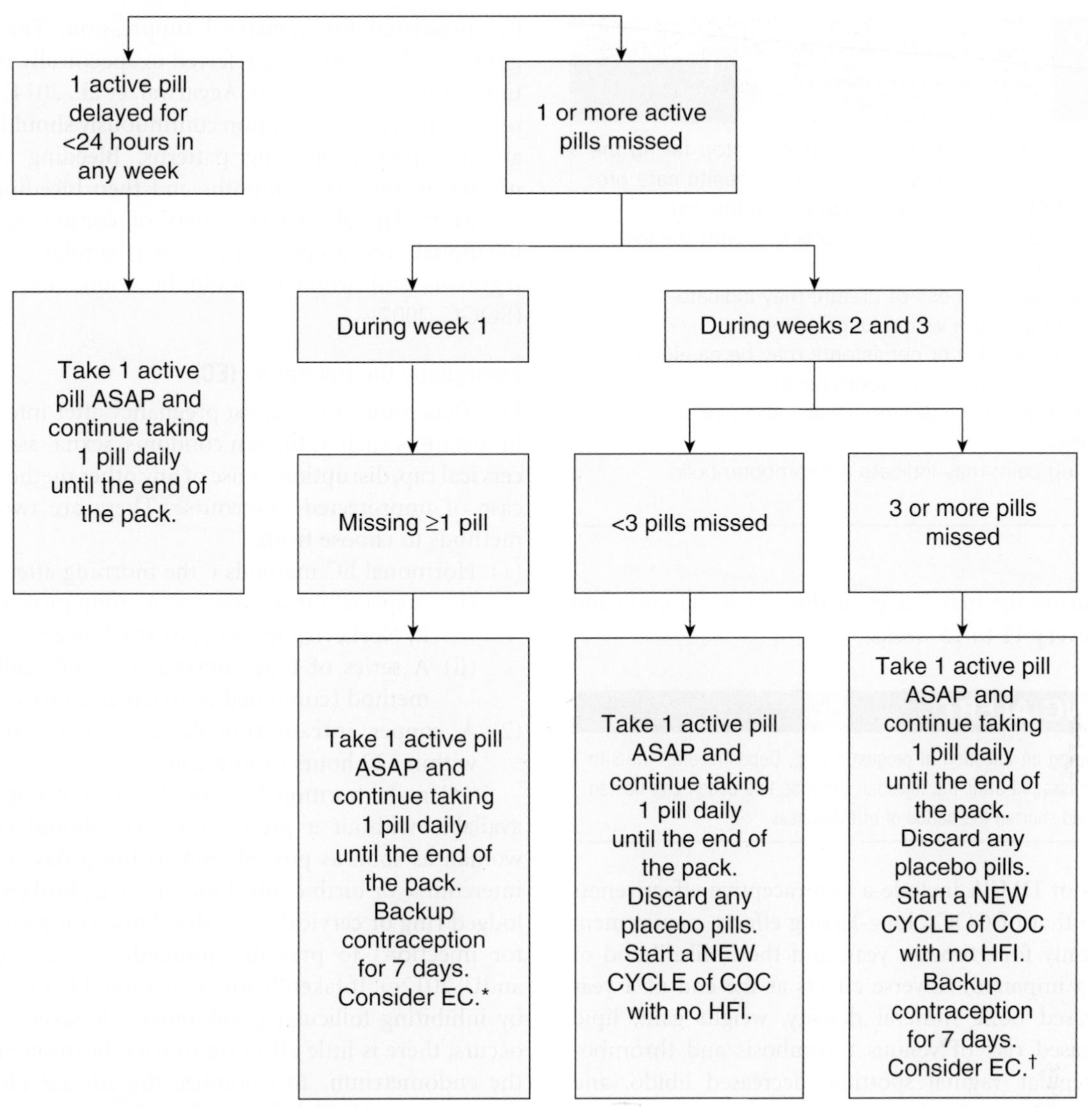

FIGURE 8-12 Flowchart for missed contraceptive pills. *ASAP*, as soon as possible; this may mean that two pills are taken on that day. *COC*, combined oral contraceptive; *EC*, emergency contraception; *HFI*, hormone-free interval. (Courtesy Society of Obstetricians and Gynaecologists of Canada [2008]. SOGC clinical practice guideline: Missed hormonal contraceptives: New recommendations. *Journal of Obstetrics and Gynaecology Canada, 30*[11], 1050–1061. Printed with permission from the SOGC.)

Progestin-only contraception. Progestin-only methods impair fertility by inhibiting ovulation, thickening and decreasing the amount of cervical mucus, thinning the endometrium, and altering cilia in the uterine tubes. Because progestin-only methods do not contain estrogen, they may be used in certain instances such as lactation, when estrogen would not be recommended.

Oral progestins (minipill). Progestin-only pills are less effective than COCs. Because minipills contain such a low dose of progestin, they must be taken at the same time every day. If the pill is taken more than 3 hours late (27 hours after the last pill), a backup contraceptive method must be initiated. Much of the contraceptive effectiveness of the minipill depends on progestin-induced changes in cervical mucus, and this effect lasts about 24 hours after oral ingestion of the pill. Users often find they have irregular vaginal bleeding. The failure rate for typical users of the minipill is approximately 8% during the first year of use. Effectiveness is increased if minipills are taken correctly. There are two instances in which the minipill is quite effective: in lactating women and women over 40. The reduced fecundity of lactation and the perimenopause period enhance the contraceptive effects of the minipill.

Injectable progestins. Depot medroxyprogesterone acetate (DMPA; Depo-Provera) is given subcutaneously or intramuscularly in the deltoid or gluteus maximus muscle. DMPA should

BOX 8-10 SIGNS OF POTENTIAL COMPLICATIONS: ORAL CONTRACEPTIVES

The woman should be alerted to immediately stop taking the pill and report the following symptoms to the health care provider. The word ACHES helps in remembering this list:

- **A**—Abdominal pain: may indicate a problem with the liver or gallbladder
- **C**—Chest pain or shortness of breath: may indicate possible clot problem within lungs or heart
- **H**—Headaches (sudden or persistent): may be caused by cardiovascular accident or hypertension
- **E**—Eye problems: may indicate vascular accident or hypertension
- **S**—Severe leg pain: may indicate a thromboembolic process

be initiated during the first 5 days of the menstrual cycle and administered every 11 to 13 weeks.

NURSING ALERT

When administering an injection of progestin (e.g., Depo-Provera), the site should not be massaged after the injection because this action can hasten the absorption and shorten the period of effectiveness.

Advantages of DMPA include a contraceptive effectiveness comparable to that of COCs, long-lasting effects, requirement of injections only four times a year, and the unlikelihood of lactation being impaired. Adverse effects at the end of a year include decreased bone mineral density, weight gain, lipid changes, increased risk of venous thrombosis and thromboembolism, irregular vaginal spotting, decreased libido, and breast changes. Other disadvantages include no protection against STIs. Return to fertility may be delayed as long as up to 18 months after discontinuing DMPA. Typical failure rate is 3% in the first year of use.

NURSING ALERT

Women who use DMPA may lose significant bone mineral density with increasing duration of use. It is unknown if this effect is reversible. It is unknown if use of DMPA during adolescence or early adulthood, a critical period of bone accretion, will reduce peak bone mass and increase the risk of osteoporotic fracture in later life. Women who receive DMPA should be counselled about vitamin D and calcium intake as well as exercise in order to protect bone health.

Continuous and extended hormonal contraception. Continuous hormonal contraception, with no breaks, is being used increasingly to suppress menstruation, for medical reasons (e.g., severe dysmenorrhea, abnormal uterine bleeding, and premenstrual dysphoric disorders—see Chapter 7) and women's preferences (vacations, sports, and special events). Women undergoing cancer treatment, those at risk for iatrogenic thrombocytopenia, and women with developmental disabilities may also be considered for menstrual suppression. The SOGC has a guideline that should be referred to specifically for these situations (Kirkham, Ornstein, Aggarwal, et al., 2014). Women who use hormonal contraception continuously should be counselled about expected bleeding patterns. Bleeding or spotting is normal in the first 3 months and then bleeding significantly decreases. The short-term safety of continuous or extended hormonal contraceptive regimens is similar to that of cyclic regimens and women should be counselled regarding this (SOGC, 2007).

Emergency Contraception (EC)

EC offers protection against pregnancy after intercourse occurs in instances such as broken condoms, sexual assault, dislodged cervical cap, disruption of use of any other method, or any other case of unprotected intercourse. There are two types of EC methods to choose from:

(1) Hormonal EC methods ("the morning after pill"):
  (i) A special formulation containing progestin only (Plan B, NorLevo, Option 2, Next Choice®)
  (ii) A series of four contraceptive pills called the Yuzpe method (combined estrogen and progestin)
(2) A copper intrauterine device (copper IUD) insertion within 120 hours of intercourse

In Canada, hormonal EC methods (morning-after pill) are available without a prescription. EC should be taken by a woman as soon as possible but within 5 days of unprotected intercourse or birth control mishap (e.g., broken condom, dislodged ring or cervical cap, missed oral contraceptive pills, late for injection) to prevent unintended pregnancy (SexualityandU, 2012c). If taken before ovulation, EC prevents ovulation by inhibiting follicular development. If taken after ovulation occurs, there is little effect on ovarian hormone production or the endometrium. To minimize the adverse effect of nausea that occurs with high doses of estrogen and progestin (Yuzpe regimen), the woman can be advised to take an over-the-counter antiemetic 1 hour before each dose. Nausea is not as common with the progestin-only regimen. If the woman vomits within 1 hour after taking the medication she will need to repeat the dose. Women with contraindications for estrogen use should use progestin-only EC. No medical contraindications for EC exist, except pregnancy and undiagnosed abnormal vaginal bleeding (Trussell & Schwarz, 2011). If the woman does not begin menstruation within 21 days after taking the pills, she should be evaluated for pregnancy (Trussell & Schwarz, 2011). EC is ineffective if the woman is pregnant as the pills do not disturb an implanted pregnancy. Risk of pregnancy is reduced by as much as 75% and 89% if the woman takes EC pills (Trussell & Schwarz, 2011). IUDs containing copper (see later discussion and Fig. 8-13, A) provide another EC option. The IUD should be inserted within 5 days of unprotected intercourse (SexualityandU, 2012c). This method is suggested only for women who wish to have the benefit of long-term contraception. The risk of pregnancy is reduced by as much as 99% with emergency insertion of the copper-releasing IUD. An IUD must be inserted by a health care provider and is only available by prescription, which makes it less

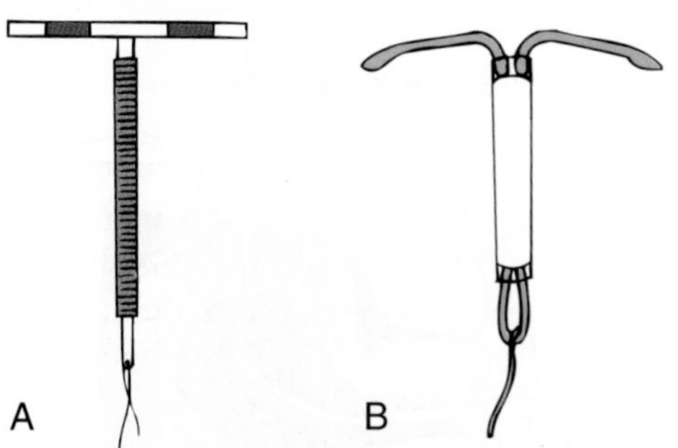

FIGURE 8-13 Intrauterine devices (IUDs) and systems (IUSs). **A:** Copper T IUD. **B:** Levonorgestrel-releasing IUS.

BOX 8-11 SIGNS OF POTENTIAL COMPLICATIONS: INTRAUTERINE DEVICES OR INTRAUTERINE SYSTEMS

Signs of potential complications related to intrauterine devices can be remembered using the PAINS mnemonic:

P—Period late, abnormal spotting or bleeding
A—Abdominal pain, pain with intercourse
I—Infection exposure, abnormal vaginal discharge
N—Not feeling well, fever, or chills
S—String missing; shorter or longer

accessible than hormonal EC methods. Research has shown that insertion of a copper IUD may be more effective than any emergency contraceptive pill. The progestin-only pill may be less effective in women with a body mass index of 25 to 29 and ineffective in women with a BMI of >30 (Health Canada, 2014). The SOGC (2014) states that until further evidence is available, women with a BMI over 30 who do not have access to or do not want a copper IUD for EC should not be discouraged from using the "morning-after pill" as it may still provide some benefit (SOGC, 2014).

Contraceptive counselling should be provided to all women requesting EC, including a discussion of modification of risky sexual behaviours to prevent STIs and unwanted pregnancy.

Intrauterine Devices (IUD)

An IUD is a small T-shaped device with bendable arms for insertion through the cervix into the uterine cavity. Two strings hang from the base of the stem through the cervix and protrude into the vagina for the woman to feel, for assurance that the device has not been dislodged (see Fig. 8-13, A). The copper IUD is made of radiopaque polyethylene and fine solid copper and provides up to 5 years of protection. The copper serves primarily as a spermicide and inflames the endometrium, preventing fertilization. Sometimes women experience an increase in bleeding and cramping within the first year after insertion, but nonsteroidal anti-inflammatory drugs (NSAIDs) can provide pain relief. The typical failure rate in the first year of use of the copper IUD is 0.8% (SexualityandU, 2012d).

The levonorgestrel intrauterine system (IUS) (Mirena) (see Fig. 8-13, B) releases levonorgestrel from its vertical reservoir. Effective for up to 5 years, it impairs sperm motility, irritates the lining of the uterus, and has some anovulatory effects. Uterine cramping and uterine bleeding are usually decreased with this device, although irregular spotting is common in the first few months following insertion. The risk of uterine perforation is a rare complication of the use of Mirena. This risk is increased in women after pregnancy, during lactation, and with abnormal uterine anatomy (Health Canada, 2010). The typical failure rate in the first year of use is 0.2% (SexualityandU, 2012d).

IUDs offers constant contraception without the need to remember to take pills each day or engage in other manipulation before or between coital acts. If pregnancy can be excluded, either device (copper IUD or levonorgestrel IUS) can be placed at any time during the menstrual cycle. These devices may be inserted shortly after childbirth or first-trimester abortion. The contraceptive effects are reversible. When pregnancy is desired, the health care provider removes the device. The SOGC now states that an IUD is a safe, effective option for contraception in an HIV-positive woman and can be considered a first-line contraceptive agent in adolescents (Caddy, Yudin, Hakim, et al., 2014).

Disadvantages of IUD use include increased risk of pelvic inflammatory disease within the first 20 days after insertion, especially if infection is present at the time of insertion. There is also a slight risk of uterine perforation. The Copper T380A is more likely to be associated with regular menses that may have heavier flow. Women who have the levonorgestrel IUS are more likely to experience scant, irregular episodes of vaginal bleeding or amenorrhea. The IUD offers no protection against STIs or HIV.

The woman should be taught to check for the presence of the IUD/IUS thread after menstruation to rule out expulsion of the device. If pregnancy occurs with the IUD/IUS in place, the system should be removed immediately in the first trimester if the strings are visible. Later in pregnancy, ultrasound examination should be used to localize the IUD/IUS and to rule out placenta previa. Retention of the IUD/IUS during pregnancy increases the risk of septic miscarriage and ectopic pregnancy. Some women allergic to copper develop a rash, necessitating removal of the copper-bearing IUD. Signs of potential complications are listed in Box 8-11.

Sterilization

Sterilization refers to surgical procedures intended to render the person infertile. Most procedures involve the occlusion of the passageways for the ova and sperm (Fig. 8-14, A). For the woman, the oviducts (uterine tubes) are occluded; for the man, the sperm ducts (vas deferens) are occluded (Fig. 8-14, B). Only surgical removal of the ovaries (oophorectomy) or uterus (hysterectomy) or both result in absolute sterility for the woman. All other sterilization procedures have a small but definite failure rate (i.e., pregnancy may result).

Female sterilization. Female sterilization (bilateral tubal ligation) may be done immediately after giving birth (within 24 to 48 hours), concomitantly with abortion, or as an interval

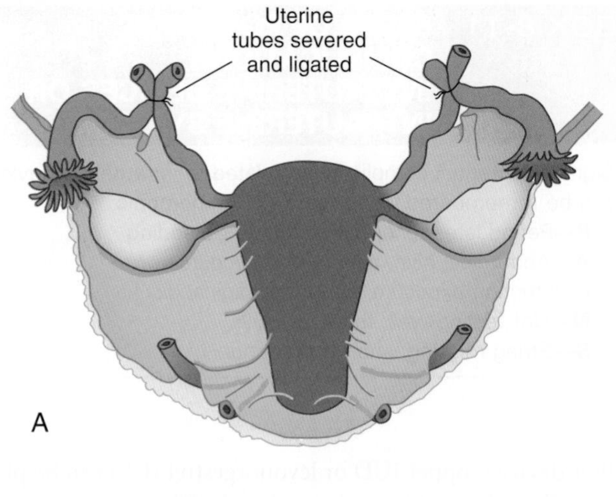

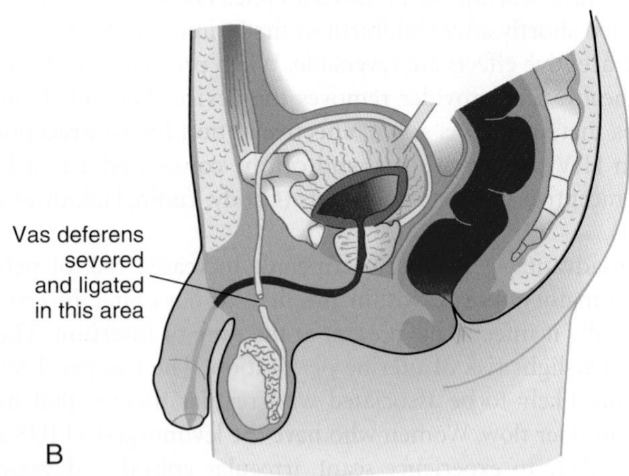

FIGURE 8-14 Sterilization. **A:** Uterine tubes ligated and severed (tubal ligation). **B:** Sperm duct ligated and severed (vasectomy).

procedure (during any phase of the menstrual cycle). Sterilization procedures can be done safely on an outpatient basis. Failure rate for methods of female sterilization vary by the method and the woman's age, but the average is 0.2 to 0.6% (SexualityandU, 2012e).

Tubal occlusion. A laparoscopic approach or a minilaparotomy may be used for tubal ligation (Fig. 8-15), tubal electrocoagulation, or the application of bands or clips. Electrocoagulation and ligation are considered to be permanent methods. Use of bands or clips has the theoretical advantage of possible removal and return of tubal patency (see Patient Teaching box).

Tubal reconstruction. Restoration of tubal continuity (reanastomosis) and function is technically feasible except after laparoscopic tubal electrocoagulation. Sterilization reversal is costly, difficult (requiring microsurgery), and uncertain. The success rate varies with the extent of tubal destruction and removal. The risk of ectopic pregnancy after tubal reanastomosis is increased by 2 to 12.5%.

Male sterilization. *Vasectomy* is the sealing, tying, or cutting of a man's vas deferens so that the sperm cannot travel from the testes to the penis. Vasectomy is the easiest and most commonly used operation for male sterilization. It can be done with local

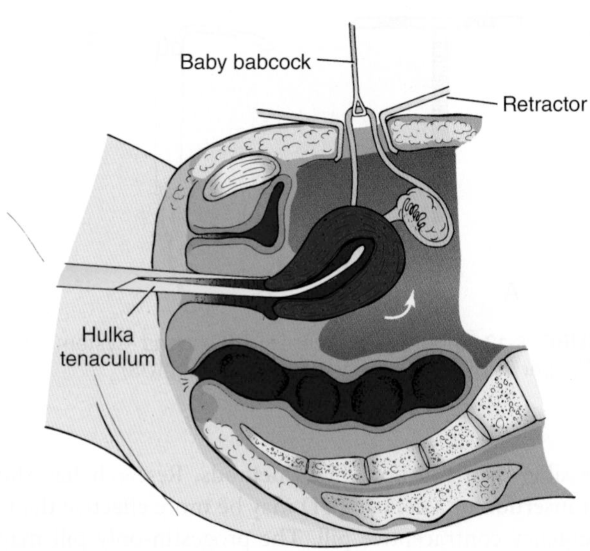

FIGURE 8-15 Use of minilaparotomy to gain access to uterine tubes for occlusion procedures. Tenaculum is used to lift uterus upward (*arrow*) toward incision.

PATIENT TEACHING

What to Expect After Tubal Ligation

- You should expect no change in hormones and their influence.
- Your menstrual period will be about the same as before the sterilization.
- You may feel pain at ovulation.
- The ovum disintegrates within the abdominal cavity.
- It is highly unlikely that you will become pregnant.
- You should not have a change in sexual functioning; you may enjoy sexual relations more because you will not be concerned about becoming pregnant.
- Sterilization offers no protection against sexually transmitted infections. Therefore, you may need to use condoms.

anaesthesia on an outpatient basis. Pain, bleeding, infection, and other postsurgical complications are considered the disadvantages to the surgical procedure.

Two methods are used for scrotal entry: conventional and no-scalpel vasectomy. The surgeon identifies and immobilizes the vas deferens through the scrotum. Then the vas is ligated or cauterized (see Fig. 8-14, B). Surgeons vary in their techniques to occlude the vas deferens: ligation with sutures, division, cautery, application of clips, excision of a segment of the vas, fascial interposition, or some combination of these methods.

Vasectomy has no effect on potency (ability to achieve and maintain erection) or volume of ejaculate. Endocrine production of testosterone continues so that secondary sex characteristics are not affected. Sperm production continues, but sperm are unable to leave the epididymis and are lysed by the immune system. Vasectomy does not change the man's transmission of the HIV virus if he is infected. He will need to be instructed to engage in a number of ejaculations until there are no viable sperm remaining above the area of the surgery. Until this occurs, as documented by semen analysis, the couple should use backup contraception.

Complications after bilateral vasectomy are uncommon and usually not serious. They include bleeding (usually external), suture reaction, and reaction to the anaesthetic agent. Men occasionally may develop a hematoma, infection, or epididymitis. Less common are painful granulomas from accumulation of sperm.

Tubal reconstruction. Microsurgery to reanastomose (restore tubal continuity) the sperm ducts can be accomplished successfully (i.e., sperm in the ejaculate) in more than 90% of cases; however, the fertility rate is only about 50%. The rate of success decreases as the time since the procedure increases. The vasectomy may result in permanent changes in the testes that leave men unable to father children. The changes are those ordinarily seen only in older men (e.g., interstitial fibrosis [scar tissue between the seminiferous tubules]). Some men develop antibodies against their own sperm (autoimmunization).

Laws and regulations. All provinces have strict regulations for informed consent. Health care providers must ensure that while obtaining informed consent there is an explanation of benefits and risks and options and determination of whether the person is competent to understand the information. Explanation must be made in the person's own language, or an interpreter must be provided to ensure that the person understands all information. Although the partner's consent is not required by law, the woman is encouraged to discuss the situation with her partner. Sterilization of minors or mentally incompetent individuals is illegal.

Nursing considerations. The nurse plays an important role in helping people with decision making so that all requirements for informed consent are met. The nurse also provides information about alternatives to sterilization such as contraception.

Information must be given about what is entailed in the various procedures, how much discomfort or pain can be expected, and what type of care is needed. Many individuals fear sterilization procedures because of the imagined effect on their sexual life. They need reassurance concerning the hormonal and psychological basis of sexual functioning. The fact that uterine tube occlusion or vasectomy has no biological sequelae in terms of sexual adequacy needs to be communicated and reinforced.

Preoperative care includes health assessment, which includes a psychological assessment, physical examination, and laboratory tests. The nurse needs to confirm the woman's understanding of printed instructions. Ambivalence and extreme fear of the procedure should be reported to the physician.

Postoperative care depends on the procedure performed (e.g., laparoscopy, laparotomy for tubal occlusion, or vasectomy). General care includes recovery after anaesthesia, vital signs, fluid–electrolyte balance (intake and output, laboratory values), prevention or early identification and treatment of infection or hemorrhage, control of discomfort, and assessment of emotional response to the procedure and recovery.

Discharge planning depends on the type of procedure performed. In general, the patient is given written instructions about observing for and reporting symptoms and signs of complications, the type of recovery to be expected, and the date and time for a follow-up appointment.

LGBTQ Issues Regarding Contraception

For transsexual men and women, it is important to discuss fertility and contraception with them prior to the use of any hormone therapy. For trans men, pregnancy is a contraindication to testosterone use and the patient must take precautions against becoming pregnant while taking it. Patients who are sexually active with people with sperm should be counselled on contraceptive options including progesterone-only oral contraception or an IUD. While many trans men have become pregnant intentionally after discontinuing testosterone to pursue pregnancy, patients may wish to consider postponing testosterone initiation if they would like to become pregnant in the future, since fertility may be permanently affected (LGBT Health Program, 2015). Transgender women should also be cautioned regarding the need for birth control if sexually active with partners who may become pregnant, since hormonal impact on fertility in trans women is also variable (LGBT Health Program, 2015).

For further information on current fertility options for trans people, see Rainbow Health Ontario's Fact Sheet "Reproductive Options for Trans People" (see Additional Resources at the end of the chapter).

ABORTION

Induced abortion is the purposeful interruption of a pregnancy before 20 weeks of gestation. (Spontaneous abortion or miscarriage is discussed in Chapter 14.) If the abortion is performed at the woman's request, the term **elective abortion** is usually used; if performed for reasons of maternal or fetal health or disease, the term **therapeutic abortion** applies. Many factors contribute to a woman's decision to have an abortion. Indications include (1) preservation of the life or health of the mother, (2) genetic disorders of the fetus, (3) rape or incest, and (4) the pregnant woman's request. The control of birth, given that it concerns human sexuality and the question of life and death, is one of the most emotional components of health care.

Abortion in Canada is safe and legal although accessibility varies between provinces. The laws for abortion in Canada have changed over the last 35 years, from being very restricted before 1969 to unrestricted in 1988. Today, Canada is one of the only countries in the world without abortion regulation. Abortion is available throughout pregnancy, although more than 90% are performed in the first trimester and only 2 to 3% are performed after 16 weeks. Hospitals maintained by Roman Catholics and some of those maintained by strict fundamentalists forbid abortion (and often sterilization) despite legal challenges.

In 2012 in Canada there were 83,700 reported induced abortions, although this number is not complete as the number of abortions done in British Columbia clinics is not captured (Canadian Institute for Health Information [CIHI], 2013). Women in Prince Edward Island must travel to another province to obtain an abortion.

Rates of biological complications after abortions, such as ectopic pregnancy, infection, or hemorrhage, tend to be low if the woman aborts during the first trimester. Psychological sequelae of induced abortion are not common but may be related to circumstances and support systems surrounding the pregnant woman, such as the attitudes reflected by friends, family, and health care workers. The woman facing an abortion is pregnant and will exhibit the emotional responses shared by all pregnant women, including the possibility of depression.

Nurses and other health care providers often struggle with the same values and moral convictions as those of the pregnant woman. The conflicts and doubts of the nurse can be readily communicated to women who are already anxious. Regardless of personal views on abortion, nurses who provide care to women seeking abortion have an ethical responsibility to counsel women about their options and to make appropriate referrals.

LEGAL TIP ***NURSES' RIGHTS AND RESPONSIBILITIES RELATED TO ABORTION***

If nurses are requested to provide care that is against their religious or moral beliefs, they must continue to provide safe, compassionate, competent, ethical care until alternative arrangements can be made. If a nurse anticipates a conflict of conscience, the nurse has an obligation to notify his or her employer so that alternative arrangements can be made. Declaring a conflict with conscience or "conscientious objection" is a serious matter that must be addressed. Nurses' rights and responsibilities related to caring for abortion patients should be protected through policies that describe how the institution will accommodate the nurse's ethical or moral beliefs and what the nurse should do to avoid patient abandonment in such situations. Nurses should know what policies are in place in their institutions and encourage such policies to be *written.*

Source: Canadian Nurses Association. (2008). *Code of ethics for registered nurses.* Ottawa: Author. Retrieved from http://www.cna-aiic.ca/CNA/documents/pdf/publications/Code_of_Ethics_2008_e.pdf

CRITICAL THINKING CASE STUDY

Termination of Pregnancy

Angelica is a 19-year-old single woman whose contraceptive failed. She is 6 weeks pregnant and is seeking termination of the pregnancy. She has many questions for the nurse in the family planning clinic: Which procedure is most likely to be chosen at this gestation? What are the risks associated with the procedure? Should her boyfriend be involved in the decision to terminate the pregnancy?

QUESTIONS

1. Evidence—Is there sufficient evidence to draw conclusions about what information the nurse should provide Angelica?
2. Assumptions—What assumptions can be made about Angelica's reaction to termination of the pregnancy?
   a. Psychological/emotional reaction and sequelae
   b. Physical response
   c. Future child-bearing
   d. Relationship with her boyfriend
3. What implications and priorities for nursing care can be drawn at this time?
4. Does the evidence objectively support your conclusion?

NURSING CARE

A thorough assessment is conducted through history, physical examination, and laboratory tests. The length of pregnancy and the condition of the woman must be determined to select the appropriate type of abortion procedure. An ultrasound examination should be performed before a second-trimester abortion is done. If the woman is Rh-negative, she is a candidate for prophylaxis against Rh isoimmunization. She should receive $Rh_o(D)$ immune globulin within 72 hours after the abortion if she is D-negative and if Coombs' test results are negative (if the woman is unsensitized or isoimmunization has not developed).

The woman's understanding of alternatives, the types of abortions, and expected recovery needs to be assessed. Misinformation and gaps in knowledge should be identified and corrected. The record is reviewed for the signed informed consent, and the woman's understanding is verified. General preoperative, operative, and postoperative assessments are performed.

Counselling about abortion includes helping the woman identify how she perceives the pregnancy, providing information about the choices available (i.e., having an abortion or carrying the pregnancy to term and then either keeping the infant or placing the baby for adoption), and informing about the types of abortion procedures (see Critical Thinking Case Study).

First-Trimester Abortion

Methods for performing early elective abortion (less than 10 weeks of gestation) include surgical (aspiration) and medical methods (mifepristone with prostaglandin and methotrexate with misoprostol). The majority of abortions that occur in Canada are performed during the first trimester (CIHI, 2013).

Surgical (Aspiration) Abortion

Aspiration (vacuum or suction curettage) is the most common procedure done in the first trimester. Aspiration abortion is usually performed under local anaesthesia in a physician's office, a clinic, or a hospital. The ideal time for performing this procedure is 8 to 12 weeks after the last menstrual period. The suction procedure for performing an early elective abortion usually requires less than 5 minutes.

A bimanual examination is done before the procedure to assess uterine size and position. A speculum is inserted, and the cervix is anaesthetized with a local anaesthetic agent. The cervix is dilated, if necessary, and a cannula connected to suction is inserted into the uterine cavity. The products of conception are evacuated from the uterus.

During the procedure, the woman is kept informed about what to expect next (e.g., menstrual-like cramping and sounds of the suction machine). The nurse needs to assess the woman's vital signs. The aspirated uterine contents must be carefully inspected to ascertain whether all fetal parts and adequate placental tissue have been evacuated. After the abortion, the woman can rest on the table until she is ready to stand. She remains in

BOX 8-12 COMPLICATIONS FROM INDUCED ABORTION

The woman should call her health care provider if she has any of the following signs:

- Fever greater than 38°C
- Chills
- Bleeding greater than two saturated pads in 2 hours or heavy bleeding lasting a few days
- Foul-smelling vaginal discharge
- Severe abdominal pain, cramping, or backache
- Abdominal tenderness (when pressure applied)

Source: Paul, M., & Stein, T. (2011). Abortion. In R. A. Hatcher, J. Trussell, & A. L. Nelson (Eds.), *Contraceptive technology* (20th ed.). Atlanta, GA: Ardent Media.

the recovery area or waiting room for 1 to 3 hours for detection of excessive cramping or bleeding, then she is discharged.

Bleeding after the operation is normally about the equivalent of a heavy menstrual period, and cramps are rarely severe. Excessive vaginal bleeding and infection such as endometritis or salpingitis are the most common complications of induced abortion. Retained products of conception are the primary cause of vaginal bleeding (Paul & Stein, 2011). Evacuation of the uterus, uterine massage, and administration of oxytocin or methylergonovine may be necessary. Prophylactic antibiotics to decrease the risk of infection are recommended. Postabortion pain can be relieved with NSAIDs such as ibuprofen.

Nursing interventions. Instructions following a surgical abortion differ among health care providers (e.g., tampons should not be used for at least 3 days or should be avoided for up to 3 weeks, and resumption of sexual intercourse may be permitted within 1 week or discouraged for 2 weeks). The woman may shower daily. She should be instructed to watch for excessive bleeding and other signs of complications (Box 8-12) and to avoid douches of any type. The woman may expect her menstrual period to resume 4 to 6 weeks after the day of the procedure. The nurse should offer information about the birth control method the woman prefers, if this has not been done during the counselling interview that usually precedes the decision to have an abortion. The woman must be strongly encouraged to return for her follow-up visit so that complications can be detected and a contraceptive method prescribed. A pregnancy test may also be performed to determine if the pregnancy has been terminated successfully.

Medical Abortion

Medical abortions are available in Canada for up to 9 weeks after the last menstrual period and should be considered in women who will be diligent with follow-up. Methotrexate, misoprostol, and mifepristone are the drugs used in the current regimens to induce early abortion.

Methotrexate is a cytotoxic drug that causes early abortion by blocking folic acid in fetal cells so they cannot divide. Misoprostol (Cytotec) is a prostaglandin analog that acts directly on the cervix to soften and dilate it and on the uterine muscle to stimulate contractions. Mifepristone, also known as RU-486, was approved by Health Canada in 2015. It works by binding to progesterone receptors and blocking the action of progesterone, which is necessary for maintaining pregnancy (Paul & Stein, 2011).

Methotrexate and misoprostol. Methotrexate can be given intramuscularly or orally (usually mixed with orange juice). Vaginal placement of misoprostol follows in 3 to 7 days. Women commonly have nausea, vomiting, and cramping after the misoprostol insertion. The woman returns for a follow-up visit to confirm that the abortion is complete. If abortion does not occur, misoprostol is repeated, or vacuum aspiration is performed. Misoprostol can also be used alone. Misoprostol 800 mcg is placed high in the vagina every 24 to 48 hours for up to three applications. Blood work at 7 days confirms whether this regimen was successful.

Mifepristone and misoprostol. Mifepristone can be taken up to 7 weeks after the last menstrual period. The Health Canada–approved regimen is that the woman takes 600 mg of mifepristone orally; 48 hours later she returns to the office and takes 400 mcg of misoprostol orally (unless abortion has already occurred and been confirmed). Two weeks after the administration of mifepristone, the woman must return to the office for a clinical examination or ultrasound to confirm that the pregnancy has been terminated. In 1 to 5% of cases the drugs do not work, and surgical abortion (aspiration) is needed (Paul & Stein, 2011).

With any medical abortion regimen, the woman usually will experience bleeding and cramping. Adverse effects of the medications include nausea, vomiting, diarrhea, headache, dizziness, fever, and chills. These are attributed to misoprostol and usually subside in a few hours after administration (Paul & Stein, 2011).

Second-Trimester Abortion

Second-trimester abortion is associated with more complications than are first-trimester abortions. Medical induction and dilation and evacuation (D&E) are both safe and effective methods for terminations in the second trimester. However, D&E is considered superior between 14 and 18 weeks' gestation (Davis, 2006). Induction of uterine contractions can also be used.

Dilation and evacuation. D&E can be performed at any point up to 20 weeks of gestation, although it is more often performed between 13 and 16 weeks (Paul & Stein, 2011). The cervix requires more dilation because the products of conception are larger. Often laminaria are inserted into the cervix several hours or several days before the procedure to assist in dilating the cervix, or misoprostol can be applied to the cervix to soften the tissue. The procedure is similar to that of vaginal aspiration, except that a larger cannula is used and other instruments may be needed to remove the fetus and placenta. Nursing care includes monitoring vital signs, providing emotional support, administering analgesics, and postoperative monitoring. Disadvantages of D&E include possible long-term harmful effects on the cervix.

Medical induction. Prior to medical induction, women may require cervical ripening with osmotic dilators, prostaglandins, or the insertion of a balloon catheter. Intra-amniotic injections of hypertonic solutions (e.g., saline) injected directly into the uterus and uterotonic agents (e.g., prostaglandin) are effective. Extra-amniotic prostaglandin can also be used. Labour may also be induced using carboprost intramuscularly, concentrated oxytocin infusion, or misoprostol (orally or vaginally). The particular method that is used should be based on the expertise of the health care provider and the wishes of the woman (Davis, 2006).

Emotional Considerations Regarding Abortion

The woman considering an abortion will need help in exploring the meaning of the various alternatives and consequences to herself and her significant others. It is often difficult for a woman to express her true feelings (e.g., what abortion means to her now and in the future and what support or regret her friends and peers may demonstrate). A calm, matter-of-fact approach from the nurse can be helpful. Clarifying, restating, and reflecting statements; open-ended questions; and feedback are communication techniques that can be used to maintain a realistic focus on the situation and bring the woman's concerns into the open. If family or friends cannot be involved, scheduling time for nursing personnel to give the necessary support is an essential component of the care plan.

Information about alternatives to abortion such as referral to adoption agencies or to support services if the woman chooses to keep her baby should be provided. If a decision is made to have an abortion, the woman must be assured of continued support. Information about what is entailed in various procedures, how much discomfort or pain can be expected, and what type of care is needed must be given. The various feelings, including depression, guilt, regret, and relief, that the woman might experience after the abortion should be discussed. Information about community resources for postabortion counselling may be needed.

After the abortion, many women report relief, but some have temporary distress or mixed emotions. Evidence of long-term depression after elective abortion has been inconclusive. Guilt and anxiety may occur more with young women, women with poor social support, multiparous women, and women with a history of psychiatric illness. Women having second-trimester abortions may have more emotional distress than women having abortions in the first trimester. Because symptoms can vary among women who have had abortions, nurses must assess women for grief reactions and facilitate the grieving process through active listening and nonjudgemental support and care.

KEY POINTS

- Infertility is the inability to conceive and carry a fetus to term gestation at a time the couple has chosen to do so.
- Infertility affects about 12 to 16% of otherwise healthy adults. It increases in women older than 35 years.
- In Canada about 40% of infertility is related to female causes, 30% to male causes, and 20% to both partners; 10% of the causes are unexplained.
- Common etiological factors of infertility include decreased sperm production, ovulation disorders, polycystic ovary syndrome, tubal occlusion, and endometriosis.
- Reproductive alternatives for family building include IVF-ET, GIFT, ZIFT, oocyte donation, embryo donation, TDI, surrogate motherhood, and adoption.
- Infertility treatment can involve emotional and monetary costs for those involved.
- A variety of contraceptive methods with various effectiveness rates, advantages, and disadvantages are available.
- Women and their partners should choose the contraceptive method(s) best suited to them.
- Effective contraceptives are available through both prescription and nonprescription sources.
- Proper concurrent use of latex condoms provides protection against STIs.
- Tubal ligations and vasectomies are permanent sterilization methods.
- Emergency contraception pills should be taken as soon as possible after unprotected intercourse but no later than 120 hours.
- Induced abortion performed in the first trimester is safer and less complex than an abortion performed in the second trimester.
- The most common complications of induced abortion include infection, retained products of conception, and excessive vaginal bleeding.

evolve WEBSITE

Visit the Evolve website for additional resources related to the content in this chapter such as Case Studies, Critical Thinking Case Study Answers, Nursing Care Plans, Nursing Processes, Nursing Skills, and Review Questions for Exam Preparation at: http://evolve.elsevier.com/Canada/Perry/maternal/

REFERENCES

Boivin, J., Griffiths, E., & Venetis, C. A. (2011). Emotional distress in infertile women and failure of assisted reproductive technologies: Meta-analysis of prospective psychosocial studies. *British Medical Journal*, 342, d223. doi:10.1136/bmj.d223.

Bushnik, T., Cook, J. L., Yuzpe, A., et al. (2012). Estimating the prevalence of infertility in Canada. *Human Reproduction*, 27(3), 738–746. doi:10.1093/humrep/der465.

Caddy, S., Yudin, M., Hakim, J., et al. (2014). SOGC clinical practice guideline: Best practices to minimize infection with intrauterine device insertion. *Journal of Obstetricians and Gynaecologists of Canada*, 36(3), 266–274.

Canadian Fertility and Andrology Society. (2013). *Human assisted reproduction 2013 live birth rates for Canada*. Montreal: Author. Retrieved from <http://www.cfas.ca/index.php?option=com_content&view=article&

id=1205%3Alive-birth-rates-2013&catid=929%3Apress-releases&Itemid=460>.

Canadian Institute for Health Information. (2013). *Induced abortions reported in Canada in 2012*. Retrieved from <https://www.cihi.ca/en/ta_11_alldatatables20140221_en.pdf>.

Cunningham, F. G., Leveno, K. J., Bloom, S. L., et al. (2014). *Williams obstetrics* (24th ed.). New York: McGraw-Hill.

CycleBeads. (2016). *The original family planning tool*. Retrieved from <http://www.cyclebeads.com/cyclebeads>.

Davis, V. (2006). SOGC clinical practice guideline: Induced abortion guidelines. *Journal of Obstetrics and Gynaecology Canada*, 28(11), 1014–1027.

D'Avanzo, C. E. (2008). *Pocket guide to cultural health assessment* (4th ed.). St. Louis: Mosby.

Government of Canada. (2004). *Assisted Human Reproduction Act*. Ottawa: Minister of Justice. Retrieved from <http://laws-lois.justice.gc.ca/eng/acts/A-13.4/>.

Government of Canada. (2013). *Fertility*. Ottawa: Author. Retrieved from <http://healthycanadians.gc.ca/healthy-living-vie-saine/pregnancy-grossesse/fert-eng.php>.

Government of Canada. (2014). *Safer condom use*. Ottawa: Author. Retrieved from <http://www.healthycanadians.gc.ca/healthy-living-vie-saine/sexual-sexuelle/condoms-eng.php>.

Health Canada. (2010). *Public communication. Health Canada endorsed important safety information on Mirena*. Retrieved from <http://www.hc-sc.gc.ca/dhp-mps/medeff/bulletin/carn-bcei_v20n4-eng.php>.

Health Canada. (2014). *Emergency contraceptive pills to carry warnings for reduced effectiveness in women over a certain body weight*. Ottawa: Author. Retrieved from <http://healthycanadians.gc.ca/recall-alert-rappel-avis/hc-sc/2014/38701a-eng.php>.

Kennedy, K., & Trussell, J. (2011). Contraceptive efficacy. In R. Hatcher (Ed.), *Contraceptive technology* (20th ed.). New York: Ardent Media.

Kirkham, Y., Ornstein, M., Aggarwal, A., et al. (2014). SOGC clinical practice guideline: Menstrual suppression in special circumstances. *Journal of Obstetricians and Gynaecologists of Canada*, 36(10), 915–924.

LGBT Health Program. (2015). *Guidelines and protocols for hormone therapy and primary health care for trans clients*. Toronto: Sherbourne Health Centre. Retrieved from <http://sherbourne.on.ca/wp-content/uploads/2014/02/Guidelines-and-Protocols-for-Comprehensive-Primary-Care-for-Trans-Clients-2015.pdf>.

LGBTQ Parenting Network. (2012). *A guidebook for lesbian, gay, bisexual, trans and queer people on assisted human reproduction in Canada*. Retrieved from <http://lgbtqpn.ca/wp-content/uploads/woocommerce_uploads/2014/08/AHRC_BOOKLET_ENGLISH.pdf>.

Okun, N., Sierra, S., Wilson, D. G., et al. (2014). SOGC clinical practice guideline: Pregnancy outcomes after assisted human reproduction. *Journal of Obstetrics & Gynaecology Canada*, 36(1), 64–83.

Paul, M., & Stein, T. (2011). Abortion. In R. A. Hatcher (Ed.), *Contraceptive technology* (20th ed.). Atlanta, GA: Ardent Media.

Reid, R., & Clinical Practice Gynaecology Committee. (2010). SOGC clinical practice guideline: Oral contraceptives and the risk of venous thromboembolism: An update. *Journal of Obstetrics and Gynaecology Canada*, 32(12), 1192–1197.

RESOLVE. (2015). *Managing infertility stress*. Retrieved from <http://www.resolve.org/support/Managing-Infertility-Stress/>.

SexualityandU. (2012a). *Natural methods*. Retrieved from <http://sexualityandu.ca/birth-control/birth_control_methods_contraception/natural_methods>.

SexualityandU. (2012b). *Non-hormonal methods*. Retrieved from <http://sexualityandu.ca/birth-control/birth_control_methods_contraception/non-hormonal-methods>.

SexualityandU. (2012c). *Emergency contraception (morning after pill)*. Retrieved from <http://sexualityandu.ca/birth-control/emergency-contraception-morning-after-pill>.

SexualityandU. (2012d). *Birth control: Hormonal methods*. Retrieved from <http://sexualityandu.ca/birth-control/birth_control_methods_contraception/hormonal-methods>.

SexualityandU. (2012e). *Permanent sterilization*. Retrieved from <http://www.sexualityandu.ca/health-care-professionals/contraceptive-methods/permanent-sterilization>.

Society of Obstetricians and Gynaecologists of Canada. (2007). Canadian consensus guideline on continuous and extended hormonal contraception 2007. *Journal of Obstetrics and Gynaecology Canada*, 27(7), S1–S32, Supplement 2.

Society of Obstetricians and Gynaecologists of Canada. (2014). *Position statement: Emergency contraception*. Retrieved from <http://sogc.org/wp-content/uploads/2013/01/gui280CPG1209ErevB.pdf>.

Trussell, J., & Schwarz, E. (2011). Emergency contraception. In R. A. Hatcher (Ed.), *Contraceptive technology* (20th ed.). Atlanta, GA: Ardent Media.

ADDITIONAL RESOURCES

Action Canada for Sexual Health & Rights: <http://www.sexualhealthandrights.ca/>.

Infertility Awareness Association of Canada: <http://www.iaac.ca>.

Infertility Network: <http://www.infertilitynetwork.org>.

Meeting the Assisted Human Reproduction (AHR) Needs of Lesbian, Gay, Bisexual, Trans and Queer (LGBTQ) People in Canada: <http://www.rainbowhealthontario.ca/wp-content/uploads/woocommerce_uploads/2014/08/AHRC_FACTSHEET_ENGLISH1.pdf>.

National Infertility Association: <http://www.resolve.org>.

Rainbow Health Ontario Fact Sheet—Reproductive Options for Trans People: <http://www.rainbowhealthontario.ca/resources/rho-fact-sheet-reproductive-options-for-trans-people/>.

SexualityandU: <http://www.sexualityandu.ca>.

SexualityandU—Choosing a Contraceptive That's Right for You: <http://sexualityandu.ca/uploads/files/refContraceptiveComparativeChartFinalENG09.pdf>.

UNIT 4

Pregnancy

CHAPTER 9

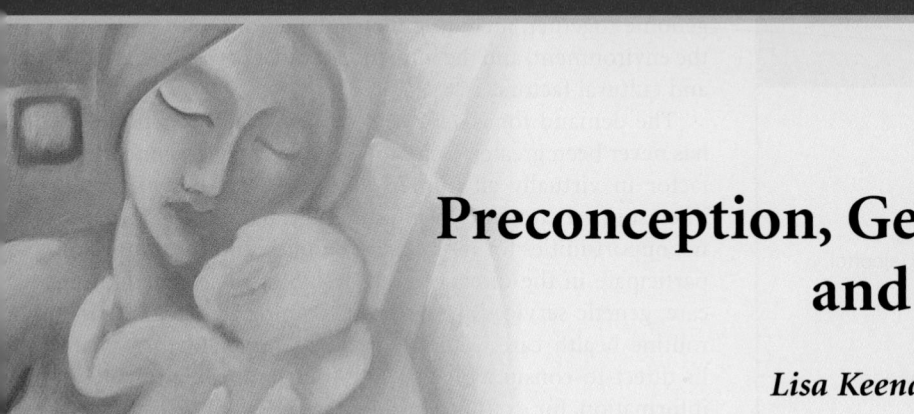

Preconception, Genetics, Conception, and Fetal Development

Lisa Keenan-Lindsay, with contributions from Shannon E. Perry

evolve WEBSITE

***Visit the Evolve website for additional resources related to the content in this chapter such as Case Studies, Critical Thinking Case Study Answers, Nursing Care Plans, Nursing Processes, Nursing Skills, and Review Questions for Exam Preparation at:** http://evolve.elsevier.com/Canada/Perry/maternal/*

OBJECTIVES

On completion of this chapter the reader will be able to:

- Discuss the importance of preconception counselling.
- Explain the key concepts of basic human genetics.
- Describe roles for nurses in genetics and genetic counselling.
- Examine ethical dimensions of genetic screening.
- Identify genetic disorders commonly tested for using prenatal testing.
- Identify the potential effects of teratogens during vulnerable periods of embryonic and fetal development.
- Summarize the process of fertilization.
- Describe the development, structure, and functions of the placenta.
- Describe the composition and functions of the amniotic fluid.
- Identify three organs or tissues arising from each of the three primary germ layers.
- Summarize the significant changes in growth and development of the embryo and fetus.

This chapter discusses the importance of preconception care and presents a brief discussion of genetics and the role of the nurse in genetics. It also provides an overview of the processes of fertilization and development of the normal embryo and fetus.

PRECONCEPTION

If women receive appropriate care prior to pregnancy, there will be improved health outcomes for both mothers and newborns. Preconception care involves identifying and modifying risk factors in women in order to improve their health. Risk factors may include medical, behavioural, and social factors, many of which may be modifiable.

The Society of Obstetricians and Gynaecologists of Canada (Wilson, Audibert, Brock, et al., 2011) suggests that during a visit to a health care provider, all women be asked the question "Are you considering pregnancy or could you possibly become pregnant?" If women state that they are considering pregnancy, then care can be focused to ensure optimum health. Women should have an evaluation of their overall health and opportunities for improving their health, and they should receive education about the effects of social, environmental, nutritional, occupational, behavioural, and genetic factors during pregnancy. Also, women at high risk for an adverse pregnancy outcome should be identified (Wilson et al., 2011). Such evaluation also involves identifying undiagnosed, untreated, or poorly controlled medical conditions. In order to make informed choices about child-bearing, all women should be counselled regarding the increased risk of infertility, pregnancy complications, and adverse pregnancy outcomes when child-bearing is delayed past the age of 35 (Johnson, Tough, et al., 2012). The goal of preconception health care is to optimize the health of every woman and fetus (Wilson et al., 2011). The components of preconception care, such as health promotion, risk assessment, and interventions, are outlined in Box 9-1.

BOX 9-1 COMPONENTS OF PRECONCEPTION CARE

Health Promotion: General Teaching

Nutrition
Healthy diet, including adequate folic acid intake
Optimum weight
Exercise and rest
Avoidance of use of certain substances (tobacco, alcohol, "recreational" drugs)
Use of risk-reducing sex practices
Attending to family and social needs
Risk of infertility with increased age (>35 years of age)

Risk Factor Assessment

Medical history
- Immune status (e.g., rubella, hepatitis B, varicella)
- Family history (e.g., genetic disorders)
- Illnesses (e.g., infections)
- Current use of medications (prescription, nonprescription)

Reproductive history
- Contraceptive
- Obstetrical

Psychosocial history
- Spouse or partner and family situation, including intimate partner violence
- Availability of family or other support systems
- Readiness for pregnancy (e.g., age, life goals, stress)

Financial resources
Environmental (home, workplace) conditions
- Safety hazards
- Toxic chemicals
- Radiation

Interventions

Anticipatory guidance and teaching
Treatment of medical conditions and results
- Medications
- Cessation of or reduction in substance use
- Immunizations (e.g., rubella, tuberculosis, hepatitis)

Nutrition, diet, and weight management
Exercise
Referral for genetic counselling
Referral to and use of
- Family planning services
- Family and social needs management

GENETICS

Genetic counselling is an important aspect of preconception and prenatal care. Recent advances in molecular biology and genomics have revolutionized the field of health care by providing the tools needed to determine the hereditary component of many diseases and improve our ability to predict susceptibility to disease, onset and progression of disease, and response to medications (Guttmacher, McGuire, Ponder, et al., 2010). With this increase in genetic knowledge, there has been a gradual shift from genetics to genomics. *Genetics* is the study of individual genes and their effect on relative rare single-gene disorders, whereas *genomics* is the study of all the genes in the human genome together, including their interactions with each other, the environment, and the influence of other psychosocial factors and cultural factors.

The demand for genetic services, especially genetic testing, has never been greater. Genetics is recognized as a contributing factor in virtually all human illnesses. With growing public interest in genetics, increasing commercial pressures, and Internet opportunities for individuals, families, and communities to participate in the direction and design of their genetic health care, genetic services are rapidly becoming an integral part of routine health care. Many individuals may have participated in direct-to-consumer genetic testing for health or ancestry information, for example at https://www.23andme.com/en-ca/. While this information is often for recreational purposes some of it can be diagnostic, and it is important that the results are conveyed in a therapeutic manner by competent health care professionals (Guttmacher et al., 2010; McGuire & Burke, 2010).

For most genetic conditions, therapeutic or preventive measures do not exist or are very limited. Consequently, the most useful means of reducing the incidence of these disorders is by preventing their transmission. It is standard practice to assess all pregnant women for heritable disorders to identify potential problems. The incidence of chromosome aberrations is estimated to be 0.5 to 0.6% in newborns. Approximately 62% of miscarriages and 5 to 7% of stillbirths and perinatal deaths are caused by chromosomal abnormalities (Groden, Gocha, & Croce, 2014).

Genetic disorders affect people of all ages, from all socioeconomic levels, and from all racial and ethnic backgrounds. They affect not only individuals but also families, communities, and society. Advances in genetic testing and genetically based treatments have altered the care provided to affected individuals. Improvements in diagnostic capability have resulted in earlier diagnosis and enabled individuals who previously would have died in childhood to survive into adulthood.

Some disorders appear more often in ethnic groups. Examples include Tay-Sachs disease in Ashkenazi Jews, French Canadians of the Eastern St. Lawrence River valley area of Québec, Cajuns from Louisiana, and the Amish in Pennsylvania; β-thalassemia in Mediterranean, Middle Eastern, Central Asian, Indian, and Far Eastern groups and in those of African heritage; sickle cell anemia in people who are Black; α-thalassemia in those from Southeast Asia, South China, the Philippine Islands, Thailand, Greece, and Cyprus; lactase deficiency in adult Chinese and Thailanders; neural tube defects in those from Ireland, Scotland, and Wales; phenylketonuria (PKU) in the Irish, Scots, Scandinavians, Icelanders, and Poles; cystic fibrosis (CF) in Whites, Ashkenazi Jews, and Latin Americans; and Niemann-Pick disease, type A, in Ashkenazi Jews (Groden et al., 2014; Wapner, 2014).

Relevance of Genetics to Nursing

Because the potential impact of genetic disease on families and the community is significant (Box 9-2), genetics must be integrated into nursing education and practice. Genetic information, technology, and testing must be incorporated into health care services.

BOX 9-2 POTENTIAL IMPACT OF GENETIC DISEASE ON FAMILY AND COMMUNITY

- Financial cost to family
- Decrease in planned family size
- Loss of geographical mobility
- Decreased opportunities for siblings
- Loss of family integrity
- Loss of career opportunities and job flexibility
- Social isolation
- Lifestyle alterations
- Reduction in contributions to their community by families
- Disruption of husband–wife or partner relationship
- Threatened family self-concept
- Coping with intolerant public attitudes
- Psychological effects
- Stresses and uncertainty of treatment
- Physical health problems
- Loss of dreams and aspirations
- Cost to society of institutionalization or home or community care
- Cost to society because of additional problems and needs of other family members
- Cost of long-term care
- Housing and living arrangement changes

From Kasper, C. E., Schneidereith, T. A., & Lashley, F. R. (2015). *Lashley's essentials of clinical genetics in nursing practice* (2nd ed.). New York: Springer.

Expanded or new roles for nurses with expertise in genetics and genomics are developing in many areas of maternity and women's health nursing. These areas include but are not limited to preconception counselling and preimplantation diagnosis for patients at risk for the transmission of a genetic disorder; prenatal screening and testing; prenatal care for women with psychiatric disorders that have a genetic component, such as bipolar disorder and schizophrenia; newborn screening and testing; the care of families who have lost a fetus or a child affected by a genetic condition; the identification and care of children with genetic conditions, and their families; and the care of women with genetic conditions who require specialized care during pregnancy, such as women with congenital heart disease, CF, Marfan syndrome, or factor V Leiden.

Although diagnosis and treatment of genetic disorders require specialized medical skills, nurses use their nursing skills as they assume important roles in counselling people about genetically transmitted or genetically influenced conditions (Box 9-3). Most diseases have a genetic component, and nurses are usually the ones who provide follow-up care and maintain contact with the patients. Community health nurses can identify groups within populations that are at high risk for illness and provide care to individuals, families, and groups. They are a vital link in follow-up for newborns who may need newborn screening.

Referral to appropriate agencies is an essential part of the follow-up management. Many organizations and foundations

BOX 9-3 NURSING SKILLS USED IN GENETIC COUNSELLING

- Taking detailed family histories
- Developing treatment plans
- Providing treatments
- Counselling patients
- Working with families
- Teaching risk reduction and health promotion
- Making referrals
- Providing follow-up
- Working in multidisciplinary teams

Source: Canadian Nurses Association. (2005). *Nursing and genetics: Are you ready?* Ottawa: Author. Retrieved from http://cna-aiic.ca/~/media/cna/page-content/pdf-en/nn_genetics_05_e.pdf

(e.g., Cystic Fibrosis Canada and Muscular Dystrophy Canada—see Additional Resources at end of the chapter) help provide services and equipment for affected children. There are also numerous parent groups in which the family can share experiences and derive mutual support from other families with similar problems.

Probably the most important of all nursing functions is providing emotional support to the family during all aspects of the counselling process. Feelings that arise under the real or imagined threat posed by a genetic disorder are as varied as the people being counselled. Responses may include a range of stress reactions such as apathy, denial, anger, hostility, fear, embarrassment, grief, and loss of self-esteem.

Gene Identification and Genetic Testing

Initial efforts to sequence and analyze the human genome have proven invaluable in the identification of genes involved in disease and in the development of genetic tests. Hundreds of genes involved in diseases such as Huntington's disease (HD), breast cancer, colon cancer, Alzheimer's disease, achondroplasia, and CF have been identified. The number of commercially available genetic tests continues to increase and can be found at GeneTests (http://www.genetests.org).

Genetic testing involves the analysis of human deoxyribonucleic acid (DNA), ribonucleic acid (RNA), **chromosomes** (threadlike packages of genes and other DNA in the nucleus of a cell; discussed later in the chapter), or proteins to detect abnormalities related to an inherited condition. Genetic tests can be used to examine directly the DNA and RNA that make up a gene (direct or molecular testing), look at markers coinherited with a gene that causes a genetic condition (linkage analysis), examine the protein products of genes (biochemical testing), or examine chromosomes (**cytogenetic** testing).

Most of the genetic tests now being offered in clinical practice are tests for single-gene disorders in patients with clinical symptoms or who have a family history of a genetic disease, although new technology can now determine if patients are getting the correct medication for their genetic makeup. Some of these genetic tests are prenatal tests, or tests used to identify the genetic status of a pregnancy at risk for a genetic condition. Current prenatal testing options include the following:

- Preimplantation genetic diagnosis (genetic profiling of embryo prior to implantation)
- First-trimester screening (nuchal translucency combined with biological markers)
- Integrated prenatal screening (a blood test combined with ultrasound examination to see if a pregnant woman is at increased risk for carrying a fetus with a neural tube defect or a chromosome abnormality, such as Down syndrome)
- Maternal blood testing for markers of certain conditions in fetus (noninvasive prenatal testing [NIPT])
- Invasive procedures (amniocentesis and chorionic villus sampling)

(See further discussion in Chapter 13.) Other tests are carrier screening tests, which are used to identify individuals who have a gene mutation for a genetic condition but do not show symptoms of the condition because it is a condition that is inherited in an autosomal recessive form (e.g., CF, sickle cell disease, Tay-Sachs disease).

Another type of genetic testing is predictive testing, which is used to clarify the genetic status of asymptomatic family members. The two types of predictive testing are presymptomatic and predispositional. Mutation analysis for HD, a neurodegenerative disorder, is an example of presymptomatic testing. If the gene mutation for HD is present, symptoms of HD are certain to appear if the individual lives long enough. Testing for a *BRCA1* gene mutation to determine breast cancer susceptibility is an example of predispositional testing. Predispositional testing differs from presymptomatic testing in that a positive result (indicating that a *BRCA1* mutation is present) does not indicate a 100% risk of developing the condition (breast cancer).

In addition to using genetic tests to test for single-gene disorders, they are being used for population-based screening (e.g., province-mandated newborn screening for PKU and other inborn errors of metabolism [IEMs]).

Factors Influencing the Decision to Undergo Genetic Testing

Decisions about genetic testing are shaped, and in many instances constrained, by factors such as social norms, cost, and where care is received. Most pregnant women in Canada now have at least one ultrasound examination and undergo some type of multiple-marker screening, and a growing number undergo other types of prenatal testing. The range of prenatal testing options available to a pregnant woman and her family may vary significantly, based on where the pregnant woman receives prenatal care. Certain types of prenatal testing may not be available in smaller communities and rural settings (e.g., chorionic villus sampling and fluorescent in situ hybridization analysis). In addition, certain types of genetic testing may not be offered in conservative medical communities (e.g., preimplantation diagnosis). NIPT may only be covered by some provincial health care plans in certain situations, so the cost must be covered by the woman and her family.

There are ethical dimensions to making the decision to be tested. The decision to undergo testing is seldom an autonomous one based solely on the needs and preferences of the individual being tested. Instead, it is often a decision based on feelings of responsibility and commitment to others. For example, a woman who has a family history of CF may decide to have genetic testing, but then decisions must be made about the outcome of the pregnancy depending on the results of the testing.

Ethical, Legal, and Social Implications

Because of widespread concern about misuse of the information gained through genetics research, the ethical, legal, and social implications (ELSIs) of genetic testing must be taken into account. The following issues must be considered:

- Privacy and fairness in the use and interpretation of genetic information
- Clinical integration of new genetic technologies
- Issues surrounding genetics research, such as possible discrimination and stigmatization
- Education for professionals and the general public about genetics, genetics health care, and the ELSIs of human genome research

Programs must address the potential that genetic information may be used to discriminate against individuals or for eugenic purposes. Informed consent is very difficult to ensure when some of the outcomes, benefits, and risks of genetic testing remain unknown. Continued awareness of and vigilance against such misuse of information is the collective responsibility of health care providers, ethicists, and society. Some ethical considerations include the following: What is normal or a disability and who decides? Are disabilities diseases that need to be prevented or cured? Who will have access to these expensive therapies? Who will pay for them?

Clinical Genetics

Genetic Transmission

Human development is a complicated process that depends on the systematic unravelling of instructions found in the genetic material of the egg and the sperm. Development from conception to birth of a normal, healthy baby occurs without incident in most cases; however, occasionally some anomaly in the genetic code of the embryo creates a birth defect or disorder. The science of genetics seeks to explain the underlying causes of congenital disorders (disorders present at birth) and the patterns in which inherited disorders are passed from generation to generation.

Genes and Chromosomes

The hereditary material carried in the nucleus of each somatic (body) cell determines an individual's physical characteristics. This material, called *DNA*, forms threadlike strands known as *chromosomes*. Each chromosome is composed of many smaller segments of DNA referred to as *genes*. Genes or combinations of genes contain coded information that determines an individual's unique characteristics. The code consists of the specific linear order of the molecules that combine to form the strands of DNA. Genes control both the types of proteins that are made and the rate at which they are produced. Genes never act in isolation; they always interact with other genes and the environment.

All normal human somatic cells contain 46 chromosomes arranged as 23 pairs of homologous (matched) chromosomes; one chromosome of each pair is inherited from each parent. There are 22 pairs of autosomes, which control most traits in the body, and one pair of sex chromosomes, which determines sex and some other traits. The larger female chromosome is called the X; the smaller male chromosome is the Y. Whereas the Y chromosome is primarily concerned with sex determination, the X chromosome contains genes that are involved in much more than sex determination. Generally the presence of a Y chromosome causes an embryo to develop as a male; in the absence of a Y chromosome, the individual develops as a female. Thus, in a normal female, the homologous pair of sex chromosomes is XX, and in a normal male, the homologous pair is XY.

Homologous chromosomes (except the X and Y chromosomes in males) have the same number and arrangement of genes. In other words, if one chromosome has a gene for hair colour, its partner chromosome also will have a gene for hair colour, and these hair colour genes will have the same loci or be located in the same place on the two chromosomes. Although both genes code for hair colour, they may not code for the same hair colour. Genes at corresponding loci on homologous chromosomes that code for different forms or variations of the same trait are called alleles. An individual with two copies of the same allele for a given trait is said to be homozygous for that trait. With two different alleles the person is heterozygous for the trait.

The term genotype typically is used to refer to the genetic makeup of an individual in the context of discussing a specific gene pair, but at times *genotype* is used to refer to an individual's entire genetic makeup or all the genes that the individual can pass on to future generations. Phenotype refers to the observable expression of an individual's genotype, such as physical features, a biochemical or molecular trait, and even a psychological trait. A trait or disorder is considered *dominant* if it is expressed or phenotypically apparent when only one copy of the gene is present. It is considered *recessive* if it is expressed only when two copies of the gene are present.

As more is learned about genetics, the concepts of dominance and recessivity have become more complex, especially in X-linked disorders. For example, traits considered to be recessive may be expressed even when only one copy of a gene located on the X chromosome is present. This occurs frequently in males because males have only one X chromosome; thus they have only one copy of the genes located on the X chromosome. Whichever gene is present on the one X chromosome determines which trait is expressed. Conversely, females have two X chromosomes; thus they have two copies of the genes located on the X chromosome. However, in any female somatic cell, only one X chromosome is functioning (otherwise there would be inequality in gene dosage between males and females). This process, known as *X-inactivation*, or the *Lyon hypothesis*, is generally a random occurrence (i.e., there is a 50:50 chance of the maternal X or the paternal X being inactivated). Occasionally, the percentage of cells that have the X with an abnormal or mutant gene is very high. This helps explain why hemophilia, an X-linked recessive disorder, can clinically manifest itself in a female known to be a heterozygous carrier (a female who has only one copy of the gene mutation). It also helps explain why traditional methods of carrier detection are less effective for X-linked recessive disorders; the possible range for enzyme activity values can vary greatly, depending on which X chromosome is inactivated.

Chromosomal Abnormalities

Chromosomal abnormalities are a major cause of reproductive loss, congenital problems, and gynecological disorders. The incidence of abnormalities is approximately 0.6% in newborns, 6% in stillbirths, and 60% in spontaneous abortions (Martin, 2008). Errors resulting in chromosome abnormalities can occur in mitosis or meiosis (see later discussion, p. 188). These errors can occur in either the autosomes or the sex chromosomes. Even without the presence of obvious structural malformations, small deviations in chromosomes can cause problems in fetal development.

The pictorial analysis of the number, form, and size of an individual's chromosomes is known as a karyotype. Cells are grown in a culture and arrested when they are in metaphase and then dropped onto a slide. The cells are stained with special stains (e.g., Giemsa stain) that create striping or "banding" patterns. These patterns aid in the analysis because they are consistent from person to person. Once the chromosome spreads are photographed or scanned by a computer, they are cut out and arranged in a specific numeric order according to their length and shape. The chromosomes are numbered from largest to smallest, 1 to 22, and the sex chromosomes are designated by the letter X or Y. Each chromosome is divided into two "arms" designated by p (short arm) and q (long arm). A female karyotype is designated as 46, XX, and a male karyotype is designated as 46, XY. Fig. 9-1 illustrates the chromosomes in a body cell and a karyotype. Karyotypes can be used to determine the sex of a child and the presence of any gross chromosomal abnormalities.

Autosomal abnormalities. Autosomal abnormalities involve differences in the number or structure of autosome chromosomes (pairs 1 to 22) resulting from unequal distribution of the genetic material during gamete (egg and sperm) formation.

Abnormalities of chromosome number. A euploid cell is a cell with the correct or normal number of chromosomes within the cell. Because most gametes are haploid (1N, 23 chromosomes) and most somatic cells are diploid (2N, 46 chromosomes), they are both considered euploid cells. Deviations from the correct number of chromosomes can be one of two types: (1) polyploidy, in which the deviation is an exact multiple of the haploid number of chromosomes, or one chromosome set (23 chromosomes), or (2) aneuploidy, in which the numeric deviation is not an exact multiple of the haploid set. A triploid (3 N) cell is an example of a polyploidy. It has 69 chromosomes. A tetraploid (4 N) cell, also an example of a polyploidy, has 92 chromosomes.

Aneuploidy is the most commonly identified chromosome abnormality in humans and the leading genetic cause of

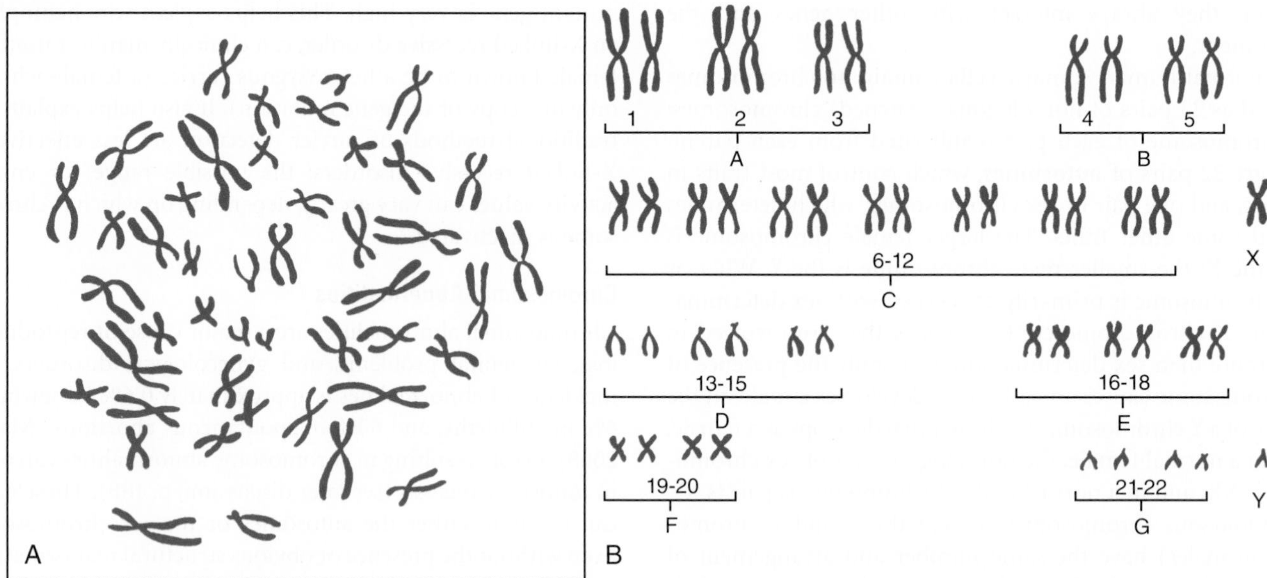

FIGURE 9-1 Chromosomes during cell division. **A:** Example of photomicrograph. **B:** Chromosomes arranged in karyotype; female and male sex-determining chromosomes.

intellectual disability. A **monosomy** is the product of the union between a normal gamete and a gamete that is missing a chromosome. Monosomic individuals have only 45 chromosomes in each of their cells. The product of the union of a normal gamete with a gamete containing an extra chromosome is a **trisomy**. The most common autosomal aneuploid conditions involve trisomies. Trisomic individuals have 47 chromosomes in most or all of their cells.

The vast majority of trisomies occur during **oogenesis** (the process by which a premeiotic female germ cell divides into a mature egg); the incidence of these types of chromosomal errors increases exponentially with advancing maternal age. Although variation exists among trisomies with regard to the parent and stage of origin of the extra chromosome, most trisomies are maternal meiosis I (MI) errors. This means that most trisomies are caused by nondisjunction during the first meiotic division. The first meiotic division involves the segregation of homologous or similar chromosomes. One pair of chromosomes fails to separate. One resulting cell contains both chromosomes, and the other contains none. The fact that most trisomies are maternal MI errors is not that surprising, because maternal MI occurs over a long time span. It is initiated in precursor cells during fetal development, but it is not completed until the time those cells undergo ovulation after menarche.

The most common trisomy abnormality is Down syndrome (DS). Approximately 1 in every 781 newborns has DS; there are over 45,000 individuals with DS living in Canada (http://www.cdss.ca). Ninety-five percent of individuals with DS have trisomy 21 (nondisjunction) or an extra chromosome 21 (47,XX+21, female with DS; or 47,XY+21, male with DS). Another type of DS, translocation, occurs when extra chromosome 21 material is present in every cell of the individual but it is attached to another chromosome. In the third type of DS, mosaicism, extra chromosome 21 material is found in some but not all of the cells.

Although the risk for having a child with DS increases with maternal age (incidence is approximately 1 in 1200 for a 25-year-old woman; 1 in 350 for a 35-year-old woman; and 1 in 30 for a 45-year-old woman), children with DS can be born to mothers of any age. Eighty percent of children with DS are born to mothers younger than 35 years (Canadian Down Syndrome Society, n.d.). Since the average age of mothers when they give birth to children with DS is about 27 years, the Society of Obstetricians and Gynaecologists of Canada (2007) recommends that all pregnant women be offered prenatal screening for DS and not just women over 35. The risk of a mother having a second child with DS is about 1% when the cause of the DS is trisomy 21 (see also Fig. 41-6 and discussion in Chapter 41).

Other autosomal trisomies that perinatal nurses might see are trisomy 18 (Edwards syndrome) and trisomy 13 (Patau syndrome). Trisomy 18 is more common than trisomy 13; it occurs in about 1 of 3000 live births versus 1 of 10,000 live births for trisomy 13. Infants with trisomy 18 and trisomy 13 usually have severe to profound intellectual disabilities. Although both conditions have a poor prognosis, with the vast majority of affected infants dying before they reach their first birthday, a growing number of infants with these trisomies are living longer and a small number are actually living into their 40s and 50s.

Nondisjunction can also occur during mitosis. If this occurs early in development, when cell lines are forming, the individual has a mixture of cells, some with a normal number of chromosomes and others either missing a chromosome or containing an extra chromosome. This condition is known as *mosaicism*. The most common form of mosaicism in autosomes is mosaic Down syndrome.

Abnormalities of chromosome structure. Structural abnormalities can occur in any chromosome. Types of structural abnormalities include translocation, duplication, deletion, microdeletion, and inversion. **Translocation** occurs when there is an exchange of chromosome material between two chromosomes. Exposure to certain drugs, viruses, and radiation can cause translocations, but often they arise for no apparent reason.

The two major types of translocation are reciprocal and robertsonian. Reciprocal translocations are the most common. In a *reciprocal* translocation, either the parts of the two chromosomes are exchanged equally (balanced translocation) or a part of a chromosome is transferred to a different chromosome, creating an unbalanced translocation because there is extra chromosomal material—extra of one chromosome but correct amount or deficient amount of the other chromosome. In a balanced translocation, the individual is phenotypically normal because there is no extra chromosome material; it is just rearranged. In an unbalanced translocation, the individual will be both genotypically and phenotypically abnormal.

In a *robertsonian* translocation, the short arms (p arms) of two different acrocentric chromosomes (chromosomes with very short p arms) break, leaving sticky ends that then cause the two long arms (q arms) to stick together. This forms a new, large chromosome that is made of the two long arms. The individual with a balanced robertsonian translocation has 45 chromosomes. Because the short arm of acrocentric chromosomes contains genes for ribosomal RNA and these genes are represented elsewhere, the individual usually does not show any symptoms. The individual may produce an unbalanced gamete (sperm or egg with too many or two few genes). This can lead to reproductive difficulties such as miscarriages or birth defects.

In *duplication*, there is an extra chromosomal segment within the same homologous or another nonhomologous chromosome. Clinical findings are highly variable and depend on which of the chromosomal segments are involved.

Deletions result in the loss of chromosomal material and partial monosomy for the chromosome involved. *Microdeletions* are deletions too small to be detected by standard cytogenetic techniques. Whenever a portion of a chromosome is deleted from one chromosome and added to another, the gamete produced may have either extra copies of genes or too few copies. The clinical effects produced may be mild or severe depending on the amount of genetic material involved. Two of the more common conditions are the deletion of the short arm of chromosome 5 (cri du chat syndrome) and the deletion of the long arm of chromosome 18.

Inversions are deviations in which a portion of the chromosome has been rearranged in reverse order. Few birth defects have been attributed to the presence of inversions, but it is suspected that inversions may be responsible for problems with infertility and miscarriages. More than 40% of inversions involve chromosome 9.

Sex chromosome abnormalities. Several sex chromosome abnormalities are caused by nondisjunction during gametogenesis in either parent. The most common deviation in females is *Turner syndrome*, or monosomy X (45,X). The affected female exhibits juvenile external genitalia with undeveloped ovaries. She is usually short in stature with webbing of the neck, a low hairline in the back, low-set ears, and lymphedema of her hands and feet. Intelligence may be impaired. Most affected embryos miscarry spontaneously. In most cases of Turner syndrome, it is the paternal X or Y that is lost.

The most common deviation in males is *Klinefelter syndrome*, or trisomy XXY. The affected male has poorly developed secondary sexual characteristics and small testes. He is infertile, usually tall, and effeminate and may be slow to learn. Males who have mosaic Klinefelter syndrome may be fertile.

Patterns of Genetic Transmission

Heritable characteristics are those that can be passed on to offspring. The patterns by which genetic material is transmitted to the next generation are affected by the number of genes involved in the expression of the trait. Many phenotypic characteristics result from two or more genes on different chromosomes acting together (referred to as *multifactorial inheritance*); others are controlled by a single gene (*unifactorial inheritance*). Specialists in genetics (e.g., geneticists, genetics counsellors, and nurses with advanced expertise in genetics) predict the probability of the presence of an abnormal gene from the known occurrence of the trait in the individual's family and the known patterns by which the trait is inherited.

Multifactorial Inheritance

Most common congenital malformations result from multifactorial inheritance, a combination of genetic and environmental factors. Examples are cleft lip, cleft palate, congenital heart disease, neural tube defects, and pyloric stenosis. Each malformation may range from mild to severe, depending on the number of genes for the defect present or the amount of environmental influence. A neural tube defect may range from spina bifida, a bony defect in the lumbar region of the vertebrae with little or no neurological impairment, to anencephaly, the absence of brain development, which is always fatal. Some malformations occur more often in one sex. For example, pyloric stenosis and cleft lip are more common in males, and cleft palate is more common in females.

Unifactorial Inheritance

If a single gene controls a particular trait, disorder, or defect, its pattern of inheritance is referred to as *unifactorial Mendelian* or *single-gene inheritance*. The number of single-gene disorders far exceeds the number of chromosomal abnormalities. Potential patterns of inheritance for single-gene disorders include autosomal dominant, autosomal recessive, and X-linked dominant and recessive modes of inheritance (Fig. 9-2).

Autosomal dominant inheritance. Autosomal dominant inheritance disorders are those in which only one copy of a variant allele is needed for phenotypic expression. The variant allele may appear as a result of a *mutation*, a spontaneous and permanent change in the normal gene structure. In this case, the disorder occurs for the first time in the family. Usually an affected individual comes from multiple generations having the disorder. An affected parent who is heterozygous for the trait has a 50% chance of passing the variant allele to each offspring (see Fig. 9-2, B and C). There is a vertical pattern of inheritance (there is no skipping of generations; if an individual has an

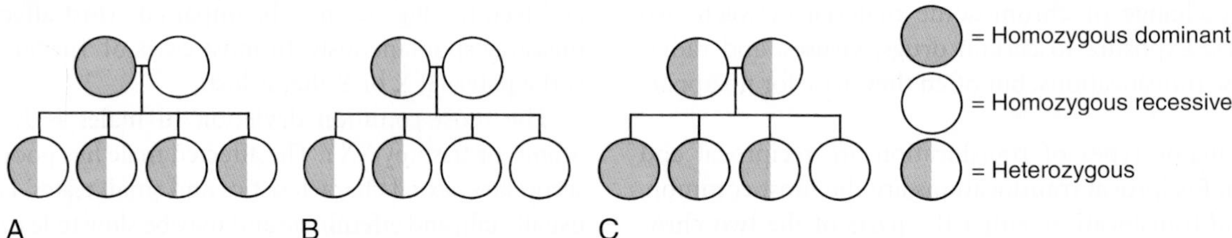

FIGURE 9-2 Possible offspring in three types of matings. **A:** Homozygous-dominant parent and homozygous-recessive parent. Children: all heterozygous, displaying dominant trait. **B:** Heterozygous parent and homozygous-recessive parent. Children: 50% heterozygous, displaying dominant trait; 50% homozygous, displaying recessive trait. **C:** Both parents heterozygous. Children: 25% homozygous, displaying dominant trait; 25% homozygous, displaying recessive trait; 50% heterozygous, displaying dominant trait.

autosomal dominant disorder such as HD, so must one of his or her parents). Males and females are affected equally.

Autosomal dominant disorders are not always expressed with the same severity of symptoms. For example, a woman who has an autosomal dominant disorder may show few symptoms and may not become aware of her diagnosis until after she gives birth to a severely affected child. The predicting of whether an offspring will have a minor or severe abnormality is not possible. Examples of autosomal dominant disorders are Marfan syndrome, neurofibromatosis, myotonic dystrophy, Stickler syndrome, Treacher Collins syndrome, and achondroplasia (dwarfism).

Autosomal recessive inheritance. Autosomal recessive inheritance disorders are those in which both genes of a pair must be abnormal for the disorder to be expressed. Heterozygous individuals have only one variant allele and are unaffected clinically because their normal gene overshadows the variant allele. They are known as *carriers* of the recessive trait. Because these recessive traits are inherited by generations of the same family, an increased incidence of the disorder occurs in consanguineous matings (closely related parents). For the trait to be expressed, two carriers must each contribute a variant allele to the offspring (see Fig. 9-2, C). The chance of the trait occurring in each child is 25%. A clinically normal offspring may be a carrier of the gene. Autosomal recessive disorders have a horizontal pattern of inheritance rather than the vertical pattern seen with autosomal dominant disorders (i.e., autosomal recessive disorders are usually observed in one or more siblings but not in earlier generations). Males and females are equally affected. Most inborn errors of metabolism, such as PKU, galactosemia, maple syrup urine disease, Tay-Sachs disease, sickle cell anemia, and CF, are autosomal recessive inherited disorders.

Inborn errors of metabolism (IEM). More than 350 IEMs have been recognized (Jorde, Carey, & Bamshad, 2015). Individually, IEMs are relatively rare, but collectively they are common (1 in 5,000 live births). IEMs occur when a gene mutation reduces the efficiency of encoded enzymes to a level at which normal metabolism cannot occur. Defective enzyme action interrupts the normal series of chemical reactions from the affected point onward. The result may be an accumulation of a damaging product, such as phenylalanine in PKU, or the absence of a necessary product, such as the lack of melanin in albinism caused by lack of tyrosinase. Diagnostic and carrier testing are available for a growing number of IEMs. In addition, many provinces in Canada have started screening for specific IEMs as part of their expanded newborn screening programs, using tandem mass spectrometry. However, many of the deaths caused by IEMs are the result of enzyme variants not currently screened for in many of the newborn screening programs (Jorde et al., 2015). (See Table 26-3 for screening tests for IEMs.) (See discussion of IEMs in Chapter 29.)

X-linked dominant inheritance. X-linked dominant inheritance disorders occur in males and heterozygous females, but because of X inactivation, affected females are usually less severely affected than affected males, and they are more likely to transmit the variant allele to their offspring. Heterozygous females (females who have one wild-type allele and one variant allele) have a 50% chance of transmitting the variant allele to each offspring. The variant allele is often lethal in affected males because, unlike affected females, they have no normal gene (wild-type allele). Mating of an affected male and an unaffected female is uncommon as a result of the tendency for the variant allele to be lethal in affected males. Relatively few X-linked dominant disorders have been identified. Two examples are fragile X syndrome and vitamin D–resistant rickets. (See discussion in Chapters 41 and 46, respectively.)

X-linked recessive inheritance. Abnormal genes for X-linked recessive inheritance disorders are carried on the X chromosome. Females may be heterozygous or homozygous for traits carried on the X chromosome because they have two X chromosomes. Males are hemizygous because they have only one X chromosome carrying genes, with no alleles on the Y chromosome. Therefore, X-linked recessive disorders are most often manifested in the male, with the abnormal gene on his single X chromosome. Hemophilia, colour blindness, and Duchenne muscular dystrophy are all X-linked recessive disorders.

The male receives the disease-associated allele from his carrier mother on her affected X chromosome. Female carriers (those heterozygous for the trait) have a 50% probability of transmitting the disease-associated allele to each offspring. An affected male can pass the disease-associated allele to his daughters but not to his sons. The daughters will be carriers of the trait if they receive a normal gene on the X chromosome from their mother. They will be affected only if they receive a

Risk Factors for Genetic Disorders

It's a good idea to review your risk factors before you see your health care provider to discuss prenatal screening and diagnostic testing. It may be helpful for you to talk with your and your partner's family members for information about diseases or conditions that run in your families.

_____What is your age?

_____What is the baby's father's age?

_____If you or the baby's father is of Mediterranean or Asian descent, do either of you or anyone in your families have thalassemia?

_____Is there a family history of neural tube defects?

_____Have you or the baby's father ever had a child with a neural tube defect?

_____Is there a family history of congenital heart defects?

_____Is there a family history of Down syndrome?

_____Have you or the baby's father ever had a child with Down syndrome?

_____If you or the baby's father is of Eastern European Jewish, French Canadian, or Cajun descent, is there a family history of Tay–Sachs disease?

_____If you or your partner is of Eastern European Jewish descent, is there a family history of Canavan disease or any other genetic disorders?

_____If you or your partner is African American, is there a family history of sickle cell disease or sickle cell trait?

_____Is there a family history of hemophilia?

_____Is there a family history of muscular dystrophy?

_____Is there a family history of Huntington disease?

_____Does anyone in your family or the family of the baby's father have cystic fibrosis?

_____Does anyone in your family or the baby's father's family have an intellectual disability? Or have they had early menopause or tremors at an early age?

_____If so, was that person tested for fragile X syndrome?

_____Do you, the baby's father, anyone in your families, or any of your children have any other genetic diseases, chromosomal disorders, or birth defects?

_____Do you have a metabolic disorder such as diabetes mellitus or phenylketonuria?

_____Do you have a history of pregnancy issues (miscarriage or ***stillbirth***)?

FIGURE 9-3 Questionnaire for identifying couples having increased risk for offspring with genetic disorders. (Reprinted with permission from American College of Obstetricians and Gynecologists. *Your pregnancy and childbirth: Month to month.* Revised 6th ed. Washington, DC: ACOG; 2016.)

disease-associated allele on the X chromosome from both their mother and their father.

Genetic Counselling

It is standard practice in perinatal care to determine whether a heritable disorder exists in a couple or in anyone in either of their families. The goal of screening is to detect or define risk for disease in low-risk populations and to identify those for whom diagnostic testing may be appropriate. A nurse can obtain a genetic history using a questionnaire or checklist such as the one in Fig. 9-3.

Genetic counselling that follows may occur in the office, or referral to a geneticist may be necessary. Health professionals should become familiar with people who provide genetic counselling and the places that offer counselling services in their area of practice (see Community Focus box).

Individuals and families seek out or are referred for genetic counselling for a wide variety of reasons and at all stages of their lives. Some seek preconception or prenatal information; others are referred after the birth of a child with a birth defect or a suspected genetic condition; still others seek information because they have a family history of a genetic condition. Regardless of the setting or the individual and family's stage of life, genetic counselling should be offered and available to all individuals and families who have questions about genetics and their health.

COMMUNITY FOCUS

Resources for Genetic Disorders

- Search the Internet for a hereditary condition (e.g., neurofibromatosis, cystic fibrosis, Marfan syndrome, Down syndrome) that has a support organization.
- Access the website for the organization. What services and resources are available for families? Are these services and resources free, or must the family pay for them? Is there a branch of the organization available in your city? If there is no branch of the organization available in your city, where could families go for information and assistance? Is preconception counselling offered?
- While reviewing the website assess the appearance, readability, and information contained in the site. Is the information available in different languages?
- For your selected genetic disorder, prepare a list of resources for families.

Estimation of Risk

Most families with a history of genetic disease want an answer to the following question: What is the chance that our future children will have this disease? Because the answer to this question may have profound implications for individual family members and the family as a whole, health care providers must be able to answer this question as accurately as they can in a timely manner.

If a couple has not yet had children but is known to be at risk for having children with a genetic disease, they will be given an *occurrence risk.* Once a couple has produced one or more children with a genetic disease, the couple will be given a *recurrence risk.* Both occurrence and recurrence risks are determined by the mode of inheritance for the genetic disease in question. For genetic diseases caused by a factor that segregates during cell division (genes and chromosomes), risk can be estimated with a high degree of accuracy by application of the Mendelian principles.

In an autosomal dominant disorder, both the occurrence and recurrence risk is 50%, or 1 in 2, that a subsequent offspring will be affected when one parent is affected and the other is not. The recurrence risk for autosomal recessive disorders is 25%, or 1 in 4, if both parents are carriers. Occasionally an individual homozygous for a recessive disease gene mates with an individual who is a carrier of the same recessive gene and in this case, the recurrence risk is 50%, or one in two. If two individuals affected by an autosomal recessive disorder mate, all of their children will be affected. For X-linked disorders, recurrence is related to the sex of the child. Translocation chromosomes have a high risk of recurrence.

A number of autosomal disorders display complex patterns of inheritance, which makes the estimation of risk more difficult. In some situations, a genetic disease may not be in a family history and may be due to a new mutation. If this occurs, the recurrence risk for the parents' subsequent children is low (1 to 2%), although not as low as for the general population. Offspring of the affected child may have a substantially elevated occurrence risk as well.

The risk of recurrence for multifactorial conditions can be estimated empirically. An empiric risk is based not on genetics theory but rather on experience and observation of the disorder in other families. Recurrence risks are determined by applying the frequency of a similar disorder in other families to the case under consideration.

An important concept that must be emphasized to families is that *each pregnancy is an independent event.* For example, in monogenic disorders in which the risk factor is 1 in 4 that the child will be affected, the risk remains the same no matter how many affected children are already in the family. Families may make the erroneous assumption that the presence of one affected child ensures that the next three will be free of the disorder. However, "chance has no memory." The risk is 1 in 4 for each pregnancy. In a family with a child who has a disorder with multifactorial causes, however, the risk increases with each subsequent child born with the disorder.

Interpretation of Risk

The guiding principle for genetics counsellors has traditionally been the principle of nondirectiveness. According to the principle of nondirectiveness, the individual who is providing genetics counselling respects the right of the individual or family being counselled to make autonomous decisions. Counsellors using a nondirective approach avoid making recommendations, and they try to communicate genetics information in an unbiased manner. The first step in providing nondirective counselling is becoming aware of one's own values and beliefs. Another important step is recognizing how one's values and beliefs can influence or interfere with the communication of genetics information.

The counsellor provides appropriate information about the nature of the disorder, the extent of the risks in the specific case, the probable consequences, and (if appropriate) alternative options available; however, the final decision to become pregnant or to continue a pregnancy must be left to the family. An important nursing role is reinforcing the information that families are given and continuing to interpret this information on their level of understanding.

Nongenetic Factors Influencing Development

Congenital disorders may be inherited or may be caused by environmental factors or by inadequate maternal nutrition. *Congenital* means that the condition was present at birth. Some congenital malformations may be the result of *teratogens,* that is, environmental substances or exposures that result in functional or structural disability. In contrast to other forms of developmental disabilities, disabilities caused by teratogens are theoretically totally preventable. Known human teratogens are drugs and chemicals, infections, exposure to radiation, and certain maternal conditions such as diabetes and PKU (Box 9-4). A teratogen has the greatest effect on the organs and parts of an embryo during its periods of rapid growth and differentiation. This occurs during the embryonic period, specifically from days 15 to 60. During the first 2 weeks of development, teratogens either have no effect on the embryo or have effects so severe that they cause miscarriage. Brain growth and

BOX 9-4 ETIOLOGY OF HUMAN MALFORMATIONS

Environmental

Maternal conditions
- Alcoholism, diabetes, endocrinopathies, phenylketonuria, smoking, nutritional deficits

Infectious agents
- Rubella, toxoplasmosis, syphilis, herpes simplex, cytomegalic inclusion disease, varicella, Venezuelan equine encephalitis

Mechanical problems (deformations)
- Amniotic band constrictions, umbilical cord constraint, disparity in uterine size and uterine contents

Chemicals, drugs, radiation, hyperthermia

Genetic

Single-gene disorders
Chromosomal abnormalities

Unknown

Polygenic or multifactorial (gene–environment interactions)
"Spontaneous" errors of development
Other unknowns

Adapted from Parikh, A. S., & Wiesner, G. L. (2011). Congenital anomalies. In R. J. Martin, A. A. Fanaroff, & M. C. Walsh (Eds.), *Fanaroff and Martin's neonatal-perinatal medicine: Diseases of the fetus and infant* (9th ed.). St. Louis: Mosby.

development continue during the fetal period, and teratogens can severely affect mental development throughout gestation (Fig. 9-4).

In addition to genetic makeup and the influence of teratogens, the adequacy of maternal nutrition influences development. The embryo and fetus must obtain the nutrients they need from the mother's diet; they cannot tap the maternal reserves. Malnutrition during pregnancy produces low-birth-weight newborns who are susceptible to infection and other conditions. Malnutrition also affects brain development during the latter half of gestation and may result in learning disabilities in the child. Inadequate folic acid is associated with neural tube defects (see Chapter 12 for more information).

PROCESS OF CONCEPTION

Cell Division

Cells are reproduced by two different methods: **mitosis** and **meiosis**. In *mitosis*, the body cells replicate to yield two cells with the same genetic makeup as the parent cell. First the cell makes a copy of its DNA, and then it divides. Each daughter cell receives one copy of the genetic material. Mitotic division facilitates growth and development or cell replacement.

Meiosis, the process by which germ cells divide and decrease their chromosome number by half, produces gametes (eggs and sperm). Each homologous pair of chromosomes contains one chromosome received from the mother and one from the father; thus meiosis results in cells that contain 1 of each of the 23 pairs of chromosomes. Because these germ cells contain 23 single chromosomes, half of the genetic material of a normal somatic cell, they are called *haploid*. When the female gamete (egg or ovum) and the male gamete (spermatozoon) unite to form the zygote, the diploid number of human chromosomes (46, or 23 pairs) is restored.

The process of DNA replication and cell division in meiosis allows different alleles (genes on corresponding loci that code for variations of the same trait) for genes to be distributed at random by each parent and then rearranged on the paired chromosomes. The chromosomes then separate and proceed to different gametes. Because the two parents have genotypes derived from four different grandparents, many combinations of genes on each chromosome are possible. This random mixing of alleles accounts for the variation of traits seen in the offspring of the same two parents.

Gametogenesis

Oogenesis, the process of egg (ovum) formation, begins during fetal life of the female. All the cells that may undergo meiosis in a woman's lifetime are contained in her ovaries at birth. The majority of the estimated 2 million primary oocytes (the cells that undergo the first meiotic division) degenerate spontaneously. Only 400 to 500 ova will mature during the approximately 35 years of a woman's reproductive life. The primary oocytes begin the first meiotic division (i.e., they replicate their DNA) during fetal life but remain suspended at this stage until puberty (Fig. 9-5, A). Then, usually monthly, one primary oocyte matures and completes the first meiotic division, yielding two unequal cells: the secondary oocyte and a small polar body. Both contain 22 autosomes and one X sex chromosome.

At ovulation, the second meiotic division begins. However, the ovum does not complete the second meiotic division unless fertilization occurs. At fertilization, a second polar body and the **zygote** (the united egg and sperm) are produced (see Fig. 9-5, C). The three polar bodies degenerate. If fertilization does not occur, the ovum also degenerates.

When a male reaches puberty, his testes begin the process of **spermatogenesis**. The cells that undergo meiosis in the male are called *spermatocytes*. The primary spermatocyte, which undergoes the first meiotic division, contains the diploid number of chromosomes. The cell has already copied its DNA before division; thus four alleles for each gene are present. Because the copies are bound together (i.e., one allele plus its copy on each chromosome), the cell is still considered diploid.

During the first meiotic division, two haploid secondary spermatocytes are formed. Each secondary spermatocyte contains 22 autosomes and one sex chromosome; one contains the X chromosome (plus its copy), and the other the Y chromosome (plus its copy). During the second meiotic division, the male produces two gametes with an X chromosome and two gametes with a Y chromosome, all of which will develop into viable sperm (see Fig. 9-5, B).

Conception

Conception, defined as the union of a single egg and sperm, marks the beginning of a pregnancy. Conception occurs not as an isolated event but as part of a sequential process. This

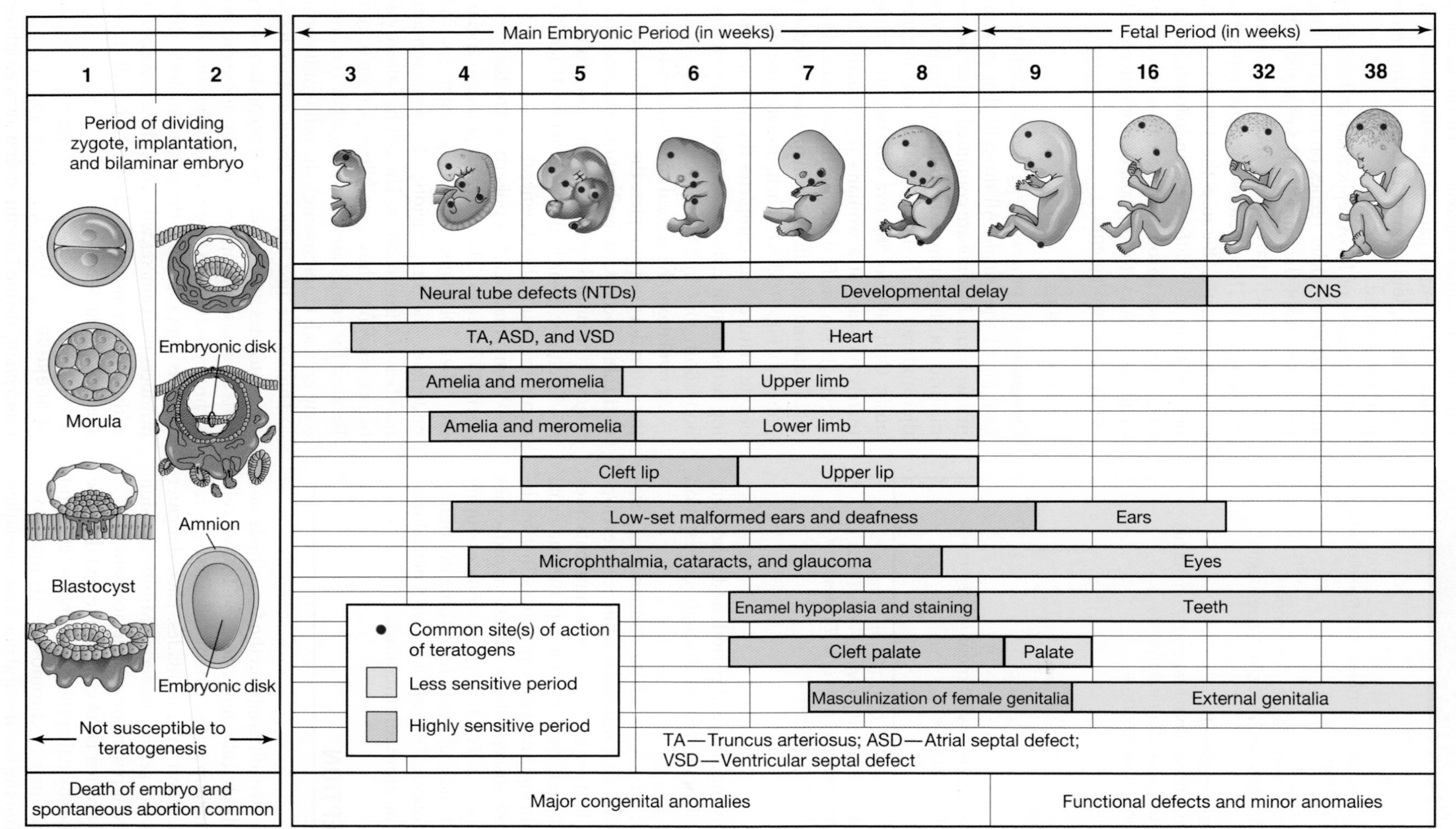

FIGURE 9-4 Sensitive, or critical, periods in human development. *Dark colour* denotes highly sensitive periods; *light colour* indicates stages that are less sensitive to teratogens. CNS, central nervous system. (From Moore, K. L., Persaud, T. V. N., & Torchia, M. G. [2013]. *Before we are born: Essentials of embryology and birth defects* [8th ed.]. Philadelphia: Saunders.)

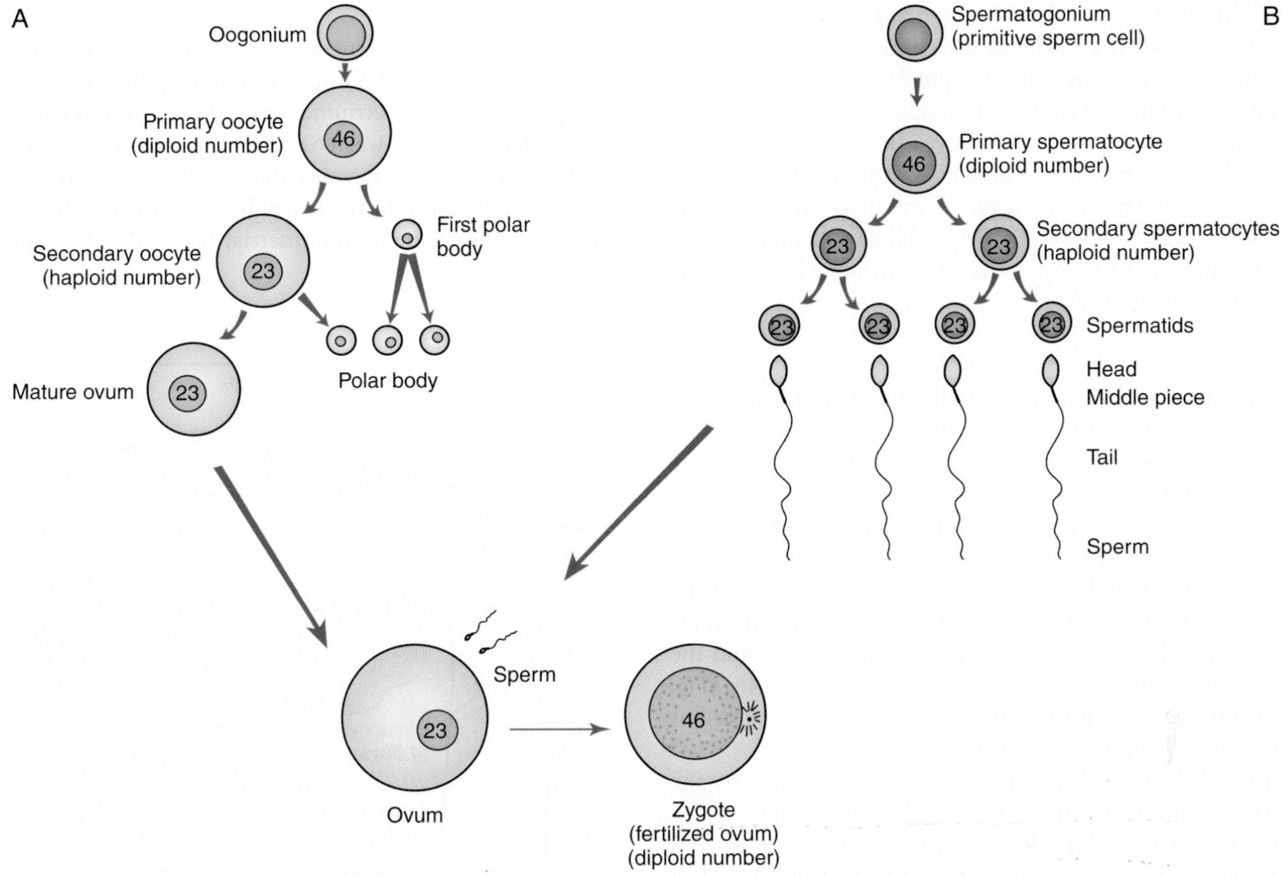

A
Oogonium
Primary oocyte (diploid number) 46
Secondary oocyte (haploid number) 23
First polar body
Polar body
Mature ovum 23

B
Spermatogonium (primitive sperm cell)
Primary spermatocyte (diploid number) 46
Secondary spermatocytes (haploid number) 23
Spermatids 23
Head
Middle piece
Tail
Sperm

C
Sperm
Ovum 23
Zygote (fertilized ovum) (diploid number) 46

FIGURE 9-5 Gametogenesis and fertilization. **A:** Oogenesis. Gametogenesis in the female produces one mature ovum and three polar bodies. Note relative difference in overall size between ovum and sperm. **B:** Spermatogenesis. Gametogenesis in the male produces four mature gametes, the sperm. **C:** Fertilization results in the single-cell zygote and restoration of the diploid number of chromosomes.

sequential process includes gamete (egg and sperm) formation, ovulation (release of the egg), union of the gametes (which results in an embryo), and implantation in the uterus.

Ovum

Meiosis occurs in the female in the ovarian follicles and produces an egg, or ovum. Each month one ovum matures with a host of surrounding supportive cells. At ovulation, the ovum is released from the ruptured ovarian follicle. High estrogen levels increase the motility of the uterine tubes so that their cilia are able to capture the ovum and propel it through the tube toward the uterine cavity. An ovum cannot move by itself.

Two protective layers surround the ovum (Fig. 9-6). The inner layer is a thick, acellular layer called the *zona pellucida.* The outer layer, called the *corona radiata*, is composed of elongated cells.

Ova are considered fertile for approximately 24 hours after ovulation. If unfertilized by a sperm, the ovum degenerates and is resorbed.

Sperm

Ejaculation during sexual intercourse normally propels about a teaspoon of semen containing as many as 200 to 500 million sperm into the vagina. The sperm swim by means of the flagellar movement of their tails. Some sperm can reach the site of fertilization within 5 minutes, but average transit time is 4 to 6 hours. Sperm remain viable within the woman's reproductive system for an average of 2 to 3 days. Most sperm are lost in the

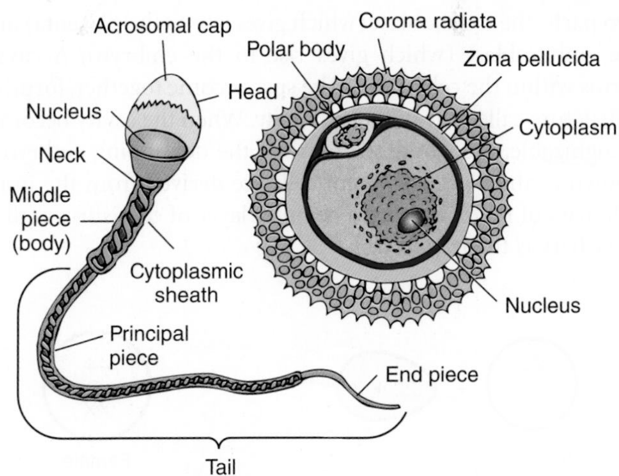

FIGURE 9-6 Sperm and ovum.

vagina, within the cervical mucus, or in the endometrium or they enter the tube that contains no ovum.

As sperm travel through the female reproductive tract, enzymes are produced to aid in their capacitation. *Capacitation* is a physiological change that removes the protective coating from the heads of the sperm. Small perforations then form in the acrosome (a cap on the sperm) and allow enzymes (e.g., hyaluronidase) to escape (see Fig. 9-6). These enzymes are necessary for the sperm to penetrate the protective layers of the ovum before fertilization.

Fertilization

Fertilization takes place in the ampulla (the outer third) of the uterine tube. When a sperm successfully penetrates the membrane surrounding the ovum, both sperm and ovum are enclosed within the membrane, and the membrane becomes impenetrable to other sperm; this process is termed the *zona reaction*. The second meiotic division of the secondary oocyte is then completed, and the ovum nucleus becomes the female pronucleus. The head of the sperm enlarges to become the male pronucleus, and the tail degenerates. The nuclei fuse, and the chromosomes combine, restoring the diploid number (46) (Fig. 9-7). Fertilization, the formation of the zygote (the first cell of the new individual), has been achieved.

Mitotic cellular replication, called *cleavage*, begins as the zygote travels the length of the uterine tube into the uterus. This voyage takes 3 to 4 days. Because the fertilized egg divides rapidly with no increase in size, successively smaller cells, called *blastomeres*, are formed with each division. A 16-cell morula, a solid ball of cells, is produced within 3 days and is still surrounded by the protective zona pellucida (Fig. 9-8, A). Further development occurs as the morula floats freely within the uterus. Fluid passes through the zona pellucida into the intercellular spaces between the blastomeres, separating them into two parts: the trophoblast (which gives rise to the placenta) and the embryoblast (which gives rise to the embryo). A cavity forms within the cell mass as the spaces come together, forming a structure called the *blastocyst cavity*. When the cavity becomes recognizable, the whole structure of the developing embryo is known as the *blastocyst*. Stem cells are derived from the inner cell mass of the blastocyst. The outer layer of cells surrounding the cavity is the *trophoblast*.

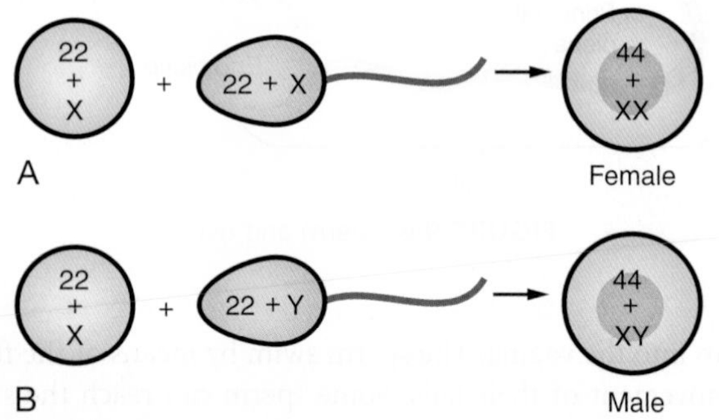

FIGURE 9-7 Fertilization. **A:** Ovum fertilized by X-bearing sperm to form female zygote. **B:** Ovum fertilized by Y-bearing sperm to form male zygote.

Implantation

The zona pellucida degenerates; the trophoblast cells displace endometrial cells at the implantation site; and the blastocyst embeds in the endometrium, usually in the anterior or posterior fundal region. Between 6 and 10 days after fertilization, the trophoblast secretes enzymes that enable it to burrow into the endometrium until the entire blastocyst is covered. This is known as *implantation*. Endometrial blood vessels erode, and

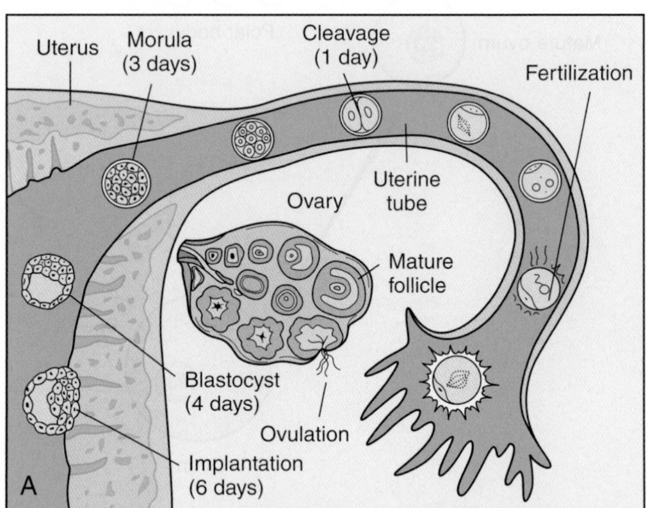

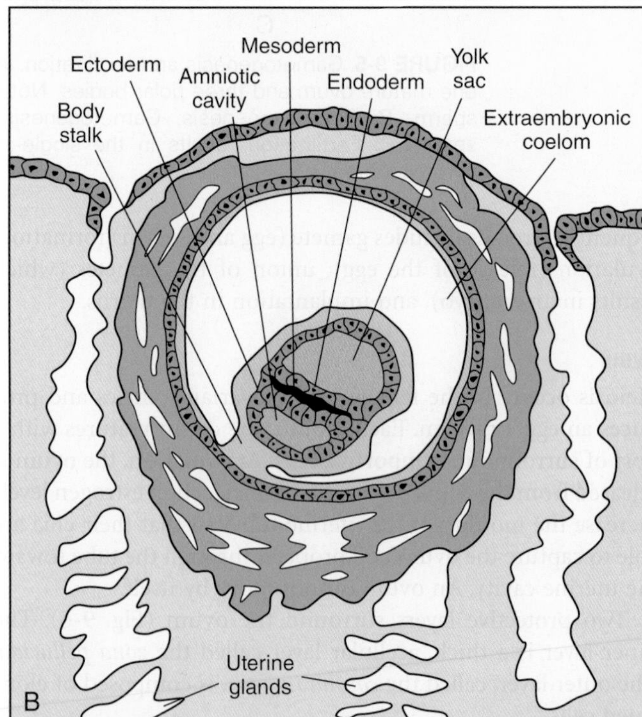

FIGURE 9-8 A: First weeks of human development. Follicular development in ovary, ovulation, fertilization, and transport of early embryo down the uterine tube and into the uterus, where implantation occurs. **B:** Blastocyst embedded in the endometrium. Germ layers are forming. (**A,** From Carlson, B. [2013]. *Human embryology and developmental biology* [5th ed.]. St. Louis: Mosby. **B,** Adapted from Langley, L., et al. [1980]. *Dynamic human anatomy and physiology* [5th ed.]. New York: McGraw-Hill.)

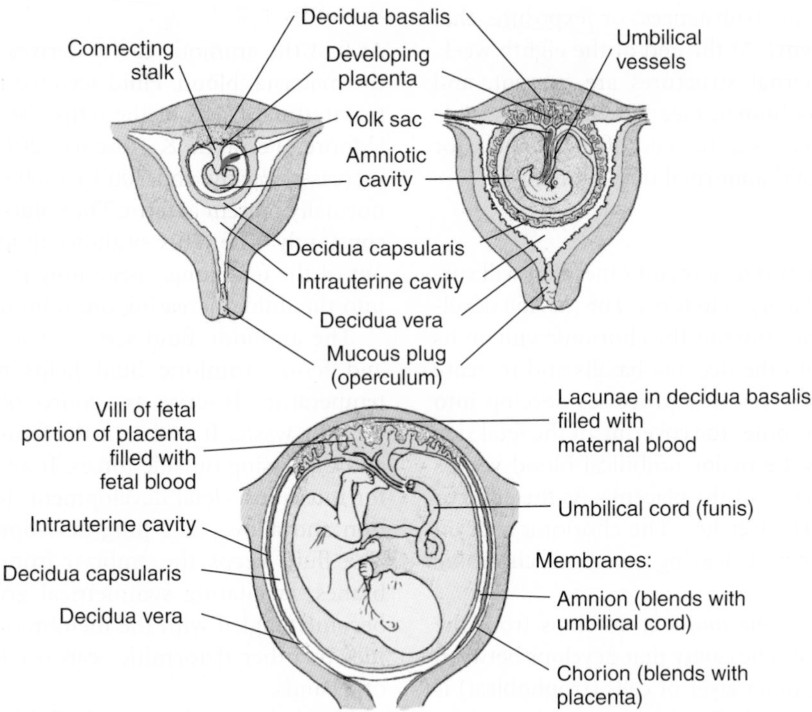

FIGURE 9-9 Development of fetal membranes. Note gradual obliteration of intrauterine cavity as decidua capsularis and decidua vera meet. Also note thinning of uterine wall. Chorionic and amnionic membranes are in apposition to each other but may be peeled apart.

some women have implantation bleeding (slight spotting and bleeding during the time of the first missed menstrual period). *Chorionic villi*, fingerlike projections, develop out of the trophoblast and extend into the blood-filled spaces of the endometrium. These villi are vascular processes that obtain oxygen and nutrients from the maternal bloodstream and dispose of carbon dioxide and waste products into the maternal blood.

After implantation, the endometrium is called the *decidua*. The portion directly under the blastocyst, where the chorionic villi tap into the maternal blood vessels, is the *decidua basalis*. The portion covering the blastocyst is the *decidua capsularis*, and the portion lining the rest of the uterus is the *decidua vera* (Fig. 9-9).

THE EMBRYO AND FETUS

Pregnancy lasts approximately 10 lunar months, 9 calendar months, 40 weeks, or 280 days. Length of pregnancy is computed from the first day of the last menstrual period (LMP) until the day of birth. However, conception occurs approximately 2 weeks after the first day of the LMP. Thus the postconception age of the fetus is 2 weeks less, for a total of 266 days, or 38 weeks. Postconception age is used in the discussion of fetal development.

Intrauterine development is divided into three stages: ovum or pre-embryonic, **embryo**, and **fetus** (see Fig. 9-4). The stage of the ovum lasts from conception until day 14. This period covers cellular replication, blastocyst formation, initial development of the embryonic membranes, and establishment of the primary germ layers.

Primary Germ Layers

During the third week after conception, the embryonic disk differentiates into three primary germ layers: the ectoderm, mesoderm, and endoderm (or entoderm) (see Fig. 9-8, B). All tissues and organs of the embryo develop from these three layers.

The *ectoderm*, the upper layer of the embryonic disk, gives rise to the epidermis, glands (anterior pituitary, cutaneous, and mammary), nails and hair, central and peripheral nervous systems, lens of the eye, tooth enamel, and floor of the amniotic cavity.

The *mesoderm*, the middle layer, develops into the bones and teeth, muscles (skeletal, smooth, and cardiac), dermis and connective tissue, cardiovascular system and spleen, and urogenital system.

The *endoderm*, the lower layer, gives rise to the epithelium lining of the respiratory and digestive tracts, including the oropharynx, liver and pancreas, urethra, bladder, and vagina. The endoderm forms the roof of the yolk sac.

Development of the Embryo

The stage of the embryo lasts from day 15 until approximately 8 weeks after conception, when the embryo measures approximately 3 cm from crown to rump. The embryonic stage is the most critical time in the development of the organ systems and the main external features. Developing areas with rapid cell division are the most vulnerable areas to malformation caused by environmental teratogens (substances or exposure that causes abnormal development). At the end of the eighth week, all organ systems and external structures are present, and the embryo is unmistakably human (see Fig. 9-4, and Visible Embryo in Additional Resources at the end of the chapter, for a pictorial view of normal and abnormal development).

Membranes

At the time of implantation, two fetal membranes that will surround the developing embryo begin to form. The *chorion* develops from the trophoblast and contains the chorionic villi on its surface. The villi burrow into the decidua basalis and increase in size and complexity as the vascular processes develop into the placenta. The chorion becomes the covering of the fetal side of the placenta. It contains the major umbilical blood vessels that branch out over the surface of the placenta. As the embryo grows, the decidua capsularis stretches. The chorionic villi on this side atrophy and degenerate, leaving a smooth chorionic membrane.

The inner cell membrane, the *amnion*, develops from the interior cells of the blastocyst. The cavity that develops between this inner cell mass and the outer layer of cells (trophoblast) is the *amniotic cavity* (see Fig. 9-8, B). As it grows larger, the amnion forms on the side opposite the developing blastocyst (see Fig. 9-8, B, and Fig. 9-9). The developing embryo draws the amnion around itself to form a fluid-filled sac. The amnion becomes the covering of the umbilical cord and covers the chorion on the fetal surface of the placenta. As the embryo grows larger, the amnion enlarges to accommodate the embryo, then fetus and the surrounding amniotic fluid. The amnion eventually comes in contact with the chorion surrounding the fetus (see Critical Thinking Case Study).

CRITICAL THINKING CASE STUDY

Ultrasound Dating of Pregnancy

Sandra believes she is 8 weeks pregnant, but her family physician believes she is closer to 12 weeks of gestation. Sandra has come to the clinic for an ultrasound examination for dating. She has many questions for the nurse: How can they tell what gestation she is? What would the fetus look like at this time if she is 8 weeks' gestation? If she is 12 weeks' gestation? What fetal structures would be apparent on ultrasound if she is 8 weeks pregnant? If she is 12 weeks pregnant? Would any structural anomalies be apparent at 8 weeks? At 12 weeks? Why is it important to date a pregnancy accurately? What information should the nurse provide Sandra?

QUESTIONS

1. Evidence—Is there sufficient evidence to draw conclusions about what information the nurse should provide to Sandra?
2. Assumptions—Describe an underlying assumption about the following factors:
   a. Sandra's motivation to learn about fetal development
   b. Sandra's understanding of fetal development
   c. Sandra's knowledge about ultrasound examinations
   d. Why dating the pregnancy is important
3. What implications and priorities for nursing care can be drawn at this time?
4. Does the evidence objectively support your conclusion?

Amniotic Fluid

At first the amniotic cavity derives its fluid by diffusion from the maternal blood. Fluid secreted by the respiratory and gastrointestinal tracts of the fetus also enters the amniotic cavity (Moore, Persaud, & Torchia, 2013). The amount of fluid increases weekly, and 700 to 1000 mL of transparent liquid is normally present at term. The volume of amniotic fluid changes constantly. The fetus swallows fluid, and fluid flows into and out of the fetal lungs. Beginning in week 11, the fetus urinates into the fluid, increasing the volume.

The amniotic fluid serves many functions for the embryo and fetus. Amniotic fluid helps maintain a constant body temperature. It serves as a source of oral fluid and as a repository for waste. It cushions the fetus from trauma by blunting and dispersing outside forces. It allows freedom of movement for musculoskeletal development. It acts as a barrier to infection and allows fetal lung development (Moore et al., 2013). The fluid keeps the embryo from tangling with the membranes, facilitating symmetrical growth. If the embryo does become tangled with the membranes, amputations of extremities or other deformities can occur from constricting amniotic bands.

The volume of amniotic fluid is an important factor in assessing fetal well-being. Having less than 300 mL of amniotic fluid (**oligohydramnios**) is associated with fetal renal abnormalities. Having more than 2 L of amniotic fluid *(polyhydramnios)* is associated with gastrointestinal and other malformations.

Amniotic fluid contains albumin, urea, uric acid, creatinine, lecithin, sphingomyelin, bilirubin, fructose, fat, leukocytes, proteins, epithelial cells, enzymes, and lanugo hair. Study of fetal cells in amniotic fluid through amniocentesis yields much information about the fetus. Genetic studies (karyotyping) provide knowledge about the sex and the number and structure of chromosomes. Other studies such as the lecithin/sphingomyelin (L/S) ratio determine the health or maturity of the fetus (see Chapter 13).

Yolk Sac

At the same time the amniotic cavity and amnion are forming, another blastocyst cavity forms on the other side of the developing embryonic disk (see Fig. 9-8, B). This cavity becomes surrounded by a membrane, forming the yolk sac. The *yolk sac* aids in transferring maternal nutrients and oxygen, which have diffused through the chorion, to the embryo. Blood vessels form to aid transport. Blood cells and plasma are manufactured in the yolk sac during the second and third weeks while uteroplacental circulation is being established and forming primitive blood cells until hematopoietic activity begins. At the end of the third week, the primitive heart begins to beat and circulate the blood through the embryo, connecting stalk, chorion, and yolk sac.

The folding in of the embryo during the fourth week results in incorporation of part of the yolk sac into the body of the embryo as the primitive digestive system. Primordial germ cells arise in the yolk sac and move into the embryo. The shrinking remains of the yolk sac degenerate (see Fig. 9-8, B), and by the fifth or sixth week the remnant has separated from the embryo.

Umbilical Cord

By day 14 after conception, the embryonic disk, amniotic sac, and yolk sac are attached to the chorionic villi by the connecting stalk. During the third week, the blood vessels develop to supply the embryo with maternal nutrients and oxygen. During the fifth week, the embryo has curved inward on itself from both ends, bringing the connecting stalk to the ventral side of the embryo. The connecting stalk becomes compressed from both sides by the amnion and forms the narrower umbilical cord (see Fig. 9-9). Two arteries carry blood from the embryo to the chorionic villi, and one vein returns blood to the embryo. Approximately 1% of umbilical cords contain only two vessels: one artery and one vein. This occurrence is sometimes associated with congenital malformations.

The cord rapidly increases in length. At term the cord is 2 cm in diameter and ranges from 30 to 90 cm in length (with an average of 55 cm). It twists spirally on itself and loops around the embryo/fetus. A true knot is rare, but false knots occur as folds or kinks in the cord and may jeopardize circulation to the fetus. Connective tissue called *Wharton's jelly* prevents compression of the blood vessels and ensures continued nourishment of the embryo and fetus. Compression can occur if the cord lies between the fetal head and the pelvis or is twisted around the fetal body. When the cord is wrapped around the fetal neck, it is called a **nuchal cord**.

Because the placenta develops from the chorionic villi, the umbilical cord is usually located centrally. The blood vessels are arrayed out from the centre to all parts of the placenta (Fig. 9-10, B). A peripheral location is less common and is known as a *battledore placenta* (see Fig. 14-14, B).

Placenta

Structure

The placenta begins to form at implantation. During the third week after conception, the trophoblast cells of the chorionic villi continue to invade the decidua basalis. As the uterine capillaries are tapped, the endometrial spiral arteries fill with maternal blood. The chorionic villi grow into the spaces with two layers of cells: the outer syncytium and the inner cytotrophoblast. A third layer develops into anchoring septa, dividing the projecting decidua into separate areas called *cotyledons*. In each of the 15 to 20 cotyledons the chorionic villi branch out, and a complex system of fetal blood vessels forms. Each cotyledon is a functional unit. The whole structure is the placenta (see Fig. 9-10).

The maternal–placental–embryonic circulation is in place by day 17, when the embryonic heart starts beating. By the end of the third week, embryonic blood is circulating between the embryo and the chorionic villi. In the intervillous spaces, maternal blood supplies oxygen and nutrients to the embryonic capillaries in the villi (Fig. 9-11). Waste products and carbon dioxide diffuse into the maternal blood.

The placenta functions as a means of metabolic exchange. Exchange is minimal at this time because the two cell layers of the villous membrane are too thick. Permeability increases as

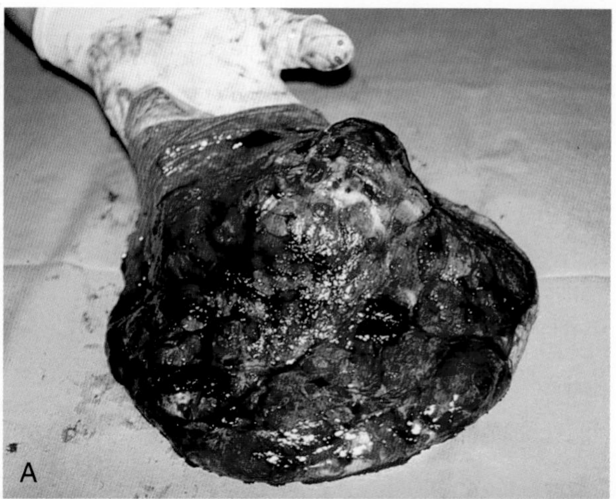

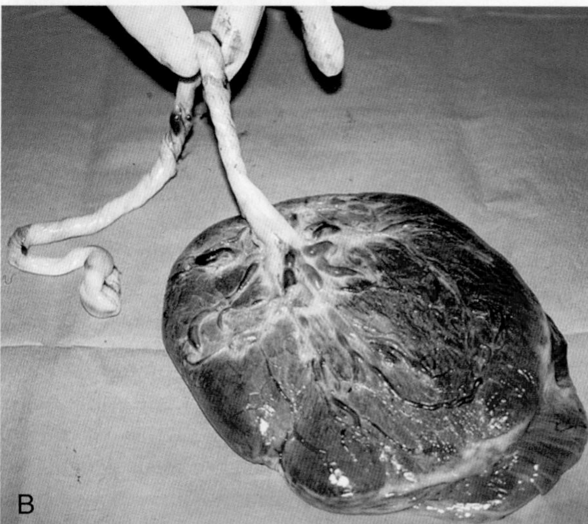

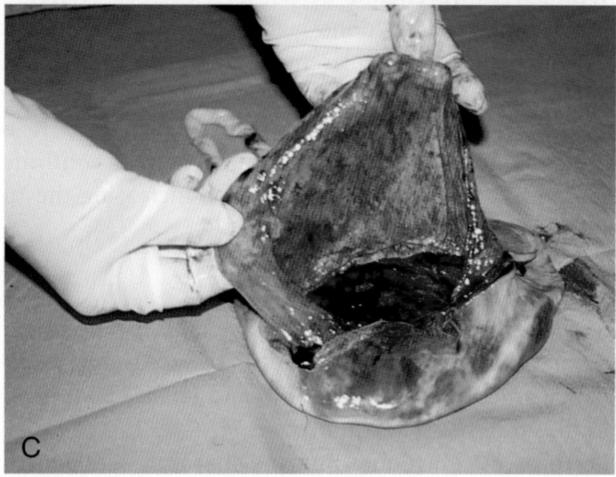

FIGURE 9-10 Full-term placenta. **A:** Maternal (or uterine) surface, showing cotyledons and grooves. **B:** Fetal (or amniotic) surface, showing blood vessels running under amnion and converging to form umbilical vessels at attachment of umbilical cord. **C:** Amnion and smooth chorion are arranged to show that they are (1) fused and (2) continuous with margins of placenta. (Courtesy Marjorie Pyle, RNC, Lifecircle.)

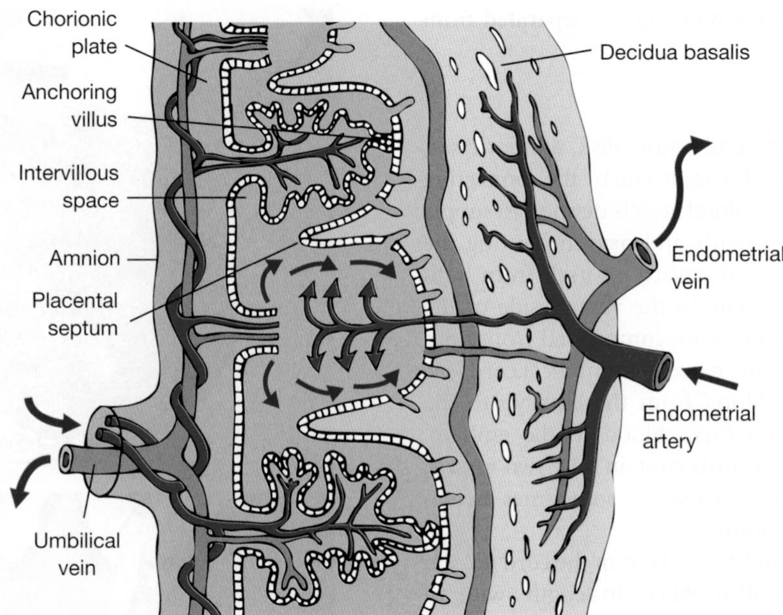

FIGURE 9-11 Schematic drawing of the placenta illustrating how it supplies oxygen and nutrition to the embryo and removes its waste products. Deoxygenated blood leaves the fetus through the umbilical arteries and enters the placenta, where it is oxygenated. Oxygenated blood leaves the placenta through the umbilical vein, which enters the fetus via the umbilical cord.

the cytotrophoblast thins and disappears; by the fifth month only the single layer of syncytium is left between the maternal blood and the fetal capillaries. The syncytium is the functional layer of the placenta. By the eighth week, genetic testing may be done on a sample of chorionic villi obtained by aspiration biopsy; however, limb defects have been associated with chorionic villi sampling done before 10 weeks (see Chapter 13). The structure of the placenta is complete by the twelfth week. The placenta continues to grow wider until 20 weeks, when it covers about half of the uterine surface. It then continues to grow thicker. The branching villi continue to develop within the body of the placenta, increasing the functional surface area.

Functions

One of the early functions of the placenta is as an endocrine gland that produces four hormones necessary to maintain the pregnancy and support the embryo and fetus. The hormones are produced in the syncytium.

The protein hormone human chorionic gonadotropin (hCG) can be detected in the maternal serum by 8 to 10 days after conception, shortly after implantation. This hormone is the basis for pregnancy tests. The hCG preserves the function of the ovarian corpus luteum, ensuring a continued supply of estrogen and progesterone needed to maintain the pregnancy. Miscarriage occurs if the corpus luteum stops functioning before the placenta can produce sufficient estrogen and progesterone. The hCG reaches its maximum level at 50 to 70 days and then begins to decrease.

The other protein hormone produced by the placenta is human chorionic somatomammotropin (hCS), or human placental lactogen (hPL). This substance is similar to a growth

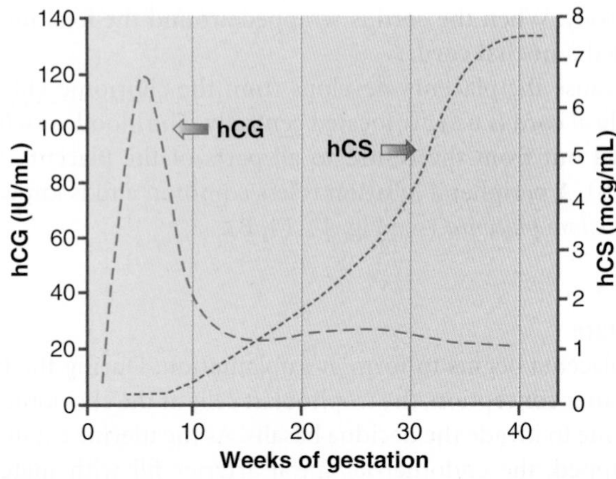

FIGURE 9-12 Distinct profile for the concentrations of human chorionic gonadotropin (hCG) and human chorionic somatomammotropin (hCS) in serum of women through normal pregnancy. *IU,* International Units. (Adapted with permission from Corton, et al., *Williams Obstetrics*, 24th ed., Copyright © 2014 by McGraw-Hill Education.)

hormone and stimulates maternal metabolism to supply needed nutrients for fetal growth. This hormone increases the resistance to insulin, facilitates glucose transport across the placental membrane, and stimulates maternal breast development to prepare for lactation (Fig. 9-12).

The placenta eventually produces more of the steroid hormone progesterone than the corpus luteum does during the first few months of pregnancy. Progesterone maintains the endometrium, decreases the contractility of the uterus, and stimulates maternal metabolism and development of breast alveoli.

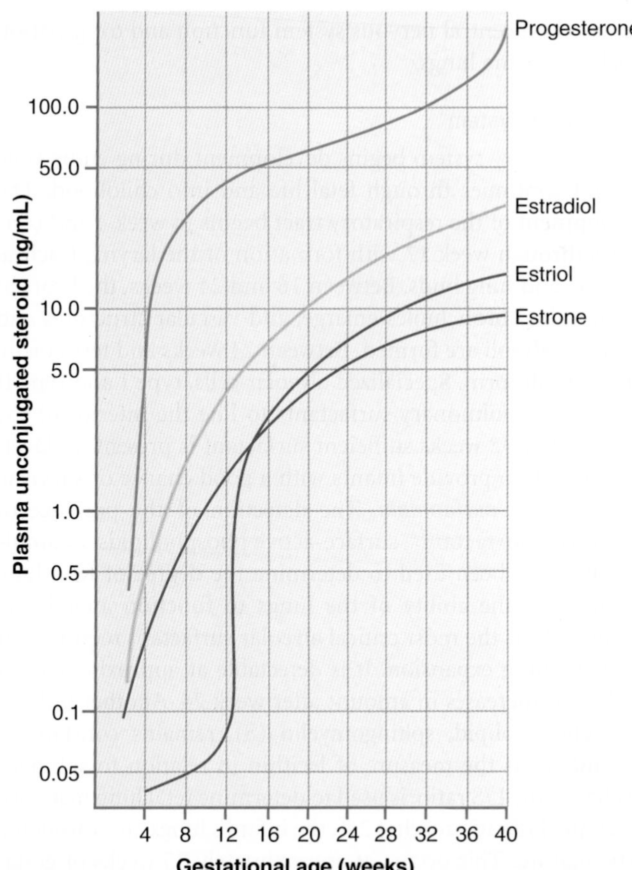

FIGURE 9-13 Plasma levels of progesterone, estradiol, estrone, and estriol in women during the course of gestation. (Adapted with permission from Corton, et al., *Williams Obstetrics*, 24th ed., Copyright © 2014 by McGraw-Hill Education. Original figure from *Yen & Jaffe's Reproductive Endocrinology*, Sam Mesiano, CHAPTER 11 The Endocrinology of Human Pregnancy and Fetoplacental Neuroendocrine Development, Pages 249–281, Copyright 2009, with permission from Elsevier.)

By 7 weeks after fertilization, the placenta is producing most of the maternal estrogens, which are steroid hormones. The major estrogen secreted by the placenta is estriol, whereas the ovaries produce mostly estradiol. Measuring estriol levels is a clinical assay for placental functioning. Estrogen stimulates uterine growth and uteroplacental blood flow. It causes a proliferation of the breast glandular tissue and stimulates myometrial contractility. Placental estrogen production increases greatly toward the end of pregnancy. One theory for the cause of the onset of labour is the decrease in circulating levels of progesterone and the increased levels of estrogen (Fig. 9-13).

The metabolic functions of the placenta are respiration, nutrition, excretion, and storage. Oxygen diffuses from the maternal blood across the placental membrane into the fetal blood, and carbon dioxide diffuses in the opposite direction. In this way, the placenta functions as a lung for the fetus.

Carbohydrates, proteins, calcium, and iron are stored in the placenta for ready access to meet fetal needs. Water, inorganic salts, carbohydrates, proteins, fats, and vitamins pass from the maternal blood supply across the placental membrane into the fetal blood, supplying nutrition. Water and most electrolytes with a molecular weight less than 500 readily diffuse through the membrane. Hydrostatic and osmotic pressures aid in the flow of water and some solutions. Facilitated and active transport assist in the transfer of glucose, amino acids, calcium, iron, and substances with higher molecular weights. Amino acids and calcium are transported against the concentration gradient between the maternal blood and fetal blood.

The fetal concentration of glucose is lower than the glucose level in the maternal blood because of its rapid metabolism by the fetus. This fetal requirement demands larger concentrations of glucose than simple diffusion can provide. Therefore, maternal glucose moves into the fetal circulation by active transport.

Pinocytosis is a mechanism used for transferring large molecules such as albumin and gamma (γ) globulins across the placental membrane. This mechanism conveys the maternal immunoglobulins that provide early passive immunity to the fetus.

Metabolic waste products of the fetus cross the placental membrane from the fetal blood into the maternal blood. The maternal kidneys then excrete them. Many viruses can cross the placental membrane and infect the fetus. Some bacteria and protozoa first infect the placenta and then infect the fetus. Drugs can also cross the placental membrane and may harm the fetus. Caffeine, alcohol, nicotine, carbon monoxide and other toxic substances in cigarette smoke, and prescription and recreational drugs (such as marijuana and cocaine) readily cross the placenta (Box 9-5).

Although no direct link exists between the fetal blood in the vessels of the chorionic villi and the maternal blood in the intervillous spaces, only one cell layer separates them. Breaks occasionally occur in the placental membrane. Fetal erythrocytes then leak into the maternal circulation, and the mother may develop antibodies to the fetal red blood cells. This is often the way the Rh-negative mother becomes sensitized to the erythrocytes of her Rh-positive fetus. (See discussion of isoimmunization in Chapter 28.)

Although the placenta and fetus are analogous to living tissue transplants, they are not destroyed by the host mother. Either the placental hormones suppress the immunological response or the tissue evokes no response.

Placental function depends on the maternal blood pressure supplying the circulation. Maternal arterial blood, under pressure in the small uterine spiral arteries, spurts into the intervillous spaces (see Fig. 9-11). As long as rich arterial blood continues to be supplied, pressure is exerted on the blood already in the intervillous spaces, pushing it toward drainage by the low-pressure uterine veins. At term gestation, 10% of the maternal cardiac output goes to the uterus.

If there is interference with the circulation to the placenta, the placenta cannot supply the embryo or fetus. Vasoconstriction such as that caused by hypertension or cocaine use diminishes uterine blood flow. Decreased maternal blood pressure or decreased cardiac output also diminishes uterine blood flow.

When a woman lies on her back with the pressure of the uterus compressing the vena cava, blood return to the right atrium is diminished. (See Fig. 17-3 and the discussion of supine hypotension in Chapter 11.) Excessive maternal exercise that diverts blood to the muscles away from the uterus compromises placental circulation. Optimum circulation is achieved

BOX 9-5 DEVELOPMENTALLY TOXIC EXPOSURES IN HUMANS

- Aminopterin
- Androgens
- Angiotensin-converting enzyme inhibitors
- Carbamazepine
- Cigarette smoking
- Cocaine
- Coumarin anticoagulants
- Cytomegalovirus
- Diethylstilbestrol
- Ethanol
- Etretinate
- Hyperthermia
- Iodides
- Ionizing radiation (>10 rads)
- Isotretinoin
- Lead
- Lithium
- Methimazole
- Methyl mercury
- Parvovirus B19
- Penicillamine
- Phenytoin
- Radioiodine
- Rubella
- Syphilis
- Tetracycline
- Thalidomide
- Toxoplasmosis
- Trimethadione
- Valproic acid
- Varicella
- Zika virus

when the woman is lying at rest on her side. Decreased uterine circulation may lead to intrauterine growth restriction of the fetus and infants who are small for gestational age.

Uterine contractions seem to enhance the movement of blood through the intervillous spaces, aiding placental circulation. However, prolonged contractions or too-short intervals between contractions during labour can reduce the blood flow to the placenta (see Chapter 20).

Fetal Maturation

The stage of the fetus lasts from 9 weeks (when the fetus becomes recognizable as a human being) until the pregnancy ends. Changes during the fetal period are not as dramatic because refinement of structure and function is taking place. The fetus is less vulnerable to teratogens, except for those that affect central nervous system functioning.

Viability refers to the capability of the fetus to survive outside the uterus. With modern technology and advances in maternal and neonatal care, infants who are 22 to 25 weeks of gestation are now considered to be on the threshold of viability (Cunningham, Leveno, Bloom, et al., 2014). The limitations on survival outside the uterus when an infant is born at this early stage are based on central nervous system function and oxygenation capability of the lungs.

Respiratory System

The respiratory system begins development during embryonic life and continues through fetal life and into childhood. The development of the respiratory tract begins in week 4 and continues through week 17 with formation of the larynx, trachea, bronchi, and lung buds. Between 16 and 24 weeks, the bronchi and terminal bronchioles enlarge, and vascular structures and primitive alveoli are formed. Between 24 weeks and term birth, more alveoli form. Specialized alveolar cells, type I and type II cells, secrete pulmonary surfactants to line the interior of the alveoli. After 32 weeks sufficient surfactant is present in developed alveoli to provide infants with a good chance of survival.

Pulmonary surfactants. The detection of the presence of pulmonary surfactants, surface-active phospholipids, in amniotic fluid has been used to determine the degree of fetal lung maturity, or the ability of the lungs to function after birth. Lecithin (L) is the most critical alveolar surfactant required for postnatal lung expansion. It is detectable at approximately 21 weeks and increases in amount after week 24. Another pulmonary phospholipid, sphingomyelin (S), remains constant in amount. Thus the measure of lecithin in relation to sphingomyelin, or the L/S ratio, is used to determine fetal lung maturity. When the L/S ratio reaches 2:1, the infant's lungs are considered to be mature. This occurs at approximately 35 weeks of gestation (Jobe & Kamath-Rayne, 2014).

Certain maternal conditions that cause decreased maternal placental blood flow, such as maternal hypertension, placental dysfunction, infection, or corticosteroid use, accelerate lung maturity. This apparently is caused by the resulting fetal hypoxia, which stresses the fetus and increases the blood levels of corticosteroids that accelerate alveolar and surfactant development.

Conditions such as gestational diabetes and chronic glomerulonephritis can delay fetal lung maturity. The use of intrabronchial synthetic surfactant in the treatment of respiratory distress syndrome in the newborn has greatly improved the chances of survival for preterm infants (see Chapter 27).

Fetal respiratory movements have been seen on ultrasound examination as early as week 11. These fetal respiratory movements may aid in development of the chest wall muscles and regulate lung fluid volume. The fetal lungs produce fluid that expands the air spaces in the lungs. The fluid drains into the amniotic fluid or is swallowed by the fetus.

Shortly before birth, secretion of lung fluid decreases. The normal birth process squeezes out approximately one third of the fluid. Infants born by Caesarean do not benefit from this squeezing process; thus they may have more respiratory difficulty at birth. The fluid remaining in the lungs at birth is usually resorbed into the infant's bloodstream within 2 hours of birth.

Circulatory System

The cardiovascular system is the first organ system to function in the developing human. Blood vessel and blood cell formation begins in the third week and supplies the embryo with oxygen and nutrients from the mother. By the end of the third week,

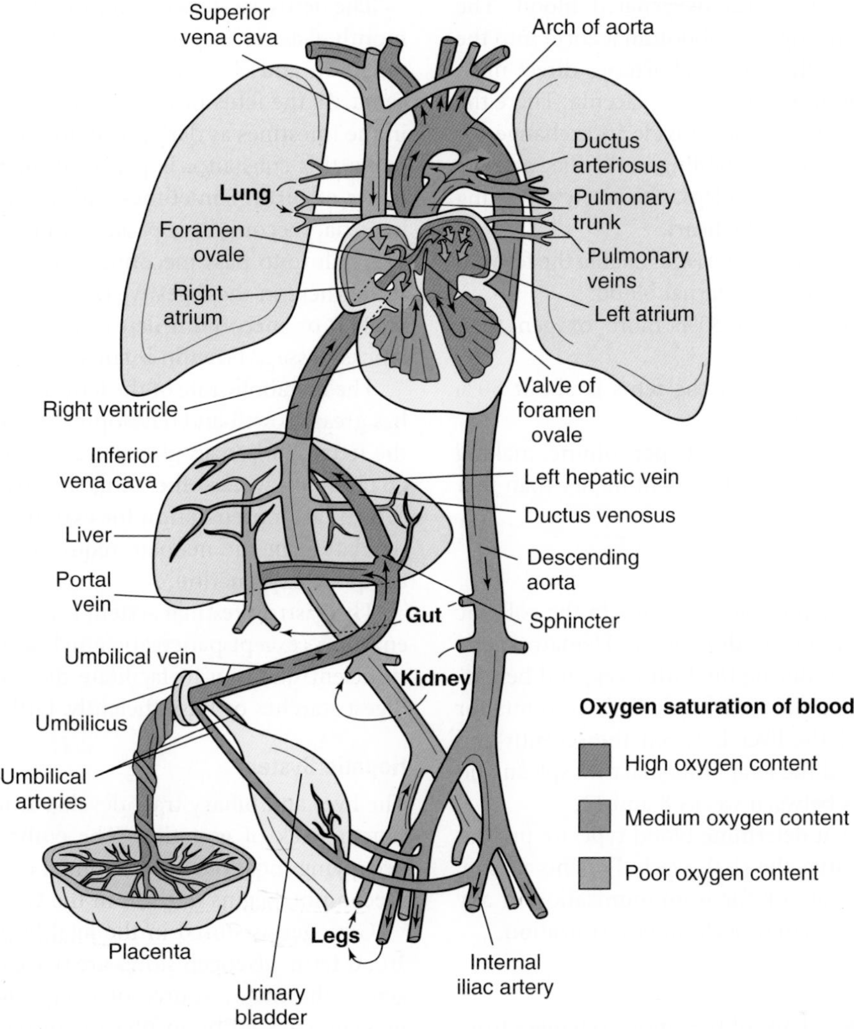

FIGURE 9-14 Schematic illustration of fetal circulation. The *colours* indicate the oxygen saturation of the blood, and the *arrows* show the course of the blood from the placenta to the heart. The organs are not drawn to scale. Observe that three shunts permit most of the blood to bypass the liver and lungs: (1) ductus venosus, (2) foramen ovale, and (3) ductus arteriosus. The poorly oxygenated blood returns to the placenta for oxygen and nutrients through the umbilical arteries. (From Moore, K. L., Persaud, T. V. N., & Torchia, M. G. [2013]. *Before we are born: Essentials of embryology and birth defects* [8th ed.]. Philadelphia: Saunders.)

the tubular heart begins to beat, and the primitive cardiovascular system links the embryo, connecting stalk, chorion, and yolk sac. During the fourth and fifth weeks, the heart develops into a four-chambered organ. By the end of the embryonic stage, the heart is developmentally complete.

The fetal lungs do not function for respiratory gas exchange; thus a special circulatory pathway, the ductus arteriosus, bypasses the lungs. Oxygen-rich blood from the placenta flows rapidly through the umbilical vein into the fetal abdomen (Fig. 9-14). When the umbilical vein reaches the liver, it divides into two branches. One branch circulates some oxygenated blood through the liver. Most of the blood passes through the ductus venosus into the inferior vena cava. There it mixes with the deoxygenated blood from the fetal legs and abdomen on its way to the right atrium. Most of this blood passes straight through the right atrium and through the foramen ovale, an opening into the left atrium. There it mixes with the small amount of deoxygenated blood returning from the fetal lungs through the pulmonary veins.

The blood flows into the left ventricle and is squeezed out into the aorta, where the arteries supplying the heart, head, neck, and arms receive most of the oxygen-rich blood. This pattern of supplying the highest levels of oxygen and nutrients to the head, neck, and arms enhances the **cephalocaudal** (head-to-rump) development of the embryo and fetus.

Deoxygenated blood returning from the head and arms enters the right atrium through the superior vena cava. This blood is directed downward into the right ventricle, where it is squeezed into the pulmonary artery. A small amount of blood circulates through the resistant lung tissue, but the majority follows the path with less resistance through the ductus arteriosus into the aorta, distal to the point of exit of the arteries supplying the head and arms with oxygenated blood. The oxygen-poor blood flows through the abdominal aorta into the internal iliac arteries, where the umbilical arteries direct most of it back through the umbilical cord to the placenta. There the blood gives up its wastes and carbon dioxide in exchange for nutrients and oxygen. The blood remaining in the iliac arteries flows through the fetal abdomen and legs, ultimately returning through the inferior vena cava to the heart.

The following three special characteristics enable the fetus to obtain sufficient oxygen from the maternal blood:

1. Fetal hemoglobin carries 20 to 30% more oxygen than maternal hemoglobin.
2. The hemoglobin concentration of the fetus is about 50% greater than that of the mother.
3. The fetal heart rate is 110 to 160 beats per minute, making the cardiac output per unit of body weight higher than that of an adult.

Hematopoietic System

Hematopoiesis, the formation of blood, occurs in the yolk sac (see Fig. 9-8, B), beginning in the third week. Hematopoietic stem cells seed the fetal liver during the fifth week, and hematopoiesis begins there during the sixth week. This accounts for the relatively large size of the liver between the seventh and ninth weeks. Stem cells seed the fetal bone marrow, spleen and thymus, and lymph nodes between weeks 8 and 11.

The antigenic factors that determine blood type are present in the erythrocytes soon after the sixth week. For this reason, the Rh-negative woman is at risk for isoimmunization in any pregnancy that lasts longer than 6 weeks after fertilization.

Gastrointestinal System

During the fourth week, the shape of the embryo changes from being almost straight to a C shape as both ends fold in toward the ventral surface. A portion of the yolk sac is incorporated into the body from head to tail as the primitive gut (digestive system).

The foregut produces the pharynx, part of the lower respiratory tract, the esophagus, the stomach, the first half of the duodenum, the liver, the pancreas, and the gallbladder. These structures evolve during the fifth and sixth weeks. Malformations that can occur in these areas include esophageal atresia, hypertrophic pyloric stenosis, duodenal stenosis or atresia, and biliary atresia (see Chapter 46).

The midgut becomes the distal half of the duodenum, the jejunum and ileum, the cecum and appendix, and the proximal half of the colon. The midgut loop projects into the umbilical cord between weeks 5 and 10. A malformation, omphalocele, results if the midgut fails to return to the abdominal cavity, causing the intestines to protrude from the umbilicus. Meckel diverticulum is the most common malformation of the midgut. It occurs when a remnant of the yolk stalk that has failed to degenerate attaches to the ileum, leaving a blind sac.

The hindgut develops into the distal half of the colon, the rectum and parts of the anal canal, the urinary bladder, and the urethra. Anorectal malformations are the most common abnormalities of the digestive system.

The fetus swallows amniotic fluid beginning in the fifth month. Gastric emptying and intestinal peristalsis occur. Fetal nutrition and elimination needs are taken care of by the placenta. As the fetus nears term, fetal waste products accumulate in the intestines as dark green–to-black, tarry meconium. Normally this substance is passed through the rectum within 24 hours of birth. Sometimes with a breech presentation or fetal hypoxia, meconium is passed in utero into the amniotic fluid. The failure to pass meconium after birth may indicate atresia somewhere in the digestive tract; an imperforate anus (see Fig. 46-11); or meconium ileus, in which a firm meconium plug blocks passage (seen in infants with CF).

The metabolic rate of the fetus is relatively low, but the infant has great growth and development needs. Beginning in week 9, the fetus synthesizes glycogen for storage in the liver. Between 26 and 30 weeks, the fetus begins to lay down stores of brown fat in preparation for extrauterine cold stress. Thermoregulation in the neonate requires increased metabolism and adequate oxygenation.

The gastrointestinal system is mature by 36 weeks. Digestive enzymes (except pancreatic amylase and lipase) are present in sufficient quantity to facilitate digestion. The neonate cannot digest starches or fats efficiently. Little saliva is produced.

Hepatic System

The liver and biliary tract develop from the foregut during the fourth week of gestation. The embryonic liver is prominent, occupying most of the abdominal cavity. Bile, a constituent of meconium, begins to form in the twelfth week.

Glycogen is stored in the fetal liver beginning at week 9 or 10. At term, glycogen stores are twice those of the adult. Glycogen is the major source of energy for the fetus and for the neonate stressed by in utero hypoxia, extrauterine loss of the maternal glucose supply, the work of breathing, or cold stress.

Iron is also stored in the fetal liver. If maternal intake is sufficient, the fetus can store enough iron to last for 6 months after birth.

During fetal life the liver does not have to conjugate bilirubin for excretion because the unconjugated bilirubin is cleared by the placenta. Therefore, the glucuronyl transferase enzyme needed for conjugation is present in the fetal liver in amounts less than those required after birth. This predisposes the neonate, especially the preterm infant, to hyperbilirubinemia.

Coagulation factors II, VII, IX, and X cannot be synthesized in the fetal liver because of the lack of vitamin K synthesis in the sterile fetal gut. This coagulation deficiency persists after birth for several days and is the rationale for the prophylactic administration of vitamin K to the newborn.

Renal System

The kidneys form during the fifth week and begin to function approximately 4 weeks later. Urine is excreted into the amniotic fluid and forms a major part of the amniotic fluid volume. Oligohydramnios is indicative of renal dysfunction. Because the placenta acts as the organ of excretion and maintains fetal water and electrolyte balance, the fetus does not need functioning kidneys while in utero. However, at birth the kidneys are required immediately for excretory and acid–base regulatory functions.

A fetal renal malformation can be diagnosed in utero. Corrective or palliative fetal surgery may treat the malformation successfully, or plans can be made for treatment immediately after birth.

At term the fetus has fully developed kidneys. However, the glomerular filtration rate (GFR) is low, and the kidneys lack the ability to concentrate urine. This makes the newborn more susceptible to both overhydration and dehydration.

Neurological System

The nervous system originates from the ectoderm during the third week after fertilization. The open neural tube forms during the fourth week. It initially closes at what will be the junction of the brain and spinal cord, leaving both ends open. The embryo folds in on itself lengthwise at this time, forming a head fold in the neural tube at this junction. The cranial end of the neural tube closes, then the caudal end closes. During week 5, different growth rates cause more flexures in the neural tube, delineating three brain areas: the forebrain, midbrain, and hindbrain.

The forebrain develops into the eyes (cranial nerve II) and cerebral hemispheres. The development of all areas of the cerebral cortex continues throughout fetal life and into childhood. The olfactory system (cranial nerve I) and thalamus also develop from the forebrain. Cranial nerves III and IV (oculomotor and trochlear) form from the midbrain. The hindbrain forms the medulla, the pons, the cerebellum, and the remainder of the cranial nerves. Brain waves can be recorded on an electroencephalogram by week 8.

The spinal cord develops from the long end of the neural tube. Another ectodermal structure, the neural crest, develops into the peripheral nervous system. By the eighth week, nerve fibres traverse throughout the body. By week 11 or 12, the fetus makes respiratory movements, moves all extremities, and changes position in utero. The fetus can suck his or her thumb, swim in the amniotic fluid pool, and turn somersaults and can occasionally tie a knot in the umbilical cord.

At term, the fetal brain is approximately one fourth the size of an adult brain. Neurological development continues. Stressors on the fetus and neonate (e.g., chronic poor nutrition or hypoxia, drugs, environmental toxins, trauma, disease) damage the central nervous system long after the vulnerable embryonic time for malformations in other organ systems. Neurological insult can result in cerebral palsy, neuromuscular impairment, intellectual disability, and learning disabilities.

Sensory awareness. Purposeful movements of the fetus have been demonstrated in response to a firm touch transmitted through the mother's abdomen. Because it can feel, the fetus requires anaesthesia when invasive procedures are done.

Fetuses respond to sound by 24 weeks. Different types of music evoke different movements. The fetus can be soothed by the sound of the mother's voice. Acoustic stimulation can be used to evoke a fetal heart rate response. The fetus becomes accustomed (habituates) to noises heard repeatedly. Hearing is fully developed at birth.

The fetus is able to distinguish taste. By the fifth month, when the fetus is swallowing amniotic fluid, a sweetener added to the fluid causes the fetus to swallow faster. The fetus also reacts to temperature changes. A cold solution placed into the amniotic fluid can cause fetal hiccups.

The fetus can see. Eyes have both rods and cones in the retina by the seventh month. A bright light shone on the mother's abdomen in late pregnancy causes abrupt fetal movements. During sleep time rapid eye movements have been observed similar to those occurring in children and adults while dreaming.

Endocrine System

The thyroid gland develops along with structures in the head and neck during the third and fourth weeks. The secretion of thyroxine begins during the eighth week. Maternal thyroxine does not readily cross the placenta; therefore, the fetus that does not produce thyroid hormones will be born with congenital hypothyroidism. If untreated, hypothyroidism can result in severe developmental delay. Screening for hypothyroidism is included in the newborn screening done after birth.

The adrenal cortex is formed during the sixth week and produces hormones by the eighth or ninth week. As term approaches, the fetus produces more cortisol. This is believed to aid in initiation of labour by decreasing the maternal progesterone and stimulating production of prostaglandins.

The pancreas forms from the foregut during the fifth through eighth weeks. The islets of Langerhans develop during the twelfth week. Insulin is produced by week 20. In infants of mothers with uncontrolled diabetes, maternal hyperglycemia produces fetal hyperglycemia, stimulating hyperinsulinemia and islet cell hyperplasia. This results in a macrosomic (large-size) fetus. The hyperinsulinemia also blocks lung maturation, placing the neonate at risk for respiratory distress and hypoglycemia when the maternal glucose source is lost at birth. Control of the maternal glucose level before and during pregnancy minimizes problems for the fetus and infant.

Reproductive System

Sex differentiation begins in the embryo during the seventh week. Female and male external genitalia are indistinguishable until after the ninth week. Distinguishing characteristics appear around the ninth week and are fully differentiated by the twelfth week. When a Y chromosome is present, testes are formed. By the end of the embryonic period, testosterone is being secreted and causes formation of the male genitalia. By week 28, the testes begin descending into the scrotum. After birth, low levels of testosterone continue to be secreted until the pubertal surge.

The female, with two X chromosomes, forms ovaries and female external genitalia. By the sixteenth week, oogenesis has been established. At birth, the ovaries contain the female's lifetime supply of ova. Most female hormone production is delayed until puberty. However, the fetal endometrium responds to maternal hormones, and withdrawal bleeding or vaginal discharge (**pseudomenstruation**) may occur at birth when these hormones are lost. The high level of maternal estrogen also stimulates mammary engorgement and secretion of fluid ("witch's milk") in newborn infants of both sexes.

Musculoskeletal System

Bones and muscles develop from somites, which are masses of mesoderm, by the fourth week of embryonic development. At that time, the cardiac muscle is already beating. The mesoderm next to the neural tube forms the vertebral column and ribs. The parts of the vertebral column grow toward each other to enclose the developing spinal cord. *Ossification*, or bone formation, begins. If there is a defect in the bony fusion, various forms of spina bifida may occur. A large defect affecting several vertebrae may allow the membranes and spinal cord to pouch out from the back, producing neurological deficits and skeletal deformity.

The flat bones of the skull develop during the embryonic period, and ossification continues throughout childhood. At birth, connective tissue sutures exist where the bones of the skull meet. The areas where more than two bones meet (called **fontanels**) are especially prominent. The sutures and fontanels allow the bones of the skull to mould, or move during birth, enabling the head to pass through the birth canal.

The bones of the shoulders, arms, hips, and legs appear in the sixth week as a continuous skeleton with no joints. Differentiation occurs, producing separate bones and joints. Ossification continues through childhood to allow growth. Beginning in the seventh week muscles contract spontaneously. Arm and leg movements are visible on ultrasound examination, although the mother usually does not perceive them until sometime between 16 and 20 weeks.

Integumentary System

The epidermis begins as a single layer of cells derived from the ectoderm at 4 weeks. By the seventh week, there are two layers of cells. The cells of the superficial layer are sloughed and become mixed with the sebaceous gland secretions to form the white, cheesy **vernix caseosa**, the material that protects the skin of the fetus. The vernix is thick at 24 weeks but becomes scant by term.

The basal layer of the epidermis is the germinal layer, which replaces lost cells. Until 17 weeks, the skin is thin and wrinkled, with blood vessels visible underneath. The skin thickens, and all layers are present at term. After 32 weeks, as subcutaneous fat is deposited under the dermis, the skin becomes less wrinkled and red in appearance.

By 16 weeks, the epidermal ridges are present on the palms of the hands, the fingers, the bottom of the feet, and the toes. These handprints and footprints are unique to that infant.

Hairs form from hair bulbs in the epidermis that project into the dermis. Cells in the hair bulb keratinize to form the hair shaft. As the cells at the base of the hair shaft proliferate, the hair grows to the surface of the epithelium. Very fine hairs, called **lanugo**, appear first at 12 weeks on the eyebrows and upper lip. By week 20 they cover the entire body. At this time, the eyelashes, eyebrows, and scalp hair are beginning to grow. By week 28, the scalp hair is longer than the lanugo, which thins and may disappear by term gestation.

Fingernails and toenails develop from thickened epidermis at the tips of the digits beginning during the tenth week. They grow slowly. Fingernails usually reach the fingertips by 32 weeks, and toenails reach toe tips by 36 weeks.

Immunological System

During the third trimester, albumin and globulin are present in the fetus. The only immunoglobulin (Ig) that crosses the placenta, IgG, provides passive acquired immunity to specific bacterial toxins. The fetus produces IgM by the end of the first trimester. This is produced in response to blood group antigens, gram-negative enteric organisms, and some viruses. IgA is not produced by the fetus; however, **colostrum**, the precursor to breast milk, contains large amounts of IgA and can provide passive immunity to the neonate who is breastfed.

The normal-term neonate can fight infection but not as effectively as an older child. The preterm infant is at much greater risk for infection.

Table 9-1 summarizes embryonic and fetal development.

Multifetal Pregnancy

Twins

The incidence of twinning is 1 in 43 pregnancies (Benirschke, 2014). The rate of multiple birth has risen from 2.8% in 2001 to 3.2% in 2010 (Public Health Agency of Canada [PHAC], 2013). This is partly attributed to delayed child-bearing. The use of artificial reproductive technologies (ARTs) such as ovulation-enhancing drugs and in vitro fertilization (IVF) if more than one embryo is implanted is another factor.

Dizygotic twins. When two mature ova are produced in one ovarian cycle, both have the potential to be fertilized by separate sperm. This results in two zygotes, or dizygotic twins (Fig. 9-15).

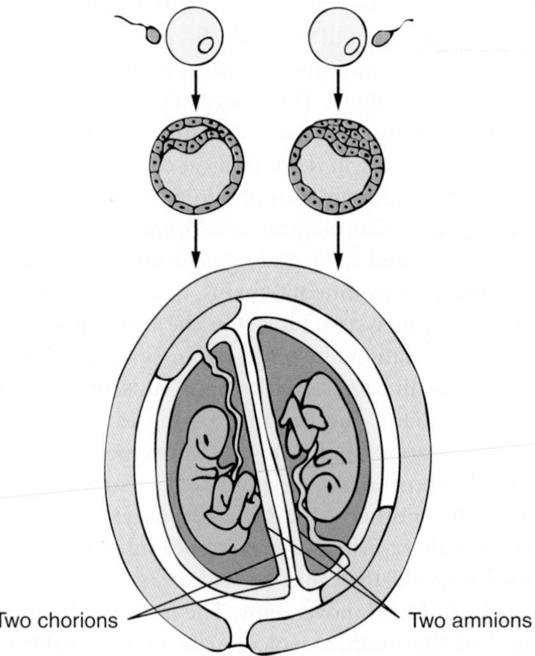

FIGURE 9-15 Formation of dizygotic twins. There is fertilization of two ova, two implantations, two placentas, two chorions, and two amnions.

TABLE 9-1 MILESTONES IN HUMAN DEVELOPMENT BEFORE BIRTH SINCE LAST MENSTRUAL PERIOD

4 WEEKS	8 WEEKS	12 WEEKS
External Appearance		
Body flexed, C-shaped; arm and leg buds present; head at right angles to body	Body fairly well formed; nose flat, eyes far apart; digits well formed; head elevating; tail almost disappeared; eyes, ears, nose, and mouth recognizable	Nails appearing; resembles a human; head erect but disproportionately large; skin pink, delicate
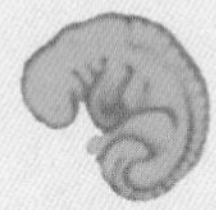	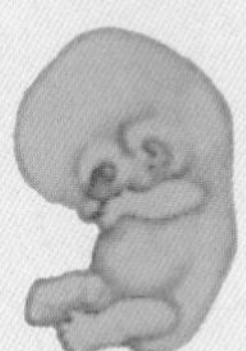	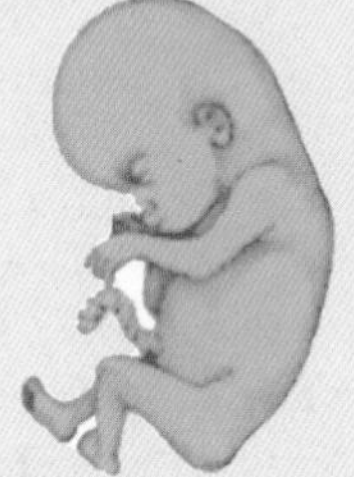
Crown-to-Rump Measurement; Weight		
0.4–0.5 cm; 0.4 g	2.5–3 cm; 2 g	6–9 cm; 19 g
Gastrointestinal System		
Stomach at midline and fusiform; conspicuous liver; esophagus short; intestine a short tube	Intestinal villi developing; small intestines coil within umbilical cord; palatal folds present; liver very large	Bile secreted; palatal fusion complete; intestines have withdrawn from cord and assume characteristic positions
Musculoskeletal System		
All somites present	First indication of ossification—occiput, mandible, and humerus; fetus capable of some movement; definitive muscles of trunk, limbs, and head well represented	Some bones well outlined, ossification spreading; upper cervical to lower sacral arches and bodies ossify; smooth muscle layers indicated in hollow viscera
Circulatory System		
Heart develops, double chambers visible, begins to beat; aortic arch and major veins completed	Main blood vessels assume final plan; enucleated red cells predominate in blood	Blood forming in marrow
Respiratory System		
Primary lung buds appear	Pleural and pericardial cavities forming; branching bronchioles; nostrils closed by epithelial plugs	Lungs acquire definite shape; vocal cords appear
Renal System		
Rudimentary ureteral buds appear	Earliest secretory tubules differentiating; bladder-urethra separates from rectum	Kidney able to secrete urine; bladder expands as a sac
Nervous System		
Well-marked midbrain flexure; no hindbrain or cervical flexures; neural groove closed	Cerebral cortex begins to acquire typical cells; differentiation of cerebral cortex, meninges, ventricular foramina, cerebrospinal fluid circulation; spinal cord extends along entire length of spine	Brain structural configuration almost complete; cord shows cervical and lumbar enlargements; fourth ventricle foramina are developed; sucking present
Sensory Organs		
Eye and ear appearing as optic vessel and otocyst	Primordial choroid plexuses develop; ventricles large relative to cortex; development progressing; eyes converging rapidly; internal ear developing	Earliest taste buds indicated; characteristic organization of eye attained
Genital System		
Genital ridge appears (fifth week)	Testes and ovaries distinguishable; external genitalia sexless but begin to differentiate	Sex recognizable; internal and external sex organs specific

Continued

TABLE 9-1 MILESTONES IN HUMAN DEVELOPMENT BEFORE BIRTH SINCE LAST MENSTRUAL PERIOD—cont'd

	16 WEEKS	20 WEEKS	24 WEEKS
External Appearance	Head still dominant; face looks human; eyes, ears, and nose approach typical appearance on gross examination; arm/leg ratio proportionate; scalp hair appears	Vernix caseosa appears; lanugo appears; legs lengthen considerably; sebaceous glands appear	Body lean but fairly well proportioned; skin red and wrinkled; vernix caseosa present; sweat glands forming
	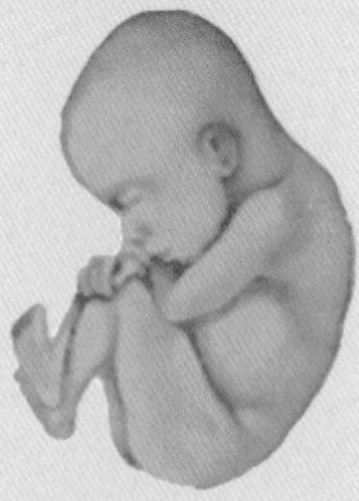	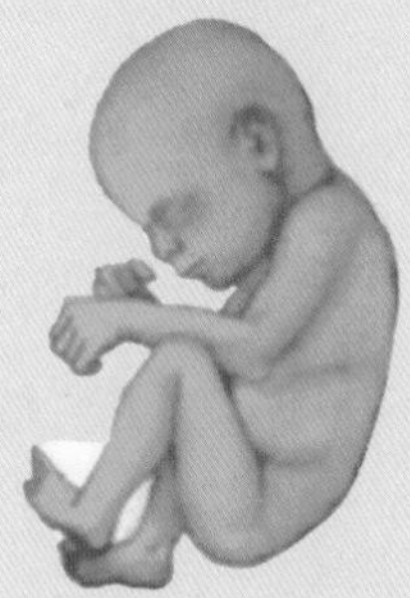	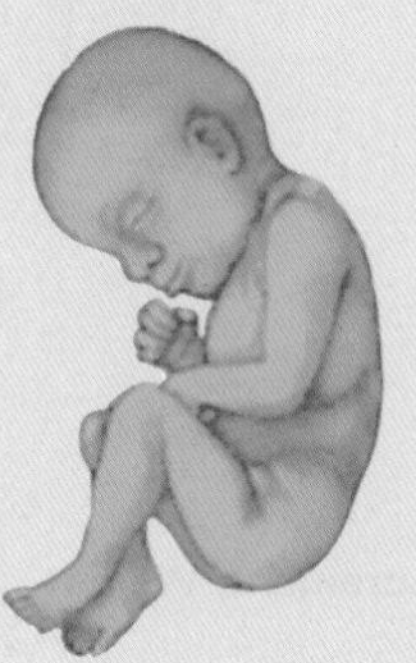
Crown-to-Rump Measurement; Weight	11.5–13.5 cm; 100 g	16–18.5 cm; 300 g	23 cm; 600 g
Gastrointestinal System	Meconium in bowel; some enzyme secretion; anus open	Enamel and dentine depositing; ascending colon recognizable	
Musculoskeletal System	Most bones distinctly indicated throughout body; joint cavities appear; muscular movements can be detected	Sternum ossifies; fetal movements strong enough for mother to feel	
Circulatory System	Heart muscle well developed; blood formation active in spleen		Blood formation increases in bone marrow and decreases in liver
Respiratory System	Elastic fibres appear in lungs; terminal and respiratory bronchioles appear	Nostrils reopen; primitive respiratory-like movements begin	Alveolar ducts and sacs present; lecithin begins to appear in amniotic fluid (wk 26–27)
Renal System	Kidney in position; attains typical shape and plan		
Nervous System	Cerebral lobes delineated; cerebellum assumes some prominence	Brain grossly formed; cord myelination begins; spinal cord ends at level of first sacral vertebra (S-1)	Cerebral cortex layered typically; neuronal proliferation in cerebral cortex ends
Sensory Organs	General sense organs differentiated	Nose and ears ossify	Can hear
Genital System	Testes in position for descent into scrotum; vagina open		Testes at inguinal ring in descent to scrotum

TABLE 9-1 MILESTONES IN HUMAN DEVELOPMENT BEFORE BIRTH SINCE LAST MENSTRUAL PERIOD—cont'd

28 WEEKS	30–31 WEEKS	36 AND 40 WEEKS
External Appearance		
Lean body, less wrinkled and red; nails appear	Subcutaneous fat beginning to collect; more rounded appearance; skin pink and smooth; has assumed birth position 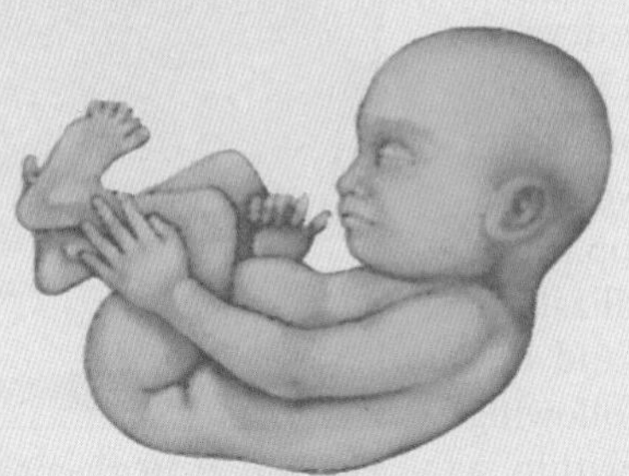	36 wk—Skin pink, body rounded; general lanugo disappearing; body usually plump 40 wk—Skin smooth and pink; scant vernix caseosa; moderate-to-profuse hair; lanugo on shoulders and upper body only; nasal and alar cartilage apparent
Crown-to-Rump Measurement; Weight		
27 cm; 1100 g	31 cm; 1800–2100 g	36 wk—35 cm; 2200–2900 g 40 wk—40 cm; 3200+ g
Musculoskeletal System		
Astragalus (talus, ankle bone) ossifies; weak, fleeting movements; minimum tone	Middle fourth phalanxes ossify; permanent teeth primordia seen; can turn head to side	36 wk—Distal femoral ossification centres present; sustained, definite movements; fair tone; can turn and elevate head 40 wk—Active, sustained movement; good tone; may lift head
Respiratory System		
Lecithin forming on alveolar surfaces	L/S ratio = 1.2 : 1	36 wk—L/S ratio ≥ 2 : 1 40 wk—Pulmonary branching only two thirds complete
Renal System		
		36 wk—Formation of new nephrons ceases
Nervous System		
Appearance of cerebral fissures, convolutions rapidly appearing; indefinite sleep–wake cycle; cry weak or absent; weak suck reflex		36 wk—End of spinal cord at level of third lumbar vertebra (L3); definite sleep–wake cycle 40 wk—Myelination of brain begins; patterned sleep–wake cycle with alert periods; cries when hungry or uncomfortable; strong suck reflex
Sensory Organs		
Eyelids reopen; retinal layers completed, light receptive; pupils capable of reacting to light	Sense of taste present; aware of sounds outside mother's body	
Genital System		
	Testes descending to scrotum	40 wk—Testes in scrotum; labia majora well developed

L/S, lecithin/sphingomyelin.

There are always two amnions, two chorions, and two placentas that may be fused together (Fig. 9-16). These dizygotic or fraternal twins may be the same sex or different sexes and are genetically no more alike than siblings born at different times. Dizygotic twinning occurs most often in families with a history of twinning. Dizygotic twinning increases in frequency with maternal age up to 35 years, with parity, and with the use of fertility drugs.

Monozygotic twins. Identical or monozygotic twins develop from one fertilized ovum, which then divides (Fig. 9-17). They are the same sex and have the same genotype. If division occurs soon after fertilization, two embryos, two amnions, two chorions, and two placentas that may be fused will develop. Most often division occurs between 4 and 8 days after fertilization; there are two embryos, two amnions, one chorion, and one placenta. Rarely division occurs after the eighth day following fertilization. In this case, there are two embryos within a common amnion and a common chorion with one placenta. This often causes circulatory problems because the umbilical cords may tangle together, and one or both fetuses may die. If division occurs very late, cleavage may not be complete and conjoined, or "Siamese," twins could result (see Fig. 9-17, C).

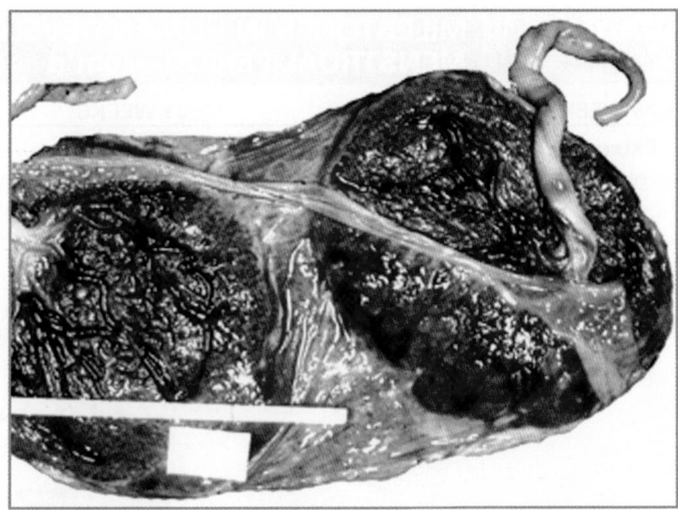

FIGURE 9-16 Diamniotic dichorionic (separate) twin placentas. (From Benirschke, K. [2014]. Multiple gestation: The biology of twinning. In R. Creasy, R. Resnik, J. Iams, et al. [Eds.], *Creasy & Resnik's maternal-fetal medicine: Principles and practice* [7th ed.]. Philadelphia: Saunders.)

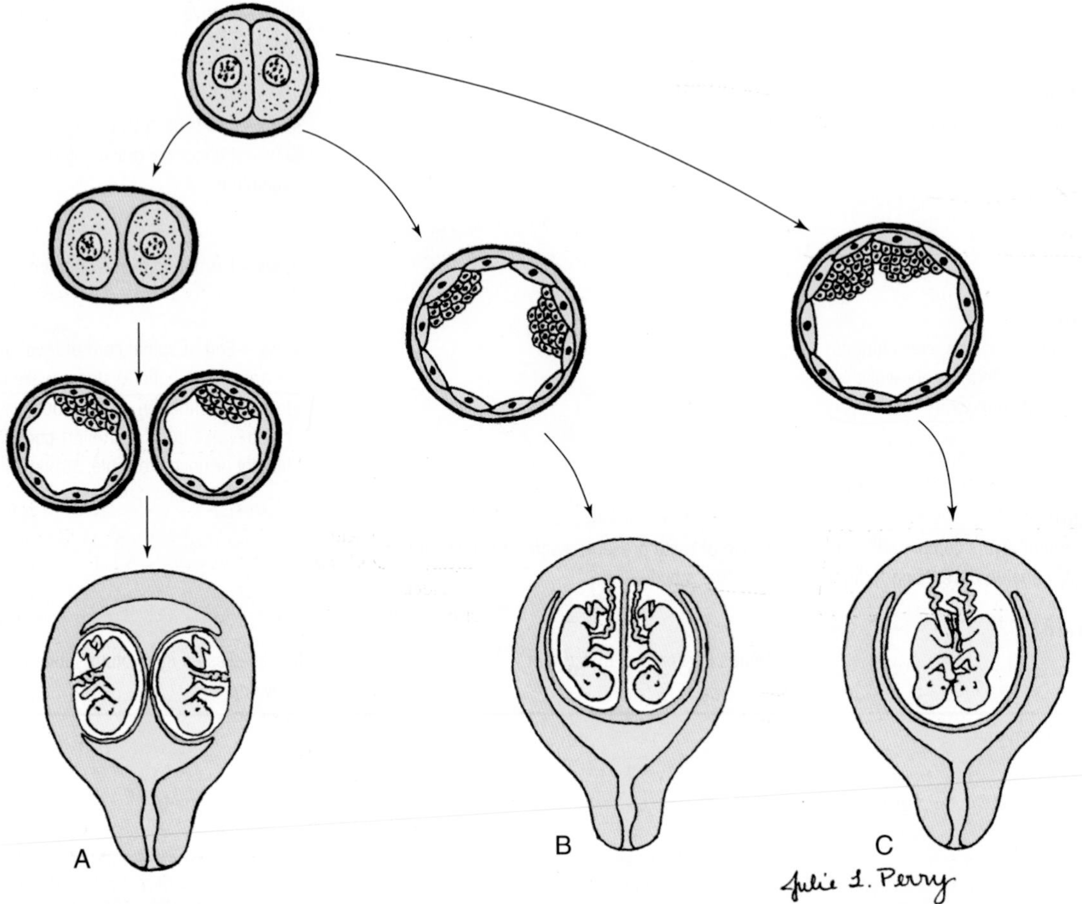

FIGURE 9-17 Formation of monozygotic twins. **A:** One fertilization: blastomeres separate, resulting in two implantations, two placentas, and two sets of membranes. **B:** One blastomere with two inner cell masses, one fused placenta, one chorion, and separate amnions. **C:** One blastomere with incomplete separation of cell mass, resulting in conjoined twins.

Monozygotic twinning occurs in approximately 3.5 to 4 per 1000 births (Benirschke, 2014). There is no association with race, heredity, maternal age, or parity. Fertility drugs also increase the incidence of monozygotic twinning.

Conjoined twins. Conjoined twins are a type of monozygotic twins in which there is incomplete embryonic division at 13 to 15 days postconception (see Fig. 9-17). The estimated frequency is 1 in 50,000 births (Malone & D'Alton, 2014). Prenatal diagnosis is possible with three-dimensional ultrasonography. Caesarean birth minimizes trauma to mother and fetuses.

Other Multifetal Pregnancies

The occurrence of multifetal pregnancies with three or more fetuses has increased with the use of fertility drugs and IVF. Triplets occur in about 1 of 1341 pregnancies (Benirschke, 2014). They can occur from the division of one zygote into two, with one of the two dividing again, producing identical triplets. Triplets can also be produced from two zygotes, one dividing into a set of identical twins and the second zygote a single fraternal sibling, or from three zygotes. Quadruplets, quintuplets, sextuplets, and so on have similar possible derivations.

KEY POINTS

- Preconception counselling is important to improve the health of all women and to ensure healthy pregnancy outcomes.
- Genetic disease affects people of all ages, from all socioeconomic levels, and from all racial and ethnic backgrounds.
- Genetic disorders span every clinical practice specialty.
- Nurses have a role to play in genetic counselling.
- Genes are the basic units of heredity responsible for all human characteristics. They comprise 23 pairs of chromosomes: 22 pairs of autosomes and one pair of sex chromosomes.
- Genetic disorders follow Mendelian inheritance patterns of dominance and segregation and an independent assortment of normal genetic transmission.
- Multifactorial inheritance includes both genetic and environmental contributions.
- Human gestation is approximately 280 days after the LMP or 266 days after conception.
- Fertilization occurs in the uterine tube within 24 hours of ovulation. The zygote undergoes mitotic divisions, creating a 16-cell morula.
- Critical periods occur in human development during which the embryo or fetus is vulnerable to environmental teratogens.
- There has been a steady rise in the incidence of multifetal pregnancies, which is partly due to ART and the increasing age at which women give birth.

evolve WEBSITE

Visit the Evolve website for additional resources related to the content in this chapter such as Case Studies, Critical Thinking Case Study Answers, Nursing Care Plans, Nursing Processes, Nursing Skills, and Review Questions for Exam Preparation at: http://evolve.elsevier.com/Canada/Perry/maternal/

REFERENCES

Benirschke, K. (2014). Multiple gestation. The biology of twinning. In R. K. Creasy, R. Resnik, J. D. Iams, et al. (Eds.), *Creasy and Resnik's maternal-fetal medicine: Principles and practice* (7th ed.). Philadelphia: Saunders.

Canadian Down Syndrome Society. (n.d.). *Celebrate being: About Down syndrome*. Retrieved from <http://www.cdss.ca/images/pdf/brochures/english/celebrate_being_about_down_syndrome_english.pdf>.

Cunningham, F., Leveno, K., Bloom, S., et al. (2014). *Williams obstetrics* (25th ed.). New York: McGraw-Hill.

Groden, J., Gocha, A., & Croce, A. (2014). Human basic genetics and patterns of inheritance. In R. K. Creasy, R. Resnik, J. D. Iams, et al. (Eds.), *Creasy & Resnik's maternal-fetal medicine: Principles and practice* (7th ed.). Philadelphia: Saunders.

Guttmacher, A., McGuire, A., Ponder, B., et al. (2010). Personalized genomic information: Preparing for the future of genetic medicine. *Nature Reviews Genetics*, *11*(2), 161–165.

Jobe, A. H., & Kamath-Rayne, B. D. (2014). Fetal lung development and surfactant. In R. K. Creasy, R. Resnik, J. D. Iams, et al. (Eds.), *Creasy & Resnik's maternal-fetal medicine: Principles and practice* (7th ed.). Philadelphia: Saunders.

Johnson, J., Tough, S., & Society of Obstetricians and Gynaecologists of Canada. (2012). SOGC committee opinion: Delayed childbearing. *Journal of Obstetrics and Gynaecology Canada*, *34*(1), 80–93.

Jorde, L., Carey, J. C., & Bamshad, M. J. (2015). *Medical genetics* (5th ed.). St. Louis: Mosby.

Malone, F., & D'Alton, M. (2014). Multiple gestation: Clinical characteristics and management. In R. K. Creasy, R. Resnik, J. D. Iams, et al. (Eds.), *Creasy & Resnik's maternal-fetal medicine: Principles and practice* (7th ed.). Philadelphia: Saunders.

Martin, R. (2008). Meiotic errors in human oogenesis and spermatogenesis. *Reproductive Biomedicine Online*, *16*(4), 523–531.

McGuire, A., & Burke, W. (2010). An unwelcome side effect of direct-to-consumer personal genome testing. *Journal of the American Medical Association*, *300*(22), 2669–2671.

Moore, K. L., Persaud, T. V. N., & Torchia, M. G. (2013). *Before we are born: Essentials of embryology and birth defects* (8th ed.). Philadelphia: Saunders.

Public Health Agency of Canada. (2013). *Perinatal health indicators for Canada 2013: A report of the Canadian Perinatal Surveillance System (Cat. No. HP7-1/2013E-PDF)*. Ottawa: Author. Retrieved from <http://publications.gc.ca/collections/collection_2014/aspc-phac/HP7-1-2013-eng.pdf>.

Society of Obstetricians and Gynaecologists of Canada. (2007). Prenatal screening for fetal aneuploidy. *Journal of Obstetrics and Gynaecology Canada*, *29*(20), 146–161.

Wapner, R. J. (2014). Prenatal diagnosis of congenital disorders. In R. K. Creasy, et al. (Eds.), *Creasy & Resnik's maternal-fetal medicine: Principles and practice* (7th ed.). Philadelphia: Saunders.

Wilson, R. D., Audibert, F., Brock, J.-A., et al. (2011). SOGC clinical practice guideline: Genetic considerations for a women's pre-conception evaluation. *Journal of Obstetrics and Gynaecology Canada*, *33*(1), 57–64.

ADDITIONAL RESOURCES

Canadian Association of Genetic Counsellors: <https://cagc-accg.ca/>.
Canadian Down Syndrome Society: <http://www.cdss.ca>.
Cystic Fibrosis Canada: <http://www.cysticfibrosis.ca/>.
Indiana University—Fetal circulatory system learning aid: <http://www.indiana.edu/~anat550/cvanim/fetcirc/fetcirc.html>.
Muscular Dystrophy Canada: <http://www.muscle.ca/>.
Society of Obstetricians and Gynaecologists of Canada: Committee Opinion—Delayed Childbearing: <http://sogc.org/guidelines/delayed-child-bearing-committee-opinion/>.
The Visible Embryo: <http://www.visembryo.com>.

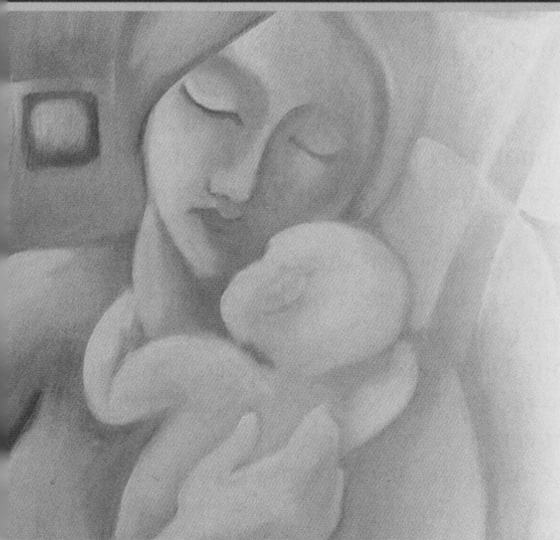

CHAPTER 10

Anatomy and Physiology of Pregnancy

Lisa Keenan-Lindsay

evolve WEBSITE

Visit the Evolve website for additional resources related to the content in this chapter such as Case Studies, Critical Thinking Case Study Answers, Nursing Care Plans, Nursing Processes, Nursing Skills, and Review Questions for Exam Preparation at: http://evolve.elsevier.com/Canada/Perry/maternal/

OBJECTIVES

On completion of this chapter the reader will be able to:

- Determine obstetrical history using the five-digit system.
- Describe the various types of pregnancy tests, including timing and interpretation of results.
- Explain the expected maternal anatomical and physiological adaptations to pregnancy.
- Differentiate among presumptive, probable, and positive signs of pregnancy.
- Identify maternal hormones produced during pregnancy, their target organs, and their major effects on pregnancy.
- Compare the characteristics of the abdomen, vulva, and cervix of the nullipara and multipara.

The goal of maternity care is a healthy pregnancy with a physically safe and emotionally satisfying outcome for mother, infant, and family. Consistent health care and surveillance are important in order to achieve this goal. However, many maternal adaptations are unfamiliar to pregnant women and their families. Helping the pregnant woman recognize the relationship between her physical status and the plan for her care can enable her to make good decisions and encourages her to participate in her care.

OBSTETRICAL TERMINOLOGY

An understanding of the following terms used to describe pregnancy and the pregnant woman (Cunningham, Leveno, Bloom, et al., 2014) is essential to the study of maternity care (Leduc, Biringer, Lee, et al., 2013; Spong, 2013):

Gravida—A woman who is pregnant

Gravidity—Pregnancy

Multigravida—A woman who has had two or more pregnancies

Multipara—A woman who has completed two or more pregnancies to 20 weeks of gestation or more

Nulligravida—A woman who has never been pregnant and is not currently pregnant

Nullipara—A woman who has not completed a pregnancy with a fetus or fetuses beyond 20 weeks of gestation

Parity—The number of pregnancies in which the fetus or fetuses have reached 20 weeks of gestation, not the number of fetuses (e.g., twins) born. Parity is not affected by whether the fetus is born alive or is stillborn (i.e., showing no signs of life at birth).

Primigravida—A woman who is pregnant for the first time

Primipara—A woman who has completed one pregnancy with a fetus or fetuses who have reached 20 weeks of gestation

Viability—Capacity to live outside the uterus, occurring about 22 to 25 weeks of gestation

Term—A pregnancy from the beginning of week 37 of gestation to the end of week 40 plus 6 days of gestation

- **Preterm**—A pregnancy that has reached 20 weeks of gestation but prior to completion of 36 weeks of gestation
- **Early Term**—A pregnancy between 37 weeks and 38 weeks 6 days

Full Term—A pregnancy between 39 weeks and 40 weeks 6 days
Late Term—A pregnancy in the 41st week
Post Term—A pregnancy after 42 weeks

Information about obstetrical history is gathered during history-taking interviews. Obtaining and documenting this information accurately is important in planning care for the pregnant woman.

The five-digit system, separated by hyphens, provides information about the woman's obstetrical history. The first digit represents gravidity (number of all pregnancies); the second digit represents the total number of term births (at 37 or more weeks' gestation); the third indicates the number of preterm births (after 20 weeks to 37 weeks' gestation); the fourth identifies the number of abortions (miscarriage or elective termination of pregnancy); and the fifth is the number of children currently living. The number of births is the actual number of children born during each pregnancy. The acronym GTPAL (gravidity, term, preterm, abortions, living children) may be helpful in remembering this system of notation. For example, if a woman who is pregnant only once gives birth at week 35 and the infant survives, the abbreviation that represents this information is "1-0-1-0-1." During her next pregnancy the abbreviation would be "2-0-1-0-1." Additional examples are given in Table 10-1.

Another system that is sometimes used is gravidity/parity, described as two digits. The first digit (G) indicates the number of pregnancies the woman has had, and the parity (P) indicates the number of pregnancies that have reached 20 weeks' gestation. It is important to remember that *para* refers to pregnancies, not fetuses. This system can be confusing and does not provide enough information about the woman, so it should not be used.

PREGNANCY TESTS

Early detection of pregnancy encourages early initiation of care. Human chorionic gonadotropin (hCG) is the earliest biological marker for pregnancy. Pregnancy tests are based on the recognition of hCG or a beta (β) subunit of hCG. Production of β-hCG begins as early as the day of implantation and can be detected as early as 7 to 10 days after conception. The level of hCG rises until it peaks at about 60 to 70 days of gestation and then declines until about 80 days of gestation. It remains stable until about 30 weeks and then gradually increases until term. Higher than normal levels of hCG may indicate ectopic pregnancy, abnormal gestation (e.g., fetus with Down syndrome), or multiple gestation; an abnormally slow increase or a decrease in hCG levels may indicate impending miscarriage (Cunningham et al., 2014).

Serum and urine pregnancy tests are performed in clinics, offices, women's health centres, public health unit clinics, and laboratory settings. Urine pregnancy tests may be performed at home (see Community Focus box). Both serum and urine tests can provide accurate results. A 7- to 10-mL sample of venous blood is collected for serum testing. Most urine tests require a first-voided morning urine specimen because it contains levels of hCG approximately the same as those in serum. Random urine samples usually have lower levels. Urine tests are less expensive and provide more immediate results than serum tests.

Many different pregnancy tests are available (Fig. 10-1). The wide variety of tests precludes discussion of each. The nurse should read the manufacturer's directions for the test that is used.

Enzyme-linked immunosorbent assay (ELISA) testing is the most popular method of testing for pregnancy. It uses a specific monoclonal antibody (anti-hCG) with enzymes that bond with hCG in urine. ELISA technology is the basis for most over-the-counter home pregnancy tests. With these one-step tests the woman usually applies urine to a strip or absorbent-tipped applicator and reads the results. The test kits come with directions for collection of the specimen, the testing procedure, and reading of results. A positive test result is indicated by a simple colour change reaction or a digital reading. The most common

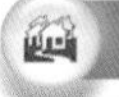

COMMUNITY FOCUS

Home Pregnancy Test Kits

Visit a pharmacy in your neighbourhood. How many different types of pregnancy home test kits are available in the pharmacy? Read the labels on three different types of pregnancy home test kits. Do the kits include material for more than one test? Are the directions printed in more than one language? After reading the directions, do you have questions about how to perform the test or how to interpret the results? If so, what does that say about the likelihood that the tests will be used correctly?

TABLE 10-1 EXAMPLES OF OBSTETRICAL HISTORY INFORMATION

	FIVE-DIGIT SYSTEM				
	G	T	P	A	L
CONDITION	GRAVIDITY	TERM BIRTH	PRETERM BIRTHS	ABORTIONS AND MISCARRIAGES	LIVING CHILDREN
Kathy is pregnant for the first time.	1	0	0	0	0
She carries the pregnancy to term, and the newborn survives.	1	1	0	0	1
She is pregnant again.	2	1	0	0	1
Her second pregnancy ends in miscarriage at 10 wk.	2	1	0	1	1
During her third pregnancy she gives birth at 36 wk to twins.	3	1	2	1	3

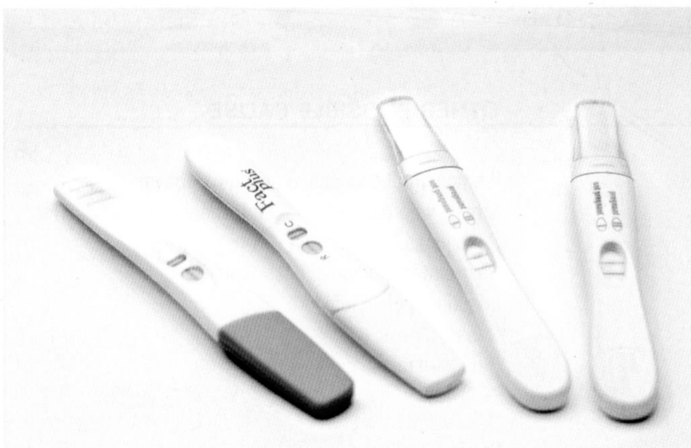

FIGURE 10-1 Many pregnancy test products are available over the counter. (THE CANADIAN PRESS/Francis Vachon.)

error in performing home pregnancy tests is doing the test too early in pregnancy before a significant rise in hCG level; this can cause a false-negative result (Pagana, Pagana, & Pike-MacDonald, 2013).

Interpreting the results of pregnancy tests requires some judgement. The type of pregnancy test and its degree of sensitivity (the ability to detect low levels of a substance) and specificity (the ability to discern the absence of a substance) must be considered in conjunction with the woman's history. This includes the date of her last normal menstrual period, her usual cycle length, and results of previous pregnancy tests. It is important to know if the woman is taking any medications or is a problematic substance user. Medications such as anticonvulsants and tranquilizers can cause false-positive results, whereas diuretics and promethazine can cause false-negative results (Pagana et al., 2013). Improper collection of the specimen, hormone-producing tumours, and laboratory errors can also cause inaccurate results.

Women who use a home pregnancy test should be advised about the variations in accuracy reporting and to use caution when interpreting results. Whenever there is any question, further evaluation or retesting may be appropriate.

CRITICAL THINKING CASE STUDY

Awareness of Physiological Changes of Pregnancy

Marlys is pregnant with her first child, and Janice is pregnant with her third child. They are both at approximately 18 weeks of gestation and have come to a prenatal appointment. While they are in the waiting room, you overhear Marlys asking Janice about the changes that she has noticed since her pregnancy and whether they are normal and will go away. Marlys says that she has not felt her baby move yet, whereas Janice says that she has been feeling fetal movement for over 2 weeks. Marlys also has questions about some of the changes in her body that she has experienced or expects to experience. Janice bases her responses on her own experience. Based on the conversation you have overheard, you identify a need to spend some time with Marlys and Janice discussing physiological changes of pregnancy.

QUESTIONS

1. Evidence—Is there sufficient evidence to draw conclusions about the normal physiological changes in pregnancy in primigravidas and multigravidas that the nurse should discuss with Marlys and Janice?
2. Assumptions—Describe an underlying assumption about each of the following topics:
   a. Differences in the normal physiological changes in pregnancy between primigravidas and multigravidas
   b. Reversibility of these physiological changes in pregnancy
   c. Information provided by the health care provider
   d. Deviations from normal in the physiological changes of pregnancy
3. What implications and priorities for nursing care can be drawn at this time?
4. Does the evidence objectively support your conclusion?

ADAPTATIONS TO PREGNANCY

Maternal physiological adaptations are attributed to the hormones of pregnancy and to mechanical pressures arising from the enlarging uterus and other tissues. These adaptations protect the woman's normal physiological functioning, meet the metabolic demands that pregnancy imposes on her body, and provide a nurturing environment for fetal development and growth (see Critical Thinking Case Study). Although pregnancy is a normal phenomenon, occasionally problems can occur.

Signs of Pregnancy

Some physiological adaptations are recognized as the signs and symptoms of pregnancy. Three commonly used categories of these signs and symptoms are as follows:

- Presumptive—those subjective changes felt by the woman (e.g., amenorrhea, fatigue, breast changes)
- Probable—those objective changes observed by an examiner (e.g., Hegar sign, ballottement, pregnancy tests)
- Positive—those signs attributed only to the presence of the fetus (e.g., hearing fetal heart tones, visualizing the fetus, palpating fetal movements)

Occasionally, these signs may mean something else besides the presence of a fetus. Table 10-2 summarizes these signs of pregnancy in relation to when they might occur and gives other possible causes for their occurrence.

Reproductive System and Breasts

Uterus

Changes in size, shape, and position. High levels of estrogen and progesterone stimulate phenomenal uterine growth in the first trimester. Early uterine enlargement results from increased vascularity and dilation of blood vessels, hyperplasia (production of new muscle fibres and fibroelastic tissue) and hypertrophy (enlargement of pre-existing muscle fibres and fibroelastic tissue), and development of the decidua. By 7 weeks of gestation the uterus is the size of a large hen's egg; by 10 weeks it is the size of an orange (twice its nonpregnant size); and by 12 weeks it is the size of a grapefruit. After the third month, uterine enlargement is primarily the result of mechanical pressure of the growing fetus.

As the uterus enlarges, it also changes in shape and position. At conception the uterus is shaped like an upside-down pear. During the second trimester, as the muscular walls strengthen

TABLE 10-2 SIGNS OF PREGNANCY

TIME OF OCCURRENCE (GESTATIONAL AGE)	SIGN	OTHER POSSIBLE CAUSE
Presumptive		
3–4 wk	Breast changes	Premenstrual changes, oral contraceptives
4 wk	Amenorrhea	Stress, vigorous exercise, early menopause, endocrine problems, malnutrition
4–14 wk	Nausea, vomiting	Gastrointestinal virus, gastroenteritis
6–12 wk	Urinary frequency	Infection, pelvic tumours
12 wk	Fatigue	Stress, illness
16–20 wk	Quickening	Gas, peristalsis
Probable		
5–6 wk	Goodell sign	Pelvic congestion
6–8 wk	Chadwick sign	Pelvic congestion
6–12 wk	Hegar sign	Pelvic congestion
4–12 wk	Positive pregnancy test (serum)	Hydatidiform mole, choriocarcinoma
6–12 wk	Positive pregnancy test (urine)	False-positive result may be caused by pelvic infection, tumours
16 wk	Braxton Hicks or prelabour contractions	Myomas, other tumours
16–28 wk	Ballottement	Tumours, cervical polyps
Positive		
5–6 wk	Visualization of fetus by real-time ultrasound examination	No other causes
6 wk	Fetal heart tones detected by ultrasound examination	No other causes
16 wk	Visualization of fetus by radiographic study	No other causes
8–17 wk	Fetal heart tones detected by Doppler ultrasound stethoscope	No other causes
17–19 wk	Fetal heart tones detected by fetal stethoscope	No other causes
19–22 wk	Fetal movements palpated	No other causes
Late pregnancy	Fetal movements visible	No other causes

and become more elastic, the uterus becomes spherical or globular. Later, as the fetus lengthens, the uterus becomes larger and more ovoid and rises out of the pelvis into the abdominal cavity.

The pregnancy may "show" after the fourteenth week, although this may depend on the woman's height and weight. Abdominal enlargement may be less apparent in the nullipara with good abdominal muscle tone (Fig. 10-2). Posture also influences the type and degree of abdominal enlargement that occurs. In normal pregnancies, the uterus enlarges at a predictable rate.

As the uterus grows, it may be palpated above the symphysis pubis sometime between the twelfth and fourteenth weeks of pregnancy (Fig. 10-3). The uterus rises gradually to the level of the umbilicus at 20 to 22 weeks of gestation and nearly reaches the xiphoid process at term. Between weeks 38 and 40, fundal height decreases as the fetus begins to descend and engage in the pelvis (**lightening**) (see Fig. 10-3, dashed line). Generally, lightening occurs in the nullipara anytime in the last 4 weeks before the onset of labour and in the multipara at the start of labour.

Uterine enlargement is determined by measuring fundal height (see Fig. 11-6). This measurement is commonly used to estimate the duration of pregnancy. However, variation in the position of the fundus or the fetus, variations in the amount of amniotic fluid present, the presence of more than one fetus, maternal obesity, and variation in examiner technique can reduce the accuracy of this estimation.

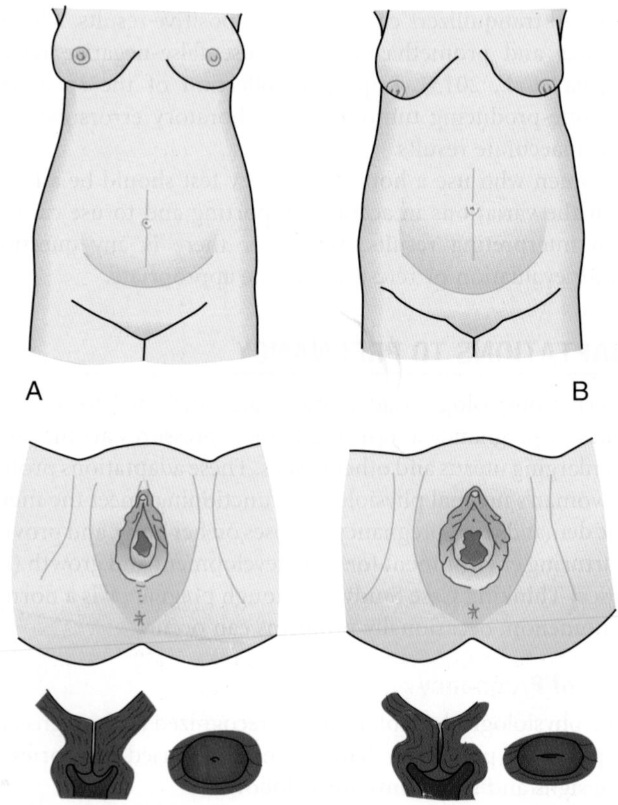

FIGURE 10-2 Comparison of abdomen, vulva, and cervix in **A,** nullipara, and **B,** multipara, at the same stage of pregnancy.

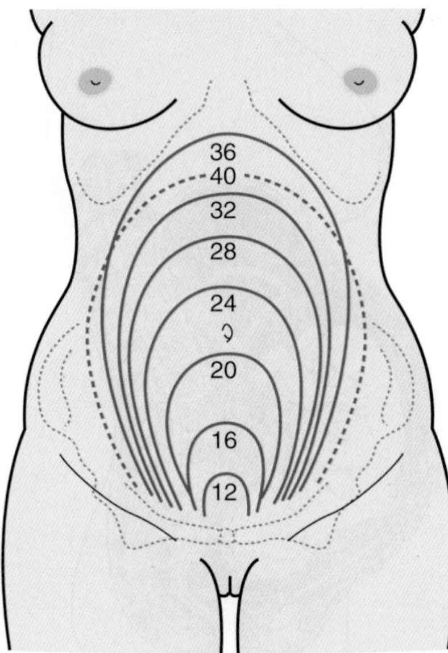

FIGURE 10-3 Height of fundus by weeks of normal gestation with a single fetus. *Dashed line*, height after lightening.

Generally, the uterus rotates to the right as it elevates, probably because of the presence of the rectosigmoid colon on the left side. However, the extensive hypertrophy (enlargement) of the round ligaments keeps the uterus in the midline. Eventually, the growing uterus touches the anterior abdominal wall and displaces the intestines to either side of the abdomen (Fig. 10-4). When a pregnant woman is standing, most of her uterus rests against the anterior abdominal wall; this can alter her centre of gravity.

At approximately 6 weeks of gestation, softening and compressibility of the lower uterine segment (uterine isthmus) occurs (**Hegar sign**) (Fig. 10-5). This results in exaggerated uterine anteflexion during the first 3 months of pregnancy. In this position, the uterine fundus presses on the urinary bladder, causing the woman to have urinary frequency.

Changes in contractility. Soon after the fourth month of pregnancy, uterine contractions can be felt through the abdominal wall. These contractions, referred to as prelabour contractions (or **Braxton Hicks contractions**), are irregular and painless contractions that occur intermittently throughout pregnancy. These contractions facilitate uterine blood flow through the intervillous spaces of the placenta and promote oxygen delivery to the fetus. Although prelabour contractions are not painful, some women are surprised by them and over time may find them to be annoying. After the twenty-eighth week, these contractions become more definite, but they usually cease with walking or exercise. Prelabour contractions can be mistaken for true labour; however, they do not increase in intensity or duration or cause cervical dilation. Conversely, premature labour contractions can be mistaken for prelabour contractions and thus lead to a delay in seeking treatment.

Uteroplacental blood flow. Placental perfusion depends on the maternal blood flow to the uterus. Blood flow increases rapidly as the uterus increases in size. Although uterine blood flow increases 20-fold, the fetoplacental unit grows even more rapidly. Consequently, more oxygen is extracted from the uterine blood during the latter part of pregnancy (Cunningham et al., 2014). In a normal term pregnancy, one sixth of the total maternal blood volume is within the uterine vascular system. The rate of blood flow through the uterus averages 450 to 650 mL/min at term, and oxygen consumption of the gravid uterus increases to meet fetal needs. Three factors known to decrease uterine blood flow are low maternal arterial pressure, contractions of the uterus, and maternal supine position. Estrogen stimulation may increase uterine blood flow. Doppler ultrasound examination can be used to measure uterine blood flow velocity, especially in pregnancies at risk due to conditions associated with decreased placental perfusion, such as hypertension, intrauterine growth restriction, diabetes mellitus, and multiple gestation (Blackburn, 2013) (see Fig. 13-14).

Using an ultrasound device or a fetal stethoscope, the examiner may hear the uterine souffle or bruit, a rushing or blowing sound of maternal blood flowing through uterine arteries to the placenta that is synchronous with the maternal pulse. The **funic souffle**, which is synchronous with the fetal heart rate and is caused by fetal blood coursing through the umbilical cord, may also be heard, as well as the actual heartbeat of the fetus (see Fig. 11-7).

Cervical changes. In a normal, unscarred cervix, a softening of the cervical tip may be observed about the beginning of the sixth week. This probable sign of pregnancy, **Goodell sign**, is brought about by increased vascularity, slight hypertrophy, and hyperplasia (increase in number of cells). The muscle and its collagen-rich connective tissue become loose, edematous, highly elastic, and increased in volume. The glands near the external os proliferate beneath the stratified squamous epithelium, giving the cervix the velvety appearance characteristic of pregnancy. Friability is increased and can result in slight bleeding after vaginal examination or after coitus with deep penetration.

Pregnancy can also cause the squamocolumnar junction, the site for obtaining cells for cervical cancer screening, to be located away from the cervix. Because of these changes, evaluation of abnormal Papanicolaou (Pap) tests during pregnancy can be complicated. However, careful assessment of all pregnant women is important—approximately 3% of all cervical cancers are diagnosed during pregnancy (Salani, Eisenhauer, & Copeland, 2012).

The cervix of the nullipara is rounded. Lacerations of the cervix almost always occur during the birth process. After childbirth, with or without lacerations, the cervix becomes more oval in the horizontal plane, and the external os appears as a transverse slit (see Fig. 10-2).

Changes related to the presence of the fetus. Passive movement of the unengaged fetus is called **ballottement** and can be identified generally between the sixteenth and eighteenth week. Ballottement is a technique of palpating a floating structure by bouncing it gently and feeling it rebound. To palpate the fetus, the examiner places a finger within the vagina and taps gently upward, causing the fetus to rise. The fetus then sinks, and a gentle tap is felt on the finger (Fig. 10-6).

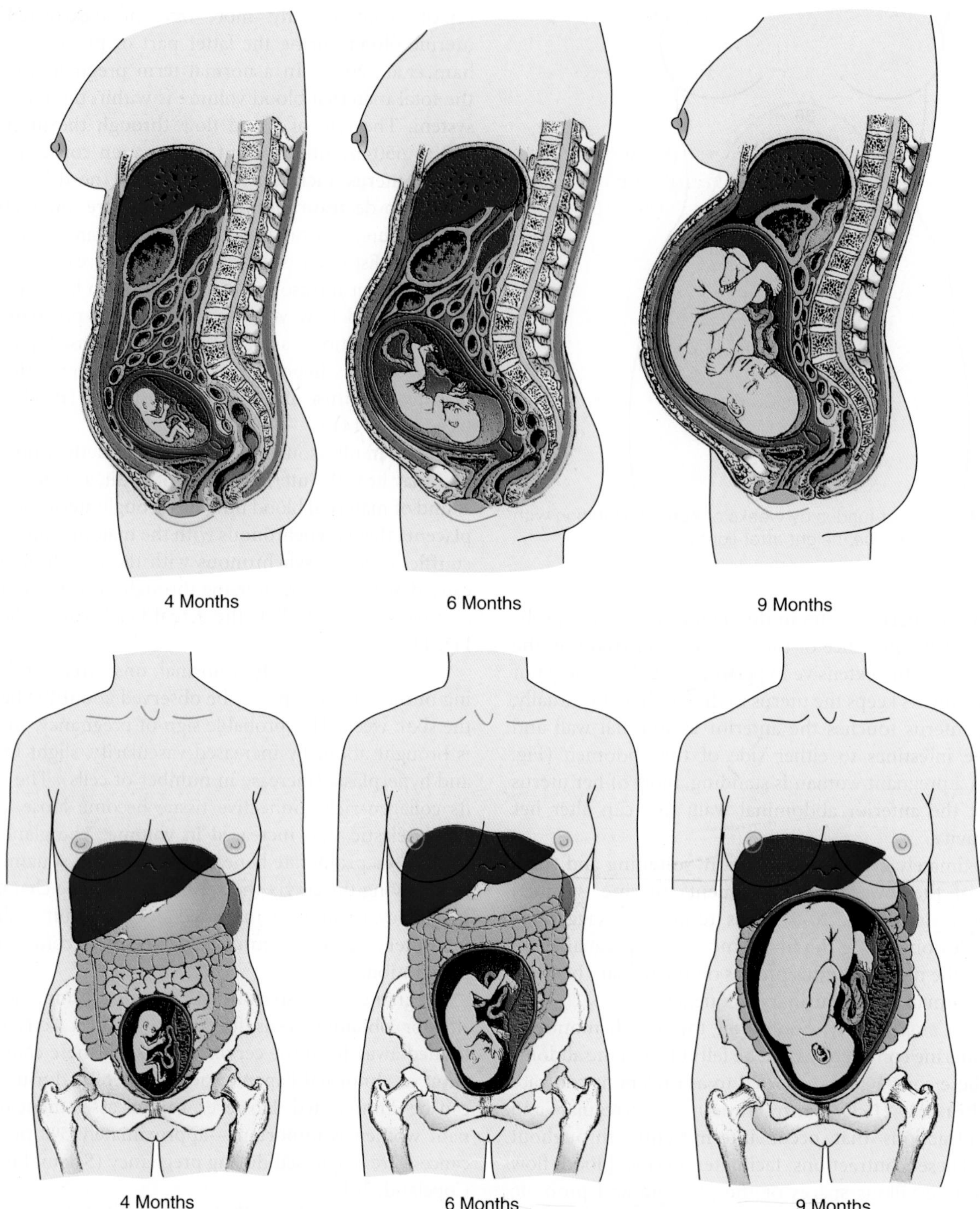

FIGURE 10-4 Displacement of internal abdominal structures and diaphragm by the enlarging uterus at 4, 6, and 9 months of gestation.

The first recognition of fetal movements, or "feeling life," may occur as early as the fourteenth week in the multiparous woman. The nulliparous woman may not notice these sensations until the eighteenth week or later. Quickening is commonly described as a flutter and is difficult to distinguish from peristalsis. Fetal movements gradually increase in intensity and frequency. The week in which quickening occurs provides a tentative clue in dating the duration of gestation.

Vagina and Vulva

Pregnancy hormones prepare the vagina for stretching during labour and birth by causing the vaginal mucosa to thicken, connective tissue to loosen, smooth muscle to hypertrophy, and the vaginal vault to lengthen. Increased vascularity results in a violet-bluish colour of the vaginal mucosa and cervix. The deepened colour, termed Chadwick sign, may be evident as early as the sixth week but is easily noted by the eighth week of pregnancy (Blackburn, 2013).

Leukorrhea is a white or slightly grey mucoid discharge with a faint musty odour. This copious mucoid fluid occurs in response to cervical stimulation by estrogen and progesterone. The fluid is whitish because of the presence of many exfoliated vaginal epithelial cells caused by the hyperplasia of normal pregnancy. This vaginal discharge is never pruritic or blood stained. The mucus fills the endocervical canal, resulting in the formation of the mucous plug (operculum) (Fig. 10-7). The operculum acts as a barrier against bacterial invasion.

During pregnancy, the pH of vaginal secretions is more acidic, ranging from about 3.5 to about 6.0 (nonpregnancy, 4.0 to 5.0), because of increased production of lactic acid (Cunningham et al., 2014). Although this acidic environment provides more protection against some organisms, the glycogen-rich environment of the vagina makes the pregnant woman more vulnerable to other infections, especially yeast infections, such as *Candida albicans* (Duff, 2014).

The increased vascularity of the vagina and other pelvic viscera results in a marked increase in sensitivity. This increased sensitivity may lead to a high degree of sexual interest and arousal, especially during the second trimester of pregnancy. The increased congestion, plus the relaxed walls of the blood vessels and the heavy uterus, may result in edema and

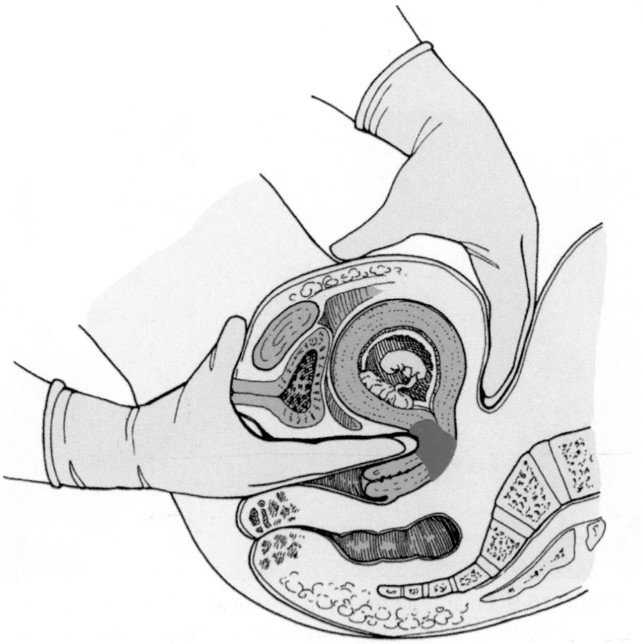

FIGURE 10-5 Hegar sign. Bimanual examination for assessing compressibility and softening of isthmus (lower uterine segment) while the cervix is still firm.

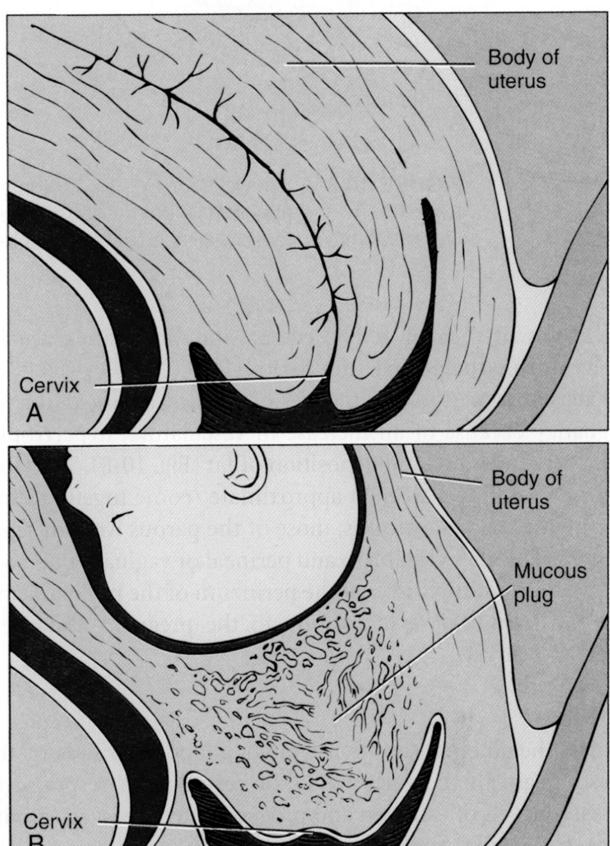

FIGURE 10-7 A: Cervix in nonpregnant woman. **B:** Cervix during pregnancy.

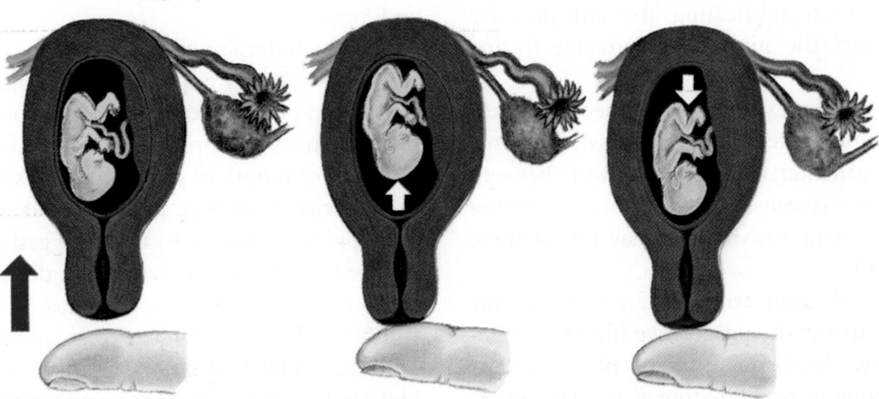

FIGURE 10-6 Internal ballottement (18 weeks).

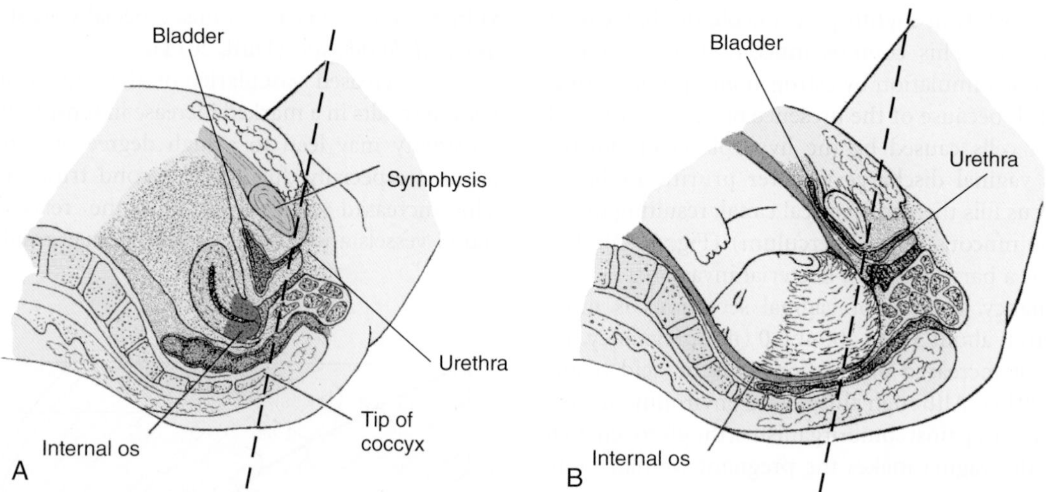

FIGURE 10-8 A: Pelvic floor in a nonpregnant woman. **B:** Pelvic floor during labour. Note marked hypertrophy and hyperplasia below dotted line joining tip of coccyx and inferior margin of symphysis. Note elongation of bladder and urethra as a result of compression. Fat deposits are increased.

varicosities of the vulva. The edema and varicosities usually resolve during the postpartum period.

External structures of the perineum are enlarged during pregnancy because of an increase in vasculature, hypertrophy of the perineal body, and deposition of fat (Fig. 10-8). The labia majora of nullipara women approximate (come together) and obscure the vaginal introitus; those of the parous woman separate and gape after childbirth and perineal or vaginal injury. See Fig. 10-2 for a comparison of the perineum of the nullipara and that of the multipara in relation to the pregnant abdomen, vulva, and cervix.

Breasts

Fullness, heightened sensitivity, tingling, and heaviness of the breasts begin in the early weeks of gestation in response to increased levels of estrogen and progesterone. Breast sensitivity varies from mild tingling to sharp pain. Nipples and areolae become more pigmented; secondary pinkish areolae develop, extending beyond the primary areolae; and nipples become more erectile. Hypertrophy of the sebaceous (oil) glands embedded in the primary areolae, called **Montgomery tubercles**, may be seen around the nipples. Within the tubercles are sebaceous and sweat glands that secrete lubricating and anti-infective substances to help protect the nipples and areolae during breastfeeding.

The richer blood supply causes the vessels beneath the skin to dilate. Once barely noticeable, the blood vessels become visible, often appearing in an intertwining blue network beneath the surface of the skin. Venous congestion in the breasts is more obvious in primigravidas. **Striae gravidarum** may appear at the outer aspects of the breasts.

During the second and third trimesters, growth of the mammary glands accounts for the progressive breast enlargement (Fig. 10-9). The high levels of luteal and placental hormones in pregnancy promote proliferation of the lactiferous ducts and lobule-alveolar tissue so that palpation of the breasts reveals a generalized, coarse nodularity. Glandular tissue displaces connective tissue, and as a result the tissue becomes softer and looser.

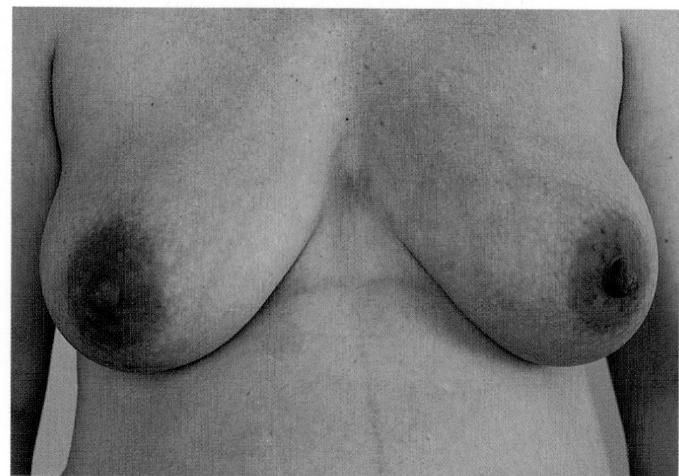

FIGURE 10-9 Enlarged breasts in pregnancy with venous network and darkened areolae and nipples. (From Seidel, H. M., Ball, J. W., Dains, J. E., et al. [2011]. *Mosby's guide to physical examination* [7th ed., p. 476]. St. Louis: Mosby.)

Although development of the mammary glands is functionally complete by midpregnancy, **lactation** is inhibited until a decrease in estrogen level occurs after birth. A thin, clear, viscous secretory material (precolostrum) can be found in the acini cells by the third month of gestation. **Colostrum**, the creamy, white-to-yellowish-to-orange premilk fluid, may be expressed from the nipples as early as 16 weeks of gestation (Lawrence & Lawrence, 2011). See Chapter 27 for a discussion of lactation.

General Body Systems

Cardiovascular System

Maternal adjustments to pregnancy involve extensive anatomical and physiological changes in the cardiovascular system.

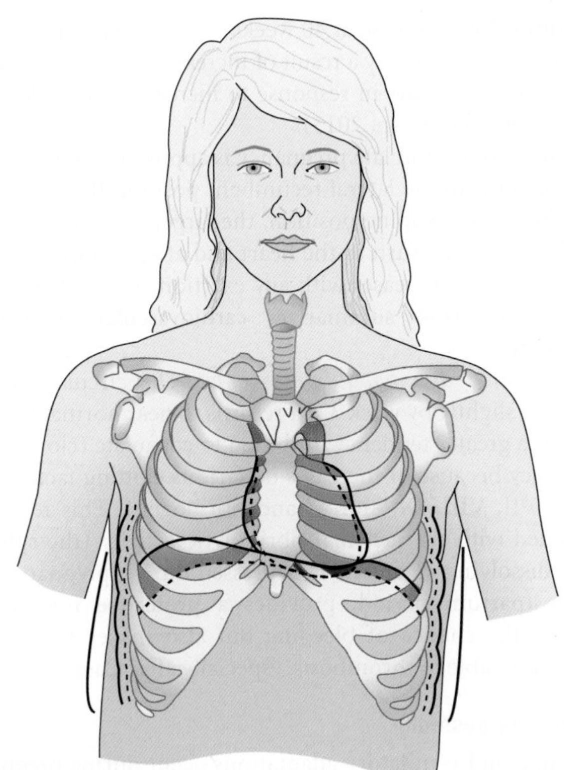

FIGURE 10-10 Changes in position of heart, lungs, and thoracic cage in pregnancy. *Broken line*, nonpregnant state; *solid line*, change that occurs in pregnancy.

Cardiovascular adaptations protect the woman's normal physiological functioning, meet the metabolic demands pregnancy imposes on her body, and provide for fetal developmental and growth needs.

Slight cardiac hypertrophy (enlargement) is probably secondary to increased blood volume and cardiac output that occurs in pregnancy. The heart returns to its normal size after childbirth. As the diaphragm is displaced upward by the enlarging uterus, the heart is elevated upward and rotated forward to the left (Fig. 10-10). The apical impulse, a point of maximal intensity, is shifted upward and laterally about 1 to 1.5 cm. The degree of shift depends on the duration of pregnancy and the size and position of the uterus.

The changes in heart size and position and the increases in blood volume and cardiac output contribute to auscultatory changes common in pregnancy. There is more audible splitting of S_1 and S_2, and S_3 may be readily heard after 20 weeks of gestation. In addition, systolic and diastolic murmurs may be heard over the pulmonic area. These changes are transient and disappear in most women shortly after they give birth (Cunningham et al., 2014).

Between 14 and 20 weeks of gestation, the pulse increases about 10 to 15 beats per minute, and this persists to term. Palpitations may occur. In twin gestations the maternal heart rate increases significantly in the third trimester (Blackburn, 2013).

The cardiac rhythm may be disturbed. The pregnant woman may experience sinus arrhythmia, premature atrial contractions, and premature ventricular systole. In the healthy woman with no underlying heart disease, no therapy is needed. Women with pre-existing heart disease need close medical and obstetrical supervision during pregnancy (see Chapter 15).

Blood pressure. Arterial blood pressure (brachial artery) varies with age, activity level, presence of health problems, pain, circadian rhythm, and use of alcohol, tobacco, or other substances. Additional factors to consider during pregnancy include maternal anxiety, maternal position, and type of blood pressure apparatus. Maternal anxiety can elevate readings. If an elevated reading is found, the woman is given time to rest and the reading is repeated.

Maternal position affects readings. Brachial blood pressure is highest when the woman is sitting, lowest when she is lying in the lateral recumbent position, and intermediate when she is supine, except for some women who experience hypotensive syndrome (see later discussion). Therefore, at each prenatal visit, the reading should be obtained in the same arm and with the woman in a seated position with her back and arm supported and her upper arm at the level of the heart. The position and arm used should be recorded along with the reading. If the blood pressure is consistently higher in one arm, the arm with the higher blood pressure should consistently be used to measure the blood pressure (Magee, Pels, Helewa, et al., 2014). The proper-size cuff is essential for accurate readings. The cuff should have a length that is 1.5 times the circumference of the arm (Magee et al., 2014). A cuff that is too small yields a falsely high reading; a cuff that is too large yields a falsely low reading.

Caution should be used when comparing auscultatory and oscillatory blood pressure readings because discrepancies can occur. Automated blood pressure monitors must be calibrated for use in women with pre-eclampsia as they may underestimate or overestimate blood pressure in those women (Magee et al., 2014).

Systolic blood pressure usually remains the same as the prepregnancy level but may decrease slightly as pregnancy advances. Diastolic blood pressure begins to decrease in the first trimester, continues to drop until 24 to 32 weeks, and gradually increases and returns to prepregnancy levels by term (Blackburn, 2013).

Some degree of compression of the vena cava occurs in all women who lie on their backs during the second half of pregnancy. Some women experience a fall of more than 30 mm Hg in their systolic pressure. After 4 to 5 minutes a reflex bradycardia is noted, cardiac output is reduced by half, and the woman feels faint. This condition is called **supine hypotensive syndrome** (Cunningham et al., 2014). (See Chapter 11, Emergency Box, p. 240.)

Compression of the iliac veins and inferior vena cava by the uterus causes increased venous pressure and reduced blood flow in the legs, except when the woman is in the lateral position. These alterations contribute to the dependent edema, varicose veins in the legs and vulva, and hemorrhoids that may develop in the latter part of term pregnancy (Fig. 10-11).

Blood volume and composition. The degree of blood volume expansion varies considerably. Blood volume increases by approximately 1500 mL, or 40 to 50% above nonpregnancy levels (Cunningham et al., 2014). This increase consists of 1000 mL of plasma plus 450 mL of red blood cells (RBCs). The

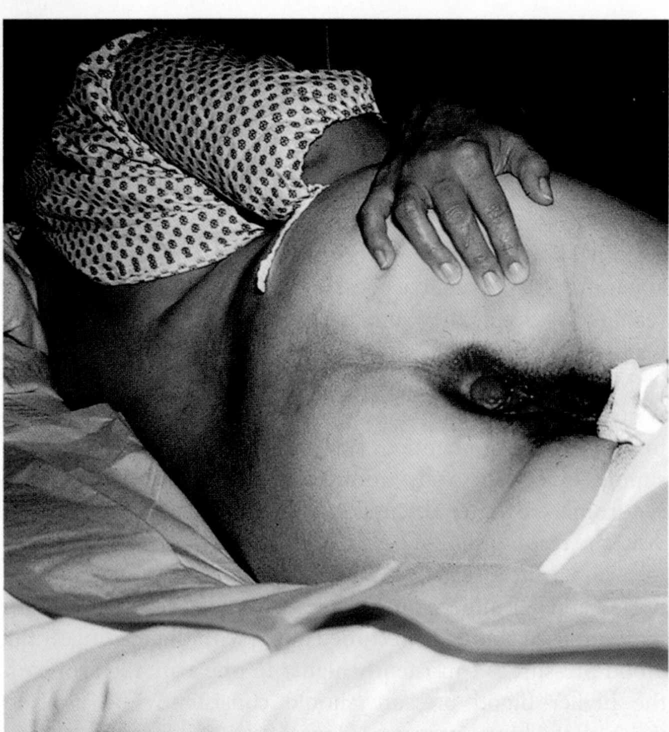

FIGURE 10-11 Hemorrhoids. (Courtesy Marjorie Pyle, RNC, Lifecircle, Costa Mesa, CA.)

increase in volume starts at weeks 10 to 12, peaks at weeks 32 to 34, and decreases slightly at week 40. The volume in a multiple gestation increases above that for a single fetus (Blackburn, 2013). Increased blood volume is a protective mechanism. It is essential for meeting the blood volume needs of the hypertrophied vascular system of the enlarged uterus, for adequately hydrating fetal and maternal tissues when the woman assumes an erect or supine position, and for providing a fluid reserve to compensate for blood loss during birth and the puerperium. Peripheral vasodilation allows for a normal blood pressure despite the increased blood volume in pregnancy.

During pregnancy, there is an accelerated production of RBCs (nonpregnant, 4.2 to 5.4 $\times 10^{12}$/L). The percentage of increase depends on the amount of iron available. The RBC mass increases by 20 to 30% (Blackburn, 2013).

Because the plasma increase is greater than the increase in RBC production, there is a decrease in normal hemoglobin values (120 to 160 g/L blood) and hematocrit values (0.37 to 0.47). This state of hemodilution is referred to as **physiological anemia**. The decrease is more noticeable during the second trimester, when rapid expansion of blood volume occurs faster than RBC production. If the hemoglobin value drops to 110 g/L or less or if the hematocrit decreases to 0.32 or less, the woman is considered anemic (Hark & Catalano, 2012).

The total white blood cell count increases during the second trimester and peaks during the third trimester. This increase is primarily in the granulocytes; the lymphocyte count stays about the same throughout pregnancy. See Table 10-3 for laboratory values during pregnancy.

Cardiac output. Cardiac output increases from 30 to 50% over the nonpregnant rate by week 32 of pregnancy; it declines to about a 20% increase at 40 weeks of gestation. This elevated cardiac output is largely a result of increased stroke volume and heart rate and occurs in response to increased tissue demands for oxygen (Blackburn, 2013).

Cardiac output in late pregnancy is appreciably higher when the woman is in the lateral recumbent position than when she is supine. In the supine position, the large, heavy uterus often impedes venous return to the heart and affects blood pressure. Cardiac output increases with any exertion such as labour and birth. Table 10-4 summarizes cardiovascular changes in pregnancy.

Circulation and coagulation times. The circulation time decreases slightly by week 32. It returns to near normal by term. There is a greater tendency for blood to coagulate (clot) during pregnancy because of increases in various clotting factors (i.e., factors VII, VIII, IX, and X, and fibrinogen). This tendency, combined with the fact that fibrinolytic activity (the splitting up or dissolving of a clot) is depressed during pregnancy and the postpartum period, provides a protective function to decrease the chance of bleeding but also makes the woman more vulnerable to thrombosis, especially after Caesarean birth.

Respiratory System

Structural and ventilatory adaptations occur during pregnancy to provide for maternal and fetal needs. Maternal oxygen requirements increase in response to the acceleration in metabolic rate and the need to add to the tissue mass in the uterus and breasts. In addition, the fetus requires oxygen and a way to eliminate carbon dioxide.

Elevated levels of estrogen cause the ligaments of the rib cage to relax, permitting increased chest expansion (see Fig. 10-10). The transverse diameter of the thoracic cage increases by about 2 cm and the circumference by 6 cm (Cunningham et al., 2014). The costal angle increases, and the lower rib cage appears to flare out. The chest may not return to its prepregnant state after birth (Seidel, Ball, Dains, et al., 2011).

The diaphragm is displaced by as much as 4 cm during pregnancy. With advancing pregnancy, chest breathing replaces abdominal breathing, and it becomes less possible for the diaphragm to descend with inspiration. Thoracic breathing is primarily accomplished by the diaphragm rather than by the costal muscles (Blackburn, 2013).

The upper respiratory tract becomes more vascular in response to elevated levels of estrogen. As the capillaries become engorged, edema and hyperemia develop within the nose, pharynx, larynx, trachea, and bronchi. This congestion within the tissues of the respiratory tract gives rise to several conditions commonly seen during pregnancy, including nasal and sinus stuffiness, epistaxis (nosebleed), changes in the voice, and marked inflammatory response to even a mild upper respiratory infection.

Increased vascularity of the upper respiratory tract also can cause the tympanic membranes and eustachian tubes to swell, giving rise to symptoms of impaired hearing, earaches, or a sense of fullness in the ears.

Pulmonary function. Respiratory changes in pregnancy are related to the elevation of the diaphragm and changes in the

TABLE 10-3 LABORATORY VALUES FOR PREGNANT AND NONPREGNANT WOMEN

VALUES	NONPREGNANT	PREGNANT
Hematological		
Complete Blood Count		
Hemoglobin, g/L	120–160*	>110
Hematocrit	0.37–0.47	>0.33
RBC volume, per millilitre	1400	1650
Plasma volume, per millilitre	2400	40–60% increase
RBC count, $\times10^{12}$/L	4.2–5.4	5–6.25
White blood cells, $\times10^{9}$/L	5–10	5–15
Neutrophils, %	55–70	60–85
Lymphocytes, %	20–40	15–40
Erythrocyte sedimentation rate (ESR), mm/hr	20	Elevated in second and third trimesters
Mean corpuscular hemoglobin concentration (MCHC), g/dL packed RBCs	32–36	No change
Mean corpuscular hemoglobin (MCH), pg/cell	27–31	No change
Mean corpuscular volume, fL	80–95	No change
Blood Coagulation and Fibrinolytic Activity*		
Factor VII	65–140	Increases in pregnancy, returns to normal in early puerperium
Factor VIII	55–145	Increases during pregnancy and immediately after birth
Factor IX	60–140	Same as factor VII
Factor X	45–155	Same as factor VII
Factor XI	65–135	Decreases in pregnancy
Factor XII	50–150	Same as factor VII
Prothrombin time, sec	11–12.5	Decreases slightly in pregnancy
Partial thromboplastin time (PTT), sec	28–35	Decreases slightly in pregnancy and decreases during second and third stage of labour (indicates clotting at placental site)
Bleeding time, min	<5 (Ivy method)	No appreciable change
Platelets, $\times10^{9}$/L	150–400	No significant change until 3–5 days after birth and then increases rapidly (may predispose woman to thrombosis) and gradually returns to normal
Fibrinolytic activity		Decreases in pregnancy and then abruptly returns to normal (protection against thromboembolism)
Fibrinogen, g/L	2–5	Levels increase late in pregnancy
Chemistry		
Mineral/Vitamin Concentrations		
Vitamin B_{12}, folic acid, ascorbic acid	Normal	Moderate decrease
Serum Proteins		
Total, g/L	64–83	55–75
Albumin, g/L	35–50	Slight increase
Globulin, total, g/L	23–34	30–40
Blood Glucose		
Fasting, mmol/L	3.3–5.8	Decreases
2-hr postprandial, mmol/L	<8.9	75 gram glucose challenge test: <5.3 initially, <10.6 at 1 hr and <9.0 at 2 hr (if 2 out of 3 are higher than normal, would be diagnosed as abnormal)
Acid–Base Values in Arterial Blood		
PO_2, mm Hg	80–100	104–108 (increased)
PCO_2, mm Hg	35–45	27–32 (decreased)
Sodium bicarbonate (HCO_3), mmol/L	21–28	18–31 (decreased)
Blood pH	7.35–7.45	7.40–7.45 (slightly increased, more alkaline)

Continued

TABLE 10-3 LABORATORY VALUES FOR PREGNANT AND NONPREGNANT WOMEN—cont'd

VALUES	NONPREGNANT	PREGNANT
Hepatic		
Bilirubin, total, mcmol/L	3.0–22	Unchanged
Serum cholesterol, mmol/L	<5.2	Increases at 16–32 wk of pregnancy; remains at this level until after birth
Serum alkaline phosphatase, U/L	30–120	Increases from wk 12 of pregnancy to 6 wk after birth
Serum albumin, g/L	35–50	Increases slightly
Renal		
Bladder capacity, mL	1300	1500
Renal plasma flow, mL/min	490–700	Increases by 25–30%
Glomerular filtration rate (GFR), mL/min	88–128	Increases by 30–50%
Blood urea nitrogen (BUN), mmol/L	2.5–8.0	Decreases
Serum creatinine, mcmol/L	44–97	Decreases
Serum uric acid, mcmol/L	180–420	Decreases but returns to prepregnancy level by end of pregnancy
Urine glucose	Negative	Present in 20% of pregnant women
Intravenous pyelogram	Normal	Slight to moderate hydroureter and hydronephrosis; right kidney larger than left kidney

Note: Abbreviations should not be used in practice.
RBC, red blood cell.
*Pregnancy represents a hypercoagulable state.
Sources: Blackburn, S. (2013). *Maternal, fetal, & neonatal physiology: A clinical perspective* (4th ed.). St. Louis: Saunders; Canadian Diabetic Association. (2013). CDA 2013 clinical practice guidelines for the prevention and management of diabetes in Canada. *Canadian Journal of Diabetes, 37*(Suppl. 1), S168–S183. Retrieved from http://guidelines.diabetes.ca/fullguidelines; Gordon, M. (2012). Maternal physiology in pregnancy. In S. G. Gabbe, J. R. Niebyl, & J. L. Simpson, et al. (Eds.), *Obstetrics: Normal and problem pregnancies* (6th ed.). Philadelphia: Saunders; Medical Council of Canada. (2013). *Clinical laboratory tests normal values.* Retrieved from http://apps.mcc.ca/Objectives_Online/objectives.pl?lang=english&loc=values; Pagana, K. D., Pagana, T. J., & Pike-MacDonald, S. A. (2013). *Mosby's Canadian manual of diagnostic and laboratory tests* (1st Canadian ed.). Toronto: Mosby; Samuels, P. (2012). Hematology complications of pregnancy. In S. G. Gabbe, J. R. Niebyl, & J. L. Simpson (Eds.), *Obstetrics: Normal and problem pregnancies* (6th ed.). Philadelphia: Saunders.

TABLE 10-4 CARDIOVASCULAR CHANGES IN PREGNANCY

PARAMETER	CHANGE
Heart rate	Increases 10–15 bpm
Blood pressure	
Systolic	Slight or no decrease from prepregnancy levels
Diastolic	Slight decrease to midpregnancy (24–32 wk) and gradual return to prepregnancy levels by end of pregnancy
Blood volume	Increases by 1500 mL or 40–50% above prepregnancy level
Red blood cell mass	Increases 17%
Hemoglobin	Decreases
Hematocrit	Decreases
White blood cell count	Increases in second and third trimesters
Cardiac output	Increases 30–50%

Data from Gordon, M. (2012). Maternal physiology. In S. G. Gabbe, J. R. Niebyl, J. L. Simpson, et al. (Eds.), *Obstetrics: Normal and problem pregnancies* (6th ed.). Philadelphia: Saunders.

chest wall. Changes in the respiratory centre result in a lowered threshold for carbon dioxide. The actions of progesterone and estrogen are presumed to be responsible for the increased sensitivity of the respiratory centre to carbon dioxide (see Table 10-5 for respiratory changes in pregnancy). Although pulmonary function is not impaired by pregnancy, diseases of the respiratory tract may be more serious during this time (Cunningham et al., 2014). One important factor related to this may be the increase in oxygen requirements.

TABLE 10-5 RESPIRATORY CHANGES IN PREGNANCY

PARAMETER	CHANGE
Respiratory rate	Unchanged or slightly increased
Tidal volume	Increased 30–40%
Vital capacity	Unchanged
Inspiratory capacity	Increased
Expiratory volume	Decreased
Total lung capacity	Unchanged to slightly decreased
Oxygen consumption	Increased 20–40%

Source: Gordon, M. (2012). Maternal physiology. In S. G. Gabbe, J. R. Niebyl, & J. L. Simpson, et al. (Eds.), *Obstetrics: Normal and problem pregnancies* (6th ed.). Philadelphia: Saunders.)

Basal metabolic rate. The basal metabolic rate (BMR) increases during pregnancy. The elevation in BMR reflects increased oxygen demands of the uterine–placental–fetal unit and greater oxygen consumption because of increased maternal cardiac work. This increase varies considerably, depending on the prepregnancy nutritional status of the woman and on fetal growth. By the third trimester, the BMR is increased by 10 to 20% over the nonpregnancy state (Cunningham et al., 2014). The BMR returns to nonpregnant levels by 5 to 6 days after birth. Peripheral vasodilation and acceleration of sweat gland activity help dissipate the excess heat resulting from the increased BMR during pregnancy. Pregnant women may experience heat intolerance. Lassitude and fatigability after only slight exertion are experienced by many women in early pregnancy. These feelings, along with a greater need for sleep, may persist and may be caused in part by the increased metabolic activity.

Acid–base balance. By about the tenth week of pregnancy, there is a decrease of about 5 mm Hg in the partial pressure of carbon dioxide (PCO_2). Progesterone may be responsible for increasing the sensitivity of the respiratory centre receptors so that tidal volume increases and PCO_2 decreases, the base excess (HCO_3, or bicarbonate) decreases, and pH increases slightly. These alterations in acid–base balance indicate that pregnancy is a state of respiratory alkalosis compensated by mild metabolic acidosis (Gordon, 2012). These changes also facilitate the transport of CO_2 from the fetus and O_2 release from the mother to the fetus.

Renal System

The kidneys are responsible for maintaining electrolyte and acid–base balance, regulating extracellular fluid volume, excreting waste products, and conserving essential nutrients.

Anatomical changes. Changes in renal structure result from hormonal activity (estrogen and progesterone), pressure from an enlarging uterus, and an increase in blood volume. As early as the tenth week of pregnancy, the renal pelvis and the ureters dilate. Dilation of the ureters is more pronounced above the pelvic brim, in part because they are compressed between the uterus and the pelvic brim. In most women the ureters below the pelvic brim are of normal size. The smooth-muscle walls of the ureters undergo hyperplasia and hypertrophy and muscle tone relaxation. The ureters elongate, become tortuous, and form single or double curves. In the latter part of pregnancy, the renal pelvis and ureter dilate more on the right side than on the left because the heavy uterus is displaced to the right by the sigmoid colon.

Because of these changes, a larger volume of urine is held in the pelvis and ureters and urine flow rate is slowed. Urinary stasis or stagnation has several consequences:

- A lag occurs between the time urine is formed and when it reaches the bladder. Therefore, clearance test results may reflect substances contained in glomerular filtrate several hours before.
- Stagnated urine is an excellent medium for the growth of microorganisms. In addition, the urine of pregnant women contains more nutrients, including glucose, that increase the pH (making the urine more alkaline). This makes pregnant women more susceptible to urinary tract infection.

Bladder irritability, nocturia, and urinary frequency and urgency (without dysuria) are commonly reported in early pregnancy. These bladder symptoms may return near term, especially after lightening occurs.

Increased urinary frequency results initially from increased bladder sensitivity and later from compression of the bladder (see Fig. 10-8). In the second trimester, the bladder is pulled up out of the true pelvis into the abdomen. The urethra lengthens to 7.5 cm as the bladder is displaced upward. The pelvic congestion that occurs in pregnancy is reflected in hyperemia of the bladder and urethra. This increased vascularity causes the bladder mucosa to be traumatized and bleed easily. Bladder tone may decrease, which increases the bladder capacity to 1500 mL. At the same time, the bladder is compressed by the enlarging uterus, resulting in the urge to void even if the bladder contains only a small amount of urine.

Functional changes. In normal pregnancy, renal function is altered considerably. Glomerular filtration rate (GFR) and renal plasma flow increase early in pregnancy (Monga & Mastrobattista, 2014). These changes are caused by pregnancy hormones; an increase in blood volume; and the woman's posture, physical activity, and nutritional intake. The woman's kidneys must manage the increased metabolic and circulatory demands of the maternal body and also the excretion of fetal waste products.

Renal function is most efficient when the woman lies in the lateral recumbent position and is least efficient when the woman assumes a supine position. A side-lying position increases renal perfusion, which increases urine output and decreases edema. When the pregnant woman is lying supine, the heavy uterus compresses the vena cava and the aorta, and cardiac output decreases. As a result, blood flow to the brain and heart is continued at the expense of other organs, including the kidneys and uterus.

Fluid and electrolyte balance. Selective renal tubular resorption maintains sodium and water balance, regardless of changes in dietary intake and losses through sweat, vomitus, or diarrhea. About 900 mEq of sodium is normally retained during pregnancy to meet fetal needs, although maternal serum levels of sodium decrease by 3 to 4 mmol/L (Gordon, 2012). To prevent excessive sodium depletion, the maternal kidneys undergo a significant adaptation by increasing tubular resorption. Because of the need for increased maternal intravascular and extracellular fluid volume, additional sodium is needed to expand fluid volume and maintain an isotonic state. As efficient as the renal system is, it can be overstressed by excessive dietary sodium intake or restriction or by the use of diuretics. Severe hypovolemia and reduced placental perfusion are two consequences of using diuretics during pregnancy.

The capacity of the kidneys to excrete water is more efficient during the early weeks than later in pregnancy. As a result, some women feel thirsty in early pregnancy because of the greater amount of water loss. The pooling of fluid in the legs in the latter part of pregnancy decreases renal blood flow and GFR. This pooling is sometimes referred to as *physiological* or *dependent edema* and requires no treatment. The normal diuretic response to the water load is triggered when the woman lies down, preferably on her side, and the pooled fluid re-enters general circulation.

Normally, the kidney resorbs almost all the glucose and other nutrients from the plasma filtrate. However, in pregnant women, tubular resorption of glucose is impaired so that glycosuria occurs at varying times and to varying degrees. Normal values range from 0 to 7.0 mmol/L, meaning that during any day, the urine is sometimes positive and sometimes negative for glucose. In nonpregnant women, blood glucose levels must be at 8.0 to 10 mmol/L or greater before glucose is "spilled" into the urine (not resorbed). During pregnancy, glucosuria occurs when maternal glucose levels are lower than 7.0 mmol/L. The reason why glucose, as well as other nutrients such as amino acids, is wasted during pregnancy is not understood, nor has the exact mechanism been discovered. Although glucosuria may be found in normal pregnancies (2+ levels may be seen with increased anxiety states), the possibility of diabetes mellitus and gestational diabetes must be considered.

Proteinuria does not usually occur in normal pregnancy except during labour or after birth (Cunningham et al., 2014). However, the increased amounts of amino acids that must be filtered may exceed the capacity of the renal tubules to absorb them, and small amounts of protein may be lost in the urine. The amount of protein excreted is not an indication of the severity of renal disease, nor does an increase in protein excretion in a pregnant woman with known renal disease necessarily indicate a progression in her disease. However, a pregnant woman with hypertension and proteinuria must be evaluated carefully because she may be at greater risk for an adverse pregnancy outcome (Gordon, 2012).

Integumentary System

Alterations in hormone balance and mechanical stretching are responsible for several changes in the integumentary system during pregnancy. Hyperpigmentation is stimulated by the anterior pituitary hormone *melanotropin*, which is increased during pregnancy. Darkening of the nipples, areolae, axillae, and vulva occurs at about the sixteenth week of gestation. Facial melasma (also called *chloasma* or *mask of pregnancy*) is a blotchy, brownish hyperpigmentation of the skin over the cheeks, nose, and forehead, especially in pregnant women with dark complexions. Chloasma appears in 50 to 70% of pregnant women, beginning after the sixteenth week and increasing gradually until term. The sun intensifies this pigmentation in susceptible women. Chloasma caused by normal pregnancy usually fades after birth but often recurs with oral contraceptive use or subsequent pregnancies (Kroumpouzos, 2012).

The linea nigra (Fig. 10-12) is a pigmented line extending from the symphysis pubis to the top of the fundus in the midline. This line is known as the linea alba before hormone-induced pigmentation. In primigravidas the extension of the linea nigra, beginning in the third month, keeps pace with the rising height of the fundus; in multigravidas the entire line often appears earlier than the third month. Not all pregnant women develop lineae nigra, and some women notice hair growth along the line with or without the change in pigmentation.

Striae gravidarum, or stretch marks (seen over the lower abdomen in Fig. 10-12), appear in 50 to 90% of pregnant women during the second half of pregnancy. These may be caused by the action of adrenocorticosteroids. Striae reflect

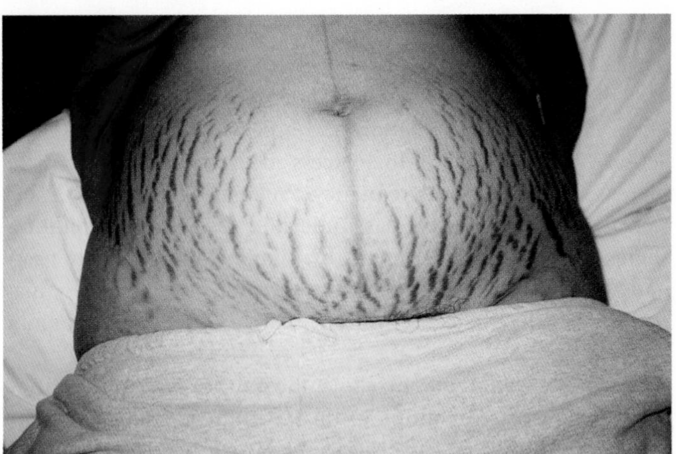

FIGURE 10-12 Striae gravidarum and linea nigra in a dark-skinned person. (Courtesy Shannon Perry, Phoenix, AZ.)

separation within the underlying connective (collagen) tissue of the skin. These slightly depressed streaks tend to occur over areas of maximum stretch (the abdomen, thighs, and breasts). The stretching sometimes causes a sensation that resembles itching. The tendency to develop striae may be familial. After birth they usually fade, although they never disappear completely. The colour of striae varies, depending on the pregnant woman's skin colour. The striae appear pinkish on a woman with light skin and are lighter than the surrounding skin in dark-skinned women. In the multipara, in addition to the striae of the present pregnancy, glistening silvery lines (in light-skinned women) or purplish lines (in dark-skinned women) are commonly seen. These represent the scars of striae from previous pregnancies.

Angiomas are commonly referred to as *vascular spiders*. These tiny, star-shaped or branched, slightly raised, and pulsating end-arterioles are usually found on the neck, thorax, face, and arms. They occur as a result of elevated levels of circulating estrogens. The spiders are bluish in colour and do not blanch with pressure. Vascular spiders appear during the second to fifth month of pregnancy in about 65% of White women and 10% of Black women. The spiders usually disappear after birth (Blackburn, 2013).

Pinkish-red diffusely mottled or well-defined blotches are seen over the palmar surfaces of the hands in about 60% of White women and 35% of Black women during pregnancy (Blackburn, 2013). These colour changes, called *palmar erythema*, are related primarily to increased estrogen levels.

! NURSING ALERT

Integumentary system changes vary greatly among women of different racial backgrounds. Therefore, when performing physical assessments, the colour of a woman's skin should be noted along with any changes that may be attributed to pregnancy.

Some dermatological conditions have been identified as unique to pregnancy or as having an increased incidence during pregnancy. Mild pruritus (pruritus gravidarum) is a relatively common dermatological symptom during pregnancy. The goal of management is to relieve the itching. Topical steroids and emollients are the usual treatment. The problem usually resolves during the postpartum period (Cunningham et al., 2014). Systemic diseases can also cause pruritus, but these causes are uncommon or rare (Box 10-1). Pre-existing skin diseases may complicate pregnancy or be improved during pregnancy. Table 11-3 discusses the discomforts and care related to pregnancy.

! NURSING ALERT

Women with severe acne taking isotretinoin (Accutane) should avoid pregnancy while receiving the treatment because it is teratogenic and associated with major fetal malformations.

BOX 10-1 PREVALENCE OF DERMATOLOGICAL DISORDERS OF PREGNANCY

Pruritic urticarial papules and plaques of pregnancy (PUPPP)—1 : 130 to 1 : 300
Prurigo of pregnancy (PP)—1 : 300 to 1 : 450
Herpes gestationis (HG)—1 : 50,000
Pruritic folliculitis of pregnancy (PFP)—Very rare; about 30 cases

Source: Kroumpouzos, G. (2012). Skin disease in pregnancy and puerperium. In S. G. Gabbe, J. R. Niebyl, J. L. Simpson, et al. (Eds.), *Obstetrics: Normal and problem pregnancies* (6th ed.). Philadelphia: Saunders.)

Gum hypertrophy may occur during pregnancy. An **epulis** (gingival granuloma gravidarum) is a red, raised nodule on the gums that bleeds easily. This lesion may develop around the third month and usually continues to enlarge as pregnancy progresses. It is usually managed by avoiding trauma to the gums (e.g., using a soft toothbrush). An epulis usually regresses spontaneously after birth.

Nail growth may be accelerated. Some women may notice thinning and softening of the nails. Oily skin and acne vulgaris may occur during pregnancy. In some women the skin clears and looks radiant. *Hirsutism*, the excessive growth of hair or growth of hair in unusual places, is commonly reported. An increase in fine hair growth may occur but tends to disappear after pregnancy. However, growth of coarse or bristly hair does not usually disappear after pregnancy. The rate of scalp hair loss slows during pregnancy; increased hair loss may be noted in the postpartum period.

Increased blood supply to the skin leads to increased perspiration. Women feel hotter during pregnancy, possibly related to a progesterone-induced increase in body temperature and the increased BMR.

Musculoskeletal System

The gradually changing body and increasing weight of the pregnant woman usually cause noticeable changes in her posture (Fig. 10-13) and in the way she walks. The great abdominal distension gives the pelvis a forward tilt, decreased abdominal muscle tone, and increased weight bearing. The woman's centre of gravity shifts forward, requiring a realignment of the spinal curvatures. An increase in the normal lumbosacral curve (lordosis) develops, and a compensatory curvature in the

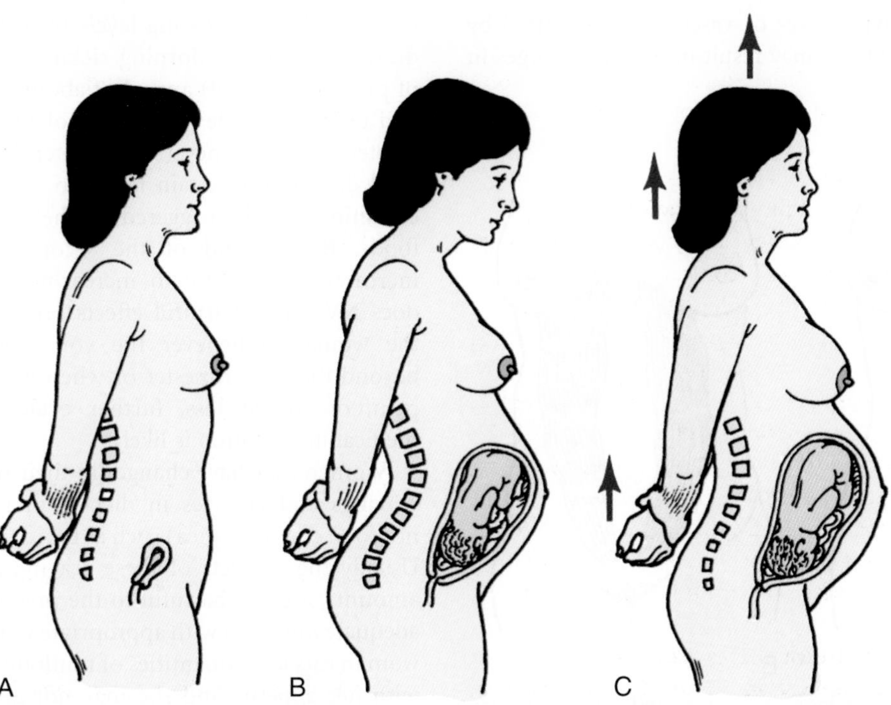

FIGURE 10-13 Postural changes during pregnancy. **A:** Nonpregnant. **B:** Incorrect posture during pregnancy. **C:** Correct posture during pregnancy.

cervicodorsal region (exaggerated anterior flexion of the head) develops to help her maintain balance. Aching, numbness, and weakness of the upper extremities may result. Large breasts and a stoop-shouldered stance further accentuate the lumbar and dorsal curves. The ligamentous and muscular structures of the middle and lower spine may be severely stressed. These and related changes often cause musculoskeletal discomfort, especially in older women or those with a back disorder or a faulty sense of balance.

Slight relaxation and increased mobility of the pelvic joints are normal during pregnancy. These adaptations permit enlargement of pelvic dimensions to facilitate labour and birth. The degree of relaxation varies, but considerable separation of the symphysis pubis and the instability of the sacroiliac joints may cause pain and difficulty in walking. A waddling gait is common. Obesity or multifetal pregnancy tends to increase the pelvic instability. Peripheral joint laxity also increases as pregnancy progresses; the cause for this is not known (Cunningham et al., 2014).

The muscles of the abdominal wall stretch and ultimately lose some tone. During the third trimester, the rectus abdominis muscles may separate (Fig. 10-14), allowing abdominal contents to protrude at the midline. The umbilicus flattens or protrudes. After birth, the muscles gradually regain tone. However, separation of the muscles (**diastasis recti abdominis**) may persist.

Neurological System

Little is known about specific alterations in function of the neurological system during pregnancy, aside from hypothalamic–pituitary neurohormonal changes. Specific physiological alterations resulting from pregnancy may cause the following neurological or neuromuscular symptoms:

- Compression of pelvic nerves or vascular stasis caused by enlargement of the uterus may result in sensory changes in the legs.

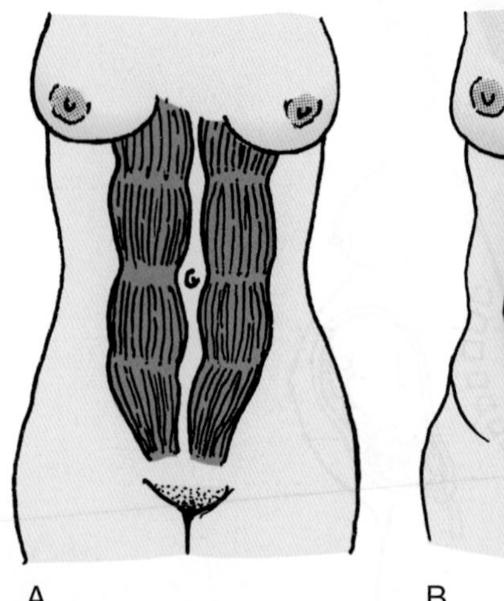

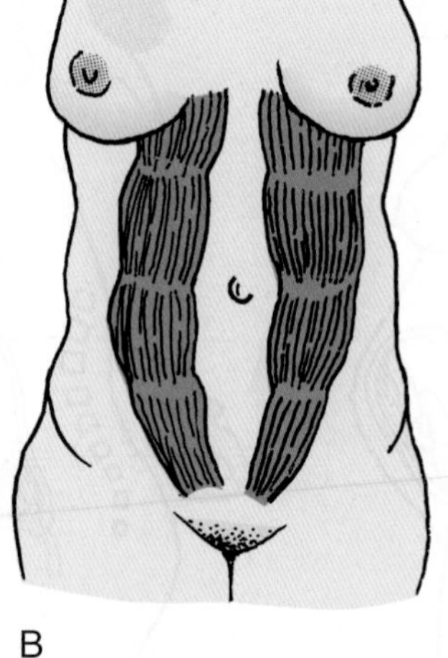

FIGURE 10-14 Possible change in rectus abdominis muscles during pregnancy. **A:** Normal position in nonpregnant woman. **B:** Diastasis recti abdominis in pregnant women.

- Dorsolumbar lordosis may cause pain because of traction on nerves or compression of nerve roots.
- Edema involving the peripheral nerves may result in **carpal tunnel syndrome** during the last trimester. The syndrome is characterized by paresthesia (abnormal sensation such as burning or tingling) and pain in the hand, radiating to the elbow. The sensations are caused by edema that compresses the median nerve beneath the carpal ligament of the wrist. Smoking and alcohol consumption can impair the microcirculation and may worsen the symptoms. The dominant hand is usually affected most, although many women report symptoms in both hands. Symptoms usually regress after pregnancy. In some cases, surgical treatment is necessary (Cunningham et al., 2014). See Table 11-3 for further discussion of discomforts of pregnancy.
- Acroesthesia (numbness and tingling of the hands) is caused by the stoop-shouldered stance (see Fig. 10-13, B) assumed by some women during pregnancy. The condition is associated with traction on segments of the brachial plexus.
- Tension headache is common when anxiety or uncertainty complicates pregnancy. However, vision problems such as refractive errors, sinusitis, or migraine may also be responsible for headaches.
- "Light-headedness," faintness, and even syncope (fainting) are common during early pregnancy. Vasomotor instability, postural hypotension, or hypoglycemia may be responsible.
- Hypocalcemia can cause neuromuscular problems such as muscle cramps or tetany.

Gastrointestinal System

Appetite. During pregnancy, the woman's appetite and food intake fluctuate. Early in pregnancy, some women have nausea with or without vomiting (morning sickness), possibly in response to increasing levels of hCG and altered carbohydrate metabolism. Morning sickness or nausea and vomiting of pregnancy (NVP) appear at about 4 to 6 weeks of gestation and usually subside by the end of the third month (first trimester) of pregnancy (see Chapter 11). Severity varies from mild distaste for certain foods to more severe vomiting. The condition may be triggered by the sight or odour of various foods. By the end of the second trimester, the appetite increases in response to increasing metabolic needs. Rarely does NVP have harmful effects on the embryo, the fetus, or the woman. Whenever the vomiting is severe or persists beyond the first trimester or when it is accompanied by fever, pain, or weight loss, further evaluation is necessary, and medical intervention is likely.

Women may have changes in their sense of taste, leading to cravings and changes in dietary intake. Some women have nonfood cravings (**pica**) such as for ice, clay, and laundry starch. Usually the subjects of these cravings, if consumed in small amounts, are not harmful to the pregnancy if the woman has adequate nutrition with appropriate weight gain; however, if the woman eats large quantities of nonfood items, this can interfere with her appetite and she may not get appropriate nutrition (Gordon, 2012). See further discussion of pica in Chapter 12, p. 281).

Mouth. The gums become hyperemic, spongy, and swollen during pregnancy. They tend to bleed easily because the increasing levels of estrogen cause selective increased vascularity and connective tissue proliferation (a nonspecific gingivitis). Epulis (discussed in the section on the integumentary system) may develop at the gum line. Some pregnant women complain of ptyalism (excessive salivation), which may be caused by the decrease in unconscious swallowing by the woman when nauseated (Cunningham et al., 2014) (see Table 11-3 for further discussion of ptyalism).

Teeth. The pregnant woman requires about 1000 mg of calcium and approximately the same amount of phosphorus every day during pregnancy. With a well-balanced diet, these requirements are satisfied. Serious dietary deficiency may deplete the mother's bony stores of these elements, but tooth calcium is stable and not available to the fetus (Russell & Mayberry, 2008). Gingivitis and poor dental hygiene may contribute to dental caries, which can lead to the loss of a tooth and during pregnancy may be a risk factor for preterm birth, low birth weight, and pre-eclampsia (Russell & Mayberry, 2008).

Esophagus, stomach, and intestines. Increased progesterone production causes decreased tone and motility of smooth muscles, resulting in esophageal regurgitation, slower emptying time of the stomach, and reverse peristalsis. As a result, the woman may experience "acid indigestion" or heartburn (pyrosis) beginning as early as the first trimester and intensifying through the third trimester.

Increased estrogen production causes decreased secretion of hydrochloric acid; this is associated with a decreased incidence of peptic ulcer disease (PUD) during pregnancy. Existing PUD tends to improve during pregnancy (Kelly & Savides, 2012).

The incidence of hiatal hernia is increased during pregnancy as a result of the upward displacement of the stomach by the enlarging uterus, which causes a widening of the hiatus of the diaphragm. Hiatal hernia occurs more often in multiparas and older or obese women.

In response to increased needs during pregnancy, iron is absorbed more readily in the small intestine. Even when the woman is deficient in iron, it will continue to be absorbed in sufficient amounts for the fetus to have a normal hemoglobin level.

Smooth muscle relaxation and reduced peristalsis caused by increased progesterone result in an increase in water absorption from the colon and may cause constipation. Constipation can also result from food choices linked to constipation, lack of fluids, iron supplementation, decreased activity level, abdominal distension by the pregnant uterus, and displacement and compression of the intestines. If the pregnant woman has hemorrhoids (see Fig. 10-11) and is constipated, the hemorrhoids can evert or bleed during straining at stool.

Gallbladder and liver. The gallbladder is often distended because of its decreased muscle tone during pregnancy. Increased emptying time and thickening of bile caused by prolonged retention are typical changes. These features, together with slight hypercholesterolemia from increased progesterone levels, may account for the development of gallstones during pregnancy.

Hepatic function is difficult to appraise during pregnancy. However, only minor changes in liver function develop. Occasionally, intrahepatic cholestasis (retention and accumulation of bile in the liver caused by factors within the liver) occurs late in pregnancy in response to placental steroids. It may result in pruritus gravidarum (severe itching) with or without jaundice. These distressing symptoms are difficult to treat during pregnancy and may be associated with fetal risk. However, symptoms subside after birth (Williamson, Mackillop, & Heneghan, 2014).

Abdominal discomfort. Intra-abdominal alterations that can cause discomfort include pelvic heaviness or pressure, round ligament tension, flatulence, distension and bowel cramping, and uterine contractions. In addition to displacement of intestines, pressure from the expanding uterus causes an increase in venous pressure in the pelvic organs. Although most abdominal discomfort is a consequence of normal maternal alterations, the health care provider must be alert to the possibility of disorders such as bowel obstruction or an inflammatory process.

Appendicitis may be difficult to diagnose in pregnancy because the appendix is displaced upward and laterally, high and to the right, away from McBurney point (Fig. 10-15).

Endocrine System

Profound endocrine changes are essential for pregnancy maintenance, normal fetal growth, and postpartum recovery. Hormones, their sources, and their effects on the pregnancy are presented in Table 10-6.

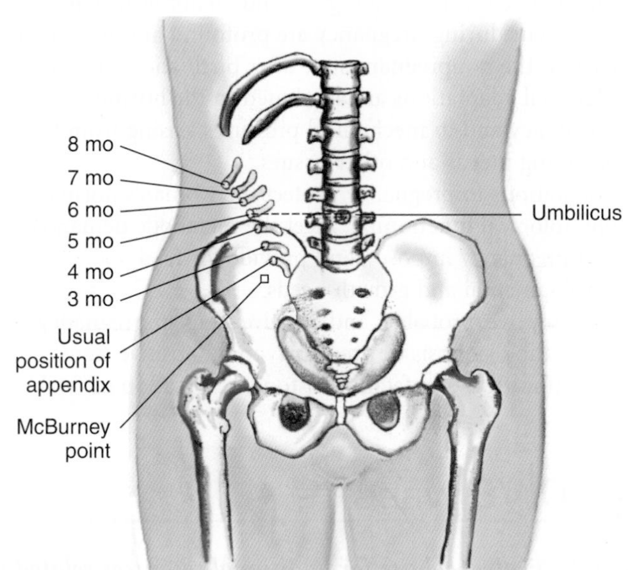

FIGURE 10-15 Change in position of appendix in pregnancy. Note McBurney point.

TABLE 10-6 HORMONES AND EFFECTS OF CHANGES DURING PREGNANCY

HORMONE	SOURCE	EFFECTS OF CHANGES DURING PREGNANCY
Human chorionic gonadotropin	Fertilized ovum and chorionic villi	Maintains corpus luteum production of estrogen and progesterone until placenta takes over the function
Progesterone	Corpus luteum until 14 wk of gestation, then the placenta	Suppresses secretion of FSH and LH by the anterior pituitary; maintains pregnancy by relaxing smooth muscles, decreasing uterine contractility; causes fat to deposit in subcutaneous tissues over the maternal abdomen, back, and upper thighs; decreases mother's ability to use insulin
Estrogen	Corpus luteum until 14 wk of gestation, then the placenta	Suppresses secretion of FSH and LH by the anterior pituitary; causes fat to deposit in subcutaneous tissues over the maternal abdomen, back, and upper thighs; promotes enlargement of genitals, uterus, and breasts; increases vascularity; relaxes pelvic ligaments and joints; interferes with folic acid metabolism; increases the level of total body proteins; promotes retention of sodium and water; decreases secretion of hydrochloric acid and pepsin; decreases mother's ability to use insulin
Serum prolactin	Anterior pituitary	Prepares breasts for lactation
Oxytocin	Posterior pituitary	Stimulates uterine contractions; stimulates milk ejection from breasts
Human chorionic somatomammotropin (previously called human placental lactogen)	Placenta	Acts as a growth hormone; contributes to breast development; decreases maternal metabolism of glucose; increases the amount of fatty acids for metabolic needs
Thyroxine-binding globulin, thyroxine, triiodothyronine	Thyroid	Causes moderate enlargement of the thyroid gland but woman remains euthyroid; possibly plays role in early neural development of the fetus
Parathyroid	Parathyroid	Controls calcium and magnesium metabolism
Insulin	Pancreas	Increases production of insulin to compensate for insulin antagonism caused by placental hormones: effect of insulin antagonists is to decrease tissue sensitivity to insulin or ability to use insulin
Cortisol	Adrenal glands	Stimulates production of insulin; increases peripheral resistance to insulin
Aldosterone	Adrenal glands	Stimulates resorption of excess sodium from the renal tubules

FSH, follicle-stimulating hormone; *LH*, luteinizing hormone.

KEY POINTS

- ELISA testing, with monoclonal antibody technology, is the most popular method of pregnancy testing and is the basis for most over-the-counter home pregnancy tests.
- The biochemical, physiological, and anatomical adaptations that occur during pregnancy are profound and most revert back to the nonpregnant state after birth and lactation.
- Maternal adaptations are attributed to the hormones of pregnancy and to mechanical pressures arising from the enlarging uterus and other tissues.
- Adaptations to pregnancy protect the woman's normal physiological functioning, meet the metabolic demands that pregnancy imposes, and provide for fetal developmental and growth needs.
- Presumptive, probable, and positive signs of pregnancy aid in the diagnosis of pregnancy; only positive signs (identification of a fetal heart tone, verification of fetal movements, and visualization of the fetus) can establish the diagnosis of pregnancy.
- Although the pH of the pregnant woman's vaginal secretions is more acidic than in the nonpregnant state, she is more vulnerable to some vaginal infections, especially yeast infections.
- Increased vascularity and sensitivity of the vagina and other pelvic viscera may lead to a high degree of sexual interest and arousal.
- Some adaptations to pregnancy result in discomforts such as fatigue, urinary frequency, nausea, constipation, and breast sensitivity.
- Balance and coordination are affected by changes in joints and in the woman's centre of gravity as pregnancy progresses.

evolve WEBSITE

Visit the Evolve website for additional resources related to the content in this chapter such as Case Studies, Critical Thinking Case Study Answers, Nursing Care Plans, Nursing Processes, Nursing Skills, and Review Questions for Exam Preparation at: *http://evolve.elsevier.com/Canada/Perry/maternal/*

REFERENCES

Blackburn, S. (2013). *Maternal, fetal, & neonatal physiology: A clinical perspective* (4th ed.). St. Louis: Saunders.

Cunningham, F., Leveno, K., Bloom, S., et al. (2014). *Williams obstetrics* (24th ed.). New York: McGraw Hill.

Duff, W. (2014). Maternal and fetal infections. In R. Resnick, R. K. Creasy, J. D. Iams, et al. (Eds.), *Creasy & Resnik's maternal-fetal medicine: Principles and practice* (7th ed.). Philadelphia: Saunders.

Gordon, M. (2012). Maternal physiology. In S. G. Gabbe, J. R. Niebyl, & J. L. Simpson (Eds.), *Obstetrics: Normal and problem pregnancies* (6th ed.). Philadelphia: Saunders.

Hark, L., & Catalano, P. M. (2012). Nutritional management during pregnancy. In S. G. Gabbe, J. R. Niebyl, J. L. Simpson, et al. (Eds.), *Obstetrics: Normal and problem pregnancies* (6th ed.). Philadelphia: Saunders.

Kelly, R. F., & Savides, T. J. (2012). Gastrointestinal disease in pregnancy. In S. G. Gabbe, J. R. Niebyl, J. L. Simpson, et al. (Eds.), *Obstetrics: Normal and problem pregnancies* (6th ed.). Philadelphia: Saunders.

Kroumpouzos, G. (2012). Skin disease in pregnancy and puerperium. In S. G. Gabbe, J. R. Niebyl, J. L. Simpson, et al. (Eds.), *Obstetrics: Normal and problem pregnancies* (6th ed.). Philadelphia: Saunders.

Lawrence, R. A., & Lawrence, R. M. (2011). *Breastfeeding: A guide for the medical profession* (7th ed.). St. Louis: Mosby.

Leduc, D., Biringer, A., Lee, L., et al. (2013). SOGC clinical practice guideline: Induction of labour at term. *Journal of Obstetrics and Gynaecology Canada, 35*(9), S1–S18.

Magee, L., Pels, A., Helewa, M., et al. (2014). SOGC clinical practice guideline: Diagnosis, evaluation and management of the hypertensive disorders of pregnancy: Executive summary. *Journal of Obstetrics and Gynaecology Canada, 36*(5), 416–438.

Monga, M., & Mastrobattista, J. (2014). Maternal cardiovascular, respiratory, and renal adaptations to pregnancy. In R. K. Creasy, R. Resnik, J. D. Iams, et al. (Eds.), *Creasy & Resnik's maternal-fetal medicine: Principles and practice* (7th ed.). Philadelphia: Saunders.

Pagana, K. D., Pagana, T. J., & Pike-MacDonald, S. A. (2013). *Mosby's Canadian manual of diagnostic and laboratory tests* (1st Canadian ed.). Toronto: Mosby.

Russell, S., & Mayberry, L. (2008). Pregnancy and oral health. *American Journal of Maternal Child Nursing, 33*(1), 32–37.

Salani, R., Eisenhauer, E., & Copeland, L. (2012). Malignant diseases and pregnancy. In S. G. Gabbe, J. R. Niebyl, J. L. Simpson, et al. (Eds.), *Obstetrics: Normal and problem pregnancies* (6th ed.). Philadelphia: Saunders.

Seidel, H., Ball, J. W., Dains, J. E., et al. (2011). *Mosby's guide to physical examination* (7th ed.). St. Louis: Mosby.

Spong, C. Y. (2013). Defining "term" pregnancy. Recommendations from the defining "term" pregnancy workgroup. *Journal of the American Medical Association, 309*(23), 2445–2446. doi:10.1001/jama.2013.6235.

Williamson, C., Mackillop, L., & Heneghan, M. A. (2014). Diseases of the liver, biliary system and pancreas. In R. K. Creasy, R. Resnik, J. D. Iams, et al. (Eds.), *Creasy & Resnik's maternal-fetal medicine: Principles and practice* (7th ed.). Philadelphia: Saunders.

CHAPTER

11

Nursing Care During Pregnancy

Nancy Watts, *with contributions from* *Kathryn R. Alden*

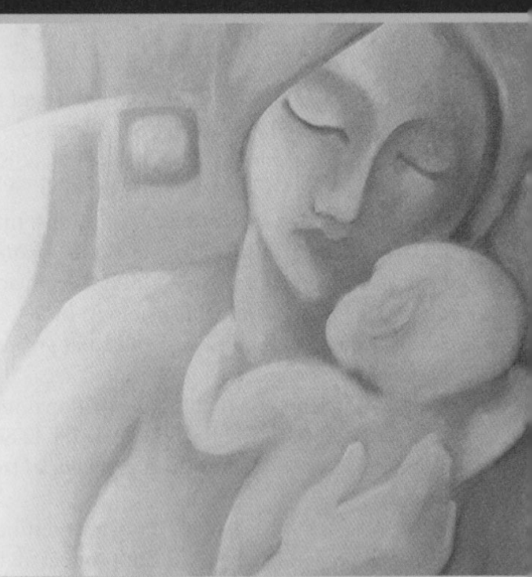

evolve WEBSITE

Visit the Evolve website for additional resources related to the content in this chapter such as Case Studies, Critical Thinking Case Study Answers, Nursing Care Plans, Nursing Processes, Nursing Skills, and Review Questions for Exam Preparation at: http://evolve.elsevier.com/Canada/Perry/maternal/

OBJECTIVES

On completion of this chapter the reader will be able to:

- Describe the processes of confirming pregnancy and estimating the date of birth.
- Summarize the physical, psychosocial, and behavioural changes that usually occur as the mother and family members adapt to pregnancy.
- Discuss the benefits of prenatal care and challenges of accessibility for some women.
- Outline the routine assessments of maternal and fetal health status at the initial and follow-up visits during pregnancy.
- Conceptualize common nursing assessments, diagnoses, interventions, and methods of evaluation in providing care for the pregnant woman and family.
- Plan education needed by pregnant women related to physical discomforts of pregnancy and recognition of the signs and symptoms of potential complications.
- Examine the effects of culture, age, parity, and number of fetuses on the response of the woman and family to the pregnancy and on the prenatal care provided.
- Compare philosophies underlying maternal choices for childbirth care.
- Describe the available options for pregnant women regarding health care providers and birth setting choices.
- Determine the options and scope of childbirth and perinatal education in the community.

The prenatal period is a time of physical and psychological preparation for birth and parenthood. Becoming a parent is a major life event that brings challenges to the woman and her family (Fowler, Reid, Minnis, et al., 2014). It is a time of intense learning and change for parents and those close to them and needs to be seen within a social context. The prenatal period provides a unique opportunity for nurses and other members of the health care team to have a positive influence on the health of all family members. During this period, healthy women seek regular care and guidance, and many are motivated to change behaviours such as eating habits, based on their pregnancy. The perinatal nurse's health promotion interventions can affect the well-being of the woman, her unborn child, and the rest of her family for many years to come.

Regular prenatal visits, ideally beginning soon after the first missed menstrual period, offer opportunities to ensure the health of the expectant mother and her infant. Care is designed to monitor the growth and development of the fetus and identify abnormalities that may interfere with the course of normal pregnancy. The woman and her family can seek support to reduce stress and learn parenting skills.

Pregnancy lasts approximately 9 calendar months. However, health care providers use the concept of lunar months, which last 28 days (or 4 weeks), to describe the duration of pregnancy or gestational age. Thus normal pregnancy lasts about 10 lunar months, that is, 40 weeks, or 280 days. Pregnancy is divided into three 3-month periods, or **trimesters**. The first trimester covers weeks 1 through 13; the second, weeks 14 through 26; and the third, weeks 27 through term gestation. The focus of this chapter is on working with the expectant family to promote a healthy pregnancy that culminates in the birth of a healthy baby.

CONFIRMATION OF PREGNANCY

Women often suspect pregnancy when they miss a menstrual period. Many women come to the first visit after a positive home pregnancy test. However, the clinical diagnosis of pregnancy before the second missed period may be challenging in some women. Factors such as physical variations, lack of abdominal muscle relaxation, obesity, or presence of fibroids may confound even the experienced examiner. Accuracy in diagnosis is important because emotional, social, or medical consequences related to an inaccurate diagnosis, either positive or negative, can be extremely serious. A correct date for the first day of the last (normal) menstrual period (LMP), the date of intercourse, and a **basal body temperature (BBT)** record may be of great value in the accurate determination of pregnancy (see Chapter 8).

Signs and Symptoms

Much variability is possible in the subjective and objective symptoms of pregnancy. Therefore, the confirmation of pregnancy may be uncertain for a time. It is based on signs and symptoms that are reported during history taking or found during physical examination. These signs and symptoms are classified as *presumptive, probable,* or *positive* (see Table 10-2, p. 210).

Estimating Date of Birth

When pregnancy is confirmed, the woman's first question usually is when will she give birth. This date is called the **estimated date of birth (EDB)**. Accurate dating of pregnancy and calculation of the EDB have implications for timing of specific prenatal screening tests, assessing fetal growth, and making critical decisions for managing pregnancy complications. Ultrasound dating of gestational age is accurate during early pregnancy.

Because the exact date of conception is usually unknown, several formulas have been suggested for calculating the EDB. None of these guides is infallible, but **Nägele's rule** is reasonably accurate and is the method used most often.

Nägele's rule is as follows: After determining the first day of the LMP, subtract 3 months, add 7 days and 1 year; or alternatively, add 7 days to the LMP and count forward 9 months. For example, if the first day of the LMP was September 10, 2015, the EDB is June 17, 2016.

Nägele's rule assumes that the woman has a 28-day menstrual cycle and that the pregnancy occurred on the fourteenth day of the cycle. An adjustment is in order if the cycle is longer or shorter than 28 days. Only about 5% of pregnant women give birth spontaneously on the EDB as determined by Nägele's rule. Most women give birth during the period extending from 7 days before to 7 days after the EDB.

ADAPTATION TO PREGNANCY

Pregnancy affects all family members, and each family member needs to adapt to the pregnancy and interpret its meaning in light of his or her own needs and circumstances. This process of family adaptation to pregnancy takes place within a cultural environment influenced by societal trends and continues for many months past the birth. Dramatic cultural and demographic changes have occurred in Western society in recent years, and the perinatal nurse must be prepared to support the diversity in family structure. Families are not limited to but may include single parents, LGBTQ families, extended families, or surrogate families.

Much of the investigation of family dynamics during pregnancy by scholars in the United States and Canada has been done with White, middle-class nuclear families; thus findings may not apply to families who do not fit this model. It is important that the nurse adapt terms in the effort to acknowledge family diversity and demonstrate cultural competence. It is helpful to ask the woman about her "family," which is whoever she may choose and their relationship to her (see Chapter 2).

Maternal Adaptation

Women of all ages use the months of pregnancy to adapt to the maternal role, a complex process of social and cognitive learning.

Pregnancy is a maturational milestone that can be stressful but also rewarding as the woman prepares for a new level of caring and responsibility. Her self-concept changes in readiness for parenthood as she anticipates her new role. She may move gradually from being self-contained and independent to being committed to a lifelong concern for another human being. This growth requires mastery of certain developmental tasks: accepting the pregnancy, identifying with the role of mother, reordering the relationships between herself and her mother and between herself and her partner, establishing a relationship with the unborn child, and preparing for the birth experience. The presence of the woman's family and emotional support are important factors in her successfully accomplishing these developmental tasks. Single women with limited support may have difficulty making this adaptation.

Accepting the Pregnancy

The first step in adapting to the maternal role is accepting the idea of pregnancy and assimilating the pregnant state into the woman's way of life. Mercer (1995) described this process as *cognitive restructuring* and credited Rubin (1975, 1984) as the nurse theorist who pioneered our understanding of maternal role attainment.

The degree of acceptance is reflected in the woman's emotional responses. Initially, many women are dismayed at finding themselves pregnant, especially if the pregnancy is unplanned or unintended. Eventual acceptance of pregnancy parallels the growing acceptance of the reality of a child. This has been described as "engagement" or an active involvement and awareness of the presence of the infant (Darvill, Skirton, & Farrand, 2010). Nonacceptance of the pregnancy should not be equated with rejection of the child. A woman may dislike being pregnant but feel love for the child to be born.

Women who are happy and pleased about their pregnancy usually have high self-esteem and tend to be confident about outcomes for themselves, their babies, and other family members. Despite a general feeling of well-being, many pregnant women are surprised to experience *emotional lability*, that is, rapid and unpredictable changes in mood. These swings in emotions and increased sensitivity to others are disconcerting to the expectant mother and those around her. Increased irritability, tears, and anger may alternate with feelings of great joy and cheerfulness. Profound hormonal changes that are part of the maternal responses to pregnancy may be responsible for these mood changes.

Many women have ambivalent feelings during pregnancy, regardless of whether the pregnancy was intended. *Ambivalence*—having conflicting feelings at the same time—is considered a normal response for people preparing for a new role. For example, during pregnancy, women may feel great pleasure that they are fulfilling a lifelong dream, but they also may feel great regret with the changes that come with parenthood.

Even women who are pleased to be pregnant may, from time to time, experience feelings of hostility toward the pregnancy or the unborn child. Negative emotions may surface with chance remarks regarding another woman's appearance or with missed employment possibilities on account of the pregnancy. Body sensations, feelings of dependence, or realization of the responsibilities of child care also can generate such feelings. Pregnancies that are the result of rape or sexual violence can be extremely difficult for women who continue them. A variety of reasons may lead them to carry out the pregnancy rather than interrupt it. When a woman who is pregnant as a result of sexual violence meets with the perinatal nurse and describes this pregnancy, it is important for the nurse to support her and to obtain additional resources for her as needed, to ensure she has coping strategies in place.

Intense feelings of ambivalence that persist through the third trimester may indicate an unresolved conflict with the motherhood role (Mercer, 1995). After the birth of a healthy child, memories of these ambivalent feelings usually are dismissed. If the child is born with a defect, a woman may look back at the times when she did not want the pregnancy and feel intense guilt. She may believe that her ambivalence caused the birth defect. She will need emotional support and information regarding actual causes for the anomaly.

Identifying With the Mother Role

The process of identifying with the mother role begins early in each woman's life, when she is being mothered as a child. Her cultural and social group's perception of what constitutes a woman's role can subsequently influence her in choosing between motherhood and a career, being married or single, being independent rather than interdependent, or being able to manage multiple roles. Practice roles such as playing with dolls, babysitting, and taking care of siblings may increase her understanding of what being a mother entails.

Many women have always wanted a baby; they like children and look forward to motherhood. Their high motivation to become a parent promotes acceptance of pregnancy and eventual prenatal and parental adaptation. Other women may not have considered in any detail what motherhood means to them. During pregnancy, these women will need to resolve conflicts such as not wanting the pregnancy and child-related or career-related decisions.

Reordering Personal Relationships

Close relationships of the pregnant woman generally undergo change as she prepares emotionally for the new role of mother. The friendship of other pregnant women or new mothers may also be important as their experience is valued (Darvill et al., 2010). Information can be passed from one woman to another that normalizes what one is feeling or doing as preparation for labour, birth, or parenting.

As family members learn their new roles, periods of tension and conflict may occur. Social support, aid, and affirmation are critical to the pregnant woman and are most often provided by her social network, extended family, and partner (Hui Choi, Lee, Chan, et al., 2012). Promoting effective communication patterns between the expectant mother and her own mother and between the expectant mother and her partner are common nursing interventions during prenatal visits.

The woman's relationship with her mother is significant in adapting to and feeling confidence in her pregnancy and motherhood. Important components in the pregnant woman's relationship with her mother are the mother's availability (past and present), her reactions to her daughter's pregnancy, respect for her daughter's autonomy, and the willingness to reminisce (Mercer, 1995). Her encouragement and support are also critical to this bond that is being strengthened during pregnancy (Darvill et al., 2010).

The mother's positive reaction to her daughter's pregnancy signifies her acceptance of the grandchild and of her daughter. If the mother is supportive, the daughter has an opportunity to discuss pregnancy and labour and her feelings of joy or ambivalence with a knowledgeable and accepting woman who is close to her (Fig. 11-1). Reminiscing about the pregnant woman's early childhood and sharing the grandmother-to-be's account of her childbirth experience can help the daughter anticipate and prepare for labour and birth.

Although the woman's relationship with her mother is significant in considering her adaptation in pregnancy, the most important person to the pregnant woman is usually the woman's partner. A woman who is nurtured by her partner during pregnancy tends to have fewer emotional and physical symptoms, reduced stress during the pregnancy, fewer labour and childbirth complications, optimal fetal growth, and an easier postpartum adjustment (Lederman & Weis, 2009). Women generally express two major needs within this relationship during pregnancy: feeling loved and valued, and having the child accepted by their partner.

In a committed relationship, the addition of a child changes forever the nature of the bond between partners. This can be a time when couples grow closer and the pregnancy has a maturing effect on the partners' relationship as they assume new roles and discover new aspects of one another. Partners who trust and support each other are able to share mutual

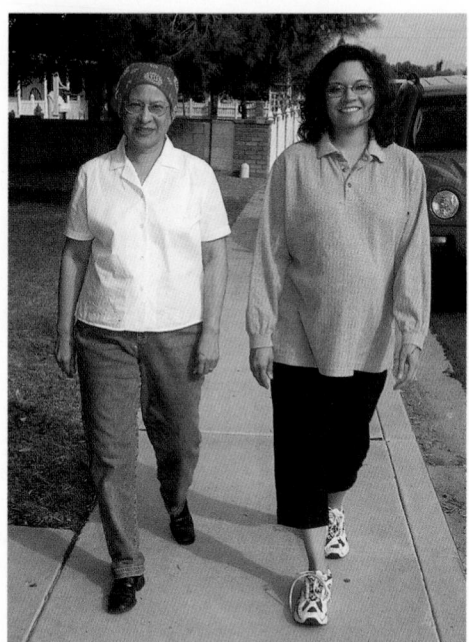

FIGURE 11-1 A pregnant woman and her mother enjoying a walk together. (Courtesy Michael S. Clement, MD.)

dependency needs (Mercer, 1995). Women who feel insecure about themselves and their new role need encouragement from their partner and families.

Sexual expression during pregnancy is highly individual. The sexual relationship is affected by physical, emotional, and interactional factors, including misinformation about sex during pregnancy, sexual dysfunction, and physical changes in the woman. An individual may inaccurately attribute anomalies, developmental disability, and other injuries to the fetus and mother to sexual relations during pregnancy. Some couples fear that the woman's genitals will be drastically changed by the birth process. Couples may not express their concerns to the health care provider because of embarrassment or because they do not want to appear foolish.

As pregnancy progresses, changes in body shape, body image, and levels of discomfort influence both partners' desire for sexual expression. During the first trimester, the woman's sexual desire may decrease, especially if she has breast tenderness, nausea, or fatigue. As she progresses into the second trimester, her sense of well-being, combined with the increased pelvic congestion that occurs at this time, may increase her desire for sexual release. In the third trimester, somatic discomforts and physical bulkiness may increase her physical discomfort and diminish her interest in sex. Partners need to feel free to discuss their sexual responses during pregnancy with each other and with their health care provider (see later discussion).

Establishing a Relationship With the Fetus

Emotional attachment—feelings of being connected through affection or love—begins during the prenatal period as women fantasize and daydream in preparing themselves for motherhood (Rubin, 1975). They think of themselves as mothers and imagine maternal qualities they would like to possess. Expectant parents wish to be warm, loving, and close to their child. They try to anticipate changes the child will bring to their lives and wonder how they will react to noise, disorder, reduced freedom, and caregiving activities. The mother–child relationship progresses through pregnancy as a developmental process that tends to unfold over three phases.

In phase 1, the woman accepts the biological fact of pregnancy. She needs to be able to state, "I am pregnant." In phase 2, the woman accepts the growing fetus as distinct from herself and as a person to nurture. She can now say, "I am going to have a baby." Attachment of a mother to her child is enhanced by experiencing a planned pregnancy, and it increases when ultrasound examination and quickening (feeling movement) confirm the reality of the fetus. During phase 3, the woman prepares realistically for the birth and parenting of the child. She expresses the thought, "I am going to be a mother," and defines the nature and characteristics of the child. For example, she may speculate about the child's sex (if she has not had an ultrasound examination that confirms the sex) and personality traits based on patterns of fetal activity.

Although the mother alone experiences the child within, both parents and siblings may believe the unborn child responds in a very individualized, personal manner. Family members may interact with the unborn child by talking to the fetus and stroking the mother's abdomen, especially when the fetus shifts position. They may sing to, play music for, or read to the fetus. The fetus may have a nickname used by family members.

Parents may occasionally show or voice disappointment over the sex of the child. The parents may experience grief and a sense of loss at birth as they release their fantasized image of the child and begin to accept the real child. However, these negative responses are usually temporary. Providing an accepting environment for parental reactions facilitates the parent's ability to move beyond disappointment to acceptance.

Preparing for Childbirth

Many women actively prepare for birth. They read books, view films, attend childbirth classes, and talk to other women. They seek the caregiver with whom they feel most comfortable for advice, monitoring, and caring. The multipara has her own history of labour and birth, which influences her approach to preparation for this childbirth experience.

Some mothers may feel anxious about safe passage—for themselves and for their child during the birth process (Mercer, 1995; Rubin, 1975). This concern may not be expressed overtly but rather through making plans for care of the new baby and other children in case "anything should happen." The nurse needs to listen for such cues of a mother's concern. These feelings can persist despite receiving statistical evidence about the safe outcome of pregnancy for mothers and their infants. Many women fear the pain of childbirth or fear mutilation; they do not understand anatomy and the birth process. Education offered by the perinatal nurse can alleviate many of these fears.

Toward the end of the third trimester, a mother's breathing can be difficult and fetal movements become vigorous enough to disturb the mother's sleep. Backaches, increased frequency and urgency of urination, constipation, and varicose veins can become troublesome. The bulkiness and awkwardness of her body interfere with the woman's ability to care for other children, perform routine work-related duties, and assume a comfortable position for sleep and rest. A strong desire to see the end of pregnancy, to be over and done with it, makes women at this stage ready to move on to childbirth.

Paternal Adaptation

The same fears, questions, and concerns of the mother may also affect her birth partner, whether the partner is a biological father or not. Birth partners need to be kept informed, supported, and included in all activities in which the mother desires the partner's participation. The nurse can do much to promote pregnancy and birth as a family experience.

Modern fatherhood is increasingly diverse, given the wide variety of family structures (Habib, 2012). The father's beliefs and feelings about the ideal mother and father and his cultural expectation of appropriate behaviour during pregnancy will affect his response to his partner's need for him. One man may engage in nurturing behaviour; another may feel lonely and alienated as the woman becomes physically and emotionally engrossed in the unborn child. The man may seek comfort and understanding outside the home or become interested in a new hobby or involved with his work. Some men view pregnancy as proof of their masculinity and their dominant role. To others, pregnancy has no meaning in terms of responsibility to either mother or child. However, for most men, pregnancy is a time of preparation for the parental role, fantasizing about being in that role, great pleasure, and intense learning (Fig. 11-2).

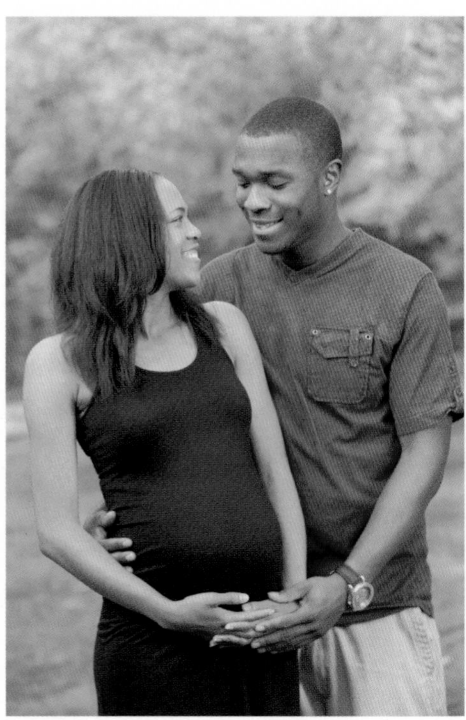

FIGURE 11-2 A prospective mother and father walk spending time together. Women respond positively to their partner's interest and concern. (Flashon Studio/Shutterstock.com.)

Accepting the Pregnancy

The ways in which fathers adjust to the parental role have been the subject of considerable research. In older societies, the man enacted the ritual couvades; that is, he behaved in specific ways and respected taboos associated with pregnancy and giving birth. In this way, the man's new status was recognized and endorsed. By contrast, some modern-day men experience pregnancy-like symptoms, such as nausea, weight gain, and other physical symptoms. This phenomenon is known as the couvade syndrome. Changing cultural and professional attitudes have encouraged fathers' participation in the birth experience; however, there are still many cultures in which pregnancy and childbirth are considered a female domain and men are not encouraged to be part of the labour and birth process. It is important that the nurse be aware and understanding of different cultural expectations.

The man's emotional response to becoming a father, his concerns, and his informational needs will change during the course of pregnancy. May (1982) described three phases characterizing the developmental tasks experienced by the expectant father:

- The *announcement phase* may last from a few hours to a few weeks. The developmental task is to accept the biological fact of pregnancy. Men react to the confirmation of pregnancy with joy or dismay, depending on whether the pregnancy is desired, unplanned, or unwanted. Ambivalence in the early stages of pregnancy is common. If pregnancy is unplanned or unwanted, some men find the alterations in life plans and lifestyles difficult to accept. Some men engage in extramarital affairs for the first time during their partner's pregnancy. Others batter their wives for the first time or escalate the frequency of battering episodes.
- The second phase, the *moratorium phase,* is the period when he adjusts to the reality of pregnancy. The developmental task is to accept the pregnancy. Men appear to put conscious thought of the pregnancy aside for a time. They become more introspective and engage in many discussions about their philosophy of life, religion, child-bearing, and child-rearing practices and their relationships with family members, particularly with their father. Depending on the man's readiness for the pregnancy, this phase may be relatively short or persist until the last trimester.
- The third phase, the *focusing phase,* begins in the last trimester and is characterized by the father's active involvement in both the pregnancy and his relationship with his child. The developmental task is to negotiate with his partner the role he is to play in labour and to prepare for parenthood. In this phase, the man concentrates on his experience of the pregnancy and begins to think of himself as a father.

These phases are not rigid, and various men will act them out to different degrees or may not go through them at all, but they can be used as a guideline.

Identifying With the Father Role

Each man brings to pregnancy attitudes that affect the way in which he adjusts to the pregnancy and parental role. His memories of the fathering he received from his own father, the experiences he has had with child care, and the perceptions of the male and father roles within his social group guide his selection of the tasks and responsibilities he will assume. Some men are highly motivated to nurture and love a child, based on modelling or perceived deficiencies in their childhood (Habib, 2012). They may be excited and pleased about the anticipated role of father. Others may be more detached or even hostile to the idea of fatherhood.

Reordering Personal Relationships

One of the partner's roles in pregnancy is to nurture and respond to the pregnant woman's feelings of vulnerability. The partner also must deal with the reality of the pregnancy. The partner's support indicates involvement in the pregnancy and preparation for attachment to the child. The father's involvement with pregnancy and the infant following birth is strongly tied to the quality of the relationship with his partner (Habib, 2012).

Some aspects of a partner's behaviour indicate rivalry. Direct rivalry with the fetus may be evident, especially during sexual activity. Men may protest that fetal movements prevent sexual gratification or that the fetus is watching them during sexual activity. Feelings of rivalry may be unconscious and not verbalized but expressed through subtle behaviours.

The woman's increased introspection may cause her partner to feel uneasy as she becomes preoccupied with thoughts of the child and of motherhood, with her growing dependence on her health care provider, and with her re-evaluation of the couple's relationship.

Establishing a Relationship With the Fetus

The father–child attachment can be as strong as the mother–child relationship, and fathers can be as competent as mothers in nurturing their infants. The father–child attachment also begins in pregnancy. A father may rub or kiss the maternal abdomen; try to listen, talk, or sing to the fetus; or play with the fetus as he notes fetal movement. Calling the unborn child by name or nickname helps to confirm the reality of pregnancy and encourage attachment.

Men prepare for fatherhood in many of the same ways that women prepare for motherhood (i.e., by reading and fantasizing about the baby). Daydreaming about their role as father is common in the last weeks before the birth; men rarely describe their thoughts unless they are reassured that such daydreams are normal. They may adjust work commitments or plan vacations so that they can spend time with their new family.

Nurses can help fathers identify concerns and prepare for the role of being a father by asking questions such as the following:

- What does the word *father* mean to you?
- How do you see yourself as a father/parent?
- What do you imagine your baby will look and act like?
- Have you thought about the baby's crying? Changing diapers? Burping the baby? Being awakened at night? Sharing your partner with the baby?

Some fathers may not wish to answer such questions when they are asked but may need time to think them through or discuss them with their partners.

As the birth day approaches, fathers may have more questions about fetal and newborn behaviours. Some fathers are shocked or amazed at the small size of the clothes and furniture for the baby. The nurse can tell the father about the unborn child's ability to respond to light, sound, and touch and encourage him to feel and talk to the fetus. Discussions with new fathers, as in childbirth classes, may be welcomed.

Preparing for Childbirth

The days and weeks immediately before the expected day of birth are characterized by anticipation and anxiety. Boredom and restlessness are common as the couple focuses on the birth process; however, during the last 2 months of pregnancy many expectant fathers experience a surge of creative energy at home and on the job. They can become dissatisfied with their present living space. They tend to act on the need to alter the environment (e.g., remodelling, painting). This activity can be overt evidence of their sharing in the child-bearing experience. They are able to channel the anxiety and other feelings experienced during the final weeks before birth into productive activities. This behaviour generally earns recognition and compliments from friends, relatives, and their partners.

Major concerns for partners are getting the mother to the birthing facility in time for the birth and not appearing ignorant. Many men want to be able to recognize labour and determine when it is appropriate to leave for the hospital or call the physician or midwife. They may imagine different situations and plan what they will do in response to them; they may rehearse taking various routes to the hospital, timing each route at different times of the day.

Some prospective fathers have questions about the birthing suite's furniture, nursing staff, and location, as well as the availability of the health care provider and anaesthesiologist. Others want to know what is expected of them when their partners are in labour. A tour of the hospital may help alleviate some of these concerns. The man may have fears concerning the safety of his partner and about the possible mutilation or death of his partner or child. It is important that he be able to express these fears; otherwise he cannot help his mate deal with her unspoken or overt apprehension.

With the exception of childbirth preparation classes, men have few opportunities to learn ways to be an involved and active participate in this rite of passage into parenthood. The tensions and apprehensions of the unprepared, unsupportive father are readily transmitted to the mother and may increase her fears.

Sibling Adaptation

Sharing the spotlight with a new brother or sister may be the first major crisis for a child. The older child often experiences a sense of loss or feels jealous at being "replaced" by the new baby. Some of the factors that influence the child's response are age, the parents' attitudes, the father's role, the length of separation from the mother, the hospital's visitation policy, and how the child has been prepared for the change.

The mother with other children needs to devote time and energy to reorganizing her relationships with these children.

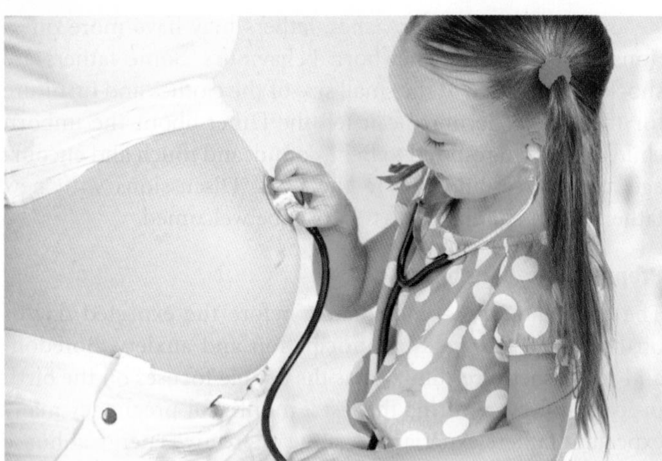

FIGURE 11-3 A 4-year-old likes to examine the pregnant abdomen of her mother. (Evgeny Atamanenko/Shutterstock.com.)

She needs to prepare siblings for the birth of the baby (Fig. 11-3 and Patient Teaching box: Tips for Sibling Preparation). She can begin the process of role transition in the family by including the children in the pregnancy and being sympathetic to older children's concerns about losing their place in the family hierarchy. No child willingly gives up a familiar position.

Sibling responses to pregnancy vary with age and dependency needs. Since a new baby spends more time interacting with sibling(s) than with anyone else, fostering a positive relationship is important to cognitive and motor development (Berger & Nuzzo, 2008). The 1-year-old infant seems largely unaware of the process, but the 2-year-old child notices the change in the mother's appearance and may comment, "Mommy's fat." The 2-year-old child's need for sameness in the environment makes the child aware of any change. Toddlers may exhibit more clinging behaviour and revert to dependent behaviours in toilet training or eating.

By age 3 or 4 years, children like to be told the story of their own beginning and accept its being compared to the present pregnancy. They like to listen to heartbeats and feel the baby moving in utero (see Fig. 11-3). Sometimes they worry about how the baby is being fed and what it wears.

School-age children take a more clinical interest in their mother's pregnancy. They may want to know in more detail "How did the baby get in there?" and "How will it get out?" Children in this age group notice pregnant women in stores, churches, and schools and sometimes seem shy if they need to approach a pregnant woman directly. On the whole, they look forward to the new baby, see themselves as "mothers" or "fathers," and enjoy buying baby supplies and readying a place for the baby. Because they still think in concrete terms and base judgements on the here and now, they respond positively to their mother's current good health.

Early and middle adolescents preoccupied with the establishment of their own sexual identity may have difficulty accepting the overwhelming evidence of the sexual activity of their parents. They reason that if they are too young for such activity, certainly their parents are too old. They seem to take on a critical parental role and may ask, "What will people think?" or "How can you let yourself get so fat?" Many pregnant women with teenage children confess that their teenagers are the most difficult factor in their current pregnancy.

Late adolescents do not appear to be unduly disturbed. They realize that they soon will be gone from home. Parents usually report that late adolescents are comforting and act more like other adults than children.

Grandparent Adaptation

Every pregnancy affects all family relationships. For expectant grandparents, a first pregnancy in a child is undeniable evidence that they are growing older. Many think of a grandparent as old, white-haired, and becoming feeble of mind and body; however, some people face grandparenthood while still in their 30s or 40s. A mother-to-be announcing her pregnancy to her mother may be greeted by a negative response, indicating that she is not ready to be a grandmother. Both daughter and mother may be startled and hurt by the response.

In some family units, expectant grandparents are nonsupportive and may inadvertently decrease the self-esteem of the parents-to-be. Mothers may talk about their terrible pregnancies; fathers may discuss the endless cost of rearing children; and a mother-in-law may complain that her son is neglecting her because his concern is now directed toward the pregnant daughter-in-law.

However, most grandparents are delighted with the prospect of a new baby in the family. It reawakens their feelings of their own youth, the excitement of giving birth, and their delight in the behaviour of the parents-to-be when they were infants. They set up a memory store of their child's first smiles, first words, and first steps that can be used later for "claiming" the newborn as a member of the family. Their satisfaction and that of the parents come with the realization that continuity between past and present is guaranteed.

The grandparent is the historian who transmits the family history, a resource person who shares knowledge based on experience, a role model, and a support person. The grandparent's presence and support can strengthen family systems by widening the circle of support and nurturance (Fig. 11-4). Other sources of information cannot replace the unique contribution that grandparents make.

NURSING CARE

The goal of prenatal care is to promote the health and well-being of the pregnant woman, her fetus, the newborn, and the family (Gregory, Niebyl, & Johnson, 2012). Major emphasis is placed on preventive aspects of care, primarily to encourage the pregnant woman to practise optimal self-management and report unusual changes early so that problems can be minimized or prevented. In holistic care, nurses provide information and guidance about not only the physical changes but also the psychosocial impact of pregnancy on the woman and members of her family. Therefore, the goals of prenatal nursing care are to foster a safe birth for the infant and mother and to promote satisfaction of the mother and family with the pregnancy and birth experience.

PATIENT TEACHING

Tips for Sibling Preparation

Prenatal

Adjust the timing and content of information about an anticipated infant to the age and understanding of the older child.

Take your child on a prenatal visit. Let the child listen to the fetal heartbeat and feel the baby move.

Involve the child in preparations for the baby, such as helping to decorate the baby's room.

Move the child to a bed (if still sleeping in a crib) at least 2 months before the baby is due or wait until a few months after the birth.

Read books, show videos, or take child to sibling preparation classes (see figure), including a hospital tour.

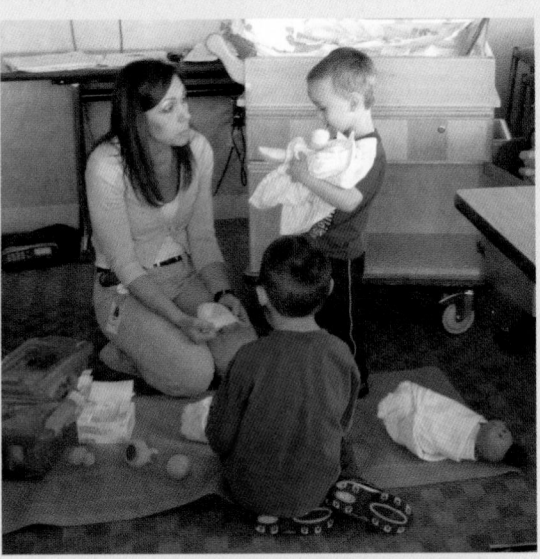

Preschoolers in a sibling class learn about childbirth and infant care using dolls. (Courtesy Julie and Darren Nelson.)

Answer your child's questions about the coming birth and what babies are like, as well as any other questions factually and at the child's level of understanding.

Take your child to the homes of friends who have babies so that the child has realistic expectations of what babies are like.

During the Hospital Stay

Have someone bring the child to the hospital to visit you and the baby (unless you plan to have the child attend the birth).

Don't force interactions between the child and the baby. Often the child will be more interested in seeing you and being reassured of your love.

Help the child explore the infant by showing how and where to touch the baby.

Give the child a gift (from you or from you, the father, and the baby).

Going Home

Leave the child at home with a relative or babysitter.

Have someone else carry the baby from the car so that you can hug the child first.

Adjustment After the Baby Is Home

Arrange for a special time with the child alone with each parent.

Don't exclude the child during infant feeding times. The child can sit with you and the baby and feed a doll or drink juice or milk with you or sit quietly with a game. Encourage others to give gifts of nutritious snacks in little gift bags to eat when feeding the baby.

Prepare small gifts for the child so that, when the baby gets gifts, the sibling won't feel left out. Praise the child for acting age appropriately (so that being a baby does not seem better than being older).

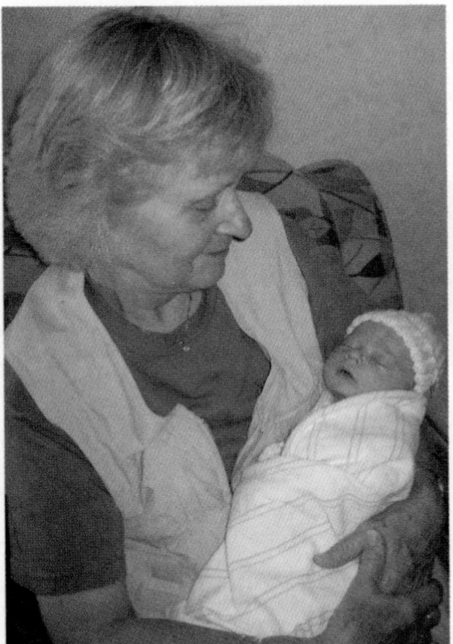

FIGURE 11-4 A grandmother relaxes with her grandson. (Courtesy Shannon Perry.)

In Canada the majority of pregnant women receive care in the first trimester (Public Health Agency of Canada [PHAC], 2009). Prenatal care is sought routinely by women of middle or high socioeconomic status. Lack of culturally sensitive care providers and barriers in communication caused by a lack of health care providers fluent in a population's language may interfere with access to care. Immigrant women from cultures in which prenatal care is not emphasized may not know to seek routine prenatal care. Thus birth outcomes in these populations are less positive, with higher rates of maternal and fetal or newborn complications. In particular, newborns with low birth weight (LBW) (less than 2500 g) and infant mortality have been associated with inadequate prenatal care (Cunningham, Leveno, Bloom, et al., 2014).

Barriers to obtaining health care during pregnancy include inadequate numbers of health care providers, unpleasant clinic facilities or procedures, inconvenient clinic hours, distance from health care facilities, lack of transportation, fragmentation of services, inadequate finances, and conflicting personal attitudes. The availability and accessibility of prenatal care may be improved by increasing the use of advanced practice nurses in collaborative practice with physicians or midwives or providing hours for clinics that accommodate working mothers. The effectiveness of a regular schedule of home visiting by nurses during pregnancy also has been validated (Agency for Healthcare Research and Quality [AHRQ] Healthcare Innovations Exchange, 2012).

The traditional model for providing prenatal care has been used for more than a century. The initial visit usually occurs in the first trimester, with monthly visits occurring through week 28 of pregnancy. Thereafter, visits are scheduled every 2 weeks until week 36 and then every week until birth.

More recently, the trend is toward individualizing the schedule of care. Women with low-risk pregnancies may have fewer routine prenatal visits, whereas those at risk for complications may be seen more frequently than the traditional schedule (American Academy of Pediatrics [AAP] Committee on Fetus and Newborn and American College of Obstetricians and Gynecologists [ACOG] Committee on Obstetric Practice, 2012).

Group prenatal care is an alternative model to traditional care during pregnancy. In group prenatal care, authority is shifted from the provider to the woman and other women who have similar due dates. The model creates an atmosphere that facilitates learning, encourages discussion, and develops mutual support. CenteringPregnancy (see Additional Resources at end of the chapter) is a well-known model of group prenatal care that involves three components: health care assessment, education, and peer support. Most care takes place in the group setting after the initial visit and continues for ten 2-hour sessions that begin at about 16 weeks. At each meeting, the first 30 to 40 minutes consists of assessments (by the woman herself and by the health care provider) and the remaining 60 to 75 minutes is spent in group discussion of specific issues such as discomforts of pregnancy and preparation for labour and birth. Families and partners are encouraged to participate. Benefits associated with group prenatal care include improved birth outcomes such as lower rates of preterm birth, increased knowledge, improved satisfaction, and higher breastfeeding initiation rates (Herrman, Rogers, & Ehrenthal, 2012; Picklesimer, Billings, Hale, et al., 2012; Robertson, Aycock, & Darnell, 2009; Rotundo, 2011).

The South Community Birth Program (SCBP) in Vancouver, British Columbia, uses a Centering Pregnancy approach called Connecting Pregnancy. Low-risk pregnant women in the underserved community of South Vancouver receive collaborative, multidisciplinary care from family physicians, midwives, community health nurses, and doulas. This is the first such multidisciplinary program of its kind in Canada in which midwives and family physicians share the care of patients (see Additional Resources at end of the chapter).

Prenatal care is ideally a multidisciplinary activity in which nurses work with midwives, nutritionists, physicians, social workers, and others. Collaboration among these individuals is necessary to provide holistic care. The case management model, which makes use of care maps and critical pathways, is one system that promotes comprehensive care with limited overlap in services. To emphasize the nursing role, care management for the initial visit and follow-up visits is organized around the central elements of the nursing process: assessment, analysis, plan of care and interventions, and evaluation.

In recent years, the concept of preconception care has been recognized as an important contributor to good pregnancy outcomes. If women can incorporate healthy lifestyle behaviours prior to conception—specifically, good nutrition, entering pregnancy with as healthy a weight as possible, adequate intake of folic acid, avoidance of alcohol and tobacco use, prevention of sexually transmitted infections (STIs) and other health hazards—a healthier pregnancy may result. Likewise, women who have health problems related to chronic diseases such as diabetes mellitus can be counselled regarding their special needs with the intent to minimize maternal and fetal complications. See Chapter 9 for further discussion of Preconception care.

Initial Visit

Once the pregnancy is confirmed and the woman's desire to continue the pregnancy has been validated, prenatal care is begun. The assessment process begins at the initial visit and is continued throughout the pregnancy. Assessment techniques include the interview, physical examination, and laboratory tests. Because the initial visit and follow-up visits are distinctly different in content and process, they are described here separately.

Interview

The pregnant woman and her partner or family members who may be present should be told that the first prenatal visit is longer and more detailed than future visits. The initial evaluation includes a comprehensive health history emphasizing the current pregnancy, previous pregnancies, the family, history of domestic violence or child abuse, a psychosocial profile, screening for mental health concerns, a physical assessment, diagnostic testing, and an overall risk assessment.

The therapeutic relationship between the nurse and the woman is established during the initial assessment interview (Fig. 11-5). Two types of data are collected: the woman's subjective appraisal of her health status and the nurse's objective observations.

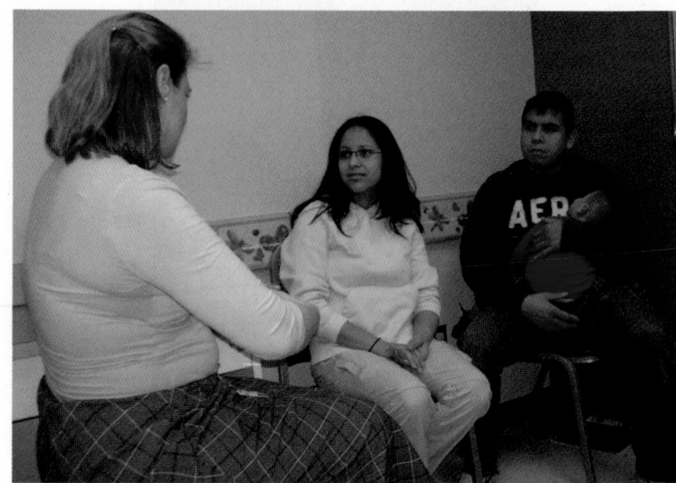

FIGURE 11-5 Prenatal interview. (Courtesy Dee Lowdermilk.)

With the woman's permission, persons accompanying her should be included in the initial prenatal interview. Observations and information about the woman's partner or family are then entered in the database. For example, if the woman is accompanied by small children, the nurse can ask about her plans for child care during the time of labour and birth. Any special needs should be noted at this time (e.g., wheelchair access, assistance in getting on and off the examining table, and cognitive deficits).

Reasons for Seeking Care

Although pregnant women are scheduled for "routine" prenatal visits, they often come to the health care provider seeking information or reassurance about a particular concern. When the woman is asked a broad, open-ended question, such as "How have you been feeling?" she may reveal problems that could otherwise be overlooked. The woman's chief concerns should be recorded in her own words to alert other personnel to the priority of needs identified by her. At the initial visit, a typical desire is for information about what is normal in the course of pregnancy. The presumptive signs of pregnancy may be of great concern to the woman. A review of symptoms she is experiencing and how she is coping with them helps establish a database for developing a plan of care. Some early teaching may be provided at this time.

Child-bearing and Female Reproductive System History

Data are gathered on the woman's age at menarche; menstrual history; contraceptive history; the nature of any infertility or gynecological conditions; history of any STIs; her sexual history; and a detailed history of all her pregnancies, including the present one, and their outcomes. The date of the last Papanicolaou (Pap) test and the result are noted. The date of her LMP is obtained to establish the EDB.

Health History

The health history includes those physical or surgical procedures that can affect the pregnancy or that can be affected by the pregnancy. For example, a pregnant woman who has diabetes or epilepsy requires special care. Because women may be anxious during the initial interview, the nurse's reference to cues such as a MedicAlert bracelet can prompt the woman to explain allergies; chronic diseases; or medications being taken, such as cortisone, insulin, or anticonvulsants.

The woman should also describe any previous surgical procedures. If a woman has had uterine surgery or extensive repair of the pelvic floor, a Caesarean birth may be necessary; previous appendectomy rules out appendicitis as a cause of right lower quadrant pain in pregnancy. Spinal surgery may contraindicate the use of spinal or epidural anaesthesia, and breast augmentation or reduction procedures may impact the breastfeeding experience. Any injury involving the pelvis should be noted.

Women may forget to mention chronic or handicapping conditions during the initial assessment because they have adapted to them. Special shoes or a limp may indicate the existence of a pelvic structural defect—an important consideration in pregnant women. The nurse who observes these special characteristics and sensitively inquires about them can obtain individualized data that will provide the basis for a comprehensive nursing care plan to help optimize pregnancy outcomes (Signore, Spong, Krotoski, et al., 2011). Observations are a vital component of the interview process because they prompt the nurse and the woman to focus on the specific needs of the woman and her family.

A detailed mental health history also needs to be completed. Whether the woman or any family member has a previous history of depression or any other mental health issues should be noted. It is important to identify these issues early in pregnancy so that prompt assessment and treatment can be implemented if concerns arise. A history of mental health concerns increases the risk for the development of further issues during pregnancy and in the postpartum period.

Nutritional History

The nutritional status of a pregnant woman has a direct effect on the growth and development of the fetus. A dietary assessment can reveal special diet practices, food allergies, eating behaviours, the practice of **pica**, and other factors related to her nutritional status (see Box 12-5). Pregnant women are usually motivated to learn about good nutrition and respond well to nutritional advice generated by this assessment. Cultural influences on diet and food selection should also be considered (see Chapter 12).

It is essential that obese women receive counselling about weight gain, nutrition, and food choices. They should also be advised about their risk for complications for themselves and increased risk for congenital abnormalities (Davies, Maxwell, McLeod, et al., 2010). Women with a history of bariatric surgery are nutritionally at risk and should be followed closely throughout pregnancy to promote maternal and fetal well-being (Magdaleno, Pereira, Chaim, et al., 2012).

History of Use of Drugs and Herbal Preparations

A woman's past and present use of substances, both prescribed or over-the-counter (OTC), and problematic (e.g., marijuana, recreational use of opioids, cocaine, nicotine, and alcohol), must be assessed because many substances cross the placenta and can harm the developing fetus. Increasing numbers of individuals, including pregnant women, are using herbal preparations. Therefore it is important for health care providers to question women regarding the use of herbal preparations and to document their responses.

It is especially important to form a relationship with women who are being treated for a history of problematic substance use, such as those in a methadone program or those who are continuing to use substances during pregnancy that will be concerning for the fetus during pregnancy or the infant at birth. Providing information about care during pregnancy and in labour and birth which is honest and transparent will help foster the therapeutic relationship needed to empower the woman and family to attend prenatal care and practise interventions required for a healthy pregnancy. Asking questions about her substance use in a nonthreatening way as well as exploring the woman's story can facilitate this relationship (Fowler et al., 2014) (see Chapter 15 for further discussion).

> **LEGAL TIP *SCREENING FOR DRUG USE***
> Hospitals must obtain informed consent from a pregnant woman before she can be tested for drug use (Wong, Ordean, & Kahan, et al., 2011). Providing the woman information about how the test will be used to provide care for her infant will help her understand the reason for the test.

Family History

The family history provides information about the woman's immediate family, including parents, siblings, and children. These data can be used to identify familial or genetic disorders or conditions that could affect the health of the woman or her fetus.

Social, Experiential, and Occupational History

Situational factors such as the family's ethnic and cultural background and socioeconomic status are assessed while the history is obtained. The following information may be gathered over several encounters. The woman's perception of this pregnancy is explored by asking her such questions as the following:

- Is this pregnancy wanted or not, planned or not?
- Is the woman or couple pleased or displeased, accepting or nonaccepting?
- What problems related to finances, career, or living accommodations may arise as a result of the pregnancy?

The family support system is determined by asking her such questions as the following:

- Who is her primary support?
- Which roles does she expect her significant other or father of the baby to play?
- Are changes needed to promote adequate support?
- What are the existing relationships among mother, father or partner, siblings, and in-laws?
- What preparations are being made for her care and that of dependent family members during labour and for the care of the infant after birth?
- Is financial, educational, or other support needed from the community?
- What are the woman's ideas about child-bearing, her expectations of the infant's behaviour, and her outlook on life and the woman's role?

Other questions that should be asked include the following:

- What does the woman think it will be like to have a baby in the home?
- How is her life going to change by having a baby?
- What plans are interrupted by having a baby at this time?

During interviews throughout the pregnancy, the nurse should remain alert for the appearance of potential parenting problems such as depression, lack of family support, and inadequate living conditions. The nurse must assess the woman's attitude toward health care, particularly during child-bearing; her expectations of health care providers; and her view of the relationship between herself and the nurse.

Coping mechanisms and patterns of interacting should also be identified. Early in the pregnancy, the nurse should determine the woman's knowledge of pregnancy, maternal changes, fetal growth, self-management, and care of the newborn, including feeding. Before planning for nursing care, the nurse needs information about the woman's decision-making abilities and living habits (e.g., exercise, sleep, diet, diversional interests, personal hygiene). Common stressors during child-bearing include the baby's welfare, the labour and birth process, the behaviours of the newborn, the relationship with the baby's father and her family, changes in body image, and physical symptoms.

Attitudes concerning the range of acceptable sexual behaviour during pregnancy can be explored by asking, for example, what the woman's family (partner, friends) have told her about sex during pregnancy. The woman's sexual self-concept can be addressed by asking such questions as: How do you feel about the changes in your appearance? How does your partner feel about your body now? How do you feel about wearing maternity clothes?

Women should be questioned regarding their occupation, past and present, since this may adversely affect maternal and fetal health. For some women, heavy lifting and exposure to chemicals and radiation may be part of their daily work, and these activities can negatively affect the pregnancy. For others, long hours of sitting at a desk working at a computer can contribute to carpal tunnel syndrome or circulatory stasis in the legs. Women also should be asked about their exposure to children, such as at a day care centre or in a school, to assess the possibility of exposure to infectious diseases such as varicella or parvovirus.

History of Physical or Sexual Abuse

All women should be assessed for a history or risk of physical or sexual abuse, particularly because the likelihood of intimate partner violence (IPV) increases during pregnancy (see Chapter 5 for a detailed discussion). A history of childhood sexual abuse also needs to be assessed, as this can have an impact on the woman's labour experience. It is essential that the screening be done in a safe, private setting with the woman alone. The nurse can ask the woman screening questions along with routine assessments during pregnancy. Examples of questions that might be asked include the following:

- Are you with a spouse or partner who threatens or physically hurts you? If yes, who?
- Within the past year or in this pregnancy, has anyone hit, slapped, kicked, or otherwise hurt you? If yes, who? Are you currently with that person?
- Has anyone forced you to have sexual activities that made you uncomfortable? If yes, who? Are you currently with that person?

Although visual cues from the woman's appearance or behaviour may suggest the possibility of abuse, no one profile of the woman who experiences IPV exists. Identification of abuse and immediate clinical intervention that includes information about safety can result in the woman taking steps that may prevent future abuse and increase the safety and well-being of the woman and her infant. During pregnancy, the target body parts tend to change during abusive episodes. Women report physical blows directed to the head, breasts, abdomen, and genitalia. Sexual assault is common.

IPV and pregnancy in teenagers constitutes a particularly difficult situation. Adolescents may be trapped in the abusive relationship because of their inexperience. Routine screening for abuse and sexual assault is recommended for pregnant adolescents. Because pregnancy in young adolescent girls may be the result of sexual abuse, the nurse should assess the girl's desire to maintain the pregnancy.

Nurses should be aware that victims of **human trafficking** may be seen in prenatal settings because of unintended pregnancy. These women or young girls are forced or deceived into commercial sex acts (prostitution) with little or no pay. They are under strict control by their traffickers. Similar to victims of IPV, these women are likely to exhibit signs of physical abuse or neglect, such as scars, bruises, burns, unusual bald patches, or tattoos that may be a sign of branding. They are likely to be accompanied by someone who never leaves them alone and speaks for them. They may not speak English and may lack identification documents. If the woman is alone, she may have her cell phone on and in speaker mode so that the person on the other end can hear everything that is said during the visit. Nurses and other health care providers must be creative in getting the woman alone for questioning. Strategies might include sending the other person to the front desk to fill out paperwork, interviewing the woman in the restroom, or telling her she needs to go for testing and cannot take her cell phone. With the consent of suspected or confirmed victims of human trafficking, intervention plans can be developed (Dovydaitis, 2010; Tracy & Konstantopoulos, 2012).

Review of Systems

During the review of systems, the woman should be asked to identify and describe pre-existing or concurrent problems in any of the body systems. Her mental status also needs to be assessed. The woman is questioned about physical symptoms she has experienced, such as shortness of breath or pain. Pregnancy affects and is affected by all body systems; therefore, information on the present status of body systems is important in planning care. For each sign or symptom described, the following additional data should be obtained: body location, quality, quantity, chronology, aggravating or alleviating factors, and associated manifestations (onset, character, and course) (Seidel, Ball, Dains, et al., 2011).

Physical Examination

The initial physical examination provides the baseline for assessing subsequent changes. The examiner should determine the woman's needs for basic information regarding reproductive anatomy and provide this information, along with a demonstration of the equipment that may be used during the examination and an explanation of the procedure itself. The interaction requires an unhurried, sensitive, and gentle approach with a matter-of-fact attitude.

The physical examination begins with assessment of vital signs, including blood pressure (BP), height, and weight (for calculation of body mass index [BMI]). The bladder should be empty before pelvic examination is done.

Each examiner develops a routine for proceeding with the physical examination; most choose the head-to-toe progression. Heart and lung sounds are evaluated and extremities examined. The skin is assessed for changes in pigmentation, rashes, and edema. Distribution, amount, and quality of body hair are of particular importance because the findings reflect nutritional status, endocrine function, and attention to hygiene. The thyroid gland is assessed carefully, as are the breasts and abdomen. The height of the fundus is noted if the first examination occurs after the first trimester of pregnancy. During the examination, the examiner must remain alert to the woman's cues that give direction to the remainder of the assessment and that indicate imminent untoward response, such as feeling light-headed or dizzy. See Chapter 6 for a detailed description of the physical examination.

Whenever a pelvic examination is performed, the tone of the pelvic musculature and the woman's knowledge of Kegel exercises should be assessed. Particular attention is paid to the size of the uterus because this is an indication of the duration of gestation. The nurse can prepare the woman prior to the examination about what she may feel and coach the woman in breathing and relaxation techniques as needed during the procedure. One vaginal examination during pregnancy is recommended; another is usually not done unless indicated for medical reasons.

Laboratory Tests

The data yielded through laboratory examination of specimens obtained during the examination add important information about the symptoms of pregnancy and the woman's health status.

Specimens are collected at the initial visit so that any abnormal findings can be treated then. Blood is drawn for a variety of tests (Table 11-1). A sickle cell screen is recommended for women of African, Asian, or Middle Eastern descent. Testing for antibody to the human immunodeficiency virus (HIV) is strongly recommended for all pregnant women. The folate level is measured when indicated. A urine specimen is collected for cultures and metabolic function tests. A purified protein derivative tuberculin test may be administered to assess exposure to tuberculosis. During the pelvic examination, cervical and vaginal smears can be obtained for cytological studies and for diagnosis of infection (e.g., chlamydia, gonorrhea).

Recognition of risk factors during pregnancy may indicate the need to repeat some tests at other times. For example, exposure to tuberculosis or an STI would necessitate repeat testing. STIs may have negative effects on the mother and fetus (see Table 7-5 on p. 133). Careful assessment and thorough screening are essential.

STI screening in pregnancy. All pregnant women should have screening for STIs done early in pregnancy. Cervical cultures for chlamydia and gonorrhea should be obtained at the first prenatal visit. All women should have serum testing for

TABLE 11-1 LABORATORY TESTS IN PRENATAL PERIOD

LABORATORY TEST	PURPOSE
Hemoglobin, hematocrit/WBC, differential	Detects anemia/detects infection
Hemoglobin electrophoresis	Identifies women with hemoglobinopathies (e.g., sickle cell anemia, β-thalassemia)
Blood type, Rh, and presence of antibodies	Identifies fetuses at risk for developing erythroblastosis fetalis or hyperbilirubinemia in neonatal period
Rubella, varicella and parvovirus B19 titre	Determines immunity to rubella, chicken pox, and parvovirus (particularly in women with a previous child or exposure to children in workplace)
Tuberculin skin testing (depending on woman's history); chest film after 20 wk of gestation in women with reactive tuberculin tests	Screens for exposure to tuberculosis
Urinalysis, including microscopic examination of urinary sediment; pH, specific gravity, colour, glucose, albumin, protein, RBCs, WBCs, casts, acetone; hCG	Identifies women with unsuspected diabetes mellitus, renal disease, hypertensive disease of pregnancy; infection; occult hematuria
Urine culture	Identifies women with asymptomatic bacteriuria
Renal function tests: BUN, creatinine, electrolytes, creatinine clearance, total protein excretion	Evaluates level of possible renal compromise in women with a history of diabetes, hypertension, or renal disease
Papanicolaou test	Screens for cervical intraepithelial neoplasia, herpes simplex type 2, and HPV
Vaginal or rectal smear for *Neisseria gonorrhoeae, Chlamydia,* HPV, GBS	Screens high-risk population for asymptomatic infection; GBS screening recommended at 35–37 wk for all women
RPR/VDRL/FTA-ABS	Identifies women with untreated syphilis
HIV antibody,* hepatitis B surface antigen, toxoplasmosis	Screens for the specific infection
1-hr glucose tolerance	Screens for gestational diabetes; done at initial visit for women with risk factors; recommended to be done at 28 wk for all pregnant women (earlier if risk factors)
2-hr glucose tolerance	Screens for diabetes in women with elevated glucose level after 1-hr test; must have two elevated readings for diagnosis (see further discussion in Chapter 14)
Cardiac evaluation: ECG, chest x-ray film, and echocardiogram	Evaluates cardiac function in women with a history of hypertension or cardiac disease

BUN, blood urea nitrogen; *ECG,* electrocardiogram; *FTA-ABS,* fluorescent treponemal antibody absorption test; *GBS,* group B streptococcus; *hCG,* human chorionic gonadotropin; *HIV,* human immunodeficiency virus; *HPV,* human papilloma virus; *RBC,* red blood cell; *RPR,* rapid plasma reagin; *VDRL,* Venereal Disease Research Laboratories; *WBC,* white blood cell.
*With patient consent following pre and post counselling.

hepatitis B virus (HBV) and syphilis at the first prenatal visit, and if they are considered to be high risk (see Box 7-3), blood testing should be repeated later in pregnancy or on admission for labour and birth (PHAC, 2013a) (see Chapter 7).

HIV in pregnancy. Testing for antibodies to the human immunodeficiency virus (HIV) is strongly recommended for all pregnant women; this testing must be voluntary and without coercion (Box 11-1). Testing should be done with the woman's understanding of the test and potential result, and documentation of the counselling and consent needs to be placed on her antenatal records. Transmission of HIV from mother to fetus can occur throughout the perinatal period. Exposure may occur to the fetus through the maternal circulation as early as the first trimester of pregnancy, to the infant during labour and birth by inoculation or ingestion of maternal blood and other infected fluids, or to the infant through breast milk (Lawrence & Lawrence, 2011; Riordan & Wambach, 2010). With identification of HIV during pregnancy, the woman can be provided with appropriate care to decrease the risk of transmission to the fetus and to the infant after birth.

Maternity nurses should be advocates for the fetus while accepting the pregnant woman's decision regarding testing, treatment, or both for HIV. Health care providers have an obligation to ensure that pregnant women are well informed about HIV symptoms, testing, and methods of decreasing maternal–fetal transmission. However, mandatory HIV screening involves ethical issues related to privacy, discrimination, social stigma, and reproductive risks to the pregnant woman. See Chapter 15 for further discussion of HIV in pregnancy.

Follow-up Visits

Monthly visits are usually scheduled during the first and second trimesters, although additional appointments may be made as the need arises. However, during the third trimester, the possibility for complications increases, and closer monitoring is warranted. Starting with week 28, visits are scheduled every 2 weeks until week 36 and then every week until birth unless the health care provider individualizes the schedule. Individual needs, complications, and risks of the pregnant woman may warrant visits more or less often. The pattern of interviewing the woman first and then assessing physical changes and performing laboratory tests is maintained.

In prenatal care models that use a reduced-frequency screening schedule or in group prenatal care models such as CenteringPregnancy, the timing of follow-up visits will be different, but assessments and care will be similar.

Interview

Follow-up visits are less intensive than the initial prenatal visit. At each of these follow-up visits, the woman is asked to summarize relevant events that have occurred since the previous visit. She is asked about her general emotional and physiologi-

BOX 11-1 HIV SCREENING FOR PREGNANT WOMEN AND THEIR INFANTS

HIV Screening in Pregnancy

All pregnant women in Canada should be offered HIV screening, with appropriate pre- and post-test counselling. Testing of women thought to be at higher risk should be offered in each trimester. Targeting only women thought to be at high risk will fail to identify all HIV-positive women, as some women do not perceive themselves to be at risk, nor do their health care providers. HIV testing must be voluntary and free from coercion. No woman should be tested without her knowledge. Women's health nurses should be advocates for the fetus while accepting of the pregnant woman's decision regarding testing or treatment for HIV.

Pregnant women should receive oral or written information that includes an explanation of HIV infection, a description of interventions that can reduce HIV transmission from mother to infant, and the meaning of positive and negative test results. They should be offered an opportunity to ask questions and to decline testing. Women should also be informed that all testing is confidential.

No additional process or written documentation of informed consent beyond that required for other routine prenatal tests should be required for HIV testing.

If a patient declines an HIV test, this decision should be documented in the medical record.

Timing of HIV Testing

Women should be tested as early as possible in pregnancy.

Rapid Testing During Labour

Any woman with undocumented HIV status at the time of labour should be screened with a rapid HIV test unless she declines. Reasons for declining a rapid test should be explored.

Immediate initiation of appropriate antiretroviral prophylaxis should be recommended to women on the basis of a reactive rapid test result without waiting for the result of a confirmatory test.

Postpartum/Newborn Testing

When a woman's HIV status is still unknown at the time of birth, she should be screened with a rapid HIV test immediately after giving birth, unless she declines.

When the mother's HIV status is unknown, rapid testing of the newborn as soon as possible after birth is recommended so that antiretroviral prophylaxis can be offered to HIV-exposed infants. Women should be informed that identifying HIV antibodies in the newborn indicates that the mother is infected.

The benefits of neonatal antiretroviral prophylaxis are best realized when it is initiated within 12 hours after birth.

Sources: Money, D., Tulloch, K., Boucoiran, I., et al. (2014). SOGC clinical practice guideline: Guidelines for the care of women living with HIV in pregnancy and interventions to reduce perinatal transmission. *Journal of Obstetrics and Gynaecology Canada, 36*(8), 721–734.

cal well-being, any concerns or problems, and questions she may have. Personal and family needs are identified and explored.

A woman's emotional state can affect her and her family's general well-being. Thus the nurse needs to ask whether the woman has had any mood swings, reactions to changes in her body image, bad dreams, anxieties, or worries. Positive feelings (her own and those of her family) are also noted. The reactions of family members to the pregnancy and the woman's progression through the developmental tasks of pregnancy are also assessed and recorded.

During the third trimester, current family situations and their effect on the woman are assessed (e.g., the response of partner, siblings, and grandparents to the pregnancy and the coming child). The nurse needs to assess the parents' understanding of the following: the warning signs that indicate emergencies such as bleeding and abdominal pain, the signs of preterm and term labour, the labour process and anxieties about labour, fetal development, and methods to assess fetal well-being. The nurse should ascertain whether the woman is planning to attend childbirth preparation classes and what she knows about the control of discomfort during labour.

A review of the woman's physical systems is appropriate at each visit, and any suggestive signs or symptoms are assessed in depth. Discomfort reflecting adaptation to pregnancy is identified. Special inquiries should be made about possible infections (e.g., genitourinary tract, respiratory tract). The woman's knowledge of and success with self-management measures are assessed, as well as outcomes of prescribed therapy.

Physical Examination

Re-evaluation is a constant aspect of a pregnant woman's care. Each woman reacts differently to pregnancy. As a result, careful monitoring of the pregnancy and her reactions to care is vital. Physiological changes are documented as the pregnancy progresses and are reviewed for possible deviations.

At each visit, physical parameters are measured. BP is taken at every visit using the same arm at the level of the heart and with the woman seated. Her weight is measured, and the appropriateness of the weight gain is evaluated in relation to her BMI. Urine may be checked by dipstick. The presence and degree of edema are noted. For examination of the abdomen, the woman lies on her back with her arms by her side and head supported by a pillow; a small wedge should be placed under her right hip to prevent supine hypotension. Supine hypotension can occur when the woman lies on her back and the weight of the abdominal contents compresses the vena cava and aorta, causing a decrease in BP and a feeling of faintness (see Emergency box). Abdominal inspection is followed by measurement of the height of the fundus (Fig. 11-6).

The findings revealed during the interview and physical examination reflect the status of maternal adaptations. When any of the findings is suspicious, an in-depth examination needs to be performed. For example, careful interpretation of BP is important in the risk-factor analysis of all pregnant women. A systolic BP (SBP) of 140 mm Hg or more and a diastolic BP (DBP) of 90 mm Hg or more, based on the average of at least two measurements, suggest the presence of hypertension (Rey, Pels, von Dadelszen, et al., 2014). See Chapter 15

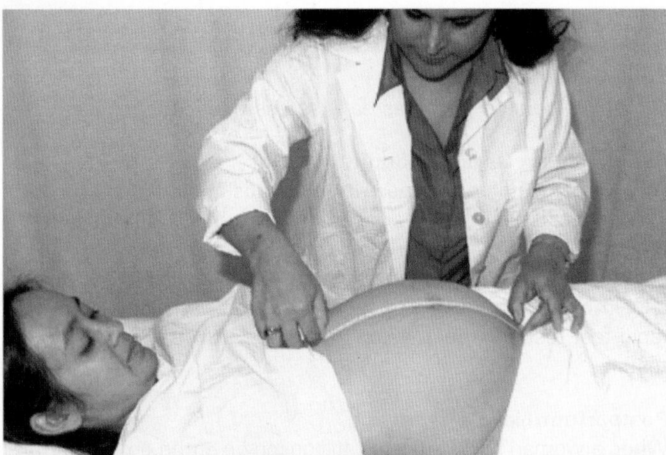

FIGURE 11-6 Measurement of fundal height from symphysis to top of fundus. Note position of hands and measuring tape. (Courtesy Chris Rozales.)

EMERGENCY

Supine Hypotension

Signs and Symptoms
Pallor
Dizziness, faintness, breathlessness
Tachycardia
Nausea
Clammy (damp, cool) skin; sweating

Intervention
Position woman on her side until her signs and symptoms subside and vital signs stabilize within normal limits.

for an in-depth discussion of problems associated with hypertension.

The pregnant woman should be monitored for a range of signs and symptoms that indicate potential complications in addition to hypertension. For example, persistent and excessive vomiting and ketonuria may indicate the development of hyperemesis gravidarum. Uterine cramping and vaginal bleeding are signs of threatened miscarriage or preterm labour. Chills and fever are symptoms of infection. Discharge from the vagina may be amniotic fluid or associated with infection (Table 11-2).

TABLE 11-2 SIGNS OF POTENTIAL COMPLICATIONS DURING THE FIRST, SECOND, AND THIRD TRIMESTERS

SIGNS AND SYMPTOMS	POSSIBLE CAUSES
First Trimester	
Severe vomiting	Hyperemesis gravidarum
Chills, fever	Infection
Burning on urination	Infection
Diarrhea	Infection
Abdominal cramping; vaginal bleeding	Miscarriage, ectopic pregnancy
Second and Third Trimesters	
Persistent, severe vomiting	Hyperemesis gravidarum, hypertension, pre-eclampsia
Sudden discharge of fluid from vagina before 37 weeks	Premature rupture of membranes
Vaginal bleeding, severe abdominal pain	Miscarriage, placenta previa, placental abruption
Chills, fever, burning on urination, diarrhea	Infection
Severe backache or flank pain	Kidney infection or stones; preterm labour
Change in fetal movements: absence of fetal movements after quickening, any unusual change in pattern or amount	Fetal position or intrauterine fetal death
Uterine contractions; pressure; cramping before 37 weeks	Preterm labour
Visual disturbances: blurring, double vision, or spots	Hypertensive conditions, pre-eclampsia
Headaches: severe, frequent, or continuous	Hypertensive conditions, pre-eclampsia
Muscular irritability or convulsions	Hypertensive conditions, pre-eclampsia
Epigastric or abdominal pain (perceived as severe stomach ache)	Hypertensive conditions, pre-eclampsia, placental abruption
Glycosuria, positive glucose tolerance test reaction	Gestational diabetes mellitus

Fetal Assessment

Toward the end of the first trimester, before the uterus is an abdominal organ, the fetal heart rate (FHR) can be heard with an ultrasound fetoscope or an ultrasound stethoscope. To hear the FHR, the instrument is placed in the midline just above the symphysis pubis and firm pressure is applied. The woman and her family should be offered the opportunity to listen to the fetal heart. The health status of the fetus is assessed at each visit for the remainder of the pregnancy.

Fundal height. During the second trimester, the uterus becomes an abdominal organ. The *fundal height*, or measurement of the height of the uterus above the symphysis pubis, is used as one indicator of fetal growth.

The measurement also provides a gross estimate of the duration of pregnancy. From gestational weeks (GW) 18 to 32, the height of the fundus in centimetres is approximately the same as the number of weeks of gestation (±2 GW) if the woman's bladder is empty at the time of measurement. As much as a 3-cm variation is possible if the bladder is full (Cunningham et al., 2014). For example, the fundal height of a woman of 28 weeks of gestation with an empty bladder would measure from 26 to 30 cm. In addition, the fundal height measurement may aid in the identification of risk factors. A stable or decreased fundal height may indicate the presence of intrauterine growth restriction (IUGR); an excessive increase could indicate the presence of multifetal gestation (more than one fetus) or polyhydramnios (excessive amniotic fluid).

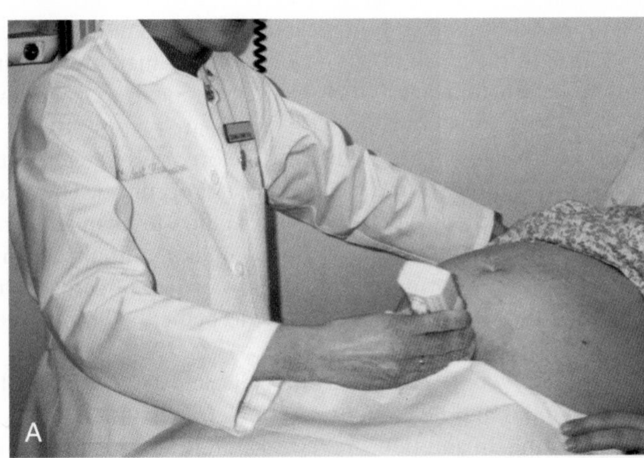
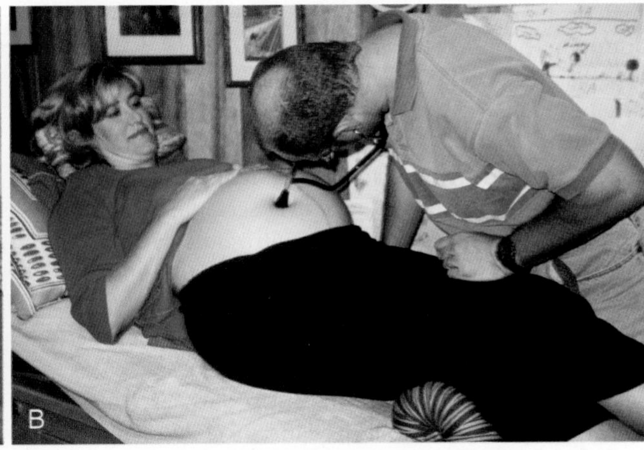

FIGURE 11-7 Detecting fetal heartbeat. **A:** Doppler ultrasound stethoscope (fetal heartbeat detectable at 12 weeks). **B:** Father can listen to the fetal heart with a fetoscope (first detectable at 18 to 20 weeks with a fetoscope). (**A**, Courtesy Shannon Perry **B**, Courtesy Dee Lowdermilk.)

A disposable paper measuring tape is preferred for measuring fundal height. To increase the reliability of the measurement, the same person examines the pregnant woman at each of her prenatal visits, although often this is not possible. All clinicians who examine a particular pregnant woman should be consistent in their measurement technique (see Fig. 11-6).

Gestational age. In an uncomplicated pregnancy, fetal gestational age is estimated after the duration of pregnancy and the EDB are determined. Fetal gestational age is determined from the menstrual history, contraceptive history, pregnancy test results, and the following findings obtained from the clinical evaluation:

- First uterine evaluation: date, size
- Fetal heart first heard: date, method (Doppler stethoscope, fetoscope)
- Date of quickening
- Current fundal height, estimated fetal weight
- Current week of gestation by history of LMP or ultrasound examination (or both)
- Ultrasound examination: date, week of gestation, biparietal diameter (if done in the first trimester, this is the ideal determination of gestational age)
- Reliability of dates

Quickening ("feeling life") refers to the mother's first perception of fetal movement. It usually occurs between weeks 16 and 20 of gestation and is initially experienced as a fluttering sensation. The mother's report should be recorded. Multiparas often perceive fetal movement earlier than primigravidas; sometimes this may occur as early as 14 weeks.

Routine ultrasound examination in early pregnancy has been recommended for fetal screening (see Chapter 13). This ultrasound may be used to establish the duration of pregnancy if the woman cannot give a precise date for her LMP or if the size of the uterus does not conform to the EDB as calculated by Nägele's rule. Ultrasound also provides information about the well-being of the fetus. It is helpful in determining the presence of postdates later in pregnancy.

Health status. The assessment of fetal health status includes consideration of fetal movement. The mother should be instructed to note the extent and timing of fetal movements and report immediately if the pattern changes or movement ceases. Regular movement has been found to be a reliable indicator of fetal health (Liston, Sawchuck, Young, et al., 2007) (see Chapter 13).

The FHR is checked on routine visits once it has been heard (Fig. 11-7). Early in the second trimester, the heartbeat may be heard with the Doppler stethoscope (see Fig. 11-7, A). To detect the heartbeat before the fetal position can be palpated by Leopold manoeuvres (see Box 17-5), the scope is moved around the abdomen until the heartbeat is audible. The heartbeat is counted for 1 minute, and the quality and rhythm are noted. Later in the second trimester, the FHR can be determined with the fetoscope (see Fig. 11-7, B). A normal rate and rhythm are other good indicators of fetal health. Once the heartbeat is noted, its absence is cause for immediate investigation.

Intensive investigation of fetal health status is initiated if any maternal or fetal complications arise (e.g., maternal hypertension, IUGR, premature rupture of membranes [PROM], irregular or absent FHR, absence of fetal movements after quickening). Careful, precise, and concise recording of patient responses and laboratory results contributes to the continuous supervision vital to ensuring the well-being of the mother and fetus.

Laboratory Tests

The number of routine laboratory tests done during follow-up visits in pregnancy is limited. A clean-catch urine specimen is obtained to test for levels of protein, nitrites, and leukocytes at each visit. Urine specimens for culture and sensitivity, and blood samples are obtained only if signs and symptoms warrant this.

First-trimester screening for chromosomal abnormalities is offered as an option between 11 and 14 weeks. This multiple marker screen includes ultrasound evaluation of nuchal translucency (NT) and biochemical markers—pregnancy-associated placental protein (PAPP-A) and free beta-human chorionic gonadotropin (β-hCG). Between 15 and 20 weeks, maternal serum alpha-fetoprotein (MSAFP) screening, the QUAD test (alpha-fetoprotein, hCG, estriol, and inhibin A), can be done to screen for neural tube defects (NTDs) and other chromosomal abnormalities. Women who had first-trimester screening need MSAFP testing after 15 weeks for NTD screening (Wilson & SOGC Genetics Committee, 2014). An ultrasound is often done at 18 to 24 weeks to survey fetal anatomy. Further discussion regarding maternal screening testing is in Chapter 13.

STIs in pregnancy. STIs in pregnancy are responsible for significant morbidity and mortality. Some consequences of maternal infection, such as infertility and sterility, last a lifetime. Congenitally acquired infection may affect a child's length and quality of life. Table 7-5 describes the effects of several common STIs on pregnancy and the fetus. It is difficult to predict these effects with certainty. Factors such as co-infection with other STIs and at what point in pregnancy the infection was treated can affect outcomes.

Testing for STIs should be repeated late in the third trimester (36 weeks) if the woman was previously positive or if she is younger than age 25, has a new sex partner, or has multiple sex partners (PHAC, 2014).

Gonococcal infections in pregnancy potentially affect both the mother and infant. Women with cervical gonorrhea may develop salpingitis in the first trimester. Perinatal complications of gonococcal infection include premature rupture of membranes, preterm birth, **chorioamnionitis**, neonatal sepsis, IUGR, and maternal postpartum sepsis. Amniotic infection syndrome—manifested by placental, fetal, and umbilical cord inflammation following premature rupture of the membranes—may result from gonorrheal infection during pregnancy.

During pregnancy, maternal infection with herpes simplex virus 2 (HSV-2) can have adverse effects on both the mother and fetus. Viremia occurs during the primary infection, and congenital infection is possible although rare. Primary infections during the first trimester have been associated with increased miscarriage rates. During pregnancy, the use of acyclovir and valacyclovir after 36 weeks' gestation may reduce the recurrence rate and thus the need for a Caesarean birth; the use of medication has not been shown to reduce the risk of maternal–child transmission (Money, Steben, & Infectious Disease Committee, 2008; PHAC, 2014). Because neonatal HSV infection is such a devastating disease, prevention is critical. (See Chapter 7 for further discussion of STIs.)

Group B streptococcus (GBS). GBS may be considered a normal vaginal flora in a woman who is not pregnant. It is present in 10 to 30% of healthy pregnant women (Money, Allen, Halifax, et al., 2013). However, GBS infection is associated with poor pregnancy outcomes. GBS infections are an important factor in perinatal and neonatal morbidity and mortality, usually resulting from vertical transmission from the birth canal of the infected mother to the infant during birth.

To decrease the risk of neonatal GBS infection, it is recommended that all women be screened at 35 to 37 weeks of gestation for GBS using a rectovaginal culture and that intravenous antibiotic prophylaxis (IAP) be offered to all who test positive. Women with planned Caesarean birth should also be swabbed because of their risk of labour or ruptured membranes earlier than the scheduled Caesarean delivery. If a culture is not available at onset of labour or if risk factors are present, IAP is also offered. IAP is not recommended before a Caesarean birth if labour or rupture of membranes has not occurred. The recommended treatment is penicillin G, 5 million units in an intravenous loading dose, and then 2.5 to 3.0 million units intravenously every 4 hours during labour. Cefazolin or clindamycin may be used in women who are allergic to penicillin (Money et al., 2013).

Other tests. Tests that are often repeated at 28 weeks include hemoglobin and hematocrit, a serological test for syphilis, and HIV testing. In addition, at 28 weeks, an Rh type and screen for antibodies is performed. If the woman is Rh negative and unsensitized, she should receive 300 mcg of Rh immune globulin (RhIG) (see Medication Guide in Chapter 22). Hematocrit testing may be repeated at 36 weeks in women with anemia and those at risk for peripartum hemorrhage (Gregory et al., 2012).

Other diagnostic tests are available to assess the health status of both the pregnant woman and the fetus. Chorionic villus sampling or amniocentesis may be needed to evaluate the fetus for genetic disorders or gestational maturity. These and other tests used to determine health risks for the mother and infant are described in Chapter 13.

Collaborative Care

After obtaining information through the assessment process, the data are analyzed to identify the unique needs of the pregnant woman and her family. Care is optimized with a collaborative approach involving the physician or midwife, nurse, other relevant health care professionals, the woman, her partner, and her family.

The nurse–patient relationship is critical in setting the tone for further interaction. The techniques of listening with an attentive expression, touching, and using eye contact have their place, as does recognizing the woman's feelings and her right to express these feelings. The interaction may occur in various formal or informal settings. A clinical setting, home visits, or telephone conversations all provide opportunities for contact and can be used effectively.

Education About Maternal and Fetal Changes

Expectant parents typically are curious about the growth and development of the fetus, the consequent changes that occur in the mother's body, and how to cope with changes. Mothers may be more tolerant of the discomforts related to the continuing pregnancy if they understand the underlying causes. The nurse who is observant, listens, and knows typical concerns of expectant parents can anticipate what questions will be asked and prompt mothers and their partners to discuss what is on their minds. The nurse can also offer printed literature to supplement the individualized teaching that he or she provides; women often avidly read books and pamphlets as well as seek Internet resources related to their own experience. When nurses read the literature before distributing it, they have an opportunity to point out areas that may not correspond with local health care practices. To be most effective, the material must reflect the pregnant woman's or couple's ethnicity, culture, and literacy level and the agency's resources. It is important to include family members in health education. Nurses can also share recommended websites from reliable sources.

Patients who receive conflicting advice or instruction are likely to grow frustrated with members of the health care team and the care provided. Several topics that may cause concern in pregnant women are discussed in the following sections.

Nutrition. Good nutrition is important in the maintenance of maternal health during pregnancy and in the provision of adequate nutrients for embryonic and fetal development. Assessing a woman's nutritional status and weight gain and providing information on nutrition are part of the nurse's responsibilities in providing prenatal care. Teaching may include discussion about foods high in iron, encouragement to take prenatal vitamins, and recommendations to limit caffeine intake. In some settings, a registered dietitian conducts classes for pregnant women on the topics of nutritional status and nutrition during pregnancy or interviews them to assess their knowledge of these topics. Nurses can refer women to a registered dietitian if a related need becomes apparent during the nursing assessment—for example, previous history of an eating disorder or nutritional deficiency. (For detailed information on maternal and fetal nutritional needs and related nursing care, see Chapter 12.)

Personal hygiene. During pregnancy, the sebaceous (sweat) glands are highly active because of hormonal influences, and women often perspire freely. They may be reassured that the increase is normal and that their previous patterns of perspiration will return after the postpartum period. Baths and warm showers can be therapeutic because they relax tense, tired muscles; help counter insomnia; and make the pregnant woman feel fresh. Tub bathing is permitted even in late pregnancy because little water enters the vagina unless under pressure. However, the temperature of the water should not be higher than 39°C as this will increase the woman's core body temperature and can cause postural hypotension. Hot tubs should also be avoided for this reason. Tub bathing after rupture of the membranes needs to be carefully monitored and may be contraindicated in some women.

Prevention of urinary tract infection. Because of physiological changes that occur in the renal system during pregnancy (see Chapter 10), infections of the lower urinary tract (acute urethritis, acute cystitis) are common. *Escherichia coli (E. coli)* is the most common causative organism for urinary tract infection (UTI) in pregnant women (Duff, 2012). Although UTIs can be asymptomatic, typical symptoms include frequency, urgency, dysuria, dribbling, and hesitancy; gross hematuria may occur. Women should be instructed to inform their health care provider if they experience these symptoms. Urinary tract infections pose a risk to the mother and fetus, mainly through increasing rates of preterm labour; thus their prevention or early treatment is essential. Oral antibiotics are commonly prescribed.

The nurse can assess the woman's understanding of appropriate hand hygiene techniques to use before and after urinating and the importance of wiping the perineum from front to back. Soft, absorbent toilet tissue, preferably white and unscented, should be used; harsh, scented, or printed toilet paper may cause irritation. Bubble bath or other bath oils should be avoided because these can irritate the urethra. Women should wear underpants and panty hose with a cotton crotch and avoid wearing tight-fitting slacks or jeans for long periods. Anything that allows a buildup of heat and moisture in the genital area can foster bacterial growth.

Some women do not consume enough fluid. After ascertaining the woman's fluid preferences, the nurse should advise the woman to drink at least 2 L (eight glasses) of liquid a day to maintain an adequate fluid intake that ensures frequent urination. Pregnant women should not limit fluids in an effort to reduce the frequency of urination. Women need to know that if urine looks dark (concentrated), they must increase their fluid intake. The consumption of yogurt and acidophilus milk can help prevent urinary tract and vaginal infections. Although drinking cranberry juice is often recommended, there is conflicting evidence regarding its effectiveness and the effective dose needed to prevent urinary tract infections.

The nurse should review healthy urination practices with the woman. Women should be told not to ignore the urge to urinate, because holding urine lengthens the time bacteria are in the bladder and allows them to multiply. Women should plan ahead when faced with situations that may normally require them to delay urination (e.g., a long car ride). They should always urinate before going to bed at night. Bacteria also can be introduced during intercourse. Therefore, women are advised to urinate before and after intercourse and to then drink a large glass of water to promote additional urination.

Kegel exercises. Kegel exercises—deliberate contraction and relaxation of the pubococcygeus muscle—strengthen the muscles around the reproductive organs and improve muscle tone. Many women are not aware of the muscles of the pelvic floor until it is pointed out that these are the muscles used during urination and sexual intercourse and that they can be consciously controlled. The pelvic floor muscles encircle the vaginal outlet, and they need to be exercised. An exercised muscle can stretch and contract readily at birth. Practice of pelvic muscle exercise during pregnancy also results in fewer concerns of urinary incontinence in late pregnancy and postpartum (see Chapter 5, Patient Teaching box, p. 72).

Preparation for breastfeeding the newborn. Pregnant women are usually eager to discuss their plans for feeding the newborn. Breast milk is the food of choice, in part because breastfeeding is associated with a decreased incidence in perinatal morbidity and mortality. The Canadian Paediatric Society recommends exclusive breastfeeding for at least 6 months with continuation to 2 years or beyond. A woman's decision about the method of infant feeding is often made before pregnancy; thus it is essential to educate women of child-bearing age about the benefits of breastfeeding. The woman and her partner are encouraged to decide what method of feeding is suitable for them; however, the benefits of breastfeeding should be emphasized. Education and support from health care providers will increase the number of women who initiate and continue with breastfeeding (Lumbiganon, Martis, Laopaiboon, et al., 2012).

Once the couple has been given information about the advantages of breastfeeding and disadvantages of formula-feeding, they can make an informed choice. Health care providers should support these decisions and provide any needed assistance.

Assessment of breasts during the prenatal period may reveal potential concerns related to breastfeeding. Scars on the breast may indicate previous breast reduction surgery, which can impact milk production. Some women may have breast implants; this may or may not affect successful breastfeeding. Examination of the breasts may reveal flat or inverted nipples, which can affect the baby's ability to successfully latch on to the breast. To determine if nipples are inverted, a woman can perform a test on her nipples to determine freedom of protrusion (Fig. 11-8). The woman places her thumb and forefinger on her areola and presses inward gently. A normal nipple will evert or stand erect while an inverted nipple will appear to withdraw (Lawrence & Lawrence, 2011).

Exercises to break the adhesions that cause the nipple to invert do not work and may cause uterine contractions (Lawrence & Lawrence, 2011). Some clinicians recommend the prenatal use of breast shells (Fig. 11-9) during the last trimester for women with flat or inverted nipples, although evidence to support their effectiveness is lacking (Lawrence & Lawrence, 2011). They can be uncomfortable and cause irritation to the nipple or areola. Breast stimulation is contraindicated in women at risk for preterm labour; therefore the decision to suggest the use of breast shells to women with flat or inverted nipples must be made judiciously (Lawrence & Lawrence, 2011; Walker, 2010).

The woman should be taught to cleanse the nipples with warm water to prevent blocking of the ducts with dried colostrum. Soap, ointments, alcohol, and tinctures should not be applied because they remove protective oils that keep nipples supple. The use of these substances may cause the nipple to crack during early lactation (Lawrence & Lawrence, 2011).

The woman who plans to breastfeed should purchase a nursing bra that will accommodate her increased breast size during the last few months of pregnancy and during lactation. If her breasts are very heavy or if the woman feels uncomfortable with the weight unsupported, the bra can be worn day and night. Some pregnant women may leak **colostrum** during the pregnancy and some may not. Whether this occurs does not relate to how much breast milk a mother will produce after the birth of the baby.

Dental health. Dental care during pregnancy is especially important because nausea during pregnancy may lead to poor oral hygiene and allow dental caries to develop. Brushing at least twice daily and flossing once in the evening can reduce the potential for caries. Inflammation and infection of the gingival and periodontal tissues may occur. There is some evidence linking periodontal infections and preterm birth (Walia & Saini, 2015). While treatment may improve dental health, it does not prevent preterm birth (Cunningham et al., 2014).

Because calcium and phosphorus in the teeth are fixed in enamel, the old adage "for every child a tooth" is not true. Diagnosis and treatment of oral health problems, including necessary

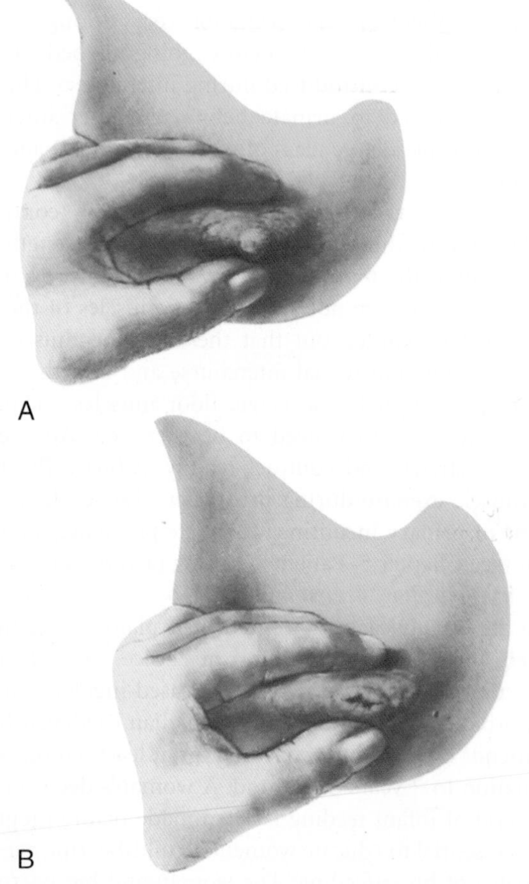

FIGURE 11-8 Pinch test. **A:** Normal nipple everts with gentle pressure. **B:** Inverted nipple inverts with gentle pressure. (Modified from Lawrence, R. A., & Lawrence, R. M. [2011]. *Breastfeeding: A guide for the medical profession* [7th ed., p. 241]. St. Louis: Mosby.)

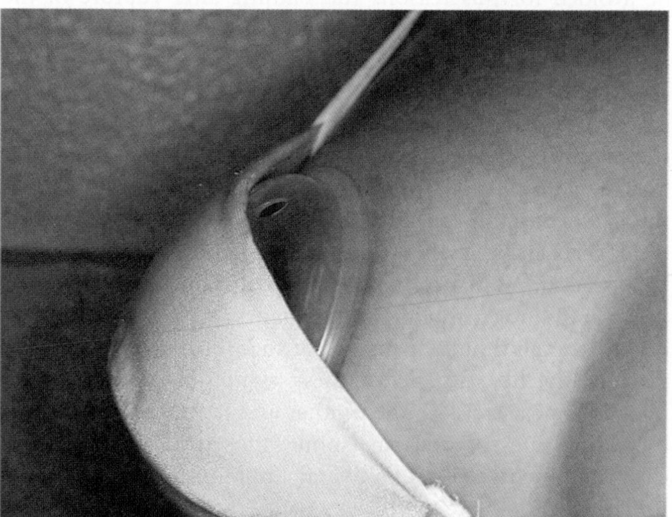

FIGURE 11-9 Breast shell in place inside bra to evert nipple. (Courtesy Michael S. Clement, MD.)

dental x-rays, are safe during pregnancy (Cunningham et al., 2014; Kumar & Samelson, 2009). Dental care and nonemergent procedures are best scheduled during the second trimester when the woman is past the stage of feeling nauseous and can sit comfortably in the dental chair. To avoid supine hypotension during dental procedures, the pregnant woman in her second or third trimester is positioned in the dental chair with a small pillow under her right hip (Kumar & Samelson, 2009). Antibacterial therapy should be considered for sepsis, especially in pregnant women who have had rheumatic heart disease or nephritis.

Physical activity. Physical activity promotes a feeling of well-being and can help reduce anxiety in the pregnant woman (see Research Focus box). It improves circulation, promotes relaxation and rest, and counteracts boredom, as it does in the nonpregnant woman. The Public Health Agency of Canada (PHAC) recommends that pregnant women engage in moderate activity for 30 minutes per day at least 5 days per week. Women who are highly active or engage in vigorous aerobic exercise can continue during pregnancy if they remain healthy and discuss with their health care provider about adjusting activity over time as needed (PHAC, 2012b). Women should be assessed using the PARmed-X for PREGNANCY, which is a guideline for health screening prior to participation in a prenatal fitness class or other exercise. See Additional Resources at end of chapter for more information.

Women should be advised that adverse pregnancy or neonatal outcomes are not increased for exercising women (Mottolo, 2011). Detailed exercise tips for pregnancy are presented in the Patient Teaching box: Exercise Tips for Pregnant Women.

RESEARCH FOCUS

Nonpharmacological Mind–Body Support Interventions for Healthy Pregnancy

—Pat Mahaffee Gingrich

Ask the Question

For pregnant women at risk for anxiety and depression, can antenatal support interventions improve health and birth outcomes?

Search for the Evidence

Search Strategies

English research–based publications on pregnancy support, anxiety, prenatal depression, and postpartum depression were included.

Databases Used

Cochrane Collaborative Database, National Guideline Clearinghouse (AHRQ), PubMed, UpToDate, CINAHL, and the professional website for AWHONN

Critically Analyze the Evidence

- A systematic review found that pregnant women who were taught guided imagery and who practised relaxation techniques experienced less anxiety during labour and decreased anxiety and depression in the immediate postpartum period (Marc, Toureche, Ernst, et al., 2011).
- For women with prenatal depression, being randomized to regular yoga or massage therapy improved scores for depression, anxiety, back and leg pain, and relationship over controls randomized to standard prenatal care. Additional benefits included greater gestational age and birth weight (Field, Diego, Hernandez-Reif, et al., 2012).
- Even brief antenatal group interventions focusing on stress management and coping skills for depressed women were able to reduce the risk of postpartum depression by as much as 18%. In addition, the group intervention reduced depression in women with poor partner support and in women experiencing unplanned pregnancy (Kozinszky, Dudas, Devosa, et al., 2012).
- For women at risk for low-birth-weight babies, additional antenatal social support did not change the birth weights, but it did reduce admissions to hospitals for pregnancy complications and Caesarean birth (Hodnett, Fredericks, & Weston, 2010).
- Exercise is a strongly recommended intervention for mental and physical well-being and weight control in pregnancy, especially for at-risk populations. Qualitative research finds that barriers to exercise for low-income women include poor motivation, misinformation, lack of affordable nearby facilities, and sociocultural barriers. Women exercised more when they were part of a group exercise class and when safe, low-cost facilities were present in their communities (Krans & Chang, 2011).

Apply the Evidence: Nursing Implications

- Women at risk for anxiety or depression may be especially vulnerable during pregnancy, when medication may not be advisable. Teaching stress management, guided imagery, and relaxation may help them cope with the changes of pregnancy and parenthood. Regular yoga and massage therapy may also provide additional benefits.
- All pregnant women benefit from social support. Some obstetrical practices have adopted group prenatal appointments to try to facilitate group support. It is important that these not only include nurse-led patient education but also allow time for social bonding and dialogue. Women at risk for depression and anxiety may benefit most.
- The nurse can also assess the community for safe, low-cost exercise opportunities and make this information readily available to local pregnant women, along with information about the benefits of exercise. Initiating a regular walking club or encouraging daily walking with partners promotes a low-cost, safer, and social activity that can improve overall pregnancy well-being. In the bigger picture, advocating for safer communities decreases stress and improves health for all.

References

Field, T., Diego, M., Hernandez-Reif, M., et al. (2012). Yoga and massage therapy reduce prenatal depression and prematurity. *Journal of Bodywork and Movement Therapies, 16*(2), 204–209.

Hodnett, E., Fredericks, S., & Weston, J. (2010). Support during pregnancy for women at increased risk of low birthweight babies. *Cochrane Database of Systematic Reviews,* (6). doi:10.1002/14651858.CD000198.pub2.

Kozinszky, Z., Dudas, R. B., Devosa, I., et al. (2012). Can a brief antepartum preventive group intervention help reduce postpartum depressive symptomatology? *Psychotherapy and Psychosomatics, 81*(2), 98–107.

Krans, E., & Chang, J. (2011). A will without a way: Barriers and facilitators to exercise during pregnancy for low-income African American women. *Women and Health, 51*(8), 777–794.

Marc, I., Toureche, N., Ernst, E., et al. (2011). Mind-body interventions during pregnancy for preventing or treating women's anxiety. *Cochrane Database of Systematic Reviews,* (7). doi:10.1002/14651858.CD007559.pub2.

PATIENT TEACHING

Exercise Tips for Pregnant Women

Participate in Aerobic and Strength-Conditioning Exercises

- You can do this as part of a healthy lifestyle during pregnancy as long as you are not considered high risk. When starting an aerobic exercise program, previously sedentary women should begin with 15 minutes of continuous exercise three times a week, increasing gradually to 150 minutes of activity per week.

Maintain a Good Fitness Level Throughout Pregnancy

- Do this in moderation; do not try to reach peak fitness or train for an athletic competition. Elite athletes who continue to train during pregnancy require supervision by an obstetrical care provider with knowledge of the impact of strenuous exercise on maternal and fetal outcomes. For very fit, medically prescreened pregnant women, the current target heart rate zones may not be appropriate and the PARmed-X for PREGNANCY should be consulted for appropriate target heart rate zones.

Perform Warm-Up and Cool-Down Exercises

- All aerobic activity should begin with a warm-up and cool-down of 5 to 10 minutes of lower intensity. After the fourth month of gestation, you should not perform exercises flat on your back.

Monitor the Intensity of Exercise

- You should be able to converse easily while exercising. If you cannot, you need to slow down.

Choose Activities That Will Minimize the Risk of Loss of Balance and Fetal Trauma

- Avoid risky activities.
- Activities such as surfing, mountain climbing, skydiving, and racquetball require precise balance and coordination and thus may be dangerous. Avoid activities that require holding your breath and bearing down (Valsalva manoeuvre). Jerky, bouncy motions also should be avoided. Stretches should be controlled.
- Avoid downhill snow skiing, because the centre of gravity changes and there is risk of falls; contact sports such as ice hockey, soccer, and basketball; and scuba diving, because the pressure from the water could put the baby at risk for decompression sickness.

Avoid Becoming Overheated for Extended Periods of Time

- Avoid hot yoga, hot pilates.
- It is best not to exercise for more than 35 minutes, especially in hot, humid weather. As your body temperature rises, the heat is transmitted to your fetus.
- Do not use hot tubs and saunas.

Drink Two or Three 250-mL Glasses of Water After You Exercise

- After you exercise you need to replace the body fluids lost through perspiration. While exercising, drink water whenever you feel the need.

Take Your Time

- This is not the time to be competitive or train for activities requiring speed or long endurance.

Wear a Supportive Bra

- Your increased breast weight may cause changes in posture and put pressure on the ulnar nerve.

Wear Supportive Shoes

- As your uterus grows, your centre of gravity shifts, and you compensate for this by arching your back. These natural changes may make you feel off balance and more likely to fall.

Stop Exercising Immediately Upon Experiencing Warning Signs

- If you experience shortness of breath, chest pain, dizziness, painful uterine contraction, vaginal bleeding, or leakage of amniotic fluid, you should stop exercising immediately and consult your health care provider.

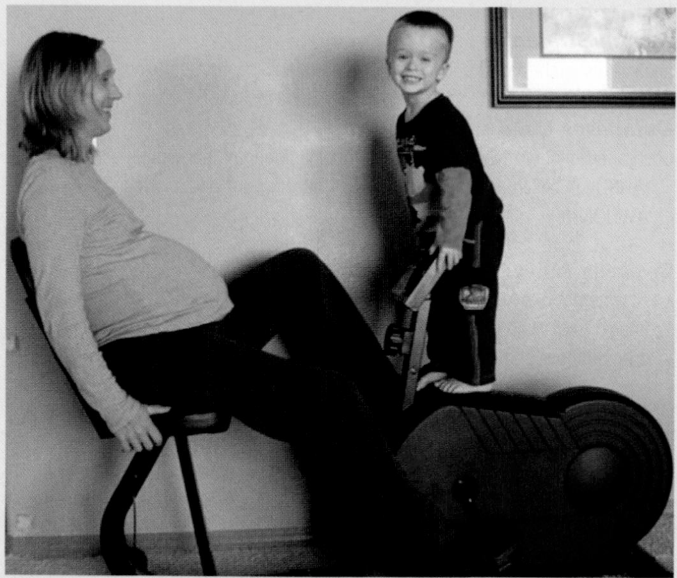

Riding a recumbent bicycle provides exercise while supplying back support. Big brother becomes involved. (Courtesy Julie Perry Nelson.)

Sources: American College of Obstetricians and Gynecologists Committee on Obstetric Practice. (2015). Committee opinion no. 650: *Physical activity and exercise during pregnancy and the postpartum period.* Retrieved from http://www.acog.org/Resources-And-Publications/Committee-Opinions/Committee-on-Obstetric-Practice/Physical-Activity-and-Exercise-During-Pregnancy-and-the-Postpartum-Period; American College of Obstetricians and Gynecologists. (2011). *Exercise during pregnancy* (FAQ 0119), www.acog.org/~/media/For%20Patients/faq119.pdf?dmc=1&ts=20120814T2219033424; Mottolo, M. (2011). *Exercise and pregnancy: Canadian guidelines for health care professionals.* Retrieved from http://sirc.ca/sites/default/files/content/docs/newsletters/archive/may12/documents/Free/guidelines.pdf.

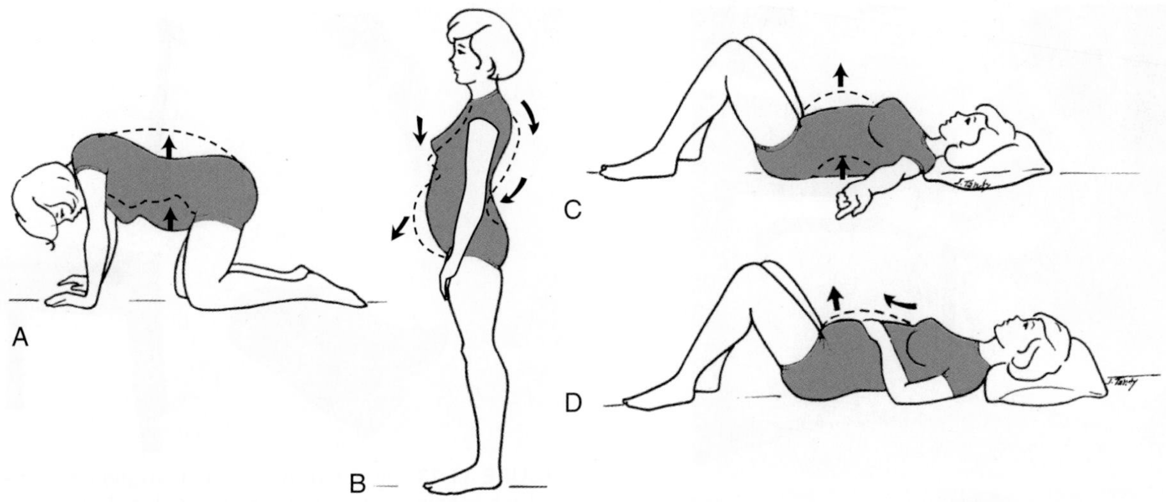

FIGURE 11-10 Exercises. **A, B** and **C:** Pelvic rocking relieves low backache (excellent for relief of menstrual cramps as well). **D:** Abdominal breathing aids relaxation and lifts the abdominal wall off the uterus.

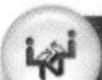

PATIENT TEACHING

Posture and Body Mechanics

To Prevent or Relieve Backache

Do pelvic tilt:

- Pelvic tilt (rock) on hands and knees (see Fig. 11-10, A) and while sitting in a straight-back chair.
- Pelvic tilt (rock) in standing position against a wall or lying on floor (see Fig. 11-10, B and C).
- Perform abdominal muscle contractions during pelvic tilt while standing, lying, or sitting to help strengthen rectus abdominis muscle (see Fig. 11-10, D).

Use good body mechanics.

- Use leg muscles to reach objects on or near floor. Bend at the knees, not the back. Knees are bent to lower body to squatting position. Keep feet shoulder-width apart to provide a solid base to maintain balance (see Fig. 11-11, A).
- Lift with the legs. To lift a heavy object (e.g., young child), place one foot slightly in front of the other and keep it flat as you lower yourself onto one knee. Lift the weight, holding it close to your body and never higher than the chest. To stand up or sit down, place one leg slightly behind the other as you raise or lower yourself (see Fig. 11-11, B).

To Restrict the Lumbar Curve

- For prolonged standing, place one foot on a low footstool or box; change positions often.
- Move car seat forward so that knees are bent and higher than hips. If needed, use a small pillow to support low back area.
- Sit in chairs low enough to allow both feet to be placed on floor, preferably with knees higher than hips.
- Use hot water bottle or ice packs intermittently on back to relieve discomfort.

Exercises that help relieve the low back pain that often arises during the second trimester because of the increased weight of the fetus are demonstrated in Fig. 11-10.

Posture and body mechanics. Skeletal, musculature, and hormonal changes (relaxin) in pregnancy can predispose the woman to backache and possible injury. As pregnancy progresses, the pregnant woman's centre of gravity changes, pelvic joints soften and relax, and stress is placed on abdominal musculature. Poor posture and body mechanics contribute to the discomfort and potential for injury. To minimize these problems, women can learn good body posture and body mechanics (Fig. 11-11). The activities described in the Patient Teaching box: Posture and Body Mechanics can also promote greater physical comfort.

Rest and relaxation. The pregnant woman is encouraged to plan regular rest periods, particularly as pregnancy advances. The side-lying position is recommended to promote uterine perfusion and fetoplacental oxygenation by eliminating pressure on the ascending vena cava and descending aorta, which can lead to supine hypotension (Fig. 11-12). Lying on the left side allows the most blood flow through the uterus, although women should be taught that it is acceptable to rest on either side. The mother should also be shown the way to rise slowly from a side-lying position, to prevent placing strain on the back and minimize the orthostatic hypotension caused by changes in position common in the latter part of pregnancy. To stretch and rest back muscles at home or at work, the woman can do the following exercises:

- While standing behind a chair, the woman supports and balances herself using the back of the chair (Fig. 11-13). She squats for 30 seconds and then stands for 15 seconds. She should repeat this six times, in several sets per day, as needed.
- While sitting in a chair, the woman lowers her head to her knees for 30 seconds and then raises her head. She should repeat this six times, several times per day, as needed.

Conscious relaxation is the process of releasing tension from the mind and body through deliberate effort and practice. The

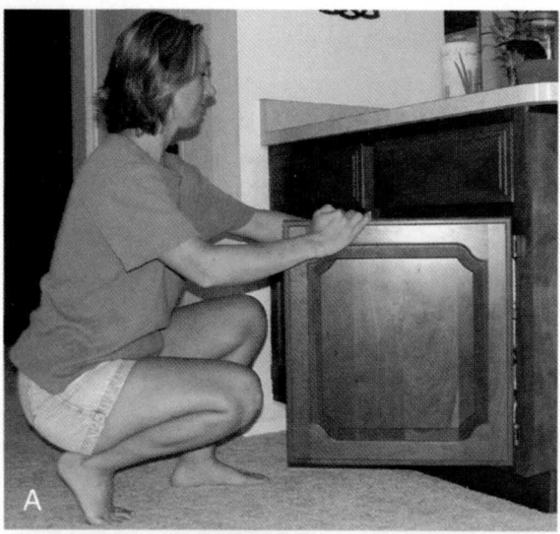

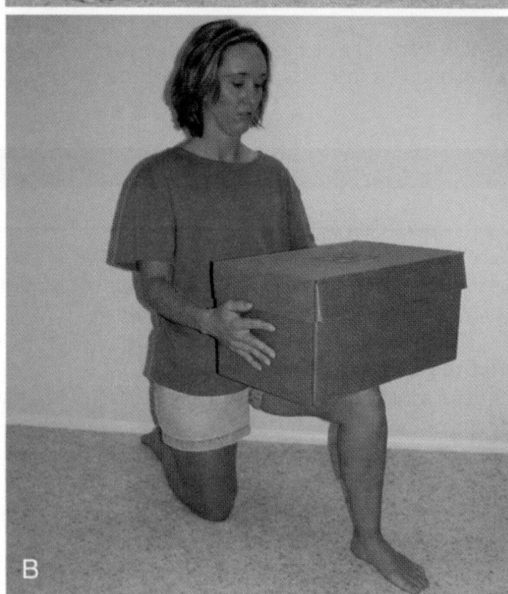

FIGURE 11-11 Correct body mechanics. **A:** Squatting. **B:** Lifting. (Courtesy Julie Perry Nelson.)

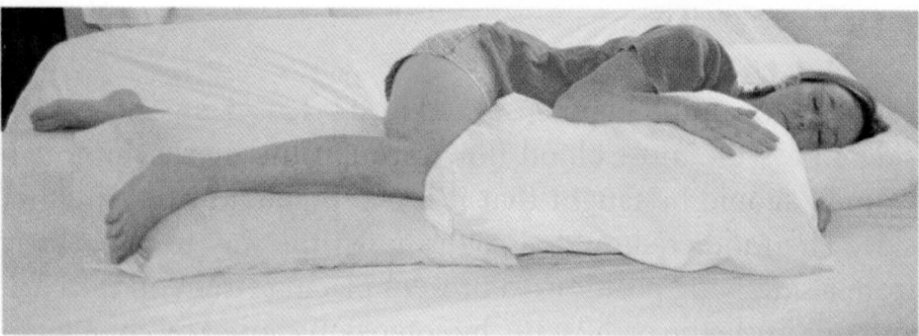

FIGURE 11-12 Side-lying position for rest and relaxation. (Courtesy Julie Perry Nelson.)

ability to relax consciously and intentionally can be beneficial for the following reasons:

- To relieve the normal discomforts related to pregnancy
- To reduce stress and diminish pain perception during the child-bearing cycle
- To heighten self-awareness and trust in one's own ability to control responses and functions
- To help cope with stress in everyday life situations, whether the woman is pregnant or not

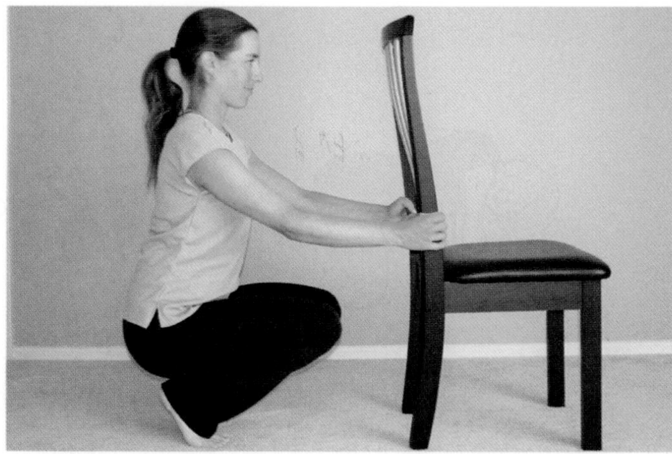

FIGURE 11-13 Squatting for muscle relaxation and strengthening and for keeping leg and hip joints flexible. (Courtesy Julie Perry Nelson.)

BOX 11-2 CONSCIOUS RELAXATION TIPS

Preparation—Loosen clothing, assume a comfortable sitting or side-lying position with all parts of body well supported with pillows. The use of soothing music is optional.

Beginning—Allow yourself to feel warm and comfortable. Inhale and exhale slowly and imagine peaceful relaxation coming over each part of the body, starting with the neck and working down to the toes. People who learn conscious relaxation often speak of feeling relaxed even if some discomfort is present.

Maintenance—Use imagery (fantasy or daydream) to maintain the state of relaxation. Using active imagery, imagine yourself moving or doing some activity and experiencing its sensations. Using passive imagery, imagine yourself watching a scene such as a lovely sunset.

Awakening—Return to the wakeful state gradually. Slowly begin to take in stimuli from the surrounding environment.

Further retention and development of the skill—Practise regularly each day (e.g., at the same hour for 10 to 15 minutes each day to feel refreshed, revitalized, and invigorated).

The techniques for conscious relaxation are numerous and varied. The guidelines given in Box 11-2 can be used by anyone.

Employment. Employment of pregnant women usually has no adverse effects on pregnancy outcomes. Job discrimination based solely on pregnancy is illegal. Unless complications occur, most women can continue working until the onset of labour. However, some job environments pose potential risk to the fetus (e.g., dry cleaning plants, chemical laboratories, and parking garages). Excessive fatigue is usually the deciding factor in the termination of employment during pregnancy. Strategies to improve safety during pregnancy are described in the Patient Teaching box: Safety During Pregnancy.

Women in sedentary jobs need to walk around at intervals to counter the sluggish circulation in the legs. They should neither sit nor stand in one position for long periods of time. They should avoid crossing their legs at the knees because this

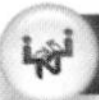

PATIENT TEACHING

Safety During Pregnancy

Changes in the body caused by pregnancy include relaxation of joints, alteration to the centre of gravity, faintness, and discomfort. Problems with coordination and balance are common. Therefore, the woman should follow these guidelines:

- Use good body mechanics.
- Use safety features on tools and vehicles (safety seat belts, shoulder harnesses, headrests, goggles, helmets) as specified.
- Avoid activities requiring coordination, balance, and concentration.
- Take rest periods; reschedule daily activities to meet rest and relaxation needs.

The developing embryo and fetus are vulnerable to environmental teratogens. Many potentially dangerous chemicals are present in the home, yard, and workplace: cleaning agents, paints, sprays, herbicides, and pesticides. The soil and water supply may be unsafe. Therefore, the woman should follow these guidelines:

- Read all labels for ingredients and proper use of a product.
- Ensure adequate ventilation with clean air.
- Dispose of wastes appropriately.
- Wear gloves when handling chemicals.
- Change job assignments or workplace as necessary.

can foster the development of varices and thrombophlebitis. Standing for long periods also increases the risk of preterm labour. The pregnant woman's chair should provide adequate back support. Use of a footstool can prevent pressure on veins, relieve strain on varicosities, minimize swelling of feet, and prevent backache.

Clothing. Some women continue to wear their usual clothes during pregnancy as long as they fit and feel comfortable. If maternity clothing is needed, outfits may be purchased new or found in good condition at thrift shops or garage sales. Comfortable, loose clothing is best. Tight bras and belts, stretch pants, garters, tight-top knee socks, body shapers, and other constrictive clothing should be avoided because tight clothing over the perineum encourages vaginitis and miliaria (heat rash), and impaired circulation in the legs can cause varicosities.

Maternity bras are constructed to accommodate the increased breast weight, chest circumference, and size of breast tail tissue (under the arm). These bras have drop-flaps over the nipples to facilitate breastfeeding. A good bra can help prevent neck ache and backache.

Maternity support (compression) hose give considerable comfort and promote greater venous emptying in women with large varicose veins. Ideally, support stockings should be put on before the woman gets out of bed in the morning. Figure 11-14 demonstrates a position for resting the legs and reducing swelling.

Comfortable shoes that provide firm support and promote good posture and balance are advisable. Very high heels and platform shoes are not recommended because of the woman's changed centre of gravity, which can cause her to lose her balance. In addition, the woman's pelvis tilts forward in the third trimester, increasing her lumbar curve. The resulting leg aches and cramps will be aggravated by shoes that do not provide good support. Figure 11-15 shows exercises to relieve leg cramps.

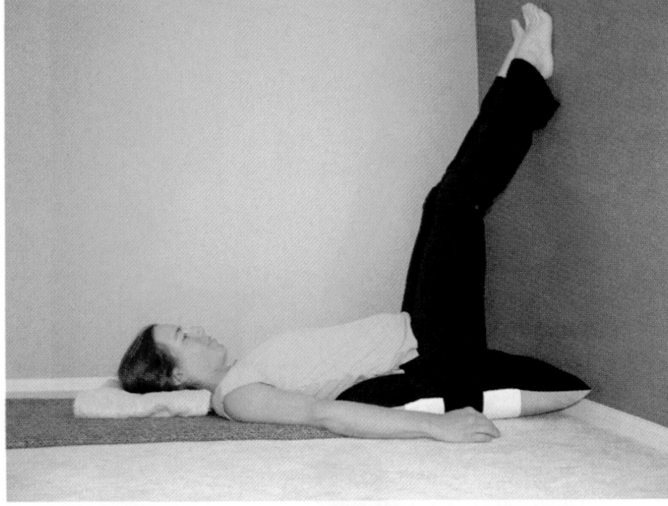

FIGURE 11-14 Position for resting legs and reducing edema and varicosities. Encourage the woman with vulvar varicosities to include a pillow under her hips. (Courtesy Julie Perry Nelson.)

Travel. Travel is not contraindicated for low-risk pregnant women. Women with high-risk pregnancies are advised to avoid long-distance travel after fetal viability has been reached, to avert the economic and psychological consequences of giving birth to a preterm infant far from home. Travel to areas where medical care is poor, water is untreated, and malaria or other communicable diseases are prevalent should be avoided if possible. Women who contemplate foreign travel should be aware that some provincial health insurance plans may not cover all expenses for birth in a foreign setting or even hospitalization for preterm labour. In addition, vaccinations for foreign travel may be contraindicated during pregnancy.

Pregnant women who travel for long distances should schedule periods of activity and rest. While sitting, the woman can practise deep breathing, foot circling, and alternately contracting and relaxing different muscle groups. She should avoid becoming fatigued. Although travel in itself is not a cause of adverse outcomes such as miscarriage or preterm labour, certain precautions are recommended when travelling in a car. For example, when riding in a car, the pregnant woman should wear a seatbelt and stop and walk every hour.

Maternal death as a result of injury is the most common cause of fetal death. The next most common cause is placental separation (**placental abruption**) due to body contours changing in reaction to the force of a collision. The uterus as a muscular organ can adapt its shape to that of the body, but the placenta is not resilient. At the impact of collision, placental separation can occur. The lap belt should be worn low across the hip bones and as snug as is comfortable (Fig. 11-16). The shoulder harness should be worn above the gravid uterus and below the neck to prevent chafing. The pregnant woman should sit upright. The headrest should be used to avoid whiplash injury. Airbags if present should remain engaged, but the steering wheel should be tilted upward away from the abdomen and the seat moved back away from the steering wheel as much as possible.

Air travel in large commercial jets usually poses little risk to the pregnant woman, although policies regarding flight by

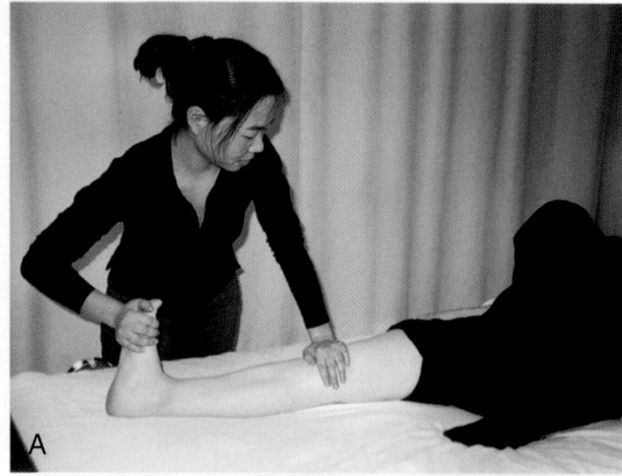
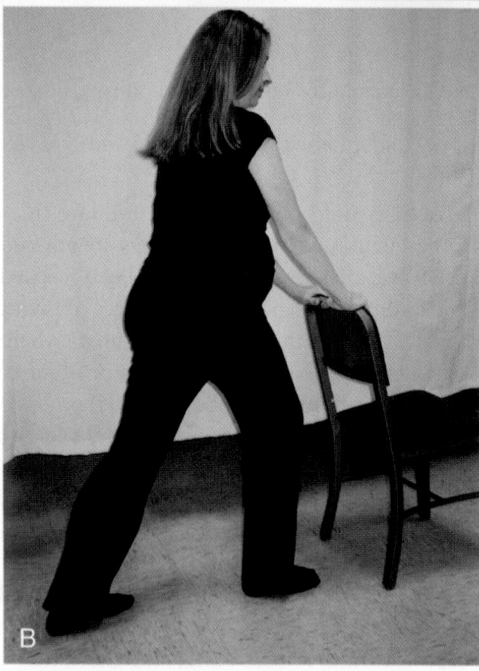

FIGURE 11-15 Relief of muscle spasm (leg cramps). **A:** Another person dorsiflexes foot with the knee extended. **B:** Woman stands and leans forward, thereby dorsiflexing foot of the affected leg. (Courtesy Shannon Perry.)

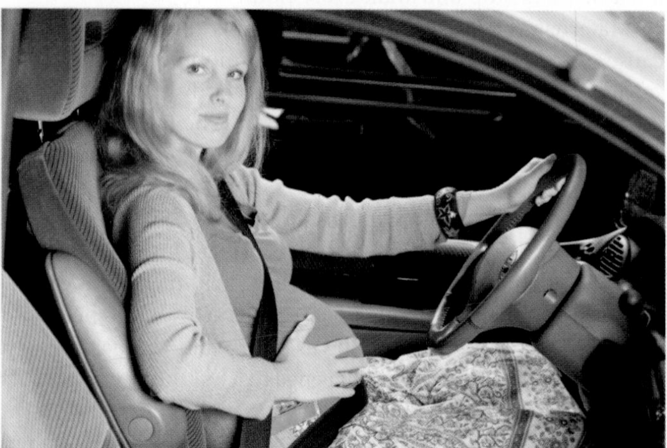

FIGURE 11-16 Proper use of seat belt and headrest. (ambrozinio/Shutterstock.com.)

pregnant women vary from airline to airline. The pregnant woman is advised to inquire about restrictions or recommendations from her carrier. Most health care providers allow air travel up to 36 weeks of gestation for women without medical or pregnancy complications. Air travel is not recommended for women with severe anemia, sickle cell disease or trait, history of thrombophlebitis, or placental abnormalities. Women at risk for preterm labour should avoid air travel (Sutton, 2012). Magnetometers (metal detectors) used at airport security checkpoints are not harmful to the fetus. The 8% humidity at which cabins are maintained in commercial airlines may result in some water loss; hydration (with water) should be maintained under these conditions. Sitting in the cramped seat of an airliner for prolonged periods may increase the risk of superficial and deep thrombophlebitis. Thus any passenger who is pregnant is encouraged to take a 15-minute walk around the aircraft during each hour of travel to minimize this risk. It is recommended that pregnant women not fly more than 200 hours during their pregnancy (Health Canada, 2007). However, women who are pilots, flight attendants, or frequent flyers may expose themselves to in-flight radiation that exceeds recommended levels. Resources from Health Canada, Radiation Protection Bureau can assist the health care provider in determining safe levels for women at high risk for radiation exposure (see Additional Resources at end of the chapter).

Medications and herbal preparations. Although much has been learned in recent years about fetal drug toxicity, the possible teratogenicity of many medications, both prescription and OTC, is still unknown. This is especially true for new medications and combinations of medications. Moreover, certain subclinical errors or deficiencies in intermediate metabolism in the fetus may cause an otherwise harmless medication to be converted into a hazardous one. The greatest danger of medication-caused developmental defects in the fetus extends from the time of fertilization through the first trimester, a time when the woman may not realize she is pregnant. Self-treatment must be discouraged. The use of all medications, including OTC medications, herbs, and vitamins, should be limited and a careful record kept of all therapeutic and nontherapeutic agents used. If women have questions regarding certain medications, they can be directed to Motherisk (see Additional Resources at end of the chapter).

The use of complementary and alternative medicine by pregnant women is widespread and is based primarily on historical use and anecdotal information. There is limited research evidence about the safety of herbal preparations, especially during pregnancy. While the use of complementary and alternative therapies is consistent with the holistic, woman-centred approach to care, caution is warranted in their use because of the lack of evidence (Hall, McKenna, & Griffiths, 2010).

SAFETY ALERT

Although some complementary and alternative medicine (CAM) may benefit the woman during pregnancy, some practices should be avoided because they may increase risk for complications. It is important to ask the woman about all medications she is taking, including OTC and herbal preparations.

Immunizations. Some concern has been raised over the safety of various immunization practices during pregnancy. Immunization with live or attenuated live virus or live bacterial vaccines is generally contraindicated during pregnancy because of potential teratogenicity. Live virus vaccines include those for measles (rubeola and rubella), chicken pox, mumps, and the Sabin (oral) poliomyelitis vaccine (no longer used in Canada). Human papilloma virus (HPV) vaccine is not recommended during pregnancy. Vaccines consisting of killed viruses that may be administered during pregnancy include tetanus, diphtheria, recombinant hepatitis B, rabies vaccines, and most influenza vaccines.

The Public Health Agency of Canada (PHAC, 2015) recommends routine administration of the tetanus, diphtheria, and acellular pertussis (Tdap) vaccine during each pregnancy. The optimal timing for the vaccine is after 26 weeks of gestation.

SAFETY ALERT

Pregnant women who become ill with seasonal respiratory influenza (flu) are more likely than other persons to develop serious complications, such as pneumonia. All women whose pregnancy will take place from November through March should be offered an influenza vaccination.

Alcohol, cigarette smoke, caffeine, and drugs. A safe level of alcohol consumption during pregnancy has not yet been established. Although the consumption of occasional alcoholic beverages may not be harmful to the mother or her developing embryo or fetus, complete abstinence is strongly advised (Senikas, Kluka, Wood, et al., 2010). Maternal **alcoholism** is associated with high rates of miscarriage and fetal alcohol spectrum disorder (FASD); the risk for miscarriage in the first trimester is dose related (three or more drinks per day). Growing evidence indicates that the pattern of drinking (frequency, timing, and duration), especially in the first trimester, is more predictive of fetal damage than the amount. FASD includes fetal alcohol syndrome (FAS), partial fetal alcohol syndrome/disorder, and alcohol-related neurodevelopmental disabilities. An estimated 9 in every 1000 children are born with FASD (PHAC, 2012a). Low birth weight, behavioural problems, and learning disabilities are some of the potential lifelong struggles facing individuals with FASD (see Chapter 29). Severe facial deformities of FASD occur at day 20 of conception, when women may not even suspect that they are pregnant.

The Society of Obstetricians and Gynaecologists of Canada (SOGC) (Senikas et al., 2010) recommends that each pregnant woman be screened for alcohol use during pregnancy. Using a harm reduction approach, they recommend that screening involve a thorough history, motivational interviewing, specific questionnaires, and diagnostic testing, bearing in mind that the woman has a right to refuse laboratory testing.

The SOGC (Senikas et al., 2010) states that one or two interview questions about alcohol use is an effective way to screen women and identify women who require further education or intervention. Questions may include the following:

- When was the last time you had a drink?
- Do you ever enjoy a drink or two?
- Do you sometimes drink beer, wine, or other alcoholic beverages?
- Do you ever use alcohol?
- In the past month or two, have you ever enjoyed a drink or two?

If a woman indicates that she does not consume alcohol, then positive reinforcement is beneficial. Research has shown that brief interventions can be very useful in helping a pregnant woman who drinks low to moderate amounts of alcohol to reduce her alcohol intake during pregnancy. If a woman identifies that she requires further intervention, a more in-depth assessment of drinking practices is necessary (Senikas et al., 2010). Several tools that are useful for this include the TWEAK, T-ACE, and CRAFFT tools (Senikas et al., 2010).

Cigarette smoking or continued exposure to secondhand smoke (even if the mother does not smoke) is associated with IUGR and an increase in perinatal and infant morbidity and mortality. Smoking is associated with an increased incidence of spontaneous abortion, ectopic pregnancy, preterm birth, PROM, placental abruption, placenta previa, and fetal death (Cunningham et al., 2014; Sidransky, Norman, McCarthy, et al., 2010). Smoking-cessation activities should be incorporated into routine prenatal care. In Canada, 10% of women reported smoking daily or occasionally during the last 3 months of pregnancy, although this varied greatly by province (PHAC, 2009). All women who smoke should be strongly encouraged to quit or at least reduce the number of cigarettes they smoke (see Critical Thinking Case Study). Pregnant women need to be told about the negative effects of secondhand smoke on the fetus and encouraged to avoid such environments. Efforts focused on preventing girls and women from beginning to smoke should be intensified.

Birth defects have not been related to caffeine consumption; however, high intake has been related to a slight decrease in birth weight and may also increase the risk of miscarriage with caffeine intake greater than 300 mg/day or fetal growth restriction with caffeine intake greater than 223 mg/day.

CRITICAL THINKING CASE STUDY

Smoking Cessation During Pregnancy

Doreen is a 25-year-old who is 8 weeks pregnant. At her first prenatal visit a history is taken; she reports that she smokes about half a pack of cigarettes a day. She says she knows that she should probably try to cut down, but she has been smoking since she was 15. She has tried to quit smoking before and has not been successful. How would you respond to her statement?

QUESTIONS

1. Evidence—Is there sufficient evidence to draw conclusions about what the nurse should say?
2. Assumptions—What assumptions can be made about the following issues?
   a. Effects of smoking on pregnancy
   b. Cessation interventions for pregnant women
3. What implications and priorities for nursing care can be made at this time?
4. Does the evidence objectively support your conclusion?

Therefore, because other effects are unknown, pregnant women are advised to limit their consumption of caffeine to less than 300 mg/day, or a little more than two 240 mL cups (PHAC, 2014). It is important for the nurse to educate the woman on the various sources of caffeine as it is found in a variety of food and drink products.

Any drug or environmental agent that enters the pregnant woman's bloodstream has the potential to cross the placenta and harm the fetus. Regarding use of recreational drugs, 6.7% of Canadian women reported using such substances in the 3 months before pregnancy, with women ages 15 to 24 years having the highest incidence of use (PHAC, 2009). It is important to note that this statistic is likely to be much higher because of underreporting by women. Marijuana, opioids for recreational use, and cocaine are common examples of such substances. Substance use in pregnancy is a major public health concern; comprehensive care of drug-addicted women can improve maternal and neonatal outcomes with increasing numbers of facilities and providers available for treatment of these women.

Normal discomforts. Pregnant women are confronted with symptoms that would be considered abnormal in the nonpregnant state. Women pregnant for the first time have a greater need for explanations of the causes of associated discomforts and advice on ways to relieve them. The discomforts are fairly specific to each trimester of pregnancy. Table 11-3 provides information about the physiology, prevention, and self care of discomforts experienced during the three trimesters. Box 11-3 lists alternative therapies used in pregnancy. Nurses can do much to allay a first-time mother's anxiety about such symptoms by telling her about them in advance, using terminology that the woman (or couple) can understand. When the woman understands the rationale for treatment, she is more likely to participate in her own care. Interventions should be individualized, with attention given to the woman's lifestyle and culture.

Recognizing potential complications. One of the most important responsibilities of health care providers is to alert the pregnant woman to signs and symptoms that indicate a potential complication of pregnancy. The woman needs to know how and to whom such warning signs should be reported (see Table 11-2). It is difficult to remember specifics when stressed by a disturbing symptom. Therefore, it is important that the woman

TABLE 11-3 DISCOMFORTS RELATED TO PREGNANCY

DISCOMFORT	PHYSIOLOGY	EDUCATION FOR SELF-CARE
First Trimester		
Breast changes, enlargement; pain, tingling, tenderness	Hypertrophy of mammary glandular tissue and increased vascularization, pigmentation, and size and prominence of nipples and areolae caused by hormonal stimulation	Wear supportive maternity bras with pads to absorb discharge (may be worn at night); wash with warm water and keep dry; breast tenderness may interfere with sexual expression and foreplay but is temporary
Urgency and frequency of urination	Vascular engorgement and altered bladder function caused by hormones; bladder capacity reduced by enlarging uterus and fetal presenting part	Empty bladder regularly; perform Kegel exercises; wear perineal pad; report pain or burning sensation to primary health care provider
Languor and malaise; fatigue (early pregnancy, most commonly)	Unexplained; may be caused by increasing levels of estrogen, progesterone, and hCG or by elevated BBT; psychological response to pregnancy and its required physical/psychological adaptations	Rest as needed; eat well-balanced diet to prevent anemia
Nausea and vomiting, morning sickness—occurs in 50–75% of pregnant women; starts between first and second missed periods and lasts until about fourth missed period; may occur any time during day; partners also may have symptoms	Cause is unknown; may result from hormonal changes, possibly hCG; may be partly emotional, related to ambivalence about pregnant state	Avoid empty or overloaded stomach (eat every 1 to 2 hours); try not to drink or eat too much at same time; don't wait to be too hungry or thirsty; keep solids and liquids separate by drinking fluids 20 to 30 minutes before and after eating (to prevent stomach from feeling too full); do not skip meals; eat dry carbohydrate on awakening; remain in bed until feeling subsides or alternate dry carbohydrate 1 hr with fluids such as hot herbal decaffeinated tea, milk, or clear coffee the next hour until feeling subsides; eat high-carbohydrate, low-fat foods and low-fat dairy products, as they are easier to digest; ensure adequate fluids (minimum 2 L/day); try adding any source of protein to each meal and snack; eat bland, dry, or salty foods; minimize or avoid spicy, fried, and/or high-fat foods; reduce strong odours (sniff lemons or limes, or get fresh air); ginger supplementation, vitamin B_6, acupuncture, or acupressure may be beneficial (Koren & Maltepe, 2013); consult primary health care provider if intractable vomiting occurs (medication may be prescribed), see Chapter 12 for further discussion
Ptyalism (excessive salivation) may occur starting 2–3 wk after first missed period	Possibly caused by elevated estrogen levels; may be related to reluctance to swallow because of nausea	Use astringent mouthwash, chew gum, eat hard candy as comfort measures

TABLE 11-3 **DISCOMFORTS RELATED TO PREGNANCY—cont'd**

DISCOMFORT	PHYSIOLOGY	EDUCATION FOR SELF-CARE
Gingivitis and epulis (hyperemia, hypertrophy, bleeding, tenderness); condition disappears spontaneously 1–2 mo after birth: often noted throughout pregnancy	Increased vascularity and proliferation of connective tissue from estrogen stimulation	Eat well-balanced diet, with adequate protein and fresh fruits and vegetables; brush teeth gently and observe good dental hygiene; avoid infection; see dentist
Nasal stuffiness; epistaxis (nosebleed)	Hyperemia of mucous membranes related to high estrogen levels	Use humidifier; avoid trauma; normal saline nose drops or spray may be used
Leukorrhea: often noted throughout pregnancy	Hormonally stimulated cervix becomes hypertrophic and hyperactive, producing abundant amount of mucus	Not preventable; do not douche; wear perineal pads; perform hygienic practices such as wiping front to back; report to primary health care provider if accompanied by pruritus, foul odour, or change in character or colour
Psychosocial dynamics, mood swings, mixed feelings; often noted throughout pregnancy	Hormonal and metabolic adaptations; feelings about female role, sexuality, timing of pregnancy, and resultant changes in life and lifestyle	Participate in pregnancy support group; communicate concerns to partner, family, and others; request referral for supportive services if needed (e.g., financial assistance)
Second Trimester		
Pigmentation deepens, acne, oily skin	Melanocyte-stimulating hormone (from anterior pituitary)	Not preventable; it usually resolves during puerperium
Spider nevi (angiomas) appear over neck, thorax, face, and arms during second or third trimester	Focal networks of dilated arterioles (end-arteries) from increased concentration of estrogens	Not preventable; they fade slowly during late puerperium but rarely disappear completely
Palmar erythema occurs in 50% of pregnant women; may accompany spider nevi	Diffuse reddish mottling over palms and suffused skin over thenar eminences and fingertips; may be caused by genetic predisposition or hyperestrogenism	Not preventable; condition fades within 1 wk after giving birth
Pruritus (noninflammatory)	Unknown cause; various types as follows: nonpapular; closely aggregated pruritic papules	Keep fingernails short and clean; contact primary health care provider for diagnosis of cause
	Increased excretory function of skin and stretching of skin possible factors	Not preventable; symptomatic; can be managed with Keri baths, mild sedation, distraction, tepid baths with sodium bicarbonate or oatmeal added to water, lotions and oils, change of soaps or reduction in use of soap, loose clothing; contact health care provider if it does not resolve with treatment
Palpitations	Unknown; should not be accompanied by persistent cardiac irregularity	Not preventable; contact primary health care provider if accompanied by symptoms of cardiac decompensation
Supine hypotension (vena cava syndrome) and bradycardia	Induced by pressure of gravid uterus on ascending vena cava when woman is supine; reduces uteroplacental and renal perfusion	Assume side-lying position or semisitting posture, with knees slightly flexed (see also Emergency box, p. 240)
Faintness and, rarely, syncope (orthostatic hypotension): may persist throughout pregnancy	Vasomotor lability or postural hypotension from hormones; in late pregnancy may be caused by venous stasis in lower extremities	Exercise moderately (deep breathing, vigorous leg movements); avoid sudden changes in position* and warm crowded areas; move slowly and deliberately; keep environment cool; avoid hypoglycemia by eating five to six small meals per day; wear compression hose; sit as necessary; if symptoms are serious, contact primary health care provider
Food cravings	Cause unknown; craving determined by culture or geographical area	Not preventable; satisfy craving unless it interferes with well-balanced diet; report unusual cravings to primary health care provider
Heartburn (pyrosis or acid indigestion): burning sensation, occasionally with burping and regurgitation of a little sour-tasting fluid	Progesterone slows GI tract motility and digestion, reverses peristalsis, relaxes cardiac sphincter, and delays emptying time of stomach; stomach displaced upward and compressed by enlarging uterus	Limit or avoid gas-producing or fatty foods and large meals; maintain good posture; drink hot herbal tea; primary health care provider may prescribe antacid between meals; contact primary health care provider for persistent symptoms
Constipation	GI tract motility slowed because of progesterone, resulting in increased reabsorption of water and drying of stool; intestines compressed by enlarging uterus; predisposition to constipation because of oral iron supplementation	Drink eight glasses of water per day; include roughage in diet; exercise moderately; maintain regular schedule for bowel movements; use relaxation techniques and deep breathing; do not take stool softener, laxatives, mineral oil, other medications, or enemas without first consulting primary health care provider
Flatulence with bloating and belching	Reduced GI motility because of hormones, allowing time for bacterial action that produces gas; swallowing air	Chew foods slowly and thoroughly; avoid gas-producing foods, fatty foods, large meals; exercise, maintain regular bowel habits

Continued

TABLE 11-3 DISCOMFORTS RELATED TO PREGNANCY—cont'd

DISCOMFORT	PHYSIOLOGY	EDUCATION FOR SELF-CARE
Varicose veins (varicosities): may be associated with aching legs and tenderness; may be present in legs and vulva; hemorrhoids are varicosities in perianal area	Hereditary predisposition; relaxation of smooth muscle walls of veins because of hormones causing tortuous dilated veins in legs and pelvic vasocongestion; condition aggravated by enlarging uterus, gravity, and bearing down for bowel movements; thrombi from leg varices are rare but may be produced by hemorrhoids	Avoid lengthy standing or sitting, constrictive clothing, and constipation and bearing down with bowel movements; exercise moderately; rest with legs and hips elevated (see Fig. 11-14); wear compression hose; thrombosed hemorrhoid may be evacuated; relieve swelling and pain with warm sitz baths; apply astringent compresses locally
Headaches (through wk 26)	Emotional tension (more common than vascular migraine headache); eye strain (refractory errors); vascular engorgement and congestion of sinuses resulting from hormone stimulation	Conscious relaxation; rest, massage, application of heat or cold; OTC analgesics (check with provider); contact primary health care provider for constant "splitting" headache to assess for pre-eclampsia
Carpal tunnel syndrome (involves thumb, second and third fingers, lateral side of little finger)	Compression of median nerve resulting from changes in surrounding tissues; pain, numbness, tingling, burning; loss of skilled movements (typing); dropping of objects	Not preventable; elevate affected arms; splinting of affected hand may help; regressive after pregnancy; surgery is curative
Periodic numbness, tingling of fingers (acrodysesthesia) occurs in 5% of pregnant women	Brachial plexus traction syndrome resulting from drooping of shoulders during pregnancy (occurs especially at night and early morning)	Maintain good posture; wear supportive maternity bra; condition will disappear if lifting and carrying baby does not aggravate it
Round ligament pain (tenderness)	Stretching of ligament caused by enlarging uterus	Not preventable; rest, maintain good body mechanics to avoid overstretching ligament; relieve cramping by squatting or bringing knees to chest; sometimes heat helps
Joint pain, backache, and pelvic pressure; hypermobility of joints	Relaxation of symphyseal and sacroiliac joints because of hormones, resulting in unstable pelvis; exaggerated lumbar and cervicothoracic curves caused by change in centre of gravity resulting from enlarging abdomen	Maintain good posture and body mechanics; avoid fatigue; wear low-heeled shoes; abdominal supports may be useful; practise conscious relaxation; sleep on firm mattress; apply local heat or ice; get back rubs; do pelvic rock exercise (see Fig. 11-10); physiotherapy; acupuncture; water gymnastics; rest; condition disappears 6–8 wk after birth
Third Trimester		
Shortness of breath and dyspnea: occur in 60% of pregnant women	Expansion of diaphragm limited by enlarging uterus; diaphragm elevated about 4 cm; some relief after lightening	Maintain good posture; sleep with extra pillows; avoid overloading stomach; stop smoking; contact health care provider if symptoms worsen, to rule out anemia, emphysema, and asthma
Insomnia (later weeks of pregnancy)	Fetal movements, muscle cramping, urinary frequency, shortness of breath, or other discomforts	Reassurance, conscious relaxation, back massage or effleurage, support of body parts with pillows, and warm milk or warm shower before bedtime are helpful
Psychosocial responses: mood swings, mixed feelings, increased anxiety	Hormonal and metabolic adaptations; feelings about impending labour, birth, and parenthood	Reassurance and support from partner and nurse, and improved communication with partner, family, and others are helpful
Urinary frequency and urgency return	Vascular engorgement and altered bladder function caused by hormones; bladder capacity reduced by enlarging uterus and fetal presenting part	Empty bladder regularly, do Kegel exercises; reassurance is helpful; wear perineal pad; contact health care provider for pain or burning sensation
Perineal discomfort and pressure	Pressure from enlarging uterus, especially when standing or walking; multifetal gestation	Rest, conscious relaxation, and good posture are helpful; contact health care provider for assessment and treatment if pain is persistent
Leg cramps (gastrocnemius spasm), especially when reclining	Compression of nerves supplying lower extremities because of enlarging uterus; reduced level of diffusible serum calcium or elevation of serum phosphorus; aggravating factors: fatigue, poor peripheral circulation, pointing toes when stretching legs or when walking, drinking more than 1 L of milk per day	Dorsiflex foot until spasm relaxes; use massage if not reddened or increased temperature at site (see Fig. 11-15, A); stand on cold surface; supplement orally with calcium carbonate or calcium lactate tablets; aluminum hydroxide gel, 30 mL, with each meal removes phosphorus by absorbing it; avoid pointing toes
Ankle edema (nonpitting) to lower extremities	Edema aggravated by prolonged standing, sitting, poor posture, lack of exercise, constrictive clothing, or hot weather	Intake ample fluid for natural diuretic effect; put on compression stockings before arising; rest periodically with legs and hips elevated (see Fig. 11-14); exercise moderately; contact health care provider if generalized edema develops; diuretics are contraindicated

BBT, basal body temperature; *GI,* gastrointestinal; *hCG,* human chorionic gonadotropin; OTC, over-the-counter.

*Caution woman to rise slowly and sit on edge of bed or to assume hands-and-knees posture before rising and to get up slowly after sitting or squatting.

Source: Koren, G., & Maltepe, C. (2013). *How to survive morning sickness successfully.* Toronto: Motherisk. Retrieved from http://www.motherisk.org/documents/BSRC_morning_sickness_EN.pdf

BOX 11-3 ALTERNATIVE THERAPIES USED IN PREGNANCY

Touch and Energetic Therapies
- Massage
- Acupressure
- Therapeutic touch
- Healing touch

Mind–Body Healing
- Imagery
- Meditation, prayer, reflection
- Biofeedback
- Aromatherapy

Other modalities that may fall outside of nurse practice guidelines unless the nurse has completed additional training or certification:
- Herbs
- Homeopathy
- Traditional Chinese medicine

and her family receive a printed form written at the appropriate literacy level listing the signs and symptoms that warrant an investigation and the phone numbers to call with questions or in an emergency.

The nurse must answer questions honestly as they arise during pregnancy. Pregnant women often have difficulty deciding when to report signs and symptoms. The mother should be encouraged to refer to the printed list of potential complications and to listen to her body. If she senses that something is wrong, she should call her care provider immediately. Several signs and symptoms must be discussed more extensively. These include vaginal bleeding, alteration in fetal movements, symptoms of pre-eclampsia, rupture of membranes, and preterm labour.

Recognizing preterm labour. Teaching each expectant mother to recognize preterm labour is necessary for early diagnosis and treatment. Preterm labour occurs after the twentieth week but before the thirty-seventh week of pregnancy. It consists of uterine contractions that, if untreated, cause the cervix to open earlier than normal, resulting in preterm birth.

Although the exact etiology of preterm labour is unknown, it is assumed to have multiple causes. While not themselves causes of preterm birth, an increased incidence is associated with sociodemographic factors such as poverty, low educational level, lack of social support, smoking, intimate partner violence, and stress. Other risk factors include a previous preterm labour, current multifetal gestation, and some uterine and cervical variations (Newnham, Dickinson, Hart, et al., 2014). The rate of preterm birth worldwide is approximately 11% and it is associated with neonatal morbidity and mortality (Newnham et al., 2014). Women with a previous preterm birth may be treated more extensively with medications such as progesterone and even be referred to a maternal fetal medicine specialist or preterm birth clinic.

If a woman knows the warning signs and symptoms of preterm labour and seeks care early enough, prevention of preterm birth may be possible, and if labour is not stopped, transport to an appropriate care facility may be planned. Warning signs and symptoms of preterm labour are given in

PATIENT TEACHING
How to Recognize Preterm Labour

Because the onset of preterm labour is subtle and often hard to recognize, it is important to know how to feel your abdomen for uterine contractions. You can feel for contractions in the following way:

- While lying down, place your fingertips on the top of your uterus. A contraction is the periodic tightening or hardening of your uterus. If your uterus is contracting, you will actually feel your abdomen get tight or hard and then feel it relax or soften when the contraction is over.
- If you think you are having any signs and symptoms of preterm labour (see below), empty your bladder, drink three to four glasses of water for hydration, lie down tilted toward your side, and place a pillow at your back for support.
- Check for contractions for 1 hour. To tell how often contractions are occurring, check the minutes that elapse from the beginning of one contraction to the beginning of the next.
- It is not normal to have frequent uterine contractions (every 10 minutes or more often for 1 hour).
- Contractions of labour are regular, frequent, and hard. They also may be felt as a tightening of the abdomen, a menstrual-like cramp, or a backache (see Fig. 11-17). This type of contraction causes the cervix to efface and dilate. Preterm labour contractions may not feel uncomfortable.
- Call your doctor, midwife, or labour and birth unit or go to the hospital if any of the following signs occur:
  - You have uterine contractions every 10 minutes or more often for 1 hour *or*
  - You feel pelvic pressure that is not relieved
  - You have any bloody spotting or leaking of fluid from your vagina
  - You feel "something is not right"
- It is often difficult to identify preterm labour. Accurate diagnosis requires assessment by the health care provider, usually in the hospital or clinic.

Adapted from Best Start. (2012). *Preterm labour signs and symptoms.* Retrieved from http://www.beststart.org/resources/rep_health/preterm/Preterm_English_2012.pdf. Adapted with permission by the Best Start Resource Centre.

the Patient Teaching box: How to Recognize Preterm Labour. Figure 11-17 shows where in the body the signs and symptoms of preterm labour may be located.

Sex Counselling

Sex counselling of expectant couples includes countering misinformation, providing reassurance of normality, and suggesting alternative sexual behaviours. The uniqueness of each couple is considered within a biopsychosocial framework (see Patient Teaching Box: Sexuality in Pregnancy). Nurses can initiate discussion about sexual adaptations that must be made during pregnancy. They need a sound knowledge base about the physical, social, and emotional responses to sex during pregnancy. Not all perinatal nurses are comfortable dealing with the sexual concerns of their patients; nurses who are aware of their personal strengths and limitations in dealing with sexual content will be better prepared to make referrals, if necessary.

Many women merely need permission to be sexually active during pregnancy. Many other women, however, need to be given information about the physiological changes that occur during pregnancy, have the myths that are associated with sex

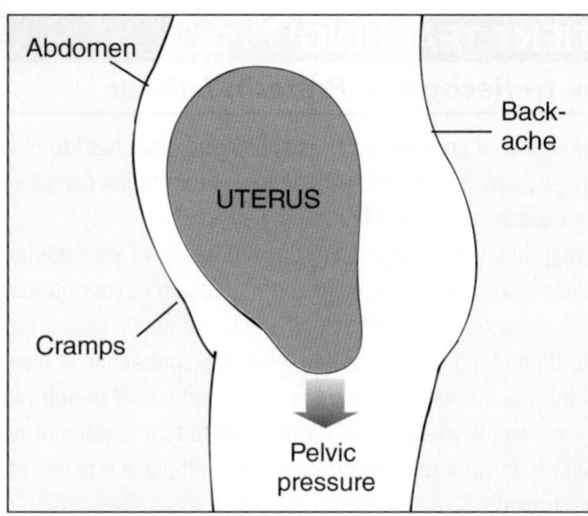

FIGURE 11-17 Symptoms of preterm labour.

PATIENT TEACHING
Sexuality in Pregnancy

- Be aware that maternal physiological changes such as breast enlargement, nausea, fatigue, abdominal changes, perineal enlargement, leukorrhea, pelvic vasocongestion, and orgasmic responses may affect sexuality and sexual expression.
- Discuss responses to pregnancy with your partner.
- Keep in mind that cultural prescriptions (do's) and proscriptions (don'ts) may affect your responses.
- Although your libido may be depressed during the first trimester, it often increases during the second trimester.
- Discuss and explore the following with your partner:
  - Alternative behaviours (e.g., mutual masturbation, foot massage, cuddling).
  - Alternative positions (e.g., female superior, side-lying) for sexual intercourse.
- Intercourse is safe as long as it is not uncomfortable. There is no correlation between intercourse and miscarriage, but observe the following precautions:
  - Abstain from intercourse if you experience uterine cramping or vaginal bleeding; report event to your health care provider as soon as possible.
  - Abstain from intercourse (or any activity that results in orgasm) if you have a history of premature dilation of the cervix until the problem is corrected or if your membranes are ruptured.
- Continue to use risk reduction behaviours. Women at risk for acquiring or conveying sexually transmitted infections are encouraged to use condoms during sexual intercourse throughout pregnancy.

during pregnancy dispelled, and participate in open discussion of positions for intercourse that decrease pressure on the gravid abdomen. Such tasks are within the purview of the perinatal nurse and should be an integral component of the health care provided.

Some couples need to be referred for sex or family therapy. Couples whose long-standing problems with sexual dysfunction are intensified by pregnancy are good candidates for sex therapy. When a sexual problem is a symptom of a more serious relationship problem, the couple may benefit from family therapy.

Using the history. The couple's sexual history provides a basis for counselling. The history also may reveal the woman's knowledge of female anatomy and physiology and her attitudes about sex during pregnancy, as well as her perceptions of the pregnancy, the health status of the couple, and the quality of their relationship.

Countering misinformation. Many myths and much of the misinformation related to sex and pregnancy are masked by seemingly unrelated issues. For example, a discussion about the baby's ability to hear and see in utero may be prompted by questions about the baby being an observer of lovemaking. The counsellor must be sensitive to the issues behind such questions when counselling in this highly charged emotional area.

Suggesting alternative behaviours. Researchers have not demonstrated that, for the obstetrically and medically healthy woman, coitus and orgasm are contraindicated at any time during pregnancy (Cunningham et al., 2014). However, women with a history of more than one miscarriage; a threatened miscarriage in the first trimester; impending miscarriage in the second trimester; or PROM, bleeding, or abdominal pain during the third trimester should use caution regarding coitus and orgasm.

Solitary and mutual masturbation and oral–genital intercourse may be used by couples as alternatives to penile–vaginal intercourse. Partners who enjoy cunnilingus (oral stimulation of the clitoris or vagina) may feel "turned off" by the normal increase in amount and odour of vaginal discharge during pregnancy. Couples who practise cunnilingus should be cautioned against the blowing of air into the vagina, particularly during the last few weeks of pregnancy, when the cervix may be slightly open. An air embolism can occur if air is forced between the uterine wall and fetal membranes and enters the maternal vascular system through the placenta.

Showing the woman or couple illustrations of the possible variations of coital position can be helpful (Fig. 11-18). The female-superior, side-by-side, rear-entry, and facing-each-other positions are alternatives to the traditional male-superior position. The woman astride (superior position) allows her to control the angle and depth of penile penetration, as well as protect her breasts and abdomen. During the third trimester, the side-by-side position or any position that places less pressure on the pregnant abdomen and requires less energy may be preferred.

Multiparous women sometimes have significant breast tenderness in the first trimester. A coital position that avoids direct pressure on the woman's breasts and decreased breast fondling during love play can be recommended to such couples. The woman should also be reassured that this condition is normal and temporary.

Some women state they have lower abdominal cramping and backache after orgasm during the first and third trimesters. A back rub can often relieve some of the discomfort and provide a pleasant experience. A tonic uterine contraction, often lasting up to a minute, replaces the rhythmic contractions of orgasm during the third trimester. Changes in FHR without fetal distress have also been reported.

The objective of risk reduction is to provide prophylaxis against the acquisition and transmission of STIs (e.g., HSV,

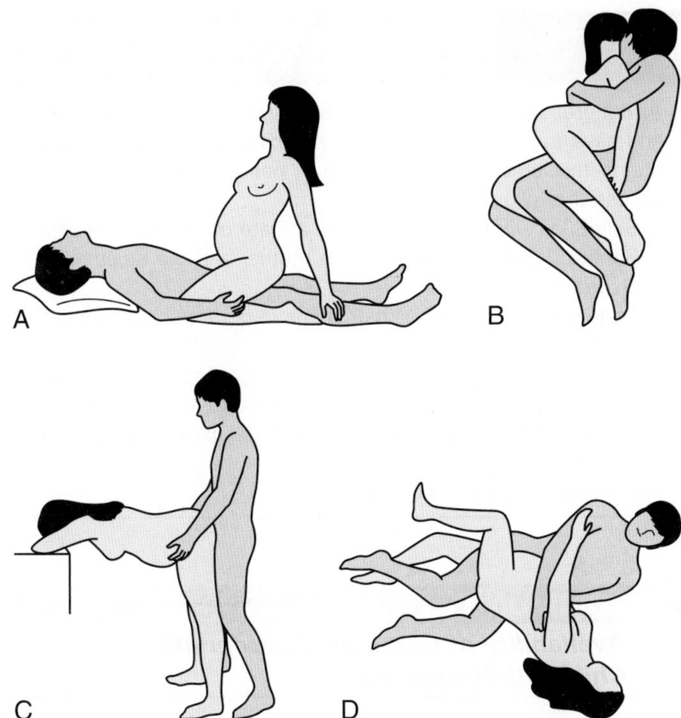

FIGURE 11-18 Positions for sexual intercourse during pregnancy. **A:** Female superior. **B:** Side by side. **C:** Rear entry. **D:** Facing each other.

HPV, and HIV). Because these diseases may be transmitted to the woman and her fetus, the use of condoms is recommended throughout pregnancy if the woman is at risk for acquiring an STI.

There is a lack of evidence regarding the safety of the use of sex toys during pregnancy. Popular pregnancy websites (e.g., http://www.baby.com; http://www.parents.com) suggest that it is generally safe to use these devices in low-risk pregnancies. However, safety practices should be followed. Sex toys must be carefully cleaned. Sex toys inserted into the anus should never be inserted into the vagina. If a vibrator or other device is made of a material that is firmer than human flesh, force should not be used when inserting it into the vagina. The use of sex toys should be discontinued if pain occurs (Quilliam, 2010). Safer sex practices to reduce the risk of STIs include using condoms and avoiding the sharing of sex toys.

Well-informed nurses who are comfortable with their own sexuality and the sex-counselling needs of expectant couples can offer information and advice in this valuable but often neglected area. They can establish an open environment in which couples can feel free to introduce their concerns about sexual adjustment and seek support and guidance. This intervention is as important for lesbian women and their partners as it is for women partnered with men.

Psychosocial Support

Respect, affection, trust, concern, consideration of cultural and religious responses, and listening are all components of the emotional support that nurses can give to the pregnant woman and her family. The woman's satisfaction with her relationships and support as well as her sense of competence and being in control are all important issues to be addressed. A discussion of fetal responses to stimuli such as sound, light, maternal posture, tension, and patterns of sleeping and waking can be helpful. Other issues that can arise for the pregnant woman and couple include fear of pain, loss of control during labour, and possible birth of the infant before reaching the hospital. Parental concerns about the responsibilities and tasks of parenthood; the safety of the mother and unborn child; siblings and their acceptance of the new baby; social and economic responsibilities; and possible conflicts in cultural, religious, or personal value systems should all be addressed. The father's or partner's commitment to the pregnancy, the couple's relationship, and their concerns about sexuality and sexual expression can emerge as issues for many expectant parents.

By providing the prospective mother and father with opportunities to discuss their concerns and validating the normality of their responses, the perinatal nurse can help them feel more at ease with the pregnancy. Nurses must also recognize that men tend to feel more vulnerable during their partner's pregnancy. Female partners may also have these feelings. Anticipatory guidance and health promotion strategies can help partners cope with their concerns. Nursing intervention may help them to deal with such concerns either directly through counselling or indirectly through the education of the mothers. Health care providers can foster and encourage open dialogue between the couple.

All women should be assessed for depression and anxiety during pregnancy, and some provinces have adapted this assessment into the routine care provided. The Edinburgh Postnatal Depression Scale (EPDS) has been found to be useful as a screening tool (see Fig. 24-9). If women are identified as having depression or anxiety during the pregnancy, it is important that they receive treatment. If left untreated, there can be serious implications for the mother, partner, and child (Denis, Michaux, & Callahan, 2012; Pires, Aracijo-Pedrosa, & Conavarro, 2014).

Variations in Prenatal Care

The course of prenatal care described thus far can seem to suggest that the experiences of child-bearing women are similar and that nursing interventions are uniform across all populations. Although typical patterns of response to pregnancy are easily recognized and many aspects of prenatal care indeed are consistent, pregnant women enter the health care system with individual concerns and needs. The nurse's ability to assess unique needs and tailor interventions to the individual is the hallmark of expertise in providing care. Factors that influence prenatal care and a woman's response to it include culture, age, and number of fetuses.

Cultural Influences

Prenatal care as we know it is a phenomenon of Western medicine. In the biomedical model of care, women are encouraged to seek prenatal care as early as possible in their pregnancy by visiting a physician, midwife, office, or clinic. This model is not only unfamiliar but may seem strange to many cultural groups.

Thus different models for providing prenatal care for women should be explored.

Many cultural variations in prenatal care exist. Even if the prenatal care described is familiar to a woman, some practices may conflict with the beliefs and practices of a subculture group to which she belongs. Because of these and other factors, such as lack of money, lack of transportation, fear of judgement, and language barriers, women from diverse cultures may not keep prenatal appointments. The nurse may misinterpret their behaviour as uncaring, lazy, or ignorant.

A concern for modesty is a deterrent to many women seeking prenatal care. For some women, exposing body parts, especially to a man, is considered a major violation of their modesty. For some women, invasive procedures such as vaginal examination may be so threatening that they cannot be discussed even with their own husbands. Thus they prefer a female health care provider. Too often, health care providers assume that women lose this modesty during pregnancy and labour, but most women value and appreciate efforts to maintain their modesty.

For many cultural groups a physician is deemed appropriate only in times of illness. Because pregnancy is considered a normal process and the woman is in a state of health, the services of a physician are considered inappropriate. Western medicine's view of problems in pregnancy may differ from that of members of other cultural groups.

Although pregnancy is considered normal by many, certain practices are expected of women of all cultures to ensure a good outcome. *Cultural prescriptions* tell women what to do, and *cultural proscriptions* establish taboos. The purposes of these practices are to prevent maternal illness caused by a pregnancy-induced imbalanced state and to protect the vulnerable fetus. Prescriptions and proscriptions regulate the woman's emotional response, clothing, physical activity and rest, sexual activity, and dietary practices. Exploration of the woman's beliefs, perceptions of the meaning of child-bearing, and health care practices may help health care providers foster her self-esteem, promote attainment of the maternal role, and positively influence her relationship with her spouse.

To provide culturally sensitive care, the nurse must be knowledgeable about specific practices and customs. Although it is not possible to know all there is to know about every culture and subculture or the many lifestyles that exist, it is important to learn about the varied cultures in the setting in which a nurse practises. By exploring and becoming knowledgeable in the cultural beliefs and practices related to child-bearing, the nurse can better support and nurture the beliefs that promote physical or emotional adaptation (Box 11-4).

Emotional response. Virtually all cultures emphasize the importance of maintaining a socially harmonious and agreeable environment for the pregnant woman (see Community Focus box). A lifestyle with minimal stress is important in ensuring a successful outcome for the mother and baby. Harmony with other people must be fostered, and visits from extended family members may be required to demonstrate pleasant and noncontroversial relationships. If discord exists in a relationship, it is usually dealt with in culturally prescribed ways.

BOX 11-4 ANTEPARTUM CULTURAL ASSESSMENT

All cultures recognize pregnancy as a special transitional period and have particular customs and beliefs that dictate behaviour during this time. In the antepartum period, the nurse should assess the following:

- Beliefs of whether pregnancy is a state of illness or health
- Behavioural expectations of the mother and the health care provider
- Dietary prescriptions or restrictions (e.g., hot/cold balance theory, pica)
- Activity restrictions or prescriptions (e.g., use of massage)
- Availability of advice (e.g., from whom and at what time advice will be sought and when prenatal care will begin [if at all])
- Considerations of modesty

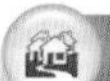

COMMUNITY FOCUS

Availability of Culturally Appropriate Childbirth Resources

Select a cultural group different from your own within your community and identify childbirth-related beliefs and practices that are unique to that group. Are there stores in the area that sell items that meet the needs of that group? Does the community centre have activities or classes that are directed toward that group? Are there outreach programs in the community that meet the cultural needs of the group? Are childbirth education programs available that provide essential information while incorporating cultural patterns? Are childbirth classes available in languages other than English? What written and online resources are available in the appropriate language and are they comprehensive? What could you, as a nurse, contribute to the community that would help meet the needs of that group?

Physical activity and rest. Norms that regulate physical activity of mothers during pregnancy vary tremendously. Many groups, including Indigenous groups as well as some Asian groups, encourage women to be active, to walk, and to engage in normal but not strenuous activities to ensure that the baby is healthy and not too large. Other groups such as Filipinos believe that any activity is dangerous, and others willingly take over the work of the pregnant woman. Some Filipinos believe that this inactivity protects the mother and child. If health care providers do not know of this belief, they could misinterpret this behaviour as laziness or noncompliance with the desired prenatal health care regimen. It is important for the nurse to find out the way that each pregnant woman views activity and rest.

Sexual activity. In most cultures, sexual activity is not prohibited until the end of pregnancy. Some Latin Americans view sexual activity as necessary to keep the birth canal lubricated. Conversely, some Vietnamese have definite proscriptions about sexual intercourse, requiring abstinence throughout the pregnancy because it is thought that sexual intercourse may harm the mother and the fetus.

Nutrition. Nutritional information given by Western health care providers may be a source of conflict for many cultural groups. Such a conflict commonly is not discovered by health care providers unless they understand the dietary beliefs and practices of the particular people for whom they are caring. For example, Muslims have strict regulations about the preparation of food; if meat cannot be prepared as prescribed, they may omit it from their diets. Many cultures permit pregnant women to eat only warm foods.

Age Differences

The age of the child-bearing couple may have a significant influence on their physical and psychosocial adaptation to pregnancy. Normal developmental processes that occur in both very young and older mothers are interrupted by pregnancy and require a different type of adaptation to pregnancy than that of the woman of typical child-bearing age. Special needs of expectant mothers 15 years of age or younger or those 35 years of age or older are summarized here.

Adolescents. Overall teenage pregnancy rates have decreased in Canada, although in 2013, the rate of adolescent pregnancies was 28.2 per 1000, which is an increase with a provincial variation (e.g., New Brunswick is slightly higher) (McKay & Sex Information and Education Council of Canada, 2012). Many of these pregnancies are unintended. Pregnancy rates are higher among teens with lower educational levels and who are economically disadvantaged. Many of these young women do not have consistent support and may not be ready for the emotional, psychosocial, and financial responsibilities of parenthood.

When adolescents become pregnant and decide to give birth, they are much less likely than older women to access adequate prenatal care, with many receiving no care at all. These young women also are more likely to smoke and less likely to gain adequate weight during pregnancy.

Delayed entry into prenatal care may be the result of late recognition of pregnancy, denial of pregnancy, or confusion about the services that are available. Such a delay in care may leave inadequate time before birth to attend to correctable problems. The very young pregnant adolescent is at higher risk for each of the confounding variables associated with poor pregnancy outcomes (e.g., socioeconomic factors) and for the conditions associated with a first pregnancy, regardless of age (e.g., gestational hypertension). However, when prenatal care is initiated early and consistently and confounding variables are controlled, very young pregnant adolescents are at no greater risk (nor are their infants) for an adverse outcome than older pregnant women. Thus the role of the nurse in reducing the risks and consequences of adolescent pregnancy is to encourage early and continued prenatal care; to provide early and ongoing education about pregnancy, birth, and parenting; and to refer the adolescent, if necessary, for appropriate social support services, which can help reverse the effects of a negative socioeconomic environment (Fig. 11-19; see Nursing Care Plan on Adolescent Pregnancy on Evolve).

Women older than 35 years of age. Two groups of older parents have emerged in the population of women having a child late in their child-bearing years. One group consists of women who have many children and who have an additional child during the menopausal period. The other group consists of women who have deliberately delayed child-bearing until their late 30s or early 40s.

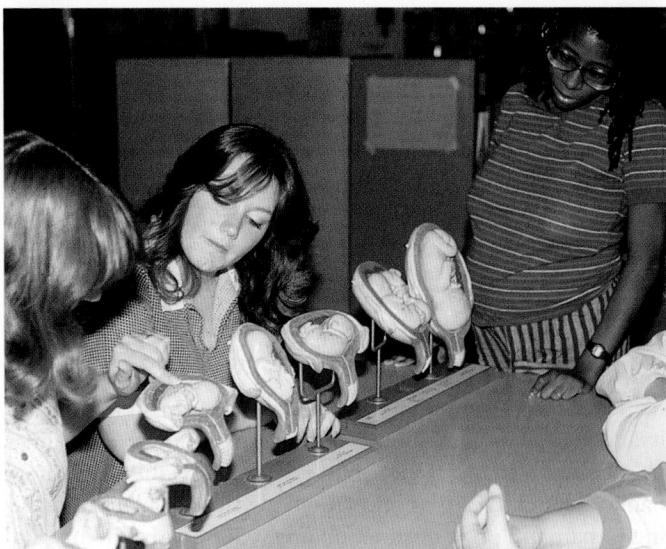

FIGURE 11-19 Pregnant adolescents review fetal development. (Courtesy Marjorie Pyle, RNC, Lifecircle.)

Multiparous women. Multiparous women may have never used contraceptives because of personal choice or a lack of knowledge about contraceptives. They also may be women who have used contraceptives successfully during the child-bearing years but, as menopause approached, ceased menstruating regularly or stopped using contraception and subsequently became pregnant. The older multiparous woman may believe that pregnancy separates her from her peer group and that her age is a hindrance to close associations with young mothers. Other parents welcome the unexpected infant as evidence of continuing maternal and paternal roles.

Nulliparous women. The number of first-time pregnancies in women between ages 35 and 40 has increased significantly over the last two decades. Currently, 11% of first births occur in women older than 35 years of age (Johnson & Tough, 2012). Seeing women in their late 30s or 40s during their first pregnancy is no longer unusual for health care providers. Reasons for delaying pregnancy include a desire to obtain advanced education, career priorities, and use of better contraceptive measures. Women who are infertile do not delay pregnancy deliberately but may become pregnant at a later age as a result of fertility studies and therapies.

These women choose parenthood. They often are established in a career and a lifestyle with a partner that includes time for self-attention, the establishment of a home with accumulated possessions, and freedom to travel. When asked the reason they chose pregnancy later in life, many reply, "Because time is running out."

The dilemma of choice includes recognition that being a parent will have both positive and negative consequences. Couples need to discuss the consequences of child-bearing and child-rearing before committing themselves to this lifelong venture. Partners in this group seem to share the preparation for parenthood, the planning for a family-centred birth, and the desire to be loving and competent parents. However, the reality of child care may prove difficult for them.

First-time mothers older than 35 years select the "right time" for pregnancy; this time is influenced by their awareness of the increasing possibility of infertility or of genetic defects in the infants of older women. Such women seek information about pregnancy from books, friends, and electronic resources. They actively try to prevent fetal disorders and are careful in searching for the best possible maternity care. They identify sources of stress in their lives. They have concerns about having enough energy and stamina to meet the demands of parenting and their new roles and relationships.

If older women become pregnant after treatment for infertility, they may suddenly have negative or ambivalent feelings about the pregnancy. They may experience a multifetal pregnancy that may create emotional and physical problems. Adjusting to parenting two or more infants requires adaptability and additional resources.

During pregnancy, parents explore the possibilities and responsibilities of changing identities and new roles. They must prepare a safe and nurturing environment during pregnancy and after birth. They must integrate the child into an established family system and negotiate new roles (parent, sibling, and grandparent roles) for family members.

Adverse perinatal outcomes are more common in older primiparas than in younger women, even when they receive good prenatal care. Women 35 years of age and older are more likely than younger primiparas to have infants with chromosomal abnormalities, LBW infants, preterm birth, placental abruption, and multiple gestation (Johnson & Tough, 2012). The incidence of malpresentation also is more common in older primiparas, and they are more likely to have a Caesarean birth. In addition, in women ages 35 years or older, there is an increased risk for maternal mortality from hemorrhage, infection, embolisms, hypertensive disorders of pregnancy, cardiomyopathy, and strokes. The occurrence of these complications is quite stressful for the new parents, thus nursing interventions that provide information and psychosocial support in addition to care for physical needs are important.

Multifetal Pregnancy

A *multifetal pregnancy*, or pregnancy with more than one fetus, increases the risk for adverse outcomes for both the mother and fetuses. The maternal blood volume is increased, resulting in an increased strain on the maternal cardiovascular system. Anemia often develops because of a greater demand for iron by the fetuses. Marked uterine distension, increased pressure on the adjacent viscera and pelvic vasculature, and diastasis of the two rectus abdominis muscles may occur. Placenta previa develops more commonly in multifetal pregnancies because of the large size or placement of the placentas. Premature separation of the placenta may occur before the second and any subsequent fetuses are born.

Twin pregnancies often end prematurely. Spontaneous rupture of membranes before term is common. Congenital malformations are twice as common in monozygotic twins as in singletons, although there is no increase in the incidence of congenital anomalies in dizygotic twins. Two-vessel cords (i.e., cords with a single umbilical artery) occur more often in twins than in singletons; this abnormality is most common in monozygotic twins. The most serious problem for the fetus is the local shunting of blood between placentas (twin-to-twin transfusion); this causes the recipient twin to be larger and the donor twin to be small, pallid, dehydrated, malnourished, and hypovolemic. However, the larger twin may develop congenital heart failure during the first 24 hours after birth.

The likelihood of a multifetal pregnancy is increased if, during a careful assessment, any one or a combination of the following factors is noted:

- History of dizygotic twins in the female lineage
- Use of fertility drugs
- More rapid uterine growth for the number of weeks of gestation
- Polyhydramnios
- Palpation of more than the expected number of small or large parts
- Asynchronous fetal heartbeats or more than one fetal electrocardiographic tracing
- Ultrasonographic evidence of more than one fetus

The diagnosis of multifetal pregnancy can come as a shock to many expectant parents, and they may need additional support and education to help them cope with the changes they face. The mother needs nutritional counselling so that she gains more weight than that needed for a singleton birth. She should be counselled that maternal adaptations will probably be more uncomfortable and be provided with information about the possibility of a preterm birth.

If the presence of more than three fetuses is diagnosed, the parents may receive counselling regarding selective reduction of the fetuses to reduce the incidence of premature birth and improve the opportunities for the remaining fetuses to grow to term gestation (Cunningham et al., 2014). This situation poses an ethical dilemma for many couples, especially those who have worked hard to overcome problems with infertility and those who harbour strong values regarding the right to life. Nurses can initiate discussions with couples to help them identify resources (e.g., a minister, priest, rabbi, or mental health counsellor) to aid in the decision-making process.

Prenatal care given to women with multifetal pregnancies includes changes in the pattern of care and modifications in other aspects such as the amount of weight gained and the nutritional intake necessary. The prenatal visits of these mothers are scheduled at least every 2 weeks in the second trimester and weekly thereafter. The recommended weight gain in twin gestations is 17 to 25 kg (37.4 to 55 lb) (Alberta Health Services, 2013). Iron and vitamin supplements are desirable. Since pre-eclampsia and eclampsia occur more commonly during multifetal pregnancies, the health care team needs to work aggressively to prevent, identify, and treat these complications of pregnancy.

The considerable uterine distension involved in a multifetal pregnancy can cause the backache commonly experienced by pregnant women to be even worse. Maternity support hose may be worn to control leg varicosities. Every multifetal pregnancy is at risk for preterm labour; thus these women need to receive education regarding the signs of preterm labour and more frequent monitoring (nonstress tests and ultrasonography). Limiting activity may be recommended beginning at 20 weeks for women carrying multiple fetuses to prevent preterm labour. Prolonged bedrest is not recommended as it does not prevent preterm labour and causes other complications. If birth is delayed until after the thirty-sixth week, the risk of morbidity and mortality decreases for the neonates.

Multiple newborns will likely place a strain on finances, space, workload, and the mother's and family's coping abilities. Lifestyle changes may be necessary. Parents will need assistance in making realistic plans for the care of the babies (e.g., how to breastfeed and whether to raise them as "alike" or as separate individuals). Parents can be referred to national organizations such as Multiple Births Canada and the La Leche League for further support (see Additional Resources at end of the chapter).

PERINATAL CARE CHOICES

Women have the option to choose from a variety of health care providers; this may include physicians, nurses, midwives, doulas, childbirth educators, and various others who may help with physical or social needs. Those caring for women during pregnancy, birth, and the early parenting period must work together to provide appropriate care for women and their families. Often the first decision the woman makes is who will be her primary health care provider for the pregnancy and birth. This decision is doubly important because it usually affects where the birth will take place. In Canada, the options for primary care during pregnancy is a physician or, in most provinces, a registered midwife. The nurse can provide information about the different types of health care providers and what kind of care to expect from each type. Women need to be provided information about choices and encouraged to ask potential care providers the following questions to ensure that they feel comfortable with the choices they make:

- Who can be with me during labour and birth?
- What happens during a normal labour and birth in your setting?
- How do you allow for differences in culture and beliefs?
- Can I walk and move around during labour? What position do you suggest for birth?
- What things do you normally do to a woman in labour?
- How do you help mothers stay as comfortable as they can be? Besides medications, how do you help relieve the pain of labour?
- What if my baby is born early or has special problems?
- What support do you have for breastfeeding mothers?

Physician Care

While specific statistics on the number of births attended by physicians are not presently collected, the Canadian Maternity Experience survey estimated that physicians (obstetricians and family practice physicians) attended approximately 94% of births in Canada in 2006 (PHAC, 2009). Physicians see both low-risk and high-risk patients. Family practice physicians may need backup from obstetricians if a specialist is needed for a problem, such as Caesarean birth. Almost all physicians manage births in a hospital setting. A woman may see one doctor for her entire pregnancy and birth or, more commonly, she may be cared for in a group practice setting, seeing multiple physicians and having the physician who is on call present at the birth.

Midwives

Registered midwives in Canada are educated through a university program as a profession distinct from nursing. Throughout history, midwives have held a holistic view of childbirth. Midwives care for low-risk obstetrical patients. Care is often noninterventionist, and the woman and her family are encouraged to be active participants in the care. Women are often cared for by one or two midwives who provide care throughout the pregnancy, birth, and postpartum period. Many women appreciate the continuity of care that this model of care provides. Midwives refer patients with complications to physicians. Births may be managed in a hospital setting, in a birth centre, or at home.

Women who are seeing a midwife may have some of their visits with the midwife at their home. The midwife will typically have one prenatal visit and several postpartum visits at the patient's home. This reduces stress on the new mother, who may find it difficult in the first few weeks after birth to get out with the baby.

In Canada, midwives are regulated by the Canadian Association of Midwives, although currently, not all provinces and territories have legislation regarding the practice of midwives. While approximately 6% of all births in Canada are attended by a midwife, this number is increasing with the greater number of available midwives (PHAC, 2009). See Chapter 4 (p. 56) for further discussion on midwifery in Canada.

Doula

A **doula** is professionally trained to provide labour support, including physical, emotional, and informational support, to the mother and her partner before, during, and just after birth, or provides emotional and practical support during the postpartum period alongside other health care providers. The doula does not become involved with clinical tasks. Birth doulas provide support during labour, and postpartum doulas provide assistance after the birth; both are part of the health care team. Doulas usually work on a fee-for-service basis, and many will offer a sliding scale for families who cannot afford to pay for their services.

Currently, many couples employ a doula for labour support. A Cochrane review found that women who had continuous labour support like that provided by doulas were more likely to have a spontaneous vaginal birth and less likely to have intrapartum analgesia or to report dissatisfaction with birth. In addition, their labours were shorter, they were less likely to have a Caesarean or instrumental vaginal birth, or a baby with a low 5-minute Apgar score. There was no apparent impact on other intrapartum interventions, maternal or neonatal complications, or breastfeeding (Hodnett, Gates, Hofmeyr, et al., 2013).

Continuous support seemed to be most effective when the provider was neither part of the hospital staff nor the woman's social network and in settings in which epidural analgesia was not routinely available.

A doula typically meets with the mother and her partner before labour to ascertain their expectations and desires for the birth experience. With this information as a guide during labour and birth, the doula works collaboratively with other health care providers and the woman's support people and focuses on assisting the woman and couple to achieve their goals. Doulas who are also trained medical interpreters can enhance the care of women with limited English proficiency (Maher, Crawford-Carr, & Neidigh, 2012).

Doulas may be found through community contacts, other health care providers, or childbirth educators; a number of organizations offer information or referral services. It is important that the expectant mother be comfortable with the doula who will be attending her. See Box 11-5 for a list of questions to ask when arranging for a doula. Doulas of North America (DONA) is one organization that certifies doulas (see Additional Resources at end of the chapter). Although the doula role originally developed as an assistant during labour, some women and their families benefit from assistance during the postpartum period. Postpartum doulas may assist with breastfeeding, teaching, and care of the mother or siblings. The postpartum doula's role is flexible, meeting the needs of the family to ensure that the mother is able to care for herself and the new baby.

Birth Setting Choices

With careful thought, the concept of family, or woman-centred maternity care can be implemented in any setting. Currently, the three primary options for birth settings are the hospital, birth centre, and home, depending on the province in which a woman lives. Women consider several factors in choosing a setting for childbirth, including where the care provider has privileges and the characteristics of the birthing unit. Approximately 98% of all births in Canada take place in a hospital setting (PHAC, 2009); the other 2% occur in homes or birthing centres. However, the types of labour and birth services vary greatly, from the traditional labour and delivery rooms with separate postpartum and newborn units to in-hospital birthing centres where all or almost all care takes place in a single unit.

BOX 11-5 QUESTIONS TO ASK WHEN CHOOSING A DOULA

To discover the specific training, experience, and services offered by anyone who provides labour support, potential patients should ask the following questions of that person:

- What training have you had?
- Tell me about your experience with birth, personally and as a doula.
- What is your philosophy about childbirth and supporting women and their partners through labour?
- May we meet to discuss our birth plans and the role you will play in supporting me and my partner through childbirth?
- May we call you with questions or concerns before and after the birth?
- When do you try to join women in labour? Do you come to our home or meet us at the hospital?
- Do you meet with us after the birth to review the labour and answer questions?
- Do you work with one or more backup doulas for times when you are not available? May we meet them?
- What is your fee?

From DONA International. (2012). *DONA International position paper: The birth doula's contribution to modern maternity care.* Retrieved from http://www.dona.org/PDF/Birth%20Position%20Paper_rev%200912.pdf

Labour, Birth, Recovery, Postpartum Rooms

Labour, birth, and recovery (LBR) and labour, birth, recovery, and postpartum (LBRP) rooms offer families a comfortable, private space for childbirth (Fig. 11-20). Women admitted to LBR units go through labour and give birth there and spend the first 1 to 2 hours postpartum there for immediate recovery, to have time with their families to bond with their newborns. After this period of recovery, the mothers and newborns are usually transferred to a mother–baby unit for the duration of their stay. In most hospitals in Canada, the same nurse provides care for both mothers and newborns (mother–baby or couplet care).

In LBRP units, total care is provided, from admission for labour through postpartum discharge, in the same room and usually by the same nursing staff. The woman and her family may stay in this unit for 6 to 48 hours after giving birth. The units are furnished in a homelike atmosphere, similar to LBR units, but have accommodations for family members to stay overnight.

Both LBR and LBRP units are equipped with fetal monitors, emergency resuscitation equipment for mother and newborn, and heated cribs or warming units for the newborn. Often this equipment is out of sight in cabinets or closets when it is not being used.

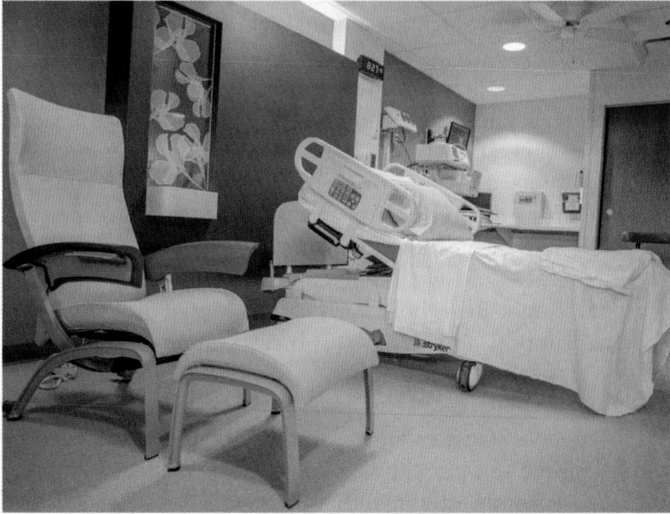

FIGURE 11-20 Labour, birth, recovery, and postpartum unit. (Courtesy Mercy Hospital.)

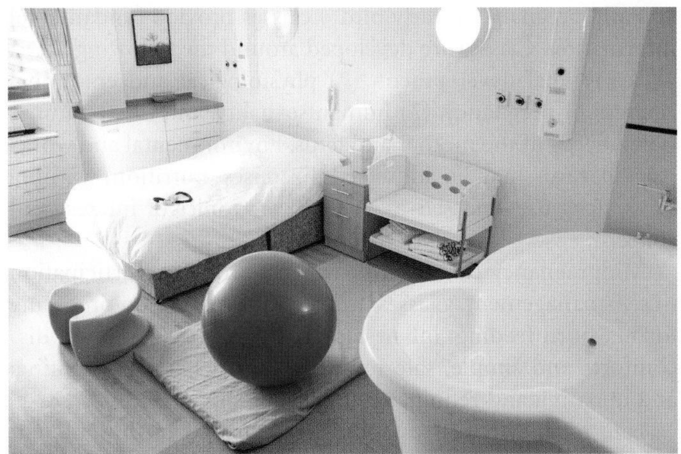

FIGURE 11-21 Birth centre. Note double bed, baby crib, and birthing stool. (Ian Hooton/Science Source.)

Birth Centres

Free-standing birth centres are usually built in locations separate from the hospital but may be located nearby, in case transfer of the woman or newborn is needed. These birth centres are intended to offer families a safe alternative to hospital or home birth. The centres are usually staffed by nurses, midwives, or physicians who also have privileges at the local hospital. Only women considered low risk are admitted for care.

Birth centres typically have homelike accommodations, including a double bed for the couple and a crib for the newborn (Fig. 11-21). Emergency equipment and medications are available but stored out of view. Private bathroom facilities are incorporated into each birth unit. There may be an early labour lounge or a living room and small kitchen. The family is admitted to the birth centre for labour and birth and will remain there until discharge, which often takes place within 6 hours of the birth.

When births occur in a birth centre or a home setting, there needs to be a plan for transfer to hospital if this becomes necessary. Ambulance service and emergency procedures must be readily available.

Home Birth

In developing countries, hospitals or adequate facilities often are unavailable to most pregnant women, and home birth is a necessity, whereas in Canada, planned home births account for approximately 1% of births and are usually attended by midwives (PHAC, 2009). Research supports the safety of planned home birth for healthy, low-risk women who are attended by registered midwives and when there is a system in place for transfer to a hospital facility (de Jonge, van der Goes, Ravelli, et al., 2009; Hutton, Reitsma, & Kaufman, 2009; Janssen, Saxell, Page, et al., 2009; McIntyre, 2012).

With a home birth, the family is in control of the experience, and the birth may be more physiologically natural in familiar surroundings (see Community Focus box). The mother may be more relaxed than she would be in the hospital environment. The family can assist in and be a part of the birth, and the mother–father or partner–infant (and sibling–infant) contact is immediate and sustained. Serious infection may be less likely (assuming aseptic principles are followed) because it is common for people to be relatively immune to the bacteria in their own home.

COMMUNITY FOCUS

Deciding About a Home Birth

Maxine, 37 years old and G1T0P0A0L0, is interested in having a home birth. She is currently 14 weeks pregnant, and her pregnancy is progressing normally. According to an ultrasound examination she has one fetus of appropriate size for gestational age with no detectable anomalies. She would like to pursue midwifery care with plans for a home birth. Explore the options for home birth in your province that are available for Maxine. What are the guidelines for midwifery care in your area? What patients are eligible for midwifery care? How many women have home births in your area and how many have hospital births? Are midwife-led birth centres available? What provisions are needed for a home birth?

CHILDBIRTH AND PERINATAL EDUCATION

The goal of childbirth and perinatal education is to assist individuals and their family members to make informed, safe decisions about pregnancy, birth, and early parenthood. It is also to assist them in comprehending the long-lasting effects that empowering birth experiences have on women and the impact of early experiences on the development of children and the family. Perinatal education ideally begins in the preconception period, when women are considering pregnancy, and continues throughout the prenatal period as nurses and other health care providers provide ongoing education for pregnant women and their partners during regular prenatal visits.

Contemporary perinatal education programs may consist of a menu of class series and activities, from preconception through pregnancy, childbirth, and the early months of parenting.

Optimally, these classes help women trust their bodies and offer them a way to take full advantage of the opportunities presented by a prepared-for and well-supported childbirth experience. Creating an environment of safety where women and their partners can ask questions as well as the opportunity to look at fears and concerns is important to learning during pregnancy and preparing for parenthood.

For the new family, prior experience related to the pregnancy and the birth of others or in the care of younger siblings or relatives is increasingly uncommon, given the small size of many North American families. Many individuals facing parenthood have little information about what to expect and do not have the important skills necessary to cope with pregnancy, childbirth, or parenthood. Perinatal education classes can partially fill this void.

All health-promoting education should be provided in a context that emphasizes the ability of a healthy body to adapt to the changes that accompany pregnancy. Without this context of health, routine care and testing for risks may foster a mindset in families that pregnancy is a pathological condition and not a healthy mind–body–spirit event.

Previous pregnancy and childbirth experiences are important elements that influence current learning needs. The woman's (and support person's) age, cultural background, personal philosophy in regard to childbirth, socioeconomic status, spiritual beliefs, and learning styles all need to be assessed when developing the best plan to help the woman meet her needs.

Most childbirth education classes are attended by the pregnant woman and her partner, although a friend, teenage daughter, sister, or parent may be the designated support person. Classes may also be held for grandparents and siblings to prepare them for their attendance at birth or the arrival of the baby. Siblings often see a film about birth and learn ways they can help welcome the baby. They also learn to cope with changes, including a reduction in parental time and attention. Grandparents learn about current child-care practices and how to help their adult children in a supportive way to adapt to parenting.

Childbirth Education

When women are prepared for childbirth and are well supported, childbirth can present a unique and powerful opportunity for women to find their core strength in a manner that forever changes their self-perception. In providing the requisite childbirth education, it is important to remember that expectant parents and their families have different interests and information needs as the pregnancy progresses.

Childbirth education classes provide important information for child-bearing families. The prenatal curriculum may include many topics (Box 11-6).

Although traditional face-to-face classes are often the preferred mode of learning, many couples are unable to commit to attending regular classes because of conflicting work schedules and long commutes. Other couples prefer to obtain their prenatal information online. To meet the needs of today's child-bearing families, many health departments have begun to offer eLearning prenatal classes. This is an excellent way of reaching pregnant women and their partners who would not have attended face-to-face prenatal classes.

Prenatal classes may be offered by other providers within the community. Hospitals often offer classes for the patients giving birth at their facility. There is usually a cost associated with these and other private classes. Many health departments offer free or fee-reduced classes.

BOX 11-6 CHILDBIRTH EDUCATION TOPICS

Physical and emotional changes during pregnancy
Breastfeeding
Nutrition during pregnancy
Working during pregnancy
Pain management strategies during labour—pharmacological and nonpharmacological
Labour and birth process
Becoming a parent
Transition to parenting
Newborn care

Early pregnancy ("early bird") classes provide fundamental information. Classes are developed around the following areas: (1) early fetal development, (2) physiological and emotional changes of pregnancy, (3) human sexuality, and (4) the nutritional needs of the mother and fetus. Environmental and workplace hazards may be addressed. Exercises, nutrition, warning signs, drug use, and self-medication are topics of interest and concern.

Midpregnancy classes emphasize the woman's participation in self-management. Classes provide information on preparing for newborn feeding; infant care; basic hygiene; common discomforts and simple, safe remedies; infant health; parenting; and updating and refining of the birth plans.

Late pregnancy classes address labour and birth. Different methods of coping with labour and birth have been developed and are often the basis for various prenatal classes. A hospital tour may be included.

Throughout the series of classes, it is important to identify support systems that people can use during pregnancy and after birth. Such support systems help parents function independently and effectively. During all the classes, members should be encouraged to openly express their feelings and concerns about any aspect of pregnancy, birth, and parenting.

Fathers or partners often worry about their role in childbirth classes and during labour and birth, as well as about the safety of their partner and baby during the birth. Many partners elect to participate actively during labour and the birth of their child. However, as noted earlier, some men, because of personal or cultural views of the father role, neither want nor intend to participate. It is important that the partners agree on each other's roles.

Current Practices in Childbirth Education

A variety of approaches to childbirth education have evolved as childbirth educators attempt to meet learning needs. In addition to classes designed specifically for pregnant adolescents, their partners, or parents, classes exist for other groups with special learning needs. These include classes for first-time mothers over age 35, single women, adoptive parents, and parents of twins.

Refresher classes for parents with children not only review coping techniques for labour and birth and address any concerns from their previous birth but also help couples prepare for sibling reactions and adjustments to a new baby. Caesarean birth classes are offered for couples who have this kind of birth scheduled because of breech position or other risk factors. Other classes focus on vaginal birth after Caesarean (VBAC), as many women successfully give birth vaginally after previous Caesarean birth.

Because of the multicultural composition of the population in Canada, there is great diversity in attitudes, expectations, and behaviours judged appropriate during pregnancy and early parenthood. No one approach can meet all needs. For example, classes for new immigrants are particularly effective when taught in their first language. For classes to be meaningful, parent educators must understand the value systems in other cultures and their influence on issues such as nutrition, exercise, valuing of early prenatal care, maternal weight gain, and infant feeding practices. Prenatal educators must establish rapport, be understood, and build on cultural practices, reinforcing the positive and promoting change only if a practice is directly harmful.

Methods of Childbirth Education

There are many different methods of childbirth education, and most educators use a combination of many techniques. The Dick-Read method focuses on the idea that pain in childbirth is socially conditioned and caused by a fear–tension–pain syndrome (see Fig. 18-3). Another option is HypnoBirthing, where pregnant women (couples) learn how the birthing muscles work when the woman is in a state of relaxation. The aim is for the woman to be relaxed and in control. The Bradley Method (see Additional Resources at end of the chapter) uses partner-coached childbirth, breath control, abdominal breathing, and general body relaxation. Working in harmony with the body is emphasized. Bradley's technique emphasizes environmental variables such as darkness, solitude, and quiet to make childbirth a more natural experience. Birthing From Within mentors (teachers) believe that childbirth is not a medical event but a profound rite of passage. Parents are taught the power of birthing-in-awareness. Mentors create a safe, nurturing class experience and help parents find their personal strength and wisdom. Birth is taught from four perspectives: mother, partner, baby, and culture. Parents are assisted in developing a pain-coping mindset. Birthing From Within advocates that parents deserve support for whatever birth option they choose.

The Childbirth and Postpartum Professional Association (CAPPA) is a nonprofit international organization that provides professional membership and training to antepartum doulas, childbirth educators, labour doulas, postpartum doulas, and lactation educators. They are proponents of evidence-informed practice in childbirth education.

Lamaze International also certifies childbirth educators. The core values, which have become an ideal for many childbirth education organizations, include that care for normal pregnancy and birth should be removed from total control of doctors, be based on the use of appropriate technology (as opposed to overuse), and be evidence informed, regionalized, multidisciplinary, holistic, family centred, and culturally appropriate. Women should be involved in decision making, and their privacy, dignity, and confidentiality should be respected. They should feel empowered to make the choices that seem right for them. Lamaze has as its foundation six care principles modified from the World Health Organization (WHO) recommendations (Box 11-7). These healthy birth practices are based on current research (see Additional Resources at end of the chapter).

Components of Perinatal Education Programs

A variety of approaches to perinatal education that go beyond preparation for birth have evolved as educators attempt to meet the learning and support needs of expectant parents and to capitalize on their openness to learning. For example, prenatal and new-mother weekly exercise classes can offer both physiological and social support for a mixture of expectant and new mothers who may also elect to stay connected by email for support between weekly classes. However, it is important that a focus on preparation for birth not become lost in all the topics that could be offered to expectant parents.

BOX 11-7 LAMAZE HEALTHY BIRTH PRACTICES

- Let labour begin on its own.
- Walk, move around, and change positions throughout labour.
- Bring a loved one, friend, or doula for continuous support.
- Avoid interventions that are not medically necessary.
- Avoid giving birth on your back, and follow your body's surges to push.
- Keep your baby with you—it's best for you, your baby, and breastfeeding.

Source: Lamaze International. (2016). Lamaze healthy birth practices. Retrieved from http://www.lamazeinternational.org/HealthyBirthPractices.

Birth plans. The birth plan is a tool with which parents can explore their childbirth options and use their plan or guide as a communication tool with their care provider to discuss their choices and preferences. The plan must be viewed as flexible and based on information that the care provider and couple have prior to labour, knowing that circumstances can change. The options of women with a high-risk pregnancy or those in whom complications develop during labour may be more limited but no less important.

It is useful for the nurse in a prenatal practice setting to initiate a discussion of choices and birth planning during the first and second prenatal visits. An early introduction to the idea of a birth plan allows the couple time to think about events or situations that could make their child-bearing experience more meaningful and those they would prefer to avoid. The nurse can think of a birth plan as a "living will" or an opportunity to express the woman's or couple's wishes about normal life events such as birthing (White-Corey, 2013). It also gives them the opportunity to express their individual needs and preferences, such as an interpreter, wishing to remain mobile as long as possible, and infant nutrition, to their health care providers.

Some maternity practices provide printed material describing available options and giving answers to commonly asked questions. The nurse can provide couples with pertinent information and make them aware of the various options for care and the advantages and consequences of each so they can begin making informed decisions. Early plans can be modified as the couple learns more details in their childbirth class.

Some health care providers provide birth plan templates, and there are numerous interactive programs on the Internet that will assist couples in creating their birth plans. Childbirth educators may provide a list of helpful websites during classes as well as topics to consider. It is important that the childbirth educator thoroughly review all resources given to potential new parents to ensure the information is appropriate and evidence-informed. Nurses have often thought of birth plans as a "curse" or "jinx" for those who complete them and bring them in. One study showed that if women have an opportunity to communicate their wishes using their plan and have choices based on their expressed wishes, they are more satisfied with their experience (than those not having this opportunity) and have no increased rate of obstetrical complications, such as Caesarean birth (White-Corey, 2013). Topics for birth plan discussion and decision making are given in Box 11-8.

Pain management. Fear of pain in labour is a key issue for pregnant women and the reason given by many for attending childbirth education classes. Numerous studies show that women who have received childbirth preparation later report no less pain but do report a greater ability to cope with the pain during labour and birth and increased birth satisfaction compared to unprepared women. Thus, although pain management strategies are an essential component of childbirth education, pain eradication is not the primary source of birth satisfaction. Control in childbirth (i.e., participation in decision making) has repeatedly been found to be the primary source of birth satisfaction. The advantages and disadvantages of all pain management strategies for coping with labour are discussed in Chapter 18 and may include relaxation, imagery and visualization, conscious breathing, biofeedback, and massage.

Preparation for Caesarean birth. Given that approximately 25 to 30% of births in Canada are by Caesarean surgery (Born, Konkin, Tepper, et al., 2014; PHAC, 2013b), this is an important topic for birth preparation education. The expectant parents can be helped to know what they can do to avoid the necessity of a Caesarean birth. Caesarean birth rates vary widely by care provider and care setting. In a setting where nursing support during labour is low and the care provider rate of Caesarean birth is high, women should be aware that their chances of a Caesarean birth are increased.

Effort can be directed at preventing the need for a subsequent Caesarean birth or preparing for it when it is inevitable or highly likely. Women who have planned Caesarean births also need to feel that they have some control over their birth experience, and it is important that this is discussed with them. Women with a prior Caesarean birth can be encouraged to explore the possibility of a vaginal birth, although this is not the case for those who have a history of classic vertical or unknown uterine incisions or those with medical contraindication. In many communities there are VBAC support groups, physicians who are known to be supportive, and special childbirth classes for those attempting a VBAC. Mothers should be prepared for the differences in postpartum recovery after a Caesarean birth. Their hospital stay will be longer, their need for assistance at home will be greater, and they may need extra support to establish breastfeeding comfortably, compared to women who have a vaginal birth.

BOX 11-8 QUESTIONS TO CONSIDER WHEN DEVELOPING A BIRTH PLAN

Partner's participation—Attend prenatal visits? Childbirth and parent education classes? Present during labour? During birth? During Caesarean birth? Cutting the umbilical cord? Skin-to-skin contact after birth if mother not able to at birth?

Birth setting—Hospital birthing room? A birthing centre? Home?

Labour management—Any culturally specific requests, such as warm water only or a female health care provider if possible? Walk around during labour? Use a rocking chair? Use a shower? Birthing ball? Use a tub if available? Intermittent or continuous use of an electronic fetal monitor? Have music or dimmed lighting? Have older children or other people present? Is telemetry monitoring available? Consider stimulation of labour? Pain management strategies?

Birth—Positions—Side-lying? On hands and knees, kneeling, or squatting? Photographing, videotaping, or recording any of the labour or birth? Who is present at birth—partner, older siblings, other family members, friends, or doula? What about the use of forceps? Episiotomies? What about delayed cord clamping?

Immediately after birth—Place the baby skin-to-skin right away? Breastfeed immediately? If wishing to do skin-to-skin or breastfeed immediately, have family members come a bit later? What is the plan for visiting? Anyone bringing in specific food for recovery?

Postpartum care—What kind of care is anticipated—labour, birth, recovery, postpartum room; mother–baby coupling? Plan to attend classes, or preference for getting such information through one-on-one discussion, DVDs, handouts, or online? On which subjects?

KEY POINTS

- The prenatal period is a preparatory one—physically, emotionally, and psychologically.
- Psychosocial aspects of care may affect pregnancy, childbirth, and the adjustment of the new family.
- The pregnant woman's readiness to learn is at a high level, making this an excellent time to help her expand her self-management skills.
- Maternal physical and familial adaptations to pregnancy generate needs that the nurse can anticipate and meet.
- Parent–child, sibling–child, and grandparent–child relationships are affected by pregnancy.
- Even with a normal pregnancy, the nurse must remain alert to hazards such as supine hypotension, warning signs and symptoms, and signs of a family having difficulty coping with the pregnancy.
- Women need to have appropriate care and screening provided throughout the pregnancy to ensure a healthy outcome.
- Each pregnant woman needs to know how to recognize and report preterm labour.
- Cultural prescriptions and proscriptions influence responses to pregnancy and to the health care delivery system.

- Childbirth education helps women to feel confident that their bodies are able to give birth and provides coping strategies that enhance their ability to give birth.
- Childbirth education is a process designed to help parents make the transition from the role of expectant parents to the role and responsibilities of parents of a new baby.

evolve WEBSITE

Visit the Evolve website for additional resources related to the content in this chapter such as Case Studies, Critical Thinking Case Study Answers, Nursing Care Plans, Nursing Processes, Nursing Skills, and Review Questions for Exam Preparation at: http://evolve.elsevier.com/Canada/Perry/maternal/

REFERENCES

Agency for Healthcare Research and Quality (AHRQ) Healthcare Innovations Exchange. (2012). *Nurse home visits improve outcomes for low-income, first-time mothers and their children*. Retrieved from <https://innovations.ahrq.gov/profiles/nurse-home-visits-improve-birth-outcomes-other-health-and-social-indicators-low-income>.

Alberta Health Services. (2013). *Nutrition guideline pregnancy*. Retrieved from <http://www.albertahealthservices.ca/assets/Infofor/hp/if-hp-ed-cdm-ns-4-1-1-pregnancy.pdf>.

American Academy of Pediatrics (AAP) Committee on Fetus and Newborn and American College of Obstetricians and Gynecologists (ACOG) Committee on Obstetric Practice. (2012). *Guidelines for perinatal care* (7th ed.). Washington, DC: Author.

Berger, S., & Nuzzo, K. (2008). Older siblings influence younger siblings' motor development. *Infant and Child Development, 17*, 607–615.

Born, K., Konkin, J., Tepper, J., & Okun, N. (2014). *Pulling back the curtain on Canada's rising C-section rate*. Retrieved from <http://healthydebate.ca/2014/05/topic/quality/c-section-variation>.

Cunningham, F., Leveno, K., Bloom, S., et al. (2014). *Williams obstetrics* (24th ed.). New York: McGraw Hill.

Darvill, R., Skirton, H., & Farrand, P. (2010). Psychological factors that impact on women's experiences of first-time motherhood: A qualitative study of the transition. *Midwifery, 26*, 357–366.

Davies, G., Maxwell, C., McLeod, L., et al. (2010). SOGC clinical practice guideline: Obesity in pregnancy. *Journal of Obstetrics and Gynaecology Canada, 32*(2), 165–173.

de Jonge, A., van der Goes, B. Y., Ravelli, A. C., et al. (2009). Perinatal mortality and morbidity in a nationwide cohort of 529,688 low-risk planned home and hospital births. *BJOG: An International Journal of Obstetrics and Gynaecology, 116*(9), 1177–1184.

Denis, A., Michaux, P., & Callahan, S. (2012). Factors implicated in moderating the risk for depression and anxiety in high risk pregnancy. *Journal of Reproductive and Infant Psychology, 30*(2), 124–134.

Dovydaitis, T. (2010). Human trafficking: The role of the health care provider. *Journal of Midwifery & Women's Health, 55*(5), 462–467.

Duff, P. (2012). Maternal and perinatal infection—bacterial. In S. G. Gabbe, J. R. Niebyl, J. L. Simpson, et al. (Eds.), *Obstetrics: Normal and problem pregnancies* (6th ed.). Philadelphia: Saunders.

Fowler, C., Reid, S., Minnis, J., & Day, C. (2014). Experiences of mothers with substance dependence: Informing the development of parenting support. *Journal of Clinical Nursing, 23*, 2835–2843.

Gregory, K. D., Niebyl, J. R., & Johnson, T. R. (2012). Preconception and prenatal care: Part of the continuum. In S. G. Gabbe, J. R. Niebyl, J. L. Simpson, et al. (Eds.), *Obstetrics: Normal and problem pregnancies* (6th ed.). Philadelphia: Saunders.

Habib, C. (2012). The transition to fatherhood: A literature review exploring paternal involvement with identity theory. *Journal of Family Studies, 18*(2/3), 103–120.

Hall, H., McKenna, L., & Griffiths, D. (2010). Complementary and alternative medicine: Where's the evidence? *British Journal of Midwifery, 18*(7), 350–358.

Health Canada. (2007). *Cosmic radiation exposure and air travel*. Ottawa: Environmental and Workplace Health, Health Canada. Retrieved from <http://www.hc-sc.gc.ca/ewh-semt/radiation/comsic-cosmique-eng.php>.

Herrman, J. W., Rogers, S., & Ehrenthal, D. B. (2012). Women's perceptions of CenteringPregnancy: A focus group study. *MCN. the American Journal of Maternal Child Nursing, 37*(1), 19–26.

Hodnett, E. D., Gates, S., Hofmeyr, G. J., & Sakala, C. (2013). Continuous support for women during childbirth. *Cochrane Database of Systematic Reviews*, (7). doi:10.1002/14651858.CD003766.pub5.

Hui Choi, W., Lee, G., Chan, C., et al. (2012). The relationships of social support, uncertainty, self-efficacy, and commitment to prenatal psychosocial adaptation. *Journal of Advanced Nursing, 68*(12), 2633–2642.

Hutton, E. K., Reitsma, A. H., & Kaufman, K. (2009). Outcomes associated with planned home and planned hospital births in low-risk women attended by midwives in Ontario, Canada, 2003–2006—a retrospective cohort study. *Birth, 36*(3), 180–189.

Janssen, P. A., Saxell, L., Page, L., et al. (2009). Outcomes of planned home birth with registered midwife versus planned hospital birth with midwife or physician. *Canadian Medical Association Journal, 181*(6–7), 377–383.

Johnson, A., & Tough, S. (2012). SOGC committee opinion: Delayed childbearing. *Journal of Obstetrics and Gynaecology Canada, 34*(1), 80–93.

Kumar, J., & Samelson, R. (2009). Oral health care during pregnancy: Recommendations for oral health professionals. *New York State Dental Journal, 75*(6), 29–33.

Lawrence, R. A., & Lawrence, R. M. (2011). *Breastfeeding: A guide for the medical profession* (7th ed.). St. Louis: Mosby.

Lederman, R., & Weis, K. (2009). *Psychosocial adaptation to pregnancy*. New York: Springer Science Business Media.

Liston, R., Sawchuck, D., Young, D., et al. (2007). SOGC clinical practice guideline: Fetal health surveillance: Antepartum and intrapartum consensus guideline. *Journal of Obstetrics and Gynaecology Canada, 29*(9), Suppl 4.

Lumbiganon, P., Martis, R., Laopaiboon, M., et al. (2012). Antenatal breastfeeding education for increasing breastfeeding duration. *Cochrane Database of Systematic Reviews*, (9). doi:10.1002/14651858.CD006425.pub3.

Magdaleno, R., Pereira, B. G., Chaim, E. A., et al. (2012). Pregnancy after bariatric surgery: A current view of maternal, obstetrical, and perinatal challenges. *Archives of Gynecology and Obstetrics, 285*(3), 559–566.

Maher, S., Crawford-Carr, A., & Neidigh, K. (2012). The role of the interpreter/doula in the maternity setting. *Nursing for Women's Health, 16*(6), 472–481.

May, K. A. (1982). Three phases of father involvement in pregnancy. *Nursing Research, 31*(6), 337–342.

McIntyre, M. (2012). Safety of non-medically led primary maternity care models: A critical review of the international literature. *Australian Health Review, 36*(2), 140–147.

McKay, A., & Sex Information and Education Council of Canada. (2012). Trends in Canadian national and provincial/territorial teen pregnancy rates: 2001–2010. *Canadian Journal of Human Sexuality, 21*(3–4), 161–175.

Mercer, R. (1995). *Becoming a mother*. New York: Springer.

Money, D., Allen, M. D., Halifax, N. S., et al. (2013). SOGC clinical practice guideline: The prevention of early-onset neonatal group B streptococcal disease. *Journal of Obstetrics and Gynaecology Canada, 35*(10), e1–e10.

Money, D., Steben, M., & Infectious Disease Committee. (2008). SOGC clinical practice guideline: Guidelines for the management of herpes simplex virus in pregnancy. *Journal of Obstetrics and Gynaecology of Canada, 30*(6), 514–519.

Mottolo, M. (2011). Exercise and pregnancy: Canadian guidelines for health care professionals. *Wellspring, 22*(4). Retrieved from <http://sirc.ca/sites/default/files/content/docs/newsletters/archive/may12/documents/Free/guidelines.pdf>.

Newnham, J., Dickinson, J., Hart, R., et al. (2014). Strategies to prevent preterm birth. *Frontiers in Immunology, 5*, 584.

Picklesimer, A. H., Billings, D., Hale, N., et al. (2012). The effect of CenteringPregnancy group prenatal care on preterm birth in a low-income population. *American Journal of Obstetrics and Gynecology, 206*(5), 415.e1–415.e7.

Pires, R., Aracijo-Pedrosa, A., & Conavarro, M. (2014). Examining the lines between perceived impact of pregnancy, depressive symptoms, and quality of life during adolescent pregnancy: The buffering role of social support. *Maternal and Child Health Journal, 18*, 789–800.

Public Health Agency of Canada. (2009). *What mothers say: The Canadian maternity experiences survey (Cat. No. HP5-74/2-2009E)*. Ottawa: Government of Canada.

Public Health Agency of Canada. (2012a). *Fetal alcohol spectrum disorder (FASD): A framework for action*. Ottawa: Author. Retrieved from <http://www.phac-aspc.gc.ca/publicat/fasd-fw-etcaf-ca/index-eng.php>.

Public Health Agency of Canada. (2012b). *The health pregnancy guide: Physical activity and pregnancy*. Ottawa: Author. Retrieved from <http://www.phac-aspc.gc.ca/hp-gs/guide/04_pa-ap-eng.php>.

Public Health Agency of Canada. (2013a). *Canadian guidelines on sexually transmitted infections: Primary care and sexually transmitted infection*. Ottawa: Author. Retrieved from <http://www.phac-aspc.gc.ca/std-mts/sti-its/cgsti-ldcits/section-2-eng.php#a4>.

Public Health Agency of Canada. (2013b). *Canadian perinatal report—2013 edition (Cat. No. HP11-12/2008E-PDF)*. Ottawa: Government of Canada. Retrieved from <http://publications.gc.ca/collections/collection_2014/aspc-phac/HP7-1-2013-eng.pdf>.

Public Health Agency of Canada. (2014). *Health pregnancy: Caffeine and pregnancy*. Ottawa: Government of Canada. Retrieved from <http://www.phac-aspc.gc.ca/hp-gs/know-savoir/caffeine-eng.php>.

Public Health Agency of Canada. (2015). *Canadian immunization guide: Immunization in pregnancy and breastfeeding*. Retrieved from <http://www.phac-aspc.gc.ca/publicat/cig-gci/p03-04-eng.php>.

Quilliam, S. (2010). Sex during pregnancy: Yes, yes, yes! *Journal of Family Planning and Reproductive Health Care, 36*(2), 97–98.

Rey, E., Pels, A., von Dadelszen, P., et al. (2014). SOGC clinical practice guideline: Diagnosis, evaluation and management of the hypertensive disorders of pregnancy: Executive Summary. *Journal of Obstetrics and Gynaecology Canada, 36*(5), 416–438.

Riordan, J., & Wambach, K. (2010). *Breastfeeding and human lactation* (4th ed.). Boston: Jones & Bartlett.

Robertson, B., Aycock, D. M., & Darnell, L. A. (2009). Comparison of CenteringPregnancy to traditional care in Hispanic mothers. *Maternal and Child Health Journal, 13*(3), 407–414.

Rotundo, G. (2011). CenteringPregnancy: The benefits of group prenatal care. *Nursing for Women's Health, 15*(6), 508–518.

Rubin, R. (1975). Maternal tasks in pregnancy. *Maternal-Child Nursing Journal, 4*(3), 143–153.

Rubin, R. (1984). *Maternity identity and the maternal experience*. New York: Springer.

Seidel, H. M., Ball, J. W., Dains, J. E., et al. (2011). *Mosby's guide to physical examination* (7th ed.). St. Louis: Mosby.

Senikas, V., Kluka, S., Wood, R., et al. (2010). SOGC clinical practice guideline: Alcohol use and pregnancy consensus clinical guideline. *Journal of Obstetrics and Gynaecology Canada, 32*(8), Suppl 3.

Sidransky, D., Norman, L. A., McCarthy, A., et al. (Eds.), (2010). *How tobacco smoke causes disease: The biology and behavioral basis for smoking attributable disease—A report of the Surgeon General*. Rockville, MD: U.S. Department of Health and Human Services.

Signore, C., Spong, C. Y., Krotoski, D., et al. (2011). Pregnancy in women with physical disabilities. *Obstetrics and Gynecology, 117*(4), 935–947.

Sutton, M. Y. (2012). Advising travelers with specific needs. In G. W. Brunette, P. E. Kozarsky, A. J. Magill, et al. (Eds.), *CDC health information for international travel*. New York: Oxford University Press.

Tracy, E. E., & Konstantopoulos, W. M. (2012). Human trafficking: A call for heightened awareness and advocacy by obstetrician-gynecologists. *Obstetrics and Gynecology, 119*(5), 1045–1047.

Walia, M., & Saini, N. (2015). Relationship between periodontal diseases and preterm birth: Recent epidemiological and biological data. *International Journal of Applied and Basic Research, 5*(1), 2–6.

Walker, M. (2010). Breast pumps and other technologies. In J. Riordan & K. Wambach (Eds.), *Breastfeeding and human lactation*. Boston: Jones & Bartlett.

White-Corey, S. (2013). Birth plans: Tickets to the OR? *American Journal of Maternal Child Nursing, 38*(5), 268–273.

Wilson, R. D., & SOGC Genetics Committee. (2014). SOGC clinical practice guideline: Prenatal screening, diagnosis and pregnancy management of fetal neural tube defects. *Journal of Obstetrics and Gynaecology Canada, 36*(10), 927–939.

Wong, S., Ordean, A., Kahan, M., et al. (2011). SOGC clinical practice guidelines: Substance use in pregnancy. *Journal of Obstetrics and Gynaecology Canada, 33*(4), 367–384.

ADDITIONAL RESOURCES

Bradley Method of childbirth preparation: <http://www.bradleybirth.com>.

Centering Healthcare Institute: <https://www.centeringhealthcare.org/>.

Doulas of North America: <http://www.dona.org>.

Health Canada Radiation Protection Bureau: <http://www.hc-sc.gc.ca/ahc-asc/branch-dirgen/hecs-dgsesc/sep-psm/rpb-br-eng.php>.

La Leche League (breastfeeding support): <http://www.lalecheleague.org>.

Lamaze International: <http://www.lamazeinternational.org>.

Motherisk: <http://www.motherisk.org/women/index.jsp>.

Motherisk—How to survive morning sickness successfully: <http://www.motherisk.org/documents/BSRC_morning_sickness_EN.pdf>.

Multiple Births Canada: <http://www.multiplebirthscanada.org>.

PARmedX for PREGNANCY: *Physical activity readiness exam* <http://www.csep.ca/cmfiles/publications/parq/parmed-xpreg.pdf>.

Peel Region Health Department: *Parenting in Peel*:

Just for Dads: <http://www.peelregion.ca/health/family-health/just-for-dad/>.

Toddlers and Preschoolers: *Jealousy and Sibling Rivalry*: <http://www.peelregion.ca/health/family-health/toddlers-and-preschoolers/behaviour/jealousy.htm>.

Perinatal Services BC—Guidelines for care: <http://www.perinatalservicesbc.ca/Documents/Guidelines-Standards/Maternal/MaternityCarePathway.pdf>.

Pregnancy after 35: *Best Start—Reflecting on the Trend: Pregnancy After 35*: <http://www.beststart.org/resources/rep_health/pdf/bs_pregnancy_age35.pdf>.

Society of Obstetricians and Gynaecologists of Canada (SOGC): <http://www.sogc.org>.

South Community Birth Program, Vancouver, BC: <http://www.scbp.ca/>.

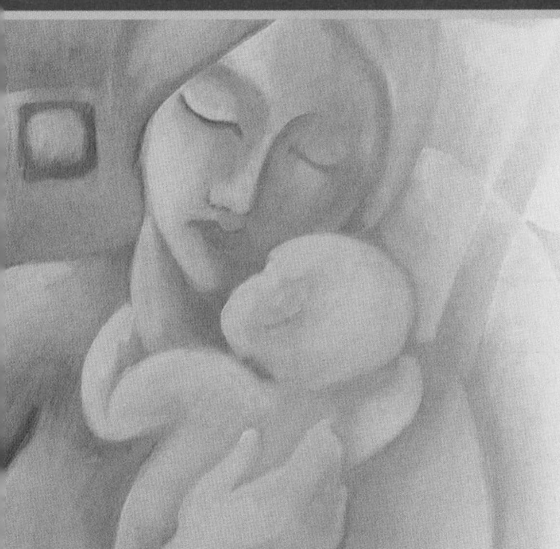

CHAPTER

12

Maternal and Fetal Nutrition

Lisa Keenan-Lindsay

evolve WEBSITE

Visit the Evolve website for additional resources related to the content in this chapter such as Case Studies, Critical Thinking Case Study Answers, Nursing Care Plans, Nursing Processes, Nursing Skills, and Review Questions for Exam Preparation at: http://evolve.elsevier.com/Canada/Perry/maternal/

OBJECTIVES

On completion of this chapter the reader will be able to:

- Explain the importance of good nutrition during the preconception period as well as prenatal period for the health of the mother and fetus.
- Explain recommended maternal weight gain during pregnancy.
- Compare the recommended levels of intake of energy sources, protein, and key vitamins and minerals during pregnancy and lactation.
- Give examples of the food sources that provide the nutrients required for optimal maternal nutrition during pregnancy and lactation.
- Examine the role of nutrition supplements during pregnancy.
- List nutritional risk factors during pregnancy.
- Compare the dietary needs of adolescent women with those of adult women.
- Analyze examples of eating patterns of women and identify potential dietary concerns.
- Assess nutritional status during pregnancy.
- Give strategies to assist with nutrition-related discomforts.

As discussed earlier, the determinants of health are important social and individual factors that influence the health of Canadians (see Table 1-1). Many of the determinants of health have an impact on the quality and amount of dietary intake that women receive, which can ultimately influence pregnancy outcomes (Fig. 12-1). Maternal nutritional status is a significant factor because it is potentially alterable and because good nutrition before and during pregnancy can help prevent a variety of problems. Inadequate nutrition for the mother can lead to an increase in the number of low-birth-weight (LBW) infants (birth weight of 2500 g or less) and preterm infants that are born. Evidence is growing that a mother's nutrition and lifestyle affect the long-term health of her children. Thus the importance of good nutrition must be emphasized to all women of childbearing potential. Key components of nutrition care during the preconception period and pregnancy include the following:

- Nutrition assessment that includes appropriate weight for height, and adequacy and quality of dietary intake and habits
- Diagnosis of nutrition-related problems or risk factors, such as diabetes, phenylketonuria (PKU), and obesity
- Intervention based on an individual's dietary goals and plan to promote appropriate weight gain, ingestion of a variety of healthy foods, appropriate use of dietary supplements, and physical activity
- Evaluation as an integral part of the nursing care provided to women during the preconception period and pregnancy, with referral to a nutritionist or dietitian as necessary (Alberta Health Services, 2013).

NUTRIENT NEEDS BEFORE CONCEPTION

A healthful diet before conception is the best way to ensure that adequate nutrients are available for the developing fetus. Maternal and fetal risks in pregnancy are increased when the mother is significantly underweight or overweight when pregnancy begins. Ideally, all women would achieve their desirable body

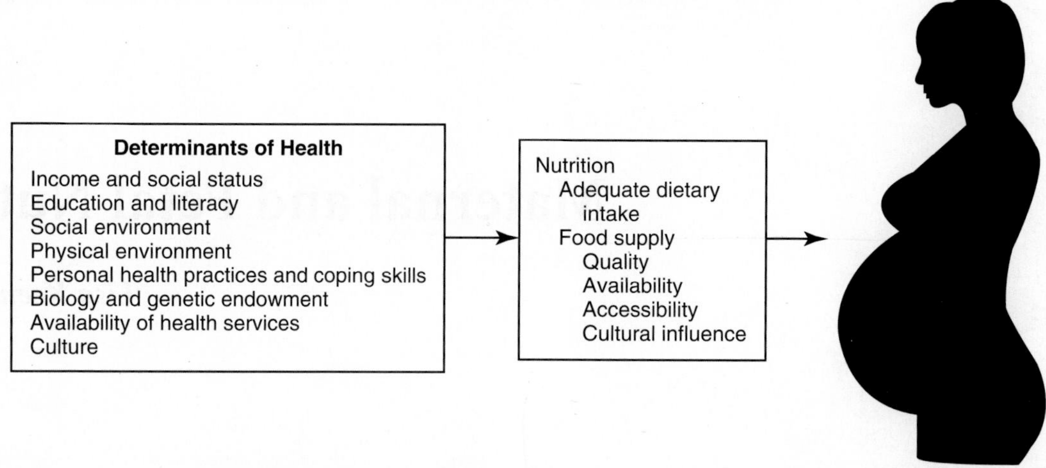

FIGURE 12-1 Determinants of health that influence nutritional status.

BOX 12-1 FOOD SOURCES OF FOLATE*

Foods Providing 500 mcg or More per Serving
- Liver: chicken, turkey, goose; cooked (75 g)

Foods Providing 200 mcg or More per Serving
- Liver: lamb, veal; cooked (75 g)
- Lentils, cooked (175 mL)
- Beans, cranberry/roman, cooked (175 mL)
- Yeast extract spread (Vegemite or Marmite) (30 mL)

Foods Providing 100 mcg or More per Serving
- Liver: beef, pork; cooked (75 g)
- Legumes, cooked (125 mL)
- Peas: (black-eyed, chickpea, garbanzo) (125 mL)
- Beans: black, kidney, pinto, red, navy, white, great northern (125 mL)
- Vegetables: edamame, okra (cooked), spinach (125 mL)
- Pasta, egg noodles, white, enriched (125 mL)
- Bagel, plain (½, 45 g)
- Sunflower seeds, without shell (60 mL)
- Soy burger/vegetarian patty (75 g)

Foods Providing 50 mcg or More per Serving
- Vegetables (125 mL): artichoke, turnip greens, collard, broccoli, asparagus, Brussels sprouts, beets
- Vegetables (250 mL): lettuce (Romaine, mesclun, escarole, endive) spinach
- Potato, with skin
- Fruits: avocado, papaya (½)
- Orange or orange juice (125 mL)
- Bread, white 1 slice (35 g)

Foods Providing 20 mcg or More per Serving
- Egg (1 large)
- Corn (125 mL)

Amounts of folate listed in food are in mcg. The amount required daily is 0.4 to 1.0 mg.
*Amounts are approximate based on Health Canada. (2010). *Canadian nutrient file. Compilation of Canadian food composition data. Users' guide.* Retrieved from http://www.hc-sc.gc.ca/fn-an/nutrition/fiche-nutri-data/index-eng.php
Source: Dieticians of Canada. (2014). *Food sources of folate.* Retrieved from http://www.dietitians.ca/Nutrition-Resources-A-Z/Factsheets/Vitamins/Food-Sources-of-Folate.aspx

weight before conception (Davies, Maxwell, McLeod, et al., 2010).

Folate or folic acid intake is of particular concern in the periconceptual period. Folate is the form in which this vitamin is found naturally in foods, and folic acid is the form used in the fortification of grain products and other foods and in vitamin supplements. *Neural tube defects* (NTD) (failure in closure of the neural tube) are more common in infants of women with poor folic acid intake. In Canada, the rate of children born with a neural tube defect has declined between 1997 and 2007 to approximately 4.0 per 10,000 births mainly due to fortification of food (Public Health Agency of Canada [PHAC], 2013). Proper closure of the neural tube is required for normal formation of the spinal cord. The neural tube begins to close within the first month of gestation, often before the woman realizes that she is pregnant. All women capable of becoming pregnant, regardless of whether or not they are considering pregnancy, should be advised during medical wellness visits (birth control renewal, Pap testing, yearly gynaecological examination) about the benefits of folic acid in a multivitamin supplement (Wilson & Genetics Committee, 2015). Women should be advised to maintain a healthy folate-rich diet (Box 12-1); however, folic acid/multivitamin supplementation also is needed to achieve the red blood cell folate levels associated with maximal protection against NTD (Health Canada, 2011a; Wilson & Genetics Committee, 2015). The amount of folic acid required depends on the risk for NTDs in the woman and partner. Women at low risk should consume 0.4 mg of folic acid in a daily multivitamin (Wilson & Genetics Committee, 2015). Women with health risks such as diabetes, epilepsy, obesity, or a first- or second-degree relative with a history of NTDs require 1.0 mg of folic acid for the 3 months prior to the pregnancy and for the first trimester, at which time their dose can be decreased to 0.4 mg. Women who have had an NTD or a previous pregnancy with an NTD require 4 mg/day at least 3 months prior to conception and through the first trimester of pregnancy, after which time they can decrease the intake to 0.4 mg daily (Wilson & Genetics Committee, 2015) (Fig. 12-2).

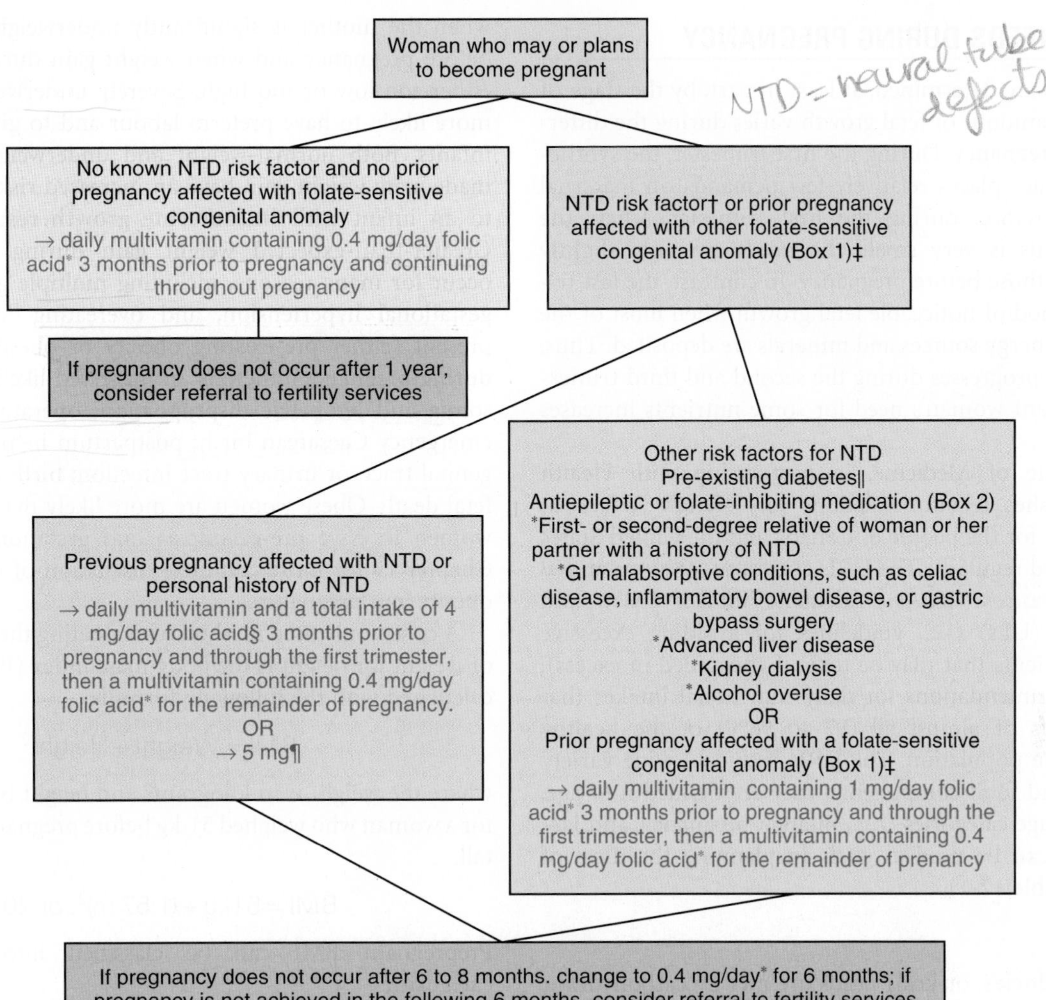

BOX 1
Congenital anomalies which may be sensitive to folate:
- Oral facial cleft (and palate)
- Certain cardiac defects
- Certain urinary tract anomalies
- Limb reduction defects

BOX 2
Practical list of folate-inhibiting medications:
- Anticonvulsant medications: phenytoin, primidone, phenobarbital, carbamazepine, valproic acid
- Metformin
- Methotrexate (a medication that is highly teratogenic to the fetus)
- Sulfasalazine
- Triamterene
- Trimethoprim (as found in cotrimoxazole)

FIGURE 12-2 Decision tree for folic acid supplementation.
*Folic acid should be taken in the form of a multivitamin containing vitamin B_{12}. Women should not take more than one multivitamin supplement each day. In large doses, some substances in multivitamins could be harmful.
†Does NOT include spina bifida occulta, as this is not a risk for NTD.
‡There are additional folate-sensitive congenital anomalies that would benefit from the folic acid levels described.
§To provide a dose of 4 mg/day folic acid, a multivitamin containing 1 mg folic acid should be consumed, with single folic acid tablets added to achieve the desired folic acid dose.
||Periconceptual glycemic control is strongly recommended to reduce the risk of a congenital anomaly in offspring of a woman with prepregnancy diabetes.
¶Folic acid intake should be at the safest and lowest effective dose; however, clinical offices that face challenges implementing recommendations for 4 mg folic acid daily because of the mode of product distribution or compliance issues with taking daily multiple oral tablets may consider the simplified regimen of one 5-mg folic acid multivitamin tablet daily.
GI: gastrointestinal; NTD: neural tube defect; RBC: red blood cells. (Reprinted from *J Obstet Gynaecol Can* 37(6), 2015. Society of Obstetricians and Gynaecologists of Canada, Pre-conception folic acid and multivitamin supplementation for the primary and secondary prevention of neural tube defects and other folic acid-sensitive congenital anomalies, pages 534–549, Copyright 2015, with permission from Elsevier.)

NUTRIENT NEEDS DURING PREGNANCY

Nutrient needs are determined, at least in part, by the stage of gestation. The amount of fetal growth varies during the different stages of pregnancy. During the first trimester, the synthesis of fetal tissues places relatively few demands on maternal nutrition. Therefore, during the first trimester, when the embryo or fetus is very small, the needs are only slightly increased over those before pregnancy. In contrast, the last trimester is a period of noticeable fetal growth when most of the fetal stores of energy sources and minerals are deposited. Thus, as fetal growth progresses during the second and third trimesters, the pregnant woman's need for some nutrients increases greatly.

The Institute of Medicine, in partnership with Health Canada, publishes recommendations for Dietary Reference Intakes (DRIs) for the people of Canada and the United States that are updated regularly. The DRIs consist of Recommended Dietary Allowances (RDAs), Adequate Intakes (AIs), and Upper Limits (ULs) (i.e., guidelines for avoiding excessive intakes of nutrients that may be toxic if consumed in excess). DRIs are recommendations for daily nutritional intakes that meet the needs of almost all (97 to 98%) of the healthy members of the population. The DRIs include a wide variety of nutrients and food components; they are divided into age, sex, and life-stage categories (e.g., infancy, pregnancy, and lactation). They can be used as goals in planning the diets of individuals (Table 12-1).

Energy Needs

Energy (kilocalories, or kcal) needs are met by carbohydrate, fat, and protein in the diet. No specific recommendations exist for the amount of carbohydrate and fat in the diet of pregnant women. However, intake of these nutrients should be adequate to support the recommended weight gain. Although protein can be used to supply energy, its primary role is to provide amino acids for the synthesis of new tissues (see discussion later in this chapter). The estimated energy expenditure for the first trimester is the same as in the prepregnant state; during the second trimester the RDA is 340 kcal greater than the prepregnancy needs, and during the third trimester it is 452 kcal more than the prepregnant needs (Health Canada, 2014a). Longitudinal assessment of weight gain during pregnancy is the best way to determine whether the kilocalorie intake is adequate; very underweight or active women may require more than the recommended increase in kilocalories to sustain the desired rate of weight gain.

Weight Gain

The recommended weight gain during pregnancy varies among women. The primary factor to consider in making a weight-gain recommendation is the prepregnancy weight for the woman's height—that is, whether the woman's weight was normal before pregnancy or whether she was underweight or overweight (Table 12-2). Whenever possible, the woman should achieve a weight in the normal range for her height before pregnancy. Maternal and fetal risks in pregnancy are increased when the mother is significantly underweight or overweight before pregnancy and when weight gain during pregnancy is either too low or too high. Severely underweight women are more likely to have preterm labour and to give birth to LBW infants. Both normal-weight and underweight women with inadequate weight gain have an increased risk for giving birth to an infant with intrauterine growth restriction (IUGR). Greater-than-expected weight gain during pregnancy may occur for many reasons, including multiple gestation, edema, gestational hypertension, and overeating. When obesity is present (either pre-existing obesity or obesity that develops during pregnancy), there is an increased likelihood of macrosomia and fetopelvic disproportion; operative vaginal birth; emergency Caesarean birth; postpartum hemorrhage; wound, genital tract, or urinary tract infection; birth trauma; and late fetal death. Obese women are more likely than normal-weight women to have pre-eclampsia and gestational diabetes. See Chapter 15 for more complete discussion of complications of obesity and pregnancy.

A commonly used method of evaluating the appropriateness of weight for height is the body mass index (BMI). The BMI is calculated with the following formula:

$$\text{BMI} = \text{Weight} \div \text{Height}^2$$

where the weight is in kilograms and height is in metres. Thus for a woman who weighed 51 kg before pregnancy and is 1.57 m tall:

$$\text{BMI} = 51\,\text{kg} \div (1.57\,\text{m})^2, \text{ or } 20.7$$

Prepregnant BMI can be classified into the following categories:

- less than 18.5, underweight or low;
- 18.5 to 24.9, normal;
- 25 to 29.9, overweight or high; and
- greater than 30, obese.

At the first health care visit, the pregnant woman should be helped to establish a weight-gain goal for pregnancy that is suited to her prepregnancy weight. Progress toward this goal should be monitored at each visit. The pregnancy weight gain calculator from Health Canada is a good resource for pregnancy women (see Additional Resources at end of the chapter).

Pattern of Weight Gain

Weight gain should take place throughout pregnancy. The optimal rate of weight gain depends on the stage of pregnancy. During the first and second trimesters, growth takes place primarily in maternal tissues; during the third trimester, growth occurs primarily in fetal tissues. During the first trimester of a singleton pregnancy, the average total weight gain is only 1 to 2 kg. Thereafter the recommended weight gain depends on the woman's BMI (see Table 12-2).

The recommended energy (kcal) intake corresponds to the recommended pattern of gain. As stated earlier, for the first trimester there is no increment; an additional 340 kcal per day and 452 kcal per day over the prepregnant intake during the second and third trimester, respectively, are recommended. These recommendations are for a singleton pregnancy and will

TABLE 12-1 **RECOMMENDATIONS FOR DAILY INTAKES OF SELECTED NUTRIENTS DURING PREGNANCY AND LACTATION**

NUTRIENT (UNITS)	RECOMMENDATION FOR NONPREGNANT WOMAN	RECOMMENDATION FOR PREGNANCY*	RECOMMENDATION FOR LACTATION*	ROLE IN RELATION TO PREGNANCY AND LACTATION	FOOD SOURCES
Energy (kilocalories [kcal] or kilojoules [kJ]†)	Variable	First trimester, same as nonpregnant; second trimester, nonpregnant needs + 340 kcal (1423 kJ); third trimester, nonpregnant needs + 452 kcal (1891 kJ)	First 6 mo, nonpregnant needs + 330 kcal (1380 kJ); second 6 mo, nonpregnant needs + 400 kcal (1674 kJ)	Growth of fetal and maternal tissues; milk production	Carbohydrate, fat, and protein
Protein (g)	46	First trimester, second and third trimesters, nonpregnant needs + 25 g‡	Nonpregnant needs + 25 g	Synthesis of the products of conception; growth of maternal tissue and expansion of blood volume; secretion of milk protein during lactation	Meats, eggs, cheese, yogurt, legumes (dry beans and peas, peanuts), nuts, grains
Water (L)	2.7 total	3 total	3.8 total	Expansion of blood volume, excretion of wastes; milk secretion	Water and beverages made with water, milk, juices; all foods, especially frozen desserts, fruits, lettuce and other fresh vegetables
Fibre (g)	25	28	29	Promotes regular bowel elimination; reduces long-term risk of heart disease, diverticulosis, and diabetes	Whole grains, bran, vegetables, fruits, nuts and seeds
Minerals					
Calcium (mg)	1300/1000	1300/1000	1300/1000	Fetal skeleton and tooth formation; maintenance of maternal bone and tooth mineralization	Milk, cheese, yogurt, sardines or other fish eaten with bones left in; deep green leafy vegetables except spinach or Swiss chard; calcium-set tofu, baked beans, tortillas
Iodine (mcg)	150	220	290	Increased maternal metabolic rate	Iodized salt, seafood, milk and milk products, commercial yeast breads, rolls, and doughnuts
Iron (mg)	15/18	27	10/9	Maternal hemoglobin formation; fetal liver iron storage	Liver§, meats, whole-grain or enriched breads and cereals, deep green leafy vegetables, legumes, dried fruits
Magnesium (mg)	360/310–320	400/350–360	360/310–320	Involved in energy and protein metabolism, tissue growth, muscle action	Nuts, legumes, cocoa, meats, whole grains
Zinc (mg)	9/8	12/11	13/12	Component of numerous enzyme systems; possibly important in preventing congenital malformations	Liver§, shellfish, meats, whole grains, milk

Continued

TABLE 12-1 RECOMMENDATIONS FOR DAILY INTAKES OF SELECTED NUTRIENTS DURING PREGNANCY AND LACTATION—cont'd

NUTRIENT (UNITS)	RECOMMENDATION FOR NONPREGNANT WOMAN	RECOMMENDATION FOR PREGNANCY*	RECOMMENDATION FOR LACTATION*	ROLE IN RELATION TO PREGNANCY AND LACTATION	FOOD SOURCES
Fat-Soluble Vitamins					
A (mcg)	700	750/770	1200/1300	Essential for cell development, tooth bud formation, bone growth	Deep green leafy vegetables, dark yellow vegetables, fruits, chili peppers, liver§, fortified margarine and butter
D (mcg)	15 (600 IU)	15 (600 IU)	15 (600 IU)	Involved in absorption of calcium and phosphorus; improves mineralization	Fortified milk and margarine, egg yolk, butter, liver§, seafood
E (mg)	15	15	19	Antioxidant (protects cell membranes from damage), especially important for preventing breakdown of RBCs	Vegetable oils, green leafy vegetables, whole grains, liver§, nuts and seeds, cheese, fish
K (mcg)	75/90	75 (14- to 18-yr-old) 90 (19- to 50-yr-old)	75 (14- to 18-yr-old) 90 (19- to 50-yr-old)	Involved in synthesis of protein, blood coagulation, and bone metabolism	Green leafy vegetables, plant oils, margarine, soybeans, lentils
Water-Soluble Vitamins					
B_6 or pyridoxine (mg)	1.2/1.3	1.9	2	Involved in protein metabolism	Meats, liver§, deep green vegetables, whole grains
B_{12} (mcg)	2.4	2.6	2.8	Production of nucleic acids and proteins; especially important in formation of RBCs and neural functioning	Milk and milk products, eggs, meats, liver§, fortified soy milk
C (mg)	65/75	80/85	115/120	Tissue formation and integrity, formation of connective tissue; enhancement of iron absorption	Citrus fruits, strawberries, melons, broccoli, tomatoes, peppers, raw deep green leafy vegetable
Folate (mcg)	400	600	500	Prevention of neural tube defects, support for increased maternal RBC formation	Fortified ready-to-eat cereals and other grain products, green leafy vegetables, oranges, broccoli, asparagus, artichokes, liver§

RBC, red blood cell.
*When two values appear, separated by a diagonal slash, the first is for females younger than 19 years, and the second is for those 19 to 50 years of age.
†The international metric unit of energy measurement is the joule (J). 1 kcal = 4.184 kJ.
‡Add an additional 25 g in twin pregnancies.
§Pregnant women should not eat liver because of a high concentration of vitamin A.
Source: Health Canada. (2010). *Dietary reference intakes tables.* Ottawa: Author. Retrieved from http://www.hc-sc.gc.ca/fn-an/alt_formats/hpfb-dgpsa/pdf/nutrition/dri_tables-eng.pdf

TABLE 12-2 RECOMMENDED RATE OF WEIGHT GAIN IN PREGNANCY

PREPREGNANCY BMI CATEGORY	MEAN† RATE OF WEIGHT GAIN IN SECOND AND THIRD TRIMESTER		RECOMMENDED RANGE OF TOTAL WEIGHT GAIN	
	kg/week	lb/week	kg	Lb
BMI <18.5 Underweight	0.5	1.0	12.5–18	28–40
BMI 18.5–24.9 Normal weight	0.4	1.0	11.5–16	25–35
BMI 25.0–29.9 Overweight	0.3	0.6	7–11.5	15–25
BMI ≥30‡ Obese	0.2	0.5	5–9	11–20

BMI, body mass index.
†Rounded values.
‡A narrower range of weight gain may be advised for women with a prepregnancy BMI of 35 or greater. Individualized advice is recommended for these women.
Source: © All rights reserved. *Prenatal nutrition guidelines for health professionals: Gestational weight gain.* Health Canada, 2010. Adapted and reproduced with permission from the Minister of Health, 2016.

need to be adjusted for multiple gestation. The amount of food providing the needed increase is not great. The additional calories can be obtained by eating two to three extra servings from *Eating Well With Canada's Food Guide* from any of the food groups (see Appendix A).

In multiple gestations, weight gain during the first half of pregnancy is important and overall weight gain should be 17 to 25 kg (Alberta Health Services, 2013). Women carrying multiples should be referred for nutrition counselling to assist with appropriate food intake and weight gain.

The reasons for an inadequate weight gain (less than 1 kg per month for normal-weight women or less than 0.5 kg per month for obese women during the last two trimesters) or excessive weight gain (more than 3 kg per month) should be evaluated thoroughly. Possible reasons for deviations from the expected rate of weight gain, besides inadequate or excessive dietary intake, include measurement or recording errors, differences in weight of clothing, time of day, and accumulation of fluids. An exceptionally high gain is likely to be caused by an accumulation of fluids; a gain of more than 3 kg in a month, especially after the twentieth week of gestation, may indicate the development of pre-eclampsia.

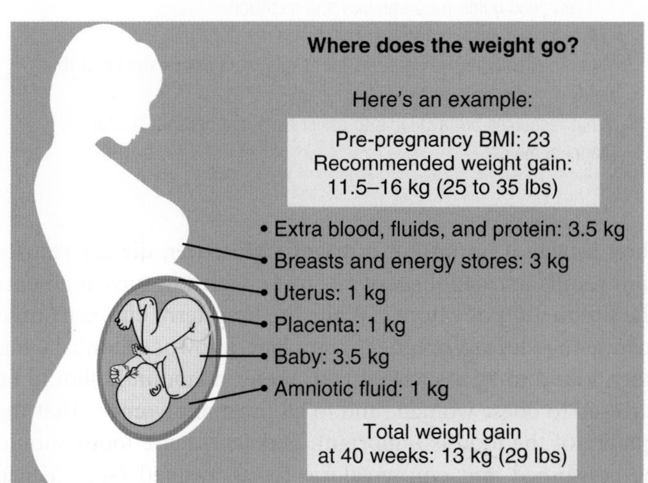

FIGURE 12-3 Distribution of weight gain in pregnancy. The numbers represent an average; variation among women is great. The component with the greatest fluctuation is the weight increase attributed to extravascular fluids (edema) and maternal reserves of fat. (Adapted from Health Canada. [2014]. *Prenatal nutrition guidelines for professionals: Gestational weight gain.* Retrieved from http://www.hc-sc.gc.ca/fn-an/nutrition/prenatal/bmi/index-eng.php.)

Hazards of Restricting Adequate Weight Gain

An obsession with thinness and dieting pervades the North American culture. Figure-conscious women may find it difficult to make the transition from guarding against weight gain before pregnancy to valuing weight gain during pregnancy. In counselling these women, the nurse can emphasize both the positive effects of good nutrition and the adverse effects of maternal malnutrition (manifested by poor weight gain) on infant growth and development. This counselling should include information on the components of weight gain during pregnancy (Fig. 12-3) and the amount of this weight that will be lost at birth. Because lactation can help reduce maternal energy stores gradually, this could be an incentive for women to breastfeed their infants and thus be an opportunity for the nurse to promote breastfeeding.

Obesity and Pregnancy

In Canada, 15 to 18% of women of child-bearing age are considered obese (Statistics Canada, 2011). Women who are obese have an increased risk of pregnancy and labour complications; these are discussed in Chapter 15, pp. 380–382. However, pregnancy is not a time for weight reduction. Even overweight or obese pregnant women need to gain at least enough weight to equal the weight of the products of conception (fetus, placenta, and amniotic fluid). If overweight women limit their energy intake to prevent weight gain, they may also excessively limit

CRITICAL THINKING CASE STUDY

Nutrition and the Overweight Pregnant Woman

Nina, age 22, of Cree descent is 3 months pregnant and comes to her initial appointment for diagnosis and care. Nina appears to be overweight for her height (167 cm, 85 kg). To provide optimal care for her, you plan to calculate her prepregnancy body mass index. When her pregnancy is confirmed, you are asked to plan a diet with Nina that meets the minimum daily requirements and allows for growth of the pregnancy. You know that it is important to include consideration of personal preferences and cultural factors in your plan. With Nina, identify barriers to implementing the plan.

QUESTIONS

1. Evidence—Is there sufficient evidence to draw conclusions about an appropriate nutrition plan, taking into consideration BMI, personal preferences, and cultural factors?
2. Assumptions—Describe underlying assumptions about each of the following issues:
   a. Dietary Reference Intakes for pregnancy and lactation
   b. Indicators of nutritional risk in pregnancy; possibility of lactose intolerance
   c. Daily food guide for pregnancy and lactation
   d. Sources of calcium for women who do not drink milk
3. What implications and priorities for nursing care can be drawn at this time?
4. What resources are available to assist Nina and her family when planning meals?

their intake of important nutrients. Moreover, dietary restriction results in catabolism of fat stores, which in turn augments the production of ketones. While the long-term effects of mild ketonemia during pregnancy are not known, ketonuria has been found to be associated with preterm labour. It should be stressed to obese women (and to all pregnant women) that the quality of the food is important: Nutrient-dense foods should be consumed and empty-calorie foods avoided (see Critical Thinking Case Study).

Excessive Weight Gain

Weight gain is important, but excessive weight gain can be detrimental. The woman should place an emphasis on the quality of her food intake as she considers her needs and those of her fetus. Excessive weight gained during pregnancy may be difficult to lose after pregnancy, contributing to chronic overweight or obesity, an etiological factor in a host of chronic diseases, including hypertension, diabetes mellitus, and arteriosclerotic heart disease. The woman who gains 18 kg or more during pregnancy is especially at risk. When counselling the woman, it is best not to focus unduly on weight gain because this could result in feelings of stress and guilt in the woman who does not follow the preferred pattern of gain.

Food energy intake, and particularly intake of fat, may be high among low-income pregnant women, as this food is less expensive.

Health Canada's *Eating Well With Canada's Food Guide* sets recommendations for daily food intake for Canadians that are based on RDAs (see Appendix A).

Protein

Protein, with its essential constituent nitrogen, is the nutrition element that is basic to growth. Adequate protein intake is essential to meet increasing physiological demands in pregnancy. These demands arise from:

- The rapid growth of the fetus
- The enlargement of the uterus and its supporting structures, the mammary glands, and the placenta
- The increase in maternal circulating blood volume and subsequent demand for increased amounts of plasma protein to maintain colloidal osmotic pressure
- The formation of amniotic fluid

Milk, meat, eggs, and cheese are **complete-protein foods** with a high biological value. Legumes (dried beans and peas), whole grains, and nuts are also valuable sources of protein. In addition, these protein-rich foods are a source of other nutrients such as calcium, iron, and B vitamins; plant sources of protein often provide needed dietary fibre. *Eating Well With Canada's Food Guide* recommends a daily food plan that would supply the quantities of protein needed (Appendix A). Pregnant adolescents and women adhering to a macrobiotic (highly restricted vegetarian) diet may need extra teaching to ensure protein intake is adequate. Food with protein can be more expensive so women with lower income may need assistance to find appropriate food sources. High-protein supplements are not recommended because they have been associated with an increased incidence of preterm birth.

Pregnant and nursing women should be especially careful when choosing fish to select those that are low in mercury. It is recommended that pregnant women consume at least 150 g of cooked fish per week, as fish contributes to a healthy pregnancy (Health Canada, 2009). Larger fish that eat smaller fish are usually higher in mercury. See Nursing Alert.

! NURSING ALERT

High levels of mercury can harm the developing nervous system of the fetus or young child. Certain fish are especially high in mercury. Women who may become pregnant, women who are pregnant or nursing, and young children need to follow some precautions: Limit consumption of fresh or frozen tuna, shark, swordfish, escolar, marlin, and orange roughy to 150 g/month, and eat as much as 75 g/week of a variety of commercially caught fish and shellfish low in mercury such as shrimp, salmon, pollock, catfish, and canned light tuna (but limit intake of albacore or "white" tuna and tuna steaks, which contain more mercury, to 300 g/week) (Health Canada, 2011b). Additional information about mercury levels in a variety of commercial fish is available in the Additional Resources.

Fluids

Water is the main substance of cells, blood, lymph, amniotic fluid, and other vital body fluids. It is essential during the exchange of nutrients and waste products across cell membranes. It also aids in maintaining body temperature. A good fluid intake promotes regular bowel function; without it, constipation can become a concern, especially during pregnancy. The recommended daily intake of liquid is 3 litres. Water, milk,

BOX 12-2 HERBAL TEAS DURING PREGNANCY

Safe (if taken in moderation, two to three cups per day): citrus peel, ginger, lemon balm, orange peel, rose hip, raspberry leaf, and peppermint

Teas to avoid: chamomiles, aloe, coltsfoot, juniper berries, pennyroyal, buckthorn bark, comfrey, Labrador tea, sassafras, duck roots, lobelia, and senna leaves

Source: Public Health Agency of Canada. (2014). *Health pregnancy: Caffeine and pregnancy.* Retrieved from http://www.phac-aspc.gc.ca/hp-gs/know-savoir/caffeine-eng.php

decaffeinated tea, and juices are good sources, although pregnant women should limit their intake of fruit juice, as it can be high in calories and therefore lead to extra weight gain. Foods in the diet should supply an additional 700 mL or more of fluid. Dehydration may increase the risk of cramping, contractions, hyperemesis gravidarium, and preterm labour.

Caffeine in moderate amounts has not been proven to cause adverse effects during pregnancy. However, women who consume more than 300 mg of caffeine daily (equivalent to a little more than 2 cups of coffee) may be at increased risk of miscarriage and giving birth to infants with IUGR. The ill effects of caffeine are thought to result from vasoconstriction of the blood vessels supplying the uterus or from interference with cell division in the developing fetus. Consequently, caffeine-containing products such as caffeinated coffee, tea, soft drinks, and cocoa beverages should be consumed only in limited quantities (300 mg daily) (PHAC, 2014). See Box 12-2 regarding the safety of herbal teas.

Artificial sweeteners commonly used in low- or no-calorie beverages and low-calorie food products have not been found to have adverse effects on the normal mother or fetus and thus are approved by Health Canada for use during pregnancy. These include Aspartame (NutraSweet, Equal), acesulfame potassium (Ace K), sucralose (Splenda), and stevioside (Stevia). It is recommended that women use artificial sweeteners in moderate amounts only. Aspartame, which contains phenylalanine, should be avoided by pregnant women with PKU (see Table 12-3).

Energy drinks claim to give people extra physical and mental energy. They are highly caffeinated beverages that also contain sugar, artificial sweeteners, amino acids, vitamins, and herbs and should be avoided during pregnancy.

SAFETY ALERT

Energy drinks are not recommended for children or for pregnant or breastfeeding women. Energy drinks contain high levels of caffeine. Some of the caffeine in energy drinks may come from herbs, such as guarana and yerba maté. The label on these energy drinks will list the herbs as ingredients, but the caffeine in the herbs may not be listed as a separate ingredient. Therefore, it is possible to unintentionally consume more caffeine than is listed on the label (Alberta Health Services, 2013; HealthLink BC, 2013).

Omega 3 Fatty Acids

Omega-3 fatty acids are important for overall health, providing benefits such as lowering the risk of heart disease. They are transferred across the placenta and play an important role in the growth and development of the infant. More of the documented health benefits of omega-3 fatty acids are from eicosapentaonoic acid (EPA) and docosahexaenoic acid (DHA) than from plant-derived alpha-linolenic acid (ALA). EPA and DHA are primarily found in fish, shellfish, fish oil supplements, and omega-3-enriched eggs. Pregnant women should be advised to consume at least two *Food Guide* servings (75 grams or 2½ ounces each) of fish each week to meet the requirement for omega-3 fatty acid (Alberta Health Services, 2013; Health Canada, 2009).

Minerals, Vitamins, and Electrolytes

In general, the nutrient needs of pregnant women, except perhaps the need for folate and iron, can be met through dietary sources. Counselling about the importance of a varied diet rich in vitamins and minerals should be a part of every pregnant woman's early prenatal care and should be reinforced throughout pregnancy.

Supplements of certain nutrients are recommended when the woman's diet is very nutritionally poor or when significant nutritional risk factors are present (Box 12-3). It is important that the pregnant woman understand that the use of a vitamin-mineral supplement does not lessen the need to consume a nutritious, well-balanced diet.

Iron

Iron is needed both to allow the transfer of adequate iron to the fetus and to permit expansion of the maternal red blood cell (RBC) mass. Poor iron status, which can result in iron-deficiency anemia, is relatively common among women in the child-bearing years. Anemic women are poorly prepared to tolerate hemorrhage at the time of birth. In addition, women who have iron deficiency anemia during early pregnancy are at increased risk for preterm birth and LBW infants. Iron deficiency during the third trimester apparently does not carry the same risk. In Canada, anemia is a common condition in approximately 25% of child-bearing–aged women. It may be caused by low intake of iron, poor absorption of iron, or blood loss. Iron-deficiency anemia is more prevalent in isolated Indigenous communities and in teenage girls of South Asian descent (British Columbia Ministry of Health, 2010).

The RDA of iron during pregnancy is 27 mg/day. Health Canada recommends that all pregnant women take a daily multivitamin with 16 to 20 mg of iron (Health Canada, 2014b). Pregnant women who are vegetarian may need an increased amount of iron. This dose is well below the level of iron supplementation that has been linked to negative side effects (reduced zinc absorption and gastrointestinal symptoms) (Alberta Health Services, 2013). Iron supplements may be poorly tolerated if a woman has significant nausea in the first trimester and may need to be started after week 12. Iron supplementation of women with iron deficiency can improve maternal hematological indices and appears to reduce the rate

TABLE 12-3 USE OF ARTIFICIAL SWEETENERS DURING PREGNANCY

SWEETENER	OTHER NAMES	COMPARISON TO SUGAR	FLAVOUR	SAFE DURING PREGNANCY AND LACTATION?	CALORIC VALUE	USES	OTHER
Acesulfame Potassium	Ace K	200× sweeter, (300× sweeter when blended with aspartame)	Bitter or metallic aftertaste in large amounts	Yes	0	Baked goods, frozen desserts, sugar-free gelatin, pudding, and beverage	Mixing with other sweeteners reduces aftertaste
Aspartame	Equal, Nutrasweet	200× sweeter (300× sweeter when blended with Ace K)	Sugar-like sweetness with no bitter aftertaste	Yes, unless woman has phenylketonuria (PKU)	4 kcal/g	Soft drinks, gelatin, desserts, pudding mixes, breakfast cereal, beverages, gum, dairy products	Has the same calories as sugar but has a much sweeter taste. Less is needed for the same sweetness.
Cyclamate	Sugar Twin	30× sweeter	Slowly gets sweeter with lasting sweet flavour	No—has been linked to cancer	0	Variety of foods, beverages, cooking and baking	Health Canada doesn't allow its addition to foods. It is approved as a table-top sweetener or for use in baking, with proper labelling.
Saccharin	Sweet'n Low, Hermesetas	300× sweeter	Bitter aftertaste in large amounts	Yes	0	Variety of foods, beverages, cooking and baking	Moderate use only is recommended by Health Canada.
Stevia	Sweet Leaf	Up to 300× sweeter	Varying reports; some report bitter or licorice aftertaste	Yes	0	Variety of foods, beverages, cooking and baking	Approved by Health Canada in 2012 for use in Canada
Sucralose	Splenda	600× sweeter	No bitter aftertaste	Yes	0	Baked goods, nonalcoholic drinks, gum, coffees/teas, frostings, fats/oils, frozen desserts, fruit juice, sweet sauce	Made from sugar itself
Sugar Alcohols	Polyols (Sorbitol, Manitol, Isomalt)	½ as sweet	Gives a cooling sensation in the mouth	Yes	~2 kcal/g	Manufactured for use in sugar-free candies, cookies, chewing gum, etc.	Does not cause cavities because it is not fermented by bacteria. May have a laxative effect with large intakes

Sources: Alberta Health Services. (2013). *Nutrition guideline pregnancy*. Retrieved from http://www.albertahealthservices.ca/assets/Infofor/hp/if-hp-ed-cdm-ns-4-1-1-pregnancy.pdf; Health Canada. (2012). *Food and nutrition: Sugar substitutes*. Retrieved from http://www.hc-sc.gc.ca/fn-an/securit/addit/sweeten-edulcor/index-eng.php

BOX 12-3 INDICATORS OF NUTRITIONAL RISK IN PREGNANCY

- Adolescence or less than 2 years postmenarche
- Frequent pregnancies: three within 2 years
- Poor fetal outcome in a previous pregnancy
- Poverty/food insecurity
- Poor diet habits with resistance to change
- Use of tobacco, alcohol, or drugs
- Weight at conception significantly under or over normal weight
- Problems with weight gain
- Any weight loss
- Weight gain of less than 1 kg/month after the first trimester
- Weight gain of more than 1 kg/week after the first trimester
- Multifetal pregnancy
- Low hemoglobin or hematocrit values (or both)
- Diabetes
- Chronic illness, including an eating disorder that affects intake, absorption, or metabolism of nutrients

PATIENT TEACHING

Iron Supplementation

- Vitamin C (in citrus fruits, tomatoes, melons, and strawberries) increases the absorption of iron; therefore, eat these foods at the same time.
- Heme iron (found in meats) is better absorbed than non-heme sources of iron (vegetable sources)
- Bran, tea, coffee, milk, oxalates (in spinach and Swiss chard), and egg yolk decrease iron absorption. Avoid consuming them at the same time as an iron source.
- Iron supplements are absorbed best if taken when the stomach is empty (i.e., take it between meals with a beverage other than tea, coffee, or milk).
- Iron supplements can be taken at bedtime if abdominal discomfort occurs when it is taken between meals.
- If an iron dose is missed, take it as soon as it is remembered if that is within 13 hours of the scheduled dose. Do not double up on the dose.
- Keep iron supplements in a childproof container and out of reach of any children in the household.
- The iron may cause stools to be black or dark green.
- Constipation is common with iron supplementation. A diet high in fibre with adequate fluid intake is recommended.

of LBW births. If maternal iron-deficiency anemia is present (preferably diagnosed by measurement of serum ferritin, a storage form of iron), increased dosages (60 to 120 mg daily) are recommended. Certain foods taken with an iron supplement can promote or inhibit absorption of iron from the supplement (e.g., tea or coffee close to meals can inhibit absorption). See the Patient Teaching box: Iron Supplementation regarding intake of iron and supplementation. Even when a woman is taking an iron supplement, she should include good food sources of iron in her daily diet (see Table 12-1).

Calcium

There is no increase in the DRI of calcium during pregnancy and lactation over that recommended for the nonpregnant woman (see Table 12-1). The DRI (1000 mg daily for women 19 years and older and 1300 mg for those younger than 19 years) appears to provide sufficient calcium for fetal bone and tooth development to proceed while maintaining maternal bone mass. Vitamin D is important for the absorption and metabolism of calcium (see discussion later in chapter).

Milk and yogurt are especially rich sources of calcium, providing approximately 300 mg per 240 mL in a serving. Nevertheless, many women either do not consume these foods or do not consume adequate amounts to provide the recommended intakes of calcium. One problem that can interfere with milk consumption is **lactose intolerance**, the inability to digest milk sugar (lactose) caused by the lack of the lactase enzyme in the small intestine. Lactose intolerance is relatively common in adults, particularly among Asians and Indigenous people. Milk consumption can cause abdominal cramping, bloating, and diarrhea in individuals with lactose intolerance, although many of these individuals can tolerate small amounts of milk without symptoms. Yogurt, sweet acidophilus milk, buttermilk, cheese, chocolate milk, and cocoa may be tolerated even when fresh liquid milk is not. Commercial lactase supplements (e.g., Lactaid) are widely available to consume with milk. Many grocery stores stock lactase-treated milk. The lactase in these products hydrolyzes, or digests, the lactose in milk, making it possible for lactose-intolerant people to drink milk.

In some cultures adults rarely drink milk. Pregnant women from these cultures may need to consume nondairy sources of calcium (Box 12-4). Vegetarian diets may also be deficient in calcium. If calcium intake appears low, a daily supplement containing 600 mg of elemental calcium may be needed.

SAFETY ALERT

Bone meal, which is sometimes used as a calcium source by pregnant women, is frequently found to be contaminated with lead. Lead freely crosses the placenta; thus regular maternal intake of bone meal may result in high levels of lead in the fetus (Shannon, 2003).

Magnesium

Magnesium is necessary for bone and tissue growth. Diets of women in the child-bearing years are likely to be low in magnesium, and as many as half of pregnant and lactating women may have inadequate intake. Adolescents and low-income women are especially at risk. Dairy products, nuts, whole grains, and green leafy vegetables are good sources of magnesium.

Sodium

During pregnancy the need for sodium increases slightly, primarily because the body water is expanding (e.g., the expanding blood volume). Sodium is essential for maintaining body water balance. In the past, dietary sodium was routinely restricted in an effort to control the peripheral edema that commonly occurs during pregnancy. It is now recognized that moderate

BOX 12-4 CALCIUM SOURCES FOR WOMEN WHO DO NOT DRINK MILK

Each of the following provides approximately the same amount of calcium as 240 mL (1 cup) of milk:

Fish
- 90 g (3-oz) can of sardines
- 150 g (4½-oz) can of salmon (if bones are eaten)

Beans and Legumes
- 750 mL (3 cups) of cooked dried beans
- 625 mL (2½ cups) of refried beans
- 500 mL (2 cups) of baked beans with molasses
- 240 mL (1 cup) of tofu (calcium is added in processing)

Greens
- 240 mL (1 cup) of collards
- 365 mL (1½ cups) of kale or turnip greens

Baked Products
- 3 pieces of cornbread
- 3 English muffins
- 4 slices of French toast
- 2 waffles (15 cm in diameter)

Fruits
- 11 dried figs
- 270 mL (1⅛ cups) of orange juice with calcium added

Sauces
- 90 mL (3 oz) of pesto sauce
- 150 g (5 oz) of cheese sauce

peripheral edema is normal in pregnancy, occurring as a response to the fluid-retaining effects of elevated levels of estrogen. Sodium is not routinely restricted in pregnancy, and restriction has not proved effective in reducing the rates of preeclampsia. Severe sodium restriction may make it difficult for pregnant women to achieve an adequate diet. Grain, milk, and meat products, which are good sources of nutrients needed during pregnancy, are significant sources of sodium. In addition, sodium restriction may stress the adrenal glands and the kidneys as they attempt to retain adequate sodium. In general, sodium restriction is necessary only if the woman has a medical condition such as renal or liver failure or hypertension that warrants such a restriction.

Excessive intake of sodium is discouraged during pregnancy, because it may contribute to the development of hypertension in salt-sensitive individuals. An adequate sodium intake for pregnant and lactating women, as well as nonpregnant women in the child-bearing years, is estimated to be 1.5 g/day, with a recommended upper limit of intake of 2.3 g/day. Table salt (sodium chloride) is the richest source of sodium, with approximately 2.3 g of sodium contained in 5 g (1 tsp) of salt. Most canned foods contain added salt unless the label states otherwise. Large amounts of sodium are also found in many processed foods, including meats (e.g., smoked or cured meats, cold cuts, and corned beef), frozen entrées and meals, baked goods, mixes for casseroles or grain products, soups, and condiments. Products low in nutritive value and excessively high in sodium include pretzels, potato and other chips (except salt-free), pickles, ketchup, prepared mustard, steak and Worcestershire sauces, some soft drinks, and bouillon. A moderate sodium intake can usually be achieved by salting food lightly during cooking; adding no additional salt at the table; and avoiding low-nutrient, high-sodium foods.

Potassium

Diets including adequate intake of potassium are associated with a reduced risk of hypertension. Potassium has been identified as one of the nutrients most likely to be lacking in the diets of women of child-bearing years. Following Canada's *Food Guide* and eating seven to eight servings of unprocessed fruits and vegetables daily, along with moderate amounts of low-fat meats and dairy products, has been effective in reducing sodium intake while providing adequate amounts of potassium.

Zinc

Zinc is a constituent of numerous enzymes involved in major metabolic pathways. Zinc deficiency is associated with malformations of the central nervous system in infants. When large amounts of iron and folic acid are consumed, the absorption of zinc is inhibited, and serum zinc levels are reduced as a result. Because iron and folic acid supplements are commonly prescribed during pregnancy, pregnant women should be encouraged to consume recommended sources of zinc daily (see Table 12-1). Women with anemia who receive high-dose iron supplements also need supplements of zinc and copper.

Fluoride

There is no evidence that prenatal fluoride supplementation reduces the child's likelihood of tooth decay during the preschool years. No increase in fluoride intake over the nonpregnant RDAs is currently recommended during pregnancy.

Fat-Soluble Vitamins

Fat-soluble vitamins—A, D, E, and K—are stored in the body tissues. These are of special concern during pregnancy because vitamin E intake is among the nutrients most likely to be lacking in the diets of women of child-bearing age, and intake of vitamins A and D is also low in the diets of some women. With chronic overdoses these vitamins can reach toxic levels. Because of the high potential for toxicity, pregnant women are advised to take fat-soluble vitamin supplements only as prescribed.

Adequate intake of vitamin A is needed so that sufficient amounts of the vitamin can be stored in the fetus. A well-chosen diet including adequate amounts of deep yellow and deep green vegetables and fruits such as leafy greens, broccoli, carrots, cantaloupe, and apricots provides sufficient amounts of carotenes that can be converted in the body to vitamin A. Congenital malformations have occurred in infants of mothers who took excessive amounts of preformed vitamin A (from supplements) during pregnancy; thus supplements are not recommended for pregnant women. Liver contains large amounts of vitamin A and is not recommended during pregnancy. Vitamin A analogs such as isotretinoin (Accutane), which are prescribed for the treatment of cystic acne, are of special concern. Isotretinoin use during early pregnancy has been associated with an increased incidence of heart malformations, facial abnormalities, cleft palate, hydrocephalus, and deafness and blindness in the infant, as well as an increased risk of miscarriage. Topical agents such as tretinoin (Retin-A, Avita) do not appear to enter the circulation in any substantial amounts, but their safety in pregnancy has not been confirmed.

Vitamin D plays an important role in the absorption and metabolism of calcium. The main food sources of this vitamin are enriched or fortified foods such as milk and ready-to-eat cereals. Vitamin D is also produced in the skin by the action of ultraviolet light (in sunlight). Severe deficiency may lead to neonatal hypocalcemia and tetany, as well as to hypoplasia of the tooth enamel. Women with lactose intolerance and those who do not include milk in their diet for any reason are at risk for vitamin D deficiency. Other risk factors for low vitamin D status include being overweight or obese, living at northern (north of 37°N) latitudes during the winter, having darker pigmented skin, or having limited exposure to direct sunlight (Alberta Health Services, 2013). Thus, Canadian women are at increased risk for having low vitamin D status.

Use of recommended amounts of sunscreen with a sun protection factor (SPF) rating of 15 or greater reduces skin vitamin D production by as much as 99%, thus regular intake of fortified foods or a supplement may be needed. All pregnant women should be advised to consume at least two servings of fish low in mercury per week and to ensure their multivitamin contains 400 IU of vitamin D.

Vitamin E is needed for protection against oxidative stress, and pregnancy is associated with increased oxidative stress. Oxidative stress above that usually associated with pregnancy has been proposed as an etiology of pre-eclampsia, although supplementation with vitamin E has not been effective in reducing rates of pre-eclampsia (see Chapter 14, p. 313, for further discussion). Vegetable oils and nuts are especially good sources of vitamin E, and whole grains and green leafy vegetables are moderate sources.

Vitamin K is involved in the synthesis of proteins needed for blood coagulation and bone metabolism. The RDA for women is 90 mcg/day. The classic sign of vitamin K deficiency is an increase in prothrombin time; severe cases result in hemorrhage. Food sources are green leafy vegetables, plant oils and margarine, and soybeans and lentils.

Water-Soluble Vitamins

Body stores of water-soluble vitamins are much smaller than those of fat-soluble vitamins. In contrast to fat-soluble vitamins, water-soluble vitamins are readily excreted in the urine. Therefore, recommended sources of these vitamins must be consumed frequently. Toxicity with overdose is less likely than with fat-soluble vitamins.

Folate or folic acid. Because of the increase in RBC production during pregnancy and the nutrition requirements of the rapidly growing cells in the fetus and placenta, pregnant women should consume about 50% more folic acid than that needed by nonpregnant women. Folic acid supplementation (0.4 mg daily) is most important preconception and during the first trimester. In Canada, all enriched grain products (which includes most white breads, flour, and pasta) must contain folic acid at a level of 0.15 mg/100 g of flour. This level of fortification is designed to supply approximately 0.1 mg of folic acid daily in the average Canadian diet and has significantly increased folic acid consumption in the population as a whole. Supplemental folic acid is usually prescribed to ensure that intake is adequate. Women who have borne a child with a neural tube defect, have diabetes or epilepsy, or are obese are advised to consume 4 mg of folic acid daily; a supplement is required for them to achieve this level of intake (see Fig. 12-2). Folic acid decreases the risk of other congenital anomalies, including congenital heart defects, urinary tract anomalies, oral facial clefts, and limb defects.

Pyridoxine. Pyridoxine, or vitamin B_6, is involved in protein metabolism. Although levels of a pyridoxine-containing enzyme have been reported to be low in women with pre-eclampsia, there is no evidence that supplementation prevents or corrects the condition. Pyridoxine has been effective in reducing the nausea and vomiting of early pregnancy in some trials.

Vitamin C. Vitamin C, or ascorbic acid, plays an important role in tissue formation and enhances the absorption of iron. The vitamin C needs of most women are readily met by a diet that includes at least one daily serving of citrus fruit or juice or another good source of the vitamin (see Table 12-1), but women who smoke need more.

Vitamin B_{12}. Vitamin B_{12} is involved in the production of nucleic acids and proteins; it is especially important in the formation of RBCs and neural functioning. It is found in milk and milk products, eggs, meats, liver, and fortified soy milk.

Other Nutritional Issues During Pregnancy

Pica and Food Cravings

Pica, the practice of consuming nonfood substances (e.g., clay, dirt, and laundry starch) or excessive amounts of foodstuffs low in nutritional value (e.g., cornstarch, ice or freezer frost, baking powder, and baking soda), is often influenced by the woman's cultural background (Fig. 12-4). Black women report practising pica more than other women, as do women from rural areas and women with a family history of pica. Regular and heavy consumption of low-nutrient products may cause more nutritious foods to be displaced from the diet, and the items consumed may interfere with the absorption of nutrients, especially minerals. As an example, cornstarch ingestion is popular among Black women. It is a source of "empty" calories; 120 mL (64 g) provides 240 kcal (57 kJ) but almost no vitamins, minerals, or protein. Overuse of cornstarch can contribute to development of gestational diabetes. Women with pica have been found to have lower hemoglobin levels than those of women without pica.

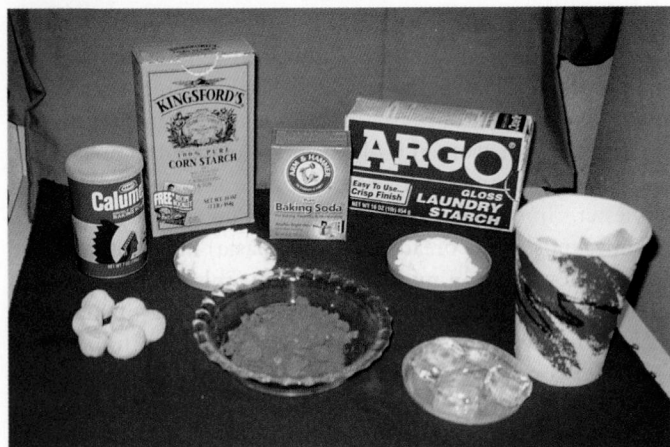

FIGURE 12-4 Nonfood substances consumed in pica: red clay from Georgia, Nzu from Eastern Nigeria, baking powder, corn starch, baking soda, laundry starch, and ice. Some individuals practise polypica (consuming more than one of these substances). (Courtesy Shannon Perry.)

Moreover, there is a risk that nonfood items are contaminated with heavy metals or other toxic substances. Among Mexican women, consumption of "tierra" includes both soil and pulverized Mexican pottery. Lead contamination of soils and soil-based products has caused high levels of lead in both pregnant women and their newborns. The possibility of pica must be considered when pregnant women are found to be anemic, and the nurse should provide counselling about the health risks associated with pica. The existence of pica and details of the types and amounts of products ingested are likely to be discovered only by the sensitive interviewer who has developed a relationship of trust with the woman.

Adolescent Pregnancy Needs

Pregnant adolescents and their infants are at increased risk of complications during pregnancy and postpartum. Dietary survey findings indicate that adolescent girls have inadequate intakes of vitamins (folate, vitamin A, E, B_6), minerals (calcium, iron, zinc), and fibre, as well as excessive intakes of total fat, saturated fat, sodium, and cholesterol (Alberta Health Services, 2013). Failure to consume an adequate diet during the adolescent period can result in delayed sexual maturation and can stop or slow linear growth.

Growth of the pelvis is delayed in comparison with growth in stature, which helps to explain why cephalopelvic disproportion and other mechanical problems associated with labour may be more common among young adolescents. Competition for nutrients between the growing adolescent and the fetus may also contribute to some of the poor outcomes apparent in teen pregnancies. Recommended weight-gain goals are not different from those of adult women. Pregnant adolescents should be encouraged to choose a weight-gain goal at the upper end of the range for their BMI. Adolescent females who have given birth have greater percentages of total fat and visceral fat (associated with the metabolic syndrome and cardiovascular disease) than those who have never given birth (Gunderson, Striegel-Moore, Schreiber, et al., 2009); thus the adolescent mother needs careful teaching regarding nutritional intake and physical activity to control body weight in the postpartum period.

Adolescents may not have adequate knowledge of nutrition, and their "present-focused" orientation may inhibit them from easily understanding how their current behaviours relate to later outcomes (Alberta Health Services, 2013). Efforts to improve the nutritional health of pregnant adolescents focus on the following:

- Improving the nutrition knowledge, meal planning, and food selection and preparation skills of young women
- Promoting access to prenatal care
- Developing nutrition interventions and educational programs that are effective with adolescents
- Striving to understand the factors that create barriers to change in the adolescent population

NURSING CARE

During pregnancy, nutrition plays a key role in achieving an optimal outcome for the mother and her unborn baby. Motivation to learn about nutrition is usually higher during pregnancy as parents strive to "do what's right for the baby." Optimal nutrition cannot eliminate all problems that may arise during pregnancy, but it does establish a good foundation for supporting the needs of the mother and her unborn baby.

Assessment

Ideally a nutritional assessment is performed before conception so that any recommended changes in diet, lifestyle, and weight can be undertaken before the woman becomes pregnant.

Information on nutrition and diet is obtained through an interview and review of the woman's health records, physical examination, and laboratory results.

Obstetrical and Gynecological Effects on Nutrition

Nutrition reserves may be depleted in the multiparous woman or one who has had frequent pregnancies (especially three pregnancies within 2 years). A history of preterm birth or the birth of an LBW or small-for-gestational-age (SGA) infant may indicate inadequate dietary intake. Birth of a large-for-gestational-age (LGA) infant often indicates the existence of maternal diabetes mellitus. Contraceptive methods also may affect reproductive health. Increased menstrual blood loss often occurs during the first 3 to 6 months after placement of an intrauterine contraceptive device; consequently the user may have low iron stores or even iron-deficiency anemia. Oral contraceptive agents are associated with decreased menstrual losses and increased iron stores; however, oral contraceptives may interfere with folic acid metabolism.

Health History

Chronic maternal illnesses such as diabetes mellitus, renal disease, liver disease, cystic fibrosis or other malabsorptive disorders, seizure disorders and the use of anticonvulsant agents, hypertension, and PKU may affect a woman's nutritional status and dietary needs. In women with illnesses that have resulted in nutrition deficits or that require dietary treatment (e.g., diabetes mellitus, PKU), it is extremely important that nutritional care be started and the condition be optimally controlled before conception. A registered dietitian can provide in-depth counselling for the woman who requires medical nutrition therapy during pregnancy and lactation.

Usual Maternal Diet

The woman's usual food and beverage intake, the adequacy of her income and other resources to meet her nutrition needs, any dietary modifications, food allergies and intolerances, all medications and nutrition supplements being taken, as well as pica and cultural dietary requirements should be ascertained. In addition, the presence and severity of nutrition-related discomforts of pregnancy such as morning sickness, constipation, and pyrosis (heartburn) should be determined (for management see Chapter 11). The nurse should be alert to any evidence of eating disorders such as anorexia nervosa, bulimia, or frequent and rigorous dieting before or during pregnancy.

The effect of food allergies and intolerances on nutritional status ranges from very important to almost nil. Lactose intolerance is of special concern in pregnant and lactating women because no other food group equals milk and milk products in terms of calcium content. If a woman has lactose intolerance, the interviewer should explore her intake of other calcium sources (see Box 12-4).

The assessment must include an evaluation of the woman's financial status and her knowledge of healthy dietary practices. The quality of the diet tends to improve with increasing socioeconomic status and educational level. Poor women may not have access to adequate refrigeration and cooking facilities and may find it difficult to obtain adequate nutritious food. Pregnancy rates can be high among homeless women, and prenatal nutrition programs may assist women in obtaining healthy food (see Community Focus box).

COMMUNITY FOCUS

Canada Prenatal Nutrition Program

The Canada Prenatal Nutrition Program (CPNP) funds community groups to develop or enhance programs for vulnerable pregnant women. Through a community development approach, the CPNP aims to reduce the incidence of unhealthy birth weights, improve the health of both infant and mother, and encourage breastfeeding.

Look for a Canada Prenatal Nutrition Program in your area. Contact the program and, if possible, visit the clinic. What services are offered by the program? Who are the clients that use this service? How difficult is it to access the services provided by the program? Does the clinic employ a dietitian or nutritionist? Are there materials and services provided in a variety of languages? Identify strengths and weaknesses of nutrition education in that setting. How do women get access to the services provided by CPNP?

Source: Public Health Agency of Canada. (2015). *Canada Prenatal Nutrition Program (CPNP)*. http://www.phac-aspc.gc.ca/hp-ps/dca-dea/prog-ini/cpnp-pcnp/index-eng.php

Box 12-5 provides a simple tool for obtaining diet history information. When potential problems are identified, they should be followed up with a careful interview.

Physical Examination

Anthropometric (body) measurements provide short- and long-term information on a woman's nutritional status and are thus essential to the assessment. At a minimum, the woman's height and weight must be determined at the time of her first prenatal visit, and her weight should be measured at each subsequent visit (see earlier discussion of BMI).

A careful physical examination can reveal objective signs of malnutrition (Table 12-4). However, it is important to note that some of these signs are nonspecific and that the physiological changes of pregnancy may complicate the interpretation of physical findings. For example, lower extremity edema often occurs in calorie and protein deficiency, but it may also be a normal finding in the third trimester of pregnancy. Interpretation of physical findings is made easier by taking a thorough health history and conducting laboratory testing, if indicated.

Laboratory Testing

The only nutrition-related laboratory testing needed by most pregnant women is a hematocrit or hemoglobin measurement to screen for the presence of anemia. Because of the physiological anemia of pregnancy, the reference values for hemoglobin and hematocrit must be adjusted during pregnancy. The lower limit of the normal range for hemoglobin during pregnancy is 110 g/L (compared with 120 g/L in the nonpregnant state). The lower limit of the normal range for hematocrit is 0.33 (compared with 0.37 in the nonpregnant state). Cut-off values for anemia are higher in women who smoke or live at high altitudes because the decreased oxygen-carrying capacity of their RBCs causes them to produce more RBCs than other women.

A woman's history or physical findings may indicate the need for additional testing. These tests might include a complete blood cell count with a differential to identify megaloblastic or macrocytic anemia and measurement of levels of specific vitamins or minerals believed to be lacking in the diet.

Nutrition Care and Teaching

For many women with uncomplicated pregnancies, the nurse can serve as the primary source of nutrition education during pregnancy (see Nursing Care Plan on Nutrition during Pregnancy on Evolve). The registered dietitian who has specialized training in evaluating diets, planning nutrition needs during illness, recognizing ethnic and cultural food patterns, and translating nutrient needs into food patterns frequently serves as a consultant. Pregnant women with serious nutrition problems, those with intervening illnesses such as diabetes (either preexisting or gestational), and any others requiring in-depth dietary counselling should be referred to the dietitian.

Nutrition teaching can take place in a one-on-one interview or in a group setting. In either case, teaching should emphasize the importance of choosing a varied diet using Canada's *Food*

BOX 12-5 FOOD INTAKE QUESTIONNAIRE

How many servings of the following did you eat or drink yesterday? If the way you ate yesterday wasn't the way you usually eat, choose a recent day that was typical for you.

Beer, wine, other alcoholic drinks _____
Tea _____
Coffee _____
Fruit drink _____
Water _____
Cheese _____
Macaroni and cheese _____
Other foods with cheese (such as lasagna, cheeseburgers) _____
Orange or grapefruit _____
Bananas _____
Peaches or apricots _____
Green salad _____
Spinach or greens _____
Green peas _____
Sweet potatoes _____
Carrots _____
Meat _____
Fish _____
Peanut butter _____
Dried beans or peas _____
Bacon or sausage _____
Bread _____
Rice _____
Spaghetti or other pasta _____
Tortillas _____
French fries _____
Orange or grapefruit juice _____
Fruit juice other than orange or grapefruit _____
Soft drinks _____
Milk _____
Cereal with milk _____
Yogurt _____
Pizza _____
Melon (such as watermelon, cantaloupe, honeydew) _____
Berries (specify kind) _____
Apples _____
Other fruit _____
Broccoli _____
Green beans _____
Potatoes (other than fried) _____
Corn _____
Other vegetables _____
Chicken or turkey _____
Eggs _____
Nuts _____
Hot dogs _____
Cold cuts (e.g., bologna) _____
Roll/bagel _____
Cereal _____
Noodles _____
Chips _____
Cake _____
Doughnuts or pastries _____
Cookies _____
Pie _____

Are you often bothered by any of the following? (Circle all that apply.)
Nausea Vomiting Heartburn Constipation

Are you on a special diet? No _____ Yes _____ If yes, what kind?

Do you try to limit the amount or kind of food you eat to control your weight? No ___ Yes ___

Do you avoid any foods for health or religious reasons?
No _____ Yes _____ If yes, what foods? _____

Do you take any prescribed drugs or medications? No _____
Yes _____ If yes, what are they? _____

Do you take any over-the-counter medications (such as aspirin, cold medicines, acetaminophen [Tylenol])? No _____
Yes _____ If yes, what are they? _____

Do you take any herbal supplements? No _____ Yes _____
If yes, what are they? _____

Do you ever have trouble affording the food you need?
No _____ Yes _____

Do you have any help getting the food you need? No _____
Yes _____ (If yes, circle all that apply.)
Prenatal Nutrition Program
School lunch or breakfast
Food from a food pantry, soup kitchen, or food bank

Guide, composed of readily available foods rather than specialized diet supplements. The importance of consuming adequate amounts from the milk, yogurt, and cheese group must be emphasized, especially for adolescents younger than 18 years of age who are still actively adding calcium to their skeletons; adolescents need at least 750 to 1000 mL (three to four glasses of milk) from the milk group daily. Good nutrition practices (and avoidance of poor practices such as smoking and alcohol or drug use) are essential content for prenatal classes designed for women in early pregnancy.

Eating Well With Canada's Food Guide can be used as a guide to making daily food choices during pregnancy, just as it is during other stages of the life cycle. Additional individualized information and resources are available from Health Canada at http://www.hc-sc.gc.ca/fn-an/food-guide-aliment/track-suivi/index-eng.php. On the website is an option for My Food Guide Servings Tracker (for Pregnancy or Lactation). *Eating Well With Canada's Food Guide* is translated into 10 different languages, including versions for First Nations, Inuit, and Métis. See Additional Resources listed at the end of the chapter.

Safe Food Preparation

Pregnant women and their unborn or newborn children are at an increased risk for foodborne illnesses because they have a weaker immune system. For example, pregnant women are

TABLE 12-4 PHYSICAL ASSESSMENT OF NUTRITIONAL STATUS

SIGNS OF GOOD NUTRITION	SIGNS OF POOR NUTRITION
General Appearance	
Alert, responsive, energetic, good endurance	Listless, apathetic, cachectic, easily fatigued, looks tired
Muscles	
Well developed, firm, good tone, some fat under skin	Flaccid, poor tone, undeveloped, tender, "wasted" appearance
Nervous System Function	
Good attention span, not irritable or restless, normal reflexes, psychological stability	Inattentive, irritable, confused, burning and tingling of hands and feet, loss of position and vibratory sense, weakness and tenderness of muscles, decrease or loss of ankle and knee reflexes
Gastrointestinal Function	
Good appetite and digestion, normal regular elimination, no palpable organs or masses	Anorexia, indigestion, constipation or diarrhea, liver or spleen enlargement
Cardiovascular Function	
Normal heart rate and rhythm, no murmurs, normal blood pressure for age	Rapid heart rate, enlarged heart, abnormal rhythm, elevated blood pressure
Hair	
Shiny, lustrous, firm, not easily plucked, healthy scalp	Stringy, dull, brittle, dry, thin and sparse, depigmented, can be easily plucked
Skin (General)	
Smooth, slightly moist, good colour	Rough, dry, scaly, pale, pigmented, irritated, easily bruised, petechiae
Face and Neck	
Skin colour uniform, smooth, pink, healthy appearance; no enlargement of thyroid gland; lips not chapped or swollen	Scaly, swollen, skin dark over cheeks and under eyes; lumpiness or flakiness of skin around nose and mouth; thyroid enlarged; lips swollen; angular lesions or fissures at corners of mouth
Oral Cavity	
Reddish pink mucous membranes and gums; no swelling or bleeding of gums; tongue healthy pink or deep red in appearance, not swollen or smooth, surface papillae present; teeth bright and clean, no cavities, no pain, no discolouration	Gums spongy, bleed easily, inflamed or receding; tongue swollen, scarlet and raw, magenta colour, beefy, hyperemic and hypertrophic papillae, atrophic papillae; teeth with unfilled caries, absent teeth, worn surfaces, mottled
Eyes	
Bright, clear, shiny, no sores at corners of eyelids, membranes moist and healthy pink colour, no prominent blood vessels or mound of tissue (Bitot's spots) on sclera, no fatigue circles beneath	Eye membranes pale, redness of membrane, dryness, signs of infection, Bitot's spots, redness and fissuring of eyelid corners, dryness of eye membrane, dull appearance of cornea, soft cornea, blue sclera
Extremities	
No tenderness, weakness, or swelling; nails firm and pink	Edema, tender calves, tingling, weakness; nails spoon-shaped, brittle
Skeleton	
No malformations	Bowlegs, knock-knees, chest deformity at diaphragm, beaded ribs, prominent scapulas

about 20 times more likely to get listeriosis than other healthy adults. Listeriosis is a rare but serious infection caused by consuming a type of bacterium called *Listeria monocytogenes* (commonly called *Listeria*) that is sometimes found in food, water, and soil. If a pregnant woman develops listeriosis during the first 3 months of her pregnancy, she may experience a miscarriage. Up to 2 weeks before a miscarriage, pregnant women may experience a mild flu-like illness with chills, fatigue, headache, as well as muscular and joint pain. Listeriosis later on in the pregnancy can result in a stillbirth or the birth of an acutely ill child (PHAC, 2012).

For safe preparation of food and to decrease the risk of contracting listeriosis or other foodborne illnesses see Patient Teaching Box.

PATIENT TEACHING

Prevention of Foodborne Illness

- Follow all food instructions on the label of the package.
- Cleanse hands frequently.
- Clean and sanitize all food preparation surfaces, knives, and utensils with a kitchen sanitizer or using a 5-mL ratio of household bleach to 750 mL of water followed by a water rinse. This is particularly important when preparing raw fish or meat.
- Clean all fruits and vegetables carefully before eating.
- Refrigerate any perishable or prepared foods at 4°C or below. The warmer the refrigerator, the higher the bacterial count will be. Keep leftovers for only 2 to 3 days and reheat to an internal temperature of 74°C.
- Defrost frozen foods in the refrigerator, in cold water, or in the microwave, but never defrost at room temperature.
- Wash and disinfect the refrigerator on a frequent basis, which decreases the risk of bacteria in food being transferred to uncontaminated food stuff.
- Avoid contact between raw meat, fish, or poultry and other foods that will not be cooked before consumption.
- Cook foods to a safe temperature.
- Avoid consumption of unpasteurized milk or products made with unpasteurized milk, including soft cheeses (Brie, Camembert); patés and meat spreads; raw eggs; raw sprouts (bean, mung); smoked seafood (unless cooked); raw seafood; hot dogs, luncheon meats, bologna and non-dried deli meats should be eaten only if they have been reheated to steaming hot.

Source: Health Canada. (2010). *Safe food handling for pregnant women.* Government of Canada. Retrieved from http://publications.gc.ca/collections/collection_2010/sc-hc/H14-55-2-2010-eng.pdf; Health Canada. (2016). *Listeria and listeriosis.* Government of Canada. Retrieved from http://healthycanadians.gc.ca/eating-nutrition/risks-recalls-rappels-risques/poisoning-intoxication/poisoning-intoxication/listeriosis-listeria-listeriose-eng.php

SAFETY ALERT

Pregnant women who contract listeriosis, a disease resulting from infection with the bacteria *Listeria,* are at increased risk for miscarriage, premature birth, and stillbirth. During pregnancy, women should not consume unpasteurized milk or products made with unpasteurized milk, including soft cheeses such as Brie and Camembert. Hot dogs, luncheon meats, bologna, and deli meats should be eaten only if they have been reheated to be steaming hot.

Medical Nutrition Therapy

During pregnancy and lactation, the food plan for women with special medical nutrition therapy may have to be modified. The registered dietitian can instruct these women about their diets and assist them in meal planning. However, the nurse should understand the basic principles of the diet and be able to reinforce the diet teaching.

The nurse should be especially aware of the dietary modifications necessary for women with diabetes mellitus (either gestational or pre-existing). This disease is relatively common, and fetal morbidity and mortality occur more often in pregnancies complicated by **hyperglycemia** or **hypoglycemia** (see discussion of diabetes in Chapter 15). Every effort should be made to maintain blood glucose levels in the normal range throughout pregnancy. The food plan of the woman with diabetes usually includes four to six meals and snacks daily, with the daily carbohydrate intake distributed fairly evenly among the meals and snacks. The complex carbohydrates—fibres and starches—should be well represented in the diet. To maintain strict control of the blood glucose level, the pregnant woman with diabetes usually must monitor her own blood glucose daily.

Gluten-Free Diet

Many women are eating gluten-free diets either due to *celiac disease*, which is a condition where the small intestine is damaged by eating foods that contain gluten, or due to personal choice. Gluten is a type of protein that is found in many grains like wheat, barley, rye, and any foods that contain these grains. A woman consuming a gluten-free diet can obtain all the necessary nutrients required for pregnancy. One concern may be the decreased intake of fibre when eating a gluten-free diet. Pregnant women should consume 28 g of fibre/day. See Table 12-1 for examples of fibre.

Vegetarian Diets

Women who consume vegetarian diets may require extra counselling to ensure all nutritional needs are met. Foods basic to almost all vegetarian diets are vegetables, fruits, legumes, nuts, seeds, and grains, but with many variations. **Lacto-vegetarians** include milk products in their diet. Lacto-ovovegetarians consume eggs and dairy products in addition to plant products. Strict vegetarians, or **vegans**, consume only plant products. All of these types of vegetarian diets, if they are well planned, can be nutritionally adequate for pregnant and lactating women (Craig & Mangels, 2009). Because vitamin B_{12} is found only in foods of animal origin, this diet is deficient in vitamin B_{12}. As a result, strict vegetarians should take a supplement or regularly consume vitamin B_{12}–fortified foods (e.g., soy milk). Vitamin B_{12} deficiency can result in megaloblastic anemia, glossitis (inflamed red tongue), and neurological deficits in the mother. Infants born to affected mothers are likely to have megaloblastic anemia and exhibit neurodevelopmental delays. The diet should be carefully planned to include adequate minerals. Iron and zinc may not be as well absorbed from plant foods as they are from meats, and calcium intake can be low if milk products are avoided. Plant proteins tend to be "incomplete," in that they lack one or more amino acids required for growth and the maintenance of body tissues. However, the daily consumption of a variety of different plant proteins—grains, dried beans and peas, nuts, and seeds—can provide all of the **essential amino acids**.

Cultural Influences

Consideration of a woman's cultural food preferences enhances the nurse's communication with the woman and provides a greater opportunity for the woman to follow necessary food requirements. Women in most cultures are encouraged to eat a diet typical for them. The nurse needs to be aware of what constitutes a typical diet for each cultural or ethnic group in the patient population. However, because several variations may occur within one cultural group, a careful exploration of individual preferences is needed. Food cravings during pregnancy are considered normal by many cultures, but the kinds of cravings often are culturally specific. In most cultures, women crave acceptable foods, such as chicken, fish, and greens.

Coping with Nutrition-Related Discomforts of Pregnancy

The most common nutrition-related discomforts of pregnancy are nausea and vomiting (or "morning sickness"), constipation, and pyrosis.

Nausea and vomiting. Nausea and vomiting are most common during the first trimester in 85% of women, and although nausea and vomiting usually cause only mild-to-moderate nutrition problems, it may be a source of substantial discomfort. Antiemetic medications, vitamin B_6, ginger, and pericardium 6 acupressure (Fig. 12-5) may be effective in reducing the severity of nausea. The pregnant woman may find the suggestions in Patient Teaching Box: Managing Nausea and Vomiting During Pregnancy helpful in alleviating the problem.

Hyperemesis gravidarium, or severe and persistent vomiting causing weight loss, dehydration, and electrolyte imbalances, occurs in about 1% of pregnant women. Intravenous fluid and electrolyte replacement, enteral tube feeding, and in some instances total parenteral nutrition have been used to nourish women with hyperemesis gravidarum. See Chapter 14, p. 326, for discussion on this condition.

Constipation. Improved bowel function generally results from increasing the intake of fibre (e.g., wheat bran and whole-wheat products, popcorn, and raw or lightly steamed vegetables) in the diet. Fibre helps retain water within the stool, creating a bulky stool that stimulates intestinal peristalsis. The recommendation for pregnant women for fibre is 28 g/day. An adequate fluid intake (at least 50 mL/kg/day) helps hydrate the fibre and increase the bulk of the stool. Warm or hot fluids may increase peristalsis more than cold fluids. Making a habit of regular exercise that uses large muscle groups (walking, swimming, cycling) also helps stimulate bowel motility. Laxatives should not be taken unless first discussed with a health care provider.

Pyrosis. Pyrosis, or heartburn, is usually caused by reflux of gastric contents into the esophagus. This condition is common in 40 to 85% of pregnant women (Koren & Maltepe, 2013). This condition can be minimized by using the following strategies:

- Eating small, frequent meals, rather than two or three larger meals, daily
- Adding a source of protein to each snack
- Avoiding drinking fluids with a meal as fluids increase the distension of the stomach
- Avoiding foods that are high in fat
- Adding probiotics (e.g., yogurt or acidophilus) or digestive enzymes may be helpful
- Avoiding lying down immediately after eating as reflux can be exacerbated by lying down

Occasionally, women may take antacids to help with heartburn. Not all antacids are safe; thus women should check with their health care provider prior to taking medication.

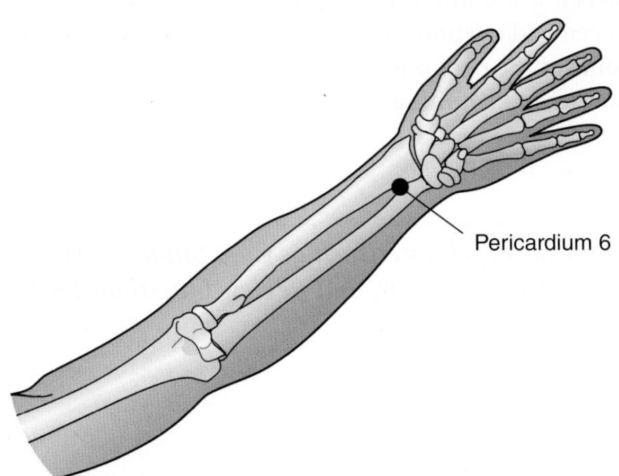

FIGURE 12-5 Pericardium 6 (P6) acupressure/acupuncture point for nausea.

NUTRIENT NEEDS DURING LACTATION

Nutrition needs during lactation are similar in many ways to those during pregnancy (see Table 12-1 and previous discussion

PATIENT TEACHING

Managing Nausea and Vomiting During Pregnancy

- Try to eat small amounts of food every 1 to 2 hours, as this will help balance blood sugar levels, and do not eat or drink too much at one time.
- Try not to mix food and drinks. Drink liquids 20 to 30 minutes before or after you eat. Do not drink alcohol at all.
- Do not skip meals.
- Try to eat high-carbohydrate, low-fat foods and low-fat dairy products, as they are easier to digest.
- Try to add any source of protein to each meal and snack.
- Try to minimize or avoid spicy, fried, or high-fat foods.
- Avoid strong odours.
- Avoid sudden movements. Get out of bed slowly and eat soon after getting out of bed.
- Try salty and tart foods (e.g., potato chips and lemonade) during periods of nausea. Sucking a lemon slice may help.
- Breathe fresh air to help relieve nausea. Keep the environment well ventilated (e.g., open a window), go for a walk outside, or decrease cooking odours by using an exhaust fan.
- Eat foods served at room or cool temperatures and foods that give off little aroma.
- Try candies, gums, and lozenges to help minimize the metallic taste in your mouth.
- Avoid brushing teeth immediately after eating.

Alternative Therapies

- Herbal teas such as those made with mint, ginger, or orange have also been used for morning sickness (see herbal teas listed earlier in the chapter, on p. 277)
- Ginger (up to 1000 mg/day)
- Vitamin B_6 (up to 200 mg/day)
- Acupuncture or acupressure

Source: Koren, G., & Maltepe, C. (2013). *How to survive morning sickness successfully.* Motherisk. http://www.motherisk.org/documents/BSRC_morning_sickness_EN.pdf

on pregnancy). Needs for energy (kilocalories), protein, calcium, iodine, zinc, the B vitamins (thiamine, riboflavin, niacin, pyridoxine, and vitamin B_{12}), and vitamin C remain greater than nonpregnant needs. The recommendations for some of these (e.g., vitamin C, zinc, and protein) are slightly to moderately higher than during pregnancy. This allowance covers the amount of the nutrients released in the milk, as well as the needs of the mother for tissue maintenance. In the case of iron and folic acid, the recommendation during lactation is lower than that during pregnancy. Both of these nutrients are essential for RBC formation and thus for maintaining the increase in the blood volume that occurs during pregnancy. With the decrease in maternal blood volume to nonpregnant levels after birth, maternal iron and folic acid needs also decrease. Many lactating women have a delay in the return of menses; this conserves blood cells and also reduces iron and folic acid needs. It is especially important that the calcium intake be adequate; if it is not, a supplement of 600 mg of calcium per day may be needed.

The recommended energy intake for the first 6 months is an increase of 330 kcal more than the woman's nonpregnant intake. This is equivalent to two to three servings from *Eating Right With Canada's Food Guide*. It is difficult to obtain adequate nutrients for maintenance of lactation if total caloric intake is less than 1800 kcal. Because of the deposition of energy stores, the woman who has gained the optimal amount of weight during pregnancy is heavier after birth than at the beginning of pregnancy. As a result of the caloric demands of lactation, the lactating mother usually experiences a gradual but steady weight loss. Most women rapidly lose several kilograms during the first month after birth, whether or not they breastfeed. After the first month, the average loss during lactation is 0.5 to 1 kg a month, and a woman who is overweight may be able to lose up to 2 kg without decreasing her milk supply.

Fluid intake must be adequate to maintain milk production; the mother's level of thirst is the best guide to the right amount. There is no need to consume more fluids than those needed to satisfy thirst.

Smoking, alcohol intake, and excessive caffeine intake should be avoided during lactation. Smoking not only may impair milk production, but it also exposes the infant to the risk of passive smoking. It is speculated that the infant's psychomotor development may be affected by maternal alcohol use, and alcoholic beverages (two drinks per day) may impair the milk ejection reflex. Caffeine intake can lead to a reduced iron concentration in milk and consequently contribute to the development of anemia in the infant. The caffeine concentration in milk is only approximately 1% of the mother's plasma level, but caffeine seems to accumulate in the infant. Breastfed infants of mothers who drink large amounts of coffee or caffeine-containing soft drinks may be unusually active and wakeful.

KEY POINTS

- A woman's nutritional status before, during, and after pregnancy contributes significantly to her well-being and that of her infant.
- A healthy diet can impact the health of the mother and fetus, and different factors can influence the ability of a pregnant woman to access a healthy diet.
- Many physiological changes occurring during pregnancy and lactation influence the need for additional nutrients and the efficiency with which the body uses them.
- Both the total maternal weight gain and the pattern of weight gain are important determinants of the outcome of pregnancy.
- The appropriateness of the mother's prepregnancy weight for height (BMI) is a major determinant of her recommended weight gain during pregnancy.
- Nutritional risk factors include adolescent pregnancy, nicotine use, alcohol or drug use, faddish food habits, a low weight for height, and frequent pregnancies.
- Iron supplementation is usually recommended during pregnancy. Other supplements may be warranted when nutritional risk factors are present.
- The nurse and the woman are influenced by cultural and personal values and beliefs that the nurse needs to take into account during nutrition counselling.
- Pregnancy complications that may be nutrition related include anemia, gestational hypertension, gestational diabetes, and intrauterine growth restriction (IUGR).
- Dietary adaptation can be an effective intervention for some of the common discomforts of pregnancy, including nausea and vomiting, constipation, and heartburn.

evolve WEBSITE

Visit the Evolve website for additional resources related to the content in this chapter such as Case Studies, Critical Thinking Case Study Answers, Nursing Care Plans, Nursing Processes, Nursing Skills, and Review Questions for Exam Preparation at: *http://evolve.elsevier.com/Canada/Perry/maternal/*

REFERENCES

Alberta Health Services. (2013). *Nutrition guideline pregnancy*. Retrieved from <http://www.albertahealthservices.ca/assets/Infofor/hp/if-hp-ed-cdm-ns-4-1-1-pregnancy.pdf>.

British Columbia Ministry of Health. (2010). *Iron deficiency: Investigation and management*. Retrieved from <http://www2.gov.bc.ca/assets/gov/health/practitioner-pro/bc-guidelines/iron_deficiency.pdf>.

Craig, W., & Mangels, A. (2009). Position of the American Dietetic Association: Vegetarian diets. *Journal of American Dietetic Association, 109*(7), 1266–1282.

Davies, G. A., Maxwell, C., McLeod, L., et al. (2010). *SOGC clinical practice guideline: Obesity in pregnancy.*

Gunderson, E., Striegel-Moore, R., Schreiber, G., et al. (2009). Longitudinal study of growth and adiposity in parous compared with nulligravid adolescents. *Archives of Pediatric & Adolescence Medicine, 163*(4), 349–356.

Health Canada. (2009). *Prenatal nutrition guidelines for health professionals: Fish and omega 3 fatty acids* (Cat. No. H164-109/4-2009E-PDF). Ottawa: Author. Retrieved from <http://www.hc-sc.gc.ca/fn-an/pubs/nutrition/omega3-eng.php>.

Health Canada (2011a). *Prenatal nutrition.* Ottawa: Author. Retrieved from <http://www.hc-sc.gc.ca/fn-an/nutrition/prenatal/index-eng.php>.

Health Canada. (2011b). *Mercury in fish: Questions and answers.* Ottawa: Author. Retrieved from <http://www.hc-sc.gc.ca/fn-an/securit/chem-chim/environ/mercur/merc_fish_qa-poisson_qr-eng.php>.

Health Canada. (2014a). *Prenatal nutrition guidelines for health professionals. Gestational weight gain.* Retrieved from <http://www.hc-sc.gc.ca/fn-an/nutrition/prenatal/ewba-mbsa-eng.php>.

Health Canada. (2014b). *Folic acid, iron and pregnancy.* Ottawa: Author. Retrieved from: <http://healthycanadians.gc.ca/healthy-living-vie-saine/pregnancy-grossesse/folic-acid-acide-folique-eng.php>.

HealthLink, B. C. (2013). *Energy drinks.* Healthlink BC, File 109. Retrieved from <http://www.healthlinkbc.ca/healthfiles/hfile109.stm>.

Koren, G., & Maltepe, C. (2013). *How to survive morning sickness successfully.* Toronto: Motherisk. <http://www.motherisk.org/documents/BSRC_morning_sickness_EN.pdf>.

Public Health Agency of Canada. (2012). *Listeria.* Retrieved from <http://www.phac-aspc.gc.ca/fs-sa/fs-fi/listerios-eng.php>.

Public Health Agency of Canada. (2013). *Congenital anomalies in Canada 2013: A perinatal health surveillance report.* Ottawa: PHAC. Cat No. HP35-40/2013E-PDF Retrieved from <http://publications.gc.ca/collections/collection_2014/aspc-phac/HP35-40-2013-eng.pdf>.

Public Health Agency of Canada. (2014). *Health and pregnancy: Caffeine and pregnancy.* Ottawa: PHAC. <http://www.phac-aspc.gc.ca/hp-gs/know-savoir/caffeine-eng.php>.

Shannon, M. (2003). Severe lead poisoning in pregnancy. *Ambulatory Pediatrics, 3*(1), 37–39.

Statistics Canada. (2011). *Overweight and obese adults (self-reported), 2010.* Ottawa: Author. Retrieved <http://www.statcan.gc.ca/pub/82-625-x/2011001/article/11464-eng.htm>.

Wilson, R. D., & Genetics Committee. (2015). Pre-conception folic acid and multivitamin supplementation for the primary and secondary prevention of neural tube defects and other folic acid-sensitive congenital anomalies. *Journal of Obstetrics & Gynaecology Canada, 37*(6), 534–549.

ADDITIONAL RESOURCES

Alberta Health Services—Nutrition Guideline Pregnancy: <http://www.albertahealthservices.ca/assets/Infofor/hp/if-hp-ed-cdm-ns-4-1-1-pregnancy.pdf>.

Canadian Consensus on Female Nutrition: Adolescence, Reproduction, Menopause and Beyond: <http://www.jogc.com/article/S1701-2163(16)00042-6/fulltext>.

Eating Well With Canada's Food Guide: First Nations, Inuit and Métis: <http://www.hc-sc.gc.ca/fn-an/pubs/fnim-pnim/index-eng.php>.

Eating Well With Canada's Food Guide: Translated Versions of the Guide (10 different languages): <http://www.hc-sc.gc.ca/fn-an/food-guide-aliment/order-commander/guide_trans-trad-eng.php>.

Eat Right Ontario: <http://www.eatrightontario.ca/en/default.aspx>.

Health Canada: Eating Well With Canada's Food Guide for Pregnancy—My Food Guide Serving Tracker: <http://www.hc-sc.gc.ca/fn-an/food-guide-aliment/track-suivi/table_female-femme_preg-ence_age19-50-eng.php>.

Health Canada: Pregnancy Weight Gain Calculator: <http://www.hc-sc.gc.ca/fn-an/nutrition/prenatal/bmi/index-eng.php>.

Health Canada—Prenatal Nutrition Guidelines for Health Professionals: Background on Canada's Food Guide: <http://www.hc-sc.gc.ca/fn-an/pubs/nutrition/guide-prenatal-eng.php>.

Health Canada—Safe fish consumption: <http://www.hc-sc.gc.ca/fn-an/securit/chem-chim/environ/mercur/cons-adv-etud-eng.php>.

Motherisk: <http://www.motherisk.org/women/index.jsp>.

CHAPTER

13

Pregnancy Risk Factors and Assessment

Nancy Watts

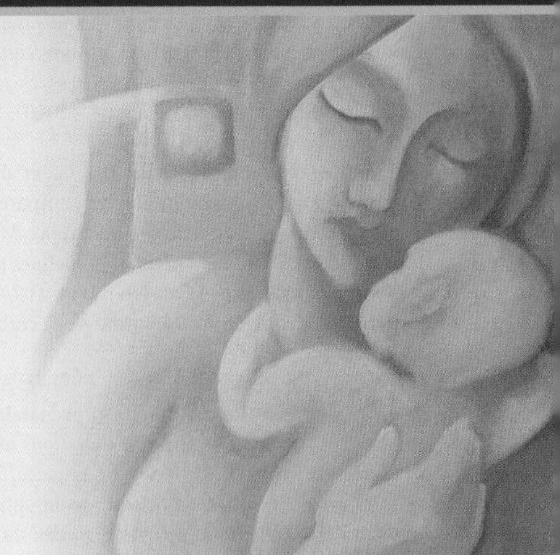

evolve WEBSITE

Visit the Evolve website for additional resources related to the content in this chapter such as Case Studies, Critical Thinking Case Study Answers, Nursing Care Plans, Nursing Processes, Nursing Skills, and Review Questions for Exam Preparation at: http://evolve.elsevier.com/Canada/Perry/maternal/

OBJECTIVES

On completion of this chapter the reader will be able to:

- Explore biophysical, psychosocial, sociodemographic, and environmental influences on high-risk pregnancy.
- Identify the determinants of health that influence pregnancy outcomes.
- Examine risk factors identified through history taking, physical examination, and diagnostic techniques.
- Differentiate among screening and diagnostic techniques, including when they are used in pregnancy and for what purpose.
- Discuss psychological considerations associated with a high-risk pregnancy diagnosis.
- Develop a teaching plan to explain screening and diagnostic techniques and the implications of findings to women and their families.

Although most pregnancies and births are considered low risk, there are pregnancies categorized as high risk due to maternal or fetal complications. Identification of the risks, together with appropriate and timely intervention during the perinatal period, can prevent morbidity and mortality among mothers and infants.

Using current Canadian demographic information, women and families can be identified as at risk on the basis of factors other than biophysical criteria. The increasing numbers of pregnant women who have limited access to prenatal care during any stage of pregnancy, as well as behaviours and lifestyles that pose a risk to the health of the mother and fetus, contribute to the increasing incidence of high-risk pregnancies. More women are presenting with mental health issues during the perinatal period, with the incidence as high as 1 in 5 reported in British Columbia for four different diagnoses contributing to increased risk in pregnancy (BC Reproductive & Mental Health Program & Perinatal Services BC, 2014; Public Health Agency of Canada [PHAC], 2012). Access to prenatal care may be challenged by language barriers, past negative experiences with health care providers, lack of transportation, and limited health care facilities available in remote or rural communities.

Care of high-risk patients requires the collaborative efforts of various health care providers. In this chapter, care of the high-risk woman and the factors associated with a diagnosis of high risk are discussed. Diagnostic techniques used to monitor the maternal–fetal unit are also outlined. Finally, psychological considerations of care of the woman experiencing a high-risk pregnancy are addressed.

DEFINITION AND SCOPE OF HIGH RISK PREGNANCY

A *high-risk pregnancy* is one in which the life or health of the mother or infant is jeopardized by a disorder coincident with or unique to pregnancy. For the mother, the high-risk status arbitrarily extends through the puerperium (approximately 6 weeks after childbirth). Postbirth maternal complications related to the pregnancy usually are resolved within 1 month of birth, but perinatal morbidity may continue for months or years. Ongoing medical challenges present before the pregnancy may have been improved or worsened during pregnancy and may take 3 to 6 months to return to prepregnancy stability.

High-risk pregnancy is a critical problem for modern medical and nursing care. The current social emphasis on quality of life and the wanted child has resulted in a reduction of family size and the number of unwanted pregnancies. At the same time, technological advances have facilitated pregnancies in previously infertile couples. As a consequence, emphasis is on the safe birth of normal infants who can develop to their potential. Scientific and technological advances have allowed perinatal health care to reach a level far beyond that previously available.

The diagnosis of high risk imposes a situational crisis on the family. These crises include, for example, loss of pregnancy before the anticipated date and a fetal or maternal diagnosis that requires decision making about whether to continue or interrupt the pregnancy or birth of a newborn who does not meet cultural, societal, or familial norms and expectations.

Determinants of Health as Risk Factors

There are many factors that contribute to high-risk pregnancies; an analysis of the determinants of health (see Table 1-1) provides a more comprehensive approach to providing care. Social and individual factors associated with high-risk childbearing include income and social status, social support networks, education, employment and working conditions, physical environment, personal health practices and coping skills, biology and genetics, availability of health services, and culture. Some personal health practices and lack of coping skills can place the mother and fetus at risk. Examples include problematic substance use, lack of prenatal care, inadequate nutritional status or dental hygiene, and psychosocial stressors (Box 13-1).

The determinants of health are interrelated and cumulative in their effects on health outcomes. The quality of the social determinants of health that Canadians experience determines the wide inequalities that exist throughout the country and for child-bearing families (Mikkonen & Raphael, 2010). A comprehensive database for pregnancy risk assessment can help ensure that appropriate resources are available. In Canada, the Canadian Perinatal Surveillance System (CPSS) provides this database (see Chapter 4, p. 51). The CPSS reports on 29 maternal, fetal, and infant health determinants and outcomes. The view is that health status is influenced by a range of factors; thus it is important to monitor not only health outcomes but also factors—such as behaviours, physical and social environments, and health services—that may affect those outcomes.

BOX 13-1 INFLUENCE OF DETERMINANTS OF HEALTH ON MATERNAL AND NEWBORN OUTCOMES

Biology and Genetic Factors

Genetic Considerations

Genetic risks include heritable factors that originate within the mother or fetus and affect the development or functioning of either or both. Genetic factors may interfere with normal fetal or newborn development, result in congenital anomalies, or create difficulties for the mother. These factors include altered genes, transmittable inherited disorders, chromosome anomalies, multiple pregnancy, large fetal size, and ABO incompatibility. A genetic risk assessment should be done to determine the family's risk (see Chapter 9).

Demographic Characteristics

Availability of Health Care

The availability and quality of prenatal care vary greatly with geographic region. Women in urban areas have more prenatal visits than women in remote and rural areas, who have fewer opportunities for specialized care because of the distance they have to travel to get to it. Women in lower socioeconomic situations are also less likely to see a specialist and more likely to wait longer for an appointment. Women who are recent immigrants to Canada may experience challenges accessing health care because they lack knowledge of the prenatal care visit schedule or have difficulty obtaining a health care provider, particularly one that is culturally competent or can provide care in their language of origin. Other women may struggle with the cost of new prescriptions if they do not have a drug plan.

Physical Environment

There may be unsafe soil and water conditions and environmental exposure to pollutants, such as paint with lead content. Many Indigenous communities have boil-water alerts to ensure that they are drinking safe water. Another example is the consumption of mercury-contaminated fish, which may pose health risks to a developing fetus.

Income and Social Status

Income may be the most important determinant of health because of its influence on living conditions, level of education, quality of diet, and extent of physical activity (Mikkonen & Raphael, 2010). A lower income level is associated with an increased risk for medical complications of pregnancy. A woman with a lower income may not have as many support people to ask for assistance, to arrange for transportation to appointments or for child care (United Nations [UN] Development Program, 2011).

Education

A woman's level of education can reflect her knowledge of the importance of prenatal care and awareness of where to receive it. Having a higher education level increases women's confidence in asking questions and making choices and has been associated with fewer adverse outcomes in pregnancy and postpartum (UN Development Program, 2011).

Social Support Networks

The increased mortality and morbidity rates for single women, including a greater risk for pre-eclampsia, are often related to inadequate prenatal care, lower socioeconomic status, lower level of education, and a younger child-bearing age. The availability of social networks and close community ties have been shown to alleviate barriers related to lower income and education (UN Development Program, 2011).

Continued

BOX 13-1 INFLUENCE OF DETERMINANTS OF HEALTH ON MATERNAL AND NEWBORN OUTCOMES—cont'd

Culture

Infant mortality rates are higher among Indigenous people. Indigenous women have described encounters with health care providers that include judgement of their lifestyle choices, racism, and discrimination. Many factors influence whether they attend prenatal care visits, including lack of transportation, complex life situations, and whether they have had experience with child protection services. Women have described their willingness to seek health care for their children but a reluctance to seek their own health care because of past negative experiences (Denison, Varcoe, & Browne, 2014; Di Lallo, 2014).

Among other cultural groups there may be cultural beliefs that do not support the prenatal care schedule used in Canada; for example, there are differences across countries as to when to initiate care. There may also be discrimination against members of marginalized communities or language barriers to receiving culturally competent prenatal care (UN Development Program, 2011).

Employment/Working Hazards

Occupational hazards can be grouped into chemical, physical, biological, and psychological hazards. The risk to the fetus depends on the timing of the exposure, the dose, and fetal and maternal susceptibility. Women who work at highly physically demanding jobs or are exposed to hazards such as industrial fumes or do shift work have higher pregnancy risks.

Personal Health Practices and Coping Skills

Substance Use

Smoking is associated with intrauterine growth restriction, preterm birth, and low birth weight. Alcohol consumption has adverse effects on the fetus, resulting in fetal alcohol spectrum disorders, which include fetal alcohol syndrome, alcohol-related neurodevelopmental disorder, and alcohol-related birth defects. Recreational or prescribed medication misuse can be teratogenic, cause metabolic disturbances, produce chemical effects, or cause depression or alteration of central nervous system function.

Nutritional Status

Adequate nutrition is one of the most important determinants of pregnancy outcome, for without it, fetal growth and development cannot proceed normally (see Fig. 12-1). Dietary deficiencies are more common among households with children that have a single parent, are part of an Indigenous area, and are receiving social assistance (Mikkonnen & Raphael, 2010). Conditions that influence nutritional status include the following: young age of the mother; three pregnancies in the previous 2 years; tobacco, alcohol, or problematic substance use; inadequate dietary intake because of chronic illness or food fads; and inadequate or excessive weight gain (see Chapter 12).

Dental Hygiene

Periodontal disease increases the risk for preterm birth and low birth weight. Women may not have adequate information about the need for ongoing dental hygiene and health promotion during pregnancy.

Psychosocial Stressors

Child-bearing triggers profound and complex physiological, psychological, and social changes; evidence suggests a relationship between emotional distress and birth complications. This risk factor includes conditions such as specific intrapsychic disturbances and addictive lifestyles; a history of child abuse or intimate partner violence (see discussion later); inadequate support systems; family disruption or dissolution; and maternal role changes or conflicts.

References

Denison, J., Varcoe, C., & Browne, A. (2014). Aboriginal women's experience of accessing healthcare when state apprehension of children is being threatened. *Journal of Advanced Nursing, 70*(5), 1105–1116.

Di Lallo, S. (2014). Prenatal care through the eyes of Canadian Aboriginal women. *Nursing for Women's Health, 18*(1), 38–46.

Mikkonen, J., & Raphael, D. (2010). *Social determinants of health: The Canadian facts.* Retrieved from <http://www.thecanadianfacts.org/the_canadian_facts.pdf>.

United Nations Development Program: Bureau for Development Policy. (2011). *Discussion paper: A social determinants approach to maternal health.* New York: Author. Retrieved from <http://www.undp.org/content/dam/undp/library/Democratic%20Governance/Discussion%20Paper%20MaternalHealth.pdf>.

Additional source: Public Health Agency of Canada. (2013). *Canadian perinatal report—2013 edition* (Cat. HP7-1/2013E-PDF). Ottawa: Government of Canada.

Regionalization of Health Care Services

Early and ongoing risk assessment is a crucial component of perinatal care. Conditions that are associated with perinatal morbidity and mortality can be prevented or treated by general perinatal health services, or they may require referral to more specialized health care providers. Factors to consider when determining a woman's risk status include resources available locally to treat the condition, availability of appropriate facilities for transport if needed, and determination of the best health care match for the woman's needs.

It is neither feasible nor reasonable for each hospital to develop and maintain the full spectrum of services required for treating high-risk perinatal patients. Consequently, health care has become regionalized, creating a system of coordinated care in which facilities within a geographic region are organized to provide different levels of care. This system also applies to preconception and ambulatory prenatal care services (see Community Focus box).

MATERNAL HEALTH PROBLEMS

The leading causes of maternal death attributable to pregnancy differ throughout the world. In general, three major causes have persisted over the last 50 years: hypertensive disorders, infection, and hemorrhage. In Canada today, the leading causes of maternal mortality are hypertensive disorders, pulmonary and amniotic embolism, hemorrhage, and other causes, such as mental illness. Factors strongly related to maternal death include age (younger than 20 years or 35 years or older), lack of prenatal

COMMUNITY FOCUS

Resources for Women Experiencing a High-Risk Pregnancy

Contact the nearest high-risk pregnancy unit to assess the resources available for women (e.g., pamphlets, websites for high-risk pregnancies) and to learn what screening is recommended during pregnancy to identify problems. For what problems is the screening conducted? What information or resources are available in your community for the problems identified? Are there specialized clinics for different populations—for example, bariatric clinics, mental health obstetrical clinics, or those for women with high-risk fetal diagnoses? How can women access the resources that are available? What geographic area does this unit serve? What determinants of health are influencing these women's lives? What is the role of the nurse in this unit?

care, and low education level. Box 13-2 lists common risk factors for several pregnancy-related problems.

In Canada in 2013, the annual **maternal mortality rate** (number of maternal deaths per 100,000 live births) was 11 (World Health Organization [WHO], 2014). Although the overall number of maternal deaths is small, maternal mortality remains a significant problem because a high proportion of these deaths are preventable, primarily through improving access to and use of prenatal care services. Nurses can be instrumental in educating the public about the importance of obtaining early and regular care during pregnancy.

Mental Health Concerns

Mental health issues may develop during the antepartum period, or they may already be present as a woman is deciding to become pregnant. Grigoriadis, VonderPorten, Mamisashvili, et al. (2013) found in a literature review that depression in mothers may have detrimental effects on perinatal outcome, such as preterm labour and lower rates of breastfeeding initiation. Depression during pregnancy is also related to poor maternal self-care, which may influence the baby's health (Dennis & Dowswell, 2013). Early education for prenatal patients and families about depression is an essential part of health promotion. Interprofessional collaboration and appropriate referrals are important interventions for the nurse to initiate when concerns regarding depression are identified.

British Columbia Mental Health Program and Perinatal Services British Columbia have developed guiding principles for the care of women with mental health issues (BC Reproductive Mental Health Program & Perinatal Services BC, 2014). The guiding principles include the following:

- All women from a variety of backgrounds (social, economic, racial, cultural) are at risk for mental health issues (as many as 1 in 5 women in the perinatal period).
- Providing services that preserve the mother–infant dyad is optimal.
- Care needs to be provided in a humane, supportive, caring environment so that women feel strengthened and supported while being treated. These women will often present in an acute state of distress, have fragile self-esteem, and experience multiple complex stressors.
- A collaborative team approach is optimal.
- Every effort should be made within communities to link services to provide support to women.

Newborns are sensitive to the emotional states of their mothers. If the mother is distressed or has a mental health issue, this can

BOX 13-2 SPECIFIC PREGNANCY PROBLEMS AND RELATED RISK FACTORS

Polyhydramnios
- Diabetes in pregnancy, with blood glucose levels beyond target levels
- Fetal congenital anomalies (e.g., gastrointestinal obstruction, twin to twin transfusion syndrome)

Intrauterine Growth Restriction

Maternal Causes
- Hypertensive disorders
- Diabetes
- Chronic renal disease
- Collagen vascular disease
- Thrombophilia
- Cyanotic heart disease
- Weight gain less than expected
- Smoking, alcohol use, problematic substance use
- Living at a high altitude

Fetoplacental Causes
- Chromosomal abnormalities
- Congenital malformations
- Intrauterine infection
- Genetic syndromes (e.g., trisomy 13, trisomy 18)
- Abnormal placental development

Oligohydramnios
- Renal agenesis (Potter syndrome)
- Preterm premature rupture of membranes
- Postdate pregnancy
- Uteroplacental insufficiency
- Severe intrauterine growth restriction (IUGR)
- Hypertensive disorders of pregnancy

Chromosomal Abnormalities
- Advanced maternal age
- Parental chromosomal rearrangements
- Previous pregnancy with autosomal trisomy
- Abnormal ultrasound findings during the current pregnancy (e.g., fetal structural anomalies, IUGR, amniotic fluid volume abnormalities)
- Increased risk, as calculated from noninvasive screening results (e.g., nuchal translucency and maternal serum analytes)

Sources: Baschat, A., Galan, H., Gabbe, S. (2012). Intrauterine growth restriction. In S. G. Gabbe, J. R. Niebyl, & J. L. Simpson, et al. (Eds.), *Obstetrics: Normal and problem pregnancies* (6th ed.). Philadelphia: Saunders; Gilbert, W. (2012). Amniotic fluid disorders: In S. G. Gabbe, J. R. Niebyl, & J. L. Simpson, et al. (Eds.), *Obstetrics: Normal and problem pregnancies* (6th ed.). Philadelphia: Saunders; Simpson, J., Richards, D., Otano, L., et al. (2012). Prenatal genetic diagnosis. In S. G. Gabbe, J. R. Niebyl, & J. L. Simpson, et al. (Eds.), *Obstetrics: Normal and problem pregnancies* (6th ed.). Philadelphia: Saunders.

lead to difficulty bonding. Therefore, it is important that mothers be identified and treated during pregnancy or in the postpartum period. The use of a screening tool, for example, the Edinburgh Postnatal Depression Scale (EPDS), anytime during the perinatal period is helpful in identifying women at risk for mental health issues. Perinatal Services BC has a number of guidelines concerning reproductive mental health issues, including specific guidelines for screening and care for various disorders, such as anxiety and bipolar (see Additional Resources at end of the chapter).

Intimate Partner Violence (IPV) During Pregnancy

Violence against women is a global public health concern, as it increases risks to their health, particularly during pregnancy. Abuse during pregnancy increases the risk for placental abruption, preterm birth, low-birth-weight infants, and infections from nonconsensual sex. Women who are in abusive situations may delay seeking health care during pregnancy or may receive inconsistent care.

During pregnancy, the perinatal nurse should assess for abuse at each prenatal visit and on admission in labour (see Box 5-10). Physically violent episodes are initiated or increase during pregnancy, for a variety of reasons: (1) the biopsychosocial stresses of pregnancy may strain the relationship beyond the couple's ability to cope, and frustration is followed by violence; (2) the partner may be jealous of the fetus, resenting the intrusion into the couple's relationship and the woman's displacement of attention; (3) the partner may be angry at the unborn child or the woman; and (4) the beating may be the partner's conscious or subconscious attempt to end the pregnancy. After birth, the mother may be so physically and emotionally drained that she has difficulty bonding with her infant. She may be at risk of becoming an abusive mother herself regardless of whether she remains in the abusive relationship. For further discussion of IPV see Chapter 5.

Abuse is about control of one person over another. In health care situations, many women can feel this same type of power imbalance with health care providers. When providing care to the woman who is a victim of IPV, it is important to give her information that can enable her to make her own decisions and have control over her decisions.

Reduction of Fetal and Newborn Health Problems

The leading causes of neonatal morbidity and mortality are preterm and multiple birth rates. Other causes of neonatal death include disorders relating to low birth weight, respiratory distress syndrome, the effects of maternal complications, and sudden infant death. Despite universal health care, the infant death rate is higher if the mother is of a lower socioeconomic status. Increased rates of survival during the newborn period have resulted largely from high-quality prenatal care and the improvement in perinatal services, including technological advances in neonatal intensive care and obstetrics.

Reducing infant mortality rates requires the removal of various barriers to care, including financial, educational, sociocultural, and logistical barriers, so that pregnant women can seek and receive appropriate health services. Commitment in this area is required at the national, provincial/territorial, and local levels. More research is needed to identify the extent to which the determinants of health, individually and collectively, affect perinatal morbidity and mortality. Ultimately, barriers to care must be removed and perinatal services modified to meet contemporary health care needs.

ANTEPARTUM TESTING IN THE FIRST AND SECOND TRIMESTER

The major expected outcome of antepartum testing is the detection of potential fetal compromise. Ideally, the technique used will identify fetal compromise before intrauterine asphyxia of the fetus occurs so that the health care provider can take measures to prevent or minimize adverse perinatal outcomes. No single test can provide this information. Assessment tests should be selected on the basis of their effectiveness, and the results must be interpreted in light of the complete clinical picture. Box 13-3 lists common maternal and fetal indications for antepartum testing that are supported by currently available evidence (Miller, Miller, & Tucker, 2013).

Prenatal Screening

First-trimester pregnancy screening for fetal aneuploidy (Down syndrome and trisomy 18) and second-trimester ultrasound examination to detect fetal anomalies should be offered to all pregnant women. Previously, women over the age of 35 were offered invasive testing, but this has been found to miss many cases of fetal anomalies. The Society of Obstetricians and Gynaecologists of Canada (SOGC) states that maternal age should be removed as an indication for invasive testing (SOGC, 2007), and with recent advances in maternal screening and ultrasound techniques, it is possible to offer all pregnant women a noninvasive method of screening. If the screening test is above a set cut-off level or if a woman is 40 years old at the time of the birth, invasive testing should be offered (amniocentesis or

BOX 13-3 COMMON MATERNAL AND FETAL INDICATIONS FOR ANTEPARTUM TESTING

- Diabetes
- Pre-existing hypertension
- Pre-eclampsia
- Systemic lupus erythematosus
- Renal disease
- Cholestasis of pregnancy
- Multiple gestation
- Oligohydramnios
- Preterm premature rupture of membranes
- Postdate or postterm gestation
- Previous stillbirth
- Fetal growth restriction
- Decreased fetal movement

From Miller, L. A., Miller, D. A., & Tucker, S. M. (2013). *Mosby's pocket guide to fetal monitoring: A multidisciplinary approach* (7th ed.). St. Louis: Mosby.

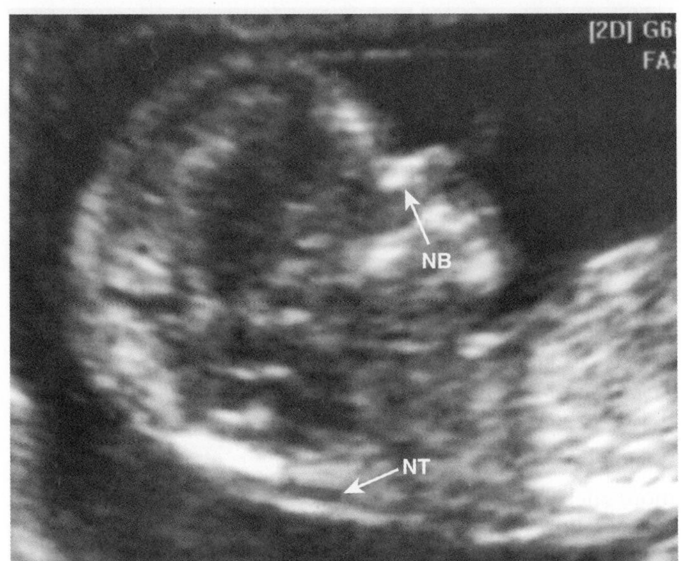

FIGURE 13-1 Midsagittal view of a 12-week fetus showing the nuchal translucency *(NT)* and nasal bone *(NB)*.

chorionic villus sampling; see discussion later in this chapter). There are regional differences across the country as to what screening tests are available, based on cost and the availability of trained ultrasound technicians. There are presently four options available for noninvasive screening.

First-Trimester Screening (FTS)

First-trimester screening (FTS) involves an ultrasound examination for nuchal translucency, combined with assessment of maternal serum biochemical markers. In *nuchal translucency* (NT) screening, ultrasound measurement of fluid in the nape of the fetal neck between 11 and 14 weeks of gestation is used to identify possible fetal abnormalities (Fig. 13-1). A finding of fluid collection that is greater than 3 mm is highly indicative of genetic disorders or physical anomalies and it is appropriate to offer the option of further diagnostic testing. A finding of 3.5 or greater increases the risk of a congenital heart defect, and a fetal echocardiogram would be recommended in the second trimester.

First-trimester maternal serum biochemical markers are pregnancy-associated plasma protein-A (PAPP-A) and free beta-human chorionic gonadotropin (ß-hCG). PAPP-A is lower in Down syndrome pregnancies and free ß-hCG is higher. FTS using all the criteria will detect 78 to 91% cases of Down syndrome, and 91 to 96% of trisomy 18 with a 5% false-positive rate (Wilson, Dzerwinski, Hoskovec, et al., 2013; Wilson & SOGC Genetics Committee, 2014). If an FTS screening test is done, it is recommended that the woman be screened for open neural tube defects (NTDs) at an 18- to 22-week ultrasound examination. A limitation of FTS is its lack of availability in some centres.

Second-Trimester Serum Screening

Maternal serum alpha-fetoprotein (MSAFP) levels are used as a screening tool for NTD in pregnancy. Through this technique, approximately 71 to 90% of all open NTDs and open abdominal wall defects can be detected early in pregnancy, although the SOGC recommends that the primary use of MSAFP for screening for open/closed NTDs be discontinued, with the limited clinical exception of pregnant women with a body mass index (BMI) > 35 or when geographic or clinical-access factors limit timely and good-quality ultrasound screening at 18 to 22 weeks' gestation (Wilson et al., 2014). A detailed second-trimester ultrasound screen is better able to detect anomalies.

AFP is produced by the fetal liver and is detectable in increasing quantities in the serum of pregnant women at 14 to 34 weeks' gestation. Although amniotic fluid AFP is diagnostic for NTD, MSAFP is a screening tool only and identifies candidates for the more definitive procedures of amniocentesis and ultrasound examination. MSAFP screening can be done with reasonable reliability any time between 15 and 20 weeks of gestation (16 to 18 weeks being ideal) (Wapner, 2014). Elevated levels are associated with other conditions such as fetal skin disorders, abdominal wall defects, fetal demise, and pregnancies at risk for placenta-related adverse events (Wilson et al., 2014).

Down syndrome—and probably other autosomal trisomies—is associated with lower than normal levels of MSAFP and amniotic fluid AFP. The triple-marker test is also performed at 16 to 18 weeks of gestation and requires the levels of three maternal serum markers: MSAFP, unconjugated estriol, and hCG, in combination with maternal age to calculate a new risk level. If a fetus has Down syndrome, the MSAFP and unconjugated estriol levels are low and the hCG level is elevated. With these two additional screening tests, approximately 72% of fetuses with Down syndrome can be identified. Testing for dimeric inhibin-A (DIA) improves the detection rate to 75 to 80%, and this is part of a quad screen (SOGC, 2007). DIA is elevated in Down syndrome and other trisomies. For more information see Nursing Care Plan, The Family with a Diagnosis of a Fetus with Down Syndrome on the Evolve website.

Integrated Prenatal Screening

The integrated prenatal screening (IPS) is a two-step process, which includes first- and second-trimester serum screening with or without NT. This screening method is superior to the other two methods, with a detection rate of 85%, a lower false-positive rate (1%), and thus a reduction in the number of invasive diagnostic procedures needed. IPS is based on the use of PAPP-A and NT in the first trimester and the quad screen in the second trimester; results are released when all the testing is completed. If NT is not available, PAPP-A is done in the first trimester and either triple or quad screening is done in the second trimester. This testing results in the detection of 83% of abnormalities (SOGC, 2007).

Noninvasive Prenatal Testing (NIPT) (Cell-Free DNA in Maternal Blood)

A new screening method for noninvasive prenatal genetic diagnosis has recently become available for use in the clinical setting. Cell-free deoxyribonucleic acid (DNA) screening already provides a definitive diagnosis noninvasively for fetal Rh status, fetal gender, and certain paternally transmitted single-gene disorders (Simpson, Richards, Otano, et al., 2012).

The method works by amplifying cell-free DNA. If the fetus has a normal karyotype, the amount of DNA is consistent with the known standard for the normal amount. For example, if more than the expected amount of chromosome 21 DNA is detected, it can then be assumed that the fetus is contributing the extra amount and therefore has trisomy 21. The same is true for trisomy 13 and 18. The test cannot actually distinguish fetal from maternal DNA, but it can accurately predict the fetal status by measuring the amount of DNA circulating in maternal blood and comparing it to known standards. The cell-free DNA screen in combination with ultrasound does not provide a definitive diagnosis for all cases of fetal trisomy 21. Women who have a positive cell-free circulating DNA test without confirming ultrasound findings or a negative blood screen with abnormal ultrasound findings require invasive diagnostic testing such as amniocentesis or chorionic villus sampling for a definitive diagnosis (Palomaki, Kloza, Lambert-Messerlian, et al., 2011).

Circulating cell-free DNA studies for the detection of fetal chromosomal abnormalities can be performed any time after 10 weeks of gestation. It is simple to perform; a sample of maternal blood is obtained by venipuncture and sent to a commercial laboratory. Results are usually available in about 10 days.

The false-positive rates are very low (<1%) and there is a very high detection rate for the three major syndromes (Down syndrome: 99–100%; trisomy 13: 79–92%; trisomy 18: 97–100%). At this time, the cost of this test is covered only upon consultation with a genetic counsellor or obstetrician and on the basis of risk factors such as a previous history of congenital anomaly or concerning test results in this pregnancy. Alternatively, women can choose to pay for this test themselves if they wish to have these results (Wilson et al., 2013).

Ultrasound

Sound is a form of wave energy that causes small particles in a medium to oscillate. The *frequency* of sound, which refers to the number of peaks or waves that move over a given point per unit of time, is expressed in hertz (Hz). Sound with a frequency of one cycle, or one peak per second, has a frequency of 1 Hz. When directional beams of sound strike an object, an echo is returned. The time delay between the emission of the sound and the return of the echo and the direction of the echo are noted. From these data, the distance and location of an object can be calculated.

Ultrasound is sound frequency higher than that detectable by humans (greater than 20,000 Hz). Diagnostic ultrasound instruments operate within a frequency range of 2 to 10 kHz, which is below the range used by sonar and radar equipment. Ultrasound images are a reflection of the strength of the sending beam, the strength of the returning echo, and the density of the medium (e.g., muscle [uterus], bone, tissue [placenta], fluid, or blood) through which the beam is sent and returned.

Diagnostic ultrasonography is an important technique in antepartum fetal surveillance (Fig. 13-2). It provides critical information to health care providers regarding fetal activity and **gestational age**, normal versus abnormal fetal growth curves, visual assistance with which invasive tests may be performed more safely, and fetal and placental anatomy early in pregnancy. Ultrasound examination done later during pregnancy is used to assess fetal well-being and will be discussed later in the chapter. Ultrasound examination can be done abdominally or transvaginally during pregnancy. Both methods produce a three-dimensional view from which a pictorial image is obtained. Abdominal ultrasonography is more useful after the first trimester when the pregnant uterus becomes an abdominal organ.

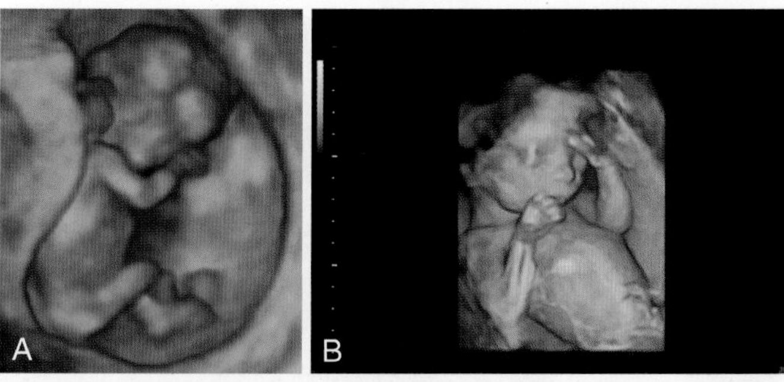

FIGURE 13-2 Fetus seen on three-dimensional ultrasound. **A:** Full body view of fetus at 11 weeks and 6 days of gestation. **B:** Close-up view of fetal face later in pregnancy. (**A**, Courtesy Shannon Perry; **B**, Courtesy Margaret Spann.)

For the procedure, the woman is usually required to have a full bladder to push the uterus up in order to get a better image of the fetus. Transmission gel is applied to the abdomen before a transducer is moved over the skin to enhance transmission and reception of the sound waves. The woman is positioned with small pillows under her head and knees. The display panel is positioned so that the woman and her partner can observe the images on the screen if they so desire.

Transvaginal Ultrasound Examination

Transvaginal ultrasound examination, in which the probe is inserted into the vagina, allows pelvic anatomy to be evaluated in greater detail and enables earlier diagnosis of intrauterine pregnancy. It is used in the first trimester to detect ectopic pregnancies, monitor the developing embryo, help identify abnormalities, and help establish gestational age. In some instances it may be used as an adjunct to abdominal scanning to evaluate preterm labour, by assessing the cervical length, in second- and third-trimester pregnancies. A transvaginal ultrasound examination is well tolerated by most women because it alleviates the need for a full bladder. It is especially useful in obese patients whose thick abdominal layers cannot be penetrated adequately with an abdominal approach.

A transvaginal ultrasound examination may be performed either with the woman in a lithotomy position or with her pelvis elevated by towels, cushions, or a folded pillow. This pelvic tilt is optimal to image the pelvic structures. A protective cover such as a condom, the finger of a clean rubber surgical glove, or a special cover provided by the manufacturer is used to cover the probe. The probe is lubricated with a water-soluble gel and placed in the vagina either by the examiner or by the woman herself. During the examination, the position of the probe or the tilt of the examining table may be changed to

BOX 13-4 MAJOR USES OF ULTRASONOGRAPHY DURING PREGNANCY

First Trimester
Confirm pregnancy
Confirm viability
Determine gestational age
Rule out ectopic pregnancy
Detect multiple gestation
Determine cause of vaginal bleeding
Use for visualization during chorionic villus sampling
Detect maternal abnormalities such as bicornuate uterus, ovarian cysts, fibroids
Assess nuchal translucency

Second Trimester
Assess fetal anatomy
Establish or confirm dates
Confirm viability
Detect polyhydramnios, oligohydramnios
Detect congenital anomalies, including neural tube defects
Detect intrauterine growth restriction (IUGR)
Assess placental placement
Assess cervical length
Use for visualization during amniocentesis

Third Trimester
Confirm viability
Detect macrosomia
Detect congenital anomalies
Detect IUGR
Determine fetal position
Detect placenta previa or placental abruption
Use for visualization during amniocentesis, external version
Biophysical profile
Assess amniotic fluid volume
Doppler flow studies
Detect placental maturity

view the complete pelvis. The procedure is not physically painful, although the woman will feel pressure as the probe is moved.

Indications for Use

Major indications for the use of obstetrical sonography are shown by trimester in Box 13-4. Ultrasonography can lead to earlier diagnoses, allowing therapy to be instituted early in pregnancy and thus in many cases decreasing the severity and duration of morbidity, both physical and emotional, for the family. For example, early diagnosis of a fetal anomaly gives the family choices, such as (1) preparation for the care of an infant with a disorder, (2) intrauterine surgery or other therapy for the fetus, or (3) termination of the pregnancy.

Fetal heart activity. Fetal heart activity can be demonstrated by about 6 weeks of gestation using transvaginal ultrasound. When the fetus is in a favourable position, good views of the fetal cardiac anatomy are possible in most patients at 13 weeks of gestation (Richards, 2012). Fetal death can be confirmed by lack of heart motion; the presence of fetal scalp edema, and maceration; and overlap of the cranial bones.

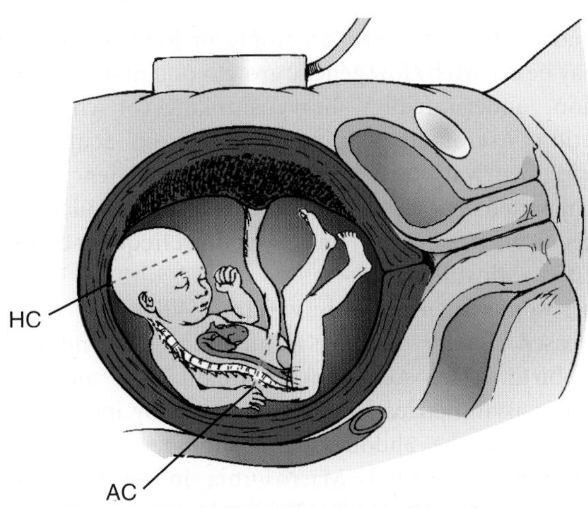

FIGURE 13-3 Appropriate planes of sections *(dotted lines)* for head circumference *(HC)* and abdominal circumference *(AC)*.

Gestational age. Gestational dating by ultrasonography is indicated for conditions such as the following: (1) uncertain dates for the last normal menstrual period, (2) recent discontinuation of oral contraceptives, (3) bleeding during the first trimester, (4) uterine size that does not agree with dates, (5) integrated prenatal screening, and (6) other high-risk conditions.

During the first 20 weeks of gestation, ultrasonography provides an accurate assessment of gestational age because most normal fetuses grow at the same rate. With increased fetal age, the accuracy of gestational-age estimates using ultrasound decreases, as fetuses grow at different rates. First-trimester dating by crown–rump length has an accuracy of plus or minus 3 to 5 days for estimating gestational age compared to the 7-day window for 18- to 22-week ultrasound and should be used whenever possible for determining gestational age (Butt, Lim, Bly, et al., 2014). A standard set of measurements has been accepted as being the most useful for determining gestational age: the crown–rump length (after 10 weeks), the biparietal diameter (BPD) (after 12 weeks), the femur length (after 12 weeks), the head circumference, and the abdominal circumference (Fig. 13-3).

Fetal growth. Fetal growth is determined by intrinsic growth potential and environmental factors that may enhance or inhibit that growth. Conditions that indicate the need for ultrasound assessment of fetal growth include the following: (1) slow maternal weight gain or pattern of weight gain, (2) previous pregnancy with intrauterine growth restriction (IUGR), (3) chronic infections, (4) ingestion of drugs (tobacco, alcohol, over-the-counter medications, and street drugs), (5) maternal diabetes mellitus, (6) hypertension, (7) multifetal pregnancy, and (8) other medical or surgical complications.

Serial evaluations of BPD, head circumference, limb length, and abdominal circumference can differentiate among size discrepancy resulting from inaccurate dates, true IUGR, and macrosomia. IUGR may be symmetrical (the fetus is small in all parameters) or asymmetrical (head and body growth vary).

Symmetrical IUGR implies a chronic or long-standing insult and may be caused by low genetic growth potential, intrauterine infection, undernutrition, heavy smoking, or chromosome aberration. Asymmetrical growth reflects an acute or late-occurring deprivation such as placental insufficiency resulting from hypertension, renal disease, or cardiovascular disease. Reduced fetal growth is still one of the most frequent conditions associated with stillbirth.

Macrosomic infants (those weighing 4000 g or more) are at increased risk for dystocia, traumatic injury, and asphyxia during birth. Macrosomia in the infant of a mother with diabetes is asymmetrical and characterized by increases in fat and muscle in the abdomen and shoulders; head circumference remains normal. Macrosomia in an infant whose mother is obese without glucose intolerance results in symmetrical changes (i.e., excessive growth of abdominal and head circumferences).

Routine assessment for fetal size has not been found to be beneficial and may increase the number of women hospitalized and requiring induction of labour without any increase in benefit. Third-trimester ultrasonography for assessment of size should only be done in women who have identified risk factors.

Fetal anatomy. Depending on the gestational age, the following structures can be identified on ultrasound scans: head (including ventricles and blood vessels), neck, spine, heart, stomach, small bowel, liver, kidneys, bladder, limbs, and umbilical cord. The SOGC recommends that all women be offered a routine second-trimester ultrasound examination between 18 and 22 weeks. Second-trimester ultrasonography is used for the detection of fetal anomalies including NTDs, assessment for multiple fetuses, location of placenta, and gestational age, and a complete anatomical scan should be performed (Cargill, Morin, Bly, et al., 2009). The SOGC recommends that second-trimester ultrasound be the primary screening tool for fetal structural abnormalities including open/closed NTDs (anencephaly, encephalocele, and spina bifida) (Wilson et al., 2014). The presence of an anomaly may influence decisions regarding where the birth takes place, whether a specialist or multidisciplinary team is needed for the rest of the pregnancy (e.g., a subspecialty centre instead of a basic care centre), and the method of birth (vaginal versus Caesarean) to optimize newborn outcomes.

Placental position and function. The pattern of uterine and placental growth and the fullness of the maternal bladder influence the apparent location of the placenta as viewed by ultrasonography. During the first trimester, differentiation between the endometrium and small placenta is difficult. By 14 to 16 weeks, the placenta is clearly defined, but its relationship to the internal cervical os can sometimes be altered dramatically by changing the degree of fullness of the maternal bladder. In approximately 4 to 6% of all pregnancies in which ultrasound scanning is performed during the second trimester, the placenta seems to be overlying the os, but at term the incidence of placenta previa is only 0.5%. Thus the diagnosis of placenta previa can seldom be confirmed before 27 weeks, primarily because of the elongation of the lower uterine segment as pregnancy advances.

Another use of ultrasonography is grading of placental maturation. Calcium and fibrin deposits in an aging placenta result in intervillous hemorrhagic infarcts. Also, as blood vessels in the placenta age and thicken, oxygen transport is affected. However, whether these placental changes adversely affect fetal outcomes in postterm pregnancies is unknown, given that most fetuses continue to grow (Gilbert, 2011).

Nursing Role

The main role of nurses in obstetrical ultrasound examination is in counselling and educating women about ultrasound scans. Providing accurate information about the procedure is imperative to allay the mother's anxiety. Although ultrasound scanning has become a widely used diagnostic tool, recommendations for the procedure are based on expectations of a fetal problem and thus may cause concern. Unlike many diagnostic tests, most women look forward to and enjoy their prenatal ultrasound. Exposure to diagnostic ultrasonography during pregnancy appears to be safe for the fetus (Richards, 2012).

Nonmedical Use of Ultrasonography During Pregnancy

In recent years the use of three- and four-dimensional ultrasonography for nonmedical purposes has become increasingly popular with pregnant women and their families. Although insurance does not cover the cost, women can make appointments to have ultrasound images made of the fetus, just as professional photographs are often taken of infants and children. Although ultrasonography is considered safe, exposure of the fetus to high-frequency sound waves without a clear medical indication for doing so should be avoided (SOGC & Canadian Association of Radiologists [CAR], 2014). In addition, casual ultrasonography performed by people who are not qualified health care professionals could give false reassurance to women or result in the discovery of abnormalities in settings that are not conducive to discussion and follow-up of findings. This technology should not be used for the sole purpose of determining fetal gender without a medical indication for that scan (SOGC & CAR, 2014).

Biochemical Assessment

Biochemical assessment involves biological examination (e.g., chromosomes in exfoliated cells) and chemical determinations (e.g., lecithin/sphingomyelin [L/S] ratio and bilirubin level) (Table 13-1). Procedures used to obtain the specimens for study include amniocentesis, percutaneous umbilical blood sampling (PUBS), chorionic villus sampling (CVS), and maternal sampling.

Coombs' Test

The indirect Coombs' test is a screening tool for Rh incompatibility. If the maternal titre for Rh antibodies is greater than 1 : 8, amniocentesis for determination of bilirubin in amniotic fluid is indicated to establish the severity of fetal hemolytic anemia. However, middle cerebral artery Doppler studies to determine the degree of fetal hemolysis have almost entirely replaced serial amniocentesis (Moise, 2012). The Coombs' test can also detect

TABLE 13-1 SUMMARY OF BIOCHEMICAL MONITORING TECHNIQUES

TEST	POSSIBLE FINDINGS	CLINICAL SIGNIFICANCE
Maternal Blood		
Coombs' test	Titre of 1:8 and rising	Significant Rh incompatibility
Amniotic Fluid Analysis		
Lung profile		
L/S ratio	2:1	Fetal lung maturity
Phosphatidylglycerol	Present	Fetal lung maturity
Creatinine	>150 mcmol/L	Gestational age >36 wk
Bilirubin (ΔOD 450 nm)*	<0.015	Gestational age >36 wk, normal pregnancy
	High levels	Fetal hemolytic disease in Rh-isoimmunized pregnancies
Lipid cells	>10%	Gestational age >35 wk
AFP	High levels after 15 wk of gestation	Open neural tube or other defect
Osmolality	Decline after 20 wk of gestation	Advancing gestational age
Genetic disorders Sex-linked Chromosomal Metabolic	Dependent on cultured cells for karyotype and enzymatic activity	Counselling possibly required

AFP, alpha-fetoprotein; *L/S*, lecithin/sphingomyelin.
*The presence of bilirubin changes the colour of amniotic fluid. The change in optical density (ΔOD) is a measure of the amount of bilirubin in the amniotic fluid.

other antibodies that may place the fetus at risk for incompatibility with maternal antigens.

Amniocentesis

Amniocentesis is performed to obtain amniotic fluid, which contains fetal cells to test for chromosomal aneuploidy. Under direct ultrasound visualization, a needle is inserted transabdominally into the uterus, amniotic fluid is withdrawn into a syringe, and various assessments are performed (Fig. 13-4). Amniocentesis is possible after week 14 of pregnancy, when the uterus becomes an abdominal organ and sufficient amniotic fluid is available for testing (see Table 13-1). Indications for the procedure include prenatal diagnosis of genetic disorders or congenital anomalies (NTDs in particular), assessment of pulmonary maturity, and rarely diagnosis of fetal hemolytic disease.

Complications in the mother and fetus occur in less than 1% of cases and include the following:

Maternal—Leakage of amniotic fluid, hemorrhage, fetomaternal hemorrhage with possible maternal Rh isoimmunization, infection, labour, placental abruption, inadvertent damage to the intestines or bladder, and amniotic fluid embolism (anaphylactoid syndrome of pregnancy)

Fetal—Death, hemorrhage, infection (amnionitis), direct injury from the needle, miscarriage, or preterm labour (0.2–0.3%)

Many of these complications have been minimized or eliminated by using ultrasound scanning to determine the exact position of the fetus, placenta, and pockets of amniotic fluid.

SAFETY ALERT

Because of the possibility of fetomaternal hemorrhage, administering RhoD immunoglobulin (e.g., WinRho) to the woman who is Rh negative is standard practice after an amniocentesis.

Indications for use

Genetic concerns. The incidence of genetic disorders is increased in women older than 35 years, those with a previous child with a chromosome abnormality, or those with a family history of chromosome anomalies. Nonetheless, the SOGC has stated that screening based on maternal age should be abandoned, except for women over the age of 40 at the time of birth, and that all women should be offered noninvasive screening for Down syndrome or trisomy 18. Older women should have the option of going automatically to CVS/amniocentesis, as should women who screen above a set risk cut-off level (SOGC, 2007).

Fetal cells can be cultured for karyotyping of chromosomes (see Chapter 9). Karyotyping also permits determination of fetal gender, which is important if a sex-linked disorder (occurring almost always in a male fetus) is suspected.

Biochemical analysis of enzymes in amniotic fluid can be used to detect inborn errors of metabolism or fetal structural anomalies. For example, AFP levels in amniotic fluid are assessed as a follow-up for elevated levels in maternal serum. High AFP levels in amniotic fluid help confirm the diagnosis of an open NTD, such as spina bifida or anencephaly, or an open abdominal wall defect, such as omphalocele. The elevation results from the increased leakage of cerebrospinal fluid into the amniotic fluid through the closure defect. AFP levels also may be elevated in a normal multifetal pregnancy and with intestinal atresia, presumably caused by lack of fetal swallowing.

A concurrent test indicating the presence of acetylcholinesterase in amniotic fluid almost always indicates a fetal defect (Wapner, 2014). In such instances, follow-up ultrasound examination is recommended.

Fetal maturity. Late in pregnancy accurate assessment of fetal lung maturity is possible by examining amniotic fluid for the presence of phosphatidylglycerol (PG) or determination of the L/S ratio (see Table 13-1).

Fetal hemolytic disease. In the past, amniocentesis was used for identification and follow-up of fetal hemolytic disease in cases of isoimmunization. Amniocentesis is now only performed for this reason in rare circumstances because of the availability of noninvasive testing. Doppler velocimetry of the fetal middle cerebral artery is now the method of choice to monitor accurately and noninvasively for fetal anemia in isoimmunized pregnancies (Moise, 2012).

Chorionic Villus Sampling

The combined advantages of earlier diagnosis and rapid results have made chorionic villus sampling (CVS) a popular technique for genetic studies with a risk of complication in 0.5

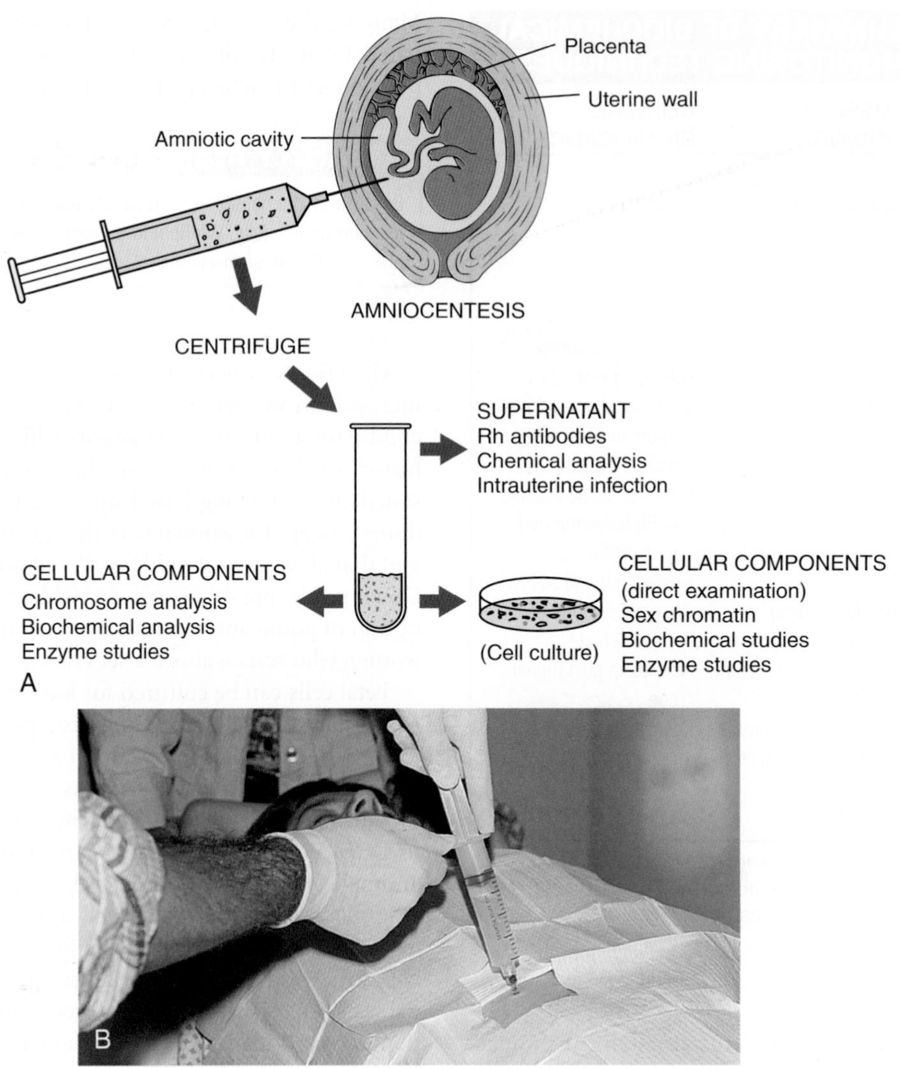

FIGURE 13-4 A: Amniocentesis and laboratory use of amniotic fluid aspirant. **B:** Transabdominal amniocentesis. (**B,** Courtesy Marjorie Pyle, RNC, Lifecircle.)

to 1%, similar to the rate for mid-trimester amniocentesis (Wilson et al., 2013). The accuracy is high because of the decreased risk of maternal cell contamination (less chance of obtaining maternal cells rather than fetal) and less chance of a mosaic result (some cells showing an abnormality and some not). CVS may be used to test for biochemical abnormalities, single-gene conditions, and collagen abnormalities. When performed after the first trimester, the procedure is better known as late CVS or placental biopsy (Simpson et al., 2012).

The procedure is usually performed between 10 and 13 weeks of gestation and involves the removal of a small tissue specimen from the fetal portion of the placenta. Because chorionic villi originate in the zygote, that tissue reflects the genetic makeup of the fetus.

CVS can be accomplished either transcervically or transabdominally. In transcervical sampling, a sterile catheter is introduced into the cervix under continuous ultrasonographic guidance, and a small portion of the chorionic villi is aspirated with a syringe (Fig. 13-5). The aspiration cannula and obturator must be placed at a suitable site, and rupture of the amniotic sac must be avoided. The transcervical procedure is contraindicated if a cervical infection such as chlamydia or herpes is present (Gilbert, 2011).

If the abdominal approach (Fig. 13-6) is used, an 18-gauge spinal needle with stylet is inserted under sterile conditions through the abdominal wall into the chorion frondosum under ultrasonographic guidance. The stylet is then withdrawn, and the chorionic tissue is aspirated into a syringe.

CVS is a relatively safe procedure. The incidence of IUGR, placental abruption, and preterm birth is no higher in women undergoing CVS than would be expected in the general population. In the early 1990s there was controversy concerning an increased risk for fetal limb reduction defects associated with CVS. However, the consensus of further studies is that, when CVS is performed after 9 completed weeks of gestation, the risk for limb reduction defects is no higher than it is in the general population (Simpson et al., 2012). See Box 13-5 regarding related fetal rights. Because of the possibility of fetomaternal hemorrhage, women who are Rh negative should receive Rh immune globulin to avoid isoimmunization.

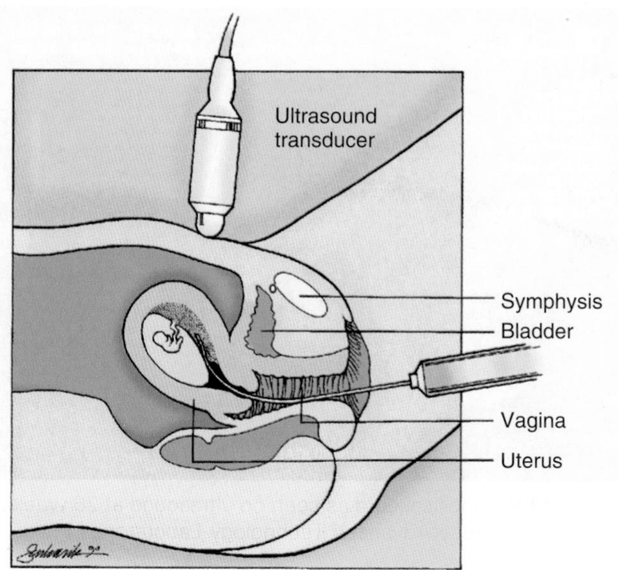

FIGURE 13-5 Transcervical chorionic villi sampling. (From Gabbe, S., Niebyl, J., Simpson, J., et al. [Eds.]. [2012]. *Obstetrics: Normal and problem pregnancies* [6th ed.]. Philadelphia: Saunders.)

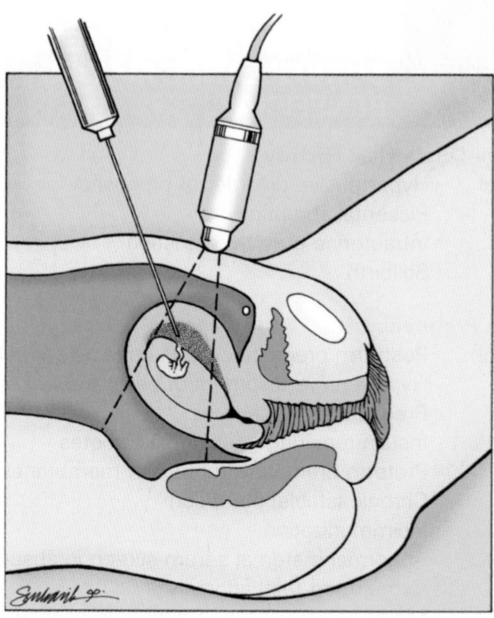

FIGURE 13-6 Transabdominal chorionic villus sampling. (From Gabbe, S., Niebyl, J., Simpson, J., et al. [Eds.]. [2012]. *Obstetrics: Normal and problem pregnancies* [6th ed.]. Philadelphia: Saunders.)

BOX 13-5 FETAL RIGHTS

Amniocentesis, percutaneous umbilical blood sampling, and chorionic villus sampling are prenatal tests used for diagnosing fetal defects in pregnancy. They are invasive and carry risks to the mother and fetus. A consideration of elective abortion is linked to the performance of these tests because there is no treatment for genetically affected fetuses. Thus, the issue of fetal rights is a key ethical concern in prenatal testing for fetal defects.

The use of amniocentesis and CVS is declining because of advances in noninvasive screening techniques. These techniques include measurement of nuchal translucency, maternal serum screening tests in the first and second trimesters, and ultrasonography in the second trimester (Wapner, 2014).

Percutaneous Umbilical Blood Sampling

Direct access to the fetal circulation during the second and third trimesters is possible through percutaneous umbilical blood sampling (PUBS) (also called cordocentesis). PUBS can be used for fetal blood sampling and transfusion. However, PUBS has been replaced in many centres by placental biopsy because it is a safer, easier, and faster alternative. Also, improvements in cytogenetic and molecular diagnostic testing have decreased the need for fetal blood samples. Many tests that were once performed using fetal blood can now be done using DNA-based analysis of chorionic villi (Simpson et al., 2012).

PUBS involves the insertion of a needle directly into the fetal umbilical vessel under ultrasonographic guidance. Ideally, the umbilical cord is punctured 1 to 2 cm from its insertion into the placenta (Fig. 13-7 and Fig. 13-8). At this point, the cord is well anchored and will not move, and the risk of maternal blood contamination (from the placenta) is slight. Generally, 1 to 4 mL of blood is removed and tested immediately by means of the Kleihauer-Betke procedure (Apt test) to ensure that it is fetal blood. Indications for the use of PUBS include prenatal diagnosis of inherited blood disorders, karyotyping of malformed fetuses, detection of fetal infection, assessment and treatment of isoimmunization, and thrombocytopenia in the fetus (Wapner, 2014). Complications that can occur include loss of the pregnancy, hematomas, bleeding from the puncture site in the umbilical cord, transient fetal bradycardia, and fetomaternal hemorrhage. Maternal complications are rare but include hemorrhage and transplacental hemorrhage (Simpson et al., 2012).

In fetuses at risk for isoimmune hemolytic anemia, PUBS enables precise identification of fetal blood type and red blood cell (RBC) count and may eliminate the need for further intervention. If the fetus is positive for the presence of maternal antibodies, a direct blood test can confirm the degree of anemia resulting from hemolysis. Intrauterine transfusion of severely anemic fetuses can be done 4 to 5 weeks earlier than through the intraperitoneal route.

Follow-up includes continuous fetal heart rate (FHR) monitoring for 1 to 2 hours after the procedure. Women should also be taught to count fetal movements at home (Gilbert, 2011).

THIRD-TRIMESTER ASSESSMENT FOR FETAL WELL-BEING

Assessment during the first and second trimesters is directed primarily at the diagnosis of fetal anomalies. The goal of third-trimester testing is to determine whether the intrauterine environment continues to be supportive to the fetus. The testing is often used to determine the timing of childbirth for patients at risk for uteroplacental insufficiency. Gradual loss of placental function results first in inadequate nutrient delivery to the fetus,

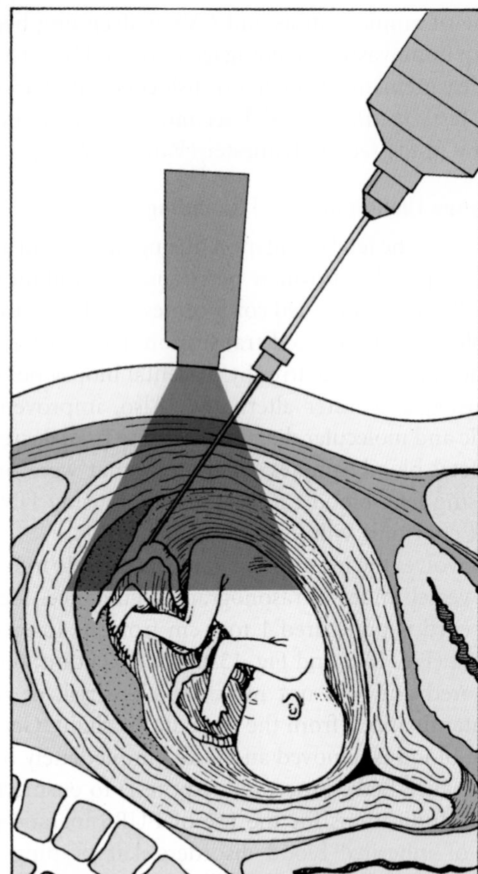

FIGURE 13-7 Technique for percutaneous umbilical blood sampling guided by ultrasonography.

leading to IUGR. Subsequently, respiratory function is compromised, resulting in fetal hypoxia. Indications for increased fetal surveillance, including fetal movement counting, nonstress test (NST), contraction stress test (CST), biophysical profile (BPP), and other ultrasound tests, are listed in Box 13-6. There is presently no evidence to suggest the use of antenatal fetal testing in uncomplicated pregnancies less than 41 weeks' gestation (Liston, Sawchuck, Young, et al., 2007).

Fetal Movement Counting

Assessment of fetal activity by the mother is a simple yet valuable method for monitoring the condition of the fetus. All women should be taught to become aware of fetal movements in the third trimester, and only if they perceive decreased movement or have risk factors should they begin daily monitoring/counting of fetal movements. Fetal movement counting (also called "kick counts") can be done at home, is simple to understand, is noninvasive, and usually does not interfere with a daily routine. The presence of movements is generally a reassuring sign of fetal health. Decreased fetal movement can be related to decreased placental perfusion and fetal acidemia.

Women should be taught the significance of the presence or absence of fetal movements, the procedure to use for counting, and when to notify their health care provider. For fetal movement counting the woman concentrates on the movements in a reclined (not supine) position. The recommended technique

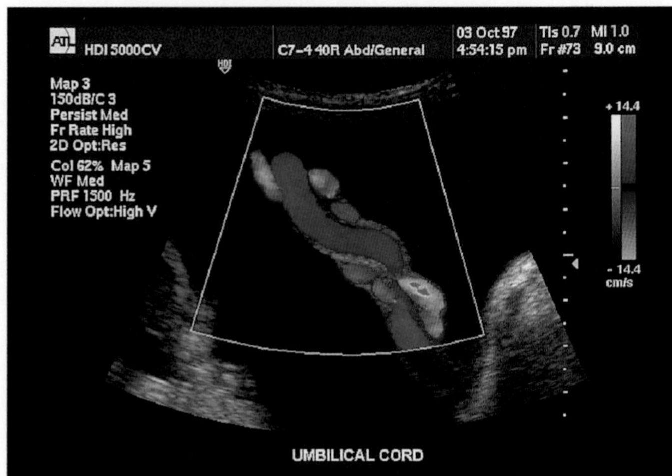

FIGURE 13-8 Umbilical cord as seen on ultrasound at 26 weeks of gestation. (Courtesy Advanced Technology Laboratories.)

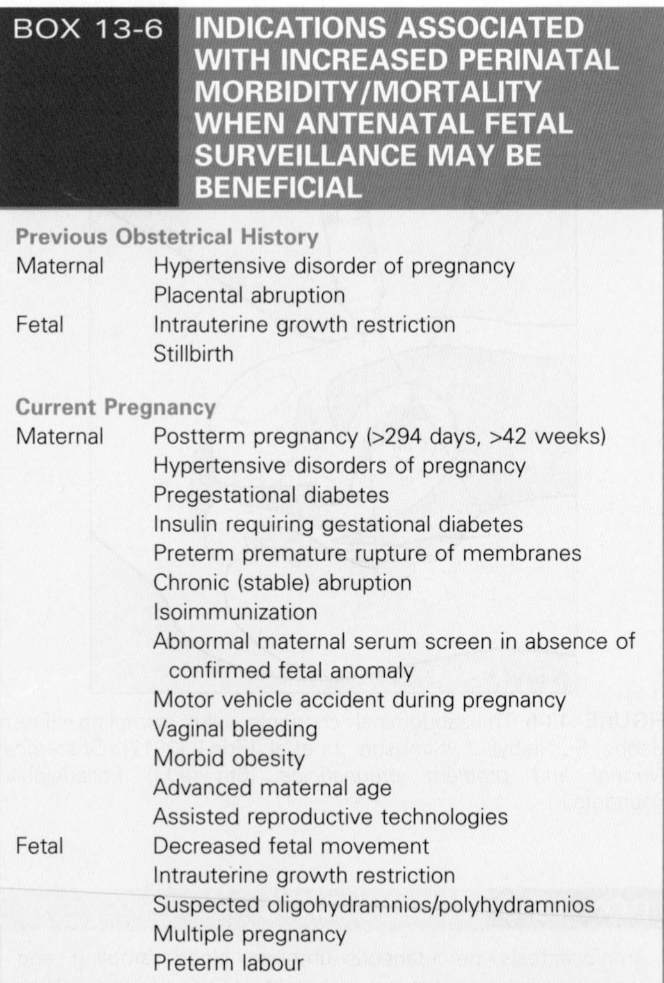

BOX 13-6 INDICATIONS ASSOCIATED WITH INCREASED PERINATAL MORBIDITY/MORTALITY WHEN ANTENATAL FETAL SURVEILLANCE MAY BE BENEFICIAL

Previous Obstetrical History

Maternal	Hypertensive disorder of pregnancy
	Placental abruption
Fetal	Intrauterine growth restriction
	Stillbirth

Current Pregnancy

Maternal	Postterm pregnancy (>294 days, >42 weeks)
	Hypertensive disorders of pregnancy
	Pregestational diabetes
	Insulin requiring gestational diabetes
	Preterm premature rupture of membranes
	Chronic (stable) abruption
	Isoimmunization
	Abnormal maternal serum screen in absence of confirmed fetal anomaly
	Motor vehicle accident during pregnancy
	Vaginal bleeding
	Morbid obesity
	Advanced maternal age
	Assisted reproductive technologies
Fetal	Decreased fetal movement
	Intrauterine growth restriction
	Suspected oligohydramnios/polyhydramnios
	Multiple pregnancy
	Preterm labour

Source: Reprinted from Liston, R., Sawchuck, D., Young, D., et al. (2007). SOGC clinical practice guideline: Fetal health surveillance: Antepartum and intrapartum consensus guideline. *Journal of Obstetrics and Gynaecology Canada, 29*(9), Suppl 4, S1–S56. Copyright 2007, with permission from Elsevier.

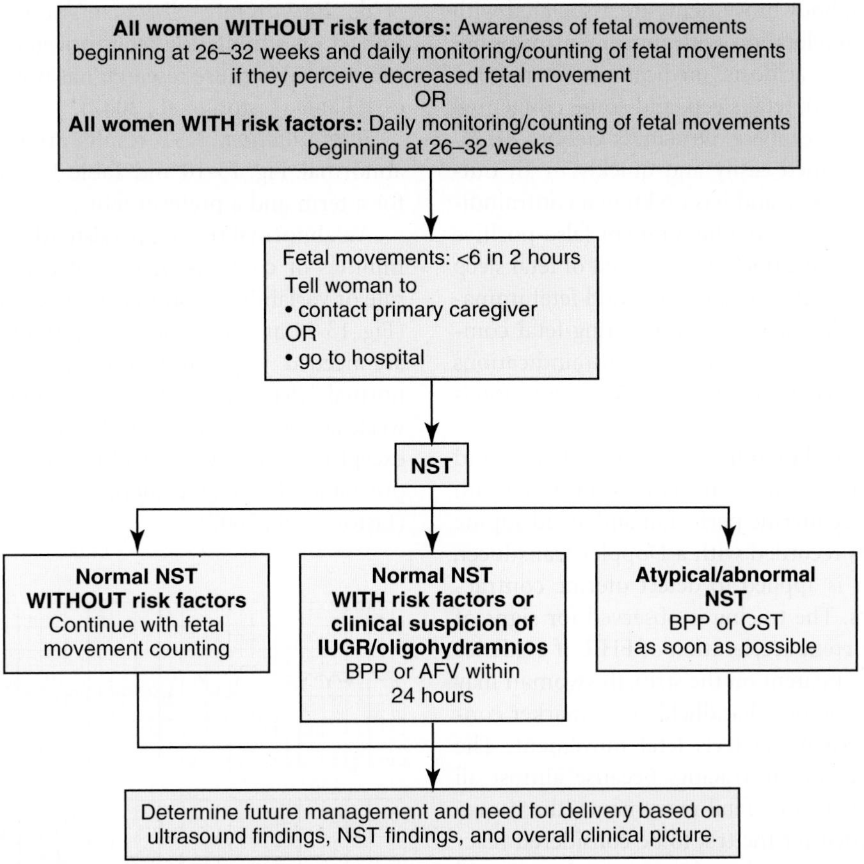

FIGURE 13-9 Fetal movement algorithm. *AFV*, amniotic fluid volume; *BPP*, biophysical profile; *CST*, contraction stress test; *IUGR*, intrauterine growth restriction; *NST*, nonstress test. (From Liston, R., Sawchuck, D., Young, D., et al. [2007]. SOGC clinical practice guideline: Fetal health surveillance: Antepartum and intrapartum consensus guideline. *Journal of Obstetricians and Gynaecologists of Canada, 29*[9], Suppl 4, S1–S23. Copyright 2007, with permission from Elsevier.)

is to count six movements. If six movements are not felt within 2 hours further evaluation of maternal and fetal status is required (Liston et al., 2007). This would initially include an NST or BPP (Fig. 13-9).

NURSING ALERT

In assessing fetal movements it is important to remember that they are usually not present during the fetal sleep cycle; they may be temporarily reduced if the woman is taking depressant medication, drinking alcohol, or smoking a cigarette. They do not decrease as the woman nears term. Obesity and an anterior placenta decrease perception of fetal movement and, consequently, the ability of the mother to count fetal movements.

Electronic Fetal Monitoring

Observable fetal responses to hypoxia or asphyxia are the clinical basis for antepartum testing with electronic fetal monitoring (EFM). Hypoxia or asphyxia elicits a number of responses in the fetus. There is a redistribution of blood flow to certain vital organs. This series of responses, including redistribution of blood flow favouring vital organs, decreased total oxygen consumption, and a switch to anaerobic glycolysis, is a temporary mechanism that enables the fetus to survive up to 30 minutes with limited oxygen supply without decompensation of vital organs. However, during more severe asphyxia or sustained hypoxemia, these compensatory responses are no longer maintained and a decrease in the cardiac output, arterial blood pressure, and blood flow to the brain and heart occurs (Nageotte, 2014), with characteristic FHR patterns reflecting these changes.

Considerable evidence supports the clinical belief that FHR variability indicates an intact nervous pathway through the cerebral cortex, midbrain, vagus nerve, and cardiac conduction system. With 98% accuracy in predicting fetal well-being, the presence of normal FHR variability is a reassuring indicator. Input from various areas of the brain decreases after cerebral asphyxia, leading to a decrease in variability after failure of the fetal hemodynamic compensatory mechanisms to maintain cerebral oxygenation (Nageotte, 2014). As a rule, normal patterns with the NST or negative results with the CST are associated with favourable outcomes.

Nonstress Test

The **nonstress test** (NST) is the most widely applied technique for antepartum evaluation of the fetus, although there is poor evidence that use of NSTs decreases perinatal morbidity or mortality. The basis for the NST is that the normal fetus produces characteristic heart rate patterns in response to fetal movement. In the healthy fetus with an intact central nervous system, 85% of gross fetal body movements are associated with FHR accelerations. The acceleration with movement response may be blunted by hypoxia, acidosis, medications (analgesics, barbiturates, and β-blockers), fetal sleep, and some congenital anomalies (Gilbert, 2011; Greenberg, Druzin, & Gabbe, 2012).

The NST can be performed easily and quickly in an outpatient setting; it is noninvasive and has no known contraindications. Disadvantages centre on the high rate of false-positive results for atypical or abnormal tracings as a result of fetal sleep cycles, chronic tobacco smoking, medications, and fetal immaturity. The test is slightly less sensitive in detecting fetal compromise than the CST or BPP. No clinical contraindications exist for the NST, but results may be inconclusive if gestation is 26 weeks or less.

Procedure. The woman should have an empty bladder and be seated in a reclining chair (or in a semi-Fowler position) with a slight left tilt, to optimize uterine perfusion and avoid supine hypotension. The FHR is recorded with a Doppler transducer, and a tocodynamometer is applied to detect uterine contractions or fetal movements. The tracing is observed for signs of fetal activity and a concurrent acceleration of FHR. If evidence of fetal movement is not apparent on the strip, the woman may be asked to depress a button on a handheld event marker connected to the monitor when she feels fetal movement. The movement is then noted on the tracing. Because almost all accelerations are accompanied by fetal movements, the movements need not be recorded for the test to be considered reactive. The test usually is completed in 20 minutes but should continue for up to 80 minutes if the response is not normal.

Administering glucose to the mother or stimulating the abdomen to encourage fetal movement is not recommended, as research has not proven either technique to be effective (Liston et al., 2007). Only vibroacoustic stimulation has had some impact on stimulating fetal movement, although it is not recommended because research has not concluded that this is safe or reliable (Liston et al., 2007).

Interpretation. NST results are either normal, atypical, or abnormal. Fig. 13-10 and Table 13-2 list criteria for the results for a term and a preterm fetus.

An abnormal tracing persistently lacks accelerations after 80 minutes or contains significant abnormality of baseline heart rate or variability or shows evidence of significant decelerations (Fig. 13-11 and see Table 13-2). In this case, further assessments are needed with ultrasonography or BPP. In most cases, a normal NST is predictive of a good perinatal outcome for 1 week as long as there are no changes to the clinical picture, except in women with insulin-dependent diabetes or postdates pregnancy. In these women, NSTs should be done twice weekly (Liston et al., 2007).

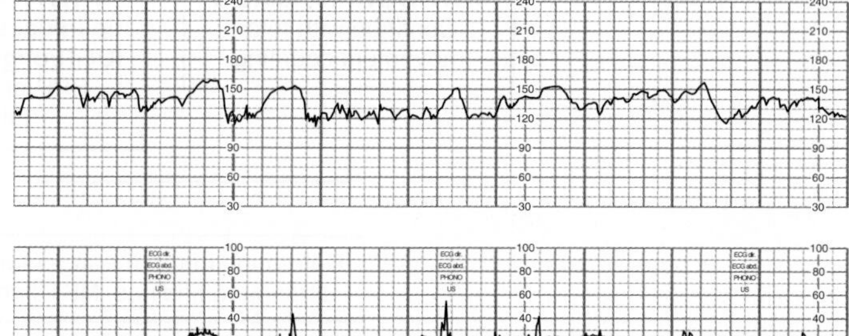

FIGURE 13-10 Normal nonstress test. Fetal heart rate accelerations with fetal movement. (From Miller L. A., Miller D. A., & Tucker, S. M. [2013]. *Mosby's pocket guide to fetal monitoring: A multidisciplinary approach* [7th ed.]. St. Louis: Mosby.)

TABLE 13-2 ANTEPARTUM CLASSIFICATION: NONSTRESS TEST

PARAMETER	NORMAL NST	ATYPICAL NST	ABNORMAL NST
Baseline	• 110–160 bpm	• 110–160 bpm • >160 bpm <30 min • Rising baseline	• Bradycardia <100 bpm • Tachycardia >160 for >30 min • Erratic baseline
Variability	• 6–25 bpm (moderate) (see Fig. 13-10) • ≤5 bpm (absent or minimal) for <40 min	• ≤ (absent or minimal) for 40–80 min (see Fig. 13-11)	• ≤5 for ≥80 min • ≥25 bpm >10 min • Sinusoidal
Decelerations	• None or occasional variable <30 sec	• Variable decelerations 30–60 sec duration	• Variable decelerations >60 sec duration • Late decelerations
Accelerations term fetus	• 2 accelerations with acme of ≥15 bpm, lasting 15 sec <40 min of testing	• ≤2 accelerations with acme of ≥15 bpm, lasting 15 sec in 40–80 min	• ≤2 accelerations with acme of ≥15 bpm, lasting 15 sec in >80 min
Preterm fetus (<32 weeks)	• ≥2 accelerations with acme of ≥10 bpm, lasting 10 sec <40 min of testing	• ≤2 accelerations with acme of ≧10 bpm, lasting 10 sec in 40–80 min	• ≤2 accelerations with acme of ≥10 bpm, lasting 10 sec in >80 min
Action	Further assessment optional, based on total clinical picture	Further assessment required	URGENT ACTION REQUIRED An overall assessment of the situation and further investigation with ultrasonography or BPP is required. Some situations will require delivery.

bpm, beats per minute; *BPP,* biophysical profile; *NST,* nonstress test.

Source: Liston, R., Sawchuck, D., Young, D., et al. (2007). SOGC clinical practice guideline: Fetal health surveillance: Antepartum and intrapartum consensus guideline. *Journal of Obstetrics and Gynaecology Canada, 29*(9), Suppl 4, S1–S56. Copyright 2007, with permission from Elsevier.

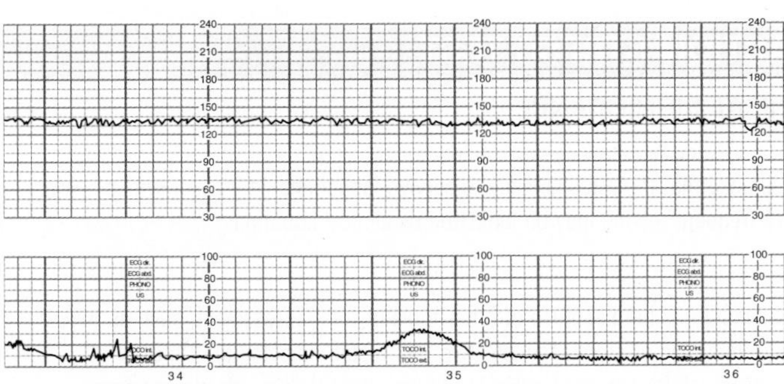

FIGURE 13-11 Atypical or Abnormal nonstress test (no fetal heart rate accelerations). (From Miller, L. A., Miller, D. A., & Tucker, S. M. [2013]. *Mosby's pocket guide to fetal monitoring: A multidisciplinary approach* [7th ed.]. St. Louis: Mosby.)

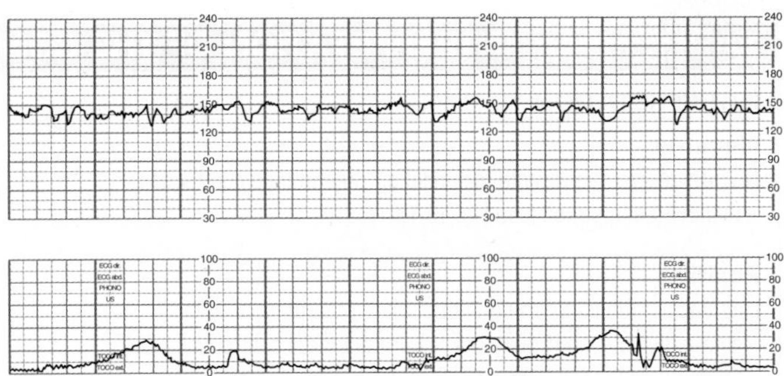

FIGURE 13-12 Negative contraction stress test (normal external fetal heart rate tracing). (From Miller, L. A., Miller, D. A., & Tucker, S. M. [2013]. *Mosby's pocket guide to fetal monitoring: A multidisciplinary approach* [7th ed.]. St. Louis: Mosby.)

Contraction Stress Test

The contraction stress test (CST) or oxytocin challenge test (OCT) was the first widely used electronic fetal assessment test. Its purpose is to evaluate the response of the fetus to induced contractions and to thus identify poor placental function (Liston et al., 2007). Uterine contractions decrease uterine blood flow and placental perfusion. If this decrease is sufficient to produce hypoxia in the fetus, a deceleration in FHR results, beginning at the peak of the contraction and persisting after its conclusion (late deceleration). CSTs are used much less frequently now, as uteroplacental function can be assessed using BPP or vascular flow measurements.

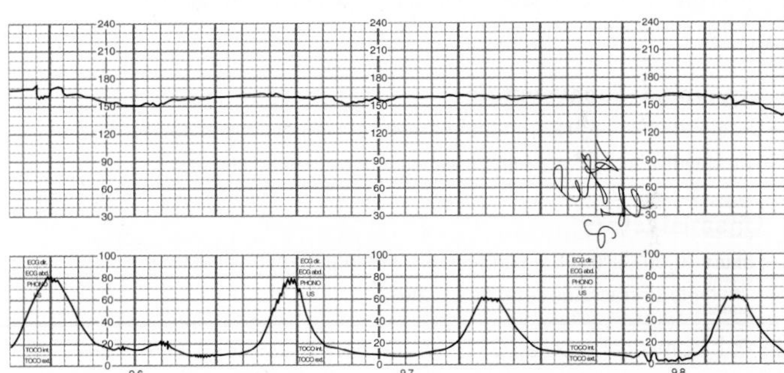

FIGURE 13-13 Positive contraction stress test (late decelerations with uterine contractions). (From Miller, L. A., Miller, D. A., & Tucker, S. M. [2013]. *Mosby's pocket guide to fetal monitoring: A multidisciplinary approach* [7th ed.]. St. Louis: Mosby.)

! NURSING ALERT

In a healthy fetoplacental unit, uterine contractions usually do not produce late decelerations; when there is underlying uteroplacental insufficiency, contractions produce late decelerations.

Procedure. The woman is placed in a semi-Fowler position or sits in a reclining chair with a slight lateral tilt, to optimize uterine perfusion and avoid supine hypotension. She is monitored electronically with the fetal ultrasound transducer and uterine tocodynamometer. The tracing is observed for 10 to 20 minutes for baseline rate, variability, and the possible occurrence of spontaneous contractions. CST should not be done in the following situations: ruptured membranes, previous classic incision for Caesarean birth, preterm labour, placenta previa, and placental abruption. Multifetal pregnancy, previous preterm labour, hydramnios, more than 36 weeks of gestation, and incompetent cervix are relative contraindications for the CST.

The goal of a CST is to induce three contractions, each lasting 1 minute within a 10-minute period so that the fetal heart response to the contractions can be evaluated (Liston et al., 2007). The CST can be done using maternal nipple stimulation or with an oxytocin infusion. Negative results for a CST are associated with favourable results.

Nipple-stimulated contraction test. Massaging the nipples causes a release of oxytocin from the posterior pituitary. The woman is instructed to stimulate one nipple through her clothing with the palmar surface of the fingers rapidly, but gently for 2 minutes, rest for 5 minutes, and repeat the cycles of massage and rest as necessary to achieve adequate uterine activity. Bilateral nipple stimulation may be considered when unable to achieve contractions while stimulating only one nipple. When adequate contractions or hyperstimulation occurs, stimulation should be stopped (Liston et al., 2007). Nipple stimulation has a shorter testing time than oxytocin infusion, although if nipple stimulation does not work, then oxytocin infusion should be considered.

Oxytocin-stimulated contraction test. Exogenous oxytocin can also be used to stimulate uterine contractions. An intravenous (IV) infusion is started and an oxytocin infusion initiated through a piggyback port into the tubing of the main IV device. An infusion pump is used to ensure accurate dosage. The oxytocin infusion usually is begun at 0.5 to 1.0 mU/minute and increased by 1.0 mU/minute at 15- to 30-minute intervals until three uterine contractions of good quality are observed within a 10-minute period. Hyperstimulation is a risk, so slowly increasing the rate of oxytocin is recommended.

Interpretation. If a normal baseline FHR tracing and no late decelerations are observed with the contractions, the findings are considered to be negative (Fig. 13-12). A CST is positive if late decelerations occur with more than 50% of the induced contractions (Fig. 13-13 and Table 13-3).

After interpretation of the FHR pattern, the oxytocin infusion is discontinued, and the maintenance IV solution is infused until the uterine activity has returned to the prestimulation

TABLE 13-3 INTERPRETATION OF THE CONTRACTION STRESS TEST

INTERPRETATION	CLINICAL SIGNIFICANCE
Negative No late decelerations, with minimum of three uterine contractions within 10-min period (see Fig. 13-12)	Reassurance that the fetus is likely to survive labour should it occur within 1 wk; more frequent testing may be indicated by clinical situation
Positive Late decelerations occurring with at least 50% or more of contractions, even if there are fewer than three contractions in 10 min (see Fig. 13-13)	Management lies between use of other tools of fetal assessment, such as BPP, and termination of pregnancy; positive test result indicates that fetus is at increased risk for perinatal morbidity and mortality; physician may perform expeditious vaginal birth after successful induction or may proceed directly to Caesarean birth; decision to intervene is determined by fetal monitoring and presence of FHR reactivity
Atypical Prolonged, variable, or late decelerations occurring with less than 50% of the contractions	NST and CST should be repeated within 24 hr; if interpretable data cannot be achieved, other methods of fetal assessment must be used*
Equivocal–Tachysystole Decelerations that occur in the presence of contractions more frequent than every 2 min or lasting longer than 90 sec	Repeat test next day
Unsatisfactory Failure to produce three contractions within a 10-min window or inability to trace the fetal heart rate	Repeat test next day

BPP, biophysical profile; *CST,* contraction stress test; *FHR,* fetal heart rate; *NST,* nonstress test.
*Applies to results noted as suspicious, hyperstimulation, or unsatisfactory.
Sources: Liston, R., Sawchuck, D., Young, D., et al. (2007). SOGC clinical practice guideline: Fetal health surveillance: Antepartum and intrapartum consensus guideline. *Journal of Obstetrics and Gynaecology Canada, 29*(9), Suppl 4; Miller, L. A., Miller, D. A., & Tucker, S. M. (2013). *Mosby's pocket guide to fetal monitoring: A multidisciplinary approach* (7th ed.). St. Louis: Mosby.

level. If the CST is negative, the IV device is removed, and the fetal monitor is disconnected. If the CST is positive, continued monitoring and further evaluation of fetal well-being are indicated. While the use of CSTs has decreased because it has been replaced by other technologies, one indication for the use of CST is to determine if a fetus that has other abnormal testing results could tolerate a vaginal birth rather than requiring a Ceasarean birth. A fetus demonstrating an atypical or abnormal NST and a positive CST is less likely to tolerate labour (Liston et al., 2007).

Ultrasound for Fetal Well-Being

Physiological parameters of the fetus that can be assessed with ultrasound scanning include amniotic fluid volume (AFV), vascular waveforms from the fetal circulation, heart motion, fetal breathing movements, fetal urine production, and fetal limb and head movements. Assessment of these parameters, singly or in combination, yields a fairly reliable picture of fetal well-being. The significance of these findings is discussed in the following sections.

Biophysical Profile (BPP)

Real-time ultrasound imaging enables detailed assessment of the physical and physiological characteristics of the developing fetus to such an extent that it is possible to examine the fetus in detail and to catalogue normal and abnormal biophysical responses to stimuli. The **biophysical profile (BPP)** is a noninvasive dynamic assessment of a fetus that is based on the assessment of acute and chronic markers of fetal disease. The BPP is used to assess current fetal well-being by observing fetal breathing movements, fetal movements, fetal tone, and AFV.

The BPP may be considered a physical examination of the fetus, including determination of vital signs. The fetus responds to central hypoxia through alteration in movement, muscle tone, breathing, and heart rate patterns. The presence of normal fetal biophysical activities indicates that the central nervous system is functional; therefore, the fetus is not hypoxemic. BPP variables and scoring are detailed in Tables 13-4 and 13-5. The BPP is done with or without an NST. If done with the NST, the score is out of 10, and if done without the NST, the score is out of 8.

The BPP is an evaluation of current fetal well-being (Liston et al., 2007). Fetal acidosis can be diagnosed early with an abnormal NST and absent fetal breathing movements. A BPP score of less than 6, or a score of 6 along with **oligohydramnios**, indicates that labour should be induced (see Table 13-5). The BPP identifies a pocket of amniotic fluid of less than 2 cm by 2 cm as oligiohydramnios. Fetal infection in women whose membranes rupture prematurely (at less than 37 weeks of gestation) can be diagnosed early by changes in biophysical activities that precede the clinical signs of infection and indicate the necessity for immediate birth. When the BPP score is normal and the risk of fetal death low, intervention is indicated only for obstetrical or maternal factors.

TABLE 13-4 SCORING THE BIOPHYSICAL PROFILE

VARIABLES	NORMAL (SCORE = 2)	ABNORMAL (SCORE = 0)
Fetal breathing movements	One or more episodes in 30 min, each lasting ≥30 sec	Episodes absent or no episode ≥30 sec in 30 min
Fetal movements	At least three trunk or limb movements in 30 min	Fewer than three episodes of body or limb movements in 30 min
Fetal tone	At least one episode of active extension with return to flexion of fetal limb or trunk; opening and closing of hand is considered normal tone	Absence of movement or slow extension/ flexion
Amniotic fluid index	At least one cord and limb-free fluid pocket that is 2 cm by 2 cm in two measurements at right angles	No single pocket of fluid that is 2 cm by 2 cm
Nonstress test—may or may not be done	Normal	Abnormal Atypical

Source: Liston, R., Sawchuck, D., Young, D., et al. (2007). SOGC clinical practice guideline: Fetal health surveillance: Antepartum and intrapartum consensus guideline. *Journal of Obstetrics and Gynaecology Canada, 29*(9), Suppl 4.

TABLE 13-5 BIOPHYSICAL PROFILE SCORE INTERPRETATION AND MANAGEMENT

SCORE	INTERPRETATION	MANAGEMENT
8–10	Normal; low risk for chronic asphyxia	Repeat testing as required based on risk factors
6 (normal fluid)	Equivocal test	Repeat testing within 24 hr
6 (abnormal fluid)	Suspect chronic asphyxia	Birth of term fetus. In fetus <34 weeks, intensive surveillance may be used and delivery considered
<6	Abnormal; suspect chronic asphyxia	Deliver for fetal indications

Source: Liston, R., Sawchuck, D., Young, D., et al. (2007). SOGC clinical practice guideline: Fetal health surveillance: Antepartum and intrapartum consensus guideline. *Journal of Obstetrics and Gynaecology Canada, 29*(9), Suppl 4.

Amniotic Fluid Volume

Abnormalities in AFV are frequently associated with fetal disorders. Subjective determinants of oligohydramnios (decreased fluid) include the absence of fluid pockets in the uterine cavity and the impression of crowding of fetal small parts. An objective criterion of decreased AFV is met if the largest pocket of fluid measured in two perpendicular planes is less than 2 cm (Kamal, 2014). Increased amniotic fluid is called *polyhydramnios* or sometimes just *hydramnios*. Subjective criteria for polyhydramnios include multiple large pockets of fluid, the impression of a floating fetus, and free movement of fetal limbs. Hydramnios is usually defined as pockets of amniotic fluid measuring more than 8 cm (Gilbert, 2012).

The total AFV can be evaluated through a method in which the depths (in centimetres) of amniotic fluid in all four quadrants surrounding the maternal umbilicus are totalled, resulting in an amniotic fluid index (AFI). A normal AFI is 10 cm or greater, with the upper range of normal being around 25 cm. AFI values between 5 and 10 cm are considered to be low normal, whereas an AFI of less than 5 cm indicates oligohydramnios. With polyhydramnios the AFI would be above 25 cm (Miller et al., 2013). There is evidence that the use of AFI, rather than pocket size, increases the rate of intervention without improving outcomes (Liston et al., 2007).

Oligohydramnios is associated with rupture of the membranes and congenital anomalies (such as renal agenesis), IUGR, and fetal distress in labour. Polyhydramnios is associated with NTDs, obstruction of the fetal gastrointestinal tract, multiple fetuses, and fetal hydrops.

Doppler Blood Flow Analysis

One of the major advances in perinatal medicine is the ability to study blood flow noninvasively in the fetus and placenta with ultrasonography. Doppler blood flow analysis is a useful adjunct in the management of pregnancies at risk due to hypertension, IUGR, diabetes mellitus, multiple fetuses, or preterm labour because it provides an indication of fetal adaptation and reserve.

When a sound wave is reflected from a moving target, there is a change in frequency of the reflected wave relative to the transmitted wave. This is called the *Doppler effect.* An ultrasound beam scattered by a group of RBCs is an example of this effect. The velocity of the RBCs can be determined by measuring the change in the frequency in the sound wave reflected off the cells.

The shifted frequencies can be displayed as a plot of velocity versus time, and the shape of these waveforms can be analyzed to give information about blood flow and resistance in a given circulation. Velocity waveforms from umbilical and uterine arteries, reported in systolic/diastolic (S/D) ratios, can be first detected at 15 weeks of pregnancy. Because of progressive decline in resistance in both the umbilical and the uterine arteries, this ratio decreases as pregnancy advances. Most fetuses achieve an S/D ratio of 3 or less by 30 weeks (Fig. 13-14). Persistent elevation of S/D ratios after 30 weeks is associated with IUGR, usually resulting from uteroplacental insufficiency. In postterm pregnancies evaluated by Doppler umbilical flow studies, an elevated S/D ratio indicates a poorly perfused placenta. Abnormal velocity study results are also seen with certain chromosome abnormalities (trisomy 13 and 18) and with lupus erythematosus in the mother. Exposure to nicotine from maternal smoking also increases the S/D ratio.

NURSING ROLE IN ANTENATAL ASSESSMENT FOR RISK

The nurse's role is that of educator and support person when the woman is undergoing examinations such as

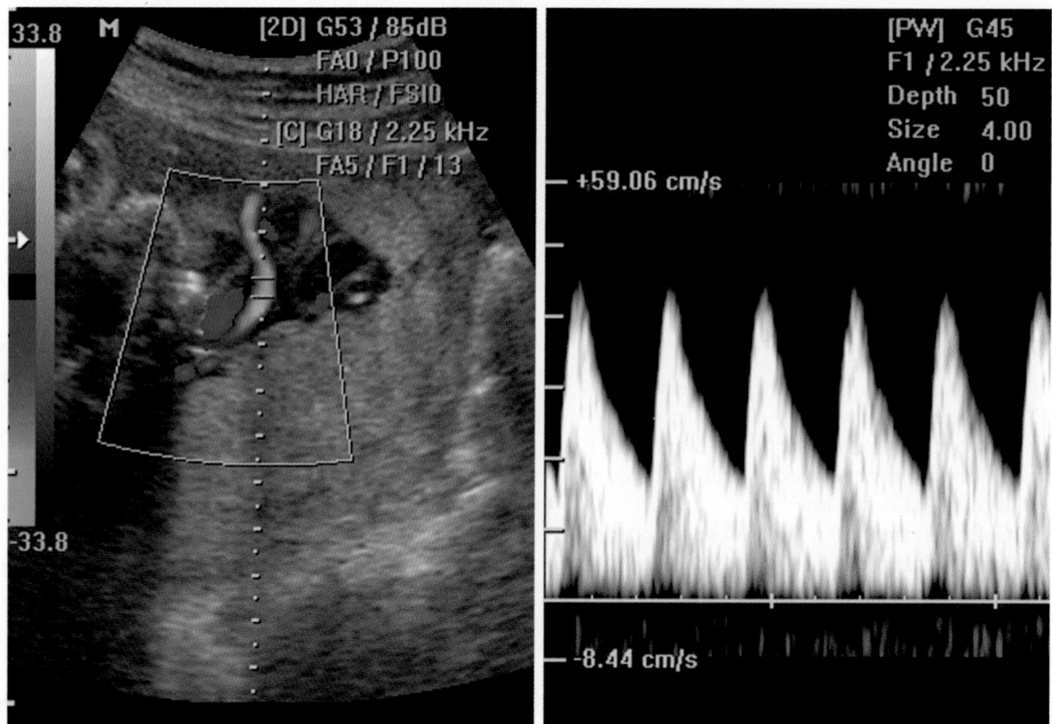

FIGURE 13-14 Colour and spectral Doppler evaluation of the umbilical artery. In the **left** panel the coiling arteries and vein are shown. *Red* indicates flow toward the transducer, and *blue* is flow away. The sample gate for the pulse Doppler is superimposed. On the **right** is the result of the pulse Doppler, depicting a normal flow velocity waveform.

ultrasonography, magnetic resonance imaging (MRI), CVS, PUBS, and amniocentesis. In some instances the nurse may assist the health care provider with the procedure. In many settings, nurses perform NSTs, CSTs, and BPPs; conduct an initial assessment; and begin necessary interventions for abnormal patterns. These nursing procedures are accomplished after additional education and training, under guidance of established protocols, and in collaboration with obstetrical providers. Patient teaching, which is an integral component of this role, involves preparing the woman for the procedure, interpreting the findings, and providing psychosocial support when needed.

Psychological Considerations

All women who undergo antenatal assessments are at risk for real and potential problems and may be anxious. In most instances, the tests are ordered because of suspected fetal compromise, deterioration of a maternal condition, or both. In the third trimester, pregnant women are most concerned about protecting themselves and their fetuses and consider themselves most vulnerable to outside influences. The label of "high risk" increases this sense of vulnerability.

When a woman is diagnosed with a high-risk pregnancy, she and her family may experience stress related to the diagnosis. The woman may exhibit various psychological responses, including anxiety, low self-esteem, guilt, frustration, and inability to function. Her perception of risk may be in the context of previous life experiences, coping strategies, and weight attached to the information provided from various sources. The development of a high-risk pregnancy also can affect parental attachment, accomplishment of the tasks of pregnancy, and family adaptation to the pregnancy.

If the woman is fearful for her own well-being, she may continue to feel ambivalence about the pregnancy and may not make regular attendance at prenatal care a priority. She may not be able to complete preparations for the baby or go to childbirth classes if she is on bedrest or hospitalized. She may also be aware of the expectations of others about her and her pregnancy that may include judgement if she is not behaving in ways perceived to reduce risks, such as continuing to smoke during pregnancy. The family may become frustrated because they cannot engage in parenting preparation or classes. Nurses should assist women in exploring their understanding of the risk associated with this pregnancy, as it is often different from that of their health care provider. Exploring this together may help the woman and family to develop questions for her health care provider regarding her care and plans for the labour and birth so that they can collaborate more effectively (Lee, Ayers, & Holden, 2012).

Antepartum hospitalization is an added stressor for the high-risk pregnant woman and her family. Emotions associated with hospitalization can include feelings of resignation; rates of depression have been reported to be as high as 15 to 25% (Denis, Michaux, & Callahan, 2012). The woman may be lonely because she is separated from her home and family. She may feel powerless and unable to make decisions for herself because her care is out of her control, including preparation for the birth process. Also, the longer the hospitalization, the greater the possibility that the mother–infant attachment process will be affected. Unexpected procedures and care for the woman or fetus may take priority over the usual birth plan and may not allow choices that would have been selected if the pregnancy had been low risk.

The nurse can help the woman and her family by encouraging her social support system—her family and friends—to visit more frequently and maintain communication. Obtaining detailed information about her care and the health of the fetus is also extremely important. While in hospital the woman may be encouraged to take part in group therapy to gain social support from others experiencing similar feelings and concerns. Providing support and encouragement, as well as opportunities for the woman to make as many choices as possible, can be helpful to this woman's care (see Community Focus box).

COMMUNITY FOCUS

Support for At-Risk Pregnant Women

At-risk pregnant women experience many stressors. Social support can relieve some of the stress, including that during labour. Nurses, social workers, and midwives, as well as trained lay persons or doulas, have all provided labour support. Investigate in your setting whether such support is available for low-income women. Is there a doula program at the hospital where you did your maternity clinical rotation or in your city? Does the program provide this service on a sliding scale for low-income women? What is the background of the doulas in your setting or city? Where do the doulas receive training? Interview a woman who has used a doula. What were the positive and negative factors associated with having a doula present during labour? Discuss your findings in a clinical conference.

KEY POINTS

- A high-risk pregnancy is one in which the life or well-being of the mother or fetus is jeopardized by a biophysical or psychosocial disorder coincident with or unique to pregnancy.
- The pregnancy, fetus, or newborn can be placed at risk through the influence of many of the determinants of health.
- Psychosocial perinatal warning indicators include characteristics of the parents, the fetus, the newborn, their support systems, and family circumstances.
- Intimate partner violence has a negative impact on pregnancy outcomes.
- There are ethnic disparities in maternal and perinatal mortality rates in Canada.
- The mortality rate decreases when risks are identified early and intensive care is applied.
- In the first and second trimester, antepartum testing is done to screen for fetal abnormalities, assess for gestational age, ensure appropriate growth, and assess placenta position.
- Biophysical assessment techniques include fetal movement counts and ultrasonography.
- Biochemical monitoring techniques include amniocentesis, PUBS, and CVS.
- Normal NSTs and negative CSTs suggest fetal well-being.
- Assessment tests may have some degree of risk for the mother and fetus and usually cause some anxiety for the woman and her family.

evolve WEBSITE

Visit the Evolve website for additional resources related to the content in this chapter such as Case Studies, Critical Thinking Case Study Answers, Nursing Care Plans, Nursing Processes, Nursing Skills, and Review Questions for Exam Preparation at: *http://evolve.elsevier.com/Canada/Perry/maternal/*

REFERENCES

BC Reproductive Mental Health Program & Perinatal Services BC. (2014). *Best practice guidelines for mental health disorders in the perinatal period.* Vancouver: Author. Retrieved from <http://www.perinatalservicesbc.ca/Documents/Guidelines-Standards/Maternal/MentalHealthDisordersGuideline.pdf>.

Butt, K., Lim, K., Bly, S., et al. (2014). SOGC clinical practice guideline: Determination of gestational age by ultrasound. *Journal of Obstetrics and Gynaecology Canada, 36*(2), 171–181.

Cargill, Y., Morin, L., Bly, S., et al. (2009). SOGC clinical practice guideline: Content of a complete routine second trimester obstetrical ultrasound examination and report. *Journal of Obstetrics and Gynaecology Canada, 31*(3), 272–275.

Chitayat, D., Langlois, S., Wilson, R. D., et al. (2007). Joint SOGC-CCMG clinical practice guideline: Screening for fetal aneuploidy in singleton pregnancies. *Journal of Obstetricians and Gynaecologists of Canada, 29*(2), 146–161.

Denis, A., Michaux, P., & Callahan, S. (2012). Factors implicated in moderating the risk for depression and anxiety in high risk pregnancy. *Journal of Reproductive and Infant Psychology, 30*(2), 124–134.

Denison, J., Varcoe, C., & Browne, A. (2014). Aboriginal women's experience of accessing healthcare when state apprehension of children is being threatened. *Journal of Advanced Nursing, 70*(5), 1105–1116.

Dennis, C. L., & Dowswell, T. (2013). Interventions (other than pharmacological, psychosocial or psychological) for treating antenatal depression. *Cochrane Database of Systematic Reviews,* (7). doi:10.1002/14651858.CD006795.pub3.

Gilbert, E. (2011). *Manual of high risk pregnancy and delivery* (5th ed.). St. Louis: Mosby.

Gilbert, W. M. (2012). Amniotic fluid disorders. In S. G. Gabbe, J. R. Niebyl, J. L. Simpson, et al. (Eds.), *Obstetrics: Normal and problem pregnancies* (6th ed.). Philadelphia: Saunders.

Greenberg, M., Druzin, M., & Gabbe, S. (2012). Antepartum fetal evaluation. In S. G. Gabbe, J. R. Niebyl, J. L. Simpson, et al. (Eds.), *Obstetrics: Normal and problem pregnancies* (6th ed.). Philadelphia: Saunders.

Grigoriadis, S., VonderPorten, E. H., Mamisashvili, L., et al. (2013). The impact of maternal depression during pregnancy on perinatal outcomes: A systematic review and meta-analysis. *Journal of Clinical Psychiatry*, *74*, e321–e341.

Kamal, A. (2014). Assessment of fetal health. In R. Resnik, R. K. Creasy, D. D. Iams, et al. (Eds.), *Creasy and Resnik's maternal–fetal medicine: Principles and practice* (7th ed.). Philadelphia: Saunders.

Lee, S., Ayers, S., & Holden, D. (2012). Risk perception of women during high risk pregnancy: A systematic review. *Health Risk & Society*, *14*(6), 511–531.

Liston, R., Sawchuck, D., Young, D., et al. (2007). SOGC clinical practice guideline: Fetal health surveillance: Antepartum and intrapartum consensus guideline. *Journal of Obstetrics and Gynaecology Canada*, *29*(9), Suppl 4.

Mikkonen, J., & Raphael, D. (2010). *Social determinants of health: The Canadian facts*. Retrieved from <http://www.thecanadianfacts.org/the_canadian_facts.pdf>.

Miller, L. A., Miller, D. A., & Tucker, S. M. (2013). *Mosby's pocket guide to fetal monitoring: A multidisciplinary approach* (7th ed.). St. Louis: Mosby.

Moise, K. (2012). Red cell alloimmunization. In S. G. Gabbe, J. R. Niebyl, J. L. Simpson, et al. (Eds.), *Obstetrics: Normal and problem pregnancies* (6th ed.). Philadelphia: Saunders.

Nageotte, M. P. (2014). Intrapartum fetal surveillance. In R. Resnik, R. K. Creasy, J. D. Iams, et al. (Eds.), *Creasy and Resnik's maternal–fetal medicine: Principles and practice* (7th ed.). Philadelphia: Saunders.

Palomaki, G. E., Kloza, E. M., Lambert-Messerlian, G. M., et al. (2011). DNA sequencing of maternal plasma to detect Down syndrome: An international clinical validation. *Genetic Medicine*, *13*(11), 913–920.

Public Health Agency of Canada. (2012). *Depression in pregnancy*. Retrieved from <http://www.phac-aspc.gc.ca/mh-sm/preg_dep-eng.php>.

Richards, D. S. (2012). Obstetrical ultrasound: Imaging, dating and growth. In S. G. Gabbe, J. R. Niebyl, J. L. Simpson, et al. (Eds.), *Obstetrics: Normal and problem pregnancies* (6th ed.). Philadelphia: Saunders.

Simpson, J., Richards, D., Otano, L., et al. (2012). Prenatal genetic diagnosis. In S. G. Gabbe, J. R. Niebyl, J. L. Simpson, et al. (Eds.), *Obstetrics: Normal and problem pregnancies* (6th ed.). Philadelphia: Saunders.

Society of Obstetricians and Gynaecologists of Canada. (2007). Clinical Practice Guideline: Screening for fetal aneuploidy. *Journal of Obstetricians and Gynaecologists of Canada*, *29*(2), 146–161. Retrieved from <http://sogc.org/guidelines/documents/187E-CPG-February2007.pdf>.

Society of Obstetricians and Gynaecologists of Canada & Canadian Association of Radiologists. (2014). Joint SOGC/CAR policy statement on non-medical use of fetal ultrasound. *Journal of Obstetricians and Gynaecologists of Canada*, *36*(2), 184–185.

Wapner, R. J. (2014). Prenatal diagnosis of congenital disorders. In R. Resnik, R. K. Creasy, J. D. Iams, et al. (Eds.), *Creasy and Resnik's maternal–fetal medicine: Principles and practice* (7th ed.). Philadelphia: Saunders.

Wilson, K., Dzerwinski, J., Hoskovec, J., et al. (2013). NSGC practice guideline: Prenatal screening and diagnostic testing options for chromosome aneuploidy. *Journal of Genetic Counselling*, *22*, 4–15.

Wilson, R. D., Audibert, F., Brock, J. A., et al. (2014). SOGC clinical practice guideline: Prenatal screening, diagnosis and pregnancy management of fetal neural tube defects. *Journal of Obstetrics and Gynaecology Canada*, *36*(10), 927–939.

World Health Organization. (2014). *Trends in maternal mortality: 1990 to 2013*. Retrieved from <http://apps.who.int/iris/bitstream/10665/112697/1/WHO_RHR_14.13_eng.pdf?ua=1>.

ADDITIONAL RESOURCES

Canadian Association of Genetic Counsellors. <https://cagc-accg.ca/>.

Perinatal Services BC Guidelines and Standards. <http://www.perinatalservicesbc.ca/health-professionals/guidelines-standards>.

Society of Obstetrician and Gynaecologists of Canada. <http://www.sogc.org>.

CHAPTER

14

Pregnancy at Risk: Gestational Conditions

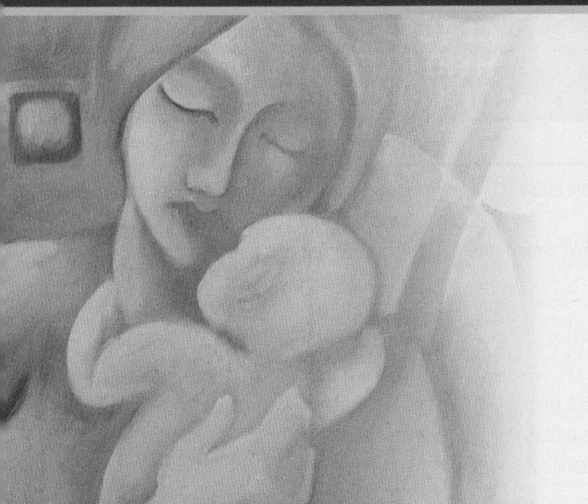

Melanie Basso

evolve WEBSITE

Visit the Evolve website for additional resources related to the content in this chapter such as Case Studies, Critical Thinking Case Study Answers, Nursing Care Plans, Nursing Processes, Nursing Skills, and Review Questions for Exam Preparation at: *http://evolve.elsevier.com/Canada/Perry/maternal/*

OBJECTIVES

On completion of this chapter, the reader will be able to:

- Differentiate gestational hypertension, pre-existing hypertension, and other hypertension.
- Describe the etiological theories and pathophysiology of pre-eclampsia.
- Compare the care management strategies for women with nonsevere pre-eclampsia and severe pre-eclampsia.
- Describe HELLP syndrome, including appropriate nursing actions.
- Understand the screening and care of a woman with gestational diabetes mellitus.
- Explain the effects of hyperemesis gravidarum on maternal and fetal well-being.
- Differentiate among causes, signs and symptoms, possible complications, and management of spontaneous abortion, ectopic pregnancy, cervical insufficiency, and hydatidiform mole.
- Compare and contrast placenta previa and placental abruption in regard to signs and symptoms, complications, and management.
- Discuss the diagnosis and management of disseminated intravascular coagulation.
- Discuss signs and symptoms, effects on pregnancy, and management of urinary tract infections.
- Explain the basic principles of care for a pregnant woman undergoing abdominal surgery.
- Discuss implications of trauma on the mother and fetus during pregnancy.
- Identify priorities in assessment and stabilization measures for the pregnant trauma victim.

Providing safe and effective care for a pregnant woman with high-risk conditions requires a multidisciplinary team working alongside the woman and her family. Each team member contributes unique knowledge and skills toward providing optimum outcomes for the mother and infant. This chapter discusses a wide range of disorders that can develop during pregnancy and place the woman and fetus at risk. Hypertensive disorders in pregnancy, gestational diabetes mellitus (GDM), hyperemesis gravidarum, hemorrhagic complications of early and late pregnancy, surgery during pregnancy, and trauma are discussed. For most conditions, management throughout the entire perinatal period (antepartum, intrapartum, and postpartum) is included; thus all information for each condition is located in one place in the text.

HYPERTENSIVE DISORDERS IN PREGNANCY

Significance and Incidence

Hypertensive disorders in pregnancy are an increasingly common and leading cause of maternal and perinatal morbidity and mortality worldwide (Magee, Pels, Helewa, et al., 2014). Approximately 5 to 10% of pregnancies are complicated by hypertensive disorders of pregnancy (Hutcheon, Lisonkova, & Joseph, 2011). Women at older ages—greater than age 40 with their first pregnancy—have the highest rates of pregnancy-related hypertension (Magee et al., 2014). Rates of development of pre-eclampsia are higher for women with a family history of pre-eclampsia and for women whose mothers had pre-eclampsia (Hutcheon et al., 2011).

Morbidity and Mortality

Maternal complications from significant hypertension include maternal death, acute renal failure, pulmonary edema, HELLP syndrome (hemolysis, elevated liver enzymes, and low platelets; see later discussion), and cerebral edema with seizures (Mehrabadi, Liu, Bartholomew, et al., 2014). Maternal deaths associated with severe hypertension result primarily from complications of hepatic rupture, placental abruption, and eclampsia (characterized by seizures) (Markham & Funai, 2013). Infants born at full term to mothers with hypertensive disorders of pregnancy have higher rates of neonatal mortality than do newborns of mothers who were not hypertensive (Hutcheon et al., 2011). The unborn fetus of the pre-eclamptic woman is at increased risk from placental abruption, preterm birth, intrauterine growth restriction (IUGR), and acute hypoxia. Clinical care goals are focused on the prevention of pre-eclampsia rather than on the prevention of complications from severe pre-eclampsia. Updates to the Society of Obstetricians and Gynaecologists of Canada (SOGC) (Magee et al., 2014) guidelines provide recommendations regarding both the prevention of pre-eclampsia and the prevention of its associated complications.

Definition of Hypertensive Disorder of Pregnancy (HDP)

Hypertension in pregnancy (HDP) is determined by an assessed blood pressure measure of systolic blood pressure (sBP) of 140 mm Hg or greater and or diastolic blood pressure (dBP) of 90 mm Hg or greater, taken at two separate measurements and at least 15 minutes apart. This level of blood pressure is associated with higher adverse perinatal outcomes. *Severe hypertension* is defined as a sBP of 160 mm Hg or greater or a dBP of 110 mm Hg, based on at least two measurements taken at least 15 minutes apart (Magee et al., 2014).

Classification

The classification of hypertensive disorders in pregnancy has been defined in three categories: pre-existing (chronic) hypertension; gestational hypertension; and other. Pre-eclampsia can occur with either category of pre-existing hypertension or gestational hypertension. Three types of "other" hypertensive effects have been introduced: transient hypertension, white-coat hypertension, and masked hypertension (Magee et al., 2014).

Pre-existing hypertension is present before pregnancy or appears prior to 20 weeks of gestation. Gestational hypertension is the development of hypertension at or after 20 weeks. For both pre-existing and gestational hypertension, there are two subgroups: (1) with comorbid conditions and (2) with evidence of pre-eclampsia. Table 14-1 presents details of the criteria for each classification. Edema and weight gain are no longer considered markers of pre-eclampsia, as neither is significantly associated with perinatal mortality and morbidity.

Pre-Existing Hypertension

Pre-existing hypertension is defined as hypertension present before the pregnancy or diagnosed before 20 weeks of gestation (Magee et al., 2014; Markham & Funai, 2013). Most women with pre-existing hypertension experience uncomplicated pregnancies; however, there is an increased risk of poor fetal growth and fetal stillbirth. Preconception counselling is recommended for these women (Magee et al., 2014).

TABLE 14-1 CLASSIFICATION OF HYPERTENSIVE DISORDERS OF PREGNANCY

DISORDER	COMMENTS
Pre-existing hypertension	Predates the pregnancy or appears before 20 weeks
A) with comorbid conditions	Comorbid conditions (pregestational type I or II diabetes mellitus or kidney disease) require tighter BP control outside of pregnancy because of their association with heightened cardiovascular risk.
B) with evidence of pre-eclampsia (onset after 20 weeks' gestation)	Also known as superimposed pre-eclampsia. One or more symptoms must be present: • Resistant hypertension (defined as need for three antihypertensive medications) or • New or worsening proteinuria or • One or more adverse conditions or • One or more severe complications
Gestational hypertension	Hypertension that appears for the first time at or beyond 20 weeks' gestation
A) with comorbid conditions	Comorbid conditions (pregestational type I or II diabetes mellitus or kidney disease) require tighter BP control outside of pregnancy because of their association with heightened cardiovascular risk.
B) with evidence of pre-eclampsia (after 20 weeks' gestation)	Defined as gestational hypertension with one or more of the following symptoms: • New or worsening proteinuria or • One or more adverse conditions or • One or more severe complications
Pre-eclampsia	May arise without previous symptoms. Defined as gestational hypertension with one or more of the following: • New or worsening proteinuria or • One or more adverse conditions or • One or more severe complications
Severe pre-eclampsia	Defined when one or more severe complications are present
Other hypertensive effects:	
Transient hypertension	Elevated BP may be due to environmental stimuli
White coat hypertension	BP that is elevated in the clinician's office (≥140/90) but is consistently normal outside of it (<135/85)
Masked hypertension	BP that is consistently normal in the clinician's office (<140/90) but is consistently higher outside of it (≥135/85)

Reprinted from Diagnosis, evaluation, and management of the hypertensive disorders of pregnancy: Executive summary, *Journal of Obstetrics and Gynaecology Canada,* 36(5), 416–438. Copyright 2014, with permission from Elsevier.

TABLE 14-2 ADVERSE CONDITIONS AND SEVERE COMPLICATIONS OF PRE-ECLAMPSIA

ORGAN SYSTEM IDENTIFIED	ADVERSE CONDITIONS (THAT INCREASE RISK OF SEVERE COMPLICATIONS)	SEVERE COMPLICATIONS (THAT WARRANT DELIVERY)
Central nervous system	Headache/visual disturbances	Eclampsia/PRES Cortical blindness or retinal detachment GCS <13 Stroke or TIA
Cardiorespiratory	Chest pain/dyspnea	Uncontrolled severe hypertension >12 hours, despite use of three antihypertensive agents
	Oxygen saturation <97%	O_2 saturation <90, need for 50% O_2 for 1 hour, intubation, pulmonary edema Positive inotropic support Myocardial ischemia or infarction
Hematological	Elevated WBC Elevated INR or aPTT Low platelets	Platelet count <50 Transfusion of any blood product
Renal	Elevated serum creatinine Elevated serum uric acid	Acute kidney injury New indication for dialysis
Hepatic	Nausea or vomiting RUQ or epigastric pain Elevated serum AST, ALT, LDH, or bilirubin Low plasma albumin	Hepatic dysfunction Hepatic hematoma or rupture
Fetoplacental	Abnormal FHR IUGR Oligohydramnios Absent or reversed end-diastolic flow by Doppler velocimetry	Abruption with evidence of maternal or fetal compromise Reverse ductus venosus A wave Stillbirth

ALT, alanine aminotransferase; *aPTT*, activated partial thromboplastin time; *AST*, aspartate aminotransferase; *DIC*, disseminated intravascular coagulation; *FHR*, fetal heart rate; *GCS*, Glasgow Coma Scale; *INR*, international normalized ratio; *IUGR*, intrauterine growth restriction; *LDH*, lactate dehydrogenase; *PRES*, posterior reversible leukoencephalopathy syndrome; *RIND*, reversible ischemic neurological deficit (<48 hr); *RUQ*, right upper quadrant; *TIA*, transient ischemic attack; *WBC*, white blood cell.

Adapted from Magee, L. A., Pels, A., Helewa, M., et al. (2014). SOGC clinical practice guideline: Diagnosis, evaluation and management of hypertensive disorders of pregnancy: Executive summary. *Journal of Obstetrics and Gynaecology Canada, 36*(5), 416–438. Copyright 2014, with permission from Elsevier.

Pre-Existing Hypertension With Superimposed Pre-Eclampsia

Approximately 25% of women with pre-existing hypertension develop pre-eclampsia or eclampsia. This disorder is associated with severe maternal and fetal complications. Pre-existing hypertension with superimposed pre-eclampsia is defined in the presence of the following findings:

- Hypertension before 20 weeks of gestation, with new or worsening proteinuria
- Both hypertension and proteinuria before 20 weeks of gestation
- A sudden increase in BP in a woman whose hypertension was previously well controlled
- Thrombocytopenia
- Elevated liver enzymes

The Link Between Hypertension and the Development of Pre-Eclampsia

Women with pre-existing hypertension and other comorbidities, such as renal disease or type 1 diabetes, are at increased risk of developing pre-eclampsia. Women who develop hypertension prior to 34 weeks are also at increased risk of developing pre-eclampsia. Certain risk factors are associated with development of the condition, such as nulliparity, family history of pre-eclampsia, multiple gestation, obesity, and chronic medical disorders (Hutcheon et al., 2011; Sibai, 2012). Some studies have shown an increased risk for pre-eclampsia in multiparous women with new partners for subsequent pregnancies (Sibai, 2012). There appears to be a paternal factor involved (i.e., men who fathered one pregnancy complicated by pre-eclampsia were nearly twice as likely to father another pre-eclamptic pregnancy in a different woman) (Sibai, 2012). Adverse conditions and severe complications of pre-eclampsia are listed in Table 14-2.

Pre-Eclampsia

Once the diagnosis of HDP has been made, women must be closely monitored for the development of pre-eclampsia, which often develops after the second trimester of pregnancy. *Pre-eclampsia* is a hypertensive disorder most commonly defined by new-onset proteinuria and, potentially, other end-organ dysfunction and may result in maternal complications or intrauterine fetal morbidity and mortality due to uteroplacental insufficiency and placental abruption. It is a multisystem, vasospastic disease process of reduced organ perfusion characterized by the presence of hypertension and proteinuria, with a clinical continuum from mild to severe (Table 14-3). It affects a myriad of maternal and fetal systems and, if not controlled, results in poor perinatal outcomes.

TABLE 14-3 DIFFERENTIATION BETWEEN NONSEVERE AND SEVERE PRE-ECLAMPSIA

MATERNAL EFFECTS	NONSEVERE PRE-ECLAMPSIA	SEVERE PRE-ECLAMPSIA
Blood pressure (BP)	BP reading of ≥140/90 mm Hg × two readings 15 minutes apart	Rise to ≥160/110 mm Hg on two separate readings 15 minutes apart
Mean arterial pressure	>105 mm Hg	>105 mm Hg
Proteinuria		
Quantitative 24-hr analysis	Proteinuria of <0.3 g in a 24-hr specimen or ≤30 mg/mmol urinary creatinine in a random urine sample	Proteinuria of >0.3 g in a 24-hr specimen or ≥30 mg/mmol urinary creatinine in a random urine sample
Qualitative dipstick	≥0.30 g/L on dipstick or 1+	2+ to 3+ protein on dipstick
Reflexes	May be normal	Hyperreflexia >3+, possible ankle clonus
Urine output	Output matching intake; ≥30 mL/hr or <650 mL/24 hr	15 mL/hr or <400 mL–500 mL/24 hr
Headache	May be present or transient	Severe
Visual problems	May be present	Blurred, photophobia, blind spots on funduscopy
Right upper quadrant or epigastric pain	May be present	Hepatic hematoma or rupture may be present
Serum creatinine	May be elevated	Elevated to > 150 mcmol/L
Thrombocytopenia	Platelets may be low	Platelets are < 50 × 10 ^{9} /L
AST, ALT, LDH, or bilirubin elevation	Elevated	Hepatic dysfunction
Fetal Effects		
Fetal heart rate	May be abnormal	May be abnormal
Placental perfusion	Reduced, oligohydramnios may be present	Decreased perfusion expressing as IUGR in fetus; FHR may show late decelerations in labour
Premature placental aging	Not apparent	At birth, placenta appearing smaller than normal for duration of pregnancy; premature aging apparent with numerous areas of ischemic necroses (white infarcts); numerous, intervillous fibrin deposition (red infarcts)

ALT, alanine aminotransferase; *AST,* aspartate aminotransferase; *FHR,* fetal heart rate; *IUGR,* intrauterine growth restriction; *LDH,* lactate dehydrogenase.
Source: Magee, L. A., Pels, A., Helewa, M., et al. (2014). SOGC clinical practice guideline: Diagnosis, evaluation and management of hypertensive disorders of pregnancy: Executive summary. *Journal of Obstetrics and Gynaecology Canada, 36*(5), 416–438.

The two key components to the diagnosis of pre-eclampsia are hypertension and new (or worsening) proteinuria. Maternal symptoms that indicate severe pre-eclampsia include presence of one or more severe complications including seizures, blindness, stroke, severe liver dysfunction, pulmonary edema, and myocardial dysfunction (see Table 14-2). While the presence of any of these symptoms alone does not indicate pre-eclampsia any one of them must be investigated immediately.

Pre-eclampsia contributes significantly to restrictions of fetal growth and the incidence of placental abruption. Impaired placental perfusion leads to early degenerative aging of the placenta. The rate of fetal complications is directly related to the severity of the disease (Magee et al., 2014; Sibai, 2012).

Possible fetal effects resulting from hypertension, which may occur independently or in conjunction with maternal symptoms, include oligohydramnios, IUGR, abnormal umbilical artery Doppler results indicating decreased blood flow to the fetus from a poorly functioning placenta, and stillbirth (Magee et al., 2014).

Proteinuria. *Proteinuria* is defined as a concentration of 0.03 g/L or more in at least two random urine specimens collected at least 6 hours apart where there is no evidence of urinary tract infection. In a 24-hour specimen, proteinuria is defined as a concentration of greater than 0.3 g/L per 24 hours (Box 14-1). The diagnosis of proteinuria should be based on the use of the urinary protein: creatinine ratio or 24-hour urine collection (Magee et al., 2014; Markham & Funai, 2013).

BOX 14-1 URINE PROTEIN VALUES

Protein readings are designated as follows:
- 0—negative
- Trace—trace
- +1—0.3 g/L
- +2—1.0 g/L
- +3—3.0 g/L
- +4—more than 10.0 g/L

Nonsevere pre-eclampsia. *Nonsevere pre-eclampsia* is defined as a combination of hypertension (sBP below 160 mm Hg and dBP below 110 mm Hg) and proteinuria, with the presence of one or more adverse conditions (see Table 14-3) which increase the risk of severe complications (Magee et al., 2014). Blood work and assessment for endothelial damage are indicated to monitor for the development of severe pre-eclampsia and the presence of one or more severe complications.

Severe pre-eclampsia. *Severe pre-eclampsia* is defined as having an sBP greater than 160 mm Hg or a dBP of at least 110 mm Hg and the presence of new proteinuria (Magee et al., 2014) and the presence of one or more severe complications.

Severe complications associated with severe pre-eclampsia include the following: oliguria; cerebral disturbances such as altered level of consciousness, confusion, or headache; eclampsia or stroke; visual disturbances such as scotoma or blurred vision; hepatic damage or rupture, including epigastric pain, right upper quadrant pain, impaired liver function, or elevated liver enzymes; thrombocytopenia with a platelet count less than 50×10^9/L; hemolytic anemia; pulmonary edema; and fetal growth restriction (see Table 14-3) (Magee et al., 2014; Markham & Funai, 2013; Sibai, 2012).

Eclampsia. Eclampsia, characterized by seizures from profound cerebral effects of pre-eclampsia, is the major maternal risk. As a rule, maternal and perinatal morbidity and mortality rates are highest when eclampsia is seen early in gestation (before 28 weeks), maternal age is greater than 40 years, the woman is a multigravida, and chronic hypertension or renal disease is present (Sibai, 2012). The incidence of eclampsia has declined dramatically, from 12.4 to 5.9 per 10,000 births in 2003 and 2009, respectively (Liu, Joseph, Liston, et al., 2011). The fetus of the eclamptic woman is at increased risk for placental abruption, preterm birth, IUGR, and acute hypoxia. Eclamptic seizures can occur before, during, or after birth. Approximately one third of eclamptic seizures occur after birth, almost always within the first 48 hours after birth (Markham & Funai, 2013).

Etiology. The etiology of pre-eclampsia is theorized to include various possibilities: abnormal prostaglandin action, endothelial cell dysfunction, coagulation abnormalities, vasoconstrictor tone, and dietary deficiencies or excesses (Fig. 14-1). Immunological factors and genetic disposition may also play an important role (Sibai, 2012). Animal studies have suggested that abnormalities of the placenta are the cause of pre-eclampsia. The trophoblast cells of the placenta usually alter the spiral arteries in the uterus to accommodate increased blood flow.

In pre-eclampsia, the vessels are abnormally thick-walled and muscular and have higher resistance. The condition also results in a distinctive lesion called *acute atherosis*, and there is greater occurrence of placental infarcts. Placental perfusion is decreased, resulting in hypoxia; this in turn causes several pathophysiological abnormalities, especially endothelial damage.

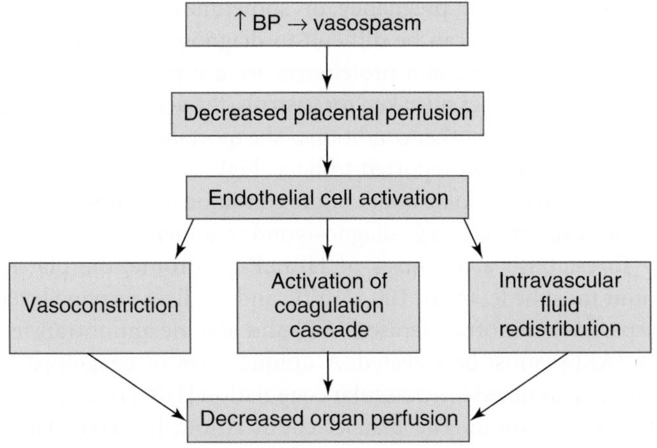

FIGURE 14-1 Etiology of pre-eclampsia. *BP*, blood pressure.

Many of these pathophysiological changes of pre-eclampsia occur before clinical symptoms develop (Sibai, 2012).

Since the etiology of pre-eclampsia is unknown, various clinical trials have attempted to correct theoretical abnormalities present in pre-eclampsia as a means of preventing pre-eclampsia. Some methods used to prevent pre-eclampsia are listed in Box 14-2.

Pathophysiology. Pre-eclampsia exists along a continuum from nonsevere disease to severe pre-eclampsia, HELLP syndrome, or eclampsia. The pathophysiology of pre-eclampsia reflects alterations in the normal adaptations of pregnancy. Normal physiological adaptations to pregnancy include increased blood plasma volume, vasodilation, decreased systemic vascular resistance, elevated cardiac output, and decreased colloid osmotic pressure. The main pathogenic factor is not an increase in BP but poor perfusion as a result of vasospasm. Arteriolar vasospasm diminishes the diameter of blood vessels, which impedes blood flow to all organs and increases BP (Magee et al., 2014; Markham & Funai, 2013) (see Community Focus box). Function in organs such as the placenta, kidneys, liver, and brain is depressed by as much as 40 to 60%. The pathophysiological sequelae are shown in Fig. 14-2.

HELLP syndrome. HELLP syndrome is a laboratory diagnosis for a variant of severe pre-eclampsia that is characterized by hemolysis (*H*), elevated liver enzymes (*EL*), and low platelets (*LP*) (American College of Obstetricians and Gynecologists [ACOG],

BOX 14-2 RECOMMENDATIONS FOR PREVENTION OF PRE-ECLAMPSIA AND IMPROVEMENT OF PREGNANCY OUTCOMES IN WOMEN AT LOW RISK OF DEVELOPING PRE-ECLAMPSIA

- Abstention from alcohol
- Smoking cessation
- Multivitamins containing folate (also to prevent neural tube defects)
- Calcium supplementation (at least 1 g/day orally) for women with low dietary intake of calcium
- Regular exercise

The following are **NOT** recommended for prevention of pre-eclampsia in low-risk women (due to insufficient evidence):

- Supplementation with magnesium or zinc
- Prostaglandin precursors such as fish and evening primrose oil
- High-protein and low-salt diet
- Calorie restriction for overweight women
- Low-dose aspirin (recommended for women at increased risk of pre-eclampsia)
- Vitamins C and E
- Thiazide diuretics
- Antihypertensive therapy (does not prevent pre-eclampsia)

Adapted from Magee, L. A., Pels, A., Helewa, M., et al. and Society of Obstetricians and Gynaecologists of Canada. (2014). SOGC clinical practice guideline: Diagnosis, evaluation and management of hypertensive disorders of pregnancy: Executive summary. *Journal of Obstetrics and Gynaecology Canada, 36*(5), 416–438.

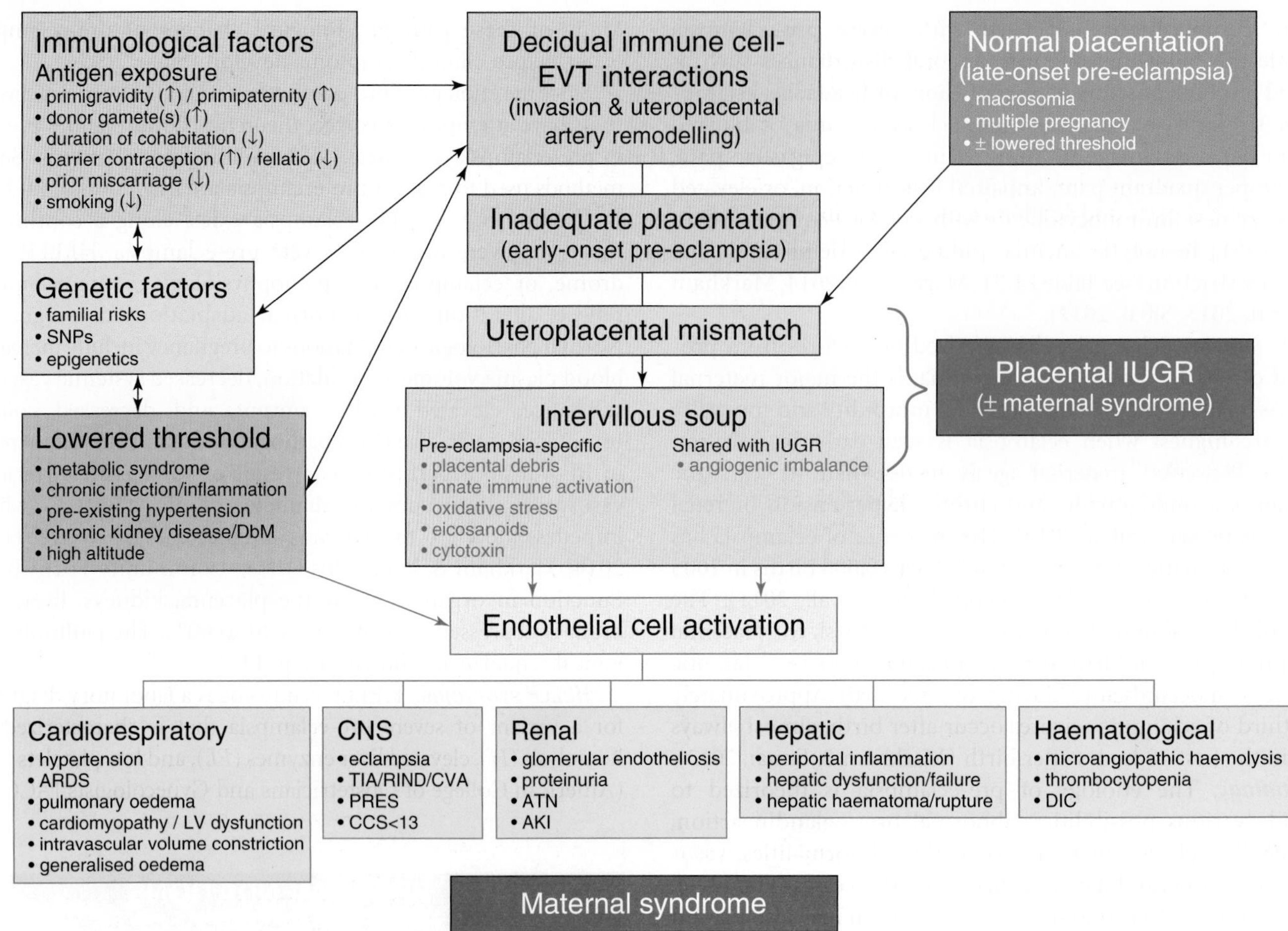

FIGURE 14-2 Pathophysiology of pre-eclampsia. AKI, acute kidney injury; ARDS, acute respiratory distress syndrome; ATN, acute tubular necrosis; CNS, central nervous system; CVA, cerebrovascular accident; DbM, diabetes mellitus; DIC, disseminated intravascular coagulation; EVT, extravillous trophoblast; GCS, Glasgow Coma Scale; IUGR, intrauterine growth restriction; LV, left ventricular; PRES, posterior reversible encephalopathy syndrome; RIND, reversible ischemic neurological deficit; SNPs, single nucleotide polymorphism; TIA, transient ischemic attack. (From Magee, L. A., Pels, A., Helewa, M., et al. (2014). SOGC clinical practice guideline: Diagnosis, evaluation and management of hypertensive disorders of pregnancy: Executive summary. *Journal of Obstetrics and Gynaecology Canada, 36*(5), 416–438. Copyright 2014, with permission from Elsevier.)

COMMUNITY FOCUS

The Woman With Pre-Eclampsia

Margie, a 25-year-old, G1T0P0A0L0, single woman who is an administrative assistant at a high school, is seen in the clinic for her routine prenatal visit at 30 weeks of gestation. On examination, you note that her blood pressure is 150/94, and on a urine dipstick she has a new finding of 1+ proteinuria.

- What is the likely diagnosis for Margie? What other signs and symptoms of this condition might you find? Develop a nursing care plan for Margie. What teaching about diet, rest, signs and symptoms to observe, and fetal assessment should be included in the plan?
- What community agencies or assistance is available to her? Develop a list of community resources for women in circumstances similar to Margie's.

2015; Magee et al., 2014; Sibai, 2012). HELLP syndrome is a life-threatening pregnancy complication usually considered to be a variant of pre-eclampsia. Both conditions usually occur during the later stages of pregnancy or sometimes after childbirth. HELLP syndrome can be difficult to diagnose, especially when high blood pressure and proteinuria are not present. Its symptoms are sometimes mistaken for gastritis, flu, acute hepatitis, gall bladder disease, or other conditions. The mortality rate of HELLP syndrome has been reported to be as high as 25%. It is critical for care providers to be aware of the condition and its symptoms so they can provide early diagnosis and treatment.

To establish a diagnosis of HELLP syndrome, the platelet count must be less than 100×10^9/L, and the liver enzyme levels (aspartate aminotransferase [AST] and alanine aminotransferase [ALT]) must be elevated. A unique form of coagulopathy (not disseminated intravascular coagulation [DIC]) occurs with HELLP syndrome. The platelet count is low, but coagulation factor assays, prothrombin time (PT), partial thromboplastin time (PTT), and bleeding time remain normal. Women who develop only one or two of the diagnostic laboratory values are diagnosed with incomplete HELLP, partial HELLP, or the ELLP syndrome (Harvey & Sibai, 2013).

The pathophysiological changes of HELLP syndrome occur as a result of arteriolar vasospasm, endothelial cell dysfunction with fibrin deposits, and adherence of platelets in blood vessels. Red blood cells are damaged as they pass through narrowed blood vessels and become hemolyzed, resulting in a decreased red blood cell and platelet count and hyperbilirubinemia. Endothelial damage and fibrin deposits in the liver lead to impaired liver function and can cause hemorrhagic necrosis. Liver enzymes are elevated when hepatic tissue is damaged (Gilbert, 2011).

HELLP syndrome appears in approximately 20% of women with severe pre-eclampsia (ACOG, 2015; Harvey & Sibai, 2013). Most commonly, HELLP syndrome is seen in older, White, multiparous women. About 90% of women report a history of malaise for several days. Many women (65%) experience epigastric or right upper quadrant abdominal pain (possibly related to hepatic ischemia), and approximately half develop nausea and vomiting. Many women with HELLP syndrome may not have signs and symptoms of severe pre-eclampsia; many are normotensive and have no proteinuria. As a result, women with HELLP syndrome are often misdiagnosed with a variety of other medical or surgical disorders (Sibai, 2012).

Recognition of the clinical and laboratory findings associated with HELLP syndrome is important if early, aggressive therapy is to be initiated to prevent maternal and newborn death. Complications reported with HELLP syndrome include renal failure, pulmonary edema, ruptured liver hematoma, DIC, and placental abruption (Gasem, al Jama, Burshaid, et al., 2009; Sibai, 2012).

Numerous clinical trials have examined various interventions to prevent pre-eclampsia, including protein or salt restriction; zinc, magnesium, fish oil, or vitamins C and E supplementation; use of diuretics or other antihypertensive medications; and use of heparin or low-dose aspirin. All of these interventions demonstrated minimal to no benefit in preventing or reducing the severity of pre-eclampsia (Sibai, 2012).

No reliable test that can be used as a routine screening tool for predicting pre-eclampsia has yet been developed. However, the search for biomarkers that can identify individual women who will develop hypertension during pregnancy is ongoing (Harvey & Sibai, 2013). For example, the tyrosine kinase (sFLt) and serum placental growth factor (PIGF) ratio at 22 to 26 weeks of gestation was shown in one study to be highly predictive of early-onset pre-eclampsia (Gilbert, 2011). An abnormal uterine artery Doppler velocimetry in the first or second trimester of pregnancy has also been suggested as a good screening test to predict pre-eclampsia (Gilbert, 2011).

Although research offers future promise, much work remains before a screening test for pre-eclampsia is available for widespread clinical use. Nurses should be aware of what strategies are being studied and use the most valid results so they can counsel pregnant women about interventions that are evidence based. Meanwhile, the best pre-eclampsia prevention methods include early prenatal care for the identification of women at risk and early detection of the disease (see Home Care box).

HOME CARE

Management of Women With Gestational or Pre-Existing Hypertension

Women with gestational or pre-existing hypertension are managed at home and are taught to assess and report clinical signs of pre-eclampsia.

Report Immediately Any Clinical Signs

- Report any increase in blood pressure, protein in urine, or decreased fetal movement.*

Take Blood Pressure With Consistency

- Take blood pressure on the same arm with the woman in a sitting position (no dangling legs) each time for consistent and accurate readings. Support the arm on a table in a horizontal position at heart level.

Dipstick Test Clean-Catch Urine Sample

- This is done to assess proteinuria; report frequency or burning on urination. Report any presence of proteinuria.

Assess Fetal Activity Daily

- Decreased activity (five or fewer movements in 2 hours) may indicate fetal compromise.

Keep Scheduled Prenatal Appointments

- Regular appointments need to be kept so that any changes in maternal or fetal condition can be detected immediately.

Keep a Daily Log or Diary

- Keep a log of assessments and bring it to prenatal visits.

*Thresholds for blood pressure, fetal movement counts, and proteinuria are set by the primary health care provider or institutional protocol.

NURSING CARE

Blood Pressure Assessment

Accurate and consistent assessment of BP is important for establishing a baseline and for monitoring subtle changes throughout the pregnancy. BP readings are affected by maternal position and measurement techniques, thus consistency must be ensured. Normally, the dBP drops an average of 10 mm Hg below nonpregnant values by midgestation and then slowly reaches nonpregnant levels in the third trimester. Evaluation of BP focuses on trends, not on a single reading (ACOG, 2015; Markham & Funai, 2013). Box 14-3 presents recommendations for standardizing this procedure.

Other Assessments

Deep tendon reflexes. Deep tendon reflexes (DTRs) are evaluated at baseline and then throughout the pregnancy to detect any changes. The biceps and patellar reflexes and ankle clonus are assessed and the findings recorded (Fig. 14-3 and Table 14-4). The evaluation of DTRs is especially important if

BOX 14-3 PROTOCOL FOR BLOOD PRESSURE MEASUREMENT

- Blood pressure (BP) should be measured with the woman in a sitting position with the arm at the level of the heart.
- Use the proper-size cuff (cuff should cover 1.5 times the circumference of the arm).
- Use Korotkoff phase V for the diastolic reading.
- If BP is consistently higher in one arm, the arm with the higher values should be used.
- Use manual sphygmomanometer, or an automated BP device that has been validated for use in pre-eclampsia.
- Women must be instructed in proper BP measurement if they are performing home BP monitoring.

Adapted from Magee, L. A., Pels, A., Helewa, M., et al. and Society of Obstetricians and Gynaecologists of Canada. (2014). SOGC clinical practice guideline: Diagnosis, evaluation and management of hypertensive disorders of pregnancy. *Journal of Obstetrics and Gynaecology Canada, 36*(5), 416–438.

TABLE 14-4 ASSESSING DEEP TENDON REFLEXES

GRADE	DEEP TENDON REFLEX RESPONSE
0	No response
1+	Sluggish or diminished
2+	Active or expected response
3+	More brisk than expected; slightly hyperactive
4+	Brisk, hyperactive, with intermittent or transient clonus

From Seidel, H. M., Ball, J. W., Dains, J. E., et al. (2011). *Mosby's guide to physical examination* (7th ed.). St. Louis: Mosby.

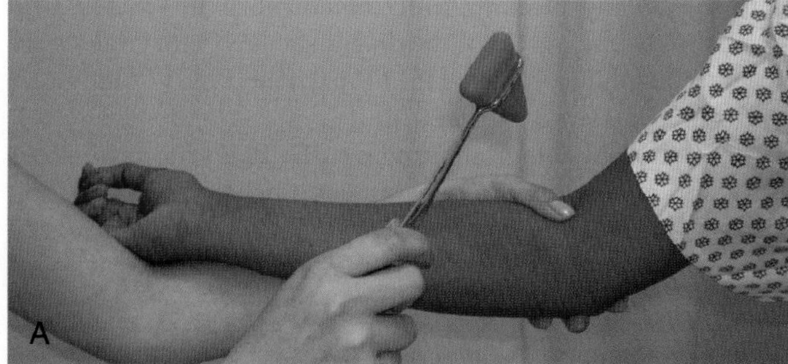

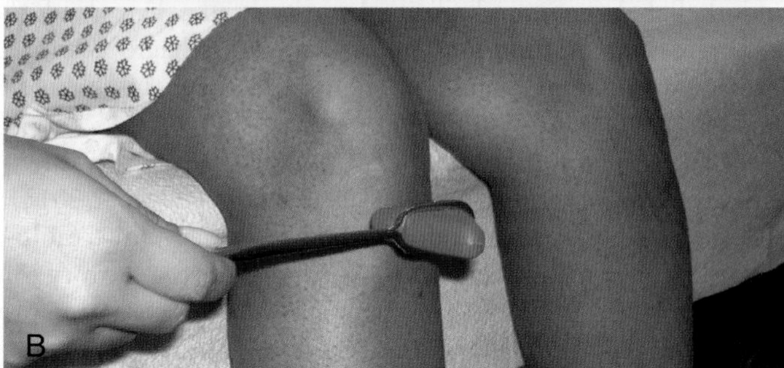

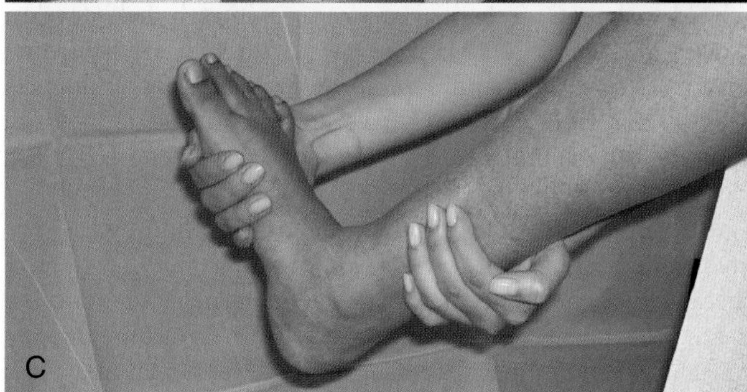

FIGURE 14-3 Deep tendon reflexes. **A:** Biceps reflex. **B:** Patellar reflex with woman's legs hanging freely over end of examining table. **C:** Test for ankle clonus. (Courtesy Shannon Perry.)

the woman is being treated with magnesium sulphate. Decreased or absent DTRs may be an indication of magnesium toxicity.

To elicit the biceps reflex, a downward blow is struck over the thumb, which is placed over the biceps tendon. Normal response is flexion of the arm at the elbow, described as a 2+ response (see Fig. 14-3, A, and Table 14-4).

The patellar reflex is elicited with the woman's legs hanging freely over the end of the examining table or with the woman lying on her side with the knee slightly flexed. A blow with a percussion hammer is dealt directly to the patellar tendon, inferior to the patella. Normal response is extension or kicking out of the leg, which is recorded as 2+ (see Fig. 14-3, B, and Table 14-4).

To assess for hyperactive reflexes (clonus) at the ankle joint, the examiner supports the leg with the knee flexed. With one hand, the examiner sharply dorsiflexes the foot, maintains the position for a moment, and then releases the foot (see Fig. 14-3, C). A normal (negative clonus) response is elicited when no rhythmic oscillations (jerks) are felt while the foot is held in dorsiflexion. When the foot is released, no oscillations are seen as the foot drops to the plantar-flexed position. An abnormal (positive clonus) response is indicated by rhythmic oscillations of one or more beats felt when the foot is in dorsiflexion and seen as the foot drops to the plantar-flexed position.

Fetal health surveillance. Uteroplacental perfusion can be decreased in women with pre-eclampsia. Fetal health surveillance, by means of such methods as the nonstress test (NST), contraction stress test (CST), biophysical profile (BPP), and serial ultrasonography, is used to assess fetal status. The fetal heart rate (FHR) is assessed for baseline rate, variability, and presence of accelerations. Abnormal baseline rate, decreased or absent variability, or late decelerations are indications of fetal intolerance to the intrauterine environment. Since the woman with pre-eclampsia is at risk for placental abruption, it is important to assess uterine tone and tenderness and check for the presence of vaginal bleeding. Doppler flow velocimetry studies can be used to evaluate uteroplacental perfusion (see Chapter 13).

! NURSING ALERT

Uterine tenderness along with increasing tone may be the earliest finding of an abruption. Idiopathic preterm contractions also may be an early sign.

An evaluation of fetal growth by ultrasonography should be obtained at diagnosis and repeated every 2 weeks. Fetal movements are counted daily (see Chapter 13, p. 302). Fetal compromise evidenced by slowed growth, abnormal FHR surveillance, or an abnormal finding during testing may necessitate immediate delivery, depending on gestational age (labour induction or Caesarean birth) (ACOG, 2015; Magee et al., 2014; Markham & Funai, 2013).

Activity Restriction

Women with pre-existing or gestational hypertension without pre-eclampsia may benefit from some bedrest in hospital in an attempt to decrease the progression to severe hypertension and preterm birth. For women with severe pre-eclampsia who are hospitalized, strict bedrest is NOT recommended, but some reduced activity may be beneficial in decreasing BP and promoting fetal growth as well as improving amniotic fluid levels. There is no evidence that bedrest alone improves pregnancy outcomes (Magee et al., 2014; Sibai, 2012). Adverse physiological outcomes related to bedrest include cardiovascular deconditioning; diuresis with accompanying fluid, electrolyte, and weight loss; muscle atrophy; and psychological stress (see Box 20-4). These changes may begin as early as the first day of bedrest and continue for the duration of therapy. Prolonged bedrest is known to increase the risk of thrombophlebitis (Sibai, 2012). Thus, strict bedrest is not recommended because of potential harmful physical, psychosocial, and financial outcomes (Magee et al., 2014).

Women with nonsevere pre-eclampsia feel reasonably well, so they often find the need for increased monitoring of their condition in hospital to be stressful. Assistance from family and friends with activities of daily living, such as grocery shopping and child care, for the family at home is helpful. Relaxation techniques can help reduce stress associated with the high-risk condition and prepare the woman for labour and the birth.

Diet

Diet and fluid recommendations are much the same as those for healthy pregnant women. Diets high in protein and low in salt are not recommended to prevent pre-eclampsia (Magee et al., 2014). The exception may be the woman with pre-existing hypertension that had been successfully controlled with a low-salt diet before the pregnancy. Adequate fluid intake helps maintain optimum fluid volume and aids in renal perfusion and bowel function (see Guidelines box).

GUIDELINES

Nutrition for Women With Pre-Eclampsia

- Eat a nutritious, balanced diet according to *Eating Well With Canada's Food Guide*. Consult with a registered dietitian on the diet best suited to the individual.
- There is no sodium restriction; however, consider limiting excessively salty foods (pretzels, potato chips, pickles, sauerkraut).
- Eat foods with roughage (whole grains, raw fruits, and vegetables).
- Drink six to eight 250-mL glasses of water per day.
- Avoid alcohol and limit caffeine intake.

Severe Pre-Eclampsia or HELLP Syndrome

Hospital care. The woman with severe pre-eclampsia or HELLP syndrome should receive appropriate treatment in a tertiary care centre from a perinatology team, including maternal–fetal medicine specialists, high-risk obstetrical nurses, internal medicine, if available, and an anaesthesiologist (see Nursing Care Plan, Severe Pre-eclampsia on Evolve). The need for tertiary care may result in the woman being transferred from her home community to a larger centre. The woman may be admitted to a high-risk antepartum or a labour and birth unit, depending on the hospital. If the woman's condition requires intensive monitoring, she may require care in an obstetrical critical care unit or a medical intensive care unit for hemodynamic monitoring. If severe pre-eclampsia is diagnosed, delivery is warranted regardless of gestational age (Magee et al., 2014). Vaginal birth is the preferred type of birth, and Caesarean birth should only be performed for obstetrical indications. For women at risk of giving birth prior to 34^{+6} weeks' gestation, corticosteroids (betamethasone) should be given to promote fetal lung maturation. The dose is 12 mg intramuscularly, repeated in 24 hours. It is ideal if the birth can be delayed for 48 hours, to provide the time for administration of steroids (see Medication Guide, Chapter 20) (Magee et al., 2014).

Recognition of the clinical and laboratory findings of severe pre-eclampsia or HELLP syndrome is important in order to prevent maternal and perinatal mortality. The woman with severe pre-eclampsia or HELLP syndrome has multisystem involvement, and nursing care must focus on both the mother and fetus. Maternal and fetal surveillance, education of the woman and her family regarding the disease process, and supportive measures should be initiated. Assessments include review of the central nervous, cardiovascular, pulmonary, and renal systems. Breath sounds are auscultated for crackles or diminished breath sounds, which may indicate pulmonary edema. An indwelling urinary catheter may be inserted to measure urinary output. An indwelling urinary catheter facilitates monitoring of renal function and effectiveness of therapy; however, the risk of urinary tract infection should be considered in the stable antepartum woman. Hemoglobin oxygen saturation can be assessed with a pulse oximeter. Baseline laboratory assessments include metabolic studies for liver enzyme (AST, ALT, lactate dehydrogenase [LDH] and bilirubin) determination, complete blood count (CBC) with platelets, coagulation profile to assess for DIC, and electrolyte studies to establish renal functioning (ACOG, 2015; Magee et al., 2014; Markham & Funai, 2013).

If there is uterine activity, vaginal examination may be done to check for cervical changes. Through abdominal palpation, uterine tonicity and fetal size, activity, and position can be determined. Assessments of fetal well-being (e.g., NST, BPP) should be ordered because of the potential for hypoxia related to uteroplacental insufficiency. Electronic monitoring to determine fetal status is initiated at least once a day with severe

BOX 14-4 HOSPITAL PRECAUTIONARY MEASURES FOR SEIZURES

- Environment
  - Quiet
  - Nonstimulating
  - Lighting subdued
  - Seizure precautions (have magnesium sulphate available)
  - Suction equipment tested and ready to use
  - Oxygen administration equipment tested and ready to use
  - Call button within easy reach
- Support for woman who may be separated from family and other children during her hospitalization
- Emergency medication tray immediately accessible
- Antihypertensive medication (labetalol, nifedipine, hydralazine) immediately available
- Calcium gluconate immediately available (if receiving magnesium sulphate)
- Emergency birth pack accessible

pre-eclampsia. The nurse's skill in implementing these techniques can be reassuring to the woman and her family. The woman's room should be close to staff and emergency medications, supplies, and equipment. Seizure precautions need to be taken (Box 14-4). Because of the risk for thromboembolism for the woman on bedrest, she may wear SCD (sequential compression device) boots while in bed or may be administered prophylactic anticoagulation. The dose may have to be withheld if delivery is imminent, to enable the provision of neuraxial analgesia.

Intrapartum nursing care of the woman with severe pre-eclampsia or HELLP syndrome involves continuous maternal and fetal assessments as labour progresses. Arterial line insertion may be useful when continuous BP monitoring is desired, in the instance of poor BP control. Central venous pressure monitoring is not routinely used, but it may be used to monitor trends over time and not absolute values (Magee et al., 2014). Invasive hemodynamic monitoring with a pulmonary artery catheter (Swan-Ganz catheter) may be required for accurate intravascular fluid volume measurement in the presence of pulmonary edema or acute renal failure (ACOG, 2015; Markham & Funai, 2013).

Magnesium sulphate. One important goal of care for the woman with pre-eclampsia is to prevent or control convulsions (eclamptic seizures). Magnesium sulphate is the medication of choice in the prevention and treatment of convulsions caused by pre-eclampsia or eclampsia. It is administered as a secondary infusion ("piggyback") to the main intravenous (IV) line by volumetric infusion pump. An initial loading dose of 4 g diluted in at least 100 mL of IV fluid per protocol or physician's order is infused over 20 to 30 minutes. This dose is followed by a maintenance dosage of magnesium sulphate diluted in an IV solution per physician's order (e.g., 20 g of magnesium sulphate in 500 mL of normal saline) and administered by infusion pump at 1 to 2 g/hr (Gilbert, 2011). Data from the MAGPIE trial indicate that at this dose there is no need to draw serial serum magnesium levels (Duley, Farrell, Sparks, et al., 2002). After the loading dose, there may be a transient lowering of the arterial BP secondary to relaxation of smooth muscle.

NURSING ALERT

The woman's BP, pulse, and respiratory rate should be monitored closely (every 5 minutes) while the loading dose of magnesium sulphate is being administered intravenously. Oxygen saturation and electronic fetal monitoring, including uterine activity, should be monitored continuously during the loading dose. Maternal vital signs, including oxygen saturation, should be monitored a minimum of hourly during the maintenance infusion or even more frequently depending on the stability of the woman's condition. Electronic fetal monitoring and uterine activity should be continuous throughout the administration of magnesium sulphate infusion.

Magnesium sulphate is rarely given intramuscularly because the absorption rate cannot be controlled, injections are painful, and tissue necrosis can occur. The intramuscular (IM) route may be used, however, with some women who are being transported to a tertiary care centre. The IM dose is 4 to 5 g given in the ventral gluteal (one on each side), for a total of 10 g (1% procaine may be ordered as an addition to the solution to reduce injection pain) and can be repeated at 4-hour intervals. Z-track technique should be used for the deep IM injection, followed by gentle massage at the site.

Magnesium sulphate interferes with the release of acetylcholine at the synapses, resulting in decreased neuromuscular irritability, depressed cardiac conduction, and decreased central nervous system (CNS) irritability. Because magnesium circulates free and unbound to protein and is excreted in the urine, accurate recordings of maternal urine output must be maintained.

Diuresis within 24 to 48 hours is an excellent prognostic sign; it is considered evidence that perfusion of the kidneys has improved as a result of relaxation of arteriolar spasm. With improved perfusion, fluid moves from interstitial spaces to the intravascular bed, and edema is reduced. Diuresis results in weight loss. Although diuresis generally indicates overall improvement, in the presence of worsening clinical status, it may indicate impending renal failure. As renal function declines and serum creatinine levels rise, renal filtration is compromised. In this situation, the woman can excrete large volumes of urine (greater than 200 mL/hr) but does not excrete magnesium sulphate.

Because magnesium sulphate is a CNS depressant, the nurse needs to assess for signs and symptoms of magnesium toxicity. This is rare with the 1 g/hr maintenance dose, and serum magnesium levels are only obtained when signs of toxicity are present. Adverse effects that are frequently experienced with magnesium sulphate include lethargy, feeling of heat or warmth, headache, or nausea (Gilbert, 2011). Early signs of toxicity include vomiting, respiratory distress, hypotension, flushing, muscle weakness, decreased reflexes, and slurred speech.

NURSING ALERT

Loss of patellar reflexes, respiratory and muscular depression, oliguria, and a decreased level of consciousness are signs of magnesium toxicity. If magnesium toxicity is suspected, the infusion should be discontinued immediately. Calcium gluconate, the antidote for magnesium sulphate, may also be ordered (10 mL of a 10% solution, or 1 g) and given by slow IV push (usually by the physician) over at least 3 minutes to avoid undesirable reactions such as dysrhythmias, bradycardia, and ventricular fibrillation, or may be given as a mini-bag infusion over 15 to 30 minutes by the nurse.

Magnesium sulphate seems to have a small negative effect on the FHR, variability, and accelerative pattern but is not sufficient clinically to warrant medical intervention (Nensi, De Silva, von Dadelszen, et al., 2014). Newborn serum magnesium levels approximate those of the mother. Doses of magnesium sulphate that prevent maternal seizures have been determined to be safe for the fetus. Toxic levels in the newborn can cause depressed respirations and hyporeflexia at birth. It is important that the neonatal team attend the birth to provide resuscitation measures as needed.

NURSING ALERT

High serum levels of magnesium can cause relaxation of smooth muscle such as the uterus. However, when administered as a 4- to 6-g loading dose followed by a 1- to 2-g/hr maintenance dose, magnesium sulphate has not been shown to significantly affect the need for oxytocin stimulation of labour. Other than a brief period of uterine muscle relaxation during and immediately after administration of the loading dose, no evidence of decreased uterine contractility has been observed (Cunningham, Leveno, Bloom, et al., 2014).

MEDICATION ALERT

Magnesium sulphate is considered a high-alert medication because it can cause patient harm when administered incorrectly. Measures to improve the safe use of this medication include developing detailed policies, procedures, protocols, and standing orders and thorough assessment and documentation. Never abbreviate magnesium sulphate as MgS04 anywhere in the medical record (Institute for Safe Medication Practices [ISMP] Canada, 2006).

Control of blood pressure. Initiation of antihypertensive therapy reduces maternal morbidity and mortality rates associated with left ventricular failure and cerebral hemorrhage; therefore, antihypertensive medications may be ordered to lower BP. Antihypertensive therapy must not decrease the arterial pressure too much or too rapidly as it will impact uteroplacental perfusion. Outcomes of the CHIPS (Control of Hypertension in Pregnancy Study) found that tight control (target diastolic BP of >85 mm Hg) versus less tight control of blood pressure (target diastolic BP >100 mm Hg) resulted in no significant differences in overall major adverse perinatal outcomes. Women in the study who were in the less tight control arm had higher rates of severe hypertension (Magee et al., 2014; Magee, von Dadelszen, Rey, et al., 2015).

Labetalol administered intravenously is the antihypertensive drug of choice for the treatment of hypertension. Nifedipine; methyldopa; other beta blockers such as acebutolol, metoprolol, pindolol, and propranolol; and hydralazine are also used (Table 14-5) (Magee et al., 2014; Markham & Funai, 2013; Sibai, 2012). The choice of medication used depends on the woman's response and physician preference.

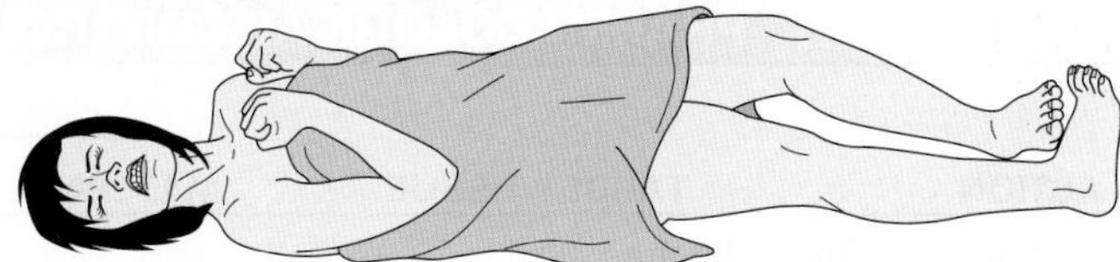

FIGURE 14-4 Eclampsia (convulsion or seizure).

NURSING ALERT

When administering antihypertensive therapy, the nurse must remember that the medication effects depend on intravascular volume. Because preeclampsia is associated with contracted intravascular volume, initial doses should be given with caution and maternal response monitored closely.

Eclampsia

Eclampsia is usually preceded by various premonitory symptoms and signs, including headache, severe epigastric pain, and hyperreflexia. However, convulsions can appear suddenly and without warning in a seemingly stable woman, with only minimum BP elevations (Sibai, 2012). Increased hypertension and tonic contraction of all body muscles (seen as arms flexed, hands clenched, legs inverted) precede the convulsions (Fig. 14-4). During this stage, muscles alternately relax and contract. Respirations are halted and then begin again with long, deep, stertorous inhalations.

Hypotension and then coma follow. Nystagmus and muscular twitching persist for a time. Disorientation and amnesia cloud the immediate recovery. Seizures may recur within minutes of the first convulsion, or the woman may never have another. During the convulsion, the pregnant woman and fetus are not receiving oxygen; thus eclamptic seizures produce a marked metabolic insult to both the woman and the fetus (Cunningham et al., 2014).

Immediate care. The immediate goal of care during a convulsion is to ensure a patent airway (see Emergency box). Time, duration, and a description of the convulsions are recorded, and any urinary or fecal incontinence is noted. Administration of magnesium sulphate is recommended to prevent recurrent seizures. Phenytoin and benzodiazapines should not be used for eclampsia prophylaxis or treatment unless magnesium sulphate is contraindicated (Magee et al., 2014). If possible, the fetus should be monitored for adverse effects; however, this task should not take precedence over other stabilizing care measures. Transient fetal bradycardia and decreased FHR variability are common.

A rapid assessment of uterine activity, cervical status, and fetal status should be performed after a convulsion. During the convulsion membranes can rupture, and the cervix can dilate because the uterus becomes hypercontractile and hypertonic; birth may be imminent. If birth is not imminent, once a

TABLE 14-5 **PHARMACOLOGICAL CONTROL OF HYPERTENSION IN PREGNANCY**

ACTION	TARGET TISSUE	ADVERSE EFFECTS: MATERNAL	ADVERSE EFFECTS: FETAL	NURSING ACTIONS
Hydralazine (Apresoline)				
Arteriolar vasodilator	Peripheral arterioles: to decrease muscle tone, decrease peripheral resistance; hypothalamus and medullary vasomotor centre for minor decrease in sympathetic tone	Headache, flushing, palpitation, tachycardia, some decrease in uteroplacental blood flow, increase in heart rate and cardiac output, increase in oxygen consumption, nausea and vomiting	Tachycardia; late decelerations and bradycardia if maternal diastolic pressure >90 mm Hg	Assess for effects of medications, alert woman (family) to expected effects of medications, assess blood pressure frequently because precipitous decrease can lead to shock and perhaps placental abruption; assess urinary output; maintain bedrest in a lateral position with side rails up; use with caution in presence of maternal tachycardia
Labetalol Hydrochloride				
β-Blocking agent causing vasodilation without significant change in cardiac output	Peripheral arterioles (see hydralazine)	Minimal: flushing, tremulousness; minimal change in pulse rate	Minimal, if any	See hydralazine; less likely to cause excessive hypotension and tachycardia; less rebound hypertension than hydralazine
Methyldopa (Aldomet)				
Maintenance therapy if needed: 250–500 mg orally every 8 hr (β_2-receptor agonist)	Postganglionic nerve endings: interferes with chemical neurotransmission to reduce peripheral vascular resistance, causes CNS sedation	Sleepiness, postural hypotension, constipation; rare: medication-induced fever in 1% of women and positive Coombs' test result in 20%	After 4 mo maternal therapy, positive Coombs' test result in infant	See hydralazine
Nifedipine				
Calcium channel blocker	Arterioles: to reduce systemic vascular resistance by relaxation of arterial smooth muscle	Headache, flushing; possible potentiation of effects on CNS if administered concurrently with magnesium sulphate, may interfere with labour	Minimal	See hydralazine; use caution if patient also receiving magnesium sulphate

CNS, central nervous system.

EMERGENCY

Eclampsia

Tonic–Clonic Convulsion Signs

- Stage of invasion—2 to 3 seconds: eyes are fixed; twitching of facial muscles occurs
- Stage of contraction—15 to 20 seconds: eyes protrude and are bloodshot; all body muscles are in tonic contraction
- Stage of convulsion—Muscles relax and contract alternately (clonic); respirations are halted and then begin again with long, deep, stertorous inhalation; coma ensues

Intervention

- Keep airway patent: turn head to one side, place pillow under one shoulder or back if possible.
- Call for assistance. Do not leave bedside.
- Protect woman from injury during seizure by having padded side rails raised and safely locked.
- Observe and record convulsion activity.

After Convulsion or Seizure

- Do not leave woman unattended until she is fully alert.
- Observe for postconvulsion coma, incontinence.
- Use suction as needed.
- Administer oxygen via face mask at 10 L/min.
- Start intravenous fluids and monitor intake.
- Give magnesium sulphate or anticonvulsant medication as ordered.
- Insert indwelling urinary catheter and monitor hourly output.
- Monitor blood pressure.
- Monitor fetal and uterine status.
- Expedite laboratory work as ordered to monitor kidney function, liver function, coagulation system, and medication levels.
- Provide hygiene and a quiet environment.
- Support woman and family and keep them informed.
- Be prepared to assist with birth when the woman is in stable condition.

woman's seizure activity and BP are controlled, a decision should be made regarding whether birth should take place. Since delivery is the definitive cure for the disease, the more serious the condition of the woman, the greater the need to proceed to the birth following the cessation of seizure activity. The means of birth (i.e., induction of labour vs. Caesarean birth) depends on maternal and fetal condition, fetal gestational age, presence of labour, and the cervical Bishop score. If fetal lungs are not mature and the birth can be delayed for 48 hours, steroids such as betamethasone can be given (Magee et al., 2014).

If the woman has been incontinent of urine and stool, or the membranes have ruptured during the convulsion, she will need assistance with hygiene and a change of gown. Oral care with a soft toothbrush may be of comfort.

! NURSING ALERT

Immediately after a seizure, the woman may be very confused and can be combative. Pad the side rails to prevent injury, and maintain a quiet, darkened environment. It may take several hours for the woman to regain her usual level of mental functioning. She should not be left alone. Provide emotional support to the family and discuss with them the seizure's management and the woman's progress.

Laboratory tests should be ordered to assess for HELLP syndrome. Blood is typed and cross-matched for administration of packed red blood cells, as needed. The eclamptic woman is at high risk for placental abruption, with accompanying hemorrhage and shock. Other tests to perform include determination of electrolyte levels; liver function; and a complete blood count and clotting profile, including platelet count and fibrin split product levels (to assess for DIC).

Aspiration is a leading cause of maternal morbidity and mortality after an eclamptic seizure. After initial stabilization and airway management, the nurse should anticipate orders for a chest x-ray film and possibly arterial blood gases to determine whether aspiration occurred.

Postpartum Nursing Care

The nursing care of the woman with hypertensive disease differs in a number of ways from that required in a normal postpartum period. After birth, the symptoms of pre-eclampsia or eclampsia resolve quickly, usually within 48 hours. However, hypertension may persist, and the woman should be monitored from days 3 to 6 after delivery. Resolution of the disease process is manifested by diuresis, which usually occurs within 24 to 48 hours after the birth. The hematopoietic and hepatic complications of HELLP syndrome may persist longer. Usually an abrupt decrease in platelet count occurs with a concomitant increase in LDH and AST levels after a trend toward normalization of values has begun. Generally, the laboratory abnormalities seen with HELLP syndrome resolve in 72 to 96 hours.

The woman will need careful assessment of her vital signs, intake and output, DTRs, level of consciousness, uterine tone, and lochia flow throughout the postpartum period. The magnesium sulphate infusion is continued 24 hours for seizure prophylaxis. Even if no convulsions occurred before the birth, they may occur during the postpartum period. The same assessments should continue until the medication is discontinued.

NURSING ALERT

The woman is at risk for a boggy uterus and a large lochia flow as a result of the muscle-relaxant effects of magnesium sulphate therapy. Uterine tone and lochial flow must be monitored closely.

The pre-eclamptic woman is usually hemoconcentrated and unable to tolerate excessive postpartum blood loss. Oxytocin or prostaglandin products are used to control bleeding. Ergot products (e.g., ergonovine and methylergonovine) are contraindicated because they increase BP. The woman should be advised to report symptoms such as headaches and blurred vision. The nurse will need to assess affect, level of consciousness, BP, pulse, and respiratory status before an analgesic is given for headache. Magnesium sulphate potentiates the action of narcotics, CNS depressants, and calcium channel blockers; thus these medications must be administered with caution. The woman may need to be restarted on antihypertensive medication if her dBP exceeds 100 mm Hg at discharge.

Postpartum recovery may be prolonged as a result of the physiological consequences of the hypertensive disease processes. The nurse should accompany the woman when she ambulates after birth and assess for weakness, dizziness, shortness of breath, and muscle soreness. Postpartum thromboprophylaxis with low molecular-weight heparin (LMWH) is not recommended for hypertension or pre-eclampsia alone but should be considered for women who have a combination of risks, including Caesarean birth or postpartum hemorrhage greater than 1 litre (Chan, Rey, & Kent, 2014).

The woman's and family's responses to the birth itself and the newborn should be monitored. Interactions and involvement in the care of the newborn can be encouraged as much as the woman and her family desire. If the pre-eclampsia was severe, the infant may be premature and in the neonatal intensive care nursery. The woman and her family may be worried about their infant's survival, and the day-to-day fluctuations in the infant's status can be emotionally draining. In addition, the woman and her family need opportunities to discuss their emotional response to complications. The primary care provider can provide information concerning the prognosis, with support from the nurses. If the outcome for the mother or baby is unfavourable, the family should be assisted in coping with their loss and grief.

Future Health Care

The recurrence risk for hypertensive disorders in subsequent pregnancy is 20.7% for pre-eclampsia; 13.8% for gestational hypertension, and 0.2% for HELLP syndrome (van Oostwaard, Langenveld, Schuit, et al., 2015). Women can be somewhat reassured that when hypertension in pregnancy does recur, it tends toward a milder response. The risk of subsequent pre-eclampsia is especially likely in women who initially developed it earlier (during the second trimester) in pregnancy (Sibai, 2012). Even if these women remain normotensive in a subsequent pregnancy, they may have a greater likelihood of an adverse pregnancy outcome such as preterm birth, small-for-gestational-age infant, and perinatal death (Sibai, 2012).

Women with pre-eclampsia (especially early-onset and severe pre-eclampsia) also have an increased risk of developing chronic hypertension and cardiovascular disease later in life and need medical follow-up. These women are also more likely to have underlying renal disease (Sibai, 2012; van Oostwaard et al., 2015). The postpartum period provides an excellent opportunity to educate women about lifestyle changes that may decrease their risk for developing future health problems (Gilbert, 2011; Sibai, 2012).

GESTATIONAL DIABETES MELLITUS (GDM)

GDM is defined as elevated glucose levels that are first recognized during pregnancy. In the first trimester of pregnancy, uncontrolled hyperglycemia can impact fetal development resulting in malformations (Thompson, Berger, Feif, et al., 2013). In Canada, the prevalence of gestational diabetes is population-specific, varying from 3.8 to 6.5% in the overall population, with higher rates reported among Indigenous, Latin American, South Asian, Asian, and African women. Women with GDM are at significant risk of developing glucose intolerance later in life; about 50% will be diagnosed as having diabetes within 5 to 10 years. Women whose GDM is diagnosed early in pregnancy and who may be obese are at increased risk of developing sustained glucose intolerance and type 2 diabetes, usually related to the degree of vascular changes that have occurred over time. Previous national guidelines suggested screening women for the presence of GDM based on risk factors. Current guidelines are based on evidence recommending universal screening of all pregnant women for the presence of hyperglycemia (Landon, Catalano, & Gabbe, 2012). Universal screening is important because hyperglycemia is difficult to detect, as it presents without symptoms. Data show that the incidence of adverse maternal and fetal outcomes increase with poorly controlled glucose levels (Gilbert, 2011; Thompson et al., 2013).

Fetal nutrient demands rise during the late second and third trimesters; maternal nutrient ingestion induces greater and more sustained levels of blood glucose. At the same time, maternal insulin resistance increases as a result of the insulin antagonistic effects of the placental hormones, cortisol and insulinase. Consequently, maternal insulin demands can rise as much as threefold. Most pregnant women are capable of increasing insulin production to compensate for the insulin resistance and maintain euglycemia. When the pancreas is unable to produce sufficient insulin or the insulin is not used effectively, GDM can result (Gilbert, 2011).

Maternal and Fetal Risks

Compared with pregnant women without GDM, women with GDM have twice the risk of developing pre-eclampsia, particularly if they have chronic hypertension already (Gilbert, 2011). They also have increased risk for fetal macrosomia, which can lead to increased rates of perineal lacerations, episiotomy, and Caesarean birth. In addition, fetal macrosomia may be associated with shoulder dystocia and birth trauma. GDM places the fetus at increased risk for hypoglycemia, IUGR (related to poor placental function), and intrauterine fetal death (Gilbert, 2011).

The overall incidence of congenital anomalies among infants of women with GDM approaches that of the general population because GDM usually develops after week 20 of pregnancy—after the critical period of organogenesis (first trimester) has passed.

Screening for Gestational Diabetes Mellitus

Thompson et al. (2013) recommend that all pregnant women be screened for the presence of GDM at 24 to 28 weeks of gestation, although some practitioners still screen on the basis of risk factors. Assessment of relevant history, clinical risk factors, and laboratory screening of blood glucose levels should be performed. If there is a high risk of GDM based on multiple clinical factors, screening should be offered at any stage in the pregnancy. Women with multiple risk factors should be screened in the first trimester to identify hyperglycemia early. If the initial screening is performed before 24 weeks of gestation and is negative, rescreening between 24 and 28 weeks of gestation is recommended.

Risk factors for GDM include the following:

- Age ≥35 years
- Previous GDM
- Prediabetes
- High-risk population among Indigenous, Latin American, South Asian, Asian, African
- Body mass index (BMI) ≥30 kg/m^2
- Polycystic ovarian syndrome
- Acanthosis nigricans
- Corticosteroid use
- History of macrosomic infant
- Current fetal macrosomia or polyhydramnios

The optimal method of screening for GDM has become a controversial topic. Testing of fasting plasma glucose (FPG) has been found to be easier and more convenient than the oral glucose tolerance test (OGTT). There are two types of screening tests that have been shown to be effective for detecting GDM: the sequential test and the one-step test. The most common test is the sequential screening test with a 50-g glucose challenge test (GCT), performed between 24 and 28 weeks' gestation (Thompson et al., 2013), followed by a diagnostic 100-g OGTT if required. The one-step approach includes a 75-g OGTT that is given to a woman between 24 and 28 weeks' gestation who has been fasting. The plasma glucose is measured within 1 to 2 hours. There has not been international support for this method of screening, as the application of blood glucose threshold values reveals up to 18% of women will be overdiagnosed with GDM. There is no clear consensus on which of the screening tests is recommended over the other. The economic analysis favours the sequential screening test. Thus the recommended "preferred" approach of the Canadian Diabetes Association Expert Committee is the sequential screening approach using

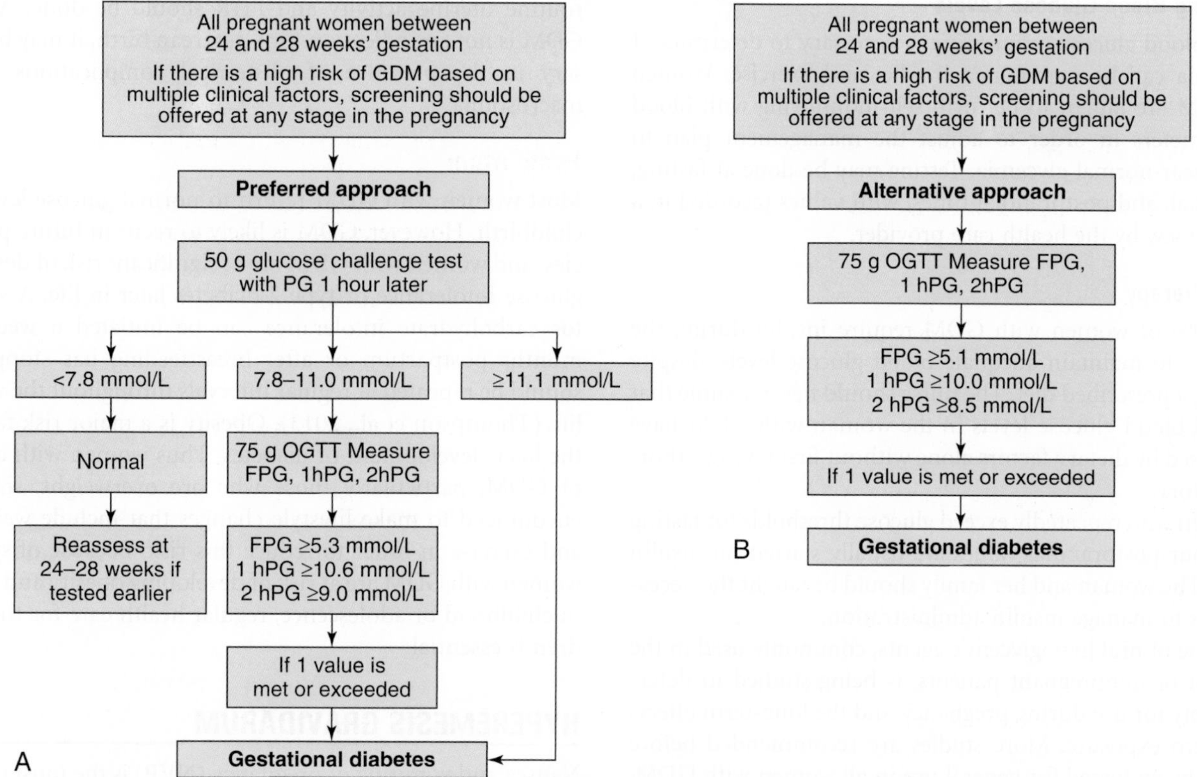

FIGURE 14-5 A. Preferred approach for screening and diagnosis of gestational diabetes. **B.** Alternative approach for screening and diagnosis of gestational diabetes. *1h PG*, 1-hour plasma glucose; *2hPG*, 2-hour plasma glucose; *FPG*, fasting plasma glucose; *GDM*, gestational diabetes mellitus; *OGTT*, oral glucose tolerance test; *PG*, plasma glucose. (From Thompson, D., Berger, H., Feif, D., et al. [2013]. Diabetes and pregnancy. *Canadian Journal of Diabetes, 37*, Supplement 1, S168–S183. Copyright 2013, with permission from Elsevier.)

the 50-g GCT, followed by a 75-g OGTT using glucose cut-off values as defined in Fig. 14-5, A (Thompson et al., 2013). The alternative approach (Figure 14-5, B) is the one-step approach of 75-g OGTT (Thompson et al., 2013).

Nursing care for the woman with GDM is basically the same as that for women with pregestational diabetes (see Chapter 15); however, the time frame for planning may be shortened with GDM because the diagnosis is usually made later in pregnancy. See the Evolve website for the Nursing Care Plan for woman with Gestational Diabetes.

NURSING CARE

Antepartum

When the diagnosis of gestational diabetes is made, treatment begins immediately, allowing little or no time for the woman and her family to adjust to the diagnosis before they are expected to participate in the treatment plan. This is in contrast to the woman with pregestational diabetes, who may have had years to learn about the disease and adapt to dietary modifications, self-monitoring of glucose, and insulin administration. With each step of the treatment plan, the nurse and other health care providers should educate the woman and her family, providing detailed and comprehensive explanations to ensure understanding of, participation in, and agreement with the necessary interventions. Potential complications should be discussed and the need for testing and maintenance of euglycemia throughout the remainder of the pregnancy reinforced. It may be reassuring for the woman and her family to know that GDM typically disappears when the pregnancy is over. (See the Nursing Care Plan: The Pregnant Woman with Gestational Diabetes on Evolve.)

As with pregestational diabetes, the aim of therapy in women with GDM is meticulous blood glucose control. Fasting (preprandial) blood glucose levels should be between 3.8 and 5.2 mmol/L; 1 hour after meals (postprandial) they should be between 5.5 and 7.7 mmol/L; and 2-hour postprandial blood levels should be between 5.0 and 6.6 mmol/L (Thompson et al., 2013).

Diet

Dietary modification is the mainstay of treatment for GDM. The woman with GDM is placed on a standard diabetic diet immediately upon diagnosis. Some authorities recommend fewer calories for overweight or morbidly obese women, believing that such a diet will cause less hyperglycemia and reduce the need for insulin (Landon et al., 2012). Dietary counselling by a dietitian is recommended.

Exercise

For women with GDM, exercise appears to be safe. It helps lower blood glucose levels and may be instrumental in eliminating the need for insulin.

Monitoring Blood Glucose Levels

Regular blood glucose monitoring is necessary to determine if euglycemia can be maintained by diet and exercise. Women with GDM are taught to perform self-monitoring with blood glucose meters in order to adjust the management plan to achieve near-normal glycemia. Testing may be done at fasting, preprandial, and postprandial times, with values recorded in a log for review by the health care provider.

Insulin Therapy

Up to 20% of women with GDM require insulin during the pregnancy to maintain adequate blood glucose levels, despite following a prescribed diet. The nurse should never assume that increased blood glucose levels in the woman with GDM have been caused by dietary factors alone without first taking a thorough history.

Women who repeatedly exceed glucose thresholds for fasting and 2-hour postprandial values are usually started on insulin therapy. The woman and her family should be taught the necessary skills to manage insulin administration.

The use of oral hypoglycemic agents, commonly used in the treatment of nonpregnant patients, is being studied to determine safety for use during pregnancy and the long-term effects of in utero exposure. More studies are recommended before they can be endorsed for general use in all women with GDM.

Fetal Surveillance

There is no standard recommendation for fetal surveillance in pregnancies complicated by GDM. Fetuses of women whose blood glucose levels are well controlled by diet are at low risk for fetal death or other fetal sequelae. Routine antepartum fetal testing on these women may not be done as long as their fasting and 2-hour postprandial blood glucose levels remain within normal limits and they have no other risk factors. Usually these women are allowed to progress to term and spontaneous labour without intervention. Once the woman reaches 40 weeks of gestation, fetal surveillance twice weekly is usually instituted (Landon et al., 2012; Liston, Sawchuck, Young, et al., 2007).

Women with GDM whose blood glucose levels are not well controlled or who require insulin therapy, have hypertension, or have a history of previous stillbirth generally receive more intensive fetal biophysical monitoring. There is no standard recommendation regarding initiation of testing. Nonstress tests and biophysical profiles are often performed weekly, beginning from 32 to 36 weeks of gestation (Liston et al., 2007) (see Chapter 13).

Intrapartum

During labour and birth, blood glucose levels are monitored at least every hour to maintain levels ideally at less than 8 mmol/L (Thompson et al., 2013). Glucose levels within this range will decrease the severity of newborn hypoglycemia. Women whose GDM has been managed on insulin can be controlled by a sliding scale of regular insulin that is titrated to blood sugars during labour. Even though IV fluids containing glucose may be given as maintenance fluids during birth, they should not be given as a bolus to the woman who has GDM. Assessment of routine uterine activity and FHR should be done. Although GDM is not an indication for Caesarean birth, it may be necessary in the presence of obstetrical complications such as macrosomia.

Postpartum

Most women with GDM return to normal glucose levels after childbirth. However, GDM is likely to recur in future pregnancies, and women with GDM are at significant risk of developing glucose intolerance or type 2 diabetes later in life. Assessment for carbohydrate intolerance can be initiated 6 weeks to 6 months postpartum or after breastfeeding has stopped and should be repeated at regular intervals throughout the woman's life (Thompson et al., 2013). Obesity is a major risk factor for the later development of diabetes. Thus women with a history of GDM, particularly those who are overweight, should be encouraged to make lifestyle changes that include weight loss and exercise in order to reduce this risk. Because offspring of women with GDM are at risk of developing obesity and diabetes in childhood or adolescence, regular health care for these children is essential.

HYPEREMESIS GRAVIDARUM

Nausea and vomiting of pregnancy (NVP) is the most common medical condition in pregnancy, affecting 50 to 90% of women (Ebrahimi, Maltepe, Bournissen, et al., 2009). It most commonly occurs between 4 and 9 weeks of gestation and usually lessens by the eighteenth week of pregnancy. In its extreme form, NVP may manifest as **hyperemesis gravidarum** (HG), a potentially life-threatening condition affecting 0.5 to 2% of pregnancies. It is characterized by protracted vomiting, retching, severe dehydration, and weight loss requiring hospitalization. HG usually begins during the first 10 weeks of pregnancy. It has been associated with women who are nulliparous, have diabetes, have increased body weight, have a history of migraines, or are pregnant with twins or have a hydatidiform mole (Gilbert, 2011; Kelly & Savides, 2014).

Although NVP may be classified as mild, moderate, or severe, the severity of nausea or vomiting may not adequately reflect the distress it causes. Vomiting may lead to dehydration, electrolyte imbalance, ketosis, and acetonuria (Kelly & Savides, 2014; Smith, Refuerzo, & Ramin, 2013). Other causes of nausea and vomiting must be ruled out, including gastrointestinal, genitourinary, central nervous system, and toxic or metabolic problems (Firoz, Maltepe, & Einearson, 2010). In addition, an interrelated psychological component has been associated with hyperemesis and must be assessed (Cunningham et al., 2014; Kelly & Savides, 2014). The effects of HG on perinatal outcome vary with the severity of the disorder.

Etiology

The etiology of HG is not well understood. Several theories have been proposed, although none of them adequately explains the disorder in all cases. HG may be related to high levels of estrogen or human chorionic gonadotropin (hCG) and associated with transient hyperthyroidism during pregnancy. Research has found that women who have severe nausea and vomiting have a 1.5-fold increased chance of carrying a female infant, supporting the association between increased estrogen exposure and HG (Cunningham et al., 2014; Kelly & Savides, 2014). Esophageal reflux, reduced gastric motility, and decreased secretion of free hydrochloric acid may contribute to the disorder.

Psychological and social factors can also play a part in the development of HG. Ambivalence toward the pregnancy and increased stress may be associated with this condition (Cunningham et al., 2014; Kelly & Savides, 2014). Women may have to take time away from work, which affects their income and can produce feelings of anxiety. Conflicting feelings about prospective motherhood, body changes, and lifestyle alterations—all normal reactions to pregnancy—may contribute to episodes of vomiting, particularly if these feelings are excessive or unresolved (Cunningham et al., 2014).

Clinical Manifestations

The woman with HG may have significant weight loss and symptoms of dehydration, such as decreased BP, increased pulse rate, and poor skin turgor. The woman is almost always unable to keep down even clear liquids taken by mouth. Laboratory tests may indicate electrolyte imbalances.

NURSING CARE

Assessment

A thorough assessment to determine the severity of the problem must be completed by the nurse. The frequency, severity, and duration of episodes of nausea and vomiting must be determined. If the woman reports vomiting, the assessment should also include the approximate amount and colour of the vomitus. Other symptoms such as diarrhea, indigestion, and abdominal pain or distension should also be identified. Assessment of sleep patterns and disruption due to vomiting is important, as sleep deprivation may contribute to how the woman is coping (Ebrahimi et al., 2009). Prepregnancy weight and documented weight gain or loss during the pregnancy are important baseline data to collect. Any effective pharmacological and nonpharmacological interventions that the woman has used should be noted. The pharmacist and dietitian can play an important role in the care of a woman with hyperemesis.

A complete physical examination, including vital signs, should be performed, with attention to signs of fluid and electrolyte imbalance and nutritional status. A urine dipstick test for ketonuria should be obtained, as ketonuria can indicate the need for IV fluids for dehydration. Other laboratory tests that may be ordered include a urinalysis, CBC, electrolytes, renal and liver function tests, assessment of thyroid function, and bilirubin levels. These tests help rule out the presence of underlying diseases, such as pyelonephritis, pancreatitis, cholecystitis, hepatitis, and thyroid dysfunction (Kelly & Savides, 2014).

Psychosocial assessment includes asking the woman about anxiety, fears, and concerns related to her own health and the effects on pregnancy outcome. Family members should be assessed for anxiety and in regard to their role in providing support for the woman.

Initial Care

Initially, if the woman can manage her symptoms with clear liquids the diet can be increased by slowly introducing small, frequent meals that are high in protein or carbohydrates but low in fat (Smith et al., 2013). The addition of a multivitamin, taken orally if tolerated, has been shown to improve a woman's status. Women should be counselled to avoid odours, tastes, or other activities that can triggers the senses and result in nausea. Examples of triggers include a stuffy room, visually stimulating lights, or strong perfumes (Smith et al., 2013). Treatment with medications is likely required to effectively control the symptoms of HG. Doxylamine succinate (Diclectin), an effective and safe treatment for nausea and vomiting in early pregnancy, is a commonly used first-line treatment that can be given as an outpatient medication. The use of alternative therapies such as ginger, acupuncture, and acupressure (see Fig. 12-5) has been shown to be beneficial to some women with nausea and vomiting (Matthews, Dowswell, Haas, et al., 2010).

If the woman is unable to maintain clear liquids by mouth, she will require IV therapy for correction of fluid and electrolyte imbalances. In the past, women needing IV therapy were admitted to the hospital. Today they often are successfully managed on an outpatient basis or at home. Antiemetic medications are introduced if nausea and vomiting are uncontrolled. Dimenhydrinate (Gravol) is given, with the addition of metoclopramide (Maxeran) if dimenhydrinate alone is not effective (Kelly & Savides, 2014). If these medications are not effective for controlling nausea and vomiting, the medication of choice is ondansetron (Zofran) (Cunningham et al., 2014). Recent concerns about the safety of this medication for use in early pregnancy arose with a reported slightly increased risk of cleft palate, but the research to date is inconclusive (Koren, 2012). Practitioners must have informed discussions with women who are experiencing severe nausea and vomiting as ondansetron may be the most effective medication to help control their symptoms, especially if other treatments have failed. Corticosteroids (methylprednisone or hydrocortisone) may be used as a fourth-line alternative to treat refractory HG, although there is little evidence that its use is effective (Cunningham et al., 2014). For women with severe HG, consultation with gastrointestinal medicine or the administration of total parenteral nutrition (TPN) may need to be considered (Kelly & Savides, 2014). Some women also benefit from psychotherapy or stress-reduction techniques.

A few women will continue to experience intractable nausea and vomiting throughout pregnancy. Rarely, it is necessary to maintain a woman on enteral nutrition, or TPN, to provide adequate nutrition for the mother and fetus. Hospitalization is often required to provide ongoing assessment and care for the woman requiring TPN.

Interventions may include initiating and monitoring IV therapy; administering antiemetics, antacids, or nutrition supplements; and monitoring the woman's response to interventions. The nurse needs to observe the woman for any signs of complications, such as metabolic acidosis, jaundice, or hemorrhage, and alert the primary care provider should these occur.

TABLE 14-6 PREGNANCY-UNIQUE QUANTIFICATION OF EMESIS (PUQE) SCALE

MOTHERISK PUQE-24 SCORING SYSTEM

In the last 24 hours, for how long have you felt nauseated or sick to your stomach?	Not at all (1)	1 hour or less (2)	2–3 hours (3)	4–6 hours (4)	More than 6 hours (5)
In the last 24 hours, have you vomited or thrown up?	7 or more times (5)	5–6 times (4)	3–4 times (3)	1–2 times (2)	I did not throw up (1)
In the last 24 hours, how many times have you had retching or dry heaves without bringing anything up?	None (1)	1–2 times (2)	3–4 times (3)	5–6 times (4)	7 or more times (5)

PUQE 24 Score: □ Mild = ≤6 □ Moderate = 7–12 □ Severe = 13–15

How many hours have you slept out of 24 hours? Why? ____________

On a scale of 0 to 10, how would you rate your well-being? ____________

0 (worst possible) – 10 (The best you felt before pregnancy)

Can you tell me what causes you to feel that way? ____________

Monitoring includes assessment of the woman's nausea, retching without vomiting, and vomiting, since the latter two symptoms, although related, are separate. A standardized assessment tool such as the Pregnancy-Unique Quantification of Emesis (PUQE) Scale allows objective quantification of the presence and severity of the nausea and vomiting and enables accurate monitoring (Table 14-6) (Ebrahimi et al., 2009). A PUQE score of 13 to 15 indicates severe symptoms; 7 to 12, moderate symptoms; and less than 6, mild symptoms. Treatment should be modified according to the score.

Accurate measurement of intake and output, including the amount of emesis, is an important aspect of nursing care. Oral hygiene while the woman is on nothing-by-mouth status and after episodes of vomiting helps allay associated discomfort. Assistance with positioning and providing a quiet, restful environment that is free from odours may give the woman some comfort. When the woman begins responding to therapy, limited amounts of oral fluids and bland foods such as crackers, toast, or baked chicken are given. The diet is progressed slowly as tolerated by the woman until she is able to consume a nutritionally sound diet. Because sleep disturbances may accompany HG, adequate rest should be promoted. The nurse can assist in coordinating treatment measures and periods of visitation so that the woman has sufficient rest periods.

Follow-Up Care

Most women are able to take nourishment by mouth after several days of treatment. They should be encouraged to eat small, frequent meals consisting of low-fat, high-protein foods; dry, bland foods; and cold foods, and to avoid greasy and highly seasoned foods (Smith et al., 2013). A snack before bedtime is also advised. They need to increase their dietary intake of potassium and magnesium. Herbal teas such as ginger, mint, and raspberry leaf may decrease nausea (Matthews et al., 2010). Taking fluids between meals rather than with them sometimes helps lessen nausea, as does drinking liquids from a cup with a lid and drinking tea or water with lemon slices (Smith et al., 2013). See Patient Teaching Box (Chapter 12, p. 287) for discussion on managing nausea and vomiting during pregnancy. Many pregnant women find that cooking odours can be nauseating; having other family members cook may decrease nausea. Women should be counselled to contact their health care provider immediately if the nausea and vomiting recur, especially if accompanied by abdominal pain, dehydration, or weight loss greater than 2.3 kg in 1 week.

The woman with HG needs calm, compassionate, and sympathetic care, with recognition that the manifestations of hyperemesis can be physically and emotionally debilitating to the woman and stressful for her family. Irritability, tearfulness, and mood changes are often consistent with this disorder. Fetal well-being is a primary concern of the woman. The nurse can provide an environment conducive to discussion of concerns and assist the woman in identifying and mobilizing sources of support. The family should be included in the plan of care whenever possible. Their participation may help alleviate some of the emotional stress associated with this disorder.

HEMORRHAGIC DISORDERS

Bleeding in pregnancy may jeopardize maternal and fetal well-being, and a multidisciplinary approach is warranted to optimize the outcome for both the mother and her fetus. Maternal blood loss decreases vital oxygen-carrying capacity and places the woman at increased risk for **hypovolemia**, anemia, infection, preterm labour, and preterm birth (Gilbert, 2011). Oxygen delivery to the fetus is compromised. Fetal risks from maternal hemorrhage include blood loss or anemia, hypoxemia, hypoxia, anoxia, preterm birth, and stillbirth.

Hemorrhagic disorders in pregnancy are medical emergencies. The incidence and type of bleeding vary by trimester. In the first trimester, most bleeding is a result of spontaneous abortion or ectopic pregnancy. Approximately 50% of bleeding in the third trimester is caused by placenta previa and placental abruption (Gilbert, 2011). Antepartum hemorrhage is a leading cause of maternal death, with ectopic pregnancy rupture, uterine rupture, and placental abruption being responsible for most maternal deaths.

With approximately 750 to 1000 mL/min (15% of maternal cardiac output) of blood flow to the uterine vasculature and placenta, disruption of vascular integrity has the potential for maternal exsanguination within 8 to 10 minutes. Prompt, expert teamwork on the part of the health care providers is essential to save the lives of the mother and fetus.

Early Pregnancy Bleeding

Bleeding during early pregnancy is alarming to the woman and of concern to health care providers. The common bleeding disorders of early pregnancy include miscarriage, premature dilation of the cervix, ectopic pregnancy, and hydatidiform mole (molar pregnancy). Bleeding can originate from the cervix, caused by sexual intercourse, or by an infection (ACOG, 2011). Women with advanced maternal age, smoking exposure, and prior preterm birth are more at risk for vaginal bleeding during pregnancy.

Pregnancy Loss

A pregnancy that ends without medical or surgical intervention prior to 20 weeks of gestation or 500-g fetal weight is defined as a *miscarriage* or *spontaneous abortion* (Cunningham et al., 2014). Therapeutic and elective abortion is discussed in Chapter 8.

Incidence and etiology. Approximately 15 to 20 % of all confirmed pregnancies end in miscarriage (ACOG, 2011; Simpson & Jauniaux, 2012). However, the true rate of early pregnancy loss is close to 50% because of the high number of pregnancies that are not recognized in the 2 to 4 weeks after conception. Most of these pregnancy failures are due to gamete failure (e.g., sperm or oocyte dysfunction) (Petrozza & Berin, 2011). The risk of spontaneous abortion is increased in obese women (Davies, Maxwell, McLeod, et al., 2010).

An early pregnancy loss is one that occurs before 12 weeks of gestation. At least 50% of all clinically recognized pregnancy losses result from chromosome abnormalities (Cunningham et al., 2014; Petrozza & Berin, 2011). More than 90% of spontaneous abortions occur before 8 weeks, and only 2 to 3% occur after 8 weeks of gestation (Simpson & Jauniaux, 2012). Possible causes of early miscarriage include endocrine imbalance (as in women who have luteal-phase defects, hypothyroidism, or diabetes mellitus with high blood-glucose levels in the first trimester), immunological factors (e.g., antiphospholipid antibodies), systemic disorders (e.g., lupus erythematosus), and genetic factors (Gilbert, 2011; Simpson & Jauniaux, 2012). Infections are not a common cause of early miscarriage (Cunningham et al., 2014), but there is an increased risk for a spontaneous abortion with varicella infection in the first trimester (Gilbert, 2011).

A late pregnancy loss occurs between 12 and 20 weeks of gestation. It usually results from maternal causes such as advancing maternal age and parity, chronic infections, premature dilation of the cervix or other anomalies of the reproductive tract, chronic debilitating diseases, inadequate nutrition, and recreational drug use (Cunningham et al., 2014). Little can be done to avoid genetic causes of pregnancy loss, but support for changes to maternal lifestyle, correction of maternal disorders, immunization against infectious diseases, adequate early prenatal care, and treatment of pregnancy complications can be effective at avoiding second-trimester pregnancy loss.

Clinical manifestations. Signs and symptoms of pregnancy loss depend on the duration of the pregnancy. The presence of uterine bleeding, uterine cramping, or low back pain is an ominous sign in early pregnancy. Assessment of beta-human chorionic gonadotropin (β-hCG) blood levels and ultrasound must be performed to confirm a viable pregnancy or pregnancy loss.

If pregnancy loss occurs prior to the sixth week of gestation, the woman may report a heavy menstrual-like flow. Miscarriage that occurs between weeks 6 and 12 of pregnancy causes moderate discomfort and blood loss. Severe cramping with heavy bleeding is often a sign of later pregnancy loss because the fetus must be expelled. The types of spontaneous abortion include threatened, inevitable, incomplete, complete, and missed (Fig. 14-6). Diagnosis of pregnancy loss is based on the signs and symptoms present (Table 14-7).

Symptoms of a *threatened pregnancy loss* (see Fig. 14-6, A) include mild to moderate spotting of blood with a closed cervical os. Mild uterine cramping may be present.

Inevitable (see Fig. 14-6, B) and *incomplete* (see Fig. 14-6, C) spontaneous abortion involve a moderate-to-heavy amount of bleeding with an open cervical os, seen on speculum exam. Tissue may be present with the bleeding. Mild-to-severe uterine cramping may be present. An inevitable pregnancy loss is accompanied by rupture of membranes (ROM) and cervical dilation with passage of the fetus and placenta together. An incomplete loss involves the expulsion of the fetus with retention of the placenta (Cunningham et al., 2014; Gilbert, 2011). Vaginal bleeding, which may be slight to heavy, is usually malodorous. Surgical evacuation may be required.

In a *complete spontaneous abortion* (see Fig. 14-6, D) all fetal tissue is passed, the cervix is closed, and there may be slight bleeding. Mild uterine cramping may be present.

The term *missed abortion* (see Fig. 14-6, E) refers to a pregnancy in which the fetus has died but the products of conception are retained in utero for up to several weeks. It may be diagnosed by ultrasonographic examination after the uterus stops increasing or even decreases in size. There may be no bleeding or cramping, and the cervical os remains closed.

Recurrent pregnancy loss is three or more consecutive pregnancy losses before 20 weeks of gestation. The etiology is often unclear but is thought to be multifactorial in nature (Petrozza & Berin, 2011). Women with a history of recurrent pregnancy loss are at increased risk for preterm birth, placenta previa, and fetal anomalies in subsequent pregnancies (Cunningham et al., 2014).

Collaborative care

Initial care. When a woman has vaginal bleeding early in pregnancy, a thorough assessment should be performed

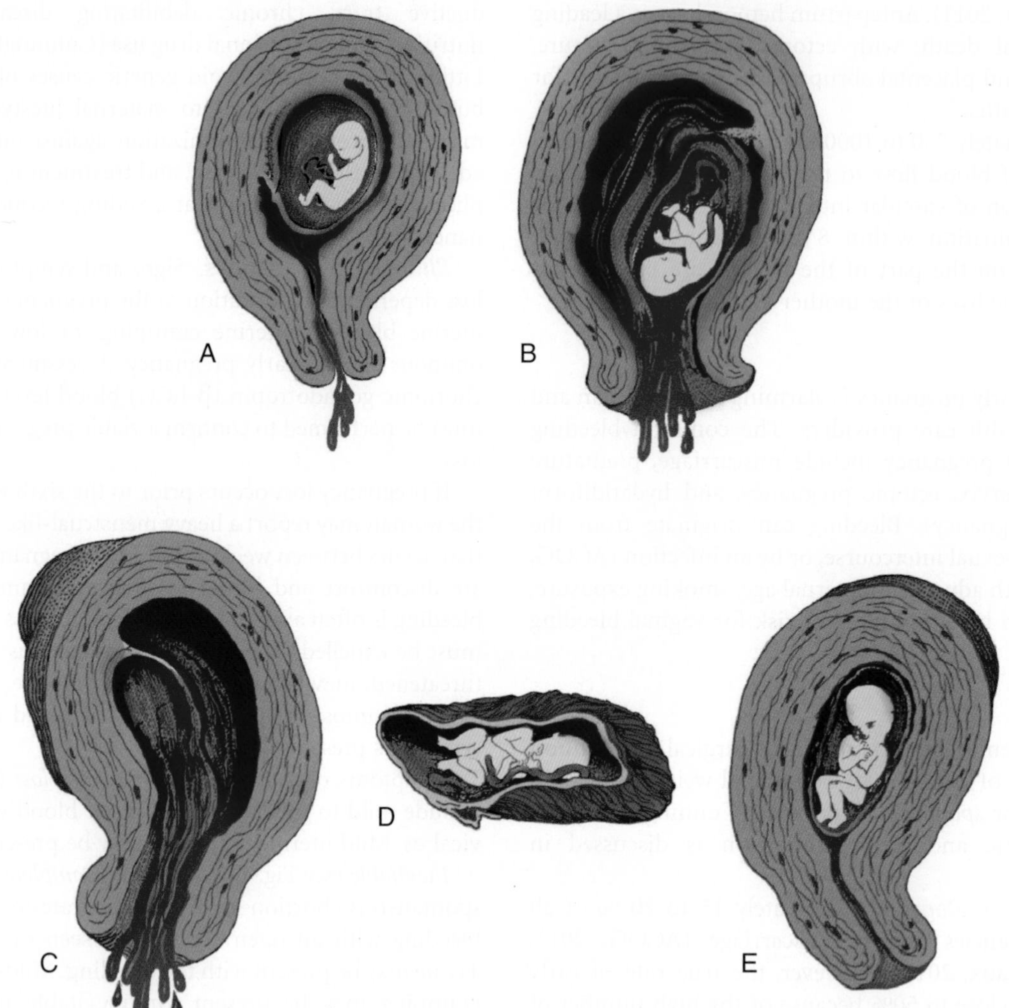

FIGURE 14-6 Types of pregnancy loss. **A:** Threatened. **B:** Inevitable. **C:** Incomplete. **D:** Complete. **E:** Missed.

(Box 14-5). It is common for the woman and her family to be anxious and fearful about what may happen to her and to her pregnancy.

Various laboratory tests are performed to determine the diagnosis of pregnancy loss, including the placental hormone β-hCG. The hormone can be detected in maternal plasma and urine 8 to 9 days after ovulation if the woman is pregnant. In early pregnancy the concentration of β-hCG should double every 1.4 to 2 days until about 60 or 70 days of gestation (Cunningham et al., 2014). Before 8 weeks of gestation, if spontaneous abortion is suspected, two serum quantitative β-hCG levels are measured 48 hours apart. If a normal pregnancy is present, the β-hCG level doubles within that time. Ultrasonography can then be used to determine the presence of a viable gestational sac. With considerable or persistent blood loss, anemia may develop. Infection is suspected if the white blood cell count is greater than 12×10^9/L. Erythrocyte sedimentation rate (ESR), typically a marker of an acute-phase response in an inflammatory process, increases in normal pregnancy and therefore is not a specific test to determine ongoing pregnancy (van den Broek & Letsky, 2001).

Medical–surgical management. Medical management of pregnancy loss (see Table 14-7) depends on the type of spontaneous abortion and its signs and symptoms. Traditionally, threatened pregnancy loss has been managed with rest, decreasing stress levels, and supportive care. However, there are no proven effective therapies for this condition, and bedrest does not prevent progression to pregnancy loss. Follow-up treatment depends on whether the threatened loss progresses to actual spontaneous abortion or symptoms subside and the pregnancy remains intact. Follow-up treatment depends on whether the threatened miscarriage progresses to actual miscarriage or symptoms subside and the pregnancy remains intact. If bleeding and infection do not occur, expectant management is a reasonable option. In approximately half of all threatened miscarriages managed in this way, the pregnancy continues (Cunningham et al., 2014).

Once the cervix begins to dilate, the pregnancy cannot continue, and miscarriage becomes inevitable. If all the products of conception are passed, no surgical intervention is necessary. However, if heavy bleeding, excessive cramping, or infection is present, the remaining embryonic, fetal, or placental tissue must

TABLE 14-7 TYPES OF SPONTANEOUS ABORTION AND USUAL MANAGEMENT

TYPE OF SPONTANEOUS ABORTION	AMOUNT OF BLEEDING	UTERINE CRAMPING	PASSAGE OF TISSUE	CERVICAL DILATION	MANAGEMENT
Threatened (Fig. 14-6, A)	Slight, spotting	Mild	No	No	Bedrest is often ordered but has not proven to be effective in preventing progression to actual miscarriage. Repetitive transvaginal ultrasounds and assessment of human chorionic gonadotropin and progesterone levels may be done to determine if the fetus is still alive and in the uterus. Further treatment depends on whether progression to actual miscarriage occurs.
Inevitable (Fig. 14-6, B)	Moderate	Mild to severe	No	Yes	Bedrest if no pain, fever, or bleeding. If rupture of membranes, bleeding, pain, or fever is present, the uterus is emptied promptly, usually by dilation and curettage.
Incomplete (Fig. 14-6, C)	Heavy, profuse	Severe	Yes	Yes, with tissue in cervix	May or may not require additional cervical dilation before curettage. Suction curettage may be performed.
Complete (Fig. 14-6, C)	Slight	Mild	Yes	No	No further intervention may be needed if uterine contractions are adequate to prevent hemorrhage and no infection is present. Suction curettage may be performed to ensure no retained fetal or maternal tissue.
Missed (Fig. 14-6, D)	None, spotting	None	No	No	If spontaneous evacuation of the uterus does not occur within 1 month, pregnancy is terminated by method appropriate to gestational age. Blood clotting factors are monitored until uterus is empty. Disseminated intravascular coagulation and incoagulability of blood with uncontrolled hemorrhage may develop in cases of fetal death after the twelfth week if products of conception are retained for longer than 5 weeks. May be treated with dilation and curettage, or misoprostol given orally or vaginally
Septic	Varies, usually malodorous	Varies	Varies	Yes, usually	Immediate termination of pregnancy by method appropriate to duration of pregnancy. Cervical culture and sensitivity studies done, and broad-spectrum antibiotic therapy (e.g., ampicillin) started. Treatment for septic shock initiated if necessary.
Recurrent	Varies	Varies	Yes	Yes, usually	Varies, depends on type. Prophylactic cerclage may be performed if premature cervical dilation is the cause. Tests of value include parental cytogenetic analysis and lupus anticoagulant and anticardiolipin antibody assays on the woman.

Adapted from Cunningham, F., Leveno, K., Bloom, S., et al. (2014). *Williams obstetrics* (24th ed.). New York: McGraw-Hill.

be removed from the uterus, usually by suction curettage. In women who are clinically stable, expectant management to allow spontaneous resolution of an incomplete miscarriage is another treatment option (Cunningham et al., 2014; Gilbert, 2011).

Most missed pregnancy losses eventually end spontaneously. Women may be offered expectant management at the time the pregnancy loss is diagnosed. Expectant management results in eventual spontaneous miscarriage in 16 to 76% of cases (Gilbert, 2011).

Dilation and curettage (D&C) is a surgical management option in which the cervix is dilated and a curette inserted to remove uterine contents. A D&C is commonly used to treat inevitable and incomplete miscarriages. The nurse provides supportive care by answering any questions or concerns and preparing the woman for surgery. Women require emotional support during this time of loss, especially if this was a wanted pregnancy.

Dilation and evacuation (D&E), performed after 16 weeks of gestation, consists of wide cervical dilation, followed by instrumental removal of the uterine contents.

Prior to either type of surgical procedure, a full history should be obtained, with both general and pelvic examinations performed. Standard preoperative and postoperative nursing

BOX 14-5 ASSESSMENT OF THREATENED PREGNANCY LOSS—EARLY AND LATE

Initial Database
Chief concern
Vital signs
Number of pregnancies, number of live births
Last menstrual period/estimated date of birth
Pregnancy history (previous and current)
Allergies
Nausea and vomiting
Pain (onset, quality, precipitating event, location)
Bleeding or coagulation problems
Level of consciousness
Emotional status and need for support

Early Pregnancy
Confirmation of pregnancy with laboratory testing
Bleeding (bright or dark, spotting or continuous)
Pain (type, intensity, location, persistence)
Vaginal discharge

Late Pregnancy
Estimated date of birth
Bleeding (amount, pinky, menstrual-like, heavy)
Pain (location, severity, intermittent, continuous)
Vaginal discharge
Amniotic membrane status
Uterine activity
Fetal heart rate present, movement felt

standards are applied in the care of the woman requiring surgical intervention for pregnancy loss. Analgesia and anaesthesia appropriate to the procedure are used.

Medical management is another treatment option if bleeding and infection are not present. Outpatient management of first-trimester pregnancy loss may be accomplished with the use of misoprostol (a synthetic prostaglandin E_1 analog) intravaginally for up to 2 days (Cunningham et al., 2014) (see Chapter 20). There has been no difference in short-term psychological outcomes between expectant and surgical management. If there is evidence of infection, unstable vital signs, or uncontrollable bleeding, a surgical evacuation is performed.

For late incomplete, inevitable, or missed pregnancy loss (16 to 20 weeks), misoprostol can be given orally or vaginally to induce labour and achieve vaginal delivery of the fetus(s). Prostaglandin (PGE_2) has been used for induction in this patient population; however, the extreme systemic adverse effects of this medication make it a less attractive option. IV oxytocin can also be used after 20 weeks' gestation when myometrial oxytocin binding sites have developed.

NURSING CARE

Nursing care is individualized depending on the type of induction (see Chapter 19). Special care may be needed for management of adverse effects of PGE_2 suppositories, such as nausea, vomiting, and diarrhea. If the fetus(es) and placenta are not passed in their entirety, the woman may be prepared for manual or surgical evacuation of the uterus.

After evacuation of the uterus, 10 to 20 units of oxytocin in 1000 mL of fluid can be given to prevent hemorrhage. For excessive bleeding, ergot products such as ergonovine or a prostaglandin derivative such as carboprost tromethamine (hemabate) can be given to contract the uterus. Antibiotics are given as necessary. Analgesics such as ibuprofen may decrease discomfort from cramping. Blood transfusion may be required for shock or anemia. The woman who is Rh negative and has not developed isoimmunization is given an IM injection of $Rh_O(D)$ immune globulin within 48 hours of the pregnancy loss.

Psychosocial aspects of care focus on what the pregnancy loss means to the woman and her family. Grief from perinatal loss is complex and is unique to each individual. The care provider and the nurse's provision of explanations of expected procedures, possible complications, and future implications for child-bearing can be helpful and reassuring to the woman and her family. Culturally sensitive education regarding recognition of grief responses and how to manage these responses effectively may also be helpful to the woman and her family (Canadian Pediatric Society, 2012; Gilbert, 2011).

The woman should be offered the choice of spending time with the fetal remains. Depending on the gestational age of the fetus, hospital disposition of the remains may be offered. If the fetus is over 20 weeks' gestation, the family will need to make arrangements for burial of fetal remains. See Chapter 24 for further discussion on grief and loss.

! NURSING ALERT

Procedures for disposition of the fetal remains vary according to gestational age from province to province. The nurse should know what the required procedures are in his or her setting.

Home care. The woman is usually discharged home after delivery or after a D&C when vital signs are stable, vaginal bleeding remains minimal, and she has recovered from anaesthesia. Discharge teaching emphasizes the need for rest. If significant blood loss has occurred, iron supplementation may be ordered. Teaching includes information about normal physical findings such as cramping and type and amount of bleeding, resumption of sexual activity, and family planning. Follow-up care is needed to assess the woman's physical and emotional recovery. Referrals to local support groups or counselling are provided as necessary (see Patient Teaching box).

Follow-up phone calls after a loss are important. The woman may appreciate a phone call on what would have been her due date. These calls acknowledge the pregnancy existed, validate the woman's experience, and provide opportunities for the woman to ask questions, seek advice, and receive information to help process her grief.

Premature Dilation of Cervix

Passive and painless dilation of the cervical os without labour or contractions of the uterus (cervical insufficiency or

PATIENT TEACHING

Discharge Teaching After Pregnancy Loss

- Advise the woman to report any heavy, profuse, or bright red bleeding to her health care provider.
- Reassure the woman that a scant, dark discharge may persist for 1 to 2 weeks.
- To reduce the risk of infection, remind the woman not to put anything into the vagina for 2 weeks or until bleeding has stopped (e.g., no tampons, no vaginal intercourse). She should take antibiotics as prescribed.
- Advise the woman to notify her health care provider if an elevated temperature or a foul-smelling vaginal discharge develops.
- Advise the woman to eat foods high in iron and protein.
- Acknowledge that the woman has experienced a loss and that she may have mood swings and depression. Talking with her family and seeking support from friends will also help her to deal with her loss.
- Refer the woman to support groups, clergy, or professional counselling, as needed.
- Advise the woman that attempts at pregnancy should be postponed for at least 2 months to allow her body to recover.

From Gilbert, E. S. (2011). *Manual of high risk pregnancy and delivery* (5th ed.). St. Louis: Mosby.

incompetent cervix) may occur in the second trimester or early in the third trimester of pregnancy; miscarriage or preterm birth may result. Current researchers contend that cervical competence is variable and exists as a continuum that is determined in part by cervical length. Other factors include composition of the cervical tissue and the individual circumstances associated with the pregnancy in terms of maternal stress and lifestyle.

Etiology. Etiological factors include a history of cervical trauma, such as lacerations during childbirth or excessive cervical dilation for curettage or biopsy. Other causes are a congenitally short cervix and cervical or uterine anomalies. Cervical insufficiency is a clinical diagnosis based on history. Short labour and recurring loss of the pregnancy at progressively earlier gestational ages are characteristics of reduced cervical competence. Transvaginal ultrasound examination is recommended to diagnose this condition objectively (Lim, Butt, Crane, et al., 2011). A short cervix (less than 25 mm in length) is indicative of reduced cervical competence. Often, but not always, the short cervix is accompanied by cervical funnelling (beaking) or effacement of the internal cervical os (Simhan, Iams, & Romero, 2012).

Collaborative care

Medical–surgical management. Conservative management consists of restricted activity and hydration. Tocolytics are not required as the woman is not experiencing contractions. A cervical cerclage such as a Shirodkar or McDonald procedure may be performed. In the Shirodkar, maternal fascia lata is threaded submucosally in the cervix anteriorly and posteriorly and tied. In the McDonald cerclage, nonabsorbable ribbon (Mersilene) is placed around the cervix beneath the mucosa to constrict the internal os of the cervix (Fig. 14-7). A cerclage procedure can be classified according to time or whether it is elective (prophylactic), urgent, or emergent (Lim et al., 2011).

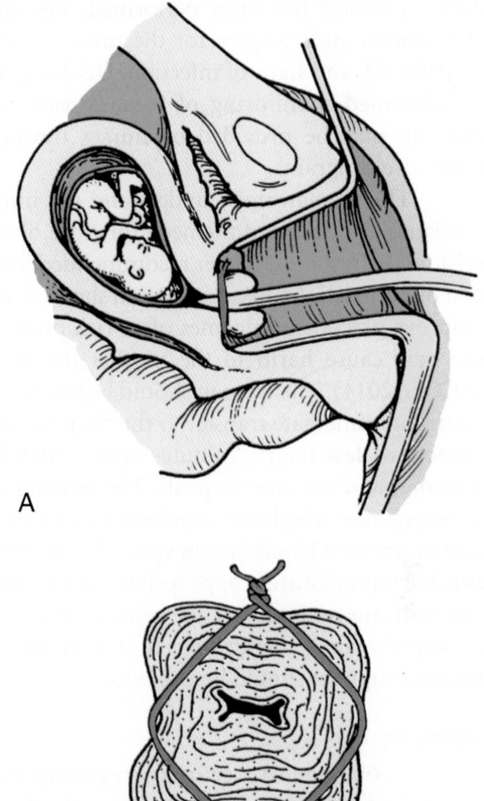

FIGURE 14-7 A: Cerclage correction of recurrent premature dilation of cervix. **B:** Cross section of closed internal os.

Prophylactic cerclage is placed at diagnosis of the shortened or dilating cervix. The woman should refrain from intercourse, prolonged (i.e., more than 90 minutes) standing, and heavy lifting (Berghella & Iams, 2014). She is monitored during the rest of her pregnancy with transvaginal ultrasound scans to assess for cervical shortening and funnelling. The cerclage is electively removed (usually an office or a clinic procedure) when the woman reaches 35 to 37 weeks of gestation, or it may be left in place and a Caesarean birth performed. Approximately 80 to 90% of pregnancies treated with cerclage result in live, viable births. A woman whose reduced cervical competence is diagnosed during the current pregnancy may undergo emergency cerclage placement. Risks of the procedure include premature rupture of membranes (PROM), preterm labour, and chorioamnionitis. Although no consensus has been reached, 24 weeks is often used as the upper gestational age limit for cerclage placement (Berghella & Iams, 2014).

NURSING CARE

The nurse needs to assess the woman's feelings about her pregnancy and her understanding of the risk for preterm birth. The woman may feel guilty or feel she is to blame for the threat to her pregnancy. Therefore, it is important to evaluate the woman's support systems. She needs the support of her family, as well as that of health care providers.

If a cervical cerclage has been performed, the nurse will monitor the woman after surgery for the presence of uterine contractions, PROM, and signs of infection. Discharge teaching focuses on continued monitoring of these aspects at home. Home follow-up may be provided by nurses through antepartum home care programs.

Home care. The woman must understand the importance of activity balance at home and the need for close observation and supervision. Bedrest is no longer recommended for women with arrested preterm labour. Recent research shows that bedrest does not improve newborn outcomes of at-risk preterm pregnancies and may cause harm to the mother due to lack of mobility (ACOG, 2014). The woman should be informed of the signs that warrant immediate transfer to the hospital, including strong contractions less than 5 minutes apart, PROM, severe perineal pressure, and an urge to push. The woman must be advised of emergency telephone numbers to call in case of sudden onset of preterm labour or unexpected imminent birth. If the fetus is born prematurely, appropriate anticipatory guidance and support are necessary. If the fetus or newborn does not survive despite management efforts to stop preterm labour, appropriate grief support should be provided.

Ectopic Pregnancy

Incidence and etiology. An ectopic pregnancy is one in which the fertilized ovum is implanted outside the uterine cavity (Fig. 14-8). It accounts for 1:7000 to 1:30,000 of spontaneously conceived pregnancies (Sepilian et al., 2011). The frequency is consistent across maternal age ranges and ethnic origins; however, the incidence is increased in women who have had assisted reproductive therapy (Gilbert, 2011). Ectopic pregnancy is responsible for 9% of pregnancy-related deaths and is the leading cause of infertility (Sepilian & Wood, 2011). Women who have been treated surgically for ectopic pregnancy have a subsequent intrauterine pregnancy rate of 50 to 80%; the recurrent ectopic pregnancy rate is up to 10 to 25% (Cunningham et al., 2014; Gilbert, 2011).

Approximately 95% of ectopic pregnancies occur in the uterine (fallopian) tube, with most located on the ampullar or largest portion of the tube. Other sites include the ovary (0.5%), abdominal cavity (1.5%), and cervix (0.3%) (Gilbert, 2011). Ectopic pregnancy is classified according to the site of implantation (e.g., tubal, ovarian). The uterus is the only organ capable of containing and sustaining a term pregnancy. However, up to 5% of abdominal pregnancies with birth by laparotomy may result in a living infant (Fig. 14-9). The risk of anomaly in these infants is as high as 40% as a result of having no amniotic fluid (severe oligohydramnios) surrounding the fetus (Gilbert, 2011). If an abdominal pregnancy is diagnosed, it is recommended that the pregnancy be terminated as a result of maternal risk of severe hemorrhage. The placenta may be adhered to one or many abdominal organs. It is recommended that the placental blood supply be ligated prior to attempting to remove the placenta. If the placenta cannot be removed safely, methotrexate may be administered. It is important to evaluate these women for the presence of infection, hemorrhage, or the risk of bowel obstruction (Gilbert, 2011).

The reported incidence of ectopic pregnancy is rising as a result of improved diagnostic techniques, such as more sensitive β-hCG assays and the availability of transvaginal ultrasonography. An increased incidence of sexually transmitted infections (STIs), better treatment of pelvic inflammatory disease (which formerly would have caused sterility), increased numbers of tubal sterilizations, and surgical reversal of tubal sterilizations also have resulted in more ectopic pregnancies (Sepilian & Wood, 2011).

Clinical manifestations. Most cases of ectopic (tubal) pregnancy are diagnosed before rupture on the basis of three classic symptoms: (1) abdominal pain, (2) delayed menses, and (3) abnormal vaginal bleeding (spotting) that occurs approximately 6 to 8 weeks after the last normal menstrual period (Gilbert, 2011). Abdominal pain occurs in almost every case. It usually begins as a dull, lower-quadrant pain on one side. The discomfort can progress from a dull to a colicky pain when the tube stretches, to sharp, stabbing pain (Cunningham et al., 2014;

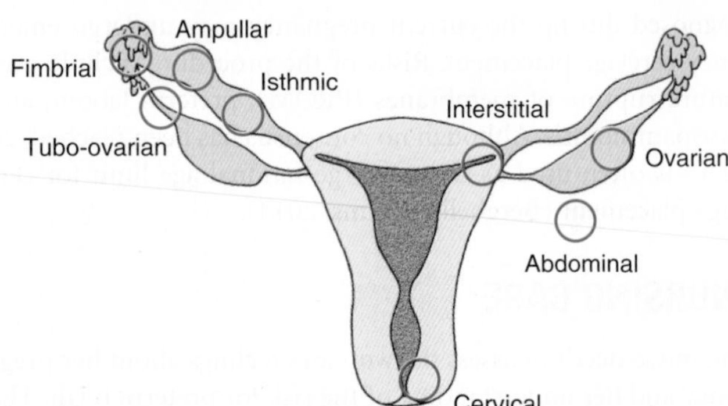

FIGURE 14-8 Sites of implantation of ectopic pregnancies. Order of frequency of occurrence is ampullar, isthmic, interstitial, fimbrial, tubo-ovarian ligament, ovarian, abdominal cavity, and cervical (external os).

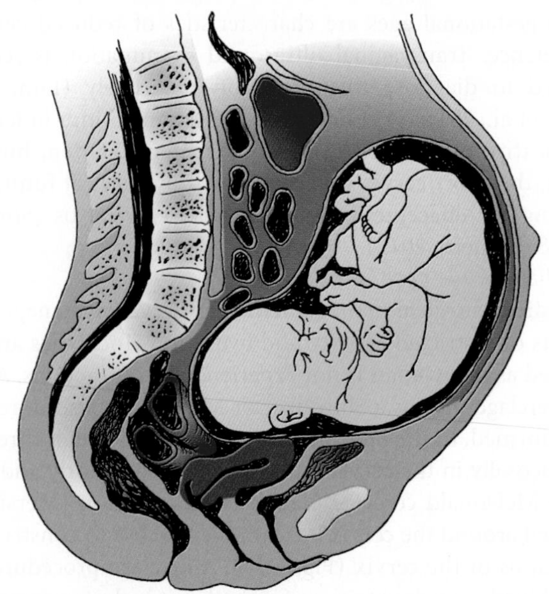

FIGURE 14-9 Ectopic pregnancy, abdominal.

Gilbert, 2011). It progresses to a diffuse, constant, severe pain that is generalized throughout the lower abdomen (Gilbert, 2011). As many as 90% of women with an ectopic pregnancy report a period that is delayed 1 to 2 weeks or is lighter than usual or an irregular period. Mild-to-moderate dark red or brown intermittent vaginal bleeding occurs in up to 80% of women (Gilbert, 2011).

If the ectopic pregnancy is not diagnosed until after rupture has occurred, referred shoulder pain may be present in addition to generalized, one-sided, or deep lower-quadrant acute abdominal pain. Referred shoulder pain results from diaphragmatic irritation caused by blood in the peritoneal cavity. The woman may exhibit signs of shock related to the amount of bleeding in the abdominal cavity and not necessarily to obvious vaginal bleeding. An ecchymotic blueness around the umbilicus (Cullen sign), indicating hematoperitoneum, may develop in an undiagnosed, ruptured intra-abdominal ectopic pregnancy.

Diagnosis. The differential diagnosis of ectopic pregnancy involves consideration of numerous disorders that share many signs and symptoms. Many of these women present to the emergency department experiencing first-trimester bleeding or pain. Miscarriage, ruptured corpus luteum cyst, appendicitis, salpingitis, ovarian cysts, torsion of the ovary, and urinary tract infection must be considered. The key to early detection of ectopic pregnancy is having a high index of suspicion for this condition. Any woman with symptoms of abdominal pain, vaginal spotting or bleeding, and a positive pregnancy test should undergo screening for ectopic pregnancy.

Laboratory screening includes determination of serum progesterone and β-hCG levels. If either of these values is lower than would be expected for a normal pregnancy, the woman should be asked to return within 48 hours for serial measurements. Transvaginal ultrasonography is done to confirm intrauterine or tubal pregnancy (Lim et al., 2011; Sepilian & Wood, 2011). Ultrasonographic identification of an intrauterine pregnancy (gestational sac plus yolk sac) rules out ectopic pregnancy in most women.

The woman should be assessed for the presence of active bleeding, which is associated with tubal rupture. If internal bleeding is present, the woman may have vertigo, shoulder pain, hypotension, and tachycardia. A vaginal examination should be performed only once, and then with great caution. Approximately half of women with tubal pregnancies have a palpable mass on examination. It is possible to rupture the mass during a bimanual examination; thus gentleness is critical.

Treatment options. Ectopic pregnancy can resolve spontaneously by tubal abortion or regression of the pregnancy from the tube. However, most ectopic pregnancies require medical or surgical management. Medical management involves giving methotrexate to dissolve the tubal pregnancy. Methotrexate is an antimetabolite and folic acid antagonist that destroys rapidly dividing cells (see Medication Guide: Methotrexate). The woman must be hemodynamically stable to be eligible for medical management. The best results following methotrexate therapy are usually obtained if the mass is unruptured and measures less than 3.5 cm in diameter by ultrasound, if no fetal cardiac activity is noted on ultrasound, and if the serum β-hCG level is less than 5000 milli-international units/mL (Cunningham et al., 2014). To be a candidate for medical management the woman must also be willing to follow post-treatment lifestyle restrictions and monitoring. Women treated with methotrexate have an intrauterine pregnancy rate of 64%; the recurrent ectopic pregnancy rate is approximately 11% (Sepilian & Wood, 2011).

Methotrexate therapy avoids surgery and is a safe and effective way of managing many cases of tubal pregnancy. The woman should be informed of how the medication works, possible adverse effects, whom to call if she has concerns or if problems develop, and the importance of follow-up care (see Patient Teaching box).

MEDICATION GUIDE

Methotrexate

Action

- Decreases action of dihydrofolic acid reductase enzyme, which stops growth of actively proliferating tissue such as a tumour or fetus; immunosuppressant

Indication

- Ectopic pregnancy, rheumatic conditions, psoriasis, chemotherapy

Pretreatment Investigations

- CBC, blood group typing and antibody screen
- Liver and renal function tests
- Serum β-hCG levels
- Transvaginal ultrasound

Dose

- 50 mg/m^2 intramuscularly: may repeat in 1 week if decrease in β-hCG is less than 25%
- Administer Rh immune globulin 300 mcg, as needed

Adverse Reactions

- Thrombocytopenia and other blood-related disorders, neurotoxicity, nausea and vomiting, fever, dizziness, diarrhea, pruritus

Nursing Considerations

Provide grief support for loss of pregnancy. Counsel woman to report increased abdominal pain, which could indicate tubal rupture. Follow-up care is needed until β-hCG levels are nondetectable. If methotrexate treatment fails, surgical intervention may be necessary.

NURSING ALERT

Women receiving methotrexate to treat an ectopic pregnancy should refrain from taking any analgesic stronger than acetaminophen. Stronger analgesics can mask symptoms of tubal rupture.

NURSING ALERT

The woman receiving methotrexate therapy who drinks alcohol and takes vitamins containing folic acid (e.g., prenatal vitamins) increases her risk of having medication adverse effects or of exacerbating the ectopic rupture.

PATIENT TEACHING

Methotrexate for Ectopic Pregnancy

- Keep all appointments (2 to 8 weeks).
- Report any vaginal bleeding or abdominal pain.
- Do not take any vitamins or folic acid.
- Do not drink any alcohol.
- Avoid prolonged sun exposure because the drug will make you more photosensitive.
- Avoid gas-forming foods.
- Put nothing in the vagina (i.e., no tampons, douches, or intercourse). Do not take any analgesics stronger than acetaminophen.
- Report to your health care provider immediately if you have severe abdominal pain, which may be a sign of impending or actual tubal rupture.

Surgical management. Surgical management depends on the location and cause of the ectopic pregnancy, the extent of tissue involvement, and the woman's desires regarding future fertility. One option is removal of the entire tube (salpingectomy). If the tube has not ruptured and the woman desires future fertility, salpingostomy may be performed instead. In this procedure an incision is made over the pregnancy site in the tube, and the products of conception are gently and very carefully removed. The incision is not sutured but left to close by secondary intention, because this method results in less scarring.

Hospital care. If surgery is planned for the woman with an ectopic pregnancy, general preoperative and postoperative care is appropriate. Vital signs (pulse, respirations, and BP) are assessed before surgery every 15 minutes or as needed, based on the severity of the bleeding and the woman's condition. Preoperative laboratory tests include determination of blood type and Rh factor, CBC, and serum quantitative β-hCG assay. Ultrasonography is used to confirm an extrauterine pregnancy. Blood replacement may be necessary. The nurse will verify the woman's Rh and antibody status and administer Rh_o(D) immune globulin, if appropriate. The woman should be encouraged to express her feelings related to the loss. Referral to community resources may be appropriate.

Future fertility should be discussed. Any woman who has had an ectopic pregnancy should be told to contact her health care provider as soon as she suspects that she might be pregnant, because of the increased risk for recurrent ectopic pregnancy. These women may need referral to grief or infertility support groups. In addition to the loss of the current pregnancy, they are faced with the possibility of future pregnancy losses and infertility.

Hydatidiform Mole (Molar Pregnancy)

Hydatidiform mole (molar pregnancy) is a benign proliferative growth of the placental trophoblast in which the chorionic villi develop into edematous, cystic, avascular transparent vesicles that hang in a grapelike cluster. Hydatidiform mole is a gestational trophoblastic disease (GTD). GTD is a group of pregnancy-related trophoblastic proliferative disorders without a viable fetus that are caused by abnormal fertilization. In addition to hydatidiform mole, GTD includes invasive mole and choriocarcinoma (DiGiulio, Wiedaseck, & Monchek, 2012).

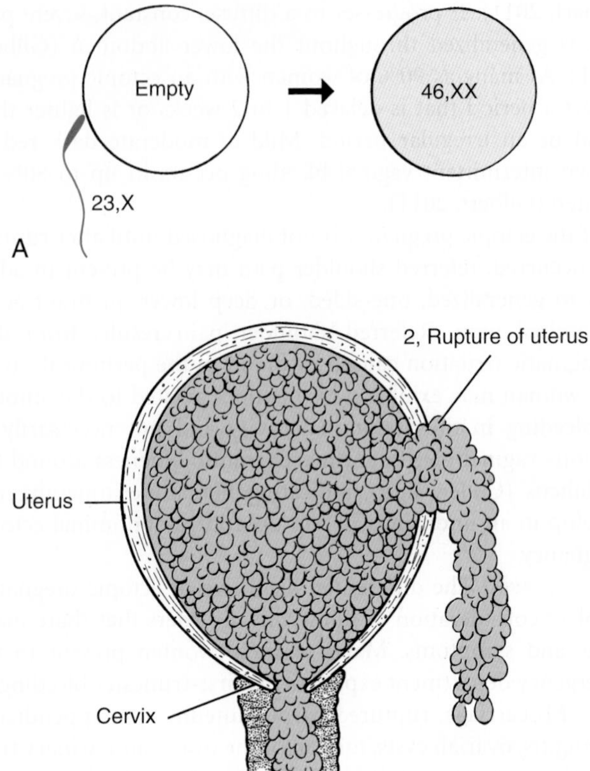

FIGURE 14-10 A: Chromosome origin of complete mole. Single sperm (in colour) fertilizes an "empty" ovum. Reduplication of the sperm's 23,X set gives completely homozygous diploid 46,XX. A similar process follows fertilization of an empty ovum by two sperm with two independently drawn sets of 23,X or 23,Y; both karyotypes of 46,XX and 46,YY can therefore result. **B:** Uterine rupture with hydatidiform mole. *1,* Evacuation of mole through cervix. *2,* Rupture of uterus and spillage of mole into peritoneal cavity (rare).

Incidence and etiology. Hydatidiform mole occurs in 1 in 1000 pregnancies (Cohn, Ramaswamy, & Blum, 2014). The etiology is unknown, although there may be an ovular defect or nutrition deficiency. Women at increased risk for hydatidiform mole formation are those who have had a prior molar pregnancy and those who are in their early teens or older than 40 years of age (DiGiulio et al., 2012).

Types. A hydatidiform mole may be further categorized as a complete or partial mole. The complete mole results from fertilization of an egg in which the nucleus has been lost or inactivated (Fig. 14-10, A). The nucleus of a sperm (23,X) duplicates itself (resulting in the diploid number 46,XX) because the ovum has no genetic material or the material is inactive. It is also possible for an "empty" egg to be fertilized by two normal sperm, thereby producing either a 46,XX or 46,XY karyotype. The mole resembles a bunch of white grapes (see Fig. 14-10, B). The hydropic (fluid-filled) vesicles grow rapidly, causing the uterus to be larger than expected for the duration of the pregnancy. Usually the complete mole contains no fetus, placenta, amniotic membranes, or fluid. Maternal blood has no placenta to receive it; therefore hemorrhage into the uterine cavity and vaginal bleeding occur. Approximately 15 to 20% of women with a complete mole have evidence of persistent GTD (Cunningham et al., 2014).

For a partial mole, chromosomal studies often show a karyotype of 69,XXY; 69,XXX; or, rarely, 69,XYY. This arrangement occurs as a result of two sperm fertilizing an apparently normal ovum. Partial moles often have embryonic or fetal parts and an amniotic sac. Congenital anomalies are usually present. The risk of persistent GTD is much less than with a complete mole. If persistent GTD does occur, it is usually not a choriocarcinoma (Cunningham et al., 2014).

Clinical manifestations. In the early stages, the clinical manifestations of a complete hydatidiform mole cannot be distinguished from those of normal pregnancy. Vaginal bleeding occurs in almost 95% of patients. The vaginal discharge may be dark brown (resembling prune juice) or bright red and either scant or profuse. It may continue for only a few days or intermittently for weeks. In early pregnancy, in about half of affected women the uterus is significantly larger than expected from menstrual dates.

Anemia from blood loss, excessive nausea and vomiting (hyperemesis gravidarum), and abdominal cramps caused by uterine distension are relatively common findings. Women may also pass vesicles, which frequently are avascular edematous villi, from the uterus. Pre-eclampsia occurs in approximately 70% of women with large, rapidly growing hydatidiform moles and occurs earlier than usual in the pregnancy. If pre-eclampsia is diagnosed before 24 weeks of gestation, hydatidiform mole should be suspected and ruled out. Hyperthyroidism is another serious complication of hydatidiform mole. Usually treatment of the hydatidiform mole restores thyroid function to normal. Partial moles cause few of these symptoms and may be mistaken for an incomplete or missed miscarriage (Cohn et al., 2014; DiGiulio et al., 2012; Nader, 2014).

Medical–surgical management. Although most moles pass spontaneously, suction curettage offers a safe, rapid, and effective method of evacuating a hydatidiform mole, if necessary (Cunningham et al., 2014; Gilbert, 2011). An alternative management plan for a woman who desires sterilization is hysterectomy. The use of oxytocic agents or prostaglandins is not recommended because of the increased risk of embolization of trophoblastic tissue. Administration of Rh_o(D) immune globulin to women who are Rh negative is needed to prevent isoimmunization.

NURSING CARE

Nursing assessments during prenatal visits should include observation for signs of molar pregnancy during the first 24 weeks. If hydatidiform mole is suspected, ultrasonography and serial β-hCG immunoassays are used to confirm the diagnosis. The sonographic pattern of a molar pregnancy is characterized by a diffuse snowstorm appearance. The β-hCG titre remains high or rises above the normal peak after the time it normally drops (i.e., 70 to 100 days).

The nurse needs to provide the woman and her family with information about the disease process, the necessity of a long course of follow-up, and the possible consequences of the disease. The nurse can help the woman understand and cope with pregnancy loss and recognize that the pregnancy was abnormal. The woman and her family should be encouraged to express their feelings, and information about support groups or counselling resources should be provided, if needed. The importance of contraceptive counselling and the need to postpone a subsequent pregnancy should also be conveyed.

! NURSING ALERT

To avoid confusion regarding rising levels of hCG that are normal in pregnancy but could indicate GTD, pregnancy should be avoided during the follow-up assessment period. Any contraceptive method, except the intrauterine device, is acceptable. Oral contraceptives are highly effective.

Home care. Follow-up management includes frequent physical and pelvic examinations along with measurement of serum β-hCG until the level drops to normal and remains normal for 3 weeks. Monthly measurements are taken for 6 months (Gilbert, 2011). The follow-up assessment period usually continues for a year. During that time a rising titre and an enlarging uterus may indicate GTD.

Late Pregnancy Bleeding

Late pregnancy bleeding disorders include placenta previa, premature separation of placenta (placental abruption or abruptio placentae), and variations in the insertion of the cord and the placenta (Fig. 14-11). When a woman presents with bleeding in pregnancy, expedient assessment for and diagnosis of the cause of bleeding is essential to reduce the risk of maternal and perinatal morbidity and mortality.

Placenta Previa

In placenta previa the placenta is implanted in the lower uterine segment such that it completely or partially covers the cervix or is close enough to the cervix to cause bleeding when the cervix dilates or the lower uterine segment effaces (Fig. 14-12).

Sonographers should report the actual distance from the placental edge to the internal cervical os by means of transvaginal sonography (TVS), using standard terminology of millimetres away from the os or millimetres of overlap. A placental edge exactly reaching the internal os is described as 0 mm. When the placental edge reaches or overlaps the internal cervical os on TVS between 18 and 24 weeks' gestation (incidence 2 to 4%), a follow-up examination for placental location in the third trimester is recommended. Overlap of more than 15 mm is associated with an increased likelihood of placenta previa at term (Oppenheimer, Armson, Farine, et al., 2007). If the placenta implants in the lower uterine segment, a diagnosis of placenta previa may be made in the second trimester. However, as uterine growth continues throughout gestation, the placenta will usually migrate from the os toward the fundus, and the lower uterine segment will develop (Hull & Resnik, 2014; Oppenheimer et al., 2007). The presence of placenta previa

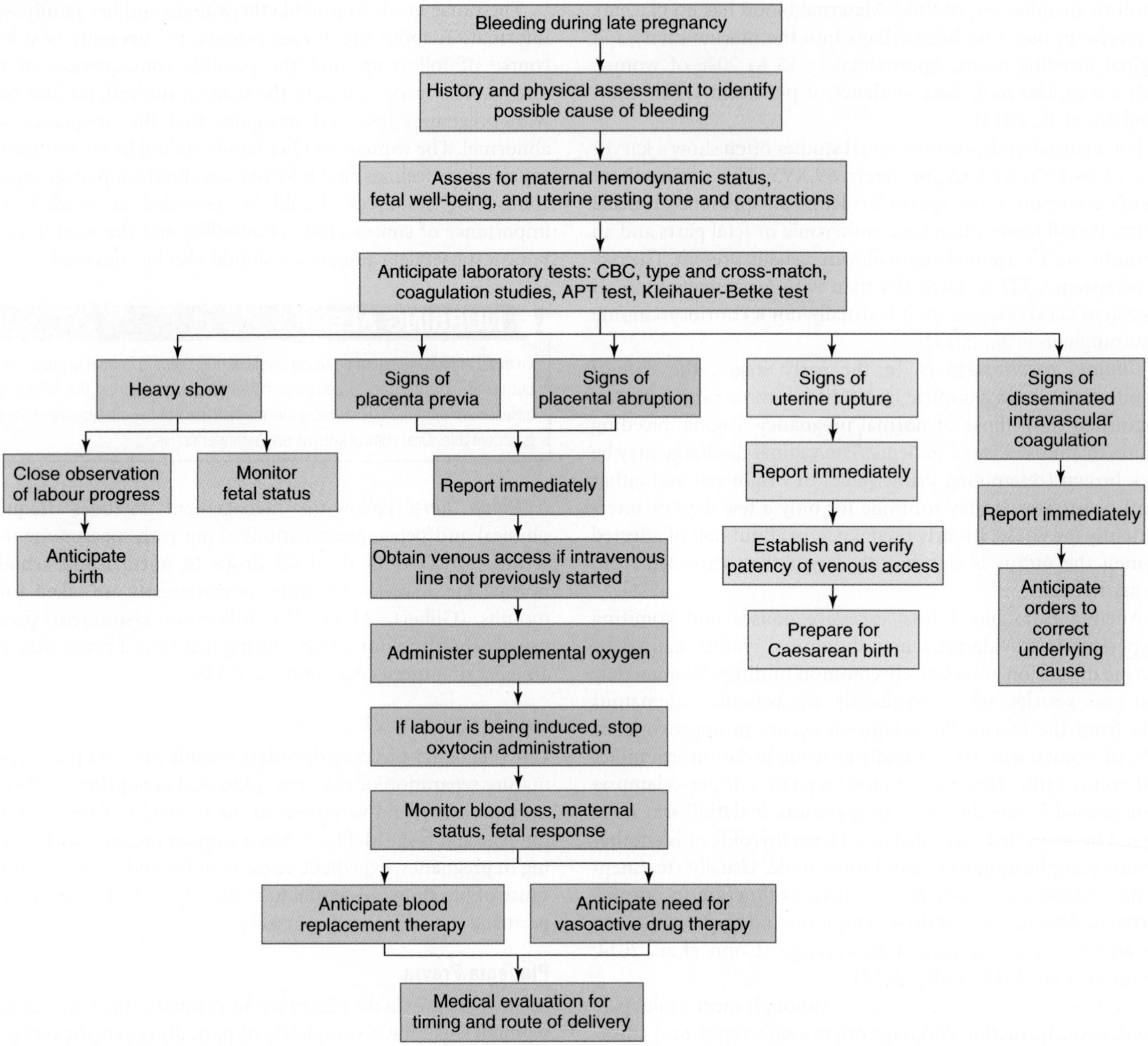

Bleeding during late pregnancy

History and physical assessment to identify possible cause of bleeding

Assess for maternal hemodynamic status, fetal well-being, and uterine resting tone and contractions

Anticipate laboratory tests: CBC, type and cross-match, coagulation studies, APT test, Kleihauer-Betke test

Heavy show
- Close observation of labour progress → Anticipate birth
- Monitor fetal status

Signs of placenta previa / Signs of placental abruption
- Report immediately
- Obtain venous access if intravenous line not previously started
- Administer supplemental oxygen
- If labour is being induced, stop oxytocin administration
- Monitor blood loss, maternal status, fetal response
- Anticipate blood replacement therapy / Anticipate need for vasoactive drug therapy
- Medical evaluation for timing and route of delivery

Signs of uterine rupture
- Report immediately
- Establish and verify patency of venous access
- Prepare for Caesarean birth

Signs of disseminated intravascular coagulation
- Report immediately
- Anticipate orders to correct underlying cause

FIGURE 14-11 Causes and treatment of bleeding during late pregnancy. *CBC,* complete blood count.

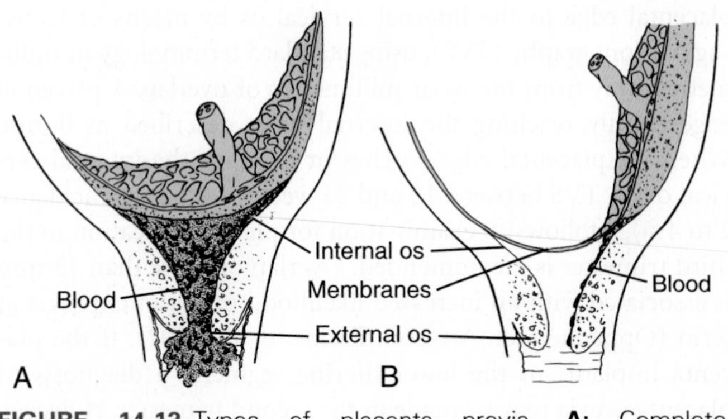

FIGURE 14-12 Types of placenta previa. **A:** Complete. **B:** Marginal.

during the second trimester is a risk factor for the development of vasa previa.

When TVS is used, the placenta is classified as a *complete placenta previa* if it covers the internal cervical os totally. In a *marginal placenta previa* the edge of the placenta is seen on transvaginal ultrasound to be 2.5 cm or closer to the internal cervical os. When the exact relationship of the placenta to the internal cervical os has not been determined or in the case of apparent placenta previa in the second trimester, the term *low-lying placenta* is used (Hull & Resnik, 2014) (see Fig. 14-12).

Incidence and etiology. Placenta previa represents a significant clinical problem because the woman may require hospitalization for observation, she may require blood transfusion, and she is at risk for premature delivery. The incidence of placenta previa is approximately 0.5% of births. The most important risk factors are previous placenta previa, previous Caesarean birth,

TABLE 14-8 SUMMARY OF FINDINGS: PLACENTAL ABRUPTION AND PLACENTA PREVIA

	PLACENTAL ABRUPTION			
	CLASS 1: MILD SEPARATION (10–20%)	CLASS 2: MODERATE SEPARATION (20–50%)	CLASS 3: SEVERE SEPARATION (>50%)	PLACENTA PREVIA
Bleeding, external, vaginal	Minimal	Absent or moderate	Absent to heavy	Minimal to severe and life threatening
Total amount of blood loss	<500 mL	1000–1500 mL	>1500 mL	Varies
Colour of blood	Dark red	Dark red	Dark red	Bright red
Shock	Rare; none	Mild shock	Common, often sudden, profound	Uncommon
Coagulopathy	Rare; none	Occasional DIC	Frequent DIC	None
Uterine tonicity	Normal	Increased; may be localized to one region or diffuse over uterus; uterus fails to relax between contractions	Tetanic, persistent uterine contraction; board-like uterus	Normal
Tenderness (pain)	Usually absent	Present (moderate to severe)	Agonizing, unremitting pain	Absent
Ultrasonographic Findings				
Location of placenta	Normal; upper uterine segment	Normal; upper uterine segment	Normal; upper uterine segment	Abnormal; lower uterine segment
Station of presenting part	Variable to engaged	Variable to engaged	Variable to engaged	High, not engaged
Fetal position	Usual distribution*	Usual distribution*	Usual distribution*	Commonly transverse, breech, or oblique
Other Findings				
Gestational or chronic hypertension	Usual distribution*	Commonly present	Commonly present	Usual distribution*
Fetal effects	Normal fetal heart rate pattern	Atypical fetal heart rate pattern	Abnormal fetal heart rate pattern; death can occur	Normal fetal heart rate pattern

DIC, disseminated intravascular coagulation.
*Usual distribution refers to the usual variations of incidence seen when there is no concurrent problem.
Adapted from Gaufberg, S. V. (2011). Emergent management of abruptio placentae. *eMedicine.* Retrieved from http://emedicine.medscape.com/article/795514-overview.

and suction curettage for miscarriage or induced abortion, possibly related to endometrial scarring. The incidence of placenta previa increases with the number of prior Caesarean births, and the incidence of placenta previa seems to be on the rise because of the increasing rate of Caesarean births. Other risk factors include multiparity, maternal age over 35 years, Black or Asian ethnicity, and smoking (Hull & Resnik, 2014). Living at a higher altitude is also a risk factor for placenta previa. Like cigarette smoking, a higher altitude causes a decrease in uteroplacental oxygenation and thus a need for increased placental surface area (Francois & Foley, 2012). Placenta previa also occurs more frequently in women carrying male fetuses. A possible explanation for this is that placental sizes are larger in pregnancies involving male fetuses. Disagreement exists regarding an increased risk for placenta previa with multiple gestations. Some studies have found a higher incidence with twins, but others have not (Francois & Foley, 2012).

Clinical manifestations. Placenta previa is typically characterized by painless bright red vaginal bleeding during the second or third trimester. In the past, placenta previa was usually diagnosed after an episode of bleeding. However, currently most cases are diagnosed by ultrasonography before significant vaginal bleeding occurs. This bleeding is associated with the disruption of placental blood vessels that occurs with stretching and thinning of the lower uterine segment (Francois & Foley, 2012). The initial bleeding is usually a small amount and stops as clots form. However, it can recur at any time (Gilbert, 2011) (Table 14-8).

Vital signs may be normal even with heavy blood loss because of the compensatory mechanisms of pregnancy, and up to 40% of blood volume can be lost without showing signs of shock. Clinical presentation and decreasing urinary output may be better indicators of acute blood loss than vital signs alone. FHR changes are not usually seen unless there is a major detachment of the placenta (Gilbert, 2011).

Abdominal examination usually reveals a soft, relaxed, nontender uterus with normal tone. The presenting part of the fetus usually remains high because the placenta occupies the lower uterine segment. Thus the fundal height is often greater than expected for gestational age. Because of the abnormally located placenta, fetal malpresentation (breech and transverse or oblique lie) is common.

Maternal and fetal outcome. The major maternal complication associated with placenta previa is hemorrhage. Another serious complication is development of an abnormal placental attachment (e.g., *placenta accreta, increta,* or *percreta*) (see discussion later in chapter). If excessive bleeding cannot be controlled, hysterectomy may be necessary (Cunningham et al.,

2014; Hull & Resnik, 2014). Because most women with placenta previa have a Caesarean birth, surgery-related trauma to structures adjacent to the uterus and anaesthesia complications are also possible. In addition, blood transfusion reactions, anemia, thrombophlebitis, and infection may occur.

The greatest risk of fetal death is caused by preterm birth. Other fetal risks include stillbirth, malpresentation, and fetal anemia. IUGR has also been associated with placenta previa. This association can be related to poor placental exchange (Gilbert, 2011). One study found an increased incidence of fetal anomalies in pregnancies complicated by placenta previa (Cunningham et al., 2014).

Diagnosis. All women with painless vaginal bleeding after 20 weeks of gestation should be assumed to have a placenta previa until proven otherwise. A transabdominal ultrasound examination should be performed initially, followed by a transvaginal scan unless the transabdominal ultrasound clearly shows that the placenta is not located in the lower uterine segment. A transvaginal ultrasound is better than a transabdominal scan for accurately determining placental location (Hull & Resnik, 2014: Orzechowski, Boeling, Baxter, et al., 2014). If ultrasonographic scanning reveals a normally implanted placenta, a speculum examination may be performed to rule out local causes of bleeding (e.g., cervicitis, polyps, carcinoma of the cervix), and a coagulation profile is obtained to rule out other causes of bleeding.

Management. Once placenta previa has been diagnosed, a management plan is developed. The woman is managed either expectantly or actively, depending on the gestational age, amount of bleeding, and fetal condition.

Expectant management. If the woman is less than 36 weeks of gestation and is not in labour and the bleeding is mild or has stopped, expectant management (i.e., reduced activity and close observation) is generally the treatment of choice to give the fetus time to mature in utero. The woman may remain in the hospital or be at home if bleeding is stable and the woman has support and lives in proximity to the hospital. Bleeding is assessed by checking the amount of bleeding on perineal pads, bed pads, and linens. Weighing of pads, although not often used, is one way to more accurately assess blood loss; 1 gram is equal to 1 mL of blood.

Ultrasound examinations may be done every 2 weeks. Fetal surveillance may include NST or BPP once or twice weekly. Serial laboratory values are evaluated for decreasing hemoglobin and hematocrit levels and changes in coagulation values. Venous access with an IV infusion or heparin lock may be placed in case blood or blood component therapy is needed. Antepartum steroids (betamethasone) may be ordered to promote fetal lung maturity if the woman is at less than 34 weeks of gestation (Goldenberg & McClure, 2015). No vaginal or rectal examinations are performed, and the woman is placed on pelvic rest (nothing in the vagina). Once she reaches 37 weeks of gestation and fetal lung maturity is documented, Caesarean birth can be scheduled.

The woman with placenta previa should always be considered a potential emergency because massive blood loss with resulting hypovolemic shock can occur quickly if bleeding resumes. The possibility always exists that she may require an emergency Caesarean birth. Placenta previa in a preterm gestation may be an indication for admission to a tertiary perinatal centre because many community hospitals are not equipped to perform emergency Caesarean births 24 hours per day, 7 days per week; nor can they provide neonatal intensive care.

If expectant management is to be implemented, a vaginal speculum examination should be postponed until fetal viability is reached (preferably after 34 weeks of gestation). If a pelvic examination is needed before that time, it is possible that an immediate Caesarean birth may be required. The woman is taken to a delivery room or an operating room set up for Caesarean birth, because profound hemorrhage can occur during the examination. This type of vaginal examination, known as the *double-setup procedure*, is not often performed.

Home care. Criteria for home care management vary among primary perinatal providers and home care agencies and are usually determined on a case-by-case basis. To be considered for home care referral, the woman must, after a period of assessment in hospital, be in stable condition with no evidence of active bleeding and must have the resources to be able to return to the hospital immediately if active bleeding resumes (Francois & Foley, 2012; Oppenheimer et al., 2007).

She must have close supervision by family or friends in the home. She should be taught how to assess fetal and uterine activity and bleeding and told to avoid intercourse, douching, and the use of enemas. She should limit her activities according to the advice of her health care provider and be advised to keep all appointments for fetal testing, laboratory assessments, and prenatal care.

Active management. If the woman is at or beyond 36 weeks of gestation or bleeding is excessive or persistent, immediate Cesaerean birth is indicated (Hull & Resnik, 2014). Expectant management is terminated as soon as the fetus is mature, if excessive bleeding develops, active labour begins, or any other obstetrical reason to end the pregnancy (e.g., chorioamnionitis) develops (Gilbert, 2011). Caesarean birth is indicated in all women with ultrasound evidence of placenta previa. Acute care of a patient with a diagnosed placenta previa should be carried out in a labour and birth unit with continuous electronic monitoring of the fetus and uterine contractions. Maternal vital signs are assessed frequently for BP changes, increasing pulse rate, changes in level of consciousness, and oliguria. The nurse should continuously assess maternal and fetal status while preparing the woman for surgery. In women with partial or marginal placenta previa (placental edge is greater than 2 mm from the cervical os) who have minimal bleeding, vaginal birth may be attempted (Francois & Foley, 2012; Hull & Resnik, 2014; Oppenheimer et al., 2007).

Blood loss may not cease with the infant's birth. The large vascular channels in the lower uterine segment may continue to bleed because of the diminished muscle content in that region. The natural mechanism to control bleeding (i.e., the interlacing muscle bundles contracting around open vessels [the "living ligature" characteristic of the upper part of the uterus]) is absent in the lower part of the uterus. Postpartum

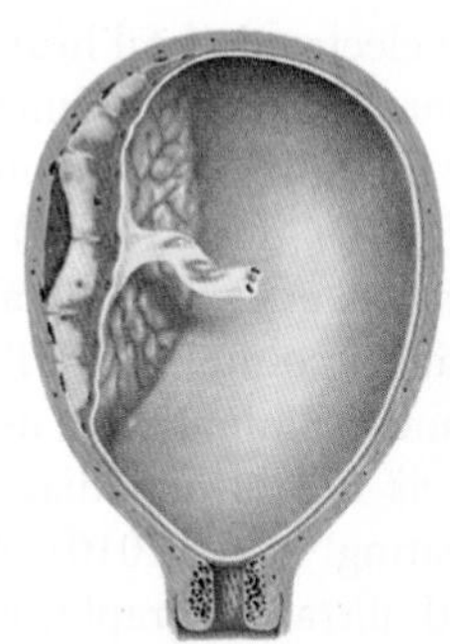
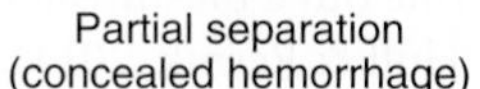

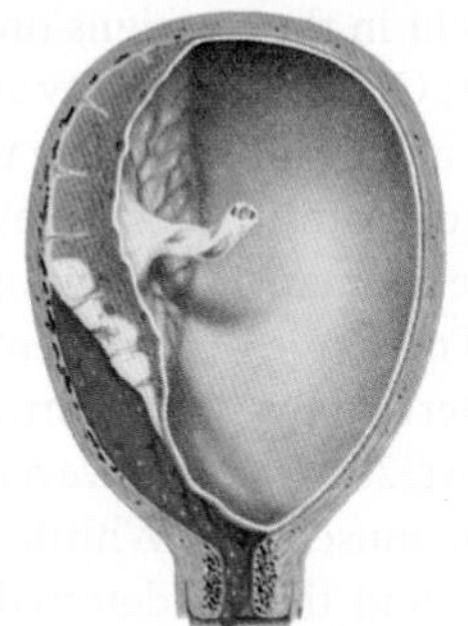

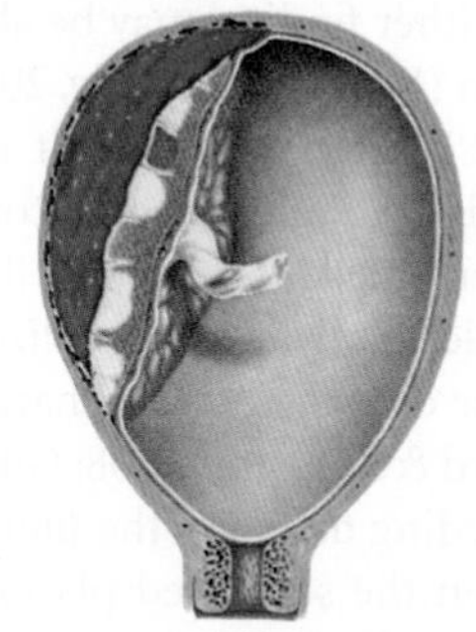

FIGURE 14-13 Placental abruption showing partial and complete placental separation.

hemorrhage may occur even if the fundus is contracted firmly (see Chapter 24).

Emotional support for the woman and her family is extremely important. The actively bleeding woman is concerned not only for her own well-being but for that of her fetus. All procedures should be explained, and a support person should be present. The woman should be encouraged to express her concerns and feelings. If the woman and her support person or family desire spiritual care support, the nurse can notify the hospital chaplain service or provide information about other supportive resources. See the Nursing Care Plan, Planeta Previa on the Evolve site.

Placental Abruption (Premature Separation of Placenta)

Premature separation of the placenta, or placental abruption (abruptio placentae), is the detachment of part or all of the placenta from its implantation site (Fig. 14-13). Separation occurs in the area of the decidua basalis after 20 weeks of pregnancy and before the birth of the baby.

Incidence and etiology. Premature separation of the placenta is a serious complication that accounts for significant maternal and fetal morbidity and mortality. Approximately 1 in 75 to 1 in 226 pregnancies is complicated by placental abruption (Francois & Foley, 2012) (see Critical Thinking Case Study).

Maternal hypertension is probably the most consistently identified risk factor for abruption. Cocaine use also is a risk factor because it causes vascular disruption in the placental bed. Blunt external abdominal trauma, most often the result of motor vehicle accidents (MVAs) or maternal battering, is another frequent cause of placental abruption (Cunningham et al., 2014; Gilbert, 2011). Other risk factors include cigarette smoking, a history of abruption in a previous pregnancy, preterm PROM, and the presence of inherited or acquired thrombophilias (e.g., factor V Leiden mutation or protein C or S deficiency) (Cunningham et al., 2014; Francois & Foley, 2012; Hull & Resnik, 2014). Abruption is more likely to occur in twin gestations than in singletons (Francois & Foley, 2012). Women who have had two previous abruptions have a recurrence risk of 25% in the next pregnancy (Hull & Resnik, 2014).

Classification systems. The most common classification of placental abruption is according to type and severity. This classification is summarized in Table 14-8.

CRITICAL THINKING CASE STUDY

Third-Trimester Vaginal Bleeding

Ashley is a 29-year-old (G7T5P0A1L5) who presents to the emergency department with heavy vaginal bleeding and contractions. She has had no prenatal care but is approximately 33 weeks of gestation by her LMP. During her medical screening examination Ashley admitted to past cocaine use and reported that her boyfriend punched her in the abdomen earlier in the day.

QUESTIONS

1. Evidence—Is there sufficient evidence to determine the cause of Ashley's bleeding?
2. Assumptions—Describe an underlying assumption about each of the following issues:
   a. Possible diagnoses for Ashley
   b. Laboratory and diagnostic tests necessary to diagnose the cause of Ashley's bleeding
   c. Management options for Ashley
   d. Need for a social work consultation regarding intimate partner violence
3. What implications and priorities for nursing care can be drawn at this time?
4. Does the evidence objectively support your argument (conclusion)?

LMP, Last menstrual period.

Clinical manifestations. The separation may be partial or complete, or only the margin of the placenta may be involved. Bleeding from the placental site may dissect (separate) the membranes from the decidua basalis and flow out through the vagina (70 to 80%), it may remain concealed (retroplacental hemorrhage) (10 to 20%), or it may do both (see Fig. 14-13) (Francois & Foley, 2012; Gilbert, 2011). Clinical symptoms vary with the degree of separation (see Table 14-8).

Minor degrees of placental abruption cause slight vaginal bleeding, vague abdominal pain, or false preterm labour. More extensive placental separation leads to acute fetal distress associated with maternal shock due to substantial revealed or concealed blood loss.

Typically, dark, vaginal nonclotting bleeding, abdominal or low back pain, "port wine" stained amniotic fluid, uterine contractions or hypertonus, uterine tenderness, and abnormal FHR patterns or fetal death are seen with placental abruption. Although abdominal pain and uterine tenderness are characteristic of abruption, either finding may be absent in the presence of a silent abruption (Baird & Kennedy, 2008; Gilbert, 2011; Hull & Resnik, 2014). Bleeding may result in maternal hypovolemia (i.e., shock, oliguria, anuria) and coagulopathy. Mild-to-severe uterine hypertonicity is present. The woman experiences pain which is mild to severe and localized over one region of the uterus or diffuse over the uterus, characterized by a "board-like" abdomen (Baird & Kennedy, 2008; Gilbert, 2011).

Extensive myometrial bleeding damages the uterine muscle. If blood accumulates between the separated placenta and the uterine wall, it may produce a Couvelaire uterus: the uterus appears purplish and copper coloured, it is ecchymotic, and contractility is lost. Shock may occur and is out of proportion to blood loss. The APT test result (for blood in amniotic fluid) is positive, hemoglobin and hematocrit levels decrease, and coagulation factor levels decrease. Clotting defects (e.g., DIC) develop in 10 to 30% of women, in most cases within 8 hours of hospital admission. A Kleihauer-Betke (KB) test may be ordered to determine the presence of fetal-to-maternal bleeding (transplacental hemorrhage), although this test appears to be of no value in the general workup of patients with placental abruption as it can take up to 45 minutes to obtain the result (Hull & Resnik, 2014; Murray & Murphy, 2008). The KB test may be useful to guide $Rh_o(D)$ immunoglobulin therapy in Rh-negative women who have had an abruption (Hull & Resnik, 2014).

Maternal, fetal, and newborn outcomes. The maternal mortality rate approaches 1% in placental abruption; this condition remains one of the leading causes of maternal death. The mother's prognosis depends on the extent of placental detachment, overall blood loss, degree of coagulopathy present, and time between placental detachment and birth. Maternal complications are associated with the abruption or its treatment. Hemorrhage, hypovolemic shock, hypofibrinogenemia, and thrombocytopenia are associated with severe abruption. Couvelaire uterus, DIC, and infection may occur. Renal failure and pituitary necrosis (Sheehan's syndrome) may result from ischemia. In rare cases, women who are Rh negative can become sensitized if fetal-to-maternal hemorrhage occurs and the fetal blood type is Rh positive.

Placental abruption accounts for about 12% of all perinatal deaths (Gilbert, 2011). Fetal complications, which include IUGR and preterm birth, are related to the severity and timing of the hemorrhage. The size of the hemorrhage is related to fetal survival. Large (greater than 60 mL) hemorrhages are associated with 50% or higher fetal mortality (Francois & Foley, 2012). Risks for neurological defects, cerebral palsy, and death from sudden infant death syndrome are greater in newborns following placental abruption (Cunningham et al., 2014; Francois & Foley, 2012).

Diagnosis. Placental abruption should be strongly suspected in the woman who has a sudden onset of intense, usually localized, uterine pain, with or without vaginal bleeding. Initial assessment is much the same as that for placenta previa. Physical examination usually reveals abdominal pain, uterine tenderness, and contractions. The fundal height may be measured over time, because increasing fundal height could indicate concealed bleeding. Approximately 60% of live fetuses exhibit abnormal signs on the electronic fetal heart monitor, such as loss of variability and late decelerations; uterine tachysystole and increased resting tone may also be noted on the monitor tracing (Francois & Foley, 2012; Gilbert, 2011). Many women demonstrate coagulopathy, as evidenced by abnormal clotting studies (fibrinogen, platelet count, PT, PTT, fibrin split products).

Ultrasound examination is used to rule out placenta previa; however, it is not always diagnostic for abruption (Walker, Whittle, Keating, et al., 2010). A retroplacental mass may be detected with ultrasonographic examination, but negative findings do not rule out a life-threatening abruption (Cunningham et al., 2014; Hull & Resnik, 2014).

Hospital care. Treatment depends on the severity of blood loss and fetal maturity and status. If the abruption is mild, expectant management is implemented if the fetus is less than 36 weeks of gestation and not in distress. The woman is hospitalized and closely observed for signs of bleeding and labour. The fetal status is monitored with intermittent FHR monitoring and NST or BPP until fetal maturity is achieved. If the woman's condition deteriorates, immediate birth is indicated. Use of corticosteroids to accelerate fetal lung maturity is appropriately included in the plan of care for the woman managed expectantly (Goldenberg & McClure, 2015; Hull & Resnik, 2014). Women who are Rh negative may be given $Rh_o(D)$ immunoglobulin if fetal-to-maternal hemorrhage occurs and the fetal blood is Rh positive.

If the mother is hemodynamically stable, a vaginal birth may be attempted if the fetus is alive and in no acute distress or if the fetus is dead. In the presence of fetal compromise, severe hemorrhage, coagulopathy, poor labour progress, or increasing uterine resting tone, a Caesarean birth is performed. At least one large-bore (16-gauge) IV line should be started. Maternal vital signs should be monitored frequently to observe for signs of declining hemodynamic status, such as increasing pulse rate and decreasing BP. Serial laboratory studies include hematocrit or hemoglobin determinations and clotting studies. Continuous electronic fetal monitoring (EFM) is mandatory. An indwelling Foley catheter can be inserted for ongoing assessment of urine output, an excellent indirect measure of maternal organ perfusion.

Blood and fluid volume replacement will most likely be ordered, with the goals of maintaining the urine output at 30 mL/hr or more and the hematocrit at 0.30 or more. If these goals are not reached despite vigorous attempts at replacement, hemodynamic monitoring may be necessary. Fresh frozen plasma or cryoprecipitate may be given to maintain the fibrinogen level at a minimum of 2.95 to 4.41 mmol/L.

Caesarean birth should be reserved for cases of abnormal EFM patterns or other obstetrical indications. Caesarean birth should not be attempted when the woman has severe and uncorrected coagulopathy because it may result in surgically uncontrollable bleeding.

Emotional support for the woman and her family is extremely important. If the woman is actively bleeding, she will be concerned not only for her own well-being but also for that of her fetus. All procedures should be explained, and a support person should be present.

Cord Insertion and Placental Variations

Placenta accreta is a serious complication of placenta previa. In this condition, trophoblastic invasion extends beyond the normal endometrial barrier. If the invasion extends into the myometrium, it is called *placenta increta. Placenta percreta* exists when the placental invasion extends beyond the uterine serosa (Hull & Resnik, 2014). Massive hemorrhage can occur with these conditions. Caesarean birth through a fundal incision, followed by total abdominal hysterectomy, may be indicated (Gagnon, Morin, Bly, et al., 2009; Hull & Resnik, 2014; Mehrabadi, Hutcheon, Liu, et al., 2015).

Velamentous insertion of the cord and vasa previa are rare placental anomalies with a higher incidence in multiple gestation and pregnancies from assisted reproductive technology (Donnolley, Halliday, & Oyelese, 2013; Murray & Murphy, 2008). Velamentous insertion of the cord occurs when the umbilical vessels begin to branch at the membranes and then course onto the placenta (Fig. 14-14, A). When the placenta is found to be low lying, further evaluation for placental cord insertion should be assessed (Gagnon et al., 2009). When some of the umbilical vessels cross the cervical os below the presenting part, vasa previa is diagnosed. ROM or traction on the cord may tear one or more of the fetal vessels. As a result, the fetus may rapidly bleed to death (Donnolley et al., 2013; Gagnon et al., 2009). Battledore (marginal) insertion of the cord (see Fig. 14-14, B) increases the risk of fetal hemorrhage, especially after marginal separation of the placenta.

Rarely, the placenta may be divided into two or more separate lobes, resulting in succenturiate placenta (see Fig. 14-14, C). Each lobe has a distinct circulation. The vessels collect at the periphery, and the main trunks eventually unite to form the vessels of the cord. Blood vessels joining the lobes may be supported only by the fetal membranes; therefore, they are in danger of tearing during labour, birth, or expulsion of the placenta. During expulsion of the placenta, one or more of the separate lobes may remain attached to the decidua basalis, preventing uterine contraction and increasing the risk of postpartum hemorrhage.

Clotting Disorders in Pregnancy

Normally, a delicate balance (homeostasis) is maintained between the opposing hemostatic and fibrinolytic systems. The hemostatic system stops the flow of blood from injured vessels, first by a platelet plug, then by formation of a fibrin clot. The coagulation process involves an interaction of the coagulation factors in which each factor sequentially activates the factor next in line—the "cascade effect" sequence. The fibrinolytic system is the process by which the fibrin is split into fibrin degradation products and circulation is restored.

A history of abnormal bleeding, inheritance of unusual bleeding tendencies, or a report of significant aberrations of laboratory findings indicates a bleeding or clotting problem. For the pregnant woman, bleeding disorders are suspected if the woman has gestational hypertension, HELLP syndrome, retained dead fetus syndrome, amniotic fluid embolism, sepsis, or hemorrhage (Romero et al., 2011). Determination of hemostasis is made by testing the usual mechanisms for the control of bleeding, the function of platelets, and the necessary clotting factors. Most clotting disorders are more a concern in the immediate postpartum period. Recognition in the antepartum period may decrease hemorrhagic problems.

Disseminated Intravascular Coagulation (DIC)

Disseminated intravascular coagulation (DIC), or consumptive coagulopathy, is a pathological form of clotting that is diffuse and consumes large amounts of clotting factors, causing

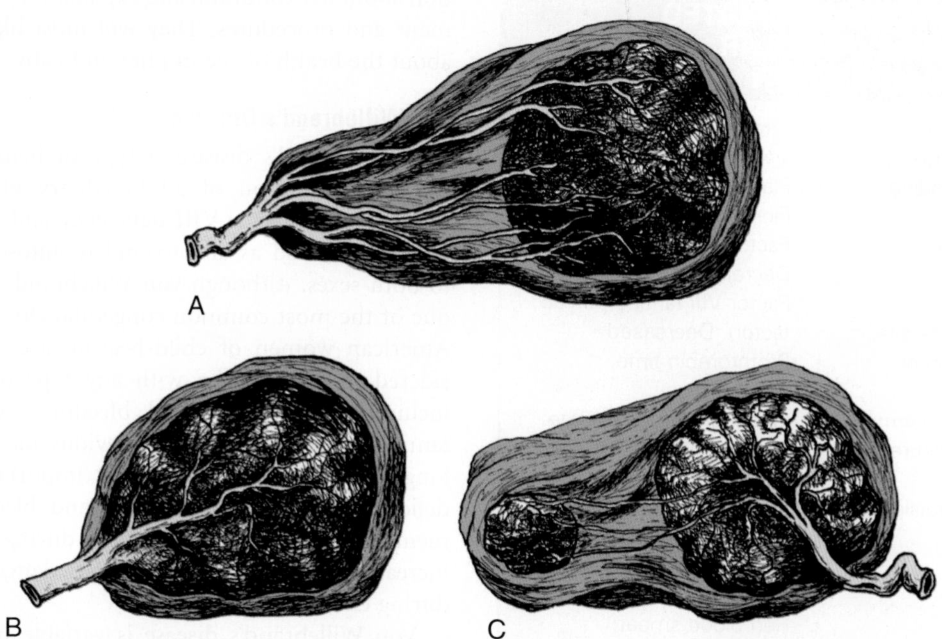

FIGURE 14-14 Cord insertion and placental variations. **A:** Velamentous insertion of cord. **B:** Battledore placenta. **C:** Succenturiate placenta.

widespread external or internal bleeding or both. DIC is an overactivation of the clotting cascade and the fibrinolytic system, resulting in the depletion of platelets and clotting factors. This results in the formation of multiple fibrin clots throughout the body's vasculature, even in the microcirculation. Blood cells are destroyed as they pass through these fibrin-choked vessels. Thus DIC results in a clinical picture of hemorrhage, anemia, and ischemia (Cunningham, et al., 2014; Moake, 2013). DIC is never a primary diagnosis. Instead, it results from some problem that triggered the clotting cascade, either extrinsically by the release of large amounts of tissue thromboplastin or intrinsically by widespread damage to vascular integrity.

In the obstetrical population DIC is most often triggered by the release of large amounts of tissue thromboplastin, which occurs in placental abruption (the most common cause of severe consumptive coagulopathy in obstetrics), retained dead fetus syndrome, and amniotic fluid embolus (anaphylactoid syndrome of pregnancy). Severe pre-eclampsia, HELLP syndrome, and gram-negative sepsis are examples of conditions that can trigger DIC because of widespread damage to vascular integrity (Cunningham et al., 2014). Clinical manifestations and laboratory test results are summarized in Box 14-6.

Medical management. The primary management of DIC involves correction of the underlying cause, which may be treatment of existing severe infection, pre-eclampsia, or eclampsia, or removal of a placental abruption or dead fetus.

Volume expansion, rapid replacement of blood products and clotting factors, optimization of oxygenation, achievement of normal body temperature, and continued reassessment of laboratory parameters are the usual forms of treatment. Vitamin K administration, recombinant activated factor VIIa, fibrinogen concentrate, and hemostatic agents should be considered as additional therapies (Francois & Foley, 2012).

BOX 14-6 CLINICAL MANIFESTATIONS AND LABORATORY SCREENING RESULTS FOR WOMEN WITH DISSEMINATED INTRAVASCULAR COAGULATION

Possible Physical Examination Findings

- Spontaneous bleeding from gums, nose
- Oozing, excessive bleeding from venipuncture site, intravenous access site, or site of insertion of urinary catheter
- Petechiae (e.g., on arm where blood pressure cuff was placed)
- Other signs of bruising
- Hematuria
- Gastrointestinal bleeding
- Tachycardia
- Diaphoresis

Laboratory Coagulation Screening Test Results

- Platelets: Decreased
- Fibrinogen: Decreased
- Factor V (proaccelerin): Decreased
- Factor VIII (antihemolytic factor): Decreased
- Prothrombin time: Prolonged
- Partial prothrombin time: Prolonged
- Fibrin degradation products: Increased
- D-dimer test (specific fibrin degradation fragment): Increased
- Red blood smear: Fragmented red blood cells

NURSING CARE

Nursing interventions include assessing for signs of bleeding (petechial, oozing from injection sites, hematuria, and hemoptysis) (see Box 14-6) and complications from the administration of blood and blood products, administering fluid or blood replacement as ordered, cardiac and hemodynamic monitoring, and protecting the woman from injury. Because acute renal failure is one consequence of DIC, urinary output needs to be carefully monitored with an indwelling Foley catheter. The goal for urine output is 30 mL/hr or greater. Vital signs should be assessed frequently.

Supportive measures include keeping the pregnant woman in a side-lying tilt to maximize blood flow to the uterus. Oxygen may be administered through a tight-fitting rebreathing mask at 8 to 10 L/min or per hospital protocol or health care provider order. To provide oxygen delivery to the tissues, blood products are usually administered. The woman should be kept warm with a forced-air warming system (e.g., Bair Hugger), which is an effective method to maintain normothermia. Other interventions include the use of warmed blankets and fluid warmers, which should be used as needed. If the woman has not yet given birth, fetal assessments by continuous EFM should be carried out. DIC is usually corrected with birth, blood and volume replacement, and resolution of the cause and as coagulation abnormalities resolve (Ramin & Ramin, 2016).

The educational and emotional needs of the woman and her family must be recognized and supported. They need information about her condition and explanations of unfamiliar equipment and procedures. They will most likely be very anxious about the health of the mother and baby.

Von Willebrand's Disease

Von Willebrand's disease, a type of hemophilia, is probably the most common of all hereditary bleeding disorders. It results from a factor VIII deficiency and platelet dysfunction. It is transmitted as an incomplete autosomal dominant trait to both sexes. Although von Willebrand's disease is rare, it is one of the most common congenital clotting defects in North American women of child-bearing age and should be considered in any woman with any type of bleeding disorder, including heavy menstrual bleeding. Symptoms include a familial bleeding tendency, previous bleeding episodes, prolonged bleeding time (the most important test), factor VIII deficiency (mild to moderate), and bleeding from mucous membranes. Factor VIII increases during pregnancy, and this increase may be sufficient to offset danger from hemorrhage during childbirth.

Von Willebrand's disease is variable in its clinical course, severity, and laboratory values; thus it is possible for this condition to go undetected throughout pregnancy until bleeding problems develop after birth. A primary treatment for many women is desmopressin, which increases levels of plasma factor VIII and von Willebrand's factor (vWF) (Rodger & Silver, 2014). If the woman is known to have von Willebrand's disease before labour, factor VIII levels should be monitored and factor VIII/vWF plasma concentrate given as needed to maintain activity at 50% of normal near-term gestation (Rodger & Silver, 2014). Hemorrhage may occur 4 or 5 days after birth. The woman should remain in the hospital for several days after birth so she can be monitored for that complication.

INFECTIONS ACQUIRED DURING PREGNANCY

Sexually Transmitted Infections

Sexually transmitted infections (STIs) in pregnancy are responsible for significant morbidity rates. Some consequences of maternal infection, such as infertility and sterility, last a lifetime. Psychosocial sequelae may include altered interpersonal relationships and lowered self-esteem. Congenitally acquired infections may affect the length and quality of a child's life. Chapter 7 discusses the diagnosis and management of STIs.

Urinary Tract Infections

Urinary tract infections (UTIs) are a common medical complication of pregnancy, occurring in approximately 20% of all pregnancies. They are also responsible for 10% of all hospitalizations during pregnancy (Duff, 2014). UTIs include asymptomatic bacteriuria, cystitis, and pyelonephritis. They are usually caused by coliform organisms that are a normal part of the perineal flora. By far the most common cause is *Escherichia coli,* a gram-negative bacterium responsible for 85% of cases. Another gram-negative bacterium that causes UTIs is *Klebsiella pneumoniae.* The gram-positive organisms group B streptococci, enterococci, and staphylococci account for approximately 3 to 7% of all infections (Gilbert, 2011).

Asymptomatic Bacteriuria

Asymptomatic bacteriuria refers to the persistent presence of bacteria within the urinary tract of women who have no symptoms. A clean-voided urine specimen containing more than 100,000 colonies per millilitre of a single organism is diagnostic. If asymptomatic bacteriuria is not treated, up to 40% of infected women will subsequently develop symptomatic infection during the pregnancy (Colombo, 2012). It is recommended that all women be screened for asymptomatic bacteriuria at their first prenatal visit (Colombo, 2012). It has been associated with preterm labour and birth and low-birth-weight infants (American Academy of Pediatrics [AAP] and ACOG, 2012; Cunningham et al., 2014).

Asymptomatic bacteriuria should be treated with an antibiotic. Antibiotics that are often prescribed include amoxicillin, ampicillin, cephalexin (Keflex), ciprofloxacin (Cipro), levofloxacin (Levaquin), nitrofurantoin (Macrodantin), and trimethoprim-sulfamethoxazole (Bactrim DS). Several different regimens, including single-dose or 3-, 7-, and 10-day treatment may be used (Cunningham et al., 2014). A repeat urine culture is usually ordered 1 to 2 weeks after completing therapy because approximately 15% of women do not respond to therapy or have a reinfection (Colombo, 2012). Women who have persistent or frequent recurrences of bacteriuria may be placed on suppressive therapy, often nitrofurantoin, each night at bedtime for the remainder of the pregnancy (Cunningham et al., 2014).

Cystitis

Cystitis (bladder infection) is characterized by dysuria, urgency, and frequency, along with lower abdominal or suprapubic pain. Usually white blood cells (WBCs) and bacteria are found in the urine. Microscopic or gross hematuria may also be present. Typically symptoms are confined to the bladder rather than becoming systemic. Cystitis is usually uncomplicated, but it may lead to ascending UTI if untreated. Approximately 40% of pregnant women with pyelonephritis experienced symptoms of bladder infection before developing pyelonephritis (Cunningham et al., 2014).

Cystitis is often treated with a 3-day course of antibiotic therapy, which is usually 90% effective in curing the infection. Antibiotics often prescribed include amoxicillin, ampicillin, cephalexin (Keflex), ciprofloxacin (Cipro), levofloxacin (Levaquin), nitrofurantoin (Macrodantin), and trimethoprim-sulphamethoxazole (Bactrim DS) (Cunningham et al., 2014). Phenazopyridine (Pyridium), a urinary analgesic, is often prescribed along with an antibiotic for relief of symptoms caused by irritation of the urinary tract. Although phenazopyridine is effective at relieving dysuria, urgency, and frequency, women should be taught that the medication colours urine and tears orange. Therefore they should be instructed to avoid wearing contact lenses while taking this medication and warned that it will stain underwear.

Pyelonephritis

Renal infection (pyelonephritis) is a common serious medical complication of pregnancy and the second most common non-birth reason for hospitalization (Cunningham et al., 2014). The most common maternal complications associated with pyelonephritis include anemia, septicemia, transient renal dysfunction, and pulmonary insufficiency. Women with pyelonephritis can develop urosepsis, sepsis syndrome, and renal dysfunction. In addition, pulmonary injury resembling acute respiratory distress syndrome (ARDS) can occur in pregnant women with acute pyelonephritis, most likely as the result of damage to alveolar tissue caused by the release of endotoxins from gram-negative bacteria (Colombo, 2012; Cunningham et al., 2014). Recurrent pyelonephritis is thought to cause fetal death and IUGR. Acute pyelonephritis is associated with preterm labour (Colombo, 2012).

Pyelonephritis develops most often during the second trimester of pregnancy and is usually caused by the *E. coli* organism. Infection develops only in the right kidney in more than half of all cases. The onset of pyelonephritis is often abrupt, with fever, shaking chills, and aching in the lumbar area of the back. Anorexia and nausea and vomiting also can be present. Usually one or both costovertebral angles are tender to palpation.

Women diagnosed with pyelonephritis are admitted to the hospital immediately. Treatment with IV antibiotics is started as soon as urine and blood samples for culture and sensitivity have been collected. Ampicillin, gentamicin, cefazolin (Ancef), or ceftriaxone (Rocephin) are often ordered initially because they are broad-spectrum antibiotics that are usually effective. The woman must be monitored closely for the possible development of sepsis (Cunningham et al., 2014).

Clinical symptoms generally resolve within a couple of days after antibiotic therapy is begun. The antibiotic may need to be changed based on the results of the initial culture and sensitivity testing or if the woman has not responded to therapy within 48 hours (Gilbert, 2011). Most women become afebrile within 72 hours. If no clinical improvement is seen within 48 to 72 hours, an ultrasound should be performed to assess for a urinary tract obstruction. Once the woman is afebrile, she is changed from IV to oral antibiotics (Cunningham et al., 2014).

Usually oral antibiotic therapy is continued for 10 to 14 days after IV therapy has been completed (Colombo, 2012). A urine culture will likely be repeated 1 to 2 weeks after antibiotic therapy has been completed. Recurrent infection develops in 30 to 40% of women after completion of treatment for pyelonephritis. Therefore, urine cultures should be obtained each trimester for the remainder of the pregnancy. Many women are maintained on a prophylactic antibiotic (often nitrofurantoin once or twice daily) for the remainder of the pregnancy (Colombo, 2012; Cunningham et al., 2014).

Patient Education

Nurses are often responsible for teaching pregnant women about taking medications safely and effectively. This education is especially important in regard to antibiotics because this type of medication is so often misused by the general public. The woman should be instructed to finish the entire course of prescribed antibiotic therapy rather than stopping the medication as soon as she feels better. Failure to complete the entire course can lead to the creation of additional drug-resistant organisms. Antibiotics should be taken on time and around the clock so medication levels in the body remain constant. Finally, many women develop a yeast infection while taking antibiotics because the medication kills normal flora in the genitourinary tract as well as pathological organisms. Therefore they should be encouraged to include yogurt, cheese, or milk containing active acidophilus cultures in their diet while on antibiotics.

The woman should also be taught simple ways to prevent future UTIs. See the Patient Teaching box in Chapter 7 on p. 132 for several suggestions.

NONOBSTETRICAL SURGERY DURING PREGNANCY

Approximately 1 in 500 women require nonobstetrical surgery during pregnancy. However, pregnancy can make the diagnosis more difficult (ACOG, 2011). An enlarged uterus and displaced internal organs may make abdominal palpation more difficult, may alter the position of an affected organ, or may change the usual signs associated with a particular disorder. The most common conditions necessitating abdominal surgery during pregnancy are appendicitis, intestinal obstruction, and gynecological problems (Abbasi, Patenaude, & Abenhaim, 2014).

Appendicitis

Appendicitis is the most common nongynecological cause of an acute surgical abdomen during pregnancy, occurring in about 1 in 1000 pregnancies (Abbasi, Patenaude, & Abenhaim, 2014). The rate of premature labour induced by nonobstetrical surgical intervention is 3.5% and occurs more often following appendectomy than with any other type of surgery. The diagnosis is often delayed because the usual signs and symptoms mimic some normal changes of pregnancy, such as nausea and vomiting and increased WBC count. As pregnancy progresses, the appendix is pushed upward and to the right from its usual anatomical location (see Fig. 10-15). Because of these changes, appendix rupture and peritonitis occur in up to 25% of pregnant women with appendicitis (Cappell, 2012).

The woman with appendicitis most commonly has right lower quadrant pain, nausea and vomiting, and loss of appetite. Approximately half of these women will have muscle guarding. Moving the uterus tends to increase the pain. Temperature may be normal or mildly increased (to 38.3°C). Because of the physiological increase in WBCs that occurs in pregnancy, laboratory findings are not helpful in the diagnosis (Kelly & Savides, 2014).

The diagnosis of appendicitis requires a high level of suspicion because the classic signs and symptoms include abdominal pain that migrates to the right lower quadrant, right lower quadrant tenderness, nausea/vomiting, and fever which may mimic other conditions, including pyelonephritis, round ligament pain, placental abruption, torsion of an ovarian cyst, cholecystitis, and preterm labour (Cunningham et al., 2014; Kelly & Savides, 2014).

Radiological imaging is necessary if appendicitis is suspected after history, physical examination, and laboratory studies have been completed. Although computed tomography (CT) is the imaging test of choice in nonpregnant patients because it is highly accurate, the use of ultrasonography during pregnancy is preferred to avoid fetal exposure to radiation from CT (Cappell, 2012). Magnetic resonance imaging (MRI) may be used if appendicitis has not been confirmed by other imaging techniques (Cappell, 2012; Kelly & Savides, 2014).

Prompt surgical intervention to remove the appendix is still the standard treatment (Kelly & Savides, 2014). Laparoscopic surgery may be performed during the first and second trimesters of pregnancy if the appendix has not ruptured or the diagnosis is uncertain. Antibiotics are often administered for uncomplicated appendicitis and are definitely necessary if rupture, abscess, or peritonitis has occurred. Clindamycin and gentamicin are often prescribed because they are considered both effective and safe. The maternal mortality rate from ruptured appendix is about 4%. The fetal mortality rate from ruptured appendix is much higher, more than 30% (Cappell, 2012).

Intestinal Obstruction

The second most common nonobstetrical abdominal emergency in pregnancy is intestinal obstruction. The incidence of intestinal obstruction during pregnancy is estimated at 1:1500

(Stukan, Kruszewski Wiesław, Dudziak, et al., 2013). Any woman with a laparotomy scar is more likely to have an intestinal obstruction (adynamic ileus) during gestation. Adhesions as a result of previous surgery or pelvic inflammatory disease, an enlarging uterus, and displacement of the intestines are etiological factors.

Symptoms of an intestinal obstruction include constipation; persistent cramp-like, abdominal pain; vomiting; auscultatory rushes within the abdomen; abdominal tenderness on palpation; and abnormal peristalsis (Stukan et al., 2013). Immediate surgical intervention is required for release of the obstruction. Pregnancy is rarely affected by the surgery, assuming the absence of complications such as peritonitis.

Cholelithiasis and Cholecystitis

Women are twice as likely to have *cholelithiasis* (presence of gallstones in the gallbladder) than men. It is hypothesized that estrogens cause increased cholesterol secretion of bile and progesterone promotes decreased gallbladder motility. Its incidence increases during pregnancy, probably because of increased hormone levels and pressure from the enlarged uterus that interferes with the normal circulation and drainage of the gallbladder. Most gallstones are asymptomatic during pregnancy. Usually the first symptom of cholelithiasis is biliary colic, epigastric, or right upper-quadrant pain that can radiate to the back or shoulders. Pain may occur spontaneously or after eating a high-fat meal. Approximately two thirds of patients with biliary colic have recurrent attacks (Cappell, 2012). Nutrition counselling is important (see Home Care box).

Cholecystitis (inflammation of the gallbladder) is usually caused when a gallstone obstructs a cystic duct and may also occur during pregnancy, due to increased pressure of the enlarged uterus interfering with the normal circulation and drainage of the gallbladder. Acute cholecystitis occurs most often in older women who have been pregnant several times and who have a history of previous attacks. As in biliary colic that occurs with cholelithiasis, epigastric or right upper-quadrant pain is present, but the pain is usually more severe and prolonged. Nausea, vomiting, and fever may also be present. Acute cholecystitis is the third most common indication for nonobstetrical surgical intervention in pregnancy, occurring in about 4 cases per 10,000 pregnancies (Cappell, 2012).

Women with acute cholecystitis usually have fatty food intolerance along with colicky abdominal pain radiating to the back or shoulder, nausea, and vomiting. Fever and an increased leukocyte count may also be present. Ultrasonography is often used to detect the presence of stones or dilation of the common bile duct.

Generally, gallbladder surgery should be postponed until the puerperium. Usually the woman can be treated with conservative medical therapy consisting of antibiotics, analgesics, IV fluids, bowel rest, and nasogastric suctioning (Chloptsios, Karanasiou, Ilias, et al., 2007). TPN can be used in some cases as an alternative to surgery. Morphine should not be used as an analgesic because it may cause ductal spasm. The woman's condition should improve significantly within 48 hours of beginning treatment. However, women with recurrent biliary colic or acute cholecystitis generally require immediate cholecystectomy. Although the second trimester has traditionally been considered the safest time for this surgery, it is increasingly performed at any time during pregnancy because of improved surgical techniques and outcomes. Both laparoscopic and open cholecystectomy procedures are acceptable during pregnancy (Cappell, 2012; Cunningham et al., 2014). Preoperative care includes IV fluids, discontinuing oral intake, analgesia, and usually antibiotics (Cappell, 2012).

HOME CARE

Nutrition Counselling for the Pregnant Woman With Cholecystitis or Cholelithiasis

- Assess diet for foods that cause discomfort and flatulence and omit foods that trigger episodes.
- Reduce dietary fat intake to 40 to 50 g/day.
- Limit protein to 10 to 12% of total calories.
- Choose foods so that most of the calories come from carbohydrates.
- Prepare food without adding fats or oils, as much as possible.
- Avoid fried foods.

Gynecological Problems

Pregnancy predisposes a woman to ovarian problems, especially during the first trimester. Ovarian cysts and twisting of ovarian cysts or adnexal tissues may occur. Other problems include retained or enlarged cystic corpus luteum of pregnancy and bacterial invasion of reproductive or other intraperitoneal organs.

Laparotomy or laparoscopy may be required to discriminate between ovarian problems and early ectopic pregnancy, appendicitis, or an infectious process.

NURSING CARE

Initial assessment of the pregnant woman requiring surgery focuses on her presenting signs and symptoms. A thorough history and physical examination should be performed. Laboratory testing includes, at a minimum, a CBC with differential and a urinalysis. FHR and activity and uterine activity should be monitored; constant vigilance is required in watching for symptoms of impending obstetrical complications. The extent of preoperative assessment is determined by the immediacy of surgical intervention and the specific condition that requires surgery.

Hospital Care

When surgery becomes necessary during pregnancy, the woman and her family will be concerned about the effects of the procedure and medication on fetal well-being and the course of pregnancy. An important part of preoperative nursing care is encouraging the woman to express her fears, concerns, and questions.

Preoperative care for a pregnant woman differs from that of a nonpregnant woman in one significant aspect: the presence of at least one other person—the fetus. Continuous FHR and uterine contraction monitoring may be performed if the fetus is considered viable. Procedures such as preparation of the operative site and time of insertion of IV lines and urinary retention catheters vary with the surgeon and the facility. However, in every instance there is total restriction of solid food and fluids or a clear specification of the type, amount, and time at which clear liquids may be taken before surgery. Some bowel preparation such as drinking clear liquids and taking laxatives may be required before surgery. Food by mouth is restricted for several hours before a scheduled procedure. If the woman experiences a prolonged nothing-by-mouth status, IV fluids with dextrose should be given. Even if she has had nothing by mouth—but more important, if surgery is unexpected—the woman is in danger of vomiting and aspirating, and special precautions are taken before the anaesthetic is administered (e.g., administering an antacid).

During surgery, perinatal nurses may collaborate with the surgical staff to meet the special needs of a pregnant woman. To improve fetal oxygenation, the woman should be positioned on the operating table with a lateral tilt, to avoid maternal compression of the vena cava. Continuous fetal and uterine monitoring during the procedure may be ordered because the risk of preterm labour is great. Depending on the surgical procedure, monitoring can be accomplished using sterile Aquasonic gel and a sterile sleeve for the transducer. Uterine contractions may be palpated manually. In the immediate recovery period, general observations and care pertinent to postoperative recovery should be initiated. Frequent assessments should be carried out for several hours after surgery. Whether the woman is cared for in the surgical postanaesthesia recovery area or in a labour and birth unit, continuous fetal and uterine monitoring will likely be initiated or resumed because of the increased risk of preterm labour. Tocolysis may be necessary if preterm labour occurs.

The use of pneumatic compression devices on all pregnant women undergoing surgery is recommended (Guyatt, Akl, Crowther, et al., 2012). The need for pharmacological thromboprophylaxis should be determined on a case-by-case basis, taking into account the expected scope and length of the procedure and whether the woman has risk factors for venous thrombosis in addition to the pregnancy (e.g., thrombophilia, prolonged immobilization, past history of venous thrombosis, malignancy, diabetes mellitus, varicose veins, paralysis, or obesity). For laparoscopic procedures (gynecological or general surgical) predicted to last greater than 45 minutes, use of LMWH is suggested; mechanical thromboprophylaxis is a reasonable alternative for shorter procedures (Guyatt et al., 2012).

Home Care

Plans for the woman's return home and for convalescent care should be completed as early as possible before discharge. The woman and other support persons must be taught signs of infection. Box 14-7 lists information that should be included in discharge teaching for the postoperative patient. The woman may also need referrals to various community agencies for evaluation of the home situation, child care, home health care, and financial or other assistance.

BOX 14-7 DISCHARGE TEACHING FOR HOME CARE

- Care of incision site
- Diet and elimination related to gastrointestinal function
- Signs and symptoms of developing complications (wound infection, thrombophlebitis, pneumonia)
- Equipment needed and technique for assessing temperature
- Recommended schedule for resumption of activities of daily living
- Treatments and medications ordered
- List of resource persons and their telephone numbers
- Schedule of follow-up visits
- If birth has not occurred:
  - Assessment of fetal activity (kick counts)
  - Signs of preterm labour

TRAUMA DURING PREGNANCY

Trauma can be a complication during pregnancy and may be caused by vehicular crashes, falls, burns, industrial mishaps, violence, gunshot wounds, and other injuries in the home and community. Treatment of pregnant trauma victims is complicated because doctors and nurses who have expertise in the care of trauma victims generally do not have similar expertise in the care of pregnant women.

Significance

Approximately 6 to 7% of pregnancies are complicated by physical trauma, which accounts for 46% of maternal mortality (Mozurkewich & Pearlman, 2012). Motor vehicle crashes are the most common cause of trauma in pregnancy, accounting for 55% of injuries. Other common causes are falls, assaults, gunshot wounds, and burns. Approximately 80% of fetal deaths associated with maternal trauma are from motor vehicle crashes (Ruth & Miller, 2013). Maternal death caused by trauma is usually the result of head injury or hemorrhagic shock. Fetal death usually occurs as a sequelae to maternal death or as a result of placental abruption.

Acts of violence are a significant health problem for pregnant women. The risk of trauma caused by abuse is increased during pregnancy, and rates of recurrence are high. The reported incidence of physical abuse during pregnancy ranges from 4 to 8% (McFarlane, 2007). As many as 45% of women subject to intimate partner violence before pregnancy continue to be abused during the pregnancy. Women who are abused during pregnancy have a threefold risk of being murdered compared with nonpregnant abused women (McFarlane, 2007).

Trauma increases the incidence of miscarriage, preterm labour, placental abruption, and stillbirth (Robbins, Martin, & Wilson, 2014). The effect of trauma on pregnancy is influenced by the length of gestation, type and severity of the trauma, and degree of disruption of uterine and fetal physiological features. Fetal death as a result of trauma is more common than the occurrence of both maternal and fetal death. Less serious trauma is associated with numerous complications in pregnancy, including fetomaternal hemorrhage, placental abruption, intrauterine fetal death, and preterm labour and birth. Careful evaluation of mother and fetus after all types of trauma is imperative.

Multisystem trauma during pregnancy is usually the result of a serious motor vehicle crash, especially if the woman is not wearing a seat belt with a shoulder harness and is ejected from the vehicle. To improve chances of survival for both mother and fetus in a potential crash, pregnant women should wear properly positioned restraints at all times when in a motor vehicle (see Fig. 11-16) (Cunningham et al., 2014).

Special considerations for the pregnant woman and her fetus are necessary when trauma occurs, because of the physiological alterations that accompany pregnancy and the presence of the fetus. Fetal survival depends on maternal survival; therefore, the pregnant woman must receive immediate stabilization and appropriate care for optimal fetal outcome.

Maternal Physiological Characteristics

Optimal care for the pregnant woman after trauma depends on having an understanding of the physiological state of pregnancy and its effects on trauma. The pregnant woman's body exhibits responses that are different from those of a nonpregnant person to the same traumatic insults. Because of the different responses to injury during pregnancy, management strategies must be adapted for appropriate resuscitation, fluid therapy, positioning, assessments, and most other interventions. Significant adaptations required for treatment of trauma in the pregnant woman are summarized in Table 14-9.

The uterus and bladder are confined to the bony pelvis during the first trimester of pregnancy and are at reduced risk for injury in cases of abdominal trauma. After pregnancy progresses beyond the fourteenth week, the uterus becomes an abdominal organ, and the risk for injury increases in cases of abdominal trauma. During the second and third trimesters, the distended bladder becomes an abdominal organ and is at increased risk for injury and rupture. Bowel injuries occur less often during pregnancy because of the protection provided by the enlarged uterus.

The elevated levels of progesterone that accompany pregnancy relax smooth muscle and profoundly affect the gastrointestinal tract. Gastrointestinal motility decreases, with a resultant increased time required for gastric emptying; the production of hydrochloric acid increases in the last trimester, and the gastroesophageal sphincter relaxes. Management of the unconscious pregnant woman's airway is of critical importance.

! NURSING ALERT

The unconscious pregnant woman is at increased risk for regurgitation of gastric contents and aspiration whenever her head is positioned lower than her stomach or if abdominal pressure is applied.

A pregnant woman has decreased tolerance for hypoxia and apnea because of her decreased functional residual capacity and increased renal loss of bicarbonate. Acidosis develops more quickly in the pregnant woman than in the nonpregnant state.

TABLE 14-9 MATERNAL ADAPTATIONS DURING PREGNANCY AND RELATION TO TRAUMA

SYSTEM	ALTERATION	CLINICAL RESPONSES
Respiratory	↑ Oxygen consumption	↑ Risk of acidosis
	↑ Tidal volume	↑ Risk of respiratory mismanagement
	↓ Functional residual capacity	
	Chronic compensated alkalosis	↓ Blood-buffering capacity
	↓ $Paco_2$	
	↓ Serum bicarbonate	
Cardiovascular	↑ Circulating volume, 1600 mL	Can lose 1000 mL of blood
	↑ Cardiac output	No signs of shock until blood loss >30% total blood volume
	↑ Heart rate	↓ Placental perfusion in supine position
	↓ Systemic vascular resistance	
	↓ Arterial blood pressure	
	Heart displaced upward to left	Point of maximal impulse, fourth intercostal space
Renal	↑ Renal plasma flow	
	Dilation of ureters and urethra	↑ Risk of stasis, infection
	Bladder displaced forward	↑ Risk of bladder trauma
Gastrointestinal	↓ Gastric motility	↑ Risk of aspiration
	↑ Hydrochloric acid production	
	↓ Competency of gastroesophageal sphincter	Passive regurgitation of stomach acids if head lower than stomach
Reproductive	↑ Blood flow to organs	Source of ↑ blood loss
	Uterine enlargement	Vena caval compression in supine position
Musculoskeletal	Displacement of abdominal viscera	↑ Risk of injury, altered rebound response
	Pelvic venous congestion	Altered pain referral
	Cartilage softened	↑ Risk of pelvic fracture
		Centre of gravity changed
	Fetal head in pelvis	↑ Risk of fetal injury
Hematological	↑ Clotting factors	↑ Risk of thrombus formation
	↓ Fibrinolytic activity	

Cardiac output increases 30 to 50% over prepregnancy values by 32 weeks of gestation and is position dependent in the third trimester. Because of compression of the inferior vena cava and descending aorta by the pregnant uterus, cardiac output decreases dramatically if the woman is placed in the supine position. Thus the supine position must be avoided, even in women with cervical spine injuries. It is of utmost importance that lateral uterine displacement be accomplished without any head movement. As soon as the neck is immobilized, the stretcher should be tilted laterally (Mozurkewich & Pearlman, 2012; Ruth & Miller, 2013).

Circulating blood volume increases 40 to 50% during gestation, and pregnant women can tolerate a 1000-mL blood loss readily without demonstrating clinical signs. Hemodynamic instability that indicates the need for transfusion may not be apparent until blood loss nears 1200 to 1500 mL (Robbins et al., 2014). Tachycardia and hypotension, typical of hypovolemic shock, may appear late in the pregnant trauma patient because of increased blood volume. Clinical signs of hemorrhage do not appear until after a 20 to 25% loss of circulating volume occurs, which will diminish uteroplacental perfusion. Although heart rate increases with pregnancy, a maternal heart rate greater than 100 beats/min should be considered abnormal. Continuous monitoring of oxygen saturation is advised, since desaturation may affect the oxygenation of the fetus and should be avoided.

Fetal Physiological Characteristics

Perfusion of the uterine arteries, which provide the primary blood supply to the uteroplacental unit, depends on adequate maternal arterial pressure because these vessels lack autoregulation. Therefore, maternal hypotension decreases uterine and fetal perfusion. Maternal shock results in splanchnic and uterine artery vasoconstriction, which decreases blood flow and oxygen transport to the fetus. EFM tracings can assist in the evaluation of fetal status after trauma to assess for hypoxia and hypoperfusion, including tachycardia or bradycardia, decreased or absent baseline variability, and late decelerations.

Careful monitoring of fetal status assists greatly in maternal assessment because the fetal monitor tracing works as an "oximeter" of internal maternal well-being. Hypoperfusion can be present in the pregnant woman before the onset of clinical signs of shock. The EFM tracings may show the first signs of maternal compromise, such as when maternal heart rate, BP, and colour appear normal yet the EFM printout shows signs of fetal hypoxia (Miller, Miller, & Tucker, 2013).

Mechanisms of Trauma

Blunt Abdominal Trauma

Blunt abdominal trauma is most commonly the result of motor vehicle crashes but also may be the result of battering or falls. Maternal and fetal morbidity and mortality rates associated with motor vehicle crashes are directly correlated with whether the mother remains inside the vehicle or is ejected. Maternal death is usually the result of a head injury or exsanguination from a major vessel rupture. Serious retroperitoneal hemorrhage after lower abdominal and pelvic trauma is reported more frequently during pregnancy. Serious maternal abdominal injuries are usually the result of splenic rupture or liver and renal injury.

In the context of maternal survival of trauma, fetal death is usually the result of placental abruption. Placental separation is thought to be a result of deformation of the elastic myometrium around the relatively inelastic placenta. Shearing of the placental edge from the underlying decidua basalis ensues and is worsened by the increased intrauterine pressure caused by the impact. It is imperative that all pregnant victims be evaluated carefully for signs and symptoms of placental abruption after even minor blunt abdominal trauma.

> **! NURSING ALERT**
>
> Signs and symptoms of placental abruption include uterine tenderness or pain, uterine irritability, uterine contractions, vaginal bleeding, leaking of amniotic fluid, or a change in FHR characteristics.

Pelvic fracture can result from severe injury and produce bladder trauma or retroperitoneal bleeding with two-point displacement of pelvic bones. One point of displacement is common at the symphysis pubis, and the second point is posterior because of the structure of the pelvis. Careful evaluation for clinical signs of internal hemorrhage is indicated.

Direct fetal injury as a complication of blunt trauma during pregnancy most often involves the fetal skull and brain. Most commonly, this injury accompanies maternal pelvic fracture in late gestation after the fetal head becomes engaged. When the force of the impact is great enough to fracture the maternal pelvis, the fetus often sustains a skull fracture. Evaluation for fetal skull fracture or intracranial hemorrhage is then indicated.

Uterine rupture as a result of trauma is rare, occurring in less than 1% of severe cases. Uterine rupture depends on numerous factors, including gestational age, the intensity of the impact, the presence of a predisposing factor such as a distended uterus caused by polyhydramnios or multiple gestation, or the presence of a uterine scar from previous uterine surgery (Cunningham et al., 2014; Gilbert, 2011). When uterine rupture occurs, the force responsible is usually a direct, high-energy blow. Fetal death is common with traumatic uterine rupture. However, maternal death occurs less frequently, in about 30% of cases (Ruth & Miller, 2013).

Thoracic Trauma

Thoracic trauma is reported to produce 25% of all trauma deaths. Pulmonary contusion results from nearly 75% of blunt thoracic trauma and is a potentially life-threatening condition. Pulmonary contusion can be difficult to recognize, especially if flail chest is also present or if there is no evidence of thoracic injury. It should be suspected in cases of thoracic injury, especially after blunt acceleration or deceleration trauma such as that occurring when a rapidly moving vehicle crashes into an immovable object.

Penetrating wounds into the chest can result in pneumothorax or hemothorax. This type of injury is usually caused by a vehicular crash that results in impalement by the steering column or a loose article in the vehicle that becomes a projectile with the force of impact.

NURSING CARE

Immediate Stabilization

Immediate priorities for stabilization of the pregnant woman after trauma should be identical to those of the nonpregnant trauma patient. Pregnancy should not result in any restriction of the usual diagnostic, pharmacological, or resuscitative procedures or manoeuvres. Fetal survival depends on maternal survival, and stabilization of the mother improves fetal chance of survival. The perinatal nurse is often called on to function collaboratively with emergency department or trauma unit staff members in providing care for the pregnant trauma victim.

NURSING ALERT

Priorities of care for the pregnant woman after trauma must be to resuscitate the woman and stabilize her condition first and then consider fetal needs.

In cases of minor trauma, the woman is evaluated for vaginal bleeding, uterine irritability, abdominal tenderness, abdominal pain or cramps, and evidence of hypovolemia. A change in or absence of FHR or fetal activity, leakage of amniotic fluid, and presence of fetal cells in the maternal circulation (Kleihauer-Betke) are also included in the assessment.

Primary Survey

The systematic evaluation begins with a *primary survey* and the initial *CABDs* of resuscitation: *compressions*, *airway*, *breathing*, and *defibrillation*. Increased oxygen needs during gestation necessitate a rapid response. The presence of a cervical spine injury is always assumed.

NURSING ALERT

Hyperextension of the neck should be avoided; instead, jaw thrust is used to establish an airway for the trauma victim.

Once an airway is established, assessment should focus on adequacy of oxygenation. The chest wall should be observed for movement. If breathing is absent, ventilations and endotracheal intubation are initiated. Supplemental oxygen should be administered with a tight-fitting, nonrebreathing face mask at 10 to 12 L/min to attempt to normalize maternal arterial oxygen tension (Pao_2 104 to 108 mm Hg) and oxygen saturation greater than 95% to optimize maternal and fetal status. The chest wall should be assessed for a penetrating chest wound or flail chest. Breathing with a flail chest will be rapid and laboured; chest wall movements will be uncoordinated and asymmetric; crepitus from bony fragments may be palpated.

Rapid placement of two large-bore (14- to 16-gauge) IV lines is necessary in most seriously injured patients. It is important to place the lines while veins are still distended. Cardiac arrest during the immediate stabilization period is usually the result of profound hypovolemia, necessitating massive fluid resuscitation. One to two litres of warmed crystalloid solutions should be infused. Ringer's solution or normal saline solution are the fluids of choice for volume resuscitation (Ruth & Miller, 2013). Because of the 50% increase in blood volume during pregnancy, published formulas for nonpregnant adults that are used for estimating crystalloid and blood replacement to counter blood loss must be adjusted upward for pregnancy.

Replacement of red blood cells and other blood components should be anticipated and blood drawn for type, cross-match, CBC, and platelet count. Infusion of type-specific packed red blood cells is usually necessary to improve fetal oxygenation status and to replace blood lost. During an extreme emergency, type O Rh-negative blood may be administered without matching.

If possible, vasopressor medications to restore maternal arterial BP should be avoided until volume replacement is administered. These medications may significantly reduce uterine blood flow and thus decrease oxygen delivery to the fetus. In addition, their use does not address the cause of the hypovolemia (Ruth & Miller, 2013).

After 20 weeks of gestation, venous return to the heart is best accomplished by positioning the uterus to one side to eliminate the weight of the uterus compressing the inferior vena cava or the descending aorta. This facilitates efforts to establish the forward flow of blood through resuscitation and stabilization. If a lateral position is not possible because of resuscitative efforts or cervical spine immobilization, the uterus can be manually deflected to the left, or a wedge can be inserted underneath the right side of the backboard or stretcher.

Signs of bleeding may be more difficult to recognize in the pregnant woman because a 30 to 35% loss of maternal blood volume may produce only a minimal change in maternal mean arterial pressure. Hypovolemia can be detrimental for the fetus because the vascular bed of the uterus is a low-resistance system that depends on adequate maternal cardiac output and arterial pressure to maintain uterine and fetal perfusion. Maternal hypovolemia can be fatal for the fetus.

Establishing a baseline neurological status (level of consciousness, pupil size, and reactivity) is essential. The Glasgow Coma Scale is commonly used at the scene of the accident to help determine the extent of the head injury.

Secondary Survey

After immediate resuscitation and successful stabilization measures, a more detailed secondary survey of the mother and fetus should be accomplished. A complete physical assessment to include all body systems is performed.

The maternal abdomen should be evaluated carefully because a large percentage of serious injuries involve the uterus, intraperitoneal structures, and retroperitoneum. The pregnant woman's stomach is assumed to be full. A nasogastric tube can be used to empty the stomach to help prevent acid aspiration syndrome. An empty stomach facilitates respiratory efforts. The uterus should be evaluated for evidence of gross deformity, tenderness, irritability, or contractions.

The greatest clinical concern after a vehicular crash is placental abruption, because as many as 40% of these women will have an abruption. If placental abruption occurs, the associated fetal mortality rate can be as high as 50 to 80% (Mozurkewich & Pearlman, 2012). Assessments should focus on recognition of this complication, with careful evaluation of fetal monitor tracings, uterine tenderness, labour, or vaginal bleeding. Ultrasonographic examination may be performed to determine gestational age, viability of fetus, and placental location. However, ultrasound studies cannot exclude placental abruption.

Peritoneal lavage for the pregnant woman after blunt abdominal trauma has proven to be a safe procedure and can be helpful in the early diagnosis of intraperitoneal injury or hemorrhage. Under direct visualization, the peritoneum is incised, and a peritoneal dialysis catheter is positioned. If aspiration yields free-flowing blood, the test is considered positive, and a laparotomy should be performed. This procedure is not necessary before laparotomy if intraperitoneal bleeding is clinically apparent. Indications for peritoneal lavage include abdominal symptoms or signs suggestive of intraperitoneal bleeding, alteration in mental status, unexplained shock, and severe multiple injuries (Cunningham et al., 2014).

If trauma is the result of a penetrating wound, the woman should be completely undressed and carefully examined for all entrance and exit wounds. Exploratory laparotomy is necessary after a gunshot wound to explore the abdominal cavity for organ damage and to repair any damage present, with careful examination of all organs, the entire bowel, and posterior vessels. If uterine injury is determined, the risks and benefits of Caesarean birth are quickly evaluated. A Caesarean birth is desirable if the fetus is alive and near term and may be necessary for the preterm fetus because of the high incidence of fetal injury in these cases. The fetus usually tolerates surgery and anaesthesia if adequate uterine perfusion and oxygenation are maintained. Tetanus prophylaxis guidelines are not changed by pregnancy.

All female trauma victims of child-bearing age should be considered pregnant until proven otherwise. Determination of the health history and a history of the events preceding the trauma are important components of care. If the pregnant woman was involved in an MVA, it should be determined whether she was the driver or a passenger and if she was ejected from the vehicle or was wearing a seatbealt and remained within the vehicle.

In addition to helping to stabilize the woman, the nurse can provide emotional support for her and her family. If the trauma is the result of an MVA, other family members may also have been critically injured or killed. The nurse should collaborate with other staff to make sure that questions are answered and consistent information given. Grief support may be necessary.

Radiation Exposure

If the pregnant woman has sustained serious injuries, any necessary radiographic examination should be performed, regardless of fetal exposure. If radiographic examination would be performed for the nonpregnant trauma victim, it also should be performed for the pregnant woman. Abdominal or pelvic CT scanning can be used to visualize extraperitoneal and retroperitoneal structures and the genitourinary tract. Radiation exposure of less than 5 rads has not been associated with fetal abnormalities or pregnancy loss, and the radiation level associated with abdominal or pelvic CT scans is far below this amount (Robbins et al., 2014). Blunt head trauma and loss of consciousness necessitate skull films and CT assessment with neurosurgical consultation. MRI can also be used safely to assess injuries because it does not produce ionizing radiation (Robbins et al., 2014).

Fetal Maternal Hemorrhage

The potential for fetal–maternal hemorrhage exists after trauma. Hemorrhage can lead to fetal anemia, distress, or even death. If the pregnant trauma victim is Rh negative, fetal–maternal hemorrhage can result in sensitization and hemolytic disease of the newborn. The KB assay is often performed in women after blunt abdominal trauma to estimate the amount of fetal blood within the maternal circulation. However, because most cases have less than 30 mL of hemorrhage, KB test results seldom alter management (Cunningham et al., 2014; Robbins et al., 2014). Usually the routine administration of 300 mcg of Rh_o(D) immunoglobulin is sufficient to protect almost all Rh-negative pregnant trauma patients from isoimmunization (Mozurkewich & Pearlman, 2012).

Ultrasound

Ultrasound after trauma is not as sensitive as EFM for diagnosing placental abruption. It may be useful to help establish gestational age, locate the placenta, evaluate cardiac activity (to determine whether the fetus is alive), and determine amniotic fluid volume. It may also be used to evaluate the presence of intra-abdominal fluid that would suggest the presence of intra-abdominal hemorrhage.

Fetal Health Surveillance

External FHR and contraction monitoring is recommended after blunt trauma in a viable gestation for a minimum of 4 hours, regardless of injury severity. Continuous EFM may show early signs of placental abruption, including a change in baseline rate, loss of accelerations, and the presence of late decelerations. If the estimated gestational age is 24 weeks or greater, fetal monitoring should be initiated soon after the woman is stable, because placental abruption usually becomes apparent shortly after the injury. Fetal monitoring should be continued and further evaluation initiated if any of these signs occur. Palpation is required to evaluate the intensity of contractions and the uterine resting tone. It is important to palpate between contractions to verify that the uterus is well relaxed. If the uterus does not relax between contractions, placental abruption could be present. Occasional uterine contractions are the most common finding with trauma during pregnancy, occurring in 40% of cases and resolving in 90% of cases with no adverse fetal outcome. The intensity and frequency of contractions are predictive of complications such as placental abruption and preterm labour. Elevated basal uterine tone also raises suspicion for traumatic placental abruption. Placental abruption occurring after trauma may be delayed for up to 48 hours after the incident.

The exact duration of FHR and contraction monitoring required after blunt abdominal trauma is not known. Monitoring should be continued indefinitely if uterine contractions, abnormal FHR characteristics, vaginal bleeding, uterine tenderness or irritability, serious maternal injury, or ruptured membranes are present. Most physicians recommend continuous monitoring for at least 24 hours. Most abruptions develop soon after the traumatic event, although in rare cases abruption has developed days afterward (Cunningham et al., 2014; Robbins et al., 2014).

Discharge Planning

Following minor trauma, the woman may be discharged home, after several hours of evaluation. Her vital signs should be stable, with no evidence of bleeding at the time of discharge. The fetal tracing should be normal before monitoring is discontinued and the woman is discharged. Education for the woman and her family is very important. She should be instructed to contact her health care provider immediately if changes in fetal movement or signs and symptoms indicative of preterm labour, PROM, or placental abruption develop. If the trauma occurred as a result of domestic violence, the woman may need information about the abuse cycle; referral to a crisis centre, law enforcement agency, or counselling centre; and help in forming a safety plan (see Chapter 5, p. 77).

Cardiopulmonary Resuscitation of the Pregnant Woman

Cardiac arrest in a pregnant woman is a rare event, most often related to events at the time of birth, such as trauma, cardiac abnormalities, embolism, eclampsia, magnesium overdose, sepsis, intracranial hemorrhage, anaesthetic complications, and uterine rupture (Robbins et al., 2014).

Various protocols exist for cardiopulmonary resuscitation (CPR) during pregnancy. The most widely used guide is the American Heart Association (AHA) advanced cardiac life support (ACLS) protocol (American Heart Association [AHA], 2010). This protocol recommends standard CPR with the uterus displaced laterally, fluid-volume restoration, and defibrillation, if indicated. The decision for Caesarean birth should be made within 4 to 5 minutes of the mother's cardiac arrest. No matter what protocol is used, nurses and other health care providers must be prepared if CPR is to be successful.

Special modifications are necessary when CPR is performed during the second half of pregnancy. In nonpregnant women chest compressions produce a cardiac output of only about 30% of normal. Cardiac output in pregnant women may be even less as a result of aortocaval compression caused by the gravid uterus. Therefore, uterine displacement during resuscitation efforts is critical (Cunningham et al., 2014). To prevent supine hypotension, the woman is placed on a flat, firm surface with the uterus displaced laterally either manually or with a wedge or rolled towel under her right hip or on her side supported by angled thighs of several rescuers or angled backs of several chairs (AHA, 2010). If a pregnant woman requires CPR outside a hospital setting, the focus of the new guidelines is C-A-B (*C*ompressions, *A*irway, *B*reathing). For untrained bystanders, the likelihood of providing CPR is greater if rescue breathing is not expected. Compressions should be provided at the depth of 5 centimetres at a rate of 100 times per minute (AHA, 2010).

Defibrillation with an automated external device (AED) is also key to increasing the chance of survival. If defibrillation is needed, the paddles, or AED pads must be placed one rib interspace higher than usual because the heart is slightly displaced by the enlarged uterus. If possible, the fetus should be monitored during the cardiac arrest. For pregnant women in hospital who require CPR, trained personnel need to tailor the sequence of rescue actions to the most likely cause of arrest. If a woman suddenly collapses, the health care provider should call for help and assess the woman for breathlessness and pulselessness prior to initiating CPR. By beginning immediate chest compressions, the delay is minimized in promoting circulation to the brain and key organs (see Emergency box).

Complications that may be associated with CPR of a pregnant woman include laceration of the liver, rupture of the uterus, hemothorax, and hemoperitoneum. Fetal complications that may occur include cardiac dysrhythmia or asystole related to maternal defibrillation and medications, CNS depression

EMERGENCY

Cardiopulmonary Resuscitation of the Pregnant Woman in the Hospital

Assessment

- Determine unresponsiveness and no breathing or no normal breathing.
- Activate emergency call system and get the emergency response cart.
- Position woman on flat, firm surface with uterus displaced laterally with a wedge if possible (e.g., a rolled towel placed under her hip).

Circulation

- Assess for the presence of a pulse by feeling carotid pulse for no longer than 10 seconds.
- If there is no pulse, begin chest compressions at rate of a minimum of 100/min at a compression depth of at least 5 cm. Allow the chest to completely recoil (re-expand) completely after compression. Chest compressions may be performed slightly higher on the sternum if the uterus is enlarged enough to displace the diaphragm into a higher position.

Airway

- Open airway with head tilt–chin lift manoeuvre.

Breathing

- Assess for presence of breathing (look, listen, feel) for no longer than 8 seconds.
- If the woman is not breathing, give two slow breaths; ensure that the chest rises with each breath.
- Rescue breathing without chest compressions should be given at a rate of 10 to 12 breaths/min.
- After five cycles of 30 compressions and two breaths (or approximately 2 minutes), check for a pulse. If pulse is not present, continue cardiopulmonary resuscitation.

Defibrillation

- Use a defibrillator according to standard protocol to analyze heart rhythm, and deliver shock if indicated.

Birth

- Consider perimortem Caesarean birth within 5 minutes if chest compressions are unsuccessful.

Continued

EMERGENCY

Cardiopulmonary Resuscitation of the Pregnant Woman in the Hospital—cont'd

Relief of Foreign-Body Airway Obstruction

- If the pregnant woman is unable to speak or cough, perform chest thrusts.
- Stand behind the woman and place your arms under her armpits to encircle her chest. Press backward with quick thrusts until the foreign body is expelled (Fig. 14-15).

Unconscious Foreign-Body Airway Obstruction

- If a pregnant woman becomes unresponsive place her on her back with a rolled blanket under her hip to ensure the uterus is displaced laterally and kneel at her side.
- Open her mouth with the tongue-jaw lift and remove the obstruction if it is visualized and can be done safely and attempt rescue breathing.
- If unable to ventilate, position hands for chest compressions. Deliver 30 chest compressions firmly, check mouth again for presence of obstruction, and attempt to provide rescue breathing. Continue sequence until the pregnant woman's airway is clear of obstruction.
- If the woman is unconscious, give chest compressions as for a woman without a pulse.

Source: American Heart Association. (2010). Guidelines for cardiopulmonary resuscitation and emergency cardiovascular care science. *Circulation, 122,* S639. Retrieved from http://circ.ahajournals.org/content/vol122/18_suppl_3/.

related to antidysrhythmic medications and inadequate utero-placental perfusion, and onset of preterm labour.

If resuscitation is successful, the woman and her fetus must receive careful monitoring. The woman remains at increased risk for recurrent pulmonary arrest and dysrhythmias (ventricular tachycardia, supraventricular tachycardia, and bradycardia). Therefore, her cardiovascular, pulmonary, and neurological status should be assessed continuously. Uterine activity and resting tone must be monitored. Fetal status and gestational age should be determined and used in decision making regarding continuation of the pregnancy or the timing and route of birth.

Another common reason for performing CPR on a pregnant woman is airway obstruction caused by choking. Clearing an airway obstruction is usually accomplished by performing abdominal thrusts. However, during the second and third trimesters of pregnancy, chest thrusts (Heimlich manoeuvre) rather than abdominal thrusts should be used (see Emergency box and Fig. 14-15).

Perimortem Caesarean Birth

In the presence of multisystem trauma, perimortem Caesarean birth may be indicated. Removal of the stressor of pregnancy early in the process of resuscitation can increase the chance for maternal survival. Fetal survival is unlikely if Caesarean birth is accomplished more than 20 minutes after maternal death. Therefore, to facilitate resuscitative efforts, consideration may be given to Caesarean birth for maternal benefit after 4 minutes of resuscitative efforts that produce no response in the mother (Mozurkewich & Pearlman, 2012; Ruth & Miller, 2013). It should be emphasized that perimortem Caesarean birth is rarely successful, especially when the maternal arrest is related to trauma (Ruth & Miller, 2013).

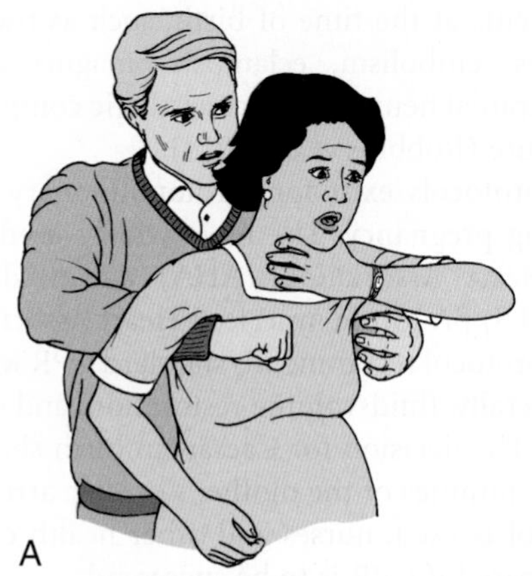

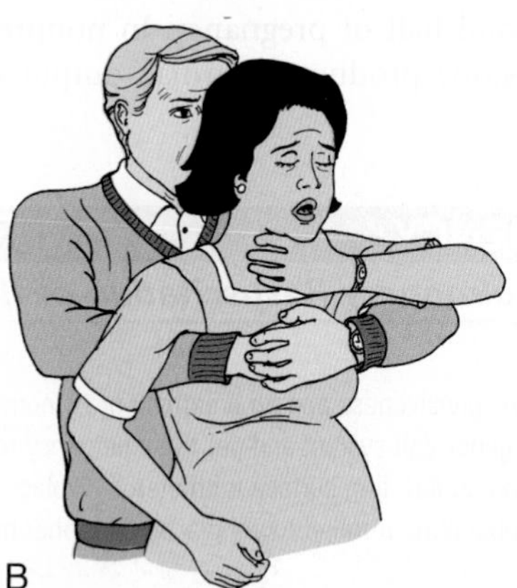

FIGURE 14-15 Heimlich manoeuvre. Clearing airway obstruction in a woman in the late stages of pregnancy. **A:** Standing behind victim, place your arms under the woman's armpits and across the chest (between nipples). Place thumb side of your clenched fist against the middle of the sternum and place other hand over fist. **B:** Perform backward chest thrusts until foreign body is expelled or woman loses consciousness.

KEY POINTS

- Hypertensive disorders of pregnancy are a leading cause of maternal and perinatal morbidity and mortality worldwide.
- The cause of pre-eclampsia is unknown, and there are no known reliable tests for predicting women at risk for developing pre-eclampsia/eclampsia.
- Pre-eclampsia/eclampsia is a multisystem disease, and the pathological changes are present long before clinical manifestations, such as hypertension, are evident.
- Once pre-eclampsia becomes clinically evident, therapeutic interventions may slow the progression of the disease, allowing the pregnancy to continue, but the underlying pathology continues.
- HELLP syndrome, which is a complication of pre-eclampsia/eclampsia, is considered life threatening.
- Magnesium sulphate, the anticonvulsant of choice for preventing or controlling eclamptic seizures, requires careful monitoring of reflexes, respirations, and renal function; its antidote, calcium gluconate, should be at the bedside.
- Intent of emergency interventions for eclampsia is to prevent self-injury, enhance oxygenation, reduce aspiration risk, and establish control with magnesium sulphate.
- Diagnosis of gestational diabetes mellitus is important to ensure glycemic control for women and thus improve perinatal outcomes.
- Ectopic pregnancy is a significant cause of maternal morbidity and mortality, even in developed countries.
- Placental abruption and placenta previa are differentiated by type of bleeding, uterine tonicity, and presence or absence of pain.
- Clotting disorders are associated with many obstetrical complications.
- The physiological adaptations of pregnancy mask warning signs and changes in vital signs during early shock state.
- Preoperative care for a pregnant woman differs from that for a nonpregnant woman in one significant aspect: the presence of the fetus.
- Trauma from accidents is the most common cause of death in women of child-bearing age.
- Fetal survival depends on maternal survival. After trauma occurs, the first priority is resuscitation and stabilization of the mother before consideration of fetal status.
- Minor trauma is associated with major complications for the pregnancy, including placental abruption, fetomaternal hemorrhage, preterm labour and birth, and fetal death.
- In the case of cardiac arrest in a pregnant woman, the advanced cardiac life support (ACLS) guidelines should be implemented without modification.

evolve WEBSITE

Visit the Evolve website for additional resources related to the content in this chapter such as Case Studies, Critical Thinking Case Study Answers, Nursing Care Plans, Nursing Processes, Nursing Skills, and Review Questions for Exam Preparation at: http://evolve.elsevier.com/Canada/Perry/maternal/

REFERENCES

Abbasi, N., Patenaude, V., & Abenhaim, H. A. (2014). Management and outcomes of acute appendicitis in pregnancy-population-based study of over 7000 cases. *BJOG: An International Journal of Obstetrics and Gynaecology*, *121*(12), 1509.

American Academy of Pediatrics (AAP) and American College of Obstetricians and Gynecologists (ACOG) (2012). *Guidelines for perinatal care* (7th ed.). Washington, DC: ACOG.

American College of Obstetricians and Gynecologists. (2011). *Bleeding in pregnancy: Frequently asked questions*. FAQ038. Retrieved from <http://www.acog.org/-/media/For-Patients/faq038.pdf?dmc=1&ts=20150312T0025158705>.

American College of Obstetricians and Gynecologists. (2014). Cerclage for the management of cervical insufficiency. *Obstetrics and Gynecology*, *123*(2 Pt. 1), 372–379. doi:10.1097/01.AOG.0000443276.68274.cc.

American College of Obstetricians and Gynecologists. (2015). Emergent therapy for acute onset severe hypertension during pregnancy and the postpartum period. Committee Opinion. Number 623. *Obstetrics and Gynecology*, *125*, 521–525. Retrieved from <http://www.acog.org/Resources-And-Publications/Committee-Opinions/Committee-on-Obstetric-Practice/Emergent-Therapy-for-Acute-Onset-Severe-Hypertension-During-Pregnancy-and-the-Postpartum-Period>.

American Heart Association. (2010). American Heart Association guidelines for cardiopulmonary resuscitation and emergency cardiovascular care science. Cardiac arrest in special situations. *Circulation*, *112*, S829–S861. Retrieved from <http://circ.ahajournals.org/cgi/content/full/122/18_suppl_3/S829>.

Baird, S. M., & Kennedy, B. B. (2008). Obstetric emergencies. In B. B. Kennedy, D. J. Ruth, & E. J. Martin (Eds.), *Intrapartum management modules: A perinatal education program*. Philadelphia: Wolters-Kluwer.

Berghella, V., & Iams, J. D. (2014). Cervical insufficiency. In R. Resnick, R. K. Creasy, J. D. Iams, et al. (Eds.), *Creasy & Resnik's maternal–fetal medicine: Principles and practice* (7th ed.). Philadelphia: Saunders.

Canadian Pediatric Society. (2012). Guidelines for health care professionals supporting families experiencing a perinatal loss. Fetus and Newborn Committee. *Paediatric and Child Health*, *6*(7), 469–477.

Cappell, M. (2012). Hepatic and gastrointestinal diseases. In S. Gabbe, J. Niebyl, J. Simpson, et al. (Eds.), *Obstetrics: Normal and problem pregnancies* (6th ed.). Philadelphia: Saunders.

Chan, W.-S., Rey, E., & Kent, N. (2014). SOGC clinical practice guideline: Venous thromboembolism and antithrombotic therapy in pregnancy. *Journal of Obstetrics Gynaecology Canada*, *36*(6), 527–553.

Chloptsios, C., Karanasiou, V., Ilias, G., et al. (2007). Cholecystitis during pregnancy: A case report and brief review of the literature. *Clinical and Experimental Obstetrics and Gynecology*, *34*(4), 250–251.

Cohn, D., Ramaswamy, B., & Blum, K. (2014). Malignancy and pregnancy. In R. Resnick, R. K. Creasy, J. Iams, et al. (Eds.), *Creasy & Resnik's maternal–fetal medicine: Principles and practice* (6th ed.). Philadelphia: Saunders.

Colombo, D. (2012). Renal disease. In S. G. Gabbe, J. R. Niebyl, H. L. Galen, et al. (Eds.), *Obstetrics: Normal and problem pregnancies* (6th ed.). New York: Saunders.

Cunningham, F., Leveno, K., Bloom, S., et al. (2014). *Williams obstetrics* (24th ed.). New York: McGraw Hill.

Davies, G., Maxwell, C., McLeod, L., et al. (2010). SOGC clinical practice guideline: Obesity in pregnancy. *Journal of Obstetrics and Gynaecology Canada*, *32*(2), 165–173.

DiGiulio, M., Wiedaseck, S., & Monchek, R. (2012). Understanding hydatidiform mole. *MCN American Journal of Maternal Child Nursing*, *37*(1), 30–34.

Donnolley, N., Halliday, L., & Oyelese, Y. (2013). Vasa previa: A descriptive review of existing literature and the evolving role of ultrasound in prenatal screening. *Australasian Journal of Ultrasound in Medicine*, *16*(2), 71–76.

Duff, P. (2014). Maternal and fetal infections. In R. Resnick, R. K. Creasy, J. Iams, et al. (Eds.), *Creasy & Resnik's maternal–fetal medicine: Principles and practice* (6th ed.). Philadelphia: Saunders.

Duley, I., Farrell, B., Sparks, P., et al. (2002). Do women with pre-eclampsia, and their babies, benefit from magnesium sulphate? The Magpie trial: A randomised placebo-controlled trial. *Lancet*, *359*, 1877–1890.

Ebrahimi, N., Maltepe, C., Bournissen, F. G., & Koren, G. (2009). Nausea and vomiting of pregnancy: Using the 24-hour Pregnancy-Unique Quantification of Emesis (PUQE-24) Scale. *Journal of Obstetrics and Gynaecology Canada*, *31*(9), 803–807.

Firoz, T., Maltepe, C., & Einarson, A. (2010). Nausea and vomiting in pregnancy is not always nausea and vomiting of pregnancy. *Journal of Obstetrics and Gynaecology Canada*, *32*(10), 970–972.

Francois, K. E., & Foley, M. R. (2012). Antepartum and postpartum hemorrhage. In S. G. Gabbe, J. R. Niebyl, & J. L. Simpson (Eds.), *Obstetrics: Normal and problem pregnancies* (6th ed.). New York: Saunders.

Gagnon, R., Morin, L., Bly, S., et al. (2009). SOGC clinical practice guideline: Guidelines for the management of vasa previa. *Journal of Obstetrics and Gynaecology Canada*, *31*(8), 748–753.

Gasem, T., al Jama, F. E., Burshaid, S., et al. (2009). Maternal and fetal outcome of pregnancy complicated by HELLP syndrome. *Journal of Maternal-Fetal & Neonatal Medicine*, *22*(12), 1140–1143.

Gilbert, E. S. (2011). *Manual of high risk pregnancy and delivery* (5th ed.). St. Louis: Mosby.

Goldenberg, R., & McClure, E. (2015). Appropriate use of antenatal corticosteroid prophylaxis. *Obstetrics and Gynecology*, *125*(2), 285–287. doi:10.1097/AOG.0000000000000655.

Guyatt, G. H., Akl, E. A., Crowther, M., et al. (2012). Executive summary: Antithrombotic therapy and prevention of thrombosis, 9th ed.: American College of Chest Physicians evidence-based clinical practice guidelines. *Chest*, *141*(2 Suppl.), 7S–47S. doi:10.1378/chest.1412S3.

Harvey, C., & Sibai, B. (2013). Hypertension in pregnancy. In N. Troiano, C. Harvey, & B. Chez (Eds.), *AWHONN's high risk and critical care obstetrics* (3rd ed.). Philadelphia: Wolters Kluwer/Lippincott Williams & Wilkins.

Hull, A. D., & Resnik, R. (2014). Placenta previa, placenta accrete, abruptio placentae, and vasa previa. In R. Resnick, R. K. Creasy, J. Iams, et al. (Eds.), *Creasy & Resnik's maternal–fetal medicine: Principles and practice* (7th ed.). Philadelphia: Saunders.

Hutcheon, J. A., Lisonkova, S., & Joseph, K. S. (2011). Epidemiology of pre-eclampsia and the other hypertensive disorders of pregnancy. *Best Practice & Research Clinical Obstetrics & Gynaecology*, *25*(4), 391–403. doi:10.1016/j.bpobgyn.2011.01.006.

Institute for Safe Medication Practices (ISMP) Canada. (2006). Eliminate use of dangerous abbreviations, symbols, and dose designations. *ISMP Canada Safety Bulletin*, *6*(4). Retrieved from <http://www.ismp-canada.org/download/safetyBulletins/ISMPCSB2006-04Abbr.pdf>.

Kelly, T. F., & Savides, T. J. (2014). Gastrointestinal disease in pregnancy. In R. Resnick, R. K. Creasy, J. Iams, et al. (Eds.), *Creasy & Resnik's maternal–fetal medicine: Principles and practice* (7th ed.). Philadelphia: Saunders.

Koren, K. (2012). Motherisk update: Is ondansetron safe for use during pregnancy? *Canadian Family Physician*, *58*(10), 1092–1093.

Landon, M. B., Catalano, P. M., & Gabbe, S. G. (2012). Diabetes mellitus complicating pregnancy. In S. G. Gabbe, J. R. Niebyl, J. L. Simpson, et al. (Eds.), *Obstetrics: Normal and problem pregnancies* (6th ed.). Philadelphia: Saunders.

Lim, K., Butt, K., Crane, J., et al. (2011). Ultrasonographic cervical length assessment in predicting preterm birth in singleton pregnancies. *Journal of Obstetrics and Gynaecology Canada*, *33*(5), 486–499.

Liston, R., Sawchuck, D., Young, D., et al. (2007). SOGC clinical practice guideline: Fetal health surveillance: Antepartum and intrapartum consensus guideline. *Journal of Obstetrics and Gynaecology Canada*, *29*(9 Suppl. 4).

Liu, S., Joseph, K. S., Liston, R. M., et al. (2011). Incidence, risk factors, and associated complications of eclampsia. *Obstetrics and Gynecology*, *118*(5), 987–994. doi:10.1097/AOG.0b013e31823311c1.

Magee, L. A., Pels, A., Helewa, M., et al. (2014). Diagnosis, evaluation, and management of the hypertensive disorders of pregnancy. *Pregnancy and Hypertension*, *4*(2), 105–145. doi:10.1016/j.preghy.2014.01.003.

Magee, L., von Dadelszen, P., Rey, E., et al. (2015). Less-tight control versus tight control of hypertension in pregnancy. *New England Journal of Medicine*, *372*(5), 407–417. doi:10.1016/j.preghy.2014.01.003.

Markham, K. B., & Funai, E. F. (2013). Pregnancy-related hypertension. In R. Resnick, R. K. Creasy, J. Iams, et al. (Eds.), *Creasy & Resnik's maternal–fetal medicine: Principles and practice* (7th ed.). Philadelphia: Saunders.

Matthews, A., Dowswell, T., Haas, D. M., et al. (2010). Interventions for nausea and vomiting in early pregnancy. *Cochrane Database of Systematic Reviews*, (9). doi:10.1002/14651858.CD007575.pub2.

McFarlane, J. (2007). Pregnancy following partner rape. What we know and what we need to know. *Trauma, Violence and Abuse*, *8*(2), 127–134.

Mehrabadi, A., Hutcheon, J., Liu, S., et al. (2015). Contribution of placenta accreta to the incidence of postpartum hemorrhage and severe postpartum hemorrhage. *Obstetrics and Gynecology*, *125*(4), 814–821. doi:10.1097/AOG.0000000000000722.

Mehrabadi, A., Liu, S., Bartholomew, S., et al. (2014). Hypertensive disorders of pregnancy and the recent increase in obstetric acute renal failure in Canada: Population based retrospective study. *BMJ (Clinical Research Ed.)*, *349*, g4731. doi:10.1136/bmj.g4731.

Miller, L. A., Miller, D. A., & Tucker, S. M. (2013). *Mosby's pocket guide to fetal monitoring: A multidisciplinary approach* (7th ed.). St. Louis: Mosby.

Moake, J. L. (2013). Disseminated intravascular coagulation. *The Merck Manual*. Retrieved from <http://www.merckmanuals.com/professional/hematology_and_oncology/coagulation_disorders/disseminated_intravascular_coagulation_dic.html>.

Mozurkewich, E., & Pearlman, M. (2012). Trauma and related surgery in pregnancy. In S. Gabbe, J. Niebyl, J. Simpson, et al. (Eds.), *Obstetrics: Normal and problem pregnancies* (6th ed.). Philadelphia: Saunders.

Murray, A., & Murphy, D. (2008). Vasa previa: Diagnosis and management. *Obstetrician and Gynecologist*, *10*(4), 217–223.

Nader, S. (2014). Thyroid disease and pregnancy. In R. Resnik, R. K. Creasy, J. Iams, et al. (Eds.), *Creasy and Resnik's maternal-fetal medicine: Principles and practice* (7th ed.). Philadelphia: Saunders.

Nensi, A., De Silva, D., von Dadelszen, P., et al. (2014). Effect of magnesium sulfate on fetal heart rate parameters: A systematic review. *Journal of Obstetrics and Gynaecology Canada*, *36*(12), 1055–1064.

Oppenheimer, L., Armson, A., Farine, D., et al. (2007). SOGC clinical practice guideline: Diagnosis and management of placenta previa. *Journal of Obstetrics and Gynaecology Canada*, *29*(3), 261–273.

Orzechowski, K., Boeling, R., Baxter, J., & Berghella, V. (2014). A universal transvaginal cervical length screening origram for preterm birth prevention. *Obstetrics and Gynecology*, *124*(3), 520–525.

Petrozza, J., & Berin, I. (2011). Recurrent early pregnancy loss. *eMedicine*. Retrieved from <http://emedicine.medscape.com/article/260495-overview>.

Ramin, S., & Ramin, K. (2016). Disseminated intravascular coagulation during pregnancy. *Up-to-Date*. Retrieved from <http://www.uptodate.com/contents/disseminated-intravascular-coagulation-during-pregnancy>.

Robbins, K. S., Martin, S. R., & Wilson, W. C. (2014). Intensive care considerations for the critically ill parturient. In R. Resnick, R. K. Creasy, J. Iams, et al. (Eds.), *Creasy & Resnik's maternal–fetal medicine: Principles and practice* (7th ed.). Philadelphia: Saunders.

Rodger, M. A., & Silver, R. M. (2014). Coagulation disorders in pregnancy. In R. Resnick, R. K. Creasy, J. Iams, et al. (Eds.), *Creasy & Resnik's maternal–fetal medicine: Principles and practice* (7th ed.). Philadelphia: Saunders.

Romero, R., Kusanovic, J., Chaiworapongsa, T., & Hassan, S. (2011). Placental bed disorders in preterm labor, preterm PROM, spontaneous abortion and abruption placentae. *Best Practice & Research Clinical Obstetrics & Gynaecology*, *25*(3), 313–327.

Ruth, D., & Miller, R. S. (2013). Trauma in pregnancy. In N. Troiano, C. Harvey, & B. Chez (Eds.), *AWHONN's high risk and critical care obstetrics* (3rd ed.). Philadelphia: Wolters Kluwer/Lippincott Williams & Wilkins.

Sepilian, V. P., & Wood, E. (2011). Ectopic pregnancy. *eMedicine*. Retrieved from <http://www.emedicine.com/med/topic3212.htm>.

Sibai, B. (2012). Hypertension. In S. G. Gabbe, J. R. Niebyl, J. L. Simpson, et al. (Eds.), *Obstetrics: Normal and problem pregnancies* (6th ed.). Philadelphia: Saunders.

Simhan, H. N., Iams, J. D., & Romero, R. (2012). Preterm birth. In S. G. Gabbe, J. R. Niebyl, & J. L. Simpson (Eds.), *Obstetrics: Normal and problem pregnancies* (6th ed.). New York: Churchill Livingstone.

Simpson, J. L., & Jauniaux, E. R. M. (2012). Pregnancy loss. In S. G. Gabbe, J. R. Niebyl, & H. L. Galen (Eds.), *Obstetrics: Normal and problem pregnancies* (6th ed.). Philadelphia: Saunders.

Smith, A., Refuerzo, J., & Ramin, S. (2013). *Patient information: Nausea and vomiting of pregnancy (beyond the basics)*. Retrieved from <http://www.uptodate.com/contents/nausea-and-vomiting-of-pregnancy-beyond-the-basics>.

Stukan, M., Kruszewski Wiesław, J., Dudziak, M., et al. (2013). Intestinal obstruction during pregnancy. *Ginekologia Polska*, *84*(2), 137–141.

Thompson, D., Berger, H., Feif, D., et al. (2013). Diabetes and pregnancy. Clinical practice guidelines for the prevention and management of diabetes in Canada. *Canadian Journal of Diabetes*, *37*(Suppl. 1), S168–S183.

Van den Broek, N. R., & Letsky, E. A. (2001). Pregnancy and the erythrocyte sedimentation rate. *BJOG: An International Journal of Obstetrics and Gynaecology*, *108*, 1164–1167. doi:10.1111/j.1471-0528.2003.00267.x.

van Oostwaard, M. F., Langenveld, J., Schuit, E., et al. (2015). Recurrence of hypertensive disorders of pregnancy: An individual patient data meta-analysis. *American Journal of Obstetrics and Gynecology*, *212*(5), 624.e15–624.e17. doi:10.1016/j.ajog.2015.01.009.

Walker, M., Whittle, W., Keating, S., & Kingdom, J. (2010). Sonographic diagnosis of chronic abruption. *Journal of Obstetrics and Gynaecology Canada*, *32*(11), 1056–1058.

ADDITIONAL RESOURCE

Society of Obstetricians and Gynaecologists of Canada. <http://sogc.org/>

CHAPTER

15

Pregnancy at Risk: Pre-Existing Conditions

Melanie Basso

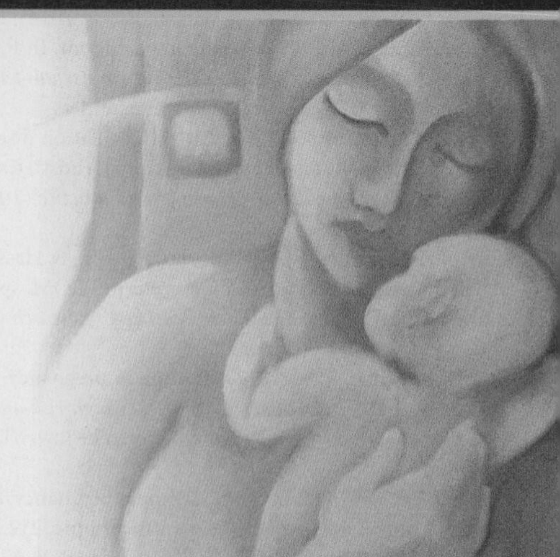

evolve WEBSITE

Visit the Evolve website for additional resources related to the content in this chapter such as Case Studies, Critical Thinking Case Study Answers, Nursing Care Plans, Nursing Processes, Nursing Skills, and Review Questions for Exam Preparation at: *http://evolve.elsevier.com/Canada/Perry/maternal/*

OBJECTIVES

On completion of this chapter the reader will be able to:

- Differentiate the types of diabetes mellitus and their respective risk factors in pregnancy.
- Compare insulin requirements during pregnancy, the postpartum period, and lactation.
- Identify maternal and fetal risks and possible complications associated with diabetes in pregnancy.
- Develop a plan of care for the pregnant woman with pregestational diabetes.
- Understand the management of hyperthyroidism and hypothyroidism in a pregnant woman.
- Differentiate the management of various cardiovascular disorders in pregnant women.
- Discuss the different types of anemia and their effects during pregnancy.
- Describe the care of pregnant women with pulmonary disorders.
- Review the effects of neurological disorders on pregnancy.
- Describe the care of women whose pregnancies are complicated by autoimmune disorders.
- Explain the effects on and the management of pregnant women with human immunodeficiency virus.
- Describe the care of the bariatric pregnant woman.
- Describe care of a pregnant woman with a spinal cord injury.
- Discuss the care of pregnant women who have issues related to substance use.

For most women, pregnancy is a normal and healthy life event. However, for some women pregnancy can be a time of significant risk due to the presence of a chronic illness. Women actively participate in self-management of their illness along with the multidisciplinary team to best manage the changes in pregnancy to promote the best pregnancy outcomes.

The goal of the health care team is to work with women to foster as normal a pregnancy experience as possible, while supporting the unique maternal and fetal needs prompted by the existence of chronic conditions. Nurses are key members of the health care team who guide and support the woman and her family in achieving optimal outcomes for both her and her fetus.

This chapter focuses on nursing care for women with metabolic disorders, including diabetes mellitus and thyroid disorders; cardiovascular disorders; selected disorders of the respiratory, gastrointestinal, integumentary, and central nervous systems; and **autoimmune disorders**. Key elements of care for women with substance use issues, human immunodeficiency virus (HIV) infection, spinal cord injury, and obesity are also discussed. For each disorder, management throughout the entire perinatal period (antepartum, intrapartum, and postpartum) is discussed; thus all the information for each condition is located in one place in the text.

METABOLIC DISORDERS

Diabetes Mellitus

Worldwide, the incidence of diabetes mellitus is increasing at a rapid rate. Diabetes mellitus is currently the most common endocrine disorder associated with pregnancy, occurring in approximately 4 to 14% of pregnant women (Gilbert, 2011). There is expected to be a marked increase in the number of women with pre-existing diabetes who will become pregnant (Moore, Hauguel-De Mouzon, & Catalano, 2014). Advances in knowledge about the effects of pregnancy on diabetes care have improved the outcomes for women. Diabetic women who are pregnant have the greatest success when they work together with a multidisciplinary team involving the obstetrician, internist or endocrinologist, pediatrician, nurse, and dietitian. These women require education regarding the effects that pregnancy can have on their diabetes management in order to prevent complications. Women with type 1 and type 2 diabetes must have frequent prenatal visits to support their knowledge about necessary changes to their diet and the importance of more frequent self-monitoring of blood glucose levels. More frequent laboratory evaluation and more intensive fetal surveillance and occasionally hospitalization to achieve optimal pregnancy outcomes may be required.

Recent studies have shown that the perinatal mortality rate for women with well-controlled diabetes, excluding major congenital malformations, is about the same as that for any other pregnancy (Landon, Catalano, & Gabbe, 2012). This is due to improvements in the understanding and management of strict maternal glucose control before conception and throughout the pregnancy. Before becoming pregnant, women with diabetes are strongly encouraged to have preconception counselling to optimize glycemic control, assess for presence of complications, review medications, and begin folate supplementation (Thompson, Berger, Feig, et al., 2013).

Nurses who provide care to pregnant women with diabetes must fully understand both the normal physiological responses to pregnancy and the physiological effects and psychosocial implications of diabetes in order to accurately assess the needs of the individual woman, help her plan for her care, and intervene, when appropriate.

Pathogenesis

Diabetes mellitus is a group of metabolic diseases characterized by **hyperglycemia** resulting from defects in insulin secretion, insulin action, or both. *Insulin*, produced by β-cells in the islets of Langerhans of the pancreas, regulates blood glucose levels by enabling glucose to enter adipose and muscle cells, where it is used for energy. Insulin stimulates protein synthesis and the storage of free fatty acids. When insulin is insufficient or ineffective in promoting glucose uptake by the muscle and adipose cells, glucose accumulates in the bloodstream, resulting in hyperglycemia. Hyperglycemia causes hyperosmolarity of the blood, which attracts intracellular fluid into the vascular system, resulting in cellular dehydration and expanded blood volume. Consequently, the kidneys function to excrete large volumes of urine (*polyuria*) in an attempt to regulate excess vascular volume and excrete the unused glucose (**glycosuria**). Polyuria and cellular dehydration cause excessive thirst (*polydipsia*).

The body compensates for its inability to convert carbohydrate (glucose) into energy by burning proteins (muscle) and fats. The end products of this metabolism are **ketones** and fatty acids, which in excess quantity produce ketoacidosis and acetonuria. Weight loss occurs because of the breakdown of fat and muscle tissue. This tissue breakdown causes a state of starvation that compels the individual to eat excessive amounts of food (*polyphagia*).

Over time, diabetes that is not well controlled causes significant changes in both the microvascular and macrovascular circulations. These structural changes affect a variety of organ systems—primarily the heart, eyes, kidneys, and nerves. Complications resulting from diabetes include premature atherosclerosis, retinopathy, nephropathy, and neuropathy.

Diabetes may be caused either by impaired insulin secretion, when the beta cells of the pancreas are destroyed by an autoimmune process, or by inadequate insulin action in target tissues at one or more points along the metabolic pathway. Both of these conditions are commonly present in the same person, and determining which, if either, abnormality is the primary cause of the disease is difficult (Thompson et al., 2013).

Classification

Diabetes during pregnancy is currently classified into two categories: pregestational diabetes and gestational diabetes. *Pregestational diabetes* applies to women with type 1 or type 2 diabetes that existed before pregnancy.

People with type 1 diabetes have an absolute insulin deficiency caused by pancreatic islet β-cell destruction, which makes them prone to ketoacidosis. Type 1 diabetes is theorized to be caused by an autoimmune process, but the cause is primarily unknown (Thompson et al., 2013).

Type 2 diabetes is the most prevalent form of the disease and affects individuals who have insulin resistance and relative (rather than absolute) insulin deficiency. Individuals may have type 2 diabetes for many years prior to diagnosis because hyperglycemia develops gradually and often is not severe enough for the person to recognize the classic signs of polyuria, polydipsia, and polyphagia. Many people who develop type 2 diabetes are obese or have an increased amount of body fat distributed primarily in the abdominal area. Other risk factors include aging, a sedentary lifestyle, hypertension, and prior gestational diabetes. Type 2 diabetes often has a strong genetic predisposition (Thompson et al., 2013).

Gestational diabetes mellitus (GDM) is the classification for women who have carbohydrate intolerance that is discovered during pregnancy. GDM is any degree of glucose intolerance with its onset or first recognition during pregnancy. This definition applies regardless of whether insulin is used for treatment or whether the diabetes persists after pregnancy. It does not exclude the possibility that glucose intolerance preceded the pregnancy. Women who experience gestational diabetes should be assessed for the presence of underlying disease 6 weeks to 6 months after the pregnancy ends (Thompson et al., 2013) (see Chapter 14 for further discussion).

Metabolic Changes Associated With Pregnancy

Normal pregnancy is characterized by complex alterations in maternal glucose metabolism, insulin production, and metabolic homeostasis. During normal pregnancy, adjustments in maternal metabolism allow for adequate nutrition for both the mother and the developing fetus. Glucose, the primary fuel used by the fetus, is transported across the placenta through the process of carrier-mediated facilitated diffusion. This means that the glucose levels in the fetus are directly proportional to maternal levels. Although glucose crosses the placenta, insulin does not. Around the tenth week of gestation, the fetus secretes its own insulin at levels adequate to use the glucose obtained from the mother. Thus, as maternal glucose levels rise, fetal glucose levels are increased, resulting in increased fetal insulin secretion.

During the first trimester and early second trimester of pregnancy, the pregnant woman's metabolic status is significantly influenced by the rising levels of estrogen and progesterone. These hormones stimulate the β-cells in the pancreas to increase insulin production, which promotes increased peripheral use of glucose and decreased blood glucose, with fasting levels reduced by approximately 10% (Fig. 15-1, A). At the same time an increase in tissue glycogen stores and a decrease in hepatic glucose production occur, which together further encourage lower fasting glucose levels. As a result of these normal metabolic changes of pregnancy, women with type 1 and type 2 diabetes are prone to **hypoglycemia** (low blood glucose) during the first trimester.

During the latter part of the second trimester and the third trimester, pregnancy exerts a **diabetogenic** effect on the maternal metabolic status. Because of the major hormonal changes, there is decreased tolerance to glucose, increased insulin resistance, decreased hepatic glycogen stores, and increased hepatic production of glucose. Increasing levels of human chorionic somatomammotropin, estrogen, progesterone, prolactin, cortisol, and insulinase increase insulin resistance through their actions as insulin antagonists. Insulin resistance is a glucose-sparing mechanism that ensures an abundant supply of glucose for the fetus. Maternal insulin requirements gradually increase from about 18 to 24 weeks of gestation to about 36 weeks of gestation, usually doubling by the end of pregnancy. During the last few weeks of pregnancy, women need to be reassured that their diabetes is not becoming worse with the increase in insulin and told that insulin requirements usually level off after 36 weeks' gestation until labour begins (see Fig. 15-1, B and C).

At birth, expulsion of the placenta prompts an abrupt decrease in levels of circulating placental hormones, cortisol, and insulinase (see Fig. 15-1, D). Maternal tissues quickly regain their prepregnancy sensitivity to insulin. For the nonbreastfeeding mother, the prepregnancy insulin–carbohydrate balance usually returns in about 7 to 10 days (see Fig. 15-1, E). Lactation uses maternal glucose; thus the breastfeeding mother's insulin requirements remain low as long as she is nursing (see Fig. 15-1, E). On completion of weaning, the mother's prepregnancy insulin requirement is re-established (see Fig. 15-1, F).

Pregestational Diabetes Mellitus

Pregestational diabetes (type 1 and type 2) has increased from 3.1 per 1000 births to 4.7 per 1000 births, primarily as a result of an increased number of women of child-bearing age with type 2 diabetes (Thompson et al., 2013). Only about 10% of pregnancies complicated by diabetes occur in women who have pre-existing disease (Landon et al., 2012). Women who have pregestational diabetes mellitus may have either type 1 or 2

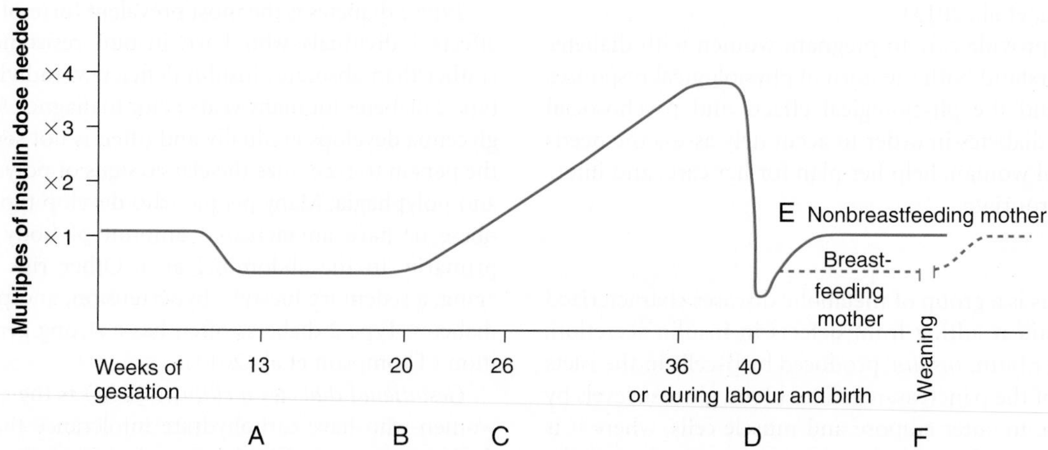

FIGURE 15-1 Changing insulin needs during pregnancy. **A:** First trimester/early second trimester: Insulin need is reduced because of increased insulin production by the pancreas and increased peripheral sensitivity to insulin; nausea, vomiting, and decreased food intake by mother and glucose transfer to the embryo or fetus contribute to hypoglycemia. **B:** Late second trimester: Insulin need increases as placental hormones, cortisol, and insulinase act as insulin antagonists, decreasing the effectiveness of insulin. **C:** Third trimester: Insulin requirements gradually increase until about 36 weeks of gestation. **D:** Day of birth: Maternal insulin requirements drop drastically to approach prepregnancy levels. **E:** Breastfeeding mother maintains lower insulin requirements, as much as 25% less than prepregnancy; insulin need of nonbreastfeeding mother returns to prepregnancy levels in 7 to 10 days. **F:** At weaning of breastfeeding infant, mother's insulin need returns to prepregnancy levels.

diabetes, which may be complicated by vascular disease, retinopathy, nephropathy, or other diabetic complications. The diabetogenic state of pregnancy imposed on the compromised metabolic system of the woman with pregestational diabetes has significant implications. The normal hormonal adaptations of pregnancy affect glycemic control, and pregnancy may accelerate the progress of vascular complications. Type 2 is a more common diagnosis than type 1. Almost all women with pregestational diabetes are insulin dependent during pregnancy.

Fetal risks for women with pregestational diabetes include perinatal mortality, congenital malformations, prematurity, macrosomia, and morbidities in the neonatal period (Thompson et al., 2013).

During the first trimester, when maternal blood glucose levels are normally reduced and the insulin response to glucose is enhanced, glycemic control is improved. The insulin dose for the woman with well-controlled diabetes may have to be reduced to prevent hypoglycemia. Nausea, vomiting, and cravings typical of early pregnancy result in dietary fluctuations that influence maternal glucose levels and may also necessitate a reduction in the insulin dose.

Because insulin requirements steadily increase after the first trimester, the insulin dose must be adjusted accordingly to prevent hyperglycemia. Insulin resistance begins as early as 14 to 16 weeks of gestation and continues to rise until it stabilizes during the last few weeks of pregnancy.

Preconception counselling. Preconception counselling is recommended by the Canadian Diabetes Association (CDA) and the Society of Obstetricians and Gynaecologists of Canada (SOGC) for all women of reproductive age with diabetes in order to support improved pregnancy outcomes (Allen, Armson, Wilson, et al., 2007; Thompson et al., 2013). Preconception care to evaluate the woman's health status, plan the optimal time for pregnancy, improve self-management of optimal glycemic control before conception, and stabilize any vascular complications of diabetes (retinopathy, nephropathy, neuropathy, and cardiovascular disease) is ideal. However, it is estimated that fewer than 50% of women with type 1 diabetes plan their pregnancies and seek preconception counselling, and this figure is even lower for women with type 2 diabetes (Thompson et al., 2013). Preconception counselling is particularly important because strict metabolic control before conception and in the early weeks of gestation during organogenesis is instrumental in decreasing the risk of congenital anomalies and spontaneous abortion (Box 15-1).

Preconception counselling includes providing information regarding medications being used for glycemic control. The use of oral antihyperglycemic medications alone during pregnancy is not recommended by the CDA; continued research is being conducted to determine their efficacy and safety before and during pregnancy (Thompson et al., 2013). Some physicians will counsel women with type 2 diabetes who are on oral hypoglycemic medications in the preconception period to start insulin as soon as the pregnancy is diagnosed (Thompson et al., 2013).

The woman's partner should be included in preconception counselling to improve the support for the woman and understanding of potential complications of pregnancy as a result of diabetes. The couple also should be informed of the anticipated alterations in the management of diabetes during pregnancy and the need for a multidisciplinary team approach to pregnancy care. Financial implications of the diabetic pregnancy and other demands related to frequent maternal and fetal surveillance should be discussed. Contraception is an important aspect of preconception counselling to assist the couple in planning the timing of pregnancy.

BOX 15-1 GOALS FOR SELF-MONITORED GLUCOSE LEVELS IN THE PRECONCEPTUAL PERIOD

Recommended glycemic targets for preconception and during pregnancy:

Prepregnancy A_{1C}	<7%*
Pregnancy A_{1C}	≤6.0%

*Ideally, A_{1C} ≤6.0% if this can be safely achieved. In some women, particularly those with type 1 diabetes, higher targets may be necessary to avoid excessive hypoglycemia. Regular measurements of glycosylated hemoglobin provide data for altering the treatment plan and lead to improvement of glycemic control. A hemoglobin A_{1C} of 6 to 7% is the desired goal, which correlates with an average glucose of 5.5 to 7.7 mmol/L (Thompson et al., 2013).

A_{1C} = glycosylated hemoglobin: With prolonged hyperglycemia, some of the hemoglobin remains saturated with glucose for the life of the red blood cell. Therefore, a test for glycosylated hemoglobin provides a measurement of glycemic control over time, specifically over the previous 8 to 12 weeks.

Maternal risks and complications. Although morbidity and mortality rates have improved significantly for pregnant women with diabetes, they remain at risk for the development of significant complications during pregnancy. Assessment of risk is best done by evaluating the woman's blood glucose control and determining the length of time since diagnosis of the woman's diabetes and whether existing diabetic complications are present. Women with poor glycemic control, longer duration of diabetes, and presence of complications typically have less than optimal pregnancy outcomes, such as perinatal mortality, congenital malformations, hypertension, preterm delivery, large-for-gestational-age infants, Caesarean birth, and neonatal morbidities (Thompson et al., 2013).

Women with pregestational diabetes who have poor glycemic control (defined as a **glycosylated hemoglobin** value greater than 7.0% around the time of conception and in the early weeks of pregnancy) have a twofold increased incidence of early pregnancy loss (28%) (Kitzmiller, Block, Brown, et al., 2008). Women with good glycemic control before conception and in the first trimester are no more likely to have a miscarriage than women without diabetes (Thompson et al., 2013) (see Research Focus box).

Poor glycemic control later in pregnancy, particularly in women without vascular disease, increases the rate of fetal macrosomia. Macrosomia has been defined as a birth weight more than 4000 to 4500 g or greater than the ninetieth percentile. It occurs in up to 50% of pregnancies in women with gestational diabetes and in 40% of pregestational diabetic pregnancies

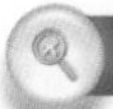

RESEARCH FOCUS

Glycemic Control and Vitamin D for Improving Pregnancy Outcomes in Patients With Diabetes

—Pat Mahaffee Gingrich

Ask the Question

For women with diabetes, which preconception and pregnancy interventions help improve fetal and maternal outcomes?

Search for the Evidence

Search Strategies

English research-based publications on diabetes in pregnancy were included.

Databases Used

Cochrane Collaborative Database, National Guideline Clearinghouse (AHRQ), CINAHL, PubMed, UpToDate, AWHONN

Critically Analyze the Evidence

- Pre-existing type 1 or 2 diabetes in pregnancy is a known risk for increased birth weight and perinatal loss. Loose glycemic control is associated with increased risk for pre-eclampsia, macrosomia, and Caesarean birth. Moderate and tight glycemic controls have improved outcomes, but tight control leads to significantly more hypoglycemia and longer hospital stays. Moderate control is recommended (Middleton, Crowther, & Simmonds, 2012).
- Vitamin D is a steroid hormone that is necessary for bone metabolism and vascular, immune, metabolic, and placental function. Vitamin D deficiency in pregnancy is associated with gestational diabetes, higher fasting blood sugar, and higher insulin levels (Poel, Hummel, Lips, et al., 2012; Senti, Thiele, & Anderson, 2012). Vitamin D deficiency may also be associated with pre-eclampsia, preterm labour, Caesarean birth, and infections. Clinical recommendations for vitamin D during pregnancy are 600 international units (IU) daily (Urrutia & Thorp, 2012).
- A meta-analysis found that preconception glycemic control in women with pre-existing diabetes leads to significantly lower hemoglobin $A1_c$ ($HgA1_c$) in the first trimester and fewer congenital anomalies, preterm births, perinatal mortality, and maternal complications (Wahabi, Alzeidan, Bawazeer, et al., 2010).

Apply the Evidence: Nursing Implications

- For women with diabetes who are contemplating pregnancy, preconception attention to glycemic control should be a part of patient education by the nurse. Women should know that lower $HgA1_c$ and moderate glycemic control before and during pregnancy are associated with significantly improved maternal and birth outcomes.
- All women need preconception information about vitamin D deficiency, which is associated with gestational diabetes. Vitamin D supplementation of 600 international units (IU) daily is recommended during pregnancy. A blood test can confirm adequate vitamin D levels.

References

Middleton, P., Crowther, C. A., & Simmonds, L. (2012). Different intensities of glycaemic control for pregnant women with pre-existing diabetes. *Cochrane Database Systematic Reviews*, (9). doi:10.1002/14651858.CD008540.pub3.

Poel, Y. H., Hummel, P., Lips, P., et al. (2012). Vitamin D and gestational diabetes: A systematic review and meta-analysis. *European Journal of Internal Medicine, 23*(5), 465–469.

Senti, J., Thiele, D. K., & Anderson, C. M. (2012). Maternal vitamin D status as a critical determinant in gestational diabetes. *Journal of Obstetric, Gynecologic, & Neonatal Nursing, 41*(3), 328–338. doi:10.1111/j.1552-6909.2012.01366.x.

Urrutia, R. P., & Thorp, J. M. (2012). Vitamin D in pregnancy: Current concepts. *Current Opinion in Obstetrics & Gynecology, 24*(2), 57–64.

Wahabi, H. A., Alzeidan, R. A., Bawazeer, G. A., et al. (2010). Preconception care for diabetic women for improving maternal and fetal outcomes: A systematic review and meta-analysis. *BMC Pregnancy and Childbirth, 10*, 63.

(Landon et al., 2012). These large infants tend to have a disproportionate increase in shoulder and trunk size; consequently, the risk of shoulder dystocia is greater in these babies than in other macrosomic infants. Thus women with type 1 and type 2 diabetes face an increased likelihood of Caesarean birth because of failure of fetal descent or labour progress or of operative vaginal birth (use of forceps or vacuum extraction).

Women with pre-existing diabetes are at risk for several obstetrical and medical complications. In general, the risk of developing these complications increases with the duration and severity of the woman's diabetes. In one study, the rates of pre-eclampsia, preterm birth, Caesarean birth, and maternal mortality were much higher in women with pre-existing diabetes than in women who did not have this disease. Approximately a third of women who have had diabetes for more than 20 years develop pre-eclampsia. Women with nephropathy and hypertension in addition to diabetes are also increasingly likely to develop pre-eclampsia. The rate of hypertensive disorders in all types of pregnancies complicated by diabetes is 15 to 30%. Chronic hypertension occurs in 10 to 20% of all pregnant women with diabetes and in up to 40% of women who have pre-existing renal or retinal vascular disease (Kitzmiller et al., 2008; Magee, Pels, Helewa, et al., 2014; Moore et al., 2014).

Preterm labour or birth is also more likely to occur, especially with more severe hypertension, chronically elevated glucose levels, and presence of genital or urinary tract infections. For these reasons, the risk for induced preterm birth is greater in women with poorly controlled pregestational diabetes (Landon et al., 2012).

Women with type 1 and type 2 diabetes should have regular testing of their eyes for retinopathy. Regular assessments by an ophthalmologist who has knowledge of diabetes is recommended preconception, during the first trimester of pregnancy, as needed within the pregnancy, and again within 1 year postpartum (Thompson et al., 2013). Women may develop retinopathy due to poor glycemic control and are at increased risk with comorbidities such as hypertension or renal disease (Thompson et al., 2013). Women with existing mild-to-moderate retinopathy who become pregnant but maintain good glycemic control are generally not at increased risk of worsening retinopathy (Thompson et al., 2013).

Women with diabetes who are contemplating a pregnancy should be screened for the presence of chronic kidney disease. During pregnancy, monitoring of renal function should occur using the protein-to-creatinine ratio (PCR) and the estimated glomerular filtration rate (eGFR) (Thompson et al., 2013). Kidney disease and microalbuminemia can be associated with poor outcomes for the mother and fetus. Pregnant women with diabetes should also be monitored for serum creatinine levels to assess for kidney status throughout the pregnancy so that deterioration in kidney function can be detected (Magee et al., 2014; Thompson et al., 2013).

Hydramnios (polyhydramnios) frequently develops during the third trimester of pregnancy in women with diabetes. While the cause is unknown, one theory is that hydramnios in women with diabetes is caused by an increased glucose concentration in amniotic fluid resulting from maternal and fetal hyperglycemia. The complications most frequently associated with hydramnios (usually defined as an amniotic fluid index [AFI] greater than 24 to 25 cm) are placental abruption, uterine dysfunction, and postpartum hemorrhage (Cunningham, Leveno, Bloom, et al., 2014).

Infections are more common and more serious in pregnant women with diabetes. Disorders of carbohydrate metabolism alter the body's normal resistance to infection. The inflammatory response, **leukocyte** function, and vaginal pH are all affected. Vaginal infections, particularly monilial vaginitis, are more common, as are urinary tract infections. Infection is serious because it causes increased insulin resistance and may result in ketoacidosis. Postpartum infection may also occur among women who have poorly controlled blood glucose.

The most common concern in pregnancy is the loss of hypoglycemic awareness. This is more common in longstanding diabetes and creates safety concerns for the mother, especially at times when concentration is required, such as driving a car. Hypoglycemic awareness may or may not return postpregnancy.

Ketoacidosis (accumulation of ketones in the blood resulting from hyperglycemia and leading to metabolic acidosis) occurs most often during the second and third trimesters, when the diabetogenic effect of pregnancy is the greatest. When the maternal metabolism is stressed by illness or infection, the woman is at increased risk for **diabetic ketoacidosis (DKA)**. Women at risk for preterm labour may be at increased risk for DKA from administration of steroids or some tocolytic medications. DKA may also occur because of the over- or under-administration of insulin.

DKA may occur with blood glucose levels barely exceeding 11 mmol/L because of an increase in the body's resistance to insulin in pregnancy; nonpregnant thresholds are higher, at 16.7 to 19.5 mmol/L. In response to stress factors such as infection or illness, hyperglycemia occurs, with a resulting increase in hepatic glucose production and decreased peripheral glucose use. The presence of nausea, vomiting, and fever can lead to ketoacidosis. Stress hormones, which can impair insulin action and further contribute to insulin deficiency, are released. Fatty acids are mobilized from fat stores into the circulation. As they are oxidized, ketone bodies are released into the peripheral circulation. The woman's buffering system is unable to compensate, and metabolic acidosis develops. The excessive blood glucose and ketone bodies result in osmotic diuresis, with subsequent loss of fluid and electrolytes, volume depletion, and cellular dehydration. Prompt treatment of DKA is necessary to avoid maternal coma or death. Ketoacidosis at any time during pregnancy can lead to intrauterine fetal death and may stimulate preterm labour. The incidence of DKA has decreased in recent years because of advances in clinical management and blood glucose monitoring (Inturrisi, Lintner, & Sorem, 2013). Currently it affects only about 1% of pregnant women with diabetes (Cunningham et al., 2014). The rate of intrauterine fetal demise (IUFD) with DKA, formerly approximately 35%, is 10% or less (Moore et al., 2014) (Table 15-1).

The risk of *hypoglycemia* (a less than normal amount of glucose in the blood) is also increased during pregnancy. Early in pregnancy, when hepatic production of glucose is diminished and peripheral use of glucose is enhanced, hypoglycemia occurs frequently, often during sleep. Later in pregnancy, hypoglycemia may also result as insulin doses are adjusted to maintain **euglycemia** (a normal blood glucose level). Women with a prepregnancy history of severe hypoglycemia are at increased risk for severe hypoglycemia during gestation. Episodic and nonsevere hypoglycemic episodes do not appear to have significant deleterious effects on fetal well-being (see Table 15-1). The long-term fetal effects of severe maternal hypoglycemia that results in ketosis may be a contributing factor in abnormal postnatal neurological development (Gilbert, 2011; Kitzmiller et al., 2008).

Fetal and neonatal risks and complications. Despite the improvements in care of pregnant women with diabetes, sudden and unexplained stillbirth is still a significant risk (Gilbert, 2011; Landon et al., 2012). Approximately 2 to 5% of all fetal deaths occur in women whose pregnancies are complicated by pre-existing diabetes. Hyperglycemia, ketoacidosis, congenital anomalies, infections, and maternal obesity are thought to be reasons for fetal death. In the third trimester fetal acidosis is the most likely cause of fetal death.

The most important cause of perinatal loss in diabetic pregnancy is congenital malformations, which account for 30 to 50% of all perinatal loss in pregnancies complicated by diabetes (Gilbert, 2011; Landon, et al., 2012). The incidence of congenital malformations is related to the severity and duration of the diabetes. Hyperglycemia during the first trimester of pregnancy, when organs and organ systems are forming, is the main cause of diabetes-associated birth defects. Central nervous system (CNS) defects (e.g., anencephaly, open spina bifida) are increased tenfold. Cardiac defects, especially ventricular septal defects (VSDs) and transposition of the great vessels, are increased fivefold (Landon et al., 2012). Caudal regression (also called caudal dysplasia or sacral agenesis) is a fetal anomaly found 200 to 400 times more often in pregnancies of mothers with diabetes (Landon et al., 2012). Infant morbidity and mortality rates associated with diabetic pregnancy are significantly reduced with strict control of maternal glucose levels before and during pregnancy.

The fetal pancreas begins to secrete insulin at 10 to 14 weeks of gestation. The fetus responds to maternal hyperglycemia by secreting large amounts of insulin (hyperinsulinism). Insulin acts as a growth hormone, causing the fetus to produce excess stores of glycogen, protein, and adipose tissue and leading to increased fetal size, or *macrosomia*. Birth injuries are more common in infants born to mothers with diabetes than in those born to mothers who do not have diabetes, and macrosomic fetuses have the highest risk for this complication. Common

TABLE 15-1 DIFFERENTIATION OF HYPOGLYCEMIA (INSULIN SHOCK) AND HYPERGLYCEMIA (DIABETIC KETOACIDOSIS)

CAUSES	ONSET	SYMPTOMS	INTERVENTIONS
Hypoglycemia (Insulin Shock)			
Excess insulin Insufficient food (delayed or missed meals) Excessive exercise or work Indigestion, diarrhea, vomiting	Rapid (regular insulin) Gradual (modified insulin or oral hypoglycemic agents)	Irritability Hunger Sweating Nervousness Personality change Weakness Fatigue Blurred or double vision Dizziness Headache Pallor; clammy skin Shallow respirations Rapid pulse Laboratory values • Urine: Negative for sugar and acetone • Blood glucose: ≤3.3 mmol/L	• Check blood glucose level when symptoms first appear. • Eat or drink 15 g fast sugar (simple carbohydrate) immediately. • 175 mL (3/4 c) unsweetened fruit juice or regular pop • 15 mL (1 tbsp) or 3 packets of table sugar dissolved in water • 5 to 6 Life Savers candies • 15 mL (1 tbsp) honey • 15 g glucose in glucose tablet form • Recheck blood glucose level in 15 minutes and eat or drink another 15 g fast sugar (simple carbohydrate) if glucose remains low. • Recheck blood glucose level in 15 minutes. • Notify primary health care provider if there is no change in glucose level. • If woman is unconscious, administer 50% dextrose IV push, 5 to 10% dextrose in water IV drip, or 1 mg glucagon subcutaneously. • Obtain blood and urine specimens for laboratory testing.
Hyperglycemia (DKA)			
Insufficient insulin Excess or wrong kind of food Infection, injuries, illness Emotional stress Insufficient exercise	Slow (hours to days)	Thirst Nausea or vomiting Abdominal pain Constipation Drowsiness Dim vision Increased urination Headache Flushed, dry skin Rapid breathing Weak, rapid pulse Acetone (fruity) breath odour Laboratory values • Urine: Positive for sugar and acetone • Blood glucose: ≥11 mmol/L	• Notify primary health care provider. • Administer insulin in accordance with blood glucose levels. • Give IV fluids such as normal saline solution or one-half normal saline solution; potassium when urinary output is adequate; bicarbonate for pH <7. • Monitor laboratory testing of blood and urine.

DKA, diabetic ketoacidosis; *IV*, intravenous.

birth injuries associated with diabetic pregnancies include brachial plexus palsy, facial nerve injury, humerus or clavicle fracture, and cephalhematoma. Most of these injuries are associated with difficult vaginal birth and shoulder dystocia (Moore et al., 2014). Hypoglycemia at birth is also a risk for infants born to mothers with diabetes. The degree of hypoglycemia is influenced by maternal glucose control during the last half of pregnancy and during labour and birth (Landon et al., 2012). (For further discussion of neonatal complications related to maternal diabetes, see Chapter 28).

NURSING CARE

Nurses play a key role in helping women who are already diabetic to understand how pregnancy may affect their management of diabetes. Women require an individualized plan of care that builds on their in-depth knowledge of their own disease management to achieve euglycemia and prevent complications (see Nursing Care Plan, Pregancy Complicated by Pregestational Diabetes on Evolve). 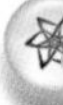 The initial prenatal visit is the optimal time to assess the woman's knowledge regarding diabetes and pregnancy, review potential maternal and fetal complications, and begin the initial plan of care with the woman and her family. In addition to the routine prenatal examination, specific efforts are made to assess the effects of the diabetes, especially retinopathy, nephropathy, peripheral and autonomic neuropathy, peripheral vascular, and cardiac involvement (Gilbert, 2011). Subsequent visits are important for monitoring a woman's progress and identifying further learning needs. Teaching should include family members.

Routine prenatal laboratory tests are performed, and baseline renal function may be assessed with a 24-hour urine collection for total protein excretion and creatinine clearance. Urinalysis and culture are performed to assess for the presence of a urinary tract infection (UTI), which is common in diabetic pregnancy. Because of the risk of coexisting thyroid disease, thyroid function tests may also be performed (see later discussion of thyroid disorders). The **glycosylated hemoglobin A1$_c$** level may be measured to assess recent glycemic control. With prolonged hyperglycemia some of the hemoglobin remains saturated with glucose for the life of the red blood cell (RBC). Therefore, a test for glycosylated hemoglobin provides a "diabetic report card," an evaluation of glycemic control over the previous 4 to 6 weeks. Hemoglobin A1$_c$ levels greater than 6 indicate elevated glucose levels during the previous 4 to 6 weeks (Gilbert, 2011). Fasting blood glucose or random (1 to 2 hours after eating) glucose levels may be assessed during antepartum visits. Self-monitoring blood glucose records may also be reviewed.

Antepartum Care

The presence of risk factors for the mother and her fetus means that the woman with diabetes is monitored more frequently than a woman with a low-risk pregnancy. During the first and second trimesters of pregnancy, her routine prenatal care visits may be scheduled every 1 to 2 weeks. In the last trimester she will likely be seen one or two times each week. Most pregnant women with diabetes are managed on an outpatient basis.

Achieving and maintaining euglycemia (normal blood glucose level; also called *normogylcemia*) with blood glucose levels in the range of 3.4 to 6.7 mmol/L (Table 15-2) is the primary goal of medical therapy for the pregnant woman with diabetes. Euglycemia is achieved through a combination of diet, insulin, exercise, and blood glucose determinations. A primary goal of nursing is to provide the woman with information on the changes to her diabetes management due to pregnancy, to help her achieve and maintain excellent blood glucose control.

Achieving euglycemia requires self-management by the woman and her family to make the necessary lifestyle adjustments, which can sometimes seem overwhelming. Maintaining tight blood glucose control is the primary goal of treatment; the woman needs to be realistic about her schedule of diet, exercise and activity, and insulin administration in order to achieve this goal. Blood glucose is measured frequently to determine how well the major components of therapy (diet, insulin, and exercise) are working together to control blood glucose levels.

Because the woman with diabetes is at risk for infections, eye problems, and neurological changes, foot care and general skin care are important. A daily bath should include good perineal and foot care. Lotions, creams, or oils can be applied to dry skin. The woman should avoid wearing tight clothing. She should always wear shoes or slippers that fit properly, preferably with socks or stockings. Feet should be inspected regularly, toenails should be cut straight across, and professional help should be sought for any foot problems. The woman needs to avoid extremes of temperature.

The woman should wear a medic alert bracelet at all times and carry her glucose meter, insulin, syringes or pens, and food to treat hypoglycemia, such as a fast-acting glucose along with a protein and a starch (see Community Focus box). The woman should be informed of how to report problems such as nausea, vomiting, and infections and should know how to reach her health care provider at all times (see Table 15-1).

Diet. The woman with pregestational diabetes has usually had previous nutrition counselling regarding the management of diabetes. The pregnant woman needs to learn to incorporate changes into dietary planning, as pregnancy precipitates special nutrition concerns and needs. Nutrition counselling is primarily provided by a registered dietitian.

Dietary management during diabetic pregnancy must be based on blood (not urine) glucose levels. The diet is individualized to allow for increased fetal and metabolic requirements, with consideration of such factors as prepregnancy weight and dietary habits, overall health, ethnic background, lifestyle, stage of pregnancy, knowledge of nutrition, and insulin therapy. The dietary goals are to have weight gain consistent with a normal pregnancy, prevent ketoacidosis, and achieve euglycemia through consistency in carbohydrate intake.

TABLE 15-2 TARGET BLOOD GLUCOSE LEVELS DURING PREGNANCY

DURING PREGNANCY	
Fasting and preprandial PG	3.8–5.2 mmol/L
1 hr postprandial PG	5.5–7.7 mmol/L
2 hr postprandial PG	5.0–6.6 mmol/L

PG, plasma glucose.
From Thompson, D., Berger, H., Feig, D., et al. (2013). Clinical practice guidelines: Diabetes and pregnancy. *Canadian Journal of Diabetes, 37*(1), S168–S183.

COMMUNITY FOCUS

Accessibility of Diabetes Supplies

It is very important that health care providers be aware of the realities of the cost and availability of diabetes equipment. Visit the local pharmacy and examine the diabetes equipment and supplies that are available. Locate glucose meters, urine test strips, insulin syringes, and insulin pens. How much does each of these items cost? Read the directions for use of each item. How easy are the instructions to follow? Could a woman with low literacy skills read and understand them? Do the directions have illustrations? Are the directions available in more than one language in addition to English? Does the pharmacy have someone who can teach women? How will this information be helpful in patient teaching?

Energy needs are usually calculated on the basis of 30 to 35 kilocalories per kilogram of ideal body weight, with the average diet including 2200 kilocalories (first trimester) to 2500 kilocalories (second and third trimesters). For obese women with a body mass index (BMI) greater than 30, experts recommend that the caloric intake total 25 kcal/kg/day (Moore et al., 2014). Total calories should be distributed among three meals and at least two snacks. Meals should be eaten on time and never skipped. Going more than 4 hours without food intake increases the risk for episodes of hypoglycemia. Snacks must be carefully planned in accordance with insulin therapy to avoid fluctuations in blood glucose levels. A large bedtime snack of at least 25 g of carbohydrate with some protein is recommended in order to help prevent hypoglycemia and starvation ketosis during the night.

In general, people with diabetes should follow the healthy diet recommended for the general population in *Eating Well With Canada's Food Guide* (see Appendix A). This involves consuming a variety of foods from the four food groups (vegetables and fruits; grain products; milk and alternatives; meat and alternatives), with an emphasis on foods that are low in energy density and high in volume to optimize satiety and discourage overconsumption. This diet will ensure an adequate intake of carbohydrate (CHO), fibre, fat and essential fatty acids, protein, vitamins, and minerals (Thompson et al., 2013) (see Patient Teaching box: Dietary management of diabetic pregnancy). Simple carbohydrates are limited. Complex carbohydrates that are high in fibre content are recommended because the starch and protein in such foods help regulate the blood glucose level by more sustained glucose release (Gilbert, 2011; Moore et al, 2014). Folic acid supplements of 4 mg/day are recommended for 3 months prior to conception and throughout the first trimester to reduce the risk of neural tube defects (Thompson et al., 2013). It is recommended that folic acid supplementation continues until 6 weeks postpartum or as long as breastfeeding continues (Thompson et al., 2013).

Exercise. Although exercise enhances the utilization of glucose and decreases insulin need in nonpregnant women with diabetes, there is limited data regarding exercise during pregnancy for the pregnant woman. Evaluation of current activity levels is done in early pregnancy to help develop a personalized activity plan for the whole pregnancy. The primary health care provider, along with a physiotherapist, will monitor and adjust activity levels to prevent complications. Blood glucose levels are also closely monitored to appropriately adjust insulin intake. For women with vasculopathy, only mild exercise is recommended because exercise causes a redistribution of blood flow, which increases the potential for ischemic injury to the placenta and already compromised organs. Women with vasculopathy typically depend completely on exogenous insulin and are at greater risk for wide fluctuations in blood glucose levels and ketoacidosis, which can be worsened by exercise.

Exercise need not be vigorous to be beneficial: 15 to 30 minutes of walking four to six times a week is satisfactory for most pregnant women. Other exercises that may be recommended include non–weight-bearing activities such as arm ergometry or use of a recumbent bicycle. Musculoskeletal concerns are addressed to enable women to actively participate in their own well-being (see also Patient Teaching box: Exercise Tips for Pregnant Women, in Chapter 11, p. 247).

The best time for exercise is after meals, when the blood glucose level is rising. To monitor the effect of insulin on blood glucose levels, the woman can measure blood glucose before, during, and after exercise.

Monitoring blood glucose levels. Blood glucose testing at home is the most important tool available for assessing the woman's degree of glycemic control. In addition, this monitoring provides feedback on how well her insulin-dose treatment is working. The data obtained facilitate interaction with the health care team in maintaining glycemic control and maximizing pregnancy outcomes (see Patient Teaching box: Testing blood glucose level).

To perform blood glucose monitoring a drop of blood is obtained, usually by means of a fingerstick, and placed on a test strip. Some newer glucose meters allow the user to obtain the blood sample from the forearm rather than a finger. After a specified amount of time the glucose level is displayed by the meter. Blood glucose levels are routinely measured at various times throughout the day, such as before breakfast, lunch, and dinner; 2 hours after meals; at bedtime; and in the middle of the night. The primary health care provider or endocrinologist determines the frequency and timing of routine blood glucose assessments for each individual woman.

PATIENT TEACHING

Dietary Management of Diabetic Pregnancy

Follow the Prescribed Diet Plan

- Practise healthy eating for pregnancy based on *Eating Well With Canada's Food Guide.*
- Divide daily food intake between three meals and two to four snacks, depending on individual lifestyle, hunger, blood glucose, ketones, insulin regime, and pregnancy-related factors, such as nausea, vomiting, heartburn, and constipation.
- Eat a substantial bedtime snack to prevent a severe drop in blood glucose level during the night.
- Limit the intake of fats if weight gain occurs too rapidly.
- Take daily vitamins and iron as prescribed by the health care provider. Folic acid supplementation should be 4 mg/day for the first trimester and then decreased to 0.4 mg/day.
- Avoid foods high in refined sugar.
- Eat at a consistent time each day; never skip meals or snacks.
- Reduce the intake of saturated fat and cholesterol.
- Eat foods high in dietary fibre.
- Avoid alcohol and limit caffeine to 300 mg/day.

NURSING ALERT

Hyperglycemia may occur in the 2-hour postprandial values because blood glucose levels peak about 2 hours after a meal.

PATIENT TEACHING

Testing Blood Glucose Level

1. Gather supplies, check expiration date, and read instructions on testing materials. Prepare glucose reflectance meter for use according to manufacturer's directions.
2. Wash hands in warm water (warmth increases circulation).
3. Select site on side of any finger (all fingers should be used in rotation).
4. Pierce site with lancet (may use automatic, spring-loaded, puncturing device). Cleaning the site with alcohol is not necessary.
5. Drop hand down to side; with the other hand, gently squeeze finger from hand to fingertip.
6. Allow blood to drop onto testing strip. Be sure to cover the entire reagent area.
7. Determine blood glucose value using the glucose reflectance meter, following manufacturer's instructions.
8. Record results.
9. Repeat as instructed by health care provider and as needed for signs of hypoglycemia or hyperglycemia.

Source: Canadian Diabetes Care Guide. (2010). *Monitoring blood glucose.* Retrieved from http://www.diabetescareguide.com

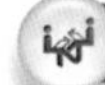

PATIENT TEACHING

What to Do When Illness Occurs

Continue to Take Insulin

- Be sure to take insulin even though appetite and food intake may be less than normal. (Insulin needs are increased with illness or infection.)

Contact Your Health Care Provider

- Call your health care provider and relay the following information:
  - Symptoms of illness (e.g., nausea, vomiting, diarrhea)
  - Fever
  - Most recent blood glucose level
  - Urine ketones
  - Time and amount of last insulin dose

Take Preventive Measures

- Increase oral intake of fluids to prevent dehydration.
- Rest as much as possible.

Seek Emergency Treatment if Needed

- If you are unable to reach your health care provider and blood glucose exceeds 11.0 mmol/L with urine ketones present, seek emergency treatment at the nearest health care facility. Do not attempt to self-treat.

Special circumstances may require more frequent testing. Women are instructed to check glucose levels at any sign of hypoglycemia or hyperglycemia. When there is any readjustment in insulin dosage or diet, more frequent measurement of blood glucose is warranted. If nausea, vomiting, or diarrhea occurs or if any illness is present, the woman will have to monitor her blood glucose levels more closely.

Target levels of blood glucose during pregnancy are lower than nonpregnant values. Acceptable fasting levels are generally between 3.8 and 5.2 mmol/L, and 2-hour postprandial levels should be less than 6.7 mmol/L (see Table 15-2) (Thompson et al., 2013). The woman should be told to report episodes of hypoglycemia (less than 3.2 mmol/L) and hyperglycemia (greater than 11 mmol/L) to her health care provider immediately so that adjustments in diet or insulin therapy can be made.

Pregnant women with diabetes are much more likely to develop hypoglycemia than hyperglycemia because the goal of therapy is to maintain the blood glucose in a narrow, low-normal range of 3.8 to 5.2 mmol/L. Although a blood glucose level greater than 6.7 mmol/L is considered too high for a pregnant woman, it will not produce the classic signs and symptoms of hyperglycemia. However, many women will have signs and symptoms of hypoglycemia with blood glucose levels below 3.8 mmol/L.

Most episodes of mild or moderate hypoglycemia can be treated with oral intake of 10 to 15 g of simple carbohydrates (see Box 15-1). If severe hypoglycemia occurs in which the woman experiences a decrease in or loss of consciousness or an inability to swallow, she will require a parenteral injection of glucagon or intravenous (IV) glucose (see Table 15-1). Because hypoglycemia can develop rapidly and impaired judgement can be associated with even moderate episodes, it is vital that family members, friends, and work colleagues be able to recognize signs and symptoms quickly and initiate proper treatment, if necessary.

Although hyperglycemia is less likely to occur, it is still a dangerous complication. Hyperglycemia can rapidly progress to DKA. Women and their family members should be alert for signs and symptoms of hyperglycemia, especially when infections or other illnesses occur (see Patient Teaching box: What to do when illness occurs).

Insulin therapy. All type 1 and almost all type 2 diabetic women will use insulin during pregnancy. Adequate insulin is the primary factor in the maintenance of euglycemia during pregnancy, thus ensuring proper glucose metabolism of the woman and fetus. Insulin requirements during pregnancy change dramatically as the pregnancy progresses, necessitating frequent adjustments in the dose.

Women with type 2 diabetes who were on oral antihyperglycemic diabetic agents must switch to insulin, as currently these agents are not recommended in pregnancy by the CDA (Thompson et al., 2013) because of an increased risk of perinatal mortality and pre-eclampsia. Insulin therapy must be individualized and adjusted to ensure proper glucose metabolism of the mother and fetus.

The goal of administration of exogenous insulin during pregnancy is to achieve diurnal glucose levels that are similar to those of a nondiabetic pregnant woman. The insulin regimen for a pregnant woman will differ from that which was effective in the nonpregnant state in combinations and timing of insulin injections (Landon et al., 2012). Thus, for the woman with type 1 pregestational diabetes who has typically been accustomed to one injection per day of intermediate-acting insulin, multiple daily injections of mixed insulin are a new experience. Many women with type 1 diabetes use insulin pumps. An insulin pump is a small device worn at waist level that has a reservoir filled with short-acting insulin. The purpose of the pump is to provide continuous adjustment to blood glucose levels and needs for insulin. Women require education to adjust their insulin dosages according to pregnancy needs.

The woman with type 2 diabetes previously treated with oral hypoglycemic agents is faced with the task of learning to self-administer injections of insulin. The nurse can be instrumental in providing education and support regarding insulin administration and the adjustment of insulin dosage to maintain euglycemia.

Since 1982 most insulin preparations have been produced by inserting portions of DNA ("recombinant DNA") into special laboratory-cultivated bacteria or yeast cells. The cells then produce synthetic human insulin (Humulin), which is less likely to cause antibody formation than animal-derived (beef or pork) insulin. More recently, insulin products called *insulin analogs,* in which the structure differs slightly from that of human insulin, have been produced. This small alteration in insulin structure results in changes in the onset and peak of action of the medication. The most commonly used insulin preparations include rapid-acting, short-acting, intermediate-acting, and long-acting (Landon et al., 2012) (Table 15-3). Mixtures of short- and intermediate-acting insulins in several proportions are also available.

Lispro (Humalog) and aspart (NovoRapid) are commonly prescribed rapid-acting insulins with a shorter duration of action than that of regular insulin. They are preferred for use during pregnancy (Landon et al., 2012). Advantages of rapid-acting insulins include convenience because they are injected immediately before mealtime, less hyperglycemia after meals, and fewer hypoglycemic episodes in some people. Because their effects last only 3 to 5 hours, most patients require a longer-acting insulin in addition to the rapid-acting insulin to maintain optimal blood glucose levels (Landon et al., 2012; Moore et al., 2014) (see Table 15-3). Glargine (Lantus) is long-acting insulin lasting approximately 24 hours. Small amounts of glargine insulin are released slowly, with no pronounced peak. This preparation is most often used in women who have insulin-resistant diabetes (type 2) requiring high doses of long-acting insulin. Glargine insulin is combined with rapid-acting insulin to prevent hypoglycemia. Glargine insulin appears to be safe for use during pregnancy. When it is administered with rapid-acting or short-acting insulin, unpredictable spikes in insulin levels and resulting hypoglycemia appear to occur less often (Landon et al., 2012) (see Table 15-3). Most women with diabetes manage their insulin with two to three injections per day. Usually, two thirds of the daily insulin dose, with longer-acting (NPH) and short-acting (regular or lispro) insulin combined in a 2 : 1 ratio, is given before breakfast. The remaining one third, again a combination of longer- and short-acting insulin, is administered in the evening before dinner. To reduce the risk of hypoglycemia during the night, separate injections are often administered, with short-acting insulin given before dinner, followed by longer-acting insulin at bedtime. An alternative insulin regimen that works well for some women is to administer short-acting insulin before each meal and longer-acting insulin at bedtime (Landon et al., 2012).

Although subcutaneous insulin injections are most commonly used, increasing numbers of pregnant women are using continuous subcutaneous insulin infusion (CSII) systems. The insulin pump is designed to mimic more closely the function of the pancreas in secreting insulin (Fig. 15-2). This portable, battery-powered device is worn like a pager during most daily activities. The pump infuses rapid-acting insulin (usually lispro) (Landon et al., 2012) at a set basal rate and has the capacity to deliver up to four different basal rates in 24 hours. It also delivers bolus doses of insulin before meals to control postprandial blood glucose levels. A fine-gauge plastic catheter is inserted into subcutaneous tissue, usually in the abdomen, and attached to the pump syringe by connecting tubing. The subcutaneous catheter and connecting tubing are changed every 2 to 3 days. Although the insulin pump is convenient and generally

TABLE 15-3 INSULIN TYPES: EXPECTED TIME OF ACTION

TYPE OF INSULIN	EXAMPLES GENERIC (TRADE) NAME	ONSET OF ACTION	PEAK OF ACTION	DURATION OF ACTION
Rapid-acting	Lispro (Humalog)	10–15 min	1–2 hr	3–5 hr
	Aspart (NovoRapid)	10–15 min	60–90 min	3–5 hr
Short-acting	Humulin R	30 min	2–3 hr	6.5 hr
	Novolin R	30 min	2.5–5 hr	6–8 hr
Intermediate-acting	Humulin N	1–3 hr	5–8 hr	Up to 18 hr
	Novolin NPH	1.5 hr	4–20 hr	24 hr
	Humulin Lente	1–3 hr	6–12 hr	18–24 hr
	Novolin L	2.5 hr	7–15 hr	22 hr
Long-acting	Humulin Ultralente	4–6 hr	8–20 hr	>36 hr
	Glargine (Lantus)	90 min	None	16–24 hr

L, Lente; *NPH* (or *N*), neutral protamine Hagedorn; *R*, regular.
Data from Thompson, D., Berger, H., Feig, D., et al. (2013). Clinical practice guidelines. Diabetes and pregnancy. *Canadian Journal of Diabetes, 37,* S168–S183.

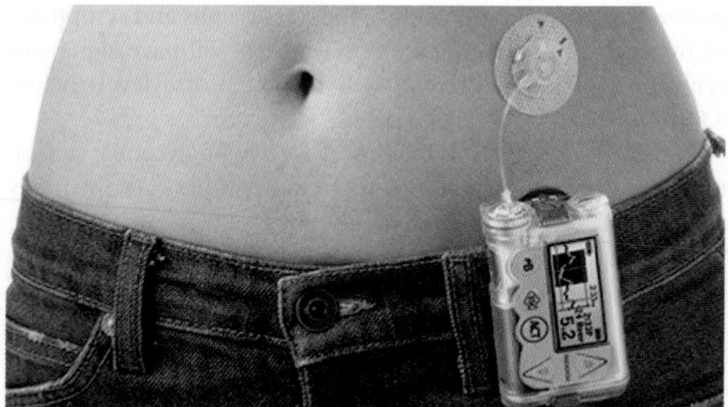

FIGURE 15-2 Insulin pump shows basal rate for pregnant women with diabetes. (MiniMed® Veo Insulin Pump and Continuous Glucose Monitoring System. © 2016 Medtronic.)

provides good glycemic control, complications such as pump failure, precipitation of insulin inside the pump mechanism, abscess formation, and poor uptake from the infusion site can still occur. Use of the insulin pump requires a knowledgeable, motivated patient; skilled health care providers; and 24-hour availability of emergency assistance (Landon et al., 2012).

Complications requiring hospitalization. Occasionally, diabetic women who are pregnant require hospitalization to regulate insulin dosage and stabilize glucose levels. Nursing care during hospitalization provides continuous support and education for regulating insulin therapy and blood glucose. Infection can lead to hyperglycemia and DKA and may require hospitalization, regardless of gestational age. Hospitalization during the third trimester for close maternal and fetal observation may be indicated for women whose diabetes is poorly controlled or who also have hypertension.

Fetal surveillance. Diagnostic techniques for fetal surveillance are often performed to assess fetal growth and well-being. The goals of fetal surveillance are to detect fetal compromise as early as possible and prevent IUFD or unnecessary preterm birth.

Early in pregnancy the estimated date of birth is determined. A baseline ultrasound is obtained during the first trimester to assess gestational age. Follow-up ultrasonography examinations are usually performed during the pregnancy (as often as every 4 to 6 weeks) to monitor fetal growth; estimate fetal weight; and detect hydramnios, macrosomia, and congenital anomalies.

Because the fetus of a woman with diabetes is at increased risk for neural tube defects (e.g., spina bifida, anencephaly, microcephaly), an integrated pregnancy screen (IPS) and detailed ultrasound is performed at 18 to 22 weeks (see Chapter 13).

Fetal echocardiography may be performed between 20 and 22 weeks of gestation to detect cardiac anomalies, especially in women who had poorer glucose control early in pregnancy, as demonstrated by a hemoglobin $A1_c$ level above 6% at the first prenatal visit (Gilbert, 2011; Moore et al., 2014). Doppler studies of the umbilical artery may be performed in women with vascular disease to detect placental compromise.

Most fetal surveillance measures are concentrated in the third trimester, when the risk of fetal compromise is greatest. The goals of antepartum testing during the third trimester are to prevent IUFD and maximize the opportunity for the woman to safely give birth vaginally. Pregnant women who are diabetic should be taught how to do daily fetal movement counts, beginning at 28 weeks of gestation (see Chapter 13) (Moore et al., 2014).

The nonstress test (NST) is the preferred primary method to evaluate fetal well-being. It is usually begun by 32 weeks of gestation and performed at least twice weekly. If the NST is abnormal, a biophysical profile or contraction stress test (oxytocin challenge test) will be performed. Testing often begins earlier, between 28 and 32 weeks of gestation, in women who have vascular disease or poor glucose control (Landon et al., 2012) (see Chapter 13).

Determination of date and mode of delivery. The majority of diabetic pregnancies progress to term (38.5 to 40 weeks of gestation), as long as good metabolic control is maintained and all parameters of antepartum fetal surveillance remain within normal limits. Reasons to consider birth before term include poor metabolic control, worsening hypertensive disorders, fetal macrosomia, prior stillbirth, or fetal growth restriction (Landon et al., 2012).

Induction of labour is often planned between 38 and 40 weeks, provided maternal glucose levels are well controlled. To confirm fetal lung maturity an amniocentesis may be performed when birth will occur before 38.5 weeks of gestation. For the pregnancy complicated by diabetes, fetal lung maturation is better predicted by the amniotic fluid phosphatidylglycerol (greater than 3%) (see Chapter 13). If the fetal lungs are still immature, birth should be postponed as long as the results of fetal assessment remain normal. Induction of labour despite fetal lung maturity may be required on the basis of assessment of fetal compromise or if severe pre-eclampsia, deteriorating vision resulting from proliferative retinopathy, or worsening renal function develops. The involvement of the obstetrical team is critical to making the best decision for each individual woman.

A planned vaginal birth is the preferred mode of birth for women with pregestational diabetes. Caesarean birth should only be performed for obstetrical reasons, such as when antepartum testing suggests a compromised fetal status. Induction of labour may be planned at term for the woman who has well-controlled blood glucose levels.

Intrapartum Care

During the intrapartum period, the woman with pregestational diabetes must be monitored closely to prevent complications related to dehydration, hypoglycemia, and hyperglycemia. Most women use large amounts of energy (kilocalories) to accomplish the work and manage the stress of labour and birth; however, this energy expenditure varies with the individual. Blood glucose levels and hydration must be controlled carefully during labour. An IV line is inserted for infusion of a maintenance fluid such as 5% dextrose in normal saline or lactated Ringer's solution. Insulin is administered by intermittent subcutaneous injection. In women who have difficulty regulating their blood glucose, a continuous insulin infusion may be required. Blood glucose levels are assessed every hour in active labour. Fluids and insulin levels are adjusted to maintain blood glucose levels at between 4 and 7 mmol/L. It is essential that these target glucose levels be maintained because hyperglycemia during labour can cause metabolic problems in the newborn, particularly hypoglycemia (Landon et al., 2012). During labour, continuous fetal heart monitoring is recommended for women who are receiving insulin (Liston, Sawchuck, Young, et al., 2007). Labouring women are encouraged to be mobile in labour; telemetry monitoring can be used to monitor the fetus remotely. Side-lying positions are preferred for the woman labouring in bed, to prevent supine hypotension due to a large fetus or polyhydramnios. Labour progresses without intervention, provided normal rates of cervical dilation, fetal descent, and fetal well-being are maintained. Epidural anaesthesia may be provided to women who require pain relief. Labour dystocia may occur because of a macrosomic infant or cephalopelvic disproportion, necessitating Caesarean birth. Labouring women with diabetes are monitored for diabetic complications, such as hyperglycemia, ketones in the urine, and ketoacidosis. During second-stage labour, the nurse should be alert for the possibility of shoulder dystocia if delivery of a macrosomic infant is attempted and should be prepared to assist with manoeuvres to free the fetal shoulder lodged behind the symphysis pubis (see Chapter 20). Depending on the gestational age of the fetus at birth, a neonatologist or pediatrician may need to be present at the birth to provide neonatal care.

If a Caesarean birth is planned, it should be scheduled in the early morning to facilitate glycemic control. Women should take their full dose of insulin the night before surgery. No morning insulin is given on the day of surgery, and the woman is given nothing by mouth. Regional anaesthesia (epidural or spinal) is recommended because hypoglycemia can be detected earlier if the woman is awake.

Postpartum Care

In the immediate postpartum period, insulin requirements decrease substantially because the major source of insulin resistance, the placenta, has been removed. Women with type 1 diabetes may require only one half the prenatal insulin dose on the first postpartum day, provided that they are eating a full diet. It takes several days after birth to re-establish carbohydrate homeostasis. Blood glucose levels are monitored in the postpartum period, and insulin dosage is adjusted accordingly. Blood glucose levels do not require such tight control after birth. Usually insulin is not given until the blood glucose level is greater than 11.0 mmol/L. Many women with type 2 diabetes do not require insulin at all for the first 1 to 2 days after giving birth, and some women require no insulin in the postpartum period and are able to maintain euglycemia through diet alone or with return to management with oral hypoglycemics (Landon et al., 2012). Women who give birth by Caesarean may require an IV infusion of glucose and insulin until they resume a regular diet (Moore et al., 2014). After birth, several days may be required to re-establish carbohydrate homeostasis (see Fig. 15-1, D and E). Blood glucose levels are monitored carefully in the postpartum period; the insulin dose is adjusted, often using a sliding scale (the amount of insulin to be administered is determined by the woman's blood glucose level at the time the dose is given).

Possible postpartum complications include pre-eclampsia or eclampsia, hemorrhage, and infection. Hemorrhage is a possibility if the mother's uterus was overdistended (by polyhydramnios or a macrosomic fetus) or overstimulated (by oxytocin induction). Postpartum infections such as endometritis are more likely to occur in a woman with diabetes.

Mothers are encouraged to breastfeed. In addition to the advantages of maternal satisfaction, breastfeeding has an anti-diabetogenic effect for the children of women with diabetes and for the women themselves (Moore et al., 2014). This effect is important because a child born to a mother with type 2 diabetes has a 70% chance of also developing type 2 diabetes later in life. In addition, children who were exposed to hyperglycemia prenatally have an increased risk for obesity in childhood (Gilbert, 2011). Infants who are exclusively breastfed are less likely to develop diabetes; exposure to artificial milk products before 8 days of age is an important risk factor for the disease. Breastfeeding has also been shown to reduce childhood obesity and may prevent the onset of type 2 diabetes (Thompson et al., 2013).

The mother may have early breastfeeding difficulties. Poor metabolic control may delay lactogenesis and contribute to decreased milk production. Initial contact and opportunity to breastfeed the infant may be delayed because of institutional practices of separating mothers and babies post-Caesarean or placing infants of mothers with diabetes in special care nurseries for observation during the first few hours after birth. Support and assistance from nursing staff and lactation specialists can facilitate the mother's early experience with breastfeeding and encourage her to continue.

Insulin requirements in breastfeeding women may be one half of prepregnancy levels because of the carbohydrate used in human milk production. Because glucose levels are lower than normal, breastfeeding women are at increased risk for hypoglycemia, especially in the early postpartum period and after breastfeeding sessions, particularly after late-night nursing (Gilbert, 2011; Moore et al., 2014). Breastfeeding mothers with diabetes may be at increased risk for **mastitis** and yeast infections of the breast. Insulin dosage, which is decreased during lactation, must be readjusted at the time of weaning (see Fig. 15-1).

The new mother needs information about family planning and contraception. While family planning is important for all women, it is essential for the woman with diabetes, to safeguard her own health and promote optimal outcomes in future pregnancies. Excellent glucose control at conception is crucial for all women with diabetes; therefore, the importance of conscientiously using a reliable contraceptive method until another pregnancy is desired should be stressed. No one best form of contraception exists for women with diabetes. Emphasis should be placed on consistent use of a reliable and effective birth control method. The risks and benefits of contraceptive methods should be discussed with the mother and her partner before discharge from the hospital.

Barrier methods are often recommended as safe, inexpensive options that have no inherent risks for women with diabetes. The intrauterine device (IUD) may also be used without concerns about an increased risk of infection (Landon et al., 2012).

The use of oral contraceptives is controversial because of the risk of thromboembolic events and vascular complications and the effect on carbohydrate metabolism. In nonsmoking women who are younger than 35 years old and do not have vascular disease, combination low-dose oral contraceptives may be prescribed. Progestin-only oral contraceptives also may be used because they affect carbohydrate metabolism minimally, if at all (Cunningham et al., 2014). Close monitoring of blood pressure and lipid levels is necessary to detect complications (Landon et al., 2012).

Opinion is divided over the use of long-acting parenteral progestins such as medroxyprogesterone (Depo-Provera). Some health care providers recommend their use, especially in women who may have difficulty with daily dosing of oral contraceptives. In contrast, other health care providers believe that this method may adversely affect glycemic control. In addition, although Depo-Provera may lower serum triglyceride and high-density lipoprotein (HDL) cholesterol levels, it does not lower total cholesterol or low-density lipoprotein (LDL) levels. For this reason it is not recommended as a first-choice method of contraception for women with diabetes (Landon et al., 2012).

The transdermal (patch) and transvaginal (vaginal ring) are newer contraceptive methods, particularly effective in women who prefer weekly or every-third-week dosing, respectively. For women weighing more than 90 kg (198 lb) the contraceptive failure rate with transdermal administration is higher than in normal-weight women. Therefore, this method would be contraindicated in obese women. Women who choose the patch as their contraceptive method should have no risk factors for cardiovascular or thromboembolic disease (Cunningham et al., 2014).

The woman and her partner should be informed that the risks associated with pregnancy increase with the duration and severity of the diabetic condition and that pregnancy may contribute to vascular changes associated with diabetes. Thus the option of tubal ligation should be discussed with the woman who has completed her family or who has significant vasculopathy.

Thyroid Disorders

Hyperthyroidism

Hyperthyroidism occurs in approximately 1 of every 1000 to 2000 pregnancies (Cunningham et al., 2014; Mestman, 2012). In 90 to 95% of pregnant women it is caused by Graves' disease or human chorionic gonadotropin (hCG)–mediated hyperthyroidism (Ross, 2014). Other rare but possible causes include functioning adenoma, toxic nodular goitre, excessive thyroid hormone intake, and thyroiditis (Inoue, Arata, Koren, et al., 2009; Mestman, 2012). Clinical symptoms of hyperthyroidism usually begin between 4 and 8 weeks of gestation and often involve severe nausea and vomiting. Because of the timing of the symptoms, hyperemesis gravidarum may be considered as the diagnosis. Careful assessment by the primary care provider is necessary, with blood work that includes thyroid levels, to get an accurate diagnosis. Other symptoms that may be associated with an increased basal metabolic rate and increased sympathetic nervous system activity include fatigue, heat intolerance, warm skin, diaphoresis, anxiety, emotional lability, and tachycardia. Because many of these symptoms are associated with pregnancy, hyperthyroidism can be difficult to diagnose. It is important to differentiate subclinical, mild hyperthyroidism from moderate to severe disease. Women with minimal or mild symptoms—low thyroid stimulating hormone (TSH) and mildly elevated thyroxine (T_4) levels—may be monitored without intervention (Stagnaro-Green, Abalovich, Alexander, et al., 2011). Signs that may help differentiate moderate to severe hyperthyroidism from normal pregnancy symptoms include unplanned weight loss, onycholysis (loose nails), and a pulse rate greater than 100 beats/min (Nader, 2014). Laboratory findings include elevated T_4 levels and triiodothyronine (T_3) levels and greatly suppressed serum TSH levels. The best possible outcomes can be achieved when hyperthyroidism is diagnosed and treated prior to pregnancy. Untreated moderate and severe hyperthyroidism can be detrimental during pregnancy, resulting in infants with low birth weight, intrauterine growth restriction (IUGR), prematurity, stillbirth, goitre, and hyper- or hypothyroidism (Mestman, 2012; Ross, 2014). However, most newborns of women with hyperthyroidism have normal thyroid function. Women with hyperthyroidism are at increased risk of developing severe pre-eclampsia, heart failure, thyroid storm, miscarriage, placental abruption, and infection (Earl, Crowther & Middleton, 2013; Mestman, 2012). Most pregnant women diagnosed with thyroid disease will have received treatment for the condition prior to conception. Generally drug therapy alone is considered for control of hyperthyroidism in pregnancy; radioiodine treatment is not used because of destruction of the fetal thyroid gland, resulting in permanent hypothyroidism in the newborn (Earl et al., 2013).

The treatment options are limited because of the fetal risks of the currently available pharmacological treatments. There are two primary choices of medications to treat hyperthyroidism, propylthiouracil (PTU) and methimazole (MM). In the past, PTU was considered the drug of choice throughout pregnancy for women with hyperthyroidism, as a result of concerns for teratogenicity of MM. More recently, reports of severe PTU-related liver failure have raised concerns about the routine use of PTU, including the use of PTU in pregnancy (Bahn, Burch, Cooper, et al., 2009). As a result, in pregnant women with hyperthyroidism, PTU use is limited to the first trimester only. The teratogenic effects of MM are to be avoided in the first trimester during fetal organogenesis. Women are directed to switch to MM after the first trimester to avoid the potential risk of longer term PTU-associated hepatotoxicity. Thyroid function testing should be performed 2 to 4 weeks after switching to MM to be sure that a euthyroid state has been maintained. Hyperthyroid women treated with MM should be switched to PTU at the time of the positive pregnancy test (Ross, 2014; Stagnaro-Green et al., 2011).

Both medications work well in and are well tolerated by most women. The most common maternal adverse effects of both PTU and MM are pruritus and skin rash. Other possible adverse effects include drug-related fever, bronchospasm, migratory polyarthritis, a lupus-like syndrome, and cholestatic jaundice (Mestman, 2012; Nader, 2014). The most severe adverse effect is agranulocytosis, which occurs rarely and usually develops only in older women and in those taking high doses of the drug. Symptoms of agranulocytosis are fever and unexpected sore throat, which should be reported immediately to the health care provider; the woman should stop taking the medication (Cunningham et al., 2014; Mestman, 2012; Nader, 2014).

Beta-adrenergic blockers such as propranolol or atenalol may be used in women with severe hyperthyroidism symptoms. Long-term use is not recommended because of the potential for IUGR and altered response to anoxic stress, postnatal bradycardia, and hypoglycemia (Ross, 2014).

If a mother taking hyperthyroid medication chooses to breastfeed, she needs to be aware that physiologically significant doses of the medication are passed to the infant through the breast milk. The infant's thyroid status should be monitored periodically so that newborn hypothyroidism can be prevented.

In severe cases, hyperthyroidism may be treated surgically with subtotal thyroidectomy during the second or third trimester. Because of the increased risk of miscarriage and preterm labour associated with major surgery, this treatment is usually reserved for women with severe disease, those for whom medication therapy proves toxic, and those who are unable to manage the prescribed medical regimen. Risks associated with the surgery are hypoparathyroidism, recurrent laryngeal nerve paralysis, and anaesthesia-related complications (Nader, 2014). Postoperative hypothyroidism is common, occurring in at least 20% of women with hyperthyroidism.

! NURSING ALERT

A serious but uncommon complication of undiagnosed or partially treated hyperthyroidism is thyroid storm, which may occur in response to stresses such as infection, pre-eclampsia, birth, or surgery. Symptoms of this rare condition include sudden fever, restlessness, tachycardia, vomiting, hypotension, or stupor. Heart failure may also occur. Prompt treatment is essential to ensure a good maternal outcome; IV fluids and oxygen are administered along with high doses of PTU. Potassium iodide, antipyretics, glucocorticoids, and beta-adrenergic blockers may also be given; sedation may be necessary for extreme restlessness (Cunningham et al., 2014; Mestman, 2012; Nader, 2014).

Hypothyroidism

Hypothyroidism is diagnosed in 2.2 to 2.5% of pregnant women. The TSH levels are high (above 6 mU/L), often caused by an underactive thyroid (hypothyroidism) (Sutander, Garcia-Bournissen, & Koren, 2007). Hypothyroidism is usually the result of Hashimoto's disease (autoimmune thyroiditis), thyroid gland ablation by radiation, previous surgery, or not taking enough antithyroid medications. Iodine deficiency in women living in developed countries is rare (Mestman, 2012; Nader, 2014), but in the rest of the world, the most common cause of thyroid problems is iodine deficiency. Symptomatic pregnant women should be screened for the presence of hypothyroidism (De Groot, Abalovich, Alexander, et al., 2012). Untreated hypothyroidism may result in poor obstetrical maternal and fetal outcomes: pre-eclampsia, low birth weight, placental abruption, spontaneous pregnancy loss, and perinatal morbidity (Sutander et al., 2007).

Characteristic symptoms of hypothyroidism include maternal fatigue, weight gain, cold intolerance, decrease in exercise capacity, constipation, cool and dry skin, coarsened hair, and muscle weakness. Laboratory findings during pregnancy include elevated levels of TSH, with or without low T_4 levels (American College of Obstetricians and Gynecologists [ACOG], 2015; Nader, 2014).

Diagnosis and treatment of pregnant women with overt hypothyroidism is important, as thyroid deficiency has been shown to cause impaired neurological development during early fetal development. The fetus is dependent on the maternal transfer of thyroid hormones, specifically T_4. If the mother is iodine deficient, fetal brain development can be impaired. Infants born to mothers with hypothyroidism may be of low birth weight and may be at risk for further cognitive deficits if born premature. Women with subclinical hypothyroidism have not been shown to have adverse pregnancy outcomes and therefore do not require treatment (ACOG, 2015).

Thyroid hormone supplements are used to treat hypothyroidism. Levothyroxine (e.g., T_4 [Synthroid]) is the treatment of choice for treatment of hypothyroidism during pregnancy (Sutander et al., 2007). Levothyroxine is considered safe and is not **teratogenic**.

As pregnancy progresses, the woman requires increased amounts of thyroid replacement hormone, usually increasing dosing up by 50% (Sutander et al., 2007). The aim of drug therapy is to maintain the TSH level at the lower end of the normal range for pregnant women. Women with little or no functioning thyroid tissue require higher doses of levothyroxine. In addition, as pregnancy progresses increased doses of thyroid hormone are usually required. This increased demand during pregnancy is probably related to increased estrogen levels (Cunningham et al., 2014; Nader, 2014). Because of increased absorption in the small intestine, taking the medication on an empty stomach is recommended. Prenatal vitamins may inhibit absorption of thyroid replacements because of the presence of iron and calcium (Sutander et al., 2007). Taking prenatal vitamins at least 4 hours after taking a thyroid replacement hormone is recommended.

! NURSING ALERT

Pregnant women should be told to take thyroid replacement hormone 4 hours before or after iron tablets because ferrous sulphate lowers the effectiveness of the medication (Nader, 2014).

The fetus depends on maternal thyroid hormones until 18 weeks of gestation, when fetal production begins. Normal maternal T_4 levels early in pregnancy are important for proper fetal brain development. Studies have shown that there may be an association between mild maternal hypothyroidism during the first trimester with impaired neurodevelopment in their children, but more research needs to be conducted on this topic (ACOG, 2015; Mestman, 2012).

NURSING CARE

A pregnant woman with thyroid dysfunction requires education to ensure the best outcomes for herself and her fetus. This education should include information about the disorder and its potential impact on her and her fetus, the medication regimen and possible adverse effects, the need for continuing medical supervision, and the importance of maintaining consistent levels of thyroid hormone. The family should be incorporated into the plan of care, to foster support among the members.

The woman often needs the nurse's help to cope with the discomforts and frustrations associated with symptoms of the disorder. For example, the woman with hyperthyroidism who has nervousness and hyperactivity along with weakness and fatigue can benefit from suggestions to channel excess energies into quiet diversional activities such as reading or crafts. Discomfort associated with hypersensitivity to heat (hyperthyroidism) or cold intolerance (hypothyroidism) can be minimized by wearing appropriate clothing, regulating environmental temperatures, and avoiding temperature extremes, when possible.

Nutrition counselling with a registered dietitian is an important component of management of symptoms. The woman with hyperthyroidism who has increased appetite and poor weight gain and the hypothyroid woman who has anorexia and lethargy need counselling to ensure adequate intake of nutritionally sound foods to meet both maternal and fetal needs.

CARDIOVASCULAR DISORDERS

The major cardiovascular changes that occur during a normal pregnancy and affect the woman with cardiac disease are increased intravascular volume, decreased systemic vascular resistance, cardiac output changes occurring during labour and birth, and the intravascular volume changes that occur just after childbirth. The strain is present during pregnancy and continues after birth. The normal heart can compensate for the increased workload so pregnancy, labour, and birth are generally well tolerated; but the diseased heart is hemodynamically challenged.

If the cardiovascular changes are not well tolerated, cardiac failure can develop during pregnancy, labour, or the postpartum period. In addition, if myocardial disease develops, valvular disease exists, or a congenital heart defect is present, cardiac decompensation (inability of the heart to maintain a sufficient cardiac output) may occur. Fever and infection are the major causes of cardiac decompensation during pregnancy (Easterling & Stout, 2012).

From 0.5 to 4% of pregnancies are complicated by heart disease. Cardiac disorders are one of the most important nonobstetrical causes of maternal mortality (Davies & Herbert, 2007a; Gaddipati & Troiano, 2013). Currently, cardiomyopathy and congenital heart disease are the major causes of cardiac disease in pregnant women (Gaddipati & Troiano, 2013). Thanks to better management of congenital heart disease in childhood, pregnancy outcomes for women with these conditions are generally positive. However, cardiac disease accounts for 15% of maternal mortality during pregnancy (Gilbert, 2011). Box 15-2 lists maternal cardiac disease risk groups and their related mortality rates. Pregnancy is not advised in women who have the following cardiac conditions: pulmonary hypertension, Marfan syndrome with aortic involvement, and Eisenmenger syndrome, because the associated maternal mortality rate is extremely high, up to 50% (Easterling & Stout, 2012; Gaddipati & Troiano, 2013).

The degree of disability experienced by the woman with cardiac disease is often more important in the treatment and

BOX 15-2 MATERNAL CARDIAC DISEASE RISK GROUPS

Group 1 (Mortality Rate <1%)
Atrial and ventricular septal defects (uncomplicated)
Patent ductus arteriosus (uncomplicated)
Corrected tetralogy of Fallot
Pulmonic/tricuspid disease
Mitral stenosis or aortic regurgitation (NYHA class I and II)
Bioprosthetic valve
Mitral valve prolapsed with regurgitation

Group II (Mortality Rate 5 to 20%)
Aortic stenosis
Coarctation of aorta without valve involvement
Artificial heart valves
Mitral stenosis (NYHA class III and IV) or with atrial fibrillation
Uncorrected tetralogy of Fallot
Previous myocardial infarction
Marfan syndrome with normal aorta

Group III (Mortality Rate 25 to 50%)
Pulmonary hypertension
Coarctation of the aorta with valvular involvement
Complicated Marfan syndrome with aortic involvement
Endocarditis
Eisenmenger Syndrome
Peripartum cardiomyopathy with persistent left ventricular dysfunction

From Gaddipati, S., & Troiano, N. H. (2013). Cardiac disorders in pregnancy. In N. H. Troiano, C. J. Harvey, & B. F. Chez (Eds.), *AWHONN's high risk and critical care obstetrics* (3rd ed.). Philadelphia: Lippincott Williams and Wilkins; Gilbert, E. S. (2011). Cardiac disease. In E. S. Gilbert (Ed.), *Manual of high risk pregnancy and delivery* (5th ed.). St. Louis: Mosby.

prognosis during pregnancy than the diagnosis of the type of cardiovascular disease. The New York Heart Association (NYHA) functional classification of heart disease is a widely accepted standard:

- Class I: Asymptomatic without limitation of physical activity
- Class II: Symptomatic with slight limitation of activity
- Class III: Symptomatic with marked limitation of activity
- Class IV: Symptomatic with inability to carry on any physical activity without discomfort

The NYHA classification system is a clear, practical guide for cardiac classification that can inform appropriate obstetrical care. Medical therapy is provided by a team approach that includes the woman, cardiologist, obstetrician, anaesthesiologist, and nurses. The functional classification may change for the pregnant woman because of the hemodynamic changes that occur in the cardiovascular system. A 30 to 45% increase in cardiac output occurs compared with nonpregnancy resting values, with most of the increase occurring in the first trimester and the peak at 20 to 26 weeks of gestation (Blanchard & Daniels, 2014). The functional classification of the disease is determined at 3 months and again at 7 or 8 months of gestation. Pregnant women may progress from class I or II to III or IV during pregnancy as cardiac output increases and more stress is placed on the heart.

Miscarriage and stillbirth both occur more often in the pregnant woman with cardiac problems than in healthy women. In addition, IUGR is common, probably because of low oxygen pressure in the mother (Blanchard & Daniels, 2014).

The two broad categories of cardiac disease are congenital and acquired. The incidence of acquired disease (e.g., rheumatic heart disease) is decreasing in developed countries. Pregnant women with congenital cardiac disease are increasing in number because of advances in childhood treatment (Davies & Herbert, 2007b).

Congenital Cardiac Diseases

Congenital heart disease is classified as acyanotic or cyanotic. Women at increased risk for a cardiac event in pregnancy include those with a prior cardiac event or arrhythmia, NYHA functional class greater than II, or cyanosis, left heart obstruction, and systemic ventricular dysfunction.

Acyanotic Cardiac Lesions

Atrial septal defect. Atrial septal defect (ASD) is an abnormal opening between the atria. It is one of the causes of a left-to-right shunt and one of the most common congenital defects seen during pregnancy (Gaddipati & Troiano, 2013). This defect may go undetected because the woman is usually asymptomatic. The pregnant woman with an ASD usually has an uncomplicated pregnancy. However, some women may develop heart failure or arrhythmias as the pregnancy progresses as a result of increased plasma volume. Another possible complication is the development of emboli (blood clots) (Gaddipati & Troiano, 2013).

Ventricular septal defect. Ventricular septal defect (VSD), an abnormal opening between the right and left ventricles, is another cause of a left-to-right shunt (see Box 47-1). It may occur as a single lesion or in combination with other cardiac anomalies such as tetralogy of Fallot. The defect is usually diagnosed and corrected early in life. As a result, a VSD is not very common in pregnancy. Women with small, uncomplicated VSDs usually do not have pregnancy complications. For women with a large VSD, there is a higher risk for heart failure or pulmonary hypertension. Medical management includes administration of anticoagulants if indicated, along with rest and decreased physical activity (Gaddipati & Troiano, 2013).

Patent ductus arteriosus. This condition is rarely seen in adults, as most people with a patent ductus arteriosus (PDA) have it corrected as a newborn or as a child (see Box 47-1). Women with a corrected PDA do well in pregnancy and women with an uncorrected PDA who have a small to moderate size ductus and who have normal pulmonary arterial pressures are likely to experience few or no complications with pregnancy related to their cardiac defect (Davies & Herbert, 2007b). However, when there is more extensive left-to-right shunting, the hemodynamic changes in pregnancy can result in Eisenmenger syndrome, which results in high morbidity and mortality for both the mother and fetus. Women in this situation are often encouraged to terminate the pregnancy.

Coarctation of the aorta. Coarctation of the aorta is a localized narrowing of the aorta near the insertion of the ductus (Box 47-2). Patients with this lesion have hypertension in their upper extremities but hypotension in the lower extremities. If at all possible, the lesion should be corrected surgically before pregnancy. However, pregnancy is usually relatively safe for the woman with uncomplicated, uncorrected coarctation. The maternal mortality rate is approximately 0 to 3% (Blanchard & Daniels, 2014). Complications that can occur include hypertension, heart failure, cerebrovascular accident (stroke), aortic dissection, and rupture of associated aneurysms (Blanchard & Daniels, 2014; Easterling & Stout, 2012), although these are rare. The mainstays of treatment for uncorrected coarctation of the aorta during pregnancy are rest and antihypertensive medications, preferably beta-adrenergic blocking agents. Some authorities recommend Caesarean birth to prevent blood pressure elevations during second-stage labour that could possibly lead to rupture of the aorta or cerebral blood vessels. However, vaginal birth is usually recommended, with Caesarean birth performed only for obstetrical indications. If bacteremia is suspected, antibiotic prophylaxis is given during labour and birth (Cunningham et al., 2014).

Marfan syndrome. Marfan syndrome is an autosomal dominant condition characterized by generalized weakness of the connective tissue, resulting in the characteristic feature of the disease, aortic wall and root dilation. Other signs and symptoms associated with Marfan syndrome include dislocation of the optic lens, deformity of the anterior thorax, scoliosis, long limbs, joint laxity, and arachnodactyly. Diagnosis is usually based on family history and physical examination, including ocular, cardiovascular, and skeletal features (Easterling & Stout, 2012).

Mortality rates for women with Marfan syndrome have been reported as high as 50%; however, women with dilation of the aortic root of 40 mm or less have a mortality rate of less than 5% (Davies & Herbert, 2007b; Easterling & Stout, 2012). Approximately 90% of these women have mitral valve prolapse, and 25% have aortic insufficiency with an increased risk of aortic dissection and rupture during pregnancy and birth. Excruciating chest pain and cardiac decompensation are the first signs of aortic rupture, which can occur primarily in the third trimester or the postpartum period.

Preconception counselling for women with Marfan syndrome is essential to make women aware of the risks of pregnancy with this disease. An accurate assessment of the aortic root using noninvasive imaging with transesophageal echocardiography, computed tomography, or magnetic resonance imaging must be obtained to assess the woman's specific risk and make management recommendations. Elective repair of the aorta is recommended when the aortic root diameter measures 5.5 to 6 cm. Therefore, women with an aortic root diameter greater than 5.5 cm should be counselled to have it repaired before becoming pregnant. On the other hand, women with an aortic root diameter less than 4 cm can attempt pregnancy with only modest risk (Easterling & Stout, 2012). Because the condition is inherited, each child born to a woman with Marfan syndrome has a 50% chance of having the disorder (Gaddipati & Troiano, 2013).

Therapy includes limiting of physical activity, prevention of hypertensive or hypotensive complications, and administration of beta-blockers as needed to maintain a resting heart rate of approximately 70 beats/min. Tachycardia should also be prevented during labour. Women with aortic root diameters less than 4 cm can give birth vaginally, reserving Caesarean birth for obstetrical indications. Some authorities believe that women with larger aortic root diameters should give birth by elective Caesarean because of concerns about increased pressure in the aorta during labour. However, data do not exist to make this a firm recommendation (Blanchard & Daniels, 2014; Easterling & Stout, 2012).

Pulmonic stenosis. Women with severe pulmonic stenosis (see Box 15-2) are encouraged to have surgical correction before pregnancy in order to improve their outcomes of pregnancy (Davies & Herbert, 2007b). As with other cardiac disorders, women with mild-to-moderate disease do well in pregnancy; however, those with severe disease have a higher risk of right-sided heart failure, resulting in higher rates of pregnancy loss and poor maternal outcomes.

Cyanotic Congenital Cardiac Lesions

Tetralogy of Fallot. Tetralogy of Fallot is by far the most common cyanotic heart disease observed during pregnancy (Blanchard & Daniels, 2014). Components of tetralogy of Fallot include a VSD; pulmonary stenosis; overriding aorta; and right ventricular hypertrophy leading to a right-to-left shunt (see Box 47-3). Women with tetralogy of Fallot are encouraged to have surgical repair preconceptionally because pregnancy does not cause a significant risk once the VSD and pulmonary stenosis have been repaired (Gaddipati & Troiano, 2013). Women with uncorrected tetralogy of Fallot experience more right-to-left shunting during pregnancy, resulting in reduced blood flow through the pulmonary circulation and increasing hypoxemia, which can cause syncope or death (Davies & Herbert, 2007b; Gaddipati & Troiano, 2013). Maintenance of venous return in women with uncorrected tetralogy of Fallot is critical. Therefore, the most dangerous time for these women is the late third trimester of pregnancy and the early postpartum period, when venous return is reduced by the large pregnant uterus and peripheral venous pooling after birth. Use of pressure-graded support hose is recommended. Blood loss during birth may also adversely affect venous return; thus blood volume must be adequately maintained. Prophylactic antibiotics should be given during the intrapartum period (Blanchard & Daniels, 2014).

As with all newborns born to mothers with congenital heart disease, they must be tested for the presence or absence of the cardiac lesion present in their mothers.

Eisenmenger syndrome. Eisenmenger syndrome is a right-to-left or bidirectional shunting that can be at the atrial or ventricular level and is combined with elevated pulmonary vascular resistance. It is associated with an underlying structural cardiac defect, either a VSD (most common) or a PDA (Blanchard & Daniels, 2014). Eisenmenger syndrome is associated with high mortality (50% in mothers and 50% in fetuses). Because of the poor pregnancy outcomes, pregnancy should be avoided by women with the syndrome. Termination may be recommended if pregnancy occurs (Gaddipati & Troiano, 2013). Although sudden death can occur at any time, the intrapartum and early postpartum periods seem to be the most dangerous (Blanchard & Daniels, 2014). Maternal morbidity is associated with right ventricular failure and associated cardiogenic shock (Cunningham et al., 2014). In women who continue pregnancy despite the risks, management includes measures to maintain pulmonary blood flow. Physical activity is strictly limited. Other interventions include the use of pressure-graded elastic support hose and oxygen therapy. Antepartal hospitalization may be necessary to provide optimal care (Blanchard & Daniels, 2014; Davies & Herbert, 2007b). During labour and birth, narcotic-based regional anaesthesia provides pain relief without causing excessive hemodynamic instability. Hypotension must be prevented at all costs because it results in more right-to-left shunting, thereby increasing hypoxemia, increasing pulmonary vascular resistance, and worsening the shunt. Volume overload or excessive systemic resistance must also be prevented because it further stresses the failing right side of the heart. Caesarean birth should be performed only for obstetrical indications and avoided whenever possible (Easterling & Stout, 2012). A team approach involving a perinatologist, skilled critical care and perinatal nurses, and cardiology and anaesthesia care providers is essential.

Primary pulmonary hypertension. Women with primary pulmonary hypertension have constriction of the arteriolar vessels in the lungs, leading to an increase in the pulmonary artery pressure. As a result of this pathology, there is right ventricular hypertension, right ventricular hypertrophy and dilation, and right ventricular failure with tricuspid regurgitation and systemic congestion. The major physiological difficulty in primary pulmonary hypertension is maintaining blood flow to the lungs. Any event that significantly decreases venous return to the heart, such as hypotension, impairs the ability of the right ventricle to pump blood through the pulmonary vessels with their high, fixed vascular resistance. Because hypotension can occur quickly and is often unresponsive to medical therapy, it must be avoided at all costs (Blanchard & Daniels, 2014).

Symptoms may be nonspecific, such as fatigue and shortness of breath. Dyspnea on exertion is the most common symptom (Cunningham et al., 2014).

Primary pulmonary hypertension is diagnosed by electrocardiography. The diagnosis is confirmed by right-sided cardiac catheterization, which may be deferred during pregnancy (Cunningham et al., 2014). Mortality rates reported during pregnancy are as high as 50%; thus pregnancy is not advised in women with this condition (Blanchard & Daniels, 2014; Davies & Herbert, 2007b). The most dangerous times for these women are the intrapartum and early postpartum periods because of increases in cardiac output and fluid shifts.

Medical management of primary pulmonary hypertension during pregnancy includes limiting activity and avoiding supine positioning. Diuretics, supplemental oxygen, and vasodilator medications are also ordered. During labour and birth, hypotension must be avoided by carefully establishing epidural analgesia and preventing blood loss (Cunningham et al., 2014).

Acquired Cardiac Disease

Mitral Valve Stenosis

Mitral stenosis is almost always caused by rheumatic heart disease (RHD), a consequence of rheumatic fever (Easterling & Stout, 2012). Rheumatic fever develops suddenly, often several symptom-free weeks after an inadequately treated group A beta-hemolytic streptococcal throat infection. Episodes of rheumatic fever create an autoimmune reaction in the heart tissue, leading to permanent damage of heart valves (usually the mitral valve) and the chordae tendineae cordis. This damage is classified as RHD. RHD may be evident during acute rheumatic fever or discovered years later. Recurrences of rheumatic fever are common, each with the potential to increase the severity of heart damage.

Mitral valve stenosis (narrowing of the opening of the mitral valve caused by stiffening of valve leaflets, thereby obstructing blood flow from the atrium to the ventricles) is the characteristic lesion often resulting from RHD. As the mitral valve narrows, cardiac output decreases and dyspnea worsens, occurring first on exertion and eventually at rest. A tight stenosis plus the increase in blood volume and required cardiac output demands of normal pregnancy and birth may cause pulmonary edema, atrial fibrillation, right-sided heart failure, ineffective endocarditis, pulmonary embolism, and massive hemoptysis (Blanchard & Daniels, 2014; Cunningham et al., 2014). Approximately 25% of women with mitral valve stenosis may become symptomatic for the first time during pregnancy. Maternal mortality is related to functional capacity. Almost all maternal deaths related to mitral stenosis occur in women who are classified as NYHA class III or IV (Cunningham et al., 2014). Women with mild-to-moderate stenosis usually tolerate pregnancy well (Davies & Herbert, 2007b).

Women with a history of RHD who are at risk for exposure to streptococcal infection should receive prophylaxis with daily oral penicillin G or monthly benzathine penicillin (Bicillin) injections. Pregnant women are usually considered at high risk for exposure because they generally live around groups of children (Easterling & Stout, 2012). Women with mitral stenosis may require diuretics such as furosemide (Lasix) to prevent pulmonary edema and beta blockers or calcium channel blockers to prevent tachycardia (Easterling & Stout, 2012). Cardioversion may be needed for new-onset atrial fibrillation, a complication associated with mitral stenosis. Women who have chronic atrial fibrillation may need digoxin or beta blockers to control the heart rate. In addition, anticoagulant therapy may be needed to prevent embolism (Blanchard & Daniels, 2014).

The care of the woman with mitral stenosis is typically managed by reducing her activity, restricting dietary sodium, and increasing bedrest, in addition to the pharmacological management discussed previously (Cunningham et al., 2014). The pregnant woman with mitral stenosis should be monitored clinically for symptoms and with echocardiography to assess the atrial and ventricular size and heart valve function. Prophylaxis for intrapartum endocarditis and pulmonary infections may be given to women at high risk (Blanchard & Daniels, 2014; Easterling & Stout, 2012).

Intrapartum care for women with severe disease includes invasive hemodynamic monitoring during labour and birth, with a goal toward maintaining adequate ventricular filling and cardiac output (Davies & Herbert, 2007c). During labour, adequate pain control is required to prevent tachycardia. Epidural analgesia for labour is preferred (Easterling & Stout, 2012). The woman should be encouraged to labour and give birth in the lateral decubitus position and avoid the supine and lithotomy positions. Shortening the second stage of labour by vacuum- or forceps-assisted birth is also important, to decrease the cardiac workload. Caesarean birth should be performed only for obstetrical indications. Aggressive diuresis is initiated immediately after birth because fluid shifts can place the woman at risk for pulmonary edema (Blanchard & Daniels, 2014; Easterling & Stout, 2012). Management by skilled providers who are alert to the signs of cardiac decompensation is critical.

For women with NYHA class III or IV cardiac disease, surgical intervention may be necessary. Valve replacement and open commissurotomy have been performed successfully during pregnancy. Currently balloon valvotomy is likely to be the procedure of choice. Surgical intervention should be considered only when symptoms cannot be controlled by medical therapy (Easterling & Stout, 2012). Balloon valvuloplasty is optimally performed after 20 weeks of gestation to decrease radiation risks to the fetus.

Aortic Stenosis

Aortic stenosis is a narrowing of the opening of the aortic valve leading to an obstruction to left ventricular ejection. It is rarely encountered as a complication of pregnancy because most women who develop this condition do so after their childbearing years are over. In the past, the maternal mortality rate was reported to be as high as 17%, but it has decreased over the last several decades (Easterling & Stout, 2012). Medical management is similar to that for mitral stenosis.

Mitral Valve Prolapse

Mitral valve prolapse (MVP) is a common, usually benign condition occurring in 1% of women (Blanchard & Daniels, 2014). In MVP the mitral valve leaflets prolapse into the left atrium during ventricular systole, allowing some backflow of blood. Midsystolic click and late systolic murmur are hallmarks of this syndrome. Most cases are asymptomatic. A few women have atypical chest pain (sharp and located in the left side of the chest) that occurs at rest, is unrelated to exercise, and does not respond to nitrates. They may have anxiety, palpitations, dyspnea on exertion, and syncope. If women are symptomatic, beta-blocking drugs are given to relieve chest pain and palpitations and reduce the risk of life-threatening arrhythmias (Cunningham et al., 2014). If symptoms are unusually severe, thyroid function should also be checked (Blanchard & Daniels, 2014). Pregnancy and its associated hemodynamic changes may change or alleviate the murmur and click of MVP as well as its symptoms. Pregnancy is usually well tolerated; but, as with RHD, antibiotic prophylaxis may be given before invasive procedures for at-risk patients and for complicated vaginal births in patients with MVP (Cunningham et al., 2014; Easterling & Stout, 2012).

Myocardial Infarction

Myocardial infarction (MI), an acute ischemic event, rarely occurs in women of child-bearing age. It is estimated to occur in only 1 of 10,000 pregnancies (Blanchard & Daniels, 2014; Davies & Herbert, 2007d). However, authorities anticipate that the incidence will rise, considering the number of women who delay child-bearing until later in life (Gaddipati & Troiano, 2013). Frequently women with coronary artery disease have classic risk factors such as diabetes, hypertension, cigarette smoking, hyperlipidemia, and obesity (Cunningham et al., 2014; Davies & Herbert, 2007d). The cardiac changes that normally occur in a pregnant woman may provoke symptoms for the first time. It is also possible for women with a history of MI to become pregnant (Gaddipati & Troiano, 2013).

MI occurs most frequently in the last trimester of pregnancy and in women older than 33 years. The maternal mortality rate from an MI during pregnancy is approximately 20%. Women are most likely to die at the time of the infarction or during labour and birth (Blanchard & Daniels, 2014). The risk of maternal death increases if the woman gives birth within 2 weeks of having an MI (Easterling & Stout, 2012). Fetal loss is also high in this population.

Medical management for pregnant women with MI is the same as that for nonpregnant women and includes the administration of morphine, nitrates, lidocaine, beta blockers, aspirin, magnesium sulphate, and calcium antagonists (Easterling & Stout, 2012). Thrombolytic agents such as urokinase, streptokinase, and tissue plasminogen activator (tPA) do not appear to cross the placenta. However, their use is considered to be relatively contraindicated in pregnancy because of the risk for subsequent maternal and fetal hemorrhage (Gaddipati & Troiano, 2013). Because pain can lead to tachycardia and increased cardiac demands, pain control during labour is crucial. The side-lying position is preferred to prevent pressure on the vena cava. Vaginal birth is preferable, with avoidance of maternal pushing and a vacuum- or forceps-assisted birth (Easterling & Stout, 2012).

Peripartum Cardiomyopathy

Peripartum cardiomyopathy (PPCM) is heart failure with cardiomyopathy. The classic criteria for the diagnosis of PPCM include development of heart failure during the last month of pregnancy or within the first 5 postpartum months; absence of heart disease before the last month of pregnancy; a left ventricular ejection fraction of less than 45%; and, most important, lack of another cause for heart failure (Sliwa, Hilfiker-Kleiner, Petrie, et al., 2010). The etiology of the disease is unknown; theories suggest genetic predisposition, autoimmunity, and viral infections.

PPCM is more common in older multiparous women, twin pregnancies, and women with pre-eclampsia (Bello, Hurtado, & Arany, 2013; Davies & Herbert, 2007d). The incidence is 1 in 3000 to 4000 live births in North America, with the maternal mortality rate estimated to be in the range of 25 to 50%; the infant mortality rate is approximately 10% (Gaddipati & Troiano, 2013; Kolte, Khera, Aronow, et al., 2014). Maternal death is usually caused by thromboembolism, arrhythmia, or progressive heart failure. Symptoms include breathlessness, dyspnea, cough, orthopnea, tachydysrhythmias, and edema, with radiological findings of cardiomegaly. The prognosis is good if cardiomegaly does not persist after 6 months postpartum. Women whose hearts remain enlarged after 6 months postpartum are highly likely to have PPCM in future pregnancies (Blanchard & Daniels, 2014; Kolte et al., 2014). Given the recurrence risk of 30 to 50%, women are counselled against subsequent pregnancies.

Medical management of cardiomyopathy during pregnancy includes treatment similar to that for heart failure and the potential for thromboembolism: diuretics, sodium restriction, afterload-reducing agents, anticoagulants, and digoxin. Anticoagulation may be necessary if the cardiac chambers are significantly dilated and contract poorly because of the increased risk for clot formation. Angiotensin-converting enzyme inhibitors, often prescribed to achieve afterload reduction, can be used only in the postpartum period because they are teratogenic agents and have been associated with severe fetal renal toxicity and stillbirth (Davies & Herbert, 2007d). During labour, epidural anaesthesia is often used for pain control to decrease the cardiac workload and reduce tachycardia. Caesarean birth should be performed only for obstetrical indications (Easterling & Stout, 2012).

Heart Surgery During Pregnancy

Ideally, a woman would have surgical correction of a cardiac lesion before pregnancy; however, pregnancy may be unplanned or the cardiac disease may be diagnosed for the first time during pregnancy. When medical therapy for a pregnant woman with cardiac disease is not sufficient to manage potentially life-threatening symptoms, cardiac surgery may be required. Early in the second trimester is the best time for surgery. The woman, fetus, and uterine activity must be monitored carefully during surgery. Closed cardiac surgery such as the release of a stenotic mitral valve can be achieved with little risk to the mother or fetus. Open heart surgery should be performed in a cardiac centre, as it requires extracorporeal circulation. Hypoxia and fetal bradycardia must be assessed, as they may occur as a result of low blood-flow rates. Periods of hypoxemia for the fetus can lead to neurological insult. An increase in flow rates on cardiopulmonary bypass may correct fetal bradycardia. Uterine contractions also increase in frequency before and during cardiopulmonary bypass and can be managed by medication.

LEGAL TIP *CARDIAC EMERGENCIES*

The management of cardiac emergencies such as maternal cardiopulmonary distress or arrest should be documented in policies, procedures, and protocols. Nursing scope of practice and independent nursing actions should be clearly identified.

Heart Transplantation

Increasing numbers of heart recipients are completing pregnancies successfully. Before conception the woman should be assessed for quality of ventricular function and potential rejection of the transplant. She should also be considered to be stabilized on her immunosuppressant regimen. Women who have no evidence of rejection and have normal cardiac function at the beginning of the pregnancy appear to do well during pregnancy, labour, and birth. Research has shown that the transplanted heart responds normally to pregnancy-related changes. Complications common in women who have had a heart transplant include hypertension and at least one episode of rejection (Cunningham et al., 2014). Conception should be postponed for at least 1 year after transplantation to prevent acute rejection episodes (Blanchard & Daniels, 2014).

NURSING CARE

The presence of cardiac disease is a significant influencing factor in the decision-making process for or against becoming pregnant. Couples planning a pregnancy must understand the risks involved in their situation. If the pregnancy is unplanned, the nurse should explore the couple's desire to continue it in light of the risks involved. Pregnancy termination is one option, depending on the severity of the cardiac defect. The family may need further information to make an informed decision regarding the future of the pregnancy.

Nursing care of the woman with a cardiovascular disorder combines routine perinatal care with care specific for the cardiac diagnosis and function. Care of these women at low, medium, and high risk requires a multidisciplinary approach. The multidisciplinary team must work with the woman and her family in an environment that has the required resources to provide appropriate maternal hemodynamic monitoring, and the woman's condition may need to be assessed as often as weekly. See the Evolve website for the Nursing Care Plan, The Pregnant Woman with Heart Disease.

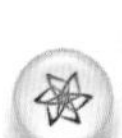

Antepartum

Nursing care for the pregnant woman with heart disease is focused on minimizing stress on the heart and ensuring that mother and fetus have a healthy outcome. Cardiac stress is greatest between 28 and 32 weeks as the hemodynamic changes reach their maximum (Pieper, 2012). The workload of the cardiovascular system is reduced by appropriate treatment of any coexisting emotional stress, hypertension, anemia, hyperthyroidism, or obesity.

Signs and symptoms of cardiac decompensation are taught at the first prenatal visit and reviewed at each subsequent visit (Box 15-3 and Patient Teaching box).

The pregnant woman with cardiovascular disease will require some modification of her activities. Reduced activity level during pregnancy affects all of the organ systems, but especially the cardiovascular and musculoskeletal systems. In addition, psychological adverse effects can be debilitating (Cunningham et al., 2014). The community health nurse, social worker, and physiotherapist or occupational therapist are key resource people whose services may be incorporated into the plan of care.

Symptoms of cardiac decompensation may appear abruptly or gradually. Medical intervention must be instituted immediately to maintain optimal cardiac status. Dyspnea, palpitations, syncope, and edema commonly occur in pregnant women and can mask the symptoms of a developing or worsening cardiovascular disorder (Pieper, 2012). A woman's sudden inability to perform activities that she previously was comfortable doing may indicate cardiovascular decompensation (see Box 15-3).

BOX 15-3 SIGNS OF POTENTIAL COMPLICATIONS: CARDIAC DECOMPENSATION

Pregnant Woman: Subjective Symptoms

- Increasing fatigue, difficulty breathing, or both with usual activities
- Feeling of smothering
- Frequent cough
- Palpitations; feeling that her heart is racing
- Generalized edema: swelling of face, feet, legs, fingers (e.g., rings do not fit anymore)

Nurse: Objective Signs

- Irregular weak, rapid pulse (100 or more beats/min)
- Progressive, generalized edema
- Crackles at base of lungs after two inspirations and exhalations that do not clear with coughing
- Orthopnea; increasing dyspnea
- Rapid respirations (25 or more breaths/min)
- Moist, frequent cough
- Cyanosis of lips and nail beds

PATIENT TEACHING

The Pregnant Woman at Risk for Cardiac Decompensation

- Instruct woman to watch for and immediately report signs of cardiac decompensation or heart failure: generalized edema, distension of neck veins, dyspnea, pulmonary crackles, cough, palpitations, sudden weight gain.
- Watch for and immediately report signs of thromboembolism: redness, tenderness, pain, or swelling in extremities or chest pain.
- Avoid constipation and straining with bowel movements (Valsalva manoeuvre) by taking in adequate fluids and fibre. A stool softener may be ordered.
- Teach importance of the following:
  - Daily weighing. Sudden weight gain indicates fluid retention.
  - Keeping all prenatal visit appointments, although they will be scheduled more frequently than for pregnant women who are not at risk.
  - Limiting activity (depending on classification of her heart disease). Patients with class I or II cardiac disease need 10 hours of sleep every night and 30 minutes of rest after meals. Patients with class III or IV cardiac disease usually need bedrest for most of each day.

Modified from Gilbert, E. S. (2011). *Manual of high risk pregnancy and delivery* (5th ed.). St. Louis: Mosby.

Intrapartum

For all pregnant women the intrapartum period is the one that evokes the most apprehension in patients and caregivers. The woman with impaired cardiac function may have increased anxiety and fear of labour because giving birth places additional stressors on her already compromised cardiovascular system, which can result in a poor maternal outcome. General intrapartum management for cardiac disease focuses on strict fluid management, preventing hypotension and maternal tachycardia (>110 beats/min), and optimizing cardiac output. A vaginal birth is preferable for women with cardiac disease. Caesearean birth should be reserved for obstetrical indications as it is associated with more blood loss and higher risks for thromboembolism and infection (Pieper, 2012).

Assessments include the routine assessments for all labouring women, as well as assessments for cardiac decompensation. In addition, arterial line placement and arterial blood gas evaluations may be needed to assess for adequate oxygenation. A pulmonary artery catheter (Swan-Ganz catheter) may be inserted to monitor hemodynamic status accurately during labour and birth. Electrocardiographic telemetry monitoring and continuous monitoring of blood pressure and pulse oximetry should be instituted for all women with cardiac issues, and the fetus should be continuously monitored electronically.

! NURSING ALERT

A pulse rate above 100 beats/min or a respiratory rate of 25 breaths/min, particularly when associated with dyspnea, may indicate impending ventricular failure (Cunningham et al., 2014). Respiratory status should be checked frequently for developing dyspnea, coughing, or crackles at the base of the lungs. The colour and temperature of the skin should also be noted. Pale, cool, clammy skin may indicate cardiac shock.

Nursing care during labour and birth focuses on the promotion of cardiac function. Anxiety is minimized by maintaining a calm atmosphere in the labour and birth rooms. The nurse can provide anticipatory guidance by keeping the woman and her family informed of labour progress and events that will probably occur and by answering any questions they have. The woman's childbirth preparation method should be supported to the degree feasible for her cardiac condition. Nursing techniques that promote comfort, such as back massage, may be used.

Cardiac function is supported by keeping the woman's head and shoulders elevated and body parts resting on pillows. The side-lying position usually facilitates hemodynamics during labour. Discomfort is relieved with medication and supportive care. Physiologically, the ideal labour for a woman with heart disease is one that is short and pain free. Therefore, use of epidural analgesia is encouraged, although care must be taken to avoid hypotension, a common adverse effect of regional anaesthesia (Easterling & Stout, 2012; Gaddipati & Troiano, 2013). The woman may require other types of medication (e.g., anticoagulants, prophylactic antibiotics). If evidence of cardiac decompensation appears, the physician may order furosemide (Lasix) for rapid diuresis and oxygen by intermittent positive pressure to decrease the development of pulmonary edema.

Spontaneous labour or planned induction of labour is the preferred method of birth for women with cardiac disease (Pieper, 2012). If there are no obstetrical interventions, a planned, vaginal birth with the woman in a side-lying position to facilitate uterine perfusion is preferred. To prevent compression of popliteal veins and an increase in blood volume in the chest and trunk as a result of the effects of gravity, stirrups are not used. The second stage is carefully managed with passive second stage (allowing the fetal head to descend without pushing), prevention of the Valsalva manoeuvre (forced expiration against a closed airway, which, when released, causes blood to rush to the heart and overload the cardiac system), open glottis pushing, and consideration for operative vaginal delivery. Oxygen via face mask is administered. Vacuum extraction or outlet forceps may be used to decrease the length and workload of the heart in second-stage labour. Caesarean birth is not routinely recommended for women who have cardiovascular disease because there is a risk of dramatic fluid shifts, sustained hemodynamic changes, and increased blood loss. Bacterial endocarditis prophylaxis is not recommended, as the risk of bacteremia is low (Allen & Canadian Paediatric Society, 2010; Wilson, Taubert, Gewitz, et al., 2007).

Dilute IV oxytocin immediately after birth may be used to prevent hemorrhage. Ergot products should not be used because they cause an increase in blood pressure. Fluid balance should be maintained and blood loss replaced. If tubal sterilization is desired, it is best to delay surgery until the woman is hemodynamically near normal, afebrile, nonanemic, and able to ambulate normally (Cunningham et al., 2014).

Postpartum

Monitoring for cardiac decompensation in the postpartum period is essential. The first 24 to 48 hours postpartum are the most hemodynamically difficult for the woman. During the immediate postpartum period, diuretic therapy may be required. Hemorrhage, infection, or both may worsen the cardiac condition. The woman with a cardiac disorder may continue to require a pulmonary artery catheter and arterial catheter for monitoring of volume status, cardiac output, blood pressure, and arterial blood gases. Discharge should be delayed up to 72 hours to allow time to assess for complications (Pieper, 2012).

NURSING ALERT

The immediate postbirth period is hazardous for a woman whose heart function is compromised. Cardiac output increases rapidly as extravascular fluid is remobilized into the vascular compartment. At the moment of birth, intra-abdominal pressure is reduced drastically; pressure on veins is removed, the splanchnic vessels engorge, and blood flow to the heart is increased. When blood flow increases to the heart, a reflex bradycardia may result.

Care in the postpartum period is tailored to the woman's functional capacity. Postpartum assessment of the woman with cardiac disease includes vital signs, oxygen saturation levels, lung and heart auscultation, presence of edema, amount and character of bleeding, uterine tone and fundal height, urinary output, pain (especially chest pain), the activity–rest pattern, dietary intake, mother–infant interactions, and emotional state. The head of the bed should be elevated and the woman encouraged to lie on her side. Progressive ambulation is encouraged as tolerated. The woman may require assistance with grooming and hygiene needs and other activities. The woman should be directed to take stool softeners and have a diet with roughage and adequate fluids to promote bowel movements without stress or strain.

The woman may need assistance from family members to help in the care of the infant. Breastfeeding is encouraged for women with acquired and congenital heart disease, but some women may not wish to nurse their infants. The woman who chooses to breastfeed requires support from her family and the nursing staff to assist in positioning herself or the infant for feeding. The infant should be brought to the mother and taken from her after the feeding to conserve her energy. Women who are breastfeeding may require less cardiac medication, especially diuretics, for the treatment of their condition. Most medications used to manage cardiac disorders are compatible with breastfeeding. However, thiazide diuretics may suppress lactation (Blanchard & Daniels, 2014). Because diuretics can cause neonatal diuresis that can lead to dehydration, lactating women must be monitored closely to determine if medication doses can be reduced and still be effective. Nurses caring for the newborn should be alerted to watch for voiding patterns and amounts and to monitor the infant closely for signs of dehydration.

Women who are too ill to care for and feed their babies should be provided with opportunities to have the baby at the bedside so they can look at and touch the baby to establish an emotional bond. Having the baby skin-to-skin with the mother gives her a powerful opportunity to get to know her baby while expending little energy. If the mother is unable to hold her infant, the nurse or a family member can hold the infant at the mother's eye level and close enough for her to touch.

Discharge should be carefully planned with the woman and family. A clear plan to support the mother's need for a balance between rest and sleep periods along with activity must be discussed. The role of relatives, friends, and others in assisting with meal preparation and household duties as well as childcare responsibilities must be addressed. The family may be referred to community resources (e.g., homemaking services) for additional support, as appropriate. Rest and sleep periods, activity, and diet must be planned. The nurse should provide information to the couple about their re-establishing sexual relations and contraception needs or answer questions about tubal ligation or vasectomy. If tubal ligation is being considered as a method of contraception, the risks of surgery, especially for the woman with class III or IV heart disease, must be discussed. Women should be counselled that oral contraceptives are contraindicated because of the risk of thromboembolism, although progestin-only pills may be used. IUDs may put the woman at increased risk for infection, especially if she has a valve replacement. Injectable progestins are an effective and safe alternative (Easterling & Stout, 2012). Both the woman and her partner should discuss the options together in order to make the best choice for their individual situation.

Medical assessment and community health nurse follow-up is important after discharge to continue monitoring for cardiac decompensation, through the first few weeks after birth, due to hormone shifts that affect hemodynamics. Few data are available regarding how quickly cardiac output returns to normal after giving birth. Older studies suggested that this occurred by 8 to 10 weeks postpartum. However, a longitudinal study that followed women before, during, and after pregnancy found that both nulliparous and multiparous women had significantly higher cardiac outputs above their prepregnancy values even at 1 year after giving birth (Katz, 2012).

Men and women with a congenital heart defect are at increased risk for having children who also have a defect. The risk for affected mothers is greater, approximately two to more than three times that of affected fathers. Children born with a congenital heart defect to parents with congenital heart defects appear to inherit the risk for cardiac maldevelopment in general rather than a specific defect because they often do not have the same defect as the parent (Easterling & Stout, 2012). Therefore, preconception and genetic counselling before a subsequent pregnancy are essential.

OBESITY

Obesity is a serious health concern that can have a profound impact on pregnancy. It is estimated that the number of obese and overweight women in Canada has risen from 9.7% in 1972 to 43.7% in 2010 (Statistics Canada, 2011). *Obesity* is defined using body mass index (BMI), which is defined as a measure of an adult's weight in kilograms divided by height in metres squared (kg/m^2) (see Table 5-1). Women with a BMI of 25 to 29.9 are considered overweight, whereas those with a BMI over 30 are considered obese. Overweight and obese women and their fetuses and infants are at increased risk of health complications (ACOG, 2013; Davies, Maxwell, & McLeod, 2010; Gunatilake & Perlow, 2011; Herring, Platek, Elliott, et al., 2010). Pregnancy can exacerbate previous health issues or initiate new health complications during and after pregnancy.

Maternal physiological changes are the product of hormonal influences and mechanical effects. In obese women, the weight of fat tissue and the subsequent added metabolic demands also affect maternal physiology. Both pregnancy and obesity cause blood volume and cardiac output to increase, and in the obese woman these levels expand in proportion to the amount of fat tissue. During labour and vaginal birth and in the immediate postpartum period, blood values and cardiac output in obese women can reach levels 80% greater than prelabour values. The enlarged uterus and abdominal fat mass also further increase the possibility of aortocaval compression.

The gastric emptying time is delayed, the tone of the cardiac sphincter is decreased, and the gastric contents are hyperacidic in all pregnant women. The obese woman is more likely to have a hiatal hernia and a marked increase in intragastric pressure and volume; therefore, these women are at great risk for regurgitation and aspiration. Comprehensive care of the bariatric patient is essential to ensure optimum outcomes for both mother and fetus.

Antepartum Risks

Obese women often have difficulty becoming pregnant and may require assisted reproductive technology. Once they are pregnant, women who are obese may have difficulty maintaining the pregnancy. There is an increased risk of spontaneous abortions, as well as increased recurrent pregnancy loss (Davies et al., 2010; Gunatilake, 2011). Increased BMI also leads to a higher risk of stillbirth; women with a BMI greater than 35 have an almost three times greater rate of stillbirth after 28 weeks (Davies et al., 2010).

It is recommended that women who are overweight or obese attempt to obtain an ideal body weight before conception, to improve their own health as well as the pregnancy outcomes (Davies et al., 2010; Walters & Taylor, 2009/2010). Once the woman is pregnant, a weight loss program is not recommended and nutritional counselling may be required. Regular exercise during pregnancy appears to decrease the risks associated with obesity.

Increasing numbers of women of reproductive age are undergoing bariatric surgery (ACOG, 2013). Women must be counselled to defer pregnancy for 12 to 18 months after bariatric surgery to preclude any surgical complications. Pregnancy outcomes are improved for women who become pregnant post–bariatric surgery, such as a reduction in pregestational diabetes and in risk of having a macrosomic infant (Gunatilake, 2011).

During pregnancy, obese women require increased surveillance and care. GDM screening should be done early in the pregnancy, as the risk for GDM and type 2 diabetes is increased in obese women (Davies et al., 2010). A dating ultrasound examination should be done because of irregular or anovulatory cycles, to confirm the estimated date of birth. During routine 18- to 22-week ultrasound examination, it can be difficult to visualize fetal structure, and repeated ultrasound scans may be required to assess fetal anatomy. This assessment is important, as infants of obese mothers have an increased rate of birth defects, including neural tube, heart, ventral wall, and possibly orofacial defects (Davies et al., 2010). Obese women also have an increased prevalence of pre-existing hypertension or risk of developing hypertensive disorder of pregnancy (Magee et al., 2014). This risk increases as BMI increases (Davies et al., 2010).

Intrapartum and Postpartum Risks

Women who are obese require care that is adapted to accommodate the challenges posed by their increased weight and size. There is an increased risk of shoulder dystocia due to fetal macrosomia (see Chapter 20). Induction of labour is more likely, as uterine contractility may be altered in obese women and higher doses of oxytocin may be required (Heavey, 2011; Zhang, Bricker, Wray, et al., 2007). Fetal monitoring poses another challenge, as there can be an inability to obtain interpretable fetal heart rate patterns or monitor uterine contractions (ACOG, 2013). The risk of Caesarean birth is increased in women who are obese; the risk is 20% for BMI less than 30 and 47.4% for BMI greater than 40 (ACOG, 2013). This increased risk could be due to a prolonged active phase of labour as well as cephalopelvic disproportion (CPD) or fetal **macrosomia**.

Care of the obese woman during labour should focus on efforts to minimize oxygen consumption and maximize pulmonary function. Monitoring by pulse oximeter has been recommended. Epidural analgesia administered during the first stage of labour can bring about decreased demand on the metabolic and respiratory systems and improved oxygenation, because pain causes the catecholamine levels to increase, which in turn causes cardiac output to increase. Effective epidural analgesia slows this increase in catecholamine levels.

Epidural administration can be difficult in the obese woman; often multiple attempts are necessary to successfully place the epidural needle. It is often difficult to locate the midline and identify the epidural space. It is also difficult to position the woman; sitting is often the best position. More than one attempt to place the epidural is needed in approximately 75% of morbidly obese women (Davies et al., 2010). There is also the risk of the epidural catheter becoming dislodged (Saravanakumar, Rao, & Cooper, 2006). The use of epidurals may require significant staff resources; thus, their use may be limited in some settings (Davies et al., 2010).

IV opioids may be used during the first stage of labour; however, the doses and effects must be monitored carefully because obese women are extremely sensitive to the respiratory depressant effects of opioids. Combined spinal epidural anaesthesia is an alternative to epidural anaesthesia. This option is now available in the morbidly obese pregnant woman because there is an appropriate long needle manufactured for this purpose.

In the obese woman who must give birth by Caesarean section, an epidural block is preferred over general anaesthesia. Problems associated with general anaesthesia in obese women include potential difficulties during intubation, a hypertensive effect of laryngoscopy and intubation, and aspiration and pulmonary complications. A spinal block may be used if there is insufficient time to induce an epidural block. Uterine displacement to prevent aortocaval compression is more difficult to achieve in the obese woman in the supine position needed for Caesarean birth. If the woman is extremely obese, a wedge may not be able to elevate one hip enough to prevent compression. In this case, it may be necessary to lift the abdominal fat pad off the abdomen manually until the peritoneal cavity has been entered.

During the postpartum period, women may have more difficulty breastfeeding and will require extra support for positioning the newborn. Wound infections are increased, as wound healing is delayed and dehiscence may occur (Heavey, 2011). There is also an increased risk for venous thromboembolism; prophylaxis with appropriate dosing low molecular-weight heparin is recommended (Chan, Rey, & Kent, 2014). The risk for postpartum hemorrhage is increased because of decreased muscle tone, decreased physical activity, and the macrosomic fetus with a corresponding large placental implantation site. During the postpartum period, it may be difficult to palpate the fundus to assess uterine contractility on account of large abdominal pannus.

NURSING CARE

Caring for the bariatric woman during the perinatal period requires a caring, knowledgeable approach (Herring et al., 2010). Appropriate-sized equipment is required. A large manual blood pressure (BP) cuff is required, as automated BP machines may not be accurate for BP assessment. It is important to have bariatric equipment such as appropriate-sized beds, operating room tables, stretchers, and wheelchairs. It is important to determine the manufacturer's weight limit on equipment prior to use. Bathrooms and shower stalls may require wider doors. It is also important to ensure that there is access to larger gowns, weight scales, and epidural needles. Nurses need to use appropriate mechanical lifts when necessary, as no patient lifting is permitted by institutional protocols and work safe procedures.

During labour, respiratory problems may occur in women who are obese, so it is necessary for nurses to monitor oxygen saturation levels along with performing thorough respiratory assessments. It may be difficult to palpate the fetus, so ultrasonographic examination may be necessary to confirm fetal position. Monitoring the fetus with electronic fetal monitoring may be difficult. When labour has progressed, it may be helpful to use an internal spiral electrode to monitor the fetal heart rate and an intrauterine pressure catheter (see Chapter 19) to monitor the contractions (Davies et al., 2010). It is important to encourage the labouring woman to reposition herself frequently in order to provide maternal comfort and promote fetal descent.

The postpartum woman requires frequent assessments to monitor bleeding and vital signs. To decrease the risk of venous thromboembolism, it is important to encourage early ambulation with the use of graduated compression stockings when walking. Women may also require prophylactic heparin therapy at appropriate dosing.

OTHER MEDICAL CONDITIONS IN PREGNANCY

Anemia

Anemia is the most common medical disorder of pregnancy, affecting 20 to 60% of pregnant women (Kilpatrick, 2014). It results in a reduction of the oxygen-carrying capacity of the blood; thus the heart tries to compensate by increasing the cardiac output. This effort increases the workload of the heart and stresses ventricular function. Therefore, anemia that occurs with any other complication (e.g., pre-eclampsia) may result in heart failure.

An indirect index of the oxygen-carrying capacity is the packed RBC volume, or hematocrit level. The normal hematocrit range in nonpregnant women is 0.37 to 0.47. Normal values for pregnant women with adequate iron stores may be as low as 0.32. This decreased level has been explained by the blood volume expansion of approximately 50% and total RBC mass expansion of approximately 25%. This *hydremia* (dilution of blood) is also called the **physiological anemia of pregnancy**.

Anemia in pregnancy is defined as a hemoglobin level of less than 110 g/L or a hematocrit of less than or equal to 0.32 (Gilbert, 2011; World Health Organization [WHO], 2012). When a woman has anemia during pregnancy, the loss of blood at birth, even if minimal, is not well tolerated. She is at increased risk for requiring blood transfusions. Women with anemia have a higher incidence of puerperal complications such as infection than do pregnant women with normal hematological values. *Severe anemia*, defined as a hemoglobin level of less than 60 g/L, has been associated with decreased fetal oxygen levels that result in abnormal fetal heart rate patterns, decreased amniotic fluid volume, and fetal death.

Nursing care of the pregnant woman with anemia requires that the nurse be able to distinguish between the normal physiological anemia of pregnancy and the disease states. About 90% of cases of anemia in pregnancy are of the iron-deficiency type. The remaining 10% embrace a considerable variety of acquired and hereditary anemias, including folic acid deficiency, sickle cell anemia, and thalassemia.

During prenatal visits, the nurse should take a diet history and provide dietary teaching as appropriate. Pregnancy may cause increased fatigue, stress, and financial difficulties for a woman with anemia as she copes with her activities of daily living. The nurse should assess the pregnant woman's needs and provide her with appropriate resources or referral.

Iron-Deficiency Anemia

Iron-deficiency anemia is by far the most common anemia of pregnancy, accounting for approximately 75% of cases. It is diagnosed by checking the woman's serum ferritin level in addition to her hemoglobin and hematocrit levels. The serum ferritin level reflects iron reserves (Samuels, 2012). Routine screening of at risk pregnant women for iron-deficiency anemia is recommended. Iron is actively transported across the placenta for fetal erythropoiesis. Ferritin levels are the primary screening tests used to diagnose iron-deficiency anemia. *Iron deficiency* is defined as serum ferritin less than 12 mcg/L, and iron-deficiency anemia is a combination of anemia (Hgb less than 110 g/L) and low serum ferritin less than 12 mcg/L (Blackburn, 2013; Haider, Olofin, Wang, et al., 2013; WHO, 2012). An association appears to exist between maternal iron-deficiency anemia, especially severe anemia, and preterm birth and low-birth-weight infants, although whether these poor pregnancy outcomes are caused by iron-deficiency anemia is uncertain (Samuels, 2012). Usually even the fetus of an anemic woman receives adequate iron stores from the mother at the cost of further depleting the mother's iron level (Blackburn, 2013).

Generally, iron-deficiency anemia is preventable or easily treated with iron supplements. Because of the increased amounts of iron needed for fetal development and maternal stores, pregnant women are often encouraged to take prophylactic iron supplementation (Blackburn, 2013; Gilbert, 2011). If iron-deficiency anemia is diagnosed, increased iron dosages are recommended (elemental iron, 60 to 120 mg/day) (WHO, 2012). Diet alone cannot replace gestational iron losses.

Inadequate nutrition without therapy will certainly mean iron-deficiency anemia during late pregnancy and the puerperium. It is important to teach the pregnant woman about the significance of iron therapy (see Table 12-1 and Patient Teaching: Iron Supplementation in Chapter 12, p. 279). In addition, the woman should be instructed to decrease the gastrointestinal adverse effects of iron therapy through diet. Those pregnant women who cannot tolerate the prescribed oral iron because of nausea and vomiting should receive parenteral iron, such as an iron–dextran complex (Imferon) or iron sucrose (Venofer) (Perelló, Masoller, Esteve, et al., 2014). Iron sucrose has been shown to be better absorbed and has a lower incidence of life-threatening anaphylaxis than iron dextran (Short & Domagalski, 2013). Blood transfusions should be considered for the woman with severe anemia to prevent fetal and maternal complications of decreased oxygen delivery.

Folic Acid–Deficiency Anemia

Folate is a water-soluble vitamin found naturally in dark green leafy vegetables, citrus fruits, eggs, legumes, and whole grains. Even in well-nourished women, folate deficiency is common. Poor diet, cooking with large volumes of water, home canning of food (especially vegetables), and increased alcohol use may contribute to folate deficiency. During pregnancy the need for folate increases, both because of fetal demands and because folate is less well absorbed from the gastrointestinal tract during gestation. Folic acid deficiency during conception and early pregnancy increases the incidence of neural tube defects, cleft lip, and cleft palate.

During pregnancy, the recommended daily intake is 0.4 mg per day of folic acid, although women who have a deficiency may need 1 mg or more per day (WHO, 2012) (see Box 12-1). Women at particular risk for folate deficiency include those who have significant hemoglobinopathies, take anticonvulsant medication, are pregnant with a multifetal gestation, or have frequent pregnancies. These women require larger than usual doses of folic acid (Samuels, 2012).

Folate deficiency is the most common cause of megaloblastic anemia during pregnancy, but a vitamin B_{12} deficiency must also be considered. Vitamin B_{12} deficiency in pregnant women is seen much more often now than in the past because of the increasing numbers of women who become pregnant after undergoing bariatric surgery (Samuels, 2012). Megaloblastic anemia rarely occurs before the third trimester of pregnancy (Kilpatrick, 2014; Samuels, 2012). Women with megaloblastic anemia caused by folic acid deficiency have the usual presenting symptoms and signs of anemia: pallor; fatigue; lethargy; and glossitis and skin roughness, which are associated specifically with megaloblastic anemia (Kilpatrick, 2014). Folate deficiency usually improves rapidly with folic acid therapy. It rarely occurs in the fetus and is not a significant cause of perinatal morbidity. Iron deficiency often occurs along with folate deficiency (Samuels, 2012).

Sickle Cell Hemoglobinopathy

Sickle cell hemoglobinopathy is a disease caused by the presence of abnormal hemoglobin in the blood. Sickle cell trait (SA hemoglobin pattern), sickling of the RBCs but with a normal RBC lifespan, usually causes only mild clinical symptoms. Sickle cell anemia (sickle cell disease) is a recessive, hereditary, familial hemolytic anemia that affects those of African or Mediterranean ancestry. These individuals usually have abnormal hemoglobin types (SS or SC), which leads to the formation of rigid and fragile sickle-shaped red cells. These cells are prone to increased breakdown, which causes hemolytic anemia, and vaso-occlusion in the small blood vessels, leading to an acute painful crisis. People with sickle cell anemia have recurrent attacks (crises) of fever and pain in the abdomen or extremities. These attacks are attributed to vascular occlusion (from abnormal cells), causing tissue ischemia and acute and chronic organ dysfunction involving the spleen, brain, lungs, and kidneys. Pain and swelling of the extremities is common and occurs as a result of aseptic necrosis of the small bones in the feet and hands. The resulting hemolysis leads to chronic anemia and predisposes the woman to aplastic crises (Langlois, Ford, & Chitayat, et al., 2008). Crises are usually triggered by dehydration, hypoxia, or acidosis (Samuels, 2012).

Population migration has resulted in sickle cell disease becoming of increasing importance worldwide. Greater numbers of affected individuals are in Europe and almost 10% of Blacks in North America have the sickle cell trait, but fewer than 1% have sickle cell anemia disease (Royal College of Obstetrics and Gynecology [RCOG], 2011). The anemia often is complicated by iron and folic acid deficiency. Iron supplementation should only be given when there is clinical evidence of anemia. Women with sickle cell trait require genetic counselling and partner testing to determine their risk of producing children with sickle cell trait or disease.

Women with sickle cell trait usually do well in pregnancy, although they are at increased risk for painful crises during pregnancy, fetal growth restriction, antepartum hospital admission, and postpartum infection (RCOG, 2011). They are also at increased risk for UTI and may be deficient in iron (Kilpatrick, 2014; Samuels, 2012). Women in impending sickle cell crisis experience painful joints (see Critical Thinking Case Study).

Pregnant women with sickle cell anemia are at risk of developing pyelonephritis, leg ulcers, bone abnormalities, strokes, cardiomyopathy, heart failure, and pre-eclampsia. Women with sickle cell are encouraged to take a low-dose aspirin following completion of the first trimester to reduce the risk of pre-eclampsia (Magee et al., 2014). The woman is monitored carefully during pregnancy for the development of UTI or pre-eclampsia. In addition, she will need serial ultrasound examinations to monitor fetal growth and will likely have antepartum fetal testing performed regularly during the third trimester. Infections are treated aggressively with antibiotics. If crises occur, they are managed with analgesia, oxygen, and hydration. Some authorities still recommend prophylactic transfusions, which replace the woman's sickle cells with normal RBCs, to improve oxygen-carrying capacity and suppress the synthesis of sickle hemoglobin. However, most clinicians believe that prophylactic transfusions do not improve fetal or neonatal

CRITICAL THINKING CASE STUDY

Sickle Cell Hemoglobinopathy

Latasha is a 23-year-old G1 T0 P0 A0 L0 with sickle cell anemia who is hospitalized with a crisis at 16 weeks of gestation. She says, "I've been in and out of the hospital all my life because of my sickle cell disease. I sure hope my baby won't have it!"

QUESTIONS

1. Evidence—Is there sufficient evidence to counsel Latasha regarding her baby's chance of having sickle cell disease?
2. Assumptions—Describe an underlying assumption about each of the following issues:
   a. The chance that Latasha's baby will inherit either sickle cell trait or sickle cell disease
   b. Pregnancy risks related to sickle cell disease
   c. Usual pregnancy management in women with sickle cell disease
3. What implications and priorities for nursing care can be drawn at this time?
4. Does the evidence objectively support your argument (conclusion)?

outcome and are not worth the associated risks of isosensitization, viral infection, transfusion reactions, and hemochromatosis (Samuels, 2012). Caesarean birth is warranted only for obstetrical indications. In the postpartum period, women with sickle cell anemia must be counselled that oral contraceptives are contraindicated because of the increased risk of thromboembolus.

SAFETY ALERT

Women with sickle cell anemia are not iron deficient. Therefore, routine iron supplementation, even that found in prenatal vitamins, should be avoided because these women can develop iron overload (Samuels, 2012).

Thalassemia

Thalassemia is a relatively common anemia in which an insufficient amount of globin is produced to fill the RBCs. It is a hereditary disorder that involves the abnormal synthesis of the alpha or beta chains of hemoglobin. Beta thalassemia is the more common variety in North America and usually occurs in persons of Mediterranean, North African, Middle Eastern, and Asian descent (Kilpatrick, 2014).

Beta thalassemia minor is the heterozygous form of this disorder. People with heterozygous beta thalassemia are carriers of the disorder and are usually asymptomatic (Samuels, 2012). Women with thalassemia minor have a mild, persistent anemia; but the RBC level may be normal or even elevated. However, no systemic problems are caused by the anemia. Women whose pregnancies are complicated by beta thalassemia minor generally do not experience associated maternal or infant complications if their condition is stable (Blackburn, 2013) and do not require antepartum fetal testing (Samuels, 2012). Thalassemia minor must be distinguished from iron deficiency anemia. Iron therapy should only be prescribed for women who are iron deficient, although folic acid supplementation is recommended for all women with beta thalassemia minor (Samuels, 2012). Current treatment procedures for beta thalassaemia are multiple blood transfusion and iron chelation therapy (treatment for removing excess iron from the blood) (RCOG, 2014). People with thalassemia minor have a normal lifespan despite a moderately reduced hemoglobin level.

The homozygous form of beta thalassemia is known as *thalassemia major*, or *Cooley's anemia* (RCOG, 2011). Persons with this form of the disease usually have hepatosplenomegaly and bone deformities caused by massive marrow tissue expansion. These individuals usually die of infection or cardiovascular complications fairly early in life. If women live to reach childbearing age, infertility is common. If women with this disorder do become pregnant, they usually experience severe anemia and heart failure, although successful full-term pregnancies have been reported. Women with beta thalassemia major are managed much like those with sickle cell anemia during pregnancy (Samuels, 2012).

If both partners are found to be carriers of thalassemia they should be referred for genetic counselling. Ideally, this should be before conception or as early as possible in the pregnancy. Additional molecular studies may be required to clarify the carrier status of the parents and thus the risk to the fetus (Langlois et al., 2008). Women who have the thalassemia trait usually have an uncomplicated pregnancy.

Pulmonary Disorders

Dyspnea is common during pregnancy, occurring by most estimates in approximately 60% of women with exertion and fewer than 20% at rest (Weinberger, Lockwood, & Barnes, 2013). The symptom is so common that it usually is referred to as physiological dyspnea. Physiological dyspnea can occur early in pregnancy and does not interfere with daily activities. Although the gravid uterus is often blamed, hyperventilation due to increased progesterone levels probably is the most important mechanism. Distinguishing this physiological dyspnea from breathlessness caused by disorders complicating pregnancy or diseases that might coexist with pregnancy is key. The presence of other symptoms and signs of cardiopulmonary disease indicates a possible pathological nature of dyspnea, and the patient should be carefully evaluated.

Asthma

Asthma is a chronic inflammatory disorder involving the tracheobronchial airways, with increased airway responsiveness to a variety of stimuli. It is characterized by periods of exacerbations and remissions. Exacerbations are triggered by allergens, marked change in ambient temperature, or emotional tension. In many cases, the cause may be unknown, although a family history of allergy is common. In response to stimuli, there is widespread but reversible narrowing of the hyperreactive airways, making it difficult to breathe. The clinical manifestations are some or all of the following: expiratory wheezing, productive cough, thick sputum, dyspnea, or any combination of these.

Approximately 4 to 8% of pregnant women have diagnosed asthma, making it the most common pulmonary disease in pregnancy (Koren, Sarkar, & Einarson, 2010; Weinberger et al.,

2013; Whitty & Dombrowski, 2012). The prevalence and morbidity rates are increasing, although the asthma-related mortality has dropped in recent years (Whitty & Dombrowski, 2012). The effect of pregnancy on asthma is unpredictable. Approximately 33% of patients improve, 33% remain stable, and 33% worsen (Madappa & Sharma, 2015; Weinberger et al., 2013; Whitty & Dombrowski, 2014). For women whose symptoms become severe in pregnancy, the challenging time is between 29 and 36 weeks of gestation (Madappa & Sharma, 2015; Weinberger et al., 2013). Asthma appears to be associated with pre-eclampsia, low birth weight or IUGR, preterm birth, and perinatal mortality (Breton, Beauchesne, Lemière, et al., 2010; Whitty & Dombrowski, 2012).

The ultimate goal of therapy for asthma is to prevent hypoxic episodes in the mother and fetus through maintaining control of asthma symptoms and prevention of acute asthma exacerbations. Achieving this goal requires monitoring lung function objectively (e.g., peak expiratory flow rate and forced expiratory volume in one second), avoiding or controlling asthma triggers (e.g., dust mites, animal dander, pollen, wood smoke), educating patients about the importance of controlling asthma during pregnancy, and drug therapy. Current drug therapy for asthma emphasizes treatment of airway inflammation to decrease airway hyperresponsiveness and prevent asthma symptoms. Decreasing airway inflammation with inhaled corticosteroids is currently the preferred treatment for managing persistent asthma during pregnancy (Whitty & Dombrowski, 2014). Respiratory infections should be treated with appropriate antibiotics, and mist or steam inhalation should be used to aid the expectoration of mucus. Pharmacotherapy to control symptoms and treat airway inflammation is safer than exacerbations of symptoms during pregnancy.

During pregnancy, women with moderate-to-severe, poorly controlled asthma need ultrasound examinations to assess fetal growth and date the pregnancy. Repeat ultrasound examinations should be performed after an asthma exacerbation to evaluate fetal activity and growth (Whitty & Dombrowski, 2012). Women with moderate or severe asthma will probably begin antepartum fetal testing by 32 weeks of gestation (Whitty & Dombrowski, 2014). Acute exacerbations may require albuterol, steroids, aminophylline, beta-adrenergic agents, and oxygen. Women with severe exacerbations unresponsive to treatment may require intubation and mechanical ventilation (Whitty & Dombrowski, 2012). Although asthma attacks during labour are rare, medications for asthma are continued during labour and the postpartum period. Women who have received systemic corticosteroids during the previous 4 weeks should be given stress doses of corticosteroids during labour and for the first 24 hours after birth (Whitty & Dombrowski, 2012). Pulse oximetry should be instituted to assess oxygenation levels during labour. Epidural analgesia reduces oxygen consumption as a result of decreased pain and the need for breathing techniques for pain relief and is an effective strategy to help prevent complications from asthma while the woman is in labour. Fentanyl, a nonhistamine-releasing narcotic, may also be used for pain control and is not associated with bronchospasm (Cunningham et al., 2014; Whitty & Dombrowski, 2014).

During the postpartum period, women who have asthma are at increased risk for hemorrhage. If excessive bleeding occurs, prostaglandin (PG)E_2 or E_1 can be given, although the patient's respiratory status should be monitored (Whitty & Dombrowski, 2012). Because carboprost (15-methyl $PGF_{2\alpha}$ [Hemabate]) and ergonovine and methylergonovine (Methergine) can cause bronchospasm, their use should be avoided (Cunningham et al., 2014). In general, only small amounts of asthma medications enter breast milk; therefore their use is not considered a contraindication to breastfeeding. However, in sensitive individuals theophylline in breast milk can cause vomiting, feeding difficulties, jitteriness, and cardiac arrhythmias in newborns (Whitty & Dombrowski, 2012). Women are encouraged to breastfeed, as it may provide protection against respiratory infections in the newborn. The woman usually returns to her prepregnancy asthma status within 3 months after giving birth (Madappa & Sharma, 2015).

Cystic Fibrosis

Cystic fibrosis is an autosomal recessive genetic disorder in which the exocrine glands produce excessive viscous secretions, causing problems with both respiratory and digestive functions. Most people with cystic fibrosis have chronic obstructive pulmonary disease, pancreatic exocrine insufficiency, and elevated sweat electrolytes. Morbidity and mortality are usually caused by progressive chronic bronchial pulmonary disease (Whitty & Dombrowski, 2014).

Despite advances in new medications and treatments to improve the symptoms management of cystic fibrosis, respiratory failure and early death (in the early 20s to 30s) may occur.

In North America approximately 4% of the Caucasian population are carriers of the cystic fibrosis gene. Cystic fibrosis occurs in 1 in 3000 live Caucasian births. People with cystic fibrosis now live much longer than they did in the past because of earlier diagnosis of the disease and advances in antibiotic therapy and nutritional support. Currently over 45% of all individuals in North America with cystic fibrosis are more than 18 years old. Men tend to live a little longer (median age of survival is 29.6 years) than women, whose median age of survival is 27.3 years. Although most men with cystic fibrosis are infertile, women with the disease are often fertile and thus able to become pregnant (Whitty & Dombrowski, 2012).

If both potential parents are identified as carriers of the cystic fibrosis gene, the SOGC recommends that cystic fibrosis carrier screening be offered to couples who are planning a pregnancy as the risk of inheriting the gene is 25% (Dahdouh, Balayla, Audibert, et al., 2015). Infertility appears to relate to changes in cervical mucus.

Pregnancy is tolerated well in women with good nutritional status, mild obstructive lung disease, and minimal impairment of lung function (Whitty & Dombrowski, 2012). In women with severe disease, the pregnancy is often complicated by chronic hypoxia and frequent pulmonary infections. Risk factors that may predict a poor pregnancy outcome are poor prepregnancy nutritional status, significant pulmonary disease with hypoxemia, pulmonary hypertension, liver disease, and diabetes mellitus (Whitty & Dombrowski, 2014). Increased maternal and perinatal mortality rates are related to severe pulmonary infection. There is an increased incidence of preterm births, IUGR, and neonatal deaths in patients with cystic fibrosis. Predictors of adverse effects to the fetus and newborn are maternal inadequate weight gain, dyspnea, and cyanosis.

Care of the pregnant woman with cystic fibrosis requires a team effort. Ideally the woman should reach 90% of her ideal body weight before becoming pregnant. A weight gain of 11 to 12 kg (24 to 26 lb) is recommended during pregnancy. Women who are unable to achieve the recommended weight gain through oral supplements may require nasogastric tube feedings at night. Pancreatic insufficiency may put the woman at risk for malnutrition because she cannot meet the increased nutritional requirements of pregnancy. If malnutrition is severe, parenteral hyperalimentation may be necessary. Fat-soluble vitamins may not be well absorbed, resulting in deficiency in those nutrients. Throughout pregnancy frequent monitoring of the woman's weight, blood glucose, hemoglobin, total protein, serum albumin, prothrombin time, and fat-soluble vitamins A and E is suggested. Pancreatic enzymes should be adjusted as necessary (Whitty & Dombrowski, 2012). Pregnant women with cystic fibrosis also may have decreased insulin secretion and increased insulin resistance, resulting in a higher incidence for the development of gestational diabetes mellitus. A glucose tolerance test should be done at 20 weeks of gestation. Pancreatic insufficiency puts the woman at risk for malnutrition because she cannot meet the increased nutrition requirements of pregnancy.

Baseline pulmonary function tests should be completed before pregnancy and continued as needed during pregnancy. Inhaled recombinant human deoxyribonuclease I may be given to improve lung function by decreasing sputum viscosity. Inhaled 7% saline is also beneficial in this regard (Cunningham et al., 2014). Early detection and treatment of infection are critical. Management of infection includes antibiotics along with chest physical therapy and bronchial drainage (Whitty & Dombrowski, 2012).

Fetal assessment is essential, given that the fetus is at risk for uteroplacental insufficiency, which can result in IUGR. Maternal nutritional status and weight gain during pregnancy significantly affect fetal growth. Fundal height should be measured routinely, and ultrasound examinations performed to evaluate fetal growth and amniotic fluid volume. Fetal movement counts are often recommended, starting at 28 weeks of gestation. NSTs should be initiated at 32 weeks of gestation or sooner if evidence of fetal compromise exists (Whitty & Dombrowski, 2012).

During labour, monitoring for fluid and electrolyte balance is required to monitor for sodium loss and hypovolemia. The increased cardiac output stresses the cardiovascular system and can lead to cardiopulmonary failure in the woman with pulmonary hypertension or cor pulmonale. These women are also more likely to develop right-sided heart failure. Epidural or local analgesia is the preferred analgesic for birth, with vaginal birth recommended. Caesarean birth should be reserved for obstetrical indications. If general anaesthesia is needed for Caesarean birth, anticholinergic medications should not be given before surgery because they tend to promote airway drying (Whitty & Dombrowski, 2012).

Oxygen should be given freely during labour, and monitoring by pulse oximetry is recommended.

Breastfeeding appears to be safe as long as the sodium content of the mother's milk is not abnormal. The milk is pumped and discarded until the sodium content has been determined. Milk samples should be tested periodically for sodium, chloride, and total fat, and the infant's growth pattern should be followed (Lawrence & Lawrence, 2011).

Integumentary Disorders

Dermatological disorders induced by pregnancy include melasma (chloasma), vascular "spiders," palmar erythema, and striae gravidarum. A number of chronic skin disorders may complicate pregnancy. These disorders may be present before pregnancy or appear for the first time during pregnancy. Their course varies during pregnancy. For example, acne may improve.

Psoriasis improves in 40% of women, remains unchanged in 40% of women, and worsens in 20% of women during pregnancy. Lesions from neurofibromatosis may increase in size and number during pregnancy (Cunningham et al., 2014). Explanation, reassurance, and commonsense measures should suffice for normal skin changes. In contrast, disease processes during and soon after pregnancy may be extremely difficult to diagnose and treat.

> **NURSING ALERT**
>
> Isotretinoin (Accutane), commonly prescribed for cystic acne, is highly teratogenic. It must be avoided under all circumstances during pregnancy. Nursing mothers also should not use Accutane. The risk of birth defects among pregnant women is extremely high. These defects include hydrocephaly (enlargement of the fluid-filled spaces of the brain) and microcephaly (small head), heart defects, facial deformities such as cleft lip and missing ears, and developmental delays.

Pruritus is a common symptom in several pregnancy-related skin diseases. *Pruritus gravidarum,* generalized itching without the presence of a rash, develops in up to 14% of pregnant women. It is often limited to the abdomen and is usually caused by skin distension and development of striae. Pruritus gravidarum is not associated with poor perinatal outcomes. It is treated symptomatically with skin lubrication, topical antipruritics, and oral antihistamines. Ultraviolet light and careful exposure to sunlight decrease itching. Pruritus gravidarum usually disappears shortly after birth but can recur in approximately half of all subsequent pregnancies (Rapini, 2014).

Pruritic Urticarial Papules and Plaques of Pregnancy

Another common pregnancy-specific cause of pruritus is pruritic urticarial papules and plaques of pregnancy (PUPPP), also known as polmorphic eruption of pregnancy (Fig. 15-3). PUPPP classically appears in primigravidas during the mid to late third trimester and occurs a bit more frequently in women carrying male fetuses. The disorder is much more commonly seen in multiple gestations than in singletons (Kroumpouzos, 2012). The abdomen is usually affected, but lesions can spread

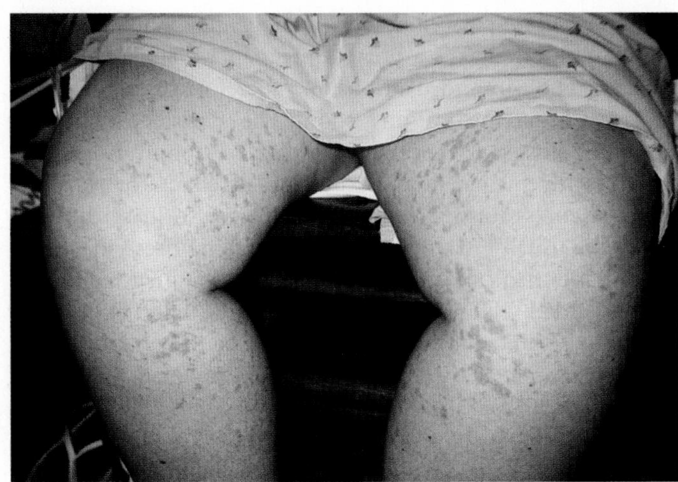

FIGURE 15-3 Woman with pruritic urticarial papules and plaques of pregnancy (PUPPP). Lesions also are present on her arms, back, abdomen, and buttocks. (Courtesy Shannon Perry.)

to the arms, thighs, back, and buttocks. PUPPP almost always causes pruritus, and the itching is severe in 80% of cases. However, it is not associated with poor maternal or fetal outcomes. Therefore, the goal of therapy is simply to relieve maternal discomfort. Antipruritic topical medications, topical steroids, and oral antihistamines usually provide relief. Women with severe symptoms may require oral prednisone. PUPPP usually resolves before birth or within several weeks after birth. However, on rare occasions it may persist or even begin after birth. PUPPP does not usually recur in subsequent pregnancies (Kroumpouzos, 2012; Rapini, 2014).

Intrahepatic Cholestasis of Pregnancy

Intrahepatic cholestasis of pregnancy (ICP) is a liver disorder unique to pregnancy that is characterized by generalized pruritus. The itching usually begins during the third trimester, most severely affects the palms and soles, and is worse at night (Cappell, 2012). ICP occurs more frequently during the winter months.

No skin lesions are present. Women with ICP have elevated serum bile acids and liver function tests. Jaundice may or may not be present. As many as one half of women with ICP develop dark urine and light-coloured stools. The cause of ICP is unknown, but approximately half of women have a family history of the disorder. Other risk factors for ICP are multiple gestations and a history of ICP in a previous pregnancy (Cappell, 2012).

Poor fetal outcomes, including meconium ileus, preterm birth, and stillbirth, are associated with ICP. The cause of these complications is likely related to increased levels of fetal serum bile levels. Treatment consists of medication, usually ursodeoxycholic acid, which effectively controls the pruritus and laboratory abnormalities associated with ICP, and continued monitoring of liver function tests and bile acids (Cappell, 2012; Williamson, Mackillop, & Heneghan, 2014). If fetal complications do not occur, birth should be considered at or near term after lung maturity has been documented. Symptoms generally disappear quickly after birth, and usually there are no long-term sequelae. However, postpartum hemorrhage is more likely in women who have had ICP, and they are also at risk to develop cholelithiasis after birth. ICP recurs in about two thirds of subsequent pregnancies (Cappell, 2012).

Neurological Disorders

Pregnant woman with neurological disorders are becoming more prevalent with the improvement of medications for treatment of these disorders. The pregnant woman with a neurological disorder must deal with potential teratogenic effects of prescribed medications, changes of mobility during pregnancy, and impaired ability to care for the baby. The nurse should be aware of all medications the pregnant woman is taking, to discuss the associated potential for producing congenital anomalies. Nurses need to counsel the pregnant woman with a neurological condition that as the pregnancy progresses, her centre of gravity shifts and causes balance and gait changes. The woman should be advised of these expected changes and provided safety measures as appropriate. Family and community resources should be explored to provide supervision for child care for the woman with neurological impairments, as she may be at risk of losing awareness of her surroundings for a time, placing her baby in danger if she is the only adult there. It is important to arrange for another person to help out until the child is a bit older.

Epilepsy

Epilepsy (often called *seizure disorder*) is a disorder of the brain, resulting in recurrent seizures; it is the most common neurological disorder accompanying pregnancy, although less than 1% of all pregnant women have a seizure disorder (Aminoff & Douglas, 2014). Seizure disorders are either acquired (less than 15% of all cases) or idiopathic (more than 85% of all cases), which means that a specific cause for the seizures cannot be identified. The majority of women with a seizure disorder who become pregnant have an uneventful pregnancy with an excellent outcome (Samuels & Niebyl, 2012).

Women with epilepsy should receive preconception counselling if at all possible. A detailed history of medication use and seizure frequency should be obtained. If the woman has frequent seizures before conception, she is likely to continue this pattern during pregnancy; therefore, achieving effective seizure control is extremely important before conception, even if changing medications is required (Samuels & Niebyl, 2012).

Seizures differ in presentation, ranging from absence seizures (brief losses of awareness without loss of consciousness) to tonic–clonic seizures (involving muscle rigidity, violent muscle contractions, and loss of consciousness). Both types of seizures are related to abnormal electrical activity in the brain. Women who have tonic–clonic seizures may experience them more frequently or have more severe complications during pregnancy, such as edema, **alkalosis**, fluid–electrolyte imbalance, cerebral hypoxia, hypoglycemia, and hypocalcemia. Seizures can also be triggered by hormonal changes, fatigue, or sleep deprivation.

NURSING ALERT

Anticonvulsants may decrease the effectiveness of oral contraceptive agents, increasing the risk of unplanned pregnancy.

The effects of pregnancy on epilepsy are unpredictable. Many women experience increased seizure frequency during pregnancy as a result of sleep deprivation or decreased dosing of their antieleptic medication due to concerns about the teratogenic effects on the developing fetus. It is important to emphasize the importance of adequate sleep, adherence to medical regimen, and minimizing stress and other factors known to precipitate seizures (Schachter, 2015). Seizure control is the primary goal in treating pregnant women with epilepsy. Pregnant women must be educated about the risks associated with uncontrolled seizures. Changes to current anticonvulsant medications may have to be made to reduce the risks of teratogenicity. The benefits of effective seizure control versus the risk of uncontrolled seizures must be discussed on an individual basis.

If anticonvulsant therapy must be adjusted or introduced as a new therapy, the lowest effective dose must be used, and monotherapy is preferable to polytherapy. Babies born to mothers exposed to anticonvulsant medications are at increased risk of congenital malformations, cognitive impairment, and fetal death (Samuels & Niebyl, 2012). Congenital anomalies associated with anticonvulsant medications include cleft lip or palate, congenital heart disease, urogenital defects, and neural tube defects. These anomalies are related to the dose, type, and number of anticonvulsant medications taken, not to epilepsy itself (Samuels & Niebyl, 2012).

Pregnant women with epilepsy are advised to take a folic acid supplement of 4 mg daily, which may decrease the incidence of neural tube defects. They are also encouraged to take a prenatal vitamin containing vitamin D daily because anticonvulsant medications can interfere with production of the active form of this vitamin (Cunningham et al., 2014; Samuels & Niebyl, 2012).

SAFETY ALERT

Carbamazepine (Tegretol) and valproate (Depakote) should be avoided if possible during pregnancy, especially during the first trimester, because their use is associated with neural tube defects in the fetus.

Several new anticonvulsant medications have been developed for use within the last decade. More information is needed regarding the fetal effects of these medications. However, any anticonvulsant medication required to achieve good seizure control in a woman with epilepsy should be used, regardless of the increased risk of fetal anomalies, because the most important goal during pregnancy is the prevention of seizures (Samuels & Niebyl, 2012).

If possible, only one anticonvulsant medication—at the lowest dose level that is effective at keeping the woman seizure free—should be prescribed during pregnancy. The increase in plasma volume that is a normal pregnancy change can affect drug metabolism and distribution. Therefore, blood levels of anticonvulsant medications should be checked, and drug dosages adjusted as necessary. With close monitoring, most women with epilepsy should experience no change or even have fewer seizures during pregnancy. An increase in seizure frequency is usually related either to not taking prescribed anticonvulsant medications or to sleep deprivation (Samuels & Niebyl, 2012). If an increase in seizure activity does occur during pregnancy, it is usually in women who had frequent seizures (more than one per month) before pregnancy (Aminoff & Douglas, 2014).

In addition to congenital anomalies, the fetus of a woman with epilepsy is at risk for IUGR. Determining an accurate gestational age as early as possible is important. This information decreases any confusion later in pregnancy regarding fetal growth issues. If the patient's weight gain and fundal height appear appropriate, serial ultrasounds for fetal weight assessment may not be necessary. Maternal serum screening around 16 weeks of gestation and detailed ultrasonography at 18 to 22 weeks of gestation should be performed to assess for the presence of a neural tube defect or other fetal anomalies. NST later in pregnancy is not necessary unless the woman has other medical or obstetrical factors that increase the risk for stillbirth (Samuels & Niebyl, 2012).

Management of anticonvulsant therapy during prolonged labour is challenging. During labour absorption of medications given orally is unpredictable, especially if vomiting occurs. Women who are maintained on phenytoin (Dilantin) or phenobarbital may be given these medications parenterally during labour. No parenteral form of carbamazepine has been developed. Oral administration of carbamazepine may be attempted; but, if the woman experiences a seizure or a preseizure aura, she may be given phenytoin intravenously instead to maintain her through labour. Vaginal birth is preferred (Samuels & Niebyl, 2012). A small risk of seizure activity exists during labour. If a woman experiences tonic–clonic seizures during pregnancy or labour, there is a threefold risk of placental abruption. Intravenous phenytoin can be administered as required.

After birth the levels of anticonvulsant medications must be monitored frequently for the first few weeks because they can rise rapidly. If medication dose levels were increased during pregnancy, they need to be reduced quickly to prepregnancy levels. All of the major anticonvulsant medications are found in breast milk, but the use of these medications is not a contraindication to breastfeeding. However, topiramate has been associated with neonatal weight loss; thus it probably should not be prescribed if the woman is breastfeeding (Samuels & Niebyl, 2012).

During the neonatal period, infants exposed in utero to phenobarbital, phenytoin, and primidone, which cause a vitamin K deficiency, can hemorrhage. However, infants who receive vitamin K at birth have not been shown to have an increased risk of bleeding. This problem is now rare, because most infants routinely receive an intramuscular injection of vitamin K immediately after birth. In addition, phenobarbital and primidone are almost never prescribed, and phenytoin is used to treat epilepsy much less often now than in the past (Samuels & Niebyl, 2012).

All methods of contraception can be used by women with an idiopathic seizure disorder. However, commonly prescribed anticonvulsant medications such as carbamazepine and phenytoin (also topiramate and oxcarbazepine at higher doses) reduce the effectiveness of oral contraceptives. Women taking low-dose oral contraceptives especially may have more breakthrough bleeding and be at risk for an unplanned pregnancy (Cunningham et al., 2014; Samuels & Niebyl, 2012).

In terms of planning for future child-bearing, couples should be informed that children born to women with a seizure disorder of unknown cause have a four times greater chance (risk of 2 to 4%) for an idiopathic seizure disorder compared to the general population. Epilepsy in the father does not appear to increase a child's risk for developing a seizure disorder (Samuels & Niebyl, 2012).

Multiple Sclerosis

Multiple sclerosis (MS), a patchy demyelinization of the spinal cord and CNS, may be a viral disorder. Onset of symptoms, which include weakness of one or both lower extremities, visual disturbances, and loss of coordination, is subtle and usually occurs between the ages of 20 and 40 years. The disease is characterized by exacerbations and remissions. Women are affected twice as often as men. MS does not affect the normal course of pregnancy or birth (Aminoff & Douglas, 2014).

Remissions during pregnancy are common. If an exacerbation occurs, it is more likely to do so during the third trimester of pregnancy or postpartum. Treatment may include corticosteroids and immunosuppressive agents along with rest. Several new drugs and biopharmaceuticals are available for treating MS. Their use in pregnancy has been limited; thus few data and no controlled studies are available. However, many consist of molecules that are too large to cross the placenta. Therefore, they may be acceptable for use during pregnancy. They do not appear to be associated with anomalies (Samuels & Niebyl, 2012). Interferon is also sometimes used to treat MS relapses during pregnancy and postpartum. Its safety for use during pregnancy has not been established, although in theory it should not cross the placenta because of its large molecular size (Stuart & Bergstrom, 2011).

Women who have become paraplegic with MS are more likely to develop UTIs during pregnancy but may feel no symptoms. Therefore they should be screened routinely. Women who have become paraplegic or have lumbosacral lesions as a result of MS may have little pain during labour. Determining when labour begins may be difficult for them. Uterine contractions occur normally, but these women may have difficulty pushing effectively during the second stage of labour. Therefore, vacuum- or forceps-assisted birth may be necessary (Samuels & Niebyl, 2012). Epidural anaesthesia can be used during labour (Stuart & Bergstrom, 2011).

Depression is common among women with MS; they should be assessed frequently for evidence of postpartum depression. Breastfeeding is encouraged, although medications that are Lactation Risk Category L5 should not be prescribed. IV immunoglobulin (IVIG) is considered safe for use during lactation; no adverse effects in infants have been reported. All hormonal contraceptives may be used by women with MS (Stuart & Bergstrom, 2011).

Bell's Palsy

Bell's palsy is an acute idiopathic facial paralysis. The clinical manifestations of Bell's palsy include the sudden development of a unilateral facial weakness, with maximum weakness within 48 hours after onset, pain surrounding the ear, difficulty closing the eye on the affected side, *hyperacusis* (abnormal acuteness of the sense of hearing), and occasionally a loss of taste (Aminoff & Douglas, 2014; Cunningham et al., 2014).

The cause is unknown, but it may be related to the reactivation of herpes virus infection or acute human immunodeficiency virus type 1 (HIV-1) retroviral infections. Bell's palsy occurs fairly often, especially in women of reproductive age. Women are affected two to four times more often than men (Cunningham et al., 2014). Pregnant women are affected three to four times more often than nonpregnant women.

The incidence usually peaks during the third trimester and the puerperium. Women who develop Bell's palsy during pregnancy have an increased risk for gestational hypertension as well (Cunningham et al., 2014).

No effects of maternal Bell's palsy have been observed in infants. Maternal outcome is generally good unless a complete block in nerve conduction occurs. Steroid therapy may improve outcome, although its benefits have not always been proven in past research studies. To be effective, steroids should be administered within the first 5 to 6 days after the paralysis develops (Aminoff & Douglas, 2014). Supportive care includes prevention of injury to the constantly exposed cornea, facial muscle massage, careful chewing and manual removal of food from inside the affected cheek, and reassurance. Although 80% of affected men and nonpregnant women recover to a satisfactory level within a year, only approximately half of women who develop the disorder during pregnancy do so (Cunningham et al., 2014).

Autoimmune Disorders

Autoimmune disorders, also called *collagen vascular diseases*, make up a large group of diseases that disrupt the function of the immune system of the body. In these types of disorders, the immune system is unable to distinguish "self" from "nonself." As a result, antibodies develop that attack its normally present antigens, causing tissue damage. Autoimmune disorders occur more frequently to women in their reproductive years; therefore, associations with pregnancy are not uncommon. Pregnancy may affect the disease process. Some disorders adversely affect the course of pregnancy or are detrimental to the fetus. Autoimmune disorders of concern in pregnancy include systemic lupus erythematosus, myasthenia gravis, antiphosopholipid syndrome, systemic sclerosis, and rheumatoid arthritis (Chin & Ware Branch, 2012; Cunningham et al., 2014).

Systemic Lupus Erythematosus

One of the most common serious disorders in women of childbearing age, systemic lupus erythematosus (SLE), is a chronic multisystem inflammatory disease characterized by autoimmune antibody production that affects the skin, joints, kidneys, lungs, serous membranes, CNS, and liver and heart. The exact cause is unknown, but probably involves the interaction of several factors, including immunological, environmental, hormonal, and genetic factors. Most cases of SLE occur in adolescence or young adulthood. Recently the incidence of SLE has nearly tripled, probably because of increased diagnosis (Chin & Ware Branch, 2012; Gilbert, 2011).

Common symptoms include myalgias, fatigue, weight change, and fevers, and these occur in nearly all women with SLE at some time during the course of the disease. Although a diagnosis of SLE is suspected on the basis of clinical signs and symptoms, it is confirmed by laboratory testing that demonstrates the presence of circulating autoantibodies. As is the case with other autoimmune diseases, SLE is characterized by a series of exacerbations (flares) and remissions (Chin & Ware Branch, 2012).

Authorities have conflicting opinions as to whether pregnancy increases the likelihood of SLE flares. However, it appears that disease activity at the beginning of pregnancy is an important predictor of exacerbations during pregnancy. Therefore, women are advised to wait until they have been in remission for at least 6 months before attempting to become pregnant (Chin & Ware Branch, 2012; Gilbert, 2011). In addition to exacerbations, other maternal risks include an increased rate of miscarriage, nephritis, and pre-eclampsia; a possible need to give birth at a preterm gestation; and an increased risk of Caesarean birth. Fetal risks include stillbirth, IUGR, and preterm birth (Chin & Ware Branch, 2012).

Medical therapy during pregnancy is kept to a minimum in women who are in remission or who have a mild form of SLE. Immunosuppressive medications should be discontinued before conception. Nonsteroidal anti-inflammatory drugs (NSAIDs) and aspirin are ordinarily the most commonly used anti-inflammatory drugs, but they are not recommended for use during pregnancy. Aspirin should not be used after 24 weeks of gestation because of an increased risk of premature closure of the fetal ductus arteriosus (Cunningham et al., 2014). Glucocorticoids such as prednisone are often used to treat SLE during pregnancy, as either maintenance therapy or short-term treatment for flares. There is a small risk for fetal cleft lip and palate if glucocorticoids are used during early pregnancy. Prolonged use of this group of medications also increases the risks for bone demineralization, gestational diabetes, pre-eclampsia, premature rupture of membranes (PROM), and IUGR. Given the significant risks associated with long-term glucocorticoid use, hydroxychloroquine, an antimalarial drug, may be the best medication for maintenance SLE therapy during pregnancy. It significantly reduces SLE disease activity and appears to cause no adverse effects on the fetus (Chin & Ware Branch, 2012).

Prenatal care otherwise focuses on close monitoring to detect common pregnancy complications such as hypertension, proteinuria, and IUGR. Ultrasound examinations are performed frequently to monitor fetal growth. Fetal assessment tests, including daily fetal movement counts and weekly or twice-weekly NSTs and amniotic fluid volume assessments or biophysical profiles, likely begin at 30 to 32 weeks of gestation (see Chapter 13). More frequent ultrasound examinations and fetal testing are necessary if the woman develops an SLE flare, antiphospholipid syndrome, hypertension, proteinuria, or evidence of IUGR (Chin & Ware Branch, 2012).

Women with SLE can develop an exacerbation during labour. Any maintenance medications should be continued throughout the intrapartum period or resumed immediately postpartum at the last pregnancy dose. Even if a flare does not occur, all women who have received chronic glucocorticoid therapy (20 mg or more of prednisone daily for at least 3 weeks) need larger (stress) doses of steroids during labour (Chin & Ware Branch, 2012). Vaginal birth is preferred, but Caesarean birth is common because of maternal and fetal complications.

Close monitoring of all women with SLE should continue after birth. Women who have more severe SLE manifestations or who had an SLE exacerbation during pregnancy are at greatest risk to experience a postpartum flare (Chin & Ware Branch, 2012). During the postpartum period, the mother should rest as much as possible to prevent an exacerbation of SLE. Breastfeeding is encouraged unless the mother is taking immunosuppressive agents. Newborns should be assessed to determine the presence of neonatal lupus, which can be a passively transferred autoimmune disease that occurs in mothers with lupus antibodies.

Women with SLE and chronic vascular or renal disease should limit their number of pregnancies because of the maternal complications associated with the illness and increased adverse perinatal outcomes (Cunningham et al., 2014; Schur & Bermas, 2014). If desired, the safest time for tubal sterilization is during the postpartum period or when the disease is in remission. Estrogen-containing oral contraceptives may increase the risk of thromboembolism (Gilbert, 2011). Progestin-only implants and injections provide effective contraception with no known effects on lupus flares (Cunningham et al., 2014). Barrier methods, in addition to progestin-only contraceptive options, are the least risky forms of contraception for women with SLE (Gilbert, 2011). Evidence does not support concerns regarding an increased risk of infection with IUDs.

Myasthenia Gravis

Myasthenia gravis (MG), an autoimmune motor (muscle) endplate disorder that involves acetylcholine use, affects the motor function at the myoneural junction. Muscle weakness results, particularly in the eyes, face, tongue, neck, limbs, and respiratory muscles. Women with MG experience symptoms of easy fatigability; intermittent double vision (diplopia); upper eyelid drooping; and difficulty speaking, swallowing, and clearing secretions. In more serious cases, upper arm weakness and breathing difficulty are seen. Because the greatest period of risk is during the first year after diagnosis, pregnancy should probably be avoided until symptomatic improvement occurs (Cunningham et al., 2014). The response of women with MG to pregnancy is unpredictable; remission, exacerbation, or continued stability during pregnancy can occur (Chaudhry, Vignarajah, & Koren, 2012).

Pregnancy does not appear to affect the overall course of MG, but as the uterus enlarges respirations may be compromised. In addition, the normal fatigue experienced by many pregnant women may be tolerated poorly by those with MG (Cunningham et al., 2014). Treatment during pregnancy is the same as for nonpregnant women. Usual medications include glucocorticoids and acetylcholinesterase inhibitors. Monitoring blood glucose values is important because hyperglycemia may result from corticosteroid therapy. Thymectomy may result in remission of the disease but is best performed before or after pregnancy if at all possible. For severe weakness plasmapheresis or IVIG therapy may be needed.

! NURSING ALERT

Magnesium sulphate must not be administered to women with MG because it inhibits the release of acetylcholine and can trigger myasthenic crisis.

Because MG does not affect smooth muscle, most women tolerate labour well. Vaginal birth is desired, but vacuum or forceps assistance may be required because of muscle weakness. Oxytocin may be given, but medications that cause muscular relaxation should be avoided if at all possible. Narcotics must be used cautiously because they may cause respiratory depression, and women with MG are already at risk for respiratory muscle weakness. Regional analgesia is preferred (Aminoff & Douglas, 2014; Chaudhry et al., 2012; Cunningham et al., 2014). After birth, women must be carefully supervised because relapses often occur during the postpartum period.

Approximately 10 to 15% of babies born to mothers with MG will develop neonatal myasthenia. This transient disorder results from the transfer of maternal antibody against acetylcholine receptors across the placenta. Symptoms, which include a poor cry, respiratory difficulties, weakness in suckling, a weak Moro reflex, and feeble limb movements, usually appear within the first 72 hours after birth. Neonatal myasthenia can be treated with anticholinesterase medications and usually resolves by 6 weeks after birth (Aminoff & Douglas, 2014).

Spinal Cord Injury

More than half of all spinal cord injuries (SCIs) occur in persons between the ages of 16 and 30, with women representing approximately 18% of cases (ACOG 2002/2014). As a result of increased survival and improved rehabilitation techniques, more women with SCIs are considering pregnancy. Chronic effects of SCI may include autonomic dysrreflexia (AD), impaired pulmonary function, chronic pulmonary or genitourinary infections, anemia, osteoporosis, and decubitus ulcers. AD is a potentially dangerous clinical syndrome that results in acute, uncontrolled hypertension. Pregnant women with SCI may also be at increased risk of deep vein thrombosis and pulmonary embolus (ACOG, 2002/2014).

Antepartum Care

Many women with disabilities identify that it is difficult to find information on pregnancy and its effects on their disability (Tarasoff, 2015). A prepregnancy assessment is preferred for women with SCI in order to determine the level of function and presence of associated medical complications. Once a woman is pregnant, it is important that antenatal visits be tailored to the disabled woman's unique needs. Frequent urine cultures and skin examination for decubitus ulcers should be conducted in addition to routine antenatal care. Anemia may be associated with an increased risk of decubitus ulcers, thus additional iron supplementation during pregnancy may be required. Women must make frequent position changes during pregnancy. Extra padding and/or refitting of wheelchairs may be necessary in later stages of pregnancy. A multidisciplinary approach is preferred for patients with SCI. Anaesthetic consultation is suggested because of the risk of AD during labour and the potential for impaired pulmonary function. Urology consultation may be considered for those with indwelling or suprapubic catheters or with evidence of impaired renal function. Physiotherapy consultation may be helpful, as mobility may become more impaired as pregnancy progresses and to assist with prevention of decubitus ulcers. Occupational therapy consultation may be helpful to optimize the patient's ability to care for her infant in her home. Rates of preterm labour, pre-eclampsia, or congenital malformation are not increased in women with SCI; however, women who have SCI related to myelomeningocele do have a risk of recurrence and should take 4.0 mg of folic acid daily for 3 months prior to conception (Wilson et al., 2011).

Collaboration among interdisciplinary team members is essential to ensure a positive perinatal experience for woman with disabilities. Perinatal care providers and those who provide disability-specific care need to practise clear communication with one another (Tarasoff, 2015). An individualized advanced care plan should be developed to ensure good communication among team members and the women's wishes for her birth.

Intrapartum Care

Vaginal birth is preferred for patients with SCI; Caesarean birth should be reserved for obstetrical indications. Induction may be considered in women who do not feel uterine activity or fetal movement, to prevent the risk of undiagnosed labour and a possible unattended birth at home. Women should be instructed that symptoms such as increased spasticity or shortness of breath may be signs of uterine contractions.

Women with spine lesions above T6 are at increased risk of AD during labour secondary to uterine contractions. Women should be cared for in a centre that is capable of invasive hemodynamic monitoring and able to provide medications for treatment of AD. The use of regional anaesthesia, such as epidural or combined spinal–epidural, preferably instituted at the onset of labour, may help to prevent or decrease the risk of AD. Foley catheters should be placed routinely in women without an indwelling catheter to avoid the need to self-catheterize during labour. Assisted vaginal birth may be necessary due to inadequate expulsive effort.

Postpartum Care

For women with SCI, special attention must be paid to bladder elimination in order to avoid urinary retention, to minimize the risk of urinary tract infection and AD. Bowel regimens should be resumed postpartum. Breastfeeding is possible and encouraged in these women, but individualized assessment is important. Women need assistance to gain independence with positioning and latching of the baby, using props to aid in their potentially limited use of gross and fine motor arm movements. Additional care must be provided to address mobility in women who have undergone Caesarean birth. An assessment of home supports and the need for extra nursing once the woman returns home should be made. Insufficient evidence exists to support routine deep vein thrombosis prophylaxis in the puerperium in women with SCI. Patients should be assessed on a case-by-case basis.

Human Immunodeficiency Virus and Acquired Immunodeficiency Syndrome

The percentage of women with HIV in Canada was 23 to 28% in 2011, with 26% of newly diagnosed cases being women (Money, Tullock, Boucoiran, et al., 2014; Public Health Agency of Canada [PHAC], 2012). Most of these women were and continue to be of child-bearing age. Antiretroviral treatment (ART) works to decrease perinatal transmission rates and the progression of AIDS-related complications. This section addresses the management of the pregnant woman who is HIV positive. See Chapter 7 for more information about the diagnosis and management of nonpregnant women with HIV and Chapter 29 for a discussion of HIV infection in infants.

Preconception Counselling

At the present time in Canada, women who are HIV positive are having successful pregnancies, resulting in noninfected, healthy newborns (Money et al., 2014). The key to optimal perinatal outcomes for women is preconception pregnancy counselling and planning. Preconception pregnancy planning should include consultation with providers specialized in the area of HIV infections and pregnancy. This assessment should include a review of the woman's HIV history, current physical status, and prenatal and HIV-specific laboratory results. The other critical component of preconception counselling is to carefully review with the woman a plan on how to decrease the risk of transmission to the child as well as decrease the pregnancy, intrapartum, and postnatal risks.

Pregnancy Risks

Pregnant women who are HIV positive need to be engaged in ongoing specialized prenatal care that involves physicians, nurses, pharmacists, nutrition counsellors, social workers, and community support to ensure healthy outcomes for both the mother and infant. Care includes strict adherence with an antiretroviral medication regime, following through with regular HIV-specific blood-level monitoring (viral plasma levels and immunological functioning), and being well informed regarding labour, birth, and postpartum. Even if a diagnosis of HIV is made late in pregnancy or during the intrapartum period, it can be treated with antiretroviral medications, thus decreasing the risk of perinatal transmission.

CRITICAL THINKING CASE STUDY

The Pregnant Woman Who Is HIV Positive

Betsy is being seen in the prenatal clinic at 34 weeks of gestation. She has been positive for the human immunodeficiency virus (HIV) for 2 years and has a past history of substance use, with a history of using intravenous cocaine and heroin for over 5 years. She has been substance free for the last 18 months. This is Betsy's first baby and it is an unplanned pregnancy. During your nursing assessment, she tells you that she was started on medication for her HIV when she was 3 months pregnant. Betsy does not seem to know the names of the pills she is taking and says she tries to remember to take them daily but sometimes misses some doses. As part of your care, you will be providing Betsy information about the importance of attending prenatal visits regularly, taking her antiretroviral medication daily, and having blood tests done monthly.

QUESTIONS

1. Evidence—Is there sufficient evidence to draw conclusions about the necessity of continued care, treatment, and support for Betsy and her infant?
2. Assumptions—What assumptions can be made about the following issues?
   a. The rationale and importance of adherence with Betsy's antiretroviral medication treatment, comprehensive prenatal care, and planning throughout her pregnancy
   b. Maternal and child HIV antiretroviral medication prophylaxis regime
   c. Risk factors for acquiring HIV infection that are in Betsy's history
   d. Review of perinatal HIV transmission prevention as you plan to provide care for Betsy and her infant
3. What implications and priorities for nursing care can be drawn at this time?
4. Does the evidence objectively support your conclusion?

HIV-positive women should be encouraged to seek prenatal care immediately if they suspect pregnancy, in order to maximize chances for a positive outcome. Pregnancy itself does not appear to significantly accelerate the progression of HIV infection. One of the most overwhelming situations for a pregnant woman is when she is newly diagnosed with a positive HIV result. This situation must be supported with intensive counselling and support for the women and often for her partner (see Critical Thinking Case Study).

Perinatal transmission. Perinatal transmission may occur to the fetus through the maternal circulation as early as the first trimester of pregnancy, to the infant during labour and birth, or to the infant through breast milk. Factors that increase the likelihood of perinatal viral transmission are listed in Box 15-4.

Identification of the HIV-positive pregnant woman is especially important because antepartum and intrapartum antiviral medication therapy has been shown to greatly decrease the risk of viral transmission to the fetus. With optimal maternal child HIV-prevention treatment available throughout Canada, the percentage of infected newborns has decreased dramatically to less than 2% (Money et al., 2014). Without treatment, the HIV perinatal transmission rate can range between 25 and 40%. Data show that almost all HIV-positive

BOX 15-4 FACTORS INCREASING THE RISK OF MOTHER-TO-CHILD PERINATAL HIV TRANSMISSION

- Lack of maternal and infant treatment with antiretroviral medications and prevention
- Maternal plasma viral level greater than 1000 copies per millilitre
- Maternal vaginal infections during pregnancy
- Amniocentesis, chorionic villus sampling, or both
- Ruptured membranes
- Presence of chorioamnionitis
- Fetal scalp monitoring and venous scalp sampling
- Interventions such as forceps, vacuum, and external cephalic version
- Breastfeeding

childhood diagnoses not attributed to mother-to-child transmission were in children from endemic countries (Forbes, Alimenti, Singer, et al., 2012).

Obstetrical complications. It is difficult to determine obstetrical risk in persons with HIV infection because so many confounding variables are often present. HIV-positive women may have lives complicated by such issues as substance use, mental health issues, poverty, poor nutrition, limited access to prenatal care, or concurrent sexually transmitted infection (STI). Many of these variables can account for a woman being at risk for preterm labour and birth, premature rupture of membranes, perinatal loss, and IUGR. The mode of birth for women who are HIV positive depends on the woman's plasma viral level and her status of labour upon admission. If a woman's plasma level is less than 1000 copies per millilitre and she has received ART, she can proceed with a vaginal birth. In women positive for HIV who are not receiving antiretrovirals and have a plasma load greater than 1000, an unknown plasma level, or antepartum bleeding, a Caesarean birth is recommended (Money et al., 2014). The postpartum period for the woman infected with HIV may be notable for infection, hemorrhage, or both. Women without symptoms may have an unremarkable postpartum course; alternatively, immunosuppressed women with symptoms may be at increased risk for postpartum UTIs, vaginitis, postpartum endometritis, and poor wound healing. HIV-related thrombocytopenia may also increase the risk of hemorrhage. It is critical that women remain on their antiretroviral medication throughout their pregnancy and into the postpartum period.

NURSING CARE

HIV counselling and testing is recommended for all pregnant women in Canada when they initially enter prenatal care. Women engaging in high-risk behaviour should be offered HIV counselling and testing at each trimester of their pregnancy. Not all HIV-positive women will be detected prenatally. Any woman whose HIV status is unknown at the time of labour or birth should be screened with a rapid HIV test, unless she declines.

HIV-infected women should also be tested for other STIs, such as gonorrhea; syphilis; chlamydia; hepatitis B, C, and D; and herpes. Cytomegalovirus and toxoplasmosis antibody testing should be done because both infections can cause significant maternal and fetal complications and can be successfully treated with antimicrobial agents. Any history of vaccination and immune status should be documented, and chicken pox (varicella) and rubella titres should be determined (Money et al., 2014). Women who are HIV positive should be vaccinated against hepatitis B, pneumococcal infection, hemophilus B influenza, and viral influenza. A tuberculin skin test should be performed; a positive test necessitates a chest x-ray film to identify active pulmonary disease. A Papanicolaou (Pap) test should also be done.

All HIV-infected women should be treated with ART during pregnancy, regardless of the CD4 counts. ART should include three drugs from at least two classes of antiretroviral medications. The major adverse effect of these medications is bone marrow suppression. Periodic hematocrit, white blood cell count, and platelet count assessments should be performed. Women with CD4 counts of less than 200 cells/mm^3 should receive prophylactic treatment for *Pneumocystis carinii* pneumonia with daily trimethoprim-sulphamethoxazole. Any other opportunistic infections should be treated with medications specific for the infection; often dosages must be higher for women with HIV infection (Money et al., 2014).

The woman who is HIV positive requires nutritional support and counselling. Weight gain or maintenance in pregnancy can be a challenge. Women need to be supported and counselled regarding safer sex practices to reduce risks for herself and her partner. Use of condoms and a spermicide is encouraged to minimize further exposure to HIV if her partner is positive.

The woman should be referred for drug rehabilitation, as necessary, to support her to discontinue the use of substances. Use of alcohol, methamphetamines ("speed," "ice"), marijuana, cocaine, nitrites ("poppers," "snappers"), or other drugs compromises the body's immune system and increases the risks of AIDS and associated conditions. It also interferes with many medical and alternative therapies for AIDS.

IV zidovudine is administered to the HIV-positive woman during the intrapartum period. A loading dose is initiated on her admission in labour, followed by a continuous maintenance dosage throughout labour (Money et al., 2014).

Every effort should be made during the birthing process to decrease the newborn's exposure to infected maternal blood and secretions if Caesarean birth is not scheduled and the woman goes into labour. If feasible, the membranes should be left intact until the birth. Increased duration of ruptured amniotic membranes has been associated with increased perinatal transmission. If rupture of membranes occurs before labour, induction of uterine contractions with oxytocin may be appropriate. Fetal scalp electrode and scalp pH sampling should be avoided because these procedures may result in inoculation of the virus into the fetus (Money et al., 2014). Operative vaginal birth (forceps or vacuum extractor) and episiotomy should also be avoided, when possible.

Immediately after birth, infants should be wiped free of all body fluids. Prior to blood testing or any injections, the skin area should be cleansed well with soap and water. All staff working with the mother or infant must adhere to routine precautions for exposure to blood and other body fluids. The infant can be placed skin-to-skin with the mother after birth, but breastfeeding is discouraged because of the risk of transmission through breast milk. Oral zidovudine treatment for the infant is initiated within 6 hours of life and continues for up 6 weeks. In the postpartum period, it is critical that women who are HIV positive be assessed for postpartum infections. Women and their infants require close postpartum follow-up by providers specialized in HIV, in the hospital and upon discharge. This will ensure that ART and maternal and infant blood work are maintained and monitored. A postpartum contraception discussion should be part of the nurse's and provider's discussion with the woman prior to discharge from the hospital.

SUBSTANCE USE

Substance use among women in Canada is recognized as an increasing concern from both a health and a social perspective (Abrahams, Mackay-Dunn, Nevmerjitskais, et al., 2010). Women are using a variety of substances, the most common being alcohol, tobacco, and mood-altering and pain-relieving prescribed medications, as well as illicit drugs such as marijuana, cocaine, heroin, crack, crystal methamphetamine, and opioids. *Substance use* or *problematic use* can be defined by compulsive drug use and loss of control over use, resulting in physical, social, and psychological consequences. Symptoms of withdrawal and tolerance can be seen in women who use substances (Wong, Ordean, & Kahan, 2011). Women who use substances have an increased incidence of unplanned pregnancies.

The damaging effects of alcohol and illicit drugs on pregnant women and their unborn babies are well documented (Gilbert, 2011; Wisner et al., 2012). Alcohol and other drugs easily pass from a mother to her baby through the placenta. Smoking during pregnancy has serious health risks, including bleeding complications, miscarriage, stillbirth, prematurity, low birth weight, and sudden unexplained infant death (Gilbert, 2011; Wisner et al., 2012). Congenital anomalies have occurred in infants of mothers who have taken drugs. The safest pregnancy is one in which the woman is drug and alcohol free, although this is not always possible for some women. For women addicted to opioids, methadone maintenance treatment is the current standard of care during pregnancy (Wisner et al., 2012).

Barriers to Treatment

Women who use substances and are pregnant often do not seek prenatal care, for many reasons. The most notable of these are guilt, stigma, and shame, as well as the fear of losing custody of a child. Pregnant women who use substances commonly have little understanding of the ways in which these substances affect them, their pregnancies, and their infants. They often delay seeking prenatal care until labour begins. Traditionally, substance use treatment programs for women have not addressed issues that affect pregnant women, such as concurrent need for obstetrical care and child care for other children. Long waiting lists and lack of women-only recovery spaces present further barriers to treatment.

Legal Considerations

Nurses who care for women who use substances in pregnancy must use a nonjudgemental and women-centred approach based on a harm reduction model of care (Abrahams et al., 2010). Women should be encouraged to attend prenatal care that is accessible for them and to participate in counselling and treatment. A flexible multidisciplinary team is invaluable when caring for women who are pregnant and using substances. It is critical that women experiencing substance use receive accessible and consistent care and support with a strong focus on their individual physical and psychosocial needs (Abrahams et al., 2010). Throughout Canada, every community needs to support policies that strengthen harm reduction practices and substance use prevention programs designed for young women and the provision of women-only treatment and recovery programs.

Drug Testing During Pregnancy

There is no legal requirement in Canada for a health care provider to test either the mother or the newborn for the presence of drugs, unless the provincial child agency requests this. However, nurses need to know the practices in the health region where they are working. In both hospitals and community health centres, it is best to consult with the facility's social workers regarding drug testing, following informed consent from the woman.

NURSING CARE

The care of the woman who is pregnant and using substances should be based on self-disclosure of her present and past use, prenatal health history, physical findings, and laboratory results. Screening questions for alcohol, tobacco, prescribed and nonprescribed medications, and illicit substance use should be included in the overall assessment of all women, regardless of socioeconomic status, at their first prenatal visit (Wong et al., 2011). Women need to be assessed for a history of violence, abuse, and mental health concerns, as well as lack of access to other determinants of health, such as poverty and lack of housing and social supports that put women at risk and can increase their substance use.

It is critical for nurses and other providers to use a nonjudgemental interview and questioning technique when gathering substance-use information from women (see Chapter 5, p. 66). Screening tools that have been developed and used in the past are not always accurate in the practice setting. Urine and toxicology testing is not recommended as a clinical screening tool for pregnant women. Testing of maternal hair and newborn meconium is also not recommended for clinical use. Maternal serum toxicology or urine testing is helpful to support a woman's self-reporting of her current substance use status. When drug testing is ordered clinically or requested by the provincial child protection agency, informed consent from the woman is mandatory. When testing is ordered in the newborn, parental or guardian informed consent is also required.

Following the initial prenatal assessment, serial ultrasound studies should be performed to confirm gestational age. Some women may have had amenorrhea as a result of substance use or may not know when their last menstrual period occurred. There is an increased risk of stillbirth and of small-for-gestational-age infants as well as the potential for perinatal hypoxia. If concerns are detected, regular ultrasound examination and fetal surveillance with monitoring should be arranged.

In planning care for a pregnant woman who uses substances, the perinatal nurse must individualize her approach, taking the women's past history and expressed needs into consideration. Although the ideal long-term outcome is total abstinence, in Canada a harm reduction philosophy of care is practised, supporting a woman's desire to stop using as well as assisting her in reducing her risks. If the woman can only reduce her use of substances, support and care are still offered. A realistic goal may be to decrease substance use, and short-term outcomes will be necessary.

A multidisciplinary team model is essential when planning care for women who use substances. Major issues that must be addressed in treatment for these women that generally are not part of treatment are low self-esteem, stigmatization, high probability of sexual abuse and physical abuse, lack of social support, need for social services and child care, need for women's health services, and need for support and education in the mothering role. Safe housing or residential supervised communities may offer an ideal route toward stabilization in a safe environment. Recovery and treatment for women must demonstrate cultural sensitivity and recognition of diversity and ethnicity as an important part of her identity. Other needs of many of these women include relationship counselling, coping skills training, and vocational and legal assistance (Wong et al., 2011).

Interventions with women who use substances need to begin with trust and communication. Women are often very receptive to learning how they can keep their growing fetus safe and healthy by stopping or reducing substance use. Women are often more receptive to making lifestyle changes during pregnancy than at any other time in their lives. The casual, experimental, or recreational drug user is often able to achieve and maintain abstinence from substances when she receives education, support, and continued monitoring throughout her pregnancy. Pregnancy presents a window of opportunity for motivating women to stop their use of substances (Abrahams et al., 2010).

Stabilization and treatment for women who use substances should be individualized for each woman, depending on the type of drug used and the frequency and amount of use.

Detoxification, short-term inpatient or outpatient treatment, long-term residential treatment, aftercare services, and self-help support groups are all possible options. Neonatal outcomes are improved among infants whose mothers received an integration of substance use treatment with prenatal care. In most communities in Canada, treatment options are limited for women, especially facilities that allow children to be with their mothers. Some women find organizations such as Alcoholics Anonymous or Narcotics Anonymous, based on the 12-step program, very helpful, and meetings can be found in almost every community. A caution for women using the 12-step program is that the program's emphasis is on powerlessness over addiction and avoidance of codependency, which some women might find disempowering and isolating.

Methadone maintenance treatment for pregnant women dependent on opiates is the current standard (Jones, Finnegan, & Kaltenback, 2012; Wisner et al., 2012). Preliminary research has found methadone treatment to have a higher patient treatment retention rate (Jones et al., 2012). Buprenorphine is a semisynthetic opioid derivative used to treat opioid addiction at higher dosages and to control moderate acute pain in non–opioid-tolerant individuals at lower dosages. Use of buprenorphine has been shown to have less neonatal abstinence syndrome (Minozzi, Amato, Bellisario, et al., 2013). Methadone and buprenorphine therapy, along with woman-focused psychosocial and behavioural counselling, has been shown to decrease the use of opiates and other drugs, reduce high-risk activity, improve birth weight, and decrease the rates of pre-eclampsia and exposure to HIV. Disadvantages of methadone therapy include fetal heart rate changes (e.g., fewer accelerations, decreased rate and variability), a decrease in fetal breathing episodes, and neonatal abstinence syndrome (Wisner et al., 2012).

Cocaine and crystal methamphetamine use during pregnancy has increased dramatically in the last few years. A number of maternal and fetal complications can occur, including placental abruption, stillbirth, prematurity, and small-for-gestational-age infants.

Because of the risks that women who use substances experience in their lives, exposure to STIs and HIV is increased. STI monitoring for gonorrhea and chlamydia infection and antibody determinations for hepatitis B and HIV counselling and testing should be offered frequently to substance-using women. A chest x-ray film may be taken to assess for pulmonary problems such as hilar lymphadenopathy, pulmonary edema, bacterial pneumonia, and foreign-body emboli. A skin test to screen for tuberculosis may also be ordered.

Nurses must understand the reasons why women use substances, the barriers to stopping use, and their life experiences. Planning the best care for women who are pregnant and use substances must be based on a women-focused framework (Box 15-5). Mother–infant attachment should be encouraged by identifying the woman's strengths and reinforcing positive maternal response and interactions. Promoting skin-to-skin contact immediately following birth and keeping mothers and their infants together has been proven to be beneficial for both members of the dyad (Abrahams et al, 2010).

Advice regarding breastfeeding must be individualized. Although all substances appear in breast milk, some in greater amounts than others, breastfeeding has many benefits. Breastfeeding should be delayed until the potential risks and benefits

BOX 15-5 PERINATAL CARE FOR WOMEN WHO USE SUBSTANCES

- Realize that the decision to stop using substances and engage in recovery can only be made by the woman herself.
- Understand that the nurse's role can be that of an advocate and facilitator for positive change in a woman's life.
- Provide education for nurses on the reasons why women use substances and the barriers to recovery in pregnancy. Know that violence, trauma, and mental health history contribute to a women's substance use and her ability to ask for help.
- Review the effects of perinatal substance use in pregnancy, intrapartum, and on the newborn infant.
- Women-centred and harm reduction practices are critical in caring for women who use substances. Respect, understanding, and choices should be key components in nursing care and planning.
- Be familiar with community resources for women, including accessible health clinics and providers; housing services, both emergency and long term; counselling and mental health supports; and substance recovery and treatment centres. Contact numbers for community services should be available in the hospital and clinic for women and their providers.

have been reviewed. Instructing and supporting women in hand expression, breast pumping, and then discarding of the expressed colostrum or breast milk is helpful for women wishing to breastfeed during this delay. Women should be encouraged to remain substance free if they are breastfeeding. Some women have no desire to breastfeed, whereas others find it provides a strong motivation to achieve and maintain their substance-free status.

Before discharge, the woman needs to have an effective and resourceful discharge plan, which should be made with the assistance of nursing and other health care providers. If the woman is unable to provide care for her infant or has chosen not to care for her infant, the infant may be placed with her family or in foster care. Support and counselling for this mother are extremely beneficial, and planning for future visits with her infant is often helpful.

Most women who have a history of substance use will require assistance in planning for hospital discharge with their infant. Adequate and safe housing, food and formula provisions, transportation supports, and recovery and parenting supports are essential services for the woman to be successful as a new parent. The hospital or community social worker, along with the provincial child agency worker, will often be involved in assessing the woman's needs and in assisting the woman to ensure that supports and resources are put in place before discharge. Often family members or friends will be asked to become actively involved with the woman and her infant before discharge. The public or community health nurse will be asked to make home visits to assist and support the women and her infant. Postpartum doula support may also be helpful at this time. Community providers will encourage the women to follow up with them soon after discharge for regular postpartum visits for herself and her infant. Primary care providers must follow up with women soon after discharge to establish regular postpartum visits for herself and the new infant.

KEY POINTS

- Careful monitoring of blood glucose levels, insulin administration, and dietary counselling are instrumental in creating a normal intrauterine environment for fetal growth and development in the pregnancy complicated by pregestational diabetes mellitus.
- Poor maternal glycemic control prior to conception and in the first trimester of pregnancy may be responsible for fetal congenital malformations and maternal complications such as miscarriage, infection, pre-eclampsia, and dystocia (difficult labour) caused by macrosomia.
- Maternal insulin requirements increase as the pregnancy progresses and may quadruple by term as a result of insulin resistance created by placental hormones, insulinase, and cortisol.
- Thyroid dysfunction during pregnancy requires close monitoring of thyroid hormone levels to regulate therapy and prevent fetal insult.
- The stress of the normal maternal adaptations to pregnancy on a women with heart disease may cause further cardiac decompensation.
- Anemia, the most common medical disorder of pregnancy, affects at least 20% of pregnant women.
- Women in their reproductive years have an increased prevalence of autoimmune disorders (e.g., systemic lupus erythematosus and myasthenia gravis); therefore, it is important for care providers to be familiar with the effects of these disorders on pregnancy.
- Women with spinal cord injuries do become pregnant and nurses need to understand the specific needs of these clients.
- Obesity in pregnancy is associated with risk factors for both mother and fetus and requires increased surveillance.
- Perinatal administration of ART is recommended to decrease perinatal transmission of HIV from mother to child. HIV testing for all pregnant women is critical, and preconception counselling is the best practice for women who are HIV positive.
- Women who use substances and are pregnant need a harm-reduction care approach, with support from a variety of sources. These supports can come from partners, family, health care providers, and the community.
- Understanding why women use substances and the barriers to recovery will assist in a woman's success with stabilization and treatment.

Evolve WEBSITE

Visit the Evolve website for additional resources related to the content in this chapter such as Case Studies, Critical Thinking Case Study Answers, Nursing Care Plans, Nursing Processes, Nursing Skills, and Review Questions for Exam Preparation at: http://evolve.elsevier.com/Canada/Perry/maternal/

REFERENCES

Abrahams, R., Mackay-Dunn, M., Nevmerjitskais, V., et al. (2010). An evaluation of rooming in among substance exposed newborns in British Columbia. *Journal of Obstetrics and Gynaecology Canada*, *32*(9), 866–871.

Allen, V., Armson, B. A., Wilson, R. D., et al. (2007). SOGC clinical practice guideline: Teratogenicity associated with pre-existing and gestational diabetes. *Journal of Obstetrics and Gynaecology Canada*, *29*(11), 927–933.

Allen, U., & Canadian Paediatric Society. (2010). Infective endocarditis: Updated guidelines. *Paediatrics & Child Health*, *15*(4), 205–208. Reaffirmed 2014.

American College of Obstetricians and Gynecologists (ACOG). (2002). Obstetric management of patient with spinal cord injuries. *ACOG*, Committee Opinion No. 275. Reaffirmed 2014.

American College of Obstetricians and Gynecologists (ACOG). (2013). Obesity in pregnancy. ACOG Committee opinion No. 549. *Obstetrics & Gynecology*, *121*(1), 213–217.

American College of Obstetricians and Gynecologists (ACOG). (2015). Thyroid disease in pregnancy. Practice bulletin No. 148. *Obstetrics & Gynecology*, *125*, 996–1005.

Aminoff, M. J., & Douglas, V. C. (2014). Neurologic disorders. In R. Resnick, R. K. Creasy, J. Iams, et al. (Eds.), *Creasy & Resnik's maternal–fetal medicine: Principles and practice* (7th ed.). Philadelphia: Saunders.

Bahn, R. S., Burch, H. S., Cooper, D. S., et al. (2009). The role of propylthiouracil in the management of Graves' disease in adults: Report of a meeting jointly sponsored by the American Thyroid Association and the Food and Drug Administration. *Thyroid*, *7*, 673.

Bello, N., Hurtado, I., & Arany, Z. (2013). The relationship between preeclampsia and peripartum cardiomyopathy: A systematic review and meta-analysis. *Journal of American College of Cardiology*, *62*(18), 1715–1723. doi:10.1016/j.jacc.2013.08.717.

Blackburn, S. (2013). *Maternal, fetal, and neonatal physiology: A clinical perspective* (4th ed.). St. Louis: Mosby.

Blanchard, D. G., & Daniels, L. B. (2014). Cardiac diseases. In R. Resnick, R. K. Creasy, J. Iams, et al. (Eds.), *Creasy & Resnik's maternal–fetal medicine: Principles and practice* (7th ed.). Philadelphia: Saunders.

Breton, M.-C., Beauchesne, M.-F., Lemière, C., et al. (2010). Risk of perinatal mortality associated with asthma during pregnancy: A 2-stage sampling cohort study. *Annals of Allergy, Asthma and Immunology*, *105*(3), 211–217.

Cappell, M. (2012). Hepatic and gastrointestinal diseases. In S. G. Gabbe, J. R. Niebyl, & J. L. Simpson (Eds.), *Obstetrics: Normal and problem pregnancies* (6th ed.). Philadelphia: Saunders.

Chan, W.-S., Rey, E., & Kent, N. (2014). Venous thromboembolism and antithrombotic therapy in pregnancy. *Journal of Obstetrics and Gynaecology Canada*, *36*(6), 527–553.

Chaudhry, S., Vignarajah, B., & Koren, G. (2012). Mothrerisk update: Myasthenia gravis during pregnancy. *Canadian Family Physician*, *58*, 1346–1349. Retrieved from <http://www.cfp.ca/content/58/12/1346.full.pdf>.

Chin, C., & Ware Branch, D. (2012). Collagen vascular diseases. In S. G. Gabbe, J. R. Niebyl, & J. L. Simpson (Eds.), *Obstetrics: Normal and problem pregnancies* (6th ed.). Philadelphia: Saunders.

Cunningham, F. G., Leveno, K., Bloom, S., et al. (2014). *Williams obstetrics* (24th ed.). New York: McGraw Hill.

Dahdouh, E. M., Balayla, J., Audibert, F., et al. (2015). SOGC technical update: Preimplantation genetic testing. *Journal of Obstetrics and Gynaecology Canada*, *37*(5), 451–463. Retrieved from <http://sogc.org/wp-content/uploads/2015/05/gui323TU1505E.pdf>.

Davies, G., & Herbert, W. (2007a). Heart disease in pregnancy 1: Assessment and management of cardiac disease in pregnancy. *Journal of Obstetrics and Gynaecology Canada*, *29*(4), 331–336.

Davies, G., & Herbert, W. (2007b). Heart disease in pregnancy 2: Congenital heart disease in pregnancy. *Journal of Obstetrics and Gynaecology Canada*, *29*(5), 409–414.

Davies, G., & Herbert, W. (2007c). Heart disease in pregnancy 3: Acquired heart disease in pregnancy. *Journal of Obstetrics and Gynaecology Canada*, *29*(6), 507–509.

Davies, G., & Herbert, W. (2007d). Heart disease in pregnancy 4: Ischemic heart disease and cardiomyopathy in pregnancy. *Journal of Obstetrics and Gynaecology Canada*, *29*(7), 575–579.

Davies, G., Maxwell, C., McLeod, L., et al. (2010). SOGC clinical practice guideline: Obesity in pregnancy. *Journal of Obstetrics and Gynaecology Canada*, *32*(2), 165–173.

De Groot, L., Abalovich, M., Alexander, E. K., et al. (2012). Management of thyroid dysfunction during pregnancy and postpartum: An Endocrine Society clinical practice guideline. *Journal of Clinical Endocrinology Metabolism*, *97*(8), 2543.

Earl, R., Crowther, C. A., & Middleton, P. (2013). Interventions for hyperthyroidism pre-pregnancy and during pregnancy. *Cochrane Database of Systematic Reviews 2013*, (11). doi:10.1002/14651858.CD008633.pub3.

Easterling, T. R., & Stout, K. (2012). Heart disease. In S. G. Gabbe, J. R. Niebyl, & J. L. Simpson (Eds.), *Obstetrics: Normal and problem pregnancies* (6th ed.). Philadelphia: Saunders.

Forbes, J. C., Alimenti, A. M., Singer, J., et al. (2012). A national review of vertical HIV transmission. *AIDS (London, England)*, *26*, 757–763.

Gaddipati, S., & Troiano, N. H. (2013). Cardiac disorders in pregnancy. In N. H. Troiano, C. J. Harvey, & B. F. Chez (Eds.), *AWHONN's high risk and critical care obstetrics* (3rd ed.). Philadelphia: Lippincott Williams and Wilkins.

Gilbert, E. S. (2011). *Manual of high risk pregnancy and delivery* (5th ed.). St. Louis: Mosby.

Gunatilake, R., & Perlow, J. (2011). Obesity and pregnancy: Clinical management of the obese gravid. *American Journal of Obstetrics and Gynecology*, *204*(2), 106–119. doi:10.1016/j.ajog.2010.10.002.

Haider, B. A., Olofin, I., Wang, M., et al. (2013). Anaemia, prenatal iron use, and risk of adverse pregnancy outcomes: A systematic review and meta-analysis. *BMJ (Clinical Research Ed)*, *346*, f3443.

Heavey, E. (2011). Obesity in pregnancy: Deliver sensitive care. *Nursing 2011*, *41*(10), 42–50. doi:10.1097/01.NURSE.0000405101.68864.19.

Herring, S. J., Platek, D. N., Elliott, P., et al. (2010). Addressing obesity in pregnancy: What do obstetric providers recommend? *Journal of Women's Health*, *19*(1), 65–70.

Inoue, M., Arata, N., Koren, G., & Ito, S. (2009). Hyperthyroidism during pregnancy. *Canadian Family Physician*, *55*, 701–703.

Inturrisi, M., Lintner, N. C., & Sorem, K. (2013). Diabetic ketoacidosis and continuous insulin infusion management in pregnancy. In N. Troiano, C. Harvey, & B. Chez (Eds.), *AWHONN's high risk and critical care obstetrics* (3rd ed.). Philadelphia: Wolters Kluwer/Lippincott Williams & Wilkins.

Jones, H., Finnegan, L., & Kaltenback, K. (2012). Methadone and buprenorphine for the management of opioid dependence in pregnancy. *Drugs*, *72*(6), 747–757.

Katz, V. (2012). Postpartum care. In S. G. Gabbe, J. R. Niebyl, & J. L. Simpson (Eds.), *Obstetrics: Normal and problem pregnancies* (6th ed.). Philadelphia: Saunders.

Kilpatrick, S. J. (2014). Anemia and pregnancy. In R. Resnick, R. K. Creasy, J. Iams, et al. (Eds.), *Creasy & Resnik's maternal–fetal medicine: Principles and practice* (7th ed.). Philadelphia: Saunders.

Kitzmiller, J. L., Block, J. M., Brown, F. M., et al. (2008). Managing preexisting diabetes for pregnancy: Summary of evidence and consensus recommendations for care. *Diabetes Care, 31*(5), 1060–1079. doi:10.2337/dc08-9020.

Kolte, D., Khera, S., Aronow, W. S., et al. (2014). Temporal trends in incidence and outcomes of peripartum cardiomyopathy in the United States: A nationwide population-based study. *Journal of the American Heart Association, 3*(3), e001056.

Koren, G., Sarkar, M., & Einarson, A. (2010). The use of Montelukast in pregnancy. *Canadian Family Physician, 56*, 881–882.

Kroumpouzos, G. (2012). Skin disease in pregnancy and puerperium. In S. G. Gabbe, J. R. Niebyl, & J. L. Simpson (Eds.), *Obstetrics: Normal and problem pregnancies* (6th ed.). Philadelphia: Saunders.

Landon, M. B., Catalano, P. M., & Gabbe, S. G. (2012). Diabetes mellitus complicating pregnancy. In S. G. Gabbe, J. R. Niebyl, & J. L. Simpson (Eds.), *Obstetrics: Normal and problem pregnancies* (6th ed.). New York: Churchill Livingstone.

Langlois, S., Ford, J., & Chitayat, D. (2008). SOGC clinical practice guideline: Carrier screening for thalassemia and hemoglobinopathies in Canada. *Journal of Obstetrics and Gynaecology Canada, 28*(4), 324–332.

Lawrence, R. A., & Lawrence, R. M. (2011). *Breastfeeding: A guide for the medical profession* (7th ed.). St. Louis: Mosby.

Liston, R., Sawchuck, D., Young, D., et al. (2007). SOGC clinical practice guideline: Fetal health surveillance: Antepartum and intrapartum consensus guideline. *Journal of Obstetrics and Gynaecology Canada, 29*(9), Suppl 4.

Madappa, T., & Sharma, S. (2015). Pulmonary disease and pregnancy. *Medscape*. Retrieved from <http://emedicine.medscape.com/article/303852-overview>.

Magee, L. A., Pels, A., Helewa, M., et al. (2014). SOGC clinical practice guideline: Diagnosis, evaluation and management of the hypertensive disorders of pregnancy: Executive Summary. *Journal of Obstetrics and Gynaecology Canada, 36*(5), 416–438.

Mestman, J. H. (2012). Thyroid and parathyroid diseases in pregnancy. In S. G. Gabbe, J. R. Niebyl, & J. L. Simpson (Eds.), *Obstetrics: Normal and problem pregnancies* (6th ed.). New York: Saunders.

Minozzi, S., Amato, L., Bellisario, C., et al. (2013). Maintenance agonist treatments for opiate-dependent pregnant women. *Cochrane Database of Systematic Reviews*, (12), CD006318.

Money, D., Tullock, K., Boucoiran, I., et al. (2014). SOGC clinical practice guideline: Guidelines for the care of pregnant women living with HIV and interventions to reduce perinatal transmission. *Journal of Obstetrics and Gynaecology Canada, 36*(8 eSuppl A), S1–S46.

Moore, T. R., Hauguel-De Mouzon, S., & Catalano, P. (2014). Diabetes in pregnancy. In R. Resnick, R. K. Creasy, J. Iams, et al. (Eds.), *Creasy & Resnik's maternal–fetal medicine: Principles and practice* (7th ed.). Philadelphia: Saunders.

Nader, S. (2014). Thyroid disease and pregnancy. In R. Resnick, R. K. Creasy, J. Iams, et al. (Eds.), *Creasy & Resnik's maternal–fetal medicine: Principles and practice* (7th ed.). Philadelphia: Saunders.

Perelló, J. L., Masoller, J., Esteve, J., & Palacioa, M. (2014). Intravenous ferrous sucrose versus placebo in addition to oral iron therapy for the treatment of severe postpartum anaemia: A randomized controlled trial. *BJOG: An International Journal of Obstetrics and Gynaecology, 121*(6), 706–713. doi:10.1111/1471-0528.12480.

Pieper, P. G. (2012). The pregnant woman with heart disease: Management of pregnancy and delivery. *Netherlands Heart Journal, 20*(1), 33–37. doi:10.1007/s12471-011-0209-y.

Public Health Agency of Canada (PHAC). (2012). *Population-specific HIV/AIDS status report: Women*. Ottawa: PHAC. Retrieved from <http://library.catie.ca/pdf/ATI-20000s/26407.pdf>.

Rapini, R. (2014). The skin and pregnancy. In R. Resnick, R. K. Creasy, J. Iams, et al. (Eds.), *Creasy & Resnik's maternal–fetal medicine: Principles and practice* (7th ed.). Philadelphia: Saunders.

Ross, D. (2014). Hyperthyroidism during pregnancy: Treatment. *UpToDate*. Retrieved from <http://www.uptodate.com/contents/hyperthyroidism-during-pregnancy-treatment>.

Royal College of Obstetrics & Gynecology. (2011). *Management of sickle cell disease in pregnancy*. Green top Guideline Number 61. Retrieved from <https://www.rcog.org.uk/globalassets/documents/guidelines/gtg_61.pdf>.

Royal College of Obstetrics & Gynecology. (2014). *Management of beta thalassemia in pregnancy*. Green Top Guideline Number 66. Retrieved from <https://www.rcog.org.uk/globalassets/documents/guidelines/gtg_66_thalassaemia.pdf>.

Samuels, P. (2012). Hematologic complications of pregnancy. In S. Gabbe, J. Niebyl, J. Simpson, et al. (Eds.), *Obstetrics: Normal and problem pregnancies* (6th ed.). Philadelphia: Saunders.

Samuels, P., & Niebyl, J. R. (2012). Neurologic disorders. In S. Gabbe, J. Niebyl, J. Simpson, et al. (Eds.), *Obstetrics: Normal and problem pregnancies* (6th ed.). Philadelphia: Saunders.

Saravanakumar, K., Rao, S., & Cooper, G. (2006). Obesity and obstetric anesthesia. *Anesthesia, 61*(1), 36–48.

Schachter, S. (2015). Management of epilepsy and pregnancy. *UpToDate*. Retrieved from <http://www.uptodate.com/contents/management-of-epilepsy-and-pregnancy>.

Schur, P., & Bermas, B. (2014). Pregnancy in women with systemic lupus erythematosus. *UpToDate*. Retrieved from <http://www.uptodate.com/contents/pregnancy-in-women-with-systemic-lupus-erythematosus?source=search_result&search=lupus+and+pregnancy&selectedTitle=1~150>.

Short, M., & Domagalski, J. (2013). Iron deficiency anemia: Evaluation and management. *American Family Physician, 87*(2), 98–104.

Sliwa, K., Hilfiker-Kleiner, D., Petrie, M. C., et al. (2010). Current state of knowledge on aetiology, diagnosis, management, and therapy of peripartum cardiomyopathy: A position statement from the Heart Failure Association of the European Society of Cardiology Working Group on peripartum cardiomyopathy. *European Journal of Heart Failure, 12*(8), 767–781. doi:10.1093/eurjhf/hfq120.

Stagnaro-Green, A., Abalovich, M., Alexander, E., et al. (2011). Guidelines of the American Thyroid Association for the diagnosis and management of thyroid disease during pregnancy and postpartum. *Thyroid, 21*(10), 1081.

Statistics Canada. (2011). *Health trends* (Statistics Canada Catalogue No. 82-213-XWE). Ottawa: Author. Retrieved from <http://www12.statcan.gc.ca/health-sante/82-213/index.cfm?Lang=ENG>.

Stuart, M., & Bergstrom, L. (2011). Pregnancy and multiple sclerosis. *Journal of Midwifery & Women's Health, 56*(1), 41–47.

Sutander, M., Garcia-Bournissen, F., & Koren, G. (2007). Hypothyroidism in pregnancy. *Journal of Obstetrics and Gynaecology Canada, 29*(4), 354–356.

Tarasoff, L. (2015). Experiences of women with physical disabilities during the prenatal period: A review of the literature and recommendations to improve care. *Health Care for Women International, 36*, 88–107.

Thompson, D., Berger, H., Feig, D., et al. (2013). Clinical practice guidelines. Diabetes and pregnancy. *Canadian Journal of Diabetes, 37*, S168–S183.

Walters, M., & Taylor, J. (2009/2010). Maternal obesity: Consequences and prevention strategies. *Nursing for Women's Health, 13*(6), 486–494.

Weinberger, S., Lockwood, C. L., & Barnes, P. (2013). Dyspnea during pregnancy. *UpToDate*. Retrieved from <http://www.uptodate.com/contents/dyspnea-during-pregnancy>.

Whitty, J., & Dombrowski, M. (2012). Respiratory diseases in pregnancy. In S. G. Gabbe, J. R. Niebyl, & J. L. Simpson (Eds.), *Obstetrics: Normal and problem pregnancies* (6th ed.). Philadelphia: Saunders.

Whitty, J. E., & Dombrowski, M. P. (2014). Respiratory diseases in pregnancy. In R. Resnick, R. K. Creasy, J. Iams, et al. (Eds.), *Creasy & Resnik's maternal–fetal medicine: Principles and practice* (7th ed.). Philadelphia: Saunders.

Williamson, C., Mackillop, L., & Heneghan, M. A. (2014). Diseases of the liver, biliary system, and pancreas. In R. Resnick, R. K. Creasy, J. Iams, et al. (Eds.), *Creasy & Resnik's maternal–fetal medicine: Principles and practice* (7th ed.). Philadelphia: Saunders.

Wilson, R. D., Audibert, F., Brock, J., et al. (2011). Genetic considerations for a woman's pre-conception evaluation. *Journal of Obstetrics and Gynaecology Canada, 33*(1), 57–64.

Wilson, W., Taubert, K. A., Gewitz, M., et al. (2007). Prevention of infective endocarditis: Guidelines from the American Heart Association. *Circulation, 116*, 1736–1754.

Wisner, K. L., Sit, D. K., Altemus, M., et al. (2012). Mental health and behavioral disorders in pregnancy. In S. G. Gabbe, J. R. Niebyl, & J. L. Simpson (Eds.), *Obstetrics: Normal and problem pregnancies* (6th ed.). Philadelphia: Saunders.

World Health Organization (WHO). (2012). *Guideline (2012): Daily iron and folic acid supplementation in pregnant women.* Geneva: Author.

Wong, S., Ordean, A., & Kahan, M. (2011). SOGC clinical practice guideline: Substance use in pregnancy. *Journal of Obstetricians and Gynaecologists Canada, 33*(4), 367–384.

Zhang, J., Bricker, L., Wray, S., & Quenby, S. (2007). Poor uterine contractility in obese women. *British Journal of Obstetrics and Gynaecology, 114*, 343–348.

ADDITIONAL RESOURCES

British Columbia Reproductive Care Program—General Clinical Management of Pregnant Substance Using Women: <http://www.perinatalservicesbc.ca/Documents/Guidelines-Standards/Maternal/ClinicalManagementSubstanceUse.pdf>.

CATIE—HIV and Pregnancy: <http://www.catie.ca/en/healthy-living/hiv#other>.

Society of Obstetricians & Gynaecologists of Canada—Substance Use in Pregnancy: <http://sogc.org/wp-content/uploads/2013/01/gui256CPG1104E.pdf>.

Spinal Cord Injury BC—Pregnancy and Spinal Cord Injury: *An information booklet for women with SCI*: <http://sexualhealth.sci-bc.ca/wp-content/uploads/2015/05/Pregnancy-and-SCI-booklet-V7.pdf>.

UNIT 5

Childbirth

CHAPTER

16

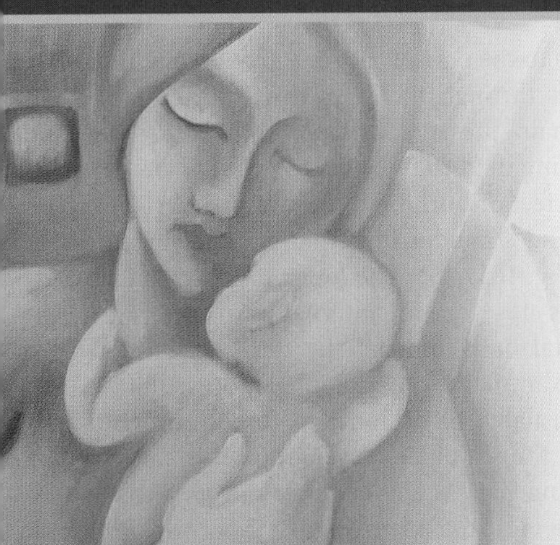

Labour and Birth Processes

Lisa Keenan-Lindsay, with contributions from Kitty Cashion

evolve WEBSITE

Visit the Evolve website for additional resources related to the content in this chapter such as Case Studies, Critical Thinking Case Study Answers, Nursing Care Plans, Nursing Processes, Nursing Skills, and Review Questions for Exam Preparation at: *http://evolve.elsevier.com/Canada/Perry/maternal/*

OBJECTIVES

On completion of this chapter the reader will be able to:

- Explain five major factors that affect the labour process.
- Describe the anatomical structure of the bony pelvis.
- Recognize the normal measurements of the diameters of the pelvic inlet, cavity, and outlet.
- Explain the significance of the size and position of the fetal head during labour and birth.
- Describe factors thought to contribute to the onset of labour.
- Summarize the cardinal movements of labour for a vertex presentation.
- Examine the maternal anatomical and physiological adaptations to labour.
- Describe fetal adaptations to labour.

During late pregnancy, the woman and fetus prepare for the labour process. The fetus has grown and developed in preparation for extrauterine life. The woman has undergone various physiological adaptations during pregnancy that prepare her for birth and motherhood. Labour and birth represent the end of pregnancy, the beginning of extrauterine life for the newborn, and a change in the lives of the family members. This chapter discusses the factors affecting labour, the processes involved, the normal progression of events, and the adaptations made by both the woman and fetus.

FACTORS AFFECTING LABOUR

At least five factors affect the process of labour and birth. These are easily remembered as the five P's: **p**assenger (fetus and placenta), **p**assageway (birth canal), **p**owers (contractions), **p**osition of the mother, and **p**sychological response. The first four factors are presented here as the basis of understanding the physiological process of labour. The fifth factor is discussed in Chapter 17. Other factors that may be a part of the woman's labour experience may be important as well. Hodnett, Gates, Hofmeyr, et al. (2012) identified external forces, including place of birth, type of provider (especially nurses), availability of labour support, and procedures. Physiology (sensations) was identified as an internal force. These factors are discussed generally in Chapter 17 as they relate to nursing care during labour.

Passenger

The movement of the passenger, or fetus, through the birth canal is determined by several interacting factors: the size of the fetal head, fetal **presentation**, fetal lie, fetal attitude, and fetal position. Because the placenta also must pass through the birth canal, it can be considered a passenger along with the fetus; however, the placenta rarely impedes the process of labour in normal vaginal birth. An exception is the case of placenta previa (see Chapter 14).

Size of the Fetal Head

Because of its size and relative rigidity, the fetal head has a major effect on the birth process. The fetal skull is composed of two

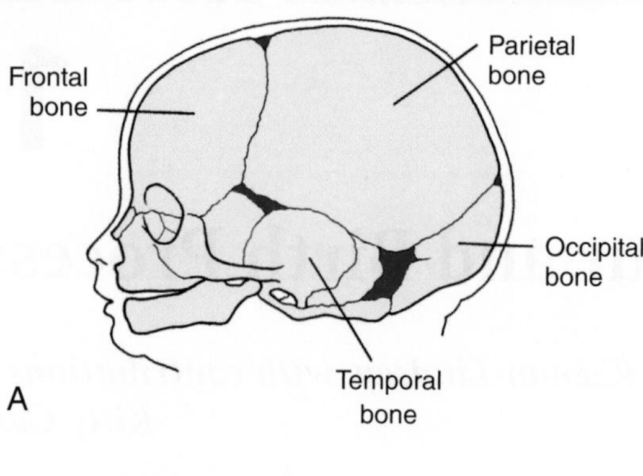

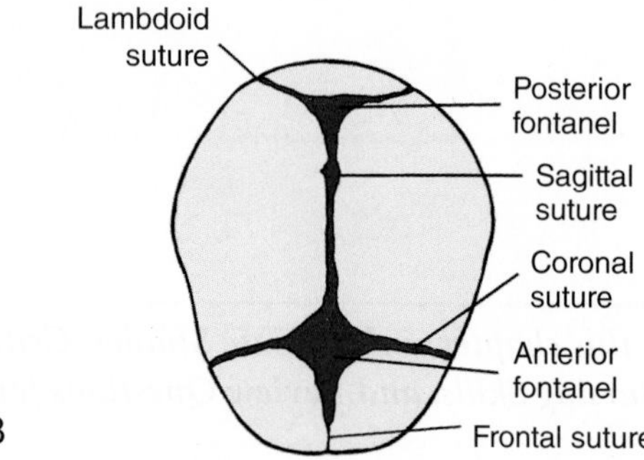

FIGURE 16-1 Fetal head at term. **A:** Bones. **B:** Sutures and fontanels.

parietal bones, two temporal bones, the frontal bone, and the occipital bone (Fig. 16-1, A). These bones are united by membranous sutures: the sagittal, lambdoidal, coronal, and frontal (see Fig. 16-1, B). Membrane-filled spaces called *fontanels* are located where the sutures intersect. During labour, after the rupture of the membranes, palpation of the fontanels and sutures during vaginal examination reveals fetal presentation, position, and attitude.

The two most important fontanels are the anterior and posterior (see Fig. 16-1, B). The larger of these, the anterior fontanel, is diamond shaped, about 3 cm × 2 cm, and lies at the junction of the sagittal, coronal, and frontal sutures. It closes by 18 months after birth. The posterior fontanel lies at the junction of the sutures of the two parietal bones and the one occipital bone, is triangular, and is about 1 cm × 2 cm. It closes 6 to 8 weeks after birth.

Sutures and fontanels make the skull flexible to accommodate the infant brain, which continues to grow for some time after birth. However, because the bones are not firmly united, slight overlapping of the bones, or moulding of the shape of the head, occurs during labour. This capacity of the bones to slide over one another also permits adaptation to the various diameters of the maternal pelvis. Moulding can be extensive, but the heads of most newborns assume their normal shape within 3 days after birth.

Although the size of the fetal shoulders may affect passage, their position can be altered relatively easily during labour so that one shoulder may occupy a lower level than the other. This creates a shoulder diameter that is smaller than the skull, facilitating passage through the birth canal. The circumference of the fetal hips is usually small enough not to create problems.

Fetal Presentation

Presentation refers to the part of the fetus that enters the pelvic inlet first and leads through the birth canal during labour at term. The three main presentations are *cephalic presentation* (head first), occurring in 96% of births (Fig. 16-2); *breech presentation* (buttocks, feet or both first), occurring in 3% of births (Fig. 16-3, A–C); and shoulder presentation, seen in less than 1% of births (see Fig. 16-3, D). The *presenting part* is that part of the fetus that lies closest to the internal os of the cervix. It is the part of the fetal body first felt by the examining finger during a vaginal examination. In a cephalic presentation, the presenting part is usually the occiput; in a breech presentation it is the sacrum; in the shoulder presentation it is the scapula. When the presenting part is the occiput, the presentation is noted as vertex (see Fig. 16-2). Factors that determine the presenting part include fetal lie, fetal attitude, and extension or flexion of the fetal head.

Fetal Lie

Lie is the relation of the long axis (spine) of the fetus to the long axis (spine) of the mother. The two primary lies are *longitudinal*, or vertical, in which the long axis of the fetus is parallel with the long axis of the mother (see Fig. 16-2); and *transverse*, horizontal, or oblique, in which the long axis of the fetus is at a right angle diagonal to the long axis of the mother (see Fig. 16-3, D). Longitudinal lies are either cephalic or breech presentations, depending on the fetal structure that first enters the mother's pelvis. Vaginal birth cannot occur when the fetus stays in a transverse lie. An *oblique lie*, one in which the long axis of the fetus is lying at an angle to the long axis of the mother, is less common and usually converts to a longitudinal or transverse lie during labour (Cunningham, Leveno, Bloom, et al., 2014).

Fetal Attitude

Attitude is the relation of the fetal body parts to one another. The fetus assumes a characteristic posture (attitude) in utero partly because of the mode of fetal growth and partly because of the way the fetus conforms to the shape of the uterine cavity. Normally, the back of the fetus is rounded so that the chin is flexed on the chest, the thighs are flexed on the abdomen, and the legs are flexed at the knees. The arms are crossed over the thorax, and the umbilical cord lies between the arms and the legs. This attitude is termed *general flexion* (see Fig. 16-2).

Deviations from the normal attitude may cause challenges for the labour and birth process. For example, in a cephalic presentation, the fetal head may be extended or flexed in a manner that presents a head diameter that exceeds the limits of the maternal pelvis, leading to prolonged labour, forceps- or vacuum-assisted birth, or Caesarean birth.

Certain critical diameters of the fetal head may be measured. The **biparietal diameter**, which is about 9.25 cm at term, is the largest transverse diameter and an important indicator of fetal head size (Fig. 16-4, B). In a well-flexed cephalic presentation, the biparietal diameter is the widest part of the head entering the pelvic inlet. Of the several anteroposterior diameters, the

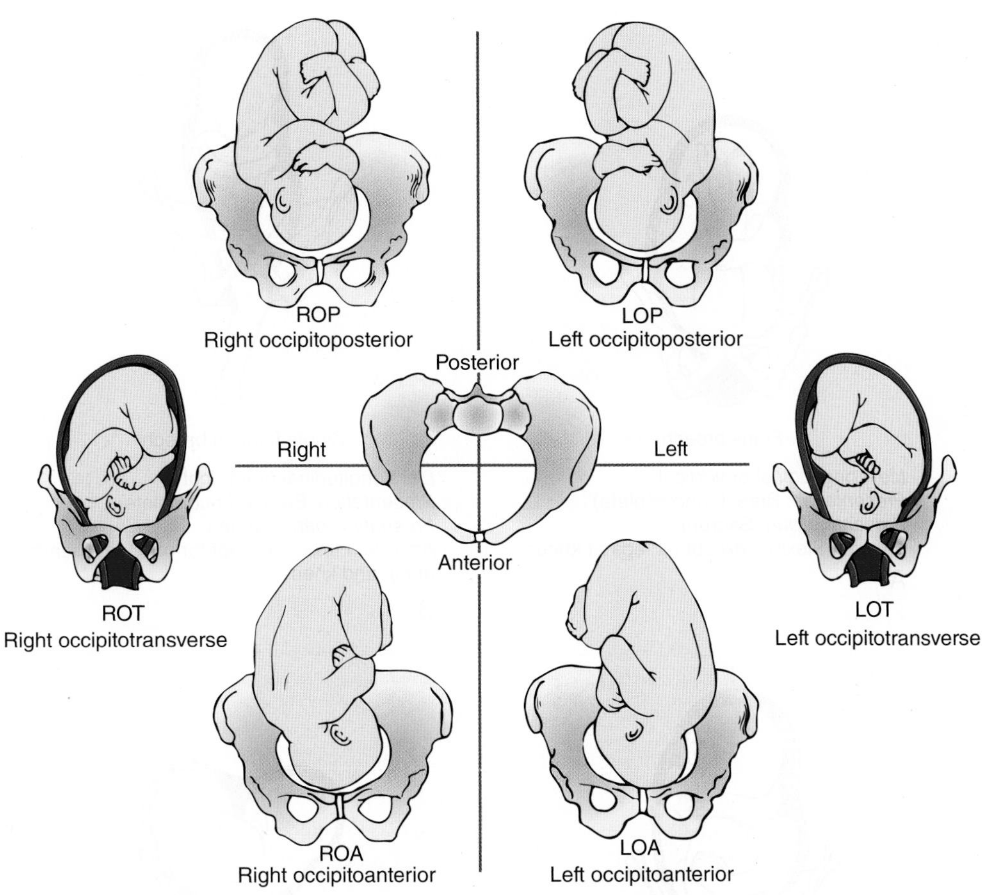

FIGURE 16-2 Examples of fetal vertex (occiput) presentations in relation to front, back, or side of the maternal pelvis.

smallest and the most critical one is the suboccipitobregmatic diameter (about 9.5 cm at term) (Fig. 16-4, A). When the head is in complete flexion, this diameter allows the fetal head to pass through the true pelvis easily (Fig. 16-5, A). As the head is more extended, the anteroposterior diameter widens, and the head may not be able to enter the true pelvis (see Fig. 16-5, B and C).

Fetal Position

The presentation or presenting part indicates the portion of the fetus that overlies the pelvic inlet. **Position** is the relationship of a reference point on the presenting part (occiput, sacrum, mentum [chin], or sinciput [deflexed vertex]) to the four quadrants of the mother's pelvis (see Fig. 16-2). Position is denoted by a three-letter abbreviation. The first letter of the abbreviation denotes the location of the presenting part in the right (R) or left (L) side of the mother's pelvis. The middle letter stands for the specific presenting part of the fetus (O for occiput, S for sacrum, M for mentum [chin], and Sc for scapula [shoulder]). The third letter stands for the location of the presenting part in relation to the anterior (A), posterior (P), or transverse (T) portion of the maternal pelvis. For example, ROA means that the occiput is the presenting part and is located in the right anterior quadrant of the maternal pelvis (see Fig. 16-2). LSP means that the sacrum is the presenting part and is located in the left posterior quadrant of the maternal pelvis (see Fig. 16-3).

Station is the relationship of the presenting fetal part to an imaginary line drawn between the maternal ischial spines and is a measure of the degree of descent of the presenting part of the fetus through the birth canal. The placement of the presenting part is measured in centimetres above or below the ischial spines (Fig. 16-6). For example, when the lowermost portion of the presenting part is 1 cm above the spines, it is noted as being minus (–) 1. At the level of the spines, the station is referred to as 0 (zero). When the presenting part is 1 cm below the spines, the station is said to be plus (+) 1. Birth is imminent when the presenting part is at +4 to +5 cm. The station of the presenting part should be determined when labour begins so that the rate of descent of the fetus during labour can be accurately determined.

Engagement is the term used to indicate that the largest transverse diameter of the presenting part (usually the biparietal diameter) has passed through the maternal pelvic brim or

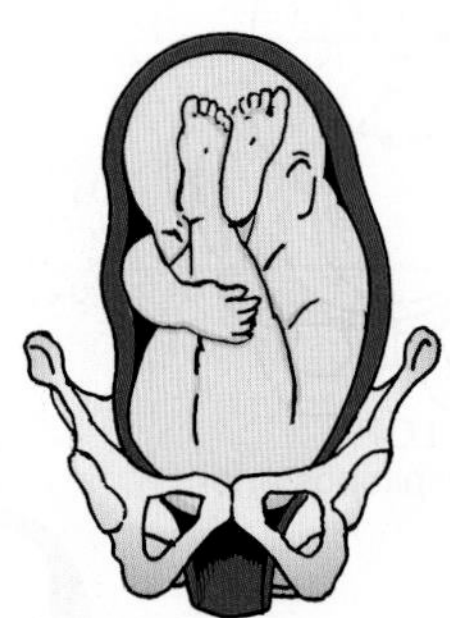

Frank breech

Lie: Longitudinal or vertical
Presentation: Breech (incomplete)
Presenting part: Sacrum
Attitude: Flexion, except for legs at knees

A

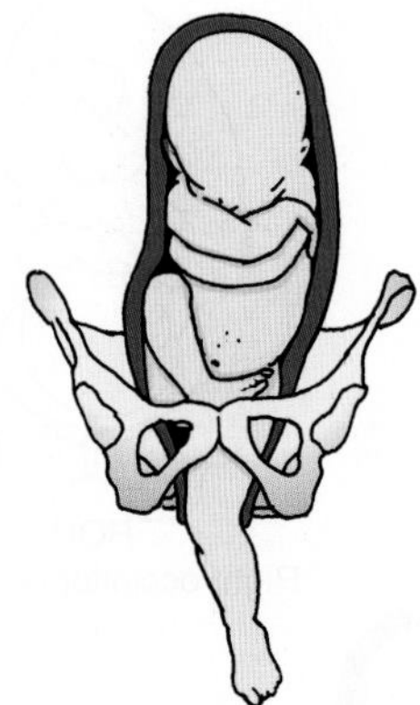

Single footling breech

Lie: Longitudinal or vertical
Presentation: Breech (incomplete)
Presenting part: Sacrum
Attitude: Flexion, except for one leg extended at hip and knee

B

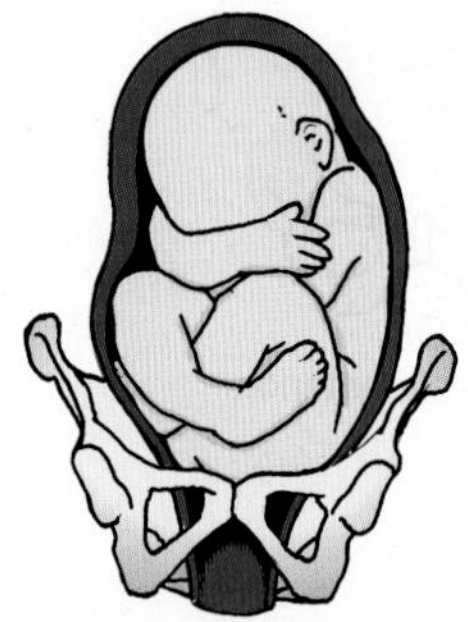

Complete breech

Lie: Longitudinal or vertical
Presentation: Breech (sacrum and feet presenting)
Presenting part: Sacrum (with feet)
Attitude: General flexion

C

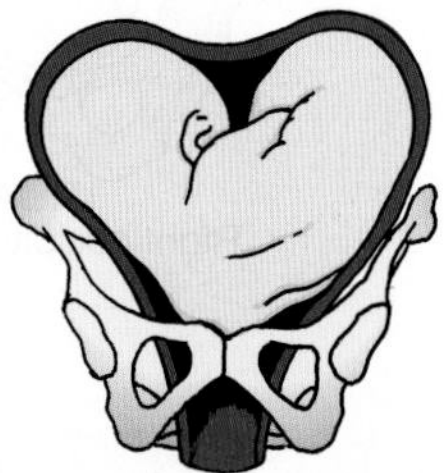

Shoulder presentation

Lie: Transverse or horizontal
Presentation: Shoulder
Presenting part: Scapula
Attitude: Flexion

D

FIGURE 16-3 Fetal presentations. **A** to **C:** Breech (sacral) presentation. **D:** Shoulder presentation.

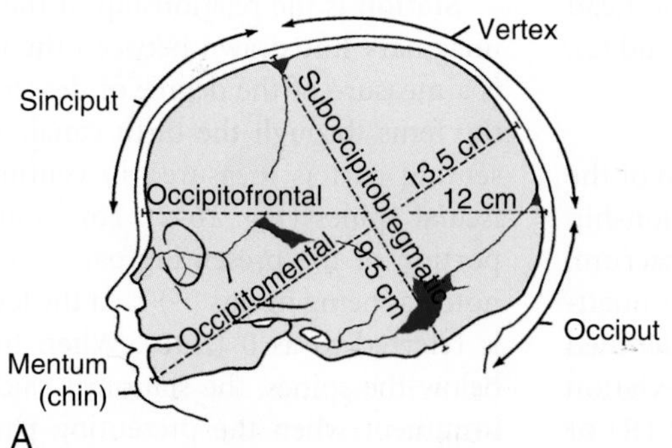

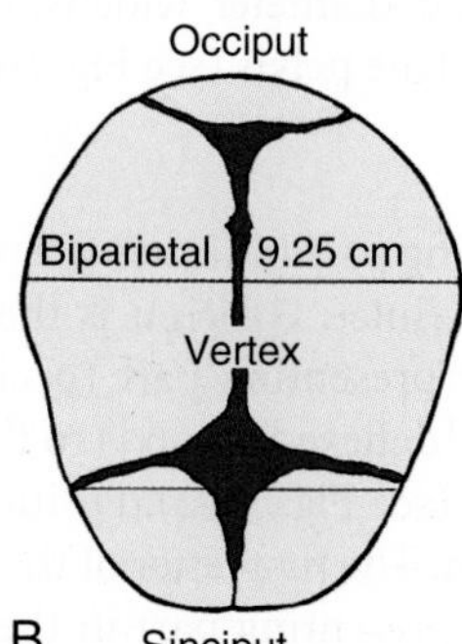

FIGURE 16-4 Diameters of the fetal head at term. **A:** Cephalic presentations: occiput, vertex, and sinciput; and cephalic diameters: suboccipitobregmatic, occipitofrontal, and occipitomental. **B:** Biparietal diameter.

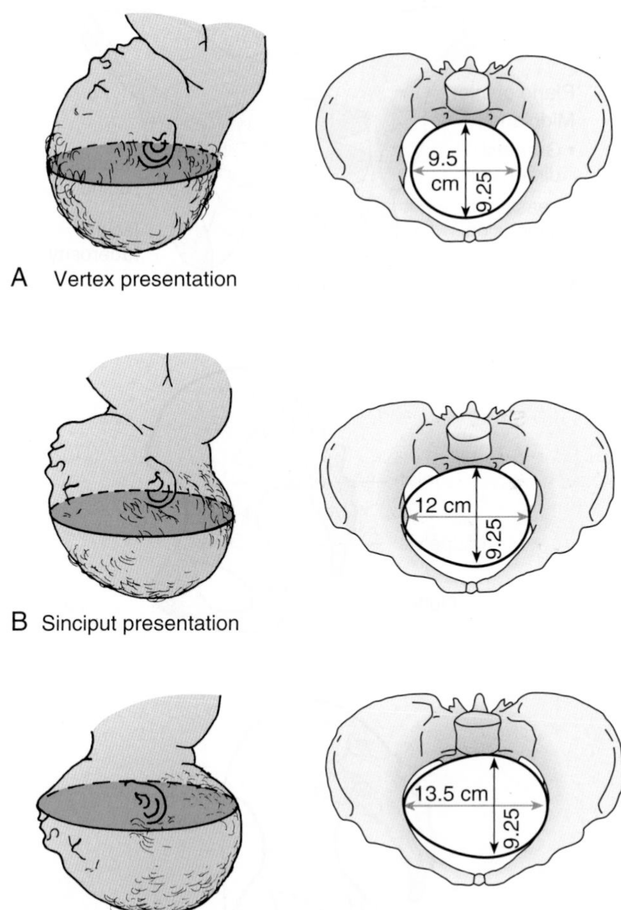

FIGURE 16-5 Head entering pelvis. Biparietal diameter is indicated with shading (9.25 cm). **A:** Suboccipitobregmatic diameter: complete flexion of head on chest so that smallest diameter enters. **B:** Occipitofrontal diameter: moderate extension (military attitude) so that large diameter enters. **C:** Occipitomental diameter: marked extension (deflection) so that the largest diameter, which is too large to permit head to enter pelvis, is presenting.

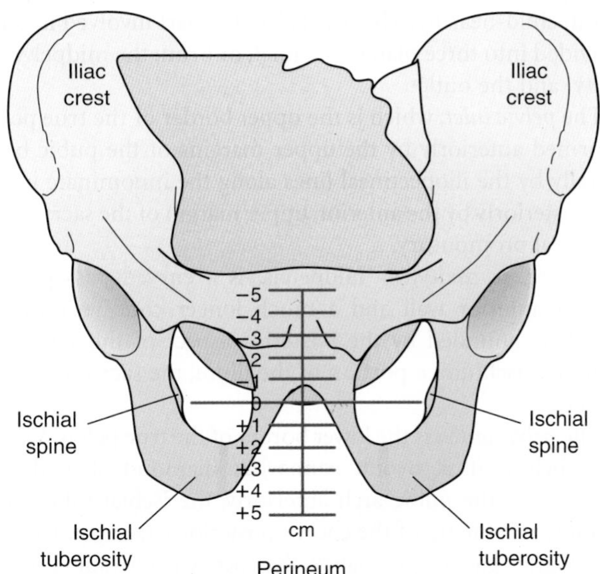

FIGURE 16-6 Stations of presenting part, or degree of descent. Lowest portion of presenting part is at level of ischial spines, station 0.

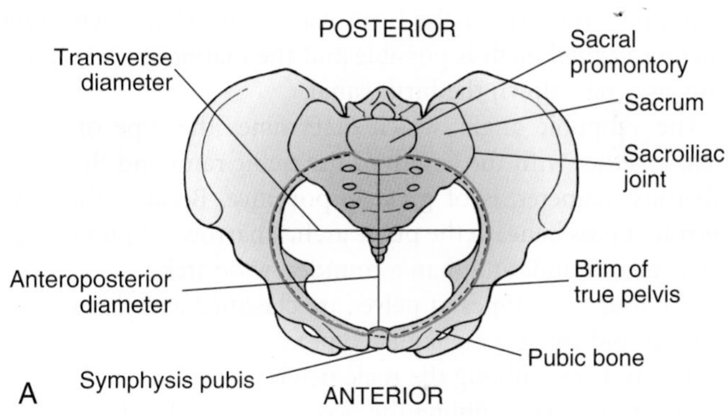

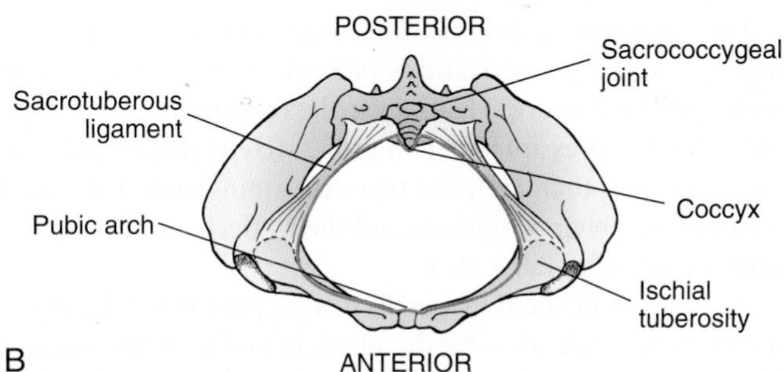

FIGURE 16-7 Female pelvis. **A:** Pelvic brim as viewed from above. **B:** Pelvic outlet from below, as seen by health care provider when the woman is lying supine.

inlet into the true pelvis and usually corresponds to station 0. Engagement often occurs in the weeks just before labour begins in nulliparas and may occur before or during labour in multiparas. Engagement can be determined by abdominal or vaginal examination.

Passageway

The *passageway*, or birth canal, is composed of the mother's rigid bony pelvis and the soft tissues of the cervix, pelvic floor, vagina, and introitus (the external opening to the vagina). Although the soft tissues, particularly the muscular layers of the pelvic floor, contribute to vaginal birth of the fetus, the maternal pelvis plays a far greater role in the labour process because the fetus must successfully accommodate itself to this relatively rigid passageway.

Bony Pelvis

The anatomy of the bony pelvis is described in Chapter 6. The following discussion focuses on the importance of pelvic configurations as they relate to the labour process. (It may be helpful to refer to Figs. 6-5 and 6-6.)

The *bony pelvis* is formed by the fusion of the ilium, ischium, pubis, and sacral bones. The four pelvic joints are the symphysis pubis, the right and left sacroiliac joints (Fig. 16-7, A), and the sacrococcygeal joint (Fig. 16-7, B). The bony pelvis is separated by the brim, or inlet, into two parts: the false pelvis and the true pelvis. The *false pelvis* is the part above the brim and plays no part in child-bearing. The *true pelvis*, the part involved in birth, is divided into three planes: the inlet, or brim; the midpelvis, or cavity; and the outlet.

The *pelvic inlet*, which is the upper border of the true pelvis, is formed anteriorly by the upper margins of the pubic bone, laterally by the iliopectineal lines along the innominate bones, and posteriorly by the anterior, upper margin of the sacrum and the sacral promontory.

The *pelvic cavity*, or midpelvis, is a curved passage with a short anterior wall and a much longer concave posterior wall. It is bounded by the posterior aspect of the symphysis pubis, the ischium, a portion of the ilium, the sacrum, and the coccyx.

The *pelvic outlet* is the lower border of the true pelvis. Viewed from below, it is ovoid; somewhat diamond shaped; and bounded by the pubic arch anteriorly, the ischial tuberosities laterally, and the tip of the coccyx posteriorly (see Fig. 16-7, B). In the latter part of pregnancy, the coccyx is movable unless it has been broken (e.g., in a fall) and has fused to the sacrum during healing.

The pelvic cavity varies in size and shape at various levels. The diameters at the plane of the pelvic inlet, midpelvis, and outlet, plus the axis of the birth canal (Fig. 16-8), determine whether vaginal birth is possible and the manner by which the fetus may pass down the birth canal.

The subpubic angle, which determines the type of pubic arch, together with the length of the pubic rami and the intertuberous diameter, is of great importance. Because the fetus must first pass beneath the pubic arch, a narrow subpubic angle is less accommodating than a rounded wide arch.

The four basic types of pelves are classified as follows:

1. Gynecoid (the classic female type)
2. Android (resembling the male pelvis)
3. Anthropoid (resembling the pelvis of anthropoid apes)
4. Platypelloid (the flat pelvis)

The gynecoid pelvis is the most common type, with major gynecoid pelvic features present in 50% of all women. Anthropoid and android features are less common, and platypelloid pelvic features are least common. Mixed types of pelves are more common than are pure types (Cunningham et al., 2014). Examples of pelvic variations and their effects on the mode of birth are given in Table 16-1.

Assessment of the bony pelvis can be performed during the first prenatal evaluation by the physician or midwife and need not be repeated if the pelvis is of adequate size and suitable shape. In the third trimester of pregnancy, the examination of the bony pelvis may be more thorough and the results more accurate because there is relaxation and increased mobility of the pelvic joints and ligaments as a result of hormonal influences. Widening of the joint of the symphysis pubis and the resulting instability may cause pain in any or all of the pelvic joints.

Because the examiner does not have direct access to the bony structures and because the bones are covered with varying amounts of soft tissue, estimates of size and shape are approximate. Precise bony pelvis measurements can be determined by use of computed tomography, ultrasonography, magnetic resonance imaging, or x-ray films. However, radiographic examination is rarely done during pregnancy because of potential damage to the developing fetus.

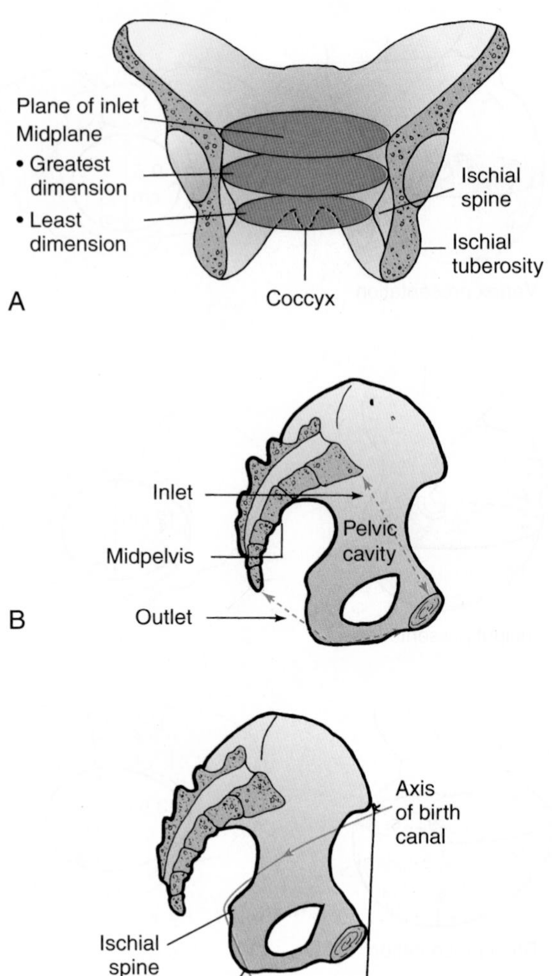

FIGURE 16-8 Pelvic cavity. **A:** Inlet and midplane. Outlet not shown. **B:** Cavity of true pelvis. **C:** Note curve of sacrum and axis of birth canal.

Soft Tissues

The soft tissues of the passageway include the distensible lower uterine segment, cervix, pelvic floor muscles, vagina, and introitus. Before labour begins, the uterus is composed of the uterine body (corpus) and cervix (neck). After labour has begun, uterine contractions cause the uterine body to have a thick and muscular upper segment and a thin-walled, passive, muscular lower segment. *A physiological retraction ring* separates the two segments (Fig. 16-9). The lower uterine segment gradually distends to accommodate the intrauterine contents as the wall of the upper segment thickens and its accommodating capacity is reduced. The contractions of the uterine body thus exert downward pressure on the fetus, pushing it against the cervix.

The cervix effaces (thins) and dilates (opens) sufficiently to allow the first fetal portion to descend into the vagina. As the

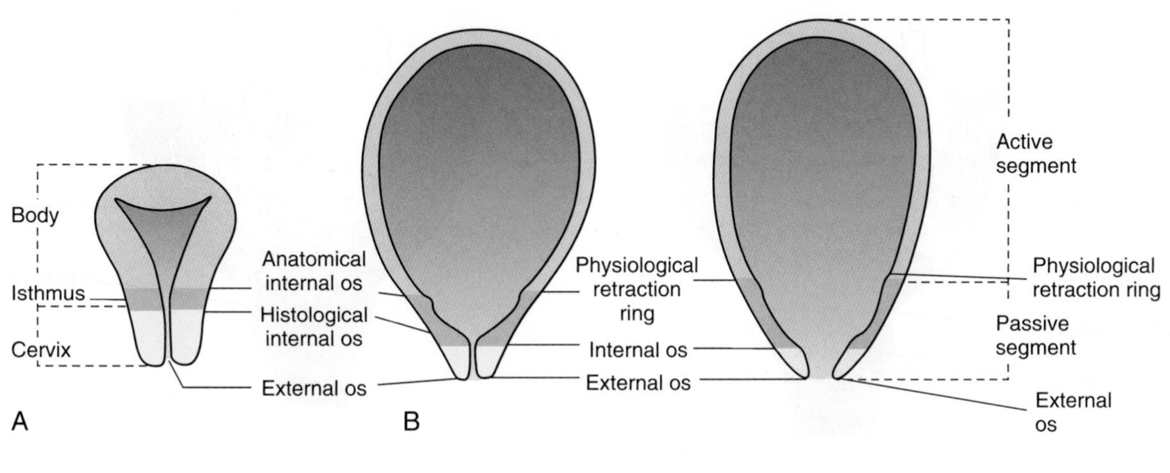

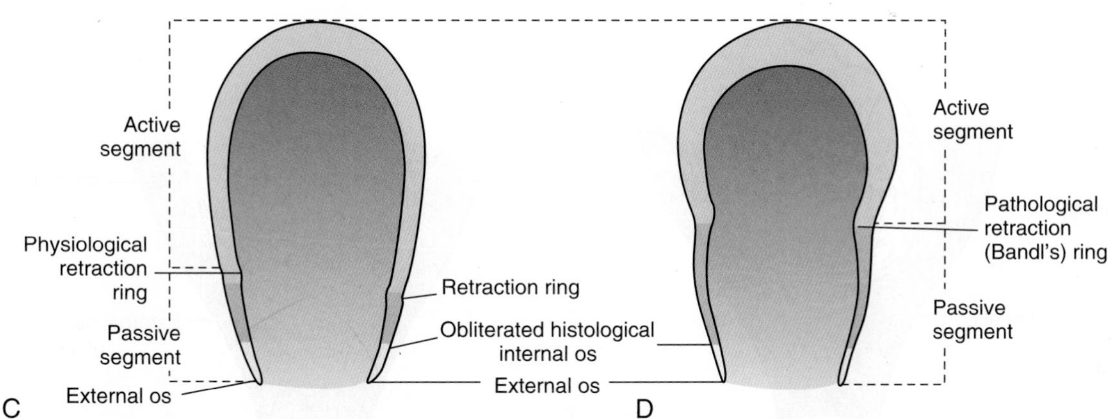

FIGURE 16-9 Uterus in normal labour. **A:** Non-pregnant uterus. **B:** In early first stage. **C:** In second stage. Passive segment is derived from lower uterine segment (isthmus) and cervix, and physiological retraction ring is derived from anatomical internal os. **D:** Uterus in abnormal labour in second-stage dystocia. Pathological retraction (Bandl's) ring that forms under abnormal conditions develops from the physiological ring.

TABLE 16-1 COMPARISON OF PELVIC TYPES

	GYNECOID (50% OF WOMEN)	ANDROID (23% OF WOMEN)	ANTHROPOID (24% OF WOMEN)	PLATYPELLOID (3% OF WOMEN)
Brim	Slightly ovoid or transversely rounded ◯ Round	Heart shaped, angulated ♡ Heart	Oval, wider anteroposteriorly 0 Oval	Flattened anteroposteriorly, wide transversely ⬭ Flat
Depth	Moderate	Deep	Deep	Shallow
Side walls	Straight	Convergent	Straight	Straight
Ischial spines	Blunt, somewhat widely separated	Prominent, narrow interspinous diameter	Prominent, often with narrow interspinous diameter	Blunt, widely separated
Sacrum	Deep, curved	Slightly curved, terminal portion often beaked	Slightly curved	Slightly curved
Subpubic arch	Wide	Narrow	Narrow	Wide
Usual mode of birth	Vaginal Spontaneous Occipitoanterior position	Caesarean Vaginal Difficult with forceps	Vaginal Forceps/spontaneous Occipitoposterior or occipitoanterior position	Vaginal Spontaneous

fetus descends, the cervix is actually drawn upward and over this first portion.

The *pelvic floor* is a muscular layer that separates the pelvic cavity above from the perineal space below. This structure helps the fetus rotate anteriorly as it passes through the birth canal. As noted earlier, the soft tissues of the vagina develop throughout pregnancy until at term the vagina can dilate to accommodate the fetus and facilitate its passage to the external world.

Powers

Involuntary and voluntary powers combine to expel the fetus and the placenta from the uterus. Involuntary uterine

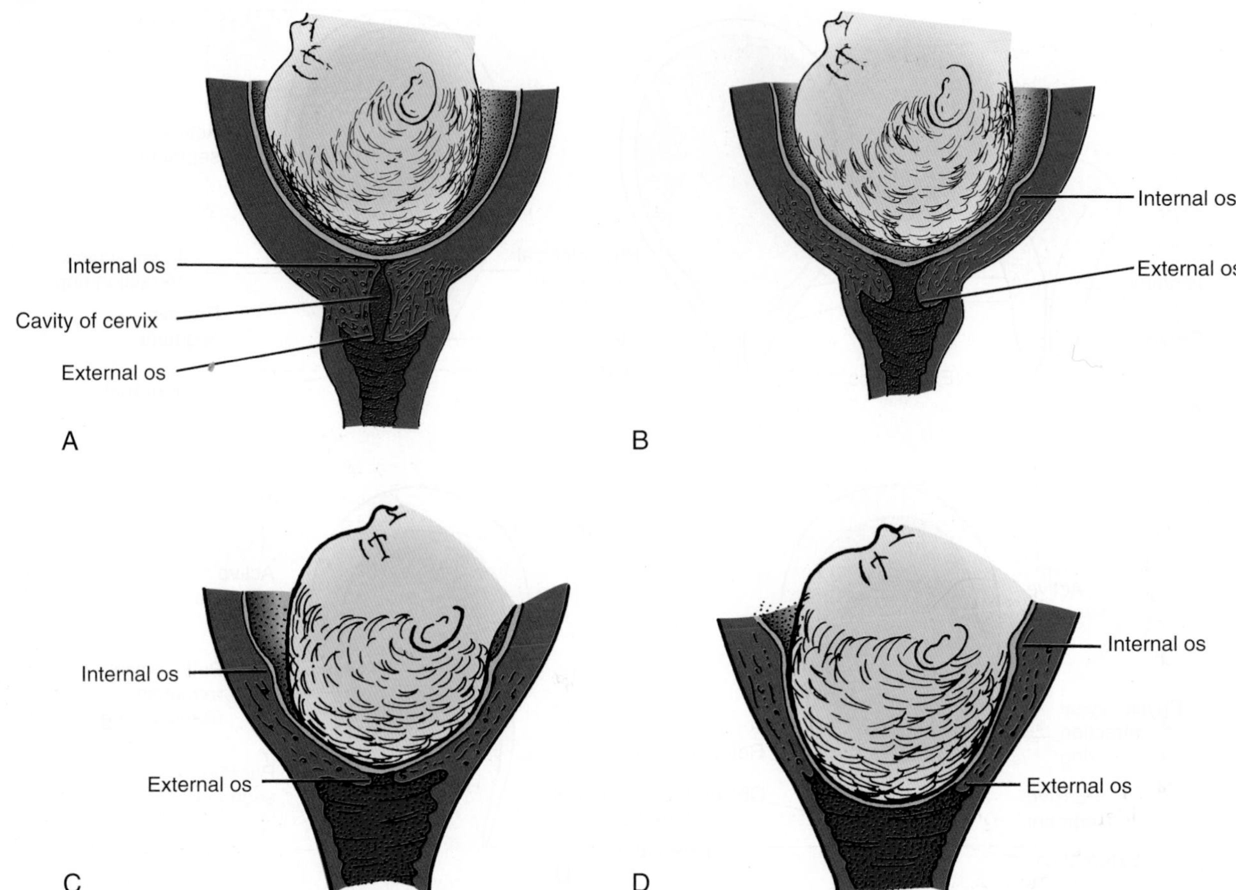

FIGURE 16-10 Cervical effacement and dilation. Note how cervix is drawn up around presenting part (internal os). Membranes are intact, and head is not well applied to cervix. **A:** Before labour. **B:** Early effacement. **C:** Complete effacement (100%). Head is well applied to cervix. **D:** Complete dilation (10 cm). Cranial bones overlap somewhat, and membranes are still intact.

contractions, called the *primary powers*, signal the beginning of labour. Once the cervix has dilated, voluntary bearing-down efforts by the woman, called the *secondary powers*, augment the force of the involuntary contractions.

Primary Powers

The involuntary contractions originate at certain pacemaker points in the thickened muscle layers of the upper uterine segment. From the pacemaker points contractions move downward over the uterus in waves, separated by short rest periods. Terms used to describe these involuntary contractions include *frequency* (the time from the beginning of one contraction to the beginning of the next), *duration* (length of contraction), and *intensity* (strength of contraction at its peak).

The primary powers are responsible for the effacement and dilation of the cervix and descent of the fetus. **Effacement** means the shortening and thinning of the cervix during the first stage of labour. The cervix, normally 2 to 3 cm long and about 1 cm thick, is obliterated or "taken up" by a shortening of the uterine muscle bundles during the thinning of the lower uterine segment that occurs in advancing labour. Only a thin edge of the cervix can be palpated when effacement is complete. Effacement generally is advanced in first-time term pregnancy before more than slight dilation occurs. In subsequent pregnancies, effacement and dilation of the cervix tend to progress together. The degree of effacement is expressed in percentages, from 0 to 100% (e.g., a cervix is 50% effaced) or in length in centimetres (Fig. 16-10, A to C).

Dilation of the cervix is the enlargement or widening of the cervical opening and the cervical canal that occurs once labour has begun. The diameter of the cervix increases from less than 1 cm to full dilation (approximately 10 cm) to allow birth of a term fetus. When the cervix is fully dilated (and completely retracted), it can no longer be palpated (see Fig. 16-10, D). Full cervical dilation marks the end of the first stage of labour.

Dilation of the cervix occurs by the drawing upward of the musculofibrous components of the cervix, caused by strong uterine contractions. Pressure exerted by the amniotic fluid while the membranes are intact or by the force applied by the presenting part can promote cervical dilation. Scarring of the cervix as a result of prior infection or surgery may slow cervical dilation.

In the first and second stages of labour, increased intrauterine pressure caused by contractions exerts pressure on the descending fetus and the cervix. When the presenting part of the fetus reaches the perineal floor, mechanical stretching of the cervix occurs. Stretch receptors in the posterior vagina cause the release of endogenous oxytocin that triggers the maternal urge to bear down, or the *Ferguson reflex*.

Uterine contractions are usually independent of external forces. For example, labouring women who are paralyzed because of spinal cord lesions above the twelfth thoracic vertebra have normal but painless uterine contractions (Cunningham et al., 2014). However, uterine contractions may decrease temporarily in frequency and intensity if narcotic analgesic medication is given early in labour. Studies of effects of epidural analgesia have demonstrated prolonged length of labour for nulliparas both in the active phase of first-stage labour and in second-stage labour (Cunningham et al., 2014).

Secondary Powers

As soon as the presenting part reaches the pelvic floor, the contractions change in character and become expulsive. The labouring woman experiences an involuntary urge to push. She uses secondary powers (bearing-down efforts) to aid in expulsion of the fetus as she contracts her diaphragm and abdominal muscles and pushes. These bearing-down efforts result in increased intra-abdominal pressure that compresses the uterus on all sides and adds to the power of the expulsive forces.

The secondary powers have no effect on cervical dilation, but they are of considerable importance in the expulsion of the infant from the uterus and vagina after the cervix is fully dilated.

When and how a woman pushes in the second stage is a much-debated topic. Studies have investigated the effects of spontaneous bearing-down efforts, directed pushing, delayed pushing, Valsalva manoeuvre (closed glottis and prolonged bearing down), and open-glottis pushing. Continued study is needed to determine the effectiveness and appropriateness of strategies that nurses use to teach pushing techniques, the suitability and effectiveness of various pushing techniques related to atypical or abnormal fetal heart patterns, and the standards for length of pushing in terms of maternal and fetal outcomes. See Chapter 17 for further discussion regarding pushing during the second stage of labour.

Position of the Labouring Woman

Position affects the woman's anatomical and physiological adaptations to labour. Frequent changes in position relieve fatigue, increase comfort, and improve circulation. Therefore, a labouring woman should be encouraged to find positions that are most comfortable to her.

An upright position (walking, sitting, kneeling, or squatting) offers a number of advantages. Gravity can promote the descent of the fetus. Uterine contractions are generally stronger and more efficient in effacing and dilating the cervix, resulting in shorter labour.

An upright position also is beneficial to the mother's cardiac output, which normally increases during labour as uterine contractions return blood to the vascular bed. The increased cardiac output improves blood flow to the uteroplacental unit and the maternal kidneys. Cardiac output is compromised if the descending aorta and ascending vena cava are compressed during labour. Compression of these major vessels may result in supine hypotension that decreases placental perfusion (see the Emergency box in Chapter 11, p. 240). With the woman in an upright position, pressure on the maternal vessels is reduced, and compression is prevented. If the woman wishes to lie down, a lateral position is suggested. The "all fours" position (hands and knees) may be used to relieve backache if the fetus is in an occipitoposterior position and may assist in anterior rotation of the fetus and in cases of shoulder dystocia. Initial research supports the use of this position even with epidural analgesia when the woman has good mobility, and it decreases the length of second stage as well as the need for assisted birth (Stremler, Halpern, Weston, et al., 2009).

Positioning for second-stage labour may be determined by the woman's preference, but it is constrained by the condition of the woman or fetus, the environment, and the health care provider's confidence in assisting in a birth in a specific position. See Chapter 17 for further discussion of positioning during birth.

PROCESS OF LABOUR

The term *labour* refers to the process of moving the fetus, placenta, and membranes out of the uterus and through the birth canal. Various changes take place in the woman's reproductive system in the days and weeks before labour begins. Labour itself can be discussed in terms of the mechanisms involved in the process and the stages the woman moves through.

Signs Preceding Labour

In first-time pregnancies, the uterus sinks downward and forward about 2 to 4 weeks before term, when the fetus's presenting part (usually the fetal head) descends into the true pelvis. This settling is called *lightening*, or "dropping," and usually happens gradually. After lightening, women breathe more easily, but usually more bladder pressure results from this shift, and consequently there is a return of urinary frequency. In a multiparous pregnancy, lightening may not take place until after uterine contractions are established and true labour is in progress.

The woman may state she feels persistent low backache and sacroiliac distress as a result of relaxation of the pelvic joints. She may identify strong, frequent, but irregular uterine (Braxton Hicks) contractions.

The vaginal mucus becomes more profuse in response to the extreme congestion of the vaginal mucous membranes. Brownish or blood-tinged cervical mucus may be passed (**bloody show**). The cervix becomes soft (ripens) and partially effaced and may begin to dilate. The membranes may rupture spontaneously.

Other phenomena are common in the days preceding labour: (1) loss of 0.5 to 1.5 kg in weight, caused by water loss resulting from electrolyte shifts that in turn are produced by changes in estrogen and progesterone levels; and (2) a surge of energy. Women speak of having a burst of energy (*nesting*) that they often use to clean the house and put everything in order. Less commonly, some women have diarrhea, nausea, vomiting, and indigestion. Box 16-1 lists signs that may precede labour.

BOX 16-1 SIGNS PRECEDING LABOUR

- Lightening
- Return of urinary frequency
- Backache
- Stronger Braxton Hicks contractions
- Weight loss of 0.5 to 1.5 kg
- Surge of energy (also called nesting)
- Flu-like symptoms
- Increased vaginal discharge; bloody show
- Cervical ripening
- Possible rupture of membranes

Onset of Labour

The onset of true labour cannot be ascribed to a single cause. Many factors, including changes in the maternal uterus, cervix, and pituitary gland, are involved. Hormones produced by the normal fetal hypothalamus, pituitary, and adrenal cortex probably contribute to the onset of labour. Progressive uterine distension and increasing intrauterine pressure seem to be associated with increasing myometrial irritability. This is a result of increased concentrations of estrogen, oxytocin, and prostaglandins and decreasing progesterone levels. The mutually coordinated effects of these factors result in the occurrence of strong, regular, rhythmic uterine contractions (Blackburn, 2013; Kilpatrick & Garrison, 2012). The outcome of these factors working together is normally the birth of the fetus and the expulsion of the placenta; however, how certain alterations trigger others and the ways in which proper checks and balances are maintained are not known.

Stages of Labour

The course of normal labour, at or near term gestation in a woman without complications and a fetus in vertex presentation, consists of (1) regular progression of uterine contractions, (2) effacement and progressive dilation of the cervix, and (3) progress in descent of the presenting part. Four stages of labour are recognized. An overview of these stages is included here. They are discussed in greater detail, along with nursing care for the labouring woman and family, in Chapter 17.

The *first stage of labour* is considered to last from the onset of regular uterine contractions to full dilation of the cervix. Commonly, the onset of labour is difficult to establish because the woman may be admitted to the labour unit just before birth, and the beginning of labour may be only an estimate. The first stage is much longer than the second and third combined. However, great variability is the rule, depending on the factors discussed previously in this chapter. Parity has a strong effect on the duration of first-stage labour. Full dilation may occur in less than 1 hour in some multiparous pregnancies. In first-time pregnancy, complete dilation of the cervix can take 18 hours or longer. Variations may reflect differences in the patient population (e.g., risk status, age) or in clinical management of the labour and birth.

The first stage of labour is divided into two phases: latent (early) and active labour (Society of Obstetricians and Gynecologists of Canada, 2016). During the latent phase, there is more progress in effacement of the cervix and little increase in descent. During the active phase, there is more rapid dilation of the cervix and increased rate of descent of the presenting part. See Chapter 17 for further discussion of the stages of labour.

The *second stage of labour* lasts from the time the cervix is fully dilated to the birth of the fetus. It is composed of two phases: the latent phase and the active pushing (descent) phase. During the latent phase the fetus continues to descend passively through the birth canal and rotate to an anterior position as a result of ongoing uterine contractions. The urge to bear down during this phase is not strong, and some women do not experience it at all. During the active pushing phase the woman has strong urges to bear down as the presenting part of the fetus descends and presses on the stretch receptors of the pelvic floor. Choosing different positions for the second stage, such as side-lying, squatting, or sitting, will shorten the second stage by increasing the efficacy of contractions, promoting uterine blood flow, and decreasing the likelihood of tears or episiotomies (Zwelling, 2010).

The *third stage of labour* lasts from the birth of the fetus until the placenta is delivered. The placenta normally separates with the third or fourth strong uterine contraction after the infant has been born. After it has separated, the placenta can be delivered with the next uterine contraction. Creating a warm environment, supporting skin-to-skin contact between mother and baby, and reducing fear and anxiety contribute to decreased catecholamine production and increased oxytocin production, which facilitate placental separation. The duration of the third stage may be as short as 3 to 5 minutes, although up to 1 hour is considered within normal limits.

The *fourth stage of labour* arbitrarily lasts about 2 hours after delivery of the placenta. It is the period of immediate recovery, when homeostasis is re-established. The fourth stage of labour is also the time when parent–child bonding and attachment begins and breastfeeding is initiated. It is an important period of observation for complications, such as abnormal bleeding (see Chapter 24).

Mechanism of Labour

As already discussed, the female pelvis has varied contours and diameters at different levels, and the presenting part of the passenger is large in proportion to the passage. Therefore, for vaginal birth to occur, the fetus must adapt to the birth canal during the descent. The turns and other adjustments necessary in the human birth process are termed the *mechanism of labour*. The seven cardinal movements of the mechanism of labour that occur in a vertex presentation are engagement, descent, flexion, internal rotation, extension, external rotation (restitution), and, finally, birth by expulsion (Fig. 16-11). Although these movements are discussed separately, in actuality a combination of movements occurs simultaneously. For example, engagement involves both descent and flexion.

Engagement

When the biparietal diameter of the head passes the pelvic inlet, the head is said to be engaged in the pelvic inlet (see Fig. 16-11,

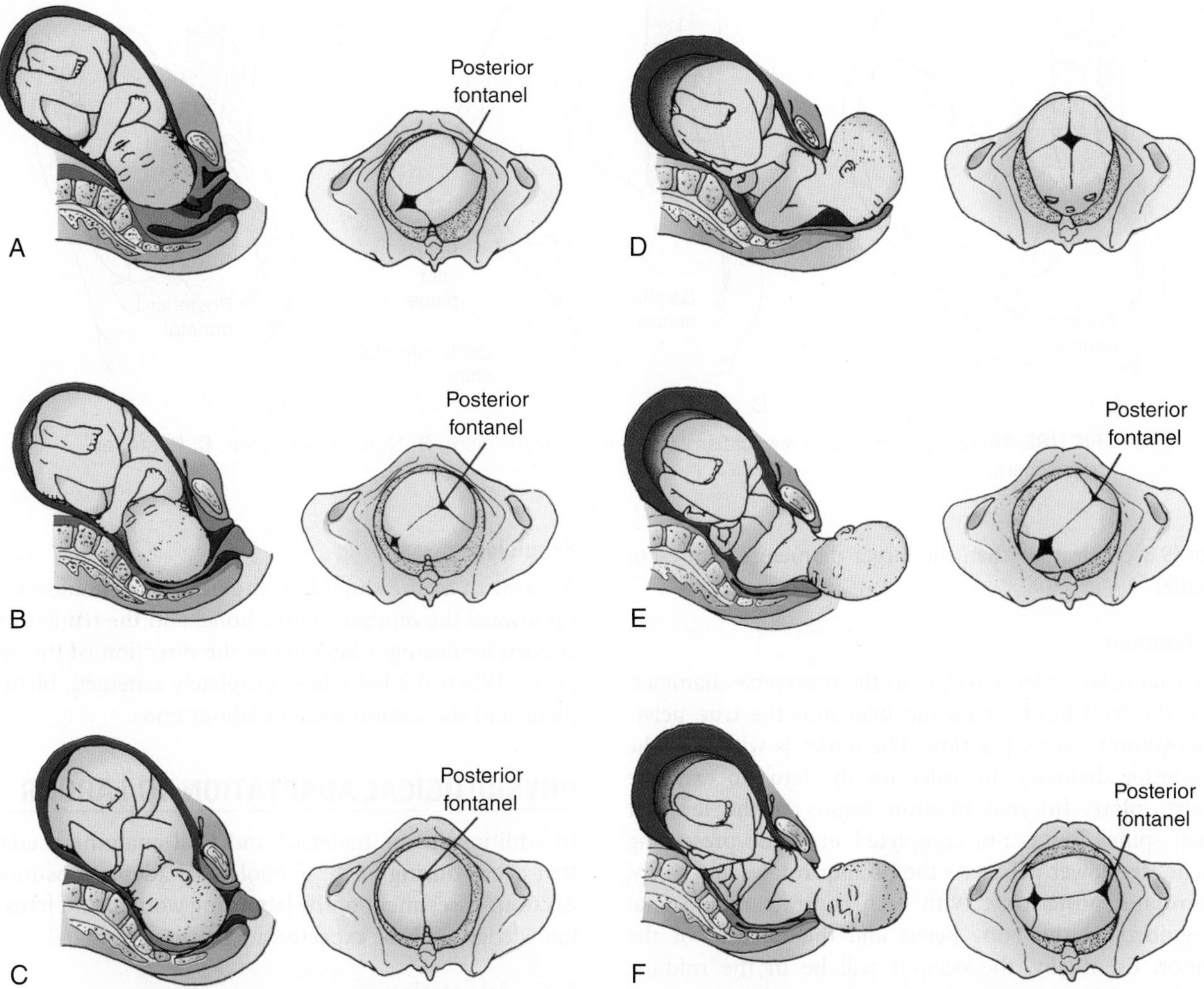

FIGURE 16-11 Cardinal movements of the mechanism of labour. Left occipitoanterior position. **A:** Engagement and descent. **B:** Flexion. **C:** Internal rotation to occipitoanterior position. **D:** Extension. **E:** External rotation beginning (restitution). **F:** External rotation.

A). In most nulliparous pregnancies, this occurs before the onset of active labour because the firmer abdominal muscles direct the presenting part into the pelvis. In multiparous pregnancies in which the abdominal musculature is more relaxed, the head often remains freely movable above the pelvic brim until labour is established.

Asynclitism. The head usually engages in the pelvis in a synclitic position (i.e., one that is parallel to the anteroposterior plane of the pelvis). Frequently, asynclitism occurs (the head is deflected anteriorly or posteriorly in the pelvis), which can facilitate descent because the head is being positioned to accommodate to the pelvic cavity (Fig. 16-12). Extreme asynclitism can cause cephalopelvic disproportion, even in a normal-size pelvis, because the head is positioned so that it cannot descend.

Descent

Descent refers to the progress of the presenting part through the pelvis. Descent depends on at least four forces: (1) pressure exerted by the amniotic fluid, (2) direct pressure exerted by the contracting fundus on the fetus, (3) force of the contraction of the maternal diaphragm and abdominal muscles in the second stage of labour, and (4) extension and straightening of the fetal body. The effects of these forces are modified by the size and shape of the maternal pelvic planes and the size of the fetal head and its capacity to mould.

The degree of descent is measured by the station of the presenting part (see Fig. 16-6). As mentioned earlier, little descent occurs during the latent phase of the first stage of labour. Descent accelerates in the active phase. It is especially apparent when the membranes have ruptured.

In a first-time labour, descent is usually slow but steady; in subsequent pregnancies, descent may be rapid. Progress in descent of the presenting part is determined by abdominal palpation and vaginal examination until the presenting part can be seen at the introitus.

Flexion

As soon as the descending head meets resistance from the cervix, pelvic wall, or pelvic floor, it normally flexes so that the chin is brought into closer contact with the fetal chest (see Fig. 16-11, B). Flexion permits the smaller suboccipitobregmatic

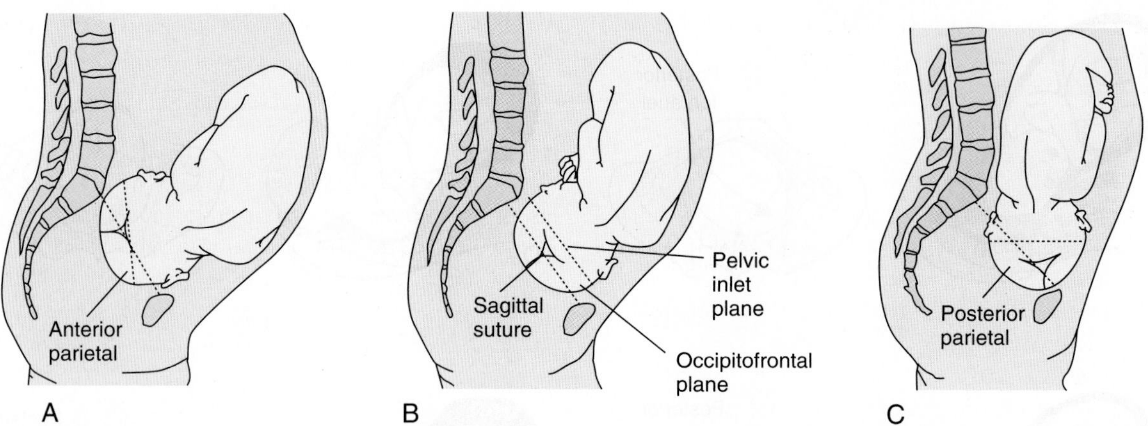

FIGURE 16-12 Synclitism and asynclitism. **A:** Anterior asynclitism. **B:** Normal synclitism. **C:** Posterior asynclitism.

diameter (9.5 cm) rather than the larger diameters to present to the outlet.

Internal Rotation

The maternal pelvic inlet is widest in the transverse diameter; therefore, the fetal head passes the inlet into the true pelvis in the occipitotransverse position. The outlet is widest in the anteroposterior diameter; in order for the fetus to exit, the head must rotate. Internal rotation begins at the level of the ischial spines but is not completed until the presenting part reaches the lower pelvis. As the occiput rotates anteriorly, the face rotates posteriorly. With each contraction the fetal head is guided by the bony pelvis and the muscles of the pelvic floor. Eventually, the occiput will be in the midline beneath the pubic arch. The head is almost always rotated by the time it reaches the pelvic floor (see Fig. 16-11, C). Both the levator ani muscles and the bony pelvis are important for achieving anterior rotation. A previous childbirth injury or regional anaesthesia may compromise the function of the levator sling.

Extension

When the fetal head reaches the perineum for birth, it is deflected anteriorly by the perineum. The occiput passes under the lower border of the symphysis pubis first, and then the head emerges by extension: first the occiput, then the face, and finally the chin (see Fig. 16-11, D).

Restitution and External Rotation

After the head is born, it rotates briefly to the position it occupied when it was engaged in the inlet. This movement is referred to as *restitution* (see Fig. 16-11, E). The 45-degree turn realigns the infant's head with her or his back and shoulders. The head can then be seen to rotate further. This external rotation occurs as the shoulders engage and descend in manoeuvres similar to those of the head (see Fig. 16-11, F). As noted earlier, the anterior shoulder descends first. When it reaches the outlet, it rotates to the midline and is delivered from under the pubic arch. The posterior shoulder is guided over the perineum until it is free of the vaginal introitus.

Expulsion

After birth of the shoulders, the head and shoulders are lifted up toward the mother's pubic bone, and the trunk of the baby is born by flexing it laterally in the direction of the symphysis pubis. When the baby has completely emerged, birth is complete, and the second stage of labour ends.

PHYSIOLOGICAL ADAPTATION TO LABOUR

In addition to the maternal and fetal anatomical adaptations that occur during birth, physiological adaptations must occur. Accurate assessment of the labouring woman and fetus requires knowledge of these expected adaptations.

Fetal Adaptation

Several important physiological adaptations occur in the fetus. These changes occur in fetal heart rate (FHR), fetal circulation, respiratory movements, and other behaviours.

Fetal Heart Rate

Fetal health surveillance (FHS) provides information about the condition of the fetus related to oxygenation. The average FHR at term is 110 to 160 beats/min. Earlier in gestation the FHR is higher, with an average of approximately 160 beats/min at 20 weeks of gestation. The rate decreases progressively as the sympathetic nervous system in the fetus matures closer to term. However, temporary accelerations and slight early decelerations of the FHR can be expected in response to spontaneous fetal movement, vaginal examination, fundal pressure, uterine contractions, abdominal palpation, and fetal head compression. Stresses to the uterofetoplacental unit result in characteristic FHR patterns (see Chapter 19 for further discussion).

Fetal Circulation

Fetal circulation can be affected by many factors, including maternal position, uterine contractions, blood pressure, and umbilical cord blood flow. Uterine contractions during labour tend to decrease circulation through the spiral arterioles and subsequent perfusion through the intervillous space. Most healthy fetuses are able to compensate for this stress and exposure to increased pressure while moving passively through the birth canal during labour. Usually the umbilical cord moves freely in the amniotic fluid. However, it can be compressed during uterine contractions (Blackburn, 2013; Lee, Sprague, Ehman, et al., 2009).

Fetal Respiration

Certain changes stimulate chemoreceptors in the aorta and carotid bodies to prepare the fetus for initiating respirations immediately after birth (Blackburn, 2013). These changes include the following:

- Fetal lung fluid is cleared from the air passages as the infant passes through the birth canal during labour and (vaginal) birth.
- Fetal oxygen pressure (Po_2) decreases.
- Arterial carbon dioxide pressure (Pco_2) increases.
- Arterial pH decreases.
- Bicarbonate level decreases.
- Fetal respiratory movements decrease during labour.

Maternal Adaptation

As the woman progresses through the stages of labour, various body system adaptations cause the woman to exhibit both objective and subjective symptoms (Box 16-2).

Cardiovascular Changes

During each contraction, an average of 400 mL of blood is emptied from the uterus into the maternal vascular system. This increases cardiac output by about 10 to 15% in the first stage. By the end of the first stage of labour, cardiac output during contractions is increased by approximately 50% above baseline pregnancy values at term. Cardiac output peaks about 10 to 30 minutes after both vaginal and Caesarean birth and returns to its prelabour baseline within the first postpartum hour.

Changes in blood pressure also occur. Blood flow, which is reduced in the uterine artery by contractions, is redirected to peripheral vessels. As a result, peripheral resistance increases and blood pressure increases. In general, both systolic and diastolic pressures increase during contractions and return to baseline levels between contractions. Systolic values increase more than diastolic values (Blackburn, 2013). Assessing blood pressure between contractions provides more accurate readings.

Supine hypotension (see Fig. 17-3, p. 424) occurs when the ascending vena cava and descending aorta are compressed. The labouring woman is at greater risk for supine hypotension if the uterus is particularly large because of multifetal pregnancy, hydramnios, or obesity or if the woman is dehydrated or hypovolemic. In addition, anxiety, pain, and some medications can cause hypotension.

The woman should be discouraged from using the Valsalva manoeuvre (holding one's breath and tightening abdominal muscles) for pushing during the second stage. This activity increases intrathoracic pressure, reduces venous return, and increases venous pressure. Cardiac output and blood pressure increase, and the pulse slows temporarily. During the Valsalva manoeuvre fetal hypoxia may occur. This process is reversed when the woman takes a breath.

The white blood cell (WBC) count can increase (Blackburn, 2013). Although the mechanism leading to this increase in WBCs is unknown, it may be secondary to physical or emotional stress or tissue trauma. Labour is strenuous, and physical exercise alone can increase the WBC count.

Some peripheral vascular changes occur, perhaps in response to cervical dilation or compression of maternal vessels by the fetus passing through the birth canal. Flushed cheeks, hot or cold feet, and eversion of hemorrhoids may result.

Respiratory Changes

Increased physical activity with greater oxygen consumption is reflected in an increase in the respiratory rate. Hyperventilation may cause respiratory *alkalosis* (an increase in pH), hypoxia, and *hypocapnia* (decrease in carbon dioxide). In the unmedicated woman in the second stage, oxygen consumption almost doubles. Anxiety also may increase oxygen consumption.

Renal Changes

During labour, spontaneous voiding may be difficult for various reasons: tissue edema caused by pressure from the presenting part, discomfort, analgesia, and embarrassment. Proteinuria up to +1 is a normal finding because it can occur in response to the breakdown of muscle tissue from the physical work of labour.

Integumentary Changes

The integumentary system changes are evident, especially in the great distensibility (stretching) in the area of the vaginal introitus. The degree of distensibility varies with the individual. Despite this ability to stretch, even in the absence of episiotomy or lacerations, minute tears in the skin around the vaginal introitus occur.

Musculoskeletal Changes

The musculoskeletal system is stressed during labour. Diaphoresis, fatigue, proteinuria (+1), and possibly an increased

BOX 16-2 MATERNAL PHYSIOLOGICAL CHANGES DURING LABOUR

- Cardiac output increases 10 to 15% in first stage; 30 to 50% in second stage.
- Heart rate increases slightly in first and second stages.
- Systolic and diastolic blood pressure increase during uterine contractions and return to baseline between contractions. Systolic values increase more than diastolic values.
- White blood cell count increases.
- Respiratory rate increases.
- Temperature may be slightly elevated.
- Proteinuria may occur.
- Gastric motility and absorption of solid food is decreased; nausea and vomiting may occur during the active phase to second-stage labour.
- Blood glucose level decreases.

temperature accompany the marked increase in muscle activity. Backache and joint ache (unrelated to fetal position) occur as a result of increased joint laxity at term. The labour process itself and the woman's pointing her toes can cause leg cramps.

Neurological Changes

Sensorial changes occur as the woman moves through phases of the first stage of labour and from one stage to the next. Initially, she may be euphoric. Euphoria gives way to increased seriousness, to amnesia between contractions during the second stage, and finally to elation or fatigue after giving birth. Endogenous *endorphins* (morphine-like chemicals produced naturally by the body) raise the pain threshold and produce sedation. In addition, physiological anaesthesia of perineal tissues, caused by pressure of the presenting part, decreases the perception of pain.

Gastrointestinal Changes

During labour, gastrointestinal motility and absorption of solid foods are decreased, and stomach-emptying time is slowed. Nausea and vomiting of undigested food eaten after onset of labour are common. Nausea and belching also occur as a reflex response to full cervical dilation. The woman may state that diarrhea accompanied the onset of labour, or the nurse may palpate the presence of hard or impacted stool in the rectum.

Endocrine Changes

The onset of labour may be triggered by decreasing levels of progesterone and increasing levels of estrogen, prostaglandins, and oxytocin. Metabolism increases, and blood glucose levels may decrease with the work of labour.

Accurate assessment of the mother and fetus during labour and birth depends on knowledge of these expected adaptations so that appropriate interventions can be implemented.

KEY POINTS

- Labour and birth are affected by the five P's: passenger, passageway, powers, position of the woman, and psychological response.
- Because of its size and relative rigidity, the fetal head is a major factor in determining the course of birth.
- The diameters at the plane of the pelvic inlet, midpelvis, and outlet, plus the axis of the birth canal, determine whether vaginal birth is possible and the manner in which the fetus passes down the birth canal.
- Involuntary uterine contractions act to expel the fetus and placenta during the first stage of labour; these are augmented by voluntary bearing-down efforts during the second stage.
- The first stage of labour lasts from the time dilation begins to the time when the cervix is fully effaced and dilated.
- The second stage of labour lasts from the time of full dilation to the birth of the infant.
- The third stage of labour lasts from the infant's birth to the expulsion of the placenta.
- The fourth stage is approximately the first 2 hours after birth.
- The cardinal movements of the mechanism of labour are engagement, descent, flexion, internal rotation, extension, restitution and external rotation, and expulsion of the infant.
- Although the events precipitating the onset of labour are unknown, many factors, including changes in the maternal uterus, cervix, and pituitary gland, are thought to be involved.
- A healthy fetus with an adequate uterofetoplacental circulation will be able to compensate for the stress of uterine contractions.
- As the woman progresses through labour, various body systems adapt to the birth process.

evolve WEBSITE

Visit the Evolve website for additional resources related to the content in this chapter such as Case Studies, Critical Thinking Case Study Answers, Nursing Care Plans, Nursing Processes, Nursing Skills, and Review Questions for Exam Preparation at: http://evolve.elsevier.com/Canada/Perry/maternal/

REFERENCES

Blackburn, S. T. (2013). *Maternal, fetal, and neonatal physiology: A clinical perspective* (4th ed.). St. Louis: Elsevier/Saunders.

Cunningham, F., Leveno, K., Bloom, S., et al. (2014). *Williams obstetrics* (24th ed.). New York: McGraw Hill.

Hodnett, E. D., Gates, S., Hofmeyr, G. J., et al. (2012). Continuous support for women during childbirth. *Cochrane Database Systems Review*, (2). doi:10.1002/14651858.CD003766.pub3.

Kilpatrick, S., & Garrison, E. (2012). Normal labor and delivery. In S. G. Gabbe, J. R. Niebyl, J. L. Simpson, et al. (Eds.), *Obstetrics: Normal and problem pregnancies* (6th ed.). Philadelphia: Saunders.

Lee, L., Sprague, A., Ehman, J., et al. (2009). *Fundamentals of fetal health surveillance* (4th ed.). Vancouver: British Columbia Perinatal Health Program; produced by the Canadian Perinatal Programs Coalition.

Society of Obstetricians and Gynecologists of Canada. (2016). *Advances in labour and risk management (ALARM) course syllabus* (23rd ed). Ottawa, ON: Author.

Stremler, R., Halpern, S., Weston, M., et al. (2009). Hands and knees positioning during labour with epidural analgesia. *Journal of Obstetrical, Gynecological and Neonatal Nursing*, *38*, 391–398.

Zwelling, E. (2010). Overcoming the challenges: Maternal movement and positioning to facilitate labour progress. *American Journal of Maternal/Child Nursing*, *35*(2), 72–78.

CHAPTER 17

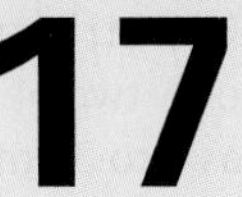

Nursing Care of the Family During Labour and Birth

Lisa Keenan-Lindsay

evolve WEBSITE

Visit the Evolve website for additional resources related to the content in this chapter such as Case Studies, Critical Thinking Case Study Answers, Nursing Care Plans, Nursing Processes, Nursing Skills, and Review Questions for Exam Preparation at: http://evolve.elsevier.com/Canada/Perry/maternal/

OBJECTIVES

On completion of this chapter the reader will be able to:

- Review the factors included in the initial assessment of the woman in labour.
- Describe the ongoing assessment of maternal progress during the first, second, third, and fourth stages of labour.
- Recognize the physical and psychosocial findings that indicate maternal progress during labour.
- Identify signs of developing complications during labour and birth.
- Incorporate evidence-informed nursing interventions into a comprehensive plan of care relevant to each stage of labour.
- Recognize the importance of support (family, partner, doula, nurse) in fostering maternal confidence and facilitating the progress of labour and birth.
- Analyze the influence of cultural and religious beliefs and practices on the process of labour and birth.
- Evaluate research findings on the importance of support from the family, partner, doula, and nurse in facilitating maternal progress during labour and birth.
- Describe the role and responsibilities of the nurse during emergency childbirth situations.
- Evaluate the impact of perineal trauma on the woman's reproductive and sexual health.

The labour process can be an exciting and anxious time for the woman and her family and support people. In a relatively short period, they experience one of the most profound changes in their lives, particularly with a first baby.

For most women, labour begins with the first uterine contraction, continues with hours of work during cervical dilation and birth, and ends as the woman and her family begin the attachment process with the newborn. Nursing care management focuses on assessment and support of the woman and her support people and family throughout labour and birth, with the goal of ensuring the best possible outcome for all involved.

Although the majority of women in Canada labour and give birth in a hospital under the care of a physician, others choose different settings and care providers. Midwifery care is available in hospitals, birth centres, or home, depending on the community (see Community Focus box).

COMMUNITY FOCUS

Availability of Alternative Childbirth Options in the Community

Consult the telephone directory and the Internet to explore options for childbearing families in your community. Is there a birthing centre in your community? Are registered midwives available? Is there an option for a home birth? For a water birth? Prepare a patient handout listing the options for childbearing families in your community. Discuss the findings from your interview with your clinical group.

FIRST STAGE OF LABOUR

The **first stage of labour** begins with the onset of regular uterine contractions and ends with complete cervical effacement and dilation. Previously the first stage of labour was divided into three phases (latent, active, and transition) but the Society of Obstetricians and Gynaecologist of Canada (2016) now identify only two phases. The first phase (latent or early labour) is defined as 0 to 3 cm dilated in a primiparous and cervical length generally less than 1 cm or 75% effaced. Active labour is defined as beginning at 4 cm dilated in a nulliparous woman (4–5 cm in a multiparous) (SOGC, 2016).

NURSING CARE

Many nulliparous women seek admission to the hospital in the latent phase because they have not experienced labour before and are unsure of the "right" time to come in. Multiparous women often do not come to the hospital until they are in the active phase.

Even though no two labours are identical, women who have given birth before often appear less anxious about the process, unless their previous experience was negative. A woman often has lingering impressions of her childbirth experiences. Satisfaction with childbirth depends on the woman's ability to maintain a sense of control. It is important that caregivers encourage a woman to be actively involved in decision making. In particular, caregivers who are respectful, supportive, available, protective, encouraging, kind, patient, professional, calm, and comforting (Registered Nurses Association of Ontario [RNAO], 2015) can help the woman remember her childbirth experiences in positive terms. A positive childbirth experience contributes to a woman's self-esteem and sense of accomplishment; this may in turn enhance the way she sees herself in her role as a mother. Frustrations that a woman feels about her childbirth experience stem from unmet expectations, loss of control, lack of knowledge, or the negative behaviours of some caregivers. A woman who perceives her childbirth to be unsatisfactory or traumatic could be at risk for post-traumatic stress disorder (PTSD) or a perinatal mood disorder, and an increased risk for Caesarean birth for a subsequent pregnancy.

Assessment

Assessment begins at the first contact with the woman, whether by telephone or in person. Many women call the hospital or birthing centre first for validation that it is all right for them to come in for evaluation or admission or that they can remain at home. However, many hospitals discourage the nurse from giving advice regarding what to do because of legal liability. Nurses are often instructed to tell women who call with questions to call their primary health care provider or to come to the hospital if they feel the need to be checked. The nature of the telephone conversation, including any advice or instructions given, should be documented in the patient's record (Gilbert, 2011).

A pregnant woman may come to the hospital while in prelabour or early in the latent phase of the first stage of labour. She may feel discouraged, angry, or confused upon learning that the contractions that feel so strong and regular to her are not true contractions because they are not causing cervical dilation or are still not strong or frequent enough for hospital admission.

PATIENT TEACHING

How to Distinguish True Labour From Prelabour

Prelabour

Contractions

- Occur irregularly or become regular only temporarily
- Often stop with walking or position change
- Can be felt in the back or abdomen above the navel
- Often can be stopped through the use of comfort measures

Cervix (by vaginal examination done by health care provider)

- May be soft, but there is no significant change in effacement or dilation or evidence of bloody show
- Is often in a posterior position

True Labour

Contractions

- Occur regularly, becoming stronger, lasting longer, and occurring closer together
- Become more intense with walking
- Usually felt in lower back, radiating to lower portion of abdomen
- Continue despite use of comfort measures

Cervix (by vaginal examination done by health care provider)

- Shows progressive change (softening, effacement, and dilation, which may be signalled by the appearance of bloody show)
- Moves to an increasingly anterior position

During the third trimester of pregnancy, women should be instructed about the stages of labour and the signs indicating its onset. They should be informed of the possibility that they may not be admitted to the hospital if they are 4 cm or less dilated. Later admission (i.e., during the active phase of labour) for low-risk women has been associated with an increased rate of spontaneous vaginal birth and fewer obstetrical interventions (see Patient Teaching box).

If the woman lives near the hospital and has adequate support and transportation, she may be asked to stay home or return home to allow labour to progress (i.e., until the contractions are more frequent and intense). The ideal setting for low-risk women in early labour is the familiar environment of her home. However, the woman who lives at a considerable distance from the hospital, who lacks adequate support and transportation, or who has a history of rapid labours in the past may be admitted in latent labour. The same measures used by the woman at home should be offered to the hospitalized woman during this stage of labour.

A warm shower or bath can be relaxing for the woman in latent labour. Soothing back, foot, and hand massages or a warm drink of preferred liquids such as tea or milk can help the woman rest and even sleep, especially if prelabour or latent labour is occurring at night. Diversional activities such as walking, reading, watching television, playing games or streaming videos on the computer, or talking with friends can reduce the perception of early discomfort, help the time pass, and reduce anxiety. Eating light snacks is also recommended.

Admission to Labour Unit

When the woman arrives at the labour unit, assessment is the top priority (Fig. 17-1). The nurse first performs a screening

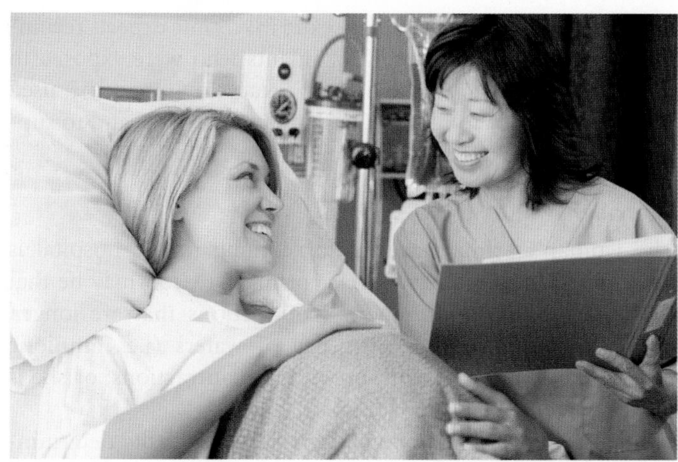

FIGURE 17-1 Woman being admitted. (Monkey Business Images/ Shutterstock.com.)

assessment, using the techniques of interview and physical assessment, and reviews laboratory and diagnostic test findings to determine the health status of the woman and her fetus and the progress of her labour. The nurse also notifies the primary health care provider, and, if the woman is admitted, a detailed systems assessment is done.

When the woman is admitted, she usually is moved from a triage area to the labour room; the labour–birth–recovery (LBR) room; or the labour–birth–recovery–postpartum (LBRP) room. Anyone coming in the room should be introduced; women often express concern about the number of people intruding on their labour experience, especially if the role of the person and purpose for his or her presence is not clearly identified.

The family-centred care approach views labour and birth as a normal, healthy life event with the woman and her support people being active participants (see Box 4-3). The woman is encouraged to have anyone she wishes present for her support. After birth, the mother, baby, and support people are permitted to stay together to celebrate the arrival of a new family member.

The woman may be asked to undress and put on her own gown or a hospital gown. An admission band is placed on the woman's wrist, as well as an allergy band (usually coloured), when relevant. Her personal belongings are put away safely or given to family members according to agency policy and her preference. Often, women who participate in prenatal education classes bring a birth bag with them that contains items to be used in labour. Tennis balls or rolling pins for counterpressure, a pillow for comfort and a reminder of home, music, an object for a focal point (e.g., meaningful picture, stuffed animal), and rice bags for warm packs may be included in her bag. This bag should be unpacked so that women will remember to use the comfort measures they brought with them.

The nurse should orient the woman and her support people to the layout and operation of the unit and room. This includes the use of the call light and telephone system, the location of personal storage areas, and how to adjust lighting in the room and positions of the bed.

The nurse needs to reassure the woman that she is in competent, caring hands and that she and her partner can ask questions related to her care and the status of herself and her fetus at any time during labour. The nurse can minimize the woman's anxiety by explaining terms commonly used during labour. The woman's interest, response, and prior experience will guide the depth of these explanations. It is most important that the nurse develop a therapeutic relationship with the woman and her family as this will enable the nurse to truly meet the woman's needs.

Admission Data

Hospital admission forms in either paper or, more commonly today, computerized format can provide guidelines for the acquisition of important assessment information when a woman in labour is being evaluated or admitted. Additional sources of data include the following: (1) antenatal record, (2) initial interview, (3) physical examination to determine baseline physiological parameters (e.g., vital signs), (4) laboratory and diagnostic test results, (5) expressed psychosocial and cultural factors, and (6) clinical evaluation of labour status.

Antenatal data. The perinatal nurse reviews the antenatal record to identify the woman's individual needs and risks. Copies of antenatal records are generally filed in the perinatal unit at some time during the woman's pregnancy (usually in the third trimester) or accessed by computer so they are readily available on admission. If the woman has had no prenatal care or her antenatal record is unavailable, certain baseline information must be obtained. If she is having discomfort, the nurse should ask questions between contractions, when she can concentrate more fully on her responses. At times, the partner or support person(s) may need to be secondary sources of essential information.

Knowing the woman's age is important so the nurse can individualize care to the needs of her age group. For example, a 14-year-old and a 40-year-old have different but specific needs, and their ages place them at risk for different problems. Accurate height and weight measurements are important to determine because a weight gain greater than that recommended may place the woman at a higher risk for Caesarean birth (Davies, Maxwell, McLeod, et al., 2010). This is especially true for women who are petite and have gained 16 kg or more. A prepregnancy body mass index (BMI) greater than 30 is also a cause for concern. Other factors to consider are the woman's general health status, current medical conditions or allergies, respiratory status, and previous surgical procedures. Questioning about physical abuse and substance use should form an integral part of the initial and ongoing assessment.

The nurse should review the woman's antenatal records carefully, taking note of her obstetrical and pregnancy history, including gravidity; parity; and problems such as history of vaginal bleeding, gestational hypertension, anemia, pregestational or gestational diabetes, infections (e.g., bacterial, viral, sexually transmitted), and immunodeficiency status. In addition, the expected date of birth (EDB) should be confirmed. Other important data found in the antenatal record include patterns of maternal weight gain; physiological measurements such as maternal vital signs (blood pressure, temperature, pulse, respirations); fundal height; baseline fetal heart rate (FHR);

and laboratory and diagnostic test results. See Table 11-1 for a list of common antenatal laboratory tests. Diagnostic and fetal assessment tests performed prenatally may include amniocentesis, nonstress test (NST), biophysical profile (BPP), and ultrasound examination. See Chapter 13 for more information.

If this is not the woman's first labour and birth experience, it is important to note the characteristics of her previous experiences. This information includes the duration of previous labours, the type of anaesthesia used, the kind of birth (e.g., spontaneous vaginal, forceps- or vacuum-assisted, or Caesarean birth), and the condition of the newborn. The woman's perception of her previous labour and birth experiences should be explored because it may influence her attitude toward her current experience.

Group B streptococcus (GBS). A woman's Group B streptococcus (GBS) status should be determined. GBS may be considered a normal vaginal flora in a woman who is not pregnant. However, GBS infection is associated with poor pregnancy outcomes and is present in 10 to 30% of healthy pregnant women (Money, Allen, Yudin, et al., 2013). These infections are an important factor in perinatal and neonatal morbidity and mortality, usually resulting from vertical transmission from the birth canal of the infected mother to the infant during birth.

Risk factors for neonatal GBS infection include positive prenatal culture for GBS in the current pregnancy, preterm birth of less than 37 weeks of gestation, prolonged rupture of membranes (ROM) (>18 hours), intrapartum maternal fever higher than 38°C (100.4°F), and a positive history for early-onset neonatal GBS (Money et al., 2013).

To decrease the risk of neonatal GBS infection, intravenous antibiotic prophylaxis (IAP) should be offered to all women who test positive. Also, if a culture is not available at the onset of labour and if risk factors are present, IAP should be offered (Money et al., 2013). Since the introduction of universal screening for GBS (rectovaginal culture at 36 to 37 weeks), the rate of GBS infection in newborns has decreased by 70% (Money et al., 2013). IAP is not recommended before a Caesarean birth if labour or rupture of membranes has not occurred. The recommended treatment is penicillin G, 5 million units in an intravenous (IV) loading dose, and then 2.5 million units intravenously every 4 hours during labour. Ampicillin, 2 g IV loading dose, followed by 1 g intravenously every 4 hours, is an alternative therapy. Therefore, the woman who is GBS positive will usually have an IV line started shortly after admission to ensure that adequate antibiotics are administered.

Herpes simplex virus (HSV). Neonatal herpes simplex virus (HSV) infection can be a devastating disease, so women need to be screened for this during labour. Current recommendations include carefully examining and questioning all women about symptoms at the onset of labour (Money, Steben, Wong, et al., 2008). If visible lesions are not present when labour begins, vaginal birth is acceptable. Caesarean birth within 4 hours after labour begins or membranes rupture is recommended if visible lesions are present. Infants who are born through an infected vagina should be carefully observed and have blood tested for the presence of HSV. Some experts recommend presumptive treatment of infants who were exposed to HSV during birth. Acyclovir and valacyclovir may be used during pregnancy to reduce the symptoms of HSV and to suppress HSV close to the time of birth (see Table 7-3).

Interview

The woman's primary reason for coming to the hospital is determined in the interview. Her primary reason may be that she is certain she is in labour (contractions that are longer, stronger, closer together); her bag of waters (i.e., amniotic membranes) ruptured, with or without contractions; or she is unsure whether she is in labour.

Even the experienced woman may have difficulty determining the onset of labour. The woman should be asked to recall the events of the previous days and to describe the following:

- Time of onset of contractions and progress in terms of intensity, frequency, and duration
- Location and character of discomfort from the contractions (e.g., back pain, abdominal or suprapubic discomfort)
- Persistence of contractions despite changes in maternal position and activity (e.g., walking or lying down)
- Presence and character of vaginal discharge or "show"
- Status of amniotic membranes such as gush or seepage of fluid (SROM [spontaneous rupture of membranes])

If there has been a discharge that may be amniotic fluid, the woman should be asked about the *C*olour, *O*dour, and *A*mount and the *T*ime (COAT) it was first noted. In many instances, a sterile speculum examination and a **nitrazine** (pH) or **fern test** can confirm that the membranes are ruptured (Box 17-1).

These descriptions can help the nurse assess the degree of progress in labour. Bloody or pink show is distinguished from bleeding in that it is pink and feels sticky because of its mucoid nature. There is very little bloody show in the beginning, but the amount increases with effacement and dilation of the cervix. A woman may report a small amount of brownish-to-bloody discharge that can be attributed to cervical trauma resulting from vaginal examination or coitus (intercourse) within the previous 48 hours.

If general **anaesthesia** is required in an emergency, it is important to assess the woman's respiratory status. The nurse can determine this by asking the woman if she has a cold or related symptoms (e.g., stuffy nose, sore throat, or cough). The nurse should recheck the status of allergies, including allergies to latex and tape. Some allergic responses cause swelling of mucous membranes of the respiratory tract, which could interfere with breathing and the administration of inhalation anaesthetics. The nurse should record the type and time of the woman's last solid food and liquid intake before coming to the hospital, as vomiting and aspiration into the respiratory tract can be a complication during an operative birth.

Any information not found in the antenatal record can be obtained during the admission assessment. Pertinent data include the **birth plan** (see Box 11-8), the choice of infant feeding method, the type of pain management preferred, and the name of the newborn's health care provider. The patient profile

BOX 17-1 PROCEDURE: TESTS FOR RUPTURE OF AMNIOTIC MEMBRANES

Nitrazine Test for pH*

Explain procedure to the woman or couple.

Procedure

Wash hands.

Use cotton-tipped applicator impregnated with Nitrazine dye or Nitrazine test paper, a dye-impregnated test paper for determining pH (differentiates amniotic fluid, which is slightly alkaline, from urine and purulent material [pus], which are acidic).

Wearing gloves, dip cotton-tipped applicator or test paper deep into vagina to pick up fluid. (The procedure may be performed during speculum examination.)

Read Results

Membranes probably intact—Identifies vaginal and most body fluids that are acidic:

Yellow	pH 5.0
Olive-yellow	pH 5.5
Olive-green	pH 6.0

Membranes probably ruptured—Identifies amniotic fluid that is alkaline:

Blue-green	pH 6.5
Blue-grey	pH 7.0
Deep blue	pH 7.5

Realize that false test results are possible because of presence of bloody show, insufficient amniotic fluid, or semen.

Provide pericare as needed.

Remove gloves and wash hands.

Document Results

Results are positive or negative.

Test for Ferning or Fern Pattern

Explain procedure to the woman or couple.

Wash hands, apply sterile gloves, obtain specimen of fluid (usually during sterile speculum examination).

Spread a drop of fluid from vagina on a clean glass slide with a sterile, cotton-tipped applicator.

Allow fluid to dry.

Examine slide under microscope. Observe for appearance of ferning (a frond-like crystalline pattern). (Do not confuse with cervical mucus test, when high levels of estrogen are responsible for causing the ferning.)

Observe for absence of ferning (alerts staff to possibility that amount of specimen was inadequate or that specimen was urine, vaginal discharge, or blood).

Provide pericare as needed.

Remove gloves and wash hands.

Document Results

Results are positive or negative.

*In some settings, the specimen is collected by the nurse or primary health care provider and sent to the laboratory for interpretation of results.

should indicate the support person or family members desired during childbirth and their availability, and ethnic or cultural expectations and needs. The woman's use of alcohol, drugs, and tobacco before or during pregnancy should be determined.

The nurse should review the birth plan. If no written plan has been prepared, the nurse can help the woman formulate a birth plan by describing options available and finding out the woman's wishes and preferences. As caregiver and advocate, the nurse integrates the woman's desires into the nursing care plan as much as possible. The nurse needs to discuss with the woman the possibility that changes may be needed in her plan as labour progresses and assure her that information will be provided so that she can make informed decisions.

The nurse should provide information about the agency's policies regarding photography and recording of the birth and under what circumstances they are allowed. Protection of privacy and safety, and infection control are major concerns for the expecting parents and the agency. To avoid future embarrassment and distress, the nurse should clarify with the woman exactly which parts of her childbirth she wishes to have photographed and the degree of detail. Remind patients and families that pictures should not be posted on social media sites without the knowledge and consent of every person who appears in the picture. The woman's record should reflect that the birth was recorded.

Psychosocial Factors

The woman's general behaviour (and that of her partner) may provide clues to the type of supportive care she will need. However, the nurse should keep in mind that general appearance and behaviour may vary, depending on the stage and phase of labour (Table 17-1 and Box 17-2).

Women with a history of sexual abuse. Labour can trigger memories of sexual abuse, especially during intrusive procedures such as vaginal examination. Monitors, IV lines, and epidurals can make the woman feel a loss of control or as if she were being confined to bed and "restrained." Being observed by students, and having intense sensations in the uterus and genital area, especially at the time when she must push the baby out, can also trigger memories. Women who are survivors of abuse may fight the labour process by reacting in panic or anger toward care providers; take control of everyone and everything related to their childbirth; surrender by being submissive and dependent; or retreat by mentally dissociating themselves from the sensations of labour and birth.

The nurse can help the abuse survivor associate the sensations she is experiencing with the process of childbirth and not with her past abuse. The nurse can help maintain the woman's sense of control by explaining all procedures to her and why they are needed, validating her needs and paying close attention to her requests. It is important to wait for the woman to give permission before touching her and accept her often extreme reactions to labour (Simpson & O'Brien-Abel, 2014). The nurse should avoid words and phrases that can cause the woman to recall the words of her abuser (e.g., "open your legs," "relax and it won't hurt so much"). The number of procedures that invade

TABLE 17-1 EXPECTED MATERNAL PROGRESS DURING FIRST STAGE OF LABOUR

CRITERION	PHASES MARKED BY CERVICAL DILATION*	
	0–3 cm (LATENT)	4–10 cm (ACTIVE)†
Duration‡	About 6–8 hr	About 3–6 hr
Contractions		
Strength	Mild to moderate	Moderate to very strong
Rhythm	Irregular	More regular
Frequency	5–30 min apart	2–5 min apart
Duration	30–45 sec	40–90 sec
Descent		
Station of presenting part	Nulliparous: 0 Multiparous: -2 cm to 0	Varies: +1 to +3 cm Varies: +1 to +3 cm
Show		
Colour	Brownish discharge, mucous plug, or pale pink mucus	Pink-to-bloody mucus
Amount	Scant	Scant to copious
Behaviour and appearance§	Excited; thoughts centre on self, labour, and baby; may be talkative or silent, calm or tense; some apprehension; alert, follows directions readily; open to instructions	Becomes more serious, doubtful of pain control, more apprehensive; desires companionship and encouragement; attention more inner directed; fatigue evidenced; malar (cheeks) flush; has some difficulty following directions Later in active phase: Pain described as moderate to severe; backache common; frustration, fear of loss of control, and irritability may be voiced; expresses doubt about ability to continue; vague in communications; amnesia between contractions; writhing with contractions; nausea and vomiting, especially if hyperventilating; hyperesthesia; perspiration of forehead and upper lips; shaking tremor of thighs; feeling of need to defecate, pressure on anus

*In the nullipara, effacement is often complete before dilation begins; in the multipara it occurs simultaneously with dilation.
†In the multipara, active labour is defined as starting at 4–5 cm.
‡Duration of each phase is influenced by such factors as parity, maternal emotions, position, level of activity, fetal size, presentation, and position. For example, the labour of a nullipara tends to last longer, on average, than the labour of a multipara. Women who ambulate and assume upright positions or change positions frequently during labour tend to experience a shorter first stage. Descent is often prolonged in breech presentations and occiput posterior positions.
§Women who have epidural analgesia for pain relief may not demonstrate some of these behaviours.

BOX 17-2 PSYCHOSOCIAL ASSESSMENT OF THE LABOURING WOMAN

Verbal Interactions
- Does the woman ask questions?
- Can she ask for what she needs?
- Does she talk to her support person(s)?
- Does she talk freely with the nurse or respond only to questions?

Body Language
- Does she change positions or lie rigidly still?
- Is she relaxed or tense?
- What is her anxiety level?
- How does she react to being touched by the nurse or support person?
- Does she avoid eye contact?
- Does she look tired? If she appears tired, ask her how much rest she has had in the past 24 hours.

Perceptual Ability
- Does she understand what the nurse says?
- Is there a language barrier?
- Are repeated explanations necessary because her anxiety level interferes with her ability to comprehend?
- Can she repeat what she has been told or otherwise demonstrate her understanding?

Discomfort Level
- To what degree does the woman describe what she is experiencing, including her pain experience?
- How does she react to a contraction?
- How does she react to assessment and care measures?
- Are any nonverbal pain messages noted?
- Can she ask for comfort measures?

her body (e.g., vaginal examinations, urinary catheter, internal monitor, forceps or vacuum extractor) should be limited as much as possible. She should be encouraged to choose a person (e.g., doula, friend, family member) to be with her during labour to provide continuous support and comfort and act as her advocate. Nurses are advised to care for all labouring women in this manner as it is not unusual for a woman to choose not to reveal a history of sexual abuse. These care measures can help a woman perceive her childbirth experience in positive terms.

Stress in Labour

The way in which women and their support person or family members approach labour is related to the manner in which they have been socialized to the child-bearing process. Their reactions reflect their life experiences regarding childbirth—physical, social, cultural, and religious. Likewise, society communicates its expectations of acceptable and unacceptable maternal behaviours that occur during labour and birth. There are thus different cultural and societal perceptions of pain in labour; these may include the following:

- Pain in childbirth is inevitable, something to be endured.
- Pain in childbirth can be avoided completely.
- Pain in childbirth is punishment for sin.
- Pain in childbirth can be managed by the woman.

It is important for the nurse to determine what beliefs the labouring woman holds as these expectations may be used by some women as the basis for evaluating their own actions during childbirth. An idealized perception of labour and birth may be a source of guilt and a sense of failure if the woman finds the process less than joyous, especially when the pregnancy is unplanned or is the product of a dysfunctional or terminated relationship. Often women have heard horror stories or seen friends or relatives go through labours that appeared anything but easy. **Multiparous** women often base their expectations of the present labour on their previous childbirth experiences.

Discuss the feelings the woman has about her pregnancy and fears regarding childbirth. This discussion is especially important if the woman is a primigravida who has not attended childbirth classes or a multiparous woman who had a previous negative childbirth experience. Women in labour usually have a variety of concerns that they will voice if asked but will rarely volunteer on their own. Major fears and concerns relate to the process and effects of childbirth, maternal and fetal well-being, and the attitude and actions of the health care staff. Unresolved fears increase a woman's stress and can slow the process of labour as a result of the inhibiting effects of catecholamines associated with the stress response on uterine contractions.

The nurse's responsibility to the woman in labour with regard to these concerns is to answer her questions or find out the answers, provide support for her and her support person and family, take care of her in partnership with the people the woman wants as her support team, and serve as their advocate. One of the most important aspects of nursing care for the labouring women is to develop a trusting relationship with the woman and her support people, as this will help the woman and her family to feel more comfortable expressing their feelings and concerns. Women can equate emotional support with information giving. Nurses are perceived as supportive when they explain things in detail by using positive terms and provide accurate information and specific directions. Women will feel empowered when they are given information they can understand and that reflects support of their efforts. This feeling of empowerment contributes to a positive perception of the birth experience. In contrast, a woman's level of anxiety and fear may increase when she does not understand what is being said or is not given adequate information.

The nurse needs to communicate to the woman that she is not expected to act in any particular way. Also, the woman's views and expectations regarding the nurse's role as caregiver should be determined. As labour progresses, the nurse–patient relationship will become increasingly important. Women need to trust in their own innate ability to give birth, and nurses need to support and protect each woman's efforts to achieve this outcome.

The partner, coach, or support person(s) also experience stress during labour. The nurse can assist and support these individuals by identifying their needs and expectations and helping to make sure these are met. The nurse can ascertain what role the support person intends to fulfill and whether he or she is prepared for that role, by making observations such as the following: Is he or she nervous, anxious, aggressive, or hostile? Does he or she look hungry, tired, worried, or confused? Does he or she watch television, sleep, or stay out of the room instead of paying attention to the woman? Does he or she touch the woman and, if so, what is the character of the touch? The nurse can also ask the support person questions regarding attendance or nonattendance of childbirth classes and the role this person expects to play during labour. The nurse should be sensitive to the needs of the support person and provide teaching and support, as appropriate. Often the support that this person is able to give to the labouring woman is in direct proportion to the support he or she receives from nurses and other health care providers.

Issues in Caring for Trans and Gender-Nonconforming Persons.

Reproductive technology has made it possible for *transmen* (a biologically female person who has transitioned to male) to give birth. If reproductive organs are still present, the person may be able to get pregnant, often with the assistance of hormone treatment. While this is rare, perinatal nurses may find themselves caring for a transman. *Gender nonconforming* (GNC) characterizes a person who does not subscribe to being either male or female (Wolfe-Roubatis & Spatz, 2015). Persons who are GNC may also make the decision to have a baby. Nurses need to be sensitive when providing care to transmen or GNC persons. It is important that the nurse develops a relationship with the patient that is based on trust and respect. Health history forms and questions nurses ask are often gender biased. Most importantly, the nurse needs to ask all patients open-ended questions, such as "How do you describe your gender identity?" (Wolfe-Roubatis & Spatz, 2015). The patient's preferred pronoun and gender identity must be documented. The patient should be referred to as "dad" instead of "mom" if this is the wish of the patient. It is ideal if these patients can meet with a nurse prior to the birth in order to develop a comprehensive birth plan. The plan should include all aspects of care, from admission, to security, to intrapartum and postpartum care, and should include discussions of all ancillary departments that will contribute to the health care of the patient (Adams, 2010). Privacy must be respected, and it is imperative that staff working in the hospital are aware of the issues with accessing records of a patient for whom they are not providing care. Most importantly, the nurse should always ask for permission prior to touching or assessing the patient and be aware that the patient may have significant concerns about being seen during labour, since the person may be conflicted about gender identity in relation to what is actually happening to their body.

Cultural Factors

Nurses need to be committed to providing culturally sensitive care and developing an appreciation of and respect for cultural diversity (Callister, 2014; Canadian Nurses Association [CNA], 2010) (see Chapter 2). For the perinatal nurse, it is important to recognize a pregnant woman's ethnic or cultural and religious values, beliefs, and practices in order to be able to anticipate nursing interventions that should be included in a mutually acceptable plan of care that fosters a sense of safety and control. The woman should be encouraged to request caregiving behaviours and practices that are important to her. If a special request contradicts usual practices in that setting, the woman or nurse can ask the woman's primary health care provider to write an order to accommodate the special request. For example, in many cultures it is unacceptable to have a male caregiver examine a pregnant woman. Most health care providers will try to accommodate this request, if possible. In some cultures it is traditional to take the placenta home; in others, the woman has only certain nourishments during labour. Some women believe that cutting her body, as with an episiotomy, allows her spirit to leave her body and that rupturing the membranes prolongs, not shortens, labour. It is important that the rationale for required care measures be carefully explained, particularly if they conflict with the woman's beliefs.

Cultural beliefs and values can influence a woman's reliance on her primary health care provider during labour and her desire to participate in making decisions about the care she receives (Callister, 2014). Indigenous women believe childbirth is a community event, one that places a high value on relationships, respect, and the collective perspective. With limited access to birthing centres, Indigenous Canadians are often moved off reserve and away from their families in late pregnancy to await labour. This may cause a disruption of the balance and harmony that are critical for a positive birth experience. Immigrants who have personally experienced or been told stories about birthing practices in other countries may be anxious about unfamiliar practices they encounter in a Canadian hospital. Health care providers can assess each patient's preferences for support and collaborate with her to meet these needs (Watts & McDonald, 2007).

Within cultures, women may learn the "right" way to behave in labour and thus react to the pain experienced in that way. These behaviours can range from total silence to moaning or screaming, but they do not necessarily indicate the degree of pain. A woman who moans with contractions may not be in as much physical pain as a woman who is silent but winces during contractions. For example, Chinese women may be stoic and quiet during labour and merely grimace during a contraction but not shout out. Rather than using pharmacological measures for pain relief, they may prefer the support of family members and nonpharmacological measures. Chinese women who believe in the balance of yin and yang view childbirth as a source of heat loss from the body. Thus, providing hot fluids and a warm shower to these women during labour could be acceptable measures of restoring the heat that is being lost.

Some women believe that screaming or crying out in pain is shameful if a man is present. If the woman's support person is her mother, she may perceive the need to "behave" more strongly than if her support person is the father of the baby. She perceives herself as failing or succeeding based on her ability to follow these "standards" of behaviour. Conversely, a woman's behaviour in response to pain may influence the support received from her support people. In some cultures, women who lose control and cry out in pain may be scolded, whereas in other cultures, support people will be more helpful.

When assessing a woman's cultural and religious preferences, the nurse can ask questions regarding the following:

- The value and meaning placed on the childbirth experience
- The view of childbirth as a wellness or illness experience and as a private or social event
- Practices regarding diet, medications, activity, and emotional and physical support
- Appropriate maternal and paternal behaviours
- Birth companions—who they should be and what they should do
- Views regarding the newborn and newborn care immediately after birth

Culture and the partner's participation. A companion is an important source of support, encouragement, and comfort to women during childbirth. The women's cultural and religious background influences her choice of a birth companion, as do trends in the society in which she lives. For example, in Western societies, the partner is viewed as the ideal birth companion. For European-North American couples, attending childbirth classes together has become a traditional, expected activity. In some other cultures, a father may be involved, but his presence in the labour and birth room with the mother may not be considered appropriate, or he may be present but resist active involvement in her care. Such behaviour could be perceived by the nursing staff as a lack of concern, caring, or interest. Women from many cultures prefer female caregivers and want to have at least one female companion present during labour and birth. They may also be very concerned about modesty. Islamic women are very modest (i.e., need to keep hair and body covered) and may not accept the presence of a man during childbirth, not even the father. In India, women are attended by other women and in rural areas by a local untrained midwife or dai. For couples from these cultures who immigrate to Canada their roles may change. The nurse needs to talk with the woman and her support people to determine the roles they will assume.

The non–English-speaking woman in labour. A woman's level of anxiety in labour increases when she does not understand what is happening to her or what is being said. Non–English-speaking women often feel a complete loss of control over their situation if there is no health care provider present who speaks their language. They can panic and withdraw or become physically abusive when someone tries to do something that they perceive might harm them or their baby. A support person is sometimes able to serve as an interpreter. However, caution is warranted in this situation because the interpreter may not be able to convey exactly what the nurse or others are saying or what the woman is saying, and this may increase the woman's stress level even more.

Ideally, a bilingual nurse will care for the woman. Alternatively, an employee or volunteer interpreter may be contacted for assistance. Preferably, the interpreter is from the woman's culture. For some women, a female interpreter may be more acceptable. If no one in the hospital is able to interpret, a translation service can be called so that an interpretation can take place over the telephone. See Chapter 2, p. 23 on how to work with an interpreter. It is important to identify the need for an interpreter early during antenatal care in order to ensure adequate time to coordinate the availability of this service when the patient arrives for labour assessment. Even when the nurse has limited ability to communicate verbally with the woman, in most instances the woman appreciates the nurse's efforts to do so. Speaking slowly and avoiding complex words and medical terms can help a woman and her partner to better understand what is happening during labour and birth. Often the woman may understand English much better than she speaks it.

Physical Examination

The initial physical examination includes a general systems assessment and an assessment of fetal status. During the examination uterine contractions are assessed and a vaginal examination is performed. The findings of the admission physical examination serve as a baseline for assessing the woman's progress from that point on and serve as the basis for determining whether the woman should be admitted and what her ongoing care should be. Expected maternal progress and minimal assessment guidelines during the first stage of labour are presented in Table 17-1 and Box 17-3.

Birth is a time when nurses and other health care providers are exposed to a great deal of maternal and newborn blood and body fluids. Therefore, routine precautions should guide all assessment and care measures (Box 17-4). Hand hygiene (e.g., washing hands with soap or application of an alcohol-based antibacterial solution) before and after assessing the woman and after providing care is a critical step in the prevention of infection transmission. The nurse should explain assessment findings to the woman and her partner. Throughout labour, accurate documentation, following agency policy, should be done as soon as possible after a procedure has been performed (Fig. 17-2).

General systems assessment. On admission the nurse should perform a brief systems assessment. This includes an assessment of the heart, lungs, and skin and an examination to determine the presence and extent of edema of the legs, face, and hands. It is also includes testing of deep tendon reflexes and for clonus if indicated. The woman's weight is also noted, as excessive size can make nursing care during labour and birth more difficult and places the woman at risk for complications such as operative birth, infection, and blood clots. See Chapter 20 for further information.

Vital signs. Vital signs (temperature, pulse, respirations, and blood pressure) are assessed on admission, and initial values are used for comparison with subsequent values. If blood pressure is elevated, it should be reassessed 30 minutes later, between contractions, after the woman has relaxed.

If the woman is in bed she should be encouraged to lie on her side to prevent supine hypotension and the resulting fetal hypoxemia (Fig. 17-3). The nurse needs to monitor the woman's temperature to identify signs of infection or a fluid deficit (e.g., dehydration associated with inadequate intake of fluids).

BOX 17-3 NURSING ASSESSMENTS IN FIRST-STAGE LABOUR

Latent Phase (if admitted to hospital)

- Assess maternal blood pressure, pulse, respirations every 30 to 60 minutes.
- Assess fetal heart rate (FHR) and pattern, uterine activity, vaginal show every 30 to 60 minutes, depending on risk status.
- Assess temperature every 4 hours until membranes rupture and then every 2 hours.
- Perform vaginal examination as needed to identify progress.
- Observe every 30 minutes: changes in maternal appearance, mood, affect, energy level, and condition of partner/support person.

Active Phase

- Assess maternal blood pressure, pulse, and respirations every 30 to 60 minutes.
- Assess FHR and pattern, uterine activity, vaginal show every 15 to 30 minutes, depending on risk status.
- Assess temperature every 4 hours until membranes rupture and then every 1 to 2 hours.
- Perform vaginal examination as needed to identify progress.
- Observe every 5 to 15 minutes: changes in maternal appearance, mood, affect, energy level, and condition of partner/coach.

! NURSING ALERT

During labour, blood pressure should be assessed with an appropriate-sized sphygmomanometer and stethoscope or a calibrated aneroid device to obtain the most accurate results. Automatic devices that measure blood pressure have been found to overestimate the systolic pressure and underestimate the diastolic pressure. Automated blood pressure machines that are used need to be validated for use in pregnant women and especially for use in women with hypertensive disorders. These devices further restrict freedom of movement and can also increase the discomfort of the woman as the cuff inflates and deflates on a regular basis. Maternal heart rate should be assessed by auscultation (i.e., apical rate) or palpation (i.e., radial pulse rate) rather than with a pulse oximeter.

Leopold manoeuvres (abdominal palpation). Leopold manoeuvres are performed with the woman briefly lying on her back (Box 17-5). These manoeuvres help to identify the (1) number of fetuses; (2) presenting part, fetal lie, and fetal attitude; (3) degree of descent of the presenting part into the

BOX 17-4 ROUTINE PRECAUTIONS DURING CHILDBIRTH

Routine precautions applicable to childbirth include the following:

- The 4 Moments of hand hygiene are implemented: (1) before initial patient/patient environment contact, (2) before aseptic procedure, (3) after body–fluid exposure risk, (4) after patient/patient environment contact. Wash hands with cleansing alcohol rub unless visibly soiled when soap and water is required.
- Wear gloves (clean or sterile, as appropriate) when performing procedures that require contact with the woman's genitalia and body fluids, including bloody show (e.g., during vaginal examination, amniotomy, hygienic care of the perineum, insertion of an internal scalp electrode and intrauterine pressure monitor, and urinary catheterization).
- Wear protective eyewear and cover gown when assisting with the birth. Masks, cap, and shoe covers are worn for Caesarean birth. Gowns worn by the primary health care provider who is attending the birth should have a waterproof front. A mask should be worn during spinal puncture or insertion of an epidural catheter.
- Wear gloves when handling the newborn immediately after birth until the first bath is completed.

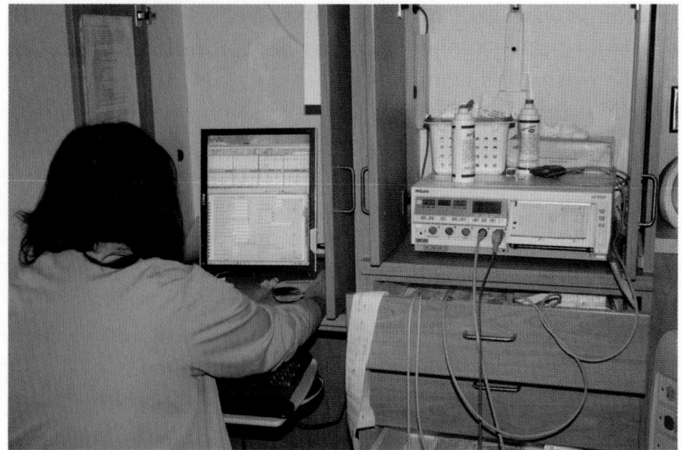

FIGURE 17-2 Nurse documenting assessment findings on computer in a labour–birth–recovery–postpartum room. (Courtesy Shannon Perry.)

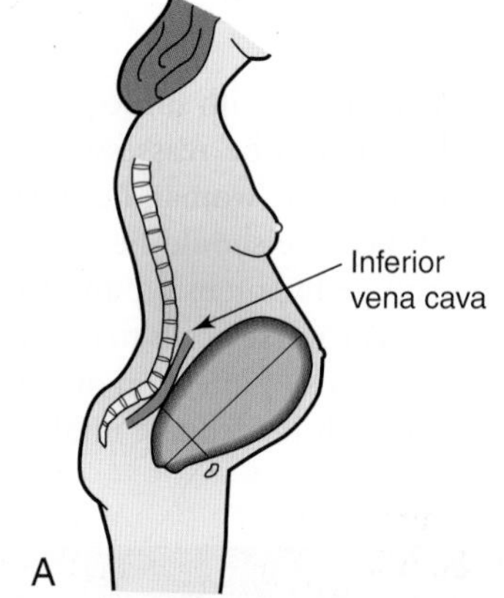

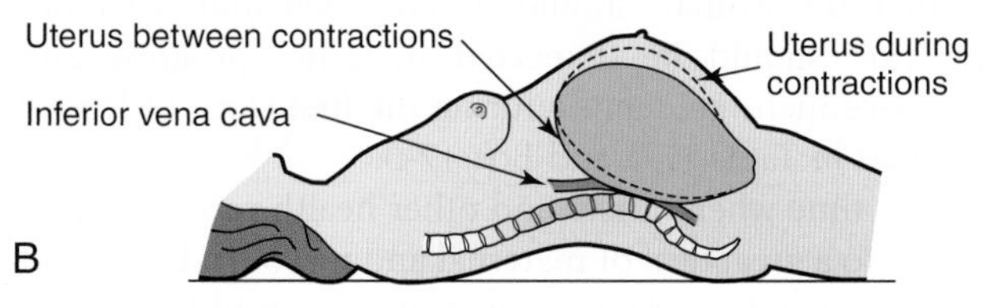

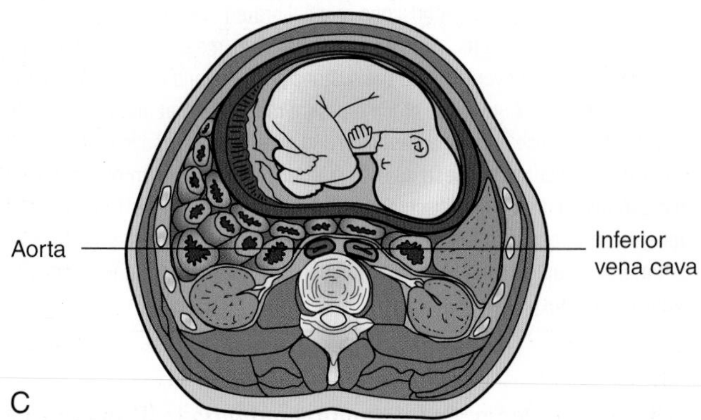

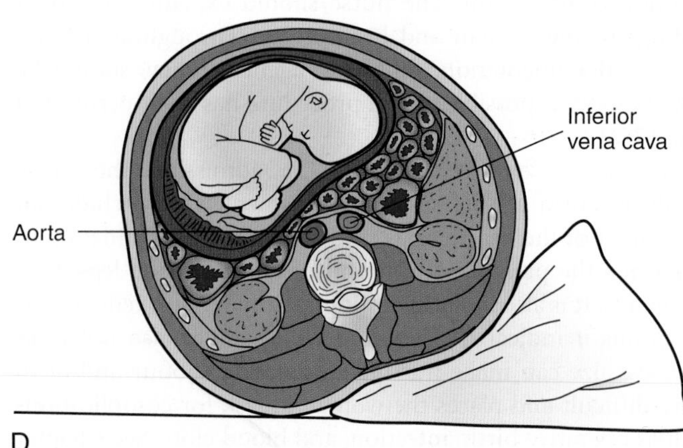

FIGURE 17-3 Supine hypotension. Note relationship of gravid uterus to ascending vena cava in standing posture **(A)** and supine posture **(B)**. **(C)** Compression of aorta and inferior vena cava with woman in supine position. **(D)** This is relieved by use of a wedge pillow placed under woman's right side.

BOX 17-5 PROCEDURE: LEOPOLD MANOEUVRES

- Wash hands.
- Ask woman to empty bladder.
- Position woman supine with one pillow under her head and her knees slightly flexed.
- Place small rolled towel under woman's right or left hip to displace uterus off major blood vessels (prevents supine hypotensive syndrome; see Fig. 17-3, D).
- If right-handed, stand on woman's right, facing her (if left-handed, stand on woman's left):

1. Identify fetal part that occupies the fundus. The head feels round, firm, freely movable, and palpable by ballottement; the breech feels less regular and softer. This manoeuvre is used to identify fetal lie (longitudinal or transverse) and presentation (cephalic or breech) (see Fig. A).
2. Using palmar surface of one hand, locate and palpate the smooth convex contour of the fetal back and the irregularities that identify the small parts (feet, hands, elbows). This manoeuvre helps identify fetal presentation (Fig. B).
3. With right hand, determine which fetal part is presenting over the inlet to the true pelvis. Gently grasp the lower pole of the uterus between the thumb and fingers, pressing in slightly (Fig. C). If the head is presenting and not engaged, determine the attitude of the head (flexed or extended).
4. Turn to face the woman's feet. Using both hands, outline the fetal head (Fig. D) with the palmar surface of the fingertips. When the presenting part has descended deeply, only a small portion of it may be outlined. Palpation of the cephalic prominence helps identify the attitude of the head. If the cephalic prominence is bound on the same side as the small parts, this means that the head must be flexed and the vertex is presenting (Fig. D). If the cephalic prominence is on the same side as the back, this indicates that the presenting head is extended and the face is presenting.
5. Document fetal presentation, position, and lie and whether presenting part is flexed or extended, engaged, or free floating. Use agency protocol for documentation (e.g., "Vtx, LOA, floating").

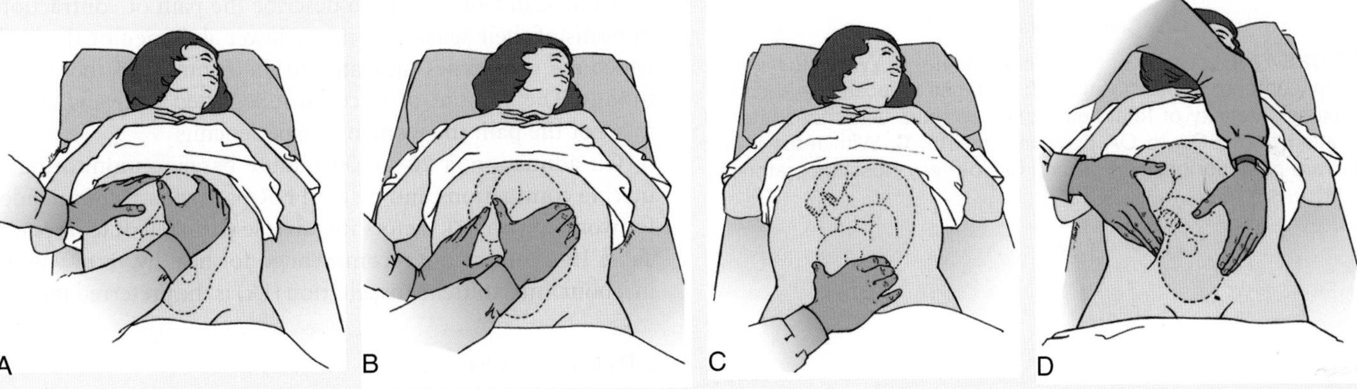

pelvis; and (4) expected location of the point of maximal intensity (PMI) of the FHR on the woman's abdomen.

Assessment of fetal heart rate and pattern. The PMI of the FHR is the location on the maternal abdomen where the FHR is heard loudest. It is usually directly over the fetal back. In a vertex presentation, FHR is usually heard below the mother's umbilicus in either the right or left lower quadrant of the abdomen. In a breech presentation, the FHR is heard above the mother's umbilicus (Fig. 17-4, A, C). As the fetus descends and rotates internally, the FHR is heard lower and closer to the midline of the maternal abdomen (see Fig. 17-4, B).

The FHR and pattern must be assessed (1) immediately after ROM, due to an increased risk for the umbilical cord to prolapse, (2) after any change in the contraction pattern or maternal status, and (3) before and after medicating the woman or performing a procedure. For a complete discussion of fetal health surveillance in labour see Chapter 19.

Assessment of uterine activity (UA). A general characteristic of effective labour is regular uterine activity (UA) (i.e., contractions becoming more frequent and of increased duration); however, UA is not directly related to labour progress. Uterine contractions are the primary powers that act involuntarily to expel the fetus and placenta from the uterus. Several methods are used to evaluate the strength of uterine contractions: the woman's subjective description, palpation and timing of the contraction by a health care provider, and internal electronic monitoring.

Each contraction exhibits a wavelike pattern. It begins with a slow increment (the "building up" of a contraction from its onset) that gradually reaches an acme (peak) and then diminishes rapidly (decrement, the "letting down" of the contraction). An interval of rest ends when the next contraction begins. The outward appearance of the woman's abdomen during and between contractions and the pattern of a typical uterine contraction are shown in Fig. 17-5.

Uterine contractions are described in terms of the following characteristics:

Frequency—How often uterine contractions occur; the time that elapses from the beginning of one contraction to the beginning of the next (in minutes)

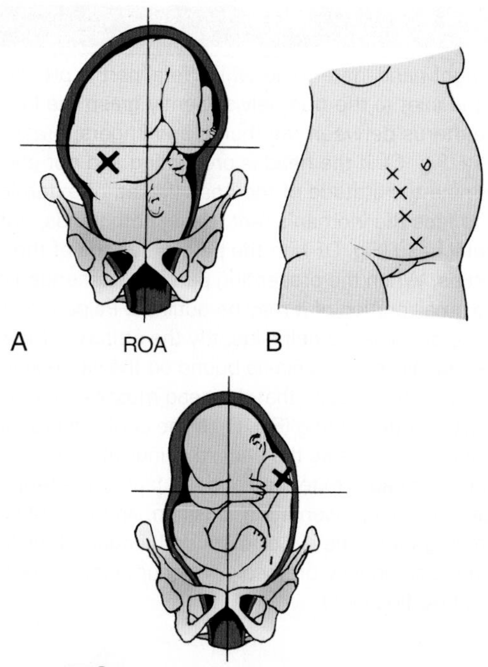

FIGURE 17-4 Location of the fetal heart rate. **A:** With fetus in right occipitoanterior (ROA) position. **B:** Changes in location of point of maximal intensity of fetal heart tones as fetus undergoes internal rotation from ROA to OA position for birth. **C:** With fetus in left sacrum posterior position. (**A** and **C**, Courtesy Ross Laboratories.)

Intensity—The strength of a contraction at its peak

Duration—The time that elapses between the onset and the end of a contraction (in seconds)

Resting tone—The tension in the uterine muscle between contractions; relaxation of the uterus

Uterine contractions are assessed by palpation or by using an external or internal electronic monitor (see Chapter 19 for further discussion). Frequency and duration can be measured by all three methods of uterine activity monitoring. Intensity can only be assessed using palpation or internal electronic monitoring. Palpation is subjective but along with the patient's report of the pain is the best way to determine the intensity of uterine contractions. The following terms are used to describe what is felt on palpation:

Mild—Slightly tense fundus that is easy to indent with fingertips (feels like touching finger to tip of nose)

Moderate—Firm fundus that is difficult to indent with fingertips (feels like touching finger to chin)

Strong—Rigid, boardlike fundus that is almost impossible to indent with fingertips (feels like touching finger to forehead)

Women in labour tend to describe the pain of contractions in terms of their sensations in the lower abdomen or the back, which are sometimes unrelated to the firmness of the uterine fundus. The amount of discomfort reported is a valid assessment of the pain the woman is experiencing.

On admission, a 20- to 30-minute baseline monitoring of uterine contractions and of the FHR pattern is recommended for women with risk factors for adverse perinatal outcomes (see Table 19-2) and is not recommended for healthy, term women in labour. Intermittent auscultation (IA) is the preferred method

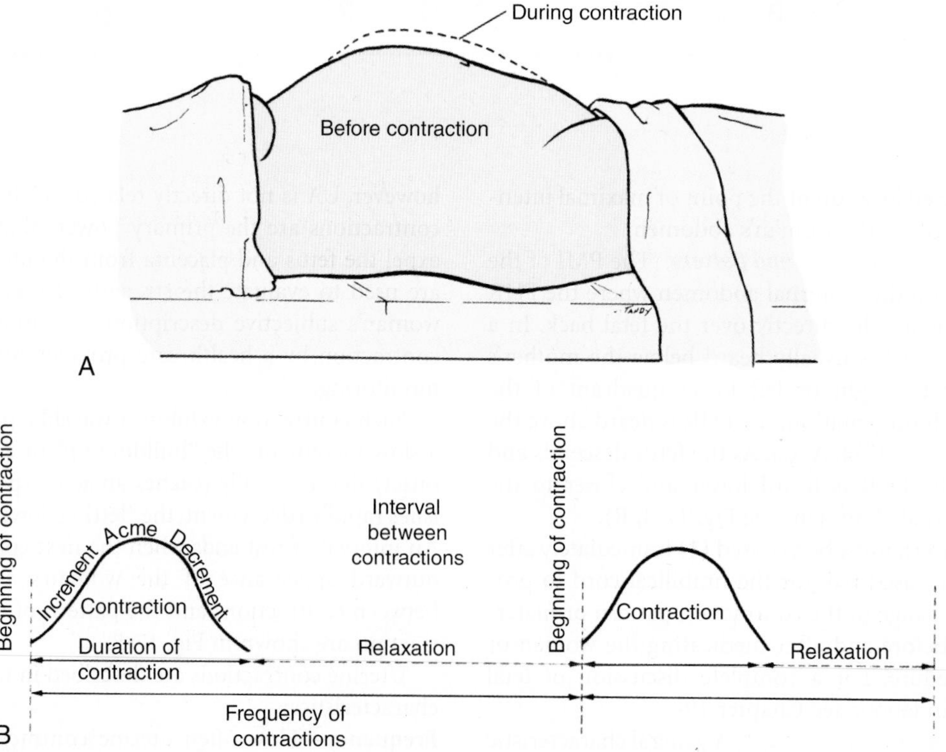

FIGURE 17-5 Assessment of uterine contractions. **A:** Abdominal contour before and during uterine contractions. **B:** Wavelike pattern of contractile activity.

for healthy women after 36 weeks' (up to 41+3 weeks) gestation in spontaneous labour in the absence of risk factors (Liston, Sawchuck, Young, et al., 2007; see Chapter 19 for more in-depth discussion).

The findings that are expected as first-stage labour progresses are summarized in Table 17-1.

The nurse's responsibility in monitoring uterine contractions is to ascertain whether they are powerful and frequent enough to accomplish the work of expelling the fetus and the placenta. UA must be considered in the context of its effect on cervical effacement and dilation and the degree of descent of the presenting part. The effect on the fetus must also be considered.

NURSING ALERT

If the characteristics of uterine activity (UA) are found to be abnormal, either exceeding or falling below what is considered acceptable in terms of the standard characteristics, the nurse should document the finding and report this finding to the primary health care provider.

NURSING ALERT

It is important for the nurse to recognize that active labour can last longer than the expected labour patterns. This finding should not be a cause for concern unless the fetus exhibits atypical or abnormal fetal heart rate (FHR) patterns or the mother has a maternal fever.

Vaginal examination. The vaginal examination reveals whether the woman is in true labour and enables the examiner to determine whether the membranes have ruptured (Fig. 17-6). Because this examination is often stressful and uncomfortable for the woman, it should be performed only when indicated by the status of the woman and her fetus. For example, a vaginal examination should be performed on admission, when significant change has occurred in UA, on maternal perception of perineal pressure or the urge to bear down, when membranes rupture, when the mother requests pain medication, or when abnormal FHR characteristics are noted. A full explanation of the examination and support of the woman are important factors in reducing the stress and discomfort associated with the examination. Vaginal examinations can reveal the amount of dilatation and effacement as well as the station and presentation of the presenting part (Box 17-6).

Laboratory and diagnostic tests

Analysis of urine specimen. A clean-catch urine specimen may be obtained to gather more data about the pregnant woman's health. Analysis of the specimen is a convenient and simple procedure that can provide information about her hydration status (e.g., by specific gravity, colour, and amount), nutritional status (e.g., ketones), infection (e.g., leukocytes), or the status of possible complications such as pre-eclampsia, shown by finding protein in the urine. The results can be obtained quickly and help the nurse to determine appropriate interventions to implement.

Blood tests. The blood tests performed vary with hospital protocol and according to the woman's health status. Blood can be obtained by a finger stick, venipuncture, or from the hub of

BOX 17-6 PROCEDURE: VAGINAL EXAMINATION OF THE LABOURING WOMAN

- Use sterile glove and antiseptic solution or soluble gel for lubrication.
- Position woman to prevent supine hypotension. Drape to ensure privacy.
- Cleanse perineum and vulva if needed.
- After obtaining the woman's permission to touch her, gently insert index and middle fingers into woman's vagina.
- Determine:
  - Cervical dilation, effacement, and position (e.g., posterior or anterior)
  - Presenting part, position, and station; moulding of head with development of caput succedaneum (may affect accuracy of determination of station)
  - Status of membranes (intact, bulging, or ruptured)
  - Characteristics of amniotic fluid (e.g., colour, clarity, and odour) if membranes are ruptured
- Explain findings of examination to woman.
- Document findings and report to primary health care provider.

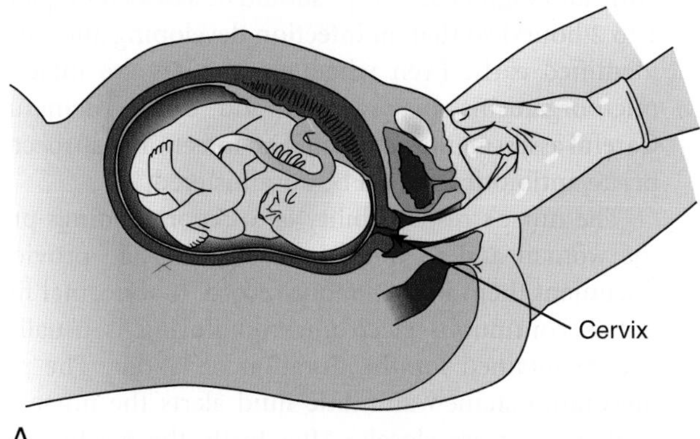

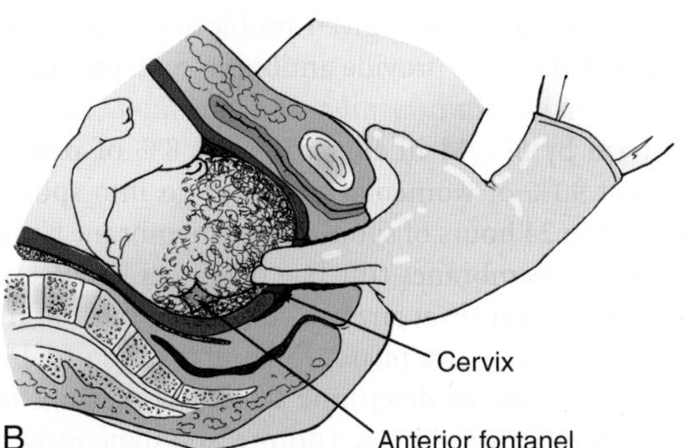

FIGURE 17-6 Vaginal examination. **A:** Undilated, uneffaced cervix; membranes intact. **B:** Palpation of sagittal suture line. Cervix effaced and partially dilated.

TABLE 17-2 ASSESSMENT OF AMNIOTIC FLUID

CHARACTERISTIC OF FLUID	NORMAL FINDING	DEVIATION FROM NORMAL FINDING	CAUSE OF DEVIATION FROM NORMAL
Colour	Pale, straw-coloured; may contain white flecks of vernix caseosa, lanugo, scalp hair	Greenish-brown colour	Hypoxic episode in fetus; meconium in fluid
		Yellow-stained fluid	May be normal finding in breech presentation as pressure is exerted on fetal abdominal wall during descent
			Fetal hypoxia ≥36 hr before ROM; fetal hemolytic disease; intrauterine infection
		Port wine–coloured	Bleeding associated with placental abruption
Viscosity and odour	Watery; no strong odour	Thick, cloudy, foul-smelling	Intrauterine infection
			Large amount of meconium can make fluid thick
Amount (normally varies with gestational age)	400 mL (20 wk of gestation) 1000 mL (36–38 wk of gestation)	≥2000 mL (32–36 wk of gestation)	Hydramnios; associated with congenital anomalies of the fetus when fetus cannot drink or fluid is trapped in the body (e.g., fetal gastrointestinal obstruction or atresias); increased risk with maternal pregestational or gestational diabetes mellitus
		≤500 mL (32–36 wk of gestation)	Oligohydramnios; associated with incomplete or absent kidney; obstruction of urethra; infant cannot secrete or excrete urine

ROM, rupture of membranes.

a catheter used to start an IV line. A complete blood count (CBC) may be ordered for women with a history of infection, anemia, gestational hypertension, or other disorders, although for most women a hematocrit is ordered. Comprehensive assessments such as white blood cell count, red blood cell count, hemoglobin level, hematocrit, and platelet values are included in the CBC. Any woman whose human immunodeficiency virus (HIV) status is undocumented at the time of labour should be screened with a rapid HIV test unless she declines (opts out of) testing.

Most hospitals require that a "type and screen" be performed on admission in order to determine the woman's blood type and Rh status. Even if these tests have already been performed during pregnancy, the hospital laboratory or blood bank must verify the results in house. If the woman had no prenatal care or if her prenatal records are not available, a prenatal screen is likely drawn on admission. The prenatal screen includes laboratory tests that would normally have been drawn at the initial prenatal visit (see Table 11-1).

Other tests. If the woman's GBS status is not known, a rapid test may be done on admission if it is available at the facility. The rapid test results are usually available within an hour and determine if the woman must be given antibiotics during labour, although this test does not provide antibiotic susceptibility.

Assessment of amniotic membranes and fluid. Labour is initiated at term by SROM in approximately 8% of pregnant women. Almost 90% of women at term will go into spontaneous labour within 24 hours of spontaneous membrane rupture (More OB, 2010). Membranes (the bag of waters [BOW]) can also rupture spontaneously at any time during labour but most commonly later in the active phase of the first stage of labour. Box 17-1 explains how to determine if membranes are ruptured. If the membranes do not rupture spontaneously, the BOW will likely be ruptured artificially at some time during labour. Artificial rupture of membranes (AROM), called an **amniotomy**, is performed by the physician or midwife using a plastic AmniHook or a surgical clamp.

Regardless of whether the membranes rupture spontaneously or artificially, the time of rupture should be recorded. Other necessary documentation includes information regarding the colour (clear or meconium-stained), estimated amount, and odour of the fluid (Table 17-2).

! NURSING ALERT

The umbilical cord may prolapse when the membranes rupture. The fetal heart rate (FHR) and pattern should be monitored closely for several minutes immediately after rupture of membranes (ROM) to ascertain fetal well-being and the findings should be documented.

Infection. After membranes rupture, microorganisms from the vagina can ascend into the amniotic sac, causing **chorioamnionitis** and placentitis to develop. The rate of infection is low, at 2.3% after 24 hours of ruptured membranes (Pintucci, Meregalli, Colombo, et al., 2014), although maternal temperature and vaginal discharge should be assessed frequently (every 1 to 2 hours) so that an infection developing after ROM can be identified early. Even when membranes are intact, however, microorganisms may ascend and cause premature ROM. Careful assessment is critical; if an infection is suspected, appropriate antibiotics should be administered.

The nurse's responsibility is to report findings promptly to the woman and to the primary health care provider and to document them in the labour record. If abnormal findings are noted, continuous electronic monitoring is usually initiated and maintained for the duration of labour. The presence of meconium-stained amniotic fluid alerts the nurse to observe fetal status more closely. After birth, the newborn may be at high risk for alteration in respiratory status if meconium is aspirated into the lungs with the first breath.

BOX 17-7 SIGNS OF POTENTIAL LABOUR COMPLICATIONS

- Contractions consistently lasting ≥90 seconds
- More than five contractions in a 10-minute period (occur more frequently than every 2 minutes)
- Relaxation between contractions lasting < 30 seconds
- Intrauterine pressure of ≥80 mm Hg (determined by intrauterine pressure catheter monitoring) or resting tone of ≥20 mm Hg
- Fetal bradycardia or tachycardia; absent or minimal variability not associated with fetal sleep cycle or temporary effects of central nervous system depressant drugs given to the woman; late, variable, or prolonged fetal heart rate decelerations (see Chapter 19)
- Irregular fetal heart rate; suspected fetal dysrhythmias
- Presence of atypical or abnormal fetal heart rate pattern (see Chapter 19)
- Appearance of meconium-stained or bloody fluid from the vagina
- Arrest in progress of cervical dilation or effacement, descent of the fetus, or both
- Maternal temperature of 38°C or more
- Foul-smelling vaginal discharge
- Persistent bright-red or dark-red vaginal bleeding

Assessment findings serve as a baseline for evaluating the woman's progress during labour. Although some problems of labour are anticipated, others may appear unexpectedly during the clinical course of labour (Box 17-7).

Nursing Care During Labour

Nurses caring for the labouring woman must use an empathic approach when providing care, which may include the following:

- Establishing rapport with the woman and her significant others
- Respecting the woman's individual needs and behaviours
- Being kind, caring, and competent when performing necessary procedures
- Explaining procedures, using words the woman can understand; repeating as necessary
- Being aware that pain and discomfort are as the woman describes them
- Carrying out appropriate comfort measures such as mouth and back care
- Including the support people in the care as desired by the woman and the support people
- Recognizing that a woman's current childbirth experience and the actions of nurses and other health care providers can have a positive or negative impact on her future childbirth experiences

The physical nursing care given to a woman in labour is also an essential component of her care. Evidence-informed practice is used to enhance the safety, effectiveness, and acceptability of the physical care measures chosen to support the woman during labour and birth. Box 17-8 lists the Lamaze Six Healthy Birth Practices, which are based on research evidence. Promoting care that is based on these birth practices will ensure that women have improved birth outcomes. The various physical needs, requisite nursing actions, and rationale for care are presented in Table 17-3 and the Nursing Care Plan: Care of Woman in Labour, available on Evolve.

BOX 17-8 LAMAZE HEALTHY BIRTH PRACTICES: DESIGNED TO PROMOTE, PROTECT, AND SUPPORT NORMAL LABOUR AND BIRTH

- Allow labour to begin on its own: Encourage spontaneous labour rather than fostering elective labour inductions.
- Encourage freedom of movement throughout labour to facilitate the progress of labour and enhance maternal comfort and control of the labour process.
- Provide labour support beginning early in labour and continuing throughout the process of childbirth to relieve maternal anxiety and stress and decrease the risk for epidural anaesthesia and Caesarean birth; support should be provided by someone not employed by the hospital (e.g., doula).
- Avoid routine implementation of interventions (e.g., intravenous fluids, oral intake restrictions, continuous electronic fetal monitoring, labour augmentation measures such as amniotomy and oxytocin administration, and epidural anaesthesia).
- Support the practice of spontaneous, nondirected pushing in nonsupine positions (e.g., lateral, squatting, standing, kneeling, and semisitting) to facilitate the progress of fetal descent and shorten the second stage of labour.
- Avoid separation of the mother from her baby after birth by encouraging skin-to-skin contact of mother and baby to keep the newborn warm, prevent newborn infection, enhance the newborn's physiological adjustment to extrauterine life, and foster early breastfeeding.

Source: Lamaze International. (2016). *Lamaze healthy birth practices.* Retrieved from http://www.lamazeinternational.org/HealthyBirthPracticesTools

General Hygiene

Nurses can offer women in labour the use of showers or warm-water baths if they are available, to enhance the feeling of well-being and minimize the discomfort of contractions. Water immersion during active labour is associated with decreases in the use of analgesia and reported maternal pain (Jones, Othman, Dowswell, et al., 2012). A Cochrane review suggested that immersion in water during the first stage of labour reduces the length of this stage and use of epidural or spinal anaesthesia during labour (Cluett & Burns, 2009). Other hygiene measures are discussed in Table 17-3.

Nutrient and Fluid Intake

Oral intake. Traditionally, the labouring woman was offered only clear liquids or ice chips or given nothing by mouth during the active phase of labour. This was to minimize the risk of anaesthesia complications and their sequelae should general

TABLE 17-3 PHYSICAL NURSING CARE DURING LABOUR

NEED	NURSING ACTIONS	RATIONALE
General Hygiene		
Showers/bed baths, Jacuzzi bath	Assess for progress in labour	Determines appropriateness of activity
	Supervise showers closely if woman is in active labour	Prevents injury from fall; labour may be accelerated
	Suggest allowing warm water to flow over back	Aids relaxation; increases comfort
Perineum	Cleanse frequently, especially after rupture of membranes and when show increases	Enhances comfort and reduces risk of infection
Oral hygiene	Offer toothbrush or mouthwash or wash the teeth with an ice-cold, wet washcloth as needed	Refreshes mouth; helps counteract dry, thirsty feeling
Hair	Brush, braid per woman's wishes	Improves morale; increases comfort
Hand washing	Offer washcloths before and after voiding and as needed	Maintains cleanliness; prevents infection
Face	Offer cool washcloth	Provides relief from diaphoresis; cools and refreshes
Gowns/linens	Change as needed	Improves comfort; enhances relaxation
Nutrient and Fluid Intake		
Oral	Offer fluids and solid foods, following orders of primary health care provider and desires of labouring woman	Provides hydration and calories; enhances positive emotional experience and maternal control
Intravenous (IV)	Establish and maintain IV line, as ordered	Maintains hydration; provides venous access for medications if required
Elimination		
Voiding	Encourage voiding at least every 2 hr	A full bladder may impede descent of presenting part; overdistension may cause bladder atony and injury and postpartum voiding difficulty
Ambulatory woman	Encourage ambulation to bathroom if woman is not on bedrest or not drowsy from medication	Reinforces normal process of urination and ambulation Precautionary measure to protect against injury
Woman on bedrest	Offer bedpan	Prevents complications of bladder distension and ambulation
	Allow tap water to run; pour warm water over vulva; give positive suggestion	Encourages voiding
	Provide privacy	Shows respect for woman
	Put up side rails on bed	Prevents injury from fall
	Place call bell within reach	Maintains cleanliness; prevents infection
	Offer washcloth for hands	Maintains cleanliness; enhances comfort; prevents infection
	Wash vulvar area	
Catheterization	Catheterize according to orders of primary health care provider or hospital protocol if measures to facilitate voiding are ineffective	Prevents complications of bladder distension
	Insert catheter between contractions	Minimizes discomfort
	Avoid force if obstacle to insertion is noted	"Obstacle" may be caused by compression of urethra by presenting part
Bowel elimination—sensation of rectal pressure	Perform vaginal examination	Prevents misinterpretation of rectal pressure from the presenting part as need to defecate Determines degree of descent of presenting part
	Help woman ambulate to bathroom or offer bedpan after careful assessment	Reinforces normal process of bowel elimination and safe care
	Cleanse perineum immediately after passage of stool	Reduces risk of infection and sense of embarrassment

anaesthesia be required in an emergency. These sequelae could include aspiration of gastric contents and resultant compromise in oxygen perfusion, which may endanger the lives of the mother and fetus. This practice is being challenged today because regional anaesthesia is used more often than general anaesthesia, even for emergency Caesarean births. Women are awake during regional anaesthesia and are able to participate in their own care and protect their airway.

A Cochrane database review of this topic concluded that there is no justification for restricting food or fluid intake during labour in women at low risk for complications (Singata, Tranmer, & Gyte, 2013). Nurses should follow the orders of the woman's primary health care provider when offering the woman food or fluids during labour. However, as advocates, nurses can facilitate change by informing others of the current research findings that support the safety and effectiveness of the oral intake of food and fluid during labour and by initiating such research themselves.

Although gastric emptying is slowed as a result of labour, stress, and the use of narcotics or sedatives, fasting does not cause gastric contents to be eliminated and may even cause them to be more acidic. In addition, fasting is identified by many labouring women as a stressor with which they must cope and a source of frustration during labour, related to a loss of control in meeting their own nourishment needs.

An adequate intake of fluids and calories is required to meet the energy demands and fluid losses associated with childbirth. The progress of labour slows, and ketosis develops if these demands are not met and fat is metabolized. Reduced energy for bearing-down efforts (pushing) increases the risk for a forceps- or vacuum-assisted birth. This is most likely to occur in women who begin to labour early in the morning after a night without caloric intake. When women are permitted to consume fluids and food freely, they typically regulate their own oral intake, eating light foods (e.g., eggs, yogurt, ice cream, dry toast and jelly, fruit) and drinking fluids during latent labour and then tapering off to an intake of clear fluid and sips of water or ice chips as labour intensifies and the second stage approaches. Women who are allowed to eat may have an enhanced sense of control and level of comfort.

Herbal teas can provide not only hydration but also other beneficial effects. Chamomile tea can enhance relaxation, lemon balm or peppermint tea can reduce nausea, and teas of ginger or ginseng root are energizing (Walls, 2009). A woman's culture may influence what she will eat and drink during labour. In addition, women who use nonpharmacological pain-relief measures and labour at home or in birthing centres are more likely to eat and drink during labour. The amount of solid and liquid carbohydrates to offer a woman in labour is still unclear. Although it is known that energy needs increase as labour becomes prolonged, there is limited evidence regarding the effect of oral carbohydrate intake in enhancing the progress of labour and reducing the risk for dystocia (Sharts-Hopko, 2010).

Intravenous intake. Fluids are administered intravenously to the labouring woman in order to maintain hydration only when the woman is unable to ingest a sufficient amount of fluid orally or if she is receiving epidural or intrathecal analgesia. While routine use of IV fluids during labour is not recommended, 17% of hospitals in Canada state they have a policy to routinely start an IV (Public Health Agency of Canada [PHAC], 2012). There is some early research that suggests increased IV fluid during labour may increase breast edema during the postpartum period that is not related to engorgement. Breast edema may lead to breastfeeding issues that may ultimately cause early weaning. Nurses need to be aware that excessive IV fluid may impact breastfeeding, although further research on this is required (Kujawa-Myles, Noel-Weiss, Dunn, et al., 2015). In most cases, an electrolyte solution without glucose is adequate and does not introduce excess glucose into the bloodstream, which results in fetal hyperglycemia and fetal hyperinsulinism. After birth, the newborn's high level of insulin will then deplete his or her glucose stores and hypoglycemia will result. Infusions containing glucose can also reduce sodium levels in the woman and fetus, leading to transient neonatal tachypnea. If maternal ketosis occurs, the primary health care provider may order an IV solution containing a small amount of dextrose to provide the glucose needed to assist in fatty acid metabolism.

NURSING ALERT

Nurses should carefully monitor the intake and output of IV fluids that labouring women receive, because these women also face an increased danger of hypervolemia as a result of the fluid retention that occurs during pregnancy.

Elimination

Voiding. A labouring woman should be encouraged to void a minimum of every 2 hours. A distended bladder may impede descent of the presenting part, slow or stop uterine contractions, and lead to decreased bladder tone or atony after birth. Women who receive epidural analgesia or anaesthesia are especially at risk for retention of urine; therefore, their need to void should be assessed more frequently.

The woman should be assisted to the bathroom to void unless the primary health care provider has ordered bedrest. She may be unable to get up to use the bathroom in some situations—for example, when the woman is receiving epidural analgesia or anaesthesia—or it may be the nurse's judgement that ambulation would compromise the status of the labouring woman or her fetus. External monitoring can be interrupted for the woman to go to the bathroom for periods of up to 30 minutes if maternal–fetal condition is stable (Liston et al., 2007).

Catheterization. If the woman is unable to void and her bladder is distended, she may need to be catheterized. Many hospitals have protocols that rely on the nurse's judgement concerning the need for catheterization. Before performing the catheterization, the vulva and perineum need to be cleaned because vaginal show and amniotic fluid may be present. An obstacle preventing advancement of the catheter is most likely the fetal presenting part. If the nurse cannot advance the catheter, the procedure should be stopped and the primary health care provider notified of the difficulty. Based on research, intermittent catheterization seems to be the preferred method of catheterization (see Research Focus box).

Bowel elimination. Most women do not have bowel movements during labour because of decreased intestinal motility. Stool that has formed in the large intestine often is moved downward toward the anorectal area by the pressure exerted by the fetal presenting part as it descends. In small numbers of women, this stool is expelled during second-stage pushing and birth. However, the passage of stool with bearing-down efforts may embarrass the woman, thereby reducing the effectiveness of these efforts. To prevent these problems, the nurse should immediately cleanse the perineal area to remove any stool, while at the same time reassuring the woman that the passage of stool at this time is a normal and expected event because the same muscles used to expel the baby also expel stool. The routine use of an enema to empty the rectum does not decrease the rate of perineal wound infections or other neonatal infection, improve women's satisfaction, or improve newborn outcomes and therefore should be discouraged (Reveiz, Gaitan, & Cuervo, 2013). In Canada, 88% of hospitals that responded to a survey stated they had a policy that stipulated that no women should receive an enema or suppository (PHAC, 2012).

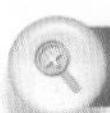

RESEARCH FOCUS

Reduction of Indwelling Urinary Catheters in Labour Patients with Epidural Anaesthesia

–Ellen Schneiderman

Ask the Question

For a labouring woman with epidural anaesthesia, does allowing her to void independently or performing intermittent catheterization versus placing an indwelling urinary catheter alter the second stage of labour and the patient's perception of her labour experience and/or reduce catheter-associated urinary tract infections (CAUTIs)?

Search for the Evidence

Search Strategies

- Search selection criteria included English-language research-based publications on catheters, urinary catheters, labour patients, maternity patients, CAUTI, and perception of birth experience without time limitation.

Databases Used

- CINAHL, UpToDate, OVID, Cochrane Database of Systematic Reviews, Joanna Briggs Institute, AHRQ

Critically Analyze the Evidence

- Indwelling urinary catheters versus intermittent catheterization did not shorten the second stage of labour. Randomized controlled study of 209 labour patients resulted in a shorter second stage for patients who were catheterized intermittently than that for women with an indwelling catheter (Evron, Dimitrochenko, Khazin, et al., 2008).
- Urinary retention is not favourably affected by the use of an indwelling catheter versus intermittent catheterization (Evron et al., 2008).
- Reducing the use of urinary catheters in labour and delivery is one way to reduce CAUTIs (Srinivas, 2008).
- Hospitals will institute evidence-informed practices to reduce CAUTIs (The Joint Commission, 2016).
- In a randomized, nonblinded trial of 146 women, bacterial urinary tract infections were found to be higher in those who were catheterized intermittently than in those who had an indwelling catheter (Millet, Shaha, & Bartholomew, 2012).
- Nurses should use as few interventions during labour as possible, to promote normal birth experiences for their patients (Romano & Lothian, 2008).
- There is no evidence to support routine labour interventions such as intravenous fluids, augmentation of labour, epidural anaesthesia, and indwelling urinary catheters. These inhibit mobility, various comfort measures, and spontaneous voiding and may increase the patient's stress level (Romano & Lothian, 2008).
- The bladder should be assessed frequently, and the patient should be given the opportunity to void independently before catheterization. The psychological effects of this procedure should not be taken lightly and can affect the woman's perception of her ability to participate and make decisions about her labour experience (DeSevo & Semeraro, 2010).
- A woman's perception of her birth experience can be affected by her ability to control her body and participate in decision making about her care during labour (Bryanton, Gagnon, Johnston, et al., 2008).
- Women should receive prenatal education regarding the effects of epidural anaesthesia as it relates to their ability to void during labour (Walsh, 2007).

Apply the Evidence: Nursing Implications

- There is sufficient evidence to support reducing the use of indwelling urinary catheters in labour patients with epidural anaesthesia (Evron et al., 2008; Srinivas, 2008; The Joint Commission, 2016). Nurses must support women in their ability to make decisions about their care during labour in order to foster the natural labour process. These decisions have been shown to make an impact on women's perception of their birth experience (Bryanton et al., 2008; Romano & Lothian, 2008).

References

Bryanton, J., Gagnon, A., Johnston, C., et al. (2008). Predictors of women's perceptions of the childbirth experience. *Journal of Obstetric, Gynecologic, and Neonatal Nursing*, 37(1), 24–34.

DeSevo, M., & Semeraro, P. (2010). Urinary catheterization during epidural anesthesia. *Nursing Women's Health*, 14(1), 11–13.

Evron, S., Dimitrochenko, V., Khazin, V., et al. (2008). The effect of intermittent versus continuous bladder catheterization on labor duration and postpartum urinary retention and infection: A randomized trial. *Journal of Clinical Anesthesia*, 20(8), 567–572.

Millet, L., Shaha, S., & Bartholomew, M. (2012). Rates of bacteriuria in laboring women with epidural analgesia: Continuous vs intermittent bladder catheterization. *American Journal of Obstetrics and Gynecology*, 206(4), 316.e1–316.e7.

Romano, J., & Lothian, J. (2008). Promoting, protecting and supporting normal birth: A look at the evidence. *Journal of Obstetric, Gynecologic, and Neonatal Nursing*, 37, 94–105.

Srinivas, S. (2008). Intermittent versus continuous bladder catheterization during labor: Does it matter? *Journal of Clinical Anesthesia*, 20(8), 565–566.

The Joint Commission. (2016). *National patient safety goals.* Oakbrook Terrace, IL: Author. Retrieved from <http://www.jointcommission.org/standards_information/npsgs.aspx>.

Walsh, D. (2007). The medicalization of bladder care. *British Journal of Midwifery*, 15(2), 1–3.

When the presenting part is deep in the pelvis, even in the absence of stool in the anorectal area, the woman may feel rectal pressure and think she needs to defecate. If the woman expresses the need to defecate, the nurse should perform a vaginal examination to assess cervical dilation and station. When a multiparous woman experiences the urge to defecate, this often means that birth will follow quickly.

Ambulation and Positioning

Freedom of maternal movement and choice of position should be encouraged throughout labour. Upright positions and mobility during labour may be more pleasant for labouring women, and these practices have been associated with improved uterine contraction intensity and shorter labours, less need for pain medications, reduced rate of operative birth (e.g., Caesarean birth, forceps- and vacuum-assisted birth), increased maternal autonomy and control, distraction from the discomforts of labour, and an opportunity for close interaction with the woman's partner and care provider as they help her assume upright positions and remain mobile (Simpson & O'Brien-Abel, 2014).

The increased use of epidurals during childbirth accompanied by multiple medical interventions (e.g., monitors, IV infusions) and reduced motor control interfere with a woman's freedom of movement. If electronic fetal monitoring (EFM) is required, many birthing areas now use wireless fetal monitors (known as **telemetry**) to allow the woman to remain mobile while continuous monitoring of the fetus takes place.

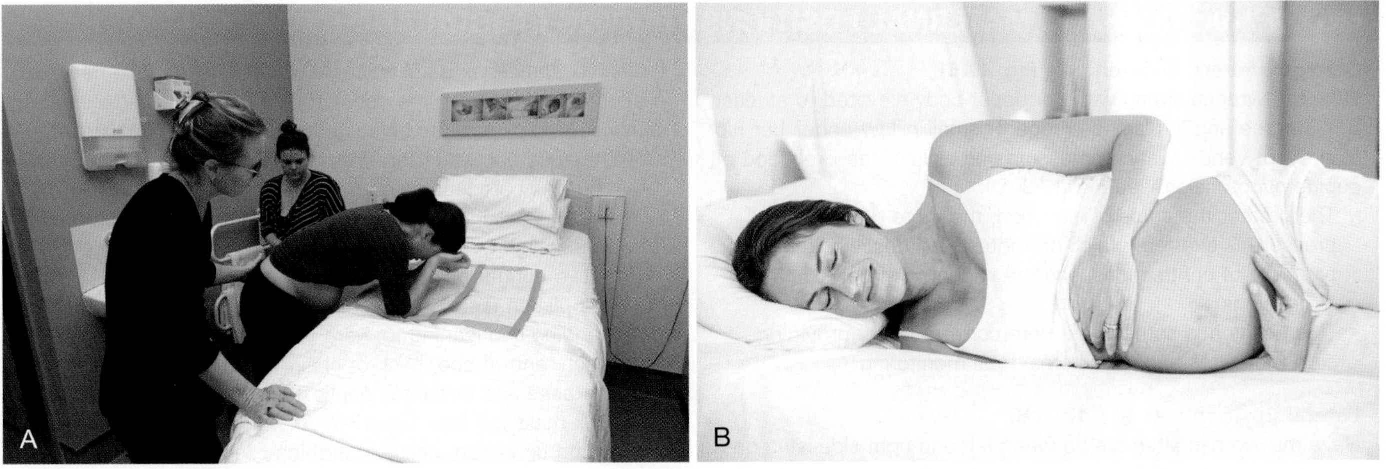

FIGURE 17-7 A: Woman standing and leaning forward with support. **B:** Lateral position. (A, Chameleons Eye/Shutterstock.com. B, wavebreakmedia/Shutterstock.com.)

Walking, sitting, or standing during early labour is more comfortable than lying down and facilitates the progress of labour. Ambulation should be encouraged if the fetal presenting part is engaged after ROM and if the woman has not received medication for pain. The woman may find it comfortable to stand and lean forward on her partner, doula, or nurse for support at times during labour (Fig. 17-7, A). At times, although rarely, ambulation is contraindicated because of maternal or fetal status.

When the woman lies in bed, she will usually change her position spontaneously as labour progresses. If she does not change position every 30 to 60 minutes, she should be assisted to do so. A variety of positions recommended for the labouring woman are described in Box 17-9 and shown in Fig. 17-8. The side-lying (lateral) position promotes optimal uteroplacental and renal blood flow and increases oxygen saturation (see Fig. 17-7, B). If the woman wants to lie supine, the nurse may place a pillow under one hip as a wedge to prevent the uterus from compressing the aorta and vena cava. Sitting is not contraindicated unless it adversely affects fetal status, which can be determined by checking the FHR and its pattern.

Occiput-posterior fetal position. If the fetus is in the occiput posterior position, it may be helpful to encourage the woman to squat during contractions because this position increases pelvic diameter, allowing the head to rotate to a more anterior position (Fig. 17-9, A). A hands-and-knees position during contractions is also recommended to facilitate the rotation of the fetal occiput from a posterior to an anterior position as gravity pulls the fetal back forward (see Fig. 17-9, B). Women with epidural anaesthesia may not be able to squat or assume a hands-and-knees position, depending on the degree of motor involvement resulting from the epidural.

These positions also provide access to the back for application of counterpressure. A support person may be taught to exert counterpressure against the woman's sacrum (see Fig. 17-9, B). The back pain is caused by the occiput pressing on spinal nerves, and counterpressure lifts the occiput off these nerves, thereby providing some relief from pain. Once counterpressure is initiated, the woman will usually ask her partner to continue doing this for each following contraction. However, the partner will need to be relieved after a while because exerting counterpressure is hard work. Application of ice packs and heat also help relieve back labour. The nurse should always ask the mother if the massages are helpful. See Box 17-10 for measures to assist a woman with a fetus that is in the occiput posterior position.

A birth ball (gymnastic ball, also used in physical therapy) can be used to support a woman's body as she assumes a variety of labour and birth positions (Fig. 17-10). The woman can sit on the ball while leaning over the bed, or she can lean over the ball to support her upper body and reduce stress on her arms and hands when she assumes a hands-and-knees position. Use of the birth ball can encourage pelvic mobility and pelvic and perineal relaxation when the woman sits on the firm yet pliable ball and rocks in rhythmic movements. Warm compresses applied to the perineum and back can maximize this relaxation effect. The birth ball should be large enough so that, when the woman sits, her knees are bent at a 90-degree angle and her feet are flat on the floor and approximately shoulder-distance apart.

Supportive Care During Labour and Birth

Support during labour and birth involves emotional support, comfort measures, and provision of information, along with physical care.

The value of the continuous supportive presence of a person (e.g., doula, childbirth educator, family member, friend, nurse, partner) during labour has long been known. Women who have continuous support beginning in early labour are less likely to use pain medication or epidurals, more likely to have a spontaneous vaginal birth, and less likely to report dissatisfaction with their birth experience. There is good evidence that labour support improves important health outcomes (Association of Women's Health, Obstetric, and Neonatal Nurses [AWHONN], 2011; Hodnett, Gates, Hofmeyr, et al., 2011).

The labouring woman should feel safe in the birthing environment and feel free to be herself and use the comfort and relaxation measures she prefers. To enhance relaxation, bright overhead lights should be turned off when not needed. Noise and intrusions should be kept to a minimum. The temperature

BOX 17-9 COMMON MATERNAL POSITIONS* DURING LABOUR AND BIRTH

Semirecumbent Position (see Fig. 17-8)

With the woman sitting with her upper body elevated to at least a 30-degree angle, place a wedge or small pillow under her hip to prevent vena caval compression and reduce the likelihood of supine hypotension (see Fig. 17-3, D).

- The greater the angle of elevation, the more gravity or pressure is exerted, which promotes fetal descent, the progress of contractions, and the widening of pelvic dimensions.
- This position is sometimes more convenient for providing care measures and for external fetal monitoring.

Lateral Position (see Fig. 17-7, B)

Have the woman alternate between left and right side-lying position and provide abdominal and back support as needed for comfort.

- Removes pressure from the vena cava and back; enhances uteroplacental perfusion and relieves backache
- Facilitates internal rotation of fetus in a posterior position to an anterior position (woman should lie on same side as fetal spine)
- Makes it easier to perform back massage or counterpressure
- Associated with less frequent but more intense contractions
- May be used as a birthing position
- Takes pressure off perineum, allowing it to stretch gradually
- Reduces risk for perineal trauma

Upright Position

The gravity effect enhances the contraction cycle and fetal descent: The weight of the fetus places increasing pressure on the cervix; the cervix is pulled upward, facilitating effacement and dilation; impulses from the cervix to the pituitary gland increase, causing more oxytocin to be secreted; and contractions are intensified, thereby applying more forceful downward pressure on the fetus, but they are less painful.

- The fetus is aligned with the pelvis, and pelvic diameters are widened slightly.
- Effective upright positions include the following:
  - Ambulation (see Fig. 17-8)
  - Standing and leaning forward with support provided by coach, end of bed, back of chair, or birth ball; relieves backache and facilitates application of counterpressure or back massage (see Fig. 17-7, A)
  - Sitting up in bed, chair, or birthing chair, on toilet or bedside commode
  - Squatting (see Fig. 17-9, A)

Hands-and-Knees Position

This position is ideal for occiput-posterior position of the presenting part (see Fig. 17-9, B; Box 17-10). The woman assumes an "all-fours" position or leans over an object (e.g., birth ball) while on her knees in bed or on a covered floor; she can also place her knees on the seat section of bed while leaning up over the back of the raised head of the bed; this allows for pelvic rocking.

- Relieves backache characteristic of back labour
- Facilitates internal rotation of the fetus by increasing mobility of the coccyx, increasing the pelvic diameters, and using gravity to turn the fetal back and rotate the head

*Assess the effect of each position on the labouring woman's comfort and anxiety level, progress of labour, and fetal heart rate and pattern. Alternate positions every 30 minutes.

should be controlled to ensure the labouring woman's comfort. The room should be large enough to accommodate a comfortable chair for the woman's partner, the monitoring equipment, and hospital personnel. Women should be encouraged to bring their own pillows to make the hospital surroundings more homelike and to facilitate position changes. This type of an environment can help women view their childbirth experience as normal and not related to illness. Environmental modifications should reflect the preferences of the woman, including the number of visitors and availability of a telephone and music. Nurses should ensure that each woman labours in an optimal birth environment. Table 17-4 lists support persons actions during the first stage of labour.

Labour Support by the Nurse

The nurse can alleviate a woman's anxiety by communicating clearly, explaining unfamiliar terms, providing information and explanations without the woman having to ask and at a level she understands, and preparing her for sensations she will experience and procedures that will follow. By encouraging the woman or couple to ask questions and by providing honest, understandable answers, the nurse can play a significant role in helping the woman achieve a satisfying birth experience.

Supportive, empathic nursing care for a woman in labour includes the following:

- Developing a trusting relationship with the woman and her support persons
- Helping the woman maintain control and participate to the extent she wishes in the birth of her infant
- Providing continuity of care that is nonjudgemental and respectful of her cultural and religious values and beliefs
- Meeting the woman's expected outcomes for her labour
- Listening to the woman's concerns and encouraging her to express her feelings
- Acting as the woman's advocate, supporting her decisions and respecting her choices as appropriate, and relating her wishes as needed to other health care providers
- Helping the woman conserve her energy and cope effectively with her pain and discomfort by using a variety of comfort measures that are acceptable to her
- Helping the woman manage her discomfort
- Acknowledging the woman's efforts during labour, including her strength and courage, as well as those of her partner, and providing positive reinforcement
- Protecting the woman's privacy and modesty
- Using touch and eye contact, if appropriate

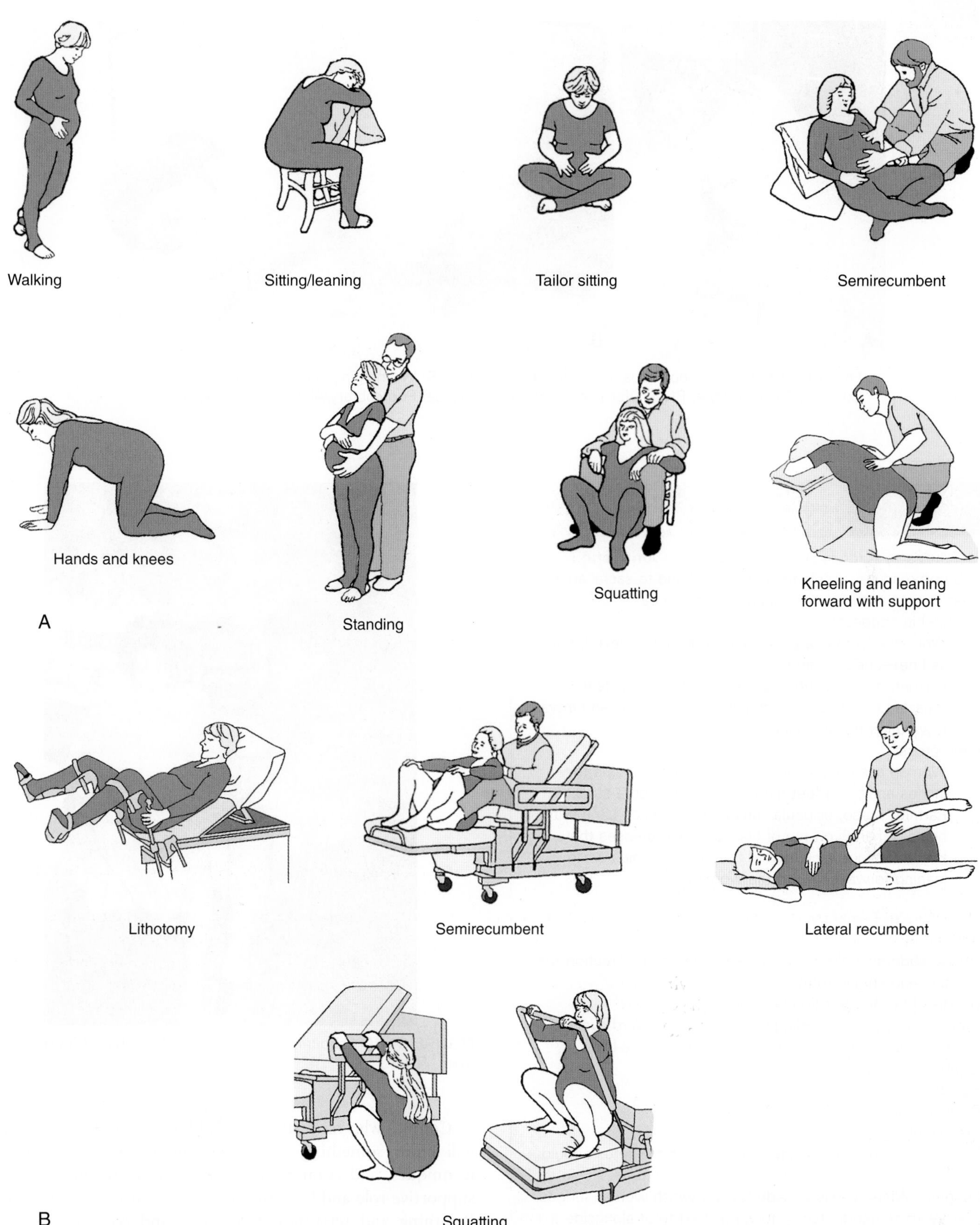

FIGURE 17-8 Positions for labour and birth. **A:** Positions for labour. **B:** Positions for birth.

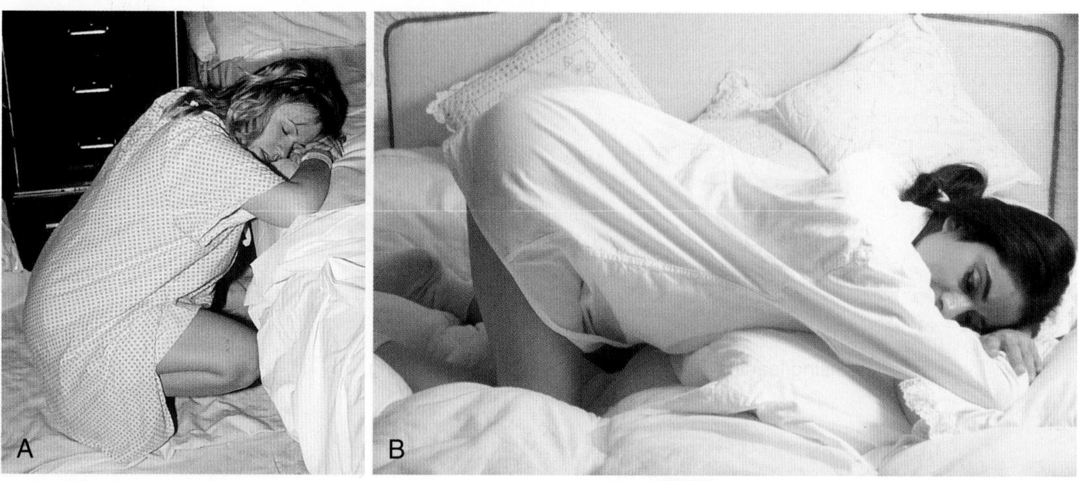

FIGURE 17-9 Maternal positions for labour. **A:** Squatting. **B:** Woman in hands-and-knees position. (A, Courtesy Marjorie Pyle, RNC, Lifecircle. B, © Janine Wiedel Photolibrary/Alamy Stock Photo.)

BOX 17-10 BACK LABOUR—OCCIPUT POSTERIOR POSITION

Measures to Reduce Back Pain During a Contraction

Counterpressure—Apply fist or heel of hand to sacral area

Heat or cold applications—Apply to sacral area

Double hip squeeze:

- Woman assumes a position with hip joints flexed, such as knee–chest position
- Partner, nurse, or doula places hands over gluteal muscles and presses with palms of hands up and inward toward centre of pelvis

Knee press:

- Woman assumes a sitting position with knees a few inches apart and feet flat on the floor or on a stool
- Partner, nurse, or doula cups a knee in each hand with heels of hands on top of tibia and then presses the knees straight back toward the woman's hips while leaning forward toward the woman

Measures to Facilitate Rotation of Fetal Head (May Also Relieve Back Pain)

Lateral abdominal stroking—Stroke abdomen in direction that fetal head should rotate

Hands-and-knees position (all-fours)—Can also be accomplished by kneeling while leaning forward over a birth ball, padded chair seat, bed, or over-the-bed table

Squatting

Pelvic rocking

Stair climbing

Lateral position—Lie on side toward which the fetus should turn

Lunges—Widen pelvis on side toward which woman lunges

- Woman stands, facing forward, next to or alongside a chair so that she can lunge toward the side the fetal back is on or in the direction of the fetal occiput
- Woman places foot on seat of chair with toes pointed toward the back of the chair and then lunges
- Alternative position for lunge is kneeling

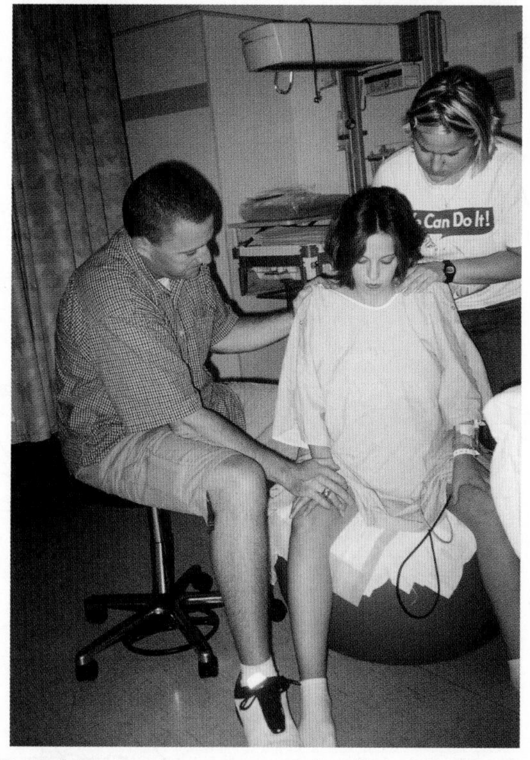

FIGURE 17-10 Labouring woman using birth ball. (Courtesy Pat Spier, RN-C.)

Couples who have attended childbirth education programs will know something about the labour process, supportive techniques, and comfort measures. The nurse should play a supportive role and keep the couple informed of the progress. Breathing and relaxation techniques and comfort measures described in Chapter 18 can be implemented.

Even when expectant parents have not attended childbirth education classes, the nurse can teach them simple breathing and relaxation techniques during the early phase of labour. In this case, the nurse may provide more of the coaching and

TABLE 17-4 WOMAN'S RESPONSES AND SUPPORT PERSON'S ACTIONS DURING FIRST STAGE OF LABOUR

WOMAN'S RESPONSES	NURSE/SUPPORT PERSON'S ACTIONS*
Dilation of Cervix 0–3 cm (Latent) (Contractions: 30–45 sec Long, 5–30 min Apart, Mild to Moderate Intensity)	
Mood: alert, happy, excited, mild anxiety Labouring at home or settles into labour room if required; selects focal point Rests or sleeps if possible Uses breathing techniques if required Uses effleurage, focusing, and relaxation techniques	Provides encouragement, feedback for relaxation, companionship Helps to cope with contractions Provides distractions Encourages use of focusing techniques Helps to concentrate on breathing techniques if required Uses comfort measures Assists woman into comfortable position Informs woman of progress; explains procedures and routines Gives praise Offers fluids, ice chips as ordered
Dilation of Cervix 4–10 cm (Active)† (Contractions: 40–90 sec Long, 2–5 Minutes Apart, Moderate to Strong in Intensity)	
Admitted to hospital when required by woman Mood: seriously labour oriented, concentration and energy needed for contractions, alert, more demanding, becomes more irritable in later stages often with intense concentration required to relax Nausea and vomiting common Continues relaxation, focusing techniques Uses breathing techniques when required and continues to use breathing techniques that are working for her Uses panting to overcome urge to push	Stays with woman; limits assessment techniques to between contractions Provides constant support Assists with contractions Encourages woman as needed to help her maintain breathing techniques • Reminds, reassures, and encourages woman to re-establish breathing pattern and concentration as needed • Alerts woman to begin breathing pattern before contraction becomes too intense if she is sedated or drowsy Uses comfort measures • Assists with frequent position changes (every 30 min), emphasizing side-lying and upright positions • Encourages voluntary relaxation of muscles of back, buttocks, thighs, and perineum; effleurage • Applies counterpressure to sacrococcygeal area; accepts irritable response to helping such as counterpressure Encourages and praises Keeps woman aware of progress Accepts woman's inability to follow instructions Assists with administration of analgesics if requested by woman (nurse only) Checks bladder; encourages her to void Gives oral care; offers fluids, ice chips as ordered Supports woman who has nausea and vomiting; gives oral care as needed; gives reassurance regarding signs of end of first stage Prompts panting respirations if woman begins to push prematurely

*Provided by nurses and support people.
†Active labour is identified as 4–5 cm in a multiparous woman.

supportive care, as some support persons may not feel able to fulfill this role.

Comfort measures vary with the situation. The nurse can draw on the couple's repertoire of comfort measures and relaxation techniques learned during the pregnancy and through life experiences. Such measures include maintaining a comfortable, calm, supportive atmosphere in the labour and birth area; using touch therapeutically (e.g., massage, heat or cold applied to the lower back in the event of back labour, a cool cloth applied to the forehead); foot or hand massage; providing nonpharmacological measures to relieve discomfort (e.g., hydrotherapy); administering analgesics when necessary; and, most important, just being there (see Tables 17-1 and 17-4). While most women in labour respond positively to touch, permission should be obtained before using any measure involving touch. See Chapter 18 for a full discussion of both pharmacological and nonpharmacological comfort measures.

The woman's perception of the soothing qualities of touch may change as labour progresses. Many women become more sensitive to touch (*hyperesthesia*) as labour progresses; this is a typical response during the active phase (see Table 17-1). They may tell their support person to leave them alone or to not touch them. The partner who is unprepared for this normal response may feel rejected and react by withdrawing active support. The nurse can reassure him or her that this response is a positive indication that the first stage is ending and the second stage is approaching. Women with increased sensitivity to touch may have a positive response when touched on surfaces of the body where hair does not grow, such as the forehead, palms of the hands, and soles of the feet.

Labour Support by the Partner

The partner is often able to provide the comfort measures and touch that the labouring woman needs. When the woman becomes focused on her pain, sometimes the partner can persuade her to try nonpharmacological variations of comfort measures. In addition, the partner may be able to interpret the woman's needs and desires to staff members.

Throughout the past 40 years, childbirth preparation education has been widely available in Canada. Initially, the partner's role was thought to be that of labour coach, and he or she was expected to actively help the woman cope with labour. However, this expectation may be unrealistic because some partners have concerns about their labour-coaching abilities. Because partners can participate in labour and birth in different ways, the nurse should encourage them to adopt the role most comfortable for them and for the woman rather than to assume an unnatural role. Participation in the birth is ego building: the partner can be of assistance and his or her presence is important (Fig. 17-11).

The feelings of a first-time parent change as labour progresses. Although the partner may be calm at the onset of labour, feelings of fear and helplessness can begin to dominate as labour becomes more active and the partner realizes that labour is more work than he or she had anticipated. A study of Swedish fathers' birth experiences found that, although about three quarters of the men reported positive or very positive experiences, less positive experiences were associated with emergency Caesarean birth, assisted vaginal birth, and dissatisfaction with their partners' medical care. The interactions of health care providers with the fathers and the fathers' perception of the health care providers' competence were also related to the fathers' birth experiences (Johansson, Rubertsson, Radestad, et al., 2012). Staff members should tell the partner that his or her presence is helpful and encourage him or her to be involved in the care of the woman to the extent to which he or she and the labouring woman are comfortable. The partner should be reassured that he or she is not assuming the responsibility for observation and management of his partner's labour but that the responsibility is to support her as the labour progresses. The nurse can suggest alternative comfort measures when those being used are no longer helpful or are rejected by the labouring woman.

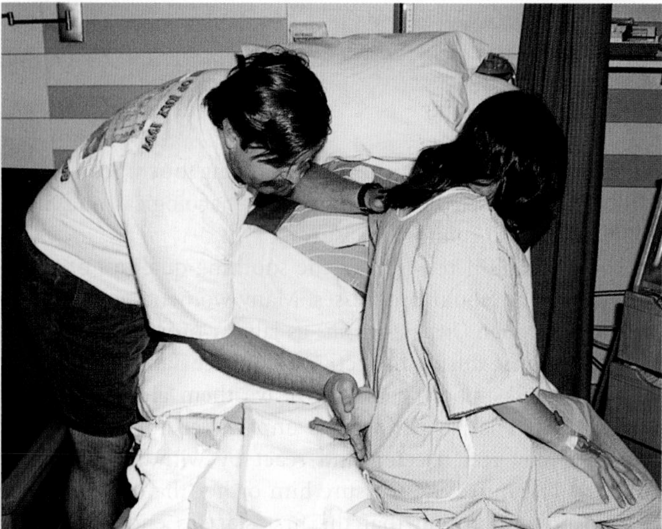

FIGURE 17-11 Partner providing comfort measures. (Courtesy Loma Linda University Medical Center.)

The first-time parent may feel excluded as birth preparations begin later during the active phase. Once the second stage begins and birth nears, the partner's focus will change from being on the woman to being on the baby who is about to be born. The partner will be exposed to many sights and smells that may never have been experienced before. Therefore, the nurse needs to tell the partner what to expect and make him or her comfortable about leaving the room to regain composure should something occur that is unexpected but make sure that someone else is available to support the woman during the absence.

Nursing actions that support the partner convey several important concepts: first, that he or she is a person of value; second, that he or she can be a partner in the woman's care; and third, that child-bearing is a team effort. Box 17-11 details ways in which the nurse can support the partner. A well-informed partner can make an important contribution to the health and well-being of the mother and child, their family interrelationship, and his or her self-esteem.

BOX 17-11 GUIDELINES FOR SUPPORTING THE PARTNER*

- Orient the partner to the labour room and the unit; explain location of the cafeteria, washroom, and waiting room, visiting hours, and names and functions of personnel present.
- Inform the partner of sights and smells he or she can expect to encounter; encourage him or her to leave the room, if necessary.
- Respect the partner's or the couple's decision about the degree of his or her involvement. Offer the partner freedom to make decisions.
- Tell the partner when his or her presence has been helpful and continue to reinforce this throughout labour.
- Offer to teach the partner comfort measures; demonstrate or role model performance of these measures.
- Inform the partner frequently of the progress of the labour and the woman's needs. Keep him or her informed about procedures to be performed.
- Prepare the partner for changes in the woman's behaviour and physical appearance.
- Remind him or her to eat; offer snacks and fluids if possible.
- Relieve the partner of the job of support person as necessary. Offer blankets if he or she is to sleep in a chair by the bedside.
- Acknowledge the stress experienced by each partner during labour and birth and identify normal responses.
- Attempt to modify or eliminate unsettling stimuli such as extra noise and extra light; create a relaxing and calm environment.

*These guidelines are appropriate for any support person or partner.

Labour Support by Doulas

Continuity of care has been cited by women as a critical component of a satisfying childbirth experience. This need can be met by a specially trained, experienced female labour attendant called a *doula*. The doula provides a continuous, one-on-one caring presence throughout the labour and birth process of the woman she is attending. Some hospitals employ doulas to work in the labour and birth unit, others have volunteer doula programs, although the majority of women who use a doula pay for the service privately. The primary role of the doula is to focus on the labouring woman and her partner and provide physical and emotional support by using soft, reassuring words, and touching, stroking, and hugging. The doula also administers comfort measures to reduce pain and enhance relaxation, walks with the woman, helps her to change positions, and encourages her bearing-down efforts. Doulas provide information and explain procedures and events. They advocate for the woman's right to participate actively in the management of her labour. These forms of caring help to reduce a woman's level of anxiety and fear, make her more confident and calm, and reduce the stress response that could inhibit the progress of labour.

The doula also supports the woman's partner, who often feels unqualified to be the sole labour support and may find it difficult to watch the woman when she is experiencing pain. The doula can encourage and praise the partner's efforts, create a partnership as caregivers, and provide respite care. Doulas also facilitate communication between the labouring woman and her partner and between the couple and the health care team (Simkin, 2012).

Doula support during labour is associated with decreased use of analgesia, decreased incidence of operative birth, increased incidence of spontaneous vaginal birth, and increased maternal satisfaction with the childbirth experience (Hodnett et al., 2011). Long-term benefits of doula care are reflected in greater success with breastfeeding, more positive maternal feelings about their parenting ability, and lower rates of postpartum mood disorders.

The roles of the nurse and the doula are complementary. They should work together as a team, recognizing and respecting the role each plays in supporting and caring for the woman and her partner during the childbirth process. The doula provides supportive nonmedical care measures, whereas the nurse provides this care and also focuses on monitoring the status of the maternal–fetal unit and implementing clinical care protocols, including pharmacological interventions, and documenting assessment findings, actions, and responses (Simkin, 2012). In the ideal world all labouring women would be offered a doula, but unfortunately this is not possible due to financial constraints or geographical locations.

Labour Support by the Grandparents

When grandparents act as a woman's labour support, it is especially important to support them and treat them with respect. They may have ways to deal with pain that are based on their experience and they should be encouraged to help. The nurse can treat grandparents with dignity and respect by acknowledging the value of their contributions to parental support and recognizing the difficulty parents have in witnessing the woman's discomfort or crisis. If they have never witnessed a birth, the nurse may need to provide explanations about what is happening. Many of the activities used to support partners also are appropriate for grandparents.

When possible, the nurse needs to offer the grandparents emotional support. A nurse can show such support by offering them liquid refreshments and initiating discussion with open-ended questions or statements, such as "It is sometimes hard to watch a daughter in labour." Nursing actions that provide support for the grandparents can have a therapeutic effect on all members of the family. In turn, a strong, supportive family unit is important for the optimal growth and development of its newest member.

Siblings During Labour and Birth

The preparation of siblings for acceptance of the new child helps promote the attachment process and may help the older children accept this change. The older child or children who know that they are important to the family become active participants. Rehearsal for the event before labour is essential.

The age and developmental level of children influence their responses to the addition of a new family member; therefore, preparation for the children to be present during labour is adjusted to meet each child's needs. The child younger than 2 years shows little interest in pregnancy and labour. However, for the older child such preparation may reduce fears and misconceptions. Parents need to be prepared for labour and birth themselves and feel comfortable about the process and the presence of their children. Most parents have a "feel" for their children's maturational level and their physical and emotional ability to observe and cope with the events of the labour and birth process.

Preparation can include a description of the anticipated sights, events (e.g., ROM, monitors, IV infusions), smells, and sounds; a labour and birth demonstration; a tour of the birthing unit; and an opportunity to be around a real newborn. Storybooks about the birth process can be read to or by children to prepare them for the event. Films are available for preparing preschool and school-age children to participate in the labour and birth experience. Children must learn that their mother will be working hard during labour and birth. She will not be able to talk to them during contractions. She may groan, scream, grunt, and pant at times and say things she would not say otherwise (e.g., "I can't take this anymore"; "Take this baby out of me"). They can be told that labour is uncomfortable but that their mother's body is made for the job.

Most agencies require that a specific person be designated to watch over the children who are participating in their mother's childbirth experience, to provide them with support, explanations, diversions, and comfort as needed. Health care providers involved in attending women during birth must be comfortable with the presence of children and the unpredictability of their questions, comments, and behaviours.

Emergency Interventions

Emergency conditions that require immediate nursing intervention can arise with startling speed.

See Chapter 19 for information on management of abnormal or atypical FHR. Management of other emergency situations, including meconium-stained amniotic fluid, shoulder dystocia, prolapsed umbilical cord, ruptured uterus, and amniotic fluid embolus, is discussed in Chapter 20.

SECOND STAGE OF LABOUR

The **second stage of labour** is the stage in which the infant is born. This stage begins with full cervical dilation (10 cm) and complete effacement (100%) and ends with the baby's birth. The force exerted by uterine contractions, gravity, and maternal bearing-down efforts facilitates achievement of the expected outcome of a spontaneous, uncomplicated vaginal birth.

The median duration of second-stage labour is 50 to 60 minutes in nulliparous women and 20 to 30 minutes in multiparous women. In addition to parity, maternal size and fetal weight, position, and descent influence the length of this stage. The use of epidural anaesthesia during labour often increases the length of the second stage of labour because the epidural blocks or reduces the woman's urge to bear down and limits her ability to attain an upright position to push.

The diagnosis of labour arrest in the second stage should not be made without pushing for at least 2 hours in multiparous women, or for at least 3 hours in nulliparous women, if maternal and fetal conditions permit (American Congress of Obstetricians and Gynecologists [ACOG], 2014). A thorough assessment of the status of the maternal fetal unit and a determination regarding the likely effectiveness and safety of further bearing-down efforts should be made (Simpson & O'Brien-Adel, 2014). Some women are still able to push after this time has been exceeded and should be allowed to continue as long as the mother and fetus are stable and allowing this may decrease the Caesarean birth rate. A prolonged second stage has been associated with increased rates of operative births and maternal morbidity. Choosing different positions for the second stage, such as side-lying, squatting, or sitting, will shorten the second stage by increasing the efficacy of contractions, promoting uterine blood flow, and decreasing the likelihood of tears or episiotomies (Zwelling, 2010).

The second stage comprises two phases: the passive phase and the active pushing (descent) phase (SOGC, 2014). These phases are characterized by maternal verbal and nonverbal behaviours, uterine activity, the urge to bear down, and fetal descent (Table 17-5).

The *passive phase* is a period of rest and relative calm (i.e., "labouring down"). During this early phase, the fetus continues to descend passively through the birth canal and rotate to an anterior position as a result of ongoing uterine contractions. The woman is quiet and often relaxes with her eyes closed

TABLE 17-5 EXPECTED MATERNAL PROGRESS AND RESPONSE DURING SECOND STAGE OF LABOUR

CRITERION	PASSIVE PHASE (AVERAGE DURATION, 10–30 MINUTES)	ACTIVE PUSHING (DESCENT) PHASE (AVERAGE DURATION VARIES)*
Contractions		
Intensity	Period of physiological lull for all criteria; period of peace and rest; "labouring down"	Significant increase becoming overwhelmingly strong and expulsive
Frequency		Every 2 to 2½ minutes progressing to every 1 to 2 minutes
Duration		90 seconds
Descent, station	0 to +2	+2 to +4; Rate of descent increases and Ferguson reflex[†] is activated; fetal head becomes visible at introitus and birth occurs
Spontaneous bearing-down efforts	Slight to absent, except at peak of strongest contractions	Increased urge to bear down; becomes stronger as fetus descends to vaginal introitus and reaches perineum
Vocalization	Quiet; concern over progress	Grunting sounds or expiratory vocalizations; announces contractions; may scream
Maternal behaviour	Experiences sense of relief that transition to second stage is finished Feels fatigued and sleepy Feels a sense of accomplishment and optimism because the "worst is over" Feels in control	Senses increased urge to push and describes increasing pain; describes *ring of fire* (burning sensation of acute pain as vagina stretches and fetal head crowns) Expresses feeling of powerlessness Shows decreased ability to listen to or concentrate on anything but giving birth Alters respiratory pattern: has short 4 to 5-second breath holds with regular breaths in between, 5 to 7 times per contraction Frequent repositioning Often shows excitement immediately after birth of head

*Duration of descent phase can vary, depending on maternal parity, effectiveness of bearing-down effort, and presence of spinal anaesthesia or epidural analgesia.

[†]Pressure of presenting part on stretch receptors of pelvic floor stimulates release of oxytocin from posterior pituitary, resulting in more intense uterine contractions.

Data from Hanson, L. (2009). Second-stage labor care. *Journal of Perinatal & Neonatal Nursing, 23*(1), 31–39. Simpson, K., Cesario, S., Morin, K., et al. (2008). *Nursing care and management of the second stage of labor: Evidence-based clinical practice guideline* (2nd ed.). Washington, DC: Association of Women's Health, Obstetric, and Neonatal Nurses.

between contractions. The urge to bear down is not strong, and some women do not experience it at all or only during the acme (peak) of a contraction. Delayed pushing has been shown to result in significant decreases in pushing time, significant increases in the duration of second-stage labour, and a reduction in the number of operative vaginal births. On the other hand, no differences in the number of Caesarean births, perineal lacerations or episiotomies, or fetal complications have been linked to delayed pushing (Kelly, Johnson, Lee, et al., 2010). In a randomized clinical trial, allowing a woman to rest during this phase and waiting until the urge to push intensifies significantly reduced the amount of time spent pushing but did not significantly increase the total length of second-stage labour. In this study maternal fatigue scores, perineal injuries, and FHR decelerations were similar in the immediate- and delayed-pushing groups (Kelly et al., 2010). Another study also found a significant decrease in pushing time in nulliparous women with epidural anaesthesia who practised delayed pushing during second-stage labour (Gillesby, Burns, Dempsey, et al., 2010).

If descent is slow and the woman becomes anxious, she should be encouraged to change positions frequently or to stand by the bedside to use the advantage of gravity and movement to facilitate descent and progress to the active pushing phase signalled by a perception of the need to bear down (Hanson, 2009).

During the phase of active pushing (descent) the woman has strong urges to bear down, as the Ferguson reflex is activated when the presenting part presses on the stretch receptors of the pelvic floor. At this point, the fetal station is usually 1+, and the position is anterior. This stimulation causes the release of oxytocin from the posterior pituitary gland, which stimulates stronger, expulsive uterine contractions. During this phase, the woman becomes more focused on bearing-down efforts, which become rhythmic. She will change positions frequently to find a more comfortable pushing position. The woman often announces the onset of contractions and becomes more vocal as she bears down. The urge to bear down intensifies as descent progresses and the presenting part reaches the perineum. The woman may be more verbal about the pain she is experiencing; she may scream or act out of control.

The nurse should encourage the woman to "listen" to and trust her body as she progresses through the phases of the second stage of labour (see Box 17-12). When a woman listens to her body to tell her when to bear down, she is using an internal locus of control and often feels more satisfied with her efforts to give birth to her baby. This enhances her sense of self-esteem and accomplishment, and her efforts become more effective. It is important to encourage the woman's trust in her own body and her ability to give birth to her baby. The nurse can validate the woman's experience of pressure, stretching, and straining as normal and as a signal that the descent of the fetus is progressing and her body is capable of withstanding birth. The nurse can honestly explain what is happening and describe the progress being made. If a woman is confined to bed, especially in a recumbent position, the rhythmic urge to bear down is delayed because gravity is not being used to press the presenting part against the pelvic floor. In this situation the woman should be encouraged to use various positions for bearing down, such as side-lying, kneeling, squatting, sitting, or standing (Fig. 17-12).

BOX 17-12 NURSING CARE IN SECOND-STAGE LABOUR

Assessment

Signs That Suggest Onset of the Second Stage

- Urge to push or feeling need to have a bowel movement
- Sudden appearance of sweat on upper lip
- An episode of vomiting
- Increased bloody show
- Shaking of extremities
- Increased restlessness; verbalization (e.g., "I can't go on.")
- Involuntary bearing-down efforts

Physical Assessment

- Perform every 5 to 30 minutes: maternal blood pressure, pulse, and respirations.
- Assess every 5 minutes: fetal heart rate and pattern.
- Assess every 10 to 15 minutes: vaginal show; signs of fetal descent; and changes in maternal appearance, mood, affect, energy level, and condition of partner/coach.
- Assess every contraction and bearing-down effort.

Interventions

Passive Phase

- Help to rest in a position of comfort; encourage relaxation to conserve energy.
- Promote progress of fetal descent and onset of urge to bear down by encouraging position changes, pelvic rock, ambulation, showering.

Active Pushing (Descent) Phase

- Help to change position and encourage spontaneous bearing-down efforts.
- Help to relax and conserve energy between contractions.
- Provide comfort and pain-relief measures as needed.
- Cleanse perineum promptly if fecal material is expelled.
- Coach to pant during contractions and to gently push between contractions when head is emerging.
- Provide emotional support, encouragement, and positive reinforcement of efforts.
- Keep woman informed regarding progress.
- Create a calm and quiet environment.
- Offer mirror to watch birth or encourage to feel top of fetal head as pushing.

NURSING CARE

The only certain objective sign that the second stage of labour has begun is the inability to feel the cervix during vaginal examination, indicating that it is fully dilated and effaced. The precise moment that this occurs is not easily determined because it depends on when a vaginal examination is performed to validate full dilation and effacement. This makes timing of the actual duration of the second stage difficult. Other signs that suggest the onset of the second stage include the urge to push or feeling the need to have a bowel movement. These signs commonly

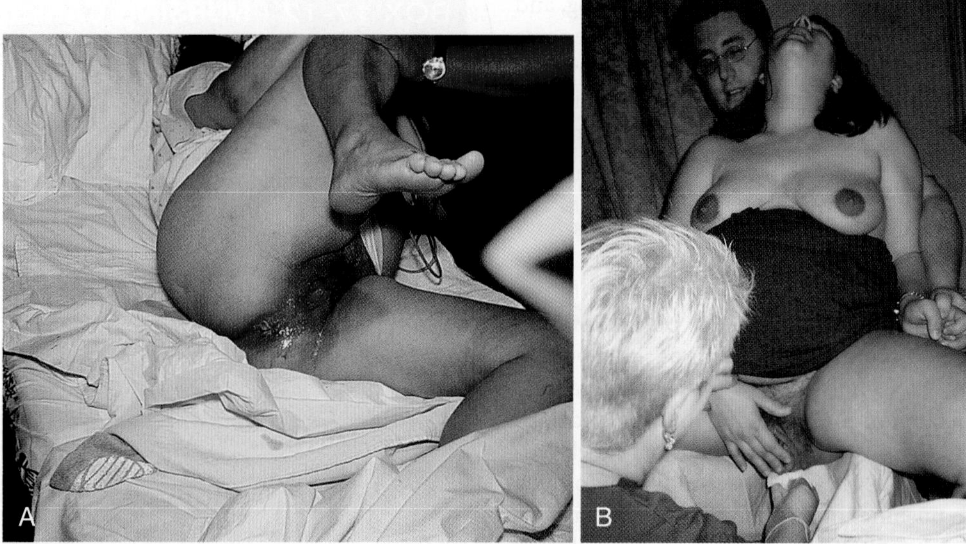

FIGURE 17-12 A, Pushing, side-lying position. Perineal bulging can be seen. **B,** Pushing, semisitting position. Midwife helps mother feel top of fetal head. (*A* Courtesy of Michael S. Clement, MD. *B* Courtesy of Roni Wernik.)

appear at the time the cervix reaches full dilation. However, they can appear earlier in labour. Women with an epidural block may not exhibit such signs.

Women can begin to experience an irresistible urge to bear down before full dilation. For some this occurs as early as 5-cm dilation. This is most often related to the station of the presenting part below the level of the ischial spines of the maternal pelvis. This occurrence creates a conflict between the woman, whose body is telling her to push, and her health care providers, who believe that pushing the fetal presenting part against an incompletely dilated cervix will result in cervical edema and lacerations and slow the labour progress. The timing of when a woman pushes in relation to dilation of her cervix should be based, however, on research evidence rather than on tradition or routine practice. Pushing with the urge to bear down at the acme of a contraction may be safe and effective for a woman if her cervix is soft, retracting, and 8 cm or more dilated and if the fetus is at +1 station and rotating to an anterior position (Hanson, 2009).

Professional standards and agency policy determine the specific type and timing of assessments and the way in which findings are documented. Signs and symptoms of impending birth (see Table 17-5) may appear unexpectedly, requiring immediate action by the nurse (Box 17-13).

The nurse continues to monitor maternal–fetal status and events of the second stage and provide comfort measures for the mother. This includes helping her change position; providing mouth care; maintaining clean, dry bedding; and keeping unnecessary noise, conversation, and other distractions (e.g., laughing, talking of attending personnel in or outside the labour area) to a minimum. The woman is encouraged to indicate other support measures she would like (see Box 17-12).

In the hospital, birth may occur in a delivery room, an LBR, or LBRP. If the mother is to be transferred to another room for birth, the nurse needs to make the transfer early enough to avoid rushing the woman. The birthing area should be readied for the birth.

Maternal Position

There is no single correct position for childbirth. Labour is a dynamic, interactive process involving the woman's uterus, pelvis, and voluntary muscles. In addition, angles between the woman's pelvis and the fetus constantly change as the infant turns and flexes down the birth canal. The woman may want to assume various positions for childbirth, and she should be encouraged and helped to attain and maintain her positions of choice (Fig 17-8, B). Supine, semirecumbent, or lithotomy positions are still widely used in Western societies despite evidence that women prefer upright positions for their bearing-down efforts and birth.

Birth attendants play a major role in influencing a woman's choice of position for birth, with midwives tending to advocate the nonlithotomy positions (e.g., upright, lateral) for the second stage of labour. An upright position (walking, sitting, kneeling, or squatting) offers a number of advantages. Gravity can promote the descent of the fetus. Uterine contractions are generally stronger and more efficient in effacing and dilating the cervix, resulting in shorter labour (Blackburn, 2013; Lawrence, Lewis, Hofmeyr, et al., 2009; Zwelling, 2010). An upright position also is beneficial to the mother's cardiac output, thereby increasing perfusion of the uterus. The use of upright and lateral positions is also associated with less pain and perineal damage, fewer episiotomies and abnormal FHR patterns, and fewer operative vaginal births (Berghella, Baxter, & Chauhan, 2008; James, 2011; Simpson, Cesario, Morin, et al., 2008; Zwelling, 2010). The benefits of upright positions may be related to the following:

- Straightening the longitudinal axis of the birth canal and improvement in the alignment of the fetus for passage through the pelvis

BOX 17-13 GUIDELINES FOR ASSISTANCE AT EMERGENCY BIRTH OF A FETUS IN THE VERTEX PRESENTATION

1. The woman usually assumes the position most comfortable for her. A lateral position is often recommended to facilitate a controlled birth of the head, thereby minimizing the risk for perineal trauma.
2. Reassure the woman that birth is usually uncomplicated in these situations. Use eye-to-eye contact and a calm, relaxed manner. If someone else is available, such as the partner, that person could help support the woman in the position, assist with coaching, and provide positive reinforcement and praise of her efforts.
3. Wash your hands and put on gloves.
4. Place under woman's buttocks whatever clean material is available.
5. Avoid touching the vaginal area to decrease the possibility of infection.
6. As the head begins to crown, perform the following tasks:
   - Tear the amniotic membranes if they are still intact.
   - Instruct the woman to pant or pant-blow, thus minimizing the urge to push.
   - Place the flat side of your hand on the exposed fetal head and apply gentle pressure toward the vagina to prevent the head from "popping out." The mother may participate by placing her hand under yours on the emerging head. Note: Rapid birth of the fetal head must be prevented because a rapid change of pressure within the moulded fetal skull follows, which may result in dural or subdural tears and cause vaginal or perineal lacerations.
7. After the birth of the head, check for the umbilical cord. If the cord is around the baby's neck, try to slip it over the baby's head or pull it gently to get some slack so that you can slip it over the shoulders.
8. Support the fetal head as external rotation occurs. With one hand on each side of the baby's head, exert *gentle* pressure downward so the anterior shoulder emerges under the symphysis pubis and acts as a fulcrum; as *gentle* pressure is exerted in the opposite direction, the posterior shoulder, which has passed over the sacrum and coccyx, emerges.
9. Be alert! Hold the baby securely because the rest of the body may emerge quickly. The baby will be slippery! Cradle the baby's head and back in one hand and the buttocks in the other and place the baby skin-to-skin on the mother's abdomen.
10. Dry the baby quickly to prevent rapid heat loss, keep the baby skin-to-skin with the mother, and cover with warm blankets (remember to keep the head warm as well). Unless immediate resuscitation is required, there is no urgency to cut the cord. There is sufficient evidence that delayed cord clamping is beneficial for the baby, especially in the preterm population.
11. When ready, double-clamp and cut the cord. Collect arterial and venous cord gases as well as cord blood if the mother is Rh negative. Compliment her (them) on a job well done and on the baby, if appropriate.
12. Wait for the placenta to separate. *Do not* tug on the cord. Note: Inappropriate traction may tear the cord, separate the placenta, or invert the uterus. Signs of placental separation include a slight gush of dark blood from the introitus, lengthening of the cord, and change in the uterine contour from a discoid to globular shape.
13. Instruct the mother to push to deliver the separated placenta. Gently ease out the placental membranes using an up-and-down motion until the membranes are removed. Check the placenta for completeness and keep the placenta until it can be inspected by the primary health provider. If birth occurs outside a hospital setting, to minimize complications, do not cut the cord without proper clamps and a sterile cutting tool. Inspect the placenta for intactness. Check the firmness of the uterus. Gently massage the fundus and demonstrate to the mother how she can massage her own fundus properly.
14. If supplies are available, clean the mother's perineal area and apply a perineal pad.
15. In addition to gentle massage of the fundus, the following measures can be taken to prevent or minimize hemorrhage:
    - Put the baby to the mother's breast as soon as possible. Sucking or nuzzling and licking the nipple stimulates the release of oxytocin from the posterior pituitary. Note: If the baby does not or cannot nurse, manually stimulate the mother's nipples.
    - Do not allow the mother's bladder to become distended. Assess the bladder for fullness and encourage her to void if fullness is found.
    - Expel any clots from the mother's uterus after ensuring that the fundus is firm.
16. Comfort or reassure the mother and her family or friends. Keep the baby skin-to-skin with mother and provide additional warmth to the mother. Give her fluids if available and tolerated.
17. If this is a multifetal birth, identify the infants in order of birth (using letters A, B, etc.).
18. Make notations regarding the following aspects of the birth:
    - Fetal presentation and position
    - Presence of cord around neck (nuchal cord) or other parts and number of times cord encircled part
    - Colour, character, and amount of amniotic fluid if rupture of membranes occurs immediately before birth
    - Time of birth
    - Estimated time of determination of Apgar score (e.g., 1 and 5 minutes after birth), resuscitation efforts implemented, and ultimate condition of baby
    - Sex of baby
    - Time of placental expulsion and the appearance and completeness of the placenta
    - Maternal condition: affect, behaviour, and demeanour, amount of bleeding, and status of uterine tonicity
    - Any unusual occurrences during the birth (e.g., maternal or paternal response, comments, or gestures in response to birth of baby).

- Application of gravity to direct the fetal head toward the pelvic inlet, thereby facilitating descent
- Enlargement of pelvic dimensions and restriction of the encroachment of the sacrum and coccyx into the pelvic inlet
- Increased uteroplacental circulation, resulting in more intense, efficient uterine contractions
- Enhancement of the woman's ability to bear down effectively, thereby minimizing maternal exhaustion

Squatting is highly effective in facilitating the descent and birth of the fetus. It is one of the best and most natural positions for the second stage of labour and has been associated with the same benefits of other upright and lateral positions (Simpson et al., 2008). Women should assume a modified, supported squat until the fetal head is engaged, at which time a deep squat can be used. A firm surface is required for this position (see Fig. 17-9, A). In a birthing bed, a squatting bar is available that she can use to help support herself (see Fig. 17-8, B). A birth ball can help a woman maintain the squatting position. The fetus will be aligned with the birth canal, and pelvic and perineal relaxation are facilitated as she sits on the ball or holds the squatting bar in front of her for support (see Box 17-9).

The predominant position in Canada is supine, followed by semisitting, with approximately 32% of women using stirrups for birth, even though research does not support this position (see Chapter 18) (PHAC, 2012). Alternative positions and position changes that result in more births over an intact perineum are more commonly used by midwives (Jacobson & Turner, 2008).

When a woman uses the supported standing position for bearing down, her weight is borne on both femoral heads, allowing the pressure in the acetabulum to increase the transverse diameter of the pelvic outlet by up to 1 cm. This can be helpful if descent of the head is delayed because the occiput has not rotated from the lateral (transverse diameter of pelvis) to the anterior position. Birthing chairs or rocking chairs may be used to provide women with a good physiological position to enhance bearing-down efforts during childbirth, although some women feel restricted by a chair. The upright position provides a potential psychological advantage in that it allows the mother to see the birth as it occurs and maintain eye contact with the attendant.

Oversized beanbag chairs and large floor pillows may be used for both labour and birth. They can mould around and support the mother in whatever position she selects. These chairs are of particular value for mothers who wish to be actively involved in the birth process. Birthing stools can be used to support the woman in an upright position similar to squatting. Some women may feel more comfortable sitting on the toilet to push because they are concerned about stool incontinence during this stage. Sitting on the toilet is similar to squatting and is an ideal position for the primiparous woman to start the pushing stage. Women must be closely monitored and removed from the toilet before birth is imminent. Because sitting on chairs, stools, toilets, or commodes can increase perineal edema and blood loss, it is important to assist the woman to change her position frequently.

The side-lying (lateral) position, with the upper part of the woman's leg held by the nurse or coach or placed on a pillow, is also an effective position for the second stage of labour (see Fig. 17-12, A). Women using the lateral position have more control over their bearing-down efforts. In addition, a slower, more controlled descent of the fetus results in a reduced risk of perineal trauma. Some women prefer a semisitting (semirecumbent) position.

If the semirecumbent position is used, the woman's legs should not be forced against her abdomen as she bears down. This position increases perineal stretching and the risk for perineal trauma and spinal and lower-extremity neurological injuries (Simpson et al., 2008).

The hands-and-knees position, along with pelvic rocking, is an effective position for birth because it enhances placental perfusion, helps rotate the fetus from a posterior to an anterior position, and may facilitate the birth of the shoulders, especially if the fetus is large (see Fig. 17-9, B). Perineal trauma may also be reduced. Women in the second stage of labour should be encouraged to change positions every 20 to 30 minutes if they are not making progress.

The birthing bed is commonly used today and can be set for different positions according to the woman's needs (Fig. 17-13). The woman can squat, kneel, sit, recline, or lie on her side, choosing the position most comfortable for her. At the same time there is exposure for examination and birth. Squatting bars, over-the-bed tables, birth balls, and pillows can be used for support. The bed can be positioned for the administration of anaesthesia and is ideal for helping women receiving an epidural to assume different positions to facilitate birth. The bed can be used to transport the woman to the operating room if a Caesarean birth is necessary.

Bearing-Down Efforts

As the fetal head reaches the pelvic floor, most women experience the urge to bear down. Reflexively, the woman will begin to exert downward pressure by contracting her abdominal muscles while relaxing her pelvic floor. This bearing down is an involuntary response to the Ferguson reflex. A strong expiratory grunt or groan (vocalization) often accompanies pushing when the woman exhales as she pushes. This natural vocalization by women during open-glottis bearing-down efforts should be encouraged by nurses.

When coaching a woman to push, the nurse should encourage her to push as she feels like pushing (instinctive, spontaneous pushing) rather than giving a prolonged push on command (directed, closed-glottis pushing). Prolonged breath-holding, or sustained, directed bearing down is still a common practice, often beginning at 10-cm dilation and before the urge to bear down is perceived. The woman is coached to hold her breath, closing her glottis, and to push while the nurse or partner counts to 10. This method of bearing down may trigger the Valsalva manoeuvre, which occurs when the woman closes her glottis (closed-glottis pushing), increasing intrathoracic and cardiovascular pressure. This reduces cardiac output and decreases perfusion of the uterus and the placenta. Adverse effects associated with prolonged breath-holding and forceful

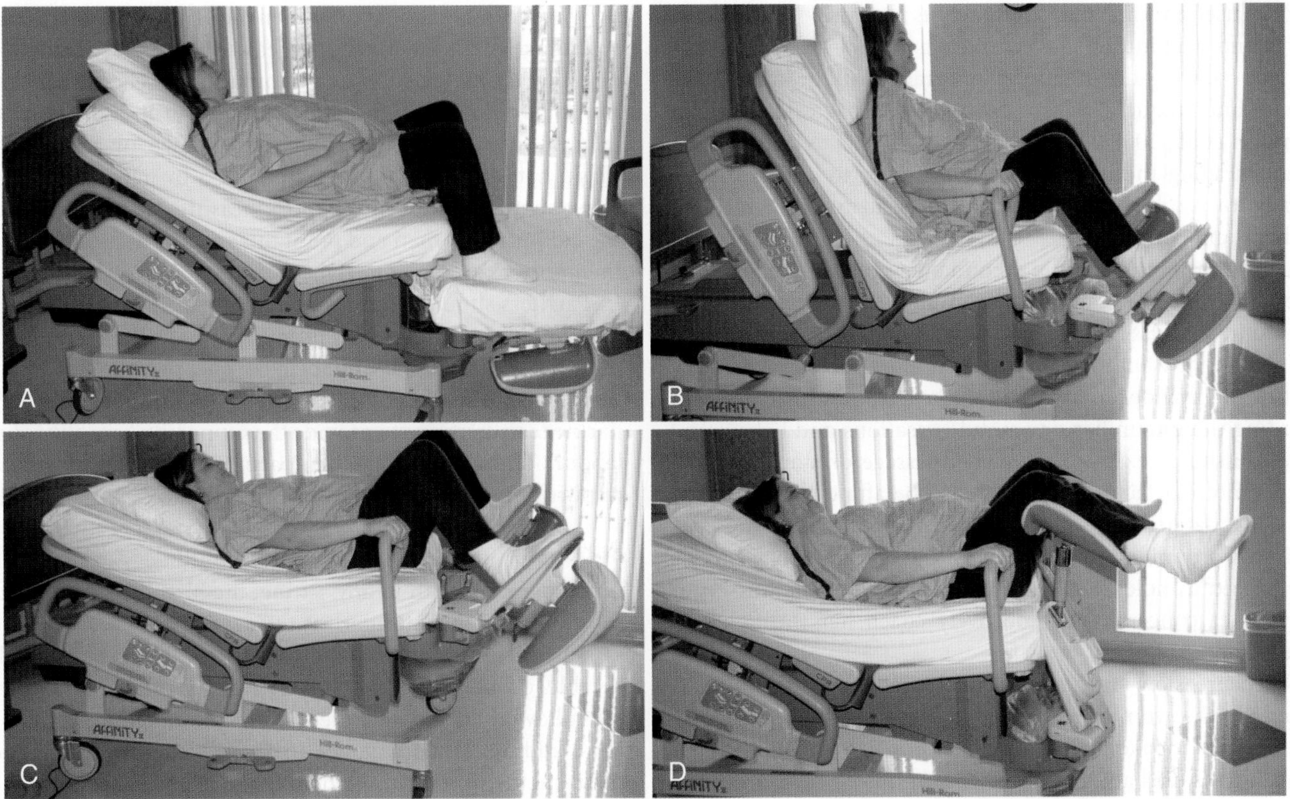

FIGURE 17-13 The versatility of today's birthing bed makes it practical in many settings. **A:** Semirecumbent (modified throne position). **B:** High Fowlers (similar to sitting or squatting position). **C:** Lithotomy with foot rests. **D:** Lithotomy with stirrups. (Courtesy Julie Perry Nelson.)

CRITICAL THINKING CASE STUDY

Delayed Pushing in Second Stage Labour

You are the nurse assigned to care for Emily, a 25-year-old G1 T0 P0 A0 L0 at 39 weeks of gestation. You have just performed a vaginal examination and found that Emily's cervix is completely dilated. She has an epidural, which is working well. Currently Emily is feeling neither pressure nor pain. On learning that Emily's cervix is completely dilated, her health care provider exclaims, "Good! Get in there and help her push so we can have this baby! I've had a long day!"

QUESTIONS

1. Evidence—Is there sufficient evidence to draw conclusions about effective management of second-stage labour?
2. Assumptions—Describe an underlying assumption about each of the following issues:
   a. Delayed pushing
   b. Positioning for pushing
   c. Spontaneous versus directed pushing efforts
3. What implications and priorities for nursing care can be drawn at this time?
4. Does the evidence objectively support your argument (conclusion)?

pushing efforts include fetal hypoxia and subsequent acidosis, increased risk for pelvic floor damage (structural and neurogenic), and perineal trauma (Blackburn, 2013; Hanson, 2009; Simpson et al., 2008). The benefits of spontaneous pushing efforts rather than sustained Valsalva pushes include less fatigue and enhanced comfort. In addition, these more effective bearing-down efforts result in less time spent actively pushing (Hanson, 2009; James, 2011). Based on this evidence it is essential that perinatal nurses advocate for the practice of delayed and spontaneous bearing-down efforts with the woman in an upright or lateral position (Hanson, 2009) (see Critical Thinking Case Study).

A woman can become confused and anxious when she is being told to do something in conflict with what her body is telling her. Using phrases such as "You are doing so well; do it again," "You are moving the baby down," and "Follow what your body is telling you," rather than "Push, push, push," encourages a woman to feel confident in her body and what she is feeling (Hanson, 2009).

The nurse should monitor the woman's breathing so that she does not hold her breath for more than 5 to 7 seconds at a time, followed by a slight exhale (a combination of open-glottis and voluntary closed-glottis pushing). Remind her to ventilate her lungs fully by taking deep, cleansing breaths before and after each contraction. Bearing down while exhaling (open-glottis pushing) and taking breaths between bearing-down efforts help to maintain adequate oxygen levels for the mother and fetus, thereby enhancing fetal well-being. Approximately five pushes occur during a contraction, with each push lasting about 5 seconds. The active pushing phase of the second stage of labour is considered to be the most physiologically stressful part of labour. Therefore, every effort should be made to ensure that women use nondirected spontaneous pushing to conserve energy and maximize the effect of each bearing-down effort. A woman's bearing-down efforts naturally will become more forceful and frequent as the second stage progresses to birth (Simpson et al., 2008).

Encouraging the mother to use a mirror to see the baby's head or to use her hand and feel the head often increases a mother's ability to push.

A woman may reach the second stage of labour and then experience a lack of readiness to complete the process and give birth to her child. She may have doubts about her readiness to be a mother or want to wait for her support person or primary health care provider to arrive. Fear, anxiety, or embarrassment regarding the unfamiliar or painful sensations and behaviours during pushing (e.g., sounds made, passage of stool) may be other inhibiting factors. She may also be afraid that the baby will be in danger once it emerges from the protective intrauterine environment. By recognizing that a woman may experience a need to hold back the birth of her baby, the nurse can address her concerns and effectively coach her through this stage of labour.

To ensure slow birth of the fetal head, the nurse should encourage the woman to control the urge to bear down, by coaching her to take panting breaths or exhale slowly through pursed lips as the baby's head crowns. At this point, the woman needs simple, clear directions from one person. Amnesia between contractions is often pronounced in the second stage, and the woman may have to be roused to participate in the bearing-down process.

Fetal Heart Rate and Pattern

Fetal heart rate assessment is done every 5 minutes during the second stage of labour. If atypical or abnormal patterns develop, prompt assessment or intervention must be initiated. The woman can be turned on her side to reduce the pressure of the uterus against the ascending vena cava and descending aorta (see Fig. 17-3), and oxygen can be administered at 8 to 10 L/min via a tight-fitting face mask (Miller, Miller, & Tucker, 2013). Often this is all that is required to restore a normal pattern. If the FHR and pattern do not become normal immediately, the primary health care provider should be notified quickly because medical intervention to hasten birth may be indicated. See Chapter 19 for more interventions related to abnormal FHR.

> **LEGAL TIP**
> ***DOCUMENTATION***
> All observations (e.g., maternal vital signs, fetal heart rate and pattern, progress of labour) and nursing interventions, including the woman's response, should be documented concurrently with care. The course of labour and maternal–fetal response may change without warning. All documentation must be accurate, complete, timely, and according to agency policy and professional standards.

Support of the Partner

During the second stage of labour, the woman needs continuous support and coaching (see Table 17-5). Because the coaching process can be physically and emotionally tiring for support people, the nurse should offer them nourishment and fluids and encourage them to take short breaks. If birth occurs in an LBR or LBRP room, the support person usually wears street clothes. The support person who attends the birth in a delivery room may be instructed to put on a cover gown or scrub clothes, mask, hat, and shoe covers as required by agency policy. The nurse should also specify support measures that can be used for the labouring woman and point out areas of the room in which the partner can move freely.

Partners should be encouraged to be present at the birth of their infants if doing so is in keeping with their cultural and personal expectations and beliefs. The presence of partners maintains the psychological closeness of the family unit, and the partner can continue to provide the supportive care given during labour. The woman and her partner need to have an equal opportunity to initiate the attachment process with the baby.

Supplies, Instruments, and Equipment

To prepare for birth in any setting, the birthing table is usually set up during the later part of the active phase.

The birthing supplies and instruments are arranged on a table or cart (Fig. 17-14). Principles of sterile technique are followed for gloving, identifying and opening sterile packages, adding sterile supplies to the table, unwrapping sterile instruments, and handing them to the primary health care provider. The crib or radiant warmer and equipment are readied for the support and stabilization of the infant, if required (Fig. 17-15).

The items used for birth may vary among different facilities; therefore, the procedure manual of each facility should be consulted to determine the protocols specific to that facility.

The nurse estimates the time until the birth will occur and notifies the primary health care provider if he or she is not in the woman's room. Even the most experienced nurse can miscalculate the time left before birth occurs; therefore, every nurse who attends a woman in labour must be prepared to assist with an emergency birth if the primary health care provider is not present (see Box 17-13).

Birth in a Delivery Room

The woman will need assistance if she needs to move from the labour bed to the delivery table (Fig. 17-16). The maternal position for birth varies from a lithotomy position with the woman's legs in stirrups or with her legs held and supported by the nurse or support person, to one in which her feet rest on footrests while she holds on to a squat bar, to a side-lying

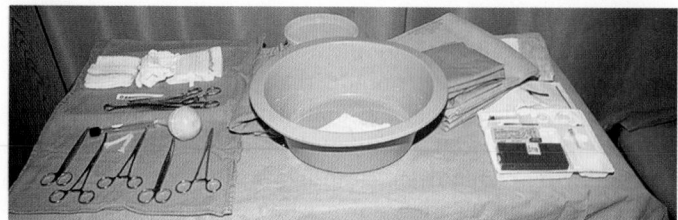

FIGURE 17-14 Instrument table. (Courtesy Marjorie Pyle, RNC, Lifecircle)

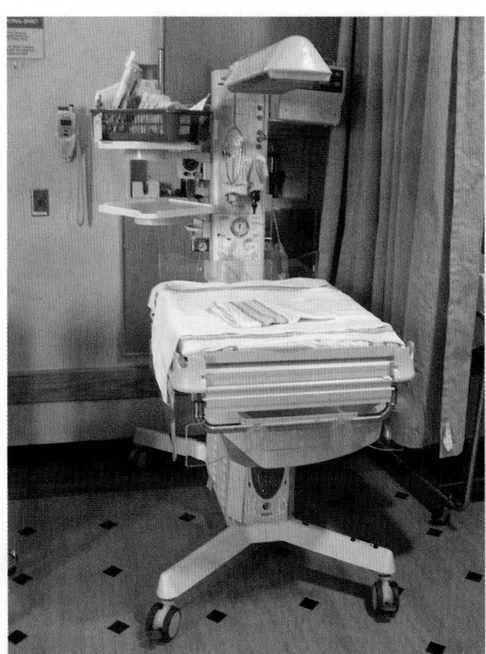

FIGURE 17-15 Radiant warmer for newborn. (Courtesy Dee Lowdermilk.)

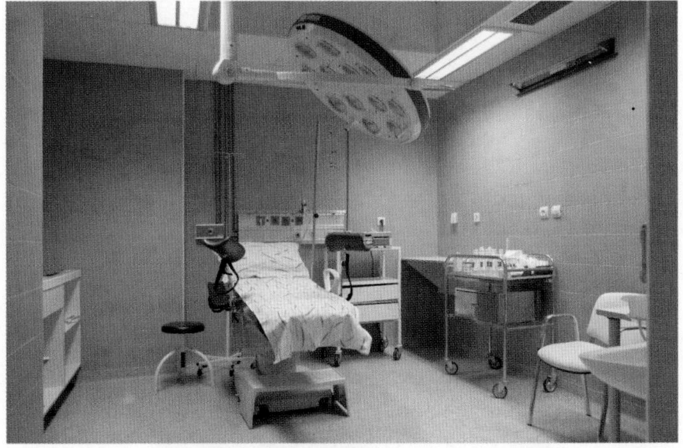

FIGURE 17-16 Delivery room. (Mirko Tabasevic/Shutterstock.com.)

position with the woman's upper leg supported by the coach, nurse, or squat bar.

Although not recommended as the ideal position for birth, the lithotomy position makes it more convenient for the primary health care provider to deal with complications that may arise. To place the woman in this position, her buttocks are brought to the edge of the table and her legs are placed in stirrups. Care must be taken to pad the stirrups, raise and place both legs simultaneously, and adjust the shanks of the stirrups so that the calves of the legs are supported. There should be no pressure on the popliteal space. If the stirrups are not the same height, ligaments in the woman's back can be strained as she bears down, leading to considerable discomfort in the postpartum period.

Once the woman is positioned, the foot of the bed may be removed so the primary health care provider attending the birth can gain better perineal access for delivering a large baby or using forceps or vacuum extractor. Alternatively the foot of the bed can be left in place and lowered slightly to form a ledge that allows access for birth and also serves as a place to lay the newborn (see Fig. 17-13, A).

The nurse needs to continue to coach and encourage the woman. The nurse should auscultate the FHR or evaluate the electronic monitor tracing every 5 minutes with active pushing and keep the primary health care provider informed of the rate and pattern of the fetal heart. An oxytocic medication such as oxytocin can be prepared so that it is ready to administer after delivery of the anterior shoulder.

If the birth is in a delivery room, the primary health care provider puts on a mask that has a shield or protective eyewear and may put on a cap and shoe covers. The provider will scrub his or her hands and put on a sterile gown (with waterproof front and sleeves) and gloves. Nurses attending the birth may also need to wear caps, protective eyewear, masks, gowns, and gloves. The woman may then be draped with sterile drapes. Birth in an LBR or LBRP usually does not require this type of protective covering but wherever the birth occurs, routine precautions need to be observed (see Box 17-4).

The nurse can maintain contact with the parents by touching and verbally comforting them, explaining the reasons for care, and sharing in the parents' joy at the birth of their child.

Mechanism of Birth: Vertex Presentation

The three phases of spontaneous birth of a fetus in a vertex presentation are (1) birth of the head, (2) birth of the shoulders, and (3) birth of the body and extremities (see Chapter 16).

With voluntary bearing-down efforts, the head appears at the introitus (Fig. 17-17, A to D). **Crowning** occurs when the widest part of the head (the biparietal diameter) distends the vulva just before birth. The mother may state that she feels a burning sensation at this time as the perineum is stretched. The birth attendant may apply oil or lubricant to the perineum and stretch it as the head is crowning. Immediately before birth, the perineal musculature becomes greatly distended. If an **episiotomy** (incision into the perineum to enlarge the vaginal outlet) is necessary, it is done at this time. Local anaesthetic should be administered before the episiotomy. Box 17-14 shows the process of normal vaginal childbirth in a series of photographs.

The physician or midwife may use a hands-on approach to control the birth of the head, believing that guarding the perineum results in a gradual birth that will prevent fetal intracranial injury, protect maternal tissues, and reduce postpartum perineal pain. This approach involves (1) applying pressure against the rectum, drawing it downward to aid in flexing the head as the back of the neck catches under the symphysis pubis; (2) applying upward pressure from the coccygeal region (modified Ritgen manoeuvre) (Fig. 17-18) to extend the head during the actual birth, thereby protecting the musculature of the perineum; and (3) assisting the mother with voluntary control of the bearing-down efforts by coaching her to pant while letting uterine forces expel the fetus.

Some health care providers use a hands-poised (hands-off) approach when attending a birth. In this approach hands are

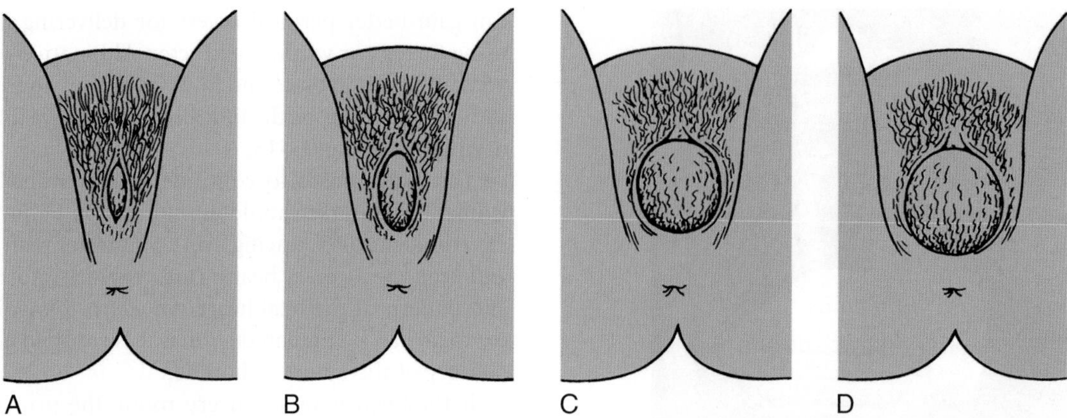

FIGURE 17-17 Beginning birth with vertex presenting. **A:** Anteroposterior slit. **B:** Oval opening. **C:** Circular shape. **D:** Crowning.

BOX 17-14 NORMAL VAGINAL CHILDBIRTH

Second Stage

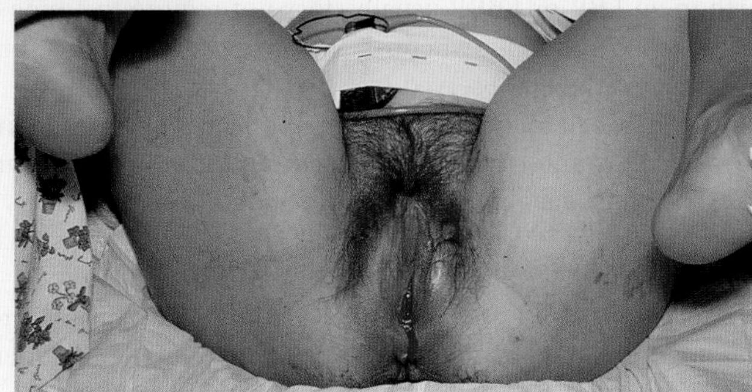

Anteroposterior slit; vertex visible during contraction.

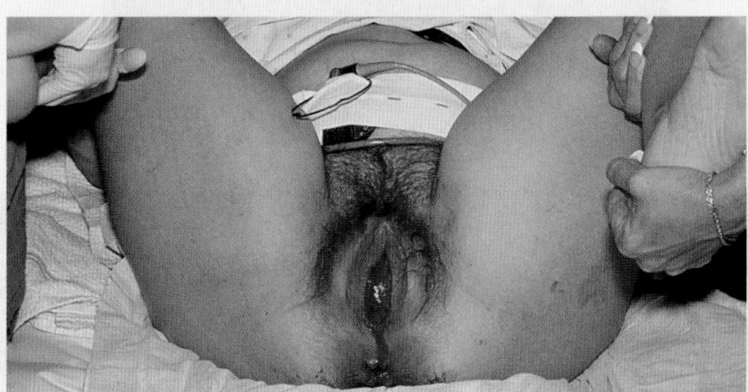

Oval opening; vertex presenting. Note: nurse (on left) is wearing gloves but support person (on right) is not.

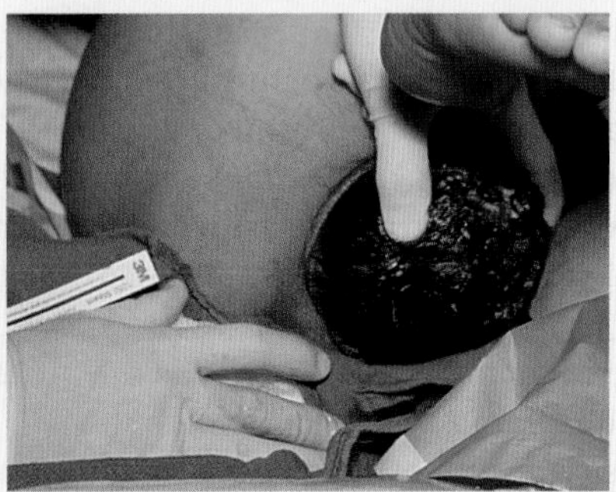

Crowning.

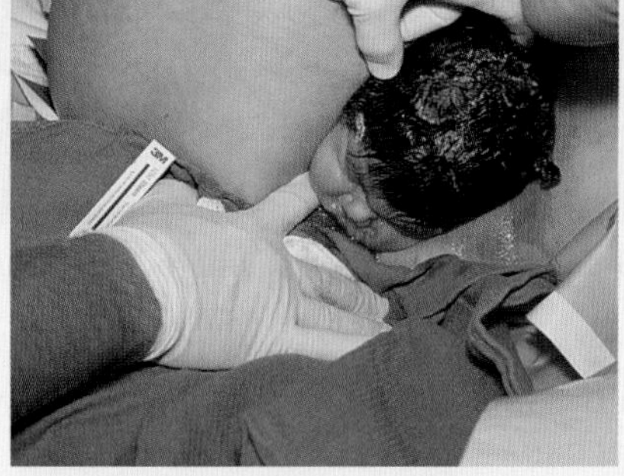

Primary care provider using Ritgen manoeuvre as head is born by extension.

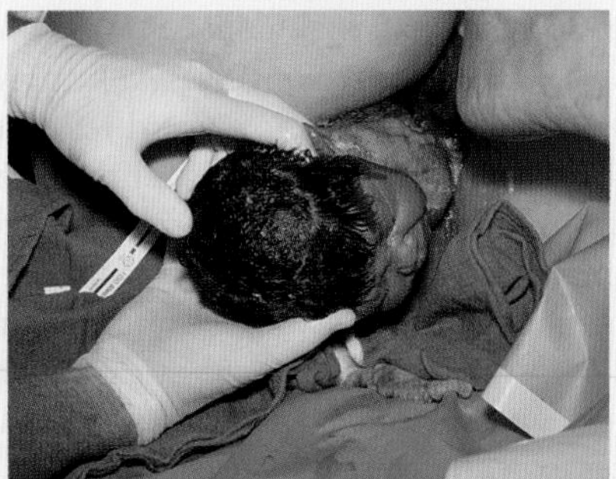

After checking for nuchal cord, the primary care provider supports head during external rotation and restitution.

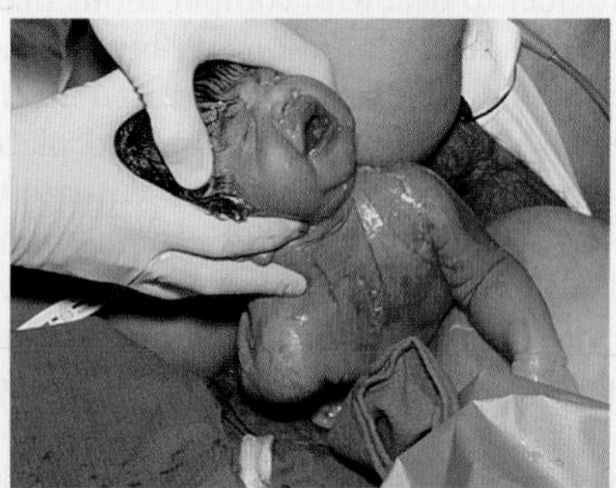

Birth of posterior shoulder.

BOX 17-14 NORMAL VAGINAL CHILDBIRTH—cont'd

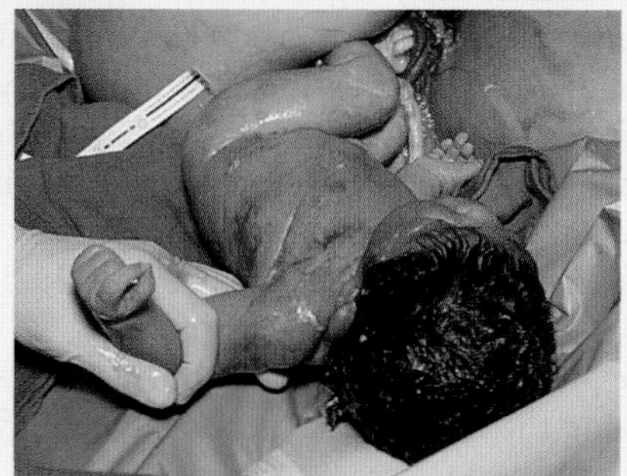
Birth of newborn by slow expulsion.

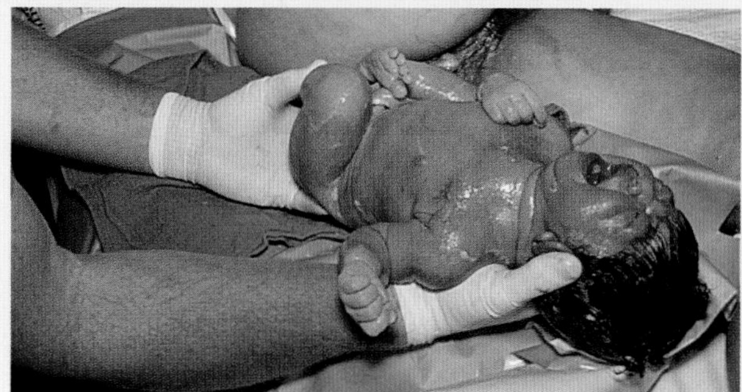
Second stage complete; note that newborn is not completely pink yet.

Third Stage

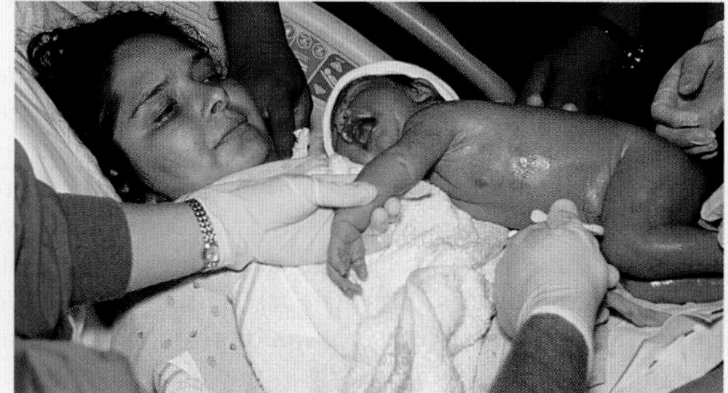
Newborn placed on mother's abdomen while cord is clamped and cut.

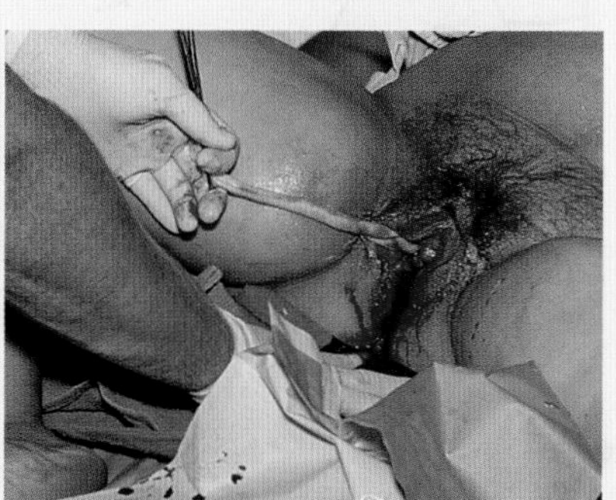
Note increased bleeding as placenta separates.

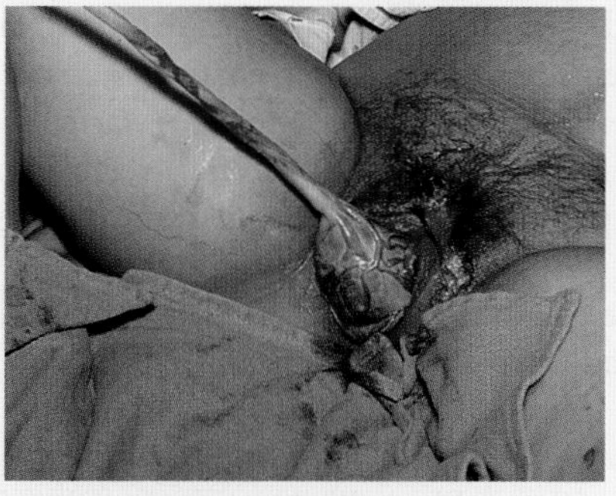
Expulsion of placenta.

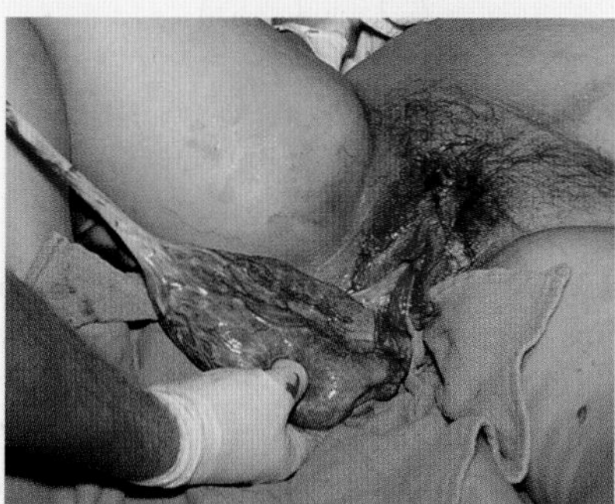
Expulsion is complete, marking the end of the third stage.

(Courtesy Michael S. Clement, MD.)

prepared to place light pressure on the fetal head to prevent rapid expulsion. They are not placed on the perineum or used to assist with birth of the shoulders and body.

The hands-on and hands-poised approaches have similar results in terms of perineal and vaginal tears, but the hands-on technique is associated with a higher incidence of third-degree tears and episiotomies. In one study the hands-poised approach resulted in fewer third-degree tears (Berghella et al., 2008). However, the hands-on approach may result in less perineal pain.

The umbilical cord often encircles the neck (**nuchal cord**) but rarely so tightly as to cause hypoxia. After the head is born, gentle palpation is used to feel for the cord. If present, the cord should be slipped gently over the head if possible. If the loop is tight or if there is a second loop, the cord is clamped twice, cut between the clamps, and unwound from around the neck before the birth is allowed to continue. Mucus, blood, or meconium in the nasal or oral passages may prevent the newborn from breathing. To eliminate this problem, moist gauze sponges may be used to wipe the nose and mouth. Rarely is suction used to aspirate the mouth or nose of the newborn.

Use of Fundal Pressure

Fundal pressure is the application of gentle, steady pressure against the fundus of the uterus to facilitate vaginal birth. Historically, it has been used when the administration of analgesia and anaesthesia decreased the woman's ability to push during

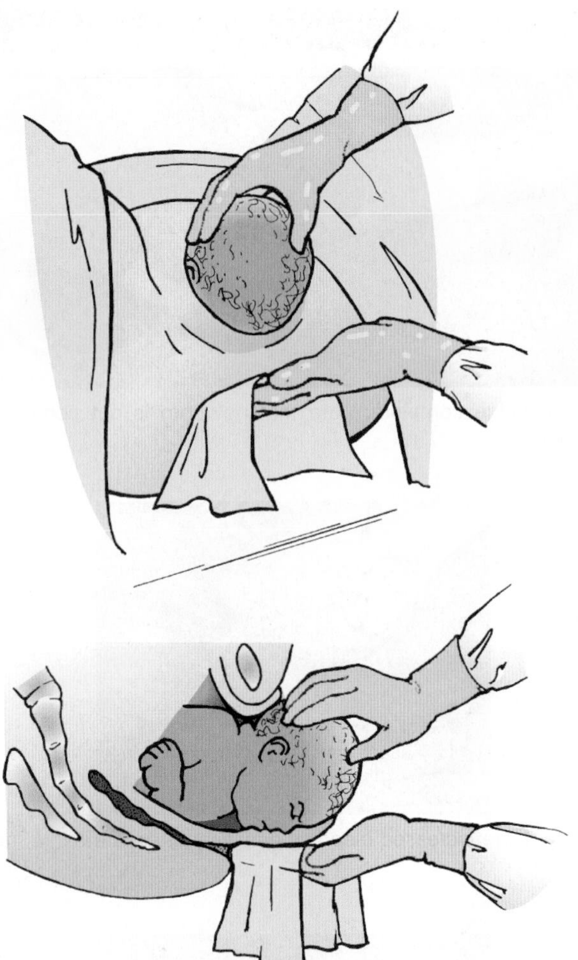

FIGURE 17-18 Birth of head with modified Ritgen manoeuvre. Note control to prevent too-rapid birth of head.

the birth, in cases of shoulder dystocia, and when second-stage fetal bradycardia or other abnormal FHR patterns were present. Use of fundal pressure by nurses is not advised because there is no standard technique available for this manoeuvre. In addition, no current legal, professional, or regulatory standards exist for its use; and no evidence related to its effectiveness in facilitating a safe vaginal birth is available (Simpson & O'Brien-Adel, 2014). The all-fours position (the Gaskin manoeuvre), suprapubic pressure, and maternal position changes are among the recommended interventions for shoulder dystocia.

Immediate Assessments and Care of the Newborn

The time of birth is the precise time when the entire body is out of the mother; this time is recorded. In the case of multiple births each birth would be noted in the same way. In most situations the newborn can be dried off and placed on the mother's chest, covered with a warm, dry blanket. Occasionally the newborn may need to be cared for on a radiant warmer until stable enough for skin-to-skin contact. The cord may be clamped at this time, and the primary health care provider may ask the woman's partner if he or she would like to cut the cord. If so, the partner is given a sterile pair of scissors and instructed to cut the cord 2.5 cm above the clamp.

Recent evidence suggests that delaying clamping of the cord for 1 to 3 minutes may significantly improve outcomes for healthy term infants. Delayed cord clamping results in higher birthweight of the newborn and increased early hemoglobin concentration and iron reserves up to 6 months after birth. These need to be balanced against a small additional risk of jaundice in newborns that requires phototherapy (Diaz-Castro, Florido, Kajarabille, et al., 2014; McDonald, Middleton, Dowswell, et al., 2013).

The care given immediately after birth focuses on assessing and stabilizing the newborn. The nurse is usually the primary person responsible for care of the infant at this time because the primary health care provider is involved with the delivery of the placenta and care of the mother. The nurse must watch the infant for any signs of distress and initiate appropriate interventions should any appear. For care of the newborn with meconium-stained amniotic fluid see Chapter 20.

A brief assessment of the newborn is performed immediately, even while the mother is holding the infant. This assessment includes assigning Apgar scores at 1 and 5 minutes after birth (see Table 26-1). Maintaining a patent airway, supporting respiratory effort, and preventing cold stress by drying and covering the newborn with a warmed blanket are the major priorities in terms of the newborn's immediate care. Further examination, identification procedures, and care can be postponed until later in the third stage of labour or early in the fourth stage.

Perineal Trauma Related to Childbirth

Most acute injuries and lacerations of the perineum, vagina, uterus, and their support tissues occur during the birth. There is evidence to suggest that alternative measures for perineal management, such as application of warm compresses and gentle antenatal perineal massage and stretching, may lessen the degree of perineal lacerations and trauma (Aasheim, Nilsen, Lukasse, et al., 2011; Beckmann & Stock, 2013).

Some degree of damage occurs to the soft tissues of the birth canal and adjacent structures during every birth. The tendency to sustain lacerations varies with each woman (i.e., the soft tissue in some women may be less distensible). Damage usually is more pronounced in nulliparous women because the tissues are firmer and more resistant than those in multiparous women. Heredity is also a factor. For example, the tissue of light-skinned women, especially those with reddish hair, is not as readily distensible as that of darker-skinned women, and healing may be less efficient. Other risk factors associated with perineal trauma include maternal position, pelvic inadequacy (e.g., narrow subpubic arch with a constricted outlet), fetal malpresentation and position (e.g., breech presentation, occiput posterior position), large (macrosomic) infants, use of forceps or vacuum to facilitate birth, prolonged second stage of labour, and rapid labour in which there is insufficient time for the perineum to stretch.

Some injuries to the supporting tissues, whether they are acute or nonacute or were repaired or not, may lead to genitourinary and sexual problems later in life (e.g., pelvic relaxation, uterine prolapse, cystocele, rectocele, dyspareunia, urinary and bowel dysfunction). Use of Kegel exercises in the prenatal and postpartum periods improves and restores the tone and strength of the perineal muscles (see Chapter 5, p. 72). Health practices, including good nutrition and appropriate hygienic measures, help maintain the integrity and suppleness of the perineal tissues, enhance healing, and prevent infection.

Perineal Lacerations

Perineal lacerations usually occur when the fetal head is being born. The extent of the laceration is defined in terms of its depth:

First degree—Laceration extends through the skin and structures superficial to muscles.

Second degree—Laceration extends through muscles of perineal body.

Third degree—Laceration continues through anal sphincter muscle.

Fourth degree—Laceration also involves the anterior rectal wall.

Perineal injury is often accompanied by small lacerations on the medial surfaces of the labia minora below the pubic rami and to the sides of the urethra (periurethral) and clitoris. Lacerations in this highly vascular area often result in profuse bleeding.

Special attention must be paid to third- and fourth-degree lacerations so that the woman retains fecal continence. Measures should be taken to promote soft stools (e.g., roughage, fluid, activity, and stool softeners) in order to increase the woman's comfort and foster healing. Antimicrobial therapy may be used in some cases. Enemas and suppositories are contraindicated for these women. Simple perineal injuries usually heal without any significant problems, regardless of whether they were repaired. However, it is easier to repair a new perineal injury to prevent sequelae than it is to correct long-term damage.

Episiotomy

An **episiotomy** is an incision made in the perineum to enlarge the vaginal outlet. Routine episiotomy is not recommended; the rate of episiotomy in Canada is nonetheless 17% as reported by hospitals (PHAC, 2012). The side-lying position for birth causes less tension on the perineum, making possible a gradual stretching of the perineum with fewer indications for episiotomies.

Different types of episiotomies are performed, depending on the site and direction of the incision (Fig. 17-19). Midline (median) episiotomy is used most commonly. It is effective, easily repaired, and generally the least painful. However, it is associated with a higher incidence of third- and fourth-degree lacerations. Sphincter tone is usually restored following primary healing and a good repair.

Mediolateral episiotomy is used in operative births when the need for posterior extension is likely. Although a fourth-degree laceration may be prevented, a third-degree laceration may occur. The blood loss is greater and the repair more difficult and painful than with midline episiotomies. It is more painful in the postpartum period and the pain lasts longer.

Currently, the practice in many settings is to manually support the perineum during birth and allow it to tear, rather than perform an episiotomy. Tears are often smaller than an episiotomy, are repaired easily or not at all, and heal quickly. Episiotomies are associated with more posterior perineal trauma, suturing and healing complications, and later pain with intercourse. The pain and discomfort resulting from episiotomies can interfere with mother–infant interaction, breastfeeding, re-establishment of the sexual relationship with her partner, and even emotional recovery after birth. The rate of episiotomies is lower when midwives rather than obstetricians attend births.

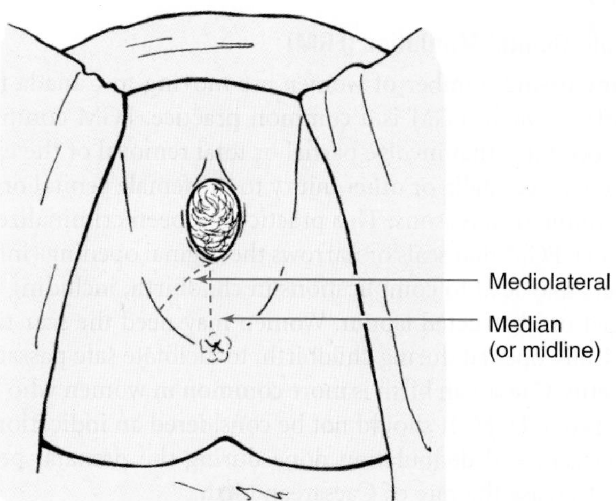

FIGURE 17-19 Types of episiotomies.

Alternative measures for perineal management such as warm compresses and massage with a lubricant (e.g., prenatal and intrapartum) may have some effectiveness in reducing perineal trauma, as they may lessen the degree of perineal lacerations. Use of Kegel exercises in the prenatal and postpartum periods improves and restores the tone and strength of the perineal muscles.

Vaginal and Urethral Lacerations

Vaginal lacerations often occur in conjunction with perineal lacerations. Vaginal lacerations tend to extend up the lateral walls (sulci) and, if deep enough, involve the levator ani. Additional injury may occur high in the vaginal vault near the level of the ischial spines. Vaginal vault lacerations may be circular and may result from use of forceps to rotate the fetal head or from rapid fetal descent or precipitous birth.

Cervical Injuries

Cervical injuries occur when the cervix retracts over the advancing fetal head. These cervical lacerations occur at the lateral angles of the external os. Most lacerations are shallow and bleeding is minimal. Larger lacerations may extend to the vaginal vault or beyond it into the lower uterine segment; serious bleeding may occur. Extensive lacerations may follow hasty attempts to enlarge the cervical opening artificially or to deliver the fetus before full cervical dilation is achieved. Injuries to the cervix can have adverse effects on future pregnancies and childbirths.

Female Genital Mutilation (FGM)

An increasing number of women are moving to Canada from countries where FGM is a common practice. FGM comprises all procedures that involve partial or total removal of the external female genitalia or other injury to the female genital organs for nonmedical reasons. This practice has been criminalized in Canada. FGM that seals or narrows the vaginal opening (infibulation) may lead to complications in childbirth, including prolonged or obstructed labour. Women may need the scar tissue surgically opened during childbirth, to facilitate safe passage of the fetus. Caesarean birth is more common in women who have undergone FGM. It should not be considered an indication for Caesarean, and defibulation done during the prenatal period may decrease the rate of Caesarean birth.

While it is not illegal to re-infubulate following childbirth according to the Canadian Criminal Code, requests for re-infibulation should be declined on medical grounds because repetitive cutting and suturing of the vulva is likely to increase scar tissue, thus causing or perpetuating dyspareunia or voiding difficulties. If incisions are made or tearing occurs during childbirth, it is reasonable to repair defects in a way that will promote good hemostasis, vaginal support, and normal appearance (Perron, Synikas, Burnett, et al., 2013). Women may be concerned about this practice and need education before the birth regarding what will occur. After the birth they may need extra care for pain management and proper wound healing.

Water Birth

There is evidence that immersion in water during first-stage labour can reduce pain and anxiety and length of labour. During the second stage of labour, immersion may increase the woman's satisfaction with the birth experience. There is no evidence of increased adverse effects to the fetus or woman from labouring in water or water birth, although further research is needed (Cluett & Burns, 2009).

If a woman wishes to have a water birth (Fig. 17-20), it usually occurs as part of a planned home birth with registered midwives, although it may occasionally occur in hospitals. The infant can be placed in the mother's arms until the cord is cut.

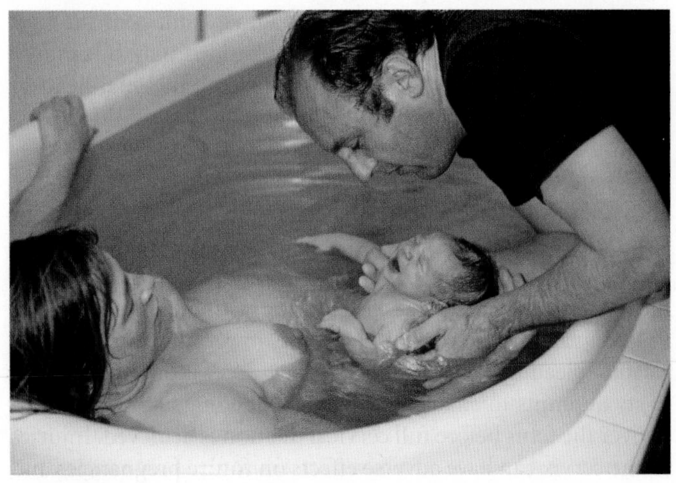

FIGURE 17-20 Water birth. (Eddie Lawrence/Science Source.)

THIRD STAGE OF LABOUR

The third stage of labour lasts from the birth of the baby until the placenta is expelled.

NURSING CARE

The goals in the management of the third stage of labour are the prompt separation and expulsion of the placenta achieved in the easiest, safest manner. Before separation of the placenta, blood is collected from the umbilical cord. Cord blood is collected for arterial and possibly venous cord gases as well as blood type, specifically if the mother is Rh negative. The third stage is generally by far the shortest stage of labour. The placenta is almost always expelled within 15 minutes after the birth of the baby. If the third stage has not been completed within 30 minutes, the placenta is considered to be retained, and interventions to hasten its separation and expulsion are usually instituted (Wing & Farinelli, 2012).

Under normal circumstances the placenta is attached to the decidual layer of the thin endometrium of the basal plate by numerous fibrous anchor villi. After the birth of the fetus strong uterine contractions and the sudden decrease in uterine size cause the placental site to shrink. This causes the anchor villi to break and the placenta to separate from its attachments. Normally the first few strong contractions that occur after the baby's birth cause the placenta to shear away from the basal plate. A placenta cannot detach itself from a flaccid (relaxed) uterus because the placental site is not reduced in size.

Placental Separation and Expulsion

Depending on the preferences of the primary health care provider, a passive (expectant) or active approach may be used to manage the third stage of labour. Passive management involves patiently watching for signs that the placenta has separated from the uterine wall spontaneously and monitoring for spontaneous expulsion. It may involve the use of gravity or nipple stimulation to facilitate separation and expulsion, but no oxytocic (uterotonic) medications are given. A quiet, relaxed environment that supports close skin-to-skin contact between mother and newborn also promotes the release of endogenous oxytocin.

In active management, placental separation and expulsion are facilitated by administration of an oxytocic medication (e.g., oxytocin) after the birth of the anterior shoulder of the fetus, clamping and cutting of the umbilical cord within 3 minutes after birth, and gently controlling cord traction following uterine contraction and separation of the placenta. Research findings and the World Health Organization recommend active management of the third stage of labour because this decreases the rate of postpartum hemorrhage caused by uterine atony (Burke, 2010; Leduc, Senikas, Lalonde, et al., 2009).

To assist in the delivery of the placenta, the woman is instructed to push when signs of separation have occurred (Fig. 17-21). If possible, the placenta should be expelled by maternal

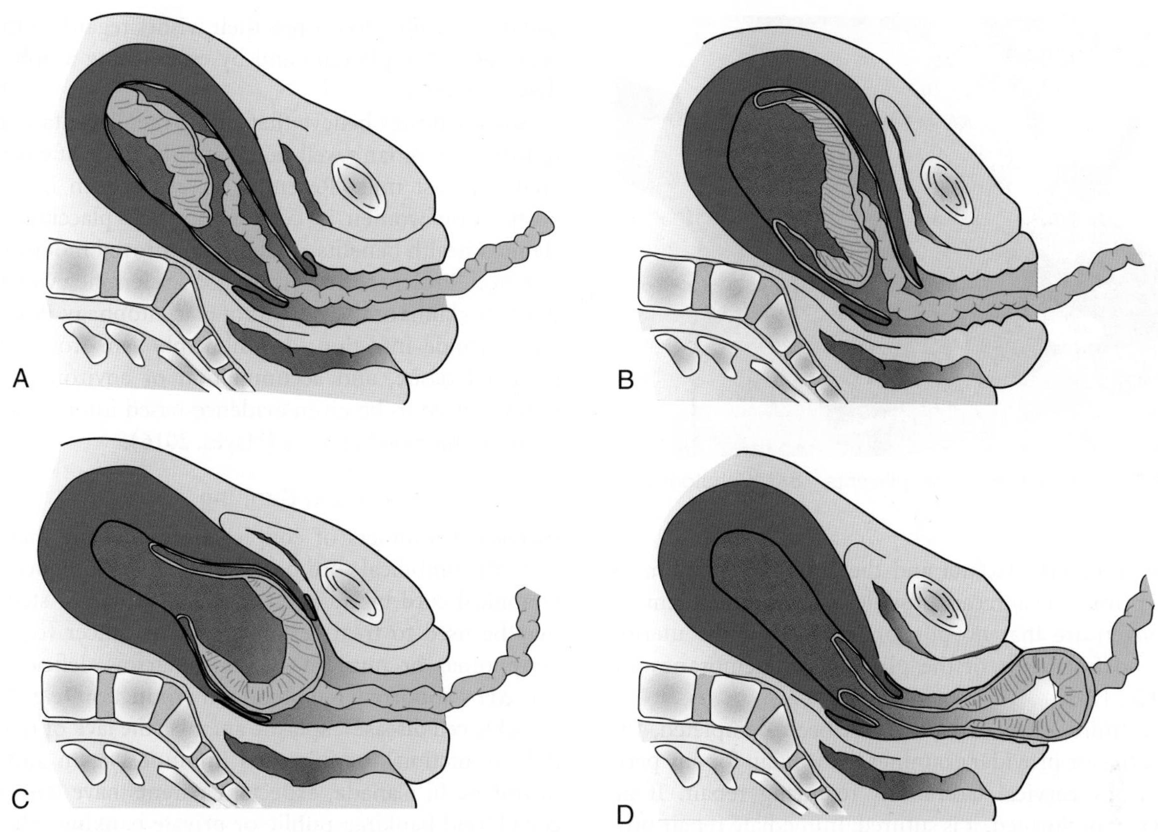

FIGURE 17-21 Third stage of labour. **A:** Placenta begins the separation process in central portion, accompanied by retroplacental bleeding. Uterus changes from discoid to globular shape. **B:** Placenta completes separation and enters lower uterine segment. Uterus is globular in shape. **C:** Placenta enters vagina, cord is seen to lengthen, and there may be increased bleeding. **D:** Expulsion (birth) of placenta and completion of third stage.

BOX 17-15 NURSING CARE IN THIRD-STAGE LABOUR

Assessment

Signs That Suggest Onset of the Third Stage

- A firmly contracting fundus
- A change in the uterus from a discoid to a globular ovoid shape as the placenta moves into the lower uterine segment
- A sudden gush of dark blood from the introitus
- Apparent lengthening of the umbilical cord as the placenta descends to the introitus
- The finding of vaginal fullness (the placenta) on vaginal examination or of fetal membranes at the introitus

Physical Assessment

- Perform every 15 minutes: maternal blood pressure, pulse, and respirations.
- Assess for signs of placental separation and amount of bleeding.
- Assess maternal and paternal response to completion of childbirth process and their reaction to the newborn.

Interventions

- Assist woman to bear down, to facilitate expulsion of the separated placenta.
- Administer an oxytocic medication as ordered to ensure adequate contraction of the uterus, thereby preventing hemorrhage.
- Provide nonpharmacological and pharmacological comfort and pain-relief measures.
- Perform hygienic cleansing measures.
- Keep woman informed of progress of placental separation and expulsion and perineal repair if appropriate.
- Explain the purpose of medications administered.
- Introduce parents to their baby and facilitate the attachment process by delaying eye prophylaxis; cover mother and baby together for skin-to-skin contact.
- Provide private time for parents to bond with their new baby.
- Encourage breastfeeding when newborn shows signs of interest.

effort during a uterine contraction. Alternate compression and elevation of the fundus plus minimal, controlled traction on the umbilical cord may be used to facilitate delivery of the placenta and amniotic membranes. Oxytocics may be administered after the placenta is removed because they stimulate the uterus to contract, thereby helping to prevent hemorrhage (Box 17-15).

Whether the placenta first appears by its shiny fetal surface (Schultze mechanism) or turns to show its dark roughened maternal surface (Duncan mechanism) is of no clinical

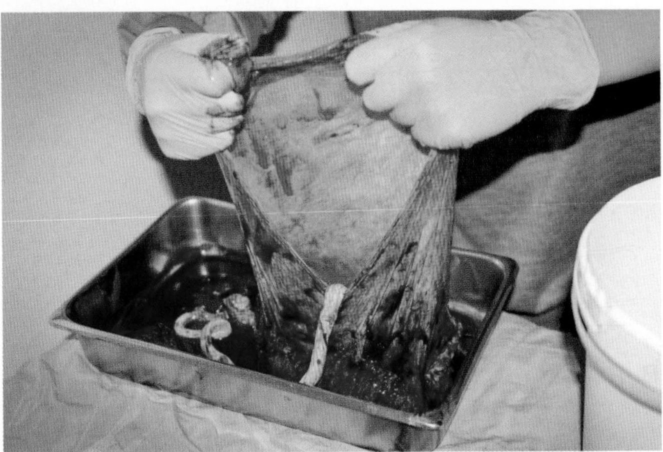

FIGURE 17-22 Examination of the placenta. (BKMCphotography/ Shutterstock.com.)

importance. After the placenta and the amniotic membranes emerge, the primary health care provider will examine them for intactness to ensure that no portion remains in the uterine cavity (i.e., no fragments of the placenta or membranes are retained) (Fig. 17-22).

When the third stage of labour has been completed, the primary health care provider examines the woman for any perineal, vaginal, or cervical lacerations requiring repair. If an episiotomy was performed, it is sutured. Immediate repair promotes healing, limits residual damage, and decreases the possibility of infection. The woman usually feels some discomfort while the primary health care provider carries out the postbirth vaginal examination. The nurse can help her use breathing and relaxation or distraction techniques for dealing with the discomfort. During this time, the nurse performs a quick assessment of the newborn's physical condition, and places matching identification bands on the baby, mother, and partner, usually while the newborn is skin-to-skin with the mother.

After any necessary repairs have been completed, the nurse cleanses the vulvar area gently and applies a perineal pad or an ice pack to the perineum. The nurse should reposition the birthing bed or table and lower the woman's legs simultaneously from the stirrups if she gave birth in a lithotomy position. The woman should be given a clean gown and blanket, which can be warmed if needed.

Some women and their families may have culturally based beliefs regarding the care of the placenta and the manner of its disposal after birth, such as viewing the care and disposal of the placenta as a way of protecting the newborn from bad luck and illness. Requests by the woman to take the placenta home and dispose of it according to her customs may be at odds with health care agency policies, especially those related to infection control and disposal of biological wastes. Many cultures follow specific rules regarding disposal of the placenta in terms of method (burning, drying, burying, or eating); site for disposal (in or near the home); and timing of disposal (immediately after birth, time of day, or by astrological signs). Disposal rituals may vary according to the gender of the child and the length of time before another child is desired. Health care providers can provide culturally sensitive health care by encouraging women and their families to express their wishes regarding the care and disposal of the placenta and by establishing a policy to fulfill these requests.

Some cultures believe that eating the placenta is a means of restoring a woman's well-being after birth or of ensuring high-quality breast milk. Recently, there has been interest among postpartum women in consuming their placentas to achieve claimed health benefits, including improved mood, energy, and lactation. Presently there is no good scientific evidence to substantiate claims of the benefits of placentophagy. Possible related risks include infection, thromboembolism from estrogens in placental tissue, and accumulation of environmental toxins. Women need to be given evidence-based information in order to make informed choices (Hayes, 2016).

Umbilical Cord Blood Banking

Increasing numbers of couples are requesting that the blood from the umbilical cord be collected and subsequently banked. Umbilical cord blood is an excellent source of stem cells that may be used to treat certain forms of cancer (e.g., leukemia, lymphomas or myelomas), bone marrow deficiency diseases caused by abnormal red blood cell production (e.g., thalassemia or sickle cell disease), aplastic anemia (the lack of normal blood cell production), or inherited immune system and metabolic disorders. In Canada, expectant parents have two options for cord blood banking: public or private banking. The Canadian Blood Services has set up the National Public Cord Blood Bank in several hospitals across the country. Currently, the woman needs to have her baby at that hospital in order to donate the cord blood. There are a few other options for public donation of cord blood in certain cities (e.g., Toronto area and Montreal/ Quebec City). Private cord banking is available in many centres throughout the country; arrangements are made prior to birth of the newborn for collection. The cost of private banking can include an initial fee of $1000 to $2000 along with an additional yearly fee. The decision to bank cord blood is a personal one made by parents, through weighing the pros and cons. Pregnant women and families should be provided with unbiased information about umbilical cord blood banking options, including the benefits and limitations of public and private banks (Armson, Allan, & Casper, 2015).

Cord blood collection is done after the birth and before delivery of the placenta. Health care providers need to be aware of the proper method of collection to ensure that the maximum amount of blood is collected and that it is collected in a sterile manner. Delayed cord clamping may decrease the amount of blood collected; parents need to be aware of this so they can make informed choices about the care they want.

FOURTH STAGE OF LABOUR

The first 1 to 2 hours after birth, sometimes called the **fourth stage of labour**, is a crucial time for the mother and her newborn. Both are not only recovering from the physical process of birth but also becoming acquainted with each other and additional family members. During this time, maternal organs undergo their initial readjustment to the nonpregnant state, and the functions of body systems begin to stabilize. Meanwhile, the newborn continues the transition from intrauterine to extrauterine existence.

NURSING CARE

In most hospitals the mother remains in the labour and birth area during this recovery time, and the labour and birth nurse cares for both the mother and newborn. When fourth-stage recovery is complete, the woman will remain in her room if she is in an LBRP unit or will be transferred via wheelchair to a room on the postpartum unit if she gave birth in an LBR or delivery room. Women who are in LBRP rooms will stay in one room from admission until discharge. Often the same nurse will care for the family through all parts of her childbirth experience.

Assessment

If the recovery nurse has not previously cared for the new mother, his or her assessment begins with an oral report from the nurse who attended the woman during labour and birth and a review of the antenatal, labour, and birth records. Of primary importance are conditions that could predispose the mother to hemorrhage, such as precipitous labour, large baby, grand multiparity (having given birth to six or more infants), induced labour, or a magnesium sulphate infusion during labour. For healthy women, hemorrhage is probably the most dangerous potential complication.

During the first hour, physical assessments of the mother are frequent. All factors except temperature are assessed every 15 minutes for 1 hour. Temperature is assessed at the beginning and end of the recovery period. After the fourth 15-minute assessment, if all parameters have stabilized within the normal range, the process is usually repeated once in the second hour. Box 17-16 describes the physical assessment of the mother during the fourth stage of labour.

Care of the New Mother

During the fourth stage of labour, many women experience intense tremors that resemble shivering from a chill. These are commonly seen and are not related to infection. Warm blankets and reassurance that the chills or tremors are common and self-limiting and last only a short while are useful interventions.

The nutritional status of the woman needs to be assessed. Restriction of food and fluid intake and the loss of fluids (blood,

BOX 17-16 ASSESSMENT DURING THE FOURTH STAGE OF LABOUR

Blood Pressure

- Measure blood pressure per assessment schedule (every 15 minutes for first hour).

Pulse

- Assess rate and regularity (every 15 minutes for the first hour).

Temperature

- Determine temperature at the beginning of the recovery period and after the first hour of recovery.

Fundus

- Position woman with knees flexed and head flat.
- Just below the umbilicus, cup hand and press firmly into the abdomen. At the same time, stabilize the uterus at symphysis with the opposite hand (see Fig. 22-3).
- If the fundus is firm (and bladder is empty), with uterus in midline, measure its position relative to the woman's umbilicus. Lay fingers flat on the abdomen under the umbilicus; measure how many centimetres (cm) fit between the umbilicus and top of the fundus. If the fundus is above the umbilicus, this is recorded as plus cm; if below, as minus cm. One fingerbreadth (fb) equals 1 cm. For example, if fundus is 1 fb or 1 cm above umbilicus, fundal height may be recorded as either +1, u+1, or 1/u. If fundus is 1 fb or 1 cm below umbilicus, fundal height may be recorded as either –1, u–1, or u/1.
- If the fundus is not firm, massage it gently to contract and expel any clots before measuring distance from the umbilicus.
- Place hands appropriately; massage gently only until firm.
- Expel clots while keeping hands placed as in Fig. 22-3. With the upper hand, firmly apply pressure downward toward the vagina; observe perineum for amount and size of expelled clots.

Bladder

- Assess distension by noting location and firmness of uterine fundus and observing and palpating the bladder. A distended bladder is seen as a suprapubic rounded bulge that is dull to percussion and fluctuates like a water-filled balloon. When the bladder is distended, the uterus is usually boggy in consistency, well above the umbilicus, and to the woman's right side.
- Assist the woman to void spontaneously. Measure amount of urine voided.
- Catheterize as necessary.
- Reassess after her voiding or catheterization to make sure that the bladder is not palpable and the fundus is firm and in the midline.

Lochia

- Observe lochia on perineal pads and on linen under the mother's buttocks. Determine amount and colour; note size and number of clots; note odour.
- Observe perineum for source of bleeding (e.g., lacerations, episiotomy).

Perineum

- Ask or assist woman to turn on her side and flex her upper leg on her hip.
- Gently lift upper buttock.
- Observe perineum in good lighting.
- Assess laceration repair or episiotomy site repair for *r*edness (erythema), *e*dema, *e*cchymosis (bruising), *d*rainage, and *a*pproximation (REEDA).
- Assess for presence of hemorrhoids.

perspiration, or emesis) during labour cause many women to express a strong desire to eat or drink soon after birth. In the absence of complications, a woman who has given birth vaginally, has recovered from the effects of the anaesthetic, and has stable vital signs, a firm uterus, and small-to-moderate lochial flow may have fluids and a regular diet, as desired. In the immediate postpartum period women who have undergone a Caesarean birth are usually restricted to clear liquids and ice chips.

Once the woman has had a chance to bond with the baby, breastfeed, and eat, most new mothers are ready for a nap or at least a quiet period of rest. Following this rest period the woman may want to shower and change clothes. Most new mothers are capable of self-care or are helped in these activities by family members or support persons.

Postanaesthesia Recovery

The woman who has given birth by Caesarean or who has received regional anaesthesia for a vaginal birth requires special attention during the recovery period. Obstetrical recovery areas are held to the same standard of care that would be expected of any other postanaesthesia recovery room. When caring for a woman recovering from anaesthesia, the nurse needs to have available cardiopulmonary support and emergency supplies. Women who are recovering from anaesthesia require further assessments every 15 minutes, including activity, respirations, oxygen saturation, level of consciousness, and colour.

NURSING ALERT

Regardless of her obstetrical status, no woman should be discharged from the recovery area until she has completely recovered from the effects of anaesthesia.

If the woman received general anaesthesia, she should be awake and alert and oriented to time, place, and person. Her respiratory rate should be within normal limits, and her oxygen saturation levels should be at least 95% as measured by a pulse oximeter. If the woman received epidural or spinal anaesthesia, she should be able to raise her legs, extended at the knees, off the bed; or flex her knees, place her feet flat on the bed, and raise her buttocks well off the bed. The numb or tingling, prickly sensation should be entirely gone from her legs. The length of time required to recover from regional anaesthesia varies greatly. Often it takes several hours for these anaesthetic effects to disappear completely.

Care of the Newborn

A brief assessment of the newborn can be performed while the baby is lying skin-to-skin on the mother. This includes checking the infant's airway and assigning the Apgar score; maintaining a patent airway; supporting respiratory effort; and preventing cold stress by drying the infant, making sure the infant maintains uninterrupted skin-to-skin contact with the mother, and covering the newborn with a warm blanket. A hat should be put on the newborn to keep the head warm. Newborns should only be brought to the radiant warmer if they

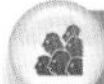

CULTURAL AWARENESS

Birth Story: The "Slimy, Wriggling" Infant

Leona moved to Canada from El Salvador several years ago, while pregnant with her second child. She spoke little English and had no family present for her labour and birth—her husband was at home with their older child. Leona explained that when her baby was born, the physician laid him on her abdomen. She took one look at the "slimy, wriggling" baby and promptly "passed out." She remembers waking up in her room some time later.

In El Salvador, she reported, a newborn is washed and wrapped in a blanket before being presented to the mother. She said the "Canadian" approach made the birthing experience much more traumatic than she had expected. Several years later, Leona was able to laugh at the memory, but she did not laugh at the time of her son's birth.

Source: Watts, N., & McDonald, C. (2007). The beginning of life: The perinatal period. In R. H. Srivastava (Ed.), *The healthcare professional's guide to clinical cultural competence*. Toronto, ON: Mosby.

require resuscitative measures. See Chapter 26 for further discussion of newborn care.

When the baby is at the breast, the nurse has an opportunity to give the newborn a vitamin K injection. There is strong evidence to support the role of breastfeeding in reducing pain in the newborn during a painful procedure (see Chapter 26). After the baby has gone to the breast, the baby can be weighed and measured, eye prophylaxis administered, and an identification bracelet applied that corresponds to the mother's identification bracelet. Once these activities are done, the baby should be given back to the mother and placed skin-to-skin to support transition of the newborn. In some agencies, the mother's partner (or another person designated by the mother) is also given a corresponding identification bracelet.

Care of the Family

Most parents enjoy being able to handle, hold, explore, and examine the baby immediately after birth. Both parents can assist with the thorough drying of the infant. Skin-to-skin contact should be encouraged based on cultural expectations (see Cultural Awareness box). Holding the newborn next to the skin of either parent helps to maintain the baby's temperature.

Many women wish to begin breastfeeding their newborns at this time, to take advantage of the infant's alert state (first period of reactivity) and stimulate the production of oxytocin that promotes contraction of the uterus and prevents hemorrhage. In most hospitals, breastfeeding is initiated within the first hour after birth. The fourth stage of labour is an excellent time to begin breastfeeding because the infant is in an alert state and ready to nurse.

Family–Newborn Relationships

The woman's reaction to the sight of her newborn may range from excited outbursts of laughing, talking, and even crying to apparent apathy. A polite smile and nod may be her only acknowledgment of the comments of nurses and the primary health care provider. Occasionally, the reaction is one of anger or indifference; the woman turns away from the baby, concentrates on her own pain, and may make hostile comments. These varied reactions can arise from pleasure, exhaustion, or deep disappointment. When evaluating parent–newborn interactions after birth, the nurse should also consider the cultural characteristics of the woman and her family and the expected behaviours of that culture. In some cultures, the birth of a male child is preferred, and women may grieve when a female child is born (Watts & McDonald, 2007).

Whatever the reaction and its cause may be, the woman needs continued acceptance and support from all staff. Notation of the parents' reaction to the newborn should be made in the recovery record. Nurses can assess this reaction by asking themselves the following questions: How do the parents look? What do they say? What do they do? Further assessment of the parent–newborn relationship can be conducted as care is given during the period of recovery. This is especially important if warning signs (e.g., passive or hostile reactions to newborn, disappointment with sex or appearance of newborn, absence of eye contact, or limited interaction of parents with each other) were noted immediately after birth. The nurse may find it helpful to discuss with the woman's primary health care provider any warning signs that may have been noted.

Siblings often experience interest and excitement when the newborn appears. They can then be encouraged to touch or hold the baby (Fig. 17-23).

Parents usually respond to praise of their newborn. Many need to be reassured that the dusky appearance of the baby's extremities immediately after birth is normal until circulation is well established. If appropriate, the nurse should explain the reason for the moulding of the newborn's head. Information about hospital routine can be communicated. However, it is important for nurses to recognize that the cultural background of the parents may influence expectations of care and handling of their newborn immediately after birth. For example, some traditional Southeast Asians believe that the head should not be touched because it is the most sacred part of a person's body. They also believe that praise of the baby is dangerous because jealous spirits may cause the baby harm or take it away (D'Avanzo, 2008).

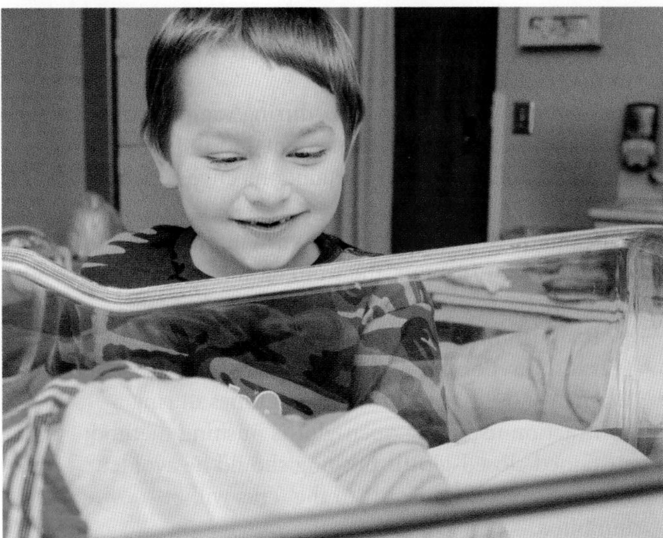

FIGURE 17-23 Big brother being introduced to baby brother. (Rob Hainer/Shutterstock.com.)

Determining a woman's satisfaction with and impressions of her childbirth experience is a critical component in the provision of high-quality maternal–newborn health care that meets the needs of women and families. Reviewing one's childbirth experience with someone who will listen, support, and explain has been found to reduce the degree of postpartum mood disorders experienced by many women during the first week or so after birth.

KEY POINTS

- The onset of labour may be difficult to determine for both nulliparous and multiparous women.
- The familiar environment of the pregnant woman's home is most often the ideal place for a woman during the latent phase of the first stage of labour.
- The nurse assumes much of the responsibility for assessing the progress of labour and keeping the primary health care provider informed about progress in labour and deviations from expected findings.
- The fetal heart rate and pattern reveal the fetal response to the stress of the labour process.
- Regardless of the actual labour and birth experience, the woman's or couple's perception of the birth experience is most likely to be positive when events and performances are consistent with expectations, especially regarding the woman maintaining control during labour and birth.
- The woman's level of anxiety may rise when she does not understand what is being said to her about her labour because of the medical terminology being used or because of a language barrier.
- Coaching, emotional support, and comfort measures help the woman to use her energy constructively in relaxing and working with the contractions.
- The progress of labour is enhanced when a woman changes her position frequently during the first stage of labour.
- Doulas provide a continuous supportive presence during labour that can have a positive effect on the process of childbirth and its outcome.
- The cultural beliefs and practices of a woman and her support people, including her partner, can have a profound influence on their approach to labour and birth.
- The quality of the nurse–patient relationship is a factor in the woman's ability to cope with the stressors of the labour process.
- Siblings present for labour and birth need preparation and support for the event.
- Women with a history of sexual abuse often experience profound stress and anxiety during childbirth.

- Assessment of the labouring woman's urinary output and bladder is critical to ensure her progress and prevent injury to the bladder.
- Inability to palpate the cervix during vaginal examination indicates that complete effacement and full dilation have occurred and is the only certain, objective sign that the second stage has begun.
- When allowed to respond to the rhythmic nature of the second stage of labour, the woman normally changes body position, bears down spontaneously, and vocalizes (open-glottis pushing) when she perceives the urge to push (Ferguson reflex).
- Women should bear down several times during a contraction using the open-glottis pushing method; sustained closed-glottis pushing should be avoided because oxygen transport to the fetus will be inhibited.
- Nurses can use the role of advocate to prevent routine use of episiotomy and reduce the incidence of lacerations by empowering women to take an active role in their childbirth and educating health care providers about approaches to managing childbirth that reduce the incidence of perineal trauma.
- Objective signs indicate that the placenta has separated and is ready to be expelled; excessive traction (pulling) on the umbilical cord, before the placenta has separated, can result in maternal injury. Most parents and families enjoy being able to handle, hold, explore, and examine the baby immediately after birth. Skin-to-skin contact between the mother or partner and baby should be encouraged.
- During the fourth stage of labour the woman's fundal tone, lochial flow, and vital signs should be assessed frequently to ensure that she is physically recovering well after giving birth.
- Women should be encouraged to initiate breastfeeding within 60 minutes of birth.
- Nurses should observe progress in the development of parent–child relationships and be alert for warning signs that may appear during the immediate postpartum period.
- Stimulation of the mothers' nipple manually or by the infant's suckling stimulates the release of oxytocin from the maternal posterior pituitary gland. Oxytocin stimulates the uterus to contract and thereby prevents hemorrhage.
- A woman who has just given birth benefits from reviewing her childbirth experience with the nurse who managed her care during the process of labour and birth.

evolve WEBSITE

Visit the Evolve website for additional resources related to the content in this chapter such as Case Studies, Critical Thinking Case Study Answers, Nursing Care Plans, Nursing Processes, Nursing Skills, and Review Questions for Exam Preparation at: *http://evolve.elsevier.com/Canada/Perry/maternal/*

REFERENCES

Aasheim, V., Nilsen, A. B. V., Lukasse, M., & Reinar, L. M. (2011). Perineal techniques during the second stage of labour for reducing perineal trauma. *Cochrane Database of Systematic Reviews*, (12). doi:10.1002/14651858.CD006672.pub2.

Adams, E. (2010). If transmen can have babies, how will perinatal nursing adapt? *MCN American Journal of Maternal/Child Nursing*, *35*(1), 26–32.

American Congress of Obstetricians and Gynecologists. (2014). Obstetric care consensus No. 1: Safe prevention of the primary cesarean delivery. *Obstetrics & Gynecology*, *123*(3), 693–711. doi:10.1097/01.AOG.0000444441.04111.1d.

Armson, A., Allan, D. S., & Casper, R. F. (2015). SOGC clinical practice guideline: Umbilical cord blood: Counselling, collection and banking. *Journal of Obstetrician and Gynaecologists of Canada*, *37*(9), 832–884.

Association of Women's Health, Obstetric, and Neonatal Nurses (AWHONN). (2011). AWHONN position statement: Nursing support of laboring women. *Journal of Obstetric, Gynecologic & Neonatal Nursing*, *40*(5), 665–666.

Beckmann, M. M., & Stock, O. M. (2013). Antenatal perineal massage for reducing perineal trauma. *Cochrane Database of Systematic Reviews*, (4). doi:10.1002/14651858.CD005123.pub3.

Berghella, V., Baxter, J., & Chauhan, S. (2008). Evidence-based labor and delivery management. *American Journal of Obstetrics and Gynecology*, *199*(5), 445–454.

Blackburn, S. T. (2013). *Maternal, fetal, and neonatal physiology: A clinical perspective* (4th ed.). St. Louis: Saunders.

Burke, C. (2010). Active versus expectant management of the third stage of labor and implementation of a protocol. *Journal of Perinatal & Neonatal Nursing*, *24*(3), 215–228. doi:10.1097/JPN.0b013e3181e8ce90.

Callister, L. C. (2014). Integrating cultural beliefs and practices when caring for childbearing women and families. In K. Rice Simpson & P. Creehan (Eds.), *AWHONN's perinatal nursing* (4th ed.). Philadelphia: Lippincott Williams & Wilkins.

Canadian Nurses Association. (2010). *Position statement: Promoting cultural competence in nursing*. Ottawa: Author. Retrieved from <https://www.cna-aiic.ca/~/media/cna/page-content/pdf-en/ps114_cultural_competence_2010_e.pdf?la=en>.

Cluett, E. R., & Burns, E. (2009). Immersion in water in labour and birth. *Cochrane Database of Systematic Reviews*, (2). doi:10.1002/14651858.CD000111.pub3.

D'Avanzo, C. E. (2008). *Mosby's pocket guide to cultural health assessment* (4th ed.). St. Louis: Mosby.

Davies, G., Maxwell, C., McLeod, L., et al. (2010). SOGC clinical practice guideline: Obesity in pregnancy. *Journal of Obstetrics and Gynaecology Canada*, *32*(2), 165–173.

Diaz-Castro, J., Florido, J., Kajarabille, N., et al. (2014). The timing of cord clamping and oxidative stress in term newborns. *Pediatrics*, *134*(2), 257–264.

Gilbert, E. (2011). *Manual of high risk pregnancy & delivery* (5th ed.). St. Louis: Mosby.

Gillesby, E., Burns, S., Dempsey, A., et al. (2010). Comparison of delayed versus immediate pushing during second stage of labor for nulliparous women with epidural anesthesia. *Journal of Obstetric, Gynecologic & Neonatal Nursing*, *39*(6), 635–643.

Hanson, L. (2009). Second-stage labor care: Challenges in spontaneous bearing down. *Journal of Perinatal & Neonatal Nursing*, *23*(1), 31–39.

Hayes, E. H. (2016). Consumption of the placenta in the postpartum period. *Journal of Obstetric, Gynecologic & Neonatal Nursing*, *45*(1), 78–89.

Hodnett, E., Gates, S., Hofmeyr, G., et al. (2011). Continuous support for women during childbirth. *Cochrane Database of Systematic Reviews*, (3).

Jacobson, P., & Turner, L. (2008). Management of the second stage of labor in women with epidural analgesia. *Journal of Midwifery & Women's Health, 53*, 82–85.

James, D. (2011). Routine obstetrical interventions: Research agenda for the next decade. *Journal of Perinatal & Neonatal Nursing, 25*(2), 148–152.

Johansson, M., Rubertsson, C., Radestad, I., et al. (2012). Childbirth—an emotionally demanding experience for fathers. *Sexual & Reproductive Health Care, 3*(1), 11–20.

Jones, L., Othman, M., Dowswell, T., et al. (2012). Pain management for women in labour: An overview of systematic reviews. *Cochrane Database of Systematic Reviews*, (3). doi:10.1002/14651858.CD009234.pub2.

Kelly, M., Johnson, E., Lee, V., et al. (2010). Delayed versus immediate pushing in second stage of labor. *MCN American Journal of Maternal/Child Nursing, 35*(2), 81–87.

Kujawa-Myles, S., Noel-Weiss, J., Dunn, S., et al. (2015). Maternal intravenous fluids and postpartum breast changes: A pilot observational study. *International Breastfeeding Journal, 10*, 18. Retrieved from <http://www.internationalbreastfeedingjournal.com/content/pdf/s13006-015-0043-8.pdf>.

Lawrence, A., Lewis, L., Hofmeyr, G. J., et al. (2009). Maternal positions and mobility during first stage labour. *Cochrane Database of Systematic Reviews*, (2).

Leduc, D., Senikas, V., Lalonde, A. B., et al. (2009). Active management of the third stage of labour: Prevention and treatment of postpartum hemorrhage. *Journal of Obstetrics and Gynaecology Canada, 31*(10), 980–993.

Liston, R., Sawchuck, D., Young, D., et al. (2007). Fetal health surveillance: Antepartum and intrapartum consensus guideline. *Journal of Obstetrics and Gynaecology Canada, 29*(9 Suppl. 4), s1–s56.

McDonald, S. J., Middleton, P., Dowswell, T., & Morris, P. S. (2013). Effect of timing of umbilical cord clamping of term infants on maternal and neonatal outcomes. *Cochrane Database of Systematic Reviews*, (7). doi:10.1002/14651858.CD004074.pub3.

Miller, L. A., Miller, D. A., & Tucker, S. M. (2013). *Pocket guide to fetal monitoring and assessment* (7th ed.). St. Louis: Mosby.

Money, D., Allen, V. M., Yudin, H., et al. (2013). SOGC clinical practice guideline: The prevention of early-onset neonatal group B streptococcal disease. *Journal of Obstetrics and Gynaecology Canada, 35*(10), e1–e10.

Money, D., Steben, M., Wong, T., et al. (2008). SOGC clinical practice guideline: Guidelines for the management of herpes simplex virus in pregnancy. *Journal of Obstetrics and Gynaecology Canada, 208*, 514–518.

More, O. B. (2010). *Management of labour*. Retrieved from <http://www.moreob.com>.

Perron, L., Synikas, V., Burnett, M., et al. (2013). SOGC clinical practice guideline: Female genital cutting. *Journal of Obstetrics and Gynaecology Canada, 35*(11), e1–e18.

Pintucci, A., Meregalli, V., Colombo, P., & Fiorilli, A. (2014). Premature rupture of membranes at term in low risk women: How long should we wait in the "latent phase"? *Journal of Perinatal Medicine, 42*(2), 189–196. doi:10.1515/jpm-2013-0017.

Public Health Agency of Canada. (2012). *Canadian hospitals' maternity policies and practices survey*. Ottawa: Author. Retrieved from <http://www.phac-aspc.gc.ca/rhs-ssg/chmpps-eppmhc-2012-eng.php>.

Registered Nurses' Association of Ontario. (2015). *Person- and family-centred care*. Toronto: Author. Retrieved from <http://rnao.ca/sites/rnao-ca/files/FINAL_Web_Version_1.pdf>.

Reveiz, L., Gaitán, H. G., & Cuervo, L. G. (2013). Enemas during labour. *Cochrane Database of Systematic Reviews*, (7). doi:10.1002/14651858.CD000330.pub4.

Sharts-Hopko, N. (2010). Oral intake during labor: A review of the evidence. *MCN: American Journal of Maternal/Child Nursing, 35*(4), 197–203.

Simkin, P. (2012). *Doulas of North America (DONA) international position paper: The birth doula's contribution to modern maternity care*. Retrieved from <http://www.dona.org/PDF/Birth%20Position%20Paper_rev%200912.pdf>.

Simpson, K. R., & O'Brien-Abel, N. (2014). Labor and birth. In K. Rice Simpson & P. A. Creehan (Eds.), *AWHONN's perinatal nursing* (4th ed.). Philadelphia: Lippincott, Williams & Wilkins.

Simpson, S., Cesario, S., Morin, K., et al. (2008). *Nursing care and management of the second stage of labor: Evidence-based clinical practice guideline* (2nd ed.). Washington, DC: Association of Women's Health, Obstetric and Neonatal Nurses.

Singata, M., Tranmer, J., & Gyte, G. M. L. (2013). Restricting oral fluid and food intake during labour. *Cochrane Database of Systematic Reviews*, (8). doi:10.1002/14651858.CD003930.pub3.

Society of Obstetricians and Gynecologists of Canada. (2016). *Advances in labour and risk management (ALARM) course syllabus* (23rd ed). Ottawa, ON: Author.

Walls, D. (2009). Herbs and natural therapies for pregnancy, birth, and breastfeeding. *International Journal of Childbirth Education, 24*(2), 29–37.

Watts, N., & McDonald, C. (2007). The beginning of life: The perinatal period. In R. H. Srivastava (Ed.), *The Healthcare professional's guide to clinical cultural competence*. Toronto, Mosby.

Wing, D., & Farinelli, C. (2012). Abnormal labor and induction of labor. In S. Gabbe, J. Niebyl, J. Simpson, et al. (Eds.), *Obstetrics: Normal and problem pregnancies* (6th ed.). Philadelphia: Saunders.

Wolfe-Roubatis, E., & Spatz, D. L. (2015). Transgender men and lactation: What nurses need to know. *MCN American Journal of Maternal/Child Nursing, 40*(1), 32–38.

Zwelling, E. (2010). Overcoming the challenges: Maternal movement and positioning to facilitate labor progress. *MCN: American Journal of Maternal/Child Nursing, 35*(2), 72–78.

ADDITIONAL RESOURCES

Association of Ontario Midwives: Tip Sheet for Providing Care to Trans Men and All "Trans Masculine Spectrum" Clients: <http://www.rainbowhealthontario.ca/wp-content/uploads/woocommerce_uploads/2014/08/Midwives%20-%20Tip%20sheet%20for%20working%20with%20trans%20clients.pdf>.

Perinatal Services BC—Core Competencies for Management of Labour: <http://www.perinatalservicesbc.ca/health-professionals/guidelines-standards/standards/core-competencies-for-management-of-labour>.

CHAPTER 18

Pain Management During Labour

France Morin, Lauren B. Rivard

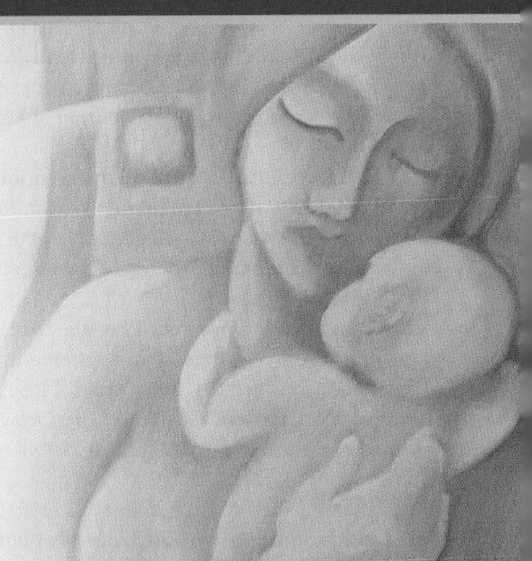

evolve WEBSITE

Visit the Evolve website for additional resources related to the content in this chapter such as Case Studies, Critical Thinking Case Study Answers, Nursing Care Plans, Nursing Processes, Nursing Skills, and Review Questions for Exam Preparation at: http://evolve.elsevier.com/Canada/Perry/maternal/

OBJECTIVES

On completion of this chapter the reader will be able to:

- Describe breathing and relaxation techniques used for each stage of labour.
- Identify nonpharmacological strategies to enhance relaxation and decrease discomfort during labour.
- Discuss types of analgesia and anaesthesia used during labour.
- Compare pharmacological methods for relief of discomfort in different stages of labour and for different methods of birth.
- Describe nursing responsibilities appropriate in providing care for a woman receiving non-pharmacological pain relief methods as well as analgesia and anaesthesia during labour.

Pain is a biological, psychological, and cultural experience that involves both physical stimuli and emotional and cognitive processing, which often occur within specific social and cultural contexts (Gibson, 2014). The International Association for the Study of Pain (IASP) defines pain as "an unpleasant sensory and emotional experience associated with actual or potential tissue damage, or described in terms of such damage" (IASP, 2012). The pain experience associated with labour is unique. Labour pain is situation specific and of limited duration and, contrary to many other sources of pain, is not indicative of underlying pathology but part of a normal physiological process. Labour pain is also a complex, multidimensional experience that is highly variable; labour pain can range from excruciating to pleasurable for different women and on different occasions (Lundgren & Dahlberg, 1998; Melzack, Kinch, Dobkin, et al., 1984). Pain is a complex phenomenon that includes sensory, cognitive, and affective components. The painful experience is the result of the interaction between these components (Fig. 18-1). The *nociceptive component* (1), purely physiological, refers to peripheral nerve activity; the *sensory-discriminative component* (2) refers to the perceived pain intensity; the *motivational-affective component* (3), under the higher nervous centres, is described by the unpleasant pain aspect, while the *cognitive-behavioural component* (4) reflects the range of behaviours related to pain. These components can exist independently or influence each other; they may also exist in the form of various combinations. Pain in labour and birth is not easily defined, nor is it simple to assess (Roberts, Gulliver, Fisher, et al., 2010).

Pregnant women commonly worry about the pain they will experience during labour and birth and how they will react to and deal with that pain. A variety of nonpharmacological and pharmacological methods can help the woman or the couple cope with the pain of labour. The methods selected depend on the situation, their availability, the health care providers' knowledge of labour pain management, and the preferences of the woman.

This chapter discusses the physiological basis for pain and factors that affect women's perception and response to pain. It will also describe pain management options and nursing care

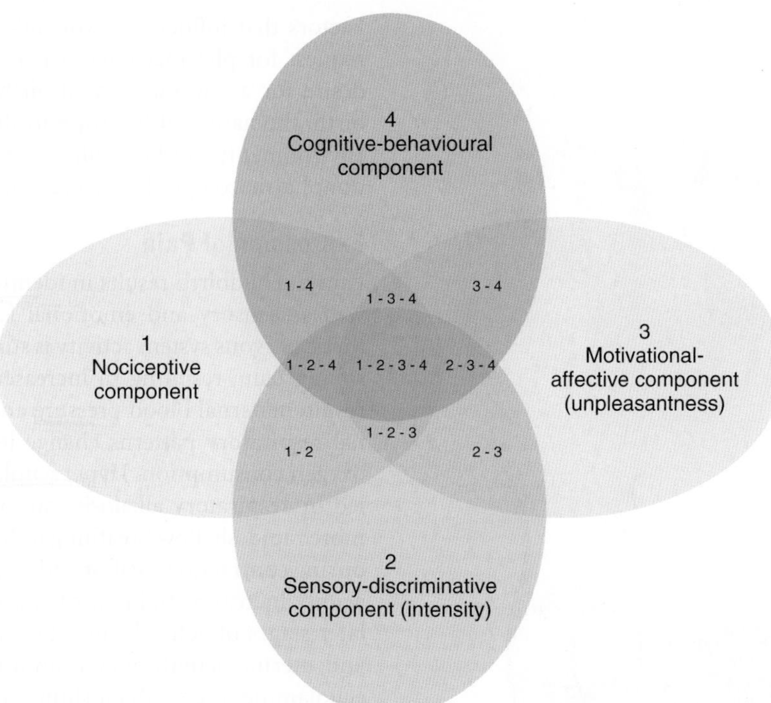

FIGURE 18-1 Circular pain model illustrating the components of pain and their interrelationships. (From Marchand, S. [2012]. *The phenomenon of pain* [p. 15]. Seattle, WA: International Association for the Study of Pain, IASP Press.)

for nonpharmacological and pharmacological methods commonly used for pain relief during labour and birth.

PAIN DURING LABOUR AND BIRTH

Neurological Origins

The pain and discomfort experienced during labour have three origins: visceral, somatic, and referred. During the first stage of labour, uterine contractions cause cervical dilation and effacement. Uterine *ischemia* (decreased blood flow and therefore local oxygen deficit) results from compression of the arteries supplying the myometrium during uterine contractions. Pain impulses during the first stage of labour are transmitted via the T10 to T12 and L1 spinal nerve segments and accessory lower thoracic and upper lumbar sympathetic nerves. These nerves originate in the uterine body and cervix (Blackburn, 2013).

The pain from distension of the lower uterine segment, stretching of cervical tissues as it effaces and dilates, pressure and traction on adjacent structures (e.g., fallopian tubes, ovaries, ligaments) and nerves, and uterine ischemia that predominates during the first stage of labour is *visceral* pain. It is located over the lower portion of the abdomen. *Referred* pain occurs when the pain that originates in the uterus radiates to the abdominal wall, lumbosacral area of the back, iliac crests, gluteal area, thighs, and lower back (Blackburn, 2013; Zwelling, Johnson, & Allen, 2006).

During the first stage of labour, the woman usually experiences pain and discomfort only during contractions and is free of pain between contractions. Some women, especially those whose fetus is in a posterior position, experience continuous contraction-related low back pain, even in the interval between contractions. As labour progresses and the pain becomes more intense and persistent, women become fatigued and discouraged, often experiencing difficulty coping with contractions (Burke, 2013; Zwelling et al., 2006).

During the second stage of labour, the woman experiences *somatic* pain, which is often described as intense, sharp, burning, and well localized. This pain results from the following:

- Distension of and traction on the peritoneum and uterocervical supports during contractions
- Pressure against the bladder and rectum
- Stretching and dissention of perineal tissues and the pelvic floor to allow passage of the fetus
- Lacerations of soft tissue (e.g., cervix, vagina, perineum)

As women concentrate on the work of bearing down to give birth to their baby, they may report a decrease in pain intensity (Blackburn, 2013; Burke, 2013). Pain impulses during the second stage of labour are carried from perineal tissues via the S2–S4 spinal nerve segments and the parasympathetic system (Blackburn, 2013).

Pain experienced during the third stage of labour and the afterpains of the early postpartum period are uterine, similar to that experienced early in the first stage of labour. Areas of discomfort during labour are illustrated in Fig. 18-2.

Perception of Pain

The pain threshold is the level at which a person physically perceives a sensation as painful (IASP, 2012). Although the pain threshold is remarkably similar in everyone regardless of gender, social, ethnic, or cultural differences, these differences play a

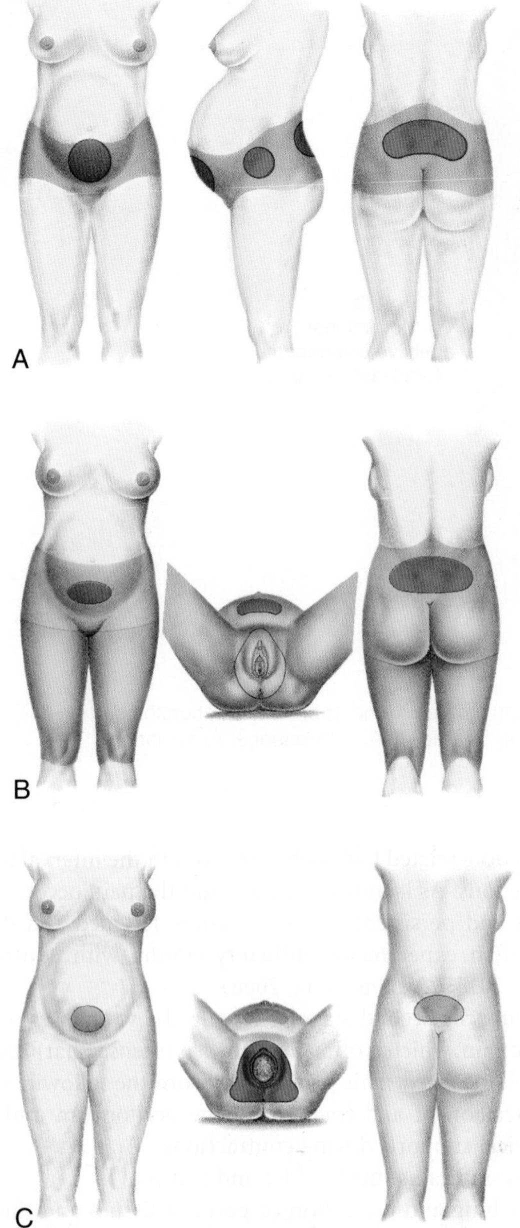

FIGURE 18-2 Discomfort during labour. **A:** Distribution of labour pain during first stage. **B:** Distribution of labour pain during later phase of first stage and early phase of second stage. **C:** Distribution of labour pain during later phase of second stage and during birth. (Grey shading indicates areas of mild discomfort; light-coloured shading indicates areas of moderate discomfort; dark-coloured shading indicates areas of intense discomfort.)

definite role in a person's perception of and behavioural responses to pain. The meaning of pain and the verbal and nonverbal expressions given to pain are apparently learned from interactions within the primary social group. Cultural influences may impose certain behavioural expectations regarding acceptable and unacceptable behaviour when one experiences pain.

Pain tolerance refers to the level of pain, in this case a labouring woman, is willing to endure (IASP, 2012). When this level is exceeded, she will seek measures to relieve the pain. Factors that influence a woman's pain tolerance level and her request for pharmacological pain relief measures include her desire for a natural, vaginal birth; her preparation for childbirth; the nature of her support during labour; the health care environment; and her willingness and ability to participate in nonpharmacological measures for comfort (Burke, 2013).

Expression of Pain

Pain in childbirth results in identifiable physiological effects as well as sensory and emotional (affective) responses. Sympathetic nervous system activity is stimulated in response to intensifying pain, resulting in increased catecholamine levels. As a result, maternal blood pressure and heart rate increase. Maternal respiratory patterns change in response to an increase in oxygen consumption. Hyperventilation, sometimes accompanied by respiratory alkalosis, can occur as pain intensifies, and more rapid, shallow breathing techniques should be encouraged during contractions. Pallor and diaphoresis may be seen. Gastric acidity increases, and nausea and vomiting are common in the later stages of active labour. Placental perfusion may decrease, and uterine activity may diminish, because of increased catecholamine levels, which shunt blood from the uterus to vital organs, potentially prolonging labour and affecting fetal well-being.

Certain emotional (affective) expressions of suffering may be seen and include increasing anxiety with lessened perceptual field, writhing, crying, groaning, gesturing (hand clenching and wringing), and excessive muscular excitability throughout the body.

Factors Influencing Pain Response

Pain during childbirth is unique to each woman. How she perceives or interprets that pain is influenced by a variety of physiological, psychological, emotional, social, cultural, and environmental factors (Zwelling et al., 2006). Women who approach pain as a challenge for which they have sufficient resources to cope effectively are unlikely to equate pain with suffering. In contrast, women without sufficient self-confidence and coping strategies may feel threatened and view their pain experience as suffering (Simkin & Bolding, 2004).

Pain is normally something most people try to avoid, but pain in labour needs to be presented as normal and having an important role in promoting labour. Women who learn to work with the pain may facilitate movement of the fetus through the birth canal. Actively responding to the pain by changing positions, rocking, or moaning may speed up the process of labour. The people supporting the woman in labour also need to understand the role of pain in normal labour and to feel comfortable watching the woman work with her pain.

Physiological Factors

A variety of physiological factors can affect the intensity of pain experienced by women during childbirth. Women with a history of dysmenorrhea may experience increased pain during childbirth as a result of higher prostaglandin levels. Back pain associated with menstruation also may increase the likelihood of contraction-related low back pain. Other physical factors that

CULTURAL AWARENESS

Some Cultural Beliefs About Pain

The following are only examples of how women of different cultural backgrounds may react to pain. Because they are generalizations, the nurse must assess each woman experiencing pain that is related to childbirth.

- Asian women may appear stoic and not exhibit reactions to pain, although it is acceptable to exhibit pain during childbirth. They consider it impolite to accept something when it is first offered; therefore, pain interventions may need to be offered more than once. Acupuncture may be used for pain relief.
- Arab or Middle Eastern women may be vocal in response to labour pain. They may prefer medication for pain relief.
- Latin American women may be stoic until late in labour, when they may become vocal and request pain relief.
- Indigenous women may use medications or remedies made from indigenous plants. They are often stoic in response to labour pain.
- Women of African descent may express pain openly. Use of medication for pain relief varies.

affect pain intensity include fatigue, the interval and duration of contractions, fetal size and position, rapidity of fetal descent, and maternal position (Zwelling et al., 2006). When upright positions are assumed during labour, they seem to result in decreased pain and an overall increase in comfort compared with that in the supine position. Women also report that being able to move freely to find a position of comfort is an important factor in reducing pain and muscle tension and in maintaining control during labour. The relation of fetal size to the dimensions of the maternal pelvis may also influence pain intensity.

Beta-endorphins are endogenous opioids secreted by the pituitary gland that act on the central and peripheral nervous systems to reduce pain. The level of beta-endorphins increases during pregnancy and birth in humans. Beta-endorphins are associated with feelings of euphoria and analgesia. The pain threshold may rise as beta-endorphin levels increase, enabling women in labour to tolerate acute pain (Blackburn, 2013).

Culture

As nurses care for women and families from a variety of cultural backgrounds, they must have knowledge and understanding of how culture mediates pain. Although all women expect to experience at least some pain and discomfort during childbirth, it is often their culture and religious belief system that determines how they will perceive, interpret, and respond to and manage the pain. For example, women with strong religious beliefs often accept pain as a necessary and inevitable part of bringing a new life into the world (Callister, Khalaf, Semenic, et al., 2003).

An understanding of the beliefs, values, expectations, and practices of various cultures will narrow the cultural gap and help the nurse to assess the labouring woman's pain experience more accurately. This will in turn enable the nurse to provide culturally sensitive care by using appropriate pain-relief measures that preserve the woman's sense of control and self-confidence (see Cultural Awareness box). It is important for the nurse to recognize that, although a woman's behaviour in response to pain may vary according to her cultural background, it may not accurately reflect the intensity of the pain she is experiencing. At the same time, each woman needs to be assessed as an individual, as each woman has a different experience of pain. The nurse must assess the woman for the physiological effects of pain and listen to the words the woman uses to describe the sensory and affective qualities of her pain (see Community Focus box).

COMMUNITY FOCUS

Culture and Pain

Talk to a man and a woman from a culture different from your own who have experienced childbirth. Ask her to describe her reactions to pain, how she sought relief of pain, the atmosphere of the childbirth setting, and the attitudes of the health care providers. Ask him if he was present for the birth and what his role in the birth was. How did his culture influence his role and reaction to childbirth? How did her culture influence her response to labour and the associated pain? What expressions of pain are "acceptable" in her culture? If he was present, how did he help her deal with the pain? What is the role of support persons in the labour process? Are the responses of the couple different from your responses to those same questions?

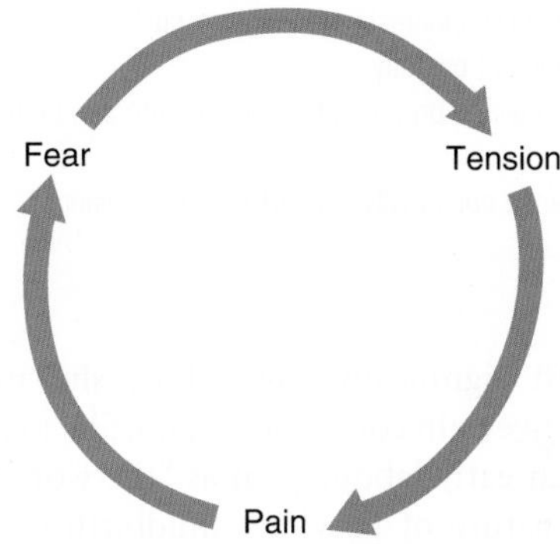

FIGURE 18-3 Fear–tension–pain cycle.

Anxiety and Fear

Anxiety and fear are commonly associated with increased pain during labour. Mild anxiety is considered normal for a woman during labour and birth. However, excessive anxiety and fear cause catecholamine secretion, resulting in more pelvic pain stimuli reaching the brain; this in turn magnifies pain perception (Fig. 18-3). As anxiety heightens, muscle tension increases, the effectiveness of the uterine contractions decreases, and the experience of discomfort increases, and a cycle of increased fear and anxiety begins (Blackburn, 2013). Ultimately, this cycle will slow the progress of labour. The woman's confidence in her ability to cope with pain will be diminished, potentially resulting in reduced effectiveness of pain-relief measures being used.

Previous Experience

Previous experience with pain and childbirth may affect a woman's description of her pain and her ability to cope with it. Childbirth for a healthy young adult woman may be her first

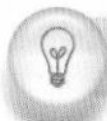

CRITICAL THINKING CASE STUDY

Anxiety in a Multipara in Active Labour

Jody was admitted in labour to a labour, birthing, and recovery (LBR) room 2 hours ago. She is 39 weeks' gestation in her second pregnancy. She is noticeably anxious and tells you that her first pregnancy ended at term but that the labour was "terrible. It was 22 hours long. I had an epidural but had to push and push to get the baby out." What interventions are appropriate?

QUESTIONS

1. Evidence—Is there sufficient evidence to draw conclusions about what intervention is needed?
2. Assumptions—Describe underlying assumptions about the following issues:
   a. Effects of anxiety on progress in labour
   b. Effect of parity on labour
   c. Effect of epidural analgesia on ability to push
   d. Education needed by Jody
3. What implications and priorities for nursing care can be made at this time?
4. Does the evidence objectively support your conclusions?

experience with significant pain; thus, she may not have developed effective pain coping strategies. She may describe the intensity of even early labour pain as "the worst pain she can imagine." The nature of previous childbirth experiences also may affect a woman's responses to pain. For women who have had a difficult and painful previous birth experience, anxiety and fear from the past experience may lead to an increased perception of pain (see Critical Thinking Case Study). Conversely, a woman who has experienced a labour and birth in which the degree of pain matched her expectations and in which her coping skills were successful may have less anxiety and feel a sense of pride in her accomplishment (Trout, 2004). However, her anxiety is likely to increase if previously successful coping skills were ineffective during a more difficult labour.

Sensory pain for **nulliparous** women is often greater than that for **multiparous** women during early latent labour (dilation less than 5 cm) because their reproductive tract structures are less supple. During the active phase of the first stage of labour and during the second stage of labour, multiparous women may experience greater sensory pain than nulliparous women because their more supple tissue increases the speed of fetal descent and thereby intensifies pain. The firmer tissue of nulliparous women results in a slower, more gradual descent. Affective pain is usually greater for nulliparous women throughout the first stage of labour but decreases for both nulliparous and multiparous women during the second stage of labour. Parity may also influence the perception of labour pain because nulliparous women often have longer labours and therefore tend to experience greater fatigue.

Fatigue and sleep deprivation magnify pain. Most women have a decrease in quality of sleep over the last few days of pregnancy, and the spontaneous onset of labour occurs most often during the night (Beebe & Lee, 2007). Thus, many women have an increased perception of the intensity of pain during labour.

Gate-Control Theory of Pain

Even particularly intense pain can at times be ignored. This is possible because certain nerve cell groupings within the spinal cord, brainstem, and cerebral cortex have the ability to modulate the pain impulse through a blocking mechanism. The gate-control theory of pain helps explain the way that hypnosis and the pain-relief techniques taught in childbirth preparation classes work to relieve the pain of labour. According to this theory, pain sensations travel along sensory nerve pathways to the brain, but only a limited number of sensations, or messages, can travel through these nerve pathways at one time. By using distraction techniques, such as massage or stroking, music, focal points, and imagery, the capacity of nerve pathways to transmit pain is reduced or completely blocked. These distractions are thought to work by closing down a hypothetical gate in the spinal cord, thus preventing pain signals from reaching the brain. The perception of pain stimuli is thereby diminished.

In addition, when the woman in labour engages in neuromuscular and motor activity, such as changing positions and walking, activity within the spinal cord itself further modifies the transmission of pain. Cognitive work involving concentration on breathing and relaxation requires selective and directed cortical activity that activates and closes the gating mechanism as well. As labour intensifies, more complex cognitive techniques are required to maintain effectiveness. Therefore, the gate-control theory underscores the need for a supportive birth setting that allows the labouring woman to relax and use various higher mental activities.

Supportive Care

Although the predominant medical approach to labour is that it is painful and the pain must be removed, an alternative view is that labour is a natural process; women can experience comfort and transcend the discomfort or pain of birth. Having needs and desires met engenders a feeling of comfort. Comfort may be viewed as strengthening. The most helpful interventions in enhancing comfort are using a caring nursing approach and providing a continuous supportive presence.

Current evidence indicates that a woman's satisfaction with her childbirth experience is determined by how well her personal expectations of childbirth were met and the quality of support and interaction she received from her caregivers (Box 18-1). In addition, her satisfaction is influenced by the degree to which she was able to stay in control of her labour and to participate in decision making regarding her labour, including the pain-relief measures used (Albers, 2007; Zwelling et al., 2006).

The value of the continuous supportive presence of a person (e.g., doulas, family members, friends, nurses, or partner) during labour who provides physical comfort, facilitates communication, and offers information and guidance to the woman in labour has long been known. Continuous support begun early in labour significantly relieves pain, improves outcomes, decreases interventions (e.g., use of pharmacological pain-relief measures) and complication rates (e.g., Caesarean rates and assisted vaginal birth) associated with labour, and enhances overall maternal satisfaction. Interestingly, in one study a more positive effect was achieved when the continuous support was

BOX 18-1 SUGGESTED MEASURES FOR SUPPORTING A WOMAN IN LABOUR

- Provide companionship and reassurance.
- Offer positive reinforcement and praise.
- Encourage participation in distracting activities and nonpharmacological measures for comfort.
- Encourage fluid intake.
- Provide nourishment if possible.
- Assist with personal hygiene.
- Offer information and advice.
- Involve the woman in decision making regarding her care.
- Interpret the woman's wishes to other health care providers and to her support group.
- Create a relaxing environment.
- Use a calm and confident approach.
- Support and encourage the woman's family members by role modelling labour support measures and providing time for breaks.

provided by people who were not part of the staff of the hospital (Hodnett, Gates, Hofmeyr, et al., 2013). The Society of Obstetricians and Gynaecologists of Canada (SOGC) recommends that all women in labour receive continuous close support from an appropriately trained person (Liston, Sawchuck, Young, et al., 2007).

Environment

The quality of the environment can influence pain perception and the labouring woman's ability to cope with her pain. Environment includes the individuals present (e.g., how they communicate, their philosophy of care, practice policies, and quality of support) and the physical space in which the labour occurs (Burke, 2013; Zwelling et al., 2006). Women usually prefer to be cared for by familiar caregivers in a comfortable, homelike setting. The environment should be safe and private, allowing a woman to feel free to be herself as she tries out different comfort measures. Stimuli such as light, noise, and temperature should be adjusted according to the woman's preferences. The environment should have space for movement, and equipment should be readily available for a variety of nonpharmacological pain-relief measures, such as birthing balls, comfortable chairs, tubs, and showers. The familiarity of the environment can be enhanced by bringing items from home, such as pillows, objects for a focal point, music, and DVDs.

ASSESSING COPING DURING LABOUR

The observant nurse will look for cues to identify the woman's desired level of control in the management of pain and its relief. Commonly, it is not the amount of pain the woman experiences but whether she meets her goals for herself in coping with the pain that influences her perception of the birth experience as "good" or "bad."

The nurse should never assume that, because a woman is in labour, her pain must be uterine in origin. Pain is a subjective phenomenon; as such, the nurse must listen to the woman's description of her pain. A self-assessment tool such as a visual analog scale allows the woman to indicate on a line how severe or intense she perceives her pain to be. Pain is rated from "no pain" to "pain as bad as it can possibly be." Self-assessment is recommended, to ensure that pain management is based on the subjective nature of the woman's pain rather than on the nurse's judgement of it. It is not unusual for a nurse to overestimate or underestimate the pain being experienced by a patient. When there are major cultural differences between the health care provider and the patient, inaccurate interpretation of pain intensity is more likely to occur.

It is critical that the nurse take note of all pain characteristics, including location, intensity, quality, frequency, duration, and effectiveness of relief measures. While pain scales may be used with the labouring woman, their use may not always be appropriate as all women cope with pain differently. Some women may find questions about their level of pain confusing or annoying (Gulliver, Fisher, & Roberts, 2008). Nurses may assume that if a woman rates her pain level as high she requires medication, but some women may be able to manage high levels of pain during labour if they have the appropriate supportive care. Open-ended questions regarding how a woman is coping with labour may be more effective in ensuring that the woman's pain management needs are met. Gulliver et al. (2008) developed a tool that assists nurses in assessing how the mother is managing pain during labour as well as providing appropriate interventions depending on the assessment (Fig. 18-4). Use of the coping algorithm enables the nurse to provide care that is appropriate to that particular woman.

By completing a thorough assessment of the labouring woman, the nurse will be able to provide the appropriate pain-relief measures required by the woman. These measures may include nonpharmacological pain relief or the use of medication.

NONPHARMACOLOGICAL MANAGEMENT OF DISCOMFORT

Minimizing pain during labour is important. Nonpharmacological measures are often simple and safe, have few if any major adverse effects, are relatively inexpensive, and can be used throughout labour. In addition, they provide the woman with a sense of control over her childbirth as she makes choices about the measures that are best for her. During the prenatal period, the woman should explore a variety of nonpharmacological measures. Techniques that she finds helpful in relieving stress and enhancing relaxation (e.g., music, meditation, massage, warm baths) may be very effective as components of a plan for managing labour pain. The woman should be encouraged to communicate to her health care providers her preferences for relaxation and pain-relief measures and to actively participate in their implementation.

The woman's perception of her behaviour during labour is of utmost importance in how she feels about her birth experience. If she has planned a nonmedicated birth but then needs and accepts medication, her self-esteem may falter. The nurse needs to provide verbal and nonverbal acceptance of her

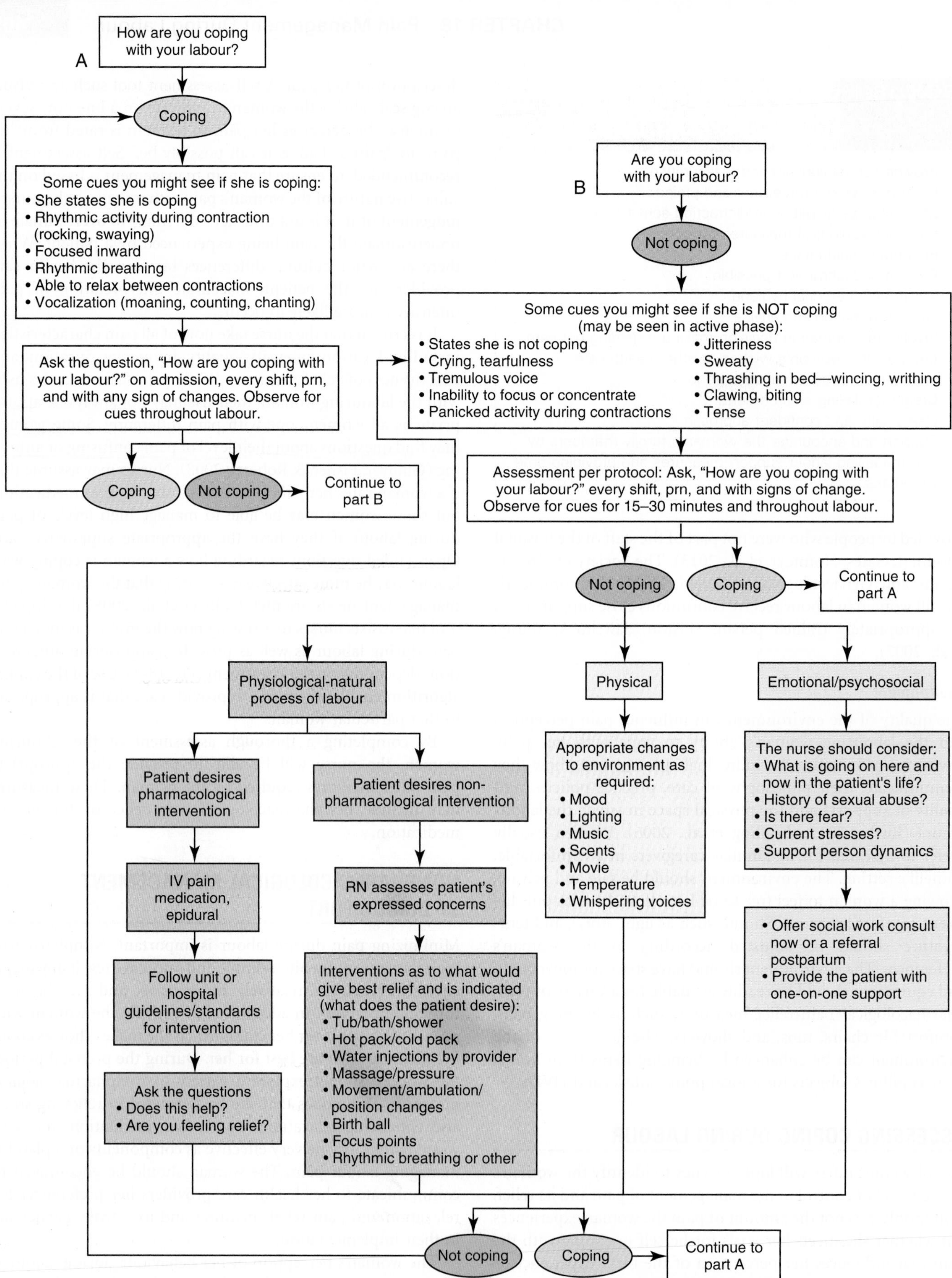

FIGURE 18-4 Coping-with-labour algorithm. **A:** How to assess coping in labour. **B:** Strategies to help labouring women who are not coping. (From Gulliver, B. G, Fisher, J., & Roberts, L. [2008]. A new way to assess pain in labouring women: Replacing the rating scale with a "coping" algorithm. *Nursing for Women's Health, 12*[5], 404–408.)

BOX 18-2 NONPHARMACOLOGICAL STRATEGIES TO ENCOURAGE RELAXATION AND RELIEVE PAIN

Cutaneous Stimulation Strategies
Counterpressure
Effleurage (light massage)
Therapeutic touch and massage
Walking
Rocking
Changing positions
Applying heat or cold
Transcutaneous electrical nerve stimulation (TENS)
Acupressure/acupuncture
Water therapy (hydrotherapy)
Intradermal water block

Sensory Stimulation Strategies
Aromatherapy
Breathing techniques
Music
Imagery
Use of focal points

Cognitive Strategies
Childbirth education
Relaxation
Hypnosis
Biofeedback

COMMUNITY FOCUS

Resources for Alternative and Complementary Methods of Pain Relief

Survey your community for services that provide pregnant women with instruction in complementary or alternative nonpharmacological methods (e.g., biofeedback, aromatherapy, yoga, transcutaneous electrical nerve stimulation, massage, hypnosis) to relieve and cope with discomforts in pregnancy and pain during labour. Create a booklet that describes each of the methods. Include the following information in the booklet:

- A description of the methods and how they work
- Evidence available to validate effectiveness of the methods
- Internet addresses for resources for the methods
- Agencies providing instruction in the methods; include contact information (address, telephone number), cost of the classes or service, and credentials of persons providing instruction
- At what point in pregnancy instruction should begin and the level of preparation and practice necessary for effective use

behaviour, as necessary, and reinforce this through discussion and reassurance after birth.

Many of the nonpharmacological methods for relief of discomfort are taught in different types of prenatal preparation classes, and the woman or couple may have read various books on the subject in advance (see Community Focus box). Many of these methods require practice for best results (e.g., hypnosis, patterned breathing, controlled relaxation techniques, and biofeedback), although the nurse may use some of them successfully without the woman or couple having prior knowledge of them (e.g., slow-paced breathing, massage and touch, effleurage, counterpressure). Women should be encouraged to try a variety of methods and to seek alternatives if the measure being used is no longer effective (Box 18-2).

Nonpharmacological methods may be used in combination with pharmacological methods, particularly as labour progresses.

With the increasing use of epidural analgesia, nurses may be less likely to encourage women to use nonpharmacological measures, in part because these methods may be viewed as more complex and time consuming than monitoring a woman receiving an epidural. In addition, new nurses may not have had the opportunity to develop skill in the implementation of these methods. It is imperative that perinatal nurses develop a commitment to and expertise in using a variety of nonpharmacological pain relief strategies in order for women in labour to be comfortable using them. Although research data to support the effectiveness of many of these nonpharmacological measures are limited, there are sufficient reports of their benefits from women and health care providers to recommend that nurses encourage their use (Burke, 2013).

Childbirth Preparation Methods

The childbirth education movement began in the 1950s. Today, most health care providers recommend or offer childbirth preparation classes to expectant parents. Historically, popular childbirth methods taught in Canada and the United States were the Dick-Read method, the Lamaze, and the Bradley (husband-coached childbirth method). Although these three organizations continue to exist, they are now less focused on a "method" approach. Rather, women are assisted to develop their birth philosophy and inner knowledge and then choose from a variety of skills to use to cope with the labour process. Few childbirth educators adhere strictly to one particular method. Instead, they incorporate a variety of strategies aimed at increasing the woman's ability to cope with labour and minimize her need for medication.

Gaining popularity are methods developed and promoted by Birthing From Within, Childbirth and Postpartum Professional Association (CAPPA), HypnoBirthing, and the Bonapace Method, to name a few (see Additional Resources at end of the chapter). These methods offer classes and other services that focus on a woman's confidence in her innate ability to give birth. The woman or couple are helped to recognize the uniqueness of their pregnancy and childbirth experience.

Most proponents of prepared childbirth agree that the major causes of pain in labour are fear and tension (see Fig. 18-2). All childbirth methods attempt to reduce these factors and eliminate pain by increasing the woman's knowledge of the labour and birth process, enhancing her self-confidence and sense of control, preparing a support person, and training the woman in physical conditioning and relaxation breathing.

In the role as advocate, the childbirth educator can let families know which care routines are ineffective or harmful and provide expectant parents ways to ask their care providers about

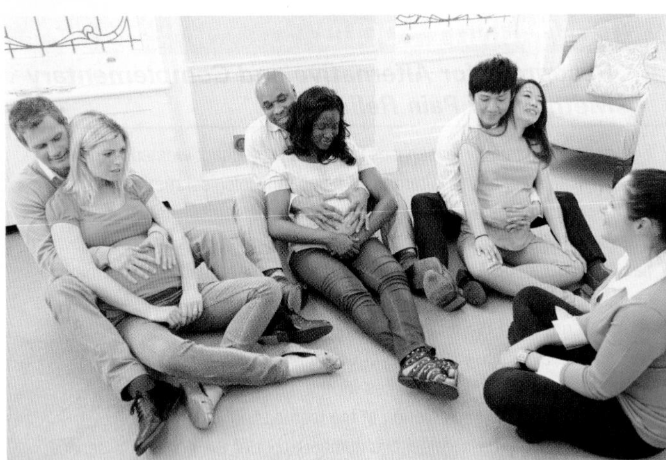

FIGURE 18-5 Expectant parents learning relaxation techniques. (From Marblehead Parenting. Retrieved from http://www.marbleheadparenting.com/prenatal1.html)

their own routine practices. These discussions might affect their choice of care provision.

Specific Nonpharmacological Comfort Strategies

Relaxation

Relaxation or reduction of body tension is a technique suggested by virtually all childbirth education organizations. Learning relaxation in childbirth education classes can help couples with the stresses of pregnancy, childbirth, and adjustment to parenting and can be a form of stress management throughout life (Fig. 18-5). Evidence suggests that relaxation may improve the management of labour pain (Jones, Othman, Dowswell, et al., 2012). Relaxation is ideally combined with activity such as walking, slow dancing, rocking, and position changes that help the baby rotate through the pelvis. Rhythmic motion stimulates mechanoreceptors in the brain, which decreases pain perception.

The nurse can assist the woman by providing a quiet and relaxed environment, offering cues as needed, and recognizing signs of tension (e.g., frowning, change in tone of voice, clenching of fists). A relaxed environment for labour is created by controlling sensory stimuli (e.g., light, noise, temperature) and reducing interruptions. Nurses should remain calm and unhurried in their approach and sit rather than stand at the bedside whenever possible (Burke, 2013).

Imagery and Visualization

Imagery and visualization are useful techniques to purposely direct thoughts to relieve stress and provide a sense of relief (Burke, 2013). Although research on their use is scant, clinical reports suggest that imagery and visualization can be used to produce a sense of well-being during pregnancy, assist with cervical dilation, and decrease the experience of pain and tension during labour. Imagery involves techniques such as imagining a walk through a peaceful garden or breathing in light, energy, and healing colour and breathing out worries and tension. Visualization of the baby coming down the birth canal during the second stage of labour can also be used effectively to enhance pushing efforts. A variety of skills taught in childbirth classes augment relaxation during pregnancy and labour. All of these can be taught as lifetime skills useful to the couple and can be used to teach their children to cope with the stresses of life.

Music

Music can provide a distraction, enhance relaxation, and lift spirits during labour, thereby reducing the woman's level of stress and anxiety and her perception of pain. It can be used to promote relaxation in early labour and to stimulate movement as labour progresses. Music can help create a more relaxed atmosphere in the birth room, leading to a more relaxed approach by health care providers (Burke, 2013; Zwelling et al., 2006). Women should be encouraged to prepare their musical preferences in advance. They should choose familiar music that is associated with pleasant memories, which can facilitate the process of guided imagery. Use of a headset or earphones may increase the effectiveness of the music because other sounds will be shut out. Live music provided at the bedside by a support person may be helpful in transmitting energy that decreases tension and elevates mood. Changing the tempo of the music to coincide with the rate and rhythm of each breathing technique may facilitate proper pacing.

Evidence is insufficient to support the effectiveness of music as a method of pain relief during labour and thus further research is recommended (Smith, Levett, Collins, et al., 2011).

Touch and Massage

Touch and massage have been an integral part of the traditional care for women in labour. A variety of massage techniques have been shown to be safe and effective during labour (Gilbert, 2011; Smith, Levett, Collins, et al., 2012).

Touch can be as simple as holding the woman's hand, stroking her body, and embracing her. When using touch to communicate caring, reassurance, and concern, it is important that the woman's preference for touch (e.g., who can touch her, where they can touch her, and how they can touch her) and responses to touch be determined. Women with a history of sexual abuse or from varying cultural backgrounds may be uncomfortable with touch. Thus it is important to ask permission before touching a woman because of the possibility of her having experienced previous sexual abuse and the potential of touch to cause flashbacks. Touch also can involve very specialized techniques that require manipulation of the human energy field.

Therapeutic touch (TT) uses the concept of energy fields within the body that are called *prana*. Prana are thought to be deficient in some people who are in pain. TT conducted by a specially trained person works to redirect disrupted energy fields associated with pain. Research has demonstrated the effectiveness of TT to enhance relaxation, reduce anxiety, and relieve pain (Aghabati, Mohammadi, & Pour Esmaiel, 2010); however, little is known about the use or effectiveness of TT for relieving labour pain.

Head, hand, back, shoulder, and foot massage may be effective in reducing tension and enhancing comfort. Some evidence

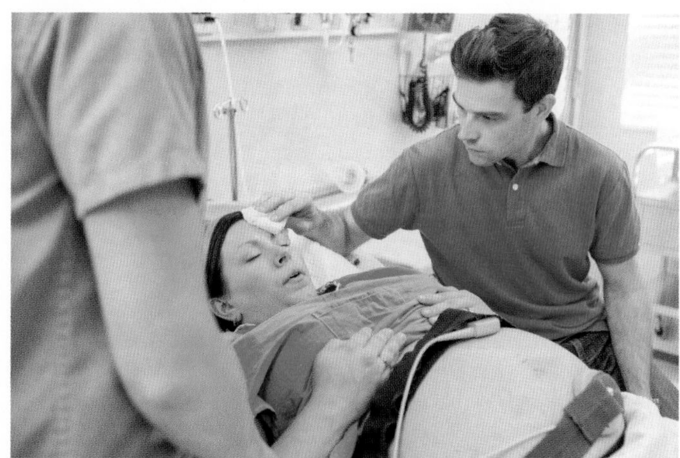

FIGURE 18-6 Labouring woman using focusing, breathing, and massage from partner during a contraction.

suggests that massage may improve management of labour pain (Jones et al., 2012; Smith et al., 2012). Hand and foot massage may be especially relaxing in advanced labour when hyperesthesia limits a woman's tolerance for touch on other parts of her body.

Breathing Techniques

Different approaches to childbirth preparation use varying breathing techniques to provide distraction, thereby reducing the perception of pain and helping the woman to maintain control throughout contractions (Fig. 18-6 and Box 18-3). Relaxed individuals automatically slow their breathing; conversely, slowing one's breathing serves to increase one's relaxation and hence may decrease the feeling of pain. All patterns begin with a deep, relaxing, cleansing breath to "greet the contraction" and end with another deep cleansing breath and subsequent exhalation to "gently blow the contraction away." These deep breaths ensure adequate oxygen for mother and baby and signal that a contraction is beginning or has ended. As the breath is exhaled, respiratory and voluntary muscles relax (Burke, 2013). During labour, nursing support includes guiding couples in applying breathing and relaxation methods, adapting methods to their particular needs, and using pushing techniques for birth that avoid breath holding. Such techniques often involve moaning or making other noises as the woman pushes without holding her breath. There is no one right way to breathe; women are encouraged to find what works for them.

The woman and her support person must be aware of and watch for symptoms of respiratory alkalosis when rapid, shallow breathing results in hyperventilation: light-headedness, dizziness, tingling of fingers, or circumoral numbness. Respiratory alkalosis may be eliminated by having the woman breathe into a paper bag held tightly around the mouth and nose. This enables her to rebreathe carbon dioxide and replace the bicarbonate ion. She can also breathe into her cupped hands if no bag is available. Maintaining a breathing rate that is not more than twice the normal rate will lessen the chances of the woman hyperventilating.

BOX 18-3 PACED BREATHING TECHNIQUES

Cleansing Breath

Relaxed breath in through the nose and out the mouth. Used at the beginning and end of each contraction.

Slow-Paced Breathing (Approximately 8 to 10 Breaths/min)

Performed at approximately half the normal breathing rate using deep breaths into the abdomen.

IN-2-3-4/OUT-2-3-4/IN-2-3-4/OUT-2-3-4

Modified-Paced Breathing (Approximately 32 to 40 Breaths/min)

Performed at about twice the normal breathing rate using shallow breathing into the upper chest. Can use the mouth or nose for breathing in and out.

IN-OUT/IN-OUT/IN-OUT ...

For more flexibility and variety, the woman may combine the slow and modified breathing by using the slow breathing for beginnings and ends of contractions and modified breathing for more intense peaks. This technique conserves energy, lessens fatigue, and reduces the risk of hyperventilation.

Patterned-Paced Breathing or Pant-Blow Breathing (Same Rate as Modified)

Enhances concentration

3:1 Patterned breathing IN-OUT/IN-OUT/IN-OUT/IN-BLOW (repeat through contractions)

4:1 Patterned breathing IN-OUT/IN-OUT/IN-OUT/IN-OUT/IN-BLOW (repeat through contractions)

Breathing During Second Stage—Pushing

Spontaneous Pushing

The urge to push is nearly involuntary. Many women hold their breath; remember to breathe.

Slow Exhalation Pushing (Open-Glottis Pushing)

Work with contraction; inhale and exhale slowly through pursed lips.

Grunting or making noise with exhalation keeps glottis open.

Directed Pushing (Closed-Glottis Pushing)

During contraction, the woman inhales and holds her breath while the support person counts to 6. She needs to exhale and inhale rapidly again, holding for another count of 6. Repeat until contraction is over.

Adapted from BirthSource. (2016). *Breathing.* Dayton, OH: Perinatal Education Associates. Retrieved from http://www.birthsource.com

Effleurage and Counterpressure

Effleurage (light massage) and counterpressure bring relief to many women during the first stage of labour. The gate-control theory may supply the reason for the effectiveness of these measures. *Effleurage* is a light stroking, usually of the abdomen, often in rhythm with breathing during contractions. It is used to distract the woman from contraction pain. The presence of monitor belts may make it difficult to perform effleurage on the abdomen; thus a thigh or the chest may be used. As labour progresses, *hyperesthesia* (hypersensitivity to touch) may make effleurage uncomfortable and thus less effective.

Counterpressure is steady pressure by a support person to the sacral area with a firm object (e.g., tennis ball) or the fist or heel of the hand. Pressure can also be applied to both hips (double hip squeeze) or to the knees (Burke, 2013). Application of counterpressure helps the woman cope with the sensations of internal pressure and pain in the lower back. It is especially helpful when back pain is caused by pressure of the occiput against spinal nerves when the fetal head is in an occiput posterior position. Counterpressure lifts the occiput off these nerves, thereby providing pain relief. The support person will need to be relieved occasionally because application of counterpressure is hard work.

Water Therapy (Hydrotherapy)

Bathing, showering, water immersion, or jet hydrotherapy (whirlpool baths) using warm water (e.g., at body temperature) are nonpharmacological measures that can promote comfort and relaxation during labour (Fig. 18-7). The warm water stimulates the release of endorphins, relaxes fibres to close the gate on pain, promotes better circulation and oxygenation, and helps soften the perineal tissues. Most women find immersion in water to be soothing, relaxing, and comforting. While immersed, they may find it easier to let go and allow labour to take its course (Gilbert, 2011). Some evidence suggests that immersion in water may improve management of labour pain (Jones et al., 2012). Numerous positive benefits of water immersion have been shown by use of hydrotherapy (Cluett & Burns, 2009) and are listed in Box 18-4.

Showers in early labour may provide relaxation and comfort through the application of heat as the handheld shower head is directed to areas of discomfort (see Fig. 18-7 A and B). The coach or partner can participate in this comfort measure by holding and directing the shower head. Sitting in a tub of body-temperature water has several immediate benefits. Buoyancy in the water results in general body relaxation and temporary relief from discomfort and pain. This reduces the woman's anxiety and enhances a feeling of well-being. Catecholamine production decreases. This triggers an increase in the levels of oxytocin (to stimulate uterine contractions) and endorphins (to reduce pain perception).

In some settings, jet hydrotherapy may need to be approved by the labouring woman's primary health care provider. The woman's vital signs must be within normal limits and fetal well-being must also be assessed regularly. To reduce the risk of a prolonged labour, hydrotherapy is usually initiated when the woman is in active labour, more than 5-cm dilation. It is at this time that she may be getting discouraged and will welcome the change that hydrotherapy offers. It is important to preserve the woman's modesty because she may be shy about the exposure of her body when getting into a tub or shower (Burke, 2013).

In addition to pain relief and relaxation, hydrotherapy offers other benefits. If a woman is having "back labour" as the result of an occiput or transverse position, assuming a hands-and-knees or a side-lying position in the tub enhances spontaneous fetal rotation to the occiput anterior position as a result of increased buoyancy. Less effort is needed to change positions while in the water, and women are encouraged to assume an upright position and to alter positions more frequently, facilitating the progress of their labour and helping them cope with labour-associated stressors (Stark, Rudell, & Haus, 2008).

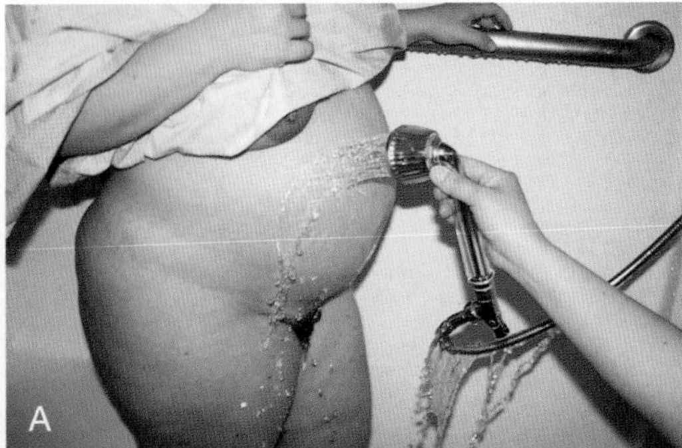

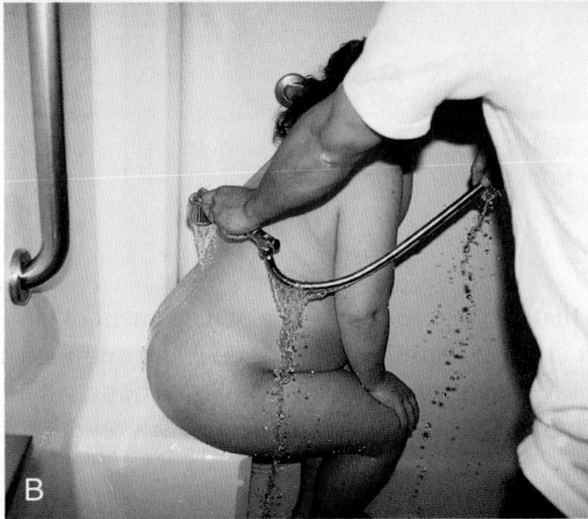

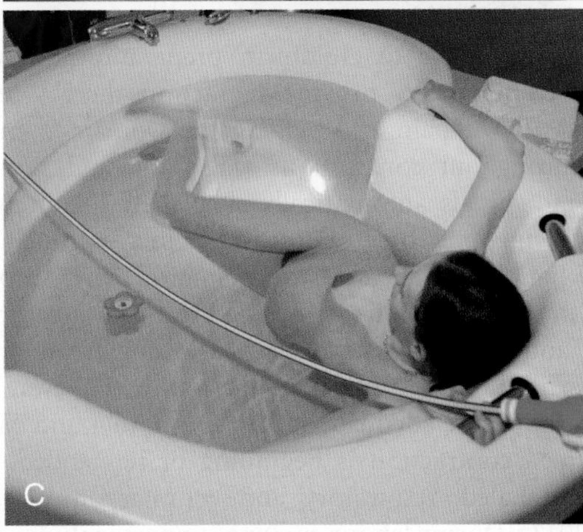

FIGURE 18-7 Water therapy during labour. **A:** Use of shower during labour. **B:** Woman experiencing back labour relaxes as partner sprays warm water on her back. **C:** Woman relaxing in Jacuzzi. (**A** and **B**, Courtesy Marjorie Pyle, RNC, Lifecircle. **C**, Courtesy Spacelabs Medical.)

When hydrotherapy is in use, fetal heart rate (FHR) monitoring can be done by means of Doppler, fetoscope, or wireless external monitoring (see Fig. 18-7, C). Placement of internal electrodes is contraindicated for jet hydrotherapy. The woman's membranes may be intact or ruptured. If the membranes are

BOX 18-4 BENEFITS OF WATER IMMERSION AND HYDROTHERAPY

- Pain and anxiety relief
- Increased diuresis
- Decreased edema
- Decreased blood pressure
- Enhanced fetal rotation due to increased buoyancy
- Faster cervical dilation
- Less use of opioids
- Less use of epidural anaesthesia
- Fewer operative births (vacuum and forceps)
- Less perineal trauma
- Fewer episiotomies

ruptured, the fluid must be clear or only lightly stained with meconium.

There is no limit to the time women can stay in the bath, and often they are encouraged to stay in it as long as desired. However, most women use hydrotherapy for 30 to 60 minutes at a time. During water immersion it is important to continue to monitor both the woman and the fetus. If the woman's temperature or the FHR increases, if the labour progress slows or the woman perceives her labour as becoming too intense, or if relief of pain is reduced, the woman should be encouraged to come out of the tub and return at a later time. Repeated baths with occasional breaks may be more effective in relieving pain during long labours than extended amounts of time in the water. The temperature of the water should not exceed 37°C, to reduce the risk of hyperthermia. Monitoring of maternal temperature every hour and offering fluids will ensure that the labouring woman's temperature remains below 37.5°C (Perinatal Services, BC, 2007).

Water birth. Emerging evidence suggests that *water birth* (process of giving birth in a tub of warm water), with careful selection criteria and experienced health care providers, does not negatively affect mothers and babies. Outcomes of water birth are comparable to those expected in any healthy childbearing population (Nutter, Meyer, Shaw-Battista, & Marovitz, 2014; Nutter, Shaw-Battista, & Marovitz, 2014). A growing number of hospitals and birthing centres in Canada are offering this birthing option. Water birth should always occur under the supervision of a qualified health care provider.

SAFETY ALERT

Be aware that warm water can cause dizziness. A shower stool should be used and the woman should be assisted when getting into and out of the tub.

Transcutaneous Electrical Nerve Stimulation

Transcutaneous electrical nerve stimulation (TENS) involves the placement of two pairs of flat electrodes on either side of the woman's lumbar and sacral spine (Fig. 18-8). These electrodes provide continuous low-voltage electrical impulses or stimuli from a handheld battery-operated device. During a contraction, the woman increases the stimulation from low to high intensity by turning control knobs on the device. High intensity should be maintained for at least 1 minute to facilitate release of endorphins. Women describe the resulting sensation as a tingling or buzzing. TENS is most useful for lower back pain during the early first stage of labour. There is limited evidence to suggest that TENS reduces pain in labour. It does not seem to have any impact on interventions and other outcomes for mother or baby, so women should be provided the opportunity to use it if they wish (Bedwell, Dowswell, Neilson, et al., 2011; Dowswell, Bedwell, Lavender, et al., 2009). No serious safety concerns are associated with the use of TENS (Hawkins & Bucklin, 2012). The nurse assists the woman in using TENS by explaining the device and its use, carefully placing and securing the electrodes, and closely evaluating its effectiveness.

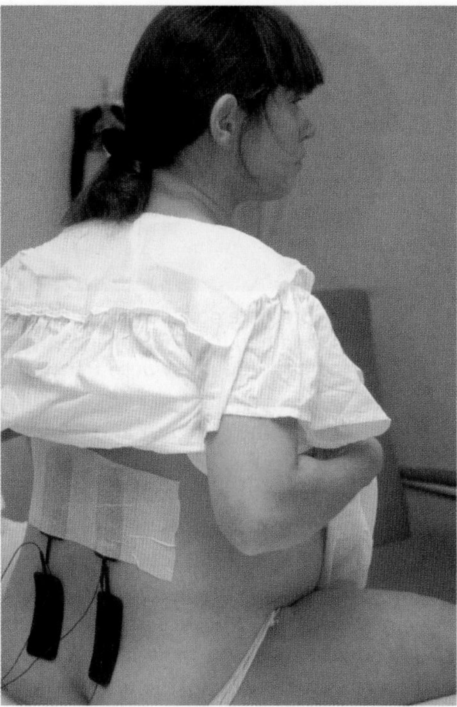
FIGURE 18-8 Placement of transcutaneous electrical nerve stimulation (TENS) electrodes on back for relief of labour pain.

Acupressure and Acupuncture

Acupressure and acupuncture can be used in pregnancy, in labour, and postpartum to relieve pain and other discomforts. Pressure, heat, or cold is applied to acupuncture points, termed *tsubos.* These points have an increased density of neuroreceptors and increased electrical conductivity. Acupressure is said to promote circulation of blood, the harmony of yin and yang, and the secretion of neurotransmitters, thus maintaining normal body functions and enhancing well-being (Tournaire & Theau-Yonneau, 2007). Acupressure is best applied over the skin without using lubricants. Pressure is usually applied with the heel of the hand, fist, or pads of the thumbs and fingers (Fig. 18-9). Tennis balls or other devices also may be used. Pressure is applied with contractions initially and then continuously as labour progresses to the later part of the active phase (Tournaire & Theau-Yonneau, 2007).

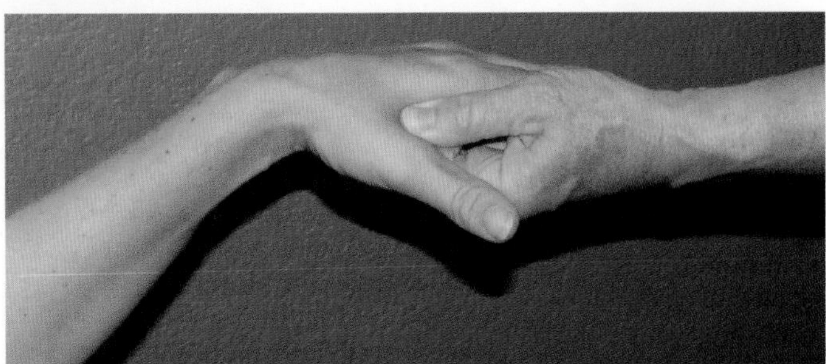

FIGURE 18-9 Ho-Ku acupressure point (back of hand where thumb and index finger come together) used to enhance uterine contractions without increasing pain. (Courtesy Julie Perry Nelson)

Synchronized breathing by the caregiver and the woman is suggested for greater effectiveness. Acupressure points are found on the neck; the shoulders; the wrists; the lower back including sacral points; the hips; the area below the kneecaps; the ankles; the nails on the small toes; and the soles of the feet.

Acupuncture is the insertion of fine needles into specific areas of the body to restore the flow of qi (energy) and decrease pain, which is thought to be obstructing the flow of energy. Effectiveness may be attributed to the alteration of chemical neurotransmitter levels in the body or to the release of endorphins as a result of hypothalamic activation. Acupuncture should be done by a trained certified therapist.

Acupuncture and acupressure may have a role in reducing pain, increasing satisfaction with pain management, and reduced use of pharmacological management. However, there is a need for further research on its use in labour (Hawkins & Bucklin, 2012; Jones et al., 2012; Smith, Collins, Crowther, et al., 2011).

Application of Heat and Cold

Warmed blankets, warm compresses, heated rice bags, a warm bath or shower, or a moist heating pad can enhance relaxation and reduce pain during labour. Heat relieves muscle ischemia and increases blood flow to the area of discomfort. Heat application is effective for back pain caused by a fetus in the occiput posterior position or for general backache from fatigue.

Cold application such as cool cloths, frozen gel packs, or ice packs applied to the back, the chest, or the face during labour may provide comfort when the woman feels warm. They may also be applied to areas of musculoskeletal pain. Cold is often more effective for back pain caused by the posterior presentation. Cooling relieves pain by lowering the muscle temperature and relieving muscle spasms (Burke, 2013). A woman's culture may make the use of cold during labour unacceptable, however.

Heat and cold may be used alternately for a greater effect. Neither heat nor cold should be applied over ischemic or anaesthetized areas because tissues can be damaged. It is important to place one or two layers of cloth between the skin and a hot or cold pack to prevent damage to the underlying skin.

Hypnosis

Hypnosis is a form of deep relaxation, similar to daydreaming or meditation (see Additional Resources at end of the chapter). While under hypnosis, the person is in a state of focused concentration and the subconscious mind can be more easily accessed. Some childbirth preparation classes offer instruction in performing self-hypnosis. Hypnosis techniques used for labour and birth place an emphasis on enhancing relaxation and diminishing fear, anxiety, and perception of pain. Women using this technique report a greater sense of control over painful contractions and a higher level of satisfaction with their childbirth experience. Because it reduces the need for pain medication, hypnosis can be helpful when used with other interventions during labour. A few negative effects of hypnosis have been reported, including mild dizziness, nausea, and headache. These negative effects seem to be associated with failure to dehypnotize the woman properly (Tournaire & Theau-Yonneau, 2007). Although hypnosis shows some promise for use in labour, further research on its use is needed (Jones et al., 2012; Madden, Middleton, Cyna, et al., 2012).

Biofeedback

Biofeedback may be useful as a relaxation technique for labour. It is based on the theory that, if a person can recognize physical signals, certain internal physiological events can be changed (i.e., whatever signs the woman has that are associated with her pain). For biofeedback to be effective, the woman must be educated during the prenatal period to become aware of her body and its responses to pain and how to relax. The woman must learn how to use thinking and mental processes (e.g., focusing) to control body responses and functions. Informal biofeedback helps couples develop awareness of their bodies and use strategies to change their responses to stress. If the woman responds to pain during a contraction with tightening of muscles, frowning, moaning, and breath holding, her partner can use verbal and touch feedback to help her relax. Formal biofeedback, which uses machines to detect skin temperature, blood flow, or muscle tension, can also prepare women to intensify their relaxation responses. Effective use of these techniques requires the strong support of caregivers (Tournaire & Theau-Yonneau, 2007). Evidence is insufficient to show that biofeedback is more effective than use of a placebo or other interventions for pain management during labour (Jones et al., 2012).

Aromatherapy

In aromatherapy, oils distilled from plants, flowers, herbs, and trees are used to promote health and to treat and balance the mind, body, and spirit. These essential oils are highly concentrated, complex essences and are mixed with lotions or creams before they are applied to the skin (e.g., for a back massage). Certain essential oils can tone the uterus, encourage contractions, reduce pain, relieve tension, diminish fear and anxiety, and enhance the feeling of well-being. Lavender, rose, and jasmine oils can promote relaxation and reduce pain. Rose oil also acts as an antidepressant and uterine tonic, whereas jasmine oil strengthens contractions and decreases feelings of panic in addition to reducing pain. Essential oils of bergamot or rosemary can be diffused or used in a massage oil to relieve exhaustion (Gilbert, 2011; Tournaire & Theau-Yonneau, 2007; Walls,

2009). Oils may also be used by adding a few drops to a warm bath, to warm water used for soaking compresses that can be applied to the body, or to an aromatherapy lamp to vapourize a room. Drops of essential oils can also be put on a pillow or on a woman's brow or palms or used as an ingredient in creating massage oil (Walls, 2009). Certain odours or scents can evoke pleasant memories and feelings of love and security. Thus the woman needs to choose the scents she will use during labour before her labour begins. There is insufficient evidence to support the effectiveness of aromatherapy for pain relief in labour, although its use has shown promising results (Jones et al., 2012; Smith, Collins, & Crowther, 2011). Hospital scent policies should be checked for women planning an in-hospital birth who wish to use aromatherapy.

SAFETY ALERT

Never apply the essential oils used for aromatherapy full strength directly to the skin. Most oils should be diluted in a vegetable oil base before use. Essential oils vary in terms of safe use during pregnancy. Inhaling vapours from the oils can lead to unpleasant adverse effects, including nausea or headaches.

Intradermal Sterile Water Block

An intradermal water block involves the injection of small amounts of sterile water (e.g., 0.05 to 0.1 mL) with a fine needle (e.g., 25-gauge) into four locations on the lower back to relieve low back pain (Fig. 18-10). It is a simple procedure to perform, with evidence of effectiveness, which is thought to relate to the gate-control mechanism (Hawkins & Bucklin, 2012). Other possible explanations for the effectiveness of intradermal water block are the mechanism of counter-irritation (i.e., reducing localized pain in one area by irritating the skin in an area nearby) and an increase in the level of endogenous opioids (endorphins) produced by the injections. Intense stinging occurs for about 20 to 30 seconds after injection, with subsequent relief of back pain for up to 2 hours. The procedure can be repeated, although the woman may find that the stinging accompanying administration creates too much discomfort (Burke, 2013).

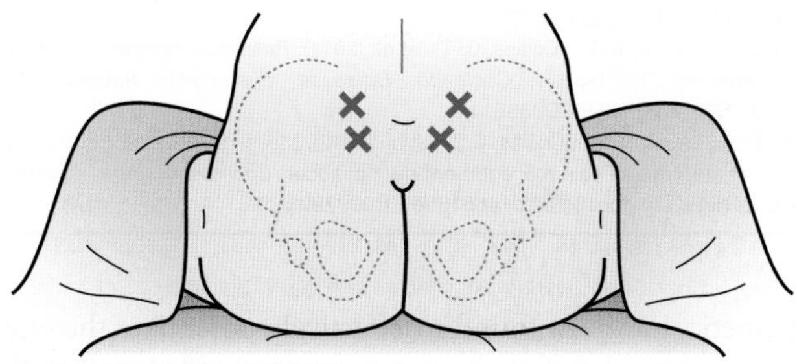

FIGURE 18-10 Intradermal injections of 0.1 mL of sterile water in the treatment of women with back pain during labour. Sterile water is injected into four locations on the lower back, two over each posterior superior iliac spine (PSIS) and two 3 cm below and 1 cm medial to the PSIS. The injections should raise a bleb on the skin. Simultaneous injections administered by two clinicians decrease the pain of injections. (From Leeman, L., Fontaine, P., King, V., et al. (2003). The nature and management of labor pain: Part I. Nonpharmacologic pain relief. *American Family Physician 68*[6], 1109–1112.)

Maternal Position and Movement

All of the comfort strategies discussed here should be combined with upright and gravity-enhancing positions, such as walking, slow dancing, and rocking. Rhythmic motion stimulates mechanoreceptors in the brain, which decrease pain perception and may enhance the labour process, as it allows the fetus to move through the birth canal more easily. Labouring women will often find a position that feels right to them, although they should be encouraged to change their position frequently during labour (Burke, 2013). Changing position in labour alters the relationship between the fetus and pelvis and may result in a more efficient labour (Cluett & Burns, 2009; Zwelling, 2010). When encouraging a woman to change position, the nurse should provide extra support and encouragement and suggest that she remain in the new position throughout several contractions before deciding whether it is comfortable.

See Research Focus box for discussion of the research behind some nonpharmacological pain management techniques. For more on nonpharmacological pain management see the Evolve website for the Nursing Care Plan, Nonpharmacological Management of Discomfort.

PHARMACOLOGICAL PAIN MANAGEMENT

When nonpharmacological pain-relief measures are no longer effective, the woman and her care provider may consider pharmacological measures for pain management. When pharmacological and nonpharmacological measures are used together, they increase the level of pain relief. Pharmacological measures for pain management can be implemented as labour becomes more active and discomfort and pain intensify and when the woman decides that nonpharmacological methods are not working for her anymore. Less pharmacological intervention often is required because nonpharmacological measures enhance relaxation and potentiate the analgesic effect. However, women are increasingly using pharmacological measures, especially epidural analgesia to relieve their pain during labour and birth.

Sedatives

Sedatives relieve anxiety and induce sleep. They may be given to a woman experiencing a prolonged latent phase of labour or when there is a need to decrease anxiety or promote sleep. They can also be given to augment analgesics and reduce nausea when an opioid is used.

Barbiturates such as secobarbital sodium (Seconal) can cause undesirable adverse effects, including respiratory and vasomotor depression affecting the woman and her fetus/newborn. Because of the potential for neonatal central nervous system (CNS) depression, barbiturates should be avoided if birth is anticipated within 12 to 24 hours. The depressant effects are increased if a barbiturate is administered with another CNS depressant such as an opioid analgesic. However, pain will be magnified if a barbiturate is given without an analgesic to women experiencing pain because normal coping mechanisms

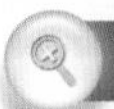

RESEARCH FOCUS

What Nonpharmacological Therapies Offer Pain Relief During Labour?

—*Pat Mahaffee Gingrich*

Ask the Question

Do women in labour have nonpharmacological therapies available that can provide safe and effective pain relief?

Search for the Evidence

Search Strategies

English research-based publications on pain, labour, nonpharmacological pain relief, and complementary and alternative therapies were included.

Database Used

Cochrane Collaborative Database

Critically Analyze the Evidence

Many women seek alternative or complementary pain relief during labour to delay or avoid pharmacological or invasive therapies. Evidence regarding their efficacy has been sparse and so they have remained underused. The Cochrane Database has recently published a series of systematic reviews of the evidence for several of the best-known therapies:

- Acupuncture was associated with less pain intensity, increased satisfaction of pain relief, decreased use of analgesia drugs, and fewer instrumental births compared with placebo control. Acupressure lessened pain intensity compared with that in placebo control (Smith, Collins, Crowther, et al., 2011).
- Relaxation techniques such as meditation, visualization, and breathing decreased pain intensity and assisted birth rates and increase satisfaction with pain relief when compared with placebo. Yoga was associated with pain relief, increased satisfaction with pain relief and birth, and reduced length of labour (Smith, Levett, Collins, et al., 2011). Evidence for music and audio analgesia was insufficient to make recommendations.
- Massage was associated with less pain and anxiety than that of control during the first stage of labour (Smith, Levett, Collins, et al., 2012). Massage was more effective than music for decreasing pain. There were no reflexology studies.
- Water immersion during labour was associated with significantly decreased use of analgesia/anaesthesia and shorter first-stage labour by a mean of 32 minutes (Cluett & Burns, 2009).
- Transcutaneous electrical nerve stimulation (TENS), which sends an electrical impulse to the back, acupuncture sites, or the cranium, may block or compete with pain pathways and is typically controlled by the patient. In labour, women using TENS reported less severe pain and said they would use it again for pain control (Dowswell, Bedwell, Lavender, et al., 2009). TENS had no effect on labour length, interventions, or maternal or infant well-being.
- Intracutaneous or subcutaneous sterile water, typically injected on four places on the back, creates stinging sensations that block or compete with pain pathways. Compared with normal saline controls, which do not sting, sterile water injections showed a nonsignificant trend toward decreased pain but did not show any differences between groups in terms of Caesarean births, rescue analgesia, timing of birth, or Apgar scores. Women reported that they would use the method in a subsequent labour (Derry, Straube, Moore, et al., 2012).
- Biofeedback involves teaching patients to control certain body signals, which are read by a machine. Small studies using a myographic machine to measure muscle tension showed some pain relief in early labour (Barragán Loayza, Solà, & Juandó Prats, 2011).
- Aromatherapy compared with control showed no difference in pain relief between groups. Evidence was insufficient to make recommendations (Smith, Collins, & Crowther, 2011).

Apply the Evidence: Nursing Implications

- Evidence is still insufficient or scanty regarding the use of various alternative or complementary therapies but does suggest that they may help and probably do not cause harm.
- Evidence is strongest for the use of acupuncture, acupressure, relaxation, yoga, and TENS. If available, they should be introduced and taught to women at prenatal visits and offered during labour.
- Less evidence is available for recommending saline injections, biofeedback, music/audio, or aromatherapy. However, they may have a complementary effect for some patients.
- Nonpharmacological methods of pain relief may be most effective in latent or early active labour. Women's needs must be continually re-evaluated, and women should know what pharmacological choices are available. Nurses should advocate for appropriate pain-relief choices during labour.

References

Barragán Loayza, I. M., Solà, I., & Juandó Prats, C. (2011). Biofeedback for pain management during labour. *Cochrane Database Systematic Review*, (6), CD006168.

Cluett, E. R., & Burns, E. (2009). Immersion in water in labour and birth. *Cochrane Database Systematic Review*, (2). doi:10.1002/14651858.CD000111.pub3.

Derry, S., Straube, S., Moore, R. A., et al. (2012). Intracutaneous or subcutaneous sterile water injections compared with blinded controls for pain management in labour. *Cochrane Database Systematic Review*, (1). doi:10.1002/14651858.CD009107.pub2.

Dowswell, T., Bedwell, C., Lavender, T., et al. (2009). Transcutaneous electrical nerve stimulation (TENS) for pain management in labour. *Cochrane Database Systematic Review*, (2). doi:10.1002/14651858.CD007214.pub2.

Smith, C. A., Collins, C. T., & Crowther, C. A. (2011). Aromatherapy for pain management in labour. *Cochrane Database Systematic Review*, (7). doi:10.1002/14651858.CD009215.

Smith, C. A., Collins, C. T., Crowther, C. A., et al. (2011). Acupuncture or acupressure for pain management in labour. *Cochrane Database Systematic Review*, (7). doi:10.1002/14651858.CD009232.

Smith, C. A., Levett, K. M., Collins, C. T., et al. (2011). Relaxation techniques for pain management in labour. *Cochrane Database Systematic Review*, (12). doi:10.1002/14651858.CD009514.

Smith, C. A., Levett, K. M., Collins, C. T., et al. (2012). Massage, reflexology and other manual methods of pain management during labour. *Cochrane Database Systematic Review*, (2). doi:10.1002/14651858.CD009290.pub2.

may be blunted. As a result of these disadvantages, barbiturates are seldom used during labour (Burke, 2013). These drugs are very rarely, if ever, used in Canada.

Phenothiazines (e.g., promethazine [Phenergan], hydroxyzine [Atarax]) do not relieve pain. In the past, promethazine was often given with opioids to enhance the analgesic effects of opioids, as well as to decrease anxiety and apprehension, increase sedation, and reduce nausea and vomiting. However, research has shown that promethazine actually impairs the analgesic efficacy of opioids. Metoclopramide (Maxeran), an antiemetic, has been found to effectively potentiate the effects of analgesics. Therefore its use is recommended, rather than promethazine (Hawkins & Bucklin, 2012).

Benzodiazepines (e.g., diazepam [Valium], lorazepam [Ativan], clonazepam [Rivotril]), when given with an opioid analgesic, seem to enhance pain relief and reduce nausea and vomiting. A major disadvantage of diazepam is that it disrupts thermoregulation in newborns, making them less able to maintain body temperature. Flumaznil (Romazicon) is a specific benzodiazepine antagonist, which can effectively reverse benzodiazepine-induced sedation and respiratory depression (Hawkins & Bucklin, 2012).

Analgesia and Anaesthesia

The ideal obstetrical analgesic or anaesthetic provides adequate pain relief to women without increasing maternal or fetal risk or affecting the progress of labour. Nursing management of obstetrical analgesia and anaesthesia combines the nurse's expertise in maternity care with a knowledge and understanding of anatomy and physiology and of medications and their therapeutic effects, adverse reactions, and methods of administration.

The term *analgesia* refers to the alleviation of the sensation of pain or the raising of the threshold for pain perception without loss of consciousness.

Anaesthesia encompasses analgesia, amnesia, relaxation, and reflex activity. Anaesthesia abolishes pain perception by interrupting the nerve impulses to the brain. The loss of sensation may be partial or complete, sometimes with the loss of consciousness.

The type of analgesic or anaesthetic chosen is determined in part by the stage of labour and the method of birth planned (Box 18-5).

Systemic Analgesia

Systemic analgesia (opioids) remains the major method of analgesia for the woman in labour when personnel trained in regional analgesia (i.e., epidural analgesia) are not available. Opioids can be administered in intermittent intravenous (IV) or intramuscular (IM) doses by health care providers or by the woman herself using patient-controlled analgesia (PCA). With PCA, the woman self-administers small doses of an opioid analgesic intravenously by using a pump programmed for dose and frequency. Overall, a lower total amount of analgesic is used. Women appreciate the sense of autonomy provided by this method of pain relief (Hawkins & Bucklin, 2012).

BOX 18-5 PHARMACOLOGICAL CONTROL OF DISCOMFORT BY STAGE OF LABOUR AND METHOD OF BIRTH

First Stage

Systemic analgesia
- Opioid agonist analgesics
- Opioid agonist–antagonist analgesics

Epidural (block) analgesia
Combined spinal–epidural (CSE) analgesia
Nitrous oxide

Second Stage

Nerve block analgesia/anaesthesia
- Local infiltration anaesthesia
- Pudendal block
- Epidural (block) analgesia and anaesthesia
- Spinal (block) anaesthesia
- CSE analgesia and anaesthesia

Nitrous oxide

Caesarean Birth

Spinal (block) anaesthesia
Epidural (block) anaesthesia
General anaesthesia

Opioids provide sedation and euphoria, but their analgesic effect in labour is limited. The pain relief they provide is incomplete, temporary, and more effective in the early part of active labour (Anderson, 2011). Prolonged gastric emptying time increases the risk for aspiration if general anaesthesia becomes necessary in a woman who has received opioids (Hawkins & Bucklin, 2012). Bladder and bower elimination may be inhibited. Maternal and fetal heart rate (e.g., bradycardia, tachycardia) and maternal blood pressure (e.g., hypotension) and respiratory effort (e.g., depression) can be adversely affected; opioid analgesics should be used cautiously in women with respiratory and cardiovascular disorders. Safety precautions should be taken after opioid administration, because several opioid side effects increase the risk for injury.

Opioids readily cross the placenta. Effects on the fetus and the newborn can be profound, including absent or minimal FHR variability during labour and significant neonatal respiratory depression requiring treatment after birth (Hawkins & Bucklin, 2012).

SAFETY ALERT

Opioids decrease maternal heart and respiratory rate and blood pressure, which affect fetal oxygenation. Therefore, maternal vital signs and FHR pattern must be assessed and documented before and after administration of opioids for pain relief.

Classifications of analgesic drugs used to relieve the pain of childbirth include opioid (narcotic) agonists and opioid (narcotic) agonist-antagonists. Choice of which medication to use often depends on the primary health care provider's preferences and the characteristics of the labouring woman. The type of systemic analgesics used therefore often varies among obstetrical units.

Opioid (narcotic) agonist analgesics. Opioid (narcotic) agonist analgesics commonly used in obstetrics include hydromorphone (Dilaudid), fentanyl (Sublimaze), sufentanil citrate (Sufenta), and morphine (Hawkins & Bucklin, 2012). As pure opioid agonists, they stimulate the major opioid receptors, mu and kappa. They have no amnesic effect but create a feeling of well-being or euphoria and enhance a woman's ability to rest between contractions. Opioids can inhibit uterine contractions; for this reason they should not be administered until labour is well established unless they are being used to enhance therapeutic rest during a prolonged latent phase of labour (Burke, 2013) (see Medication Guide).

Meperidine hydrochloride (Demerol) used to be the most commonly used opioid agonist analgesic for women in labour, but it is no longer recommended because other medications have fewer adverse effects. Its use in labour is becoming more controversial because of undesirable adverse effects, particularly in the newborn (Anderson, 2011). Both meperidine and normeperidine, an active metabolite of meperidine, cross the

MEDICATION GUIDE

Hydromorphone Hydrochloride (Dilaudid)

Classification
Opioid agonist analgesic

Action
Opioid agonist analgesic stimulates mu- and kappa-opioid receptors to decrease transmission of pain impulses.

Indication
Moderate-to-severe labour pain and postoperative pain after Caesarean birth

Dosage and Route
IV: 1 mg every 3 hours as needed
IM: 1 to 2 mg every 3 to 6 hours as needed; or 3 to 4 mg every 4 to 6 hours as needed

Adverse Effects
Nausea and vomiting, sedation, confusion, drowsiness, tachycardia or bradycardia, hypotension, dry mouth, pruritus, urinary retention, respiratory depression (woman and newborn), decreased fetal heart rate (FHR) variability, decreased uterine activity if given in early labour

Nursing Considerations
Assess maternal vital signs, degree of pain, FHR and pattern, and uterine activity before and after administration. Observe for respiratory depression, notifying primary health care provider if maternal respirations are 12 breaths/min or less. Encourage voiding every 2 hours and palpate for bladder distension. Administer with a phenothiazine or benzodiazepine, if ordered, to potentiate the analgesic effect, enhance sedation, and decrease nausea and vomiting. If birth occurs within 1 to 4 hours of dose, observe newborn for respiratory depression; have naloxone available as antidote. Implement safety measures as appropriate, including use of side rails and assistance with ambulation. Continue use of nonpharmacological pain-relief measures.

MEDICATION GUIDE

Fentanyl (Sublimaze) and Sufentanil (Sufenta)

Classification
Opioid agonist analgesic

Action
Potent opioid agonist analgesics that stimulates both mu- and kappa-opioid receptors to decrease the transmission of pain impulses. Has a rapid onset of action with short duration (0.5 to 1 hour IV; 1 to 2 hours IM)

Indication
Moderate to severe labour pain and postoperative pain after Caesarean birth

Dosage and Route
Fentanyl
IV: 50 to 100 mcg every hour
IM: 50 to 100 mcg every hour

Sufentanil
Epidural: 1 mcg with 0.125% bupivacaine at rate of 10 mL/hr

Adverse Effects
Sedation, respiratory depression, nausea and vomiting, urinary retention

Nursing Considerations
Assess for respiratory depression; naloxone should be available as an antidote. Implement safety measures as appropriate, including use of side rails and assistance with ambulation; continue use of nonpharmacological pain relief measures. Given its short duration of action, frequent dosing will be necessary when given intravenously. Maximum total dose for fentanyl for labour is usually 500 to 600 mcg.

Source: Anderson, D. (2011). A review of systemic opioids commonly used for labor pain relief. *Journal of Midwifery and Women's Health, 56*(3), 222–239.

placenta and cause prolonged neonatal sedation and neurobehavioural changes. These metabolite-related effects cannot be reversed with naloxone (Anderson, 2011). Both meperidine and normeperidine have long half-lives, thus the neonatal effects can persist for the first 2 to 3 days of life (Hawkins & Buckin, 2012).

Fentanyl citrate (Sublimaze) and sufentanil citrate (Sufenta) are potent, short-acting opioid agonist analgesics (see Medication Guide). Sufentanil use is increasing because it has a more potent analgesic action than that of fentanyl when given via epidural. In addition, less sufentanil crosses the placenta, resulting in reduced fetal exposure. Fentanyl rapidly crosses the placenta so is present in fetal blood within 1 minute after IV maternal administration (Anderson, 2011). As compared with meperidine, fentanyl provides equivalent analgesia with fewer neonatal effects and less maternal sedation and nausea. Fentanyl and sufentanil are used as labour analgesics because of the rapid onset of action, short half-life, and lack of a metabolite (Anderson, 2011). A disadvantage of sufentanil and fentanyl is that more frequent dosing is required because of its relatively short duration of action (Hawkins & Bucklin, 2012). As a result, these medications are most commonly administered by PCA pump, intrathecally, epidurally, alone, or in combination with a local anaesthetic agent.

Opioid (narcotic) agonist–antagonist analgesics. An agonist is an agent that activates or stimulates a receptor to act; an antagonist is an agent that blocks a receptor or a medication designed to activate a receptor. Nalbuphine (Nubain) is a commonly used opioid (narcotic) agonist–antagonist analgesics (Hawkins & Buckin, 2012). In the doses used during labour, nalbuphine provides adequate analgesia without causing significant respiratory depression in the mother or the newborn. The major advantage of these drugs is their ceiling effect for respiratory depression, meaning higher doses do not produce additional risk of respiratory depression. They are less likely to cause nausea and vomiting, but sedation may be as great as or greater than that of pure opioid agonists (Anderson, 2011; Hawkins & Buckin, 2012). As a result of these effects, parental opioid agonist–antagonist analgesics are used more commonly during labour than the opioid agonist analgesics. IM, subcutaneous (SC), and IV routes of administration can be used, but the IV route is preferred. This classification of opioid analgesics, especially nalbuphine, is not suitable for women with an opioid dependence because the antagonist activity could precipitate withdrawal symptoms (abstinence syndrome) in both the mother and her newborn (Hawkins & Bucklin, 2012) (see Medication Guide: Nalbuphine Hydrochloride [Nubain] and Box 18-6).

Opioid (narcotic) antagonists. Opioids such as hydromorphone and fentanyl can cause excessive CNS depression in the mother, the newborn, or both. However, the current practice of giving lower doses of opioids intravenously has reduced the incidence and severity of opioid-induced CNS depression. *Opioid antagonists* such as naloxone (Narcan) can promptly reverse the CNS depressant effects, especially respiratory depression, in most situations. As stated earlier, however, naloxone cannot reverse the effects of normeperidine, an active metabolite of meperidine. In addition, the antagonist counters the effect of stress-induced levels of endorphins. An opioid antagonist is especially valuable if labour is more rapid than expected and birth occurs when the opioid is at its peak effect. The antagonist may be given intravenously, or it can be administered intramuscularly (see Medication Guide: Naloxone Hydrochloride [Narcan]). The woman should be told that the pain that was relieved with the use of the opioid analgesic will return with the administration of the opioid antagonist.

BOX 18-6 SIGNS OF POTENTIAL COMPLICATIONS—MATERNAL OPIOID ABSTINENCE SYNDROME (OPIOID/NARCOTIC WITHDRAWAL)

- Yawning, rhinorrhea (runny nose), sweating, lacrimation (tearing), mydriasis (dilation of pupils)
- Anorexia
- Irritability, restlessness, generalized anxiety
- Tremors
- Chills and hot flashes
- Piloerection ("goose bumps")
- Violent sneezing
- Weakness, fatigue, and drowsiness
- Nausea and vomiting
- Diarrhea, abdominal cramps
- Bone and muscle pain, muscle spasm, kicking movements

MEDICATION GUIDE

Nalbuphine Hydrochloride (Nubain)

Classification
Opioid agonist–antagonist analgesic

Action
Mixed agonist–antagonist analgesic that stimulates kappa-opioid receptors and blocks or weakly stimulates mu-opioid receptors, resulting in good analgesia but with less respiratory depression and nausea and vomiting than with opioid agonist analgesics

Indication
Moderate to severe labour pain or postoperative pain after Caesarean birth

Dosage and Route
IV: 10 mg every 3 hours as needed
IM: 10 to 20 mg every 3 hours as needed

Adverse Effects
Sedation, drowsiness, nausea, vomiting, dizziness, respiratory depression, transient sinusoidal-like fetal heart rate (FHR) pattern

Nursing Considerations
Nalbuphine may precipitate withdrawal symptoms in opioid-dependent women and their newborns. Assess maternal vital signs, degree of pain, FHR, and uterine activity before and after administration. Observe for maternal respiratory depression and notify the primary care provider if maternal respirations are ≤12 breaths/min. Encourage voiding every 2 hours and palpate for bladder distension. If birth occurs within 1 to 4 hours of dose administration, observe newborn for respiratory depression. Implement safety measures as appropriate, including use of side rails and assistance with ambulation. Continue use of nonpharmacological pain relief measures.

Source: Anderson, D. (2011). A review of systemic opioids commonly used for labor pain relief. *Journal of Midwifery and Women's Health 56*(3), 222–239.

NURSING ALERT

Although adults and newborns receive the same medication, the dosage is different for naloxone. It is important to ensure that the correct dose is given.

MEDICATION GUIDE

Naloxone Hydrochloride (Narcan)

Classification
Opioid antagonist

Action
Blocks both mu- and kappa-opioid receptors from the effects of opioid agonists

Indication
Reverses opioid-induced respiratory depression in woman or newborn; may be used to reverse pruritus from epidural opioids

Dosage and Route
Adult
Opioid overdose: 0.4 to 2 mg IV, may repeat IV at 2- to 3-minute intervals until a maximum of 10 mg has been given; if IV route unavailable, IM or SC administration may be used

Newborn
Opioid-induced depression: Initial dose is 0.1 mg/kg; preferred route is IV but may be administered IM

Adverse Effects
Maternal hypotension and hypertension, tachycardia, hyperventilation, nausea and vomiting, sweating and tremulousness

Nursing Considerations
The woman should delay breastfeeding until the medication is out of her system. Do not give to the mother or newborn if the woman is opioid dependent—this may cause abrupt withdrawal in the woman and newborn. If given to the woman for reversal of respiratory depression caused by opioid analgesic, pain will return suddenly. The duration of action of naloxone is shorter than that of most opioids. Therefore, monitor the patient closely for the return of opioid-induced respiratory depression when the effects of naloxone are gone. Additional doses of naloxone may be necessary to maintain reversal.

MEDICATION ALERT

An opioid antagonist is contraindicated for an infant of an opioid-dependent woman because it may precipitate neonatal abstinence syndrome (withdrawal symptoms). For the same reason, opioid agonist–antagonist analgesics such as nalbuphine (Nubain) should not be given to opioid-dependent women (see Box 18-5).

Nerve Block Analgesia and Anaesthesia

A variety of local anaesthetic agents are used in obstetrics to produce regional analgesia (some pain relief and motor block) and regional anaesthesia (complete pain relief and motor block). Most of these agents are related chemically to cocaine and end with the suffix *-caine.* This helps to identify a local anaesthetic.

The principal pharmacological effect of local anaesthetics is the temporary interruption of the conduction of nerve impulses, notably pain. Examples of common agents given are lidocaine (Xylocaine), bupivacaine (Marcaine), chloroprocaine (Nesacaine), and ropivacaine (Naropin).

Rarely, people are sensitive (allergic) to one or more local anaesthetics. Such a reaction may include respiratory depression, hypotension, and other serious adverse effects. Epinephrine, antihistamines, oxygen, and supportive measures should reverse these effects. Sensitivity may be identified by administering tiny amounts of the medication to test for an allergic reaction.

Local infiltration anaesthesia. Local infiltration anaesthesia may be used when an episiotomy is to be performed or when lacerations must be sutured after birth in a woman who does not have regional anaesthesia. Rapid anaesthesia is produced by injecting approximately 5 to 15 mL of 1% lidocaine into the skin and then subcutaneously into the region to be anaesthetized. Epinephrine often is added to the solution to localize and intensify the anaesthesia to the region and to prevent excessive bleeding and systemic absorption by constricting local blood vessels. Injections can be repeated to keep the woman comfortable while post-birth repairs are completed.

Pudendal nerve block. Pudendal nerve block, administered late in the second stage of labour, is useful if an episiotomy is to be performed or if forceps or a vacuum extractor is to be used to facilitate birth (in a woman without an epidural). It can also be administered during the third stage of labour if an episiotomy or lacerations need to be repaired. Its use has declined as a result of the increased use of epidural anaesthesia. A pudendal nerve block is considered to be reasonably effective for pain relief, simple to perform, and very safe (Cunningham, Leveno, K., Bloom, et al., 2014; Hawkins & Bucklin, 2012). Although a pudendal nerve block does not relieve pain from uterine contractions, it does relieve pain in the lower vagina, vulva, and perineum (Fig. 18-11, A). A pudendal nerve block must be administered 10 to 20 minutes before perineal anaesthesia is needed.

The pudendal nerve traverses the sacrosciatic notch just medial to the tip of the ischial spine on each side. Injection of an anaesthetic solution at or near these points anaesthetizes the pudendal nerves peripherally (Fig. 18-12). The transvaginal approach is generally used because it is less painful for the woman, has a higher rate of success in blocking pain, and tends to cause fewer fetal complications. This technique can provide pain relief within 2 to 10 minutes after administration that lasts for approximately 1 hour (Jackson, Jarvie, & Smith, 2015). Pudendal block does not change maternal hemodynamic or respiratory functions, vital signs, or FHR. However, the bearing-down reflex may be lessened or lost completely.

Spinal anaesthesia. In spinal anaesthesia (block), an anaesthetic solution containing a local anaesthetic alone or in combination with an opioid is injected through the third, fourth, or fifth lumbar interspace into the subarachnoid space (Fig. 18-13, A and B), where the anaesthetic solution mixes with cerebrospinal fluid (CSF). Low spinal anaesthesia (block) may be used for vaginal birth, but it is not suitable for labour. Spinal anaesthesia (block) used for Caesarean birth provides anaesthesia from the nipple (T6) to the feet. If it is used for vaginal birth,

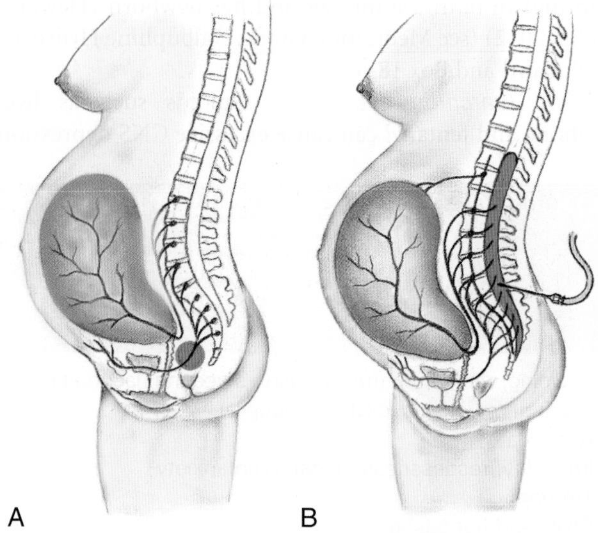

FIGURE 18-11 Pain pathways and sites of pharmacological nerve blocks. **A:** Pudendal block; suitable during second and third stages of labour and for repair of episiotomy. **B:** Epidural block; suitable during all stages of labour and for repair of episiotomy.

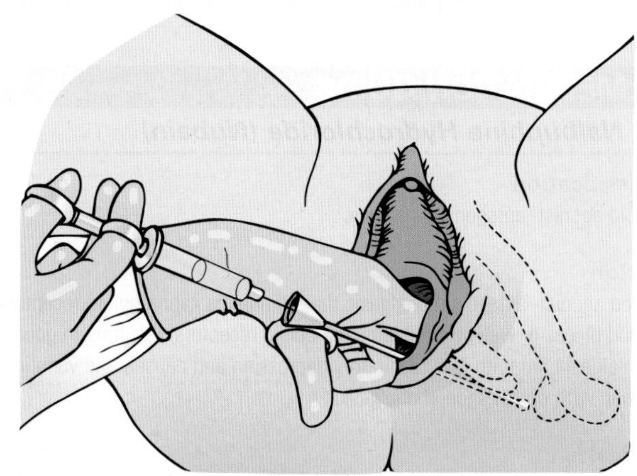

FIGURE 18-12 Pudendal block. Use of needle guide ("Iowa trumpet") and Luer-Lok syringe to inject medication.

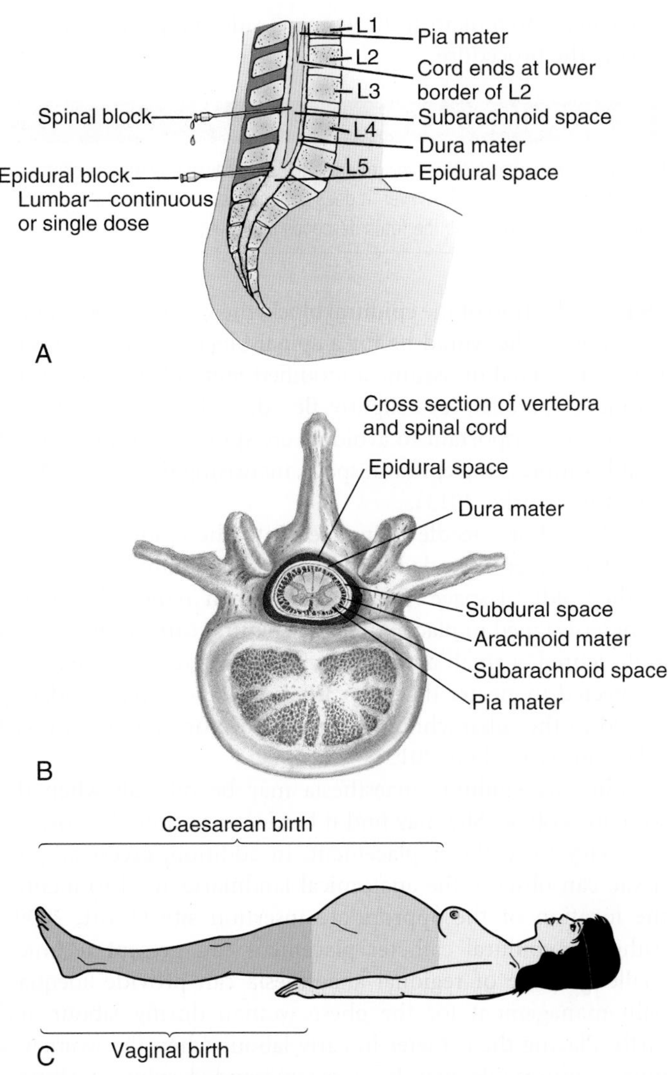

FIGURE 18-13 A: Membranes and spaces of spinal cord and levels of sacral, lumbar, and thoracic nerves. **B:** Cross section of vertebra and spinal cord. **C:** Levels of anaesthesia necessary for Caesarean and vaginal births.

the anaesthesia level is from the hips (T10) to the feet (see Fig. 18-13, C).

For spinal anaesthesia (block), the woman sits or lies on her side (e.g., modified Sims position) with her back curved to widen the intervertebral space; this position facilitates insertion of a small-gauge spinal needle and injection of the anaesthetic solution in the spinal canal. The nurse supports the woman and encourages her to use breathing and relaxation techniques in order to help her remain still during placement of the spinal needle. The needle is inserted and the anaesthetic injected between contractions. After the anaesthetic solution has been injected, the woman may be positioned upright to allow the heavier (hyperbaric) anaesthetic solution to flow downward to obtain the lower level of anaesthesia suitable for a vaginal birth. To obtain the higher level of anaesthesia desired for Caesarean birth, she is positioned supine with head and shoulders slightly elevated. To prevent supine hypotensive syndrome, the uterus is displaced laterally by tilting the operating table or placing a

EMERGENCY

Maternal Hypotension With Decreased Placental Perfusion

Signs/Symptoms

Maternal hypotension (20% drop from preblock baseline level or less than 100 mm Hg systolic)
Fetal bradycardia
Absent or minimal fetal heart rate (FHR) variability

Interventions

Turn woman to lateral position or place pillow or wedge under hip (see Fig. 18-3, D) to displace uterus.
Maintain intravenous (IV) infusion at rate specified, or increase administration per hospital protocol.
Administer oxygen by non-rebreather face mask at 10 to 12 L/min or per protocol.
Elevate woman's legs.
Notify the primary health care provider and anaesthesiologist.
Administer IV vasopressor (e.g., ephedrine 5 to 10 mg or phenylephrine 50 to 100 mcg) as per primary health care provider's order if previous measures are ineffective.
Remain with the woman; continue to monitor maternal blood pressure and FHR every 5 minutes until her condition is stable.

wedge under one of her hips. Usually the level of the block will be complete and fixed within 5 to 10 minutes after the anaesthesic solution is injected, but it can continue to creep upward for 20 minutes or longer (Hawkins & Bucklin, 2012). The anaesthetic effect will last 1 to 3 hours, depending on the type and amount of agent used.

SAFETY ALERT

To reduce the risk for transmission of pathogens, it is recommended that (1) the patient's back is cleansed before the procedure and (2) during the induction of spinal and epidural anaesthesia/analgesia, the anaesthesia care provider removes jewellery, washes hands, and wears sterile gloves and a face mask.

Marked hypotension, impaired placental perfusion, and an ineffective breathing pattern may occur during any spinal anaesthesia. Before induction of the spinal anaesthetic, maternal vital signs are assessed and the FHR is evaluated. In addition, the woman's fluid balance should be assessed, and IV fluid is usually administered to decrease the potential for hypotension caused by *sympathetic blockade* (vasodilation with pooling of blood in the lower extremities decreases cardiac output). If a bolus is given, the fluid should not contain dextrose, which could contribute to neonatal hypoglycemia (Hawkins & Bucklin, 2012).

After induction of the anaesthetic, maternal blood pressure, pulse, and respirations and FHR and pattern must be checked and documented every 5 to 10 minutes. If signs of serious maternal hypotension (e.g., the systolic blood pressure drops to 100 mmHg or less or the blood pressure falls 20% or more below the baseline) or abnormal FHR patterns (e.g., bradycardia, minimal or absent variability, late decelerations) develop, emergency care must be given (Burke, 2013) (see Emergency box).

Given the nature of spinal anaesthesia, the woman may be unable to sense her contractions; thus she must be instructed when to bear down during a vaginal birth. Use of a combination of local anaesthetic agent and an opioid reduces the degree of motor function loss, enhancing a woman's ability to push effectively. If the birth occurs in a delivery room (rather than a labour–birth–recovery room), the woman will need assistance in the transfer to a recovery bed after expulsion of the placenta and perineal repair, if required.

Advantages of spinal anaesthesia include ease of administration and absence of fetal hypoxia with maintenance of maternal blood pressure within normal range. Maternal consciousness is maintained, excellent muscular relaxation is achieved, and blood loss is not excessive.

Disadvantages of spinal anaesthesia include potential medication reactions (e.g., allergy), hypotension, and the risk of a high spinal leading to respiratory depression or a sense of not being able to breathe effectively despite having oxygen saturation levels well within the normal parameters. In the rare event that a high spinal does occur, causing respiratory depression, cardiopulmonary resuscitation may be required. When a spinal anaesthetic is given, the need for operative birth (e.g., episiotomy, forceps- or vacuum-assisted birth) tends to increase because voluntary expulsive efforts are reduced or eliminated. After birth, the incidence of bladder and uterine atony, as well as postdural puncture headache, is higher.

Epidural anaesthesia or analgesia (block). Relief from the pain of uterine contractions and birth (vaginal and Caesarean) can be achieved by injecting a suitable local anaesthetic agent (e.g., bupivacaine, ropivacaine), an opioid analgesic (e.g., fentanyl, sufentanil), or both into the epidural space. Injection is made between the fourth and fifth lumbar vertebrae for a lumbar epidural block (see Figs. 18-10, B, and 18-12, A). Depending on the type, amount, and number of medications used, an anaesthetic or analgesic effect will occur with varying degrees of motor impairment. The combination of an opioid with the local anaesthetic agent reduces the dose of anaesthetic required, thereby preserving a greater degree of motor function.

Epidural anaesthesia and analgesia is the most effective pharmacological pain-relief method for labour currently available. As a result, it is the most commonly used method for relieving pain during labour in Canada. In 2014-2015, epidural rates varied among the provinces. About two thirds of vaginal births in Quebec (71.9%) and Ontario (64.9%) were preceded by an epidural—nearly double the rates of Manitoba (39.7%) and British Columbia (36.2%) (Canadian Institute of Health Information [CIHI], 2016).

For relieving the discomfort of labour and vaginal birth, a block from T10 to S5 is required. For Caesarean birth, a block from at least T8 to S1 is essential (see Fig. 18-12, C). The diffusion of epidural anaesthesia depends on the location of the catheter tip, the dose and volume of the anaesthetic agent used, and the woman's position (e.g., horizontal or head-up position). The women must maintain her position without moving during the insertion of the epidural catheter to prevent misplacement, neurological injury, or hematoma formation. The nurse needs to remain at the woman's side and provide support during the procedure.

NURSING ALERT

Epidural anaesthesia effectively relieves the pain caused by uterine contractions for most women. However, it does not completely remove the pressure sensations that occur as the fetus descends in the pelvis.

For induction of the epidural block, the woman is positioned the same as she would be for a spinal block. She may sit with her back curved or assume a modified Sim's position with her shoulders parallel, legs slightly flexed, and back arched (Fig. 18-14). It is important to avoid severe spinal flexion because it could compress the epidural space, increasing the risk for dural puncture (Burke, 2013).

A large-bore needle is inserted into the epidural space. A catheter is then threaded through the needle until its tip rests in the epidural space. The needle is then removed, and the catheter is taped in place. After the epidural catheter is inserted and secured, a small amount of medication, called a *test dose,* is injected to ensure that the catheter has not been accidently placed in the subarachnoid (spinal) space or in a blood vessel (Hawkins & Bucklin, 2012).

Initiating epidural anaesthesia may be difficult when the woman is obese. She may find it harder to assume the position necessary for catheter placement. In addition, excess adipose tissue can obscure the anatomical landmarks used to identify the location of the appropriate insertion site (Jevitt, 2009). Although epidural catheter placement can present technical challenges, use of regional anaesthesia can provide adequate pain management for the obese woman during labour and birth. Placing the catheter in early labour when the woman is more comfortable may be a recommended solution (Burke, 2013). Early placement of a functioning epidural may reduce the risk of requiring intubation and the potential complications associated with intubation during an emergent delivery. Note that epidural anaesthesia presents less risk for the obese woman than does general anaesthesia (see further discussion in Chapter 15, p. 381).

After the epidural has been initiated, the woman is positioned preferably on her side; this is done so that the uterus does not compress the ascending vena cava and descending aorta, which can impair venous return, reduce cardiac output and blood pressure, and decrease placental perfusion. Her position should be alternated from side to side at minimum every hour. Upright position and ambulation may be possible, depending on the degree of motor impairment. Oxygen should be available if hypotension occurs despite maintenance of hydration with IV fluid and displacement of the uterus to the side. Blood pressure should be monitored every 5 to 10 minutes for the first 30 minutes after insertion. Ephedrine or phenylephrine (vasopressors used to increase maternal blood pressure) and increased IV fluid infusion may be needed (see Emergency box). The FHR, contraction pattern, and progress in labour must be monitored carefully because the woman may not be aware of changes in strength of uterine contractions or

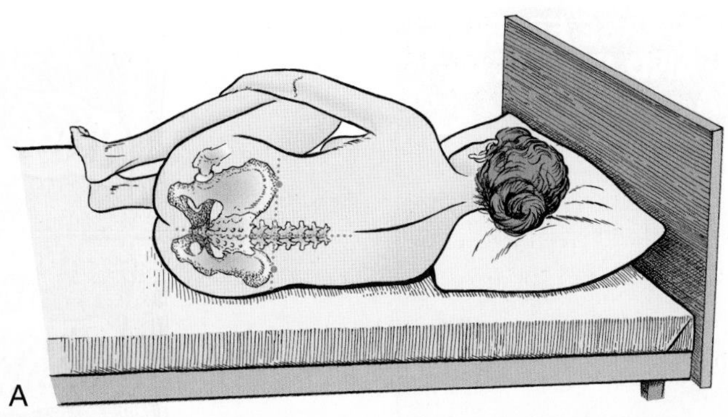

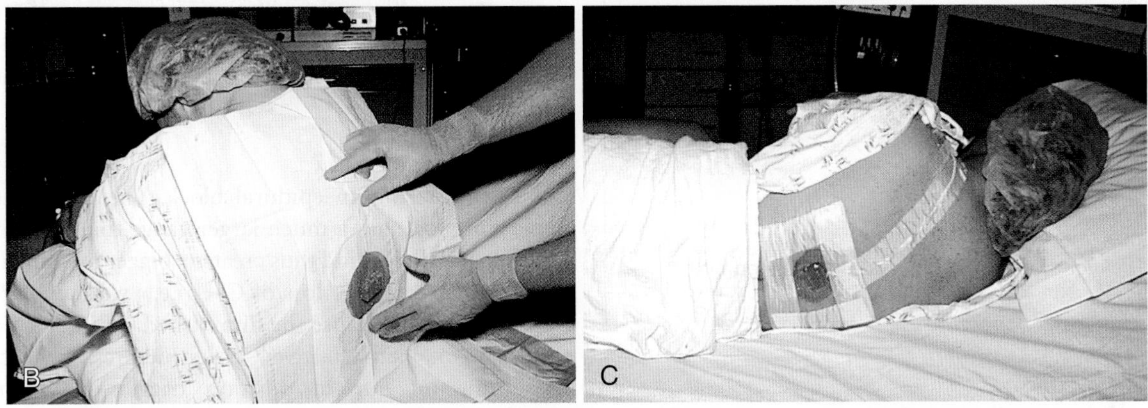

FIGURE 18-14 Position for spinal and epidural blocks. **A:** Lateral position. **B:** Upright position. **C:** Catheter is taped to woman's back with port segment located near her shoulder. (**B** and **C**, Courtesy Michael S. Clement, MD.)

the descent of the presenting part. There is no evidence to support the use of continuous electronic fetal monitoring for women who have received epidural anaesthesia; intermittent auscultation is appropriate in many situations; and the decision on how to monitor a woman in labour who has an epidural must take into account the entire clinical picture (Liston et al., 2007).

Several methods can be used for an epidural block. An intermittent block is achieved by using repeated injections of anaesthetic solution; it is the least common method because of the inconsistent nature of the pain relief provided from this method. The most common method is the continuous epidural infusion, achieved by using a pump to infuse the anaesthetic solution through an indwelling plastic catheter. Patient-controlled epidural analgesia (PCEA) involves an indwelling catheter and a programmed pump that allows the woman to control the dosing. PCEA can be used either with or without a basal infusion rate. This method enhances a woman's sense of control over her labour and has been found to decrease the total amount of medication used.

The advantages of an epidural block are numerous:

- The woman remains alert and is more comfortable and remains able to participate in the birth.
- Good relaxation is achieved.
- Airway reflexes remain intact.
- Mild motor paralysis may develop.
- Gastric emptying is not delayed.

Fetal complications are rare but may occur in the event of rapid absorption of the medication or marked maternal hypotension. The dose, volume, type, and number of medications used can be modified (1) to allow the woman to push, to assume upright positions, and even to walk; (2) to produce perineal anaesthesia; and (3) to permit forceps-assisted, vacuum-assisted, or Caesarean birth if required (Cunningham et al., 2014).

The disadvantages of an epidural block are also numerous. Length of labour may be longer and there may be increased requirement for oxytocin (Kukulu & Demirok, 2008). The woman's ability to move freely and maintain control of her labour is limited, related to the use of numerous medical interventions (e.g., an IV infusion, electronic monitoring, bladder catheterization) and the occurrence of orthostatic hypotension and dizziness, sedation, and weakness of the legs. CNS effects (Box 18-7) can occur if a solution containing a local anaesthetic agent is accidentally injected into a blood vessel or if excessive amounts of local anaesthetic are given.

High spinal or "total spinal" anaesthesia, resulting in respiratory arrest, can occur if the relatively high dosage used with an epidural block is accidentally injected into the subarachnoid space. Women who receive an epidural have a higher rate of fever (i.e., intrapartum temperature of 38°C or higher), especially when labour lasts longer than 12 hours; temperature elevation is most likely related to thermoregulatory changes, although infection cannot be ruled out. The elevation in temperature can result in fetal tachycardia and subsequent neonatal

BOX 18-7 POTENTIAL ADVERSE EFFECTS OF EPIDURAL AND SPINAL ANAESTHESIA

Hypotension
Local anaesthetic toxicity
Lightheadedness
Dizziness
Tinnitus (ringing in the ears)
Metallic taste
Numbness of the tongue and mouth
Bizarre behaviour
Slurred speech
Convulsions
Loss of consciousness
High or total spinal anaesthesia
Fever
Urinary retention
Pruritus (itching)
Limited movement
Longer second-stage labour
Increased use of oxytocin
Increased likelihood of forceps- or vacuum-assisted birth
Postdural punctural headache

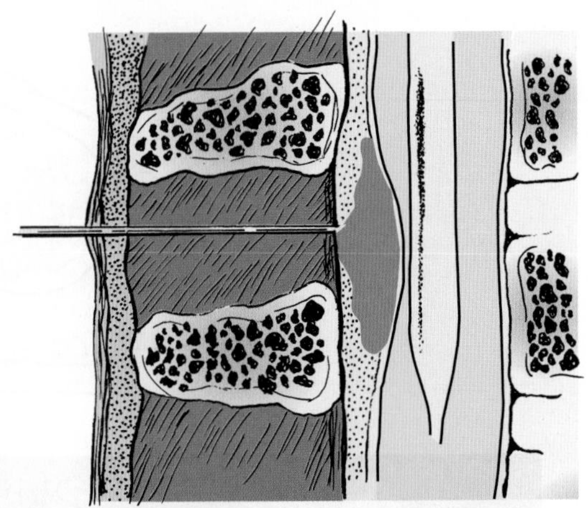

FIGURE 18-15 Blood-patch therapy for spinal headache.

workup for sepsis, regardless of whether or not signs of infection are present (see Box 18-7).

Hypotension as a result of sympathetic blockade can occur in about 10 to 30% of women who receive regional (spinal or epidural) anaesthesia during labour (Witcher & McLendon, 2013) (see Emergency box). Hypotension can result in a significant decrease in uteroplacental perfusion and oxygen delivery to the fetus (Anim-Somuah, Smyth, & Jones, 2011). Urinary retention and stress incontinence can occur in the immediate postpartum period. This temporary difficulty in urinary elimination could be related not only to the effects of the epidural block and the need for catheterization but also to the increased duration of labour and need for forceps- or vacuum-assisted birth associated with the block. **Pruritus** (itching) is an adverse effect that often occurs with the use of an opioid, especially fentanyl and morphine. A relationship between epidural analgesia and longer second-stage labour, increased incidence of fetal malposition, use of oxytocin, and forceps- or vacuum-assisted birth has been documented. Research findings have been unable to demonstrate a significant increase in Caesarean birth associated with epidural analgesia (Anim-Somuah et al., 2011; Hawkins & Bucklin, 2012). For some women, the epidural block is not effective and a second form of analgesia is required to establish effective pain relief. When women progress rapidly in labour, pain relief may not be obtained before birth occurs.

Postdural puncture headache (PDPH). Inadvertent puncture of the dura mater may cause leakage of CSF from the site of puncture of the dura mater (membranous covering of the spinal cord). This is thought to be the major causative factor in *postdural puncture headache* (PDPH), commonly referred to as a *spinal headache*. Spinal headache is most likely to occur when the dura is accidentally punctured during the process of administering an epidural block. The needle used for an epidural block has a much larger gauge than the one used for spinal anaesthesia and thus creates a bigger opening in the dura, resulting in a greater loss of CSF (i.e., "wet tap"). Presumably, postural changes cause the diminished volume of CSF to exert traction on pain-sensitive CNS structures. Characteristically, assuming an upright position triggers or intensifies the headache, whereas assuming a supine position achieves relief (Hawkins & Bucklin, 2012). The resulting headache and auditory problems (e.g., tinnitus) and visual problems (e.g., blurred vision, photophobia) begin within 2 days of the puncture and may persist for days or weeks.

The likelihood of headache after dural puncture can be reduced if the anaesthesiologist uses a small-gauge spinal needle and avoids making multiple punctures of the meninges. If a dural puncture is suspected, passing an epidural catheter through the dural opening at the time of puncture to provide continuous spinal anaesthesia, with removal of the catheter 24 hours later, may help prevent spinal headache. Injecting preservative-free saline through the spinal catheter before removing it may also decrease the incidence of headache. Hydration and bedrest in the prone position have been recommended as preventive measures but have not been proven to be of much value (Arevalo-Rodriguez, Ciapponi, Munoz, et al., 2013; Hawkins & Bucklin, 2012).

Conservative management for PDPH usually includes administration of oral analgesics and methylxanthines (e.g., caffeine or theophylline) (Basurto Ona, Martínez García, Solà, et al., 2011). Methylxanthines cause constriction of cerebral blood vessels and may provide symptomatic relief. An autologous epidural blood patch is the most rapid, reliable, and beneficial relief measure for PDPH. The woman's blood (i.e., 10 to 20 mL) is injected slowly into the lumbar epidural space, creating a clot that patches the tear or hole in the dura mater around the spinal cord. Treatment with a blood patch is considered if the headache is severe or debilitating or does not resolve after conservative management. The blood patch is remarkably effective and is nearly complication free (Hawkins & Bucklin, 2012) (Fig. 18-15).

The woman should be observed for alteration of vital signs, pallor, clammy skin, and leakage of CSF for 1 to 2 hours after the blood patch is performed. If no complications occur, she may then resume normal activity. She should, however, be instructed to avoid coughing or straining the first day after the blood patch (Hawkins & Bucklin, 2012). She is also taught to avoid analgesics that affect platelet aggregation (e.g., nonsteroidal anti-inflammatory drugs [NSAIDs]) for 2 days, drink plenty of fluids, and observe for signs of infection at the site and for neurological symptoms such as pain, numbness, and tingling in legs and difficulty with walking or elimination.

Combined spinal–epidural analgesia. In the combined spinal–epidural (CSE) analgesia technique, an epidural catheter is inserted into the epidural space in the same manner of a conventional epidural; however, before the epidural catheter is placed, a smaller-gauge spinal needle is inserted through the bore of the epidural needle into the subarachnoid space. A small amount of opioid or combination of opioid and local anaesthetic is then injected intrathecally to rapidly provide analgesia. Afterward, the epidural catheter is inserted as usual. The CSE technique is an increasingly popular approach that can be used to block pain transmission without compromising motor ability. The concentration of opioid receptors is high along the pain pathway in the spinal cord, in the brainstem, and in the thalamus. These receptors are highly sensitive to opioids; as a result a small quantity of an opioid agonist analgesic produces marked pain relief lasting for several hours. If additional pain relief is needed, medication can be injected through the epidural catheter. The most common adverse effects of CSE are pruritus, urinary retention, immediate or delayed respiratory depression, and nausea. Naloxone can be given intravenously to manage these adverse effects without decreasing the degree of analgesia achieved (Cunningham et al., 2014; Hawkins & Bucklin, 2012). CSE analgesia is also associated with a greater incidence of FHR abnormalities than with epidural analgesia alone, necessitating close assessment of FHR and pattern (Cunningham et al., 2014).

Although women can walk with CSE, they often choose not to do so because of sedation and fatigue, abnormal sensations in and weakness of the legs, and a feeling of insecurity. Often health care providers are reluctant to encourage or assist these women to ambulate for fear of injury. However, women can be assisted to change positions and use upright positions during labour and birth.

Epidural and intrathecal (spinal) opioids. Opioids can be used alone, eliminating the effect of a local anaesthetic altogether. The use of epidural or intrathecal (spinal) opioids without the addition of a local anaesthetic agent during labour has several advantages. Opioids administered in this manner do not cause maternal hypotension or affect vital signs. The woman feels contractions but not pain. Her ability to bear down during the second stage of labour is preserved because the pushing reflex is not lost and her motor power remains intact.

Fentanyl, sufentanil, or preservative-free morphine may be used. Fentanyl and sufentanil produce short-acting analgesia (i.e., 1.5 to 3.5 hours), and morphine may provide pain relief for 4 to 7 hours. Morphine may be combined with fentanyl or sufentanil. Using short-acting opioids with multiparous women and morphine with nulliparous women or women with a history of long labour is appropriate. For most women, intrathecal opioids alone usually do not provide adequate analgesia; they are most often given in combination with a local anaesthetic such as bupivicaine (Cunningham et al., 2014). A more common indication for the administration of epidural or intrathecal analgesics is the relief of postoperative pain. For example, a woman who gives birth by Caesarean can receive fentanyl or morphine through a catheter. The catheter can then be removed, and the woman is usually free of pain for 24 hours. Occasionally, the catheter is left in place in the epidural space in case another dose is needed.

Women who receive epidurally administered morphine after Caesarean birth can ambulate sooner than women who do not. The early ambulation and freedom from pain also facilitate bladder functioning, enhance peristalsis, and prevent clot formation (e.g., thrombophlebitis) in the lower extremities. Woman may require additional medication for breakthrough pain during the first 24 hours after surgery. If so, they will usually be given an NSAID such as ibuprofen (Motrin) or naproxen rather than a narcotic.

Adverse effects of opioids administered by the epidural and intrathecal routes include nausea, vomiting, diminished peristalsis, pruritus, urinary retention, and delayed respiratory depression. These effects are more common when morphine or fentanyl is administered. Antiemetics, antipruritics, and opioid antagonists are used to relieve these symptoms. For example, naloxone (Narcan), promethazine (Phenergan), diphenhydramine (Benadryl), or metoclopramide (Maxeran) may be administered. Hospital protocols should provide specific instructions for treatment of these adverse effects. Use of epidural opioids is not without risks. Respiratory depression is a serious concern; for this reason, the woman's respiratory rate should be assessed and documented every hour for 24 hours or as designated by hospital protocol. Naloxone should be readily available for use if the respiratory rate decreases to less than 10 breaths/min or if the oxygen saturation rate decreases to less than 89%. Administration of oxygen by non-rebreather face mask may also be initiated, and the anaesthesia care provider should be notified.

Contraindications to subarachnoid and epidural blocks. Contraindications to epidural analgesia (Burke, 2013; Cunningham et al., 2014; Hawkins & Bucklin, 2012) include the following:

- Active or anticipated maternal hemorrhage. Acute hypovolemia leads to increased sympathetic tone to maintain the blood pressure. Any anaesthetic technique that blocks the sympathetic fibres can produce significant hypotension that can endanger the mother and baby.
- Significant maternal hypotension
- Coagulopathy. If a woman is receiving anticoagulant therapy (e.g., last dose of low-molecular-weight heparin within 12 hours) or has a bleeding disorder, injury to a blood vessel may cause the formation of a hematoma that may compress the cauda equina or the spinal cord and lead to serious CNS complications.

- Infection at or near the injection site. Infection can be spread through the peridural or subarachnoid spaces if the needle traverses an infected area.
- Increased intracranial pressure caused by a mass lesion
- Allergy to the anaesthetic drug
- Maternal refusal or inability to assist with insertion
- Some types of maternal cardiac conditions

With an increase in the number of women who have body art and specifically low-back tattoos, there has been some concern over whether it is safe to give an epidural through a tattoo. The present recommendation is that an epidural should not be denied to someone with a low-back tattoo, although direct tattoo puncture should be avoided, if possible, as there is potential for the epidural not to be effective (Mercier & Bonnet, 2009).

Epidural block effects on newborn. Analgesia or anaesthesia during labour and birth has little or no lasting effect on the physiological status of the newborn, although further research needs to be done on the immediate effects of the medications on the newborn, specifically related to breastfeeding. There is no evidence that the administration of maternal analgesic or anaesthesic agents during labour and birth has a significant effect on the child's later mental and neurological development (American Academy of Pediatrics [APA] and American Congress of Obstetricians and Gynecologists [ACOG] 2012).

Nitrous oxide for analgesia. Nitrous oxide administered as Entonox (a 50/50 oxygen: nitrous oxide mixture) is a CNS depressant thought to alter pain stimuli, resulting in a decreased perception of pain (Rooks, 2012). This form of analgesia is widely used in Canada as well as in the United Kingdom, Australia, and Finland. It can be used during the first and second stages of labour and can be used in combination with other nonpharmacological and pharmacological measures for pain relief.

Nitrous oxide is self-administered by women with a face mask or mouthpiece. The maximum therapeutic effect occurs approximately 50 seconds after continuous inhalation is commenced; therefore, beginning the inhalation process 30 seconds before the onset of a contraction (if regular) or as soon as a contraction begins (if irregular) provides the best pain relief (Jackson et al., 2015). When the woman inhales, a valve opens and the gas is released. She should continue to inhale the gas slowly and deeply until the contraction starts to subside. When inhalation stops, the valve closes. Between contractions, the woman should remove the device and breathe normally.

The nurse should observe the woman for adverse effects such as nausea and vomiting, drowsiness, dizziness, hazy memory, and loss of consciousness. Loss of consciousness is more likely to occur if opioids are used with the nitrous oxide. The use of nitrous oxide does not appear to depress uterine contractions or cause adverse reactions in the fetus and newborn. Its ease of use, rapid onset, and rapid termination of action make nitrous oxide a good option for labour analgesia (Rooks, 2011).

General anaesthesia. *General anaesthesia* rarely is used for uncomplicated vaginal birth. It is often the anaesthesia method of choice when rapid anaesthesia is needed in an emergency childbirth situation or when a spinal or epidural block is contraindicated (Witcher & McLendon, 2013). In addition, being awake and aware during major surgery may be unacceptable for some women having a Caesarean birth. The major risks associated with general anaesthesia are difficulty with or inability to intubate and aspiration of gastric contents (Cunningham et al., 2014; Hawkins & Bucklin, 2012). Anaesthesiologists are more likely to encounter difficulty with intubating morbidly obese patients, especially in an emergency situation, than with women of normal weight (Witcher & McLendon, 2013).

If general anaesthesia is being considered, the woman will have nothing by mouth and an IV infusion is put into place. If time allows, the woman will be premedicated with a nonparticulate (clear) oral antacid (e.g., sodium citrate/citric acid) to neutralize the acidic contents of the stomach. Aspiration of highly acidic gastric contents will damage lung tissue. Administration of a histamine (H_2)-receptor blocker such as famotidine (Pepcid) or ranitidine (Zantac) to decrease the production of gastric acid and metoclopramide (Reglan) to accelerate gastric emptying may also be ordered (Hawkins & Bucklin, 2012). Before the anaesthesia is given, a wedge should be placed under one of the woman's hips to displace the uterus. Uterine displacement prevents compression of the aorta and vena cava, which maintains cardiac output and placental perfusion (Hawkins & Bucklin, 2012).

Before the induction of anaesthesia, the woman will be preoxygenated with 100% oxygen by non-rebreather face mask for 2 to 3 minutes. This is especially important in pregnant women, who are more likely than other adults to rapidly become hypoxemic if there is a delay in successful intubation. Propofol, a short-acting barbiturate, or ketamine is administered intravenously to render the woman unconscious. Next, succinylcholine, a muscle relaxant, is administered to facilitate passage of an endotracheal tube (Cunningham et al., 2014; Hawkins & Bucklin, 2012). Sometimes the nurse is asked to assist with applying cricoid pressure—*the Sellick manoeuvre*—before intubation as the woman begins to lose consciousness. This manoeuvre blocks the esophagus and prevents aspiration should the woman vomit or regurgitate (Fig. 18-16). Pressure is released once the endotracheal tube is securely in place.

After the woman is intubated, a 50:50 mixture of nitrous oxide and oxygen is administered. A low concentration of a volatile halogenated agent (e.g., isoflurane) may also be administered to increase pain relief and to reduce maternal awareness and recall (Cunningham et al., 2014; Hawkins & Bucklin, 2012). In low concentrations, these agents do not relax the uterus, so bleeding should not increase because of their use (Hawkins & Bucklin, 2012). In higher concentrations, isoflurane or methoxyflurane relaxes the uterus quickly and facilitates intrauterine manipulation, version, and extraction. However, at higher concentrations, these agents cross the placenta readily and can produce narcosis in the fetus and could reduce uterine tone after birth, increasing the risk for hemorrhage. Given the risk for neonatal narcosis, it is critical that the baby be delivered as soon as possible after the induction of the anaesthetic to reduce the degree of fetal exposure to the anaesthetic agents and the CNS depressants administered.

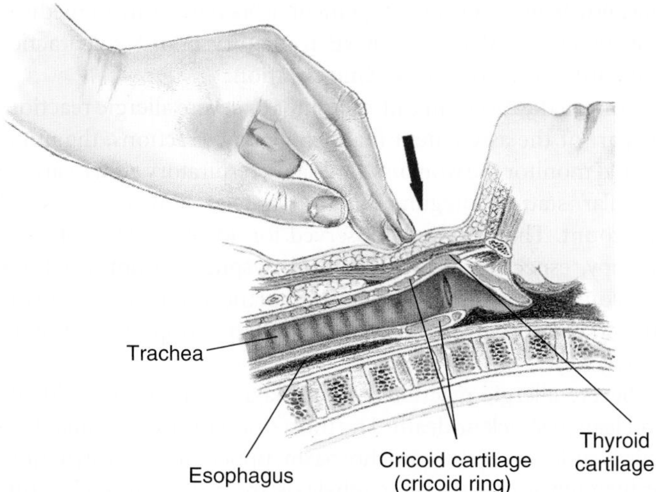

FIGURE 18-16 Technique of applying pressure on cricoid cartilage to occlude esophagus to prevent aspiration of gastric contents during induction of general anaesthesia.

Priorities for recovery room care are to maintain an open airway and cardiopulmonary function and to prevent postpartum hemorrhage. Women who had surgery under general anaesthesia will require pain medication soon after regaining consciousness. Routine postpartum care is organized to facilitate parent–infant attachment as soon as possible and to answer the mother's questions. The nurse needs to assess the mother's readiness to see her baby, as well as her response to the anaesthesia and to the event that necessitated general anaesthesia (e.g., emergency Caesarean birth when vaginal birth was anticipated).

NURSING CARE

The choice of pain relief depends on a combination of factors, including the woman's special needs and wishes, the availability of the desired method(s), the knowledge and expertise in nonpharmacological and pharmacological methods of the health care providers involved in the woman's care, and the phase and stage of labour (see Critical Thinking Case Study).

Informed Consent

Pregnant women have the right to be active participants in determining the best pain care approach to use during their labour and birth. The primary health care provider and anaesthesia care provider are responsible for fully informing women of the alternative methods of pharmacological pain relief available in the hospital. A description of the various anaesthetic techniques and what they entail is essential to informed consent, even if the woman received information about analgesia and anaesthesia earlier in her pregnancy. The initial discussion of pain management options ideally should take place in the third trimester so that the woman has time to consider an alternative. Nurses play a part in the informed consent process by clarifying and describing procedures or by acting as the woman's advocate by asking the primary health care provider for further explanations (Box 18-8).

BOX 18-8 DO WOMEN HAVE A CHOICE FOR LABOUR ANALGESIA?

A technological birthing model that uses labour induction, epidural analgesia, continuous electronic fetal monitoring, and Caesarean birth increasingly dominates labour and birth wards in industrialized countries. It is unknown whether the use of epidural analgesia by women in labour in Canada is a true preference or if it is selected because the only other choice is parenteral opioids. The rate of use of epidural analgesia is high in highly technological teaching hospitals. There is ample evidence of the benefits of the use of doulas and continuous support in labour, yet many women are not offered these options. Do women really have choices for pain management if they are not offered alternative pain management strategies? Research is needed to discover which pain-relief methods women would choose if they were offered a wide range of options.

CRITICAL THINKING CASE STUDY

Pain Management

You are assigned to care for a 17-year-old, single, nulliparous woman in active labour who is thrashing about in her bed and requesting something for "this terrible pain." She did not attend childbirth preparation classes and is alone for labour. She has the PRN orders for pain that are routine on your unit. She can ambulate and has intermittent auscultation as appropriate for her stage of labour.

QUESTIONS

1. Evidence—Is there sufficient evidence to draw conclusions about what nonpharmacological and pharmacological pain-relief techniques can be instituted?
2. Assumptions—What assumptions can be made about the following issues?
   a. Reactions to pain of a young, single woman who lacks support in labour
   b. Degree of pain relief expected by the woman
   c. Degree of pain relief expected by the nurse
   d. Nonpharmacological measures that are effective
3. What implications and priorities for nursing care can be drawn at this time?
4. Does the evidence objectively support your conclusion?

LEGAL TIP

INFORMED CONSENT FOR ANAESTHESIA

The woman receives (in an understandable manner) all of the following:

- Explanation of the alternative methods of analgesia and anaesthesia available
- Description of anaesthetic, including its effects and procedure for its administration
- Description of the benefits, discomfort, risks, and consequences for the mother and the fetus
- Explanation of how complications can be treated
- Information that the anaesthetic is not always effective
- Indication that the woman may withdraw consent at any time
- Opportunity to have any questions answered
- Opportunity to have components of the consent explained in the woman's own words

NURSING ALERT

In some cultures, the husband must consent to procedures performed on the wife. Although in Canada the woman is the person who gives consent and signs the necessary forms, she may not be willing to do so unless her husband also approves.

Timing of Administration

Accurate monitoring of the progress of labour and assessment of the labouring woman's level of coping assist the nurse in helping the woman decide when it is appropriate to start pharmacological control of discomfort. It is often the nurse who notifies the primary health care provider when the woman requests pharmacological measures to relieve her discomfort. Orders are often written for the administration of pain medication as needed by the woman and are based on the nurse's clinical judgement. In the past, pharmacological measures for pain relief were not implemented until labour had advanced to the active phase of the first stage of labour and the cervix had dilated approximately 4 to 5 cm, to avoid suppressing the progress of labour. However, it is now known that epidural anaesthesia in early labour does not increase the rate of Caesarean birth. Whereas it may shorten the duration of the first stage of labour in some women, epidural anaesthesia lengthens it in others (Hawkins & Bucklin, 2012). It is no longer recommended that women in labour reach a certain level of cervical dilation or fetal station before receiving epidural anaesthesia (APA & ACOG, 2012; Cunningham et al., 2014). It is, however, still recommended that the administration of systemic opioid analgesics be delayed until labour is well established (Burke, 2013). Nonpharmacological measures can be used to relieve pain and stress and enhance progress at any time in labour.

Preparation for Procedures

The methods of pain relief available to the woman are reviewed and information is clarified as necessary. The procedure and what should be expected of the woman (e.g., to maintain flexed position during insertion of epidural needle) must be explained.

The woman can also benefit from knowing the way the medication will be given, the degree of discomfort to expect from administration of the medication, the interval before the medication takes effect, and the expected pain relief from the medication. Skin-preparation measures are described and an explanation is given for the need to empty the bladder before the analgesic or anaesthetic is administered and the reason for keeping the bladder empty. When an indwelling catheter is to be threaded into the epidural space, the woman should be told that she may experience a momentary twinge down her leg, hip, or back and that this feeling is not a sign of injury.

A long needle is used for pudendal blocks (see Fig. 18-11). The sight of this needle may be frightening; the woman should be reassured that only the tip of the needle will be inserted.

Administration of Medication

It is essential for nurses to have current and accurate information about medications used during childbirth. They must have the knowledge, skill, and judgement needed to perform medication practices safely. Provincial regulatory bodies set practice standards for medication administration.

Any medication can cause a minor or severe allergic reaction. As part of the assessment for such allergic reactions, the nurse should monitor the woman's vital signs, respiratory effort, cardiovascular status, integument, and platelet and white blood cell count. The woman is observed for adverse effects of drug therapy, especially drowsiness and dyspnea. Minor reactions can consist of rash, rhinitis, fever, shortness of breath, or pruritus. Management of the less acute allergic response is not an emergency.

Severe allergic reactions (anaphylaxis) may occur suddenly and lead to shock or death. The most dramatic form of anaphylaxis is sudden, severe bronchospasm, upper airway obstruction, or hypotension. Signs of anaphylaxis are largely caused by contraction of smooth muscles and may begin with irritability, extreme weakness, nausea, and vomiting. This may lead to dyspnea, cyanosis, convulsions, and cardiac arrest. Anaphylaxis must be diagnosed and treated immediately. Initial treatment usually consists of placing the woman in a supine position, injecting epinephrine intramuscularly as per the primary health care provider's order, administering fluid intravenously, securing and supporting the airway with ventilation if necessary, and giving oxygen. If response to these measures is inadequate, IV epinephrine should be given. Cardiopulmonary resuscitation may be necessary (see Chapter 14).

Intravenous route. The preferred route of administration of medications such as fentanyl and nalbuphine is through IV tubing, administered into the port nearest the port insertion of the infusion (proximal port). The medication is given slowly and in small increments during a contraction. It may be given over a period of three to five consecutive contractions if needed to complete the dose. It is given during contractions to decrease fetal exposure to the medication because uterine blood vessels are constricted during contractions and the medication stays within the maternal vascular system for several seconds before the uterine blood vessels reopen. The IV infusion is then restarted slowly to prevent a bolus of medication from being administered. IV medications may be administered by a physician in some hospitals. With this method of injection, the amount of medication crossing the placenta to the fetus is minimized. With decreased placental transfer, the mother's degree of pain relief is maximized. The IV route has the following advantages:

- Onset of pain relief is rapid and more predictable.
- Pain relief is obtained with small doses of the drug.
- Duration of effect is more predictable.

Intramuscular route. Although analgesics are still given intramuscularly, this is not the preferred route of administration for the woman in labour. The advantages of using the IM route are quick administration and no need to start an IV line.

Disadvantages of the IM route include the following:

- Onset of pain relief is delayed.
- Higher doses of medication are required.
- Medication is released at an unpredictable rate from the muscle tissue and is available for transfer across the placenta to the fetus.

The maternal medication levels (after IM injections) are unequal because of uneven distribution (maternal uptake) and metabolism. IM injections given in the upper portion of the arm (deltoid muscle) seem to result in more rapid absorption and higher blood levels of the medication than when administered in other sites.

Regional (epidural or spinal) anaesthesia. The registered nurse is permitted to monitor the status of the woman, the fetus, and the progress of labour; replace empty infusion syringes or bags with the same medication and concentration; stop the infusion and initiate emergency measures if the need arises; and remove the catheter if properly educated to do so. In some institutions the registered nurse may also alter the rate of medication infusion. Only qualified care providers (a physician in Canada) are permitted to insert a catheter and initiate epidural anaesthesia, verify catheter placement, and inject medication through the catheter.

SAFETY ALERT

Safe regional anaesthesia administration requires specialized education, experience, and competence. There is potential for significant maternal or fetal morbidity and mortality associated with some obstetrical anaesthesia complications. Therefore a licensed, credentialled anaesthesia care provider should manage regional anaesthesia and analgesia during labour and birth and be readily available to manage obstetrical anaesthesia-related emergencies (AWHONN, 2015).

Spinal nerve blocks can reduce bladder sensation, resulting in difficulty in voiding, thus the woman should be encouraged to empty her bladder before the induction of the block and should be encouraged to void at least every 2 hours thereafter. The nurse should palpate for bladder distension and measure urinary output to ensure that the bladder is being completely emptied. A distended bladder can inhibit uterine contractions and fetal descent, resulting in a slowing of the progress of labour. If a woman is unable to empty her bladder, a catheter may be necessary. An intermittent catheter is the preferred method, although occasionally an indwelling catheter may be inserted and left in place for the remainder of the first stage of labour. The status of the maternal–fetal unit and the progress of labour must be established before the block is performed. The nurse must assist the woman to assume and maintain the correct position for induction of epidural and spinal anaesthesia (see Fig. 18-15).

Depending on the level of motor blockage, the woman should be assisted to remain as mobile as possible. When in bed, her position should be alternated side to side at minimum every hour to ensure adequate distribution of the anaesthetic solution and to maintain circulation to the uterus and placenta.

SAFETY ALERT

After receiving an epidural block or opioid intravenously for pain, the woman should not be allowed to ambulate alone. She must either remain in bed or request assistance before attempting to get out of bed. The nurse assesses the woman for signs of orthostatic hypotension and return of sensation and motor function of the lower extremities before ambulation.

After a woman receives a spinal nerve block, she may not require massage and assistance with breathing but she will still need emotional support, reassurance, and information from the nurse. It is important to ensure that she receives reassurance and reminders that labour is still progressing. Having the woman feel the contractions with her hand will remind her of what is happening in her body. Some women may feel disappointed in themselves for requiring pain medication, and they need to be reassured regarding their decision.

Health care providers should be aware that effective epidural anaesthesia prolongs the second stage of labour by 15 to 30 minutes. A delay in the second stage of labour does not negatively affect maternal or fetal outcome, however, as long as the FHR tracing is normal, maternal hydration and analgesia are adequate, and there is ongoing progress in the descent of the fetal head. Therefore, operative interventions (e.g., the use of forceps or vacuum) to hasten the birth solely because the second stage is prolonged are unnecessary. Reducing the density of the epidural block during the second stage of labour, delaying pushing until the woman feels the urge to do so, and avoiding arbitrary definitions for the "normal" duration of second-stage labour are suggested as interventions to decrease the risk of operative vaginal birth (Hawkins & Bucklin, 2012). (See Chapter 17 for a full discussion of second-stage labour management.) Box 18-9 summarizes the nursing interventions for women receiving epidural or spinal anaesthesia.

Safety and General Care

The nurse monitors and records the woman's response to nonpharmacological pain-relief methods and to medication(s). This includes the degree of pain relief, the level of apprehension, the return of sensations and perception of pain, and allergic or adverse reactions (e.g., hypotension, respiratory depression, fever, pruritus, nausea and vomiting). The nurse continues to monitor maternal vital signs and FHR and pattern at frequent intervals, the strength and frequency of uterine contractions, changes in the cervix and station of the presenting part, the presence and quality of the bearing-down reflex, bladder filling, and state of hydration. Determining the fetal response after the administration of analgesia or anaesthesia is vital. The woman should be asked if she (or the family) has any questions. The nurse also assesses the woman's and her family's understanding of the need to ensure her safety (e.g., keeping side rails up, calling for assistance as needed).

The time that elapses between the administration of an opioid and the baby's birth should be documented. Medication given to the newborn to reverse opioid effects are also recorded. After birth, the woman who has had spinal, epidural, or general anaesthesia is assessed for return of sensory and motor function in addition to the usual postpartum assessments. Both the nurse and the anaesthesiologist are responsible for documenting assessments and care in relation to regional (epidural or spinal) anaesthesia.

BOX 18-9 NURSING INTERVENTIONS FOR THE WOMAN RECEIVING EPIDURAL OR SPINAL ANAESTHESIA

Prior to the Block

- Assess the woman's level of coping, using Fig. 18-4.
- Assist primary health care provider or anaesthesia care provider with explaining the procedure and obtaining the woman's informed consent.
- Assess maternal vital signs, level of hydration, labour progress, and fetal heart rate (FHR) and pattern.
- Insert an intravenous (IV) line and infuse a bolus of fluid (Ringer's lactate or normal saline) if ordered (e.g., 500 to 1000 mL 15 to 30 minutes before induction of the anaesthesia).
- Obtain laboratory results (hematocrit or hemoglobin level, other tests as ordered). Assist the woman to void.

During Initiation of the Block

- Assist the woman with assuming and maintaining proper position.
- Verbally guide the woman through the procedure, explaining sounds and sensations as she experiences them.
- Assist the anaesthesia care provider with documentation of vital signs, time and amount of medications given, etc.
- Monitor maternal vital signs (especially blood pressure) and FHR as ordered.
- Have oxygen and suction readily available.
- Monitor for signs of local anaesthetic toxicity (see Box 18-7) as the test dose of medication is administered.

While the Block Is in Effect

- Continue to monitor maternal vital signs and FHR as ordered (continuous monitoring of maternal heart rate [electrocardiogram (ECG)] and blood pressure may be ordered to monitor for accidental intravenous injection of medication).
- Continue to assess the woman's level of coping.
- Monitor for bladder distension:
  - Assist with spontaneous voiding on bedpan or toilet.
  - Insert urinary catheter if necessary.
- Encourage or assist the woman to change positions from side to side every 30 to 60 minutes.
- Promote safety:
  - Keep side rails up on the bed.
  - Place telephone and call light within easy reach.
  - Instruct woman not to get out of bed without help.
  - Make sure there is no prolonged pressure on anaesthetized body parts.
  - Keep the epidural catheter insertion site clean and dry.
  - Continue to monitor for anaesthetic side effects (see Box 18-7).

While the Block Is Wearing off After Birth

- Assess regularly for the return of sensory and motor function.
- Continue to monitor maternal vital signs as ordered.
- Monitor for bladder distension:
  - Assist with spontaneous voiding on bedpan or toilet.
  - Insert urinary catheter if necessary.
- Promote safety:
  - Keep side rails up on the bed.
  - Place telephone and call light within easy reach.
  - Instruct woman not to get out of bed without help.
  - Make sure there is no prolonged pressure on anaesthetized body parts.
  - Keep the epidural catheter insertion site clean and dry.
  - Continue to monitor for anaesthetic side effects (see Box 18-7).

KEY POINTS

- Nonpharmacological pain and stress management strategies are valuable for managing labour discomfort on their own or in combination with pharmacological methods.
- Women need to be supported during labour by health care providers who feel comfortable assessing a woman's level of coping during labour and providing the appropriate support based on the woman's needs.
- The gate-control theory of pain and the stress response form the basis for many of the nonpharmacological methods of pain relief.
- The type of analgesic or anaesthetic to be used is determined by maternal and health care provider preference, the stage of labour, and the method of birth.
- Sedatives may occasionally be used for women in prolonged early labour when there is a need to decrease anxiety or promote sleep or therapeutic rest.The use of opioid agonist–antagonist analgesics in women with pre-existing opioid dependence may cause symptoms of abstinence syndrome (opioid withdrawal).
- Naloxone (Narcan) is an opioid (narcotic) antagonist that can reverse narcotic effects, especially respiratory depression.
- Pharmacological control of pain during labour requires collaboration among the health care providers and the labouring woman.
- The nurse must understand medications, their expected effects, potential adverse effects, and methods of administration.
- Maintenance of maternal fluid balance is essential during spinal and epidural nerve blocks.
- Maternal analgesia or anaesthesia potentially affects neonatal neurobehavioural response.
- Epidural anaesthesia and analgesia is the most effective pharmacological pain relief method for labour that is available.
- General anaesthesia is rarely used for vaginal birth but may be used for Caesarean birth or whenever rapid anaesthesia is needed in an emergency childbirth situation.

evolve WEBSITE

Visit the Evolve website for additional resources related to the content in this chapter such as Case Studies, Critical Thinking Case Study Answers, Nursing Care Plans, Nursing Processes, Nursing Skills, and Review Questions for Exam Preparation at: *http://evolve.elsevier.com/Canada/Perry/maternal/*

REFERENCES

Aghabati, N., Mohammadi, E., & Pour Esmaiel, Z. (2010). The effect of therapeutic touch on pain and fatigue of cancer patients undergoing chemotherapy. *Evidence-based Complementary and Alternative Medicine, 7*(3), 375–381. doi:10.1093/ecam/nen006.

Albers, L. (2007). The evidence for physiologic management of the active phase of the first stage of labor. *Journal of Midwifery Women's Health, 52*(3), 207–215.

American Academy of Pediatrics (AAP), & American College of Obstetricians and Gynecologists (ACOG). (2012). *Guidelines for perinatal care* (7th ed.). Washington, DC: ACOG.

Anderson, D. (2011). A review of systemic opioids commonly used for labor pain relief. *Journal of Midwifery and Women's Health, 56*(3), 222–239.

Anim-Somuah, M., Smyth, R., & Jones, L. (2011). Epidural versus no epidural or no analgesia in labour. *Cochrane Database of Systematic Reviews*, (12). doi:10.1002/14651858.

Arevalo-Rodriguez, I., Ciapponi, A., Munoz, L., et al. (2013). Posture and fluids for preventing post-dural puncture headache. *Cochrane Database of Systematic Reviews*, (7). doi:10.1002/14651858.CD009199.pub2.

Association of Women's Health, Obstetric and Neonatal Nurses (AWHONN). (2015). Role of the registered nurse in the care of the pregnant woman receiving analgesia and anesthesia by catheter techniques. *Journal of Obstetric, Gynecologic, & Neonatal Nursing, 44*(1), 151–154. doi:10.1111/1552-6909.12532.

Basurto Ona, X., Martínez García, L., Solà, I., & Bonfill Cosp, X. (2011). Drug therapy for treating post-dural puncture headache. *Cochrane Database of Systematic Reviews*, (8). doi:10.1002/14651858.CD007887.pub2.

Bedwell, C., Dowswell, T., Neilson, J. P., & Lavender, T. (2011). The use of transcutaneous electrical nerve stimulation (TENS) for pain relief in labour: A review of the evidence. *Midwifery, 27*(5), e141–e145. doi:10.1016/j.midw.2009.12.004.Epug2010Feb18.

Beebe, K. R., & Lee, K. (2007). Sleep disturbance in late pregnancy and early labour. *Journal of Perinatal & Neonatal Nursing, 21*(2), 103–108.

Blackburn, S. T. (2013). *Maternal, fetal, and neonatal physiology: A clinical perspective* (4th ed.). St. Louis: Saunders.

Burke, C. (2013). Pain relief and comfort measures in labor. In K. Rice Simpson & P. Creehan (Eds.), *AWHONN's perinatal nursing* (4th ed.). Philadelphia: Lippincott Williams & Wilkins.

Callister, L. C., Khalaf, I., Semenic, S., et al. (2003). The pain of childbirth: Perceptions of culturally diverse women. *Pain Management Nursing, 4*(4), 145–154.

Canadian Institute of Health Information (CIHI). (2016). *Childbirth indicators by place of residence*. Retrieved from <http://apps.cihi.ca/mstrapp/asp/Main.aspx?Server=apmstrextprd_i&project=Quick+Stats&uid=pce_pub_en&pwd=&evt=2048001&visualizationMode=0&documentID=029DB170438205AEBCC75B8673CCE822>.

Cluett, E. R., & Burns, E. (2009). Immersion in water in labour and birth. *Cochrane Database of Systematic Reviews*, (2). doi:10.1002/14651858.CD000111.pub3.

Cunningham, F., Leveno, K., Bloom, S., et al. (2014). *Williams obstetrics* (24th ed.). New York: McGraw Hill.

Dowswell, T., Bedwell, C., Lavender, T., & Neilson, J. P. (2009). Transcutaneous electric nerve stimulation (TENS) for pain relief in labour. *Cochrane Database of Systematic Reviews*, (2). doi:10.1002/14651858.CD007214.pub2.

Gibson, E. (2014). Women's expectations and experiences with labour pain in medical and midwifery models of birth in the United States. *Women and Birth, 27*(3), 185–189.

Gilbert, E. S. (2011). *Manual of high risk pregnancy & delivery*. St. Louis: Mosby.

Gulliver, B. G., Fisher, J., & Roberts, L. (2008). A new way to assess pain in labouring women: Replacing the rating scale with a "coping" algorithm. *Nursing for Women's Health, 12*(5), 404–408.

Hawkins, J., & Bucklin, B. (2012). Obstetrical anesthesia. In S. Gabbe, J. Niebyl, H. Galan, et al. (Eds.), *Obstetrics: Normal and problem pregnancies* (6th ed.). Philadelphia: Saunders.

Hodnett, E. D., Gates, S., Hofmeyr, G., & Sakala, C. (2013). Continuous support for women during childbirth. *Cochrane Database of Systematic Reviews*, (7). doi:10.1002/14651858.CD003766.pub5.

International Association for the Study of Pain. (2012). *IASP taxonomy*. Retrieved from <http://www.iasp-pain.org/Taxonomy?navItemNumber=576#Pain>.

Jackson, K. T., Jarvie, L., & Smith, J. K. (2015). Pharmacologic pain management of labour. In R. Evans, M. K. Evans, & Y. M. R. Brown (Eds.), *Canadian maternity, newborn & women's health nursing* (2nd ed., p. 683). New York: Wolters Kluwer.

Jevitt, C. (2009). Pregnancy complicated by obesity: Midwifery management. *Journal of Midwifery & Women's Health, 54*(6), 445–451.

Jones, L., Othman, M., Dowswell, T., et al. (2012). Pain management for women in labour: An overview of systematic reviews. *Cochrane Database of Systematic Reviews*, (3). doi:10.1002/14651858.CD009234.pub2.

Kukulu, K., & Demirok, H. (2008). Effects of epidural anesthesia on labor progress. *Pain Management Nursing, 9*(1), 10–16.

Liston, R., Sawchuck, D., Young, D., et al. (2007). Fetal health surveillance: Antepartum and intrapartum consensus guideline. SOGC clinical practice guideline No. 197. *Journal of Obstetrics and Gynaecologists of Canada, 29*(9), s1–s56.

Lundgren, L., & Dahberg, K. (1998). Women's experience of pain during childbirth. *Midwifery, 14*, 105–110.

Madden, K., Middleton, P., Cyna, A. M., et al. (2012). Hypnosis for pain management during labour and childbirth. *Cochrane Database of Systematic Reviews*, (11). doi:10.1002/14651858.CD009356.pub2.

Marchand, S. (2012). *The phenomenon of pain*. Seattle, WA: International Association for the Study of Pain, IASP Press.

Melzack, R., Kinch, R., Dobkin, P., et al. (1984). Severity of labour pain: Influence of physical as well as psychologic variables. *Canadian Medical Association Journal, 130*, 579–584.

Mercier, F., & Bonnet, M. P. (2009). Tattooing and various piercing: Anaesthetic considerations. *Current Opinions in Anaesthesiology, 22*(3), 436–441.

Nutter, E., Meyer, S., Shaw-Battista, J., & Marowitz, A. (2014). Waterbirth: An integrative analysis of peer-reviewed literature. *Journal of Midwifery & Women's Health, 59*(3), 286–319. doi:10.1111/jmwh.12194.

Nutter, E., Shaw-Battista, J., & Marwitz, A. (2014). Waterbirth fundamentals for clinicians. *Journal of Midwifery & Women's Health, 59*(3), 350–354. doi:10.1111/jmwh.12193.

Perinatal Education Associates. (2016). *Breathing*. Retrieved from <http://www.birthsource.com/scripts/article.asp?articleid=211>.

Perinatal Services BC. (2007). *Pain management options during labour*. Retrieved from <http://www.perinatalservicesbc.ca/Documents/Guidelines-Standards/Maternal/PainManagementGuideline.pdf>.

Roberts, L., Gulliver, B., Fisher, J., & Cloyes, K. G. (2010). The coping with labor algorithm: An alternative pain assessment tool for laboring woman. *Journal of Midwifery & Women's Health*, *55*(2), 107–116. doi:10.1016/j.jmwh.2009.11.002.

Rookes, J. (2011). Safety and risks of nitrous oxide labor analgesia: A review. *Journal of Midwifery & Women's Health*, *56*(6), 557–565.

Rookes, J. (2012). Labor pain management other than neuraxial: What do we know and where do we go next? *Birth (Berkeley, Calif.)*, *39*(4), 318–322. doi:10.1111/birth.12009.EpubNov5.Review.

Simkin, P., & Bolding, A. (2004). Update on nonpharmacologic approaches to relieve labour pain and prevent suffering. *Journal of Midwifery & Women's Health*, *49*(6), 489–504.

Smith, C. A., Collins, C. T., & Crowther, C. A. (2011). Aromatherapy for pain management in labour. *Cochrane Database of Systematic Reviews*, (7). doi:10.1002/14651858.CD009215.

Smith, C. A., Collins, C. T., Crowther, C. A., & Levett, K. M. (2011). Acupuncture or acupressure for pain management in labour. *Cochrane Database of Systematic Reviews*, (7). doi:10.1002/14651858.CD009232.

Smith, C., Collins, C. T., Cyna, A. M., & Crowther, C. A. (2006). Complementary and alternative therapies for pain management in labour. *Cochrane Database of Systematic Reviews*, (4). doi:10.1002/14651858.CD003521.pub2.

Smith, C. A., Levett, K. M., Collins, C. T., & Crowther, C. A. (2011). Relaxation techniques for pain management in labour. *Cochrane Database of Systematic Reviews*, (12). doi:10.1002/14651858.CD009514.

Smith, C. A., Levett, K. M., Collins, C. T., & Jones, L. (2012). Massage, reflexology and other manual methods for pain management in labour. *Cochrane Database of Systematic Reviews*, (2). doi:10.1002/14651858.CD009290.pub2.

Stark, M., Rudell, B., & Haus, G. (2008). Observing position and movements in hydrotherapy: A pilot study. *Journal of Obstetric Gynecologic & Neonatal Nursing*, *37*(1), 116–122.

Tournaire, M., & Theau-Yonneau, A. (2007). Complementary and alternative approaches to pain relief during labor. *Evidenced-Based Complementary Alternative Medicine*, *4*(4), 409–417.

Trout, K. (2004). The neuromatrix theory of pain: Implications for selected nonpharmacologic methods of pain relief for labour. *Journal of Midwifery & Women's Health*, *49*(6), 482–488.

Walls, D. (2009). Herbs and natural therapies for pregnancy, birth, and breastfeeding. *International Journal of Childbirth Education*, *24*(2), 29–37.

Witcher, P., & McLendon, K. (2013). Anesthesia emergencies in the obstetric setting. In N. Troian, C. Harvey, & B. Chez (Eds.), *AWHONN's high risk and critical care obstetrics* (3rd ed.). Philadelphia: Wolters Kluwer/Lippincott Williams & Wilkins.

Zwelling, E. (2010). Overcoming the challenges: Maternal movement and positioning to facilitate labor progress. *MCN: American Journal of Maternal/Child Nursing*, *35*(2), 72–78. doi:10.1097/NMC.0b013e3181caeab3.

Zwelling, E., Johnson, K., & Allen, J. (2006). How to implement complementary therapies for laboring women. *MCN: American Journal of Maternal/Child Nursing*, *31*(6), 364–372.

ADDITIONAL RESOURCES

Bonapace Childbirth Training Program: <http://www.bonapace.com>.

Childbirth and Postpartum Professional Association (CAPPA) Canada: <http://www.cappacanada.ca/>.

Hypnobirthing: <http://www.hypnobirthingcanada.com/>.

International Childbirth Educators Association: <http://www.icea.org/>.

Lamaze International: <http://www.lamazeinternational.org>.

Registered Nurses' Association of Ontario (2013)—Assessment and Management of Pain (3rd ed.): <http://rnao.ca/sites/rnao-ca/files/AssessAndManagementOfPain_15_WEB-_FINAL_DEC_2.pdf>.

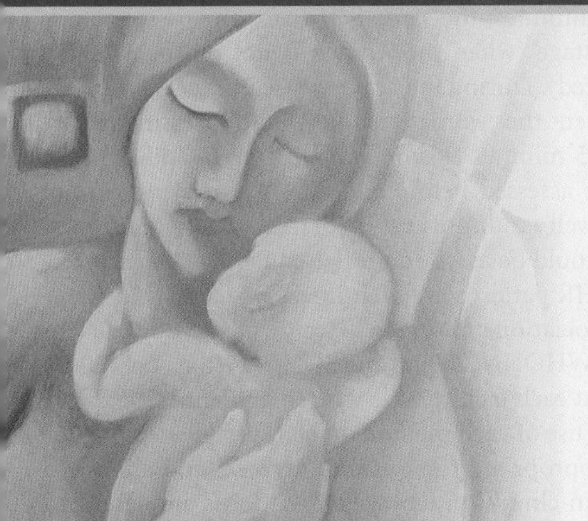

CHAPTER

19

Fetal Health Surveillance During Labour

Lauren B. Rivard, France Morin

evolve WEBSITE

***Visit the Evolve website for additional resources related to the content in this chapter such as Case Studies, Critical Thinking Case Study Answers, Nursing Care Plans, Nursing Processes, Nursing Skills, and Review Questions for Exam Preparation at:** http://evolve.elsevier.com/Canada/Perry/maternal/*

OBJECTIVES

On completion of this chapter the reader will be able to:

- Explain baseline fetal heart rate (FHR) and identify accelerations and decelerations of the FHR.
- Identify signs of normal, atypical, and abnormal FHR patterns.
- Describe nursing measures that can be used to maintain FHR patterns within normal limits and interventions used to manage atypical and abnormal FHR patterns.
- Compare FHR monitoring done by intermittent auscultation with electronic methods.
- Review the frequency and documentation of the monitoring process during labour.

FETAL HEALTH SURVEILLANCE

The ability to assess the fetus by auscultation of the fetal heart was initially described more than 300 years ago. With the advent of the fetoscope and stethoscope after the turn of the twentieth century, the listener could hear clearly enough to count the fetal heart rate (FHR). Electronic fetal monitoring (EFM) was introduced in the 1960s and was meant to be used primarily with high-risk women in labour. The Society of Obstetricians and Gynaecologists of Canada (SOGC) has published the Canadian guidelines for antepartum and **intrapartum** fetal surveillance that are used in obstetrical practice throughout Canada (Liston, Sawchuck, Young, et al., 2007). This chapter discusses the basis for fetal health surveillance during labour, the types of monitoring used, and nursing assessment and management of FHR findings.

When EFM was first introduced, it was anticipated that its use would decrease the rate of cerebral palsy (CP) and be more sensitive than auscultation in predicting and preventing fetal compromise (Garite, 2012). Consequently, the use of EFM rapidly expanded. However, research has shown that EFM has not reduced the incidence of CP. Furthermore, rates of CP are less likely to decline now as more preterm infants survive (Gilbert, 2011). Rising Caesarean birth rates have also been attributed to increased EFM use. The rate of Caesarean birth rates in Canada was 27.5% in 2014–2015 (Canadian Institute for Health Information [CIHI], 2016), representing a 46% increase from the previous decade. While the SOGC recommends **intermittent auscultation** (IA) for healthy term women in spontaneous labour and reserves the use of EFM for pregnancies at risk of adverse perinatal outcomes, the predominant method of fetal surveillance during labour, as reported by Canadian women, remains EFM (Public Health Agency of Canada [PHAC], 2009).

BASIS FOR MONITORING

Fetal Response

Labour is a period of physiological stress for the fetus; as such, monitoring of fetal status is an essential part of nursing care throughout labour. The fetal oxygen supply must be maintained during labour to prevent fetal compromise and promote newborn health after birth. Maternal, uteroplacental, and fetal factors may reduce the oxygen supply to the fetus; these are included in Box 19-1.

BOX 19-1 FACTORS THAT MAY AFFECT FETAL OXYGENATION IN LABOUR

Maternal Factors

- Decreased maternal arterial oxygen tension
  - Respiratory disease
  - Hypoventilation, seizure, trauma
  - Smoking
  - Obesity (BMI >35–40)
- Decreased maternal oxygen-carrying capability
  - Significant anemia (e.g., iron deficiency, hemoglobinopathies)
  - Carboxyhemoglobin (smokers)
- Decreased uterine blood flow
  - Hypotension (e.g., blood loss, sepsis)
  - Regional anaesthesia
  - Maternal positioning
- Chronic maternal conditions
  - Vasculopathies (e.g., systemic lupus erythematosus, type I diabetes, chronic hypertension)
  - Antiphospholipid syndrome
  - Cyanotic heart disease
  - Chronic obstructive pulmonary disease

Uteroplacental Factors

- Excessive uterine activity
  - Tachysystole secondary to oxytocin, prostaglandins (PGE_2), or spontaneous labour
  - Placental abruption
- Uteroplacental dysfunction
  - Placental abruption
  - Placental infarction—dysfunction marked by IUGR, oligohydramnios, or abnormal Doppler studies
  - Chorioamnionitis
  - Uterine rupture

Fetal Factors

- Cord compression
  - Oligohydramnios
  - Cord prolapse or entanglement
- Decreased fetal oxygen carrying capability
  - Significant anemia (e.g., isoimmunization, maternal–fetal bleed, ruptured vasa previa)
  - Carboxyhemoglobin (if mother is a smoker)

BMI, body mass index; IUGR, intrauterine growth restriction.
Adapted from Liston, R., Sawchuck, D., Young, D., et al. (2007). SOGC clinical practice guideline: Fetal health surveillance: Antepartum and intrapartum consensus guideline. *Journal of Obstetrics and Gynaecologists of Canada, 29*(9), s1–s56, p. S25.

FHR and uterine activity must both be assessed together and interpretation of the results should be based on the total clinical picture. Standards have been established for how frequently the FHR should be assessed, based on the clinical picture and the stage of labour. The SOGC recommends that the FHR be assessed and interpreted hourly in the latent stage of labour (if the woman is admitted to hospital) or when a significant change occurs (e.g., spontaneous rupture of the amniotic membrane). In active labour, the FHR should be assessed and interpreted every 15 to 30 minutes; the same is true for the passive phase of the second stage (when the women is not pushing despite being fully dilated). During the active phase of the second stage of labour (when the woman is pushing), assessments are required every 5 minutes (Liston et al., 2007). In addition, the FHR should be assessed before and after artificial rupture of membranes as well as administration of medications and anaesthesia, and it should be assessed more frequently when atypical or abnormal FHR patterns are identified.

Both the Association of Women's Health, Obstetric and Neonatal Nurses (AWHONN, 2009a) and SOGC (Liston et al., 2007) recommend that each facility have written guidelines regarding the appropriate use of each method of fetal surveillance, including clinically appropriate responses to atypical and abnormal FHR findings. In clinical practice, FHR patterns are described as normal with no intervention required, or as atypical or abnormal which require various interventions (Liston et al., 2007). It is the responsibility of the perinatal nurse to document the FHR, method of monitoring it, and interpretation of the FHR according to institutional policies and guidelines.

Uterine Activity

Uterine activity (UA) is assessed by palpation; additional assessment methods used include an external tocotransducer or an internal intrauterine pressure catheter (IUPC) (both generally used in conjunction with the EFM) (see discussion later in chapter). The following components should be included in a complete assessment of uterine activity: frequency, duration, intensity, and resting tone (Fig. 19-1). The type of information obtained depends on the type of monitoring method selected.

- *Frequency* is measured in minutes, from the beginning of one contraction to the beginning of the next contraction. Contraction frequency generally ranges from two to five contractions per 10 minutes during labour, with lower frequencies seen in the first stage of labour and higher frequencies seen during the second stage of labour (Miller, Miller, & Tucker, 2013).
- *Duration* is measured in seconds, from the beginning to the end of the contraction. Contraction duration remains fairly stable throughout first and second stages of labour, ranging from 45 to 80 seconds. *A contraction should last no longer than 90 seconds* (Miller et al., 2013).
- *Intensity* may be determined by palpation or by IUPC. If palpation is the method of assessment, the contractions are described as mild, moderate, or strong. If an IUPC is in place, intensity is measured in mmHg.
- *Resting tone* is the degree of muscular tension and is assessed between contractions. Average resting tone during labour is 10 mmHg; if assessed by palpation, it is usually described as soft or relaxed (AWHONN, 2009b).

A normal UA pattern in labour is characterized by contractions occurring no more than every 2 minutes (maximum of five contractions in 10 minutes) and lasting less than 90 seconds, with a minimum of 30 seconds of rest period between contractions. Ideal contractions are moderate to strong in intensity (assessed by palpation) and allow for uterine relaxation to be detected between them.

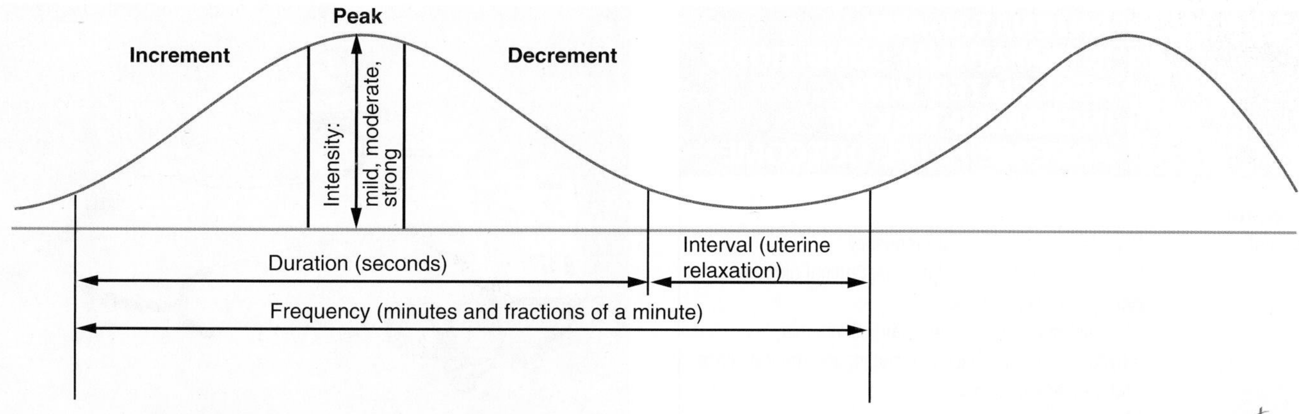

FIGURE 19-1 Components of uterine activity during labour. (From Murray, S. S., & McKinney, E. S. [2010]. *Foundations of maternal-newborn nursing* [5th ed.]. St. Louis: Saunders).

It is essential to document the UA in conjunction with the FHR assessment.

UA can be described as follows:

Normal—≤5 contractions in 10 minutes, averaged over a 30-minute window

Tachysystole—>5 contractions in 10 minutes, averaged over a 30-minute window

- Tachysystole should always be qualified by presence or absence of associated FHR changes.
- Tachysystole may occur in both spontaneous and stimulated labour.

Fetal Assessment

The goal of intrapartum fetal surveillance is to identify potential fetal decompensation, allowing for timely and effective interventions to prevent perinatal morbidity or mortality (Liston et al., 2007). UA is always assessed in association with the FHR. Components of a normal intrapartum fetal surveillance assessment are given in Table 19-1. The types of fetal monitoring (IA and EFM) are discussed later in the chapter.

TABLE 19-1 NORMAL INTRAPARTUM FETAL SURVEILLANCE FINDINGS

	IF USING IA	IF USING EFM
Baseline FHR	110–160 bpm	110–160 bpm
Rhythm	Regular (e.g., no skipped beats)	Not used with EFM
Variability	Not used with IA	Moderate (range of 6–25 bpm in FHR) Minimal or absent (range of ≤5 bpm in FHR) for <40 min
Deceleration	None heard	None or occasional uncomplicated variables or early decelerations
Accelerations	May be heard	Spontaneous accelerations may be present; accelerations occur with fetal scalp stimulation

bpm, beats per minute; *EFM*, electronic fetal monitoring; *FHR*, fetal heart rate; *IA*, intermittent auscultation.

Adapted from Liston, R., Sawchuck, D., Young, D., et al. (2007). SOGC clinical practice guideline: Fetal health surveillance: Antepartum and intrapartum consensus guideline. *Journal of Obstetrics and Gynaecologists of Canada, 29*(9 Suppl 4), S16.

MONITORING TECHNIQUES

The ideal method of fetal assessment during labour continues to be debated. Research indicates that IA of the FHR and EFM are associated with similar fetal outcomes in low-risk intrapartum patients (Gilbert, 2011). The use of EFM has been shown to increase the rate of intervention during labour, including Caesarean birth, operative vaginal births, and greater use of analgesia and anaesthesia. Given these findings, use of EFM is recommended for pregnancies at risk for adverse perinatal outcomes but not for low-risk women (Alfirevic, Devane, & Gyte, 2013; Liston et al., 2007). See Table 19-2 for antenatal and intrapartum conditions that are associated with adverse fetal outcomes which are considered high risk.

Despite the recommendation that EFM be used only for high-risk pregnancies, the use of EFM remains high, perhaps because of the following:

- Lack of nursing staff to provide one-to-one supportive care
- Caregiver skill and comfort with IA
- False belief that EFM will prevent all bad outcomes
- False caregiver belief that an EFM record will prevent medical legal actions

Regardless of the method used, there should be discussion with the women about benefits, risks, and limitations of IA and EFM (Liston et al., 2007).

Intermittent Auscultation

Intermittent auscultation (IA) involves listening to fetal heart sounds at periodic intervals in order to assess the FHR. IA of the fetal heart can be performed with a Pinard stethoscope (Fig. 19-2), Doppler ultrasound (doptone), an ultrasound stethoscope, or a DeLee-Hillis fetoscope (Fig. 19-3). The doptone, which is used most frequently for IA of the FHR, transmits ultra-high-frequency sound waves reflecting movement of the fetal heart and converts these sounds into an electronic signal that can be counted (see Fig. 19-3, A). The technique used for auscultation is described in Box 19-2.

TABLE 19-2 ANTENATAL AND INTRAPARTUM CONDITIONS ASSOCIATED WITH INCREASED RISK OF ADVERSE FETAL OUTCOME

Antenatal	
Maternal	Hypertensive disorders of pregnancy
	Pre-existing diabetes mellitus/gestational diabetes
	Antepartum hemorrhage
	Maternal medical condition: cardiac, anemia, hyperthyroidism, vascular disease, and renal disease
	Maternal MVA/trauma
	Morbid obesity
Fetal	Intrauterine growth restriction (IUGR)
	Prematurity
	Oligohydramnios
	Abnormal umbilical artery Doppler velocimetry
	Isoimmunization
	Multiple pregnancy
	Breech presentation
Intrapartum	
Maternal	Vaginal bleeding in labour
	Intrauterine infection/chorioamnionitis
	Previous Caesarean birth
	Prolonged membrane rupture >24 hours at term
	Induced labour
	Augmented labour
	Hypertonic uterus
	Preterm labour
	Postterm labour (>42 weeks)
Fetal	Meconium staining of the amniotic fluid
	Abnormal fetal heart rate on auscultation

MVA, motor vehicle accident.
Reprinted from Liston, R., Sawchuck, D., Young, D., et al. (2007). SOGC clinical practice guideline: Fetal health surveillance: Antepartum and intrapartum consensus guideline. *Journal of Obstetrics and Gynaecologists of Canada, 29*(9 Suppl 4), s1–s56. Copyright 2007, with permission from Elsevier.

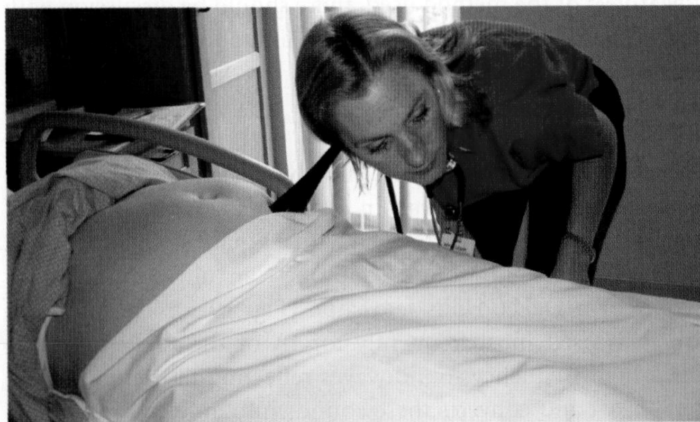

FIGURE 19-2 Pinard stethoscope. NOTE: Hands should not touch stethoscope while nurse is listening. (Courtesy Julie Perry Nelson.)

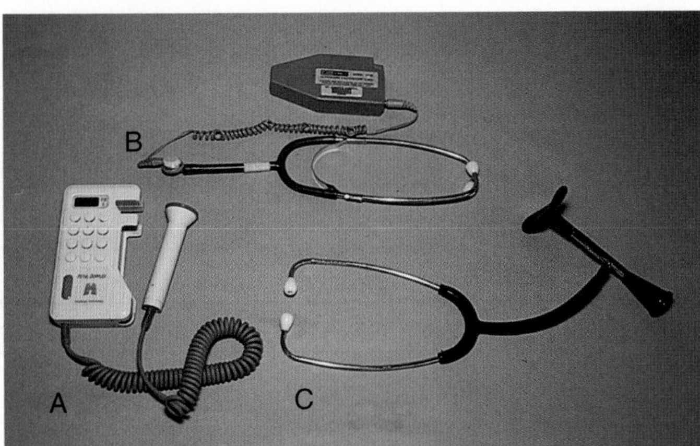

FIGURE 19-3 A: Doptone (ultrasound fetoscope). **B:** Ultrasound stethoscope. **C:** DeLee-Hillis fetoscope. (Courtesy Michael S. Clement, MD.)

BOX 19-2 INTERMITTENT AUSCULTATION PROCEDURE

Auscultation is performed as follows:

1. Explain the procedure to the woman and her support person(s).
2. Perform Leopold manoeuvres (see Box 17-5) by palpating the maternal abdomen to identify fetal presentation and position.
3. Palpate the uterus for the absence of uterine activity (UA) so that the fetal heart rate (FHR) is assessed between contractions.
4. Place the listening device over the area of maximal intensity, usually the fetal back, to obtain the clearest and loudest sound. Apply ultrasound gel to Doppler ultrasound device if used.
5. Assess the maternal radial pulse at the same time as listening to the FHR to differentiate it from the fetal rate.
6. Listen to the FHR for 60 seconds immediately after uterine contractions to identify the baseline rate (this rate can only be obtained between uterine contractions). There is no clear evidence about the best way to count to determine the baseline rate. The most accurate rate would be assessed by counting the FHR for 60 consecutive seconds, excluding any periodic changes noted in the heart rate. Others count for 30 seconds and multiply by 2 to obtain the beats per minute. And still others may count during a few consecutive 15-second intervals, multiplying each by 4 to obtain an approximate baseline and to determine the presence of variations within the rate (Feinstein, Sprague, & Trepanier, 2008). The FHR obtained is recorded as a single number or as a range if counted over short time intervals.
7. To clarify FHR accelerations (increases) or decelerations (decreases), counting for multiple, consecutive 6-second periods and multiplying by 10 may be helpful.
8. After each auscultation, interpret FHR findings and document the following:
   - Baseline FHR
   - Rhythm (regular or irregular)
   - Presence of accelerations or decelerations
   - Categorization of the FHR as normal or abnormal
9. Make a decision for ongoing care based on the findings (see Fig. 19-4).

NURSING ALERT

Nurses may use the electronic transducer from the EFM to listen to the FHR using IA protocols; however, if the EFM is connected to an archived central monitoring system, it should not be used for IA.

IA is easy to use, inexpensive, and less invasive than EFM. It is more comfortable for the woman and gives her more freedom of movement. Other care measures such as ambulation and the use of baths or showers are more easily carried out when IA is used. IA is recommended for healthy women at term in whom adverse perinatal outcomes are not expected (Liston et al., 2007).

When the FHR is auscultated, it should be described as a baseline number or range and as having a regular or irregular rhythm. The presence or absence of accelerations (increases) and decelerations (decreases) from the baseline rate should be noted (Liston et al., 2007; Miller et al., 2013). If the FHR is assessed as normal, then IA should continue to be used. If an abnormal FHR is detected, the nurse should auscultate the FHR immediately after the next contraction, assess potential causes, and intervene in order to eliminate or reduce the effects of the problem(s) or causes. Initiation of EFM may be considered at this time, depending on the findings of the subsequent auscultation of the FHR, clinicians experience, and the total clinical picture (Fig. 19-4).

NURSING ALERT

It is always important to assess the maternal pulse at the same time as listening to the FHR with IA to ensure that the identified FHR is not in fact a maternal heart rate.

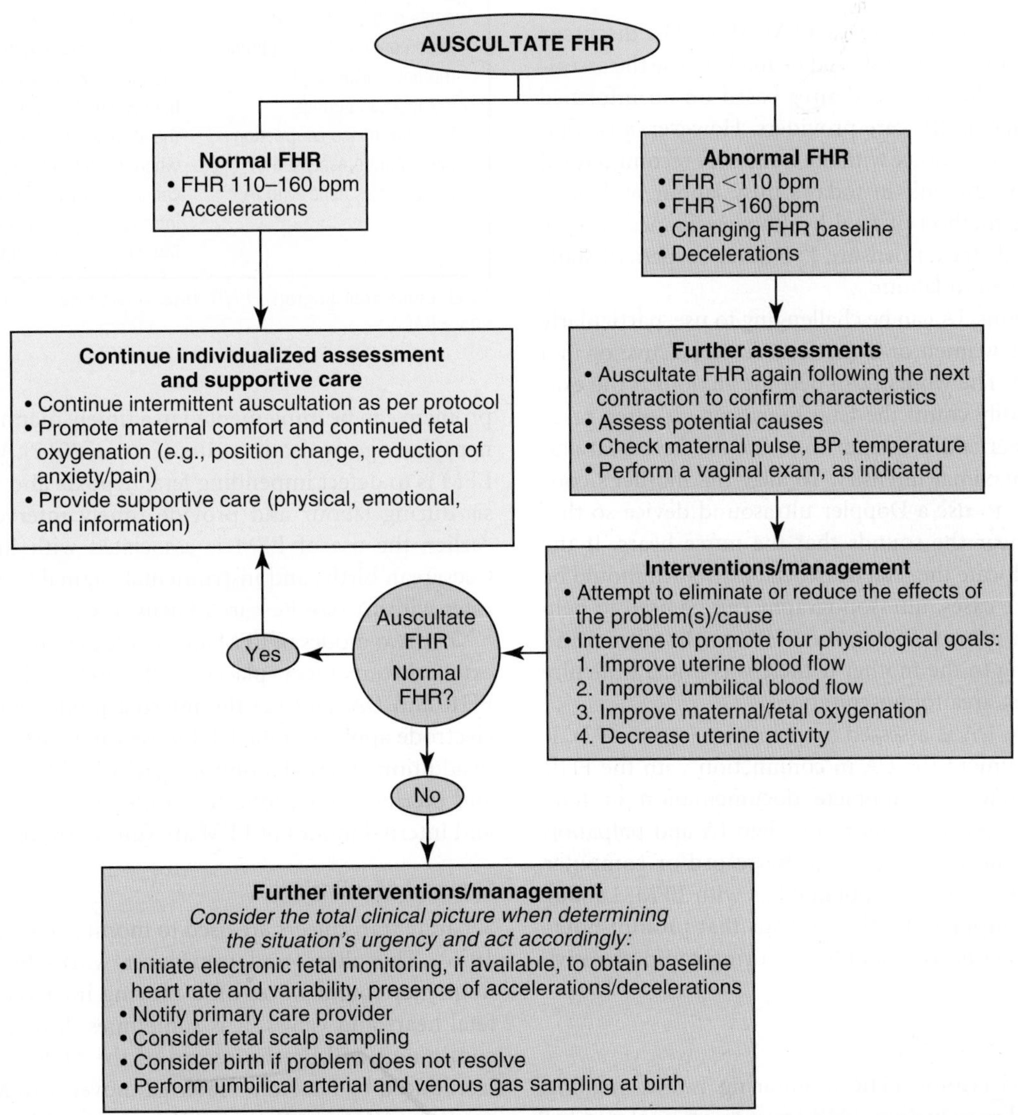

FIGURE 19-4 Decision support tool for intermittent auscultation. *bpm*, beats per minute. (Reprinted from Liston, R., Sawchuck, D., Young, D., et al. [2007]. SOGC clinical practice guideline: Fetal health surveillance: Antepartum and intrapartum consensus guideline. *Journal of Obstetrics and Gynaecologists of Canada, 29*[9], s1–s56. Copyright 2007, with permission from Elsevier.)

Frequency of Intermittent Auscultation

The recommended frequency of IA depends on the stage of labour that the woman is in. Women in the latent phase of labour are often at home, so they do not need frequent assessments. If they are hospitalized, IA should be done at the time of assessment and approximately every hour. Once a woman is in the active phase of the first stage of labour, IA is done every 15 to 30 minutes. During the active phase of the second stage of labour (when the woman is pushing), the frequency of IA increases to every 5 minutes (Liston et al., 2007).

! NURSING ALERT

When the FHR is auscultated and documented, it is inappropriate to use the descriptive terms associated with EFM (e.g., *moderate variability, variable deceleration*) because these terms are visual descriptions of the patterns produced on the monitor tracing. However, terms that are numerically defined, such as *bradycardia* and *tachycardia*, can be used.

Fetal assessment methods (IA vs. EFM) should be discussed with each woman. Every effort should be made to use the assessment method that the woman desires based on an informed discussion with her health care providers. However, auscultation of the FHR in accordance with the frequency recommended may sometimes be difficult in today's busy labour and birth units. Despite the method of fetal health surveillance chosen, all hospitals should strive to ensure 1 : 1 nurse-to-patient staffing ratios for women in labour.

In some situations, IA can be challenging to use, particularly in morbidly obese women or if the fetus is very active or in a posterior position. The woman can become anxious if the examiner cannot readily count the fetal heartbeats. It often takes time for the inexperienced listener to locate the heartbeat and find the area of maximal intensity. To allay the mother's concerns, it is helpful to use a Doppler ultrasound device so that the mother can hear the sounds that the nurse hears. If the examiner cannot locate the fetal heartbeat, assistance should be requested. In some cases, ultrasonography can be used to help locate the fetal heartbeat. Seeing the FHR on the ultrasound screen is reassuring to the mother if there was initial difficulty in locating the best area for auscultation.

When using IA, UA is assessed by palpation (see p. 492). It is essential to document the UA in conjunction with the FHR assessment. Accurate and complete documentation of fetal status and UA is especially important when IA and palpation are being used because no paper tracing record or computer storage of these assessments is obtained as with EFM. Labour flow records or computer charting systems that prompt notations of all assessments are useful for ensuring comprehensive documentation.

Electronic Fetal Monitoring

The purpose of electronic FHR monitoring is the ongoing assessment of fetal oxygenation. FHR tracings are analyzed for characteristic patterns that suggest fetal hypoxic events and metabolic acidosis during labour. When hypoxia or metabolic acidosis is suspected in labour, interventions to resolve the problem can be implemented in a timely manner before permanent damage or death occurs (Garite, 2012). While the goal of EFM is to detect impending fetal hypoxia and metabolic acidosis during labour and provide timely intervention, as stated earlier, the use of EFM is associated with increased rates of Caesarean births and instrumental vaginal births, compared to rates with IA (see Research Focus box).

The two modes of EFM are (1) the external mode, which uses external **transducers** placed on the maternal abdomen to assess FHR and UA, and (2) the internal mode, which uses a spiral electrode applied to the fetal presenting part to assess the FHR; in addition, internal monitoring may include IUPC to assess UA and uterine resting tone. The differences between the external and internal modes of EFM are summarized in Table 19-3.

TABLE 19-3 EXTERNAL AND INTERNAL MODES OF MONITORING

EXTERNAL MODE	INTERNAL MODE
Fetal Heart Rate	
Ultrasound transducer: High-frequency sound waves reflect mechanical action of the fetal heart; noninvasive, does not require rupture of membranes or cervical dilation; used during both the antepartum and intrapartum periods.	*Spiral electrode:* Converts fetal ECG as obtained from the presenting part to the FHR via a cardiotachometer; can be used only when membranes are ruptured and the cervix is sufficiently dilated during the intrapartum period; electrode penetrates into the fetal presenting part by 1.5 mm and must be attached securely to ensure a good signal.
Uterine Activity	
Tocotransducer: Monitors frequency and duration of contractions by means of a pressure-sensing device applied to the maternal abdomen; used during both the antepartum and intrapartum periods. Strength of the contraction must still be assessed by palpation as done with IA.	*Intrauterine pressure catheter (IUPC):* Monitors the frequency, duration, and intensity of contractions; two types of IUPCs: fluid-filled system and solid catheter; both measure intrauterine pressure at the catheter tip and convert the pressure into millimetres of mercury (mm Hg) on the uterine activity panel of the strip chart; both can be used only when membranes are ruptured and the cervix is sufficiently dilated during the intrapartum period. The IUPC is used in few hospitals in Canada.

ECG, electrocardiogram; *FHR*, fetal heart rate; *IA*, intermittent auscultation.

External Monitoring

Separate transducers are used to monitor the FHR and UA (Fig. 19-5). The ultrasound transducer works by reflecting high-frequency sound waves off a moving interface, in this case the fetal heart and valves. It is sometimes difficult to reproduce a continuous and precise record of the FHR because of artifact introduced by fetal and maternal movement. Maternal obesity, occiput posterior position of the fetus, and anterior attachment of the placenta can cause weak or absent signals (AWHONN, 2009b). Once the area of maximal intensity of the FHR has been located, conductive gel is applied to the surface of the

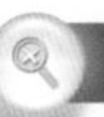

RESEARCH FOCUS

Fetal Monitoring

—*Pat Gingrich*

Ask the Question

What are the optimal methods of assessing fetal well-being during labour?

Search for Evidence

Search Strategies

Professional organization guidelines, meta-analyses, systematic reviews, randomized controlled trials, nonrandomized prospective studies, and retrospective studies since 2006

Databases Searched

CINAHL, Cochrane, Medline, National Guideline Clearinghouse, TRIP Database Plus, and the websites for the American Congress of Obstetricians and Gynecologists (ACOG), Association of Women's Health, Obstetric and Neonatal Nurses (AWHONN), Society of Obstetricians and Gynaecologists of Canada (SOGC), and National Institute of Health and Clinical Excellence (NICE)

Critically Analyze the Evidence

Electronic fetal heart monitoring (EFM; also known as cardiotocography [CTG]) has become standard practice in the labour and birth setting for many decades, especially in North America. It has been suggested that such monitoring is not necessary for the low-risk labour patient and may even present a risk of false abnormal readings, leading to high rates of Caesarean births.

A meta-analysis of trials measuring fetal outcomes and use of EFM showed that there was no significant change in Apgar scores for women who had EFM on admission for labour compared to women who were not monitored at admission. However, there was a statistically increased risk for Caesarean birth in the monitored women (Gourounti & Sandall, 2007).

The SOGC has issued professional guidelines for intrapartum care that do not recommend EFM for the low-risk labouring patient (Liston, Sawchuck, Young, et al., 2007). EFM should be used for high-risk women, along with fetal scalp blood pH testing if abnormal patterns arise. The guidelines do not recommend the routine use of fetal pulse oximetry. Similar clinical practice guidelines from NICE recommend intermittent auscultation (IA) at admission and during labour with a stethoscope or Doppler study.

Use of continuous EFM should be initiated in the presence of postterm pregnancy (≥42 weeks' gestation), induction of labour, meconium, antepartum or intrapartum bleeding, abnormal fetal heart rate (FHR) heard on auscultation (less than 110 beats per minute [bpm] or more than 160 bpm or decelerations heard), oxytocin use, or patient request (Alfirevic, Devane, & Gyte, 2013; Liston et al., 2007; NICE, 2008).

Implications for Practice

EFM is here to stay, but it is only a tool. Women and providers have come to expect the constant feedback that EFM provides. In addition, busy nurses have come to rely on the remote monitoring screens as they move from room to room. However, the risk of false alarms and the legal vulnerability of ambiguous patterns may be contributing to the soaring Caesarean rate, which carries its own risks. Continuous monitoring of low-risk women restricts patient mobility, potentially prolonging labour and increasing discomfort. In high-risk situations, EFM can be a valuable tool for identifying atypical and abnormal FHR patterns indicative of fetal decompensation; however, the tracings may also be inaccurate and ambiguous, causing needless anxiety. Women who expect routine monitoring need information about the risks and benefits of continuous monitoring in comparison to those with IA. This information can enable them to make informed decisions about their preference for monitoring their baby's heart rate in labour. The health care team may also need to become more proficient and familiar with auscultation as an assessment tool, and they must consider the information obtained as only one part of the total clinical picture.

References

Alfirevic, Z., Devane, D., & Gyte, G. M. L. (2013). Continuous cardiotocography (CTG) as a form of electronic fetal monitoring (EFM) for fetal assessment during labour. *Cochrane Database of Systematic Reviews*, (5). doi:10.1002/14651858.CD006066.pub2.

Gourounti, K., & Sandall, J. (2007). Admission cardiotocography versus intermittent auscultation of fetal heart rate: Effects on neonatal Apgar score, on the rate of Caesarean sections, and on the rate of instrumental delivery—a systematic review. *International Journal of Nursing Studies, 44*(6), 1029–1035.

Liston, R., Sawchuck, D., Young, D., et al. (2007). SOGC clinical practice guideline: Fetal health surveillance: Antepartum and intrapartum consensus guideline. *Journal of Obstetrics and Gynaecology Canada, 29*(9 Suppl. 4), s1–s56.

National Institute for Health and Clinical Excellence (NICE). (2008). *Intrapartal care: Care for healthy women and their babies during childbirth. NICE clinical guideline 55.* London: Author. Retrieved from <www.nice.org.uk/nicemedia/pdf/IPCNICEGuidance.pdf>

ultrasound transducer, and the transducer is then positioned over this area and held securely in place using an elastic belt. The FHR is printed on specially formatted monitor paper. The most common paper speed in Canada is 3 cm/min; however, some provinces use 1 or 2 cm/min. It is important to determine the paper speed prior to interpreting the EFM tracing.

The tocotransducer (tocodynamometer) measures UA transabdominally. The device is placed on the fundus above the umbilicus and held securely in place with an elastic belt (see Fig. 19-5, B). UA or fetal movements depress a pressure-sensitive surface on the side next to the abdomen. The tocotransducer can measure and record the frequency and approximate duration of contractions but not their intensity. If the woman is obese, the tocotransducer may be unable to detect the exact frequency and duration of UA.

The tocotransducer of most electronic fetal monitors is designed for assessing UA in term pregnancy, and for this reason, it may not be sensitive enough to detect preterm UA. When monitoring the woman in preterm labour, it is important to remember that the fundus may be located below the level of the umbilicus. The nurse may need to rely on the woman to indicate when UA is occurring and to use palpation as an additional way of assessing contraction frequency and validating the monitor tracing. The strength of the contractions is always determined by palpation, unless an IUPC is in place.

The external transducers are applied easily by the nurse but must be repositioned at least every hour and as the woman or fetus changes position. The use of an external monitor confines the woman to a bed or chair. Portable telemetry monitors are becoming more widely available and allow observation of the FHR and UC patterns by means of centrally located electronic display stations. These portable units provide opportunity for women to remain mobile while still receiving continuous EFM monitoring.

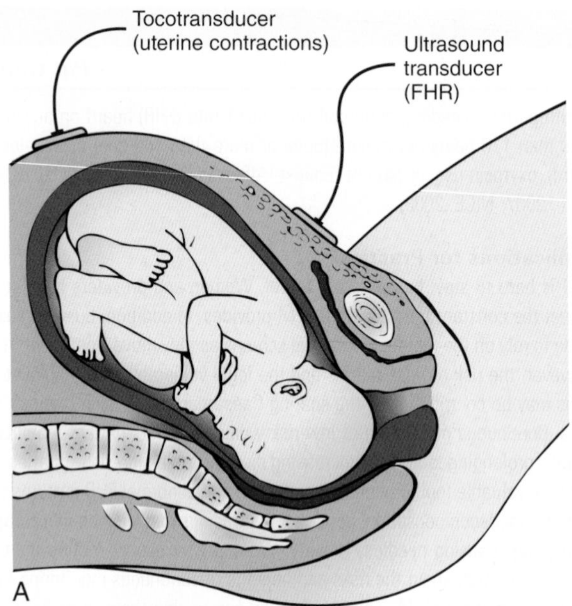

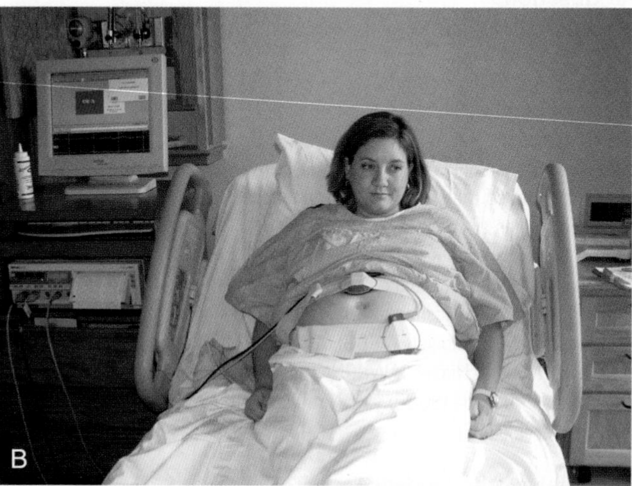

FIGURE 19-5 A: External noninvasive fetal monitoring with tocotransducer and ultrasound transducer. *FHR*, fetal heart rate. **B:** Ultrasound transducer is placed over the area where fetal heart rate is best heard, and tocotransducer is placed on uterine fundus. (**B**, Courtesy Julie Perry Nelson.)

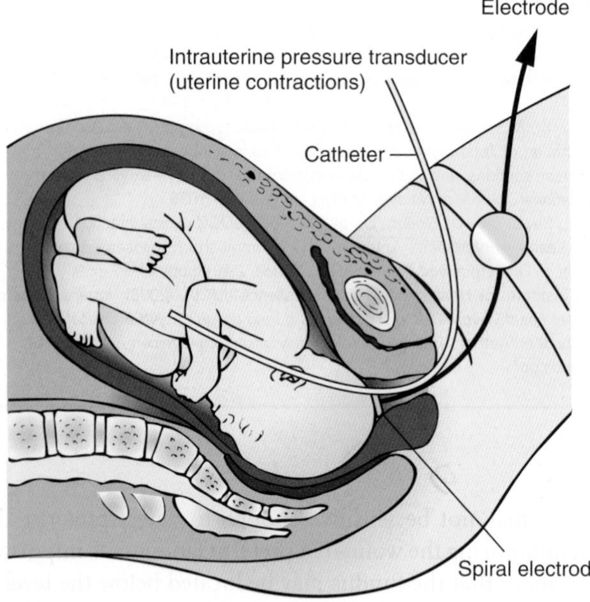

FIGURE 19-6 Diagrammatic representation of internal invasive fetal monitoring with intrauterine pressure catheter and spiral electrode in place (membranes ruptured and cervix dilated).

Internal Monitoring

The technique of continuous internal FHR or UA monitoring provides a more accurate appraisal of fetal well-being during labour than external monitoring because it is not interrupted by fetal or maternal movement or affected by maternal size (Fig. 19-6). For this type of monitoring, the membranes must be ruptured and the cervix sufficiently dilated (at least 2 to 3 cm) and the presenting part low enough to allow placement of the spiral electrode, IUPC, or both. Internal and external modes of monitoring may be combined (i.e., internal FHR with external UA or external FHR with internal UA) without difficulty.

Internal monitoring of the FHR is accomplished by attaching a small spiral electrode to the presenting part. To monitor UA internally, an IUPC is introduced into the uterine cavity. The catheter has a pressure-sensitive tip that measures changes in intrauterine pressure. As the catheter is compressed during a contraction, pressure is placed on the pressure transducer. This pressure is then converted into a pressure reading in millimetres of mercury (mm Hg). The IUPC can objectively measure the frequency, duration, and intensity of UCs as well as uterine resting tone.

The precise measurement of UCs measured by an IUPC can be used to assess the adequacy of contractions for achieving progress in labour. Montevideo units (MVUs) are calculated by subtracting the baseline uterine pressure from the peak contraction pressure for each contraction that occurs in a 10-minute window and then adding together the pressures for each contraction that occurs during that period of time (Cunningham, Leveno, Bloom, et al., 2014; Miller et al., 2013).

MVUs usually range from 100 to 250 in the first stage of labour; they may rise to 300 to 400 in the second stage. Contraction intensities of 40 mmHg or more and MVUs of 80 to 120 are generally sufficient to initiate spontaneous labour. MVUs are only used with IUPC monitoring of contractions in labour.

The FHR and UA are displayed on the monitor paper or computer screen, with the FHR in the upper section and UA in the lower section. Fig. 19-7 contrasts the internal and external modes of electronic monitoring. Note that each small square on the monitor paper or screen horizontally represents 10 seconds; each larger box of six squares equals 1 minute (when paper is moving through the monitor at the rate of 3 cm/min).

Admission Fetal Monitor Strips

There has been much debate over the routine use of admission electronic fetal monitor strips. Although it is common practice in many hospitals to perform a 20-minute monitor strip on admission, this is not supported by evidence or recommended for low-risk women (Liston et al., 2007). The SOGC states that women who are at risk for adverse outcomes (see Table 19-2) should have an admission FHR tracing completed, but for women with low risk there is no evidence showing any benefit. Admission FHR tracings should not be used to determine whether a woman is in labour. Palpation along with IA is an effective method to determine the status of labour and the fetus.

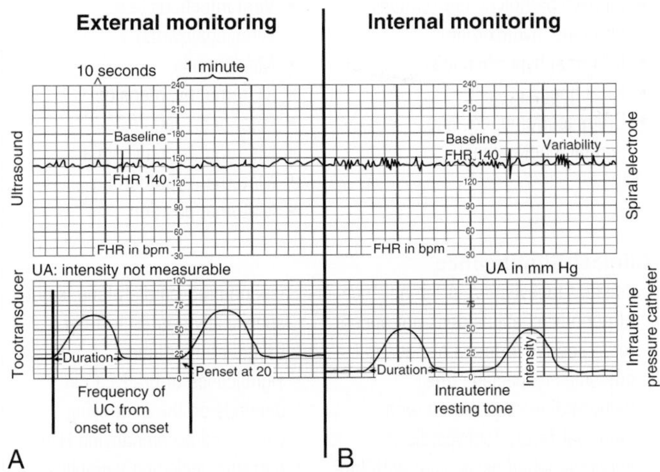

FIGURE 19-7 Display of fetal heart rate and uterine activity on monitor paper. **A:** External mode with ultrasound and tocotransducer as signal source. **B:** Internal mode with spiral electrode and intrauterine catheter as signal source. Frequency of contractions is measured from the beginning of one contraction to the beginning of the next. *BPM,* beats per minute; *FHR,* fetal heart rate; *UA,* uterine activity; *UC,* uterine contractions. (From Miller, L. A., Miller, D. A., & Tucker, S. M. [2013]. *Mosby's pocket guide to fetal monitoring: A multidisciplinary approach* [7th ed.]. St. Louis: Mosby.)

FETAL HEART RATE PATTERNS

Characteristic FHR patterns are associated with fetal and maternal physiological processes; these patterns have been identified for many years. However, because EFM was introduced into clinical practice before consensus was reached regarding standardized terminology, variations in the description and interpretation of common FHR patterns were often great. In 1997, the National Institute of Child Health and Human Development (NICHD) published a proposed nomenclature system for EFM interpretation, with standardized definitions for FHR monitoring. In 2007, the SOGC introduced a three-tier system of FHR interpretation and categorization when using EFM (Table 19-4). This change in nomenclature provides care providers with clear and concise guidelines to communicate changes in FHR patterns.

The FHR must be assessed systematically, including all key components (baseline FHR, variability, and accelerations or decelerations) and must include interpretation of uterine activity. Standard terminology should be used when describing the FHR tracing.

Baseline Fetal Heart Rate

The intrinsic rhythmicity of the fetal heart, the central nervous system (CNS), and the fetal autonomic nervous system control the FHR. An increase in sympathetic response results in acceleration of the FHR, whereas an increase in parasympathetic response produces a slowing of the FHR. Usually, a balanced increase of sympathetic and parasympathetic response occurs during contractions, with no observable change in the baseline FHR.

Baseline FHR is the approximate mean FHR rounded to increments of 5 bpm during a 10-minute tracing segment; it excludes accelerations, decelerations, and periods of marked variability (Liston et al., 2007; Macones et al., 2008; Miller et al., 2013). The baseline FHR must be present for at least 2 minutes in any 10-minute segment or the baseline for that time period is indeterminate (Cunningham et al., 2014; Macones, Hankins,

TABLE 19-4 FETAL HEART RATE INTERPRETATION SYSTEM WHEN USING ELECTRONIC FETAL MONITORING

	NORMAL	ATYPICAL	ABNORMAL
Baseline	• 110–160 bpm	• FHR 100–110 bpm • FHR >160 bpm for >30 min to <80 min • Rising baseline	• FHR <100 bpm • FHR >160 bpm for >80 min • Erratic baseline
Variability	• 6–25 bpm (moderate) • <5 bpm for <40 min	• ≤5 bpm for 40–80 min	• ≤5 bpm for >80 min • ≥25 bpm for >10 min • Sinusoidal
Decelerations	• None or occasional uncomplicated variables or early decelerations	• Repetitive (≥3) uncomplicated variable decelerations • Occasional late decelerations • Single prolonged deceleration >2 min but <3 min	• Repetitive (≥3) complicated variable decelerations • Late deceleration >50% of contractions • Single prolonged deceleration >3 min but <10 min
Accelerations	• Spontaneous accelerations present • Accelerations present with fetal scalp stimulation	• Absence of acceleration with fetal scalp stimulation	• Usually absent*

*Usually absent, but if accelerations are present, this does not change the classification of the tracing. *bpm,* beats per minute; *FHR,* fetal heart rate. From Liston, R., Sawchuck, D., Young, D., et al. (2007). SOGC clinical practice guideline: Fetal health surveillance: Antepartum and intrapartum consensus guideline. *Journal of Obstetrics and Gynaecologists of Canada, 29*(9 Suppl 4), s1–s56. Copyright 2007, with permission from Elsevier.

Song, et al., 2008; Miller et al., 2013). The baseline rate can be recorded as a range or as a single number (Liston et al., 2007). For example, if the FHR varies between 130 and 140 bpm over a 10-minute period, the baseline FHR could be recorded as 135 bpm or 130 to 140 bpm. Recording practices should be determined on an individual organization level, communicated with staff and written in organizational policies and procedures. The normal range at term is 110 to 160 bpm. In the preterm fetus, the baseline rate is slightly higher.

Tachycardia

Fetal **tachycardia** is a baseline FHR greater than 160 bpm (Miller et al., 2013). Tachycardia is labelled as either "atypical" or "abnormal," depending on the length of time it occurs (see Table 19-4). It can be considered an early sign of fetal hypoxemia, especially when associated with late decelerations and minimal or absent variability. Fetal tachycardia most commonly occurs as a result of maternal fever. Other causes of fetal tachycardia include maternal or fetal infection, maternal hyperthyroidism, fetal anemia, and maternal administration of medications (e.g., atropine, hydroxyzine) or illicit drugs (e.g., cocaine, methamphetamines). Table 19-5 lists causes, clinical significance, and nursing interventions for fetal tachycardia.

Bradycardia

Fetal **bradycardia** is a baseline FHR less than 110 bpm (Miller et al., 2013). In the presence of possible fetal bradycardia, it is essential to confirm the maternal pulse to differentiate it from the FHR. True bradycardia occurs rarely and is not specifically related to fetal oxygenation. It is critical to distinguish true bradycardia from a prolonged deceleration, since the causes and management of these two conditions are very different. Bradycardia is often caused by some type of fetal cardiac problem, such as structural defects involving the pacemakers or conduction system or fetal heart failure. Other causes of bradycardia include viral infections (e.g., cytomegalovirus), maternal hypoglycemia, and maternal hypothermia. The clinical significance of the bradycardia depends on the underlying cause and accompanying FHR patterns, including variability and the presence of accelerations or decelerations (Miller et al., 2013). Table 19-5 lists causes, clinical significance, and nursing interventions for bradycardia.

TABLE 19-5 FETAL TACHYCARDIA AND BRADYCARDIA AND NURSING IMPLICATIONS

	TACHYCARDIA	BRADYCARDIA
Definition	FHR >160 bpm lasting >10 min	FHR <110 bpm lasting >10 min
Possible Causes	• Early fetal hypoxemia • Fetal cardiac arrhythmias or congenital anomalies • Maternal fever • Infection (including chorioamnionitis) • Parasympatholytic medications (atropine, hydroxyzine) • Maternal hyperthyroidism • Fetal anemia • Drugs (caffeine, cocaine, methamphetamines)	• Fetal hypoxia/acidosis • AV dissociation (heart block)—may be related to maternal connective tissue disease (e.g., lupus) • Structural defects • Viral infections (e.g., cytomegalovirus) • Medications • Maternal hypotension • Fetal heart failure • Maternal hypoglycemia • Maternal hypothermia • Maternal position
Clinical Significance	Persistent tachycardia in the absence of periodic changes does not appear to be serious in terms of neonatal outcomes (especially true if tachycardia is associated with maternal fever); tachycardia is abnormal when associated with late decelerations, complicated variable decelerations, or absent variability.	Baseline bradycardia alone is not specifically related to fetal oxygenation. Clinical significance of bradycardia depends on the underlying cause and accompanying FHR patterns, including variability, accelerations, or decelerations.
Nursing Interventions	• Confirm maternal vital signs • Notify the primary care provider and carry out health care provider's orders based on alleviating cause—this may include antipyretics, antibiotics, and cooling measures; fluid bolus; and scalp pH sampling • Intrauterine resuscitation if thought due to hypoxia (see Box 19-8)	• Confirm maternal pulse as different from FHR • Consider vaginal examination to rule out cord prolapse • May consider scalp stimulation or scalp pH sampling • Other interventions, dependent on cause

AV, atrioventricular; *bpm*, beats per minute; *FHR*, fetal heart rate.

Fetal Heart Rate Variability

Baseline variability of the FHR can be described as fluctuations in the baseline FHR that are determined in a 10-minute segment, excluding accelerations and decelerations. Fluctuations are irregular in amplitude and frequency and are visually quantified as the amplitude of the peak to trough in bpm (AWHONN, 2009b; Liston et al., 2007; Miller et al., 2013). Distinctions are no longer made between short-term (beat-to-beat) or long-term variability because in actual practice they are visually determined as a unit (Miller et al., 2013).

Variability is classified as follows:

- Absent: amplitude range is undetectable (0 to 2 bpm)
- Minimal: amplitude range is detectable but ≤5 bpm
- Moderate: amplitude range is 6 to 25 bpm
- Marked: amplitude range is >25 bpm

Minimal or absent FHR variability (Fig. 19-8, A and B) can result from fetal hypoxemia and metabolic acidemia. Other conditions potentially associated with minimal or absent variability include fetal sleep, fetal tachycardia, medications, prematurity, congenital anomalies, fetal anemia, cardiac arrhythmias, infection, and pre-existing neurological injury (Miller et al., 2013). Table 19-6 contrasts key differences between increased and decreased variability and the clinical implications of each.

Moderate variability is considered normal (see Fig. 19-8, C). Its presence is highly predictive of a normal fetal acid–base balance (absence of fetal metabolic acidemia). Moderate variability indicates that FHR regulation is not affected significantly

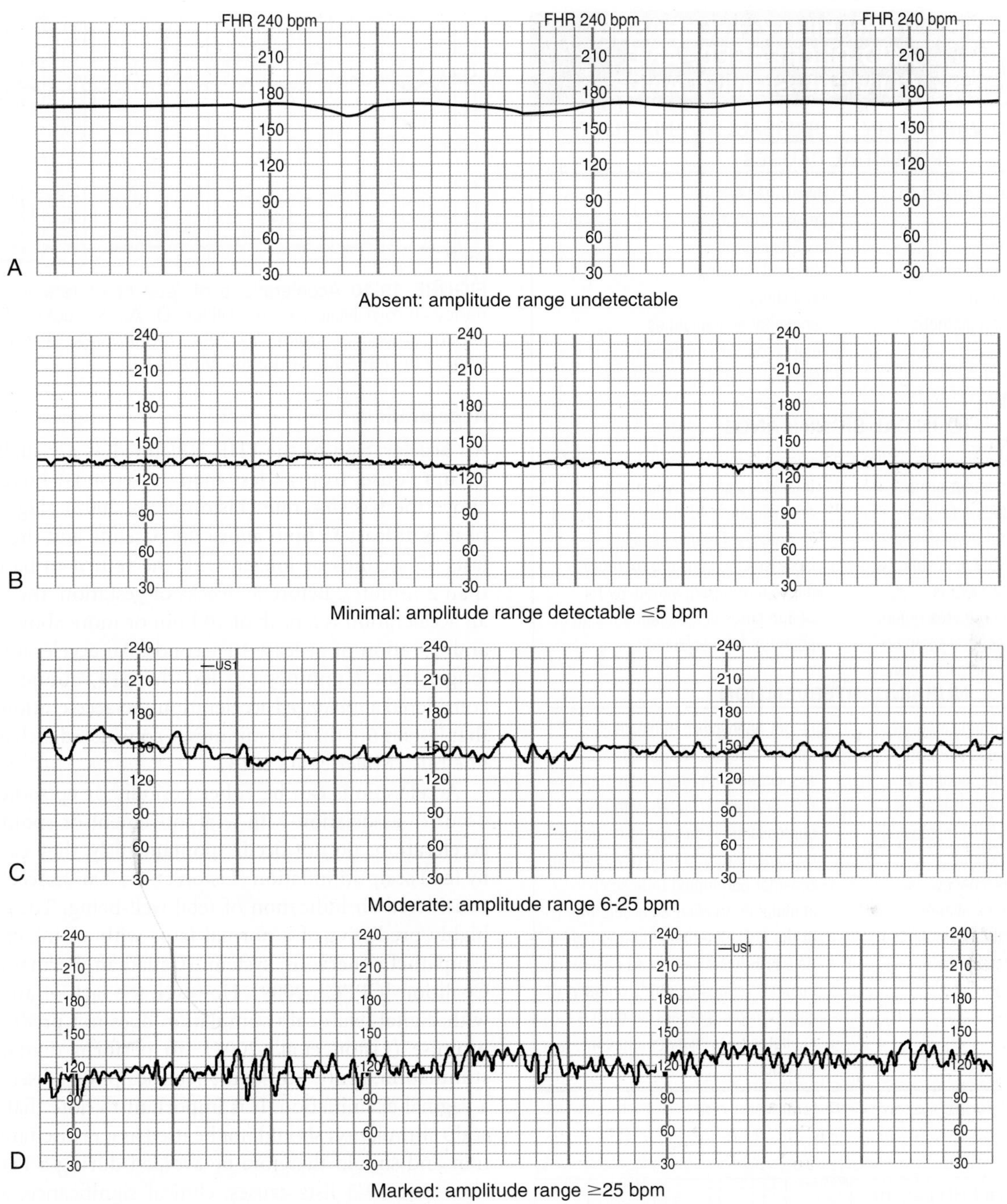

FIGURE 19-8 Fetal heart rate variability. **A,** Absent: amplitude range undetectable. **B,** Minimal: amplitude range detectable ≤5 beats/min. **C,** Moderate: amplitude range 6–25 beats/min. **D,** Marked: amplitude range ≥25 beats/min. *FHR,* fetal heart rate. (From Miller, L. A., Miller, D. A., & Tucker, S. M. [2013]. *Mosby's pocket guide to fetal monitoring: A multidisciplinary approach* [7th ed.]. St. Louis: Mosby.)

by fetal sleep cycles, tachycardia, prematurity, congenital anomalies, pre-existing neurologic injury, or CNS depressant medications (Macones et al., 2008; Miller et al., 2013).

The significance of marked variability (see Fig. 19-8, D) is unclear. Possible explanations include a normal variant or an exaggerated autonomic response to interruption of fetal oxygenation (Macones et al., 2008; Miller et al., 2013).

A sinusoidal FHR pattern is not included in the definition of FHR variability. A sinusoidal FHR pattern is a smooth, wave-like undulating pattern of the FHR with a cycle frequency of 3 to 5 waves/min that persists for 20 minutes or more (Fig. 19-9). This uncommon pattern classically occurs with severe fetal anemia. Variations of the sinusoidal pattern have been described in association with chorioamnionitis, fetal sepsis, and administration of opioids (Miller et al., 2013).

Periodic and Episodic Changes in Fetal Heart Rate

Changes in FHR from baseline are categorized as periodic or episodic. *Periodic* changes are those that occur with uterine contractions. *Episodic* changes are those that are not associated with uterine contractions. These patterns include accelerations and decelerations (Macones et al., 2008).

TABLE 19-6 VARIABILITY: INCREASED AND DECREASED, AND CLINICAL SIGNIFICANCE

INCREASED VARIABILITY	DECREASED VARIABILITY
POTENTIAL CAUSES	
Hypoxic events (e.g., uterine tachysystole) Hyperoxygenation Fetal cardiac dysrhythmias Normal maturation Increased parasympathetic activity Illicit drug use Fetal stimulation	Hypoxia/acidosis Severe fetal anemia CNS depressants Maternal smoking Fetal sleep cycles Congenital abnormalities Fetal cardiac dysrhythmias Maternal temperature elevation Hypovolemia
CLINICAL SIGNIFICANCE	
Significance of marked variability not known; rule out artifact; if thought to be due to hypoxia maximize fetal oxygenation. Marked variability persisting for 10 minutes or more is abnormal and requires urgent action such as fetal scalp pH sampling or emergent delivery.	Benign when associated with periodic fetal sleep states, which last approximately 40 minutes; if caused by drugs, variability usually increases as drugs are excreted; minimal or absent variability for >80 minutes is considered a sign of potential fetal acidemia.
NURSING INTERVENTION	
If delivery is not indicated, continuously observe FHR tracing for other abnormal characteristics that may develop, including increasing baseline, prolonged decelerations, changes in variability to minimal or absent, and the development of complicated variable decelerations or late decelerations.	Rule out nonhypoxic etiologies; intervention not warranted if associated with fetal sleep states or temporarily associated with CNS depressants; if thought to be due to hypoxia, maximize fetal oxygenation, consider performing fetal scalp stimulation to elicit an acceleration of the FHR, determine duration of time FHR has experienced absent or minimal variability, notify primary care provider, prepare for birth if indicated by primary health care provider.

CNS, central nervous system; *FHR*, fetal heart rate.

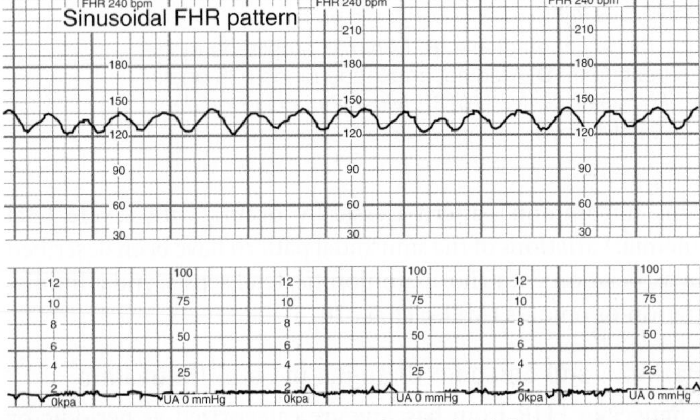

FIGURE 19-9 Sinusoidal pattern. *FHR,* fetal heart rate. (From Miller, L. A., Miller, D. A., & Tucker, S. M. [2013]. *Mosby's pocket guide to fetal monitoring: A multidisciplinary approach* [7th ed.]. St. Louis: Mosby.)

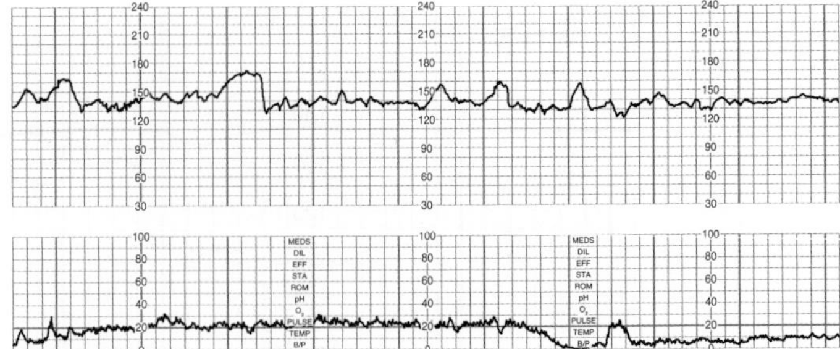

FIGURE 19-10 Accelerations of fetal heart rate in a term pregnancy. (From Miller, L. A., Miller, D. A., & Tucker, S. M. [2013]. *Mosby's pocket guide to fetal monitoring: A multidisciplinary approach* [7th ed.]. St. Louis: Mosby.)

Accelerations

An **acceleration** of the FHR is defined as a visually apparent, abrupt (onset to peak less than 30 seconds) increase in FHR above the baseline rate (Liston et al., 2007) (Fig. 19-10). The peak is at least 15 bpm above the baseline and the acceleration lasts 15 seconds or longer, with the return to baseline in less than 2 minutes. Before 32 weeks of gestation, the definition of an acceleration is a peak of 10 bpm or more above the baseline and duration of at least 10 seconds. An acceleration that lasts longer than 2 minutes but less than 10 minutes in length is considered a *prolonged* acceleration. An acceleration of the FHR that lasts more than 10 minutes is considered a change in baseline rate (Miller et al., 2013).

Accelerations can be either periodic or episodic. They may occur in association with fetal movement or spontaneously. If accelerations do not occur spontaneously, they can be elicited by fetal scalp stimulation (Liston et al., 2007). Accelerations are considered an indication of fetal well-being. Their presence is highly predictive of a normal fetus with an intact oxygenated sympathetic nervous system (Canadian Perinatal Programs Coalition [CPPC], 2009). However, the lack of an acceleration with digital fetal scalp stimulation does not predict fetal compromise (Liston et al., 2007). To perform digital fetal scalp stimulation, gently stroke the fetal scalp for 15 seconds during a vaginal examination. It is important to note that digital fetal scalp stimulation should not be used as a resuscitative intervention and should therefore be avoided during a FHR deceleration. Box 19-3 lists causes, clinical significance, and nursing interventions for accelerations.

Decelerations

A deceleration (caused by dominance of a parasympathetic response) may be benign or abnormal. FHR decelerations are categorized as early, variable, late, or prolonged. They are described by their visual relation to the onset and end of a contraction and by their general shape. In the SOGC guideline, "repetitive" decelerations are defined as greater than three decelerations (Liston et al., 2007). In the 2008 (NICHD) Workshop on EFM documentation, decelerations are defined as "recurrent" if they occur with ≥50% of uterine contractions in any 20-minute window (Macones et al., 2008).

Early decelerations. An **early deceleration** of the FHR is a visually apparent, usually symmetrical, gradual decrease (onset to

BOX 19-3 ACCELERATIONS

Cause

Spontaneous fetal movement
Vaginal examination
Electrode application
Fetal scalp stimulation
Fetal reaction to external sounds
Uterine contractions
Fundal pressure
Abdominal palpation
Brief occlusion of umbilical vein only

Clinical Significance

Normal pattern: Acceleration with fetal movement signifies fetal well-being, representing fetal alertness or arousal states.

Nursing Interventions

None required

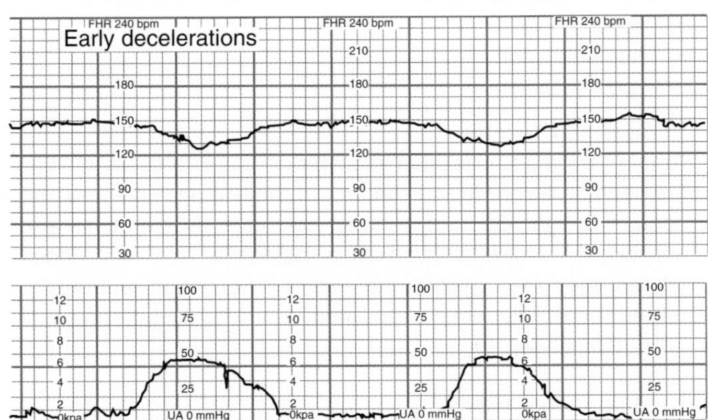

FIGURE 19-11 Electronic fetal monitor tracing showing early decelerations. *FHR,* fetal heart rate; *UA,* uterine activity. (From Miller, L. A., Miller, D. A., & Tucker, S. M. [2013]. *Mosby's pocket guide to fetal monitoring: A multidisciplinary approach* [7th ed.]. St. Louis: Mosby.)

lowest point [nadir] ≥30 seconds) in the FHR and return to baseline associated with a UC (Fig. 19-11 and Fig. 19-12) (CPPC, 2009). They are thought to be caused by transient fetal head compression and are considered normal and generally benign (Macones et al., 2008; Miller et al., 2013). The onset, **nadir**, and recovery of the deceleration usually correspond to the beginning, peak, and end of the contraction. For this reason an early deceleration is sometimes referred to as the "mirror image" of a contraction.

Although uncommon, when early decelerations are present, they usually occur during the first stage of labour when the cervix is dilated 4 to 7 cm. However, they are sometimes seen during the second stage when the woman is pushing.

Early decelerations are thought to be benign, thus interventions are not necessary. Identifying early decelerations is valuable so the clinician can distinguish them from late or variable decelerations, which may lead to atypical or abnormal FHR patterns and for which interventions are appropriate. Box 19-4

BOX 19-4 EARLY DECELERATIONS

Cause

Head compression resulting from the following:

- Uterine contractions
- Malposition
- Unengaged presenting part
- Vaginal examination
- Fundal pressure
- Placement of internal spiral electrode
- Cephalopelvic disproportion (CPD); usually seen early in labour

Clinical Significance

Normal pattern: not associated with fetal hypoxemia, acidemia, or low Apgar scores. If thought to be due to CPD, monitor labour progress. If seen in association with atypical or abnormal baseline features, early decelerations may have acid–base implications for the fetus.

Nursing Interventions

None required

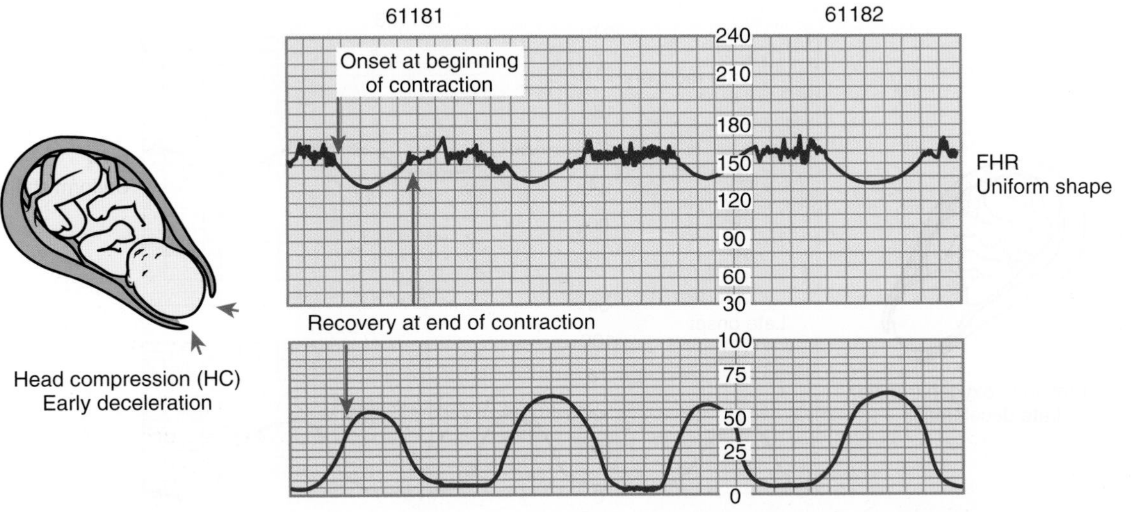

FIGURE 19-12 Line drawing illustrating early decelerations. *FHR,* fetal heart rate. (From Tucker, S. M. [2004]. *Pocket guide to fetal monitoring and assessment* [5th ed.]. St. Louis: Mosby.)

lists causes, clinical significance, and nursing interventions for early decelerations.

Late decelerations. A late deceleration of the FHR is a visually apparent gradual (onset to nadir ≥30 seconds) decrease in and return to baseline FHR associated with uterine contractions (Liston et al., 2007; Macones et al., 2008). In most cases, the onset, nadir, and recovery of the deceleration occur after the beginning, peak, and ending of the contraction, respectively. The deceleration begins after the contraction has started, and the lowest point of the deceleration occurs after the peak of the contraction. The deceleration usually does not return to baseline until after the contraction is over (Fig. 19-13 and 19-14). Traditionally, late decelerations have been attributed to uteroplacental insufficiency. However, in reality a number of factors can disrupt oxygen transfer to the fetus, even with mild UCs and a normally functioning placenta (Miller et al., 2013). Potential causes, clinical significance, and nursing interventions for late decelerations are described in Box 19-5.

Rarely, fetal oxygenation can be interrupted sufficiently to result in metabolic acidemia. For that reason, persistent and repetitive late decelerations should be considered an ominous sign when they are uncorrectable, especially if they are associated with absent or minimal variability and tachycardia (Liston et al., 2007; Miller et al., 2013).

Variable decelerations. Variable decelerations are the most common type of deceleration seen in labour. They are defined

BOX 19-5 LATE DECELERATIONS

Cause

Uteroplacental insufficiency caused by the following:

ACUTE CONDITIONS	CHRONIC CONDITIONS
• Uterine tachysystole • Maternal hypotension related to epidural or spinal anaesthesia • Maternal supine positioning • Reduced maternal P_{O_2} • Acute placental disruption (i.e., abruption, previa) • Intra-amniotic infection • Vasoconstriction • Maternal hypo/hyperventilation	• Maternal comorbidities (e.g., diabetes, collagen disease, hypertensive disorders) • Postdates or postterm pregnancy • Reduced maternal P_{O_2} • Poor placental development/malformation • Premature placental aging (i.e., intrauterine growth restriction)

Clinical Significance

An FHR tracing is classified as atypical if the late decelerations are seen occasionally and abnormal if the late decelerations are occurring with >50% of contractions. Late decelerations are associated with fetal hypoxemia, acidemia, and low Apgar scores; they are considered ominous if persistent and uncorrected, especially when associated with fetal tachycardia and loss of variability.

Nursing Interventions

When occasional late decelerations are detected, change maternal position (lateral), check maternal vital signs, and continue to observe closely. When late decelerations are repetitive, intrauterine resuscitation should be initiated (see Box 19-8).

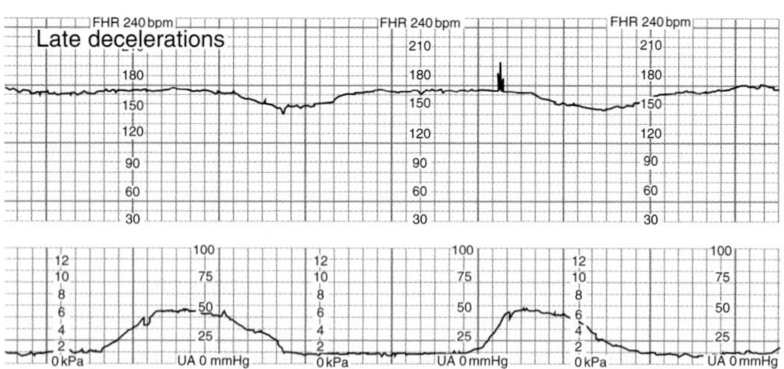

FIGURE 19-13 Electronic fetal monitor tracing showing late decelerations. *FHR,* fetal heart rate; *UA,* uterine activity. (From Miller, L. A., Miller, D. A., & Tucker, S. M. [2103]. *Mosby's pocket guide to fetal monitoring: A multidisciplinary approach* [7th ed.]. St. Louis: Mosby.)

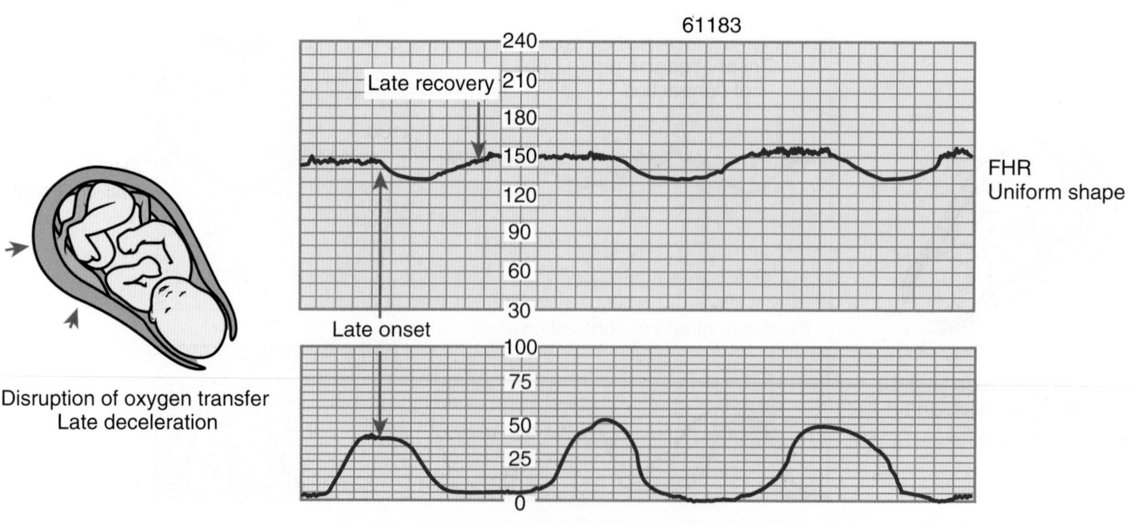

FIGURE 19-14 Line drawing illustrating late decelerations. *FHR,* fetal heart rate. (Modified from Tucker, S. M. [2004]. *Pocket guide to fetal monitoring and assessment* [5th ed.]. St. Louis: Mosby.)

as a visually abrupt (onset to nadir <30 seconds) decrease in the FHR below the baseline. The FHR decreases at least 15 bpm below the baseline and the deceleration lasts for at least 15 seconds but less than 2 minutes from the time of onset (Fig. 19-15 and 19-16). They can occur during or between contractions (CPPC, 2009; Macones et al., 2008).

Variable decelerations are thought to be a response to umbilical cord compression (Garite, 2012). Box 19-6 lists causes, clinical significance, and nursing interventions for variable decelerations.

The appearance of variable decelerations differs from those of early and late decelerations, which closely approximate the shape of the corresponding uterine contraction. Instead, variable decelerations often have a U, V, or W shape, are characterized by a rapid descent to the nadir of the deceleration, and return to the FHR baseline (see Fig. 19-16). Variable decelerations are further classified as uncomplicated and complicated variable decelerations.

Uncomplicated variable decelerations are spiky in appearance. Their shape may often be accompanied by an acceleration prior to and immediately following the deceleration of the

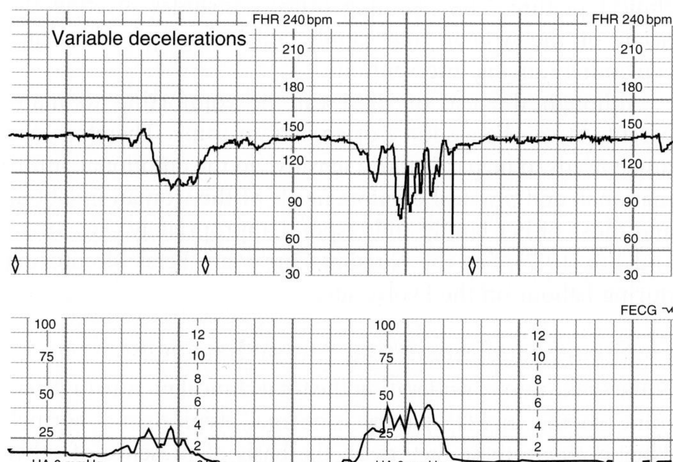

FIGURE 19-15 Electronic fetal monitor tracing showing variable decelerations. *FHR,* fetal heart rate; *FECG,* fetal electrocardiogram. (From Miller, L. A., Miller, D. A., & Tucker, S. M. [2013]. *Mosby's pocket guide to fetal monitoring: A multidisciplinary approach* [7th ed.]. St. Louis: Mosby.)

BOX 19-6 VARIABLE DECELERATIONS

Cause

Umbilical cord compression caused by the following:

- Oligohydramnios
- Maternal position with cord between fetus and maternal pelvis (occult umbilical cord prolapse)
- Cord around fetal neck (nuchal cord), arm, leg, or other body part
- Short cord
- Knot in cord
- Prolapsed umbilical cord
- Decreased amniotic fluid

Clinical Significance

Variable decelerations occur in most labours and are usually correctable. Complicated variable decelerations require critical analysis and timely decision making, including intrauterine resuscitation and confirmation of fetal well-being, either directly or indirectly (fetal scalp stimulation or fetal scalp blood sampling for pH) (Liston et al., 2007). Preparation for an expeditious birth may be necessary.

Nursing Interventions

- Change maternal position (side to side, knee chest).
- Consider need for intrauterine resuscitation (particularly if variables are complicated) (see Box 19-8).
- Notify primary care provider.
- Assess for possible cord prolapse.
- Assist with scalp stimulation, scalp pH, or amnioinfusion (see discussion later in chapter), if ordered.
- Alter pushing technique (e.g., open glottis, shorter pushes).
- Assist with birth (vaginal assisted or Caesarean) if pattern cannot be corrected.

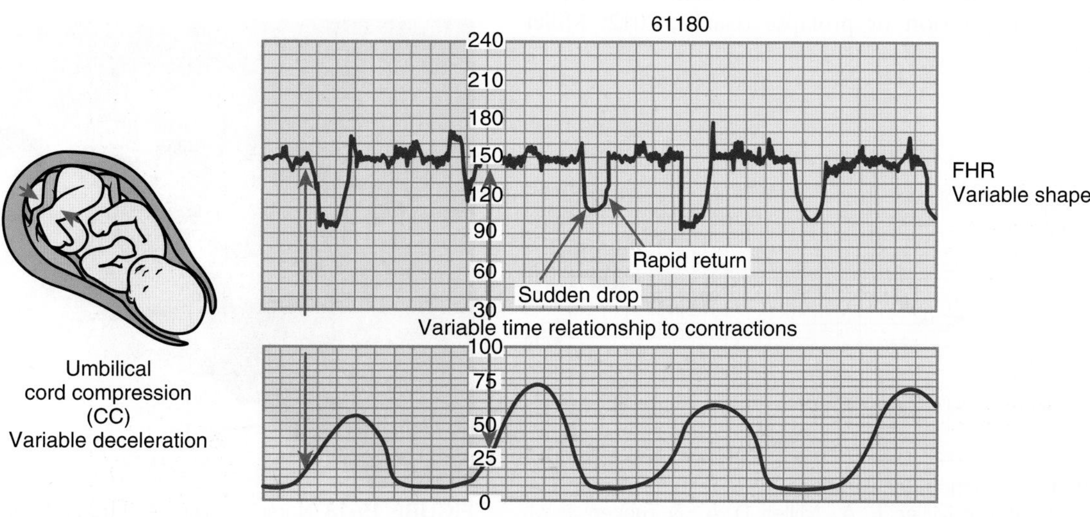

FIGURE 19-16 Line drawing illustrating variable decelerations. *FHR,* fetal heart rate. (From Tucker, S. M. [2004]. *Pocket guide to fetal monitoring and assessment* [5th ed.]. St. Louis: Mosby.)

FHR—these accelerated portions of the fetal heart tracing are part of the deceleration and are commonly called "shoulders." The accelerations or "shoulders" are a compensatory response to compression of the umbilical vein. Uncomplicated variable decelerations rarely alter the fetal pH and have little clinical significance. When uncomplicated variable decelerations are present in the FHR tracing, it may be classified as either normal, atypical, or abnormal depending on the frequency of the decelerations and other characteristics of the FHR baseline.

Complicated variables are more likely to affect fetal well-being, and the FHR tracing is classified as abnormal if the decelerations are repetitive (≥3) (Liston et al., 2007). These decelerations can deplete the fetal reserve and lead to fetal hypoxemia. Complicated variable decelerations include the following:

- Deceleration to <70 bpm lasting >60 seconds
- Loss of variability in the baseline FHR and in the trough of the deceleration
- Biphasic deceleration (W shape)
- Prolonged secondary acceleration or overshoot of 20 bpm increase or lasting more than 20 seconds
- Slow return to baseline
- Continuation of baseline rate at lower level than before the deceleration
- Presence of fetal tachycardia or bradycardia

Prolonged decelerations. A *prolonged deceleration* is a visually apparent decrease (may be either gradual or abrupt) of at least 15 bpm below the baseline and lasting more than 2 minutes but less than 10 minutes from onset to return to baseline (Fig. 19-17). A deceleration lasting more than 10 minutes is considered a baseline change (Macones et al., 2008). Prolonged decelerations occur when the mechanisms responsible for late or variable decelerations last for an extended period (more than 2 minutes). Examples of conditions that can cause an interruption in the fetal oxygen supply long enough to produce a prolonged deceleration include maternal hypotension, cervical examination, uterine tachysystole or rupture, extreme placental insufficiency, cord entanglement, and prolonged cord compression or prolapse (Garite, 2012; Miller et al., 2013).

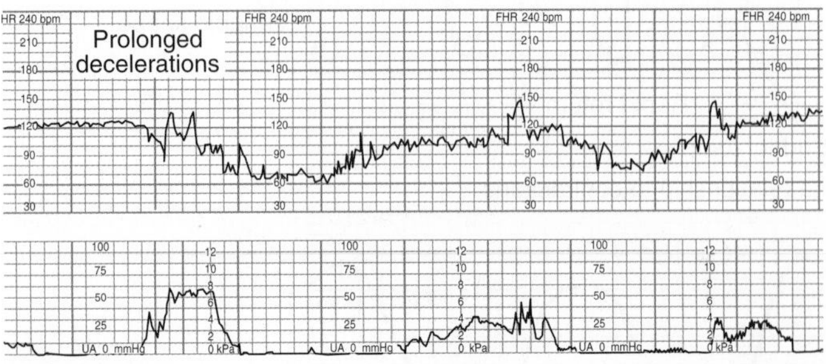

FIGURE 19-17 Prolonged decelerations. *FHR,* fetal heart rate; *UA,* uterine activity. (From Miller, L. A., Miller, D. A., & Tucker, S. M. [2013]. *Mosby's pocket guide to fetal monitoring: A multidisciplinary approach* [7th ed.]. St. Louis: Mosby.)

The presence and severity of hypoxia are thought to correlate with the depth and duration of the prolonged deceleration, how long it takes for the FHR to return to the baseline, how much variability is lost during the deceleration, and whether or not rebound tachycardia and decreased variability are seen following the deceleration (Garite, 2012).

! NURSING ALERT

Nurses should notify the primary care provider immediately and initiate appropriate intrauterine resuscitation when they see a prolonged deceleration.

NURSING CARE

The primary goals of obstetrical nursing care are to have healthy fetal and maternal outcomes. Knowledge of fetal status and standards for care determine the interventions implemented. All planning and interventions must take into account the total clinical picture. The planning process includes meeting the needs of the woman and family, answering questions, and explaining nursing interventions.

Although the use of EFM can be comforting to many parents, it can be a source of anxiety to some. Therefore, the nurse needs to be particularly sensitive to the emotional, informational, and physical comfort needs of the woman in labour and those of her family and respond appropriately (Fig. 19-18 and Box 19-7). See the Nursing Care Plan, Fetal Monitoring during Labour on the Evolve site.

Electronic Fetal Monitoring Pattern Recognition

Nurses take into consideration the total clinical picture to determine whether an FHR pattern is normal, atypical, or abnormal. They evaluate these factors on the basis of presence of other obstetrical complications, progress in labour, and use of analgesia or anesthesia. They also need to consider the estimated time to birth. Considering these factors, the nurse must determine which interventions are appropriate, based on sound clinical judgements of a complex, integrated process.

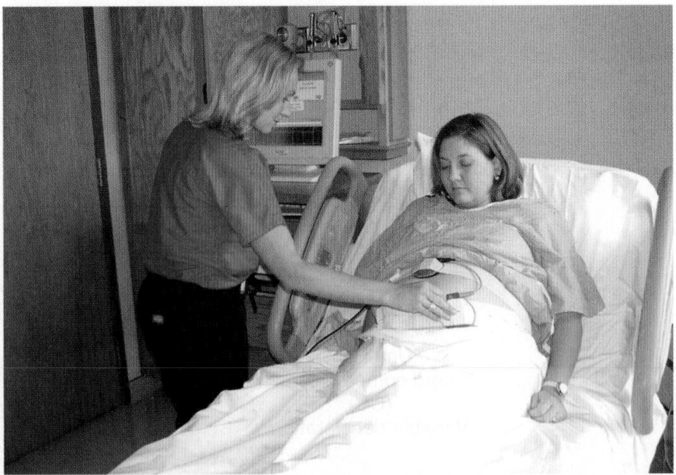

FIGURE 19-18 Nurse explains electronic fetal monitoring as ultrasound transducer monitors the fetal heart rate. (Courtesy Julie Perry Nelson.)

BOX 19-7 PATIENT AND FAMILY TEACHING WHEN INTERMITTENT AUSCULTATION OR ELECTRONIC FETAL MONITOR IS USED

The following guidelines relate to patient teaching:

- Explain the purpose of monitoring to identify fetal well-being in labour.
- Explain each procedure.
- Provide the rationale for maternal position other than supine.
- Explain that fetal status can be assessed safely using intermittent auscultation (IA) or explain the need for electronic fetal monitoring (EFM) if there are risk factors for adverse perinatal outcomes.
- If using EFM, explain that the lower tracing on the monitor strip paper shows uterine activity (UA); the upper tracing shows the fetal heart rate (FHR).
- Reassure the woman and her partner that prepared childbirth techniques can be implemented without difficulty.
- Using palpation, note peak of contraction; knowing that contraction will not get stronger and is half over is usually helpful. Note diminishing intensity.
- Reassure the woman and her partner that the use of internal monitoring does not restrict movement unless medically indicated. Portable telemetry monitors allow the FHR and uterine contraction patterns to be monitored and may increase ambulation during labour.
- Reassure the woman and her partner that the use of monitoring does not imply fetal jeopardy.

- *Normal*—Characteristics are within normal parameters.
- *Atypical*—Further vigilant assessment is required, especially when combined features are present. This may involve the correction of a reversible cause for compromise, intrauterine fetal resuscitation, or further fetal evaluation (scalp stimulation and/or blood sampling if >34 weeks, ultrasound).
- *Abnormal*—Action is required: Review the overall clinical situation; intrauterine resuscitation and prompt operative delivery (vaginal or Caesarean birth) are indicated unless there is evidence of normal oxygenation by scalp pH assessment.

LEGAL TIP *FETAL MONITORING STANDARDS*

Nurses who care for women during childbirth are legally responsible for maintaining an interpretable monitor strip, correctly interpreting FHR patterns, initiating appropriate nursing interventions based on those patterns, and documenting the outcomes of those interventions. Perinatal nurses are responsible for the timely notification of the primary care provider in the event of atypical or abnormal FHR patterns or contraction patterns (i.e., patterns that indicate the need for intervention or expedited birth). Perinatal nurses also are responsible for initiating the institutional chain of command should differences in opinion arise among health care providers about the interpretation of the FHR pattern and the intervention required.

BOX 19-8 MANAGEMENT OF ATYPICAL OR ABNORMAL FETAL HEART RATE PATTERN

Intrauterine resuscitation:
- Stop or decrease oxytocin.
- Change maternal position (to left or right lateral).
- Improve maternal hydration with an IV fluid bolus.
- Perform vaginal examination to assess progress in labour or relieve pressure of presenting part on the cord.
- Consider administration of oxygen (8 to 10 L/min) by mask, although there is little evidence to evaluate its effectiveness when used in the management of suspected fetal compromise.
- Prolonged maternal oxygen administration may have negative implications on fetal cord blood gas samples at the time of birth and as such should be used cautiously as part of intrauterine resuscitation (Fawole & Hofmeyr, 2012; Liston et al., 2007).
- Consider amnioinfusion (see discussion later in chapter) if variable decelerations are present.

Reduce maternal anxiety (to lessen catecholamine impact).

Coach woman to modify breathing or pushing techniques during second stage:
- Use open-glottis rather than Valsalva-style pushing.
- Use fewer pushing efforts during each contraction or make individual pushing efforts shorter.
- Push only with every second or third contraction.
- Push only with contractions (with use of regional anaesthesia) or the urge to push.

Notify primary health care provider.

From Liston, R., Sawchuck, D., Young, D., et al. (2007). SOGC clinical practice guideline: Fetal health surveillance: Antepartum and intrapartum consensus guideline. *Journal of Obstetrics and Gynaecologists of Canada, 29*(9 Suppl 4), s1–s56, p. 37.

Nursing Management of Atypical or Abnormal Patterns

The five essential components of the FHR tracing that must be evaluated regularly are baseline, baseline variability, accelerations, decelerations, and changes or trends over time. Whenever one of these five essential components of the FHR tracing is assessed as atypical or abnormal, corrective measures must be taken immediately. The purpose of these actions is to improve fetal oxygenation (Miller et al., 2013). The term *intrauterine resuscitation* is sometimes used to refer to specific interventions initiated when an atypical or abnormal FHR pattern is noted. Basic corrective measures include instituting maternal position changes, increasing intravenous fluid administration, and potentially administering supplemental oxygen. These interventions are implemented to improve uterine and intervillous space blood flow and increase maternal oxygenation and cardiac output (Miller et al., 2013). Box 19-8 lists basic interventions to improve maternal and fetal oxygenation status.

Nurses must assign priorities to interventions in order to maximize the efficacy of the intrauterine resuscitation. The first priority is to open the maternal and fetal vascular systems; the second priority is to increase blood volume; and the third priority is to optimize oxygenation of the circulating blood volume.

Some interventions are specific to the FHR pattern. Nursing interventions appropriate for the management of tachycardia and bradycardia are given in Table 19-5, and those appropriate for the management of increased or decreased variability are given in Table 19-6. No specific nursing interventions are required for the management of FHR accelerations or early decelerations (see Boxes 19-3 and 19-4). However, late and some types of variable FHR decelerations require aggressive intervention (see Boxes 19-5 and 19-6). Based on the FHR response to these interventions, the primary health care provider decides whether additional interventions should be instituted or whether immediate vaginal or Caesarean birth should be performed.

Additional Methods of Assessment and Intervention

A major shortcoming of EFM is its high rate of false-positive results. Even the most abnormal patterns are poorly predictive of neonatal morbidity. Therefore, other methods of assessment have been developed to evaluate fetal status and intervene as warranted. Fetal scalp blood sampling is sometimes employed to evaluate the fetus further; amnioinfusion is sometimes used to decrease the physiological stress of uterine activity that has resulted in an atypical or abnormal FHR pattern. Umbilical cord blood acid–base determination is a postpartum assessment technique that is useful as an adjunct to the Apgar score in assessing the immediate condition of the newborn.

Fetal scalp blood sampling. Fetal scalp blood sampling involves obtaining a capillary fetal blood sample in a fetus >34 weeks' gestation. It is obtained through a small incision in the fetal scalp taken through the dilated cervix after the membranes have ruptured. It is an adjunct to EFM when the pattern is difficult to interpret or is atypical or abnormal and birth is not imminent. The capillary sample is tested for pH. Results will guide the primary care provider on whether to expedite delivery, reassess within 30 minutes, or allow labour to continue. If the pH is 7.20 or less, delivery is indicated because of the risk of fetal acidemia; pH greater than 7.20 requires further surveillance and reassessment in 30 minutes, especially if the atypical or abnormal EFM persists (Liston et al., 2007). Fetal scalp blood sampling is limited by many factors, including the requirement for cervical dilation and ruptured membranes, technical difficulty of the procedure, and the need for repetitive pH determinations. There is some evidence that scalp lactate levels may also be used to determine fetal status with similar outcomes as fetal scalp pH (Royal College of Obstetricians and Gynaecologists, 2015). The blood may be easier to obtain, as only a very small sample is required. The guideline for determination of fetal status is determined by the type of meter used, although lactate levels <4.2 probably indicate a healthy fetus; 4.2 to 4.8 requires continued monitoring and further testing in 30 minutes; >4.8 indicates immediate birth is required (Wiberg-Itzel, Lipponer, Norman, et al., 2008).

Amnioinfusion. Amnioinfusion is infusion of room or body (in the case of preterm labour) temperature isotonic fluid (usually normal saline or lactated Ringer's solution) into the uterine cavity when the volume of amniotic fluid is low. Without the buffer of amniotic fluid, the umbilical cord can easily become compressed during contractions or fetal movement, diminishing the flow of blood between the fetus and placenta. The purpose of amnioinfusion is to relieve intermittent umbilical cord compression that results in variable decelerations and transient fetal hypoxemia by restoring the amniotic fluid volume to a normal or near-normal level (Miller et al., 2013).

Women with an abnormally small amount of amniotic fluid (*oligohydramnios*) or no amniotic fluid (*anhydramnios*) are candidates for this procedure. Conditions that can result in oligohydramnios or anhydramnios include uteroplacental insufficiency, premature rupture of membranes, or spontaneous or artificial rupture of membranes at term.

Routine amnioinfusion for meconium-stained amniotic fluid without the presence of variable decelerations is no longer recommended. Very few centres in Canada use amnioinfusion as a choice for treatment.

Risks of amnioinfusion include overdistension of the uterine cavity and increased uterine tone. Fluid is administered through an IUPC by either gravity flow or an infusion pump. Usually a bolus of fluid is administered over 20 to 30 minutes; then the infusion is slowed to a maintenance rate. Likely no more than 1000 mL of fluid will need to be administered. The fluid can be warmed for the preterm fetus by infusing it through a blood warmer (Miller et al., 2013).

Intensity and frequency of UCs should be assessed continually during the procedure. The recorded uterine resting tone during amnioinfusion appears higher than normal because of resistance to outflow and turbulence at the end of the catheter. Uterine resting tone should not exceed 40 mm Hg during the procedure. The amount of fluid return must be estimated and documented during amnioinfusion to prevent overdistension of the uterus. The volume of fluid returned should be approximately the same as the amount infused (Miller et al., 2013).

Umbilical cord acid–base determination. In assessing the immediate condition of the newborn after birth, a sample of cord blood is a useful adjunct to the Apgar score. The SOGC strongly recommends that both umbilical arterial and venous cord gases be measured after all births, as they may help in providing appropriate care to the newborn and in planning in subsequent management (Liston et al., 2007). Umbilical arterial values reflect fetal condition and thus are considered by some as most relevant; umbilical venous blood values reflect placental function (Miller et al., 2013). Umbilical cord gas measurements reflect the acid–base status of the newborn at birth, a measurement not reflected in the Apgar score (Table 19-7). If only one sample is possible, it should be arterial since arterial samples are the best indicator of fetal oxygenation at birth. If acidemia is present, the type—respiratory, metabolic, or mixed—is determined by analyzing the blood gas values (Table 19-8).

Patient and Family Teaching

Part of the perinatal nurse's role includes acting as a partner with the woman and her family to achieve a high-quality birthing experience (see Community Focus box). In addition to providing teaching and support for the woman and her family

TABLE 19-7 APPROXIMATE NORMAL VALUES FOR CORD BLOOD

CORD BLOOD	pH	PCO_2 (mm Hg)	HCO_3 (MMOL/L)	BASE EXCESS (MMOL/L)
Artery	7.20–7.34	39.2–61.4	18.4–25.6	−5.5–0.1
Vein	7.28–7.40	32.8–48.6	18.9–23.9	−4.4–0.4

From Liston, R., Sawchuck, D., Young, D., et al. (2007). SOGC clinical practice guideline: Fetal health surveillance: Antepartum and intrapartum consensus guideline. *Journal of Obstetrics and Gynaecology Canada* 29(9 Suppl 4), s1–s56.

TABLE 19-8 TYPES OF ACIDEMIA

	RESPIRATORY	METABOLIC	MIXED
pH	<7.20	<7.20	<7.20
PCO_2	Elevated	Normal	Elevated
Base deficit	<12 mmol/L (normal)	≥12 mmol/L (Elevated)	≥12 mmol/L (Elevated)

Adapted from Miller, L. A., Miller, D. A., & Tucker, S. M. (2013). *Mosby's pocket guide to fetal monitoring: A multidisciplinary approach* (7th ed.). St. Louis: Mosby.

COMMUNITY FOCUS

Education About Electronic Fetal Monitoring

Interview childbirth educators from two different types of childbirth preparation classes regarding what they teach expectant parents about electronic fetal monitoring. Do the educators regard it to be "normal"? Do they discuss its advantages and disadvantages, or do they just describe it as a usual intervention? Do they discuss choice in labour (i.e., are parents able to select auscultation rather than electronic monitoring)? Intermittent rather than continuous monitoring? What implications does this information have for your practice as a labour and birth nurse?

or support people regarding the labour and birth process, breathing techniques, use of equipment, and pain management techniques, the nurse can help with two factors that have an effect on fetal status: pushing and positioning.

Maternal Positioning

Maternal supine hypotensive syndrome is caused by the weight and pressure of the gravid uterus on the ascending vena cava when the woman is in a supine position. The supine position decreases venous return to the woman's heart and cardiac output and subsequently reduces her blood pressure. Low maternal blood pressure decreases intervillous space blood flow during uterine contractions and results in fetal hypoxemia. This is reflected on the fetal monitor as an atypical or abnormal FHR pattern; usually this begins with variable decelerations, followed by decreasing variability, and ultimately may result in late decelerations. The nurse should instruct the woman to avoid using the supine position, if possible. She should be encouraged to maintain an upright, side-lying, or semi-Fowler position with a lateral tilt to the uterus. Either the right or left lateral maternal position effectively enhances uteroplacental blood flow.

Discouraging the Valsalva Manoeuvre

The Valsalva manoeuvre can be described as the process of making a forceful bearing-down attempt while holding one's breath with a closed glottis and tightening the abdominal muscles. This process stimulates the parasympathetic division of the autonomic nervous system, producing a vagal response, and results in the decrease of maternal heart rate and blood pressure. Prolonged pushing in this manner can decrease placental blood flow, alter maternal and fetal oxygenation, decrease the fetal pH and PO_2, increase the fetal PCO_2, and increase the likelihood of fetal hypoxemia, as reflected in FHR pattern changes.

During the second stage of labour, when the woman needs to push, an alternative to breath holding with a closed glottis is to perform the open-mouth and open-glottis breathing-pushing technique. The nurse can instruct the woman to keep her mouth and glottis open and let air escape from the lungs during the pushing process. This may result in an audible grunting sound and will prevent the Valsalva manoeuvre (see Chapter 17, p. 444).

Documentation

Clear and complete documentation in the woman's medical record is essential. As recommended by the SOGC, all fetal health assessments, the plan of action, and the clinical actions taken must be accurately documented (Liston et al., 2007). When describing FHR tracings, it is important to document the contraction pattern, the baseline FHR, variability, and the presence of accelerations and decelerations. In addition to this description, it is also important to provide an interpretation, such as normal or abnormal IA, or normal, atypical, or abnormal tracing, and any clinical action taken. It is also recommended to document maternal and fetal response to any interventions. FHR data and interpretation should be documented at least hourly in the latent phase of the first stage of labour (every 15 minutes if oxytocin infusing), every 15 to 30 minutes in the active phase of the first stage of labour, and every 5 minutes in the active phase of the second stage of labour (Liston et al., 2007). More and more hospitals are moving to use of the electronic medical record and computer charting. With computerized charting, each required component usually appears on the screen so that it will be addressed routinely. Computerized charting often includes forced choices that greatly increase the use of standardized FHR terminology by all members of the health care team. Electronic documentation also has space for comments on the EFM record, which are archived with the medical record (Fig. 19-19). As much as possible, duplicate documentation should be avoided. The nurse needs to follow the documentation standards for fetal surveillance as outlined by the hospital. Regardless of the documentation method, it is important that the time on the fetal monitor and the time the nurse uses to chart progress notes or other documentation are synchronous.

An important point in fetal surveillance documentation is that caregivers use proper descriptive terminology. It is important to avoid such terms as *asphyxia*, *hypoxia*, and *fetal distress*, as these terms are imprecise and nonspecific and lack standard definitions (CPPC, 2009).

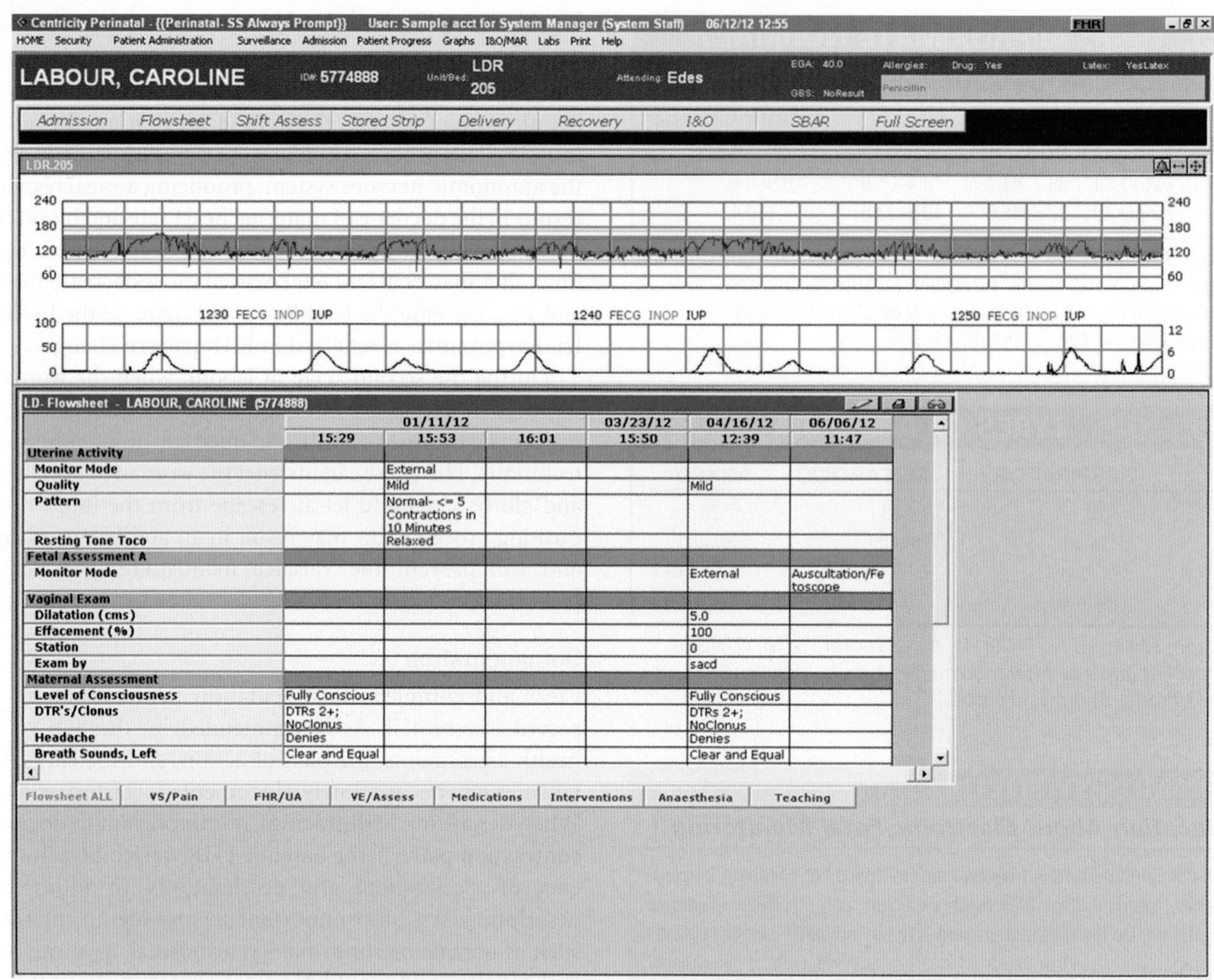

FIGURE 19-19 With integration of the fetal monitor tracing into the electronic medical record, the nurse can view the fetal tracing while charting. (Courtesy General Electric Healthcare Technologies, Barrington, IL.)

KEY POINTS

- Fetal well-being during labour is gauged by the response of the FHR to UCs.
- Essential components of the FHR tracing are the contraction pattern, baseline FHR, variability, accelerations, decelerations, and changes or trends over time.
- FHR cannot be accurately assessed without accurate knowledge of UA assessed through palpation or an IUPC.
- The monitoring of fetal well-being includes FHR assessment, watching for meconium-stained amniotic fluid, and assessment of maternal vital signs and UA.
- It is the responsibility of the nurse to assess FHR and patterns, implement independent nursing interventions, and report atypical and abnormal patterns to the primary care provider.
- The SOGC has established and published health care provider standards and guidelines for fetal heart monitoring.
- The emotional, informational, and comfort needs of the woman and her family must be addressed when the mother and her fetus are being monitored.
- Documentation is initiated and updated according to institutional protocol.

evolve WEBSITE

Visit the Evolve website for additional resources related to the content in this chapter such as Case Studies, Critical Thinking Case Study Answers, Nursing Care Plans, Nursing Processes, Nursing Skills, and Review Questions for Exam Preparation at: *http://evolve.elsevier.com/Canada/Perry/maternal/*

REFERENCES

Alfirevic, Z., Devane, D., & Gyte, G. M. L. (2013). Continuous cardiotocography (CTG) as a form of electronic fetal monitoring (EFM) for fetal assessment during labour. *Cochrane Database of Systematic Reviews*, (5). doi:10.1002/14651858.CD006066.pub2.

Association of Women's Health, Obstetric and Neonatal Nurses (AWHONN). (2009a). *Antepartum and intrapartum fetal heart rate monitoring: Clinical competencies and education guide* (5th ed.). Dubuque, IA: Kendall/Hunt.

Association of Women's Health, Obstetric and Neonatal Nurses (AWHONN). (2009b). *Fetal heart rate monitoring: Principles and practice*. Dubuque, IA: Kendall/Hunt.

Canadian Institute for Health Information (CIHI). (2016). *Childbirth indicators by place of residence*. Retrieved from <http://apps.cihi.ca/mstrapp/asp/Main.aspx?Server=apmstrextprd_i&project=Quick+Stats&uid=pce_pub_en&pwd=&evt=2048001&ßvisualizationMode=0&documentID=029DB170438205AEBCC75B8673CCE822>.

Canadian Perinatal Programs Coalition (CPPC). (2009). *Fundamentals of fetal health surveillance: A self learning manual* (4th ed.). Vancouver: British Columbia Perinatal Health Program.

Cunningham, F. G., Leveno, K. J., Bloom, S. L., et al. (Eds.), (2014). *Williams obstetrics* (24th ed.). New York: McGraw Hill.

Fawole, B., & Hofmeyr, G. J. (2012). Maternal oxygen administration for fetal distress. *Cochrane Database of Systematic Reviews*, (12). doi:10.1002/14651858.CD000136.pub2.

Feinstein, N. F., Sprague, A., & Trepanier, M. J. (2008). *Fetal heart rate auscultation* (2nd ed.). Washington, DC: AWHONN.

Garite, T. J. (2012). Intrapartum fetal evaluation. In S. Gabbe, J. Niebyl, J. Simpson, et al. (Eds.), *Obstetrics: Normal and problem pregnancies* (6th ed.). Philadelphia: Saunders.

Gilbert, E. (2011). *Manual of high risk pregnancy & delivery* (5th ed.). St. Louis, MO: Mosby.

Liston, R., Sawchuck, D., Young, D., et al. (2007). Fetal health surveillance: Antepartum and intrapartum consensus guideline. *Journal of Obstetrics and Gynaecology Canada*, *29*(9 Suppl. 4), s1–s56.

Macones, G. A., Hankins, G. D., Spong, C. Y., et al. (2008). The 2008 National Institute of Child Health and Human Development workshop report on electronic fetal monitoring: Update on definitions, interpretation, and research guidelines. *Journal of Obstetric, Gynecologic, and Neonatal Nursing*, *37*(5), 510–515. doi:10.1097/AOG.0b013e3181841395.

Miller, L., Miller, D., & Tucker, S. M. (2013). *Mosby's pocket guide to fetal monitoring: A multidisciplinary approach* (7th ed.). St. Louis: Mosby.

Public Health Agency of Canada. (2009). *What mothers say: The Canadian maternity experiences survey (Cat. No. HP5-74/2-2009E-PDF)*. Ottawa: Author.

Royal College of Obstetricians and Gynaecologists. (2015). *Is it time for UK obstetricians to accept fetal scalp lactate as an alternative to scalp pH?* Retrieved from <https://www.rcog.org.uk/globalassets/documents/guidelines/scientific-impact-papers/sip_47.pdf>.

Wiberg-Itzel, E., Lipponer, C., Norman, M., et al. (2008). Determination of pH or lactate in fetal scalp blood in management of intrapartum fetal distress: Randomised controlled multicentre trial. *British Medical Journal*, *336*(7656), 1284–1287.

ADDITIONAL RESOURCES

SOGC Fetal Health Surveillance: Antepartum and Intrapartum Consensus Guideline: <http://www.sogc.org/guidelines/documents/gui197CPG0709.pdf>

CHAPTER

20

Labour and Birth at Risk

Shelly Petruskavich

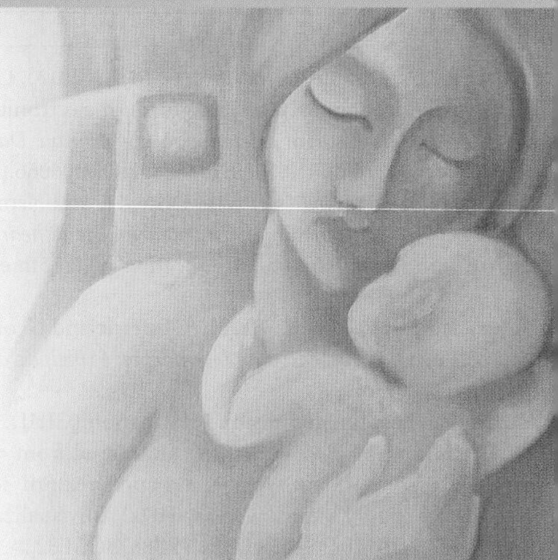

Evolve WEBSITE

Visit the Evolve website for additional resources related to the content in this chapter such as Case Studies, Critical Thinking Case Study Answers, Nursing Care Plans, Nursing Processes, Nursing Skills, and Review Questions for Exam Preparation at: http://evolve.elsevier.com/Canada/Perry/maternal/

OBJECTIVES

On completion of this chapter the reader will be able to:

- Differentiate between preterm birth and low birth weight.
- Identify major risk factors associated with preterm labour.
- Analyze current interventions to prevent spontaneous preterm labour.
- Discuss the use of tocolytics and antenatal glucocorticoids in preterm labour.
- Design a nursing care management plan for women with preterm premature rupture of the membranes (PPROM).
- Describe the care of a woman experiencing postterm pregnancy.
- Identify the care of a woman who experiences labour dystocia.
- Summarize the nursing care management for a trial of labour, induction and augmentation of labour, forceps- and vacuum-assisted birth, a Caesarean birth, and vaginal birth after a Caesarean birth.
- Discuss obstetrical emergencies and their appropriate management.

When complications arise during labour and birth, perinatal morbidity and mortality risks increase. Some complications may be anticipated, especially if the woman is identified as high risk during the antepartum period; others are unexpected or unforeseen. It is crucial for nurses to understand the normal birth process in order to prevent and detect deviations from normal labour and birth and promptly implement nursing measures when complications arise. Optimum care of the labouring woman, the fetus, or both, as well as of the family, is possible only when the perinatal nurse and other members of the obstetrical team use their knowledge and skills in a concerted effort to provide competent and compassionate care. This chapter focuses on the problems of preterm labour and birth, dystocia, postterm pregnancy, and obstetrical emergencies.

PRETERM LABOUR AND BIRTH

Preterm labour is defined as cervical changes and regular uterine contractions occurring between 20 and 37 weeks of pregnancy. **Preterm birth** is any birth that occurs before the completion of 37 weeks of pregnancy. Complications related to preterm birth account for more newborn and infant deaths than any other cause (Simhan, Iams, & Romero, 2012). In 2010, the overall preterm birth rate for Canada was 7.7%, although the rate of births that occur before the completion of 32 weeks of pregnancy was only 1.2% (Public Health Agency of Canada [PHAC], 2013).

The majority of all preterm births are termed **late preterm** because they occur between 34 and 37 weeks of gestation. Late preterm infants are at increased risk for early death and long-term health problems when compared with infants who are born full term. Although late preterm babies do experience significant problems, the great majority of infant deaths and the most serious morbidity occur among the 16% of all preterm infants who are born before 32 weeks of gestation (*very preterm birth*) (Simhan, Berghella, & Iams, 2014).

Preterm Birth Versus Low Birth Weight

Although they have distinctly different meanings, the terms *preterm birth* or *prematurity* and *low birth weight* are often used interchangeably. *Preterm birth* describes length of gestation (i.e., less than 37 weeks regardless of the weight of the infant), whereas *low birth weight* describes only weight at the time of birth (i.e., 2500 g or less). Because birth weight is far easier to determine than gestational age, in many settings and publications low birth weight has been used as a substitute term for preterm birth. Preterm birth, however, is a more dangerous health condition for an infant because less time in the uterus correlates with immaturity of body systems. Low-birth-weight infants can be preterm but are not necessarily preterm. Low birth weight can be caused by conditions other than preterm birth, such as intrauterine growth restriction (IUGR), a condition of inadequate fetal growth not necessarily correlated with initiation of labour. Pregnant women who have various complications of pregnancy that interfere with uteroplacental perfusion, such as gestational hypertension or poor nutrition, may give birth to a baby at term who is at low birth weight because of IUGR. However, infants born at a preterm gestation can weigh more than 2500 g at birth, such as infants born to women with diabetes who have poorly controlled blood glucose levels. Today, thanks to advances in pregnancy dating, outcomes related to gestational age can be distinguished with greater frequency from outcomes related to birth weight (Simhan et al., 2014).

The incidence of preterm birth in Canada is increasing, with rates higher among socially disadvantaged populations, single women, women with low levels of education, and women who receive late or no prenatal care. The preterm birth rate is higher among women younger than 18 years of age or older than 35 years (Lim, Butt, Crane, et al., 2011). Multifetal pregnancy from infertility treatment also is associated with an increase in preterm births.

Spontaneous Versus Indicated Preterm Birth

Preterm birth is divided into two categories: spontaneous and indicated. *Spontaneous preterm birth* occurs after an early initiation of the labour process and comprises nearly 75% of all preterm births in North America. Conditions such as preterm labour with intact membranes, preterm premature rupture of membranes (preterm PROM), cervical insufficiency, or amnionitis often result in preterm birth (Simhan et al., 2014).

Indicated preterm birth occurs as a means to resolve maternal or fetal risk related to continuing the pregnancy. About 25% of all preterm births in North American are indicated because of medical or obstetrical conditions that affect the mother, the fetus, or both. An increase in the number of indicated preterm births between 34 and 36 weeks of gestation accounts for much of the recent rise in late preterm births (Simhan et al., 2012, 2014). Box 20-1 lists some common causes of indicated preterm births.

The remainder of this section deals with spontaneous preterm labour and birth.

Spontaneous Preterm Labour and Birth Risk Factors

Major risk factors for spontaneous preterm birth are listed in Box 20-2. Many of the social determinants of health, including poverty, lack of education, living in a disadvantaged geographical area, and lack of access to prenatal care, have been identified as risk factors. In addition, the risk for preterm birth appears to be genetically related. For example, women who were themselves born prematurely have an increased risk for giving birth prematurely (Simhan, Iams, & Romero, 2012). Researchers have developed many risk scoring systems in an attempt to determine which women might go into labour prematurely. No risk scoring system has been very successful in lowering the preterm birth rate, however, because at least 50% of all women who ultimately give birth prematurely have no identifiable risk factors (Simhan et al., 2014; Simhan et al., 2012). Therefore, it is important that all women be educated about prematurity, not only in early pregnancy but also in the preconception period.

BOX 20-1 COMMON CAUSES OF INDICATED PRETERM BIRTH

- Pre-existing or gestational diabetes
- Chronic hypertension
- Pre-eclampsia
- Obstetrical disorders or risk factors in the current or a previous pregnancy
- Placental disorders
- Medical disorders
- Seizures
- Thromboembolism
- Maternal HIV or herpes infection
- Obesity
- Advanced maternal age
- Fetal disorders
- Chronic (IUGR) or acute (abnormal NST or BPP) fetal compromise
- Excessive or inadequate amount of amniotic fluid
- Birth defects

BPP, biophysical profile; *HIV,* human immunodeficiency virus; *IUGR,* intrauterine growth restriction; *NST,* nonstress test.
Data from Simhan, H., Iams, J., & Romero, R. (2012). Preterm birth. In S. Gabbe, J. Niebyl, J. Simpson, et al. (Eds.), *Obstetrics: Normal and problem pregnancies* (6th ed.). Philadelphia: Saunders.

BOX 20-2 RISK FACTORS FOR SPONTANEOUS PRETERM LABOUR

- History of previous spontaneous preterm birth
- Family history of preterm labour
- African race
- Genital tract infection
- Multifetal gestation
- Second-trimester bleeding
- Low prepregnancy weight
- Low socioeconomic status
- Lack of access to prenatal care

Data from Simhan, H., Berghella, V., & Iams, J. (2014). Preterm labor and birth. In R. Creasy, R. Resnik, J. Iams, et al. (Eds.), *Creasy and Resnik's maternal-fetal medicine: Principles and practice* (7th ed.). Philadelphia: Saunders; Simhan, H., Iams, J., & Romero, R. (2012). Preterm birth. In S. Gabbe, J. Niebyl, J. Simpson, et al. (Eds.), *Obstetrics: Normal and problem pregnancies* (6th ed.). Philadelphia: Saunders.

Unless all women are included in prevention efforts, a widespread reduction in preterm birth rates cannot be expected.

Infection is definitely associated with preterm labour. Women in spontaneous preterm labour with intact membranes commonly have organisms that are normally found in the lower genital tract present in their amniotic fluid, placenta, and membranes. Clinical and laboratory evidence of infection is more common when birth occurs earlier than 30 to 32 weeks of gestation than closer to term. Urinary tract and intra-abdominal (e.g., appendicitis) infections have also been related to preterm birth (Simhan et al., 2012). Women with periodontal disease have been shown to have an increased risk for preterm birth. However, the risk is not reduced by periodontal care, which suggests that the link between periodontal disease and preterm birth is not a cause-and-effect relationship (American College of Obstetricians and Gynecologists [ACOG], 2013; Simhan et al., 2012). Recommendations for all pregnant women include regular dental care before and during pregnancy, oral assessment as part of prenatal health care, and good oral hygiene measures.

Another proposed cause of preterm labour and birth is bleeding at the site of placental implantation in the uterus in the first or second trimester of pregnancy. The resulting uteroplacental ischemia or hemorrhage at the decidual layer of the placenta may somehow activate the preterm labour process. Intrauterine inflammation is associated with infection, uterine vascular compromise, and decidual hemorrhage and may contribute to preterm labour. Maternal and fetal stress, uterine overdistension, allergic reaction, and a decrease in progesterone are other factors that may play a part in initiating preterm labour. It has becoming increasingly clear that preterm labour is caused by multiple pathological processes that eventually result in uterine contractions, cervical changes, and membrane rupture (Romero & Lockwood, 2014; Simhan et al., 2014).

Fetal Fibronectin Test

Fetal fibronectin (FFN) is a biochemical marker that may be used as a diagnostic test for preterm labour. It is a glycoprotein "glue" found in plasma and produced during fetal life. FFN normally appears in cervical and vaginal secretions early in pregnancy and then again in late pregnancy. The test is performed by collecting fluid from the woman's vagina using a swab during a speculum examination. The presence of FFN during the late second and early third trimesters of pregnancy may be related to placental inflammation, which is thought to be one cause of spontaneous preterm labour. However, the presence of FFN is not very sensitive as a predictor of preterm birth. Before 35 weeks of gestation, a positive FFN test predicts preterm birth only about 25% of the time. The test's sensitivity may be better earlier in pregnancy. In one study, the FFN test predicted 65% of preterm births occurring before 28 weeks when it was performed between 22 and 24 weeks. Often the test is used to predict who will *not* go into preterm labour because preterm labour is very unlikely to occur in women with a negative result. In one study in Ontario, it was determined there was a small but statistically significant reduction in the rate of hospital admissions for preterm labour following the introduction of FFN testing. In most cases, women with a negative FFN test can be monitored as outpatients, avoiding unnecessary interventions, hospitalizations, or maternal transport to a hospital with a higher level of neonatal care (Fell, Sprague, Grimshaw, et al., 2014).

Cervical Length

Another possible predictor of imminent preterm labour is endocervical length. Changes in cervical length occur before uterine activity, so cervical measurement can identify women in whom the labour process has begun. However, because preterm cervical shortening occurs over a period of weeks, neither digital nor ultrasound cervical examination is very sensitive at predicting imminent preterm birth (Simhan et al., 2014). Women whose cervical length is greater than 30 mm are unlikely to give birth prematurely even if they have symptoms of preterm labour (Simhan et al., 2012, 2014).

NURSING CARE

Prenatal care should focus on performing ongoing holistic risk assessment, encouraging women to participate in health-promoting activity (e.g., good nutrition, exercise, stress management), and implementing appropriate medical and psychosocial interventions. The onset of preterm labour is often insidious and can be easily mistaken for normal discomforts of pregnancy. Nursing diagnoses, expected outcomes of care, and evidence-informed interventions should be established for each woman on the basis of her assessment findings (see Nursing Care Plan: Women at Risk for Preterm Labour, available on Evolve).

Prevention

Primary prevention strategies that address risk factors associated with preterm labour and birth are less costly in human and financial terms than the high-tech and often lifelong care required by preterm infants and their families. Programs aimed at health promotion and disease prevention that encourage healthy lifestyles for the population in general and women of child-bearing age in particular should be developed to prevent preterm labour and birth. Preconception counselling and care for women, especially those with a history of preterm birth, may help in identifying correctable risk factors and provide a means to encourage women to participate in health-promoting activities. Smoking cessation, for example, has been shown to prevent preterm labour and birth (Simhan et al., 2014).

Preterm birth can be prevented in some women by administering prophylactic progesterone supplementation. Both daily vaginal suppositories or creams and weekly intramuscular injections of 17-alpha hydroxyprogesterone caproate have been shown to decrease the rate of preterm birth by about 40% in women with a history of prior preterm birth or with a short (less than 15 mm to 20 mm length) cervix before 24 weeks of gestation. Supplementation begins at 16 weeks and continues until 36 weeks of gestation. Progesterone supplementation is not recommended for use in nulliparous women and does not affect the rate of preterm birth in women with multiple gestations. Exactly how progesterone works to prevent preterm

BOX 20-3 SIGNS AND SYMPTOMS OF PRETERM LABOUR

Uterine Activity
- Uterine contractions more frequent than every 10 minutes, persisting for 1 hour or more
- Uterine contractions painful or painless

Discomfort
- Lower abdominal cramping similar to gas pains; may be accompanied by diarrhea
- Dull, intermittent low back pain (below the waist)
- Painful, menstrual-like cramps
- Suprapubic pain or pressure
- Pelvic pressure or heaviness; feeling that "baby is pushing down"
- Urinary frequency

Vaginal Discharge
- Change in character and amount of usual discharge: thicker (mucoid) or thinner (watery), bloody, brown or colourless, increased amount, odour
- Rupture of amniotic membranes

PATIENT TEACHING

What to Do If Symptoms of Preterm Labour Occur

- Empty your bladder.
- Drink two to three glasses of water or juice.
- Lie down on your side for 1 hour.
- Palpate for contractions.
- If symptoms continue, call your health care provider or go to the hospital.
- If symptoms go away, resume light activity but not what you were doing when the symptoms began.
- If symptoms return, call your health care provider or go to the hospital.
- If any of the following symptoms occur, call your health care provider or go to the hospital immediately:
  - Uterine contractions every 10 minutes or less for 1 hour or more
  - Vaginal bleeding
  - Fluid leaking from the vagina

birth is unclear (Brizot, Hernandez, Liao, et al., 2015; Simhan et al., 2012).

One of the most important nursing interventions aimed at preventing preterm birth is the education of pregnant women about the early symptoms of preterm labour so that, if symptoms occur, the woman can be referred promptly to her care provider for more intensive care (Box 20-3). Nurses can provide patient education regarding symptoms of regular contractions or cramping between 20 and 37 weeks of gestation and should inform the woman that these symptoms are not normal discomforts of pregnancy and that contractions, cramping, or back pain that does not go away, becomes regular in timing, or increases in intensity should prompt the woman to contact her primary health care provider. Women also must be taught the significance of these symptoms of preterm labour and what to do should they occur (see Patient Teaching box). Waiting too long to see a health care provider could result in inevitable preterm birth without the benefit of treatments that may improve outcomes.

Early Recognition and Diagnosis

Although preterm birth often is not preventable, early recognition of preterm labour is still essential to implement interventions that have been demonstrated to reduce neonatal and infant morbidity and mortality. These interventions include the following (ACOG, 2012; Simhan et al., 2012):

- Transferring the mother before birth to a hospital equipped to care for her preterm infant
- Giving antibiotics during labour to prevent neonatal group B streptococcal infection
- Administering corticosteroids to women in labour to prevent or reduce neonatal and infant morbidity and mortality from health problems including respiratory distress syndrome, intraventricular hemorrhage, and necrotizing enterocolitis
- Administering magnesium sulphate to women giving birth before 32 weeks of gestation, to reduce the incidence of cerebral palsy in their infants
- Administering tocolytic therapy for short-term prolongation of pregnancy (up to 48 hours) to allow for administration of antenatal steroids

Although maternal transport helps ensure a better health outcome for the mother and the baby, it also has a downside. Women may be transported to tertiary centres far from home, making visits by family and friends difficult and increasing the anxiety of the woman and her family. Attention to the needs of the woman and her family before, during, and after the transport is essential to comprehensive nursing care.

The diagnosis of preterm labour is based on three major diagnostic criteria:

1. Gestational age between 20 and 37 weeks
2. Uterine activity (contractions)
3. Progressive cervical change (e.g., cervical effacement of 80% or cervical dilation of 2 cm or greater)

If the presence of FFN is used as another diagnostic criterion, a sample of cervical mucus for testing should be obtained before doing an examination for cervical changes, because the lubricant used to examine the cervix can reduce the accuracy of the test for FFN. The presence of vaginal bleeding or ruptured membranes or a history of intercourse within the past 24 hours can also reduce the accuracy of the test results.

The pregnant woman at 30 weeks of gestation with an irritable uterus but no documented cervical change is not in preterm labour, although she should be carefully evaluated during follow-up care to determine whether she has progressed to active preterm labour (e.g., effacement, dilation, or both). Misdiagnosis of preterm labour can lead to inappropriate use of pharmacological agents that can be dangerous to the health of the woman, the fetus, or both.

Lifestyle Modifications

Activity Restriction

Activity restriction, including bedrest and limited work, was a commonly prescribed intervention for the prevention of

BOX 20-4 ADVERSE EFFECTS OF BEDREST

Maternal Effects (Physical)
- Weight loss; indigestion; loss of appetite
- Muscle wasting, weakness; aching muscles
- Potential for thrombus formation and thromboembolism
- Bone demineralization and calcium loss
- Decreased plasma volume and cardiac output
- Increased clotting tendency; risk for thrombophlebitis
- Alteration in bowel function; constipation
- Sleep disturbance, fatigue
- Prolonged postpartum recovery

Maternal Effects (Psychosocial)
- Loss of control associated with role reversals
- Dysphoria—anxiety, depression, hostility, and anger
- Guilt associated with difficulty complying with activity restriction and inability to meet role responsibilities
- Boredom, loneliness
- Emotional lability (mood swings); difficulty concentrating
- Increased stress

Effects on Support System
- Stress associated with role reversals, increased responsibilities, and disruption of family routines
- Financial strain associated with loss of maternal income
- Fear and anxiety regarding well-being of the mother and fetus

preterm birth. Bedrest, however, is not a benign intervention, and there is no evidence in the literature to support the effectiveness of this intervention in reducing preterm birth rates (ACOG, 2012; Simhan et al., 2012). Research indicates that bedrest causes adverse physical effects, including risk for thrombus formation, muscle atrophy, osteoporosis, and cardiovascular deconditioning. In many instances, these symptoms are not resolved by 6 weeks postpartum. In addition, bedrest affects women and their families psychologically, emotionally, socially, and financially. Box 20-4 lists adverse effects of bedrest. Many health care providers now recommend only modified activity restriction, if at all.

Restriction of Sexual Activity

Restriction of sexual activity is frequently recommended for women at risk for preterm birth. This intervention has not been shown to be effective at preventing preterm birth. However, sexual abstinence has not been studied in women with specific risk factors for preterm birth, such as a short cervix. Therefore, more research is indicated (Simhan et al., 2014). If, however, symptoms of preterm labour occur after sexual activity, then that activity may need to be curtailed until 37 weeks of gestation.

Suppression of Uterine Activity

Should preterm labour occur, women are usually admitted to the hospital for assessment; fetal monitoring; cervical and vaginal cultures; and assessment of cervical status, amniotic fluid leakage, and maternal temperature (an increase can be an early sign of chorioamnionitis). The initiation of tocolytic therapy might be considered at this time; however, once the pregnancy has progressed beyond 34 weeks of gestation, the benefits of prolonging the pregnancy do not justify its risk to the woman.

BOX 20-5 CONTRAINDICATIONS TO TOCOLYSIS

Maternal
Severe pre-eclampsia or severe gestational hypertension
Significant vaginal bleeding
Intrauterine infection (chorioamnionitis)
Cardiac disease
Medical or obstetrical condition that contraindicates continuation of pregnancy

Fetal
Gestational age of 37 weeks or more
Fetal demise
Lethal fetal anomaly
Evidence of acute or chronic fetal compromise

Data from Simhan, H., Iams, J., & Romero, R. (2012). Preterm birth. In S. Gabbe, J. Niebyl, J. Simpson, et al. (Eds.), *Obstetrics: Normal and problem pregnancies* (6th ed.). Philadelphia: Saunders.

Tocolytics

Tocolytics are medications given to arrest labour after uterine contractions and cervical change have occurred. No medications have been approved for use as tocolytics in Canada. Drugs marketed for other purposes, such as for treatment of asthma or hypertension or as anti-inflammatory or analgesic agents, are used on an "off-label" basis (i.e., drugs known to be effective for a specific purpose though not specifically developed and tested for this purpose) to suppress preterm labour (ACOG, 2012; Simhan et al., 2014). No tocolytic has been shown to reduce the rate of preterm birth. Rather, the rationale for giving these medications is to delay birth long enough to allow time for maternal transport and for corticosteroids to reach maximum benefit to reduce neonatal morbidity and mortality. Studies of individual drugs used for tocolysis rarely contain information about whether delaying birth improved infant outcomes (Simhan et al., 2012). Maternal and fetal contraindications to tocolytic therapy are listed in Box 20-5. Box 20-6 describes nursing care for women receiving tocolytic therapy.

! NURSING ALERT

To date, there are no medications approved by the Health Protection Branch of Health Canada to arrest preterm labour, although some medications are prescribed for this purpose. Nurses need to be aware of the use of off-label medications.

In Canada, the medications most commonly used for arrest of labour are nifedipine (Adalat), indomethacin (Indocin), and nitroglycerin. Prostaglandin inhibitors and calcium channel blockers have the highest probability of delaying birth and

BOX 20-6 NURSING CARE FOR WOMEN RECEIVING TOCOLYTIC THERAPY

- Explain to the woman and her family the purpose and adverse effects of the tocolytic medication(s) ordered.
- Position woman on her side to enhance placental perfusion and reduce pressure on the cervix.
- Monitor maternal vital signs, including lung sounds and respiratory effort, fetal heart rate and pattern, and labour status according to hospital protocol and professional standards.
- Assess mother and fetus for signs of adverse reactions related to the tocolytic medication(s) being administered (see Medication Guide).
- Determine maternal fluid balance by measuring intake and output.
- Provide psychosocial support to the woman and her family as well as opportunities for them to express feelings and concerns.
- Offer comfort measures as required.
- Encourage diversional activities and relaxation techniques.

improving neonatal and maternal outcomes (Haas, Caldwell, Kirkpatrick, et al., 2012).

Nifedipine (Adalat), a calcium channel blocker, is a tocolytic agent that can suppress contractions. Because of its ease of administration and low incidence of significant maternal and fetal adverse effects, the use of nifedipine is increasing and is usually the first choice of tocolytic. The drug is rapidly absorbed after oral administration. Maternal adverse effects, which include headache, flushing, dizziness, and nausea, are generally mild and relate primarily to the hypotension and reflex tachycardia that occur with administration. The decrease in blood pressure that occurs may be helpful for women who are also diagnosed with gestational hypertension or pre-eclampsia (see Medication Guide).

Indomethacin (Indocin), a nonsteroidal anti-inflammatory drug (NSAID), has been shown in some trials to suppress preterm labour by blocking the production of prostaglandins. Serious maternal adverse effects are uncommon, and indomethacin is usually well tolerated. However, four serious fetal or neonatal adverse effects have caused major concerns about its use as a tocolytic; these effects include constriction of the ductus arteriosus, oligohydramnios, necrotizing enterocolitis, and neonatal pulmonary hypertension. Therefore, limiting the

MEDICATION GUIDE

Tocolytic Therapy for Preterm Labour

Action	Dosage and Route	Adverse Effects	Nursing Considerations
Nifedipine (Adalat)* Calcium channel blocker; relaxes smooth muscles, including the uterus, by blocking calcium entry	Loading dose: 20 mg PO Maintenance dosage: 10–20 mg PO 3 to 4 times daily adjusted according to uterine activity (however, the ideal dose has not been established)	**Maternal (most effects are mild)** • Hypotension • Dizziness • Headache • Nausea • Flushing **Fetal** • No known adverse effects	• Do not use sublingual route. • Use with caution with antihypertensives because severe hypotension can result. • Assess woman and fetus according to agency protocol, being alert for adverse reactions. • Contraindicated in women with preload-dependent cardiac lesion (e.g., aortic insufficiency). • Long-acting formulations decrease incidence of adverse effects
Indomethacin* Relaxes uterine smooth muscle by inhibiting prostaglandins	Loading dose: 50 mg rectally or 50–100 mg PO; then 25–50 mg PO q6h for 48 hr	**Maternal (common)** • Nausea and vomiting • Heartburn **Less common, but more serious** • GI bleeding • Prolonged bleeding time • Thrombocytopenia • Asthma in aspirin-sensitive patients **Fetal** • Constriction of ductus arteriosus • Oligohydramnios, caused by reduced fetal urine production • Neonatal pulmonary hypertension • Necrotizing enterocolitis **Maternal** • Severe hypotension • Headaches (usually transient) • Tachycardia • Postural hypotension	• Used only if gestational age is less than 32 wk • Administer for 48 hr or less. • Do not use in women with renal or hepatic disease, active peptic ulcer disease, poorly controlled hypertension, asthma, or coagulation disorders. • Can mask maternal fever • Assess woman and fetus according to agency policy; be alert for adverse effects. • Determine amniotic fluid volume and function of fetal ductus arteriosus before initiating therapy and within 48 hr of discontinuing therapy; assessment is critical if therapy continues for more than 48 hr. • Administer with food to decrease GI distress. • Monitor for signs of postpartum hemorrhage. • Should be used with caution in women who are volume depleted or who are already hypotensive.

Continued

MEDICATION GUIDE

Tocolytic Therapy for Preterm Labour—cont'd

Action	Dosage and Route	Adverse Effects	Nursing Considerations
Nitroglycerin* Vasodilating agent, relaxes vascular smooth muscle	Transdermal patch—applied, and if patient's contractions persist after 1 hr, a second patch is applied. Keep both patches on and remove at 24 hr.	Nitroglycerin can cause severe hypotension.	• Monitor vital signs closely to ensure vital signs remain at a normal level. • Headaches can be treated with acetaminophen. • Transdermal patch should be applied to non-hairy skin.
Magnesium Sulphate CNS depressant; relaxes smooth muscles including uterus	IV fluid should contain 40 g in 1000 mL, piggyback to primary infusion, and administer using pump. Loading dose: 4 g over 30 min Maintenance dose: 1 g/hr Use for stabilization only. Discontinue within 24–48 hr at the maintenance dose or if intolerable adverse effects occur.	**Maternal** • Hot flushes, sweating, burning at IV insertion site, nausea and vomiting, dry mouth, drowsiness, blurred vision, diplopia, headache, ileus, generalized muscle weakness, lethargy, dizziness • Hypocalcemia • SOB • Transient hypotension • Some reactions may subside when loading dose is completed **Intolerable** • Respiratory rate fewer than 12 breaths/min • Pulmonary edema • Absent DTRs • Chest pain • Severe hypotension • Altered level of consciousness • Extreme muscle weakness • Urine output less than 25–30 mL/hr or less than 100 mL/4 hr **Fetal (uncommon)** • Decreased breathing movement • Reduced FHR variability • Abnormal NST	• Assess woman and fetus to obtain baseline before beginning therapy and then before and after each incremental change; follow frequency of agency protocol. • Discontinue infusion and notify physician if intolerable adverse effects occur. • Ensure that calcium gluconate 1 g (10 mL of 10% solution) or calcium chloride (normal dose is 500 mg IV infused over 30 min) is available for emergency administration to reverse magnesium sulphate toxicity. • Should not be given to women with myasthenia gravis • Total IV intake should be limited to 125 mL/hr.

DTR, deep tendon reflex; *FHR*, fetal heart rate; *GI*, gastrointestinal; *IV*, intravenous; *NST*, nonstress test; *PO*, by mouth; *SOB*, shortness of breath.

***Caution:** Not approved by Health Canada for preterm labour (off-label use).

use of indomethacin to a short duration of treatment in women with preterm labour at less than 32 weeks of gestation is recommended (ACOG, 2013; Simhan et al., 2012) (see Medication Guide).

Nitroglycerin works to dilate blood vessels, predominantly those in venous vascular beds, as well as relax smooth muscles. An adverse effect of nitroglycerin is the decrease in blood pressure that it can cause. Women need to be monitored closely for postural hypotension and blood pressure that is too low to perfuse the fetus. Nitroglycerin appears to decrease the rate of preterm labour, although maternal adverse effects are greater (Shaikh, Shaikh, Akhter, et al., 2012).

Magnesium sulphate inhibits uterine contractions and decreases intracellular calcium levels (Simhan et al., 2012). Magnesium sulphate produces few serious maternal or neonatal complications, and clinicians are familiar with its use. However, although magnesium sulphate is still frequently used, a recent meta-analysis of tocolytic agents found that it is not effective when given for tocolysis and is used more appropriately for fetal neuroprotection (see Medication Guide and discussion below) (Simhan et al., 2012).

SAFETY ALERT

Because using a calcium channel blocker can result in orthostatic hypotension and dizziness, it is essential to instruct women taking this type of drug to slowly change position from supine to upright and then sit before standing until any dizziness disappears. In addition, it is important to maintain adequate fluid balance to reduce the drop in blood pressure that can occur with the drug-related vasodilation.

Promotion of Fetal Lung Maturity

Antenatal Glucocorticoids

Antenatal glucocorticoids are given as intramuscular injections to the mother to accelerate fetal lung maturity by stimulating fetal surfactant production. They are now considered one of the most effective and cost-efficient interventions for preventing morbidity and mortality associated with preterm labour. Antenatal glucocorticoids have been shown to significantly reduce the incidence of respiratory distress syndrome, intraventricular hemorrhage, necrotizing enterocolitis, and death in newborns without increasing the risk for infection in either mothers

MEDICATION GUIDE

Antenatal Glucocorticoid Therapy With Betamethasone, Dexamethasone

Action*
- Stimulates fetal lung maturation by promoting release of enzymes that induce production or release of lung surfactant.

Indication
- To prevent or reduce the severity of neonatal respiratory distress syndrome by accelerating lung maturity in fetuses between 24 and 34 weeks of gestation. Infants born to women who received antenatal glucocorticoids are also less likely to experience intraventricular hemorrhage, necrotizing enterocolitis, or neonatal death.

Dosage and Route
- Betamethasone: 12 mg intramuscular (IM) for two doses 24 hours apart
- Dexamethasone: 6 mg IM for four doses 12 hours apart

Maternal Effects
- Transient (lasting 72 hours) increase in white blood cell (WBC) count
- Hyperglycemia

Fetal Effects
- Transient (lasting 72 hours) decrease in fetal breathing and body movements

Nursing Considerations
- Give deep IM in ventral gluteal or vastus lateralis muscle.
- Medication *must* be given by intramuscular injection; oral administration is *not* an acceptable alternative.
- Injection is painful.
- Medication should *not* affect maternal blood pressure.
- Assess blood glucose levels. Women with diabetes whose blood sugar levels have previously been well controlled may require increased insulin doses for several days.

*__Note:__ Health Canada has not approved these medications for this use (i.e., this is an unlabelled use for obstetrics).
Data from Simhan, H., Iams, J., & Romero, R. (2012). Preterm birth. In S. Gabbe, J. Niebyl, J. Simpson, et al. (Eds.), *Obstetrics: Normal and problem pregnancies* (6th ed.). Philadelphia: Saunders.

or newborns (Mercer, 2014a). The National Institutes of Health (NIH) consensus panel recommended that all women between 24 and 34 weeks of gestation be given a single course of antenatal glucocorticoids when preterm birth is threatened, unless evidence indicates that glucocorticoids will have an adverse effect on the mother or birth is imminent. In general, women who are candidates for tocolytic therapy are also candidates for antenatal glucocorticoids (ACOG, 2013; Lee & Guinn, 2015; Mercer, 2014a). The regimen for administration of antenatal glucocorticoids is given in the Medication Guide.

NURSING ALERT

All women between 24 and 34 weeks of gestation who are at risk for preterm birth within 7 days should receive treatment with a single course of antenatal glucocorticoids. Because optimal benefit to the fetus begins 24 hours after the first injection, timely administration is essential.

Management of Inevitable Preterm Birth

When preterm birth appears inevitable, magnesium sulphate may be administered to reduce or prevent neonatal neurological morbidity (e.g., cerebral palsy). Current recommendations are that magnesium sulphate for neuroprotection be given to women who are at least 24 but less than 32 weeks of gestation at the time birth is expected to occur. How magnesium sulphate works to provide neuroprotection is not well understood. Although it is likely that the neuroprotective effects are the result of residual concentrations of the medication in the newborn's system, data are insufficient to determine the precise maternal dose necessary to confer the benefit (Simhan et al., 2012). Currently, the dose of magnesium sulphate administered for neuroprotection is the same as that given for tocolysis (see Medication Guide on pp. 517–518). If antenatal magnesium sulphate has been started for fetal neuroprotection, tocolysis should be discontinued. Magnesium sulphate should be discontinued if delivery is no longer imminent or a maximum of 24 hours of therapy has been administered (Magee, Sawchuck, Synnes, et al., 2011).

Labour that has progressed to a cervical dilation of 4 cm is likely to lead to inevitable preterm birth. If birth appears imminent, preparations to care for a small, immature newborn should be made. Women in preterm labour may rapidly progress to birth and a very small fetus may be born through a partially dilated cervix. Also, malpresentation (e.g., breech presentation) occurs much more frequently in preterm than in term fetuses. Therefore, nurses must be prepared to handle the emergency birth of a preterm infant, from either cephalic or breech presentation, without the woman's primary health care provider being present. Personnel skilled in neonatal resuscitation should be present at the time of birth. Equipment, supplies, and medications used for neonatal resuscitation should be gathered in advance and prepared for immediate use. If birth occurs in a hospital that is not prepared to provide continuing care for a preterm newborn, plans should be made for transfer of the baby to a higher level of care as soon as possible after stabilization.

Fetal and Early Neonatal Loss

Preterm birth or the presence of congenital anomalies or genetic disorders incompatible with life are major reasons for intrauterine fetal demise (stillbirth) or early neonatal death. In many of these situations, the parents will have already been told that the fetus has died or that the baby has a condition that is incompatible with life and will most likely die very soon after birth. Sometimes, however, the fetal death will be unexpected, diagnosed only after the woman has been admitted to the labour and birth unit. Whatever the case, labour and birth nurses must be prepared to provide sensitive care to these women and their families.

If fetal or early neonatal death is expected, the parents and members of the health care team need to discuss the situation before the birth and decide on a management plan that is acceptable to everyone. Despite counselling about the likelihood of a poor outcome, some parents want "everything possible," including Caesarean birth for an abnormal fetal heart rate (FHR) tracing, done for the baby. If such intervention is not desired, usually the FHR will not be monitored during labour.

Another major decision is whether to attempt neonatal resuscitation and to what lengths resuscitation should go. Sometimes the feasibility of neonatal resuscitation cannot be determined until the baby's size and physical appearance have been assessed. If the baby is too small, too immature, or too malformed for effective resuscitation, comfort care can be provided instead. The baby is kept warm and comfortable, either at the mother's bedside or in the nursery, depending on the parents' desires, until death occurs. Parents can choose to view and hold the baby as they wish.

After the birth, the woman should be given the opportunity to decide if she wants to stay on the maternity unit or be moved to another hospital unit. She may prefer to be away from the sound of crying babies and exposure to other families who have had healthy infants. However, postpartum care and grief support may not be as good on another hospital unit where the staff are not experienced in postpartum and bereavement care.

Whether death occurs in utero or after birth, parents are faced with the same needs. See Chapter 24 for additional information on providing care families experiencing a perinatal loss.

BOX 20-7 RISK FACTORS FOR PRETERM PREMATURE RUPTURE OF MEMBRANES (PRETERM PROM)

- History of prior preterm birth, especially if associated with preterm PROM
- History of cervical conization or cerclage
- Urinary or genital tract infection
- Short cervical length in the second trimester
- Preterm labour in the current pregnancy
- Uterine overdistension
- Second- and third-trimester bleeding
- Pulmonary disease
- Connective tissue disorders
- Low socioeconomic status
- Low body mass index
- Nutritional deficiencies (copper and ascorbic acid)
- Cigarette smoking

Data from Mercer, B. (2012). Premature rupture of the membranes. In S. Gabbe, J. Niebyl, J. Simpson, et al. (Eds.), *Obstetrics: Normal and problem pregnancies* (6th ed.). Philadelphia: Saunders.

PREMATURE RUPTURE OF MEMBRANES

Premature rupture of membranes (PROM) is the spontaneous rupture of the amniotic sac and leakage of amniotic fluid beginning before the onset of labour at any gestational age. **Preterm premature rupture of membranes (preterm PROM)** (i.e., membranes rupture before the completion of 37 weeks of gestation) is associated with approximately 10% of all preterm births. The frequency of preterm PROM appears to have decreased over the past decade (Mercer, 2012). Preterm PROM most likely results from pathological weakening of the amniotic membranes, caused by inflammation, stress from uterine contractions, or other factors that cause increased intrauterine pressure. Infection of the urogenital tract is a major risk factor associated with preterm PROM (Mercer, 2012, 2014b); Box 20-7 lists other risk factors. PROM or preterm PROM is diagnosed after the woman reports either a sudden gush of fluid or a slow leak of fluid from the vagina.

Chorioamnionitis is the most common maternal complication of preterm PROM, making it a major complication of pregnancy (see later discussion). Other less common but serious maternal complications include placental abruption, retained placenta and hemorrhage requiring dilation and curettage (D&C), sepsis, and death. Fetal complications from preterm PROM are related primarily to intrauterine infection, cord prolapse, umbilical cord compression associated with oligohydramnios, and placental abruption. Another possible fetal complication when preterm PROM occurs before 20 weeks of gestation is pulmonary hypoplasia (Mercer, 2012, 2014b).

NURSING CARE

Management of PROM is determined for each woman on the basis of an assessment of the estimated risk for maternal, fetal, and neonatal complications if pregnancy is allowed to continue or immediate labour and birth are attempted. At term, because infection is the greatest maternal, fetal, and neonatal risk, birth is the best option. Labour will most likely be induced if it does not begin spontaneously soon after PROM occurs, although some women are given the option of waiting 24 hours to determine if labour will begin on its own (Mercer, 2012, 2014b).

Preterm PROM (occurring at or after 23 weeks of gestation) is often managed expectantly or conservatively if the risks to the fetus and newborn associated with preterm birth are considered to be greater than the risks of infection. Women with preterm PROM are usually hospitalized for conservative management in an attempt to prolong the pregnancy and allow additional time for fetal maturation, unless intrauterine infection, significant vaginal bleeding, placental abruption, advanced labour, or atypical or abnormal fetal assessment is assessed (Mercer, 2012). Nursing support of the woman and her family is critical at this time. They are often anxious about the health of the baby, and the woman may fear that she was responsible in some way for the membrane rupture. The nurse can reassure the woman that in most cases the cause of PROM is unknown (Gilbert, 2011). Other nursing interventions include encouraging expression of feelings and concerns, providing information, and making referrals as needed.

Frequent **biophysical profiles (BPP)** should be performed to determine fetal health status and estimate amniotic fluid volume (AFV) (see Chapter 13). The woman with PROM also should be taught how to count fetal movements daily, because a slowing of fetal movement has been shown to be a precursor to severe fetal compromise. Most women should feel six movements in 2 hours; if they do not, further antenatal testing (nonstress test [NST], BPP, or both) is required (Liston, Sawchuck, Young, et al., 2007). Antenatal glucocorticoids may be administered to women who are less than 32 weeks of gestation, because they have been proven to decrease the risk for several neonatal complications. Also, a 7-day course of broad-spectrum antibiotics (e.g., ampicillin, erythromycin) will be administered. Antibiotic treatment has been shown to prolong the time between membrane rupture and birth; decrease maternal chorioamnionitis and postpartum endometritis; and prevent sepsis, pneumonia, and intraventricular hemorrhage in the newborn (Mercer, 2012; Yudin, van Schalwyk, Van Eyk, et al., 2009).

Vigilance for signs of infection is a major part of nursing care and patient education after preterm PROM. The woman must be taught how to keep her genital area clean and that nothing should be introduced into her vagina. Signs of infection (e.g., fever, foul-smelling vaginal discharge, maternal and fetal tachycardia) should be reported immediately to the primary health care provider. If chorioamnionitis develops, labour will be induced. Should preterm labour occur, tocolytic medications may be administered in an attempt to gain time for transporting the woman to a hospital capable of providing care to a preterm infant or for antenatal corticosteroids or antibiotics to reach effective levels (Gilbert, 2011). Magnesium sulphate may also be administered for fetal neuroprotection.

CHORIOAMNIONITIS

Chorioamnionitis, bacterial infection of the amniotic cavity, is a major cause of complications for both mothers and newborns at any gestational age. It occurs in approximately 1 to 5% of term births but in as many as 25% of preterm births (Duff, 2012). Other terms for this condition include *clinical chorioamnionitis, amnionitis, intrapartum infection, amniotic fluid infection,* and *intra-amniotic infection.* Chorioamnionitis is usually diagnosed by the clinical findings of maternal fever, maternal and fetal tachycardia, uterine tenderness, and foul odour of amniotic fluid (Duff, 2014).

Chorioamnionitis most often occurs after membranes rupture or labour begins, as organisms that are part of the normal vaginal flora ascend into the amniotic cavity. Many of the risk factors for chorioamnionitis are associated with a long labour, such as prolonged membrane rupture, multiple vaginal examinations, and use of internal FHR and contraction monitoring modes (Duff, 2014). Other risk factors include young maternal age, low socioeconomic status, nulliparity, and pre-existing infections of the lower genital tract (Duff, 2012).

Women with chorioamnionitis can develop bacteremia. They are also more likely to have labour dystocia, which can result in the need for Caesarean birth (see later discussion). If Caesarean birth is necessary, wound infection or pelvic abscess is a possible complication. Neonatal risks include pneumonia, bacteremia, and sepsis. Death is more likely to occur in preterm than in term infants (Duff, 2012, 2014). An association between chorioamnionitis and long-term neurological development in the newborn, including cerebral palsy, has been reported (Duff, 2014).

To prevent maternal and neonatal complications, prompt treatment with intravenous broad-spectrum antibiotics and birth of the fetus are necessary. Ampicillin or penicillin and gentamicin are the antibiotics most often used to treat chorioamnionitis during labour. After Caesarean birth, an antibiotic that provides coverage for anaerobic organisms, such as clindamycin or metronidazole (Flagyl), should be added. Antibiotics can usually be discontinued soon after birth (Duff, 2012).

The increased use of intrapartum antibiotic prophylaxis during labour in women who are group B streptococci positive has decreased the incidence of chorioamnionitis. Other measures that have proven to be effective in decreasing the frequency of chorioamnionitis are active management of labour (see later discussion) and induction of labour, rather than expectant management, after rupture of membranes at term (Duff, 2014).

POSTTERM PREGNANCY, LABOUR, AND BIRTH

A *postterm* or *postdate pregnancy* is one that extends beyond the end of week 42 of gestation, or more than 294 days from the first day of the last menstrual period (LMP). The rate of postterm pregnancies in Canada has decreased; in 2010 it was 0.61 per 100 live births (PHAC, 2013). Many pregnancies are misdiagnosed as prolonged. The use of first-trimester ultrasound for pregnancy dating has confirmed that the first day of the LMP, traditionally used for pregnancy dating, is much less reliable as a predictor of true gestational age. Therefore use of the LMP alone for pregnancy dating tends to greatly overestimate the number of postterm gestations (Rampersad & Macones, 2012). Ideally, every pregnant woman should be offered a first-trimester dating ultrasound; however, if the availability of obstetrical ultrasound is limited, it is reasonable to use a second-trimester scan to assess gestational age (Butt & Lim, 2014).

The exact cause of postterm pregnancy is still unknown. However, it is clear that the timing of labour is determined by complex interactions among the fetus, the placenta and membranes, the uterine myometrium, and the cervix. For example, congenital primary fetal adrenal hypoplasia and placental sulphatase deficiency cause low estrogen production. Low levels of estrogen may result in a decrease in prostaglandin precursors, thereby preventing normal cervical ripening (softening and thinning), reducing the formation of oxytocin receptors in the myometrium, and delaying the onset of labour. Although postterm pregnancy is more common in primiparous women, a woman who experiences one postterm pregnancy is more likely to experience it again in subsequent pregnancies (Rampersad & Macones, 2012).

Clinical manifestations of postterm pregnancy include maternal weight loss and decreased uterine size (related to decreased amniotic fluid), meconium in the amniotic fluid, and advanced bone maturation of the fetal skeleton with an exceptionally hard fetal skull (Gilbert, 2011).

Maternal and Fetal Risks

Maternal risks include increased risk for perineal injury related to fetal macrosomia. Risk for hemorrhage and infection is higher. Interventions such as induction of labour with prostaglandins or oxytocin, forceps- or vacuum-assisted birth, and Caesarean birth are more likely to be necessary. Each of these interventions, of course, carries its own set of risks. The woman also may experience fatigue, physical discomfort, and psychological reactions such as depression, frustration, and feelings of inadequacy as she passes her estimated date of birth. Relationships with close friends and family members may become strained, and the woman's negative feelings about herself may be projected as feelings of resentment toward the fetus (Gilbert, 2011).

Another complication associated with postterm pregnancy is abnormal fetal growth. Although the risk for having a small-for-gestational-age infant is increased, only 10 to 20% of postterm fetuses are undernourished. Macrosomia (birth weight more than 4000 g) occurs far more often. Macrosomia occurs when the placenta continues to provide adequate nutrients to support fetal growth after 40 weeks of gestation. Macrosomic infants have an increased risk for birth injuries caused by difficult forceps-assisted births and shoulder dystocia.

Other fetal risks associated with postterm gestation are related to the intrauterine environment. After 43 to 44 weeks of gestation, the placenta begins to age. Enlarging areas of infarction and increased deposition of calcium and fibrin in its tissue decrease the placenta's reserve and may affect its ability to oxygenate the fetus. Decreased amniotic fluid (less than 400 mL), **oligohydramnios**, is the complication most frequently associated with postterm pregnancy. Because of the decreased amount of amniotic fluid, there is a potential for cord compression and resulting hypoxemia (Gilbert, 2011). Other potential complications include meconium-stained amniotic fluid, increased chance of meconium aspiration, and low Apgar scores. Oligohydramnios magnifies the effect of meconium staining. Having less than the normal amount of amniotic fluid available to dilute it makes the meconium thicker and stickier than it would otherwise be (Gilbert, 2011).

Postmaturity syndrome occurs in about 20% of newborns born after postterm pregnancies. Postmaturity syndrome is characterized by dry, cracked, peeling skin; long nails; meconium staining of skin, nails, and umbilical cord; and perhaps loss of subcutaneous fat and muscle mass (Gilbert, 2011).

Collaborative Care

Women should be offered induction of labour between 41 and 42 weeks, as this intervention may reduce perinatal mortality and meconium aspiration syndrome without increasing the Caesarean birth rate (Leduc, Biringer, Lee, et al., 2013). Women who choose to delay induction past 41 weeks should undergo twice-weekly assessment for fetal well-being (Leduc et al., 2013).

Antepartum assessments for postterm pregnancy may include daily fetal movement counts, NSTs, AFV assessments, contraction stress tests, BPPs, and Doppler flow measurements (see Chapter 13). The woman and her family should be fully informed about the tests, including why they are being performed and the meaning of the results obtained in terms of the health of the mother and fetus.

An amniotic fluid index (AFI) of less than 5 has been associated with an increased risk of Caesarean birth for an abnormal fetal status and an Apgar score of less than 7 at 5 minutes. The BPP may be the best way of gauging fetal well-being because it combines nonstress testing with real-time ultrasound scanning to assess fetal movements, fetal breathing movements, and AFV.

> **PATIENT TEACHING**
> ***Postterm Pregnancy***
>
> - Perform daily fetal movement counts.
> - Assess for signs of labour.
> - Call your primary health care provider if your membranes rupture or if you perceive a decrease in or no fetal movement.
> - Keep appointments for fetal assessment tests or cervical checks.
> - Go to the hospital soon after labour begins.

Ideally, the AFI should be greater than 8, with at least one pocket of amniotic fluid greater than 2 cm, and amniotic fluid should be present throughout the uterine cavity (Gilbert, 2011).

During the postterm period, the woman should be encouraged to assess fetal activity daily, assess for signs of labour, and keep appointments with her primary health care provider (see Patient Teaching box). The woman and her family should be encouraged to express their feelings about the prolonged pregnancy (e.g., frustration, anger, impatience, fear) and reassured that these feelings are normal. At times, the emotional and physical strain of a postterm pregnancy may seem overwhelming.

If the woman's cervix is favourable, expectant management can be followed, but labour is usually induced with oxytocin. If the cervix is not favourable, fetal surveillance is continued, and a cervical ripening agent (e.g., prostaglandin E_2) may be administered, followed by oxytocin induction (Gilbert, 2011).

During labour, the fetus of a woman with a postterm pregnancy should be continuously monitored electronically for a more accurate assessment of the FHR and pattern. Inadequate fluid volume leads to compression of the cord, which results in a transient fetal hypoxia that is reflected in variable or prolonged deceleration patterns. If oligohydramnios is present, **amnioinfusion** may be performed to restore AFV, to maintain a cushioning of the cord. See Chapter 19, p. 508, for additional information on amnioinfusion, and see Research Focus box.

DYSTOCIA

Dystocia is defined as abnormally slow progress of labour; it is caused by various conditions related to the five P's of labour (*p*assenger, *p*assageway, *p*owers, *p*osition of the mother, and *p*sychological response) (see Chapter 16). *Dystocia* is defined as greater than 4 hours of less than 0.5 cm per hour of cervical dilation in active labour or greater than 1 hour of active pushing with no descent of the presenting part (Society of Obstetricians and Gynaecologists of Canada [SOGC], 1995). Dystocia is a common reason for Caesarean birth (Gilbert, 2011). Dystocia can be caused by any of the following:

- Hypotonic, uncoordinated, or infrequent uterine contractions or ineffective maternal bearing-down efforts (the powers); the most common cause of dystocia
- Alterations in the pelvic structure (the passage way)
- Fetal causes, including abnormal presentation or position, anomalies, excessive size, and number of fetuses (the passenger)

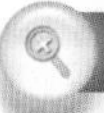

RESEARCH FOCUS

Amnioinfusion in Labour

—Pat Mahaffee Gingrich

Ask the Question

Is amnioinfusion a safe and effective intervention or treatment for certain complications of labour?

Search for the Evidence

Search Strategies

English research-based publications on amnioinfusion, labour, meconium, oligohydramnios, and rupture of membranes were included.

Databases Used

Cochrane Collaborative Database, National Guideline Clearinghouse (AHRQ), CINAHL, PubMed, UpToDate, and the professional website for AWHONN

Critically Analyze the Evidence

- Oligohydramnios, or low amniotic fluid level, may occur as a result of ruptured membranes or fetal abnormality. Some fetuses show signs of distress, which may be caused by pressure on the umbilical cord, leading to fetal hypoxia and acidosis. This stress may in turn lead to fetal passing of meconium, increasing the risk for meconium aspiration and respiratory distress at birth.
- Amnioinfusion is the instillation of normal saline or lactated Ringer's solution into the uterus via the cervix or transabdominally to relieve the pressure on the fetus and cord. For potential or suspected cord compression, amnioinfusion is associated with fewer Caesarean births, fewer 5-minute Apgar scores less than 7, less meconium below the vocal cords, less postpartum maternal endometritis, improved pH, and decreased hospital stay (Hofmeyr & Lawrie, 2012).
- The American College of Obstetricians and Gynecologists (ACOG) states that the highest level of evidence recommends amnioinfusion as a treatment for fetal heart rate (FHR) tracing of absent or minimal variability and recurrent variable decelerations (ACOG, 2010).
- Another possible benefit of amnioinfusion is the dilution of meconium. Amnioinfusion is associated with fewer Caesarean births, a decreased rate of meconium aspiration syndrome, less meconium below the vocal cords, less use of neonatal ventilation, fewer neonatal intensive care unit (NICU) admissions, and a trend toward lower perinatal mortality (Hofmeyr & Xu, 2010). It is not clear if the benefits are from the relief of oligohydramnios or dilution of meconium. Amnioinfusion is recommended for facilities where babies are at risk because of limited fetal monitoring.
- In the case of preterm premature rupture of membranes, four small trials showed improved umbilical arterial pH, decreased persistent variable decelerations for transcervical amnioinfusion, and fewer perinatal deaths, less neonatal sepsis, and decreased rate of pulmonary hypoplasia (small lungs) and less maternal sepsis with transabdominal amnioinfusion (Hofmeyr, Essilfie-Appiah, & Lawrie, 2011). However, the evidence is not sufficient to recommend amnioinfusion routinely for this purpose.

Apply the Evidence: Nursing Implications

- In labour, it is usually the nurses who monitor the electronic FHR and patterns. Abnormal FHR patterns that include absent baseline variability plus recurrent late or recurrent variable decelerations, bradycardia, or sinusoidal pattern require consultation with the medical team.
- A known rupture of membranes or oligohydramnios demonstrated by an ultrasound amniotic fluid index of less than 5 cm, plus an atypical or abnormal FHR, requires medical decision making regarding improving fetal well-being. An order for amnioinfusion may be one of the interventions. The nurse is often responsible for setting this up as well as communicating with the patient and family.
- Other supportive nursing therapy that can increase uteroplacental oxygenation includes maternal repositioning, supplemental oxygen, and intravenous access for increasing fluids. Modifying or stopping oxytocin in the presence of abnormal FHR is also a nursing judgement.
- Any sign of meconium staining in amniotic fluid requires planning for specialized attention to the newborn at birth to prevent as much as possible the complications of meconium aspiration.

References

American College of Obstetricians and Gynecologists (ACOG). (2010). *Management of intrapartum fetal heart rate tracings* (ACOG Practice Bulletin No. 16). National Guidelines Clearinghouse, NGC: 008177.

Hofmeyr, G. J., Essilfie-Appiah, G., & Lawrie, T. A. (2011). Amnioinfusion for preterm premature rupture of membranes. *Cochrane Database Systematic Review,* (12). doi:10.1002/14651858.CD000942.pub2.

Hofmeyr, G. J., & Lawrie, T. A. (2012). Amnioinfusion for potential or suspected umbilical cord compression in labour. *Cochrane Database Systematic Review,* (1). doi: 10.1002/14651858.CD000013.pub2.

Hofmeyr, G. J., & Xu, H. (2010). Amnioinfusion for meconium-stained liquor in labour. *Cochrane Database Systematic Review,* (1). doi:10.1002/14651858.CD000014.pub3.

- Maternal position during labour and birth
- Psychological responses of the mother to labour that are related to past experiences, preparation, culture and heritage, and support system

These five factors are interdependent. In assessing the woman for labour dystocia, the nurse must consider the ways in which they interact and influence labour progress. Dystocia should be suspected when there is an alteration in the characteristics of uterine contractions, a lack of progress in the rate of cervical dilation, or a lack of progress in fetal descent and expulsion.

Gilbert (2011) cited several factors that seem to increase a woman's risk for uterine dystocia, including the following:

- Overweight
- Short stature
- Advanced maternal age
- Infertility difficulties
- Prior external cephalic version
- Uterine abnormalities (i.e., congenital malformations; overdistension, as with multiple gestation or polyhydramnios)
- Malpresentations and positions of the fetus
- Cephalopelvic disproportion (CPD)
- Uterine overstimulation with oxytocin
- Maternal fatigue, dehydration and electrolyte imbalance, and fear
- Inappropriate timing of analgesic or use of continuous epidural analgesia

Abnormal Uterine Activity (Alteration in Power)

Dystocia can occur due to abnormal uterine contractions that prevent the normal progress of cervical dilation, effacement (primary powers), or descent (secondary powers).

Dysfunction of uterine contractions can be further described as being *hypertonic* or *hypotonic*.

Hypertonic Uterine Dysfunction

The woman experiencing hypertonic uterine dysfunction often is an anxious first-time mother who is having painful and frequent contractions that are ineffective in causing cervical dilation or effacement to progress. These contractions usually occur in the latent stage (cervical dilation of less than 5 cm) and are usually uncoordinated. The force of the contraction may be in the midsection of the uterus rather than in the fundus; therefore, the uterus is unable to apply downward pressure to push the presenting part against the cervix. The uterus may not relax completely between contractions (Gilbert, 2011).

Women with hypertonic uterine dysfunction may be exhausted and express concern about loss of control because of the intense pain they are experiencing and the lack of progress. Therapeutic rest, which is achieved with a warm bath or shower and the administration of analgesics such as morphine to inhibit uterine contractions, reduce pain, and encourage sleep, is usually prescribed for the management of hypertonic uterine dysfunction (Gilbert, 2011). After a 4- to 6-hour rest, these women are likely to awaken in active labour with a normal uterine contraction pattern.

Hypotonic Uterine Dysfunction

The second and more common type of uterine dysfunction is hypotonic uterine dysfunction, or secondary uterine inertia. The woman initially makes normal progress into the active stage of labour, then the contractions become weak and inefficient or stop altogether. The uterus is easily indented, even at the peak of contractions. Intrauterine pressure during the contraction is insufficient for progress of cervical effacement and dilation (Gilbert, 2011). CPD and malposition are common causes of this type of uterine dysfunction.

A woman with hypotonic uterine dysfunction may become exhausted and be at increased risk for infection. Management usually consists of ruling out CPD, assessing the FHR and pattern, characteristics of amniotic fluid if membranes are ruptured, and maternal well-being. If findings are normal, measures such as ambulation, hydrotherapy, stripping or rupture of membranes, nipple stimulation, and oxytocin infusion can be used to augment labour.

Alteration in Secondary Powers

Secondary powers, or bearing-down efforts, are compromised when large amounts of analgesic medications are given. Anaesthesia may also block the bearing-down reflex and, as a result, alter the effectiveness of voluntary bearing-down efforts. Exhaustion resulting from lack of sleep or long labour and fatigue resulting from inadequate hydration and food intake reduce the effectiveness of the woman's voluntary bearing-down efforts. Maternal position can work against the forces of gravity and decrease the strength and efficiency of the contractions.

Table 20-1 summarizes the characteristics of dystocia related to ineffective contractions (power).

Abnormal Labour Patterns

Six abnormal labour patterns were identified and classified by Friedman (1989) according to the nature of cervical dilation and fetal descent. These patterns are (1) prolonged latent phase, (2) protracted active-phase dilation, (3) secondary arrest: no change, (4) protracted descent, (5) arrest of descent, and (6) failure of descent. Table 20-2 further describes these abnormal labour patterns. These abnormal patterns may result from a variety of causes, including ineffective uterine contractions, pelvic contractures, CPD, abnormal fetal presentation or position, early use of analgesics, nerve block analgesia or anaesthesia, and anxiety and stress. Progress in either the first or second stage of labour can be protracted (prolonged) or arrested (stopped).

Abnormal progress can be identified by plotting cervical dilation and fetal descent on a labour graph (partogram) at various intervals after the onset of labour and comparing the resulting curve with the expected labour curve for a nulliparous or multiparous labour. If a woman exhibits an abnormal labour pattern, the primary health care provider should be notified.

Health care providers must be careful when diagnosing a labour pattern as prolonged and when intervening on the basis of this diagnosis. Criteria defining the differences between prelabour, latent, and active labour should be established. Evaluation of a woman's labour status in the hospital or unit admission areas is helpful in preventing the premature implementation of labour interventions such as administration of systemic opioid analgesics or induction of epidural analgesia or anaesthesia. If a woman is found to be in prelabour or latent (early) labour, she can be sent home or remain in the admission area until labour becomes active. If possible, women should not be admitted to the labour and birth unit until they are in active labour.

Alterations in Pelvic Structure (Passageway)

Pelvic Dystocia

Pelvic dystocia can occur whenever there are contractures of the pelvic diameters that reduce the capacity of the bony pelvis, including the inlet, midpelvis, outlet, or any combination of these planes. Pelvic contractures may be caused by congenital abnormalities, maternal malnutrition, neoplasms, or lower spinal disorders. An immature pelvic size predisposes some adolescent mothers to pelvic dystocia. Pelvic deformities may also be the result of automobile or other accidents or trauma.

Soft Tissue Dystocia

Soft tissue dystocia results from obstruction of the birth passage by an anatomical abnormality other than that involving the bony pelvis. The obstruction may result from placenta previa that partially or completely obstructs the internal os of the cervix. Other causes such as leiomyomas (uterine fibroids) in the lower uterine segment, ovarian tumours, and a full bladder or rectum may prevent the fetus from entering the pelvis. Occasionally, cervical edema occurs during labour when the cervix is caught between the presenting part and the

TABLE 20-1 DYSTOCIA RELATED TO INADEQUATE PRIMARY AND SECONDARY POWERS

PRIMARY POWERS (ABNORMAL UTERINE ACTIVITY)		SECONDARY POWERS
HYPERTONIC UTERUS	**HYPOTONIC UTERUS**	**INADEQUATE VOLUNTARY EXPULSIVE FORCES**
Description		
Usually occurs before 5 cm dilation; cause unknown, may be related to fear and tension	Cause is usually cephalopelvic disproportion or fetal malposition	Involves abdominal and levator ani muscles Occurs in second stage of labour; cause may be related to nerve block anaesthetic, analgesia, exhaustion
Change in Pattern of Progress		
Pain is out of proportion to intensity of contractions and to effectiveness of contractions in effacing and dilating the cervix. Contractions increase in frequency and are uncoordinated. Uterus is contracted between contractions, cannot be indented.	Contractions decrease in frequency and intensity. Uterus is easily indented even at peak of contractions. Uterus is relaxed between contractions (normal).	No voluntary urge to push or bear down or inadequate or ineffective pushing
Potential Maternal Effects		
Loss of control related to intensity of pain and lack of progress Exhaustion Fear regarding unexpected nature of labour	Infection Exhaustion Stress regarding change in progress	Spontaneous vaginal birth prevented; assisted birth possible
Potential Fetal Effects		
Fetal asphyxia with meconium aspiration	Fetal infection Fetal and neonatal death	Fetal asphyxia
Care Management		
Initiate therapeutic rest measures. Administer analgesic (e.g., morphine) if membranes are intact and pelvic adequacy is confirmed. Relieve pain to permit mother to rest. Assist with measures to enhance rest and relaxation (e.g., hydrotherapy, massage, music, distracting activities).	Rule out cephalopelvic disproportion. Augment labour with oxytocin. Perform amniotomy. Assist with measures to enhance the progress of labour (e.g., position changes, ambulation, hydrotherapy).	Encourage mother to bear down with contractions; assist with relaxation between contractions. Position mother in favourable position for pushing. Reduce epidural infusion rate. Assist with forceps- or vacuum-assisted birth. Prepare for Caesarean birth if abnormal fetal status occurs.

symphysis pubis or when the woman begins bearing-down efforts prematurely, inhibiting complete dilation. Sexually transmitted infections (e.g., human papillomavirus) can alter cervical tissue integrity and thus interfere with adequate effacement and dilation.

Bandl's ring, a pathological retraction ring that forms between the upper and lower uterine segments (see Fig. 16-9, C), is associated with prolonged rupture of membranes, protracted labour, and increased risk of uterine rupture (Cunningham, Leveno, Bloom, et al., 2014).

Fetal Causes (Passenger)

Dystocia of fetal origin may be caused by anomalies, excessive fetal size and malpresentation, malposition, or multifetal pregnancy. Complications associated with dystocia of fetal origin include neonatal asphyxia, fetal injuries or fractures, and maternal vaginal lacerations. Although spontaneous vaginal birth is possible in these instances, a forceps-assisted, vacuum-assisted birth or Caesarean birth often is necessary.

Anomalies

Gross ascites, large tumours, and open neural tube defects such as myelomeningocele and hydrocephalus are fetal anomalies that can cause dystocia. The anomalies affect the relationship of the fetal anatomy to the maternal pelvic capacity, with the result that the fetus is unable to descend through the birth canal.

Cephalopelvic Disproportion

Cephalopelvic disproportion (CPD), also called *fetopelvic disproportion*, is disproportion between the size of the fetus and the size of the mother's pelvis. With CPD, the fetus cannot fit through the maternal pelvis to be born vaginally. Although CPD is often related to excessive fetal size, or macrosomia (i.e., 4000 g or more), the problem in many cases is malposition of the fetal presenting part rather than true CPD (Wing & Farinelli, 2012). Fetal macrosomia is associated with maternal diabetes mellitus, obesity, multiparity, or the large size of one or both parents. If the maternal pelvis is too small or abnormally shaped, CPD may be of maternal origin. In this case, the fetus may be of average size or even smaller. CPD cannot be accurately predicted (Wing & Farinelli, 2012).

Malposition

The most common fetal malposition is persistent occipitoposterior position (i.e., right occipitoposterior [ROP] or left occipitoposterior [LOP]) (see Fig. 16-2), occurring in about 15% of all labours during the latent phase of the first stage of labour. About 5% of all fetuses are in this position at birth (Gilbert, 2011). Labour, especially the second stage, is prolonged; the woman typically feels severe back pain from the pressure of the fetal head (occiput) pressing against her sacrum. See Box 17-10 for suggested measures to relieve back pain and promote rotation of the fetal occiput to an anterior position, which will facilitate birth.

Malpresentation

Malpresentation (the fetus presentation is something other than cephalic, or head first) is another commonly reported complication of labour and birth. Breech presentation is the most common form of malpresentation, occurring in approximately 3 to 4% of all labours (Lanni & Seeds, 2012). The three types of breech presentation are (Gilbert, 2011) (Fig. 20-1):

- Frank breech (thighs flexed, knees extended)
- Complete breech (thighs and knees flexed)
- Footling breech (when one foot [single footling] or both feet [double footling] present before the buttocks)

Breech presentations are associated with multifetal gestation, preterm birth, fetal and maternal anomalies, hydramnios, and oligohydramnios. High rates of breech presentation are also noted in fetuses with certain genetic disorders (e.g., trisomies 13, 18, and 21; Potter's syndrome [renal agenesis]; and myotonic dystrophy). Fetuses with neuromuscular disorders have a high rate of breech presentation, perhaps because they are less capable of movement within the uterus. Abnormal amniotic fluid volume (both increased and decreased) also contributes to more breech presentations because it affects fetal mobility. Breech presentation is diagnosed by abdominal palpation (e.g., Leopold manoeuvres; see Box 17-5) and vaginal examination and usually is confirmed by ultrasound scan (Lanni & Seeds, 2012; Thorp & Laughon, 2014).

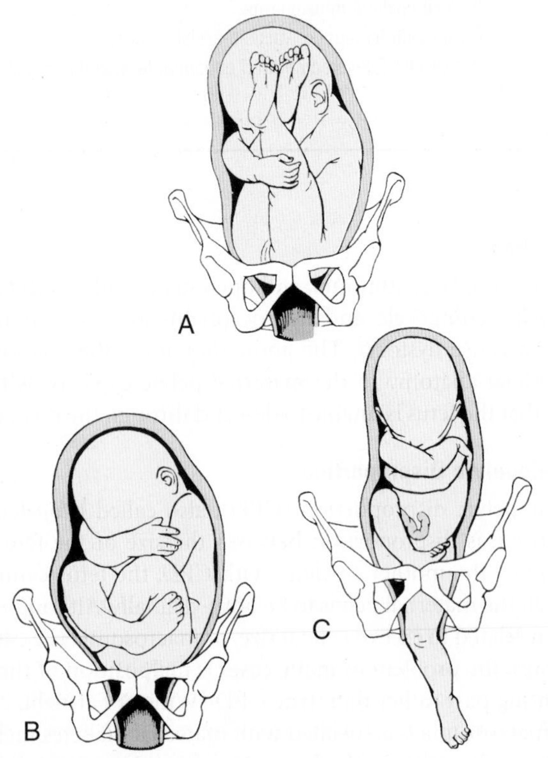

FIGURE 20-1 Breech presentation. **A:** Frank breech. **B:** Complete breech. **C:** Single footling breech. (From Gilbert, E. [2011]. *Manual of high risk pregnancy & delivery* [5th ed.]. St. Louis: Mosby.)

During labour, fetal descent may be slow because the breech is not as effective a dilating wedge as the fetal head. There is risk of prolapse of the umbilical cord if the membranes rupture in early labour. The presence of meconium in amniotic fluid is not necessarily a sign of fetal compromise because it results from pressure on the fetal abdominal wall as it traverses the birth canal. Assessment of FHR and pattern should be used to determine whether the passage of meconium is an expected finding associated with breech presentation or is an abnormal sign associated with fetal hypoxia. The fetal heart tones of infants in a breech position are best heard at or above the maternal umbilicus.

Vaginal birth is accomplished by mechanisms of labour that manipulate the buttocks and lower extremities as they emerge from the birth canal (Fig. 20-2). Risks associated with vaginal birth from a breech presentation include prolapse of the umbilical cord (especially in single or double footling breech presentations) and trapping of the after-coming fetal head (especially with preterm infants). Safe vaginal birth from a breech presentation largely depends on the experience, judgement, and skill of the health care provider who assists the birth. Criteria for attempting a vaginal birth from a breech presentation are as follows (Thorp & Laughon, 2014):

- Frank or complete breech presentation
- Estimated fetal weight between 2000 and 3800 g
- Normal (gynecoid) maternal pelvis
- Flexed fetal head

A woman who labours with a fetus in a breech presentation needs to be assessed frequently for adequate progress in labour. Although Caesarean birth reduces the risks to the fetus, the maternal risks are increased. Women whose breech presentation occurs late in pregnancy need to be informed about the options for birth, including the risks associated with each option (Kotaska, Menticoglou, Gagnon, et al., 2009). External cephalic version (ECV) (see later discussion) may be tried to turn the fetus to a vertex presentation.

Face and brow presentations are uncommon and are associated with fetal anomalies, pelvic contractures, and CPD. Vaginal birth is possible if the fetus flexes to a vertex presentation, although forceps often are used. Caesarean birth is indicated if the presentation persists, if there is an abnormal FHR and pattern, or if labour stops progressing.

Caesarean birth is usually necessary for a fetus in a transverse lie (i.e., shoulder) presentation, although ECV may be attempted after 36 to 37 weeks of gestation (Thorp & Laughon, 2014).

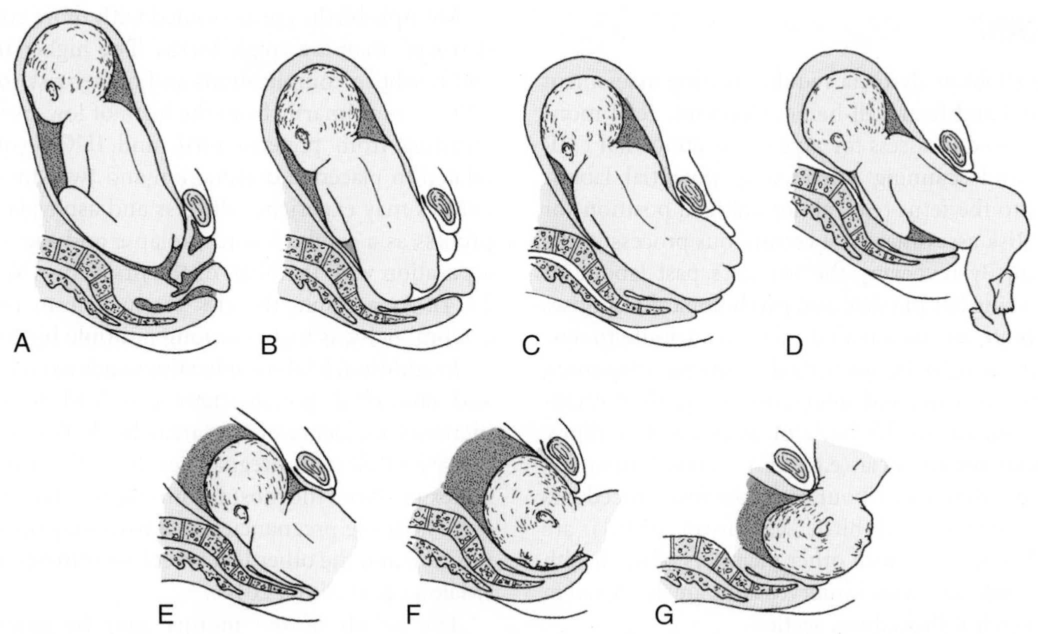

FIGURE 20-2 Mechanism of labour in breech presentation. **A:** Breech before onset of labour. **B:** Engagement and internal rotation. **C:** Lateral flexion. **D:** External rotation or restitution. **E:** Internal rotation of shoulders and head. **F:** Face rotates to sacrum when occiput is anterior. **G:** Head is born by gradual flexion during elevation of fetal body.

TABLE 20-2 LABOUR PATTERNS IN NORMAL AND ABNORMAL LABOUR

NORMAL LABOUR

Dilation: continues
Latent phase: <5 cm and low slope
Active phase: >5 cm or high slope
Deceleration phase: ≥9 cm
Descent: active at ≥9 cm dilation

ABNORMAL LABOUR

PATTERN	NULLIPARAS	MULTIPARAS
Prolonged latent phase	>20 hr	>14 hr
Protracted active phase dilation	<1.2 cm/hr	<1.5 cm/hr
Secondary arrest: no change	≥2 hr	≥2 hr
Protracted descent	<1 cm/hr	<2 cm/hr
Arrest of descent	≥1 hr	≥ ½ hr
Failure of descent	No change during deceleration phase and second stage	
Precipitous labour	>5 cm/hr	10 cm/hr

Position of the Woman

The functional relationships among the uterine contractions, the fetus, and the mother's pelvis are altered by the maternal position. The position can provide a mechanical advantage or disadvantage to the mechanisms of labour by altering the effects of gravity and the body-part relationships that are important to the progress of labour. For example, the hands-and-knees position facilitates rotation from a posterior occiput position more effectively than does the lateral position (Lawrence, Lewis, Hofmeyr, et al., 2013). Upright positions such as sitting and squatting facilitate fetal descent during pushing and shorten the second stage of labour (Gupta, Hofmeyr, & Shehmar, 2012). See Box 17-9 for suggested positions to enhance fetal descent. Limiting maternal movement or restricting labour to the recumbent or lithotomy position may compromise progress. The incidence of dystocia in women confined to these positions is increased, resulting in increased need for augmentation of labour, the use of forceps, and incidence of vacuum-assisted or Caesarean birth.

Psychological Responses

Hormones and neurotransmitters released in response to stress (e.g., catecholamines) can cause dystocia. Sources of stress vary for each woman, although pain and the absence of a support person are two recognized factors. Confinement to bed and restriction of maternal movement can be a source of psychological stress that compounds the physiological stress caused by immobility in the unmedicated labouring woman. When anxiety is excessive, it can inhibit cervical dilation and result in prolonged labour and increased pain perception. Anxiety also causes increased levels of stress-related hormones (e.g., beta-endorphin, adrenocorticotropic hormone, cortisol, and epinephrine). These hormones act on the smooth muscles of the uterus; increased levels can cause dystocia by reducing uterine contractility. The continuous supportive presence of a nurse or doula may help to decrease the stress felt by the labouring woman.

NURSING CARE

Women who have labour dystocia require nursing assessment to ensure maternal and fetal well-being. Electronic fetal monitoring should be used to assess for atypical or abnormal FHR patterns. Ultrasound scanning can identify potential labour problems related to the fetus (e.g., abnormal fetal position) or maternal pelvis. Risk assessment is a continuous process in the labouring woman. By reviewing the woman's past labour or labours and observing her physical and psychological responses to the current labour, any factors that might contribute to dysfunctional labour should be identified. Nursing diagnoses, expected outcomes of care, and interventions are then established for each woman on the basis of assessment findings. Many interventions for dystocia (e.g., ECV, cervical ripening, induction or augmentation of labour, and operative procedures [forceps- or vacuum-assisted birth, Caesarean birth]) are implemented collaboratively with other members of the health care team. Commonly performed interventions are discussed in detail in the Obstetrical Procedures section.

When providing care for a woman who is experiencing labour or birth complications, all members of the health care team are responsible for complying with professional standards of care.

LEGAL TIP *STANDARD OF CARE—LABOUR AND BIRTH COMPLICATIONS*

- Document all assessment findings, interventions, and the woman's responses in the medical record according to unit protocols, procedures, and policies and professional standards.
- Assess whether the woman (and her family, if appropriate) is fully informed about the procedures for which she is consenting.
- Provide full explanations regarding what is happening and what needs to be done to help her and her baby.
- Maintain safety in administering medications and treatments correctly.
- Have telephone orders signed as soon as possible.
- Provide care at the acceptable standard (e.g., according to unit protocols and professional standards).
- Continue maternal and fetal monitoring until birth according to the policies, procedures, and protocols of the birthing facility, even after a decision to carry out Caesarean birth is made.

MULTIFETAL PREGNANCY

Multifetal pregnancy is the gestation of twins, triplets, quadruplets, or more infants. Multiple gestations accounted for 3.2% of all live births in Canada in 2010 (PHAC, 2013). The increasing incidence of twin gestations has been attributed to the use of fertility-enhancing medications and procedures and the older age of child-bearing women. Compared with younger women, those age 35 years and older are more likely to have a multifetal pregnancy. The rate of triplet and higher-order multiple pregnancies has been steadily declining, likely due to refinements in the treatments used for infertility, particularly limiting the number of embryos transferred during in vitro fertilization (IVF) procedures (Malone & D'Alton, 2014; Newman & Unal, 2012).

Multiple births are associated with more complications (i.e., dystocia) than are single births. The higher incidence of fetal and newborn complications and higher risk for perinatal mortality stem primarily from the birth of low-birth-weight infants resulting from preterm birth and IUGR (or both), in part related to placental dysfunction and twin-to-twin transfusion. Fetuses may experience distress and asphyxia during the birth process as a result of cord prolapse and the onset of placental separation with the birth of the first fetus (Malone & D'Alton, 2014). As a result, the risk for long-term problems, such as cerebral palsy, is higher among multiple births.

In addition, fetal complications such as congenital anomalies and abnormal presentations can lead to dystocia and an increased incidence of Caesarean birth. For example, in only 40 to 45% of all twin pregnancies do both fetuses present in the vertex position, the most favourable one for vaginal birth. In 35 to 40% of the pregnancies, one twin may present in the vertex position and the other in a breech or transverse lie presentation (Malone & D'Alton, 2014).

The health of the mother may be compromised by an increased risk for hypertension, anemia, and hemorrhage associated with uterine atony, placental abruption, and multiple or adherent placentas. Duration of the phases and stages of labour may vary from that experienced with singleton births.

Teamwork and planning are essential in the management of childbirth in multiple pregnancies, especially those of the higher-order multiples. The perinatal nurse plays a key role in coordinating the activities of the highly skilled health care providers involved. Early detection and effective care of maternal, fetal, and newborn complications associated with multiple births are essential to achieving a positive outcome for mothers and babies. Maternal positioning and active support are used to enhance labour progress and placental perfusion. Stimulation of labour with oxytocin, epidural anaesthesia, forceps and vacuum assistance, and internal or external cephalic version may be used to accomplish the vaginal birth of twins. Caesarean birth is most likely with higher-order multiple births. Each infant may have its own team of health care providers present at the birth. Emotional support that includes expression of feelings and full explanations of events as they occur and of the status of the mother and the fetuses and newborns is important for reducing the anxiety and stress that the mother and her family can experience. See Additional Resources at the end of the chapter for websites that may be helpful for families having a multiple birth.

PRECIPITOUS LABOUR

Precipitous labour is defined as labour that lasts less than 3 hours from the onset of contractions to the time of birth. This abnormal labour pattern occurs in approximately 2% of all births. Precipitous birth alone is usually not associated with significant maternal or infant morbidity or mortality (Wing & Farinelli, 2012).

Precipitous labour may result from hypertonic uterine contractions that are tetanic in intensity. Conditions often associated with this type of uterine contractions include placental abruption, uterine tachysystole, and recent cocaine use (Wing & Farinelli, 2012). Maternal complications can include uterine rupture, lacerations of the birth canal, amniotic fluid embolus (anaphylactoid syndrome of pregnancy), and postpartum hemorrhage. Fetal complications include shoulder dystocia (Wing & Farinelli, 2012), hypoxia caused by decreased periods of uterine relaxation between contractions, and, in rare instances, intracranial trauma related to rapid birth (Cunningham et al., 2014).

Women who have experienced precipitous labour often describe feelings of disbelief that their labour began so quickly, alarm that their labour progressed so rapidly, panic about the possibility that they would not make it to the hospital on time to give birth, and, finally, relief when they arrived at the hospital. In addition, women have expressed frustration when nurses would not believe them when they reported their readiness to push. Progress can be so rapid in some women that they may have difficulty remembering the details of their childbirth. They should be provided with an opportunity to discuss their labour and birth with caregivers who were present.

OBSTETRICAL PROCEDURES

Version

Version is the turning of the fetus from one presentation to another. It may be performed externally or internally by the physician.

External Cephalic Version

External cephalic version (ECV) is used in an attempt to turn the fetus from a breech or shoulder presentation to a vertex presentation for birth. This is done by a physician. It is typically performed as an elective procedure in a labour and birth setting of a nonlabouring women at or near term to improve their chances of having a vaginal cephalic birth. ECV is accomplished by the exertion of gentle, constant pressure on the abdomen (Fig. 20-3). Before ECV is attempted, ultrasound scanning is done to:

- Determine the fetal position
- Locate the umbilical cord
- Rule out placenta previa
- Evaluate the adequacy of the maternal pelvis
- Assess the amount of amniotic fluid, the gestational age, and the presence of any anomalies

A nonstress test (NST) is performed to confirm fetal well-being, or the FHR and pattern are monitored for a period of time (10 to 20 minutes). Informed consent needs to be obtained. Contraindications to ECV include (Cunningham et al., 2014; Hofmeyr, 2015; Lanni & Seeds, 2012):

- Uterine anomalies
- Third trimester bleeding
- Multiple gestation
- Oligohydramnios
- Evidence of uteroplacental insufficiency
- A nuchal cord (identified by ultrasound)
- Obvious CPD

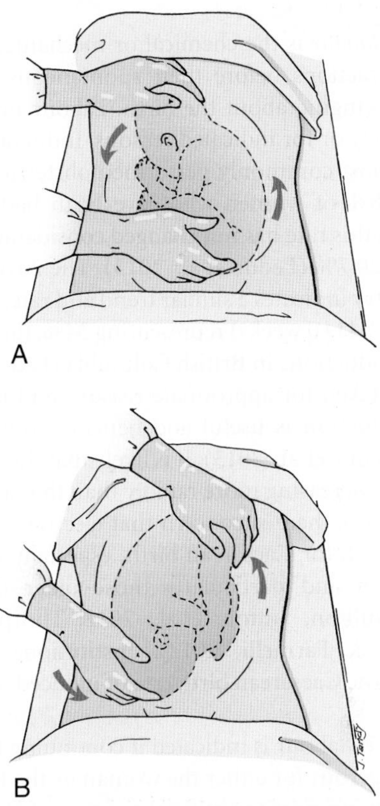

FIGURE 20-3 External version of fetus from breech to vertex presentation. This must be achieved without force. **A:** Breech is pushed up out of pelvic inlet while the head is pulled toward inlet. **B:** The head is pushed toward inlet while breech is pulled upward.

ECV is most successful in a multiparous woman who has a normal amount of amniotic fluid and whose fetus is not yet engaged in the pelvis (Cunningham et al., 2014). ECV performed at term to avoid breech birth is a beneficial form of care and may decrease the use of Caesarean birth.

During an attempted ECV, the nurse continuously monitors the FHR and pattern, especially for bradycardia and variable decelerations; checks the maternal vital signs; and assesses the woman's level of comfort because the procedure may cause discomfort. After the procedure is completed, the nurse continues to monitor maternal vital signs and uterine activity to assess for vaginal bleeding until the woman's condition is determined to be stable. FHR and pattern monitoring should continue for at least 1 hour. Women who are Rh negative should receive Rh immune globulin because the manipulation can cause fetomaternal bleeding (Thorp & Laughon, 2014) (see Medication Guide, p. 577, Chapter 22).

Internal Version

With internal version, the fetus is turned by the care provider, who inserts a hand into the uterus and changes the presentation to cephalic (head) or podalic (foot). Internal version is rarely used, most often in twin gestations to assist with birth of the second fetus. The safety of this procedure has not been documented; maternal and fetal injuries are possible. The nurse's role is to monitor the status of the fetus and support the woman.

Induction of Labour

Induction of labour is the chemical or mechanical initiation of uterine contractions before their spontaneous onset for the purpose of bringing about the birth. Labour may be induced either electively or for indicated reasons. Induction of labour is one of the most commonly performed obstetrical procedures. In 2005, 21.8% of women who gave birth had their labours induced, and this rate has not changed considerably since 1996, when it was 20.7% (Leduc et al., 2013). The 2010 BC Perinatal Health Registry indicates a similar trend and rate, with postterm pregnancies (>41+0 weeks) representing 34%, the largest group, of the total inductions in British Columbia (Leduc et al., 2013). When undertaken for appropriate reasons and by appropriate methods, induction is useful and benefits both mothers and newborns (Leduc et al., 2013). It is likely that the rate of elective inductions is increasing more rapidly than the rate of indicated inductions. Also, there is concern that elective inductions may increase the risk for Caesarean birth, especially among primigravid women and particularly those older than 35 years (Martin, Hamilton, Sutton, et al., 2012; Thorp & Laughon, 2014; Wing & Farinelli, 2012). Institutional factors may play a role in the Caesarean birth rate of induced labours (Leduc et al., 2013).

Induction of labour is indicated if continuing the pregnancy could be dangerous for either the woman or the fetus and if no contraindications exist to artificial rupture of the membranes (amniotomy) or augmenting uterine contractions with oxytocin. Before labour induction, gestational age should be determined and any potential risks to mother and fetus evaluated. Women must be fully counselled regarding risks, benefits, and alternatives of labour stimulation methods as part of the process for informed consent (ACOG, 2009; Thorp & Laughon, 2014). Box 20-8 lists indications and contraindications for labour induction.

BOX 20-8 INDICATIONS AND CONTRAINDICATIONS FOR LABOUR INDUCTION

High Priority

- Pre-eclampsia >37 weeks
- Significant maternal disease not responding to treatment
- Significant but stable antepartum hemorrhage
- Chorioamnionitis
- Suspected fetal compromise
- Term prelabour rupture of membranes (PROM) with maternal group B streptococcus (GBS) colonization

Other Indications

- Postdates (>41+0 weeks) or postterm (>42+0 weeks) pregnancy
- Uncomplicated twin pregnancy >38 weeks
- Diabetes mellitus (glucose control may dictate urgency)
- Alloimmune disease at or near term
- Intrauterine growth restriction
- Oligohydramnios
- Gestational hypertension >38 weeks
- Intrauterine fetal death
- PROM near or at term (GBS negative)
- Logistical problems (history of fast labour, distance from the hospital)
- Intrauterine device in prior to pregnancy (to allay anxiety)

Unacceptable Indications

- Suspected fetal macrosomia
- Absence of fetal or maternal indication
- Caregiver or patient convenience

Source: Leduc, D., Biringer, A., Lee, L., et al., (2013). SOGC clinical practice guideline: Induction of labour. *Journal of Obstetrics & Gynaecology Canada, 35*(9), S1–S20.

TABLE 20-3 BISHOP SCORE

	SCORE			
	0	1	2	3
Dilation (cm)	Closed	1–2	3–4	≥5
Effacement (%)	0–30	40–50	60–70	≥80
Station (cm)	−3	−2	−1, 0	+1, +2
Cervical consistency	Firm	Medium	Soft	
Cervix position	Posterior	Midposition	Anterior	

Elective Induction of Labour

An elective induction is one in which labour is initiated without a medical indication. Methods to ripen the cervix (e.g., application of prostaglandins or intracervical insertion of a balloon catheter) enhance the likelihood of successful induction. Therefore, they have been a factor in the use of elective induction as an option for managing childbirth rather than waiting for labour to begin spontaneously. Many of these elective inductions are purely for the convenience of the woman or her primary health care provider. At times, however, labour may be electively induced to allay maternal fears and anxieties associated with prior perinatal losses or to ensure that experienced multispecialty personnel are available to handle anticipated maternal or neonatal complications immediately after birth (Wing & Farinelli, 2012).

The major risks associated with elective labour induction at term are increased rates of Caesarean birth, neonatal morbidity, and cost (Wing & Farinelli, 2012). The SOGC strongly recommends not inducing women unless there is a medical indication or until they are at least 41 weeks' gestation without any other indications. The Association of Women's Health, Obstetric and Neonatal Nurses (AWHONN) has created an informational campaign to educate pregnant women and their families about the dangers of early term births (see Additional Resources at end of the chapter).

Chemical, mechanical, physical, and alternative methods are used to ripen the cervix and induce labour. Intravenous oxytocin and amniotomy are the most common methods used to induce labour. Success rates for induction of labour are higher when the condition of the cervix is favourable, or inducible. Cervical ripeness is the most important predictor of successful induction. A rating system such as the Bishop score (Table 20-3) can be used to evaluate inducibility. For example, a score of 8 or more on this 13-point scale indicates that the cervix is soft, anterior, 50% or more effaced, and dilated 2 cm or more and that the presenting part is engaged. When the Bishop score totals 7 or more, induction of labour is usually successful (Gilbert, 2011; Leduc et al., 2013). The Bishop score should be documented before the use of methods to ripen the cervix or induce labour.

Cervical Ripening Methods

Chemical agents. Preparations of prostaglandins E_1 (PGE_1) and E_2 (PGE_2) have been shown to be effective when used before induction to ripen the cervix (see Medication Guides) (Hill & Harvey, 2013). In some cases, women spontaneously begin labouring after the administration of prostaglandin, thereby eliminating the need to administer oxytocin to induce labour. Additional advantages of prostaglandin use for cervical ripening include decreased oxytocin induction time and a decrease in the amount of oxytocin required for successful induction (Gilbert, 2011). PGE_1 (Misoprostol) has been found to be an effective agent for cervical ripening and labour induction. Many randomized trials have been conducted to study its efficacy and safety (Leduc et al., 2013). The benefits of PGE_1 include its stability at room temperature, rapid onset of action, multiple potential routes of administration, and low cost. These potential benefits make it an attractive alternative to PGE_2.

Although the drug's manufacturer has acknowledged for several years that PGE_1 is effective for cervical ripening and labour induction, it has not yet been approved by Health Canada for these uses (Leduc et al., 2013; Thorp & Laughon, 2014). PGE_2 in the form of a vaginal insert (dinoprostone [Cervidil]), although more expensive than PGE_1, has the major advantage of easy removal should adverse reactions, including uterine tachysystole, occur (Moleti, 2009).

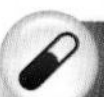

MEDICATION GUIDE

Prostaglandin E_2 (PGE_2): Dinoprostone (Cervidil Insert; Prepidil Gel)

Action

- PGE_2 ripens the cervix, making it softer and causing it to begin to dilate and efface; it stimulates uterine contractions. Dinoprostone is the only Health Canada–approved medication for cervical ripening or labour induction.

Indications

- PGE_2 is used for preinduction cervical ripening (to ripen cervix before oxytocin induction of labour when the Bishop score is 6 or less) and to induce labour or abortion (abortifacient agent).
- It is not recommended for use if the woman has a history of previous Caesarean birth or other major uterine surgery.

Dosage and Route

Cervidil Insert

- Dosage is 10 mg of dinoprostone, designed to be gradually released over 12 hours. Insert is placed transvaginally into the posterior fornix of the vagina. The insert is removed after 12 hours or at the onset of active labour or earlier if tachysystole or abnormal FHR and patterns occur.

Prepidil Gel

- Dosage is 0.5 mg of dinoprostone in a 2.5-mL syringe. Gel is administered through a catheter attached to the syringe into the cervical canal just below the internal cervical os. Dose may be repeated every 6 hours as needed for cervical ripening up to a maximum cumulative dose of 1.5 mg (3 doses) in a 24-hour period.

Adverse Effects

- Potential adverse reactions include headache, nausea and vomiting, diarrhea, fever, hypotension, tachysystole (10 or more uterine contractions in 20 minutes with or without alteration of FHR or pattern), and fetal passage of meconium.

Nursing Considerations

- Explain the procedure to the woman and her family. Ensure that informed consent has been obtained per agency policy.
- Assess the woman and fetus before each insertion and during treatment following agency protocol for frequency. Assess maternal vital signs and health status, FHR and pattern, and status of pregnancy, including indications for cervical ripening or induction of labour, signs of labour or impending labour, and the Bishop score. Recognize that an abnormal FHR and pattern; maternal fever, infection, vaginal bleeding, or hypersensitivity; and regular, progressive uterine contractions contraindicate the use of dinoprostone.
- Avoid use in women with asthma, glaucoma, and hypotension or hypertension.
- Use with caution if the woman has cardiac, renal, or hepatic disease, anemia, jaundice, diabetes, epilepsy, or genitourinary infections.
- Bring the gel to room temperature just before administration. Do not force the warming process by using a warm-water bath or other source of external heat such as microwave because heat may cause inactivation.
- Keep the insert frozen until just before insertion. No warming is needed.
- Have the woman void before insertion.
- Assist the woman in maintaining a supine position with lateral tilt or a side-lying position for at least 30 minutes after insertion of gel or for 2 hours after placement of insert.
- Allow the woman to ambulate after a recommended period of bedrest and observation.
- Prepare to pull the string to remove the insert if significant adverse effects occur. There is no effective way to remove the gel from the vagina if uterine tachysystole occurs.
- Delay initiation of oxytocin for induction of labour for 6 hours after last instillation of gel or at least 30 to 60 minutes after removal of the insert. Follow agency protocol for induction if ripening has occurred and labour has not begun.
- Document all assessment findings and administration procedures.

FHR, fetal heart rate.

Data from Hill, W., & Harvey, C. (2013). Induction of labor. In N. Troiano, C. Harvey, & B. Chez, (Eds.), (2013). *AWHONN's high risk & critical care obstetrics* (3rd ed.). Philadelphia: Wolters Kluwer/Lippincott Williams & Wilkins; Leduc, D., Biringer, A., Lee, L., et al. (2013). SOGC clinical practice guideline: Induction of labour. *Journal of Obstetrics and Gynaecology Canada, 35*(9), S1–S18; Moleti, C. (2009). Trends and controversies in labor induction. *MCN: American Journal of Maternal Child Nursing, 34*(1), 40–47.

MEDICATION GUIDE

Prostaglandin E_1 (PGE_1): Misoprostol

Action

- PGE_1 ripens the cervix, making it softer and causing it to begin to dilate and efface; it stimulates uterine contractions.

Indications

- PGE_1 is used for preinduction cervical ripening (ripen the cervix before oxytocin induction of labour when the Bishop score is 4 or less) and for inducement of labour or abortion (abortifacient agent); it has not yet been approved by Health Canada for cervical ripening or labour induction (i.e., this is an unlabelled use for obstetrics).
- It should not be used if the woman has a history of previous Caesarean birth or other major uterine surgery.

Dosage and Administration

- Misoprostol is available either as a 100-mcg or a 200-mcg tablet. Therefore, tablets must be broken to prepare the correct dose. This preparation should take place in the pharmacy to ensure accurate doses.
- Initial dose is 50 mcg orally with a drink of water (ensure that it is swallowed quickly to avoid sublingual absorption) or 25 mcg vaginally. Insert intravaginally into the posterior vaginal fornix using the tips of index and middle fingers, without the use of a lubricant. Repeat every 4 hours up to 6 doses in a 24-hour period or until an effective contraction pattern is established (three or more uterine contractions in 10 minutes), the cervix ripens (Bishop score of 8 or greater), or significant adverse effects occur.

Adverse Effects

- Higher doses (e.g., 50 mcg every 6 hours) are more likely to result in adverse reactions such as nausea and vomiting, diarrhea, fever, uterine tachysystole with or without an abnormal FHR and pattern, or fetal passage of meconium. The risk for adverse reactions is reduced with lower dosages and longer intervals between doses.

Nursing Considerations

- Explain the procedure to the woman and her family; ensure that informed consent has been obtained as per agency policy.
- Assess the woman and fetus before each insertion and during treatment following agency protocol for frequency. Assess maternal vital signs and health status, FHR and pattern, and status of pregnancy, including indications for cervical ripening or induction of labour, signs of labour or impending labour, and the Bishop score. Recognize that an atypical or abnormal FHR and pattern; maternal fever, infection, vaginal bleeding, or hypersensitivity; and regular, progressive uterine contractions contraindicate the use of misoprostol.
- Avoid giving aluminum hydroxide and magnesium-containing antacids along with misoprostol.
- Use with caution in women with renal failure because the medication is eliminated through the kidneys.
- Contraindicated in women with previous Caesarean birth due to increased risk of uterine rupture.
- Have the woman void before insertion.
- Assist the woman in maintaining a supine position with a lateral tilt or a side-lying position for 30 to 40 minutes after vaginal insertion.
- Prepare to swab the vagina to remove unabsorbed vaginal medication using a saline-soaked gauze wrapped around fingers if significant adverse effects occur.
- Initiate oxytocin for induction of labour no sooner than 4 hours after the last dose of misoprostol was administered, following agency protocol, if ripening has occurred and labour has not begun.
- Document all assessment findings and administration procedures.

FHR, fetal heart rate.

Data from Hill, W., & Harvey, C. (2013). Induction of labor. In N. Troiano, C. Harvey, & B. Chez, (Eds.), (2013). *AWHONN's high risk & critical care obstetrics* (3rd ed.). Philadelphia: Wolters Kluwer/Lippincott Williams & Wilkins; Leduc, D., Biringer, A., Lee, L., et al. (2013). SOGC clinical practice guideline: Induction of labour. *Journal of Obstetrics and Gynaecology Canada, 35*(9), S1–S18; Moleti, C. (2009). Trends and controversies in labor induction. *MCN: American Journal of Maternal Child Nursing, 34*(1), 40–47; Thorp, J. M., & Laughon, K. (2014). Clinical aspects of normal and abnormal labor. In R. Creasy, R. Resnik, J. Iams, et al. (Eds.), *Creasy and Resnik's maternal-fetal medicine: Principles and practice* (6th ed.). Philadelphia: Saunders.

Mechanical and physical methods. Mechanical dilators ripen the cervix by stimulating the release of endogenous prostaglandins. Balloon catheters (e.g., Foley catheter) can be inserted through the intracervical canal to ripen and dilate the cervix and are often used in women attempting a trial of labour following a previous Caesarean birth. Simplicity of use, potential for reversibility, reduction in certain side effects such as excessive uterine activity, and low cost are advantages to using a mechanical dilator (Leduc et al., 2013). For a single balloon catheter, a number 18 Foley catheter is introduced under sterile technique into the intracervical canal past the internal os. The bulb is then inflated with 30 to 60 mL of water. This process results in pressure and stretching of the lower uterine segment and the cervix, as well as the release of endogenous prostaglandins. It is especially helpful for women who cannot receive exogenous prostaglandins for cervical ripening. The balloon will fall out when cervical dilation reaches approximately 3 cm or is removed after 24 hours have elapsed. Evidence supports the insertion of a balloon catheter as a cervical ripening method because of its low cost compared with that of prostaglandins, stability at room temperature, and reduced risk for uterine tachysystole with or without FHR changes (ACOG, 2009; Hill & Harvey, 2013; Leduc et al., 2013; Simpson, 2013).

Low-lying placenta is an absolute contraindication to the use of a Foley catheter. Relative contraindications include antepartum hemorrhage, rupture of membranes, and evidence of lower tract genital infection (Leduc et al., 2013).

Hygroscopic dilators (substances that absorb fluid from surrounding tissues and enlarge) also can be used for cervical ripening. Laminaria tents (natural cervical dilators made from desiccated seaweed) and synthetic dilators containing magnesium sulphate (Lamicel) are inserted into the endocervix without rupturing the membranes. As they absorb fluid, they expand and cause cervical dilation and the release of endogenous prostaglandins. These dilators are left in place for 6 to 12 hours before being removed to assess cervical dilation. Fresh dilators are inserted if further cervical dilation is necessary. Synthetic dilators swell faster than natural dilators and become larger with less discomfort. When compared with prostaglandins, these mechanical methods achieved a lower rate of birth within 24 hours but resulted in no change in the Caesarean birth rate. Also, they were less likely to cause uterine tachysystole with or without changes in the FHR (ACOG, 2009; Thorp & Laughon, 2014).

Hydroscopic dilators compare favourably with prostaglandins in terms of their effectiveness in ripening the cervix but are associated with increased discomfort at insertion and during expansion and with a higher incidence of postpartum maternal and newborn infections. They are a reliable alternative when prostaglandins are contraindicated or are unavailable. Nursing responsibilities for women who have dilators inserted include the following (Gilbert, 2011):

- Documenting the number of dilators and sponges inserted during the procedure, as well as the number removed
- Assessing for urinary retention, rupture of membranes, uterine tenderness or pain, contractions, vaginal bleeding, infection, and fetal distress

Amniotic membrane stripping or sweeping is a method of inducing labour through the release of prostaglandins and oxytocin. The procedure involves separation of the membrane from the wall of the cervix and lower uterine segment by inserting a finger into the internal cervical os and rotating it 360 degrees. Membrane stripping seems to work best when the woman is a primigravida at term with an unripe cervix and with the vertex well applied to the cervix. The procedure is uncomfortable and increases the risk for infection, rupture of membranes, bleeding, and precipitous labour and birth (Wing & Farinelli, 2012).

Routine membrane stripping is not recommended because there is no evidence that this practice improves maternal or fetal outcome. However, weekly membrane stripping at term shortens the time interval to the onset of spontaneous labour and may decrease the need for labour induction using chemical or mechanical methods (Wing & Farinelli, 2012).

Physical methods such as sexual intercourse (prostaglandins in the semen and stimulation of contractions with orgasm), nipple stimulation (release of endogenous oxytocin from the pituitary gland), and walking (gravity applies pressure to the cervix, which stimulates the secretion of endogenous oxytocin) may be used by women to "self-induce" labour in an effort to "get it over with." Breast (nipple) stimulation has been shown to initiate or enhance labour, especially the latent phase of labour. Although orgasm does stimulate uterine contractions, it is unclear whether sexual intercourse enhances cervical ripening (Leduc et al., 2013). Ambulation is an effective measure to augment labour (Moleti, 2009).

Alternative methods. A variety of alternative methods have been used by women to stimulate cervical ripening and the onset of labour. For example, some women may take blue cohosh and castor oil for labour-stimulation effects and black cohosh and evening primrose oil to ripen the cervix. Although the effects of these alternative methods are not well researched, nurses must be knowledgeable about these preparations and ask about their use when assessing women during prenatal visits and on admission during labour. Women may accidentally take too much of the preparation or use it incorrectly. Also, these preparations may potentiate the effect of pharmacological methods to stimulate cervical ripening and uterine contractions, thereby increasing the potential for tachysystole and precipitous labour and birth (Gilbert, 2011; Moleti, 2009).

Acupuncture has been used effectively to induce labour and has been found, in several studies, to reduce the duration of labour, the use of oxytocin, and the rate of Caesarean birth. Specific points have been identified to stimulate uterine contractions or to facilitate cervical dilation. More than one treatment may be required to establish labour (Gilbert, 2011; Moleti, 2009).

Amniotomy

Amniotomy (i.e., artificial rupture of membranes [AROM]) can be used to induce labour when the condition of the cervix is favourable (ripe) or to augment labour if progress begins to slow. Labour usually begins within 12 hours of the rupture. Amniotomy can decrease the duration of labour by up to 2 hours, even without oxytocin administration. However, if amniotomy does not stimulate labour, the resulting prolonged rupture may lead to intra-amniotic infection. Variable FHR deceleration patterns can occur as a result of cord compression associated with umbilical cord prolapse or decreased amniotic fluid. Once an amniotomy is performed, the woman is committed to giving birth with an unknown outcome for how and when she will give birth. For this reason, amniotomy often is used in combination with oxytocin induction. Evidence from controlled trials clearly demonstrates that amniotomy combined with oxytocin for induction is more effective than either amniotomy or oxytocin alone (Leduc et al., 2013).

! NURSING ALERT

An amniotomy is performed by the primary health care provider (physician or midwife).

Before the procedure, the woman should be told what to expect; she should also be assured that the actual rupture of membranes is painless for her and the fetus, although she may experience some discomfort when the Amnihook is inserted through the vagina and cervix (Box 20-9). The presenting part of the fetus should be engaged and well applied to the cervix to reduce the risk of cord prolapse (Wing & Farinelli, 2012). The woman should be free of active infection of the genital tract (e.g., herpes) and should be human immunodeficiency virus (HIV) negative or have a viral load low enough that vaginal birth is acceptable. After rupture the amniotic fluid is allowed to drain slowly. The fluid is assessed for colour, odour, amount, and consistency (i.e., for the presence or absence of meconium or blood). The time of rupture and characteristics of the fluid are recorded.

BOX 20-9 PROCEDURE: ASSISTING WITH AMNIOTOMY

Procedure

Explain to the woman what will be done.

Assess fetal heart rate and pattern before procedure begins, to obtain a baseline reading.

Place several underpads under the woman's buttocks to absorb fluid.

Position the woman on a padded bed pan, fracture pan, or rolled-up towel to elevate her hips as needed.

Assist the health care provider who is performing the procedure by providing sterile gloves and lubricant for the vaginal examination.

Unwrap sterile package containing Amnihook or Allis clamp and pass instrument to the primary health care provider, who inserts it alongside the fingers and then hooks and tears the membranes.

Reassess fetal heart rate and pattern.

Assess colour, consistency, amount, and odour of fluid.

Assess the woman's temperature every 2 hours or per protocol.

Evaluate the woman for signs and symptoms of infection.

Documentation

Record the following:

- Indication for amniotomy
- Time of rupture
- Colour, odour, amount, consistency, and clarity of fluid
- Fetal heart rate and pattern before and after procedure
- Maternal status and how well procedure was tolerated

BOX 20-10 INDICATIONS AND CONTRAINDICATIONS FOR USE OF OXYTOCIN FOR INDUCTION OR AUGMENTATION OF LABOUR

The indications for oxytocin induction or augmentation of labour may include but are not limited to the following:

- Suspected fetal jeopardy (e.g., intrauterine growth restriction)
- Inadequate uterine contractions; dystocia
- Prelabour rupture of membranes
- Postterm pregnancy
- Chorioamnionitis
- Maternal medical problems (e.g., woman with severe Rh isoimmunization, inadequately controlled diabetes, chronic renal disease, or chronic pulmonary disease)
- Gestational hypertension (e.g., pre-eclampsia, eclampsia)
- Fetal death

The management of stimulation of labour is the same, regardless of indication. Because of the potential dangers associated with the injection of oxytocin in the prenatal and perinatal periods, there are contraindications to its use.

Contraindications to oxytocic stimulation of labour include but are not limited to the following:

- Cephalopelvic disproportion, prolapsed cord, transverse lie
- Abnormal fetal heart rate
- Placenta previa or vasa previa
- Prior classic uterine incision or other uterine surgery
- Active genital herpes infection
- Invasive cancer of the cervix
- Previous uterine rupture

! NURSING ALERT

The FHR is assessed before and immediately after the amniotomy to detect any changes (transient tachycardia is common, but bradycardia and variable decelerations are not), which may indicate cord compression or prolapse.

The woman's temperature should be checked at least every 2 hours after rupture of membranes and more frequently if signs or symptoms of infection are noted. If her temperature is 38°C (100.4°F) or greater, the primary health care provider should be notified. The nurse needs to assess for other signs and symptoms of infection, such as maternal chills, fetal tachycardia, uterine tenderness on palpation, and foul-smelling vaginal drainage. Comfort measures such as frequently changing the woman's underpads and perineal cleansing need to be implemented.

Oxytocin

Oxytocin is a hormone normally produced by the posterior pituitary gland. It stimulates uterine contractions and aids in milk let-down. A synthetic version of this hormone may be used to either induce labour or augment (speed up) a labour that is progressing slowly because of inadequate uterine contractions.

See Box 20-10 for indications and contraindications for oxytocin induction or augmentation. Although certain maternal and fetal conditions are not contraindications to the use of oxytocin to stimulate labour, they do require special caution during its administration. These conditions include the following:

- Multifetal presentation
- Breech presentation
- Presenting part above the pelvic inlet
- Atypical FHR and pattern not requiring emergency birth
- Polyhydramnios
- Grand multiparity
- Previous Caesarean birth
- Maternal cardiac disease; hypertension

Oxytocin is the drug most commonly associated with adverse events during childbirth. The most common errors involving oxytocin administration during labour are dose related (Clark, Simpson, Knox, et al., 2009; Simpson & Knox, 2009).

SAFETY ALERT

Oxytocin was added to the Institute for Safe Medication Practices' list of high-alert medications in 2007 because it has the potential to cause significant harm when used inappropriately (Simpson, 2011).

Oxytocin use can present hazards to the mother and fetus. Maternal hazards include placental abruption, uterine rupture, unnecessary Caesarean birth because of abnormal FHR and patterns, postpartum hemorrhage, and infection. When placental perfusion is diminished by contractions that are too frequent or prolonged, the fetus can experience hypoxemia and acidemia, which eventually results in late decelerations and minimal or absent baseline variability. The goal of oxytocin use is to produce contractions of normal intensity, duration, and frequency while using the lowest dose of medication possible (Simpson & Knox, 2009).

The primary health care provider writes the order for the induction or augmentation of labour with oxytocin. The nurse implements the order by initiating the primary intravenous infusion and administering the oxytocin solution through a secondary line. The nurse's actions related to assessment and care of a woman whose labour is being induced are guided by hospital protocol and professional standards. The ideal dosing regimen of oxytocin is not known and there are both low-dose and high-dose protocols (see Medication Guide). Continuous electronic fetal monitoring is recommended with the use of oxytocin (Fig. 20-4).

Nursing considerations. An evidence-informed written protocol for the preparation and administration of oxytocin should be established by the obstetrical department (physicians, midwives, nurses) in each institution.

NURSING ALERT

Oxytocin is decreased or discontinued and the health care provider notified if tachysystole resulting in an abnormal FHR or pattern occurs. Other nursing interventions, such as administering 8 to 10 L oxygen by nonrebreather mask, positioning the woman on her side, and administering an intravenous fluid bolus, are independent nursing interventions and are implemented immediately (see Emergency Measures in Medication Guide). Based on the status of the maternal–fetal unit, the primary health care provider may order the infusion to be restarted once the FHR and uterine activity return to acceptable levels. Depending on the FHR and pattern assessment and the length of time the infusion was discontinued, the oxytocin may be restarted at half the rate that resulted in tachysystole (e.g., discontinued for 10 to 20 minutes) or at the same rate as the initial rate (e.g., discontinued for more than 30 to 40 minutes) (Simpson, 2013).

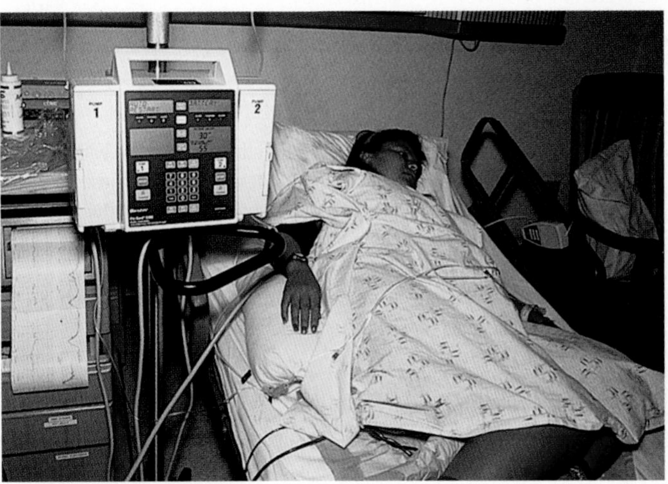

FIGURE 20-4 Woman in side-lying position being monitored with continuous electronic fetal monitoring and receiving oxytocin. (Courtesy Michael S. Clement, MD.)

Augmentation of Labour

Augmentation of labour is the stimulation of uterine contractions after labour has started spontaneously but progress has been unsatisfactory. Augmentation is usually implemented for the management of hypotonic uterine dysfunction resulting in a slowing of labour (protracted active phase). Common augmentation methods include oxytocin infusion and amniotomy. Noninvasive methods such as emptying the bladder, ambulation, position changes, relaxation measures, nourishment, hydration, and hydrotherapy can be attempted before invasive interventions are initiated. The procedures and nursing assessments are similar to those used for oxytocin induction of labour (see Medication Guide). See Evolve for Nursing Care Plan on Woman with Hypotonic Uterine Dysfunction.

Some physicians advocate *active management of labour,* that is, augmentation of labour to establish efficient labour with the aggressive use of oxytocin so that the woman gives birth within 12 hours of admission to the labour unit. Advocates of active

MEDICATION GUIDE

Oxytocin

Action

- Oxytocin is a hormone produced in the posterior pituitary gland that stimulates uterine contractions and aids in milk let-down. Syntocinon is a synthetic form of this hormone.

Indications

- Oxytocin is used primarily for labour induction and augmentation. It is also used to control postpartum bleeding.

Dosage

- The IV solution containing oxytocin should be mixed in a standard concentration. Concentrations often used are 10 units in 1000 mL of fluid, 20 units in 1000 mL of fluid, or 30 units in 500 mL of fluid.
- Isotonic IV solutions (e.g., 0.9% sodium chloride, lactated Ringer's) are used to avoid electrolyte imbalance.
- Oxytocin is administered intravenously through a secondary line connected to the main line at the proximal port (connection closest to the IV insertion site). Oxytocin is always administered by pump.
- Oxytocin administration is started at a low-dose or high-dose regimen (see below). Dosage is increased per protocol until an adequate contraction pattern is established.
- The goal of oxytocin administration is to produce acceptable uterine contractions as evidenced by a consistent pattern of one contraction every 2 to 3 minutes, lasting 80 to 90 seconds, and strong to palpation.
- Once labour is established, oxytocin is maintained at or decreased to a rate adequate for continued labour progress.
- If a dose of 30 mU/min is reached the woman needs to be reassessed.

Continued

MEDICATION GUIDE

Oxytocin—cont'd

Adverse Effects

- Possible maternal adverse effects include uterine tachysystole with or without FHR changes, placental abruption, uterine rupture, unnecessary Caesarean birth caused by abnormal FHR and patterns, postpartum hemorrhage, infection, and death from water intoxication (e.g., severe hyponatremia).
- Possible fetal adverse effects include hypoxemia and acidosis, eventually resulting in abnormal FHR and patterns.

Nursing Considerations

- Patient and partner teaching and support:
  - Reasons for use of oxytocin (e.g., to start or improve labour)
  - Reactions to expect concerning the nature of contractions: the intensity of the contraction increases more rapidly, holds the peak longer, and ends more quickly; contractions will come regularly and more often
- Continue to keep woman and her partner informed regarding progress.
- Remember that women vary greatly in their response to oxytocin; some require only very small amounts of medication to produce adequate contractions, whereas others need larger doses.
- Continue to provide labour support techniques, such as use of the birth ball or a rocking chair.
- Assess level of maternal discomfort and pain and the effectiveness of pain management.
- Encourage change in position every 20 to 30 minutes; encourage walking or standing, if possible.
- Observe emotional responses of the woman and her partner.

Assessment

- Fetal status using electronic fetal monitoring: Evaluate tracing every 15 minutes and with every change in dose during the first stage of labour and every 5 minutes during the active pushing phase of the second stage of labour.
- Monitor the contraction pattern and uterine resting tone every 15 minutes and with every change in dose during the first stage of labour and every 5 minutes during the second stage of labour.
- Monitor blood pressure, pulse, and respirations every 30 to 60 minutes and with every change in dose.
- Assess intake and output; limit IV intake to 1000 mL in 8 hours; urine output should be 120 mL or more every 4 hours.
- Perform vaginal examination as indicated.
- Monitor for adverse effects, including nausea, vomiting, headache, hypotension.
- Observe emotional responses of woman and her partner.
- The rate of oxytocin infusion should be continually titrated to the lowest dose that achieves acceptable labour progress. Usually the oxytocin dose can be decreased or discontinued after rupture of membranes and in the active phase of first-stage labour.

Reportable Conditions

- Uterine tachysystole (with or without FHR changes)
- Abnormal FHR and pattern (absent baseline variability and any of the following: [1] recurrent late decelerations, [2] recurrent variable decelerations, [3] bradycardia, or [4] prolonged decelerations)
- Suspected uterine rupture
- Inadequate uterine response at 30 mU/min

Emergency Measures

Discontinue use of oxytocin per hospital protocol and notify primary care provider immediately:

- Turn woman on her side.
- Give IV bolus of at least 500 mL lactated Ringer's solution.
- If there is an indeterminate or abnormal FHR pattern, consider giving the woman oxygen by nonrebreather face mask at 8 to 10 units/min or per protocol or primary health care provider's order.
- Prepare to administer nitroglycerine, if ordered, to decrease uterine activity.
- Continue monitoring FHR and pattern and uterine activity.

Documentation

- The time the oxytocin infusion is begun, and each time the infusion is increased, decreased, or discontinued
- Assessment data as described above
- Interventions for uterine tachysystole and abnormal FHR and patterns and the response to the interventions
- Notification of the primary health care provider and that person's response

Low-Dose Protocol

Initial dose: 1–2 mU/min
Increase interval: 30 minutes
Dosage increment: 1–2 mU/min
Usual dose for adequate labour: 8–12 mU/min
Maximum dose before reassessment: 30 mU/min
Benefits: less risk of tachysystole; overall use of a smaller dose

High-Dose Protocol

Initial dose: 4–6 mU/min
Increase interval: 15–30 minutes
Dosage increment: 4–6 mU/min
Usual dose for adequate labour: 8–12 mU/min
Maximum dose before reassessment: 30 mU/min
Benefits: reduced length of labour with no appreciable increase in neonatal morbidity
Risks: associated with an increase in uterine tachysystole with associated FHR changes

ALERT: Because mixing methods may vary, *the rate of infusion should always be documented in mU/min* rather than mL/hr.

FHR, fetal heart rate; *IV,* intravenous.

Data from American College of Obstetricians and Gynecologists (ACOG). (2009). *Induction of labor* (ACOG Practice Bulletin No. 107). Washington, DC: Author; Clark, S., Simpson, K., Knox, G., et al. (2009). Oxytocin: new perspectives on an old drug. *American Journal of Obstetrics & Gynecology, 200*(1), 35, e1–e6; Hill, W., & Harvey, C. (2013). Induction of labor. In N. Troiano, C. Harvey, & B. Chez (Eds.), *AWHONN's high risk & critical care obstetrics* (3rd ed.). Philadelphia: Wolters Kluwer/Lippincott Williams & Wilkins; Leduc, D., Biringer, A., Lee, L., et al. (2013). SOGC clinical practice guideline: Induction of labour. *Journal of Obstetricians and Gynaecologists of Canada, 35*(9), S1–S18; Mahlmeister, L. (2008). Best practices in perinatal care: Evidence-based management of oxytocin induction and augmentation of labor. *Journal of Perinatal & Neonatal Nursing, 22*(4), 259–263; Simpson, K. (2008). Labor and birth. In K. Simpson & P. Creehan (Eds.), *AWHONN's perinatal nursing* (3rd ed.). Philadelphia: Lippincott Williams & Wilkins; Simpson, K., & Knox, G. (2009). Oxytocin as a high-alert medication: Implications for perinatal patient safety. *MCN: American Journal of Maternal Child Nursing, 34*(1), 8–15.

management believe that intervening early (as soon as a nulliparous labour is not progressing at least 1 cm/hr) with use of higher (pharmacological) oxytocin doses administered at frequent increment intervals shortens labour (Gilbert, 2011).

Additional components of the active management of labour include the following:

- Strict criteria to diagnose that the woman is indeed in active labour with 100% effacement
- Amniotomy within 1 hour of admission of a woman in labour if spontaneous rupture of the membranes has not occurred
- Continuous presence of a nurse who provides one-on-one care for the woman while she is in labour

Many health care providers emphasize using high-dose oxytocin protocols but do not implement all the other components of active management. At least one review of published studies on the effectiveness of active management of labour protocols concluded that the presence of a nurse who provides constant emotional and physical one-on-one support is the only component associated with shorter labours and lower rates of Caesarean birth (Clark et al., 2009; Gilbert, 2011).

The original active management of labour protocols were written for nulliparous women who began labouring spontaneously. However, active management of labour protocols has been implemented by some providers on women who were not appropriate candidates (Mahlmeister, 2008).

OPERATIVE VAGINAL BIRTHS

Operative vaginal births are performed using either forceps or vacuum extractor. The use of both devices has continued to decline. Indications and prerequisites for the use of both instruments are similar. The decision to use forceps or vacuum is based on the experience and personal preference of the physician performing the procedure. There are several types of operative vaginal births.

Forceps-Assisted Birth

A forceps-assisted vaginal birth is one in which an instrument with two curved blades is used to assist in the birth of the fetal head. The cephalic-like curve of the forceps commonly used is similar to the shape of the fetal head, with a pelvic curve to the blades conforming to the curve of the pelvic axis. The blades are joined by a pin, screw, or groove arrangement. These locks prevent the forceps from compressing the fetal skull (Fig. 20-5). There are several types of forceps-assisted births, defined primarily by the station and position of the fetal head in relationship to the maternal pelvis (Table 20-4) (American Academy of Pediatrics [AAP] and ACOG, 2012).

Maternal indications for forceps-assisted birth include a prolonged second stage of labour and the need to shorten the second stage of labour for maternal reasons (e.g., maternal exhaustion or maternal cardiopulmonary or cerebrovascular disease) (Nielsen & Galan, 2012). Fetal indications include an abnormal FHR tracing or certain abnormal presentations; arrest of rotation; or extraction of the head in a breech presentation (Nielsen & Galan, 2012; Thorp & Laughon, 2014).

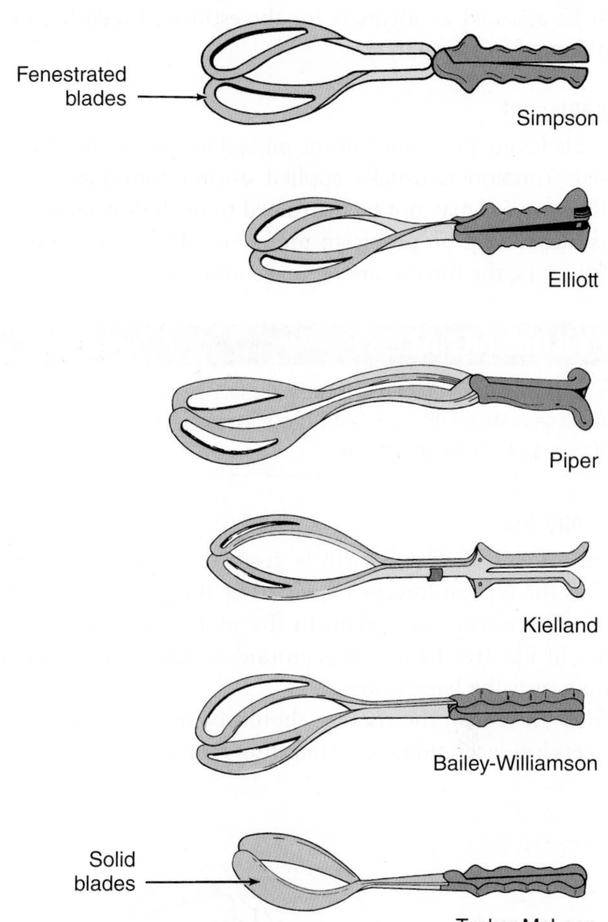

FIGURE 20-5 Types of forceps. Piper forceps are used to assist birth of the head in a breech birth.

TABLE 20-4 DEFINITIONS FOR FORCEPS- AND VACUUM-ASSISTED BIRTHS

Outlet	Fetal scalp is visible on the perineum without manually separating the labia
Low	Fetal head is at least at the +2 station
Midpelvis	Fetal head is engaged (no higher than 0 station) but above the +2 station

Data from American Academy of Pediatrics (AAP) and American College of Obstetricians and Gynecologists (ACOG). (2012). *Guidelines for perinatal care* (7th ed.). Elk Grove Village, IL: AAP.

The use of forceps during childbirth has been decreasing; in 2014–2015, the forceps-assisted delivery rate was 3.3% (Canadian Institute for Health Information [CIHI], 2016). Certain conditions are required for a forceps-assisted birth to be successful. The woman's cervix must be fully dilated to prevent lacerations and hemorrhage. The bladder should be empty. The presenting part must be engaged—vertex presentation is desired. Membranes must be ruptured so the position of the fetal head can be determined precisely and the forceps can grasp the head firmly during birth (Fig. 20-6). The size of the maternal pelvis must be assessed as adequate for the estimated fetal head circumference and weight.

Management

Both blades are positioned by the physician, and the handles are locked. Traction is usually applied during contractions. The mother may or may not be instructed to push during contractions, depending on physician preference. If a decrease in the FHR occurs, the forceps are removed and reapplied.

> **! NURSING ALERT**
>
> Because compression of the cord between the fetal head and the forceps will cause a decrease in FHR, the FHR is assessed, reported, and recorded before and after application of the forceps.

Nursing Care

When a forceps-assisted birth is deemed necessary, the nurse obtains the type of forceps requested by the physician (see Fig. 20-5). The nurse can explain to the mother that the forceps blades fit like two tablespoons around an egg, with the blades coming over the baby's ears.

After the birth, the mother should be assessed for vaginal and cervical lacerations (e.g., bleeding that occurs even with a contracted uterus); urine retention, which may result from bladder injuries or urethral injuries; and hematoma formation in the pelvic soft tissues, which may result from blood vessel damage. The infant should be assessed for bruising or abrasions at the site of the blade applications, facial palsy resulting from pressure of the blades on the facial nerve (cranial nerve VII), and subdural hematoma. Newborn and postpartum caregivers should be told that the birth was forceps assisted.

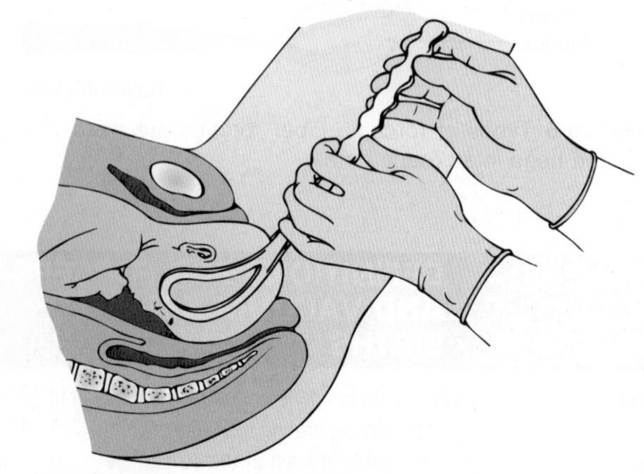

FIGURE 20-6 Outlet forceps-assisted extraction of the head.

Vacuum-Assisted Birth

Vacuum-assisted birth, or vacuum extraction, is a birth method involving the attachment of a vacuum cup to the fetal head, using negative pressure to assist in the birth of the head (Fig. 20-7). It is generally not used to assist birth before 34 weeks of gestation. Indications for use are similar to those for outlet forceps. Prerequisites for use include a completely dilated cervix, ruptured membranes, engaged head, vertex presentation, and no suspicion of CPD (Cunningham et al., 2014). The types of vacuum-assisted births are defined the same as for forceps-assisted births—by the station and position of the fetal head in relation to the maternal pelvis (see Table 20-4) (AAP & ACOG, 2012). The rate of vacuum-assisted birth in Canada in 2014–2015 was 9.3% (CIHI, 2016). Advantages of vacuum-assisted birth over forceps-assisted birth are the ease with which the vacuum can be placed and the need for less anaesthesia. Also, it is far easier to learn the skills necessary to safely use the vacuum than to gain a similar level of skill with forceps (Thorp & Laughon, 2014).

Management

The vacuum cup is applied to the fetal head by the physician. Basically two types of vacuum devices are in use. One is a self-contained unit, which allows the physician to both position the cup on the baby's head and generate the desired amount of negative pressure to create a vacuum. With other type of vacuum device, the physician applies the cup to the baby's head, then the nurse connects the suction tubing attached to the cup to wall suction or a separate hand pump and generates the amount of pressure requested by the physician. With both devices, a caput develops inside the cup as the pressure is initiated (see Fig. 20-7, B). The woman is encouraged to push as

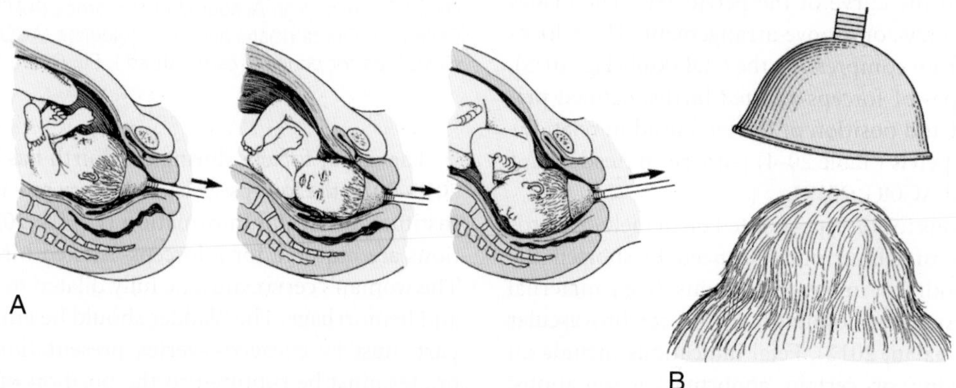

FIGURE 20-7 Use of vacuum extraction to rotate fetal head and assist with descent. **A:** *Arrow* indicates direction of traction on the vacuum cup. **B:** Caput succedaneum formed by the vacuum cup.

traction is applied by the physician. The vacuum cup is released and removed after birth of the head. If vacuum extraction is not successful, a forceps-assisted or Caesarean birth is performed.

Risks to the newborn include **cephalhematoma**, scalp lacerations, and subdural hematoma. Fetal complications can be reduced by adhering strictly to the manufacturer's recommendations for method of application, degree of suction, and duration of application. Maternal complications are uncommon but can include perineal, vaginal, and cervical lacerations and soft tissue hematomas.

Nursing Care

The nurse's role for the woman who has a vacuum-assisted birth is primarily one of support and educator. The nurse can prepare the woman for birth and encourage her to remain active in the birth process through her pushing during contractions. The FHR should be assessed frequently during the procedure. After birth, the newborn should be observed for signs of trauma at the application site and for cerebral irritation (e.g., poor sucking or listlessness). Documentation includes the time and number of applications, any "pop-offs," the number of pulls, and the maximum amount of suction used.

Neonatal caregivers should be told that the birth was vacuum assisted. After birth, the newborn must be observed for signs of trauma and infection at the application site and for cerebral irritation (e.g., poor sucking or listlessness). The newborn may also be at risk for hyperbilirubinemia and neonatal jaundice as bruising resolves. The parents may need to be reassured that the caput succedaneum usually disappears in 3 to 5 days (see Fig. 20-7, B) (Gilbert, 2011).

Caesarean Birth

Caesarean birth is the birth of a fetus through a transabdominal incision of the uterus. Whether Caesarean birth is planned (scheduled) or unplanned, the loss of the experience of giving birth to a child in the traditional manner may have a negative effect on a woman's self-esteem. Thus it is important to maintain the focus on the birth of the baby rather than on the operative procedure.

The purpose of Caesarean birth is to preserve the life or health of the mother, her fetus, or both; it may be the best choice when there is evidence of maternal or fetal complications. Since the advent of modern surgical methods and care and the use of antibiotics, maternal and fetal morbidity and mortality rates have decreased. In addition, incisions are made into the lower uterine segment rather than into the muscular body of the uterus and thus promote more effective healing. However, despite these advances, Caesarean birth still poses threats to the health of both the mother and infant.

The incidence of Caesarean births has increased, from 17.6% in 1993 to 27.5% in 2014–2015 (CIHI, 2016). Part of the reason for this increase is that a number of common risk factors for Caesarean birth are increasing, such as fetal macrosomia, advanced maternal age, obesity, gestational diabetes, and multifetal pregnancy (Thorp & Laughon, 2014). Other factors cited include the increase in primary elective Caesarean births and a decline in the rate of **vaginal birth after Caesarean (VBAC)**. This decline may be the result of risks of VBAC (e.g., uterine rupture), legal pressures, conservative practice guidelines, and debate over the relative benefits and risks of Caesarean versus vaginal route for births. Although some women desire elective Caesarean birth, fewer than 10% of all North American women prefer a Caesarean birth, based solely on their request (Berghella & Landon, 2012).

Approaches for the management of labour and birth in order to reduce the rate of Caesarean births while increasing the rate of VBACs are presented in Box 20-11. These approaches involve the combined efforts of health care providers and pregnant women and their families. The labour management approach that most consistently reduces the risk for a Caesarean birth outcome is continuous, early support of the labouring woman that is provided by another woman (e.g., doula, relative, friend, nurse, or midwife). When this woman is not a member of the labour unit staff and is thus able to spend all of her time providing physical and emotional support, the risk for Caesarean birth is further reduced (Hodnett, Gates, Hofmeyr, et al., 2013).

The type of nursing care given also may influence the rate of Caesarean births. A labour management approach that uses one-to-one support and emphasizes ambulation, maternal position changes, relaxation measures, oral fluids and nutrition, hydrotherapy, and nonpharmacological pain relief can facilitate the progress of labour and reduce the incidence of dystocia.

Indications

Few absolute indications exist for Caesarean birth. Currently, most are performed for conditions that might pose a threat to both the mother and the fetus if vaginal birth occurred, such as placenta previa or placental abruption (Berghella & Landon, 2012). Box 20-12 lists common indications for Caesarean birth.

Elective Caesarean Birth

Elective Caesarean birth, sometimes referred to as *Caesarean on request* or *Caesarean on demand,* refers to a primary Caesarean birth without medical or obstetrical indication. Reasons given for elective Caesarean birth include fear of the pain of childbirth and the belief that the surgery will prevent future problems with pelvic support, bladder and bowel incontinence, or sexual dysfunction. Although some nulliparous women may fear the pain of labour because of no firsthand experience, multiparous women may request a Caesarean birth after a previous traumatic vaginal birth. Other women desire an elective Caesarean birth because of the convenience of planning a date or having control and choice about when to give birth. At this time, evidence is insufficient to recommend elective Caesarean birth to prevent urinary or fecal incontinence later in life (Collard, Diallo, Habinsky, et al., 2008/2009; Roberts & Mangan, 2009; Thorp & Laughon, 2014).

Potential risks of Caesarean birth on request include the following:

- Higher rates of endometritis, blood transfusion, and venous thrombosis
- A longer hospital stay and recovery time for the woman

BOX 20-11 SELECTED MEASURES TO REDUCE CAESAREAN BIRTH RATE AND INCREASE RATE OF VAGINAL BIRTHS AFTER CAESAREAN

Educate Women Regarding
- Advantages and safety of the home environment for early or latent labour.
- Indicators for hospital admission.
- Management techniques to use during labour to enhance progress.
- Nonpharmacological measures to reduce pain and discomfort and enhance relaxation.
- Safety and effectiveness of TOL and VBAC.

Establish Admission Criteria for Women in Labour That
- Distinguish clinical manifestations for false labour, latent (early) labour, and active labour.
- Conduct admission assessments in a separate admissions area.
- Send women in false or latent (early) labour home or keep them in the admissions area.
- Admit women in active labour to the labour and birth unit.

Use Appropriate Assessment Techniques To
- Determine status of the woman and fetus.
- Establish an individualized rationale for initiating labour interventions such as epidural anaesthesia, induction/augmentation, amniotomy, and Caesarean birth.

Initiate a Doula Program That
- Provides one-to-one support for women in labour.

Develop a Philosophy of Labour Management That
- Supports admission during active labour.
- Uses measures that promote, support, and encourage normal spontaneous labour.
- Avoids automatic interventions such as routine induction for spontaneous rupture of membranes at term or postterm pregnancy and Caesarean birth for breech presentation, twin gestation, genital herpes (unless active), or failure to progress.
- Relies on assessment findings reflective of the status of the woman and fetus rather than strict adherence to set ranges for the duration of the stages and phases of labour.
- Uses intermittent rather than continuous electronic fetal monitoring of low-risk pregnant women.
- Focuses on measures known to enhance the progress of labour, such as one-to-one support, ambulation, upright positions, maternal position changes, oral nutrition and hydration, relaxation techniques, and hydrotherapy.
- Emphasizes nonpharmacological measures to relieve pain.
- Establishes criteria for elective Caesarean birth and TOL.
- Encourages women who have had a previous Caesarean birth to participate in a TOL in order to attempt a vaginal birth.

TOL, trial of labour; *VBAC*, vaginal birth after Caesarean.

BOX 20-12 INDICATIONS FOR CAESAREAN BIRTH

Maternal
- Specific cardiac disease (e.g., Marfan syndrome, unstable coronary artery disease)
- Specific respiratory disease (e.g., Guillain-Barré syndrome)
- Conditions associated with increased intracranial pressure
- Mechanical obstruction of the lower uterine segment (tumours, fibroids)
- Mechanical vulvar obstruction (e.g., extensive condylomata)
- History of two or more previous Caesarean births
- Elective Caesarean birth (Caesarean on maternal request)

Fetal
- Abnormal fetal heart rate (FHR) or pattern
- Malpresentation (e.g., breech or transverse lie)
- Active maternal herpes lesions
- Maternal human immunodeficiency virus (HIV) with a viral load of more than 1000 copies/mL
- Congenital anomalies

Maternal–Fetal
- Dysfunctional labour (e.g., cephalopelvic disproportion, "failure to progress" in labour)
- Placental abruption
- Placenta previa

Data from Berghella, V., & Landon, M. (2012). Cesarean delivery. In S. Gabbe, J. Niebyl, J. Simpson, et al. (Eds.), *Obstetrics: Normal and problem pregnancies* (6th ed.). Philadelphia: Saunders; Duff, P. (2014). Maternal and fetal infections. In R. Creasy, R. Resnik, J. Iams, et al. (Eds.), *Creasy and Resnik's maternal-fetal medicine: Principles and practice* (7th ed.). Philadelphia: Saunders; Thorp, J. M., & Laughon, K. (2014). Clinical aspects of normal and abnormal labor. In R. Creasy, R. Resnik, J. Iams, et al. (Eds.), *Creasy and Resnik's maternal-fetal medicine: Principles and practice* (7th ed.). Philadelphia: Saunders.

- An increased risk for respiratory problems for the baby
- Greater complications in subsequent pregnancies, including uterine rupture and placental implantation problems

Caesarean birth on request should not be performed unless a gestational age of 39 weeks has been accurately determined. Also, the procedure is not recommended for women who desire several additional children, because the risks for placenta previa, placenta accreta, and Caesarean hysterectomy increase with each Caesarean birth (Berghella & Landon, 2012).

The Society of Obstetricians and Gynaecologists of Canada (SOGC) does not promote Caesarean on demand and promotes vaginal childbirth but believes that the final decision as to the safest route for childbirth rests with the woman and her health care provider (SOGC, 2004). It is essential that women be fully informed about the risks and benefits of Caesarean birth when they consider requesting elective Caesarean birth.

Scheduled Caesarean Birth

Caesarean birth is scheduled or planned if:
- Labour and vaginal birth is contraindicated (e.g., complete placenta previa, active genital herpes, positive HIV status with a high viral load)

- Birth is necessary but labour is not inducible (e.g., hypertensive states that cause an intrauterine environment that threatens the health of the fetus)
- This course of action has been chosen by the primary health care provider and the woman (e.g., a repeat or elective Caesarean birth).

Women who are scheduled for a Caesarean birth have time to prepare for it psychologically. However, the psychological responses of these women may vary. Those having a repeat Caesarean birth can have disturbing memories of the conditions preceding the initial (primary) Caesarean birth and their experiences in the postoperative recovery period. They may be concerned about the added burden of caring for an infant and perhaps other children while recovering from a surgical operation. Others may feel glad to have been relieved of the uncertainty about the date and time of birth and to be free from the pain of labour.

Unplanned Caesarean Birth

The psychosocial outcomes of unplanned or emergency Caesarean birth are usually more pronounced and negative in nature than the outcomes associated with a scheduled or planned Caesarean birth. Women and their families experience abrupt changes in their expectations for birth, postpartum care, and the care of the new baby at home. This may be a traumatic experience for all involved.

The woman may approach the procedure tired and discouraged after a difficult labour. She may worry about her own safety and well-being and that of her fetus. She may be dehydrated, with low glycogen reserves. Because preoperative procedures must be done quickly and competently, the time available for explanation of the procedures and operation is often short. Maternal and family anxiety levels tend to run high at this time, so much of what is said may be forgotten or misunderstood. The woman may experience feelings of anger or guilt in the postpartum period. Fatigue is often noticeable in these women, and they need much supportive care.

After surgery, it is important to spend time with the woman reviewing the events preceding the operation and the operation itself to ensure that she understands what has happened and that gaps in her recollections are filled. This approach will help create more realistic memories of the childbirth experience and can thus leave a more positive impression for future pregnancies and labours.

Forced Caesarean Birth

A woman's refusal to undergo a Caesarean birth required for fetal reasons is often described as having a maternal–fetal conflict. Health care providers are ethically obliged to protect the well-being of both the mother and the fetus; a decision for one affects the other. If a woman refuses a Caesarean birth that is recommended because of fetal jeopardy, health care providers must make every effort to find out why she is refusing and provide clear information to ensure that she is making an informed decision. If the woman continues to refuse surgery, the health care providers must decide if it is ethical to get a court

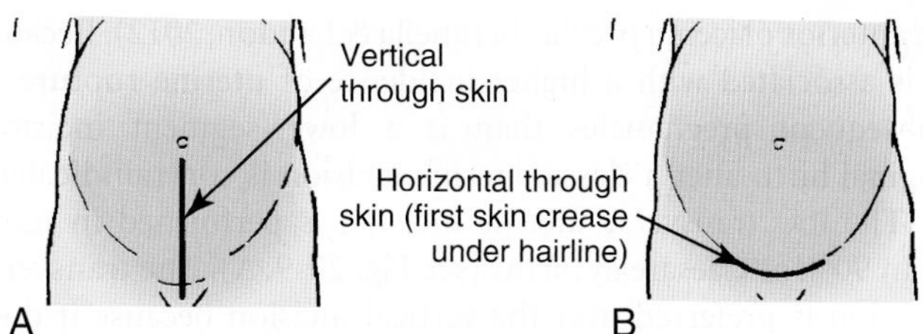

FIGURE 20-8 Skin incisions for Caesarean birth. **A:** Vertical. **B:** Horizontal (Pfannenstiel).

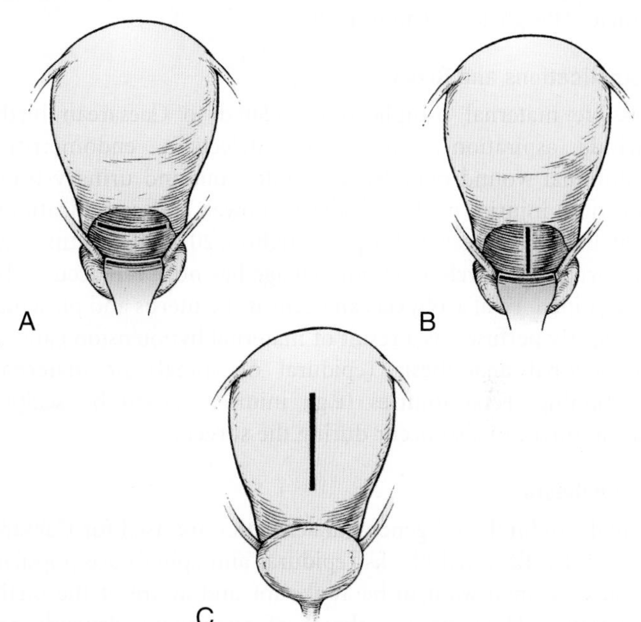

FIGURE 20-9 Uterine incisions for Caesarean birth. **A:** Low transverse incision. **B:** Low vertical incision. **C:** Classic incision. (From Gabbe, S. G., Niebyl, J., Simpson, J., et al. (2012). *Obstetrics: Normal and problem pregnancies* (6th ed.). Philadelphia: Saunders.)

order for the surgery; however, every effort should be made to avoid this legal step.

Surgical Techniques

The skin incision used is either vertical, extending from near the umbilicus to the mons pubis, or transverse (Pfannenstiel) in the lower abdomen (Fig. 20-8). The transverse incision, sometimes referred to as the "bikini" incision, is performed more often. The type of skin incision is generally determined by the urgency of the surgery and the presence of any prior skin incisions (Berghella & Landon, 2012). The type of skin incision does *not* necessarily indicate the type of uterine incision.

The two main types of uterine incision are the low transverse incision (Fig. 20-9, A) and the vertical incision, which may be either low or classic (see Fig. 20-9, B and C). Ideally, the vertical incision is contained entirely within the lower uterine segment, but extension into the contractile portion of the uterus (e.g., a classic incision) can occur (Berghella & Landon, 2012). Indications for a vertical incision include an underdeveloped lower uterine segment, a transverse lie or preterm breech presentation, certain fetal anomalies such as massive hydrocephalus, and an anterior placenta previa (Berghella & Landon, 2012). Because it is associated with a higher incidence of uterine rupture in subsequent pregnancies than is a lower-segment incision, vaginal birth after a classic uterine incision is contraindicated.

The low transverse uterine incision is performed in more than 90% of Caesarean births (see Fig. 20-9, A). The transverse incision is preferred over the vertical incision because it does not compromise the upper uterine segment, is easier to perform and repair, and is associated with less blood loss. It also provides for the option of trial of labour and VBAC in subsequent pregnancies (Berghella & Landon, 2012).

Complications and Risks

Possible maternal complications related to Caesarean birth include aspiration, hemorrhage, atelectasis, endometritis, abdominal wound dehiscence or infection, and urinary tract infection; injuries to the bladder or bowel; and complications related to anaesthesia (Thorp & Laughon, 2014). The fetus may be born prematurely if gestational age has not been accurately determined. Fetal asphyxia can occur if the uterus and placenta are poorly perfused as a result of maternal hypotension caused by regional anaesthesia (epidural or spinal) or maternal positioning. Fetal injuries (e.g., injuries caused by scalpel lacerations) can also occur during the surgery.

Anaesthesia

Spinal, epidural, and general anaesthetics are used for Caesarean births. Regional blocks (epidural and spinal) are popular because women want to be awake for and aware of the birth experience. However, the choice of anaesthetic depends on several factors. The mother's medical history or present condition, such as a spinal injury, hemorrhage, or coagulopathy, may rule out the use of regional anaesthesia. In the case of an emergency and the mother's or infant's life being at risk, general anaesthesia will most likely be used unless an epidural is already in place. The woman herself is a factor. She may not know all the options or may have fears about "a needle in her back" or of being awake and feeling pain. She needs to be fully informed about the risks and benefits of the different types of anaesthesia so that she can participate in the decision whenever there is a choice to be made. See Chapter 18 for further discussion.

Prenatal Preparation

A discussion of Caesarean birth should be included in all childbirth preparation classes. No woman can be guaranteed a vaginal birth, even if she is in good health and no indication of danger to the fetus exists before the onset of labour. Therefore, every woman needs to be aware of and prepared for the possibility of having a Caesarean birth.

Childbirth educators should emphasize the similarities and differences between a Caesarean and a vaginal birth. Most hospitals permit fathers and other partners and family members to share in these births as they do in vaginal births. Women who have undergone Caesarean birth agree that the continued presence and support of their partners helped them respond more positively to the entire experience. In addition, hospitals are moving toward practices in the operating room, such as skin-to-skin, that help normalize the birth process for the mother and the baby. See Additional Resources for video resource on breastfeeding after Caesarean birth.

Childbirth educators should prepare women for the possibility of Caesarean birth, but more importantly they should empower women to believe in their ability to give birth vaginally and to seek care measures during labour that will enhance the progress of their labours and reduce their risk for Caesarean birth.

NURSING CARE

Preoperative Care

Family-centred care is the goal for the woman who is to undergo Caesarean birth and for her family. The preparation of the woman for Caesarean birth is the same as that for other elective or emergency surgery. The primary health care provider discusses with the woman and her family the need for the Caesarean birth and the prognosis for mother and infant. The anaesthesiologist assesses the woman's cardiopulmonary system and describes the options for anaesthesia. Women who are scheduled for an elective Caesarean are often told to remain NPO (nothing by mouth) for at least 8 hours before the surgery. Informed consent is obtained for the procedure.

Blood and urine tests are usually done within a week before a planned Caesarean birth or on admission to the labour unit. Laboratory tests, most commonly ordered to establish baseline data, include a complete blood cell count, blood typing, and possibly a urinalysis. Maternal vital signs and blood pressure and FHR and pattern continue to be assessed per hospital routine until the operation begins. Intravenous fluids are started to maintain hydration and to provide an open line for the administration of medications and for blood, if needed. Other physical preoperative preparation usually includes inserting a retention (Foley) catheter to keep the bladder empty (this should be done after administration of anaesthetic, if possible) and administering prescribed preoperative medications. In the rare instance that an abdominal-mons shave or a clipping of pubic hair is ordered by the primary health care provider, this is performed in the operating room just before making the incision because shaving can result in injury of the integument, thereby increasing the risk for infection. Often TED hose and SCD boots will be placed on the woman's legs to prevent blood clot formation, especially if she is determined to be at risk for development of a thrombophlebitis. An antacid is often administered orally to neutralize gastric secretions in case of aspiration. Removal of contact lenses, dentures, nail polish, and jewellery may be optional, depending on hospital policies and type of anaesthesia used. If the woman wears glasses and is going to be awake, the nurse should make sure that her glasses accompany her to the operating room so she can see her infant.

During preoperative preparation, the support person is encouraged to remain with the woman as much as possible to provide continuing emotional support (if this is culturally acceptable to the woman and support person). The nurse needs to provide essential information about the preoperative procedures during this time. Although nursing actions may have to be carried out quickly if a Caesarean birth is unplanned, verbal communication, particularly explanations, is important. Silence and lack of information can be frightening to the woman and her support person. The nurse's use of touch (if culturally appropriate) can communicate feelings of care and concern for the woman. The nurse can assess the woman's and her partner's perceptions about Caesarean birth. As the woman expresses her feelings, the nurse may identify possible self-concept concerns that may need to be addressed during the postpartum period. If there is time before the birth, the nurse can teach the woman about postoperative expectations and pain relief, turning, coughing, and deep-breathing measures.

Intraoperative Care

Caesarean births occur in operating rooms in the surgical suite or in the labour and birth unit. Once the woman has been taken to the operating room, her care becomes the responsibility of the obstetrical team, surgeon, anaesthesiologist, and surgical nursing staff (Fig. 20-10). If possible, the partner or another person, dressed appropriately for the operating room, accompanies the mother to the surgical unit and remains close to her so that continued support and comfort can be provided. In an unplanned Caesarean birth, the nurse who cared for the woman during labour should be part of the interprofessional care team in the operating room, if possible.

The nurse who is circulating can assist with positioning the woman on the birth (surgical) table. It is important to position her so that the uterus is displaced laterally, to prevent compressing the inferior vena cava, which causes decreased placental perfusion. This is usually accomplished by placing a wedge under the hip. The woman's legs should be strapped to the table to ensure proper positioning during the surgery. A Foley catheter is inserted into the bladder at this time if one is not already in place.

If the partner either is not allowed or has chosen not to be present in the operative suite, the nurse can stay in communication with him or her and give progress reports whenever possible. If the mother is awake during the birth, the nurse or anaesthetist can tell her what is happening and provide support. The mother may be anxious about the sensations she is experiencing, such as the coldness of solutions used to prepare the abdomen and pressure or pulling during the actual birth of the infant. She also may be apprehensive because of the bright lights or the presence of unfamiliar equipment and masked and gowned personnel in the room. Explanations by the nurse can help decrease the woman's anxiety.

Care of the infant usually is delegated to a nurse or other care provider skilled in neonatal resuscitation. If risk factors are present, a pediatrician may also be present. An infant warmer with resuscitation equipment is readied before surgery. Those responsible for care are expert not only in resuscitative techniques but also in the ability to detect normal and abnormal infant responses. After birth, if the infant's condition permits and the mother is awake, the baby may be placed skin-to-skin on the mother or her partner or can be given to the woman's partner to hold (Fig. 20-11). The infant whose condition is compromised is transported after initial stabilization to the nursery for observation and the implementation of appropriate interventions. In some institutions, the partner may accompany the infant; if not, personnel should keep the family informed of the infant's progress, and parent–infant contacts are initiated as soon as possible.

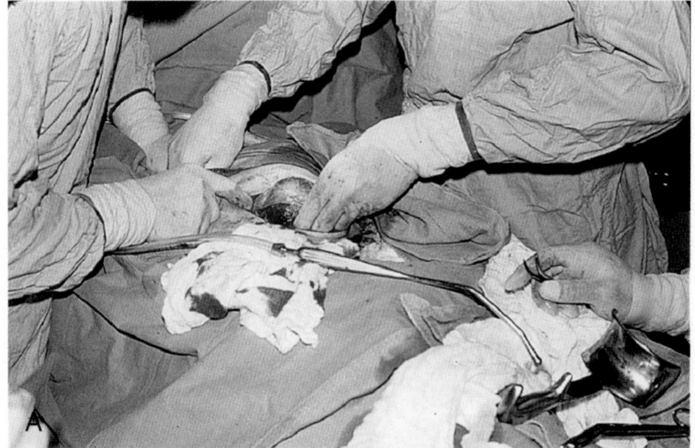

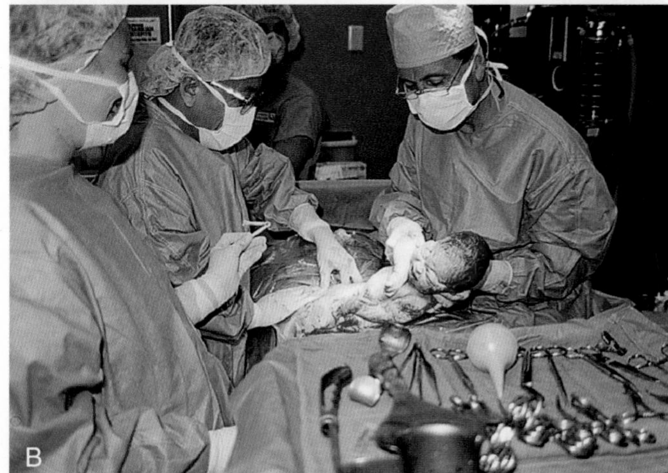

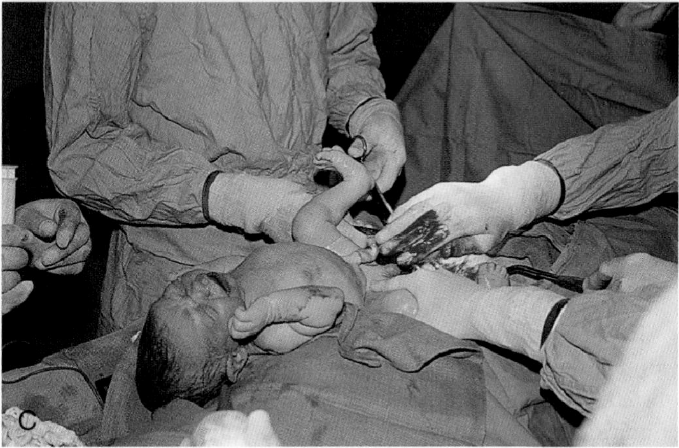

FIGURE 20-10 Caesarean birth. **A:** "Bikini" incision has been made, the muscle layer is separated, the abdomen is entered, the uterus has been exposed and incised. Note small amount of bleeding. **B:** The newborn's birth through the uterine incision is nearly complete. **C:** A quick assessment is performed; note significant moulding of head resulting from cephalopelvic disproportion. (Courtesy Marjorie Pyle, RNC, Lifecircle.)

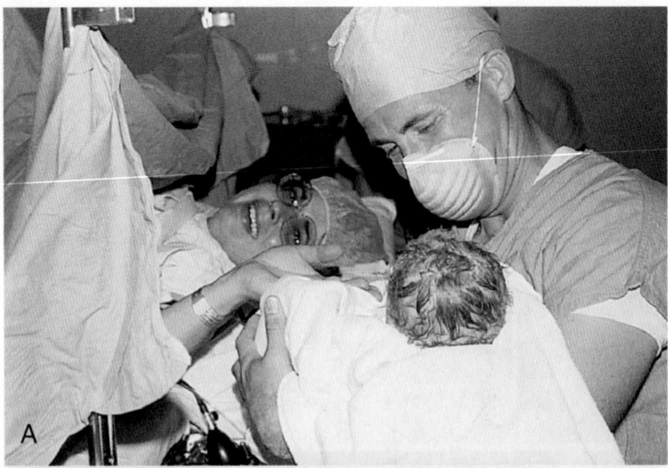

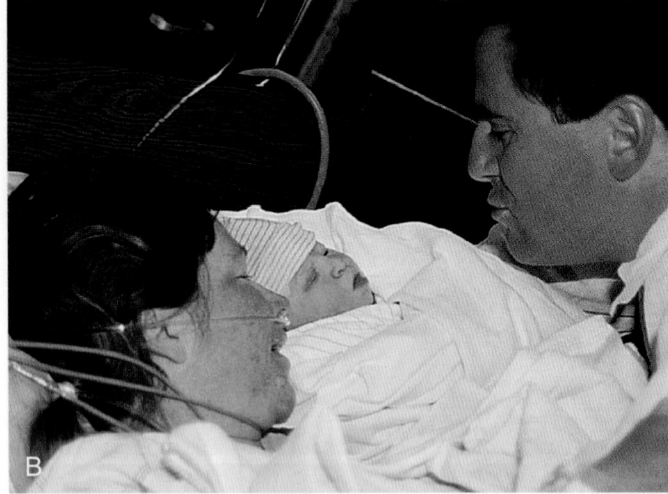

FIGURE 20-11 **A:** Parents and their newborn. The physician manually removes the placenta; suctions the remaining amniotic fluid and blood from the uterine cavity; and closes the uterine incision, peritoneum, muscle layer, fatty tissue, and, finally, the skin while the new family shares some private time. **B:** Parents become better acquainted with their newborn while mother rests after surgery. (Courtesy Marjorie Pyle, RNC, Lifecircle.)

If the family cannot (or does not want to) accompany the woman during surgery, they are directed to the surgical or obstetrical waiting room. The physician then reports on the condition of the mother and child to family members after the birth is completed. Family members may accompany the infant if he or she needs to be transferred to the nursery, giving them an opportunity to see the new baby.

Immediate Postoperative Care

Once surgery is completed, the mother is transferred to a recovery room or back to her labour room. Women who undergo a Caesarean birth have both postoperative and postpartum needs that must be addressed. They are surgical patients, as well as new mothers. Nursing assessments in this immediate postbirth period follow agency protocol and include degree of recovery from the effects of anaesthesia, postoperative and postbirth status, and degree of pain. If general anaesthesia was administered, it is essential that a patent airway be maintained and that the woman be positioned to prevent possible aspiration until she is fully alert and responsive (see Chapter 18, p. 484). Vital signs should be taken every 15 minutes for 1 to 2 hours or until stable. The condition of the incisional dressing, the fundus, and the amount of lochia need to be assessed, as well as intravenous intake and urine output through the Foley catheter. Oxytocin is usually added to at least the first litre of the intravenous infusion to ensure that the fundus remains firmly contracted, thereby reducing blood loss. The woman should be helped to turn and do coughing, deep-breathing, and leg exercises. Medications for pain relief should be administered before postoperative pain becomes severe.

Routine postpartum care is organized to facilitate parent–infant interaction as soon as possible and to answer the mother's questions. When appropriate, the nurse should assess the mother's readiness to see the baby, as well as her response to the anaesthesia and to the event that may have necessitated general anaesthesia (e.g., emergency Caesarean birth when vaginal birth was anticipated). If the baby is present, the mother and her partner should be given some time alone with the baby to facilitate bonding and attachment. Newborns should be placed skin-to-skin with the mothers as soon as possible, and breastfeeding can be initiated when the mother feels like trying, preferably within the first 30 to 60 minutes. If the woman is in a recovery area or her labour room, she usually is transferred to the postpartum unit after 1 to 2 hours or once her condition is stable and the effects of anaesthesia have worn off (i.e., she is alert, oriented, and able to feel and move extremities).

Postoperative or Postpartum Care

The attitude of the nurse and other health team members can influence the woman's perception of herself after a Caesarean birth. The caregivers should stress that the woman is a new mother first and a surgical patient second. This attitude helps the woman perceive herself as having the same problems and needs as those of other new mothers while at the same time requiring supportive postoperative care.

The woman's physiological concerns for the first few days may be dominated by pain at the incision site and pain resulting from intestinal gas, thus the need for pain relief. For the first 24 hours after surgery, pain relief can be provided by epidural opioids, patient-controlled analgesia (PCA), or intravenous or intramuscular injections. The most commonly used analgesics include opioids (e.g., hydromorphone or morphine sulphate) and NSAIDs (e.g., naproxen). If opioids are used, an antiemetic (e.g., promethazine [Phenergan], ondansetron [Zofran]) is often ordered to be administered either as needed by the woman or around the clock as long as the opioid is used. Palpation of the fundus with the possibility of massage should be performed after an analgesic is given to decrease pain. By 24 hours after surgery, women are generally given oral analgesics. Other comfort measures such as position changes, splinting the incision with pillows, and relaxation and breathing techniques may be implemented. Women are often the best judge of what their bodies need and can tolerate, including the postoperative ingestion of foods and fluids. Because most women have an epidural or spinal anaesthetic for surgery, most health care providers

PATIENT TEACHING

Postpartum Pain Relief After Caesarean Birth

Incisional Pain

- Splint incision with a pillow when moving or coughing.
- Use relaxation techniques such as music, breathing, and dim lights.

Intestinal Gas

- Walk as often as you can.
- Do not eat or drink gas-forming foods, carbonated beverages, or whole milk.
- Do not use straws for drinking fluids.
- Take antiflatulence medication if prescribed.
- Lie on your left side to expel gas.
- Rock in a rocking chair.

allow the early introduction of solid food if desired and tolerated. Some health care providers may order clear fluids until bowel sounds return, but research does not support this practice for gynecological surgery (Charoenkwan & Matovinovic, 2014). Intravenous fluids are usually continued until the woman is tolerating fluids orally. Ambulation and rocking in a rocking chair may relieve gas pains. Women should be taught to avoid gas-forming foods, ice chips, carbonated beverages, and using a straw to drink beverages, to help limit gas formation and thereby minimize the severity of gas pains (see Patient Teaching box).

Nurses must be alert to the woman's physiological needs, managing care to ensure adequate rest and pain relief. Mother–baby care (couplet care) for a Caesarean birth mother can be modified according to her physiological limitations as a surgical patient.

Daily care includes perineal care and routine hygienic care, including showering after the dressing has been removed (if showering is acceptable according to the woman's cultural beliefs and practices). The indwelling (Foley) catheter is also usually removed on the first postpartum day (usually within 8 to 12 hours). The woman is encouraged to be out of bed and ambulating several times each day as soon as the urinary catheter is removed. Use of TED hose or SCD boots should continue as long as the woman remains in bed. They may be removed when she begins ambulating. The nurse assesses the woman's vital signs, incision, fundus, and lochia according to hospital policies, procedures, or protocols. Breath sounds, bowel sounds, circulatory status of lower extremities, and urinary and bowel elimination also are assessed. It is important to note maternal emotional status and progress of attachment to her baby.

SAFETY ALERT

The woman should be taught to seek assistance initially when getting out of bed, especially when an intravenous line and catheter are still in place. Thereafter, when rising from a supine position, she should sit on the side of the bed first to determine if dizziness will occur, then stand at the bedside, and finally ambulate.

During the postpartum period, the nurse can provide care that meets the psychological and learning needs of mothers who have had Caesarean births. The nurse should explain postpartum procedures to help the woman participate in her recovery from surgery. Also, the nurse can help the woman plan care and visits from family and friends that allow for adequate rest periods. Information and assistance with infant care can facilitate adjustment to her role as a mother. The woman needs to be supported as she breastfeeds her baby, receiving individualized assistance to comfortably hold and position the baby at her breast. The side-lying position or football hold and the use of pillows to support the newborn can enhance comfort and facilitate successful breastfeeding.

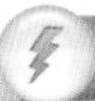

SAFETY ALERT

When holding her baby or breastfeeding, a woman may become drowsy and even fall asleep because of the sedation that occurs with the use of analgesics. It is important that someone be with her during these times.

Whether a Caesarean birth is planned (scheduled) or unplanned (emergency or determined to be necessary during labour), the loss of the experience of giving birth to an infant in the traditional manner may have a negative effect on a woman's self-confidence. She may feel frustration at losing control, disappointment, anger, and loss of self-esteem. These feelings are related to a change in body image and perceived inability to give birth as she had expected and hoped. Often women experience a delay in the ability to interact with their newborn after a Caesarean birth. They are less likely to breastfeed and may even have difficulty expressing positive feelings about their newborn for some time after birth. They often are less satisfied with their childbirth experience and report more fatigue and poor physical functioning during the first few weeks after discharge.

Success at mothering and in the recovery process can do much to restore the self-esteem of these women. Some women see the scar as mutilating, and worries about sexual attractiveness may surface. Some men are fearful of resuming intercourse because of the fear of hurting their partner. Parents may wonder if a Caesarean birth was absolutely necessary, and such feelings may surface even years later. A clear explanation should be given to the woman and her family regarding the necessity of the Caesarean birth. They should also be given opportunities to discuss the childbirth, in an effort to resolve concerns that may arise after the birth.

Discharge after Caesarean birth is usually by the second or third postoperative day. The woman's predominant needs at home are for rest and sleep; relief of pain and discomfort; and assistance with household chores, infant care and feeding, and self-care. The nurse must provide discharge teaching in the limited time the woman is in the hospital, while ensuring that the woman is comfortable and able to rest. The nurse should assess the woman's information needs and coordinate the health care team's efforts to meet them.

PATIENT TEACHING

Signs of Postoperative Complications After Discharge Following Caesarean Birth

Report the following signs to your health care provider:
- Temperature exceeding 38°C (100.4°F)
- Urination; painful urination, urgency, cloudy urine
- Lochia: a heavier than normal menstrual period, clots, odour
- Caesarean incision: redness, swelling, bruising, foul-smelling discharge or bleeding, wound separation
- Severe, increasing abdominal pain

Discharge teaching and planning should include information about the following:
- Nutrition
- Measures to relieve pain and discomfort
- Exercise and specific activity restrictions
- Time management that includes periods of uninterrupted rest and sleep
- Hygiene, breast, and incision care
- Timing for resumption of sexual activity and contraception
- Signs of complications (see Patient Teaching box)
- Infant care

The woman's family and friends should be educated about her needs during the recovery process, and their assistance should be coordinated before discharge. Referrals to community agencies may be indicated to further promote the recovery process. A postdischarge program of telephone follow-up and home visits can facilitate the woman's full recovery after Caesarean birth.

Trial of Labour

A *trial of labour* (TOL) is the observance of a woman and her fetus for a reasonable period of spontaneous active labour to assess the safety of vaginal birth for both. TOL may be initiated if the mother's pelvis is of questionable size or shape, if she wishes to have a vaginal birth after a previous Caesarean birth, or if the fetus is in an abnormal presentation. A woman who has had a previous low-segment Caesarean birth may be a candidate for a TOL. The cervix must be ripe (soft and dilatable). During a TOL, the woman is evaluated for the occurrence of active labour, including adequate contractions, engagement and descent of the presenting part, and effacement and dilation of the cervix.

The perinatal nurse assesses maternal vital signs and FHR and pattern and should be alert for signs of potential complications. If complications develop, the nurse is responsible for initiating appropriate actions, including notifying the primary health care provider, and for evaluating and documenting the maternal and fetal responses to the interventions. Supporting and encouraging the woman and her partner and providing information on progress can reduce stress, enhance the labour process, and facilitate a successful outcome.

BOX 20-13 SELECTION CRITERIA FOR VAGINAL BIRTH AFTER CAESAREAN

- One or two previous low-transverse Caesarean births
- Clinically adequate pelvis
- No other uterine scars or history of previous rupture
- Physicians available throughout active labour capable of monitoring labour and performing an emergency Caesarean birth if necessary

Data from American College of Obstetricians and Gynecologists (ACOG). (2010). *Vaginal birth after previous cesarean delivery* (ACOG Practice Bulletin No. 115), Washington, DC: Author.

CRITICAL THINKING CASE STUDY

Trial of Labour for Vaginal Birth After Caesarean (TOL/VBAC)

Heather, a 28-year-old G2T1P0A0L, gave birth by Caesarean during her last pregnancy. During her routine prenatal visit at 32 weeks of gestation, Heather tells the nurse that she really wants to have a vaginal birth this time. Heather asks, "What do you think? Can I try for a VBAC?"

QUESTIONS

1. Evidence—Is there sufficient evidence to advise Heather about the safety and feasibility of a trial of labour (TOL) for vaginal birth after Caesarean (VBAC)?
2. Assumptions—Describe an underlying assumption about each of the following issues:
   a. Risks that Heather faces if she chooses a TOL for VBAC
   b. Criteria that must be met for Heather to attempt a TOL for VBAC
   c. Labour management practices that facilitate a successful VBAC
3. What implications and priorities for nursing care can be drawn at this time?
4. Does the evidence objectively support your argument (conclusion)?

Vaginal Birth After Caesarean (VBAC)

Indications for primary Caesarean birth such as dystocia, breech presentation, or abnormal FHR pattern often are nonrecurring. Therefore, a woman who has had a Caesarean birth and subsequently becomes pregnant may not have any contraindications to labour and vaginal birth in that pregnancy and may choose to attempt a VBAC. Box 20-13 lists selection criteria suggested by the ACOG for identifying candidates for VBAC. Women who succeed in having a VBAC and thus avoid major abdominal surgery have less hemorrhage, fewer infections, and a shorter recovery period than do women who give birth by repeat Caesarean (ACOG, 2010). The major risk associated with VBAC is uterine rupture (Berghella & Landon, 2012). Other maternal risks include operative injury, blood transfusion, hysterectomy, endometritis, and maternal death (ACOG, 2010) (see Critical Thinking Case Study).

The overall VBAC success rate is approximately 60 to 80%. The strongest predictors for a successful VBAC are a prior vaginal birth and spontaneous (rather than induced or augmented) labour (ACOG, 2010). Women whose first Caesarean birth was performed because of a nonrecurring indication (e.g., breech presentation) also are likely to have a successful VBAC (Berghella & Landon, 2012). Women with the following characteristics are less likely to have a successful VBAC (ACOG, 2010):

- Recurrent indication (e.g., labour dystocia) for initial Caesarean birth
- Increased maternal age
- Non-White race or ethnicity
- Gestational age >40 weeks
- Maternal obesity
- Pre-eclampsia
- Short interpregnancy interval
- Increased neonatal birth weight

Women are most often the primary decision makers with regard to choice of birth method. During the antepartum period, the woman should be given information about VBAC and encouraged to choose it as an alternative to a repeat Caesarean, as long as no contraindications exist. VBAC support groups (see Additional Resources at end of the chapter) and prenatal classes can help prepare the woman psychologically for labour and vaginal birth. Women need to believe not only that their efforts during a TOL will be successful but also that they are fully capable of doing what is necessary to give birth vaginally. They must be given the opportunity to discuss their previous labour experience, including feelings of failure and loss of control, and to express concern they may have about how they will manage during their upcoming labour and birth. Not everyone is enthusiastic about TOL and VBAC. After being fully informed about the benefits and risks, more than 25% of potential candidates choose to have a repeat Caesarean birth instead (Thorp & Laughon, 2014).

There is conflicting evidence that administering oxytocin to induce or augment labour increases the risk of uterine rupture. If oxytocin is used for the TOL, caution and close monitoring of the labouring woman are urged. However, use of prostaglandins to ripen the cervix or induce labour is not recommended because they have been associated with an increased risk for uterine rupture.

If a woman chooses TOL, attention should be given to her psychological as well as physical needs during the TOL. Anxiety increases the release of catecholamines and can inhibit the release of oxytocin, delaying the progress of labour and possibly leading to a repeat Caesarean birth. To alleviate anxiety, the nurse can encourage the woman to use breathing and relaxation techniques and change position to promote labour progress. The woman's partner can be encouraged to provide comfort measures and emotional support. Collaboration among the woman in labour, her partner, the nurse, and other health care providers often results in a successful VBAC. If a TOL does not proceed to vaginal birth, the woman will need support and encouragement to express her feelings about having another Caesarean birth. It is important that this outcome not be labelled a failed VBAC.

Many women who are appropriate candidates for TOL and VBAC lack access to providers and health care facilities that are able and willing to offer this option. Because resources for immediate Caesarean birth may not be available in all birthing facilities, the best alternative in some situations may be to refer interested women to other facilities that have the obstetrical, anaesthetic, pediatric, and surgical staff necessary to offer TOL and VBAC (Berghella & Landon, 2012).

OBSTETRICAL EMERGENCIES

Meconium-Stained Amniotic Fluid

Meconium-stained amniotic fluid indicates that the fetus has passed meconium (first stool) before birth. Meconium-stained amniotic fluid is green. The consistency of the amniotic fluid is often described as either thin (light) or thick (heavy), depending on the amount of meconium present. Three possible reasons for the passage of meconium are as follows:

- It is a normal physiological function that occurs with maturity (meconium passage being infrequent before weeks 23 or 24, with an increased incidence after 38 weeks) or with a breech presentation.
- It is the result of hypoxia-induced peristalsis and sphincter relaxation.
- It may be a sequel to umbilical cord compression–induced vagal stimulation in mature fetuses.

The major risk associated with meconium-stained amniotic fluid is the development of **meconium aspiration syndrome (MAS)** in the newborn. MAS causes a severe form of aspiration pneumonia that occurs most often in term or postterm infants who have passed meconium in utero. MAS most likely results from a long-standing intrauterine process rather than from aspiration immediately after birth as respirations are initiated (Rozance & Rosenberg, 2012).

Collaborative Care

The presence of a team skilled in neonatal resuscitation is required at the birth of any infant with meconium-stained amniotic fluid. To address occurrence of meconium-stained amniotic fluid, the Canadian Paediatric Society along with the American Academy of Pediatrics and the AHA Neonatal Resuscitation Program no longer recommends routine suctioning of the newborn's mouth and nose on the perineum (after the head is out but before the rest of the baby is born) followed by endotracheal suctioning after birth. Instead, management of a newborn with meconium-stained amniotic fluid is based only on assessment of the baby's condition at birth. No clinical studies warrant basing tracheal suctioning guidelines simply on meconium consistency (AAP & AHA, 2011). See the Emergency box for specific interventions.

SAFETY ALERT

Every birth should be attended by at least one person whose only responsibility is the baby and who is capable of initiating resuscitation. Either that person or someone else who is immediately available should have the skills required to perform a complete resuscitation, including endotracheal suctioning to remove meconium, if necessary.

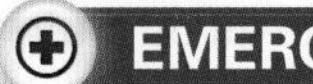

EMERGENCY

Immediate Management of the Newborn With Meconium-Stained Amniotic Fluid

Before Birth

- Assess the amniotic fluid for the presence of meconium after rupture of membranes.
- If the amniotic fluid is meconium stained, gather equipment and supplies that might be necessary for neonatal resuscitation.
- Have at least one person capable of performing endotracheal intubation on the baby present at the birth.

Immediately After Birth

- Assess the baby's respiratory efforts, heart rate, and muscle tone.
- Consider suctioning only the baby's mouth and nose if the baby has:
  - Strong respiratory efforts
  - Good muscle tone
  - Heart rate >100 beats/min
- Suction the trachea using an endotracheal tube connected to a meconium aspiration device and suction source to remove any meconium present before many spontaneous respirations have occurred or assisted ventilation has been initiated if the baby has:
  - Depressed respirations
  - Decreased muscle tone
  - Heart rate <100 beats/min

Data from American Academy of Pediatrics (AAP) and American Heart Association (AHA). (2011). *Textbook of neonatal resuscitation* (6th ed.). Elk Grove Village, IL: AAP.

Shoulder Dystocia

Shoulder dystocia is an uncommon obstetrical emergency that increases the risk for fetal or neonatal and maternal morbidity and mortality during the attempt to deliver the fetus vaginally. It is a condition in which the head is born but the anterior shoulder cannot pass under the pubic arch. It is estimated that 0.6 to 1.4% of all vaginal births are complicated by shoulder dystocia (Cunningham et al., 2014). The incidence of shoulder dystocia has increased in recent years, perhaps because of larger birth weights or simply because more attention is now paid to documenting the condition (Cunningham et al., 2014).

Fetopelvic disproportion caused by excessive fetal size (greater than 4000 g) or maternal pelvic abnormalities may be a cause of shoulder dystocia, although up to half of all cases of shoulder dystocia occur with smaller fetuses (Lanni & Seeds, 2012; Thorp & Laughon, 2014). Other risk factors for shoulder dystocia include maternal diabetes (risk for macrosomia) and a history of shoulder dystocia with a previous birth. In half of all cases of shoulder dystocia, however, no risk factors are identified (Thorp & Laughon, 2014). Shoulder dystocia cannot be accurately predicted or prevented (Cunningham et al., 2014). Retraction of the fetal head against the perineum immediately after its emergence (turtle sign), however, is an early warning sign that birth of the shoulders may be difficult (Thorp & Laughon, 2014).

Fetal injuries are usually caused either by asphyxia related to the delay in completing the birth or by trauma from the manoeuvres used to accomplish the birth. Complications related to trauma include brachial plexus and phrenic nerve injuries and fracture of the humerus or clavicle. The most serious complication is brachial plexus injury (Erb palsy), which occurs in 10 to 20% of infants born following shoulder dystocia (Thorp & Laughon, 2014). Evidence now exists that brachial plexus injuries may result from intrauterine forces during the second stage of labour rather than from the manoeuvres used to accomplish birth (Lanni & Seeds, 2012). If brachial plexus injuries are recognized early and treated properly, 80 to 90% heal completely. Therefore, permanent neurological injury is rare. The major maternal complications associated with shoulder dystocia are postpartum hemorrhage and rectal injuries (Thorp & Laughon, 2014).

Collaborative Care

Many manoeuvres, such as suprapubic pressure and maternal position changes, have been suggested and tried to free the anterior shoulder. Suprapubic pressure can be applied to the anterior shoulder using the Mazzanti or Rubin technique (Fig. 20-12) in an attempt to push the shoulder under the symphysis pubis.

In the McRoberts manoeuvre (Fig. 20-13), the woman's legs are flexed apart with her knees on her abdomen. This manoeuvre causes the sacrum to straighten, and the symphysis pubis rotates toward the mother's head; the angle of pelvic inclination is decreased, freeing the shoulder. Suprapubic pressure can be applied at this time. The McRoberts manoeuvre is the preferred method when a woman is receiving epidural anaesthesia.

Having the woman move to a hands-and-knees position (the Gaskin manoeuvre), a squatting position, or a lateral recumbent position also has been used to resolve cases of shoulder dystocia. However, the Gaskin manoeuvre requires that the woman be mobile with no significant loss of motor function caused by regional anaesthesia. Also, a wide and stable surface must be available (Lanni & Seeds, 2012).

Fundal pressure as a method of relieving shoulder dystocia should be avoided. Its use has been associated with neurological complications (Gilbert, 2011).

When shoulder dystocia is diagnosed, the nurse should stay calm and immediately call for additional assistance. The nurse then helps the woman assume the position(s) that may facilitate birth of the shoulders, assist the primary health care provider with these manoeuvres, and monitor the fetal response. The nurse should also provide encouragement and support to reduce anxiety and fear.

Newborn assessment should include examination for fracture of the clavicle or humerus, brachial plexus injuries, and asphyxia. Maternal assessment should focus on early detection of hemorrhage and trauma to the soft tissue of the birth canal.

Prolapsed Umbilical Cord

Prolapse of the umbilical cord occurs when the cord lies below the presenting part of the fetus. Umbilical cord prolapse may be occult (hidden, not visible) at any time during labour, regardless of whether or not membranes are ruptured (Fig. 20-14, A and B). It is most common to see frank (visible) prolapse directly after rupture of membranes, when gravity washes

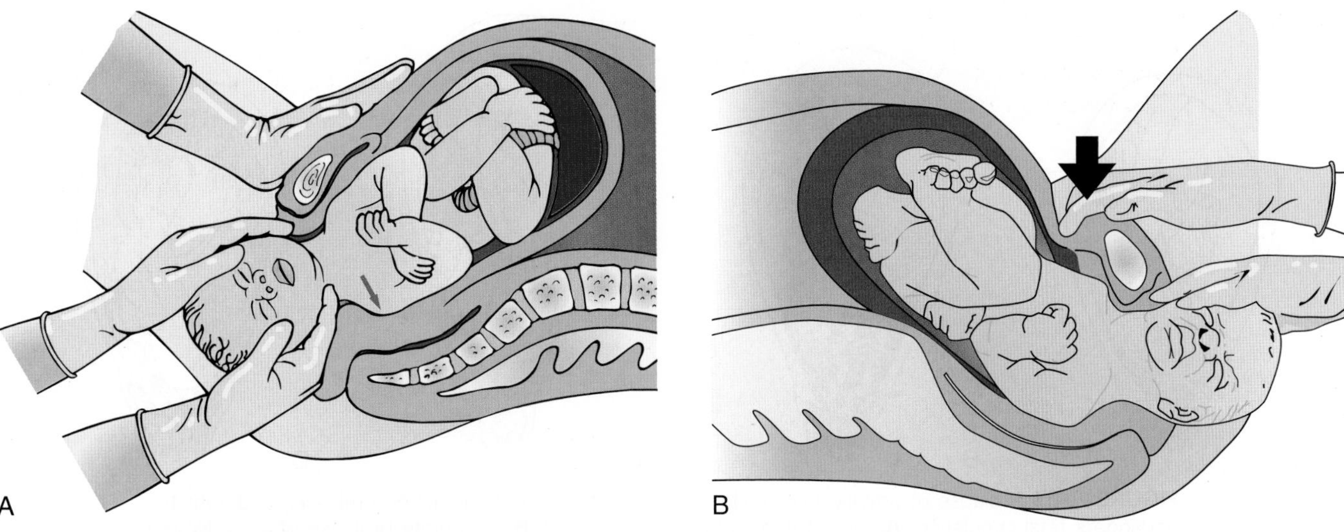

FIGURE 20-12 Application of suprapubic pressure. **A:** Mazzanti technique: Pressure is applied directly posteriorly and laterally above the symphysis pubis. **B:** Rubin technique: Pressure is applied obliquely posteriorly against the anterior shoulder.

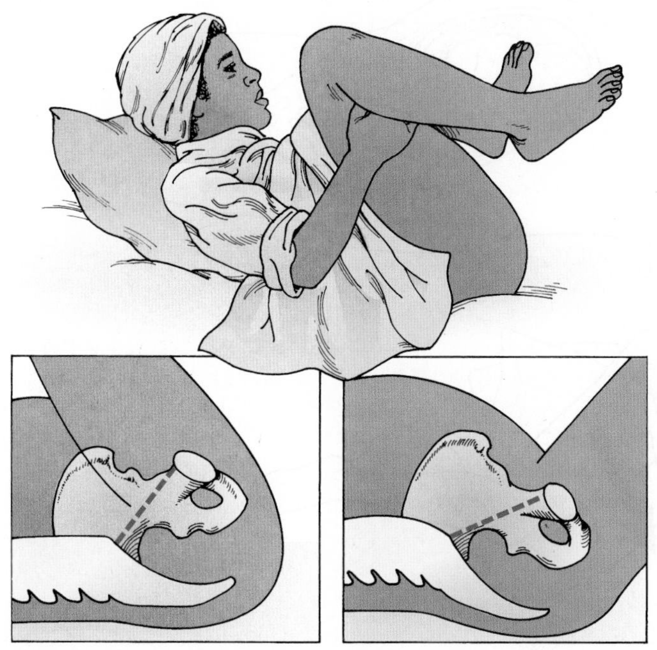

FIGURE 20-13 McRoberts manoeuvre. (Adapted from Lanni, S. M., & Seeds, J. W. [2007]. Malpresentations. In S. G. Gabbe, J. R. Niebyl, & J. L. Simpson [Eds.], *Obstetrics: Normal and problem pregnancies* [5th ed.]. New York: Churchill Livingstone.)

the cord in front of the presenting part (see Fig. 20-14, C and D). Contributing factors are a long cord (longer than 100 cm), malpresentation (breech or transverse lie), or unengaged presenting part.

If the presenting part does not fit snugly into the lower uterine segment, as in polyhydramnios, when the membranes rupture, a sudden gush of amniotic fluid may cause the cord to be displaced downward. Similarly, the cord may prolapse during amniotomy if the presenting part is high. A small or preterm fetus may not fit snugly into the lower uterine segment; as a result, cord prolapse is more likely to occur.

Collaborative Care

Prompt recognition of a prolapsed cord is important because fetal hypoxia resulting from prolonged cord compression (i.e., occlusion of blood flow to and from the fetus for more than 5 minutes) can occur and potentially lead to fetal hypoxia, newborn asphyxia, neurological brain injury, or death of the fetus. Pressure on the cord may be relieved by the examiner putting a sterile gloved hand into the vagina and holding the presenting part off of the umbilical cord (Fig. 20-15, A and B). The woman should be assisted into a position such as a modified Sims' (see Fig. 20-15, C), Trendelenburg, or knee–chest (see Fig. 20-15, D) position, in which gravity keeps the presenting part off the cord. If the cervix is fully dilated, a forceps- or vacuum-assisted birth can be performed for the fetus in a cephalic presentation; otherwise, emergent Caesarean surgery is likely to be performed. Abnormal FHR and pattern (e.g., bradycardia, absent or minimal variability, and variable or prolonged decelerations), inadequate uterine relaxation, and bleeding also can occur as a result of a prolapsed umbilical cord. Indications for immediate interventions are presented in the Emergency box. Ongoing assessment of the woman and her fetus is critical to determine the effectiveness of each action taken. The woman and her family are often aware of the seriousness of the situation; therefore, the nurse must provide support by giving explanations for the interventions being implemented and their effect on the status of the fetus.

Rupture of the Uterus

Rupture of the uterus, in which there is complete nonsurgical disruption of all uterine layers, is a rare but very serious obstetrical injury that occurs in 1 in 2000 births (Francois & Foley, 2012). During labour and birth, the major risk factor for uterine rupture is a scarred uterus as a result of previous Caesarean birth or other uterine surgery. Rupture usually occurs during a TOL for VBAC; symptomatic rupture is rarely observed in planned, repeat Caesarean births. The likelihood of uterine

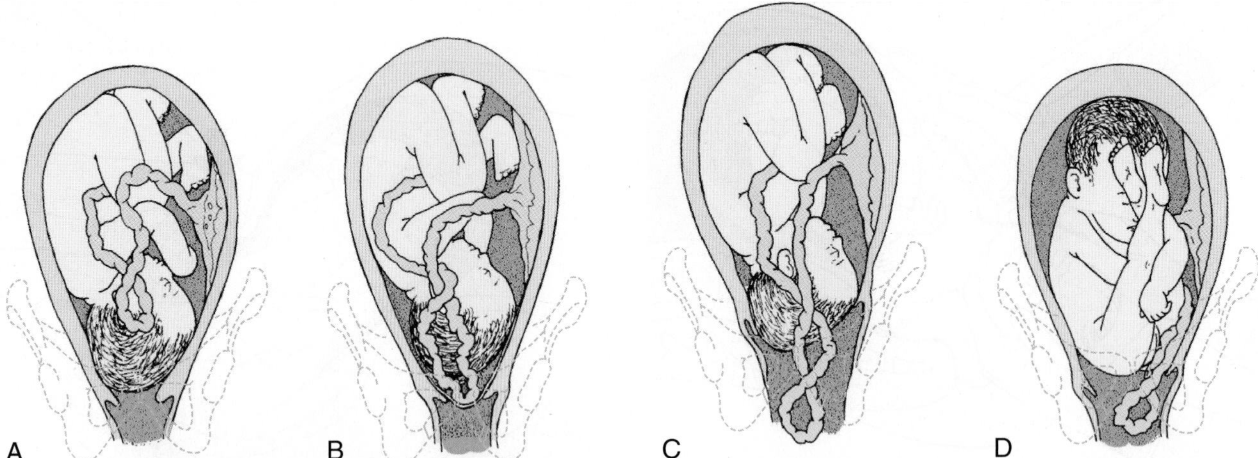

FIGURE 20-14 Prolapse of umbilical cord. Note pressure of presenting part on umbilical cord, which endangers fetal circulation. **A:** Occult (hidden) prolapse of cord. **B:** Complete prolapse of cord. Note that membranes are intact. **C:** Cord presenting in front of fetal head may be seen in vagina. **D:** Frank breech presentation with prolapsed cord.

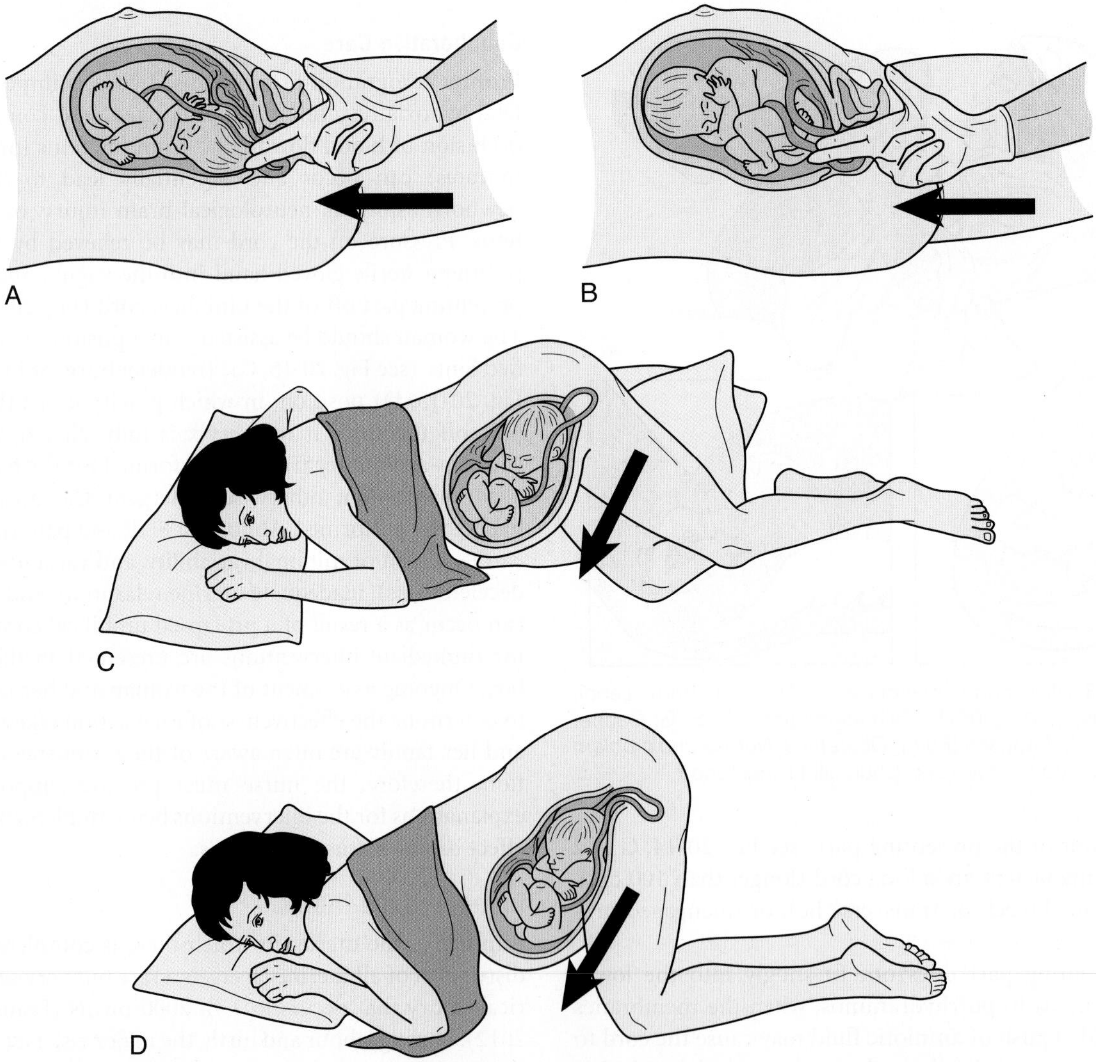

A

B

C

D

FIGURE 20-15 *Arrows* indicate direction of pressure against presenting part to relieve compression of prolapsed umbilical cord. Pressure exerted by examiner's fingers in **A:** vertex presentation, and **B:** breech presentation. **C:** Gravity relieves pressure when woman is in modified Sims' position with hips elevated as high as possible with pillows. **D:** Knee–chest position.

EMERGENCY

Prolapsed Cord

Signs

- Variable or prolonged deceleration during uterine contraction.
- Woman reports feeling the cord after membranes rupture.
- Cord is seen or felt in or protruding from the vagina.

Interventions

- Call for assistance. Do not leave woman alone.
- Have someone notify the primary health care provider immediately.
- Glove the examining hand quickly and insert two fingers into the vagina to the cervix. With one finger on either side of the cord or both fingers to one side, exert upward pressure against the presenting part to relieve compression of the cord (see Fig. 20-15, A and B). Do not move your hand. Another person may place a rolled towel under the woman's right or left hip.
- Place woman into the extreme Trendelenburg or a modified Sims' position (see Fig. 20-15, C), or a knee–chest position (see Fig. 20-15, D).
- If cord is protruding from the vagina, wrap it loosely in a sterile towel saturated with warm, sterile, normal saline solution. Do not attempt to replace cord into cervix.
- Administer oxygen to the woman by mask at 8 to 10 L/min until birth is accomplished.
- Start intravenous fluids or increase existing drip rate.
- Continue to monitor fetal heart rate continuously.
- Explain to woman and support person what is happening and the management plan.
- Prepare for immediate vaginal birth if the cervix is fully dilated or for Caesarean birth if it is not.

rupture varies, depending on the type and location of the previous uterine incision. Uterine rupture occurs most often with a previous classic incision. Other factors that increase the risk for uterine rupture include multiple prior Caesarean births, no previous vaginal births, induced or augmented labour, term gestation, multifetal gestation, fetal macrosomia, post-Caesarean birth infection, and short interpregnancy interval (Berghella & Landon, 2012; Francois & Foley, 2012).

Uterine dehiscence, sometimes called *incomplete uterine rupture,* is separation of a prior scar. It may go unnoticed unless the woman undergoes a subsequent Caesarean birth or other uterine surgery. The potential for maternal or fetal complications as a result of uterine dehiscence is negligible because separation of a prior scar does not result in hemorrhage (Berghella & Landon, 2012).

Signs and symptoms vary with the extent of the uterine rupture. The most common finding is an abnormal FHR tracing, particularly variable or prolonged decelerations or bradycardia. A loss of fetal station may also occur. The woman may experience constant abdominal pain, uterine tenderness, a change in uterine shape, and cessation of contractions (Berghella & Landon, 2012; Francois & Foley, 2012). She may also exhibit signs of hypovolemic shock caused by hemorrhage (i.e., hypotension, tachypnea, pallor, and cool, clammy skin). If the placenta separates, the FHR will be absent. Fetal parts may be palpable through the abdomen.

Collaborative Care

Prevention is the best treatment. Women at risk for uterine rupture should be assessed closely during labour. Women whose labours are induced with oxytocin or prostaglandin (especially if their previous birth was Caesarean) should be monitored for signs of uterine tachysystole with or without FHR changes because this can precipitate uterine rupture. If tachysystole occurs, the oxytocin infusion is discontinued or decreased, and a tocolytic medication may be given to decrease the intensity of uterine contractions. After giving birth, women should be assessed for excessive bleeding, especially if the fundus is firm and signs of hemorrhagic shock are present.

If rupture occurs, the type of medical management depends on its severity. A small rupture may be managed with a laparotomy and birth of the infant, repair of the laceration, and blood transfusions, if needed. Hysterectomy and blood replacement are the usual treatments for a complete rupture.

The nurse's role may include starting intravenous fluids, transfusing blood products, administering oxygen, and assisting with preparation for immediate surgery. Supporting the woman's family and providing information about the treatment are important during this emergency. The associated fetal mortality rate is high (approximately 50 to 70%). Maternal morbidity and mortality can also be substantial (Cunningham et al., 2014). Providing information about spiritual support services or suggesting that the family contact their own support system may be warranted.

Amniotic Fluid Embolism

Amniotic fluid embolism (AFE), also known as **anaphylactoid syndrome of pregnancy**, is a rare but devastating complication of pregnancy characterized by the sudden, acute onset of hypoxia, hypotension, cardiovascular collapse, and coagulopathy. The incidence is estimated at 1 in 8000 to 1 in 30,000 births. The true incidence is unknown because of the difficulty in confirming the diagnosis and inconsistent reporting of nonfatal cases (Jones & Clark, 2013).

AFE occurs during labour, during birth, or within 30 minutes after birth. This combination of sudden respiratory and cardiovascular collapse, along with coagulopathy, is similar to that observed in patients with anaphylactic or septic shock. In both conditions, a foreign substance is introduced into the circulation, resulting in disseminated intravascular coagulation, hypotension, and hypoxia (Robbins, Martin, & Wilson, 2014).

In AFE, the foreign substance that initiates the condition is presumed to be present in amniotic fluid that is introduced into the maternal circulation. However, the exact factor that initiates AFE has not been identified. In the past, particles of fetal debris (e.g., vernix, hair, skin cells, or meconium) found in amniotic fluid were thought to be responsible for initiating the syndrome; however, fetal debris can be found in the pulmonary circulation of most normal labouring women. Also, fetal debris is identified in only 78% of women diagnosed with AFE. Therefore, AFE is diagnosed clinically (Jones & Clark, 2013; Robbins et al., 2014). Although AFE is rare, the mortality rate is 61% or higher (Robbins et al., 2014). Neonatal outcome in cases of AFE is poor. If the event occurs before birth, the neonatal survival rate is approximately 80%. However, only half of these fetuses survive neurologically intact (Jones & Clark, 2013).

Maternal risk factors for AFE include advanced age, non-White race, placenta previa, pre-eclampsia, and forceps-assisted or Caesarean birth. Other factors commonly associated with the development of AFE are rapid labour and meconium staining (Cunningham et al., 2014). Previously it was thought that the hypertonic uterine contractions that often accompany AFE actually caused the event. Instead, it appears that the physiological response to AFE produces the hypertonic contractions (Jones & Clark, 2013).

Collaborative Care

The immediate interventions for AFE are summarized in the Emergency box. Care must be instituted immediately. Cardiopulmonary resuscitation is often necessary. If cardiopulmonary arrest occurs, for optimal fetal survival, a perimortem Caesarean birth should be accomplished within 5 minutes (Robbins et al., 2014). The nurse's immediate responsibility is to assist with the resuscitation efforts.

If the woman survives, she is usually moved to a critical care unit. Additional interventions will likely include replacing blood and clotting factors and maintaining adequate hydration and blood pressure. The woman is usually placed on mechanical ventilation. Invasive hemodynamic monitoring may also be required (Robbins et al., 2014).

Support of the woman's partner and family is needed; they will be anxious and distressed. Brief explanations of what is happening are important during the emergency and can be reinforced after the immediate crisis is over. If the woman dies and the infant survives, grieving, anger, and blame may interfere with parent–infant attachment. When both the mother and infant die, it is important that the family has the opportunity to spend time with them. Emotional support and involvement of the perinatal loss support team or other resource for grief counselling, including the spiritual care team, are needed (see Box 24-7). Referral to grief and loss support groups is appropriate. The nursing staff also may need help in coping with emotions that result from a maternal death.

EMERGENCY

Amniotic Fluid Embolism (Anaphylactoid Syndrome of Pregnancy)

Signs

- Respiratory distress
- Restlessness
- Dyspnea
- Cyanosis
- Pulmonary edema
- Respiratory arrest
- Circulatory collapse
- Hypotension
- Tachycardia
- Shock
- Cardiac arrest
- Hemorrhage
- Coagulation failure: bleeding from incisions, venipuncture sites, trauma (lacerations); petechiae, ecchymoses, purpura
- Uterine atony

Interventions

Oxygenate.

- Administer oxygen by nonrebreather face mask (10 L/min) or resuscitation bag delivering 100% oxygen.
- Prepare for intubation and mechanical ventilation.
- Initiate or assist with cardiopulmonary resuscitation (see Chapter 14, p. 353). Tilt pregnant woman 30 degrees to side to displace uterus.
- Maintain cardiac output and replace fluid losses.
- Position woman on her side.
- Administer intravenous fluids.
- Administer blood: packed cells, fresh frozen plasma.
- Insert in-dwelling catheter and measure hourly urine output.

Correct coagulation failure.

Monitor fetal and maternal status.

Prepare for emergency birth once woman's condition has stabilized.

Provide emotional support to the woman, her partner, and her family.

KEY POINTS

- *Preterm labour* is defined as uterine contractions leading to cervical change occurring between 20 and 37 completed weeks of pregnancy; *preterm birth* is any birth that occurs before the completion of 37 weeks of pregnancy.
- The cause of preterm labour is unknown and is assumed to be multifactorial.
- Bedrest, a commonly prescribed intervention for preterm labour, has many deleterious adverse effects and has never been shown to decrease preterm birth rates.
- Preterm birth that occurs in a tertiary care centre leads to better neonatal and maternal outcomes.
- Vigilance for signs of infection is a major part of the care for women with PPROM.
- Dystocia results from differences in the normal relationships among any of the five factors affecting labour.
- Dystocia due to uterine contractions occurs as a result of hypertonic uterine dysfunction, hypotonic uterine dysfunction, or inadequate voluntary expulsive forces.
- The functional relationships among the uterine contractions, the fetus, and the mother's pelvis are altered by maternal positioning.
- Uterine contractility is increased by oxytocin and prostaglandin and decreased by tocolytic drugs.
- Cervical ripening using chemical or mechanical measures can increase the success of labour induction.

- Expectant parents benefit from learning about operative obstetrics (e.g., forceps- or vacuum-assisted birth, Caesarean birth) during the prenatal period.
- The basic purpose of Caesarean birth is to preserve the life and health of the mother and her fetus.
- Unless contraindicated, a vaginal birth may be possible after a previous Caesarean birth.
- Labour management that emphasizes one-to-one support of the labouring woman by another woman (doula, nurse, or midwife) can reduce the rate of Caesarean birth and increase the rate of VBACs.
- Obstetrical emergencies (e.g., shoulder dystocia, prolapsed cord, rupture of the uterus, and amniotic fluid embolism) occur rarely but require immediate intervention.
- The perinatal loss support team or other resource for grief counselling, including the spiritual care team, provides support for families experiencing death of the mother, the infant, or both.

evolve WEBSITE

Visit the Evolve website for additional resources related to the content in this chapter such as Case Studies, Critical Thinking Case Study Answers, Nursing Care Plans, Nursing Processes, Nursing Skills, and Review Questions for Exam Preparation at: *http://evolve.elsevier.com/Canada/Perry/maternal/*

REFERENCES

American Academy of Pediatrics (AAP) & American Heart Association (AHA). (2011). *Textbook of neonatal resuscitation* (6th ed.). Elk Grove Village, IL: AAP.

American College of Obstetricians and Gynecologists (ACOG). (2009). *Induction of labor* (ACOG Practice Bulletin No. 107). Washington, DC: Author.

American College of Obstetricians and Gynecologists (ACOG). (2010). *Vaginal birth after previous Cesarean delivery* (ACOG Practice Bulletin No. 115). Washington, DC: Author.

American College of Obstetricians and Gynecologists (ACOG). (2012). Management of preterm labor. ACOG Practice Bulletin No. 127. *Obstetrics and Gynecology*, *119*(6), 1308–1317.

American College of Obstetricians and Gynecologists (ACOG). (2013). Oral health care during pregnancy and throughout the lifespan. Committee opinion No. 569. *Obstetrics and Gynecology*, *122*, 417–422. Retrieved from <http://www.acog.org/~/media/Committee%20Opinions/Committee%20on%20Health%20Care%20for%20Underserved%20Women/co569.pdf?dmc=1&ts=20130724T0816301062>.

Berghella, V., & Landon, M. (2012). Cesarean delivery. In S. Gabbe, J. Niebyl, J. Simpson, et al. (Eds.), *Obstetrics: Normal and problem pregnancies* (6th ed.). Philadelphia: Saunders.

Brizot, M. L., Hernandez, W., Liao, A. W., et al. (2015). Vaginal progesterone for the prevention of preterm birth in twin gestations: A randomized placebo-controlled double-blind study. *American Journal of Obstetrics & Gynecology*, *213*(1), 82, e81–89.

Butt, K., & Lim, K. (2014). SOGC clinical practice guideline: Determination of gestational age by ultrasound. *Journal of Obstetrics and Gynecology Canada*, *36*(2), 171–181.

Canadian Institute for Health Information (CIHI). (2016). *Caesarean section rate*. Retrieved from <http://indicatorlibrary.cihi.ca/display/HSPIL/Caesarean+Section+Rate>.

Charoenkwan, K., & Matovinovic, E. (2014). Early versus delayed oral fluids and food for reducing complications after major abdominal gynaecologic surgery. *The Cochrane Database of Systematic Reviews*, (12). doi: 10.1002/14651858.CD004508.pub4.

Clark, S., Simpson, K., Knox, G., et al. (2009). Oxytocin: New perspectives on an old drug. *American Journal of Obstetrics & Gynecology*, *200*(1), 35e1–e6.

Collard, T., Diallo, H., Habinsky, A., et al. (2008/2009). Elective Cesarean section: Why women choose it and what nurses need to know. *Nursing for Women's Health*, *12*(6), 480–488.

Cunningham, F., Leveno, K., Bloom, S., et al. (2014). *Williams obstetrics* (24th ed.). New York: McGraw Hill.

Duff, P. (2012). Maternal and perinatal infection—bacterial. In S. Gabbe, J. Niebyl, J. Simpson, et al. (Eds.), *Obstetrics: Normal and problem pregnancies* (6th ed.). Philadelphia: Saunders.

Duff, P. (2014). Maternal and fetal infections. In R. Creasy, R. Resnik, J. Iams, et al. (Eds.), *Creasy and Resnik's maternal-fetal medicine: Principles and practice* (7th ed.). Philadelphia: Saunders.

Fell, D. B., Sprague, A. E., Grimshaw, J. M., et al. (2014). Evaluation of the impact of fetal fibronectin test implementation on hospital admissions for preterm labour in Ontario: A multiple baseline time-series design. *British Journal of Obstetrics & Gynecology*, *121*(4), 438–446. doi:10.1111/1471-0528.12511.

Francois, K. E., & Foley, M. R. (2012). Antepartum and postpartum hemorrhage. In S. Gabbe, J. Niebyl, J. Simpson, et al. (Eds.), *Obstetrics: Normal and problem pregnancies* (6th ed.). Philadelphia: Saunders.

Friedman, E. (1989). Normal and dysfunctional labour. In W. Cohen, D. B. Acker, E. A. Friedman, et al. (Eds.), *Management of labour* (2nd ed.). Rockville, MD: Aspen.

Gilbert, E. S. (2011). *Manual of high risk pregnancy and delivery* (5th ed.). St. Louis: Mosby.

Gupta, J. K., Hofmeyr, G. J., & Shehmar, M. (2012). Position in the second stage of labour for women without epidural anaesthesia. *The Cochrane Database of Systematic Reviews*, (5). doi:10.1002/14651858.CD002006.pub3.

Haas, D. M., Caldwell, D. M., Kirkpatrick, P., et al. (2012). Tocolytic therapy for preterm delivery: Systematic review and network meta-analysis. *British Medical Journal*, *345*, e6226. doi:10.1136/bmj.e6226.

Hill, W., & Harvey, C. (2013). Induction of labor. In N. Troiano, C. Harvey, & B. Chez (Eds.), *AWHONN's high risk & critical care obstetrics* (3rd ed.). Philadelphia: Wolters Kluwer/Lippincott Williams & Wilkins.

Hodnett, E. D., Gates, S., Hofmeyr, G. J., & Sakala, C. (2013). Continuous support for women during childbirth. *The Cochrane Database of Systematic Reviews*, (7). doi:10.1002/14651858.CD003766.pub5.

Hofmeyr, G. J. (2015). External cephalic version. *UptoDate*. Retrieved from <http://www.uptodate.com/contents/external-cephalic-version>.

Jones, R., & Clark, S. (2013). Amniotic fluid embolus (anaphylactoid syndrome of pregnancy). In N. Troiano, C. Harvey, & B. Chez (Eds.), *AWHONN's high risk & critical care obstetrics* (3rd ed.). Philadelphia: Wolters Kluwer/Lippincott Williams & Wilkins.

Kotaska, A., Menticoglou, S., Gagnon, R., et al. (2009). SOGC clinical practice guideline: Vaginal delivery of breech presentation. *Journal of Obstetrics and Gynaecology Canada*, *31*(6), 557–566.

Lanni, S., & Seeds, J. (2012). Malpresentations and shoulder dystocia. In S. Gabbe, J. Niebyl, J. Simpson, et al. (Eds.), *Obstetrics: Normal and problem pregnancies* (6th ed.). Philadelphia: Saunders.

Lawrence, A., Lewis, L., Hofmeyr, G. J., & Styles, C. (2013). Maternal positions and mobility during first stage labour. *The Cochrane Database of Systematic Reviews*, (10). doi:10.1002/14651858.CD003934.pub4.

Leduc, D., Biringer, A., Lee, L., et al. (2013). SOGC clinical practice guideline: Induction of labour. *Journal of Obstetrics and Gynaecology Canada, 35*(9), S1–S18.

Lee, M., & Guinn, D. (2015). Antenatal corticosteroid therapy for reduction of neonatal morbidity and mortality from preterm delivery. *UpToDate.* Retrieved from <http://www.uptodate.com/contents/antenatal-corticosteroid-therapy-for-reduction-of-neonatal-morbidity-and-mortality-from-preterm-delivery>.

Lim, K., Butt, K., Crane, J. M., et al. (2011). SOGC clinical practice guideline: Ultrasonographic cervical length assessment in predicting preterm birth in singleton pregnancies. *Journal of Obstetrics and Gynaecology Canada, 33*(5), 486–499.

Liston, R., Sawchuck, D., Young, D., et al. (2007). Fetal health surveillance: Antepartum and intrapartum consensus guideline. *Journal of Obstetrics and Gynaecology Canada, 29*(9 Suppl. 4), s1–s56.

Magee, L., Sawchuck, D., Synnes, A., et al. (2011). Magnesium sulphate for fetal neuroprotection. *Journal of Obstetrics and Gynaecology Canada, 33*(5), 516–529.

Mahlmeister, L. (2008). Best practices in perinatal care: Evidence-based management of oxytocin induction and augmentation of labor. *Journal of Perinatal & Neonatal Nursing, 22*(4), 259–263.

Malone, F. D., & D'Alton, M. E. (2014). Multiple gestation. Clinical characteristics and management. In R. K. Creasy, R. Resnick, J. Iams, et al. (Eds.), *Creasy & Resnik's maternal–fetal medicine: Principles and practice* (7th ed.). Philadelphia: Saunders.

Martin, J., Hamilton, B., Sutton, P., et al. (2012). Births: Final data for 2010. *National Vital Statistics Report, 61*(1), 1–100.

Mercer, B. M. (2012). Premature rupture of membranes. In S. G. Gabbe, J. R. Niebyl, J. L. Simpson, et al. (Eds.), *Obstetrics: Normal and problem pregnancies* (6th ed.). New York: Saunders.

Mercer, B. (2014a). Assessment and induction of fetal pulmonary maturity. In R. K. Creasy, R. Resnick, J. Iams, et al. (Eds.), *Creasy & Resnik's maternal–fetal medicine: Principles and practice* (7th ed.). Philadelphia: Saunders.

Mercer, B. (2014b). Premature rupture of the membranes. In R. K. Creasy, R. Resnick, J. Iams, et al. (Eds.), *Creasy & Resnik's maternal–fetal medicine: Principles and practice* (7th ed.). Philadelphia: Saunders.

Moleti, C. (2009). Trends and controversies in labor induction. *MCN: American Journal of Maternal Child Nursing, 34*(1), 40–47.

Newman, R., & Unal, E. (2012). Multiple gestations. In S. G. Gabbe, J. R. Niebyl, J. L. Simpson, et al. (Eds.), *Obstetrics: Normal and problem pregnancies* (6th ed.). New York: Saunders.

Nielsen, P., & Galan, H. (2012). Operative vaginal delivery. In S. G. Gabbe, J. R. Niebyl, J. L. Simpson, et al. (Eds.), *Obstetrics: Normal and problem pregnancies* (6th ed.). New York: Saunders.

Public Health Agency of Canada. (2013). *Perinatal health indicators for Canada 2013: A report of the Canadian perinatal surveillance system* (Cat. No. HP7-1/2013E-PDF). Ottawa, ON: Author.

Rampersad, R., & Macones, G. (2012). Prolonged and postterm pregnancy. In S. G. Gabbe, J. R. Niebyl, J. L. Simpson, et al. (Eds.), *Obstetrics: Normal and problem pregnancies* (6th ed.). New York: Saunders.

Robbins, K. S., Martin, S., & Wilson, W. (2014). Intensive care considerations of the critically ill parturient. In R. K. Creasy, R. Resnick, J. Iams, et al. (Eds.), *Creasy & Resnik's maternal–fetal medicine: Principles and practice* (7th ed.). Philadelphia: Saunders.

Roberts, C., & Mangan, S. (2009). Special delivery: Know the risks of Cesarean section. *OR Nurse, 3*(2), 22–30.

Romero, R., & Lockwood, C. (2014). Pathogenesis of spontaneous preterm labor. In R. K. Creasy, R. Resnick, J. Iams, et al. (Eds.), *Creasy & Resnik's maternal–fetal medicine: Principles and practice* (7th ed.). Philadelphia: Saunders.

Rozance, P., & Rosenberg, A. (2012). The neonate. In S. Gabbe, J. Niebyl, J. Simpson, et al. (Eds.), *Obstetrics: Normal and problem pregnancies* (6th ed.). Philadelphia: Saunders.

Shaikh, S., Shaikh, A. H., Akhter, S., & Isran, B. (2012). Efficacy of transdermal nitroglycerine in idiopathic pre-term labour. *Journal of Pakistan Medical Association, 62*(1), 47–50.

Simhan, H., Iams, J., & Romero, R. (2012). Preterm birth. In S. Gabbe, J. Niebyl, J. Simpson, et al. (Eds.), *Obstetrics: Normal and problem pregnancies* (6th ed.). Philadelphia: Saunders.

Simhan, H. N., Berghella, V., & Iams, J. D. (2014). Preterm labour and birth. In R. K. Creasy, R. Resnick, J. Iams, et al. (Eds.), *Creasy & Resnik's maternal–fetal medicine: Principles and practice* (7th ed.). Philadelphia: Saunders.

Simpson, K. (2011). Clinicians' guide to the use of oxytocin for labor induction and augmentation. *Journal of Midwifery & Women's Health, 56*(3), 214–221.

Simpson, K. R. (2013). Labor and birth. In K. Simpson & P. Creehan (Eds.), *AWHONN's perinatal nursing* (4th ed.). Philadelphia: Lippincott Williams & Wilkins.

Simpson, K., & Knox, G. (2009). Oxytocin as a high-alert medication: Implications for perinatal patient safety. *MCN: American Journal of Maternal Child Nursing, 34*(1), 8–15.

Society of Obstetricians and Gynaecologists of Canada. (1995). *Management of dystocia. Policy statement 40.* Ottawa: Author.

Society of Obstetricians and Gynaecologists of Canada. (2004). News: C-sections on demand—SOGC's position. *Birth (Berkeley, Calif.), 31*(2), 154.

Thorp, J. M., & Laughon, K. (2014). Clinical aspects of normal and abnormal labour. In R. K. Creasy, R. Resnick, J. Iams, et al. (Eds.), *Creasy & Resnik's maternal–fetal medicine: Principles and practice* (7th ed.). Philadelphia: Saunders.

Wing, D., & Farinelli, C. (2012). Abnormal labor and induction of labor. In S. Gabbe, J. Niebyl, J. Simpson, et al. (Eds.), *Obstetrics: Normal and problem pregnancies* (6th ed.). Philadelphia: Saunders.

Yudin, M. H., van Schalwyk, J., Van Eyk, N., et al. (2009). SOGC clinical practice guideline: Antibiotic therapy in preterm premature rupture of membranes. *Journal of Obstetrics and Gynecology Canada, 31*(9), 863–867.

ADDITIONAL RESOURCES

AWHONN—40 Reasons to Go the Full 40. <http://www.health4mom.org/zones>.

Multiple-birth resources for parents. <http://www.multiplebirthscanada.org> and <http://www.tripletconnection.org>.

Trillium Health Partners—Breastfeeding Your Baby After a Caesarean Birth. <http://trilliumhealthpartners.ca/patientservices/womens/Pages/breastfeeding-after-caesarean-birth.aspx>.

Vaginal birth after Caesarean (VBAC) support groups. <http://www.vbac.com> and <http://www.ican-online.org>.

UNIT 6

Postpartum Period

CHAPTER

21

Maternal Physiological Changes

Lisa Keenan-Lindsay, with contributions from Kathryn R. Alden

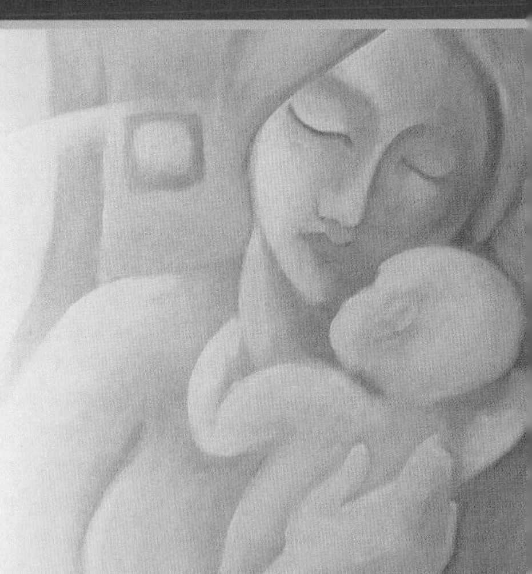

evolve WEBSITE

Visit the Evolve website for additional resources related to the content in this chapter such as Case Studies, Critical Thinking Case Study Answers, Nursing Care Plans, Nursing Processes, Nursing Skills, and Review Questions for Exam Preparation at: http://evolve.elsevier.com/Canada/Perry/maternal/

OBJECTIVES

On completion of this chapter the reader will be able to:

- Describe the anatomical and physiological changes that occur during the postpartum period.
- Apply assessment techniques for uterine involution and lochial flow.
- List expected values for vital signs and blood pressure, deviations from normal findings, and probable causes of the deviations.

The postpartum period is the interval between the birth of the newborn and the return of the reproductive organs to their normal nonpregnant state. This period is sometimes referred to as the **puerperium**, or **fourth trimester** of pregnancy, and is considered to last approximately 6 weeks. The physiological changes that occur during the reversal of the processes of pregnancy are distinctive, but they are normal. To provide care during the recovery period that is beneficial to the mother, her infant, and her family, the nurse needs to synthesize knowledge of maternal anatomy and physiology of the recovery period, the newborn's physical and behavioural characteristics, infant care activities, and the family response to the birth of the infant. This chapter focuses on anatomical and physiological changes that occur in the mother during the postpartum period.

REPRODUCTIVE SYSTEM AND ASSOCIATED STRUCTURES

Uterus

Involution Process

The return of the uterus to a nonpregnant state following birth is called **involution**. This process begins immediately after expulsion of the **placenta** with contraction of the uterine smooth muscle.

At the end of the third stage of labour the uterus is in the midline, approximately 2 cm below the level of the umbilicus, with the **fundus** resting on the sacral promontory. At this time, the uterus weighs approximately 1000 g (Cunningham, Leveno, Bloom, et al., 2014).

Within 12 hours, the fundus may rise to approximately 1 cm above the umbilicus (Fig. 21-1). By 24 hours after birth, the uterus is about the same size as it was at 20 weeks of gestation. Involution progresses rapidly during the next few days. The fundus descends 1 to 2 cm every 24 hours. By the sixth postpartum day, the fundus is normally located halfway between the umbilicus and the symphysis pubis. The uterus should not be palpable abdominally after 2 weeks.

The uterus, which at full term weighs approximately 11 times its prepregnancy weight, involutes to approximately 500 g by 1 week after birth and to 350 g by 2 weeks after birth. At 6 weeks postpartum it weighs 60 to 80 g.

Increased estrogen and progesterone levels are responsible for stimulating the massive growth of the uterus during pregnancy. Prenatal uterine growth results from both *hyperplasia*, an increase in the number of muscle cells, and *hypertrophy*, an enlargement of the existing cells. After birth, the decrease in these hormones causes *autolysis*, the self-destruction of excess hypertrophied tissue. The additional cells laid down during

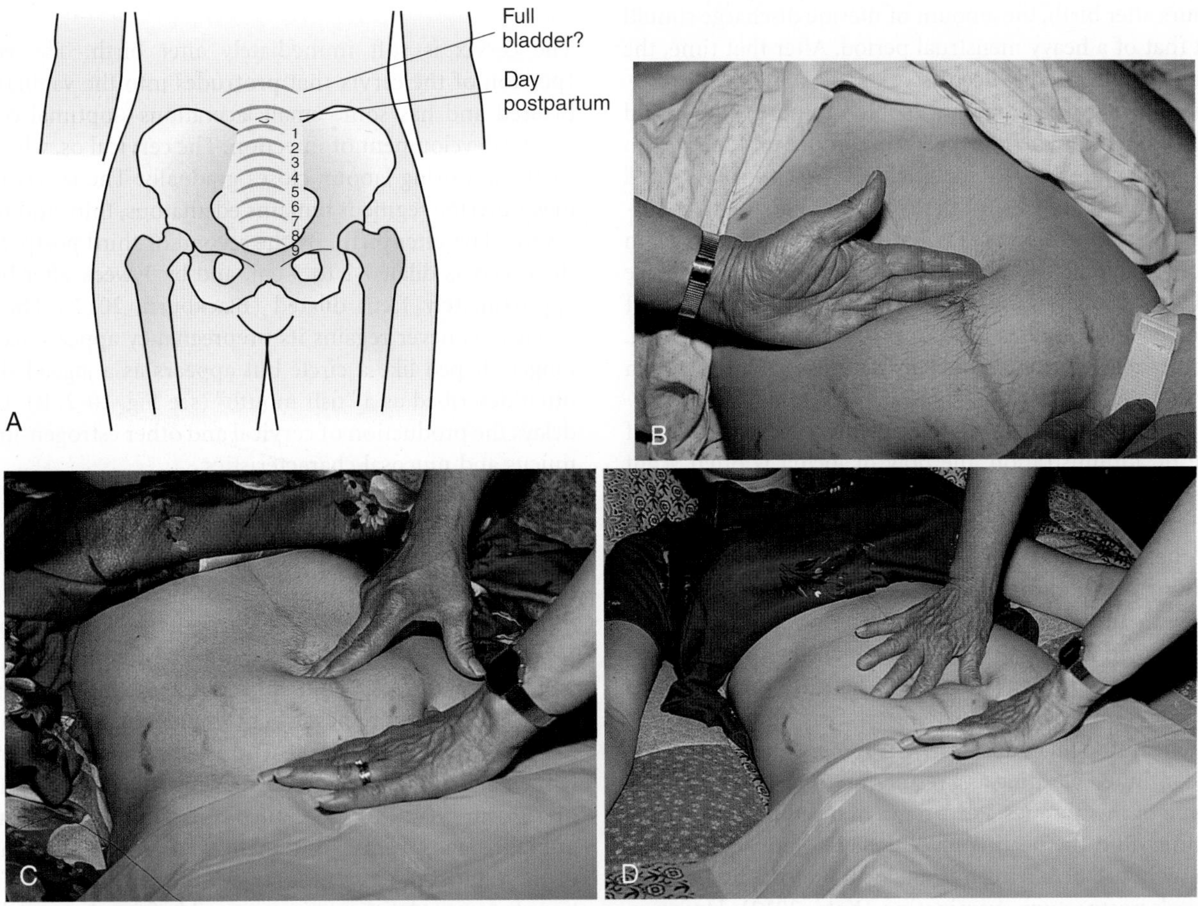

FIGURE 21-1 Assessment of involution of uterus after childbirth. **A:** Normal progress, days 1 through 9. **B:** Size and position of uterus 12 hours after childbirth. **C:** Two days after childbirth. **D:** Four days after childbirth. (**B** through **D,** courtesy Marjorie Pyle, RNC, Lifecircle.)

pregnancy remain and account for the slight increase in uterine size after each pregnancy.

Subinvolution is the failure of the uterus to return to a nonpregnant state. The most common causes of subinvolution are retained placental fragments and infection (see Chapter 22).

Contractions

Postpartum hemostasis is achieved primarily by compression of intramyometrial blood vessels as the uterine muscle contracts rather than by platelet aggregation and clot formation. The hormone oxytocin, released from the pituitary gland, strengthens and coordinates these uterine contractions, which compress blood vessels and promote hemostasis. During the first 1 to 2 postpartum hours, uterine contractions may decrease in intensity and become uncoordinated. Because it is vital that the uterus remain firm and well contracted, exogenous oxytocin is usually administered intravenously or intramuscularly immediately after expulsion of the placenta. The uterus is very sensitive to oxytocin during the first week or so after birth. Breastfeeding immediately after birth and in the early days postpartum increases the release of oxytocin, which decreases blood loss and reduces the risk for postpartum hemorrhage.

Afterpains. In first-time mothers uterine tone is good, the fundus generally remains firm, and the woman usually perceives only mild uterine cramping. Periodic relaxation and vigorous contractions are more common in subsequent pregnancies and may cause uncomfortable cramping called afterpains (afterbirth pains), which persist throughout the early puerperium. Afterpains are more noticeable after births in which the uterus was overdistended (e.g., large baby, multifetal gestation, polyhydramnios). Breastfeeding and exogenous oxytocic medication usually intensify these afterpains because both stimulate uterine contractions.

Placental Site

Immediately after the placenta and membranes are expelled, vascular constriction and thromboses reduce the placental site to an irregular nodular and elevated area. Upward growth of the endometrium causes sloughing of necrotic tissue and prevents the scar formation characteristic of normal wound healing. This unique healing process enables the endometrium to resume its usual cycle of changes and permit implantation and placentation in future pregnancies. Endometrial regeneration is completed by postpartum day 16, except at the placental site. Regeneration at the placental site usually is not complete until 6 weeks after birth (Blackburn, 2013).

Lochia

Postbirth uterine discharge, commonly called lochia, initially is bright red (lochia rubra) and may contain small clots. For the first 2 hours after birth, the amount of uterine discharge should be about that of a heavy menstrual period. After that time, the lochia flow should steadily decrease.

Lochia rubra consists mainly of blood and decidual and trophoblastic debris. The flow pales, becoming pink or brown (lochia serosa) after 3 to 4 days. **Lochia serosa** consists of old blood, serum, leukocytes, and tissue debris. The median duration of lochia serosa discharge is 22 to 27 days (Katz, 2012). In most women about 10 days after childbirth the drainage becomes yellow to white (lochia alba). **Lochia alba** consists of leukocytes, decidua, epithelial cells, mucus, serum, and bacteria. Lochia can persist for approximately 4 to 8 weeks after birth (Cunningham et al., 2014).

If the woman receives an oxytocic medication, regardless of the route of administration, the flow of lochia is often scant until the effects of the medication wear off. The amount of lochia is usually less after a Caesarean birth because the surgeon suctions the blood and fluids from the uterus or wipes the uterine lining before closing the incision. Flow of lochia usually increases with ambulation. Lochia tends to pool in the vagina when the woman is lying in bed; the woman then may experience a gush of blood when she stands. This gush should not be confused with hemorrhage.

Persistence of lochia rubra early in the postpartum period suggests continued bleeding as a result of retained fragments of the placenta or membranes. Recurrence of bleeding 7 to 14 days after birth is from the healing placental site. About 10 to 15% of women will still be having normal lochia serosa discharge at their 6-week postpartum examination (Katz, 2012). However, in some women, the continued flow of lochia serosa or lochia alba by 3 to 4 weeks after birth can indicate endometritis, particularly if fever, pain, or abdominal tenderness is associated with the discharge. Lochia should smell like normal menstrual flow; an offensive odour usually indicates infection.

Not all postpartal vaginal bleeding is lochia; vaginal bleeding after birth may be caused by unrepaired vaginal or cervical lacerations. Box 21-1 lists factors used to distinguish between lochial and nonlochial bleeding.

BOX 21-1 LOCHIAL AND NONLOCHIAL BLEEDING

Lochial Bleeding

- Lochia usually trickles from the vaginal opening. The steady flow is greater as the uterus contracts.
- A gush of lochia may result as the uterus is massaged. If it is dark in colour, it has been pooled in the relaxed vagina, and the amount soon lessens to a trickle of bright red lochia (in the early puerperium).

Nonlochial Bleeding

- If the bloody discharge spurts from the vagina, there may be cervical or vaginal tears in addition to the normal lochia.
- If the amount of bleeding continues to be excessive and bright red, a tear may be the source.

Cervix

The cervix is soft immediately after birth. The ectocervix (portion of the cervix that protrudes into the vagina) appears bruised and has some small lacerations—optimal conditions for the development of infection. The cervical os, which dilated to 10 cm during labour, closes gradually. The cervix up to the lower uterine segment remains edematous, thin, and fragile for several days after birth. By the second or third postpartum day, the cervix is dilated 2 to 3 cm, and by 1 week after birth, it is approximately 1 cm dilated (Blackburn, 2013). The external cervical os never regains its prepregnancy appearance; it is no longer shaped like a circle but appears as a jagged slit that is often described as a "fish mouth" (see Fig. 10-2, B). **Lactation** delays the production of cervical and other estrogen-influenced mucus and mucosal characteristics.

Vagina and Perineum

Postpartum estrogen deprivation is responsible for the thinness of the vaginal mucosa and the absence of **rugae**. The greatly distended, smooth-walled vagina gradually decreases in size and regains tone, although it never completely returns to its prepregnancy state (Cunningham et al., 2014). Rugae reappear within 3 weeks, but they are never as prominent as they are in the nulliparous woman. Most rugae are permanently flattened. The hymen remains as small tags of tissue that scar and form the myrtiform caruncles. The mucosa remains atrophic in the lactating woman, at least until menstruation resumes. Thickening of the vaginal mucosa occurs with the return of ovarian function. Estrogen deficiency is responsible for a decreased amount of vaginal lubrication. Localized dryness and coital discomfort (**dyspareunia**) may persist until ovarian function returns and menstruation resumes. The use of a water-soluble lubricant to reduce discomfort during sexual intercourse is usually recommended.

Immediately after birth, the introitus is erythematous and edematous, especially in the area of the **episiotomy** or laceration repair. Within 2 weeks, it is barely distinguishable from that of a nulliparous woman if lacerations and an episiotomy have been carefully repaired, hematomas are prevented or treated early, and the woman practises good hygiene.

Most episiotomy or laceration repairs are visible only if the woman is lying on her side with her upper buttock raised or if she is placed in the lithotomy position. A good light source is essential for visualization of some repairs. Healing of an episiotomy or laceration is the same as that of any surgical incision. Signs of infection (pain, redness, warmth, swelling, or discharge) or loss of approximation (separation of the edges of the incision) may occur. Initial healing occurs within 2 to 3 weeks, but 4 to 6 months can be required for the repair to heal completely (Blackburn, 2013). If forceps were used for the birth, the woman may have experienced vaginal or cervical lacerations; hematomas of the pelvic soft tissues can also occur with forceps-assisted birth (see Chapter 20).

Hemorrhoids (anal varicosities) are commonly seen (see Fig 10-11). Internal hemorrhoids may evert while the woman is pushing during birth. Women often experience associated symptoms such as itching, discomfort, and bright red bleeding upon defecation. Hemorrhoids usually decrease in size within 6 weeks of childbirth.

Pelvic Muscular Support

The supporting structure of the uterus and vagina can be injured during childbirth and can contribute to later gynecological problems. Supportive tissues of the pelvic floor that are torn or stretched during childbirth may require up to 6 months to regain tone. Kegel exercises, which help strengthen perineal muscles and encourage healing, are recommended after childbirth (see Patient Teaching box in Chapter 5, p. 72). Later in life, women can experience *pelvic relaxation*—the lengthening and weakening of the fascial supports of pelvic structures. These structures include the uterus, upper posterior vaginal wall, urethra, bladder, and rectum. Although relaxation can occur in any woman, it is commonly a direct but delayed complication of childbirth.

Abdomen

When the woman stands during the first days after birth, her abdomen protrudes and gives her a still-pregnant appearance. During the first 2 weeks after birth, the abdominal wall is relaxed. It takes about 6 weeks for the abdominal wall to return almost to its prepregnancy state (Fig. 21-2). The skin regains most of its previous elasticity, but some striae may persist. The return of muscle tone depends on previous tone, proper exercise, and the amount of adipose tissue. Occasionally, with or without overdistension because of a large fetus or multiple fetuses, the abdominal wall muscles separate, a condition termed diastasis recti abdominis (see Fig. 10-14, B). Persistence of this separation may be disturbing to the woman, but surgical correction rarely is necessary. With time, the separation becomes less apparent.

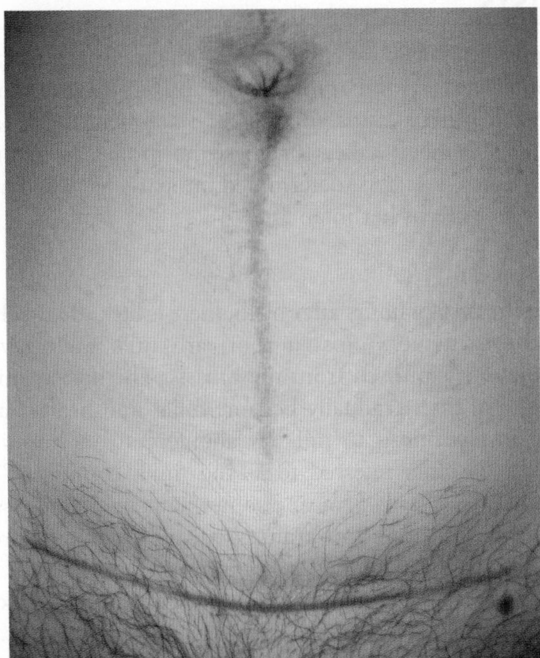

FIGURE 21-2 Abdominal wall 7 weeks after Caesarean birth is almost back to prepregnancy appearance. Note that the linea nigra is still visible. (Azoreg. This file is licensed under the Creative Commons Attribution-Share Alike 3.0 Unported license, https://creativecommons.org/licenses/by-sa/3.0/deed.en.)

ENDOCRINE SYSTEM

Placental Hormones

Significant hormonal changes occur during the postpartum period. Expulsion of the placenta results in dramatic decreases of the hormones produced by that organ. Decreases in human chorionic somatomammotropin (also called human placental lactogen), estrogens, cortisol, and the placental enzyme insulinase reverse the diabetogenic effects of pregnancy, resulting in significantly lower blood sugar levels in the immediate puerperium. Mothers with type 1 diabetes will likely require much less insulin for several days after birth. Because these normal hormonal changes make the puerperium a transitional period for carbohydrate metabolism, it is more difficult to interpret glucose tolerance tests at this time.

Estrogen and progesterone levels drop markedly after expulsion of the placenta and reach their lowest levels 1 week after birth. Decreased estrogen levels are associated with diuresis of excess extracellular fluid accumulated during pregnancy. In nonlactating women, estrogen levels begin to increase by 2 weeks after birth and by postpartum day 17 are higher than in women who breastfeed (Katz, 2012).

Human chorionic gonadotropin (hCG) disappears fairly quickly from maternal circulation. However, because removing hCG from the extravascular and intracellular spaces takes additional time, the hormone can be detected in the maternal system for 3 to 4 weeks after birth (Blackburn, 2013).

Pituitary Hormones and Ovarian Function

Prolactin levels in blood rise progressively throughout pregnancy. After birth, as levels of estrogen and progesterone decrease, prolactin levels increase more. In women who breastfeed, prolactin levels are highest during the first month after birth and remain elevated above nonpregnant levels as long as the woman is breastfeeding. Serum prolactin levels are influenced by the frequency of breastfeeding, the duration of each feeding, and the degree to which supplementary feedings are used. Individual differences in the strength of an infant's sucking stimulus probably also affect prolactin levels. In nonlactating women, prolactin levels decline after birth and reach the prepregnant range by the third postpartum week (Katz, 2012).

Lactating and nonlactating women differ considerably in the timing of their first ovulation and when menstruation resumes. Ovulation occurs as early as 27 days after birth in nonlactating women, with a mean time of about 7 to 9 weeks. About 70% of nonbreastfeeding women resume menstruating by 12 weeks after birth. The mean time to ovulation in women who breastfeed is about 6 months (Katz, 2012). The persistence of elevated serum prolactin levels in breastfeeding women appears to be responsible for suppressing ovulation. In lactating women, both the resumption of ovulation and the return of menses are determined in large part by breastfeeding patterns. For example, ovulation is delayed longer in women who breastfeed exclusively than in women who breastfeed and offer supplemental infant formula to their infants. Because of the uncertainty about the return of ovulation and menstruation, the woman needs to consider contraceptive options early in the postpartum period. The first menstrual flow after childbirth is usually heavier than normal. Within three or four cycles the amount of menstrual flow returns to the woman's prepregnancy volume.

URINARY SYSTEM

The hormonal changes of pregnancy (i.e., high steroid levels) contribute to an increase in renal function; diminishing steroid levels after childbirth may partly explain the reduced renal function that occurs during the puerperium. Kidney function returns to normal within 1 month after birth. About 6 weeks are required for the pregnancy-induced hypotonia and dilation of the ureters and renal pelves to return to the nonpregnant state (Cunningham et al., 2014). In a small percentage of women, dilation of the urinary tract may persist for 3 months or longer, increasing the chances of developing a urinary tract infection.

Urine Components

The renal glycosuria induced by pregnancy disappears by 1 week postpartum, but lactosuria may occur in lactating women. The blood urea nitrogen increases during the puerperium as autolysis of the involuting uterus occurs. Pregnancy-associated proteinuria resolves by 6 weeks after birth (Blackburn, 2013). Ketonuria may occur in women with an uncomplicated birth or after a prolonged labour with dehydration.

Postpartal Fluid Loss

Within 12 hours of birth, women begin to lose excess tissue fluid accumulated during pregnancy. Profuse diaphoresis often occurs, especially at night, for the first 2 or 3 days after childbirth. Postpartal diuresis, caused by decreased estrogen levels, removal of increased venous pressure in the lower extremities, and loss of the remaining pregnancy-induced increase in blood volume, also aids the body in ridding itself of excess fluid. Fluid loss through perspiration and increased urinary output accounts for a weight loss of approximately 2.25 kg during the puerperium.

Urethra and Bladder

Birth-induced trauma, increased bladder capacity following childbirth, and the effects of conduction anaesthesia (epidural or spinal) combine to cause a decreased urge to void. In addition, pelvic soreness caused by the forces of labour, vaginal lacerations, or the episiotomy reduces or alters the voiding reflex. Decreased voiding combined with postpartal diuresis may result in bladder distension.

Immediately after birth, excessive bleeding can occur if the bladder becomes distended because it pushes the uterus up and to the side and prevents it from contracting firmly. Later in the puerperium, overdistension can make the bladder more susceptible to infection and impede the resumption of normal voiding (Cunningham et al., 2014). With adequate emptying of the bladder, bladder tone is usually restored by 5 to 7 days after childbirth.

GASTROINTESTINAL SYSTEM

Appetite

The mother is often hungry shortly after birth and usually can tolerate a regular diet. Requests for extra portions of food and frequent snacks are not uncommon.

Bowel Evacuation

A spontaneous bowel evacuation may not occur for 2 to 3 days after childbirth. This delay can be explained by decreased muscle tone in the intestines during labour and the immediate puerperium, prelabour diarrhea, lack of food, or dehydration. The mother often anticipates discomfort during the bowel movement because of perineal tenderness as a result of episiotomy, lacerations, or hemorrhoids and may resist the urge to defecate. Women need to be encouraged to increase fluid and fibre intake to prevent constipation and discomfort. Regular bowel habits should be re-established when bowel tone returns. Occasionally stool softeners may be required.

Operative vaginal birth (forceps or vacuum use) and anal sphincter lacerations are associated with an increased risk of postpartum anal incontinence. Women with this problem are more often incontinent of flatus than of stool. If anal incontinence lasts more than 6 months, studies should be conducted to determine the specific cause and appropriate treatment (Katz, 2012).

Women who have had a Caesarean birth may have problems with abdominal pain due to a buildup of flatus. Women need to be encouraged to move as much as possible to enhance movement of the intestinal system.

BREASTS

Promptly after birth there is a decrease in the concentrations of hormones (i.e., estrogen, progesterone, hCG, prolactin, cortisol, and insulin) that stimulated breast development during pregnancy. The time it takes for these hormones to return to prepregnancy levels is determined in part by whether the mother breastfeeds her infant.

Breastfeeding Mothers

During the first 24 hours after birth, there is little, if any, change in the breast tissue. Colostrum, or early milk, a clear, yellow fluid, may be expressed from the breasts. The breasts initially feel soft and then gradually become fuller and heavier as the colostrum transitions to milk by about 72 to 96 hours after birth; this is often referred to as the "milk coming in." The breasts may feel warm, firm, and somewhat tender. Bluish-white milk with a skim-milk appearance (true milk) can be expressed from the nipples. As milk glands and milk ducts fill with milk, breast tissue may feel somewhat nodular or lumpy. Unlike the lumps associated with fibrocystic breast disease or cancer (which can be palpated consistently in the same location), the nodularity associated with milk production tends to shift in position. Some women experience engorgement, but with frequent breastfeeding and proper care this is a temporary condition that typically lasts only 24 to 48 hours (see Chapter 27).

Nonbreastfeeding Mothers

The breasts generally feel nodular in contrast to the granular feel of breasts in nonpregnant women. The nodularity is bilateral and diffuse. Prolactin levels drop rapidly. Colostrum is present for the first few days after childbirth. Palpation of the breast on the second or third day as milk production begins may indicate tissue tenderness in some women. On the third or fourth postpartum day engorgement may occur. The breasts are distended (swollen), firm, tender, and warm to the touch. Breast distension is caused primarily by the temporary congestion of veins and lymphatics rather than by an accumulation of milk. Milk is present but should not be expressed. Axillary breast tissue (the tail of Spence) and any accessory breast or nipple tissue along the milk line can be involved. Engorgement resolves spontaneously, and discomfort decreases usually within 24 to 36 hours. A breast binder or well-fitted supportive bra, ice packs, fresh cabbage leaves, or mild analgesics may be used to relieve discomfort. Nipple stimulation should be avoided. If suckling is never begun (or is discontinued), lactation ceases within a few days to a week.

CARDIOVASCULAR SYSTEM

Blood Volume

Changes in blood volume after birth depend on several factors, such as blood loss during childbirth and the amount of extravascular water (physiological edema) mobilized and excreted.

Pregnancy-induced hypervolemia (an increase in blood volume of 40 to 45% over prepregnancy values near term) (Cunningham et al., 2014) allows most women to tolerate considerable blood loss during childbirth. The average blood loss for a vaginal birth of a single fetus ranges from 300 mL to 500 mL (10% of blood volume). The typical blood loss for women who give birth by Caesarean is 500 mL to 1000 mL (15 to 30% of blood volume). During the first few days after birth, the plasma volume decreases further as a result of diuresis (Blackburn, 2013).

The woman's response to blood loss during the early puerperium differs from that in a nonpregnant woman. Three postpartum physiological changes protect the woman by increasing the circulating blood volume: (1) elimination of uteroplacental circulation reduces the size of the maternal vascular bed by 10 to 15%; (2) loss of placental endocrine function removes the stimulus for vasodilation; and (3) mobilization of extravascular water stored during pregnancy occurs. By the third postpartum day, the plasma volume has been replenished as extravascular fluid returns to the intravascular space (Katz, 2012) (see Critical Thinking Case Study).

Cardiac Output

Pulse rate, stroke volume, and cardiac output increase throughout pregnancy. Cardiac output remains increased for at least 48 hours after birth because of an increase in stroke volume. This increased stroke volume is caused by the return of blood to the maternal systemic venous circulation, a result of rapid decrease in uterine blood flow and mobilization of extravascular fluid (Monga & Mastrobattasta, 2014). Stroke volume,

CRITICAL THINKING CASE STUDY

Maternal Postpartum Blood Loss and Fatigue

You are caring for four women on the postpartum unit, two of whom had vaginal births and two who had Caesarean births. Each of the women has stated she is feeling tired and has expressed concern about the amount of blood she lost during birth. Before providing patient education related to fatigue after birth and blood loss, you review the patient records with attention to estimated blood loss, and hemoglobin and hematocrit values, intake and output, and nursing notes.

QUESTIONS

1. Evidence—Is there sufficient evidence to draw conclusions about the relation between tiredness (fatigue) after birth and blood loss?
2. Assumptions—What assumptions can be made about the following factors?
   a. Comparison of amount of blood loss between women who give birth vaginally and by Caesarean
   b. Postpartum norms for hematocrit and hemoglobin for women who give birth vaginally and by Caesarean
   c. Causes of fatigue after birth
   d. Interventions to alleviate fatigue and replace blood lost at birth
3. What implications and priorities for nursing care can be drawn at this time?
4. Does the evidence objectively support your conclusion?

cardiac output, end-diastolic volume, and systemic vascular resistance remain elevated over nonpregnant values for 12 weeks after birth and may not stabilize until 24 weeks after birth (Monga & Mastrobattasta, 2014).

Vital Signs

Few alterations in vital signs are seen under normal circumstances. Heart rate and blood pressure return to nonpregnant levels within a few days (Katz, 2012) (Table 21-1). Respiratory function rapidly returns to nonpregnant levels after birth. After the uterus is emptied, the diaphragm descends, the normal cardiac axis is restored, and the point of maximal impulse and the electrocardiogram are normalized.

Blood Components

Hematocrit and hemoglobin. In women with an average blood loss during birth, the hematocrit level drops moderately for 3 to 4 days, then begins to increase, and reaches nonpregnant levels by 8 weeks postpartum (Katz, 2012). A postpartum hematocrit can be lower than normal if the blood loss was increased or if the hypervolemia of pregnancy was less than normal.

White blood cell count. Normal leukocytosis of pregnancy averages approximately 12×10^9/L. During the first 10 to 12 days after childbirth, values between 20 and 25×10^9/L are common. Neutrophils are the most numerous white blood cells. Leukocytosis, coupled with the normal increase in erythrocyte sedimentation rate, may obscure the diagnosis of acute infections at this time.

Coagulation factors. Clotting factors and fibrinogen are normally increased during pregnancy and remain elevated in the immediate puerperium. When combined with vessel damage

TABLE 21-1 VITAL SIGNS AFTER CHILDBIRTH

NORMAL FINDINGS	DEVIATIONS FROM NORMAL FINDINGS AND PROBABLE CAUSES
Temperature	
During the first 24 hours temperature may increase to 38°C as a result of dehydrating effects of labour. After 24 hours the woman should be afebrile.	A diagnosis of puerperal sepsis is suggested if an increase in maternal temperature to 38°C is noted after the first 24 hours after childbirth and recurs or persists for 2 days. Other possibilities are mastitis, endometritis, urinary tract infections, and other systemic infections.
Pulse	
Pulse, along with stroke volume and cardiac output, remains elevated for the first hour or so after childbirth. It then begins to decrease at an unknown rate to a nonpregnant rate.	A rapid pulse rate or one that is increasing may indicate hypovolemia as a result of hemorrhage or an increased temperature.
Respirations	
The respiratory rate should rapidly decrease to within the woman's normal prebirth range.	Hypoventilation (respiratory depression) may occur after an unusually high subarachnoid (spinal) block or epidural narcotic after a Caesarean birth.
Blood Pressure	
Blood pressure is altered slightly, if at all. Orthostatic hypotension, as indicated by feelings of faintness or dizziness immediately after standing up, can develop in the first 48 hours as a result of the splanchnic engorgement that may occur after birth.	A low or decreasing blood pressure may indicate the existence of hypovolemia secondary to hemorrhage; however, it is a late sign, and other symptoms of hemorrhage are usually seen first. An increased reading may result from excessive use of vasopressor or oxytocic medications. Because gestational hypertension can persist into or occur first in the postpartum period, routine evaluation of blood pressure is needed. If a woman states she has a headache, hypertension must be ruled out as a cause before analgesics are administered.

and immobility, this hypercoagulable state causes an increased risk of thromboembolism, especially after a Caesarean birth. Women need to be encouraged to move around as soon as possible after birth to prevent thromboembolism and some women may require anticoagulants. Fibrinolytic activity also increases during the first few days after childbirth (Katz, 2012). Factors I, II, VIII, IX, and X decrease to nonpregnant levels within a few days. Fibrin split products, probably released from the placental site, can also be found in maternal blood.

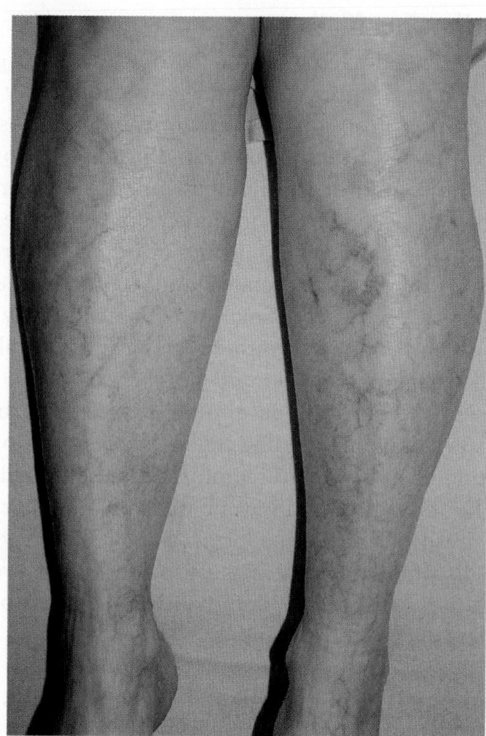

FIGURE 21-3 Varicosities in legs. (Courtesy Cheryl Briggs, BSN, RNC-NIC.)

Varicosities

Varicosities (varices) of the legs and around the anus (hemorrhoids) are common during pregnancy (Fig. 21-3). All varices, even the less common vulvar varices, regress (empty) rapidly immediately after childbirth. Total or nearly total regression of varicosities is expected after childbirth.

RESPIRATORY SYSTEM

When birth occurs, there is an immediate decrease in intra-abdominal pressure, which allows for greater excursion of the diaphragm. With decreased pressure on the diaphragm and reduced pulmonary blood flow, chest wall compliance increases. Rib cage elasticity can take months to return to a prepregnancy state. The costal angle that was increased during pregnancy may not completely return to the prepregnancy level. The decline in progesterone that occurs with loss of the placenta causes $Paco_2$ levels to rise (Blackburn, 2013). The basal metabolic rate gradually returns to prepregnancy levels, usually within 1 to 2 weeks after birth.

NEUROLOGICAL SYSTEM

Neurological changes during the puerperium are those that result from a reversal of maternal adaptations to pregnancy and those resulting from trauma during labour and childbirth.

Pregnancy-induced neurological discomforts disappear after birth. Elimination of physiological edema through the diuresis that follows childbirth relieves carpal tunnel syndrome by easing compression of the median nerve. The periodic numbness and tingling of fingers that afflict 5% of pregnant women usually disappear after the birth, unless lifting and carrying the baby aggravates the condition.

Headache requires careful assessment. Postpartum headaches may be caused by various conditions, including postpartum-onset pre-eclampsia, stress, and leakage of cerebrospinal fluid into the extradural space during placement of the needle for administration of epidural or spinal anaesthesia (see Postdural Puncture Headache, Chapter 18, p. 482).

MUSCULOSKELETAL SYSTEM

Adaptations of the mother's musculoskeletal system that occur during pregnancy are reversed in the puerperium. These adaptations include the relaxation and subsequent hypermobility of the joints and the change in the mother's centre of gravity in response to the enlarging uterus. The joints are completely stabilized by 6 to 8 weeks after birth. Although all other joints return to their normal prepregnancy state, those in the parous woman's feet do not. The new mother may notice a permanent increase in her shoe size.

INTEGUMENTARY SYSTEM

Melasma (chloasma or "mask of pregnancy") usually disappears in the postpartum period but persists in about 30% of women (Kroumpouzos, 2012). Hyperpigmentation of the areolae and linea nigra may not regress completely after childbirth. Some women will have permanent darker pigmentation of those areas. **Striae gravidarum** (stretch marks) (Fig. 10-12) on the breasts, abdomen, and thighs may fade but usually do not disappear.

Vascular abnormalities such as spider angiomas (nevi), palmar erythema, and epulis generally regress in response to the rapid decline in estrogens after the end of pregnancy. For some women, spider nevi persist indefinitely.

Hair growth slows during the postpartum period. Some women may experience hair loss because the amount of hair lost is temporarily more than the amount regrown. The abundance of fine hair seen during pregnancy usually disappears after giving birth; however, any coarse or bristly hair that appears during pregnancy usually remains. Fingernails return to their prepregnancy consistency and strength.

IMMUNE SYSTEM

In the postpartum period, the woman's immune system, which was mildly suppressed during pregnancy, gradually returns to its prepregnant state, although the exact timeline is unclear (Blackburn, 2013). This rebound of the immune system can trigger flare-ups of autoimmune conditions such as multiple sclerosis or lupus erythematosus (Katz, 2012).

KEY POINTS

- The uterus involutes rapidly after birth and returns to the true pelvis within 2 weeks and resumes normal size and position by 6 weeks.
- The rapid decrease in estrogen and progesterone levels after expulsion of the placenta is responsible for triggering many of the anatomical and physiological changes in the puerperium.
- Assessment of lochia and fundal height is essential to monitor the progress of normal involution and to identify potential problems.
- The return of ovulation and menses is determined in part by whether the woman breastfeeds her infant.
- Few alterations in vital signs are seen after birth under normal circumstances.
- Hypercoagulability, vessel damage, and immobility predispose the woman to thromboembolism.
- Marked diuresis, decreased bladder sensitivity, and overdistension of the bladder can lead to problems with urinary elimination.
- Pregnancy-induced hypervolemia, combined with several postpartum physiological changes, allows the woman to tolerate considerable blood loss at birth.

evolve WEBSITE

Visit the Evolve website for additional resources related to the content in this chapter such as Case Studies, Critical Thinking Case Study Answers, Nursing Care Plans, Nursing Processes, Nursing Skills, and Review Questions for Exam Preparation at: *http://evolve.elsevier.com/Canada/Perry/maternal/*

REFERENCES

Blackburn, S. T. (2013). *Maternal, fetal, and neonatal physiology* (4th ed.). St. Louis: Saunders.

Cunningham, F., Leveno, K. J., Bloom, S. L., et al. (2014). *Williams obstetrics* (24th ed.). New York: McGraw Hill.

Katz, V. (2012). Postpartum care. In S. G. Gabbe, J. R. Niebyl, J. L. Simpson, et al. (Eds.), *Obstetrics: Normal and problem pregnancies* (6th ed.). Philadelphia: Saunders.

Kroumpouzos, G. (2012). Skin disease in pregnancy and puerperium. In S. G. Gabbe, J. R. Niebyl, J. L. Simpson, et al. (Eds.), *Obstetrics: Normal and problem pregnancies* (6th ed.). Philadelphia: Saunders.

Monga, M., & Mastrobattasta, J. M. (2014). Maternal cardiovascular, respiratory, and renal adaptation to pregnancy. In R. K. Creasy, R. Resnick, J. Iams, et al. (Eds.), *Creasy & Resnik's maternal-fetal medicine: Principles and practice* (7th ed.). Philadelphia: Saunders.

CHAPTER

22

Nursing Care of the Family During the Postpartum Period

Lisa Keenan-Lindsay

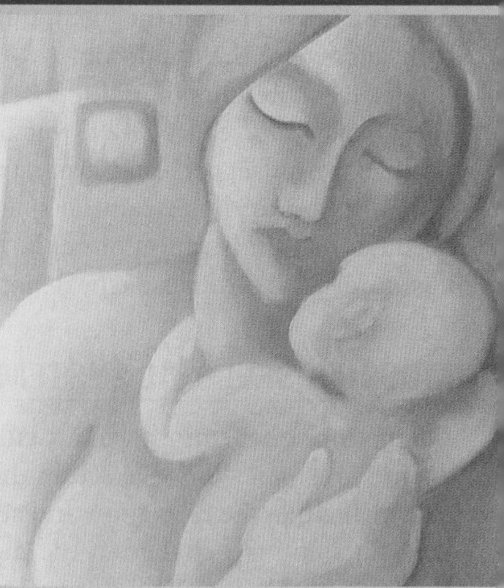

evolve WEBSITE

Visit the Evolve website for additional resources related to the content in this chapter such as Case Studies, Critical Thinking Case Study Answers, Nursing Care Plans, Nursing Processes, Nursing Skills, and Review Questions for Exam Preparation at: *http://evolve.elsevier.com/Canada/Perry/maternal/*

OBJECTIVES

On completion of this chapter the reader will be able to:

- Describe components of a systematic postpartum assessment.
- Recognize signs of potential complications in the postpartum woman.
- Identify criteria for postpartum discharge.
- Formulate a nursing care plan for a woman in the postpartum period.
- Explain the influence of cultural beliefs and practices on postpartum care.
- Identify psychosocial needs of the woman in the early postpartum period.
- Prepare a plan for postpartum teaching for a new mother's self-management.
- Describe the nurse's role in these postpartum follow-up strategies: home visits, telephone follow-up, warm lines and help lines, support groups, and referrals to community resources.

At no other time is family-centred maternity care more important than in the postpartum period. Nursing care is provided in the context of the family unit and focuses on assessment and support of the woman's physiological and emotional adaptation after birth. During the early postpartum period, components of nursing care include assisting the mother with rest and recovery from the process of labour and birth, assessing her physiological and psychological adaptation after birth, preventing complications, educating her about self-care and infant care, and supporting the mother and her partner during the initial transition to parenthood. In addition, the nurse considers the needs of other family members and includes strategies in the nursing care plan to help the family adjust to the new baby.

The approach to the care of women after birth is wellness oriented. In Canada most women remain hospitalized no more than 1 or 2 days after vaginal birth and 2 to 4 days for a Caesarean birth. Because so much important information needs to be shared with these women in a very short time, their care must be thoughtfully planned and provided. This chapter discusses nursing care of the woman and her family in the postpartum period extending into the fourth trimester.

TRANSFER FROM THE RECOVERY AREA

After the initial recovery period of about 1 to 2 hours, has been completed, the woman may be transferred to a postpartum room in the same or another nursing unit. In facilities with labour, birth, recovery, and postpartum (LBRP) rooms, the woman labours, gives birth, recovers, and spends the postpartum period in the same room, and the nurse who provides care during the recovery period may continue to care for the woman. In many settings women who have received general or regional anaesthesia must be cleared for transfer from the recovery area by a member of the anaesthesia care team. In other settings a nurse makes this determination. In preparing the transfer report, the nurse caring for the woman during the recovery period uses information from the records of admission, birth record, and recovery. Information communicated to

TABLE 22-1 RECOVERY NURSE'S REPORT

ITEM	EXAMPLE OF DOCUMENTATION OF MOTHER	EXAMPLE OF DOCUMENTATION OF NEWBORN
Type of labour and birth; unusual observations, if any, of the placenta	Spontaneous or assisted (forceps, vacuum extraction) vaginal birth; vertex presentation; time of ROM	Spontaneous or assisted (forceps) vaginal birth; vertex presentation; time of ROM
GTPAL, age	G1T0P0A0L0, age 22 yr; 39 wk of gestation	G1T0P0A0L0, age 22 yr; 39 wk of gestation
Anaesthesia and analgesia used	None; epidural, spinal, local	None; epidural, spinal, local
Condition of perineum	Episiotomy; lacerations; repaired; intact	
Events since birth	Vital signs, BP, fundus, lochia, intake and output, medications (dosage, time of administration, and results); length of time newborn was skin-to-skin and with whom; response to newborn; observation of family interactions, including siblings, if present	Vital signs, blood glucose level (if assessed), nursed at breast for ____ min Voided × 1; meconium stool × 1 Eye prophylaxis given Vitamin K injection given Skin-to-skin for ____ min Held by siblings who are happy (or have other response to newborn)
Condition and sex of newborn; other information	Time of birth; weight; whether breastfeeding or bottle-feeding; sex of the baby	Time of birth; Apgar at 1 and 5 min; sex; weight; name of health care provider; breastfeeding or bottle-feeding; mother's hepatitis B status and GBS status; whether mother received magnesium sulphate; time of last systemic analgesia; whether mother received adequate antibiotic prophylaxis for GBS
Relevant information from prenatal record	Need for rubella vaccination; presence of infections; hepatitis B status; HIV status; blood type; Rh status; GBS status and treatment if positive	Unremarkable pregnancy
Miscellaneous information: IV drip	If IV drip is infusing, rate of infusion, medications added (e.g., oxytocin), whether to keep open or discontinue after completion of bag that is hung	
Social factors	If woman is releasing baby for adoption, whether she wants to see baby, breastfeed, or allow visitors, or other preferences she may have	Baby up for adoption

BP, blood pressure; *GBS*, group B streptococcus; *HIV*, human immunodeficiency virus; *IV*, intravenous; *NBN*, newborn nursery; *ROM*, rupture of membranes.

the postpartum nurse includes identity of the health care provider; obstetrical history; age; anaesthetic used; any medications given; duration of labour and time of rupture of membranes; whether labour was induced or augmented; type of birth and repair; blood type and Rh status; group B streptococcus status; status of rubella immunity; hepatitis serology test results; intravenous infusion of any fluids; physiological status since birth; description of fundus, lochia, bladder, and perineum; sex and weight of infant; time of birth; name of the newborn's care provider; chosen method of feeding; any abnormalities noted; and assessment of initial parent–infant interactions. In addition, specific information should be provided regarding the infant's Apgar scores (see Chapter 26), voiding, and stooling and whether the infant has been fed since birth. Nursing interventions that have been completed (e.g., eye prophylaxis and vitamin K injection) also must be recorded. Table 22-1 gives examples for documenting this information before the transfer of the woman from the recovery area.

PLANNING FOR DISCHARGE

From their initial contact with the labouring woman, nurses prepare the new mother for the time when she will return home. Planning for discharge begins with the first interaction between the nurse, the woman, and her family and continues until they leave the hospital or birthing facility.

The length of stay after giving birth depends on many factors, including the physical condition of the mother and the newborn, emotional status of the mother, social support at home, patient education needs for self-care and infant care, and financial constraints.

Women who give birth in birthing centres and in hospital may be discharged within a few hours, after the woman's and infant's conditions are stable, although most mothers and newborns who have no complications are discharged from the hospital within 24 to 36 hours after vaginal birth.

Before discharge the nurse needs to ensure that the health of the mother and her newborn is stable and that the mother is able and confident to provide care for her infant; there should be adequate support systems in place and access to follow-up care. It is essential that the nurse consider the individual needs of the woman and her newborn and provide care that is coordinated to meet these needs, to provide timely physiological interventions and treatment that can prevent morbidity and hospital readmission. Hospital-based maternity nurses continue to play invaluable roles as caregivers, teachers, and advocates for mothers, newborns, and families in developing and implementing effective home-care strategies. With predetermined criteria for identifying low risk in mothers and newborns (Box 22-1), the length of hospitalization can be based on medical need for care in an acute care setting or in consideration of ongoing care needed in the home. Postpartum order sets and maternal teaching checklists (Fig. 22-1) can be used to accomplish patient care tasks and educational outcomes. Nurses must also provide discharge teaching related to the newborn. With coordination, clinical care and education can be planned and provided throughout pregnancy, during the hospital stay, and in the home after discharge to promote and support the family's continued well-being. Community-based postpartum care programs are key to reducing readmission of newborns. Mothers should be contacted and, if needed, seen by a skilled caregiver within 24 to 48 hours after discharge to ensure that newborn health issues are identified (e.g., jaundice, dehydration).

LEGAL TIP *EARLY DISCHARGE*

Whether or not the woman and her family have chosen early discharge, the nurse and the primary health care provider are responsible for ensuring that the woman is not discharged before her condition has stabilized within normal limits.

NURSING CARE

The nursing plan of care includes both the postpartum woman and her infant. It is also family centred, considering the needs and concerns of the family and focusing on family unity (Waller-Wise, 2012). In most hospitals in Canada, combined care (also called *single-room maternity care*) is practised. Nurses in these settings have been educated in both mother and infant care and function as primary nurses for the mother and infant.

Ongoing Physical Assessment

Ongoing assessments are performed throughout hospitalization. In addition to vital signs, physical assessment of the postpartum woman focuses on evaluation of the breasts, uterine fundus, lochia, perineum, bladder and bowel function, vital signs, and legs, using the acronym BUBBLLEE. See Table 22-2 for normal findings.

- B = **Breasts** (firmness) and nipples
- U = **Uterine** fundus (location; consistency)
- B = **Bladder** function (amount; frequency)
- B = **Bowel** function (passing gas or bowel movement)
- L = **Lochia** (amount; colour)
- L = **Legs** (peripheral edema)
- **E = Episiotomy/Laceration or Caesarean birth incision** (perineum: discomfort; condition of repair, if done)
- E = **Emotional status** (mood, fatigue)

Routine Laboratory Tests

Several laboratory tests may be performed in the immediate postpartum period. Hemoglobin and hematocrit values may be evaluated on the first postpartum day to assess blood loss during birth, especially after Caesarean birth. In addition, if the woman's rubella and Rh status are unknown, tests to determine

BOX 22-1 CRITERIA FOR DISCHARGE

Mother

Perineum is healing with appropriate care provided.
There are no intrapartum or postpartum complications that require ongoing treatment or observation.
The mother is mobile with adequate pain control.
Bladder and bowel functions are adequate (although she will probably not have had a bowel movement).
The mother has received Rh immune globulin, if appropriate.
The mother has demonstrated ability to feed the infant—i.e., the infant has demonstrated adequate latch.
Contraception advice has been provided.
The care provider for ongoing care has been identified and notified of discharge.
The community liaison nurse is aware of discharge and has access to the patient's contact information for postdischarge follow-up (if appropriate).
Appointments are made for follow-up and the mother understands the necessity for and timing of newborn health checks.
If the home environment is not adequate, community resources are in place to support the new mother and infant.
The mother is aware of community resources and how and when to access these resources.
The mother has received rubella immunization if she is not immune.

Infant

The infant is a term infant (37 to 42 weeks) with weight appropriate for gestational age.
There is normal cardiorespiratory adaptation to extrauterine life.
Temperature, respirations, and heart rate are within normal limits and stable. At least two successful feedings have been completed (normal sucking and swallowing).
Urination and stooling have occurred at least once.
There is no evidence of significant jaundice in the first 24 hours after the birth.
There is no evidence of sepsis.
There is no evidence of bleeding from circumcision for ≥2 hours (if procedure is performed prior to discharge).
Metabolic screening tests have been performed according to provincial policies; tests should be repeated at the follow-up visit if done before the infant is 24 hours old.
Newborn hearing screening test is completed before discharge; if not, alternative arrangements have been made for testing.
The mother is able to provide newborn care and recognizes signs of illness or concerns related to her newborn.
Arrangements have been made for assessment and evaluation of the newborn within 48 hours of discharge, i.e., with a community health nurse, physician, or midwife.
Initial hepatitis B vaccine has been given or scheduled for the first follow-up visit if required by provincial guidelines.

Summary, Education/Anticipatory Guidance

☐ Interpretation req'd Language ____________________

EDUCATION/ANTICIPATORY GUIDANCE	INITIALS	INITIALS	N/A	COMMENTS
1. Breast, nipple care, management of engorement				
2. Knows how to hand express milk				
3. Recognizes and responds to infant feeding cues, behaviours				
4. Recognizes effective feeding and milk transfer				
5. For infants fed breastmilk substitute: appropriate formula, preparation, and storage				
6. Normal physiological change/care, fundus & flow, incision				
7. Voiding & bowel patterns				
8. Self-care hygiene, pericare				
9. Pain management/options				
10. S &S for follow-up (e.g., fever, infection, overly drowsy)				
11. Community and Admission medications reviewed. Discharge prescription written and given to patient. Patient teaching complete.				
Discharge prescription given to patient and patient teaching complete.				
12. Activity and rest				
13. Healthy eating				
14. Postpartum blues/depression				
15. Family planning/sexuality				
16. Support systems in place				
17. Access to *Baby's Best Chance* Parents' Handbook				
18. Tests and procedures Rubella status _______ MMR given: Date _______ Initials _______ Rh immune globulin given: Date _______ Time _______ Initials _______ Other: ____________________ ____________________				
19. Tobacco cessation/exposure to second-hand smoke				
20. Review of communicable diseases				
21. Knows who primary health care provider (PHCP) is, how to access & when to contact				
22. Aware of PHN contact/role/community resources				
23. Ready for hospital discharge, discharge order				

Variances - Plan(s) including referrals

____

5 Discharge Postpartum hours/days at discharge: ____________ ☐ Home with Baby ☐ Liaison completed

Hospital discharge: Date ______________ Time __________ RN Signature ____________________

PSBC 1592 – JANUARY 2011 V2 ©Perinatal Services BC

FIGURE 22-1 Maternal teaching and discharge plan. *MMR*, measles, mumps, and rubella; *N/A*, not applicable; *PHN*, public health nurse; *RN*, registered nurse; *S&S*, signs and symptoms. (Printed with permission from Perinatal Services BC.)

TABLE 22-2 POSTPARTUM ASSESSMENT AND SIGNS OF POTENTIAL COMPLICATIONS

ASSESSMENT	NORMAL FINDINGS	SIGNS OF POTENTIAL COMPLICATIONS
Blood pressure (BP)	Consistent with BP baseline during pregnancy; can have orthostatic hypotension for 48 hours	Hypertension: anxiety, pre-eclampsia, essential hypertension Hypotension: hemorrhage
Temperature	36.2°–38° C (97.2°–100.4° F)	>38° C (100.4° F) after 24 hours: infection
Pulse	60–100 beats/min	Tachycardia: pain, fever, dehydration, hemorrhage
Respirations	16–24 breaths/min	Bradypnea: effects of narcotic medications Tachypnea: anxiety; may be sign of respiratory disease
Breath sounds	Clear to auscultation	Crackles: possible fluid overload
Breasts	Days 1–2: soft Days 2–3: filling Days 3–5: full, soften with breastfeeding (milk is "in")	Firmness, heat, pain: engorgement Redness of breast tissue, heat, pain, fever, body aches: mastitis
Nipples	Skin intact; no soreness reported	Redness, bruising, cracks, fissures, abrasions, blisters: usually associated with latching problems
Uterus (fundus)	Firm, midline; first 24 hours at level of umbilicus; involutes ≈1–2 cm/day	Soft, boggy, higher than expected level: uterine atony Lateral deviation: distended bladder
Bladder	Able to void spontaneously by 8 hours; no distension; able to empty completely; no dysuria Diuresis begins ≈12 hours after birth; can void 3000 mL/day	Overdistended bladder possibly causing uterine atony, excessive lochia Dysuria, frequency, urgency: infection
Bowels and abdomen	Bowel movement by day 2 or 3 after birth Abdomen soft, active bowel sounds in all quadrants (assessed if Caesarean birth)	No bowel movement by day 3 or 4: constipation; diarrhea
Lochia	Days 1–3: rubra (dark red) Days 4–10: serosa (brownish red or pink) After 10 days: alba (yellowish white) Amount: scant to moderate Few clots Fleshy odour	Large amount of lochia: uterine atony, vaginal or cervical laceration Foul odour: infection
Swelling (legs)	Peripheral edema possibly present	Redness, tenderness, pain, venous thromboembolism (VTE)
Perineum/Incision	Minimal edema Laceration or episiotomy: edges approximated Caesarean: incision dressing clean and dry; suture line intact	Pronounced edema, bruising, hematoma Redness, warmth, drainage: infection Abdominal incision—redness, edema, warmth, drainage: infection
Rectal area	No hemorrhoids; if hemorrhoids are present, soft and pink	Discoloured hemorrhoidal tissue, severe pain: thrombosed hemorrhoid
Emotional status/ Energy level	Able to care for self and infant; able to sleep Excited, happy, interested or involved in infant care Sad and tearful on day 3–14: postpartum blues	Lethargy, extreme fatigue, difficulty sleeping: postpartum depression Sad, tearful, disinterested in infant care: postpartum mood disorder

her status and need for possible treatment should be performed at this time.

Nursing Interventions

Based on the available data (e.g., medical record) and assessment findings, the nurse plans with the woman which nursing measures are appropriate and which are to be given priority. The nursing plan of care includes periodic assessments to detect deviations from normal physical changes, measures to relieve discomfort or pain, safety measures to prevent injury or infection, and teaching and counselling measures designed to promote the woman's feelings of competence in self-care and newborn care. The spouse or partner as well as other family members who are present can be included in the teaching. The nurse evaluates continuously and is ready to change the plan, if indicated. Almost all hospitals use standardized care plans or care maps as a base. Nurses individualize care of the postpartum woman and newborn according to their specific needs (see Nursing Care Plan: Postpartum Care—Vaginal Birth, available on Evolve). Signs of potential problems that may be identified during the assessment process are listed in Table 22-2.

Nurses assume many roles while implementing the nursing plan of care. They provide direct physical care, teach mother and baby care, and provide anticipatory guidance and counselling. Perhaps most important of all, they nurture the woman by providing encouragement and support as she begins to assume the many tasks of motherhood. Nurses who take the time to "mother the mother" do much to increase feelings of self-confidence in new mothers. Nurses need to be careful to include the woman's partner and other primary support persons in education and counselling.The woman and her family need to be oriented to their surroundings. Familiarity with the postpartum unit, routines, resources, and personnel reduces one potential source of anxiety—the unknown. The mother can be reassured through knowing whom and how she can call for assistance and what she can expect in the way of supplies and services. If the woman's usual daily routine before admission differs from the routine of the facility, the nurse should work with the woman to develop a mutually acceptable routine. The nurse must also confirm the woman's identity, by checking her wristband. At the same time, the infant's identification number is matched with the corresponding band on the mother's wrist and, in some instances, the partner's wrist. The nurse should determine how the mother wishes to be addressed and note her preference in her record.

While infant abduction from hospitals in Canada is rare, hospital staff should be alert and prepared for such an event. The mother should be taught to check the identity of any person who comes to remove the baby from her room; hospital personnel wear picture identification badges. On some units all staff members wear matching scrubs or special badges. Other units use closed-circuit television, computer monitoring systems, or fingerprint identification pads. Many hospitals have systems to prevent infant abduction that involve attaching a security tag to the infant's ankle. This will cause an alarm to sound or doors to lock when the infant is close to a unit exit. Patients and nurses must work together to ensure the safety of newborns in the hospital environment.

SAFETY ALERT

Nurses play a critical role in educating parents about measures to prevent infant abduction. Parents should be instructed how to identify legitimate hospital personnel, to never leave the newborn in the hospital room without direct supervision, and to request a second staff member to verify the identity of any questionable person who wants to take the baby from the mother's room. Parents should be instructed to use caution when posting photos of the new baby on the Internet and publishing public notices about the birth (Vincent, 2009).

Prevention of Infection

Nurses in the postpartum setting are acutely aware of the importance of preventing infection in their patients. One important means of preventing infection is maintaining a clean environment. Bed linens should be changed as needed. Disposable pads should be changed frequently. Women should wear shoes when walking about to avoid picking up bacteria from the floor and contaminating the linens when they return to bed. Personnel must be conscientious about their hand hygiene to prevent cross-infection. Routine precautions must be practised. Staff members with colds, coughs, or skin infections (e.g., a cold sore on the lips [herpes simplex virus type I]) must follow hospital protocol when in contact with postpartum patients. In many hospitals, staff with open herpetic lesions, strep throat, conjunctivitis, upper respiratory infections, or diarrhea are encouraged to avoid contact with mothers and infants by staying home until the condition is no longer contagious. Visitors with signs of illness should not be permitted to enter the postpartum unit.

Perineal lacerations and episiotomies can increase the risk of infection through interruption in skin integrity. Proper perineal care helps prevent infection in the genitourinary area and aids the healing process. Nurses should teach the woman to wipe from front to back (urethra to anus) after voiding or defecating in order to prevent infection. In many hospitals, a squeeze bottle (peri bottle) filled with warm water is used after each voiding to cleanse the perineal area. The woman should change her perineal pad from front to back each time she voids or defecates and wash her hands thoroughly before and after doing so (Box 22-2).

Prevention of Excessive Bleeding

The most frequent cause of excessive bleeding after childbirth is uterine **atony**, or failure of the uterine muscle to contract firmly. The two most important interventions for preventing excessive bleeding are maintaining good uterine tone and preventing bladder distension. If uterine atony occurs, the relaxed uterus distends with blood and clots, blood vessels in the placental site are not clamped off, and excessive bleeding results.

One reason for uterine atony can be retained placental fragments. Excessive blood loss after childbirth can also be caused by vaginal or vulvar hematomas or by unrepaired lacerations of the vagina or cervix. These potential sources might be suspected if excessive vaginal bleeding occurs in the presence of a firmly contracted uterus. See discussion of postpartum hemorrhage (PPH) in Chapter 24 for more information on reasons for excessive bleeding.

NURSING ALERT

A perineal pad saturated in 15 minutes or less or pooling of blood under the buttocks is an indication of excessive blood loss requiring immediate assessment, intervention, and notification of the primary health care provider.

Accurate visual estimation of blood loss is an important nursing responsibility. Blood loss is usually described subjectively as scant, light, moderate, or heavy (profuse). Fig. 22-2 shows examples of perineal pad saturation corresponding to each of these descriptions.

Although postpartal blood loss may be estimated by observing the amount of staining on a perineal pad, it is difficult to judge the amount of lochial flow based only on observation of perineal pads. More objective estimates of blood loss include measuring serial hemoglobin or hematocrit values, weighing blood clots and items saturated with blood (1 g equals 1 mL), and establishing the millilitres it takes to saturate perineal pads being used. See Additional Resources at the end of the chapter for a video developed by the Association of Women's Health, Obstetrical and Neonatal Nurses (AWHONN) that discusses estimation of blood loss.

Any estimation of lochial flow is inaccurate and incomplete without consideration of the time factor. The woman who saturates a perineal pad in 1 hour or less is bleeding much more heavily than the woman who saturates a perineal pad in 8 hours.

Nurses in general tend to overestimate rather than underestimate blood loss. Also, different brands of perineal pads vary in their saturation volume and soaking appearance. For example, blood placed on some brands tends to soak down into the pad,

BOX 22-2 INTERVENTIONS FOR EPISIOTOMY, LACERATIONS, AND HEMORRHOIDS

Explain both the procedure and rationale before implementation.

Cleansing

Teach the woman to:

- Wash hands before and after cleansing perineum and changing pads.
- Wash perineum with mild soap and warm water at least once daily.
- Cleanse from symphysis pubis to anal area.
- Apply peripad from front to back, protecting inner surface of pad from contamination.
- Wrap soiled pad and place in covered waste container.
- Change pad with each void or defecation or at least four times per day.
- Assess amount and character of lochia with each pad change.

Ice Pack (for First 24 Hours)

Apply a covered ice pack to perineum from front to back:

- During first 2 hours to decrease edema formation and to increase comfort
- After the first 2 hours following the birth to provide anaesthetic effect

Squeeze Bottle (Peri Bottle)

Demonstrate use and assist woman.

Fill bottle with tap water warmed to approximately 38°C (comfortably warm on the wrist).

Instruct woman to position nozzle between her legs so that squirts of water reach perineum as she sits on toilet seat. Explain that it will take the whole bottle of water to cleanse the perineum.

Teach her to blot dry with toilet paper or clean wipes.

Remind her to avoid contamination from anal area.

Apply clean pad.

Peri bottle. (Courtesy of Lunapads.)

Sitz Bath: Disposable

Encourage woman to use at least twice a day for 20 minutes, if required.

Place call bell within easy reach.

Clamp tubing and fill bag with warm water.

Raise toilet seat and place bath in bowl with overflow opening directed toward back of toilet.

Place container above toilet bowl.

Attach tube into groove at front of bath.

Loosen tube clamp to regulate rate of flow; fill bath to about one-half full.

Teach woman to sit on sitz bath by first tightening gluteal muscles and keeping them tightened and then relaxing them after she is on the sitz bath.

Place dry towels within reach.

Ensure privacy.

Check woman in 15 minutes.

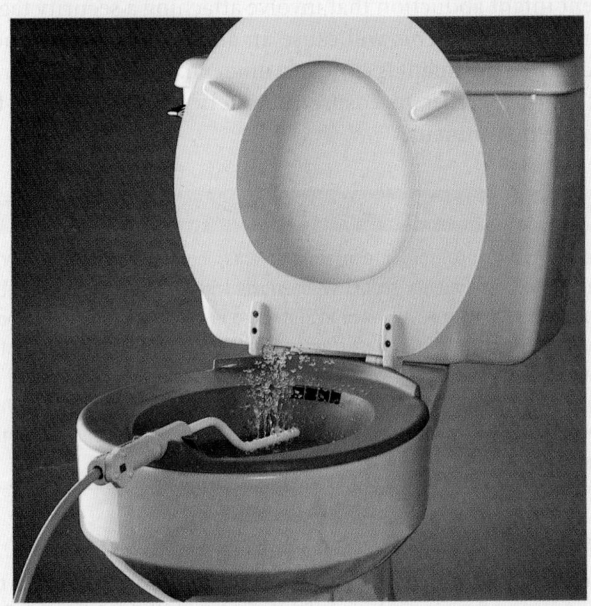

Sitz bath. (Leifer, G. [2015]. *Introduction to maternity and pediatric nursing* [7th ed.]. St. Louis: Saunders.)

Topical Applications

Apply anaesthetic cream or spray: use sparingly three to four times per day, if required.

Offer witch hazel pads (Tucks) for after voiding or defecating; woman pats perineum dry from front to back and then applies witch hazel pads.

Apply hemorrhoidal cream as ordered to anal area after cleansing.

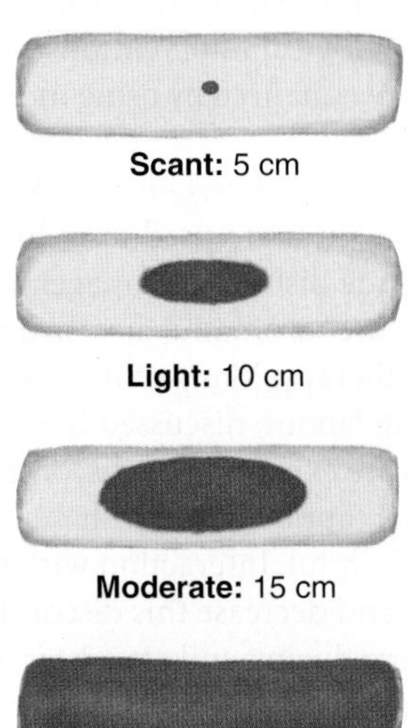

FIGURE 22-2 Blood loss after birth is assessed by the extent of perineal pad saturation as (from top to bottom) scant, light, moderate, or heavy (one pad saturated within 2 hours). (From Leifer, G. [2015]. *Introduction to maternity and pediatric nursing*, [7th ed.]. St. Louis: Saunders.)

whereas on other brands it tends to spread outward. Nurses should determine saturation volume and soaking appearance for the perineal pad brands used in their institution to improve accuracy of blood loss estimation.

NURSING ALERT

The nurse should always check under the mother's buttocks. Although the amount on the perineal pad may be slight, blood may flow between the buttocks onto the linens under the mother. When this happens, excessive bleeding goes undetected.

When excessive bleeding occurs, vital signs need to be monitored closely. Blood pressure is not a reliable indicator of impending shock from early hemorrhage because compensatory mechanisms prevent a significant drop in blood pressure until the woman has lost 30 to 40% of her blood volume. Respirations, pulse, skin condition, urinary output, and level of consciousness are more sensitive means of identifying hypovolemic shock. The frequent physical assessments performed during the fourth stage of labour (see Box 17-16, p. 455) are designed to provide prompt identification of excessive bleeding (see Emergency box).

Maintenance of Uterine Tone

A major intervention to restore good uterine tone is stimulation, by gently massaging the fundus until firm (Fig. 22-3). Fundal massage can cause a temporary increase in the amount of vaginal bleeding seen as pooled blood leaves the uterus. Clots can be expelled. The uterus may remain boggy even after massage and expulsion of clots.

Fundal massage can be a very uncomfortable procedure. Communicating the causes and dangers of uterine atony and the purpose of fundal massage to the woman can help her understand the reason for the procedure and tolerate it. Teaching the woman to massage her own fundus enables her to maintain some control and can decrease her anxiety.

When uterine atony and excessive bleeding occur, additional interventions likely to be used are administration of intravenous fluids and uterotonic medications (drugs that stimulate contraction of the uterine smooth muscle). See the Medication Guide, Chapter 24 (p. 610) for information about common uterotonic medications.

Prevention of Bladder Distension

Uterine atony and excessive bleeding after birth can be the result of bladder distension. A full bladder causes the uterus to be displaced above the umbilicus and well to one side of the midline in the abdomen. It also prevents the uterus from contracting normally.

Women can be at risk of bladder distension resulting from urinary retention, based on intrapartum factors. These risk factors include epidural anaesthesia, extensive vaginal or perineal lacerations, episiotomy, instrument-assisted birth, or prolonged labour. Women who have had in-dwelling catheters can

EMERGENCY

Hypovolemic Shock

Signs and Symptoms

Persistent significant bleeding: Perineal pad is soaked within 15 minutes; initially it may not be accompanied by a change in vital signs or maternal colour or behaviour.
Woman states she feels weak, light-headed, "funny," or "nauseated" or "sees stars."
Woman appears anxious or exhibits air hunger.
Skin colour turns ashen or greyish.
Skin feels cool and clammy.
Pulse rate increases.
Blood pressure declines.

Interventions

Notify primary health care provider.
If uterus is atonic, massage gently and expel clots to cause uterus to contract.
Administer utertonic medications (e.g., oxytocin, prostaglandins) as ordered to increase uterine tone.
Give oxygen by nonrebreather face mask or nasal prongs at 8 to 10 L/min.
Tilt woman to her side or elevate the right hip; elevate her legs to at least a 30-degree angle.
Provide additional or maintain existing IV infusion of lactated Ringer's solution or normal saline solution to restore circulatory volume (the woman should have two patent IV lines: insert second IV infusion using 16- to 18-gauge IV catheter).
Administer blood or blood products as ordered.
Monitor vital signs.
Insert an in-dwelling urinary catheter to monitor perfusion of kidneys.
Administer emergency medications as ordered.
Prepare for possible surgery or other emergency treatments or procedures.
Record incident, medical and nursing interventions instituted, and woman's response to interventions.

IV, intravenous.

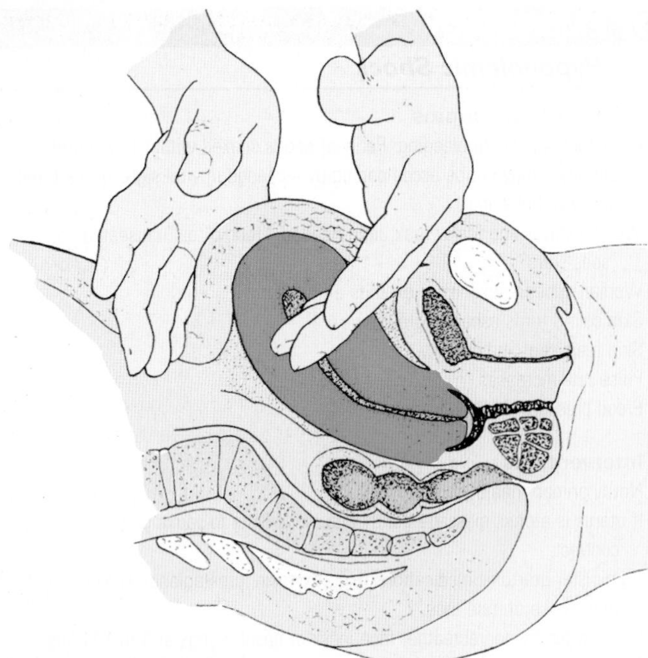

FIGURE 22-3 Palpating and massaging fundus of uterus. Note that upper hand is cupped over fundus; lower hand dips in above symphysis pubis and supports uterus while it is massaged gently.

experience some difficulty, as they initially attempt to void after the catheter is removed. Nurses aware of these risk factors can be proactive in preventing complications.

Nursing interventions focus on helping the woman empty her bladder spontaneously as soon as possible. The first priority is to assist the woman to the bathroom or onto a bedpan if she is unable to ambulate. Having her listen to running water, placing her hands in warm water, or pouring water from a squeeze bottle over her perineum may stimulate voiding. Assisting the woman into the shower or sitz bath and encouraging her to void can be effective. Administering analgesics, if ordered, may be indicated because some women anticipate pain and thus fear voiding. If these measures are unsuccessful, a sterile catheter can be inserted to drain the urine.

Promotion of Comfort

Most women experience some degree of discomfort during the postpartum period. Common causes of discomfort include afterbirth pains (afterpains), perineal laceration or episiotomy, hemorrhoids, sore nipples, and breast engorgement. The woman's description of the type and severity of her pain is the best guide in choosing an appropriate intervention. To confirm the location and extent of discomfort, the nurse needs to inspect and palpate areas of pain, as appropriate, for redness, swelling, discharge, and heat and observe for body tension, guarded movements, and facial tension. Blood pressure, pulse, and respirations may be elevated in response to acute pain. Diaphoresis may accompany severe pain. A lack of objective signs does not necessarily mean there is no pain because there may also be a cultural component to the expression of pain. Nursing interventions are intended to eliminate the pain sensation entirely or reduce it to a tolerable level that allows the woman to care for herself and her baby. Nurses may use both nonpharmacological and pharmacological interventions to promote comfort. Pain relief is generally enhanced by using more than one method or route.

Nonpharmacological interventions. A variety of nonpharmacological measures are used to reduce postpartum discomfort. These include distraction, imagery, therapeutic touch, relaxation, acupressure, aromatherapy, hydrotherapy, massage therapy, and music therapy. Many of these measures are similar to those used during labour, discussed in Chapter 18.

For women who are experiencing discomfort associated with uterine contractions, applying warmth (e.g., heating pad) or lying prone may be helpful. Interaction with the infant may also provide distraction and decrease this discomfort. Because afterpains are more severe during and after breastfeeding, interventions are planned to provide the most timely and effective relief. Administering pain medication about 30 minutes before breastfeeding can help minimize afterpains that are caused by breastfeeding.

Simple interventions that can decrease the discomfort associated with an episiotomy or perineal lacerations include encouraging the woman to lie on her side whenever possible. Other interventions include application of an ice pack (for first 24 hours); topical medication (if ordered); heat; cleansing with a squeeze bottle; and a cleansing shower, tub bath, or sitz bath. Many of these interventions, especially ice packs, sitz baths, and topical applications (e.g., witch hazel pads), are also effective for hemorrhoids (see Box 22-2).

Sore nipples in breastfeeding mothers are most likely related to ineffective latch technique. Assessment of and assistance with feeding are most important in helping the mother establish an effective technique. To ease discomfort associated with sore nipples, the mother may apply: expressed colostrum or breastmilk, topical preparations such as purified lanolin or hydrogel pads (see Chapter 27).

Breast engorgement can occur whether the woman is breastfeeding or formula-feeding. The discomfort associated with engorged breasts may be reduced by applying ice packs or cabbage leaves (or both) (see further discussion below, p. 575) to the breasts and wearing a well-fitted support bra. Anti-inflammatory medications can also help relieve some of the discomfort. Decisions about specific interventions for engorgement are based on whether the woman chooses breastfeeding or bottle-feeding.

Pharmacological interventions. Pharmacological interventions are commonly used to relieve or reduce postpartum discomfort. Most health care providers routinely order a variety of analgesics to be administered as needed, including both opioid and nonopioid (e.g., nonsteroidal anti-inflammatory drugs [NSAIDs]) medications. Topical application of antiseptic or anaesthetic ointments or spray can be used for perineal pain. Patient-controlled analgesia (PCA) pumps and epidural analgesia are commonly used to provide pain relief after Caesarean birth.

! NURSING ALERT

The nurse should monitor all women receiving opioids carefully because respiratory depression and decreased intestinal motility are adverse effects.

Many women want to participate in decisions about using analgesia. If an analgesic is to be given, the nurse must, in conjunction with the mother, make a clinical judgement of the type, dosage, and frequency from the medications ordered. The woman should be informed of the prescribed analgesic and its common adverse effects; this teaching should be documented. Many hospitals offer self-medication packages for postpartum women. These packages have the medications that a woman might require in the immediate postpartum period. Women are given instructions regarding the medications and administration and to take them when necessary, documenting when they take the medication.

If acceptable pain relief has not been obtained within 1 hour and there has been no change in the initial assessment, the nurse can contact the primary care provider for additional pain-relief orders or further directions. Unrelieved pain results in fatigue, anxiety, and a worsening perception of the pain. It can also indicate the presence of a previously unidentified or untreated problem.

Breastfeeding mothers often have concerns about the effects of an analgesic on the infant. Although nearly all medications present in maternal circulation are also found in breast milk, many analgesics commonly used during the postpartum period are considered relatively safe for breastfeeding mothers. Non-opioid analgesics are preferred for pain management in postpartum breastfeeding women because they do not alter maternal or infant alertness (Lawrence & Lawrence, 2011). Timing of medication administration can be adjusted to minimize infant exposure. A mother may be given pain medication immediately after breastfeeding so that the interval between medication administration and the next nursing period is as long as possible. The decision to administer medications of any type to a breastfeeding mother must always be made by carefully weighing the woman's need against actual or potential risks to the infant. Resources are readily accessible for nurses and health care providers to examine the safety of medications for breastfeeding mothers (see Additional Resources at the end of the chapter).

Promotion of Rest

Fatigue is common in the early postpartum period and involves both physiological and psychological components. Physical fatigue or exhaustion can be associated with long labours or Caesarean birth; hospital routines and infant care demands, such as breastfeeding, also contribute to maternal fatigue. It can also be associated with anemia, infection, or thyroid dysfunction. The excitement and exhilaration experienced after the birth of the infant make resting difficult. Physical discomfort can interfere with sleep. Well-intentioned visitors can interrupt periods of rest in the hospital and at home.

Postpartum fatigue. *Postpartum fatigue (PPF)* is more than just feeling tired; it is a complex phenomenon affected by a combination of physiological, psychological, and situational variables (Volrathongchai, Neelasmith, & Thinkhamrop, 2013). Symptoms of PPF and depressive symptoms are interrelated (Doering Runquist, Morin, & Stetzer, 2009; Song, Chang, Park, et al., 2010), yet each has distinct patterns (Kuo, Yang, Kuo, et al., 2012). Depressive symptoms can affect fatigue, whereas fatigue can lead to depressive symptoms. Depression-related PPF can be differentiated from nondepression-related PPF on the basis of whether or not depressive symptoms are reduced when fatigue is decreased (Runquist, 2007).

Fatigue is likely to worsen over the first 6 weeks after birth, often because of situational factors. After discharge from the hospital, fatigue increases as the woman provides care and feeding for the newborn in combination with other family and household responsibilities, such as caring for other children, preparing meals, and doing laundry. Many women have partners, family members, or friends to provide much-needed assistance, whereas others can be without any help at all. The nurse needs to inquire about resources available to the woman after discharge and help her plan accordingly.

Interventions are planned to meet the woman's individual needs for sleep and rest while she is in the hospital. Back rubs and other comfort measures may be necessary. The side-lying position for breastfeeding minimizes fatigue in nursing mothers. Support and encouragement of mothering behaviours can help reduce anxiety. Hospital and nursing routines can be adjusted to meet the needs of individual mothers. In addition, the nurse can help the family limit visitors and provide a comfortable chair or bed for the partner or other family member staying with the new mother.

Because PPF can be very debilitating, follow-up after hospital discharge is important. Screening for PPF can be accomplished with a nurse-initiated telephone call at 2 weeks postpartum and at the routine 6-week postpartum visit with the health care provider. Nurses in the pediatric care provider's office or clinic should also be alert for signs of PPF, as they often see the mother before she sees her obstetrical care provider.Physiological factors contributing to PPF are amenable to intervention and may be identified even before birth. Women with sleeping problems during pregnancy, anemia, infection or inflammation, or thyroid dysfunction can be identified as having increased risk for PPF. Other physical conditions and psychological or situational factors that might contribute to PPF can be identified during the prenatal period. The medical records of women with known risk factors can be flagged to alert hospital staff to their special needs (see Critical Thinking Case Study).

Promotion of Ambulation

Early ambulation is successful in reducing the incidence of venous thromboembolism (VTE); it also promotes the return of strength. Free movement should be encouraged once anaesthesia wears off, unless an opioid analgesic has been administered. After the initial recovery period is over, the mother should be encouraged to ambulate frequently.

In the early postpartum period women can feel light-headed or dizzy upon standing. The rapid decrease in intra-abdominal pressure after birth results in a dilation of blood vessels supplying the intestines (splanchnic engorgement) and causes blood to pool in the viscera. This condition contributes to the development of orthostatic hypotension and can occur when the woman who has recently given birth sits or stands, first

CRITICAL THINKING CASE STUDY

Fatigue and Rest After Childbirth

Patricia gave birth to her third baby; she has two children at home, ages 3 years and 18 months. Her husband travels frequently with his job. She is breastfeeding the baby without difficulty but is concerned about how she will care for all three of her children, stating, "I remember how tired I was after my last baby. I'm not sure I can manage with three children since my husband is gone so much. Do you have any suggestions to help me?"

QUESTIONS

1. Evidence—Is there sufficient evidence to draw conclusions about whether support would be helpful for Patricia?
2. Assumptions—What assumptions can be made about the following factors?
   a. The relation between breastfeeding and fatigue
   b. Support in the postpartum period
   c. The role of sleep and rest in relation to fatigue and depression
   d. Spacing of pregnancies and fatigue
3. What implications and priorities for nursing care can be drawn at this time?
4. Does the evidence objectively support your conclusion?

ambulates, or takes a warm shower or sitz bath. The nurse must consider the baseline blood pressure; amount of blood loss; and type, amount, and timing of analgesic or anaesthetic medications administered when assisting a woman to ambulate.

Women who have had epidural or spinal anaesthesia may have slow return of sensory and motor function in their lower extremities, increasing the risk of falls with early ambulation. Careful assessment by the postpartum nurse can prevent falls. Factors that the nurse should consider are the time lapse since the medication was given; the woman's ability to bend both knees, place both feet flat on the bed, and lift buttocks off the bed without assistance; medications since birth; vital signs; and estimated blood loss with birth. Before allowing the woman to ambulate the nurse should assess her ability to stand unassisted beside her bed: the woman should simultaneously bend both knees slightly and then stand with knees locked. If the woman is unable to balance herself, she can be eased back into bed safely (Frank, Lane, & Hokanson, 2009).

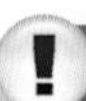

NURSING ALERT

To promote patient safety and prevent injury, it is important to have hospital personnel present at least the first time the woman gets out of bed after birth, because she can feel weak, dizzy, faint, or light-headed. The woman should be instructed to call for assistance before getting out of bed the first time and any time thereafter if she feels dizzy or weak. The partner or family members who are present should be instructed to call for help as well.

Prevention of VTE is important. Women who must remain in bed after giving birth are at increased risk. Antiembolic stockings (TED hose) or a sequential compression device (SCD) boots may be ordered prophylactically, especially after Caesarean birth. If a woman remains in bed longer than 8 hours (e.g., for postpartum magnesium sulphate therapy for pre-eclampsia), exercise to promote circulation in the legs is indicated, using the following routine:

- Alternate flexion and extension of feet.
- Rotate ankles in circular motion.
- Alternate flexion and extension of legs.
- Press back of knee to bed surface; relax.

If the woman is susceptible to thromboembolism, she should be encouraged to walk about actively and discouraged from sitting immobile in a chair. Women with increased risk for thromboembolism include those who are obese (body mass index [BMI] >40), had an unexpected Caesarean birth, are over 35 years of age, and had VTE during pregnancy. These women should be offered low molecular-weight heparin during the postpartum period. The length of time required for the prophylaxis ranges from 7 days to 8 weeks and depends on the number of risk factors (Royal College of Obstetricians and Gynaecologists, 2009). (See discussion in Chapter 24, p. 614.)

Women with varicosities are advised to wear support hose. If a thrombus is suspected, as evidenced by warmth, redness, or tenderness in the suspected leg, the primary health care provider should be notified immediately; meanwhile the woman should be confined to bed with the affected limb elevated on pillows.

Promotion of Exercise

Most women who have just given birth are interested in regaining their nonpregnant figures. Postpartum exercise can begin soon after birth, although the woman should be encouraged to start with simple exercises and gradually progress to more strenuous ones. Fig. 22-4 illustrates a number of exercises appropriate for the new mother. Abdominal exercises are postponed until about 4 weeks after Caesarean birth. It often takes several months for the body to return to prepregnancy weight and shape, and nurses should provide new mothers with realistic information regarding this.

Kegel exercises to strengthen muscle tone are extremely important, particularly after vaginal birth. Kegel exercises help women regain the muscle tone that is often lost as pelvic tissues are stretched and torn during pregnancy and birth. Women who maintain muscle strength may benefit years later by maintaining urinary continence.

It is essential that women learn to perform Kegel exercises correctly (see Patient Teaching box in Chapter 5, p. 72). Some women perform them incorrectly and can increase their risk of incontinence, which can occur when inadvertently bearing down on the pelvic floor muscles, thrusting the perineum outward. The woman's technique can be assessed during the pelvic examination at her checkup by inserting two fingers intravaginally and checking whether the pelvic floor muscles correctly contract and relax.

Promotion of Nutrition

During the hospital stay, most women have a good appetite and eat well; nutritious snacks are usually welcomed. Women may request that family members bring to the hospital favourite or culturally appropriate foods. Cultural dietary preferences must be respected. An example is that some Asian women may only eat hot food after birth and will avoid anything cold. This interest in

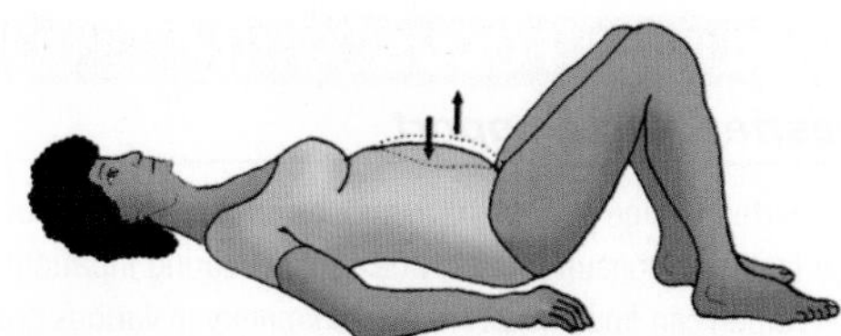

Abdominal Breathing. Lie on back with knees bent. Inhale deeply through nose. Keep ribs stationary and allow abdomen to expand upward. Exhale slowly but forcefully while contracting the abdominal muscles; hold for 3 to 5 seconds while exhaling. Relax.

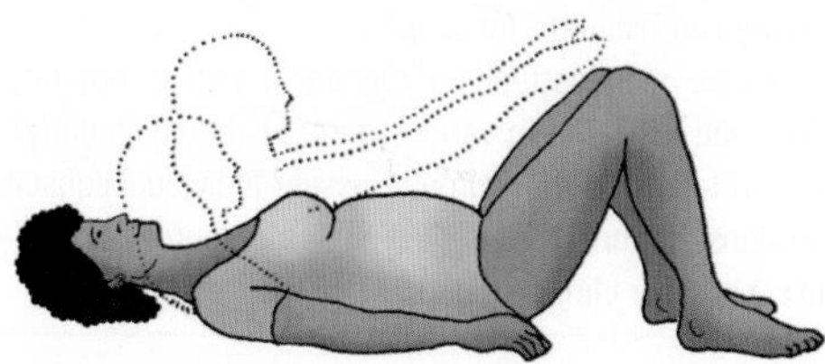

Reach for the Knees. Lie on back with knees bent. While inhaling, deeply lower chin onto chest. While exhaling, raise head and shoulders slowly and smoothly and reach for knees with arms outstretched. The body should rise only as far as the back will naturally bend while waist remains on floor or bed (about 6 to 8 inches). Slowly and smoothly lower head and shoulders back to starting position. Relax.

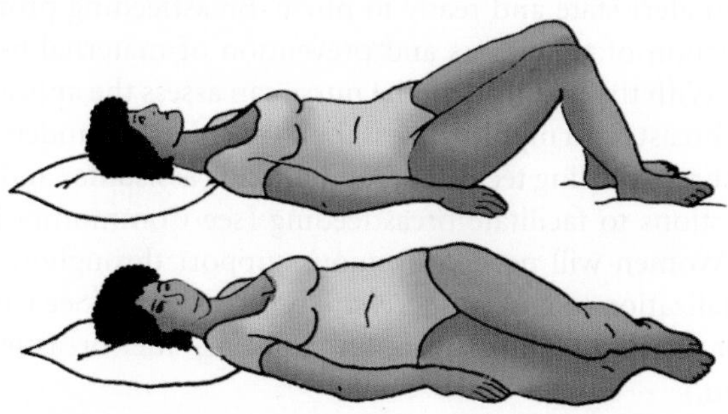

Double Knee Roll. Lie on back with knees bent. Keeping shoulders flat and feet stationary, slowly and smoothly roll knees over to the left to touch floor or bed. Maintaining a smooth motion, roll knees back over to the right until they touch floor or bed. Return to starting position and relax.

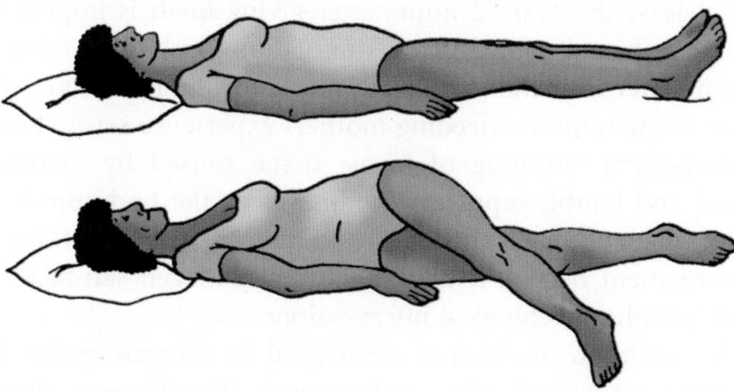

Leg Roll. Lie on back with legs straight. Keeping shoulders flat and legs straight, slowly and smoothly lift left leg and roll it over to touch the right side of floor or bed and return to starting position. Repeat, rolling right leg over to touch left side of floor or bed. Relax.

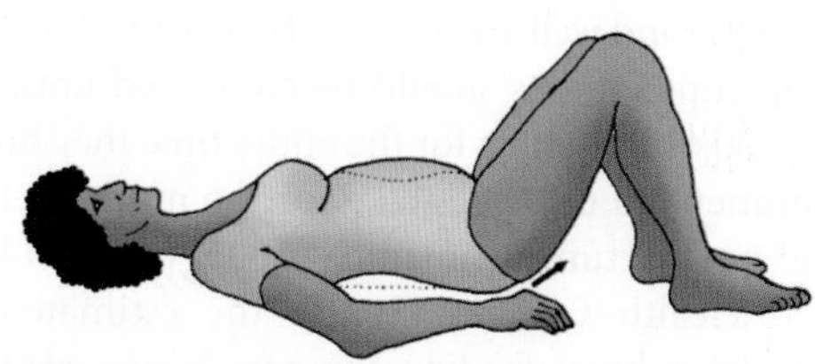

Combined Abdominal Breathing and Supine Pelvic Tilt (Pelvic Rock). Lie on back with knees bent. While inhaling deeply, roll pelvis back by flattening lower back on floor or bed. Exhale slowly but forcefully while contracting abdominal muscles and tightening buttocks. Hold for 3 to 5 seconds while exhaling. Relax.

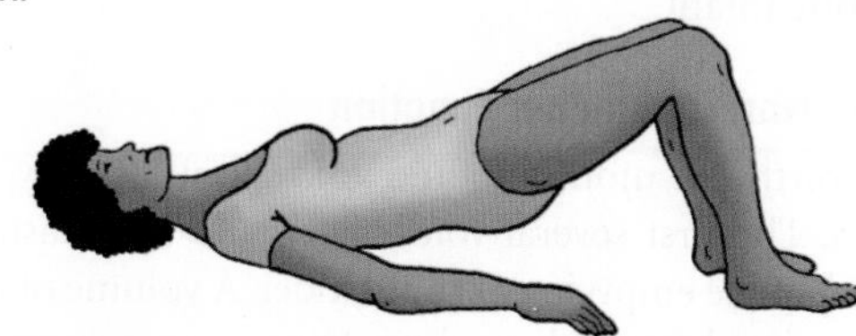

Buttocks Lift. Lie on back with arms at sides, knees bent, and feet flat. Slowly raise buttocks and arch back. Return slowly to starting position.

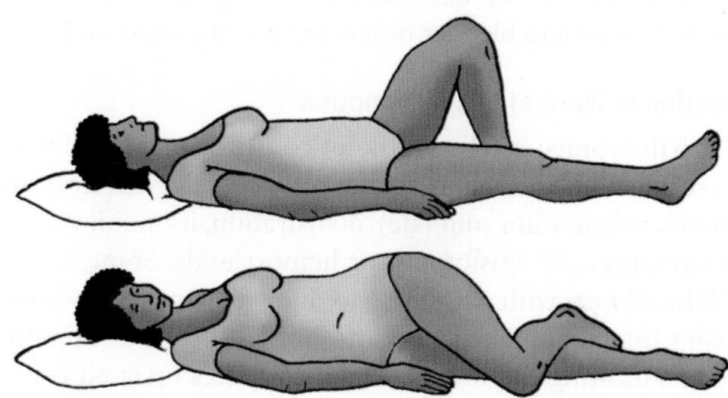

Single Knee Roll. Lie on back with right leg straight and left leg bent at the knee. Keeping shoulders flat, slowly and smoothly roll left knee over to the right to touch floor or bed and then back to starting position. Reverse position of legs. Roll right knee over to the left to touch floor or bed and return to starting position. Relax.

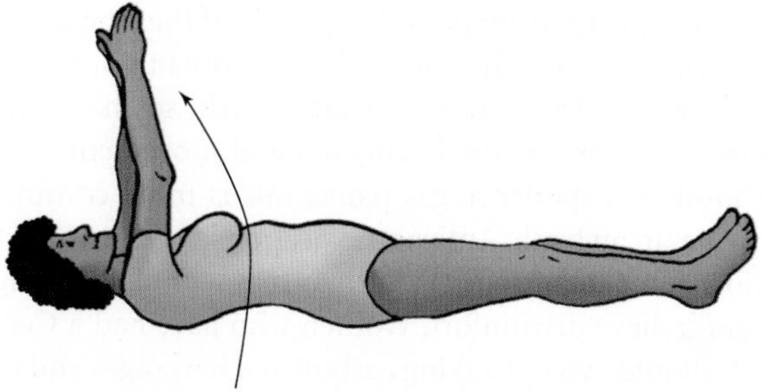

Arm Raises. Lie on back with arms extended at 90-degree angle from body. Raise arms so they are perpendicular and hands touch. Lower slowly.

FIGURE 22-4 Postpartum exercise should begin as soon as possible. The woman should start with simple exercises and gradually progress to more strenuous ones.

food presents an ideal opportunity for nutrition counselling on dietary needs after pregnancy, such as for breastfeeding, preventing constipation and anemia, promoting weight loss, and promoting healing and well-being (see Chapter 12). Prenatal vitamins and iron supplements should be continued until 6 weeks after birth or for some women for the entire time they breastfeed.

The recommended caloric intake for the moderately active, nonlactating postpartum woman is 1800 to 2200 kcal/day. According to Health Canada (2010), the estimated energy requirement for a breastfeeding woman is an extra 350 to 400 kcal/day, which is an extra two to three servings, based on *Canada's Food Guide* (see Appendix A). Higher-than-normal caloric intake is recommended for women who are underweight or who exercise vigorously and those who are breastfeeding more than one infant.

Promotion of Normal Bladder Function

After giving birth, the mother should void spontaneously within 6 to 8 hours. The first several voidings should be measured to document adequate emptying of the bladder. A volume of at least 150 mL is expected for each voiding. Some women experience difficulty in emptying the bladder, possibly as a result of diminished bladder tone, edema from trauma, use of epidural or spinal anaesthetic, or fear of discomfort. Nursing interventions for inability to void and bladder distension are discussed on p. 572.

Promotion of Normal Bowel Function

After birth, women can be at risk for constipation related to the adverse effects of medications (e.g., opioid analgesics, iron supplements, magnesium sulphate), dehydration, immobility, perineal lacerations or episiotomy, or hemorrhoids. Some women fear discomfort with straining to have a bowel movement. Nursing interventions to promote normal bowel elimination include educating the woman about measures to avoid constipation. These interventions include consuming adequate roughage, increasing fluid intake, and ambulating. Alerting the woman to adverse effects of medications such as opioid analgesics (decreased gastrointestinal tract motility) may encourage her to implement measures to reduce the risk of constipation. Occasionally, stool softeners or laxatives may be necessary during the early postpartum period, especially if the woman has extensive perineal repairs. It is normal for a woman not to have a bowel movement for 2 to 3 days after birth, so many new mothers may be home before having a bowel movement.

Some mothers experience gas pains; this is more common following Caesarean birth. Antigas medications may be ordered. Ambulation or rocking in a rocking chair may stimulate passage of flatus and relieve discomfort. Women who have had a Caesarean birth should avoid drinking carbonated beverages and the use of straws, as this promotes gas formation.

! NURSING ALERT

Rectal suppositories and enemas should not be administered to women with third- or fourth-degree perineal lacerations. These measures to treat constipation can be very uncomfortable and can cause hemorrhage or damage to the suture line.

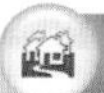

COMMUNITY FOCUS

Breastfeeding Support

Women breastfeed longer if they have support in their breastfeeding efforts. Nurses and lactation consultants provide support during inpatient stays after childbirth. Women can find support in the community in various groups. Social support interventions that include peer support are successful in increasing the duration of exclusive breastfeeding and satisfaction with breastfeeding. In discharge planning, nurses can refer breastfeeding mothers to community groups for support. Community health nurses can facilitate breastfeeding efforts through organizing or facilitating support groups. Mothers experienced in breastfeeding can facilitate these efforts.

Identify sources of breastfeeding support in your community. Are these resources free and available in various parts of the community? What form does the support take? Are there group classes? Individual consultation? Who provides the consultation? Make a list of the resources you identified and share the list with your clinical group.

Promotion of Breastfeeding

The ideal time to initiate breastfeeding is within the first 1 to 2 hours after childbirth. Baby-Friendly hospitals mandate that the infant be put to breast within the first hour after birth (Breastfeeding Committee for Canada, 2012). At this time, the infant is in an alert state and ready to nurse. Breastfeeding promotes contraction of the uterus and prevention of maternal hemorrhage. With the first feeding the nurse can assess the appearance of the breasts and nipples, assess the woman's basic understanding of breastfeeding technique, and provide assistance and basic instructions to facilitate breastfeeding (see Community Focus box). Women will need continuous support throughout their hospitalization to ensure successful breastfeeding. (See Chapter 27 for further information on assisting the breastfeeding woman.)

Suppression of Lactation

Suppression of lactation is necessary when the woman has decided not to breastfeed or in the case of neonatal death. Wearing a well-fitted support bra or breast binder continuously for at least the first 72 hours after giving birth is important. Women should avoid breast stimulation, including running warm water over the breasts, newborn suckling, or expressing milk. Some nonbreastfeeding mothers experience severe breast engorgement (swelling of breast tissue caused by increased blood and lymph supply to the breasts as the body produces milk, which occurs at about 72 to 96 hours after birth). If breast engorgement occurs, it usually can be managed satisfactorily with nonpharmacological interventions.

Ice packs to the breasts are helpful in decreasing the discomfort associated with engorgement. The woman should use a 15-minutes-on, 45-minutes-off schedule (to prevent the rebound swelling that can occur if ice is used continuously). Some women use cabbage leaves to help relieve the engorgement, although there are differing opinions as to whether this works. The woman who has chosen to formula-feed can place cold raw cabbage leaves over her breasts insider her bra. The leaves are replaced each time they wilt. A mild analgesic or anti-inflammatory medication can reduce discomfort associated with engorgement and help the mother through this uncomfortable time. Medications that were once prescribed for lactation suppression (estrogen, estrogen and testosterone, and bromocriptine) are no longer used.

Health Promotion for Planning Future Pregnancies and Children

Rubella vaccination. For women who have not had rubella or women who are serologically not immune (titre of 1:8 or enzyme immunoassay level less than 0.8), a subcutaneous injection of rubella vaccine is recommended in the immediate postpartum period to prevent the possibility of contracting rubella in future pregnancies. Seroconversion occurs in approximately 90% of women vaccinated after birth. The live attenuated rubella virus is not communicable; therefore, breastfeeding mothers can be vaccinated (Gruslin, Steben, Halperin, et al., 2009). However, because the virus is shed in urine and other body fluids, the vaccine should not be given if the mother or other household members are immunocompromised. Rubella vaccine is made from duck eggs; thus, women who have allergies to these eggs may develop a hypersensitivity reaction to the vaccine, for which they will need adrenaline. A transient arthralgia or rash is common in vaccinated women. Because the vaccine may be teratogenic, women must be informed about this fact.

> **LEGAL TIP *RUBELLA VACCINATION***
>
> Informed consent for rubella vaccination in the postpartum period includes information about possible adverse effects and the risk of teratogenic effects. Women need to understand that they must practise contraception for 1 month after being vaccinated to avoid pregnancy.

Prevention of Rh isoimmunization. Injection of Rh immune globulin (a solution of gamma-globulin that contains Rh antibodies) within 72 hours after birth prevents sensitization in the Rh-negative woman who has had a fetomaternal transfusion of Rh-positive fetal red blood cells (RBCs) (see Medication Guide). Rh immune globulin promotes lysis of fetal Rh-positive blood cells before the mother forms her own antibodies against them.

> **! NURSING ALERT**
>
> After birth, Rh immune globulin is administered to all Rh-negative, antibody (Coombs' test)–negative women who give birth to Rh-positive infants. Rh immune globulin is administered to the mother intramuscularly or intravenously. It should never be given to an infant.

The administration of 300 mcg of Rh immune globulin is usually sufficient to prevent maternal sensitization. However, if a large fetomaternal transfusion is suspected, the dosage needed should be determined by performing a Kleihauer-Betke test, which detects the amount of fetal blood in the maternal circulation. If more than 15 mL of fetal blood is present in maternal circulation, the dosage of Rh immune globulin must be increased.

Because Rh immune globulin is considered a blood product, precautions similar to those used for transfusing blood are necessary when it is given. The identification number on the woman's hospital wristband should correspond to the identification number found on the laboratory slip. The nurse must also check to see that the lot number of the laboratory slip corresponds to the lot number on the vial. Finally, the expiration date on the vial should be checked to ensure that it is a usable product.

Rh immune globulin suppresses the immune response. Therefore, the woman who receives both Rh immune globulin and a live virus immunization such as rubella must be tested in 3 months to see if she has developed immunity. If not, the woman will need another dose of the vaccine.

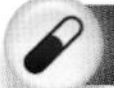

MEDICATION GUIDE

Rh Immune Globulin

Action

Suppression of immune response in nonsensitized women with Rh-negative blood who receive Rh-positive blood cells because of fetomaternal hemorrhage, transfusion, or accident

Indications

Routine antepartum prevention at 26 to 28 weeks of gestation in women with Rh-negative blood; suppress antibody formation after birth, miscarriage, pregnancy termination, abdominal trauma, ectopic pregnancy, amniocentesis, version, or chorionic villi sampling

Dosage/Route

Standard dose: 1 vial (300 mcg) IM in deltoid or ventrogluteal muscle
Microdose: 1 vial (50 mcg) IM in deltoid or ventrogluteal muscle
Rh_o(D) immune globulin can be given IM or IV

Adverse Effects

Myalgia, lethargy, localized tenderness and stiffness at injection site, mild and transient fever, malaise, headache; rarely nausea, vomiting, hypotension, tachycardia, and allergic response can occur.

Nursing Considerations

Give a standard dose to the mother at 28 weeks of gestation as prophylaxis or after an incident or exposure risk that occurs after 28 weeks of gestation (e.g., amniocentesis, second-trimester miscarriage or abortion, after external version) and within 72 hours after birth if the baby is Rh positive.

- Give microdose for first-trimester miscarriage or abortion, ectopic pregnancy, or chorionic villi sampling.
- Verify that the woman is Rh negative and has not been sensitized; if postpartum that Coombs' test is negative; and that baby is Rh positive. Provide explanation to the woman about the procedure, including the purpose, possible adverse effects, and the effect on future pregnancies. Have the woman sign a consent form if required by the agency. Verify correct dosage and confirm the lot number and woman's identity before giving the injection (verify with another nurse or by other procedure per agency policy); document administration per agency policy. Observe the patient for at least 20 minutes after administration for allergic response.
- Document lot number and expiration date in the patient record.
- The medication is made from human plasma (a consideration if the woman is a Jehovah's Witness). Women receiving this medication must be informed about the risks and benefits, and the nurse needs to document this discussion and the patient's understanding before administering the medication. The risk of transmitting infectious agents, including viruses, cannot be completely eliminated.

IM, intramuscularly; *IV*, intravenously.

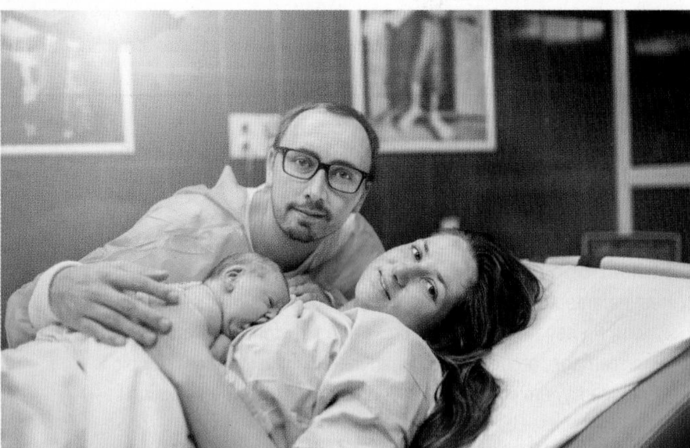

FIGURE 22-5 Parents getting acquainted with their new son. (Halfpoint/Shutterstock.com.)

Ongoing Psychosocial Assessment and Care

Meeting the psychosocial needs of new parents involves assessing their reactions to the birth experience, their feelings about themselves, and their interactions with the new baby (Fig. 22-5) and other family members. Specific interventions are then planned in order to increase the parents' knowledge and self-confidence as they assume the care and responsibility of the new baby and integrate this new member into their existing family structure in a way that meets their cultural expectations.

Taking time to assess maternal emotional needs and concerns before discharge can promote better psychological health and adjustment to parenting. Ongoing support for postpartum women is also needed. Issues such as fatigue that often appear during the hospital stay tend to continue after discharge and can intensify. Postpartum support is especially beneficial to at-risk populations, such as low-income primiparas, women who lack adequate support because of isolation (e.g., physical or language), those at risk for family dysfunction and child abuse, and those at risk for perinatal mood disorders (PMD) (see Chapter 24).

Sometimes the findings of the psychosocial assessment indicate serious actual or potential problems that must be addressed. Box 22-3 identifies psychosocial characteristics and behaviours that may warrant ongoing evaluation after hospital discharge. Women exhibiting these needs should be referred to appropriate community resources for assessment and management.

Cultural issues must be considered when planning care, as childbirth occurs within a sociocultural context. The nurse must take time to interact with the woman and her extended family in order to learn and understand which practices need to be followed regarding the new mother and her newborn infant. Recognizing the importance of family and community in relation to the woman and her infant is integral to providing culturally appropriate care.

Impact of the Birth Experience

Many women indicate a need to examine the birth process itself and look at their own behaviour during labour in retrospect. Their partners may express similar desires. If their birth experience was quite different from the one they had planned (e.g., induction, epidural anaesthesia, Caesarean birth), both partners may need to mourn the loss of their expectations before they can adjust to the reality of their actual birth experience. Inviting them to review the events and describe how they feel helps the nurse assess how well they understand what happened and how well they have been able to put their childbirth experience into perspective.

BOX 22-3 SIGNS OF POTENTIAL PSYCHOSOCIAL COMPLICATIONS

The following signs in the mother can suggest potentially serious complications and should be reported to the health care provider or clinic (these may be noticed by the partner or other family members):

- Unable or unwilling to discuss labour and birth experience
- Refers to self as ugly and useless
- Excessively preoccupied with self (body image)
- Markedly depressed
- Lacks social support
- Partner or other family members react negatively to baby
- Refuses to interact with or care for baby (e.g., does not name baby, does not want to hold or feed baby, is upset by vomiting and wet or dirty diapers) (cultural appropriateness of actions must be considered)
- Expresses disappointment over baby's sex
- Sees baby as messy or unattractive
- Baby reminds mother of family member or friend she doesn't like
- Has difficulty sleeping
- Experiences loss of appetite

Maternal Self-Image

An important assessment concerns the woman's self-concept, body image, and sexuality. How this new mother feels about herself and her body during the **postpartum period** may affect her behaviour and adaptation to parenting. The woman's self-concept and body image may also affect her sexuality.

Adaptation to Parenthood and Parent–Infant Interactions

The psychosocial assessment includes evaluating adaptation to parenthood as evidenced by the mother's and partner's reactions to and interactions with the new baby. Clues indicating successful adaptation begin to appear early in the postbirth period as parents react positively to the newborn infant and continue the process of establishing a relationship with their child.

Parents are adapting well to their new roles when they exhibit a realistic perception and acceptance of their newborn's needs and his or her limited abilities, immature social responses, and helplessness. Examples of positive parent–infant interactions include taking pleasure in the infant and the tasks done for and with him or her; understanding the infant's emotional states and providing comfort; and reading the infant's cues for new experiences and sensing his or her fatigue level (see Chapter 23).

If these indicators are missing, the nurse must investigate further in an attempt to identify what is hindering the normal adaptation process. The nurse can ask several questions, such as "Tell me how you are feeling?" or "What are your concerns about being a parent?"; these will help determine if the woman is experiencing the normal "baby blues" or if there is a more serious underlying condition (i.e., PMD).

Postpartum Blues

The period surrounding the first day or two after birth is characterized by heightened joy and feelings of well-being. This is often followed by a "blue" period. Approximately 50 to 80% of women of all ethnic and racial groups experience the postpartum blues or "baby blues." During this period, women are emotionally labile and often cry easily for no apparent reason. This lability seems to peak around the fifth day and subside by the tenth day. Other symptoms of postpartum blues include depression, a let-down feeling, restlessness, fatigue, insomnia, headache, anxiety, sadness, and anger. Postpartum blues are transient, mild, and time limited and do not require treatment other than reassurance. Biochemical, psychological, social, and cultural factors have been explored as possible causes of the postpartum blues; however, the etiology remains unknown. Because the postpartum blues occur in up to 80% of women, all women must be taught about the symptoms of the blues and that this is a normal postpartum occurrence.

Whatever the cause, the early postpartum period appears to be one of emotional and physical vulnerability for new mothers who may be psychologically overwhelmed by the reality of parental responsibilities. The mother may feel deprived of the supportive care she received from family members and friends during pregnancy. Some mothers regret the loss of the mother–unborn child relationship and mourn its passing. Still others have a let-down feeling when labour and birth are complete. Most women experience fatigue after childbirth, which is compounded by the around-the-clock demands of the new baby and can accentuate the feelings of depression. Symptoms of depression can have a negative effect on women's development of a maternal role. To help mothers cope with postpartum blues, nurses can suggest various strategies (see Patient Teaching box).

Although the postpartum blues are usually mild and short-lived, approximately 15% of women experience a PMD (see Chapter 24). PMD symptoms can range from mild to severe, with women having good and bad days. It can go undetected because new parents generally do not voluntarily admit to this kind of emotional distress out of embarrassment, guilt, or fear. Nurses must include teaching about the normality of the blues as well as how to differentiate symptoms of the blues and those of PMD and urge parents to report depressive symptoms promptly if they do occur (see Box 24-4). For further discussion of PMD and how to screen for it, see Chapter 24.

Family Structure and Functioning

A woman's adjustment to her role as mother is affected greatly by her relationships with her partner, her mother and other relatives, and any other children (Fig. 22-6). Nurses can help ease the new mother's return home by identifying possible conflicts among family members and helping the woman plan strategies for dealing with these problems before discharge. Such a conflict could arise when couples have very different ideas about parenting. Dealing with the stresses of sibling rivalry and unsolicited grandparent advice can also affect the woman's transition to motherhood. Only by asking about other nuclear and extended family members can the nurse discover potential problems in such relationships and help plan workable solutions for them.

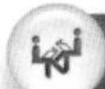

PATIENT TEACHING

Coping With Postpartum Blues

It is important to teach this information to all new mothers.

- Remember that the blues are normal.
- Get plenty of rest; nap when the baby does, if possible. Go to bed early and let friends know when to visit.
- Use relaxation techniques learned in childbirth classes (or ask the nurse to teach you and your partner some techniques).
- Do something for yourself. Take advantage of the time when your partner or family members care for the baby—soak in the tub or go for a walk.
- Plan a day out of the house—go to the mall with the baby, being sure to take a stroller or carriage, or go out to eat with friends without the baby. Many communities have churches or other agencies that provide child care programs, such as Mothers' Morning Out.
- Share your feelings with your partner. For example, talk about feeling tied down, if applicable; how the birth met your expectations; and things that will help you.
- If you are breastfeeding, give yourself and your baby time to learn.
- Monitor yourself closely for signs of depression, anxiety, and psychosis.
- Seek out and use community resources, such as La Leche League or community mental health centres.

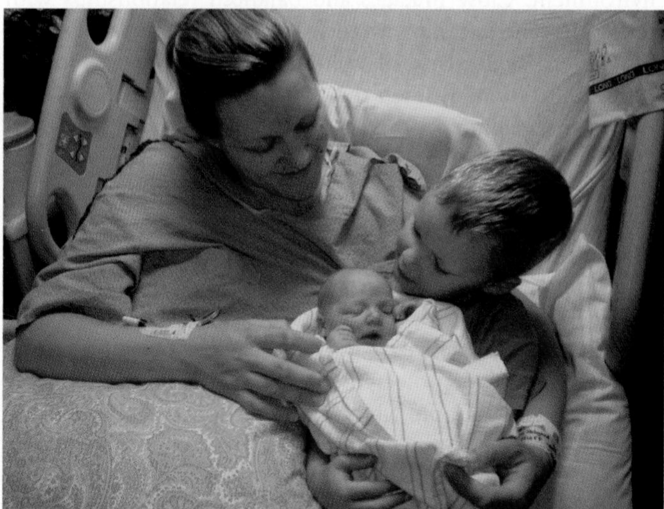

FIGURE 22-6 Older sibling cuddles with mother and new baby. (Courtesy of Jennifer Hobgood.)

Impact of Cultural Diversity

The final component of a complete postpartum psychosocial assessment is the woman's cultural beliefs and values. Much of a woman's behaviour during the postpartum period is strongly influenced by her cultural background. Nurses are likely to come into contact with women from many different countries and cultures. All cultures have developed safe and satisfying methods of caring for new mothers and babies. The nurse can identify some cultural beliefs and practices through observation and interaction with the mother and her family. Asking questions of the mother and her family about their cultural practices can provide useful information to help the nurse provide optimal care. Only by understanding and respecting the values and beliefs of each woman can the nurse design a plan of care to meet individual needs.

Many traditional health beliefs and practices exist among the various cultures within the North American population. Traditional health practices used to maintain health or avoid illnesses deal with the whole person (body, mind, and spirit) and tend to be culturally based. Women from various cultures may view health as a balance between opposing forces (e.g., cold versus hot, yin versus yang), being in harmony with nature, or just "feeling good." Indigenous beliefs are holistic and encompass a balance between physical, emotional, mental, and spiritual elements. The importance of balance also extends beyond the individual to include the family, the community, and the environment. Close linkages and balanced relationships with land, water, and ice and with their communities and their societies govern their sense of well-being and may be expressed among Indigenous women through distinct cultural practices in relation to labour, birth, and postpartum periods (Best Start Resource Centre, 2013; Wilson, de la Ronde, Brascoupé, et al., 2013). Traditional practices among some cultures may include the observance of certain dietary restrictions, wearing certain clothing, or taboos for balancing the body; participation in certain activities such as sports and art for maintaining mental health; and use of silence, prayer, or meditation for developing spiritually. Some practices (e.g., using religious objects or eating garlic) are used to protect the person from illness and may involve avoiding people who are believed to create hexes and spells or who have an "evil eye." Restoration of health may involve a person accessing alternative and complementary health models (e.g., herbs, animal substances) or using a traditional healer.

Birth occurs within this sociocultural context. Rest, seclusion, dietary restraints, and ceremonies honouring the mother are all common traditional practices that are followed for the promotion of the health and well-being of the mother and baby.

During the postpartum period there are several common traditional health practices used and beliefs held by women and their families. For example, in Southeast Asia, pregnancy is considered to be a "hot" state, and childbirth results in a sudden loss of this state. Therefore, balance needs to be restored by increasing the return of the hot state, which is present physically or symbolically in hot food, hot water, and warm air. Women may wish to stay warm and avoid bathing, exercising, and hair washing for 7 to 30 days after childbirth. They may also prefer not to give their babies colostrum.

Another common belief is that the mother and baby remain in a weak and vulnerable state for a period of several weeks following birth. During this time, the mother may remain in a passive role, take no baths or showers, and stay in bed to prevent cold air from entering her body.

It is important that nurses consider all cultural aspects when planning care and not use their own cultural beliefs as the framework for that care. Although the beliefs and behaviours of other cultures may seem different or strange, they should be encouraged as long as the mother wants to conform to them and she and the baby have no ill effects. The nurse must determine whether a woman is using complementary medication during the postpartum period because active ingredients in some herbal remedies can have adverse physiological effects on the woman when ingested with prescribed medicines. Also, women who have immigrated to Western nations without their extended families may not have much help at home, making it difficult for them to observe these activity restrictions. Many young women who are first- or second-generation Canadians may feel conflicted about following their cultural traditions and need to be supported in the decisions they make.

Discharge Teaching

Discharge planning begins at the time of admission to the unit and should be reflected in the nursing care plan developed for each woman. The nurse functions primarily as teacher, encourager, and supporter rather than doer, while implementing the plan of care for a postpartum woman. Implementation of this care plan involves carrying out specific activities to achieve the expected outcome of care planned for each woman. The goal is for all women to be capable of providing basic care for themselves and their infants at the time of discharge. Topics that should be included are promotion of parenting skills and adjustment of family members to the newborn infant, self-care, and sexual activity and contraception.

Because of the limited time available for teaching, nurses must target their teaching on the woman's expressed needs. Giving the woman a list of topics and asking her to indicate her teaching needs will help the nurse maximize teaching efforts and can increase the woman's retention of information. Using "teachable moments" (i.e., when the topic arises during the daily routine) enhances the mother's learning. It is also important that teaching be provided when the mother is ready to learn and not distracted by pain, visitors, or a crying baby. Providing written materials on postpartum self-care, breastfeeding, and infant care that the woman can consult after discharge may be helpful. See Chapter 5 for more information on health teaching.

Just before the time of discharge, the nurse should review the woman's chart to check that laboratory reports, medications, signatures, and other items are in order. Some hospitals use a checklist to be completed before the woman's discharge. The nurse should also verify that the infant is ready to be discharged.

Self-Care and Signs of Complications

Every woman must be taught to recognize physical and psychological signs and symptoms that might indicate problems and how to obtain advice and assistance quickly if these signs appear. Table 22-2 and Box 22-3, respectively, list several common indications of maternal physical and psychosocial problems in the postpartum period. (See Chapter 24 for more information on postpartum complications.) Before discharge, women need basic instruction regarding a variety of self-care topics such as nutrition, exercise, family planning, the resumption of sexual intercourse, prescribed medications, and routine mother–baby follow-up care. No medication that would make the mother sleepy should be administered if she is the one who will be holding the baby on the way out of the hospital. In some instances, the woman is seated in a wheelchair and given the baby to hold. Some families leave unescorted and ambulatory, depending on hospital protocol. The woman's possessions are gathered and taken out with her and her family. The woman's and the baby's identification bands are carefully checked. In most hospitals, nurses must ensure that the parents are able to properly secure the baby in a car seat for the drive home (see Fig. 26-23).

Sexual Activity and Contraception

Feelings related to sexual adjustment after childbirth are often a cause of concern for new parents. Women who have recently given birth may be reluctant to resume sexual intercourse for fear of pain or worry that coitus could damage healing perineal tissue. Because many new parents are anxious for information but reluctant to bring up the subject, postpartum nurses should matter-of-factly include the topic of postpartum sexuality during their routine physical assessment. For example, while examining a perineal laceration or episiotomy site the nurse can say, "I know you're sore right now, but it probably won't be long until you (or you and your partner) are ready to make love again. Do you have any questions about resuming sex?" This approach assures the woman and her partner that resuming sexual activity is a legitimate concern for new parents and indicates the nurse's willingness to answer questions and share information.

Discussing sexual activity with the woman and her partner is important before they leave the hospital, because many couples resume sexual activity before the traditional postpartum checkup 6 weeks after childbirth (see Research Focus box). For most women the risk of hemorrhage or infection is minimal by approximately 2 weeks after birth. The nurse needs to discuss the physical and psychological effects that giving birth can have on sexual activity (see Home Care box).

Contraceptive options should be discussed with women (and their partners if present) before discharge so that they can make informed decisions about fertility management before resuming sexual activity. Waiting to discuss contraception at the 6-week checkup may be too late. Ovulation can occur as soon as 1 month after birth, particularly in women who formula-feed. Breastfeeding mothers should be taught about appropriate birth control methods that include the lactational amenorrhea method (see p. 158) or condoms. Hormonal methods of birth control (e.g., oral contraceptives) may be used once breastfeeding is well established. Contraceptive options are discussed in detail in Chapter 8.

Prescribed Medications

Women should continue to take their prenatal vitamins for the first 6 weeks after birth. Breastfeeding mothers may be instructed to continue prenatal vitamins for the duration of breastfeeding. Supplemental iron can be prescribed for mothers with lower-than-normal hemoglobin levels. Women with extensive episiotomies or perineal lacerations (third or fourth degree) are usually prescribed stool softeners to take at home. Pain medications (analgesics or NSAIDs) may be prescribed, especially for women who had Caesarean birth. The nurse should make certain that the woman knows the route, dosage, frequency, and common adverse effects of all ordered medications. Written information about the medications is usually included in the discharge instructions.

Dealing With Visitors

A newborn in the family or neighbourhood draws visitors. The nurse can help the parents explore ways in which they can assert their needs in such situations. When family or friends ask what they can do to help, the family can respond with "Please bring us a casserole or a meal" or "Could you please pick up some items at the grocery store?" The couple can work out a signal for alerting the partner that the new mother is becoming tired or uncomfortable and needs to have the partner invite the visitors into another part of the house. Some new mothers have found that if they remain in their robes and do not appear ready for company, visitors stay for a shorter time. A "Please Do Not Disturb" sign on the front door may be useful when the mother is resting.

Follow-up After Discharge

Routine Mother and Baby Checkups

Women who have experienced uncomplicated vaginal births are still commonly scheduled for the traditional 6-week postpartum examination. Women who have had a Caesarean birth are often seen in the health care provider's office or clinic within 2 weeks after hospital discharge. The date and time for the follow-up appointment should be included in the discharge instructions. If an appointment is not made before the woman leaves the hospital, she should be encouraged to call the health care provider's office or clinic to schedule one.

Parents who have not already done so need to make plans for newborn follow-up at the time of discharge. Most offices and clinics like to see newborns for an initial examination within 3 to 5 days after birth or 48 to 72 hours after hospital discharge. If an appointment for a specific date and time was not made for the infant before leaving the hospital, the parents should be encouraged to call the office or clinic right away.

Telephone Follow-up

Many local health departments have implemented postpartum telephone follow-up calls to women for assessment, health teaching, and identification of complications to effect timely intervention and referrals. Telephonic nursing assessments may also be used after a postpartum home care visit to reassess a woman's knowledge about the signs and symptoms of adequate intake by the breastfeeding infant or, after initiating home

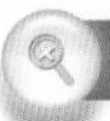

RESEARCH FOCUS

Perineal Trauma and Postpartum Sexual Function

—Pat Mahaffee Gingrich

Ask the Question

Which perinatal interventions for perineal trauma minimize pain and prevent sexual dysfunction?

Search for the Evidence

Search Strategies

English research-based publications on perineal trauma, birth, postpartum, sexual were included.

Databases Used

Cochrane Collaborative Database, National Guideline Clearinghouse (AHRQ), CINAHL, PubMed, and UpToDate

Critically Analyze the Evidence

- Sexual dysfunction can affect more than half of all women at 2 to 3 months after birth. One major cause is dyspareunia (painful intercourse) after perineal trauma, especially third- and fourth-degree lacerations requiring repair. Other causes can include decreased libido and lower estrogen resulting from breastfeeding, a postpartum mood disorder, and fatigue.
- Both episiotomy and second-degree lacerations with repair are associated with lower libido, orgasm, sexual satisfaction, and greater dyspareunia than in women with an intact perineum (Rathfisch, Dikencik, Beji, et al., 2010). Routine episiotomy and fundal pressure during birth are not recommended.
- Warm compresses and perineal massage during first- and second-stage birth significantly decrease third- and fourth-degree tears (Aasheim, Nilsen, Lukasse, et al., 2011).
- Evidence is still mixed regarding whether to suture or not suture first- and second-degree lacerations. Although small studies have found little difference between groups for pain and wound complications, despite slower wound healing the unsutured group still experienced greater satisfaction than the sutured group (Elharmeel, Chaudhary, Tan, et al., 2011).

Apply the Evidence: Nursing Implications

Women can be embarrassed to discuss sexual function with their partners and with their health care team. Nurses are ideally placed to initiate and keep the dialogue going throughout child-bearing. Leeman and Rogers (2012) recommend the following clinical approach for assessing and preventing postpartum sexual dysfunction:

- Discussion of anatomy, physiology, and sexual function should begin in early pregnancy and continue throughout the postpartum period, including a brief valid and reliable sexual function survey.
- Antenatal perineal massage should be taught to minimize perineal damage.
- Perineal management at birth should include limited use of instrumental delivery, especially forceps, and avoidance of episiotomy, along with careful assessment and repair of anal sphincter lacerations with synthetic, absorbable sutures.
- Before hospital discharge, discussions regarding pain, dyspareunia, resumption of intercourse, and contraception should be initiated with the woman and her partner. Women should know the hypoestrogenic and sensitivity changes that they can experience as a result of breastfeeding and the need for additional vaginal lubrication.
- At postpartum visits urine, bowel, and sexual function should be assessed and perineum inspected; mood and intimacy challenges need to be assessed and discussed, such as fatigue and timing issues. Alternative positions can be suggested, to help increase comfort during intercourse. Satisfaction with the chosen contraceptive method should be evaluated.

References

Aasheim, V., Nilson, A. B., Lukasse, M., et al. (2011). Perineal techniques during the second stage of labour for reducing perineal trauma. *Cochrane Database Systematic Reviews*, (12). doi:10.1002/14651858.

Elharmeel, S. M., Chaudhary, Y., Tan, S., et al. (2011). Surgical repair of spontaneous perineal tears that occur during childbirth versus no intervention. *Cochrane Database Systematic Reviews*, (8). doi:10.1002/14651858.

Leeman, L. M., & Rogers, R. G. (2012). Sex after childbirth. *Obstetrics & Gynecology, 119*(3), 647–655.

Rathfisch, G., Dikencik, B. K., Beji, N. K., et al. (2010). Effects of perineal trauma on postpartum sexual function. *Journal of Advanced Nursing, 66*(12), 2640–2649.

HOME CARE

Resumption of Sexual Intercourse

- Unless your health care provider indicates otherwise, you can safely resume sexual activity (intercourse) by the second to fourth week after birth, when bleeding has stopped and the perineum is healed. Many women resume sexual activity by 5 to 6 weeks after birth, although this varies and is often related to perineal discomfort. Perineal lacerations or episiotomy increases the chances of discomfort with intercourse. For the first 6 weeks to 6 months, vaginal lubrication can be decreased, especially among breastfeeding women.
- Your physiological reactions to sexual stimulation for the first 3 months after birth will be slower and less intense. The strength of the orgasm is reduced.
- A water-soluble gel, or contraceptive cream or jelly might be recommended for lubrication. If some vaginal tenderness is present, your partner can be instructed to insert one or more clean, lubricated fingers into the vagina and rotate them to help the vagina relax and identify possible areas of discomfort. A position in which you have control of the depth of the insertion of the penis also is useful. The side-by-side or female-on-top position may be more comfortable than other positions.
- The presence of the baby influences postbirth lovemaking. Parents hear every sound made by the baby; conversely, you may be concerned that the baby hears every sound you make. In either case, any phase of the sexual response cycle may be interrupted by hearing the baby cry or move, leaving both of you frustrated and unsatisfied. In addition, the amount of psychological energy you expend in child care activities may lead to fatigue. Newborns require a great deal of attention and time.
- Some women have reported feeling sexual stimulation and orgasms when breastfeeding their babies. Some breastfeeding mothers often are interested in returning to sexual activity before nonbreastfeeding mothers are, although some breastfeeding mothers may find their interest in sexual relations is decreased, as they may feel their breasts are for feeding the baby and may not find sexual stimulation desirable.
- You should be instructed to correctly perform the Kegel exercises to strengthen your pubococcygeal muscle. This muscle is associated with bowel and bladder function and with vaginal feeling during intercourse.

phototherapy, to assess the caregiver's knowledge regarding equipment complications.

Home Visits

Community health nurse visits to new mothers and babies can help bridge the gap between hospital care and routine visits to health care providers. Nurses are able to assess the mother, infant, and home environment; answer questions and provide education; and make referrals to community resources, if necessary. Home visits reduce the need for more expensive health care, such as emergency department visits and rehospitalization. They can also help to improve the overall quality of care provided to infants and their parents. Ideally, immediate follow-up contact and home visits should be available 7 days a week.

The support provided by nurses and other trained community health workers can enhance parent–infant interaction and parenting skills; home visits also help to promote mutual support between the mother and her partner (De La Rosa, Perry, & Johnson, 2009). Breastfeeding outcomes can be enhanced through home visitation programs.

Community nursing care may not be available, even if needed, because of funding issues, but in most provinces mothers receive a phone call within the first week after discharge. Women who are assessed to be high risk may then receive a home visit from a community health nurse to assist with the new mother's concerns, depending on the practice of the local health department.

During the home visit, the nurse conducts an assessment of the mother and newborn to determine physiological adjustment, identify any existing complications, and answer any questions the mother has about herself or newborn care. Conducting the assessment in a separate room provides private time for the mother to ask questions on topics such as breast care, family planning, and constipation. The assessment should also include the mother's emotional adjustment and her knowledge of self-care and infant care. During the newborn assessment, the nurse can demonstrate and explain normal newborn behaviour and capabilities and encourage the mother and family to ask questions or express concerns they may have. See Chapter 38 for more information on home visiting.

Warm Lines

The warm line is another type of telephone link between the new family and concerned caregivers or experienced parent volunteers. A *warm line* is a helpline or consultation service, not a crisis intervention line. The warm line is appropriately used for dealing with less extreme concerns that can seem urgent at the time the call is placed but are not actual emergencies. Calls to warm lines commonly relate to infant feeding, prolonged crying, sibling rivalry, or perinatal mood disorder concerns. Warm-line services can extend beyond the fourth trimester. Families need to call when concerns arise and should be given telephone numbers for easy access to answers to their questions.

Support Groups

The woman adjusting to motherhood sometimes seeks a special group experience. Postpartum women who have met earlier in prenatal clinics or on the hospital unit can begin to associate for mutual support. Members of childbirth preparation classes who attend a postpartum reunion can decide to extend their relationship during the fourth trimester.

A postpartum support group enables mothers and partners to share with and support each other as they adjust to parenting. Many new parents find it reassuring to discover that they are not alone in their feelings of confusion and uncertainty. An experienced parent can often impart concrete information to other members. Inexperienced parents can find themselves imitating the behaviour of others in the group whom they perceive to be particularly capable.

Referral to Community Resources

In order to develop an effective referral system, it is important that the nurse have a clear understanding of the needs of the woman and family and of the organization and community resources available for meeting those needs. Locating and compiling information about available community services contributes to the development of a referral system. It is important for the nurse to develop his or her own resource file of local and national services that are frequently useful to postpartum families.

KEY POINTS

- Postpartum care is modelled on the concept of health.
- Postpartum nursing care is influenced by knowledge of antepartum and intrapartum care.
- Cultural beliefs and practices affect the patient's response to the puerperium.
- The nursing care plan includes assessments to detect deviations from normal comfort measures for relieving discomfort or pain and safety measures for preventing infection.
- A postpartum assessment includes a review of breasts, uterus, bladder elimination, bowel elimination, amount and colour of lochia, swelling of legs, condition of episiotomy or laceration, and emotional status.
- Teaching and counselling measures are designed to promote the woman's feelings of competence in self-management and baby care.
- Common nursing interventions in the postpartum period include evaluating and treating the boggy uterus and the full urinary bladder; providing for nonpharmacological and pharmacological relief of pain and discomfort associated with the episiotomy, lacerations, afterbirth pains, or breastfeeding; and instituting measures to promote or suppress lactation.
- Meeting the psychosocial needs of new mothers involves taking into consideration the composition and functioning of the entire family as well as an understanding of different cultural beliefs and practices.

- Many mothers may exhibit signs of postpartum blues (baby blues).
- Postpartum teaching includes self-care needs, warning signs, exercise, and sexuality and resumption of sexual relations.
- Telephone follow-up, home visits, warm lines, and support groups are effective means of facilitating physiological and psychological adjustments in the postpartum period.

evolve WEBSITE

Visit the Evolve website for additional resources related to the content in this chapter such as Case Studies, Critical Thinking Case Study Answers, Nursing Care Plans, Nursing Processes, Nursing Skills, and Review Questions for Exam Preparation at: *http://evolve.elsevier.com/Canada/Perry/maternal/*

REFERENCES

Best Start Resource Centre. (2013). *Pimotisiwin: A good path for pregnant and parenting Aboriginal teens.* Toronto: Author. Retrieved from <http://www.beststart.org/resources/rep_health/pimotosiwin_oct.pdf>.

Breastfeeding Committee for Canada. (2012). *Integrated 10 steps and WHO code practice outcome indicators for hospitals and community health services: Summary.* Drayton Valley, AB: Author. Retrieved from <http://breastfeedingcanada.ca/documents/2012-05-14_BCC_BFI_Ten_Steps_Integrated_Indicators_Summary.pdf>.

De La Rosa, I., Perry, J., & Johnson, V. (2009). Benefits of increased home-visitation services: Exploring a case management model. *Family & Community Health, 32*(10), 58–75.

Doering Runquist, J. J., Morin, K., & Stetzer, F. C. (2009). Severe fatigue and depressive symptoms in lower-income urban postpartum women. *Western Journal of Nursing Research, 31*(5), 599–612.

Frank, B., Lane, C., & Hokanson, H. (2009). Designing a postepidural fall risk assessment score for the obstetric patient. *Journal of Nursing Care Quality, 24*(1), 50–54.

Gruslin, A., Steben, M., Halperin, S., et al. (2009). SOGC clinical practice guideline: Immunization in pregnancy. *Journal of Obstetricians and Gynaecologists of Canada, 31*(11), 1085–1092.

Health Canada. (2010). *Prenatal nutrition guidelines for health professionals–Background on Canada's food guide.* Ottawa: Author. Retrieved from <http://www.hc-sc.gc.ca/fn-an/pubs/nutrition/guide-prenatal-eng.php>.

Kuo, S., Yang, S., Kuo, P., et al. (2012). Trajectories of depressive symptoms and fatigue among postpartum women. *Journal of Obstetrical, Gynecological & Neonatal Nursing, 41*(2), 216–226.

Lawrence, R. A., & Lawrence, R. M. (2011). *Breastfeeding: A guide for the medical profession* (7th ed.). St. Louis: Mosby.

Royal College of Obstetricians and Gynaecologists. (2009). *Reducing the risk of thrombosis and embolism during pregnancy and the puerperium (Green-top guideline No. 37a).* London: Author. Retrieved from <http://www.rcog.org.uk/womens-health/clinical-guidance/reducing-risk-of-thrombosis-greentop37a>.

Runquist, J. J. (2007). A depressive symptoms responsiveness model for differentiating fatigue from depression in the postpartum period. *Archives of Women's Mental Health, 10*(6), 267–275.

Song, J. E., Chang, S. B., Park, S. M., et al. (2010). Empirical test of an explanatory theory of postpartum fatigue in Korea. *Journal of Advanced Nursing, 66*(12), 2627–2639.

Vincent, J. L. (2009). Infant hospital abduction: Security measures to aid in prevention. *MCN American Journal of Maternal Child Nursing, 34*(3), 179–183.

Volrathongchai, K., Neelasmith, S., & Thinkhamrop, J. (2013). Non-pharmacological interventions for women with postpartum fatigue. *The Cochrane Database of Systematic Reviews,* (3). doi:10.1002/14651858.CD010444.

Waller-Wise, R. (2012). Mother-baby care: The best for patients, nurses, and hospitals. *Nursing for Women's Health, 16*(4), 273–278.

Wilson, D., de la Ronde, S., Brascoupé, S., et al. (2013). SOGC consensus clinical practice guideline: Health professionals working with First Nations, Inuit, and Métis consensus guideline. *Journal of Obstetricians and Gynaecologists of Canada, 35*(6 eSuppl), S1–S52.

ADDITIONAL RESOURCES

Association of Women, Obstetrical and Neonatal Nurses (AWHONN)—Video on estimation of postpartum blood loss. <https://www.youtube.com/watch?v=F_ac-aCbEn0&list=UUPrOhL3Od7ZeFDq27ycS00g>.

LactMed—Provides information about medication use while breastfeeding: <http://toxnet.nlm.nih.gov/cgi-bin/sis/htmlgen?LACT>.

Motherisk—Information on medications during pregnancy and lactation: <http://www.motherisk.org/>.

Perinatal Services BC: *Postpartum Nursing Care Pathway:* <http://www.perinatalservicesbc.ca/NR/rdonlyres/EF4F92F4-5BFF-461E-8B0C-9E8B9EDCF2AD/0/ToolkitOBGuideline20PPNursingCarePathway.pdf>.

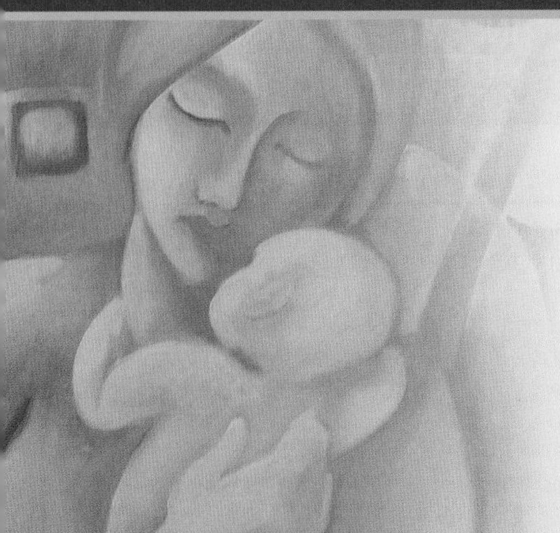

CHAPTER

23

Transition to Parenthood

Lisa Keenan-Lindsay

evolve WEBSITE

Visit the Evolve website for additional resources related to the content in this chapter such as Case Studies, Critical Thinking Case Study Answers, Nursing Care Plans, Nursing Processes, Nursing Skills, and Review Questions for Exam Preparation at: *http://evolve.elsevier.com/Canada/Perry/maternal/*

OBJECTIVES

On completion of this chapter the reader will be able to:

- Identify parental and infant behaviours that facilitate and those that inhibit parental attachment.
- Describe sensual responses that strengthen attachment.
- Examine the process of becoming a mother.
- Compare maternal and paternal adjustments to parenthood.
- Describe ways in which the nurse can facilitate parent–infant adjustment.
- Examine the effects of the following on parenting responses and behaviour: parental age (i.e., adolescence and older than 35 years), same-sex parenting, social support, culture, socioeconomic conditions, personal aspirations, and sensory impairment.
- Describe sibling adjustment.
- Describe grandparent adaptation.

Becoming a parent creates a period of change and instability for men and women who decide to have children. This period occurs whether parenthood is biological or adoptive and whether the parents are husband–wife couples, cohabiting couples, single mothers, single fathers, lesbian couples with one woman as biological mother, gay male couples who adopt a child, or transgendered couples. Parenting is a process of role attainment and role transition. The transition is an ongoing process as the parent(s) and infant develop and change.

A thorough understanding of the process parents go through during their transition to parenthood guides the nurse in helping family members adapt. Family-centred care supports the family as the primary source of knowledge about what is best for them as they work in collaboration with health care providers to plan care. This chapter reviews the transition to parenthood, including the parenting process and the adjustment of all family members.

PARENTAL ATTACHMENT, BONDING, AND ACQUAINTANCE

The process by which a parent comes to love and accept a child and a child comes to love and accept a parent is known as **attachment**. Using the terms *attachment* and **bonding**, Klaus and Kennell (1976) originally proposed that there is a sensitive period during the first few minutes or hours after birth when mothers and fathers must have close contact with their infants to optimize the child's later development. Klaus and Kennel (1982) later revised their theory of parent–infant bonding, modifying their claim of the critical nature of immediate contact with the infant after birth. They acknowledged the adaptability of parents, stating that it took longer than minutes or hours for parents to form an emotional relationship with their infants. The terms *attachment* and *bonding* continue to be used interchangeably.

Attachment is developed and maintained through proximity and interaction with the infant as the parent becomes acquainted

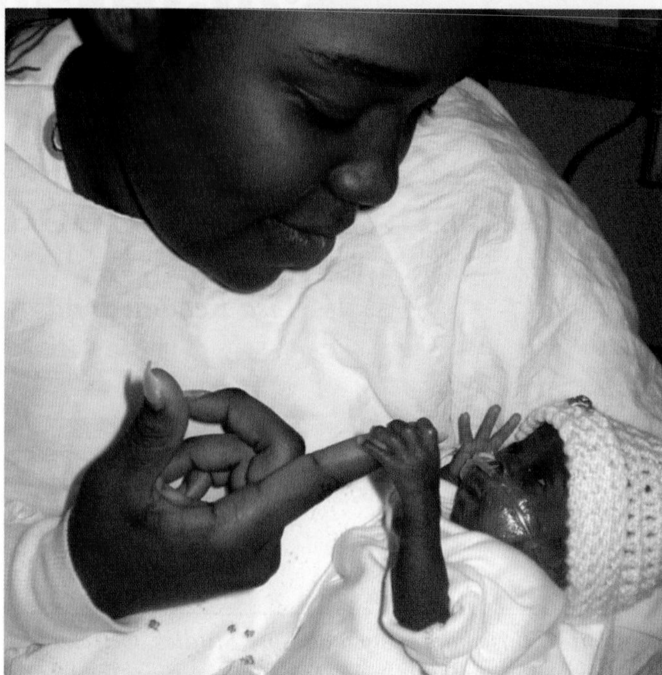

FIGURE 23-1 Grasping. (Courtesy Cheryl Briggs, BSN, RNC-NIC.)

with the infant, identifies the infant as an individual, and claims the infant as a member of the family. Attachment is facilitated by positive feedback (i.e., social, verbal, and nonverbal responses, whether real or perceived, that indicate acceptance of one partner by the other). Attachment occurs through a mutually satisfying experience. One mother commented on her daughter's grasp reflex, noting, "I put my finger in her hand, and she grabbed right on. It's just a reflex, I know, but it felt good anyway" (Fig. 23-1).

The concept of attachment includes mutuality (i.e., the infant's behaviours and characteristics elicit a corresponding set of parental behaviours and characteristics). The infant displays signalling behaviours such as crying, smiling, and cooing that initiate the contact and bring the caregiver to the child. These behaviours are followed by behaviours such as rooting, grasping, and postural adjustments that maintain the contact. Most caregivers are attracted to an alert, responsive, cuddly infant and repelled by an irritable, apparently disinterested infant. Attachment occurs more readily with the infant whose temperament, social capabilities, appearance, and sex fit the parent's expectations. If the child does not meet these expectations, the parent's disappointment can delay the attachment process. Table 23-1 presents a comprehensive list of classic infant behaviours affecting parental attachment. Table 23-2 presents a corresponding list of parental behaviours that affect infant attachment.

An important part of attachment is acquaintance. Parents use eye contact (Fig. 23-2), touching, talking, and exploring to become acquainted with their infant during the immediate postpartum period. Adoptive parents undergo the same process when they first meet their new child. During this period, families engage in the *claiming process*, which is the identification of the new baby. The child is first identified in terms of likeness to other family members, then in terms of differences, and finally in terms of "uniqueness." The unique newcomer is thus incorporated into the family. Parents examine their infant carefully and point out characteristics that the child shares with other family members and that are indicative of a relationship between them. The claiming process is revealed by maternal comments such as the following: "David held him close and said, 'He's the image of his father,' but I found one part like me—his toes are shaped like mine."

Conversely, some mothers react negatively. They "claim" the infant in terms of the discomfort or pain the baby causes. The mother interprets the infant's normal responses as being negative toward her and reacts to her child with dislike or indifference. She does not hold the child close or touch the child to be comforting; for example, "The nurse put the baby into Marie's arms. She promptly laid him across her knees and glanced up at the television. 'Stay still until I finish watching—you've been enough trouble already.'"

Nurses play an important role in facilitating parental attachment. They can enhance positive parent–infant contacts

TABLE 23-1 INFANT BEHAVIOURS AFFECTING PARENTAL ATTACHMENT

FACILITATING BEHAVIOURS	INHIBITING BEHAVIOURS
Visually alert; eye-to-eye contact; tracking or following of parent's face	Sleepy; eyes closed most of the time; gaze averted
Appealing facial appearance; randomness of body movements reflecting helplessness	Resemblance to person parent dislikes; hyperirritability or jerky body movements when touched
Smiles	Bland facial expression; infrequent smiles
Vocalization; crying only when hungry or wet	Crying for hours on end; colicky
Grasp reflex	Exaggerated motor reflex
Anticipatory approach behaviours for feedings; sucks well; feeds easily	Feeds poorly; regurgitates; vomits often
Enjoys being cuddled, held	Resists being held and cuddling by crying, stiffening body
Easily consolable	Inconsolable; unresponsive to parenting, caretaking tasks
Activity and regularity somewhat predictable	Unpredictable feeding and sleeping schedule
Attention span sufficient to focus on parents	Inability to attend to parent's face or offered stimulation
Differential crying, smiling, and vocalizing; recognizes and prefers parents	Shows no preference for parents over others
Approaches through locomotion	Unresponsive to parent's approaches
Clings to parent; puts arms around parent's neck	Seeks attention from any adult in room
Lifts arms to parents in greeting	Ignores parents

From Gerson, E. (1973). *Infant behavior in the first year of life*. New York: Raven Press.

TABLE 23-2 PARENTAL BEHAVIOURS AFFECTING INFANT ATTACHMENT

FACILITATING BEHAVIOURS	INHIBITING BEHAVIOURS
Looks; gazes; takes in physical characteristics of infant; assumes en face position; eye contact	Turns away from infant; ignores infant's presence
Hovers; maintains proximity; directs attention to and points to infant	Avoids infant; does not seek proximity; refuses to hold infant when given opportunity
Identifies infant as unique individual	Identifies infant with someone parent dislikes; fails to discern any of infant's unique features
Claims infant as family member; names infant	Fails to place infant in family context or identify infant with family member; has difficulty naming
Touches; progresses from fingertip to fingers to palms to encompassing contact	Fails to move from fingertip touch to palmar contact and holding
Smiles at infant	Maintains bland countenance or frowns at infant
Talks to, coos, or sings to infant	Wakes infant when infant is sleeping; handles roughly; hurries feeding by moving nipple continuously
Expresses pride in infant	Expresses disappointment, displeasure in infant
Relates infant's behaviour to familiar events	Does not incorporate infant into daily life
Assigns meaning to infant's actions and sensitively interprets infant's needs	Makes no effort to interpret infant's actions or needs
Views infant's behaviours and appearance in positive light	Views infant's behaviour as exploiting, deliberately uncooperative; views appearance as distasteful, ugly

From Mercer, R. (1983). Parent–infant attachment. In L. Sonstegard, K. Kowalski, & B. Jennings (Eds.), *Women's health. Vol. 2: Childbearing*. New York: Grune & Stratton.

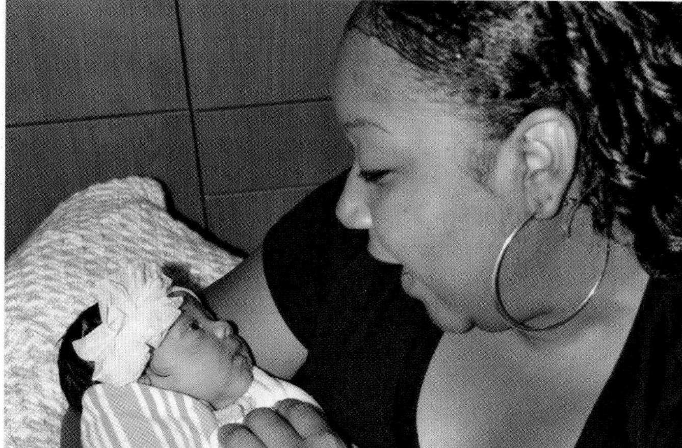

FIGURE 23-2 Eye-to-eye contact. (Courtesy Cheryl Briggs, BSN, RNC-NIC.)

by heightening parental awareness of an infant's responses and ability to communicate. As the parent attempts to become competent and loving in that role, nurses can bolster the parent's self-confidence and ego. Nurses are in prime positions to identify actual and potential problems and to collaborate with other health care providers who will care for the parents after discharge. Nursing interventions related to the promotion of parent–infant attachment are numerous and varied (Table 23-3).

Assessment of Attachment Behaviours

One of the most important areas of assessment is careful observation of behaviours thought to indicate the formation of emotional bonds between the newborn and family, especially the mother. Unlike physical assessment of the newborn, which has concrete guidelines to follow, assessment of **parent–infant attachment** relies more on skillful observation and interviewing. Rooming-in of mother and infant and liberal visiting privileges for the partner, siblings, and grandparents can help nurses identify behaviours that demonstrate positive or negative attachment. An excellent opportunity exists during infant feeding sessions. Box 23-1 presents guidelines for assessment of attachment behaviours.

During pregnancy and often even before conception, parents develop an image of the "ideal" or "fantasy" infant. At birth, the fantasy infant becomes the real infant. How closely the dream child resembles the real child influences the bonding process. Assessing such expectations during pregnancy and at the time of the infant's birth enables identification of discrepancies in the parents' view of the fantasy child and the real child.

The labour process significantly affects the immediate attachment of mothers to their newborn infants. Factors such as a long labour, feeling tired or "drugged" after birth, problems with breastfeeding (Tharner, Luijk, Raat, et al., 2012), premature birth, and being separated from the infant at birth (Flacking, Lehtonen, Thomson, et al., 2012; Hoffenkamp, Tooten, Hall, et al., 2012) can delay the development of initial positive feelings toward the newborn. Nurses providing breastfeeding support and referrals to groups such as La Leche League Canada or Postpartum Support International (see Additional Resources at the end of the chapter) can be useful.

PARENT–INFANT CONTACT

Early Contact

Early close contact may facilitate the attachment process between parent and child. Although a delay in contact does not necessarily mean that attachment will be inhibited, additional psychological energy may be necessary to achieve the same effect. To date, no scientific evidence has demonstrated that immediate contact after birth is essential for the parent–child relationship.

Early skin-to-skin contact between the mother and newborn, such as immediately after birth and during the first hour, facilitates maternal affection and attachment behaviours (Flacking et al., 2012; Hung & Berg, 2011; Moore, Anderson, Bergman, et al., 2012). The newborn is placed in the prone position on

TABLE 23-3 EXAMPLES OF PARENT–INFANT ATTACHMENT INTERVENTIONS

INTERVENTION LABEL AND DEFINITION	ACTIVITIES
Attachment Promotion	
Facilitating the development of an affective, enduring relationship between infant and parent	Discuss with patient culture-based expressions of attachment before and after birth. Place newborn skin-to-skin with parent immediately after birth (if mother wishes this). Provide opportunity for parent or parents to see, hold, and examine newborn immediately after birth (i.e., delay unnecessary procedures and provide privacy). Discuss infant behavioural characteristics with parent. Assist parent of multiples in recognizing individuality of each infant. Instruct parent on attachment development, emphasizing its complexity, ongoing nature, and opportunities.
Family Integrity Promotion: Child-Bearing Family	
Facilitation of the growth of individuals or families who are adding an infant to family unit	Respect and support family's cultural value system. Assist family in developing adaptive coping mechanisms to deal with the transition to parenthood. Prepare parent(s) for expected role changes involved in becoming a parent. Prepare parent(s) for responsibilities of parenthood. Reinforce positive parenting behaviours. Identify effect of newborn on family dynamics and equilibrium.
Lactation Counselling	
Assisting in the establishment and maintenance of successful breastfeeding	Correct misconceptions, misinformation, and inaccuracies about breastfeeding. Provide mother the opportunity to breastfeed after birth, when possible. Instruct on infant's feeding cues (e.g., rooting, sucking, and quiet alertness). Determine frequency of normal feeding patterns, including cluster feedings and growth spurts. Discuss strategies aimed at optimizing milk supply (e.g., breast massage, frequent milk expression, complete emptying of breasts, kangaroo care, and medications). Instruct on signs and symptoms warranting reporting to a health care practitioner or lactation consultant.
Parent Education: Infant	
Instruction on nurturing and physical care needed during the first year of life	Determine parent's (or both parents') knowledge and readiness and ability to learn about infant care. Provide anticipatory guidance about developmental changes during first year of life. Teach parent(s) skills to care for newborn. Demonstrate ways in which parent(s) can stimulate infant's development. Discuss infant's capabilities for interaction. Demonstrate quieting techniques.
Risk Identification: Child-Bearing Family	
Identification of individual or family likely to experience difficulties in parenting, and prioritization of strategies to prevent parenting problems	Ascertain understanding of English or other language used in community. Determine developmental stage of parent or parents. Review prenatal history for factors that predispose patient to complications. Monitor parent–infant interactions, noting behaviours thought to indicate attachment. Plan for risk-reduction activities, in collaboration with the individual or family. Refer to the appropriate community agency for follow-up if risk for parent problems or a lag in attachment has been identified.

Data from Bulechek, G., Butcher, H., Dochterman, J., et al. (2013). *Nursing interventions classification (NIC)* (6th ed.). St. Louis: Mosby.

the mother's bare chest; the baby and mother's chest are covered with a warm, dry blanket (Fig. 23-3). This practice promotes early and effective breastfeeding and increases breastfeeding duration. It is also associated with less infant crying, improved thermoregulation (especially in low-birth-weight infants), and improved cardiorespiratory stability in late preterm infants (Moore et al., 2012; Thukral, Sankar, Agarwal, et al., 2012).

Parents who cannot have early contact with their newborn (i.e., the infant was transferred to the intensive care nursery) can be reassured that such contact is not essential for optimal parent–infant interactions. Otherwise, adopted infants would not form ties of affection with their parents. Nurses need to stress that the parent–infant relationship is a process that develops over time.

Nurses can facilitate skin-to-skin contact in most birth settings, whether the infant is preterm or term or birthed vaginally or by Caesarean, and with fathers or partners and mothers.

Extended Contact

Rooming-in ensures that the infant stays in the room with the mother and is the norm in Canadian hospitals. In most facilities, the newborn never leaves the mother's presence; nurses perform the initial and ongoing assessments and care in the room with the parents. Nurses should encourage the partner to

BOX 23-1 ASSESSING ATTACHMENT BEHAVIOURS

- When the infant is brought to the parents, do they reach out for the infant and call him or her by name? (Recognize that in some cultures parents may not name the infant in the early newborn period.)
- Do the parents speak about the infant in terms of identification—whom the infant resembles, and what appears special about their infant over other infants?
- When parents are holding the infant, what kind of body contact is seen—do parents feel at ease in changing the infant's position, are fingertips or whole hands used, and does the infant have parts of the body they avoid touching or parts of the body they investigate and scrutinize?
- When the infant is awake, what kinds of stimulation do the parents provide—do they talk to the infant, to each other, or to no one? How do they look at the infant—using direct visual contact, avoiding eye contact, or looking at other people or objects?
- How comfortable do the parents appear in terms of caring for the infant? Do they express any concern regarding their ability or disgust for certain activities, such as changing diapers?
- What types of affection do they demonstrate to the newborn, such as smiling, stroking, kissing, or rocking?
- If the infant is fussy, what kinds of comforting techniques do the parents use, such as rocking, talking, or stroking?

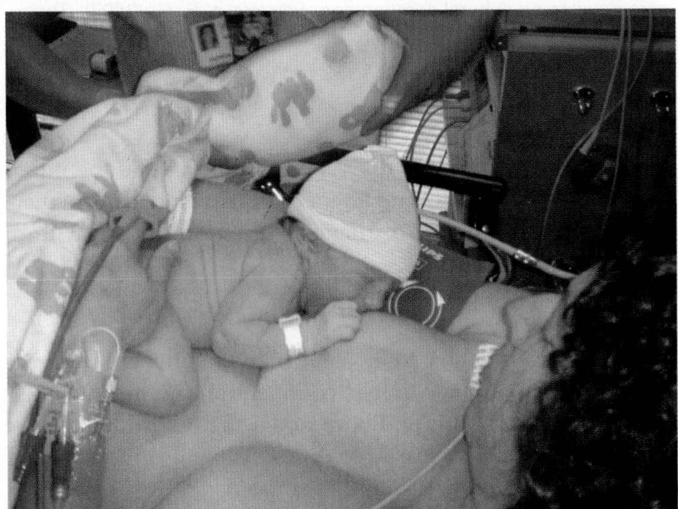

FIGURE 23-3 Placing the naked infant on the bare chest of the mother encourages both breastfeeding and bonding. (Leifer, G. [2015]. *Introduction to maternity and pediatric nursing* [7th ed.]. St. Louis: Saunders.)

participate in caring for the infant in as active a role as desired (Fig. 23-4). They can also encourage siblings and grandparents to visit and become acquainted with the infant.

Extended contact with the infant should be available for all parents but especially for those at risk for parenting difficulties, such as adolescents and those with low social and financial support. Perinatal nurses need to consider and encourage activities that optimize family-centred care (Welch, Hofer, Brunelli, et al., 2012). Baby Friendly status for a hospital is one means to promote family-centred care (Jaafar, Lee, & Ho, 2012; Perrine, Scanlon, Li, et al., 2012; Smith, Moore, & Peters, 2012; Vasquez & Berg, 2012). See more discussion on the Baby Friendly Hospital Initiative in Chapter 27.

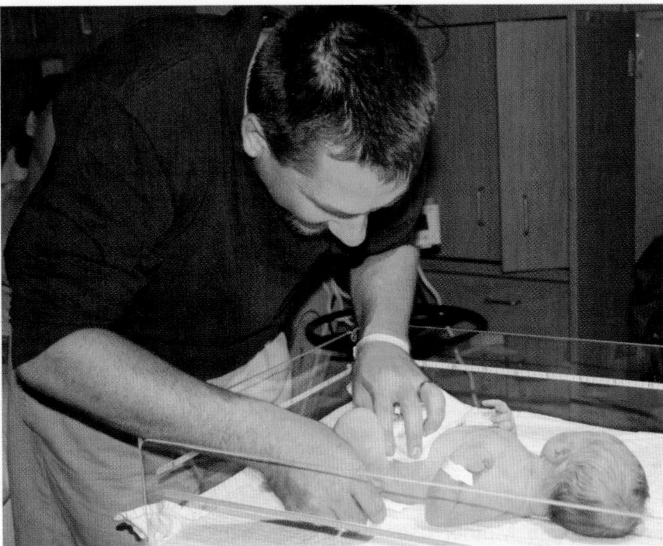

FIGURE 23-4 Father changes diaper of his newborn son. (Courtesy Darren Nelson.)

COMMUNICATION BETWEEN PARENT AND INFANT

The parent–infant relationship is strengthened through the use of sensual responses and abilities by both partners in the interaction. The nurse should keep in mind that there may be cultural variations in these interactive behaviours.

The Senses

Touch

Touch, or the tactile sense, is used extensively by parents as a means of becoming acquainted with the newborn. Many mothers reach out for their infants as soon as they are born. Mothers lift their infants to their breasts, enfold them in their arms, and cradle them. Once the infant is close, the mother begins the exploration process with her fingertips, one of the most touch-sensitive areas of the body (Fig. 23-5). Within a short period of time, she uses her palm to caress the baby's trunk and eventually enfolds the infant. Gentle, stroking motions are used to soothe and quiet the infant. Patting or gently rubbing the infant's back is a comfort after feedings. Infants also pat the mother's breast as they nurse. Both seem to enjoy sharing each other's body warmth. Parents seem to have an innate desire to touch, pick up, and hold the infant. They comment on the softness of the baby's skin and note details of the baby's appearance. As parents become increasingly sensitive to the infant's like or dislike of different types of touch, they draw closer to their baby.

Variations in touching behaviours have been noted in mothers from different cultural groups. For example, minimal touching and cuddling is a traditional Southeast Asian practice

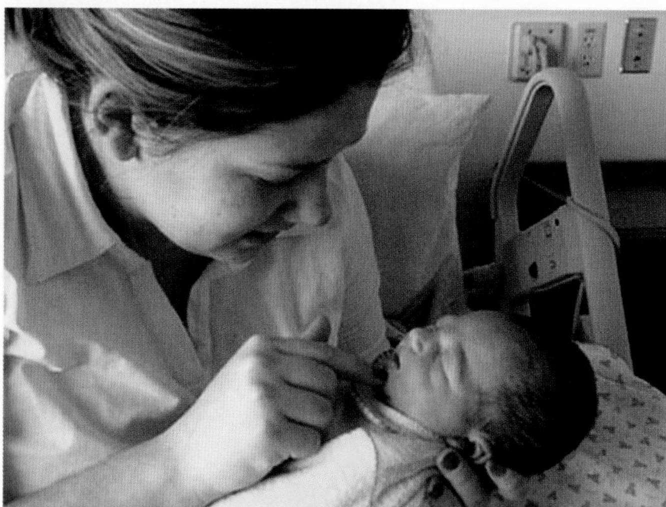

FIGURE 23-5 Mother uses fingertip to explore infant. (Courtesy Rebekah Vogel.)

thought to protect the infant from evil spirits. Because of tradition and spiritual beliefs, women in India and Bali have practised infant massage since ancient times (Waugh, 2011).

Eye Contact

Parents repeatedly demonstrate interest in having eye contact with the baby. Some mothers remark that, once their babies have looked at them, they feel much closer to them. Parents spend much time getting their babies to open their eyes and look at them. In North American culture, eye contact appears to reinforce the development of a trusting relationship and is an important factor in human relationships at all ages (see Fig. 23-2). In other cultures, eye-to-eye contact may be perceived differently (see Cultural Awareness box). For example, in Mexican culture, sustained direct eye contact is considered to be rude and immodest and even dangerous for some individuals. This danger may arise from the *mal ojo* (evil eye), resulting from excessive admiration. Women and children are thought to be more susceptible to the *mal ojo* (D'Avanzo, 2008).

As newborns become functionally able to sustain eye contact with their parents, time is spent in mutual gazing, often in the en face position. In this position, the parent's face and the infant's face are approximately 20 cm apart and on the same plane (see Fig. 23-2).

Nurses and other obstetrical health care providers can facilitate eye contact immediately after birth by positioning the infant on the mother's abdomen or breasts with the mother's and the infant's faces on the same plane. Dimming the lights encourages the infant's eyes to open. To promote eye contact, instillation of prophylactic antibiotic ointment in the infant's eyes can be delayed until the infant and parents have had some time together in the first 2 hours after birth.

Voice

The shared response of parents and infants to each other's voices is also remarkable. Parents wait tensely for the first cry. Once that cry has reassured them of the baby's health, they begin comforting behaviours. As the parents speak, the infant is alerted and turns toward them. Infants respond to higher-pitched voices and can distinguish the mother's voice from others soon after birth.

Odour

Another behaviour shared by parents and infants is a response to each other's odour. Mothers comment on the smell of their babies when first born and have noted that each infant has a unique odour. Infants learn rapidly to distinguish the odour of their mother's breast milk.

Entrainment

Newborns move in time with the structure of adult speech, which is termed entrainment. They wave their arms, lift their heads, and kick their legs, seemingly "dancing in tune" to a parent's voice. Culturally determined rhythms of speech are ingrained in the infant long before he or she uses spoken language to communicate. This shared rhythm also gives the parent positive feedback and establishes a positive setting for effective communication.

Biorhythmicity

The fetus is in tune with the mother's natural rhythms, or *biorhythmicity*, such as her heartbeat. After birth, the mother's

CULTURAL AWARENESS

Fostering Bonding: Women of Varying Ethnic and Cultural Groups

Canadian women, families, and health care workers are made up of different races, socioeconomic backgrounds, sexual orientations, and ethnic groups. Child-bearing practices and rituals may be incongruent with Anglo-Canadian standards. For example, Chinese families traditionally use extended family members to care for the newborn so that the mother can rest and recover, especially after a Caesarean birth. Some Asian and Latin American women do not initiate breastfeeding until their breast milk comes in. Indigenous persons consciously place long silences in conversation for reflection and engage in minimal eye contact. It would be easy for Anglo-Canadian health care workers to perceive this as disrespect and indifference.

Nurses must become knowledgeable about child-bearing beliefs and practices of diverse cultural and ethnic groups. They must also develop cultural sensitivity and use relevant cultural resources. The Registered Nurses' Association of Ontario has an excellent resource that recommends the development of cultural competency through knowledge as well as self-awareness and communication skills, to promote and embrace diversity. Because individual cultural variations exist within groups, nurses need to clarify with the patient and family members or friends the cultural norms that the patient follows. Incorrect judgements may be made about mother–infant bonding if nurses do not practise culturally sensitive care.

Adapted from D'Avanzo, C. (2008). *Mosby's pocket guide to cultural health assessment* (4th ed.). St. Louis: Mosby; Registered Nurses' Association of Ontario. (2007). *Embracing cultural diversity in health care: Developing cultural competence.* Toronto: Author. Retrieved from http://rnao.ca/bpg/guidelines/embracing-cultural-diversity-health-care-developing-cultural-competence; Srivastava, R. H. (2007). *The healthcare professional's guide to cultural competence.* Toronto: Elsevier Canada.

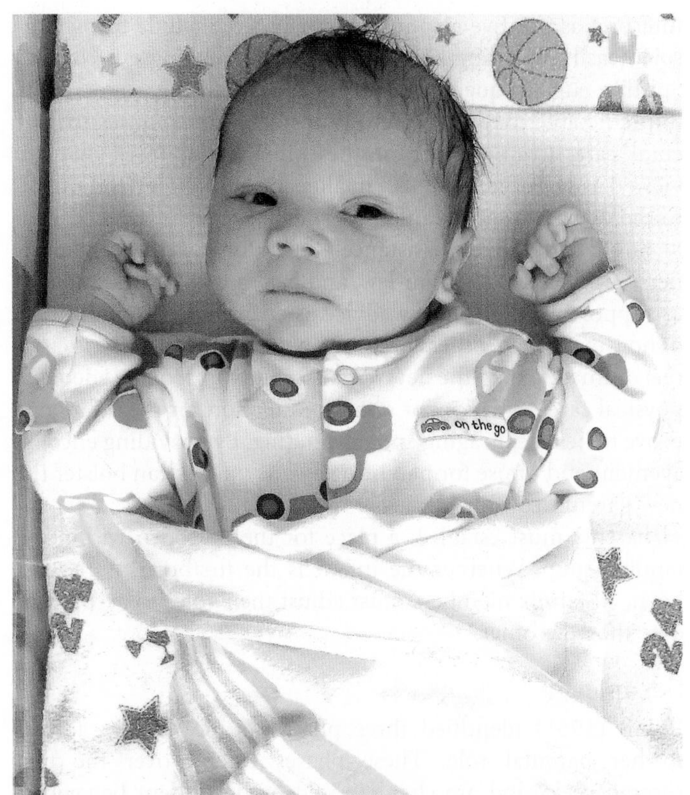

FIGURE 23-6 Infant in alert state. (Courtesy Cheryl Briggs, BSN, RNC-NIC.)

heartbeat or a recording of a heartbeat can sooth a crying infant. One task of the newborn is to establish a personal biorhythm. Parents can help in this process by giving consistent loving care and using their infant's alert state to develop responsive behaviour and increase social interactions and opportunities for learning (Fig. 23-6). The more quickly parents become competent in child care activities, the more quickly their psychological energy can be directed toward observing the communication cues that the infant gives them.

Reciprocity and Synchrony

Reciprocity is a type of body movement or behaviour that provides the observer with cues. The observer or receiver interprets those cues and responds to them. Reciprocity often takes several weeks to develop with a new baby. For example, when the newborn fusses and cries, the mother responds by picking up and cradling the infant; the baby becomes quiet and alert and establishes eye contact; and the mother verbalizes, sings, and coos while the baby maintains eye contact. As the baby habituates to the stimulus, the infant's responses stop, the baby then averts the eyes and yawns; and the mother decreases her active response. If the parent continues to stimulate the infant, the baby may become fussy.

Synchrony refers to the fit between the infant's cues and the parent's response. When parent and infant have a synchronous interaction, it is mutually rewarding (Fig. 23-7). Parents need time to learn to interpret the infant's cues correctly. For example, the infant develops a specific cry in response to different situations, such as boredom, loneliness, hunger, and discomfort. The parent may need assistance in interpreting these cries, along with trial-and-error interventions, before synchrony develops.

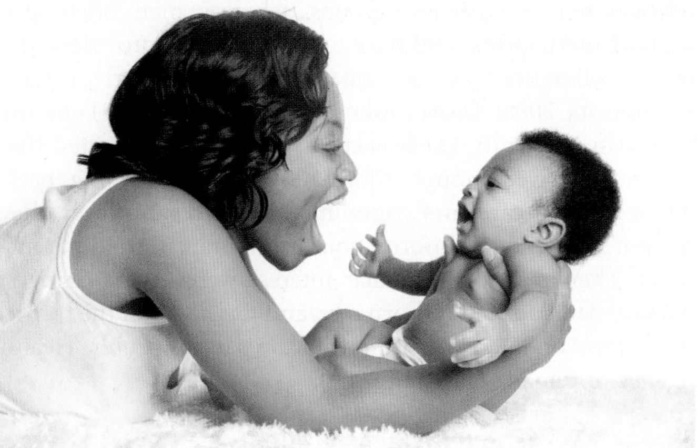

FIGURE 23-7 Sharing a smile; an example of synchrony. (Kim Ruoff/Shutterstock.com.)

PARENTAL ROLE AFTER BIRTH

Adaptation involves stabilizing tasks and coming to terms with commitments. Parents demonstrate growing competence in child care activities and become increasingly attuned to their infant's behaviour. The period from the decision to conceive through the first months of having a child is termed the *transition to parenthood.*

Transition to Parenthood

Historically, the transition to parenthood was viewed as a crisis; however, the current perspective is that for most families parenthood is a developmental transition rather than a major life crisis. The transition to parenthood is described as a time of disorder and disequilibrium, as well as satisfaction, for mothers and their partners. Usual methods of coping may seem ineffective during this time. Some parents can be so distressed that they are unable to be supportive of each other. Because men often identify their spouses as their primary or only source of support, the transition can be harder for fathers. They often feel deprived when the mothers, who are also experiencing stress, cannot provide their usual level of support. Many parents are unprepared for the strong emotions that can develop, such as the helplessness, inadequacy, and anger that arise when dealing with a crying infant. However, parenthood allows adults to develop and display a selfless, warm, and caring side that may not be expressed in other adult roles.

For most mothers and their partners, the transition to parenthood is an opportunity rather than a time of danger. Parents try new coping strategies as they work to master their new roles and reach new developmental levels. As they work through the transition, they often find personal strength and resourcefulness.

Some parents have limited knowledge of what being a parent entails. These parents can benefit from more information on child care, changes in relationships, and differing views of parenting held by partners. Women have more support from female relatives and postpartum groups, whereas men often lack support mechanisms and have only health care providers and work colleagues for information and support (Deave & Johnson, 2008; Deave, Johnson, & Ingram, 2008). In the Canadian Maternity Experience Survey, women reported that they had received enough information on breastfeeding, basic infant and self-care, and community resources; however, they did not have enough information on the transition to parenthood. The topics of particular interest were sexual changes, physical demands of newborn care, and the effects of the transition period on the relationship with the partner (Public Health Agency of Canada [PHAC], 2009).

Parental Tasks and Responsibilities

Parents need to reconcile the actual child with the fantasy and dream child. This means coming to terms with the infant's physical appearance, sex, innate temperament, and physical status. If the real child differs greatly from the fantasy child, parents may delay acceptance of the child. In some instances, they may never accept the child.

Many parents know the sex of the infant before birth because of ultrasonographic assessments. For those who do not have this information, disappointment over the sex can take time to resolve. The parents can provide adequate physical care but find it difficult to be sincerely involved with the infant until this internal conflict has been resolved. See Cultural Awareness box.

The normal appearance of the newborn—size, colour, moulding of the head, or bowed appearance of the legs—is startling for some parents. Nurses can encourage parents to examine their babies and to ask questions about newborn characteristics.

Parents need to become adept in the care of the infant, including caregiving activities, noting the communication cues the infant gives to indicate needs and responding appropriately to those needs. Self-esteem grows with competence. Breastfeeding helps mothers feel they are contributing in a unique way to the welfare of the infant. The parent may interpret the infant's response to his or her parental care and attention as a comment on the quality of that care. Infant behaviours that parents interpret as positive responses to their care include being consoled easily, enjoying being cuddled, and making eye contact. Spitting up frequently after feedings, crying, and being unpredictable may be perceived as negative responses to parental care. Continuation of these infant responses that are viewed as negative can result in alienation of parent and infant, to the detriment of the infant.

Some people view assistance—including advice from partners, mothers, mothers-in-law, and health care professionals—as supportive. Others view advice as criticism or an indication of how inept these others judge the new parents to be. Criticism, real or imagined, of the new parents' ability to provide adequate physical care, nutrition, or social stimulation for the infant can prove to be discouraging and devastating. By providing encouragement and praise for parenting efforts, nurses can bolster the new parents' confidence.

Parents must establish a place for the newborn within the family group. Whether the infant is the firstborn or the last born, all family members must adjust their roles to accommodate the newcomer.

CULTURAL AWARENESS

Birth Story: It's a Girl (Again)!

Faduma is a midwife from Saudi Arabia who faced a difficult situation while assisting a woman who desperately wanted her baby to be a boy because she already had several little girls.

When the patient gave birth to yet another baby girl, Faduma says, she set the newborn aside for as long as she could and kept telling the woman she had given birth to a "beautiful, healthy baby." She shared that the baby was a girl only when the patient pressed her for the information. Her reasons for doing this were to give the mother time to stabilize physically before she received what she would consider disappointing news. Faduma reported that this was common practice among midwives in her country.

From Watts, N., & McDonald, C. (2007). The beginning of life (the perinatal period). In R. Srivastava (Ed.). *The healthcare professional's guide to clinical cultural competence.* Toronto: Elsevier.

Becoming a Mother

Rubin (1961) identified three phases as the mother adjusts to her parental role. These phases extend over the first several weeks and are characterized by dependent behaviour, dependent–independent behaviour, and interdependent behaviour (Table 23-4). Rubin's research was conducted when the

TABLE 23-4 PHASES OF MATERNAL POSTPARTUM ADJUSTMENT

PHASE	CHARACTERISTICS
Dependent: taking-in phase	First 24 hr (range of 1–2 days) Focus: self and meeting of basic needs • Reliance on others to meet needs for comfort, rest, closeness, and nourishment • Excited and talkative • Desire to review birth experience
Dependent–independent: taking-hold phase	Starts second or third day; lasts 10 days to several weeks Focus: care of baby and competent mothering • Desire to take charge • Nurturing and acceptance by others still important • Eagerness to learn and practise—optimal period for teaching by nurses • Handling of physical discomforts and emotional changes • Possible experience with postpartum blues (see Chapter 22, p. 579)
Interdependent: letting-go phase	Focus: forward movement of family as unit with interacting members • Reassertion of relationship with partner • Resumption of sexual intimacy • Resolution of individual roles

From Rubin, R. (1961). Basic maternal behavior. *Nursing Outlook, 9,* 683–686.

length of stay in the hospital was for a longer period of time (3 to 5 or more days). With today's early discharge, women seem to move through the phases faster.

Mercer (2004) has suggested that the concept of maternal-role attainment introduced by Rubin in 1967 be replaced with *becoming a mother*, to signify the transformation and growth of the mother identity. Becoming a mother implies more than attaining a role; it includes her learning new skills and increasing her confidence in herself as she meets new challenges in caring for her child or children.

Mercer (2004) identified four stages in the process of becoming a mother (Mercer & Walker, 2006):

1. Commitment, attachment to the unborn baby, and preparation for birth and motherhood during pregnancy
2. Acquaintance/attachment to the infant, learning to care for the infant, and physical restoration during the first 2 to 6 weeks following birth
3. Moving toward a new normal
4. Achievement of a maternal identity through redefining self to incorporate motherhood (around 4 months)

The time of achievement of the stages varies, and the stages may overlap. Achievement is influenced by mother and infant variables and the social environment.

Maternal sensitivity or maternal responsiveness is an important determinant of the maternal–infant relationship. It can be defined as the quality of a mother's sensitive behaviours that are based on her awareness, perception, and responsiveness to infant cues and behaviours. Maternal sensitivity significantly influences the infant's physical, psychological, and cognitive development. Maternal qualities inherent to this sensitivity include awareness and responsiveness to infant cues, affect, timing, flexibility, acceptance, and conflict negotiation. Maternal sensitivity is dynamic and develops over time in a reciprocal give-and-take with the infant (Shin, Park, Ryu, et al., 2008).

Not all mothers experience the transition to motherhood in the same way. For some women, becoming a mother entails multiple losses. For example, for some single women there may be a loss of the family of origin when they do not accept her decision to have the child. There may be loss of a relationship with the father of the baby, with friends, and with their own sense of self. Women describe a loss of dreams, including loss of job, financial security, and a future profession.

More reality-based perinatal education programs are needed, to better prepare mothers and decrease their anxiety. Classes allow time for questions to be answered and for mothers to lend support to one another. These classes can be provided in person or online, through Skype or video chat. Mothers need to know during the first months of parenthood that it is common to feel overwhelmed and insecure and to experience physical and mental fatigue. They need to be assured that this situation is temporary and that 3 to 6 months may be needed to become comfortable in caregiving and in being a mother. Maternal support by professionals should not end with hospital discharge but extend over the next 4 to 6 months; long-term interventions tend to be more successful than one-time encounters. Nurses can advocate for the extension of such support services well into the postpartum period (Shapiro, Nahm, Gottman, et al., 2011).

During pregnancy and after birth, nurses can discuss the usual postpartum concerns that mothers experience. They can provide anticipatory guidance on coping strategies, such as resting when the infant sleeps and planning with an extended family member or friend to do the housework for the first week or two after the baby is born. In some provinces, once a mother is home, she will receive a phone call and, if needed, a visit from a community health nurse. Nurses should plan additional supportive counselling for first-time mothers inexperienced in child care, women whose careers had provided outside stimulation, women who lack friends or family members with whom to share delights and concerns, and adolescent mothers. Whenever possible, postpartum home visits should be included in the plan of care.

Becoming a Father

The realities of the first few weeks at home with a newborn cause fathers to change their expectations, set new priorities, and redefine their role. They develop strategies for balancing work, their own needs, and the needs of their partner and infant. Men usually become increasingly more comfortable with infant care. During this time, they may struggle for recognition and positive feedback from their partner, the infant, and others. They may feel excluded from support and attention by health care providers. The final phase of becoming an involved father is one of reaping rewards, the most significant being reciprocity from the infant, such as a smile. This phase typically occurs around 6 weeks to 2 months. Increased sociability of the infant enhances the father–infant relationship (Table 23-5).

First-time fathers tend to perceive the first 4 to 10 weeks of parenthood in much the same way that mothers do. It is a period characterized by uncertainty, increased responsibility, disruption of sleep, and inability to control the time needed to care for the infant and re-establish the relationship with their partner (Yu, Hung, Chan, et al., 2012). Fathers express concerns about decreased attention from their partners relative to their

TABLE 23-5 EARLY DEVELOPMENT OF THE INVOLVED FATHER ROLE

PHASE	CHARACTERISTICS
Expectations and intentions	Desire for emotional involvement and deep connection with infant
Confronting reality	Dealing with unrealistic expectations, frustration, disappointment, feelings of guilt, helplessness, and inadequacy
Creating the role of involved father	Altering expectations, establishing new priorities, redefining role, negotiating changes with partner, learning to care for infant, increasing interaction with infant, struggling for recognition
Reaping rewards	Infant smile, sense of meaning, completeness and immortality

Data from Goodman, J. (2005). Becoming an involved father of an infant. *Journal of Obstetrics, Gynecology, & Neonatal Nursing, 34*(2), 190–200.

personal relationship, the mother's lack of recognition of the father's desire to participate in decision making for the infant, and limited time for establishing a relationship with their infants (de Montigny, Lacharité, & Devault, 2012). These concerns can precipitate feelings of jealousy of the infant. The father should discuss his individual concerns and needs with his partner and become more involved with the infant. This can help alleviate feelings of jealousy.

Concerns of fathers are often not addressed adequately in prenatal or postnatal education. The father's relationship with the child is fostered by time alone with the child. Health professionals must address the father's needs to assist in infant care in his transition to parenthood (Premberg, Hellström, & Berg, 2008). An excellent resource for fathers is *The New Fathers Guide*, as well the Region of Peel Health Department's website (see Additional Resources).

Father–Infant Relationship

As in many other cultures, in North American culture, newborns have a powerful impact on their fathers, who can become intensely involved with their babies. The term used for the father's absorption, preoccupation, and interest in the infant is **engrossment**. Characteristics of engrossment include some of the sensual responses relating to touch and eye-to-eye contact that were discussed earlier (see The Senses, p. 589) and the father's keen awareness of features both unique and similar to himself that validate his claim to the infant. An outstanding response is one of strong attraction to the newborn. Fathers spend considerable time "communicating" with the infant and taking delight in the infant's responses to them (Fig. 23-8). Fathers often experience increased self-esteem and a sense of pride and of being more mature and older after seeing their baby for the first time.

In male–female partnerships, fathers tend to spend less time with infants than do mothers, and fathers' interactions with their infants tend to be characterized by stimulating social play rather than caretaking. The subtle and more obvious differences in stimulation from the mother and father provide a wider social experience for the infant.

Fathers receive less interpersonal and professional support than do mothers and can feel excluded from antenatal appointments and prenatal classes (Steen, Downe, Bamford, et al., 2012). They need information and encouragement during pregnancy and in the postnatal period related to infant care, parenting, and relationship changes. During the postpartum hospital stay, nurses can arrange to teach infant care when the father is present and provide anticipatory guidance for fathers about the transition to parenthood. Mothers need to be made aware that fathers may take more time to learn certain skills and that this is normal; the father needs support and encouragement from the mother, not criticism. Separate prenatal and parenting classes and parenting support groups for fathers can provide them with an opportunity to discuss their concerns and enhance their knowledge of the transition to parenting. Postpartum phone calls and home visits by a nurse should include time for assessment of the father's adjustment and needs.

Parenting Among LGBTQ Couples

Although same-sex marriage has been legal in Canada since 2003, the transition to parenting for same-sex couples can still present unique challenges. Whether the couple consists of two women (Fig. 23-9), two men, or a transgender parent, issues such as lack of family acceptance and support, public ignorance, and social invisibility can influence their ability to adapt as new parents. The health care environment is heteronormative; for example, most educational materials for new parents include information for mothers and fathers, and photos depict the traditional heterosexual couple (Röndahl, Bruhner, & Lindhe, 2009). Attitudes of health care professionals can affect the care provided to same-sex couples either positively or negatively.

The decision for lesbian couples to conceive is intentional. Factors that influence the decision include the age, health, infertility, and career considerations of each partner.

Several pathways are available for two women in a lesbian relationship who wish to become parents. The couple may decide for one of the women to conceive a child who is genetically related to her; this is usually done through donor insemination. Alternatively, the fertilized egg of one partner can be

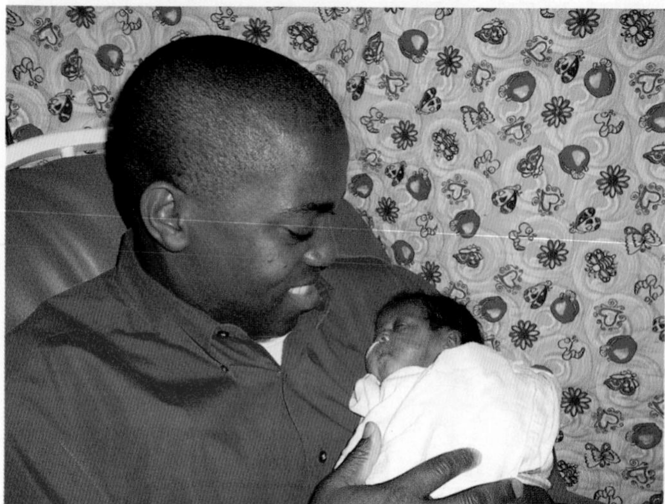

FIGURE 23-8 Father interacts with his newborn son. (Courtesy Cheryl Briggs, BSN, RNC-NIC.)

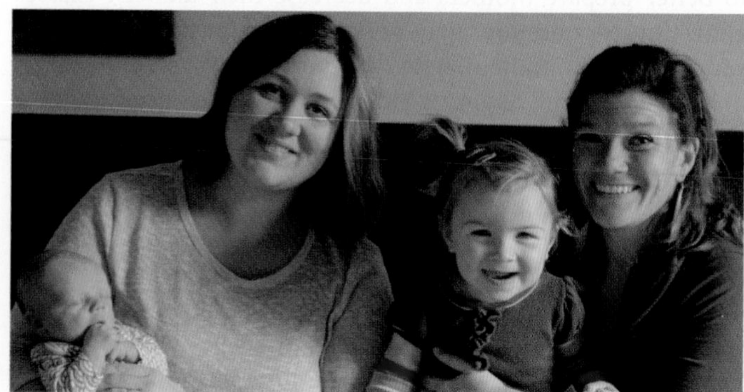

FIGURE 23-9 Lesbian couple and their daughter welcoming a new member of the family. (Courtesy Elliana Gilbert Photography.)

implanted into the uterus of the other partner, who carries the pregnancy. In some cases, a woman is implanted with the fertilized egg from a donor so the child is not biologically related to either partner. Another option is for a lesbian couple to adopt an infant born to a surrogate mother. They can also choose to adopt an infant through an adoption agency or by private arrangement.

Health care professionals demonstrate a variety of reactions to lesbian couples, ranging from rejection and exclusion to complete acceptance and inclusion. Some couples attempt to hide their relationship because they fear a homophobic response (Goldberg, Ryan, & Sawchyn, 2009). Judgemental attitudes, confusion, or lack of understanding can affect the quality of care provided to these families. Although the traditional roles of the mother and father in heterosexual relationships are well recognized, the role of the lesbian non-birth parent can be questioned, misunderstood, and ignored by society and by health care providers. Intentionally or accidentally, health care providers can exclude partners or fail to acknowledge their roles in pregnancy, birth, and parenting. Integration of the non-birth parent into care includes offering opportunities afforded male partners of heterosexual women, such as cutting the cord and rooming in with the mother and baby during hospitalization.

An option not available to male partners is to actually breastfeed the infant. The non-birth female partner can stimulate milk production through induced lactation using medications and regular pumping. A supplemental feeding device containing expressed breast milk or formula can be used to provide additional milk to the breastfeeding infant. Women who choose not to induce lactation yet desire to have the breastfeeding experience can put the baby to breast using a supplemental feeding device containing formula or expressed breast milk (Riordan & Wambach, 2010).

Similar to heterosexual parents, lesbian couples face challenges in adjusting to life with a new baby. After birth, the birth mother tends to be the one most responsible for child care because she is likely to be working fewer hours than her partner. As in heterosexual relationships, tensions can arise between the partners in relation to their roles. This can be compounded by the lack of a formal, recognized relationship between the non-birth parent and the infant and issues surrounding her legal rights in relation to her partner and the infant (Abelsohn, Epstein, & Ross, 2013).

Men in same-sex relationships, or gay couples, can become parents by adoption or by impregnating a surrogate by artificial insemination or sexual intercourse. Same-sex male couples face the same social sanctions regarding pregnancy and parenting that lesbian couples encounter. Both lesbian and gay couples may have children from previous heterosexual relationships.

Nurses are likely to encounter gay couples in the hospital setting if they are present for birth by a surrogate or if they are adopting a newborn and visit the hospital to spend time with the infant and learn about infant care. Nurses can help these men locate support groups that will address their needs. They need to ensure that these families receive effective health care. Data on gay parenting are limited and focus more on developmental outcomes of the children than on parenting styles or parental caregiving. Research is needed to identify the needs of gay parents and ways to support them in their parenting.

Male transgender individuals who have not gone through a transition may also decide to become pregnant. These men require respectful, supportive care and the appropriate space to feel comfortable.

Non-birth parents deserve to have their unique experiences validated and celebrated in their personal relationships and social networks, through accessible and appropriate resources that address their health and wellness needs, and through policies that respect the creation of their families and facilitate a supportive legal environment in which to do so (Abelson et al., 2013).

In situations in which family support is limited or absent, the nurse can help LGBTQ couples locate supportive social groups.

Adjustment for the Couple

The transition to parenthood brings about changes in the relationship between the mother and her partner. A strong, healthy couple relationship is the best foundation for parenthood, although even the best relationships are often shaken with the addition of a baby. During the first few weeks after birth, parents experience a plethora of emotions. Even though they may feel an overwhelming love and a sense of amazement toward their newborn, they also feel a great responsibility. Even if the mother and her partner have attended prenatal classes, read books, or sought advice from family or friends, they are usually surprised by the realities of life with a new baby and the changes in their relationship. Because men and women experience pregnancy and birth differently, the expectation is that they will also vary in their adjustment to parenthood.

Common issues that couples face as they become parents include changes in their relationship with one another, division of household and infant care responsibilities, financial concerns, balancing work and parental responsibilities, and social activities (Menéndez, Hidalgo, Jiménez, et al., 2011). To assist new parents in their transition, nurses can encourage them during pregnancy and in the postpartum period to share personal expectations with each other and to assess their relationship periodically. Couples need to schedule time into their busy lives for one-on-one conversation and try to have regular "dates" or time apart from the infant. The mother and her partner need to express appreciation for one another as well as for their baby. Support from family, friends, and community health professionals should be identified early and used as needed during pregnancy and in the postpartum period and beyond. The couple who is willing to experiment with new approaches to their lifestyle and habits may find the transition to parenthood less difficult. Nurses can provide opportunities for parents to discuss concerns and ask questions about resuming sexual intimacy. Sexual intimacy enhances the adult aspect of the family, and the adult pair share a closeness denied to other family members. Changes in a woman's sexuality after childbirth are related to hormonal shifts, increased breast size, uneasiness with a body that has yet to return to a prepregnant size, fatigue related to sleep deprivation, and physical exhaustion. The resumption of sexual intimacy seems to bring the parents' relationship back into focus (see Home Care box in Chapter 22, p. 582). Before and after birth, nurses should review with new parents their plans for other pregnancies and their preferences for contraception.

Infant–Parent Adjustment

Newborns participate actively in shaping their parents' reaction to them. Behavioural characteristics of the infant influence parenting behaviours. The infant and parent each have unique rhythms, behaviours, and response styles that are brought to every interaction. Infant–parent interactions can be facilitated in at least three ways: (1) modulation of rhythm, (2) modification of behavioural repertoires, and (3) mutual responsivity. Nurses can teach parents about these three aspects of infant–parent interaction through discussions, written materials, and video recordings describing infant capabilities. A creative approach is to record the parent–infant pair during an interaction and then use the individualized recording to discuss the pair's rhythm, behavioural repertoire, and responsivity.

Rhythm

To modulate rhythm, both parent and infant must be able to interact. Therefore, the infant must be in the quiet alert state, one of the most difficult of the sleep–wake states to maintain. The alert state (Fig. 23-10) occurs most often during a feeding or in face-to-face play. The parent must work hard to help the infant maintain the alert state long enough and often enough for interactions to take place. The en face position is usually assumed (see Fig. 23-10, B–E). Multiparous mothers in particular are very sensitive and responsive to the infant's feeding rhythms. Mothers learn to reserve stimulation for pauses in sucking activity and not to talk or smile excessively while the infant is sucking because the baby will stop feeding to interact with her. With maturity, the infant can sustain longer interactions by modulating activity rhythms (i.e., limb movement, sucking, gaze alternation, and habituation). Meanwhile, the parent becomes more attuned to the infant's rhythms and learns to modulate the rhythms, facilitating a rhythmic turn-taking interaction.

Behavioural Repertoires

Both the infant and the parent have a repertoire of behaviours they can use to facilitate interactions. Fathers and mothers engage in these behaviours, depending on the extent of their contact with the infant and their caregiving.

The infant's behavioural repertoire includes gazing, vocalizing, and facial expressions. The infant is able to focus and follow the human face from birth and to alternate the gaze voluntarily, looking away from the parent's face when understimulated or overstimulated (see Fig. 23-10, F). Parents need to learn to be sensitive to the infant's capacity for attention and inattention and to recognize the states and signs of overstimulation (see Family-Centred Teaching box on p. 669). Developing this sensitivity is especially important when interacting with preterm infants.

Body gestures form a part of the infant's early language. Babies greet parents with waving hands (see Fig. 23-10, E) or a reaching out of hands. They can raise an eyebrow or soften their expression to elicit loving attention. Game playing can stimulate them to smile or laugh. Pouting or crying, arching of the back, and general squirming usually signal the end of an interaction.

The parents' repertoire includes various types of interactive behaviours, such as constantly looking at the infant and noting

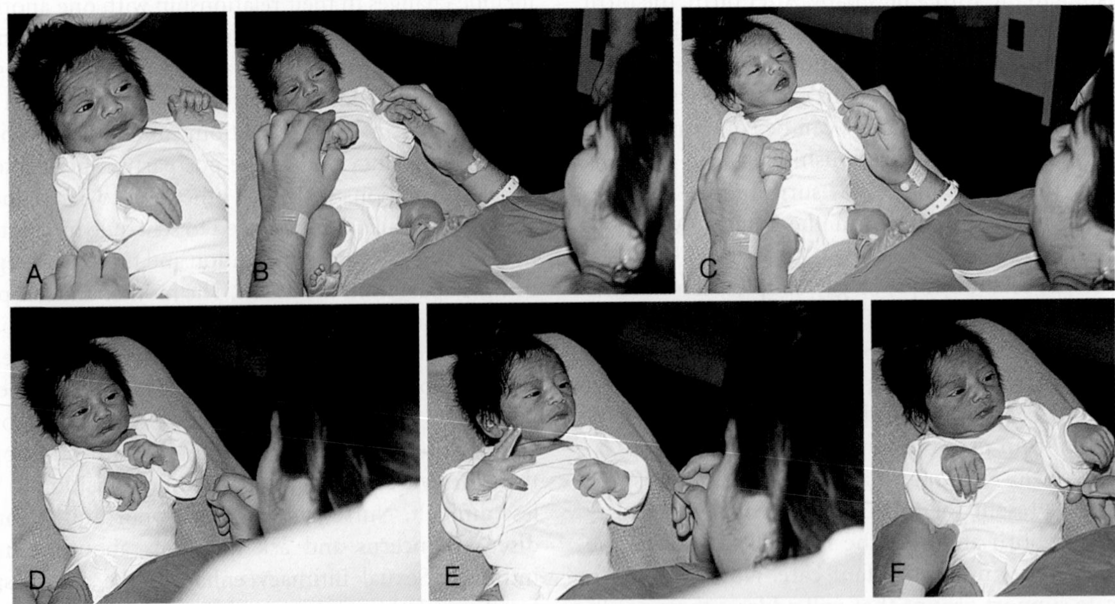

FIGURE 23-10 Holding newborn in en face position, a mother works to alert her daughter, 6 hours old. **A:** Infant is quiet and alert. **B:** Mother begins talking to daughter. **C:** Infant responds, opens mouth like her mother. **D:** Infant gazes at her mother. **E:** Infant waves hand. **F:** Infant glances away, resting. Hand relaxes. (Courtesy Marjorie Pyle, RNC, Lifecircle.)

the infant's response. New parents often remark that they are exhausted from looking at the baby and smiling. Adults also "infantilize" their speech to help the infant listen. They do this by slowing the tempo, speaking loudly and rhythmically, and emphasizing key words. Phrases are repeated frequently. Infantilizing does not mean using baby talk, which involves distortion of sounds.

To communicate emotions to the infant, parents often use facial expressions such as slow and exaggerated looks of surprise, happiness, and confusion. Games such as "peek-a-boo" and imitation of the infant's behaviours are other means of interaction. For example, if the baby smiles, so does the parent; if the baby frowns, the parent responds in kind.

Responsivity

Contingent responses (responsivity) are those that occur within a specific time and are similar in form to a stimulus behaviour. The adult has the feeling of having an influence on the interaction. Infant behaviours such as smiling, cooing, and sustained eye contact, usually in en face position, are viewed as contingent responses. The infant's responses act as rewards to the initiator and encourage the adult to continue with the game when the infant responds positively. When the adult imitates the infant, the infant appears to enjoy it. A progression occurs in the types of behaviours that parents present for the baby to imitate; for example, in early interactions the parent will grimace rather than laugh, which is in keeping with the infant's developmental level. Such behaviours sustain interactions and promote harmony in the relationship.

NURSING CARE

Numerous changes occur during the first weeks of parenthood. Nursing care should be directed toward helping parents cope with infant care, role changes, altered lifestyle, and change in family structure resulting from the addition of a new baby. Developing skill and confidence in caring for an infant can be anxiety provoking. Anticipatory guidance can help prevent or minimize parents' shock of reality in the transition from hospital or birthing centre to home that might negate the parents' joy or cause them undue stress.

Through education, support, and encouragement, nurses are instrumental in assisting mothers and their partners in the transition to parenthood, whether they are first-time parents or parents of several other children. Early and ongoing assessment and intervention promote positive outcomes for parents, infants, and family members (see Community Focus box). (See also Nursing Care Plan: Home Care Follow-up: Transition to Parenthood, available on Evolve.)

DIVERSITY IN TRANSITIONS TO PARENTHOOD

Various factors, including age (adolescent or older than 35 years), social support networks, culture, socioeconomic conditions, and personal aspirations for the future, influence how parents respond to the birth of a child. Cultural beliefs and practices also affect parenting behaviours.

COMMUNITY FOCUS

Identifying Parenting Resources on the Web

- Visit the website of a hospital that provides maternity services in your community. Does the hospital offer childbirth education, parenting, sibling, or infant/child cardiopulmonary resuscitation (CPR) classes? Are group tours of the birthing centre provided for expectant parents?
- Visit a local health department website. Look for information for parents about pregnancy, parenting, and children's health. Review the information about postpartum emotional health, causes and treatments of baby blues, and baby blues versus postpartum mood disorder. Is there adequate information there for new families?
- Research the availability of support groups for parents in your community.

CRITICAL THINKING CASE STUDY

Postpartum Adjustment for the Adolescent and the Older Mother

You are a community health nurse and have had two patients referred to you. Carol is a 15-year-old first-time mother of a 5-day-old girl; she lives with her mother. The father of the baby, Robert, is 17 years old and attended childbirth education classes with Carol. She is breastfeeding the baby but says that the baby sucks too slowly and takes too much time to eat. She says she thinks the baby should know enough to sleep longer at night. Robert would like to feed the baby some cereal since he heard that solid food will make a baby sleep longer at night.

Audrey is a 36-year-old lawyer who has been practising law for 7 years. She just gave birth to her first baby; she and her husband delayed parenting by choice until their careers were well established. She had an uneventful pregnancy, labour, and birth. During a telephone call 48 hours after discharge, when she was asked how things were going, Audrey burst into tears and said, "I didn't expect it to be like this! Nothing is going right."

QUESTIONS

1. Evidence—Is there sufficient evidence to draw conclusions about what teaching and care these new parents need?
2. Assumptions—What assumptions can be made about the following factors:
   a. The relationship of maternal age and postpartum adjustment
   b. The need for social support in the postpartum period
   c. The need for perinatal education
   d. Long-term prognosis for positive outcomes
3. What implications and priorities for nursing care can be drawn at this time?
4. Does the evidence objectively support your conclusion?

Age

Maternal age has a definite effect on the outcome of pregnancy. The mother and fetus are at highest risk when the mother is an adolescent or is more than 35 years old (see Critical Thinking Case Study).

The Adolescent Mother

Although becoming a parent is biologically possible for the adolescent female, her egocentricity and concrete thinking can interfere with her ability to parent effectively. Adolescent mothers are more likely to give birth to preterm or low-birth-weight infants (Kochanek, Kirmeyer, Martin, et al., 2012).

Mortality rates are higher among infants of adolescent mothers. This can be related to inherent problems associated with preterm birth or other conditions, but it is also influenced by the mother's inexperience, lack of knowledge, and immaturity. Nevertheless, in most instances, with adequate support and developmentally appropriate teaching, adolescents can learn effective parenting skills. Strong social and functional support promotes positive outcomes for adolescent mothers.

Contrary to popular beliefs regarding the detrimental effects of adolescent pregnancy, research evidence suggests that the life course for adolescent mothers is similar to that of their socioeconomic peers (Beers & Hollo, 2009). In some families or communities, adolescent parenthood is considered a normal or positive life event. Even so, adolescent pregnancy and parenting are important public health concerns.

The transition to parenthood can be difficult for adolescent parents. Because many adolescents have their own unmet developmental needs, coping with the developmental tasks of parenthood is often difficult. Some young parents experience difficulty accepting a changing self-image and adjusting to new roles related to the responsibilities of infant care. Adolescent mothers are at increased risk for postpartum mood disorders; this is often associated with a lack of social support and poor relations with their partner (Beers & Hollo, 2009; Molborn & Jacobs, 2011). As adolescent parents move through the transition to parenthood, they may feel "different" from their peers, excluded from "fun" activities, and prematurely forced to enter an adult social role. The conflict between their own desires and the infant's demands, in addition to the low tolerance for frustration that is typical of adolescence, further contribute to the normal psychosocial stress of childbirth and parenting. Maintaining a relationship with the baby's father is beneficial for the teen mother and her infant, although adolescent pregnancy often heralds the departure of the young father from the relationship.

Adolescent mothers provide warm and attentive physical care; however, they use less verbal interaction than older parents, and adolescents tend to be less responsive to and interact less positively with their infants than older mothers. Interventions emphasizing verbal and nonverbal communication skills between mother and infant are important. Such strategies must be concrete and specific to match the cognitive level of adolescents. In comparison with adult mothers, teenage mothers have a limited knowledge of child development. They tend to expect too much of their children too soon and often characterize their infants as being fussy. This limited knowledge may cause teenagers to respond to their infants inappropriately.

Many young mothers pattern their maternal role on what they themselves experienced. Therefore, nurses need to determine the kind of support that people close to the young mother are able and prepared to give, as well as the kinds of community assistance available to supplement this support. Many teen mothers can identify a source of social support, the predominant source being their own mothers.

Continued assessment of the new mother's parenting abilities during this postbirth period is essential. Continued support should be provided by involving grandparents and other family members and through home visits and group sessions for discussion of infant care and parenting concerns. Community-based programs for pregnant adolescents and adolescent parents improve access to health care, education, and other support services. Outreach programs addressing self-management, parent–child interactions, and child injuries, in addition to programs that provide prompt and effective community intervention, can prevent serious problems from occurring. As the adolescent performs her mothering role within the framework of her family, she may need to address dependence and independence issues. The adolescent's family members also may need help adapting to their new roles.

The Adolescent Father

The adolescent father and mother face immediate developmental crises, which include completing the developmental tasks of adolescence, making a transition to parenthood, and sometimes adapting to marriage. These transitions can be stressful. The nurse can initiate interaction with the adolescent father if he is present during prenatal visits or if he is with his partner during labour and birth. During the hospital stay, the nurse can include the adolescent father in teaching sessions about infant care and parenting. The nurse can ask him to be present during postpartum home visits and to accompany the mother and baby to well-baby checkups at the clinic or health care provider's office. With the adolescent mother's agreement, the nurse may contact the father directly.

Adolescent fathers need support to discuss their emotional responses to the pregnancy, birth, and fatherhood. The nurse needs to be aware of the father's feelings of guilt, powerlessness, or bravado because these feelings may have negative consequences for both the parents and the child. Counselling of adolescent fathers needs to be reality oriented and should include topics such as finances, child care, parenting skills, and the father's role in the birth experience. Teenage fathers also need to know about reproductive physiology, birth control options, as well as sex practices that lower the risk for pregnancy and sexually transmitted infections.

The adolescent father may or may not continue to be involved in an ongoing relationship with the young mother and his baby. If he does, he can play an important role in the decisions about child care and raising the child. He may need help to develop realistic perceptions of his role as "father to a child" and should be encouraged to use coping mechanisms that are not harmful to his own, his partner's, or his child's well-being. The nurse can enlist support systems, parents, and professional agencies on his behalf.

Maternal Age Greater Than 35 Years

Women older than 35 years of age continue their child-bearing either by choice or because of a lack or failure of contraception during the perimenopausal years. Added to this group are women who have postponed pregnancy because of careers or for other reasons, as well as women of infertile couples who finally become pregnant with the aid of reproductive technology.

Support from partners aids in the adjustment of older mothers to changes involved in becoming a parent and seeing themselves as competent. Support from other family members and friends is also important for positive self-evaluation of parenting, a sense of well-being and satisfaction, and help in dealing with stress. Women who are older can experience social isolation. Older mothers may have less family and social support than that of younger mothers. They are less likely to live near family, and their own parents, if still living, may be unable to provide assistance or support because of age or health issues. These mothers are often caught in the "sandwich generation," taking on responsibility for care of aging parents while parenting young children. Social support may be lacking because their peers are busy with their careers and have limited time to help. Their friends are likely to have older children and have less in common with the new mother.

Changes in the sexual aspect of a relationship can create a stressor for new midlife parents. Mothers report that it is difficult to find time and energy for any romance. They attribute much of this difficulty to the reality of caring for an infant, but the decreasing libido that normally accompanies getting older also contributes.

Work and career issues are sources of conflict for older mothers. Conflicts emerge over being disinterested in work, worrying about giving enough attention to work with the distractions of a baby, and anticipating what it will be like to return to work. Child care is a major factor in causing stress about work.

Another major issue for older mothers with careers is the perception of loss of control. Mothers older than 35 are at a different stage in their careers than younger mothers, often having attained high levels of education, career, and income. The loss of control experienced when going from the consistency of a work role to the inconsistency of the parent role comes as a surprise to many. Helping the older mother have realistic expectations of herself and parenthood is essential.

New mothers who are also perimenopausal may have difficulty understanding that fatigue, loss of sleep, decreased libido, or other physiological symptoms are the causes of the change in their sex drive. Although many women view menopause as a natural stage of life, for midlife mothers this cessation of menstruation coincides with the state of parenthood. The changes of midlife and menopause can add more emotional and physical stress to older mothers' lives because of the time- and energy-consuming aspects of raising a young child. An excellent resource for women who are over 35 years is available from Best Start Ontario (see Additional Resources at the end of the chapter).

Paternal Age Greater Than 35 Years

Although many older fathers describe their experience of midlife parenting as wonderful, they also recognize the drawbacks. Positive aspects of parenthood in older years include increased love and commitment between the two parents, a reinforcement of why one married in the first place, a feeling of being complete, experiencing "the child" in oneself again, more financial stability than in younger years, and more freedom to focus on parenting rather than on career. Drawbacks of midlife parenting include having a young child and not being physically fit to participate in activities, being much older than other fathers, and the change it makes in the relationship with their partner.

Social Support

Social support is strongly related to positive adaptation by new parents, especially adolescent parents, during the transition to parenthood. Social support is multidimensional and includes the number of members in a person's social network, the types of support, perceived general support, actual support received, and satisfaction with support available and received. Partner support in pregnancy can decrease emotional distress in the postpartum period (Goldberg & Smith, 2011; Stapleton, Schetter, Westling, et al., 2012). The type and satisfaction of support appear to be more important than the total number of support network members.

Across cultural groups, families and friends of new parents form an important dimension of the parents' social network. Through seeking help within the social network, new mothers learn culturally valued practices and develop competency in their role as mother.

While social networks provide a support system on which parents can rely for assistance, they also can be a source of conflict. Sometimes a large network can cause problems because it results in conflicting advice coming from numerous people. Grandparents or in-laws are most appreciated when they assist with household responsibilities and do not intrude on the parents' privacy or judge them critically.

Because of the extent of restructuring and reorganization that occurs in a family with the birth of a child, the mother's moods and fatigue in the postpartum period can be helped more by situation-specific support from family and friends than by general support. General support addresses feeling loved, respected, and valued. Situation-specific support relates to practical concerns, such as physical needs and child care. For example, the practical support of a grandparent bathing the infant can help lessen a second-time mother's feelings of loss by providing her time to be with her firstborn child.

Culture

Cultural beliefs and practices are important determinants of health for the mother and infant and also influence parenting behaviours. Culture influences interactions with the baby and the parents' or family's caregiving style. For example, providing for a period of rest and recuperation for the mother after birth is prominent in several cultures. Asian mothers are encouraged to remain at home with the baby up to 30 days after birth and are not supposed to engage in household chores, including care of the baby. Often, the grandmother takes over the baby's care immediately, even before discharge from the hospital. Jordanian mothers have a 40-day lying-in after birth, during which their mothers or sisters care for the baby (D'Avanzo, 2008). Japanese mothers rest for the first 2 months after childbirth. Latin Americans may practise an intergenerational family ritual, *la cuarentena*: for 40 days after birth, the mother is expected to recuperate and get acquainted with her infant. Traditionally, this involves many restrictions concerning food (spicy or cold foods, fish, pork, and citrus are avoided; tortillas and chicken soup are encouraged); exercise; and activities, including sexual intercourse. Many women avoid bathing and washing their hair. Traditional Latin American husbands do not expect to see their wives or infants until both have been cleaned and dressed after birth. The practice of *la cuarentena* incorporates individuals into the family, instills parental responsibility, and integrates the family during a critical life event (D'Avanzo, 2008).

All cultures place importance on desiring and valuing children. In Asian families, children are a source of family strength and stability, are perceived as wealth, and are objects of parental love and affection. Infants almost always are given an affectionate cradle name that is used during the first years of life (e.g., a Filipino girl might be called "Bong-Bong" and a boy "Ling-Ling").

Differing cultural values can influence parents' interactions with health care providers. For example, Asians are taught to be humble and obedient; to be outspoken is frowned upon. They are brought up to refrain from questioning authority figures (such as a nurse), to avoid confrontation, and to respect the yin/yang balance in nature. Because of these learned values, an Asian mother might not confront the nurse about the length of time it has taken to receive the medication requested for her perineal pain. A mother may nod and say "Yes" in response to the nurse's directions for using an iced sitz bath but then will not use the sitz bath. The "yes" in this case is a gesture of courtesy, meaning "I'm listening"; it is not an indication of agreement with the plan.

Knowledge of cultural beliefs can help the nurse make more accurate assessments and diagnoses of observed parenting behaviours. For example, nurses may become concerned when they observe cultural practices that appear to reflect poor maternal–infant bonding. Algerian mothers may not unwrap and explore their infants as part of the acquaintance process because in Algeria babies are wrapped tightly in swaddling clothes to protect them physically and psychologically (D'Avanzo, 2008). A Vietnamese woman may give minimal care to her infant and refuse to cuddle or further interact with her baby. This apparent lack of interest in the newborn is this cultural group's attempt to ward off evil spirits and actually reflects an intense love and concern for the infant (Galanti, 2015). An Asian mother might be criticized for almost immediately relinquishing the care of the infant to the grandmother and not attempting to hold her baby when it is brought to her room; in Asian extended families, members show their support for a new mother's need for rest and recuperation by assisting with the care of the baby. Contrary to the guidance given to new mothers in Canada to watch for breastfeeding difficulties when using a mix of breastfeeding and bottle-feeding initially, this mix of feeding is standard practice for Japanese mothers. This tradition is related to concern for the mother's rest during the first 2 to 3 months and does not usually lead to any problems with lactation; breastfeeding is widespread and successful among Japanese women.

Cultural beliefs and values give perspective to the meaning of childbirth for a new mother. Nurses can provide an opportunity for a new mother to talk about her perception of the meaning of child-bearing. In helping new families adjust to parenthood, nurses must provide culturally competent care by following principles that facilitate nursing practice within transcultural situations. At the same time, because not all members of a cultural group adhere to traditional practices, nurses need to validate which cultural practices are important to individual parents.

Indigenous Families

Given the legacy of residential schools in the Indigenous community, there continue to be parents who have difficulty being effective parents to their children (see Chapter 1, p. 6). One of the greatest impacts of residential schools is the breakdown of family relationships, as families were separated for months or years. Children were deprived of the positive family environment necessary for the transmission of parenting knowledge and skills. Survivors describe being removed from loving families into situations that were deplorable and "loveless" (Truth and Reconciliation Commission, 2012). The impact of this institutionalization and separation continues to be seen to this day and is evidenced in high rates of child apprehensions by social services and Indigenous youth involvement in crime. The Truth and Reconciliation Commission (TRC) (2015) has recommended that families not be separated, if possible, and that adequate housing, addiction resources, and educational supports for parents be provided to help overcome some of the negative impact of residential schools.

Nurses should be aware of the potential impact of residential schools on any Indigenous family and be able to incorporate this knowledge into the care provided. Nurses can also work with partner groups to develop culturally appropriate early-childhood and parent programs that assist young parents and families affected by the impact of residential schools and historic policies of cultural oppression in the development of parental understanding and skills (TRC, 2015). See Additional Resources at the end of the chapter for resources for caring Indigenous families.

Socioeconomic Conditions

Socioeconomic conditions, a key determinant of health, often determine access to available resources. Parents who have low socioeconomic status may find childbirth complicated by concern for their own health and a sense of helplessness. Serious financial problems may override any desire for mothering the infant. Similarly, fathers who are overwhelmed with financial stresses may lack effective parenting skills and behaviours. Families who have limited access to social support and financial resources may require extra education and support to access necessary supports.

Personal Aspirations

For some women, parenthood may interfere with their plans for personal freedom or advancement in their careers. Unresolved resentment can affect caregiving activities and adjustment to parenting. This situation may result in indifference and neglect of the infant or in excessive concerns; the mother may set impossibly high standards for her own behaviour or the child's performance.

Nursing interventions include providing opportunities for mothers to express their feelings freely to an objective listener, discuss measures to enable personal growth, and learn about the care of their infant. Referring the woman to a support group of other mothers who are in similar circumstances may also be helpful.

Nurses also can be proactive in influencing changes in work policies related to work sharing and to promoting family-friendly work environments. Some corporations already structure their workplace to support new mothers (e.g., by providing on-site day care facilities and lactation rooms).

PARENTAL SENSORY IMPAIRMENT

In the early interactions between parent and child, each uses all senses—sight, hearing, touch, taste, and smell—to initiate and sustain the attachment process. A parent who has an impairment of one of the senses needs to maximize use of the remaining senses. Mothers with disabilities tend to value performing parenting tasks in a way perceived as culturally normative. It is important for nurses and other health care providers to remember that these individuals are parents living with a disability, not disabled parents. Most provinces now have legislation to ensure that people with disabilities have access to required resources.

Visually Impaired Parent

Visual impairment alone does not appear to have a negative effect on parents' early parenting experiences. These parents, just as sighted parents, express the wonders of parenthood, and they encourage other visually impaired persons to become parents.

Although visually impaired mothers initially feel pressure to conform to traditional, sighted ways of parenting, they soon adapt these ways and develop methods better suited to themselves. For example, visually impaired parents may prepare the infant's nursery, clothes, and supplies in a way that is different from a sighted person's routine. Some parents put an entire clothing outfit together and hang it in the closet rather than keeping the items separate in drawers. Some develop a labelling system for the infant's clothing and put diapering, bathing, and other care supplies where these will be easy to locate. A strength that visually impaired parents have is a heightened sensitivity to other sensory outputs. A visually impaired parent can tell when their infant is facing them because they can feel the baby's breath on the face.

One of the major difficulties that visually impaired parents experience is the skepticism, open or hidden, of health care providers. Visually impaired people may sense reluctance on the part of others to acknowledge that they have a right to be parents. All too often, health care providers lack the experience to deal with the child-bearing and child-rearing needs of visually impaired parents and those of parents with other disabilities (such as the hearing impaired, physically impaired, and mentally challenged). The nurse's best approach here is to assess the parent's capabilities. From that basis the nurse can make plans to assist the parent, often in much the same way as for a parent with sight. Visually impaired mothers have made suggestions for providing care to women such as themselves during child-bearing (Box 23-2). The nurse can use such approaches to help a parent avoid feeling increased vulnerability.

BOX 23-2 NURSING APPROACHES FOR WORKING WITH VISUALLY IMPAIRED PARENTS

- Parents who are visually impaired need oral teaching by health care providers because pregnancy and childbirth information is usually not accessible to visually impaired people.
- A visually impaired parent needs an orientation to the hospital room that enables the parent to move about the room independently; for example, "Go to the left of the bed and trail the wall until you feel the first door. That is the bathroom."
- Parents who are visually impaired need explanations of routines.
- Parents who are visually impaired need to feel devices (e.g., portable sitz bath equipment, breast pump) and to hear descriptions of the devices.
- Visually impaired parents need a chance to ask questions.
- Visually impaired parents need the opportunity to hold and touch the baby after birth.
- Nurses need to demonstrate baby care by touch and to follow with "Now show me how you would do it."
- Nurses need to give instructions, such as "I'm going to give you the baby. The head is to your left side."

Eye contact with others is considered important in North American culture. With a parent who is visually impaired, this critical factor in the parent–child attachment process is obviously missing. However, the visually impaired parent who may never have experienced this method of strengthening relationships does not miss it. The infant will need other sensory input from that parent. An infant looking into the eyes of a mother who is visually impaired may not be aware that the eyes are unseeing. Other people in the newborn's environment can participate in active eye-to-eye contact to supply this need. A problem may arise, however, if the visually impaired parent has an impassive facial expression. The infant, making repeated unsuccessful attempts to engage in face play with the mother, will abandon the behaviour with her and intensify it with the father or other persons in the household. Nurses can provide anticipatory guidance regarding this situation and help the mother learn to nod and smile while talking and cooing to the infant.

Hearing-Impaired Parent

A parent who has a hearing impairment faces challenges in caregiving and parenting, particularly if the deafness dates from birth or early childhood. Whether one or both parents are hearing impaired, they are likely to have established an independent household. Devices that transform sound into light flashes can be fitted into the infant's room to enable immediate detection of crying. Even if the parent is not speech trained, vocalizing can serve as both a stimulus and a response to the infant's early vocalizing. Deaf parents can provide additional vocal training by use of recordings and television so that from birth the child is aware of the full range of the human voice. Young children acquire sign language readily, and the first sign used is as varied as the first word.

Hospitals and other institutions use various communication techniques and resources with the hearing-impaired, including having staff members or certified interpreters who are proficient in sign language. For example, providing written materials with demonstrations and having nurses stand where the parent can read their lips (if the parent practises lip-reading) are two techniques that can be used. A creative approach is for the nursing unit to develop movies in which information on postpartum care, infant care, and parenting issues is signed by an interpreter and spoken by a nurse or that has closed-captioning. Many resources are available to the deaf parent via the Internet (see Additional Resources at the end of the chapter). Box 23-3 lists suggestions for working with hearing-impaired parents.

SIBLING ADAPTATION

Because the family is an interactive, open unit, the addition of a new family member affects everyone in the family. Siblings have to assume new positions within the family hierarchy. Parents often face the task of caring for a new child while not neglecting the others and need to distribute their attention equitably. When the newborn was born prematurely or has special needs, this can be difficult.

Reactions of siblings result from temporary separation from the mother, changes in the mother's or father's behaviour, or the infant coming home. Positive behavioural changes of siblings include interest in and concern for the baby and increased independence. Regression in toileting and sleep habits, aggression toward the baby, and increased seeking of attention and whining are examples of behaviours that are normal. Parents should be taught that punishing the child for these behaviours is not the best strategy but rather diverting the child's attention is often more effective.

The parents' attitudes toward the arrival of the baby can set the stage for the other children's reactions. Because the baby absorbs the time and attention of the important people in the other children's lives, jealousy (**sibling rivalry**) is to be expected once the initial excitement of having a new baby in the home is over. See the Region of Peel: Parenting in Peel website for more resources for parents on sibling rivalry (see Additional Resources at the end of the chapter).

Parents, especially mothers, spend much time and energy promoting sibling acceptance of a new baby. If sibling preparation classes are available, participation in these classes can help prepare older children to understand what life may be like with a new baby and may make a difference in the ability of parents to cope with their behaviour. Older children are actively involved in preparing for the infant, and this involvement intensifies after the birth of the child. Parents have to manage their feelings of guilt that the older children are being deprived of parental time and attention. They have to monitor the behaviour of older children toward the more vulnerable infant and divert aggressive behaviour. Strategies that parents have used to facilitate siblings' acceptance of a new baby are presented in the Family-Centred Teaching box.

Siblings demonstrate acquaintance behaviours with the newborn. The acquaintance process depends on the information given to the child before the baby is born and on the child's cognitive development level. The initial behaviours of siblings with the newborn include looking at the infant and touching the head. The adjustment of older children to a newborn takes time, and children should be allowed to interact at their own pace rather than forcing them to interact. To expect a young child to accept and love a rival for the parents' affection assumes an unrealistic level of maturity. The bond between siblings involves a secure base in which one child provides support for the other, is missed when absent, and is looked to for comfort and security.

BOX 23-3 NURSING APPROACHES FOR WORKING WITH HEARING-IMPAIRED PARENTS

- Before initiating communication, be aware of the parents' preferences and capabilities: Do they wear a hearing aid? Do they read lips? Do they wish to have an interpreter?
- Make certain that the parent(s) sees you approaching to avoid startling the parent.
- Before speaking, be directly in front of the parent and have that person's full attention.
- When speaking, face the parent directly and be at the same level.
- Avoid standing in front of a light or a window while speaking to the parent.
- Keep your hands away from your face while speaking, to minimize distractions.
- If the parent relies on lip-reading, sit close enough so that the parent can easily see your lip movements.
- Speak clearly with a regular voice volume and lip movements, while maintaining eye contact.
- Speak in short, simple sentences to facilitate understanding.
- If the parent does not understand something, it is better to find a different way to say what needs to be communicated rather than repeating the same words over and over.
- Written messages aid in communication. A small white or black erasable board can be useful.
- Give educational materials to hearing-impaired parents and ask them to read the materials before doing parent teaching. They can refer to the materials after discharge.
- Use visual aids such as pictures, diagrams, or other devices when doing parent teaching.
- When doing parent teaching, it is helpful for a hearing person (partner or family member) to be present.
- Allow ample time to communicate with the hearing-impaired parent; being in a rush can evoke stress and create barriers to effective communication.

GRANDPARENT ADAPTATION

Becoming a grandparent is usually associated with great joy and happiness. Yet it is a time of transition as roles and relationships are changing and new opportunities arise. Emotions are varied and can change from day to day; feelings of joy, anticipation,

FAMILY-CENTRED TEACHING

Strategies for Facilitating Sibling Acceptance of a New Baby

- Take your older child (or children) on a tour of your hospital room and point out similarities between this birth and his or her birth; for example, "This is like the room I was in with you, and the baby is in the same kind of bassinet that you were in."
- Have a small gift from the baby to give to your older child each day he or she visits in the hospital.
- Give the older child a T-shirt that says, "I'm a big brother" (or "sister").
- Arrange for your children to be among the first to see the newborn. Let them hold the baby in the hospital.
- When the older child visits for the first time, make sure you are not holding the new baby. Your arms need to be open and available for the older child. Instruct the person accompanying the older child to call ahead or give a warning knock to give you time to lay the baby down or have someone else hold the baby.
- Plan individual time with each child. The father or partner can spend time with the older siblings while the mother is taking care of the baby and vice versa. Siblings like to have time and attention from both parents.
- Give preschool and early school-age siblings a newborn doll as "their baby." Give the sibling a photograph of the new baby to take to school to show off "his" or "her" baby. Older siblings may enjoy the responsibility of helping care for the newborn, such as learning how to change a diaper. Remember to supervise interactions between the siblings and new baby.

and excitement are often intermingled with some degree of anxiety and uncertainty. Circumstances surrounding the pregnancy and birth influence the feelings, reactions, and responses of grandparents.

Pregnancy and birth necessitate redefining intergenerational roles and relationships within the family. A primary role of the grandparents is to support, nurture, and empower their child in his or her parenting role. Grandparents must acknowledge that things have changed since they first became parents as they deal with changes in practices and attitudes toward childbirth and child-rearing. The degree to which grandparents understand and accept current practices can influence how supportive they are to their adult children.

At the same time that they are adjusting to grandparenthood, the majority of grandparents are experiencing normative middle- and old-age life transitions, such as retirement and a move to smaller housing, and they may need support from their adult children. Some may feel regret about their limited involvement because of poor health or geographic distance.

The extent of involvement of grandparents in the care of the newborn depends on many factors—for example, the willingness of the grandparents to become involved, the proximity of the grandparents, and ethnic and cultural expectations of their role (Fig. 23-11). If the new parents live in Canada and the grandparents do not, they may be asked to come to Canada to care for the baby and mother after birth. Many Canadian-born paternal grandparents, in contrast to those in other cultures, consider themselves secondary to the maternal grandparents. Less seems expected of them and they are initially less involved. Nevertheless, these grandparents are often eager to help and express great pleasure in their son's fatherhood and his involvement with the baby.

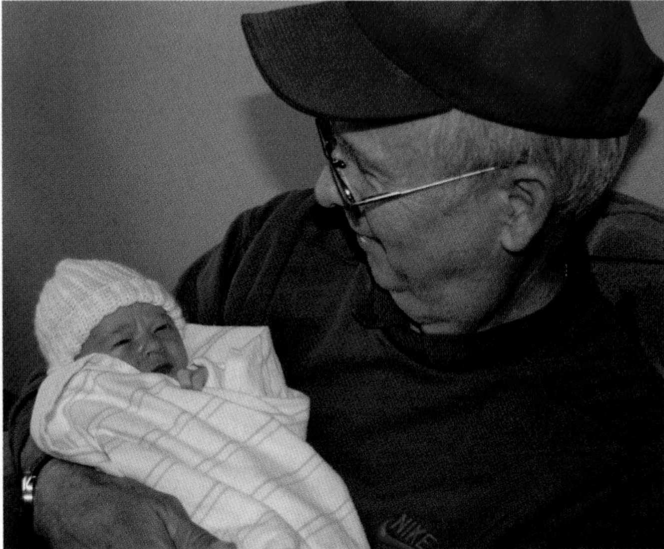

FIGURE 23-11 Grandfather and new grandson get acquainted. (Courtesy William Perry.)

COMMUNITY FOCUS

Helping Grandparents Bridge the Generation Gap

Interview a grandfather and grandmother about their experiences with childbirth and infant care. Prepare a "letter to new parents" (written from the grandparents' perspective), which can be included in prenatal kits distributed in childbirth preparation classes and made available to all family members on the postpartum unit. Include how the birth of their adult child occurred, how things are different now, what role the grandparent can play in helping the new parents adjust to home and child care, and what the grandparent might contribute to the family in memories.

Relationships between grandparents and parents may change with the birth of a new baby. For first-time parents, pregnancy and parenthood can reawaken old issues related to dependence versus independence. Couples often do not plan on their parents' help immediately after the baby arrives. They want time "to be a family," implying a couple–baby unit, not the intergenerational family network. Intergenerational help may be perceived as interference. Contrary to their expectations, however, most new parents do call on their parents for help, especially the maternal grandmother. Many grandparents are aware of their adult children's wishes for autonomy, respect these wishes, and remain available to help, when asked.

Grandparents' classes can be used to bridge the generation gap and to help the grandparents understand their adult children's parenting concepts. The classes include information on up-to-date child-bearing practices; family-centred care; infant care, feeding, and safety (car seats); and exploration of roles that grandparents can play in the family unit (see Community Focus box).

Increasing numbers of grandparents are providing permanent care to their grandchildren as a result of divorce, substance use, child abuse or neglect, abandonment, teenage pregnancy, death, human immunodeficiency virus and acquired immunodeficiency syndrome, incarceration, and mental health problems. Educational and financial considerations must be addressed and available support systems identified for these families.

KEY POINTS

- The birth of a child necessitates changes in the existing interactional structure of a family.
- Attachment is the process by which the parent and infant come to love and accept each other.
- Attachment is strengthened through the use of sensual responses or interactions by both partners in the parent–infant interaction.
- Women go through stages in becoming a mother.
- Fathers and non-birth parents experience emotions and adjustments during the transition to parenthood that are similar to and also distinctly different from those of mothers.
- LGBTQ families require respectful support when becoming parents, as they may face different challenges, including legal aspects of parenting.
- Modulation of rhythm, modification of behavioural repertoires, and mutual responsivity facilitate infant–parent adjustment.
- Many factors (e.g., age, culture, socioeconomic level, and expectations of what the child will be like) influence adaptation to parenthood.
- Sibling adjustment to a new baby requires creative parental interventions.
- Grandparents can have a positive influence on the postpartum family.

evolve WEBSITE

Visit the Evolve website for additional resources related to the content in this chapter such as Case Studies, Critical Thinking Case Study Answers, Nursing Care Plans, Nursing Processes, Nursing Skills, and Review Questions for Exam Preparation at: *http://evolve.elsevier.com/Canada/Perry/maternal/*

REFERENCES

Abelsohn, K. A., Epstein, R., & Ross, L. E. (2013). Celebrating the "other" parent: Mental health and wellness of expecting lesbian, bisexual, and queer non-birth parents. *Journal of Gay & Lesbian Mental Health*, *17*(4), 387–405. doi:10.1080/19359705.2013.771808.

Beers, L., & Hollo, R. (2009). Approaching the adolescent-headed family: A review of teen parenting. *Current Problems in Pediatric and Adolescent Health Care*, *39*(9), 216–233.

D'Avanzo, C. (2008). *Mosby's pocket guide to cultural health assessment* (4th ed.). St. Louis: Mosby.

Deave, T., & Johnson, D. (2008). The transition to parenthood: What does it mean for fathers? *Journal of Advanced Nursing*, *63*(6), 626–633.

Deave, T., Johnson, D., & Ingram, J. (2008). Transition to parenthood: The needs of parents in pregnancy and early parenthood. *BMC Pregnancy and Childbirth*, *8*, 30. Retrieved from <http://bmcpregnancychildbirth.biomedcentral.com/articles/10.1186/1471-2393-8-30>.

de Montigny, F., Lacharité, C., & Devault, A. (2012). Transition to fatherhood: Modeling the experience of fathers of breastfed infants. *Advances in Nursing Science*, *35*(3), E11–E22.

Flacking, R., Lehtonen, L., Thomson, G., et al. (2012). Closeness and separation in neonatal intensive care. *Acta Paediatrica*, *101*(10), 1032–1037.

Galanti, G. (2015). *Caring for patients from different cultures* (5th ed.). Philadelphia: University of Pennsylvania Press.

Goldberg, A. E., & Smith, J. Z. (2011). Stigma, social context, and mental health: Lesbian and gay couples across the transition to adoptive parenthood. *Journal of Counseling Psychology*, *58*(1), 139–150.

Goldberg, L., Ryan, A., & Sawchyn, J. (2009). Feminist and queer phenomenology: A framework for perinatal nursing practice, research, and education for advancing lesbian health. *Health Care for Women International*, *30*(6), 536–549.

Hoffenkamp, H. N., Tooten, A., Hall, R. A., et al. (2012). The impact of premature childbirth on parental bonding. *Evolutionary Psychology*, *10*(3), 542–561.

Hung, K. J., & Berg, O. (2011). Early skin-to-skin after Cesarean to improve breastfeeding. *MCN American Journal of Maternal Child Nursing*, *36*(5), 318–324, quiz 325–326.

Jaafar, S. H., Lee, K. S., & Ho, J. J. (2012). Separate care for new mother and infant versus rooming-in for increasing the duration of breastfeeding. *Cochrane Database Systematic Review*, (9), CD00641.

Klaus, M., & Kennell, J. (1976). *Maternal–infant bonding*. St. Louis: Mosby.

Klaus, M., & Kennell, J. (1982). *Parent–infant bonding* (2nd ed.). St. Louis: Mosby.

Kochanek, K. D., Kirmeyer, S. E., Martin, J. A., et al. (2012). Annual summary of vital statistics: 2009. *Pediatrics*, *129*(2), 338–348.

Menéndez, S., Hidalgo, M. V., Jiménez, L., et al. (2011). Father involvement and marital relationship during transition to parenthood: Differences between dual and single-earner families. *Spanish Journal of Psychology*, *14*(2), 639–647.

Mercer, R. T. (2004). Becoming a mother versus maternal role attainment. *Journal of Nursing Scholarship*, *36*(3), 226–232.

Mercer, R. T., & Walker, L. O. (2006). A review of nursing interventions to foster becoming a mother. *Journal of Obstetric, Gynecologic, and Neonatal Nursing*, *35*(5), 568–582.

Molborn, S., & Jacobs, J. (2011). "We'll figure a way": Teenage mothers' experiences in shifting social and economic contexts. *Qualitative Sociology*, *35*(1), 23–46.

Moore, E., Anderson, G., Bergman, N., et al. (2012). Early skin-to-skin contact for mothers and their healthy newborn infants. *Cochrane Database Systematic Review*, (5), CD003519, pub3. doi: 10.1002/14651858..

Perrine, C. G., Scanlon, K. S., Li, R., et al. (2012). Baby-friendly hospital practices and meeting exclusive breastfeeding intention. *Pediatrics, 130*(1), 54–60.

Premberg, A., Hellström, A. L., & Berg, H. (2008). Experiences of the first year as father. *Scandinavian Journal of Caring Sciences, 22*(1), 56–63.

Public Health Agency of Canada. (2009). *What mothers say: The Canadian maternity experiences survey* (Cat. No. HP5-74/2-2009E-PDF). Ottawa: Author.

Riordan, J., & Wambach, K. (2010). *Breastfeeding and human lactation* (4th ed.). Sudbury, MA: Jones & Bartlett.

Röndahl, G., Bruhner, E., & Lindhe, J. (2009). Heteronormative communication with lesbian families in antenatal care, childbirth and postnatal care. *Journal of Advanced Nursing, 65*(11), 2337–2344.

Rubin, R. (1961). Basic maternal behaviour. *Nursing Outlook, 9*, 683–686.

Shapiro, A. F., Nahm, E. Y., Gottman, J. M., et al. (2011). Bringing baby home together: Examining the impact of a couple-focused intervention on the dynamics within family play. *American Journal of Orthopsychiatry, 81*(3), 337–350.

Shin, H., Park, Y. J., Ryu, H., et al. (2008). Maternal sensitivity: A concept analysis. *Journal of Advanced Nursing, 64*(3), 304–314.

Smith, P. B., Moore, K., & Peters, L. (2012). Implementing baby-friendly practices: Strategies for success. *MCN: American Journal of Maternal Child Nursing, 37*(4), 228–233, quiz 234–235.

Stapleton, L. R., Schetter, C. D., Westling, E., et al. (2012). Perceived partner support in pregnancy predicts lower maternal and infant distress. *Journal of Family Psychology, 26*(3), 453–463.

Steen, M., Downe, S., Bamford, N., et al. (2012). Not-patient and not-visitor: A metasynthesis fathers' encounters with pregnancy, birth and maternity care. *Midwifery, 28*(4), 362–371.

Tharner, A., Luijk, M. P., Raat, H., et al. (2012). Breastfeeding and its relation to maternal sensitivity and infant attachment. *Journal of Developmental and Behavioral Pediatrics, 33*(5), 396–404.

Thukral, A., Sankar, M. J., Agarwal, R., et al. (2012). Early skin-to-skin contact and breast-feeding behavior in term neonates: A randomized controlled trial. *Neonatology, 102*(2), 114–119.

Truth and Reconciliation Commission. (2012). *Truth and Reconciliation Commission of Canada: Interim report*. Winnipeg: Government of Canada. Retrieved from <http://www.myrobust.com/websites/trcinstitution/File/Interim%20report%20English%20electronic.pdf>.

Truth and Reconciliation Commission. (2015). *Truth and Reconciliation Commission of Canada: Calls to action*. Winnipeg: Government of Canada. Retrieved from <http://www.trc.ca/websites/trcinstitution/File/2015/Findings/Calls_to_Action_English2.pdf>.

Vasquez, M. J., & Berg, O. R. (2012). The baby-friendly journey in a US public hospital. *Journal of Perinatal and Neonatal Nursing, 26*(1), 37–46.

Waugh, L. J. (2011). Beliefs associated with Mexican immigrant families' practice of la cuarentena during postpartum recovery. *Journal of Obstetrics, Gynecology & Neonatal Nursing, 40*(6), 732–741.

Welch, M. G., Hofer, M. A., Brunelli, S. A., et al. (2012). Family Nurture Intervention (FNI) Trial Group: Family nurture intervention (FNI): Methods and treatment protocol of a randomized controlled trial in the NICU. *BMC Pediatrics, 12*, 14.

Yu, C. Y., Hung, C. H., Chan, T. F., et al. (2012). Prenatal predictors of father–infant attachment after childbirth. *Journal of Clinical Nursing, 21*(11–12), 1577–1583.

ADDITIONAL RESOURCES

Best Start—What to expect in the first 3 months: Information for new parents. <http://www.beststart.org/resources/hlthy_chld_dev/K82-E-hospitalhandout.pdf>.

Best Start—Resources for Aboriginal Families. <http://www.beststart.org/resources/aboriginal/TCoOC.pdf>.

Best Start—Father Resources. <http://www.beststart.org/resources/hlthy_chld_dev/BSRC_Daddy_and_Me_EN.pdf>.

La Leche League Canada—Breastfeeding support: <http://www.lllc.ca>.

LGBTQ Parenting Network: <http://lgbtqpn.ca/>.

March of Dimes—Infant States: <http://www.marchofdimes.com/nursing/modnemedia/othermedia/states.pdf>.

Parenting in Peel—Health after Pregnancy: <http://www.peelregion.ca/health/family-health/after-pregnancy/>.

Postpartum Support International: <http://postpartum.net>.

Region of Peel—Sibling Rivalry: <http://www.peelregion.ca/health/family-health/toddlers-and-preschoolers/behaviour/jealousy.htm>.

Silent Voice—Deaf parenting programs: <http://silentvoice.ca/deaf-adult-programs/deaf-parenting-program-and-services/>.

Truth and Reconciliation Commission (2015) Call to Action: <http://www.trc.ca/websites/trcinstitution/File/2015/Findings/Calls_to_Action_English2.pdf>.

Truth and Reconciliation Commission (2012) Interim Report: <http://www.myrobust.com/websites/trcinstitution/File/Interim%20report%20English%20electronic.pdf>.

Waiting for Baby: Pregnancy After Age 35—Best Start Ontario: <http://www.beststart.org/resources/rep_health/pdf/pregnancy35plus_12pg_book.pdf>.

Fathering Resources

Canadian Father Involvement Network: <http://www.candads.ca/>.

Dad Central Ontario—The New Fathers Guide: <http://dadcentral.ca/>.

Region of Peel Health Department—Just for Dads: <http://www.peelregion.ca/health/family-health/just-for-dad/>.

CHAPTER

24

Postpartum Complications

Janet Andrews

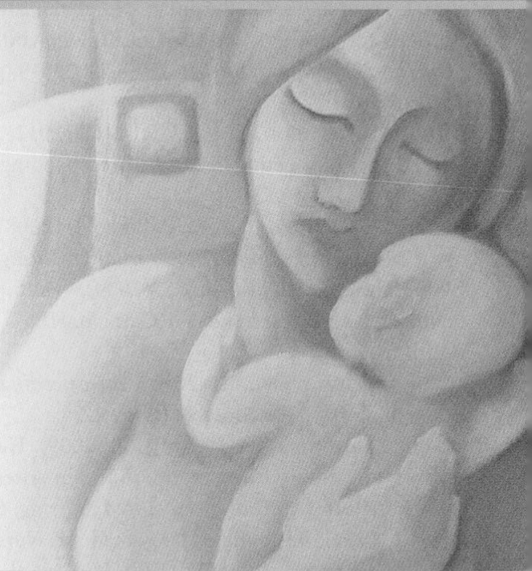

evolve WEBSITE

Visit the Evolve website for additional resources related to the content in this chapter such as Case Studies, Critical Thinking Case Study Answers, Nursing Care Plans, Nursing Processes, Nursing Skills, and Review Questions for Exam Preparation at: http://evolve.elsevier.com/Canada/Perry/maternal/

OBJECTIVES

On completion of this chapter the reader will be able to:

- Identify causes, signs and symptoms, possible complications, and medical and nursing management of postpartum hemorrhage.
- Describe hemorrhagic shock (hypovolemic shock) as a complication of postpartum hemorrhage, including collaborative management.
- Identify causes, signs and symptoms, possible complications, and medical and nursing management of postpartum infection.
- Describe thromboembolic disorders, including incidence, etiology, signs and symptoms, and management.
- Describe structural disorders of the uterus and vagina that can result from child-bearing.
- Differentiate among perinatal mood disorders, including incidence, risk factors, signs and symptoms, severity, and management.
- Describe the nurse's role in assisting families who are grieving from perinatal loss.

Providing safe and effective care to women and their families experiencing postpartum physical and psychological complications, sequelae of childbirth trauma, or grief related to perinatal loss requires a collaborative effort from all members of the health care team. Whenever possible the mother–baby dyad must be supported to remain together. Involvement of partners and families in caring for mom and baby is important in the face of postpartum complications. This chapter focuses on the postpartum complications of hemorrhage and infection, sequelae of childbirth trauma, psychological complications, and loss and grief.

POSTPARTUM HEMORRHAGE

Definition and Incidence

Postpartum hemorrhage (PPH) is among the leading causes of maternal death worldwide. It is a life-threatening event that can occur with little warning and is often unrecognized until the mother has profound symptoms. It is preventable in more than half of cases (Della Torre, Kilpatrick, Hibbard, et al., 2011). PPH occurs in 5% of births worldwide (Society of Obstetricians and Gynaecologists of Canada [SOGC], 2014). Traditionally, PPH has been defined as the loss of more than 500 mL of blood during a vaginal birth and more than 1000 mL of blood during a Caesarean birth, but definitions have changed in that any blood loss that has the potential to cause hemodynamic instability should be considered PPH (SOGC, 2014).

PPH is classified as primary or late with respect to the birth. Early, acute, or primary PPH occurs within 24 hours of the birth. Late or secondary PPH occurs more than 24 hours but less than 6 weeks after the birth and is due to retained products, infection, or both (Francois & Foley, 2012). Due to shortened hospital stays after birth, the potential for acute episodes of PPH to occur outside the traditional hospital or birth centre setting has increased.

Risk factors for and causes of PPH are listed in Box 24-1. It is common to look at the etiology of PPH within four

BOX 24-1 RISK FACTORS AND CAUSES OF POSTPARTUM HEMORRHAGE

Tone: Uterine Atony
- Overdistended uterus—Large fetus, multiple fetuses, hydramnios, distension with clots
- Anaesthesia and analgesia—Conduction anaesthesia
- Previous history of uterine atony
- High parity
- Prolonged labour, oxytocin-induced labour
- Magnesium sulphate administration during labour or postpartum period
- Chorioamnionitis
- Uterine subinvolution

Trauma
- Lacerations of the birth canal
- Trauma during labour and birth—Forceps-assisted birth, vacuum-assisted birth, Caesarean birth
- Ruptured uterus
- Inversion of the uterus
- Manual removal of a retained placenta

Tissue
- Retained placental fragments
- Placenta accreta, increta, percreta
- Placental abruption
- Placenta previa

Thrombin
- Coagulation disorders

categories: tone, tissue, trauma, and thrombin. These are referred to as the four T's of PPH.

Tone (Uterine Atony)

Uterine atony is marked hypotonia (relaxation) of the uterus. Normally, placental separation and expulsion are facilitated by contraction of the uterus, which also prevents hemorrhage from the placental site. The uterine corpus is in essence a basket weave of strong, interlacing smooth-muscle bundles through which many large maternal blood vessels pass (see Fig. 6-3). The pregnant uterus processes 500 mL of blood per minute. Therefore it is essential for the myometrium to contract particularly after the expulsion of the placenta. If the uterus is flaccid after detachment of all or part of the placenta, brisk venous bleeding occurs, and normal coagulation of the open vasculature is impaired and continues until the uterine muscle is contracted.

Uterine atony is the leading cause of early PPH. It is associated with high parity, polyhydramnios, fetal macrosomia, and multifetal gestation. In such conditions, the uterus is "overstretched" and contracts poorly after birth. Other causes of atony include traumatic birth, use of halogenated anaesthetic (e.g., halothane), magnesium sulphate, rapid or prolonged labour, chorioamnionitis, use of oxytocin for labour induction or augmentation, and uterine atony in a previous pregnancy (Francois & Foley, 2012).

Late postpartum bleeding may occur as a result of subinvolution of the uterus (delayed return of the enlarged uterus to normal size and function). Recognized causes of subinvolution include retained placental fragments (discussed below, in the section Tissue) and pelvic infection. Signs and symptoms include prolonged lochial discharge, foul odour, pain, fever, irregular or excessive bleeding, and sometimes hemorrhage. A pelvic examination usually reveals a larger-than-normal uterus that may be boggy. The woman is often at home when the symptoms occur. Discharge teaching should emphasize the signs of normal involution, potential complications, and the importance of prompt assessment by a health care provider in the event of PPH.

Trauma

Any lacerations of the genital tract, extensions or lacerations during Caesarean birth, uterine rupture, and uterine inversion are all considered trauma and can cause PPH. Lacerations of the perineum are the most common of all injuries in the lower portion of the genital tract. These are classified as first, second, third, and fourth degree (see Chapter 17, p. 451). An **episiotomy** may extend to become either a third- or fourth-degree laceration.

Hemorrhage related to lacerations should be suspected if bleeding continues despite a firm, contracted uterine fundus. This bleeding can be a slow trickle, an oozing, or frank hemorrhage.

Factors that influence the causes and incidence of obstetrical lacerations of the lower genital tract include operative birth, precipitous birth, congenital abnormalities of the maternal soft parts, and contracted pelvis. Size, abnormal presentation, and position of the fetus; relative size of the presenting part and the birth canal; and deep engagement in the pelvis prior to Caesarean birth may all lead to tissue trauma.

Hematomas

Although rarely causing hemodynamic instability, bleeding may spread into connective tissues, remaining concealed. Pelvic hematomas (i.e., a collection of blood in the connective tissue) may be vulvar, vaginal, or retroperitoneal in origin. Vulvar hematomas are the most common. Pain is the most common symptom, and most vulvar hematomas are visible. Vaginal hematomas occur more commonly in association with a forceps-assisted birth, an episiotomy, or primigravidity (Francois & Foley, 2012).

Retroperitoneal hematomas are least common but may be life threatening. They are caused by laceration of one of the vessels attached to the hypogastric artery, usually associated with rupture of a Caesarean scar during labour. During the postpartum period, if the woman reports a persistent perineal or rectal pain or a feeling of pressure in the vagina, a careful examination is made. However, a retroperitoneal hematoma may cause minimal pain, and the initial symptoms may be signs of shock (Francois & Foley, 2012).

Hematomas are usually surgically evacuated. Once the bleeding has been controlled, usual postpartum care is provided with attention to pain relief, monitoring of the amount of bleeding, replacement of fluids, and review of laboratory results (hemoglobin and hematocrit).

Inversion of the Uterus

Uterine inversion (turning inside out) after birth is a potentially life-threatening complication. It occurs in approximately 1 in 25,000 births (SOGC, 2014) and can recur with a subsequent birth. Uterine inversion may be incomplete, complete, or prolapsed. Incomplete inversion cannot be seen; a smooth mass can be palpated through the dilated cervix. In complete inversion the lining of the fundus crosses through the cervical os and forms a mass in the vagina. Prolapsed inversion of the uterus is obvious; a large, red, rounded mass (perhaps with the placenta attached) protrudes 20 to 30 cm outside the introitus.

Factors contributing to uterine inversion include fundal implantation of the placenta, vigorous fundal pressure, excessive traction applied to the cord, fetal macrosomia, short umbilical cord, tocolysis, prolonged labour, uterine atony, nulliparity, and abnormally adherent placental tissue (Francois & Foley, 2012). The primary presenting signs of uterine inversion are sudden and include hemorrhage, shock, and pain. The uterus is not palpable abdominally. The uterus must be replaced into its proper position by the obstetrical health care provider.

Prevention—always the easiest, cheapest, and most effective therapy—is especially appropriate for uterine inversion. The umbilical cord should not be pulled unless the placenta has definitely separated.

Uterine inversion is an emergency situation requiring immediate interventions that include maternal fluid resuscitation, repositioning of the uterus within the pelvic cavity, and correction of associated clinical conditions. Tocolytics or halogenated anaesthetics may be given to relax the uterus before attempting replacement (Francois & Foley, 2012). Oxytocic agents are given after the uterus is repositioned; broad-spectrum antibiotics should be initiated. The woman's response to treatment should be observed closely to prevent shock or fluid overload. If the uterus has been repositioned manually, care must be taken to avoid aggressive fundal massage.

Tissue

Delivery of the placenta occurs in the third stage of labour. Uterine involution and the prevention of PPH rely on expulsion of the entire placenta. Retained placental segments (tissue) may result from partial separation of a normal placenta, the existence of an additional succenturiate lobe, entrapment of the partially or completely separated placenta by an hourglass constriction ring of the uterus, mismanagement of the third stage of labour, or abnormal adherence of the entire placenta or a portion of the placenta to the uterine wall.

Nonadherent retained placenta is managed through manual separation and removal by the obstetrical care provider. Supplementary anaesthesia is usually not needed for women who have had regional anaesthesia for birth. For other women, administration of light nitrous oxide and occasionally general anaesthetic is required for uterine exploration and placental removal. After the removal, the woman is at continued risk for PPH and infection. Dilation and curettage (D&C) may be needed in order to remove retained placental fragments or debride the placental site.

In rare instances there is abnormal adherence of the placenta to the myometrium. Although the cause is unknown, this condition is thought to result from zygote implantation in an area of defective endometrium, resulting in no zone of separation between the placenta and the decidua. Attempts to remove the placenta in the usual manner are unsuccessful, and laceration or perforation of the uterine wall can result, putting the woman at great risk for severe PPH and infection (Francois & Foley, 2012).

Unusual placental adherence can be partial or complete. The following degrees of attachment are recognized:

- **Placenta accreta**—Slight penetration of myometrium
- **Placenta increta**—Deep penetration of myometrium
- **Placenta percreta**—Perforation of uterus

Placenta accreta can be diagnosed before birth using ultrasonography and magnetic resonance imaging (MRI), but often it is not recognized until there is excessive bleeding after birth. Bleeding with complete or total placenta accreta may not occur unless separation of the placenta is attempted. With more extensive involvement, bleeding becomes profuse when delivery of the placenta is attempted. Less blood is lost if the diagnosis is made antenatally and no attempt is made to manually remove the placenta. Treatment includes blood component replacement therapy. Hysterectomy can be indicated if bleeding is uncontrolled (Cunningham, Leveno, Bloom, et al., 2014; SOGC, 2014).

Thrombin (Coagulopathies)

The final T in the etiology of PPH stands for thrombin, or coagulopathies. When bleeding is continuous and there is no identifiable source, a coagulopathy may be the cause. The woman's coagulation status must be assessed quickly and continuously. Abnormal results depend on the cause and may include increased prothrombin time, increased partial thromboplastin time, decreased platelets, decreased fibrinogen level, increased fibrin degradation products, and prolonged bleeding time. Causes of coagulopathies may be pre-existing or pregnancy related, such as idiopathic or immune thrombocytopenic purpura (ITP), von Willebrand disease, thrombocytopenia with pre-eclampsia, or disseminated intravascular coagulation (DIC). Coagulopathies may also develop as a result of fetal demise, severe infection, or amniotic fluid embolus (SOGC, 2014).

Idiopathic Thrombocytopenic Purpura (ITP)

Idiopathic thrombocytopenic purpura (ITP) is an autoimmune disorder in which antiplatelet antibodies decrease the lifespan of the platelets. Thrombocytopenia, capillary fragility, and increased bleeding time are diagnostic findings. ITP may cause severe hemorrhage after Caesarean birth or from cervical or vaginal lacerations. The incidence of postpartum uterine bleeding and vaginal hematomas is also increased.

Medical management focuses on control of platelet stability. If ITP was diagnosed during pregnancy, the woman likely was treated with corticosteroids or IV immune globulin. Platelet transfusions are usually given when there is significant bleeding.

A splenectomy may be needed if the ITP does not respond to medical management (Cunningham et al., 2014).

von Willebrand Disease (vWD)

von Willebrand disease (vWD), a type of hemophilia, is probably the most common of all hereditary bleeding disorders. Although vWD is rare, it is among the most common congenital clotting defects in North American women of child-bearing age. It results from a deficiency or defect in a blood-clotting protein called *von Willebrand factor (vWF)*. There are as many as 20 variations of vWD, most of which are inherited as autosomal dominant traits—types I and II are the most common ones (Cunningham et al., 2014). Symptoms include recurrent bleeding episodes, such as nosebleeds or after tooth extraction, bruising easily, heavy menstrual bleeding, prolonged bleeding time (the most important test), factor VIII deficiency (mild to moderate), and bleeding from mucous membranes. Although factor VIII increases during pregnancy, a risk for PPH still exists as levels of vWF begin to decrease (Cunningham et al., 2014).

The woman may be at risk for bleeding for up to 4 weeks after birth. The treatment of choice is administration of desmopressin, which promotes the release of vWF and factor VIII. It can be given nasally, intravenously, or orally. Transfusion therapy with plasma products that have been treated for viruses and contain factor VIII and vWF also may be used. Concentrates of antihemophiliac factor (Humate) may be used (Cunningham et al., 2014).

Disseminated Intravascular Coagulation (DIC)

Disseminated intravascular coagulation (DIC), also known as *consumptive coagulopathy*, is an imbalance between the body's clotting and fibrinolytic systems. It is a pathological form of clotting that is diffuse and consumes large amounts of clotting factors, including platelets, fibrinogen, prothrombin, and factors V and VII. Widespread external bleeding, internal bleeding, or both can result. DIC also causes vascular occlusion of small vessels that results from small clots forming in the microcirculation. In the obstetrical population, DIC may occur as a result of acute antepartum hemorrhage or PPH, placental abruption, amniotic fluid embolism, dead fetus syndrome (i.e., fetus dies but is retained in utero for at least 6 weeks), severe pre-eclampsia, sepsis, saline abortion, and acute fatty liver of pregnancy (Francois & Foley, 2012).

The diagnosis of DIC is made according to clinical findings and laboratory markers. Physical examination reveals unusual bleeding; spontaneous bleeding from the woman's gums or nose may be noted. Petechiae may appear around a blood pressure cuff placed on the woman's arm. Excessive bleeding may occur from the site of a slight trauma (e.g., venipuncture sites, intramuscular or subcutaneous injection sites, nicks from shaving abdomen, and injury from insertion of a urinary catheter). Hypotension is out of proportion to the observed blood loss. Other symptoms include tachycardia and diaphoresis. Laboratory tests reveal decreased levels of platelets, fibrinogen, proaccelerin, antihemophiliac factor, and prothrombin (the factors consumed during coagulation). Fibrinolysis is increased at first but is later severely depressed. Degradation of fibrin leads to the accumulation of fibrin split products in the blood; these have anticoagulant properties and prolong the prothrombin time. Bleeding time is normal, coagulation time shows no clot, clot-retraction time shows no clot, and partial thromboplastin time is increased. DIC must be distinguished from other clotting disorders before therapy is initiated.

Primary medical management in all cases of DIC involves correction of the underlying cause (e.g., removal of the dead fetus, treatment of existing infection or of pre-eclampsia or eclampsia, or removal of a placental abruption). Volume replacement, blood component therapy, optimization of oxygenation and perfusion status, and continued reassessment of laboratory parameters are the usual forms of treatment. Resolution of DIC usually begins with the birth of the newborn (Francois & Foley, 2012; SOGC, 2014).

Nursing interventions include assessing for signs of bleeding, administering fluid or blood replacement as ordered, observing for signs of complications from the administration of blood and blood products, and protecting the woman from injury. Because renal failure is one consequence of DIC, urinary output is monitored, usually by insertion of an in-dwelling urinary catheter. Urinary output must be maintained at more than 30 mL/hr.

The woman and her family will be anxious or concerned about her condition and prognosis. The nurse should offer explanations about care and provide emotional support to them throughout this critical time.

Collaborative Care

Early recognition and treatment of PPH are critical to care management. The first step is to evaluate the contractility of the uterus. If the uterus is hypotonic, management is directed toward increasing contractility and minimizing blood loss.

If the uterus is firmly contracted and bleeding continues, the source of bleeding still must be identified and treated. Assessment may include visual or manual inspection of the perineum, vagina, uterus, cervix, or rectum and laboratory studies (e.g., hemoglobin, hematocrit, coagulation studies, platelet count). Treatment depends on the source of the bleeding.

The Society of Obstetricians and Gynaecologists of Canada (SOGC) recommends active management of the third stage of labour in order to prevent PPH, where possible (Senikas, Leduc, Lalonde, et al., 2009). This involves administering oxytocin after the delivery of the anterior shoulder, considering delayed cord clamping, gentle cord traction, and immediate fundal massage after the complete birth. If it takes longer than 30 minutes to deliver the placenta, the risk of PPH increases sixfold (More^OB, 2010).

The initial management of excessive postpartum bleeding due to uterine atony is firm massage of the uterine fundus. Expression of any clots in the uterus, elimination of bladder distension, and continuous intravenous (IV) infusion of 10 to 40 units of oxytocin in 1000 mL of Ringer's lactate or normal saline solution are also primary interventions. If the uterus fails to respond to oxytocin, other uterotonic medications are administered. Misoprostol (Cytotec), a synthetic prostaglandin E_1 analog, is often used. An advantage is that it can be given by

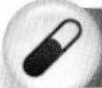

MEDICATION GUIDE

Uterotonic Drugs Used to Manage Postpartum Hemorrhage

Drug	Action	Adverse Effects	Contradictions	Dosage and Route	Nursing Considerations
Oxytocin (Syntocinon)	Contraction of uterus; decreases bleeding	Infrequent: water intoxication, nausea and vomiting	None for PPH	20–40 units/L diluted in lactated Ringer's solution or normal saline at 125 to 200 milliunits/min IV; or 10 to 20 units IM	Continue to monitor vaginal bleeding and uterine tone
Misoprostol (Cytotec)*	Contraction of uterus	Headache, nausea, vomiting, diarrhea, fever, chills	Do not use if history of allergy to prostaglandins	600 to 1000 mcg rectally once or 400 mcg sublingual or PO once	Continue to monitor vaginal bleeding and uterine tone
Methylergonovine; Ergonovine Maleate	Contraction of uterus	Hypertension, hypotension, nausea, vomiting, headache	Hypertension, pre-eclampsia, cardiac disease	0.2 mg IM every 2 to 4 hr up to five doses; may also be given intrauterine or orally	Check blood pressure before giving, and do not give if >140/90 mm Hg; continue monitoring vaginal bleeding and uterine tone
Carboprost tromethamine (Hemabate)	Contraction of uterus	Headache, nausea, vomiting, diarrhea, fever, chills, tachycardia, hypertension	Avoid with asthma or hypertension	0.25 mg IM or intrauterine every 15 to 90 min up to eight doses	Continue to monitor vaginal bleeding and uterine tone
Tranexamic acid (Cyclokapron)	For blood clotting and to stop prolonged bleeding	Nausea, vomiting, diarrhea, dizziness	History of blood clots or taking any anticoagulant	10mg/kg IV	Often given to prevent PPH in someone with a bleeding disorder

*Off-label use; research reports vary in conclusions about dosage and efficacy of use in comparison to other medications used to manage postpartum hemorrhage.
IM, intramuscular; *IV*, intravenous; *PO*, by mouth; *PPH*, postpartum hemorrhage.

more than one route. Common dosages of misoprostol are 600 to 1000 mcg rectally or 400 mcg sublingually. A 0.2-mg dose of ergonovine may be given intramuscularly to produce sustained uterine contractions; this can be repeated every 2 to 4 hours. A 0.25-mg dose of a derivative of prostaglandin $F_2\alpha$ (carboprost tromethamine [Carboprost; Hemabate]) may be given intramuscularly. It can also be given intramyometrially at Caesarean birth or intra-abdominally after vaginal birth. Carboprost can be repeated in recurrent doses of 0.25 mg every 15 to 90 minutes, up to eight doses. Women with a history of asthma should not receive this medication because it can cause bronchoconstriction (Francois & Foley, 2012) (see the Medication Guide for a comparison of uterotonic drugs used to manage PPH). In addition to the medications used to contract the uterus, rapid administration of crystalloid solutions or blood, blood products, or both will be needed to restore the woman's intravascular volume (Francois & Foley, 2012). (See Research Focus box.)

Oxygen can be given by nonrebreather face mask to enhance oxygen delivery to the cells. An in-dwelling urinary catheter is usually inserted to monitor urine output as a measure of intravascular volume and to keep the bladder empty. Laboratory studies usually include a complete blood count with platelet count, fibrinogen, fibrin split products, prothrombin time, and partial thromboplastin time. Blood type and antibody screen are done if not previously performed (Cunningham et al., 2014; SOGC, 2014).

If bleeding persists, bimanual compression may be performed by an obstetrical health care provider. This procedure involves inserting a fist into the vagina and pressing the knuckles against the anterior side of the uterus and then placing the other hand on the abdomen and massaging the posterior uterus with it. If the uterus still does not become firm, the physician or midwife performs manual exploration of the uterine cavity for retained placental fragments. If the preceding procedures are ineffective, surgical management is needed. Surgical management options include uterine tamponade (uterine packing or an intrauterine tamponade balloon), bilateral uterine artery ligation, ligation of utero-ovarian arteries and infundibulopelvic vessels, and selective arterial embolization. Uterine compression suturing (using, for example, B-Lynch or Hayman vertical sutures) may be performed and is sometimes combined with a tamponade balloon. If other treatment measures are ineffective, hysterectomy will likely be needed (Cunningham et al., 2014; Francois & Foley, 2012).

! NURSING ALERT

Use of ergonovine or methylergonovine is contraindicated in the presence of hypertension or cardiovascular disease.

Herbal Remedies

Herbal remedies have been used, with some success, to control PPH after the initial management and control of bleeding.

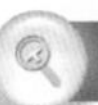

RESEARCH FOCUS

Active Third-Stage Labour Management for Preventing Postpartum Hemorrhage

—*Pat Mahaffee Gingrich*

Ask the Question

For third-stage labour, what management techniques are most effective for prevention of postpartum hemorrhage (PPH)?

Search for the Evidence

Search Strategies

English-language research-based publications on uterotonics, postpartum hemorrhage (or haemorrhage), labour bleeding, cord clamping, active management, oxytocin, prostaglandins were included.

Databases Used

Cochrane Collaborative Database, National Guideline Clearinghouse (AHRQ), CINAHL, PubMed, UpToDate

Critically Analyze the Evidence

PPH is still a major cause of maternal death, especially in low- and middle-income countries.

- In third-stage labour, uterine contractions expel the placenta and constrict the blood vessels of the uterine wall. To prevent PPH, health care providers actively manage third-stage labour by clamping the cord before pulsations have stopped, administering uterotonics to increase uterine contractions, and providing steady traction on the cord and counterpressure on the fundus, causing earlier expulsion of the placenta.
- Maternal effects: When compared with expectant management, the active-management protocol results in less maternal blood loss and less maternal anemia (Begley, Gyte, Devane, et al., 2011). Adverse effects of active management include adverse effects of the uterotonics and uterine pressure: higher maternal diastolic pressure, pain requiring analgesia, nausea and vomiting. Active management is also more likely to result in readmission for bleeding, for unknown reasons.
- Effects on the newborn: Birth weight is less when the cord was clamped before cessation of pulsing, because there is less transfer of blood volume to the newborn. However, there are no differences in the number of neonatal intensive care unit (NICU) admissions nor the occurrences of neonatal jaundice (Begley et al., 2011).
- Uterotonics stimulate smooth muscle contraction of the uterus. Intravenous carbetocin, when compared with oxytocin, results in less need for uterine massage and use of other uterotonics, but no difference in occurrence of PPH. When compared with ergometrine-oxytocin, carbetocin is associated with less blood loss and fewer adverse effects of nausea, vomiting, and postpartum hypertension (Su, Chong, & Samuel, 2012).
- Prostaglandins are also uterotonic. Oral or sublingual misoprostol is better than placebo for preventing blood loss and need for blood transfusion but causes dose-related shivering, increased temperature, and diarrhea.
- Conventional injectable uterotonics such as intramuscular (IM) ergot alkaloids are the drugs of choice for preventing PPH, but prostaglandins may be useful in low-resource areas (Tunçalp, Hofmeyr, & Gülmezoglu, 2012).

Apply the Evidence: Nursing Implications

- Active management of third-stage labour is beneficial and recommended. However, it may be possible to individualize the protocol. Women should be educated before labour on their options for third-stage management and the risks and benefits of uterotonics.
- Some women request that the cord clamping be delayed until pulsations have ceased. This may benefit the newborn without significantly increasing the woman's risk for PPH.
- Nurses need to carefully assess the fundus and bleeding while recovering the immediate postpartum woman and are frequently the first to notice PPH.
- A protocol for PPH should be made clear to all staff. All staff should be able to identify when bleeding is too heavy and know the correct steps of emptying the bladder, uterine massage, and whom to call immediately.

References

Begley, C. M., Gyte, G. M., Devane, D., et al. (2011). Active versus expectant management for women in the third stage of labour. *Cochrane Database Systematic Review*, (11). doi:10.1002/14651858.CD007412.pub3.

Su, L., Chong, Y., & Samuel, M. (2012). Carbetocin for preventing postpartum haemorrhage. *Cochrane Database Systematic Review*, (4). doi:10.1002/14651858.CD005457.pub4.

Tunçalp, Ö., Hofmeyr, G. J., & Gülmezoglu, A. M. (2012). Prostaglandins for preventing postpartum haemorrhage. *Cochrane Database Systematic Review*, (8). doi:10.1002/14651858.CD000494.pub4.

Some herbs have homeostatic actions, whereas others work as oxytocic agents to contract the uterus. However, published evidence of the safety and efficacy of herbal therapy is lacking. Evidence from well-controlled studies is needed before recommendations for their use can be made.

NURSING CARE

The nurse must be alert to the symptoms of hemorrhage and hypovolemic shock and be prepared to act quickly to minimize blood loss (Fig. 24-1). Astute assessment of circulatory status can be done with noninvasive monitoring (Box 24-2). Frequent monitoring of the woman and encouraging her to empty her bladder are important nursing interventions for treatment and prevention of PPH. Interventions are based on the cause of PPH, as previously discussed. Nurses must be able to quantify blood loss accurately. The American Association of Women, Obstetrical and Neonatal Nurses (AWHONN) (2015) states that visual estimation of blood loss can be inaccurate, with underestimates of 33 to 55%, which can delay life-saving treatment. Weighing is a much more accurate method of determining blood loss and is recommended by AWHONN. See Additional Resources at the end of the chapter for a video on how to quantify blood loss.

The woman and her family will be anxious about her condition. The nurse can intervene by calmly providing explanations about interventions being performed and the need to act quickly.

Once the woman's condition is stabilized, preparations for discharge can be made. Discharge instructions for a woman who has experienced PPH are similar to those for any postpartum woman. In addition, the woman should be told that she will probably feel fatigue, even exhaustion, and will need to limit her physical activities to conserve her strength. She may need instructions in increasing her dietary iron and protein intake as well as using iron supplementation to rebuild lost red

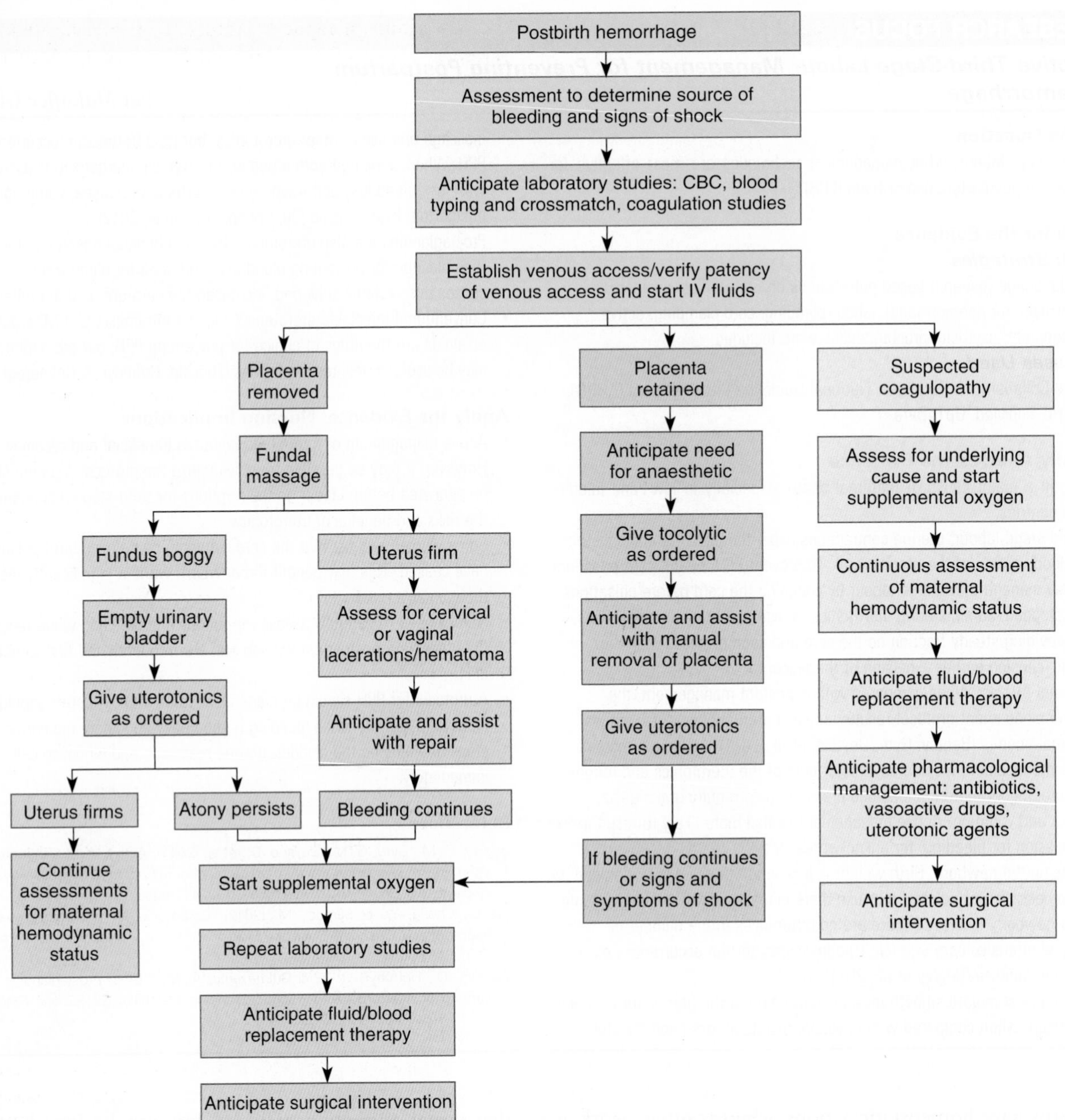

FIGURE 24-1 Nursing assessments for postpartum bleeding. *CBC,* complete blood count; *IV,* intravenous; *tocolytics,* medications to relax the uterus; *uterotonics,* medications to contract the uterus.

BOX 24-2 NONINVASIVE ASSESSMENTS OF CIRCULATORY STATUS IN POSTPARTUM WOMEN WHO ARE BLEEDING

Palpation of Pulses (Rate, Quality, Equality)
- Arterial

Inspection
- Skin colour, temperature, turgor
- Level of consciousness
- Capillary refill
- Neck veins
- Mucous membranes

Auscultation
- Heart sounds/murmurs
- Breath sounds

Observation
- Presence or absence of anxiety, apprehension, restlessness, disorientation

Measurement
- Blood pressure
- Pulse oximetry
- Urinary output

EMERGENCY

Hemorrhagic Shock

Assessment	Characteristics
Respirations	Rapid and shallow
Pulse	Rapid, weak, irregular
Blood pressure	Decreasing (late sign)
Skin	Cool, pale, clammy
Urinary output	Decreasing
Level of consciousness	Lethargy → coma
Mental status	Anxiety → coma
Central venous pressure	Decreased

Interventions

Summon assistance and equipment.
Start intravenous infusion per standing orders.
Ensure patent airway; administer oxygen.
Continue to monitor status.

blood cell (RBC) volume. She may need assistance with infant care and household activities until she has regained strength. Some women have problems with delayed lactation or insufficient milk production and develop a perinatal mood disorder (PMD). Referrals for home care follow-up or to community resources may be needed (see Nursing Care Plan: Postpartum Hemorrhage, available on Evolve).

Hemorrhagic (Hypovolemic) Shock

Hemorrhage may result in **hemorrhagic (hypovolemic) shock**. Shock is an emergency situation in which the perfusion of body organs may become severely compromised; death may occur. Physiological compensatory mechanisms are activated in response to hemorrhage. The adrenal glands release catecholamines, causing arterioles and venules in the skin, lungs, gastrointestinal tract, liver, and kidneys to constrict. The available blood flow is diverted to the brain and heart and away from other organs, including the uterus. If shock is prolonged, the continued reduction in cellular oxygenation results in an accumulation of lactic acid and acidosis (from anaerobic glucose metabolism). Acidosis (lowered serum pH) causes arteriolar vasodilation; venule vasoconstriction persists. A circular pattern is established (i.e., decreased perfusion, increased tissue anoxia and acidosis, edema formation, and pooling of blood further decrease the perfusion). Cellular death occurs. See the Emergency box for assessment of and interventions for hemorrhagic shock.

Collaborative Care

Vigorous treatment is necessary to prevent adverse outcomes. Management of hypovolemic shock involves restoring circulating blood volume and eliminating the cause of the hemorrhage (e.g., lacerations, uterine atony, or inversion). Critical to successful management of the woman with a hemorrhagic complication is establishment of venous access, preferably with a large-bore IV catheter. The use of two IV lines facilitates fluid resuscitation. Fluid resuscitation includes the administration of crystalloids (lactated Ringer's, normal saline solution), colloids (albumin), blood, and blood components. To restore circulating blood volume, a rapid IV infusion of crystalloid solution is given at a rate of 3 mL infused for every 1 mL of estimated blood loss (e.g., 3000 mL infused for 1000 mL of blood loss). Packed RBCs are usually infused if the woman is still actively bleeding and no improvement in her condition is noted after the initial crystalloid infusion. Infusion of fresh frozen plasma may be needed if clotting factors and platelet counts are below normal values (Cunningham et al., 2014; Francois & Foley, 2012; SOGC, 2014).

Hemorrhagic shock can occur rapidly, but the classic signs of shock may not appear until the postpartum woman has lost 30 to 40% of her blood volume. The nurse must continue to reassess the woman's condition as evidenced by the degree of measurable and anticipated blood loss and mobilize appropriate resources.

Most interventions are instituted to improve or monitor tissue perfusion. Fluid resuscitation must be monitored carefully because fluid overload can occur. Intravascular fluid overload occurs most often with colloid therapy.

Transfusion reactions can follow administration of blood or blood components, including cryoprecipitates. Even in an emergency, each unit of blood or blood products should be carefully checked per hospital protocol. Complications of fluid or blood replacement therapy include hemolytic reactions, febrile reactions, allergic reactions, circulatory overloading, and air embolism.

LEGAL TIP *STANDARD OF CARE FOR BLEEDING EMERGENCIES*

The standard of care for obstetrical emergency situations such as PPH or hypovolemic shock is that provision should be made for the nurse to implement nursing actions independently. Policies, procedures, standing orders or protocols, and clinical guidelines should be established by each health care facility in which births occur and should be agreed on by health care providers involved in the care of obstetrical patients.

The nurse continues to monitor the woman's pulse and blood pressure. If invasive hemodynamic monitoring is ordered, the nurse may assist with placement of a central venous pressure (CVP) or pulmonary artery (Swan-Ganz) catheter. The nurse then monitors CVP, pulmonary artery pressure, or pulmonary artery wedge pressure as ordered.

Additional assessments to be made include evaluation of skin temperature, colour, and turgor and assessment of the woman's mucous membranes. Breath sounds should be auscultated before fluid volume replacement to provide a baseline for future assessment. Inspection for oozing at the sites of incisions or injections and assessment of the presence of petechiae or ecchymosis in areas not associated with surgery or trauma are critical in the evaluation for DIC.

Oxygen is administered, preferably by a nonrebreathing face mask, at 10 to 12 L/min to maintain oxygen saturation. Oxygen saturation should be monitored with a **pulse oximeter**, although measurements may not always be accurate in a patient with hypovolemia or decreased perfusion. Level of consciousness is assessed frequently and provides additional indications of blood volume and oxygen saturation (Gilbert, 2011). In early stages of decreased blood flow, the woman may report "seeing stars" or feeling dizzy or nauseated. She may become restless and orthopneic. As cerebral hypoxia increases, she may become confused and react slowly to stimuli or not at all. Some women state they have headaches. An improved sensorium is an indicator of improved perfusion.

Continuous electrocardiographic monitoring may be indicated for the woman who is hypotensive or tachycardic, continues to bleed profusely, or is in shock. A Foley catheter with a urometer is inserted to allow hourly assessment of urine output. The most objective and least invasive assessment of adequate organ perfusion and oxygenation is a urine output of at least 30 mL/hr (Cunningham et al., 2014). Hemoglobin and hematocrit levels, platelet count, and coagulation studies need to be closely monitored.

VENOUS THROMBOEMBOLIC DISORDERS

Venous thromboembolism (VTE) results from the formation of a blood clot or clots inside a blood vessel and is caused by inflammation (thrombophlebitis) or partial obstruction of the vessel. Three thromboembolic conditions are of concern in the postpartum period:

- **Superficial venous thrombosis**—Involvement of the superficial saphenous venous system
- **Deep venous thrombosis (DVT)**—Involvement varies but can extend from the foot to the iliofemoral region
- **Pulmonary embolism (PE)**—Complication of deep venous thrombosis occurring when part of a blood clot dislodges and is carried to the pulmonary artery, where it occludes the vessel and obstructs blood flow to the lungs

Incidence and Etiology

Pregnant women have a four to five times increased risk of thromboembolism, and it is one of the leading causes of death in the postpartum period. The incidence of VTE, which includes DVT and PE, is 4.3 per 10,000 pregnancies postpartum (Chan, Rey, Kent, et al., 2014). VTE can occur in any trimester of pregnancy or during the postpartum period. DVT occurs most often during pregnancy, although it can occur up to 3 weeks postpartum, and PE is more common in the postpartum period. The incidence of VTE in the postpartum period has declined in the last 30 years because early ambulation after childbirth, a preventive measure, has become standard practice. However, PE is a major cause of maternal death (Chan et al., 2014; Pettker & Lockwood, 2012). The major causes of thromboembolic disease are venous stasis and hypercoagulation, both of which are present in pregnancy and continue into the postpartum period. Caesarean birth nearly doubles the risk for VTE; other risk factors include operative vaginal birth; history of venous thrombosis, PE, or varicosities; obesity; maternal age over 35; multiparity; and smoking (Pettker & Lockwood, 2012).

The SOGC recommends that each woman be evaluated for risk, and consideration for thromboprophylaxis should be individualized (Chan et al., 2014). Women who are at risk for VTE should have TED stockings applied soon after birth. If compression stockings do not fit, then a sequential compression device (SCD) should be used (Royal College of Obstetricians and Gynaecologists, 2009).

Clinical Manifestations

Superficial venous thrombosis is the most common form of postpartum thrombophlebitis. It is characterized by pain and tenderness in the lower extremity. Physical examination may reveal warmth; redness; and an enlarged, hardened vein over the site of the thrombosis. DVT is more common in pregnancy and is characterized by unilateral leg pain, calf tenderness, and swelling. Physical examination may reveal redness and warmth, but women may also have a large clot with few symptoms.

Acute PE usually results from dislodged deep vein thrombi. Presenting symptoms are dyspnea and tachypnea (more than 20 breaths/min). Other signs and symptoms frequently seen include tachycardia (more than 100 beats/min), apprehension, pleuritic chest pain, cough, hemoptysis, elevated temperature, and syncope (Cunningham et al., 2014; Pettker & Lockwood, 2012).

Physical examination is not a sensitive diagnostic indicator for thrombosis. Venous ultrasonography with or without colour Doppler is the most commonly used diagnostic test. MRI and D-dimer assays may also be used (Chan et al., 2014). With PE, echocardiographic abnormalities may be seen in right ventricular size or function. Pregnancy limits the usefulness of arterial blood gases and oxygen saturation in diagnosis. A ventilation-perfusion scan, spiral computed tomography scan, magnetic resonance angiography, and pulmonary arteriogram may be used for diagnosis (Chan et al., 2014; Pettker & Lockwood, 2012).

Collaborative Care

Anticoagulant therapy is the treatment of choice for superficial VTE, DVT, and PE. Superficial venous thrombosis is also treated with analgesia (nonsteroidal anti-inflammatory medications), rest with elevation of the affected leg, and elastic compression stockings (Cunningham et al., 2014). DVT is initially treated with anticoagulant therapy (usually continuous IV heparin), bedrest with the affected leg elevated, and analgesia. After the symptoms have decreased, the woman may be fitted with elastic compression stockings to use when she is allowed to ambulate. Anticoagulant therapy involves a combination of IV, oral, and subcutaneous injections and may require prolonged therapy.

Acute pulmonary embolus is an emergent situation that requires prompt treatment. Massive pulmonary emboli can lead to pulmonary hypertension and right ventricular dysfunction; mortality is increased to 25% in these cases (Cunningham et al., 2014). Immediate treatment of PE is anticoagulant therapy. Continuous IV heparin therapy is used for PE until symptoms have resolved. Intermittent subcutaneous heparin or oral anticoagulant therapy is often continued for up to 6 months (Pettker & Lockwood, 2012).

In the hospital, nursing care of the woman with a thrombosis consists of continued assessments: inspection and palpation of the affected area; palpation of peripheral pulses; measurement and comparison of leg circumferences; inspection for signs of bleeding; monitoring for signs of PE, including chest pain, coughing, dyspnea, and tachypnea; and checking respiratory status for presence of crackles. Laboratory reports are monitored for prothrombin or partial thromboplastin times. The woman and her family are assessed for their level of understanding about the diagnosis and their ability to cope during the unexpected extended period of recovery.

Interventions include explanations and education about the diagnosis and treatment. The woman will need assistance with personal care as long as she is on bedrest. The family should be encouraged to participate in her care if she and they wish. While the woman is on bedrest, she should be encouraged to change positions frequently but not to place the knees in a sharply flexed position that could cause pooling of blood in the lower extremities. She should also be cautioned not to rub the affected areas, because rubbing could cause the clot to dislodge. Once the woman is allowed to ambulate, she should be taught how to prevent venous congestion by putting on the elastic stockings before getting out of bed.

Medications used vary by hospital and physician. All anticoagulant therapies require monitoring of clotting times. The physician should be notified if clotting times are outside the therapeutic level. If the woman is breastfeeding, she should consult with the lactation consultant.

Pain can be managed with a variety of measures. Changing of positions, elevation of the leg, and application of moist heat may decrease discomfort. It may be necessary to administer analgesics and anti-inflammatory medications.

! NURSING ALERT

Medications containing aspirin are not given to women on anticoagulant therapy because aspirin inhibits synthesis of clotting factors and can lead to prolonged clotting time and increased risk of bleeding.

The woman and her family must be taught how to administer subcutaneous injections and about site rotation. They should also be given information about safe care practices to prevent bleeding and injury while she is on anticoagulant therapy, such as using a soft toothbrush and an electric razor. She will need information about follow-up with her health care provider for monitoring of clotting times and ensuring that the correct dosage of anticoagulant therapy is maintained.

POSTPARTUM INFECTIONS

Postpartum infection or puerperal infection is any clinical infection of the genital canal that occurs within 28 days after miscarriage, induced abortion, or birth. The definition of postpartum infection is the presence of a fever of 38° C (100.4° F) or more on 2 successive days of the first 10 postpartum days (not counting the first 24 hours after birth) (Katz, 2012). In North America it occurs after approximately 2% of vaginal births and 10 to 15% of Caesarean births (Katz, 2012). Common postpartum infections include endometritis, wound infections, mastitis, urinary tract infections (UTIs), and respiratory tract infections.

The most common infecting organisms are the numerous streptococcal and anaerobic organisms. *Staphylococcus aureus*, gonococci, coliform bacteria, and Clostridia are less common but serious pathogenic organisms that can cause puerperal infection. Postpartum infections are more common in women who are obese, have concurrent medical or immunosuppressive conditions, or who had a Caesarean or other operative birth. Intrapartal factors such as prolonged rupture of membranes, prolonged labour, and internal maternal or fetal monitoring also increase the risk of infection (Cunningham et al., 2014). Factors that predispose the woman to postpartum infection are listed in Box 24-3.

BOX 24-3 PREDISPOSING FACTORS FOR POSTPARTUM INFECTION

Preconception or Antepartal Factors

- History of previous venous thrombosis, urinary tract infection, mastitis, pneumonia
- Diabetes mellitus
- Alcoholism
- Substance use
- Immunosuppression
- Anemia
- Malnutrition
- Obesity

Intrapartal Factors

- Caesarean birth
- Prolonged rupture of membranes
- Chorioamnionitis
- Prolonged labour
- Bladder catheterization
- Internal fetal or uterine pressure monitoring
- Multiple vaginal examinations after rupture of membranes
- Epidural anaesthesia
- Retained placental fragments
- Postpartum hemorrhage
- Episiotomy or lacerations
- Hematomas

Endometritis

Endometritis (infection of the lining of the uterus) is the most common postpartum infection. It usually begins as a localized infection at the placental site but can spread to the entire endometrium. Incidence is higher after Caesarean birth. Signs of endometritis include fever (usually greater than 38°C); increased pulse; chills; anorexia; nausea; fatigue and lethargy; pelvic pain; uterine tenderness; and foul-smelling, profuse lochia. Leukocytosis and a markedly increased RBC sedimentation rate are typical laboratory findings of postpartum infections. Anemia may also be present. Blood cultures or intracervical or intrauterine bacterial cultures (aerobic and anaerobic) should reveal the offending pathogens within 36 to 48 hours (Cunningham et al., 2014).

Wound Infections

Wound infections are common postpartum infections that often develop after the woman is at home. Sites of infection include the Caesarean incision and repaired laceration or episiotomy site. Predisposing factors are similar to those for endometritis (see Box 24-3). Signs of wound infection include erythema, edema, warmth, tenderness, seropurulent drainage, and wound separation. Fever and pain may also be present. In order to decrease the risk of wound infections in women who have a Caesarean birth, the SOGC recommends that all women undergoing elective or emergency Caesarean section receive antibiotic prophylaxis. The timing of the antibiotic should be 15 to 30 minutes before the skin incision (van Schalkwyk, Van Eyk, Yudin, et al., 2010). Prophylactic antibiotics may also be considered for women who have third- and fourth-degree perineal injury, and the dose may be doubled for women who are morbidly obese (body mass index [BMI] >35) (van Schalkwyk et al., 2010).

Treatment of wound infections may involve combined antibiotic therapy with wound debridement. Wounds can be opened and drained. Nursing care includes frequent assessments of the wound and vital signs and wound care. Comfort measures are sitz baths, warm compresses, and perineal care. The woman should be taught good hygiene techniques (e.g., changing perineal pads front to back, hand hygiene before and after perineal care), self-care measures, and the signs of worsening conditions to watch for and report to the primary health care provider. The woman is usually discharged home for self-care or home nursing care after treatment is initiated in the inpatient setting.

Urinary Tract Infections

UTIs occur in 2 to 4% of postpartum women. Risk factors include urinary catheterization, frequent pelvic examinations, epidural anaesthesia, genital tract injury, history of UTI, and Caesarean birth. Signs and symptoms include dysuria, frequency and urgency, low-grade fever, urinary retention, hematuria, and pyuria. Costovertebral angle tenderness or flank pain may indicate an upper UTI. The most common infecting organism is *Escherichia coli*, although other Gram-negative aerobic bacilli also may cause UTIs.

Medical management for UTIs consists of antibiotic therapy, analgesia, and hydration. Postpartum women are usually treated on an outpatient basis; therefore teaching should include instructions on how to monitor temperature, bladder function, and appearance of urine. The woman should also be taught about signs of potential complications and the importance of taking all antibiotics as prescribed. Other suggestions for prevention of UTIs include proper perineal care, wiping from front to back after urinating or having a bowel movement, and increasing fluid intake.

Mastitis

Mastitis, or breast infection, affects 2 to 10% of women soon after childbirth. Mastitis is almost always unilateral and develops well after the flow of milk has been established (Fig. 24-2). The infecting organism generally is the hemolytic *S. aureus*. An infected nipple fissure usually is the initial lesion, followed by ductal system involvement. Inflammatory edema and engorgement of the breast obstruct the flow of milk in a lobe; regional, then generalized, mastitis follows. If treatment is not prompt, mastitis may progress to a breast abscess.

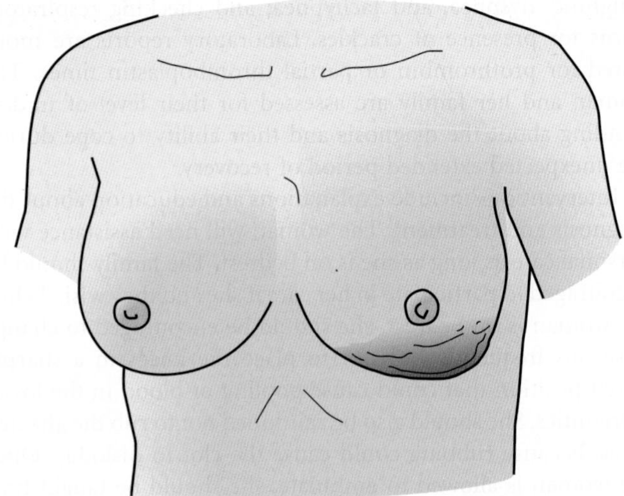

FIGURE 24-2 Mastitis.

Symptoms rarely appear before the end of the first postpartum week and are more common in the second to fourth weeks. Chills, fever, malaise, and local breast tenderness are noted first. Localized breast tenderness, pain, swelling, redness, and axillary adenopathy may also occur. Antibiotics are prescribed for treatment. Lactation can be maintained by emptying the breasts every 2 to 4 hours by breastfeeding, manual expression, or a breast pump.

Because mastitis rarely occurs before the postpartum woman is discharged, she should be taught in hospital about its warning signs and receive counselling about prevention of cracked nipples. Management includes intensive antibiotic therapy (e.g., cephalosporins and vancomycin, which are particularly useful in staphylococcal infections), support of breasts, local heat or cold, adequate hydration, and analgesics.

Almost all instances of acute mastitis can be avoided by using proper breastfeeding technique to prevent cracked nipples. Missed feedings, waiting too long between feedings, and abrupt weaning may lead to clogged nipples and mastitis. Cleanliness practised by all who have contact with the newborn and new mother also reduces the incidence of mastitis. See also Chapter 27.

NURSING CARE

Women with factors predisposing to postpartum infection (see Box 24-3) should be assessed carefully. Nurses need to assess for relevant signs and symptoms, discussed here earlier, that can accompany each infection. Elevation of temperature, redness, and swelling are common signs. The woman may also state she has chills, fever, localized tenderness, or pain. Depending on the type of infection, laboratory tests usually performed include a complete blood count, venous blood cultures, urine cultures, and uterine tissue cultures. Review of the woman's history and the laboratory results should be included in the assessment.

The most effective and least expensive treatment of postpartum infection is prevention. Preventive measures include

COMMUNITY FOCUS

Prevention of Postpartum Infection

After giving birth, many women are discharged home before an infection can develop. Prepare a "Fact Sheet About Postpartum Infection" that could be distributed to postpartum women on discharge from the hospitals or birth centres in your community. Include signs and symptoms, and phone numbers and addresses of health care providers who could be contacted. Many Canadian communities have large populations who do not speak English, and this must be considered when teaching and producing handout information.

good prenatal nutrition to control anemia and intrapartal hemorrhage. Good maternal perineal hygiene with thorough hand hygiene should be emphasized. Use of aseptic techniques by all health care personnel during childbirth and the postpartum period is very important.

Postpartum women are usually discharged home before 48 hours after birth, which is often before signs of infection are evident. Nurses in birth centres and hospital settings need to be able to identify women at risk for postpartum infection and provide anticipatory teaching and counselling before the woman's discharge (see Community Focus box). After discharge, telephone follow-up, hot lines, support groups, lactation consultants, home visits by a community health nurse, and teaching materials (movies, written materials, apps) are all interventions that can be implemented to decrease the risk of postpartum infections. Nurses working in the community must be able to recognize signs and symptoms of postpartum infection and convey these to the woman so that she knows when to contact her primary health care provider. Community nurses must also be able to provide the appropriate nursing care for women who need follow-up home care.

STRUCTURAL DISORDERS OF THE VAGINA AND UTERUS RELATED TO CHILD-BEARING

Women are at risk for problems related to the reproductive system from the age of menarche through menopause and the older years. These problems, which include structural disorders of the uterus and vagina related to pelvic relaxation and urinary incontinence (UI), are often the delayed but direct result of child-bearing.

With fetopelvic disproportion, prolonged labour, or a precipitous birth, structures of the vesical and vaginal walls are stretched and may be injured. The bladder neck and urethra may be compressed between the presenting part and the pubic bones or forced downward ahead of the presenting part. Since soft tissue damage usually occurs behind an intact vaginal epithelium, there is nothing visible to repair. However, defects may also occur in women who have never been pregnant.

Structural disorders can have far-reaching effects for the woman and her family. Beyond the obvious physiological alterations, the woman can also experience threats to her self-image and her ability to cope. A woman's concept of herself as a sexual being may also be affected. Her partner and family may need support as well.

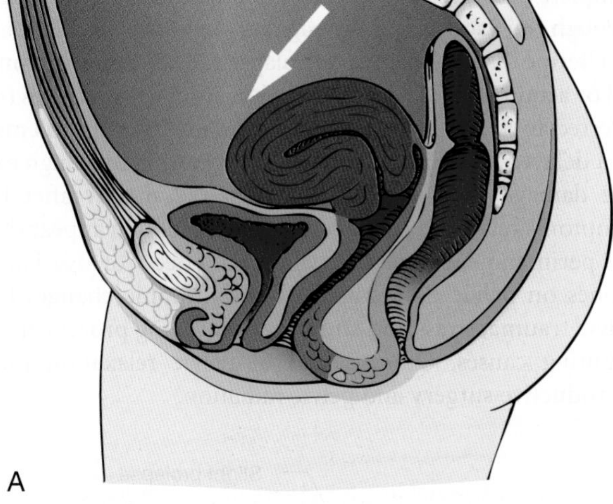

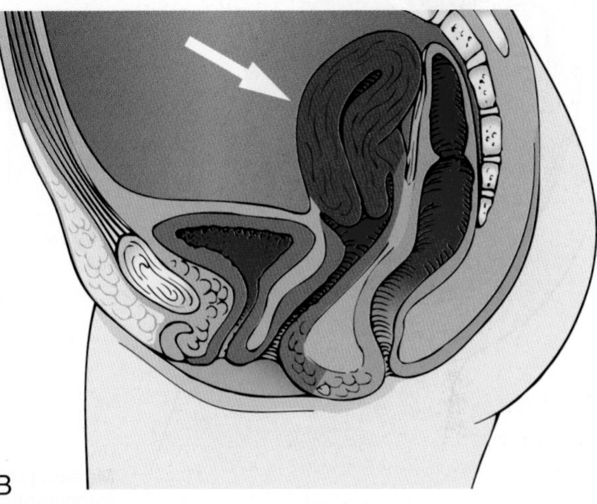

FIGURE 24-3 Types of uterine displacement. **A:** Anterior displacement. **B:** Retroversion (backward displacement).

Uterine Displacement and Prolapse

Normally, the round ligaments hold the uterus in anteversion, and the uterosacral ligaments pull the cervix backward and upward. **Uterine displacement** is a variation of this normal placement (Fig. 24-3). The most common type of displacement is posterior displacement, or retroversion, in which the uterus is tilted posteriorly and the cervix rotates anteriorly. Other variations include retroflexion and anteflexion.

By 2 months postpartum, the ligaments should return to normal length, but in about one third of women the uterus remains retroverted. This condition is rarely symptomatic, but conception may be difficult because the cervix points toward the anterior vaginal wall and away from the posterior fornix, where seminal fluid pools after coitus. If symptoms occur, they may include pelvic and low back pain, dyspareunia, and exaggeration of premenstrual symptoms.

Uterine prolapse is a more serious type of displacement. Degrees of prolapse can vary from mild to complete. In complete prolapse, the cervix and body of the uterus protrude through the vagina, and the vagina is inverted (Fig. 24-4).

Uterine displacement and prolapse can be caused by congenital or acquired weakness of the pelvic support structures (often referred to as **pelvic relaxation**). In many cases, problems can be a delayed but direct result of child-bearing. Although extensive damage may be noted and repaired shortly after birth, symptoms related to pelvic relaxation most often appear during the perimenopausal period, when the effects of ovarian hormones on pelvic tissues are lost and atrophic changes begin. Pelvic trauma, stress and strain, and the aging process are contributing causes. Other causes of pelvic relaxation include reproductive surgery and pelvic radiation.

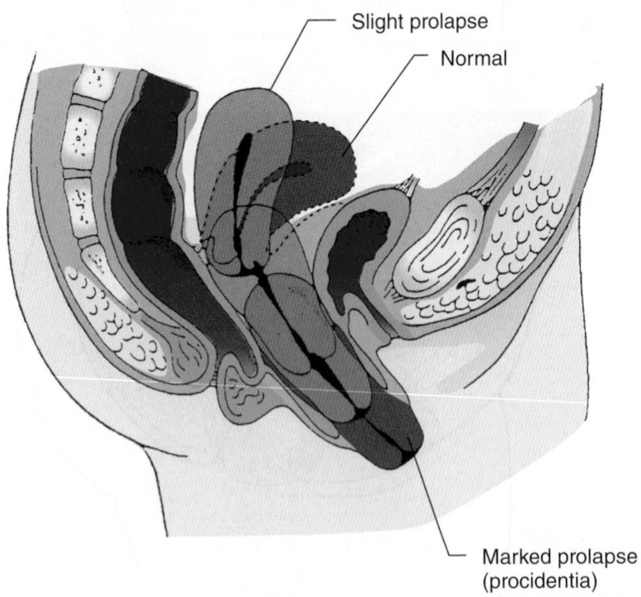

FIGURE 24-4 Prolapse of uterus.

In general, symptoms of pelvic relaxation relate to the structure involved: urethra, bladder, uterus, vagina, cul-de-sac, or rectum. The most common discomforts are pulling and dragging sensations, pressure, protrusions, fatigue, and low backache. Symptoms may be worse after prolonged standing or deep penile penetration during intercourse. Urinary incontinence may also occur.

Collaborative Care

If discomfort related to uterine displacement is a problem, several interventions can be implemented to treat uterine displacement. Kegel exercises can be performed several times a day to increase muscular strength. A knee–chest position performed for a few minutes several times a day can correct a mildly retroverted uterus. A pessary is another noninvasive option which immediately eliminates symptoms. It is a silicone device placed into the vagina to support the prolapsing vagina wall or to provide urinary continence (Fig. 24-5). Usually a pessary is used for only a short time because it can lead to pressure necrosis and vaginitis. Good hygiene is important; some women are taught to remove the pessary at night, cleanse it, and replace it in the morning. If the pessary is always left in place, regular douching with commercially prepared solutions or weak vinegar solutions (e.g., 15 mL to 1 litre) to remove increased secretions and keep the vaginal pH at 4.0 to 4.5 is suggested. After a period of treatment, most women are free of symptoms and do not require the pessary. Surgical correction is rarely indicated.

Treatment for uterine prolapse depends on the degree of prolapse. Pessaries can be useful for mild prolapse. Estrogen therapy may be used in the older woman to improve tissue tone. If these conservative treatments do not correct the problem or the degree of prolapse is significant, abdominal or vaginal hysterectomy is usually recommended.

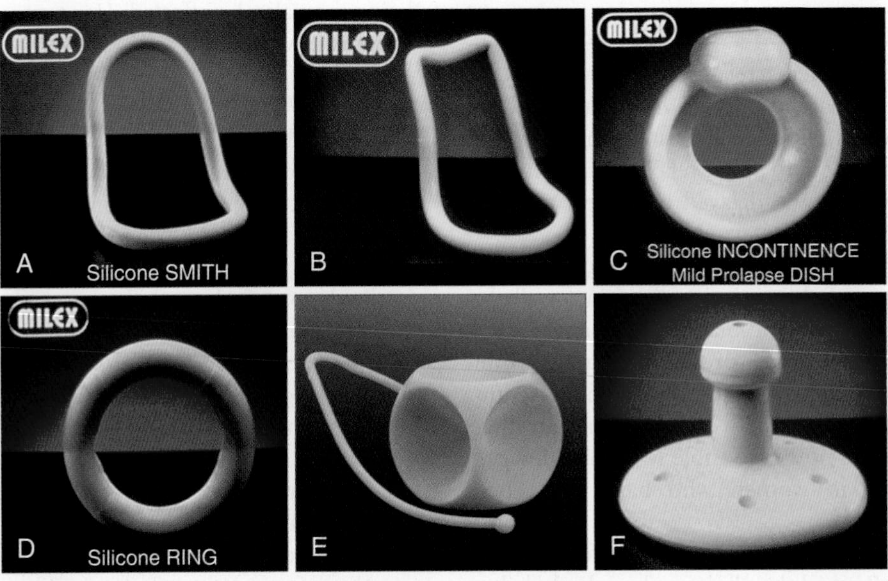

FIGURE 24-5 Examples of pessaries. **A:** Smith. **B:** Hodge without support. **C:** Incontinence dish with support. **D:** Ring without support. **E:** Cube. **F:** Gellhorn. (Courtesy Milex Products, Inc., a division of CooperSurgical, Trumbull, CT.)

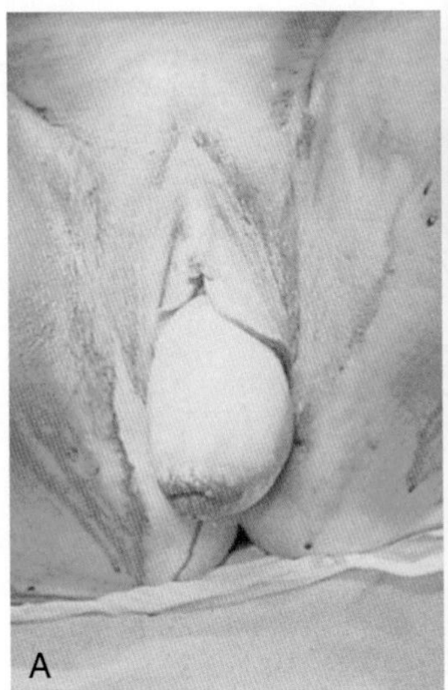

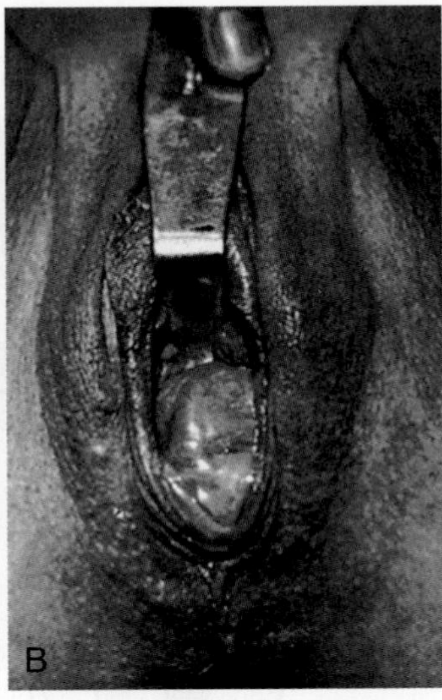

FIGURE 24-6 Views of **A:** cystocele; **B:** rectocele. (From Jarvis, C. [2008]. *Physical assessment and health assessment* [1st Canadian ed.]. Toronto: Saunders Canada.)

Cystocele and Rectocele

Cystocele and rectocele often occur with uterine prolapse (although they can occur independently), causing the uterus to sag even further backward and downward into the vagina. Cystocele (Fig. 24-6, A) is the protrusion of the bladder downward into the vagina that develops when supporting structures in the vesicovaginal septum are injured. Anterior wall relaxation develops gradually over time as a result of congenital defects of support structures, child-bearing, obesity, or advanced age. When the woman stands, the weakened anterior vaginal wall cannot support the weight of the urine in the bladder; the vesicovaginal septum is forced downward, the bladder is stretched, and its capacity is increased. With time, the cystocele enlarges until it protrudes into the vagina. Complete emptying of the bladder is difficult because the cystocele sags below the bladder neck. Rectocele is the herniation of the anterior rectal wall through the relaxed or ruptured vaginal fascia and rectovaginal septum; it appears as a large bulge that may be seen through the relaxed introitus (see Fig. 24-6, B).

Cystoceles and rectoceles often are asymptomatic. When symptoms of cystocele are present, they may include a bearing-down sensation or the feeling that "something is in my vagina." Other symptoms are urinary frequency, retention, incontinence, and possible recurrent cystitis and UTIs. On pelvic examination, there is a bulging of the anterior wall of the vagina when the woman is asked to bear down. Unless the bladder neck and urethra are damaged, urinary continence is unaffected. Women with large cystoceles state they have to push upward on the sagging anterior vaginal wall in order to be able to void.

Rectoceles may be small and produce few symptoms, but some are so large that they protrude outside of the vagina when the woman stands. Symptoms are absent when the woman is lying down. A rectocele causes a disturbance in bowel function, a sensation of bearing down, or a sensation that the pelvic organs are falling out. With a very large rectocele it may be difficult to have a bowel movement. Each time the woman strains during bowel evacuation, the feces are forced against the thinned rectovaginal wall, stretching it even more. Some women facilitate evacuation by applying digital pressure vaginally to hold up the rectal pouch.

Collaborative Care

Treatment for a cystocele includes use of a vaginal pessary or surgical repair. Pessaries may not be effective. An anterior repair (colporrhaphy) is the most common surgical procedure and is usually done for large symptomatic cystoceles. This involves a surgical shortening of pelvic muscles to provide better support for the bladder. An anterior repair is often combined with a vaginal hysterectomy.

Small rectoceles may not need treatment. The woman with mild symptoms may get relief from a high-fibre diet and adequate fluid intake, stool softeners, or mild laxatives. Vaginal pessaries usually are not effective. Large rectoceles causing significant symptoms are usually repaired surgically with a posterior repair (colporrhaphy). This surgery is performed vaginally and involves shortening the pelvic muscles to provide better support for the rectum. Anterior and posterior repairs can be performed at the same time and with vaginal hysterectomy.

Genital Fistulas

Genital fistulas are abnormal passageways between genital tract organs. Most occur between the bladder and the genital tract (e.g., vesicovaginal), between the urethra and the vagina (urethrovaginal), and between the rectum or sigmoid colon and the vagina (rectovaginal) (Fig. 24-7). Genital fistulas may also be a result of a congenital anomaly, gynecological surgery, obstetrical trauma, cancer, radiation therapy, gynecological trauma, or infection (e.g., in the episiotomy). Fistulas are more common in women who have given birth to many children or have had obstructed labours with minimal access to appropriate care, as in developing countries.

Collaborative Care

Management of genital fistulas depends on their location. Surgical repair is the usual treatment; however, it may not be successful.

Nursing care of the woman with a fistula requires great sensitivity because the woman's reactions are often intense. She can become withdrawn or hostile because of embarrassment about odours and soiling of her clothing that are beyond her control. Her sexuality can be threatened; her partner may refuse sexual intimacy.

The nurse can tactfully suggest hygiene practices that reduce odour. Commercial deodorizing douches are available, or noncommercial solutions such as diluted chlorine (e.g., 5 mL of chlorine household bleach to 1 L of water) may be used. The chlorine solution is also useful for external perineal irrigation. Sitz baths and thorough washing of the genitalia with unscented, mild soap and warm water are helpful measures. Sparse dusting with deodorizing powders can be useful.

If a rectovaginal fistula is present, enemas given before leaving the house may provide temporary relief from oozing of fecal material until corrective surgery is performed. Irritated

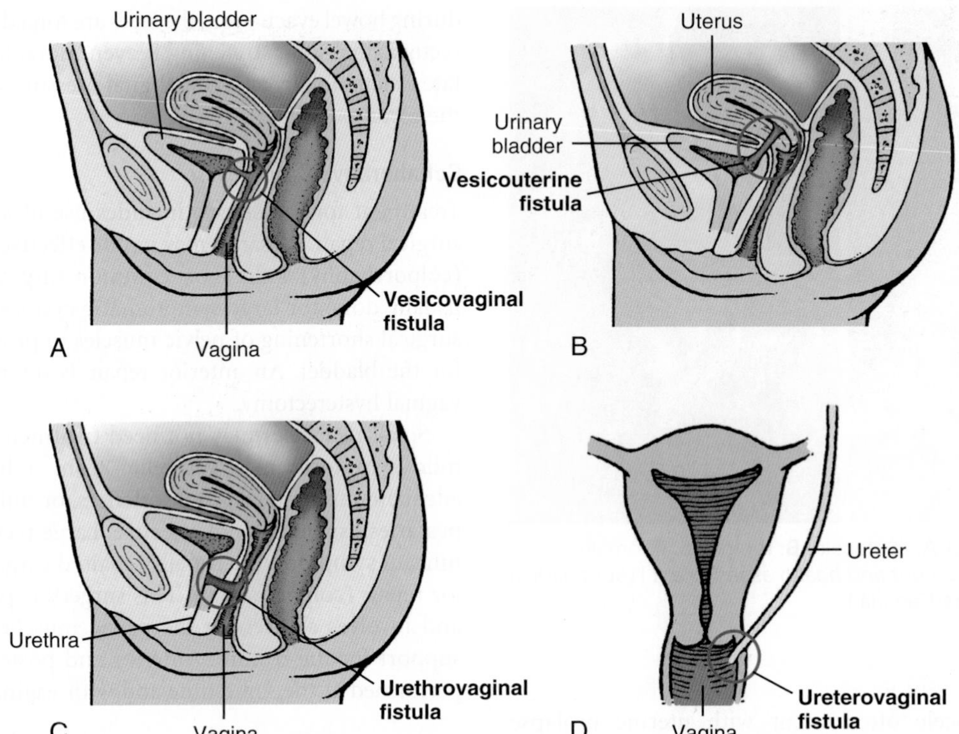

FIGURE 24-7 Types of genitourinary fistulas. **A:** Vesicovaginal (bladder to vagina). **B:** Vesicouterine (bladder to uterus). **C:** Urethrovaginal (urethra to vagina). **D:** Ureterovaginal (ureter to vagina). Fistulas range in size from tiny and difficult to locate to large, disfiguring the base of the bladder. (From Monahan, F. D., et al. [2007]. *Phipps' medical-surgical nursing: Health and illness perspectives* [8th ed., p. 1696]. St. Louis: Mosby.)

skin and tissues may benefit from exposure to a heat lamp or application of an emollient. Hygienic care is time consuming and may need to be repeated frequently throughout the day; the woman may need to wear protective pads or pants. All of these activities can be demoralizing to the woman and frustrating to her and her family.

Urinary Incontinence

Urinary incontinence (UI) affects young and middle-age women, with the prevalence increasing as the woman ages. The main symptom is involuntary leaking of urine, especially during coughing, laughing, or exercising. Research suggests that a significant number of women have undiagnosed UI (Wallner, Porten, Meenan, et al., 2009).

Although nulliparous women can have UI, the incidence is higher among women who have given birth and increases with parity. Women who are overweight and those who have had a hysterectomy are also at increased risk (Sung & Hampton, 2009). Conditions that disturb urinary control include the following:

- Stress incontinence, caused by sudden increases in intra-abdominal pressure (e.g., caused by sneezing or coughing)
- Urge incontinence, caused by disorders of the bladder and urethra (e.g., urethritis, urethral stricture, trigonitis, and cystitis)
- Neuropathies (e.g., multiple sclerosis, diabetic neuritis, and pathological conditions of the spinal cord)
- Congenital and acquired urinary tract abnormalities

Stress UI may follow injury to bladder neck structures. A sphincter mechanism at the bladder neck compresses the upper urethra, pulls it upward behind the symphysis, and forms an acute angle at the junction of the posterior urethral wall and the base of the bladder (Fig. 24-8). To empty the bladder, the sphincter complex relaxes, and the trigone contracts to open the internal urethral orifice and pull the contracting bladder wall upward, forcing urine out. The angle between the urethra and the base of the bladder is lost or increased if the supporting pubococcygeus muscle is injured; this change, coupled with a urethrocele, causes incontinence. Urine spurts out when the woman is asked to bear down or cough while she is in the lithotomy position.

Collaborative Care

Mild to moderate UI can be significantly decreased or relieved in many women through bladder training and pelvic muscle (Kegel) exercises (Dumoulin & Hay-Smith, 2010). Other management strategies include pelvic-flow support devices (i.e., pessaries), vaginal estrogen therapy, serotonin–norepinephrine reuptake inhibitors, electrical stimulation, insertion of an artificial urethral sphincter, and surgery (e.g., anterior repair) (Tarnay & Bhatia, 2010).

NURSING CARE

Assessment for problems related to structural disorders of the uterus and vagina focuses primarily on the genitourinary tract,

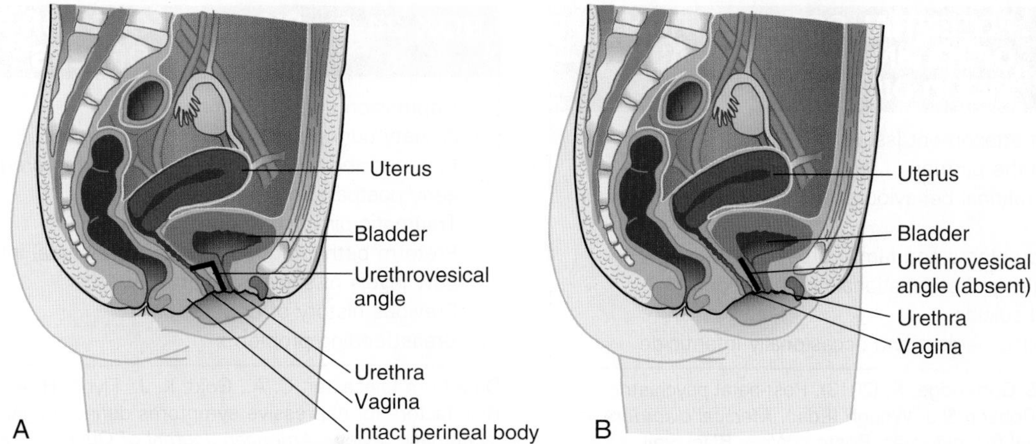

FIGURE 24-8 Urethrovesical angle. **A:** Normal angle. **B:** Widening (absence) of angle.

the reproductive organs, bowel elimination, and psychosocial and sexual factors. A complete health history, a physical examination, and laboratory tests are done to support the appropriate medical diagnosis. The nurse must assess the woman's knowledge of the disorder, its management, and possible prognosis. Assessment for depression that can result from decreased quality of life and functional status is also important.

In general, nurses working with women with structural disorders can provide information and self-care education to prevent problems before they occur, manage or reduce symptoms and promote comfort and hygiene if symptoms are already present, and recognize when further intervention is needed. For example, women may need guidance about changes in lifestyle (e.g., losing weight) and education about pelvic muscle exercises (Sung, West, Hernandez, et al., 2009). This information can be part of all postpartum discharge teaching or provided at postpartum follow-up visits in clinics or physician or midwife offices, during postpartum home visits, or during gynecological health examinations. Information on how to prevent or recognize problems can be provided at workshops for women or at health fairs in community settings.

When surgery is required, the nurse will focus care on preparing the woman for surgery and her postoperative care. Preoperative teaching involves the primary nurse, operating room nurse, surgeon, and anaesthesiologist. Postoperative nursing care focuses on prevention of infection and helping the woman avoid putting stress on the surgical site. The nurse in the health-promotion setting is usually most aware of the woman's living circumstances, physical limitations, and social problems and therefore may be best suited to coordinate continuity of care after discharge.

POSTPARTUM PSYCHOLOGICAL COMPLICATIONS

For many women the weeks after birth are a time of vulnerability to psychological complications, causing significant distress for the mother, disrupting family life, and, if prolonged, negatively affecting the child's emotional and social development. **Perinatal mood disorders**, which includes anxiety or major and minor depressive episodes that occur during pregnancy or in the first 12 months after delivery, is one of the most common medical complications during pregnancy and the postpartum period, affecting one in seven women. It is important to identify pregnant and postpartum women with a mood disorder because untreated perinatal depression and other mood disorders can have devastating effects on women, infants, and families (ACOG, 2015). Pre-existing mood and anxiety disorders are particularly likely to recur or worsen during these weeks. Because birth is usually thought to be a happy event, a new mother's emotional distress can puzzle and immobilize family and friends. Nurses can offer anticipatory guidance, assess the mental health of new mothers, offer therapeutic interventions, and make referrals, when necessary. Failure to do so can result in tragic consequences. Mood disorders are the predominant mental health disorder in the postpartum period.

Perinatal Mood Disorders (PMD)

Perinatal mood disorders (PMD) have traditionally been called postpartum mood disorders, but the terminology has been revised to perinatal mood disorders because these mental health issues may affect women any time during pregnancy and in the first year after the birth of the baby, although they most commonly begin within the first 12 weeks postpartum. These affective disorders range in severity from "the blues" to depression, anxiety, obsessive-compulsive disorder, bipolar disorder, and psychosis.

Up to 80% of women experience a mild depression or "baby blues" after the birth of a child; however, functioning of the woman is usually not impaired. Baby blues are characterized by mood swings; feelings of sadness, anxiety, or both; crying; difficulty sleeping; and loss of appetite. The symptoms are normal, resolve within a few days, and treatment is not needed. See Chapter 22, p. 579, for further discussion of postpartum blues.

Serious mood disorders, experienced by 10 to 15% of postpartum women, can eventually incapacitate them to the point of being unable to care for themselves or their babies (Sadock, Sadock, & Ruiz, 2009). PMD affects women from all cultures, although the manifestations vary. The incidence of mental health issues in some cultures is underreported because of its

BOX 24-4 POTENTIAL COMPLICATIONS OF HAVING A PERINATAL MOOD DISORDER

- Mother–infant attachment issues
- Depression in the partner
- Long-term emotional behavioural and cognitive problems in the child
- Relationship problems and family breakdown
- Social, financial, and occupational complications
- Self-harm and suicide
- Infant and sibling neglect and occasionally infanticide

From Lazarus, R., & Gutteridge, K. (2013). Post-natal psychiatric disorders. In S. E. Robson & J. Wough (Eds.), *Medical disorders in pregnancy: A manual for midwives.* Boston: Wiley Blackwell.

stigma and the hesitancy to seek professional help (Callister, Beckstrand, & Corbett, 2011; Goyal, Wang, Shen, et al., 2012). PMD affects parental infant attachment and the quality of parenting, and children are at increased risk of developing mental, social, and behavioural difficulties (Dennis, 2014). The complications of having a PMD are listed in Box 24-4.

Some women have more serious mood disorders that can eventually incapacitate them to the point of being unable to care for themselves or their babies. The cause of a PMD can be biological, psychological, situational, or multifactorial. Estrogen fluctuations and postpartum hypogonadism (the change from the high levels of estrogen and progesterone at the end of pregnancy to the much lower levels of both hormones that are present after birth) are important etiological factors. Women at greatest risk for PMD are those with a history of anxiety or depression and especially those who have had a previous episode of major depressive disorder (MDD), including during or after pregnancy (Cunningham et al., 2014; Davey, Tough, Adair, et al., 2011). Other risk factors include younger age, unintended pregnancy, personal history of severe premenstrual dysphoria, family history of mood disorder, unmarried status, marital discord, lack of social support, lower socioeconomic status, lower education level, substance use, and stressful life events in the year before the pregnancy (Cunningham et al., 2014; Le Strat, Dubertret, & Le Foll, 2011). Women facing multiple or severe psychosocial problems or chronic interpersonal difficulties are at increased risk for a major depressive episode. Dennis (2014) concluded that women who have feelings of incompetence, a loss of self, and loneliness are also at risk.

Complications of pregnancy and birth increase the risk for PMD (Blom, Jansen, Verhulst, et al., 2010). Having a preterm, low-birth-weight, and ill neonate is associated with higher rates of depression (Vigod, Villegas, Dennis, et al., 2010). Women who are victims of intimate partner violence are also at increased risk for depression (Beydoun, Beydoun, Kaufman, et al., 2012; Cerulli, Talbor, Tang, et al., 2011; Woolhouse, Gartland, Hegarty, et al., 2012). Cultural practices can positively or negatively affect the development of PMD. Women facing multiple or severe psychosocial problems or chronic interpersonal difficulties are at increased risk for experiencing a major depressive episode. Box 24-5 lists common risk factors for PMD.

BOX 24-5 RISK FACTORS FOR PERINATAL MOOD DISORDERS

- Depression during pregnancy
- Anxiety during pregnancy
- Experiencing stressful life events during pregnancy or the early postpartum period
- Traumatic birth experience
- Preterm birth/infant admission to neonatal intensive care
- Low levels of social support
- Previous history of depression
- Breastfeeding problems

Data from Lancaster, C. A., Gold, K. J., Flynn, H. A., et al. (2010). Risk factors for depressive symptoms during pregnancy: A systematic review. *American Journal of Obstetrics and Gynecology, 202,* 5–14; Robertson, E., Grace, S., Wallington, T., & Stewart, D. E. (2004). Antenatal risk factors for postpartum depression: A synthesis of recent literature. *General Hospital Psychiatry, 26,* 289–295.

Paternal Mood Disorder

Often, women are not alone in their experience of a mood disorder; partners may have depression or anxiety as well. The incidence is unclear, with reports varying from 10% to more than 50% (Letourneau, Tryphonopoulos, Duffett-Leger, et al., 2012; Paulson & Bazemore, 2010). The best predictor of paternal depression is having a partner with postpartum depression. According to Dennis (2010), maternal postpartum depression increases the incidence of paternal depression to 25 to 50%. Men may not exhibit classic symptoms of PMD but are likely to display fatigue, frustration, anger, irritability, indecisiveness, and withdrawal from social situations, usually between 3 and 6 months postpartum (Paulson & Bazemore, 2010). Lone-parent mood disorders as well as dual-partner mood disorders significantly affect development of the children; further studies are required to develop intervention strategies.

Postpartum Anxiety Disorders

Anxiety disorders include generalized anxiety disorder, obsessive-compulsive disorder, panic disorder and panic attacks, specific phobias, social anxiety disorder, and post-traumatic stress disorder. Common characteristics of these disorders are irrational fear, worry, and tension; physical symptoms such as trembling, nausea and vomiting, dizziness, dyspnea, and insomnia are often seen (Cunningham et al., 2014).

Women who have obsessive-compulsive disorder (OCD) often report worsening of their symptoms during pregnancy and in the postpartum period (Forray, Focseneanu, Pittman, et al., 2010). Onset of OCD can occur after birth. Compulsive checking on the sleeping baby and repetitive ritualistic washing are common. Obsessions are usually focused and specific and associated with fear of consequences (Speisman, Storch, & Abramowitz, 2011).

It is very important to distinguish between the symptoms of OCD in the postpartum woman and those of postpartum psychosis, because either can involve ideation regarding harming the newborn (Speisman et al., 2011). Delusions and hallucinations are typical in psychosis and have implications for infant safety, but these are not found in OCD. Aggressive thoughts of women with psychoses are not distressing to them, whereas women with OCD find their obsessive thoughts are very disturbing (Speisman et al., 2011).

Panic attacks are discrete periods of sudden onset of intense apprehension, fearfulness, or terror (American Psychiatric Association [APA], 2013). During these attacks, symptoms such as shortness of breath, palpitations, chest pain, choking, smothering sensations, and fear of losing control are present. Women with panic attacks have reported having intrusive thoughts about terrible injury done to the infant, such as stabbing or burns, sometimes by themselves. Rarely do these women harm their baby. Nurses need only to listen to a mother with such attacks to hear symptoms of panic disorder. Usually these women are so distraught that they will share their thoughts with whoever will listen. Often the family has tried to tell them that what they are experiencing is normal; however, they know that their symptoms are not normal. These women need to have their feelings validated, and they need monitoring or treatment.

Collaborative care. There are effective treatments for anxiety disorders; this fact should be communicated to affected women. Cognitive-behavioural therapy (CBT) is an option that is limited in duration, does not expose the infant to medications, and has proven durability of effect. For pharmacological therapy, the effectiveness of treatment, widespread availability, and ease of administration make selective serotonin reuptake inhibitors (SSRIs) an appealing and popular option (Cunningham et al., 2014; Speisman et al., 2011). Medications should be prescribed with careful consideration of safety for the breastfeeding infant. Each woman should be approached on an individualized basis: the severity of her symptoms needs to assessed, her history and response to any previous treatments should be obtained, her preferences need to be acknowledged, and the potential benefits and risks of each treatment must be conveyed. Treatment is usually a combination of medications, education, psychotherapy, and CBT, along with an attempt to identify any medical or physiological contributors.

Education is a crucial nursing intervention. New mothers should be provided with anticipatory guidance concerning the possibility of anxiety disorders during the postpartum period. Preparing for the attacks can help offset their unexpected, terrifying nature. Women can be reassured that it is common to feel a sense of impending doom and fear of insanity during panic attacks. Nurses can help women identify panic triggers that are particular to their own lives. Keeping a diary can help in identifying such triggers.

Family and social supports are helpful. The new mother needs to be encouraged to put usual chores on hold and to ask for and accept help. Support groups can help these mothers experience some comfort in seeing others in similar circumstances.

A variety of other treatment options can be recommended for women with anxiety disorders. These include sensory interventions such as music therapy and aromatherapy, behavioural interventions such as breathing exercises and progressive muscle relaxation, cognitive interventions such as positive self-talk training, and exercise.

Postpartum Depression

Postpartum depression can be mild to severe. It is characterized by low mood and lack of interest in activities that would normally be of interest to the person. In addition, the depressed person often has low energy, a general lack of enjoyment, and labile mood swing. Whereas postpartum blues affects 50 to 80% of women, with similar symptoms of irritability, tearfulness, and low mood, it is transient. Depression, by contrast, is more serious and persistent than postpartum blues and often includes reduced concentration and self-esteem as well as feelings of hopelessness and guilt. Women often describe alterations in sleep patterns and appetite and, in severe cases, suicidal ideation (Lazarus & Gutteridge, 2013). These symptoms rarely disappear without outside help (Dennis, 2010). Most of these mothers seek help only after reaching a "crisis point" (McCarthy & McMahon, 2008). The occurrence of this type of depression is higher among younger women and those with less education. Mothers who have no one to talk to about their problems after giving birth tend to have a high rate of depression and a low rate of seeking help. This situation can be a concern for newly immigrated women who have difficulty with language and limited social support. Having established and supportive relationships facilitates seeking of care, as does outreach and follow-up (Sword, Busser, Ganann, et al., 2008).

The symptoms of postpartum major depression do not differ from those of nonpostpartum depression except that the mother's ruminations of guilt and inadequacy feed her worries about being an incompetent and inadequate parent. New mothers report an increased yearning for sleep, sleeping heavily but awakening instantly with any infant noise, and an inability to go back to sleep after infant feedings. Determining difficulty falling asleep is a relevant screening question to ascertain risk for depression.

A distinguishing feature of major depression is irritability. These episodes of irritability may flare up with little provocation and may sometimes escalate to violent outbursts or dissolve into uncontrollable sobbing. Many of these outbursts are directed against significant others ("He never helps me") or the baby ("She cries all the time, and I feel like hitting her"). Postpartum women with major depressive episodes often have spontaneous crying long after the usual duration of baby blues.

Many women feel especially guilty about having depressive feelings at a time when they believe they should be happy. They may be reluctant to discuss their symptoms or their negative feelings toward the infant. A prominent feature of depression is rejection of the infant, often caused by abnormal jealousy. The mother may be obsessed by the notion that the baby may take her place in her partner's affections. Attitudes toward the infant may include disinterest, annoyance with care demands, and blaming because of her lack of maternal feeling. The mother may appear awkward in her responses to the baby. Obsessive thoughts about harming the infant are very frightening to her. Often she does not share these thoughts because of embarrassment; when she does, other family members can become very frightened.

Collaborative care. The natural course is one of gradual improvement over the 6 months after birth, although 50% of women will remain clinically depressed at 6 months with approximately 25% continuing beyond the first year if they remain untreated (Dennis, 2010). Often supportive treatment alone is not efficacious for major depression. Pharmacological intervention is often required. Treatment options include antidepressants, antianxiety drugs, and electroconvulsive therapy. Alternative therapies such as herbs, dietary supplements, massage, aromatherapy, and acupuncture may be helpful. Psychotherapy for the depressed postpartum mother focuses on her fears and concerns regarding her new responsibilities and roles, and monitoring for suicidal or homicidal thoughts. For some women, hospitalization is necessary.

Postpartum Psychosis

The most severe of the perinatal mood disorders, **postpartum psychosis**, is rare, affecting approximately 0.1 to 0.2% of postpartum women (Sadock et al., 2009). Once a woman has had one episode of postpartum psychosis, there is a 30 to 50% likelihood of recurrence with each subsequent birth (APA, 2013). This disorder tends to show onset within 2 weeks postpartum; however, it can present later in the course of the illness as a depression (Sadock et al., 2009).

Episodes of postpartum psychosis are typified by auditory or visual hallucinations, paranoid or grandiose delusions, elements of delirium or disorientation, and extreme deficits in judgement accompanied by high levels of impulsivity that can contribute to increased risks of suicide or infanticide (in 5% of psychotic women) (Sadock et al., 2009). Characteristically, the woman has fatigue, insomnia, and restlessness and may have episodes of tearfulness and emotional lability. The woman may state she has the inability to move, stand, or work. Later, suspiciousness, confusion, incoherence, irrational statements, and obsessive concerns about the baby's health and welfare may be present. Delusions may occur in 50% of all women with postpartum psychosis, and hallucinations in about 25%. Auditory hallucinations that command the mother to kill the infant can also occur in severe cases. When delusions are present, they are often related to the infant. The mother may think the infant is possessed by the devil, has special powers, or is destined for a terrible fate (APA, 2013). Grossly disorganized behaviour may be manifested as a disinterest in the infant or an inability to provide care. Some affected mothers insist that something is wrong with the baby or accuse nurses or family members of hurting or poisoning their child. Nurses are advised to be alert for mothers who are agitated, overactive, confused, or suspicious.

Postpartum psychosis is most commonly associated with the diagnosis of bipolar (or manic-depressive) disorder (Sadock et al., 2009; Sharma, Burt, & Ritchie, 2009). This mood disorder is defined by the presence of one or more episodes of abnormally elevated energy levels, cognition, and mood and one or more depressive episodes. The elevated moods are clinically referred to as *mania*. Clinical manifestations of a manic episode include at least three of the following: grandiosity, decreased need for sleep, pressured speech, flight of ideas, distractibility, psychomotor agitation, and excessive involvement in pleasurable activities without regard for negative consequences (APA, 2013). While in a manic state, mothers need constant supervision when caring for their infant. Usually, however, they are too preoccupied to provide child care. Individuals who experience manic episodes also commonly experience depressive episodes or symptoms or mixed episodes, in which features of both mania and depression are present at the same time. These episodes are usually separated by periods of "normal" mood, but in some individuals, depression and mania may rapidly alternate. These rapid changes in mood are known as *rapid cycling*.

Collaborative care. Postpartum psychosis carries a relatively good prognosis with early detection and aggressive treatment; however, if left untreated, it can progress to the second postpartum year and become more refractory to treatment (Sadock et al., 2009). Postpartum psychosis is a psychiatric emergency, and the mother will probably need inpatient psychiatric care. Antipsychotics and mood stabilizers such as lithium are the treatments of choice (Tables 24-1 and 24-2). Antidepressants should be used very cautiously in treating postpartum psychosis, even when depressive symptoms are present, because of the risk for precipitating rapid cycling. Because of potential risks to the breastfeeding infant, informed consent regarding the risks and benefits of exposing the newborn to a psychotropic agent and maternal mental illness must be discussed and documented (see additional discussion of lactation and psychotropic medications later in this chapter). Electroconvulsive therapy (ECT), especially when bilaterally administered, has also been shown to be highly effective in the treatment of postpartum psychosis. It is usually advantageous for the mother to have contact with her baby if she so desires, but visits must be

TABLE 24-1 MOOD STABILIZERS

MOOD STABILIZERS	PREGNANCY RISK CATEGORY	LACTATION RISK CATEGORY
Carbamazepine (Tegretol)	C	L2
Clonazepam (Klonopin, Rivotril)	C	L3
Gabapentin	C	L3
Lamotrigine (Lamictal)	C	L3
Lithium carbonate (Carbolith, Lithane)	C	L4
Topiramate (Topamax)	C	L3
Valproic acid (Depakene, Epival ECT)	D	L2

C, animal studies show adverse effects on fetus but no controlled studies in pregnant women, or no studies available; *D*, positive evidence of human fetal risk; *L2*, medication studied in limited number of breastfeeding women with no adverse effects in infant, or evidence is remote; *L3*, no controlled studies, or studies show minimal nonthreatening effects; *L4*, possibly hazardous.

Sources: Hale, T. (2012). *Medications and mother's milk* (15th ed.), Amarillo, TX: Pharmasoft; Schatzberg, A., Cole, J. O., & DeBattista, C. (Eds.). (2010). *Manual of clinical psychopharmacology* (7th ed.), Arlington, VA: American Psychiatric Publishing.

TABLE 24-2 ANTIPSYCHOTIC MEDICATIONS

ANTIPSYCHOTIC MEDICATIONS	PREGNANCY RISK CATEGORY	LACTATION RISK CATEGORY
Traditional Antipsychotics		
Chlorpromazine hydrochloride	C	L3
Fluphenazine hydrochloride; fluphenazine deconate (Modecate Concentrate)	C	L3
Haloperidol	C	L2
Perphenazine	C	L3
Thioridazine	C	L4
Trifluoperazine	Unknown	Unknown
Atypical Antipsychotics		
Aripiprazole (Abilify)	C	L3
Clozapine (Clozaril)	C	L3
Loxapine (Loxitane)	C	L4
Olanzapine (Zyprexa)	C	L2
Quetiapine (Seroquel)	C	L4
Risperidone (Risperdal)	C	L3
Ziprasidone (Zeldox)	C	L4

C, Animal studies show adverse effects on fetus but no controlled studies in pregnant women, or no studies available; *L2,* medication studied in limited number of breastfeeding women with no adverse effects in infant, or evidence is remote; *L3,* no controlled studies, or studies show minimal nonthreatening effects; *L4,* possibly hazardous. Sources: Hale, T. (2012). *Medications and mother's milk* (15th ed.), Amarillo, TX: Pharmasoft; Schatzberg, A., Cole, J. O., & DeBattista, C. (Eds.). (2010). *Manual of clinical psychopharmacology* (7th ed.), Arlington, VA: American Psychiatric Publishing.

closely supervised. Psychotherapy is indicated after the period of acute psychosis has passed.

NURSING CARE

Nurses can also assist women by teaching them self-care, especially the symptoms and risk factors for PMD; helping them to feel safe and empowered in discussing their mental and social health; and facilitating adequate social and partner support. Women and their families should be given written resources in their native language and emergency numbers to call. Last but not least, follow-up is a powerful tool for detection and deterrence of PMD. In practice it is the responsibility of all who are in contact with the woman to provide screening, assessment, and education to facilitate early detection and treatment.

Even though the prevalence of PMD is fairly well established, women may be unlikely to seek help from a mental health care provider. This can be related to social stigma of mental illness, cultural beliefs, lack of knowledge, or fear of child custody implications (Yonkers, Vigod, & Ross, 2011). Primary health care providers can usually recognize severe depression or postpartum psychosis but may miss milder forms; even if it is recognized, the woman may be treated inappropriately or subtherapeutically. Nurses should be strategically positioned to offer anticipatory guidance, assess the mental health of new mothers, offer therapeutic interventions, and make referrals when necessary. Failure to do so may result in tragic consequences. Identification and treatment of PMD must be continued beyond the immediate postbirth period to prevent negative effects of maternal mood disorders on the children of these mothers. To recognize symptoms of PMD as early as possible, the nurse should be an active listener and demonstrate a caring attitude. Nurses cannot depend on women to volunteer unsolicited information about their mental health or ask for help. Examples of ways to initiate conversation include the following: "Now that you've had your baby, how are things going for you? Have you had to change many things in your life since having the baby?" and "How much time do you spend crying?" If the nurse assesses that the new mother is depressed, the nurse must ask if the mother has thought about hurting herself or the baby. The woman may be more willing to answer honestly if the nurse says, "Many women feel depressed after having a baby, and some feel so bad that they think about hurting themselves or the baby. Have you had these thoughts?"

! NURSING ALERT

Because mothers with postpartum psychosis may harm their infants, extra precaution is needed in assessment and intervention. The nurse needs to ask specifically if the mother has had thoughts about harming her baby.

Screening for Perinatal Mood Disorders

When PMD is identified early, it is highly treatable. Screening for anxiety or depression during pregnancy and the postpartum period aids in prevention and early intervention for PMD. Women at risk should be identified (see Box 24-4), although all women should be screened during pregnancy and postpartum (ACOG, 2015).

The Registered Nurses' Association of Ontario (RNAO) Best Practice Guideline: Interventions for Postpartum Depression recommends use of the Edinburgh Postnatal Depression Scale (EPDS) as the screening tool of choice (RNAO, 2005). The EPDS is a self-report assessment designed specifically to identify women experiencing PMD (Fig. 24-9). It has been used and validated in studies in numerous cultures and is viewed as a valid screening tool throughout pregnancy and postpartum for PMD. The assessment tool asks the woman to respond to 10 statements about the common symptoms of depression. The woman is asked to choose the response that is closest to describing how she has felt for the past week. A maximum score on the EPDS is 30; women with scores of 13 or greater on the EPDS and those who have a history of depression or anxiety require more intensive postpartum follow-up. Women who answer "yes" to the question about the thought of hurting themselves need immediate care.

Screening for PMD can be done before women are discharged from the hospital although this may be too early and while the screening may identify some who are at risk, it is important that follow-up screening is also done. PMD is most

Edinburgh Postnatal Depression Scale (EPDS)

Name: ______________________ Address: ______________________

Your Date of Birth: ______________ Baby's Date of Birth: ______________ Phone: ______________

As you are pregnant or have recently had a baby, we would like to know how you are feeling. Please check the answer that comes closest to how you have felt IN THE PAST 7 DAYS, not just how you feel today.

Here is an example, already completed.

I have felt happy:

- ☐ Yes, all the time
- ☒ Yes, most of the time
- ☐ No, not very often
- ☐ No, not at all

(This would mean: "I have felt happy most of the time" during the past week.)

Please complete the other questions in the same way.

1. I have been able to laugh and see the funny side of things.
   - ☐ As much as I always could
   - ☐ Not quite so much now
   - ☐ Definitely not so much now
   - ☐ Not at all

2. I have looked forward with enjoyment to things.
   - ☐ As much as I ever did
   - ☐ Rather less than I used to
   - ☐ Definitely less than I used to
   - ☐ Hardly at all

*3. I have blamed myself unnecessarily when things went wrong.
   - ☐ Yes, most of the time
   - ☐ Yes, some of the time
   - ☐ Not very often
   - ☐ No, never

4. I have been anxious or worried for no good reason.
   - ☐ No, not at all
   - ☐ Hardly ever
   - ☐ Yes, sometimes
   - ☐ Yes, most of the time

*5. I have felt scared or panicky for no good reason.
   - ☐ Yes, quite alot
   - ☐ Yes, sometimes
   - ☐ No, not much
   - ☐ No, not at all

*6. Things have been getting on top of me.
   - ☐ Yes, most of the time I have not been able to cope at all
   - ☐ Yes, sometimes I have not been able to cope as well as usual
   - ☐ No, most of the time I have coped quite well
   - ☐ No, I have been coping as well as ever

*7. I have been so unhappy that I have had difficulty sleeping.
   - ☐ Yes, most of the time
   - ☐ Yes, sometimes
   - ☐ Not very often
   - ☐ No, not at all

*8. I have felt sad or miserable.
   - ☐ Yes, most of the time
   - ☐ Yes, quite often
   - ☐ Not very often
   - ☐ No, not at all

*9. I have been so unhappy that I have been crying.
   - ☐ Yes, most of the time
   - ☐ Yes, quite often
   - ☐ Only occasionally
   - ☐ No, never

*10. The thought of harming myself has occurred to me.
   - ☐ Yes, quite often
   - ☐ Sometimes
   - ☐ Hardly ever
   - ☐ Never

Administered/Reviewed by: ______________________

SCORING

QUESTIONS 1, 2, & 4 (without an *)

Are scored 0, 1, 2 or 3 with top box scored as 0 and the bottom box scored as 3.

QUESTIONS 3, 5–10

(marked with an *)

Are reverse scored, with the top box scored as a 3 and the bottom box scored as 0.

Maximum score: 30

Possible Depression: 10 or greater

Always look at item 10 (suicidal thoughts)

Instructions for using the Edinburgh Postnatal Depression Scale:

1. The mother is asked to check the response that comes closest to how she has been feeling in the previous 7 days.
2. All the items must be completed.
3. Care should be taken to avoid the possibility of the mother discussing her answers with others. (Answers come from the mother or pregnant woman.)
4. The mother should complete the scale herself, unless she has limited English or has difficulty with reading.

FIGURE 24-9 Edinburgh Postnatal Depression Scale (EPDS). (© 1987 The Royal College of Psychiatrists. Cox, J. L., Holden, J. M., & Sagovsky, R. [1987]. Detection of postnatal depression: Development of the 10-item Edinburgh Postnatal Depression Scale. *British Journal of Psychiatry, 150,* 782–786. Written permission must be obtained from the Royal College of Psychiatrists for copying and distribution to others or for republication [in print, online or by any other medium]. Translations of the scale, and guidance as to its use, may be found in Cox, J. L., Holden, J., & Henshaw, C. [2014]. *Perinatal mental health: The Edinburgh Postnatal Depression Scale (EPDS) manual* [2nd Ed.]. London: RCPsych Publications. http://www.rcpsych.ac.uk/usefulresources/publications/books/rcpp/9781909726130.aspx.)

likely to occur around 4 weeks after birth. Follow-up assessments for risks and signs of PMD can be done by primary care providers during pediatric care visits for the infant and during postpartum follow-up visits for the mother. Women with a positive screen should be referred appropriately for evaluation and treatment.

On the Postpartum Unit

The postpartum nurse must observe the new mother carefully for any signs of tearfulness and conduct further assessments as necessary. Nurses must discuss PMD to prepare all new parents for potential problems in the postpartum period and discuss ways to help prevent a PMD (see Patient Teaching box). The family must be able to recognize the symptoms and know where to go for help. Printed materials that explain what the woman can do to prevent a mood disorder can be used as part of discharge education (Logsdon, Tomasulo, Eckert, et al., 2012).

Mothers are often discharged before the blues or depression occurs. If the postpartum nurse is concerned about the mother, a mental health consult should be requested before the mother leaves the hospital. The family must be able to recognize the symptoms and know where to go for help. Written materials that explain what the woman can do to prevent depression are useful.

NURSING ALERT

Because the newborn may be scheduled for a checkup before the mother's 6-week checkup, nurses in well-baby clinics or physician offices should be alert for signs of PMD in new mothers and be knowledgeable about community referral resources.

PATIENT TEACHING

Preventing a Perinatal Mood Disorder

- Share knowledge about postpartum emotional problems with close family and friends.
- At least once each day or every other day, purposely relax for 15 minutes, using deep breathing or meditating or by taking a hot bath.
- Take care of yourself: eat a balanced diet.
- Exercise on a regular basis, at least 30 minutes a day.
- Sleep as much as possible; make a promise to yourself to try to sleep when the baby sleeps.
- Get out of the house: try to leave home for 30 minutes a day; take a walk outdoors or walk at the mall.
- Share your feelings with someone close to you; don't isolate yourself at home with the TV.
- Don't overcommit yourself or feel like you need to be a superwoman. Ask for help from family and friends.
- Don't place unrealistic expectations on yourself; you don't need to be a perfect mother.
- Be flexible with your daily activities.
- Go to a new mothers' support group: for example, take a postpartum exercise class or attend a breastfeeding support group.
- Don't be ashamed of having emotional problems after your baby is born. It happens to approximately 15 to 20% of women.

In the Home and Community

Postpartum home visits can reduce the incidence of or complications from PMD. A brief home visit or phone call at least once a week until the new mother returns for her postpartum visit may save the life of a mother and her infant; however, home visits may not be feasible or available. Some provinces have mandatory telephone follow-up of all new mothers after the birth, and women who are identified as high risk should receive more comprehensive follow-up. Supervision of the mother with emotional complications may become a prime concern. Because PMD can greatly interfere with her mothering functions, family and friends may need to participate in the infant's care. This is a time for extended family and friends to determine what they can do to help; the nurse can work with them to ensure adequate supervision and their understanding of the woman's mental illness.

When the woman has a PMD, a partner often reacts with confusion, shock, denial, and anger and feels neglected and blamed. The nurse can provide nonjudgemental opportunities for the partner to express feelings and concerns, help the partner identify positive coping strategies, and be a source of encouragement for the partner to continue supporting the woman. Suggestions for partners of women with PMD include helping around the house, setting limits with family and friends, going with her to doctor's appointments, educating himself or herself about PMD, writing down concerns and questions to take to the primary care provider or therapist, and just being with her—sitting quietly, hugging her, and demonstrating concern and compassion. Both the woman and her partner need an opportunity to express their needs, fears, thoughts, and feelings in a nonjudgemental environment.

Even if the woman is severely depressed, hospitalization can be avoided if adequate resources can be mobilized to ensure safety for both mother and infant. The community health nurse will need to make frequent phone calls or home visits for assessment and counselling. Community resources that may be helpful are temporary child care or foster care, homemaker service, meals on wheels, parenting guidance centres, mother's-day-out programs, and telephone support groups such The Pacific Post Partum Support Society and The Peel Postpartum Mood Disorder Program (see Additional Resources at the end of the chapter).

Referral

Women with moderate to severe cases of PMD should be referred to a mental health professional such as an advanced-practice psychiatric nurse or psychiatrist for evaluation and therapy. Inpatient psychiatric hospitalization may be necessary. This decision is made when the safety of the mother or child is threatened.

Providing Safety

If delusional thinking about the baby is suspected, the nurse should ask, "Have you thought about hurting your baby?" When PMD is suspected, the nurse asks, "Have you thought about hurting yourself?" Four criteria measure the seriousness of a suicidal plan: method, availability, specificity, and lethality.

Has the woman specified a method? Is the method of choice available? How specific is the plan? If the method is concrete and detailed, with access to it right at hand, the suicide risk is increased. How lethal is the method? The most lethal method is shooting, with hanging being a close second. The least lethal method is slashing one's wrists. Medication overdose with tricyclic antidepressants (TCAs) causes death. Use of TCAs in suicidal women should be avoided because of the danger of overdose.

! NURSING ALERT

Suicidal thoughts or attempts are among the most serious symptoms of PMD and require immediate assessment and intervention.

Psychiatric Hospitalization

Women with postpartum psychosis have a psychiatric emergency and must be referred immediately to a psychiatrist who is experienced in working with women with psychosis, can prescribe medication and other forms of therapy, and can assess the need for hospitalization.

LEGAL TIP *COMMITMENT FOR PSYCHIATRIC CARE*

If a woman with PMD is experiencing active suicidal ideation or harmful delusions about the baby and is unwilling to seek treatment, legal intervention may be necessary to commit the woman to an inpatient setting for treatment.

Within the hospital setting, the reintroduction of the baby to the mother can occur at the mother's own pace. A schedule is set for increasing the number of hours during which the mother cares for the baby over several days, culminating in the infant staying overnight in the mother's room. This enables the mother to experience meeting the infant's needs and giving up sleep for the baby, a situation that is difficult for new mothers even under ideal conditions. The mother's readiness for discharge and caring for the baby should be assessed. Her interactions with her baby should also be carefully supervised and guided. A postpartum nurse may be asked to assist the psychiatric nursing staff in assessment of the mother–infant interactions.

Nurses need to observe the mother for signs of bonding with the baby. Attachment behaviours are defined as eye-to-eye contact; physical contact that involves holding, touching, cuddling, and talking to the baby and calling the baby by name; and the initiation of appropriate care. A staff member should be assigned to keep the baby in sight at all times. Indirect teaching, praise, and encouragement are designed to bolster the mother's self-esteem and self-confidence.

Psychotropic Medications

If a woman is diagnosed with depression, antidepressant medications will often be used. If the woman is not breastfeeding, antidepressants can be prescribed without special precautions.

A variety of medications can be prescribed for these women, including tricyclic antidepressants (TCAs), selective serotonin reuptake inhibitors (SSRIs), serotonin/norepinephrine reuptake inhibitors (SNRIs), monoamine oxidase inhibitors (MAOIs), mood stabilizers, and antipsychotic medications.

MAOIs may be used for women with major depression who are not responsive to other medications and for women with panic disorder and bipolar disorder. Hypertensive crisis is the main reason that MAOIs are not prescribed more frequently than other psychotropic medications. The woman should be taught to watch for signs of hypertensive crisis—a throbbing occipital headache, stiff neck, chills, nausea, flushing, retro-orbital pain, apprehension, pallor, sweating, chest pain, and palpitations. This crisis is brought on by the woman taking any of a large variety of over-the-counter medications or eating foods that contain tyramine, which normally is broken down by the enzyme *monoamine oxidase.* The nurse must give extensive teaching about absolute avoidance of foods and medications that contain tyramine such as pseudoephedrine-containing medications, aged cheese, red wine, fava or Italian green beans, brewer's yeast, smoked fish, chicken or beef livers, and preserved meats (Hadley, Albanese, & Rochester, 2012).

The woman taking mood stabilizers (see Table 24-1) must be taught about the many adverse effects, and especially for those taking lithium, the need to have serum lithium levels determined every 6 months. Women with severe psychiatric syndromes such as schizophrenia, bipolar disorder, or psychotic depression will probably require antipsychotic medications (see Table 24-2). Most of these antipsychotic medications can cause sedation and orthostatic hypotension—both of which can interfere with the mother being able to care safely for her baby. They also can cause peripheral nervous system (PNS) effects such as constipation, dry mouth, blurred vision, tachycardia, urinary retention, weight gain, and agranulocytosis. Central nervous system (CNS) effects may include akathisia, dystonias, parkinsonian-like symptoms, tardive dyskinesia (irreversible), and neuroleptic malignant syndrome (potentially fatal). Medication education is especially important when caring for women who are taking antipsychotic medications. The nurse should use discretion in selecting the content to be shared because of the women's altered thought processes and the large number of adverse effects. The nurse may choose to provide more extensive education to a close family member. The newer, atypical antipsychotic medications such as aripiprazole, olanzapine, quetiapine, risperidone, and ziprasidone are usually safer and have fewer adverse effects than the older, more traditional antipsychotics. Their safety in breastfeeding women, however, has not been established.

Psychotropic Medications and Lactation

Use of any psychotropic medication in a breastfeeding mother is done with consideration of risks and benefits. The risk of not treating the mother versus not breastfeeding the infant prompts providers to prescribe medications that reduce maternal symptoms without harming the infant. Concerns about many psychotropic drugs are related to the long-term use and potential effects on the infant (Lawrence & Lawrence, 2011).

Factors that affect the passage of a medication through breast milk include the size of the molecule, the solubility in lipids and water, the protein-binding capacity, the drug's pH,

CRITICAL THINKING CASE STUDY

Perinatal Mood Disorder

Jenna, 31, gave birth to a 3400-g boy 4 weeks ago. She has been diagnosed with depression, and an SSRI (sertraline [Zoloft]) medication has been prescribed. Jenna is breastfeeding and has concerns about taking the medication.

QUESTIONS

1. Evidence—Is there sufficient evidence regarding the safety of psychotropic medications and lactation?
2. Assumptions—What assumptions can be made about the following?
   a. Lactation risk categories of SSRI medications
   b. Timing of feeding and medication administration
   c. Risks of discontinuing medications while breastfeeding
3. What is the nursing priority in this situation?
4. Does the evidence objectively support your conclusion?

SSRI, selective serotonin reuptake inhibitor.

and the rate of diffusion. Infant factors to consider relate to the gestational and chronological age of the infant, weight, health, and frequency and amount of feeding (Lawrence & Lawrence, 2011). To minimize the infant's exposure to maternal medication, the mother should avoid breastfeeding when the blood levels of the medication are peaking.

SSRIs are the most common treatment for postpartum depression; they are also prescribed for anxiety disorders. Research has shown that the majority of the SSRIs taken by breastfeeding mothers pass through the milk to the infant in small amounts and have no untoward effects on the infant (Kendall-Tackett & Hale, 2010). Paroxetine, sertraline, and nortriptyline provide less infant exposure than fluoxetine and citalopram. All breastfeeding mothers who take SSRIs should be taught to monitor their infants for signs of irritability, poor feeding, and alterations in sleep pattern (Kendall-Tackett & Hale, 2010) (see Critical Thinking Case Study).

Benzodiazepines, mood stabilizers, and antipsychotic medications are all used frequently in the treatment of postpartum psychiatric disorders despite the lack of research in this population. No long-term effects have been reported in exclusively breastfed infants whose mothers were taking benzodiazepines on a regular basis. The shorter-acting agents (alprazolam, lorazepam) are favoured over those with longer half-lives (clonazepam, diazepam) (Lawrence & Lawrence, 2011).

Mood-stabilizing medications are present in the breast milk of women who take these drugs. Lithium has been the most extensively studied. Lithium has been linked to several serious adverse effects in breastfeeding infants, including hypotonia, hypothermia, cyanosis, and electrocardiogram abnormalities. Therefore, its use is not recommended in breastfeeding mothers. Valproic acid and carbamazepine are considered reasonably safe for use while breastfeeding, although careful monitoring for infant hepatotoxicity is recommended. The benefits of breastfeeding and the potential risks must be carefully considered before using lithium or other mood stabilizers.

In summary, all psychotropic medications studied to date are excreted in breast milk. The best psychotropic medications for breastfeeding women are those with the greatest documentation of prior use, lower Hale risk category, few or no metabolites, and fewer adverse effects (Hale, 2012).

When breastfeeding women have emotional complications and need psychotropic medications, referral to a mental health care provider who specializes in postpartum disorders is preferred. The woman should be informed of the risks and benefits to her and her infant of the medications to be taken. Depressed women will need the nurse to reinforce the importance of taking antidepressants as ordered. Because antidepressants usually do not exert any significant effect for approximately 2 weeks and usually do not reach full effect for 4 to 6 weeks, many women discontinue taking the medication on their own. Patient and family teaching should reinforce the schedule for taking medications until therapeutic effects are present and for as long as prescribed by the health care provider.

Other Treatments for Perinatal Mood Disorders

Other treatments for PMD include hormone therapy (often combined with antidepressant medication), complementary or alternative therapies (e.g., yoga, massage, relaxation techniques), ECT, and psychotherapy. ECT may be used for women with depression who have not improved with antidepressant therapy. Psychotherapy in the form of group therapy or individual (interpersonal) therapy has been used with positive results alone and in conjunction with antidepressant therapy; however, more studies are needed to determine what types of professional support are most effective. Repetitive transcranial magnetic stimulation is a new therapy for depression, but more studies need to be done to demonstrate the efficacy (Garcia, Flynn, Pierce, et al., 2010). Alternative therapies may be used alone but often are used with other treatments for PMD. Safety and efficacy studies of these alternative therapies are needed to ensure that care and advice are based on evidence.

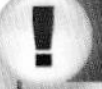

NURSING ALERT

St. John's wort is often used to treat depression. It has not been proven safe for women who are breastfeeding.

LOSS AND GRIEF

Situational life crises can be superimposed on the experiences of child-bearing. Examples may include infertility, premature labour or premature birth, a Caesarean birth, any perception of loss of control during the birthing experience, the birth of a boy when the parents wanted a girl or vice versa, the birth of a child with a handicap, a maternal death, or fetal or neonatal death (see Community Focus box). All of these situations have a common denominator: they are losses of what was hoped for, dreamed about, and planned.

These crises vary in degree, and every situation requires empathy, knowledge, and compassion from the health care provider. At the birth, the patient, partner, and family may be mourning instead of celebrating life.

Infant mortality rates continue to decrease in Canada, with a rate of 5 deaths per 1000 live births in 2009, and 75% of these

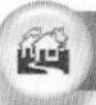

COMMUNITY FOCUS

Community Resources for Loss and Grief

Investigate what resources and support groups exist in your community to assist parents who have experienced a maternal death; birth of a child with physical or intellectual challenges; a Caesarean birth if they hoped for vaginal; or the death of a baby through miscarriage, stillbirth, or newborn death. Are resources available? Are there groups available for people who speak a language other than English? Are there enough of these resources to assist parents? How difficult was it for you to identify these resources? What could you do to make resources more known to bereaved parents and families?

being within the first 1 month after birth (Public Health Agency of Canada [PHAC], 2013). The leading cause of death is prematurity (PHAC, 2013). Infants may die in the early postpartum period from prematurity, birth defects, birth trauma, or other acute illnesses. Thus, parents can experience grief before or during the child-bearing experience.

The focus of this section is to prepare the nurse to provide sensitive, supportive, and therapeutic interventions to parents and families experiencing perinatal loss in a variety of settings. An overview of the grief process is presented as a guide for assessing and understanding the responses of bereaved women, men, and their families. Guidelines for intervention are given, and specific intervention approaches are discussed.

Grief Responses

Grief is the process of recovering from a loss, and in that process individuals experience many emotional, cognitive, behavioural, and physical responses. Grief is a normal process that can be facilitated or complicated by other life events, as well as by interactions with health care practitioners. Parental grief responses occur in four overlapping phases. According to Wilke and Limbo (2012) there is an early period of acute distress, shock, and numbness which is most intense for the first 2 weeks. From the second week to the fourth month the phase is characterized by searching and yearning. From the fifth through the ninth month, the third phase is defined as disorientation. The final phase, reorganization or resolution, may be reached in the tenth through the twenty-fourth month when parents return to their usual level of functioning in society, although the pain associated with the death remains. The duration of grief varies with the individual, but there is general agreement that grief is a long-term process that can extend for months and years. With a very close relationship such as with one's baby, some aspects of grief never truly end.

Phase One: Shock and Numbness

The loss of a pregnancy or death of an infant is an acute and distressing experience for mothers and partners who planned for and expected a normal healthy infant as the outcome. The loss encompasses a loss of their identity as a mother or partner and of their many dreams related to parenthood. The immediate reaction to news of a perinatal loss or infant death is a period of acute distress. Parents generally are in a state of shock and numbness. They may feel a sense of unreality, loss of innocence, and powerlessness, as though they were in a bad dream or in a fog or trancelike state. Disbelief and denial can occur. Sadness, devastation, depression, and intense outbursts of emotion and crying are common. Individuals describe feeling stunned, having a short attention span, and an inability to concentrate or make decisions. In contrast, lack of affect, euphoria, and calmness may occur and may reflect numbness, denial, or a personal way of coping with stress.

Much of the attention during the time of a loss is on the mother. The response of partners may vary more than that of mothers and depends on the level of identification with the pregnancy. Partners may be profoundly affected and grieve deeply for a perinatal loss, and it is important that they are supported in their grief as well as the mother.

Partners are often distressed by the grief of the mother and may feel helpless in comforting her with the intense pain. Some partners may appear stoic and unemotional to maintain the societal expectation that they be "strong" for the mother and other family members. Because many men do not easily share their feelings or ask for help, special efforts may be needed to help them acknowledge these feelings and realize that they, too, have a right to support from others in their pain.

During this time of acute distress, parents face the first task of grief: accepting the reality of the loss. The pregnancy has ended, or the baby has died, and their lives have changed. Although parents are often required to make many decisions such as having an autopsy, naming the infant, and making funeral arrangements, normal functioning is impeded, and decisions are difficult to make. Grandparents, friends, clergy, or other relatives may be available to help the couple cope. However, it is important that the mother and her partner ultimately make the decisions that are right for them.

Phase Two: Searching and Yearning

The phase of intense grief encompasses many difficult emotions as the parents work through their pain and adjust to life without the wished-for child. In the early months after the loss, parents often experience feelings of loneliness, emptiness, and yearning. The mother may report that her arms ache to hold or nurse her baby and that she wakes to the sound of a baby crying. Both the mother and her partner may be preoccupied with thoughts about the wished-for child. Some parents cope with these feelings by avoiding memories and not talking about the baby, whereas others want to reminisce and discuss their loss over and over.

Deciding what to do about the nursery and baby clothes is particularly difficult during this period. Some women want the room taken down before they go home, whereas others want the room left intact until they have had time to grieve their loss. It is not unusual for a grandparent or other family member to want to rush home to take down the nursery, thinking that they would be sparing additional grief. In fact, their actions might only complicate the grief if the parents were not involved in the decision. The bereaved parents must go through these types of experiences in their own time frame so that healing can take place.

During this phase of intense grief, guilt may emerge from the deep feelings of helplessness in not somehow preventing the pregnancy loss or the death of the infant. Mothers are particularly vulnerable to feeling guilt because of their sense of responsibility for the well-being of the fetus and baby. With many perinatal losses, there is no clear cause of the event, leaving the woman to speculate about what she might have done or not done to bring about the loss. Guilt may be intense if the mother thinks she is being punished for some unrelated event, such as having had a prior induced abortion. Many women describe feeling tortured by "self-blame" and they need repeated emotional reassurance that they are not at fault.

Other common responses during this phase are anger, resentment, bitterness, and irritability. Anger may be focused on the health care team who failed to save the pregnancy or infant; toward a God who allowed the loss to occur; or toward family, friends, or peers when they do not provide the support the bereaved parents need and want. Some parents focus their resentment on parents who do not appreciate their children or neglect and abuse them. A sense of bitterness or generalized irritability rather than frank anger may be another response. Physical symptoms of grief may include fatigue, headaches, palpitations, and lack of strength.

During the grief process, fear and anxiety can occur as a profound worry that something else bad might happen to another pregnancy. Some parents, especially mothers, are almost obsessed with the desire to become pregnant again; others struggle with whether they can cope with the possibility of another loss.

Phase Three: Disorientation

Deep sadness and depression can arise when the parent has full awareness of the loss. This often occurs several months after a perinatal loss and can continue for some time. Sadness and depression can be accompanied by disorganization and problems with cognitive processing, memory, and organization. This coupled with insomnia, social withdrawal, and lack of energy leads to behavioural changes, such as difficulty in getting things done, an inability to concentrate, restlessness, confused thought processes, difficulty solving problems, and poor decision making. Disorganization, feelings of failure, and depression often cause difficulties in keeping up with work and family expectations. In addition, parents returning to work face issues such as handling well-meaning but painful comments or the silence of coworkers.

Physical symptoms of grief include fatigue, headaches, dizziness, and altered appetite and exhaustion. Parents are at risk for developing health problems and chronic undefined feelings of illness. It may be difficult to sleep; appetite may be depressed or voracious. Lack of sleep and inadequate nutrition and fluids can complicate other grief responses.

Grief responses are very personal, ongoing, and difficult to handle. Some parents may suppress or deny their feelings because of perceived societal indifference toward pregnancy loss and infant death. On the surface, suppression of feelings may be more socially acceptable. However, denying the pain of grief may lead to eventual physical and emotional distress or illness. Although bereaved parents have many ups and downs for many months and even years after a child's death, few parents actually become mentally ill or commit suicide. Knowing that these feelings are normal and that others have had similar feelings can be helpful to them. The grief process during this phase is often difficult for partners. Some may continue to have difficulty sharing their feelings. A rift can occur if one parent, usually the mother, wants to talk about the loss and pain, and the other parent—often, but not always, the partner—withdraws. Other signs of problems include reliance on alcohol and drugs, extramarital affairs, prolonged hours at work, and over-involvement in activities outside the home as an escape.

Phase Four: Reorganization and Resolution

According to Wilke and Limbo (2012), reorganization and resolution continue beyond 24 months for many parents. From the time of the pregnancy loss or infant death, parents attempt to understand why this happened. This leads to a long and intense search for meaning. At first the "why" is focused on the cause of death, which is often never determined. Finding few good answers, parents next focus on "why me, why mine?" These questions can lead some parents into an existential search about the meaning of life and death. This search continues into the phase of reorganization and may lead to profound changes in the parents' view of the fragility of life.

Time helps to slowly ease the painful feelings of grief. Reorganization occurs when parents are better able to function at home and work, experience a return of self-esteem and confidence, can cope with new challenges, and have placed the loss in perspective. Reorganization begins to peak sometime after the first year, as parents begin to achieve the task of moving on with their lives as they feel renewed energy and a sense of release. Enjoying the simple pleasures of life without feeling guilty, nurturing self and others, developing new interests, and re-establishing relationships are all signs of moving on. For some women and families, another pregnancy and the birth of a subsequent child are important steps in moving on with their lives; however, the term *recovery* is used because the grief related to perinatal loss can continue to varying degrees throughout life.

Parents who have suffered a pregnancy loss or infant death have shared that they will never forget the baby who died and they are not the same people as before the loss (Box 24-6). The term *bittersweet grief* refers to the grief response that occurs with reminders of the loss. This typically happens on birthdays, death days, and anniversaries; at school events; during changes in the seasons; and during the time of the year when the loss occurred. Grief feelings also can be triggered during subsequent pregnancies and after birth.

Resumption of the couple's sexual relationship is an important aspect of recovery but can be very complicated. Many parents are comforted by the belief that their babies were conceived in love, lived in love, and died in love. Their love and intimacy created this child, and parents may believe that they may never experience joy and closeness again. Some couples may have an increased need for sexual activity in an attempt for closeness and healing, whereas others have a decreased desire for sexual intimacy.

BOX 24-6 I AM STRONG

I am strong.

I am strong because at my 38 week OB appointment, I listened to a strong heartbeat and the doctor said everything was great.

I am strong because she told me I was 3 cm dilated and labour could begin at any time.

I am strong because I left the office, completely excited and happy and couldn't wait to be able to meet my new love shortly!

I am strong because the next day at 1130 pm labour and contractions began. They weren't very strong or close together yet at that point.

I am strong because the following morning at 9 am the contractions began to get closer together so I slipped into the tub to relax just a bit.

I am strong because by 930 am contractions became so strong and frequent, I got out of the tub and called the hospital triage.

I am strong because they told me to make my way over to the hospital.

I am strong because, although I was in an amazing amount of pain, and contractions were now just under 2 minutes apart, I was so excited. I had arrived at labour and delivery around 10 am.

I am strong because they took me into the triage room and began the routine.

I am strong because I immediately knew there was a problem when the nurse seemed to be having a hard time locating the heartbeat.

I am strong because she called in the doctor on call who tried to locate a heartbeat also.

I am strong because he gave us the news, news no parent should ever have to hear, "I'm so sorry, but the baby doesn't have a heartbeat."

I am strong because I cried.

I am strong because I then had to make a decision, to deliver my sleeping baby or proceed with a Caesarean section.

I am strong because I choose to continue with the labour and contractions, I wanted to deliver this baby. I am strong because I was planning a VBAC and I wanted it to be that way.

I am strong because I laboured for hours and at 6 pm I delivered my baby.

I am strong because I had a son, a beautiful baby boy, 3500 gm.

I am strong because we named him Matteo.

I am strong because the nurse cleaned up my baby and brought him over to me. I am strong because I had the opportunity to hold, cuddle and kiss my sleeping, stillborn son.

I am strong because I cried.

I am strong because my husband and my daughter were able to hold their baby son and baby brother.

I am strong because my family was able to come and meet my new baby.

I am strong because I knew he wouldn't be coming home.

I am strong because at midnight I had to let him go.

I am strong because I cried.

I am strong because the next day I was discharged and was able to go home. I sobbed as my husband wheeled me out of the room and down the hall.

I am strong because I had to leave the hospital, after a day of labour, contractions, pains and sadness without my baby.

I am strong because I cried.

I am strong because we then had to go about and make arrangements for the baby boy I wasn't able to take home.

I am strong because we chose a spot for him amongst other sleeping babies, he could sleep with them, under a large green tree.

I am strong because I chose a cozy little pajama with elephants for my baby to sleep in and a soft warm blanket for him to snuggle in.

I am strong because I cried.

I am strong because one week later, my husband, daughter, sleeping baby and myself, were allowed to be in a room together for one last time.

I am strong because this is where I held his tiny hand in my fingers, I am strong because I was able to kiss his tiny nose, his perfect lips. I am strong because I spoke to him softly.

I am strong because this is where we had to say goodbye to baby Matteo.

I am strong because I cried.

I am strong because we proceeded to the cemetery where we had a simple, sweet ceremony for our baby.

I am strong because we all cried.

I am strong because I watched as he was buried. I am strong because my sweet baby, my son was buried.

I am strong because I cried.. I cried.. we all cried..

I am strong because I have the hope that we will see our baby Matteo again, soon.

I am strong because I believe he now won't have to live in a world of sin, pain and suffering, and I am strong because I know I will hold and cuddle him again, and he will be safe in my arms.

I am strong because every day I think about him.

I am strong because every day I want him back.

I am strong because I am a mommy of two beautiful children. I am strong because I am only currently a parent to one of them.

I am strong because of my daughter, although only 3 years old, she's strong too.

I am strong because, although every day I may be sad, I am also happy.

I am strong because I am able to cry and I am strong because I am able to smile.

I am strong because of all the blessings I have been given, including my beautiful sleeping baby.

(Used with permission of Author.) VBAC, vaginal birth after caesarean.

Sexuality also brings with it decisions about a future pregnancy. Some couples are eager to have another child, although this child cannot replace the one who died and the grief will continue despite another pregnancy. Other parents have a deep fear of experiencing the pain of loss again, which can make the resumption of sexual activity difficult. These ambivalent feelings are normal, and couples can find themselves moving back and forth between the emotions of exhilaration and fear. The excitement that many other parents experience with a pregnancy is very different for previously bereaved parents. For some, this emotional distress can affect maternal attachment to the new baby. In one study, mothers who became pregnant again within 6 months after a stillbirth had fewer depressive symptoms at a 3-year follow-up than those who did not have a subsequent pregnancy (Surkan, Rådestad, Cnattinguis, et al., 2008).

Couples often mark the progress of the pregnancy in terms of fetal development, waiting anxiously until the number of weeks of the previous loss is passed. In some cases, the fear of repeated loss, especially after a stillbirth, is so great that induction of labour may be considered if the fetus is mature. Support groups are important in helping women through pregnancies after loss of a fetus or infant.

Family Aspects of Grief

Grandparents and Siblings

It is extremely important for the nurse taking care of women who have experienced a loss to keep in mind that they have an entire family to care for, including grandparents and siblings. Grandparents have hopes and dreams for a grandchild; these have been shattered. The grief of grandparents is often complicated by the fact that they are experiencing intense emotional pain by witnessing and feeling the immense grief of their own child. It is extremely difficult to watch their son or daughter experience unimaginable emotional trauma, with very few ways to comfort them and end their pain. As a result, the grief response may be complicated or delayed for grandparents. On occasion, some grandparents experience immense survivor guilt because they are alive and their grandchild has died.

The siblings of the expected infant also experience a profound loss. Most children have been prepared for having another child in the family, once the pregnancy is confirmed. These children's ages and stages of development must be considered in understanding how they view the event and experience the loss. A young child responds more to the response of his or her parents, picking up on the fact that they are behaving differently and are extremely sad. This can cause clinging, altered eating and sleeping patterns, or acting-out behaviours; and it is a time when parents have limited patience for responding to and meeting the needs of the child. Older children have a more complete understanding of the loss. School-age children may be frightened by the entire event, whereas teens may understand fully but feel awkward in responding.

Older siblings need to be included in grieving rituals, to the extent that the parents and the child feel comfortable. They may need to see the baby to realize the loss. Nurses need to have a basic understanding of how children view death and grief in order to reach out to siblings in an appropriate and sensitive manner. Nurses also need to help parents recognize and be sensitive to the grief of siblings, include them in family rituals, and keep the baby alive in the family memory.

NURSING CARE

Nursing care of mothers and partners experiencing a perinatal loss begins the first time they are faced with the potential loss of their pregnancy or death of their infant. Assessment is as important for families experiencing a miscarriage or ectopic pregnancy as it is for those experiencing stillbirth or neonatal loss. Supportive interventions are important at the time of the loss and after the parents have returned home.

Parents often cannot recall details of their experiences at the time of the child's death, but they may recall vividly a minor event that was perceived as particularly painful or particularly helpful. The interventions provided below are general ideas about what may be helpful to parents. However, care must be individualized for each parent and family. Cultural and spiritual beliefs and practices of individual parents and families must also be considered.

Communicating and Caring Techniques

Mothers, partners, and extended families look to the medical and nursing staff for support and understanding during the time of loss. Therapeutic communication and counselling techniques help the mother, partners, and other family members express their feelings and emotions, understand their responses to the loss, and make decisions.

The nurse should listen patiently while people tell their story of loss and grief. It may be necessary to ask questions that help people talk about their grief and the experiences surrounding the loss. However, grief responses in the initial days of crisis make it difficult for individuals to concentrate on what is being asked, think about what a question means, and respond to a question. The use of silence often gives the bereaved person the opportunity to collect thoughts and respond to questions. The nurse should resist the temptation to give advice or use clichés in offering support (Box 24-7).

Nurses need to become comfortable with their own feelings of grief and loss to effectively support and care for the bereaved. It is appropriate to express feelings with the bereaved families and share the moment with them. The nurse might use some of the lines in Box 24-7 in helping the family share and express their grief.

Help Mother, Partners, and Other Family Members Actualize the Loss

When a loss or death occurs, the nurse should be sure that parents have been honestly told about the situation by their primary health care provider or others on the health care team. It is important for their nurse to be with the parents during this time. With early pregnancy loss, it is recommended that the term *miscarriage* be used consistently. With infant death, caregivers should use the words "dead" and "died," rather than "lost" or "gone" to assist the bereaved in accepting this reality. One

BOX 24-7 WHAT TO SAY AND WHAT NOT TO SAY TO BEREAVED PARENTS

What to Say

"I'm sad for you."
"How are you doing with all of this?"
"This must be hard for you."
"What can I do for you?"
"I'm sorry."
"I'm here, and I want to listen."

What Not to Say

"God had a purpose for her."
"Be thankful you have another child."
"The living must go on."
"I know how you feel."
"It's God's will."
"You have to keep on going for her sake."
"You're young; you can have others."
"We'll see you back here next year, and you'll be happier."
"Now you have an angel in heaven."
"This happened for the best."
"Better for this to happen now, before you knew the baby."
"There was something wrong with the baby anyway."

Used with permission of Gundersen Lutheran Medical Foundation, Inc., La Crosse, WI.

way of actualizing the loss is to tell the parents the sex of the baby and give them the option of naming the fetus or help them name an infant who has died. Choosing a name helps make the baby a member of their family, so that the baby can be remembered in a special way.

NURSING ALERT

A caution about naming is important to note. Naming is an individual decision that should never be imposed on parents. Beliefs and needs vary widely across individuals, cultures, and religions. Cultural taboos and rules in some religious faiths prohibit the naming of an infant who has died.

On the basis of vast clinical experience with parents, many professionals believe that seeing the dead fetus or baby helps parents face the reality of the loss, reduces painful fantasies, and offers an opportunity for continued parenting. Many parents relish the memory of parenting their deceased baby by holding, bathing, and dressing him or her. However, parents should never be made to feel that they should see or hold their baby when this is something they do not want to do. It is good policy for the nurse to first tell them about this option and then give them time to think about it. The nurse can ask a question such as "Some parents have found it helpful to see their baby. Would you like time to consider this?" Later the nurse can return and ask each parent individually what he or she has decided. Because the need or willingness to see the child also may vary between the mother and her partner, it is important to determine what each parent really wants. This should not be a joint decision made by one person or a decision made for the parents by grandparents or others.

In preparation for the visit with the baby, parents appreciate explanations about what to expect. A description of how their baby looks is important. For example, babies may have red, peeling skin like a bad sunburn, dark discolouration similar to bruises, moulding of the head that makes the head look soft and swollen, or birth defects. The nurse should make the baby look as normal as possible and remember that parents see their baby with different eyes from those of health care professionals. Bathing the baby, applying lotion to the baby's skin, combing hair, placing identification bracelets on the arm and leg, dressing the baby in a diaper and special outfit, sprinkling powder in the baby's blanket, and wrapping the baby in a pretty blanket conveys to the parents that their baby has been cared for in a special way. Many parents participate in these activities. If the baby has been in the morgue, he or she can be placed underneath a warmer for 20 to 30 minutes and wrapped in a warm blanket before being brought to the parents. Cold cream rubbed over stiffened joints can help in positioning the baby. The use of powder and lotion stimulates the parents' senses and can help provide pleasant memories of their baby.

When bringing the baby to the parents, it is important to treat the baby as one would a live baby. Holding the baby close, touching a hand or cheek, using the baby's name, and talking with the parents about the special features of their baby convey that it is all right for them to do likewise. If a baby has a congenital anomaly, the nurse can focus on aspects of the baby that are normal. Nurses can help parents explore the baby's body as they desire. Parents often seek to identify family resemblance. A good question might be: "Who in your family does your baby resemble?"

Some families may like to have the opportunity to bathe and dress their baby. Although the skin may be fragile, parents can still apply lotion with cotton balls; sprinkle powder; tie ribbons; fasten the diaper; and place amulets, medallions, rosaries, or special toys or mementos in their baby's hands or next to their baby. Volunteer women in communities across the country often make special burial clothes to give parents at this difficult time. Parents may want to perform other parenting activities, such as combing the baby's hair, dressing the baby in a special outfit, wrapping the baby in a blanket, or placing the baby in a crib.

Parents need to be offered time alone with their baby if they wish. They also need to know when the nurse will return and how to call if they should need anything. If at all possible, the family should be placed in a private room, and the room should have a rocking chair for the parents to sit in when holding their baby. This offers the mother and partner special time together with their baby and with other family members (Fig. 24-10). Marking the door to the room with a special card can be helpful in reminding staff that this family has experienced a loss (Fig. 24-11).

Sensitivity to parental needs in actualizing the loss and coping with the reality of the death is essential for their healing. Grandparents should be offered the same opportunities to hold,

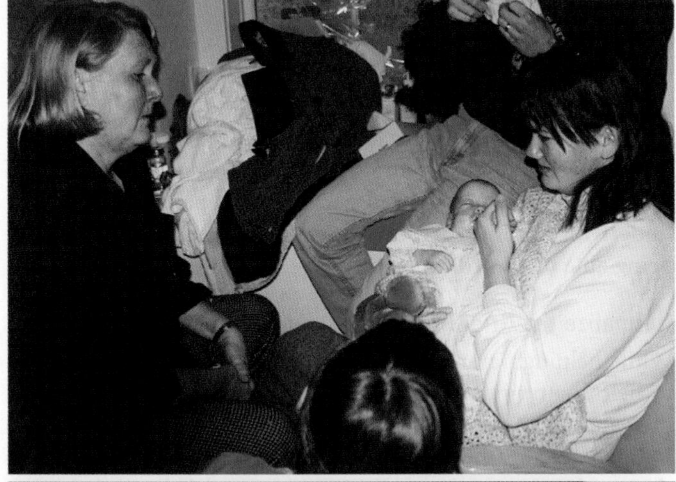

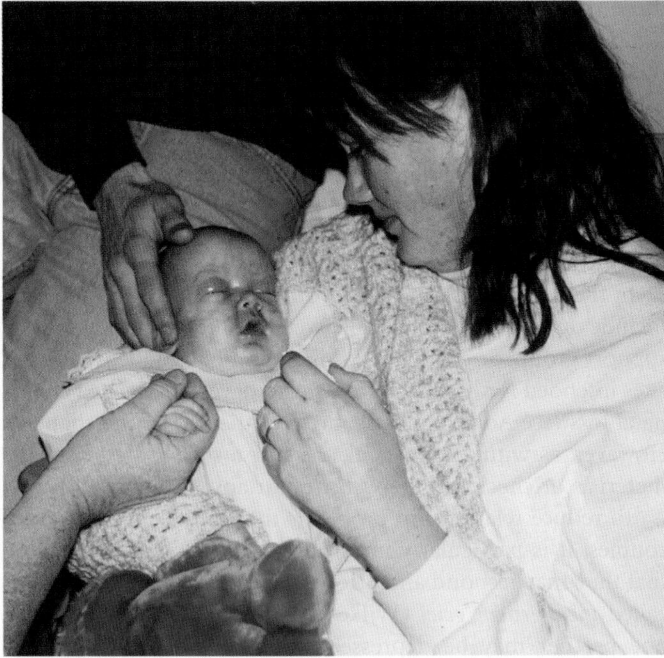

FIGURE 24-10 Laura's family members say a special good-bye. (Courtesy Amy and Ken Turner, Cary, NC.)

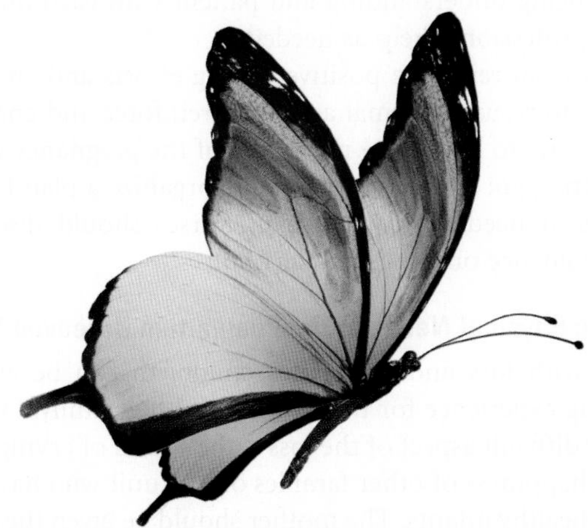

FIGURE 24-11 Door card for room of mother who has experienced perinatal loss. (suns07butterfly/Shutterstock.com.)

rock, swaddle, and love their grandchildren so that their grief is started in a healthy way.

Help Parents With Decision Making

At a time when parents are experiencing the great distress of a perinatal loss, and especially if the loss was of an infant, these parents have many decisions to make. Mothers, partners, and extended families look to the medical and nursing staff for guidance in knowing what decisions they must and can make and in understanding the options related to those decisions. It is a primary responsibility of the nurse to help them and to advocate for them, because decisions made during the time of their loss will provide memories for a lifetime.

One decision might be related to conducting an autopsy. An autopsy can be very important in answering the question "why" if there is a chance that the cause of death can be determined. This information can be helpful in processing grief and perhaps in preventing another loss. Some parents may believe that their baby has been through enough and prefer not to have further information about the cause of death. Some religions prohibit autopsy or limit the choice to instances in which autopsy may help prevent another loss. Options for the type of autopsy, such as excluding the head, should be made available to parents. Parents may need time to make this decision. There is no need to rush them unless there was evidence of contagious disease or maternal infection at the time of death.

Organ donation can be an aid to grieving and an opportunity for the family to see something positive associated with their experience. The most common donation is of corneas; donation of corneas from a baby can occur if the baby was born alive at 36 weeks of gestation or later.

Another important decision relates to spiritual rituals that may be helpful and important to parents. Support from clergy is an option that should be offered to all parents. Parents may wish to have their own pastor, priest, rabbi, or spiritual leader contacted; or they may wish to see the hospital's chaplain. They may choose to do neither. Clergy persons may offer the parents the opportunity for baptism, when appropriate. Other rituals that may be important include a blessing, a naming ceremony, anointing, ritual of the sick, memorial service, or prayer.

One of the major decisions that parents must make has to do with disposition of the body. Parents should be given information about the choices for the final disposition of their baby, regardless of gestational age. However, nurses must be aware of cultural and spiritual beliefs that may dictate the choices of parents, as well as the cost of burial, alternatives to burial, and provincial laws related to burial. A fetus younger than 20 weeks of gestation that weighs less than 500 g is considered a miscarriage; embryos, uterine tubes removed with an ectopic pregnancy, and tissue from a pregnancy obtained during a D&C are all considered tissue. Many hospitals will make arrangements for the cremation of these fetuses or tissue. The nurse should know the hospital's policies and procedures about burial and cremation and answer the parents' questions honestly. In Canada, if a fetus is greater than or equal to 20 weeks of gestational age or is born alive, it is the parents' responsibility to make the final arrangements for their baby.

LEGAL TIP ***LAWS REGARDING LIVE BIRTH***

Laws in all provinces govern what constitutes a live birth. In most provinces, a live birth is considered to be any products of conception expelled from a woman that show any signs of life. Signs of life are considered to be any muscle irritability, respiratory effort, or heart rate, regardless of gestational age. All nurses should be knowledgeable about the provincial laws regarding what constitutes a live birth and the forms that must be completed and filed in the case of fetal death, stillbirth, or newborn death.

In making final arrangements for their baby, parents may want a special service. They may choose to have a service in the hospital chapel, visitation at a funeral home or their own home, a funeral service, or a graveside service. Parents can make any of these services as special, personal, and memorable as they like. They can choose special music, poetry, or prose written by themselves or others.

The timing for actions such as naming the baby, seeing and holding the baby, creating mementos (e.g., pictures and footprint moulds), disposition of the body, and funeral arrangements should never be rushed. In some cases, the mother may be discharged home before these decisions are made. Then the family can think about them in the comfort of their home and contact the hospital in the following days to give their answers.

Help Bereaved to Acknowledge and Express Feelings

One of the most important goals of the nurse is to validate the experience and feelings of the parents, by encouraging them to tell their stories and by listening with care. Because nurses tend to be very focused on the physical and emotional needs of the mother, it is especially important to ask the partner directly about his or her views of what happened and the feelings of loss.

Bereaved parents have many questions surrounding the event of their loss, and some questions can leave them feeling guilty. This is particularly true for mothers. Such questions include "What did I do?" "What caused this to happen?" "What do you think I should have, could have done?" Part of the grief process for bereaved parents is figuring out what happened, their role in the loss, why it happened to them, and why it happened to their baby. The nurse should recognize that these questions must be answered by the bereaved themselves; it is part of their healing. For example, a bereaved mother might ask, "Do you think that this was caused by painting the baby's room?" An appropriate response might be, "I understand you need to find an answer for why your baby died, but we really don't know why she died. What are some of the other things you have been thinking about?" Trying to give bereaved parents answers when there are no clear answers or trying to squelch their guilt feelings by telling them they should not feel guilty does not help them process their grief. In reality, many times there are no definite answers to the question of why this terrible thing has happened to them. However, factual information such as data about the frequency of miscarriages in pregnant women or the fact that there usually is no clear cause of a stillbirth can be helpful.

Feelings of anger, guilt, and sadness can occur immediately but often become more problematic in the early days and months after a loss. When a bereaved person expresses feelings of anger, it can be helpful to identify the feeling by simply saying, "You sound angry," or "You look angry." The nurse's willingness to sit down and listen to these surface feelings of anger can help the bereaved person move past them into the underlying feelings of powerlessness and helplessness in not being able to control the many aspects of the situation.

Normalize the Grief Process and Facilitate Positive Coping

While helping parents share their feelings of pain, it is critical to help them understand their grief responses and know that they are not alone in these painful responses. Most parents are not prepared for the raw feelings they experience or the fact that these painful, complex feelings and related behavioural reactions continue for many weeks or months. Thus, reassuring them of the normality of their responses and preparing them for the length of their grief is important.

The nurse can help the parent be prepared for the emptiness, loneliness, and yearning; for the feelings of helplessness that can lead to anger, guilt, and fear; and for the disorganization, difficulty making decisions, and sadness and depression that are part of the grief process.

In the initial days after a loss, other useful nursing strategies include follow-up phone calls, referrals to a perinatal grief support group, or providing books, pamphlets, videos, or websites intended for helping parents who have experienced a perinatal loss (see Additional Resources at the end of the chapter). However, as with any referral, the nurse should first read the materials or check out the websites for applicability.

To reduce relationship problems that can occur in grieving couples, it is particularly important to help them understand that they may respond and grieve in very different ways. This is called *incongruent grief* (Wilke & Limbo, 2012). For example, one partner may be depressed and have no energy and be unable to work, while the other partner may cope by going back to work and working long hours. The differences in grieving can lead to serious relationship problems and be a risk factor for complicated bereavement. Remind the couple of the importance of being understanding and patient with each other and seeking professional help as needed.

Nurses can reinforce positive coping efforts and encourage attempts to resume normal activities; reinforce and encourage positive ways to hold onto memories of the pregnancy or baby while letting go; and help the parents organize a plan for daily activities, if needed. In particular, nurses should discourage overdependence on drugs and alcohol.

Meet the Physical Needs of the Postpartum Bereaved Mother

Coping with loss and grief after childbirth can be an overwhelming experience for the woman and her family. One particularly difficult aspect of the loss is the sound of crying babies and the happiness of other families on the unit who have given birth to healthy infants. The mother should be given the opportunity to decide if she wants to remain on the maternity unit or be moved to another hospital unit. She also should be helped to understand the pluses and minuses of each choice. Postpartum care and grief support may not be as good on another hospital unit where the staff are not experienced in postpartum and bereavement care.

The physical needs of a bereaved mother are the same as those of any woman who has given birth. The cruel reality for many bereaved mothers is that their milk can come in with no baby to nurse, their afterpains remind them of their emptiness, and gas pains feel as though a baby is still moving inside. The nurse should ensure that the mother receives appropriate medications to reduce these physical symptoms. Adequate rest, diet, and fluids must be offered to replenish her physical strength.

Mothers need postpartum care instructions on discharge. They also need ideas about how to cope with sleep problems, such as decreasing food or fluids that contain caffeine, limiting alcohol and nicotine consumption, exercising regularly, using strategies for rest, taking a warm bath or drinking warm milk before bedtime, doing relaxation exercises, listening to restful music, or a getting a massage. Furthermore, the couple needs to be encouraged and supported in maintaining their relationship and keeping open channels of communication. They also need to be prepared for some of the issues related to resuming sexual relations after perinatal loss.

Create Memories for Parents to Take Home

Parents may want tangible mementos of their baby to help them actualize the loss. Some may want to bring in a previously purchased baby book. Special memory books, cards, and information on grief and mourning are often available to give to parents (Fig. 24-12).

The nurse can provide information about the baby's weight, length, and head circumference to the family. Footprints and handprints can be taken and placed with the other information on a special card or in a memory or baby book. Sometimes it is difficult to obtain good handprints or footprints. Application of alcohol or acetone on the palms or soles can help the ink adhere to make the prints clearer, especially for small babies. When making prints, it is helpful to have a hard surface underneath the paper to be printed. The baby's heel or palm should be placed down first and the foot or hand rolled forward, keeping the toes or fingers extended. It may be helpful to have assistance in this procedure. If the print does not turn out, the nurse can trace around the baby's hands and feet, although this distorts the actual size. Moulds can also be used to make an imprint of the baby's hand or foot.

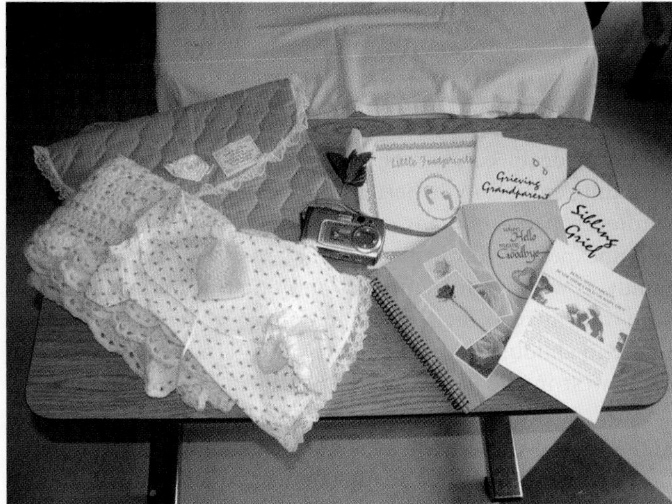

FIGURE 24-12 Memory kit assembled at John C. Lincoln Hospital, Phoenix, AZ. Memory kits may include pictures of the infant, clothing, death certificate, footprints, ID bands, and ultrasound picture. (Courtesy Julie Perry Nelson.)

Parents often appreciate articles that were in contact with or used in caring for the baby. This might include the tape measure used to measure the baby, baby lotions, combs, clothing, hats, blankets, crib cards, and identification bands. The identification band helps the parents remember the size of the baby and personalizes the mementos. The nurse should ask parents if they wish to have these articles. A lock of hair may be another important keepsake. Parents must be asked for permission before cutting a lock of hair, which can be removed from the nape of the neck where it is not noticeable.

For some parents, pictures are the most important memento. Photographs are generally taken whenever there is an identifiable baby and when it is culturally acceptable to the family to take photos. It does not matter how tiny the baby is, what the baby looks like, or how long the baby has been dead. Pictures should include close-ups of the baby's face, hands, and feet and photos of the baby clothed and wrapped in a blanket and unclothed. If there are any congenital anomalies, close-ups of these also should be taken. Flowers, blocks, stuffed animals, or toys can be placed in the background to make the picture more special. Parents may want their pictures taken holding the baby. Keeping a camera nearby and taking pictures when parents are spending special time with their baby can provide special memories. Some parents may have their own camera, video camera, or smartphone and ask the nurse to record them as they bathe, dress, hold, or diaper their baby. An organization called Now I Lay Me Down to Sleep provides a professional photographer to take pictures for families at no cost. Their website can be consulted to determine if there is a photographer within the geographical location.

Cultural and Spiritual Needs of Parents

Many of the responses to perinatal loss and suggested interventions described in this section are based on middle-class European-American views. Although there may be no particular differences in individual, intrapersonal experiences of grief based on culture, ethnicity, or religions, there are complex differences in the meaning of children and parenthood, the role of women and men, the beliefs and knowledge about modern medicine, views about death, mourning rituals and traditions, and behavioural expressions of grief. Thus, nurses must be sensitive to the responses and needs of parents from various cultural backgrounds and religious groups. Nurses need to be aware of their own values and beliefs and acknowledge the importance of understanding and accepting the values and beliefs of others that are different or even in conflict with theirs. Further, it is critical to understand that the individual and unique responses of parents to a perinatal loss cannot be entirely predicted by their cultural or spiritual backgrounds. Each mother and partner must be approached first as an individual needing support during a profoundly difficult and distressing life experience.

Provide Postmortem Care

Preparation of the baby's body and transport to the morgue depend on the procedures and protocols developed by individual hospitals. Nurses should use a sensitive and respectful approach when taking the fetus or infant to the morgue. Postmortem care can be an emotional and sometimes difficult task for the nurse. Nurses and organizations are encouraged to facilitate perinatal bereavement training for all involved in perinatal loss (see Additional Resources at the end of the chapter). Nurses may experience compassion fatigue and are encouraged to seek assistance in the form of debriefs, support from colleagues, and seeking professional guidance when needed.

Documentation

Many hospitals have a checklist that is used in providing care, mobilizing members of the multidisciplinary health care team, communicating options that the family has chosen, and keeping track of all the details in meeting the needs of bereaved parents. The checklist may or may not be a permanent part of the chart. Documentation in the nursing notes of primary concerns, grief responses, health teaching, health care advice, and referrals of the mother or any other family members is essential to ensure continuity and consistency of care.

Provide Sensitive Care at and After Discharge

Leaving the hospital can be a devastating experience for the mother who has had a pregnancy loss, as not carrying a baby in her arms is a very empty and painful experience. It is especially difficult if others are seen leaving with babies; thus, the discharge of mothers and partners who have suffered a perinatal loss should be done with great sensitivity to their feelings (i.e., they should not be discharged at a time when other mothers with live babies are leaving). Giving the mother a special flower to carry in her arms can be a thoughtful gesture.

The grief of the mother and her family does not end with discharge; it really begins once they return home, attend the funeral, and start to live their lives without their baby. There are numerous models for providing follow-up care to parents after discharge. Although there is no solid evidence from sound clinical trials regarding the benefit of these programs, nonexperimental studies and clinical evaluations suggest that these programs are helpful. Such programs include hospital-based bereavement teams who provide support during hospitalization and follow-up contacts and memorial services.

Phone calls from hospital staff after a loss may be helpful to some parents; however, it must be determined which parents do not want them. Follow-up calls let the parents know that someone still thinks and cares about them. The calls are made at predictably difficult times, such as the first week at home, 1 month to 6 weeks later, 4 to 6 months after the loss, and at the anniversary of the death. Families who have experienced a miscarriage, ectopic pregnancy, or death of a preterm baby may appreciate a phone call on the estimated due date. Such calls provide an opportunity for parents to ask questions, share their feelings, seek advice, and receive information to help them process their grief.

A grief conference can be planned when parents return for an appointment with their doctor, nurses, and other health care providers. At the conference, the loss or death of the infant is discussed in detail, parents are given information about the baby's autopsy report and genetic studies, and they have the opportunity to ask questions that have arisen since their baby's death. Parents appreciate the opportunity to review the events of hospitalization, go over the baby's and mother's chart with their primary health care provider, and talk with those who cared for them and their baby during hospitalization. This is an important time to help parents understand the cause of the loss or accept the fact that the cause will forever be unknown. This meeting also gives health care providers the opportunity to assess how the family is coping with their loss and to offer additional information and education on grief.

Some parents are very interested in finding a perinatal or parent grief support group. Talking with others who have been through similar experiences, sharing memories of the pregnancy and the baby, and gaining an understanding of the normality of the grief process generally have been found to be supportive. Over time, it may be the only place where bereaved parents can talk about the wished-for child and their grief. However, not all parents find such groups helpful.

When referring parents to a group, it is important to know something about the group and how it operates. For example, if a group has a religious base for their interventions, a nonreligious parent would not likely find the group to be helpful. If parents experiencing a perinatal loss are referred to a general parental grief group, they might feel overwhelmed with the grief of parents whose older children have died of cancer, suicide, or homicide. In addition, the grief of parents following a perinatal loss might be minimized by other parents. Thus, the needs of the parents must be matched with the focus of the group.

MATERNAL DEATH

Maternal death can be caused by a variety of complications, including embolism, hypertension, hemorrhage, infection, and cardiomyopathy. In many cases, the death of a mother is sudden and unexpected. Any instance of maternal death is tragic for the family as well as for the nurses and other health professionals who were involved in her care. In Canada it is rare for a woman to die in childbirth; the incidence of maternal deaths is one of the lowest in the world: in 2010–2011 it was 6.1 per 100,000 (PHAC, 2013).

When a woman dies of a complication related to childbearing, the husband or partner and extended family are faced with mourning the death of a wife or partner and mother. The loss and grief are greatly compounded when there is also the death of a fetus or neonate. When the infant survives, the husband or partner is faced with parenting a baby without a surviving mother. The responsibilities of infant care can be overwhelming during this time of intense loss and grief.

Because most maternal deaths are unexpected, the grief that follows a maternal death is sudden. This differs from anticipatory grief in which the loss is expected, such as with cancer. The shock and disbelief associated with unplanned grief can be engulfing and debilitating, overwhelming the normal coping abilities and creating difficulties with everyday functioning and decision making.

Nurses and other health care professionals working with families who experience maternal loss need to consider the context and the implications of the maternal death for the remaining family members. Young parents may never have experienced a significant personal loss or tragedy; in many cases, their parents and grandparents are still living. Cultural beliefs and customs surrounding death can influence a family's response to maternal death (Hill, 2012). The grief response of each family member will vary; grief is an individual response, and the grieving process does not always proceed in a predictable manner.

Families who experience maternal loss are at risk for developing complicated bereavement and altered parenting of the surviving infant and other children in the family. A referral to social services to help the family mobilize support systems and for counselling can help combat potential problems before they develop and can be beneficial not only at the time of the loss but also in the future. Follow-up care for grieving families is essential as they progress through the stages of grief and adjust to life without the mother.

The emotional toll that a maternal death can take on the nursing and medical staff must also be addressed. Guilt, anger, fear, sadness, and depression are all common responses to a maternal death. The staff may want to participate in a debriefing session in which they can review the situation surrounding the events, their participation in caring for the mother, and their response to the death. Attending memorial or funeral services may benefit staff and family. Follow-up conferences with a social worker or grief counsellor can help staff members work through their grief.

KEY POINTS

- PPH is the most common and most serious type of excessive obstetrical blood loss.
- Hemorrhagic (hypovolemic) shock is an emergency situation in which the perfusion of body organs may become severely compromised and death may ensue.
- The potential hazards of therapeutic interventions can further compromise the woman with hemorrhagic disorders.
- Postpartum infection is a major cause of maternal morbidity and mortality throughout the world.
- Postpartum UTIs are common during the postpartum period.
- Breast infection affects about 1% of women soon after childbirth.
- Structural disorders of the uterus and vagina related to pelvic relaxation are often the delayed but direct result of child-bearing.
- Perinatal mood disorders (PMD) account for most mental health disorders in the postpartum period.
- Suicidal thoughts or attempts are among the most serious symptoms of postpartum psychosis.
- Treatment of PMD requires a combination of medication, education, supportive measures, and psychotherapy.
- Antidepressant medications are the usual treatment for PMD; however, specific precautions are needed for breastfeeding women.
- An understanding of grief responses and the bereavement process is fundamental in implementation of the nursing process.
- Therapeutic communication and counselling techniques can help families identify their feelings and feel comfortable in expressing their grief.
- Follow-up after discharge is an essential component to providing care to families who have experienced a loss.
- Nurses need to be aware of their own feelings of grief and loss to provide a nonjudgemental environment of care and support for bereaved families.

evolve WEBSITE

***Visit the Evolve website for additional resources related to the content in this chapter such as Case Studies, Critical Thinking Case Study Answers, Nursing Care Plans, Nursing Processes, Nursing Skills, and Review Questions for Exam Preparation at:** http://evolve.elsevier.com/Canada/Perry/maternal/*

REFERENCES

American Association of Women, Obstetrical and Neonatal Nurses (AWHONN). (2015). Quantification of blood loss: AWHONN practice brief number 1. *Journal of Obstetric, Gynecologic, & Neonatal Nursing, 44*, 158–160.

American College of Obstetricians and Gynecologists, Committee on Obstetric Practice. *Committee opinion: Screening for perinatal depression.* (2015). Retrieved from: <http://www.beststart.org/resources/hlthy_chld_dev/BSRC_Daddy_and_Me_EN.pdf>.

American Psychiatric Association. (2013). *Diagnostic and statistical manual of mental disorders* (5th ed.). Washington, DC: American Psychiatric Association Press.

Beydoun, H. A., Beydoun, M. A., Kaufman, J. S., et al. (2012). Intimate partner violence against adult women and its association with major depressive disorder, depressive symptoms and postpartum depression: A systematic review and meta-analysis. *Social Science and Medicine, 75*(6), 959–975.

Blom, E. A., Jansen, P. W., Verhulst, F. C., et al. (2010). Perinatal complications increase the risk of postpartum depression: The Generation R study. *BJOG: An International Journal of Obstetrics and Gynaecology, 117*(11), 1390–1398.

Callister, L. C., Beckstrand, R. L., & Corbett, C. (2011). Postpartum depression and help-seeking behaviors in immigrant Hispanic women. *Journal of Obstetrics, Gynecology, and Neonatal Nursing, 40*(4), 440–449.

Cerulli, C., Talbor, N. L., Tang, W., et al. (2011). Co-occurring intimate partner violence and mental health diagnoses in perinatal women. *Journal of Women's Health, 20*(12), 1797–1803.

Chan, W., Rey, E., Kent, N. E., & SOGC VTE in Pregnancy Guideline Working Group. (2014). SOGC clinical practice guideline: Venous thromboembolism and antithrombotic therapy in pregnancy. *Journal of Obstetrics and Gynaecology of Canada, 36*(6), 527–553.

Cunningham, F., Leveno, K., Bloom, S., et al. (2014). *Williams obstetrics* (24th ed.). New York: McGraw Hill.

Davey, H. L., Tough, S. C., Adair, C. E., et al. (2011). Risk factors for sub-clinical and major postpartum depression among a community cohort of Canadian women. *Maternal and Child Health Journal, 15*(7), 866–875.

Della Torre, M., Kilpatrick, S. J., Hibbard, J. U., et al. (2011). Assessing preventability for obstetric hemorrhage. *American Journal of Perinatology, 28*(10), 753–760.

Dennis, C. (2010). Postpartum depression peer support: Maternal perceptions from a randomized controlled trial. *International Journal of Nursing Studies, 47*, 560–568.

Dennis, C. (2014). Psychosocial interventions for the treatment of perinatal depression. *Best Practice & Research Clinical Obstetrics & Gynecology, 28*, 97–111.

Dumoulin, C., & Hay-Smith, E. (2010). Pelvic floor muscle training versus no treatment, or inactive control treatments, for urinary incontinence in women. *Cochrane Database of Systematic Reviews 2010*, (1), CD005654.

Forray, A., Focseneanu, M., Pittman, B., et al. (2010). Onset and exacerbation of obsessive-compulsive disorder in pregnancy and the postpartum period. *Journal of Clinical Psychiatry, 71*(8), 1061–1068.

Francois, K. E., & Foley, M. R. (2012). Antepartum and postpartum hemorrhage. In S. G. Gabbe, J. R. Niebyl, & J. L. Simpson (Eds.), *Obstetrics: Normal and problem pregnancies* (6th ed.). New York: Saunders.

Garcia, K. S., Flynn, P., Pierce, K. J., et al. (2010). Repetitive transcranial magnetic stimulation treats postpartum depression. *Brain Stimulation, 3*, 36–41.

Gilbert, E. (2011). *Manual of high risk pregnancy & delivery* (5th ed.). St. Louis: Mosby.

Goyal, D., Wang, E. J., Shen, J., et al. (2012). Clinically identified postpartum depression in Asian American women. *Journal of Obstetrics, Gynecology, and Neonatal Nursing, 41*(3), 408–416.

Hadley, D. E., Albanese, W. P., & Rochester, C. D. (2012). Psychiatric drug interactions explored: From the literature to clinical practicality. *Pharmacy Practice News*. Retrieved from <www.pharmacypracticenews.com/download/ppn0212_ER_WM.pdf>.

Hale, T. (2012). *Medications and mother's milk* (15th ed.). Amarillo, TX: Pharmasoft.

Hill, P. E. (2012). Support and counseling after maternal death. *Seminars in Perinatology, 36*(1), 84–88.

Katz, V. (2012). Postpartum care. In S. G. Gabbe, J. R. Niebyl, J. L. Simpson, et al. (Eds.), *Obstetrics: Normal and problem pregnancies* (6th ed.). Philadelphia: Saunders.

Kendall-Tackett, K., & Hale, T. W. (2010). Review: The use of antidepressants in pregnant and breastfeeding women: A review of recent studies. *Journal of Human Lactation, 26*(2), 187–195.

Lawrence, R. A., & Lawrence, R. M. (2011). *Breastfeeding: A guide for the medical profession* (7th ed.). St. Louis: Mosby.

Lazarus, R., & Gutteridge, K. (2013). Post-natal psychiatric disorders. In S. E. Robson & J. Wough (Eds.), *Medical disorders in pregnancy: A manual for midwives*. Boston: Wiley Blackwell.

Le Strat, Y., Dubertret, C., & Le Foll, B. (2011). Prevalence and correlates of major depressive episode in pregnant and postpartum women in the United States. *Journal of Affective Disorders, 135*(1–3), 128–138.

Letourneau, N., Tryphonopoulos, P. D., Duffett-Leger, L., et al. (2012). Support intervention needs and preferences of fathers affected by postpartum depression. *Journal of Perinatal and Neonatal Nursing, 26*(1), 69–80.

Logsdon, M. C., Tomasulo, R., Eckert, D., et al. (2012). Identification of mothers at risk for postpartum depression by hospital-based perinatal nurses. *MCN: The American Journal of Maternal Child Nursing, 37*(4), 218–225.

McCarthy, M., & McMahon, C. (2008). Acceptance and experience of treatment for postnatal depression in a community mental health setting. *Health Care for Women International, 29*(6), 618–637.

More[OB]. (2010). *Postpartum hemorrhage*. Retrieved from <http://www.Moreob.com>.

Paulson, J. F., & Bazemore, S. D. (2010). Prenatal and postpartum depression in fathers and its association with maternal depression: A meta-analysis. *JAMA: The Journal of the American Medical Association, 303*(19), 1961–1969. doi:10.1001/jama.2010.605.

Pettker, C. M., & Lockwood, C. J. (2012). Thromboembolic disorders. In S. G. Gabbe, J. R. Niebyl, & J. L. Simpson (Eds.), *Obstetrics: Normal and problem pregnancies* (6th ed.). New York: Saunders.

Public Health Agency of Canada. (2013). *Perinatal health indicators for Canada 2013: A report of the Canadian Perinatal Surveillance System*. Cat. No. HP7-1/2013E-PDF. Ottawa: Author.

Registered Nurses' Association of Ontario. (2005). *Interventions for postpartum depression*. Toronto: Author. Retrieved from <http://rnao.ca/sites/rnao-ca/files/Interventions_for_Postpartum_Depression.pdf>.

Royal College of Obstetricians and Gynaecologists. (2009). *Reducing the risk of thrombosis and embolism during pregnancy and the puerperium (Green-top guideline No. 37a)*. London: Author. Retrieved from <http://www.rcog.org.uk/womens-health/clinical-guidance/reducing-risk-of-thrombosis-greentop37a>.

Sadock, B., Sadock, V., & Ruiz, P. (2009). *Kaplan & Sadock's comprehensive textbook of psychiatry* (9th ed., Vol. 2). Philadelphia: Lippincott Williams & Wilkins.

Senikas, V., Leduc, D., Lalonde, A., et al. (2009). SOGC clinical practice guideline: Active management of the third stage of labour: Prevention and treatment of postpartum hemorrhage. *Journal of Obstetrics and Gynaecology of Canada, 31*(10), 980–993.

Sharma, V., Burt, V., & Ritchie, H. (2009). Bipolar II postpartum depression: Detection, diagnosis, and treatment. *American Journal of Psychiatry, 166*(11), 1201–1204.

Society of Obstetricians and Gynaecologists of Canada. (2014). *Advances in labour and risk management (ALARM) course syllabus* (21st ed.). Ottawa: Author.

Speisman, B. B., Storch, E. A., & Abramowitz, J. S. (2011). Postpartum obsessive-compulsive disorder. *Journal of Obstetrics, Gynecology, and Neonatal Nursing, 40*(6), 680–690.

Sung, V., & Hampton, B. (2009). Epidemiology of pelvic floor dysfunction. *Obstetrics and Gynecology Clinics of North America, 36*(3), 421–443.

Sung, V., West, D., Hernandez, A., et al. (2009). Association between urinary incontinence and depressive symptoms in overweight and obese women. *American Journal of Obstetrics and Gynecology, 200*(5), 557.e1–e5.

Surkan, P. J., Rådestad, I., Cnattinguis, S., et al. (2008). Events after stillbirth in relation to maternal depressive symptoms: A brief report. *Birth (Berkeley, Calif.), 35*(2), 153–157.

Sword, W., Busser, D., Ganann, R., et al. (2008). Women's care-seeking experiences after referral for postpartum depression. *Qualitative Health Research, 18*(9), 1161–1173.

Tarnay, C., & Bhatia, N. (2010). Genitourinary dysfunction: Pelvic organ prolapse, urinary incontinence, and infection. In N. Hacker, J. Gambone, & C. Hobel (Eds.), *Hacker and Moore's essentials of obstetrics and gynecology* (5th ed.). Philadelphia: Saunders.

van Schalkwyk, J., Van Eyk, N., Yudin, M., et al. (2010). SOGC clinical practice guideline: Antibiotic prophylaxis in obstetric procedures. *Journal of Obstetrics and Gynaecology Canada, 32*(9), 878–884.

Vigod, S. N., Villegas, L., Dennis, C. L., et al. (2010). Prevalence and risk factors for postpartum depression among women with preterm and low-birth-weight infants: A systematic review. *British Journal of Obstetrics and Gynecology*, *117*(5), 540–550.

Wallner, L., Porten, S., Meenan, R., et al. (2009). Prevalence and severity of undiagnosed urinary incontinence in women. *American Journal of Medicine*, *122*(11), 1037–1042.

Wilke, J., & Limbo, R. (2012). *Resolve through training: Gundersen Health System. Bereavement training in perinatal death* (8th ed.). LaCrosse, WI: Gundersen Lutheran Medical Foundation Inc.

Woolhouse, H., Gartland, D., Hegarty, K., et al. (2012). Depressive symptoms and intimate partner violence in the 12 months after childbirth: A prospective pregnancy cohort study. *British Journal of Obstetrics and Gynecology*, *119*(3), 315–323.

Yonkers, K. A., Vigod, S., & Ross, L. E. (2011). Diagnosis, pathophysiology and management of mood disorders in pregnant and postpartum women. *Obstetrics and Gynecology*, *117*(4), 961–977.

ADDITIONAL RESOURCES

ACOG Depression and Postpartum: Depression Resource Overview: <http://www.acog.org/Womens-Health/Depression-and-Postpartum-Depression>.

AWHONN Postpartum Hemorrhage Project: <http://www.pphproject.org/resources.asp>.

AWHONN Quantification of Blood Loss: <https://www.youtube.com/watch?v=F_ac-aCbEn0&list=UUPrOhL3Od7ZeFDq27ycS00g>.

Bereaved Families of Ontario: <http://www.bereavedfamilies.net/>.

Edinburgh Postnatal Depression scale in different languages: <http://www.rikshandboken-bhv.se/Dokument/Edingburgh%20Depression%20Scale%20Translated%20Gov%20Western%20Australia%20Dept%20Health.pdf>.

Pacific Post Partum Support Society: <http://www.postpartum.org>.

Peel Postpartum Mood Disorder Program: <http://www.pmdinpeel.ca>.

Perinatal Bereavement Documentaries: <http://www.bereavementdocumentaries.ca/>.

Registered Nurses' Association of Ontario—Interventions for Postpartum Depression: <http://rnao.ca/bpg/guidelines/interventions-postpartum-depression>.

UNIT 7

Newborn

CHAPTER

25

Physiological Adaptations of the Newborn

Pat O'Flaherty

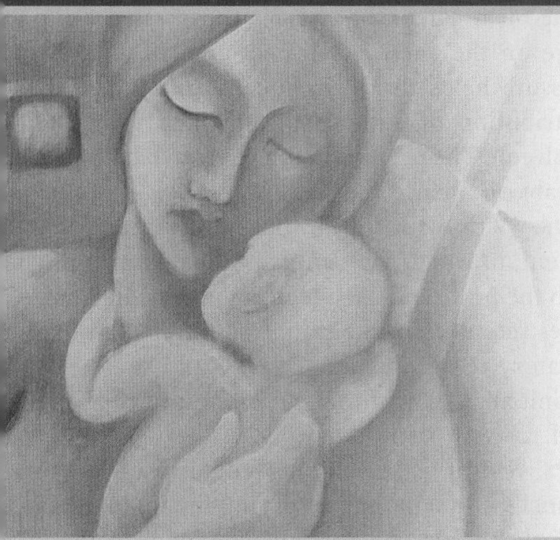

evolve WEBSITE

Visit the Evolve website for additional resources related to the content in this chapter such as Case Studies, Critical Thinking Case Study Answers, Nursing Care Plans, Nursing Processes, Nursing Skills, and Review Questions for Exam Preparation at: *http://evolve.elsevier.com/Canada/Perry/maternal/*

OBJECTIVES

On completion of this chapter the reader will be able to:

- Describe the physiological adaptations the newborn must make during the period of transition from intrauterine to extrauterine environment.
- Describe the behavioural adaptations that are characteristic of the newborn during the transition period.
- Explain the mechanisms of thermoregulation in the newborn and the potential consequences of hypothermia and hyperthermia.
- Recognize newborn reflexes and differential characteristic responses from abnormal responses.
- Discuss the sensory and perceptual function of the newborn.
- Identify signs that the newborn is at risk related to problems with each body system.

The newborn period includes the time from birth through day 28 of life. During this time, the newborn must make many physiological and behavioural adaptations to extrauterine life. Tasks of physiological adjustment are those that involve (1) establishing and maintaining respirations; (2) adjusting to circulatory changes; (3) regulating temperature; (4) ingesting, retaining, and digesting nutrients; (5) eliminating waste; and (6) regulating weight. Behavioural tasks include (1) establishing a regulated behavioural tempo independent of the mother, which involves self-regulating arousal, self-monitoring changes in state, and patterning sleep; (2) processing, storing, and organizing multiple stimuli; and (3) establishing a relationship with caregivers and the environment. The term newborn usually makes these adjustments with little or no difficulty.

TRANSITION TO EXTRAUTERINE LIFE

The major adaptations associated with transition from intrauterine to extrauterine life occur during the first 6 to 8 hours after birth. The predictable series of events during transition are mediated by the sympathetic nervous system and result in changes that involve heart rate, respirations, temperature, and gastrointestinal function. This transition period represents a time of vulnerability for the newborn and warrants careful observation by nurses. To detect disorders in adaptation soon after birth, nurses must be aware of normal features of the transition period.

In their classic work on newborn adaptation to extrauterine life, Desmond, Rudolph, and Phitaksphraiwan (1966) proposed three stages termed the *transition period.* The stages are still considered valid today.

The first phase of the transition period lasts up to 30 minutes after birth and is called the *first period of reactivity.* The newborn's heart rate increases rapidly to 160 to 180 beats per minute (bpm) but gradually falls by 30 minutes of age to a baseline rate between 100 and 160 bpm. Respirations may be irregular, with variation in the rate between 60 and 80 breaths/min. Fine crackles may be present on auscultation; audible grunting, nasal flaring, and retractions of the chest may also be noted, but these should resolve within the first hour of birth. The infant is alert and may have spontaneous startles, tremors, crying, and movement of the head from side to side. Bowel sounds are audible, and meconium may be passed.

After the first period of reactivity, the newborn either sleeps or has a marked decrease in motor activity. This *period of decreased responsiveness* lasts from 60 to 100 minutes. During this time the infant is pink and respirations may be rapid and shallow (up to 60 breaths/min) but not laboured.

The *second period of reactivity* occurs roughly between 2 and 8 hours after birth and lasts from 10 minutes to several hours. Brief periods of tachycardia and tachypnea occur, associated with increased muscle tone, skin colour changes, and mucus production. Meconium is commonly passed during this phase. Most healthy newborns experience this transition regardless of type of birth; very preterm infants do not because of physiological immaturity.

PHYSIOLOGICAL ADJUSTMENTS

Respiratory System

When the umbilical cord is clamped, the newborn undergoes rapid and complex physiological changes. The most critical and immediate adjustment is the establishment of respirations. Most newborns breathe spontaneously after birth and are able to maintain adequate oxygenation. Preterm infants often encounter respiratory difficulties related to immaturity of the lungs and gestational age.

Initiation of Breathing

During intrauterine life oxygenation of the fetus occurs through transplacental gas exchange. However, at birth the lungs must be established as the site of gas exchange. In utero, fetal blood was shunted away from the lungs, but when birth occurs the pulmonary vasculature must be fully perfused for this purpose. Clamping the umbilical cord causes a rise in blood pressure (BP), which increases circulation and lung perfusion.

It has been recognized that there is no single trigger for newborn respiratory function. The initiation of respirations in the newborn is the result of a combination of chemical, mechanical, thermal, and sensory factors.

Chemical factors. The activation of chemoreceptors in the carotid arteries and aorta results from the relative state of hypoxia associated with labour. With each labour contraction there is a temporary decrease in uterine blood flow and transplacental gas exchange, resulting in transient fetal hypoxia and hypercarbia. Although the fetus is able to recover between contractions, there appears to be a cumulative effect that results in progressive decline in Po_2, increased Pco_2, and lowered blood pH. Decreased levels of oxygen and increased levels of carbon dioxide are involved in initiating newborn breathing by stimulating the respiratory centre in the medulla. Another chemical factor may also play a role: it is thought that, as a result of clamping the cord, there is a drop in levels of a prostaglandin that can inhibit respirations.

Mechanical factors. Respirations in the newborn can be stimulated by changes in intrathoracic pressure resulting from compression of the chest during vaginal birth. As the infant passes through the birth canal, the chest is compressed. With birth this pressure on the chest is released, and the negative intrathoracic pressure helps draw air into the lungs. Crying increases the distribution of air in the lungs and promotes expansion of the alveoli. The positive pressure created by crying helps to keep the alveoli open.

Thermal factors. With birth the newborn enters the extrauterine environment, in which the temperature is significantly lower. Exposure to the profound change in environmental temperature stimulates receptors in the skin, resulting in stimulation of the respiratory centre in the medulla. Cold stress may be important for initializing breathing but prolonged exposure should be avoided.

Sensory factors. Sensory stimulation occurs in a variety of ways with birth, such as in handling or drying the infant. Pain associated with birth can also be a factor. The lights, sounds, and smells of the new environment can also be involved in stimulation of the respiratory centre.

At term the lungs hold approximately 20 mL of fluid per kilogram. Air must be substituted for the fluid that filled the fetal respiratory tract. Previously it had been thought that the thoracic squeeze occurring during normal vaginal birth resulted in significant clearance of lung fluid, but now it appears that this event plays a minor role. In the days preceding labour there is reduced production of fetal lung fluid and concomitant decreased alveolar fluid volume. Shortly before the onset of labour there is a catecholamine surge that appears to promote fluid clearance from the lungs, which continues during labour (Goldsmith, 2011). The movement of lung fluid from the air spaces takes place through active transport into the interstitium, with drainage occurring through the pulmonary circulation and lymphatic system. Retention of lung fluid can interfere with the infant's ability to maintain adequate oxygenation, especially if other factors (e.g., meconium aspiration, congenital diaphragmatic hernia, esophageal atresia with fistula, choanal atresia, congenital cardiac defect, immature alveoli) that compromise respirations are present. Infants born by Caesarean when labour did not occur before birth can experience some lung fluid retention, although it typically clears without deleterious effects on the infant. These infants are also more likely to develop **transient tachypnea of the newborn (TTNB)** caused by the lower levels of catecholamines (Abu-Shaweesh, 2011).

The alveoli of the term infant's lungs are lined with two types of alveolar epithelium, named alveolar type I and type II cells. Type I alveolar cells comprise approximately 95% of the alveolar surface, with type II alveolar cells making up the remaining 5%. The type II cells make and produce surfactant, a group of phospholipids that reduce the alveolar surface tension. Subsequently, with lower surface tension the pressure required to keep the alveoli open with inspiration is reduced, which prevents total alveolar collapse on exhalation, thereby maintaining alveolar stability. The decreased surface tension results in increased lung compliance, helping to establish the functional residual capacity of the lungs. With absent or decreased surfactant, more pressure must be generated for inspiration, which can soon tire or exhaust preterm or sick term infants.

Breathing movements that began in utero as intermittent become continuous after birth, although the mechanism for this is not well understood. Once respirations are established, breaths are shallow and irregular, ranging from 30 to 60 breaths/min, with periods of breathing that include pauses in respirations lasting less than 20 seconds. These episodes of periodic breathing occur most often during the active (rapid eye movement [REM]) sleep cycle and decrease in frequency and duration with age. Apneic periods longer than 20 seconds indicate a pathological process and should be evaluated.

! NURSING ALERT

Newborn infants are by preference nose breathers. The reflex response to nasal obstruction is to open the mouth to maintain an airway. This response is not present in most infants until 3 weeks after birth; therefore, cyanosis or asphyxia can occur with nasal blockage or stenosis and requires immediate intervention to support adequate ventilation and oxygenation.

In most newborn infants auscultation of the chest reveals loud, clear breath sounds that seem very near because little chest tissue intervenes. Breath sounds should be clear and equal bilaterally. The ribs of the infant articulate with the spine at a horizontal rather than a downward slope; consequently, the rib cage cannot expand with inspiration as readily as that of an adult. Because newborn respiratory function is largely a matter of diaphragmatic contraction, abdominal breathing is characteristic of infants. The newborn infant's chest and abdomen rise simultaneously with inspiration. Characteristics of the respiratory system of the newborn and the effects of these characteristics on respiratory function are listed in Table 25-1.

Signs of Respiratory Distress

Signs of respiratory distress may include nasal flaring, intercostal or subcostal retractions (i.e., drawing in of tissue between the ribs, or below the rib cage), or grunting with respirations. Suprasternal or subclavicular retractions with stridor or gasping most often represent an upper airway obstruction (Askin, 2009a). Seesaw or paradoxical respirations (exaggerated rise in abdomen, with respiration, as chest falls) instead of abdominal respirations are abnormal and should be reported. A respiratory rate less than 30 or greater than 60 breaths/min with the infant at rest must be carefully evaluated. The respiratory rate can be negatively influenced (slowed, depressed, or absent) by analgesics or anaesthetics administered to the mother during birth. Apneic episodes may be related to a number of events (rapid increase in body temperature, hypothermia, hypoglycemia, and sepsis) that require careful evaluation. Tachypnea may result from inadequate clearance of lung fluid, or it may be an indication of newborn respiratory distress due to sepsis, pneumonia, or surfactant deficiency. Respiratory scoring may be done to evaluate the degree of respiratory distress (ACoRN Editorial Board, 2012) and is helpful in evaluating the degree of respiratory insufficiency.

Changes in the infant's colour can indicate respiratory distress. Acrocyanosis, the bluish discolouration of hands and feet, is a normal finding in the first 7 to 10 days after birth (Fig. 25-1). Transient periods of duskiness while crying are not uncommon immediately after birth; however, central cyanosis is abnormal and signifies hypoxemia. With central cyanosis the lips and mucous membranes are bluish. It can be the result of inadequate delivery of oxygen to the alveoli, poor perfusion of the lungs that inhibits gas exchange, or cardiac dysfunction. Because central cyanosis is a late sign of distress, newborns usually have significant hypoxemia when cyanosis appears (Askin, 2009b).

Infants who experience mild TTNB often have signs of respiratory distress during the first 1 to 2 hours after birth as they transition to extrauterine life. Tachypnea with rates up to 100

TABLE 25-1 CHARACTERISTICS OF THE RESPIRATORY SYSTEM OF THE NEWBORN

CHARACTERISTIC	EFFECT ON FUNCTION
Immature alveoli; decreased size and number of alveoli	Risk of respiratory insufficiency, inadequate oxygenation and ventilation
Thicker alveolar wall; decreased alveolar surface area	Less efficient gas transport and exchange; poor alveolar compliance
Continued development of alveoli until childhood	Possible opportunity to reduce effects of chronic lung disease
Decreased lung elastic tissue and recoil	Decreased lung compliance requiring higher pressures and more work to expand; increased risk of atelectasis
Reduced diaphragm movement and maximal force potential	Less effective respiratory movement; difficulty generating negative intrathoracic pressures; risk of atelectasis
Tendency to nose breathe; altered position of larynx and epiglottis	Enhanced ability to synchronize swallowing and breathing; risk of airway obstruction; possibly more difficult to intubate
Small compliant airway passages with higher airway resistance; immature reflexes	Risk of airway obstruction and apnea
Increased pulmonary vascular resistance with sensitive pulmonary arterioles	Risk of ductal shunting and hypoxemia with events such as hypoxia, acidosis, hypothermia, hypoglycemia, and hypercarbia
Increased oxygen consumption	Increased respiratory rate and work of breathing; risk of hypoxia; risk of retinopathy of prematurity
Increased intrapulmonary right–left shunting	Increased risk of atelectasis with ineffective ventilation; risk of persistent pulmonary hypertension; lower P_{CO_2}
Immaturity of pulmonary surfactant system in immature infants	Increased risk of atelectasis and respiratory distress syndrome; increased work of breathing
Immature respiratory control	Irregular respirations with periodic breathing; risk of apnea; inability to rapidly alter depth of respirations

P_{CO_2}, partial pressure of carbon dioxide.
From Blackburn, S. (2013). *Maternal, fetal, and neonatal physiology: A clinical perspective* (4th ed.). St. Louis: Saunders. P. 338, Table 10–12, Adapted from Blackburn, S. (1992). Alterations in the respiratory system in the neonate: Implications for practice. *J Perinat Neonatal Nurs* 6, 46.

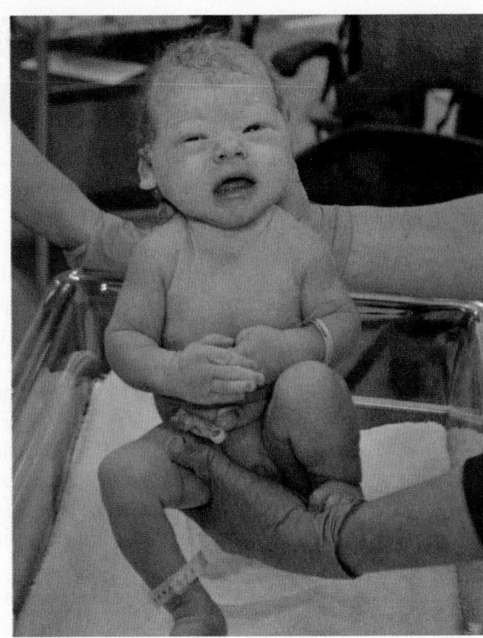

FIGURE 25-1 Newborn infant with acrocyanosis of upper and lower extremities. (Courtesy Barbara Wilson.)

breaths/min can be present along with intermittent grunting, nasal flaring, and mild retractions. Supplemental oxygen or noninvasive ventilator support may be needed.

In newborns with more serious respiratory problems, symptoms of distress are more pronounced and tend to last beyond the first 2 hours after birth. Respiratory rates can exceed 120 breaths/min. Moderate-to-severe retractions, grunting, pallor, and central cyanosis can occur. The respiratory symptoms can be accompanied by hypotension, temperature instability, hypoglycemia, acidosis, and signs of cardiac problems. Common respiratory complications affecting newborns include respiratory distress syndrome (RDS), meconium aspiration, pneumonia, and persistent pulmonary hypertension of the newborn (PPHN) (Askin, 2009b) (see Chapters 28 and 29).

Cardiovascular System

The cardiovascular system changes significantly after birth. The infant's first breaths, combined with increased alveolar capillary distension, inflate the lungs and reduce pulmonary vascular resistance to pulmonary blood flow from the pulmonary arteries. Pulmonary artery pressure drops, and pressure in the right atrium declines. Increased pulmonary blood flow from the left side of the heart increases pressure in the left atrium, which causes a functional closure of the foramen ovale (see Chapter 47). During the first few days of life, crying may temporarily reverse the flow through the foramen ovale and lead to mild cyanosis.

In utero, fetal Po_2 is 20–30 mm Hg. After birth, when the Po_2 level in the arterial blood approximates 50 mm Hg, the ductus arteriosus constricts in response to increased oxygenation. Circulating hormone prostaglandin (PGE_2) levels also have an important role in closure of the ductus arteriosus. In term infants it functionally closes within the first hours after birth; permanent closure usually occurs within 3 to 4 weeks, and the ductus arteriosus becomes a ligament. The ductus arteriosus can open in response to low oxygen levels in association with hypoxia, asphyxia, or prematurity. With auscultation of the chest a patent ductus arteriosus can be detected as a heart murmur.

The umbilical vein and arteries constrict rapidly within the first 2 minutes after birth. It is thought that this is related to exposure of the cord to the cooler extrauterine environment and to increased oxygenation as the infant begins to breathe. With the clamping and severing of the cord, the umbilical arteries, the umbilical vein, and the ductus venosus are functionally closed; they are converted into ligaments within 2 to 3 months. The hypogastric arteries also occlude and become ligaments. Table 25-2 summarizes the cardiovascular changes at birth.

Heart Rate and Sounds

The newborn heart rate averages 110 to 160 bpm at birth, with variations noted during sleep and wake states. The range of the heart rate in the term infant can be as low as 90 to 100 bpm during deep sleep and can increase to 180 bpm or higher when the infant cries. A heart rate that is either high (more than 160 bpm) or low (fewer than 110 bpm) should be re-evaluated within 30 minutes to 1 hour or when the activity of the infant changes. Immediately after birth the heart rate can be palpated by grasping the base of the umbilical cord.

The apical impulse (point of maximal impulse [PMI]) in the newborn is at the fourth intercostal space and to the left of the midclavicular line. The PMI is often visible and easily palpable because of the thin chest wall; this is also called *precordial activity*.

Apical pulse rates should be obtained on all newborn infants. Auscultation should be for a full minute, preferably when asleep. An irregular heart rate in newborns is not uncommon in the first few hours of life. After this time, an irregular heart rate not attributed to changes in activity or respiratory pattern should be further evaluated. Heart sounds during the newborn period are of higher pitch, shorter duration, and greater intensity than during adult life. The first sound (S_1) is typically louder and duller than the second sound (S_2), which is sharp. The third and fourth heart sounds are not auscultated in newborns. Most heart murmurs heard during infancy have no pathological significance, and more than half of the murmurs disappear by 6 months. However, the presence of a murmur and accompanying signs such as poor feeding, apnea, cyanosis, or pallor is considered abnormal and should be further investigated. There can be significant cardiac defects without symptoms in the early newborn period. This reinforces the importance of ongoing assessment (Sadowski, 2015).

Blood Pressure (BP)

Values for newborn BP vary with gestational age and weight. The term newborn infant's average systolic BP is 60 to 80 mm Hg, and average diastolic BP is 40 to 50 mm Hg. The number of weeks of gestation can be used as a guide for the mean arterial pressure (MAP). While not exact, it is a useful guide; for example, an infant born at 40 weeks of gestation

TABLE 25-2 CARDIOVASCULAR CHANGES AT BIRTH

PRENATAL STATUS	POSTBIRTH STATUS	ASSOCIATED FACTORS
Primary Changes		
Pulmonary Circulation		
High pulmonary vascular resistance, increased pressure in right ventricle and pulmonary arteries	Low pulmonary vascular resistance; decreased pressure in right atrium, ventricle, and pulmonary arteries	Expansion of collapsed fetal lung with air; assume responsibility for adequate gas exchange
Systemic Circulation		
Low pressures in left atrium, ventricle, and aorta	High systemic vascular resistance; increased pressure in left atrium, ventricle, and aorta	Loss of placental blood flow
Secondary Changes		
Umbilical Arteries		
Patent, carrying of blood from hypogastric arteries to placenta	Functionally closed at birth; obliteration by fibrous proliferation possibly taking 2 to 3 months, distal portions becoming lateral vesicoumbilical ligaments, proximal portions remaining open as superior vesicle arteries	Closure preceding that of umbilical vein, probably accomplished by smooth muscle contraction in response to thermal and mechanical stimuli and alteration in oxygen tension Mechanically severed with cord at birth
Umbilical Vein		
Patent, carrying of blood from placenta to ductus venosus and liver	Closed; becoming ligamentum teres hepatis after obliteration	Closure shortly after umbilical arteries; hence blood from placenta possibly entering newborn for short period after birth Mechanically severed with cord at birth
Ductus Venosus		
Patent, connection of umbilical vein to inferior vena cava	Closed; becoming ligamentum venosum after obliteration	Loss of blood flow from umbilical vein
Ductus Arteriosus		
Patent, shunting of blood from pulmonary artery to descending aorta	Functionally closed almost immediately after birth; anatomical obliteration of lumen by fibrous proliferation requiring 1 to 3 months, becoming ligamentum arteriosum	Increased oxygen content of blood in ductus arteriosus creating vasospasm of its muscular wall High systemic resistance increasing aortic pressure; low pulmonary resistance reducing pulmonary arterial pressure
Foramen Ovale		
Formation of a valve opening that allows blood to flow directly to left atrium (shunting of blood from right to left atrium)	Functionally closed at birth; constant apposition gradually leading to fusion and permanent closure within a few months or years in most persons	Increased pressure in left atrium and decreased pressure in right atrium, causing closure of valve over foramen

Data from Blackburn, S. (2013). *Maternal, fetal, and neonatal physiology: A clinical perspective* (4th ed.). St. Louis: Saunders.

should have a MAP of at least 40. The BP increases by the second day of life, with minor variations noted during the first month of life. A drop in systolic BP (about 15 mm Hg) in the first hour of life is common. Crying and movement usually cause increases in the systolic BP. The measurement of BP is best accomplished with an oscillometric device while the infant is at rest. A correctly sized cuff with proper placement must be used for accurate measurement of an infant's BP.

Unless there is a specific indication, BP is not routinely measured in the healthy newborn. In the presence of cardiovascular symptoms such as tachycardia, murmur, abnormal pulses, poor perfusion, or abnormal precordial activity, four extremity BP and preductal and postductal oxygen saturation levels may be taken. If the systolic pressure is more than 10 mm Hg higher in the upper extremities than in the lower extremities, further diagnostic testing may be needed (Kenney, Hoover, Williams, et al., 2011).

Blood Volume

Blood volume in the newborn is about 80 to 100 mL/kg of body weight. Immediately after birth, the total blood volume averages 300 mL, but this volume can increase by as much as 100 mL, depending on the length of time to cord clamping and cutting. The infant born prematurely has a relatively greater blood volume than the term newborn because the preterm infant has a proportionately greater plasma volume, not a greater red blood cell (RBC) mass.

Early or delayed clamping of the cord changes circulatory dynamics of the newborn. Late clamping expands the blood volume from the so-called placental transfusion of blood to the newborn. Delayed cord clamping (≥2 minutes after birth) has been reported to have some advantages in healthy term infants, such as higher birth weight, improved hematocrit and iron status, and decreased anemia; such benefits can last up to 6 months (Andersson, Lindquist, Lindgren, et al., 2015; Arca,

Botet, Palacio, et al., 2010; McDonald, Middleton, Dowswell, et al., 2013). Delayed cord clamping has also been associated with improved fine motor skills at 4 years of age (Andersson et al., 2015). Polycythemia that occurs with delayed clamping is usually not harmful, although there can be an increased risk of jaundice that requires phototherapy.

Signs of Cardiovascular Problems

Close monitoring of the newborn's vital signs is important for early detection of impending problems. Persistent tachycardia (more than 160 bpm) can be associated with anemia, hypovolemia, hyperthermia, or sepsis. Persistent bradycardia (less than 100 bpm) can be a sign of a congenital heart block, hypoxemia, normal sinus bradycardia, or hypothermia.

The newborn's skin colour can reflect cardiovascular problems. Pallor in the immediate postbirth period is often symptomatic of underlying problems such as anemia or marked peripheral vasoconstriction as a result of intrapartum asphyxia, difficult assisted delivery, or sepsis. Any central or prolonged cyanosis can indicate respiratory or cardiac problems and requires immediate investigation and evaluation.

Congenital heart defects are the most common type of congenital malformations (see Chapter 47). Although the more serious defects of cyanotic heart defects, such as transposition of the great arteries, tricuspid atresia, and tetralogy of Fallot, are likely to have clinical manifestations such as cyanosis, dyspnea, and hypoxia, others, such as small ventricular septal defects, can be asymptomatic. The prenatal history can provide information regarding risk factors for congenital heart defects, alerting the nurse to watch for symptoms. Maternal illness such as rubella, metabolic disease such as diabetes, and drug ingestion are associated with an increased risk of cardiac defects.

Hematopoietic System

The hematopoietic system of the newborn exhibits certain variations from that of the adult. Levels of RBCs and leukocytes differ, but platelet levels are relatively the same.

Red Blood Cells and Hemoglobin

Because fetal circulation is less efficient at oxygen exchange than the lungs, the fetus needs additional RBCs for transport of oxygen in utero. Therefore, at birth, the average levels of RBCs and hemoglobin (fetal hemoglobin is predominant) are higher than those in the adult; these levels fall slowly over the first month. At birth the RBC count ranges from 4.8 to 7.1×10^{12}/L (Blackburn, 2013). The term newborn can have a hemoglobin concentration of 137 to 201 g/L at birth, decreasing gradually to 120 to 200 g/L during the first 2 weeks (Pagana, Pagana, & MacDonald, 2013). Hematocrit levels at birth range from 0.51 to 0.56, increase slightly in the first few hours or days as fluid shifts from intravascular to interstitial spaces (Blackburn, 2013), and by 8 weeks are between 0.39 and 0.59 (Pagana et al., 2013). Polycythemia (central venous hematocrit greater than 65%) can occur in term and preterm infants as a result of delayed cord clamping, maternal hypertension or diabetes, or intrauterine growth restriction.

The source of the sample is a significant factor in levels of RBCs, hemoglobin, and hematocrit because capillary blood yields higher values than venous blood. The timing of blood sampling is also significant; the slight rise in RBCs after birth is followed by a substantial drop. At birth, the infant's blood contains an average of 70% fetal hemoglobin, but because of the shorter lifespan of the cells containing fetal hemoglobin, the percentage falls to 55% by 5 weeks and to 5% by 20 weeks. Iron stores generally are sufficient to sustain normal RBC production for 4 to 5 months in the term infant, at which time a transient physiological anemia can occur.

Leukocytes

Leukocytosis, with a white blood cell (WBC) count of approximately 18×10^9/L (range 9 to 30×10^9/L), is normal at birth (Pagana et al., 2013). The number of WBCs increases to 23 to 24×10^9/L during the first day after birth. The initial high WBC count of the newborn decreases rapidly, and a stable level of 12×10^9/L is normally maintained during the newborn period. Serious infection is not well tolerated by the newborn; leukocytes are slow to recognize foreign protein and to localize and fight infection early in life. Sepsis may be accompanied by a concomitant rise in granulocytes (neutrophilia); however, some infants may initially be seen with clinical signs of sepsis without a significant elevation in WBCs. In addition, events other than infection—prolonged crying, maternal hypertension, asymptomatic hypoglycemia, hemolytic disease, meconium aspiration syndrome, labour induction with oxytocin, surgery, difficult labour, high altitude, and maternal fever—may cause neutrophilia in the newborn (Weinberg & Powell, 2011).

Platelets

Platelet count ranges between 150 and 300×10^9/L and is essentially the same in newborns as in adults (Pagana et al., 2013). The levels of factors II, VII, IX, and X, found in the liver, are decreased during the first few days of life because the newborn cannot synthesize vitamin K. However, bleeding tendencies in the newborn are uncommon, and unless the vitamin K deficiency is great, clotting is sufficient to prevent hemorrhage.

Blood Groups

The infant's blood group is genetically determined and established early in fetal life. However, during the neonatal period, there is a gradual increase in the strength of the agglutinogens present in the RBC membrane. Cord blood samples may be used to identify the infant's blood type and Rh status. This is of particular significance when evaluating the infant presenting with hyperbilirubinemia or identifying the at-risk infant antenatally.

Thermogenic System

Next to establishing respiration and adequate circulation, heat regulation is most critical to the newborn's survival. During the first 12 hours after birth the infant attempts to achieve thermal balance in adjusting to the extrauterine environmental temperature. **Thermoregulation** is the maintenance of balance between heat loss and heat production. Newborns attempt to stabilize their core body temperatures within a narrow range. Hypothermia from excessive heat loss is a common and dangerous problem in newborns.

Anatomical and physiological characteristics of newborns place them at risk for heat loss. Infants have a thin layer of subcutaneous fat. The blood vessels are close to the surface of the skin.

Changes in environmental temperature alter the temperature of the blood, thereby influencing temperature regulation centres in the hypothalamus. Newborns have larger body surface–to–body weight (mass) ratios than do children and adults (Blackburn, 2013).

Heat Loss

The body temperature of newborn infants depends on the heat transfer between the infant and the external environment. Factors that influence heat loss to the environment include the temperature and humidity of the air, the flow and velocity of the air, and the temperature of surfaces in contact with and around the infant. The goal of care is to maintain a neutral thermal environment for the newborn in which heat balance is maintained. The neutral thermal environment is the ideal environmental temperature that allows the infant to maintain a normal body temperature to minimize oxygen and glucose consumption. Heat loss in the newborn occurs by four modes (Fig. 25-2):

1. Convection is the flow of heat from the body surface to cooler ambient air. Because of heat loss by convection, the ambient temperature in the nursery is kept at approximately 24°C and newborns in open bassinets are wrapped to protect them from the cold. A cap may be worn to decrease heat loss from the infant's head.
2. Radiation is the loss of heat from the body surface to a cooler solid surface not in direct contact but in relative proximity. To prevent this type of loss, cribs and examining tables are placed away from outside windows and care providers need to avoid exposing the infant to direct air drafts.
3. Evaporation is the loss of heat that occurs when a liquid is converted to a vapour. In the newborn, heat loss by evaporation occurs as a result of vaporization of moisture from the skin. This heat loss is intensified by failing to dry the newborn directly after birth or by drying the infant too slowly after a bath. The less mature the newborn, the more severe the evaporative heat loss. Evaporative heat loss, as a component of insensible water loss, is the most significant cause of heat loss in the first few days of life.
4. Conduction is the loss of heat from the body surface to cooler surfaces in direct contact. The scales used for weighing the newborn should have a protective cover to minimize conductive heat loss.

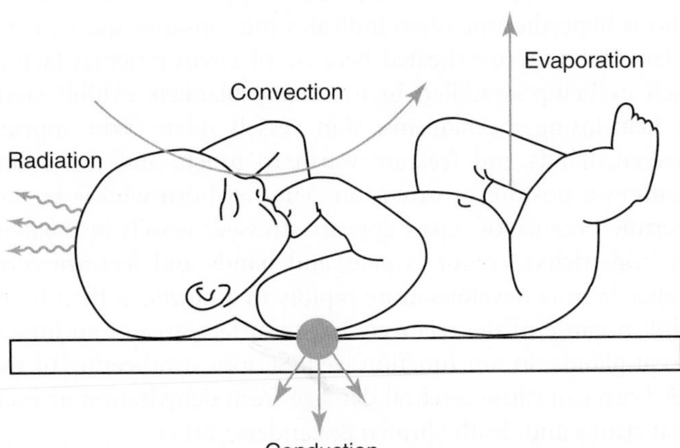

FIGURE 25-2 Heat loss in the newborn occurs in four ways: convection, radiation, evaporation, and conduction. (From WHO [1997]. *Safe motherhood: Thermal protection of the newborn, a practical guide.* Retrieved from http://apps.who.int/iris/bitstream/10665/63986/1/WHO_RHT_MSM_97.2.pdf.)

Skin-to-Skin Contact

Loss of heat must be controlled to protect the infant. Control of such modes of heat loss is the basis of caregiving policies and techniques. One method for promoting maternal–newborn interaction is to place the naked, healthy dried newborn next to the mother's skin and to cover both with a blanket (Fig. 25-3). This skin-to-skin contact reduces conductive and radiant heat loss and enhances newborn temperature control and maternal–infant interaction. Newborns who are placed skin-to-skin remain warmer than newborns held swaddled in their mother's arms. If the mother is unavailable, then the father or another significant person in the room could hold the newborn skin-to-skin.

Thermogenesis

In response to cold the newborn attempts to generate heat (thermogenesis) by increasing muscle activity. Cold infants

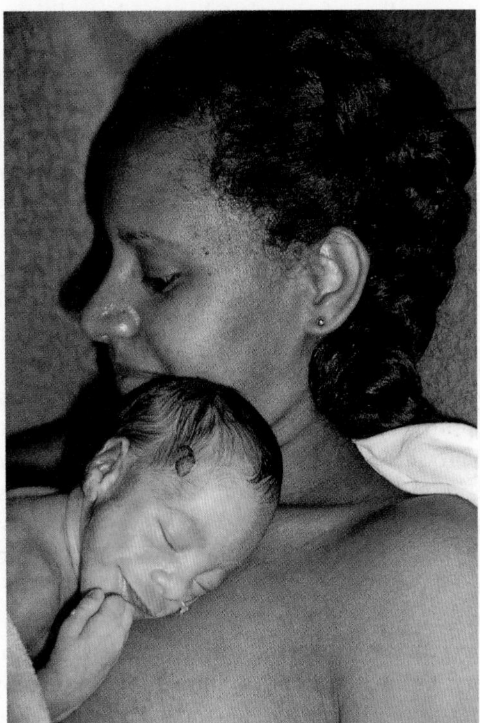

FIGURE 25-3 Infant in skin-to-skin contact with mother. (Courtesy Cheryl Briggs, BSN, RNC-NIC.)

may cry and appear restless. Because of vasoconstriction the skin can feel cool to touch, and acrocyanosis can be present. There is an increase in cellular metabolic activity, primarily in the brain, heart, and liver; this also increases oxygen and glucose consumption.

In an effort to conserve heat, term newborns assume a position of flexion that helps guard against heat loss because it diminishes the amount of body surface exposed to the environment. Infants also can reduce the loss of internal heat through the body surface by constricting peripheral blood vessels.

Adults are able to produce heat through shivering; however, the shivering mechanism of heat production is rarely operable in the newborn unless there is prolonged cold exposure (Blackburn, 2013). Newborns produce heat through **nonshivering thermogenesis**. This is accomplished primarily by metabolism of **brown fat**, which is unique to the newborn, and secondarily by increased metabolic activity in the brain, heart, and liver. Brown fat is located in superficial deposits in the interscapular region and axillae and in deep deposits at the thoracic inlet, along the vertebral column, and around the kidneys. Brown fat has a richer vascular and nerve supply than ordinary fat. Heat produced by intense lipid metabolic activity in brown fat can warm the newborn by increasing heat production as much as 100%. Reserves of brown fat, usually present for several weeks after birth, are rapidly depleted with cold stress. The amount of brown fat reserve increases with the weeks of gestation. A full-term newborn has greater stores than those of a preterm infant.

Cold Stress

Cold stress imposes metabolic and physiological demands on all infants, regardless of gestational age and condition. The respiratory rate increases in response to the increased need for oxygen. In the cold-stressed infant oxygen consumption and energy are diverted from maintaining normal brain and cardiac function and growth to thermogenesis for survival. If the infant cannot maintain an adequate oxygen tension, vasoconstriction follows and jeopardizes pulmonary perfusion. As a consequence the Po_2 is decreased, and the blood pH drops. These changes can prompt a transient respiratory distress or aggravate existing RDS. Moreover, decreased pulmonary perfusion and oxygen tension can maintain or reopen the right-to-left shunt across the ductus arteriosus.

The basal metabolic rate increases with cold stress. If cold stress is protracted, anaerobic glycolysis occurs, resulting in increased production of acids. Metabolic acidosis develops, and, if an alteration in respiratory function is present, respiratory acidosis also develops (Fig. 25-4). Excessive fatty acids can displace the bilirubin from the albumin-binding sites and exacerbate hyperbilirubinemia.

Hypoglycemia is another metabolic consequence of cold stress. The process of anaerobic glycolysis uses approximately three to four times the amount of blood glucose, thereby depleting existing stores. If the infant is sufficiently stressed and low glucose stores are not replaced, hypoglycemia, which can be asymptomatic in the newborn, can develop.

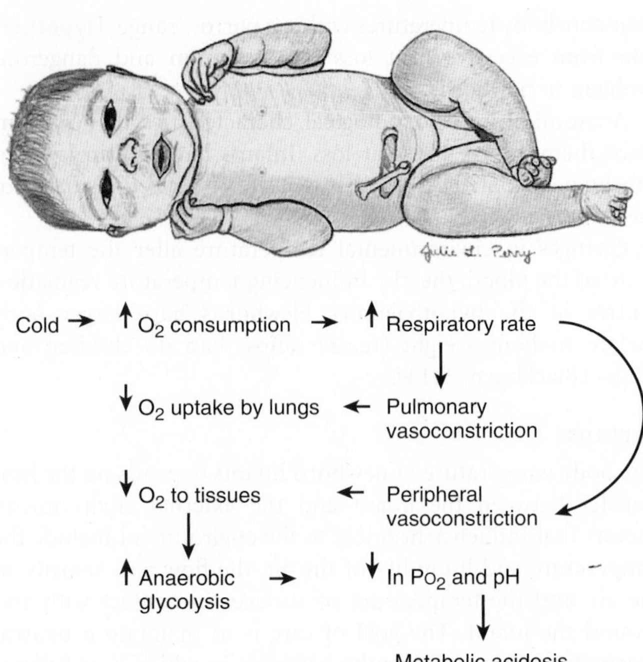

FIGURE 25-4 Effects of cold stress. When an infant is stressed by cold, oxygen consumption increases and pulmonary and peripheral vasoconstriction occur, thereby decreasing oxygen uptake by the lungs and oxygen to the tissues; anaerobic glycolysis increases; and there is a decrease in Po_2 and pH, leading to metabolic acidosis.

Hyperthermia

Although occurring less frequently than hypothermia, **hyperthermia** can occur and must be corrected. A body temperature greater than 37.5° C (99.5° F) is considered to be abnormally high and is typically caused by excess heat production related to sepsis or a decrease in heat loss. Hyperthermia can result from the inappropriate use of external heat sources such as radiant warmers, phototherapy, sunlight, increased environmental temperature, and use of excessive clothing or blankets (Brown & Landers, 2011). The clinical appearance of the infant who is hyperthermic often indicates the causative mechanism. Infants who are overheated because of environmental factors such as being swaddled in too many blankets exhibit signs of heat-losing mechanisms: skin vessels dilate, skin appears flushed, hands and feet are warm to touch, and the infant assumes a posture of extension. The newborn who is hyperthermic because of sepsis appears stressed: vessels in the skin are constricted, colour is pale, and hands and feet are cool. Hyperthermia develops more rapidly in a newborn than in an adult because of the relatively larger surface area of an infant. Sweat glands do not function well. Serious overheating of the newborn can cause cerebral damage from dehydration or even heat stroke and death (Brown & Landers, 2011).

Renal System

At term, the kidneys occupy a large portion of the posterior abdominal wall. The bladder lies close to the anterior abdominal wall and is an abdominal as well as a pelvic organ. In the newborn, almost all palpable masses in the abdomen are renal in origin.

At birth, a small quantity (approximately 40 mL) of urine is usually present in the bladder of a full-term newborn. Many newborns void at the time of birth, although this is easily missed and may not be recorded. During the first few days term infants generally excrete 15 to 60 mL/kg; output gradually increases over the first month (Blackburn, 2013). The frequency increases with age of the infant. At 1 day of age, a minimum of one void is expected. This increases one void per day for the first 5 days. At 1 week of age, about six to eight voidings per day of pale straw-coloured urine are indicative of adequate fluid intake.

! NURSING ALERT

Noting and recording the first voiding are important. An infant who has not voided by 24 hours should be assessed for adequacy of fluid intake, bladder distension, restlessness, and symptoms of pain. The pediatric health care provider should be notified.

Full-term newborns have limited capacity to concentrate urine; therefore, the specific gravity ranges from 1.001 to 1.020 (Pagana et al., 2013). The ability to concentrate urine fully is attained by about 3 months of age. After the first voiding, the infant's urine may appear cloudy (because of mucus content) and have a much higher specific gravity. This decreases as fluid intake increases. Normal urine during early infancy is usually straw coloured and almost odourless. Sometimes pink-tinged uric acid crystal stains appear on the diaper; these stains are normal, although they can be misinterpreted as blood. Loss of fluid through urine, feces, lungs, increased metabolic rate, and limited fluid intake results in a 5 to 10% loss of the birth weight. See Chapter 27 for discussion on how to determine weight loss. This weight loss usually occurs over the first 3 to 5 days of life. If the mother is breastfeeding and her milk supply has not come in yet (which occurs by the third or fourth day after birth), the newborn is somewhat protected from dehydration by its increased extracellular fluid volume. Most newborns should regain the birth weight within the first week of life to 10 days, depending on the feeding method (breast or bottle).

Fluid and Electrolyte Balance

In the term newborn approximately 75% of body weight consists of total body water (extracellular and intracellular). A reduction in extracellular fluid occurs with diuresis during the first few days after birth. The weight loss experienced by most newborns during the first few days after birth is caused primarily by extracellular water loss (Dell, 2011).

The daily fluid requirement for newborns weighing more than 1500 g is 60 to 80 mL/kg/day during the first 2 days of life, and from 3 to 7 days the requirement is 100 to 150 mL/kg/day (Dell, 2011).

At birth the glomerular filtration rate (GFR) of a newborn is approximately 30 to 50% that of the adult. This results in a decreased ability to remove nitrogenous and other waste products from the blood. The GFR rapidly increases during the first month of life as a result of postnatal physiological changes, including decreased renal vascular resistance, increased renal blood flow, and increased filtration pressure.

Sodium reabsorption is decreased as a result of a lowered sodium- and potassium-activated adenosine triphosphate activity. The decreased ability to excrete excessive sodium results in hypotonic urine, leading to a higher concentration of sodium, phosphates, chloride, and organic acids and a lower concentration of bicarbonate ions. The infant has a higher renal threshold for glucose than adults.

Bicarbonate concentration and buffering capacity are decreased. This can lead to acidosis and electrolyte imbalance.

Signs of Renal System Problems

The renal system has a wide range of functions. Dysfunction resulting from physiological abnormalities can range from the lack of a steady stream of urine to anomalies such as hypospadias and exstrophy of the bladder, which can be identified at birth (see Chapter 49). Enlarged or cystic kidneys can be identified as masses during abdominal palpation. Some kidney anomalies also can be detected by ultrasound examination during pregnancy.

Gastrointestinal System

The full-term newborn is capable of swallowing, digesting, metabolizing, and absorbing proteins and simple carbohydrates, and emulsifying fats. With the exception of pancreatic amylase, the characteristic enzymes and digestive juices are present even in low-birth-weight infants.

In the adequately hydrated infant, the mucous membrane of the mouth is moist and pink; the hard and soft palates are intact. The presence of moderate to large amounts of mucus is common in the first few hours after birth. Small whitish areas (Epstein pearls) may be found on the gum margins and at the juncture of the hard and soft palates. The cheeks are full because of well-developed sucking pads. These, like the labial tubercles (sucking calluses) on the upper lip, disappear around the age of 12 months, when the sucking period is over.

Even though in utero sucking motions occur as early as 15 to 16 weeks, as recorded by ultrasonography, these motions are not coordinated with swallowing in any infant born before 32 to 33 weeks of gestation. Sucking behaviour is influenced by neuromuscular maturity, maternal medications received during labour and birth, and the type of initial feeding. Sucking takes place in small bursts of 3 or 4 and up to 8 to 10 sucks at a time, with a brief pause between bursts. The infant is unable to move food from the lips to the pharynx; therefore, placing the nipple (breast or bottle) well inside the baby's mouth is necessary. Peristaltic activity in the esophagus is uncoordinated in the first few days of life. It quickly becomes a coordinated pattern in healthy full-term infants, and they swallow easily.

Teeth begin developing in utero, with enamel formation continuing until about 10 years of age. Tooth development is influenced by newborn illnesses and medications, and by illnesses of or medications taken by the mother during pregnancy. The fluoride level in the water supply also influences tooth development. Occasionally a newborn may be born with one or more teeth. These natal teeth have poorly formed roots and as they loosen place the infant at risk of aspiration. Therefore they are usually extracted.

Bacteria are not present in the newborn's gastrointestinal tract at birth. Soon after birth, oral and anal orifices permit entrance of bacteria and air. Generally, the highest bacterial concentration is found in the lower portion of the intestine, particularly in the large intestine. Normal colonic bacteria are established within the first week after birth, and normal intestinal flora help synthesize vitamin K, folate, and biotin. Bowel sounds can usually be heard shortly after birth.

Stomach capacity varies, from 30 mL on day 1 (5–10 mL/kg) to more than 90 mL by the end of the first week of life, depending on the infant's size. After birth the newborn stomach becomes increasingly more compliant and relaxed to accommodate larger volumes. Several factors such as time and volume of feedings or type and temperature of food may affect the emptying time. The cardiac sphincter and nervous control of the stomach are immature, so some regurgitation may occur.

Digestion

The infant's ability to digest carbohydrates, fats, and proteins is regulated by the presence of certain enzymes. Most of these are functional at birth except for pancreatic amylase and lipase. Amylase is produced by the salivary glands after about 3 months and by the pancreas at about 6 months of age. This enzyme is necessary to convert starch into maltose and occurs in high amounts in colostrum. The other exception is lipase, which is also secreted by the pancreas; it is necessary for the digestion of fat. Thus, the normal newborn is capable of digesting simple carbohydrates and proteins but has a limited ability to digest fats. Mammary lipase in human milk aids in digestion of fats by the newborn.

Lactase levels in newborns are higher than in older infants. This enzyme is necessary for digestion of lactose, the major carbohydrate in human milk and commercial infant formula.

Stools

At birth, the lower intestine is filled with meconium. Meconium is formed during fetal life from the amniotic fluid and its constituents, intestinal secretions (including bilirubin), and cells (shed from the mucosa). Meconium is greenish black and viscous and contains occult blood. The first meconium passed is usually sterile, but within hours all meconium passed contains bacteria. Most healthy term infants pass meconium within 12 to 24 hours of life, and almost all do so by 48 hours. The number of stools passed varies during the first week, being most numerous between the third and sixth days. Newborns fed early pass stools sooner. Progressive changes in the stool pattern indicate a properly functioning gastrointestinal tract (Box 25-1 and Fig. 25-5).

Signs of Gastrointestinal Problems

The time, colour, and character of the infant's first stool should be noted. Failure to pass meconium can indicate bowel obstruction related to conditions such as malrotation, small or large bowel atresia, an inborn error of metabolism (e.g., cystic fibrosis), or a congenital disorder (e.g., Hirschsprung disease or an imperforate anus). An active rectal "wink" reflex (contraction of the anal sphincter muscle in response to touch) is a sign of good sphincter tone.

Fullness of the abdomen above the umbilicus can be caused by problems such as hepatomegaly, duodenal atresia, or distension. Abdominal distension at birth usually indicates a serious disorder, such as a ruptured viscus (from abdominal wall defects). Distension that occurs later can be the result of overfeeding or failure to pass stool or signal gastrointestinal disorders. A scaphoid (sunken) abdomen, with bowel sounds heard in the chest and signs of respiratory distress, indicate a diaphragmatic hernia. Fullness below the umbilicus can indicate a distended bladder.

Some infants are intolerant of certain commercial infant formulas. If an infant is allergic or unable to digest a formula, the stools can become very soft with a high water content that is signalled by a distinct water ring around the stool on the diaper. Forceful ejection of stool and a water ring around the stool are signs of diarrhea. Care must be taken to avoid misinterpreting transitional stools for diarrhea. The loss of fluid in diarrhea can rapidly lead to fluid and electrolyte imbalance. Passage of meconium from the vagina or urinary meatus is a sign of a possible fistulous tract from the rectum.

The amount and frequency of regurgitation ("spitting up") after feedings should be documented. Colour change, gagging, and projectile (very forceful) vomiting occur in association with esophageal and tracheoesophageal anomalies (Chapter 46). Bilious emesis is always considered a serious condition until proven otherwise (volvulus, malrotation).

BOX 25-1 CHANGES IN STOOLING PATTERNS OF NEWBORNS

Meconium

- Meconium is the infant's first stool, composed of amniotic fluid and its constituents, intestinal secretions, shed mucosal cells, and possibly blood (ingested maternal blood or minor bleeding of alimentary tract vessels) (Fig. 25-5, A).
- Passage of meconium should occur within the first 24 to 48 hours, although it may be delayed up to 7 days in very-low-birth-weight infants.

Transitional Stools

- Transitional stools usually appear by the third day after initiation of feeding.
- They are greenish brown to yellowish brown, are thin and less sticky than meconium, and may contain some milk curds (Fig. 25-5, B).

Milk Stool

- Milk stool usually appears by the fourth day.
- *Breastfed infants:* Stools yellow to golden, pasty in consistency, resemble a mixture of mustard and cottage cheese, with an odour similar to sour milk (Fig. 25-5, C).
- *Formula-fed infants*: Stools pale yellow to light brown, have firmer consistency, with an odour more characteristic of a normal stool.

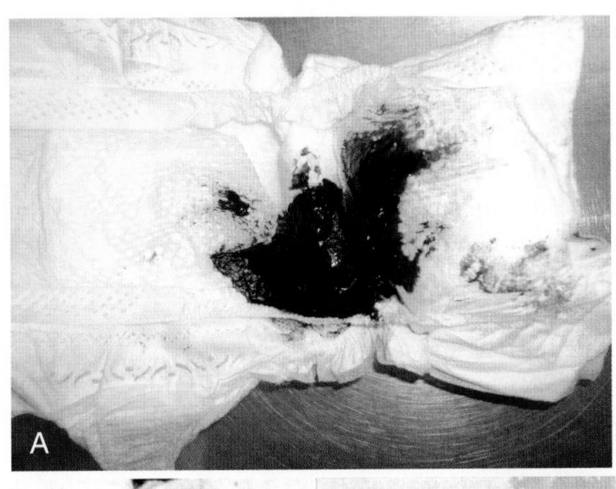

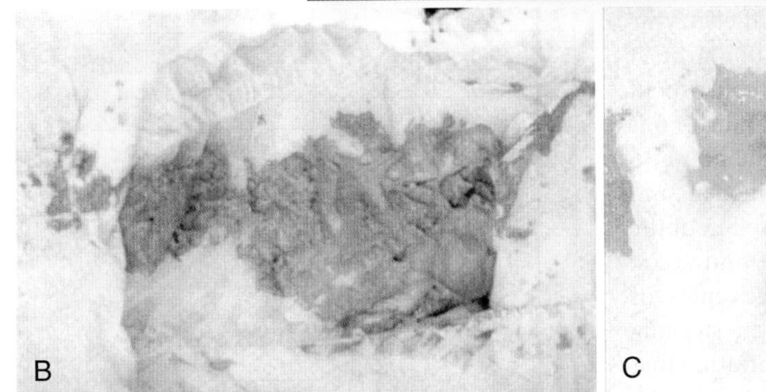

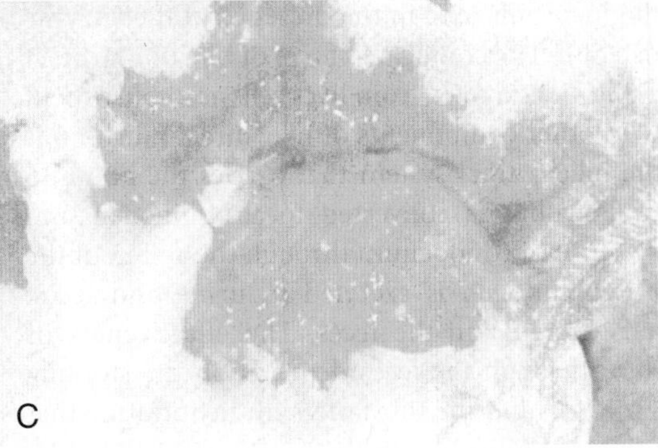

FIGURE 25-5 Breastfed newborn stools. **A:** Meconium. **B:** Transition stool. **C:** Milk stool. (**A,** Courtesy Janet Andrews. **B, C,** Courtesy Connie Livingstone.)

Hepatic System

The liver and gallbladder are formed by the fourth week of gestation. In the newborn, the liver can be palpated about 1 to 2 cm below the right costal margin because it is enlarged and occupies about 40% of the abdominal cavity. The infant's liver plays an important role in iron storage, carbohydrate metabolism, conjugation of bilirubin, and coagulation.

Iron Storage

The fetal liver, which serves as the site for production of hemoglobin after birth, begins storing iron in utero. The infant's iron store is proportional to total body hemoglobin content and length of gestation. At birth, the term newborn has an iron store sufficient to last 4 to 6 months.

Iron stores of preterm and small-for-gestational-age infants are often lower and are depleted sooner than in healthy term infants. Although both breast milk and cow's milk contain iron, the bioavailability of iron in breast milk is far superior. Exclusive breastfeeding during the first 6 months is accepted as the nutrition standard for infants according to the Dietary Reference Intakes and is promoted by the World Health Organization (WHO) as a global public health recommendation. Current opinion suggests that iron supplements are not generally needed for breastfed infants during the first 6 months. Infants with lower iron stores are at higher risk of iron deficiency, and supplementation with oral iron drops should be prescribed when appropriate. Formula-fed infants should receive a formula that contains supplemental iron (Baker, Greer, & the Committee on Nutrition, 2010).

Carbohydrate Metabolism

In utero the glucose concentration in the umbilical vein is approximately 80% of the maternal level. At birth the newborn is cut off from its maternal glucose supply and as a result experiences an initial decrease in serum glucose levels. Glucose levels reach a low point between 30 and 90 minutes after birth and then rise gradually. In most healthy term newborns blood glucose levels stabilize at 2.5 to 3.0 mmol/L during the first several hours after birth; by the third day of life, the blood glucose levels should be approximately 4.0 to 6.0 mmol/L.

The initiation of feedings helps to stabilize the newborn's blood glucose levels. Colostrum contains high amounts of glucose, thus also assisting in the stabilization of blood glucose levels in breastfed newborns. In general, blood glucose levels less than 2.2 mmol/L are considered abnormal and may require intervention (see further discussion in Chapter 26, p. 696). The hypoglycemic infant can display the classic symptoms of jitteriness, lethargy, apnea, feeding problems, or seizures; or the infant can be asymptomatic. Hypoglycemia in the initial newborn period is most often transient and easily corrected through feeding. Persistent or recurrent hypoglycemia necessitates intravenous glucose therapy and possible pharmacological intervention.

Conjugation of Bilirubin and Newborn Jaundice

Jaundice, the visible yellowish colour of the skin and sclera, is caused by elevated serum levels of unconjugated (indirect) bilirubin. The liver is responsible for the conjugation of bilirubin, which results from the breakdown of RBCs. When RBCs reach the end of their lifespan, their membranes rupture, and hemoglobin is released. The hemoglobin is phagocytosed by macrophages; it then splits into heme and globin. The heme is broken down by the reticuloendothelial cells, converted to bilirubin, and released in an unconjugated form. The unconjugated (indirect) bilirubin is relatively insoluble and almost entirely bound to circulating albumin, a plasma protein. The unbound bilirubin can leave the vascular system and permeate other extravascular tissues (e.g., skin, sclera, and oral mucous membranes). It can also cross the blood-brain barrier and cause neurotoxicity.

The unconjugated bilirubin must be conjugated so it becomes soluble and excretable. In the liver the unbound bilirubin is conjugated with glucuronic acid in the presence of the enzyme glucuronyl transferase. The conjugated form of bilirubin (direct bilirubin) is soluble and excreted from liver cells as a constituent of bile. Along with other components of bile, direct bilirubin is excreted into the biliary tract system that carries the bile into the duodenum. Bilirubin is converted to urobilinogen and stercobilinogen within the duodenum through the action of the bacterial flora. Urobilinogen is excreted in urine and feces; stercobilinogen is excreted in the feces. The effectiveness of bilirubin excretion through the feces depends on the stooling pattern of the newborn and the substances in the intestine that break down conjugated bilirubin. In the newborn intestine the enzyme beta-glucuronidase is able to convert conjugated bilirubin into the unconjugated form, which is subsequently reabsorbed by the intestinal mucosa and transported to the liver; this is called *enterohepatic circulation*. Feeding is important in reducing serum bilirubin levels because it stimulates peristalsis and produces more rapid passage of meconium, thus diminishing the amount of reabsorption of unconjugated bilirubin. Feeding also introduces bacteria to aid in the reduction of bilirubin to urobilinogen. Colostrum, a natural laxative, facilitates the passage of meconium (Fig. 25-6).

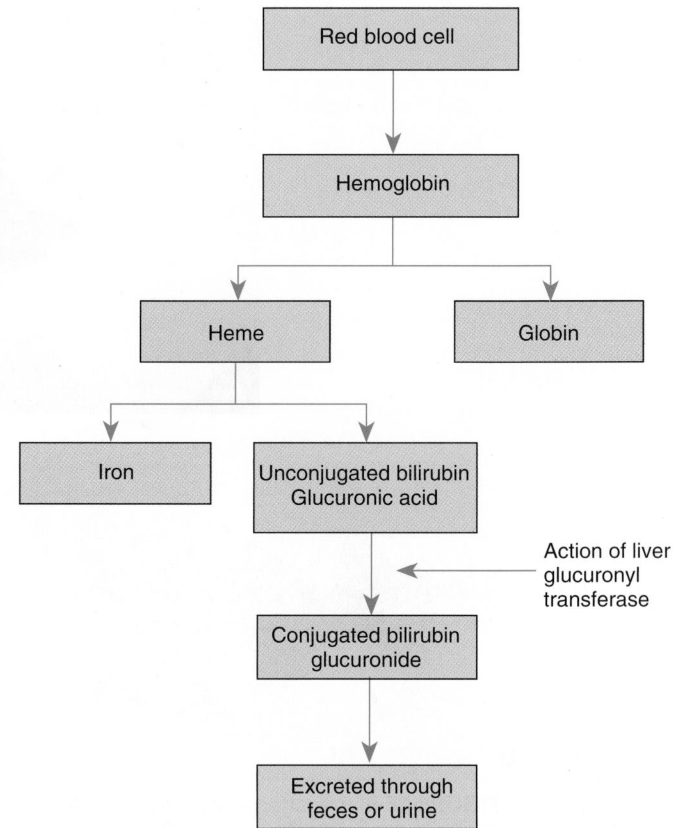

FIGURE 25-6 Formation and excretion of bilirubin.

When levels of unconjugated bilirubin exceed the ability of the liver to conjugate it, plasma levels of bilirubin increase and jaundice appears. Jaundice is generally noticeable first in the head, especially in the sclera and mucous membranes, and progresses gradually to the thorax, abdomen, and extremities. The degree of jaundice is determined by serum total bilirubin measurements. Jaundice is likely to appear when bilirubin levels exceed 85 to 102 mcmol/L (Blackburn, 2013).

The newborn is at risk for hyperbilirubinemia because of distinctive aspects of normal neonatal physiology. The higher RBC mass at birth and shorter lifespan of neonatal RBCs mean that greater bilirubin synthesis is needed. The ability of the liver to conjugate bilirubin is reduced during the first few days after birth; it can metabolize and excrete only about two thirds of the circulating bilirubin. In addition, there are fewer bilirubin binding sites because newborns have lower serum albumin levels. In the intestines, conjugated bilirubin becomes unconjugated and recirculated through the enterohepatic circulation, which increases serum bilirubin levels (Blackburn, 2013).

Traditionally, newborn jaundice has been categorized as either *physiological* or *pathological* (nonphysiological), depending primarily on the time it appears and on serum bilirubin levels. Controversy surrounds the definitions of normal or physiological ranges of total serum bilirubin. Total serum bilirubin levels in newborns are affected by variables such as length of gestation, age, weight, race, blood group, nutritional status, and mode of feeding (Blackburn, 2013). The time of onset of jaundice is a key factor in evaluating its cause and determining if treatment is needed. *Early-onset jaundice* is usually related to increased bilirubin production; *late-onset jaundice* is most often related to delayed elimination of bilirubin, with or without increased production (Kamath, Thilo, & Hernandez, 2011). Table 25-3 lists the varying causes of neonatal hyperbilirubinemia.

Among the factors that increase the risk of hyperbilirubinemia, prematurity is the most significant one. Prematurity affects liver and brain metabolism and albumin binding sites, placing preterm and late preterm infants at greater risk for hyperbilirubinemia. Infants of Asian and Indigenous ethnicity have higher bilirubin levels. Breastfeeding infants are at greater risk of hyperbilirubinemia (see later discussion).

Although there is no consistent definition for neonatal hyperbilirubinemia, the Canadian Paediatric Society suggests that an unconjugated hyperbilirubinemia greater than 340 mcmol/L in the first 28 days of life constitutes hyperbilirubinemia (Barrington, Sankaran, & Canadian Paediatric Society, 2007/2011). Conjugated hyperbilirubinemia is rare; it is defined as direct bilirubin levels greater than 26 mcmol/L (Kaplan, Wong, Sibley, et al., 2011).

TABLE 25-3 CAUSES OF NEONATAL INDIRECT HYPERBILIRUBINEMIA

BASIS	CAUSES
Increased Production of Bilirubin	
Increased hemoglobin destruction	Fetomaternal blood group incompatibility (Rh, ABO) Congenital red blood cell abnormalities Congenital enzyme deficiencies (G6PD, galactosemia) Sepsis Enclosed hemorrhage (cephalhematoma, bruising)
Increased amount of hemoglobin	Polycythemia (maternal–fetal or twin–twin transfusion, SGA) Delayed cord clamping
Increased enterohepatic circulation	Delayed passage of meconium, meconium ileus, or plug Fasting or delayed initiation of feeding Intestinal atresia or stenosis
Altered Hepatic Clearance of Bilirubin	
Alteration in uridine diphosphoglucuronyl transferase production or activity	Immaturity Metabolic or endocrine disorders (e.g., Criglar-Najjar syndrome, hypothyroidism, disorders of amino acid metabolism)
Alteration in hepatic function and perfusion (and thus conjugating ability)	Sepsis (also causes inflammation) Asphyxia, hypoxia, hypothermia, hypoglycemia Medications and hormones
Hepatic obstruction (associated with direct hyperbilirubinemia)	Congenital anomalies (biliary atresia, cystic fibrosis) Biliary stasis (hepatitis, sepsis) Excessive bilirubin load (often seen with severe hemolysis)

G6PD, glucose-6-phosphate dehydrogenase; *SGA*, small for gestational age.
From Blackburn, S. T. (2013). *Maternal, fetal, and neonatal physiology: A clinical perspective* (4th ed.). St. Louis: Saunders.)

Physiological jaundice. Physiological or nonpathological jaundice occurs in approximately 60% of newborn infants born at term and 80% of preterm infants (Kaplan et al., 2011). It appears after 24 hours of age and usually resolves without treatment.

Two phases of physiological jaundice have been identified in full-term infants. In the first phase, bilirubin levels gradually increase to approximately 85 to 100 mcmol/L by 60 to 72 hours of life, then decrease to a plateau of 35 to 50 mcmol/L by the fifth day (Blackburn, 2013). In Asian infants, levels may reach a peak of 170 to 240 mcmol/L around the third to fifth day of life; the levels gradually fall to 35 to 50 mcmol/L by the seventh to tenth day. Bilirubin levels maintain a steady plateau state in the second phase without increasing or decreasing until approximately 12 to 14 days, at which time levels decrease to the normal adult value of 17 mcmol/L (Blackburn, 2013). This pattern varies according to racial group, method of feeding (breast versus bottle), and gestational age. In preterm formula-fed infants, serum bilirubin levels may peak as high as 170 to 200 mcmol/L at 5 to 6 days of life and decrease slowly over a period of 2 to 4 weeks (Kaplan et al., 2011).

! NURSING ALERT

The appearance of jaundice during the first 24 hours of life or persistence beyond the ages previously delineated usually indicates a potential pathological process that requires investigation.

Pathological jaundice. Although physiological jaundice is usually considered benign, unconjugated bilirubin (indirect) can accumulate to hazardous levels and lead to a pathological condition. Pathological or nonphysiological jaundice is unconjugated hyperbilirubinemia that is either pathological in origin or severe enough to warrant further evaluation and treatment (see Chapter 26). Jaundice is usually considered pathological or nonphysiological if it appears within 24 hours of birth, if total serum bilirubin levels increase by more than 100 mcmcol/L in 24 hours, and if the serum bilirubin level exceeds 256 mcmol/L at any time (Blackburn, 2013). High levels of unconjugated bilirubin are usually caused by excessive production of bilirubin through hemolysis. Hemolytic disease of the newborn caused by maternal/newborn blood group incompatibility is the most common cause of hyperbilirubinemia. It can also be caused by glucose-6-phosphate dehydrogenase (G6PD) deficiency, a genetic disorder that is more common among Asian and Indigenous populations. Other causes are listed in Table 25-3.

If increased levels of unconjugated bilirubin are left untreated, neurotoxicity can result as bilirubin is transferred into the brain cells. **Acute bilirubin encephalopathy** refers to the acute manifestations of bilirubin toxicity that occur during the first weeks after birth. This can include a range of symptoms, such as lethargy, hypotonia, irritability, seizures, coma, and death. **Kernicterus** refers to the irreversible, long-term consequences of bilirubin toxicity, such as hypotonia, delayed motor skills, hearing loss, cerebral palsy, and gaze abnormalities.

Jaundice related to breastfeeding. Two forms of breastfeeding-related jaundice are recognized: *breastfeeding-associated jaundice* and *breast milk jaundice*. These typically occur in otherwise healthy infants. Both types can occur in the same infant and are not easily differentiated (Blackburn, 2013).

Breastfeeding-associated jaundice (early-onset jaundice) begins at 2 to 5 days of age. Breastfeeding does not cause the jaundice; rather it is a lack of effective breastfeeding that contributes to the hyperbilirubinemia. If the infant is not feeding effectively, there is less caloric and fluid intake and possible dehydration. Hepatic clearance of bilirubin is reduced. With less intake, there are fewer stools. As a result, bilirubin is reabsorbed from the intestine back into the bloodstream and must be conjugated again so it can be excreted (Blackburn, 2013; Lawrence & Lawrence, 2011).

Breast milk jaundice (late-onset jaundice) usually occurs at 5 to 10 days of age. Infants are usually feeding well and gaining weight appropriately. Rising levels of bilirubin peak during the second week and gradually diminish. Despite high levels of bilirubin that may persist for 3 to 12 weeks, these infants have no signs of hemolysis or liver dysfunction. The etiology of breast milk jaundice is uncertain. However, it seems to be related to factors in the breast milk (e.g., pregnanediol, fatty acids, and beta-glucuronidase) that either inhibit the conjugation or decrease the excretion of bilirubin (Blackburn, 2013). (See Chapter 27 for a discussion of these conditions in relation to newborn nutrition.)

Coagulation. The liver plays an important role in blood coagulation. Coagulation factors, which are synthesized in the liver, are activated by vitamin K. The lack of intestinal bacteria needed to synthesize vitamin K results in transient blood coagulation deficiency between the second and fifth days of life. The levels of coagulation factors slowly increase to reach adult levels by age 9 months. The administration of intramuscular vitamin K shortly after birth helps prevent clotting problems. Any bleeding problems noted in the newborn should be reported immediately and tests for clotting ordered (Manco-Johnson, Rodden, & Hays, 2011).

Immune System

Beginning early in gestation, the immune system of the fetus is developing the capacity to respond to foreign antigens. The development of the immune system is necessary to equip the newborn to meet the numerous environmental challenges (e.g., microorganisms) associated with life in the extrauterine world.

At birth, most of the circulating antibodies in the newborn are immunoglobulin (Ig) G antibodies that were transported across the placenta from the maternal circulation. IgG is key to immunity to bacteria and viruses. This transfer of antibodies from the mother begins as early as 14 weeks of gestation and is greatest during the third trimester. By term the IgG levels in the cord blood of the infant are higher than those in maternal blood. The passive immunity afforded the infant through the placental transfer of IgG usually provides sufficient antimicrobial protection during the first 3 months of life. Production of adult concentrations of IgG is reached by 4 to 6 years of age (Kapur, Yoder, & Polin, 2011).

The fetus is capable of producing IgM by the eighth week of gestation, and low levels are present at term (less than 10% of adult levels). IgM is important for immunity to bloodborne infections and is the major Ig synthesized during the first month. By the age of 2 years, IgM reaches adult levels. The production of IgA, IgD, and IgE is much more gradual, and maximal levels are not attained until early childhood (Kapur et al., 2011).

Natural barrier mechanisms such as the acidity of the stomach and the production of pepsin and trypsin, which maintain sterility of the small intestine, are not fully developed until ages 3 to 4 weeks.

The membrane-protective IgA is missing from the respiratory and urinary tracts, and, unless the newborn is breastfed, it also is absent from the gastrointestinal tract. Breast milk provides the newborn with important immunity. The secretory IgA in human milk acts locally in the intestines to neutralize bacterial and viral pathogens. It may also lessen the risk of allergy and food intolerance through modulation of exposure to foreign milk protein antigens.

The newborn is capable of producing a protective immune response to vaccines, given as early as a few hours after birth. For example, when hepatitis B vaccine is administered at birth to the infant born to a mother with hepatitis B, there is an excellent immune response. This holds true even if the infant does not receive additional hepatitis B Ig.

The WBCs of the newborn display a delayed response to invading bacteria. The influx of phagocytic cells to areas of inflammation is somewhat slowed, although the ability of these cells to attack and destroy bacteria is equivalent to that of adults (Kapur et al., 2011).

The newborn who is breastfed receives significant passive immunity through the colostrum and breast milk.

Risk for Infection

All newborns, and preterm newborns especially, are at high risk for infection during the first several months of life. During this period infection is one of the leading causes of morbidity and mortality. The newborn cannot limit the invading pathogen to the portal of entry because of the generalized hypofunctioning of the inflammatory and immune mechanisms.

Early signs of infection must be recognized so that prompt diagnosis and treatment can occur. Temperature instability or hypothermia can be symptomatic of serious infection; newborns do not typically exhibit fever, although hyperthermia can occur (temperature greater than 38°C or 100.4° F). Lethargy, irritability, poor feeding, vomiting or diarrhea, decreased reflexes, and pale or mottled skin colour are some of the clinical signs that suggest infection. Respiratory symptoms such as apnea, tachypnea, grunting, or retracting can be associated with infection such as pneumonia (Lott, 2015). The greatest risk factor for neonatal infection is prematurity because of immaturity of the immune system. Other risk factors include premature rupture of membranes, chorioamnionitis, maternal fever, antenatal or intrapartal asphyxia, invasive procedures, stress, and congenital anomalies (Lott, 2015). Hand hygiene is key to prevention of serious infections.

Integumentary System

All skin structures are present at birth. The epidermis and dermis are loosely bound and extremely thin. After 35 weeks' gestation the skin is covered by **vernix caseosa** (a cheeselike whitish substance) that is fused with the epidermis and serves as a protective covering. Vernix caseosa is a complex substance that contains sebaceous gland secretions. It has emollient and antimicrobial properties and prevents fluid loss through the skin; it also has antioxidant properties. Removal of the vernix is followed by desquamation of the epidermis in most infants. There is evidence that leaving residual vernix intact after birth has positive benefits for neonatal skin, such as decreasing the skin pH, decreasing skin erythema, and improving skin hydration (Visscher, Utturkar, Pickens, et al., 2011). The infant's skin is sensitive and can be easily damaged.

The term infant has erythematous (red) skin for a few hours after birth, after which it fades to its normal colour. The skin often appears blotchy or mottled, especially over the extremities. The hands and feet appear slightly cyanotic (**acrocyanosis**);

this is caused by vasomotor instability and capillary stasis. Acrocyanosis is normal and appears intermittently over the first 7 to 10 days, especially with exposure to cold (see Fig. 25-1).

The healthy term newborn usually has a plump appearance because of large amounts of subcutaneous tissue and extracellular water content. Subcutaneous fat accumulated during the last trimester acts as insulation. Fine lanugo hair may be noted over the face, shoulders, and back. Edema of the face and ecchymosis (bruising) may be noted as a result of face presentation, forceps-assisted birth, or vacuum extraction.

Creases can be found on the palms of the hands. The simian line, a single palmar crease, is often found in Asian infants or in infants with Down syndrome. The soles of the feet should be inspected for the number of creases during the first few hours after birth; as the skin dries, more creases appear. Increasing numbers of creases correlate with a greater maturity rating. Premature newborns have few if any creases.

Sweat Glands

Distended, small, white sebaceous glands noticeable on the newborn face are known as milia. Although sweat glands are present at birth, term infants usually do not sweat for the first 24 hours. By day 3, sweating begins on the face and later progresses to the palms. Infants can sweat as a function of body or environmental temperature; there can also be emotional sweating from crying or pain (Hoath & Narendran, 2011).

Desquamation

Desquamation (peeling) of the skin of the term infant does not occur until a few days after birth. Large generalized areas of skin desquamation present at birth may be an indication of postmaturity.

Mongolian Spots (Congenital Dermal Melancytosis)

Mongolian spots, bluish black areas of pigmentation, may appear over any part of the exterior surface of the body, including the extremities. They are more commonly noted on the back and buttocks (Fig. 25-7). These pigmented areas are most frequently noted in newborns whose ethnic origins are in the Mediterranean area, Latin America, Asia, or Africa (Blackburn, 2013). They fade gradually over months or years.

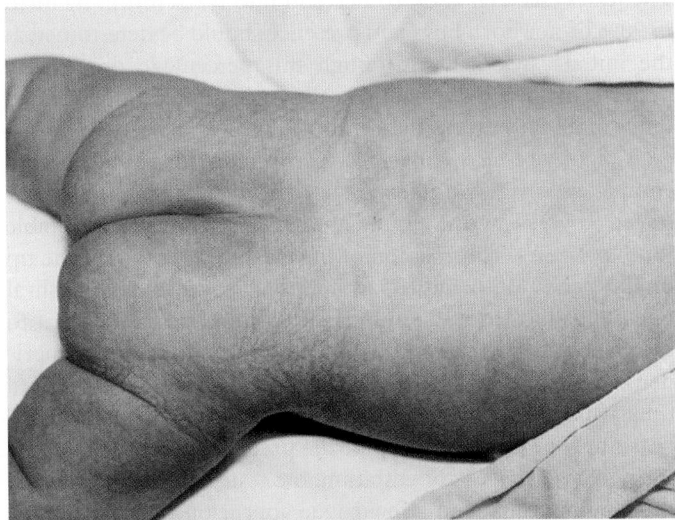

FIGURE 25-7 Mongolian spot.

Nevi

Nevus simplex, also known as *salmon patches, telangiectatic nevi, "stork bites,"* or *"angel kisses,"* are flat, pink capillary hemangiomas that are easily blanched (Fig. 25-8, A). They appear on the upper eyelids, nose, upper lip, lower occiput bone, and nape of the neck. They have no clinical significance and fade between the first and second years of life. Facial lesions fade between the first and second years of life, whereas neck lesions can be visible into adulthood.

A nevus vasculosus, or strawberry hemangioma, is a common type of capillary hemangioma. It consists of dilated, newly formed capillaries occupying the entire dermal and subdermal layers with associated connective tissue hypertrophy. The typical lesion is a raised, sharply demarcated, bright or dark red, rough-surfaced swelling. These are rarely seen at birth, although 90% become visible in the neonatal period. Strawberry hemangiomas tend to grow rapidly during the first years and usually fade or shrink with time (Habif, 2009).

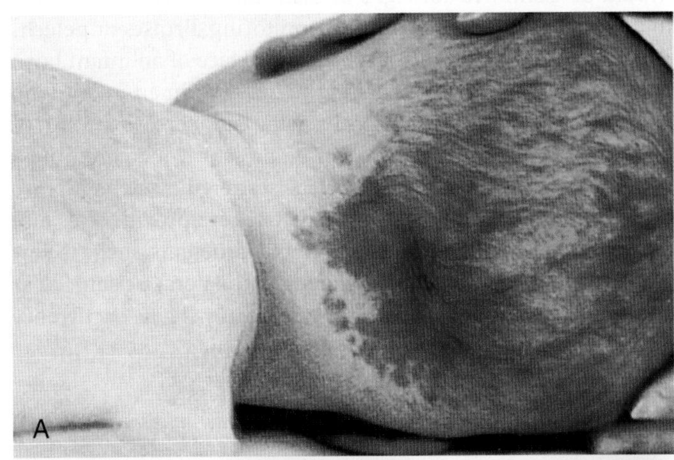

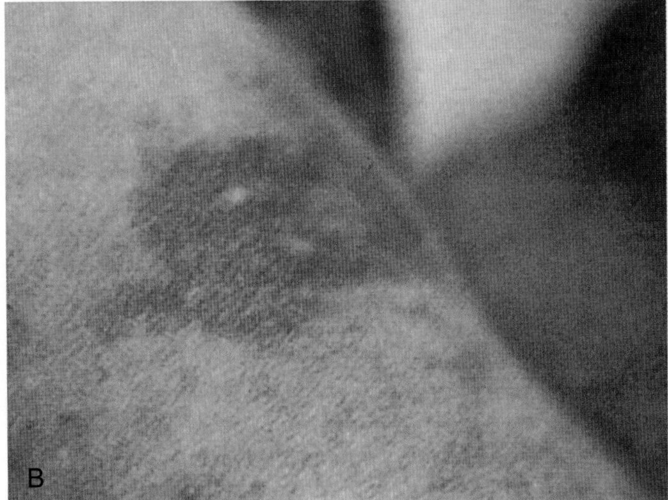

FIGURE 25-8 A: Telangiectatic nevi (stork bite). **B:** Erythema toxicum. (Courtesy Mead Johnson & Co., LLC.)

A port-wine stain, or **nevus flammeus**, is usually visible at birth and is composed of a plexus of newly formed capillaries in the papillary layer of the corium. It is red to purple; varies in size, shape, and location; and is not elevated. True port-wine stains do not blanch on pressure or disappear. They are most commonly found on the face and neck.

Erythema Toxicum

Erythema toxicum, a transient rash, is also called *erythema neonatorum*, or *newborn rash*. It first appears in term newborns during the first 24 to 72 hours after birth and can last up to 3 weeks of age. It has lesions in different stages: erythematous macules, papules, and small vesicles (see Fig. 25-8, B). The lesions may appear suddenly anywhere on the body. The rash is thought to be an inflammatory response. Eosinophils, which help decrease inflammation, are found in the vesicles. Although the appearance is alarming, the rash has no clinical significance and requires no treatment.

Signs of Integumentary Problems

Close observation of the newborn's skin colour can lead to early detection of potential problems. Any pallor, plethora (deep purplish colour from increased circulating RBCs), petechiae, central cyanosis, or jaundice should be noted and described. The skin should be examined for signs of birth injuries, such as forceps marks and lesions related to fetal monitoring. Bruises or petechiae may be present on the head, neck, and face of an infant born with a nuchal cord (cord around the neck) or in an infant who had a face presentation at birth. Bruising can increase the risk of hyperbilirubinemia. Petechiae can be present if increased pressure was applied to an area. Petechiae scattered over the infant's body should be reported to the pediatric care provider because their presence can indicate underlying problems such as low platelet count or infection. Unilateral or bilateral periauricular papillomas (skin tags) occur fairly frequently. Their occurrence is usually a family trait and of no consequence.

Reproductive System

Female

At birth, the ovaries contain thousands of primitive germ cells. These represent the full complement of potential ova; no oogonia form after birth in term infants. The ovarian cortex, which is made up primarily of primordial follicles, occupies a larger portion of the ovary in the female newborn than in the adult. From birth to sexual maturity, the number of ova decreases by approximately 90%.

An increase in estrogen during pregnancy, followed by a drop after birth, results in a mucoid vaginal discharge and some slight bloody spotting (**pseudomenstruation**). External genitalia (i.e., labia majora and minora) are usually edematous, with increased pigmentation. In term newborns, the labia majora and minora cover the vestibule (Fig. 25-9, A). In preterm infants, the clitoris is prominent and the labia majora are small and widely separated. Vaginal or hymenal tags are common findings and have no clinical significance. Vernix caseosa may be present between the labia and should not be forcibly removed during bathing.

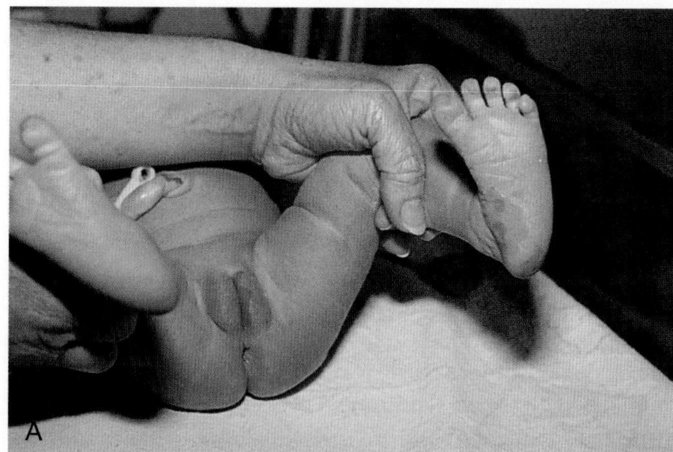

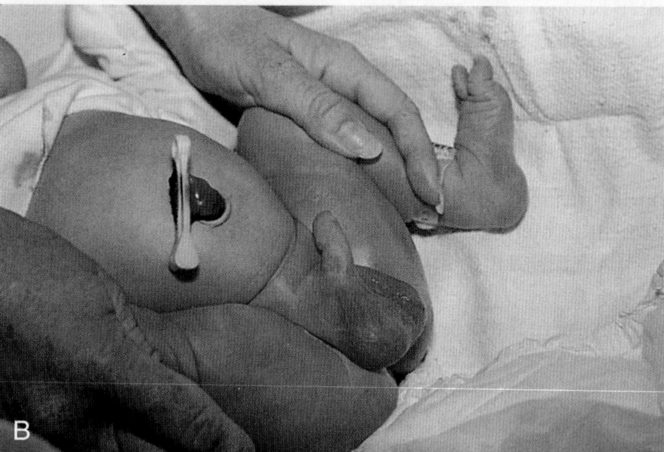

FIGURE 25-9 External genitalia. **A:** Genitalia in female term infant. **B:** Genitalia in uncircumcised male infant. Rugae cover scrotum, indicating term gestation. (Courtesy Marjorie Pyle, RNC, Lifecircle.)

If the girl was born in the breech position, the labia may be edematous and bruised. The edema and bruising resolve in a few days; no treatment is necessary.

Male

The testes (see Fig. 25-9, B) descend into the scrotum by birth in 90% of newborn boys and presence should be determined at the initial assessment. Although this percentage drops with preterm birth, by 1 year of age the incidence of undescended testes in all boys is less than 1%.

A tight **prepuce** (foreskin) is common in newborns and completely covers the glans. The urethral opening may be completely covered by the prepuce, which may not be retractable for 3 to 4 years. The position of the urethra should be at the tip of the penis. With **hypospadius**, or **epispadias**, the urethral opening is located in an abnormal position, on or adjacent to the glans, although it can be placed on the penile shaft or perineum. Smegma, a white, cheesy substance, is commonly found under the foreskin. Small, white, firm cysts called *epithelial pearls* may be seen at the tip of the prepuce.

By 28 to 36 weeks of gestation, the testes can be palpated in the inguinal canal and a few **rugae** appear on the scrotum. At 36 to 40 weeks of gestation, the testes are palpable in the upper scrotum and rugae appear on the anterior portion. After 40 weeks, the testes can be palpated in the scrotum and rugae cover the scrotal sac. The postterm newborn has deep rugae and a pendulous scrotum. The scrotum is usually more deeply pigmented than the rest of the skin, a difference that is especially apparent in darker-skinned infants. This pigmentation is a response to maternal estrogen. A hydrocele, caused by an accumulation of fluid around the testes, may be found. This can be transilluminated with a light and usually decreases in size without treatment.

If the male infant is born in a breech presentation, the scrotum is edematous and may be bruised (Fig. 26-6). The swelling and discolouration subside within a few days.

Swelling of Breast Tissue

Swelling of the breast tissue in term infants of both sexes is caused by the hyperestrogenism of pregnancy. In a few infants a thin discharge ("witch's milk") can be seen. This finding has no clinical significance, requires no treatment, and subsides within a few days as the maternal hormones are eliminated from the infant's body.

The nipples should be symmetrical on the chest. Breast tissue and areola size increase with gestation. The areola appears slightly elevated at 34 weeks of gestation. By 36 weeks, a breast bud of 1 to 2 mm is palpable; this increases to 12 mm by 42 weeks.

Signs of Reproductive System Problems

The newborn must be inspected closely for ambiguous genitalia and other abnormalities. Normally, in a female newborn the urethral opening is located behind the clitoris. Any deviation from this can incorrectly suggest that the clitoris is a small penis, which can occur in conditions such as adrenal hyperplasia. Nearly all female newborns are born with hymenal tags; absence of such tags can indicate vaginal agenesis. Fecal discharge from the vagina indicates a rectovaginal fistula. Any of these findings must be reported to the pediatric health care provider for further evaluation.

Hypospadias or epispadias, undescended or maldescended testes, and other abnormalities of the male genitalia must be reported. Circumcision is contraindicated in the presence of hypospadias or epispadias since the foreskin is used in repair of these anomalies.

Inguinal hernias can be present and become more obvious when the infant cries.

Skeletal System

The infant's skeletal system undergoes rapid development during the first year of life. At birth, more cartilage is present than ossified bone. Because of cephalocaudal (head-to-rump) development, the newborn looks somewhat out of proportion.

The head at term is one fourth of the total body length. The arms are slightly longer than the legs. In the newborn, the legs are one third of the total body length but only 15% of the total body weight. As growth proceeds, the midpoint in head-to-toe measurements gradually descends from the level of the umbilicus at birth to the level of the symphysis pubis at maturity.

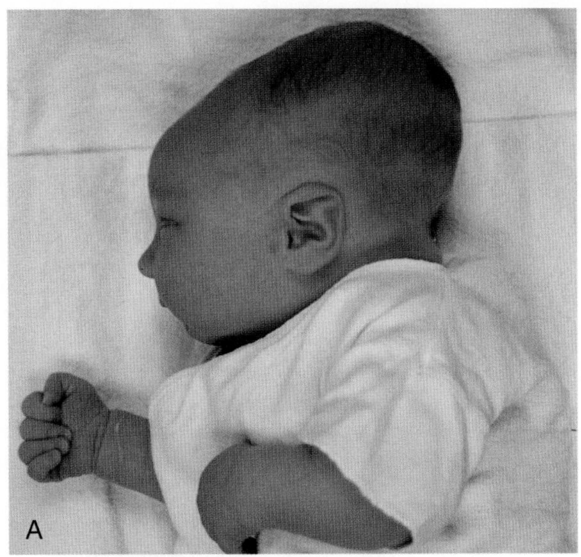

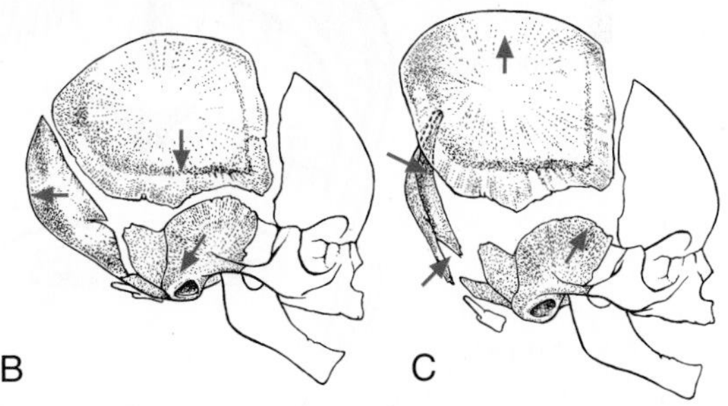

FIGURE 25-10 Moulding. **A:** Significant moulding after vaginal birth. **B:** Schematic of bones with no moulding. **C:** Schematic of bones with moulding. (**A,** Courtesy Kim Molloy.)

The face appears small in relation to the skull. The skull appears large and heavy. Cranial size and shape can be distorted by moulding (the shaping of the fetal head through overlapping of the cranial bones to facilitate movement through the birth canal during labour) (Fig. 25-10).

Caput Succedaneum

Caput succedaneum is a generalized, easily identifiable edematous area of the scalp, most commonly found on the occiput (Fig. 25-11, A). The sustained pressure of the presenting vertex against the cervix results in compression of local vessels, thereby slowing venous return. The slower venous return causes an increase in tissue fluids within the skin of the scalp, and an edematous swelling develops. This edematous swelling, present at birth, extends across the suture lines of the skull and disappears spontaneously within 3 to 4 days. Infants who are born with the assistance of vacuum extraction usually have a caput in the area where the cup was applied.

Cephalhematoma

Cephalhematoma is a collection of blood between a skull bone and its periosteum. Thus, a cephalhematoma does not cross a

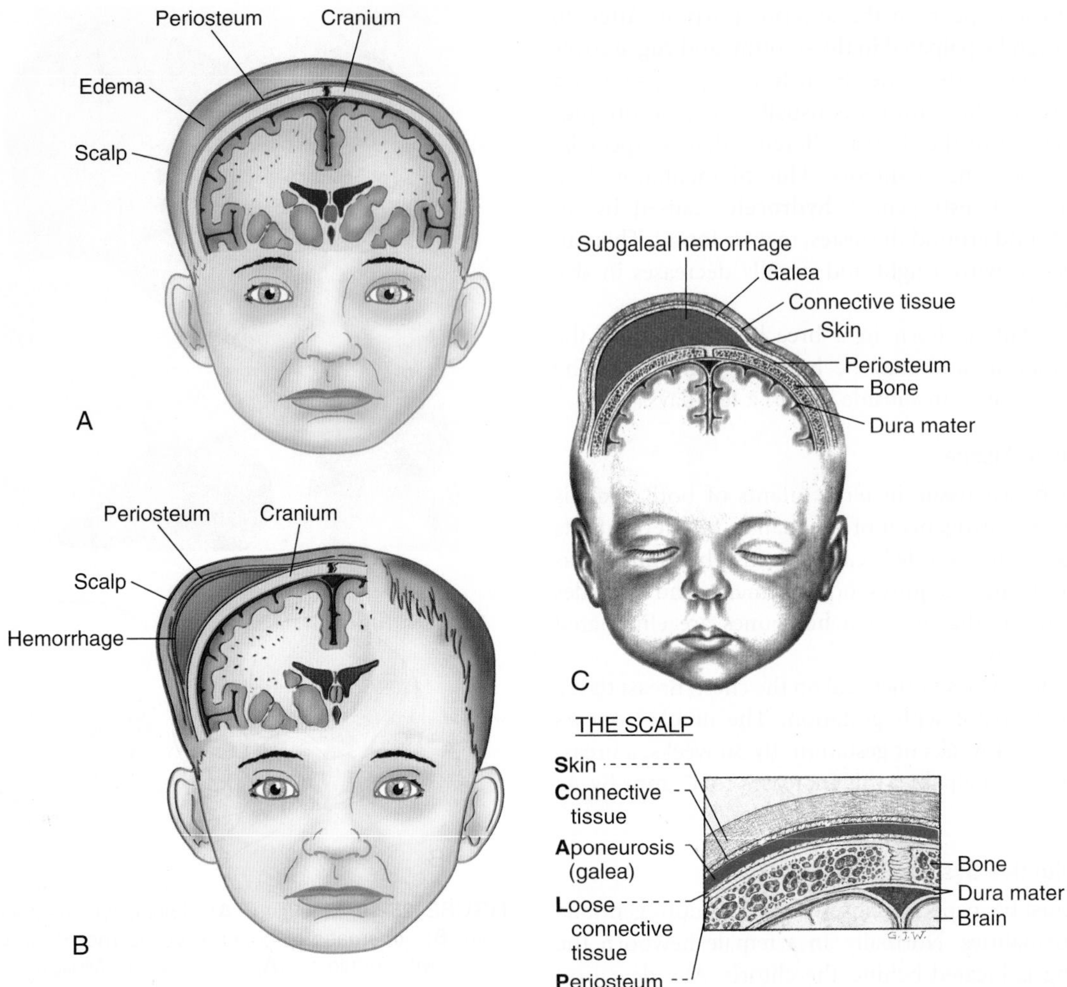

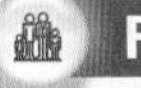

FIGURE 25-11 **A:** Caput succedaneum. **B:** Cephalhematoma. **C:** Subgaleal hemorrhage. (**A** and **B** from Seidel, H. M., Stewart, R. W., Ball, J. W., et al. (2006). *Mosby's guide to physical examination* (6th ed.). St. Louis: Mosby.)

cranial suture line (see Fig. 25-11, B). Often caput succedaneum and cephalhematoma occur simultaneously.

Bleeding may occur with spontaneous birth from pressure against the maternal bony pelvis. Low forceps birth and difficult forceps rotation and extraction may also cause bleeding. This soft, fluctuating, irreducible fullness does not pulsate or bulge when the infant cries. It appears several hours or the day after birth and may not become apparent until a caput succedaneum is absorbed. A cephalhematoma is usually largest on the second or third day, by which time the bleeding stops (see Family-Centred Teaching box). The fullness of a cephalhematoma spontaneously resolves in 3 to 6 weeks. It is not aspirated because infection may develop if the skin is punctured. As the hematoma resolves, hemolysis of RBCs occurs and jaundice may result. Hyperbilirubinemia and jaundice may occur from a cephalhematoma after the newborn is discharged home.

Subgaleal Hemorrhage

Subgaleal hemorrhage is bleeding into the subgaleal compartment (see Fig. 25-11, C). The subgaleal compartment is a potential space that contains loosely arranged connective tissue; it is located beneath the galea aponeurosis, the tendinous sheath that connects the frontal and occipital muscles and forms the inner surface of the scalp. Subgaleal hemorrhage is commonly associated with difficult operative vaginal birth, especially vacuum extraction. With the vacuum extractor the scalp is pulled away from the bony calvarium; the vessels are torn, and blood collects in the subgaleal space. Blood loss can be severe, resulting in hypovolemic shock, disseminated intravascular coagulation (DIC), and death.

FAMILY-CENTRED TEACHING

Swelling on the Scalp

A 2-day-old healthy newborn has a "bump" on the left side of the head. The mother is concerned that the baby may have somehow fallen out of the crib and injured the head. Nursing assessment findings are that the scalp swelling is raised and soft to the touch but does not cross cranial suture lines; there is no apparent bruising or discolouration. The neurological assessment reveals no significant findings, and the newborn's behaviour appears to be that of a healthy term infant. How could the nurse explain the condition and reassure the mother that her newborn has a common finding rather than an abnormal condition requiring immediate medical attention?

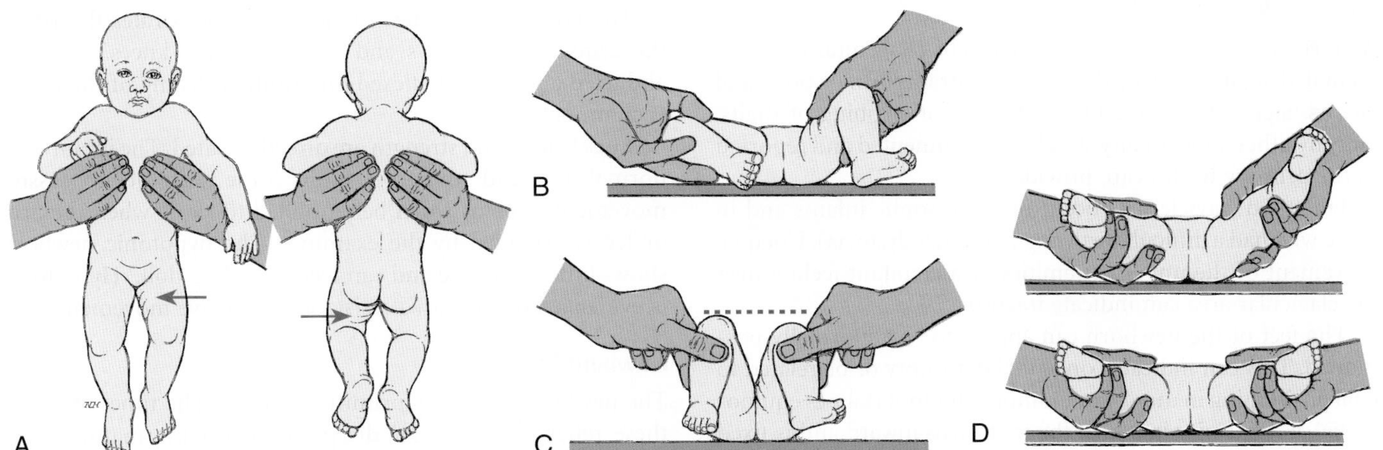

FIGURE 25-12 Signs of developmental dysplasia of the hip. **A:** Asymmetry of gluteal and thigh folds with shortening of the thigh (Galeazzi sign). **B:** Limited hip abduction, as seen in flexion (Ortolani test). **C:** Apparent shortening of the femur, as indicated by the level of the knees in flexion (Allis sign). **D:** Ortolani test with femoral head moving in and out of acetabulum (in infants 1 to 2 months old). (From Hockenberry, M. J., & Wilson, D. [2013]. *Wong's essentials of pediatric nursing* [9th ed.]. St. Louis: Mosby.)

Early detection of the hemorrhage is vital; serial head circumference measurements and inspection of the back of the neck for increasing edema and a firm mass are an essential aspect of assessment of newborns who are delivered via a vacuum extractor. A boggy scalp, pallor, tachycardia, and increasing head circumference may also be early signs of a subgaleal hemorrhage. Computed tomography (CT) or magnetic resonance imaging (MRI) is useful in confirming the diagnosis. Replacement of lost blood and clotting factors is required in acute cases of hemorrhage. Another possible early sign of subgaleal hemorrhage is a forward and lateral positioning of the newborn's ears, because the hematoma extends posteriorly. Monitoring the infant for changes in level of consciousness and decreases in hematocrit is also key to early recognition and management (Mangurten & Puppala, 2011).

Spine

The bones in the vertebral column of the newborn form two primary curvatures—one in the thoracic region and one in the sacral region. Both are forward, concave curvatures. As the infant gains head control at approximately age 3 months, a secondary curvature appears in the cervical region. The newborn's spine appears straight and can be flexed easily. The newborn can lift the head and turn it from side to side when prone. The vertebrae should appear straight and flat. If a pilonidal dimple is noted, further inspection is required to determine whether a sinus is present. A pilonidal dimple, especially with a sinus and nevus pilosis (hairy nevus), is significant because it can be associated with spina bifida.

Extremities

The infant's extremities should be symmetrical and of equal length. Fingers and toes should be equal in number (five fingers on each hand and five toes on each foot) and should have nails present. Digits may be missing (**oligodactyly**). Extra digits (**polydactyly**) are sometimes found on hands or feet. Fingers or toes may be fused (**syndactyly**). In some newborn infants, there is a significant separation of the knees when the ankles are held together, resulting in an appearance of bowlegs. At birth, there is no apparent arch to the foot.

The infant is examined for **developmental dysplasia of the hip (DDH)**. In newborns with DDH the affected hip is unlikely to be dislocated at birth; instead it is easily dislocatable. Postnatal factors determine whether the hip dislocates, subluxates, or remains stable. DDH occurs more often in female infants, in breech presentations (Fig. 25-12), and in infants with a family history of DDH (Cooperman & Thompson, 2011).

Signs of DDH are asymmetrical gluteal and thigh skinfolds, uneven knee levels, a positive Ortolani test, and a positive Barlow test. The hips are inspected for symmetry. Gluteal and thigh skin folds should be equal and symmetrical, and legs should be of equal length (Fig. 25-12, A). The level of the knees in flexion should be equal (see Fig. 25-12, C). Hip integrity is assessed by using the Barlow test and the Ortolani manoeuvre. For the Barlow test the examiner places the middle finger over the greater trochanter and the thumb along the midthigh. The hip is flexed to 90 degrees and adducted, followed by gentle downward pushing of the femoral head. If the hip can be dislocated with this manoeuvre, the femoral head moves out of the acetabulum, and the examiner feels a "clunk." The hip is then checked to determine if the femoral head can be returned into the acetabulum using the Ortolani test. As the hip is abducted and upward leverage is applied, a dislocated hip returns to the acetabulum with a clunk that is felt by the examiner (see Fig. 25-12, B and D).

SAFETY ALERT

Only expert examiners (physicians, nurse practitioners) should perform the Barlow test and Ortolani manoeuvre to assess for developmental dysplasia of the hip. An unskilled examiner can cause injury to the newborn.

Signs of Skeletal Problems

Abnormalities of the skeletal system can be congenital, developmental, drug induced, or the result of intrapartum or postnatal factors. Signs of DDH, additional digits or webbing of digits, and any other abnormality should be documented and reported to the primary health care provider.

Fractured clavicle may occur in macrosomic infants and in those who had a difficult birth (e.g., shoulder dystocia). Unequal movement of the upper extremities or a crepitant feeling over the clavicular area can indicate fracture.

The feet of the newborn can appear to be abnormally positioned. This can indicate congenital deformity or be related to fetal positioning in utero. For example, clubfoot (talipes equinovarus), a deformity in which the foot turns inward and is fixed in a plantar-flexion position, is a congenital condition that warrants attention. If the foot is turned inward in the plantar-flexion position but can be moved into the normal position, it is likely caused by fetal positioning and should gradually resolve.

Neuromuscular System

The neuromuscular system is almost completely developed at birth. The term newborn is a vital, responsive, and reactive being with a remarkable capacity for social interaction and self-organization.

Growth of the brain after birth follows a predictable pattern of rapid growth during infancy and early childhood; growth becomes more gradual during the remainder of the first decade and minimal during adolescence. The cerebellum ends its growth spurt, which began at about 30 gestational weeks, by the end of the first year.

The brain requires glucose, as a source of energy, and a relatively large supply of oxygen for adequate metabolism. Such requirements signal a need for careful assessment of the infant's respiratory status. The necessity for glucose requires attentiveness to those newborns who are at risk for hypoglycemia (e.g., infants of diabetic mothers; infants who are **macrosomic** or small for gestational age; and newborns experiencing prolonged birth, hypoxia, or preterm birth).

Spontaneous motor activity may be seen as transient tremors of the mouth and chin, especially during crying episodes, and of the extremities, notably the arms and hands. Transient tremors are normal and can be observed in nearly every newborn. These tremors should not be present when the infant is quiet and should not persist beyond 1 month of age. Persistent tremors or tremors involving the entire body may indicate pathological conditions. Normal tremors, tremors of hypoglycemia, and central nervous system (CNS) disorders need to be differentiated so that corrective care can be instituted as necessary.

> **! NURSING ALERT**
>
> To differentiate between tremors or jitteriness and seizure activity, consider the following signs (Verklan & Lopez, 2011):
>
> - Tremors and jitteriness are easily elicited by motions or voice and cease with gentle restraint of the body part, whereas seizure activity continues.
> - Seizure activity is associated with ocular changes (eyes deviating or staring) and autonomic changes (apnea, tachycardia, pupil changes, increased salivation); these signs are not associated with jitteriness or tremors.

The posture of the term newborn demonstrates flexion of the arms at the elbows and the legs at the knees. Hips are abducted and partially flexed. Intermittent fisting of the hands is common.

Muscle tone and strength are directly related. The infant with normal tone and strength exhibits some resistance to passive movement, such as when being pulled to sit or when the arm or leg is extended by the examiner. The hypotonic newborn shows little resistance and can feel like a "rag doll." Hypertonia is evidenced by increased resistance to passive movement.

Newborn Reflexes

The newborn has many primitive reflexes. The times at which these reflexes appear and disappear reflect the maturity and intactness of the developing nervous system. Primary reflexes reflect normal brainstem activity. CNS depression should be suspected if they cannot be elicited or they are persistent beyond a certain age; this suggests damage of cortical functioning. The most common reflexes found in the normal newborn are described in Table 25-4.

BEHAVIOURAL CHARACTERISTICS

The healthy newborn must accomplish behavioural and biological tasks to develop normally. Behavioural characteristics form the basis of the infant's social capabilities. Newborns progress through a hierarchy of developmental challenges as they adapt to their environment and caregivers. They must first be able to regulate their physiological or autonomic system, including involuntary physiological functions such as heart rate, respiration, and temperature. The next level is motor organization, in which infants regulate or control their motor behaviour. This includes controlling random movements, improving muscle tone, and reducing excessive activity. The third level of behaviour is state regulation, which refers to the ability to modulate the state of consciousness. The infant develops predictable sleep and wake states and is able to react to stress through self-regulation or through communicating with the caregiver by crying and then being consoled. Finally, the infant reaches the fourth level of attention and social interaction. He or she is able to attend to visual and auditory stimulation, stay alert for long periods, and engage in social interaction (Brazelton & Nugent, 2011).

This progression in behaviour is the basis for the Brazelton Neonatal Behavioral Assessment Scale (NBAS) (Brazelton & Nugent, 2011). The NBAS is an interactive examination that assesses the infant's response to 28 areas organized according to the clusters in Box 25-2. It is generally used as a research or diagnostic tool and requires special training. The NBAS helps the practitioner identify where the infant falls along the continuum of behaviours and determine the type of support needed.

The Newborn Behavioral Observations (NBO) system, based on the NBAS, is a tool that is used in clinical settings to help parents identify, understand, and respond to newborn behaviour (Nugent, Keefer, Minear, et al., 2007). Karl and Keefer (2011) developed a training program using the NBO system to educate clinicians about newborn behaviour, self-regulation skills, and social interaction capabilities. A major benefit of this program is that nurses and other clinicians can use the information to educate parents and help them interpret newborn cues and respond appropriately, which promotes attachment (Karl & Keefer, 2011). See Chapter 23 for further discussion of attachment.

Sleep–Wake States

Healthy newborns differ in their activity levels, feeding patterns, sleeping patterns, and responsiveness. Parents' reactions to their newborns are often determined by these differences. Showing parents the unique characteristics of their infant helps them develop a more positive perception of the newborn and promotes increased interaction between infant and parent. Newborn responses to environmental stimuli and to their caregivers depend on the newborn's state or state of consciousness.

In the early newborn period infants tend to alternate periods of sleep and wakefulness that resemble their fetal inactivity and activity patterns. Variations in the state of consciousness of infants are called **sleep–wake states**. The six states form a continuum from deep sleep to extreme irritability (Fig. 25-13): two sleep states (deep sleep and light sleep) and four wake states

TABLE 25-4 ASSESSMENT OF NEWBORN REFLEXES

REFLEX	ELICITING THE REFLEX	CHARACTERISTIC RESPONSE	COMMENTS
Sucking and rooting	Touch infant's lip, cheek, or corner of mouth with nipple or finger.	Infant turns head toward stimulus and opens mouth.	Response is difficult if not impossible to elicit after infant has been fed. Parental guidance: Avoid trying to turn head toward breast or nipple; allow infant to root; response disappears after 3–4* mo but may persist up to 1 yr. A weak or absent response can indicate prematurity or neurological deficit.
Swallowing	Feed infant; swallowing usually follows sucking and obtaining fluids.	Swallowing is usually coordinated with sucking and breathing and usually occurs without gagging, coughing, apnea, or vomiting.	If response is weak or absent, this may indicate preterm birth, effects of maternal analgesics, or illness that needs investigation. Sucking, swallowing, and breathing are often uncoordinated in a preterm infant.
Grasp			
Palmar	Place finger in palm of hand.	Infant's fingers curl around examiner's fingers.	Palmar response lessens by 3–4 mo; parents enjoy this contact with infant.
Plantar	Place finger at base of toes.	Toes curl downward.	Plantar response lessens by 8 mo.

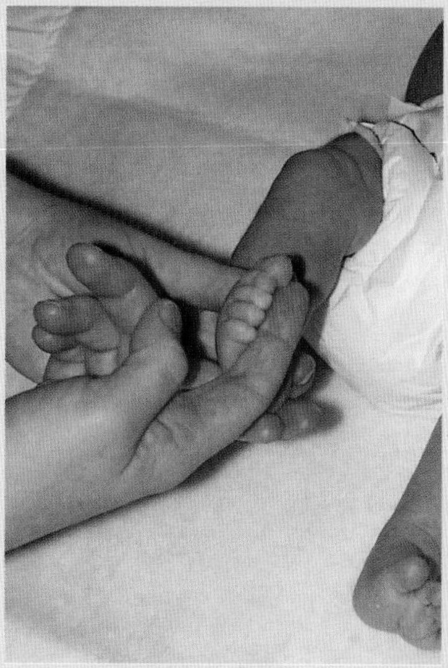

Plantar grasp reflex. (From Zitelli, B. J., & Davis, H. W. (2007). *Atlas of pediatric physical diagnosis* (5th ed.). St. Louis: Mosby.)

*All durations for persistence of reflexes are based on time elapsed after 40 weeks of gestation; that is, if newborn was born at 36 weeks of gestation, add 1 month to all time limits given.

Continued

TABLE 25-4 ASSESSMENT OF NEWBORN REFLEXES—cont'd

REFLEX	ELICITING THE REFLEX	CHARACTERISTIC RESPONSE	COMMENTS
Extrusion	Touch or depress tip of tongue.	Newborn forces tongue outward.	Response disappears at about fourth to fifth month.
Glabellar (Myerson)	Tap over forehead, bridge of nose, or maxilla of newborn whose eyes are open.	Newborn blinks for first four or five taps.	Continued blinking with repeated taps is consistent with extrapyramidal signs.
Tonic neck or "fencing"	With infant in a supine neutral position, turn head quickly to one side.	With infant facing left side, arm and leg on that side extend; the opposite arm and leg flex (turn head to right, and extremities assume opposite postures).	Responses in leg are more consistent. Complete response disappears by 3–4 mo; incomplete response may be seen until third or fourth year. After 6 wk, persistent response is a sign of an abnormality.
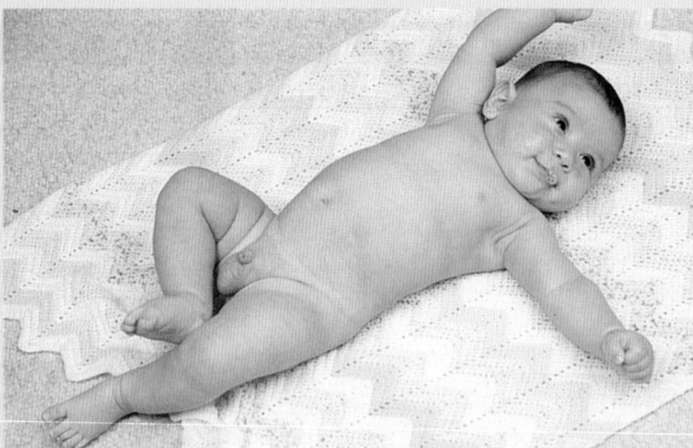 Classic pose in tonic neck reflex. (Courtesy Marjorie Pyle, RNC, Lifecircle.)			
Moro (or startle)	Hold infant in semisitting position, allowing head and trunk to fall backward (with support). Place infant supine on flat surface; make a loud, abrupt noise.	Symmetrical abduction and extension of arms are seen; fingers fan out and form a *C* with thumb and forefinger; slight tremor may be noted; arms are adducted in embracing motion and return to relaxed flexion and movement. A cry may accompany or follow motor movement. Legs may follow similar pattern of response. Preterm infants do not complete "embrace"; instead, their arms fall backward because of weakness.	Response is present at birth; complete response may be seen until 8 wk; body jerk only is seen between 8 and 18 wk; response is absent by 6 mo if neurological maturation is not delayed; response may be incomplete if infant is in deep sleep state; give parental guidance about normal response. Asymmetrical response may connote injury to brachial plexus, clavicle, or humerus. Persistent response after 6 mo indicates possible neurological abnormality.
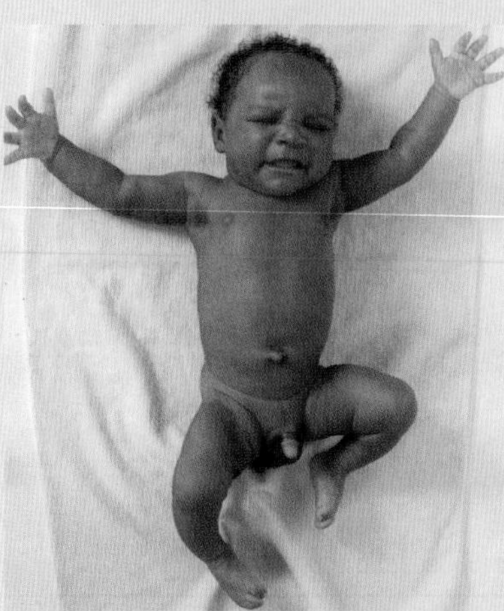 Moro reflex. (Courtesy Paul Vincent Kuntz, Texas Children's Hospital.)			

TABLE 25-4 ASSESSMENT OF NEWBORN REFLEXES—cont'd

REFLEX	ELICITING THE REFLEX	CHARACTERISTIC RESPONSE	COMMENTS
Stepping or "walking"	Hold infant vertically under arms or on trunk, allowing one foot to touch table surface.	Infant will simulate walking, alternating flexion and extension of feet; term infants walk on soles of their feet, and preterm infants walk on their toes.	Response is normally present for 3–4 wk.

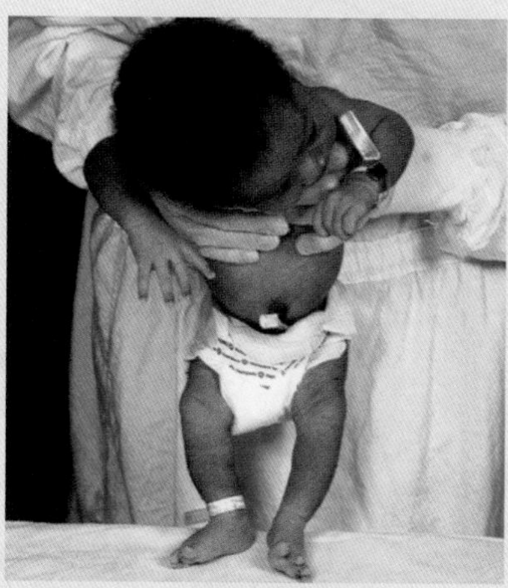

Stepping reflex. (From Dickason, E. J., Silverman, B. L., & Kaplan, J. A. [1998]. *Maternal–infant nursing care* [3rd ed.]. St. Louis: Mosby.)

REFLEX	ELICITING THE REFLEX	CHARACTERISTIC RESPONSE	COMMENTS
Crawling	Place newborn on abdomen.	Newborn makes crawling movements with arms and legs.	Response should disappear at about 6 wk of age.

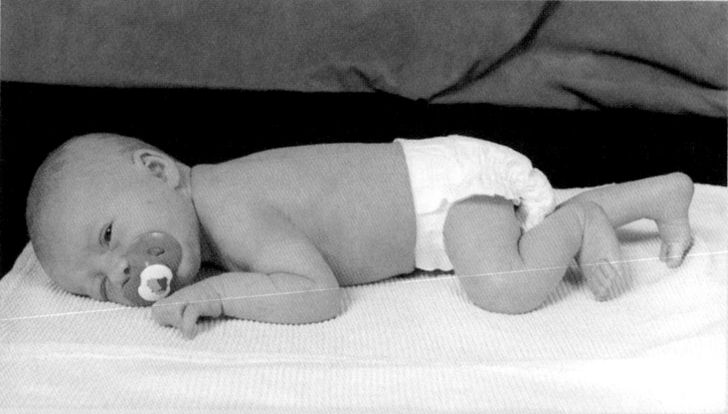

Crawling reflex. (Courtesy Paul Vincent Kuntz, Texas Children's Hospital)

REFLEX	ELICITING THE REFLEX	CHARACTERISTIC RESPONSE	COMMENTS
Deep tendon	Use finger instead of percussion hammer to elicit patellar, or knee jerk, reflex; newborn must be relaxed.	Reflex jerk is present; even with newborn relaxed, nonselective overall reaction may occur.	
Crossed extension	With infant in supine position, examiner extends one leg of infant and presses down knee. Stimulation of sole of foot of fixated limb should cause free leg to flex, adduct, and extend as if attempting to push away stimulating agent.	Opposite leg flexes, adducts, and then extends.	This reflex should be present during newborn period.

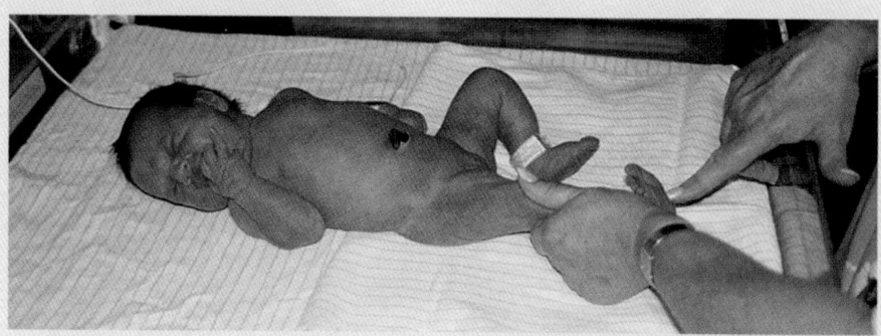

Crossed extension reflex. (Courtesy Marjorie Pyle, RNC, Lifecircle.)

Continued

TABLE 25-4 ASSESSMENT OF NEWBORN REFLEXES—cont'd

REFLEX	ELICITING THE REFLEX	CHARACTERISTIC RESPONSE	COMMENTS
Babinski (plantar)	On sole of foot, beginning at heel, stroke upward along lateral aspect of sole, then move finger across ball of foot.	All toes hyperextend, with dorsiflexion of big toe—recorded as a positive sign.	Absence requires neurological evaluation, should disappear after 1 yr of age. Response depends on infant's general muscle tone, maturity, and condition.
Pull-to-sit (traction response); postural tone	Pull infant up by wrists from supine position with head in midline.	Head lags until infant is in upright position; then head is held in same plane with chest and shoulder momentarily before falling forward; infant attempts to right head.	Response depends on general muscle tone and maturity and condition of infant.
Truncal incurvation (Galant)	Place infant prone on flat surface; run finger down back about 4–5 cm lateral to spine, first on one side and then down the other.	Trunk is flexed and pelvis is swung toward stimulated side.	Response disappears by fourth week. Response varies but should be obtainable in all infants, including preterm ones. Absence suggests general depression of central nervous system. With transverse lesions of cord, no response below the level of lesion is present.

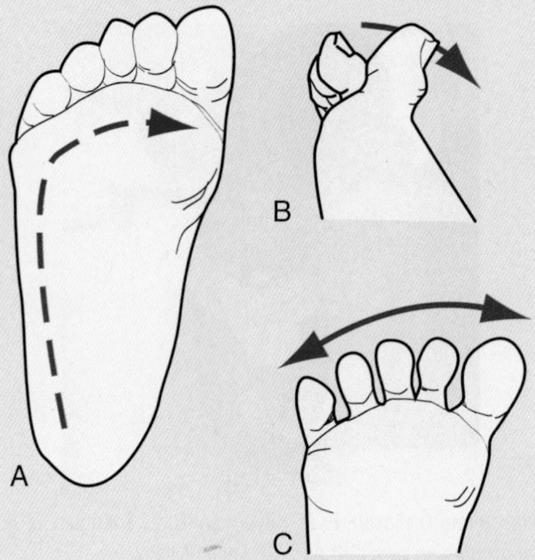

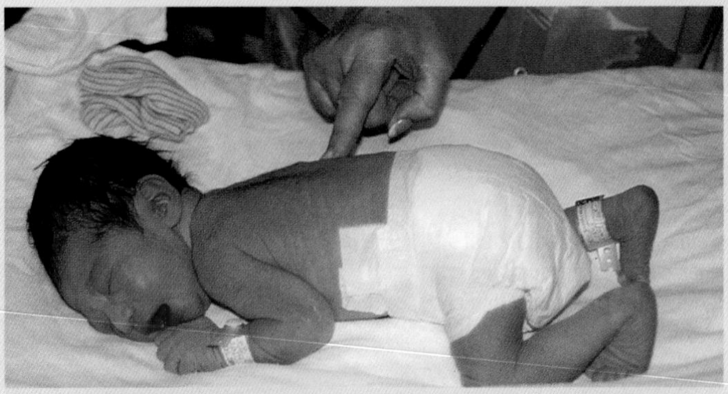

Babinski reflex. **A:** Direction of stroke. **B:** Dorsiflexion of big toe. **C:** Fanning of toes. (From Hockenberry, M. J., & Wilson, D. [2013]. *Wong's nursing care of infants and children* [9th ed.]. St. Louis: Mosby.)

Trunk incurvation reflex. (Courtesy Marjorie Pyle, RNC, Lifecircle.)

TABLE 25-4 ASSESSMENT OF NEWBORN REFLEXES—cont'd

REFLEX	ELICITING THE REFLEX	CHARACTERISTIC RESPONSE	COMMENTS
Magnet	Place infant in supine position, partially flex both lower extremities, and apply light pressure with fingers to soles of feet (Fig. A). Normally, while examiner's fingers maintain contact with soles of feet, lower limbs extend.	Both lower limbs should extend against examiner's pressure (Fig. B).	Absence suggests damage to central nervous system. Weak reflex may be seen after breech presentation without extended legs or may indicate sciatic nerve stretch syndrome. Breech presentation with extended legs may evoke exaggerated response.

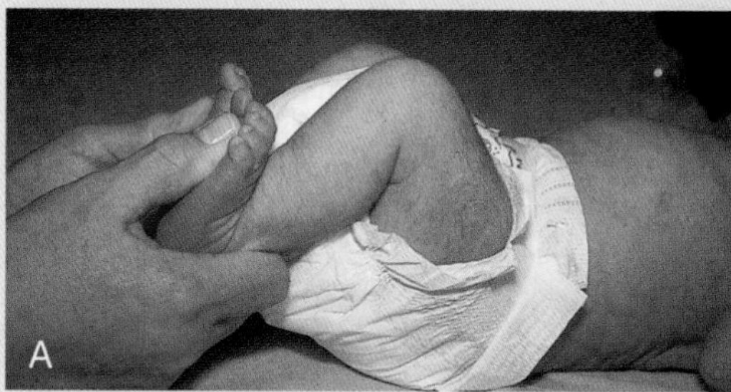

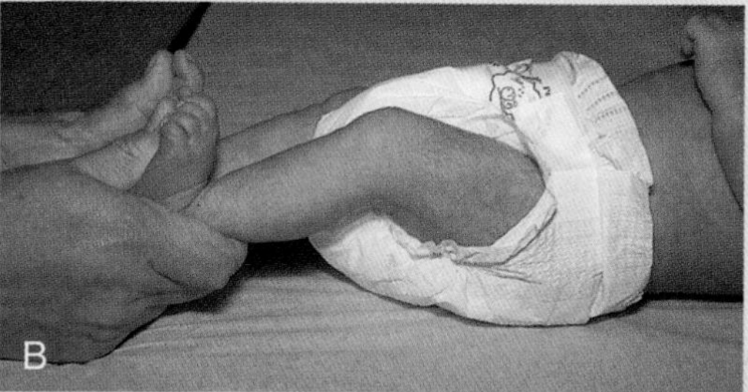

Magnet reflex. (Courtesy Michael S. Clement, MD.)

REFLEX	ELICITING THE REFLEX	CHARACTERISTIC RESPONSE	COMMENTS
Additional newborn responses: yawn, stretch, burp, hiccup, sneeze	These are spontaneous behaviours.	They may be slightly depressed temporarily because of maternal analgesia or anaesthesia, fetal hypoxia, or infection.	Parental guidance: Most of these behaviours are pleasurable to parents. Parents need to be assured that behaviours are normal. Sneeze is usually a response to mucus in nose and not an indicator of a cold (upper respiratory tract infection). No treatment is needed for hiccups; sucking may help. In the preterm infant, these are signs of neurodevelopmental immaturity and physiological stress.

BOX 25-2 CLUSTERS OF NEONATAL BEHAVIOURS IN BRAZELTON NEONATAL BEHAVIOURAL ASSESSMENT SCALE

- Habituation—Ability to respond to and then inhibit responding to discrete stimulus (e.g., light, rattle, bell, pinprick) while asleep
- Orientation—Quality of alert states and ability to attend to visual and auditory stimuli while alert
- Motor performance—Quality of movement and tone
- Range of state—Measure of general arousal level or arousability of newborn
- Regulation of state—How newborn responds when aroused
- Autonomic stability—Signs of stress (e.g., tremors, startles, skin colour) related to homeostatic (self-regulator) adjustment of the nervous system
- Reflexes—Assessment of several neonatal reflexes

From Brazelton, T., & Nugent, J. (2011). *Neonatal behavioural assessment scale* (4th ed.). London: MacKeith.

(drowsy, quiet alert, active alert, and crying) (Brazelton & Nugent, 2011). Each state has specific characteristics and state-related behaviours. The optimal state of arousal is the quiet alert state. During this state newborns smile, vocalize, move in synchrony with speech, watch their parents' faces, and respond to people talking to them. They respond to internal and external environmental factors by controlling sensory input and regulating the sleep–wake states; the ability to make smooth transitions between states is called *state modulation.* The ability to regulate sleep–wake states is essential in the newborn's neurobehavioural development. As infants approach term gestation, they are better able to cope with external or internal factors that affect the sleep–wake patterns.

Newborns use purposeful behaviour to maintain the optimal arousal state as follows: (1) actively withdrawing by increasing physical distance, (2) rejecting by pushing away with hands and feet, (3) decreasing sensitivity by falling asleep or breaking eye contact by turning the head, or (4) using signalling behaviours such as fussing and crying. These behaviours permit the newborn to quiet self and reinstate readiness to interact.

The first 6 weeks of life involve a steady decrease in the proportion of active REM sleep to total sleep. A steady increase in the proportion of quiet sleep to total sleep also occurs. Periods of wakefulness increase. For the first few weeks the wakeful

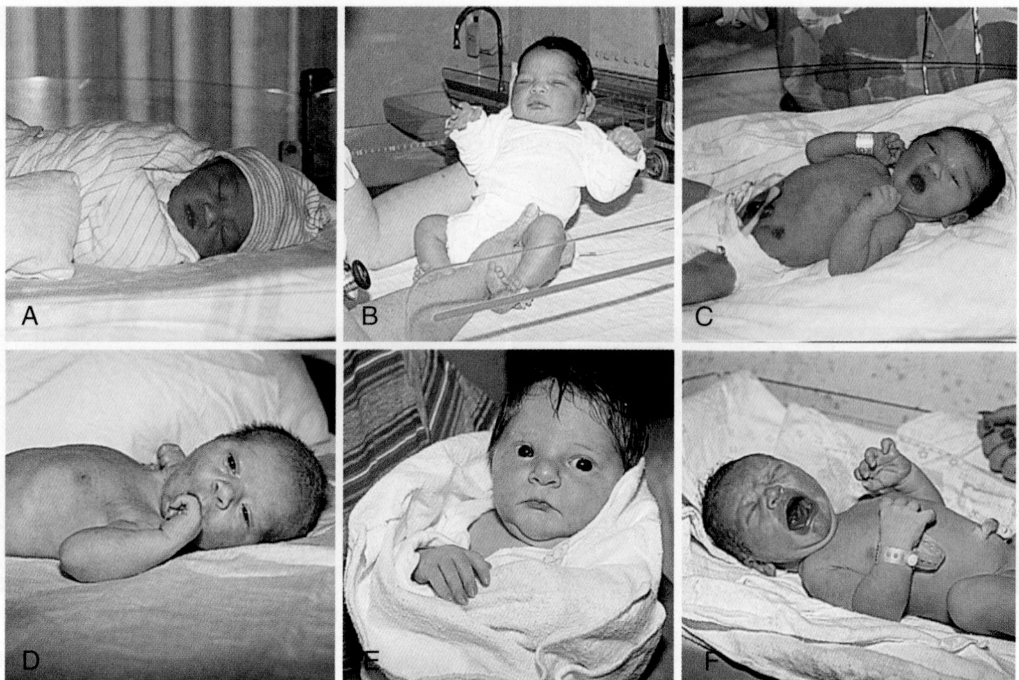

FIGURE 25-13 Newborn sleep–wake states. **A:** Deep sleep. **B:** Light sleep. **C:** Drowsy. **D:** Quiet alert. **E:** Active alert. **F:** Crying. (Courtesy Marjorie Pyle, RNC, Lifecircle.)

periods seem dictated by hunger, but soon a need for socializing appears. The newborn sleeps on average approximately 17 hours a day, with periods of wakefulness gradually increasing. By the fourth week of life some newborns stay awake from one feeding to the next.

Other Factors Influencing Behaviour of Newborns

Gestational Age

Postnatal gestational age assessment is unreliable in infants that are premature or postterm. The most common techniques for determining gestational age in the immediate postnatal period include assessment and the Ballard score to determine neuromuscular and physical maturity (see Chapter 26 for further discussion).

Stimuli

Environmental events and stimuli affect newborns' behavioural responses. The newborn responds to animate and inanimate stimuli. Nurses in intensive care nurseries have observed that newborns respond to loud noises, bright lights, monitor alarms, and tension in the unit.

Medication

No conclusive evidence exists regarding the effects of maternal analgesia or anaesthesia during labour on neonatal behaviour. Researchers who have studied the effects of epidural medications on breastfeeding behaviours have been unable to show a cause-and-effect relationship (Hoyt, 2011).

Sensory Behaviours

From birth, newborns possess sensory capabilities that indicate a state of readiness for social interaction. Newborns effectively use behavioural responses in establishing their first dialogues. These responses, coupled with the newborns' "baby appearance" (e.g., facial proportions of forehead and eyes larger than the lower part of the face) and their small size and helplessness, evoke feelings of wanting to hold and protect them and to interact with them.

Vision

At birth, the eye is structurally incomplete and the muscles are immature. The process of accommodation is not present at birth but improves over the first 3 months of life. The pupils react to light, the blink reflex is easily stimulated, and the corneal reflex is activated by light touch. Term newborns can see objects as far away as 50 cm. The clearest visual distance is 17 to 20 cm, which is about the distance the newborn's face is from the mother's face as she breastfeeds or cuddles. Newborns are sensitive to light; they will frown if a bright light is flashed in their eyes and will turn toward a soft, red light. If the room is darkened, they will open their eyes wide and look about. By 2 months of age, they can detect colour; but at 5 days of age and younger, they seem more attracted by black-and-white patterns.

Response to movement is noticeable. If a bright light is shown to newborns (even at 15 minutes of age), they will follow it visually; some will even turn their heads to do so. Because human eyes are bright, shiny objects, newborns will track their parents' eyes. Parents often comment on how exciting this behaviour is. The development of eye-to-eye contact is important for parent–infant attachment. Children of blind parents and parents who have blind children must circumvent this obstacle to form a relationship. See discussion on p. 601.

Visual acuity is surprising; even at 2 weeks of age, newborns can distinguish patterns with stripes 3 mm apart. By 6 months their vision is as acute as that of an adult. They prefer to look at patterns rather than plain surfaces, even if the latter are brightly coloured. Newborns prefer more complex patterns to simple ones. They prefer novelty (changes in pattern) by 2 months of age. The infant of a few weeks of age is thus capable of responding actively to an enriched environment.

Hearing

As soon as the amniotic fluid drains from the ears, the newborn's hearing is similar to that of an adult. Loud sounds of about 90 decibels cause the newborn to react with a Moro reflex. The newborn responds to low-frequency sounds such as a heartbeat or lullaby by decreasing motor activity or stopping crying. High-frequency sound elicits an alerting response.

The newborn responds readily to the mother's voice. Studies indicate a selective listening to maternal voice sounds and rhythms during intrauterine life that prepares newborns for recognition of and interaction with their primary caregivers—their mothers. Newborns are accustomed to hearing the regular rhythm of the mother's heartbeat. As a result, they respond by relaxing and ceasing to fuss and cry if a regular heartbeat simulator is placed in their cribs. Hearing is integral to bonding and attachment and may be more important than vision (Gardner & Goldson, 2011).

Routine hearing screening is recommended for all newborns before hospital discharge, although it is not mandatory in all provinces. See Chapter 26 for a discussion about screening of newborn hearing.

Smell

Newborns have a highly developed sense of smell and can detect and discriminate distinct odours. It has been shown that preterm infants as early as 28 weeks are capable of reacting to odours. They react to strong odours, such as alcohol or vinegar, by turning their heads away but are attracted to sweet smells. Breastfed infants are able to smell breast milk and can differentiate their mother from other lactating women by the smell (Lawrence & Lawrence, 2011).

Taste

The newborn can distinguish among tastes, and various types of solutions elicit differing facial expressions. A tasteless solution produces no response, a sweet solution elicits eager sucking, a sour solution causes puckering of the lips, and a bitter liquid produces a grimace.

Young infants are particularly oriented toward the use of their mouths, both for meeting their nutritional needs for rapid growth and for releasing tension through sucking. The early development of circumoral sensation, muscle activity, and taste would seem to be preparation for survival in the extrauterine environment.

Touch

The newborn is responsive to touch on all parts of the body. The face (especially the mouth), hands, and soles of the feet appear to be the most sensitive. Reflexes can be elicited by stroking the infant. The newborn's responses to touch suggest that this sensory system is well prepared to receive and process tactile messages. Touch and motion are essential to normal growth and development, and infant massage is a way to increase tactile stimulation. However, each infant is unique, and variations can be seen in newborns' responses to touch (see Family-Centred Teaching box). Birth trauma or stress and depressant medications taken by the mother decrease the infant's sensitivity to touch or painful stimuli. Multiple studies demonstrate the benefits of skin-to-skin care immediately after birth.

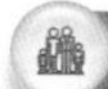

FAMILY-CENTRED TEACHING

Newborn Behaviour

A first-time single mother asks the nurse about her newborn's activity. She voices concern that the newborn cries when she changes his diaper. "He sleeps a lot and only wakes up to eat or when I change his diaper. Is that normal?" Develop a short parent teaching lesson to present newborn behaviour and care in relation to the following: sleep–wake states, newborn activities and relationship to crying behaviours in the first few days of life, and how to comfort and console the newborn.

Response to Environmental Stimuli

Habituation

Habituation is a protective mechanism that allows the newborn to become accustomed to environmental stimuli. Habituation is a psychological and physiological phenomenon in which the response to a constant or repetitive stimulus is decreased.

The ability to habituate allows the healthy term newborn to select stimuli that promote continued learning about the social world, thus avoiding overload. The intrauterine environment appears to have programmed the newborn to be especially responsive to human voices, soft lights, soft sounds, and sweet tastes.

The newborn quickly learns the sounds in the home environment and is able to sleep in their midst. The selective responses of the newborn indicate cerebral organization capable of memory and making choices. The ability to habituate depends on the state of consciousness, hunger, fatigue, and temperament. These factors also affect consolability, cuddliness, irritability, and crying.

Consolability

Newborns vary in the ability to console themselves or be consoled. In the crying state most newborns initiate one of several ways to reduce their distress. Hand-to-mouth movements with or without sucking and being alert to voices, noises, or visual stimuli are common. Some infants are consoled only if they are held and rocked (Brazelton & Nugent, 2011).

Cuddliness

Cuddliness is especially important to parents because they often gauge their ability to care for the child by the child's responses to their actions. The degree to which newborns mould into the contours of the person holding them varies. One extreme is the infant who always resists being held with thrashing and stiffening of the body. This is in contrast to the infant who immediately relaxes when held and moulds to the body of the person. Less extreme behaviour is demonstrated by infants who are passive when held and those who gradually mould after being held for a while (Brazelton & Nugent, 2011).

Irritability

Some newborns cry longer and harder than others. For some, the sensory threshold seems low. They are readily upset by unusual noises, hunger, wetness, or new experiences and thus respond intensely. Others with a high sensory threshold require a great deal more stimulation and variation to reach the active, alert state.

Crying

Crying is the language a newborn uses most often to communicate needs. It may signal hunger, discomfort, pain, desire for attention, or fussiness. Infants may cry in response to environmental stimuli such as cold, being overstimulated, or being held by multiple persons. Responsiveness of the caregiver to the crying creates trust as the newborn learns to associate the caregiver with comfort.

The amount and tone of crying vary based on gestational age, weight, and the reason for the cry (e.g., hunger, pain). A high-pitched cry can be a sign of a neurological disorder. Some mothers state that they learn to distinguish among the cries. The breastfeeding mother's body responds physiologically to infant crying by stimulating the milk-ejection reflex ("let-down") (Gardner & Goldson, 2011).

The duration of crying also varies greatly in each infant; newborns may cry for as little as 5 minutes or as much as 2 hours or more per day. The amount of crying peaks in the second month and then decreases. There is a diurnal rhythm of crying, with more crying occurring in the evening hours.

Parents need to learn that most crying is normal and a way for the newborn to communicate his or her needs. Some parents who are exhausted and overwhelmed can become frustrated with a baby who cries excessively. Parents need to be taught to recognize when they have reached their limit and that if this occurs, it is important to put the newborn in a safe place and take a few minutes away from the baby. See further discussion on interpretation of crying in Chapter 26.

KEY POINTS

- By full term, the newborn's various anatomical and physiological systems have reached a level of development and functioning that permits a physical existence apart from the mother.
- The newborn's most critical adaptation to extrauterine life is to establish effective respirations.
- Heat loss in the healthy term newborn may exceed the capacity to produce heat; this can lead to metabolic and respiratory complications that threaten the newborn's well-being.
- Physiological jaundice occurs in 60% of term infants and 80% of preterm infants.
- The appearance of jaundice during the first day of life or persistence of jaundice beyond 7 to 10 days may indicate a pathological process that requires further investigation.
- Some reflex behaviours are important for the newborn's survival.
- The healthy newborn has sensory abilities that indicate a state of readiness for social interaction. Sleep–wake states and other factors influence the newborn's behaviour.
- Newborn behaviour progresses from self-regulation of autonomic processes to social interaction.
- Each full-term newborn has a predisposed capacity to handle the multitude of stimuli in the external world.

evolve WEBSITE

Visit the Evolve website for additional resources related to the content in this chapter such as Case Studies, Critical Thinking Case Study Answers, Nursing Care Plans, Nursing Processes, Nursing Skills, and Review Questions for Exam Preparation at: *http://evolve.elsevier.com/Canada/Perry/maternal/*

REFERENCES

Abu-Shaweesh, J. M. (2011). Respiratory disorders in preterm and term infants. In R. J. Martin, A. A. Fanaroff, & M. C. Walsh (Eds.), *Fanaroff and Martin's neonatal-perinatal medicine: Diseases of the fetus and infant* (9th ed.). St. Louis: Mosby.

ACoRN Editorial Board. (2012). *Acute care of at-risk newborns*. Vancouver: Author.

Andersson, O., Lindquist, B., Lindgren, M., et al. (2015). Effect of delayed cord clamping on neurodevelopment at 4 years of age. *JAMA Pediatrics, 169*(7), 631–638. doi:10.1001/jamapediatrics.2015.0358.

Arca, G., Botet, F., Palacio, M., et al. (2010). Timing of umbilical cord clamping: New thoughts on an old discussion. *Journal of Maternal-Fetal and Neonatal Medicine, 23*(11), 1274–1285.

Askin, D. F. (2009a). Chest and lungs assessment. In E. P. Tappero & M. E. Honeyfield (Eds.), *Physical assessment of the newborn* (4th ed.). Petaluma, CA: NICU Ink.

Askin, D. F. (2009b). Fetal-to-neonatal transition—what is normal and what is not? Part II: Red flags. *Neonatal Network, 28*(3), e37–e40. Retrieved from <http://www.metapress.com/content/V471277271677852>.

Baker, R. D., Greer, F. R., & Committee on Nutrition. (2010). Diagnosis and prevention of iron deficiency and iron-deficiency anemia in infants and young children (0–2 years of age). *Pediatrics, 126*(5), 1040–1050.

Barrington, K. J., Sankaran, K., & Canadian Paediatric Society. (2007). Guidelines for detection, management and prevention of hyperbilirubinemia in term and late term newborn infants [35 or more weeks gestation]. *Paediatric Child Health, 12*(Suppl. B), 1B–12B. Reaffirmed 2011.

Blackburn, S. T. (2013). *Maternal, fetal, and neonatal physiology: A clinical perspective* (4th ed.). St. Louis: Saunders.

Brazelton, T., & Nugent, J. (2011). *Neonatal behavioural assessment scale* (4th ed.). London: MacKeith.

Brown, V. D., & Landers, S. (2011). Heat balance. In S. L. Gardner, B. S. Carter, M. Enzman-Hines, et al. (Eds.), *Merenstein & Gardner's handbook of neonatal intensive care* (7th ed.). St. Louis: Mosby.

Cooperman, D. R., & Thompson, G. H. (2011). Musculoskeletal disorders. In R. J. Martin, A. A. Fanaroff, & M. C. Walsh (Eds.), *Fanaroff and Martin's neonatal-perinatal medicine: Diseases of the fetus and infant* (9th ed.). St. Louis: Mosby.

Dell, K. M. (2011). Fluids, electrolytes, and acid-base homeostasis. In R. J. Martin, A. A. Fanaroff, & M. C. Walsh (Eds.), *Fanaroff and Martin's neonatal-perinatal medicine: Diseases of the fetus and infant* (9th ed.). St. Louis: Mosby.

Desmond, M., Rudolph, A., & Phitaksphraiwan, P. (1966). The transitional care nursery: A mechanism for preventive medicine in the newborn. *Pediatric Clinics of North America, 13*(3), 651–668.

Gardner, S. L., & Goldson, E. (2011). The neonate and the environment: Impact on development. In S. L. Gardner, B. S. Carter, M. Enzman-Hines, et al. (Eds.), *Merenstein & Gardner's handbook of neonatal intensive care* (7th ed.). St. Louis: Mosby.

Goldsmith, J. P. (2011). Delivery room resuscitation of the newborn. In R. J. Martin, A. A. Fanaroff, & M. C. Walsh (Eds.), *Fanaroff and Martin's neonatal-perinatal medicine: Diseases of the fetus and infant* (9th ed.). St. Louis: Mosby.

Habif, T. P. (2009). Vascular tumors and malformations. In T. P. Habif (Ed.), *Clinical dermatology* (5th ed.). Philadelphia: Mosby.

Hoath, S. B., & Narendran, V. (2011). The skin. In R. J. Martin, A. A. Fanaroff, & M. C. Walsh (Eds.), *Fanaroff and Martin's neonatal-perinatal medicine: Diseases of the fetus and infant* (9th ed.). St. Louis: Mosby.

Hoyt, M. R. (2011). Anesthetic options for labor and delivery. In R. J. Martin, A. A. Fanaroff, & M. C. Walsh (Eds.), *Fanaroff and Martin's neonatal-perinatal medicine: Diseases of the fetus and infant* (9th ed.). St. Louis: Mosby.

Kamath, B. D., Thilo, E. H., & Hernandez, J. A. (2011). Jaundice. In S. L. Gardner, B. S. Carter, M. Enzman-Hines, et al. (Eds.), *Merenstein & Gardner's handbook of neonatal intensive care* (7th ed.). St. Louis: Mosby.

Kaplan, M., Wong, R. J., Sibley, E., et al. (2011). Neonatal jaundice and liver disease. In R. J. Martin, A. A. Fanaroff, & M. C. Walsh (Eds.), *Fanaroff and Martin's neonatal-perinatal medicine: Diseases of the fetus and infant* (9th ed.). St. Louis: Mosby.

Kapur, R., Yoder, M. C., & Polin, R. A. (2011). Developmental immunology. In R. J. Martin, A. A. Fanaroff, & M. C. Walsh (Eds.), *Fanaroff and Martin's neonatal-perinatal medicine: Diseases of the fetus and infant* (9th ed.). St. Louis: Mosby.

Karl, D. J., & Keefer, C. H. (2011). Use of the behavioral observation of the newborn educational trainer for teaching newborn behavior. *Journal of Obstetrics, Gynecological & Neonatal Nursing (JOGNN), 40*(1), 75–83.

Kenney, P. M., Hoover, D., Williams, L. C., et al. (2011). Cardiovascular diseases and surgical interventions. In S. L. Gardner, B. S. Carter, M. Enzman-Hines, et al. (Eds.), *Merenstein & Gardner's handbook of neonatal intensive care* (7th ed.). St. Louis: Mosby.

Lawrence, R. A., & Lawrence, R. M. (2011). *Breastfeeding: A guide for the medical profession* (7th ed.). St. Louis: Mosby.

Lott, J. W. (2015). Immunology and infectious disease. In M. T. Verklan & M. Walden (Eds.), *Core curriculum for neonatal intensive care nursing* (5th ed.). St. Louis: Saunders.

Manco-Johnson, M., Rodden, D. J., & Hays, T. (2011). Newborn hematology. In S. L. Gardner, B. S. Carter, M. Enzman-Hines, et al. (Eds.), *Merenstein & Gardner's handbook of neonatal intensive care* (7th ed.). St. Louis: Mosby.

Mangurten, H. H., & Puppala, B. L. (2011). Birth injuries. In R. J. Martin, A. A. Fanaroff, & M. C. Walsh (Eds.), *Fanaroff and Martin's neonatal-perinatal medicine: Diseases of the fetus and infant* (9th ed.). St. Louis: Mosby.

McDonald, S. J., Middleton, P., Dowswell, T., & Morris, P. S. (2013). Effect of timing of umbilical cord clamping of term infants on maternal and neonatal outcomes. *The Cochrane Database of Systematic Reviews,* (7). doi:10.1002/14651858.CD004074.pub3.

Nugent, J. K., Keefer, C. H., Minear, S., et al. (2007). *Understanding newborn behavior and early relationships: The newborn behavioral observations (NBO) system handbook.* Baltimore: Brookes Publishing.

Pagana, K. D., Pagana, T. J., & MacDonald, S. (2013). *Mosby's Canadian manual of diagnostic and laboratory tests.* Toronto: Mosby.

Sadowski, S. (2015). Cardiovascular disorders. In M. T. Verklan & M. Walden (Eds.), *Core curriculum for neonatal intensive care nursing* (5th ed.). St. Louis: Saunders.

Verklan, M. T., & Lopez, S. M. (2011). Neurologic disorders. In S. L. Gardner, B. S. Carter, M. Enzman-Hines, et al. (Eds.), *Merenstein & Gardner's handbook of neonatal intensive care* (7th ed.). St. Louis: Mosby.

Visscher, M. O., Utturkar, R., Pickens, W. L., et al. (2011). Neonatal skin maturation—vernix caseosa and free amino acids. *Pediatric Dermatology, 28*(2), 122–132.

Weinberg, J. A., & Powell, K. R. (2011). Laboratory aids for diagnosis of neonatal sepsis. In J. S. Remington, J. O. Klein, C. B. Wilson, et al. (Eds.), *Infectious diseases of the fetus and newborn infant* (7th ed.). Philadelphia: Elsevier.

ADDITIONAL RESOURCE

Provincial Council of Maternal Child Health: <http://www.pcmch.org>.

CHAPTER

26

Nursing Care of the Newborn and Family

Ileen Gladding

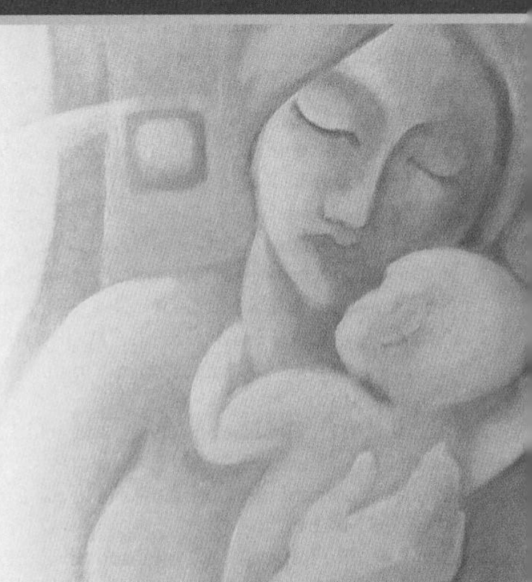

evolve WEBSITE

***Visit the Evolve website for additional resources related to the content in this chapter such as Case Studies, Critical Thinking Case Study Answers, Nursing Care Plans, Nursing Processes, Nursing Skills, and Review Questions for Exam Preparation at:** http://evolve.elsevier.com/Canada/Perry/maternal/*

OBJECTIVES

On completion of this chapter the reader will be able to:

- Explain the purpose and components of the Apgar score.
- Provide nursing care to assist the newborn to transition to extrauterine life.
- Describe a systematic approach to assessment of the newborn.
- Describe how to perform a gestational age assessment of a newborn.
- Compare the characteristics of preterm, late preterm, term, and postterm newborns.
- Explain the elements of a providing a safe environment for a newborn.
- Discuss jaundice and phototherapy and the guidelines for teaching parents about this condition and treatment.
- Explain the purposes and methods of circumcision, the postoperative care of the circumcised infant, and parent teaching information regarding care of the circumcised or uncircumcised penis.
- Review the procedures for performing an intramuscular injection, performing a heel stick, collecting urine specimens, and venipuncture.
- Evaluate pain in the newborn based on physiological changes and behavioural observations and provide pain management strategies.
- Review anticipatory guidance that nurses provide parents before discharge.

Although most infants make the necessary biopsychosocial adjustment to extrauterine existence without undue difficulty, their well-being depends on the care they receive from others. This chapter describes the assessment and care of the infant from immediately after birth until discharge, as well as important anticipatory guidance related to ongoing infant care. A discussion of pain in the newborn and its management is included.

BIRTH THROUGH THE FIRST 2 HOURS

NURSING CARE

Care begins immediately after birth and focuses on assessing and stabilizing the newborn's condition. The nurse works alongside the primary health care provider to be alert for any signs of distress and initiate appropriate interventions.

The foundation for providing comprehensive, family-centred newborn care is awareness of the mother's preconception and prenatal history as well as intrapartal events. Recognition of risk factors (Box 26-1) enables the nurse to be more astute in observations and assessments and more likely to identify early signs of complications. This allows for earlier intervention and promotes positive outcomes.

Immediate Care After Birth

The primary goal of care in the first moments after birth is to assist the newly born infant to transition to extrauterine life by establishing effective respirations. If the infant is at term, is crying or breathing, and has good muscle tone, routine care can

BOX 26-1 ASSESSMENT OF PRECONCEPTION, PRENATAL, AND INTRAPARTUM RISK FACTORS

Preconception
- Maternal age
- Pre-existing medical conditions: Diabetes, hypertension, cardiac disease, anemia, thyroid disorder, renal disease, obesity
- Genetic factors: Family history
- Obstetrical history: Gravidity, parity, number of living children and their ages, history of stillbirth, previous infant with congenital anomalies, recurrent abortions, use of assisted-reproductive technology, interpregnancy spacing

Prenatal
- Prenatal care: When started
- Nutrition: Weight gain, diet, obesity, eating disorders
- Health-compromising behaviours: Smoking, alcohol or substance use
- Blood group or Rh sensitization
- Medications: Prescription, over-the-counter, and complementary/alternative medications
- History of infection: Sexually transmitted infections, TORCH infections,* group B streptococci status

Intrapartum
- Length of gestation: Preterm, late preterm, term, or postterm
- First stage of labour: Length, electronic fetal monitoring—internal or external, rupture of membranes (time, presence of meconium), signs of fetal distress, labour complications (bleeding [placental abruption or placenta previa]), maternal analgesia or anaesthesia
- Group B streptococci status: Treatment during labour
- Second stage of labour: Length, vaginal or Caesarean, instrument assisted—forceps or vacuum extractor, complications (e.g., shoulder dystocia, cord prolapse)

*TORCH is the collective name for *t*oxoplasmosis, *o*ther infections (e.g., hepatitis), *r*ubella virus, *c*ytomegalovirus (CMV), and *h*erpes simplex virus (see further discussion in Chapter 29).
Adapted from Broussard, A. B., & Hurst, H. M. (2010). Antepartum-intrapartum complications. In T. M. Verklan & M. Walden (Eds.), *AWHONN core curriculum for neonatal intensive care nursing* (4th ed.). St. Louis: Saunders.

begin (Kattwinkel, Perlman, Aziz, et al., 2010). The infant is placed prone on the mother's chest, and the nurse assesses the airway. Drying the infant with vigorous rubbing removes moisture to prevent evaporative heat loss and provides tactile stimulation to stimulate respiratory effort. The mother and her newborn are covered with a warm blanket (Niermeyer & Clarke, 2011).

The heart rate is quickly assessed by palpating the base of the cord or by auscultating the left chest with a stethoscope. The heart rate should be greater than 100 beats per minute (bpm). The newborn's trunk and lips should be pink; acrocyanosis is a normal finding (see Fig. 25-1) (Niermeyer & Clarke, 2011).

TABLE 26-1 APGAR SCORE

	SCORE		
SIGN	**0**	**1**	**2**
Heart rate	Absent	Slow (<100 beats/min)	≥100 beats/min
Respiratory rate	Absent	Slow (hypoventilation), weak cry	Good, crying
Muscle tone	Flaccid	Some flexion of extremities	Well flexed
Reflex irritability	No response	Grimace	Cry or active withdrawal
Colour	Blue, pale	Body pink, extremities blue	Completely pink

All newborns require the initial steps of resuscitation, drying, and stimulating after birth. If the newborn does not respond to initial measures or requires more aggressive respiratory or circulatory support, the nurse and other members of the health care team (e.g., attending physician or midwife, pediatrician, respiratory therapist) will perform interventions as outlined in systematic algorithms (Finan, Aylward, Aziz, et al., 2011).

As soon as possible after birth the nurse places identically numbered bands on the infant, the mother, and often on the partner. With the possibility of transmission of viruses such as hepatitis B virus and human immunodeficiency virus (HIV) via maternal blood and blood-stained amniotic fluid, the newborn must be considered a potential contamination source until proved otherwise. As part of routine precautions, nurses should wear gloves when handling the newborn until blood and amniotic fluid are removed by bathing; gloves should be worn when conducting physical assessments, when in contact with breast milk, during routine diaper changes, and at any time contact with body fluids may be evident.

Apgar Scoring

The Apgar score enables a rapid assessment of the newborn's transition to extrauterine existence on the basis of five signs indicating his or her physiological state: (1) heart rate, based on **auscultation** with a stethoscope or **palpation** of the umbilical cord; (2) respiratory rate, based on observed movement or auscultation of respiratory efforts; (3) muscle tone, based on degree of flexion and movement of the extremities; (4) reflex irritability, based on response to stimulation; and (5) generalized skin colour, described as pallid, cyanotic, or pink (Table 26-1). Evaluations are made at 1 and 5 minutes after birth and can be done by the nurse or birth attendant. Scores of 0 to 3 indicate severe distress, scores of 4 to 6 indicate moderate difficulty, and scores of 7 to 10 indicate that the infant is having minimal or no difficulty adjusting to extrauterine life. The Apgar score is reassessed at 10 and 20 minutes if the score is less than 7 at 5 minutes. Apgar scores do not predict future neurological outcome but are useful for describing the newborn's transition to the extrauterine environment. If resuscitation is required, it must be initiated after initial drying and before the 1-minute Apgar score (American College of Obstetricians and Gynecologist [ACOG] Committee on Obstetric Practice, 2006/2010).

BOX 26-2 INITIAL PHYSICAL ASSESSMENT OF INFANT BY BODY SYSTEM

General Appearance

Colour: □ pink
□ acrocyanosis

□ Alert
□ Active

Central Nervous System

□ Infant moves all four extremities; flexion, muscle tone appropriate
□ Symmetrical features, movement
□ Moro, suck, rooting, and grasp reflexes present
□ Anterior fontanel soft and flat

Cardiovascular System

□ Heart auscultation, regular in rate and rhythm
□ No murmurs heard
□ Pulses strong, equal bilaterally
□ Capillary refill less than 3 seconds centrally and in peripheral tissues (not nail beds)

Respiratory System

□ Lungs auscultated, clear bilaterally with minimal fine crackles shortly after birth
□ Respiratory rate less than 60 breaths/min
□ Respiratory effort nonlaboured
□ Chest expansion symmetrical
□ Absence of nasal flaring, grunting, retractions

Skin

□ Skin lesions or abrasions documented
□ Birthmarks documented
□ Caput/moulding
□ Other ________

Eyes, Ears, Nose, and Throat

□ Eyes clear
□ Palates intact
□ Nares patent
□ Ears in place; correct alignment

Genitourinary System

□ Male: Urethral opening at tip of penis, testes descended bilaterally
□ Female: Labia minora and majora intact, hymenal tag may be visible

Gastrointestinal System

□ Abdomen soft, no visible distension
□ Cord attached and clamped
□ Anus patent

Initial Physical Assessment

The nurse will complete a brief physical examination shortly after birth (Box 26-2). The first assessment can often be done while the newborn is skin-to-skin with the mother. If the baby is vigorous, Apgar scoring and further assessments can be conducted without breaking this intimate time. Skin-to-skin contact enhances the newborn's transition to extrauterine life and initial bonding. Breastfeeding should begin shortly after birth (World Health Organization [WHO], 2009a). If the mother is not able to be present, the newborn can be placed skin-to-skin with the father or partner (Fig. 26-1). Healthy newborns should remain with their parent(s) throughout the hospital stay, although some infants who require extra care may be admitted to a nursery.

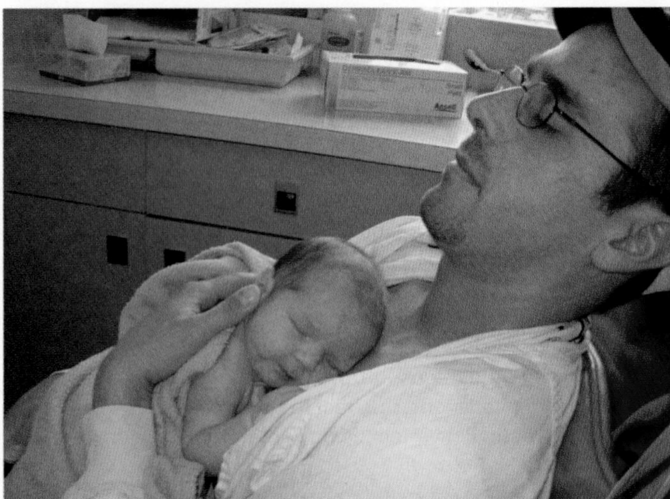

FIGURE 26-1 Father and newborn skin-to-skin. (Courtesy Fraser Health.)

Early contact between mother and newborn can be important in developing their and the child's future relationships. It also has a positive effect on breastfeeding. Physiological benefits of early mother–infant contact include increased oxytocin and prolactin levels in the mother and initiation of suckling activity in the infant. The process of developing active immunity begins as the infant ingests flora from the mother's colostrum.

Interventions

Changes can occur rapidly in the newborn immediately after birth. Assessment must be followed by implementation of appropriate care.

Airway Maintenance

Generally, the healthy term infant born vaginally has little difficulty clearing the airway. Most secretions are moved by gravity and brought by the cough reflex to the oropharynx to be drained or swallowed and suctioning is rarely necessary. The infant who has difficulty clearing mucus from the airway may initially be placed in a side-lying position (head stabilized, not in Trendelenburg position) until secretions are cleared, and then placed supine. It is important to explain to parents why the side-lying position is being used and that this is only a temporary measure until the mucus has cleared. Parents must be instructed that newborns are normally placed on their backs when sleeping.

The infant who is choking on secretions should be supported with the head to the side or by initiating the first steps in infant cardiopulmonary resuscitation (CPR), by tapping between the baby's shoulders while holding firmly in a slightly downward motion to optimize gravity for the expulsion of mucus. The mouth is suctioned first to prevent the infant from inhaling pharyngeal secretions when gasping, as newborns are obligatory nose breathers. The centre of the infant's mouth should be avoided to prevent stimulation of the gag reflex. The nasal passages are suctioned one nostril at a time. It is important that hospital rooms have suctioning equipment available for use.

The nurse should listen to the infant's respirations and lung sounds with a stethoscope to determine whether there are crackles, rhonchi, or inspiratory stridor. Fine crackles may be auscultated for several hours after birth. If air movement is adequate, suctioning is rarely necessary. If mucus is interfering with respiratory effort, mechanical suctioning may be necessary. If the newborn has an obstruction that is not cleared with suctioning, the pediatric care provider should be notified for further investigation to determine whether there is a mechanical defect (e.g., tracheoesophageal fistula, choanal atresia) causing the obstruction.

Deeper suctioning may be necessary to remove mucus from the infant's nasopharynx or posterior oropharynx; however, this should be performed only after assessment of the risks involved. Proper catheter insertion and suctioning for 5 seconds or less per catheter insertion help prevent vagal stimulation and hypoxia. If wall suction is used, the pressure should be adjusted to less than 80 mm Hg. After the catheter is properly placed, suction is created by placing one's thumb over the control as the catheter is carefully rotated and gently withdrawn. This procedure may need to be repeated until the infant has a clear airway.

Four conditions are essential for maintaining an adequate oxygen supply:

1. A clear airway
2. Effective establishment of respirations
3. Adequate circulation, adequate perfusion, and effective cardiac function
4. Adequate thermoregulation (exposure to cold stress increases oxygen and glucose needs). Signs of potential complications related to abnormal newborn breathing are listed in Box 26-3.

BOX 26-3 SIGNS OF POTENTIAL COMPLICATIONS: ABNORMAL NEWBORN BREATHING

Bradypnea—Respirations (less than 30 breaths/min)
Tachypnea—Respirations (60 breaths/min or more)
Abnormal breath sounds—Crackles (fine crackles may be heard in first few hours after birth), wheezing, rhonchi, expiratory grunting, stridor, diminished or absent air movement
Respiratory distress—Nasal flaring, retractions (substernal or intercostals), stridor, gasping, apnea lasting 20 seconds or longer
Seesaw or paradoxical respirations
Skin colour: Cyanosis, mottling
Pulse oximetry value <95%

Maintaining Body Temperature

Effective neonatal care includes maintenance of an optimal thermal environment (see Chapter 25, pp. 648–650). Cold stress increases the need for oxygen and may deplete glucose stores. The infant may react to exposure to cold by increasing the respiratory rate and may become cyanotic. The ideal way of promoting warmth and maintaining neonatal body temperature is for the infant to have early skin-to-skin contact with the mother or partner. The naked infant is placed prone directly on the mother's or partner's chest and covered with a warm blanket (see Fig. 26-1). Early skin-to-skin contact has distinct short- and long-term benefits, including temperature stabilization, reduced crying, improved breastfeeding initiation and duration, and infant–maternal attachment (Bramson, Lee, Moore, et al., 2010; Gabriel, Martin, Escobar, et al., 2010; Moore, Anderson, Bergman, et al., 2012). Other interventions to promote warmth include keeping the head well covered and keeping the ambient temperature of the nursery or mother's room at 22° to 26°C (72° to 78°F).

Newborns should not be separated from their mother, but if they are, for instance because of a medical condition, the nurse should place the thoroughly dried newborn under a radiant warmer or in a warm isolette until the body temperature stabilizes. The infant's skin temperature is used as the point of control when using a warmer with a servocontrolled mechanism. The control panel usually is kept at between 36° and 37°C. This setting should maintain the healthy term infant's skin temperature at around 36.5° to 37°C. A thermistor probe (automatic sensor) is usually placed on the upper quadrant of the abdomen immediately below the right or left costal margin (never over a bone); a reflector adhesive patch may be used over the probe to provide adequate warming. This probe is designed to detect minor temperature changes resulting from external environmental factors or neonatal factors (peripheral vasoconstriction, vasodilation, or increased metabolism) before a dramatic change in core body temperature develops. The servocontroller adjusts the warmer temperature to maintain the infant's skin temperature within the preset range. The sensor needs to be checked periodically to ensure that it is securely attached to the infant's skin. The newborn's axillary temperature should be checked every hour (or more often as needed) until his or her temperature stabilizes. The length of time required to stabilize and maintain body temperature varies; each newborn should be allowed to achieve thermal regulation as necessary, and care should be individualized.

During all procedures, heat loss must be avoided or at least minimized for the newborn. The initial bath should be postponed until the newborn's skin temperature is stable and can adjust to heat loss from a bath. For every infant, the optimal timing of the bath varies and should be individualized according to the infant's ability to maintain a stable body temperature, which can often takes 8 hours or more.

Even a healthy term infant can become hypothermic: birth in a car on the way to the hospital, a cold birthing room, or inadequate drying and wrapping immediately after birth may cause the infant's temperature to fall below normal range (**hypothermia**). Warming the hypothermic newborn should be

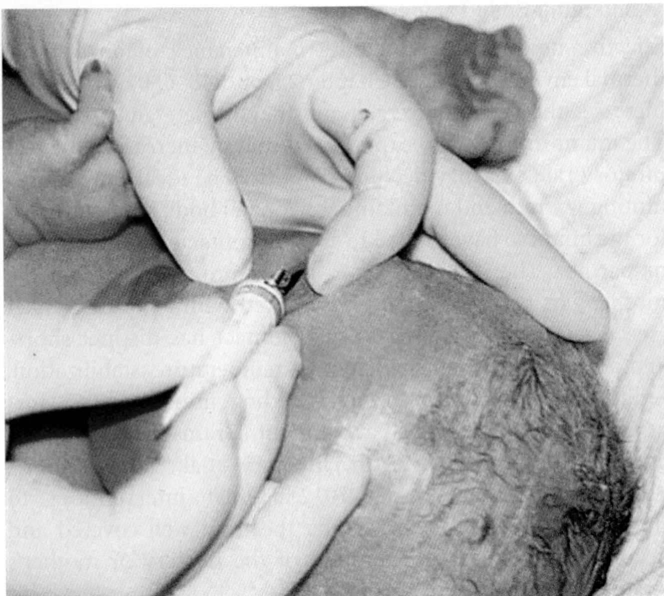

FIGURE 26-2 Instillation of medication into eye of newborn. The thumb and forefinger are used to open the eye; medication is placed in the lower conjunctiva from the inner to outer canthus. (Courtesy Marjorie Pyle, RNC, Lifecircle.)

accomplished with care, as rapid warming may cause apnea and acidosis in an infant. The warming process needs to be monitored to progress slowly over a period of 2 to 4 hours.

Eye Prophylaxis

Instillation of a prophylactic agent in the eyes (Fig. 26-2) to prevent **ophthalmia neonatorum** is presently recommended for all newborns and is mandatory by law in some provinces and territories. A recent position statement from the Canadian Paediatric Society (CPS), however, recommends discontinuing this practice, on the basis of new research (Moore, MacDonald, & CPS, 2015) although the practice has not changed significantly at this point in time. Ophthalmia neonatorum is an inflammation of the eyes from gonorrheal or chlamydial infection, contracted by the newborn during passage through the mother's birth canal. The agent used for prophylaxis varies according to hospital protocols, but usual agents include forms of erythromycin or tetracycline. Instillation of eye prophylaxis may be delayed until 2 hours after birth, to facilitate eye contact and parent–infant attachment and bonding (see Medication Guide). Topical antibiotics such as tetracycline and erythromycin, and a 2.5% povidone-iodine solution are not effective in the treatment of chlamydial conjunctivitis. A 14-day course of oral erythromycin or an oral sulphonamide can be given for chlamydial conjunctivitis (American Academy of Pediatrics [AAP] Committee on Infectious Diseases, 2012).

Vitamin K Prophylaxis

Administration of vitamin K intramuscularly is routine in the newborn period to prevent hemorrhagic disease of the newborn (HDN). A single injection of 1.0 mg of vitamin K for babies weighing greater than or equal to 1500 g and 0.5 mg for those less than 1500 g is given within 6 hours after birth (Canadian Paediatric Society & College of Family Physicians of Canada [CPS & CFPC], 1997/2014). Oral vitamin K is not recommended; however, if parents refuse an intramuscular injection, an oral dose of 2.0 mg vitamin K can be given at the first feeding. Parents should be advised of the importance of the baby receiving follow-up doses and be cautioned that their infant remains at increased risk of late HDN (including the potential for intracranial hemorrhage) with oral dosing (CPS & CFPC, 1997/2014). Vitamin K is synthesized by intestinal flora, which are not present at birth. The introduction of bacteria begins with the first feedings; by day 7, healthy newborns are able to produce their own vitamin K (see Medication Guide).

MEDICATION GUIDE

Eye Prophylaxis With Erythromycin Ophthalmic Ointment 0.5% and Tetracycline Ophthalmic Ointment 1%

Action

Erythromycin and tetracycline antibiotic ointments are both bacteriostatic and bactericidal. They provide prophylaxis against ophthalmia neonatorum.

Indication

These medications are presently used for the prevention of ophthalmia neonatorum in newborns of mothers who are infected with gonorrhea and chlamydia although recent research may not support this practice (Moore, MacDonald, & CPS, 2015).

Neonatal Dosage

Apply a 1- to 2-cm ribbon of ointment to the lower conjunctival sac of each eye; the medicines may also be used in drop form.

Adverse Reactions

They may cause chemical conjunctivitis that lasts 24 to 48 hours; vision may be blurred temporarily.

Nursing Considerations

Administer within 2 hours of birth. Wear gloves. Cleanse eyes if necessary before administration. Open eyes by putting a thumb and finger at the corner of each lid and gently pressing on the periorbital ridges. Squeeze the tube and spread the ointment from the inner canthus of the eye to the outer canthus. Do not touch the tube to the eye. After 1 minute, excess ointment may be wiped off. Observe eyes for irritation. Explain treatment to parents.

NURSING ALERT

Vitamin K is never administered via intravenous route for prevention of hemorrhagic disease of the newborn except in some cases of a preterm infant who has no muscle mass. In such cases, the medication should be diluted and given over 10 to 15 minutes. The infant should be closely monitored with a cardiorespiratory monitor as rapid bolus administration of vitamin K may cause cardiac arrest.

CARE OF THE NEWBORN FROM 2 HOURS AFTER BIRTH UNTIL DISCHARGE

NURSING CARE

Most hospitals have adopted variations of either labour-birth-recovery (LBR) or labour-birth-recovery-postpartum (LBRP)

MEDICATION GUIDE

Vitamin K: Phytonadione

Action

This intervention provides vitamin K; the newborn does not have the intestinal flora to produce this vitamin in the first week after birth. Vitamin K also promotes formation of clotting factors (II, VII, IX, and X) in the liver.

Indication

Vitamin K is used for prevention and treatment of hemorrhagic disease in the newborn.

Neonatal Dosage

Administer a 1.0-mg dose of vitamin K for babies weighing greater than or equal to 1500 g, and 0.5-mg dose for those less than 1500 g, intramuscularly within 6 hours of birth; the dose may be repeated if the newborn shows bleeding tendencies. The oral dose recommendation is 2.0 mg vitamin K at the time of the first feeding. The parenteral form of vitamin K for oral administration is all that is currently available. This should be repeated at 2 to 4 weeks and 6 to 8 weeks of age. Parents should be advised of the importance of the baby receiving follow-up doses.

Adverse Reactions

Edema, erythema, and pain at the injection site may occur rarely; hemolysis, jaundice, and hyperbilirubinemia have been reported, particularly in preterm infants.

Nursing Considerations

Wash hands prior to putting on gloves. If an oral dose is given, ensure that parents know the importance of follow-up and that the newborn is at increased risk for hemorrhagic disease of the newborn (HDN).

Intramuscular Injection

Follow procedure for intramuscular injection on p. 701.

rooms. One nurse provides care for both the mother and baby (couplet). The nurse caring for the mother–baby couplet is responsible for ongoing assessment and care of the newborn. Astute assessment skills and appropriate interventions promote positive outcomes, especially for newborns who experience any problems before going home. Newborn care is family centred, as the nurse provides education and support for the new parents throughout the hospital stay and assists them in preparing for hospital discharge. See Evolve for Nursing Care Plan of Healthy Newborn.

Physical Assessment

Although the initial assessment after birth can reveal significant anomalies, birth injuries, and cardiopulmonary problems that have immediate implications, a more detailed, thorough physical examination should follow within 12 to 18 hours after birth (see Guidelines Box and Table 26-2). The parents' presence during this and other examinations encourages discussion of their concerns and actively involves them in the health care of their infant from birth. It also gives the nurse an opportunity to observe parental interactions with the infant. The findings provide a database for nurses to plan appropriate care for newborns and give anticipatory guidance for the parents. Ongoing assessments are made throughout the hospital stay.

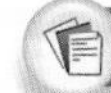

GUIDELINES

Physical Examination of the Newborn

Provide a normothermic and nonstimulating examination area.
Check that equipment and supplies are working properly and are accessible.
Undress only the body area to be examined to prevent heat loss.
Proceed in an orderly sequence (usually head to toe), with the following exceptions:

- Perform all procedures that require quiet first, such as observing position, skin colour, tone, and condition.
- Next auscultate the lungs, heart, and abdomen.
- Perform more disturbing procedures, such as taking temperature and testing reflexes, last.
- Measure head circumference and length as a baseline for further comparison as needed.

Proceed quickly to avoid stressing the infant.
Comfort the infant during and after examination; involve parents in the following:

- Talking softly to the infant
- Holding the infant's hands against the chest
- Holding the infant
- Giving the infant a gloved finger to suck

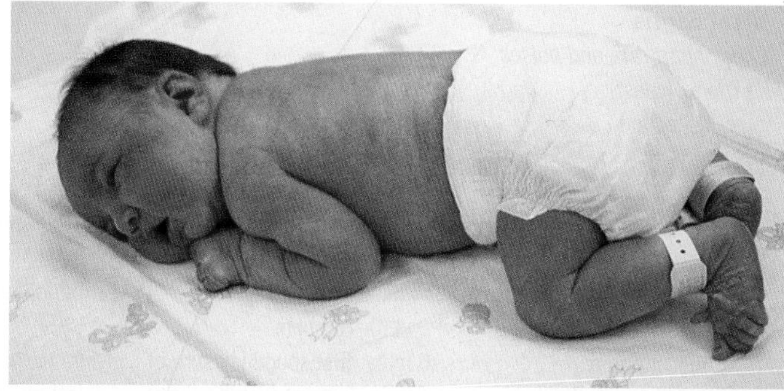

FIGURE 26-3 Newborn in position of flexion in prone position while awake. (From Hockenberry, M. J., et al. [2007]. *Wong's nursing care of infants and children* [8th ed., p. 274]. St. Louis: Mosby.)

General Appearance

The newborn's maturity level can be gauged by assessment of general appearance. Features to assess in the general survey include posture, activity, any overt signs of anomalies that may cause initial distress, presence of bruising or other consequences of birth, and state of alertness. The normal resting position of the newborn is one of general flexion (Fig. 26-3).

Vital Signs

The temperature, heart rate, and respiratory rate are always obtained. BP is not routinely assessed unless cardiac problems are suspected. An irregular, very slow, or very fast heart rate may indicate a need for further evaluation of circulatory status, including BP measurement.

The axillary temperature is a safe, accurate measurement of temperature. Electronic thermometers have expedited this task and provide a reading within 1 minute. Temporal artery, tympanic, and oral routes for measuring temperature in the

Text continued on p. 688

TABLE 26-2 PHYSICAL ASSESSMENT OF NEWBORN NORMAL FINDINGS

AREA ASSESSED AND APPRAISAL PROCEDURE	NORMAL FINDINGS		DEVIATIONS FROM NORMAL RANGE—POSSIBLE PROBLEMS (ETIOLOGY)
	AVERAGE FINDINGS	NORMAL VARIATIONS	
Posture			
Inspect newborn before disturbing for assessment. Refer to maternal chart for fetal presentation, position, and type of birth (vaginal, surgical), since newborn readily assumes in utero position.	Vertex: arms, legs in moderate flexion; fists clenched Resistance to having extremities extended for examination or measurement, crying possible when attempted Cessation of crying when allowed to resume curled-up fetal position (lateral) Normal spontaneous movement bilaterally asynchronous (legs flex and extend in alternating fashion) but equal extension in all extremities	Frank breech: legs straighter and stiff, newborn assuming intrauterine position in repose for a few days Prenatal pressure on limb or shoulder possibly causing temporary facial asymmetry or resistance to extension of extremities	Hypotonia, relaxed posture while awake (preterm or hypoxia in utero, maternal medications, neuromuscular disorder such as spinal muscular atrophy) Hypertonia (chemical dependence, CNS disorder) Limitation of motion in any of extremities
Vital Signs			
Check heart rate and pulses:			
Thorax (chest):			
Inspection	Visible pulsations in left midclavicular line, fifth intercostal space		
Palpation	Apical pulse, fourth intercostal space, midclavicular region, 110–160 bpm	80–100 bpm (sleeping) to 180 bpm (crying); possibly irregular for brief periods, especially after crying	Tachycardia: persistent, ≥180 bpm (RDS, pneumonia, fever) Bradycardia: persistent, ≤80 bpm (congenital heart block, maternal lupus)
Auscultation Apex: mitral valve Second interspace, left of sternum: pulmonic valve Second interspace, right of sternum: aortic valve Junction of xiphoid process and sternum: tricuspid valve	Quality: first sound (closure of mitral and tricuspid valves) and second sound (closure of aortic and pulmonic valves) sharp and clear	Murmur, especially over base or at left sternal border in interspace 3–4 (foramen ovale anatomically closing at about 1 yr	Murmur (possibly functional) Arrhythmias: irregular rate Sounds: Distant (pneumopericardium) Poor quality Extra (S_3, S_4) Heart on right side of chest (dextrocardia), often accompanied by reversal of intestines
Peripheral pulses: femoral, brachial, popliteal, posterior tibial	Peripheral pulses equal and strong		Weak or absent peripheral pulses (decreased cardiac output, thrombus, possible coarctation of aorta if weak on left and strong on right) Bounding
Obtain temperature:			
Axillary: method of choice Temporal and intra-auricular thermometers: not proved effective in measuring newborn temperature	Axillary: 37°C (98.6°F) Temperature stabilized by 8–10 hr of age	36.5°–37.5°C (97.7°–100°F) Heat loss from evaporation, conduction, convection, radiation (see Fig. 25-2)	Subnormal (preterm birth, infection, low environmental temperature, inadequate clothing, dehydration) Increased (infection, high environmental temperature, excessive clothing, proximity to heating unit or in direct sunshine, chemical dependence, diarrhea and dehydration) Temperature not stabilized by 8–10 hr after birth (if mother received magnesium sulphate, newborn less able to conserve heat by vasoconstriction; maternal analgesics possibly reducing thermal stability in newborn)

TABLE 26-2 **PHYSICAL ASSESSMENT OF NEWBORN NORMAL FINDINGS—cont'd**

AREA ASSESSED AND APPRAISAL PROCEDURE	NORMAL FINDINGS		DEVIATIONS FROM NORMAL RANGE—POSSIBLE PROBLEMS (ETIOLOGY)
	AVERAGE FINDINGS	NORMAL VARIATIONS	
Observe and monitor respiratory rate and effort:			
Observe respirations when infant is at rest. Observe respiratory effort. Count respirations for a full minute. Auscultate breath sounds. Listen for sounds audible without stethoscope.	30–60 breaths/min Tendency to be shallow and irregular in rate, rhythm, and depth when infant is awake Crackles may be heard after birth. No adventitious sounds audible on inspiration and expiration Breath sounds: bronchial: loud, clear	Short periodic breathing episodes and no evidence of respiratory distress or apnea (>20 seconds); periodic breathing First period (reactivity): 50–60 breaths/min Second period: 50–70 breaths/min Stabilization (1–2 days): 30–40 breaths/min Crackles (fine)	Apneic episodes: >20 sec (preterm infant: rapid warming or cooling of infant; CNS or blood glucose instability) Bradypnea: <30 breaths/min (maternal narcosis from analgesics or anaesthetics, birth trauma) Tachypnea: >60 breaths/min (RDS, transient tachypnea of the newborn, congenital diaphragmatic hernia) Breath sounds: Crackles (coarse), rhonchi, wheezing Expiratory grunt (narrowing of bronchi) Distress evidenced by nasal flaring, grunting, retractions, laboured breathing Stridor (upper airway occlusion)
Obtain blood pressure (BP) (usually not done in normal term infant):			
Check oscillometric monitor BP cuff: BP cuff width affects readings; use appropriately sized cuff and palpate brachial, popliteal, or posterior tibial pulse (depending on measurement site).	60–80/40–50 mm Hg (approximate ranges) At birth: Systolic: 60–80 mm Hg Diastolic: 40–50 mm Hg At 2 weeks: Systolic: 68–80 mm Hg Diastolic: 40–60 mm Hg	Variation with change in activity level: awake, crying, sleeping	Difference between upper and lower extremity pressures (coarctation of aorta) Hypotension (sepsis, hypovolemia) Hypertension (coarctation of aorta, renal involvement, thrombus)
Weight*			
Put protective liner cloth or paper in place and adjust scale to 0 g. Protect newborn from heat loss.	Female: 3400 g Male: 3500 g Regaining of birth weight within first 2 wk	2500–4000 g Acceptable weight loss: 10% or less in first 3–5 days Second baby weighs more than first (on average)	Weight ≤2500 g (preterm, small for gestational age, rubella syndrome) Weight ≥4000 g (large for gestational age, maternal diabetes, heredity—normal for these parents) Weight loss 10–15% (growth failure, dehydration); assess breastfeeding success, latch-on

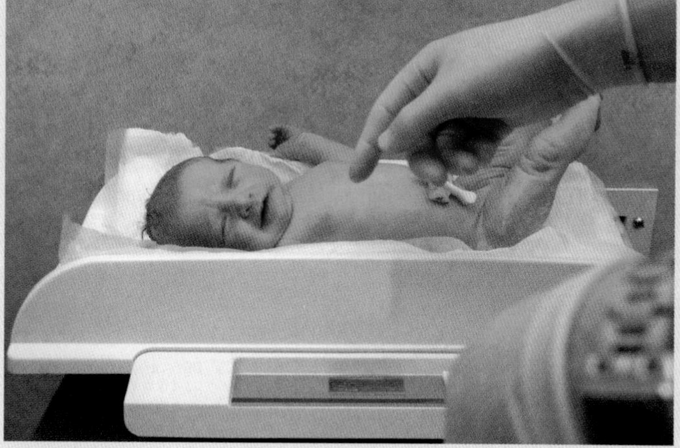

Weighing the infant. Note that a hand is held over the infant as a safety measure. The scale is covered to protect against cross-infection and heat loss. (Francois Etienne du Plessis/Shutterstock.com.)

Continued

TABLE 26-2 PHYSICAL ASSESSMENT OF NEWBORN NORMAL FINDINGS—cont'd

AREA ASSESSED AND APPRAISAL PROCEDURE	NORMAL FINDINGS: AVERAGE FINDINGS	NORMAL FINDINGS: NORMAL VARIATIONS	DEVIATIONS FROM NORMAL RANGE—POSSIBLE PROBLEMS (ETIOLOGY)
Length*			
Measure length from top of head to heel. Measuring is difficult in term infants because of moulding and incomplete extension of knees. Ideally this should be done using a length board.	45–55 cm		<45 cm or >55 cm (chromosomal abnormality, heredity—normal for these parents); some syndromes result in shorter-than-average limb length (skeletal dysplasias, achondroplasia)
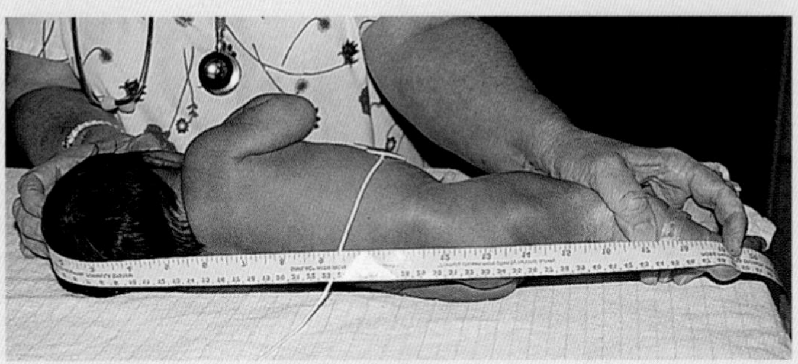 Length, crown to heel. To determine total length, include length of legs. (Courtesy Marjorie Pyle, RNC, Lifecircle.)			
Head Circumference*			
Measure head at greatest diameter: occipitofrontal circumference May need to remeasure on second or third day after resolution of moulding and caput succedaneum	33–35 cm Circumference of head and chest approximately the same for first 1 or 2 days after birth; chest circumference rarely measured on routine basis	32–36.8 cm	Microcephaly: head ≤32 cm (maternal rubella, toxoplasmosis, cytomegalovirus, Zika virus, fused cranial sutures [craniosynostosis]) Hydrocephaly: sutures widely separated, circumference ≥4 cm more than chest circumference (infection) Increased intracranial pressure (hemorrhage, space-occupying lesion)
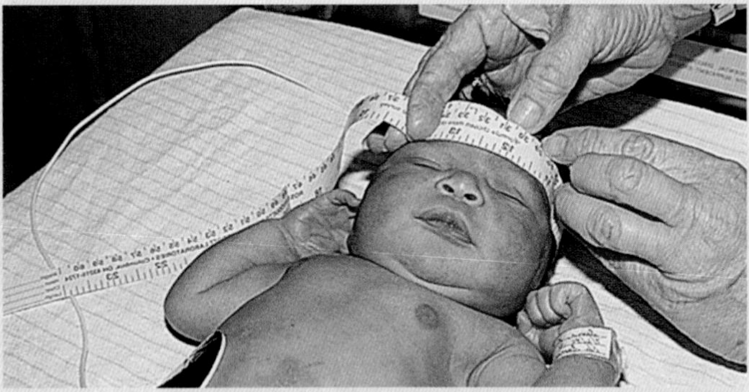 Circumference of head. (Courtesy Marjorie Pyle, RNC, Lifecircle.)			
Skin			
Check colour. Inspect and palpate: Inspect semi-naked newborn in well-lit, warm area without drafts; natural daylight is best. Inspect newborn when quiet and alert.	Generally pink Varying with ethnic origin; skin pigmentation beginning to deepen right after birth in basal layer of epidermis Acrocyanosis common after birth	Mottling Harlequin sign Plethora Telangiectases ("stork bites" or capillary hemangiomas) (see Fig. 25-8, A) Erythema toxicum neonatorum ("newborn rash") (see Fig. 25-8, B) Milia Petechiae over presenting part Ecchymoses from forceps in vertex births or over buttocks, genitalia, and legs in breech births	Dark red (preterm, polycythemia) Grey (hypotension, poor perfusion) Pallor (cardiovascular problem, CNS damage, blood dyscrasia, blood loss, twin-to-twin transfusion, infection) Cyanosis (hypothermia, infection, hypoglycemia, cardiopulmonary diseases, neurological, or respiratory malformations) Generalized petechiae (clotting factor deficiency, infection) Generalized ecchymoses (hemorrhagic disease)

*Weight, length, and head circumference should all be close to the same percentile for any child.

TABLE 26-2 PHYSICAL ASSESSMENT OF NEWBORN NORMAL FINDINGS—cont'd

AREA ASSESSED AND APPRAISAL PROCEDURE	NORMAL FINDINGS		DEVIATIONS FROM NORMAL RANGE—POSSIBLE PROBLEMS (ETIOLOGY)
	AVERAGE FINDINGS	NORMAL VARIATIONS	
Observe for jaundice.	None at birth	Physiological jaundice in up to 60% of term infants in first week of life	Jaundice within first 24 hr (pathological jaundice) (increased hemolysis, Rh isoimmunization, ABO incompatibility)
Observe for birthmarks or bruises: Inspect and palpate for location, size, distribution, characteristics, and colour, if obstructing airway or oral cavity.		Mongolian spot (see Fig. 25-7) in infants of African, Asian, or other ethnicities with darker-coloured skin	Hemangiomas Nevus flammeus: port-wine stain Nevus vasculosus: strawberry hemangioma Cavernous hemangioma
Check skin condition: Inspect and palpate for intactness, smoothness, texture, edema, pressure points if ill or immobilized.	Eyelid edema (result of eye prophylaxis) Opacity: few large blood vessels visible indistinctly over abdomen	Possibly puffy Slightly thick; superficial cracking, peeling, especially of hands, feet No visible blood vessels, a few large vessels clearly visible over abdomen Some fingernail scratches	Edema on hands, feet; pitting over tibia; periorbital (overhydration; hydrops) Texture thin, smooth, or of medium thickness; rash or superficial peeling visible (preterm, postterm) Numerous vessels very visible over abdomen (preterm) Texture thick, parchment-like; cracking, peeling (postterm) Skin tags, webbing Papules, pustules, vesicles, ulcers, maceration (impetigo, candidiasis, herpes, diaper rash)
Weigh infant as per routine.		Normal weight loss after birth: up to 10% of birth weight	
Gently pinch skin between thumb and forefinger over abdomen and inner thigh to check for turgor.	After pinch is released, skin returns to original state immediately.	Dehydration: loss of weight is best indicator	Loose, wrinkled skin (prematurity, postmaturity, dehydration: fold of skin persisting after release of pinch) Tense, tight, shiny skin (edema, extreme cold, shock, infection)
Note presence of subcutaneous fat deposits (adipose pads) over cheeks and buttocks.		Variation in amount of subcutaneous fat	Lack of subcutaneous fat, prominence of clavicle or ribs (preterm, malnutrition)
Observe for vernix caseosa: Observe colour, amount, and odour before bath or removing clothing.	Whitish, cheesy, odourless	Usually more found in creases, folds	Absent or minimal (postterm) Abundant (preterm) Green colour (possible in utero release of meconium or presence of bilirubin) Odour (possible intrauterine infection)
Assess lanugo: Inspect for fine, downy hair, amount and distribution.	Over shoulders, pinnae of ears, forehead	Variation in amount	Absent (postterm) Abundant (preterm, especially if lanugo abundant, long, and thick over back)
Head			
Palpate head		Caput succedaneum, possibly showing some ecchymosis (see Fig. 25-12, A)	Cephalhematoma (see Fig. 25-12, C)
Inspect shape and size.	Making up one fourth of body length Moulding (see Fig. 25-11)	Slight asymmetry from intrauterine position Lack of moulding (preterm, breech presentation, Caesarean birth)	Severe moulding (birth trauma) Indentation (fracture from trauma)
Palpate, inspect, and note status of fontanels (open vs. closed).	Anterior fontanel 5-cm diamond, increasing as moulding resolves Posterior fontanel triangle, smaller than anterior	Variation in fontanel size with degree of moulding Difficulty in feeling fontanels possible because of moulding	Fontanels: Full, bulging (tumour, hemorrhage, infection) Large, flat, soft (malnutrition, hydrocephaly, delayed bone age, hypothyroidism) Depressed (dehydration)
Palpate sutures.	Palpable and separated sutures	Possible overlap of sutures with moulding	Sutures: Widely spaced (hydrocephaly) Premature closure (fused) (craniosynostosis)

Continued

TABLE 26-2 PHYSICAL ASSESSMENT OF NEWBORN NORMAL FINDINGS—cont'd

AREA ASSESSED AND APPRAISAL PROCEDURE	NORMAL FINDINGS		DEVIATIONS FROM NORMAL RANGE—POSSIBLE PROBLEMS (ETIOLOGY)
	AVERAGE FINDINGS	NORMAL VARIATIONS	
Inspect pattern, distribution, and amount of hair; feel texture.	Silky, single strands lying flat; growth pattern toward face and neck	Variation in amount	Fine, woolly (preterm) Unusual swirls, patterns, or hairline; or coarse, brittle (endocrine or genetic disorders)
Eyes			
Check placement on face.	Eyes and space between eyes each one-third the distance from outer (left) to outer (right) canthus	Epicanthal folds (upward sloping): characteristic in some ethnicities	Epicanthal folds when present with other signs (chromosomal disorders such as Down, cri-du-chat syndromes)
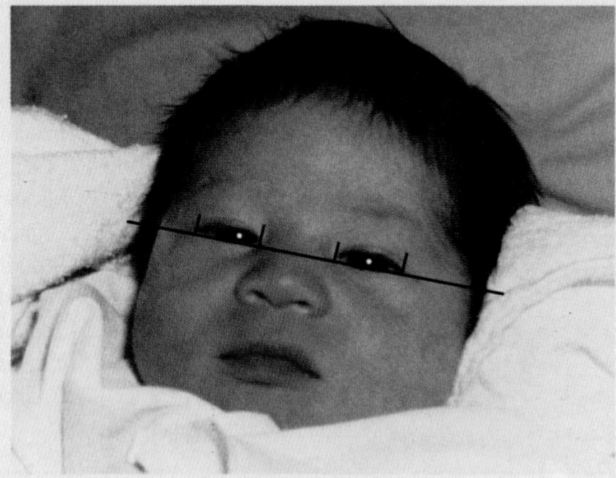 In pseudostrabismus, inner epicanthal folds cause the eyes to appear misaligned; however, corneal light reflexes are perfectly symmetrical. Eyes are symmetrical in size and shape and are well placed.			
Check for symmetry in size and shape.	Symmetrical in size, shape		
Check eyelids for size, movement, and blink.	Blink reflex	Edema if eye prophylaxis ointment instilled	
Assess for discharge.	None No tears	Occasional presence of some tears	Discharge: purulent (infection) Chemical conjunctivitis from eye medication is common—requires no treatment
Evaluate eyeballs for presence, size, and shape.	Both present and of equal size, both round, firm	Subconjunctival hemorrhage	Agenesis or absence of one or both eyeballs Lens opacity or absence of red reflex (congenital cataracts, possibly from rubella, retinoblastoma [cat's eye reflex]) Lesions: coloboma, absence of part of iris (congenital) Pink colour of iris (albinism) Jaundiced sclera (hyperbilirubinemia)
Check pupils.	Present, equal in size, reactive to light Physician or nurse practitioner will evaluate red reflex.		Pupils: unequal, constricted, dilated, fixed (intracranial pressure, medications, tumour)
Evaluate eyeball movement.	Random, jerky, uneven, focus possible briefly, following to midline	Transient strabismus or nystagmus until third or fourth month	Persistent strabismus Doll's eyes (increased intracranial pressure) Sunset (increased intracranial pressure)
Assess eyebrows: amount of hair, pattern.	Distinct (not connected in midline)		Connection in midline (Cornelia de Lange syndrome)

TABLE 26-2 PHYSICAL ASSESSMENT OF NEWBORN NORMAL FINDINGS—cont'd

AREA ASSESSED AND APPRAISAL PROCEDURE	NORMAL FINDINGS		DEVIATIONS FROM NORMAL RANGE—POSSIBLE PROBLEMS (ETIOLOGY)
	AVERAGE FINDINGS	NORMAL VARIATIONS	
Nose			
Observe shape, placement, patency, and configuration.	Midline Some mucus but no drainage Preferential nose breather Sneezing to clear nose	Slight deformity (flat or deviated to one side) from passage through birth canal	Copious drainage (rarely, congenital syphilis) Blockage—membranous or bone with cyanosis at rest and return of pink colour with crying (choanal atresia) Malformed (congenital syphilis, chromosomal disorder) Flaring of nares (respiratory distress)
Ears			
Observe size, placement on head, amount of cartilage, open auditory canal.	Correct placement: line drawn through inner and outer canthi of eyes reaching to top notch of ears (at junction with scalp) Well-formed, firm cartilage	Size: small, large, floppy Darwin's tubercle (nodule on posterior helix)	Agenesis Lack of cartilage (preterm) Low placement (chromosomal disorder, cognitive impairment, kidney disorder) Preauricular tag or sinus Size: possibly overly prominent or protruding ears
Assess hearing.	Responds to voice and other sounds	State (e.g., alert, asleep) influencing response	Lack of response to loud noise should not imply deafness.
Ensure newborn hearing screening is completed to identify deficits (in some provinces) (see Fig. 26-12).	Both ears pass.		One or both ears fail.
Face			
Observe overall appearance and symmetry of face.	Rounded and symmetrical; influenced by birth type or any moulding	Positional deformities associated with intrauterine positioning, cranial moulding	Asymmetrical facial features may be accompanied by other characteristics, such as low-set ears, absence of outer ear, or other structural disorders (hereditary, chromosomal aberration).
Mouth			
Inspect and palpate. Assess buccal mucosa: Dry or moist Pink Status intact Assess lips for colour, configuration, and movement.	Symmetry of lip movement	Transient circumoral cyanosis	Gross anomalies in placement, size, shape (cleft lip or palate, gums) Cyanosis, circumoral pallor (respiratory distress, hypothermia) Asymmetry in movement of lips (seventh cranial nerve paralysis)
Check gums.	Pink gums	Inclusion cysts (Epstein pearls—Bohn nodules, whitish, hard nodules on gums or roof of mouth)	Teeth: predeciduous or deciduous (hereditary)

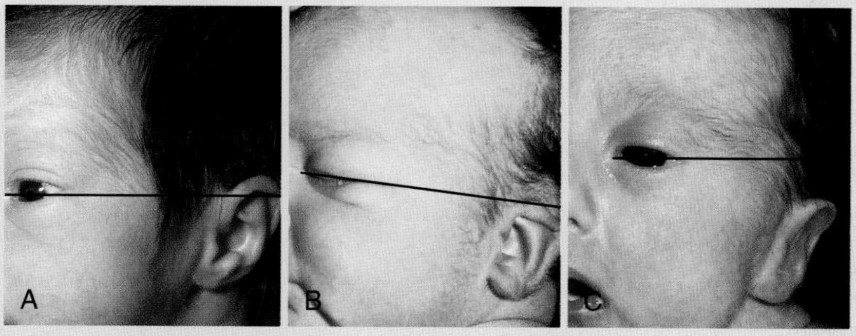

Placement of ears on the head in relation to a line drawn from the inner to outer canthus of the eye. **A:** Normal position. **B:** Abnormally angled ear. **C:** True low-set ear. (Courtesy Mead Johnson Nutritionals, Evansville, IN.)

Continued

TABLE 26-2 PHYSICAL ASSESSMENT OF NEWBORN NORMAL FINDINGS—cont'd

AREA ASSESSED AND APPRAISAL PROCEDURE	NORMAL FINDINGS		DEVIATIONS FROM NORMAL RANGE—POSSIBLE PROBLEMS (ETIOLOGY)
	AVERAGE FINDINGS	NORMAL VARIATIONS	
Assess tongue for colour, mobility, movement, and size.	Tongue not protruding; freely movable; symmetrical in shape, movement Sucking pads inside cheeks	Short lingual frenulum (ankyloglossia-tongue-tie)	Macroglossia (preterm, chromosomal disorder) Thrush: white plaques on cheeks or tongue that bleed if touched (*Candida albicans*)
Assess palate (soft, hard): Arch Uvula	Soft and hard palates intact Uvula in midline	Anatomical groove in palate to accommodate nipple, disappearance by 3–4 yr of age Epstein pearls	Cleft hard or soft palate
Assess chin.	Distinct chin		Micrognathia—recessed chin with prominent overbite (Pierre Robin sequence or other syndrome)
Evaluate saliva for amount and character.	Mouth moist, pink		Excessive salivation and choking or turning blue (esophageal atresia, tracheoesophageal fistula)
Check reflexes: Rooting, sucking, extrusion (See Table 25-4)	Reflexes present	Reflex response dependent on state of wakefulness and hunger	Absent (preterm)
Neck			
Inspect and palpate for movement, flexibility, masses, and bruising.	Short, thick, surrounded by skin folds; no webbing		Webbing (Turner syndrome)
Check sternocleidomastoid muscles, movement and position of head.	Head held in midline (sternocleidomastoid muscles equal), no masses Freedom of movement from side to side and flexion and extension; no movement of chin past shoulder	Transient positional deformity apparent when newborn is at rest; passive movement of head possible	Restricted movement, holding of head at angle (torticollis [wryneck], opisthotonos) Absence of head control (preterm birth, Down syndrome, hypotonia [spinal muscular atrophy])
Assess trachea for position and thyroid gland.	Thyroid not palpable		Mass (enlarged thyroid, cystic hygroma) Distended veins (cardiopulmonary disorder) Skin tags
Chest			
Inspect and palpate: Shape	Almost circular, barrel shaped	Tip of sternum possibly prominent	Bulging of chest, unequal movement (pneumothorax, pneumomediastinum) Malformation (funnel chest—pectus excavatum)
Observe respiratory movements.	Symmetrical chest movements, chest and abdominal movements synchronized during respirations	Occasional retractions, especially when crying	Retractions with or without respiratory distress (preterm, RDS) Paradoxical breathing
Evaluate clavicles.	Clavicles intact		Fracture of clavicle (trauma); crepitus
Assess ribs.	Rib cage symmetrical, intact; moves with respirations		Poor development of rib cage and musculature (preterm)
Assess nipples for size, placement, and number.	Nipples prominent, well formed, symmetrically placed		Nipples: Supernumerary, along nipple line Malpositioned or widely spaced
Check breast tissue.	Breast nodule: approximately 6 mm in term infant	Breast nodule: 3–10 mm Secretion of *witch's milk*	Lack of breast tissue (preterm) Sounds: bowel sounds may be heard in diaphragmatic hernia (see Abdomen, below)
Abdomen			
Inspect and palpate umbilical cord.	Two arteries, one vein Whitish grey Definite demarcation between cord and skin; no intestinal structures within cord Dry around base, drying Odourless Cord clamp may be in place	Reducible umbilical hernia	One artery (renal anomaly) Meconium stained (intrauterine distress) Bleeding or oozing around cord (hemorrhagic disease) Redness or drainage around cord (infection, possible persistence of urachus) Hernia: herniation of abdominal contents through cord opening (e.g., omphalocele); defect covered with thin, friable membrane, possibly extensive

TABLE 26-2 PHYSICAL ASSESSMENT OF NEWBORN NORMAL FINDINGS—cont'd

AREA ASSESSED AND APPRAISAL PROCEDURE	NORMAL FINDINGS: AVERAGE FINDINGS	NORMAL FINDINGS: NORMAL VARIATIONS	DEVIATIONS FROM NORMAL RANGE—POSSIBLE PROBLEMS (ETIOLOGY)
Inspect size of abdomen and palpate contour.	Rounded, prominent, dome shaped because abdominal musculature not fully developed Liver possibly palpable 1–2 cm below right costal margin No other masses palpable No distension Few visible veins on abdominal surface	Some diastasis recti (separation) of abdominal musculature	Gastroschisis: herniation of abdominal contents to the side or above the cord; contents not covered by membranous tissue and may include liver Distension at birth (ruptured viscus, genitourinary masses or malformations: hydronephrosis, teratomas, abdominal tumours): Mild (overfeeding, high gastrointestinal tract obstruction) Marked (lower gastrointestinal tract obstruction, anorectal malformation, anal stenosis), often with bilious emesis Intermittent or transient (overfeeding) Partial intestinal obstruction (stenosis of bowel) Visible peristalsis (obstruction) Malrotation of bowel or adhesions Sepsis (infection)
Auscultate bowel sounds and note number, amount, and character of stools.	Sounds present within minutes after birth in healthy term infant Meconium stool passing within 24–48 hr after birth		Scaphoid, with bowel sounds in chest and severe respiratory distress (congenital diaphragmatic hernia)
Assess colour.		Linea nigra possibly apparent and caused by hormone influence during pregnancy	
Observe movement with respiration.	Respirations primarily diaphragmatic, abdominal and chest movement synchronous		Decreased or absent abdominal movement with breathing (phrenic nerve palsy, congenital diaphragmatic hernia)
Genitalia			
Female (see Fig. 25-9, A)			
Inspect and palpate			
General appearance		Increased pigmentation caused by pregnancy hormones	Ambiguous genitalia—wide variation (small phallus not well distinguished from enlarged clitoris)
Clitoris	Usually edematous		Virilized female—extremely large clitoris (congenital adrenal hyperplasia)
Labia majora	Usually edematous, covering labia minora in term newborns	Edema and ecchymosis after breech birth Some vernix caseosa between labia possible	
Labia minora	Possible protrusion over labia majora		Enlarged clitoris with urinary meatus on tip, absent scrotum, micropenis, fused labia Stenosed meatus Labia majora widely separated and labia minora prominent (preterm)
Discharge	Smegma	Blood-tinged discharge from pseudomenstruation caused by pregnancy hormones	Fecal discharge (fistula)
Vagina	Open orifice Mucoid discharge Hymenal/vaginal tag		Absence of vaginal orifice
Urinary meatus	Beneath clitoris, difficult to see		Bladder exstrophy (bladder outside abdominal cavity and turned inside out)
Check urination.	Voiding 1 void per day for each day of life until fifth day and then 6–8 wet diapers	Rust-stained urine (uric acid crystals)	No void within first 24 hours (renal agenesis; Potter syndrome)

Continued

TABLE 26-2 PHYSICAL ASSESSMENT OF NEWBORN NORMAL FINDINGS—cont'd

AREA ASSESSED AND APPRAISAL PROCEDURE	NORMAL FINDINGS		DEVIATIONS FROM NORMAL RANGE—POSSIBLE PROBLEMS (ETIOLOGY)
	AVERAGE FINDINGS	NORMAL VARIATIONS	
Male (see Fig. 25-9, B)			
Inspect and palpate:			
General appearance		Increased size and pigmentation caused by pregnancy hormones Wide variation in size of genitalia	Ambiguous genitalia Micropenis
Penis:			
Urinary meatus appearance Prepuce (foreskin)—do not forcibly retract foreskin if uncircumcised	Foreskin covers glans (if uncircumcised), meatus at tip of penis	Prepuce removed if circumcised	Urinary meatus not on tip of glans penis (hypospadias, epispadias, foreskin may be retracted or absent); chordee (ventral curvature) Round meatal opening
Scrotum: Rugae (wrinkles)	Large, edematous, pendulous in term infant; covered with rugae	Scrotal edema and ecchymosis if breech birth Hydrocele, small, noncommunicating	Scrotum smooth and testes undescended (preterm, cryptorchidism) Bifid scrotum Hydrocele Inguinal hernia
Testes	Palpable on each side	Bulge palpable in inguinal canal	Undescended (preterm)
Check reflexes: Cremasteric	Testes retracted, especially when newborn is chilled		
Check urination.	Voiding within 24 hr, stream adequate, amount adequate Voiding 1 void per day for each day of life until fifth day and then 6–8 wet diapers	Rust-stained urine (uric acid crystals)	No void in first 24 hr Renal agenesis: Potter syndrome
Extremities			
Make a general check.	Assuming of position maintained in utero	Transient positional deformities	Limited motion (malformations)
Inspect and palpate: Degree of flexion Range of motion Symmetry of motion Muscle tone	Attitude of general flexion Full range of motion, spontaneous movements		Poor muscle tone (preterm, maternal medications, CNS anomalies)
Check arms and hands. Inspect and palpate: Colour Intactness Appropriate placement	Longer than legs in newborn period Contours and movements symmetrical	Slight tremors sometimes apparent Some acrocyanosis	Asymmetry of movement (fracture or crepitus, brachial nerve trauma, malformations) Asymmetry of contour (malformations, fracture) Amelia or phocomelia (teratogens) Palmar creases Simian line with short, incurved little fingers (Down syndrome)
Count number of fingers	Five on each hand Fist often clenched with thumb under fingers		Webbing of fingers: syndactyly Absence or excess of fingers Strong, rigid flexion; persistent fists; positioning of fists in front of mouth constantly (CNS disorder) Yellowed nail beds (meconium staining)
Evaluate joints: Shoulder Elbow Wrist Fingers	Full range of motion, symmetrical contour		Increased tonicity, clonus, prolonged tremors (CNS disorder)

TABLE 26-2 **PHYSICAL ASSESSMENT OF NEWBORN NORMAL FINDINGS—cont'd**

AREA ASSESSED AND APPRAISAL PROCEDURE	NORMAL FINDINGS: AVERAGE FINDINGS	NORMAL FINDINGS: NORMAL VARIATIONS	DEVIATIONS FROM NORMAL RANGE—POSSIBLE PROBLEMS (ETIOLOGY)
Check reflex: grasp (palmar and plantar)	Palmar: Infant's fingers flex tightly around examiner's finger when palm is stimulated Plantar: Infant's toes flex tightly around examiner's finger when base of toes on sole of foot is stimulated	Spontaneous grasp responses during sucking	Weak or absent reflexes can indicate CNS depression.
Observe legs and feet. Inspect and palpate: Colour Intactness Length in relation to arms and body and to each other	Appearance of bowing because lateral muscles more developed than medial muscles	Feet appearing to turn in but can be easily rotated externally, positional defects tending to correct while infant is crying Acrocyanosis	Amelia, phocomelia (chromosomal defect, teratogenic effect) Clubfoot Temperature of one leg differing from that of the other (circulatory deficiency, CNS disorder) Webbing, syndactyly (chromosomal defect)
Count number of toes	Five toes on each foot		Absence or excess of digits (chromosomal defect, familial trait)
Femur	Intact femur		Femoral fracture (difficult breech birth)
Head of femur as legs are flexed and abducted, placement in acetabulum (see Fig. 25-13)			Developmental dysplasia of the hip (DDH)
Major gluteal folds	Major gluteal folds even		Gluteal folds uneven: DDH
Soles of feet	Soles well lined (or wrinkled) over two thirds of foot in term infants Plantar fat pad giving flat-footed effect		Soles of feet: Few creases (preterm) Covered with creases (postterm)
Evaluate joints: Hip Knee Ankle Toes	Full range of motion, symmetrical contour		Hypermobility of joints (Down syndrome)
Check reflexes (see Table 25-4)			Asymmetrical movement (trauma, CNS disorder)
Back			
Assess anatomy. Inspect and palpate: Spine, shoulders, scapulae, iliac crests	Spine straight and easily flexed Infant able to raise and support head momentarily when prone Shoulders, scapulae, and iliac crests lining up in same plane	Temporary minor positional deformities; correction with passive manipulation	Limitation of movement (fusion or deformity of vertebra)
Base of spine—pilonidal dimple or sinus			Meningocele, myelomeningocele (spina bifida cystica) Pigmented nevus with tuft of hair, located anywhere along the spine, often associated with spina bifida occulta Sinus (opening to spinal cord)
Check reflexes (spinal related): Test trunk incurvation reflex (see Table 25-4)	Trunk flexed and pelvis swings to stimulated side	May not be apparent in first few days but is usually present in 5–6 days	If transverse lesion is present, no response below lesion; absence of response: CNS abnormality or CNS depression
Test magnet reflex.	Lower limbs extend as pressure applied to feet with legs in semiflexed position	Weak or exaggerated response with breech presentation	Absence suggestive of CNS damage or malformation

Continued

TABLE 26-2 PHYSICAL ASSESSMENT OF NEWBORN NORMAL FINDINGS—cont'd

AREA ASSESSED AND APPRAISAL PROCEDURE	NORMAL FINDINGS		DEVIATIONS FROM NORMAL RANGE—POSSIBLE PROBLEMS (ETIOLOGY)
	AVERAGE FINDINGS	NORMAL VARIATIONS	
Anus			
Inspect and palpate: Placement Patency	One anus with good sphincter tone Passage of meconium within 24 hr after birth = patent	Passage of meconium within 48 hr after birth	Imperforate anus without fistula Rectal atresia and stenosis Absence of anal opening; drainage of fecal material from vagina in female or urinary meatus in male (rectal fistula) or along perineal raphe (midline area between base of penis and anus) (anorectal malformation)
Test for sphincter response (active "wink" reflex).	Anal "wink" present, anal opening patent		
Observe for the following: Abdominal distension Passage of meconium from anal opening Fecal drainage from perineum, penis, vagina			
Stools			
Observe frequency, colour, and consistency.	Meconium followed by transitional and soft yellow stool (Fig. 25-5)		No stool (obstruction), dehydration Frequent watery stools (infection, phototherapy)

bpm, beats per minute; *CNS*, central nervous system; *RDS*, respiratory distress syndrome.

newborn are not considered accurate (Brown & Landers, 2011). Taking an infant's temperature may cause the infant to cry and struggle against the placement of the thermometer in the axilla. Before taking the temperature, the examiner may determine the apical heart rate and respiratory rate while the infant is quiet and at rest. The normal axillary temperature averages 37°C (98.6°F) with a range from 36.5° to 37.5°C (97.7° to 99.5°F).

SAFETY ALERT

Rectal temperatures should not be done on a newborn because of the risk for perforation.

The respiratory rate varies with the state of alertness and activity after birth. Respirations are abdominal and can be counted by observing or by lightly feeling the rise and fall of the abdomen while listening to air entry. Newborn respirations are shallow and irregular. It is important to count the respirations for a full minute to obtain an accurate count as there can be episodes of periodic breathing during which respirations may cease for up to 20 seconds and then resume again. The examiner should also observe for symmetry of chest movement. The average respiratory rate is between 30 and 60 breaths/min or may be higher than 60 breaths/min if the newborn is very active or crying.

An apical pulse rate should be obtained on all newborns. Auscultation should be for a full minute, preferably when the infant is asleep or in a quiet alert state. The infant may need to be held and comforted during assessment. Heart rate may range from 110 to 160 bpm. It is common to detect brief irregularities in the heart rate. Heart rate varies with the newborn's behavioural state. Bradycardia is a heart rate less than 100 bpm. However, a term infant in deep sleep may have a heart rate in the 80s or 90s; the rate should increase when the infant awakens. Tachycardia is defined as a sustained heart rate exceeding 160 bpm. It is not unusual for a crying infant to have a heart rate greater than 160; the heart rate should decrease when the crying ceases (Furdon & Benjamin, 2010). Brachial and femoral pulses should be assessed for equality and strength.

If BP is measured, an oscillometric monitor calibrated for neonatal pressures is preferred. An appropriate-sized cuff (width-to-arm or calf ratio of 0.45 to 0.70, or approximately ½ to ¾) is essential for accuracy. Neonatal BP usually is highest immediately after birth and falls to a minimum by 3 hours after birth. It then begins to rise steadily and reaches a plateau between 4 and 6 days after birth. This measurement is usually equal to that of the immediate postbirth BP. The BP varies with the newborn's activity; accurate measurement is best obtained while the newborn is at rest. BP varies with gestational age and chronological age. Systolic pressure in a term newborn averages 60 to 80 mm Hg; diastolic pressure averages 40 to 50 mm Hg. The mean arterial pressure should approximate the newborn's week of gestation. According to agency protocol, four extremity blood pressures may be assessed routinely or only when a murmur is auscultated. If the upper extremity pressures are more than 10 mm Hg greater than those in the lower extremities, the infant may have a cardiac defect such as coarctation of the aorta (Furdon & Benjamin, 2010). Peripheral pulses are also palpated as part of the assessment in any infant with a heart murmur. A baseline pulse oximetry measurement may be obtained along with palpation of peripheral pulses (brachial, femoral, pedal) before the infant's discharge, especially if there is concern for a congenital cardiac defect (see Chapter 29).

Baseline Measurements of Physical Growth

Baseline measurements are taken and recorded to help assess the progress and determine the growth patterns of the newborn. These may be recorded on growth charts. The following measurements are made when the newborn is assessed.

Weight. The newborn is usually weighed shortly after birth. Care must be taken to ensure that the scales are balanced. The totally unclothed newborn is placed in the centre of the scale, which is usually covered with a disposable pad or cloth to prevent heat loss via conduction and prevent cross-infection. The nurse should place one hand over (but not touching) the newborn to prevent the infant from falling off the scale. Most newborns need to be weighed only at birth and at discharge, although newborns who are small for gestational age or who are not feeding well may require daily weighing. This should be done at the same time every day during the hospital stay. Birth weight of a term infant typically ranges from 2500 to 4000 g.

Head circumference and length. The head is measured at the widest part, which is the occipitofrontal diameter. The tape measure is placed around the head just above the infant's eyebrows. The term newborn's head circumference ranges from 32 to 36.8 cm (12.6 to 14.5 in).

The length may be difficult to obtain because of the flexed posture of the newborn. The examiner places the newborn on a flat surface and extends the leg until the knee is flat against the surface. Placing the head against a perpendicular surface and extending the leg may assist with this measurement. In the term newborn, head-to-heel length ranges from 45 to 55 cm (17.7 to 21.7 in.).

Neurological Assessment

The physical assessment includes a neurological assessment of newborn reflexes (see Table 25-4). This assessment provides useful information about the infant's nervous system and state of neurological maturation. Many reflex behaviours (e.g., sucking and rooting) are important for proper development. Other reflexes such as gagging and sneezing act as primitive safety mechanisms. The assessment needs to be carried out as early as possible because abnormal signs present in the early neonatal period may require further investigation before the newborn is discharged home.

Gestational-Age Assessment

Assessment of gestational age is important because perinatal morbidity and mortality rates are related to gestational age and birth weight. A frequently used method of determining gestational age is the New Ballard score, which can be used to measure gestational ages of infants as young as 20 weeks of gestation (Fig. 26-4, A). It assesses six external physical and six neuromuscular signs. Each sign has a number score, and the cumulative score correlates with a maturity rating (gestational age). See Additional Resources for video on how to complete the scoring.

The examination of infants with a gestational age of 26 weeks or less should be performed at a postnatal age of less than 12 hours. For infants with a gestational age of at least 26 weeks, the examination can be performed up to 96 hours after birth. However, it is recommended that the initial examination be performed within the first 48 hours of life. Neuromuscular adjustments after birth in extremely immature newborns require that a follow-up examination be performed to further validate neuromuscular criteria. Box 26-4 highlights specific manoeuvres used in gestational-age assessment.

Classification of Newborns by Gestational Age and Birth Weight

Classification of infants at birth by both birth weight and gestational age is a more satisfactory method for predicting mortality risk and providing guidelines for management of the newborn than estimating gestational age or birth weight alone. The infant's birth weight, length, and head circumference are plotted on standardized graphs that identify normal values for gestational age. A normal range of birth weights exists for each gestational week (see Fig. 26-4, B).

Intrauterine growth curves have been used to classify infants according to birth weight and gestational age. Canadian data suggest that infants born to parents of East Asian and South Asian ancestry may be of lower birth weight than those of European descent. Using traditional newborn birth weight curves, some Canadian newborns of East Asian and South Asian ancestry may be misclassified as small for gestational age (SGA), while they are actually normal in birth weight if compared to other East Asian and South Asian infants (Ray, Jiang, Sgro, et al., 2009). Nurses should access and use the most current intrauterine growth chart specific to the population being evaluated, especially when considering multiples such as twins. See Additional Resources at the end of the chapter for birth-weight curves that have been developed on the basis of maternal ancestry.

The infant whose weight is appropriate for gestational age (AGA) (between the tenth and ninetieth percentiles) can be presumed to have grown at a normal rate regardless of the length of gestation—preterm, term, or postterm. The infant who is large for gestational age (LGA) (above the ninetieth percentile) can be presumed to have grown at an accelerated rate during fetal life; the SGA infant (below the tenth percentile) can be presumed to have grown at a restricted rate during intrauterine life. When gestational age is determined according to the Ballard scale, the newborn will fall into one of the following nine possible categories for birth weight and gestational age: AGA—term, preterm, postterm; SGA—term, preterm, postterm; or LGA—term, preterm, postterm. Birth weight influences mortality: the lower the birth weight, the higher the mortality rate. The same is true for gestational age: the lower the gestational age, the higher the mortality rate (Gardner & Hernandez, 2011).

Infants may also be classified in the following ways according to gestation:

- Preterm or premature—born before completion of 37 weeks of gestation, regardless of birth weight
- Late preterm—born between 34 0/7 and 36 6/7 weeks
- Early term—born between 37 and 38+6 weeks gestation
- Full term—born between the beginning of week 39 and the end of week 40+6 of gestation
- Late term—born in the forty-first week of gestation

ESTIMATION OF GESTATIONAL AGE BY MATURITY RATING

NEUROMUSCULAR MATURITY

	−1	0	1	2	3	4	5
Posture							
Square Window (wrist)	> 90∞	90∞	60∞	45∞	30∞	0∞	
Arm Recoil		180∞	140∞–180∞	110∞–140∞	90∞–110∞	< 90∞	
Popliteal Angle	180∞	160∞	140∞	120∞	100∞	90∞	< 90∞
Scarf Sign							
Heel to Ear							

PHYSICAL MATURITY

	−1	0	1	2	3	4	5
Skin	Sticky friable transparent	Gelatinous red, translucent	Smooth pink, visible veins	Superficial peeling&/ or rash, few veins	Cracking pale areas rare veins	Parchment deep cracking no vessels	Leathery cracked wrinkled
Lanugo	None	Sparse	Abundant	Thinning	Bald areas	Mostly bald	
Plantar Surface	Heel-toe 40–50 mm:−1 <40 mm: −2	>50 mm no crease	Faint red marks	Anterior transverse crease only	Creases ant. 2/3	Creases over entire sole	
Breast	Imperceptible	Barely perceptible	Flat areola no bud	Stippled areola1–2 mm bud	Raised areola 3–4 mm bud	Full areola 5–10 mm bud	
Eye/Ear	Lids fused loosely: −1 tightly: −2	Lids open pinna flat stays folded	Slightly curved pinna; soft; slow recoil	Well-curved pinna; soft but ready recoil	Formed firm instant recoil	Thick cartilage ear stiff	
Genitals (male)	Scrotum flat, smooth	Scrotum empty faint rugae	Testes in upper canal rare rugae	Testes descending few rugae	Testes down good rugae	Testes pendulous deep rugae	
Genitals (female)	Clitoris prominent labia flat	Prominent clitoris small labia minora	Prominent clitoris enlarging minora	Majora minora equally prominent	Majora large minora small	Majora cover clitoris minora	

MATURITY RATING

Score	Weeks
−10	20
−5	22
0	24
5	26
10	28
15	30
20	32
25	34
30	36
35	38
40	40
45	42
50	44

A

FIGURE 26-4 Estimation of gestational age. **A:** New Ballard scale for newborn maturity rating. Expanded scale includes extremely preterm infants and has been refined to improve accuracy in more mature infants. See Box 26-3 for explanation of assessments of neuromuscular maturity.

- Postterm (postdate)—born after completion of week 42 of gestation
- Postmature—born after completion of week 42 of gestation and showing the effects of progressive placental insufficiency

Early Term Infant

Experts have proposed another category to classify newborns. "Early term" describes infants born from 37 0/7 to 38 6/7 weeks of gestation (Fleischman, Oinuma, & Clark, 2010). A recent increase in the number of early term infants is associated with elective inductions and elective Caesarean births that are scheduled before 39 weeks. Compared with full-term infants, early term infants are at greater risk for short-term and long-term health problems. Birth at 37 to 38 weeks is associated with higher incidence of breastfeeding difficulties and respiratory problems such as respiratory distress syndrome (RSD) and transient tachypnea of the newborn (TTNB) (Bates, Rouse, Chapman, et al., 2010). These infants are also at increased risk for long-term problems such as learning difficulties (e.g., attention deficit hyperactivity disorder [ADHD]) (Lindstrom, Lindblad, & Hjern, 2011). Early term infants have higher neonatal, postnatal, and infant mortality rates (Reddy, Bettegowda, Dias, et al., 2011). Nurses and other health care providers need to be aware of the vulnerability of this population of newborns and monitor them closely (Craighead, 2012).

Late Preterm Infant

Much attention has been focused on infants who are considered "late preterm"; they are often the size and weight of term infants

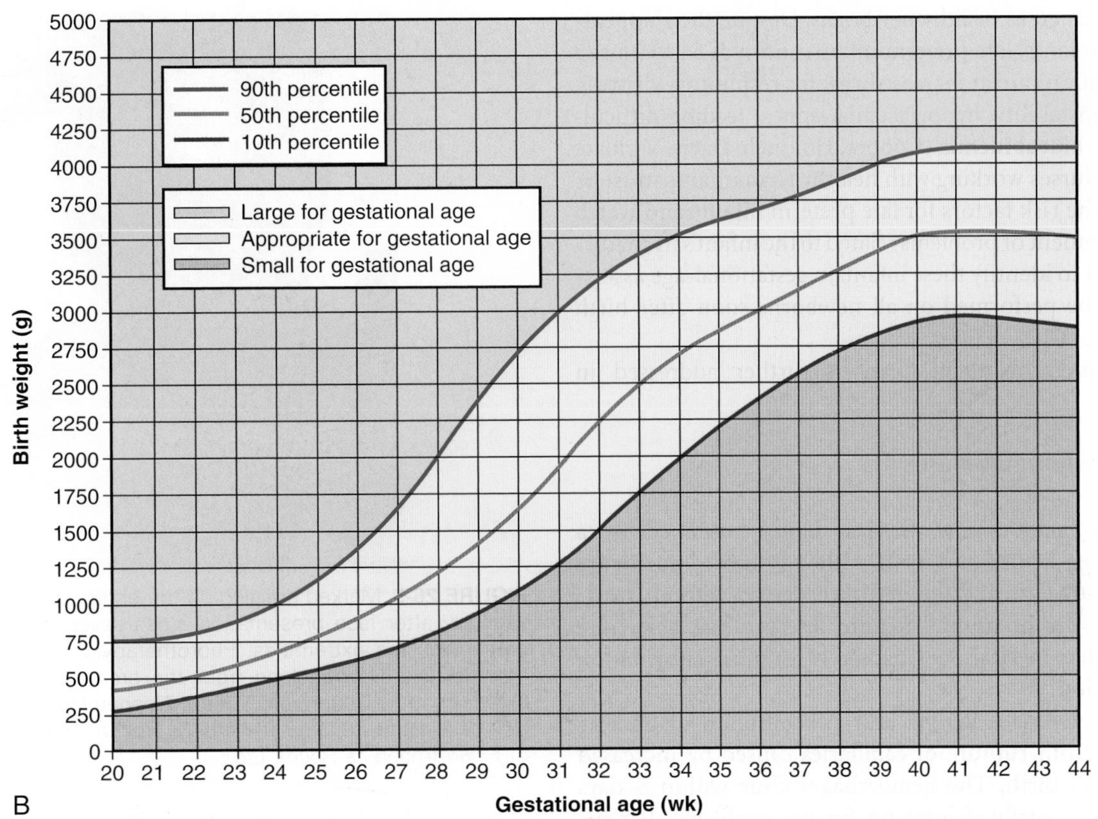

FIGURE 26-4, cont'd B: Intrauterine growth: birth weight percentiles based on live single births at gestational ages 20 to 44 weeks. (**A,** Reprinted from Ballard, J., Khoury, J. C., Wedig, K., et al. [1991]. New Ballard score, expanded to include extremely premature infants. *Journal of Pediatrics, 119*[3], 417. Copyright 1991, with permission from Elsevier. **B,** Data from Alexander, G. R., Himes, J. H., Kaufman, R. B., et al. [1996]. A United States national reference for fetal growth. *Obstetrics and Gynecology, 87*[2], 163–168.)

BOX 26-4 TECHNIQUES USED IN ASSESSING GESTATIONAL AGE

Posture
With infant quiet and in a supine position, observe degree of flexion in arms and legs. Muscle tone and degree of flexion increase with maturity. Full flexion of the arms and legs = score 4.*

Square Window
With thumb supporting back of arm below the wrist, apply gentle pressure with index and third fingers on dorsum of hand without rotating infant's wrist. Measure angle between base of thumb and forearm. Full flexion (hand lies flat on ventral surface of forearm) = score 4.

Arm Recoil
With infant supine, fully flex both forearms on upper arms and hold for 5 seconds; pull down on hands to fully extend and rapidly release arms. Observe rapidity and intensity of recoil to a state of flexion. A brisk return to full flexion = score 4.

Popliteal Angle
With infant supine and pelvis flat on a firm surface, flex lower leg on thigh and then flex thigh on abdomen. While holding knee with thumb and index finger, extend lower leg with index finger of the other hand. Measure degree of angle behind knee (popliteal angle). An angle of less than 90 degrees = score 5.

Scarf Sign
With infant supine, support head in midline with one hand; use the other hand to pull infant's arm across the shoulder so that infant's hand touches shoulder. Determine location of elbow in relation to midline. Elbow does not reach midline = score 4.

Heel to Ear
With infant supine and pelvis flat on a firm surface, pull foot as far as possible up toward ear on same side. Measure distance of foot from ear and degree of knee flexion (same as popliteal angle). Knees flexed with a popliteal angle of less than 10 degrees = score 4.

*See Fig. 26-4 for scale and interpretation of scores.
From Hockenberry, M. J., & Wilson, D. (2015). *Wong's nursing care of infants and children* (10th ed.). St. Louis: Mosby.

and may be treated as healthy newborns. Despite their appearance as term infants, late preterm infants (born at 34 to 36-6/7 weeks of gestation) are at increased risk for respiratory distress, temperature instability, hypoglycemia, apnea, feeding difficulties, and hyperbilirubinemia (Cooper, Holditch-Davis, Verklan, et al., 2012). Nurses working with healthy term infants must be cognizant of the risk factors for late preterm infants and watch for the development of problems related to the infant's immaturity. In an effort to identify these infants, a gestational-age assessment should be performed on all newborns soon after birth (Cooper et al., 2012).

The late preterm infant's care is further addressed in Chapter 28.

Common Newborn Concerns

Birth Injuries

Birth trauma includes any physical injury sustained by a newborn during labour and birth. Although most injuries are minor and resolve during the newborn period without treatment, some types of trauma require intervention; a few are serious enough to be fatal. See Chapter 29 for more information on birth injuries.

Soft-tissue injuries. Retinal and subconjunctival hemorrhages result from rupture of capillaries caused by increased pressure during birth. The hemorrhages clear within 5 days after birth and usually present no further problems. Parents need explanation about them and reassurance that these injuries are harmless.

Erythema, ecchymoses, petechiae, abrasions, lacerations, or edema of buttocks and extremities may be present. Localized discolouration can appear over a presenting part as a result of forceps or vacuum-assisted birth. Ecchymoses and edema can appear anywhere on the body. *Petechiae*, or pinpoint hemorrhagic areas, acquired during birth may extend over the upper trunk and face. These lesions are benign if they disappear within 2 or 3 days of birth and no new lesions appear. Ecchymoses and petechiae may be signs of a more serious disorder, such as thrombocytopenic purpura. To differentiate hemorrhagic areas from a skin rash or discolouration, the nurse can apply pressure to the skin with two fingers. Petechiae and ecchymoses do not blanch because extravasated blood remains within the tissues, whereas skin rashes and discolourations do blanch.

Trauma can occur during labour and birth to the presenting part. Caput succedaneum and cephalhematoma are normal and are discussed in Chapter 25 (see Fig. 25-10). Forceps injury and bruising from the vacuum cup occur at the site of application of the instruments. A forceps injury commonly produces a linear mark across both sides of the face in the shape of the blades of the forceps, with rarely skin integrity being compromised. These injuries usually resolve spontaneously within several days with no specific therapy. If small abrasions are evident the area should be kept clean to minimize the risk of infection. A topical ointment may be ordered by the primary health care provider to optimize healing. With increased use of the vacuum extractor, the incidence of these lesions has been significantly reduced.

Bruises over the face may be the result of face presentation (Fig. 26-5). In a breech presentation, bruising and swelling may

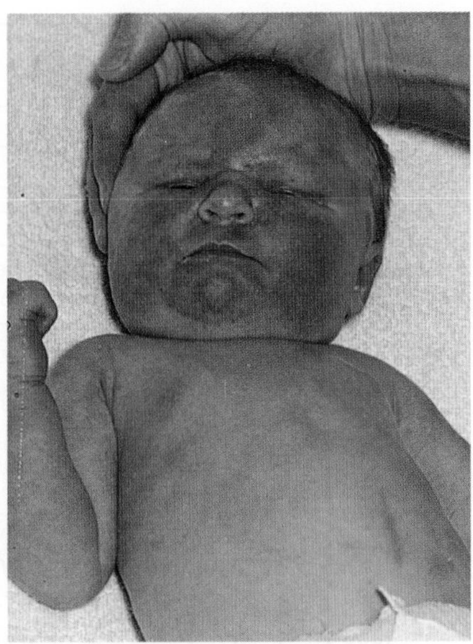

FIGURE 26-5 Marked bruising on the entire face of an infant born vaginally after face presentation. Less severe ecchymoses were present on the extremities. Phototherapy was required for treatment of jaundice resulting from the breakdown of accumulated blood. (From O'Doherty, N. [1986]. *Neonatology: Micro atlas of the newborn.* Nutley, NJ: Hoffmann–La Roche. Used with permission of F. Hoffmann-La Roche Ltd.)

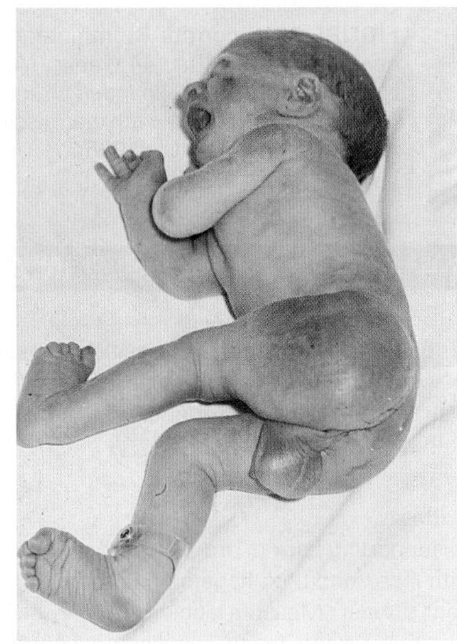

FIGURE 26-6 Swelling of genitalia and bruising of the buttocks after a breech birth. (From O'Doherty, N. [1986]. *Neonatology: Micro atlas of the newborn.* Nutley, NJ: Hoffmann–La Roche. Used with permission of F. Hoffmann-La Roche Ltd.)

be seen over the buttocks or genitalia (Fig. 26-6). The skin over the entire head may be ecchymotic and covered with petechiae caused by a tight nuchal cord or a precipitous delivery. If the hemorrhagic areas do not disappear spontaneously in 2 days or if the infant's condition changes, the primary health care provider should be notified.

Accidental lacerations can be inflicted with a scalpel during a Caesarean birth. These cuts may occur on any part of the body but are most often found on the scalp, buttocks, and thighs. Usually they are superficial and only need to be kept clean. If skin closure is needed, an adhesive substance or strips may be applied. Rarely are sutures needed.

Physiological Problems

Jaundice. Approximately 60% of all full-term newborns are visibly jaundiced (yellow) by the second through fifth day of life (Barrington, Sankaran, & CPS, 2007/2016). In most cases it is *physiological jaundice*, caused by increased levels of unconjugated bilirubin; physiological jaundice is usually self-limiting, requires no treatment, and resolves in a few days. Physiological jaundice or neonatal hyperbilirubinemia occurs in 80% of preterm newborns. The incidence of physiological jaundice is increased in Asian and Indigenous infants. It must be differentiated from pathological jaundice, or hyperbilirubinemia, which is associated with higher levels of unconjugated bilirubin. This type of jaundice can appear in the first 24 hours and often requires phototherapy to resolve. (See Chapter 25, pp. 653–655 for further discussion on pathophysiology of jaundice.)

Every newborn should be assessed for jaundice; this can be easily done when vital signs are assessed. Jaundice is generally first noticed in the head, especially the sclera and mucous membranes, and then progresses gradually to the thorax, abdomen, and extremities. Visual assessment of jaundice alone does not provide an accurate assessment of the level of serum bilirubin, especially in dark-skinned newborns; only 50% of babies with a total serum bilirubin (TSB) concentration greater than 128 mcmol/L appear jaundiced (Barrington et al., 2007/2016). To differentiate cutaneous jaundice from normal skin colour, the nurse applies pressure with a finger over a bony area (e.g., the nose, forehead, sternum) for several seconds to empty all the capillaries in that spot. If jaundice is present, the blanched area will look yellow before the capillaries refill. The conjunctival sacs and buccal mucosa are also assessed, especially in darker-skinned infants. Assessing for jaundice in natural light is recommended because artificial lighting and the reflection from walls can distort the actual skin colour.

Noninvasive monitoring of bilirubin via cutaneous reflectance measurements (transcutaneous bilirubinometry [TcB]) allows for repetitive estimations of bilirubin; however, there are limitations to the use of TcB monitors (Fig. 26-7). They are more accurate at lower TSB levels, are not accurate once phototherapy is initiated, and may be unreliable with changes in skin colour and thickness. TcB monitors may be used to screen clinically significant jaundice and decrease the need for serum bilirubin measurements (Barrington et al., 2007/2016). The CPS recommends monitoring healthy newborns at 35 weeks of gestation or greater before discharge from the hospital using hour-specific serum bilirubin levels to determine the infant's risk for development of hyperbilirubinemia requiring medical treatment or closer screening (Barrington et al., 2007/2016). Use of a nomogram (see Fig. 26-8) with three levels (high, intermediate, or low risk) of rising TSB values assists in the determination of newborns that might need further evaluation after discharge. Universal bilirubin screening based on hour-specific TSB may be done at the same time as the routine newborn profile (phenylketonuria [PKU], galactosemia, and others) (Barrington et al., 2007/2016).

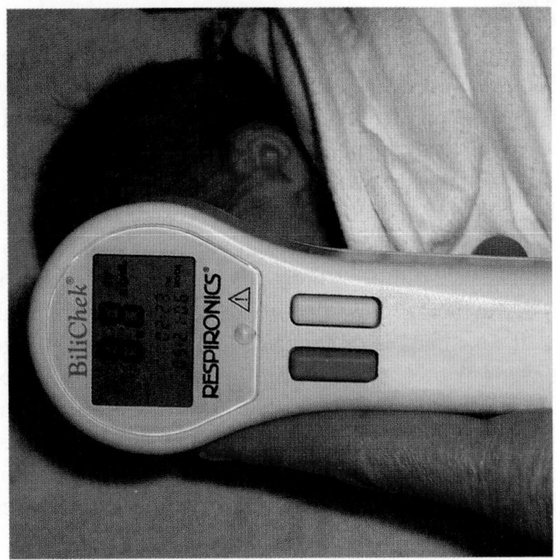

FIGURE 26-7 Transcutaneous monitoring of bilirubin with a transcutaneous bilirubinometry (TcB) monitor. (Courtesy Cheryl Briggs, BSN, RNC-NIC.)

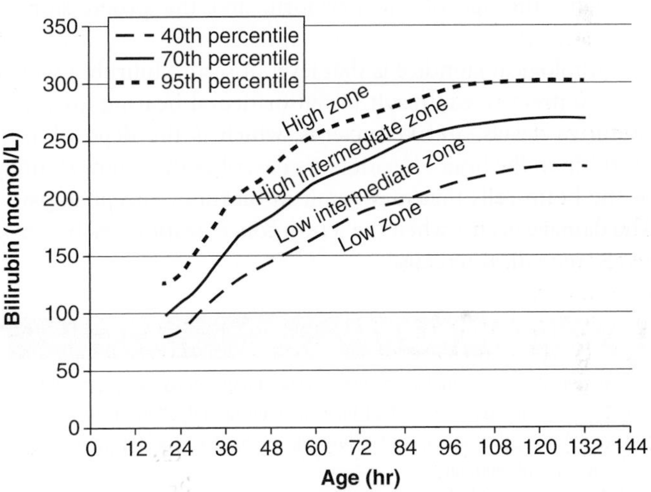

FIGURE 26-8 Nomogram for evaluation of screening total serum bilirubin (TSB) concentration in term and late preterm infants, according to the TSB concentration obtained at a known postnatal age in hours. (From Barrington, K. J., Sankaran, K., & Canadian Paediatric Society. [2007/2016]. Guidelines for detection, management and prevention of hyperbilirubinemia in term and late term newborn infants [35 or more weeks gestation]. *Paediatric Child Health, 12*[Suppl B], 1B–12B. Figure reproduced and adapted with permission from *Pediatrics, 114,* 297–316. Copyright © 2004 by the AAP.)

Risk factors that place infants in the high-risk category include gestational age 35 to 38 weeks, exclusive breastfeeding not well established and excessive weight loss, a sibling who had neonatal jaundice, visible bruising, cephalohematoma, DAT+ or other known hemolytic disease, G6PD deficiency (diagnosed at birth), ethnic background (East Asian), asphyxia (Apgar 0–3 beyond 5 minutes and cord PH less than 7), acidosis (ph less than 7 beyond initial cord sample), albumin less than 30 g/L, sepsis currently treated, temperature instability, and significant lethargy/poor feeding (Barrington et al., 2007/2016; Provincial Council for Maternal & Child Health [PCMCH] & Ministry of Health and Long-term Care, 2013). It is recommended that healthy infants (35 weeks or greater) receive assessment of bilirubin between 24 and 72 hours of life. If intervention is not required, further follow-up will depend on individual risk factors. If an infant is discharged before 24 hours of age, the infant needs further review within 24 hours by someone experienced in newborn care and with access to testing (Barrington et al., 2007/2016). Close follow-up of infants at risk for severe hyperbilirubinemia is essential; parents should be educated about the symptoms and encouraged to follow postdischarge recommendations.

If an infant is jaundiced in the first 24 hours of life, a TcB or TSB level should be measured and results interpreted on the basis of the newborn's age in hours according to the hour-specific nomogram for infants born at 35 weeks of gestation or later. Repeat testing is based on the risk level (low, intermediate, or high), the age of the newborn, and the progression of jaundice.

Pathological jaundice is that level of serum bilirubin which, if left untreated, can result in sensorineural hearing loss, mild cognitive delays, and kernicterus, which is the deposition of bilirubin in the brain. **Kernicterus** describes the yellow staining of the brain cells that may result in bilirubin encephalopathy. The damage occurs when the serum concentration reaches toxic levels, regardless of cause.

! NURSING ALERT

Breastfeeding is essential in preventing hyperbilirubinemia. Newborns should breastfeed early (within the first hour after birth) and often (at least 8–12 times/24 hr). Colostrum acts as a laxative to promote stooling, which helps rid the body of bilirubin.

Therapy for hyperbilirubinemia. The best therapy for hyperbilirubinemia is prevention. Because bilirubin is excreted in meconium, prevention can be facilitated by early and frequent feeding, which stimulates passage of meconium. However, despite early passage of meconium, some term infants may have trouble conjugating the increased amount of bilirubin derived from disintegrating fetal red blood cells (RBCs). As a result, the serum levels of unconjugated bilirubin may rise beyond normal limits, causing hyperbilirubinemia. The goal of treatment of hyperbilirubinemia is to help reduce the newborn's serum levels of unconjugated bilirubin. There are two ways to reduce unconjugated bilirubin levels: **phototherapy** and **exchange blood transfusion**.

Phototherapy. The purpose of phototherapy is to reduce the level of circulating unconjugated bilirubin or to keep it from increasing. Phototherapy uses light energy to change the shape and structure of unconjugated bilirubin and convert it to molecules that can be excreted. The dose and effectiveness of phototherapy are affected by the source of light. Phototherapy units vary in the spectrum of light they deliver and in the filters that are used. The most effective therapy is achieved with special blue fluorescent tubes or a specially designed light-emitting diode (LED). Phototherapy lights do not emit significant ultraviolet radiation; the small amount that is emitted does not cause erythema. Most of the ultraviolet light is absorbed by the glass wall of the fluorescent tube and by the plastic cover of the light (Kamath, Thilo, & Hernandez, 2011). Phototherapy is usually effective for treatment of hyperbilirubinemia that has not reached levels associated with acute bilirubin encephalopathy or kernicterus.

The effectiveness of phototherapy is related to the distance between the light and the newborn and on the area of skin that is exposed. During phototherapy, the unclothed infant is placed under a bank of lights approximately 45 to 50 cm from the light source. Research suggests that the newborn be placed supine for maximum exposure to the light source (Bhethanabhotia, Thurak, Sankar, et al., 2013). Phototherapy can be used for the infant in an isolette (Fig. 26-9) or in an open crib. The distance varies according to unit protocol and type of light used. The lamp's energy output should be monitored routinely with a photometer during treatment to ensure efficacy of therapy. Phototherapy is used until the infant's serum bilirubin level decreases to within an acceptable range. The decision to discontinue therapy is based on the observation of a definite downward trend in bilirubin values.

The infant's eyes must be protected by an opaque mask to prevent overexposure to the light. The eye shield should cover the eyes completely but not occlude the nares. Before the mask is applied, the infant's eyes should be closed gently to prevent excoriation of the corneas. The mask should be removed periodically and during infant feedings so that the eyes can be

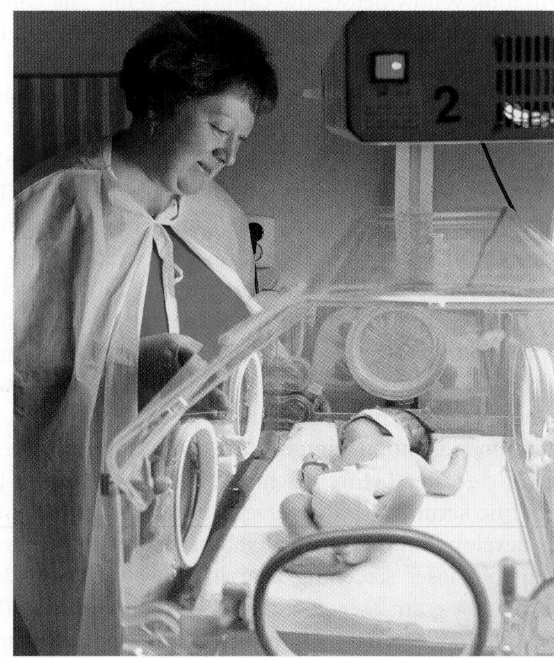

FIGURE 26-9 Infant under phototherapy lights while in isolette. (Olesia Bilkei/Shutterstock.com.)

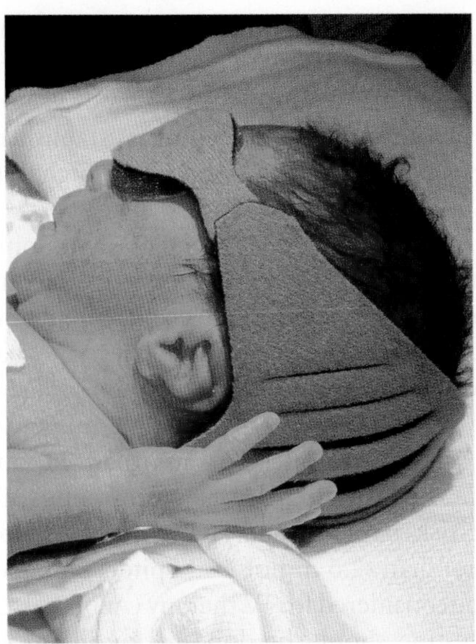

FIGURE 26-10 Infant with eyes covered while receiving phototherapy. (Courtesy Cheryl Briggs, BSN, RNC-NIC.)

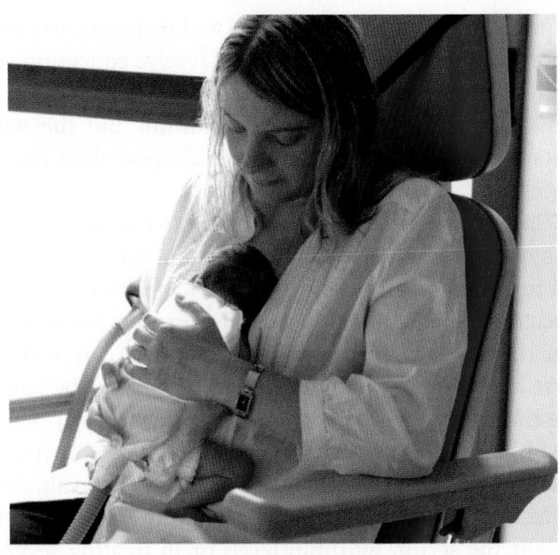

FIGURE 26-11 A mother can put her newborn skin-to-skin without interrupting phototherapy when a fibre-optic blanket is used. (Courtesy Mother and Childcare, Phillips Healthcare.)

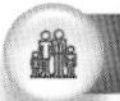

FAMILY-CENTRED CARE

Phototherapy and Parent–Infant Interaction

The traditional use of phototherapy has evoked concerns regarding a number of psychobehavioural issues, including parent–infant separation, potential social isolation, decreased sensorineural stimulation, altered biological rhythms, altered feeding patterns, and activity changes. Parental anxiety is greatly increased, particularly at the sight of the newborn blindfolded and under special lights. The interruption of breastfeeding for phototherapy is a potential deterrent to successful maternal–infant attachment and interaction. Because research has demonstrated that bilirubin catabolism occurs primarily within the first few hours of the initiation of phototherapy, there is increased support for the removal of the infant from treatment for feeding and holding. Intermittent phototherapy may be just as effective as continuous therapy when used correctly.

checked and cleansed with water and the parents can have visual contact with the infant (see Family-Centred Care box and Fig. 26-10).

Phototherapy may cause changes in the infant's temperature, depending partially on the bed used: bassinet, isolette, or radiant warmer. When under a phototherapy light, infants are usually clothed only with a diaper. The infant's temperature should be closely monitored at least every 2 hours. Phototherapy lights can increase the rate of insensible water loss, which contributes to fluid loss and dehydration. Therefore, it is important that the infant be adequately hydrated. The healthy newborn is kept hydrated with human milk or infant formula; there is no advantage or benefit to administering oral glucose or plain water because these do not promote excretion of bilirubin in stools and may in fact perpetuate enterohepatic circulation, thus delaying bilirubin excretion.

It is important to closely monitor urinary output as an indicator of hydration status while the infant is receiving phototherapy. Urine output can be decreased or unaltered; the urine can have a dark gold or brown appearance.

The number and consistency of stools should also be monitored. Bilirubin breakdown increases gastric motility, which results in loose stools that can cause skin excoriation and breakdown. The infant's buttocks must be cleaned after each stool to maintain skin integrity. A fine maculopapular rash may appear during phototherapy, but this is transient.

Additional systems used for phototherapy include a bassinet system that provides special blue light above and beneath the infant. Another phototherapy device is a fibre-optic blanket that is connected to a light source (see Fig. 26-11). The blanket is flexible and can be placed around the infant's torso or underneath the infant in the bassinet. There are also bilirubin beds with LED lights in a pad that covers the surface of the bassinet. The LED lights do not produce heat and can be used with radiant warmers. These devices are usually less effective when used alone than with conventional phototherapy lights. They can be very useful in combination with overhead phototherapy lights. In certain instances, the infant's bilirubin levels increase rapidly and intensive phototherapy is required; this situation involves the use of a combination of conventional lights and fibre-optic blankets to maximize bilirubin reduction. Although fibre-optic lights do not produce heat as conventional lights do, staff should ensure that a covering pad is placed between the infant's skin and the fibre-optic device to prevent skin burns, especially in preterm infants. The newborn can remain in the mother's room in an open crib or in her arms during treatment. The use of eye patches depends on whether the devices are used alone or in combination with phototherapy lights.

Home phototherapy. The use of home phototherapy should be reserved for healthy term infants with bilirubin levels in the "optional phototherapy" range according to the nomogram. The concern is that home phototherapy units do not provide the same level of irradiance or body surface coverage as phototherapy devices used in the hospital.

Follow-up. Serum levels of bilirubin in the newborn continue to rise until the fifth day of life. Many parents leave the hospital within 24 hours of birth, and some as early as 6 hours after birth. Therefore, parents must receive education regarding jaundice and its treatment. They should have written instructions for assessing the infant's condition and the name of a contact person to whom they should report their findings and concerns.

Close follow-up is needed for infants who have been treated for hyperbilirubinemia. Repeat testing of serum bilirubin levels and follow-up visits with the pediatric health care provider are expected. When follow-up serum bilirubin levels are needed after discharge from the hospital, a health care technician or nurse may draw the blood for the specimen or the parents may take the baby to a laboratory to have blood drawn for a serum bilirubin. In some cases, parents take the newborn to an outpatient clinic or to the physician's office to be evaluated.

Exchange transfusion. When phototherapy is not effective in reducing serum bilirubin levels or in treating severe hyperbilirubinemia such as in hemolytic disease, exchange transfusion may be needed. This procedure is done in an intensive care setting. The infant's blood is replaced with a combination of blood products such as RBCs mixed with 5% albumin or fresh frozen plasma (Kaplan, Wong, Sibley, et al., 2011). This invasive procedure is rarely done and can be minimized by early management and treatment (see discussion in Chapter 29).

Hypoglycemia. Hypoglycemia during the early newborn period of a term infant is defined as a blood glucose concentration less than that needed to support adequate neurological, organ, and tissue function; however, there is a lack of consensus regarding the precise level at which this concentration occurs.

At birth, the maternal source of glucose is cut off with the clamping of the umbilical cord. Most healthy term newborns experience a transient decrease in glucose levels to as low as 1.7 mmol/L during the first 1 to 2 hours after birth, with a subsequent mobilization of free fatty acids and ketones to help maintain adequate glucose levels (Blackburn, 2013). Infants who are asphyxiated or have other physiological stress may experience hypoglycemia as a result of a decreased glycogen supply, inadequate gluconeogenesis, or overutilization of glycogen stored during fetal life. There is concern about neurological injury as a result of severe or prolonged hypoglycemia, especially in combination with ischemia (Kalhan & Devaskar, 2011).

There is no need to routinely assess glucose levels of healthy term infants (Aziz, Dancey, & CPS, 2004/2014). Breastfeeding early and often helps these newborns maintain adequate glucose levels.

Glucose levels should be measured in newborns at 34 weeks of gestation or more if risk factors or clinical manifestations of hypoglycemia are present. In infants who are at risk for altered metabolism as a result of maternal illness factors (diabetes, gestational hypertension) or newborn factors (perinatal hypoxia, infection, hypothermia, polycythemia, congenital malformations, hyperinsulinism, SGA, LGA, fetal hydrops), close observation and monitoring of blood glucose levels within 2 hours of birth, after an initial feeding, are recommended. The frequency of glucose testing is determined by the risk factors for each individual newborn. Infants of diabetic mothers should undergo glucose screening before feedings for at least the first 12 hours after birth; further testing is done if glucose levels are less than 2.6 mmol/L. However, preterm and SGA infants may be vulnerable up to 36 hours of age so should be screened until 36 hour of age if feeding is established and blood glucose is maintained at 2.6 mmol/L or higher (Aziz et al., 2004/2014).

The CPS recommendations state that asymptomatic, at-risk babies should receive at least one effective feeding before a blood glucose check at 2 hours of age and should be encouraged to feed regularly thereafter. At-risk babies who have a blood glucose of less than 1.8 mmol/L at 2 hours of age despite one feeding (breastfeeding or approximately 5 mL/kg to 10 mL/kg of formula or glucose water) or less than 2.0 mmol/L after subsequent feeding should receive an intravenous (IV) dextrose infusion. At-risk babies who repeatedly have blood glucose levels of less than 2.6 mmol/L despite subsequent feeding should also be considered for IV therapy (Aziz et al., 2004/2014).

Glucose testing should be done in any infant with clinical signs of hypoglycemia. The clinical signs can be transient or recurrent and include jitteriness, lethargy, poor feeding, abnormal cry, hypotonia, temperature instability (hypothermia), respiratory distress, apnea, and seizures (Kalhan & Devaskar, 2011). It is important to remember that hypoglycemia can be present in the absence of clinical manifestations.

Hypoglycemia in the low-risk term infant is usually eliminated by feeding the infant a source of carbohydrate (i.e., preferably human milk) and putting the newborn skin-to-skin with a parent. Occasionally, the IV administration of glucose is required for infants with persistently high insulin levels or in those with depleted stores of glycogen.

> **! NURSING ALERT**
>
> Late preterm infants are at increased risk for hypoglycemia. They have decreased glycogen stores and lack hepatic enzymes for gluconeogenesis and glycogenolysis. Their hormonal regulation and insulin secretion are immature. The increased risk of cold stress and feeding difficulties adds to the risk for hypoglycemia (Cooper, Holditch-Davis, Verklan, et al., 2012).

Hypocalcemia. Hypocalcemia in infants is defined as serum calcium levels less than 2 mmol/L in the term infant and slightly lower (1.75 mmol/L) in the preterm infant. Hypocalcemia is common in critically ill newborns but also can occur in infants of mothers with diabetes or in those who experienced perinatal asphyxia or trauma and in low-birth-weight and preterm infants. Infants born to mothers treated with anticonvulsants during pregnancy are also at risk (Rigo, Mohamed, & De Curtis, 2011). Early-onset hypocalcemia usually occurs within the first 24 to 48 hours after birth. Signs of hypocalcemia include jitteriness, tremors, twitching, high-pitched cry, irritability, apnea, and laryngospasm, although some infants may be asymptomatic. Jitteriness is a symptom of both hypoglycemia and hypocalcemia; therefore, hypocalcemia must be considered if the therapy for hypoglycemia proves ineffective.

In most instances, early-onset hypocalcemia is self-limiting and resolves within 1 to 3 days. Treatment usually includes early feeding of an appropriate source of calcium, such as fortified human milk or a preterm infant formula (Jones, Hayes, Starbuck, et al., 2011). In some cases (e.g., the medically unstable, extremely low-birth-weight infant) the administration of IV elemental calcium and phosphorus may be necessary.

Laboratory and Screening Tests

Because newborns experience many transitional events in the first 28 days of life, laboratory samples are often gathered to determine adequate physiological adaptation and to identify disorders that may adversely affect the child's life beyond the neonatal period. Most laboratory tests for newborn screening may be obtained from the newborn with a heel puncture, also known as a heel stick. Tests that may be performed include bilirubin levels, blood glucose, newborn screening tests (e.g., PKU, hypothyroidism [T_4], sickle cell disease, and galactosemia), and drug serum levels. Box 26-5 lists standard laboratory values in a term newborn.

Universal Newborn Screening

Newborn genetic screening is an important public health program aimed at early detection of genetic diseases that result in severe health problems if not treated early. As many as 40 conditions may be screened. Earlier identification of genetic conditions may prevent further developmental delays and morbidities in affected children. The majority of disorders included in the screening are not symptomatic at birth.

All provinces have programs for newborn screening, but the number of conditions screened for varies by province. Newborn screening is considered the standard of care, and specific consent from the parents is not required, although parents can decline the testing. If this occurs, it is important to ensure that they understand the importance of screening. Information about which tests are performed in each province can be obtained from provincial and territorial health departments. Some of the major disorders for which infants are screened are described in Table 26-3.

Blood samples are obtained from newborn infants using a heel stick; blood is collected on a special filter paper and sent to a designated provincial/territorial laboratory for analysis. Newborn screening is done between 24 and 48 hours of age, although if a newborn is discharged prior to 24 hours it is recommended that the blood work be done before discharge and then again within 2 weeks (Perinatal Services BC, 2010).

Nurses can provide education for parents regarding the purpose of the screening, the procedure for blood sampling, when to expect results, and the importance of follow-up (Araia, Wilson, Chakraborty, et al., 2012).

BOX 26-5 STANDARD LABORATORY VALUES IN A TERM NEWBORN

Hemoglobin	140–240 g/L
Hematocrit	0.47–0.48
Glucose	1.7–3.3 mmol/L
Leukocytes (white blood cells)	9–30 × 10^9/L
Bilirubin, total serum	<30 mcmol/L
Blood Gases	
Arterial	pH 7.32–7.49
	PCO_2 26–41 mm Hg
	PO_2 60–70 mm Hg
Venous	pH 7.31–7.41
	PCO_2 40–50 mm Hg
	PO_2 40–50 mm Hg

PCO_2, partial pressure of carbon dioxide; *PO_2*, partial pressure of oxygen.

Data from Hockenberry, M. J., & Wilson, D. (2011). *Wong's nursing care of infants and children* (9th ed.). St. Louis: Mosby; Pagana, K., Pagana, T., & Pike-MacDonald, S. (2013). *Mosby's Canadian manual of diagnostic and laboratory tests* (1st Canadian ed.). St. Louis: Mosby.

Newborn Hearing Screening

Hearing loss is one of the most common congenital disorders, with approximately 1 to 3 in 1000 newborns having permanent hearing loss (Patel, Feldman, & CPS, 2011/2014). In Canada, newborn hearing screening has been an established routine practice in most provinces, but not all. This screening offers a potentially critical sequelae of tests to establish that the newborn is able to hear and will be aware of the early engagement in sound and language. If testing points to a hearing loss, interventions can be implemented early to mitigate the potential for complex social barriers (Patel et al., 2011/2014). Through early hearing detection and intervention programs, the outcome for infants who are deaf or hard of hearing can be maximized.

Using noninvasive technology, newborn hearing screening provides information about the pathways from the external ear to the cerebral cortex. Two tests commonly are used to assess hearing function in the newborn: initial screening is done with the evoked otoacoustic emissions (EOAE) test, and the auditory brainstem response (ABR) test is used as follow-up if the initial screening is abnormal. Neither test is definitive in diagnosing hearing loss; they are used to determine whether further, more accurate hearing testing is needed through audiological evaluation. For the EOAE test, a soft rubber earpiece that makes a soft clicking noise is placed in the baby's outer ear (Fig. 26-12, A). A healthy ear will "echo" the click sound back to a microphone inside the earpiece that is in the baby's ear. The ABR test is performed by attaching sensors to the baby's forehead and behind each ear. An earphone is placed in the baby's outer ear and sends a series of quiet sounds into the sleeping baby's ear (Fig. 26-12, B). The sensors measure the responses of the baby's acoustic nerve. The responses are recorded and stored in a computer.

Newborns who do not pass the initial screening test should have the hearing screening test repeated as part of follow-up care. If the infant still does not pass the test, a comprehensive audiological evaluation should be done by 3 months of age.

Collection of Specimens

Ongoing evaluation and screening of a newborn often requires obtaining blood by heel stick or venipuncture or the collection of a urine specimen. Laboratory tests may be ordered routinely

TABLE 26-3 SELECTED DISORDERS FROM UNIVERSAL NEWBORN SCREENING

DISORDER AND EVIDENCE	SYMPTOMS	SCREENING INCIDENCE	TREATMENT
PKU (classic) Elevated phenylalanine plasma concentrations	Severe cognitive impairment if early detection and treatment not started, eczema, seizures, behaviour disorders, decreased pigmentation, distinctive musty or mouselike odour	1 : 16,000 More common in White and First Nations, Métis, and Inuit	Lifelong dietary management with low-phenylalanine diet; possible tyrosine supplementation
Congenital hypothyroidism (primary) Low T_4, elevated TSH	Asymptomatic at birth; cognitive and motor delays (although neonatal detection and treatment have decreased incidence of cognitive impairment); short stature; coarse, dry skin and hair; hoarse cry; constipation	1 : 3000 with some ethnic variation	Maintain l-thyroxine levels in upper half of normal range; periodic bone age testing to monitor growth
Galactosemia (transferase deficiency) Elevated galactose; low or absent fluorescence	Hypotonia, lethargy, vomiting, diarrhea, metabolic acidosis, *Escherichia coli* sepsis, liver dysfunction, cognitive impairment, jaundice, blindness, cataracts, long-term behavioural problems, neurological impairment	1 : 60,000	Eliminate galactose and lactose from the diet (breastfeeding is contraindicated); use soy formulas in infancy; lactose-free solid foods
Maple syrup urine disease (MSUD) Elevated leucine	Poor feeding; lethargy; hypotonia; vomiting; ketoacidosis; seizures; sweet maple syrup odour in urine, cerumen, or sweat	1 : 185,000; Higher in certain Mennonites (Older Order, 1 : 358) and those of French Canadian ancestry	Branched-chain amino acid–free formula with added protein-based formula; thiamine supplement in some individuals; lifelong treatment and monitoring necessary
Homocystinuria Elevated methionine and homocysteine	Infancy: nonspecific growth failure; developmental delay; more commonly diagnosed around age 3 yr Cognitive impairment, seizures, behavioural disorders, early-onset thromboses, dislocated lenses, tall lanky body habitus	1 : 200,000 to 1 : 350,000; more prevalent in Irish, Danish, German, and Australian populations (1 : 60,000)	Methionine-restricted diet; vitamin B_6 supplement if responsive
Congenital adrenal hyperplasia (CAH) Elevated 24-hydroxyprogesterone; abnormal electrolytes	Hyponatremia, hyperkalemia, hypoglycemia, dehydration; weight loss; hypotension; shock in "salt wasting" type; female virilization; progressive virilization in both sexes	1 : 15,000 to 1 : 20,000; less common in those of African descent (1 : 42,000)	Reduce excessive corticotropins; replace glucocorticoids and mineralocorticoids; corrective surgery for ambiguous genitalia (intersex assignment is controversial)
Sickle cell/hemoglobin SC (thalassemias)	Repeated infections, growth failure, pallor, hemolytic anemia; sickle cell crisis	Sickle cell anemia more common in African, Mediterranean, Middle Eastern, and Asian communities: 1 : 400 individuals from Caribbean and parts of Africa	Preventive care: treatment of meningococcal and pneumococcal infections; hydroxyurea (antisickling agent); prevent human parvovirus B19 infection (limits production of reticulocytes)
Biotinidase deficiency Deficient or absent activity of biotinidase on colorimetric assay	Myoclonic seizures, hypotonia, feeding difficulties, organic aciduria, fungal infections, ataxia, skin rash, hearing loss, alopecia, optic nerve atrophy, developmental delay, coma, death	1 : 60,000	5–20 mg biotin daily; less with partial deficiency

PKU, phenylketonuria; *SC*, sickle cell; *T_4*, thyroxine; *TSH*, thyroid-stimulating hormone.

Data from DeBaun, M. R., Frei-Jones, M., & Vichinsky, E. (2016). Hemoglobinopathies. In R. Kliegman, B. Stanton, J. St. Geme, et al. (Eds.), *Nelson textbook of pediatrics* (20th ed.). Philadelphia: Saunders; Kishnani, P. S., & Chen, Y. (2016). Defects in metabolism of carbohydrates. In R. Kliegman, B. Stanton, J. St. Geme, et al. (Eds.), *Nelson textbook of pediatrics* (20th ed.). Philadelphia: Saunders; LaFranchi, S. & Huang, S.A. (2016). Hypothyroidism. In R. Kliegman, B. Stanton, J. St. Geme, et al. (Eds.), *Nelson textbook of pediatrics* (20th ed.). Philadelphia: Saunders; Rezvani, I. & Ficicioglu, C.H. (2011). Defects in metabolism of amino acid. In R. Kliegman, B. Stanton, J. St. Geme, et al. (Eds.), *Nelson textbook of pediatrics* (20th ed.). Philadelphia: Saunders; White, P. (2016). Congenital adrenal hyperplasia and related disorders. In R. Kliegman, B. Stanton, J. St. Geme, et al. (Eds.), *Nelson textbook of pediatrics* (20th ed.). Philadelphia: Saunders.

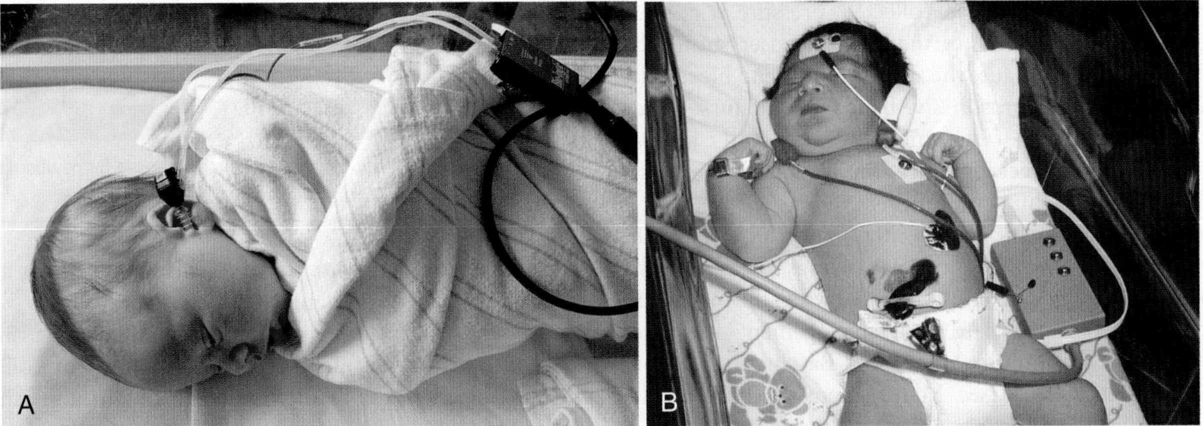

FIGURE 26-12 Newborn hearing screening. **A:** Evoked otoacoustic emissions (EOAE) test. **B:** Auditory brain response (ABR) test. (**A**, Courtesy Julie and Darren Nelson. **B**, Courtesy Dee Lowdermilk.)

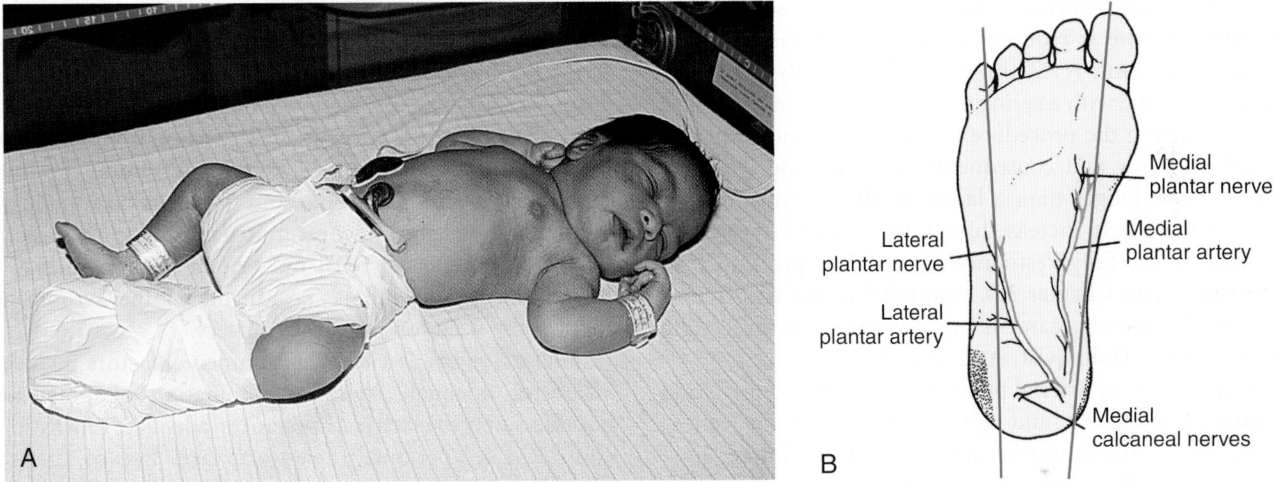

FIGURE 26-13 Heel stick. **A:** Newborn with foot wrapped for warmth to increase blood flow to extremity before heel stick. **B:** Heel stick sites (shaded areas) on infant's foot for obtaining samples of capillary blood. (**A,** Courtesy Marjorie Pyle, RNC, Lifecircle.)

(e.g., newborn screening) or for a specific purpose as directed by the health care provider.

Heel stick. Some blood specimens may be drawn by laboratory technicians. However, nurses generally have established a relationship with the family and are able to perform heel sticks at the bedside to obtain blood for glucose monitoring or newborn screening or other tests.

! NURSING ALERT

Blood samples should be collected in a manner that minimizes pain and trauma to the infant and maximizes the accuracy of test results. If a laboratory technician is collecting the specimen, the nurse assists as needed to maximize safety and infant comfort.

It is often helpful to warm the heel before the sample is taken; application of heat for 5 to 10 minutes helps dilate the blood vessels in the area. A cloth soaked with warm water (not hot) and wrapped loosely around the foot provides effective warming (Fig. 26-13, A). Disposable heel warmers are available from a variety of companies; they should be used with care to prevent burns. Nurses should wear gloves when collecting any specimen. The nurse cleanses the area with an appropriate skin antiseptic, allows the area to dry, restrains the infant's foot with a free hand, and then punctures the site. A spring-loaded automatic puncture device causes less pain and requires fewer punctures than a manual lance blade; therefore, manual lance blades should not be used on newborns.

The most serious complication of infant heel stick is necrotizing osteochondritis from lancet penetration of the bone. To prevent this, the penetration should be made at the outer aspect of the heel and should be no deeper than 2.4 mm. To identify the appropriate puncture site, the nurse should draw an imaginary line running from between the fourth and fifth toes and parallel to the lateral aspect of the foot to the heel where the puncture is made; a second line can be drawn from the great toe to the medial aspect of the heel (see Fig. 26-13, B). Repeated trauma to the walking surface of the heel can cause fibrosis and scarring that may lead to problems with walking later in life.

After the specimen has been collected, pressure is applied with a dry gauze square. No further skin cleanser should be applied because this will cause the site to continue to bleed. The site is then covered with an adhesive bandage. The nurse needs to ensure proper disposal of equipment used, review the laboratory requisition for correct identification, and check the specimen for adequate labelling and routing.

A heel stick is traumatic for the infant and causes pain. To reassure the infant and to promote feelings of safety, the newborn should be cuddled and comforted when the procedure is complete, and appropriate pain management measures should be taken to minimize the pain (Barrington, Batton, Finley, et al., 2007/2015) (see Management of Pain in the Newborn, p. 705).

Venipuncture. Occasionally, laboratory tests are ordered that require larger samples of blood than can be collected with a heel stick. Venous blood samples can be drawn from antecubital, saphenous, superficial wrist, and rarely, scalp veins. When venipuncture is required, positioning of the needle is extremely important. A 23- or 25-gauge butterfly needle or hypodermic needle with a syringe is used (Fig. 26-14). Patience is required during the procedure because the blood return in small veins is slow and consequently the small needle must remain in place longer than a larger needle. A tourniquet is optional but can help increase blood flow with venipuncture. The infant is carefully restrained during the procedure to prevent injury (see Chapter 39). Pain relief is also a key component to the nursing care in any venipuncture procedure (Gradin, Erikson, Holmqvist, et al., 2014).

If venipuncture or arterial puncture is performed for blood gas studies, crying, fear, and agitation will affect the values; therefore, every effort must be made to keep the infant quiet during the procedure. Pressure must be maintained over an arterial or femoral vein puncture with a dry gauze square for 3 to 5 minutes to prevent bleeding from the site.

For an hour after any venipuncture, the nurse should observe the infant frequently for evidence of bleeding or hematoma formation at the puncture site. The infant should be cuddled and comforted when the procedure is completed, and appropriate pain management measures taken. The nurse assesses and documents the infant's tolerance of the procedure.

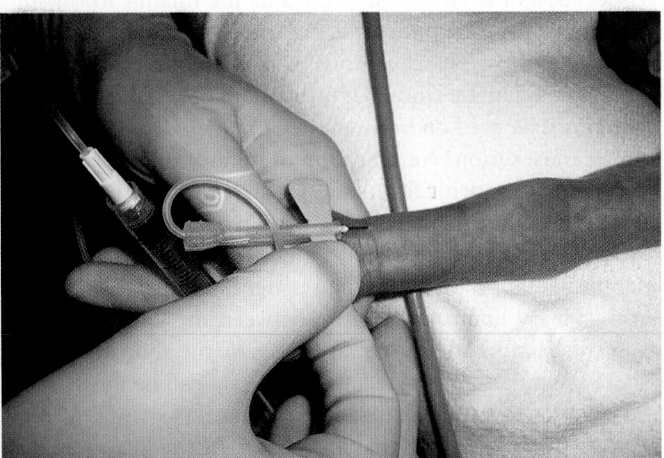

FIGURE 26-14 Venipuncture using a butterfly needle. (Courtesy Cheryl Briggs, BSN, RNC-NIC.)

NURSING ALERT

Only venous or capillary blood samples may be used for newborn screening and genetic studies; cord blood is not used for these samples.

Obtaining a urine specimen. Analysis of urine is a valuable laboratory tool for infant assessment; the way in which the specimen is collected can influence the results. The urine sample should be fresh and analyzed within 1 hour of collection. A urine collection bag is often used to obtain a specimen (see Chapter 44 for more information about the procedure for collecting a urine specimen from an infant).

Interventions

Protective Environment

The provision of a protective environment is basic to the care of the newborn. Hospital personnel develop their own policies and procedures for protecting the newborns under their care. Prescribed standards cover areas such as environmental factors, measures to control infection, and safety factors.

Current health care trends and the focus on nonseparation of mothers and babies have prompted most hospitals to abandon having a separate newborn nursery. In the mother/baby care model of care, the infant stays in the mother's room, which reduces the need for a separate nursery.

Environmental factors. Environmental factors include provision of adequate lighting, elimination of potential fire hazards, safety of electrical appliances, adequate ventilation, and controlled temperature (i.e., warm and free of drafts) and humidity.

Measures to control infection. Measures to control infection include adequate floor space for positioning bassinets at least 90 cm apart in all directions if in a newborn nursery, hand hygiene facilities, and areas for cleaning and storing equipment and supplies. Only those personnel directly involved in the care of mothers and infants are allowed in these areas, thereby reducing opportunities for the introduction of pathogenic organisms.

NURSING ALERT

Proper hand hygiene is essential to preventing the spread of health care–associated infections (HAI).

Personnel should wash hands with soap and water or use an alcohol-based hand rub in accordance with hospital infection control policies. Hand hygiene should be performed before and after touching the infant, before an invasive procedure or medication administration, after contact with potentially contaminated objects (e.g., computer keyboards, telephone, countertop surfaces), and after removing sterile or nonsterile gloves (WHO, 2009b).

Health care workers must wear gloves when handling the infant before blood and amniotic fluid have been removed from the infant's skin, when drawing blood (e.g., heel stick), when caring for a fresh wound (e.g., circumcision), when assisting with breastfeeding, and during diaper changes.

Visitors and health care providers, including nurses, physicians, parents, siblings, and grandparents, are expected to wash their hands before having contact with infants or equipment. Individuals with infectious conditions, including upper respiratory tract or gastrointestinal tract infections and infectious skin conditions, should be excluded from contact with newborns or must take special precautions when working with infants.

Safety factors. Personnel caring for newborns must be clearly identified by photo identification, and parents must be educated about measures to prevent abduction from the mother's room (i.e., be certain they know the identity of anyone who cares for the infant and never release the infant to anyone who is not wearing the appropriate identification) (Vincent, 2009). Other measures include placing matching identification bracelets on newborns and their parents and using identification bands with radiofrequency transmitters that set off an alarm if the bracelet is removed or if a certain threshold is crossed (doorway to exit building or floor).

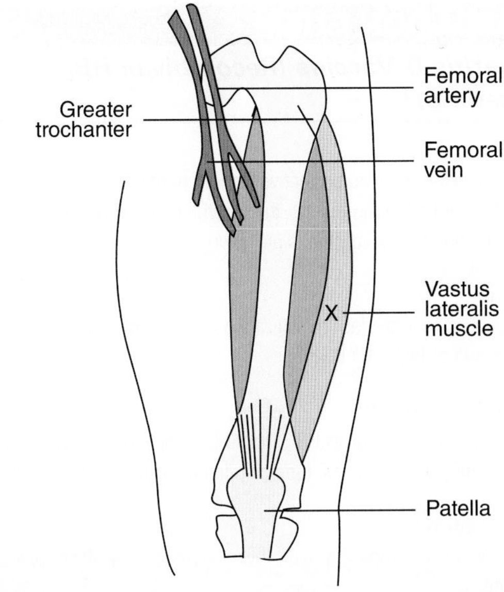

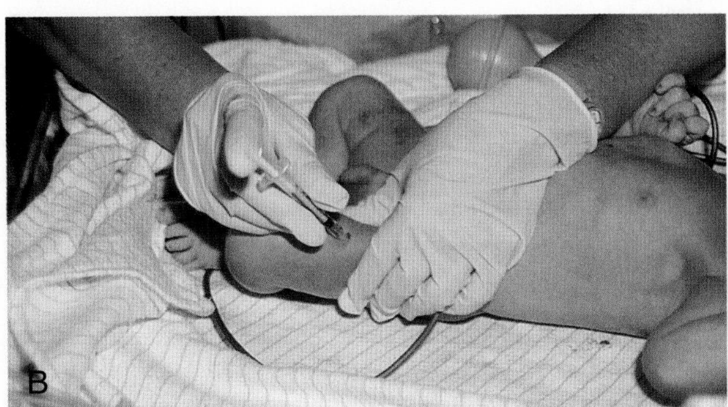

FIGURE 26-15 Intramuscular injection. **A:** Acceptable intramuscular injection site (X) for newborn infant. **B:** Infant's leg being stabilized for intramuscular injection. The nurse is wearing gloves to give the injection. (**B,** Courtesy Marjorie Pyle, RNC, Lifecircle.)

Therapeutic and Surgical Procedures

Intramuscular injection. Newborns routinely receive intramuscular injections before discharge. A single dose of vitamin K is administered shortly after birth and hepatitis B (HepB) vaccine may be administered before discharge. Under specific circumstances, other intramuscular injections may be ordered, such as a dose of hepatitis B immunoglobulin (HBIG) for infants born to mothers who are positive for hepatitis B.

Selection of the appropriate equipment and site for intramuscular injection is important. In most cases, a 25-gauge, ⅝-inch (16 mm) to 7/8-inch (22-mm) needle is used. Injections must be given in muscles large enough to accommodate the medication, and major nerves and blood vessels must be avoided. The muscles of newborns may not tolerate more than 0.5 mL per intramuscular injection. The preferred injection site for newborns is the vastus lateralis (Fig. 26-15). The dorsogluteal muscle is very small, poorly developed, and dangerously close to the sciatic nerve, which occupies a proportionately larger area in infants than in older children. Therefore, it is not recommended as an injection site in small children. The newborn's deltoid muscle has an inadequate amount of muscle for intramuscular administration. A key factor in preventing and minimizing local reaction to intramuscular injections is adequate deposition of the medication deep within the muscle; therefore, muscle size, needle length, and amount of medication injected should be carefully considered.

The nurse wears nonsterile gloves when administering an injection. The newborn's leg should be stabilized. The nurse cleanses the injection site with an appropriate skin antiseptic and then stabilizes the infant's muscle between the thumb and forefinger. The needle is inserted into the vastus lateralis at a 90-degree angle. The medication is injected slowly. After the medication is injected, the nurse withdraws the needle quickly and places a dry gauze pad over the site, applying gentle pressure to minimize pain and bleeding.

The nurse needs to comfort the infant after an injection and discard equipment properly. Needles are never recapped but are properly discarded in an appropriate safety container. The name of the medication, date and time, amount, route, and site of injection are documented in the newborn's record.

Immunizations. In some provinces the hepatitis B vaccine is given at birth, whereas in others it is given before the child is a preteen. If not routinely given at birth, hepatitis B vaccination is recommended for infants at highest risk of contracting hepatitis B. This includes newborns born to women who have hepatitis B or whose hepatitis B status is unknown or if another family member who lives in the home has hepatitis B. If the infant is born to an infected mother or to a mother who is a chronic carrier, hepatitis B vaccine and HBIG should be given within 12 hours of birth (see Medication Guides). Go to the Public Health Agency of Canada website to see the schedule for different provinces (see Additional Resources at the end of the chapter). The hepatitis B vaccine is given in one site, and the HBIG in another. Parental consent must be obtained before administering these medications.

Circumcision. Circumcision is the removal of all or part of the foreskin (prepuce) of the penis. Usually it is performed during the first week of life, but is sometimes done at a later time for preterm or ill newborns or for religious or cultural reasons. The most recent reported rate of newborn male

MEDICATION GUIDE

*Hepatitis B Vaccine (Recombivax HB, Engerix-B)**

Action
Hepatitis B vaccine induces protective anti–hepatitis B antibodies in 95 to 99% of healthy infants who receive the recommended three doses. The duration of protection of the vaccine is unknown.

Indication
Hepatitis B vaccine provides immunization against infection caused by all known subtypes of hepatitis B virus.

Neonatal Dosage
The usual dosage is Recombivax HB 5 mcg/0.5 mL or Engerix-B 10 mcg/0.5 mL at birth, 1 month, and 6 months. (See also Immunizations, Chapter 35.)

Adverse Reactions
Common adverse reactions are rash, fever, erythema, swelling, and pain at injection site.

Nursing Considerations
Parental consent must be obtained before administration. Follow proper procedure for administration of intramuscular (IM) injection (see p. 701). If infant also needs hepatitis B immune globulin (HBIG), use separate sites for the two injections.

For infants born to hepatitis B surface antigen (HBsAg)–positive mothers: administer HepB vaccine and HBIG within 12 hours after birth.

Document immunization administration on a vaccination card for parent(s) to have a record.

***Note:** The combination vaccines containing hepatitis B are not recommended for the birth (first) dose.

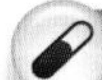

MEDICATION GUIDE

Hepatitis B Immune Globulin

Action
Hepatitis B immunoglobulin (HBIG) provides a high titre of antibody to hepatitis B surface antigen (HBsAg).

Indication
The HBIG vaccine provides prophylaxis against infection in infants born to HBsAg-positive mothers.

Neonatal Dosage
Administer one 0.5-mL dose intramuscularly within 12 hours of birth.

Adverse Reactions
Hypersensitivity may occur.

Nursing Considerations
The vaccine must be given within 12 hours of birth. Follow proper procedure for administration of intramuscular injection (see p. 701). The HBIG vaccine may be given at the same time as hepatitis B vaccine, but at a different site. Document immunization administration on a vaccination card for parent(s) to have a record.

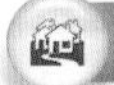

COMMUNITY FOCUS

Newborn Circumcision

Prepare a poster presentation to provide parents information on newborn circumcision. Because circumcision is considered an optional surgical procedure, it may not be performed until after the infant is discharged home. Include in your display the advantages and disadvantages of circumcision, as well as the care of the uncircumcised penis in infants and young children.

circumcision (NMC) in Canada was in 2007 and was 32%; the rates are highest in Alberta (44%) and Ontario (43%) and below 10% in Northwest Territories and Nova Scotia (Public Health Agency of Canada [PHAC], 2009). All provincial health insurance plans have removed nontherapeutic NMC from the schedule of procedures covered under provincial health care plans. This factor, and possibly a wider movement to holistic health, has led to a decline in the rate of NMC in Canada ("Rates of Circumcision," 2006). Circumcision of male infants is usually performed within the first few weeks of life and may occur before the newborn is discharged from the hospital, or it may be done as an outpatient procedure.

In 2015, the CPS issued a new policy statement regarding NMC stating that NMC may have some health benefits, including prevention of urinary tract infection in male infants younger than 1 year, reduced risk for penile cancer, and reduced risk for heterosexual acquisition of sexually transmitted infections, particularly HIV (Sorokan, Finlay, Jefferies, et al., 2015). Despite the scientific evidence of potential medical benefits of circumcision for some boys in high-risk populations, the CPS has stated that the data are not sufficient to recommend routine circumcision (Sorokan et al., 2015). The World Health Organization (WHO) (2012) recognizes male circumcision as an important intervention in reducing the risk for heterosexually acquired HIV in men.

Circumcision is a matter of personal parental choice. Parents usually decide to have their newborn circumcised on the basis of one or more of the following factors: religious conviction, tradition, culture, social norms, or perceived hygiene. Parents need to make an informed choice regarding newborn circumcision based on the most current evidence and recommendations. Health care providers and nurses who care for child-bearing families can help parents make an informed choice about newborn circumcision by providing factual, unbiased, evidence-informed information. They can provide opportunities for discussion about the benefits and risks of the procedure (see Community Focus box).

Procedure. Circumcision involves removal of the **prepuce** (foreskin) of the glans. The procedure is not usually done immediately after birth because of the danger of cold stress and decreased clotting factors, but it may be performed in some hospitals before the infant's discharge. The circumcision of a Jewish boy is performed on the eighth day after birth and is done at home in a ceremony called a *bris*. The timing is logical from a physiological standpoint because clotting factors drop somewhat immediately after birth and do not return to prebirth levels until the end of the first week.

Feedings are usually withheld up to 2 to 3 hours before the circumcision to prevent vomiting and aspiration, although in some hospitals, infants are allowed to breastfeed until the time they are taken for the procedure. To prepare the infant for the circumcision, he is positioned on a plastic restraint form (Fig. 26-16) and the penis is cleansed with soap and water or other prep solution such as povidone-iodine. The infant is draped to provide warmth and a sterile field, and the sterile equipment is readied for use.

In the hospital setting, newborn circumcision is usually performed using the Gomco (Yellen) or Mogen clamp or the Plasti-Bell device. The technique is usually based on health care provider training and preference. The procedure takes only a few minutes to perform. Use of the Gomco or Mogen clamp involves surgical removal of the foreskin. The clamp technique minimizes blood loss (Fig. 26-17). After it is completed, a small petrolatum gauze dressing or a generous amount of petrolatum or A&D ointment may be applied to the penis for the first few days to prevent the diaper from adhering to the site. With the PlastiBell technique, the plastic bell is first fitted over the glans, a suture is tied around the rim of the bell, and excess foreskin is cut away. The plastic rim remains in place for about a week; it falls off after healing has taken place, usually within 5 to 7 days (Fig. 26-18). Petrolatum is not usually needed when the bell is used.

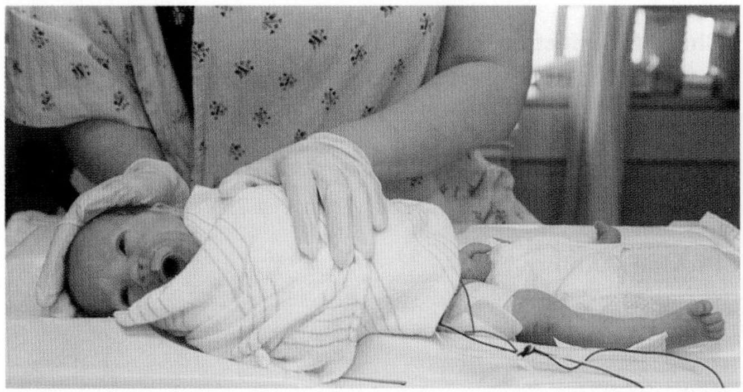

FIGURE 26-16 Proper positioning of infant in Circumstraint. (Courtesy Paul Vincent Kuntz, Texas Children's Hospital.)

Procedural pain management. Circumcision is painful. The pain is manifested by both physiological and behavioural changes in the infant (see discussion on newborn pain that follows). Four types of anaesthesia and analgesia are used in newborns undergoing circumcision: ring block, dorsal penile nerve block (DPNB), topical anaesthetic such as eutectic mixture of lidocaine and prilocaine (EMLA) (prilocaine-lidocaine), and concentrated oral sucrose. Nonpharmacological methods such as non-nutritive sucking and swaddling may be used to enhance pain management.

The Cochrane Group exploring pain relief for newborn circumcision found that DPNB was the most effective intervention for decreasing the pain of circumcision. A DPNB includes subcutaneous injections of buffered lidocaine at the 2 o'clock and 10 o'clock positions at the base of the penis. A ring block is the injection of buffered lidocaine administered subcutaneously on

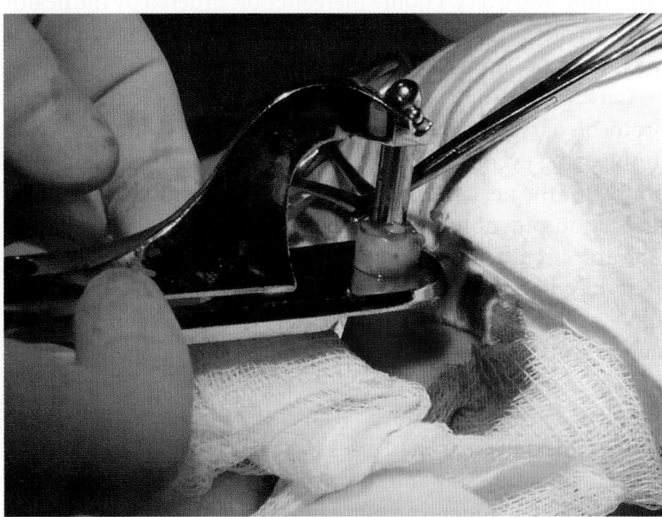

FIGURE 26-17 Circumcision with Gomco (Yellen) clamp. After hemostasis occurs, the foreskin (over the metal dome) is cut away. (Courtesy Cheryl Briggs, BSN, RNC-NIC.)

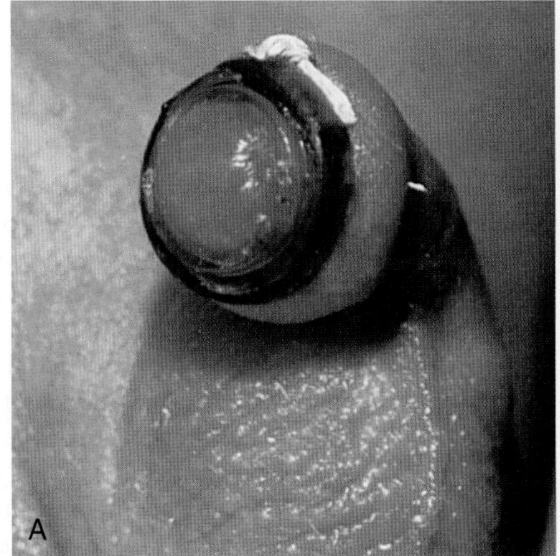

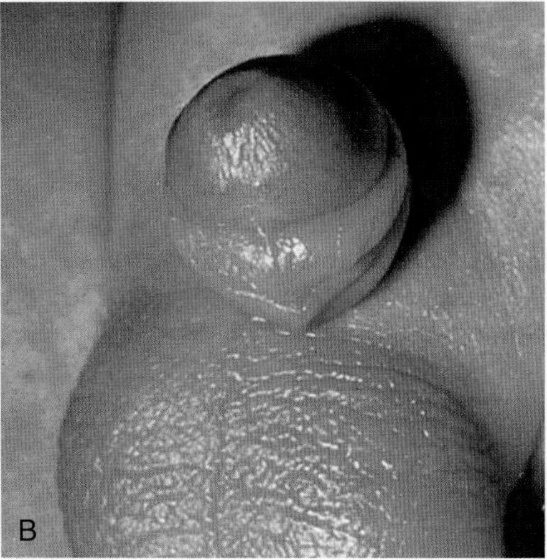

FIGURE 26-18 Circumcision using Hollister PlastiBell. **A:** Suture around rim of PlastiBell controls bleeding. **B:** Plastic rim and suture drop off in 7 to 10 days. (Owned by Briggs Healthcare.)

each side of the penile shaft. The circumcision should not be performed for at least 5 minutes after these injections.

A topical anaesthetic cream (eutectic mixture of local anaesthetic [EMLA]) can be applied to the penis at least 1 hour before the circumcision. The area where the prepuce attaches to the glans is well coated with 1 g of the cream and then covered with a transparent occlusive dressing or finger cot. Just before the procedure, the cream is removed. Blanching or redness of the skin can occur.

After the circumcision, the infant should be comforted until he is quieted. If the parents were not present during the procedure, the infant should be returned to them. The baby should be positioned to breastfeed, or put skin-to-skin with mother or other care provider. Afterwards, the infant may be fussy for several hours and may have disturbed sleep–wake states and disorganized feeding behaviours. Some infants will go into a deep sleep after circumcision until they are awakened for feeding. Oral acetaminophen may be administered before the procedure and every 4 hours thereafter (as ordered by the health care provider) for a maximum of five doses in 24 hours or a maximum of 75 mg/kg/day.

Care of the newly circumcised infant. Postcircumcision protocols vary. In many settings, the circumcision site is assessed for bleeding every 15 to 30 minutes for the first hour and then hourly for the next 4 to 6 hours. The nurse monitors the infant's urinary output, noting the time and amount of the first voiding after the circumcision.

If bleeding occurs from the circumcision site, the nurse applies gentle pressure with a folded sterile gauze pad. A hemostatic agent such as Gelfoam® powder or sponge can be applied to help control bleeding. If bleeding is not easily controlled, a blood vessel may need to be ligated. In this event, one nurse notifies the physician and prepares the necessary equipment (i.e., circumcision tray and suture material) while another nurse maintains intermittent pressure until the physician arrives.

Nurses provide education for parents related to care of the circumcised infant, which includes observing for complications such as bleeding or infection (see Patient Teaching box). Parents need support and encouragement as they perform postcircumcision care. Newborns typically cry when the diaper is changed and when petrolatum gauze is removed and reapplied. This can make new parents feel anxious because they do not want to inflict pain on the infant. Nurses can inform parents that the discomfort is usually temporary and will soon subside.

Nursing actions can help prevent infection. Prepackaged commercial wipes are not used because they can contain alcohol, which delays healing and causes discomfort. Instead, the nurse washes the penis gently with water to remove urine and feces and, if necessary, applies fresh petrolatum around the glans after each diaper change. The glans penis, normally dark red during healing, becomes covered with a yellow exudate within 24 hours. This is part of normal healing, not an infective process. No attempt should be made to remove the exudate, which persists for 2 to 3 days. Parents should be taught to fanfold the diaper so that it does not press on the circumcised area. They should be encouraged to change the diaper at least every 4 hours to prevent it from sticking to the penis.

PATIENT TEACHING

Care of the Circumcised Newborn at Home

Wash hands before touching the newly circumcised penis.

Check for Bleeding

- Check circumcision for bleeding with each diaper change.
- If bleeding occurs, apply gentle pressure with a folded sterile gauze square. If bleeding does not stop with pressure, notify the primary health care provider.

Observe for Urination

- Check to see that the infant urinates after being circumcised.
- Infant should have wet diapers appropriate for age (see Elimination, p. 711).

Keep Area Clean

- Change diaper and inspect circumcision at least every 4 hours.
- Wash penis gently with warm water to remove urine and feces. Apply petrolatum liberally to the glans with each diaper change (omit petrolatum if PlastiBell was used). Do not use baby wipes because they can contain alcohol.
- Do not wash the penis with soap until the circumcision is healed (5 to 6 days).
- Sponge bath only until circumcision heals.
- Apply the diaper loosely over the penis to prevent pressure on the circumcised area.

Check for Infection

- Glans penis is dark red after circumcision, then becomes covered with yellow exudate in 24 hours. This is normal and will persist for 2 to 3 days. Do not attempt to remove it.
- Redness, swelling, or discharge indicates infection. Notify the primary health care provider if you think the circumcision area is infected.

Provide Comfort

- Circumcision is painful. Handle the area gently.
- Provide acetaminophen as required and ordered by the health care provider.
- Provide comfort measures such as holding the baby skin-to-skin, cuddling, rocking, and giving opportunities for non-nutritive sucking for a day or two.

Pain in the Newborn

Newborn Responses to Pain

While pain in the newborn and pain in later life can be qualitatively different, research has substantiated that newborns do experience pain (Blackburn, 2013). This counters previous thinking that the immaturity of the nervous system prevented or blunted pain sensation and that newborns were incapable of remembering painful experiences.

Pain has physiological and psychological components. Its psychological component and the diffuse total body response to pain exhibited by the newborn led many health care providers in the past to believe that infants, especially preterm infants, do not experience pain. The central nervous system is well developed, however, as early as 24 weeks of gestation. The peripheral and spinal structures that transmit pain information are present and functional between the first and second trimesters.

The pituitary–adrenal axis is also well developed at this time, and a fight-or-flight reaction is observed in response to the catecholamines released in response to stress.

The physiological response to pain in newborns can be life threatening. Pain response can decrease tidal volume, increase demands on the cardiovascular system, increase metabolism, and cause neuroendocrine imbalance. The hormonal–metabolic response to pain in a term infant has greater magnitude and shorter duration than that in adults. The newborn's sympathetic response to pain is less mature and therefore less predictable than an adult's.

Pain response is influenced by a variety of factors such as characteristics of the painful stimulus, gestational age, biological factors, and behavioural state. The source, location, and timing of the pain affect the response; newborns respond differently to acute pain than to prolonged or recurrent pain. In general, infants of younger gestational ages seem to display less vigorous pain responses. There can be genetic differences in pain responses related to the amount and type of neurotransmitters and receptors available to mediate pain. The behavioural state of the newborn also affects the pain response. Those who are more awake tend to have more robust pain responses than those in sleep states (Gardner, Enzman-Hines, & Dickey, 2011).

The most common behavioural sign of pain is a vocalization or crying, ranging from a whimper to a distinctive high-pitched, shrill cry. Facial expressions include grimacing, eye squeeze, brow contraction, deepened nasolabial furrows, a taut and quivering tongue, and an open mouth (Fig. 26-19) (Harrison, Bueno, & Reszel, 2015). The infant will flex and adduct the upper body and lower limbs in an attempt to withdraw from the painful stimulus. The preterm infant has a lower-than-normal threshold for initiation of this flex response.

Pain can result in significant changes in heart rate, BP (increased or decreased), intracranial pressure, vagal tone, respiratory rate, and oxygen saturation. Newborns respond to painful stimuli with release of epinephrine, norepinephrine, glucagon, corticosterone, cortisol, 11-deoxycorticosterone, lactate, pyruvate, and glucose (Blackburn, 2013) (Box 26-6).

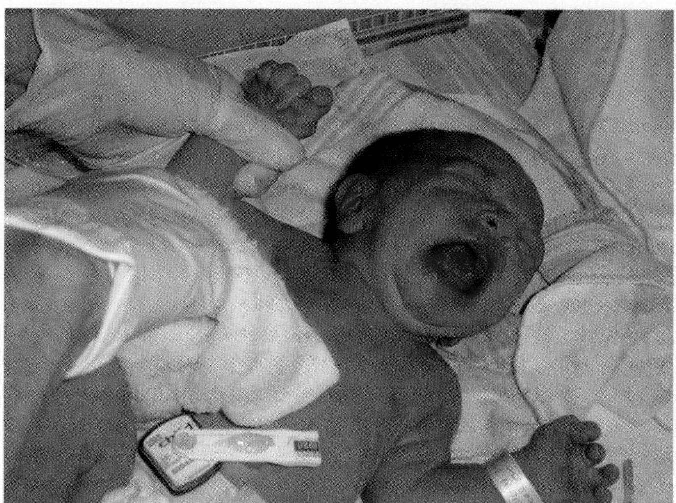

FIGURE 26-19 Signs of discomfort: note eye squeeze, brow bulge, nasolabial furrow, and wide-spread mouth. (Courtesy Kathryn Alden.)

Assessment of Pain in the Newborn

In assessing pain, the nurse needs to consider the health of the newborn, the type and duration of the painful stimulus, environmental factors, and the infant's state of alertness. For example, severely compromised newborns may be unable to generate a pain response although they are, in fact, experiencing pain.

Pain should be assessed and documented on a regular basis for all newborns, and a pain management plan should be developed if required.

Pain assessment tools include the following:

- Neonatal Infant Pain Scale (NIPS) (Lawrence, Alcock, McGrath, et al., 1993)
- Premature Infant Pain Profile (PIPP) (Stevens, Johnston, Petryshen, et al., 1996)
- Neonatal Pain Agitation and Sedation Scale (NPASS) (Hummel, Puchalski, Creech, et al., 2008)

A pain assessment tool used by nurses in some neonatal intensive care units (NICUs) is CRIES (Krechel & Bildner, 1995) (Table 26-4). This tool was developed for use by nurses who work with preterm and term infants. CRIES is an acronym for the physiological and behavioural indicators of pain used in the tool: **c**rying, **r**equiring increased oxygen, **i**ncreased vital signs, **e**xpression, and **s**leeplessness. Each indicator is scored from 0 to 2. The total possible pain score, which represents the worst pain, is 10. A pain score greater than 4 should be considered significant. This tool can be used on infants between 32 weeks of gestation and 20 weeks after birth.

Healthy term newborns are exposed to fewer sources of pain than preterm infants in an NICU where painful procedures are inherent to care management. Even in low-risk newborns, nurses need to assess for signs of discomfort as part of routine assessments, especially during and after routine procedures such as heel sticks, injections, and circumcision.

Management of Pain in the Newborn

The goals of the management of neonatal pain are to (1) minimize the intensity, duration, and physiological cost of the pain; and (2) maximize the newborn's ability to cope with and recover from the pain. Nonpharmacological and pharmacological strategies are used. It is important to note that despite research evidence, policies, and standards of practice focused on assessing and managing pain in newborns, acute infant pain remains undermanaged and, in some cases, unmanaged (Gardner et al., 2011; Taddio, Appleton, Bortolussi, et al., 2010).

Nonpharmacological management. A variety of nonpharmacological pain management techniques are used with newborns. Nurses and parents may combine two or more techniques as they seek to promote infant comfort and reduce pain. In a recent study of nonpharmacological techniques targeting preterm infants, the authors concurred that providing relief from repetitious painful stimuli enhances the experience of the newborn, particularly in their response to the next blood draw (Bergomi, Chieppi, Maini, et al., 2014).

BOX 26-6 MANIFESTATIONS OF ACUTE PAIN IN THE NEWBORN

Physiological Responses

Vital signs—Observe for variations.
- Increased heart rate
- Increased blood pressure
- Rapid, shallow respirations

Oxygenation
- Decreased transcutaneous oxygen saturation ($tcPo_2$)
- Decreased arterial oxygen saturation (Sao_2)

Skin—Observe colour and character.
- Pallor or flushing
- Diaphoresis
- Palmar sweating

Laboratory evidence of metabolic or endocrine changes
- Hyperglycemia
- Lowered pH
- Elevated corticosteroids

Other observations:
- Increased muscle tone
- Dilated pupils
- Decreased vagal nerve tone
- Increased intracranial pressure

Behavioural Responses

Vocalizations—Observe quality, timing, and duration.
- Crying
- Whimpering
- Groaning

Facial expression—Observe characteristics, timing, orientation of eyes and mouth.
- Grimaces
- Brow furrowed
- Chin quivering
- Eyes tightly closed
- Mouth open and squarish

Body movements and posture—Observe type, quality, and amount of movement or lack of movement; relationship to other factors.
- Limb withdrawal
- Thrashing
- Rigidity
- Flaccidity
- Fist clenching

Changes in state—Observe sleep, appetite, activity level.
- Changes in sleep–wake cycles
- Changes in feeding behaviour
- Changes in activity level
- Fussiness, irritability
- Listlessness

Modified from Blackburn, S. (2013). *Maternal, fetal, and neonatal physiology: a clinical perspective* (4th ed.). St Louis: Mosby; Gardner, S. L., Enzman-Hines, M., & Dickey, L. A. (2011). Pain and pain relief. In S. L. Gardner, B. S. Carter, M. Enzman-Hines M, et al. (Eds.), *Merenstein & Gardner's handbook of neonatal intensive care* (7th ed.). St. Louis: Mosby.

TABLE 26-4 CRIES NEONATAL POSTOPERATIVE PAIN SCALE*

	0	1	2
Crying	No	High pitched	Inconsolable
Requires oxygen for saturation >95%	No	<30%	>30%
Increased vital signs	Heart rate and blood pressure equal to or less than preoperative state	Heart rate and blood pressure <20% of preoperative state	Heart rate and blood pressure >20% of preoperative state
Expression	None	Grimace	Grimace and grunt
Sleepless	No	Wakes at frequent intervals	Constantly awake

Coding Tips for Using CRIES

Crying
- The characteristic cry of pain is high pitched.
- If no cry or cry that is not high pitched, score 0.
- If cry is high pitched but infant is easily consoled, score 1.
- If cry is high pitched and infant is inconsolable, score 2.

Requires oxygen for saturation >95%
Look for changes in oxygenation. Infants experiencing pain manifest decreases in oxygenation as measured by total carbon dioxide or oxygen saturation. (Consider other causes of changes in oxygenation, such as atelectasis, pneumothorax, oversedation.)
If no oxygen is required, score 0.
If <30% oxygen is required, score 1.
If >30% oxygen is required, score 2.

Increased vital signs
Note: Measure blood pressure last because this may wake the infant, causing difficulty with other assessments. Use baseline preoperative parameters from a nonstressed period.
Multiply baseline heart rate (HR) × 0.2; then add this to baseline HR to determine the HR that is 20% over baseline. Do likewise for blood pressure (BP). Use mean BP.
If HR and BP are both unchanged or less than baseline, score 0.
If HR or BP is increased but increase is <20% of baseline, score 1.
If either one is increased >20% over baseline, score 2.

Expression
The facial expression most often associated with pain is a grimace.
This may be characterized by brow lowering, eyes squeezed shut, deepening of the nasolabial furrow, open lips and mouth.
If no grimace is present, score 0.
If grimace alone is present, score 1.
If grimace and noncry vocalization grunt is present, score 2.

Sleepless
This is scored based on the infant's state during the hour preceding this recorded score.
If the child has been continuously asleep, score 0.
If he or she has awakened at frequent intervals, score 1.
If he or she has been awake constantly, score 2.

*Neonatal pain assessment tool developed at the University of Missouri–Columbia.

From Krechel, S. W., & Bildner, J. (1995). CRIES: A new neonatal postoperative pain measurement score. Initial testing of validity and reliability. *Paediatric Anaesthesia, 5*(1), 53–61. Copyright © 1995, John Wiley and Sons.

Non-nutritive sucking on a pacifier is a common comfort measure used with newborns. Oral sucrose in small amounts given with a syringe with or without a pacifier for sucking is safe and effective in reducing neonatal pain during single events (Bueno, Yamada, Harrison, et al., 2013; Cignacco, Sellam, Stoffel, et al., 2012; Kassab, Roydhouse, Fowler, et al., 2012; Riddell, Racine, Turcotte, et al., 2011). Oral sucrose and non-nutritive sucking given a few minutes before a painful procedure may help reduce the discomfort (Liaw, Zeng, Yang, et al., 2011).

Skin-to-skin contact with the mother, also known as *kangaroo care,* during a painful procedure can help reduce pain (Chermont, Falcão, de Sousa Silva, et al., 2009; Harrison et al., 2015; Riddell et al., 2011). Breastfeeding helps reduce pain during heel lancing and blood collection (Cong, Ludington-Hoe, Vazquez, et al., 2013; Leite, Linhares, Lander, et al., 2009; Weissman, Aranovitch, Blazer, et al., 2009). Many health care providers have integrated breastfeeding into their routine when taking blood work from the baby as an effective and readily available method of decreasing pain. Other nonpharmacological measures for reducing pain in newborns include touch, massage, rocking, holding, and environmental modification (e.g., low noise and lighting). Combining these nonpharmacological methods results in more effective pain reduction. Distraction with visual, oral, auditory, or tactile stimulation can be helpful in managing pain in term newborns or older infants (see Research Focus).

Pharmacological management. Pharmacological agents are used to alleviate pain in newborns associated with procedures. Local anaesthesia is routinely used during procedures such as circumcision and chest tube insertion. Topical anaesthesia is

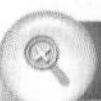

RESEARCH FOCUS

Nonpharmacological Pain Relief for Newborns

—Pat Mahaffee Gingrich and Lisa Keenan-Lindsay

Ask the Question

For term newborns, what complementary or alternative pain relief is effective for minor painful procedures, such as heel stick?

Search for the Evidence

Search Strategies

English-language research-based publications on newborn, pain, breastfeeding, heel stick, and sucrose were included.

Databases Used

Cochrane Collaborative Database, National Guidelines Clearinghouse (AHRQ), CINAHL, PubMed, and UpToDate

Critically Analyze the Evidence

- Pain scores in newborns assess physical changes to determine pain levels. Term newborns have lower pain scores during minor painful procedures when they use sucking-related interventions and are held and rocked. Preterm newborns 30 to 36 weeks of gestation benefit from kangaroo care (being carried bundled skin-to-skin upright on the caregiver's chest), sucking-related interventions, and swaddling (Riddell, Racine, Turcotte, et al., 2011).
- Breastfeeding is the first choice for single painful procedures, for the multisensorial and synergistic comfort it brings. It also provides the parents a caregiving role (Academy of Breastfeeding Medicine [ABM] Protocol Committee, 2010).
- Skin-to-skin contact, along with 24% sucrose or 25 to 50% glucose administered via pacifier, dropper, syringe, or finger, provides significant pain relief (ABM Protocol Committee, 2010; Johnston, Campbell-Yeo, Fernandes, et al., 2014; Kassab, Roydhouse, Fowler, et al., 2012).
- Preterm babies are at risk for more painful procedures. If breastfeeding is not possible, sucking-related interventions with sucrose decrease pain scores. However, there is concern that prolonged sucrose exposures in premature infants may lead to delays in motor skills and attention scores (ABM Protocol Committee, 2010).
- Infants in a Canadian neonatal intensive care unit whose mothers were present during a painful procedures were more likely to receive effective pain management strategies than those infants whose mothers were not present, indicating that parents may have a positive influence on pain management in their children (Johnson, Barrington, Taddio, et al., 2011).
- For term infants, sensory saturation uses multiple senses to diminish minor pain. A protocol of simultaneously massaging the infant's face, speaking to the infant, and instilling a sweet solution into the infant's mouth is more effective for relieving pain than the sweet solution alone (Bellieni, Tei, Coccina, et al., 2012).

Apply the Evidence: Nursing Implications

- Nonpharmacological pain relief methods for newborns are based on the gate-control theory to distract the newborn's attention, by using strong single or multisensorial stimulation. Warmth, touch, auditory and visual attention, and sucking a sweet solution decrease pain scores.
- Sensory saturation can be easily accomplished in the nursery. Parents who are taught this technique become active participants in their newborn's procedural care. However, they need clear education that using sucrose is not an appropriate long-term strategy for use at home.
- Parents need to be educated and involved in pain management strategies for their newborns (Johnston et al., 2011).
- Although skin-to-skin contact, breastfeeding, and human milk are not well researched as pain relief interventions for preterm newborns, the ABM (2010) recommends that parents be allowed to try these measures.
- Comfort measures usually work best when initiated a few minutes before the procedure to allow the newborn time to relax and reorganize (Kassab et al., 2012).
- Procedures other than single heel sticks or needlestick should be evaluated for pharmacological analgesia. Sucrose is not sufficient pain relief for circumcisions.

References

Academy of Breastfeeding Medicine (ABM) Protocol Committee. (2010). Clinical protocol #23: Non-pharmacologic management of procedure-related pain in the breastfeeding infant. *Breastfeeding Medicine, 5*(6), 315–319.

Bellieni, C. V., Tei, M., Coccina, F., et al. (2012). Sensorial saturation for infants' pain. *Journal of Maternal-Fetal & Neonatal Medicine, 25*(Suppl. 1), 79–81.

Johnston, C., Barrington, K. J., Taddio, A., et al. (2011). Pain in Canadian NICUs: have we improved over the past 12 years? *The Clinical Journal of Pain, 27*(3), 225–232.

Johnston, C., Campbell-Yeo, M., Fernandes, A., et al. (2014). Skin-to-skin care for procedural pain in neonates. *The Cochrane Database of Systematic Reviews,* (1), CD008435.

Kassab, M. I., Roydhouse, J. K., Fowler, C., et al. (2012). The effectiveness of glucose in reducing needle-related procedural pain in infants. *Journal of Pediatric Nursing, 27*(1), 3–17.

Riddell, R. P., Racine, N. M., Turcotte, K., et al. (2011). Non-pharmacological management of infant and young child procedural pain. *Cochrane Database Systematic Review,* (10). doi:10.1002/14651858.CD006275.pub2.

used for circumcision, lumbar puncture, venipuncture, and heel sticks. Nonopioid analgesia (oral liquid acetaminophen) is effective for mild to moderate pain from inflammatory conditions. Morphine and fentanyl are the most widely used opioid analgesics for pharmacological management of newborns' pain. Continuous or bolus IV infusion of opioids provides effective and safe pain control. Other methods for managing newborns' pain are epidural infusion, local and regional nerve blocks, and intradermal or topical anaesthetics (Gardner et al., 2011).

Promoting Parent–Infant Interaction

Nurses play an important role in promoting early social interaction between parents and their newborn infant. From birth throughout the hospital stay, nurses assess attachment behaviours (see Chapter 23) and provide support and education to parents as they become acquainted with the newborn. Nurses working in outpatient settings or home care provide follow-up assessments and care related to parent–child interactions. By teaching parents to recognize infant cues and respond appropriately, the nurse facilitates development of the parents' confidence in meeting the needs of their newborn (see Family-Centred Teaching box).

The sensitivity of the parent to social responses of the infant is basic to development of a mutually satisfying parent–child relationship (van der Voort, Juffer, Bakermans-Kranenburg, 2014). Sensitivity increases over time as parents become more aware of their infant's social capabilities. In supporting parents, nurses need to consider cultural beliefs and traditions that influence parenting behaviours and infant care practices (see Cultural Awareness box).

FAMILY-CENTRED TEACHING

Helping Parents Recognize, Interpret, and Respond to Newborn Behaviours

Learning to read a baby's body language can enable parents to be more effective in preventing and solving problems around the infant's sleeping, eating, and crying and enhances parent–infant interaction. Nurses can teach new parents the following:

1. Identify three newborn "zones," traditionally referred to as newborn states.
   "Resting zone": also known as sleep states
   - Still/deep sleep: Baby is completely still. Breathing is regular. No spontaneous activity. No movement of eyes, and eyelids stay shut. No vocalizing. Muscles are totally relaxed.
   - Active/light sleep: Baby may wiggle or vocalize. Eyes may flash open. Baby may make sucking movements—but still be asleep.

   "Ready zone": alert state
   - Baby's eyes are bright. Baby can focus on an object or person. Baby reacts to stimulation. Motor activity is minimal.

   "Rebooting zone": fussy/crying state
   - Baby's motor activity increases and is jerky. Baby is less responsive and moves from fussing to crying.
2. Identify signs of stress.
   When babies are stressed or overstimulated they show changes in their body and behaviour. These changes are called SOSs (Signs of Over-Stimulation), traditionally referred to as a baby's stress response.
   - Body SOSs: changes in colour (becoming more red or pale); changes in breathing (becoming more irregular or choppy); changes in movement (becoming jerky or having more tremors)
   - Behavioural SOSs: "spacing out" (going from an alert state to a drowsy state); "switching off" (gaze aversion, or looking away from parent); "shutting down" (going from drowsy to a sleep state)

   When baby shows an SOS, parents should decrease stimulation and increase support by doing one or several of the following:
   - Quiet one's voice
   - Glance away from baby
   - Encourage baby to suck on a finger or mother's breast
   - Place baby skin-to-skin
3. Help baby sleep well.
   Distinguish active/light sleep from still/deep sleep.
   Parent's care:
   - Prepare baby to sleep: feed in quiet, dark room at night and active, light environment during day.
   - Get baby to sleep: put baby down for sleep while he or she is still awake.
   - Help baby stay asleep: don't pick up during active/light sleep.
   - After breastfeeding is well established, notice when sleeping baby moves into active/light sleep. Wait and see if baby will transition from active/light sleep back to deep/still sleep—and sleep a bit longer.
4. Help baby eat well.
   - Recognize early signs of hunger during the first few weeks: wiggling, making sucking movements, bringing hand to mouth.
   - Notice if a fragile baby "spaces out" or "shuts down" when trying to eat. Bring this baby skin-to-skin and decrease stimulation before resuming feeding.
   - If a parent needs to wake a fragile or small baby to eat, do so from active/light sleep, not from still/deep sleep.
5. Help crying baby: Consider what "TO DO."
   - T: Talk quietly to baby in sing-song voice.
   - O: Observe to see if baby takes self-calming actions: brings hand to his or her mouth, making sucking movements, or moves into the fencing reflex position.
   - DO: Bring baby's hands to his or her chest; encourage sucking; make gentle "shooshing" sounds; and/or bring baby skin to skin.
6. Play with baby so he or she can learn and grow.
   - Demonstrate baby's ability to look at a parent's face, watch a toy move, or turn to parent's voice.
   - Watch for an SOS during play. If an SOS occurs, decrease stimulation and increase support as described earlier in box.
   - Observe baby's developing process of interaction: first, getting quiet and still; second, turning toward parent; third, turning toward and looking at parent.
   - Reinforce benefits of sensitive, face-to-face parent interaction with baby.

Data from Tedder, J. L. (2008). Give them the HUG: An innovative approach to helping parents understand the language of their newborn. *Journal of Perinatal Education, 17*(2), 14–20; Tedder, J. L. (n.d.) *H.U.G.: Help-understanding-guidance for young families*. Retrieved from http://www.hugyourbaby.org.

The activities of daily care during the newborn period are the best times for infant and family interactions. While caring for their newborn, the mother and father or partner (or other family member) can talk to the infant, play baby games, caress and cuddle the baby, and perhaps use infant massage. Feeding is an optimal time for interaction because the infant is usually awake and alert, at least at the beginning of the feeding. Too much stimulation should be avoided after feeding and before a sleep period. In Fig. 26-20 a great-grandmother and infant are shown engaging in arousal, imitation of facial expression, and smiling. Older children's contact with a newborn is encouraged and should be supervised according to the developmental level of the child (Fig. 26-21). Parents often keep memento books that record the birth, the hospital stay, and their infant's progress.

Discharge Planning and Teaching

Providing infant care can cause much anxiety for the new parent. Support from nursing staff can be an important factor in determining whether new mothers seek and accept help in the future. The nurse should try to avoid covering all the content at one time because the parents can be overwhelmed by too much information and become anxious. However, because new mothers go home quickly from the hospital, it is difficult for nurses to teach all the content that is necessary. It is important to start teaching on admission to the hospital. Community health nurses may visit families after birth and provide teaching, but this is not a standard practice across the country.

To set priorities for teaching, the nurse should follow parental cues. Learning needs should be identified before beginning to teach. Normal growth and development and the changing needs of the infant (e.g., for personal interaction and stimulation, growth milestones, exercise, injury prevention, and social contacts), as well as the topics that follow, should be included during discharge planning with parents. Safety issues should also be addressed (see Home Care box).

CULTURAL AWARENESS

Cultural Beliefs and Practices Regarding Newborns

Nurses working with child-bearing families from cultures and ethnic groups other than their own must be aware of cultural beliefs and practices that are important to individual families. People with a strong sense of heritage may hold on to traditional health beliefs long after adopting other Canadian lifestyle practices. These health beliefs may involve practices regarding the newborn. For example, some Asians, Latin Americans, and Eastern Europeans delay breastfeeding because they believe that colostrum is "bad." Some Latin Americans and Africans place a belly band over the infant's navel. The birth of a male child is generally preferred by Asians and Indians, and some Asians and Haitians delay naming their infant. East Indians may want to put something sweet on the newborn's lips right after birth.

Temperature

Parents need to understand practical information related to thermoregulation. The nurse should discuss the following topics in parent teaching:

- The causes of elevation in body temperature (e.g., overwrapping, cold stress with resultant vasoconstriction, or response to infection) and the body's response to extremes in environmental temperature
- Ways to promote normal body temperature, such as dressing the infant appropriately for the environmental air temperature and protecting the infant from exposure to direct sunlight, and how to assess whether the infant is hot or cold by feeling the back of the neck
- Use of warm wraps or extra blankets in cold weather
- Technique for taking the newborn's axillary temperature, and normal values for axillary temperature
- Signs to be reported to the primary health care provider, such as high or low temperatures with accompanying fussiness, lethargy, irritability, poor feeding, and excessive crying

Respirations

The nurse can provide information to parents regarding the normal characteristics of newborn respirations, emergency

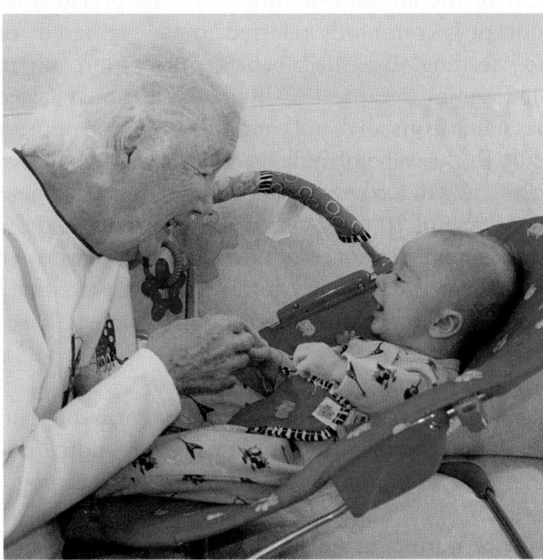

FIGURE 26-20 Great-grandmother and infant enjoying social interaction. (Courtesy Freida Belding.)

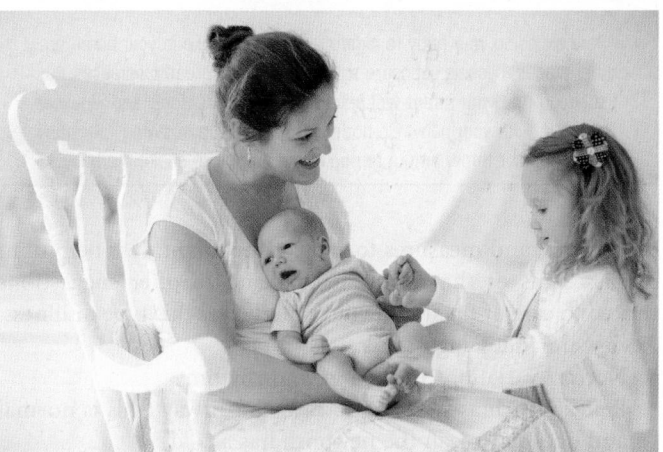

FIGURE 26-21 Mother supervising contact of older sibling with newborn. (FamVeld/Shutterstock.com.)

HOME CARE

Infant Safety

- Never leave your baby alone on a bed, couch, or table. Even newborns can move enough to eventually reach the edge and fall off.
- Never put your baby on a cushion, pillow, beanbag, or waterbed to sleep. Your baby may suffocate. Also, do not keep pillows, large floppy toys, or loose plastic sheeting in the crib.
- Always lay the baby flat in bed on his or her back for sleep. Do not place your infant on the abdomen or side for sleep.
- When using an infant carrier, place the carrier on the floor in a place where you can see the baby. It should never be on a high place, such as a table, couch, or store counter.
- Infant carriers do not keep your baby safe in a car. Always place your baby in an approved car safety seat when travelling in a motor vehicle (car, truck, bus, or van). Car safety seats are recommended for travel on trains and airplanes as well. Use the car safety seat for *every* ride. Your baby should be in a rear-facing infant car safety seat from birth until at minimum 1 year or until exceeding the car seat's limits for height and weight. Do not be in a rush to turn the car safety seat to the forward-facing position. The car safety seat should be in the back seat of the car (see Fig. 26-23). This precaution is especially important in vehicles with front passenger air bags because when air bags inflate, they can be fatal for infants and toddlers. If an infant must ride in the front seat, disable the air bag.
- When bathing your baby, never leave him or her alone. Newborns and infants can drown in 2 to 5 cm of water.
- Be sure that your hot water heater is set at 49°C (120°F) or less. Always check bath-water temperature with your elbow before putting your baby in the bath.
- Do not tie anything around your baby's neck. Pacifiers, for example, tied around the neck with a ribbon or string can strangle your baby.
- Check your baby's crib for safety. Slats should be no more than 5.7 cm apart. The space between the mattress and sides should be less than two fingerwidths. The bedposts should have no decorative knobs.
- There should be no bumper pads, blankets, stuffed toys, or other items in the baby's crib because of the risk for suffocation.
- Keep the crib or playpen away from window blind and drapery cords; your baby could strangle on them.
- Keep the crib and playpen well away from radiators, heat vents, and portable heaters. Linens in the crib or playpen can catch fire if they come into contact with these heat sources.
- Install smoke detectors on every floor of your home. Check them once a month to be sure they are working properly. Change batteries twice a year.
- Avoid exposing your baby to cigarette or cigar smoke in your home or other places. Passive exposure to tobacco smoke greatly increases the likelihood that your infant will have respiratory symptoms and illnesses.
- Be gentle with your baby. Do not pick your baby up or swing your baby by the arms or throw him or her up in the air. Never shake the baby.

procedures, and measures to protect the infant. It is helpful to discuss signs of the common cold and to offer suggestions related to care of the infant who experiences this type of illness. Review the following points:

- Normal variations in the rate and rhythm
- Reflexes such as sneezing to clear the airway (this is normal and does not mean the newborn has a cold)
- Steps to take if the infant appears to be choking
- The need to protect the infant from the following:
  - Exposure to people with upper respiratory tract infections and respiratory syncytial virus
  - Exposure to second-hand and third-hand tobacco smoke
  - Suffocation from loose bedding, water beds, and beanbag chairs; drowning (in bath water); entrapment under excessive bedding or in soft bedding; anything tied around the infant's neck; blind cords near cribs; poorly constructed playpens, bassinets, or cribs
- Sleep position—on back when put to sleep
- Avoid the use of baby powder, which is a commonly aspirated substance. Whenever a powder is used, it should be placed in the caregiver's hand and then applied to the skin. It is kept away from the infant's face.
- Notify the health care provider if the infant develops symptoms such as difficulty breathing or swallowing, nasal congestion, excess drainage of mucus, coughing, sneezing, decreased interest in feeding, or fever.
- If the infant has a respiratory illness such as the "common cold," the following suggestions can be helpful:
  - Feed smaller amounts more often to prevent overtiring the infant.
  - Hold the baby in an upright position to feed.
  - For sleeping, raise the infant's head and chest by raising the mattress 30 degrees. (Do not use a pillow.)
  - Avoid drafts; do not overdress the baby.
  - Use only medications prescribed by a physician. Do not use over-the-counter medications without health care provider approval.
  - Use nasal saline drops in each nostril and suction well with bulb syringe to decrease and relieve secretions.

Feeding Patterns

Nurses instruct parents about infant feeding and provide assistance based on whether they have chosen breastfeeding or formula feeding. The infant should be put to breast ideally within the first hour after birth. Newborns should be allowed to feed when they awaken and demonstrate typical hunger cues, regardless of the amount of time since the previous feeding. This concept is commonly referred to as "cue-based" or "on-demand" feeding. Breastfed babies nurse more often than bottle-fed babies because breast milk is digested faster than formulas made from cow's milk and the stomach empties sooner as a result. Exclusively formula feeding newborns will typically awaken and cue to feed every 3 to 4 hours. Breastfed newborns feed an average of 10 to 12 times per day. Water and dextrose water supplements are not recommended in the newborn period since these have the tendency to decrease breastfeeding. For a thorough discussion of infant feeding, see Chapter 27.

Elimination

Awareness of the normal elimination patterns of newborns helps parents recognize problems related to voiding or stooling. The following points are included in teaching about elimination:

- Colour of normal urine and number of voidings to expect each day; one wet diaper for each day of life until fifth to sixth day; then 6 to 10 per day (see Fig. 27-9)

- Changes to be expected in the colour of the stool (i.e., meconium to transitional to soft yellow or golden yellow) and the number of bowel evacuations, plus the odour of stools for breastfed or formula-fed infants (see Box 25-1 and Fig. 25-5)
- Formula-fed infants may have as few as one stool every other day after the first few weeks of life; stools are pasty to semiformed.
- Breastfed infants should have at least three stools every 24 hours for the first few weeks. The stools are looser and resemble mustard mixed with cottage cheese.

Prevention of Sudden Infant Death Syndrome (SIDS)

By definition, sudden infant death syndrome (SIDS) is the sudden death of an infant under the age of 1 year. Current evidence explains SIDS as a disorder arising from a combination of environmental, genetic, and metabolic factors (PHAC et al., 2012). The rate of SIDS in Canada is 1 in every 3000 babies; the rate is higher among Indigenous infants (PHAC et al., 2012). The PHAC guideline recommends placing the infant to sleep in the supine position to prevent SIDS. The prone position has been associated with an increased incidence of SIDS (see Critical Thinking Case Study). Other recommendations for preventing SIDS include ensuring a smoke-free environment (before and after birth), providing a safe crib environment (no toys or loose bedding), room sharing for 6 months, avoiding instances of the infant being overheated, and no sleeping in waterbeds or on sofas (PHAC et al., 2012). Breastfeeding and pacifier use may also decrease the rate of SIDS (Leduc, Côté, Woods, et al., 2004/2014). In addition, co-bedding practices may contribute to unintentional suffocation caused by entrapment or overlaying, often occurring when the infant is sharing a sleep surface with an adult or another child (PHAC et al., 2012).

Anatomically, the infant's shape—a barrel chest and flat, curve-less spine—makes it easy for the infant to roll from the side to the prone position; thus, the side-lying position for sleep is not recommended. When the infant is awake, "tummy time" can be provided under parental supervision so that the infant may begin to develop appropriate muscle tone for eventual crawling; this tummy time is also effective in the prevention of a misshaped head (positional **plagiocephaly**). Newborns should be placed on their stomach several times per day for increasing lengths of time but always when they are awake and supervised by an adult (Cummings & CPS, 2011/2014).

Care must also be taken to prevent the infant from rolling off flat, unguarded surfaces. When an infant is on such a surface, the parent or nurse who must turn away from the infant even for a moment should always keep one hand placed securely on the infant. The infant should always be held securely with his or her head supported because newborns are unable to maintain an erect head posture for more than a few moments. Fig. 26-22 illustrates holding an infant with adequate support.

Rashes

Diaper rash. Most infants develop a diaper rash at some time. This dermatitis or skin inflammation appears as redness, scaling, blisters, or papules. Various factors contribute to diaper rash, including infrequent diaper changes, diarrhea, use of plastic pants to cover the diaper, or a change in the infant's diet, such as when solid foods are added.

Parents are instructed in measures to help prevent and treat diaper rash. Diapers should be checked often and changed as soon as the infant voids or stools. Plain water with mild soap is used to cleanse the diaper area; if baby wipes are used, they should be unscented and contain no alcohol. The infant's skin should be allowed to dry completely before applying another diaper. Because bacteria thrive in moist, dark areas, exposing the skin to dry air decreases bacterial proliferation. Zinc oxide

CRITICAL THINKING CASE STUDY

Late Preterm Infant, Sudden Infant Death Syndrome, and Infant Sleep Position

Mary gave birth to a 35-week, 2250-g female infant whom she named Delilah. This is her third baby; the other children are 18 and 20 years old. Mary and Delilah are being discharged today.

The nurse has given her instructions about placing Delilah on her back for sleep. Mary says that she remembers her other two children slept best when they were on their "tummies" for sleep. When Mary was in college, she worked as a unit secretary in a newborn nursery and she recalls that when babies were on their backs, they tended to "spit up" and turn blue. Recently, her sister had a baby who had to be under bilirubin lights and the nurses turned the baby on her abdomen sometimes for sleep. Mary voices concerns to the nurse about putting Delilah down to sleep on her back at home. How should the nurse respond to Mary's concerns?

QUESTIONS

1. Evidence—Is there sufficient evidence to draw conclusions about the safety and efficacy of the supine position for sleep for the late preterm infant in reducing the incidence of sudden infant death syndrome (SIDS)?
2. Assumptions—What assumptions can be made about the following factors related to infant positioning?
   a. Risk for aspiration
   b. Sleep position in the hospital versus sleep position at home
   c. Sleep position for late preterm versus term infants
3. What implications and priorities for nursing care can be drawn at this time?
4. Does the evidence objectively support your conclusion?

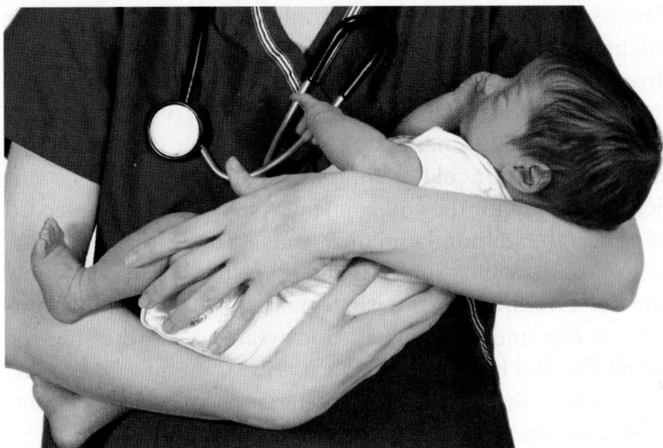

FIGURE 26-22 Holding baby securely with support for the head. (Duplass/Shutterstock.com.)

ointments can be used to protect the infant's skin from moisture and further excoriation if a rash develops.

Although diaper rash can be alarming to parents and annoying to babies, most cases resolve within a few days with simple home treatments. There are instances when diaper rash is more serious and requires medical treatment.

The warm, moist atmosphere in the diaper area provides an optimal environment for *Candida albicans* growth; dermatitis appears in the perianal area, inguinal folds, and lower abdomen. The affected area is intensely erythematous with a sharply demarcated, scalloped edge, often with numerous satellite lesions that extend beyond the larger lesion. The usual source of infection is from handling by persons who do not practise adequate hand hygiene. It may also appear 2 to 3 days after an oral infection (thrush). Therapy consists of applications of an anticandidal ointment, such as clotrimazole or miconazole, with each diaper change. Sometimes the infant also is given an oral antifungal preparation such as nystatin or fluconazole to eliminate any gastrointestinal source of infection.

Other rashes. A rash on the cheeks may result from the infant's scratching with long unclipped fingernails or from rubbing the face against the crib sheets, particularly if regurgitated stomach contents are not washed off promptly. The newborn's skin begins a natural process of peeling and sloughing after birth. Dry skin may be treated with a neutral-pH lotion, but this should be used sparingly. Newborn rash, erythema toxicum, is a common finding and needs no treatment.

Clothing

Parents commonly ask how warmly they should dress their infant. A simple rule of thumb is to dress the child as they would dress themselves, adding or subtracting clothes and wraps for the child as necessary. Feeling the temperature of the skin at the back of the infant's neck is often an indicator of whether the child is too hot or cold. A cotton shirt and diaper may be sufficient clothing for the young infant. A hat or bonnet is needed to protect the scalp and minimize heat loss if the weather is cool, or to protect against sunburn and shade the eyes if it is sunny and hot. Overdressing in warm temperatures can cause discomfort, as can underdressing in cold weather. Overdressing the infant has also been associated with SIDS. Parents are encouraged to dress the infant in flame-retardant clothing. Infant sunglasses are available to protect the eyes when outdoors.

Safety: Use of Car Seat

Infants should travel only in federally approved, rear-facing safety seats secured in the rear seat (Fig. 26-23). The safest area of the car is in the middle of the back seat. A car seat that faces the rear gives the best protection for the infant's disproportionately weak neck and heavy head. In this position, the force of a frontal crash is spread over the head, neck, and back; the back of the car seat supports the spine. Car seats have expiration dates on them as well as Canadian Standards Association stickers, and parents need to ensure the car seat they are using is safe. A car seat that has been in a previous car accident should not be used. See Additional Resources for more information on car seat installation.

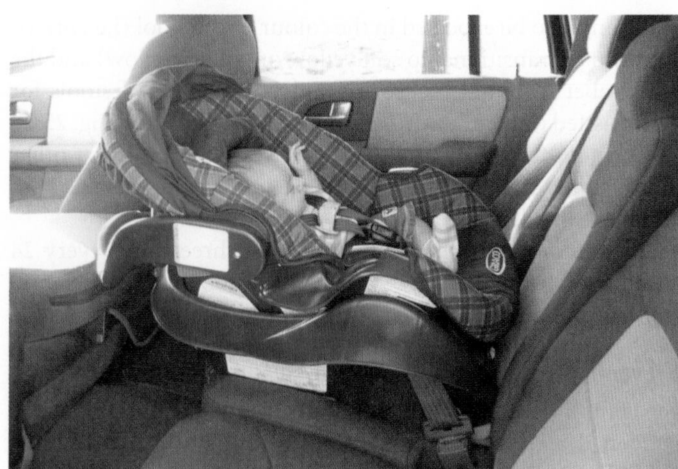

FIGURE 26-23 Rear-facing infant seat in rear seat of car. Infant is placed in seat when going home from the hospital. (Courtesy Brian and Mayannyn Sallee.)

> **! NURSING ALERT**
>
> Infants should use a rear-facing car seat from birth to 10 kg (22 lb), and the child must be able to walk unassisted. If the child meets these criteria and is under 1 year of age, they should remain in a rear-facing car seat. It is advisable to keep a child in a rear-facing car seat even after these criteria have been met.

To secure the infant in the rear-facing car safety seat, shoulder harnesses are placed in the slots at or below the level of the infant's shoulders. The harness is snug, and the retainer clip is placed at the level of the infant's armpits as opposed to on the abdomen or neck area. The car seat is secured by using the vehicle seat belts.

> **NURSING ALERT**
>
> In cars equipped with air bags, rear-facing infant seats should not be placed in the front seat unless the air bag has been deactivated. Serious injury can occur if the air bag inflates because these types of infant seats fit closer to the dashboard than a passenger does.

Non-Nutritive Sucking

Sucking is the infant's chief pleasure. However, sucking needs may not be satisfied by breastfeeding or bottle-feeding alone. In fact, sucking is such a strong need that infants who are deprived of sucking, such as those with a cleft lip, will suck on their tongues. Some newborns are born with sucking pads on their fingers or lips that developed during in utero sucking. Several benefits of non-nutritive sucking have been demonstrated, such as an increased weight gain in preterm infants, greater ability to maintain an organized state, and less crying.

Problems arise when parents are concerned about the sucking of fingers, thumbs, or pacifiers and try to restrain this natural tendency. Before giving advice, nurses should investigate the parents' feelings and base the guidance they give on the information solicited. For example, some parents may see no problem with the use of a finger but may find the use of a pacifier objectionable. In general, there is no need to restrain either practice, unless thumb sucking persists past 4 years of age or past the time when the permanent teeth erupt. Parents are advised to consult with their health care provider on this topic.

There is compelling evidence that pacifiers help prevent SIDS. It is suggested that parents consider offering a pacifier for naps and bedtime (AAP Task Force on Sudden Death Syndrome, 2011; Ponti & CPS, 2003/2014). The pacifier should be used when the infant is placed supine for sleep, and it should not be reinserted once the infant falls asleep. No infant should be forced to take a pacifier. Pacifiers should be cleaned often and replaced regularly and should not be coated with any type of sweet solution. Pacifier use for breastfeeding infants should be delayed for 3 to 4 weeks to ensure that breastfeeding is well established.

A parent's excessive use of the pacifier to calm the child should also be explored, however. It is not unusual for parents to place a pacifier in the infant's mouth as soon as he or she begins to cry, thus reinforcing a pattern of distress-relief.

If parents choose to let their child use a pacifier, they need to be aware of certain safety considerations before purchasing one. Homemade, improvised, or poorly designed pacifiers can be dangerous because the entire object may be aspirated if it is small, or a portion may become lodged in the pharynx. Safe pacifiers are made of one piece that includes a shield or flange large enough to prevent entry into the mouth and a handle that can be grasped (Fig. 26-24).

Bathing and Umbilical Cord Care

Bathing. Bathing serves a number of purposes. It provides opportunities for (1) completely cleansing the infant, (2) observing the infant's condition, (3) promoting comfort, and (4) parent–child–family interaction.

An important consideration in skin cleansing is preservation of the skin's acid mantle, which is formed from the uppermost horny layer of the epidermis, sweat, superficial fat, metabolic products, and external substances such as amniotic fluid and microorganisms. To protect the newborn's skin, a cleanser with a neutral pH should be used.

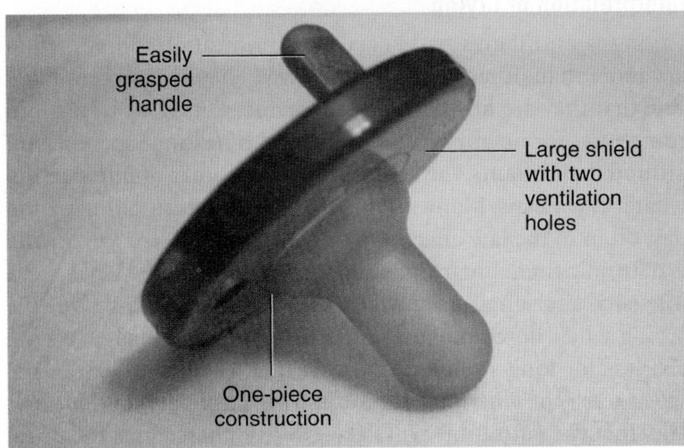

FIGURE 26-24 Design of a safe pacifier. (Courtesy Julie Perry Nelson.)

Although the sponging technique may be used, bathing the newborn by immersion results in less heat loss and less crying and is thus recommended even with the umbilical cord still intact. It is recommended that the water is deep enough to cover the newborn's shoulders to ease discomfort from being cold (Association of Women's Health, Obstetrical and Neonatal Nurses [AWHONN], 2013). Immersion bathing is considered a safe alternative to sponge bathing provided the infant's condition is stable (no temperature instability or respiratory or cardiac illness) and he or she is dried off immediately afterward and kept warm (AWHONN, 2013). A daily bath is not necessary for achieving cleanliness and may do more harm by disrupting the integrity of the newborn's skin; cleansing the perineum after a soiled diaper and daily cleansing of the face may suffice. Until the initial bath is completed, hospital personnel must wear gloves to handle the newborn.

The infant bath time provides a wonderful opportunity for parent–infant social interaction. While bathing the baby, parents can talk to the infant, caress and cuddle the infant, and engage in arousal and imitation of facial expressions and smiling. Parents can pick a time for the bath that is easy for them and when the baby is awake, usually before a feeding.

Umbilical cord care. The goal of care is to prevent or decrease the risk for hemorrhage or infection. The umbilical cord stump is an excellent medium for bacterial growth and can become infected. Hospital protocol determines the technique for routine cord care. The current recommendations for cord care by the Association of Women's Health, Obstetric and Neonatal Nurses (AWHONN, 2013) include cleaning the cord with water (and cleanser if needed to remove debris) during the initial bath and subsequently cleaning with plain water if the umbilical stump is soiled with urine or stool. Evidence does not support the routine use of antiseptic or antimicrobial preparations for cord care (Lund & Durand, 2011).

The stump and base of the cord should be assessed for edema, erythema, and drainage with each diaper change. The area should be kept clean and dry and open to air or loosely covered with clothing. If soiled, the area is cleansed with plain water and dried with clean absorbent gauze. The diaper is folded down and away from the stump (AWHONN, 2013). The umbilical cord begins to dry, shrivel, and blacken by the second or third day of life. The stump deteriorates through the process of dry gangrene; thus, odour alone is not a positive indicator of *omphalitis* (infection of the umbilical stump).

The umbilicus should be inspected often for signs of infection (e.g., foul odour, redness, and purulent discharge), granuloma (i.e., small, red, raw-appearing polyp where the umbilical cord separates), bleeding, and discharge. The cord clamp may be removed when the cord is dry, in about 24 to 36 hours, although this is not routine practice in all hospitals (Fig. 26-25). Some institutions send the newborn home with the clamp still in place and it will fall off when the cord falls off. It is important to ensure that if a cord clamp remover is used, it is disinfected between uses.

Cord separation time is influenced by several factors, including type of cord care, type of birth, and other perinatal events. The average cord separation time is 10 to 14 days, although it can take up to 3 weeks for this to occur. Some dried blood may

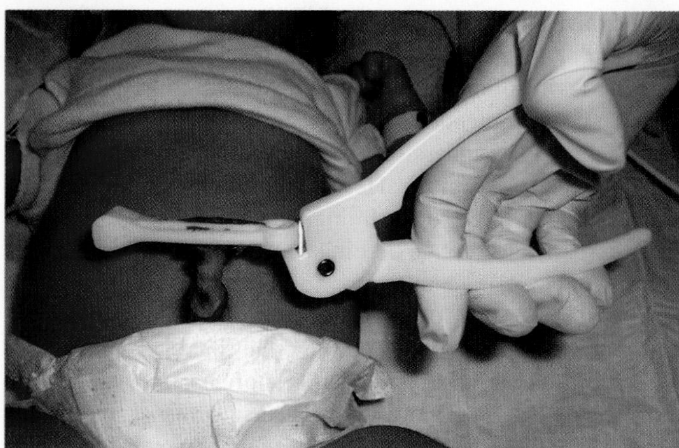

FIGURE 26-25 Using special scissors, remove clamp after cord begins drying (about 24 hours). (Courtesy Cheryl Briggs, BSN, RNC-NIC.)

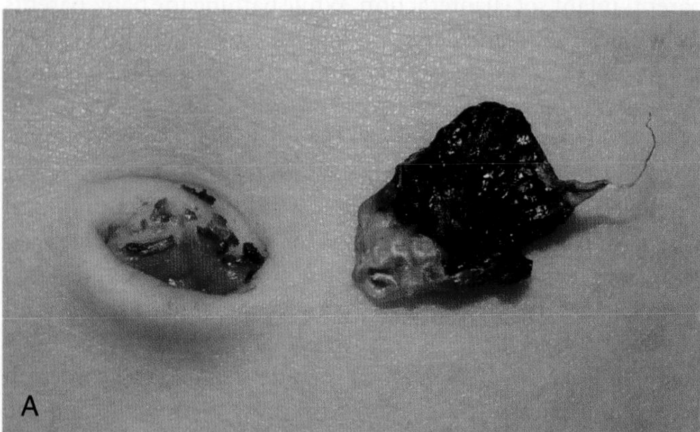

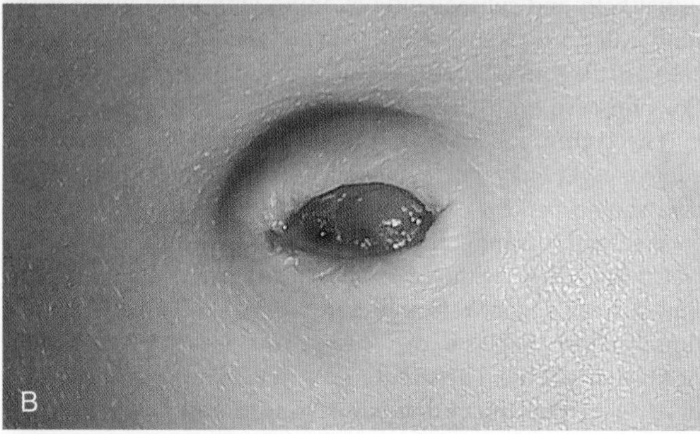

FIGURE 26-26 Cord separation. **A:** Cord separated with some dried blood still in the umbilicus. **B:** Umbilicus cleansed and beginning to heal. (Courtesy Cheryl Briggs, BSN, RNC-NIC.)

be seen in the umbilicus at separation (Fig. 26-26). Parents should be instructed in appropriate home cord care and the expected time of cord separation.

See the Home Care box for information regarding tub and sponge bathing, skin care, cord care, trimming nails, and dressing the infant.

Infant Follow-Up Care

With shorter hospital stays, the focus and site of infant care are changing. Across the country varying methods of early follow-up health care visits have been implemented, including follow-up by a visiting nurse or community health team, and home visits by midwives and community health nurses to assess and support breastfeeding and wellness.

Parents should plan for their child's routine follow-up health care at the following ages: within 2 or 3 days to check for status of jaundice, feeding, and elimination; at 2 to 4 weeks of age; then every 2 months until 6 to 7 months of age; then every 3 months until 18 months; at 2 years; at 3 years; at preschool; and every 2 years thereafter.

Cardiopulmonary Resuscitation

All personnel working with infants must have current neonatal **resuscitation** (NRP). Parents should be encouraged to receive instruction in relieving airway obstruction and in CPR. Classes are often offered in hospitals and clinics during the prenatal period or to parents of newborns. Such instruction is especially important for parents whose infants were preterm or had cardiac or respiratory problems.

Practical Suggestions for the First Weeks at Home

Numerous changes occur during the first weeks of parenthood. Nursing care should be directed toward helping parents cope with infant care, role changes, altered lifestyle, and changes in family structure resulting from the addition of a new baby. Developing skill and confidence in caring for an infant can be especially challenging. The nurse's anticipatory guidance can help ease the transition home and decrease stress that might otherwise negate the parents' joy or cause them undue stress. For example, the nurse can teach parents several strategies that help quiet a fussy baby, prevent crying, and induce quiet attention or sleep. This is especially important for first-time parents. Even the simplest strategies can provide enormous support. Printed materials reinforcing education topics are helpful, as is a list of available community resources, both local and national, and websites that provide reliable information about child care. Classes in the prenatal period or during the postpartum stay are helpful. Instructions for the first days at home include relevant topics such as activities of daily living, dealing with visitors, and activity and rest.

Interpretation of Crying

Crying is an infant's first social communication. Some babies cry more than others, but all babies cry. They cry to communicate that they are hungry, uncomfortable, wet, ill, or bored and sometimes for no apparent reason at all. The longer parents are around their infants, the easier the task becomes of interpreting what a cry means. Many infants have a fussy period during the day, often in the late afternoon or early evening when everyone is naturally tired. Environmental tension adds to the length and intensity of crying spells. Babies also have periods of vigorous crying when no comforting can help. These periods of crying can last for long stretches until the infants seem to cry themselves to sleep. The nurse should inform new parents that time and infant maturation will take care of these types of cries. Many hospitals distribute a DVD on infant crying to new parents. *The Period of PURPLE Crying* is an example (see

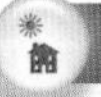

HOME CARE

Newborn Bath

Timing

- Newborns do not need a bath every day. Every 2 to 3 days is often enough.
- Fit bath time into the family's schedule.
- Give a bath at any time convenient to you but not immediately after a feeding period because the increased handling can cause regurgitation.

Prevent Heat Loss

- The temperature of the room should be no cooler than 24°C (75°F), and the bathing area should be free of drafts.
- Control heat loss during the bath to conserve the infant's energy. Bathing the infant quickly, exposing only what is being washed, and thoroughly drying the infant are all important parts of the bathing technique.

Gather Supplies and Clothing Before Starting

- Clothing suitable for wearing indoors: diaper, shirt; sleeper or nightgown optional
- Towels for drying infant and a clean washcloth
- Receiving blanket
- Tub or sink for water
- Unscented, mild soap; with a neutral pH
- Diaper

Bathe the Baby

- Bring infant to the bathing area when all supplies are ready.
- Never leave the infant alone on the bath table or in bath water, not even for a second! If you have to leave, take the infant with you or put the infant back into the crib.
- Fill the tub to try to cover as much of the infant's body as you feel comfortable. Infants like to have as much of their body under water as possible (preferably to cover shoulders).
- Test temperature of the water. It should feel pleasantly warm to the elbow 38.0° to 40.0°C (100° to 104°F).
- Do not hold infant under running water—water temperature may change, and the infant may be scalded or chilled rapidly.
- If sponge bathing is to be performed (usually only necessary if circumcision is healing), undress the baby and wrap in a towel with the head exposed. Uncover the parts of the body you are washing, taking care to keep the rest of the baby covered as much as possible to prevent heat loss.
- Always work from clean to dirty. Start with the face, neck, and ears first. Do not use soap on the face. Cleanse the eyes from the inner canthus outward, using separate parts of a clean washcloth for each eye. For the first 2 or 3 days, there may be a discharge resulting from the reaction of the conjunctiva to the ointment used as a prophylactic measure against infection. Any discharge should be considered abnormal and reported to the health care provider.
- Cleanse ears and nose with twists of moistened cotton or a corner of the washcloth. Do not use cotton-tipped swabs because they may cause injury.
- Creases under the chin and arms and in the groin may need daily cleansing. The crease under the chin may be exposed by elevating the infant's shoulders 5 cm and letting the head drop back.
- When washing the infant's hair, hold the baby in a football hold. Wash infant's hair before or after body to prevent heat loss from prolonged exposure to cold (scalp loses heat rapidly because of size). Wash the scalp with warm water and mild soap; dry thoroughly. Scalp desquamation, called *cradle cap*, often can be prevented by removing any scales with a fine-toothed comb or brush after washing. If the condition persists, notify the health care provider.
- Wash the body with mild soap (pH neutral); rinse and dry to decrease heat loss. Place your hand under the baby's shoulders and lift gently to expose the neck, lift the chin, and wash the neck, taking care to cleanse between the skin folds. Wash between the fingers and toes, and then rinse and dry thoroughly. Wash the genital area last. Pat dry gently.

Skin Care

- The skin of a newborn is sensitive and should be cleaned only with water between baths. Soap has drying properties, and its use is limited to bathing. Creams, lotions, ointments, or powders are not recommended. If the skin seems excessively dry during the first 2 to 3 weeks after birth, an unscented, non–alcohol-based lotion may be used; checking with the pediatric health care provider for suggestions on skin care products is best. Experts advise that baby clothes be laundered using a mild laundry detergent.
- The fragile skin can be injured by too vigorous cleansing. If stool or other debris has dried and caked on the skin, soak the area to remove it. Do not attempt to rub it off because abrasion may result. Gentleness, patting dry rather than rubbing, and using a mild soap without perfumes or colouring are recommended. Chemicals in the colouring and perfume can cause rashes on sensitive skin.
- Babies are very prone to sunburn and should be kept out of direct sunlight. Use of sunscreens should be discussed with the health care provider but are not recommended for the first 6 months of life.
- Babies often develop rashes that are normal. Neonatal acne resembles pimples and can appear at 2 to 4 weeks of age, resolving without treatment by 6 to 8 months. Heat rash is common in warm weather, which appears as a fine red rash around creases or folds where the baby sweats.

Cord Care

- Cleanse with plain water around base of the cord where it joins the skin. Notify the health care provider of any odour, discharge, or skin inflammation (redness) around the cord. The clamp may be removed when the cord is dry (approximately 24 to 48 hours after birth). The diaper should not cover the cord because a wet or soiled diaper will slow or prevent drying of the cord and foster infection. When the cord drops off after 10 to 14 days, a few small drops of blood may be seen. If there is active bleeding, notify the pediatric health care provider.

Nail Care

- Use caution cutting the nails—use blunt scissors, or a nail file. The nails have to grow out far enough from the skin so that the skin is not cut by mistake. Nails should be kept short so infants do not scratch themselves. Covering hands with mitts may frustrate infants who wants to suck on them, so it is better to keep nails short. The ideal time to trim the nails is when the infant is sleeping. Soft emery boards may be used to file the nails.

Continued

HOME CARE

Newborn Bath—cont'd

Genital Care

- Cleanse the infant's genitalia daily and after voiding or defecating.
- For girls, the genitalia may be cleansed by separating the labia slightly and gently washing from the pubic area to the anus.
- For uncircumcised boys, wash and rinse the penis with soap and warm water. Do not attempt to retract the foreskin. In most newborns, the inner layer of the foreskin adheres to the glans and the foreskin cannot be retracted. By age 3 years in 90% of boys, the foreskin can be retracted easily without causing pain or trauma. For others, the foreskin is not retractable until adolescence. As soon as the foreskin is partly retractable and the child is old enough, he can be taught self-care. Once healed, the circumcised penis does not require any special care other than cleansing with diaper changes.
- The infant's skin should be allowed to dry completely before applying another diaper. Exposing the buttocks to air can help dry up diaper rash. Zinc oxide ointments can be used to protect the infant's skin from moisture and further excoriation.

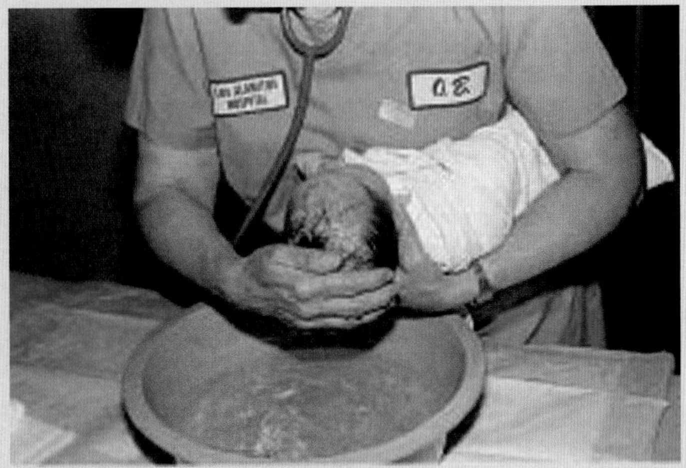

Wash hair with baby wrapped to prevent heat loss from wet scalp using the football hold. (Courtesy Marjorie Pyle, RNC, Lifecircle.)

FAMILY-CENTRED TEACHING

The Period of PURPLE Crying®

The Period of PURPLE Crying is a program to educate new parents about infant crying and the dangers of shaking a baby. Each letter in the acronym "PURPLE" represents key concepts:

P = Peak of crying. Your baby may cry more each week—the most at 2 months, then less at 3 to 5 months.
U = Unexpected. Crying can come and go and you don't know why.
R = Resists soothing. Your baby may not stop crying, no matter what you try.
P = Pain-like face. Crying babies may look like they are in pain, even when they are not.
L = Long lasting. Crying can last as much as 5 hours a day, or more.
E = Evening. Your baby may cry more in the later afternoon and evening.

From National Center on Shaken Baby Syndrome, PURPLEcrying.info.

Family-Centred Teaching box). It is intended to help parents understand that crying is normal and help them cope with infant crying. If parents have greater understanding of infant crying, they may be less likely to inflict harm such as occurs with "shaken-baby" syndrome.

Recognizing signs of illness

In addition to explaining the need for well-baby follow-up visits, the nurse should discuss with parents the signs of illness in newborns (see Patient Teaching box). Of particular importance is the parents' assessment of jaundice in newborns discharged early. Parents should be advised to call their pediatric care provider immediately if they notice increasing jaundice or signs of illness and to ask about over-the-counter medications, such as acetaminophen for infants, to keep at home.

PATIENT TEACHING

Signs of Illness

Notify the pediatric health care provider if any of these signs occur:

- Fever: temperature above 38°C (100.4°F) axillary; also a continual rise in temperature (**Note:** Tympanic [ear] thermometers are not recommended for infants younger than 3 months.)
- Hypothermia: temperature below 36.5°C (97.7°F) axillary and not able to increase temperature by putting on an extra layer of clothing or putting skin-to-skin
- Poor feeding or little interest in food: refusal to eat for two feedings in a row
- Vomiting: more than one episode of forceful vomiting or frequent vomiting (over a 6-hr period)
- Diarrhea: two consecutive green, watery stools (**Note:** Stools of breastfed infants are normally looser than stools of formula-fed infants. Diarrhea will leave a water ring around the stool, whereas breastfed stools will not.)
- Decreased bowel movement: in a breastfed infant, fewer than three stools per day; in a formula-fed infant, fewer than one stool every other day
- Decreased urination: fewer than six to eight wet diapers per day after 5 days of age
- Breathing difficulties: laboured breathing with flared nostrils or absence of breathing for more than 20 seconds (**Note:** A newborn's breathing is normally irregular and between 30 and 60 breaths/min. Count the breaths for a full minute but only if concerned.)
- Cyanosis (bluish skin colour) whether accompanying a feeding or not
- Lethargy: sleepiness, difficulty waking, or periods of sleep longer than 6 hours (most newborns sleep for short periods, usually from 1 to 4 hours, and wake to be fed)
- Inconsolable crying (attempts to quiet not effective) or continuous high-pitched cry
- Bleeding or purulent (yellowish) drainage from umbilical cord or circumcision; foul odour or redness at the site
- Drainage from the eyes

KEY POINTS

- Assessment of the newborn requires data from the prenatal, intrapartum, and postnatal periods.
- The immediate assessment of the newborn includes Apgar scoring and a general evaluation of physical status.
- Knowledge of biological and behavioural characteristics is essential for guiding assessment and interpreting data.
- Gestational-age assessment provides important information for predicting risks and guiding care management.
- Nursing care immediately after birth includes maintaining an open airway, preventing heat loss, and promoting parent–infant interaction.
- Providing a protective environment is a key responsibility of the nurse and includes such measures as careful identification procedures, support of physiological functions, and ways to prevent infection.
- The newborn has social and physical needs.
- Newborns require careful assessment for physiological and behavioural manifestations of pain.
- Nonpharmacological and pharmacological measures are used to reduce infant pain.
- Before hospital discharge, nurses provide anticipatory guidance for parents regarding feeding and elimination patterns; positioning and holding; comfort measures; car seat safety; bathing, skin care, cord care, and nail care; and signs of illness.

evolve WEBSITE

Visit the Evolve website for additional resources related to the content in this chapter such as Case Studies, Critical Thinking Case Study Answers, Nursing Care Plans, Nursing Processes, Nursing Skills, and Review Questions for Exam Preparation at: *http://evolve.elsevier.com/Canada/Perry/maternal/*

REFERENCES

American Academy of Pediatrics (AAP) Committee on Infectious Diseases. (2012). *Red book: 2012 report of the Committee on Infectious Diseases* (29th ed.). Elk Grove Village, IL: Author.

American Academy of Pediatrics (AAP) Task Force on Sudden Infant Death Syndrome. (2011). SIDS and other sleep-related infant deaths: Expansion of recommendations for a safe infant sleeping environment. *Pediatrics, 128*(5), e1341–e1367.

American College of Obstetricians and Gynecologists (ACOG) Committee on Obstetric Practice. (2006). Committee opinion no. 333: The Apgar score. *Obstetrics & Gynecology, 107*, 1209–1212. Reaffirmed 2010.

Araia, M. H., Wilson, B. J., Chakraborty, P., et al. (2012). Factors associated with knowledge of and satisfaction with newborn screening education: A survey of mothers. *Genetics in Medicine, 14*(12), 963–970.

Association of Women's Health, Obstetric and Neonatal Nurses (AWHONN). (2013). *Neonatal skin care: Evidence-based clinical practice guideline* (3rd ed.). Washington, DC: Author.

Aziz, K., Dancey, P., & Canadian Paediatric Society. (2004). Screening guidelines for newborns at risk for low blood glucose. *Paediatrics & Child Health, 9*(10), 723–729. Reaffirmed February 1, 2014.

Barrington, K. J., Batton, D. G., Finley, G. A., et al. (2007). Prevention and management of pain in the neonate: An update. A joint statement with the American Academy of Pediatrics. *Paediatrics & Child Health, 12*(2), 137–138. Reaffirmed 2015.

Barrington, K. J., Sankaran, K., & Canadian Paediatric Society. (2007). Guidelines for detection, management and prevention of hyperbilirubinemia in term and late term newborn infants [35 or more weeks gestation]. *Paediatrics & Child Health, 12*(Suppl. B), 1B–12B. Reaffirmed 2016.

Bates, E., Rouse, D., Chapman, V., et al. (2010). Fetal lung maturity testing before 39 weeks and neonatal outcomes. *Obstetrics & Gynecology, 116*(6), 1288–1295.

Bergomi, P., Chieppi, M., Maini, A., et al. (2014). Nonpharmacological techniques to reduce pain in preterm infants who receive heel-lance procedure: A randomized controlled trial. *Research and Theory for Nursing Practice, 28*(4), 335–348.

Bhethanabhotia, S., Thurak, A., Sankar, M., & Paul, V. (2013). Effect of position of infant during phototherapy in management of hyperbilirubinemia in late preterm and term neonates: A randomized control trial. *Journal of Perinatology, 33*(10), 795–799.

Blackburn, S. T. (2013). *Maternal, fetal, and neonatal physiology: A clinical perspective* (4th ed.). St. Louis: Saunders.

Bramson, L., Lee, J. W., Moore, E., et al. (2010). Effect of early skin-to-skin mother-infant contact during the first 3 hours following birth on exclusive breastfeeding during the maternity hospital stay. *Journal of Human Lactation, 26*(2), 130–137.

Brown, V. D., & Landers, S. (2011). Heat balance. In S. L. Gardner, B. S. Carter, M. Enzman-Hines, et al. (Eds.), *Merenstein & Gardner's handbook of neonatal intensive care* (7th ed.). St. Louis: Mosby.

Bueno, M., Yamada, J., Harrison, D., et al. (2013). A systematic review and meta-analyses of non-sucrose sweet solutions for pain relief in neonates. *Pain Research & Management, 18*(3), 153–161.

Canadian Paediatric Society & College of Family Physicians of Canada. (1997). Routine administration of vitamin K to newborns. *Paediatrics & Child Health, 2*(6), 429–431. Reaffirmed 2014.

Chermont, A., Falcão, L., de Souza Silva, E., et al. (2009). Skin-to-skin contact and/or oral 25% sucrose for procedural pain relief for term newborn infants. *Pediatrics, 124*(6), e1102–e1107.

Cignacco, E. L., Sellam, G., Stoffel, L., et al. (2012). Oral sucrose with facilitated tucking is effective pain control for preterm infants: A randomized control trial. *Pediatrics, 129*(2), 299–308.

Cong, X., Ludington-Hoe, S., Vazquez, V., et al. (2013). *Neonatal Network, 32*(5), 353–357.

Cooper, B. M., Holditch-Davis, D., Verklan, M. T., et al. (2012). Newborn clinical outcomes of the AWHONN late preterm infant research-based practice project. *Journal of Obstetric, Gynecologic, & Neonatal Nursing, 41*(6), 774–785.

Craighead, D. V. (2012). Early term birth: Understanding the health risks to infants. *Nursing for Women's Health, 16*(2), 136–145.

Cummings, C., & Canadian Paediatric Society. (2011). Positional plagiocephaly. *Paediatrics & Child Health, 16*(8), 493–494. Reaffirmed February 1, 2014.

Finan, E., Aylward, D., Aziz, K., & Canadian Paediatric Society. (2011). Neonatal resuscitation guidelines update: A case-based review. *Paediatrics*

& Child Health, 16(5), 289–291. Retrieved from <http://www.cps.ca/en/documents/position/neonatal-resuscitation-guidelines>.

Fleischman, A. R., Oinuma, M., & Clark, S. L. (2010). Rethinking the definition of "term pregnancy". *Obstetrics & Gynecology, 116*(1), 136–139.

Furdon, S. A., & Benjamin, K. (2010). Physical assessment. In M. T. Verklan & M. Walden (Eds.), *Core curriculum for neonatal intensive care nursing* (4th ed.). St. Louis: Saunders.

Gabriel, M. M., Martin, K. L., Escobar, A. L., et al. (2010). Randomized controlled trial of early skin-to-skin contact: Effects on the mother and the newborn. *Acta Paediatrica, 99*(11), 1630–1634.

Gardner, S. L., Enzman-Hines, M., & Dickey, L. A. (2011). Pain and pain relief. In S. L. Gardner, B. S. Carter, M. Enzman-Hines, et al. (Eds.), *Merenstein & Gardner's handbook of neonatal intensive care* (7th ed.). St. Louis: Mosby.

Gardner, S. L., & Hernandez, J. A. (2011). Initial nursery care. In S. L. Gardner, B. S. Carter, M. Enzman-Hines, et al. (Eds.), *Merenstein & Gardner's handbook of neonatal intensive care* (7th ed.). St. Louis: Mosby.

Gradin, M., Erikson, M., Holmqvist, G., et al. (2014). Pain reduction at venipuncture in newborns: Oral glucose compared with local anesthetic cream. *Pediatrics, 110*(6), 1053–1057.

Harrison, D., Bueno, M., & Reszel, J. (2015). Prevention and management of pain and stress in the neonate. *Research and Reports in Neonatology, 5*, 9–16. doi:10.2147/RRN.S52378.

Hummel, P., Puchalski, M., Creech, S. D., et al. (2008). Clinical reliability and validity of the N-Pass: Neonatal pain, agitation, and sedation scale with prolonged pain. *Journal of Perinatology, 28*(1), 55–60.

Jones, J. E., Hayes, R. D., Starbuck, A. L., et al. (2011). Fluid and electrolyte management. In S. L. Gardner, B. S. Carter, M. Enzman-Hines, et al. (Eds.), *Merenstein & Gardner's handbook of neonatal intensive care* (7th ed.). St. Louis: Mosby.

Kalhan, S. C., & Devaskar, S. U. (2011). Disorders of carbohydrate metabolism. In R. J. Martin, A. A. Fanaroff, & M. C. Walsh (Eds.), *Fanaroff and Martin's neonatal-perinatal medicine: Diseases of the fetus and infant* (9th ed.). St. Louis: Mosby.

Kamath, B. C., Thilo, E. H., & Hernandez, J. A. (2011). Jaundice. In S. L. Gardner, B. S. Carter, M. Enzman-Hines, et al. (Eds.), *Merenstein & Gardner's handbook of neonatal intensive care* (7th ed.). St. Louis: Mosby.

Kaplan, M., Wong, R. J., Sibley, E., et al. (2011). Neonatal jaundice and liver disease. In R. J. Martin, A. A. Fanaroff, & M. C. Walsh (Eds.), *Fanaroff and Martin's neonatal-perinatal medicine: Diseases of the fetus and infant* (9th ed.). St. Louis: Mosby.

Kassab, M. I., Roydhouse, J. K., Fowler, C., et al. (2012). The effectiveness of glucose in reducing needle-related procedural pain in infants. *Journal of Pediatric Nursing, 27*(1), 3–17.

Kattwinkel, J., Perlman, J. M., Aziz, K., et al. (2010). Part 15: Neonatal resuscitation: 2010 American Heart Association guidelines for cardiopulmonary resuscitation and emergency cardiovascular care. *Circulation, 122*(Suppl. 3), S909–S919.

Krechel, S. W., & Bildner, J. (1995). CRIES: A new neonatal postoperative pain measurement score. Initial testing of validity and reliability. *Paediatric Anaesthesia, 5*(1), 53–61.

Lawrence, J., Alcock, D., McGrath, P., et al. (1993). The development of a tool to assess neonatal pain. *Neonatal Network, 12*(6), 59–66.

Leduc, D., Côté, A., Woods, S., & Canadian Paediatric Society. (2004). Recommendations for safe sleeping environments for infants and children. *Paediatrics & Child Health, 9*(9), 659–663.

Leite, A., Linhares, M., Lander, J., et al. (2009). Effects of breastfeeding on pain relief in full-term newborns. *Clinical Journal of Pain, 25*(9), 827–832.

Liaw, J., Zeng, W., Yang, L., et al. (2011). Nonnutritive sucking and oral sucrose relieve neonatal pain during intramuscular injection of hepatitis vaccine. *Journal of Pain Management, 42*(6), 918–930.

Lindstrom, K., Lindblad, F., & Hjern, A. (2011). Preterm birth and attention-deficit/hyperactivity disorder. *Pediatrics, 127*(5), 858–865.

Lund, C. H., & Durand, D. J. (2011). Skin and skin care. In S. L. Gardner, B. S. Carter, M. Enzman-Hines, et al. (Eds.), *Merenstein & Gardner's handbook of neonatal intensive care* (7th ed.). St. Louis: Mosby.

Moore, D. S., MacDonald, N., & Canadian Paediatric Society, Infectious Diseases and Immunization Committee. (2015). Preventing opthalmia neonatorum. *Paediatrics & Child Health, 20*(2), 93–96.

Moore, E. R., Anderson, G. C., Bergman, N., et al. (2012). Early skin-to-skin contact for mothers and their healthy newborn infants. *Cochrane Database Systematic Review*, (5), CD003519.

Niermeyer, S., & Clarke, S. B. (2011). Delivery room care. In S. L. Gardner, B. S. Carter, M. Enzman-Hines, et al. (Eds.), *Merenstein & Gardner's handbook of neonatal intensive care* (7th ed.). St. Louis: Mosby.

Patel, H., Feldman, M., & Canadian Paediatric Society Community Paediatrics Committee. (2011). Universal newborn hearing screening. *Paediatrics & Child Health, 16*(5), 301–305. Reaffirmed 2014.

Perinatal Services BC. (2010). *Neonatal guideline 9: Newborn screening*. Retrieved from <http://www.perinatalservicesbc.ca/Documents/Guidelines-Standards/Newborn/NewbornScreeningGuideline.pdf>.

Ponti, M., & Canadian Paediatrics Society. (2003). Recommendations for the use of pacifiers. *Paediatrics & Child Health, 8*(8), 515–519. Reaffirmed February 1, 2014.

Provincial Council for Maternal & Child Health (PCMCH) & Ministry of Health and Long-term Care. (2013). *Quality based procedures clinical handbook for hyperbilirubinemia in term and late pre-term infants (>35 weeks)*. Retrieved from <http://www.health.gov.on.ca/en/pro/programs/ecfa/docs/qbp_jaundice.pdf>.

Public Health Agency of Canada. (2009). *What mothers say: The Canadian maternity experiences survey (Cat No: HP5-74/2-2009E)*. Ottawa: Author.

Public Health Agency of Canada, Canadian Paediatric Society, Canadian Foundation for Study of Infant Deaths, Canadian Institute for Child Health & Health Canada. (2012). *Joint statement on safe sleep: Preventing sudden infant deaths in Canada*. Ottawa: PHAC. Retrieved from <http://www.phac-aspc.gc.ca/hp-ps/dca-dea/stages-etapes/childhood-enfance_0-2/sids/pdf/jsss-ecss2011-eng.pdf>.

Rates of circumcision slashed in past 30 years. *The Gazette*, Montreal, Thursday, March 23, 2006: A13.

Ray, J. G., Jiang, D., Sgro, M., et al. (2009). Thresholds for small for gestational age among newborns of East Asian and South Asian ancestry. *Journal of Obstetrics and Gynaecology Canada, 31*, 322–330.

Reddy, U. M., Bettegowda, V. R., Dias, T., et al. (2011). Term pregnancy: A period of heterogenous risk for infant mortality. *Obstetrics & Gynecology, 117*(6), 1279–1287.

Riddell, R. P., Racine, N. M., Turcotte, K., et al. (2011). Non-pharmacological management of infant and young child procedural pain. *Cochrane Database Systematic Review*, (10), CD006275.

Rigo, J., Mohamed, M. W., & De Curtis, M. (2011). Disorders of calcium, phosphorus, and magnesium metabolism. In R. J. Martin, A. A. Fanaroff, & M. C. Walsh (Eds.), *Fanaroff and Martin's neonatal-perinatal medicine: Diseases of the fetus and infant* (9th ed.). St. Louis: Mosby.

Sorokan, S. T., Finlay, J. C., Jefferies, A. L., et al. (2015). Newborn male circumcision. *Paediatric & Child Health, 20*(6), 311–315.

Stevens, B., Johnston, C., Petryshen, P., et al. (1996). Premature infant pain profile: Development and initial validation. *Clinical Journal of Pain, 12*(1), 13–22.

Taddio, A., Appleton, M., Bortolussi, R., et al. (2010). Reducing the pain of childhood vaccination: An evidence-based clinical practice guideline (summary). *Canadian Medical Association Journal, 182*(18), 1989–1995.

van der Voort, A., Juffer, F., & Bakermans-Kranenburg, M. (2014). Sensitive parenting is the foundation for secure attachment relationships and positive social-emotional development of children. *Journal of Children's Services, 9.2*, 176–185.

Vincent, J. L. (2009). Infant hospital abduction: Security measures to aid in prevention. *MCN American Journal of Maternal/Child Nursing, 34*(3), 179–183.

Weissman, A., Aranovitch, M., Blazer, S., et al. (2009). Heel-lancing in newborns: Behavioral and spectral analysis assessment of pain control methods. *Pediatrics, 124*(5), e921–e926.

World Health Organization. (2009a). *Infant and young child feeding: Model chapter for textbooks for medical students and allied health professionals.*

Geneva: WHO Press. Retrieved from <http://whqlibdoc.who.int/publications/2009/9789241597494_eng.pdf>.
World Health Organization (WHO). (2009b). *WHO guidelines on hand hygiene in health care: A summary*. Geneva: WHO Press.
World Health Organization (WHO). (2012). *Voluntary medical male circumcision for HIV prevention*. Retrieved from <http://www.who.int/hiv/topics/malecircumcision/fact_sheet/en/index.html>.

ADDITIONAL RESOURCES

Baby's Breath: <www.babysbreathcanada.ca>.
Birth weight curves based on maternal ancestry: <http://www.stmichaelshospital.com/birthweights.php>.
City of Brampton, Fire and Emergency Services—Is Your Child Safe and Secure? (information on car seats): <http://www.brampton.ca/en/residents/fire-emergency-services/Fire-Safety/Pages/Child-Safe-and-Secure.aspx>.
New Ballard Score Maturational Assessment of Gestational Age video: <http://www.ballardscore.com/Pages/videos.aspx>.
Ontario Newborn Screening—Fact sheets for parents (in many different languages): <www.newbornscreening.on.ca/bins/content_page.asp?cid=6-14&lang=1>.
Perinatal Services BC Newborn Guidelines: <http://www.perinatalservicesbc.ca/Guidelines/Guidelines/newborn/default.htm>.
Public Health Agency of Canada—Immunization schedule: <http://www.phac-aspc.gc.ca/im/ptimprog-progimpt/table-1-eng.php>.
Public Health Agency of Canada—Safe Sleep for Your Baby: <http://www.phac-aspc.gc.ca/hp-ps/dca-dea/stages-etapes/childhood-enfance_0-2/sids/index-eng.php>.
Transport Canada—Keep Kids Safe (car seat information): <http://www.tc.gc.ca/eng/roadsafety/safedrivers-childsafety-car-time-stages-1083.htm>.

CHAPTER

27

Newborn Nutrition and Feeding

Maureen White

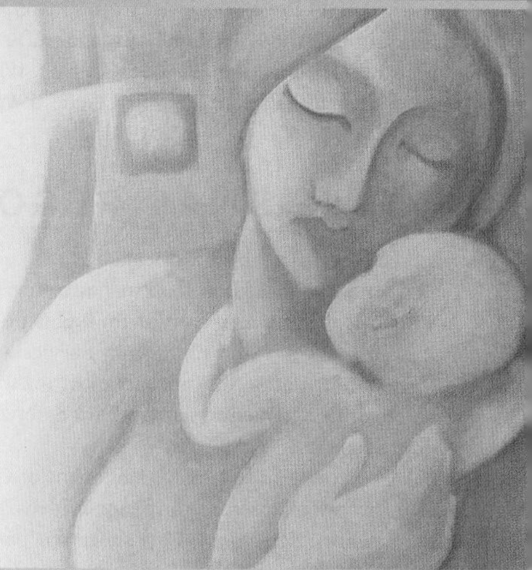

Evolve WEBSITE

Visit the Evolve website for additional resources related to the content in this chapter such as Case Studies, Critical Thinking Case Study Answers, Nursing Care Plans, Nursing Processes, Nursing Skills, and Review Questions for Exam Preparation at: *http://evolve.elsevier.com/Canada/Perry/maternal/*

OBJECTIVES

On completion of this chapter the reader will be able to:

- Describe current recommendations for infant feeding.
- Explain the nurse's role in helping families choose an infant feeding method.
- Discuss the importance of breastfeeding for infants, mothers, families, and society.
- Describe the nutritional needs of newborns.
- Describe the anatomy and physiology of breastfeeding.
- Recognize newborn feeding-readiness cues.
- Explain maternal and infant indicators of effective breastfeeding.
- Examine nursing interventions to facilitate and promote successful breastfeeding.
- Analyze common problems associated with breastfeeding and interventions to help resolve them.
- Compare powdered, concentrated, and ready-to-use forms of commercial infant formula.
- Discuss patient teaching for the family who is formula-feeding their newborn.

Good nutrition in infancy fosters optimal growth and development. Infant feeding is more than the provision of nutrition; it represents an opportunity for social and psychological interaction between parent and infant. It can also establish a basis for developing good eating habits and influence lifelong health habits.

Through preconception and prenatal education and counselling, nurses play an instrumental role in helping parents make an informed decision about infant feeding. Scientific evidence is clear that human milk provides the best nutrition for infants, and parents should be strongly encouraged to choose breastfeeding. Although many consider commercial infant formula to be equivalent to breast milk, this belief is erroneous. Human milk is the gold standard for infant nutrition. It is species specific, uniquely designed to meet the needs of human infants. The composition of human milk changes to meet the nutritional needs of growing infants. It is highly complex, with anti-infective and nutritional components combined with growth factors, enzymes that aid in digestion and absorption of nutrients, and fatty acids that promote brain growth and development. Infant formulas are usually adequate in providing nutrition to maintain infant growth and development within normal limits, but they are not equivalent to human milk.

Breastfeeding is defined as the transfer of human milk from the mother to the infant; the infant receives milk directly from the mother's breast. *Exclusive breastfeeding* means that the infant receives no other liquid or solid food (Health Canada, Canadian Paediatric Society [CPS], Dietitians of Canada and Breastfeeding Committee for Canada [BCC], 2012). If the infant is fed expressed breast milk from the mother or a donor milk bank, it is called *human milk feeding*.

Whether the parents choose breastfeeding, human milk feeding, or formula-feeding, nurses provide support and ongoing education. Parent education and care management are necessarily based on current research findings and standards of practice. Nurses and **lactation consultants** (who are often nurses) provide education, assistance, and support for mothers, infants, and families. After hospital discharge, nurses and lactation consultants in primary care and community health settings provide ongoing support and assistance to promote optimal feeding practices and positive health outcomes.

This chapter focuses on meeting the nutritional needs for normal growth and development from birth to 6 months of age, with an emphasis on the newborn period, when feeding practices and patterns are established. Both breastfeeding and formula-feeding are addressed. Information on breastfeeding is focused on the direct transfer of milk from mother to infant.

RECOMMENDED INFANT NUTRITION

The World Health Organization (WHO), Health Canada, Canadian Paediatric Society (CPS), Dieticians of Canada, and Breastfeeding Committee for Canada recommend exclusive breastfeeding for the first 6 months of life for healthy, term infants (Health Canada et al., 2012; WHO, 2011). Breast milk is recognized as the normal and optimal food for infants. Nutrient-rich complementary foods, with particular attention to iron, should be introduced at 6 months with continued partial breastfeeding for 2 years or longer. Breastfed babies should also receive a daily vitamin D supplement until their diet provides a reliable source or until they reach 1 year of age. If weaned before 12 months, infants should receive iron-fortified infant formula (Health Canada et al., 2012).

Breastfeeding Rates

The rate of breastfeeding initiation in Canada has increased from 84.6% in 2003 to 90.3% in 2012 (Statistics Canada, 2014). The rate of women who exclusively breastfeed (no water, other liquids, or solid food) for 6 months or longer has increased from 16.8% in 2003 to 24.4% in 2012 (Statistics Canada, 2014).

Although there are reports that breastfeeding is low among Indigenous families (Best Start Resource Centre, 2013), in some Indigenous communities 43% of children were breastfed longer than 6 months (UNICEF, 2009). Breastfeeding patterns vary across Canada and across communities, with a trend toward higher initiation rates in the west and among women over 25 years of age (Public Health Agency of Canada [PHAC], 2013).

Benefits of Breastfeeding

Human milk is designed specifically for human infants and is nutritionally superior to any alternative. Breast milk is considered a living tissue because it contains almost as many live cells as blood. It is bacteriologically safe and is always fresh. The nutrients in breast milk are more easily absorbed than those in formula.

Benefits of breastfeeding for the infant include the following:

- Breast milk enhances maturation of the gastrointestinal tract and contains immune factors that contribute to a lower incidence of gastroenteritis, necrotizing enterocolitis in preterm infants, childhood obesity as well as obesity in adolescence and adulthood, Crohn's disease, and celiac disease (Oddy, 2012; Pound, Unger, & CPS, 2012/2015).
- Breastfed infants receive specific antibodies and cell-mediated immunological factors that help protect against otitis media, respiratory illnesses such as respiratory syncytial virus and pneumonia, urinary tract infections, bacteremia, and bacterial meningitis (Denne, 2015; Pound et al., 2012/2015).
- There is a lower incidence of certain allergies among breastfed infants, particularly for families at high risk. Allergic manifestations occur at a greater rate and are more severe in formula-fed infants (Iyengar & Walker, 2012).
- Breastfed infants are less likely to die from sudden infant death syndrome (SIDS) (Pound et al., 2012/2015).
- Breast milk may have a protective effect against childhood lymphoma and type 1 and type 2 diabetes mellitus (Geddes & Prescott, 2013; Horta & Victora, 2013).
- Breast milk may enhance cognitive development for term and preterm infants (Horta & Victora, 2013; Kramer, Aboud, Mironova, et al., 2008).
- Breastfeeding has been shown to provide pain relief for newborns undergoing painful procedures such as venipuncture and heel stick (Johnston, Campbell-Yeo, Fernandes, et al., 2014; Shah, Herbozo, Aliwalas, et al., 2012).

Maternal benefits include the following:

- Women who have breastfed have a decreased risk of ovarian cancer, uterine cancer, breast cancer, rheumatoid arthritis, type II diabetes, hypertension hypercholesterolemia, and cardiovascular disease (Pikwer, Bergström, Nilsson, et al., 2009; Pound et al., 2012/2015; Stuebe & Swartz, 2010).
- Breastfeeding promotes uterine involution and is associated with a decreased risk of postpartum hemorrhage (Lawrence & Lawrence, 2011).
- Mothers who are breastfeeding tend to return to their prepregnancy weight more quickly (Pound et al., 2012/2015).
- Breastfeeding may provide some protection against the development of osteoporosis and risk for hip fractures (Chapman, 2012).
- Breastfeeding provides a unique bonding experience, enhances development of the maternal role, and may provide protection against postpartum depression, when breastfeeding difficulties are appropriately addressed (Kendall-Tackett, 2007, 2015; Lawrence & Lawrence, 2011).

Benefits to families and society include the following:

- Breastfeeding is convenient; there are no bottles or other equipment to purchase, clean, or dispose of (a benefit to the community by not having to dispose of formula bottles and equipment used in manufacture).
- Breastfed babies are portable; when travelling, there are fewer supplies to take along.
- Parental absenteeism from work is decreased (Abdulwadud & Snow, 2012).
- Breastfeeding saves money. The cost of formula far exceeds the cost of extra food for the lactating mother. Because breastfed babies have a lower incidence of illness and infection, health care costs are lower for families and for federal and provincial governments (Pound et al., 2012/2015).

Contraindications to Breastfeeding

Contraindications to breastfeeding include the following (Lawrence & Lawrence, 2015; Pound et al., 2012/2015; WHO, 2015):

- Maternal cancer therapy or diagnostic and therapeutic radioactive isotopes
- Active tuberculosis not under treatment in the mother
- Human immunodeficiency virus (HIV) infection in the mother, in high-income countries
- Maternal herpes simplex lesion on a breast
- Galactosemia (classic) in the infant
- Maternal substance use (e.g., cocaine, methamphetamines, marijuana)
- Maternal human T-cell leukemia virus type 1
- Some medications (although rare) that may exert an untoward effect on the breastfeeding infant; use of these requires consultation of the practitioner and available references such as Hale and Rowe (2014) or Motherisk (http://www.motherisk.org)

Conditions that are not considered contraindications to breastfeeding are as follows (Lawrence & Lawrence, 2015; Pound et al., 2012/2015):

- Maternal infection with hepatitis A or C
- Hepatitis B surface antigen (HBsAg)–positive status
- Maternal fever
- Mothers who are cytomegalovirus (CMV) positive

Baby-Friendly Hospital Initiative

All parents are entitled to a birthing environment in which breastfeeding is promoted and supported. To that end, the Baby-Friendly Hospital Initiative (BFHI) is a joint effort of the WHO and the United Nations Children's Fund (UNICEF) to promote and support worldwide breastfeeding as the model for optimum infant nutrition, through the Ten Steps to Successful Breastfeeding.

The Breastfeeding Committee for Canada (BCC) is the national authority for the BFHI in Canada, which is called the Baby-Friendly Initiative (BFI). To reflect the continuum of care between hospitals and communities, the BCC describes the international standards within the Canadian context and has developed a set of 10 practice outcome indicators (Box 27-1). These integrated steps are the basis for the process by which hospitals and communities can achieve the Baby-Friendly™ designation, an internationally recognized accomplishment confirming that the 10 BFHI outcomes have been achieved and that there is adherence to the WHO International Code of Marketing of Breastmilk Substitutes (BCC, 2012).

The number of BFI-designated facilities in Canada is steadily increasing. The BCC 2014 annual report noted that the BFI designation has been achieved by 10 hospitals, 7 birthing centres, 109 Community Health Services, and 1 Indigenous health centre across the provinces of British Columbia, Saskatchewan, Manitoba, Ontario, and Quebec (BCC, 2014). The BFI is an important step toward re-establishing a culture that supports breastfeeding in Canada. Meanwhile, the BFI requires time and resources to implement and is not without its critics. Some women may not be willing or able to breastfeed and may experience pressure to conform to the new breastfeeding norms. Some health providers interpret the BFI as eliminating discussions with families about formula and the practicalities of formula-feeding. One of the key messages of the BFI, however, is that health care providers have the responsibility to inform parents of safe and alternative feeding methods when a baby needs to be supplemented or when an informed decision to use infant formula has been made (Best Start Resource Centre & Baby-Friendly Initiative Ontario, 2013). Application of the BFI 10 steps involves using effective communication skills in a supportive and nonjudgemental manner to promote informed decision making about infant feeding. Nursing care includes respecting parents' feeding choices and supporting their learning about responding to infant needs.

BOX 27-1 TEN STEPS TO BABY-FRIENDLY DESIGNATION

Step 1. Have a written breastfeeding policy that is routinely communicated to all health care providers and volunteers.

Step 2. Ensure that all health care providers have the knowledge and skills necessary to implement the breastfeeding policy.

Step 3. Inform pregnant women and their families about the importance and process of breastfeeding.

Step 4. Place babies in skin-to-skin contact with their mothers immediately following birth for at least an hour or until completion of the first feeding or as long as the mother wishes; encourage mothers to recognize when their babies are ready to feed, offering help as needed.

Step 5. Assist mothers in breastfeeding and maintaining lactation should they face challenges, including separation from their infants.

Step 6. Infants are not offered food or drink other than human milk for the first 6 months, unless *medically* indicated.

Step 7. Facilitate 24-hour rooming-in for all mothers; mothers and infants remain together.

Step 8. Encourage baby-led or cue-based breastfeeding. Encourage sustained breastfeeding beyond 6 months with appropriate introduction of complementary foods.

Step 9. Support mothers to feed and care for their breastfeeding babies without the use of artificial teats or pacifiers (dummies or soothers).

Step 10. Provide a seamless transition between the services provided by the hospital, community health services, and peer support programs.

From Breastfeeding Committee for Canada. (2010). *Summary: Integrated 10 steps practice outcome indicators for hospitals and community health services.* Retrieved from <http://www.breastfeedingcanada.ca/BFI.aspx>.

CHOOSING AN INFANT FEEDING METHOD

For most women there is a clear choice to either breastfeed or formula-feed. In some cases women decide to combine breastfeeding and formula-feeding. However, this practice may be associated with a shorter duration of breastfeeding (Holmes,

Auinger, & Howard, 2011). In some instances women want their infants to receive breast milk but prefer not to feed directly from their breasts.

Choosing to Breastfeed

Women most often choose to breastfeed because they are aware of the benefits to the infant (Nelson, 2012). This reinforces the importance of prenatal education about the numerous benefits of breastfeeding. Breastfeeding is a natural extension of pregnancy and childbirth; it is much more than simply a means of supplying nutrition for infants. Many women seek the unique bonding experience between mother and infant that is characteristic of breastfeeding. The support of the partner and family is a major factor in a mother's decision to breastfeed and in her ability to do so successfully. Women who perceive their partners to prefer breastfeeding are more likely to breastfeed. Women are more likely to breastfeed successfully when partners and family members have a positive view of breastfeeding and have the skills to support it. Ideally, prenatal preparation includes the woman's partner, who needs information about the benefits of breastfeeding and how he or she can participate in infant care and nurturing.

There appears to be a correlation between maternal weight and infant feeding decisions: women who are overweight or obese are less likely to breastfeed than women who are underweight or of average weight (Mehta, Siega-Riz, Herring, et al., 2011). Also, women tend to select the same method of infant feeding for each of their children. If the first child was breastfed, subsequent children will likely also be breastfed.

The decision to breastfeed exclusively is related to the mother's knowledge about the health benefits to the infant and her comfort level with breastfeeding in social settings (Stuebe & Bonuck, 2011). The likelihood that women will breastfeed exclusively may be greater if they made the decision to do so during pregnancy (Tenfelde, Finnegan, & Hill, 2011). In a meta-synthesis of 14 qualitative studies about decision making regarding infant feeding, Nelson (2012) reported that common barriers to breastfeeding included lack of comfort or uneasiness with breastfeeding, pain, lifestyle incompatibility, discomfort with public breastfeeding, and a lack of formal support.

Individualized, needs-based prenatal breastfeeding education has been used effectively to encourage the intention to breastfeed (Best Start Resource Centre, 2015; Dyson, McCormick, & Renfrew, 2005). Each encounter with an expectant parent is an opportunity to dispel myths, clarify misinformation, and address personal concerns. Connecting expectant mothers with women who are breastfeeding or who have successfully breastfed and are from similar backgrounds may be helpful for all involved. Peer counselling programs, such as those instituted by La Leche League, are beneficial, particularly in low socioeconomic groups, where formula-feeding is common. To provide effective support for the mother, health care providers must be knowledgeable about the benefits of breastfeeding, the basic process of breastfeeding, breastfeeding management, and interventions for common concerns (Box 27-2).

BOX 27-2 GUIDELINES FOR BREASTFEEDING SUPPORT

During pregnancy, perform an assessment that includes intent to breastfeed, breastfeeding history, access to breastfeeding support, a breast examination, and a medication use history.

Develop a prenatal care plan to prepare the woman for lactation.

Inform the mother and her family of the importance of early and frequent skin-to-skin contact after birth.

After birth, the nurse

- Encourages the mother to position her baby skin-to-skin on the mother's chest as soon as possible and until after the first feeding unless medically contraindicated.
- Assists with recognition of early feeding cues, latch-on, and positioning, as needed.
- Reinforces the need for frequent feedings of breast milk—at least 8–12 times per day (without supplementation).
- Encourages keeping mothers and infants in the same room during the entire postpartum stay.
- Gives discharge instructions emphasizing signs of successful breastfeeding.
- Provides information about community resources for breastfeeding support.
- Encourages breastfeeding, especially for preterm and low-birth-weight infants.
- Reinforces the recommendation for exclusive breastfeeding for the first 6 months, with the introduction of complementary foods at 6 months and continued breastfeeding up to 2 years and beyond.

Adapted from International Lactation Consultant Association. (2014). *Clinical guidelines for the establishment of exclusive breastfeeding* (3rd ed.). Morrisville, NC: Author; Registered Nurses' Association of Ontario (RNAO). (2003). *Breastfeeding best practice guidelines for nurses.* Toronto: Author; RNAO (2007). *Breastfeeding best practice guidelines revision supplement.* Toronto: Author. Retrieved from <http://rnao.ca/bpg/guidelines/breastfeeding-best-practice-guidelines-nurses>.

Choosing to Formula-Feed

Parents who choose to formula-feed often make this decision without complete information and understanding of the benefits of breastfeeding. Even women who are educated about the advantages of breastfeeding may still decide to formula-feed. Cultural beliefs and myths and misconceptions about breastfeeding influence women's decision making. Many women see bottle-feeding as more convenient or less embarrassing than breastfeeding. Some view formula-feeding as a way to ensure that the father, partner, or other family members, and day care providers can feed the baby. Some women lack confidence in their ability to produce breast milk of adequate quantity or quality. Women who have had previous unsuccessful breastfeeding experiences may choose to formula-feed subsequent infants. Some women see breastfeeding as incompatible with an active social life, or they think that it will prevent them from going back to work. Modesty issues and societal barriers exist against breastfeeding in public. A major barrier for many women is the influence of family and friends (Nelson, 2012).

Cultural Influences on Infant Feeding

Cultural beliefs and practices are significant influences on infant feeding methods. Many regional and ethnic cultures are found within Canada. Nurses need to be knowledgeable about and sensitive to the various cultural factors influencing infant feeding practices among their patients. At the same time, they must not assume that generalized observations about any cultural group hold true for all members of that group.

Breastfeeding beliefs and practices vary across cultures. For example, generally the historical tradition among Indigenous people was to only breastfeed infants until they were able to digest other food sources. These traditional practices shifted to bottle-feeding in the 1950s when infant formula was introduced to these communities. Since then the incidence of breastfeeding among this population had remained somewhat lower than that for the general population in Canada: however, there now appears to be a trend toward increased breastfeeding among Indigenous populations (UNICEF, 2009). Among Indigenous peoples are communities unique in culture, language, and history; thus, their breastfeeding practices and beliefs vary. For instance, among the Cree women of Northern Quebec, breastfeeding is the norm and is considered good for the health of the baby. These women accept the traditional view that, in order to make milk, they must eat a large amount and expect to have difficulty losing their pregnancy weight. The Cree concept of *miyupimaatisiiun*, or "being alive well," which places emphasis on quality of life rather than on aspects of the physical body, has been a starting point for community-based programs that support breastfeeding while addressing issues of obesity in this population. Current recommendations for promotion and support of breastfeeding for Indigenous women include careful attention to the social determinants of breastfeeding experiences and attitudes toward breastfeeding in communities (Best Start Resource Centre & Baby-Friendly Initiative Ontario, 2013; Eni, Phillips-Beck, & Mehta, 2014).

Because of beliefs about the harmful nature or inadequacy of colostrum, some cultures apply restrictions on breastfeeding for a period of days after birth. Such is the case for many cultures in Southern Asia, the Pacific Islands, and parts of sub-Saharan Africa. Before the mother's milk is deemed to be "in," babies are fed prelacteal food such as honey or clarified butter in the belief that these substances will help clear out meconium. Other cultures begin breastfeeding immediately after birth and offer the breast each time the infant cries.

A common practice among Mexican women is *las dos cosas* ("both things"). This refers to combining breastfeeding and commercial infant formula. It is based on the belief that, by combining the two methods, the mother and infant receive the benefits of breastfeeding, and the infant receives the additional vitamins from infant formula (Bartick & Reyes, 2012; Rios, 2009). This practice can result in problems with milk supply and babies refusing to latch on to the breast, which can lead to early termination of breastfeeding.

Some cultures have specific beliefs and practices related to the mother's intake of foods that foster milk production. Korean mothers often eat seaweed soup and rice to enhance milk production. Hmong women believe that boiled chicken, rice, and hot water are the only appropriate nourishments during the first postpartum month. The balance between energy forces, hot and cold, or yin and yang is integral to the diet of the lactating mother. Latin Americans, Vietnamese, Chinese, East Indians, and Arabs often use this principle in choosing foods for particular conditions. "Hot" foods are considered best for new mothers. This belief does not necessarily relate to the temperature or spiciness of foods; for example, chicken and broccoli are considered "hot," whereas many fresh fruits and vegetables are considered "cold." Families often bring desired foods into the health care setting.

Faith-based breastfeeding traditions are also evident in some cultures. For example, Muslim and Jewish cultures value breastfeeding of infants (Rassin, Klug, Nathanzon, et al., 2009). Some Muslim women practise the tradition of a 40-day rest period, during which the woman is relieved of housekeeping duties and other women help care for her. During this time, the mother may exclusively breastfeed. Breastfeeding for 2 years is recommended in the Qur'an; however, Muslim women typically cease exclusive breastfeeding early in infancy due to the cultural custom of prelacteal feedings (Jessri, Farmer, & Olson, 2013). For many Jewish women, breastfeeding is perceived as being important, but its practice is highly influenced by maternal education level, assimilated cultural values depending on geographic region of origin, and previous breastfeeding experience. The Talmud endorses the value of human milk and of breastfeeding for 2 to 4 years.

Cultural attitudes regarding modesty and breastfeeding are important considerations in whether a woman breastfeeds her baby. Language barriers may also prevent successful breastfeeding and counselling when women cannot connect with resources in their language. With the large percentage of immigrants in Canada, it is incumbent on nurses to consider the range of cultural values related to infant feeding and perceptions of the benefits of breastfeeding so that the mother can make an informed decision based on both knowledge and an approach that is personally acceptable. Breastfeeding support services need to be provided in a culturally sensitive manner and, where possible, in the family's native language. One of the goals of the Canada Prenatal Nutrition Program (CPNP) is to provide long-term funding to community groups to develop or enhance programs for breastfeeding education and support (PHAC, 2015).

Sociocultural values may preclude the mother from receiving adequate information on breastfeeding; for example, if the family is strongly patriarchal and the father is the only English-speaking person in the family and acts as translator, the necessary information being conveyed to the mother by the health care provider may not be correctly translated. Persons immigrating to North America often tend to acquire the local customs of their new home; although breastfeeding may have been common in their own country, they may abandon the practice in their new country, considering it "outdated."

Nurses need to be aware that many parenting and breastfeeding challenges are common across cultures for heterosexual and same-sex or queer families. At the same time, members of LGBTQ communities may have specific parenting and infant feeding questions and concerns related to co-nursing and induced lactation, chest-feeding versus breastfeeding, or breastfeeding after breast augmentation (transgender women). In feeding discussions with and physical examination of transgendered individuals, the nurse needs to be sensitive to the potential for processes of pregnancy and lactation to effect *gender dysphoria* (when an individual feels discomfort about parts of the body not matching the person's gender) (Farrow, 2015). Detailed information on LGBTQ breastfeeding concerns is available from Rainbow Health Ontario and Milk Junkies (see Additional Resources at the end of the chapter).

Overall, most parents want what is best for their children. This desire provides a focus for nursing discussions on infant feeding. Nurses need to clarify individual parental expectations of infant feeding and collaborate with parents to meet their goals.

Nutrient Needs

Fluids

During the first 2 days of life the fluid requirement for healthy infants (more than 1500 g) is 60 to 80 mL of water per kilogram of body weight per day. From day 3 to 7 the requirement is 100 to 150 mL/kg/day; from day 8 to day 30 it is 120 to 180 mL/kg/day (Dell, 2011). In general, neither breastfed nor formula-fed infants need to be given water, not even those living in very hot climates. Breast milk contains 87% water, which easily meets the infant's fluid requirements. Feeding water to infants can decrease caloric consumption at a time when they are growing rapidly.

Infants have room for little fluctuation in fluid balance and should be monitored closely for fluid intake and water loss. They lose water through excretion of urine and insensibly through respiration. Under normal circumstances they are born with some fluid reserve, and some of the weight loss during the first few days is related to fluid loss. However, in some cases they do not have this fluid reserve, possibly because of inadequate maternal hydration during labour or birth.

Juices are not necessary for proper nutrient intake. There is no evidence that juice intake provides better nutrients than human milk or fortified formula; on the contrary, there are data indicating that excess juice consumption may replace essential elements, leading to nutritional deficits (Health Canada et al., 2012). Juices may also cause significant dental decay, especially when consumed from a bottle.

Energy

Infants require adequate caloric intake to provide energy for growth, digestion, physical activity, and maintenance of organ metabolic function. Energy needs vary according to age, maturity level, thermal environment, growth rate, health status, and activity level. For the first 3 months, the infant needs 110 kcal/kg/day. From 3 months to 6 months, the requirement decreases to approximately 100 kcal/kg/day. This level decreases slightly to 95 kcal/kg/day from 6 to 9 months, and increases to 100 kcal/kg/day from 9 months to 1 year (American Academy of Pediatrics, Committee on Nutrition, 2009).

Human milk provides an average of 67 kcal/100 mL or 20 kcal/30 mL. The fat portion of the milk provides the greatest amount of energy. Infant formulas are made to simulate the caloric content of human milk. Usually a standard formula contains 20 kcal/30 mL, although the composition differs among brands.

Carbohydrates

According to the Institute of Medicine (2005), the recommended Adequate Intake (AI) for carbohydrates in the first 6 months of life is 60 g/day and 95 g/day for the second 6 months. Because newborns have only small hepatic glycogen stores, carbohydrates should provide at least 40 to 50% of the total calories in the diet. Moreover, newborns may have limited ability for gluconeogenesis (formation of glucose from amino acids and other substrates) and ketogenesis (formation of ketone bodies from fat), the mechanisms that provide alternative sources of energy.

As the primary carbohydrate in human milk and commercially prepared formula, lactose is the most abundant carbohydrate in the diet of infants up to 6 months of age. Lactose provides calories in an easily available form. Its slow breakdown and absorption probably also increase calcium absorption. Corn syrup solids or glucose polymers are added to infant formulas to supplement the lactose in cow's milk and provide sufficient carbohydrates.

Oligosaccharides, another form of carbohydrate found in breast milk, are critical in the development of microflora in the intestinal tract of the newborn. These prebiotics promote an acidic environment in the intestines, preventing the growth of Gram-negative and other pathogenic bacteria, thus increasing the infant's resistance to gastrointestinal (GI) illness.

Fat

Fats provide a major source of energy for infants, supplying as much as 50% of the calories in breast milk and formula. The recommended AI of fat for infants younger than 6 months is 31 g/day (Institute of Medicine, 2005). The fat content of human milk is composed of lipids, triglycerides, and cholesterol; cholesterol is an essential element for brain growth. Human milk contains the essential fatty acids (EFAs) linoleic acid and linolenic acid and the long-chain polyunsaturated fatty acids arachidonic acid (ARA) and docosahexaenoic acid (DHA). Fatty acids are important for growth, neurological development, and visual function. Cow's milk contains fewer of the EFAs and no polyunsaturated fatty acids. Most formula companies add DHA to their products, although there is a lack of evidence supporting the benefit (Lawrence & Lawrence, 2011).

Modified cow's milk is used to make most infant formulas, but the milk fat is removed and replaced by another fat source, such as corn oil, that can be more easily digested and absorbed by the infant. If whole milk or evaporated milk without added carbohydrate is fed to infants, the resulting fecal loss of fat (and therefore loss of energy) may be excessive because the milk moves through the infant's intestines too quickly for adequate absorption to take place. This can lead to poor weight gain. There is evidence that whole milk may also increase the infant's chances for developing allergies from exposure to cow's milk protein.

Protein

High-quality protein from breast milk, infant formula, or other complementary foods is necessary for infant growth. The protein requirement per unit of body weight is greater in the newborn than at any other time of life. For infants younger than 6 months the recommended AI for protein is 9.1 g/day (Institute of Medicine, 2005).

Human milk contains the two proteins whey and casein in a ratio of approximately 70:30, compared with the ratio of 20:80 in most cow's milk–based formula (Blackburn, 2013). This whey/casein ratio in human milk makes it more easily digestible and produces the soft stools seen in breastfed infants. The primary whey protein in human milk is alpha-lactalbumin; this protein is high in essential amino acids needed for growth. The whey protein lactoferrin in human milk has iron-binding capabilities and bacteriostatic properties, particularly against Gram-positive and Gram-negative aerobes, anaerobes, and yeasts. The casein in human milk enhances the absorption of iron, thus preventing iron-dependent bacteria from proliferating in the GI tract (Lawrence & Lawrence, 2015). The amino acid components of human milk are uniquely suited to the newborn's metabolic capabilities. For example, cystine and taurine levels are high, whereas phenylalanine and methionine levels are low.

Vitamins

With the exception of vitamin D, human milk contains all of the vitamins required for infant nutrition, with individual variations based on maternal diet and genetic differences (Kim & Froh, 2012). Vitamins are added to cow's-milk formulas to resemble levels found in breast milk. Although cow's milk contains adequate amounts of vitamin A and B complex, vitamin C (ascorbic acid), vitamin E, and vitamin D must be added.

Vitamin D facilitates intestinal absorption of calcium and phosphorus, bone mineralization, and calcium resorption from bone. Canadian recommendations regarding vitamin D supplementation are based on Canada's northern geographic latitude, current practices related to protection from the sun, prevalence of vitamin D–deficiency rickets, and history of safe use of vitamin D supplementation. Health Canada recommends that all breastfed, healthy term infants in Canada receive a daily vitamin D supplement of 10 mcg (400 IU). Supplementation should begin at birth and continue until the infant's diet includes at least 10 mcg (400 IU) per day of vitamin D from other dietary sources or until the breastfed infant reaches 1 year of age (Health Canada et al., 2012).

Vitamin K, required for blood coagulation, is produced by intestinal bacteria. However, the gut is relatively sterile at birth, and a few days are needed for intestinal flora to become established and to produce vitamin K. To prevent hemorrhagic problems in the newborn, an injection of vitamin K is routinely given within the first 6 hours after birth, following initial stabilization of the baby and family–baby interaction (McMillan, CPS, & College of Family Physicians of Canada, 1997/2016) (see Chapter 26, Medication Guide on vitamin K, p. 677).

The breastfed infant's vitamin B_{12} intake depends on the mother's dietary intake and stores. Mothers who are on strict vegetarian (vegan) diets and those who consume few dairy products, eggs, or meat are at risk for vitamin B_{12} deficiency. Breastfed infants of vegan mothers should be supplemented with vitamin B_{12} from birth.

Minerals

The mineral content of commercial infant formula is designed to reflect that of breast milk. Whole cow's milk is much higher in mineral content than human milk, which also makes it unsuitable for infants in the first year of life. Minerals are typically highest in human milk during the first few days after birth and decrease slightly throughout lactation.

The ratio of calcium to phosphorus in human milk is 2:1, an optimal proportion for bone mineralization. Although cow's milk is high in calcium, the calcium/phosphorus ratio is low, resulting in decreased resorption. Consequently, young infants (less than 12 months) fed whole cow's milk are at risk for hypocalcemia, tetany, and seizures. The calcium/phosphorus ratio in commercial infant formulas is between the ratios of human and cow's milk.

Milk of all types is low in iron; however, iron from human milk is better absorbed than that from cow's milk, iron-fortified formula, or infant cereals. Breastfed infants draw on iron reserves deposited in utero and benefit from the high lactose and vitamin C levels in human milk that facilitate iron absorption. The infant who is totally breastfed normally maintains adequate hemoglobin levels for at least the first 6 months of life. After that time, meat, meat alternatives, iron-fortified cereals, and other iron-rich foods may be added to the diet. Infants weaned from the breast before 6 months of age and all formula-fed infants should receive an iron-fortified commercial infant formula until 12 months of age. Infants should not be given low-iron formula (Health Canada et al., 2012).

Fluoride levels in human milk and commercial formulas are low. This mineral, which is important in the prevention of dental caries, can cause staining of the permanent teeth (fluorosis) in excess amounts. Fluoride supplementation should be considered for any child over age 6 months whose drinking water is deficient in fluoride or if other factors put the child at high risk for developing dental caries (Canadian Dental Association, 2012; Health Canada et al., 2012).

OVERVIEW OF LACTATION

Breast Anatomy

Each female breast is composed of approximately 15 to 20 segments (lobes) embedded in fat and connective tissues and well supplied with blood vessels, lymphatic vessels, and nerves (Fig. 27-1). Within each lobe is glandular tissue consisting of alveoli, the milk-producing cells, surrounded by myoepithelial cells that

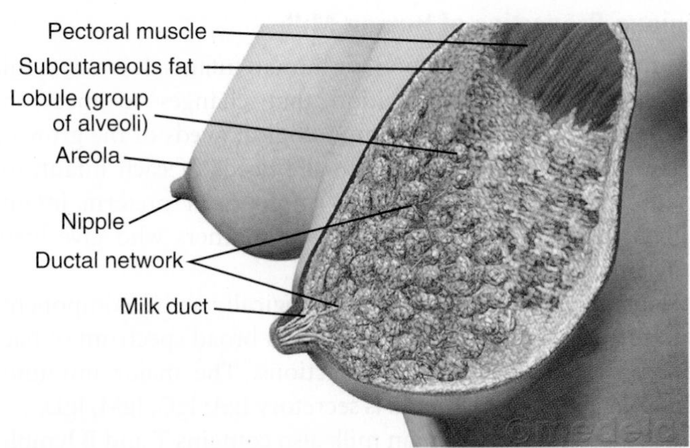

FIGURE 27-1 Anatomy of the lactating breast. (Copyright © 2013 Medela.)

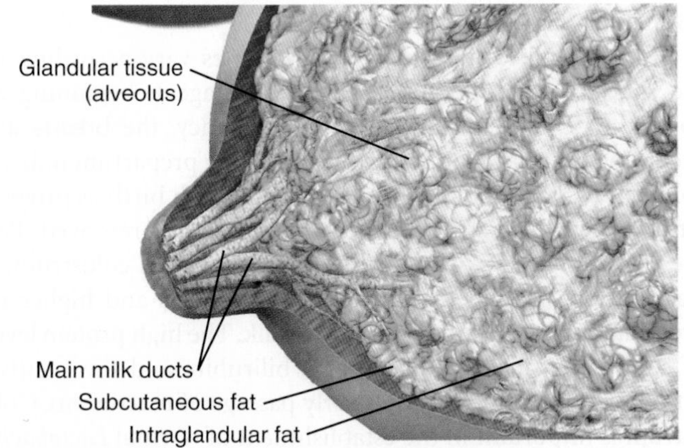

FIGURE 27-2 Enhanced view of milk glands and ducts. (Copyright © 2013 Medela.)

contract to send the milk forward to the nipple during milk ejection. Each nipple has multiple pores that transfer milk to the suckling infant. The ratio of glandular to adipose tissue in the lactating breast is approximately 2 : 1, compared with a 1 : 1 ratio in the nonlactating breast. Within each breast is a complex, intertwining network of milk ducts that transport milk from the alveoli to the nipple. The milk ducts dilate and expand at milk ejection (Riordan & Wambach, 2010a). Previous thinking held that the milk ducts converged behind the nipple in lactiferous sinuses, which acted as reservoirs for milk. However, research based on ultrasonography of lactating breasts has shown that these sinuses do not exist and, in fact, glandular tissue can be found directly beneath the nipple (Geddes, 2007; Ramsay, Kent, Hartmann, et al., 2005) (Fig. 27-2). The nipple and areola are very elastic so that they can be drawn fully into the infant's mouth for deep latch-on (Lawrence & Lawrence, 2015).

The size and shape of the breast are not accurate indicators of its ability to produce milk. Although nearly every woman can lactate, a small number have insufficient glandular development to breastfeed their infants exclusively. Typically these women experienced few breast changes during either puberty or early pregnancy. In some cases they are still able to produce some breast milk, although the quantity is not likely to be sufficient to meet the nutritional needs of the infant. These mothers can offer supplemental nutrition to support optimal infant growth. Devices are available to allow mothers to offer supplements while the baby is nursing at the breast.

Lactogenesis

After the mother gives birth, a precipitous fall in progesterone triggers the release of **prolactin** from the anterior pituitary. During pregnancy, prolactin prepares the breasts to secrete milk and during lactation to synthesize and secrete milk. Prolactin levels are highest during the first 10 days after birth, gradually declining over time but remaining above baseline levels for the duration of lactation. Prolactin is produced in response to infant suckling and emptying the breasts (lactating breasts are never completely empty; milk is constantly being produced by the alveoli as the infant feeds) (Fig. 27-3, A). Milk production is a *supply-meets-demand system* (i.e., as milk is removed from the breast, more is produced). Incomplete removal of milk from the breasts can lead to decreased milk production.

Oxytocin is another hormone essential to lactation. As the nipple is stimulated by the suckling infant, the posterior pituitary is prompted by the hypothalamus to produce oxytocin. This hormone is responsible for the **milk ejection reflex (MER)**, or *let-down reflex* (see Fig. 27-3, B). The myoepithelial cells surrounding the alveoli respond to oxytocin by contracting and sending the milk forward through the ducts to the nipple. The MER is triggered multiple times during a feeding session. Thoughts, sights, sounds, or odours that the mother associates with her baby (or other babies), such as hearing the baby cry, can trigger the MER. Many women report a tingling "pins and needles" sensation in the breasts as milk ejection occurs, although some mothers can detect milk ejection only by observing the sucking and swallowing of the infant. The MER also can occur during sexual activity because oxytocin is released during orgasm. The reflex can be inhibited by fear, stress, and alcohol consumption.

> **! NURSING ALERT**
>
> Be cautious in referring to the MER as "let-down." Some women may interpret let-down as being associated with feelings of depression.

Oxytocin is the same hormone that stimulates uterine contractions during labour. Consequently, the MER can be triggered during labour, as evidenced by leakage of colostrum. This reflex readies the breasts for immediate feeding by the infant after birth. Oxytocin has the important function of contracting the mother's uterus after birth to control postpartum bleeding and promote uterine involution. Thus, mothers who breastfeed are at decreased risk for postpartum hemorrhage. Uterine contractions that occur with breastfeeding can be painful during and after the feeding for the first 3 to 5 days. These "after-pains" are more common in multiparas and tend to resolve completely within 1 week after birth.

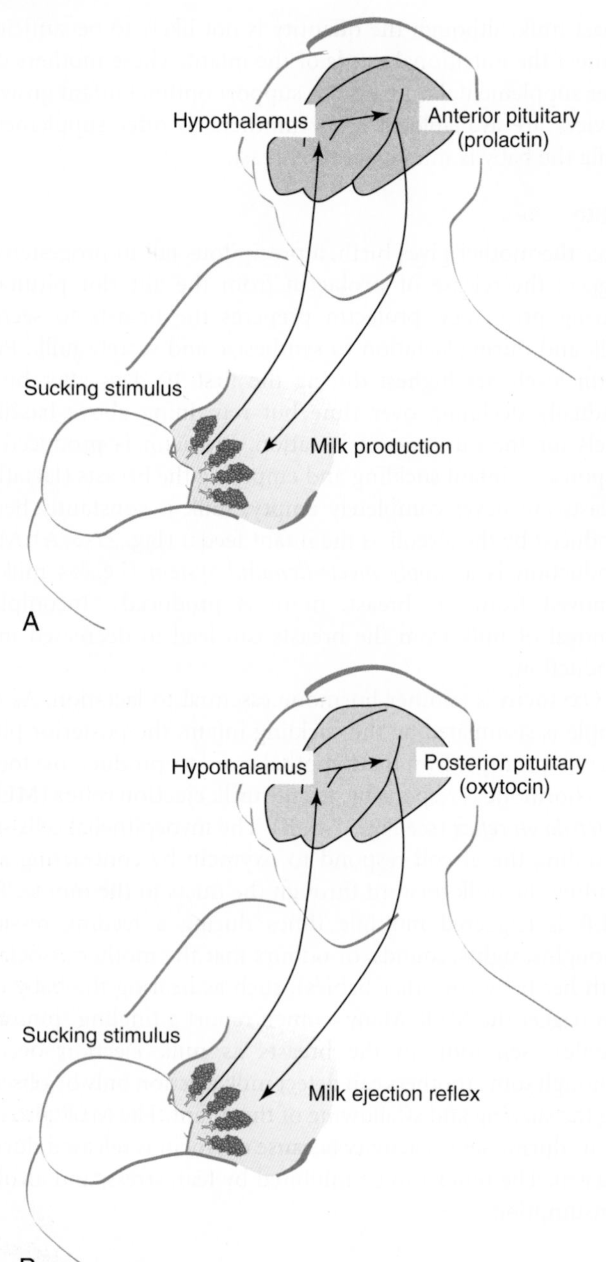

FIGURE 27-3 Maternal breastfeeding reflexes. **A:** Milk production. **B:** Milk ejection reflex (Let-down).

Prolactin and oxytocin have been referred to as the *mothering hormones* because they affect the postpartum woman's emotions as well as her physical state. Many women report feeling thirsty or relaxed during breastfeeding, probably as a result of these hormones.

The nipple-erection reflex is an integral part of lactation. When the infant cries, suckles, or rubs against the breast, the nipple becomes erect, which aids in the propulsion of milk through the ducts to the nipple pores. Nipple sizes, shapes, and ability to become erect vary with individuals. Some women have flat or inverted nipples that do not become erect with stimulation; these women may need assistance to achieve an effective latch. Their infants should not be offered bottles or pacifiers until breastfeeding is well established.

Unique Properties of Human Milk

Human milk is the ideal food for human infants. It is a dynamic substance with a composition that changes to meet the changing nutritional and immunological needs of the growing infant. Breast milk is specific to the needs of each infant; for example, the milk produced by mothers of preterm infants differs in composition from that of mothers who give birth at term.

Human milk contains immunologically active components that provide some protection against a broad spectrum of bacterial, viral, and protozoan infections. The major immunoglobulin (Ig) in human milk is secretory IgA; IgG, IgM, IgD, and IgE are also present. Human milk also contains T and B lymphocytes, epidermal growth factor, cytokines, interleukins, bifidus factor, complement (C3 and C4), and lactoferrin, all of which have a specific role in preventing localized and systemic bacterial and viral infections (Lawrence & Lawrence, 2015; Lönnerdal, 2014).

Human milk composition and volumes vary according to the stage of lactation. In **lactogenesis** stage I, beginning at approximately 16 to 18 weeks of pregnancy, the breasts are preparing for milk production by producing prepartum milk or **colostrum**. Stage II of lactogenesis begins with birth as progesterone levels drop sharply when the placenta is removed. For the first 2 to 3 days after birth, the baby receives colostrum, a clear, yellowish fluid that is rich in antibodies and higher in protein but lower in fat than mature milk. The high protein level of colostrum facilitates binding of bilirubin, and the laxative action of colostrum promotes early passage of meconium. Colostrum is important in the establishment of normal *Lactobacillus bifidus* flora in the infant's digestive tract. It gradually changes to transitional milk. By 3 to 5 days after birth the woman experiences a noticeable increase in milk production. This is often referred to as *the milk coming in*. Breast milk continues to change in composition for approximately 10 days, when the mature milk is established. This is stage III of lactogenesis (Lawrence & Lawrence, 2011).

The composition of human milk changes over time as the infant grows and develops. Fat is the most variable component of human milk with changes in concentration over a feeding, over a 24-hour period, and across time. Variations in fat content exist between breasts and among individuals (Lawrence & Lawrence, 2015). During each feeding the concentration of fat gradually increases from the lower fat foremilk (provides primarily lactose, protein, and water soluble vitamins) to the richer hindmilk. The hindmilk contains the denser calories from fat necessary for ensuring optimal growth and contentment between feedings. The hindmilk is usually let down 10 to 20 minutes into the feeding, although it may occur sooner. Because of this changing composition of human milk during each feeding, it is important to breastfeed the infant long enough to supply a balanced feeding.

Milk production gradually increases as the baby grows. Infants have fairly predictable **growth spurts** (at approximately 10 days, 3 weeks, 6 weeks, 3 months, and 6 months), when more frequent feedings stimulate increased milk production. These growth spurts usually last 24 to 48 hours, after which the infants resume their usual feeding pattern as the mother's milk supply increases.

NURSING CARE

Supporting Breastfeeding Mothers and Infants

The key to encouraging mothers to breastfeed is education and anticipatory guidance, beginning as early as possible during and even before pregnancy. Each encounter with an expectant mother and her family is an opportunity to educate, dispel myths, clarify misinformation, and address concerns. Prenatal education and preparation for breastfeeding influence feeding decisions, breastfeeding success, and the amount of time that women breastfeed. Prenatal preparation ideally includes the father of the baby, partner, or another significant support person and provides information about benefits of breastfeeding and how he or she can participate in infant care and nurturing.

Connecting expectant mothers with women from similar backgrounds who are breastfeeding or have successfully breastfed is often helpful. Nursing mothers' support groups such as La Leche League provide information about breastfeeding along with opportunities for breastfeeding mothers to talk with one another and share concerns.

For some women the postpartum period may provide the first opportunity for education about breastfeeding. Even women who have indicated the desire to formula-feed can benefit from information about the benefits of breastfeeding. In offering these women the chance to try breastfeeding with the assistance of a nurse or lactation consultant they may change their infant feeding practices. Learning along with other new mothers can be encouraging (Fig. 27-4).

Promoting feelings of competence and confidence in the breastfeeding mother and reinforcing the unequalled contribution she is making toward the health and well-being of her infant are the responsibility of the nurse and other health care providers. The first 2 weeks of breastfeeding can be the most challenging, as mothers are adjusting to life with a newborn, the baby is learning to latch on and feed effectively, and the mother may be experiencing nipple or breast discomfort. This is a time when support is critical. Primiparous women are most likely to experience early breastfeeding problems, which often result in less exclusive breastfeeding and shorter duration of breastfeeding (Chantry, 2011). Anticipatory guidance during the prenatal period and especially during the hospital stay after birth can provide the mother with information and increase her confidence in her ability to successfully breastfeed her infant. New mothers need access to lactation support following discharge through primary care offices, health departments, or outpatient lactation services. Peer support is also helpful.

The most common reasons for breastfeeding cessation are insufficient milk supply, painful nipples, and problems getting the infant to feed (Lauwers & Swisher, 2011; Lawrence & Lawrence, 2015). Early and ongoing assistance and support from health care providers to prevent and address problems with breastfeeding can help promote a successful and satisfying breastfeeding experience for mothers and infants. Many health care agencies have certified lactation consultants on staff. These consultants, who are often nurses, have specialized training and experience in helping breastfeeding mothers and infants.

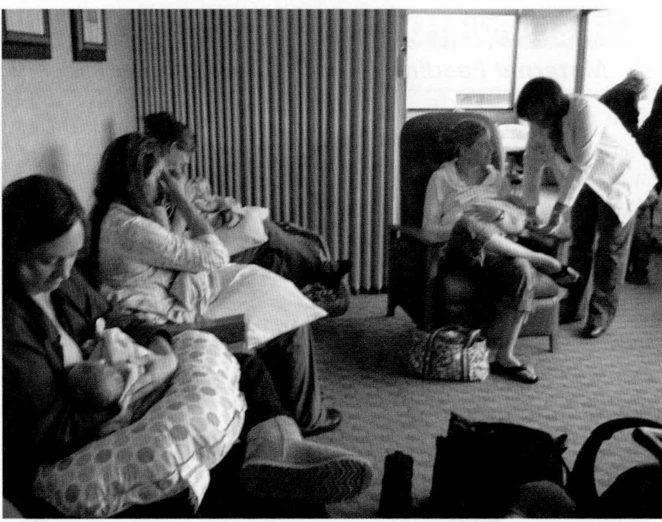

FIGURE 27-4 Breastfeeding mothers' support group with lactation consultant. (Courtesy Shannon Perry.)

Care of the breastfeeding mother and infant requires that nurses and other health care providers be knowledgeable about the benefits and basic anatomical and physiological aspects of breastfeeding. They also need to know how to help the mother with feedings and discuss interventions for common problems. Ongoing support of the mother enhances her self-confidence and promotes a satisfying and successful breastfeeding experience. Mothers should be encouraged to ask for help with breastfeeding, especially while they are in the hospital. Primiparas are likely to need the most assistance and in many facilities are routinely seen by lactation consultants. The mother needs to understand infant behaviours in relation to breastfeeding and recognize signs that the baby is ready to feed. Infants exhibit **feeding-readiness cues** or early signs of hunger. Instead of waiting to feed until the infant is crying in a distraught manner or withdrawing into sleep, the mother should attempt to breastfeed when the baby exhibits feeding cues. Feeding cues are often easiest to recognize when the newborn is held skin-to-skin (see Research Focus box). Common newborn hunger cues are as follows:

- Hand-to-mouth or hand-to-hand movements
- Sucking motions
- *Rooting reflex*—infant moves toward whatever touches the area around the mouth and attempts to suck
- Mouthing
- Flexed arms and legs with clenched fists held over chest and tummy (sometimes called *hunger posture*)

In the postpartum period interventions focus on helping the mother and the newborn initiate successful breastfeeding. An important goal is to build maternal confidence in breastfeeding. Interventions to promote successful breastfeeding include educating and assisting mothers and their partners with basics such as latch-on and positioning, cue-based feeding, signs of adequate

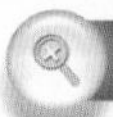

RESEARCH FOCUS

Maternal Feeding Styles and Childhood Obesity

—Pat Mahaffee Gingrich

Ask the Question

Does caregiver responsiveness to infant feeding cues have an impact on overweight in early childhood and beyond?

Search for the Evidence

Search Strategies

English-language research-based publications on infant, feeding, satiety, breastfeeding, overweight, and obesity were included.

Databases Used

Cochrane Collaborative Database, National Guidelines Clearinghouse (AHRQ), CINAHL, PubMed, UpToDate

Critically Analyze the Evidence

- Childhood obesity can have its roots in the feeding patterns established in infancy. This research field for primary prevention of obesity is new, and many infant feeding studies are currently ongoing.
- Overfeeding can impair the infant's ability to self-regulate. Infants whose caregivers are responsive to an infant's hunger and satiety (full) cues are significantly less likely to be overweight (DiSantis, Hodges, Johnson, et al., 2011).
- Discordant responsiveness occurs when the caregiver perceives that the infant cannot recognize hunger or satiety. Restrictive feeding style is associated with maternal fear of causing obesity. Pressuring feeding style is associated with caregiver concern that the infant has poor appetite and will be underweight (Gross, Mendelsohn, Fierman, et al., 2011).
- In a Latin American population a pressuring feeding style emerged as a result of belief that all infant crying or hand sucking is caused by hunger and that babies should always finish their bottles. Pressuring style is more likely in foreign-born women and women with less than a high-school education (Gross, Fierman, Mendelsohn, et al., 2010).
- Low-income, food-insecure mothers are more likely to be discordant, either restrictive or pressuring, than food-secure mothers (Gross, Mendelsohn, Fierman, et al., 2012).

Apply the Evidence: Nursing Implications

- Parental education about infant hunger and satiety cues ideally should begin in prenatal education classes and be reinforced intensively during the postpartum period. The nurse should point out the infant cues and praise the parents for appropriate responsiveness.
- Videos and printed material and warm lines should be made available to new parents. Specific suggestions about how much formula to feed initially and how voiding and stool patterns and weight gain reflect adequate nutrition can provide education guidelines.
- Assessing for familial and cultural beliefs enables the nurse to address parental and extended-family concerns. The nurse can address how the new mother might respond to well-meaning but incorrect comments from family and strangers.
- Education regarding the various newborn cries and their possible causes can reassure parents and their extended families that feeding should not be the first and only option.
- Breastfeeding is the gold standard for infant feeding because it is more difficult to overfeed.
- Nurses can advocate on a local and national level to eliminate food insecurity.

References

DiSantis, K. I., Hodges, E. A., Johnson, S. L., et al. (2011). The role of responsive feeding in overweight during infancy and toddlerhood: A systematic review. *International Journal of Obesity (London), 35*(4), 480–492.

Gross, R. S., Fierman, A. H., Mendelsohn, A. L., et al. (2010). Maternal perceptions of infant hunger, satiety, and pressuring feeding styles in an urban Latina WIC population. *Academic Pediatrics, 10*(1), 29–35.

Gross, R. S., Mendelsohn, A. L., Fierman, A. H., et al. (2011). Maternal controlling feeding styles during early infancy. *Clinical Pediatrics, 50*(12), 1125–1133.

Gross, R. S., Mendelsohn, A. L., Fierman, A. H., et al. (2012). Food insecurity and obesogenic maternal infant feeding styles and practices in low-income families. *Pediatrics, 130*(2), 254–261.

feeding, and self-care measures such as prevention of engorgement. It is important to provide the parents with a list of resources that they can contact after discharge from the hospital.

The ideal time to begin breastfeeding is within the first hour after birth, when the infant is in the quiet, alert state (WHO, 2010). Newborns without complications should be allowed to remain in direct skin-to-skin contact with the mother until the baby is able to breastfeed for the first time (Pound et al., 2012/2015). This is true both for mothers who gave birth by Caesarean and for those who gave birth vaginally. Early skin-to-skin holding and delay of infant bathing for 12 to 24 hours after birth have both been linked to the successful initiation of breastfeeding and longer exclusive breastfeeding (Bramson, Lee, Moore, et al., 2010; Moore, Anderson, Bergman, et al., 2012; Preer, Pisegna, Cook, et al., 2013). Routine procedures such as vitamin K injection, eye prophylaxis, and weighing should be delayed until the newborn has completed the first feeding.

During feeding, the infant is assessed by direct observation for feeding cues, latch-on, position and alignment, and suckling and swallowing. A breastfeeding assessment tool known as LATCH was developed by Jensen, Wallace, and Kelsey in 1994. Subsequent research has demonstrated that early LATCH scores are linked to breastfeeding success at 6 weeks of age (Kumar, Mooney, Wieser, et al., 2006; Mannel, 2011). Higher LATCH scores have been linked to higher milk intake (Altuntas, Kocak, Akkurt, et al., 2015). The tool involves assessing for the following:

L (characteristics of latch-on)
A (degree of audible swallowing)
T (type of nipple)
C (maternal comfort)
H (holding skills)

Systematic assessment of these five aspects can assist the mother and nurse to focus together on what is needed for extra support.

Positioning

For the initial feedings it can be advantageous to encourage and assist the mother to breastfeed in a semi-reclining position with the newborn lying prone, skin-to-skin on the mother's bare chest. Her body supports the baby. The mother is more relaxed, nipple pain is reduced or eliminated, and the mother has more freedom of movement to use her hands. The baby is able to use

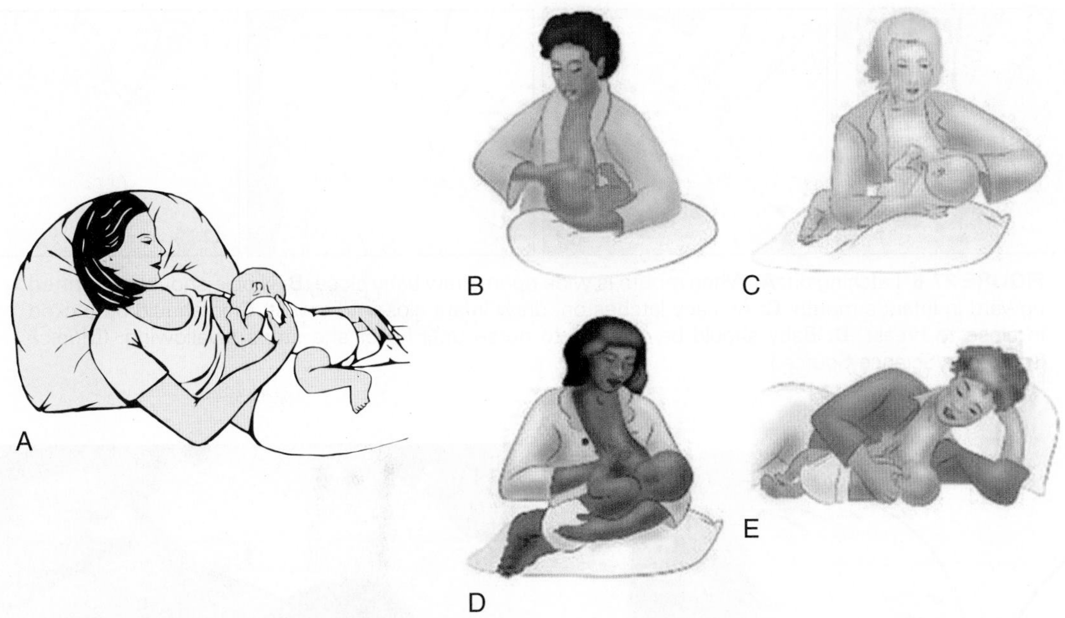

FIGURE 27-5 Breastfeeding positions. **A:** Laid-back breastfeeding (biological nurturing). **B:** Football hold. **C:** Cross-cradle. **D:** Cradling. **E:** Side-lying position. (Reprinted with permission by the Best Start Resource Centre.)

inborn reflexes to latch on to the breast and feed effectively. This approach to breastfeeding is based on the concept of "biological nurturing" (BN) (Colson, 2010, 2012). BN is described as a neurobehavioural approach to initiating breastfeeding (Colson, 2012; La Leche League International, 2014). There is no one "correct" position for BN: the mother assumes a comfortable semi-reclining position and the baby lies prone on top of the mother so that every part of the baby is facing and close to the mother; thus the term *laid-back breastfeeding* is sometimes applied to this approach (Fig. 27-5, A). Stimulation of primitive newborn reflexes occurs with this posture, aiding suckling. With BN, mothers are encouraged to be comfortable with responding to their own and their baby's natural breastfeeding instincts.

The four other positions for breastfeeding are the football or clutch hold (under the arm), cross-cradle or across the lap, cradle, and side-lying. The mother should be encouraged to use the position that most easily facilitates latch while allowing maximal comfort. The football or clutch hold is often recommended for early feedings because the mother can see the baby's mouth easily as she guides the infant on to the nipple.

Mothers who gave birth by Caesarean often prefer the football or clutch hold (Fig. 27-5, B). The cross-cradle or across-the-lap position works well for early feedings, especially with smaller babies (Fig. 27-5, C). The side-lying position allows the mother to rest while breastfeeding and is often preferred by women experiencing perineal pain and swelling (Fig. 27-5, E). Cradling is the most common breastfeeding position for infants who have learned to latch on easily and feed effectively (Fig. 27-5, D). Before discharge from the birth institution, the nurse can help the mother try all of the positions so that she will feel confident in her ability to vary positions at home.

During breastfeeding the mother should be as comfortable as possible. After arranging for privacy, the nurse might suggest that she empty her bladder and attend to other needs before starting to feed the newborn. The nurse who is assisting with breastfeeding should be at the mother's eye level. The mother holds the infant securely at the level of the breast, supported by firm pillows or folded blankets, facing toward her ("belly-to-belly"). The newborn's nose should be pointing toward the mother's nipple, avoiding "centring" the mouth over the nipple. The mother should support the baby's neck and shoulders with her hand and not push on the occiput. The baby's body is held in alignment (ears, shoulders, and hips are in a straight line) during latch and feeding.

Latch

Latch, or latch-on, is defined as placement of the infant's mouth over the nipple, areola, and breast, making a seal between the mouth and breast to create adequate suction for milk removal. In preparation for latch during early feedings it may be helpful for the mother to manually express a few drops of colostrum or milk to spread over the nipple. This lubricates the nipple and may entice the baby to open the mouth as the milk is tasted.

To facilitate latch when in an upright position, the mother may support her breast in one hand with the thumb on top and four fingers underneath at the back edge of the areola; this may be called the *C hold* (Fig. 27-6, A). She may also compress the breast slightly so that an adequate amount of breast tissue is taken into the mouth with latch. Some mothers need to support the breast during feeding for at least the first few days until the infant is adept at feeding.

The mother holds the baby close to the breast and lightly touches the infant's upper lip with her nipple, stimulating the mouth to open (rooting reflex). When the mouth is open wide and the tongue is down, the mother brings the baby in close (Fig. 27-6, B), with the head slightly tilted so that the chin touches the breast first; if the infant does not move forward

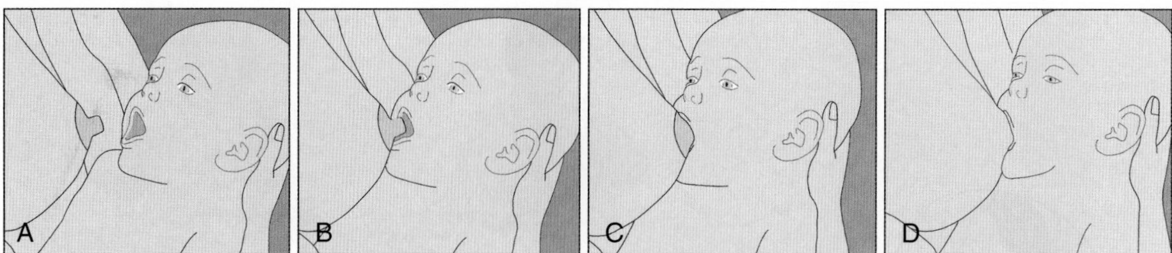

FIGURE 27-6 Latching on. **A:** When mouth is wide open, draw baby close. **B:** Nipple should be centred upward in infant's mouth. **C:** As baby latches on, draw infant closer to breast. Chin should be tucked in close to breast. **D:** Baby should be allowed to nurse until he or she stops swallowing. (Monica Schroeder/Science Source.)

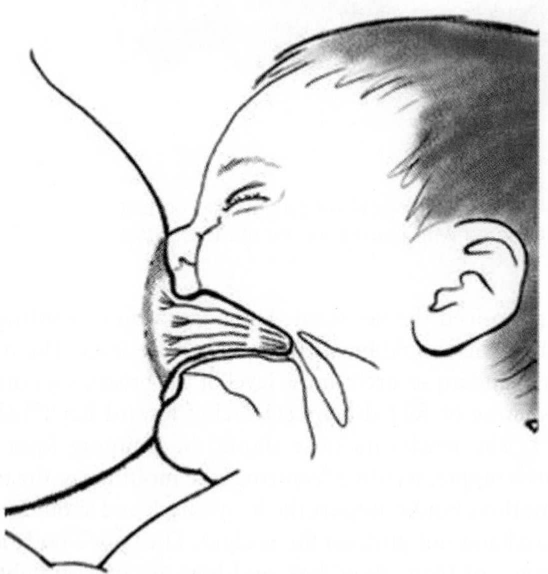

FIGURE 27-7 Correct attachment (latch-on) of infant at breast. (Courtesy Cumberland Health Authority.)

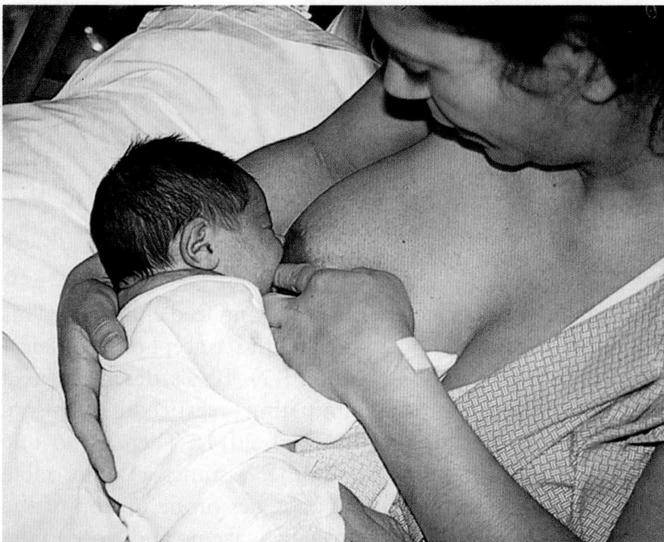

FIGURE 27-8 Removing infant from the breast. (Courtesy Marjorie Pyle, RNC, Lifecircle.)

independently, she can quickly pull the infant onto the nipple (Fig. 27-6, C). She should bring the infant to the breast, not the breast to the infant. If the breast is pushed into the infant's mouth, the infant often closes the mouth too soon and does not latch on.

The amount of the areola in the newborn's mouth with latch depends on the size of the newborn's mouth and the size of the areola and nipple. In general, the infant's mouth should cover the nipple and areola, with more of the areola visible above the baby's upper lip than below the lower lip (Fig. 27-7).

When the newborn is latched on effectively, the chin should be pressed into the breast, and the cheeks and nose may be lightly touching the breast. The mother should not pull the nipple out of the mouth when trying to create a breathing space for the newborn's nose. Depressing the breast tissue around the newborn's nose is not necessary. If the mother is worried about the infant's breathing, she can raise the newborn's hips slightly to change the angle of the infant's head at the breast. If the newborn cannot breathe, reflexes will prompt the newborn to move the head and pull back to breathe.

Once the newborn is latched on and sucking, there are signs that the feeding is going well: (1) the mother reports a firm tugging sensation on her nipple, but feels no pinching or pain; (2) the baby sucks with cheeks rounded, not dimpled; (3) the baby's jaw glides smoothly with sucking; and (4) swallowing is usually audible. Sucking creates a vacuum in the intraoral cavity as the breast is compressed between the tongue and the palate. When the infant is latched on and sucking correctly, breastfeeding is not painful. If the mother feels pinching or pain after the initial sucks or does not feel a strong tugging sensation on the nipple, the latch and positioning are evaluated. If breastfeeding is painful, the baby likely has not taken enough of the breast into the mouth, and the tongue is pinching the nipple. Repositioning usually alleviates this problem. For a small number of infants *ankyloglossia* ("tongue-tie") may lead to difficulty latching effectively, resulting in low milk intake and maternal nipple pain and trauma.

Any time the signs of adequate latch and sucking are not present, the newborn should be taken off the breast and latch attempted again. To prevent nipple trauma as the newborn is taken off the breast, the mother is instructed to break the suction by inserting her finger in the side of the infant's mouth between the gums and keeping it there until the nipple is completely out of the newborn's mouth (Fig. 27-8) (see Nursing

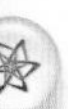

Care Plan: Breastfeeding and Infant Nutrition, available on Evolve).

Milk Ejection, or Let-Down

As the newborn begins suckling on the nipple, the milk ejection, or let-down, reflex is stimulated. Two to three "let-downs" can occur with each feeding session. The following signs indicate that milk ejection has occurred:

- The mother may feel a tingling sensation in the nipples and breasts, although some women never feel when milk ejection (let-down) occurs.
- The newborn's suck changes from quick, shallow sucks to a slower, deeper, more drawing sucking pattern.
- Audible swallowing is present as the baby sucks.
- The mother may feel thirsty and relaxed or drowsy during feedings.
- In the early days the mother feels uterine cramping.
- The opposite breast may leak milk.

Frequency of Feedings

Babies normally consume small amounts of colostrum with frequent feedings during the first 3 days of life. As the mother's transitional milk is followed by mature milk, the baby adjusts to extrauterine life, and the digestive tract is cleared of meconium, the baby's fluid intake gradually increases. Feeding patterns vary because every mother–infant dyad is unique. Breastfeeding frequency is influenced by a variety of factors, including the infant's age and weight, the infant's stomach capacity and gastric emptying time, and the storage capacity of the breast (i.e., the milk available when the breast is full).

The feeding pattern should include cue-based feedings without time restrictions, on average at least 8 to 12 times per 24 hours (International Lactation Consultant Association [ILCA], 2014; Registered Nurses' Association of Ontario [RNAO], 2003) (see Critical Thinking Case Study). Some infants breastfeed every 2 to 3 hours throughout a 24-hour period. Others cluster-feed, breastfeeding every hour or so for three to five feedings and then sleeping for 3 to 4 hours between clusters. During the first 24 to 48 hours after birth, most newborns do not awaken this often to feed. Parents need to understand that they should awaken the sleepy infant to feed at least every 3 hours during the day and at least every 4 hours at night during the first few weeks of life. Feeding frequency is determined by counting from the beginning of one feeding to the beginning of the next. Once the newborn is feeding well and gaining weight adequately, going to *demand feeding* is appropriate, in which case the infant determines the frequency of feedings. With demand feeding the infant should still receive at least eight feedings in 24 hours.

Parents should be cautioned about attempting to place newborn infants on strict feeding schedules. Infants should be fed whenever they exhibit feeding cues such as hand-to-mouth movements, rooting, and mouth and tongue movements. Crying is a late sign of hunger, and infants may become frantic when they have to wait too long to feed. Some infants will shut down or go into a deep sleep when their needs are not met. Understanding and responding to an infant's states and cues (see Chapter 25) is essential to the infant feeding interaction.

Frequent skin-to-skin holding helps mothers to notice state changes and early hunger cues and thus provide the frequent feedings required at the breast in the first few days (see Research Focus box). One recommendation is that mother and breastfeeding infant sleep in close proximity (in the same room but not in the same bed) to promote breastfeeding. The issue of bed sharing has raised concerns because of the association between a higher incidence of SIDS and bed sharing with an adult. Health Canada recommends that the safest place for any infant to sleep is in a crib within arm's reach of where the parents sleep. This practice allows for more convenient breastfeeding and at the same time prevents continuous bed sharing (Health Canada, 2010). Room sharing is recommended for at least the first 6 months. (See Chapter 26 for more discussion on SIDS.)

Duration of Feedings

The duration of breastfeeding sessions is highly variable, as the timing of milk transfer differs for each mother–baby pair. The average time for early feedings is 30 to 40 minutes, or approximately 20 minutes per breast, although instructing mothers to feed for a set number of minutes is inappropriate. It is more effective to teach mothers how to determine when an infant has finished a feeding: the infant's suck-swallow pattern has slowed, and the newborn appears content and may fall asleep or release the nipple. Other, more subtle, satiation cues include extended and relaxed fingers, arms and legs extended, back arching, or pushing away (Spietz, Johnson-Crowley, Summer, et al., 2008). As infants grow they become more efficient at breastfeeding

CRITICAL THINKING CASE STUDY

Newborn Breastfeeding

Neide is a 27-year-old married woman from Costa Rica who recently moved to Canada and has a 5-day-old, 3180 g male infant. His birth weight was 3540 g. She is being seen in the clinic for a follow-up consultation on breastfeeding and jaundice. On examination the infant is alert, fussy, and visibly jaundiced. Neide states that breastfeeding has not been going as well and she is not certain the infant is receiving enough milk. She states, in tears, that all the baby does is cry and fuss when she places him to the breast, and she wants to try formula. She recalls that yesterday the baby had one or two greenish stools and three wet diapers.

1. Evidence—Is there sufficient evidence to draw conclusions about the effectiveness of the infant's breastfeeding pattern?
2. Assumptions—What assumptions can be made about the following factors?
   a. The infant's ability to latch on
   b. Adequacy of breast milk intake
   c. The need for additional infant assessments
   d. The mother's desire to give the infant formula
   e. The mother's physical and emotional status
3. What implications and priorities for nursing care can be drawn at this time?
4. Does the evidence objectively support your conclusion?

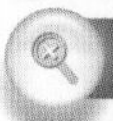

RESEARCH FOCUS

Skin-to-Skin Contact for Full-Term Newborns

—Maureen White

Ask the Question

What is the evidence for recommending skin-to-skin (STS) contact for full-term newborns?

Search for Evidence

Search Strategies

Randomized controlled trials, meta-analyses, systematic reviews, experimental research, prospective studies, and guidelines from professional and international health organizations since 2008

Databases Searched

MedLine, PubMed, Ovid CINAHL, Cochrane, and websites for the Canadian Paediatric Society (CPS), Association of Women's Health, Obstetric and Neonatal Nurses (AWHONN), Association of Breastfeeding Mothers (ABM), World Health Organization (WHO), Breastfeeding Committee for Canada (BCC), World Alliance for Breastfeeding Action (WABA)

Critically Analyze the Evidence

Health care research concerning STS contact increased in the 1970s following "kangaroo mother care" (KMC) interventions with premature infants in Bogota, Colombia. Subsequent evidence for clinical, physiological, and psychological advantages of KMC led to KMC being regarded as safe and superior care for vulnerable infants worldwide. The term *KMC* is now used chiefly to describe a method of intensive care for preterm and very-low-birth-weight infants that involves extended STS, exclusive breastfeeding, and support of the mother–infant dyad. Recent research also focuses on the impact of STS contact on full-term newborns and their parents. STS contact involves holding the baby naked in a prone position against the skin of the mother's (or partner's) chest between the breasts. The baby wears only a diaper and, if needed, a hat. A blanket or shirt can cover baby and parent.

A 2012 Cochrane Database Systematic Review examined 34 studies involving 2177 healthy mother–infant dyads and concluded that, for full-term infants, STS contact with their mothers in the first 24 hours of life had a significant positive impact on breastfeeding initiation and duration for 1 to 4 months, improved cardiorespiratory stability, and less crying, with no short- or long-term negative effects (Moore, Anderson, Bergman, et al., 2012).

Several studies concluded that longer periods of STS contact lead to increased positive impact on breastfeeding for full-term infants. STS contact in the first 3 hours of life contributes to effective suckling and increased exclusive breastfeeding rates in hospitals (Bramson, Lee, Moore, et al., 2010; Cantrill, Creedy, Cooke, et al., 2014). In addition to breastfeeding outcomes, recent studies show that STS can be an effective means of maintaining the newborn's temperature, regulating sleep–wake cycles, and minimizing the impact of painful procedures. Parents report high levels of satisfaction with STS contact, and some evidence is emerging that parent–child interaction is enhanced by STS contact (Moore et al., 2012; Saloojee, 2008). Further research is required to examine more outcome measures and best practices in STS care.

Implications for Practice

There is compelling evidence to warrant giving support to breastfeeding families in initiating STS contact following birth and encouraging frequent and prolonged STS holding in the newborn period. Such support can be achieved through education of health care providers, discussion of STS care prenatally with expectant parents, and implementation of supportive policies. In hospitals, policies should include initiating STS contact as soon as possible after each birth and limiting unnecessary interruptions for care activities—for example, delaying infant weighing and the first newborn bath.

Studies show benefits of STS care across cultures and settings; in practice, nurses need to attend to the individual responses of parents related to modesty, culture, and personal feelings (Saloojee et al., 2008). Promoting discreet ways to manage STS contact and offering practical help in positioning the baby can increase the practice of STS care.

Caesarean birth is a common barrier to initiation of STS holding within the first hour following birth because of traditional operating room practices, although many institutions are changing practice so the newborn can be placed STS with the mother or her partner. While it is important to promote early STS contact and breastfeeding for the postoperative or ill mother, when feasible, encouraging her partner to hold the newborn STS can promote stabilization of infant temperature and parental attachment. Most studies focus on breastfeeding outcomes; however, the benefits of STS contact are not limited to breastfeeding families (Erlandsson, Dsilna, Fagerberg, et al., 2007; Gouchon, Gregori, Picotto, et al., 2010). Nurses should encourage parents who are formula-feeding to practise frequent STS holding so that parents and their infants have more opportunities for attachment and to promote stable infant physiological and behavioural states.

References

Bramson, L., Lee, J. W., Moore, E., et al. (2010). Effect of early skin-to-skin mother–infant contact during the first 3 hours following birth on exclusive breastfeeding during the maternity hospital stay. *Journal of Human Lactation, 26*(2), 130–137. doi:10.1177/0890334409355779.

Cantrill, R. M., Creedy, D. K., Cooke, M., & Dykes, F. (2014). Effective suckling in relation to naked maternal-infant body contact in the first hour of life: An observation study. *BMC Pregnancy and Childbirth, 14*, 20. doi:10.1186/1471-2393-14-20.

Erlandsson, K., Dsilna, A., Fagerberg, I., & Christensson, K. (2007). Skin-to-skin care with the father after Cesarean birth and its effect on newborn crying and prefeeding behaviour. *Birth (Berkeley, Calif.), 34*(2), 105–114.

Gouchon, S., Gregori, D., Picotto, A., et al. (2010). Skin-to-skin contact after Cesarean delivery: An experimental study. *Nursing Research, 59*(2), 78–84. doi:10.1097/NNR.0b013e3181d1a8bc.

Moore, E. R., Anderson, G. C., Bergman, N., & Dowswell, T. (2012). Early skin-to-skin contact for mothers and their healthy newborn infants. *The Cochrane Database of Systematic Reviews*, (5), doi:10.1002/14651858.CD003519.pub3.

Saloojee, H. (2008). *Early skin-to-skin contact for mothers and their healthy newborn infants: RHL commentary. WHO Reproductive Health Library*. Geneva: World Health Organization. Retrieved from <http://apps.who.int/rhl/archives/hsguide2/en/index.html>.

and, consequently, the length of feedings decreases. The amount of time an infant spends breastfeeding is not a reliable indicator of the amount of milk the infant consumes because some of the time at the breast is spent in non-nutritive sucking.

The amount of intake with each feeding reflects the size of the infant's stomach; approximate increases in stomach capacity for term infants are 5 to 7 mL on day 1; 22 to 27 mL on day 3; and 60 to 81 mL on day 10. Comparing these volumes to a cherry, a walnut, and a hen's egg is one way to help parents visualize the sizes (Fig. 27-9).

If a baby seems to be feeding effectively and the urine output is adequate but the weight gain is not satisfactory, the mother may be switching to the second breast too soon. Feeding on the first breast until it softens ensures that the baby receives the higher-fat hindmilk, which usually results in increased weight gain.

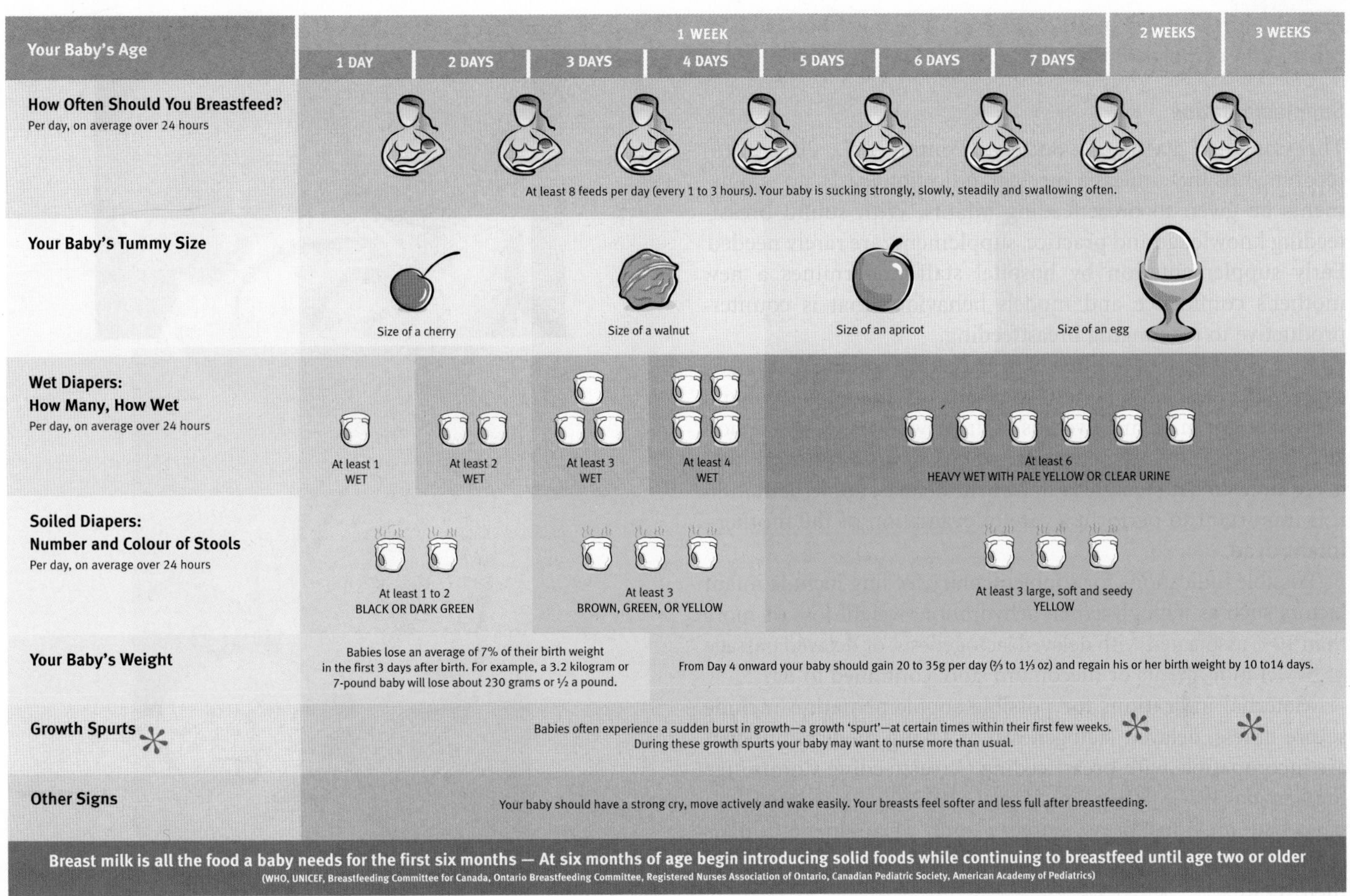

FIGURE 27-9 Guidelines for nursing mothers regarding how often to feed and how to know the baby is getting enough to eat. (Courtesy Best Start, http://beststart.org/resources/breastfeeding/pdf/breastfdeskref09.pdf. Reprinted with permission by the Best Start Resource Centre.)

Indicators of Effective Breastfeeding

One of the most common concerns of breastfeeding mothers is how to determine if the baby is getting enough milk. In the newborn period, when breastfeeding is becoming established, parents should be taught about the signs that breastfeeding is going well. Awareness of these signs helps them recognize when problems arise so they can seek appropriate assistance (see Fig. 27-9).

During the early days of breastfeeding, keeping a feeding diary can be helpful, recording the time and length of feedings and infant urine output and bowel movements. The data from the diary provide evidence of the effectiveness of breastfeeding and are useful to health care providers in assessing adequacy of feeding. Parents are instructed to take this feeding diary to the follow-up visit with the pediatric care provider.

The infant's output is highly indicative of feeding adequacy. It is important that parents are aware of the expected changes in the characteristics of urine output and bowel movements during the early newborn period. As the volume of breast milk increases, urine becomes more dilute and should be light yellow; dark, concentrated urine can be associated with inadequate intake and possible dehydration. (**Note**: Infants with jaundice often have darker urine as bilirubin is excreted.) Infants should have at least six sufficiently wet diapers (light yellow urine) every 24 hours after day 5. The first 1 to 2 days after birth newborns pass meconium stools, which are greenish black, thick, and sticky. By day 3 the stools become greener, thinner, and less sticky. If the mother's mature milk has come in by day 3 or 4, the stools start to appear greenish yellow and are looser. By the end of the first week breast milk stools are yellow, soft, and seedy (they resemble a mixture of mustard and cottage cheese) (see Fig. 25-5). If an infant is still passing meconium stool by day 3 or 4, breastfeeding effectiveness and milk transfer should be assessed.

Infant should have at least three stools (quarter-size or larger) per day for the first month. Some babies stool with every feeding. The stooling pattern gradually changes; breastfed infants can continue to stool more than once per day or they may stool only every 2 or 3 days or even longer. As long as the baby continues to gain weight and appears healthy, this decrease in the number of bowel movements is normal.

Other factors to assess include the presence of jaundice, weight loss greater than 10%, and whether the infant has regained birth weight by 10 to 14 days of age. See Box 28-2 for calculation of weight loss.

Supplementation

The Canadian Paediatric Society (Pound et al., 2012/2015) recommends that, unless a medical indication exists, no supplements be given to breastfeeding infants. With sound breastfeeding knowledge and practice, supplements are rarely needed. Early supplementation by hospital staff undermines a new mother's confidence and models behaviour that is counterproductive to prolonging breastfeeding.

If a supplement is deemed necessary, giving the baby expressed breast milk is best. Mothers can be taught to hand express breast milk and give this to the newborn (see discussion later in chapter). A small amount of colostrum is often all that is required to supplement a newborn. Before supplementation it is important to perform a careful evaluation of the mother–infant dyad.

Possible indications for supplementary feeding include infant factors such as hypoglycemia, dehydration, weight loss of more than 10% associated with delayed lactogenesis, or delayed passage of bowel movements or meconium stool continued to day 5.

Maternal indications for possible supplementation include severe illness, delayed lactogenesis, or taking medications that are incompatible with breastfeeding (Breastfeeding Committee for Canada [BCC], 2012; Pound et al., 2012/2015). Women who have had previous breast surgery such as augmentation or reduction may need to provide supplementary feedings for their infants.

Supplemental feedings may contribute to "nipple confusion" (i.e., difficulty knowing how to latch on to the breast or preferring the easy flow from an artificial nipple) and to low milk supply because the baby becomes overly full and does not breastfeed often enough. Supplementation interferes with the supply-meets-demand cycle of milk production. The parents may interpret the newborn's willingness to take a bottle to mean that the mother's milk supply is inadequate. They need to know that a newborn will automatically suck from a bottle, as the artificial nipple triggers the suck-swallow reflex.

Bottles and Pacifiers

Newborns may become confused going from breast to bottle or bottle to breast when breastfeeding is first initiated. Breastfeeding and bottle-feeding require different oral motor skills. The ways newborns use their tongues, jaw, and lips, as well as the swallowing patterns, are very different. It is recommended that parents avoid giving bottles until breastfeeding is well established, usually at least after 3 to 4 weeks.

If supplemental feeding is needed, nurses or lactation consultants can help parents use supplemental nursing devices. This allows the baby to be supplemented with expressed breast milk or infant formula while still breastfeeding (Fig. 27-10). Infants can also be fed with a spoon, dropper, cup, or syringe. If parents choose to use bottles, a slow-flow nipple is recommended. Although some parents combine breastfeeding and bottle-feeding, many babies never take a bottle and go directly from the breast to a cup.

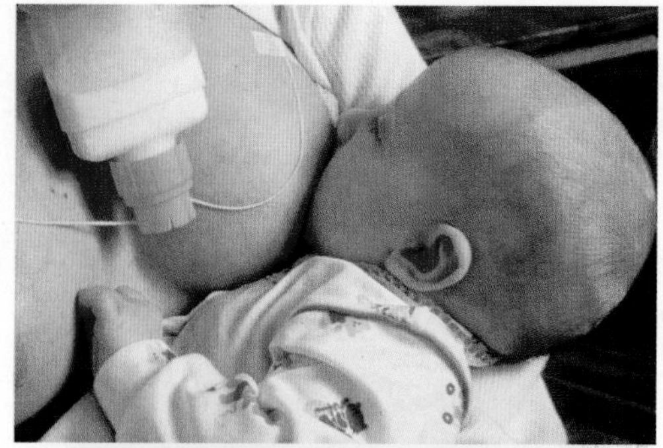

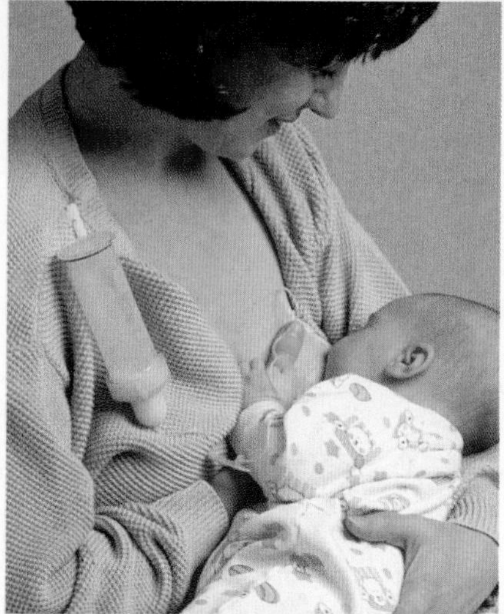

FIGURE 27-10 Supplemental nursing device. (Copyright © 2013 Medela.)

The Canadian Paediatric Society (Ponti & CPS, 2003/2016) recommends that health care providers recognize pacifier use as a parental choice determined by the needs of their child and that pacifier use be delayed until breastfeeding is established. Pacifier use should not replace actual feeding or suckling. Prohibiting early pacifier use will not ensure an increase in the length of breastfeeding, but it may help with promoting milk production (Jaafar, Jahanfar, Angolkar, et al., 2012). The emphasis should be on allowing the infant to control the pace, frequency, and termination of feeding, instead of allowing the pacifier (or anything else) to become the focus of the interaction. The CPS recommends that pacifiers not be routinely discouraged, as the current evidence suggests a decreased risk of SIDS associated with their use (Ponti & CPS, 2003/2016). The American Academy of Pediatrics (2011/2015) recommends that parents consider offering a pacifier at nap time and bedtime, as there is reported to be a protective effect against the incidence of SIDS that persists through the sleep period even if the pacifier falls out of the infant's mouth.

Special Considerations

Sleepy newborn. During the first few days of life, some newborns need to be awakened for feedings. If the infant is awakened from a sound sleep, attempts at feeding are more likely to be unsuccessful. Babies are more likely to feed if they are awakened from a light or active sleep state. Signs that the

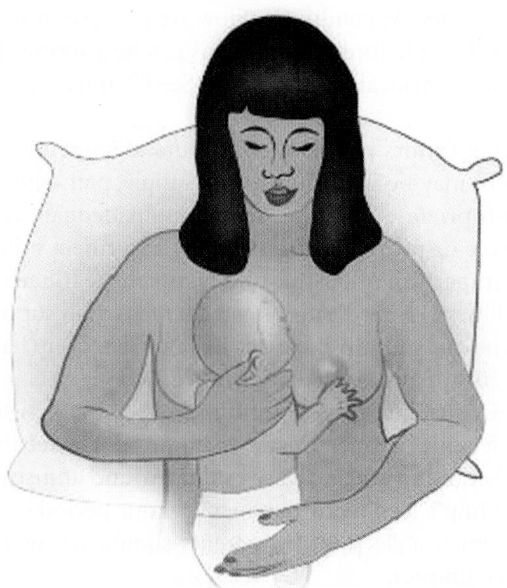

FIGURE 27-11 Infant and mother skin-to-skin. Infant is placed between the mother's breasts. (Reprinted with permission by the Best Start Resource Centre.)

infant is in this sleep state are movements of the eyelids, body movements, and making sounds while sleeping. Unwrapping or undressing the newborn, changing the diaper, sitting the infant upright, talking to the newborn with variable pitch, gently massaging the infant's chest or back, and stroking the arms, legs, palms, or soles may bring the newborn to an alert state. Placing the sleeping infant skin-to-skin with the mother's chest may also stimulate a state change; she can move the infant to the breast when feeding-readiness cues are apparent (Fig. 27-11).

Fussy newborn. In the early days at home some babies start crying soon after they are put in their beds and are asking to be comforted (see Patient Teaching box). Other infants sometimes awaken from sleep crying frantically. Although they may be hungry, they cannot focus on feeding until they are calmed. Calming techniques include holding him or her close, talking soothingly, and allowing the infant to suck on a clean finger until calm enough to latch on to the breast. Placing the baby skin-to-skin with the mother can be very effective in calming a fussy infant. Fussiness during feeding can be the result of birth injury, such as bruising of the head or fractured clavicle. Changing the feeding position can help alleviate this problem.

Infants who were suctioned extensively or intubated at birth can demonstrate an aversion to oral stimulation. The baby may scream and stiffen if anything approaches the mouth. Parents need to spend time holding and cuddling the baby before attempting to breastfeed.

An infant can become fussy and appear discontented when sucking if the nipple does not extend far enough into the mouth. The feeding can begin with well-organized sucks and swallows, but the infant soon begins to pull off the breast and cry. The mother should support her breast throughout the feeding so the nipple stays in the same position as the feeding proceeds and the breast softens.

PATIENT TEACHING

Baby's Second Night

You've made it through your first 24 hours as a new mom. Maybe you have other children, but you are a new mom all over again ... and now it's your baby's second night.

All of a sudden, your little one discovers that he's no longer back in the warmth and comfort—though a bit crowded—womb where he spent the last 9 months—and it is SCARY out here! He isn't hearing your familiar heartbeat, the swooshing of the placental arteries, the soothing sound of your lungs, or the comforting gurgling of your intestines. Instead, he's in a crib, swaddled in a diaper, a tee-shirt, a hat, and a blanket. All sorts of people have been handling him, and he's not yet become accustomed to the new noises, lights, sounds, and smells. He has found one thing though, and that's his voice ... and you find that each time you take him off the breast, where he comfortably drifted off to sleep, and put him in the bassinet—he protests, loudly!

In fact, each time you put him back on the breast he nurses for a little bit and then goes to sleep. As you take him off and put him back to bed—he cries again ... and starts rooting around, looking for you. This goes on—seemingly for hours. A lot of moms are convinced it is because their milk isn't "in" yet, and the baby is starving. However, it isn't that, but the baby's sudden awakening to the fact that the most comforting and comfortable place for him to be is at the breast. It's the closest to "home" he can get. It seems that this is pretty universal among babies; lactation consultants all over the world have noticed the same thing.

So, what do you do? When he drifts off to sleep at the breast after a good feed, break the suction and take your nipple gently out of his mouth. Don't move him except to gently slide him into an upright neutral position with his head to the side. Don't try and burp him—just snuggle with him until he falls into a deep sleep where he won't be disturbed by being moved. Babies go into a light sleep state (REM) first, and then cycle in and out of REM and deep sleep about every half-hour or so. If he starts to root and act as though he wants to go back to breast, that's fine—this is his way of settling and comforting. During deep sleep, the baby's breathing is very quiet and regular, and there is no movement beneath his eyelids.

Another helpful hint: his hands were his best friends in utero ... he could suck on his thumb or his fingers anytime he was the slightest bit disturbed or uncomfortable. And all of a sudden he's had them taken away from him and someone has put mittens on him! He has no way of soothing himself with those mittens on. Babies need to touch—to feel—and even his touch on your breast will increase your oxytocin levels, which will help boost your milk supply! So take the mittens off and loosen his blanket so he can get to his hands. He might scratch himself, but it will heal very rapidly—after all, he had fingernails when he was inside you, and no one put mittens on him then!

By the way—this might happen every once in a while at home too, particularly if you've changed his environment, such as going to the doctor's, to church, to the mall, or to the grandparents! Don't let it throw you—sometimes babies just need some extra snuggling at the breast, because for the baby, the breast is "home."

Fussiness may be related to GI distress (i.e., cramping and gas pains). It can occur in response to an occasional feeding of infant formula or be related to something the mother ingested. Most mothers are able to eat a normal diet without causing GI distress to the breastfeeding baby. Persistent crying or refusing

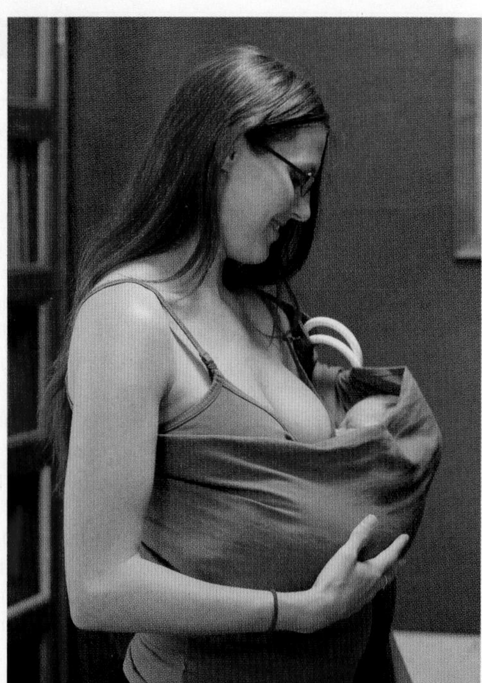

FIGURE 27-12 Baby breastfeeding while in sling. (Courtesy Julie Perry Nelson.)

to breastfeed can indicate illness. Parents should be instructed to notify the health care provider if either circumstance occurs (see Family-Centred Teaching box in Chapter 26, "The Period of PURPLE Crying®", p. 716).

Some mothers find that their babies are less fussy when placed in a sling or carrier. Some slings make it easy to breastfeed without removing the baby from the sling (Fig. 27-12).

Slow weight gain. Newborns may lose up to 10% of their birth weight during the first 3 to 5 days after birth; this is mostly water weight acquired in utero. Thereafter, they should begin to gain weight at the rate of 110 to 200 g/week, or 20 to 28 g/day. The breastfed infant who loses more than 10% of birth weight requires careful assessment regarding feeding behaviours and maternal milk supply. The infant who continues to lose weight after 5 days, does not regain birth weight by 2 weeks, or whose weight is below the tenth percentile by 1 month should be evaluated and closely monitored by a health care provider.

At times, slow weight gain is related to inadequate breastfeeding. Feedings can be short or infrequent, or the infant may be latching on incorrectly or sucking ineffectively or inefficiently. Other causes are illness, infection, malabsorption, or circumstances that increase the newborn's energy needs, such as congenital heart disease, cystic fibrosis, or simply being small for gestational age. However, newborns gain weight in differing patterns, and one should not assume that the newborn is ill just because weight gain is not the same as that of another breastfed or bottle-fed infant. Breastfed infants and formula-fed infants have different patterns of growth in the first year. Use of the WHO growth charts is recommended for appropriate growth monitoring (Denne, 2015; Health Canada et al., 2012) (see Appendix C). Slow weight gain must be differentiated from failure to thrive; this can be a serious problem that warrants medical intervention. (See Chapter 35, Failure to thrive.)

Maternal factors may also contribute to slow infant weight gain. There may be inadequate milk supply, pain with feeding, or inappropriate timing of feedings. Inadequate glandular breast tissue or previous breast surgery may affect milk supply. Severe intrapartum or postpartum hemorrhage (Sheehan's syndrome), illness, or medications can decrease milk supply. Stress and fatigue also negatively affect milk production (Lauwers & Swisher, 2011; Lawrence & Lawrence, 2015).

In most instances the solution to slow weight gain is to increase feeding frequency and to improve the feeding technique. Positioning and latch are evaluated, and adjustments are made. Adding a feeding or two in a 24-hour period can help. If the problem is a sleepy baby, parents should be instructed in waking techniques.

Using alternate breast massage during feedings can help increase the amount of milk going to the infant. With this technique, the mother massages her breast from the chest wall to the nipple whenever the baby has sucking pauses. This technique also can increase the fat content of the milk, which aids in weight gain.

When newborns are calorie deprived and need supplementation, the extra breast milk or formula can be given with a spoon or cup, syringe, a supplemental nursing device (see Fig. 27-10), or a bottle. If there are latch-on problems, it is best to avoid bottles and pacifiers. In most cases, supplementation is needed only for a short time until the newborn gains weight and is feeding adequately. Most breastfeeding problems require simple solutions; a lactation consultant can help by developing a feeding plan with the mother.

Jaundice. **Jaundice** and **hyperbilirubinemia** in the newborn are discussed in detail in Chapter 26. Breastfeeding infants can develop *early-onset jaundice* or *breastfeeding-associated jaundice,* which is associated with insufficient feeding and infrequent stooling. Colostrum has a natural laxative effect and promotes early passage of meconium. Bilirubin is excreted from the body primarily through the intestines. Infrequent stooling allows bilirubin in the stool to be resorbed into the infant's system, thus increasing bilirubin levels (Blackburn, 2013). To prevent early-onset, breastfeeding-associated jaundice, newborns should be breastfed frequently during the first several days of life. Increased frequency of feedings is associated with decreased bilirubin levels.

To treat early-onset jaundice, breastfeeding is evaluated in terms of frequency and length of feedings, positioning, latch, and milk transfer. Factors such as a sleepy or lethargic infant or maternal breast engorgement can interfere with effective breastfeeding and should be corrected. If the infant's intake of milk needs to be increased, a supplemental feeding device can deliver additional breast milk or formula while the infant is nursing. Bilirubin levels should be closely monitored (see Chapter 26).

Late-onset jaundice or *breast milk jaundice* affects a small number of breastfed infants and develops between 5 and 10 days of age. Affected infants are typically thriving, gaining weight, and stooling normally; all pathological causes of jaundice have been ruled out. In the presence of other risk factors, hyperbilirubinemia can be severe enough to require phototherapy. In most cases of breast milk jaundice no intervention is necessary.

Any breastfeeding infant who develops jaundice should be evaluated carefully for weight loss greater than 7%, decreased milk intake, infrequent stooling (fewer than three stools per day by day 4), and decreased urine output (fewer than four to six wet diapers per day). Bilirubin levels should be assessed by serum testing or transcutaneous monitoring. The CPS recommendations on management of hyperbilirubinemia include professional breastfeeding support and continued exclusive breastfeeding during phototherapy treatment (Barrington, Sankaran, & CPS, 2007/2016) (see Chapter 26).

Preterm infants. Human milk is the ideal food for preterm infants, with benefits that are unique to the individual preterm infant in addition to those received by healthy term infants. Breast milk enhances retinal maturation in the preterm infant and improves neurocognitive outcomes; it also decreases the risk of necrotizing enterocolitis. Greater physiological stability occurs with breastfeeding than with bottle-feeding (Lawrence & Lawrence, 2015).

Initially, breast milk for preterm infants contains higher concentrations of energy, protein, sodium, chloride, potassium, iron, and magnesium than term milk. It is more similar to term milk by approximately 4 to 6 weeks. Depending on gestational age and physical condition, many preterm infants are capable of breastfeeding for at least some feedings each day. Mothers of preterm infants who are not able to breastfeed their infants should begin pumping their breasts as soon as possible after birth with a hospital-grade electric pump (Fig. 27-13). Pumping frequency depends on the mother's breastfeeding goals but may be recommended 8 to 10 times every 24 hours to establish the milk supply. These women must be taught proper handling and storage of breast milk to minimize bacterial contamination and growth. Kangaroo care (skin-to-skin contact) is advised until the baby is able to breastfeed and while breastfeeding is established because it enhances milk production (Hurst & Meier, 2010; Lauwers & Swisher, 2011).

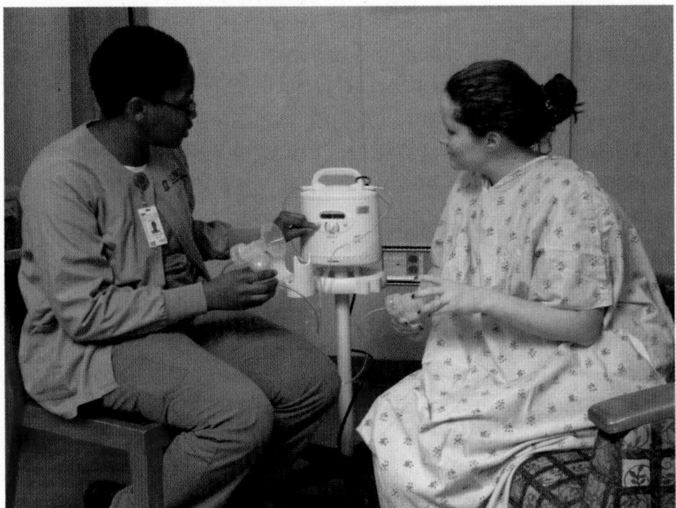

FIGURE 27-13 Nurse explains use of hospital-grade electric breast pump to new mother. (Courtesy Kathryn Alden.)

Mothers of preterm infants often receive specific emotional benefits in breastfeeding or providing breast milk for their babies. They find reward in knowing that they can provide the healthiest nutrition for the infant and experience enhanced feelings of closeness to the infant through breastfeeding.

Late preterm infants. Newborns born at 34 0/7 to 36 6/7 weeks of gestation are categorized as *late preterm infants.* These newborns are at risk for feeding difficulties because of their low energy stores and high energy demands (ABM Protocol Committee, 2011a; Cooper, Holditch-Davis, Verklan et al., 2012). They tend to be sleepy, with minimal and short wakeful periods. Late preterm infants often tire easily while feeding and have a weak suck and low tone; these factors can contribute to inadequate milk intake. Early and extended skin-to-skin contact promotes breastfeeding and helps prevent hypothermia. Because these infants are more prone to positional apnea than term infants, mothers are advised to use the clutch (under the arm or football) hold for feeding and avoid flexing the head, which can impede breathing. Often supplementation is needed; expressed breast milk is the optimal supplement, preferably at the breast using a supplemental feeding device (see Fig. 27-10) (Cleveland, 2010).

Breastfeeding multiple infants. Breastfeeding is especially beneficial to twins, triplets, and other higher-order multiples because of the immunological and nutritional advantages and the opportunity for the mother to interact with each baby frequently. Most mothers are capable of producing an adequate milk supply for multiple infants. Parenting multiples can be overwhelming; mothers and their husbands or partners need extra support and help to learn how to manage feedings (Fig. 27-14).

Caring for twins takes planning and organization, but with breastfeeding feedings are always ready and no one has to wash bottles and prepare formula; some mothers can feed both babies at once. The mother with twins will need extra nourishment for herself (200 to 500 kcal/day for each infant).

A typical pattern is that each newborn feeds from one breast per feeding, usually for about 20 to 30 minutes. Some mothers assign each newborn a breast; others switch infants from one breast to the other, either on a schedule or randomly. The mother may find it easiest to use a modified demand feeding schedule; that is, feeding the first infant who wakes up and then waking the second infant for feeding.

During the early weeks, parents may find it helpful to keep a record of feeding times and of which breast was used first by which infant. If one twin nurses more vigorously than the other, that infant should be alternated between breasts to equalize breast stimulation.

If the mother wants to feed the newborns simultaneously, she may wish to experiment with positions. For example, one newborn can be held in the football hold and the other in the cradle hold, or the newborns can each be held in the football

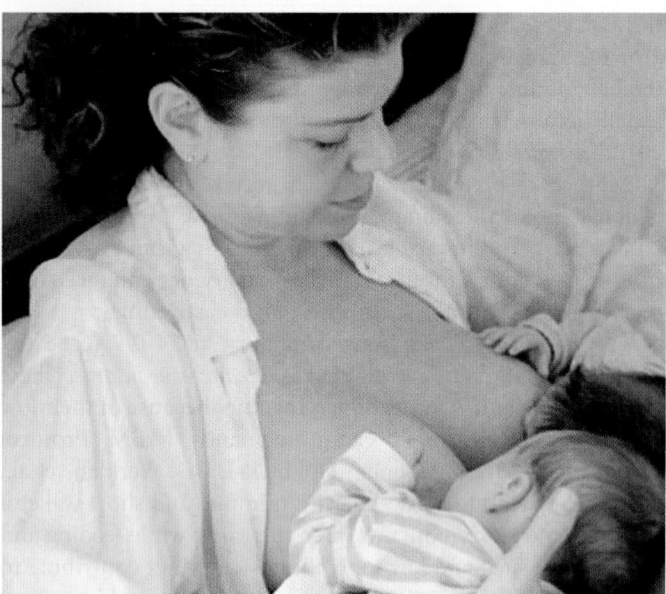

FIGURE 27-14 Breastfeeding twins. (© Beth Dixson/Alamy Stock Photo.)

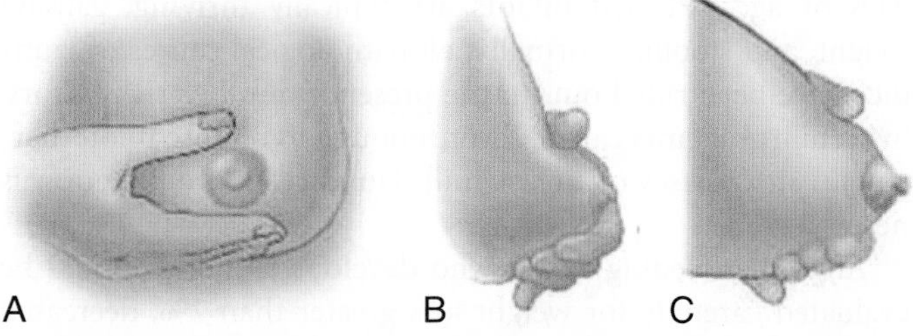

FIGURE 27-15 Hand expression. **A:** One hand is placed on breast with thumb above and fingers below. Press back toward chest. **B:** Gently compress the breast while rolling thumb and fingers forward. Maintain steady, light pressure while milk is flowing. **C:** Relax. Rotate hand to all sections of breast. (Reprinted with permission by the Best Start Resource Centre.)

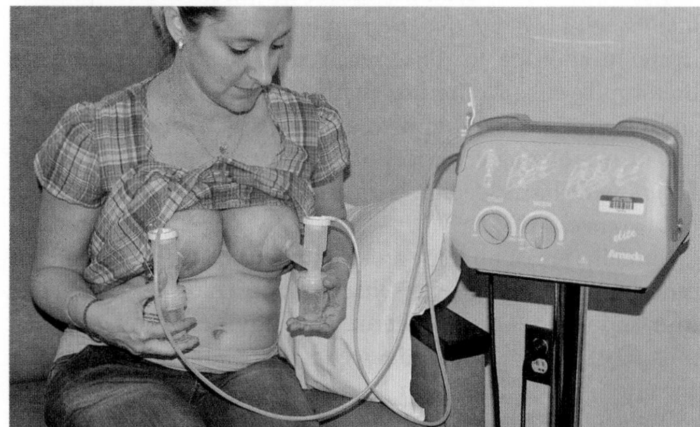

FIGURE 27-16 Bilateral breast pumping. (Courtesy Cheryl Briggs, BSN, RNC-NIC.)

position. Each infant can be supported on firm pillows while in the football hold.

Expressing and Storing Breast Milk

Breast milk expression is a common practice, typically performed to obtain breast milk for someone other than the mother to feed to the baby. It is most often associated with maternal employment. In some situations expression of breast milk is necessary or desirable, such as when engorgement occurs, when the mother's nipples are sore or damaged, when the mother and baby are separated as in the case of a preterm infant who remains in the hospital after the mother is discharged, or when the mother leaves the infant with a caregiver and will not be present for feeding. Some women express milk to have an emergency supply. Some women choose to pump exclusively, providing breast milk for their infants but never allowing the baby to suckle at the breast. Because pumping and hand expression are rarely as effective as an infant in removing milk from the breast, the milk supply should never be judged on the basis of volume expressed.

Hand expression. All mothers should be instructed in hand expression. After thoroughly washing her hands, the mother places one hand on her breast at the edge of the areola (Fig. 27-15, A). With her thumb above and fingers below, she presses in toward her chest wall and gently compresses the breast while rolling her thumb and fingers forward (Fig. 27-15, B). She repeats these motions rhythmically until the milk begins to flow. The mother simply maintains a steady, light pressure while the milk is flowing easily (Fig. 27-15, C). The thumb and fingers should not pinch the breast or slip down to the nipple. The hand should be rotated to reach all sections of each breast. After expressing milk from the second breast, she should return to the first breast and then repeat the procedure until all readily available milk is expressed. Applying warm moist towels to the breasts and gently massaging can aid in stimulating the MER (Riordan & Hoover, 2010).

Mechanical milk expression (pumping). For most women it is recommended that pumping be initiated only after the milk supply is well established and the infant is latching and breastfeeding well. However, when breastfeeding is delayed after birth, such as when babies are ill or preterm, mothers should begin pumping with an electric breast pump as soon as possible and continue to pump regularly until the infant is able to breastfeed effectively.

There are numerous ways to approach pumping. Some women pump when they first wake up in the morning or after feedings. Others choose to pump one breast while the baby is feeding from the other; this is usually done if the baby typically feeds from only one breast at each feeding. Double pumping (pumping both breasts at the same time) saves time and can stimulate the milk supply more effectively than single pumping (Fig. 27-16). The amount of milk obtained when pumping depends on the type of pump being used, the time of day, the time since the baby breastfed, the mother's milk supply, how practiced she is at pumping, and her comfort level (pumping is

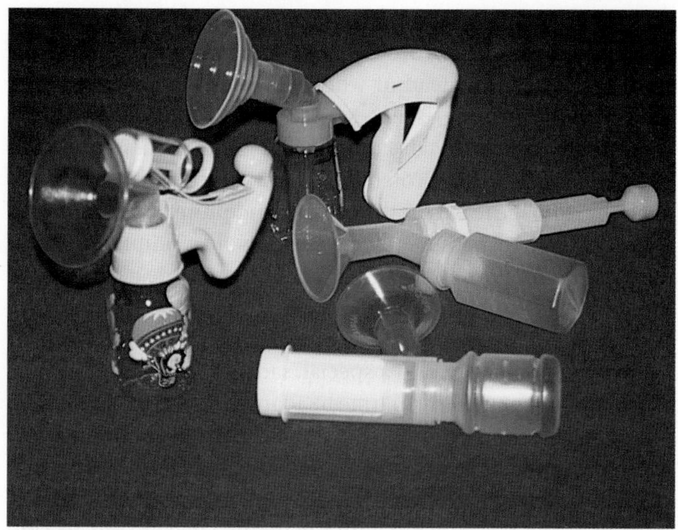

FIGURE 27-17 Manual breast pumps. (Courtesy Marjorie Pyle, RNC.)

PATIENT TEACHING

Breast Milk Storage Guidelines for Home Use for Full-Term Infants

- Before expressing or pumping breast milk, wash your hands.
- Containers for storing milk should be washed in hot, soapy water and rinsed thoroughly; they can also be washed in a dishwasher. If the water supply may not be clean, boil containers after washing. Plastic bags designed specifically for breast milk storage can be used for short-term storage (<72 hours).
- Write the date of expression on container before storing milk. A waterproof label is best.
- Store milk in serving sizes of 60 to 120 mL to prevent waste.
- Storing breast milk in the refrigerator or freezer with other food items is acceptable.
- When storing milk in a refrigerator or freezer, place containers in the middle or back of the freezer, not on the door.
- When filling a storage container that will be frozen, fill only three-quarters full, allowing space at the top of the container for expansion.
- To thaw frozen breast milk, place container in the refrigerator for gradual thawing or under warm, running water for quicker thawing. Never boil or microwave.
- Milk thawed in the refrigerator can be stored for 24 hours.
- Thawed breast milk should never be refrozen.
- Shake milk container before feeding baby and test the temperature of the milk on the inner aspect of your wrist.
- Any unused milk left in the bottle after feeding is discarded.

Human Milk Storage Guidelines for Full-Term Infants

Location of Storage	Temperature	Recommended Safe Duration for Storage
Room temperature	16–29°C (60–85°F)	3–4 hours optimal 6–8 hours acceptable*
Refrigerator	4°C (39°F) or lower	72 hours optimal 5–8 days acceptable*
Freezer	Less than −4°C (24°F)	2 weeks in a freezer compartment inside a refrigerator 6 months optimal in a freezer with separate door 12 months acceptable

*Under very clean conditions.

Modified from Academy of Breastfeeding Medicine Protocol Committee. (2010). ABM clinical protocol no. 8: Human milk storage information for home use for full-term infants, *Breastfeeding Medicine, 5*(3), 127–130.

uncomfortable for some women). Breast milk may vary in colour and consistency, depending on the time of day, the infant's age, and foods the mother has eaten.

Types of pumps. Many types of breast pumps are available, varying in price and effectiveness. Before purchasing or renting a breast pump, the mother will benefit from counselling by a nurse or lactation consultant to determine which pump best suits her needs. The flange (funnel-shaped device that fits over the nipple or areola) should fit the nipple to prevent nipple pain, trauma, and possible reduction in milk supply. Mothers are advised to use the lowest suction setting on electric pumps, increasing gradually if needed. Breast massage before and during pumping can increase the amount of milk obtained.

Manual or hand pumps are the least expensive pumps and can be the most appropriate when portability and quietness of operation are important (Fig. 27-17).

Full-service electric pumps, or hospital-grade pumps, have similar sucking action and pressure to that of the breastfeeding infant. When breastfeeding is delayed after birth (e.g., the infant is preterm or ill), or when mother and baby are separated for lengthy periods, these pumps are most appropriate (see Fig. 27-13). Electric, self-cycling double pumps are efficient and easy to use. Because hospital-grade breast pumps are very heavy and expensive, portable versions of these pumps are available to rent for home use.

Electric self-cycling double pumps are efficient and easy to use. They are designed for working mothers. Some of these pumps come with carry bags containing coolers to store pumped milk.

Smaller electric or battery-operated pumps are typically used when pumping is performed occasionally, but some models are satisfactory for working mothers or others who pump on a regular basis.

Storage of breast milk. Mothers who express and feed breast milk to their infants need to be educated about safe practices for handling, storing, and feeding milk. Attention to hand hygiene and proper cleaning of equipment can reduce the risk of bacterial contamination. This is especially important when mothers are providing milk for preterm or ill newborns (Hurst & Meier, 2010; Labiner-Wolfe & Fein, 2013). Guidelines for storing expressed breast milk for a healthy term infant are listed in the Patient Teaching box.

The preferred containers for long-term storage of breast milk have hard sides, such as hard plastic or glass with an air-tight seal. Flexible polyethylene bags are not recommended for long-term milk storage (>72 hours) because there is a greater chance of leakage and loss of immune cells (Tully & Jones, 2010).

SAFETY ALERT

Breast milk is never thawed or heated in a microwave oven. Microwaving does not heat evenly and can cause encapsulated boiling bubbles to form in the centre of the liquid, which may not be detected when drops of milk are checked for temperature. Babies have sustained severe burns to the mouth, throat, and upper GI tract as a result of microwaved milk. In addition, microwaving significantly decreases the anti-infective properties and vitamin C content. The safety of low-temperature microwaving is questionable (Lawrence & Lawrence, 2015).

Being Away From the Infant

Many women successfully combine breastfeeding with employment, school, or other commitments. If feedings are missed, the milk supply may be affected. Some women's bodies adjust the milk supply to the times she is with the infant for feedings. Other mothers must pump while away or their supply diminishes rapidly. Mothers should be encouraged to set realistic goals for employment and breastfeeding. Many mothers find that a program of breast pumping when away from home and bottle-feeding the infant the expressed milk with or without formula supplementation is successful. Although feeding the infant at home may occur on a demand basis, pumping milk away from home may be needed every 3 to 4 hours to maintain an adequate supply. Lactation rooms that provide space and privacy for pumping are available at many worksites and on college and university campuses.

In addition to efficient breast pumping, mothers also need child care by a trusted individual or agency and support and assistance from significant others. As with all breastfeeding mothers, these women must have proper nutrition and rest for adequate lactation. Careful planning, flexibility, and employer support are key to successful breastfeeding by employed mothers. Canadian maternity benefits permit a new mother who has been employed to have up to 50 weeks of paid leave. Some provinces extend these benefits to self-employed mothers.

Weaning

Weaning is initiated when babies are introduced to foods other than breast milk and concludes with the last breastfeeding. Gradual weaning over weeks or months is easier for mothers and infants than abrupt weaning. Abrupt weaning is likely to be distressing for mother and baby and physically uncomfortable for the mother.

Weaning is initiated by either the infant or the mother. With infant-led weaning the infant moves at his or her own pace in omitting feedings, which usually facilitates a gradual decrease in the mother's milk supply. Mother-led weaning means that the mother decides which feedings to drop. This approach is most easily undertaken by omitting the feeding of least interest to the baby or the one through which the infant is most likely to sleep. Every few days thereafter the mother drops another feeding until the infant is gradually weaned from the breast (Lauwers & Swisher, 2011).

Infants can be weaned directly from the breast to a cup. If the infant is weaned before 1 year of age, iron-fortified formula should be offered instead of whole cow's milk.

If abrupt weaning is necessary, breast **engorgement** often occurs. To relieve the discomfort the mother can take mild analgesics such as ibuprofen, wear a supportive bra, apply ice packs or cabbage leaves to the breasts, and pump small amounts if needed. When possible, it is best to avoid pumping because the breasts should remain full enough to promote a decrease in the milk supply (Lauwers & Swisher, 2011).

Weaning is often a very emotional time for mothers; many believe that it is the end to a special, satisfying relationship with the infant and benefit from time to adapt to the changes. Sudden weaning can evoke feelings of guilt and disappointment. Some women go through a grieving period after weaning. Nurses and others can help the mother by discussing other ways to continue this nurturing relationship with the infant, such as skin-to-skin contact while bottle-feeding or holding and cuddling the baby. Support from the father or partner and other family members is essential at this time.

Milk Banking

For those infants who cannot be breastfed but who also cannot survive except on human milk, banked donor milk is critically important. Because of the anti-infective and growth-promoting properties of human milk, as well as its superior nutrition, donor milk is used in many neonatal intensive care units for preterm or sick infants when the mother's own milk is not available. Donor milk is also used therapeutically in other situations, such as for infants with short gut syndrome, infants with IgA deficiency who are not breastfed, and older children or adults with IgA deficiency (Tully & Jones, 2010).

Pasteurized donor milk is recommended for preterm infants if the mother's own milk is not available despite substantial lactation support (AAP Section on Breastfeeding, 2012). The value of donor milk is further emphasized by the ABM in their recommendation of pasteurized donor milk for the healthy term and preterm infant when the mother's milk is not available (ABM Protocol Committee, 2009).

The Human Milk Banking Association of North America (HMBANA) (see Additional Resources at the end of the chapter) has established annually reviewed guidelines for the operation of donor human milk banks. The milk banks collect, screen, process, and distribute milk donated by lactating mothers. All donors are screened both by interview and serologically for communicable diseases. Donor milk is stored frozen until it is heat processed to kill potential pathogens; it is then refrozen for storage until it is dispensed for use. The heat processing adds a level of protection for the recipient that is not possible with any other donor tissue or organ. Banked milk is dispensed only by prescription. A fee is charged by the bank for processing, but the HMBANA guidelines prohibit payment to donors. At the present time, there are four human milk banks in Canada, which are located in Vancouver, Calgary, Montreal, and Toronto (Héma-Québec, 2014; HMBANA, 2016). The CPS is advocating for more centres to open across the country, as the health benefits, especially for the very preterm baby, are considerable.

Care of the Mother

Nutrition. In general, the breastfeeding mother should eat a healthy, well-balanced diet. Caloric intake during lactation should be sufficient to achieve the goal of balancing energy intake and expenditure. Most women are able to achieve that balance by adding 350 to 500 calories per day, which is equivalent to approximately two to three extra servings from *Eating Well With Canada's Food Guide* (see Appendix A). Even with the increased caloric intake, women who are breastfeeding tend to lose weight more quickly than those who are formula-feeding.

Medications or diets that promote weight loss are not recommended for breastfeeding mothers. Rapid loss of large amounts of weight can be detrimental, given that fat-soluble contaminants to which the mother has been exposed are stored in body fat reserves and these can be released into the breast milk. Another potential consequence of weight loss is reduced milk production. For most women a weight loss of 1 to 2 kg (2.2 to 4.4 lb) per month is safe; however, if weight loss exceeds this amount, careful evaluation of infant weight and feeding pattern is recommended. The mother's diet is also evaluated. See Chapter 12 for further discussion regarding nutrition during lactation.

No specific foods that the breastfeeding mother must consume or avoid have been identified. In most cases the woman can consume a normal diet, according to her personal preferences and cultural practices. Women may be advised to continue taking their prenatal vitamins as long as they are breastfeeding.

It is recommended that breastfeeding mothers consume 200 to 300 mg of the ω-3 long-chain polyunsaturated fatty acids (DHA) daily. A DHA supplement and a multivitamin may be needed for women who are undernourished and those on vegan diets (AAP Section on Breastfeeding, 2012).

Mothers are encouraged to drink fluids in response to thirst (women often report feeling thirsty when they are breastfeeding). If her urine appears light yellow (like lemonade), she is probably consuming adequate fluids. Increased consumption of water or other fluids by the mother does not increase milk supply, and overhydration can actually decrease milk production.

Exercise. There is no reason for a breastfeeding woman to restrict her physical activity. Women continue activities such as hiking, jogging, swimming, and aerobics with no detrimental effect on milk supply or composition. Women often find that they are more comfortable if they engage in exercise soon after breastfeeding, when their breasts are as empty as possible. Wearing a well-designed, supportive bra may also help.

Rest. The breastfeeding mother should rest as much as possible, especially in the first 1 to 2 weeks after birth. Fatigue, stress, and worry may interfere with milk production and ejection (let-down). The nurse can encourage the mother to sleep when the baby sleeps. Breastfeeding in a side-lying or laid-back position promotes rest for the mother. Household chores and care for other children can be done by the partner, grandparents or other relatives, and friends.

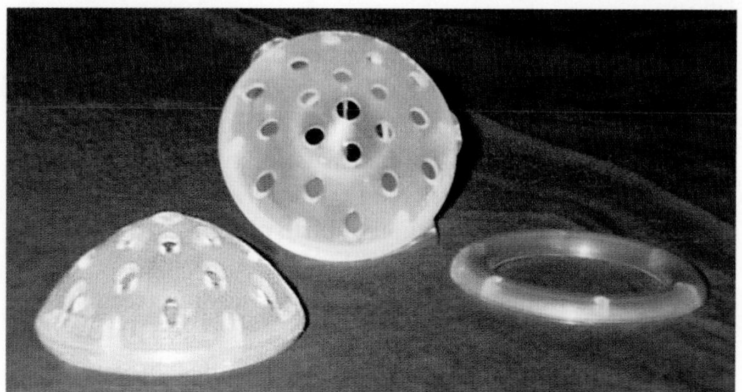

FIGURE 27-18 Breast shells.

Breast care. The breastfeeding mother's normal bathing routine is all that is required to keep her breasts clean. Soap can have a drying effect on nipples, so she should be instructed to avoid washing the nipples with soap. The small amount of soap that runs down her breasts while washing her face and neck or shampooing her hair is of no concern.

Breast creams should not be used routinely because they may block the natural oil secreted by Montgomery's glands on the areola. The mother with flat or inverted nipples may benefit from wearing breast shells in her bra, although there is a lack of evidence to support the effectiveness of doing so. It is thought that these hard plastic devices exert mild pressure around the base of the nipple to encourage nipple eversion. Breast shells are also useful for sore nipples, to keep the mother's bra or clothing from touching the nipples (Fig. 27-18).

If a mother needs breast support, she will be more comfortable wearing a bra, since the ligament that supports the breast (Cooper's ligament) will otherwise stretch and be painful. If she is comfortable without a bra, there is no reason for her to wear one. If a woman prefers to wear a bra, it should fit well, offer nonbinding support, and feel comfortable. Underwire bras or improperly fitting bras may contribute to clogged milk ducts.

If milk leakage between feedings is a problem, mothers can wear breast pads (disposable or washable) inside the bra. Plastic-lined breast pads are not recommended because they trap moisture and can contribute to sore nipples. To stop leakage, the mother can be alert to any sensation, such as tingling, that her milk is letting down. If this happens, she can usually stop the let-down by pressing straight back on her nipples. In public, the mother can fold her arms across her chest to apply pressure unobtrusively.

Effect of menstruation. The return of menstrual periods varies among lactating women. Most women will resume menstruation by 6 months postpartum, although for some women this may not occur until lactation has ceased. Menstruation has no effect on breastfeeding. There are no hormonal effects on the infant, although some babies may seem fussy for the first day. The quality of milk is not affected (Lawrence & Lawrence, 2015).

Sexual sensations. Some women experience rhythmic uterine contractions during breastfeeding. Such sensations are not unusual because uterine contractions and milk ejection are both triggered by oxytocin, but they may be disturbing to some mothers who perceive them to be similar to orgasm.

Breastfeeding and contraception. Breastfeeding may confer a period of infertility for up to 6 months. Breastfeeding delays the return of ovulation and menstruation; however, ovulation may occur before the first menstrual period after birth. The lactational amenorrhea method of birth control can be a highly effective temporary method of birth control for the first 6 months if the woman is exclusively breastfeeding (see Chapter 8, p. 158).

The contraceptive methods least likely to affect breastfeeding and milk production are the lactational amenorrhea method, natural family planning, barrier methods (diaphragm/cap, spermicides, condoms), and intrauterine devices. Hormonal contraceptives containing estrogen, including combined estrogen-progesterone pills or injectables, are not recommended for breastfeeding mothers because of the potential for reducing milk supply. Progestin-only contraceptives (pill, injection, or implant) are better options for breastfeeding mothers, although their use is not recommended during the first 4 weeks after birth (Centers for Disease Control and Prevention, 2010) (see Chapter 8).

Breastfeeding during pregnancy. It is possible for a breastfeeding woman to conceive and continue breastfeeding throughout the subsequent pregnancy if there are no medical contraindications (e.g., risk of preterm labour). For pregnant women who are breastfeeding, adequate nutrition is especially important to promote normal fetal growth.

Nipple tenderness associated with early pregnancy can cause discomfort when nursing the older child. The taste and composition of breast milk are altered during pregnancy, which can prompt some children to self-wean (Lawrence & Lawrence, 2015).

When the second baby is born, colostrum is produced. The practice of breastfeeding a newborn and an older child is called *tandem nursing*. The nurse should remind the mother to always feed the newborn first, to ensure that the newborn is receiving adequate nutrition. The supply-meets-demand principle works just as with breastfeeding multiple babies.

Diabetic mother. The mother with type 2 diabetes is encouraged to breastfeed. In addition to benefits for the infant and maternal satisfaction, breastfeeding has an antidiabetogenic effect. Blood glucose levels and insulin requirements are lower because of the carbohydrate used in milk production. During lactation, the diabetic woman may be able to eat more food and still take less insulin. However, insulin dosage must be adjusted as the infant is weaned. Some diabetic women are at increased risk for sore nipples caused by monilial infections and may have an increased risk for mastitis (Lawrence & Lawrence, 2015).

Breastfeeding after breast surgery. Previous breast surgery can affect the ability to produce breast milk and transfer it to the infant. Before undergoing breast surgery all women should discuss their lactation potential with their surgeon. Surgical procedures can damage nerves and interrupt milk ducts. Women who have had augmentation mammoplasty (breast implants) should be able to breastfeed successfully. However, if the procedure was done because of hypoplastic or asymmetrical breasts, there can be concerns about adequate milk production. Reduction mammoplasty is more likely to cause problems with the ability to successfully lactate because of interference with milk ducts, removal of glandular tissue, and nerve damage. Even so, many women are still able to breastfeed completely or partially. Mothers with a history of breast surgery are instructed to monitor their infants carefully for signs of adequate feeding.

It is possible for some women with a history of breast cancer to breastfeed. However, treatment for breast cancer (surgery, radiation, chemotherapy) can result in reduced milk supply or absence of lactation in the affected breast.

Breastfeeding and obesity. Women who are overweight or obese are more likely to experience delayed onset of lactogenesis stage II and reduced milk production compared with women of average weight. Breastfeeding duration tends to be shorter among this population of mothers (Lepe, Bacardí Gascón, Castañeda-González et al., 2011; Turcksin, Bel, Galjaard, et al., 2014; Wojcicki, 2011).

For women who have had bariatric surgery and plan to breastfeed, it is important to know when the surgery was performed. Nutrient and weight losses tend to stabilize approximately 12 to 18 months following the procedure. If the mother is consuming at least 1800 kcal/day and her weight has stabilized, her milk supply may be adequate. Breastfeeding mothers who have had a malabsorptive procedure such as a Roux-en-Y gastric bypass should take daily dietary supplements, including a prenatal vitamin, vitamin B_{12}, and iron with vitamin C (to maximize absorption).

It is important to monitor infant weight gain. Vitamin B_{12} deficiency or decreased milk production can cause failure to thrive. In addition, vitamin B_{12} deficiency can result in infant anemia, developmental delays, and neurological problems (Lamb, 2011).

Medications, alcohol, smoking, and caffeine. Despite much concern about the compatibility of medications and breastfeeding, in fact, few medications are contraindicated during lactation. Considerations in evaluating the safety of a specific medication during breastfeeding include the pharmacokinetics of the drug in the maternal system and the absorption, metabolism, distribution, storage, and excretion in the infant. The gestational and chronological age of the infant, body weight, and breastfeeding pattern are also considered. In general, any medication that is given to an infant routinely is safe for a mother who is breastfeeding. Breastfeeding mothers should be cautioned about taking any medications except those that are deemed essential. They are advised to check with their health care provider before taking any medication. Current, reliable online information about the safety of medications and breastfeeding can be accessed through LactMed, a website provided by National Library of Medicine or Motherisk which is an educational resource for families and professionals with evidence-based information for mothers and infants, provided by the Hospital for Sick Children in Toronto (see Additional Resources at the end of the chapter).

Drugs that are absolutely contraindicated for breastfeeding mothers include antimetabolite and cytotoxic medications and drugs of misuse, such as cocaine, heroin, amphetamines, and phencyclidine. Other medications that are generally contraindicated are amiodarone, chloramphenicol, doxepin, lithium, and radiopharmaceuticals (Hale & Rowe, 2014).

It is recommended that women who have been stable on a methadone maintenance program be allowed to breastfeed. Their infants may have decreased severity of neonatal abstinence symptoms when they are receiving breast milk (Lawrence & Lawrence, 2015).

Certain medications can reduce maternal milk production and should be avoided. These include ergot alkaloids (bromocriptine, cabergoline, ergotamine) and pseudoephedrine (Hale & Rowe, 2014).

As the use of antidepressant medications rises among childbearing women, there are increasing concerns about the effects of these medications on breastfeeding infants. A review of psychotropic medications indicates that the safest antidepressant drugs for breastfeeding mothers are sertraline, paroxetine, and fluvoxamine because there is minimal transfer into human milk. Antidepressants that are contraindicated while breastfeeding include citalopram, escitalopram, and fluoxetine because of the high levels excreted in breast milk, their long half-life, and adverse effects on the infant (Fortinguerra, Clavenna, & Bonati, 2009).

Alcohol consumption by breastfeeding mothers requires special caution. Although there is no standard recommendation about avoiding alcohol use when breastfeeding, it is important for mothers to be aware of potential risks. Health Canada et al. (2012) recommends that alcohol intake by breastfeeding women be minimal. Alcohol passes freely from the blood into breast milk, with peak levels occurring in 30 to 60 minutes on an empty stomach and 60 to 90 minutes when consumed with food. The MER and milk production can be adversely affected by maternal alcohol intake. If a breastfeeding mother chooses to have one or two drinks, she should not breastfeed for at least 2 hours. Contrary to popular belief, pumping and discarding milk does not accelerate removal of alcohol from the milk (Lawrence & Lawrence, 2015).

Breastfeeding mothers should be advised to stop or reduce smoking (Health Canada et al., 2012). It can impair milk production; it also exposes the infant to the risks of secondhand smoke. Nicotine is transferred to the infant in breast milk, whether the mother smokes or uses a nicotine patch, although the effect on the infant is uncertain. If a mother continues to smoke, she should be advised that breastfeeding remains important for her infant's health and may mitigate some of the negative effects of exposure to tobacco smoke on the infant. Lactating mothers who continue to smoke should be advised not to smoke within 2 hours before breastfeeding, and they along with other family members who smoke should go outside to smoke.

Moderate intake of caffeine by breastfeeding mothers appears to pose no risk to normal full-term infants. Minimal amounts of caffeine pass through to the infant in the breast milk. However, caffeine does accumulate in infants, especially if they are preterm (Lawrence & Lawrence, 2015).

Herbal preparations. Herbs and herbal preparations such as teas are often recommended for breastfeeding women, especially when there is a need to increase milk supply. Although some are considered safe, others contain pharmacologically active compounds that may have detrimental effects, particularly on the newborn. Although these herbal preparations may seem to be effective for some women, the recommendations are based on anecdotal information and there is a lack of evidence related to the prevalence, effectiveness, and safety of herbs during breastfeeding (ABM Protocol Committee, 2011b; Mortell & Mehta, 2013). A thorough history should include noting the composition of any herbal remedies (Amer, Cipriano, Venci, et al., 2015). Each remedy should then be evaluated for its compatibility with breastfeeding. Herbal teas considered safe during lactation include rose hips, orange spice, chicory, peppermint, raspberry, and red bush tea (Lawrence & Lawrence, 2015). The regional poison control centre or Motherisk can provide information on the active properties of herbs.

SPECIAL CONSIDERATIONS

The breastfeeding mother may experience some common concerns. In most cases complications are preventable if the mother receives appropriate education about breastfeeding. Early recognition and resolution of problems is important in order to prevent interruption of breastfeeding and promote the mother's comfort and sense of well-being. Emotional support provided by the nurse or lactation consultant is essential to help allay frustration and anxiety and to prevent early cessation of breastfeeding.

Engorgement

Mild engorgement is a common postpartum response of the breasts to the sudden change in hormones and the increased volume of milk. It usually occurs on the second to fifth day postpartum when the mature milk comes in, and it lasts about 24 hours. Painful distension can often be prevented by frequent feedings in the first 48 hours. Intense engorgement can result from accumulation of milk and from the naturally increasing blood supply to the breasts, causing swelling of tissues surrounding the milk ducts. The ducts may be pinched shut, so that the milk does not flow. The breasts become firm, tender, swollen, and hot, and appear shiny and red. The tenderness and swelling may extend into the axilla. With engorgement the areolae can become firm and the nipples may flatten, making it difficult for the newborn to latch on. Back pressure on full milk glands inhibits milk production if the milk is not removed from the breasts, and the milk supply may diminish (see Critical Thinking Case Study).

When mild engorgement occurs, the nurse should assure the mother that this is usually a temporary condition that resolves within 24 hours. To avoid more severe engorgement a mother should be instructed to feed frequently (every 2–3 hours), softening at least one breast, and pumping the other breast to soften. Pumping during engorgement will not cause a problematic increase in milk supply.

A variety of interventions are used to treat engorgement, although there is a lack of research evidence confirming the effectiveness of any specific intervention. Frequently used

CRITICAL THINKING CASE STUDY

Breastfeeding: Engorgement and Nipple Soreness

The home care nurse visits Mary, a 35-year-old primipara who was discharged from the hospital 24 hours after giving birth to Matthew, a 3400 g baby boy who is now 3 days old. When Mary answers the door, she is tearful and appears very tired. Mary's mother is holding the baby, who is asleep in her arms. Mary tells the nurse that, when she awakened this morning, her breasts were very firm and "achy." She tried to latch the baby on to the breast, but the nipple was too flat, and he could not get it in his mouth; he was crying so hard that her mother gave him some formula. Mary's nipples appear irritated and cracked; she says "it hurts too much to feed him anyway." The baby has had only two wet diapers and no bowel movements in the last 24 hours. Mary says he cries much of the time and never seems to settle down to sleep for very long. Mary states, "I think it would be easier if I switch to formula."

1. Evidence—Does the nurse have enough evidence at this time to draw conclusions about the feeding difficulties experienced by this mother and infant?
2. Assumptions—What assumptions can be made about the following issues?
   a. Mary's milk supply
   b. Mary's sore nipples
   c. Matthew's urinary output and bowel elimination pattern
   d. Mary's commitment to breastfeeding
3. What implications and priorities for nursing care can be identified at this time?
4. Does the evidence objectively support your conclusion?

treatments for engorgement include the use of cold (ice packs, gel packs, cold compresses, chilled cabbage leaves) after breastfeeding, warmth (warm compresses, warm showers) before breastfeeding, anti-inflammatory medications, breast massage, and pumping.

Because of the swelling of breast tissue surrounding the milk glands' ducts, ice packs can be used in a rotation of 15 to 20 minutes on, 45 minutes off between feedings. The ice packs should cover both breasts. Large bags of frozen peas or corn make easy packs and can be refrozen between uses. Research shows some association between application of cold to the breasts and improvement in the symptoms of engorgement (Mangesi & Dowswell, 2010).

Anti-inflammatory medications such as ibuprofen may help reduce pain and swelling associated with engorgement. Mothers often have an elevated temperature and experience achiness in their breasts; ibuprofen can help remedy this.

Because heat increases blood flow, application of heat to an already congested breast is usually counterproductive. Occasionally, however, standing in a warm shower will start the milk leaking, or the mother may be able to manually express enough milk to soften the areola sufficiently to allow the baby to latch and breastfeed.

When engorgement occurs as a result of excessive intravenous fluids during labour, the nipple and areola can become distended, making it difficult for the newborn to latch successfully. This can also occur in mothers who have received oxytocin for labour induction or augmentation. A technique called *reverse pressure softening* is used to manually displace the areolar interstitial fluid inward, softening the areola and making it easier for the infant's mouth to grasp the nipple and areola with latch (Kujawa-Myles, Noel-Weiss, Dunn, et al., 2015; Lauwers & Swisher, 2011).

Sore Nipples

Many women expect breastfeeding to be painful, based on stories they have heard from family and friends; however, breastfeeding is not supposed to be painful. While mild nipple discomfort at the beginning of feedings is common, severe soreness and abraded, cracked, or bleeding nipples are not normal and most often result from poor positioning, incorrect latch, improper suck, or infection.

Severe nipple pain can be related to vasospasm or Raynaud's phenomenon (Lawrence & Lawrence, 2015). The key to preventing sore nipples is correct breastfeeding technique. Limiting the time at the breast does not prevent sore nipples; instead, they are often the result of the mother allowing the baby to latch on to the breast before the mouth is open wide.

For the first few days after birth, the nursing mother may experience some mild discomfort with the infant's initial sucks. This should quickly dissipate as the milk begins to flow and acts as a lubricant. To make the initial sucks less painful, the mother can express a few drops of milk to moisten the nipple and areola before latch. If the mother continues to experience nipple pain or discomfort after the first few sucks, the nurse or lactation consultant can help her evaluate the latch and baby's position at the breast. If the nipple pain continues, the mother needs to remove the baby from the breast, breaking suction with her finger in the baby's mouth. Repositioning the mother or infant may be helpful in resolving the nipple discomfort. The mother then proceeds to attempt latch again, making sure that the baby's mouth is open wide before latching him or her on to the breast (see Fig. 27-6).

The infant's suck can be assessed by a lactation consultant or a nurse who is specially trained, by inserting a clean gloved finger in the newborn's mouth and stimulating the newborn to suck. If the newborn is not extruding the tongue over the lower gum and the mother reports pain or pinching with sucking, the newborn may have a short frenulum (commonly referred to as being "tongue-tied"). In some cases, ankyloglossia is corrected surgically to free the tongue for less painful, more effective breastfeeding (Powers, 2010; Rowan-Legg & CPS, 2015).

The treatment for sore nipples is first to identify the cause and then attempt to correct the problem. Early assessment and intervention are essential to increase the likelihood that the mother will continue to breastfeed. Once the problem is identified and corrected, sore nipples should heal within a few days, even though the baby continues to breastfeed regularly. When sore nipples occur, the woman is advised to start the feeding on the least sore nipple. It is important to assess the nipples for cracking or other damage to the skin integrity, which increases the risk of infection. If there is any break in the skin, the mother is advised to wipe the nipples with water after feeding to remove the baby's saliva. A thin coating of a topical antibiotic may help reduce the risk of infection and promote healing (the antibiotic cream or ointment should be removed before breastfeeding).

Sore nipples should be open to air as much as possible. To promote comfort, breast shells may be worn inside the bra; these devices allow air to circulate while keeping clothing off sore nipples (see Fig. 27-18).

Rapid healing of sore nipples is critical to relieve the mother's discomfort, maintain breastfeeding, and prevent mastitis. Although numerous creams, ointments, gels, and gel pads have been used to treat sore nipples, there is a lack of conclusive evidence related to the effectiveness of any particular method (Dennis, Jackson, & Watson, 2014). However, because they have not been shown to cause harm, many health care providers recommend their use. Some women report increased comfort for sore nipples with the application of purified lanolin or hydrogel pads (Smith & Riordan, 2010). Lanolin is made from sheep's wool and is not appropriate for use with women who have wool allergies. Lanolin is not recommended if it is suspected that nipple soreness may be due to a monilial infection. Antifungal creams are used to treat yeast infections on nipples. Antiseptic sprays and premoistened towelettes containing alcohol are not recommended.

NURSING ALERT

Nurses must assess women's allergies prior to applying lanolin ointment. Lanolin is made from sheep's wool so must not be used on women who have a wool allergy.

If nipples are extremely sore or damaged and if the mother cannot tolerate breastfeeding, she may need to use an electric breast pump for 24 to 48 hours to allow the nipples to begin healing before resuming breastfeeding. She should use a pump that effectively empties the breasts.

NURSING ALERT

The mother who has a sudden onset of sore nipples or experiences sore nipples after days or weeks of comfortable breastfeeding likely has some type of nipple infection, most often bacterial or fungal (candidiasis). Other possible causes are skin problems such as psoriasis, allergic reactions, or vasospasm. Careful assessment and referral for treatment are needed (Smith & Riordan, 2010).

Silicone (flexible) nipple shields may be helpful for a mother with flat or inverted nipples and particularly for preterm babies who have trouble latching and maintaining suction and for babies who develop a preference for a bottle nipple and refuse the breast (Riordan & Wambach, 2010b). While nipple shields help protect abraded, sore nipples, the cause of the pain must be determined and remedied promptly. The shield should be applied on the nipple areola area just before putting the baby on the breast: the brim of the shield is flipped up, the shield placed directly over the nipple, and the brim gently patted down. Nipple shields should be used for a short time only, or the baby may become so accustomed to them that he or she refuses the breast. In addition, lactation consultants should closely monitor the infant's growth and intake of milk.

Monilial infections. Sore nipples that occur after the newborn period are often due to a *Candida* or monilial (yeast) infection. The mother usually reports severe nipple pain and tenderness, burning, or stinging, and she may have sharp, shooting, burning pains in the breasts during and after feedings. The nipples appear somewhat pink and shiny or may be scaly or flaky; there may be a visible rash, small blisters, or thrush. Most often, the pain is out of proportion to the appearance of the nipple. Yeast infections of the nipples and breast can be excruciatingly painful and can lead to early cessation of breastfeeding if not recognized and treated promptly.

Infants may or may not exhibit symptoms of monilial infection. Oral thrush and a red, raised diaper rash are common indications of a yeast infection. An affected infant is often fussy and gassy. When feeding, the infant is likely to pull off the breast soon after starting to feed, crying with apparent pain. The infant may be biting or gumming at the breast.

The most common predisposing factors for yeast infections of the breast include previous antibiotic use, vaginal yeast infections, and nipple damage.

Mothers and infants must be treated simultaneously, even if the infant has no visible signs of infection. Treatment for the mother is typically an antifungal cream applied to the nipples after feedings and, in some cases, a systemic antifungal medication such as fluconazole. Most physicians prescribe an oral antifungal medication, such as nystatin or fluconazole, for infants. Treatment should continue for at least 14 days even after symptoms begin to improve in 1 to 2 days (Lawrence & Lawrence, 2015). Good hand hygiene is essential to prevent the spread of yeast.

Insufficient Milk Supply

A major reason that women stop breastfeeding is perceived or actual insufficient milk supply (Brand, Kothari, & Stark, 2011; Lauwers & Swisher, 2011). Careful evaluation of the mother–infant dyad is needed, including assessment of infant weight gain or loss, feeding technique, and milk transfer and consideration of possible medical causes for low supply (e.g., medications, glandular insufficiency, previous breast surgery). Stress and fatigue can cause decreased milk production.

Interventions for increasing milk supply are based on causative factors. In many cases the mother is instructed to spend time with the baby skin-to-skin, increase feeding frequency, express milk using an electric pump, rest as much as possible, consume a healthy diet, and reduce stress. If nonpharmacological measures to increase milk supply are not effective, pharmaceutical galactogogues (medications used to increase milk supply) may be prescribed by the health care provider. Metoclopramide and domperidone are the most commonly prescribed medications; both are dopamine antagonists typically used to treat gastroesophageal reflux. They also increase prolactin levels, which enhances milk production. Metoclopramide has unpleasant adverse effects such as fatigue, irritability, and depression; there is a risk of severe allergic reaction. Domperidone is often prescribed for lactating women in Canada (Flanders, Lowe, Kramer, et al., 2012). Health Canada has issued a warning about the use of domperidone, although it is based on very few studies and it is still being recommended as a medication to increase milk production (Bozzo, Koren, & Ito, 2012).

Plugged Milk Ducts

A milk duct can become plugged or clogged, causing an area of the breast to become swollen and tender. This area typically does not empty or soften with feeding or pumping. A small white pearl may be visible on the tip of the nipple; this pearl is the curd of milk blocking the flow. The mother is afebrile and has no generalized symptoms.

Plugged milk ducts are most often the result of inadequate emptying of the breast, which can be caused by clothing that is too tight, a poorly fitting or underwire bra, or always using the same position for feeding. Application of warm compresses to the affected area and to the nipple before feeding helps promote emptying of the breast and release of the plug.

Frequent feeding is recommended, with the infant beginning the feeding on the affected side in order to foster more complete emptying. The mother is advised to massage the affected area while the infant nurses or while she is pumping. Varying feeding positions and feeding without wearing a bra may be useful in resolving a plugged duct (Riordan & Wambach, 2010b).

Plugged milk ducts can increase susceptibility to breast infection. For recurrent plugged ducts, taking lecithin, a fat emulsifier, may be useful for the mother (Lawrence & Lawrence, 2015).

Mastitis

Although the term mastitis means inflammation of the breast, it is most often used to refer to infection of the breast. It is characterized by the sudden onset of flu-like symptoms, including fever, chills, body aches, and headache. The woman usually has localized breast pain and tenderness and a hot, reddened area on the breast. Mastitis most commonly occurs in the upper outer quadrant of the breast; one or both breasts can be affected. Most cases occur during the first 6 weeks of breastfeeding, but mastitis can occur at any time (Lawrence & Lawrence, 2015).

Certain factors may predispose a woman to mastitis. Inadequate emptying of the breasts is common, related to engorgement, plugged ducts, a sudden decrease in the number of feedings, abrupt weaning, or wearing underwire bras. Sore, cracked nipples may lead to mastitis by providing a portal of entry for the causative organism (staphylococci, streptococci, and *E. coli* are most common). Stress and fatigue, maternal illness, ill family members, breast trauma, and poor maternal nutrition also are predisposing factors for mastitis (Lauwers & Swisher, 2011; Lawrence & Lawrence, 2015). Breastfeeding mothers should be taught the signs of mastitis before they are discharged from the hospital, and they need to know to call the health care provider promptly if the symptoms occur. Treatment includes antibiotics such as cephalexin or dicloxacillin for 10 to 14 days and analgesic and antipyretic medications such as ibuprofen. The mother is advised to rest as much as possible and breastfeed the baby or pump frequently, striving to empty the affected side adequately. Warm compresses to the breast before feeding or pumping can be useful. Adequate fluid intake and a balanced diet are important for the mother with mastitis (Lauwers & Swisher, 2011).

Complications of mastitis include breast abscess, chronic mastitis, and fungal infections of the breast. Most complications can be prevented by early recognition and treatment.

Follow-Up After Hospital Discharge

Concerns such as infant feeding patterns, jaundice, or breast discomfort may occur after discharge. Thus, it is the hospital nurse's role to educate the mother about potential problems she may encounter once she is home. It is critical that the mother receive a list of resources for help with breastfeeding concerns and that she knows who and when to call for assistance. Community resources for breastfeeding mothers include lactation consultants, physicians, nurses in pediatric or obstetrical offices, community health nurses, and peer support groups.

Telephone follow-up by hospital, office, or community health nurses within the first day or two after discharge can provide a means of identifying any problems and offering needed advice and support. Infants discharged should meet specific criteria for physiological stability and safety (including successful feedings) and have arrangements to be seen by a health care provider, usually within 48 hours. Late preterm infants require careful assessment of effective feeding and adequate thermoregulation before discharge (AAP, 2010; Whyte & CPS, 2010/2015). In some settings and circumstances, home care follow-up is available for mothers after hospital discharge.

FORMULA-FEEDING

Parent Education

Some parents choose formula-feeding instead of breastfeeding, others combine the two methods. If the infant is weaned from breastfeeding before the first birthday, iron-fortified infant formula should be given.

Parents who choose to formula-feed need clear, evidence-based guidance on best practices. Since the vast majority of women in Canada initiate breastfeeding, nurses may be less familiar with providing guidance for families using formula. However, nurses are in an ideal position to provide individualized education to parents about infant feeding. It is also important to determine if breastfeeding families intend to use formula at home, so that best practices can be discussed before discharge (Hancock & Brown, 2010). Mothers have reported that they do not get sufficient information from health care providers about formula-feeding (Lakshman, Ogilvie, & Ong, 2009). Because of the lack of clear information about the practical aspects of formula-feeding, parents often rely on advice from friends and family. If that advice is incorrect and the parents use unsafe practices for formula preparation and feeding, the infant is at risk for foodborne illness and burns.

Readiness for Feeding

The first feeding of formula is ideally given after the initial transition to extrauterine life. Feeding readiness cues include stability of vital signs, bowel sounds, an active sucking reflex, an effective breathing pattern, and hunger cues (clenched hands to mouth, licking, and sucking). Crying is a late hunger cue. If the baby is frequently held skin-to-skin, subtle hunger cues will be more obvious to the parents.

Feeding Patterns

In the first 24 to 48 hours of life, a newborn typically consumes 10 to 30 mL of formula at a feeding. Intake gradually increases during the first week of life as the capacity of the stomach increases to 60 to 90 mL by the end of the first week. The newborn infant should be fed in response to hunger and satiation cues or at least every 3 to 4 hours, even if that requires waking the newborn for the feedings; however, rigid feeding schedules are not recommended. The infant showing an adequate weight gain can be allowed to sleep at night and be fed only on awakening. Most newborns need six to eight feedings in 24 hours, and the number of feedings decreases as the infant matures. Usually by 3 to 4 weeks after birth a fairly predictable feeding pattern has developed. Scheduling feedings arbitrarily at predetermined intervals may not meet a newborn's needs, but initiating feedings at convenient times often moves the newborn's feedings to times that work for the family.

Mothers will usually notice an increase in the infant's appetite at ages 7 to 10 days, 3 weeks, 6 weeks, 3 months, and 6 months. These appetite spurts correspond to growth spurts. The amount of formula per feeding should be increased by about 30 mL at these times to meet the baby's needs.

Feeding Techniques

During feedings, parents should be encouraged to sit comfortably, holding the infant closely in a semi-upright position. Feedings provide opportunities for interaction and cognitive growth, as well as to bond with the infant through touching, talking, singing, or reading aloud. Parents should consider feedings, whether breast or bottle, as a time of peaceful relaxation with their newborn (Fig. 27-19).

The bottle should never be propped with a pillow or other inanimate object and left with the infant. Likewise, small children should not be given charge of bottle-feeding the infant unless there is close adult supervision. This practice may result in choking, and it deprives the infant of important interaction during feeding. Moreover, propping the bottle has been implicated in causing nursing-bottle caries, or decay of the first teeth, resulting from continuous bathing of the teeth with carbohydrate-containing fluid as the infant sporadically sucks the nipple.

Newborns must learn to coordinate sucking, swallowing, and breathing as they feed. The typical fast flow of milk from bottles can create difficulty for an infant trying to learn to feed. A slow-flow nipple is often used for the first few weeks.

Traditionally, parents are told to position the infant in a semi-reclining position and to hold the bottle so that fluid fills the nipple and none of the air in the bottle is allowed to enter it (Fig. 27-19, A). A more physiological approach to bottle-feeding is called *paced bottle-feeding*. With this method of feeding the bottle is held at more of a horizontal angle; when the baby pauses between bursts of sucking, the parent withdraws the nipple, allowing it to rest on the baby's lip until he or she is ready to resume sucking (Lauwers & Swisher, 2011). This position slows the flow of milk from the bottle so the infant is more in control. Paced bottle-feeding works well for infants who are primarily breastfeeding but are occasionally fed from a bottle (see Patient Teaching box on p. 752 and Fig. 27-19, B).

If the infant falls asleep or ceases to suck, it usually indicates that he or she has consumed enough formula to feel satiated. Parents need to be taught to look for these cues and avoid overfeeding, which can contribute to obesity.

Parents should be instructed to observe the infant for signs of stress during feeding, including turning the head, arching the back, choking, sputtering, changing colour, moving the arms,

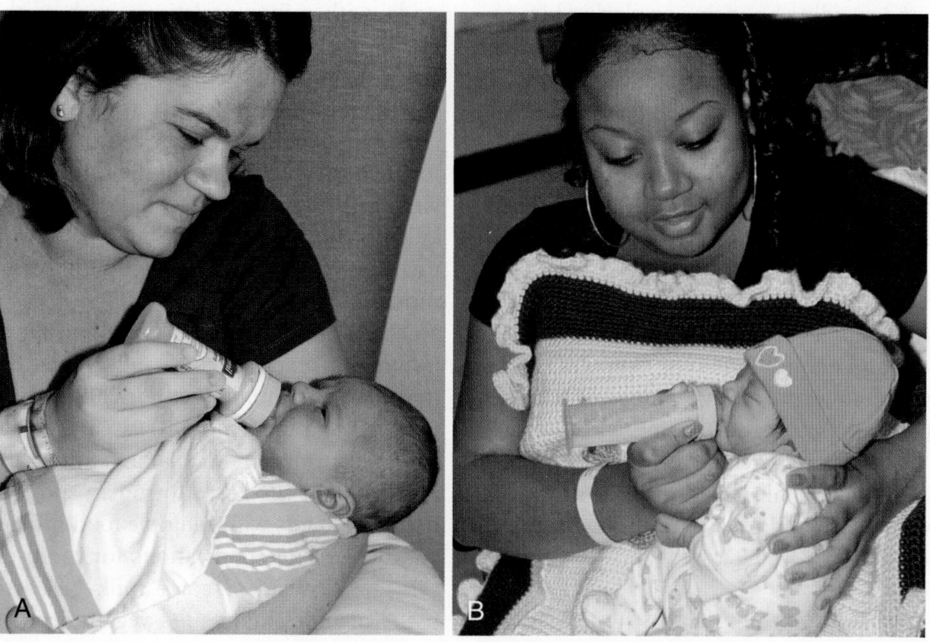

FIGURE 27-19 A: Bottle-feeding: traditional technique with infant semi-reclining. **B:** Paced bottle-feeding: infant is more upright. (Courtesy Cheryl Briggs, BSN, RNC-NIC.)

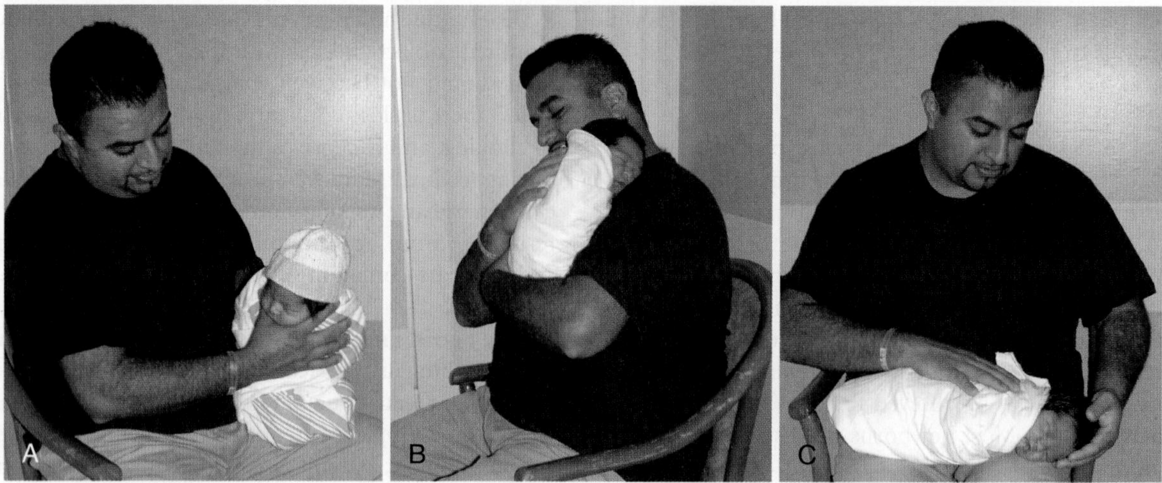

FIGURE 27-20 Positions for burping an infant. **A:** Sitting. **B:** On shoulder. **C:** Across lap. (Courtesy Julie Perry Nelson.)

and tensing fists (Lauwers & Swisher, 2011). When these signs occur, the parent should stop feeding and attempt to calm the infant before resuming. The signs can indicate that the infant is finished with the feeding and does not want to drink any more.

Most infants swallow air when fed from a bottle and need a chance to burp several times during a feeding. Parents are taught various positions that can be used for burping (Fig. 27-20).

Common Concerns

Parents need to know what to do if the infant spits up. They may need to decrease the amount of feeding or feed smaller amounts more frequently. Burping the infant several times during a feeding such as when the infant's sucking slows down or stops can decrease spitting. Holding the baby upright for 30 minutes after feeding and avoiding bouncing or placing him or her on the abdomen soon after the feeding is finished can also help. Spitting can be a result of overfeeding, or it can be symptomatic of gastroesophageal reflux. Parents should report vomiting of one third or more of the feeding at most feeding sessions or projectile vomiting to the health care provider and should be cautioned to refrain from changing the infant's formula without consulting the health care provider.

Bottles and Nipples

Many styles of bottles and nipples are available. Most babies will feed well with any bottle and nipple. The bottles, nipples, rings, and caps should be washed in warm, soapy water using a bottle and nipple brush to facilitate thorough cleansing. Most household dishwashers use hot water and are safe for cleaning bottles and nipples. Boiling of bottles and nipples is not always needed. It is best to check with the local Public Health Department regarding recommendations.

Infant Formulas

Commercial infant formulas are designed to resemble human milk as closely as possible, although none has ever duplicated it. The exact composition of infant formula varies with the manufacturer, but all must meet specific standards.

Infants who are not breastfed should be given commercial iron-fortified formulas. If this is too expensive, the family may be eligible for services through various income assistance programs.

Commercially prepared formulas are cow's milk–based formulas that have been modified to closely resemble the nutritional content of human milk. The caloric content of standard infant formula is 20 kcal/30 mL. These formulas are altered from cow's milk by removing butterfat, decreasing the protein content, and adding vegetable oil and carbohydrate. Some have demineralized whey added to yield a whey/casein ratio of 60:40. Regardless of the commercial brand, the standard cow's milk–based formulas have essentially the same compositions of vitamins, minerals, protein, carbohydrates, and essential amino acids, with minor variations, such as the source of carbohydrate; nucleotides to enhance immune function; and long-chain polyunsaturated fatty acids (DHA and ARA), which are thought to improve visual and cognitive function. The composition, processing, packaging, and labelling of all infant formula is regulated under the Canadian Food and Drug Regulations to ensure product safety and quality (Health Canada et al., 2012). Iron-fortified cows' milk formulas are designed to meet the nutritional requirements of infants until 9 to 12 months of age.

Four main categories of commercially prepared infant formulas are available: (1) cow's milk–based formulas; (2) soy-based formulas, commonly used for children who are lactose or cow's milk–protein intolerant; (3) casein- or whey-hydrolysate formulas, used primarily for children who cannot tolerate or digest cow's milk or soy-based formulas; and (4) amino acid formulas, used for infants with multiple food protein intolerances.

There are few indications for the use of soy protein–based formulas instead of cow's milk–based formulas. Appropriate usage includes infants fed vegan diets and infants with galactosemia (Health Canada et al., 2012). Infants with documented IgE allergies caused by cow's milk should be fed an extensively hydrolyzed protein formula because about 10 to 14% of infants with cow's milk–based formula intolerance will also have a soy protein allergy. Soy protein–based formulas have not been proved to be effective in preventing colic or allergy in healthy or high-risk infants.

Alternative milk sources such as goat's milk; skim or low-fat milk; condensed milk; or raw, unpasteurized milk from any animal source should not be fed to infants because they are inadequate to support growth and can contain excess protein or an inadequate calcium/phosphorus ratio, which can cause seizures.

SAFETY ALERT

Because of concerns about potential harmful effects of bisphenol A (BPA), parents should be cautioned about using hard plastic polycarbonate baby bottles or containers. BPA is a chemical that is used to harden plastics, prevent bacterial contamination of foods, and prevent can rusting. It is in many food and liquid containers, including baby bottles. In order to avoid exposure to BPA, parents are advised to look for BPA-free bottles or to use glass bottles as an alternative, but parents must be aware of the risk for injury if a glass bottle is dropped or broken. Because heat can cause the release of BPA from plastic, polycarbonate bottles should never be boiled, heated in the microwave, or washed in a dishwasher.

Formula Preparation

Commercial formulas are available in three forms: powder, concentrate, and ready-to-feed. All are equivalent in nutritional content (20 kcal/30 mL or 68 kcal/100 mL), but they vary considerably in price.

- Ready-to-feed formula is the most expensive but easiest one to use. The desired amount is poured into the bottle. The opened can is refrigerated safely for 48 hours. This type of formula can be purchased in individual disposable bottles for the most convenient feeding.
- Concentrated formula is less expensive than ready-to-feed formula. It is diluted with equal parts of water and can be stored in the refrigerator for 48 hours after opening.
- Powdered formula is the least expensive formula. It is easily mixed by using one scoop for every 60 mL of water. Powdered formula is not recommended for premature or low-birth-weight infants for at least 2 months after birth. It is recommended that they be fed liquid formula.

The commercial infant formula must include label directions for preparation and use of the formula with pictures and symbols for the benefit of individuals who cannot read. Some manufacturers translate the directions into many languages, such as French, Chinese, Punjabi, and Vietnamese, to prevent misunderstanding and errors in formula preparation. The water used to mix either powdered or concentrated liquid formula need not contain any fluoride, especially in the first 6 months of life. Excess fluoride can permanently stain the teeth once they appear. Parents must be taught that it is extremely important that formula not be diluted with more water than recommended, in an effort to try to save money. A thorough assessment of parents' formula preparation and of any concerns may indicate a family's financial need and further support and referral may be required.

SAFETY ALERT

An important aspect to impress on families is that the proportions must not be altered (i.e., neither diluted to extend the amount of formula nor concentrated to provide more calories). The newborn's kidneys are immature; giving the infant overly concentrated formula can provide protein and minerals in amounts that exceed the excretory ability of the kidneys. In contrast, if the formula is diluted too much (sometimes done to save money), the infant does not consume sufficient calories and grow appropriately.

Sterilization of formula rarely is recommended when families have access to a safe public water supply. Instead, formula is prepared with attention to cleanliness. When water from a private well is used, parents should be advised to contact the health department to have a chemical and bacteriological analysis of the water performed before using the water in formula preparation. The presence of nitrates, excess fluoride, or bacteria may be harmful to the infant.

It is usually safe to mix infant formula with cold tap water that has been boiled for 1 to 2 minutes and allowed to cool (Health Canada et al., 2012). Bottled water that is labelled as "sterile" is safe for mixing formula. However, nonsterile bottled water should be boiled for 1 to 2 minutes and cooled.

If the conditions in the home appear unsanitary, it may be better to recommend the use of ready-to-feed formula or to teach the mother to sterilize the formula. The two traditional methods for sterilization are terminal heating and the aseptic method. In the terminal heating method, the prepared formula is placed in the bottles, which are topped with the nipples placed upside down and covered with the caps, and then sealed loosely with the rings. The bottles are then boiled together in a water bath for 25 minutes. In the aseptic method, the bottles, rings, caps, nipples, and any other necessary equipment, such as a funnel, are boiled separately, after which the formula is poured into the bottles. Any formula left in the bottle after the feeding should be discarded because the infant's saliva has mixed with it. (Instructions for formula preparation and feeding are provided in the Patient Teaching box.)

Vitamin and Mineral Supplementation

Commercial iron-fortified formula contains all the nutrients needed by the infant for the first 6 months of life. After 6 months, fluoride supplementation of 0.25 mg/day is required if the local water supply is not fluoridated. Vitamin D supplementation is discussed earlier in this chapter.

Weaning

The bottle-fed infant will gradually learn to use a cup, and the parents will find that they are preparing fewer bottles. Commonly, the feeding before bedtime is the last one to remain. Infants have a strong need to suck, and the infant who has had the bottle taken away too early or abruptly will compensate with non-nutritive sucking on his or her fingers, thumb, a pacifier, or even the tongue. Therefore, weaning from a bottle should be attempted gradually because the infant has learned to rely on the comfort that sucking provides.

PATIENT TEACHING

Formula Preparation and Feeding

Formula Preparation

- Using warm soapy water, wash your hands, arms, and under your nails; rinse well. Clean and sanitize the surface where you will be preparing the bottles.
- Thoroughly wash bottles, nipples, rings, caps, can opener, and other preparation utensils in hot soapy water and rinse thoroughly. Squeeze water through nipples to make sure that the holes are open.
- Place bottles, nipples, rings, and caps in a pot and cover with water; boil for 5 minutes; remove items from pot with sanitized tongs and allow them to air dry. (Do this at least before using items the first time; thereafter washing in the dishwasher or hot soapy water is sufficient.)
- Note the expiration date on the formula container. It should be used before the expiration date. Any unopened expired formula should be returned to the place of purchase.
- Read the label on the container of formula and mix it exactly according to the directions.
- Mix formula with tap water deemed safe by the local health department. Allow cold water to run for 2 minutes before collecting it. Then bring it to a rolling boil and continue boiling for 1 to 2 minutes. If using bottled water, make sure that it is labelled as "sterile"; unsterile bottled water must be boiled. After boiling, allow water to cool before mixing the formula but not for longer than 30 minutes.
- If using a can of ready-to-feed or concentrated formula, wash the top of the can with hot soapy water and rinse well. Shake the can before opening.

Mixing Formula

- *Ready-to-feed:* No mixing is needed; do not add water. Pour desired amount of formula into clean bottle; add nipple and ring.
- *Concentrate:* Pour desired amount of formula into clean bottle and add equal amount of cooled boiled water. Add nipple and ring and shake well.
- *Powder:* When first opening the container of powder, write the date on the lid. Using the scoop from the container, add 1 scoop of powdered formula for each 60 mL of boiled, cooled water in a clean bottle. For example, if 180 mL of water is in the bottle, add three scoops of powder. Add nipple and ring and shake well.
- If preparing multiple bottles at the same time, place nipple right side up on each bottle and cover with a clean nipple cap. Use bottles within 48 hours.
- Opened cans of ready-to-feed or concentrated formula should be covered and refrigerated. Any unused portions must be discarded after 48 hours.
- Bottles or cans of unopened formula can be stored at room temperature.
- If the formula is refrigerated, warm it by placing the bottle in a pan of hot water. Never use a microwave to warm any food to be given to a baby. Test the temperature of the formula by letting a few drops fall on the inside of your wrist. If the formula feels comfortably warm to you, the temperature is correct.

Feeding Techniques and Tips

- Newborns should be fed on demand usually every 2½ to 3 hours and should never go longer than 4 hours without feeding until a satisfactory pattern of weight gain is established. This period can be as long as 2 weeks. If a baby cries or fusses between feedings, check to see if the diaper should be changed and if the baby needs to be picked up and cuddled. If the baby continues to cry and acts hungry, feed him or her. Babies do not get hungry on a regular schedule.
- Infants gradually increase the amount of milk they drink with each feeding. The first day or so most newborns consume 15 to 30 mL with each feeding. This amount increases as the infant grows. If any formula remains in the bottle as the feeding ends, it must be thrown away because saliva from the baby's mouth can cause the formula to spoil.
- Keep a feeding diary, writing down the amount of formula the infant drinks with each feeding for approximately the first week. Also record the wet diapers and bowel movements the baby is having. Take this diary with you when you take the baby for the first follow-up visit with the primary health care provider.
- For feeding, hold the infant close in a semi-reclining position. Talk to him or her during the feeding. This time is ideal for social interaction and cuddling.
- Place the nipple in the infant's mouth on the tongue. It should touch the roof of the mouth to stimulate the baby's sucking reflex. Hold the bottle like a pencil. Keep it tipped so the nipple stays filled with milk and the baby does not suck in air.
- Taking a few sucks and then pausing briefly before continuing to suck again is normal for infants. Some infants take longer to feed than others. Be patient. Keep the baby awake; encouraging sucking may be necessary. Moving the nipple gently in the infant's mouth may stimulate sucking.
- Another technique that can be used for bottle-feeding is *paced bottle-feeding.* The infant is placed in a more upright position, and the bottle is held at a more horizontal angle. When the baby pauses between bursts of sucking, withdraw the nipple and allow it to rest on the baby's lip until he or she is ready to resume sucking. This slows the flow of milk from the bottle so the infant is more in control. Paced bottle-feeding works well for infants who are primarily breastfeeding but are occasionally fed from a bottle.
- Newborns are apt to swallow air when sucking. Give the infant opportunities to burp several times during a feeding. As he or she gets older, you will know better when to stop for burping.
- After the first 2 or 3 days the stools of a formula-fed infant are yellow and soft but formed. The infant may have a stool with each feeding in the first 2 weeks, although this amount can decrease to one or two stools each day. It is not abnormal for formula-fed infants to have a stool every other day.

Safety Tips

- Infants should be held and never left alone while feeding. Never prop the bottle. The infant might inhale formula or choke on any that was spit up. Infants who fall asleep with a propped bottle of milk or juice can be prone to cavities when the first teeth come in.
- Know how to use the bulb syringe and help an infant who is choking.

COMPLEMENTARY FEEDING: INTRODUCING SOLID FOODS

Complementary feedings are defined as foods or liquids given to the infant in addition to breast milk or formula. Health Canada et al. (2012) recommend introducing solid foods after 6 months of age. Traditionally, the recommended first foods were single-grain cereals, followed by vegetables and fruits. However, breastfeeding infants in particular can benefit from a source of iron, such as iron-fortified cereal, meat, or meat alternatives; these are recommended to be the first solid foods introduced. Fruits and vegetables should be offered to infants daily, starting by at least 8 months. Fruit juices are not recommended before 6 months of age because it is possible that the infant who drinks juice will consume less breast milk or formula. Consumption of low-nutrient foods such as fatty or sugary foods or restaurant foods should be limited. There is no evidence that the order in which solid foods are introduced to older infants affects their risk of developing a food allergy (Health Canada et al., 2012). If a parent is worried about food allergies, it is recommended that only one new food that may cause an allergy be given per day and to wait at least 2 days before another food allergen is introduced. See Chapter 35 for further discussion on introducing solids to infants.

In spite of the recommendations from Health Canada, many parents begin complementary feedings earlier than 6 months. The notion that the feeding of solids helps the infant sleep through the night is not true. Parents should not put cereal into the infant's bottle. Introduction of solid foods before the infant is 6 months of age can result in overfeeding and decreased intake of breast milk or formula.

Nurses and other health care providers educate parents regarding complementary feedings. This most often occurs during well-baby supervision visits with the pediatric health care provider. Early feeding practices have implications for long-term dietary patterns; therefore, it is essential to teach parents about proper nutrition.

KEY POINTS

- Human milk is species specific and is the recommended form of nutrition for infants. It provides immunological protection against many infections and diseases.
- During the prenatal period, parents should be informed of the importance of breastfeeding for infants, mothers, families, and society.
- Breast milk changes in composition with each stage of lactation, during each feeding, and as the infant grows.
- Infants should be breastfed as soon as possible after birth and at least 8 to 12 times per day thereafter.
- Nurses play a key role in helping mothers to ensure that newborns latch on to the breast effectively.
- There are objective, measurable indicators that the infant is breastfeeding effectively.
- Breast milk production is based on a supply-meets-demand principle; the more the infant nurses, the greater the milk supply.
- Commercial infant formulas can provide satisfactory nutrition for most infants.
- Infants should be held for all feedings.
- Parents should be instructed about the types of commercial infant formulas, safe preparation for feeding, and correct feeding technique.
- Unmodified (whole) cow's milk is not appropriate for feeding the infant during the first year of life.

evolve WEBSITE

Visit the Evolve website for additional resources related to the content in this chapter such as Case Studies, Critical Thinking Case Study Answers, Nursing Care Plans, Nursing Processes, Nursing Skills, and Review Questions for Exam Preparation at: http://evolve.elsevier.com/Canada/Perry/maternal/

REFERENCES

Abdulwadud, O., & Snow, M. (2012). Interventions in the workplace to support breastfeeding for women in employment. *The Cochrane Database of Systematic Reviews*, (10), CD006177, doi:10.1002/14651858.CD006177.pub3.

Academy of Breastfeeding Medicine (ABM) Protocol Committee. (2009). ABM clinical protocol #3: Hospital guidelines for the use of supplementary feedings in the healthy term breastfed infant. *Breastfeeding Medicine*, *4*(3), 175–182.

Academy of Breastfeeding Medicine (ABM) Protocol Committee. (2011a). ABM clinical protocol #10: Breastfeeding the late preterm infant. *Breastfeeding Medicine*, *5*(3), 127–130.

Academy of Breastfeeding Medicine (ABM) Protocol Committee. (2011b). ABM clinical protocol #9: Use of galactogogues in initiating or augmenting the rate of maternal milk secretion. *Breastfeeding Medicine*, *6*(1), 41–49.

Altuntas, N., Kocak, M., Akkurt, S., et al. (2015). LATCH scores and milk intake in preterm and term infants: A prospective comparative study. *Breastfeeding Medicine*, *10*(2), 96–101. doi:10.1089/bfm.2014.0042.

Amer, M., Cipriano, G., Venci, J., & Gandhi, M. (2015). Safety of popular herbal supplements in lactating women. *Journal of Human Lactation*, *31*(3), 348–353. doi:10.1177/0890334415580580.

American Academy of Pediatrics. (2010). Policy statement: Hospital stay for healthy term infants. *Pediatrics*, *125*(2), 405–409. doi:10.1542/peds.2009-3119.

American Academy of Pediatrics. (2011). Policy statement: SIDS and other sleep-related infant deaths: Expansion of recommendations for a safe infant sleeping environment. *Pediatrics*, *135*(4), e1105–e1106. doi:10.1542/peds.2015-0339.

American Academy of Pediatrics (AAP) Committee on Nutrition. (2009). *Pediatric nutrition handbook* (6th ed.). Elk Grove Village, IL: Author.

American Academy of Pediatrics (AAP) Section on Breastfeeding. (2012). Breastfeeding and the use of human milk—policy statement. *Pediatrics*, *129*(3), e827–e841.

Barrington, K. J., Sankaran, K., & Canadian Paediatric Society Fetus and Newborn Committee. (2007). Position statement: Guidelines for detection, management and prevention of hyperbilirubinemia in term and late preterm newborn infants. *Paediatric & Child Health*, *12*(Suppl. B), 1B–12B. Retrieved from <http://www.cps.ca/documents/position/hyperbilirubinemia-newborn>. Reaffirmed 2016.

Bartick, M., & Reyes, C. (2012). Las dos cosas: An analysis of attitudes of Latina women on non-exclusive breastfeeding. *Breastfeeding Medicine*, *7*(1), 19–24.

Best Start Resource Centre. (2013). *Breastfeeding for the health and future of our nation: A guide for Aboriginal families and communities in Ontario, Canada*. Toronto: Author. Retrieved from <http://beststart.org/resources/breastfeeding/BFHFN_sept26.pdf>.

Best Start Resource Centre. (2015). *Populations with lower rates of breastfeeding: A summary of findings*. Toronto: Author. Retrieved from <http://www.beststart.org/resources/breastfeeding/BSRC_Breastfeeding_Summary_EN_fnl.pdf>.

Best Start Resource Centre & Baby-Friendly Initiative Ontario. (2013). *The Baby-Friendly Initiative: Evidence-informed key messages and resources*. Toronto. Retrieved from <http://www.beststart.org/resources/breastfeeding/Baby_Friendly_Resource_linked_final.pdf>.

Blackburn, S. T. (2013). *Maternal, fetal, and neonatal physiology* (4th ed.). St. Louis: Saunders.

Bozzo, P., Koren, G., & Ito, S. (2012). Health Canada advisory on domperidone. *Canadian Family Physician, 58*(9), 952–953.

Bramson, L., Lee, J. W., Moore, E., et al. (2010). Effect of early skin-to-skin mother–infant contact during the first 3 hours following birth on exclusive breastfeeding during the maternity hospital stay. *Journal of Human Lactation, 26*(2), 130–137. doi:10.1177/0890334409355779.

Brand, E., Kothari, C., & Stark, M. A. (2011). Factors related to breastfeeding discontinuation between hospital discharge and 2 weeks' postpartum. *The Journal of Perinatal Education, 20*(1), 36–44.

Breastfeeding Committee for Canada. (2012). *BFI integrated 10 steps practice outcome indicators for hospitals and community health services*. Retrieved from <http://www.breastfeedingcanada.ca/documents/2012-05-14_BCC_BFI_Ten_Steps_Integrated_Indicators.pdf>.

Breastfeeding Committee for Canada. (2014). *Annual report*. Retrieved from <http://www.breastfeedingcanada.ca/documents/BCC%20AGM%20 2015%20final%20reportsEN.pdf>.

Canadian Dental Association. (2012). *CDA position on use of fluorides in caries prevention*. Retrieved from <http://www.cda-adc.ca/_files/position_statements/fluoride.pdf>.

Centers for Disease Control and Prevention. (2010). US medical eligibility criteria for contraceptive use, 2010: Adapted from the World Health Organization medical eligibility criteria for contraceptive use. *MMWR. Morbidity and Mortality Weekly Report, 59*(RR4), 1–86.

Chantry, C. J. (2011). Supporting the 75%: Overcoming barriers after breastfeeding initiation. *Breastfeeding Medicine, 6*(5), 337–339.

Chapman, D. J. (2012). Research spotlight: Longer cumulative breastfeeding duration associated with improved bone strength. *Journal of Human Lactation, 28*(1), 18–19. doi:10.1177/0890334411433573.

Cleveland, K. (2010). Feeding challenges in the late preterm infant. *Neonatal Network, 29*(1), 37–41.

Colson, S. (2010). What happens to breastfeeding when mothers lie back? *Clinical Lactation, 1*, 9–12.

Colson, S. (2012). The laid-back breastfeeding revolution. *Midwifery Today, 101*, 9–11, 66.

Cooper, B. M., Holditch-Davis, D., Verklan, M. T., et al. (2012). Newborn clinical outcomes of the AWHONN late preterm infant research-based practice project. *Journal of Obstetric, Gynecologic, and Neonatal Nursing, 41*(6), 774–785.

Dell, K. M. (2011). Fluid, electrolytes, and acid-base homeostasis. In R. J. Martin, A. A. Fanaroff, & M. C. Walsh (Eds.), *Fanaroff and Martin's neonatal-perinatal medicine: Diseases of the fetus and infant* (9th ed.). St. Louis: Mosby.

Denne, S. C. (2015). Neonatal nutrition. *Pediatric Clinics of North America, 62*(2), 427–438. doi:10.1016/j.pcl.2014.11.006.

Dennis, C. L., Jackson, K., & Watson, J. (2014). Interventions for treating painful nipples among breastfeeding women. *The Cochrane Database of Systematic Reviews*, (12), CD007366, doi:10.1002/14651858.CD007366.pub2.

Dyson, L., McCormick, F. M., & Renfrew, M. J. (2005). Interventions for promoting the initiation of breastfeeding. *The Cochrane Database of Systematic Reviews*, (2), CD001688, doi:10.1002/14651858.CD001688.pub2.

Eni, R., Phillips-Beck, W., & Mehta, P. (2014). At the edges of embodiment: Determinants of breastfeeding for First Nations women. *Breastfeeding Medicine, 9*(4), 203–214. doi:10.1089/bfm.2013.0129.

Farrow, A. (2015). Lactation support and the LGBTQI community. *Journal of Human Lactation, 31*(1), 26–28. doi:10.1177/0890334414554928.

Flanders, D., Lowe, A., Kramer, M., et al. (2012). *A consensus statement on the use of domperidone to support lactation*. Canadian Lactation Consultant Association. Retrieved from <http://rcp.nshealth.ca/sites/default/files/Domperidone_Consensus_Statement_May_11_2012.pdf>.

Fortinguerra, F., Clavenna, A., & Bonati, M. (2009). Psychotropic drug use during breastfeeding: A review of the evidence. *Pediatrics, 124*(4), e547–e556.

Geddes, D. (2007). Inside the lactating breast: The latest anatomy research. *Journal of Midwifery & Women's Health, 52*(6), 556–563.

Geddes, D. T., & Prescott, S. L. (2013). Developmental origins of health and disease: The role of human milk in preventing disease in the 21st century. *Journal of Human Lactation, 29*(2), 123–127. doi:10.1177/0890334412474371.

Hale, T. W., & Rowe, H. E. (2014). *Medications and mothers' milk* (16th ed.). Amarillo, TX: Hale.

Hancock, M., & Brown, J. (2010). Formula-feeding safety: What nurses need to teach parents who choose to formula-feed. *Nursing for Women's Health, 14*(4), 303–309. doi:10.1111/j.1751-486X.2010.01560.x.

Health Canada. (2010). *Safe sleep tips*. Ottawa: Author. Retrieved from <http://www.phac-aspc.gc.ca/hp-ps/dca-dea/stages-etapes/childhood-enfance_0-2/sids/pdf/jsss-ecss2011-eng.pdf>.

Health Canada, Canadian Paediatric Society, & Dietitians of Canada and Breastfeeding Committee for Canada. (2012). *Nutrition for healthy term infants: Birth to six months*. Ottawa: Health Canada. Retrieved from <http://www.hc-sc.gc.ca/fn-an/nutrition/infant-nourisson/recom/index-eng.php>.

Héma-Québec. (2014). *Public mothers milk bank*. Retrieved from <http://www.hema-quebec.qc.ca/lait-maternel/donneuses-lait/banque-publique-lait-maternel.en.html>.

Holmes, A. H., Auinger, P., & Howard, C. R. (2011). Combination feeding of breast milk and formula: Evidence for shorter breast-feeding duration from the National Health and Nutrition Examination Survey. *The Journal of Pediatrics, 159*(2), 186–191.

Horta, B. L., & Victora, C. G. (2013). *Long-term effects of breastfeeding: A systematic review*. Geneva: World Health Organization. Retrieved from <http://www.who.int/maternal_child_adolescent/documents/breastfeeding_long_term_effects/en/>.

Human Milk Banking Association of North America (HMBANA). (2016). *Locations*. Retrieved from <https://www.hmbana.org/locations>.

Hurst, N. M., & Meier, P. P. (2010). Breastfeeding the preterm infant. In J. Riordan & K. Wambach (Eds.), *Breastfeeding and human lactation* (4th ed.). Sudbury, MA: Jones and Bartlett.

Institute of Medicine. (2005). *Dietary reference intakes for energy, carbohydrate, fiber, fatty acids, cholesterol, protein, and amino acids*. Washington, DC: Food and Nutrition Board, Institute of Medicine, National Academies Press.

International Lactation Consultant Association (ILCA). (2014). *Clinical guidelines for the establishment of exclusive breastfeeding* (3rd ed.). Morrisville, NC: Author.

Iyengar, S. R., & Walker, W. A. (2012). Immune factors in breast milk and the development of atopic disease. *Journal of Pediatric Gastroenterology and Nutrition, 55*(6), 641–647. doi:10.1097/MPG.0b013e3182617a9d.

Jaafar, S. H., Jahanfar, S., Angolkar, M., & Ho, J. J. (2012). Effect of restricted pacifier use in breastfeeding term infants for increasing duration of breastfeeding. *The Cochrane Database of Systematic Reviews*, (7), CD007202, doi:10.1002/14651858.CD007202.pub3.

Jessri, M., Farmer, A. P., & Olson, K. (2013). Exploring Middle-Eastern mothers' perceptions and experiences of breastfeeding in Canada: An ethnographic study. *Maternal & Child Nutrition, 9*, 41–56. doi:10.1111/j.1740-8709.2012.00436.x.

Johnston, C., Campbell-Yeo, M., Fernandes, A., et al. (2014). Skin-to-skin care for procedural pain in neonates. *The Cochrane Database of Systematic Reviews*, (1), CD008435, doi:10.1002/14651858.CD008435.pub2.

Kendall-Tackett, K. (2007). A new paradigm for depression in new mothers: The central role of inflammation and how breastfeeding and anti-inflammatory treatments protect maternal health. *International Breastfeeding Journal, 2*, 2–6. doi:10.1186/1746-4358-2-2.

Kendall-Tackett, K. (2015). The new paradigm for depression in new mothers: Current findings on maternal depression, breastfeeding and resiliency across the lifespan. *Breastfeeding Review, 1*, 7–10.

Kim, J. H., & Froh, E. B. (2012). What nurses need to know regarding nutritional and immunobiological properties of human milk. *Journal of Obstetric, Gynecologic, and Neonatal Nursing, 4*(1), 122–137. doi:10.1111/j.1552-6909.2011.01314.x.

Kramer, M. S., Aboud, F., Mironova, E., et al. (2008). Breastfeeding and child cognitive development: New evidence from a large randomized trial. *Archives of General Psychiatry, 65*(5), 578–584.

Kujawa-Myles, S., Noel-Weiss, J., Dunn, S., et al. (2015). Maternal intravenous fluids and postpartum breast changes: A pilot observational study. *International Breastfeeding Journal, 10*, 18.

Kumar, S. P., Mooney, R., Wieser, L. J., & Haystad, S. (2006). The LATCH scoring system and prediction of breastfeeding duration. *Journal of Human Lactation, 22*(4), 391–396. doi:10.1177/0890334406293161.

Labiner-Wolfe, J., & Fein, S. B. (2013). How US mothers store and handle their expressed breast milk. *Journal of Human Lactation, 29*(1), 54–58.

Lakshman, R., Ogilvie, D., & Ong, K. (2009). Mothers' experiences of bottle-feeding: A systematic review of qualitative and quantitative studies. *Archives of Disease in Childhood, 94*(8), 596–601.

La Leche League International. (2014). *How do I position my baby to breastfeed?* Retrieved from <http://www.llli.org/faq/positioning.html>.

Lamb, M. (2011). Weight-loss surgery and breastfeeding. *Clinical Lactation, 2*(2–3), 17–21.

Lauwers, J., & Swisher, A. (2011). *Counseling the nursing mother: A lactation consultant's guide* (5th ed.). Sudbury, MA: Jones and Bartlett.

Lawrence, R. A., & Lawrence, R. M. (2015). *Breastfeeding: A guide for the medical profession* (8th ed.). Elsevier: Mosby.

Lawrence, R. M., & Lawrence, R. A. (2011). Breastfeeding: More than just good nutrition. *Pediatrics in Review, 32*(7), 267–280.

Lepe, M., Bacardí Gascón, M., Castañeda-González, L. M., et al. (2011). Effect of maternal obesity on lactation: Systematic review. *Nutrición Hospitalaria, 26*(6), 1266–1269.

Lönnerdal, B. (2014). Infant formula and infant nutrition: Bioactive proteins of human milk and implications for composition of infant formulas. *The American Journal of Clinical Nutrition, 99*(3), 712S–717S. doi:10.3945/ajcn.113.071993.

Mangesi, L., & Dowswell, T. (2010). Treatments for breast engorgement during lactation. *The Cochrane Database of Systematic Reviews*, (9), CD006946, doi:10.1002/14651858.CD006946.pub2.

Mannel, R. (2011). Defining lactation acuity to improve patient safety and outcomes. *Journal of Human Lactation, 27*(2), 163–170. doi:10.1177/0890334410397198.

McMillan, D., & Canadian Paediatric Society, & College of Family Physicians of Canada. (1997). Routine administration of vitamin K to newborns. *Paediatric & Child Health, 2*(6), 429–431. Retrieved from <http://www.cps.ca/documents/position/administration-vitamin-K-newborns>. Reaffirmed 2016.

Mehta, U. J., Siega-Riz, A. M., Herring, A. H., et al. (2011). Maternal obesity, psychological factors, and breastfeeding duration. *Breastfeeding Medicine, 6*(6), 369–376.

Moore, E. R., Anderson, G. C., Bergman, N., et al. (2012). Early skin-to-skin contact for mothers and their healthy newborn infants. *The Cochrane Database of Systematic Reviews*, (5), CD003519, doi:10.1002/1465158.CD003519.pub3.

Mortell, M., & Mehta, S. D. (2013). Systematic review of the efficacy of herbal galactogogues. *Journal of Human Lactation, 29*(2), 154–162. doi:10.1177/0890334413477243.

Nelson, A. M. (2012). A meta-synthesis related to infant feeding decision making. *MCN: American Journal of Maternal Child Nursing, 37*(4), 247–252.

Oddy, W. H. (2012). Infant feeding and obesity risk in the child. *Breastfeeding Review, 20*(2), 7–12.

Pikwer, M., Bergström, U., Nilsson, J. A., et al. (2009). Breast-feeding, but not oral contraceptives, is associated with a reduced risk of rheumatoid arthritis. *Annals of Rheumatic Disease, 68*(4), 526–530. doi:10.1136/ard.2007.084707.

Ponti, M., & Canadian Paediatric Society, Community Paediatrics Committee. (2003). Position statement: Recommendations for the use of pacifiers. *Paediatrics & Child Health, 8*(8), 515–519. Retrieved from <http://www.cps.ca/documents/position/pacifiers>. Reaffirmed 2016.

Pound, C. M., Unger, S. L., & Canadian Paediatric Society, Nutrition and Gastroenterology Committee. (2012). Position statement: The Baby-Friendly Initiative: Protecting, promoting and supporting breastfeeding. *Paediatrics & Child Health, 17*(6), 317–321. Retrieved from <http://www.cps.ca/documents/position/baby-friendly-initiative-breastfeeding>. Reaffirmed 2015.

Powers, N. G. (2010). Low intake in the breastfed infant: Maternal and infant considerations. In J. Riordan & K. Wambach (Eds.), *Breastfeeding and human lactation* (4th ed.). Sudbury, MA: Jones and Bartlett.

Preer, G., Pisegna, J., Cook, J., et al. (2013). Delaying the bath and in-hospital breastfeeding rates. *Breastfeeding Medicine, 8*(6), 485–490. doi:10.1089/bfm.2012.0158.

Public Health Agency of Canada. (2013). *Perinatal health indicators for Canada 2013: A report of the Canadian Perinatal Surveillance System.* Cat. No. HP7-1/2013E-PDF. Ottawa: Author.

Public Health Agency of Canada. (2015). *Canada Prenatal Nutrition Program (CPNP).* Retrieved from <http://www.phac-aspc.gc.ca/hp-ps/dca-dea/prog-ini/cpnp-pcnp/index-eng.php>.

Ramsay, D., Kent, J., Hartmann, R., et al. (2005). Anatomy of the lactating human breast redefined with ultrasound imaging. *Journal of Anatomy, 206*(6), 525–534.

Rassin, M., Klug, E., Nathanzon, H., et al. (2009). Cultural differences in child delivery: Comparisons between Jewish and Arab women in Israel. *International Nursing Review, 56*(1), 123–130. doi:10.1111/j.1466-7657.2008.00681.x.

Registered Nurses' Association of Ontario. (2003). *Breastfeeding best practice guidelines for nurses.* Toronto: Author. Retrieved from <http://rnao.ca/sites/rnao-ca/files/Breastfeeding_Best_Practice_Guidelines_for_Nurses.pdf>.

Riordan, J., & Hoover, K. (2010). Perinatal and intrapartum care. In J. Riordan & K. Wambach (Eds.), *Breastfeeding and human lactation* (4th ed.). Sudbury, MA: Jones and Bartlett.

Riordan, J., & Wambach, K. (2010a). *Breastfeeding and human lactation* (4th ed.). Sudbury, MA: Jones & Bartlett Publishers.

Riordan, J., & Wambach, K. (2010b). Breast-related problems. In J. Riordan & K. Wambach (Eds.), *Breastfeeding and human lactation* (4th ed.). Sudbury, MA: Jones and Bartlett.

Rios, E. (2009). Promoting breastfeeding in the Hispanic community. *Breastfeeding Medicine, 4*(Suppl. 1), S69–S70.

Rowan-Legg, A., & Canadian Paediatric Society, Community Paediatrics Committee. (2015). Position statement: Ankyloglossia and breastfeeding. *Paediatrics & Child Health, 20*(4), 209–213. Retrieved from <http://www.cps.ca/en/documents/position/ankyloglossia-breastfeeding>.

Shah, P. S., Herbozo, C., Aliwalas, L. L., & Shah, V. S. (2012). Breastfeeding or breast milk for procedural pain in neonates. *The Cochrane Database of Systematic Reviews*, (12), CD004950, doi:10.1002/14651858.CD004950.pub3.

Smith, L., & Riordan, J. (2010). Postpartum care. In J. Riordan & K. Wambach (Eds.), *Breastfeeding and human lactation* (4th ed.). Sudbury, MA: Jones and Bartlett.

Spietz, A., Johnson-Crowley, N., Summer, G., & Bernard, K. (2008). *Keys to caregiving: Study guide* (revised). Seattle, WA: NCAST (Nursing Child Assessment Satellite Training), University of Washington School of Nursing.

Statistics Canada. (2014). *Health trends: Breastfeeding initiation.* Statistics Canada Catalogue No. 82-213-XWE. Ottawa: Author. Retrieved from <http://www.statcan.gc.ca/pub/82-624-x/2013001/article/11879-eng.htm>.

Stuebe, A., & Bonuck, K. (2011). What predicts intent to breastfeed exclusively? Breastfeeding knowledge, attitudes, and beliefs in a diverse urban population. *Breastfeeding Medicine, 6*(6), 413–420.

Stuebe, A., & Swartz, E. (2010). The risks and benefits of infant feeding practices for women and their children. *Journal of Perinatology, 30*, 155–162. doi:10.1038/jp.2009.107.

Tenfelde, S., Finnegan, L., & Hill, P. D. (2011). Predictors of breastfeeding exclusivity in a WIC sample. *Journal of Obstetric, Gynecologic, and Neonatal Nursing, 40*(2), 179–189.

Tully, M., & Jones, F. (2010). Donor milk banking. In J. Riordan & K. Wambach (Eds.), *Breastfeeding and human lactation* (4th ed.). Sudbury, MA: Jones and Bartlett.

Turcksin, R., Bel, S., Galjaard, S., et al. (2014). Maternal obesity and breastfeeding intention, initiation, intensity and duration: A systematic review. *Maternal & Child Nutrition, 10*(2), 166–183. doi:10.1111/j.1740-8709.2012.00439.x.

UNICEF. (2009). *Canadian supplement to the state of the world's children 2009. Aboriginal children's health: Leaving no child behind.* Retrieved from <http://www.nccah.ca/docs/child%20and%20youth/Report%20 Summary%20Leaving%20no%20child%20behind.pdf>.

Whyte, R. K., & Canadian Paediatric Society, Fetus and Newborn Committee. (2010). Position statement: Safe discharge of the late preterm infant. *Paediatrics & Child Health, 15*(10), 655–660. Reaffirmed 2015.

Wojcicki, J. M. (2011). Maternal prepregnancy body mass index and initiation and duration of breastfeeding: A review of the literature. *Journal of Women's Health, 20*(3), 341–347.

World Health Organization. (2010). *Combined hormonal contraceptive use during the postpartum period.* Geneva: Author. Retrieved from <http://www.who.int/reproductivehealth/publications/family_planning/rhr_10_15/en/>.

World Health Organization. (2011). *Exclusive breastfeeding.* Geneva: Author. Retrieved from <http://www.who.int/nutrition/topics/exclusive_breastfeeding/en/>.

World Health Organization. (2015). *Mother-to-child transmission of HIV.* <http://www.who.int/hiv/topics/mtct/en/>.

ADDITIONAL RESOURCES

AVERT—Pregnancy, Childbirth & Breastfeeding and HIV: <http://www.avert.org/hiv-and-breastfeeding.htm>.

Best Start—Breastfeeding Guidelines for Consultants: <http://www.beststart.org/resources/breastfeeding/pdf/breastfdeskref09.pdf>.

Best Start: Breastfeeding Matters—An Important Guide to Breastfeeding for Women and Their Families: <https://www.beststart.org/resources/breastfeeding/pdf/BreastfeedingMatters_2013_low_rez_reference.pdf>.

Breastfeeding in Peel (Region of Peel Health Department)—Multilingual resources for new parents, including videos: <http://www.peelregion.ca/health/family-health/breastfeeding/>.

INFACT Canada—Infant feeding action coalition: <http://www.infactcanada.ca/>.

Lactmed—Information on safety of medications and breastfeeding: <http://toxnet.nlm.nih.gov/cgi-bin/sis/htmlgen?LACT>.

La Leche League Canada—Breastfeeding education and mother–mother support: <http://www.lllc.ca/>.

LGBTQ health in Canada: <http://www.rainbowhealthontario.ca/>.

Milk Junkies—A resource for transgendered people who want to breastfeed: <http://www.milkjunkies.net/>.

Motherisk: <http://www.motherisk.org>.

Public Health Agency of Canada—Ten Valuable Tips for Successful Breastfeeding: <http://www.phac-aspc.gc.ca/hp-ps/dca-dea/stages-etapes/childhood-enfance_0-2/nutrition/tips-cons-eng.php>.

Registered Nurses' Association of Ontario—Breastfeeding Best Practice Guidelines: <http://rnao.ca/bpg/guidelines/breastfeeding-best-practice-guidelines-nurses>.

Human Milk Banking Information

Héma Québec—Mother's Milk: <http://www.hema-quebec.qc.ca/lait-maternel/index.en.html>.

Human Milk Banking Association of North America (HMBANA): <https://www.hmbana.org/hmbana-about>.

CHAPTER

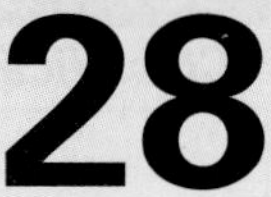

Infants With Gestational Age–Related Problems

Deborah Aylward

evolve WEBSITE

***Visit the Evolve website for additional resources related to the content in this chapter such as Case Studies, Critical Thinking Case Study Answers, Nursing Care Plans, Nursing Processes, Nursing Skills, and Review Questions for Exam Preparation at:** http://evolve.elsevier.com/Canada/Perry/maternal/*

OBJECTIVES

On completion of this chapter the reader will be able to:

- Compare and contrast the physical characteristics of preterm, term, and postterm neonates.
- Discuss respiratory distress syndrome and approaches to treatment.
- Compare methods of oxygen therapy for the high-risk infant.
- Describe nursing interventions for nutritional care of the preterm infant.
- Describe management of the infant with meconium aspiration.
- Describe risk factors associated with the birth and transition of an infant of a diabetic mother.
- Plan developmentally appropriate care for the high-risk infant.
- Develop a plan to address the unique needs of parents of high-risk infants.

Modern technology, interprofessional collaboration, and expert nursing care have made important contributions to improving the health and survival of high-risk infants. However, infants who are born considerably before term and survive are particularly susceptible to the development of sequelae related to their preterm birth. This chapter focuses on care of the preterm infant as well as care of other high-risk infants with gestational age–related problems, such as near-term and postterm infants. Infants born to mothers with diabetes are included because such infants may experience problems that place them at risk for altered development and transition.

High-risk infants are most often classified according to birth weight, gestational age, and common pathophysiological problems (Box 28-1). Intrauterine growth rates are not the same for all infants, and other factors (e.g., heredity, placental insufficiency, and maternal disease) influence intrauterine growth and birth weight.

THE PRETERM INFANT

Preterm infants, those born before 37 completed weeks of gestation, are at increased risk for health problems because their organ systems are immature and they lack adequate physiological reserves to function in the extrauterine environment. Morbidity and mortality rates vary among preterm infants. Despite advances in technology and management strategies, the lower the birth weight and the gestational age, the lower the chances of survival among infants born preterm. Preterm birth is responsible for almost 40% of infant deaths (Public Health Agency of Canada [PHAC], 2013).

The cause of preterm birth is multifactorial (see Box 20-2). Factors such as poverty (which can contribute to suboptimal health care and prenatal diet), maternal infections, previous preterm birth, multiple pregnancies, pregnancy-induced hypertension, and placental problems that interrupt the normal course of gestation before completion of fetal development are responsible for a large number of preterm births. According to 2013 data, 7.7% of infants born in Canada were preterm, 8.3% were small for gestational age (SGA) (PHAC, 2013), and approximately 6% were low birth weight (LBW) (Statistics Canada, 2012). The incidence of preterm birth is highest among low socioeconomic groups (Canadian Institute for Health Information [CIHI], 2009; Räisänen, Gissler, Saari, et al., 2013). This is likely a result of the lack of comprehensive prenatal

BOX 28-1 CLASSIFICATION OF HIGH-RISK INFANTS

Classification According to Size

Low-birth-weight (LBW)—An infant whose birth weight is less than 2500 grams (g), regardless of gestational age

Very-low-birth-weight (VLBW)—An infant whose birth weight is less than 1500 g

Extremely-low-birth-weight (ELBW)—An infant whose birth weight is less than 1000 g

Appropriate for gestational age (AGA)—An infant whose birth weight falls between the tenth and ninetieth percentiles on intrauterine growth charts

Small for gestational age (SGA) or small-for-dates (SFD)—An infant whose rate of intrauterine growth was slowed and whose birth weight falls below the tenth percentile on intrauterine growth charts

Intrauterine growth restriction (IUGR)—Found in infants whose growth in utero does not meet norms for gestational age and sex and is usually less than the third percentile.

Symmetrical IUGR—Growth restriction in which the weight, length, and head circumference are all affected

Asymmetrical IUGR—Growth restriction in which the head circumference remains within normal parameters as does length, while birth weight falls below the tenth percentile

Large for gestational age (LGA)—An infant whose birth weight falls above the ninetieth percentile on intrauterine growth charts

Classification According to Gestational Age*

Gestational age is the interval, in completed weeks, between the first day of a woman's last menstrual period and the day of birth.

Preterm (premature) infant—An infant born before 37 completed weeks of gestation, regardless of birth weight

Late preterm infant—An infant born between 34 0/7 and 36 6/7 weeks of gestation, regardless of birth weight*

Term infant—An infant born between the beginnings of 38 through 42 completed weeks of gestation, regardless of birth weight

Postterm (postmature) infant—An infant born after 42 completed weeks of gestation regardless of birth weight

Classification According to Mortality

Live birth—Birth in which the neonate manifests any heartbeat, breathes, or displays voluntary movement, regardless of gestational age. In Canada, an infant born less than 20 weeks' gestation who dies within the first few minutes after birth may be registered as a live birth and then as an infant death.

Fetal death—Death of the fetus, at any gestational age, before birth, with absence of any signs of life after birth. Only fetal deaths where the product of conception has a birth weight of 500 g or more or the duration of pregnancy is 20 weeks or longer are registered in Canada.

Neonatal death—Death that occurs in the first 28 days of life; early neonatal death occurs in the first week of life; late neonatal death occurs at 7 to 28 days.

Perinatal mortality—Total number of fetal and early neonatal deaths per 1000 live births

*Note: Definitions of late preterm vary among experts.

From Sauve, R., & McCourt, C. (2009). Infant mortality in Canada. *Journal of Obstetrics and Gynaecology Canada, 31*(4), 351–352; Statistics Canada. (2013). *Table 102-4514—Fetal deaths (20 weeks or more of gestation) and late fetal deaths (28 weeks or more of gestation)*, Canada, provinces and territories, annual (number), CANSIM (database). Ottawa: Ministry of Industry.

health care. Although SGA rates have decreased in the past few decades, the issue is still a cause for concern.

Opinions vary about the practical and ethical dimensions of resuscitation of extremely-low-birth-weight (ELBW) infants. Ethical issues associated with resuscitation of these infants include whether to resuscitate; who should make that decision; whether the cost of resuscitation is justified; and whether the benefits of technology outweigh the burdens on the infant, family, and society in relation to the infant's quality of life.

Late Preterm Infant

There has been increased interest in late preterm infants of 34 to 36 6/7 weeks of gestation who may receive the same treatment as term infants. Late preterm infants often experience morbidities similar to those of preterm infants, including respiratory distress, hypoglycemia requiring treatment, temperature instability, poor feeding, jaundice, and discharge delays as a result of illness (Whyte & Canadian Paediatric Society [CPS], 2010/2015). Talge, Holzman, Wang, and colleagues (2010) found that late preterm birth was associated with cognitive (lower IQ) and behavioural problems at follow-up in children at 6 years of age. It is estimated that late preterm infants represent 70% of the total preterm infant population. The morbidity and mortality rate for this group is significantly higher than that of term infants (Teune, Bakhuizen, Bannerman, et al., 2011; Whyte et al., 2010/2015). Because late preterm infants may be cared for in the same manner as healthy term infants, risk factors specific to late preterm infants may be overlooked. Late preterm infants are often discharged early from the hospital and have a significantly higher rate of rehospitalization than that of term infants (Lain, Roberts, Bowen, et al., 2015; Whyte et al., 2010/2015). See Table 28-1 for risk factors and nursing interventions for late preterm infants.

NURSING CARE

For the high-risk infant, an accurate assessment of gestational age (see Chapter 26, p. 689) is critical in helping the nurse to identify the potential problems that the newborn is likely to experience. The response of the preterm infant to extrauterine life is different from that of the term infant. By understanding the physiological basis of these differences, the nurse, as a member of an interprofessional care team, can assess these infants, determine the appropriate response of the preterm infant, and discern which potential problems are most likely to occur.

TABLE 28-1 LATE PRETERM INFANT ASSESSMENT AND INTERVENTIONS

RISK FACTORS	ASSESSMENT	INTERVENTIONS*
Respiratory distress	Assess for signs of respiratory distress (nasal flaring, grunting, tachypnea, central cyanosis, retractions) and presence of apnea.	Perform gestational age assessment. Observe for signs of respiratory distress; monitor oxygenation by pulse oximetry; provide supplemental oxygen as ordered.
Thermal instability	Monitor axillary temperature every 30 min immediately postpartum until stable; then every 1–4 hr depending on gestational age and ability to maintain thermal stability.	Provide skin-to-skin care in immediate postpartum period for stable infant. Implement measures to avoid excess heat loss (adjust environmental temperature, avoid drafts). Bathe only after thermal stability has been maintained for 1 hr.
Hypoglycemia	Monitor for signs and symptoms of hypoglycemia. Assess feeding ability (latch, suck and swallow reflexes). Monitor bedside glucose in infants with additional risk factors (IDM, prolonged labour, respiratory distress, poor feeding).	Initiate early feedings of human milk or, when medically indicated, formula. Avoid dextrose water or water feedings. Provide IV dextrose as necessary for hypoglycemia.
Jaundice	Observe for jaundice in first 24 hr. Evaluate maternal–fetal history for additional risk factors that may cause increased hemolysis and circulating levels of unconjugated bilirubin (Rh, ABO, spherocytosis, bruising). Assess feeding method and intake and voiding and stooling patterns.	Monitor bilirubin [transcutaneous and/or serum] and note risk zone on hour-specific nomogram (see Fig. 26-8).
Feeding problems	Assess ability to coordinate suck–swallow and breathing. Assess for respiratory distress, hypoglycemia, and thermal stability. Assess latch, milk transfer, and maternal comfort with feeding method. Determine weight loss (should be ≤10% of birth weight).	Initiate early feedings (human milk or, when medically indicated, formula). Ensure maternal knowledge of feeding method and of signs of inadequate feeding (sleepiness, lethargy, colour changes during feeding, apnea during feeding, decreased or absent urine output).
Neurodevelopmental problems	Assess for respiratory distress, neonatal jaundice, hypoglycemia, and thermal instability. Assess neurological status. Assess for seizure activity.	Perform newborn screening, including hearing test. Implement individualized developmental care. Encourage parents to keep follow-up appointments with primary care provider for evaluation of growth and development (including cognitive function and achievement of appropriate milestones).
Infection	Evaluate maternal–fetal history for risk factors that may contribute to neonatal septicemia. Assess for signs and symptoms of neonatal infection (see Box 28-3).	Use routine practices, especially hand hygiene between infants and after contact with surfaces that may harbour bacteria (e.g., keyboards, telephones). Maintain thermal stability. Administer hepatitis B vaccine if required. Encourage breastfeeding and assist mother and baby with breastfeeding. Encourage parents to decrease infant exposure to respiratory viruses after discharge and to obtain vaccines as appropriate to prevent development of respiratory viruses (e.g., influenza).

IDM, infant of diabetic mother; *IV,* intravenous.
*This is not an exhaustive list of nursing interventions; additional interventions include those discussed under the care of the high-risk infant in this chapter.
Portions adapted from Association of Women's Health, Obstetric and Neonatal Nurses (AWHONN). (2010). *Assessment and care of the late preterm infant: Evidence-based clinical practice guideline.* Washington, DC: Author.

The best environment for fetal growth and development is the uterus of a healthy, well-nourished woman. The goal of care for the preterm infant is to provide an extrauterine environment that approximates a healthy intrauterine environment in order to promote optimal growth and development. Medical and nursing personnel, respiratory therapists, occupational therapists and physiotherapists, dieticians, social workers, case managers, and pharmacists must work as a team and with parents to provide the intensive care needed. The admission of a preterm infant to the intensive care nursery is usually an emergent situation, and many members of the interprofessional team may be involved. A rapid initial assessment must be performed to determine the infant's need for stabilization and life-saving treatment.

When required, resuscitation is started in the birthing unit and the infant is supported en route to the nursery, where additional resuscitative and stabilization measures are implemented.

Respiratory Support

The preterm infant is likely to have difficulty making the pulmonary transition from intrauterine to extrauterine life. Numerous problems may affect the respiratory system of preterm infants, including the following:

- Decreased number of functional alveoli
- Deficient surfactant levels
- Smaller airway lumen
- Decreased tracheal cartilage
- Obstruction of respiratory passages
- Insufficient calcification of the bony thorax
- Circulating hormones (prostaglandins) that may affect cardiovascular function
- Immature and fragile pulmonary vasculature
- Greater distance between functional alveoli and capillary bed, especially in ELBW infants

In combination, these deficits hinder the infant's respiratory efforts and can produce respiratory distress or respiratory failure. Clinical tools have been developed to facilitate an objective assessment of the severity of respiratory compromise (Acute Care of at-Risk Newborns [ACoRN], 2012). Early signs of respiratory distress include tachypnea, nasal flaring, and expiratory grunting. Depending on the severity of respiratory distress and its cause, retractions may begin as subcostal, intercostal, or suprasternal. Increasing respiratory effort (e.g., paradoxical breathing patterns, retractions, nasal flaring, expiratory grunting, tachypnea, or apnea) indicates increasing distress. As a result of pulmonary immaturity very-low-birth-weight (VLBW) and ELBW infants may progress rapidly from respiratory distress to complete respiratory failure. Initially, a compromised infant's colour may be cyanotic centrally or pale. Acrocyanosis is a normal finding in the neonate; however, central cyanosis indicates poor oxygenation.

Periodic breathing is a respiratory pattern commonly seen in preterm infants and is manifested by 5- to 10-second respiratory pauses followed by 10 to 15 seconds of compensatory rapid respirations. Periodic breathing should not be confused with *apnea*—a cessation of respirations for 20 seconds or more associated with hypoxia, bradycardia, or both. The nurse must be prepared to respond to an apneic infant by providing stimulation (e.g., gentle rubbing of back), ventilation, and supplemental oxygen as necessary.

Oxygen therapy. The goals of oxygen therapy are to provide adequate oxygen to the tissues, prevent lactic acid accumulation resulting from hypoxia, and avoid the potentially negative effects of oxygen and barotrauma. Numerous methods are available to improve oxygenation. All require that the oxygen be warmed and humidified before entering the respiratory tract. If the infant does not require intubation and mechanical ventilation, oxygen can be supplied by nasal cannula or via nasal prongs in conjunction with continuous positive airway pressure (CPAP). If oxygen saturation of the blood cannot be maintained at a satisfactory level and the carbon dioxide level ($PaCo_2$) rises, infants require ventilatory assistance. Because oxygen therapy has inherent risks, each infant must be carefully monitored to prevent hyperoxemia and hypoxemia.

Infants who require oxygen should have frequent assessments of respiratory status and oxygenation; the timing of assessments is based on the infant's status. Oxygenation assessment includes continuous pulse oximetry and arterial blood gases (ABGs), as ordered. Vital signs should be monitored to ensure adequacy of respiratory function, circulation, and perfusion of tissues.

Studies of the resuscitation of compromised newborns with 21% oxygen, rather than 100% oxygen, have demonstrated no significant neurological morbidities at 18 to 24 months in newborns resuscitated with 21% oxygen. Room air resuscitation has been associated with fewer complications related to oxidative stress and hyperoxemia (Dawson, Vento, Finer, et al., 2012; Paul, 2015; Vento & Saugstad, 2011). Current resuscitation guidelines advocate the use of room air, as the initial gas, for term infants and judicious use of oxygen when resuscitating preterm infants. The goal is to minimize oxygen free radicals and avoid both hyperoxia and hypoxia (Paul, 2015; Perlman, Wyllie, Kattwinkel, et al., 2010). A review of several studies indicates that neonatal mortality is reduced by 30 to 40% when room air is used, instead of 100% oxygen, for neonatal resuscitation; rates of retinopathy of prematurity (ROP) and bronchopulmonary dysplasia (BPD) are lower in infants whose saturation (SaO_2) is kept between 93 and 95%. Fluctuations in oxygen saturation are also deemed harmful. It is recommended that for ELBW infants oxygen saturations be maintained at 90 to 95% (Saugstad & Aune, 2014). Whenever supplemental oxygen is used, continuous pulse oximetry should be used to monitor the infant's oxygenation status and to guide the titration of oxygen being delivered.

Nasal cannula. Low-flow oxygen can be administered by nasal cannula, sometimes called *nasal prongs* (Fig. 28-1). A *nasal cannula* consists of the tubing that connects to the gas source as well as the prongs that are inserted into the nares and is used for infants who require low concentrations of supplemental oxygen; it is often used during the weaning process and for home oxygen administration. The infant receives supplemental oxygen without compromising positioning, vision, or parental holding. Infants can also breast- or bottle-feed while receiving oxygen by this method. The nasal prongs must be inspected often to ensure that they remain in place, are patent, and do not cause skin irritation or excoriation.

Continuous distending pressure. Infants who are unable to maintain adequate oxygenation (Pao_2) despite the administration of oxygen by nasal cannula may require the use of continuous positive airway pressure (CPAP). CPAP delivers a preset pressure of oxygen (21% or more) (Fig. 28-2) using nasal prongs, nasopharyngeal tube, or face mask. Use of nasal prongs is a common method of CPAP delivery. CPAP increases the functional residual capacity, improves the diffusion of pulmonary gases, and can decrease pulmonary vascular resistance and

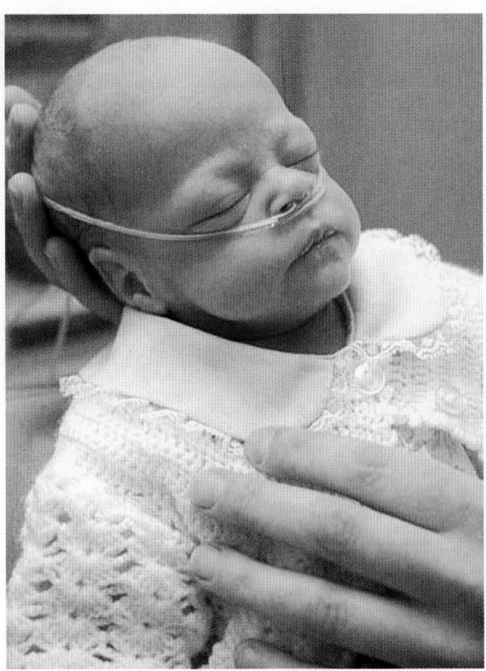

FIGURE 28-1 Infant with nasal cannula. (© Angela Hampton Picture Library/Alamy Stock Photo.)

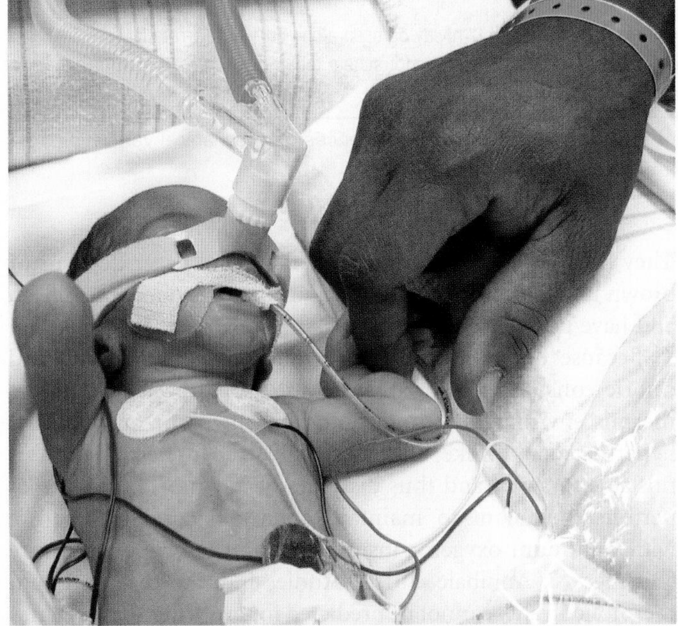

FIGURE 28-2 Infant on nasal continuous positive airway pressure (CPAP) with father's finger in hand. (Courtesy E. Jacobs, Texas Children's Hospital.)

intrapulmonary shunting. If implemented early enough, CPAP may eliminate the need for mechanical ventilation. CPAP is the preferred mode for infants who require minor distending pressure, as it avoids the trauma associated with endotracheal intubation and its inherent complications (Gardner, Enzman-Hines, & Dickey, 2011). The infant with a nasal CPAP device must be monitored closely for signs of nasal damage and skin breakdown (Squires & Hyndman, 2009). An orogastric tube may be needed to decompress the stomach during the use of CPAP.

Mechanical ventilation. Mechanical ventilation must be implemented if other methods of therapy cannot correct abnormalities in oxygenation. Its use is indicated whenever blood gas values reveal severe hypoxemia or severe hypercapnia. Mechanical ventilation may be required for the infant with apnea, meconium aspiration syndrome (MAS), respiratory distress syndrome (RDS), or congenital defects. Ventilator settings are individualized: the ventilator is set to provide a predetermined amount of oxygen during spontaneous respirations and to provide assisted ventilation in the absence of spontaneous respirations. Newer technologies allow oxygen to be delivered at lower pressures and in assist modes. This decreases barotrauma and associated complications such as pneumothorax and pulmonary interstitial emphysema (Wheeler, Klingenberg, McCallion, et al., 2010). Table 28-2 outlines the types of mechanical ventilation used in newborns.

High-frequency ventilation. Other modes of ventilator therapy include high-frequency oscillator ventilation and jet ventilation (see Table 28-2). These methods of high-frequency ventilation work by providing smaller volumes of oxygen at a significantly more rapid rate (more than 300 breaths/min) than that of traditional mechanical ventilators. As a result, the intrathoracic pressure and the risk of barotrauma are decreased.

Weaning from ventilatory support. The infant is ready to be weaned from ventilatory support when acid–base balance, ABGs, and oxygen saturation are maintained within normal limits. A spontaneous, adequate respiratory effort must be present, and the infant must show sustained muscle tone during spontaneous respirations. Weaning is done in a stepwise, gradual manner. The infant may be extubated, placed on nasal CPAP, and then weaned to oxygen alone. Throughout the weaning process, the infant's oxygen levels are monitored by pulse oximetry, ABGs, or both.

Some infants are not able to be weaned from oxygen by the time of discharge and may require home oxygen therapy. Parents need to be given consistent information and be reassured about the infant's respiratory progress. Decisions regarding the nature of interventions should be included in an interprofessional care plan, and the management strategy should be explained frequently to the family.

Frequent skin care assessments are essential when the infant is receiving supplemental oxygen with any of the methods described here, particularly in infants with poor perfusion and in those requiring equipment that comes in continuous contact with the infant's skin (e.g., nasal CPAP, nasal cannula, pulse oximetry probes).

Cardiovascular Support

Evaluation of heart rate and rhythm, skin colour, blood pressure, perfusion, peripheral pulses, oxygen saturation, and acid–base status provides information on cardiovascular status. The nurse must be prepared to intervene if symptoms of hypovolemia, shock, or both are found. These symptoms include prolonged capillary refill (longer than 3 seconds), pale colour (pallor), poor muscle tone, lethargy, initial tachycardia then bradycardia, and continued respiratory distress despite the

TABLE 28-2 COMMON METHODS FOR ASSISTED VENTILATION IN NEONATAL RESPIRATORY DISTRESS*

METHOD	DESCRIPTION	HOW PROVIDED
Conventional Methods		
Continuous positive airway pressure (CPAP)	Provides constant distending pressure to airway in a spontaneously breathing infant	Nasal cannula, face mask attached to flow-inflating bag or T-piece resuscitator
Intermittent mandatory ventilation (IMV)	Allows infant to breathe spontaneously at own rate but provides mechanical cycled respirations and pressure at regular preset intervals	Endotracheal intubation and ventilator
Synchronized intermittent mandatory ventilation (SIMV)	Mechanically delivered breaths are synchronized to the onset of spontaneous patient breaths Assist/control (A/C) mode facilitates full inspiratory synchrony; involves signal detection of onset of spontaneous respiration from abdominal movement, thoracic impedance, and airway pressure or flow changes Pressure support ventilation provides inspiratory pressure assistance when spontaneous breathing is detected to decrease infant's work of breathing.	Patient-triggered infant ventilator with signal detector and A/C mode; endotracheal tube
Volume guarantee ventilation	Delivers a predetermined volume of gas using inspiratory pressure that varies according to the infant's lung compliance (often used in conjunction with SIMV)	Volume guarantee ventilator with flow sensor; endotracheal tube
Alternative Methods		
High-frequency oscillation (HFO)	Application of high-frequency, low-volume, sine-wave flow oscillations to airway at rates between 480 and 1200 breaths/min	Variable-speed piston pump (or loudspeaker, fluidic oscillator); endotracheal tube
High-frequency jet ventilation (HFJV)	Uses a separate, parallel, low-compliant circuit and injector port to deliver small pulses or jets of fresh gas deep into airway at rates between 250 and 900 breaths/min	May be used alone or with low-rate IMV; endotracheal tube

*This is not a comprehensive list of available ventilation modes. For more information, consult specific references on mechanical ventilation, such as Gardner, Enzman-Hines, and Dickey (2011), and Wheeler, Klingenberg, McCallion, et al. (2010).

provision of adequate oxygen and ventilation. Hypotension may initially be present or may occur in some infants as a late sign of shock.

Blood pressure is monitored routinely in the sick neonate by either internal or external means. Direct recording with arterial catheters is often used but carries the risks inherent in any procedure in which a catheter is introduced into an artery. An umbilical venous catheter may also be used to monitor the neonate's central venous pressure. Oscillometry is a noninvasive, effective means for detecting alterations in systemic blood pressure (hypotension or hypertension) and implementing appropriate therapy to maintain cardiovascular function.

Thermoregulation

After or concurrent with the establishment of respiration, the most crucial need of LBW infants is application of external warmth. Preventing heat loss in distressed infants is absolutely essential for survival, and maintaining a **neutral thermal environment (NTE)** is a challenging aspect of neonatal intensive nursing care. Heat production is a complicated process that involves the cardiovascular, neurological, and metabolic systems; immature neonates have all of the problems related to heat production that are faced by full-term infants (see Thermogenic System, Chapter 25, p. 648). However, LBW infants are placed at further disadvantage by a number of additional problems. They have an even smaller muscle mass and fewer deposits of brown fat for producing heat, lack insulating subcutaneous fat, and have poor reflex control of skin capillaries.

Because overheating produces an increase in oxygen and calorie consumption, infants are also jeopardized in a hyperthermic environment. Apnea and flushed colour may indicate hyperthermia. Unlike an older child, the preterm infant is not able to sweat and thus dissipate heat. An NTE is one that permits the infant to maintain a normal core temperature with minimum oxygen consumption and calorie expenditure (Bissinger & Annibale, 2010). Studies indicate that optimum thermoneutrality cannot be predicted for every high-risk infant's needs. In healthy term infants it is recommended that axillary temperatures be maintained at 36.5° to 37.5°C (97.7° to 99.5°F). Normal axillary temperatures in the preterm or at-risk newborn may range between 36.3° and 37.2°C (ACoRN, 2012; Brown & Landers, 2011). Guidelines for maintaining an NTE in the LBW infant are published; however, further research is needed to define an NTE for the ELBW infant (Brown & Landers, 2011).

VLBW and ELBW infants, with thin skin and almost no subcutaneous fat, can control body heat loss or gain only within a limited range of environmental temperatures. In these infants heat loss from radiation, evaporation, and transepidermal water loss is three to five times greater than in larger infants, and a decrease in body temperature is associated with an increase in mortality. Extremely premature infants may require environmental temperatures equal to or greater than skin and core temperature to achieve thermoneutrality (ACoRN, 2012).

The consequences of cold stress that produce additional hazards to neonates are (1) hypoxia, (2) metabolic acidosis, and (3) hypoglycemia. Increased metabolism in response to chilling creates a compensatory increase in oxygen and calorie consumption. If available oxygen is not increased to accommodate this need, arterial oxygen tension is decreased. This is further complicated by a smaller lung volume in relation to the metabolic rate, which creates diminished oxygen in the blood and concurrent pulmonary disorders. A small advantage is gained by the presence of fetal hemoglobin because its increased capacity to carry oxygen allows the infant to exist for longer periods in conditions of lowered oxygen tension.

High-risk infants may need an external heat source to achieve an NTE. A probe applied to the infant is attached to the external heat source supplied by a radiant warmer or a servocontrolled isolette. To delay or prevent the effects of cold stress, at-risk newborns are placed in a prewarmed isolette immediately after birth, where they remain until they are able to maintain thermal stability (i.e., the capacity to balance heat production and conservation with heat dissipation). ELBW infants may be placed in a food-grade polyethylene bag (or wrap) to decrease heat and water loss during resuscitation and the immediate postpartum period. Skin-to-skin contact between the preterm infant and parent can help maintain body temperature.

Care of the hypothermic infant. Rapid changes in body temperature may cause apnea and acidosis in the neonate. Therefore, warming a hypothermic infant should occur gradually, over a period of hours. Rapid rewarming may cause apnea; too slow rewarming increases metabolic distress and oxygen consumption. Rewarming can proceed at a rate of 1° to 2°C per hour. Rewarming should be individualized for each infant and a servocontrolled environment (radiant warmer or isolette) used. If the infant's condition allows, skin-to-skin contact is an effective method to regulate or increase body temperature.

Transition from the isolette. Infants who are medically stable and gaining weight, tolerate enteral feedings, and weigh 1300 to 1500 g may be transitioned from the isolette. The following guidelines may be followed to wean the infant from the isolette:

- Disconnect the servocontrol probe (if still in use).
- Dress the infant in a diaper, shirt, and cap.
- Lower the isolette temperature no more than 0.5°C every 2 hours.
- Record the temperature of the infant, the air, and the isolette.
- Assess the infant's responses to the changes every hour until four stable readings are obtained.
- Monitor the infant's temperature and other vital signs.

This procedure is repeated until the isolette temperature is the same as the room temperature and the infant's body temperature consistently remains within normal limits. The infant is then placed in an open bassinet (away from any drafts) and reassessed during routine care. If the infant is unable to maintain his or her temperature, the infant is returned to the isolette and the weaning process restarted once the infant is able to regulate his or her temperature. Consistent weight gain and absence of any clinical distress signs (poor feeding, respiratory distress and temperature instability) are measures of effective weaning to an open bassinet.

Neurological Support

The preterm infant's central nervous system (CNS) is susceptible to injury as a result of the following:

- Birth trauma with damage to immature intracranial structures
- Bleeding from fragile capillaries
- Impaired coagulation process, including prolonged prothrombin time
- Recurrent hypoxic and hyperoxic episodes
- Predisposition to hypoglycemia
- Fluctuating systemic blood pressure with concomitant variation in cerebral blood flow and pressure

In the preterm neonate, neurological function depends on gestational age, illness factors, and predisposing factors (i.e., intrauterine asphyxia). Clinical signs of neurological dysfunction may be subtle, nonspecific, or specific. A neurological assessment should be completed and include an assessment of tone, symmetry and quality of movements, reflexes, and cranial nerves (Blackburn, 2009a, 2009b; Heaberlin, 2014). Preterm infants should be evaluated for seizure activity, hyperirritability, CNS depression, elevated intracranial pressure, and abnormal movements. Primary and tendon reflexes are generally present in preterm infants by 28 weeks of gestation and should be part of the neurological examination.

Nutritional Support

Optimum nutrition is critical in the management of LBW and preterm infants, yet providing for their nutritional needs is difficult. The various systems and mechanisms for ingestion and digestion of foods are not fully developed; the more immature the infant, the greater the challenge. In addition, the nutritional requirements for this group of infants are not known with certainty. Preterm infants are at risk for nutritional compromise because of poor nutritional stores as well as physical (immaturity of the gastrointestinal tract) and developmental characteristics (lack of coordinated suck, swallow, and breathe reflexes).

Although some sucking and swallowing activities are demonstrated in utero in preterm infants, coordination of these mechanisms does not occur until approximately 32 to 34 weeks of gestation and these activities are not fully synchronized until 36 to 37 weeks. Initial sucking is not accompanied by swallowing and esophageal contractions are uncoordinated. The gag reflex may not be developed until 36 weeks. Consequently, preterm infants are prone to aspiration and complications thereof. As infants mature, the suck–swallow–breathe pattern develops, but it is a slow process and infants may become easily exhausted if overtaxed.

The amount and method of feeding are determined by the infant's size and condition. Nutrition can be provided by either the parenteral or enteral route or by a combination of the two. ELBW, VLBW, or critically ill infants are often initially fed exclusively via the parenteral route because of their inability to digest and absorb enteral nutrition. Organ immaturity and conditions resulting in hypoxia further preclude the use of enteral feeding until the infant's condition has stabilized. Necrotizing enterocolitis (NEC) has been associated with enteral feedings in acutely ill or distressed infants (see p. 778). Total parenteral nutrition (TPN) support of acutely ill infants may be accomplished with commercially available intravenous (IV) solutions of protein, amino acids, trace minerals, vitamins, carbohydrates (dextrose), and fat (lipid emulsion). There is evidence to support early (within hours of birth) introduction of parenteral nutrition with the introduction of minimal enteral feedings within the first 5 days of life.

Early introduction of small amounts of enteral feedings in metabolically stable preterm infants is beneficial and has been shown to stimulate the infant's gastrointestinal tract, preventing mucosal atrophy and subsequent enteral feeding difficulties; improve developmental outcome; and prevent growth failure (American Academy of Pediatrics [AAP], 2014; Anderson, Wood, Keller, et al., 2011). Minimal feedings, as little as 0.1 to 4 mL/kg of breast milk or preterm formula, may be given by gavage as early as the first or second postnatal day (Morgan, Young, & McGuire, 2014). Parenteral hydration and nutrition continue until the infant is able to tolerate an amount of enteral feeding sufficient to sustain growth. A systematic review of the literature did not find evidence that early trophic feeds were associated with an increase in the incidence of NEC in very preterm infants (Morgan, Bombell, & McGuire, 2013). Support for initiating minimal enteral feedings includes increased mineral absorption, increased serum calcium and alkaline phosphatase activity, and a substantial decrease in the incidence of bilious gastric residuals and feeding intolerance in preterm infants (Donovan, Puppala, Angst, et al., 2006; Prince & Groh-Wargo, 2013).

Type of nourishment. The types of formulas used, method and volume of feeding, and the infant's feeding schedule are based on assessment of the following variables:

- Weight of the infant
- Pattern of weight gain or loss (Infants <1500 g require more energy for growth and thermoregulation.)
- Presence or absence of suck and swallow reflexes
- Behavioural readiness for oral feedings
- Physical condition (presence or absence of bowel sounds, abdominal distension, bloody stools, respiratory distress, and apnea)
- Residual from previous feeding, if being gavage fed
- Malformations (especially gastrointestinal defects)
- Renal function (urine output) and laboratory values (e.g., electrolyte balance, glucose level)

Human milk is the best source of nutrition for term and preterm infants. Studies indicate that even small preterm infants are able to breastfeed, if they have adequate sucking and swallowing reflexes and no other contraindications. Mothers who wish to breastfeed their preterm infants are encouraged to pump their breasts until their infants are stable enough to tolerate breastfeeding. Guidelines for the storage of expressed mother's milk should be followed to decrease the risk of milk contamination and destruction of its beneficial properties (see Chapter 27). Because of the significant breastfeeding attrition rates, mothers of preterm or unwell infants need additional support and frequent encouragement to continue pumping until their infant is able to nurse.

Preterm infants may be able to successfully breastfeed earlier than previously believed (28 to 36 weeks). Breastfed preterm infants have fewer desaturations; warmer skin temperature; and better coordination of breathing, sucking, and swallowing than their bottle-fed counterparts (Gardner & Lawrence, 2011).

Commercially available preterm formulas are cow's milk based and whey predominant with a higher concentration of protein, calcium, and phosphorus than term formulas in order to meet the unique needs of the preterm infant (AAP, 2014). Most preterm formulas are either 22 or 24 kcal/30 mL. The preparation of powdered formula for preterm infants should be performed under strict aseptic technique, preferably in a pharmacy, and the formula properly refrigerated to prevent infection (Health Canada, 2010). Preterm infants fed human milk with fortifier (protein, phosphorus, and calcium) have increased weight gain and improved bone mineralization; therefore, human milk fortifier is recommended for LBW preterm infants (Lawrence & Lawrence, 2015). Supplementation with iron, vitamin D, and multivitamins may be considered in exclusively breastfed LBW infants.

! NURSING ALERT

In the hospital, contamination of powdered infant formula with *Enterobacter sakazakii* has been associated with serious neonatal infections, NEC, and death (Health Canada, 2010). When possible, alternatives to powdered formula (i.e., liquid or concentrate) should be chosen; otherwise, such formula should be carefully mixed in a pharmacy or designated formula preparation room using aseptic technique. Continuous infusion of powdered formula should not exceed 4 hours.

Gavage feeding. Gavage feeding is a method of providing breast milk or formula through a nasogastric or orogastric tube (Fig. 28-3). It can be done either intermittently (bolus) or continuously through an in-dwelling feeding tube. Human milk or formula can be supplied intermittently using a syringe with gravity-controlled flow or can be given continuously using an infusion pump. The type and amount of fluid are recorded with every feed or syringe change. The volume of the continuous feedings is recorded hourly, and gastric aspirates are checked every 2 to 4 hours. When bolus feeding, residuals are measured before each feed. Residuals of less than 25% of a feeding can usually be refed to the infant. It is important to follow unit protocol for specifics and further guidance. Feeding may be stopped if the residual is greater than 2 to 4 mL/kg or more than a 1-hour volume of a continuous feed. Feeding is not resumed until the infant can be assessed for a possible feeding intolerance (Anderson et al., 2011).

Theoretically, the orogastric route for gavage feedings may be preferred, as most infants are preferential nose breathers, but this does not seem to be borne out in practice. A study in Canada found no consensus on the use of orogastric versus

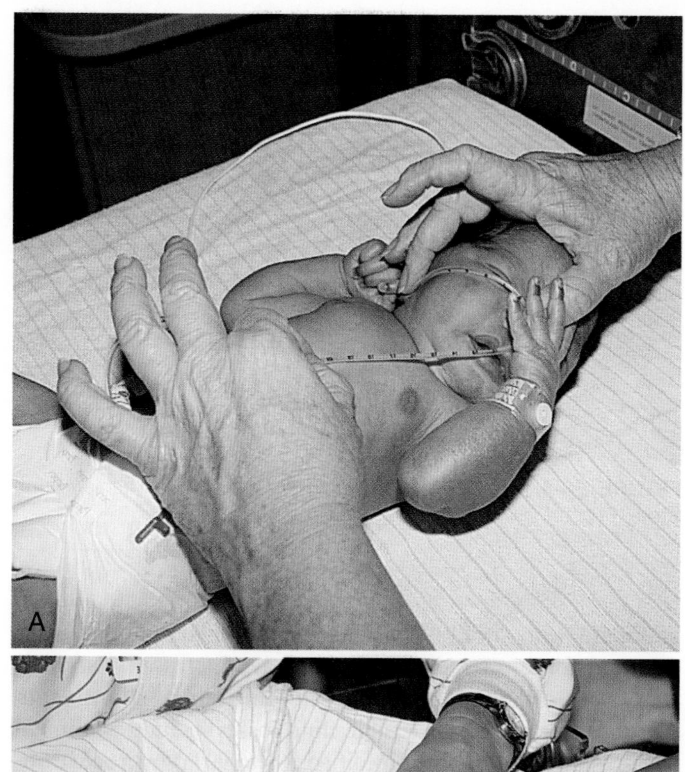

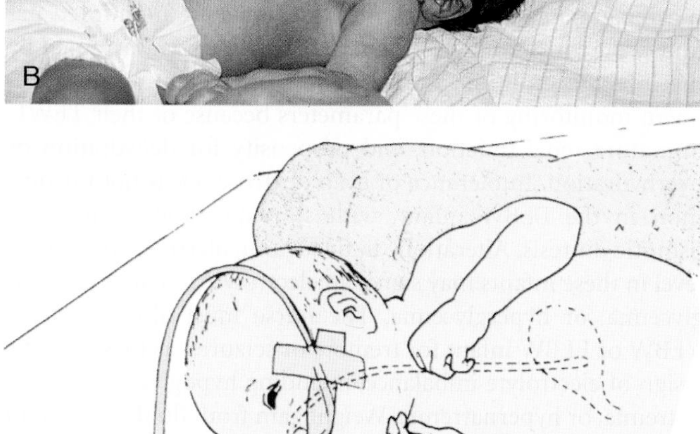

FIGURE 28-3 Gavage feeding. **A:** Measurement of gavage feeding tube from tip of nose to earlobe and to midpoint between end of xiphoid process and umbilicus. Tape may be used to mark correct length on tube. **B:** Insertion of gavage tube using orogastric route. **C:** In-dwelling gavage tube, nasogastric route. After feeding by orogastric or nasogastric tube, the infant is propped on right side or placed prone (preterm infant) for 1 hour to facilitate emptying of the stomach into the small intestine. Note rolled towel for support. (**A** and **B,** Courtesy Marjorie Pyle, RNC, Lifecircle.)

nasogastric tubes. Most of the 28 centres (75%) surveyed used nasogastric tubes the vast majority (more than 90%) of the time (Birnbaum & Limperopoulos, 2009). Smaller flexible feeding tubes (e.g., 5 Fr) may be inserted via the nasal route without interfering with the infant's breathing. The procedure for inserting a gavage feeding tube is described below and shown in Fig. 28-3. Complications of in-dwelling tubes include aspiration, obstructed nares, mucus plugs, purulent rhinitis, epistaxis, infection, and possible stomach perforation. Current best practice dictates a radiograph as the only certain way to determine nasogastric tube placement in the stomach. Methods such as auscultation of an air bubble, neck-ear-xiphoid (NEX) measurements for insertion depth, or pH measurements are considered imprecise when used as the only method for determination of placement of feeding tubes in infants (de Boer, Smit, & Mainous, 2009; Farrington, Lang, Cullen, et al., 2009; Freeman, Saxton, & Holberton, 2012; Quandt, Schraner, Ulrich Bucher, et al., 2009; Renner, 2010). Ellett, Cohen, Perkins, et al. (2011) developed an age-related, height-based regression equation for determining adequate gastric tube insertion length for use in neonates less than 1 month old (corrected age). Others have developed guidelines for correct nasogastric tube insertion and placement in LBW and term infants based on the infant's weight (Freeman et al., 2012). Further research is needed to determine optimal positioning of feeding tubes in high-risk infants on intermittent bolus or continuous gavage feedings.

To begin the feeding, the nurse connects the barrel of a syringe to the gavage tube. While clamping (or pinching) the feeding tube, the nurse pours the specified amount of breast milk or formula into the syringe. The clamp is then released and the feeding allowed to flow by gravity at a rate that approximates that of an oral feeding (about 1 mL/min). The infant may be held during gavage feedings by the caregiver or parent. If necessary, oxygen may be supplied via nasal cannula to facilitate handling. It is not recommended that the infant be removed from a primary source of oxygen for feedings because doing so decreases oxygen availability.

Once the prescribed volume has been delivered, the tube is clamped or pinched and the syringe either removed or left in place. If the gavage tube is to be left in situ, it is flushed with sterile water (1–2 mL) or air. If it is to be discontinued, the gavage tube is capped (or the nurse continues to pinch it) and is removed in one steady motion. Capping or pinching the tube prevents breast milk or formula from leaking from the tube and being aspirated during removal of the tube.

Documentation of the procedure includes size of the feeding tube, amount and quality of the residual from the previous feeding, type and quantity of fluid instilled, and the infant's tolerance of the procedure.

Gastrostomy feeding. Gastrostomy feeding involves the surgical placement of a tube through the skin of the abdomen into the stomach. With percutaneous gastrostomy insertion, feedings are often started within hours of insertion. Feedings by gravity are done slowly over 20 to 30 minutes, depending on the volume. Special care must be taken to avoid a rapid bolus of the fluid because this may lead to respiratory compromise,

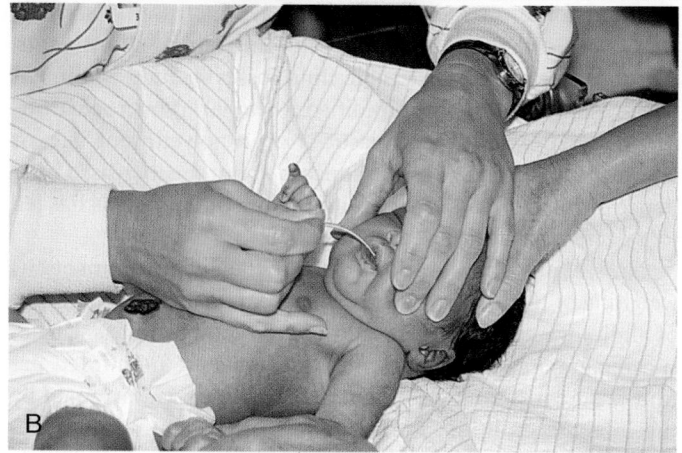

abdominal distension, reflux into the esophagus, or diarrhea with malabsorption. Meticulous skin care at the tube insertion site is necessary to prevent skin breakdown and infection. Intake and output should be carefully monitored to ensure adequate fluid and calorie intake and adequate renal function. Non-nutritive sucking should be offered with feeds to help the infant associate satiation with suckling.

Advancing infant feedings. Feedings are advanced from passive (parenteral and gavage) to active (nipple and breast-feeding) on the basis of the infant's readiness for and ability to tolerate feedings. The infant's sucking patterns and demonstration of a quiet, alert state can also be used to determine readiness to nipple feed.

The infant receiving parenteral nutrition is gradually weaned off this type of nutrition. The nourishment given by gavage feedings is increased as tolerated by the infant, and the parenteral fluids are decreased. Feedings are advanced slowly and cautiously; if feedings are advanced too rapidly, apnea, abdominal distension, vomiting, and diarrhea may result.

Gavage feedings then progress to nipple feedings (breast or bottle). Gavage feedings are decreased as the infant's ability to suckle improves. Often the infant is fed by both nipple and gavage feeding during this transition; this ensures intake of the prescribed volumes of both fluid and nutrients. The parents should be encouraged to interact by holding, making eye contact, and talking to the infant during feedings.

Because preterm infants may be discharged weighing as little as 1500 g, the need to closely monitor nutritional intake and growth continues after discharge. A recent review of feeding practices in preterm infants following discharge was inconclusive as to best practice and did not recommend the use of nutrient-enriched formula for feeding preterm infants (Garg & Gupta, 2013).

Non-nutritive sucking. For the infant who requires gavage or parenteral feedings, non-nutritive sucking on a pacifier during the procedure may improve oxygenation and facilitate earlier transition to nipple feeding (Fig. 28-4). Mothers of preterm infants should be encouraged to let their infant start sucking at the breast during kangaroo care; some infants may have coordinated suck and swallow reflexes as early as 32 weeks of gestation. Proposed benefits of non-nutritive sucking include improved weight gain, improved milk intake, more stable heart rate and oxygen saturation, earlier age at full oral feeds, and improved behavioural state.

Hydration

High-risk infants often receive supplemental parenteral fluids to supply additional calories, electrolytes, or water. Adequate hydration is particularly important in preterm infants because their extracellular water content is higher (70% in term infants and up to 90% in preterm infants), their body surface is larger, their skin barrier is immature and unable to prevent trans-epidermal water loss (TEWL) losses, and glomerular immaturity decreases the ability to concentrate urine. Therefore, preterm infants are vulnerable to fluid depletion, fluid volume overload, and electrolyte abnormalities.

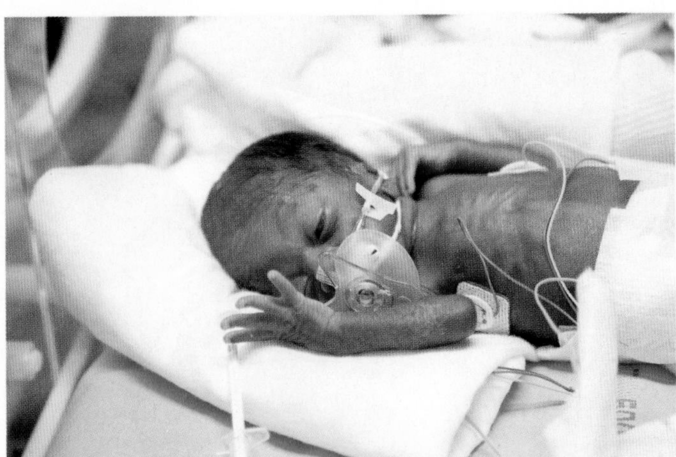

FIGURE 28-4 Non-nutritive sucking by infant. (© Phanie/Alamy Stock Photo.)

Infants who are ELBW, tachypneic, receiving phototherapy, or cared for on a radiant warmer have increased insensible water losses that require fluid administration adjustments. Methods to decrease insensible fluid losses include placement of the infant in a highly humidified (60 to 90%) microenvironment (isolette) and use of plastic wrap, a polyethylene bag, or emollient to decrease TEWL. Concern about the increased incidence of infection associated with the use of emollients has led to a decrease in their use.

Nurses must monitor fluid status with daily (or more often) weighing of the infant and ensuring accurate intake and output of all fluids, including medications and blood products. Urine-specific gravity and dipstick measurements are monitored per unit protocol. Serum electrolytes are obtained as warranted by the infant's condition. ELBW infants often require more frequent monitoring of these parameters because of their TEWL, immature renal function, and propensity for dehydration or overhydration. Intolerance of even dextrose 5% is not uncommon in the ELBW infant, with subsequent glycosuria and osmotic diuresis. Alterations in behaviour, alertness, or activity level in these infants may signal an electrolyte imbalance, hypoglycemia, or hyperglycemia. The nurse must also assess the VLBW or ELBW infant for tremors or seizures, as these may be a sign of electrolyte imbalance, including hypoglycemia, hyponatremia, or hypernatremia. Weight gain from fluid overload in the sick preterm infant may occur as a result of fluid retention (renal failure), inappropriate fluid administration (parenteral), or heart failure. An increased fluid gain may result in the opening of a previously closed patent ductus arteriosus (PDA), thus exacerbating associated illness. Growing preterm infants, especially those with BPD and those on oral electrolyte supplements, should be carefully monitored for rapid weight gain that may result in pulmonary congestion, PDA, and electrolyte imbalance. See Box 28-2 for calculation of a weight loss or gain.

Renal Support

The preterm infant's immature renal system is unable to (1) adequately excrete metabolites and drugs; (2) concentrate urine;

BOX 28-2 CALCULATION OF A WEIGHT LOSS OR GAIN

Net Weight Gain/Loss	Percentage Weight Gain/Loss
Current weight – previous weight = net weight gain (+) or weight loss (–)	$\frac{\text{Net weight gain or loss}}{\text{previous weight}} \times 100$ = percentage weight gain (+) or loss (–)
Example 1	
Weight day 1 = 1750 g (birth weight)	–70 g/1750 g
Weight day 2 = 1680 g	–.04 × 100 (%) = 4.0% weight loss
Net gain/**loss**: 1680 – 1750 = –70g	
Example 2	
Weight day 3 = 1680 g	
Weight day 4 = 1720 g	40 g/1680 g
Net **gain**/loss: 1720 – 1680 = 40 g	0.24 × 100 = 2.4% weight gain

or (3) maintain acid–base, fluid, or electrolyte balance. Therefore, intake and output, as well as specific gravity, must be assessed. Laboratory tests must be performed to assess acid–base and electrolyte balance. Medication levels (e.g., gentamycin) are also monitored in preterm infants because metabolism via renal and hepatic routes is often hindered. Because of great variability in drug metabolism, serum levels are obtained to ensure adequate therapeutic range for treatment and to prevent toxicity.

Hematological Support

The preterm infant is predisposed to hematological problems because of the following conditions:

- Increased capillary fragility
- Increased tendency to bleed (prolonged prothrombin time and partial thromboplastin time)
- Decreased production of red blood cells (RBCs) resulting from physiological rapid decrease in erythropoiesis after birth
- Large amount of fetal hemoglobin (up to 80% of total volume)
- Loss of blood attributable to frequent blood sampling for laboratory tests
- Decreased RBC survival related to the increased size of the RBC and its increased permeability to sodium and potassium
- Decreased levels of circulating albumin

The nurse needs to assess infants for any evidence of bleeding from puncture sites, the gastrointestinal tract, and pulmonary system. Infants should also be examined for signs of anemia (e.g., decreased hemoglobin and hematocrit levels, pale skin or pallor, apnea, lethargy, tachycardia, and poor weight gain). In high-risk infants, the amount of blood withdrawn for laboratory testing should be monitored and documented.

Protection From Infection

While protection from infection is an integral part of all newborn care, preterm and sick infants are particularly susceptible to infectious organisms. As with all aspects of care, strict hand hygiene is the single most important measure to prevent health care–associated infections. Personnel with known infectious disorders should be excluded from the unit until they are no longer infectious. Routine practices need to be instituted in all nursery areas as a method of infection control to protect the infants and staff.

Neonates are highly susceptible to infection as a result of diminished nonspecific (inflammatory) and specific (humoral) **immunity** and impaired phagocytosis, delayed chemotactic response, decreased complement levels, and minimal or absent immune globulins (Ig) A and M. Because of the infant's poor response to pathogenic agents, there is usually no local inflammatory reaction at the portal of entry to signal an infection, and symptoms tend to be vague and nonspecific. Consequently, diagnosis and treatment may be delayed. Preterm and term infants exhibit various nonspecific signs and symptoms of infection (Box 28-3). Early identification and treatment of sepsis are essential.

Skin Care

The skin of preterm infants is immature relative to that of term infants. In most preterm infants the skin barrier properties resemble those of the term infant by 2 to 4 weeks' postnatal age, regardless of gestational age at birth. Because of its increased sensitivity and fragility, no alkaline-based soap that might destroy the acid mantle of the skin is used. The increased permeability of the skin facilitates absorption of ingredients. All skin products (e.g., alcohol, chlorhexidine, povidone-iodine) should be used with caution; the skin is rinsed with water afterward because these substances may cause severe irritation and chemical burns in VLBW and ELBW infants.

The skin is easily excoriated and denuded; care must be taken to avoid damage to the delicate structure. The total skin is thinner than that of full-term infants and lacks rete pegs, appendages that anchor the epidermis to the dermis. Therefore, there is less cohesion between the thinner skin layers. The use of adhesive tape or bandages may excoriate the skin or adhere to the skin surface so well that the epidermis can be separated from the dermis and pulled away with the tape, thus altering skin barrier function. Pectin barriers and hydrocolloid adhesives may be useful because these products mould well to skin contours and adhere in moist conditions. Recommendations for protecting the integrity of the skin of preterm infants include minimal use of adhesive tape, backing the tape with cotton, and delaying adhesive and pectin barrier removal until adherence is reduced (Lund & Kuller, 2013). Emollients such as Eucerin or Aquaphor have been used to promote skin integrity and prevent dry, cracking, and peeling skin in infants at risk for skin breakdown. Emollients may also reduce TEWL and protect infants from health care–associated infection (Polin, Denson, Brady, et al., 2012). However, in some studies these agents have been shown to increase the risk for coagulase-negative infections in preterm infants and therefore should be used with caution. The

BOX 28-3 SIGNS AND SYMPTOMS OF NEONATAL INFECTION

Signs and symptoms are subtle and nonspecific and include the following:

Temperature instability
- Hypothermia—most common
- Hyperthermia—rarely

Central nervous system changes
- Lethargy
- Irritability
- Altered level of consciousness

Changes in colour
- Cyanosis, pallor
- Mottling
- Jaundice

Cardiovascular instability
- Poor perfusion
- Prolonged capillary refill (>3 seconds)
- Hypotension
- Bradycardia or tachycardia

Respiratory distress
- Tachypnea or bradypnea
- Apnea
- Retractions, nasal flaring, grunting
- Gastrointestinal problems
- Feeding intolerance, increased residuals (when gavage fed)
- Abdominal distension
- Vomiting
- Diarrhea
- Bloody stools (frank or occult positive)
- Metabolic instability
- Glucose instability
- Metabolic acidosis

Other
- Electrolyte imbalance
- Decreased urine output

use and effectiveness of emollients in high-risk neonates is controversial, and further studies are needed (Telofski, Morello, Mack Correa, et al., 2012).

It is unsafe to use scissors to remove dressings or tape from the extremities of very small and immature infants because it is easy to snip off tiny extremities or nick loosely attached skin. Solvents used to remove tape should be avoided because they tend to dry and burn the skin.

Guidelines for skin care are listed in the Guidelines box. It is recommended that a validated skin assessment tool such as the Braden Q Scale or Neonatal Skin Condition Score be used once daily to evaluate the high-risk infant's skin condition in order to implement interventions aimed at minimizing skin breakdown (see Additional Resources).

Environmental Concerns

Infants in neonatal intensive care units (NICUs) are exposed to high levels of auditory input from the various machine alarms

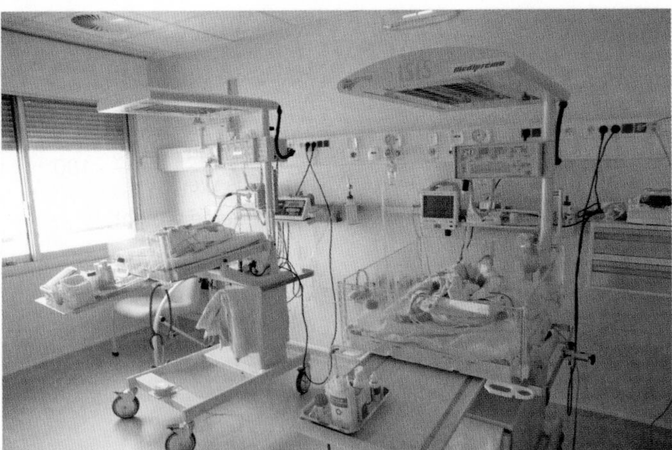

FIGURE 28-5 Neonatal intensive care unit (NICU) equipment, although necessary, contributes to environmental noise. Note radiant warmer, gas outlets, suction apparatus, monitor, ventilator, and pumps, all of which contribute to the auditory environment of the NICU. (Chassenet/Science Source.)

(Fig. 28-5), which can have adverse effects. Continuous noise levels of 45 to 85 decibels (dB) are common in the NICU. An isolette produces a constant noise level of approximately 60 dB (Thomas & Uran, 2007); each piece of life-support equipment adds to the background noise. The infant's hearing may be damaged if exposed to a constant decibel level of 90 dB or frequent decibel levels higher than 110 dB.

The noise level from monitoring equipment, alarms, and general unit activity has been correlated with the incidence of intracranial hemorrhage, especially in the ELBW or VLBW infant. Personnel should reduce noise-generating activities, such as slamming doors (including isolette portholes), listening to radios, talking loudly, and handling equipment (e.g., trash containers). Monitoring sound levels in the nursery has been shown to reduce ambient noise (Almadhoob & Ohlsson, 2015; Wang, Aubertin, Barrowman, et al., 2014).

Twenty-four-hour surveillance of sick infants requires appropriate visibility and often bright lights. Units should establish a night–day sleep pattern by either darkening the room, covering cribs with blankets, or placing eye patches over the infants' eyes at night. Infants need scheduled rest periods during which the lights are dimmed, the isolettes are covered with blankets, and the infants are not disturbed for handling of any kind (Fig. 28-6) (Holditch-Davis & Blackburn, 2013). Sleep periods should be undisturbed for at least 50 minutes to allow complete sleep cycles. Infants' eyes should be shielded from bright lights (e.g., procedure lighting) to prevent potential harm. Many experts suggest that the human face, especially the parent's, is the best visual stimulus and that other visual stimuli be kept to a minimum early in development.

Effects of environmental hazards can be potentiated by some medications used for infant therapy. Diuretics (especially furosemide [Lasix]), ototoxic antibiotics such as gentamycin and kanamycin, and antimalarial agents can potentiate noise-induced hearing loss. Routine hearing screening should be performed on all infants before discharge.

GUIDELINES

Neonatal Skin Care

General Skin Care

Assessment

- Assess skin frequently for redness, dryness, flaking, scaling, rashes, lesions, excoriation, or breakdown. An ideal time to assess the skin integrity and condition is during the bath and with diaper changes, but assessment can be performed during taking of vital signs and repositioning.
- Identify risk factors for skin injury: gestational age less than 30 weeks, unwell infants, intravenous and/or adhesive use, assisted ventilation devices, medications that compromise tissue perfusion (i.e., vasopressors).
- Use a valid assessment tool to provide reliable and objective measurement of skin condition (e.g., Braden Q Scale or Neonatal Skin Condition Score; see Additional Resources at end of chapter).
- Evaluate and report abnormal skin findings and assess for possible causes.
- Intervene according to cause or health care provider order.

Bathing

Initial Bath

- Assess for stable temperature a minimum of 2 to 4 hours before the first bath.
- Use cleansing agents with neutral pH. Avoid agents with dyes or scents.
- Use routine practices; wear gloves.
- Do not completely remove vernix; allow vernix to wear off with care and handling.
- Use warm water only to bathe preterm infants (less than 32 weeks gestation) for the first week.

Routine

- Decrease frequency of baths to every second or third day; continue daily cleansing of eyes, mouth, diaper areas, and pressure points, if present.
- Use cleanser or soaps no more than two or three times a week.
- Avoid rubbing skin during bathing or drying.
- Immerse stable infants fully (except head) in an appropriate-sized tub.
- Use swaddled immersion bathing technique: slow unwrapping after gently lowering into water for infants needing assistance with motor system reactivity.

Emollients

- Apply sparingly to dry, flaking, fissured areas as needed.
- Choose petrolatum-based products that are free of preservatives, dyes, and fragrances.
- Observe neonates who weigh less than 750 g receiving emollient therapy for increased risk of coagulase-negative *Staphylococcus* infections.
- Use emollients from the hospital pharmacy that are dispensed in a unit dose or patient-specific container. Follow hospital protocol or consider applying emollient as needed to infants older than 32 weeks for dry, flaking skin.

Adhesives

- Decrease use as much as possible.
- Use semipermeable transparent adhesive dressings to secure intravenous lines (IVs), nasogastric or orogastric tubes, silicone catheters, and central lines.
- Use hydrogel or limb electrodes.
- Consider pectin barriers beneath adhesives to protect skin.
- Secure pulse oximeter probe or electrodes with elasticized dressing material (carefully to avoid restricting blood flow).
- Do not use adhesive remover, solvents, or bonding agents.
- Avoid removing adhesives for at least 24 hours after application.
- Facilitate adhesive removal using water, mineral oil, or petrolatum.
- Remove adhesives or skin barriers slowly, supporting the skin underneath with one hand and gently peeling away the product from the skin with the other hand.*

Antiseptic Agents

- Apply before invasive procedures.
- Consider the potential for skin breakdown or irritation with disinfectant.
- No specific disinfectant is recommended for all neonates; remove completely with sterile water or saline after use. Follow instructions for use of chosen disinfectant.
- Avoid use of isopropyl alcohol for skin preparation or removal of other disinfectants.

Transepidermal Water Loss

Minimize TEWL and heat loss in preterm infants less than 29 weeks of gestation by doing the following:

- Apply an occlusive food-grade polyethylene bag or wrap at delivery; remove it once the infant's temperature is stable.
- Supply and measure ambient humidity during the first weeks of life (isolette).
- Maintain the humidity in the microenvironment (isolette) between 60 and 90% for first 7 days and at 50% for the first 28 days (or according to hospital policy).
- Use supplemental conductive heat and reduce radiant heat source.
- Apply semipermeable transparent dressings to skin surfaces on the infant's chest, abdomen, and back.

Skin Breakdown

Prevention

- Decrease pressure from externally applied forces using water, air, or gel mattresses; sheepskin; or cotton bedding.
- Provide adequate nutrition, including protein, fat, and zinc.
- Apply transparent adhesive dressings to protect arms, elbows, and knees from friction injury.
- Use tracheostomy and gastrostomy dressings for drainage and relief of pressure from a tracheostomy or gastrostomy tube.
- Use emollient in the diaper area (groin and thighs) to reduce urine irritation.

Treating Skin Breakdown

- Irrigate wound gently every 4 to 8 hours with warm, half-strength normal saline.
- Culture wound and treat if signs of infection are present (excessive redness, swelling, pain on touch, heat, or resistance to healing).
- Use a transparent adhesive dressing for uninfected wounds.
- Apply hydrogel with or without antibacterial or antifungal ointments (as ordered) for infected wounds.
- Use hydrocolloid for deep, uninfected wounds (leave in place for 5 to 7 days) or as an ostomy barrier and to improve appliance adhesion: warm barrier in your hand for several minutes to soften it before applying it to the skin.
- Avoid use of antiseptic solutions for wound cleansing (use for intact skin only).

Treating Diaper Dermatitis

- Maintain clean, dry skin; use absorbent diapers and change them often.
- If mild irritation occurs, use petrolatum barrier.

Continued

GUIDELINES

Neonatal Skin Care—cont'd

- For dermatitis, apply a generous quantity of zinc-oxide barrier; when cleaning, remove only the soiled layer of barrier as excessive friction can cause skin irritation and hinder healing.
- For severe dermatitis, identify the cause and treat (e.g., frequent stooling from spina bifida, severe opiate withdrawal, malabsorption syndrome).
- Treat *Candida albicans* with antifungal ointment or cream.
- Avoid use of powders and antibiotic ointments. (See Chapter 26, Bathing and Umbilical Cord Care and Care of the Newly Circumcised Infant.)

Other Skin Care Concerns

Use of Substances on Skin

- Evaluate all substances that come in contact with infant's skin.
- Before using any topical agent, analyze its components and
  - Use sparingly and only when necessary.
  - Confine use to the smallest possible area.
  - Whenever possible and appropriate, wash off with water.
  - Monitor infant carefully for signs of toxicity and systemic effects.

Use of Thermal Devices

- Avoid use of heat lamps because of the increased potential for burns. If needed, measure temperature of the exposed skin every 15 minutes.
- When using heated mattresses,
  - Refer to the manufacturer's instruction manual for proper use.
  - Change the infant's position every 15 minutes initially and then every 1 to 2 hours.
  - Preset temperature of the mattress to less than 40°C.
- When using transcutaneous electrodes, set at the lowest possible temperature.
  - Change the location of the probe frequently.
  - Use pulse oximetry rather than transcutaneous monitoring whenever possible.
- If prewarming the infant's heel before phlebotomy, avoid temperatures over 40°C.
- Provide warm ambient humidity, directed away from infant; use aerosolized sterile water and maintain ambient temperature so as to not exceed 40°C.
- Document use and temperature, if known, of all heating devices.

Use of Fluid Therapy and Hemodynamic Monitoring

- Be certain that fingers or toes are visible whenever an extremity is used for peripheral IV or arterial line.
- Secure catheter or needle with transparent dressing and tape for easy visualization of site.
- Assess site hourly for signs of ischemia, infiltration, and inadequate perfusion (check capillary refill, pulses, colour).
- Avoid use of restraints (e.g., arm boards); if used, ensure that they are secured safely and not restricting circulation or movement (check for pressure areas).
- Use commercial IV protector (e.g., I.V. House) with minimal tape.

IV, intravenous; *TEWL*, transepidermal water loss.

*Caution: Scissors should be used with caution for tape or dressing removal because of the hazard of cutting skin or amputating tiny digits.

Data from Association of Women's Health, Obstetric and Neonatal Nursing (AWHONN). (2013). *Neonatal skin care: Evidence-based clinical practice guideline* (3rd ed.). Washington, DC: Author; Taquino, L. T. (2000). Promoting wound healing in the neonatal setting: Process versus protocol. *Journal of Perinatal and Neonatal Nursing, 14*(1), 108–118.

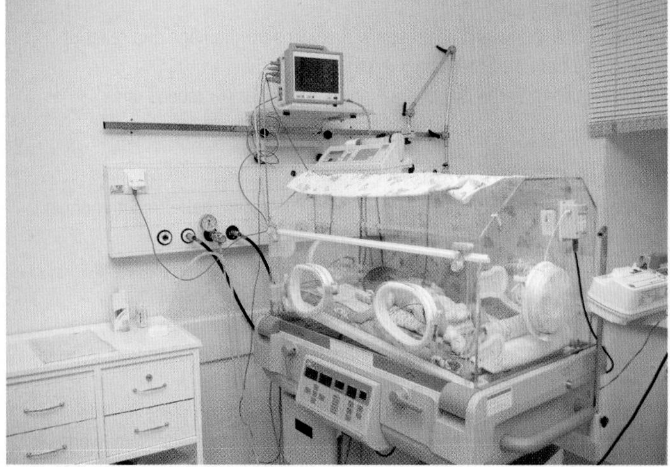

FIGURE 28-6 Infant in double-walled isolette with a blanket as a light shield. (Fanfo/Shutterstock.com.)

Nurses can modify the environment to provide a neurodevelopmentally supportive milieu. In that way, the infant's neurobehavioural and physiological needs can be better met, the infant's developing organization can be supported, and growth and development can be fostered.

Developmental Care

Much attention has been focused on the effects of early developmental intervention on both term and preterm infants. Infants experience and respond to a great variety of stimuli. As stated earlier, the atmosphere and activities of the NICU are overstimulating and can be harmful to infants in the NICU. Nursing care activities, such as taking vital signs, weighing, repositioning, and changing diapers, have been associated with periods of hypoxia, oxygen desaturation, and elevated intracranial pressure. The more immature the infant, the less able he or she is to habituate to a single procedure without becoming overstimulated. The caregiver needs to use the infant's own behavioural and physiological responses as the basis for planning care and providing interventions. Through observation, caregivers can identify the infant's strengths, thresholds for disorganization, and areas of vulnerability.

Developmental care should be tailored to each infant on the basis of a comprehensive behavioural assessment. During the early stages of development (especially before 33 weeks' gestation), external stimulation produces uncoordinated, random activity (jerky limb extension, hyperflexion) and irregular vital signs. At this stage, the infant needs to have minimal environmental stimulation. Using the developmental model of supportive care, the nurse can closely monitor physiological and behavioural signs to foster organization and well-being of the high-risk infant during handling. Softly calling the infant by name and then gently placing a hand on the body signal that care is beginning. The infant should be handled with slow, controlled movements. The infant's random movements should be controlled and limbs held flexed close to the infant's body during turning or other position changes. This containment or facilitated tucking may also be used before doing invasive procedures, such as a heel stick, to alleviate distress. Blanket swaddling and nesting or containment has been shown to decrease physiological and behavioural stress during routine care procedures. A nest constructed by placing blanket rolls underneath the bed sheet helps the infant maintain flexion when prone or side lying.

Skin-to-skin contact (kangaroo care) and short periods of gentle massage can help reduce stress in preterm infants, although such contact must be assessed and implemented individually. Regular skin-to-skin contact between parents and LBW infants has been shown to alleviate stress (Fig. 28-7). The undressed (except for diaper) infant is placed in a vertical position on the parent's bare chest to permit direct eye contact, skin-to-skin sensations, and close proximity. In addition to being a safe and effective method for infant–parent acquaintance, skin-to-skin contact between parent and infant can have a positive healing effect for the mother with a high-risk pregnancy. Mothers may experience psychological healing and regain the mothering role through early skin-to-skin contact with their VLBW infants. Additional benefits of skin-to-skin care include earlier contact for mechanically ventilated infants, maintenance of neonatal thermal stability and oxygen saturation, increased feeding ability and tolerance, maintenance of organized state, and decreased pain perception during heel sticks (Conde-Agudelo, Belizan, & Diaz-Rossello, 2011). In term and preterm newborns, skin-to-skin contact has a strong analgesic effect during procedures such as heel lance (Johnston, Campbell-Yeo, Fernandes, 2014). LBW infants receiving skin-to-skin contact maintain higher oxygen saturation and are less likely to have desaturations below 90%. In addition, their mothers are more likely to continue breastfeeding both in the hospital and for 1 month after discharge. Kangaroo care of preterm infants fosters neurobehavioural development by promoting stability of cardiac and respiratory function, minimizing purposeless movements, offering maternal proximity, improving the infant's behavioural state, and permitting self-regulating behaviours (Johnston et al., 2014).

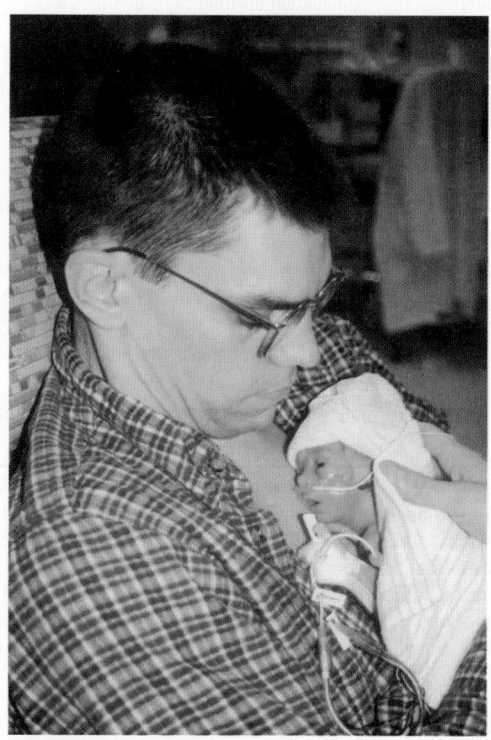

FIGURE 28-7 Father providing kangaroo care. (Courtesy Judy Meyr.)

Cobedding of twins (or multiples) is another developmental intervention that has been implemented in NICUs and newborn nurseries to provide a better environment for neonatal growth and development. Cobedding involves placing twins or other multiples together in the same crib or isolette. Preliminary data from a multicentre study indicate that twins who were cobedded had improved thermoregulation, significantly fewer apnea and bradycardia episodes, more rapid weight gain, and shorter length of hospital stay than their single-bedded counterparts. Parental satisfaction was also significantly greater with cobedded newborns. One major concern with cobedding is cross-transmission of infection between the neonates, but increased infection rates have not occurred with cobedding (LaMar & Dowling, 2006).

Studies have confirmed the beneficial effects of developmental care with preterm infants. In addition to requiring fewer days of mechanical ventilation, preterm infants who received individualized developmental care had shorter hospital stays; a significant decrease in complications (i.e., intraventricular hemorrhage [IVH] and BPD); less need for sedation when critically ill; improved neurodevelopmental scores at 9, 18, and 36 months of life; and a decrease in feeding intolerance (Westrup, Sizun, & Lagercrantz, 2007).

Developmental care for preterm infants has expanded to use of a wide variety of interventions, such as infant massage, playing of soothing soft music, recordings of parents reading stories, positioning to enhance self-regulatory abilities, enhancement of hand-to-mouth activities, uninterrupted sleep periods, and minimizing environmental light and noise. These interventions may also lead parents to perceive the NICU environment as less threatening. Active participation in providing a developmentally supportive environment for their infant involves the parents in daily caregiving activities when the newborn is critically ill and cannot be fed or held.

When infants have reached sufficient developmental organization and stability, interventions need to be designed and implemented to support their growing abilities. Nurses and parents must become adept at learning to read the infant's behavioural cues and supplying appropriate interventions

(Table 28-3). Cues include both approach and avoidance behaviours. Approach behaviours that are supported and enhanced include tongue extension, hand clasp, hand-to-mouth movements, sucking, looking, and cooing. Signs of stress or fatigue that signal the infant's need for "time-out" are described in Table 28-3.

When an infant is medically stable and on room air or minimal amounts of oxygen, ongoing assessment and documentation of his or her behavioural state organization and ability to self-regulate should be continued. Activities need to be individualized according to each infant's cues, temperament, state, behavioural organization, and particular needs. Intervention periods must be short (e.g., 2 to 3 minutes of voices, 5 minutes of quiet music). Auditory and vestibular interventions should be initiated earlier than visual stimulation. Interventions should be introduced one at a time and the infant's tolerance to each assessed and documented. An intervention program for a convalescing infant includes parents and siblings being present early in the infant's hospitalization; teaching parents to be responsive to the infant's individual cues is an important function of the NICU nurse. Parents, siblings, and health care providers should be advised to adhere to the established developmental care plan in order to avoid disruption in the infant's sleep–wake cycles and minimize inappropriate stimuli.

Growth and Development Potential

The corrected gestational age of a preterm newborn is calculated by subtracting the number of weeks born before 40 weeks of gestation from the chronological age. For example, a 6-month-old (chronological age) infant born at 32 weeks of gestation would have a corrected age of 4 months (6 months–8 weeks). The infant's responses are evaluated against the norms expected for a 4-month-old infant. For preterm infants, chronological age is not equal to corrected age. Growth and development milestones (e.g., motor milestones, vocalization) are corrected for gestational age until the child is approximately 3 years of age.

An effective discharge plan should include outpatient follow-up visits with a primary care practitioner and a developmental specialist for monitoring growth and achievement of appropriate developmental milestones.

Family Support and Involvement

Professional health care workers often are so absorbed in the life-saving physical aspects of care that they ignore the emotional needs of infants and their families. The significance of early parent–child interaction and infant stimulation has been documented by reliable research. Nurses must be aware of these infant and family needs and incorporate activities that facilitate family interaction into the nursing care plan.

The birth of a preterm infant is an unexpected and stressful event for which families are emotionally unprepared. They find themselves simultaneously coping with their own needs, the needs of their infant, and the needs of their family (especially when they have other children). To compound the situation, their infant's precarious condition engenders an atmosphere of

TABLE 28-3 SIGNS OF STRESS OR FATIGUE IN NEONATES

SUBSYSTEM	SIGNS OF STRESS
Autonomic	Physiological instability
Respiratory	Tachypnea, pauses, gasping, sighing
Colour	Mottled, flushed, dusky, pale or grey
Visceral	Hiccups, gagging, choking, spitting up, grunting and straining as if having a bowel movement, coughing, sneezing, yawning
Autonomic	Tremors, startles, twitches
Motor	Fluctuating tone; lack of control over movement, activity, and posture
Flaccidity	Low tone in trunk; limp, floppy upper and lower extremities; limp, drooping jaw (gape face)
Hypertonicity	Arm or leg extensions, arm(s) outstretched with fingers splayed in salute gesture, fingers stiffly outstretched, trunk arching, neck hyperextended
Hyperflexion	Trunk, extremities, fisting
Activity	Squirming; frantic, diffuse activity or little or no activity or responsiveness
State	Disorganized quality to state behaviours, including available states, maintenance of state control, and transition from one state to another
Sleep	Whimpering sounds, facial twitching, irregular respirations, fussing, grimacing, restless appearance
Awake	Glazed, unfocused look; staring; worried or pained expression; hyperalert or panicked appearance; eye roving; crying; cry-face; actively averting gaze or closing eyes; irritability; prolonged awake periods; inconsolability; frenzy
	Abrupt or rapid state changes
Other state-related behaviours and attention interaction	Efforts to attend to and interact with environmental stimulation eliciting signs of stress and disorganized subsystem functioning
Autonomic	Physiological instability of varying degrees with autonomic, respiratory, colour, and visceral responses
Motor	Fluctuating tone, increased motor activity; progressively frantic diffuse activity if stimulation continues
State	Roving eyes; gaze averting; glazed, unfocused look or worried, panicked expression; weak cry; cry-face; irritability
	Closed eyes and sleeplike withdrawal
	Abrupt state changes
	Signs of stress when presented with more than one type of stimulus at a time

Data from Als, H. (1982). Toward a synactive theory of development: Promise for the assessment and support of infant individuality, *Infant Mental Health Journal, 3*(4), 229–243; Als, H. (1986). A synactive model of neonatal behavior organization: Framework for the assessment of neurobehavioral development in the premature infant and for support of infants and parents in the neonatal intensive care environment. *Physical & Occupational Therapy in Pediatrics, 6*, 3–55; Hunter, J. G. (2001). The neonatal intensive care unit. In J. Case-Smith, A. S. Allen, & P. N. Pratt, (Eds.), *Occupational therapy for children* (4th ed.). St. Louis: Mosby.

apprehension and uncertainty. They are faced with multiple crises and overwhelming feelings of responsibility, helplessness, and frustration.

All parents have some anxieties about the outcome of a pregnancy, but after a preterm birth the concern is heightened regarding both the viability and normalcy of their infant. Mothers may see their infant only briefly before the newborn is removed to the NICU or even to another hospital, leaving them with just the recollection of the infant's very small size and unusual appearance. They often feel alone or lost on the mother-baby unit, belonging neither with mothers who have lost their infants nor with those who have delivered healthy, full-term infants. The staff and physicians are often guarded in discussing the infant's condition; mothers are continually expecting to hear that their infant has died, and they are sensitive to the anxieties of other mothers and staff members. Going home without their infant only compounds their feelings of disappointment, failure, and deprivation. See Transfer to a Regional Centre on page 784 for care of family when infant is transported to another hospital.

Parents need to be informed of their infant's progress and reassured that he or she is receiving proper care. They need to understand the smallest aspects of the infant's condition and treatment. Parents need a realistic, honest, and direct assessment of the situation. Using nonmedical terminology, moving at a pace that is comfortable for parents to assimilate the information, and avoiding lengthy technical explanations facilitate communication with family members. Psychological tasks that must be accomplished by parents during their infant's care are presented in Box 28-4. See Family-Centred Teaching box.

Facilitating parent–infant relationships. Because of their physiological instability, infants are separated from their mothers immediately and surrounded by a complex, impenetrable barrier of glass windows, mechanical equipment, and special caregivers. There is some evidence indicating that the emotional separation that accompanies the physical separation of mothers and infants may interfere with the normal mother–infant attachment process discussed in Chapter 23. Maternal attachment is a cumulative process that begins before conception, strengthens by significant events during pregnancy, and matures through mother–infant contact during the neonatal period and infancy.

When an infant is sick, the necessary physical separation appears to be accompanied by an emotional estrangement by the parents, which may seriously damage the capacity for parenting their infant. This detachment is further hampered by the tenuous nature of the infant's condition. When survival is in doubt, parents may be reluctant to establish a relationship with their infant. They prepare themselves for the infant's death while continuing to hope for recovery. This **anticipatory grief** and hesitancy to embark on a relationship are evidenced by behaviours such as delay in giving the infant a name, reluctance in visiting the nursery (or when they do visit, focusing on equipment and treatments rather than on their infant), and hesitancy to touch or handle the infant when given the opportunity.

BOX 28-4 PSYCHOLOGICAL TASKS OF PARENTS OF A HIGH-RISK INFANT

- Work through the events surrounding labour and birth.
- Acknowledge that the infant's life is endangered and begin the anticipatory grieving process.
- Confront and recognize feelings of inadequacy and guilt in not delivering a healthy child.
- Adapt to the neonatal intensive care environment.
- Resume parental relationships with the sick infant and initiate the caregiving role.
- Prepare to take the infant home.

Modified from Siegel, R., Gardner, S. L., & Dickey, L. A. (2011). Families in crisis: Theoretical and practical considerations. In S. L. Gardner, B. S. Carter, M. Enzman-Hines, et al. (Eds.), *Merenstein and Gardner's handbook of neonatal intensive care* (7th ed.). St. Louis: Mosby.

FAMILY-CENTRED TEACHING

Preterm Infant

A multiparous, single woman had a preterm infant born at 28 weeks' gestation and the neonate was subsequently transported to an NICU in a city 125 kilometres away from her home town. The mother is to be discharged tomorrow. The infant will likely require a stay in the NICU for at least 6 to 8 weeks. What information should the transport team provide the mother? What methods of assistance will this mother need now? Identify resources in the community that have services of potential benefit to the woman. Use your community or town as a guide to such resources.

Family-centred care of high-risk newborns includes encouraging and facilitating parental involvement rather than isolating parents from their infant and associated care. This is particularly important for mothers; to reduce the effects of physical separation, mothers are united with their newborn at the earliest opportunity.

Preparing the parents to see their infant for the first time is an important nursing responsibility. The nurse prepares them for their infant's appearance, the equipment attached to the child, and the general atmosphere of the unit. The initial encounter with the NICU is a stressful experience; and the frightening array of people, equipment, and activity is likely to be overwhelming. A book of photographs or pamphlets describing the NICU environment (infants in isolettes or under radiant warmers, monitors, mechanical ventilators, and IV equipment) provides a useful and nonthreatening introduction to the NICU.

Parents are encouraged to visit their infant as soon as possible. Even if they saw the infant at the time of transport or shortly after birth, he or she may have changed considerably, especially if a number of medical and equipment requirements are associated with the hospitalization. At the bedside the nurse should explain the function of each piece of equipment and the role it plays in facilitating recovery. Explanations may often need to be patiently repeated because parents' anxiety over the infant's condition and the surroundings may prevent them from really "hearing" what is being said. When possible, some items related to therapy can be removed (e.g., phototherapy can be discontinued temporarily, and eye patches removed to permit eye-to-eye contact).

Parents appreciate the support of a nurse during the initial visit with their infant, but they may also appreciate some time alone with the infant for a short while. It is important during the early visits to emphasize the positive aspects of their infant's behaviour and development so the parents can focus on their child as an individual rather than on the equipment that surrounds him or her. For example, the nurse may describe the infant's spontaneous behaviours during care, such as the grasp reflex and spontaneous movement, or make comments about the infant's biological functions. Most institutions have open visiting policies so that parents and siblings may visit their infant as often as they wish.

Parents vary greatly in the degree to which they are able to interact with their infant. Some may wish to touch or hold him or her during the first visit, but others may not feel comfortable enough to even enter the nursery. These reactions depend on a variety of prenatal and postnatal factors, such as the parity of the mother and her preparation before birth; the infant's size, condition, and physical appearance; and the type of treatment the infant is receiving. It is essential to recognize that the individualized pacing and quality of the interactions are more important than an early onset of these interactions. Parents may not be receptive to early and extended infant contact because they need time to adjust to the impact of an infant with birth problems and must be helped to grieve before they can accept the child.

One recent study of fathers with an infant in the NICU found that common barriers to paternal involvement included the infant's small size and fragile health status, perceived infant feedback (negative), nurses' attitudes toward paternal involvement, and conflict over the demands of home, work responsibilities, and care of other children. Facilitators of paternal involvement included the support of family and friends, perceived positive infant responses, maternal encouragement, and nurses' encouraging attitudes (Feeley, Waitzer, Sherrard, et al., 2013). The study concluded that NICU nurses have a strong positive or negative influence on the father's involvement with infant care and his perception of his ability to care for the infant.

The parents' inability to focus on their infant is a clue for the nurse to help them express and deal with feelings of guilt, anxiety, helplessness, inadequacy, anger, and ambivalence. Nurses can help them recognize that these are normal responses shared by other parents. It is important to point out and reinforce the positive aspects of parents' behaviour and interactions with their infant.

Most parents feel shaky and insecure about initiating interaction with their infant. Nurses can sense parents' level of readiness and offer encouragement in these initial efforts. Parents of preterm infants follow the same acquaintance process as that of parents of term infants. They may quickly proceed through the process or may require several days or even weeks to complete it. They begin by touching their infant's extremities with their fingertips and poking the infant tenderly and then proceed to caresses and fondling (Fig. 28-8). Touching is the first act of communication between parents and child. Parents need to be prepared for their infant's exaggerated and generalized startle responses to touch so they do not interpret these as negative reactions to their overtures. It may be necessary to limit tactile stimuli when the infant is critically ill and labile, but the nurse can offer other options, such as speaking softly or sitting at the bedside.

Parents of acutely ill preterm infants may express feelings of helplessness and lack of control. Involving the parent in some type of caregiving activity, no matter how minor it may seem to the nurse, enables the parent to "take on" a more active role. Examples of such caregiving for an acutely ill infant who cannot be held and is seemingly not responding positively

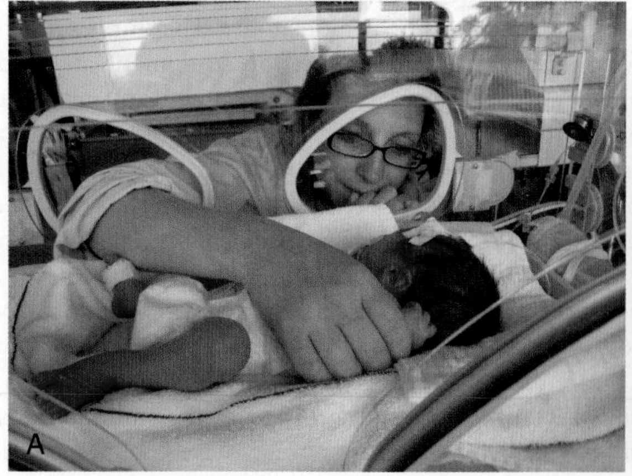

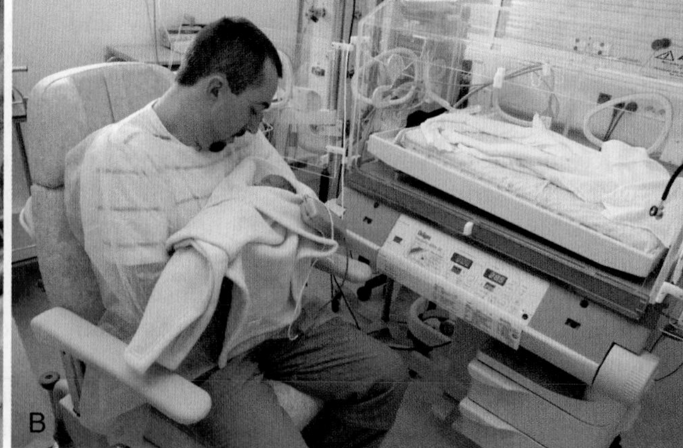

FIGURE 28-8 A: Mother interacts with her preterm infant by touch. **B:** Father interacts with his newborn by stroking and touching the infant with his fingertips. (A, iStock.com/metinkiyak. B, BSIP/ Science Source.)

include moistening the infant's lips with a small amount of sterile water on a cotton-tipped swab or pumping and storing breast milk.

Eventually, parents begin to endow their infant with an identity—as part of the family. When an infant no longer appears as a foreign object and begins to take on aspects of family members, such as the father's chin or the sister's nose, nurses can facilitate this incorporation. Parents are encouraged to bring in clothes, a toy, a stuffed animal, or a family snapshot for their infant; and the nurse can help them set goals for themselves and the child. Parents may become involved by reading a children's storybook or nursery rhymes in a soft, soothing voice. Some families record the parents' voices telling or reading stories and play the recordings when the infant is able to cope with such stimuli. The nurse must discuss feeding schedules, and parents are encouraged to visit at times when they can become involved in the care of their infant. Throughout the parent–infant acquaintance process, the nurse needs to listen carefully to what the parents say to assess their concerns and their progress toward incorporating their infant into their lives. The manner in which parents refer to their infant and the questions they ask will reveal their worries and feelings and can serve as valuable clues to future relationships with the child. The alert nurse is attuned to these subtle indications of parents' needs, which provide guidelines for nursing intervention. Often all that they need is reassurance that they will have the support of the nurse during caregiving activities and that the behaviours about which they are concerned are normal reactions and will disappear as the infant matures.

Parents need guidance in their relationships with their infant and help in their efforts to meet the child's physical and developmental needs. The nursing staff must help parents understand that their preterm infant will offer few behavioural rewards and show them how to accept small rewards. The infant's reactions and behaviours are explained to parents, who may take their infant's jerky, rejective behaviour personally. They need reassurance that these behaviours are not a reflection on their parenting skills. Parents are taught to recognize their infant's cues regarding stimulation, handling, and other interaction, especially aversive behaviours that indicate a need for rest. Nurses need to include parents in planning their infant's care and sensory stimulation materials, such as a music box or recording.

Above all, nurses and other members of the interprofessional care team must encourage and reinforce parents during their caregiving activities and interactions with their infant to promote healthy parent–child relationships. It is also helpful for the parents to have contact and communication with a consistent group of nurses. This decreases the amount of different information given to them and often instills confidence that, although they cannot be at their infant's bedside 24 hours a day, there are competent and caring nurses whom they may call to inquire about the infant's status. Periodic parent conferences involving the staff caring for the child serve to clarify misunderstandings or problems related to the infant's condition.

Support groups for parents of infants in intensive care nurseries are often a source of comfort and support for parents who may feel isolated from peers because of the birth of the preterm infant. These groups can encourage parents experiencing anxiety and grief to share their feelings. A parent with NICU experience often makes contact with a new member and provides additional support. These parents support the new NICU parent through hospital visits, phone contact, email or video conference, and home visits.

Some high-risk infants may be discharged earlier than expected. Criteria for early discharge require the infant to be physiologically stable, receive and ingest adequate nutrition, consistently gain weight, and maintain a stable body temperature in an open bassinet. In addition, screening for hyperbilirubinemia, newborn metabolic and hematological conditions, safe transportation, and hearing should occur before the preterm infant's discharge. An evaluation of the home environment and family resources, and arrangements for appropriate medical follow-up are essential. The parents or other caregivers must exhibit physical, emotional, and educational readiness to assume care of the infant. The parents need to show that they know how to take the infant's temperature, recognize signs and symptoms of illness, and understand the infant's dietary needs (Jefferies & Canadian Paediatric Society [CPS] Fetus and Newborn Committee, 2014; Whyte et al., 2010).

Parent Education

Sudden infant death syndrome (SIDS) is more likely to occur in preterm infants than in term infants. Infants discharged from an NICU are almost twice as likely to die unexpectedly during the first year of life as infants in the general population. Instruction in **cardiopulmonary resuscitation (CPR)** is essential for parents of all infants but especially for parents of infants at risk for life-threatening events. Risk factors include preterm birth, apnea or bradycardia spells, neurological immaturity, and the tendency to choke. All parents should be encouraged to obtain instruction in CPR at the hospital, local Red Cross, or other community agency. It should be emphasized that CPR knowledge does not preclude the need for proper positioning of the infant in the crib (i.e., supine, unless otherwise directed by the primary care provider) when put to sleep. In addition, the bed should have a firm mattress and be free of extra blankets and stuffed animals or toys, which may cause the infant to become entangled and subsequently smothered.

Complications of Prematurity

Respiratory Distress Syndrome

Respiratory distress is a name applied to respiratory dysfunction in neonates and is primarily a disease related to developmental delay in lung maturation. Respiratory distress syndrome (RDS) is a lung disorder usually affecting preterm infants, although a small percentage of term or late preterm infants may also be affected. The incidence and severity of RDS increase as gestational age decreases. Perinatal asphyxia, hypovolemia, male gender, Caucasian race, maternal diabetes, second-born twin, familial predisposition, Caesarean birth without labour, hydrops fetalis, and third-trimester bleeding are factors that place an infant at increased risk for RDS (Gardner et al., 2011). Alternatively, conditions associated with a decrease in the incidence and severity of RDS include female gender, maternal steroid (betamethasone) therapy, intrauterine growth restriction (IUGR), and stressors such as maternal hypertension (gestational), maternal drug use, chronic placental abruption, and prolonged rupture of membranes.

Preterm infants are born before the lungs are fully prepared to serve as efficient organs for gas exchange. This appears to be a critical factor in the development of RDS. The effects of lung immaturity are compounded by the presence of more cartilage in the chest wall, leading to increased compliance of the chest wall, which collapses inward in response to less compliant (stiffer) lung tissue.

There is evidence of fetal respiratory activity before birth. The lungs make feeble respiratory movements, and fluid is excreted through the alveoli. Because the final unfolding of the alveolar septa, which increases the surface area of the lungs, occurs during the last trimester of pregnancy, preterm infants are born with numerous underdeveloped and many uninflatable alveoli. Pulmonary blood flow is limited as a result of the collapsed state of the fetal lungs, particularly poor vascular development in general, and an immature capillary network. Because of increased pulmonary vascular resistance (PVR), the major portion of fetal blood is shunted from the lungs by way of the ductus arteriosus and foramen ovale.

At birth infants must initiate breathing and keep the previously fluid-filled lungs inflated with air. At the same time the pulmonary capillary blood flow must be increased approximately 10-fold to provide for adequate lung perfusion and alter the intracardiac pressure that closes the fetal cardiac structures. Most full-term infants successfully accomplish these adjustments, but preterm infants with respiratory distress are unable to do so. Although numerous factors are involved, immaturity of the surfactant system plays a central role.

The diagnosis of RDS is made on the basis of clinical manifestations (Box 28-5) and radiographic studies. Radiographic findings characteristic of RDS include (1) a diffuse granular pattern over both lung fields that closely resembles ground glass and represents alveolar atelectasis, and (2) dark streaks, or bronchograms, within the ground-glass areas that represent dilated, air-filled bronchioles. It is often difficult to distinguish between RDS and pneumonia in infants with respiratory distress. The extent of respiratory function and acid–base balance is determined by blood gas analysis. Pulse oximetry, carbon dioxide monitoring, and pulmonary function studies help to differentiate pulmonary and extrapulmonary illness and are used in the management of RDS.

The treatment of RDS involves immediate establishment of adequate oxygenation and ventilation, supportive care and measures required for any preterm infant, and those instituted to prevent further complications associated with preterm birth (see Evolve for Nursing Care Plan).

BOX 28-5 CLINICAL MANIFESTATIONS OF RESPIRATORY DISTRESS SYNDROME

- Tachypnea (≥60 breaths/min) initially*
- Dyspnea
- Pronounced intercostal or substernal retractions
- Fine inspiratory crackles
- Audible expiratory grunt
- Flaring of the external nares
- Cyanosis or pallor
- Apnea
- With progression of condition, deteriorating vital signs, including blood pressure, apnea, body temperature instability

*Not all infants born with respiratory distress syndrome manifest these characteristics; very-low-birth-weight and extremely-low-birth-weight infants may have respiratory failure and shock at birth because of physiological immaturity.

The supportive measures most crucial to a favourable outcome are to

- Maintain adequate ventilation and oxygenation.
- Maintain acid–base balance.
- Maintain a neutral thermal environment.
- Maintain adequate tissue perfusion and oxygenation.
- Prevent hypotension.
- Maintain adequate hydration and electrolyte status.

Nipple and gavage feedings are contraindicated in any situation that creates a marked increase in respiratory rate because of the greater hazards of aspiration. Nutrition is provided by parenteral therapy during the acute stage of the disease, and minimal enteral feeding is provided to enhance maturation of the neonate's gastrointestinal system.

Respiratory distress, nonpulmonary in origin, may also be caused by sepsis, cardiac defects (structural or functional), exposure to cold, airway obstruction (atresia), IVH, hypoglycemia, metabolic acidosis, acute blood loss, and certain medications. Bacterial or viral pneumonia in the neonatal period may manifest as respiratory distress and may occur alone or as a complication of RDS.

Surfactant replacement therapy. Surfactant is a surface-active phospholipid secreted by the alveolar epithelium. Surfactant acts much like a detergent and reduces the surface tension of fluids that line the alveoli and respiratory passages. This results in uniform expansion and maintenance of lung expansion at low intra-alveolar pressure. Immature lung development and surfactant deficiency can seriously compromise respiratory efficiency. Deficient surfactant production causes unequal inflation of alveoli on inspiration and the collapse of alveoli on expiration. Without surfactant, infants are unable to keep their lungs inflated and thus exert a great deal of effort to re-expand the alveoli with each breath. As infants tire, they are able to open fewer and fewer alveoli. This inability to maintain lung expansion produces widespread atelectasis.

A lack of alveolar stability (normal functional residual capacity) and progressive atelectasis cause PVR to increase. As a result, there is decreased pulmonary blood flow and hypoperfusion of the lung tissue occurs. The increase in PVR can cause a partial reversion to the fetal circulation, with right-to-left shunting of blood through the persisting fetal communications—the ductus arteriosus and foramen ovale. Inadequate ventilation and reduced pulmonary perfusion produce hypoxemia and hypercapnia. Pulmonary arterioles, with their thick muscular layer, are highly reactive to diminished oxygen concentration. Decreased oxygen tension causes vasoconstriction in the pulmonary arterioles. Vasoconstriction leads to hypoxemia, which is exacerbated by a decrease in blood pH. Vasoconstriction contributes to a significant increase in PVR. In contrast, during normal transition, with adequate ventilation and increasing oxygen concentration, the ductus arteriosus constricts and the pulmonary vessels dilate to decrease PVR.

Surfactant can be administered as an adjunct to oxygen and ventilation therapy. Generally, infants born before 32 weeks of gestation do not have adequate amounts of pulmonary surfactant. In many centres the use of surfactant is reserved for infants at greatest risk for RDS, those between 29 and 32 weeks of gestation (Bahadue & Soll, 2012; Gardner et al., 2011; Rojas-Reyes, Morley, & Soll, 2012). Exogenous surfactant is manufactured synthetically or extracted from bovine, porcine, or calf lung extract. A course of one or two doses is given through an endotracheal tube (Fig. 28-9). The infant must be monitored for potential adverse effects (apnea, bradycardia, desaturation, plugging of the endotracheal tube, pulmonary hemorrhage). Surfactant has been associated with a significant decrease in duration mechanical ventilation and oxygen therapy. Despite an increased survival rate in preterm infants, surfactant has not significantly decreased the incidence of BPD, IVH, or patent ductus arteriosus (PDA) in extremely immature infants.

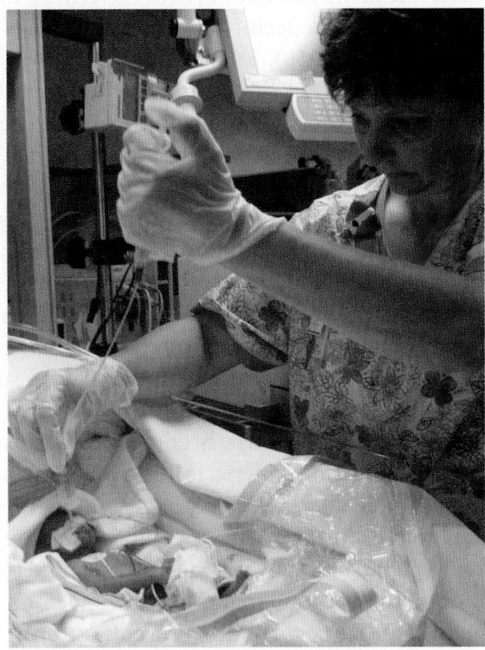

FIGURE 28-9 Exogenous surfactant administration via endotracheal tube. (Courtesy E. Jacobs, Texas Children's Hospital.)

When comparing the effects of natural versus synthetic surfactant, studies have shown rapid improvement of respiratory status, less ROP and BPD, lower mortality, and decreased incidence of pneumothorax in infants who received natural surfactant (Davis, Barrington, & Canadian Paediatric Society, et al., 2005/2015; Gardner et al., 2011). However, newer synthetic surfactant products may be equally effective.

Early versus rescue administration of surfactant is recommended (Davis et al., 2005/2015; Stevens, Blennow, Myers, et al., 2007) for infants with or at risk for RDS, especially ELBW infants and those not exposed to maternal antenatal steroids. The administration of antenatal steroids and surfactant replacement has decreased the incidence of RDS and concomitant morbidities. A multicentre, randomized trial found that CPAP may be a reasonable alternative to intubation and surfactant administration (Finer & the SUPPORT Study Group, 2010).

Inhaled nitric oxide (INO) and extracorporeal membrane oxygenation (ECMO). Inhaled nitric oxide (INO) and extracorporeal membrane oxygenation (ECMO) are additional therapies used in the treatment of severe respiratory distress and respiratory failure in neonates. INO is used in term and late preterm infants with persistent pulmonary hypertension of the newborn (PPHN), MAS, pneumonia, sepsis, and congenital diaphragmatic hernia to decrease or reverse pulmonary hypertension and vasoconstriction, acidosis, and hypoxemia. Nitric oxide is a colourless, highly diffusible gas that is administered blended with oxygen, through the ventilator circuit. INO therapy may be used in conjunction with surfactant replacement therapy, high-frequency ventilation, or ECMO. INO has been proved to be significantly effective in decreasing RDS and in improving survival rates in preterm infants (Donohue, Gilmore, Cristofalo, et al., 2011), but it has not been shown to prevent BPD (Kinsella, Cutter, Steinhorn, et al., 2014). Clinical trials have demonstrated that the use of INO improved ventilatory status in infants with pulmonary hypertension, decreased requirements for ventilatory support (Barrington & Finer, 2010), and decreased the need for ECMO (Field, Elbourne, Hardy, et al., 2007).

ECMO may also be used in the management of term infants with acute severe respiratory failure for the same conditions as those mentioned for INO. This therapy involves a modified heart-lung machine, although with ECMO the heart is not stopped and blood does not entirely bypass the lungs. Blood is shunted from a catheter in the right atrium or right internal jugular vein by gravity to a servo-regulated roller pump, pumped through a membrane lung where it is oxygenated, through a small heat exchanger where it is warmed, and then returned to the systemic circulation via a major artery (carotid) to the aortic arch. ECMO provides oxygen to the circulation, allowing the lungs to "rest," and decreases pulmonary hypertension and hypoxemia seen with PPHN, congenital diaphragmatic hernia (CDH), sepsis, MAS, and severe pneumonia. ECMO is not used in infants less than 34 weeks' gestation because the anticoagulant therapy required in the pump and circuits may increase the potential for IVH in these infants. In some centres, the success of high-frequency ventilation and INO has greatly decreased the demand for ECMO.

Patent Ductus Arteriosus

The ductus arteriosus is a muscular contractile structure in the fetus connecting the left pulmonary artery and the dorsal aorta. The ductus constricts after birth as oxygenation increases. Other factors that promote ductal closure include catecholamines, low pH, bradykinin, and acetylcholine. When the fetal ductus arteriosus fails to close after birth, a patent ductus arteriosus (PDA) occurs. Ductal closure usually occurs within hours or days in the term infant but may be delayed in preterm infants as a result of oxygenation and circulating **hormones** (prostaglandins).

The clinical presentation of an infant with a PDA includes systolic murmur, active precordium, bounding peripheral pulses, tachycardia, tachypnea, crackles, and hepatomegaly. The systolic murmur is heard best at the second or third intercostal space at the upper left sternal border. An active precordium is caused by an increased left ventricular stroke volume. A widened pulse pressure may result in bounding peripheral pulses.

Radiographic studies of infants with a large shunting PDA typically show cardiac enlargement and pulmonary edema; with a smaller PDA, the radiograph may appear normal for the infant's age (Kenney, Hoover, Williams, et al., 2011). ABG findings reveal hypercarbia and metabolic acidosis. A colour flow Doppler echocardiograph can demonstrate a PDA and be used to identify the direction of the shunting (left to right, right to left, or both) and quantify the amount of blood shunting across the PDA.

A PDA can be managed medically or surgically. Medical management consists of ventilatory support, fluid restriction, diuretics, and nonsteroidal anti-inflammatory drugs (NSAIDs), such as indomethacin or ibuprofen. Indomethacin is a prostaglandin synthetase inhibitor that blocks the effect of the arachidonic acid products on the ductus and causes the PDA to constrict. Ibuprofen administered orally reportedly has fewer adverse effects than indomethacin, yet a recent Cochrane review reports that they are equally effective (Ohlsson, Walia, & Shah, 2015).

Ventilatory support is adjusted on the basis of ABG levels. Fluid restriction and diuretic therapy are implemented to decrease cardiovascular volume overload. Surgical ligation is performed when PDA is clinically significant and medical management has failed. Nursing care of the infant with PDA focuses on supportive care. The infant needs an NTE, adequate oxygenation, and meticulous fluid balance. Parental support is imperative.

Periventricular-Intraventricular Hemorrhage

Periventricular-intraventricular hemorrhage (PV-IVH) is one of the more common types of neurological injuries that occurs in neonates and is among the most severe in both short- and long-term outcomes. While the true incidence of PV-IVH is unknown, a general estimate is 15% in infants less than 32 weeks of gestation or under 1500 g (Volpe, 2008). PV-IVH occurs in approximately 3.5 to 5% of term infants, with 50% of those cases caused by asphyxia or trauma. Research has shown that contributing events may occur antenatally and postnatally (Carlo & Ambalavanan, 2016).

The pathogenesis of PV-IVH includes intravascular factors (e.g., fluctuating or increasing cerebral blood flow, increased cerebral venous pressure, and coagulopathy), vascular factors, extravascular factors (hypoglycemia, acidosis), and routine medical care (rapid volume expansion, blood transfusion). The developing preterm infant's brain has highly vascularized areas with fragile blood vessels that are prone to bleeding when homeostasis is not maintained; the most commonly affected area is in and around the subependymal germinal matrix. PV-IVH events typically occur within the first 72 hours of birth. PV-IVH is classified according to severity, which informs long-term neurodevelopmental outcomes.

Nursing care focuses on recognition of factors that increase the risk of PV-IVH, interventions to decrease the risk of bleeding, and supportive care to infants who have bleeding episodes. The infant should be positioned with his or her head in midline and the head of the bed elevated slightly to prevent or minimize fluctuations in intracranial blood pressure. NTE is maintained, as well as oxygenation. Rapid infusions of fluids should be avoided. Blood pressure should be monitored closely for fluctuations. The infant must be monitored for signs of pneumothorax because it often precedes PV-IVH.

Necrotizing Enterocolitis

Necrotizing enterocolitis (NEC) is an acute inflammatory disease of the bowel with increased incidence in preterm infants. The precise cause of NEC is still uncertain, but it appears to occur in infants whose gastrointestinal tracts have experienced vascular compromise. Intestinal ischemia of unknown etiology, immature gastrointestinal host defences, bacterial proliferation, and feeding substrate (formula) are now believed to have a multifactorial role in the etiology of NEC. Preterm birth remains the most prominent risk factor in the development of NEC (Maheshwari & Carlo, 2016).

The damage to mucosal cells lining the bowel wall may be significant. Diminished blood supply to these cells causes their death in large numbers; they stop secreting protective, lubricating mucus; and the thin, unprotected bowel wall is attacked by proteolytic enzymes. Thus the bowel wall continues to swell and break down; it is unable to synthesize protective IgM; and the mucosa is permeable to macromolecules (e.g., exotoxins), which further hampers intestinal defences. Gas-forming bacteria invade the damaged areas to produce **pneumatosis intestinalis**, the presence of gas in the submucosal or subserosal surfaces of the bowel.

A consistent relationship has been observed between the development of NEC and enteric feeding of hypertonic substances (e.g., formula, hyperosmolar medications). It is unclear whether this connection is a result of the formula imposing a stress on an ischemic bowel or serving as a substrate for bacterial growth or possibly a combination of these factors.

Treatment of NEC begins with prevention. Oral feedings may be withheld for at least 24 to 48 hours from infants who are believed to have experienced birth asphyxia. Breast milk is the preferred enteral nutrient because it confers some passive immunity (IgA), macrophages, and lysozymes. Breast milk banks may be able to provide donated breastmilk for preterm infants which may help to decrease the risk of NEC (see Milk banking, Chapter 27, p. 742). The early clinical signs of NEC are subtle and nonspecific and may often be overlooked for other conditions; the earliest clinical signs include lethargy, abdominal distension, and high gastric residuals (Kastenberg & Sylvester, 2013).

With early recognition and treatment, medical management has become increasingly successful. If there is progressive deterioration or evidence of perforation, surgical resection and anastomosis may be performed. Extensive involvement may necessitate surgical intervention and establishment of an ileostomy, jejunostomy, or colostomy. Sequelae include short-bowel syndrome, colonic stricture with obstruction, fat malabsorption, and failure to thrive secondary to intestinal dysfunction. Various surgical interventions for NEC are available and depend on the extent of bowel necrosis, associated illness factors, and infant stability. Intestinal transplantation has been successful in a small number of infants with NEC-associated short-bowel syndrome and life-threatening TPN-related complications. Bowel-lengthening procedures and intestinal transplantation may be life-saving options for infants who previously faced high morbidity and mortality (King, Carlson, Khalil, et al., 2013). Therapy may be prolonged and recovery may be delayed by adhesions, complications of bowel resection, short-bowel syndrome (especially if the ileocecal valve is removed), and intolerance of oral feedings.

The onset of NEC in the term infant, although rare, usually occurs between 4 and 10 days after birth. In the preterm infant the onset may be delayed for up to 30 days. Signs of NEC are nonspecific, a characteristic of many neonatal disease processes. Some general signs include decreased activity, hypotonia, pallor, recurrent apnea and bradycardia, respiratory distress, metabolic acidosis, **oliguria**, hypotension, decreased perfusion, temperature instability, and cyanosis. Gastrointestinal symptoms include abdominal distension, increasing or bile-stained gastric aspirates, vomiting (bile or blood), grossly bloody stools, abdominal tenderness, and erythema of the abdominal wall (Lovvan, Glenn, Pacetti, et al., 2011).

Diagnosis of NEC is confirmed by radiographic examination that reveals bowel loop distension, pneumatosis intestinalis, pneumoperitoneum, portal air, or a combination of these findings. The abnormal findings are caused by NEC-associated bacterial colonization of the gastrointestinal tract, resulting in an ileus. Pneumatosis intestinalis, pneumoperitoneum, and portal air are caused by gas produced by the bacteria that invade the wall of the intestines and escape into the peritoneum and portal system when perforation occurs. Laboratory evaluation includes a complete blood count (CBC) with differential, blood culture, coagulation studies, ABG analysis, and serum electrolyte levels. The white blood cell count may be either increased or decreased. The platelet count and coagulation studies may be abnormal, with thrombocytopenia and evidence of DIC. Electrolyte levels may be abnormal, related to leaking capillary beds and fluid shifts seen with the infection.

Treatment of infants with NEC is supportive and preventive for bowel perforation. Feedings should be discontinued to rest the gastrointestinal tract. A nasogastric tube is inserted and placed to low intermittent suction to provide gastric decompression, and parenteral therapy (often TPN) is initiated. NEC is an infectious disease; control of infection is imperative, with an emphasis on careful hand hygiene before and after infant contact. Systemic antibiotic therapy should be instituted.

THE POSTTERM INFANT

Postterm (or postmature) infants are those whose gestation is prolonged beyond 42 weeks, regardless of birth weight. These infants may be large or small for gestational age, but most often their weight is appropriate for gestational age. The rate of infants born postterm has been declining, and in 2010 it was 0.61% (PHAC, 2013). The cause of prolonged pregnancy is unknown. **Postmaturity** can be associated with placental insufficiency, resulting in a newborn that has a thin, emaciated appearance *(dysmature)* at birth because of loss of subcutaneous fat and muscle mass. Not all postterm infants show signs of dysmaturity. There may be meconium staining of the fingernails, the hair and nails may be long, and vernix may be absent. The skin may also peel off.

Perinatal mortality is significantly higher in the postterm infant. During labour and birth, increased oxygen demands of the postterm fetus may not be met. Insufficient gas exchange in the postterm placenta increases the likelihood of intrauterine hypoxia. This may result in the passage of meconium in utero and the risk for meconium aspiration syndrome (MAS). In one study, postterm infants were found to have a mortality rate almost three times higher than that of a control group of term infants (Carlo, 2016).

Meconium Aspiration Syndrome

Meconium-staining of the amniotic fluid can be indicative of atypical or abnormal fetal heart rate status and stress in utero. It appears in 10 to 15% of all births, primarily in term and postterm births. Many infants with meconium staining exhibit no signs of depression at birth; however, the presence of meconium in the amniotic fluid necessitates careful supervision of labour and close monitoring of fetal well-being. The presence of a team skilled in neonatal resuscitation is required at the birth of any infant with meconium-stained amniotic fluid (Fig. 28-10). The infant's mouth and nares are no longer routinely suctioned on the perineum before the infant's first breath. There seems to be no difference in outcomes between infants who are suctioned and those who are not. Current resuscitation guidelines (Perlman et al., 2010) assert that there is not enough evidence to change the current practice of intubation and suctioning below the cords for nonvigorous infants. More research is recommended.

If meconium is not removed from the airway at birth, it can migrate down to the terminal airways, causing mechanical obstruction and leading to MAS. The fetus may aspirate meconium in utero, causing a chemical pneumonitis. These infants may develop persistent pulmonary hypertension of the

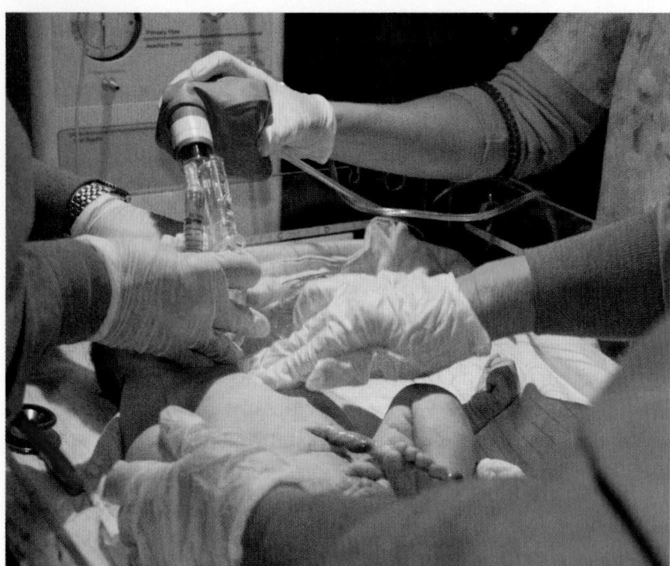

FIGURE 28-10 Infant being resuscitated at birth. Note presence of meconium on abdomen and umbilical cord. (Courtesy Shannon Perry.)

newborn, further complicating their management. Exogenous surfactant, INO, or ECMO may be used for treatment.

Persistent Pulmonary Hypertension of the Newborn

Persistent pulmonary hypertension of the newborn (PPHN) is a term applied to the combined findings of pulmonary hypertension, right-to-left shunting, and a structurally normal heart. PPHN may manifest either as a single entity or a sequela of MAS, CDH, RDS, hyperviscosity syndrome, neonatal pneumonia, or sepsis. PPHN is also called *persistent fetal circulation* because the syndrome involves reversion to fetal pathways of blood flow.

A brief review of fetal blood flow can help in visualization of the problems with PPHN (see Fig. 9-14). In utero, oxygen-rich blood leaves the placenta via the umbilical vein, goes through the ductus venosus, and enters the inferior vena cava. From there it empties into the right atrium and is mostly shunted across the foramen ovale to the left atrium, effectively bypassing the lungs. This blood enters the left ventricle, leaves through the aorta, and preferentially perfuses the carotid and coronary arteries—the heart and brain receive the most oxygenated blood. Blood drains from the brain into the superior vena cava, re-enters the right atrium, proceeds to the right ventricle, and exits through the main pulmonary artery. The lungs, a high-pressure circuit, need only enough perfusion for growth and nutrition. The ductus arteriosus (connecting the main pulmonary artery and the aorta) is the path of least resistance for the blood leaving the right side of the fetal heart and shunts most of the cardiac output away from the lungs and toward the systemic system. This right-to-left shunting is the key to fetal circulation.

After birth, both the foramen ovale and the ductus arteriosus close in response to biochemical processes, pressure changes within the heart, and dilation of the pulmonary vessels. This dilation allows virtually all of the cardiac output to enter the lungs, become oxygenated, and provide oxygen-rich blood to the tissues. Any process that interferes with this transition from fetal to neonatal circulation may precipitate PPHN. PPHN characteristically proceeds into a downward spiral of increasing hypoxia and pulmonary vasoconstriction. Prompt recognition and aggressive intervention are required to reverse this process.

The infant with PPHN is typically born at term or postterm and exhibits tachycardia and cyanosis that, within minutes or hours, progresses to severe respiratory compromise with concomitant acidosis, further compromising pulmonary perfusion and oxygenation. Management depends on the underlying cause of the persistent pulmonary hypertension. The use of INO and ECMO has improved survival in some of these infants.

Another mode of treatment for PPHN and other respiratory disorders is high-frequency ventilation, an assisted-ventilation method that delivers small volumes of gas at high frequencies and limits the development of high airway pressure, thus theoretically reducing barotrauma.

OTHER PROBLEMS RELATED TO GESTATION

Small-for-Gestational-Age Infants and Intrauterine Growth Restriction

Infants who are SGA or IUGR are considered high risk, with a perimortality rate 5 to 20 times greater than that for normal term infants (Kliegman, 2014).

Conditions occurring in the first trimester (e.g., infections, teratogens, chromosomal abnormalities) can affect all aspects of fetal growth. Extrinsic conditions early in pregnancy can also result in symmetrical IUGR (i.e., head circumference, length, and weight are all less than the tenth percentile). Infants with symmetrical growth restriction have a smaller head circumference and concomitant reduced brain growth. Growth restriction during later stages of pregnancy, due to maternal or placental factors, results in asymmetrical growth restriction—weight will be less than the tenth percentile, whereas length and head circumference will be greater than the tenth percentile, possibly within normal limits. Infants with asymmetrical IUGR have the potential for normal growth and development.

Care of the SGA infant is guided by the accompanying clinical problems and is comparable to the care provided to preterm infants with similar problems. Gas exchange is supported by maintaining a clear airway and preventing cold stress. Hypoglycemia is treated with oral feedings (e.g., breast, formula) or IV dextrose as the infant's condition warrants. An external heat source (radiant warmer or isolette) should be used until the infant is able to maintain an adequate body temperature. Nursing support of parents is the same as that given to parents of preterm infants.

Common problems that affect SGA or IUGR infants are perinatal asphyxia, meconium aspiration (discussed previously), immunodeficiency, hypoglycemia, polycythemia, and temperature instability.

Hypoglycemia and Hyperglycemia

All high-risk infants are at risk for hypoglycemia. Infants who experience physiological stress may experience hypoglycemia as a result of a decreased glycogen supply, inadequate gluconeogenesis, or overutilization of glycogen stored during fetal and postnatal life. Preterm infants may also become hypoglycemic as a result of inadequate intake and increased metabolic demands due to illness (see Chapter 26, p. 696, for discussion of hypoglycemia). The SGA infant, not unlike the preterm infant, is at higher risk for hypoglycemia as a result of decreased fetal stores and decreased rate of gluconeogenesis.

Hyperglycemia is defined as a blood glucose level greater than 6.9 mmol/L (whole blood) or plasma glucose of 8.0 to 8.3 mmol/L (Blackburn, 2012). Hyperglycemia may be just as harmful to the preterm infant as hypoglycemia. Increased circulating levels of glucose may lead to osmotic changes, increased urine output, and fluid shifts in the already compromised CNS of the preterm infant. The net result of hyperglycemia may be cellular dehydration and IVH. Preterm infants undergoing stress (i.e., surgery) may also become hyperglycemic with increased catecholamine release, which inhibits insulin release and glucose utilization (Blackburn, 2012). In summary, ELBW and VLBW infants should be monitored closely for both hypoglycemia and hyperglycemia.

Heat Loss

SGA infants are particularly susceptible to temperature instability as a result of decreased brown fat deposit, decreased adipose tissue, large body surface exposure, inability to accomplish flexed position due to poor muscle tone, and decreased glycogen storage in major organs such as the liver and heart. Close attention must be given to maintenance of a neutral thermal environment.

Large-for-Gestational-Age Infants

An infant is considered large for gestational age (LGA) when the weight is above the ninetieth percentile on growth charts or 2 standard deviations above the mean weight for gestational age. The LGA infant is at greater risk for morbidity than the SGA and preterm infant; such infants have a higher incidence of birth injuries, asphyxia, and congenital anomalies such as heart defects. In Canada the rate of infants born who were LGA was 10.4% in 2010 (PHAC, 2013).

LGA newborns may be preterm, term, or postterm; they may be infants of diabetic mothers. Each of these problems carries special concerns. Regardless of coexisting potential problems, the LGA infant is at risk by virtue of size alone.

The nurse needs to assess the LGA infant for hypoglycemia and trauma resulting from vaginal or Caesarean birth. Any specific birth injuries should be identified and treated appropriately.

Infants of Diabetic Mothers

Before insulin therapy, few women with diabetes were able to conceive; for those who did, the mortality rate for both the mother and infant was high. The morbidity and mortality of infants of diabetic mothers (IDMs) have been reduced significantly as a result of effective control of maternal diabetes and an increased understanding of fetal disorders. Because infants born to women with gestational diabetes mellitus (DM) are at risk for the same complications as IDMs, the following discussion of IDMs includes infants born to women with gestational DM.

The severity of maternal diabetes affects infant survival. It is determined by the duration of the disease before pregnancy; age of onset; extent of vascular complications; and abnormalities of the current pregnancy, such as pyelonephritis, diabetic ketoacidosis, pregnancy-induced hypertension, and inability to follow treatment regimen. The single most important factor influencing fetal well-being is the euglycemic status of the mother. It has been found that reasonable metabolic control that begins before conception and continues during the first weeks of pregnancy can prevent malformation in an IDM. Elevated levels of hemoglobin A1c during the periconception period appear to be associated with a higher incidence of congenital malformations (see Chapter 15). In the case of gestational diabetes, macrosomia is the most common finding; serious complications are rare (Mitanchez, 2010).

Hypoglycemia may appear a short time after birth and in IDMs is associated with increased insulin activity in the blood. The serum glucose level that corresponds to clinical hypoglycemia has not been well defined, but the Canadian Paediatric Society recommends that serum glucose levels be maintained at 2.6 mmol/L. At-risk infants with glucose levels less than 1.8 mmol/L on one occasion (assuming one effective feed), or repeatedly less than 2.6 mmol/L, require intervention. Symptomatic infants should be treated immediately for blood glucose levels less than 2.6 mmol/L; there should be concurrent investigation and management of the underlying cause (Aziz, Dancy, & Canadian Paediatric Society, 2004/2014).

Hypoglycemia in IDMs is related to hypertrophy and hyperplasia of the pancreatic islet cells and thus is a transient state of hyperinsulinism. High maternal blood glucose levels during fetal life provide a continual stimulus to the fetal islet cells for insulin production (glucose easily passes the placental barrier from maternal to fetal side; however, insulin does not cross the placental barrier). Historically, maternal hyperglycemia was believed to contribute to fetal macrosomia. However, Hay (2012) has suggested that maternal hyperlipidemia and increased lipid transfer to the fetus are responsible for the excessive weight gain and fat deposition seen in such infants (Hay, 2012). IDMs are more likely to have disproportionately large abdominal circumferences and shoulders, leading to an increased risk of shoulder dystocia and birth injury (Dailey & Coustan, 2010). When the newborn's glucose supply is removed abruptly at the time of birth, the continued production of insulin soon depletes the blood of circulating glucose, creating a state of hyperinsulinism and hypoglycemia within 0.5 to 4 hours, especially in infants of mothers with poorly controlled diabetes. Precipitous drops in blood glucose levels can cause serious neurological damage or death.

IDMs have a characteristic appearance (Box 28-6 and Fig. 28-11). Infants of mothers with advanced diabetes may be

BOX 28-6 CLINICAL MANIFESTATIONS OF INFANTS OF DIABETIC MOTHERS

- Large for gestational age
- Very plump and full faced
- Abundant vernix caseosa
- Plethora
- Listless and lethargic
- Possibly meconium stained at birth
- Hypotonia

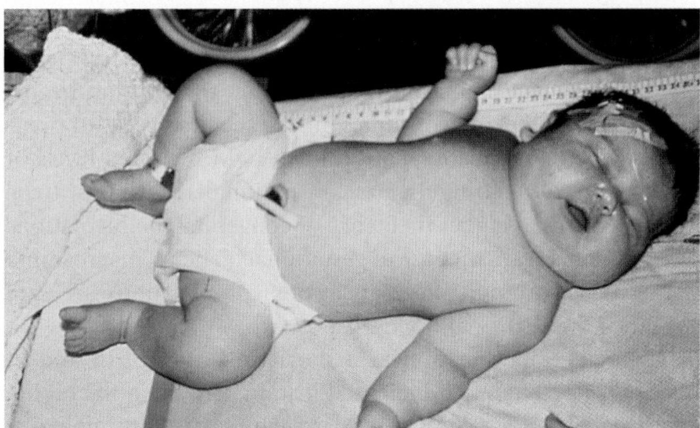

FIGURE 28-11 Large-for-gestational-age infant. This infant of a diabetic mother weighed 5 kg (11 lbs) at birth and exhibits the typical round facies. (From Zitelli, B. J., & Davis, H. W. (2007). *Atlas of pediatric physical diagnosis* (5th ed.). Philadelphia: Mosby.)

SGA, have IUGR, or be the appropriate size for gestational age because of the maternal vascular (placental) involvement. There is an increase in congenital anomalies in IDMs in addition to a high susceptibility to hypoglycemia, hypocalcemia, hypomagnesemia, polycythemia, hyperbilirubinemia, cardiomyopathy, and RDS (Dailey and Coustan, 2010). CNS anomalies such as anencephaly, spina bifida, and holoprosencephaly occur at rates 10 times higher than in any other population of mothers. Cardiac anomalies such as ventriculoseptal defects and coarctation of the aorta are increased five-fold in IDMs, and sacral agenesis and caudal regression occur almost exclusively in IDMs (Landon, Capalano, & Gabbe, 2012). Hyperinsulinemia and hyperglycemia in the diabetic mother may be factors in reducing fetal surfactant synthesis, thus contributing to the development of RDS. Although large, these infants may be delivered before term as a result of maternal complications or increased fetal size.

Congenital hyperinsulinism is a condition that causes neonatal macrosomia, and profound hypoglycemia is often present in the neonatal period. However, this condition is usually not associated with maternal DM, but appears to have a genetic etiology; the condition is also associated with syndromes such as Beckwith-Wiedemann syndrome (Sperling, 2016).

Some IDMs are also at increased risk for deep vein thrombosis, with renal vein thrombosis and hematuria being the most common presentation (Hay, 2012). Additional problems in IDMs include perinatal iron deficiency and neurological impairments (seizures, lethargy, jitteriness, and changes in tone) (Hay, 2012).

The most important management of IDMs is careful monitoring of serum glucose levels and observation for accompanying complications such as RDS and cardiac anomalies. The infants are examined for the presence of any anomalies or birth injuries, and blood studies for determination of glucose, calcium, hematocrit, and bilirubin are obtained on a regular basis.

Because the hypertrophied pancreas is so sensitive to blood glucose concentrations, the administration of oral glucose may trigger a massive insulin release, resulting in rebound hypoglycemia. Therefore, feedings of breast milk or formula begin within the first hour after birth, provided that the infant's cardiorespiratory condition is stable. Approximately half of these infants do well and adjust without complications. Infants born to mothers with poorly controlled diabetes may require IV dextrose infusions. Studies confirm the importance of maintaining serum glucose levels above 2.8 mmol/L in hyperinsulinemic infants with hypoglycemia to prevent serious neurological sequelae (Aziz et al., 2004/2014). Enteral supplementation may be used in asymptomatic infants with blood glucose levels of 1.8 mmol/L to 2.5 mmol/L to augment caloric intake. It is recommended that symptomatic, hypoglycemic infants (and asymptomatic infants who have failed to respond to enteral supplementation) be treated with intravenous dextrose solution. Consider investigation, consultation, and pharmacological intervention if target blood glucose levels are not achieved by intravenous dextrose (Aziz et al., 2004/2014).

Oral and IV intake may be titrated to maintain adequate blood glucose levels. Frequent blood glucose determinations are needed for the first 2 to 4 days of life to assess the degree of hypoglycemia present at any given time. Testing blood taken from the heel with calibrated portable reflectance meters (e.g., glucometers) is a simple and effective screening evaluation that can then be confirmed by laboratory examination (see Heel stick, Chapter 26, p. 699).

NURSING CARE

The nursing care of IDMs involves early examination for congenital anomalies, signs of possible respiratory or cardiac problems, maintenance of adequate thermoregulation, early introduction of carbohydrate feedings as appropriate, and monitoring of serum blood glucose levels. The latter is of particular importance because many infants with hypoglycemia may remain asymptomatic. Symptomatic IDMs who are unable to feed should be started on a continuous IV infusion of 10% dextrose at 4 to 6 mg/min/kg unless blood glucose is below 1.1 mmol/L. In such cases a one-time bolus infusion of 10% dextrose (200 mg/kg) should be given over 2 to 4 minutes, followed by a constant IV infusion of 10% dextrose and water as noted previously (Hay, 2012). IV glucose infusion requires careful monitoring of the site and the newborn's reaction to therapy; high glucose concentrations (≥12.5%) should be infused via a central line instead of a peripheral site.

IDMs also need to be monitored for hypocalcemia and hypomagnesemia. Signs of hypocalcemia are similar to those of hypoglycemia, but they occur within the first 24 hours of age. Infants also need to be monitored closely for hyperbilirubinemia.

Because macrosomic infants are at risk for problems associated with a difficult birth, they are monitored for birth injuries such as brachial plexus injury and palsy, fractured clavicle, and phrenic nerve palsy. Additional monitoring of the infant for problems associated with this condition (polycythemia, hypocalcemia, poor feeding, and hyperbilirubinemia) is also a vital nursing function.

Some evidence indicates that IDMs have an increased risk of acquiring type 2 diabetes and metabolic syndrome in childhood or early adulthood (Hay, 2012); therefore, nursing care should also focus on healthy lifestyle and prevention later in life with IDMs. See the Nursing Care Plan, The Infant of Mother With Diabetes Mellitus on the Evolve site.

DISCHARGE PLANNING AND TRANSPORT

Discharge Planning

Discharge planning for the high-risk newborn begins early in the hospitalization. Throughout the infant's hospitalization, the nurse must gather information from the health care team members and the family. This information is used to determine the infant's and family's readiness for discharge.

As the nurse assesses the discharge needs of the infant's parents, he or she needs to take steps to eliminate any knowledge deficits. Discharge teaching for the high-risk newborn's family is extensive, requires time and planning, and cannot be accomplished on the day of discharge alone. Information should be provided about infant care, especially as it pertains to the infant's particular needs (e.g., supplemental oxygen, gastrostomy feedings, follow-up medical visits). Parent education includes having them give return demonstrations of their infant care skills to show whether they are becoming increasingly independent in providing care for their infant. Parents of a preterm infant or one with special needs should be given the opportunity to room in and spend a night or two providing care for their infant away from the NICU. This affords them the opportunity to become more aware of the necessary care and to have transition time during which to ask questions regarding home care. Additional parent teaching should include bathing and skin care; requirements for meeting nutritional needs after discharge; safety in the home, including supine sleep position and prevention of infection (e.g., respiratory syncytial virus); and medication administration.

Medical equipment and supplies required for care of the infant in the home should be delivered to the home before discharge; parents and care providers should have education and ample practice in its use. Parents of an infant being discharged with special needs (i.e., gavage or gastrostomy feedings, oxygen, tracheostomy, or colostomy) should receive several days of carefully planned education in the various procedures before discharge.

Car seat safety is an essential aspect of discharge planning. Parents should obtain an age-appropriate car seat before discharge and demonstrate its use with the infant. Previously it was recommended that all infants less than 37 weeks should have an infant car seat challenge testing done prior to discharge. The CPS latest recommendation states that while it is clear that infants placed in a car seat are more likely to experience oxygen desaturation or bradycardia than when they are supine, this does not predict an adverse neurodevelopmental outcome or mortality post-discharge, therefore routine use of the infant car seat challenge as part of discharge planning for preterm infants is no longer recommended (Narvey & CPS Fetus and Newborn Committee, 2016).

Preterm infants have a high rate of readmission to hospital and emergency department visits. It is imperative that the family have a health care provider they can contact for questions regarding infant care and behaviour once they are home.

Before discharge, all high-risk or preterm infants should receive the appropriate immunizations, metabolic screening, hematology assessment (bilirubin risk as appropriate), and evaluation of hearing and for ROP (Jefferies & CPS Fetus and Newborn Committee, 2010). Successful discharge of a high-risk infant requires an interprofessional and family-centred approach. Medical, nursing, social services, and other professionals (physiotherapy, occupational therapy, developmental follow-up specialist) are crucial to the smooth transition of these infants and their families to the community and home. If the infant is retrotransferred to a facility providing less acute care, interfacility communication is essential to continuity of care.

Discharge to home for high-risk infants does not mean they can be treated like healthy term newborns. Follow-up by a practitioner familiar with the issues common to the high-risk newborn is essential. Further follow-up of specific complications by qualified specialists and referral to centres for developmental interventions can help ensure the best outcome possible for these infants.

Referrals for appropriate community resources also need to be made for infants with developmental disabilities or those at risk for further problems (e.g., preterm infants). Social-service involvement is especially important for young or psychosocially high-risk parents (e.g., parents with a history of substance use or child maltreatment).

For the family of the child who is technology dependent, special education needs should be discussed before discharge. For further discussion of home care, see Chapter 42.

Transport to a Regional Centre

If a hospital is not equipped to care for a high-risk mother and fetus or a high-risk infant, transfer to a specialized perinatal or regional tertiary care centre is arranged. Maternal transport that occurs with the fetus in utero and this has two distinct advantages: (1) neonatal morbidity and mortality are decreased, and (2) the mother and infant are not separated at birth.

For a variety of reasons, it is not always possible to transport the mother before the birth. Therefore, physicians and nurses in all facilities must have the skills and equipment necessary for making an accurate diagnosis and implementing emergency interventions to stabilize the infant's condition until transport can occur (Rojas, Shirley, & Rush, 2011). The goal of these interventions is to maintain the infant's condition within the normal physiological range. Specific attention should be given to vital signs, oxygenation and ventilation, thermoregulation, acid–base balance, fluid and electrolyte status, blood glucose, and developmental interventions.

Arrangements for transport to a tertiary centre should be made as soon as the high-risk infant is identified (see Community Focus box) and best done by a specially trained neonatal transport team. The infant must be kept warm and adequately oxygenated (including intubation and surfactant replacement as indicated); have vital signs and oxygen saturation monitored; and, when indicated, receive an IV infusion. The infant must be transported in a specially designed isolette containing a complete life support system and other emergency equipment that can be carried by ambulance, helicopter, or a fixed-wing aircraft (Fig. 28-12).

The transport team may consist of physicians, nurse practitioners, nurses, and respiratory therapists or paramedics. The team must have experience in resuscitation, stabilization, and provision of critical care during the transport. When an infant is to be transported from the hospital, the parents need a description of the facility where the infant is going. They need to know the location, reputation, and nature of the facility and the care that the infant is expected to receive. The name of the infant's physician and the telephone number of the nursery should be given to them, and unfamiliar terms such as *neonatologist*, *ventilator*, *infusion*, and *isolette* should be explained. Explanations should be kept simple, and parents should be given the opportunity to ask questions. If booklets and a website are available that describe the facility, they are given to the family.

Perhaps most important, the parents should have some contact with the infant before the transport. Being able to see, touch, and (if possible) hold their infant may help decrease parents' anxiety. Often a photograph or even a video recording of their infant can serve as tangible evidence of the newborn's existence until the parents are able to travel to the regional facility. When possible, it is often advisable to transfer the mother to the same institution as her infant.

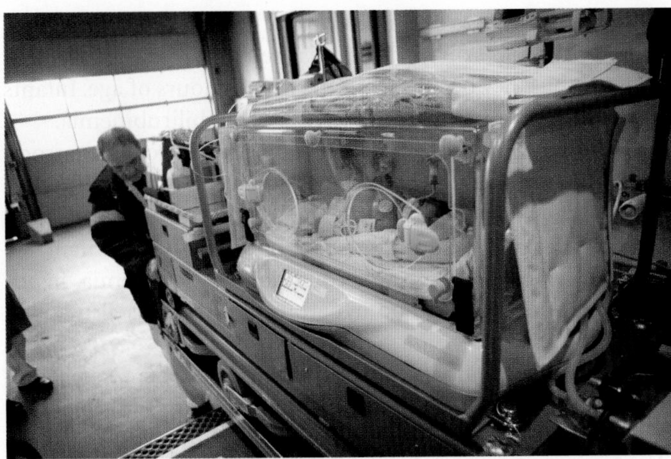

FIGURE 28-12 Total life support system for transport of high-risk newborns. (© BSIP SA/Alamy Stock Photo.)

COMMUNITY FOCUS

Neonatal Transport

During a scheduled clinical experience in the nursery at a community hospital, observe a neonatal transport team working to stabilize an infant before transport to the tertiary centre. Who are the transport team members? What are their roles and responsibilities? What equipment have they brought with them? How was the referral made? What communication links exist between the community hospitals and the tertiary centre's NICU? What communication links exist between the NICU and the transport team when they are stabilizing and transporting the sick infant? To whom does the transport team report? How are the parents kept informed of the infant's condition?

KEY POINTS

- Preterm infants are at risk for problems related to the immaturity of their organ systems.
- Late preterm infants are at higher risk for feeding problems, respiratory distress, jaundice, poor neurodevelopment, hypoglycemia, infection, and thermoregulation than their term counterparts.
- RDS, ROP, and chronic lung disease (BPD) are associated with preterm birth.
- High-risk infants must be observed for respiratory distress and other early signs of physiological distress.
- The adaptation of parents to preterm or high-risk infants differs from that of parents of term infants.
- Infants born to diabetic mothers (gestational or otherwise) are at risk for hypoglycemia, RDS, and birth asphyxia and trauma.
- Metabolic abnormalities of diabetes mellitus in pregnancy adversely affect embryonic and fetal development.
- SGA infants are considered to be at risk because of fetal growth restriction.
- Health concerns of postterm infants are related to the progressive placental insufficiency that can occur in a postterm pregnancy.
- Parents need special instruction (e.g., CPR, oxygen therapy, suctioning, developmental care) before they take a high-risk infant home.
- Specially trained nurses may transport high-risk infants to and from special care units.

evolve WEBSITE

Visit the Evolve website for additional resources related to the content in this chapter such as Case Studies, Critical Thinking Case Study Answers, Nursing Care Plans, Nursing Processes, Nursing Skills, and Review Questions for Exam Preparation at: http://evolve.elsevier.com/Canada/Perry/maternal/

REFERENCES

ACoRN Editorial Board. (2012). *Acute care of at-risk newborns*. Vancouver: Author. Retrieved from <http://www.cps.ca/en/acorn>.

Almadhoob, A., & Ohlsson, A. (2015). Sound reduction management in the neonatal intensive care unit for preterm or very low birth weight infants. *The Cochrane Database of Systematic Reviews*, (1), CD010333. doi:10.1002/14651858.CD010333.pub2.

American Academy of Pediatrics. (2014). *Pediatric nutrition handbook* (7th ed.). Elk Grove Village, IL: Author.

Anderson, M. S., Wood, L. L., Keller, J. A., & Hay, W. W., Jr. (2011). Enteral nutrition. In S. L. Gardner, B. S. Carter, M. Enzman-Hines, & J. A. Hernandez (Eds.), *Merenstein & Gardner's handbook of neonatal intensive care* (7th ed., pp. 398–433). St. Louis: Mosby.

Aziz, K., Dancy, P., & Canadian Paediatric Society, Fetus and Newborn Committee. (2004). Screening guidelines for newborns at risk for low blood glucose. *Paediatrics and Child Health*, *9*(10), 723–729. Reaffirmed 2014.

Bahadue, F. L., & Soll, R. (2012). Early versus delayed selective surfactant treatment for neonatal respiratory distress syndrome. *The Cochrane Database of Systematic Reviews*, (11), CD001456. doi:10.1002/14651858.CD001456.pub2.

Barrington, K. J., & Finer, N. (2010). Inhaled nitric oxide for respiratory failure in preterm infants. *The Cochrane Database of Systematic Reviews*, (12), CD000509. doi:10.1002/14651858.CD000509.pub4.

Birnbaum, R., & Limperopoulos, C. (2009). Nonoral feeding practices for infants in the neonatal intensive care unit. *Advances in Neonatal Care*, *9*(4), 180–184. doi:10.1097/ANC.0b013e3181aa9c65.

Bissinger, R. L., & Annibale, D. J. (2010). Thermoregulation in very low–birth-weight infants during the golden hour: Results and implications. *Advances in Neonatal Care*, *10*(5), 230–238.

Blackburn, S. T. (2009a). Central nervous system vulnerabilities in preterm infants, part I. *Journal of Perinatal and Neonatal Nursing*, *23*(1), 12–14. doi:10.1097/JPN.0b013e31819685cc.

Blackburn, S. T. (2009b). Central nervous system vulnerabilities in preterm infants, part II. *Journal of Perinatal and Neonatal Nursing*, *23*(2), 108–110. doi:10.1097/JPN.0b013e3181a3924b.

Blackburn, S. T. (2012). *Maternal, fetal, and neonatal physiology: A clinical perspective* (4th ed.). St. Louis: Saunders.

Brown, W. D., & Landers, S. (2011). Heat balance. In S. L. Gardner, B. S. Carter, M. Enzman-Hines, & J. A. Hernandez (Eds.), *Merenstein & Gardner's handbook of neonatal intensive care* (7th ed., pp. 113–133). St. Louis: Mosby.

Canadian Institute for Health Information (CIHI). (2009). *Too early, too small: A profile of small babies across Canada*. Ottawa: Author. Retrieved from <https://secure.cihi.ca/free_products/too_early_too_small_en.pdf>.

Carlo, W. A. (2016). The high-risk infant. In R. M. Kliegman, B. F. Stanton, J. St. Geme, et al. (Eds.), *Nelson textbook of pediatrics* (20th ed.). Philadelphia: Saunders.

Carlo, W. A., & Ambalavanan, N. (2016). Intracranial-intraventricular hemorrhage and periventricular leukomalacia. In R. M. Kliegman, B. F. Stanton, J. St. Geme, et al. (Eds.), *Nelson textbook of pediatrics* (20th ed.). Philadelphia: Saunders.

Conde-Agudelo, A., Belizan, J. M., & Diaz-Rossello, J. (2011). Kangaroo mother care to reduce morbidity and mortality in low birthweight infants. *The Cochrane Database of Systematic Reviews*, (3), CD002771. doi:10.1002/14651858.CD002771.pub2.

Dailey, T. L., & Coustan, D. R. (2010). Diabetes in pregnancy. *NeoReviews*, *11*(11), e619–e625.

Davis, D. J., Barrington, K. J., & Canadian Paediatric Society, Fetus and Newborn Committee. (2005). Recommendations for neonatal surfactant therapy. *Paediatrics and Child Health*, *10*(2), 109–116. Reaffirmed 2015.

Dawson, J., Vento, M., Finer, N. N., et al. (2012). Managing oxygen therapy during delivery room stabilization of preterm infants. *Journal of Pediatrics*, *160*(1), 158–161.

de Boer, J. C., Smit, B. J., & Mainous, R. O. (2009). Nasogastric tube position and intragastric air collection in a neonatal intensive care population. *Advances in Neonatal Care*, *9*(6), 293–298.

Donohue, P. K., Gilmore, M. M., Cristofalo, E., et al. (2011). Inhaled nitric oxide in preterm infants: A systematic review. *Pediatrics*, *127*(2), e414–e422.

Donovan, R., Puppala, B., Angst, D., & Coyle, B. W. (2006). Outcomes of early nutrition support in extremely low-birth-weight infants. *Nutrition in Clinical Practice*, *21*, 395–400. doi:10.1177/0115426506021004395.

Ellett, M. L., Cohen, M. D., Perkins, S. M., et al. (2011). Predicting the insertion length for gastric tube placement for neonates. *Journal of Obstetrics Gynecology & Neonatal Nursing*, *40*(4), 412–421.

Farrington, M., Lang, S., Cullen, L., et al. (2009). Nasogastric tube placement verification in pediatric and neonatal patients. *Pediatric Nursing*, *35*(1), 17–24.

Feeley, N., Waitzer, E., Sherrard, K., et al. (2013). Fathers' perceptions of the barriers and facilitators to their involvement with their newborn hospitalized in the neonatal intensive care unit. *Journal of Clinical Nursing*, *22*(3–4), 521–530.

Field, D., Elbourne, D., Hardy, P., et al. on behalf of the INNOVO Trial Collaborating Group. (2007). Neonatal ventilation with inhaled nitric oxide vs. ventilatory support without inhaled nitric oxide for infants with severe respiratory failure born at or near term: The INNOVO multicenter randomised controlled trial. *Neonatology*, *91*(2), 73–82. doi:10.1542/peds.2004-1209.

Finer, N. N., & the SUPPORT Study Group. (2010). Early CPAP versus surfactant in extremely preterm infants. *New England Journal of Medicine*, *362*, 1970–1979.

Freeman, D., Saxton, V., & Holberton, J. (2012). A weight-based formula for the estimation of gastric tube insertion length in newborns. *Advances in Neonatal Care*, *12*(3), 179–182.

Gardner, S., Enzman-Hines, M., & Dickey, L. A. (2011). Respiratory diseases. In S. L. Gardner, B. S. Carter, M. Enzman-Hines, & J. A. Hernandez (Eds.), *Merenstein & Gardner's handbook of neonatal intensive care* (7th ed., pp. 581–677). St. Louis: Mosby.

Gardner, S. L., & Lawrence, R. A. (2011). Breastfeeding the neonate with special needs. In S. L. Gardner, B. S. Carter, M. Enzman-Hines, & J. A. Hernandez (Eds.), *Merenstein & Gardner's handbook of neonatal intensive care* (7th ed., pp. 434–481). St. Louis: Mosby.

Garg, B. S., & Gupta, S. S. (2013). Nutrient-enriched formula versus standard term formula for preterm infants following hospital discharge: RHL commentary. *The WHO Reproductive Health Library*. Geneva: World Health Organization.

Hay, W. W. (2012). Care of the infant of the diabetic mother. *Current Diabetes Report*, *12*(1), 4–15.

Heaberlin, P. D. (2014). Neurologic assessment. In E. P. Tappero & M. E. Honeyfield (Eds.), *Physical assessment of the newborn: A comprehensive approach to the art of physical examination* (5th ed.). Santa Rosa, CA: NICU Ink.

Health Canada. (2010). *Recommendations for the preparation and handling of powdered infant formula (PIF)*. Retrieved from <http://www.hc-sc.gc.ca/fn-an/nutrition/infant-nourisson/pif-ppn-recommandations-eng.php>.

Holditch-Davis, D., & Blackburn, S. T. (2013). Neurobehavioral development. In C. Kenner & W. J. Lott (Eds.), *Comprehensive neonatal care* (5th ed.). St. Louis: Saunders.

Jefferies, A. L., & Canadian Paediatric Society, Fetus and Newborn Committee. (2010). Retinopathy of prematurity: Recommendations for screening. *Paediatrics and Child Health, 15*(10), 667–670.

Jefferies, A. L., & Canadian Paediatric Society, Fetus and Newborn Committee. (2014). Position statement: Going home: Facilitating discharge of the preterm infant. *Paediatrics and Child Health, 19*(1), 31–36.

Johnston, C., Campbell-Yeo, M., Fernandes, A., et al. (2014). Skin to-skin care for procedural pain in neonates. *The Cochrane Database of Systematic Reviews*, (1), CD008435. doi:10.1002/14651858.CD008435.pub2.

Kastenberg, Z. J., & Sylvester, K. G. (2013). The surgical management of necrotizing enterocolitis. *Clinical Perinatology, 40*(1), 135–148.

Kenney, P. M., Hoover, D., Williams, L. C., & Iskersky, V. (2011). Cardiovascular diseases and surgical interventions. In S. L. Gardner, B. S. Carter, M. Enzman-Hines, & J. A. Hernandez (Eds.), *Merenstein & Gardner's handbook of neonatal intensive care* (7th ed., pp. 678–716). St. Louis: Mosby.

King, B., Carlson, G., Khalil, B. A., & Morabito, A. (2013). Intestinal bowel lengthening in children with short bowel syndrome: Systematic review of the Bianchi and STEP procedures. *World Journal of Surgery, 37*(3), 694–704.

Kinsella, J. P., Cutter, G. R., Steinhorn, R. H., et al. (2014). Noninvasive inhaled nitric oxide does not prevent bronchopulmonary dysplasia in premature newborns. *Journal of Pediatrics, 165*(6), 1104–1108.

Kliegman, R. M. (2014). Intrauterine growth restriction. In R. J. Martin, A. A. Fanaroff, & M. C. Walsh (Eds.), *Fanaroff & Martin's neonatal–perinatal medicine: Diseases of the fetus and infant* (10th ed.). Philadelphia: Mosby.

Lain, S. J., Roberts, C. L., Bowen, J. R., & Nassar, N. (2015). Early discharge of infants and risk of readmission for jaundice. *Pediatrics, 135*(2), 314–321. doi:10.1542/peds.2014-2388.

LaMar, K., & Dowling, D. A. (2006). Incidence of infection for preterm twins cared for in cobedding in the neonatal intensive-care unit. *Journal of Obstetric, Gynecologic, and Neonatal Nursing, 35*(2), 193–198. doi:10.1111/j.1552-6909.2006.00025.x.

Landon, M. B., Catalano, P. M., & Gabbe, S. G. (2012). Diabetes mellitus. In S. G. Gabbe, J. R. Niebyl, & J. L. Simpson (Eds.), *Obstetrics: Normal and problem pregnancies* (6th ed.). Philadelphia: Saunders.

Lawrence, R. A., & Lawrence, R. M. (2011). *Breastfeeding: A guide for the medical profession* (7th ed.). Philadelphia: Mosby.

Lovvan, H. N., III, Glenn, J. B., Pacetti, A. S., & Carter, B. S. (2011). Neonatal surgery. In S. L. Gardner, B. S. Carter, M. Enzman-Hines, & J. A. Hernandez (Eds.), *Merenstein & Gardner's handbook of neonatal intensive care* (7th ed., pp. 812–848). St. Louis: Mosby.

Lund, C. H., & Kuller, J. M. (2013). Integumentary system. In C. Kenner & J. W. Lott (Eds.), *Comprehensive neonatal care* (5th ed.). St. Louis: Saunders.

Maheshwari, A., & Carlo, W. A. (2016). Digestive system disorders. In R. M. Kliegman, B. F. Stanton, J. St. Geme, et al. (Eds.), *Nelson textbook of pediatrics* (20th ed.). Philadelphia: Saunders.

Mitanchez, D. (2010). Foetal and neonatal complications in gestational diabetes: Perinatal mortality, congenital malformations, macrosomia, shoulder dystocia, birth injuries, neonatal complications. *Diabetes & Metabolism Journal, 36*(6 Pt 2), 617–627.

Morgan, J., Bombell, S., & McGuire, W. (2013). Early trophic feeding versus enteral fasting for very preterm or very low birth weight infants. *The Cochrane Database of Systematic Reviews*, (3), CD000504. doi:10.1002/14651858.CD000504.pub4.

Morgan, J., Young, L., & McGuire, W. (2014). Delayed introduction of progressive enteral feeds to prevent necrotizing enterocolitis in very low birth weight infants. *The Cochrane Database of Systematic Reviews*, (12), CD001970. doi:10.1002/14651858.CD001970.pub5.

Narvey, M. R., & Canadian Paedatric Society, Fetus and Newborn Committee. (2016). Assessment of cardiorespiratory stability using the infant car seat challenge before discharge in preterm infants (<37 weeks' gestational age). *Paediatric & Child Health, 21*(3), 155–158. Retrieved from <http://www.cps.ca/en/documents/position/infant-car-seat-challenge>.

Ohlsson, A., Walia, R., & Shah, S. S. (2015). Ibuprofen for the treatment of patent ductus arteriosus in preterm or low birth weight (or both) infants. *Cochrane Database of Systematic Reviews Issue*, (2), CD003481, doi:10.1002/14651858.CD003481.pub6.

Paul, M. (2015). Oxygen administration to preterm neonates in the delivery room. Minimizing oxidative stress. *Advances in Neonatal Care, 15*(2), 94–103.

Perlman, J. M., Wyllie, J., Kattwinkel, J., et al. on behalf of the Neonatal Resuscitation Chapter Collaborators. (2010). Part 11: Neonatal resuscitation: 2010 international consensus on cardiopulmonary resuscitation and emergency cardiovascular care science with treatment recommendations. *Circulation, 122*(Suppl. 2), S516–S538. doi:10.1161/CIR.0b013e3181fdf77e.

Polin, R. A., Denson, S., Brady, M. T., et al. (2012). Strategies for prevention of health care–associated infections in the NICU. *Pediatrics, 129*(4), e1085–e1093.

Prince, A., & Groh-Wargo, S. (2013). Nutrition management for the promotion of growth in very low birth weight premature infants. [Review]. *Nutrition in Clinical Practice, 28*(6), 659–668.

Public Health Agency of Canada (PHAC). (2013). *Perinatal health indicators for Canada 2013. A report of the Canadian Perinatal Surveillance System.* Ottawa: Author. Retrieved from <http://www.phac-aspc.gc.ca/rhs-ssg/phi-isp-2013-eng.php>.

Quandt, D., Schraner, T., Ulrich Bucher, H., et al. (2009). Malposition of feeding tubes in neonates: Is it an issue? *Journal of Pediatric Gastroenterology and Nutrition, 48*(5), 608–611.

Räisänen, S., Gissler, M., Saari, J., et al. (2013). Contribution of risk factors to extremely, very and moderately preterm births—Register-based analysis of 1,390,742 singleton births. *PLoS ONE, 8*(4), e60660. doi:10.1371/journal.pone.0060660.

Renner, M. (2010). Far from reliable: pH testing in the neonatal intensive care unit. *Journal of Pediatric Nursing, 25*(6), 580–583.

Rojas, M. A., Shirley, K., & Rush, M. G. (2011). Perinatal transport and levels of care. In S. L. Gardner, B. S. Carter, M. Enzman-Hines, & J. A. Hernandez (Eds.), *Merenstein & Gardner's handbook of neonatal intensive care* (7th ed., pp. 39–51). St. Louis: Mosby.

Rojas-Reyes, M., Morley, C. J., & Soll, R. (2012). Prophylactic versus selective use of surfactant in preventing morbidity and mortality in preterm infants. *The Cochrane Database of Systematic Reviews*, (3), CD000510. doi:10.1002/14651858.CD000510.pub2.

Saugstad, O. D., & Aune, D. (2014). Optimal oxygenation of extremely low birth weight infants: A meta-analysis and systematic review of oxygen saturation target studies. *Neonatology, 105*(1), 55–63. doi:10.1159/000356561.

Sperling, M. A. (2016). Hypoglycemia. In R. M. Kliegman, B. F. Stanton, J. St. Geme, et al. (Eds.), *Nelson textbook of pediatrics* (20th ed.). Philadelphia: Saunders.

Squires, A. J., & Hyndman, M. (2009). Prevention of nasal injuries secondary to NCPAP application in the ELBW infant. *Neonatal Network, 28*(1), 13–27.

Statistics Canada. (2012). *Live birth, by birth weight (less than 2,500 grams) and sex, Canada, provinces and territories, annual* (CANSIM Table 102-4005). Ottawa: Author. Retrieved from <http://www5.statcan.gc.ca/cansim/a26?lang=eng&id=1024509>.

Stevens, T. P., Blennow, M., Myers, E. H., & Soll, R. (2007). Early surfactant administration with brief ventilation vs. selective surfactant and continued mechanical ventilation for preterm infants with or at risk for respiratory distress syndrome. *The Cochrane Database of Systematic Reviews*, (4), CD003063. doi:10.1002/14651858.CD003063.pub3.

Talge, N. M., Holzman, C., Wang, J., et al. (2010). Late-preterm birth and its association with cognitive and socioemotional outcomes at 6 years of age. *Pediatrics, 126*, 1124–1131. doi:10.1542/peds.2010-1536.

Telofski, L. S., Morello, A. P., Mack Correa, M. C., et al. (2012). The infant skin barrier: Can we preserve, protect, and enhance the barrier? *Dermatology Research & Practice*, 198789. doi:10.1155/2012/198789.

Teune, M. J., Bakhuizen, S., Bannerman, C. G., et al. (2011). A systematic review of severe morbidity in infants born late preterm. *American Journal of Obstetrics & Gynecology*, *205*(374), e1–e9. doi:10.1016/j.ajog.2011.07.015.

Thomas, K. A., & Uran, A. (2007). How the NICU environment sounds to a preterm infant. *MCN: American Journal of Maternal/Child Nursing*, *32*(4), 250–253. doi:10.1097/01.NMC.0000281966.23034.e9.

Vento, M., & Saugstad, O. D. (2011). Oxygen supplementation in the delivery room: Updated information. *Journal of Pediatrics*, *158*(2) Supplement 1, e5–e7.

Volpe, J. J. (2008). *Neurology of the newborn* (5th ed.). Philadelphia: Saunders.

Wang, D., Aubertin, C., Barrowman, N., et al. (2014). Reduction of noise in the neonatal intensive care unit using sound-activated noise meters. *Archives of Disease in Childhood. Fetal and Neonatal Edition*, *99*(6), F515–F516.

Westrup, B., Sizun, J., & Lagercrantz, H. (2007). Family-centered developmental supportive care: A holistic and humane approach to reduce stress and pain in neonates. *Journal of Perinatology*, *27*(Suppl. 1), S12–S18. doi:10.1038/sj.jp.7211724.

Wheeler, K., Klingenberg, C., McCallion, N., et al. (2010). Volume-targeted versus pressure-limited ventilation in the neonate. *The Cochrane Database of Systematic Reviews*, (11), CD003666. doi:10.1002/14651858.CD003666.pub3.

Whyte, R. K., & Canadian Paediatric Society, Fetus and Newborn Committee. (2010). Safe discharge of the late preterm infant. *Paediatrics and Child Health*, *15*(10), 655–660. Reaffirmed 2015.

ADDITIONAL RESOURCES

AWHONN Neonatal Skin Condition Score: <http://www.awhonn.org/awhonn/content.do?name=03_JournalsPubsResearch%2F3G4_NeonatalSkinCare.htm>.

Fenton Preterm Growth Charts: <http://www.ucalgary.ca/fenton/2013chart>.

Therapy B. C. *Modified Braden Q Scale*: <http://www.therapybc.ca/eLibrary/docs/Resources/Braden%20Q%20scale%20for%20paeds.pdf>.

CHAPTER

29

The Newborn at Risk: Acquired and Congenital Problems

Deborah Aylward

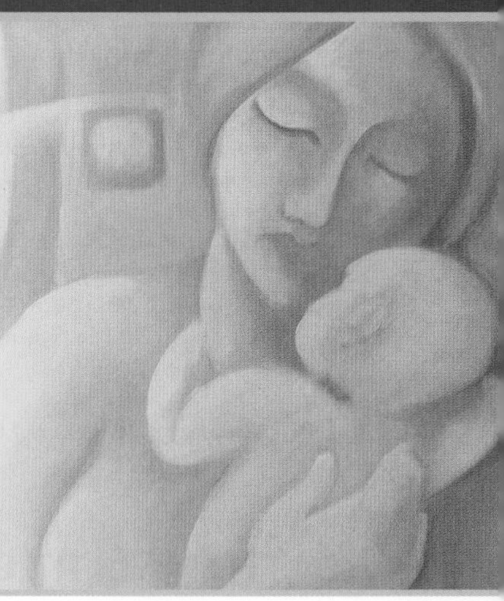

evolve WEBSITE

Visit the Evolve website for additional resources related to the content in this chapter such as Case Studies, Critical Thinking Case Study Answers, Nursing Care Plans, Nursing Processes, Nursing Skills, and Review Questions for Exam Preparation at: http://evolve.elsevier.com/Canada/Perry/maternal/

OBJECTIVES

On completion of this chapter the reader will be able to:

- Summarize assessment and care of the newborn that has soft-tissue, skeletal, and neurological injuries due to birth trauma.
- Identify maternal conditions that place the newborn at risk for infection.
- Identify clinical signs of infection in the newborn.
- Describe the nurse's role in the diagnosis and care of neonatal sepsis.
- Identify the effects of maternal use of alcohol, heroin, methadone, marijuana, methamphetamine, cocaine, and tobacco on the fetus and newborn.
- Describe the assessment of a newborn exposed to harmful drugs in utero.
- Compare characteristics of neonatal Rh and ABO incompatibility.
- Describe preoperative and postoperative nursing care of the newborn.
- Describe congenital disorders and identify nursing care for infants with a congenital condition.

The birth of an at-risk or high-risk infant is a challenge for health care providers as transition to extrauterine life is complicated by additional conditions or circumstances. The infant may be considered high risk because of antenatal, intrapartum, or neonatal conditions such as maternal substance use, birth trauma, infection, or congenital anomalies. Birth trauma includes physical injuries a newborn sustains during labour and birth.

At times, the nurse can anticipate problems, such as when a woman is admitted in preterm labour or a congenital anomaly is diagnosed in the antenatal period. At other times, the birth of a high-risk infant is unanticipated. In either case, the personnel and equipment necessary for immediate care of the infant must be available.

BIRTH TRAUMA

Birth trauma (injury) is physical injury sustained by a newborn during labour and birth. It remains an important source of neonatal morbidity. Most birth injuries are avoidable, especially with careful assessment of risk factors and appropriate planning of the birth. The use of fetal ultrasonography allows antepartum diagnosis of certain fetal conditions that may be treated in utero or shortly after birth. Elective Caesarean birth can be chosen for some pregnancies to prevent significant birth injury. A small percentage of significant birth injuries caused by prolonged labour or an abnormal fetal presentation are unavoidable despite skilled and competent obstetrical care. Emergency Caesarean birth may improve outcome in some circumstances, but in others the injury may be unavoidable.

Many injuries are minor and resolve without treatment in the newborn period. Others require some degree of intervention; few are serious enough to be fatal. The nurse's contributions to the newborn's welfare begin with early observation of the infant's transition. Prompt recognition and reporting of signs that indicate deviations from normal facilitate early

TABLE 29-1 TYPES OF BIRTH INJURIES

SITE OF INJURY	TYPE OF INJURY
Scalp	Subgaleal hemorrhage (see Fig. 25-11, C)
Skull	Linear fracture
	Depressed fracture
	Occipital osteodiastasis (abnormal separation of adjacent bones)
Intracranial	Epidural hematoma
	Subdural hematoma (laceration of falx, tentorium, or superficial veins)
	Subarachnoid hemorrhage
	Cerebral contusion
	Cerebellar contusion
	Intracerebellar hematoma
Spinal cord (cervical)	Vertebral artery injury
	Intraspinal hemorrhage
	Spinal cord transection or injury
Plexus	Erb palsy
	Klumpke paralysis
	Total (mixed) brachial plexus injury
	Horner syndrome
	Diaphragmatic (phrenic nerve) paralysis
	Lumbosacral plexus injury
Cranial and peripheral nerve	Radial nerve palsy
	Medial nerve palsy
	Sciatic nerve palsy
	Laryngeal nerve palsy
	Diaphragmatic paralysis
	Facial nerve palsy

From Verklan, M. T., & Lopez, S. M. (2011). Neurologic disorders. In S. L. Gardner, B. S. Carter, M. Enzman-Hines, & J. A Hernandez (Eds.), *Merenstein & Gardner's handbook of neonatal intensive care* (7th ed., pp. 748–786). St. Louis: Mosby.

initiation of appropriate therapy. Table 29-1 provides an overview of birth injuries and the sites in which they occur.

NURSING CARE

When the infant is born, the nurse performs a rapid inspection and physical assessment to determine whether there are any life-threatening conditions requiring immediate medical or surgical attention. A comprehensive physical assessment of the newborn is performed after the parents have had the opportunity to interact with their new baby. Because some birth injuries may not be immediately apparent, ongoing assessment is necessary and should occur during each interaction with the infant.

Soft-tissue injuries that commonly occur at birth (i.e., caput succedaneum and cephalohematoma) are discussed in Chapter 25.

Skeletal Injuries

The newborn's immature, flexible skull can withstand a great degree of deformation (moulding) before fracture results. Considerable force is required to fracture the newborn's skull. Two types of skull fractures typically occur: linear fractures and depressed fractures. The location of the fracture and involvement of underlying structures determine its significance.

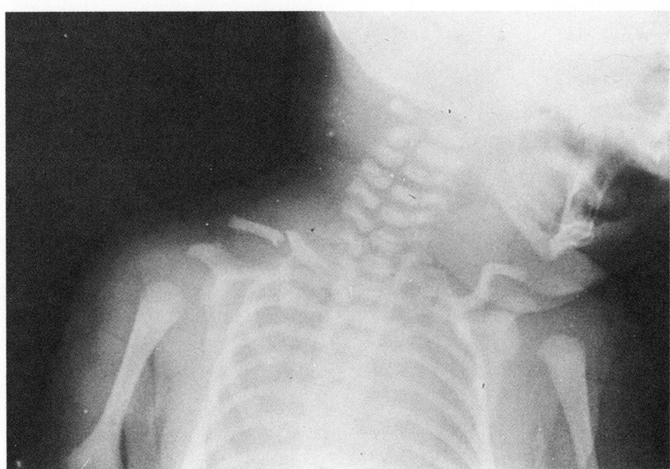

FIGURE 29-1 Fractured clavicle after shoulder dystocia. (O'Doherty, N. [1986]. *Neonatology: Micro atlas of the newborn.* Nutley, NJ: Hoffman-La Roche. Used with permission of F. Hoffmann-La Roche Ltd.)

If an artery lying in a groove on the undersurface of the skull is torn as a result of the fracture, increased intracranial pressure (ICP) will result. Unless a blood vessel is involved, linear fractures, which account for 70% of all fractures in this age group, heal without special treatment. The infant's skull may become indented without laceration of either the skin or the dural membrane. Depressed fractures, or ping-pong ball indentations, may occur during a difficult birth from pressure of the head on the bony pelvis. They also can occur as a result of injudicious application of forceps.

The clavicle is the bone most often fractured during birth as a result of shoulder dystocia. Generally, the break is in the middle third of the bone (Fig. 29-1). Limited arm motion, crepitus over the bone, and absence of the Moro reflex on the affected side are often present. Except for use of gentle rather than vigorous handling and containment of the limb against the chest, no accepted treatment for fractured clavicle of the newborn exists, and the prognosis is good. The humerus and femur are other bones that may be fractured during a difficult birth. Fractures in newborns generally heal rapidly. Immobilization is accomplished with slings, splints, swaddling, and other immobilization devices.

The parents need support when handling their infant with a skeletal injury because they often are fearful of hurting the baby. Nurses can encourage and offer support to parents as they handle, change, and feed their infant. This increases parental knowledge and confidence and facilitates attachment.

Peripheral Nervous System Injuries

Plexus injury results from forces that alter the normal position and relationship of the arm, shoulder, and neck. Erb palsy (Erb-Duchenne paralysis) is caused by damage to the upper plexus and usually results from a stretching or pulling away of the shoulder from the head. Erb palsy may occur with shoulder dystocia or with a difficult vertex or breech delivery. Klumpke

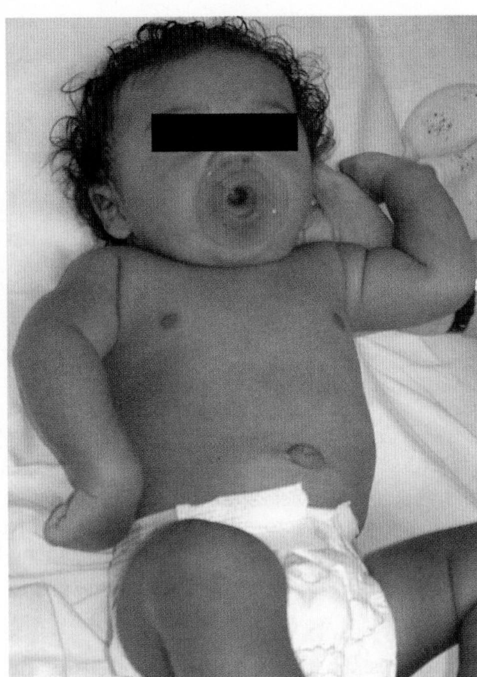

FIGURE 29-2 Erb-Duchenne paralysis in newborn infant. Moro reflex is absent in right upper extremity. Recovery was complete. (From Chung, K. C., Yang, L. J.-S., & McGillicuddy, J. E. [2012]. *Practical management of pediatric and adult brachial plexus palsies.* Philadelphia: Saunders.)

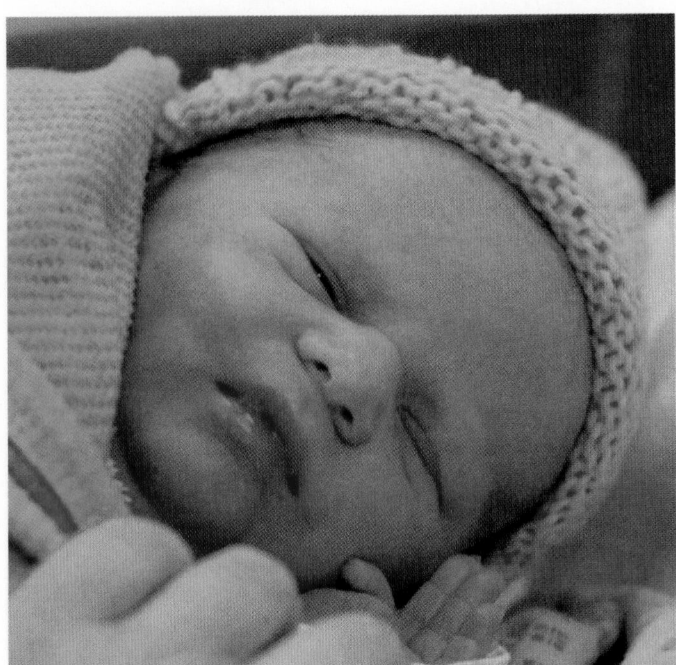

FIGURE 29-3 Facial paralysis (palsy). Absence of movement on the affected side is especially noticeable when the infant cries. (Courtesy of Facial Palsy UK.)

palsy, a less common lower plexus palsy, results from severe stretching of the upper extremity while the trunk is relatively less mobile.

The clinical manifestations of Erb palsy are related to the paralysis of the affected extremity and muscles. The arm hangs limply alongside the body. The shoulder and arm are adducted and internally rotated; the elbow is extended, and the forearm is pronated, with the wrist and fingers flexed. Despite this paralysis, a grasp reflex may be present because finger and wrist movement remains normal (Nelson, 2016) (Fig. 29-2). In lower plexus palsy, the muscles of the hand are paralyzed, with resultant wrist drop and relaxed fingers. In a third and more severe form of brachial palsy, the entire arm is paralyzed and hangs limply and motionless at the infant's side. The Moro reflex is absent on the affected side in all forms of brachial palsy. Total plexus is the second most common type of plexus injury.

The goal of treatment for any of the palsies described above is twofold: prevention of contractures, and maintenance of correct placement of the humeral head within the glenoid fossa of the scapula. Complete recovery from stretched nerves usually takes 3 to 6 months. However, avulsion (disconnection) of the nerves of the ganglia from the spinal cord results in permanent damage. For those injuries that do not improve by 3 to 6 months, surgical intervention may be needed to relieve pressure on the nerves or to repair the nerves with grafting (Nelson, 2016).

Nursing care of the newborn with brachial palsy is concerned primarily with proper positioning of the affected arm: it should be abducted 90 degrees with external shoulder rotation, forearm supination, and extension at the wrist with the palm facing the infant's face. Passive range-of-motion exercises of the shoulder, wrist, elbow, and fingers are initiated in the latter part of the first week. Wrist flexion contractures may be prevented with the use of a wrist splint with padding in the fist. In dressing the infant, preference is given to the affected arm. Undressing begins with the unaffected arm, and redressing begins with the affected arm to prevent unnecessary manipulation and stress on the paralyzed muscles. Parents need to be taught to use the football position when holding the infant and to avoid picking the child up from under the axillae or by pulling on the arms.

Pressure on the facial nerve (cranial nerve VII) during birth may result in injury to it. The primary clinical manifestations are loss of movement on the affected side, such as an inability to completely close the eye, drooping of the mouth, and absence of wrinkling of the forehead and nasolabial fold (Fig. 29-3). Facial palsy or paralysis is most noticeable when the infant cries. The mouth is drawn to the unaffected side, wrinkles are deeper on the normal side, and the eye on the involved side remains open. Often the condition is temporary, resolving within hours or days of birth. Permanent paralysis is rare unless the nerve fibres were torn, in which case surgical intervention may be necessary.

Nursing care of the infant with facial nerve paralysis involves assisting the infant to suck and helping the mother with feeding techniques. The infant may require gavage feeding to prevent aspiration. Breastfeeding is not contraindicated, but the mother may need additional assistance to help the infant latch on to the breast.

If the eyelid on the affected side does not close completely, artificial tears can be instilled daily to prevent drying of the conjunctiva, sclera, and cornea. The lid is often taped shut to prevent accidental injury. If eye care is needed at home, the parents should be taught to administer eye drops before discharge.

Phrenic nerve paralysis results in diaphragmatic paralysis as found on ultrasonography, which shows paradoxical chest movement and an elevated diaphragm. An elevated diaphragm may not be obvious if the newborn is receiving positive-pressure ventilation. This injury sometimes occurs in conjunction with brachial palsy. Respiratory distress is the most common and important sign of injury. Because injury to the phrenic nerve is usually unilateral, the lung on the affected side does not expand and respiratory efforts are ineffective. The infant needs to be positioned on the affected side to facilitate maximum expansion of the uninvolved lung. Breathing is primarily thoracic, and cyanosis, tachypnea, or complete respiratory failure may be seen. Pneumonia and atelectasis on the affected side may also occur.

The infant with phrenic nerve paralysis requires the same nursing care as that for any infant with respiratory distress. As with other birth injuries, the family's emotional needs are similar to those discussed for soft-tissue injury. Follow-up is essential because of the extended length of recovery.

Neurological Injuries

Neurological injury in newborn infants is common with the increased survival of low-birth-weight (LBW) and very-low-birth-weight (VLBW) infants; in addition, the lower the gestational age, the higher the risk for certain neurological injuries. Such infants are particularly vulnerable to ischemic injury caused by variable (both increased and decreased) cerebral blood flow subsequent to asphyxia; preterm infants, with a fragile cerebrovascular network, are highly prone to periventricular or intraventricular hemorrhage. Fragility and increased permeability of capillaries and prolonged prothrombin time predispose preterm infants to trauma when delicate structures are subjected to the forces of labour. The more common cerebral complications and nursing care are outlined in Table 29-2.

The highest incidence of abnormal neurological findings occurs in VLBW infants and those with intracranial hemorrhage (ICH). Major neurological problems such as cerebral palsy, seizures, and hydrocephalus are usually diagnosed in the first 2 years of life. Less severe deficits such as learning disorders, attention deficit hyperactivity disorder (ADHD), and fine- and gross-motor incoordination may not be diagnosed until preschool or even school age. Cerebral palsy is one of the most common neurological deficits in survivors of preterm birth (see Chapter 54).

Research has shown that therapeutic hypothermia provided by cooling either the infant's head or the whole body reduces the severity of the neurological damage in hypoxic ischemic encephalopathy (HIE) when it is applied in the early stages of injury (first 6 hours after birth) in infants with a gestational age of 35 to 36 weeks or more (Azzopardi, Strohm, Edwards, et al., 2009; Edwards, Brocklehurst, Gunn, et al., 2010; Jacobs, Hunt, Tarnow-Mordi, et al., 2007; Laptook, 2009).

Many types of ICH occur in newborns. ICH as a result of birth trauma is more likely to occur in the full-term macrosomic infant. In the newborn, more than one type of hemorrhage can and does commonly occur (Table 29-2). The nursing care of an infant with ICH is supportive and includes monitoring of neurological signs, observation and management of seizures, prevention of increased ICP, and intravenous (IV) therapy.

Spinal cord injuries may result from complicated breech births, especially difficult ones in which version and extraction are used. Clinical manifestations include respiratory failure and flaccid extremities.

NEONATAL INFECTIONS

Sepsis

Sepsis (the presence of microorganisms or their toxins in the blood or other tissues) continues to be one of the most significant causes of neonatal morbidity and mortality. Perinatally acquired infections may cause miscarriage, stillbirth, intrauterine infection, congenital malformations, and acute neonatal disease. Maternal immune globulin M (IgM) does not cross the placenta. IgG levels in term infants are equal to maternal levels; however, in preterm infants the amount of IgG is directly proportional to gestational age. Neonatal neutrophils are present in term infants but have decreased functional capabilities; response to infections is sluggish. Phagocytosis is less efficient. Serum complement levels are low in term infants and even lower in the preterm infant; serum complement (C1 through C6) is involved in immunological reactions, some of which kill or lyse bacteria and enhance phagocytosis. The gut mucosal barrier is initially immature in both term and preterm infants; this barrier is enhanced by the ingestion of human colostrum, which contains anti-infective properties. Dysmaturity seen with intrauterine growth restriction (IUGR) and preterm and post-date birth further compromises the immune system of the neonate.

Table 29-3 outlines risk factors for neonatal sepsis. Precautions for preventing infection, as well as prompt recognition when it occurs, are necessary for optimum newborn care. Neonatal infections may be acquired in utero, at birth, or shortly thereafter and as a health care–associated infection (HAI).

Neonatal bacterial infection is classified into two categories according to the time of presentation—early onset and late onset. Early-onset (congenital) sepsis usually manifests within 24 to 48 hours of birth, progresses more rapidly than later-onset infection, and carries a mortality rate as high as 50%. Early-onset sepsis is acquired in the perinatal period; infection can occur from direct contact with organisms from the maternal gastrointestinal and genitourinary tracts. The most common organism in preterm infants is *Escherichia coli*; in term infants, the most common organism is group B streptococci (GBS), although screening has decreased the incidence of early-onset disease (Stoll, Hansen, Sánchez, et al., 2011). *E. coli*, which may be present in the vagina, accounts for approximately half of all cases of sepsis caused by Gram-negative organisms. GBS is an extremely virulent organism in neonates, with a high (50%) mortality rate in affected infants (see discussion on p. 801).

TABLE 29-2 NEUROLOGICAL COMPLICATIONS

DESCRIPTION	CLINICAL MANIFESTATIONS	THERAPEUTIC MANAGEMENT	CARE MANAGEMENT
Hypoxic-Ischemic Brain Injury			
Nonprogressive neurological (brain) impairment caused by intrauterine or postnatal asphyxia resulting in hypoxemia or cerebral ischemia Hypoxic-ischemic encephalopathy—the resultant cellular damage that causes the clinical manifestations	Appears within first 6–12 hr after hypoxic episode Seizures Abnormal muscle tone (usually hypotonia) Disturbance of sucking and swallowing Apneic episodes Stupor or coma Muscular weakness in hips and shoulders (full term), lower-limb weakness (preterm)	Prevent hypoxia. Provide supportive care. Provide adequate ventilation. Maintain cerebral perfusion. Prevent cerebral edema. Treat underlying cause. Administer antiseizure drugs. Initiate therapeutic hypothermia if criteria met (see Neurological Injuries).	Observe for signs that indicate cerebral hypoxia. Monitor ventilatory and intravenous therapy. Observe for and manage seizures. Support family. Provide guidelines for family management of potential mild-to-severe neurological damage.
Germinal Matrix or Intraventricular Hemorrhage			
Hemorrhage into and around ventricles caused by ruptured vessels as a result of an event that increases cerebral blood flow to area	Sudden deterioration in condition if bleed is large Most bleeds initially asymptomatic Tense, bulging anterior fontanel Neurological signs: • Twitching • Stupor • Apnea • Seizures Evident on cranial ultrasonography or magnetic resonance imaging	Provide supportive care. Provide ventilatory support. Maintain oxygenation. Regulate fluid, electrolytes, acid–base balance. Suppress or prevent seizures. Provide ventricular shunting or drainage.	Prevent increased cerebral blood pressure. Avoid events that may increase or decrease cerebral blood flow (e.g., pain, unnecessary stimulation, endotracheal suctioning, hypoxia, hyperosmolar drugs, rapid volume expansion). Elevate head of bed 20–30 degrees; keep head in midline. Support family. Monitor for posthemorrhagic hydrocephalus after diagnosis. Provide developmental care and enhancement.
Intracranial Hemorrhage			
Subdural Subarachnoid Intracerebellar	Sudden decrease in hematocrit Change in sensorium Poor feeding See Chapter 50.	See Chapter 50.	Same as for germinal matrix or intraventricular hemorrhage

Other bacteria noted to cause early-onset infection include *Haemophilus influenzae*, *Citrobacter* and *Enterobacter* organisms, coagulase-negative staphylococci, and *Streptococcus viridans*. Other pathogens that are harboured in the vagina and may infect the infant include gonococci, *Candida albicans*, herpes simplex virus (HSV type 2), and chlamydia. Early-onset sepsis is associated with a history of obstetrical events such as preterm labour, prolonged rupture of membranes (more than 18 hours), maternal fever during labour, and chorioamnionitis (Venkatesh, Adams, & Weisman, 2011). Early-onset infection is also inversely related to infant birth weight (Polin & American Academy of Pediatrics [AAP] Committee on Fetus and Newborn, 2012).

Late-onset sepsis, usually occurring between 7 and 30 days of age, is considered to be primarily an infection acquired in the hospital or community. The offending organisms include staphylococci, *Klebsiella* organisms, enterococci, *E. coli*, and *Pseudomonas* or *Candida* species (Stoll & Shane, 2016). Coagulase-negative staphylococci, considered to be a contaminant in older children and adults, are commonly found to be the cause of septicemia in extremely-low-birth-weight (ELBW) and VLBW infants. Additional infections of concern include methicillin-resistant *Staphylococcus aureus* (MRSA), vancomycin-resistant enterococci (VRE), and multidrug-resistant Gram-negative pathogens (Stoll & Shane, 2016). Bacterial invasion can occur through the umbilical stump; the skin; mucous membranes of the eye, nose, pharynx, and ear; as well as the respiratory, nervous, urinary, and gastrointestinal systems.

Viral infections such as respiratory syncytial virus (RSV), rotavirus, herpes, influenza, and varicella may occur in the neonatal intensive care unit (NICU). These pathogens may also cause chronic infection, with subtle manifestations that may be recognized only after a prolonged period. It is important to recognize the manifestations of infections in the neonatal period so that the acute infection can be treated, HAIs in other

TABLE 29-3 RISK FACTORS FOR NEONATAL SEPSIS

SOURCE	RISK FACTORS
Maternal	Low socioeconomic status
	Poor prenatal care
	Poor nutrition
	Substance use
	Sexually transmitted infections
Intrapartum	Premature rupture of fetal membranes
	Maternal fever
	Chorioamnionitis
	Prolonged labour
	Rupture of membranes >18 hr
	Premature labour
	Maternal urinary tract infection
Neonatal	Twin or multiple gestation
	Male infant
	Birth asphyxia
	Meconium aspiration
	Congenital anomalies of skin or mucous membranes
	Galactosemia
	Absent spleen
	Low birth weight or prematurity
	Malnourishment
	Prolonged hospitalization
	Multiple interventions

TABLE 29-4 SIGNS OF SEPSIS*

SYSTEM	SIGNS
Respiratory	Apnea, bradycardia
	Tachypnea
	Grunting, nasal flaring
	Retractions
	Decreased oxygen saturation
Cardiovascular	Decreased cardiac output
	Tachycardia
	Hypotension
	Decreased perfusion
	Metabolic acidosis
Central nervous	Temperature instability
	Lethargy
	Hypotonia
	Irritability, seizures
Gastrointestinal	Feeding intolerance (increasing residuals)
	Abdominal distension
	Vomiting, diarrhea
Integumentary	Jaundice
	Pallor
	Petechiae
	Mottling

*Laboratory findings include neutropenia, increased bands, hypoglycemia or hyperglycemia, metabolic acidosis, and thrombocytopenia.

Modified from Askin, D. F. (1995). Bacterial and fungal sepsis in the neonate. *Journal of Obstetric, Gynecologic, and Neonatal Nursing, 24*(7), 635–643.

infants are prevented, and effects on the infant's subsequent growth and development can be anticipated.

Pneumonia, the most common form of neonatal infection, is one of the leading causes of perinatal death. Bacterial meningitis occurs in approximately 0.2 to 0.4 cases per 1000 live births, with a higher rate in preterm infants. Gastroenteritis is sporadic, depending on epidemic outbreaks. Fungal infections are of greatest concern in the immunocompromised or preterm infant. Occasionally, fungal infections, such as thrush, are found in otherwise healthy term infants. Infection by any pathogen continues to be a significant factor in fetal and neonatal morbidity and mortality in Canada.

NURSING CARE

The antenatal record should be reviewed for risk factors associated with infection and the signs and symptoms suggestive of infection. Maternal vaginal or perineal infection may be transmitted directly to the infant during passage through the birth canal. Psychosocial history and history of sexually transmitted infections (STIs) may indicate possible human immunodeficiency virus (HIV), hepatitis B virus (HBV), herpes (type 2), or cytomegalovirus (CMV) infection.

Perinatal events should also be reviewed. Premature rupture of membranes (PROM) may be caused by maternal or intrauterine infection. Ascending infection may occur after prolonged PROM, prolonged labour, or intrauterine fetal monitoring. In some cases infection may occur with intact membranes or contribute to early rupture. A maternal history of fever during labour or the presence of foul-smelling amniotic fluid may also indicate infection. Antibiotic therapy initiated during labour should be noted. The neonate's gestational age, birth weight, and gender all affect the incidence and severity of infection. Sepsis occurs about twice as often and results in a higher mortality in male infants than in female infants. The neonate needs to be assessed for respiratory distress, skin abscesses, petechial rashes, and other indications of infection.

During the postnatal period, the time of onset of suspicious signs needs to be noted. Onset within the first 48 hours of life is more often associated with prenatal or perinatal predisposing factors; onset after 2 or 3 days more often reflects an HAI.

The earliest clinical signs of neonatal sepsis are characterized by a lack of specificity. The nonspecific signs include lethargy, poor feeding, poor weight gain, and irritability. The nurse or parent may simply note that the infant is not doing as well as before. Differential diagnosis may be difficult because signs of sepsis are similar to signs of noninfectious neonatal problems such as hypoglycemia and respiratory distress. Additional clinical and laboratory information, including cultures, will substantiate the findings described. Table 29-4 outlines the clinical signs associated with neonatal sepsis.

Laboratory studies are important in assessing for neonatal infection. Specimens for cultures include blood, cerebrospinal fluid (CSF), stool, and urine. A complete blood cell count

(CBC) with differential should be performed to determine the presence of bacterial infection or increased or decreased white blood cell count (the latter is an ominous sign). The total neutrophil count, immature to total neutrophil (I/T) ratio, absolute neutrophil count (ANC), and C-reactive protein may be used to determine the presence of sepsis. It is important to note that these tests are often adjuncts for the confirmation of neonatal sepsis; a combination of these tests and clinical signs often alert the practitioner to the need for treatment. Additional diagnostic tests that may be used to identify or exclude neonatal sepsis include sedimentation rate, interleukins (IL-8, IL-2, IL-6, and IL-1β), and nucleic acid amplification testing (NAAT). Antepartum infection can now be treated successfully with a number of antiviral medications to decrease viral replication and fetal transmission of disease; neonates may also be treated with antiviral medications such as acyclovir and ganciclovir. In high-risk infants with significant illness, antiviral or antibiotic treatment may begin once cultures are obtained. Once the pathogen is identified, antibiotic, antiviral, or antifungal therapy may be modified.

Vigilant assessment needs to continue during and after treatment. Prolonged administration of antibiotics to ELBW neonates without positive cultures in the first week of life is associated with an increased incidence of necrotizing enterocolitis (NEC), mortality, and late-onset infection; therefore, careful use of antibiotics and close observation of such infants are recommended (Cotten, Taylor, Stoll, et al., 2009; Kuppala, Meinzen-Derr, Morrow, et al., 2011). The newborn continues to be assessed for sequelae to septicemia, which include meningitis, disseminated intravascular coagulation (DIC), pneumonia, and septic shock. Septic shock results from the toxins released into the bloodstream. The most common signs of septic shock include decreasing oxygen saturation, poor perfusion (prolonged capillary refill, cool extremities, mottling), tachycardia, respiratory distress, and hypotension.

Breastfeeding (medically stable infants) or feeding the newborn expressed breast milk from the mother is encouraged. Breast milk provides protective mechanisms. Colostrum contains IgA, which offers protection against infection in the gastrointestinal tract. Human milk contains iron-binding protein that exerts a bacteriostatic effect on *E. coli.* Human milk also contains macrophages and lymphocytes. The vulnerability of infants to common mucosal pathogens such as RSV may be reduced by passive transfer of maternal immunity in the colostrum and breast milk. There is evidence that early enteral feedings with human milk are beneficial in establishing a natural barrier to infection in ELBW and VLBW infants. Human milk is also thought to provide some degree of protection from NEC (Rodriguez & Caplan, 2015).

Administering medications, taking precautions when performing treatments, and following isolation procedures are also interventions to consider in the prevention and treatment of neonatal sepsis.

Monitoring an IV infusion and administering antibiotics are important nursing responsibilities. It is important to administer the prescribed dose of antibiotic within 1 hour after it is prepared in order to avoid loss of drug stability. If the IV fluid that the infant is receiving contains electrolytes, vitamins, or other medications, the nurse should check with the hospital pharmacy before adding antibiotics. The antibiotic (or other medication) may be deactivated or may form a precipitate when combined with other medications.

Care must be taken in suctioning secretions from any newborn's oropharynx or trachea. Routine suctioning is not recommended and may further compromise the infant's immune status, cause hypoxia, and increase ICP. Efforts should also be taken to prevent ventilator-associated pneumonia in infants on mechanical ventilation (see Chapter 45). Isolation procedures are implemented as indicated according to hospital policy. Isolation protocols change rapidly, and the nurse is urged to participate in continuing education and in-service programs to remain up to date.

Prevention

Nurses, as key members of the interprofessional team, are responsible for minimizing or eliminating environmental sources of infectious agents in the nursery. Measures to be taken include routine practices, careful and thorough cleaning of contaminated equipment, frequent replacement of used equipment (e.g., changing IV and nasogastric tubing per hospital protocol; cleaning resuscitation and ventilation equipment, IV pumps, and isolettes), and appropriate disposal of contaminated linens and diapers. Overcrowding must be avoided in nurseries. Guidelines regarding infection control, space, and visitation in areas where newborns receive care have been established and should be followed (Public Health Agency of Canada [PHAC], 2010).

Infants cared for in NICUs are at high risk for infection. In a study of infants admitted at less than 4 days of age to 1 of 17 NICUs in the Canadian Neonatal Network, 23.5% of infants with a birth weight less than 1500 g developed an HAI, as did 2.5% of infants with a birth weight greater than 1500 g. Infection rates varied considerably between facilities, with 6.7 to 74.5% of infants having one episode of confirmed infection (Aziz, McMillan, Andrews, et al., 2005). While hand hygiene is the single most effective measure to reduce infection, the rate of compliance with standards for hand hygiene is only 22%. The combined use of hand hygiene and gloves is even more effective in reducing the incidence of infection (Coffin, 2014). It is incumbent on caregivers to strictly adhere to recommended guidelines for hand hygiene.

The skin, its secretions, and normal flora are natural defences that protect against invading pathogens, thus care practices that preserve this protection should be used. Warm water may be used to remove blood and meconium from the neonate's face, head, and body. A mild nonmedicated soap (in single-use container) can be used with careful water rinsing. Vernix caseosa should not be scrubbed vigorously for removal, since this further disrupts the skin barrier properties. No single method of cord care has been shown to be more effective in the promotion of drying, separating, and preventing colonization. Nurses must follow agency protocols for cord care and can advocate for revision of protocols based on research (see also Chapter 26, Umbilical Cord Care, p. 713).

NURSING ALERT

Artificial and natural long fingernails worn by nurses have been associated with serious neonatal infection and morbidity from *Pseudomonas aeruginosa* and *Klebsiella* organisms in the NICU. Therefore, nurses caring for neonates should keep their fingernails short.

MATERNAL INFECTIONS

The range of pathological conditions produced by infectious agents is large, and the difference between the maternal and fetal effects caused by any one agent is also great. Some maternal infections, especially during early gestation, can result in fetal loss or malformations because the fetus's ability to handle infectious organisms is limited and the fetal immunological system is unable to prevent the dissemination of infectious organisms to the various tissues.

Not all prenatal infections produce teratogenic effects. Furthermore, the clinical picture of disorders caused by transplacental transfer of infectious agents is not always well defined. Some viral agents can cause remarkably similar manifestations, and it is common to test for all of them when a prenatal infection is suspected. This is the so-called TORCH complex, an acronym for:

- *T*—Toxoplasmosis
- *O*—Other (e.g., HBV, parvovirus, HIV, West Nile)
- *R*—Rubella
- *C*—CMV infection
- *H*—Herpes simplex

To determine the causative agent in a symptomatic infant, tests are performed to rule out each of these infections. The *O* category may involve testing for several viral infections (e.g., HBV, varicella zoster, measles, mumps, HIV, syphilis, and human parvovirus). Bacterial infections are not included in the TORCH workup because they are usually identified by clinical manifestations and readily available laboratory tests. Gonococcal conjunctivitis (ophthalmia neonatorum) and chlamydial conjunctivitis have been reduced significantly by prophylactic measures at birth (see Critical Thinking Case Study and Chapter 26, p. 676). The major maternal infections, their possible effects, and specific nursing considerations are outlined in Table 29-5.

Human Immunodeficiency Virus (Type 1)

It is estimated that globally, in 2013, 3.2 million children under the age of 15 years were infected with HIV; the vast majority of those children lived in developing countries (UNICEF, 2015). In Canada, the number of infants perinatally exposed to the virus has increased over recent years, yet the number of infants with confirmed HIV infection has decreased since the advent of antiretroviral therapy (ART), from approximately 25% in the 1990s to less than 1% in 2013. A critical factor in perinatal transmission is the maternal viral load; a high viral load (especially more than 100,000 copies/mL) creates a greater chance (up to 40%) for perinatal transmission of the virus. See Table 29-5 for further discussion of HIV infection in the newborn.

CRITICAL THINKING CASE STUDY

Neonate With Chlamydia

An 8-day-old male infant is brought to the pediatric urgent care centre on a Sunday morning by Maggie, an 18-year-old single mother, with a eye drainage for 2 days. Maggie is breastfeeding and states that she was diagnosed and partially treated for a couple of sexually transmitted infections in late gestation; she does not remember the name but says one started with a "C." The medications made her stomach sick, so she quit taking them after 2 days. The practitioner examines the infant, who has a purulent yellowish discharge from both eyes but otherwise appears healthy; she suspects chlamydial conjunctivitis and orders cultures of the eye drainage. The retrieved medical record from the infant's birth indicates that eye prophylaxis with erythromycin ophthalmic ointment was administered.

1. Evidence—Is there sufficient evidence to draw conclusions about the cause of the infant's eye drainage?
2. Assumptions—What assumptions can be made about the following factors:
   a. Treatment for neonatal chlamydia infection.
   b. Sequelae of inadequate chlamydia treatment in newborn.
   c. The mother's health status and possible treatment (she is not allergic to penicillin).
3. What implications and priorities for nursing care can be drawn at this time?
4. Does the evidence objectively support your conclusion?

Although it is rare for an infant to be born with symptoms of HIV infection, all infants born to seropositive mothers should be presumed to be HIV positive until proven otherwise. Management begins by implementing routine practices. Measures should also be taken to protect the infant from further exposure to maternal blood and body fluids.

Varicella Zoster

The varicella zoster virus responsible for chickenpox and shingles is a member of the herpes family. About 90% of women in their child-bearing years are immune; therefore, the risk of infection in pregnancy is low (Yudin, Koren, Farine, et al., 2012). When maternal infection occurs in the last few days of pregnancy or the first postpartum days, up to 30% of infants will develop clinical varicella (PHAC, 2012a). See Table 29-5 for more information.

Chlamydia Infection

Chlamydia trachomatis is an intracellular bacterium that causes neonatal conjunctivitis and pneumonia. Chlamydia infection is the most common reportable disease in Canada; the rate of this STI is increasing (PHAC, 2014). Pregnant women should be screened for chlamydia early in pregnancy; women who are positive or high risk for reinfection should be rescreened during the third trimester (PHAC, 2013a). Conjunctivitis, with minimal watery discharge, develops 5 days to 2 weeks after birth. The organism may spread to the lungs from nasal secretions if left untreated, causing chlamydia pneumonia in about 33% of infected infants, with symptoms of a repetitive staccato cough, tachypnea, rales, hyperinflation, and bilateral diffuse infiltrates on radiography examination.

Text continued on p. 800

TABLE 29-5 INFECTIONS ACQUIRED FROM THE MOTHER BEFORE, DURING, OR AFTER BIRTH*

FETAL OR NEWBORN EFFECT	TRANSMISSION	NURSING CONSIDERATIONS†
Human Immunodeficiency Virus (HIV)		
No significant difference between infected and uninfected infants at birth in some instances Embryopathy reported by some observers: • Depressed nasal bridge • Mild upward or downward obliquity of eyes • Long palpebral fissures with blue sclerae • Patulous lips • Ocular hypertelorism • Prominent upper vermilion border See also Chapter 48	Transplacental; during vaginal birth; potentially in breast milk	Administer combination antiretroviral prophylaxis to HIV-positive mother; prophylaxis to prevent perinatal transmission may begin after first trimester. Choice of regimens is determined by examining a number of factors, including mother's current treatment. Detailed recommendations can be obtained from the SOGC (Boucoiran, Tulloch, Caddy, et al., 2014) and Panel on Treatment of HIV-Infected Pregnant Women and Prevention of Perinatal Transmission (2015). During labour *ZDV is recommended for all HIV-infected pregnant women, regardless of the antepartum treatment regimen.* HIV-exposed newborns (regardless of maternal antiretroviral dosing) should receive a 6-week course of ZDV starting as soon after birth as possible but preferably within 6 to 12 hours; nevirapine may also be given in 3 doses during the first week of life. ZDV dosing varies according to infant gestational age and route of administration. Vaginal birth is acceptable on basis of viral load and needs to be discussed with the health care provider. HIV-positive mothers in developed countries should avoid breastfeeding. Exclusive breastfeeding for 12 months is acceptable for infants with HIV-positive mothers in developing countries where infant food supply is not readily available or has a greater chance of contamination (poor sanitary conditions, water supply) (World Health Organization, 2010). For chemoprophylaxis against *Pneumocystis carinii* pneumonia in HIV-exposed infants, the drug of choice is trimethoprim-sulphamethoxazole (Bactrim, Septra). Documented routine HIV education and routine testing with consent are recommended for all pregnant women in Canada.
Chickenpox (Varicella-Zoster Virus [VZV])		
Intrauterine exposure—congenital varicella syndrome: limb dysplasia, microcephaly, cortical atrophy, chorioretinitis, cataracts, cutaneous scars, other anomalies, auditory nerve palsy, motor and cognitive delays Severe symptoms (rash, fever) and higher mortality in infant whose mother develops varicella 5 days before to 2 days after birth	First trimester (fetal varicella syndrome); perinatal period (infection)	Use varicella zoster immune globulin or IVIG to treat infants born to mothers with onset of disease within 5 days before or 2 days after birth. Healthy term infants exposed postnatally to varicella (especially if mother's rash does not appear until after 48 hours after birth) should not receive varicella zoster immune globulin. Infection should be mild (American Academy of Pediatrics [AAP] Committee on Infectious Diseases, 2012). Institute isolation precautions in newborn born to mother with varicella up to 21–28 days (latter time if newborn received varicella zoster immune globulin or IVIG after birth (if hospitalized).†
Chlamydia Infection (*Chlamydia trachomatis*)		
Conjunctivitis, pneumonia	Last trimester or postpartum period	Standard ophthalmic prophylaxis for gonococcal ophthalmia neonatorum (topical erythromycin or tetracycline) is *not effective* in treatment or prevention of chlamydial ophthalmia. Treat with oral erythromycin or oral sulfonamide for 14 days; a second course of erythromycin may be required, and follow-up of exposed infant is recommended (see Critical Thinking Case Study p. 795).
Coxsackievirus (Group B Enterovirus-Nonpolio, Parechovirus)		
Poor feeding, vomiting, diarrhea, fever; cardiac enlargement, arrhythmias, heart failure; lethargy, seizures, meningoencephalitis, pneumonitis Mimics bacterial sepsis	Peripartum	Treatment is supportive. Provide IVIG in neonatal infections.

TABLE 29-5 INFECTIONS ACQUIRED FROM THE MOTHER BEFORE, DURING, OR AFTER BIRTH—cont'd

FETAL OR NEWBORN EFFECT	TRANSMISSION	NURSING CONSIDERATIONS†
Cytomegalovirus (CMV)		
Variable manifestation from asymptomatic to severe Microcephaly, cerebral calcifications, chorioretinitis Jaundice, hepatosplenomegaly Petechial or purpuric rash (Fig. 29-4) Neurological sequelae—seizure disorders, sensorineural hearing loss, cognitive impairment	Throughout pregnancy	Infection acquired at birth, shortly thereafter, or via human milk is not associated with clinical illness in term infants. Exposed preterm infants may have systemic infection, including interstitial pneumonia. Affected individuals excrete virus. Virus is detected in urine or tissue by electron microscopy. Pregnant women should avoid close contact with known cases. To treat infection administer antivirals such as IV ganciclovir or oral valganciclovir for 6 weeks to newborn (AAP Committee on Infectious Diseases, 2012).
Parvovirus B19 (Erythema Infectiosum)		
Fetal hydrops and death from anemia and heart failure with early exposure Anemia with later exposure No teratogenic effects established Ordinarily low risk of adverse effect to fetus	Transplacental	First-trimester infection has most serious effects. Perform serial ultrasonography for fetus who is exposed to assess hydrops. Conduct cordocentesis to determine need for intrauterine transfusion if hydrops is present (Crane & SOGC Maternal Fetal Medicine and Infectious Diseases Committees, 2014). Aggressive cardiovascular and respiratory support is required in newborns with hydrops. Pregnant health care workers should not care for patients who might be highly contagious (e.g., child with sickle cell anemia, aplastic crisis). Routine exclusion of pregnant women from workplace where disease is occurring is not recommended.

Continued

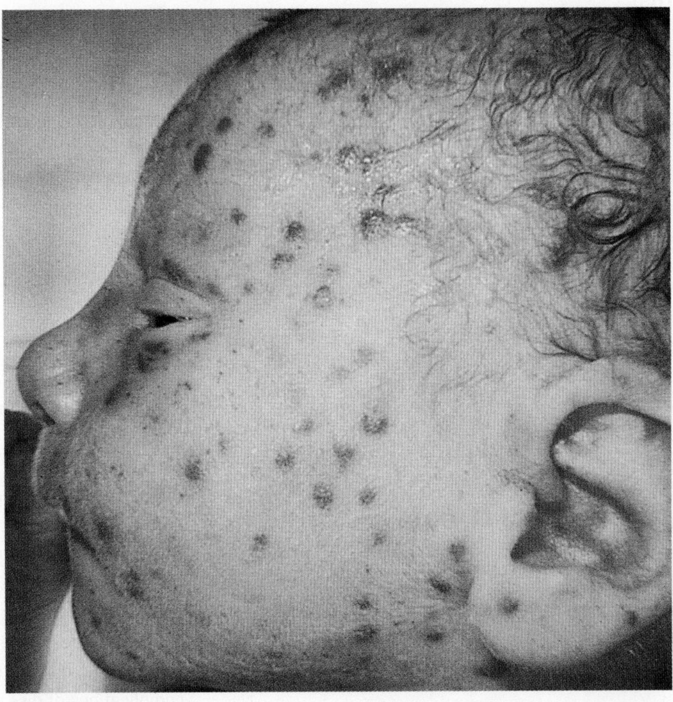

FIGURE 29-4 Neonatal cytomegalovirus infection. Shown here is a typical rash in a severely affected infant.

TABLE 29-5 INFECTIONS ACQUIRED FROM THE MOTHER BEFORE, DURING, OR AFTER BIRTH—cont'd

FETAL OR NEWBORN EFFECT	TRANSMISSION	NURSING CONSIDERATIONS†
Gonorrhea (*Neisseria gonorrhoeae*)		
Ophthalmitis Neonatal gonococcal arthritis, septicemia, meningitis	Last trimester or postpartum period	Routine prophylactic medication to eyes at time of birth is questioned as useful (Moore, MacDonald, Canadian Paediatric Society [CPS], 2015). Infant with confirmed ophthalmia, scalp abscess, or disseminated infection should be hospitalized and cultures obtained to determine antimicrobial treatment. Consider testing infant for *Chlamydia*, HIV, and syphilis. Irrigate infant's eyes with saline until discharge is eliminated. Obtain smears for culture. To treat ophthalmia and nondisseminated infection (in infants born to mothers who were not treated, even if healthy at birth), administer IV or IM ceftriaxone once. Disseminated disease requires cefotaxime treatment for 1 week (Moore et al., 2015).
Hepatitis B Virus (HBV)		
May be asymptomatic at birth; more than 90% of infants infected perinatally develop chronic HBV infection Clinical hepatitis, jaundice, changes in liver function; possible fulminant hepatitis (mortality rate of 75%) Increased risk for preterm birth	Transplacental; contaminated maternal fluids or secretions during birth	Administer HBIG to all infants of HBsAG-positive mothers within 12 hours of birth; in addition, administer HepB vaccine at separate site. Infant will receive two more doses at 1 month and 6 months of age. Prevention—Screen all pregnant women. Infants born to HBsAG-positive mothers and weighing <2000 g (4 lbs 7 oz) should receive 3-dose vaccine series *in addition* to birth dose (See Immunizations, Chapter 35.)
Listeriosis (Listeria monocytogenes)		
Maternal infection associated with spontaneous abortion, preterm birth, and fetal death Preterm birth, sepsis, and pneumonia seen in early-onset disease; late-onset disease usually manifests as meningitis	Transplacental by ascending infection or exposure at birth	Hand hygiene is essential to prevent health care–associated infection. Treat infected newborn with antibiotics—ampicillin and an aminoglycoside such as gentamicin (14- to 21-day treatment is recommended for meningitis).
Rubella, Congenital (Rubella Virus)		
Congenital rubella syndrome Eyes—retinopathy, cataracts (unilateral or bilateral), microphthalmia, retinitis, glaucoma CNS signs—microcephaly, seizures, severe cognitive impairment Congenital heart defects—patent ductus arteriosus Auditory defects—sensorineural hearing loss Dermal erythropoiesis—blueberry muffin lesions IUGR—hyperbilirubinemia, meningitis, thrombocytopenia, hepatomegaly	First trimester; early second trimester	Pregnant women should avoid contact with all affected persons, including infants with rubella syndrome. Emphasize vaccination of all unimmunized prepubertal children, susceptible adolescents, and women of child-bearing age (nonpregnant). Caution women against becoming pregnant for at least 28 days after vaccination.
Syphilis, Congenital *(Treponema pallidum)*		
Stillbirth, prematurity, hydrops fetalis May be asymptomatic at birth and in first few weeks of life or may have multisystem manifestations: hepatosplenomegaly, lymphadenopathy, hemolytic anemia, pneumonia, and thrombocytopenia Copper-coloured maculopapular cutaneous lesions (Fig. 29-5) (usually after first few weeks of life), mucous membrane patches, hair loss, nail exfoliation, snuffles (syphilitic rhinitis), profound anemia, poor feeding, pseudoparalysis of one or more limbs, dysmorphic teeth (older child)	Transplacental; can be anytime during pregnancy or at birth	This is the most severe form of syphilis. Prevention—routine screening of all pregnant women. Treatment consists of IV aqueous penicillin or IM procaine penicillin for 10 days. Diagnostic evaluation depends on maternal serology testing, maternal therapy and response, maternal and infant serology titres, results of nontreponemal infant tests, and infant physical examination (including ophthalmological examinations and long-bone radiographs) and laboratory examination results (e.g., LFTs, CBC, platelets, CSF protein and cell count). Monitor closely for development of complications of disease during first year of life.

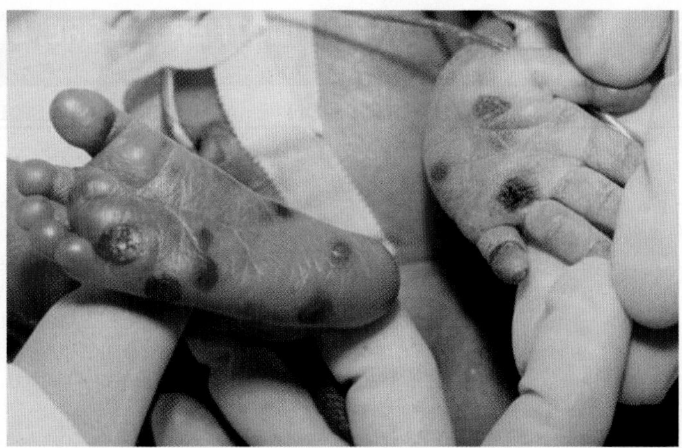

FIGURE 29-5 Neonatal syphilis lesions on hands and feet.

TABLE 29-5 INFECTIONS ACQUIRED FROM THE MOTHER BEFORE, DURING, OR AFTER BIRTH—cont'd

FETAL OR NEWBORN EFFECT	TRANSMISSION	NURSING CONSIDERATIONS†
Toxoplasmosis, Congenital *(Toxoplasma gondii)*		
May be asymptomatic at birth (70–90% of cases) or have maculopapular rash, lymphadenopathy, hepatosplenomegaly, jaundice, thrombocytopenia In some cases severely infected fetus may die in utero or shortly after birth (10–15%) Preterm birth is common. Later developments— hydrocephaly, cerebral calcifications, chorioretinitis (classic triad), microcephaly, seizures, cognitive impairment, deafness, encephalitis, myocarditis, hepatosplenomegaly, anemia, jaundice, diarrhea, vomiting, purpura	Throughout pregnancy, although first-trimester exposure is more serious Predominant host for organism is cats May be transmitted through cat feces or poorly cooked or raw infected meats	Caution pregnant women to avoid contact with cat feces (e.g., emptying cat litter boxes). Administer sulphadiazine (with folinic acid) and pyrimethamine (Daraprim). Spiramycin and cotrimaxazole may be administered to infected pregnant female to reduce transmission to fetus but have no effect if fetal infection has occurred (Valentini, Buonsenso, Barone, et al., 2015).
Herpes Simplex Virus (HSV)		
Neonatal herpes manifests in one of three ways: (1) with SEM involvement; (2) as localized CNS disease; or (3) as disseminated disease involving multiple organs. In skin and eye disease rash appears as vesicles or pustules on erythematous base. Clusters of lesions are common. Lesions ulcerate and crust over rapidly (Fig. 29-6). Ophthalmological clinical findings include chorioretinitis and microphthalmia; neurological involvement such as microcephaly and encephalomalacia may also develop. Disseminated infections may involve virtually every organ system, but liver, adrenal glands, and lungs are most commonly affected. In HSV meningitis, infants develop multiple lesions of cortical hemorrhagic necrosis. It can occur alone or with SEM lesions. Presenting symptoms, which may occur in second to fourth weeks of life, include lethargy, poor feeding, irritability, and local or generalized seizures. Neonatal HSV has high mortality rate.	Transplacental, although 86 to 90% of cases transmitted at birth (Allen & CPS, 2014) Direct transmission from infected personnel or family	Absence of skin lesions in neonate exposed to maternal herpes virus does not indicate absence of disease. Contact precautions (in addition to routine precautions) should be instituted. It is recommended that swabs of mouth, nasopharynx, conjunctivae, rectum, and any skin vesicles be obtained from exposed neonate; in addition, urine, stool, blood, and CSF specimens should be obtained for culture. Therapy with IV acyclovir is initiated if culture results are positive or if there is strong suspicion of herpes virus infection. Treatment is for 14 days if limited to SEM and 21 days if CNS involvement; ophthalmic treatment (e.g., 1% trifluridine or 3% vidarabine) is required for ocular involvement in addition to acyclovir. Therapy with oral acyclovir for 6 months is recommended for neonates with HSV CNS disease (AAP Committee on Infectious Diseases, 2012; Allen & CPS, 2014). Breastfeeding is encouraged if there are no lesions on the mother's breast.

Continued

TABLE 29-5 INFECTIONS ACQUIRED FROM THE MOTHER BEFORE, DURING, OR AFTER BIRTH—cont'd

FETAL OR NEWBORN EFFECT	TRANSMISSION	NURSING CONSIDERATIONS†
Group B Streptococcus		
Early-onset infection (first 7 days of life)—pneumonia, respiratory distress, shock, apnea, and meningitis Late-onset infection (7 days to 3 months of age)—bacteremia or meningitis; may occur later in LBW infants Significant mortality rate	Acquired perinatally; intrapartum antibiotics decrease early-onset but not late-onset disease Risk factors include preterm birth, maternal GBS (untreated), previous birth of GBS-infected newborn, maternal chorioamnionitis	Offer screening to all pregnant women at 35–37 weeks of pregnancy (see Chapter 11). Administer ampicillin plus an aminoglycoside such as gentamicin in infant with presumptive GBS infection; in infant with positive GBS, administer penicillin G. Observe routine precautions, including strict hand hygiene for handling of all infants.

CBC, complete blood count; *CNS,* central nervous system; *CSF,* cerebrospinal fluid; *GBS,* group B streptococcus; *HBIg,* hepatitis B immunoglobulin; *HBsAG,* hepatitis B surface antigen; *IUGR,* intrauterine growth restriction; *IM,* intramuscular; *IV,* intravenous; *IVIG,* intravenous immunoglobulin; *LBW,* low-birth-weight; *LFT,* liver function test; *SEM,* skin, eye, and mouth; *SOGC,* Society of Obstetricians and Gynaecologists of Canada; *ZDV,* zidovudine.

*This table is not an exhaustive representation of all perinatally transmitted infections. For further information regarding specific diseases or treatment not listed here, refer to American Academy of Pediatrics (AAP) Committee on Infectious Diseases, Pickering, L. (Ed.). (2012). *2012 Red book: Report of the Committee on Infectious Diseases* (29th ed.). Elk Grove Village, IL, 2012, AAP.

†Isolation precautions depend on institutional policy.

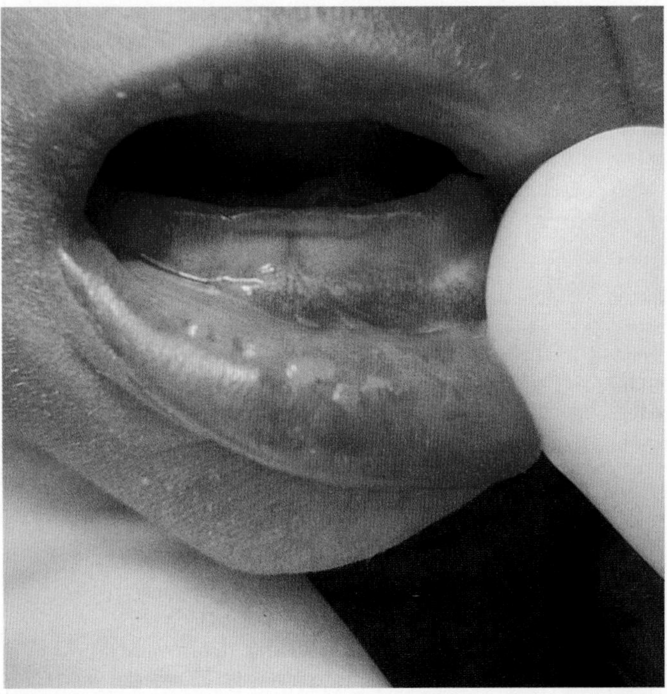

FIGURE 29-6 Herpes simplex virus oral lesions. (Courtesy David A. Clarke.)

Erythromycin administration in infants younger than 6 weeks has been associated with an increased risk of infantile hypertrophic pyloric stenosis; therefore, parents should be educated regarding the symptoms of the condition (feeding intolerance, projectile vomiting, and abdominal distension) (PHAC, 2013a).

Cytomegalovirus Infection

CMV infection during pregnancy may result in miscarriage, stillbirth, or congenital illness. It is the most common cause of congenital viral infections in North America (Yinon, Farine, & Yudin, 2010). Most (90 to 95%) of the infected infants are asymptomatic at birth. Antenatally infected infants who are asymptomatic at birth are at risk for late sequelae. Hearing loss may not be apparent until after the first year of life (Goderis, De Leenheer, Smets, et al., 2014). Chorioretinitis, microcephaly, cognitive impairment, and neuromuscular deficits may occur by 2 years of age. Some children are at risk for a defect in tooth enamel, resulting in severe caries. See Table 29-5 for further discussion of CMV.

Parvovirus B19

Parvovirus B19 is well known in older children as fifth disease or "slapped cheek illness" because of the characteristic facial appearance of the affected child. The estimated risk of transplacental transmission is approximately 30%, and fetal death may occur in about 9% of those affected.

Gonorrhea

In Canada, the overall rate of reported cases of gonorrhea increased by 40.8% between 2002 and 2011 (PHAC, 2014). The incidence of gonococcal infection in pregnant women ranges from 2.5 to 7.3%. After rupture of membranes, ascending *Neisseria gonorrhoeae* infection can be transmitted to the fetus, although this is infrequent (Moore et al., 2015). The organism may invade mucosal surfaces such as the conjunctiva (ophthalmia neonatorum), rectal mucosa, and pharynx.

Eye prophylaxis with erythromycin ointment, administered within the first 2 hours after birth, has been the accepted practice in Canada, although recent recommendations question the utility of this practice and no longer support routine use of ocular prophylaxis, although the legislation in many provinces has not yet changed (Moore et al., 2015).

Hepatitis B Virus

The transmission rate of HBV to the newborn ranges from 70 to 90% when the mother is seropositive for both hepatitis B surface antigen (HBsAg) and hepatitis B e antigen (HBeAg) (AAP Committee on Infectious Diseases, 2012). Infants are most commonly infected during birth or in the first few days of life. The rate of transmission is highest when the mother contracts the virus immediately before birth. These mothers will be positive for HBsAg. Transmission may occur through breast milk, but antigens also develop in formula-fed infants at the same or higher rate. Diagnosis is made by viral culture of amniotic fluid and by the presence of HBsAg and IgM in the cord blood or newborn's serum.

HBV vaccine should protect the child for up to 9 years. Breastfeeding may be initiated prior to receiving the vaccine. Vaccination for infants not exposed to maternal HBV is provided in some provinces before discharge from the hospital.

Rubella Infection

Since rubella vaccination was begun in 1983, cases of congenital rubella have been reduced from 5300 (1971–1982) to 30 cases (1998–2004) to approximately 5 cases/year between 2006 and 2010 (PHAC, 2012b); however, it is still seen very occasionally in the newborn. Vaccination failures, failure to complete recommended vaccination schedule, and the immigration of unimmunized persons result in periodic outbreaks of rubella, also known as German, or 3-day measles.

The risk for congenital anomalies varies with the fetus's gestational age at the time maternal infection occurs. Abnormalities are most severe if the mother contracts the virus during the first trimester, with occurrence of congenital defects as high as 85% in the first 12 weeks of gestation; infection during this time may also result in miscarriage or stillbirth (PHAC, 2012b).

More than two-thirds of infected infants have no symptoms apparent at birth, but sequelae may develop years later, such as diabetes mellitus. Hearing loss, a common finding, appears to be progressive after birth. The rubella virus has been cultured in infants for up to 18 months after their birth. These infants are a serious source of infection to susceptible individuals, particularly women in the child-bearing years. Extended pediatric isolation is mandatory until the noncontagious stage of rubella has been reached (i.e., the infant should be isolated until pharyngeal mucus and the urine are free of virus). See Table 29-5 for further discussion.

Syphilis

Congenital and neonatal syphilis have re-emerged in recent years as significant health problems (PHAC, 2013a; Robinson & CPS Infectious Diseases and Immunization Committee, 2009). It is estimated that for every 100 women diagnosed with primary or secondary disease, 2 to 5 infants will contract congenital syphilis. If syphilis (primary or secondary) during pregnancy is left untreated, 70 to 100% of neonates born to these women will have symptomatic congenital syphilis. In approximately 40% of pregnancies, fetal demise may occur (Robinson et al., 2009).

The most severely affected infants are born to untreated mothers. The newborn may be hydropic (edematous) and anemic, with enlarged liver and spleen. Hepatosplenomegaly likely results from extramedullary hematopoietic activity stimulated by the severe anemia. In some infants, signs of congenital syphilis do not appear until late in the neonatal period. See Table 29-5 for further discussion.

! NURSING ALERT

The infant with congenital syphilis may be entirely asymptomatic until after discharge from the birth hospital. It is therefore imperative that caregivers use routine precautions with all newborns.

Group B Streptococcus

Historically, GBS was one of the more common causes of neonatal sepsis and meningitis in North America; however, antepartum maternal screening and administration of penicillin have significantly decreased the incidence of GBS. As a result of screening and intrapartum prophylaxis, the incidence of neonatal GBS in North America decreased from 1 to 3 per 1000 in the early 1990s to 0.35 to 0.5 per 1000 since adoption and implementation of screening (Centers for Disease Control and Prevention [CDC], 2010; Money, Dobson, & Society of Obstetricians and Gynaecologists of Canada [SOGC], Infectious Disease Committee, 2013).

In the newborn with presumed or confirmed GBS infection, ampillicin or penicillin and an aminoglycoside are the therapy of choice (AAP Committee on Infectious Diseases, 2012; Barrington & CPS Fetus and Newborn Committee, 2007/2011). The newborn born to a mother who did not receive complete intrapartum prophylaxis is observed for 24 to 48 hours before discharge (Barrington et al., 2007/2011; CDC, 2010).

Other Infections

Tuberculosis

The incidence of tuberculosis (TB), which is caused by *Mycobacterium tuberculosis*, is increasing in Canada; most cases observed in children under 14 are in international adoptees, foreign-born immigrants, and Indigenous children (Health Canada, 2012). Congenitally acquired TB, although rare, can cause otitis media, pneumonia, hepatosplenomegaly, enlarged lymph glands, or disseminated disease. After birth, exposed infants contract TB through droplets expelled by infected individuals, which results in pneumonia and necrosis of lung tissue. Untreated neonatal tuberculosis is almost always fatal.

Candidiasis

Candida infections, formerly known as moniliasis, may occur in the newborn. *C. albicans*, the organism usually responsible, may cause disease in any organ system. It is a yeastlike fungus (producing yeast cells and spores) that can be acquired from a maternal vaginal infection during birth, by person-to-person transmission or from contaminated hands, bottles, nipples, or other articles. It usually is a benign disorder in the newborn, often confined to the oral and diaper regions. Diaper dermatitis caused by *Candida* organisms manifests as a moist, erythematous eruption with small white or yellow pebbly pustules. Small areas of skin erosion may also be seen.

Candidal diaper dermatitis appears on the perianal area, inguinal folds, and lower portion of the abdomen. The affected area is intensely erythematous, with a sharply demarcated, scalloped edge, often with numerous satellite lesions that extend beyond the larger lesion. The source of the infection can be through the gastrointestinal tract or caretakers' hands.

Topical application of 1 mL nystatin (Mycostatin) over the surfaces of the oral cavity four times a day (every 6 hours) is usually sufficient to prevent spread of the disease and limit its course. Several other medications may be used, including amphotericin B, clotrimazole (Canesten), fluconazole (Diflucan), or miconazole (Monistat, Micatin) given intravenously, orally, or topically. To prevent relapse, therapy should be continued for at least 2 days after the lesions disappear (Lawrence & Lawrence, 2015). Gentian violet solution may be used in addition to one of the antifungal medications in chronic cases of oral thrush; however, the former does not treat gastrointestinal candida and may irritate the oral mucosa.

! NURSING ALERT

Nystatin is best absorbed when given either 1 hour before feeding or after a feeding. Using a needleless syringe or medicine dropper, apply the medication to each side of the infant's mouth for optimal absorption.

Oral candidiasis (thrush or mycotic stomatitis) is characterized by white plaques on the oral mucosa, gums, and tongue. The white patches are easily differentiated from milk curds; the patches cannot be removed and tend to bleed when touched. In most cases the infant does not seem to be in discomfort from the infection; however, some will pull away from the breast or bottle and cry. The child may be seen by the primary care provider because of poor oral intake.

Infants who are sick, debilitated, or receiving prolonged antibiotic therapy are more susceptible to thrush. Those with conditions such as cleft lip or palate, neoplasms, and hyperparathyroidism seem to be more vulnerable to mycotic infection.

The objectives of management are to eradicate the causative organism and to control exposure to *C. albicans*. Interventions include maintenance of scrupulous cleanliness (by nursing staff, parents, and others) to prevent reinfection. Good hand hygiene is always essential. Clean surfaces should be provided for changing neonates' diapers. Diaper dermatitis is treated with a topical fungicide at each diaper change. For the infant who is prone to diaper dermatitis, a barrier cream such as zinc oxide may be helpful, provided there is not already an infection. Diaper dermatitis that is not caused by *Candida* organisms may require treatment with a mild topical hydrocortisone ointment. When possible, exposing the perineal area to dry air is recommended because yeast prefers a moist environment. Other measures to control thrush include rinsing the infant's mouth with plain water after each feeding before applying the medication, and boiling reusable nipples and bottles for at least 20 minutes after a thorough washing (spores are heat resistant). Pacifiers should be boiled for at least 20 minutes once daily, and the nipples of breastfeeding mothers should be treated with an antifungal to prevent reinfection.

Infants who are breastfed may acquire thrush from the mother. If the mother is colonized, treatment for mother and infant is recommended. There is no need to stop breastfeeding even if the mother is receiving systemic antifungal medications (Lawrence & Lawrence, 2015).

NURSING CARE

One of the major goals in the care of infants suspected of having an infectious disease is identification of the causative organism. Routine precautions are implemented according to institution policy. Pregnant health care personnel are cautioned to avoid contact with infants with suspected CMV and rubella infections. HSV is easily transmitted from one infant to another; therefore, the risk of cross-contamination is reduced or eliminated by wearing gloves for patient contact. The *2012 Red Book: Report of the Committee on Infectious Diseases* (AAP Committee on Infectious Diseases, 2012) provides guidelines for the type and duration of precautions for most bacterial and viral exposures. Careful hand hygiene is the most important nursing intervention in reducing the spread of any infection.

Specimens need to be obtained for laboratory examinations, and the infant and parents need to be prepared for diagnostic procedures. When possible, long-term disabilities are prevented by early evaluation and implementation of therapy. The family is taught any special handling techniques needed for the care of their infant and signs of complications or possible sequelae. If sequelae are inevitable, the family needs assistance in determining how they can best cope with the problems, such as assistance with home care, referral to appropriate agencies, or placement in an institution for care. The major goal of nursing care is prevention of these disorders, through provision of adequate prenatal care for the expectant mother and precautions regarding exposure to teratogenic infections.

DRUG-EXPOSED INFANTS

Maternal habits hazardous to the fetus and neonate include problematic drug use, smoking, and alcohol use. (Unless otherwise noted, the information presented throughout this section refers to drug-exposed neonates in general, regardless of the drug to which they have been exposed.) Occasional withdrawal reactions have been reported in neonates of mothers who use to excess such drugs as barbiturates, alcohol, amphetamines, or antidepressants. Serious reactions are seen in neonates whose mothers use psychoactive drugs or are treated with methadone. In the context of substance use, the term *addiction* is often associated with behaviours in which an individual seeks drug(s) to experience a "high," achieve euphoria, escape from reality, or satisfy a personal need. Newborns that have been exposed to drugs in utero are not addicted in a behavioural sense, yet they may experience mild to strong physiological signs of addiction as a result of the exposure. Thus, to say that an infant born to a mother who uses substances is addicted is incorrect; *drug-exposed newborn*, which implies intrauterine drug exposure, is a better term. In North America, the number of newborns that have experienced intrauterine drug exposure has increased dramatically over the last 10 years. In 2011, over 1000 babies were born in Canada with neonatal abstinence syndrome (NAS). According to the Canadian Institute for Health Information (CIHI) this represents an 18% increase from the preceding year (Paperny, 2012).

The adverse effects of fetal exposure to drugs are varied and include transient changes, such as differences in fetal breathing movements to irreversible effects, such as IUGR, structural malformations, and fetal death. Determining the specific effects of individual drugs on an individual fetus is made difficult by polydrug use, which is common; errors or omissions in reporting drug use; and variations in the strength, purity, and types of additives found in street drugs. Maternal conditions such as poverty, malnutrition, and comorbid conditions such as STIs further compound the difficulty in identifying the presence and consequences of intrauterine drug exposure. Most infants who are exposed to drugs in utero may demonstrate no immediate untoward effects and appear normal at birth. The use of prescription painkillers, also called opioids, has also increased for pregnant women, including drugs such as hydrocodone (Vicodin), oxycodone (Oxycontin), codeine, and morphine (Patrick, Dudley, Martin, et al., 2015).

Neonatal abstinence syndrome (NAS) is the term used to describe the set of behaviours exhibited by infants exposed to narcotics in utero (Dow, Ordean, Murphy-Oikonen, et al., 2012; Logan, Brown & Hayes, 2013). Infants exposed only to heroin may begin to exhibit signs of drug withdrawal within 12 to 24 hours. If mothers have been taking methadone, the signs appear somewhat later (i.e., anywhere from 1 or 2 days to 2 to 3 weeks or more after birth). The clinical manifestations may fall into any one or all of the following categories: CNS, gastrointestinal, respiratory, and autonomic nervous system signs. The manifestations become most pronounced between 48 and 72 hours of age and may last from 6 days to 8 weeks, depending on the severity of the withdrawal (Box 29-1). Although these infants suck avidly on fists and display an exaggerated rooting reflex, they are poor feeders with uncoordinated and ineffectual sucking and swallowing reflexes.

Some effects may not be identified until after the newborn period, possibly not until school entry, and include cognitive and motor delay as well as behavioural problems. Critical determinants of the drug's effect on the fetus depend on the specific drug, the dosage, the route of administration, the genotype of the mother or fetus, and the timing of the drug exposure. Table 29-6 summarizes the effects of commonly used substances on the fetus and neonate.

BOX 29-1 SIGNS OF WITHDRAWAL IN NEONATES

NEUROLOGICAL
- Irritability
- Seizures
- Hyperactivity
- High-pitched cry
- Tremors
- Exaggerated Moro reflex
- Hypertonicity of muscles

AUTONOMIC
- Diaphoresis
- Fever
- Mottled skin
- Nasal stuffiness

GASTROINTESTINAL
- Poor feeding
- Diarrhea
- Dehydration
- Vomiting
- Frantic, uncoordinated sucking
- Gastric residuals

MISCELLANEOUS
- Disrupted sleep patterns
- Diaphoresis
- Tachypnea (>60 breaths/min)
- Excoriations (knees, face)
- Temperature instability

TABLE 29-6 SUMMARY OF NEONATAL EFFECTS OF COMMONLY USED SUBSTANCES

SUBSTANCE	NEONATAL EFFECTS
Alcohol	*Fetal alcohol syndrome (FAS)*—Craniofacial features varied and may include short eyelid opening, flat midface, flat upper lip groove, thin upper lip; also may involve microcephaly, hyperactivity, developmental delays, attention deficits *Alcohol-related neurodevelopmental disorder (ARND)*—Varying forms of FAS; cognitive, behavioural, and psychosocial problems without typical physical features
Cocaine	Preterm birth, small for gestational age, microcephaly, poor feeding, irregular sleep patterns, diarrhea, visual attention problems, hyperactivity, difficult to console, hypersensitivity to noise and external stimuli, irritability, developmental delays, congenital anomalies such as prune belly syndrome (i.e., distended, flabby, wrinkled abdomen caused by lack of abdominal muscles)
Heroin	Low birth weight, small for gestational age, irritability, tachypnea, feeding difficulties, vomiting, high-pitched cry, seizures
Methamphetamine	Small for gestational age, preterm birth, poor weight gain, lethargy, abnormal sleep patterns, agitation, poor feeding and state disorganization, behavioural problems later in childhood (higher-order functioning), cleft lip and palate, cardiac defects (Pitts, 2010)
Tobacco	Preterm birth, low birth weight, increased risk for sudden infant death syndrome, increased risk for bronchitis, pneumonia, developmental delays, orofacial clefts
Marijuana	Possible neonatal tremors, low birth weight, growth restriction, attention problems (Marroun, Hudziak, Tiemeier, et al., 2011)
Selective serotonin reuptake inhibitors	Hypertonia, tremulousness, wakefulness, high-pitched crying, feeding problems

BOX 29-2 CHARACTERISTICS FOR DIAGNOSING FETAL ALCOHOL SYNDROME (FAS)

Facial Dysmorphia

Despite consideration of racial norms (i.e., those appropriate for a person's race), the person exhibits all three of the following characteristic facial features:

1. Smooth philtrum (University of Washington Lip-Philtrum Guide* rank 4 or 5*)
2. Thin vermillion border (University of Washington Lip-Philtrum Guide rank 4 or 5)
3. Small palpebral fissures (≤10th percentile)

Growth Problems

Confirmed, documented prenatal or postnatal height, weight, or both below the tenth percentile, adjusted for age, sex, gestational age, and race or ethnicity

Central Nervous System Abnormalities

Structural

Head circumference ≤10th percentile, adjusted for age and sex

Clinically meaningful brain abnormalities observable through imaging (e.g., reduction in size or change in shape of the corpus callosum, cerebellum, or basal ganglia)

Neurological

Neurological problems (e.g., motor problems or seizures) not resulting from sepsis, metabolic disturbances, postnatal insult, or other soft neurological signs outside normal limits

Functional

Test performance substantially below that expected for a person's age, schooling, or circumstances as evidenced by either:

1. Global cognitive or intellectual deficits representing multiple domains of deficit (or substantial developmental delay in younger children) with performance below the third percentile (i.e., 2 standard deviations below the mean for standardized testing); or
2. Functional deficits below the sixteenth percentile (i.e., 1 standard deviation below the mean for standardized testing) in at least three of the following domains:
   - Cognitive or developmental deficits or discrepancies
   - Executive functioning deficits
   - Motor functioning delays
   - Problems with attention or hyperactivity
   - Social skills
   - Other (e.g., sensory problems, pragmatic language problems or memory deficits)

Maternal Alcohol Exposure

Confirmed prenatal exposure to alcohol

Unknown prenatal exposure to alcohol

Criteria for FAS Diagnosis

Diagnosis requires all three of the following findings:

1. Documentation of all three facial abnormalities listed above
2. Documentation of growth problems
3. Documentation of central nervous system abnormality

*Astley, S. J. (2004). *Diagnostic guide for fetal alcohol spectrum disorders: The four-digit diagnostic code* (3rd ed.). Seattle: University of Washington.

Adapted from Bertrand, J., Floyd, R. L., Weber, M. K., et al. (2004). *Fetal alcohol syndrome: Guidelines for referral and diagnosis.* Atlanta, GA: Centers for Disease Control and Prevention; Chudley, A. E., Conry, J., Cook, J. L., et al. (2005). Fetal alcohol spectrum disorder: Canadian guidelines for diagnosis. *Canadian Medical Association Journal 172*(5 Suppl), S1–S21.

Alcohol Exposure

Alcohol is a teratogen that produces CNS effects that may not be evident for years. Maternal ethanol use during pregnancy can lead to a range of effects known as *fetal alcohol spectrum disorder* (FASD) and may include fetal alcohol syndrome (FAS), alcohol-related birth defects (ARBD), or neurobehavioural and cognitive problems that may be identified only by maternal history and behavioural characteristics. The incidence of FASD in Canada has been estimated at approximately 9 per 1000 live births (Schröter & CPS, First Nations, Inuit, and Métis Health Committee, 2010). FAS is diagnosed in the presence of confirmed alcohol exposure in utero along with the following features: (1) midfacial dysmorphisms, (2) growth restriction, and (3) evidence of neurological impairment in 3 or more cognitive domains (Schröter et al., 2010) (see Box 29-2). Any single or multiple combinations of these may be present in addition to confirmed or unknown history of maternal alcohol consumption. The diagnosis of FAS is complicated by the absence of a specific single biological marker and by manifestations that are often seen in other childhood conditions.

FAS is recognized as the leading cause of cognitive impairment (Interagency Coordinating Committee on Fetal Alcohol Spectrum Disorders [ICCFASD], 2011; Schröter et al., 2010). Alcohol (ethanol and ethyl alcohol) interferes with normal fetal development; the effects on the fetal brain are permanent, and even moderate use of alcohol during pregnancy may cause long-term postnatal difficulties, including impaired maternal–infant attachment.

Fetal abnormalities are not related to the amount of the mother's alcohol intake per se, but to the amount consumed in excess of the liver's ability to detoxify it. The liver's capacity to detoxify alcohol is limited and inflexible; when the liver receives more alcohol than it is able to handle, the excess is continually recirculated until the organ is able to reduce it to carbon dioxide and water. This circulating alcohol has a special affinity for brain tissue. Poor nutritional state, smoking, polydrug intake, and infrequent or lack of prenatal care may compound the problem of alcohol use during pregnancy (May, Blankenship, Marais, et al., 2013).

Cognitive and motor delays, hearing disorders, and a variety of defects in craniofacial development are prominent features (Fig. 29-7) and Box 29-2. Magnetic resonance imaging (MRI) studies of children with diagnosed FAS have revealed structural anomalies, including alteration in the midbrain anomalies, particularly microencephaly (Guerri, Bazinet, & Riley, 2009; Norman, Crocker, Mattson, et al., 2009). Some affected infants

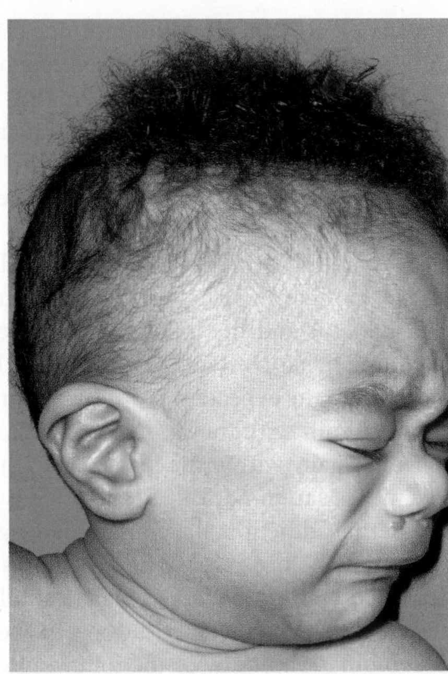

FIGURE 29-7 Child with fetal alcohol syndrome. (© Alamy Stock Photo.)

display physical features of the syndrome; behaviours, however, are nonspecific in newborns and may thus pass undetected. These features include difficulty in establishing respiration, irritability, lethargy, poor suck reflex, and abdominal distension.

Infants who do not display the signs of FAS but are born to mothers who are also heavy alcohol drinkers have significantly more tremors, hypertonia, restlessness, excessive mouthing movements, crying, and inconsolability than infants of substance-using mothers who do not consume alcohol during pregnancy.

Nursing care of affected infants involves the same assessment and observations employed for any high-risk infant. Poor feeding is characteristic of infants with FAS and can be a significant problem throughout infancy. The provision of individualized developmental care is paramount and includes reduction of noxious environmental stimuli and helping the infant achieve self-regulation. Special emphasis is placed on monitoring weight gain, assessing feeding behaviours, and devising strategies to promote nutritional intake. Early diagnosis and intervention are reported to be beneficial for reducing the effects of alcohol exposure on the growing child. Therefore, nurses should be actively involved in identifying and referring children exposed to alcohol prenatally.

When possible, long-term disabilities may be mitigated through early evaluation and implementation of therapy. The family should be taught any special techniques needed for the care of their infant and the signs of complications or possible sequelae. When sequelae are inevitable, the family will need assistance in determining how to best cope, such as with home care assistance or referral to appropriate agencies.

Tobacco Exposure

Cigarette smoking during pregnancy is associated with birth weight deficits of up to 250 g for a full-term newborns (Reed, Aranda, & Hales, 2014). Passive exposure to second-hand smoke by a pregnant woman may also result in the birth of an LBW infant. The many effects of tobacco on a fetus are listed in Table 29-6. Nicotine and cotinine, the two pharmacologically active substances in tobacco, are found in higher concentrations in infants whose mothers smoke. These substances can be secreted in breast milk for up to 2 hours after the mother has smoked. Further, cigarette smoke contains more than 2000 compounds, including carbon monoxide, dioxin, cyanide, and cadmium. Deficits in growth, intellectual and emotional development, poor auditory responsiveness, increased fine motor tremors, hypertonicity, and decreased verbal comprehension have been observed in infants exposed to smoke. There is also a positive dose–response relationship between the amount of tobacco exposure and newborn neurobehaviour; increased tobacco exposure in utero is related to more negative neurobehavioural effects. In addition, it is now recognized that neonates may experience withdrawal symptoms following exposure to nicotine.

Pregnant women must be informed about the harmful effects of smoking on their unborn baby's health. Smoking cessation during pregnancy greatly decreases the chance of fetal complications; thus, women should be counselled regarding smoking cessation programs (see Chapter 5). All individuals should refrain from smoking near an infant; the house and car should be smoke-free zones for infants and children. Some Canadian provinces have laws that make it illegal for anyone to smoke in a vehicle with children under the age of 18.

Marijuana Exposure

Marijuana has replaced cocaine as the more common illicit drug used by women ages 18 to 44 years (nonpregnant and pregnant) in North America (Kuczkowski, 2007). Marijuana crosses the placenta; however, specific effects on the fetus have been difficult to determine. Some studies have reported an association between the chronic use of marijuana and a decrease in fetal growth and infant birth weight and length (Kuczkowski, 2007); however, this finding is confounded by cigarette smoking (Bandstra & Accornero, 2014). More subtle effects of major exposure such as an increase in attention problems have also been identified (Marroun et al., 2011) (see Table 29-6). Compounding the issue of the effects of marijuana, especially among women ages 18 to 30 years (Kuczkowski, 2007), is multidrug use, which combines the harmful effects of marijuana, tobacco, alcohol, opiates, and cocaine. Long-term follow-up studies on exposed infants are needed.

Cocaine Exposure

Cocaine is a CNS stimulant and peripheral sympathomimetic. Legally it is classified as a narcotic, but it is not an opioid. The effects on the fetus are secondary to maternal effects of increased blood pressure, decreased uterine blood flow, and increased vascular resistance. Consequently, the fetus suffers decreased blood flow and oxygenation as a result of placental and fetal vasoconstriction. The difficulties encountered by cocaine-exposed infants are compounded by maternal polydrug use (see Table 29-6). A woman's lack of prenatal care, poor nutrition, and use of tobacco, alcohol, and other drugs during pregnancy add to the effects of cocaine exposure in the infant. Infants may appear normal or may show neurological problems at birth that may continue during the newborn period. In much of the research literature these findings were transient, and evidence demonstrating permanent sequelae has varied. Either of two types of behaviour may emerge as a result of the effects of cocaine on fetal development: neurobehavioural depression or excitability. The behaviours of a depressed infant include lethargy, poor suck, hypotonia, a weak cry, and difficulty in arousing. The behaviours of an excitable neonate may include a high-pitched cry, hypertonicity, rigidity, irritability, an inability to be consoled, and an intolerance to changes in routine (Chiriboga, Kuhn, & Wasserman, 2007).

Sequelae of prenatal cocaine exposure include preterm birth, a smaller head circumference, decreased birth length, and decreased weight. Head growth may be one of the best predictors of long-term development. Early studies of cocaine exposure identified an increased incidence of gastroschisis, genitourinary anomalies, and periventricular and intraventricular hemorrhage; however, meta-analyses have not confirmed these complications (Bandstra et al., 2010). Heavy cocaine exposure has been shown to result in elevated heart rate and irregular respirations after birth.

Long-term sequelae for newborns exposed to cocaine include lower language, motor, and cognitive scores and an increased risk for learning disabilities. In a study that controlled for other prenatal drug exposures, a dose-related effect of cocaine was found on expressive, receptive, and total language scores at 3, 5, and 12 years of age (Bandstra et al., 2011). Other investigators have found that the subtle effects of cocaine on school performance are moderated by the child's environment (Ackerman, Riggins, & Black, 2010). Studies using the Brazelton Neonatal Assessment Scale have again shown inconsistent results, with subtle abnormalities in neurobehavioural clusters varying in timing of severity and according to levels of exposure (Bandstra et al., 2010).

Nursing care of cocaine-exposed infants is the same as that for other drug-exposed infants. Because they have increased flexor tone, these infants respond to swaddling in a semiflexed position (Pitts, 2010). Positioning, infant massage, and limited tactile stimulation have been shown to be effective interventions. Significant amounts of cocaine have been found in breast milk; mothers should be cautioned about this hazard to their infants.

Referral to early intervention programs, including child health care, parental drug treatment, individualized developmental care, and parenting education, is essential in promoting optimum outcome for these children. Because they often live in impoverished environments, they are at high risk for cognitive delays, lack of child health care, and inadequate nutrition and benefit from early intervention programs.

Heroin Exposure

Heroin crosses the placenta and often results in IUGR. Heroin may have a direct growth-inhibiting effect on the fetus, but the exact mechanisms of growth inhibition are not clear. Among mothers who use heroin there is an increased rate of stillbirths but not of congenital anomalies in their infants. Additional neonatal effects include meconium aspiration, increased neonatal death, microcephaly, neurobehavioural problems, and a 74-fold increase in SIDS (Minozzi, Amato, Vecchi, et al., 2008) (see Table 29-6).

Many of the medical complications attributed to heroin ingestion result from preterm birth. Other risks include physical dependence in the fetus and the increased risk of exposure to infections, including hepatitis B and C virus and HIV.

Drug withdrawal in the expectant mother is accompanied by fetal withdrawal. Heroin withdrawal occurs in infants born to addicted mothers, usually within the first 24 to 72 hours of life (Finnegan, Pacini, & Maremmani, 2010). The signs depend on the length of maternal addiction, the amount of drug taken, and the time of injection before birth. The symptoms of infants whose mothers used heroin or methadone are similar. Initially the infant may be depressed. The withdrawal syndrome may manifest as a combination of any of the following signs:

- The infant may be jittery and hyperactive.
- Cry is shrill and persistent.
- The infant may yawn or sneeze frequently.
- Tendon reflexes are increased; Moro reflex is decreased.
- The infant may exhibit poor feeding and sucking, tachypnea, vomiting, diarrhea, hypothermia, or hyperthermia and sweating.
- The infant may exhibit an abnormal sleep cycle, with absence of quiet sleep and disturbance of active sleep.

The risk of SIDS is higher for infants with significant withdrawal problems than for infants in the general population. If withdrawal is not treated, vomiting, diarrhea, dehydration, apnea, and seizures may develop. Death may follow.

Therapy needs to be individualized. Dehydration and electrolyte imbalance should be prevented or treated. Usually the following drugs are given, singly or in combination: phenobarbital, diluted tincture of opium (paregoric), methadone, and morphine.

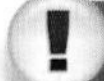
NURSING ALERT

The use of naloxone (Narcan) is contraindicated in infants born to women addicted to narcotics or on methadone therapy because it may exacerbate neonatal abstinence syndrome (NAS) and cause seizures.

Methadone Exposure

Methadone, a synthetic opiate, has been the therapy of choice for heroin addiction since 1965. Methadone crosses the placenta. An increasing number of infants have been born to methadone-maintained mothers, women who seem to have better prenatal care and a somewhat better lifestyle than those taking heroin.

Some question exists concerning the benefits of methadone therapy during pregnancy because of its effect on the fetus. Methadone withdrawal in infants resembles heroin withdrawal but tends to be more severe and prolonged. Signs of methadone withdrawal include tremors, irritability, state lability, hypertonicity, hypersensitivity, vomiting, mottling, and nasal stuffiness. These infants exhibit a disturbed sleep pattern similar to that seen in heroin withdrawal. They have a higher birth weight than those infants in heroin withdrawal and usually are appropriate for gestational age. No increased incidence of congenital anomalies is seen. Women in a methadone treatment program are encouraged to breastfeed, regardless of the methadone treatment dosage (Finnegan et al., 2010). Follow-up counselling and monitoring of the mother and infant are recommended. The few available follow-up studies of these infants indicate a high incidence of hyperactivity, learning and behaviour disorders, and poor social adjustment.

Late-onset withdrawal occurs at age 2 to 4 weeks and may continue for weeks or months. A higher incidence of SIDS also has been reported in these infants (Burns, Conroy, & Mattick, 2010). This risk factor is important for perinatal nurses to recognize as they coordinate the follow-up care for the infant and provide education for the mother or other caregivers. Community health nurses must know about the potential for withdrawal symptoms.

Therapy for methadone withdrawal is similar to that for heroin withdrawal. Buprenorphine, an opioid analgesic, has gained acceptance in the treatment of opioid addiction. Preliminary studies indicate that this medication may have advantages over methadone in relation to neonatal outcomes. Offspring of mothers treated with buprenorphine had higher birth weights than those exposed to methadone, had shorter hospital stays, and had lower NAS scores (Kakko, Heilig, & Sarman, 2008).

Methamphetamine Exposure

The fetal and neonatal effects of maternal use of methamphetamines in pregnancy are not well known, and findings are often confounded by polydrug use and the effects of the newborn or child's environment. LBW, preterm birth, and anomalies such as cleft lip and palate and cardiac defects have been reported in infants exposed to methamphetamines in utero (Pitts, 2010).

Study reports vary in the time of clinical manifestations of withdrawal from this drug; one study did not identify any signs of withdrawal in the first 3 days after birth, but long-term data were not collected (Smith, Yonekura, Wallace, et al., 2003). A study of infants exposed to methamphetamine in utero showed that such infants had significantly smaller head circumferences and birth weights than those not exposed; in addition, the exposed infants exhibited withdrawal signs of agitation, vomiting, and tachypnea, which were not observed in the unexposed infants (Chomchai, Na Manorom, Watanarungasan, et al., 2004). After birth infants may experience abnormal sleep patterns, agitation, poor feeding, and state disorganization (Pitts, 2010).

The long-term effects of methamphetamine exposure on children remain unclear; however, some studies have shown problems with mathematics and language skills. It is postulated that, similar to cocaine, methamphetamine exposure may affect areas of the brain responsible for higher-order functioning, with effects more likely to be manifest when the child reaches school age (Lester & Lagasse, 2010).

Selective Serotonin Reuptake Inhibitors

Studies estimate that between 15 and 25% of pregnant women experience major depression (Cantor Sackett, Weller, & Weller, 2009). For many of these women selective serotonin reuptake inhibitors (SSRIs) provide an important therapeutic benefit; however, these drugs may result in adverse effects in their newborns. Signs of withdrawal are present in up to one-third of infants exposed to SSRIs in utero (Burgos & Burke, 2009). Findings include hypertonia, tremulousness, wakefulness, high-pitched crying, and feeding problems. An increased risk of persistent pulmonary hypertension has been reported in neonates exposed to SSRIs early in pregnancy (Cantor Sackett et al., 2009); however, this finding has not been reported consistently (Wilson, Zelig, Harvey, et al., 2011). Some SSRIs are transferred into breast milk. Breastfeeding infants whose mothers are taking SSRIs should be monitored for sleep disturbances, irritability, and poor feeding.

NURSING CARE

One of the key factors in the treatment of drug-exposed newborns is early identification of substance use in the pregnant woman so treatment can be initiated and side effects minimized. This is especially problematic from a social and legal standpoint because the pregnant woman is often aware of the consequences of admitting to substance use and therefore may be less likely to readily admit to the problem for fear of social and legal repercussions. If the mother has had good prenatal care, the practitioner is aware of the problem and may have instituted therapy before birth. However, a number of mothers deliver their infants without the benefit of adequate care, and the condition is unknown to health care personnel at the time of birth.

The degree of withdrawal is closely related to the amount of drug the mother has habitually taken, the length of time she has been taking the drug, and her drug level at the time of birth. The most severe symptoms are observed in the infants of mothers who have taken large amounts of drugs over a long period. In addition, the nearer to the time of birth that the mother takes the drug, the longer it takes the child to develop withdrawal, and the more severe the manifestations. The infant may not exhibit withdrawal symptoms until 7 to 10 days after birth, by which time most newborns have been discharged from the birth centre, and caregivers are less likely to recognize signs of irritability and poor feeding as withdrawal, thus predisposing the newborn to abuse or neglect and growth failure (failure to thrive). The infant may be at further risk for subsequent abuse or neglect because of home conditions that preclude adequate newborn care and follow-up. Newborn urine, hair, or meconium sampling may be required to identify drug exposure and to implement appropriate early interventional therapies aimed at minimizing the consequences of intrauterine drug exposure (Koren, Hutson, & Gareri, 2008), although parental consent is required to obtain these specimens. Methamphetamine may be found in fetal hair samples when intrauterine exposure occurs. Meconium sampling for fetal drug exposure is reported to provide more screening accuracy than urine, since drug metabolites accumulate in meconium. Urine toxicology screening has less accuracy because it reflects only recent substance intake by the mother. Meconium testing for drug metabolites has the advantage of being easy to collect, noninvasive, and more accurate.

Caring for the infant born to a substance-using mother presents a challenge to the health care team. The mother needs to be included in planning for the newborn's care and encouraged to plan for her own care. It is important that newborns be able to room in with the mother, if possible, as this facilitates skin-to-skin contact, breastfeeding, and maternal–infant bonding. The Fir Square Combined Care Unit in Vancouver, the first of its kind in Canada, provides care to substance-exposed infants and their mothers in a single unit. The mother–infant dyad is preserved whenever possible and both mother and baby receive specialized services as they stabilize and withdraw from substances and transition to home. Fir Square models the interprofessional approach needed to care for these women and infants and includes physicians, nurses, social workers, addictions counsellors, nutritionists, and life skills/parenting counsellors (BC Women's Hospital, 2013). Community resource personnel (e.g., regulatory agencies such as child protective services) may also be involved in providing care. Education and social support to prevent use of drugs is the ideal approach. However, given the scope of the drug use problem, total prevention may be unrealistic.

The Neonatal Abstinence Scoring System or Finnegan tool (Fig. 29-8) was developed to monitor infants in an objective manner and evaluate their response to clinical and pharmacological interventions (Finnegan, 1985). This system is also designed to help nurses and other health care workers evaluate the severity of infants' withdrawal symptoms.

The Neonatal Intensive Care Unit Network Neurobehavioral Scale (NNNS) is a comprehensive neurological and behavioural assessment tool that may be used to identify newborns at risk as a result of intrauterine drug exposure. The tool measures stress or abstinence, state, neurological status, and muscle tone in the context of the newborn's medical condition at the time of examination. The NNNS may be used for medically stable newborns who are at least 30 weeks of gestation and up to 48 weeks of corrected or conceptional age.

Pharmacological treatment is based on the severity of withdrawal symptoms, as determined by an assessment tool (such as the Finnegan tool). An evaluation of NAS is recommended within 2 hours of the newborn's admission to the nursery and every 4 hours thereafter. A score of 8 or higher requires more frequent assessment. With three consecutive scores of 8 or more, pharmacological interventions are recommended (Weiner & Finnegan, 2011). A number of medications have been used to decrease the adverse effects of withdrawal in the newborn, including phenobarbital, morphine, diluted tincture of opium (paregoric), methadone, and buprenorphine in conjunction with naloxone (Wiegand, Stringer, Stuebe, et al., 2015). A recent study demonstrated a decrease in neonatal abstinence when narcotic tapering began during pregnancy (Dooley, Dooley, Antone, et al., 2015). When NAS is identified in an infant, nursing care is directed toward treating the presenting signs, decreasing stimuli that may precipitate hyperactivity and irritability (e.g., dimming the lights, decreasing noise levels), providing adequate nutrition and hydration, and promoting positive maternal–infant relationships (promoting skin-to-skin contact). Appropriate individualized developmental care should be implemented to facilitate the infant's self-consoling and self-regulating behaviours. Irritable and hyperactive infants have been found to respond to physical comforting, movement, and close contact. Wrapping infants snugly and rocking and holding them tightly limit their ability to self-stimulate. The infant's arms should remain flexed with hands in close proximity of the mouth for sucking, as sucking on fingers or hands is a form of self-control and comfort. Organizing of nursing activities and clustering of care reduce the amount of handling and help decrease exogenous stimulation. Infants should be offered a pacifier for characteristic frantic, excessive sucking, and it is important not to overfeed infants who demand frequent sucking as part of the withdrawal process. Specific suggestions for providing care to infants experiencing withdrawal are listed in the Patient Teaching box.

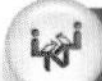

PATIENT TEACHING

Care of the Infant Experiencing Withdrawal

- Place the infant in a side-lying position with the spine and legs flexed when awake.
- Position the infant's hands in midline with the arms at the side.
- Carry the infant in a flexed position.
- When interacting with the infant, introduce one stimulus at a time. Interaction should occur when the infant is in a quiet, alert state. Watch for time-out or distress signals (e.g., gaze aversion, yawning, sneezing, hiccups, arching, mottled colour).
- When the infant is distressed, swaddle in a flexed position and rock in a slow, rhythmic fashion.
- Put the infant in a sitting position with chin tucked down for feeding.

Loose stools, poor intake, and regurgitation after feeding predispose these infants to malnutrition, dehydration, and electrolyte imbalance. Careful monitoring of intake and output as well as of electrolytes, additional caloric supplementation, and daily weighing may be necessary. These infants have a tendency to burn up additional energy as a result of continuous activity and have increased oxygen consumption at the cellular level. It takes considerable time and patience to ensure that they receive a sufficient caloric and fluid intake.

In addition, these infants must be protected from skin abrasions on the knees, toes, and cheeks caused by rubbing on bed linens while in a prone position. The incidence of SIDS is high, and parents should be reminded that the supine position for sleep is preferred. Monitoring and recording the infant's tolerance for routine activities (feeding, diaper changes) and preventing complications are important nursing functions.

Breastfeeding is encouraged for mothers who are not using illicit substances, are negative for HIV infection, and are following a methadone program. Breastfeeding promotes

NEONATAL ABSTINENCE SCORING SYSTEM

System	Signs and Symptoms	Score	AM	PM	Comments
Central Nervous System Disturbances	Excessive high-pitched (or other) cry	2			Daily weight:
	Continuous high-pitched (or other) cry	3			
	Sleeps <1 hour after feeding	3			
	Sleeps <2 hours after feeding	2			
	Sleeps <3 hours after feeding	1			
	Hyperactive Moro reflex	2			
	Markedly hyperactive Moro reflex	3			
	Mild tremors disturbed	1			
	Moderate-severe tremors disturbed	2			
	Mild tremors undisturbed	3			
	Moderate-severe tremors undisturbed	4			
	Increased muscle tone	2			
	Excoriation (specific area)	1			
	Myoclonic jerks	3			
	Generalized convulsions	5			
Metabolic/Vasomotor/Respiratory Disturbances	Sweating	1			
	Fever 37.2–38.2°C	1			
	Fever > 38.4°C	2			
	Frequent yawning (>3 or 4 times/interval)	1			
	Mottling	1			
	Nasal stuffiness	1			
	Sneezing (>3 or 4 times/interval)	1			
	Nasal flaring	2			
	Respiratory rate >60/min	1			
	Respiratory rate >60/min with retractions	2			
Gastrointestinal Disturbances	Excessive sucking	1			
	Poor feeding	2			
	Regurgitation	2			
	Projectile vomiting	3			
	Loose stools	2			
	Watery stools	3			
	Total Score				
	Initials of Scorer				

FIGURE 29-8 Neonatal Abstinence Scoring (NAS) system, developed by L. Finnegan. (From Nelson, N. [1990]. *Current therapy in neonatal-perinatal medicine* [2nd ed.]. St. Louis: Mosby.)

maternal–infant bonding, and the small amount of methadone passed through breast milk has not proved to be harmful to the neonate (Hale & Rowe, 2014; Lefevere & Allegaert, 2015). Lawrence and Lawrence (2015) suggest, however, that maternal methadone regimens of 100 mg/day or more may cause increased withdrawal in infants, requiring paregoric for 6 to 8 weeks. Because many new medications are being manufactured, the reader is advised to consult with updated references regarding the safety of medications for breastfeeding. It is important to teach pregnant women the effects of the recreational drugs discussed earlier. (See Nursing Care Plan on Evolve.)

HEMOLYTIC DISORDERS

Hyperbilirubinemia in the first 24 hours of life is most often the result of hemolytic disease of the newborn (HDN) (erythroblastosis fetalis), an abnormally rapid rate of red blood cell (RBC) destruction. Anemia caused by this destruction stimulates the production of RBCs, which in turn provides increasing numbers of cells for hemolysis. Major causes of increased erythrocyte destruction are isoimmunization (primarily Rh) and ABO incompatibility.

Blood Incompatibility

The membranes of human blood cells contain a variety of antigens, also known as agglutinogens, substances capable of producing an immune response if recognized by the body as foreign. The reciprocal relationship between antigens on RBCs and antibodies in the plasma causes agglutination (clumping). In other words, antibodies in the plasma of one blood group (except the AB group, which contains no antibodies) produce agglutination when mixed with antigens of a different blood group. In the ABO blood group system, the antibodies occur naturally. In the Rh system the person must be exposed to the Rh antigen before significant antibody formation takes place and causes a sensitivity response known as isoimmunization.

Rh Incompatibility (Isoimmunization)

The Rh blood group consists of several antigens (with D being the most prevalent). For simplicity, only the terms *Rh positive* (presence of antigen) and *Rh negative* (absence of antigen) are used in this discussion. The presence or absence of the naturally occurring Rh factor determines the blood type.

Ordinarily, no problems are anticipated when the Rh blood types are the same in both the mother and the fetus or when the mother is Rh positive and the infant is Rh negative. Difficulty may arise when the mother is Rh negative and the infant is Rh positive. Although the maternal and fetal circulations are separate, there is evidence of a bidirectional trafficking of fetal RBCs and cell-free DNA to the maternal circulation (Moise, 2012). However, more commonly, fetal RBCs enter into the maternal circulation at the time of birth. The mother's natural defence mechanism responds to these alien cells by producing anti-Rh antibodies.

Under normal circumstances, this process of isoimmunization has no effect during the first pregnancy with an Rh-positive fetus because the initial sensitization to Rh antigens rarely occurs before the onset of labour. However, with the increased risk of fetal blood being transferred to the maternal circulation during placental separation, maternal antibody production is stimulated. During a subsequent pregnancy with an Rh-positive fetus, these previously formed maternal antibodies to Rh-positive blood cells may enter the fetal circulation, where they attack and destroy fetal erythrocytes (Fig. 29-9). Multiple gestations, placental abruption, placenta previa, manual removal of the placenta, and Caesarean birth increase the incidence of transplacental hemorrhage and subsequent isoimmunization (Diehl-Jones & Fraser Askin, 2010).

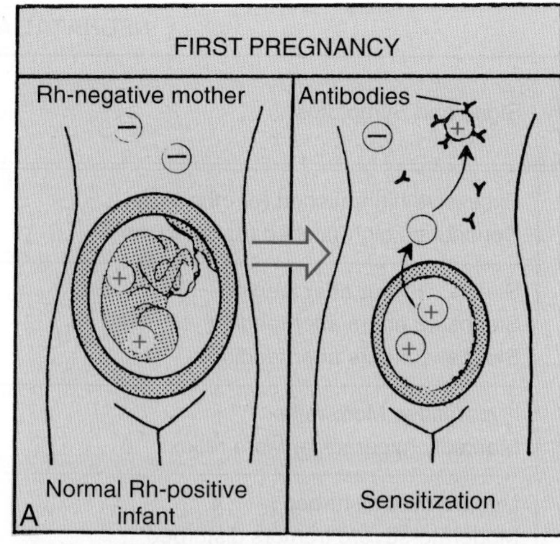

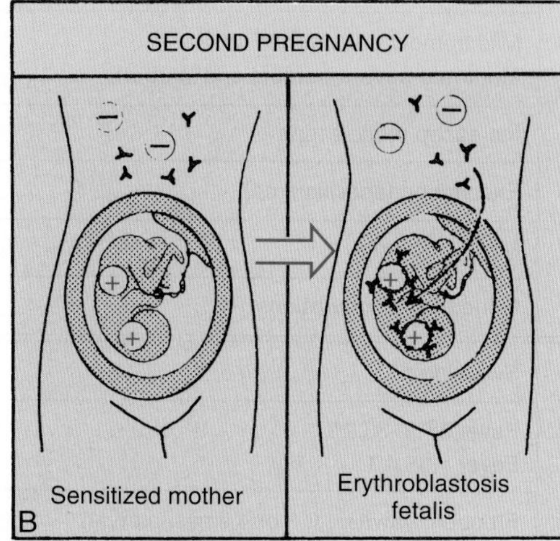

FIGURE 29-9 Development of maternal sensitization to Rh antigens. **A:** Fetal Rh-positive erythrocytes enter the maternal system. Maternal anti-Rh antibodies are formed. **B:** Anti-Rh antibodies cross the placenta and attack fetal erythrocytes.

Because the condition begins in utero, the fetus attempts to compensate for the progressive hemolysis and anemia by accelerating the rate of erythropoiesis. As a result, immature RBCs (erythroblasts) appear in the fetal circulation, thus the term **erythroblastosis fetalis**.

There is wide variability in the development of maternal sensitization to Rh-positive antigens. Sensitization may occur during the first pregnancy if the woman had previously received an Rh-positive blood transfusion. No sensitization may occur in situations in which a strong placental barrier prevents transfer of fetal blood into the maternal circulation. In approximately 10 to 15% of sensitized mothers there is no hemolytic reaction in the newborn. In addition, some Rh-negative women, even though exposed to Rh-positive fetal blood, are immunologically unable to produce antibodies to the foreign antigen.

In the most severe form of erythroblastosis fetalis, **hydrops fetalis**, the progressive hemolysis causes fetal hypoxia; cardiac failure; generalized edema (anasarca); and fluid effusions into the pericardial, pleural, and peritoneal spaces (hydrops). The fetus may be delivered stillborn or in severe respiratory distress. Maternal Rh immune globulin (RhIG) administration, early intrauterine detection of fetal anemia by ultrasonography (serial Doppler assessment of the peak velocity in the fetal middle cerebral artery), and subsequent treatment by fetal blood transfusions or high-dose IVIG have dramatically improved the outcome of affected fetuses (Moise & Argoti, 2012).

ABO Incompatibility

Hemolytic disease can also occur when the major blood group antigens of the fetus are different from those of the mother.

The major blood groups are A, B, AB, and O. The presence or absence of antibodies and antigens determines whether agglutination will occur. Antibodies in the plasma of one blood group (except the AB group, which contains no antibodies) produce agglutination (clumping) when mixed with antigens of a different blood group. Naturally occurring antibodies in the recipient's blood cause agglutination of a donor's RBCs. The agglutinated donor cells become trapped in peripheral blood vessels, where they hemolyze, releasing large amounts of bilirubin into the circulation.

The most common blood group incompatibility in the neonate is between a mother with O blood group and an infant with A or B blood group (see Table 29-7 for possible ABO incompatibilities). Naturally occurring anti-A or anti-B antibodies already present in the maternal circulation cross the placenta and attack the fetal RBCs, causing hemolysis. Usually the hemolytic reaction is less severe than in Rh incompatibility; however, rare cases of hydrops have been reported (Black & Maheshwari, 2009). Unlike the Rh reaction, ABO incompatibility may occur in the first pregnancy. The risk of significant hemolysis in subsequent pregnancies is higher when the first pregnancy is complicated by ABO incompatibility.

Jaundice may appear shortly after birth (during the first 24 hours) in newborns affected by HDN, and serum levels of unconjugated bilirubin rise rapidly. Anemia results from the hemolysis of large numbers of erythrocytes, and hyperbilirubinemia and jaundice result from the inability of the liver to conjugate and excrete the excess bilirubin. Most newborns with HDN are not jaundiced at birth. However, hepatosplenomegaly and varying degrees of hydrops may be evident. If the infant is severely affected, signs of anemia (notably marked pallor) and hypovolemic shock are apparent. Hypoglycemia may occur as a result of pancreatic cell hyperplasia.

TABLE 29-7 POTENTIAL MATERNAL–FETAL ABO INCOMPATIBILITIES

MATERNAL BLOOD GROUP	INCOMPATIBLE FETAL BLOOD GROUP
O	A or B
B	A or AB
A	B or AB

Early identification and diagnosis of Rh(D) sensitization are important in the management and prevention of fetal complications. A maternal antibody titre (indirect Coombs' test) should be drawn at the first prenatal visit. Genetic testing allows early identification of paternal zygosity at the Rh(D) gene locus, thus allowing earlier detection of the potential for isoimmunization and avoiding further maternal or fetal testing (Moise, 2008). Amniocentesis can be used to test the fetal blood type of a woman whose antibody screen result is positive; the use of polymerase chain reaction (PCR) may determine the fetal blood type and presence of maternal antibodies. The fetal hemoglobin and hematocrit can also be measured. Chorionic villus sampling has drawbacks that preclude its use, including possible spontaneous abortion of the fetus and fetomaternal hemorrhage, which would essentially make the situation worse. With either method, if the fetus is found to be Rh negative, no further treatment is required. The detection of cell-free fetal DNA in the maternal plasma of Rh(D)-negative women to detect an Rh(D)-positive fetus has been used successfully in Europe. Such testing usually negates the necessity of amniocentesis for fetal blood type (Moise & Argoti, 2012).

Ultrasonography is considered an important adjunct in the detection of isoimmunization; alterations in the placenta, umbilical cord, and amniotic fluid volume and the presence of fetal hydrops can be detected with high-resolution ultrasonography and allow early treatment before the development of erythroblastosis. Doppler ultrasonography of fetal middle cerebral artery peak velocity has been used to detect and measure fetal hemoglobin and, subsequently, fetal anemia (Moise & Argoti, 2012). Erythroblastosis fetalis caused by Rh incompatibility can also be monitored by evaluating rising anti-Rh antibody titres in the maternal circulation or testing the optical density of amniotic fluid (delta OD450 test) because bilirubin discolours the fluid.

The disease in the newborn is suspected on the basis of the timing and appearance of jaundice and can be confirmed postnatally by detecting antibodies attached to the circulating erythrocytes of affected infants (direct Coombs' test or direct antiglobulin test). The Coombs' test may be performed on umbilical cord blood samples from infants born to Rh-negative mothers if there is a history of incompatibility or further investigation is warranted.

The primary aim of therapeutic management of isoimmunization is prevention. Postnatal therapy is usually phototherapy for mild cases of hemolysis and exchange transfusion for more severe forms. Although phototherapy may control bilirubin levels in mild cases, the hemolytic process may continue, causing severe anemia between 7 and 21 days of life.

Other Hemolytic Disorders

It is not within the scope of this text to discuss the many potential causes of hemolytic jaundice in childhood. However, in some populations there is a high incidence of glucose-6-phosphate dehydrogenase deficiency (G6PD), which may cause an exaggerated jaundice in a newborn within 24 to 48 hours of birth. G6PD red cells hemolyze at a greater rate than healthy red cells, thus overwhelming the immature neonatal liver's ability to conjugate the indirect bilirubin. Some of the triggers that potentiate hemolysis include vitamin K, acetaminophen, aspirin, sepsis, and exposure to certain chemicals. Hereditary spherocytosis may also cause serious neonatal hemolytic anemia as a result of high quantities of fetal hemoglobin; jaundice may develop rapidly and require phototherapy (Segel & Casey, 2016). Treatment is the same as for any newborn with rapidly rising serum bilirubin levels.

Other metabolic and inherited conditions that increase hemolysis and may cause jaundice in the infant include galactosemia, Crigler-Najjar disease, and hypothyroidism.

Prevention

The administration of RhIG, a human gamma globulin concentrate of anti-D, to all unsensitized Rh-negative mothers after birth or abortion of an Rh-positive infant or fetus prevents the development of maternal sensitization to the Rh factor. The injected anti-Rh antibodies are thought to destroy (by subsequent phagocytosis and agglutination) fetal RBCs passing into the maternal circulation before they can be recognized by the mother's immune system. Because the immune response is blocked, anti-D antibodies and memory cells (which produce the primary and secondary immune responses, respectively) are not formed (Blackburn, 2013). The inhibition of memory cell formation is especially important because memory cells provide long-term immunity by initiating a rapid immune response after the antigen is reintroduced (McCance & Huether, 2014).

To be effective, RhIG (e.g., WinRho) must be administered to unsensitized mothers within 72 hours (but possibly as long as 3 to 4 weeks) after the first birth or abortion and repeated after subsequent pregnancies or losses. The administration of RhIG at 26 to 28 weeks of gestation further reduces the risk of Rh isoimmunization. RhIG is not effective against existing Rh-positive antibodies in the maternal circulation.

Studies have demonstrated the effectiveness of IVIG at decreasing the severity of RBC destruction (hemolysis) in HDN and subsequent development of neonatal jaundice (Elalfy, Elbarbary, & Abaza, 2011). IVIG administered to the neonate is believed to attack the maternal cells that destroy neonatal RBCs, slowing the progression of bilirubin production. This therapy, often used in conjunction with phototherapy, may decrease the necessity for exchange transfusion. Maternal administration of high-dose IVIG, alone or in combination with plasmapheresis, decreases the fetal effects of Rh(D) isoimmunization (Moise, 2008; Urbaniak, 2008).

Intrauterine transfusion. Infants of mothers already sensitized may be treated by intrauterine transfusion, which consists of infusing blood into the umbilical vein of the fetus. The need for therapy is based on the antenatal diagnosis of fetal anemia by serial Doppler assessments of peak systolic velocity of the middle cerebral artery (Moise & Argoti, 2012). With the advance of ultrasound technology, fetal transfusion may be accomplished directly via the umbilical vein, infusing type O Rh-negative packed RBCs to raise the fetal hematocrit to 40 to 50%; fetal movement and transfusion risks are minimized by administering vecuronium bromide for temporary fetal paralysis. The frequency of intrauterine transfusions may vary according to institution and fetal hydropic status, but one recommendation is for intervals of 10 days, 2 weeks, and then 3 weeks for subsequent procedures until the fetus reaches pulmonary maturity at approximately 37 to 38 weeks of gestation (Moise, 2008; Moise & Argoti, 2012). Intraperitoneal blood transfusions are used less commonly for isoimmunization because of higher associated fetal risks; however, they may be used when intravascular access is impossible.

Exchange transfusion. Exchange transfusions are needed infrequently because of the decrease in the incidence of severe hemolytic disease in newborns resulting from isoimmunization. Exchange transfusion is a standard mode of therapy for treatment of severe hyperbilirubinemia and is the treatment of choice for hyperbilirubinemia and hydrops caused by Rh incompatibility. Exchange transfusion removes the sensitized erythrocytes, lowers the serum bilirubin level to prevent bilirubin encephalopathy, corrects the anemia, and prevents cardiac failure. Indications for exchange transfusion in full-term infants may include a rapidly increasing serum bilirubin level and hemolysis despite intensive phototherapy. The criteria for exchange transfusions in preterm infants vary according to associated illness factors. Other factors must be considered, particularly the infant's clinical condition, because it is a procedure with potential complications. Guidelines for the initiation of exchange transfusion for infants 35 weeks of gestation or greater have been developed by the Canadian Paediatric Society (Barrington, Sankaran, & CPS, Fetus and Newborn Committee, 2007/2011).

Exchange transfusion is accomplished by alternately removing a small amount of the infant's blood and replacing it with an equal amount of donor blood. If the infant has Rh incompatibility, type O Rh-negative blood is used for transfusion, so the maternal antibodies still present in the infant do not hemolyze the transfused blood. Depending on the infant's size, gestational age, and condition, 5 to 20 mL of the infant's blood is removed at one time and replaced with an equal amount of warmed donor blood. Preservatives in donor blood lower the infant's serum calcium level; therefore, calcium gluconate is often given during the exchange transfusion. The neonate is monitored closely for signs of a blood transfusion reaction as well as hypotension, temperature instability, and cardiorespiratory compromise.

NURSING CARE

The initial nursing responsibility is recognizing jaundice in the newborn at risk. The possibility of hemolytic disease can be anticipated from the prenatal and perinatal history. Prenatal evidence of incompatibility and a positive Coombs' test result are cause for increased vigilance for early signs of jaundice in an infant. Data indicate that the hour-specific bilirubin nomogram can be used in infants born at 35 weeks or more with ABO incompatibility and a positive Coombs' test result to follow the infant's serum bilirubin to determine the need for additional follow-up after hospital discharge (Schutzman, Sekhon, & Hundalani, 2010). (See Fig. 26-8.)

If an exchange transfusion is required, the nurse prepares the infant and the family and assists the practitioner with the procedure. The infant receives nothing by mouth (NPO) during the procedure; therefore, a peripheral infusion of dextrose and electrolytes is established. The nurse documents the blood volume exchanged, including the amount of blood withdrawn and infused, the time of each procedure, and the cumulative record of the total volume exchanged. Vital signs monitored electronically are evaluated frequently and correlated with the removal and infusion of blood. If signs of cardiac or respiratory problems occur, the procedure is stopped temporarily and resumed after the infant's cardiorespiratory function stabilizes. The nurse also observes for signs of blood transfusion reaction and maintains the infant's blood glucose levels and fluid balance.

Throughout the procedure attention must be given to the infant's thermoregulation. Hypothermia increases oxygen and glucose consumption, causing metabolic acidosis. Not only do these consequences hinder the infant's overall physical ability to withstand the long procedure, but they also inhibit the binding capacity of albumin and bilirubin and the hepatic enzymatic reactions, thus increasing the risk of kernicterus. Conversely, hyperthermia damages the donor erythrocytes, elevating the free potassium content and predisposing the infant to cardiac arrest.

The exchange transfusion is performed with the infant in a radiant warmer. However, the infant is usually covered with sterile drapes that may prevent the radiant heat from sufficiently warming the skin. The blood may also be warmed (using specially designed blood warming devices only) before infusion.

After the procedure is completed, the nurse inspects the umbilical site for evidence of bleeding. The catheter may remain in place in case repeated exchanges are required.

CONGENITAL ANOMALIES

Major congenital anomalies are reported to occur in 3 to 5% of newborn infants and account for 8 to 10% of stillbirths (PHAC, 2013b). Major congenital defects are a leading cause of death in infants, second only to prematurity, younger than 1 year of age in Canada and account for almost 24% of neonatal deaths (PHAC, 2013b).

The most common major congenital anomalies that cause serious problems in the neonate are congenital heart disease, abdominal wall defects, imperforate anus, neural tube defects (NTDs), cleft lip or palate, clubfoot, and developmental dysplasia of the hip. These are thought to result from the interaction of multiple genetic and environmental factors.

Ways of detecting and preventing some of these anomalies are being improved continuously, as are some surgical techniques for the care of the fetus with certain anomalies. Promoting the availability of these services to populations at risk can challenge community health care systems. An interdisciplinary team approach is vital for providing holistic care: the surgical treatment, rehabilitation, and education of the child, as well as psychosocial and financial assistance for the parents. Parental disappointment and disillusion add to the complexity of the nursing care needed for these infants.

A number of congenital anomalies are discussed in the following pediatric systems and conditions chapters (Part 3):

- Cleft lip and palate, Chapter 46
- Esophageal atresia and tracheoesophageal fistula, Chapter 46
- Omphalocele and gastroschisis, Chapter 46
- Congenital cardiac defects, Chapter 47
- Congenital diaphragmatic hernia and choanal atresia, Chapter 45
- Neural tube defects and myelomeningocele, Chapter 54
- Developmental dysplasia of the hip and clubfoot, Chapter 53
- Hypospadias, disorders of sex development, and bladder exstrophy, Chapter 49

Newborn Screening for Disease

A number of genetic disorders can be detected in the newborn period. There is no national policy for such detection in Canada; therefore, the extent of neonatal screening is determined by provincial and territorial guidelines (see Table 26-3). Most provinces require screening for phenylketonuria (PKU), congenital hypothyroidism (CH), galactosemia, and hemoglobin defects such as sickle cell disease; screening for congenital hearing loss is recommended to be done at the same time as disease screening.

The use of pulse oximetry to screen for critical congenital heart disease in healthy term infants has been endorsed by the Canadian Paediatric Society and is being implemented in numerous hospitals; it has been suggested that screening for critical congenital heart disease be incorporated into the routine newborn screening panel (Bradshaw & Martin, 2012; Mahle, Martin, Beekman, et al., 2012). When performing cardiac screening on term newborns, one should:

- Screen term newborns after 24 hours of life or as close to discharge from the birth hospital as possible.
- Use a motion-tolerant pulse oximeter.
- Avoid false-positive results by screening while the infant is alert.
- Obtain pulse oximeter readings from the right hand and one foot.

The response to cardiac screening varies with the saturation values that are obtained and are outlined below:

- Saturations ≥95% in the right hand or foot and ≤3% difference between the two extremities is a negative screen (no further testing is required).
- Saturations of ≤90% in right hand or foot is considered a positive screening, and additional evaluation is warranted (e.g., echocardiogram).
- Saturations between 90 and 95% in the right hand or foot or >3% difference between the two extremities warrants a repeat test in 1 hour. If screening values remain the same as

those from the first screen, consider repeating the screen in 1 hour. If parameters remain unchanged after the second screen, repeat a third time. If unchanged, consider it a positive screen (Kemper, Mahle, Martin, et al., 2011).

Inborn Errors of Metabolism

Inborn errors of metabolism (IEM) is the term applied to a large group of disorders caused by a metabolic defect that results from the absence of or change in a protein, usually an enzyme, and mediated by the action of a certain gene. These defects can involve any substrate produced from protein, carbohydrate, or fat metabolism. IEMs are recessive disorders and an individual must receive a defective gene from each parent for them to occur. The parents usually are unaffected because their dominant gene directs the synthesis of sufficient protein to meet their metabolic needs under normal circumstances.

With the advent of new biochemical techniques, it is now possible to detect the gene responsible for causing an increasing number of these disorders early in the newborn period so that appropriate therapies to prevent further morbidity may be implemented. Tandem mass spectrometry has the potential for identifying up to as many as 40 IEMs. With tandem mass spectrometry, earlier identification of IEMs may prevent further developmental delays and morbidities in affected children.

Phenylketonuria. Phenylketonuria (PKU), an IEM inherited as an autosomal recessive trait (the *PAH* gene is located on chromosome 12q24), is caused by a deficiency or absence of the enzyme needed to metabolize the essential amino acid phenylalanine. Classic PKU is at one end of a spectrum of conditions known as hyperphenylalaninemia. Within the spectrum of hyperphenylalaninemia are conditions with varying degrees of severity, depending on the degree of enzyme deficiency. Because rarer forms are a result of a deficiency in other enzymes and are diagnosed and treated differently, the following discussion of PKU is limited to the severe, classic form.

In PKU the hepatic enzyme phenylalanine hydroxylase, which normally controls the conversion of phenylalanine to tyrosine, is deficient. This results in the accumulation of phenylalanine in the bloodstream and urinary excretion of abnormal amounts of its metabolites, the phenyl acids. One of these phenylketones, phenylacetic acid, gives urine the characteristic musty odour associated with the disease. Another is phenylpyruvic acid, which is responsible for the term *phenylketonuria*.

Tyrosine, the amino acid produced by the metabolism of phenylalanine, is absent in PKU. Tyrosine is needed to form the pigment melanin and the hormones epinephrine and T_4. Decreased melanin production results in similar phenotypes of most individuals with PKU, which is blond hair, blue eyes, and fair skin that is particularly susceptible to eczema and other dermatological problems. Children with a genetically darker skin colour may be red haired or brunette.

Clinical manifestations in untreated PKU include failure to thrive (growth failure); frequent vomiting; irritability; hyperactivity; and unpredictable, erratic behaviour. Cognitive impairment is thought to be caused by the accumulation of phenylalanine and presumably by decreased levels of the neurotransmitters dopamine and tryptophan, which affect the normal development of the brain and CNS, resulting in defective myelinization, cystic degeneration of the grey and white matter, and disturbances in cortical lamination. Older children commonly display bizarre or schizoid behaviour patterns such as fright reactions, screaming episodes, head banging, arm biting, disorientation, failure to respond to strong stimuli, and catatonia-like positions.

The objective in diagnosing and treating the disorder is to prevent cognitive impairment. Every newborn should be screened for PKU. The test for PKU is not reliable until the newborn has ingested an ample amount of the amino acid phenylalanine, a constituent of both human and cow's milk. The nurse must document the initial ingestion of milk and perform the test at least 24 hours after that time. The current trend toward early infant discharge from the hospital has the potential to cause neonates with a disorder such as PKU not to be adequately screened. A number of agencies have developed guidelines to minimize the risk of this happening and recommend the following:

- Obtain a subsequent sample by 2 weeks of age if the initial specimen is collected before the newborn is 24 hours old.
- Designate a primary care provider for all newborns before discharge for adequate newborn screening follow-up.
- Collect the initial specimen as close as possible to discharge and no later than 7 days after birth (Newborn Screening Ontario, n.d.; Perinatal Services BC, 2010).

! NURSING ALERT

Avoid "layering" the blood specimen on the special Guthrie paper. Layering is placing one drop of blood on top of the other, or overlapping the specimen. This practice results in a falsely high reading, or false positive, which will lead the newborn screening department to call the family and health care provider to arrange for a diagnostic blood phenylalanine test to determine whether the newborn truly has PKU. Best results are obtained by collecting the specimen with a pipette from the heel stick and spreading the blood uniformly over the blot paper.

If the infant is found to have PKU, a diet low in phenylalanine is begun soon after birth. A new medication, sapropterin dihydrochloride, has been approved for use in persons with PKU; the drug acts to decrease blood phenylalanine levels in persons with hyperphenylalaninemia (Stokowski, 2008). Breastfeeding or partial breastfeeding may be possible for some infants if the phenylalanine levels are monitored carefully and remain within acceptable limits (Lawrence & Lawrence, 2015). Many affected children have some intellectual impairment. Successful management and outcome are largely dependent on early identification of the condition, modification of the diet, and compliance with the treatment regimen throughout the entire life.

Galactosemia. Galactosemia is a rare autosomal recessive disorder that results from various gene mutations leading to three distinct enzymatic deficiencies. The most common type of galactosemia (classic galactosemia) results from a deficiency of a hepatic enzyme, galactose 1-phosphate uridyltransferase (GALT), and affects approximately one in 50,000 births. The other two varieties of galactosemia involve deficiencies in the enzymes galactokinase (GALK) and galactose 4′-epimerase (GALE); these are extremely rare disorders. All three enzymes (GALT, GALK, and GALE) are involved in the conversion of galactose into glucose.

As galactose accumulates in the blood, several organs are affected. Hepatic dysfunction leads to cirrhosis, resulting in jaundice in the infant by the second week of life. The spleen subsequently becomes enlarged as a result of portal hypertension. Cataracts are usually recognizable by 1 or 2 months of age; cerebral damage, manifested by the symptoms of lethargy and hypotonia, is evident soon afterward. Infants with galactosemia appear normal at birth, but within a few days of ingesting milk (which has a high lactose content) they begin to experience vomiting and diarrhea, leading to weight loss. *E. coli* sepsis is also a common presenting clinical sign. Death during the first month of life is frequent in untreated infants. Occasionally, classic galactosemia is seen with milder, chronic manifestations, such as growth failure, feeding difficulty, and developmental delay.

Diagnosis is made on the basis of the infant's history, physical examination, galactosuria, increased levels of galactose in the blood, and decreased levels of GALT activity in erythrocytes. The infant may display characteristics of malnutrition (i.e., hypoglycemia, jaundice, hepatosplenomegaly, sepsis, cataracts, and decreased muscle tone).

During infancy treatment consists of eliminating all milk and lactose-containing formula, including breast milk. Traditionally, lactose-free formulas are used, with soy-protein formula being the feeding of choice; however, some research suggests that elemental formula (galactose-free) may be more beneficial than soy formulas (Zlatunich & Packman, 2005). As the infant progresses to solids, only foods low in galactose should be consumed. Certain fruits are high in galactose, and some dietitians recommend that they be avoided. Food lists should be given to the family to ensure that appropriate foods are chosen.

If galactosemia is suspected, supportive treatment and care are implemented, including monitoring for hypoglycemia, liver failure, bleeding disorders, and *E. coli* sepsis.

Nursing interventions are similar to those for PKU, except that dietary restrictions are easier to maintain because many more foods are allowed. However, reading food labels carefully for the presence of any form of lactose, especially dairy products, is mandatory. Many drugs, such as some of the penicillin preparations, contain lactose as filler and also must be avoided. Unfortunately, lactose is an unlabelled ingredient in many pharmaceuticals. Therefore, parents need to be instructed to ask their local pharmacist about galactose content of any over-the-counter or prescription medication.

Congenital hypothyroidism. CH may have a number of causes and can be either permanent or transient. Transient CH is frequently associated with maternal Graves' disease that was treated with antithyroid drugs. Most cases are sporadic (nonhereditary), but approximately 15% of all cases are transmitted as an autosomal dominant trait. The most common pathogenesis is thyroid dysgenesis, mostly with unknown causes. Worldwide, the most common cause of CH resulting in hypothyroidism is iodine deficiency. However, no matter what the cause, the manifestations (Box 29-3) and management are similar. In some conditions, the thyroid deficiency is severe, and manifestations develop early; in others, the symptoms may be delayed for months or years. Early detection and prompt initiation of treatment are essential because their delay results in various degrees of cognitive impairment.

BOX 29-3 CLINICAL MANIFESTATIONS OF CONGENITAL HYPOTHYROIDISM

Birth*

- Poor feeding
- Lethargy
- Prolonged jaundice (>2 weeks)
- Respiratory difficulties
- Cyanosis
- Constipation
- Bradycardia
- Hoarse cry
- Large anterior and posterior fontanels
- Postterm
- Birth weight over 4000 g (8 lbs 13 oz)

Older Child

- Short stature
- Obesity
- Varying degrees of intellectual deficits
- Abnormal tendon reflexes
- Slow, awkward movements

Ages 6 to 9 Weeks†

- Depressed nasal bridge
- Short forehead
- Puffy eyelids
- Large tongue
- Thick, dry, mottled skin
- Coarse, dry, lustreless hair
- Abdominal distension
- Umbilical hernia
- Hyporeflexia
- Bradycardia
- Hypothermia
- Hypotension
- Anemia
- Widely patent cranial sutures

*Clinical manifestations may not be obvious at birth, possibly because of maternal transfer of thyroid hormone to the fetus. Manifestations may be delayed in infants with certain types of familial hypothyroidism and in breastfed infants (may show after weaning).

†If untreated, classical features.

Results of screening tests indicate that CH occurs in approximately 1 in 3000 to 1 in 4000 newborns (Kaye & AAP Committee on Genetics, 2006; Ontario Newborn Screening Program, 2006). A higher incidence of other congenital abnormalities has been observed in infants with CH. Many preterm infants have transient hypothyroidism (hypothyroxinemia) at birth as a result of hypothalamic and pituitary immaturity. Infants born before 28 weeks of gestation may require temporary thyroid hormone replacement.

Because CH is one of the most common preventable causes of cognitive impairment, early diagnosis and treatment of this disease are essential interventions. Neonatal screening consists of an initial filter paper blood spot T_4 measurement followed by measurement of thyroid-stimulating hormone (TSH) in specimens with low T_4 values.

All provinces in Canada routinely screen for hypothyroidism. Although a heel stick blood sample for the test is best obtained between 2 and 6 days of age, specimens are usually taken within the first 24 to 48 hours or before discharge as part of a concurrent screening for other metabolic defects. At this time, the normally expected increase in thyroxine (T_4) would be lacking in newborns with hypothyroidism. Early screening can result in overdiagnosis (false positives) but is preferable to missing the diagnosis. In the newborn, thyroid function studies are elevated in comparison with values in older children; therefore, it is important to document the timing of the tests. In preterm and sick full-term infants thyroid function tests are usually lower than in the healthy full-term infant. A repeat test for T_4 and TSH may be evaluated after 30 weeks (corrected age) in newborns born before that time and after resolution of the acute illness in the sick full-term infant.

Treatment involves lifelong thyroid hormone replacement therapy as soon as possible after diagnosis to abolish all signs of hypothyroidism and re-establish normal physical and mental development. The drug of choice is synthetic levothyroxine sodium (Synthroid, Levothroid). Optimum dosage of L-thyroxine should be able to maintain blood TSH concentration between 0.5 and 2 mU/L during the first 3 years of life. Regular measurement of T_4 levels is important to ensure optimum treatment. Bone age surveys are also performed to ensure optimum growth.

The most important nursing objective is early identification of the disorder. Nurses caring for newborns must be certain that screening is performed, especially in infants who are preterm, discharged early, or born at home. Approximately 10% of cases are detected only by a second screening at 2 to 6 weeks of age. Nurses in community health need to be aware of the earliest signs of the disorder. Parental remarks about an unusually "quiet and good" baby and demonstrated symptoms such as prolonged jaundice, constipation, and umbilical hernia should lead to a suspicion of hypothyroidism, which requires a referral for specific tests.

After the diagnosis is confirmed, parents need an explanation of the disorder and the necessity of lifelong treatment. The child should be referred to a pediatric endocrinologist for care. The importance of compliance with the drug regimen for the child to achieve normal growth and development must be stressed (Kaye & AAP Committee on Genetics, 2006). Because the drug is tasteless, it can be crushed and added to formula, water, or food. If a dose is missed, twice the dose should be given the next day. Unless there are maternal contraindicative factors, breastfeeding is acceptable and encouraged in infants with hypothyroidism (Lawrence & Lawrence, 2015). Parents also need to be aware of signs indicating overdose, such as a rapid pulse, dyspnea, irritability, insomnia, fever, sweating, and weight loss. Ideally, they should know how to count the pulse and be instructed to withhold a dose and consult their health care provider if the pulse rate is above a certain value. Signs of inadequate treatment are fatigue, sleepiness, decreased appetite, and constipation.

Genetic Evaluation and Counselling

Genetic counselling addresses the problems associated with the occurrence or risk of occurrence of a genetic disorder in a family. It involves the relaying of information about the diagnosis, treatment options, recurrence risk, and availability of prenatal diagnosis. It is essential that nurses understand basic principles of heredity, understand how heredity contributes to disorders, and be aware of the types of genetic testing available (see Chapter 9).

Nurses frequently encounter children with a genetic disorder, including an IEM, as well as families in which there is a risk that a disorder may be transmitted to or occur in an offspring. It is the nurse's responsibility to be alert to situations in which persons could benefit from genetic evaluation and counselling. Nurses also need to be aware of the local genetic resources, aid the family in finding related services, and offer support and care for children and families affected by genetic conditions.

NURSING CARE

Newborn

A collaborative health team approach that includes specialists and community service representatives is needed in the care of the infant with a congenital anomaly. Surgical intervention in the neonatal period may be necessary for the infant requiring either immediate correction or a palliative procedure to relieve the symptoms of the anomaly until definitive correction can be done. There is higher morbidity and mortality in neonates than in older children or adults undergoing similar procedures. However, despite the problems unique to neonates, advances in surgical techniques, fluid and electrolyte management, anaesthesia, pain management, and the nursing care given in intensive care nurseries have together been responsible for decreasing the risk of surgery in neonates.

The health care team must be highly skilled to meet the infant's needs. These needs are similar to those of other high-risk infants. In addition to stabilization of the infant's condition (oxygenation and perfusion of tissues), other preoperative interventions, such as nasogastric tube placement for abdominal decompression, pain management, and the maintenance of fluid and electrolyte balance, are implemented to manage specific problems.

Postoperatively, the infant is often returned to the intensive care nursery, where he or she needs to be closely monitored. The infant's respiratory efforts need to be supported; this often requires mechanical ventilation. Constant surveillance is necessary to detect any respiratory complications resulting from the anaesthesia. A pulse oximeter is attached to measure the oxygen saturation and oxygen is provided as needed. An in-dwelling gastric catheter may be placed to remove gastric secretions, thereby preventing aspiration and abdominal distension. The infant's fluid, electrolyte, and acid–base balance should be monitored and adjusted as needed. Urine output is also monitored and should equal 1 to 2 mL/kg/hr. Other nursing interventions include assessment and care of the surgical site, thermoregulation, pain management, and promotion of comfort.

Parents and Family

While the infant is receiving care, the parents also have needs that must be met as they deal with the crisis of having an infant with an abnormal condition. Their reactions should be carefully assessed and are likely to be those typical of a grief response. Facilitating their understanding of the information given them about their infant's condition is a vital nursing intervention. A newly diagnosed disorder often implies the need for the implementation of a therapeutic regimen. For example, the disorder may be an IEM, such as PKU, which requires consistent and rigid adherence to a diet. The family may need help securing the required formula and may require counselling from a clinical dietician. The importance of maintaining the diet, keeping an adequate supply of special preparations, and avoiding the use of unauthorized substitutions must be impressed upon the family. These conditions often require a drastic change in family lifestyle and functioning; families often depend on others for assistance. Family coping skills and resources may be stretched thin with a diagnosis such as PKU or galactosemia.

Referral to appropriate agencies is another essential component of the follow-up management, and the nurse should make the parents aware of all possible sources of aid, including pertinent literature, parent groups, and national organizations. Many organizations and foundations (e.g., Canadian Organization of Rare Disorders) provide services and counselling for families of affected children. Numerous parent support groups are also available, where they can share experiences and derive mutual support in coping with problems similar to those of other group members. Nurses must be familiar with the services available in their community that provide assistance and education to families with these particular needs.

A major nursing role is the provision of emotional support during all phases of care to the family of an infant with an anomaly or disorder. The feelings that stem from the real or imagined threat posed by a congenital anomaly are as varied as the people being counselled. Responses may include apathy, denial, anger, hostility, fear, embarrassment, grief, and loss of self-esteem.

Parents may benefit from seeing before-and-after pictures of other babies born with the same defect. In addition to verbal and nonverbal supportive care, this visual reassurance may be effective in allaying their concerns.

Families need much information, guidance, and support as they make decisions regarding their infant's care. Once parents have been given the facts, possible consequences, and any assistance they need in problem solving, the final decision regarding a course of action must be their own. It is then incumbent on health care providers to support the family's decision.

KEY POINTS

- The identification of maternal and fetal risk factors in the antepartum and intrapartum periods is vital for planning adequate care of high-risk infants.
- A small percentage of significant birth injuries may occur despite skilled and competent obstetrical care.
- Infection in the newborn may be acquired in utero, at birth, in breast milk, or from within the nursery.
- The most common maternal infections during early pregnancy that are associated with various congenital malformations include toxoplasmosis, herpes, CMV, rubella, parvovirus B19, and varicella.
- HIV transmission from mother to infant occurs transplacentally at various gestational ages, perinatally by maternal blood and secretions, and postnatally through breast milk.
- The nurse often is the first person to observe signs of newborn drug withdrawal (NAS) and then acquires additional information from the maternal history.
- Maternal–fetal Rh and ABO incompatibility may cause significant hemolysis and jaundice in the neonatal period.
- The injection of Rho(D) immune globulin in Rh-negative and Coombs' test–negative women minimizes the possibility of isoimmunization.
- Congenital defects are now the leading cause of death in the first year of life.
- The supportive care given to the parents of infants with a congenital anomaly or inborn error of metabolism must begin at birth or at the time of diagnosis and continue for years.

evolve WEBSITE

Visit the Evolve website for additional resources related to the content in this chapter such as Case Studies, Critical Thinking Case Study Answers, Nursing Care Plans, Nursing Processes, Nursing Skills, and Review Questions for Exam Preparation at: http://evolve.elsevier.com/Canada/Perry/maternal/

REFERENCES

Ackerman, J. P., Riggins, T., & Black, M. M. (2010). A review of the effects of prenatal cocaine exposure among school-aged children. *Pediatrics, 125*(3), 554–565.

Allen, U., & Canadian Paediatric Society, Infectious Diseases and Immunization Committee. (2014). Prevention and management of neonatal herpes simplex virus infections. *Paediatrics and Child Health, 19*(4), 201–206.

American Academy of Pediatrics, Committee on Infectious Diseases. (2012). *Red book: 2012 report of the committee on infectious diseases* (29th ed.). Elk Grove Village, IL: Author.

Aziz, K., McMillan, D., Andrews, W., et al. (2005). Variations in rates of nosocomial infection among Canadian neonatal intensive care units may be practice-related. *BMC Pediatrics, 5*, 22. doi:10.1186/1471-2431-5-22.

Azzopardi, D. V., Strohm, B., Edwards, D., et al. (2009). Moderate hypothermia to treat perinatal asphyxial encephalopathy. *New England Journal of Medicine, 361*(14), 1349–1358.

Bandstra, E. S., & Accornero, V. H. (2014). Infants of substance abusing mothers. In R. J. Martin, A. A. Fanaroff, & M. C. Walsh (Eds.), *Fanaroff and Martin's neonatal-perinatal medicine: Diseases of the fetus and infant* (10th ed.). Philadelphia: Mosby.

Bandstra, E. S., Morrow, C. E., Accornero, V. H., et al. (2011). Estimated effects of in utero cocaine exposure on language development through early adolescence. *Neurotoxicology & Teratology, 33*(1), 25–3511.

Bandstra, E. S., Morrow, C. E., Mansoor, E., et al. (2010). Prenatal drug exposure: Infant and toddler outcomes. *Journal of Addictive Diseases, 29*(2), 245–258.

Barrington, K. J., & Canadian Paediatric Society, Fetus and Newborn Committee. (2007). Management of the infant at increased risk for sepsis. *Paediatrics and Child Health, 12*(10), 893–898. Reaffirmed 2011.

Barrington, K., Sankaran, K., & Canadian Paediatric Society, Fetus and Newborn Committee. (2007). Guidelines for detection, management and prevention of hyperbilirubinemia in term and late preterm newborn infants (35 or more weeks' gestation). *Paediatrics and Child Health, 12*(5), 1B–12B. Reaffirmed 2011.

BC Women's Hospital. (2013). *Pregnancy, Drugs & Alcohol.* Retrieved from <http://www.bcwomens.ca/services/pregnancybirthnewborns/hospitalcare/substanceusepregnancy.htm>.

Black, L. V., & Maheshwari, A. (2009). Disorders of the fetomaternal unit: Hematologic manifestations in the fetus and neonate. *Seminars in Perinatology, 33*(1), 12–19.

Blackburn, S. (2013). *Maternal, fetal, and neonatal physiology: A clinical perspective* (4th ed.). St. Louis: Saunders.

Boucoiran, I., Tulloch, K., Caddy, S., & Money, D. (2014). SOGC clinical practice guidelines: Guidelines for the care of pregnant women living with HIV and interventions to reduce perinatal transmission. *Journal of Obstetrics and Gynaecology Canada, 36*(8e Suppl. A), S1–S46.

Bradshaw, E. A., & Martin, G. R. (2012). Screening for critical congenital heart disease: Advancing detection in the newborn. *Current Opinions in Pediatrics, 24*(5), 603–608.

Burgos, A. E., & Burke, B. L. (2009). Neonatal abstinence syndrome. *NeoReviews, 10*(5), e222–e228.

Burns, L., Conroy, E., & Mattick, R. P. (2010). Infant mortality among women on a methadone program during pregnancy. *Drug and Alcohol Review, 29*(5), 551–556. doi:10.1111/j.1465-3362.2010.00176.x.

Cantor Sackett, J., Weller, R. A., & Weller, E. B. (2009). Selective serotonin reuptake inhibitor use during pregnancy and possible neonatal complications. *Current Psychiatry Reports, 11*(3), 253–257.

Centers for Disease Control and Prevention. (2010). Prevention of perinatal group B streptococcal disease. *MMWR. Morbidity and Mortality Weekly Report, 59*(RR10), 1–32. Retrieved from <http://www.cdc.gov/mmwr/preview/mmwrhtml/rr5910a1.htm>.

Chiriboga, C. A., Kuhn, L., & Wasserman, G. A. (2007). Prenatal cocaine exposures and dose-related cocaine effects on infant tone and behavior. *Neurotoxicology & Teratology, 29*(3), 323–330.

Chomchai, C., Na Manorom, N., Watanarungasan, P., et al. (2004). Methamphetamine abuse during pregnancy and its impact on neonates born at Siriraj Hospital, Bangkok, Thailand. *Southeast Asian Journal of Tropical Medicine & Public Health, 35*(1), 228–231.

Coffin, S. E. (2014). Fighting infections in the neonatal intensive care unit: Gloves on or off? *JAMA Pediatrics, 168*(10), 885–887. doi:10.1001/jamapediatrics.2014.1269.

Cotten, C. M., Taylor, S., Stoll, B., et al. (2009). Prolonged duration of initial empirical antibiotic treatment is associated with increased rates of necrotizing enterocolitis and death for extremely low–birth-weight infants. *Pediatrics, 123*(1), 58–66.

Crane, J., & Society of Obstetricians and Gynaecologists of Canada, Maternal Fetal Medicine and Infectious Diseases Committees. (2014). Parvovirus B19 infection in pregnancy. *Journal of Obstetrics and Gynaecology Canada, 36*(12), 1107–1116.

Diehl-Jones, W. L., & Fraser Askin, D. (2010). Hematologic disorders. In M. T. Verklan & M. Walden (Eds.), *Core curriculum for neonatal intensive care nursing* (4th ed.). St. Louis: Saunders.

Dooley, R., Dooley, J., Antone, I., et al. (2015). Narcotic tapering in pregnancy using long-acting morphine: An 18-month prospective cohort study in northwestern Ontario. *Canadian Family Physician, 61*(2), e88–e95.

Dow, J., Ordean, A., Murphy-Oikonen, J., et al. (2012). Neonatal abstinence syndrome clinical practice guidelines for Ontario. *Journal of Population Therapeutics & Clinical Pharmacology, 19*(3), e488–e506.

Edwards, A. D., Brocklehurst, P., Gunn, A. J., et al. (2010). Neurological outcomes at 18 months of age after moderate hypothermia for perinatal hypoxic ischaemic encephalopathy: Synthesis and meta-analysis of trial data. *British Medical Journal, 340*, c.363.

Elalfy, M. S., Elbarbary, N. S., & Abaza, H. W. (2011). Early intravenous immunoglobulin (two-dose regimen) in the management of severe Rh hemolytic disease of newborn—a prospective randomized controlled trial. *European Journal of Pediatrics, 170*(4), 461–467.

Finnegan, L. P. (1985). Neonatal abstinence. In N. Nelson (Ed.), *Current therapy in neonatal perinatal medicine*. Toronto: Decker.

Finnegan, L., Pacini, M., & Maremmani, I. (2010). Methadone treatment for pregnant heroin addicted women. *Heroin Addiction and Related Clinical Problems, 12*(2), 29–36.

Goderis, J., De Leenheer, E., Smets, K., et al. (2014). Hearing loss and congenital CMV infection: A systematic review. *Pediatrics, 134*(5), 972–982. doi:10.1542/peds.2014-1173.

Guerri, C., Bazinet, A., & Riley, E. P. (2009). Fetal alcohol spectrum disorders and alterations in brain and behaviour. *Alcohol and Alcoholism, 44*(2), 108–114. doi:10.1093/alcalc/agn105.

Hale, T. W., & Rowe, H. E. (2014). *Medications and mothers' milk* (16th ed.). Amarillo, TX: Pharmasoft Medical.

Health Canada. (2012). *First Nations and Inuit health. Tuberculosis.* Retrieved from <http://www.hc-sc.gc.ca/fniah-spnia/diseases-maladies/tuberculos/index-eng.php>.

Interagency Coordinating Committee on Fetal Alcohol Spectrum Disorders (ICCFASD). (2011). *Consensus statement: Recognizing alcohol-related neurodevelopmental disorder (ARND) in primary health care of children.* Rockville, MD: Author.

Jacobs, S., Hunt, R., Tarnow-Mordi, W., et al. (2007). Cooling for newborns with hypoxic ischaemic encephalopathy. *Cochrane Database System Reviews*, (4), CD003311.

Kakko, J., Heilig, M., & Sarman, I. (2008). Buprenorphine and methadone treatment of opiate dependence during pregnancy: Comparison of fetal growth and neonatal outcomes in two consecutive case series. *Drug and Alcohol Dependence, 96*(1–2), 69–78. doi:10.1016/j.drugalcdep.2008.01.025.

Kaye, C. I., & American Academy of Pediatrics, Committee on Genetics. (2006). Newborn screening fact sheets. *Pediatrics, 118*(3), e934–e963. doi:10.1542/peds.2006-1783.

Kemper, A. R., Mahle, W. T., Martin, G. R., et al. (2011). Strategies for implementing screening for critical congenital heart disease. *Pediatrics, 128*(5), e1259–e1267.

Koren, G., Hutson, J., & Gareri, J. (2008). Novel methods for the detection of drug and alcohol exposure during pregnancy: Implications for maternal and child health. *Clinical Pharmacology and Therapeutics, 83*, 631–634. doi:10.1038/sj.clpt.6100506.

Kuczkowski, K. M. (2007). The effects of drug abuse on pregnancy. *Current Opinions in Obstetrics & Gynecology, 19*(6), 578–585.

Kuppala, V. S., Meinzen-Derr, J., Morrow, A. L., et al. (2011). Prolonged initial empirical antibiotic treatment is associated with adverse outcomes in premature infants. *Journal of Pediatrics, 159*(5), 720–725.

Laptook, A. R. (2009). Use of therapeutic hypothermia for term infants with hypoxic-ischemic encephalopathy. *Pediatrics Clinics of North America, 56*(3), 601–616.

Lawrence, R. M. & Lawrence, R. A. (2015). *Breastfeeding: A guide for the medical profession* (8th ed.). St. Louis: Elsevier.

Lefevere, J., & Allegaert, K. (2015). Is breastfeeding useful in the management of neonatal abstinence syndrome? *Archives of Disease in Childhood, 100*(4), 414–415.

Lester, B. M., & Lagasse, L. L. (2010). Children of addicted women. *Journal of Addictive Diseases, 29*(2), 259–276.

Logan, B. A., Brown, M. S., & Hayes, M. J. (2013). Neonatal abstinence syndrome: Treatment and pediatric outcomes. *Clinical Obstetrics and Gynecology, 56*(1), 186–192. doi:10.1097/GRF.0b013e31827feea4.

Mahle, W. T., Martin, G. R., Beekman, R. H., et al. (2012). Endorsement of Health and Human Services recommendation for pulse oximetry screening for critical congenital heart disease. *Pediatrics, 129*(1), 190–192.

Marroun, H. E., Hudziak, J. J., Tiemeier, H., et al. (2011). Intrauterine cannabis exposure leads to more aggressive behavior and attention problems in 18-month-old girls. *Drug & Alcohol Dependence, 118*(2–3), 470–474.

May, P. A., Blankenship, J., Marias, G., et al. (2013). Maternal alcohol consumption producing fetal alcohol spectrum disorders (FASD): Quantity, frequency, and timing of drinking. *Drug and Alcohol Dependence, 133*(2), 502–512.

McCance, K., & Huether, S. (2014). *Pathophysiology: The biological basis for disease in infants and children* (7th ed.). St. Louis: Mosby.

Minozzi, S., Amato, L., Vecchi, S., & Davoli, M. (2008). Maintenance agonist treatments for opiate dependent pregnant women. *The Cochrane Database of Systematic Reviews*, (2), CD006318, doi:10.1002/14651858.CD006318.pub2.

Moise, K. J. (2008). Management of rhesus alloimmunization in pregnancy. *Obstetrics & Gynecology, 112*(1), 164–176.

Moise, K. J. (2012). Red cell alloimmunization. In S. G. Gabbe, J. R. Niebyl, H. L. Galan, et al. (Eds.), *Obstetrics: Normal and problem pregnancies* (6th ed.). Philadelphia: Saunders.

Moise, K. J., & Argoti, P. S. (2012). Management and prevention of red cell alloimmunization in pregnancy: A systematic review. *Obstetrics & Gynecology, 120*(5), 1132–1139.

Money, D., Dobson, S., & Society of Obstetricians and Gynaecologists of Canada Infectious Disease Committee. (2013). SOGC clinical practice guideline: The prevention of early-onset neonatal group B streptococcal disease. *Journal of Obstetrics and Gynaecology Canada, 26*(9), 826–832.

Moore, D. L., MacDonald, N. E., & Canadian Paediatric Society, Infectious Diseases and Immunization Committee. (2015). Preventing ophthalmia neonatorum. *Pediatrics and Child Health, 20*(2), 93–96.

Nelson, M. R. (2016). Birth brachial plexus palsy. In R. M. Kliegman, B. F. Stanton, J. W. St. Geme, & N. F. Schor (Eds.), *Nelson textbook of pediatrics* (20th ed.). Philadelphia: Saunders.

Newborn Screening Ontario. (n.d.). *Information for health care providers*. Retrieved from <http://www.newbornscreening.on.ca/bins/content_page.asp?cid=7-272>.

Norman, A. L., Crocker, N., Mattson, S. N., & Riley, E. P. (2009). Neuroimaging and fetal alcohol spectrum disorders. *Developmental Disabilities Research Reviews, 15*(3), 209–217. doi:10.1002/ddrr.72.

Ontario Newborn Screening Program. (2006). *Congenital hypothyroidism (CH)—Endocrine disorder*. Ottawa: Author. Retrieved from <http://www.newbornscreening.on.ca/data/1/rec_docs/529_fs_ch.pdf>.

Panel on Treatment of HIV-Infected Pregnant Women and Prevention of Perinatal Transmission. (2015). *Recommendations for use of antiretroviral drugs in pregnant HIV-infected women for maternal health and interventions to reduce perinatal HIV transmission in the United States*, Washington, DC: National Institutes of Health, pp. 1–207. Retrieved from <https://aidsinfo.nih.gov/contentfiles/lvguidelines/perinatalgl.pdf>.

Paperny, A. M. (2012, January 6). Treating the tiny victims of Canada's fastest-growing addiction. *The Globe and Mail*. Retrieved from <http://www.theglobeandmail.com/life/health-and-fitness/health/conditions/treating-the-tiny-victims-of-canadas-fastest-growing-addiction/article547509/>.

Patrick, S. W., Dudley, J., Martin, P., et al. (2015). Prescription opioid epidemic and infant outcomes. *Pediatrics, 135*(5), 842–850. doi:10.1542/peds.2014-3299.

Perinatal Services BC. (2010). *Neonatal guideline 9: Newborn screening*. Retrieved from <http://www.perinatalservicesbc.ca/Documents/Guidelines-Standards/Newborn/NewbornScreeningGuideline.pdf>.

Pitts, K. (2010). Perinatal substance abuse. In M. T. Verklan & M. Walden (Eds.), *Core curriculum for neonatal intensive care nursing* (4th ed.). St. Louis: Saunders.

Polin, R. A., & American Academy of Pediatrics, Committee on Fetus and Newborn. (2012). Management of neonates with suspected or proven early-onset bacterial sepsis. *Pediatrics, 129*(5), 1006–1015. doi:10.1542/peds.2012-0541.

Public Health Agency of Canada. (2010). *Essential resources for effective infection prevention and control programs: A matter of patient safety—A discussion paper*. Ottawa: Author. Retrieved from <http://www.phac-aspc.gc.ca/nois-sinp/guide/ps-sp/partII-eng.php#b61>.

Public Health Agency of Canada. (2012a). *Varicella (Chickenpox)*. Retrieved from <http://www.phac-aspc.gc.ca/im/vpd-mev/varicella-eng.php>.

Public Health Agency of Canada. (2012b). *Canadian immunization guide. Part 4: Active vaccines*. Ottawa: Author. Retrieved from <http://www.phac-aspc.gc.ca/publicat/cig-gci/p04-eng.php>.

Public Health Agency of Canada. (2013a). *Canadian guidelines on sexually transmitted infections. Section 5—Management and treatment of specific infections*. Ottawa: Author. Retrieved from <http://www.phac-aspc.gc.ca/std-mts/sti-its/cgsti-ldcits/section-5-10-eng.php>.

Public Health Agency of Canada. (2013b). *Congenital anomalies in Canada 2013: A perinatal health surveillance report*. Ottawa: Author. Retrieved from <http://publications.gc.ca/collections/collection_2014/aspc-phac/HP35-40-2013-eng.pdf>.

Public Health Agency of Canada. (2014). *Executive summary—Report on sexually transmitted infections in Canada: 2011*. Retrieved from <http://www.phac-aspc.gc.ca/sti-its-surv-epi/rep-rap-2011/index-eng.php>.

Reed, M. D., Aranda, J. V., & Hales, B. F. (2014). Developmental pharmacology. In R. J. Martin, A. A. Fanaroff, & M. C. Walsh (Eds.), *Fanaroff and Martin's neonatal-perinatal medicine: Diseases of the fetus and infant* (10th ed.). St. Louis: Mosby.

Robinson, J. L., & Canadian Paediatric Society, Infectious Diseases and Immunization Committee. (2009). Congenital syphilis: No longer just of historical interest. *Paediatrics & Child Health, 14*(5), 337.

Rodriguez, N. A., & Caplan, M. S. (2015). Oropharyngeal administration of mother's milk to prevent necrotizing enterocolitis in extremely low-birth-weight infants. Theoretical perspectives. *Journal of Perinatal and Neonatal Nursing, 29*(1), 81–90. doi:10.1097/JPN.0000000000000087.

Schröter, H., & Canadian Paediatric Society, First Nations, Inuit and Métis Health Committee. (2010). Fetal alcohol spectrum disorder: Diagnostic update. *Paediatrics & Child Health, 15*(7), 455–456.

Schutzman, D. L., Sekhon, R., & Hundalani, S. (2010). Hour-specific bilirubin nomogram in infants with ABO incompatibility and direct Coombs-positive results. *Archives of Pediatric & Adolescent Medicine, 164*(12), 1158–1164.

Segel, G. B., & Casey, D. (2016). Hereditary spherocytosis. In R. M. Kliegman, B. F. Stanton, J. St. Geme, & N. F. Schor (Eds.), *Nelson textbook of pediatrics* (20th ed.). Philadelphia: Saunders.

Smith, L., Yonekura, M. L., Wallace, N., et al. (2003). Effects of prenatal methamphetamine exposure on fetal growth and drug withdrawal symptoms in infants born at term. *Journal of Development and Behavior in Pediatrics, 24*(1), 17–23.

Stokowski, I. A. (2008). Noteworthy professional news: Drug to treat phenylketonuria approved. *Advances in Neonatal Care, 8*(3), 139–140. doi:10.1097/01.ANC.0000324334.56228.14.

Stoll, B. J., Hansen, N. I., Sánchez, P. J., et al. (2011). Early onset neonatal sepsis: The burden of group B streptococcal and *E. coli* disease continues. *Pediatrics, 127*(5), 817–826. doi:10.1542/peds.2010-2217.

Stoll, B. J., & Shane, A. L. (2016). Infections in the neonatal infant. In R. M. Kliegman, B. F. Stanton, J. St. Geme, & N. Schor (Eds.), *Nelson textbook of pediatrics* (20th ed.). Philadelphia: Saunders.

UNICEF. (2015). *The AIDS epidemic continues to take a staggering toll, especially in sub-Saharan Africa.* Retrieved from <http://data.unicef.org/hiv-aids/global-trends.html>.

Urbaniak, S. J. (2008). Noninvasive approaches to the management of RhD hemolytic disease of the fetus and newborn. *Transfusion, 48*(1), 12–19.

Valentini, P., Buonsenso, D., Barone, G., et al. (2015). Spiramycin/cotrimoxazole versus pyrimethamine/sulfonamide and spiramycin alone for the treatment of toxoplasmosis in pregnancy. *Journal of Perinatology, 35*(2), 90–94.

Venkatesh, M., Adams, K. M., & Weisman, L. E. (2011). Infection in the neonate. In S. L. Gardner, B. S. Carter, M. Enzman-Hines, & J. A. Hernandez (Eds.), *Merenstein & Gardner's handbook of neonatal intensive care* (7th ed.). St. Louis: Mosby.

Weiner, S. M., & Finnegan, L. P. (2011). Drug withdrawal in the neonate. In S. L. Gardner, B. S. Carter, M. Enzman-Hines, & J. A. Hernandez (Eds.), *Merenstein & Gardner's handbook of neonatal intensive care* (7th ed.). St. Louis: Mosby.

Wiegand, S. L., Stringer, E. M., Stuebe, A. M., et al. (2015). Buprenorphine and naloxone compared with methadone treatment in pregnancy. *Obstetrics & Gynecology, 125*(2), 363–368. doi:10.1097/AOG.0000000000000640.

Wilson, K. L., Zelig, C. M., Harvey, J. P., et al. (2011). Persistent pulmonary hypertension of the newborn is associated with mode of delivery and not with maternal use of selective serotonin reuptake inhibitors. *American Journal of Perinatology, 28*(1), 19–24.

World Health Organization. (2010). *Guidelines on HIV and infant feeding: Principles and recommendations for infant feeding in the context of HIV and a summary of evidence.* Geneva: Author. Retrieved from <http://whqlibdoc.who.int/publications/2010/9789241599535_eng.pdf>.

Yinon, Y., Farine, D., & Yudin, M. H. (2010). SOGC clinical practice guideline: Cytomegalovirus infection in pregnancy. *Journal of Obstetrics and Gynaecology Canada, 32*(4), 348–354.

Yudin, M., Koren, G., Farine, D., & Shrim, A. (2012). SOGC clinical practice guideline: Management of varicella infection (chicken pox) in pregnancy. *Journal of Obstetrics and Gynaecology Canada, 34*(3), 287–292.

Zlatunich, C. O., & Packman, S. (2005). Galactosaemia: Early treatment with an elemental formula. *Journal of Inherited Metabolic Disease, 28*, 163–168.

PART 3

Pediatric Nursing

8. Children, Their Families, and the Nurse
9. Assessment of the Child and Family
10. Health Promotion and Special Health Problems
11. Special Needs, Illness, and Hospitalization
12. Health Problems of Children

UNIT 8

Children, Their Families, and the Nurse

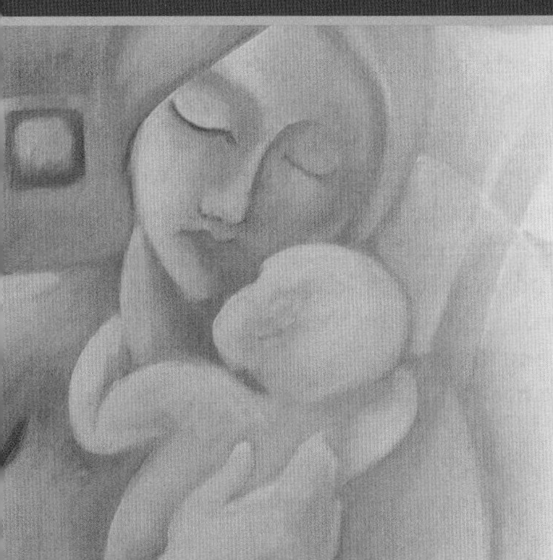

CHAPTER

30

Pediatric Nursing in Canada

Cheryl Sams

evolve WEBSITE

Visit the Evolve website for additional resources related to the content in this chapter such as Case Studies, Critical Thinking Case Study Answers, Nursing Care Plans, Nursing Processes, Nursing Skills, and Review Questions for Exam Preparation at: *http://evolve.elsevier.com/Canada/Perry/maternal/*

OBJECTIVES

On completion of this chapter the reader will be able to:

- Identify at least two ways in which knowledge of mortality and morbidity can improve child health.
- List three major causes of death during infancy, early childhood, later childhood, and adolescence.
- List two major causes of illness during childhood.
- Describe five broad functions of the pediatric nurse in promoting the health of children.
- Define the term *critical reasoning.*
- Identify the five steps of the nursing process.
- Define the term *nursing diagnosis.*
- Define *evidence-informed practice.*

HEALTH PROMOTION FOR CHILDREN

The pediatric nurse has a very important role in helping children and their families achieve optimum health. The major goal of pediatric nursing is to improve the quality of health care for children. When providing nursing care to children, it is essential that the pediatric nurse do so in the context of the family. To provide effective care, the pediatric nurse must develop a trusting and collaborative relationship with the child and family. Respect for social and cultural differences and beliefs is the cornerstone of high-quality pediatric care. Pediatric nursing is a challenging and rewarding career path. The practice of a pediatric nurse is based on both the science and art of nursing. Evidence-informed nursing care provides the scientific base, whereas the art of pediatric nursing care requires a strong sense of compassion and caring for children of all ages and stages and for their families. The qualities of an excellent pediatric nurse include creativity, effective communication skills, playfulness, patience, and resilience.

In 2011 there were approximately 5,607,345 children under the age of 14 living in Canada (Statistics Canada, 2012). The health of Canadian children has steadily improved over time with improvements such as the development of new vaccines, decreased tobacco smoking, and improved child health outcomes. For example, hospitalization rates for all causes for males and females 0 to 19 years of age declined between 2001/2002 and 2010/2011. For males there was a 15% decrease and for females a 16.1% decrease. Advancements in the quality of care and approaches to care, as well as health care reform, contributed to the decrease in hospitalizations (Canadian Institute of Child Health, 2015). The Canadian Institute of Child Health (CICH) (2015) reported that while Canadian children have relatively good health compared to children in other countries in the world, they still confront challenges to their health and well-being. These challenges differ according to gender and age group. In 2012 as in previous years, infants had the highest death rate among children and youth. Male infants had a higher death rate (5.1/1000) than that of female infants (4.6/1000) (Statistics Canada, 2015a). Between the ages of 1 and 14 years, death rates were consistently low and did not vary significantly between age groups. For youth 15 to 19 years of age, death rates were slightly higher, which is in part due to the rise in deaths caused by injuries in this age group (Statistics Canada, 2015a). Many factors, discussed in this and subsequent chapters, have played a role in this improvement and explain why more Canadian children are healthier.

In today's world, there are a myriad of technological advances that have helped to improve the health of children and their families. For example, researchers have significantly decreased mortality rates of childhood cancer and increased the survival rates of infant heart transplants. At the same time, this new technological world has also created many challenges that can have a negative impact on the health of children and their families. For example, global warming from increased industrialization has thinned the ozone layer, leading to a significant increase in the rate of skin cancer. Another example is higher levels of sedentary activity, related to an increase in the use of electronic devices (e.g., watching television, playing video games, surfing the Web); this trend has contributed to the higher rates of obesity and type 2 diabetes among children.

Another factor that affects children's health is family income level. The Canadian government has identified income level and socioeconomic status as having the greatest impact on health, with poverty having a significant detrimental effect on children's health. When children live in poverty they have less access to quality health care, live with food and housing insecurity, and receive inadequate maternal nutrition and prenatal care, resulting in a delay in early childhood development (Mikkonen & Raphael, 2010). While Canada's child poverty rate fell more than the poverty rate for the population as a whole during the past recession, in the 1990s until 2008, children in Canada remained more likely to be poor than the population as whole. The total population poverty rate remained at 18%. It was 5 points lower than the rate for child poverty in 2008 (23%), and in 2011 was still 2 points lower than that for child poverty (21%) (UNICEF Canada, 2014). Poverty levels are highest in the Indigenous and new immigrant populations of Canada.

In Canada, the medicare system provides health care for all of its legal residents (see Chapter 1). The government is gradually shifting the emphasis in health care from treatment of illnesses to health promotion and prevention. In order to promote good health, the many, complex influences on health need to be investigated and understood. To this end, the federal government has outlined the *social determinants of health* (see Table 1-1). These determinants provide a blueprint for health care policies and help direct population health research with the goal of improving health for its citizens (Public Health Agency of Canada [PHAC], 2011). Understanding of these health determinants is continuing to evolve as researchers discover more evidence to add to the Canadian health database.

In this third part of the textbook, we focus on the complex factors that influence health in the Canadian pediatric population, from the infant to the adolescent. The chapters in Part 3 provide foundational knowledge on how the determinants of health affect each age group. Topics addressed include assessment of the family and the child; health promotion and special health problems; special needs, illness, and hospitalization; and health problems of children. All of these topics are discussed in the context of pediatric nursing.

Health Promotion

The World Health Organization (WHO), Health and Welfare Canada, and the Canadian Public Health Agency (1986) developed the Ottawa Charter of Health Promotion in order to provide a health prevention focus for health care in Canada. The Charter defines *health promotion* as the process of enabling people to increase control over and improve their health. To reach a state of complete physical, mental, and social well-being, an individual or group must be able to identify and to realize goals, satisfy needs, and change or cope with the environment. Health promotion and disease prevention are important to optimizing the health of children and their families. Nurses who work with children and their families in a variety of health care settings promote health through teaching, modelling, and programming.

Many of the leading causes of death, disease, and disability—including cardiovascular disease, cancer, chronic lung diseases, depression, violence, substance use, injuries, nutritional deficiencies, and human immunodeficiency virus/acquired immunodeficiency syndrome (HIV/AIDS)—can be significantly reduced in children and adolescents through the prevention of six categories of behaviour (WHO, 2015):

1. Tobacco use
2. Behaviour that results in injury and violence
3. Alcohol and substance use
4. Dietary and hygienic practices that cause disease
5. Sedentary lifestyle
6. Sexual behaviour that causes unintended pregnancy and disease

Child health promotion opens up opportunities to reduce differences in health status among members of various groups and helps ensure that all children have equal opportunities and resources to achieve their fullest health potential.

Nutrition

Nutrition is an essential component for healthy growth and development, and its promotion begins at birth. Health Canada, the Canadian Paediatric Society (CPS), Dietitians of Canada, and Breastfeeding Committee for Canada (2015) recommend human milk as the preferred form of nutrition for all infants up to 2 years of age; other foods can be introduced at the 6-month mark. Breastfeeding provides the infant with micronutrients, immunological properties, and several enzymes that enhance digestion and absorption of these nutrients (see Chapter 27). There has been a resurgence in breastfeeding due to education of mothers and fathers regarding its benefits. Nonetheless, although not recommended, some mothers wean their infants early to avoid breast pumping during the workday and return to work early. Not all mothers can afford to take the 12-month government maternity leave.

Young children tend to establish eating habits during the first 2 to 3 years of life. The nurse can be instrumental in guiding parents in the selection of nutritious foods. During childhood, eating preferences and attitudes related to food habits are established by family influences and culture. During adolescence, parental influence diminishes as the adolescent makes food choices related to peer acceptability and sociability. Many current food choices are leading to an increased prevalence of chronic illnesses in childhood, such as diabetes, hypertension, and heart or renal disease. These diseases are occurring in higher numbers of children than ever before.

Given the scarcity of resources, children in families living in poverty are at most risk for experiencing unhealthy nutrient deficiencies, developmental and growth delays, depression, hunger, and behavioural problems. Fresh fruits and vegetables, milk, and other proteins are important nutritional resources that can be difficult for this population to obtain. For example, two Canadian groups at risk for food inadequacies are children in families without a home and families living in isolated Indigenous villages.

Dental Care

Oral health is an essential element of overall health. Dental caries is the single most common chronic disease of childhood (Rowan-Legg & CPS, 2013/2016). *Early childhood caries (ECC)* is defined as the occurrence of one or more decayed, missing (due to caries), or filled tooth surfaces in any primary tooth in a preschool-age child (Canadian Dental Association, 2010). Canadian children continue to have a high level of dental disease, which disproportionately affects lower socioeconomic groups, particularly Indigenous and new immigrant populations, who may have lower incomes (Rowan-Legg & CPS, 2013/2016). ECC in preschool children in some Indigenous communities exceeds 90% (Schroth, Harrison, & Moffatt, 2009).

Dental pain can have can have a destructive impact on children, including lost sleep, poor growth, behavioural concerns, and poor learning. Poor dental health also affects development of communication, socialization, and self-esteem (Rowan-Legg & CPS, 2013/2016). Dental complications are related to a significant decrease in school attendance and parent working days. The WHO has linked oral disease with the four leading chronic diseases: cardiovascular disease, cancer, chronic respiratory disease, and diabetes (WHO, 2012).

Since dental caries is a preventable disease, nursing plays an essential role in the promotion of early tooth care. Nurses can instruct children and their parents in dental hygiene, before the first tooth eruption; encourage them to drink fluoridated water, including bottled water; and promote early dental preventive care.

Dental care is not covered under the Canadian medicare program. However, individual provinces and territories have variable plans to cover dental care for families with low incomes. Indigenous peoples have federal government coverage for dental care which is determined on an individual basis, according to current oral health status, recipient history, and availability of treatment alternatives (Health Canada, 2014).

Immunizations

The two public health interventions that have had the greatest impact on world health are clean drinking water and vaccines. The Public Health Agency of Canada (PHAC) (2015a) has identified vaccination as one of the most important public health interventions provided to Canadians. Yet only 85% of Canada's children are vaccinated (UNICEF Canada, 2014). The PHAC (2015b) has sought to address the public's concerns about immunization myths and tracks outbreaks of vaccinated conditions. At each clinic visit a child's immunization record should be reviewed and parents should be instructed to keep immunizations current. Children's vaccines are generally paid for by the Canadian provincial and territorial governments (PHAC, 2012). The immunization schedule and types of vaccines vary between province and territories (see Additional Resources at the end this chapter).

CHILDHOOD HEALTH PROBLEMS

The health of Canada's children continues to improve in many areas, such as a decrease in pregnancy rates for adolescents and expanded vaccine coverage. However, changes in contemporary society, including disruptive social and economic influences on the family, and the increase in sedentary activity associated with use of current technologies, such as watching video games for long periods of time, are contributing to significant medical problems that affect the health of children. There is a large body of research indicating that a reduction in any type of sedentary time is related to a reduction in health risks in 5- to 17-year-olds (Tremblay, LeBlanc, Kho, et al., 2011). The researchers reported that daily TV viewing in excess of 2 hours is related to reduced physical and psychosocial health and that decreasing sedentary time results in a decrease in body mass index (BMI) (Tremblay et al., 2011).

Recent concern has focused on specific groups of children who tend to have increased morbidity: homeless and immigrant children; children living in poverty; Indigenous peoples; children in care of child services; low-birth-weight (LBW) children; children with chronic illnesses; and immigrant adopted children. A number of factors identified as determinants of health (PHAC, 2011), such as lower income and socioeconomic status, lack of social support networks, lack of education, environmental contaminants, and decreased access to health care (see Table 1-1), place these groups at risk for poor health. Also, while infants of very low birth weight (VLBW) have improved survival over that of previous decades, these children are twice as prone to having chronic lifelong health problems as children of normal weight (PHAC, 2011).

In addition to disease and injury, children face behavioural, social (family), and educational problems, referred to as the *new morbidity* or *pediatric social illness*. These adversities, such as poverty, violence, aggression, school failure, and adjustment to divorce or bereavement, can interfere with children's social and academic development. In addition, mental health issues cause challenges in childhood and adolescence. Examples of challenges to pediatric health that are on the rise include obesity, type 2 diabetes, injuries, violence, and substance use.

Obesity and Type 2 Diabetes

Childhood obesity is the most common nutritional problem among Canadian children and is increasing at epidemic proportions, as is type 2 diabetes. The WHO has ranked Canada 27th in childhood obesity (Health Canada, 2009).

The rate of childhood obesity in Canada has tripled since 1975 (Ontario Ministry of Health Promotion and Sport, 2010).

TABLE 30-1 CHILDREN'S PERCENTILE AND WEIGHT CATEGORY

PERCENTILE	WEIGHT CATEGORY
For Children Aged 2–4 Years	
Below third percentile	Risk for underweight
Third percentile to below 85th percentile	Healthy weight
85th to 97th percentile	Risk for overweight
Above the 97th to 99.9th percentile	Overweight
Above the 99.9th percentile	Obese
For 5- to 19-Year-Olds	
Below third percentile	Risk for underweight
Third percentile to below 85th percentile	Healthy weight
85th to 97th percentile	Overweight
Above the 97th percentile to 99.9th percentile	Obese
Above the 99.9th percentile	Severely Obese

Adapted from Dietitians of Canada. (2015). *BMI for children/teens.* Retrieved from http://www.dietitians.ca/Your-Health/Assess-Yourself/Assess-Your-BMI/BMI-Children.aspx

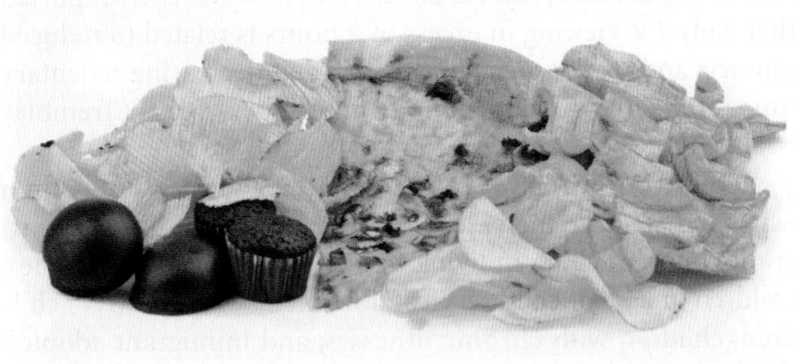

FIGURE 30-1 The Canadian cultural tendency toward excessive intake of high-caloric, fatty foods contributes to obesity in children. (Anidimi/Shutterstock.com.)

In Canada, children's basal metabolic index and rate of growth are measured using growth charts developed by the WHO, CPS, and the Canadian Dietitians of Canada (Dietitians of Canada, 2015) (see Appendix C for measurement charts). These growth charts are gender and age specific and are used because they measure the changes in the amount of body fat as children grow (Table 30-1).

The levels of obesity vary across the different ethnic groups. Research has shown that Indigenous populations have the highest level of obesity among all ethnicities in Canada for child and adult age groups (Katzmarzyk, 2008).

Preventing obesity is an important focus for Health Canada and its Healthy Canadians program (Fig. 30-1). Statistics Canada (2015b) reports that WHO and Canadian guidelines recommend that, for health benefits, children (aged 5 to 11) and youth (aged 12 to 17) accumulate at least 60 minutes of moderate-to-vigorous-intensity activity daily. Just under 7% of Canadian children and youth achieve the guideline of 60 minutes of moderate to vigorous physical activity per day at least 6 days a week. Significantly higher percentages accumulate 30 minutes per day on at least 6 days a week, and these averages increase significantly for activity at least 3 days a week (Statistics Canada, 2015b). One factor that contributes to obesity among children is the lack of outdoor physical activity because neighbourhood environments are unsafe and facilities for activities are in inconvenient locations. Another is the easy access to video games and television within the home and lack of viewing limits. The CPS recommends that electronic media time be limited to 2 hours per day for older children. Canadian children watch television, talk online, or play virtual games for about 6 hours every weekday and 7 hours on the weekend (Ontario Ministry of Health Promotion and Sport, 2010). Nurses can play an important role in prevention of obesity as they can teach health promotion strategies to families and their children to help reduce the number of overweight children.

Childhood Injuries

Injuries are the most common cause of death and disability among children in Canada (Pike, Richmond, & Rothman, et al., 2015). Unintentional injuries are the leading cause of death for Canadian children ages 1 to 14; injury accounts for more deaths than all other causes combined. See Table 30-2 for the rates and causes of injuries and hospitalizations among Canadian children. Indigenous people have a 26% injury mortality rate for all age groups compared to 6% for the rest of the country (Banerji & CPS First Nations, Inuit and Métis Health Committee, 2012/2015). While the major causes of injury-related deaths in children aged 0 to 14 years are mostly preventable, Canada still does not have a national injury prevention strategy for children and youth, which could help reduce childhood injuries (Health Canada, 2009).

The WHO has reported that rates of unintentional injuries are high across the world. According to Health Canada (2009), Canada ranks twenty-second out of 29 Organization for Economic Co-operation and Development (OECD) nations when it comes to preventable childhood injuries and deaths. The WHO (2008) has indicated that if high-income countries were to plan and implement programs using proven effective strategies that addressed the special vulnerabilities of children, more than a thousand children's lives would be saved each day.

The type of injury and the circumstances surrounding it are closely related to normal growth and developmental behaviour. As children develop, their innate curiosity impels them to investigate activities and to mimic the behaviour of others. While it is essential to acquire competency in this trait as an adult, it predisposes children to numerous hazards. Injury prevention through different ages will be discussed in the chapters on developmental stages.

The pattern of deaths caused by unintentional injuries, especially from motor vehicles, drowning, and burns, is remarkably consistent in most Western societies. Fortunately, prevention strategies such as the use of car restraints, bicycle helmets, and smoke and carbon monoxide detectors have resulted in a significant decrease in fatalities among children. The Government of Canada has enacted safety regulations for motor vehicles and booster seat safety that require manufacturers to modify car seats and booster seats to improve the safety level. When used correctly, child car seats reduce the risk of fatal injury by 71%

TABLE 30-2 MAJOR CAUSES OF UNINTENTIONAL INJURY DEATHS AND HOSPITALIZATION AMONG CANADIAN CHILDREN AGES 0–19 YEARS, 2007–2009

LEADING CAUSES OF UNINTENTIONAL INJURY DEATHS FOR 2007 BY AGE GROUP				
UNDER 1 YEAR	**1 TO 4 YEARS**	**5 TO 9 YEARS**	**10 TO 14 YEARS**	**15 TO 19 YEARS**
Threat to breathing (54%)	Motor vehicle traffic crash (22%)	Motor vehicle traffic crash (58%)	Motor vehicle traffic crash (55%)	Motor vehicle traffic crash (71%)
Motor vehicle traffic crash (18%)	Drowning (21%)	Drowning, fall, fire/flame (6% each)	Drowning (13%)	Poisoning (7%)
Drowning (15%)	Threat to breathing (19%)	Threat to breathing (5%)	Fall (7%)	Drowning (6%)
LEADING CAUSES OF UNINTENTIONAL INJURY HOSPITALIZATIONS FOR 2008/2009 BY AGE GROUP				
UNDER 1 YEAR	**1 TO 4 YEARS**	**5 TO 9 YEARS**	**10 TO 14 YEARS**	**15 TO 19 YEARS**
Fall (46%)	Fall (39%)	Fall (56%)	Fall (39%)	Fall (24%)
Threat to breathing, Fire/Hot object/substance (6% each)	Poisoning (15%)	Struck by/against an obstacle, Pedal cyclist non-traffic (7% each)	Struck by/against an obstacle (15%)	Motor vehicle traffic crash (21%)
Poisoning (5%)	Fire/Hot object/substance (7%)	Motor vehicle traffic crash (7%)	Motor vehicle traffic crash, Pedal cyclist non-traffic (8% each)	Struck by/against an obstacle (14%)

Source: Yanchar, N. L., Warda, L. J., Fuselli, P., Canadian Paediatric Society, et al. (2012). Child and youth injury prevention: A public health approach. *Paediatric & Child Health 17*(9), 511. Retrieved from http://www.cps.ca/documents/position/child-and-youth-injury-prevention

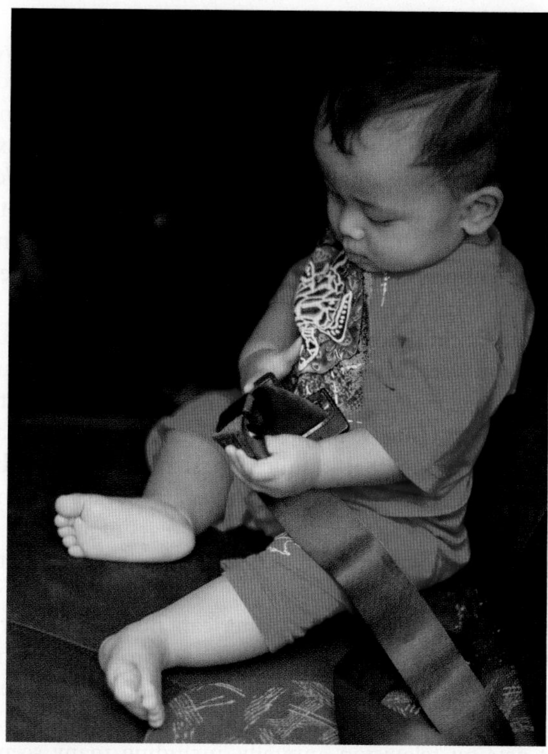

FIGURE 30-2 Motor vehicle injuries are the leading cause of death in children older than 1 year of age. Despite mandatory-seatbelt legislation, some children still remain unrestrained and are at higher risk of injuries. (manzrussali/Shutterstock.com.)

and the risk of serious injury by 67% (Van Schaik & CPS Injury Prevention Committee, 2008) (Fig. 30-2). Transport Canada's National Collision Database (NCDB) indicated that in 2013 the number of fatalities, serious injuries, and total injuries decreased and that in 2013 the lowest counts for all three of these casualty groups were recorded since these data were first collected in the early 1970s (Transport Canada, 2013). For more information regarding car seat safety tips and legislation see Additional Resources at the end of the chapter and the developmental stages chapters.

Pedestrian injuries among children account for significant numbers of motor vehicle–related deaths. Most pedestrian injuries occur at midblock, at intersections, in driveways, and in parking lots. Driveway injuries typically involve small children and large vehicles backing up. Parents may not be alert to the dangers leading to such injuries and consequently fail to protect their children.

Bicycle injuries are another significant cause of childhood deaths. Children ages 5 to 9 years are at greatest risk of bicycling fatalities. Most bicycling deaths are from head injuries. Helmet use reduces the risk of head injury by 85% (Rivara & Grossman, 2015). Community-wide bicycle helmet use campaigns and mandatory-use laws have resulted in significant increases in helmet use. Still, issues such as stylishness, comfort, and social acceptability remain important factors in whether children will actually wear a helmet. Children ages 10 to 14 are those most likely not to wear helmets (Parachute, n.d.).

Nurses can educate children and their families about pedestrian and bicycle safety. In particular, community nurses can promote helmet wearing and encourage peer leaders to act as role models. When parents wear helmets, their children are more likely to wear them (Parachute, n.d.).

Drowning, suffocation, and burns are also leading causes of death throughout childhood (Fig. 30-3). During infancy, more males succumb to death from aspiration or suffocation than do females (Fig. 30-4). The leading cause of unintentional poisoning in children under 5 years of age is medication **ingestion**, although household cleaners and personal care products are also ingested (Government of Canada, 2014) (Fig. 30-5). The Canadian Association of Poison Control Centres reports that

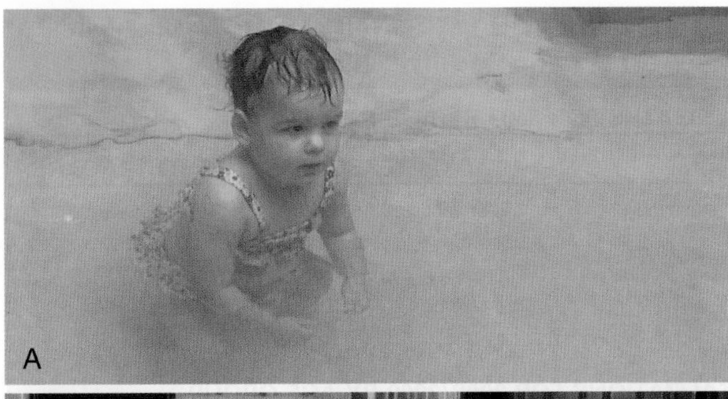

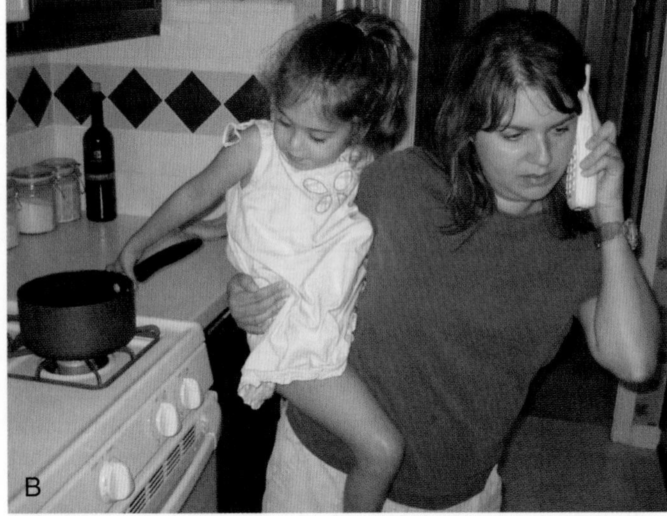

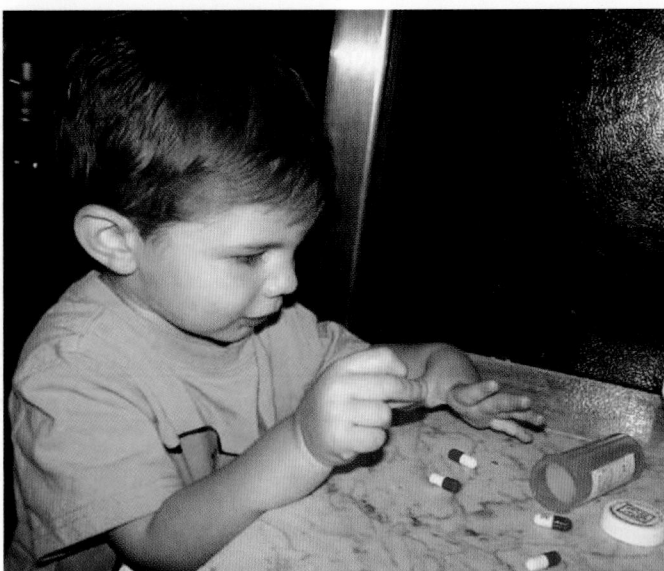

FIGURE 30-3 **A:** Drowning is one of the leading causes of death among children. Children left unattended are unsafe even in shallow water. **B:** Burns are among the top three leading causes of death from injury in children ages 1 to 14 years.

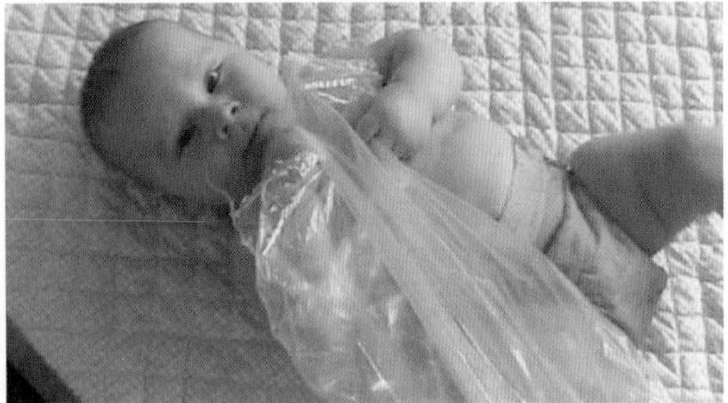

FIGURE 30-4 Suffocation is the leading cause of death from injury in infants.

FIGURE 30-5 Poisoning causes a considerable number of injuries in children under 4 years of age. Prescription medications should never be left where young children can reach them.

their centres receive thousands of calls regarding unintentional poisonings every year.

Violence

Children are one of the more vulnerable populations in the context of violence. Violence against children most commonly occurs within the family. In 2008, there were 236,842 child maltreatment and neglect investigations carried out by children's services in Canada. From 1998 to 2003, there was an increase of 100,000 investigations; this rate then levelled off, without a further increase between 2003 and 2008. The major reasons for these investigations were neglect (34%) and exposure to domestic violence (34%) (Canadian Child Welfare Research Portal, 2011). Indigenous children continue to be overrepresented in Canadian child services organizations, as found in a comparison study of Indigenous and non-Indigenous children (MacLaurin, Trocmé, Fallon, et al., 2011).

In Canada, child homicides rates are on the decline. In 2009, 34 homicides were committed against children and youth under 18 years of age, compared to 20 homicides in 2013 (Statistics Canada, 2011). Usually, physical force such as strangulation, beating, or shaking that resulted in shaken baby syndrome was used against children under 6 years of age. Homicide victims in the older age group of 7 to 17 years of age were most frequently killed by a weapon (e.g., knife or firearm) (Statistics Canada, 2011).

Violence permeates North American households through the violent images portrayed in television programs, commercials, video games, and movies, which tend to desensitize children toward violence. The average Canadian child sees 12,000 violent acts on television annually, including many scenes of murder and rape. Canada was one of the first countries to research this issue; Canadian researchers identified that children's exposure to media violence early in the school year predicted higher verbally aggressive behaviour, higher relationally aggressive behaviour, higher physically aggressive behaviour, and less prosocial behaviour later in the school year (Gentile, Coyne, & Walsh, 2011).

The number of Canadian young offenders (ages 12 to 17) has declined by 23% since 2002/2003. Youth courts in Canada processed 48,000 cases in 2011/2012, which is down 10% from the previous year and marks the lowest number of cases completed in youth courts since data were collected nationally in 1991/1992. All types of completed youth court cases declined in 2011/2012. Some of the largest declines were for theft, breaking and entering, and major assault cases. There was an increase in drug possession and in other drug crimes involving theft (Statistics Canada, 2013).

This decrease in the number of youth offenders has taken place since enactment of the *Youth Criminal Justice Act*, which diverts minor crimes away from the criminal court system and usually involves community service for the young offender found guilty (Statistics Canada, 2013). Despite this decrease in the youth crime rate, however, assessment of high-risk behaviours in youth must continue to be a major focus of health promotion.

Pediatric nurses can assess children and adolescents for risk related to violence. For instance, families that own firearms must be educated about their safe use and storage. A home with a gun is five times more likely to be a scene of a suicide than a home without a gun and increases the risk of homicide (Canada Safety Council, 2011). The suicide risk is higher in Indigenous communities, where there are more firearms in homes (Health Canada, 2010). In Canada, suicide prevention experts have emphasized the importance of stronger gun laws, which have successfully reduced suicide rates overall, particularly those for youth (Gagné, 2008). Canadian gun law efforts have focused on preventing specific groups, such as felons and children, from having access to firearms (Canada Safety Council, 2011). Technological changes such as childproof safety devices, safer storage, and loading indicators could improve the safety of firearms.

Substance Use

Risk-taking behaviours, particularly among males, tend to begin in the first decade of life and continue into adolescence with drinking of alcohol while driving, speeding, or using illicit drugs. In children and young adults, alcohol and illicit drug use occurs most commonly between ages 12 and 24 and is associated with violence and injury. In a 2008 survey, the age of first use of alcohol was 15.6 years of age and those under age 25 had five times the number of heavy drinking episodes in the 25 or older age group. The average age of starting to use cannabis was 15.5 years and those under age 25 were much heavier users than the 25-year-olds (Narconon International, 2015). Recent surveys indicate that over one-third of Canadian students in grades 7 to 9 had binged on alcohol. Over 40% of 15- to 19-year-olds had binged on alcohol at least once in the past year and had binged 12 or more times in the past year. While tobacco smoking rates among adolescents have decreased, cannabis rates still remain high. Nonetheless, in grades 5 to 9, 19% of students had tried smoking a cigarette, and 2% smoked daily (Narconon International, 2015).

Substance use is a major health problem in Canada. Early substance use and hazardous drug ingestion during adolescence can lead to the development of serious long-term problems in adulthood, such as **addiction**. Evolving research in this age group suggests that some adolescents use substances to help cope with difficult environments, untreated trauma, and underlying psychological conditions. Alcohol, tobacco, and cannabis are most commonly used. Hallucinogenic drugs such as psilocybin and mescaline are next in line, with 10% of middle- and high-school students reporting use. Among Western nations, Canada has the highest rates of alcohol and cannabis use in the 12- to 24-year-old age groups (United Nations Office on Drugs and Crime, 2011). Alcohol is the most commonly used substance and is a major factor in causing injury and death, such as in motor vehicle accidents.

Mental Health Concerns

There are many children and youth in Canada who have mental health problems; as many as 15%, or 1.2 million, Canadian children are affected by anxiety, attention deficit, depression, addiction, autism spectrum disorders, behavioural disorders, eating disorders, and schizophrenia, as well as other mental health issues. Mental illness in this age group is often the beginning of an adult mental illness. Mental health issues, such as developmental, emotional, and behavioural disorders, have a direct and significant impact on families and caregivers. Nurses play an important role in helping children and their families identify early signs of mental illness and psychological stressors. Teaching the child and the family resiliency strategies can help them deal with some of the stress. Unfortunately, there are many gaps in service and long waits for services for this population (Zayed, Davidson, Nadeau, et al., 2016). Canada needs a national program to coordinate the various mental health services.

Suicide among children and youth remains a serious issue in Canada. Suicide is the second leading cause of death among youth in Canada and one of the top three causes of death among youth worldwide. Each year, 2 out of every 100,000 children aged 10 to 14 years commit suicide. For adolescents aged 15 to 19 years, the rate increases to 10 of every 100,000 children, with substantial variation across provinces and territories (Kutcher & Szumilas, 2008). These statistics mean that 256 young Canadians die every year from suicide. In addition to these children, there are many more individuals in these age groups who contemplate or attempt suicide. Untreated mental disorder, the most important risk factor for suicide, is present in as many as 90% of adolescent suicide victims (Kutcher & Szumilas, 2008). Depression is one of the more common factors and occurs in 60% of suicides and in 40 to 80% of adolescents who have suicidal ideation or have attempted suicide (Renaud, Séguin, Lesage, et al., 2014). Substance use and conduct disorder are often present in youth suicides, particularly among boys (Kutcher & Szumilas, 2008). In order to reduce the suicide rate in this young population, it is important to treat and prevent mental health disorders. Another cause of adolescent suicide is bullying. Health Canada provides bullying prevention programs (see Additional Resources at the end of this chapter).

In British Columbia and Ontario, the Indigenous suicide rate varies from 5 to 20 times higher than that of the general population. Researchers found that some of the Indigenous bands had rates as high as 800 times the national average, but more than half had no youth suicides between 1987 and 2000. The research showed that strong cultural continuity of the band, including women leaders; pursuit of land claims; culture-designated buildings; and community control of child services, lowering of fostering rates, band school, band health, and fire and police services protected the band from youth suicide (Chandler & Lalonde, 2009). Lesbian, gay, bisexual, and transgender youth face 14 times the risk for suicide and have higher rates of suicidality according to the Canadian Mental Health Association (n.d.).

Suicide is a preventable occurrence, placing a heavy burden on nurses to identify the at-risk child or adolescent who may display mental health and emotional problems. More completely integrated medical and mental health services for children and adolescents are needed. Early identification and treatment of mental illness are important ways in which to assist in suicide prevention (Korczak & CPS, 2015). Mental health issues affecting youth will be covered in more detail in Chapters 38, 39, and 50.

Childhood Mortality

Figures describing rates of occurrence of events such as death among children are referred to as *vital statistics*. *Mortality statistics* describe the incidence, or number of individuals who have died over a specific period. These statistics are usually presented as rates per 1000 and are calculated from a sample of death certificates. Statistics Canada, under the auspices of the federal government, is responsible for the collection, analysis, and dissemination of data on the health of the Canadian people.

Over the past 50 years, the mortality rate for children that die before reaching the age of 5 has significantly decreased in Canada. In 1960, the mortality rate for this group was 32.6 per 1000, and from 2011 to 2015 it dropped to 6.1 per 1000 (World Bank, 2016).

From a worldwide perspective, however, Canada lags behind other nations in reducing infant mortality. In 2014, Canada had the forty-second lowest **infant mortality rate** out of 222 nations. The top three ranked countries with the three lowest rates are Monaco, Japan, and Bermuda (Index Mundi, 2015). Researchers suggest that Canada has had an increase in higher-risk births because of success in delivery of early **preterm infants** and more multiple births occurring from fertility programs. There is also variation in how countries define the parameters of low birth weight and in registration of births and deaths (Conference Board of Canada, 2011). Overall, the rate of infant mortality has remained stable and has remained very low (five deaths per thousand live births) over the past decade (PHAC, 2014).

Birth weight is considered the major determinant of newborn death in technologically developed countries; there is a definite relationship between birth weight and infant morbidity and mortality. Access to and use of high-quality prenatal care is the single most important preventive strategy to decrease early delivery and infant mortality rates.

Many of the leading causes of death during infancy are due to issues that occur during the perinatal period. Congenital anomalies and preterm birth are the first two causes of infant death. The overall Canadian birth **congenital** anomaly prevalence rate between 1998 and 2009 has decreased from 451 to 385 per 10,000 births while the number of preterm births has increased (PHAC, 2013).

This decline in anomalies is likely due to increased prenatal diagnosis and subsequent pregnancy termination; implemented measures such as folic acid fortification in food; and changes in health behaviours and practices to reduce the risk for some congenital anomalies (e.g., tobacco smoking cessation and multivitamin use). The report also points to maternal obesity as an important emerging risk factor for some congenital anomalies, while noting that alcohol use and smoking during pregnancy remain key risks that require ongoing public health measures for prevention and prevalence reduction of such anomalies.

Childhood Morbidity

Measurements of the prevalence of specific illnesses in the population at a particular time are known as *morbidity statistics*, generally presented as rates per 1000 population because of their **frequency** of occurrence. Unlike mortality, morbidity is difficult to define and may denote acute illness, chronic disease, or disability. Sources of data for morbidity statistics include documented reasons for visits to physicians, recorded diagnoses qualifying for hospital admission, and household interviews. Unlike death rates, which are updated annually, morbidity statistics are revised less frequently and may not represent actual prevalence of specific illnesses in the general population.

Acute illness is defined as symptoms severe enough to limit activity or require medical attention. Respiratory illness accounts for the majority of all acute conditions; infections, parasitic disease, and injuries are also leading causes of disease. The common cold is the illness that occurs most frequently.

The types of diseases that children contract during childhood vary according to age. For example, incidence of upper respiratory tract infections and diarrhea decreases with age, but other disorders such as acne and headaches increase in occurrence. Children who have had a particular type of problem are more likely to have that problem again. Morbidity is not distributed randomly among children.

THE ART OF PEDIATRIC NURSING

Philosophy of Care

Pediatric nursing in Canada follows the practice guidelines and standards set by the Canadian Nurses Association (CNA) and the individual provincial and territorial regulatory bodies.

The Hospital for Sick Children (Sick Kids) (2011) in Toronto is an example of a tertiary pediatric centre that has developed a pediatric nursing philosophy that integrates Canadian nursing practice standards, as follows:

- Staff are committed to achieving the highest level of nursing care for children and their families.
- The diversity of the community and uniqueness of each individual child and family are recognized and respected.
- Through partnerships and collaboration, nurses strive to promote and restore optimal health and to assist children and families to effectively adjust to health challenges.

- A work environment is fostered in which excellence and innovation in practice, education, and research are valued.
- Nursing knowledge, skills, and judgement are used to provide safe, competent, and high-quality care.
- The Centre for Nursing (CFN) fosters a world-class environment for nursing excellence through its leadership, professional support, spirit of inquiry, and innovation. The CFN is dedicated to providing world-class leadership in nursing practice, education, research, and technology.

Family-Centred Care

The philosophy of family-centred care recognizes the family as the one constant in a child's life. The core concepts of family-centred care include supporting, respecting, encouraging, and enhancing the family's strength and competence by developing a collaborative and information-sharing partnership with parents. Nurses support families in their natural caregiving and decision-making roles by building on families' unique strengths and acknowledging their expertise in caring for their child both within and outside the hospital setting. The needs of all family members, not just the child's, are considered (Box 30-1). Family-centred care addresses the diversity among family structures and backgrounds; family goals, dreams, strategies, and actions; and family support, service, and information needs. It is essential that the pediatric nurse work within the framework of family-centred care. See Additional Resources on family-centred care at the end of the chapter.

The two outcomes favoured in family-centred care are enabling and empowerment. Health care providers enable families by creating opportunities for all family members to carry out their current abilities and competencies and to acquire new ones that are necessary for meeting the needs of the child and family. Empowerment involves interaction of health care providers with families in a way that assists families to maintain or acquire a sense of control over their lives and make positive changes through the fostering of their own strengths, abilities, and actions (Institute for Patient- and Family-Centered Care, 2011).

BOX 30-1 KEY ELEMENTS OF FAMILY-CENTRED CARE

Incorporating into policy and practice the recognition that the family is the constant in a child's life while the service systems and support personnel within those systems fluctuate

Facilitating family–provider collaboration at all levels of hospital, home, and community care:
- Care of an individual child
- Program development, implementation, and evaluation
- Policy formation

Exchanging complete and unbiased information between family members and health care providers in a supportive manner at all times

Incorporating into policy and practice the recognition and honouring of cultural diversity, strengths, and individuality within and across all families, including ethnic, racial, spiritual, social, economic, educational, and geographical diversity

Recognizing and respecting different methods of coping and implementing comprehensive policies and programs that provide developmental, educational, emotional, environmental, and financial support to meet the diverse needs of families

Encouraging and facilitating family-to-family support and networking

Ensuring that home, hospital, and community service and support systems for children needing specialized health and developmental care and their families are flexible, accessible, and comprehensive in responding to diverse family-identified needs

Appreciating families as families and children as children, recognizing that they possess a wide range of strengths, concerns, emotions, and aspirations beyond their need for specialized health and developmental services and support

From Shelton, T. L., & Stepanek, J. S. (1994). *Family-centred care for children needing specialized health and developmental services.* Bethesda, MD: Association for the Care of Children's Health.

Critical Thinking

A systematic thought process is essential to the nursing profession. It assists the professional in meeting the patient's needs. *Critical thinking* is purposeful, goal-directed thinking that assists individuals in making judgements based on evidence rather than on guesswork (Alfaro-LeFevre, 2005). It is based on the scientific method of inquiry, which is also the root of the nursing process. Critical thinking and the nursing process are considered crucial to professional nursing in that they constitute a holistic approach to problem solving.

Critical thinking is a complex developmental process based on rational and deliberate thought. In becoming a critical thinker one has a common denominator for knowledge that exemplifies disciplined and self-directed thinking. The knowledge is acquired, assessed, and organized by thinking through the clinical situation and developing an outcome focused on optimum patient care. The cognitive skills used in high-quality thinking include intellectual discipline, self-evaluation, creativity, persistence, risk taking, and intuition (Ignatavicius, 2001). Critical thinking transforms the way in which individuals view themselves, understand the world, and make decisions.

Evidence-Informed Practice

Evidence-informed practice (EIP) is the collection, interpretation, and integration of valid, important, and applicable patient-reported, nurse-observed, and research-derived information. Evidence-informed nursing practice combines knowledge with clinical experience and intuition. It provides a rational approach to decision making that facilitates best practice. EIP is an important tool that complements the nursing process by using critical thinking skills to make decisions based on existing knowledge. The traditional nursing process approach to patient care (discussed further in the next section) can be used to conceptualize the essential components of evidence-informed nursing.

During the assessment and diagnostic (first and second) phases of the nursing process, the nurse establishes important clinical questions and completes a critical review of existing knowledge. EIP also begins with identification of the problem. The nurse asks clinical questions in a concise, organized way that elicits clear answers. Once the specific questions are identified, extensive searching for the best information to answer the question begins. The nurse evaluates clinically relevant research, analyzes findings from the history and physical examinations, and reviews the specific pathophysiology of the defined problem. The third step in the nursing process is to develop a care plan. In evidence-informed nursing practice, the care plan is established after a critical appraisal of what is known and not known about the defined problem. Next, in the traditional nursing process, the nurse implements the care plan. By integrating evidence with clinical expertise, the nurse focuses care on the patient's unique needs. The final step in EIP is consistent with the final phase of the nursing process: evaluating the effectiveness of the care plan.

Nursing Process

The *nursing process* is a method of problem identification and problem solving that describes what the nurse actually does. The five-step nursing process model involves assessment, diagnosis (problem identification), planning (with outcome development), implementation, and evaluation. Although documentation is not one of the five steps of the nursing process, it is essential for evaluation. All of these activities will be discussed in detail as they are practised in pediatric nursing care for specific disorders presented in subsequent chapters.

Atraumatic Care

Atraumatic care is the provision of therapeutic care in settings, by personnel, and through the use of interventions that eliminate or minimize the psychological and physical distress experienced by children and their families in the health care system. *Therapeutic care* encompasses the prevention, diagnosis, treatment, and palliation of chronic or acute conditions. *Setting* refers to whatever place in which care is given—the home, the hospital, or any other health care setting. *Personnel* include anyone directly involved in providing therapeutic care. *Interventions* range from psychological approaches, such as preparing children for procedures, to physical interventions, such as providing space for a parent to room in with a child. *Psychological distress* may include anxiety, fear, anger, disappointment, sadness, shame, or guilt. *Physical distress* may range from sleeplessness and immobilization to disturbing sensory stimuli such as pain, temperature extremes, loud noises, bright lights, or darkness. Thus atraumatic care is concerned with the who, what, when, where, why, and how of any procedure performed on a child, for the purpose of preventing or minimizing psychological and physical stress.

The overriding goal in providing atraumatic care is first, *do no harm*. Three principles constitute the framework for achieving this goal: (1) prevent or minimize the child's separation from the family; (2) promote a sense of control; and (3) prevent or minimize bodily injury and pain. Examples of atraumatic care include fostering the parent–child relationship during hospitalization, preparing the child before any unfamiliar treatment or procedure, controlling pain, allowing the child privacy, providing play activities for expression of fear and aggression, offering choices to children, and respecting cultural differences.

Role of the Pediatric Nurse

Pediatric nurses are involved in every aspect of a child's and family's growth and development. Nursing functions vary according to regional job structures, individual education and experience, and personal career goals. Just as patients (children and their families) have unique backgrounds, each nurse brings an individual set of variables that affect the nurse–patient relationship. No matter where pediatric nurses practise, their primary concern is the welfare of the child and family.

Therapeutic Relationship

The establishment of a therapeutic relationship is the essential foundation for providing high-quality nursing care. Pediatric nurses need to have meaningful relationships with the children and families they encounter and yet remain separate enough to distinguish their own feelings and needs. In a therapeutic relationship, caring, well-defined boundaries separate the nurse from the child and family. These boundaries are positive and professional and promote the family's control over the child's health care. For effective family advocacy to occur, these boundaries need to be established and therapeutic relationships promoted. Both the nurse and the family are empowered, and open communication is maintained. In a nontherapeutic relationship, these boundaries are blurred, and many of the nurse's actions may serve personal needs, such as a need to feel wanted and involved, rather than the family's needs.

Exploring whether relationships with patients are therapeutic or nontherapeutic can help nurses identify problem areas early in their interactions with children and families. Although questions for exploring types of involvement can be labelled negative or positive, no one action makes a relationship therapeutic or nontherapeutic. For example, nurses may spend additional time with the family but still recognize their own needs and maintain professional separateness. An important clue to nontherapeutic relationships is the staff's concerns about their peer's actions with the family. See Guidelines box for building relationships with children and families.

Family Advocacy and Caring

Although nurses are responsible to themselves, the profession, and the institution of employment, their primary responsibility is to the consumer of nursing services—the child and the family. The nurse must work with family members, identify their goals and needs, and plan interventions that meet the defined problems. As an advocate, the nurse assists children and their families in making informed choices and acting in the child's best interest. Advocacy involves ensuring that families are aware of all available health services, informed of treatments and procedures, involved in the child's care, and encouraged to change or support existing health care practices. The United Nations

GUIDELINES

Building Your Relationships With Children and Families

To foster therapeutic relationships with children and families, you must first become aware of your caregiving style, including how effectively you take care of yourself. The following questions should help you understand the therapeutic quality of your professional relationships.

Negative Actions

- Are you overinvolved with children and their families?
- Do you work overtime to care for the family?
- Do you spend off-duty time with children's families, either in or out of the hospital?
- Do you call frequently (either the hospital or home) to see how the family is doing?
- Do you show favouritism toward certain patients?
- Do you buy clothes, toys, food, or other items for the child and family?
- Do you compete with other staff members for the affection of certain patients and families?
- Do other staff members comment to you about your closeness to the family?
- Do you attempt to influence families' decisions rather than facilitate their informed decision making?
- Are you underinvolved with children and families?
- Do you restrict parent or visitor access to children, using excuses such as the unit is too busy?
- Do you focus on the technical aspects of care and lose sight of the person who is the patient?
- Are you overinvolved with children and underinvolved with their parents?
- Do you become critical when parents do not visit their children?
- Do you compete with parents for their children's affection?

Positive Actions

- Do you strive to empower families?
- Do you explore families' strengths and needs in an effort to increase family involvement?
- Have you developed teaching skills to instruct families rather than doing everything for them?
- Do you work with families to find ways to decrease their dependence on health care providers?
- Can you separate families' needs from your own needs?
- Do you strive to empower yourself?
- Are you aware of your emotional responses to different people and situations?
- Do you seek to understand how your own family experiences influence reactions to patients and families, especially as they affect tendencies toward overinvolvement or underinvolvement?
- Do you have a calming influence, not one that will amplify emotionality?
- Have you developed interpersonal skills in addition to technical skills?
- Have you learned about ethnic and religious family patterns?
- Do you communicate directly with persons with whom you are upset or take issue?
- Are you able to "step back" and withdraw emotionally, if not physically, when emotional overload occurs, yet remain committed?
- Do you take care of yourself and your needs?
- Do you periodically interview family members to determine their current issues (e.g., feelings, attitudes, responses, wishes), communicate these findings to peers, and update records?
- Do you avoid relying on initial interview data, assumptions, or gossip regarding families?
- Do you ask questions if families are not participating in care?
- Do you assess families for feelings of anxiety, fear, intimidation, worry about making a mistake, a perceived lack of competence to care for their child, or fear of health care providers overstepping their boundaries into family territory, or vice versa?
- Do you explore these issues with family members and provide encouragement and support to enable families to help themselves?
- Do you keep communication channels open among self, family, physicians, and other care providers?
- Do you resolve conflicts and misunderstandings directly with those who are involved?
- Do you clarify information for families or seek the appropriate person to do so?
- Do you recognize that from time to time a therapeutic relationship can change to a social relationship or an intimate friendship?
- Are you able to acknowledge the fact when it occurs and understand why it happened?
- Can you ensure that there is someone else who is more objective who can take your place in the therapeutic relationship?

Declaration of the Rights of the Child (Box 30-2) provides guidelines for nursing practice that can be used to ensure that every child receives optimum care. The nurse can use this knowledge to adapt care for the child's physical and emotional well-being.

As nurses care for children and families, they must demonstrate caring, compassion, and empathy for others. Aspects of caring embody the concepts of atraumatic care and the development of a therapeutic relationship with patients. Parents perceive caring as a sign of high-quality nursing care, which is often focused on the nontechnical needs of the child and family. Parents describe "personable" care as actions by the nurse that include acknowledging the parents' presence, listening, making the parents feel comfortable, involving both the parents and the child in care, showing interest and concern for their welfare, showing affection and sensitivity to the parent and child, communicating with them, and individualizing the nursing care. Parents perceive personable nursing care as an integral part of a positive relationship.

Disease Prevention and Health Promotion

Every nurse involved with child care must understand the importance of disease prevention and health promotion. A nursing care plan must include a thorough assessment of all aspects of child growth and development, including nutrition, immunizations, safety, dental care, socialization, discipline, and education. If problems are identified, the nurse can intervene directly or refer the family to other health care providers or agencies.

The best approach to prevention is education and anticipatory guidance. An appreciation of the hazards or conflicts of each developmental period enables the nurse to guide

BOX 30-2 UNITED NATIONS DECLARATION OF THE RIGHTS OF THE CHILD

All children need:
- To be free from discrimination
- To develop physically and mentally in freedom and dignity
- To have a name and nationality
- To have adequate nutrition, housing, recreation, and medical services
- To receive special treatment, if handicapped
- To receive love, understanding, and material security
- To receive an education and to develop their abilities
- To be the first to receive protection in disaster
- To be protected from neglect, cruelty, and exploitation
- To be brought up in a spirit of friendship among people

parents regarding child-rearing practices aimed at preventing potential problems. One of the most significant examples is safety. Because each age group is at risk for special types of injuries, preventive teaching can significantly reduce the rate of injuries, in turn lowering permanent disability and mortality rates.

Prevention also involves less obvious aspects of care. In addition to preventing physical disease or injury, the nurse should also promote mental health. For example, it is not sufficient to administer immunizations without regard to the psychological trauma associated with the procedure. The nurse and all other health care providers must ensure that humane care is provided.

Health Teaching

Health teaching is inseparable from family advocacy and prevention. Health teaching may be the nurse's direct goal, such as during parenting classes, or may be indirect, such as by:

- Helping parents and children understand a diagnosis or treatment
- Encouraging children to ask questions about their bodies
- Referring families to health-related professional or lay groups
- Supplying appropriate literature
- Providing anticipatory guidance

Health teaching is one area in which nurses often need preparation and practice with competent role models as it involves the transmission of information at the child's and family's levels of understanding and desire for information. As an effective educator, the nurse focuses on providing the appropriate health teaching along with generous feedback and evaluation to promote learning.

Support and Counselling

Attention to emotional needs requires support and sometimes counselling. The role of child advocate or health teacher requires an individualized approach. The nurse can offer support by listening, touching, and being physically present. Touching and physical presence are helpful to use with children because these interventions facilitate nonverbal communication.

Counselling involves a mutual exchange of ideas and opinions that provides the basis for mutual problem solving. It involves supporting, teaching, fostering expression of feelings or thoughts, and helping families cope with stress. Optimally, counselling not only helps resolve a crisis or problem but also enables the family to attain a higher level of functioning, greater **self-esteem**, and closer relationships. Although counselling is often the role of nurses in specialized areas, some counselling techniques are discussed in various sections of this text to help students and nurses cope with immediate crises and refer families for additional professional assistance.

Coordination and Collaboration

As a member of the health care team, the nurse collaborates and coordinates nursing services with the activities of other health care providers. Working in isolation does not serve the child's best interest. The concept of holistic care can only be realized through a unified interdisciplinary approach. Being aware of individual contributions and limitations to the child's care, the nurse collaborates with other specialists to provide high-quality health services. Failure to recognize one's limitations can be nontherapeutic and perhaps destructive. For example, the nurse who feels competent in counselling but who is really inadequate in this area may not only not prevent the child from dealing with a crisis but may also impede future success with a qualified professional.

Health Care Planning

The nurse's role has expanded beyond the nucleus of the family to include the community-based, health-driven system. Traditionally, nurses were involved in public health either on a continuous or an episodic basis. Nurses were less frequently involved in health care planning at a political or legislative level. Future nurses will need to incorporate a political component into their professional identity in the attempt to influence the decision-making arm of government to support health-promoting legislation. Some Canadian professional nursing organizations provide organizational mechanisms to respond to political issues.

As the largest health care profession, nursing has a valuable voice, especially as a family and consumer advocate. Nurses must become aware of community needs, be interested in the formulation of bills, and be supportive of politicians to ensure passage (or rejection) of significant legislation. Nurses also need to become actively involved with groups dedicated to the welfare of children (e.g., professional nursing societies, parent–teacher organizations, parent support groups, and volunteer organizations).

Health care planning involves not only providing new services to children and their families but also promoting the highest quality in existing services. In the past, pediatric nursing had no national or international standards of care or education. Most pediatric nurses merged pediatrics with other specialties within nursing and followed the Standards of Maternal-Child Health Nursing or the standards of several of the pediatric specialties, such as pediatric oncology nursing or school nursing. However, as a profession, pediatric nursing is increasing in momentum in Canada. For example, the CNA offers the Critical Care Pediatric Certificate, and the British Columbia Institute of Technology offers the Pediatric Nursing Specialty Option.

The highest standards of nursing practice are reflected in the emphasis on thorough assessment, the focus on scientific rationale as the basis for care, the summary of nursing care goals and responsibilities, and the comprehensive discussion of growth and development.

Future Trends

The current shift from treatment of disease to promotion of health has expanded nurses' roles in ambulatory care and highlighted the prevention and health-teaching aspects of nursing practice. The need for home care and community health services requires nurses to be more independent and to acquire skills useful in settings beyond the hospital. As changing social policy shapes the expanding health care arena, the focus of nursing care has shifted from what nurses do *for* families to what nurses do *in partnership with* them. The philosophy of family-centred care is no longer an option but a mandate.

Changing demographics will also influence pediatric nursing. The adult population is growing faster than the pediatric population. Statistics Canada (2015c) reports that the number of children (aged 0 to 14) is estimated at 16.2% of the population, which is down 5.8 percentage points from 1982 (22.0%). At the same time, the number of individuals aged 65 and over represents 14.9% of the Canadian population. Consequently, the decrease in the number of children means fewer hospitalized children and less need for pediatric beds. As well, medical innovations shorten hospital stays for children and there is an increase in children being treated medically at home rather than in the hospital. Pediatric units may amalgamate with obstetrical units, creating maternal child nursing units. Because older adults make up a larger percentage of the population, health care dollars will be split between the youngest and oldest groups, with shrinking resources available to meet the needs of both. Cost containment will present an ever-present challenge to providing high-quality care.

As the Canadian population becomes more diverse, nurses will need to continually adapt their care to the cultural milieu in which they practise. Finally, with the general trend of increasing complexity in pediatric medicine, nurses will need to be aware of developments in this field.

KEY POINTS

- The *Healthy Canadians* government program broadened the health care objectives of the past and shifted the focus to prevention as the method to accomplish health goals.
- While the infant mortality rate in Canada is at an all-time low, it continues to be higher than that in other major countries.
- LBW, which is closely related to early gestational age, is a leading cause of neonatal death in Canada.
- Injuries are the leading cause of death in children over age 1 year, with the majority being motor vehicle injuries.
- Childhood morbidity encompasses acute illness, chronic disease, and disability.
- The *new morbidity* refers to behavioural, social, and educational problems that can significantly alter a child's health.
- Developmental stage and environment are important factors in the prevalence of injuries at every age and should guide injury prevention measures.
- The philosophy of family-centred care recognizes the family as the constant in a child's life and that service systems and personnel must support, respect, encourage, and enhance the family's strength and competence.
- Evidence-informed practice is the collection, interpretation, and integration of valid, important, and applicable patient-reported, nurse-observed, and research-derived information.
- Atraumatic care is the provision of therapeutic care in settings, by personnel, and through the use of interventions that eliminate or minimize the psychological and physical distress experienced by children and their families in the health care system.
- Roles of the pediatric nurse include establishing a therapeutic relationship, advocating for families, preventing disease and promoting health, providing health teaching, providing support and counselling, coordinating and collaborating on care, making ethical decisions, and doing research.
- With the shift in focus from treatment of disease to promotion of health, nurses' roles have expanded beyond working in traditional health care facilities to providing care in ambulatory care centres, schools, the family's home, and the community.
- The process of nursing for children and families includes accurate and complete assessment, analysis of assessment data to arrive at a nursing diagnosis, planning of care, implementation of the plan, evaluation of interventions, and documentation.

evolve WEBSITE

Visit the Evolve website for additional resources related to the content in this chapter such as Case Studies, Critical Thinking Case Study Answers, Nursing Care Plans, Nursing Processes, Nursing Skills, and Review Questions for Exam Preparation at: *http://evolve.elsevier.com/Canada/Perry/maternal/*

REFERENCES

Alfaro-LeFevre, R. (2005). *Applying nursing process: A tool for critical thinking* (6th ed.). Philadelphia: Lippincott.

Banerji, A., & Canadian Paediatric Society, First Nations, Inuit and Métis Health Committee. (2012). Preventing unintentional injuries in indigenous children and youth in Canada. *Paediatric Child Health, 17*(7), 393. Reaffirmed 2015. Retrieved from <http://www.cps.ca/documents/position/unintentional-injuries-indigenous-children-youth>.

Canada Safety Council. (2011). *Unload and lock your firearms, store them safely!* Retrieved from <http://canadasafetycouncil.org/news/unload-and-lock-your-firearms-store-them-safely>.

Canadian Child Welfare Research Portal. (2011). *Child abuse & neglect.* Retrieved from <http://cwrp.ca/child-abuse-neglect>.

Canadian Dental Association. (2010). *CDA position on early childhood caries.* Retrieved from <http://www.cda-adc.ca/_files/position_statements/earlyChildhoodCaries.pdf>.

Canadian Institute of Child Health. (2015). *The health of Canada's children and youth: A CICH profile.* Retrieved from <http://profile.cich.ca/en/index.php/chapter1/1.3-health-outcomes/96>.

Canadian Mental Health Association: Ontario. (n.d.). *Lesbian, gay, bisexual, trans & queer identified people and mental health.* Retrieved from <http://ontario.cmha.ca/mental-health/lesbian-gay-bisexual-trans-people-and-mental-health/>.

Chandler, M. J., & Lalonde, C. E. (2009). Cultural continuity as a moderator of suicide risk among Canada's First Nations. In L. J. Kirmayer & G. Valaskakis (Eds.), *Healing traditions: The mental health of Aboriginal peoples in Canada* (pp. 221–248). Vancouver: UBC Press.

Conference Board of Canada. (2011). *Infant mortality.* Retrieved from <http://www.conferenceboard.ca/hcp/details/health/infant-mortality-rate.aspx>.

Dietitians of Canada. (2015). *BMI for children/teens.* Retrieved from <http://www.dietitians.ca/Your-Health/Assess-Yourself/Assess-Your-BMI/BMI-Children.aspx>.

Gagné, M.-P. (2008). *L'effet des législations canadiennes entourant le contrôle des armes à feu sur les homicides et les suicides* [The effect of Canadian laws surrounding gun control on homicide and suicide]. M.Sc. Thesis, Université de Montréal.

Gentile, D. A., Coyne, S., & Walsh, D. A. (2011). Media violence, physical aggression, and relational aggression in school age children: A short-term longitudinal study. *Aggressive Behavior, 37*(2), 193–206. doi:10.1002/ab.20380.

Government of Canada. (2014). *Government of Canada reminds Canadians how to protect children from dangerous household chemicals—Products should be locked out of sight and out of reach.* Retrieved from <http://news.gc.ca/web/article-en.do?nid=826029&_ga=1.249383950.868197850.1432519476>.

Health Canada. (2009). *Reaching for the top: A report by the Advisor on Healthy Children and Youth.* Retrieved from <http://www.hc-sc.gc.ca/hl-vs/pubs/child-enfant/advisor-conseillere/index-eng.php>.

Health Canada. (2010). *Acting on what we know: Preventing youth suicide in First Nations.* Retrieved from <http://www.hc-sc.gc.ca/fniah-spnia/pubs/promotion/_suicide/prev_youth-jeunes/index-eng.php#s21>.

Health Canada. (2014). *First Nations & Inuit health: Dental benefits.* Retrieved from <http://www.hc-sc.gc.ca/fniah-spnia/nihb-ssna/benefit-prestation/dent/index-eng.php>.

Health Canada, Canadian Paediatric Society, Dietitians of Canada, & Breastfeeding Committee for Canada. (2015). *Nutrition for healthy term infants: Recommendations from 6 to 24 months.* Retrieved from <http://www.hc-sc.gc.ca/fn-an/nutrition/infant-nourisson/recom/recom-6-24-months-6-24-mois-eng.php>.

Hospital for Sick Children. (2011). *Nursing.* Retrieved from <http://www.sickkids.ca/Nursing/index.html>.

Ignatavicius, D. (2001). Critical thinking skills for at the bedside success. *Nursing Management, 32*(1), 37–39.

Index Mundi. (2015). *Canada infant mortality rate.* Retrieved from <http://www.indexmundi.com/canada/infant_mortality_rate.html>.

Institute for Patient- and Family-Centered Care. (2011). *Advancing the practice of patient- and family-centered care in hospitals. How to get started …* Retrieved from <http://www.ipfcc.org/pdf/getting_started.pdf>.

Katzmarzyk, P. (2008). Obesity and physical activity among Aboriginal Canadians. *Obesity, 16,* 184–190. doi:10.1038/oby.2007.51.

Korczak, D. L., & Canadian Paediatric Society, Mental Health and Developmental Disabilities Committee. (2015). Suicidal ideation and behaviour. *Paediatric Child Health, 20*(5), 257–260.

Kutcher, R., & Szumilas, M. (2008). Youth suicide prevention. *Canadian Medical Association Journal, 178*(3), 282–285. doi:10.1503/cmaj.071315.

MacLaurin, B., Trocmé, N., Fallon, B., et al. (2011). *A comparison of First Nations and non-Aboriginal children investigated for maltreatment in Canada in 2003.* Retrieved from <http://www.cecw-cepb.ca/publications/537>.

Mikkonen, J., & Raphael, D. (2010). *Social determinants of health: The Canadian facts.* Toronto: York University School of Health Policy and Management. Retrieved from <http://www.thecanadianfacts.org/the_canadian_facts.pdf>.

Narconon International. (2015). *Canada drug abuse.* Retrieved from <http://www.narconon.org/drug-information/canada-drug-abuse.html>.

Ontario Ministry of Health Promotion and Sport. (2010). *Active living: Help your kids get active.* Retrieved from <http://www.mhp.gov.on.ca/en/healthy-ontario.asp?utm_campaign=jan2011>.

Parachute. (n.d.). *Wheeled activities.* Retrieved from <http://www.parachutecanada.org/injury-topics/topic/C108>.

Pike, I., Richmond, S., Rothman, L., & Macpherson, A. (Eds.). (2015). *Canadian injury prevention resource: An evidence-informed guide to injury prevention in Canada.* Toronto: Parachute. Retrieved from <http://www.parachutecanada.org/downloads/research/Canadian_Injury_Prevention_Resource.pdf>.

Public Health Agency of Canada. (2011). *What determines health?* Retrieved from <http://www.phac-aspc.gc.ca/ph-sp/determinants/index-eng.php>.

Public Health Agency of Canada. (2012). *Where can I get vaccinated, and do I have to pay.* Retrieved from <http://phac-aspc.gc.ca/im/vs-sv/vs-faq17-eng.php>.

Public Health Agency of Canada. (2013). *Congenital anomalies in Canada: A perinatal health surveillance report.* Retrieved from <http://publications.gc.ca/collections/collection_2014/aspc-phac/HP35-40-2013-eng.pdf>.

Public Health Agency of Canada. (2014). *Maternal and infant health: Canadian perinatal system surveillance (CPSS).* Retrieved from <http://www.phac-aspc.gc.ca/rhs-ssg/index-eng.php>.

Public Health Agency of Canada. (2015a). *Vaccine safety.* Retrieved from <http://www.phac-aspc.gc.ca/im/safety-securite-eng.php>.

Public Health Agency of Canada. (2015b). *Immunizations and vaccines.* Retrieved from <http://www.phac-aspc.gc.ca/im/index-eng.php>.

Renaud, J., Séguin, M. J., Lesage, A. D., et al. (2014). Service use and unmet needs in youth suicide: A study of trajectories. *Canadian Journal of Psychiatry, 59*(10), 523–530.

Rivara, F. P., & Grossman, D. C. (2015). Injury control. In R. M. Kliegman, B. F. Stanton, J. W. St. Geme, & N. Schor (Eds.), *Nelson textbook of pediatrics* (20th ed.). Philadelphia: Saunders.

Rowan-Legg, A., & Canadian Paediatric Society, Community Paediatrics Committee. (2013). Oral health care for children—a call for action. *Paediatric Child Health, 18*(1), 37–43. Reaffirmed 2016. Retrieved from <http://www.cps.ca/en/documents/position/oral-health-care-for-children>.

Schroth, R. J., Harrison, R. L., & Moffatt, M. E. (2009). Oral health of indigenous children and the influence of early childhood caries on childhood health and well-being. *Pediatric Clinics of North America, 56*(6), 1481–1499.

Statistics Canada. (2011). *Family violence in Canada: A statistical profile.* Retrieved from <http://www.statcan.gc.ca/pub/85-224-x/85-224-x2010000-eng.pdf>.

Statistics Canada. (2012). *2011 Census of population*. Ottawa: Author. Retrieved from <http://www12.statcan.gc.ca/census-recensement/index-eng.cfm>.

Statistics Canada. (2013). *Youth court statistics, 2011/2012*. Retrieved from <http://www.statcan.gc.ca/daily-quotidien/130613/dq130613d-eng.htm>.

Statistics Canada. (2015a). *Infant mortality rates by province and territory*. Retrieved from <http://www.statcan.gc.ca/tables-tableaux/sum-som/l01/cst01/health21a-eng.htm>.

Statistics Canada. (2015b). *Physical activity levels of Canadian children and youth, 2007 to 2009*. Retrieved from <http://www.statcan.gc.ca/pub/82-625-x/2011001/article/11553-eng.htm>.

Statistics Canada. (2015c). *Section 2: Population by age and sex*. Retrieved from <http://www.statcan.gc.ca/pub/91-215-x/2012000/part-partie2-eng.htm>.

Transport Canada. (2013). *Canadian motor vehicle traffic collisions, 2013*. Retrieved from <http://www.tc.gc.ca/media/documents/roadsafety/cmvtcs2013_eng.pdf>.

Tremblay, M. S., LeBlanc, A. G., Kho, M. E., et al. (2011). Systematic review of sedentary behaviour and health indicators in school-aged children and youth. *International Journal of Behavioral Nutrition and Physical Activity*, *8*, 98. doi:10.1186/1479-5868-8-98.

UNICEF Canada. (2014). *UNICEF report card 12: Children of the recession—Canadian companion*. Toronto: Author. Retrieved from <http://www.unicef.ca/sites/default/files/imce_uploads/images/reports/rc12_canadian_companion_en_2810.pdf>.

United Nations Office on Drugs and Crime. (2011). *World drug report: 2011*. Vienna: United Nations Office on Drugs and Crime. Retrieved from <http://www.unodc.org/documents/data-and-analysis/WDR2011/World_Drug_Report_2011_ebook.pdf>.

Van Schaik, C., & Canadian Paediatric Society, Injury Prevention Committee. (2008). Transportation of infants and children in motor vehicles. *Pediatric Child Health*, *13*(4), 313–318. Retrieved from <http://www.cps.ca/documents/position/car-seat-safety>.

World Bank. (2016). *Mortality rate under 5*. Retrieved from <http://data.worldbank.org/indicator/SH.DYN.MORT>.

World Health Organization. (2008). *World report on child injury prevention*. Retrieved from <http://www.who.int/violence_injury_prevention/child/injury/world_report/report/en/index.html>.

World Health Organization. (2012). *Oral health*. Retrieved from <http://www.who.int/mediacentre/factsheets/fs318/en/>.

World Health Organization. (2015). *School health promotion*. Retrieved from <http://www.who.int/topics/school_health_promotion/en/>.

World Health Organization, Health and Welfare Canada, & Public Health Agency of Canada. (1986). *Ottawa Charter for health promotion*. Retrieved from <http://www.phac-aspc.gc.ca/ph-sp/docs/charter-chartre/pdf/charter.pdf>.

Zayed, R., Davidson, B., Nadeau, L., et al. (2016). Canadian rural/remote primary care physicians' perspectives on child/adolescent mental health care service delivery. *Journal of Canadian Academy of Child and Adolescent Psychiatry*, *25*(1), 24–34.

ADDITIONAL RESOURCES

About Kids Health: <http://www.aboutkidshealth.ca/Default.aspx>.

Canadian Association of Poison Control Centres—Contact information for individual provincial and territorial poison control centres: <http://www.capcc.ca/>.

Canadian Family Violence Initiative under the Department of Justice—Information on family violence and child maltreatment in Canada: <http://justice.gc.ca/eng/fund-fina/cj-jp/fv-vf.html>.

Canadian Task Force on Preventive Health Care—Youth Suicide Report (2015): <http://canadiantaskforce.ca/>.

Caring for Kids: <http://www.caringforkids.cps.ca/>.

Government of Canada: Provincial and Territorial Immunization Information: <http://healthycanadians.gc.ca/healthy-living-vie-saine/immunization-immunisation/children-enfants/schedule-calendrier-eng.php>.

Healthy Canadians—Bullying prevention programs: <http://healthycanadians.gc.ca/healthy-living-vie-saine/bullying-intimidation/index-eng.php>.

Healthy Canadians—Information on childhood obesity in Canada: <http://www.healthycanadians.gc.ca/healthy-living-vie-saine/obesity-obesite/index-eng.php>.

Institute for Patient- and Family-Centred Care: <http://www.ipfcc.org>.

Kids' Help Line: 1-800-668-6868 (gives children a way to seek help when experiencing violence).

Parachute Canada: <http://www.parachutecanada.org/thinkfirstcanada>.

Transport Canada—Information on car seat safety tips and legislation: <http://www.tc.gc.ca/eng/motorvehiclesafety/safedrivers-childsafety-car-time-stages-1083.htm>.

CHAPTER

31

Family, Social, Cultural, and Religious Influences on Children's Health

Helen Edwards

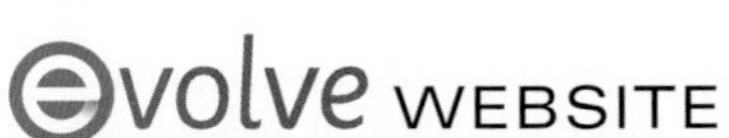

Visit the Evolve website for additional resources related to the content in this chapter such as Case Studies, Critical Thinking Case Study Answers, Nursing Care Plans, Nursing Processes, Nursing Skills, and Review Questions for Exam Preparation at: http://evolve.elsevier.com/Canada/Perry/maternal/

OBJECTIVES

On completion of this chapter the reader will be able to:

- Discuss the relationship that the nurse builds with the child and family.
- Discuss role transitions experienced by new parents.
- Explain various parenting behaviours, such as parenting styles, disciplinary patterns, and communication skills.
- Demonstrate an understanding of special parenting situations, such as adoption, divorce, lone parenting, parenting in reconstituted families, and LGBTQ parenting, and how these situations affect the child.
- Identify child maltreatment in the form of physical abuse or neglect, emotional abuse or neglect, or sexual abuse and the characteristics or circumstances that may predispose children to maltreatment.
- Discuss key influences that parents have on their children's socialization.
- Identify key social determinants of health and be able to describe the influences of socioeconomic status, culture, religion, peer groups, and schools on child development.
- Demonstrate an understanding of health and religious beliefs and practices that can have an impact on a family's view of their child's illness and treatment-seeking behaviours.

PEDIATRIC NURSING AND THE FAMILY

Nurses must be aware of the various family structures and functions within a family. Once a child is brought into a new family, the nurse needs to understand how this changes the family dynamics. The nurse can provide guidance for directing family-oriented interventions as needed and how to care for children in the context of individual families (Kaakinen, Hanson, & Denham, 2010).

Family Nursing Interventions

In working with children, nurses must include family members in their care plan. To discover family dynamics, strengths, and weaknesses, a thorough family assessment is necessary (see Chapters 2 and 33). For example, family systems theory is a common approach that nurses use to understand and assess families as a whole, as well as in understanding and assessing the individuals that make up that whole, by using concepts that help one to think about the family as a system. The various theories and assessment models that are relevant to family nursing practice are summarized in Table 2-2. When working with families, the nurse's choice of interventions depends on the theoretical family model that is used (Box 31-1).

Nurses need to be cautious not to rely too heavily on one specific theoretical framework when working in diverse settings, as a broad knowledge base is required in order to adequately assess and act on challenging health issues faced by families (Kaakinen & Hanson, 2010).

Families' Roles, Relationships, and Strengths

Each family also has its own traditions and values and sets its own standards for interaction within and outside the group. Each family decides and influences the experiences their children should have, those they are to be shielded from, and how

BOX 31-1 FAMILY NURSING INTERVENTIONS

- Behaviour modification
- Case management and coordination
- Collaborative strategies
- Contracting
- Counselling, including support, cognitive reappraisal, and reframing
- Empowering families through active participation
- Environmental modification
- Family advocacy
- Family crisis intervention
- Networking, including use of self-help groups and social support
- Providing information and technical expertise
- Role modelling
- Role supplementation
- Teaching strategies, including stress management, lifestyle modifications, and anticipatory guidance

From Friedman, M. M., Bowden, V. R., & Jones, E. G. (2003). *Family nursing: Research theory and practice* (5th ed.). Upper Saddle River, NJ: Pearson Education.

each of these experiences meets the needs of family members. When family ties are strong, social control is highly effective, and most members conform to their roles willingly and with commitment. Conflicts arise when people do not fulfill their roles in ways that meet other family members' expectations, either because they are unaware of the expectations, they choose not to meet them, or they are incapable of meeting them. Knowledge of characteristics that help families function effectively can help the nurse throughout the nursing process, to predict ways that families may cope and respond to a stressful event, such as a child's illness. It is important for the nurse to provide individualized support that builds on family strengths and unique functioning style and to assist family members in obtaining requisite resources. Family strengths and their unique ways of functioning are significant resources that nurses can use to meet family needs. By building on qualities that make a family work well and including supportive family resources, the family unit can become even stronger, taking into account that all families have strengths as well as vulnerabilities (Kaakinen et al., 2010). It is important for the nurse to remember that the family has a crucial impact on the well-being of a child. For example, a child with a chronic illness such as cystic fibrosis requires a significant amount of time and commitment from family members to optimize the child's well-being; a specific diet, chest physiotherapy, medication administration, and physical activity are only some of the tasks to be carried out by family members to meet the child's needs.

Parental Roles

Historically, the family was headed by socially recognized and sanctioned roles of father (male) and mother (female). These traditional roles modelled what were considered appropriate sexual behaviour and family responsibilities, including child-rearing. The behaviours these gender roles served were intended to provide stability and prolonged care for children.

Parental roles have changed and continue to change significantly as a result of the changing economy, increased opportunities for women, evolving gender roles within family structures, and greater variety in family configurations. Women have and continue to achieve equality with men in education, more women have entered the workforce, and the number of women who choose to have fewer children or none at all is increasing. As the role of women has changed, the complementary role of men has also changed. Many fathers are taking a more active role in child-rearing and household tasks. In Canada, new family structures such as lone-parent families and families with same-sex or transgender parents have also redefined traditional gender roles. Role conflicts in families may still occur because of a cultural lag of persisting traditional role definitions assumed by some of the family members.

Role Learning

Roles are learned through the socialization process. During all stages of **development**, children learn and practise, through interaction with others and in their play, a set of social roles and characteristics of other roles. They behave in patterned and more or less predictable ways because they learn roles that define mutual expectations in typical social relationships. Although role definitions are changing, the basic determinants of parenting remain the same. Several determinants of parenting infants and young children are parental personality and mental well-being, systems of support, and child characteristics. These determinants have been used as consistent measurements to determine a person's success in fulfilling the parental role.

Parents, peers, and authority figures (such as care providers and teachers), who use positive and negative sanctions to ensure conformity, transmit role conceptions to children. Role behaviours positively reinforced by rewards, such as love, affection, friendship, and honours, are strengthened. Negative reinforcement can take the form of ridicule, withdrawal of love, expressions of disapproval, or banishment.

In some cultures, the role behaviour expected of children conflicts with desirable adult behaviour. For example, in some North American families, children are expected to be submissive in childhood but dominant as adults. This conflict of expectations is known as *role discontinuity*. Other cultures value the same behaviours, such as courage and assertiveness, in both children and adults; this provides *role continuity*.

One responsibility of the family is to develop culturally appropriate role behaviour in children. Children learn to perform in expected ways that are consistent with their position in the family and culture. The observed behaviour of each child is a single manifestation—a combination of social influences and individual psychological processes. In this way, the uniting of the child's intrapersonal system (the self) with the family's interpersonal system is simultaneously understood as the child's conduct.

Role structuring initially takes place within family units, in which children fulfill a set of roles and respond to the roles of their parents and other family members. Children's roles are shaped primarily by their parents, who apply direct or indirect pressure to induce or force children into desired patterns of behaviour or direct their efforts toward modification of the child's role responses on a mutually acceptable basis. Children respond to life situations according to behaviours learned in reciprocal transactions. As they acquire important role-taking skills, their relationships with others change. For instance, when a teenager is also a mother but lives in a household with her grandmother, the teenager may be viewed more as an adolescent than as a mother. Children become proficient at understanding others as they acquire the ability to discriminate their own perspectives from those of others. Children who get along well with others and attain status in the peer group have well-developed role-taking skills.

The ability of parents to provide optimal care and support is dependent on having an adequate structure for healthy growth and development, a safe family environment, appropriate housing, adequate nutrition, opportunities to participate in recreational activities, and timely health care, as well as on using noncoercive discipline (Kaakinen et al., 2010; McNeill, 2010).

Family Size and Configuration

Parenting practices differ between small and large families. In small families, generally more emphasis is placed on the individual development of children. Children's development and achievement are measured against those of other children in the neighbourhood and social class. In small families, there tends to be more democratic participation by the children than in larger families. Adolescents in small families often identify more strongly with their parents and rely more on parental advice. They have well-developed, autonomous inner controls as contrasted with adolescents from larger families, who may rely more on adult authority.

Children in a large family are generally able to adjust to a variety of changes and crises. There is often more emphasis on the group and less on the individual. Cooperation is essential, often because of economic necessity. The large number of people sharing a limited amount of space requires a greater degree of organization, administration, and authoritarian control. A dominant family member (a parent or older child) wields control and discipline. The number of children can reduce the intimate, one-to-one contact between the parent and any individual child. Consequently, children turn to each other for what they cannot get from their parents. The reduced parent–child contact encourages individual children to adopt specialized roles to gain recognition in the family. Siblings are usually attuned to what constitutes misbehaviour. Sibling disapproval or ostracism is frequently a more meaningful disciplinary measure than parental interventions. In situations such as death or illness of a parent, an older sibling often assumes responsibility for the family at considerable personal sacrifice. Large families generate a sense of security in the children that is fostered by sibling support and cooperation.

Sibling Interactions

Spacing of children. Age differences between siblings affect the childhood environment, but to a lesser extent than does the sex of the sibling. The arrival of a sibling is often difficult for toddlers and preschool children, especially between the ages of 2 and 3 years old. At this age, they are still attached to their parents and do not understand the concept of sharing. An older child is able to understand the situation and is less likely to see the newcomer as a threat (Fig. 31-1), although the child does feel the loss of the only-child status. In general, the narrower the spacing between siblings, the more the children influence one another, especially in emotional characteristics. The wider the spacing, the greater the influence of the parents.

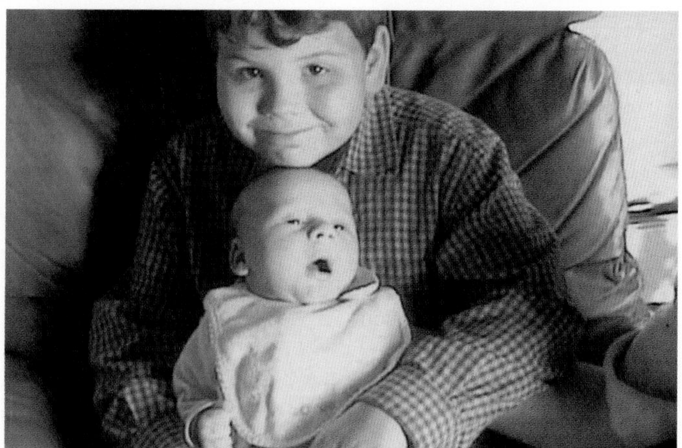

FIGURE 31-1 Older school-age children often enjoy taking responsibility for the care of a younger sibling.

Sibling functions. The sibling relationship's most unique feature is its duration. The longest relationship one will share with another human being is usually the sibling relationship, which lasts through a lifetime (often 50 to 80 years), compared to a parent relationship of approximately 30 to 50 years.

Siblings exert power, exchange services, and express feelings in reciprocal ways that are often not revealed in the presence of the parents. They see themselves in their brother or sister, experience life vicariously through their sibling's behaviour, and begin to expand on their own possibilities. Siblings can also be touchstones for what the other would not like to be, and they use each other as yardsticks for comparison. They provide a sounding board for each other and offer a safe forum for experimenting with new behaviours and roles. Brothers and sisters provide each other with tangible services (e.g., lending money, clothing, toys, or sports equipment; teaching a skill), help each other with childhood problems, provide support in dealing with parents or others outside the family, and provide introductions to new friendship groups.

Children learn to negotiate and bargain, and sometimes to manipulate, from their siblings. Their interactions with each other provide opportunities for conflict and conflict resolution. They protect one another from parental-executive abuse of power and can form a coalition to deal with issues of authority, power, and emotional support. Negotiating with parents is stronger when siblings act together rather than singly.

Siblings interpret the outside world for each other and perform educative functions for the parents. A related function is *pioneering*, in which one sibling initiates a process, thereby giving the others permission to follow, such as breaking explicit family rules, taking new pathways, or adopting different moral or political codes and lifestyles.

Tattling can be an important lever in sibling interactions. There can also be a conspiracy of silence among siblings, leaving the parents feeling isolated and excluded. A willingness to maintain each other's privacy often serves as a powerful bond of loyalty that distinguishes the relationship between siblings from that between friends.

More active sibling relationships. Sibling relationships vary among cultures. Also, some social factors give the sibling relationship greater significance in North American families than in the past. The current trends of shrinking family size, longer lifespans, divorce and remarriage, geographic mobility, maternal employment, alternative sources of child care, competitive pressures, stress, and sometimes parental insufficiency may be propelling siblings into greater contact with each other and emotional interdependence than ever before. Siblings often join forces to confront the trauma of divorce, and they frequently rely on each other for support when parents remarry. With the increased prevalence of both parents working outside the home, young siblings can have significant amounts of time when a caring adult is not available to provide direct supervision, resulting in more children at home alone for longer periods of time. In a worried, mobile, small-family, high-stress, fast-paced, parent-absent society, children often turn to a brother or sister to meet their needs for contact, constancy, and permanency.

Ordinal Position

Researchers have observed that the birth position of children can affect their personalities. Parents treat children differently, and sibling interactions are different, depending on the child's position within the family. Power is unequally distributed among siblings. Older siblings may attempt to dominate younger ones; younger siblings tend to develop interpersonal skills, learn the ability to negotiate, and accept unfavourable outcomes to a greater extent than older siblings. Later-born children are obliged to interact with other siblings from birth and seem to be more outgoing and make friends more easily than firstborns. General characteristics of children according to their ordinal position in the family are presented in Box 31-2. It is important to bear in mind, however, that children vary tremendously, and such generalizations do not always apply to individuals.

The only child. Only children tend to strongly resemble firstborn children in respects such as higher educational goals. Only children perform better on cognitive tests, are more mature and socially sensitive, and demonstrate superiority in language facility.

Only children enjoy the advantage of having parents who can devote more time to them, talk to them, and stimulate them in intellectual activities. Parents also exert greater pressure for mature behaviour at an early age and for achievement. Relative isolation from peers contributes to intellectual pursuits and encourages a rich fantasy life, independence, and originality.

BOX 31-2 INFLUENCE OF ORDINAL POSITION ON CHILDREN

Firstborn Children
- Are more achievement oriented
- Are more dominant
- Receive more physical punishment
- Have stronger consciences; are more self-disciplined and inner directed
- Are more socially anxious
- Are prone to feelings of guilt
- Identify more with parents than with peers
- Are more conservative
- Are subject to greater parental expectations
- Begin to speak earlier in life
- Demonstrate higher intellectual achievement
- Plan better and experience fewer frustrations

Middle Children
- Have more demands made on them for household help
- Are praised less often
- Receive less of parents' time
- Learn to compromise and be adaptable
- Are less stimulated toward achievement
- Are more difficult to characterize because of having a variety of positions in the family

Youngest Children
- Are less dependent than firstborn children
- Are less tense, more affectionate, and more good-natured
- Tend to identify more with a peer group than with parents
- Are more flexible in their thinking
- Have fewer demands placed on them for household help

Only Children
- Resemble firstborn children
- Are more mature and cultivated
- Experience greater parental pressure for mature behaviour and achievement
- Demonstrate superiority in language facility
- Rarely develop into the stereotype of a spoiled, selfish child
- Often enjoy a rich fantasy life as a result of isolation

Multiple Births

Multiple births occur with variable frequency. While twins are not uncommon in the population, triplets are rare, and quadruplets or quintuplets are extremely unusual. Statistics Canada reported the incidence of multiple births for 2011 as 12,543 (Statistics Canada, 2013a). The rate of multiple births increased between 1995 and 2008 due to an increased use of reproductive technologies, but this trend has slowed over recent years (1 in 31 in 2011) because of improvements in fertility treatments that have reduced the occurrence of multiple births (Multiple Births Canada, 2011).

Twins are of two distinct types: *identical*, or *monozygotic* (MZ), and *fraternal*, or *dizygotic* (DZ). A special kind of sibling relationship is observed in twins, although getting along with each other and quarrelling are not much different from the behaviours observed for any other two siblings, especially if they are different-sex fraternal twins. Twins tend to work out a relationship that is reasonably satisfactory to both and demonstrate early independence from parental attention. They develop a remarkable capacity for cooperative play and considerable loyalty and generosity toward each other. It is not uncommon for a private language to evolve between the twins that may interfere with the development of the family language.

In a twinship, one member of the pair, to a greater or lesser extent, is more dominant, outgoing, and assertive than the other, often to the parents' consternation. The seemingly more passive twin is nonetheless able to accomplish as much and get his or her way as frequently as the more assertive twin.

There can be differences in the behaviours between identical and fraternal twins. There is near-unison in the actions of identical twins (although they alternate in assuming the leadership), but fraternal twins, even of the same sex, do not display this quality. Sibling rivalry can be pronounced in fraternal twins, especially in different-sex twins.

Identical twins also differ in their response to the tendency of some parents to treat twins exactly alike. The present philosophy is to determine the degree to which the children demonstrate an inclination toward togetherness. Some twins thrive best when they are constantly in each other's company; others prefer more individuality and separateness. The conservative approach is to allow the children to follow their natural inclinations. Early years of togetherness are often the basis of the children's security, and separating them too early may produce unnecessary stress. Fostering individual differences as they become evident could ease the process of separation, when it becomes advisable.

Parental adjustment. The entrance of any new member into a household creates stress, but with multiple births, two or more new members must be incorporated into the family at the same time. The problems are obvious: two or more infants must be provided with physical care, including feeding and diapering, and all of the purchasing and preparation that accompanies the care of any infant is multiplied. Scheduling becomes crucial, and advancement in development brings new problems and adjustments (e.g., space and sleeping arrangements, selection of a stroller and other equipment). Toys must be selected carefully. As play becomes a serious business, some toys that would be safe and appropriate for a single child can become weapons when two infants share the play space. It is a good idea to select different toys for each child as they grow older and to encourage sharing.

Special Parenting Situations

Parenting is a demanding task under ideal circumstances, but when parents and children face challenges then the potential for family disruption is increased. Situations that are encountered frequently are divorce, lone parenthood, blended families, adoption, and dual-career families. In addition, as cultural diversity increases in our communities, many immigrants are making the transition to parenthood and a new country, culture, and language simultaneously. Other situations that create unique parenting challenges are parental alcoholism, homelessness, and incarceration. Although these topics are not addressed here, the reader may wish to investigate them further.

Parenting the Adopted Child

While adoption laws in Canada vary among provinces and territories, in general they follow similar requirements and guidelines from child protection legislation, defining *parent* as anyone who has decision-making authority over a child and assumes all the rights, duties, obligations, and responsibilities of the child. Certain adoption agencies may have specific requirements for adoptive parents, but in general anyone who is over 18 years of age and is a Canadian citizen without a criminal record is eligible to adopt a child (Government of Canada Department of Justice, 2015a).

Adoption establishes a legal relationship between a child and parents who are not related by birth but who have the same rights and obligations that exist between children and their biological parents. In the past, the biological mother alone made the decision to relinquish the rights to her child. In recent years, the courts have acknowledged the legal rights of the biological father regarding this decision. Concerned child advocates have questioned whether decisions that honour the father's rights are in the child's best interests. As the rights of the child have become recognized, older children have successfully dissolved their legal bond with their biological parents to pursue adoption by adults of their choice. Furthermore, there is a growing demand among gay, lesbian, bisexual, transgender, and queer (LGBTQ) adults to adopt.

Unlike biological parents, who prepare for their child's birth with prenatal classes and the support of friends and relatives, adoptive parents have few sources of support and preparation for the new addition to their family. Nurses can provide the information, support, and reassurance needed to reduce parental anxiety regarding the adoptive process and can refer adoptive parents to parental support groups. Such resources can be contacted through a department of health or provincial or territorial social services office.

Most problems faced by adoptive parents are not different from those encountered by birth parents, but the desire to be a good parent is often intensified in adoptive parents. Some adoptive parents may actually need less assistance than biological parents because adoptive parents have made the decision to become parents, they have had a relatively long period of time to prepare for parenting, and adoption generally requires maturity.

The sooner infants enter their adoptive home, the better the chances of parent–infant attachment. The more caregivers the infant had before adoption, the greater the risk for attachment problems. The infant must break the bond with the previous caregiver and form a new bond with the adoptive parents. Difficulties in forming an attachment depend on the amount of time infants have spent with earlier caregivers (e.g., birth mother, nurse, adoption agency personnel).

Siblings, adopted or biological, who are old enough to understand should be included in decisions regarding the commitment to adopt, with reassurance that they are not being

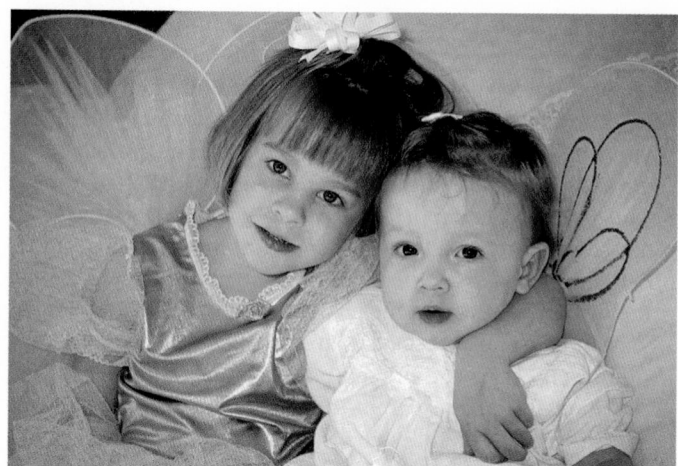
FIGURE 31-2 An older sister lovingly embraces her adopted sister.

replaced. Ways in which the siblings can interact with the adopted child should be stressed (Fig. 31-2).

Issues of origin. The task of telling children that they are adopted can be a cause of deep concern and anxiety. There are no clear-cut guidelines for parents to follow in determining when and at what age children are ready for the information. Parents are naturally reluctant to present children with such potentially unsettling news. It is important that parents not withhold knowledge of the adoption from the child, since it is an essential component of the child's identity.

The timing arises naturally, as parents become aware of the child's readiness. Most authorities believe that children should be informed at an age young enough so that, as they grow older, they do not remember a time when they did not know they were adopted. The time is highly individual but must be right for parents and the child. It may be when children ask where babies come from, at which time children can also be told the facts of their adoption. If they are told in a way that conveys the idea that they were active participants in the selection process, they will be less likely to feel that they were abandoned, helpless victims. For example, parents can tell children that their personal qualities drew the parents to them. It is wise for parents to tell children that they are adopted before the children enter school, to avoid having them hear it from third parties. Complete honesty between parents and children strengthens the relationship.

Parents should anticipate behaviour changes after disclosure, especially in older children. Children who are struggling with the revelation that they are adopted may benefit from individual and family counselling. Children may use the fact of their adoption as a weapon to manipulate and threaten parents. Statements such as "My real mother would not treat me like this" or "You don't love me as much because I'm adopted" can hurt parents and increase their feelings of insecurity. Such statements may also cause parents to become overpermissive. Adopted children need the same undemanding love, combined with firm discipline and limit setting, as any other child.

Cross-racial and international adoption. Since 1993, Canadian parents considering international adoption must follow the laws of the adopting countries, which are governed by the Hague Convention. The Hague Convention on Protection of Children and Co-operation in Respect of Intercountry Adoption's main goals are to (1) protect the best interests of adopted children, (2) standardize the process between countries, and (3) prevent child abuse and child trafficking.

In 2009, 2127 international adoptions were reported in Canada, with the majority of children being welcomed from China, followed by the United States, Ethiopia, Vietnam, and Haiti. Canadian law offers parents seeking international adoptions two avenues: (1) the citizenship process, which makes the child a Canadian citizen, or (2) the immigration process, which makes the child a permanent resident (Government of Canada Immigration and Citizenship, 2016a).

Adoption of children of a racial background different from that of the family is commonplace. In addition to the problems faced by adopted children in general, children of a cross-racial adoption must deal with physical and sometimes cultural differences. It is advised that parents who adopt such children do everything possible to preserve the adopted children's cultural heritage.

! NURSING ALERT

As a health care provider, it is important not to ask insensitive questions, such as the following: "Is she yours?" "Is she adopted?" "What do you know about the 'real' mother?" "Do they have the same father?" "How much did it cost to adopt him?" "Your children look so different, which one is yours?"

Although cross-racial adopted children are full-fledged members of an adopting family and citizens of the adopted country, if they have a strikingly different appearance from other family members or exhibit distinct racial or ethnic characteristics, challenges may be encountered outside the family. Strangers may make thoughtless comments and talk about the children as though they were not members of the family. It is vital that family members declare to others that this is their child and a cherished member of the family. It may help to have a response already prepared in anticipation of insensitive remarks.

In international adoptions the medical information that parents receive may be incomplete or inaccurate; weight, height, and head circumference are often the only objective information present in the child's medical record. There are potential health risks for children who are being adopted internationally and the prevalence of these risks depends on the child's country of origin as well as the child's individual health patterns. Adoptive children come from many different parts of the world, and countries often open and then close the option of allowing international adoptions. International children may be healthy and are well cared for while others may have received very little medical care. Children who come from institutions such as orphanages may be more prone to developmental delays or behavioural problems (Canadian Paediatric Society [CPS], 2011). Some children have serious or multiple health problems that can be stressful for the parents.

Nurses frequently are required to collect personal information about children and their family members as part of a comprehensive assessment. Often the child's adoption is revealed when asking about birth or family history, but if the child is unaware of the adoption the parents might deflect the questions to a later time so they can provide the information without the child learning of their adoption.

Adolescence. Adolescence may be an especially trying time for parents of adopted children. Whether adopted children have more adjustment issues than nonadopted children is debatable; more evidence-informed research on this area needs to be done in Canada. The normal confrontations of adolescents and parents can assume more painful aspects in adoptive families. Adolescents may use their adoption to defy parental authority or as a justification for aberrant behaviour. As they attempt to master the task of identity formation, the feeling of abandonment by their biological parents can come into awareness and may be intensified. Gender differences in reacting to adoption may surface.

Adopted children can fantasize about their biological parents and may feel the need to discover their parents' identity to define themselves and their own identity. It is important for parents to keep the lines of communication open and to reassure their child that they understand the need to search for their identity. Access to biological birth certificates differs from province to province. Some provinces and territories make them legally available to adopted children when they come of age, while others require court orders to have the original birth record released. Adoptive parents should be honest with questioning adolescents and tell them of this possibility (the parents themselves are unable to obtain the birth certificate; it is the children's responsibility if they desire it).

Parenting and Divorce

Since the introduction of the divorce laws in 1968, there has been a steady increase in the Canadian divorce rate. However, since the 1990s, the divorce rate has remained relatively stable, with a less than 2% increase per year. The divorce rate is approximately 21.1 per 10,000 population (Statistics Canada, 2011). The process of divorce begins with a period of marital conflict of varying length and intensity, followed by a separation, the actual legal divorce, and re-establishment of different living arrangements. Because a function of parenthood is to provide for the security and emotional welfare of children, disruption of the family structure often engenders strong feelings of guilt in the divorcing parents.

During a divorce, parents' coping abilities may be compromised. The parents may be preoccupied with their own feelings, needs, and life changes and unable to be available and supportive to their children. Newly employed parents, usually mothers, are likely to leave children with new caregivers, in strange settings, or alone after school. The parent may also spend more time away from home, searching for or establishing new relationships. Sometimes, the adults feel frightened and alone and begin to depend on children as a substitute for the absent parent, which places an enormous burden on the child.

Impact of divorce on children. Numerous studies indicate that divorce has a profound effect on children. Many youngsters suffer for years from psychological and social difficulties associated with continuing or new stresses in the post-divorce family. Even when a divorce is amicable and open, children recall parental separation with the same emotions felt by victims of a natural disaster: loss, grief, and vulnerability to forces beyond their control. Children may also exhibit physiological symptoms as a result of the stress related to the changes caused by the divorce. It is important for the nurse in any setting (hospital, community health care facility, home, etc.) to include observations and assessments in order to accurately determine if the divorce is affecting the child.

The impact of divorce on children depends on several factors, including children's age and sex, parental interaction or conflict, and the quality of the parent–child relationship and parental care during the years following the divorce. Family characteristics are more crucial to the child's well-being than specific child characteristics, such as age or gender. High levels of ongoing family conflict are related to problems of social development, emotional stability, and cognitive skills for the child.

Complications associated with divorce include efforts on the part of one parent to subvert the child's loyalties to the other, abandonment to other caregivers, and adjustment to a stepparent. A major problem occurs when children are "caught in the middle" between divorced parents. They become message bearers between parents, are often quizzed about activities of the other parent, and have to listen to one parent criticize the other. A nurse may be able to intercede by helping the child get out of the middle by using "I messages" based on the formula of "I feel … (state the feeling) when you … (state the source). I would like it if you. …" This approach enables children to feel in control. An example of an "I message" is as follows: "I do not feel comfortable when you ask me questions about Mom; maybe you could ask her yourself."

Feelings of children toward divorce vary with age (Box 31-3). Some children feel a sense of shame and embarrassment about the family situation. Some feelings cause children to see themselves as different, inferior, or unworthy of love, especially if they feel responsible for the family dissolution. Although the social stigma attached to divorce no longer produces the emotions it did in the past, such feelings may still exist in small towns or in some cultural groups and can reinforce children's negative self-image. Lasting effects of divorce depend on the children's and parents' adjustment to the transition from an intact family to a lone-parent family and, often, to a reconstituted family.

Although most studies have concentrated on the negative effects of divorce on youngsters, some positive outcomes of divorce have been reported. A successful post-divorce family, either a lone-parent or a reconstituted family, can improve the quality of life for adults and children. If conflict is resolved, a better relationship with one or both parents may result, and some children may have less contact with a disturbed parent. Greater stability in home settings and the removal of arguments between parents at home can be a positive outcome for children's long-term well-being.

Previously, it was believed that divorce had a greater impact on younger children, but recent observations indicate that divorce constitutes a major disruption for children of all

BOX 31-3 CHILDREN'S FEELINGS AND BEHAVIOURS RELATED TO DIVORCE

Infants
- Effects of reduced mothering or lack of mothering
- Increased irritability
- Disturbance in eating, sleeping, and elimination
- Interference with attachment process

Early Preschool Children (Ages 2 to 3 Years)
- Frightened and confused
- Blame themselves for the divorce
- Fear of abandonment
- Increased irritability, whining, tantrums
- Regressive behaviours (e.g., thumb sucking, loss of elimination control)
- Separation anxiety

Later Preschool Children (Ages 3 to 5 Years)
- Fear of abandonment
- Blame themselves for the divorce; decreased self-esteem
- Bewilderment regarding all human relationships
- Become more aggressive in relationships with others (e.g., siblings, peers)
- Engage in fantasy to seek understanding of the divorce

Early School-Age Children (Ages 5 to 6 Years)
- Depression and immature behaviour
- Loss of appetite and sleep disorders
- May be able to verbalize some feelings and understand some divorce-related changes
- Increased anxiety and aggression
- Feelings of abandonment by departing parent

Middle School-Age Children (Ages 6 to 8 Years)
- Panic reactions
- Feelings of deprivation—loss of parent, attention, money, and secure future
- Profound sadness, depression, fear, and insecurity
- Feelings of abandonment and rejection
- Fear about the future
- Difficulty expressing anger at parents
- Intense desire for reconciliation of parents
- Impaired capacity to play and enjoy outside activities
- Decline in school performance
- Altered peer relationships—become bossy, irritable, demanding, and manipulative
- Frequent crying, loss of appetite, sleep disorders
- Disturbed routine, forgetfulness

Later School-Age Children (Ages 9 to 12 Years)
- More realistic understanding of divorce
- Intense anger directed at one or both parents
- Divided loyalties
- Ability to express feelings of anger
- Ashamed of parental behaviour
- Desire for revenge; may wish to punish the parent they hold responsible
- Feelings of loneliness, rejection, and abandonment
- Altered peer relationships
- Decline in school performance
- May develop somatic complaints
- May engage in aberrant behaviour such as lying, stealing
- Temper tantrums
- Dictatorial attitude

Adolescents (Ages 12 to 18 Years)
- Able to disengage themselves from parental conflict
- Feelings of a profound sense of loss—of family, childhood
- Feelings of anxiety
- Worry about themselves, parents, siblings
- Expression of anger, sadness, shame, embarrassment
- May withdraw from family and friends
- Disturbed concept of sexuality
- May engage in acting-out behaviours

ages. While feelings and behaviours of children may be different for various ages and genders, all children suffer stress second only to the stress produced by the death of a parent. Although considerable research has looked at gender differences in children's adjustments to divorce, the findings are not conclusive.

Telling the children. Parents are understandably hesitant to tell children about their decision to divorce. Most parents neglect to discuss either the divorce or its inevitable changes with their preschool child. Without preparation, even children who remain in the family home are confused by parental separations. Frequently, children are already experiencing vague, uneasy feelings that are more difficult to cope with than being told the truth about the situation. If possible, the initial disclosure should include both parents and siblings, followed by individual discussions with each child. Sufficient time should be set aside for these discussions in a period of calm, not after an argument, and include reasons for the divorce (if age appropriate) and reassurance that the divorce is not the children's fault.

Parents should not fear crying in front of the children because their crying gives the children permission to cry also. Children may feel guilt, a sense of failure, or that they are being punished for misbehaviour. They normally feel anger and resentment and should be allowed to communicate these feelings without punishment. They need consistency and order in their lives. They want to know where they will live, who will take care of them, if they will be with their siblings, and if there will be enough money to live on. Children fear that if their parents stopped loving each other, they could stop loving them. Their need for love and reassurance is tremendous at this time. Children may also wonder what will happen on special days such as birthdays and holidays, whether both parents will come to school events, and whether they will still have the same friends.

Custody and parenting partnerships. In the past, when parents separated, mothers were given custody of the children, with visitation agreements for fathers. Now both parents and the courts are seeking alternatives. Current belief is that neither fathers, partners, nor mothers should be awarded custody automatically. Custody should be awarded to parents who are best able to provide for the children's welfare. In some cases, children experience severe stress when living or spending time with a parent.

Two other types of custody arrangements are divided custody and joint custody. *Divided*, or *split, custody* means that each parent is awarded custody of one or more of the children, thereby separating siblings. For example, sons might live with the father and daughters with the mother.

Joint custody takes one of two forms. In *joint physical custody*, the parents alternate the physical care and control of the children on an equitable basis while maintaining shared parenting responsibilities legally. This custody arrangement works well for families who live close to each other and whose occupations permit an active role in the care and rearing of the children. In *joint legal custody*, children reside with one parent but both parents are the children's legal guardians and participate in child-rearing.

Co-parenting offers substantial benefits for the family: children can be close to both parents, and life with each parent can be more normal (as opposed to having, for instance, a disciplinarian mother and a recreational father). To be successful, parents in these arrangements must place high value on the commitment to provide normal parenting and to separate their marital conflicts from their parenting roles. The primary consideration is the welfare of the children.

Common characteristics in the custodial household after separation and divorce include coercive types of control, inflammable tempers in parents and children, reduced parental competence, a greater sense of parental helplessness, poorly enforced discipline, and diminished regularity in enforcing household routines. Noncustodial parents are seldom prepared for the role of visitor, may assume the role of recreational and "fun" parent, and may not have a residence suitable for children's visits. They may also be concerned about maintaining the arrangement over the years to follow.

The nurse providing care to a child of divorced parents must be aware of the family situation and of the details regarding custody. Depending on the details of the custody, one of the parents or both if they have joint custody have the legal right to make decisions about the child's health treatment. It is important to ask the parent for the details about custody and to document them in the child's health record to ensure that all health care providers caring for the child are aware of the situation. Although one parent might have legal custody, it is not uncommon for both parents to participate in decision making regarding their children, especially in the matter of health. Nurses have a unique role in supporting the child and family through an illness, but if custody issues are complex or if challenges arise, the nurse should involve others who can assist with moving the family forward toward resolution—this could include social workers and hospital legal counsel.

Lone Parenting

An individual may become a lone parent as a result of divorce, separation, death of a spouse, or birth or adoption of a child. Although divorce rates have stabilized, the number of lone-parent households continues to rise. In 2011, these families accounted for 16.3% of all Canadian families, with almost 80% being headed by women (Statistics Canada, 2015). It is estimated that at least half of the children born during the early part of the twenty-first century will spend part of their life in a family headed by a divorced, separated, widowed, or never-married mother. Although some women are lone parents by choice, most never planned on being parents on their own, and many feel pressure to marry or remarry.

Managing shortages of money, time, and energy is a major concern for lone parents. The stigma of poverty may be more keenly felt than the discrimination associated with being a lone parent. These families are often forced by their financial status to live in communities with inadequate housing and personal safety concerns. Lone parents are singly responsible for ensuring the financial viability of the family. This can lead to long hours away from the home, relying on other caregivers or their adolescents to provide care to the younger children. This can result in lone parents feeling guilty about the time spent away from their children and the burden they may feel they are placing on others.

Teen mothers are typically lone parents, with all the associated burdens, plus the additional challenges faced when trying to further their education, establish long-term relationships, and provide for their child over the short and long term. Teenage pregnancy rates have been steadily declining in Canada (McKay & Barrett, 2010); in the 20 years between 1991 and 2011 the rate dropped almost 50% (Statistics Canada, 2013b). Teen mothers should be encouraged to seek out programs that enable them to finish high school while still caring for their child. These programs typically exist within high schools and include services such as case management services, collaboration with community agencies designed to support teenage mothers, on-site child care, and on-site counselling, academic support services that also assist with career preparation (Van Pelt, 2012).

Fathers and partners who have custody of their children face many of the same challenges that single mothers do. They feel overburdened by the responsibility, depressed, and concerned about their ability to cope with the emotional needs of their children. Some partners find it difficult at first to coordinate household tasks, school visits, and other activities. Fathers often demand more assistance with household tasks and more independence from their children than custodial mothers do and are likely to make use of alternative care-giving and support systems.

Parenting in Reconstituted Families

In North America, many of the children living in homes where parents have divorced will experience another major change in their lives, such as the addition of a stepparent or new siblings. The Canadian 2011 census revealed 12.6% of total families are stepfamilies, the first time a census has considered this family configuration (Statistics Canada, 2015). The entry of a stepparent into an existing family requires adjustments for all family members. Some obstacles to the role adjustments and family problem solving include disruption of previous lifestyles and interaction patterns, complexity in the formation of new ones, and lack of social supports.

Cooperative parenting relationships can allow more time for each set of parents to be alone to establish their own relationship with the children. Under ideal circumstances, power conflicts between the two households can be reduced, and tension and anxiety can be lessened for all family members. In addition, the children's self-esteem can be increased, and there is a greater likelihood of continued contact with grandparents. Flexibility, mutual support, and open communication are critical to forming successful relationships in stepfamilies. Unfortunately, stepfamilies usually do not seek help to prevent problems. Typically, information and counselling are sought only when problems have surfaced and can no longer be ignored.

LGBTQ Marriages and Parenting

In Canada, same-sex marriage became legal in 2005. The 2011 census reported 0.8% same-sex couple families, an increase of more than 42% from the 2006 census. Among married same-sex men, 3.4% had children in their home; and of married same-sex women, 16.5% had children in their home (Statistics Canada, 2015). Little research exists on the effects of LGBTQ parents on socialization and social competence of children. The studies that do exist indicate that more research is required, thus conclusions should not be drawn from the limited data that are available, as sample sizes are typically small. The cultural and legal conflicts that drive many of the concerns for children of LGBTQ married parents have become less pronounced as LGBTQ family living arrangements have become more commonplace. This shift in perspective may result in sample sizes and comparative groups becoming more plentiful, inspiring researchers to develop better tools that can more accurately measure outcomes (Eggeben, 2012). See Additional Resources for information on working with LGBTQ families.

Foster Parenting

Foster care is defined as placement in an approved living situation away from the family of origin. The living situation may be an approved foster home, possibly with other children, or a preadoptive home. The 2011 census indicated that there are more than 29,000 children aged 14 years and under living in 17,410 foster households across Canada (Statistics Canada, 2015). The Child Welfare Services from each province and territory offer training and ongoing education for foster parents. Each province and territory has guidelines regarding the relative health of the prospective foster parents and their families, background checks regarding legal issues for the adults, personal interviews, and a safety inspection of the residence and surroundings.

Children in foster care tend to have a higher-than-normal incidence of acute and chronic health problems and may experience feelings of isolation or confusion (Annie E. Casey Foundation, 2012). Foster children are often at risk because of their previous caregiving environment. Nurses should strive to implement strategies to improve the health care for this group of children. In particular, assessment and case management skills are required to involve other disciplines in meeting their needs.

CHILD MALTREATMENT

The broad term *child maltreatment* includes intentional physical abuse or neglect, emotional abuse or neglect, and sexual abuse of children, usually by adults. It is one of the most significant social problems affecting children around the world. In 2008, there were an estimated 235,842 Canadian children maltreatment-related investigations by Child Welfare Services. Eighteen percent of these investigations had more than one category of maltreatment. Male and female maltreatment numbers were equal. Of the confirmed cases, 20% were physical abuse, 3% were sexual abuse (does not include all nonrelated abusers), 34% showed neglect, and 9% were emotional abuse; 34% had exposure to intimate partner violence. In 2008, two children in Canada died as a result of child maltreatment (Public Health Agency of Canada [PHAC], 2008). Indigenous children were identified as a key at-risk group because they are overrepresented in foster care and have four times the maltreatment rate for non-Indigenous children (PHAC, 2008). Reported statistics only partially represent the actual incidence of child maltreatment, since many cases likely go unreported.

Child Neglect

Child neglect is the most common form of maltreatment. *Neglect* is generally defined as the failure of a parent or other person legally responsible for the child's welfare to provide for the child's basic needs and an adequate level of care.

Important factors contributing to child neglect are lack of knowledge of child's needs, lack of resources, and caretaker substance use. For example, neglectful parents often demonstrate poor parenting skills. They may be unaware that an infant needs to be fed on demand, may not know what to feed the child, and may have insufficient funds to buy food. Another serious lack of knowledge is failure to recognize emotional nurturing as an essential need of children. (See also Chapter 35, Growth Failure [Failure to Thrive].)

Types of Neglect

Neglect takes many forms and can be classified broadly as physical or emotional maltreatment. *Physical neglect* involves the deprivation of necessities, such as food, clothing, shelter, supervision, medical care, and education. *Emotional neglect* generally refers to failure to meet the child's needs for affection, attention, and emotional nurturance.

Neglect may also include lack of intervention for or fostering of maladaptive behaviour, such as delinquency or substance use. Emotional abuse, an even more difficult aspect of maltreatment to define, refers to the deliberate attempt to destroy or significantly impair a child's self-esteem or competence. Emotional abuse may take the following forms: rejecting, isolating, terrorizing, ignoring, corrupting, verbally assaulting, or overpressuring the child.

Physical Abuse

The Justice Department of Canada defines *child abuse* as violence, mistreatment, or neglect that a child or adolescent may experience while in the care of someone they trust or depend on, such as a parent, sibling, or relative, caregiver, or guardian. Abuse may take place anywhere and may occur, for example, within the child's home or that of someone known to the child (PHAC, 2008). Legal steps to address child abuse in Canada include mandatory reporting laws, creation of child abuse registries, changes to the Criminal Code and the *Canada Evidence Act*, extended time limits for filing charges in child sexual abuse cases, and establishment of child protection agencies run by Indigenous peoples (PHAC, 2008). Minor physical injury is responsible for more reported cases of maltreatment than major physical injury, but major physical abuse causes more deaths. In total, police reported just over 18,300 child victims of family-related violence in 2011. This represented a rate of 267 child victims of family violence for every 100,000 Canadians under the age of 18 (Sinha & Statistics Canada, 2015).

NURSING ALERT

Nurses have a mandatory legal and professional ethical responsibility to report suspected cases of child maltreatment to Child Welfare Services. Every new abuse incident must be reported.

Factors Predisposing to Physical Abuse

The causes of child abuse are multifaceted. Child maltreatment occurs across all socioeconomic, religious, cultural, racial, and ethnic groups. Three risk factors are commonly identified in child abuse: parental characteristics, characteristics of the child, and environmental characteristics. However, no single factor or group of factors is predictive of abuse. Rather, the interaction of these factors is thought to increase the risk of abuse occurring in a particular family.

Parental characteristics. Certain identified characteristics occur more frequently in parents who abuse their children and are therefore considered risk factors. Younger parents more often are abusers of their children. Lone-parent families are at higher risk for abuse, and in lone-parent families that include an unrelated partner, the partner is sometimes the abuser, although a biological parent is most commonly the perpetrator.

Abusive families are often more socially isolated and have fewer supportive relationships. These parents are often from low-income circumstances, with little education. Parents with substance use problems pose a greater risk for abuse and neglect because of a variety of factors. The additional stressors of substance use with the demands of normal care of children create situations in which abuse and neglect can occur because these parents have impaired judgement and may react with violence while under the influence of drugs or alcohol (Wells, 2009). With little or no available support system and concurrent stressors imposed by the child or environment, these parents are vulnerable to additional crises of any nature and may strike out at the child as a method of releasing their increasing frustration and anxiety.

Other factors identified in abusive parents include low self-esteem and little knowledge of appropriate parenting skills. Parenting skills are learned behaviours, and parents who grew up with poor parental role models may have difficulty parenting their own children. Approximately one third of parents who were maltreated as children will subject their children to similar maltreatment (Gara, Allen, Herzog, et al., 2000). More research is needed to study the long-term effects of child maltreatment to determine if children who are abused have an increased propensity for becoming abusers.

Characteristics of the child. The onus for child abuse is always on the abuser; however, children who are abused do have some common characteristics. Children from birth to 3 years of age are at the highest risk for being abused (PHAC, 2008). Infants and small children require constant attention and must have all of their needs met by others. This can result in parental or caretaker fatigue with resultant striking out at the child with physical force, shaking the child, or ignoring the child's needs. Shaking the child can result in a serious head injury (see Chapter 50 for information on shaken baby syndrome).

The physical and emotional demands placed on the parents or caretaker of an unwanted, brain-damaged, hyperactive, or physically disabled child may overwhelm them, resulting in abuse. Children with disabilities may not understand that abusive behaviours are not appropriate; thus they may not tell others or defend themselves. Preterm infants may be at risk for maltreatment because of failure of parent–child bonding during early infancy, increased physical needs, or irritability. One child in the family may be singled out in an abusive family. Removing that child from the home often places the other siblings at risk for abuse. Therefore, no child is safe if left in the abusive environment unless the parents can be helped to learn new parenting skills, meet the children's needs, and release their frustration through alternatives other than attacking their children.

Environmental characteristics. Environment is a significant part of the potentially abusive situation. A typical environment is one of chronic stress, including problems of divorce, poverty, unemployment, poor housing, frequent relocation, and substance use issues. Increased exposure between children and parents, such as that which occurs in crowded living conditions, also increases the likelihood of abuse.

Although most reporting of abuse has been from populations of lower socioeconomic status, as stated previously, child abuse is not a problem of any one societal group. Stresses imposed by poverty predispose low-income families to abusive situations, and abuse in these groups is more apt to be reported. However, concealed crises may also be present in upper-income families. Families who have substitute caregivers such as day care providers and babysitters may also be at risk for child abuse, especially if the family has not fully evaluated the caregiver. Nurses need to be aware of all these factors to identify the less obvious examples of child abuse and neglect.

Sexual Abuse

Sexual abuse is one of the most devastating types of child maltreatment. No universal definition for sexual abuse exists.

Definitions cover a range of acts, including involvement of children in sexual acts they do not understand, to which they cannot give consent, or that violate social taboos. Sexual abuse and exploitation in Canada involves using a child for sexual purposes. Estimates of sexual abuse indicate that it has increased significantly during the past decade (PHAC, 2016). It is difficult to estimate the number of children in Canada who are sexually abused, as assaults are underreported and there is no nationwide reporting system. The number of estimated sexual assaults and exploitations, however, is very concerning. In 2011, children and youth were far more likely to be victims of sexual offences, with police-reported rates five times higher than among adults (207 victims per 100,000 versus 41 victims per 100,000). This was true for all types of sexual assaults, as well as other sexual offences. Included in the latter category are those violations specific to children, such as sexual interference, invitation to sexual touching, luring a child via a computer, sexual exploitation, and corrupting children (Sinha & Statistics Canada, 2015).

Some of the apparent increase can be attributed to increased awareness. These trends in sexual assault do not include child-specific sexual offences, such as luring a child over the Internet and invitation to sexual touching, which have generally increased in recent years (PHAC, 2016).

To further protect children from sexual abuse, the Criminal Code has been changed to create new criminal offences relating to child sexual assault, to include female genital mutilation as sexual abuse (see Chapter 5, p. 74, for more information), and to amend provisions on child sex tourism to make it easier to prosecute offenders. Bill C-15 (Parliament of Canada, 2002), which became law in 2002, aims to protect children from sexual exploitation by criminalizing actions such as luring children via the Internet to meet them somewhere in person; transmitting, making available, or exporting child pornography; or accessing child pornography on the Internet. Sentencing provisions are also strengthened.

Sexual abuse includes the following types of sexual maltreatment (PHAC, 2016):

- *Incest*—Any physical sexual activity between family members; blood relationship is not required (abusers can include stepparents, unrelated siblings, grandparents, uncles, and aunts); does not include sexual relations between legally sanctioned partners such as spouses
- *Molestation*—Vague term that includes "indecent liberties" such as touching, fondling, kissing, single or mutual masturbation, or oral–genital contact
- *Exhibitionism*—Indecent exposure, usually exposure of the genitalia by an adult man to children or women
- *Child pornography*—Arranging and photographing, in any media, sexual acts involving children, alone or with adults or animals, regardless of consent by the child's legal guardian; also may denote distribution of such material in any form with or without profit
- *Child prostitution*—Involving children in sex acts for profit and usually with changing partners
- *Pedophilia*—Literally means "love of child" and does not denote a type of sexual activity but rather the preference of an adult for prepubertal children as the means of achieving sexual excitement

Human trafficking often involves some form of coerced sexual activity and thus sexual abuse that may also often involve physical and mental abuse. Many victims of human trafficking are females under the age of 18 years who are forced to perform sexual acts for the monetary profit of the perpetrators. One form of sex trafficking called "sex tourism" involves adult men travelling to developing nations to have sex with young children (Sabella, 2011). Nurses may encounter victims of sex trafficking and subsequent sexual and physical abuse who are seeking medical care in outpatient and emergent health care settings for many different health problems (sexually transmitted infections [STIs], bruises, wound infections, post-traumatic stress disorder [PTSD], suicidal ideation, and addiction). However, nurses may not be aware of the victim's plight unless he or she delves further into the person's history and background (Sabella, 2011).

Characteristics of Abusers and Victims

Anyone, including siblings and mothers, can be sexual abusers, but a typical abuser is a man whom the victim knows. Offenders come from all levels of society. Adults make up 80% of offenders of sexual abuse, with the remaining 20% being adolescents and preadolescents. Many offenders hold full-time jobs and are active in community affairs, and they may not have prior criminal records. Offenders often are employed in or volunteer for positions that will bring them into contact with young girls and boys, such as teachers or coaches. Approximately 44% of sexual assaults against children and youth were carried out by nonparental family members, 29% of abusers were friends or acquaintances, and only 2% were strangers (PHAC, 2016). Child and youth victims of violence most often know the abuser. About one quarter (26%) of those accused of violence against children and youth were family members, including a parent, stepparent, foster parent, sibling, grandparent, or extended family member, while another 53% were either acquaintances or friends of the child or youth (Sinha & Statistics Canada, 2015). The abusers who were family members were equally likely to be a biological father or stepfather and less apt to be a biological mother or foster or adoptive parent (PHAC, 2016). Offenders may commit many assaults before being caught.

Incestuous relationships between father or stepfather and daughter are generally prolonged, and the victims are usually reluctant to report the situation because of fear of retaliation and fear that they will not be believed. Typically, incestuous relationships begin later than other forms of child abuse. The eldest daughter is usually abused, but in her absence another sister may be substituted. Sibling incest may also occur. Sexual abuse by relatives with a strong emotional bond with the victim is the most devastating to the child.

Boys are also victims of both intrafamilial and extrafamilial abuse. Male victims are much less likely to report abuse, and they may suffer much greater emotional harm from incestuous relationships. Boys are likely to be subjected to anal penetration and oral–genital contact. They often have subtle physical findings and are abused by a father, stepfather, or mother's boyfriend.

Children who have a disability or a limiting health condition are at higher risk of sexual assault (Kaufman & CPS, 2011). A 2008 British Columbia study reported that these children were three times more likely than nondisabled children to be both physically and sexually abused (Smith, Stewart, Peled, et al., 2009).

The number of sexual assaults among Indigenous children is uncertain. There are wide differences in reported statistics, ranging from high to low numbers of assault. Child protection agencies report that the rate of sexual abuse among Indigenous children and youth is lower than that for the general population, at 0.53 per 1000 versus 0.62 per 1000 (Collin-Vézina, Dion, & Trocmé, 2009). However, there may be significant underreporting in the Indigenous populations, and more research is required. Significant risk factors for child sexual abuse include parental unavailability, lack of emotional closeness and flexibility, social isolation, emotional deprivation, and communication difficulties.

Initiation and Perpetuation of Sexual Abuse

The cycle of sexual abuse often starts insidiously unless it involves an isolated attack, such as rape. Often offenders spend time with the victims to gain their trust before initiating any sexual contact. Most victims are then pressured into being an accessory to the sexual activity through various means (Box 31-4) and may be unaware that sexual activity is part of the offer. Children may not reveal the truth for fear that their parents would not believe them if told, especially if the offender is a trusted member of the family. Some fear that they will be blamed for the situation, and many young children with limited vocabulary have difficulty describing the activity when they do have the courage or opportunity to reveal the abuse.

Incest most frequently occurs between fathers and daughters, but may be between grandfather and granddaughter or brother and sister. Brother–sister incest can be just as damaging as father–daughter abuse. Victims may take years to disclose this abuse. However, not all incestuous relationships follow a pattern of silence. Reports of father–daughter incest during child custody conflicts have become more common and have raised serious concerns regarding the possibility of false accusation. Rather than tolerating or denying the child's sexual abuse, the other parent (usually the mother) is typically the chief accuser.

BOX 31-4 METHODS USED TO PRESSURE CHILDREN INTO SEXUAL ACTIVITY

- The child is offered gifts or privileges.
- The adult misrepresents moral standards by telling the child that it is "okay to do."
- Isolated and emotionally and socially impoverished children are enticed by adults who meet their needs for warmth and human contact. The offender asks the child for help in finding a favourite pet or object with which the child can easily identify.
- The successful sex offender pressures the victim into secrecy regarding the activity by describing it as a "secret between us" that other people may take away if they find out.
- The offender plays on the child's fears, including fear of punishment by the offender, fear of repercussions if the child tells, and fear of abandonment or rejection by the family.

NURSING CARE

Identification and Assessment of Child Abuse

A critical responsibility of health care providers is identifying abusive situations as early as possible. The characteristics that may predispose members of some families to commit abuse can serve as a framework for assessing vulnerability but are never predictive of actual abuse. A careful, detailed history and interview combined with a thorough physical examination are the diagnostic tools needed to identify abuse. Nurses have a special role in identifying abuse, because they may be the first person to see the child and parent and are the consistent caregivers if the child is hospitalized (see Guidelines box).

During the interview with the child and family, the nurse must be careful to avoid biasing the child's retelling of the events. Some experts suggest that health care providers limit the interview to the child's physical and mental health concerns and leave topics of the family's social, legal, or other problems to the police or Child Protection Services (Kellogg, 2005). If this is not possible, an effort should be made to coordinate the interview process so that all pertinent health care providers can be present.

Recognition of abuse or neglect necessitates a familiarity with both the physical and behavioural signs that suggest maltreatment (Box 31-5). No one indicator can be used to diagnose maltreatment. It is a pattern or combination of indicators that should arouse suspicion and further investigation. Some situations may be misinterpreted as abuse, such as bleeding disorders, osteogenesis imperfecta, sudden infant death syndrome, and cultural practices such as cupping or coin rubbing that may mimic physical abuse (see Health Practices, below). Unintentional injuries, such as burns from metal buckles on car seats,

GUIDELINES

Talking With Children Who Reveal Abuse

- Provide a private time and place to talk.
- Do not promise not to tell; tell them that you are required by law to report the abuse.
- Do not express shock or criticize their family.
- Use their vocabulary to discuss body parts.
- Avoid using any leading statements that can distort their report.
- Reassure them that they have done the right thing by telling you.
- Tell them that the abuse is not their fault, that they are not bad or to blame.
- Determine their immediate need for safety.
- Let the child know what will happen when you report the incident.

BOX 31-5 WARNING SIGNS OF ABUSE

- Physical evidence of abuse or neglect, including previous injuries
- Conflicting stories about the "accident" or injury from the parents or others
- Cause of injury blamed on sibling or other party
- An injury inconsistent with the history, such as a concussion and broken arm from falling off a bed
- History inconsistent with child's developmental level, such as a 6-month-old turning on the hot water
- A health concern other than the one associated with signs of abuse (e.g., a chief health concern of a cold when there is evidence of first- and second-degree burns)
- Inappropriate response of caregiver, such as an exaggerated or absent emotional response, refusal to sign for additional tests or to agree to necessary treatment, excessive delay in seeking treatment, or absence of parents for questioning
- Inappropriate response of child, such as little or no response to pain, fear of being touched, excessive or lack of separation anxiety, indiscriminate friendliness to strangers
- Child's report of physical or sexual abuse
- Previous reports of abuse in the family
- Repeated visits to emergency facilities with injuries
- Parent or caregiver report of being gone and finding the child unresponsive, indicating absence during the supposed event that resulted in harm

bruising from seat belts, or spiral fractures from a twist and fall injury, may also be wrongly diagnosed as abuse. Normal variants, such as Mongolian spots and congenital anomalies of genitalia, can also be mistaken for abuse.

Caregiver–Child Interaction

The nurse can use the initial contact with the family to assess the interaction between the caregiver and the child. Observations of the caregivers should include emotional support for the child, attentiveness to his or her needs, and concern for his or her injury. Although caregivers and children may vary in responses to a stressful event, an unusual caregiver–child relationship should be noted and factored into the overall evaluation of the child.

Certain behavioural responses of the parents to their child and to the interviewer should alert the nurse to the possibility of maltreatment. Abusive parents may have difficulty showing concern toward their child. They may be unable or unwilling to comfort the child. Abusers may blame the child for the injuries or belittle them for being "clumsy" or "stupid." When interacting with health care providers the parent may become hostile or uncooperative. During the child's hospitalization they may not participate in the child's care and may show little concern for his or her progress, eventual discharge, or need for follow-up care.

Abused children's responses to their parents or the injury may also support the suspicion of abuse. Although no one pattern is typical, extremes of behaviour may be observed. Children may be unresponsive to the parent or excessively clinging and intolerant of separation. They may be overly attached to the abusive parent, possibly in the hope of preventing any upset that may precipitate anger and another attack. During care of the injury, children may be passive and accepting of the discomfort or uncooperative and fearful of any physical contact. They may avoid eye contact. Some children maintain a wary watchfulness of all strangers; some shy away from strangers as if frightened; others are unusually affectionate and outgoing.

History and Interview

Child physical abuse. It is often difficult to distinguish child maltreatment from accidental injuries. Caregivers whose history of events may be deceptive or incomplete and children who are nonverbal may make the assessment more complex. A purposeful, skilled history and appropriate interview questions will help the nurse to ensure the right course of action. Knowledge of the mechanism of injury and child development is essential. Cases of abuse are often detected by inconsistencies in child or caregiver history of events compared with physical findings. Children who are verbal can often give a history of the injury. Separating the child from the caregiver may provide a more reliable history. It is important to ask nonleading, open-ended questions. The history should include a narrative of the injury from both the caregiver and child (if verbal). Date, time, and location where injury took place, along with who was present at the time of the injury, are essential questions. Family history for bleeding or bone disorders is important. Box 31-6 outlines areas of the history that are of concern for potential abuse.

Neglect and emotional abuse. Each child may manifest different responses to neglect depending on the situation and the child's developmental age. The goal of the interview is to determine whether the child is in a safe environment and whether the caregiver has the skills and resources to care for the child. It is often difficult to determine whether the circumstances constitute poor parenting skills or true neglect. Warning signals of behaviours to look for are found in Box 31-5.

Sexual abuse. An essential component to identifying sexual abuse is the interview. Several dynamics may impede the child's revelation of sexual abuse. Child sexual abuse is often perpetrated by someone known to the child, including family members. In some cases, the children may have been sworn to secrecy. They may have been told that no one will believe them or their family would be harmed if they tell someone about the abuse. The nurse must be able to recognize normal, age-related sexual curiosity and self-stimulating behaviours; typically, children do not act out specific details of the sexual act or perform intrusive acts on others unless they have sexual knowledge beyond their normal age-related development.

Children's reports of sexual abuse may vary from contradictory stories to unwavering versions of the experience. Stories that sound contradictory may reflect the child's experiences in several instances of abuse. In addition, children who repeatedly tell identical facts may have been prompted to do so.

Increasing evidence suggests that the types of interrogation that children are exposed to after reports of sexual abuse shape their thinking. To avoid biasing the interaction, nurses must be

BOX 31-6 CLINICAL MANIFESTATIONS OF POTENTIAL CHILD MALTREATMENT

Physical Neglect

Suggestive Physical Findings

Failure to thrive (growth failure)
Signs of malnutrition, such as thin extremities, abdominal distension, lack of subcutaneous fat
Poor personal hygiene
Unclean or inappropriate dress
Evidence of poor health care, such as delayed immunization, untreated infections, frequent colds
Frequent injuries from lack of supervision

Suggestive Behaviours

Dull and inactive affect; excessively passive or sleepy
Self-stimulatory behaviours, such as finger sucking or rocking
Begging for or stealing food
Absenteeism from school
Child's substance use
Vandalism or shoplifting

Emotional Abuse and Neglect

Suggestive Physical Findings

Failure to thrive
Eating or feeding disorder
Enuresis
Sleep disorder

Suggestive Behaviours

Self-stimulatory behaviours, such as biting, rocking, sucking
During infancy, lack of social smile, and anxiety toward strangers
Withdrawal from environment and people
Unusual fearfulness
Antisocial behaviour, such as destructiveness, stealing, or cruelty toward animals or people
Extremes of behaviour, such as being overcompliant and passive, or aggressive and demanding
Lags in emotional and intellectual development, especially language
Suicide attempts or attempts to harm self

Physical Abuse

Suggestive Physical Findings

Bruises and welts
- On face, lips, mouth, back, buttocks, thighs, or areas of torso
- Regular patterns descriptive of object used, such as belt buckle, hand, wire hanger, chain, wooden spoon; squeeze or pinch marks
- May be present in various stages of healing

Burns
- On soles of feet, palms of hands, back, or buttocks
- Patterns descriptive of object used, such as round cigar or cigarette burns; sharply demarcated areas from immersion in scalding water; rope burns on wrists or ankles from being bound; burns in the shape of an iron, radiator, or electric stove burner
- Absence of "splash" marks and presence of symmetrical burns
- Stun gun injury: lesions circular, fairly uniform (up to 0.5 cm), and paired about 5 cm apart

Fractures and dislocations
- Skull, nose, or facial structures
- Injury denoting type of abuse, such as spiral fracture or dislocation from twisting of an extremity or whiplash from shaking the child
- Multiple new or old fractures in various stages of healing

Lacerations and abrasions
- On backs of arms, legs, torso, face, or external genitalia
- Unusual symptoms, such as abdominal swelling, pain, and vomiting from punching
- Descriptive marks such as from human bites or pulling out of hair

Chemical
- Unexplained repeated poisoning, especially drug overdose
- Unexplained sudden illness, such as hypoglycemia from insulin administration

Suggestive Behaviours

Wary of physical contact with adults
Apparent fear of parents or of going home
Lying very still while surveying environment
Inappropriate reaction to injury, such as failure to cry from pain
Lack of reaction to frightening events
Apprehension when hearing other children cry
Indiscriminate friendliness and displays of affection
Superficial relationships
Acting-out behaviour, such as aggression, to seek attention
Withdrawal behaviour

Sexual Abuse

Suggestive Physical Findings

Bruises, bleeding, lacerations, or irritation of external genitalia, anus, mouth, or throat
Torn, stained, or bloody underclothing
Pain on urination or pain, swelling, and itching of genital area
Penile discharge
Sexually transmitted infection, nonspecific vaginitis, or venereal warts
Difficulty in walking or sitting
Unusual odour in the genital area
Recurrent urinary tract infections
Presence of sperm
Pregnancy in young adolescent

Suggestive Behaviours

Sudden emergence of sexually related problems, including excessive or public masturbation, age-inappropriate sexual play, promiscuity, or overtly seductive behaviour
Withdrawn behaviour, excessive daydreaming
Preoccupation with fantasies, especially in play
Poor relationships with peers
Sudden changes, such as anxiety, weight loss or gain, clinging behaviour
In incestuous relationships, excessive anger at mother for not protecting daughter
Regressive behaviour, such as bed-wetting or thumb-sucking
Sudden onset of phobias or fears, particularly fears of the dark, men, strangers, or particular settings or situations (e.g., undue fear of leaving the house or staying at the day care centre or the babysitter's house)
Running away from home
Substance use, particularly of alcohol or mood-elevating drugs
Profound and rapid personality changes, especially extreme depression, hostility, and aggression (often accompanied by social withdrawal)
Rapidly declining school performance
Suicidal attempts or ideation

skillful interviewers when questioning children who may be victims of abuse. Medical records should include verbatim statements made by the child and the interviewer that reflect appropriate nonleading questions and statements. The child may not be emotionally ready to discuss the abuse. Establishing rapport with the child is essential to gaining his or her trust. Interviews should not be rushed. Engaging the child in play activities while encouraging conversation may help the child discuss the abuse. It may take several interviews or psychological counselling for the child to be forthcoming about the abuse.

Information regarding the last sexual contact is important because it determines the need for a forensic evaluation.

Unfortunately, there is no typical profile of the victim, and there must be a high index of suspicion to identify these children. Physical signs vary and may include any of those listed for sexual abuse. The victim may exhibit various behavioural manifestations, none of which is diagnostic. When abused children exhibit these behaviours, the signs may be incorrectly attributed to the normal stresses of childhood, especially in older school-age children or adolescents. Even signs considered most predictive of sexual abuse, such as certain genital findings, sexually inappropriate behaviour for age, enactment of adult sexual activity, and intense focus on sexual activity (e.g., masturbation), do not always indicate that sexual abuse has occurred. Conversely, abused children may not demonstrate more knowledge of sexual activity than nonabused children. However, one difference in the abused children's explanation of sexual activity may be unusual affective responses. For example, abused children may have an increased incidence of sleep disorders, temper tantrums, and depression.

> **! NURSING ALERT**
>
> When children report potentially sexually abusive experiences, their reports need to be taken seriously but also with caution, to avoid alarming the child or falsely accusing someone.

Munchausen syndrome by proxy. Munchausen syndrome by proxy (MSBP) is a rare but serious form of child abuse in which caretakers deliberately exaggerate or fabricate histories and symptoms or induce symptoms. Alternative names have been suggested and include pediatric condition falsification, factitious disorder (illness) by proxy, child abuse in the medical setting, and medical child abuse. It is a form of child maltreatment that may include physical, emotional, and psychological abuse for the gratification of the caretaker. In most cases the perpetrator is the biological mother, with some degree of health care knowledge and training. Health care providers can become easily misled and unknowingly enable the perpetrator (Flaherty & Macmillan, 2013). Because of the history of symptoms provided by the caretaker, the child endures painful and unnecessary medical testing and procedures. Common symptoms are seizures, nausea and vomiting, diarrhea, and altered mental status; these symptoms are usually witnessed only by the perpetrator. Considerations when determining whether a child is a victim of MSBP include the following:

- Is the child's condition consistent with the reported history?
- Does the diagnostic evidence support the reported history?
- Has anyone other than the caretaker witnessed the symptoms?
- Is treatment being provided primarily because of the caretaker's demands?

The resolution of symptoms after separation from the perpetrator confirms the diagnosis.

Physical Assessment

Child physical abuse. The goal of the physical assessment for child physical abuse is identification of all injuries. A systems approach ensures that the whole body is evaluated. In instances of severe abuse and injuries, the assessment should begin with a rapid assessment of airway, breathing, circulation (ABC) and of neurological systems. A systematic head-to-toe examination follows. Attention to areas often overlooked, such as the scalp, behind the ears, and the lingual frenulum, is essential. The child's exterior genitalia and posterior surface should be completely examined. The location and a detailed description of all injuries should be recorded. Colour, size, and location of all bruising need to be noted. Burn documentation should include location, pattern, demarcation lines, and presence of eschar or blisters. Diagrams of the injuries using a body diagram form are helpful. If available, photographs of the injuries using a measurement tool should be obtained.

Not all forms of physical abuse have obvious signs. Intra-abdominal organ injury from blunt trauma to the abdomen can occur without signs of external abdominal bruising. Nurses should consider intra-abdominal injury in infants and children who have any other signs of abuse.

> **! NURSING ALERT**
>
> Incompatibility between the history and the injury is probably the most important criterion on which to base the decision to report suspected abuse.

Neglect and emotional abuse. Neglect from deprivation of necessities is easier to identify than emotional neglect or abuse because physical signs are usually evident. Assessment of the child's height, weight, nutritional status, hygiene, and age-appropriate interactions is important for the overall picture of potential neglect. Emotional maltreatment may be readily suspected, but it is difficult to substantiate. Physical signs are often nonspecific, and nurses must rely on behavioural indicators, which range from depression to acting-out behaviour, to help identify a possibly abusive situation. Any persistent and unexplained change in the child's behaviour is an important clue to possible emotional abuse.

Sexual abuse. Identifying instances of sexual abuse is particularly difficult because often, few if any obvious physical indications of the activity exist. Physical signs vary and may include any of those listed in Box 31-6 for sexual abuse. The goal of the physical examination is to document genital findings. In most cases the genital examination is normal, which does not mean that sexual abuse did not occur. Fondling or genital-to-genital contact without penetration may leave no physical findings. Forensic-evidence collection should be considered for any child with known or suspected sexual contact within 72 hours. Forensic evidence obtained directly from a prepubertal victim's body diminishes greatly after 24 hours, with the best chance for evidence collection coming from bed linens or the child's underwear.

The female genital examination should include a description of the vulva, hymen, and surrounding tissue. Abnormal findings of concern are injuries to the posterior vulva or the lower half of the hymenal ring, or abrasions, bruising, or bleeding of the genital or anal tissue. It is often helpful to use a magnifying instrument (colposcope) to detect subtle injuries. There are many variants of normal findings for female genital anatomy, so it is recommended that the examination be done by a practitioner experienced with these types of cases. Contrary to popular myth, the size of the hymenal opening is not predictive of the likelihood of sexual abuse. For male victims, presence of swelling, abrasions, or bruising of the genital tissue is of concern for abuse. The anal area should be examined for symmetry, tone, fissures, or scars.

Genital tissue heals quickly and most often without scars. Therefore, unless seen within a few days of injury, the genital tissue may appear normal. In addition, the vaginal and anal mucosa is elastic; therefore, penetration without disruption of tissue is possible. This defies another myth that there is always evidence of female virginity. Consider the collection of specimens for determining the presence of STIs, which may have been contracted during the sexual contact.

Protecting the Child From Further Abuse

Initially, identification of instances of suspected abuse or neglect is essential. The nurse may come in contact with abused children in an emergency department, practitioner's office, home, day care centre, or school.

NURSING ALERT

The priority is to remove the child from the abusive situation to prevent further injury.

All provinces have laws of mandatory reporting of child maltreatment. Suspected child abuse is reported to the local Child Welfare Agency. After a referral has been made, a caseworker is assigned to investigate the report. Based on the findings, the child is left in the home or removed temporarily.

A court proceeding may be necessary before the child can be placed outside the home or when parental rights are to be terminated. When the courts are involved, they usually require firsthand testimony by the referring parties. Nurses may be subpoenaed to appear in court, or their notes may be introduced as evidence in court hearings. Accurate and factual documentation is essential. Behaviours need to be described, not interpreted, and recorded daily to establish a progress record (see Guidelines box). Conversations among the nurse, child, and parent should be recorded verbatim as much as possible.

GUIDELINES

Recording Assessment Data in Suspected Abuse

History of Injury

- Date, time, and place of occurrence
- Sequence of events with recorded times
- Presence of witnesses, especially person caring for child at time of incident
- Time lapse between occurrence of injury and initiation of treatment
- Interview with child, when appropriate, including verbal quotations and information from drawing or other play activities, such as using a doll to represent the body to demonstrate what happened, which decreases anxiety
- Interview with parent, witnesses, or other significant persons, including verbal quotations
- Description of parent–child interactions (verbal interactions, eye contact, touching, parental concern)
- Name, age, and condition of other children in home (if possible)

Physical Examination

- Nursing physical examination to be done with permission from the child or parent(s)
- Location, size, shape, and colour of bruises; approximate location, size, and shape on drawing of body outline
- Distinguishing characteristics, such as a bruise in the shape of a hand, or a round burn (possibly caused by cigarette)
- Symmetry or asymmetry of injury; presence of other injuries
- Ophthalmic exam for intraocular bleeds
- Degree of pain; any bone tenderness
- Evidence of past injuries; general state of health and hygiene
- Digital photographs with date and time stamp should be taken if there is evidence on the child's body for physical abuse, sexual abuse, or neglect (there may no specialized team outside of urban centres that can do the photography)
- Developmental level of child; perform screening test (see Developmental Assessment, Chapter 33)

Support Child

Children suspected of being abused are often hospitalized for medical management of their injuries and to allow further assessment of their safety needs. The needs of these children are the same as those of any hospitalized child. The child should be treated as a child with the usual physical needs, developmental tasks, and play interests—not as a victim of abuse. The goal of the nurse–child relationship is to provide a role model for the parents in helping them relate positively and constructively to their child and to foster a therapeutic environment for the child in his or her reprieve from the abusing situation.

Support Family

The nurse also needs to encourage the child's relationship with the nonoffending parent. The nurse does not become a substitute parent, but rather acts as a role model for parents in helping them to relate positively and constructively to their child. When parental ignorance of child-rearing practices has played a part in the abuse, the nurse can educate the parent about children's physical and emotional needs. Because of the parents' own child-rearing, they may not be aware of nonviolent methods of discipline, such as timeout. They may also need help in dealing with their frustration so that they do not vent anger on the child. Because these parents may be sensitive to criticism or perceptions of domination, teaching is best implemented through demonstration and example rather than through lecturing. Any competent parenting abilities they demonstrate should be praised to promote their sense of parental adequacy.

Family members should be advised to encourage the child to resume normal activities and to observe the child for signs of distress. Children express their feelings primarily through behaviour. Parents should be alert for changes in behaviour that indicate distress resulting from the incident, such as remaining in the house, refusing to go to school, changing sleeping patterns, and having more frequent dreams and nightmares. Children should be encouraged to talk about these feelings and nightmares, because the more they talk about the experience, the more they are able to gain control over it.

Referral to appropriate social service agencies is also essential. Some abusive parents live in poverty, and the daily stresses imposed by their circumstances are overwhelming. Resources for financial aid, improved housing, and child care should be sought. Self-help groups can also provide important services. Groups such as Parents Anonymous (a group for parents who have abused or fear that they may abuse their child, but only in terms of physical abuse, not sexual abuse) and Parents United International, Inc. (a group devoted to helping sexually abused families) are accepting and nonjudgemental (see Additional Resources at the end of this chapter).

Plan for Discharge

Discharge planning should begin as soon as the legal disposition for placement has been decided, which may be temporary foster home placement, return to the parents, or permanent termination of parental rights. The latter is the most drastic solution but is necessary in situations of life-threatening abuse. Whenever children are sent to a foster home they must be allowed an opportunity to express their feelings. No matter how severe the abuse, they usually mourn the loss of their parents. They need help in understanding why they must not return home and that this new home is in no way a punishment. Whenever possible, foster parents should be encouraged to visit the child in the hospital, and the nurse should take an active role in helping these new parents understand the child and his or her health care needs, because studies have shown that the health care needs of children in foster care often go unmet (Mekonnen, Noonan, & Rubin, 2009).

Prevent Abuse

Prevention of child maltreatment has been an extremely difficult goal. Programs aimed at identifying potential abusers and instituting supportive intervention before the occurrence of an abusive act have met with variable success. However, nurses have played an important role in such programs. For example, home visits by nurses to primiparas who were either teenagers or of low socioeconomic status have been noted to be an effective preventive measure. The nurses provided information on normal child growth and development and routine health care needs, served as informal support persons, and referred families to appropriate services when a need for assistance was identified (Donelan-McCall, Eckenrode, & Olds, 2009).

Such programs provide models that can be used to reduce factors that increase the risk of abuse. Nurses in a variety of settings can implement similar activities. For example, nurses in prenatal clinics can prepare expectant families for adjustment to parenthood. Postpartum nurses can foster the attachment process by encouraging parents to hold and look at their infant and practise skin-to-skin-contact, as well as by teaching coping mechanisms for prolonged crying. Nurses in neonatal intensive care units can minimize the effects of separation by encouraging parents to visit the infant and can help parents become comfortable caring for their child. Nurses in ambulatory settings can teach parents appropriate methods of bathing, feeding, toileting, disciplining, and preventing injuries, while stressing the normal needs and developmental characteristics of children. Nurses must be sensitive to parental needs for attention, reassurance, and reinforcement and refer parents to community services and self-help groups when needed.

Unlike preventive efforts for neglect and physical abuse, which are aimed at the potential offender, prevention of child sexual abuse centres on education of children to protect themselves. Materials are available for parents that describe sexual abuse and its prevention (see Additional Resources at the end of the chapter). Supporting parental qualities of respect, affection, empathy, and ability to set boundaries and providing high-quality child care and education represent the true preventive approach to sexual abuse. Helpful games such as "What if the babysitter wants to wrestle and hug but tells you to keep it a secret?" can be used to explore dangerous situations in advance and help children learn the importance of saying "no." They need reassurance that no matter what the other person says or does, the parents want to know about it and will not punish them. Even if children participate in the activity before telling the parents, they must be reassured that it was not their fault.

It is equally important to teach children safety in terms of potential risk situations. Several suggestions for parents regarding protecting and educating children against possible molestation are presented in the Family-Centred Teaching box. The nurse is frequently in a position to discuss the topic of abuse with parents and to provide guidelines.

SOCIAL, CULTURAL, AND RELIGIOUS FACTORS THAT IMPACT HEALTH

The health of Canadians is not dependent primarily on the health care provided but rather by access to the social determinants of health, or broadly speaking, the living conditions to which people are subjected. Since the mid-1800s the importance of living conditions on health has been recognized, and since the 1970s it has been embedded in Canadian government policy (Mikkonen & Raphael, 2010). Social determinants of health exist at an individual as well as a population level, and they affect the degree to which each person has the necessary

FAMILY-CENTRED TEACHING

Preventing or Dealing With Sexual Abuse of Children

Sexual assault of children is much more common than most people realize. It may be preventable if children have good preparation. To provide protection and preparation, the following measures can be taken:

- Pay careful attention to who is around children. (Unwanted touch may come from someone liked and trusted.)
- Back up a child's right to say "no."
- Encourage communication by taking seriously what children say.
- Take a second look at signals of potential danger.
- Refuse to leave children in the company of those not trusted.
- Include information about sexual assault when teaching about safety.
- Provide specific definitions and examples of sexual assault.
- Remind children that even "nice" people sometimes do mean things.
- Urge children to tell about anybody who causes them to be uncomfortable.
- Prepare children to deal with bribes, threats, and possible physical force.
- Virtually eliminate secrets between children and parents.
- Teach children how to say "no," ask for help, and control who touches them and how.
- Model self-protective and limit-setting behaviour for children.

Should it ever become necessary to help a child recover from a sexual assault:

- Listen carefully to understand children.
- Support the child for telling through praise, belief, sympathy, and lack of blame.
- Know local resources and choose help carefully.
- Provide opportunities to talk about the assault.
- Provide opportunities for the entire family to go through a recovery process.

Sexual assault affects everyone. To help deal with this social problem:

- Provide care and support to those who have been victimized.
- Recognize that offenders do not change without intervention.
- Organize neighbourhood programs to support each other's efforts to protect children.
- Encourage schools to provide information about sexual assault as a problem of health and safety.
- Organize community groups to support educational treatment and law enforcement programs.

resources to meet their daily needs and achieve their goals. The key determinants that are generally accepted as impacting the health of Canadians are listed in Table 1-1.

Key Social Determinant Influences

There is strong evidence that social factors are interconnected and complex and that they have a significant influence on health. Health is a developmental process, a product of interactions among personal, physical, and environmental factors. Children are particularly sensitive to social determinants, especially in their younger years; the first 3 years of life present a crucial period during which they are susceptible to both negative and positive influences. If the exposure to negative influences outweighs that to positive ones, their adaptation can be compromised, setting the stage for greater problems later in life. While very young children are dependent on supportive caregiving for healthy development, older children are more dependent on relationships with peers and on school, neighbourhood, and community environments (Halfon, Larson, & Russ, 2010; Viner, Ozer, Denny, et al., 2012).

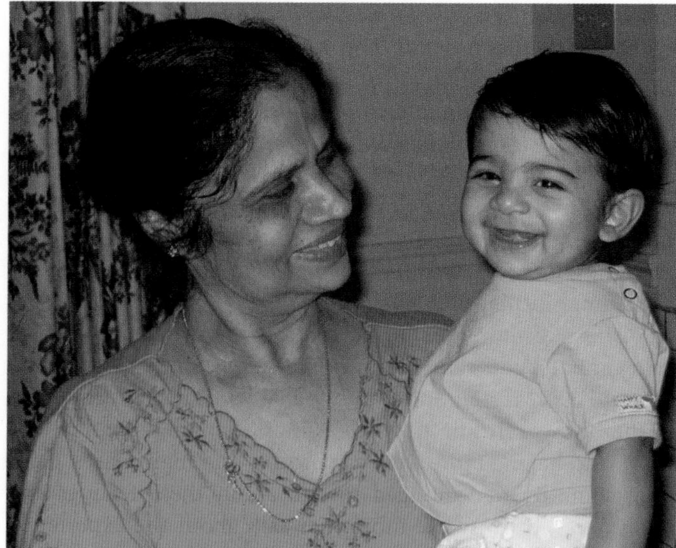

FIGURE 31-3 Children grow up within a shared cultural, social, and linguistic heritage.

Culture

Society reflects the collective success of families to prepare their children for their future, and it also reflects how the decisions made by government and other institutions shape the social environment in which the families live (McNeill, 2010).

Children interact within a cultural context every day and are impacted by its influences. Social values and beliefs differ among cultures, and children learn directly through the teachings of their families and indirectly through the behaviours around them. Children learn and apply the values and beliefs common to their culture; for example, in some cultures, competition and individual achievement are highly valued, whereas in other cultures collaboration and working with others are highly valued (Copple & Bredekamp, 2009; Kostelnik, Whiren, Soderman, et al., 2014).

Except in rare situations, children grow and develop in a blend of cultures and subcultures (Fig. 31-3). In a large, complex society such as that of Canada, different groups have their own sets of standards, values, and expectations within the collective ways of the larger culture. Although many cultural differences are related to geographic boundaries, subcultures are not always restricted by location.

Culture also influences health and illness, as there are differences in the way people of diverse cultures conceptualize sickness, seek health care, relate to health care providers, and accept treatments. Children are dependent on their adult caregivers (typically parents) for survival since in the early stages of language development they are not able to clearly communicate symptoms of an illness. Health care providers must rely on parents to speak for their child and describe the illness the child is suffering from. If the adults have their own cultural biases or interpretations about illness and appropriate treatments, their description and management of the illness may be shaped and altered by these beliefs and understandings (Tseng & Streltzer, 2008).

Social roles. Family roles, like cultural beliefs and values, are learned and transmitted through generations. A role prohibits some behaviours and allows others. Much of children's self-concept is derived from their ideas about their family and social roles. Parents use praise, punishment, and role modelling to teach children culturally acceptable roles. Because roles are shaped and clarified according to the prevailing culture, it has a significant influence on the development of children's self-concept (i.e., attitudes and beliefs they have about themselves).

A social group consists of a system of roles carried out in primary and secondary groups. A *primary group* is characterized by intimate, continued, face-to-face contact; mutual support of members; and the ability to order or constrain a considerable proportion of individual members' behaviour. Two such groups are the family and the peer group, both of which exert a great deal of influence on the child.

Secondary groups are groups that have limited, intermittent contact and in which there is generally less concern about members' behaviour. These groups offer little in terms of support or pressure toward conformity except in rigidly limited areas. Examples of secondary groups are church organizations, Girl Guides and Boy Scouts, sports organizations, and formal recreational children's play groups (also considered in relation to subgroups). The child-rearing orientation in a secondary group environment, such as urban communities, differs considerably from that of a primary group community. An urban community is dynamic and rapidly changing; thus many of the traditional behaviours and values do not meet its needs. Consequently, parents are often uncertain about what to teach their children. They may wish to raise their children with values consistent with their own, but the differences in experience between the generations are too great. As a result, they often grant their children autonomy in some areas of decision making early in the developmental process, and other secondary groups assume a greater influence. The children are exposed to an assortment of social groups with diverse sets of values and expectations. None of the groups is highly dominant in its influence; children are exposed to an eclectic set of values, some in agreement and some in conflict with the others. From these they must ultimately select those values that they determine to be best for them and adopt them to form a consistent set of roles and behaviours to be incorporated into their self-concept.

Self-esteem. Culture influences a child's sense of self-esteem, often referred to as self-view or self-evaluation. People from different cultures share a common motivation to be a good person—to live up to the standards of what is perceived to be appropriate and significant in the context of their own culture. But these perceptions vary greatly across cultures. In North America, a highly individualistic environment, the most valued attributes are those associated with self-evaluation of competence, talent, independence, and risk-taking to achieve success. But in East Asia, it is how others perceive an individual's competence and success and their ability to apply the criticisms to self-improvement that dictate self-esteem. In other cultures, it is the achievements and successes of group efforts that lead to more positive self-esteem.

For children, school experiences that focus on personal achievement may promote positive self-esteem in some children but not in others who are more dependent on the success of a whole family or peer group. A child's sense of control may not come from individual self-reliance but rather from a feeling of worthiness in his or her family or community.

Families and culture also influence the criteria that children use to evaluate their own abilities. Additionally, cultures vary in the degree to which they instill an internal locus of control (a belief in the ability to regulate one's own life). Effects on self-esteem are minimal if these beliefs are directed by parents and are in accordance with cultural customs. What is damaging to emotional health is the helplessness that can stem from prejudice. Ethnic pride has helped individuals maintain a positive self-image and protect against the damage that prejudice can cause (Becker, Vignoles, Owe, et al., 2014; Falk & Heine, 2015).

Socioeconomic Status

Socioeconomic status relates to a family's economic and education levels. As a determinant of health, the influence of socioeconomic class cannot be overlooked; the most overwhelming adverse influence on health is low socioeconomic status. At any one time, a higher percentage of low-income individuals suffers from some health problem than any other group (see Chapter 1, Fig. 1-1).

The number of children living in poverty has continued to increase into the twenty-first century. The child poverty rate in Canada is among the highest in the developed world. In 2013, an average of 19% of children were living in poverty, despite the continued economic growth in Canada and the introduction of a Canadian Child Tax Benefit and National Child Benefit Supplement for lower-income families (Campaign 2000, 2015). Large urban centres have child poverty rates as high as 29% (McNeill, 2010). Persistent poverty puts children at risk for suffering health problems, including infant mortality, asthma, obesity, poor literacy, developmental delays, and behavioural and mental health difficulties. These children also tend to attain lower levels of education and are more likely to live in poverty as adults (Fleury, 2008).

Families living in poverty struggle to provide health care for themselves and for their children. Travel to health care facilities often requires finding money for public transit or a taxi, borrowing a car, or seeking other means of transportation. They must find care for dependents, such as other infants and small children, or have them accompany them when taking the child for care. Families tend to delay preventive care indefinitely unless health services are relatively accessible. They are more likely to consult traditional practitioners or other persons within their community. Day-to-day needs of food, clothing, and lodging take precedence over health care as long as the ailing person feels able to perform activities of daily living.

One of the more pressing problems in Canada is the growing number of homeless families. Homeless children experience all of the health problems associated with poverty, as well as other types of disorders. Most of these children experience poor health. They may not have a regular source of health care, and the focus of their care may not be preventive. Their care is likely fragmented, crisis oriented, and often sought in emergency departments of hospitals. Another group of homeless children are the "runaway" adolescents, who are at risk for violence, victimization, STIs, and substance use (Employment and Social Development Canada, 2015).

School

Next to family, schools are a major force in providing continuity between generations, by conveying a vast amount of culture from older members of society to the young. In this way, children are prepared to carry out the traditional social roles expected of them as adults in society. School rules and regulations regarding attendance, authority relationships, and the system of sanctions and rewards based on achievement transmit to the child the behavioural expectations of the adult world of employment and relationships. School is often the only institution in which children systematically learn about the negative consequences of behaviours that deviate from societal expectations. Teachers are expected to stimulate and guide the intellectual development of children and their sense of aesthetics and to foster their capacity for creative problem solving. Access to education is an important determinant of health. Through education, individuals of lower socioeconomic status are offered the opportunity and capacity to move up in the social strata.

Traditionally, the socialization process of school began when the child entered kindergarten or first grade. Today, with almost 70% of mothers whose youngest child is aged 3 to 5 years old working outside the home, this socialization process begins much earlier for a significant number of children in a variety of child care settings. This statistic increases to more than 78% for mothers whose youngest child is 6 to 15 years old (Ferrao, 2010). For adolescents, close school connectedness and socialization has been linked with fewer health risk behaviours and better long-term health outcomes (Viner et al., 2012).

Community

The child's or adolescent's community is made up of the family, school, neighbourhood, youth organizations, and other members. These all contribute to the young person's experience within any culture (Search Institute, 2016). Studies of students in grades 6 through 12 have shown that those who experience a higher number of relationships, opportunities, and personal qualities, or assets that they need to thrive in their lives, are more likely to make healthy choices and avoid high-risk behaviours. These assets offer a framework for positive child and adolescent development (Viner et al., 2012).

Four categories of external assets that youth receive from the community are as follows (Search Institute, 2016):

1. **Support**—Young people need to feel support, care, and love from their families, neighbours, and others. They also need organizations and institutions that offer positive, supportive environments.
2. **Empowerment**—Young people need to feel valued by their community and be able to contribute to others. They need to feel safe and secure.
3. **Boundaries and expectations**—Young people need to know what is expected of them and what actions and behaviours are within the community boundaries and what are outside of them.
4. **Constructive use of time**—Young people need opportunities for growth through constructive, enriching opportunities and quality time at home.

Internal assets must also be nurtured in the community's younger members. These internal qualities guide choices and create a sense of centredness, purpose, and focus. The four categories of internal assets are as follows (Search Institute, 2016):

1. **Commitment to learning**—Young people need to develop a commitment to education and life-long **learning**.
2. **Positive values**—Youth need to have a strong sense of values that direct their choices.
3. **Social competencies**—Young people need competencies that help them make positive choices and build relationships.
4. **Positive identity**—Young people need a sense of their own power, purpose, worth, and promise.

Peer Groups

The aspects of everyday life that are most important to people are typically family life, time with friends, school, work, and play—all involving relationships with other humans. From birth, humans are social beings who spend their lifetime actively engaging with others in small and large groups. Children belong to some groups that they have not joined voluntarily—most specifically their families, day cares and school classrooms. Through social interactions children gain a sense of belonging, companionship, social stimulation; they learn about themselves and how the world works. Personal and interpersonal skills are developed and children learn what is expected of them and about the values inherent in the society in which they live. The lessons learned in early life about how to behave and interact with others set the foundations for adolescent and adult life. Navigating the social environment is such an important aspect of human experience that it is a primary focus of growth and development (Kostelnik et al., 2014).

Children are active learners, not waiting for others to provide information or opportunities for learning. They make sense of social experiences through observing, experimenting in situations, interacting with other people, and reflecting on what happens. Through these activities they form ideas about how their social world works, gradually adjusting their thinking and constructing new ideas about codes of behaviour and strategies to use.

As children interact with peer groups in day care, school, or neighbourhood settings, a significant amount of socialization occurs. Groups are regarded differently by younger and older children, and group concepts change as children age—the younger the child, the less sense he or she has of group awareness, while adolescents typically define themselves through their group memberships.

Peer groups provide natural opportunities for social learning as children are able to practise and receive feedback about skills (e.g., sharing) rather than just hearing or talking about skills and behaviours. The social negotiation that occurs helps children learn to understand others' thoughts, emotions, and intentions and results in better understanding about consequences of their behaviours both for themselves and for others.

The value systems that children are exposed to can vary greatly as they grow. Their family, social class, and ethnic group provide some value constancy from a young age, while peer groups typically provide a diverse set of values. These peer group values can compel children to change their own values, since acceptance to the group is largely based on conformity. If there is a fair degree of similarity between the values of the peer group and those of family and teachers, the small difference creates the separation between children and the adults in their lives, strengthening the bond with their peers.

The kind of socialization that occurs in peer groups can be dependent on the type of group and its members—the backgrounds of the members, the capabilities of its individual members, and the reason that they are brought together (Fig. 31-4). Scholastic groups and sports team members focus on educational or athletic achievements, while other less goal-oriented peer groups might focus on less productive goals. Although peer groups do not have the same formal authority that parents or schools do, they convey significant amounts of information and a significant degree of influence (Kostelnik et al., 2014; Rubin & Bukowski, 2011).

The Child and Family in North America

The frontier background of North American culture has contributed to the overall orientation toward life and child-rearing. There has always been a basic optimistic view of the world, a belief that things can be better and that the children can and will be better off than their parents. This hopeful outlook and a general future orientation, together with the possibility of upward social mobility, have created a pervasive attitude of optimism. Increasing development of self-confidence and autonomy in children is fostered and encouraged. Children in North America are generally permitted a greater degree of freedom than in some more tradition-oriented cultures, where individuals remain in one class for life.

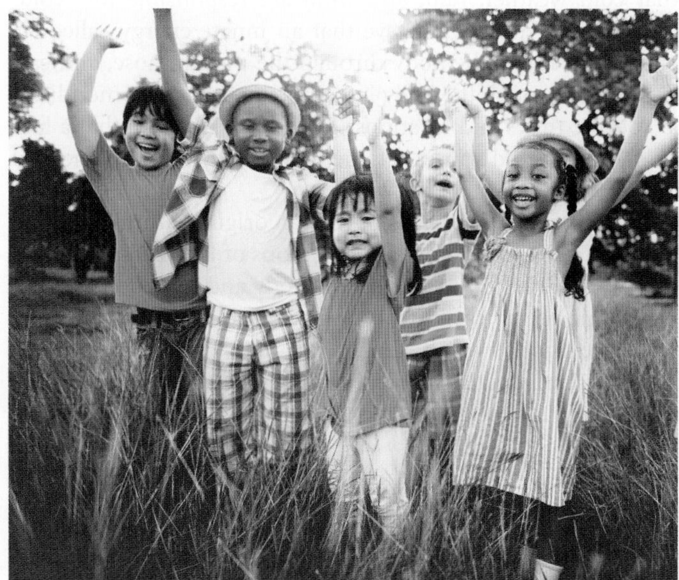

FIGURE 31-4 Youngsters from different cultural backgrounds interact within the larger culture. (Rawpixel.com/Shutterstock.com.)

Family life in North America is characterized by increasing geographic and economic mobility. There is less reliance on tradition, families are fragmented, and there may be fewer opportunities to transmit and acquire traditional and accepted customs of a culture. Consequently, young adults rely to a greater extent on professed experts, peers, and mass media for acquisition of acceptable patterns of behaviour, including child-rearing practices. Conflicting information can be a source of confusion and frustration as parents attempt to determine the comparatively stable, essential components of the culture and transmit these to their children.

In Canada, diversity is embraced and valued. People of all races and ethnicities need to be respected and children encouraged to feel secure and confident in their racial or ethnic identity. As with all children, the most important influences on development of a positive self-image are warm, understanding parents who take an active interest in fostering their children's growth. Parents who have established a healthy and loving relationship with their children and react positively will help their children develop feelings of self-worth, self-esteem, and self-acceptance. The more adequate children feel, the more positive their attitudes will be toward children of all backgrounds. Parents who have not established a close relationship with their children and who treat them in nonsupportive ways put their children at risk of acting aggressively and bullying others, particularly those who appear or act differently (Pepler, German, Craig, et al., 2011).

Indigenous Peoples

Indigenous peoples is the name given for the original peoples of North America. In Canada, the Constitution recognizes three groups of Indigenous people: First Nations (made up of more than 615 bands across the country), Métis (European–First Nation ancestry), and Inuit (Arctic-situated Indigenous peoples). These three peoples have distinct histories, languages, cultural practices, and spiritual beliefs (Fig. 31-5).

Unlike the rest of Canada's population, Indigenous youth under 25 years of age make up over 50% of the Indigenous populations. This population is growing twice as fast as the general Canadian population, with the largest increase occurring in families living on reserve (Indigenous and Northern Affairs Canada, 2015).

Indigenous peoples tend to experience health problems that are common to people living in poverty, related largely to the position they have historically held in Canadian society. The health of Indigenous children under 16 years of age lags behind that of other Canadian children. Infant mortality rates are three times higher, immunization rates are lower, and infectious diseases continue to be a key factor of morbidity for Indigenous children. The rates of diabetes in adolescents are higher, and the number of deaths related to injuries (motor vehicle accidents, fires, self-harm, and harm to others) is four times higher than that for the overall Canadian population. In addition, the suicide rate is almost four times higher than the national

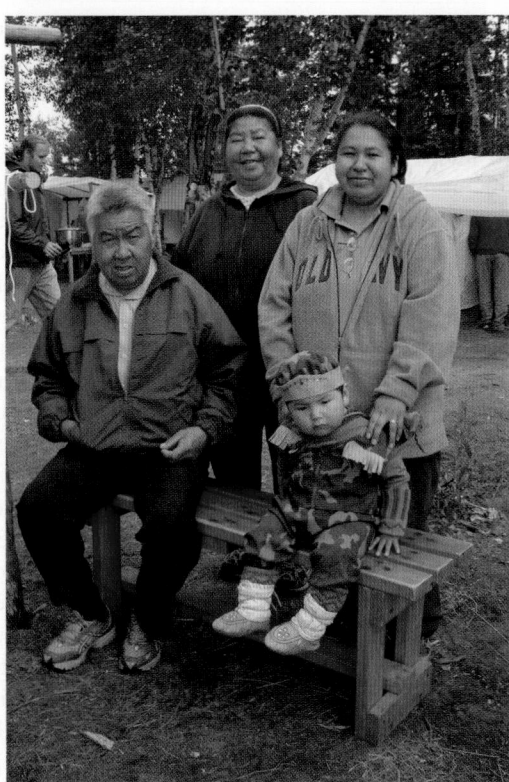

FIGURE 31-5 This Eabametoong First Nation family represents a subculture that interrelates with the larger Canadian culture. (© Megapress/Alamy Stock Photo.)

average, and suicide frequently occurs in clusters. The most common reasons for poorer health status among Indigenous peoples are lower incomes, a higher jobless rate, poor shelter, lower education level, inadequate water and sewage systems, and living in remote communities (see discussion in Chapter 1, p. 6) (Postl, Cook, & Moffatt, 2010).

Immigrant Families

Immigration to Canada has been on the rise over the past two decades. In the 2006 census, immigrants made up 19.8% of the population, up from 17.4% in 1996 (Barozzino, 2010). In 2009, more than 250,000 people immigrated to Canada, with just over 50,000, or 20%, being children under the age of 15 years (Government of Canada, Immigration and Citizenship, 2016a). In 2016 alone Canada welcomed over 26,000 new immigrants from Syria (Government of Canada, Immigration and Citizenship, 2016b).

For decades it was generally accepted that immigrants to Canada arrived with a variety of health issues and were in need of health care that was absent in their countries of origin. More recent research and observations have indicated that new immigrants arrive with relatively better overall health (lower chronic disease and mortality rates) than that of their Canadian-born counterparts (with the exception of HIV/AIDS and tuberculosis) and maintain this health for 5 to 10 years—this is termed the *healthy migrant effect* (Barozzino, 2010).

Social determinants of health are thought to affect immigrants to Canada more significantly than native-born Canadians, leading to a phenomenon known as *immigrant overshoot*, where immigrants' health not only deteriorates to the Canadian average but also may get worse as a result of the impact of the social determinants of health that affect immigrants more powerfully (Barozzino, 2010). Immigrant families face unique challenges, including language barriers, lack of recognition of their skills and credentials, lack of access to affordable housing and to appropriate community and settlement supports, limited health care coverage until provincial or territorial health insurance is arranged, limited access to and navigation of the health care system, and health care providers who lack any significant knowledge of and sensitivity to their diverse health care needs.

Health Beliefs

Generally speaking, health care providers in North America and many other parts of the world believe that illness is a result of a biological cause and use scientific methods and processes to diagnose and address health issues. A family's cultural heritage fundamentally shapes their beliefs related to the cause of illness and the maintenance of health. These beliefs can be closely linked with religious beliefs and influence the way families cope with illness and respond to health care providers. Families can assign meaning to illnesses and believe that the illness is a result of some wrongdoing on their part or the part of the child. Predominant among many cultures are beliefs related to natural forces, supernatural forces, and imbalance between forces. Because families are such an important part of the care process, it is therefore important to understand their health beliefs in developing and carrying out a child's plan of care.

Natural Forces

The most common natural forces held responsible for ill health are cold air entering the body and impurities in the air; if the body is not adequately protected, illness can ensue. For example, a Chinese mother may overdress her infant in an effort to keep cold wind from entering the child's body. The Chinese believe that cold weather, rain, and wind are responsible for "cold" conditions. They also believe that an innate energy called *chi* enters and leaves the body through the mouth, nose, and ears and flows through the body in definite pathways, or meridians, at specific times and locations. The Chinese believe that a lack of chi and blood causes fatigue, low energy, and a variety of ailments.

Among some Canadians of African origin, natural phenomena such as phases of the moon, seasons of the year, and planet positions are believed to affect the body and its processes; thus health maintenance is strongly associated with the ability to read "the signs."

Most Indigenous people consider health to be a state of harmony with nature and the universe.

Supernatural Forces

Evil influences such as voodoo, witchcraft, or evil spirits are viewed in some cultures as causes of adverse health, especially those illnesses that cannot be explained by other means. A health belief common among some people from Central America, the Middle East, the Mediterranean, and some Asian and African societies is the concept of the evil eye (Spector, 2009). Strength and power are associated with the evil eye; therefore, as long as an individual's strength and weakness remain in balance, he or she is unlikely to become a victim of the evil eye. Weaknesses are not necessarily physical. For example, an excess of some emotion, such as envy, can create weakness. Infants and small children, because of immature development of their internal strength–weakness states, are especially vulnerable to the gaze of the evil eye. Consequently, the evil eye serves to rationalize an inexplicable onset of illness in children who display symptoms such as restlessness, crying, diarrhea, vomiting, and fever. Because this belief is seldom expressed to health care providers, they may not be aware of its influence on parents' understanding of their child's illness.

Imbalance of Forces

The concept of balance or equilibrium is widespread throughout the world. One of the most common imbalances is that which exists between "hot" and "cold." This belief derived from the ancient Greek concept of body humours (Andrews & Boyle, 2008), which states that illness is caused by an imbalance of the four humours: phlegm, blood, black bile, and yellow bile. These are balanced in healthy people and out of balance in those with illnesses. Such imbalance is thought to cause internal damage or altered function. Treatment of the illness is directed at restoring balance. The hot and cold understanding of disease is based in this concept. Diseases, areas of the body, foods, and illnesses are classified as either "hot" or "cold." Foods and beverages are designated hot or cold based on the effect they exert, not their actual temperature. In Chinese health belief, the forces are termed *yin* (cold) and *yang* (hot) (Spector, 2009; Tseng & Streltzer, 2008).

Illness is treated by restoring normal balance through the application of appropriate "hot" or "cold" remedies. A "cold" condition such as a respiratory disease is believed to be caused by exposure to cold weather, rain, or cold wind entering the body; it is treated by administration of "hot" foods, herbs, or drugs. Menstruation is considered a "hot" condition; therefore women are cautioned against ingesting "hot" foods, which might increase menstrual flow or produce cramping. Ingesting too much of either "hot" or "cold" foods can also be interpreted as a cause of illness.

Health care workers who are aware of this belief are better able to understand why some persons refuse to eat certain foods. It is often useful to discuss the diet with the family to determine their beliefs regarding food choices. The nurse can help families devise a diet that contains the necessary balance of basic food groups prescribed by the medical subculture while continuing to maintain the beliefs of the ethnic subculture.

Culturally Competent Nursing Care

In order to provide culturally competent and culturally sensitive care, nurses must be aware of the need to consider cultural differences among patients. An understanding of the various beliefs regarding the causation of illness and disease, as well as traditional health practices, is essential to successful intervention. The more nurses know about the values, beliefs, and customs of various ethnic groups, the better they will be able to meet the needs of families and work together to plan care. Nurses must first relate to the family's perceptions and interpretations of experiences from the family's background and cultural belief system before they can effectively intervene. It is important that health care providers are conscious that even within an identified particular ethnic group many heterogeneous subgroups exist and that there are many people with mixed ethnic backgrounds associated with interethnic marriages. In addition, there can be wide individual variations within groups, so ethnic stereotyping must be avoided (Tseng & Streltzer, 2008).

A model for learning about health traditions that differ from the Western, or modern, health care system is based on three dimensions:

1. What are the physical aspects of caring for the body (e.g., are there special clothes, foods, medicines)?
2. What are the mental parts of caring for health (e.g., feelings, attitudes, rituals, actions)?
3. What are the spiritual aspects of health (who I am, spiritual customs, prayers, healers)?

For each of these dimensions, one must consider the cultural traditions used to maintain health, protect health, and restore health (Spector, 2009).

In some cultures, the child's gender may determine the opportunities for access to and use of health information, care, and services. For example, in some cultures, boys are held in higher esteem than girls. This could result in boys receiving better health care and more food because they are expected to take care of their parents in old age (Low & Low, 2012).

Perceptions of disease or signs and symptoms of illness are also influenced by culture. Some cultures, for example, see diarrhea as a cleansing of the body that is essential for health maintenance and prevention or cure of illness. Furthermore, signs or symptoms resulting from diarrhea and ensuing dehydration, such as malaise, fever, anorexia, and irritability, may be viewed as separate illness entities.

Nurses can often recognize a family's health-related cultural perceptions and interpretations through discussion and observation. Implications of these perceptions should be explored with the family and considered when planning culturally appropriate interventions. Complementary treatments the family would like employed need to be documented on the child's health plan to ensure consistent approaches among members of the health care team. Family roles differ by culture as well. Authority figures in a family may be a mother, father, or grandparent and may change depending on the circumstance and whether in public or in the home. Decision making may involve the extended family, with women being subordinate to men and young people to older people, even including the extended family (Tseng & Streltzer, 2008).

Nurses who are members of a majority culture may encounter tension and distrust in a child from a minority culture as a result of the child's learned perception of or relationships with other persons in the majority group. On the basis of these biases, such children may suspect that nurses have hostile feelings toward them and may fear ill treatment. When these children are hospitalized (Fig. 31-6) this feeling compounds the

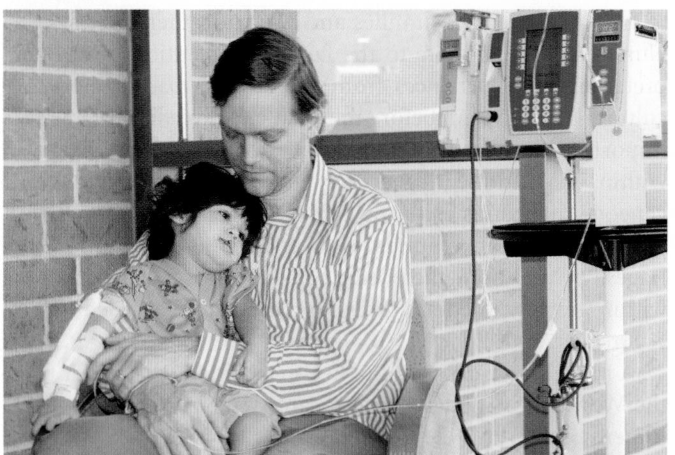

FIGURE 31-6 A father with his hospitalized child. (aren Jai Wicklund/Shutterstock.com.)

feelings of loneliness and helplessness, which accompany frightening experiences and separation from families. The reverse situation may be encountered by a nurse from a minority culture attempting to meet the needs of a child who has been conditioned to view the nurse's culture, ethnic group, or gender as inferior.

NURSING ALERT

In working with families, it is essential for nurses to identify key members of the family. Failure to include these significant individuals in communication or teaching can seriously hinder working together to achieve the care plan.

Communication

Communication may be a source of distress and misunderstanding between persons from different ethnic groups, especially if the languages are different. Lack of interpreter services and linguistically appropriate health education materials is associated with patient dissatisfaction, poor understanding and adherence to treatment, and lower-quality health care (see discussion in Chapter 2, p. 22).

Some persons with poor or limited language comprehension may simply smile and nod in agreement if they do not understand the questions or directives. It is vital that the family fully understand all implications of a child's care and management before they sign permissions for special procedures or assume responsibility for the child's care. It is not uncommon for a Vietnamese or a Japanese family to indicate "yes" in order to avoid social disharmony, when in fact they mean "no". They tend to use indirectness rather than confrontation and may become evasive when direct questioning makes them uncomfortable.

It is not uncommon for health care providers to request that an English-speaking relative accompany the patient and family to an appointment. Although family members might have knowledge of the patient's concerns and backgrounds, they might make incorrect assumptions and might hold back information that they feel would upset the family, particularly if a child is asked to interpret. Comprehensive planning prior to a patient or family appointment is essential to acquire the appropriate interpretation services in order to prevent miscommunication, misdiagnosis, and ineffective treatment. Trained medical interpreters are sensitive to the cultural nuances of communication as well as the language and can guide the health care provider in how best to approach the visit. This can include identifying any issues with relation to cultures that have distinct boundaries between the genders and planning the health assessment to move from the more superficial to more sensitive questions in order to gain trust. It is very important to explain why the questions are being asked as part of the health assessment and that the information obtained will be kept confidential (Tseng & Streltzer, 2008).

Many Indigenous people practise nonverbal communication and are highly sensitive to body language. They use periods of silence to formulate thoughts in preparation for speech and often remain silent after listening to statements by others in order to properly assimilate what has been said. They can view speaking too quickly or too loudly as a sign of disrespect.

Families may be reluctant to question or otherwise initiate contact with health care providers. In Asian cultures, for example, it is considered a sign of disrespect to question those who are viewed as persons of authority. A Japanese family may wait silently rather than ask questions or question decisions being made. They believe that health care providers know best and will meet their needs without their being asked. It is also important to avoid criticism. Criticism can cause some Asians to "lose face," or feel ashamed, which is highly undesirable.

Health care providers generally ask questions and use handouts, booklets, and—particularly with children—dolls and pictures as communication aids. This practice is uncommon in some cultures. For example, Indigenous healers ask few questions and do not use forms. Nurses need to consider both verbal and nonverbal communication techniques to interact effectively with children and their families from cultures different from their own (Tseng & Streltzer, 2008).

Food Customs

Children may have a number of food restrictions. Some have a physiological origin, such as lack of dairy foods in the diets of some persons of African or Asian ancestry, in whom a hereditary lactase deficiency prevents digestion of foods containing lactose. Others have religious restrictions, such as kosher foods and restrictions on food preparation according to the Orthodox Jewish faith; avoidance of pork by persons of Islamic faith; and the lacto-ovo-vegetarian diet of Seventh-Day Adventists.

Children in a strange environment, such as the hospital, feel much more comfortable when they are served familiar foods (Fig. 31-7). Hospital food often tastes strange and bland. The family may be concerned that their child is not receiving foods appropriate to their culture and beliefs. When possible, it is advisable to provide children foods that are familiar to them or to allow families to bring favourite foods. Concern for differences in food habits and patterns conveys an attitude of respect for the family's ethnic or religious heritage.

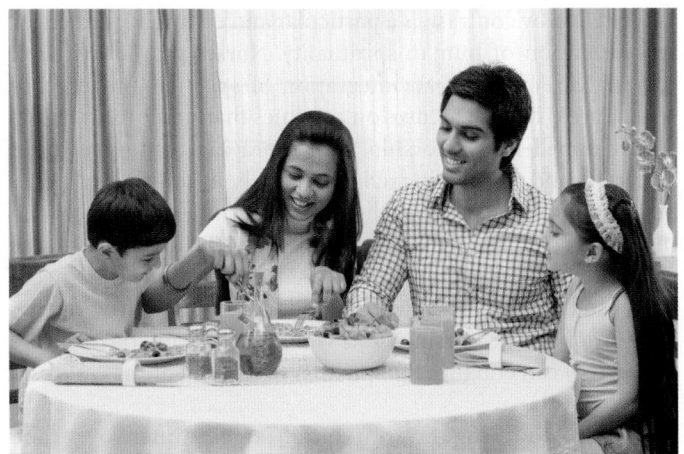

FIGURE 31-7 Food customs outside the home can differ significantly from traditional cultural practices. (India Picture/ Shutterstock.com.)

Health Practices

There are numerous similarities among cultures regarding prevention and treatment of illness. All cultures have some types of home remedies that are applied before seeking help from other persons. Within some ethnic communities, traditional healers who are endowed with the ability to treat maladies are sought for special situations or when home remedies are unsuccessful. Chinese traditional medicine has a very long history and is commonly used. Asian families frequently consult herbalists, who are knowledgeable in herbal remedies and tonics, or ethnic practitioners experienced in Asian therapies, including acupuncture (insertion of needles), acupressure (application of pressure), and moxibustion (application of heat). These traditional remedies are frequently applied in addition to Western medical treatments. Indigenous peoples may consult a variety of traditional healers with specific skills and knowledge. The Truth and Reconciliation Commission (2015) has recommended that health care providers work with traditional healers when caring for Indigenous people. Specialized healers diagnose illness, provide nonsacred treatments (usually by way of massage and herbs), and care for souls. Other specialists perform services or affect cures through spiritual means.

Traditional healers are powerful and respected persons in their community. They "speak the language" of the family who seeks help and often combine their rituals and potions with prayer and entreaties to God. They also are able to create an atmosphere conducive to successful management and often can acquire important information about the illness without asking too many probing questions. Furthermore, they exhibit a sincere interest in the family and their problem.

Practices that do no harm should be respected. Overcoming the effect of the evil eye usually requires specialized rituals conducted by the appropriate practitioner. Sometimes the faith in the traditional practitioner results in a delay in obtaining needed medical treatment, although the practitioner will usually suggest medical care if his or her ministrations are unsuccessful.

Health practices of different cultures may also present problems in assessment and interpretation. For example, certain cultural practices or remedies can be misdiagnosed as evidence of child abuse by uninformed professionals (Box 31-7). Health care providers need to be aware of the practices so they do not misinterpret symptoms, such as red welts from coining. Families need to understand how such practices can place them in jeopardy with child protective services. For example, female genital mutilation is by law considered to be child maltreatment and a crime under the Criminal Code of Canada. Canadians who take children to other countries for this practice will be charged under Canadian law. Nurses and all other citizens are required legally to report this practice to child protection services (Government of Canada Department of Justice, 2015b). See discussion of child maltreatment in an earlier section for further information.

Faith healing and religious rituals are closely allied with many traditional healing practices. The wearing of amulets, medals, and other religious relics believed by the culture to protect the individual and facilitate healing is a common practice. It is important for health workers to recognize the value of this practice and keep the items where the family has placed them or nearby. It offers comfort and support and rarely impedes medical and nursing care. If an item must be removed during a procedure, it should be replaced, if possible, when the procedure is completed. The reason for its temporary removal

BOX 31-7 CULTURAL PRACTICES POSSIBLY CONSIDERED ABUSIVE BY THE DOMINANT CULTURE

Coin rubbing or spooning—An Asian practice of repeated pressured strokes with the smooth edge of a coin, cup, or other object with a smooth edge over skin lubricated with water or oil to rid the body of a disease (Ravanfar & Dinulos, 2010).

Cupping—Practised by a variety of cultures, including Egyptian, Chinese, Greek, Middle-Eastern and some European countries, cupping is the practice of heating a cup or other vessel over an open flame and placing it over the skin. As the air inside the cup cools, a vacuum is created and the skin is drawn into the cup, leaving bruise-like lesions. Cupping is thought to rid the body of evil spirits or disease (Ravanfar & Dinulos, 2010).

Burning—A practice of some Southeast Asian groups whereby small areas of skin are burned with specific herbs to treat enuresis and temper tantrums.

Female genital mutilation (female circumcision)—Removal of or injury to any part of the female genital organ; practised in some parts of Africa (Tseng & Streltzer, 2008).

Forced kneeling—A discipline measure of some Caribbean groups in which a child is forced to kneel for long periods of time.

Topical garlic application—A practice of Yemenite Jews in which crushed garlic cloves or garlic–petroleum jelly plaster is applied to the wrists to treat infectious disease. The practice can result in blisters or garlic burns.

Traditional remedies that contain lead—*Greta* and *azarcon* (Mexico; used for digestive problems), *paylooah* (Southeast Asia; used for rash or fever), and *surma* (India; used as a cosmetic to improve eyesight).

should be explained to the family, and they should be reassured that their wishes will be respected.

Nurses can be most effective by operating from a multicultural perspective. This means using appropriate aspects of each culture's orientation toward health in developing culturally acceptable health care interventions (see Cultural Awareness box).

> **! NURSING ALERT**
>
> Avoid directly criticizing traditional cultural health beliefs and practices as wrong or harmful or implying that biomedical measures are uniformly correct and effective and the only way to prevent illness or treat sickness. Such criticisms usually result in rejection of both biomedical health care practitioners and their health teaching. When traditional practices do not interfere with the patient's welfare, they do not need to be discouraged. Often a compromise can be reached that accomplishes the nurse's goal while maintaining the dignity and self-esteem of the child and family.

Religious Beliefs and Practices

Religious and spiritual dimensions are among the most important influences in many people's lives. The terms *religion* and *spirituality* are often used interchangeably, but they mean different things. Spirituality is "concerned with the deepest levels of human experiencing, the places of deepest ... meaning in and for our lives" (Mercer, 2006). For children in particular, spirituality possesses a relational consciousness; it concerns the child in relation to the source of power (God, Allah) that gives meaning to the relationship, other people, the surrounding world, and within oneself.

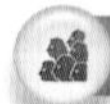

> **CULTURAL AWARENESS**
>
> ***Being Culturally Mindful***
>
> Three-year-old Han is in the Respiratory Clinic with her parents, who emigrated to Ontario from Vietnam less than a year ago. Han has been treated for asthma since her arrival in Canada and was hospitalized once for a short period when her asthma flared as a result of a respiratory illness. Han and her family live with her maternal grandparents. When entering Han's examination room the nurse notes that the parents appear quite tentative. They speak little English and have some difficulty answering the health care provider's initial questions. The nurse knows that it is important that the health care provider have a thorough understanding of how Han has been doing and if they are having any challenges with her medication regime (inhalers and steroids), so the nurse asks their permission to contact an interpreter through a telephone interpretation service. The nurse gives the family sufficient time to answer the questions through the interpreter, keeping a calm and steady voice. The nurse understands that in the Vietnamese culture, being loud or appearing in a rush is considered impolite. The nurse ensures that the interpreter stays on the line while the nurse performs a physical assessment and also when the health care provider is in the examination room so that any additional information can be relayed immediately. Toward the end of the visit, the family appears significantly more relaxed, and through the interpreter they ask if the nurse and health care provider could assist them by providing information that would help the grandfather understand how his smoking might be negatively impacting Han's asthma, as they are concerned that if she gets another respiratory infection she might need hospitalization again, a very distressing event for them.

Religion, by contrast, is a particular and culturally influenced representation of human spirituality. Nurses promote holistic nursing care through an integration of spiritual and psychosocial care. The care focuses on activities that support a person's system of beliefs and worship, such as praying, reading religious materials, and performing religious rituals. In addition, it means being attentive and open to the unique spiritual experiences and insights of children. Whereas meeting the spiritual needs of the child and family can provide strength, unmet spiritual needs can result in spiritual distress and debilitation. In practice, application of the nursing process for religious or spiritual care (Box 31-8) can enhance the spiritual well-being of the child and family.

Culture and religion are typically tightly interwoven and work together to affect the way in which people interpret and respond to illness. Among many groups, illness, injury, or death is believed to be sent by God as a punishment for sin. Some may believe that health workers will be unable to help a person whom God is punishing and may express a fatalistic attitude toward treatment, stating it is "the will of God." Others view it as a test of strength, like the testing of Job in the Bible, and strive to remain faithful and overcome the conflicts.

Many immigrants came to Canada for religious freedom and established a religious and moral atmosphere that persists today. At the same time, individual differences are also part of the general culture. Many religions are practised in Canada, such as Judaism, Christianity, and Islam; because of recent immigration patterns, there has been an increase in religious diversity in Canada.

The family's religious orientation can dictate a code of morality and influence the family's attitudes toward education, male

> **BOX 31-8 GUIDELINES FOR INTEGRATING SPIRITUAL OR RELIGIOUS CARE INTO PEDIATRIC NURSING PRACTICE**
>
> - Respect the child's and family's religious beliefs and practices.
> - Consider the child's development when talking about spiritual concerns.
> - Contact the institution's chaplaincy department for patients and families who have symptoms of spiritual distress or ask for specific religious rituals.
> - Become knowledgeable about the religious worldviews of cultural groups found in the patients you care for.
> - Encourage visitation with family members, members of the patient's spiritual community, and spiritual leaders.
> - Allow children and families to teach you about the specifics of their religious beliefs.
> - Develop awareness of your own spiritual perspective.
> - Listen for understanding rather than agreement or disagreement.

Adapted from Barnes, L., Plotnikoff, G., Fox, K, et al. (2000). Spirituality, religion, and pediatrics: Intersecting worlds of healing. *Pediatrics, 106*(Suppl 4), 899–908; Brooks, B. (2004). Spirituality. In N. Kline (Ed.), *Essentials of pediatric oncology nursing: A core curriculum* (2nd ed.). Glenview, IL: Association of Pediatric Oncology Nurses.

and female role identity, and beliefs regarding their ultimate destiny. Religion may also be a factor in determining the school that children attend, the companions with whom they associate, and, often, their mate selection. In a few instances, such as in Mennonite and Amish communities, religion is the basis for a common way of life that determines both where children are reared and their lifestyle. It is also important to remember that families who do not subscribe to a particular religion or who are atheist also have beliefs and convictions about family, the surrounding world, and life in general that influence children in these families.

Religious affiliation has implications for many health-related functions and procedures. It can be comforting for the family of an ill child to have this need recognized and respected. Nurses need to determine whether there are any special considerations, including dietary restrictions, related to spiritual practices that are important to the family. Family members should be asked whether they want a clergy member present and whether they prefer hospital staff to call the clergy person or prefer to do this on their own.

It is also important to determine the wishes of the family regarding baptism, rites or practices related to death, and other religious rituals (such as circumcision, communion, or use of amulets or icons). Religion, which offers families understanding and spiritual support, is a valuable asset to health care (Fig. 31-8). Characteristics of selected religions with beliefs that affect health care are outlined in Table 31-1.

Cultural and Religious Awareness

Cultural and religious rituals are important practices among families from various cultures. Rather than attempting to change longstanding beliefs, it is beneficial to adapt a family's ethnic practices to their health needs. In the effort to understand and respect the cultural beliefs of families, nurses need to develop knowledge of how cultural groups understand life processes, define health and illness, and view the causes of illness. Nurses need to combine their cross-cultural knowledge with excellent communication skills to learn from the individual patient and family about issues important to their care. As an example, hair-cutting holds special significance for certain cultures. As part of a Jewish boy's third birthday celebration, an *upsherenish* ceremony is held where he has his first haircut. Indigenous peoples often cut their hair to represent the extent of their grief, with the haircut "resetting" their spiritual button. Any procedure requiring haircutting, such as placement of an intravenous line in a scalp vein, must be discussed with parents first to obtain their permission. Not doing so could be misinterpreted as disrespectful and even offensive.

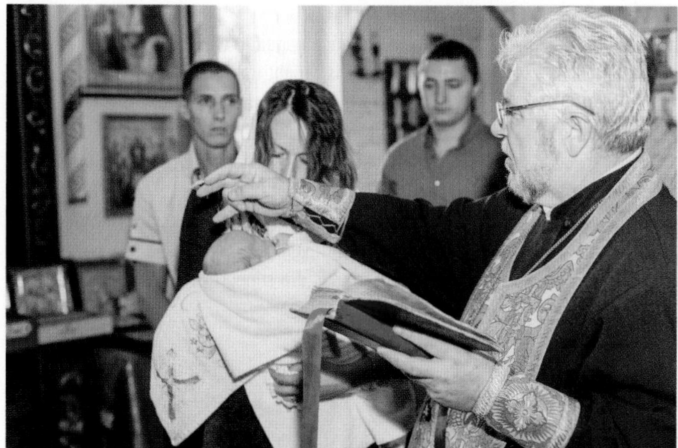

FIGURE 31-8 Many families have a special religious ceremony soon after an infant is born. (Andrii_K/Shutterstock.com.)

Nurses must assess the cultural and religious practices of families to identify how these practices are similar to and different from those of their own cultural and religious backgrounds. At the same time, they must remember to treat each patient as an individual, not simply as a member of a particular group.

Concepts that come from medical anthropology can provide a framework for addressing health care issues. These concepts can have a direct impact on patient care. They lead the nurse away from an ethnocentric or medicocentric view of the health care encounter into the health care reality as constructed by the patient and family. It is also important for nurses to recognize that disease and illness are distinct entities. Clinicians diagnose and treat diseases—that is, abnormalities in the structure and function of body organs and systems. Illness and disease are not interchangeable; illness may occur even when disease is not present, and the course of a disease may vary substantially from the experience of illness. Illness is culturally constructed; an individual's culture influences how a sickness is perceived, labelled, and explained. Culture also influences the meaning assigned to the illness, the role the individual with the sickness adopts, and the response of the family and community to the sickness.

Tension may arise when the perception of the illness and disease varies widely among the patient, family, and health care team. Failure of health care providers to recognize these disparities may be partially to blame in cases of difficulty carrying out proposed treatment, delivery of inadequate care, and patient or family dissatisfaction. To begin addressing these issues, it is important for nurses to understand the various domains of health care in which individuals operate in Canadian society, including professional (health care providers and institutions), popular (family, community, and lay literature), and folk (nonprofessional healers). Each domain possesses a method for defining and explaining the sickness and what should be done to address it. The challenge for nurses and other health care providers is to address the tensions that may exist in understanding these domains with families and develop mutually agreed-upon goals. Nurses are in a prime position to assume this role because understanding the human response to disease is central to their role. In addition, collaboration with the child and family is central to the role of the pediatric nurse.

One method of addressing families and beginning the process of collaboration is by understanding the family's explanatory model of illness. The questions in Box 31-9 aim to elicit an individual's beliefs about illness, the meaning that is attached to it, goals and expected outcomes, and the roles of health care providers. Nurses can use these questions to

TABLE 31-1 RELIGIOUS BELIEFS THAT MAY AFFECT NURSING CARE

BIRTH AND DEATH	DIET AND FOOD PRACTICES	MEDICAL CARE
Buddhism		
Birth—No baptism Infant presentation **Death**—Last rite chanting is often practised at bedside soon after death; the deceased's family or Buddhist priest should be contacted. **Organ donation/transplantation**—Organ donation is a matter of individual conscience. Brain death is not accepted by all, therefore organ donation requires sensitive dialogue.	Restrictions on some foods (e.g., "the 5 pungent spices" and food combinations; extremes must be avoided. Some sects are strictly vegetarian. Use of alcohol and drugs is discouraged.	Illness is believed to be a trial to aid development of the soul; illness results from Karmic causes. Surgery is permitted, but extreme measures are avoided. Cleanliness is of great importance. Family, community, and a Buddhist priest are supportive visitors.
Church of Christ, Scientist (Christian Science)		
Birth—No baptism **Death**—No last rites; autopsy is not permitted except in cases of sudden death; individuals can choose burial or cremation. **Organ donation/transplantation**—The church takes no specific position on transplantation as distinct from other medical or surgical procedures. Individuals decide on organ donation.	Abstain from alcohol and some forms of tea and coffee	Oppose human intervention with medications or other therapies; however, may accept legally required immunizations. Accept physical and moral healing. Family, friends, and members of the spiritual community may visit.
Church of Jesus Christ of Latter-Day Saints (Mormon)		
Birth—No baptism practiced is at birth. Infant is blessed by a church official at first opportunity after birth (in church). Baptism is by full water immersion at 8 years of age. **Death**—Believe that it is proper to bury the dead in the ground; cremation is discouraged. **Organ donation/transplantation**—Individuals can choose whether to donate organs to be used in transplants.	Prohibit caffeine — coffee, tea (unless herbal), and some avoid chocolate as well. Alcohol is prohibited. Fasting for 24 hours each month	Devout adherents believe in divine healing. Medical therapy is not prohibited. **Spiritual items**—A "garment" (type of underwear) that is considered sacred; the person may not want to remove it. Family, friends, and church members are supportive visitors.
Hindu		
Birth—No baptism **Death**—Certain prescribed rites are followed after death; a priest may tie a thread around the neck or wrist to signify blessing; the family will wash the body and are particular about who touches the dead; bodies are to be cremated. **Organ donation/transplantation**—No religious laws prohibit donation; this is an individual decision.	Many dietary restrictions Eating meat and eggs is forbidden; lactovegetarian diets are followed. There are many days of fasting in the calendar with additional food restrictions.	With an amputation, loss of a limb is believed to represent sins committed in a previous life. Accept most modern medical practices; some belief in faith healing **Spiritual items**—Person may wear a thread around the wrist or body; it should not be removed. Family, community members, and the priest are supportive visitors.
Islam (Muslim)		
Birth—At birth, the first words said to the infant in his or her right ear are *Allah-o-Akbar* (Allah is great), and the remainder of the Call for Prayer is recited. An *Aqeeqa* (party) to celebrate the birth of the child is arranged by the parents. Male children are circumcised. **Death**—At the time of death, specific rituals (e.g., bathing, wrapping the body in cloth) must be done by a same-sex Muslim. Before moving and handling the body, it is preferable to contact someone from the person's mosque or the local Islamic Society to perform these rituals. **Organ donation/transplantation**—Individual decides on organ donation/transplantation. Brain death is not accepted by all, therefore organ donation requires sensitive dialogue.	Halal restrictions are followed, including meat being slaughtered under Halal guidance. All pork products and alcohol are prohibited. Fasting is practised during the ninth month of the Islamic year (Ramadan).	Believers are encouraged in the Qu'ran to seek treatment. It is taught that only Allah cures; however, Muslims are taught not to refuse treatment in the belief that Allah will take care of them because he also chooses at times to work through the efforts of humans. **Other practices**—Right hand is used for eating; left hand is for hygiene. Family and friends are supportive visitors.

TABLE 31-1 RELIGIOUS BELIEFS THAT MAY AFFECT NURSING CARE—cont'd

BIRTH AND DEATH	DIET AND FOOD PRACTICES	MEDICAL CARE
Jehovah's Witnesses		
Birth—No baptism **Death**—No official last rites are practised when death occurs. **Organ donation/transplantation**—Organ donation is forbidden.	No tobacco; moderate alcohol use is permissible.	Blood or blood products are not allowed; volume expanders are permissible if not derived from blood.
Judaism (Orthodox and Conservative)		
Birth—No baptism Ritual circumcision of male infants occurs on the eighth day; performed by a mohel (ritual circumciser familiar with Jewish law and aseptic technique). **Death**—According to tradition, during last moments of life, relatives and close friends remain with the deceased and do not leave the body unattended until burial. Amputated limbs or surgically removed tissues should be made available to the family for burial. Cremation is not allowed. Burial usually occurs quickly. **Organ donation/transplantation**—Organ transplantation/donation is a complex issue. Donating organs that can be extracted while alive (e.g., kidney) is acceptable, but after death may not be accepted by all.	Numerous dietary kosher laws exist; followers are allowed only meat from animals that are vegetable eaters and are ritually slaughtered; predatory fowl, shellfish, and pork are prohibited. Milk products served first can be followed by meat in a few minutes, but milk may not be consumed for several hours after eating meat. Fasting is part of Yom Kippur observance. Matzo replaces leavened bread during Passover week.	May resist surgical procedures during Sabbath, which extends from sundown Friday until sundown Saturday. Illness is grounds for violating dietary laws. **Spiritual items**—Men may wear a prayer shawl, yarmulka (cap), or both while praying. Family, friends, and the rabbi are supportive visitors.
Roman Catholicism		
Birth—Infant baptism; this is especially urgent if there is a poor prognosis, when it may be performed by anyone. **Death**—Sacrament of the Sick is performed if prognosis is poor while patient is alive. **Organ donation/transplantation**—Transplantation of organs is ethically and morally acceptable to the Vatican; organ donation is viewed as an act of charity.	Abstaining from meat is practised on Ash Wednesday, Good Friday, and Fridays during Lent (as a rule).	Encourage anointing of the sick **Spiritual items**—Rosary beads, crucifix Traditional church teaching does not approve of contraceptives or abortion.
Indigenous		
Most Indigenous peoples practise some form of Christianity, along with the traditional spiritual beliefs and practices that are primarily passed from generation to generation orally. **Birth**—Viewed as a sacred event experienced by the whole family **Death**—Typically, practices of the Christian religion are followed, but may include traditional rituals, such as family members cutting their hair or lighting ceremonial fires.	Fasting is common in order to participate in certain spiritual experiences. Specific foods may be used as symbols during ceremonies or rituals—these foods differ from area to area.	Follow practices of Christianity. Individuals may burn sweetgrass, tobacco, sage, or other sacred herbs to aid in healing.

Data from Galanti, G. (2004). *Caring for patients from different cultures* (3rd ed.). Philadelphia: University of Pennsylvania Press; Lipson, J. G., Dibble, S. L., & Minarik, P. A. (2005). *Culture and clinical care: A pocket guide.* San Francisco: UCSF Nursing Press; Purnell, L. D., & Paulanka, B. J. (2003). *Transcultural health care: A culturally competent approach.* Philadelphia: Davis; Spector, R. E. (2009). *Cultural diversity in health and illness* (7th ed.). Upper Saddle River, NJ: Prentice Hall; National Defence and the Canadian Forces. (2009). *Religions in Canada: Native spirituality.* Ottawa: Government of Canada; Srivastava, R. (2007). *The healthcare professional's guide to clinical cultural competence.* Toronto: Elsevier Canada; Tseng, W. S., & Streltzer, J. (2008). *Cultural competence in health care: A guide for professionals.* New York: Springer Science and Business Media.

BOX 31-9 **EXPLORING A FAMILY'S CULTURE, ILLNESS, AND CARE**

Significant understanding can be gained by asking the family straightforward questions, such as:

- What do you think is causing your child's illness?
- Why do you think it started when it did?
- How severe do you think your child's illness is, and do you think it will be a short or long illness?
- How do you think this illness affects the rest of the family?
- What are the major problems this illness has caused?
- What have you done for the illness until now?
- What kind of treatment do you think your child should receive?
- What are the most important results you hope to receive from your child's treatment?
- What do you fear most about your child's illness?

Adapted from Kleinman, A., Eisenberg, L., & Good, B. (1978). Culture, illness, and care: Clinical lessons from anthropologic and cross-cultural research. *Annals of Internal Medicine,* 88, 251–258.

discern areas of discrepancy for further dialogue, negotiation, and collaboration. This discussion, when conducted with a genuine interest in the family's and child's perspective, is a significant step toward building trusting relationships, promoting adherence, decreasing disparities, and increasing health care satisfaction.

Nurses are frequently asked by family members to provide advice about or assistance with employing traditional health practices, including practices that seem extraordinary or abusive. The nurse needs to ensure that personal feelings are not used to guide the interaction; the focus should be instead on attempting to understand the meaning of the practice. For example, if asked about how to arrange for the excision of female genitalia (a practice most common in Africa, Asia, and the Middle East), the nurse should explore fully with the family what their motivation is and provide information on the potential health risks and the illegal nature of the practice in Canada. Through an open and sincere approach the nurse has the ability to help the family find alternative options toward achieving their goal (College of Nurses of Ontario, 2009).

KEY POINTS

- Because there is no agreement on the definition of family, a family is what an individual considers it to be.
- Three areas of special concern to adoptive families include the initial attachment process, the task of telling children that they are adopted, and identity formation during adolescence.
- Marital factors within the home significantly influence a child's development. The impact of divorce on a child depends on the child's age, the outcome, and the quality of the parent–child relationship and parental care following the divorce.
- Lone parenting and stepparenting create adjustment difficulties and add stress to the already demanding parental role. Significant numbers of children will live in a lone-parent or reconstituted family at some point.
- Child maltreatment may take the form of physical abuse or neglect, emotional abuse or neglect, or sexual abuse.
- Parental, child, and environmental characteristics are criteria that may predispose children to maltreatment.
- Identification of abuse entails securing evidence of maltreatment, taking a history pertaining to the incident, and assessing parental and child behaviours.
- Culture is the pattern of assumptions, beliefs, and practices encompassing other products of human work and thoughts specific to members of an intergenerational group, community, or population.
- Nurses have a responsibility to continually develop cultural competence. This includes understanding and respecting the influence of culture, race, and ethnicity on the development of social and emotional relationships, child-rearing practices, and attitudes toward health.
- A child's self-concept evolves from ideas about his or her social roles.
- Socioeconomic influences play a major role in opportunities for health promotion and wellness.
- Groups of children suffering from greater physical and mental health issues are those living in poverty; those who are homeless; Indigenous peoples; and those who are recent immigrants to Canada.
- Because verbal and nonverbal communication is an important cultural consideration, nurses need to acknowledge and respect their patients' communication practices in order for productive interaction to occur.
- Religious practices greatly influence health-promotion beliefs in families.
- Cultural and religious beliefs related to the cause of illness and maintenance of health may focus on natural forces, supernatural forces, or imbalance of forces.
- In planning and implementing patient care, nurses need to strive to adapt ethnic practices to the family's health needs rather than attempt to change longstanding beliefs.
- No cultural group is homogeneous; every racial and ethnic group contains great diversity.
- Culturally competent care is family-centred care, as it focuses on exploring the child's and family's meaning of illness, preferences, and needs.
- The practice of cultural humility is continual and an important concept in the nursing process. Nurses can facilitate this process by recognizing cultural differences, integrating cultural knowledge, being aware of their own beliefs and practices, and acting in a culturally appropriate manner.

evolve WEBSITE

Visit the Evolve website for additional resources related to the content in this chapter such as Case Studies, Critical Thinking Case Study Answers, Nursing Care Plans, Nursing Processes, Nursing Skills, and Review Questions for Exam Preparation at: http://evolve.elsevier.com/Canada/Perry/maternal/

REFERENCES

Andrews, M., & Boyle, J. (2008). *Transcultural concepts in nursing care* (5th ed.). Philadelphia: Lippincott.

Annie E. Casey Foundation. (2012). *Stepping up for kids: What government and communities should do to support kinship families.* Retrieved from <https://www.ncfr.org/sites/default/files/downloads/news/steppingupforkidspolicyreport2012.pdf>.

Barozzino, T. (2010). Immigrant health and the children and youth of Canada: Are we doing enough? *Healthcare Quarterly, 14*, 52–59.

Becker, M., Vignoles, V., Owe, E., et al. (2014). Cultural bases for self-evaluation: Seeing oneself positively in different cultural contexts. *Personality and Social Psychology Bulletin, 40*(5), 657–675. doi:10.1177/0146167214522836.

Campaign 2000. (2015). *2015 Report card on child and family poverty in Canada: Let's end child poverty for good.* Family Service Toronto. Retrieved from <http://www.campaign2000.ca/reportcards.html>.

Canadian Paediatric Society. (2011). *International adoption: Health issues for families.* Retrieved from <http://www.caringforkids.cps.ca/handouts/international_adoption>.

Coehlo, D., & Manoogian, M. (2010). Culturally sensitive nursing care of families. In J. Kaakinen, V. Gedaly-Duff, D. Coehlo, et al. (Eds.), *Family health care nursing: Theory, practice and research* (4th ed., pp. 151–174). Philadelphia: F.A. Davis Company.

College of Nurses. (2009). *Practice guideline: Culturally sensitive care.* Retrieved from <http://www.cno.org/globalassets/docs/prac/41040_culturallysens.pdf>.

Collin-Vézina, D., Dion, J., & Trocmé, N. (2009). Sexual abuse in Canadian Aboriginal communities: A broad review of conflicting evidence. *Journal of Aboriginal and Indigenous Community Health, 7*, 27–47. Retrieved from <http://www.pimatisiwin.com/online/?page_id=609>.

Copple, C., & Bredekamp, S. (2009). *Developmentally appropriate practice in early childhood programs serving children from birth through age 8.* Washington, DC: National Association for the Education of Young Children.

Donelan-McCall, N., Eckenrode, J., & Olds, D. L. (2009). Home visiting for the prevention of child maltreatment: Lessons learned during the past 20 years. *Pediatric Clinics of North America, 56*(2), 389–403. doi:10.1016/j.pcl.2009.01.002.

Eggeben, D. (2012). What can we learn from studies of children raised by gay or lesbian parents? *Social Science Research, 41*, 775–778.

Employment and Social Development Canada. (2015). *Homelessness strategy.* Retrieved from <http://www.hrsdc.gc.ca/eng/homelessness/index.shtml>.

Falk, C., & Heine, S. (2015). What is implicit self-esteem, and does it vary across cultures? *Personality and Social Psychology Review, 19*(2), 177–198. doi:10.1177/1088868314544693.

Ferrao, V. (2010). *Paid work. Women in Canada: A gender-based report* (Cat. No. 89-503-X). Retrieved from <http://www.statcan.gc.ca/pub/89-503-x/2010001/article/11387-eng.pdf>.

Flaherty, E. G., & Macmillan, H. L. (2013). Caregiver-fabricated illness in a child: A manifestation of child maltreatment. *Pediatrics, 132*(3), 590–597. doi:10.1542/peds.2013-2045.

Fleury, D. (2008). Low-income children. *Perspectives on Labour and Income 9(5) (Cat. No. 75-001-X).* Statistics Canada.

Gara, M., Allen, L. A., Herzog, E. P., et al. (2000). The abused child as parent: The structure and content of physically abused mothers' perceptions of their babies. *Child Abuse and Neglect, 24*(5), 627–639.

Government of Canada, Department of Justice. (2015a). *An analysis of options for changes in the legal regulation of child custody and access: Adoption.* Retrieved from <http://www.justice.gc.ca/eng/rp-pr/fl-lf/parent/2001_2b/implic3.html>.

Government of Canada, Department of Justice. (2015b). *Child abuse is wrong: What can I do?* Retrieved from <http://www.justice.gc.ca/eng/rp-pr/cj-jp/fv-vf/caw-mei/p11.html>.

Government of Canada, Immigration and Citizenship. (2016a). *Home page.* Retrieved from <http://www.cic.gc.ca/english/index.asp>.

Government of Canada, Immigration and Citizenship. (2016b). *#WelcomeRefugees: Canada's plan to resettle 25,000 Syrian refugees.* Retrieved from <http://www.cic.gc.ca/english/refugees/welcome/>.

Halfon, N., Larson, K., & Russ, S. (2010). Why social determinants? *Healthcare Quarterly, 14*, 9–20.

Indigenous and Northern Affairs Canada. (2015). *Aboriginal peoples and communities.* Retrieved from <https://www.aadnc-aandc.gc.ca/eng/1100100013785/1304467449155>.

Kaakinen, J., & Hanson, S. (2010). Theoretical foundations for the nursing of families. In J. Kaakinen, V. Gedaly-Duff, D. Coehlo, & S. Hanson (Eds.), *Family health care nursing: Theory, practice and research* (4th ed., pp. 3–33). Philadelphia: F.A. Davis Company.

Kaakinen, J., Hanson, S., & Denham, S. (2010). Family health care nursing: An introduction. In J. Kaakinen, V. Gedaly-Duff, D. Coehlo, & S. Hanson (Eds.), *Family health care nursing: Theory, practice and research* (4th ed., pp. 63–102). Philadelphia: F.A. Davis Company.

Kaufman, M., & Canadian Paediatric Society. (2011). *The sexual abuse of young people with a disability or chronic health condition.* Retrieved from <http://www.cps.ca/documents/position/sexual-abuse-youth-disability-chronic-condition>.

Kellogg, N. (2005). The evaluation of sexual abuse in children. *Pediatrics, 116*(2), 506–512.

Kostelnik, M., Whiren, A., Soderman, A., et al. (2014). *Guiding children's social development and learning* (8th ed.). Stamford, CT: Cengage Learning.

Low, M., & Low, B. (2012). Health determinants. In S. Loue & M. Sajatovic (Eds.), *Encyclopedia of immigrant health* (pp. 65–74). New York: Springer.

McKay, A., & Barrett, M. (2010). Trends in teen pregnancy rates from 1996 to 2006: A comparison of Canada, Sweden, U.S.A., and England/Wales. *Canadian Journal of Human Sexuality, 19*(1/2), 43–52.

McNeill, T. (2010). Family as a social determinant of health. *Healthcare Quarterly, 14*, 60–67.

Mekonnen, R., Noonan, K., & Rubin, D. (2009). Achieving better health care outcomes for children in foster care. *Pediatric Clinics of North America, 56*(2), 405–415. doi:10.1016/j.pcl.2009.01.005.

Mercer, J. (2006). Children as mystics, activists, sages, and holy fools: Understanding the spirituality of children and its significance for clinical work. *Pastoral Psychology, 54*(5), 497–515.

Mikkonen, J., & Raphael, D. (2010). *Social determinants of health: The Canadian facts.* Toronto: York University School of Health Policy and Management.

Multiple Births Canada. (2011). *Multiple birth facts and figures.* Retrieved from <http://multiplebirthscanada.org/mbc_factsheets/FS-MF_FactsFigures.pdf>.

Parliament of Canada. (2002). *Bill C-15A: An act to amend the Criminal Code and to amend other acts.* Retrieved from <http://www.parl.gc.ca/About/Parliament/LegislativeSummaries/bills_ls.asp?ls=C15A&Parl=37&Ses=1#2.%C2%A0%20Child>.

Pepler, D., German, J., Craig, W., et al. (2011). Why worry about bullying? *Healthcare Quarterly, 14*, 72–79.

Postl, B., Cook, C., & Moffatt, M. (2010). Aboriginal child health and the social determinants: Why are these children so disadvantaged? *Healthcare Quarterly, 14*, 42–51.

Public Health Agency of Canada. (2008). *Canadian incidence study of reported child abuse and neglect—2008*. Retrieved from <http://www.phac-aspc.gc.ca/cm-vee/csca-ecve/2008/cis-eci-04-eng.php>.

Public Health Agency of Canada. (2016). *Stop family violence*. Retrieved from <http://www.phac-aspc.gc.ca/sfv-avf/index-eng.php>.

Ravanfar, P., & Dinulos, J. (2010). Cultural practices affecting the skin of children. *Current Opinion in Pediatrics, 22*(4), 423–431. doi:10.1097/MOP.0b013e32833bc352.

Rubin, K., & Bukowski, W. (2011). *Handbook of peer interactions, relationships, and groups*. New York: Guildford Press.

Sabella, D. (2011). The role of the nurse in combating human trafficking. *American Journal of Nursing, 111*(2), 28–37. doi:10.1097/01.NAJ.0000394289.55577.b6.

Search Institute. (2016). *Developmental assets tools: Preparing young people for success*. Retrieved from <http://www.search-institute.org/what-we-study/developmental-assets>.

Sinha, M., & Statistics Canada. (2015). *Section 4: Family violence against children and youth*. Retrieved from <http://www.statcan.gc.ca/pub/85-002-x/2013001/article/11805/11805-4-eng.htm#a>.

Smith, A., Stewart, D., Peled, M., et al. (2009). *A picture of health: Highlights of the 2008 British Columbia adolescent health survey*. Vancouver: McCreary Centre Society. Retrieved from <http://www.mcs.bc.ca/pdf/AHSIV_APictureOfHealth.pdf>.

Spector, R. E. (2009). *Cultural diversity in health and illness* (7th ed.). Upper Saddle River, NJ: Prentice-Hall.

Statistics Canada. (2011). *Marital status: Overview, 2011*. Retrieved from <http://www.statcan.gc.ca/pub/91-209-x/2013001/article/11788-eng.htm>.

Statistics Canada. (2013a). *Table 102-4515: Live births and fetal deaths by type, Canada, provinces and territories*. Retrieved from <http://www5.statcan.gc.ca/cansim/a26?lang=eng&id=1024515>.

Statistics Canada. (2013b). *Table 102-4503: Live births, by age of mother, Canada, provinces and territories*. Retrieved from <http://www5.statcan.gc.ca/cansim/a26?lang=eng&id=1024503>.

Statistics Canada. (2015). *Portrait of families and living arrangements in Canada: Table 1*. Retrieved from <http://www12.statcan.ca/census-recensement/2011/as-sa/98-312-x/2011001/tbl/tbl1-eng.cfm>.

Truth and Reconciliation Commission of Canada. (2015). *Calls to action*. Retrieved from <http://www.trc.ca/websites/trcinstitution/File/2015/Findings/Calls_to_Action_English2.pdf>.

Tseng, W. S., & Streltzer, J. (2008). *Cultural competence in health care: A guide for professionals*. New York: Springer Science and Business Media.

Van Pelt, J. (2012). Keeping teen moms in school—A school social work challenge. *Social Work Today, 12*(2), 24. Retrieved from <http://www.socialworktoday.com/archive/031912p24.shtml>.

Viner, R., Ozer, E., Denny, S., et al. (2012). Adolescence and the social determinants of health. *Lancet, 379*, 1641–1652.

Wells, K. (2009). Substance abuse and child maltreatment. *Pediatric Clinics of North America, 56*(2), 345–362. doi:10.1016/j.pcl.2009.01.006.

ADDITIONAL RESOURCES

Canadian Institute of Child Health: <http://www.cich.ca/about.html>

Child Abuse Is Wrong: What Can I Do?: <http://www.justice.gc.ca/eng/rp-pr/cj-jp/fv-vf/caw-mei/toc-tdm.html>

Key Assets—The Fostering Process: <http://www.keyassets.ca/want-to-foster/the-fostering-process/>

Rainbow Health Ontario Resource Database—Reliable, up-to-date health resources to LGBTQ communities, service providers, and others with an interest in LGBTQ health: <http://www.rainbowhealthontario.ca/resource-search/>

Service Canada for Families and Children: <http://www.servicecanada.gc.ca/eng/audiences/families/index.shtml>

CHAPTER

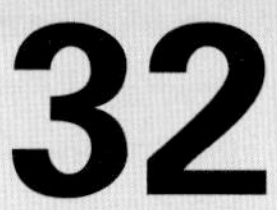

Developmental Influences on Child Health Promotion

Cheryl Sams

evolve WEBSITE

Visit the Evolve website for additional resources related to the content in this chapter such as Case Studies, Critical Thinking Case Study Answers, Nursing Care Plans, Nursing Processes, Nursing Skills, and Review Questions for Exam Preparation at: *http://evolve.elsevier.com/Canada/Perry/maternal/*

OBJECTIVES

On completion of this chapter the reader will be able to:

- Describe major trends in growth and development.
- Explain the alterations in the major body systems that take place during the process of growth and development.
- Discuss the development and relationships of personality, cognition, language, morality, spirituality, and self-concept.
- Describe the role of play in the growth and development of children.
- Demonstrate an understanding of the role of innate and environmental factors in the physical and emotional development of children.
- Describe the influence of mass media on children and how parents can help children to understand the media's impact.

GROWTH AND DEVELOPMENT

Foundations of Growth and Development

Growth and development, usually referred to as a unit, express the sum of the numerous changes that take place during the lifetime of an individual. The entire course is a dynamic process that encompasses several interrelated dimensions:

Growth—An increase in the number and size of cells as they divide and synthesize new proteins; results in increased size and weight of the whole or any of its parts

Development—A gradual change and expansion; advancement from lower to more advanced stages of complexity; the emerging and expanding of the individual's capacities through growth, maturation, and learning

Maturation—An increase in competence and adaptability; aging; usually used to describe a qualitative change; a change in the complexity of a structure that makes it possible for that structure to begin functioning; to function at a higher level

Differentiation—Processes by which early cells and structures are systematically modified and altered to achieve specific and characteristic physical and chemical properties; development from simple to more complex activities and functions

All of these processes are interrelated, simultaneous, and ongoing; none occurs apart from the others. The processes depend on a sequence of endocrine, genetic, constitutional, environmental, and nutritional influences (Ball, Dains, Flynn, et al., 2014). The child's body becomes larger and more complex; the personality simultaneously expands in scope and complexity. Very simply, *growth* can be viewed as a quantitative change, and *development* as a qualitative change.

Stages of Development

Most authorities in the field of child development conveniently categorize child growth and behaviour into approximate age stages or in terms that describe the features of an age group. The age ranges of these stages are admittedly arbitrary and, because they do not take into account individual differences, cannot be applied to all children with any degree of precision. However, categorization affords a convenient means to describe the characteristics associated with the majority of children at

BOX 32-1 DEVELOPMENTAL AGE PERIODS

Prenatal Period—Conception to Birth

Germinal—Conception to approximately 2 weeks
Embryonic—2 to 8 weeks
Fetal—8 to 40 weeks (birth)

A rapid growth rate and total dependency make this one of the most crucial periods in the developmental process. The relationship between maternal health and certain manifestations in the newborn emphasizes the importance of adequate prenatal care to the health and well-being of the infant.

Infancy Period—Birth to 12 Months

Newborn—Birth to 27 or 28 days
Infancy—1 month to approximately 12 months

The infancy period is one of rapid motor, cognitive, and social development. Through mutuality with the caregiver (parent), the infant establishes a basic trust in the world and the foundation for future interpersonal relationships. The critical first month of life, although part of the infancy period, is often differentiated from the remainder because of the infant's major physical adjustments to extrauterine existence and the parent's psychological adjustment.

Early Childhood—1 to 6 Years

Toddler—1 to 3 years
Preschool—3 to 6 years

This period, which extends from the time children attain upright locomotion until they enter school, is characterized by intense activity and discovery. It is a time of marked physical and personality development. Motor development advances steadily. Children at this age acquire language and wider social relationships, learn role standards, gain self-control and mastery, develop increasing awareness of dependence and independence, and begin to develop a self-concept.

Middle Childhood—6 to 10 Years

Frequently referred to as the school age, this period of development is one in which the child is directed away from the family group and centred on the wider world of peer relationships. There is steady advancement in physical development and sexual maturity, which is measured by the Tanner stages of development tool (see Chapter 39 for more information). Mental and social development is occurring with emphasis on developing skill competencies. Social cooperation and early moral development take on more importance with relevance for later life stages. This is a critical period in the development of a self-concept.

Later Childhood—10 to 18 Years

Prepubertal—10 to 13 years
Adolescence—13 to approximately 18 years

The tumultuous period of rapid maturation and change known as adolescence is considered to be a transitional period that begins at the onset of puberty and extends to the point of entry into the adult world—usually high school graduation. Biological and personality maturation are accompanied by physical and emotional turmoil, and there is redefining of the self-concept. In the late adolescent period, the young person begins to internalize all previously learned values and to focus on an individual, rather than a group, identity.

periods when distinctive developmental changes appear and specific developmental tasks must be accomplished. (A **developmental task** is a set of skills and competencies peculiar to each developmental stage that children must accomplish or master in order to deal effectively with their environment.) It is also significant for nurses to know that there are characteristic health problems peculiar to each major phase of development. The sequence of descriptive age periods and subperiods that are used here and elaborated on in subsequent chapters is listed in Box 32-1.

Patterns of Growth and Development

There are definite and predictable patterns in growth and development that are continuous, orderly, and progressive. While these patterns, or trends, are universal and basic to all human beings, each person accomplishes these in a manner and time unique to that individual.

Directional trends. Growth and development proceed in regular, related directions, or gradients, and reflect the physical development and maturation of neuromuscular functions (Fig. 32-1). The first pattern is the *cephalocaudal*, or head-to-tail, direction. The head end of the organism develops first and is large and complex, whereas the lower end is small and simple and takes shape at a later period. While the physical evidence of this trend is most apparent during the period before birth, it also applies to postnatal behaviour development. Infants achieve structural control of the head before they have control of the

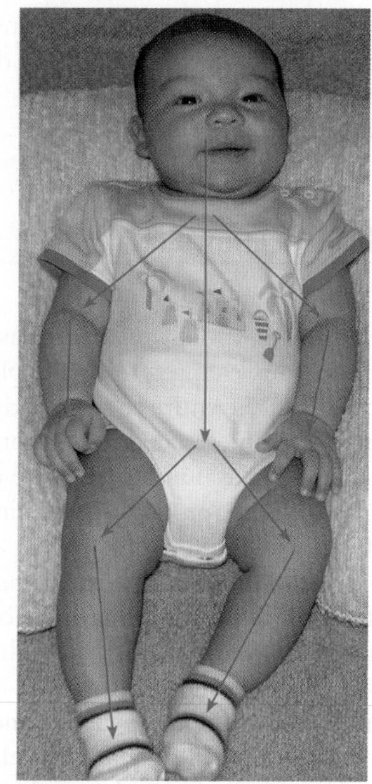

FIGURE 32-1 Directional trends in growth.

trunk and extremities, hold their back erect before they stand, use their eyes before their hands, and gain control of their hands before they have control of their feet.

The second pattern, the **proximodistal**, or near-to-far, trend, applies to midline-to-peripheral development. A conspicuous illustration is the early embryonic development of limb buds, which is followed by rudimentary fingers and toes. In the infant, shoulder control precedes mastery of the hands, the whole hand is used as a unit before the fingers can be manipulated, and the central nervous system develops more rapidly than the peripheral nervous system.

These trends or patterns are bilateral and appear symmetrical (i.e., each side develops in the same direction and at the same rate as the other). For some of the neurological functions, this symmetry is only external because of unilateral differentiation of function at an early stage of postnatal development. For example, by the age of approximately 5 years, the child has demonstrated a decided preference for the use of one hand over the other, even though previously either one had been used.

The third trend, *differentiation*, describes development from simple operations to more complex activities and functions. From broad, global patterns of behaviour, more specific, refined patterns emerge. All areas of development (physical, mental, social, and emotional) proceed in this direction. Through the process of development and differentiation, early embryonal cells with vague, undifferentiated functions progress to an immensely complex organism composed of highly specialized and diversified cells, tissues, and organs. Generalized development precedes specific or specialized development; gross, random muscle movements take place before fine muscle control.

Sequential trends. In all dimensions of growth and development there is a definite, predictable sequence, with each child normally passing through every stage. Children crawl before they creep, creep before they stand, and stand before they walk. Later facets of the personality are built on the early foundation of **trust**. The child babbles, then forms words and, finally, sentences; writing emerges from scribbling.

Developmental pace. Although development has a fixed, precise order, it does not progress at the same rate or pace in each child. There are periods of accelerated growth and periods of decelerated growth in both total body growth and the growth of subsystems. Not all areas develop at the same pace. When a spurt occurs in one area such as gross motor, minimal advances may take place in language, fine motor, or social skills. Once the gross motor skill has been achieved, then development will shift to another area. The rapid growth before and after birth gradually levels off throughout early childhood. Growth is relatively slow during middle childhood, markedly increases at the beginning of adolescence, and levels off in early adulthood. Each child grows at his or her own pace. Distinct differences are observed between children as they reach developmental milestones.

Sensitive periods. There are limited times during the process of growth when the organism will interact with a particular environment in a specific manner. Periods termed *critical*, *sensitive*, *vulnerable*, and *optimal* are those times in the life of an organism when it is more susceptible to positive or negative influences.

The quality of interactions during these sensitive periods determines whether the effects on the organism will be beneficial or harmful. For example, physiological maturation of the central nervous system is influenced by adequacy and timing of contributions from the environment, such as stimulation and nutrition. The first 3 months of prenatal life are sensitive periods for physical growth of the fetus. Children are increasingly exposed to environmental exposures during critical periods of growth. For example, infants, toddlers, and preschoolers are engaged in a lot of hand-to-mouth activities and those closer to the ground, which can expose them to an increased levels of toxins such as garden pesticides and new carpet toxins. It is also a time of rapidly dividing cells and active development, and exposure to toxins can have a detrimental effect. For example, lead exposure from lead paint on toys and furniture can have a negative impact on a child's intelligence quotient. See Unit 10 for specific age groups and the impact of environmental toxins.

Psychological development also appears to have sensitive periods when an environmental event has maximal influence on the developing personality. For example, primary socialization occurs during the first year, when the infant makes the initial social attachments and establishes a basic trust in the world. A close relationship with a parent figure is fundamental to a healthy personality. The same concept might be applied to readiness for learning skills such as toilet training or reading. In these instances, there appears to be an opportune time when the skill is best learned.

Individual Differences

Each child grows in his or her own unique and personal way. Great individual variation exists in the age at which developmental milestones are reached. The sequence is predictable; the exact timing is not. Rates of growth vary, and measurements are defined in terms of ranges, to allow for individual differences. Some children are fast growers, others are moderate, and some are slower to reach maturity. Periods of fast growth, such as the pubescent growth spurt, may begin earlier or later in some children than in others. Children may grow fast or slowly during the spurt and may finish sooner or later than other children. Gender is an influential factor; girls seem to be more advanced in physiological growth at all ages.

Biological Growth and Physical Development

As children grow, their external dimensions change. These changes are accompanied by corresponding alterations in structure and function of internal organs and tissues that reflect the gradual acquisition of physiological competence. Each part has its own rate of growth, which may be directly related to alterations in the child's size (e.g., the heart rate). Skeletal muscle growth approximates whole-body growth; brain, lymphoid, adrenal, and reproductive tissues follow distinct and individual patterns (Fig. 32-2). When growth deficiency has a secondary cause, such as severe illness or acute malnutrition, recovery from the illness or establishment of an adequate diet will

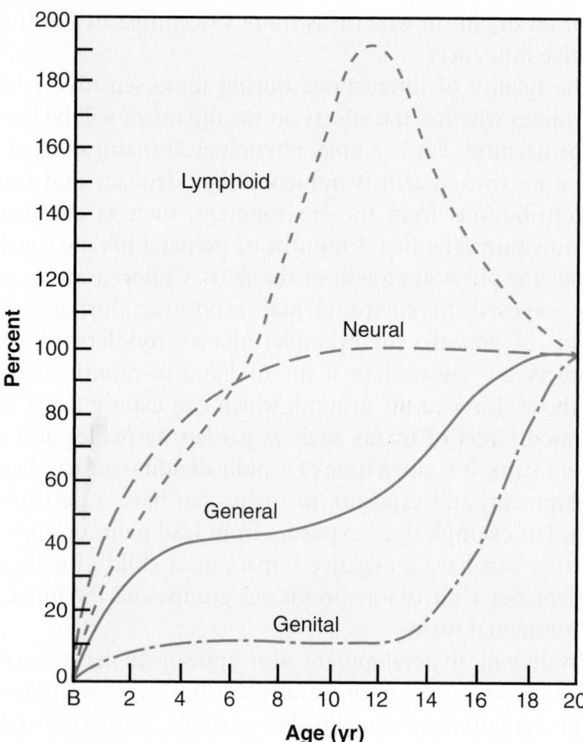

FIGURE 32-2 Growth rates for the body as a whole and examples of some specific tissue growth patterns. Lymphoid: thymus, lymph nodes, and intestinal lymph masses. Neural: brain, dura, spinal cord, optic apparatus, and head dimensions. Genital: reproductive tissues. General: body as a whole; external dimension; and respiratory, digestive, renal, circulatory, and musculoskeletal systems. *B*, birth. (From Jackson, J. A., Patterson, D. G., & Harris, R. E. [1930]. *The measurement of man.* Minneapolis: University of Minnesota Press.)

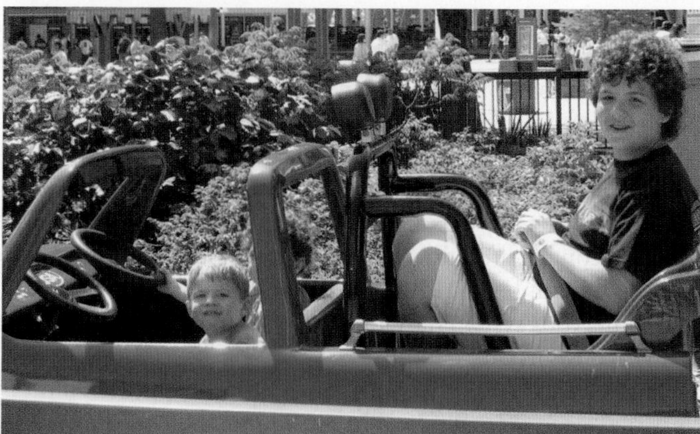

FIGURE 32-3 Changes in body proportions occur dramatically during childhood.

produce a dramatic acceleration of the growth rate that usually continues until the child's individual growth pattern is resumed.

External Proportions

Variations in the growth rate of different tissues and organ systems produce significant changes in body proportions during childhood. The cephalocaudal trend of development is most evident in total body growth as indicated by these changes. During fetal development, the head is the fastest-growing body part, and at 2 months of gestation the head constitutes 50% of total body length. During infancy, growth of the trunk predominates; the legs are the most rapidly growing part during childhood; in adolescence, the trunk once again elongates. In the newborn infant, the lower limbs are one third the total body length but only 15% of the total body weight; in the adult, the lower limbs constitute one half of the total body height and 30% or more of the total body weight. As growth proceeds, the midpoint in head-to-toe measurements gradually descends from a level even with the umbilicus at birth to the level of the symphysis pubis at maturity.

Biological Determinants of Growth and Development

The most prominent feature of childhood and adolescence is physical growth (Fig. 32-3). Throughout development various tissues in the body undergo changes in size, composition, and structure. In some tissues the changes are continuous (e.g., bone growth and dentition); in others, significant alterations occur at specific stages (e.g., appearance of secondary sex characteristics). When these measurements are compared with standardized norms, a child's developmental progress can be determined with a high degree of confidence. The Canadian pediatric growth charts have been developed jointly by the Canadian Paediatric Society (CPS), Dietitians of Canada, the College of Family Physicians of Canada, Community Health Nurses of Canada, and the Canadian Pediatric Endocrine Group (Marchand et al., 2010/2016) and are based on the 2007 World Health Organization (WHO) reference growth charts. These charts are based on the child's gender, height, weight, body mass index (BMI), and head circumference. The charts define growth norms and obesity levels for Canadian children. See Appendix C to access the growth charts. Some pediatric illnesses will lead to slower growth patterns. Pediatric disorders of genetic, developmental, intellectual, or other types have growth patterns that are different from the standard growth charts (Marchand et al., 2010/2016). For example, children with Down syndrome have a lower growth velocity. A Down syndrome growth chart, developed to help monitor growth patterns more accurately in this population (Myrelid, Gustafsson, Ollars, et al., 2002), was developed from very small samples and relatively old data and may be out of date in terms of current nutritional care. The CPS recommends that such adapted growth charts may be useful but should be used with caution and in conjunction with the current Canadian 2014 growth charts (Marchand et al., 2010/2016).

Linear growth, or height, occurs almost entirely as a result of skeletal growth and is considered a stable measurement of general growth. Growth in height is not uniform throughout life but ceases when maturation of the skeleton is complete. The maximum rate of growth in length occurs before birth, but the newborn continues to grow at a rapid, though slower, rate.

At birth, weight is more variable than height and is, to a greater extent, a reflection of the intrauterine environment. The average newborn weighs from 3175 to 3400 g. In general, the birth weight doubles by 4 to 7 months of age and triples by

BOX 32-2 FORMULA FOR PREDICTING ADULT HEIGHT

A common method for predicting an adult height is to double the child's height at the age of 2 years to estimate how tall he or she may be as an adult. However, it is very difficult to predict height because of differences in individual growth velocities. A kinesiology research group from Saskatchewan has developed a more accurate method to predict children's adult heights (Sherar, Mirwald, Baxter-Jones, et al., 2005). This formula can be found at http://taurus.usask.ca/growthutility.

the end of the first year. By the age of 2 to 2½ years the birth weight usually quadruples. After this point the "normal" rate of weight gain, just as the growth in height, assumes a steady annual increase of approximately 2 to 2.75 kg per year until the adolescent growth spurt. See Box 32-2 for discussion of how to predict adult height.

Both bone age determinants and state of dentition are used as indicators of development. These indicators are discussed elsewhere in the text (see next section for bone age; see also Chapters 35 and 37 for dentition).

Skeletal Growth and Maturation

The most accurate measure of general development is skeletal or bone age, the radiological determination of osseous maturation. Skeletal age appears to correlate more closely with other measures of physiological maturity (such as onset of menarche) than with chronological age or height. Bone age is determined by comparing the mineralization of ossification centres and advancing bony form to age-related standards.

Bone formation begins during the second month of fetal life when calcium salts are deposited in the intercellular substance (matrix) to form calcified cartilage first and then true bone. In small bones, the bone continues to form in the centre and cartilage continues to be laid down on the surfaces. In long bones, the ossification begins in the *diaphysis* (the long central portion of the bone) and continues in the *epiphysis* (the end portions of the bone). Between the diaphysis and the epiphysis an epiphyseal cartilage plate (or growth plate) unites with the diaphysis by columns of spongy tissue, the *metaphysis*. Active growth in length takes place in the epiphyseal growth plate. Interference with this growth site by trauma or infection can result in deformity.

The first centres of ossification appear in the 2-month-old embryo, and at birth the number is approximately 400, about half the number at maturity. New centres appear at regular intervals during the growth period and represent bone age. Postnatally the earliest centres to appear (at 5 to 6 months of age) are those of the capitate and hamate bones in the wrist. Therefore, radiographs of the hand and wrist provide the most useful areas for screening to determine skeletal age, especially before age 6 years. These centres appear earlier in girls than in boys.

Nurses must understand that the growing bones of children possess many unique characteristics. Bone fractures occurring at the growth plate may be difficult to discover and may significantly affect subsequent growth and development. Factors that may influence skeletal muscle injury rates and types in children and adolescents include the following (Caine, DiFiori, & Maffulli, 2006):

- Not enough protective sports equipment being used
- Less emphasis placed on conditioning, especially flexibility
- In adolescents, fractures are more common than ligamentous ruptures because of the rapid growth rate of the physeal (segment of tubular bone that is concerned mainly with growth) zone of hypertrophy.

Neurological Maturation

In contrast to other body tissues, which grow rapidly after birth, the nervous system grows proportionately more rapidly before birth. Two periods of rapid brain cell growth occur during fetal life: a dramatic increase in the number of neurons between 15 and 20 weeks of gestation and another increase at 30 weeks, which extends to 1 year of age. The rapid growth of infancy continues during early childhood and then slows to a more gradual rate during later childhood and adolescence.

Postnatal growth consists of increasing the amount of cytoplasm around the nuclei of existing cells, increasing the number and intricacy of communications with other cells, and advancing their peripheral axons to keep pace with expanding body dimensions. This allows for increasingly complex movement and behaviour. Neurophysiological changes also provide the foundation for language, learning, and behaviour development. Neurological or electroencephalographic development is sometimes used as an indicator of maturational age in the early weeks of life.

Lymphoid Tissues

Lymphoid tissues contained in the lymph nodes, thymus, spleen, tonsils, adenoids, and blood lymphocytes follow a growth pattern unlike that of other body tissues. These tissues are small in relation to total body size, but they are well developed at birth. A fetus depends on the mother's immune system for protection from infections before birth. Once born, a newborn's lymphatic system begins to respond to the frequent exposure to new organisms and diseases. They increase rapidly to reach adult dimensions by 6 years of age and continue to grow. At about age 10 to 12 years, they reach a maximum development that is approximately twice their adult size. This is followed by a rapid decline to stable adult dimensions by the end of adolescence. For example, children are constantly fighting off new organisms and infections and their lymphatic system quickly responds to fight these antigens. Because of this response, it is quite common for children to have slightly enlarged lymph nodes in certain areas of the body some of the time. However, changes in the lymph nodes can also indicate certain conditions or diseases that need special treatment (Ball et al., 2014).

Development of Organ Systems

All tissues and organ systems undergo changes during development. Some are striking; others are subtle. Many have implications for assessment and care. Because the major importance of these changes relates to their dysfunction, the developmental characteristics of various systems and organs are discussed throughout the book as they relate to these areas. Physical characteristics and physiological changes that vary with age are included in age group descriptions; see Unit 10.

Physiological Changes

Physiological changes that take place in all organs and systems are discussed in this book as they relate to dysfunction (see Unit 12). Other changes such as pulse and respiratory rates and blood pressure are an integral part of physical assessment (see Chapter 33). In addition, changes occur in basic functions, including metabolism, temperature, and patterns of sleep and rest.

Metabolism

The rate of metabolism when the body is at rest (basal metabolic rate [BMR]) demonstrates a distinctive change throughout childhood. Highest in the newborn infant, the BMR closely relates to the proportion of surface area to body mass, which changes as the body increases in size. In both sexes the proportion decreases progressively to maturity. The BMR is slightly higher in boys at all ages and further increases during pubescence over that in girls.

The rate of metabolism determines the child's caloric requirements. The basal energy requirement is about 108 kcal/kg of body weight in infancy and decreases to 40 to 45 kcal/kg at maturity. Water requirements throughout life remain at approximately 1.5 mL/calorie of energy expended. Children's energy needs vary considerably at different ages and with changing circumstances. The energy requirement to build tissue steadily decreases with age, following the general growth curve; however, energy needs vary with the individual child and may be considerably higher. For short periods (e.g., during strenuous exercise) and more prolonged periods (e.g., illness), the needs can be very high.

Temperature

Body temperature, reflecting metabolism, decreases over the course of development. Thermoregulation is one of the most important adaptation responses of the infant during the transition from intrauterine to extrauterine life (see Chapter 25, p. 648). In the healthy newborn, hypothermia can result in several negative metabolic consequences, such as hypoglycemia, elevated bilirubin levels, and metabolic acidosis (see Fig. 25-4). Skin-to-skin care is an effective way to prevent hypothermia in infants (see Chapter 27, Research Focus box on skin-to-skin contact). Unclothed, diapered infants are placed on the parent's bare chest after birth, promoting thermoregulation and attachment (Jefferies & CPS Fetus and Newborn Committee, 2012/2015). After the unstable regulatory ability in the newborn period, heat production steadily declines as the infant grows into childhood. Individual differences of 0.7 of a Celsius degree are normal, and occasionally a child will normally display an unusually high or low temperature. Beginning at approximately 12 years of age, girls' temperature remains relatively stable, whereas the temperature in boys continues to fall for a few more years. Females maintain a temperature slightly above that of males throughout life.

Even with improved temperature regulation, infants and young children are highly susceptible to temperature fluctuations. Body temperature responds to changes in environmental temperature and is increased with active exercise, crying, and emotional stress. Infections can cause a higher and more rapid temperature increase in infants and young children than in older children. In relation to body weight, an infant produces more heat per unit than adolescents. Consequently, during active play or when heavily clothed, an infant or small child is likely to become overheated.

Sleep and Rest

Sleep, a protective function in all organisms, allows for repair and recovery of tissues after activity. As in most aspects of development, there is wide variation among individual children in the amount and distribution of sleep at various ages. As children mature, the total time they spend in sleep and the amount of time they spend in deep sleep change.

Newborn infants sleep much of the time. As infants grow older, the total sleep time gradually decreases, they remain awake for longer periods, and they sleep longer at night. The average sleep patterns for different age groups are as follows:

- Newborns may sleep as much as 16 hours for 3 to 4 hours at a time.
- Babies aged 2 to 6 months sleep 14 to 16 hours and after 3 months have more regular nap routines. By 4 months, most babies nap three times a day.
- Babies aged 6 months to 1 year sleep 14 hours and have two longer naps.
- Toddlers aged 1 to 3 years sleep 10 to 13 hours and after 2 years will go to one nap per day.
- Preschoolers aged 3 to 5 years sleep 10 to 12 hours and often give up daytime naps.
- School children aged 5 to 10 years sleep 10 to 12 hours (CPS, 2012).
- Adolescents sleep longer with pubertal spurts.

The quality of sleep changes as children mature. As children develop through adolescence, their need for sleep does not decline, but their opportunity for sleep may be affected by social activity and academic schedules. The time spent in deep, restful sleep increases from 50% in infancy to 80% in the older child.

Nutrition

Nutrition is probably the single most important influence on growth. Dietary factors regulate growth at all stages of development, and their effects are exerted in numerous and complex ways. During the rapid prenatal growth period, poor nutrition may influence development from the time of implantation of the ovum until birth (see Chapter 12). During infancy and childhood, the demand for calories is relatively great, as evidenced by the rapid increase in both height and weight. At this time, protein and caloric requirements are higher than at almost any period of postnatal development. As the growth rate slows, with its concomitant decrease in

COMMUNITY FOCUS

Healthy Food Choices

Research indicates that new lower-fat recipes in school lunch programs are well accepted by children (Matvienko, 2007). However, less-healthy foods are still more available than more-healthy foods in our nation's schools. Because students consume about 30% of their daily food at school, this situation can contribute to a higher rate of obesity. Indeed, obesity is on the increase in the pediatric population in Canada, which can have a long-term negative impact on health. The Dietitians of Canada (2016) support healthy nutrition programs in day care centres and schools across Canada, with the goal of children developing lifelong healthy eating habits. This group has been involved with school policies regarding the provision of healthier food choices. Many provinces and territories, such as Manitoba, British Columbia, and Ontario, along with multiple school districts, have tried to improve food options in cafeterias and vending machines. One unexpected outcome, however, is that some students go outside the school to buy unhealthy food at fast-food outlets. This pattern can decrease the income of food delivery companies as well as the income of schools, which share in the food profits (Finkelstein, 2009). More research is needed and strategic planning required to encourage lower-fat and low-salt food options. For example, a study was done to look at out-of-school snack programs. The research showed that children chose sliced fruit over whole fruit. Fruit was chosen over unflavoured grain product. However, fruit was rarely chosen over sugar-sweetened and salty snacks (6% vs. 58%). Snack policies that want to serve fruit need to limit less-healthful snack options simultaneously (Beet, Tilley, Kyryliuk, et al., 2014). The provision of healthier choices in food delivery in schools remains a challenge.

BOX 32-3 ATTRIBUTES OF TEMPERAMENT

Activity—Level of physical motion during activity such as sleep, eating, play, dressing, and bathing

Rhythmicity—Regularity in the timing of physiological functions such as hunger, sleep, and elimination

Approach–withdrawal—Nature of initial responses to new stimuli such as people, situations, places, foods, toys, and procedures (*Approach* responses are positive and are displayed by activity or expression; *withdrawal* responses are negative expressions or behaviours.)

Adaptability—Ease or difficulty with which the child adapts or adjusts to new or altered situations

Threshold of responsiveness (sensory threshold)—Amount of stimulation, such as sounds or light, required to evoke a response in the child

Intensity of reaction—Energy level of the child's reactions, regardless of quality or direction

Mood—Amount of pleasant, happy, friendly behaviour compared with unpleasant, unhappy, crying, unfriendly behaviour exhibited by the child in various situations

Distractibility—Ease with which a child's attention or direction of behaviour can be diverted by external stimuli

Attention span and persistence—Length of time a child pursues a given activity (attention) and the continuation of an activity in spite of obstacles (persistence)

metabolism, there is a corresponding reduction in caloric and protein requirements.

Growth is uneven during the periods of childhood between infancy and adolescence, when there are plateaus and small growth spurts. The child's appetite fluctuates in response to these variations until the turbulent growth spurt of adolescence, when adequate nutrition is extremely important but may be subject to numerous emotional influences. Adequate nutrition is closely related to good health throughout life, and an overall improvement in nourishment is evidenced by the gradual increase in size and early maturation of children in this century (see Community Focus box).

Eating Well with Canada's Food Guide has been developed to meet nutrient standards (Dietary Reference Intakes [DRI] for vitamins, elements [minerals], and macronutrients) and to be consistent with evidence linking diet to a reduced risk of chronic diseases. The food intake pattern describes the types and amounts of foods that should be eaten at various ages, including for children (Health Canada, 2007). See Appendix A to review the *Food Guide.*

Temperament

Temperament is defined as "the manner of thinking, behaving, or reacting characteristic of an individual" (Chess & Thomas, 1999) and refers to the way in which a person deals with life. From the time of birth, children exhibit marked individual differences in the way they respond to their environment and the way that others, particularly the parents, respond to them and their needs. A genetic basis has been suggested for some differences in temperament. Nine characteristics of temperament have been identified through interviews with parents (Box 32-3). Temperament refers to behavioural tendencies, not to discrete behavioural acts; there are no implications of good or bad. Most children can be placed into one of three common categories based on their overall pattern of temperamental attributes:

1. **The easy child**—Easy-going children are even tempered, are regular and predictable in their habits, and have a positive approach to new stimuli. They are open and adaptable to change and display a mild to moderately intense mood that is typically positive. Approximately 40% of children fall into this category.
2. **The difficult child**—Difficult children are highly active, irritable, and irregular in their habits. Negative withdrawal responses are typical, and they require a more structured environment. These children adapt slowly to new routines, people, or situations. Mood expressions are usually intense and primarily negative. They exhibit frequent periods of crying, and frustration often produces violent tantrums. This group represents about 10% of children.
3. **The slow-to-warm-up child**—Slow-to-warm-up children typically react negatively and with mild intensity to new stimuli and, unless pressured, adapt slowly with repeated contact. They respond with only mild but passive resistance to novelty or changes in routine. They are inactive and moody but show only moderate irregularity in functions. Approximately 15% of children demonstrate this temperament pattern.

Roughly 35% of children either have some, but not all, of the characteristics of one of the categories or are inconsistent in their behavioural responses. Many children demonstrate this wide range of behavioural patterns.

Significance of Temperament

Observations indicate that children who display the difficult or slow-to-warm-up patterns of behaviour are more vulnerable to the development of behavioural problems in early and middle childhood. Any child can develop behavioural problems if there is dissonance between the child's temperament and the environment. Demands for change and adaptation that are in conflict with the child's capacities can become excessively stressful. However, authorities emphasize that it is not the children's temperament patterns that place them at risk; it is the degree of fit between children and their environment, specifically their parents, that determines the degree of vulnerability. The potential for optimal development exists when environmental expectations and demands fit with the individual's style of behaviour and the parents' ability to navigate this period (Chess & Thomas, 1999) (see Chapter 35, Growth Failure [Failure to Thrive]).

Early identification of temperament provides a useful tool for caregivers in anticipating probable areas of difficulty or risk associated with development. For example, "difficult" children may be prone to colic in infancy, active children require more vigilance to prevent injury, and school entry requires different approaches for children with different temperaments.

Research indicates that irritable and uncooperative infants can raise doubts in mothers about the mother's competence. Additional research indicates that a child's temperament can affect parent–child interactions and influence the parents' self-esteem, marital harmony, mood, and overall satisfaction as parents. Studies on the relationship between temperament and the ability to perform a task successfully (mastery motivation) have found that infants with high mastery are more easy-going (Morrow & Camp, 1996). Activities that parents can use to promote their infants' mastery of performing tasks are listed in Box 32-4.

Some parents and their children have a low degree of "fit" with their child's temperament. For parents in this situation, they may have difficulty understanding their child's temperament and might not know how to resolve the conflicts that can arise from their differences. Pediatric nurses play an important role in helping parents understand the normal growth and development of their children. The nurse can use anticipatory guidelines that are age specific to help parents develop tools and techniques for managing their child's behaviour in a preventative, positive way. For example, some children with attention deficit hyperactivity disorder (ADHD) may be considered to have "difficult" temperaments. These children are usually in a high activity mode and may have trouble understanding and following through with instructions. This behaviour can be very challenging for parents. The Family-Centred Teaching box has anticipatory guidance steps from the Child Development Institute to help parents manage children with ADHD (Child Development Institute, 2015).

BOX 32-4 ACTIVITIES TO PROMOTE MASTERY MOTIVATION IN INFANTS

- Provide inconspicuous assistance during play.
- Share pleasure with infant in accomplishments.
- Do not give immediate assistance during tasks.
- Do not interrupt infant during tasks.
- Let infant initiate activities.
- Limit controlling feedback during play.
- Provide audio and visually responsive toys.
- Provide early kinesthetic stimulation (picking up, rocking).

From Morrow, J. D., & Camp, B. W. (1996). Mastery motivation and temperament of 7-month-old infants. *Pediatric Nursing, 22*(3), 211–217.

FAMILY-CENTRED TEACHING
Parenting Tips for Child With ADHD

There are some straightforward strategies that can help you and your family adapt your lifestyle to assist your child with attention deficit hyperactivity disorder (ADHD).

- Set up a written home schedule with specific times for activities such as waking up, eating meals, doing household chores, completing homework, watching television, or playing computer games. Organize the schedule with your child and prepare the child for any changes in the schedule.
- Establish written house rules on the schedule that are short and clear. Describe the consequences of the child following the rules or if the child breaks the rules. The child's consequences for not following the rules need to be consistent, fair, and quickly follow the rule-breaking behaviour.
- Use a positive reward for good behaviour and praise the smallest positive behaviour. A child with ADHD often receives negative comments throughout the day.
- Let your child know what your positive expectations are with direct eye contact in a calm voice with short and clear instructions. Have the child repeat the instructions back to you. Praise your child as each step is achieved.
- Follow through with consistent consequences and warn only once in a calm voice when the child breaks the rules. It is important not to use physical punishment, which can make the situation worse.
- Provide adult supervision for your child because of the tendency of children with ADHD to behave impulsively.
- Select playmates with comparable language and social skills. It can be difficult for your child with ADHD to learn social skills and rules. Limit the number to one or two friends at a time and give positive reinforcement for good play behaviours.
- Set up a homework schedule at a standard location that is away from potential distractions. Build in short homework times and then put in break times for snacks or play activities. It is important to encourage your child and to not do the homework yourself. Positive rewards for good marks also encourage a child.

Adapted from Child Development Institute. (2015). *Parenting your ADHD child—Easy techniques that work!* Retrieved from http://childdevelopmentinfo.com/add-adhd/parenting-adhd-child-easy-techniques-work/

TABLE 32-1 SUMMARY OF PERSONALITY, COGNITIVE, AND MORAL DEVELOPMENT THEORIES

PSYCHOSEXUAL (FREUD)	PSYCHOSOCIAL (ERIKSON)	COGNITIVE (PIAGET)	MORAL JUDGEMENT (KOHLBERG)	SPIRITUAL (FOWLER)
I. Infancy—Birth to 1 Yr				
Oral-sensory	Trust vs. mistrust	Sensorimotor (birth–2 yr)		Undifferentiated
II. Toddlerhood—1 to 3 Yr				
Anal-urethral	Autonomy vs. shame and doubt	Preoperational thought, preconceptual phase (transductive reasoning [e.g., specific to specific]) (2–4 yr)	Preconventional (premoral) level Punishment and obedience orientation	Intuitive-projective
III. Early Childhood—3 to 6 Yr				
Phallic-locomotion	Initiative vs. guilt	Preoperational thought, intuitive phase (transductive reasoning) (4–7 yr)	Preconventional (premoral) level Naive instrumental orientation	Mythical-literal
IV. Middle Childhood—6 to 12 Yr				
Latency	Industry vs. inferiority	Concrete operations (inductive reasoning and beginning logic) (7–11 yr)	Conventional level Good-boy, nice-girl orientation Law-and-order orientation	Synthetic-convention
V. Adolescence—12 to 18 Yr				
Genitality	Identity vs. role confusion	Formal operations (deductive and abstract reasoning) (11–15 yr)	Postconventional or principled level Social-contract orientation Universal ethical principle orientation	Individuating-reflexive

DEVELOPMENT OF PERSONALITY AND MENTAL FUNCTION

Personality and cognitive skills develop in much the same manner as biological growth—new accomplishments build on previously mastered skills. Many aspects depend on physical growth and maturation. The following discussion acts as an introduction to the multiple facets of personality and behaviour development; many aspects of this development are also integrated into the book's later discussion of children's emotional and social development at various ages (see Unit 10). Table 32-1 summarizes some of the relevant developmental theories.

Theoretical Foundations of Personality Development

Psychosexual Development (Freud)

According to Freud (1923/1961), all human behaviour is energized by psychodynamic forces, and this psychic energy is divided among three components of personality: the id, the ego, and the superego. The *id*, the *unconscious mind*, is the inborn component that is driven by instincts (Freud, 1923/1961). The id obeys the pleasure principle of immediate gratification of needs, regardless of whether the object or action can actually do so. The *ego*, the *conscious mind*, serves the reality principle. It functions as the conscious or controlling self that is able to find realistic means for gratifying the instincts while blocking the irrational thinking of the id. The *superego*, the *conscience*, functions as the moral arbitrator and represents the ideal. It is the mechanism that prevents individuals from expressing undesirable instincts that might threaten the social order.

Freud considered the sexual instincts to be significant in the development of the personality. However, he used the term *psychosexual* to describe any sensual pleasure. During childhood, certain regions of the body assume a prominent psychological significance as the source of new pleasures and new conflicts gradually shifts from one part of the body to another at particular stages of development:

Oral stage (birth to 1 year)—During infancy, the major source of pleasure seeking is centred on oral activities such as sucking, biting, chewing, and vocalizing. Children may prefer one of these over the others, and the preferred method of oral gratification can provide some indication of the personality they develop.

Anal stage (1 to 3 years)—Interest during the second year of life centres on the anal region as sphincter muscles develop and children are able to withhold or expel fecal material at will. At this stage, the climate surrounding toilet training can have lasting effects on children's personalities.

Phallic stage (3 to 6 years)—During the phallic stage, the genitalia become an interesting and sensitive area of the body. Children recognize differences between the sexes and become curious about the dissimilarities. This is the period around which the controversial issues of the Oedipus and Electra complexes, penis envy, and castration anxiety are centred.

Latency period (6 to 12 years)—During the latency period, children elaborate on previously acquired traits and skills. Physical and psychic energy are channelled into acquisition of knowledge and into vigorous play.

Genital stage (age 12 and older)—The last significant stage begins at puberty with maturation of the reproductive system and production of sex hormones. The genital organs become the major source of sexual tensions and pleasures, but energies are also invested in forming friendships and preparing for marriage.

Psychosocial Development (Erikson)

The most widely accepted theory of personality development is that advanced by Erikson (1963). Although built on Freudian theory, it is known as *psychosocial* development and emphasizes a healthy personality as opposed to a pathological approach. Erikson also uses the biological concepts of critical periods and epigenesis, describing key conflicts or core problems that the individual strives to master during critical periods in personality development. Successful completion or mastery of each of these core conflicts is built on the satisfactory completion or mastery of the previous stage.

Each psychosocial stage has two components—the favourable and the unfavourable aspects of the core conflict—and progress to the next stage depends on resolution of this conflict. No core conflict is ever mastered completely but remains a recurrent problem throughout life. No life situation is ever secure. Each new situation presents the conflict in a new form. For example, when children who have satisfactorily achieved a sense of trust encounter a new experience (e.g., hospitalization), they must again develop a sense of trust in those responsible for their care in order to master the situation. Erikson's lifespan approach to personality development consists of eight stages; however, only the first five relating to childhood are included here:

1. **Trust versus mistrust (birth to 1 year)**—The first and most important attribute to develop for a healthy personality is basic *trust*. Establishment of basic trust dominates the first year of life and describes all of the child's satisfying experiences at this age. Corresponding to Freud's oral stage, it is a time of "getting" and "taking in" through all the senses. It exists only in relation to something or someone; therefore, consistent, loving care by a mothering person is essential for development of trust. *Mistrust* develops when trust-promoting experiences are deficient or lacking or when basic needs are inconsistently or inadequately met. Although shreds of mistrust are sprinkled throughout the personality, from a basic trust in parents stems trust in the world, other people, and oneself. The result is faith and optimism.
2. **Autonomy versus shame and doubt (1 to 3 years)**—Corresponding to Freud's anal stage, the problem of *autonomy* can be symbolized by the holding on and letting go of the sphincter muscles. The development of autonomy during the toddler period is centred on children's increasing ability to control their bodies, themselves, and their environment. They want to do things for themselves, using their newly acquired motor skills of walking, climbing, and manipulating and their mental powers of selecting and decision making. Much of their learning is acquired by imitating the activities and behaviour of others. Negative feelings of *doubt* and *shame* arise when children are made to feel small and self-conscious, when their choices are disastrous, when others shame them, or when they are forced to be dependent in areas in which they are capable of assuming control. The favourable outcomes are *self-control* and *willpower*.

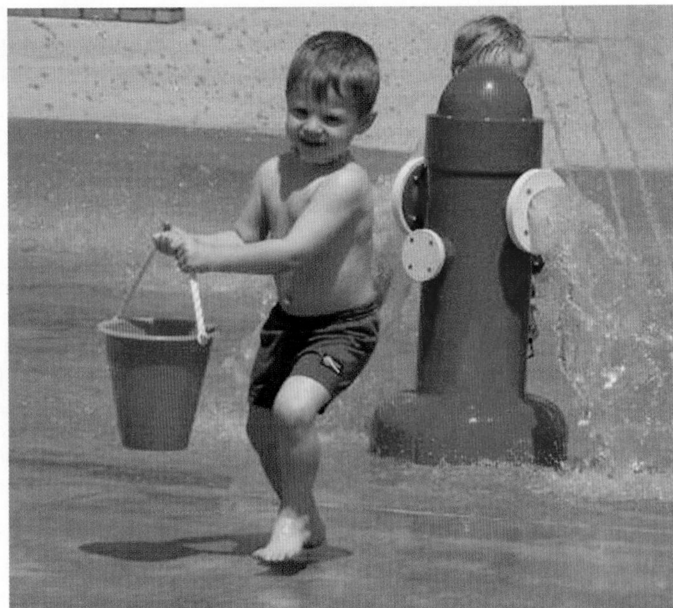

FIGURE 32-4 The stage of initiative is characterized by physical activity and imagination while children explore the physical world around them.

3. **Initiative versus guilt (3 to 6 years)**—The stage of *initiative* corresponds to Freud's phallic stage and is characterized by vigorous, intrusive behaviour; enterprise; and a strong imagination. Children explore the physical world with all their senses and powers (Fig. 32-4). They develop a conscience. No longer guided only by outsiders, they have an inner voice that warns and threatens. Children sometimes undertake goals or activities that are in conflict with those of parents or others, and being made to feel that their activities or imaginings are bad produces a sense of guilt. Children must learn to retain a sense of initiative without impinging on the rights and privileges of others. The lasting outcomes are *direction* and *purpose*.
4. **Industry versus inferiority (6 to 12 years)**—The stage of *industry* is the latency period of Freud. Having achieved the more crucial stages in personality development, children are ready to be workers and producers. They want to engage in tasks and activities that they can carry through to completion; they need and want real achievement. Children learn to compete and cooperate with others, and they learn the rules. It is a decisive period in their social relationships with others. Feelings of *inadequacy* and *inferiority* may develop if too much is expected of them or if they believe that they cannot measure up to the standards set for them by others. The ego quality developed from a sense of industry is competence.
5. **Identity versus role confusion (12 to 18 years)**—Corresponding to Freud's genital period, the development of *identity* is characterized by rapid and marked physical

changes. Previous trust in their bodies is shaken, and children become overly preoccupied with the way they appear in the eyes of others as compared with their own self-concept. Adolescents struggle to fit the roles they have played and those they hope to play with the current roles and fashions adopted by their peers, to integrate their concepts and values with those of society, and to come to a decision regarding an occupation. Inability to solve the core conflict results in *role confusion*. The outcome of successful mastery is *devotion* and *fidelity* to others and to values and ideologies.

Cognitive Development (Piaget)

The term *cognition* refers to the process by which developing individuals become acquainted with the world and the objects it contains. Children are born with inherited potentials for intellectual growth, but they must develop that potential through interaction with the environment. By assimilating information through the senses, processing it, and acting on it, they come to understand relationships between objects and between themselves and their world. With cognitive development, children acquire the ability to reason abstractly, to think in a logical manner, and to organize intellectual functions or performances into higher-order structures. Language, morals, and spiritual development emerge as cognitive abilities advance. Cognitive development consists of age-related changes that occur in mental activities. The best-known theory regarding children's thinking, and a more comprehensive developmental theory than those already described, was developed by the Swiss psychologist Jean Piaget (1969). According to Piaget, intelligence enables individuals to make adaptations to the environment that increase the probability of survival, and through their behaviour individuals establish and maintain equilibrium with the environment.

Piaget (1969) proposed three stages of reasoning: (1) intuitive, (2) concrete operational, and (3) formal operational. When children enter the stage of concrete logical thought at about age 7 years, they are able to make logical **inferences**, classify, and deal with quantitative relationships about concrete things. Not until adolescence are they able to reason abstractly with any degree of competence. Each stage is derived from and builds on the accomplishments of the previous stage in a continuous, orderly process. The course of intellectual development is both maturational and invariant and is divided into the following stages (ages are approximate):

- **Sensorimotor (birth to 2 years)**—The sensorimotor stage of intellectual development consists of six substages (see Chapter 36 for more in-depth discussion) that are governed by sensations in which simple learning takes place. Children progress from reflex activity through simple repetitive behaviours to imitative behaviour. They develop a sense of cause and effect as they direct behaviour toward objects. Problem solving is primarily by trial and error. They display a high level of curiosity, experimentation, and enjoyment of novelty and begin to develop a sense of self as they are able to differentiate themselves from their environment. They become aware that objects have permanence—that an object exists even though it is no longer visible. Toward the end of the sensorimotor period, children begin to use language and representational thought. For example, a child pulls a string to keep a toy train in motion or shakes a rattle to make a noise.
- **Preoperational (2 to 7 years)**—The predominant characteristic of the preoperational stage of intellectual development is **egocentrism**, which in this sense does not mean selfishness or self-centredness but the inability to put oneself in the place of another. Children interpret objects and events not in terms of general properties but in terms of their relationships or their use to them. They are unable to see things from any perspective other than their own; they cannot see another's point of view, nor can they see any reason to do so (see Chapter 37, Cognitive Development). Preoperational thinking is concrete and tangible. Children cannot reason beyond the observable, and they lack the ability to make deductions or generalizations. Thought is dominated by what they see, hear, or otherwise experience. However, they are increasingly able to use language and symbols to represent objects in their environment. Through imaginative play, questioning, and other interactions, they begin to elaborate concepts and to make simple associations between ideas. In the latter stage of this period, their reasoning is intuitive (e.g., the stars have to go to bed just as children do), and they are only beginning to deal with problems of weight, length, size, and time. Reasoning is also transductive—because two events occur together, they cause each other, or knowledge of one characteristic is transferred to another (e.g., all women with big bellies have babies).
- **Concrete operations (7 to 11 years)**—At this age, thought becomes increasingly logical and coherent. Children are able to classify, sort, order, and otherwise organize facts about the world to use in problem solving. They develop a new concept of permanence—**conservation** (see Chapter 38, Cognitive Development [Piaget]); that is, they realize that physical factors such as volume, weight, and number remain the same even though outward appearances are changed. They are able to deal with a number of different aspects of a situation simultaneously. They do not have the capacity to deal in abstraction; they solve problems in a concrete, systematic fashion based on what they can perceive. Reasoning is inductive. Through progressive changes in thought processes and relationships with others, thought becomes less self-centred. They can consider points of view other than their own. Thinking has become socialized. For example, a child can classify objects according to several features, such as choose dolls with blond hair and blue eyes and put the dolls in order along a single dimension such as size.
- **Formal operations (11 to 15 years)**—Formal operational thought is characterized by adaptability and flexibility. Adolescents can think in abstract terms, use abstract symbols, and draw logical conclusions from a set of observations. For example, they can solve the following question: If A is larger than B, and B is larger than C, which symbol is the largest? (The answer is A.) They can make hypotheses and test them; they can consider abstract, theoretical, and philosophical

matters. Although they may confuse the ideal with the practical, most contradictions in the world can be dealt with and resolved.

Moral Development (Kohlberg)

Children also acquire moral reasoning in a developmental sequence. Moral development, as described by Kohlberg (1968), is based on cognitive developmental theory and consists of the following three major levels, each of which has two stages:

1. **Preconventional level**—The preconventional level of moral development parallels the preoperational level of cognitive development and intuitive thought. Culturally oriented to the labels of good/bad and right/wrong, children integrate these in terms of the physical or pleasurable consequences of their actions. At first, children determine the goodness or badness of an action in terms of its consequences. They avoid punishment and obey without question those who have the power to determine and enforce the rules and labels. They have no concept of the basic moral order that supports these consequences. Later, children determine that the right behaviour consists of that which satisfies their own needs (and sometimes the needs of others). Although elements of fairness, give and take, and equal sharing are evident, they are interpreted in a practical, concrete manner without loyalty, gratitude, or justice.
2. **Conventional level**—At the conventional stage, children are concerned with conformity and loyalty. They value the maintenance of family, group, or community expectations regardless of consequences. Behaviour that meets with approval and pleases or helps others is considered good. One earns approval by being "nice." Obeying the rules, doing one's duty, showing respect for authority, and maintaining the social order are the correct behaviours. This level is correlated with the stage of concrete operations in cognitive development.
3. **Postconventional, autonomous, or principled level**—At the postconventional level, the individual has reached the cognitive stage of formal operations. Correct behaviour tends to be defined in terms of general individual rights and standards that have been examined and agreed on by the entire society. Although procedural rules for reaching consensus become important, with emphasis on the legal point of view, there is also emphasis on the possibility for changing law in terms of societal needs and rational considerations.

The most advanced level of moral development is one in which self-chosen ethical principles guide decisions of conscience. These are abstract and ethical but universal principles of justice and human rights with respect for the dignity of persons as individuals. Kohlberg believed that few persons reach this stage of moral reasoning.

Spiritual Development (Fowler)

Spiritual beliefs are closely related to the moral and ethical portion of the child's self-concept and, as such, must be considered as part of the child's basic needs assessment. Children need to have meaning, purpose, and hope in their lives. Also, the need for confession and forgiveness is present, even in very young children. Extending beyond religion (an organized set of beliefs and practices), spirituality affects the whole person: mind, body, and spirit. Fowler (1981) has identified six stages in the development of faith, four of which are closely associated with and parallel cognitive and psychosocial development in childhood:

Stage 0: Undifferentiated—This stage of development encompasses the period of infancy, during which children have no concept of right or wrong, no beliefs, and no convictions to guide their behaviour. However, the beginnings of a faith are established with the development of basic trust through their relationships with the primary caregiver.

Stage 1: Intuitive-projective—Toddlerhood is primarily a time of imitating the behaviour of others. Children imitate the religious gestures and behaviours of others without comprehending any meaning of or significance to the activities. During the preschool years, children assimilate some of their parents' values and beliefs. Parental attitudes toward moral codes and religious beliefs convey to children what they consider to be good and bad. Children still imitate behaviour at this age and follow parental beliefs as part of their daily lives rather than through an understanding of their basic concepts.

Stage 2: Mythic-literal—Through the school-age years, spiritual development parallels cognitive development and is closely related to children's experiences and social interaction. Most have a strong interest in religion during the school-age years. They accept the existence of a deity, and petitions to an omnipotent being are important and expected to be answered; good behaviour is rewarded, and bad behaviour is punished. Their developing conscience bothers them when they disobey. They have a reverence for thoughts about spiritual matters and are able to articulate their faith. They may even question its validity.

Stage 3: Synthetic-conventional—As children approach adolescence, however, they become increasingly aware of spiritual disappointments. They recognize that prayers are not always answered (at least on their own terms), and they may begin to abandon or modify some religious practices. They begin to reason, to question some of the established parental religious standards, and to drop or modify some religious practices.

Stage 4: Individuative-reflective—Adolescents become more skeptical and begin to compare their parents' religious standards with those of others. They attempt to determine which to adopt and incorporate into their own set of values. They also begin to compare religious standards with a scientific viewpoint. It is a time of searching rather than reaching conclusions. Adolescents are uncertain about many religious ideas but will not achieve profound insights until late adolescence or early adulthood.

Language Development

Children are born with the mechanism and capacity to develop speech and language skills. However, they do not speak spontaneously. The environment must provide a means for them to acquire these skills. Speech requires intact physiological structure and function (including respiratory, auditory, and cerebral) plus intelligence, a need to communicate, and stimulation.

The rate of speech development varies from child to child and is directly related to neurological competence and cognitive development. Gesture precedes speech, and in this way a small child communicates satisfactorily. As speech develops, gesture recedes but never disappears entirely. Research suggests that infants can learn sign language before vocal language and that it may enhance the development of vocal language (Thompson, Cotnoir-Bichelman, McKerchar, et al., 2007). At all stages of language development, children's comprehension vocabulary (what they understand) is greater than their expressed vocabulary (what they can say), and this development reflects a continuing process of modification that involves both the acquisition of new words and the expansion and refinement of word meanings previously learned. By the time they begin to walk, children are able to attach a name to objects and persons.

The first parts of speech used are nouns, sometimes verbs (e.g., "go"), and combination words (such as "bye-bye"). Responses are usually structurally incomplete during the toddler period, although the meaning is clear. Next they begin to use adjectives and adverbs to qualify nouns, followed by adverbs to qualify nouns and verbs. Later, pronouns and gender words are added (such as "he" and "she"). By the time children enter school, they are able to use simple, structurally complete sentences that average five to seven words.

Babies and children have the capability to learn more than one language at a very young age. It should not be assumed that a language delay is caused by exposure to two languages. When raising a child bilingually, parents should be encouraged to make sure the child has sufficient exposure in both languages. Referral to speech-language pathologist should be encouraged if a simultaneous-bilingual child is not achieving major communication milestones on time (Staniforth, n.d.).

If parents are concerned that their child's speech or language is delayed, they need to speak with their health care provider. The child may be then referred to a speech-language pathologist, who is a health professional trained to evaluate and treat people with speech or language disorders for an evaluation. A hearing test and other testing may be done (National Institute on Deafness and Other Communication Disorders, 2014).

Development of Self-Concept

Self-concept is how an individual describes himself or herself. The term *self-concept* includes all the beliefs and convictions that constitute an individual's self-knowledge and that influence relationships with others. It develops gradually as a result of unique experiences within the self, with significant others, and with the realities of the world. However, an individual's self-concept may or may not reflect reality.

In infancy the self-concept is primarily an awareness of one's independent existence learned in part as a result of social contacts and experiences with others. The process becomes more active during toddlerhood as children explore the limits of their capacities and the nature of their impact on others. School-age children are more aware of differences among people, are more sensitive to social pressures, and become more preoccupied with issues of self-criticism and self-evaluation. During early adolescence, children focus more on physical and emotional changes taking place and on peer acceptance. Self-concept is crystallized during later adolescence as young people organize their self-concept around a set of values, goals, and competencies acquired throughout childhood.

Body Image

A vital component of self-concept, *body image* refers to the subjective concepts and attitudes that individuals have toward their own bodies. It consists of the physiological (the perception of one's physical characteristics), psychological (values and attitudes toward the body, abilities, and ideals), and social nature of one's image of self (the self in relation to others). All three components interrelate with one another. Body image is a complex phenomenon that evolves and changes during the process of growth and development. Any actual or perceived deviation from the "norm" (no matter how this is interpreted) is cause for concern and is influenced by the attitudes and behaviour of those around them.

The significant others in children's lives exert the most important and meaningful impact on children's body image. Labels that are attached to them (such as "skinny," "pretty," or "fat") or body parts (such as "ugly mole," "bug eyes," or "yucky skin") are incorporated into the body image. Because they lack the understanding of deviations from the physical standard or norm, children notice prominent differences in others and unwittingly make rude or cruel remarks about such minor deviations as large or widely spaced front teeth, large or small eyes, moles, or extreme variations in height.

Infants receive input about their bodies through self-exploration and sensory stimulation from others. As they begin to manipulate their environment, they become aware of their bodies as separate from others. Toddlers learn to identify the various body parts and are able to use symbols to represent objects. Preschoolers become aware of the wholeness of their bodies and discover the genitalia. Exploration of the genitalia and the discovery of differences between the sexes become important.

School-age children begin to learn about internal body structure and function and become aware of differences in body size and configuration. They are highly influenced by the cultural norms of society and current fads. Children whose bodies deviate from the norm are often criticized or ridiculed. Adolescence is the age when children become most concerned about the physical self. The unfamiliar body changes, and the new physical self must be integrated into the self-concept. Adolescents face conflicts over what they see and what they visualize as the ideal body structure. Body image formation during adolescence is a crucial element in the shaping of identity, the psychosocial crisis of adolescence.

Self-Esteem

Self-esteem is the value that an individual places on himself or herself and refers to an overall evaluation of oneself. *Self-esteem* is described as the affective component of the self, whereas *self-concept* is the cognitive component; however, the two terms are almost indistinguishable and are often used interchangeably.

The term *self-esteem* refers to a personal, subjective judgement of one's worthiness derived from and influenced by the social groups in the immediate environment and individuals' perceptions of how they are valued by others. Self-esteem changes with development. Highly egocentric toddlers are unaware of any difference between competence and social approval. By contrast, preschool and early school-age children are increasingly aware of the discrepancy between their competencies and the abilities of more advanced children. Being accepted by adults and peers outside the family group becomes more important to them. Positive feedback enhances their self-esteem; they are vulnerable to feelings of worthlessness and are anxious about failure.

As children's competencies increase and they develop meaningful relationships, their self-esteem rises. Their self-esteem is again at risk during early adolescence when they are defining an identity and sense of self in the context of their peer group. Unless children are continually made to feel incompetent and of little worth, a decrease in self-esteem during vulnerable times is only temporary. Children assess the following aspects of themselves in forming an overall evaluation of their self-esteem:

Competence—How adequate are my cognitive, physical, and social skills?

Sense of control—How well can I complete tasks needed to produce desired actions? Are my successes or failures due to someone or something specific or is it due to luck?

Moral worth—How well do my actions and behaviours meet moral standards that have been set?

Worthiness of love and acceptance—How worthy am I of love and acceptance from parents, other significant adults, siblings, and peers?

Factors that influence the formation of a child's self-esteem include (1) the child's temperament and personality, (2) abilities and opportunities available to accomplish age-appropriate developmental tasks, (3) how significant others interact with the child, and (4) social roles assumed and the expectations surrounding these roles (see also Chapter 33, Psychosocial History).

ROLE OF PLAY IN DEVELOPMENT

Through the universal medium of play, children learn what no one can teach them. They learn about their world and how to deal with this environment of objects, time, space, structure, and people. They learn about themselves operating within that environment—what they can do, how to relate to things and situations, and how to adapt themselves to the demands society makes on them. Play is the work of the child. In play, children continually practise the complicated, stressful processes of living, communicating, and achieving satisfactory relationships with other people.

Classification of Play

From a developmental point of view, patterns of children's play can be categorized according to content and social character. In both there is an additive effect; each builds on past accomplishments, and some element of each is maintained throughout life.

Content of Play

The content of play involves primarily the physical aspects of play, although social relationships cannot be ignored. Play follows the simple to the complex:

Social-affective play—Play begins with social-affective play, in which infants take pleasure in relationships with people. As adults talk to, touch, and nuzzle an infant and in various ways elicit a response from an infant, the infant soon learns to provoke parental emotions and responses with such behaviours as smiling, cooing, or initiating games and activities. The type and intensity of the adult behaviour with children vary among cultures.

Sense-pleasure play—Sense-pleasure play is a nonsocial stimulating experience that originates from without. Objects in the environment—light and colour, tastes and odours, textures and consistencies—attract children's attention, stimulate their senses, and give them pleasure. Pleasurable experiences are derived from handling raw materials (water, sand, food), from body motion (swinging, bouncing, rocking), and from other uses of senses and abilities (smelling, humming) (Fig. 32-5).

Skill play—After infants have developed the ability to grasp and manipulate, they persistently demonstrate and exercise their newly acquired abilities through skill play, repeating an action over and over. The element of sense-pleasure play is often evident in practising a new ability, but frequently the determination to conquer the elusive skill produces pain and frustration (e.g., learning to get onto a play motorcycle) (Fig. 32-6).

Unoccupied behaviour—In unoccupied behaviour, children are not playful but focusing their attention momentarily on anything that strikes their interest. Children daydream,

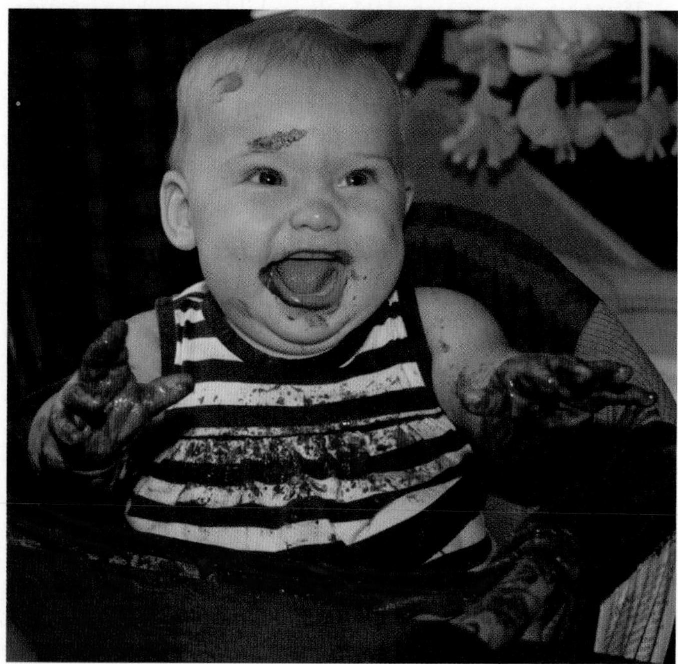

FIGURE 32-5 Children derive pleasure from handling raw materials. (Paints in this picture are nontoxic.)

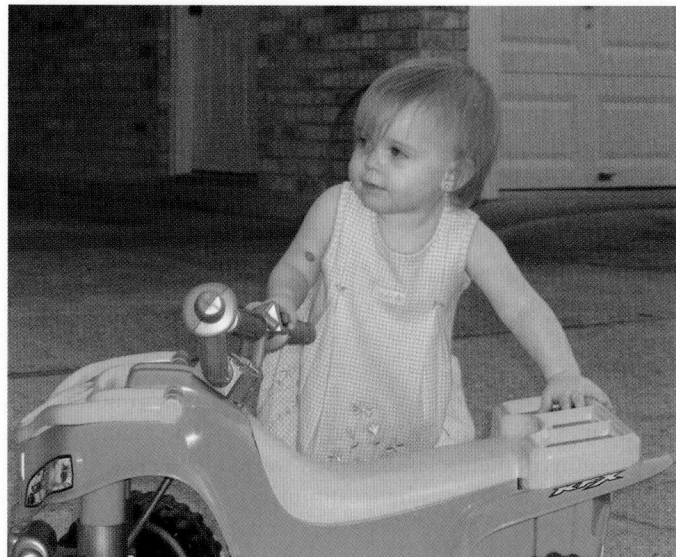

FIGURE 32-6 After infants develop new skills to grasp and manipulate, they begin to conquer new abilities, such as getting on a play motorcycle.

fiddle with clothes or other objects, or walk aimlessly. This role differs from that of onlookers, who actively observe the activity of others.

Dramatic, or pretend, play—One of the vital elements in children's process of identification is dramatic play, also known as symbolic or pretend play. It begins in late infancy (11 to 13 months) and is the predominant form of play in the preschool child. After children begin to invest situations and people with meanings and to attribute affective significance to the world, they can pretend and fantasize almost anything. By acting out events of daily life, children learn and practise the roles and identities modelled by the members of their family and society. Children's toys, replicas of the tools and pastimes of society, provide a medium for learning about adult roles and activities that may be puzzling and frustrating to them. Interacting with the world is one way children get to know it. The simple, imitative, dramatic play of the toddler, such as using the telephone or computer, driving a car, or rocking a doll, evolves into more complex, sustained dramas of the preschooler, which extend beyond common domestic matters to the wider aspects of the world and the society, such as playing police officer, storekeeper, teacher, or nurse. Older children work out elaborate themes, act out stories, and compose plays.

Games—Children in all cultures engage in games alone and with others. Solitary activity involving games begins as very small children participate in repetitive activities and progress to more complicated games that challenge their independent skills, such as puzzles, solitaire, and computer or video games. Very young children participate in simple, imitative games, such as pat-a-cake and peek-a-boo. Preschool children learn and enjoy formal games, beginning with ritualistic, self-sustaining games, such as ring-around-a-rosy and London Bridge. With the exception of some simple board games, preschool children do not engage in competitive games. Preschoolers hate to lose and will try to cheat, want to change rules, or demand exceptions and opportunities to change their moves. School-age children and adolescents enjoy competitive games, including computer or smartphone video games, cards, chess, and physically active games such as baseball.

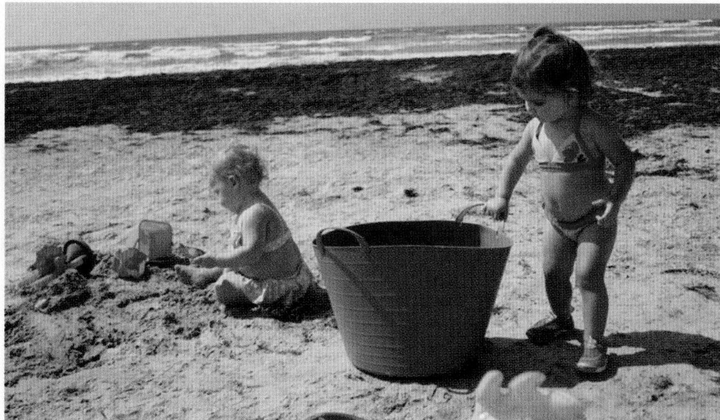
FIGURE 32-7 Parallel play at the beach.

Social Character of Play

The play interactions of infancy are between the child and an adult. Children continue to enjoy the company of adults but are increasingly able to play alone. As children grow, interaction with age-mates increases in importance and becomes an essential part of the socialization process. Through interaction, highly egocentric infants, unable to tolerate delay or interference, ultimately acquire concern for others and the ability to delay gratification or even to reject gratification at the expense of another. A pair of toddlers will engage in considerable combat because their personal needs cannot tolerate delay or compromise. By the time they reach age 5 or 6 years, children are able to arrive at a compromise or make use of arbitration, usually after they have attempted but failed to gain their own way. Through continued interaction with peers and the growth of conceptual abilities and social skills, children are able to increase participation with others in the following types of play:

Onlooker play—During onlooker play, children watch what other children are doing but make no attempt to enter into the play activity. There is an active interest in observing the interaction of others but no movement toward participating. Watching an older sibling bounce a ball is a common example of the onlooker role.

Solitary play—During solitary play, children play alone with toys different from those used by other children in the same area. They enjoy the presence of other children but make no effort to get close to or speak to them. Their interest is centred on their own activity, which they pursue with no reference to the activities of the others.

Parallel play—During parallel activities, children play independently but among other children. They play with toys similar to those that the children around them are using but as each child sees fit, neither influencing nor being influenced by the other children (Fig. 32-7). There is no group association. Parallel play is the characteristic of toddlers, but it may occur at other ages. Individuals who are involved in a creative craft

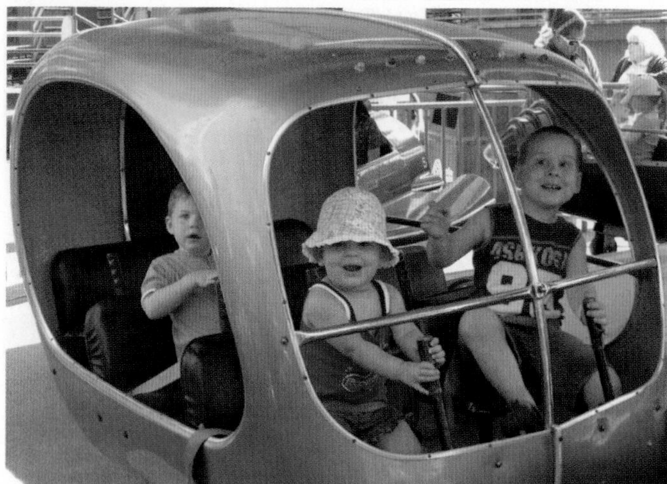

FIGURE 32-8 Associative play.

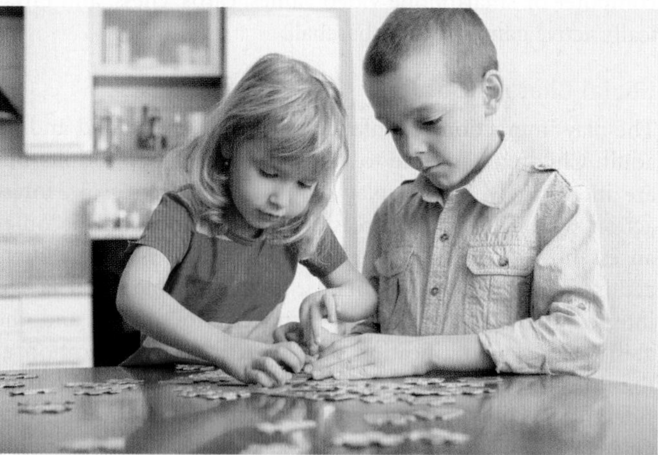

FIGURE 32-9 Cooperative play. (Gladskikh Tatiana/Shutterstock .com.)

with each person separately working on an individual project are engaged in parallel play.

Associative play—In associative play, children play together and are engaged in a similar or even identical activity, but there is no organization, division of labour, leadership assignment, or mutual group goal. Children borrow and lend play materials, follow each other with wagons and tricycles, and sometimes attempt to control who may or may not play in the group. Each child acts according to his or her own wishes; there is no group goal (Fig. 32-8). For example, two children play with dolls, borrowing articles of clothing from each other and engaging in similar conversation, but neither directs the other's actions or establishes rules regarding the limits of the play session. There is a great deal of behavioural contagion: when one child initiates an activity, often, the entire group follows the example.

Cooperative play—Cooperative play is organized, and children play in a group with other children (Fig. 32-9). They discuss and plan activities for the purposes of accomplishing an end—to make something, to attain a competitive goal, to dramatize situations of adult or group life, or to play formal games. The group is loosely formed, but there is a marked sense of belonging or not belonging. The goal and its attainment require organization of activities, division of labour, and role playing. The leader–follower relationship is definitely established, and the activity is controlled by one or two members who assign roles and direct the activity of the others. The activity is organized to allow one child to supplement another's function to complete the goal.

Functions of Play

Sensorimotor Development

Sensorimotor activity is a major component of play at all ages and is the predominant form of play in infancy. Active play is essential for muscle development and serves a useful purpose as a release for surplus energy. Through sensorimotor play, children explore the nature of the physical world. Infants gain impressions of themselves and their world through tactile, auditory, visual, and kinesthetic stimulation. Toddlers and preschoolers revel in body movement and exploration of objects in space. With increasing maturity, sensorimotor play becomes more differentiated and involved. Whereas very young children run for the sheer joy of body movement, older children incorporate or modify the motions into increasingly complex and coordinated activities, such as racing, playing games, skateboarding, and bicycle riding.

Intellectual Development

Through activities involving exploration and manipulation of objects, children learn colours, shapes, sizes, textures, and the significance of objects. They learn the significance of numbers and how to use them; they learn to associate words with objects; and they develop an understanding of abstract concepts and spatial relationships, such as *up*, *down*, *under*, and *over*. Activities such as puzzles and games help them develop problem-solving skills. Books, stories, films, and collections expand knowledge and provide enjoyment as well. Play provides a means to practise and expand language skills. Through play, children continually rehearse past experiences to assimilate them into new perceptions and relationships. Play helps children comprehend the world in which they live and distinguish between fantasy and reality.

Socialization

From very early infancy children show interest and pleasure in the company of others. Their initial social contact is with the mothering person, but through play with other children they learn to establish social relationships and solve the problems associated with these relationships. They learn to give and take, which is more readily learned from critical peers than from more tolerant adults. They learn the sex role that society expects them to fulfill and approved patterns of behaviour and deportment. Closely associated with socialization is development of moral values and ethics. Children learn right from wrong, the standards of the society, and to assume responsibility for their actions.

Creativity

In no other situation is there more opportunity to be creative than in play. Children can experiment and try out their creative ideas in play through every medium at their disposal, including raw materials, fantasy, and exploration. Creativity is stifled by pressure toward conformity; therefore, striving for peer approval may inhibit creative endeavours in the school-age or adolescent child. Creativity is primarily a product of solitary activity, yet creative thinking is often enhanced in group settings where listening to others' ideas stimulates further exploration of one's own ideas. After children feel the satisfaction of creating something new and different, they transfer this creative interest to situations outside the world of play.

Self-Awareness

Beginning with active explorations of their bodies and awareness of themselves as separate from the mother, the process of developing a self-identity is facilitated through play activities. Children learn who they are and their place in the world. They become increasingly able to regulate their own behaviour, to learn what their abilities are, and to compare their abilities with those of others. Through play, children are able to test their abilities, to assume and try out various roles, and to learn the effect their behaviour has on others. They learn the gender role that society expects them to fulfill, as well as approved patterns of behaviour and deportment.

Therapeutic Value

Play is therapeutic at any age (Fig. 32-10). In play, children can express emotions and release unacceptable impulses in a socially acceptable fashion. Children are able to experiment and test fearful situations and can assume and vicariously master the roles and positions that they are unable to perform in the world of reality. Children reveal much about themselves in play. Through play, children are able to communicate to the alert observer the needs, fears, and desires that they are unable to express with their limited language skills. Throughout their play, children need the acceptance of adults and their presence to help them control aggression and channel their destructive tendencies.

Moral Value

Although children learn at home and at school those behaviours considered right and wrong in the culture, the interaction with peers during play contributes significantly to their moral training. Nowhere is the enforcement of moral standards as rigid as in the play situation. If they are to be members of the group, children must adhere to the accepted codes of behaviour of the culture (e.g., fairness, honesty, self-control, consideration for others). Children soon learn that their peers are less tolerant of violations than are adults and that to maintain a place in the play group, they must conform to the group's standards.

Toys

The type of toys chosen by or provided for children can support and enhance the child's development in the areas just described. Although no scientific evidence shows that any toy is necessary for optimal learning, toys offer an opportunity to bring the child and parent together. Toys that are small replicas of the culture and its tools help children assimilate into their culture. Toys that require pushing, pulling, rolling, and manipulating teach them about physical properties of the items and help develop muscles and coordination. Rules and the basic elements of cooperation and organization are learned through board and some video games.

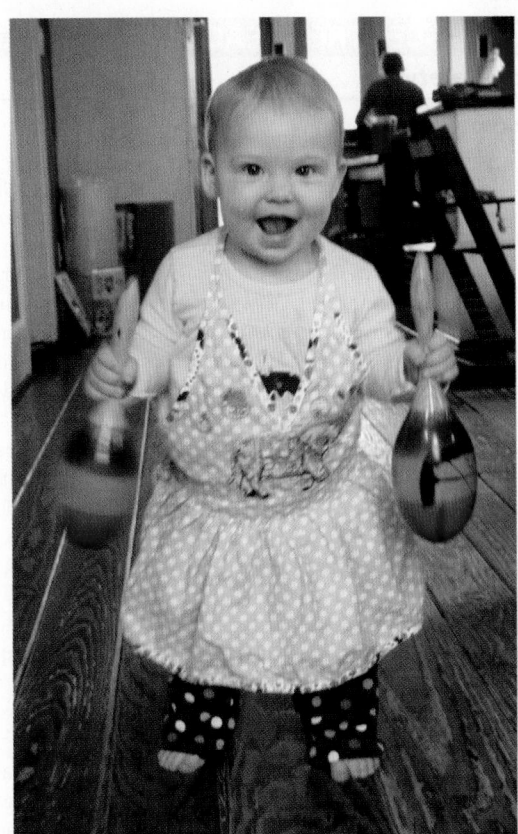

FIGURE 32-10 Play is therapeutic at any age and provides a means for release of tension and stress.

Because they can be used in a variety of ways, raw materials allow children to exercise their own creativity and imagination and are sometimes superior to ready-made items. For example, building blocks can be used to construct a variety of structures, to count, and to learn shapes and sizes.

Toy Safety

While selection of toys and play equipment is a joint effort between parents and children, evaluation of their safety is the adult's responsibility. Government agencies do not inspect and police all toys on the market. Thus, adults who purchase toys, supervise purchases, or allow children to use play equipment need to evaluate such equipment for its safety and age appropriateness. This includes toys that are gifts or those that are purchased by the children themselves (see Family-Centred Teaching box).

Parents should also be alert to notices of toys determined to be defective and recalled by the manufacturers. Parents and health care workers can obtain information on a variety of recalled products and can report potentially dangerous toys and

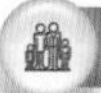

FAMILY-CENTRED TEACHING

Toy Safety

Selection

Select toys that suit the skills, abilities, and interests of children.

Select toys that are safe for the specific child; look for a label that indicates the intended age group. Toys that are safe for one age may not be safe for another.

For infants, toddlers, and all children who still mouth objects, avoid toys with small parts that may pose a fatal choking or aspiration hazard. A choke tube tester such as a cardboard toilet paper roll (diameter 3 cm) can be used to see if a toy fits inside the tube and will be a choking hazard for children under 3 years of age (Parachute, n.d.). Toys in this category are usually labelled "Not recommended for children under 3 years."

For infants, avoid toys with strings or cords that are 18 cm or longer because they may cause strangulation. Remove all crib toys strung across the crib as soon as the infant starts to push up on hands or knees or is 5 months old (whichever comes first).

For all children younger than 8 years, avoid electric toys with heating elements.

For children younger than 5 years, avoid arrows or darts.

Check for clear safety labels such as "flame retardant" or "flame resistant" and that toys are nontoxic.

Select toys durable enough to survive rough play; look for sturdy construction, such as tightly secured eyes, nose, or any small parts.

Select toys light enough that they will not cause harm if one falls on a child.

Look for toys with smooth, rounded edges. Avoid toys with sharp edges that can cut or that have sharp points. Points on the inside of the toy can puncture the skin if the toy is broken.

Avoid toys with any shooting or throwing objects that can injure eyes. This includes toys with which other missiles such as sticks or pebbles might be used as substitutes for the intended projectiles.

Arrows and darts used by children should have blunt tips and be manufactured from resilient materials; make certain the tips are securely attached.

Avoid toys that make loud noises that might damage a child's hearing. Even some squeaking toys are too loud when held close to the ear.

Discourage toys that promote violence, such as guns and violent video games.

If selecting caps for cap guns, look for the label on boxes or packages of caps which states: "Warning—Do not fire closer than 30 cm to the ear. Do not use indoors."

If selecting a toy gun, be certain that the barrel or the entire gun is brightly coloured, to avoid being mistaken for a real gun.

BB guns or pellet rifles should not be given to children under the age of 16.

Toys with magnets are a significant swallowing risk for the under-6 age group, which can lead to serious gastrointestinal complications. The magnet toy must contain a warning label on it with an alert symbol (/!\) and "WARNING!"

Battery-operated toys must be in good condition and the batteries not in reach of children. Button-type batteries, when swallowed, can cause internal poisoning or chemical burns.

Supervise children who are playing with balloons. Throw away immediately any pieces of the balloon that are broken. Use Mylar (foil) balloons because latex balloons pose a choking and allergy hazard.

Do not let children chew on metal jewellery. Some jewellery can contain large levels of lead, which can lead to serious illness in children.

Do not use baby walkers that allow young babies to move quickly, as babies may then fall down stairs or get burned from pulling hot objects or liquid onto themselves.

Never use baby rings or bath seats as they can tip over and cause young children to drown or nearly drown.

Do not put stuffed toys in an infant's crib, as they can pose a suffocation hazard. Secure televisions with brackets or straps to prevent them from toppling onto children; this can cause serious injuries.

Supervision

Maintain a safe play environment.

Remove and discard plastic wrappings on toys immediately; they could suffocate a child.

Remove large toys, bumper pads, and boxes from playpens; an adventuresome child can use such items as a means of climbing or falling out.

Set ground rules for play.

Supervise young children closely during play.

Teach children how to use toys properly and safely.

Instruct older children to keep their toys away from younger brothers, sisters, and friends.

Keep children who are playing with riding toys away from stairs, hills, traffic, and swimming pools.

Establish and enforce rules regarding protective gear.

- Insist that children wear helmets when using bicycles, skateboards, skis, or in-line skates.
- Insist that children wear gloves and wrist, elbow, and knee pads when using skateboards or in-line skates.

Instruct children on electrical safety and how to properly unplug an electric toy—pull on the plug.

- Teach children to beware of electric appliances and even electrically operated playthings; often children are unfamiliar with the hazards of electricity in association with water.
- Teach children the safe use of utensils or other items that under certain circumstances can cause injury—scissors, knives, needles, heating elements, loops, long string, or cord.

Maintenance

Inspect old and new toys regularly for breakage, loose parts, and other potential hazards.

Look for jagged or sharp edges or broken parts that might constitute a choking hazard.

Check movable parts to make certain they are attached securely to the toys; sometimes pieces that are safe when attached to the toy become a danger when detached.

Examine all outdoor toys regularly for rust and weak or sharp parts that could become a danger to a child.

Check electrical cords and plugs for cracked or fraying parts.

Maintain toys in good repair, without signs of possible hazards such as sharp edges, splinters, weak seams, or rust.

Make repairs immediately, or discard out of reach of children.

Sand sharp wooden toys or splintered surfaces so they are smooth.

Use only paint labelled "nontoxic" to repaint toys, toy boxes, or children's furniture.

Storage

Provide a place for children to store toys safely to prevent accidental injury from stepping, tripping, or falling on a toy.

Select a toy chest or toy box that is ventilated and is free of self-locking devices that could entrap or suffocate a child inside. It must have a spring-loaded lid support, designed not to pinch a child's fingers or fall on a child's head.

Playthings meant for older children and adults should be safely stowed away in areas unavailable to younger children.

Adapted from Parachute. (n.d.). *Home safety: Playtime.* Retrieved from http://www.parachutecanada.org/injury-topics/item/home-safety-play-time

child products to Health Canada, Consumer Product Safety (see Additional Resources at the end of this chapter). The Canadian federal government has passed a new toy safety *Consumer Product Safety Act* that is intended to deal quickly with any toy safety issues. For example, Canada was the first country in the world to ban the importation, advertisement, and sale of wheeled baby walkers.

SELECTED FACTORS THAT INFLUENCE DEVELOPMENT

Heredity

Inherited characteristics have a profound influence on development. The child's sex, determined by random selection at the time of conception, directs both the pattern of growth and the behaviour of others toward the child. In all cultures, attitudes and expectations are shaped by the child's sex. Sex and other hereditary determinants strongly affect the progress and end result of growth. There is a high correlation between parent and child with regard to traits such as height, weight, and rate of growth. Most physical characteristics, including shape and form of features, body build, and physical peculiarities, are inherited and can influence the way in which children grow and interact with their environment. Many dimensions of personality, such as temperament, activity level, responsiveness, and a tendency toward shyness, are believed to be inherited.

Differences in children's health and vigour may be attributed to hereditary traits. An inherited physical or mental disorder will alter or modify a child's physical or emotional growth and interactions.

Altered growth and development are one of the clinical manifestations in a number of hereditary disorders. Growth impairment is particularly marked in skeletal disorders, such as the various forms of dwarfism and at least one of the chromosomal anomalies (Turner's syndrome). Many of the disorders of metabolism, such as vitamin D–resistant rickets, the mucopolysaccharidoses, and the numerous endocrine disorders, interfere with the normal growth pattern. In other disorders (e.g., Klinefelter's and Marfan syndromes) the tendency is toward the upper percentile of height.

Many chronic illnesses associated with varying degrees of growth failure are congenital cardiac anomalies, chronic renal disease, and respiratory disorders, such as cystic fibrosis. Any disorder characterized by the inability to digest and absorb body nutrients will have an adverse effect on growth and development.

Genes, Genetics, and Genomics

Nurses and other health care providers are increasingly needing to incorporate genetic and genomic information into their practice. In earlier times, human diseases were thought to be either clearly genetic or typically environment. However, the observation that some genetic disorders are congenital (present at birth) but others are expressed later in life has led scientists to conclude that many, if not most, diseases are caused by a genetic predisposition that can be activated by an environmental trigger. Examples of such interactions are found in single-gene disorders such as phenylketonuria (PKU) and sickle cell disease and in multifactorial conditions such as cancer and neural tube defects (NTDs). PKU is as disorder resulting from (genetically determined) absence of an enzyme that metabolizes the amino acid phenylalanine. However, the deleterious effects in the infant are expressed only after sufficient ingestion of phenylalanine-containing substances such as milk (environmental trigger). Even in the case of a classic genetic condition such as sickle cell disease, its acute symptoms are precipitated by certain conditions, such as lowered oxygen tension, infection, or dehydration.

Evidence is growing that genes play an important role in human susceptibility and resistance to infection, even in cases with a clear environmental cause of the infectious disease. Evidence for this genetic element in resistance gained heightened recognition during the first decade of the acquired immunodeficiency syndrome (AIDS) epidemic. Researchers discovered that adults with a specific deletion in both copies of the *CCR5* genes did not become infected with human immunodeficiency virus (HIV) despite repeated exposures. Later it was discovered that children exposed in utero to HIV typically had a significantly delayed onset of disease if at least one of their *CCR5* genes had the specific mutation (McLaren & Carrington, 2015).

All nurses need to be prepared to use genetic and genomic information and technology when providing care. Often the nurse is the first one to recognize the need for genetic evaluation by identifying an inherited disorder in a family history or noting physical, cognitive, or behavioural abnormalities when performing a nursing assessment.

Neuroendocrine Factors

The hypothalamic–pituitary axis produces a number of releasing and inhibitory hormones that influence growth. Probably all hormones affect growth in some fashion. Three hormones—growth hormone, thyroid hormone, and androgens—when given to persons deficient in these hormones, stimulate protein anabolism and thereby produce retention of elements essential for building protoplasm and bony tissue. It appears that each of the hormones that has a significant influence on growth manifests its major effect at a different period of growth (see Chapter 51).

Interpersonal Relationships

Relationships with significant others play a critical role in development, particularly in emotional, intellectual, and personality development. Not only do the quality and quantity of contacts with other persons exert an influence on the growing child, but the widening range of contacts is essential to learning and developing a healthy personality.

The mothering person is unquestionably the single most influential person during early infancy who meets the infant's basic needs of food, warmth, comfort, and love. He or she stimulates the child's senses and facilitates his or her expanding capacities. Through this person the child learns to trust the world and feel secure to venture in increasingly wider relationships.

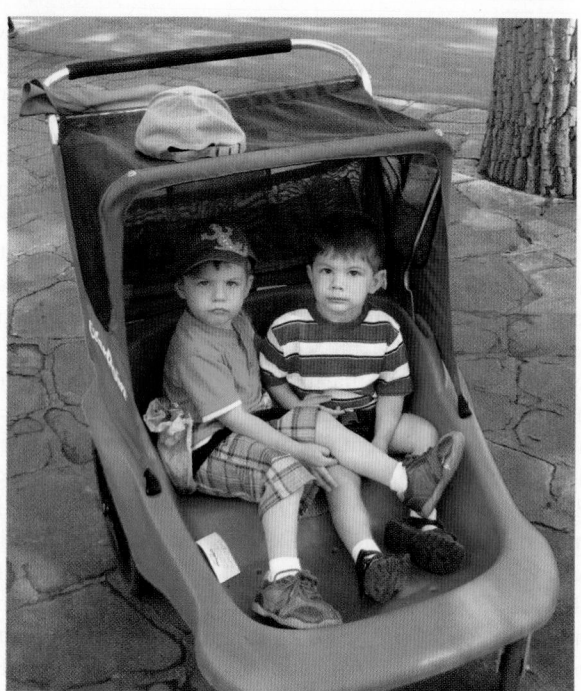

FIGURE 32-11 Peers become increasingly important as children develop friendships outside the family group.

Generally, the parents are most influential in helping the child to assume sex-role identification. Parents define and reinforce acceptable sex-role behaviour and provide sex-appropriate role models for the child. In the absence of a same-sex role model in the family setting, the child may adopt some characteristics of the opposite-sex parent or sibling. Frequently, the child identifies with a teacher or other significant person of the same sex.

Siblings are children's first peers, and the way in which they learn to relate to each other affects later interactions with peers outside the family group. The sphere of persons from whom children seek approval widens to include other members of their family, their peers, and, to a lesser extent, other authority figures (e.g., teachers) (Fig. 32-11). The increasing importance of the peer group in determining the behaviour of school-age children and adolescents is well documented.

When children fail to have high-quality interpersonal relationships with mothering persons they experience *emotional deprivation*. The most prominent feature of emotional deprivation, particularly during the first year, is developmental delays. Much of the information regarding the adverse effects of interpersonal influences on development has been acquired through retrospective studies of gross deprivation and trauma. The most notable instances involved homeless infants who were placed in institutions for care (Bowlby, 1951). Those infants who did not receive consistent mothering care failed to gain weight even with an adequate diet; were pale, listless, and immobile; and were unresponsive to stimuli such as smiling or cooing that usually elicit a response from the normal infant. If emotional deprivation continues for a sufficient length of time, the child may not survive infancy. The term *masked deprivation* has been used to describe children reared in homes in which there is a distorted parent–child relationship or otherwise disordered home environment. Infants do not thrive if the caregiving person is hostile, fearful of handling them, or indifferent to them and their needs. Such children exhibit poor growth even though they are apparently free of physical disease. Growth delays in these children are believed to be caused by a psychologically induced endocrine imbalance that interferes with growth. These same infants and children display "catch-up" growth in a changed environment, however (see Chapter 35, Growth Failure [Failure to Thrive]). Le Mare and Audet (2006) studied adoptees from Romanian orphanages, where the children received minimal mothering care, who were adopted by Canadians. These researchers discovered that all of the adoptees had growth delays when they first arrived in Canada but then thrived and achieved normal growth patterns after 10.5 years.

Socioeconomic Level

The families' socioeconomic level can have a significant impact on children's growth and development. At all ages, children from upper- and middle-class families are taller than comparative children of families in the lower socioeconomic strata. The cause of these differences is less definite, although the poorer health and nutrition of children in lower socioeconomic levels are probably significant factors. Nutritious food sources (especially proteins) tend to be scarce, and other factors, such as larger family size and irregularity in eating, sleeping, and exercise, may also play a role.

Families from lower socioeconomic groups may lack the knowledge or resources needed to provide the safe, stimulating, and enriched environment that fosters optimum development for children. They may be unable to move from unsafe neighbourhoods where drug traffic and drive-by shootings are common. The effects on the emotional development of children living under these conditions have been compared with those experienced by children living in war zones.

Canadian researchers studied the impact of living in poor neighbourhoods on families' health. Some of the parents in these neighbourhoods had poorer mental health and more strained family relations compared with parents in higher-income neighbourhoods and used more punitive parenting (Kohen, Leventhal, Dahinten, et al., 2008), which can put children at risk for behavioural and emotional problems.

Environmental Hazards

Hazards in the environment, another determinant of health, are a source of concern to health care providers and others interested in health and safety. Physical injuries are the most prevalent consequences of environmental dangers; these are discussed extensively throughout the Pediatric Nursing section (Part 3) of this book in relation to age, specific hazards, and selected physical disabilities.

Children are at a high risk for harm resulting from the chemical residues present in the environment. The hazards of these chemical residues relate to their potential carcinogenicity, enzymatic effects, and accumulation. The harmful agents most often associated with health risks are chemicals and radiation, including sun exposure (see Community Focus box). Water, air,

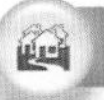

COMMUNITY FOCUS

Sun Protection Basics

The incidence of skin cancer is increasing in children, accounting for about 4% of pediatric malignancies. A resource to use for protecting children from harmful sun exposure is the Environment Canada UV (ultraviolet) Index level, with a scale from 1 to 11, which has associated precautions, including sunglasses, sunscreens, sun-protective clothing, and sun avoidance. Environment Canada predicts the maximum daily UV index levels, which measure the sun's burning UV rays on a daily basis, countrywide. This information is available on the Government of Canada's website at https://weather.gc.ca/forecast/public_bulletins_e.html?Bulletin=fpcn48.cwao. Following are some practices to protect children from harmful UV exposure:

- Children's sunglasses must absorb at least 99% of UV radiation. Sunglasses with the label "Blocks 99% of UV rays" should be used. The glasses must have unbreakable plastic lenses with a wrap-around style that closely fits, to maximize UV and light protection. The glasses should be worn on cloudy as well as sunny days.
- Children should be allowed to choose their sunglasses. A child who wears prescription glasses should also wear prescription sunglasses.
- Avoid sun exposure between 10 A.M. and 2 P.M. High altitude, sand, concrete, snow, and water increase UV exposure.
- Wear wide-brim hats and sun-protective clothing.
- Apply an adequate layer of sunscreen, preferably waterproof or water resistant, and reapply at regular intervals.

Sources: Maguire-Eisen, M., Rothman, K., & Demierre, M. (2005). The ABC's of sun protection. *Dermatology Nursing, 17*(6), 419–433; Government of Canada. (2015). *Sun safety tips for parents.* Retrieved from http://healthycanadians.gc.ca/healthy-living-vie-saine/environment-environnement/sun-soleil/tips-parent-conseils-eng.php

and food contamination from a variety of sources are well documented. Significant means of exposure are substances such as asbestos and lead being present in the immediate environment; secretion of chemicals in breast milk (especially prescribed drugs and nicotine); and contamination within well-insulated homes (especially from disinfectants or burning of substances that produce toxic fumes) (Newman, 2009). Passive inhalation of tobacco smoke by infants and children is a hazard at all stages of development. The harmful effects of large doses of radiation are unquestioned, although the effects of low-dose or short-term radiation are debatable, as are the dosage levels that are considered safe or harmful.

Stress in Childhood

Defined from both a physiological and an emotional point of view, *stress* is "an imbalance between environmental demands and a person's coping resources that … disrupts the equilibrium of the person" (Masten, Garmezy, Tellegan, et al., 1988). Although all children experience stress, some youngsters appear to be more vulnerable than others and are affected by age, temperament, life situation, and state of health in their reactions and ability to handle stress. Also, the responses to a stressor can be behavioural, psychological, or physiological. It is impossible and undesirable to protect children from stress, but providing them with interpersonal security helps them develop coping strategies for dealing with stress. The concept of an *emotional bank*, in which "deposits" and "withdrawals" can be made, can help parents and caregivers maintain a proper perspective on the effects of stress and coping. Children with a good, positive balance in the account can tolerate significant withdrawal experiences. For children with a low balance, even a minor withdrawal may bankrupt the account, causing it to be overdrawn.

Parents and other caregivers can try to recognize signs of stress to help children deal with stressors before they become overwhelming. Signs of stress take many forms but are typically the same ones seen in children who are abused (see Chapter 31) or depressed (see Chapter 38). If a number of stressors are imposed on children at the same time, the children are more vulnerable. When a succession of stressors produces an excessive stress load, children may experience a serious change in health or behaviour.

It is important that parents and persons working with children understand the nature of childhood stress and ways in which it can be recognized or anticipated. Caregivers must listen to children so that they are aware of children's fears and concerns. They need to let children know that they are important and that what they say matters. Physical contact is usually comforting and reassuring to children. Simply holding, touching, or hugging children can be both relaxing and comforting and facilitate communication. Spending unhurried time with children, taking family outings or vacations, and exposing children to positive influences can help build children's strength and security. Supportive interpersonal relationships are essential to children's psychological well-being.

Coping

Coping refers to a special class of individual reactions to stressors—specifically, a reaction to a stressor that resolves, reduces, or replaces the affective state classified as stressful. *Coping strategies* are the specific ways in which children cope with stressors, as distinguished from *coping styles*, which are relatively unchanging personality characteristics or outcomes of coping. As children age, they tend toward a more internal locus of control and use more vigilant modes of coping. Children, like adults, respond to everyday stress by trying to change the circumstances or trying to adjust to circumstances the way they are. Any strategy that provides relaxation is effective in reducing stress, and most children have their own natural methods of dealing with stress, such as withdrawing, engaging in physical activity, reading, listening to music, working on a project, or taking a nap. Some turn to parents to solve their problems, or they may develop socially unacceptable strategies, such as cheating, stealing, or lying.

Children can be taught stress-reduction techniques to use in coping. First, they must be helped to recognize signs of tension in themselves. Then they can be taught any of a variety of appropriate strategies—special exercises, relaxation and breathing, mental imagery, and numerous other simple activities. Also, parents and other caregivers can anticipate possible stress-provoking events and prepare children for coping by role playing a scenario or "talking it through" so that they can learn how to solve problems. When children can view any new situation as a problem to be solved and an opportunity to learn, they are not vulnerable to the control of others. It provides them with a sense of mastery over their own lives and reinforces the fact that they have within themselves the ability and information to handle whatever comes their way. Problem-solving skill gives them the confidence to know where and how to seek help when they need it.

Mass Media

The media can have an enormous influence on the developing child. There is no doubt that the media provide children with a means of extending their knowledge about the world in which they live and have helped narrow the differences between classes. However, there is growing concern about the enormous influence that the media can have on the developing child because of the large number of hours that children spend watching media, such as movies, video games, and television shows. The portable technology of hand-held electronic devices has given children even more access to the multitude sources of media. For instance, the images of risky behaviour presented in the media may establish or reinforce teenagers' perceptions of their social environment.

Children may identify closely with and be influenced by people or characters portrayed in reading materials, movies, video games, and television programs and commercials. Ways in which children respond to behaviours depicted in media and positive ways in which parents can help children work through media influences are presented in Box 32-5.

Most researchers have concluded that protracted television viewing can have detrimental effects on children. For example, in one study, television viewing was implicated as contributing to irregular sleep schedules in children under 3 years of age (Thompson & Christakis, 2005). Recognizing the negative effects of television viewing, the Canadian Paediatric Society (2003/2011) has recommended that children under age 2 not participate in screen-based activities and that older children watch no more than 1 to 2 hours of high-quality television a day. However, this warning has not been heeded, with approximately 40% of infants already watching television by 3 months of age and the number increasing to 90% by age 24 months. Parents reported three primary reasons for allowing their infants to watch television: 1) they thought it was educational for their children, 2) they thought it was entertaining, and 3) the parents needed time to get other things done. Parents did watch television with their infants more than half the time (Zimmerman, Christakis, & Meltzoff, 2007).

It is especially important to identify at-risk children and control their viewing. These children include those left without adult supervision, emotionally disturbed children, children with learning disabilities, children who are abused by their parents, and children in families in distress (CPS, 2003/2011). For all children, house rules that specify the type and amount of television help children understand limits, and recorded selections of appropriate programs can be substituted for less desirable offerings. Parents need to carefully monitor cable and other pay-television programming. Lockboxes, V-chips, and blocking devices are available for cable receivers to prevent children from viewing uncensored programs when unsupervised.

Like movies, some television programs and commercials contain many implicit and explicit messages that promote consumerism, alcohol consumption, smoking, violence, and promiscuous or unsafe sexual activity. There is evidence, although limited, documenting a relationship between viewing these activities on television and the actual use of alcohol or tobacco, exposure to violence, and aggressive behaviour (Mitrofan, Paul, Weich, et al., 2014). Children are vulnerable to advertising, which can encourage unhealthy habits, such as asking parents for sugary, low-fibre cereals.

Parents can help children evaluate violence on television by pointing out the subtleties that children miss, such as the aggressor's motives and intentions and the unpleasant consequences that the perpetrators suffer as a result of their aggressive acts. Often the consequence is separated from the act by a commercial, thus children cannot make the correlation. Parents need to point out that conflicts can be resolved without resorting to violent behaviour. They can also stress the program's purpose—primarily entertainment—and explain why they like or dislike something on television (e.g., "This show is trying to tell you that crime does not pay and that if people do wrong, they will go to jail"). Explanations and discussions can take place between shows (with the volume turned down), and young children can learn from both older children and adults. These discussions can be effective when begun early and carried out consistently.

Television is the medium by which most children learn of a natural disaster or act of terrorism. For example, there was extensive media coverage in Canada of the September 11, 2001, terrorist attacks. Research on the effects of these terrorist attacks

BOX 32-5 FACTORS THAT ENCOURAGE LEARNING BASED ON BEHAVIOURS PRESENTED ON MASS MEDIA

Age—Younger children focus on behaviours rather than on motives or consequences. They view alternatives in a concrete manner, and they are unable to differentiate between central and peripheral plot information.

Identification with characters or situations—Children often imitate behaviours of persons in situations similar to those in their own lives.

Reward and punishment syndrome—Children imitate behaviours they see rewarded or not punished when that is expected. They are less likely to repeat an act they see punished; their attention is immediately attracted when they see an act committed that they know should be punished but is not.

Opportunity to reproduce behaviours—Children imitate behaviours when given the right environment or when violence seems an accepted solution. When children see a situation on television, they use this information when they encounter a similar situation that requires a solution.

Motivation to reproduce behaviours—Children imitate behaviour when given the appropriate incentives: expectation of reward or lack of punishment. Some children have self-control; others do not.

suggests that post-traumatic stress reactions increase with greater exposure to media coverage. Reading about the event rather than watching it on television may produce less traumatic associations of the experience (Hamblen & Dart Center for Journalism and Trauma, 2016). In addition, parents should limit the exposure to media coverage of traumatic events, talk to their child about the event, and maintain daily routines as much as possible. With regard to television news coverage, while there are no Canadian statistics available on this topic, the Media Smarts group has expressed concern about television news programs having increased crime coverage, which can frighten children and exaggerate the actual risk (see Additional Resources at the end of this chapter for information on media's impact on children).

Television has been shown, however, to have a positive influence on children's abilities to deal with a variety of social issues, such as divorce, the arrival of a new baby, discrimination, honesty, and helpfulness. Children who view educational programming for an extended period tend to become more affectionate, considerate, cooperative, and helpful toward their playmates. A systematic review of preschoolers who watched television found that educational viewing can increase their knowledge, positively affect their attitudes toward racial difference, and increase their imaginative behaviour (Thakkar, Garrison, & Christakis, 2006). The ways in which non-White characters and those of various ethnicities are portrayed on television can have an impact on the ways in which the predominantly White culture views non-White persons and on the self-image of non-White children. The impact can be positive or negative, depending on whether the characters are treated with respect or discrimination.

In short, parents need to supervise the amount and type of media programs their children watch and to teach their children how to watch media (Box 32-6 and Family-Centred Care box). As the CPS (2003/2011) recommends, parental role modelling may have a more positive influence on the child's behaviour than media programming. The CPS recommends that parents watch media with their child and that parents help him or her understand the difference between the child's life and habits and those of persons represented on television.

Nurses and parents can be powerful forces in influencing the media. They can watch closely for an increase in violence and other undesirable programming and express their concerns to sponsors and television stations if they believe it is not appropriate. Good programming can be both educational and entertaining.

Internet

The use of computers and personal tablets in both the classroom and home has affected childhood learning and development. Many schools offer computer programs and use digital devices that enable children of all ages to research a range of topics and broaden their world view. These technologies can be used for interactive learning, and their use can improve hand–eye coordination. Parents have a wide variety of computer software to choose from for their children's learning and gaming.

The Internet and email have made correspondence and information available to children from around the world in seconds. Social networking sites (e.g., Twitter, Facebook, Tumblr, Instagram, Kik Messenger, Snapchat) provide opportunities for children and adolescents to express themselves through blogs, music, pictures, and videos, and the overwhelming majority of adolescents use these sites responsibly (Holloway, Dunlap, Del Pino, et al., 2014; Steeves, 2015).

Although computer and digital technology has enhanced many forms of learning and recreation, there are potential dangers to children. The negative aspects of television and video games also apply to the Internet. It is important for parents to be aware of the websites that their children access, as they are vulnerable to exposure to pornographic sites. Children can also be lured into interactions with pedophiles. Locks that block certain websites should be considered. Children can also spend too much time sitting in front of a computer screen. With excessive use of digital devices such as smartphones they can also develop repetitive-use injuries.

BOX 32-6 FIVE IMPORTANT IDEAS TO TEACH CHILDREN AND ADOLESCENTS ABOUT MASS MEDIA

1. You are smarter than what you see on your media devices.
2. The media world is not real.
3. Media teach that some people are more important than others.
4. Media keep showing the same things over and over again.
5. Somebody is always trying to make money through media.

Modified from Davis, J. (1992). Five important ideas to teach your children about TV. *Media Values, 59/60*, 10–14.

FAMILY-CENTRED TEACHING
Media Viewing

Provide a positive role model by developing media substitutes such as reading, athletics, physical conditioning, and hobbies.

Together with your child, construct a time chart of activities (homework, media viewing, scheduled and other outside activities, playing with a friend).

Require that the child choose doing something from this list before watching media.

Limit the child's viewing to 2 hours or less per day.

Rule out media viewing at specific times (e.g., mealtimes, before breakfast, or on school nights).

Discuss the purpose of a program and of commercial content with the child:

- Distinguish between the real and the unreal.
- Correlate consequences with actions.
- Point out subtle messages.
- Explore alternatives to aggressive conflict resolution.

Remove televisions and hand-held electronic devices from children's bedrooms.

Limit use of media viewing as a distraction to potentially stressful times (e.g., keeping the children occupied while the parent gets organized after a difficult day).

Nurses should encourage parents to be knowledgeable of their children's Internet activities and to provide appropriate learning activities unique to computers and digital devices. One helpful strategy is to locate the computer in a public area of the home, such as the kitchen or family room, to enable parents to easily monitor its use. Nurses can engage parents in conversations about the negative and positive consequences of watching too much television and of their child viewing shows that are inappropriate for his or her age. In hospitals, many bedsides have a television or computer and videogames with Wi-Fi available for children to use. Nurses can help to set limits on viewing and encourage other activities for these children.

KEY POINTS

- Growth describes a change in quantity and occurs when cells divide and synthesize new proteins.
- Maturation, a qualitative change, describes the aging process or an increase in competence and adaptability.
- Differentiation refers to biological processes by which early cells and structures are modified and altered to achieve specific and characteristic physical and chemical properties.
- Development involves change from a lower to a more advanced stage of complexity.
- The five major developmental periods are prenatal, infancy, early childhood, middle childhood, and later childhood (pubescence and adolescence).
- Growth and development proceed in predictable patterns of direction, sequence, and pace.
- The directional trends in growth and development are cephalocaudal, proximodistal, and mass to specific.
- Physical development includes increase in height and weight and changes in body proportion, dentition, and some body tissues.
- The three broad classifications of child temperament are the easy child, the difficult child, and the slow-to-warm-up child.
- The developmental theories most widely used in explaining child growth and development are Freud's psychosexual stages, Erikson's stages of psychosocial development, Piaget's stages of cognitive development, Kohlberg's stages of moral development, and Fowler's stages of spiritual development.
- To develop a positive self-concept, children need recognition for their achievements and the approval of others.
- Through play, children learn about their world and how to relate to objects, people, and situations.
- Play provides a means of development in the areas of sensorimotor and intellectual progress, socialization, creativity, self-awareness, and moral behaviour; it serves as a means for the release of tension and expression of emotions.
- Growth and development are affected by a variety of conditions and circumstances, including heredity, physiological function, gender, disease, physical environment, nutrition, and interpersonal relationships.
- All nurses should be familiar with genetic or genomics information as it relates to their patient's care.
- Children's vulnerability and reaction to stress depend to a large extent on their age, coping behaviours, and support systems.
- Mass media can be influential in children's learning and behaviour.

evolve WEBSITE

Visit the Evolve website for additional resources related to the content in this chapter such as Case Studies, Critical Thinking Case Study Answers, Nursing Care Plans, Nursing Processes, Nursing Skills, and Review Questions for Exam Preparation at: *http://evolve.elsevier.com/Canada/Perry/maternal/*

REFERENCES

Ball, J. W., Dains, J. E., Flynn, J. E., et al. (2014). *Seidel's guide to physical examination* (8th ed.). St. Louis: Mosby.

Beet, M. W., Tilley, F., Kyryliuk, R., et al. (2014). Children select unhealthy choices when given a choice among snack offerings. *Journal of Academy of Nutrition and Dietetics, 114*(9), 1440–1446. doi:10.1016/j.jand.2014.04.022.

Bowlby, J. (1951). *Maternal care and mental health*. Geneva: World Health Organization.

Caine, D., DiFiori, J., & Maffulli, N. (2006). Physeal injuries in children's and youth sports: Reasons for concern? *British Journal of Sports Medicine, 40*(9), 749–760. doi:10.1136/bjsm.2005.017822.

Canadian Paediatric Society. (2003). Impact of media use on children and youth. *Paediatrics and Child Health, 8*(5), 301–306. Reaffirmed 2011.

Canadian Paediatric Society. (2012). *Healthy sleep for your baby and child*. Retrieved from <http://www.caringforkids.cps.ca/handouts/healthy_sleep_for_your_baby_and_child>.

Chess, S., & Thomas, A. (1999). *Goodness of fit: Clinical applications from infancy through adult life*. London: Routledge.

Child Development Institute. (2015). *Parenting your ADHD child—Easy techniques that work!* Retrieved from <http://childdevelopmentinfo.com/add-adhd/parenting-adhd-child-easy-techniques-work/>.

Dietitians of Canada. (2016). *School nutrition*. Retrieved from <http://www.dietitians.ca/Dietitians-Views/Children-and-Teens/School-Nutrition.aspx>.

Erikson, E. H. (1963). *Childhood and society* (2nd ed.). New York: Norton.

Finkelstein, P. (2009). School nutrition: Are we failing Canadian kids? *Best Health Magazine*, March/April. Retrieved from <http://

www.besthealthmag.ca/eat-well/nutrition/school-nutrition-are-we-failing-canadas-kids>.

Fowler, J. (1981). *Stages of faith: The psychology of human development and the quest for meaning*. New York: HarperCollins.

Freud, S. (1961). *The ego and the id*. In J. Strachey (Ed. and Trans.), *The standard edition of the complete psychological works of Sigmund Freud* (Vol. 19, pp. 3–66). London: Hogarth Press. (Original work published 1923).

Hamblen, J., & Dart Center for Journalism and Trauma. (2016). *Media coverage of traumatic events: Research on effects*. Retrieved from <http://www.ptsd.va.gov/professional/trauma/basics/media-coverage-traumatic-events.asp>.

Health Canada. (2007). *Canada's food guide*. Retrieved from <http://hc-sc.gc.ca/fn-an/food-guide-aliment/context/evid-fond-eng.php>.

Holloway, I. W., Dunlap, S., Del Pino, H. E., et al. (2014). Online social networking, sexual risk and protective behaviors: Considerations for clinicians and researchers. *Current Addiction Reports*, *1*(3), 220–228.

Jefferies, A. L., & Canadian Paediatric Society, Fetus and Newborn Committee. (2012). Kangaroo care for the preterm infant and family. *Paediatrics & Child Health*, *17*(3), 141–143. Retrieved from <http://www.cps.ca/documents/position/kangaroo-care-for-preterm-infant>. Reaffirmed 2015.

Kohen, D. E., Leventhal, T., Dahinten, V. S., & McIntosh, C. N. (2008). Neighborhood disadvantage: Pathways of effects for young children. *Child Development*, *79*(1), 156–169. doi:10.1111/j.1467-8624.2007.01117.x.

Kohlberg, L. (1968). Moral development. In D. L. Sills (Ed.), *International encyclopedia of the social sciences*. New York: Macmillan.

Le Mare, L., & Audet, K. (2006). A longitudinal study of the physical growth and health of postinstitutionalized Romanian adoptees. *Paediatrics & Child Health*, *11*(2), 85–91.

Marchand, V., & Canadian Paediatric Society, Dietitians of Canada, College of Family Physicians of Canada, & Community Health Nurses of Canada. (2010). Promoting optimal monitoring of child growth in Canada: Using the new WHO growth charts—Executive summary. *Paediatrics & Child Health*, *15*(2), 77–79. Retrieved from <http://www.cps.ca/documents/position/child-growth-charts>. Reaffirmed 2016.

Masten, A. S., Garmezy, N., Tellegan, A., et al. (1988). Competence and stress in school children: Moderating effects of individual and family qualities. *Journal of Child Psychology and Psychiatry*, *29*, 747–764.

Matvienko, O. (2007). Impact of a nutrition education curriculum on snack choices of children ages six and seven years. *Journal of Nutrition Education & Behavior*, *39*(5), 281–285. doi:10.1016/j.jneb.2007.01.004.

McLaren, P. J., & Carrington, M. T. (2015). The impact of host genetic variation on infection with HIV-1. *Nature Immunology*, *16*(6), 577–583. doi:10.1038/ni.3147.

Mitrofan, B., Paul, M., Weich, S., & Spencer, N. (2014). Aggression in children with behavioural/emotional difficulties: Seeing aggression on television and video games. *BioMed Central Psychiatry*, *14*, 287.

Morrow, J. D., & Camp, B. W. (1996). Mastery motivation and temperament of 7-month-old infants. *Pediatric Nursing*, *22*(3), 211–217.

Myrelid, A., Gustafsson, J., Ollars, B., & Annerén, G. (2002). Growth charts for Down's syndrome from birth to 18 years of age. *Archives of Disease in Childhood*, *87*(2), 97–103.

National Institute on Deafness and Other Communication Disorders. (2014). *Speech and language developmental milestones*. Retrieved from <http://www.nidcd.nih.gov/health/voice/pages/speechandlanguage.aspx>.

Newman, J. (2009). *Canadian Breast Feeding Foundation: Toxins and infant feeding*. Retrieved from <http://www.canadianbreastfeedingfoundation.org/basics/toxins.shtml>.

Parachute. (n.d). *Home safety: Playtime*. Retrieved from <http://www.parachutecanada.org/injury-topics/item/home-safety-play-time>.

Piaget, J. (1969). *The theory of stages in cognitive development*. New York: McGraw-Hill.

Sherar, L. B., Mirwald, R. L., Baxter-Jones, A., et al. (2005). Prediction of adult height using maturity-based cumulative height velocity curves. *Journal of Pediatrics*, *147*(4), 508–514.

Staniforth, C. (n.d.) *Child language development in bilingual and multilingual environments*. Retrieved from <http://www.beststart.org/events/detail/bsannualconf09/webcov/presentations/B5-Staniforth.pdf>.

Steeves, V. (2015). *Young Canadians in a wired world, phase III: Trends and recommendations*. Ottawa: MediaSmarts. Retrieved from <http://mediasmarts.ca/sites/mediasmarts/files/publication-report/full/ycwwiii_trends_recommendations_fullreport.pdf>.

Thakkar, R., Garrison, M., & Christakis, D. (2006). A systematic review for the effects of television viewing by infants and preschoolers. *Pediatrics*, *118*(5), 2025–2031. doi:10.1542/peds.2006-1307.

Thompson, D. A., & Christakis, D. A. (2005). The association between television viewing and irregular sleep schedules among children less than 3 years of age. *Pediatrics*, *116*(4), 851–856. doi:10.1542/peds.2004-2788.

Thompson, R., Cotnoir-Bichelman, N., McKerchar, P., et al. (2007). Enhancing early communication through infant sign training. *Journal of Applied Behavior Analysis*, *40*(1), 15–23. doi:10.1901/jaba.2007.23-06.

Zimmerman, F., Christakis, D., & Meltzoff, A. (2007). Television and DVD/video viewing in children younger than 2 years. *Archives of Pediatric and Adolescent Medicine*, *161*, 473–479.

ADDITIONAL RESOURCES

Dietitians of Canada—A comprehensive resource for healthy nutrition programs and safe food supplies; a tracking system is available that can help individuals make healthy choices: <http://www.dietitians.ca>.

Government of Canada—Sun Safety Tips: <http://healthycanadians.gc.ca/healthy-living-vie-saine/environment-environnement/sun-soleil/tips-parent-conseils-eng.php>.

Government of Canada—The Ultraviolet Index and Your Local Forecast: <http://healthycanadians.gc.ca/healthy-living-vie-saine/environment-environnement/sun-soleil/index-uv-indice-eng.php>.

Health Canada—Consumer Product Safety: <http://www.hc-sc.gc.ca/cps-spc/index-eng.php>.

MediaSmarts: Canada's Centre for Digital and Media Awareness (formerly Media Awareness Network) <http://www.mediasmarts.ca/>.

Motion Picture Association—Movie rating categories: <http://www.mpaa.org>.

University of Saskatchewan adult height prediction formula: <http://kinesiology.usask.ca/growthutility>.

UNIT 9

Assessment of the Child and Family

CHAPTER

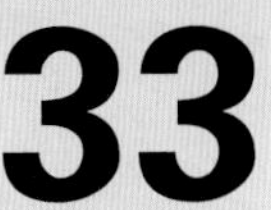

Communication, History, Physical, and Developmental Assessment

Cheryl Sams

evolve WEBSITE

Visit the Evolve website for additional resources related to the content in this chapter such as Case Studies, Critical Thinking Case Study Answers, Nursing Care Plans, Nursing Processes, Nursing Skills, and Review Questions for Exam Preparation at: http://evolve.elsevier.com/Canada/Perry/maternal/

OBJECTIVES

On completion of this chapter the reader will be able to:

- Identify communication strategies for interviewing parents.
- Identify communication strategies for communicating with children of different age groups.
- Describe four communication techniques that are useful with children.
- State the components of a complete health history.
- List three areas that are evaluated as part of a nutritional assessment.
- Identify developmental assessment tools that can be used to perform a developmental assessment.
- Prepare a child for a physical examination based on his or her developmental needs.
- Perform a comprehensive physical examination in a sequence appropriate to the child's age.
- Recognize expected findings for children at various ages.
- Record the physical examination according to the head-to-toe format.

COMMUNICATING WITH FAMILIES AND CHILDREN

Communication is the cornerstone of providing nursing care to children and their families. When a nurse meets a child and the family, she or he is starting the process of building a relationship with all of the individuals involved. It essential that the nurse be able to develop a rapport and a sense of trust with the family in order to encourage the child and the family to share information relevant to the child's care. By sharing information this will help in obtaining an accurate history and health assessment of the child. The most widely used method by nurses to communicate with parents and children on a professional basis is the interview process. Unlike social conversation, interviewing is a specific form of goal-directed communication. As nurses converse with children and adults, they focus on the individuals to determine their usual mode of handling problems, whether help is needed, and the way they react to counselling. Developing interviewing skills requires time and practice, but following some guiding principles can facilitate this process. An organized approach is most effective when using interviewing skills in patient teaching.

Establishing a Setting for Communication

Appropriate Introduction

When first meeting a patient and his or her family, the nurse needs to introduce herself or himself to the family members and ask each person's name. Parents and other adults should be addressed by their appropriate titles, such as "Mr.," "Mrs.," or "Ms.," unless they specify a preferred name. The nurse should record the preferred name on the medical record. Using formal address or their preferred names, rather than using first names or "mother" or "father" conveys respect for the parents or other caregivers (Ball, Dains, Flynn, et al., 2014).

At the beginning of the visit, to establish rapport, children should be included in the interaction, by asking them their name, age, grade, and favourite activities. Nurses often direct all questions to adults, even when children are old enough to speak for themselves, which can exclude a valuable source of

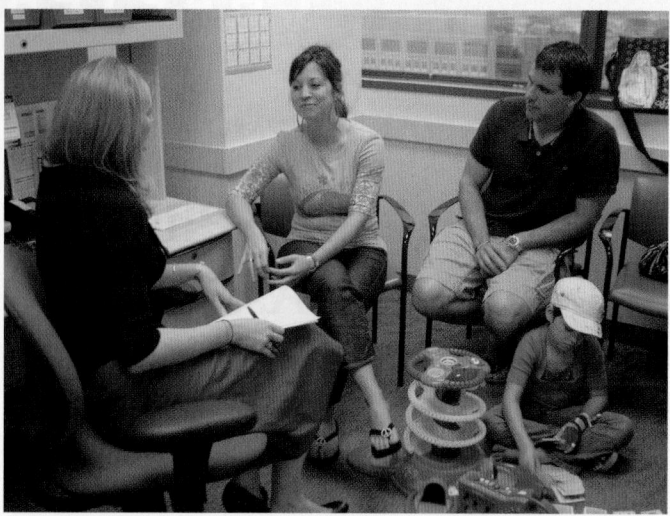

FIGURE 33-1 A child plays while the nurse interviews the parents.

information: the patient. When the child is a participant in the interview, the nurse should use the general rules for communicating with children that are given in the Guidelines box on p. 900.

Assurance of Privacy and Confidentiality

The place where the interview is conducted is almost as important as the interview itself. The physical environment should allow for as much privacy as possible, with distractions, such as interruptions, noise, or other visible activity, kept to a minimum. If young children are present, the environment should have some toys, to keep them occupied during the parent–nurse interview (Fig. 33-1). Parents who are constantly interrupted by their children are unable to concentrate fully and may give brief answers in order to finish the interview as quickly as possible.

Confidentiality is another essential component of the interview. One of the primary nursing values of the Canadian Nurses Association (CNA) (2008) is recognizing the importance of privacy and confidentiality; the nurse needs to protect personal, family, and community information obtained within the framework of a professional relationship. Since the interview is usually shared with other members of the health team care or possibly with a teacher (in the case of students), it is imperative to inform the family of the limits regarding confidentiality. If confidentiality is a concern in a particular situation, such as when talking to a parent suspected of child abuse or a teenager contemplating suicide, this should be dealt with directly and the person informed that in such instances confidentiality cannot be ensured.

> **! NURSING ALERT**
>
> In Canada, the *Privacy Act of 1985* is the law that protects the privacy of individuals with respect to personal information held by a government institution and that provides individuals with a right to access to that information. The *Personal Information Protection and Electronic Documents Act (PIPEDA)* protects the privacy and confidentiality of an individual's personal information within the private and health care sectors and applies in jurisdictions that have not adopted similar legislation, such as Quebec, Alberta, and Ontario (Office of the Privacy Commissioner of Canada, 2015) (see Additional Resources at the end of the chapter).

Communicating With Parents

When providing nursing care for children, the nurse's relationship with the child is frequently mediated by the parent, particularly for younger children. For the most part, information about the child is acquired by direct observation or is communicated to the nurse by the parents. Usually it can be assumed that, because of the parent's close contact with the child, the parent is giving reliable information. To make an assessment of the child the nurse needs input from the child (verbal and nonverbal), information from the parent(s), and the nurse's own observations of the child and interpretation of the relationship between the child and parent(s). Counselling and guidance must be directed to the caregiver of infants and small children; when children are old enough to be active participants in their own health maintenance, the parent becomes a collaborator in health care.

Encouraging Parents to Talk

Interviewing parents provides the opportunity to not only determine the child's health and developmental status but also to obtain information about factors that influence the child's well-being. Whatever the parent sees as a problem should be a concern for the nurse. Such issues are not always easy to identify, thus nurses need to be alert for clues and signals by which a parent communicates worries and anxieties. Careful phrasing with broad, open-ended questions, such as "What is Jack eating now?" provides more information than several single-answer questions, such as "Is Jack eating what the rest of the family eats?" Sometimes the parent will take the lead without prompting. At other times it may be necessary to direct another question on the basis of an observation, such as "Angelica seems unhappy today" or "How do you feel when Jamil cries?" If the parent appears to be tired or distraught, consider asking, "What do you do to relax?" or "What help do you have with the children?" A comment such as "You handle the baby very well. What kinds of experience have you had with babies?" to new parents who appear comfortable with their first child gives positive reinforcement and provides an opening for any questions they might have regarding the infant's care. Often all that is required to maintain communication is a nod or saying "yes" or "uh-huh."

When attempting to elicit feelings or information regarding issues more difficult for parents to address, closed-ended questions that begin with "Does … ," "Did … ," or "Is … ," should be avoided as these usually require only a single response. Asking questions such as "Does your son have any problems at school?" subtly implies a lack of parental skills and can evoke defensiveness. Instead, use questions that begin with "What … ," "How … ," or "Tell me about … ," and encourage elaboration with phrases like "You were saying …" or "You say that … " or by reflecting back a key word. Open-ended questions are nonthreatening and encourage description.

Directing the Focus

The ability to direct the focus of the interview while allowing for maximum freedom of expression is one of the most difficult goals in effective communication. One approach is the use of open-ended or broad questions, followed by guiding statements. For example, if the parent proceeds to list the other children by name, say, "Tell me their ages, too." If the parent continues to describe each child in depth, which is not the purpose of the interview, redirect the focus by stating, "Let's talk about the other children later. You were beginning to tell me about Olivia's activities at school." This approach conveys interest in the other children but focuses the assessment on the patient.

Listening and Cultural Awareness

Listening is the most important component of effective communication. When listening is truly aimed at understanding the patient, it is an active process that requires concentration and attention to all aspects of the conversation—verbal, and nonverbal. Major blocks to listening are environmental distraction and premature judgement.

The nurse's attitudes and feelings are easily injected into an interview. Often nurses' perceptions of a parent's behaviour are influenced by their own perceptions, prejudices, and **assumptions**, which may include racial, religious, and cultural stereotypes. What may be interpreted as a parent's passive hostility or lack of interest may be shyness or an expression of anxiety. For example, in Western cultures, eye contact and directness are signs of paying attention. However, in many non-Western cultures, including some First Nations, Métis, and Inuit cultures, directness, such as looking someone in the eye, is considered rude. Children are taught to avert their gaze and to look down when being addressed by an adult, especially one with authority (Ball et al., 2014). Therefore, judgements about listening and verbal interactions need to be made with an appreciation of cultural differences (see Chapter 31).

The nurse's minimal speaking, along with active listening, can facilitate parents' involvement. While it is tempting to spend time explaining, describing, and interpreting health information when the opportunity presents itself, it is possible to provide effective health education by timing the information properly and presenting only as much as is necessary at the moment.

Careful listening relies on the use of clues, verbal leads, or signals from the interviewee to move the interview along. Frequent references to an area of concern, repetition of certain key words, or special emphasis on something or someone can serve as cues to the interviewer for directing the inquiry. Concerns and anxieties are often mentioned in a casual, offhand manner; however, they are nonetheless important and deserve careful scrutiny to identify problem areas. For example, a parent who is concerned about a child's habit of bed-wetting may casually mention that the child's bed was "wet this morning."

Providing Anticipatory Guidance

The ideal way to handle a situation is to deal with it *before* it becomes a problem. In nursing the best preventive measure is anticipatory guidance. Traditionally, anticipatory guidance has focused on providing families with information on children's growth and development. Parents who are unprepared for their child's development can be disturbed by many normal developmental changes, such as a toddler's diminished appetite, negativism, altered sleeping patterns, and anxiety toward strangers. (See Chapters 35–39 for informing parents about pediatric health promotion according to developmental age.) Anticipatory guidance also includes nurturing child-rearing practices that promote the health of the child, for example, injury prevention. Beginning prenatally, parents need specific instructions on home safety. As the child's developmental skills mature and change, so too should home safety measures be implemented to minimize risks to the child. However, anticipatory guidance should extend beyond giving general information during health care visits; families should also be encouraged to use the information as a means of building competence in their parenting abilities. To achieve this level of anticipatory guidance, the nurse should do the following:

- Base interventions on needs identified by the family, not by the health care provider.
- View the family as competent or as having the ability to be competent.
- Provide opportunities for the family to achieve competence.

Avoiding Blocks to Communication

A number of blocks or hindrances to communication can adversely affect the quality of the helping relationship. Often the interviewer unwittingly introduces some of these blocks, such as giving unrestricted advice or forming prejudged conclusions. Sometimes interviewees experience information overload when presented with too much information or information that is overwhelming and will demonstrate signs of increasing anxiety or decreasing attention. Such signals should alert the interviewer to give less information or to clarify what has been said. Box 33-1 lists some of the more common blocks to communication, including signs of information overload.

BOX 33-1 BLOCKS TO COMMUNICATION

Communication Barriers (Nurse)

- Socializing
- Giving unrestricted and sometimes unasked-for advice
- Offering premature or inappropriate reassurance
- Giving over-ready encouragement
- Defending a situation or opinion
- Using stereotyped comments or clichés
- Limiting expression of emotion by asking directed, closed-ended questions
- Interrupting and finishing the person's sentence
- Talking more than the interviewee
- Forming prejudged conclusions
- Deliberately changing the focus

Signs of Information Overload (Patient)

- Long periods of silence
- Wide eyes and fixed facial expression
- Constant fidgeting or attempting to move away
- Nervous habits, such as tapping, playing with hair
- Sudden disruptions, such as asking to go to the bathroom
- Looking around
- Yawning, eyes drooping
- Frequently looking at a watch or clock
- Attempting to change the topic of discussion

Communicating With Families Through an Interpreter

Sometimes communication is impossible because the health care provider and the patient speak different languages. In this case, it is necessary to obtain information through a third party, the interpreter. When an interpreter is used, the same interviewing guidelines as those used without an interpreter apply. Specific guidelines for using an adult interpreter are presented in Box 2-4.

It is important to choose the translator carefully and provide time for the interpreter and family to establish rapport. Communicating with families through an interpreter requires sensitivity to cultural, legal, and ethical considerations. For example, in obtaining informed consent through an interpreter, the nurse needs to ensure that the family is fully informed of all aspects of the particular procedure to which they are consenting. Because of increased sensitivity to patient rights and confidentiality, many institutions now require consent forms to be produced in the patient's primary language.

> **NURSING ALERT**
>
> When using translated materials, such as a health history form, be certain the informant is literate in the foreign language.

Communicating With Children

Although the greatest amount of verbal communication is usually carried out with the parent, the child should not be excluded during the interview. Infants and younger children can be observed through play; occasionally, younger children can answer questions or respond to remarks. Older children should be included as active participants in the interview.

In communication with children of all ages, the nonverbal components of the communication process convey the most significant messages (Fig. 33-2). It is difficult to disguise feelings, attitudes, and anxiety when relating to children. They are alert to surroundings and attach meaning to every gesture and move that is made; this is particularly true of very young children.

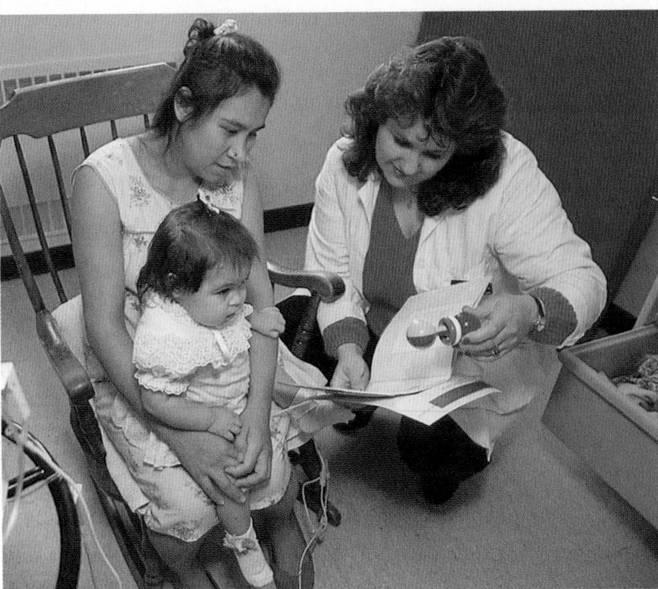

FIGURE 33-2 Nurse assumes position at child's level.

Active attempts to make friends with children before they have had an opportunity to evaluate an unfamiliar person tend to increase their anxiety. It is helpful to continue to talk to the child and parent but go about activities that do not involve the child directly, thus allowing the child to observe from a safe position. If the child has a special toy or doll, the nurse can "talk" to the doll first. Simple questions such as "Does your teddy bear have a name?" can be asked to ease the child into conversation. Other guidelines for communicating with children are presented in the Guidelines box.

Communication and Development of Thought Processes

The normal development of language and thought in children offers a frame of reference for communicating with children. Thought processes progress from sensorimotor to perceptual to concrete and, finally, to abstract, formal operations. An understanding of the typical characteristics of these stages provides the nurse with a framework to facilitate social communication (Box 33-2).

Infancy. Because infants are unable to use words, they primarily use and understand nonverbal communication. Infants communicate their needs and feelings through nonverbal behaviours and vocalizations that can be interpreted by someone who is around them for a sufficient time. Infants smile and coo when content and cry when distressed. Crying is provoked by unpleasant stimuli from inside or outside, such as hunger, pain, body restraint, or loneliness. Adults interpret this to mean that an infant needs something and consequently try to alleviate the discomfort and reduce tension. Crying (or the desire to cry) persists as a part of everyone's communication repertoire.

Infants respond to adults' nonverbal behaviours. They become quiet when they are cuddled, are patted, or receive other forms of gentle physical contact. They derive comfort from the sound of a voice, even though they do not understand the words spoken. Until infants reach the age at which they experience stranger anxiety, they readily respond to any firm,

> **GUIDELINES**
>
> ***Communicating With Children***
>
> - Allow children time to feel comfortable.
> - Avoid sudden or rapid advances, broad smiles, extended eye contact, or other gestures that may be seen as threatening.
> - Talk to the parent if the child is initially shy.
> - Communicate through transition objects such as dolls, puppets, and stuffed animals before questioning a young child directly.
> - Give older children the opportunity to talk without the parents present.
> - Assume a position that is at eye level with the child (see Fig. 33-2).
> - Speak in a quiet, unhurried, and confident voice.
> - Speak clearly, be specific, and use simple words and short sentences.
> - State directions and suggestions positively.
> - Offer a choice only when one exists.
> - Be honest with children.
> - Allow them to express their concerns and fears.
> - Use a variety of communication techniques.

BOX 33-2 DEVELOPMENT OF COMMUNICATION IN YOUNG CHILDREN

Perlocutionary Stage (0 to 8–9 Months)

Child is reflexive to stimuli.

- Crying provides air movement across vocal cords to experience sound and experience a change in breathing patterns.
- Progressive suck–swallow development
- Makes noncrying speech sounds, often while feeding, such as cooing
- Makes babbling sounds that are consonant-vowel combinations

Child shows increasing purpose in action, such as pointing to an object.

Emerging Illocutionary Stage (8–9 to 12–15 Months)

Child communicates intentionally with signals and gestures.

- Responds more consistently to speech
- Begins to look at objects when they are named
- Babbling, jargon, and phonetically consistent forms emerge
- Echolalic speech may emerge, which is infant's repetition of sounds made by others

Conventional Illocutionary—Emerging Locutionary Stage (12–15 to 18–24 Months)

Child communicates intentionally with gestures, vocalizations, and verbalizations.

- Language development moves beyond single words
- Development of both lexicon (personal vocabulary) and word combinations
- Use of 50 verbs at 18 months; most have same consonants used in babbling, such as "ma" or "no" or reduplicated such as "bye-bye"
- Likes rhymes, songs, and fingerplays
- Decrease in use of jargon and babbling (but still remains)

Modified from Hoge, D. R., & Parette, H. P. (1995). Facilitating communicative development in young children with disabilities. *Transdisciplinary Journal, 5*(2), 113–130.

gentle handling and quiet, calm speech. Loud, harsh sounds and sudden movements are frightening to infants.

Early childhood. Children younger than 5 years of age are egocentric. They see things only in relation to themselves and from their point of view. Therefore, communication needs to be focused on them. They should be told what they can do or how they will feel. Experiences of others are of no interest to them. It is futile to use another child's experience in an attempt to gain the cooperation of small children. During the health assessment they should be allowed to touch and examine articles that will come in contact with them. A stethoscope bell will feel cold; palpating a neck might tickle. Although they have not yet acquired sufficient language skills to express their feelings and wants, toddlers are able to communicate effectively with their hands to transmit ideas without words. For example, they will push an unwanted object away, pull another person to show them something, point, and cover the mouth or ears when they wish to not say or hear something.

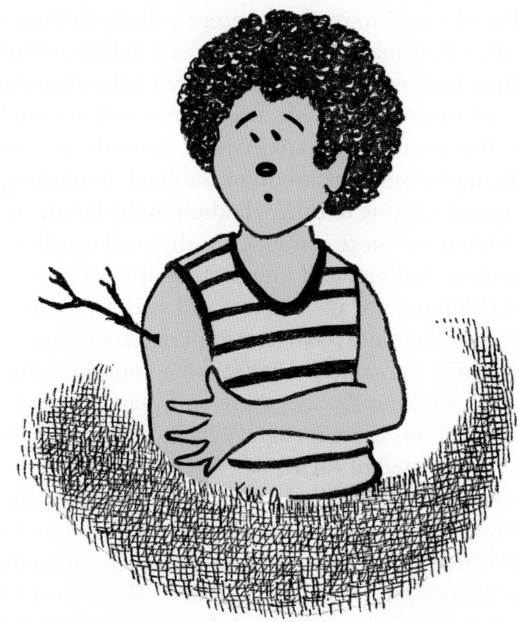

FIGURE 33-3 A young child may take the expression "a little stick in the arm" literally.

Everything is direct and concrete to small children. They are unable to work with abstractions and interpret words literally. Analogies escape them because they are unable to separate fact from fantasy. For example, they attach literal meaning to such common phrases as "two-faced," "sticky fingers," or "coughing your head off." Children who are told they will get "a little stick in the arm" may not be able to envision an injection (Fig. 33-3). Therefore, avoid using a phrase that might be misinterpreted by a small child.

Young children assign human attributes to inanimate objects. Consequently, they fear that objects may jump, bite, cut, or pinch all by themselves. Children do not know that these devices are unable to perform without human direction. To minimize their fear, unfamiliar equipment should be kept out of view until it is needed.

School-age years. Younger school-age children rely less on what they see and more on what they know, when faced with new problems. They want explanations and reasons for everything but require no verification beyond that. They are interested in the functional aspect of all procedures, objects, and activities. They want to know why an object exists, why it is used, how it works, and the intent and purpose of its user. They need to know what is going to take place and why it is being done to them specifically. For example, to explain a procedure such as taking blood pressure (BP), the child should be shown how squeezing the bulb pushes air into the cuff and makes the "silver" in the tube go up. The child should be allowed to operate the bulb. An explanation for the procedure might be as simple as "I want to see how far the silver goes up when the cuff squeezes your arm." The child then becomes an enthusiastic participant.

School-age children have a heightened concern about body integrity. Because of the special importance they place on their body, they are sensitive to anything that constitutes a threat or suggestion of injury to it. This concern extends to their possessions, so that they may appear to overreact to loss or threatened loss of treasured objects. Helping children voice their concerns enables the nurse to provide reassurance and to implement activities that reduce their anxiety. For example, if a shy child dislikes being the centre of attention, the child should be ignored, by talking and relating to other children in the family or group. When children feel more comfortable, they will usually interject personal ideas, feelings, and interpretations of events.

Older children have an adequate and satisfactory use of language. They still require relatively simple explanations, but their ability to think concretely can facilitate communication and explanation. Commonly, they have sufficient experience with health care workers to understand what is transpiring and what is generally expected of them.

Adolescence. As children move into adolescence, they fluctuate between child and adult thinking and behaviour. They are riding a current that is moving them rapidly toward a maturity that may be beyond their coping ability. Thus when tensions arise, they may seek the security of the more familiar and comfortable expectations of childhood. Anticipating these shifts in identity allows the nurse to adjust the course of interaction to meet the needs of the moment. No single approach can be relied on consistently; one can expect to encounter cooperation, hostility, anger, bravado, and a variety of other behaviours and attitudes. It is as much a mistake to regard the adolescent as an adult with an adult's wisdom and control as it is to assume that the teenager has the concerns and expectations of a child.

Frequently, adolescents are more willing to discuss their concerns with an adult outside the family, and they often welcome the opportunity to interact with a nurse outside the presence of their parents. They are usually accepting of anyone who displays a genuine interest in them. However, adolescents are quick to reject persons who attempt to impose their values on them, whose interest is feigned, or who appear to have little respect for who they are and what they think or say.

Interviewing the adolescent presents some special issues. The first may be whether to talk with the adolescent alone or with the adolescent and parents together. Of course, if the parent is not there, the only question is whether to suggest to the teenager that the parents be interviewed at another time. If the parents and teenager are together, talking with the adolescent first has the advantage of immediately identifying with the young person, thus fostering the relationship. However, talking with the parents initially may provide insight into the family dynamics. In either case, both parties should be given an opportunity to be included in the interview. If there are time constraints, such as during history taking, this should be clarified at the outset, to avoid the appearance of "taking sides" by talking more with one person than with the other.

Confidentiality is of great importance when interviewing adolescents. Parents and teenagers need to have the limits of confidentiality explained to them, specifically that young persons' disclosures will not be shared unless they indicate a need for intervention, as in the case of suicidal behaviour.

Another dilemma in interviewing adolescents is that two views of a problem frequently exist—the teenager's and the parents'. However, providing both parties an opportunity to discuss their perceptions in an open and unbiased atmosphere can, by itself, be therapeutic. The demonstration of positive communication skills can help families communicate more effectively (see Guidelines box).

GUIDELINES

Communicating With Adolescents

Build a Foundation

- Spend time together.
- Encourage expression of ideas and feelings.
- Respect their views.
- Tolerate differences.
- Praise good points.
- Respect their privacy.
- Set a good example.

Communicate Effectively

- Give undivided attention.
- Listen, listen, listen.
- Be courteous, calm, and open-minded.
- Try not to overreact. If you do, take a break.
- Avoid judging or criticizing.
- Avoid the "third degree" of continuous questioning.
- Choose important issues when taking a stand.
- After taking a stand:
  - Think through all options.
  - Make expectations clear.

Communication Techniques

Nurses use a variety of verbal techniques to encourage communication. In addition to such conventional interviewing methods as reflection and open-ended questions, a number of techniques encourage family members to express their thoughts and feelings in a less directive and confrontational manner. However, for many children and adults, talking about feelings is difficult, and verbal communication may be more stressful than supportive. In such instances, several nonverbal techniques can be used to encourage communication.

Box 33-3 describes both verbal and nonverbal communication techniques used with children. Because of the importance of play in communicating with children, play is discussed more extensively in Chapter 32. Any of the verbal or nonverbal techniques can give rise to strong feelings that surface unexpectedly. The nurse should be prepared to handle them or to recognize when issues go beyond his or her ability to deal with them. At that point, an appropriate referral can be considered.

Telephone Triage and Counselling

Nurses are increasingly responsible for assessing children's symptoms and providing clinical judgement regarding further medical care (triage) by means of telephone report. Most often, health problems are assessed and prioritized according to urgency, and treatment is judiciously provided via telephone services. The goal of telephone triage care management is to provide access to high-quality health care services and to increase patient satisfaction. Successful outcomes are based on the

BOX 33-3 CREATIVE COMMUNICATION TECHNIQUES WITH CHILDREN

Verbal Techniques

"I" Messages

Relate a feeling about a behaviour in terms of "I."

Describe the effect that the behaviour had on the person.

Avoid use of "you;" "you" messages are judgemental and provoke defensiveness.

Example—"You" message: "You are being uncooperative about doing your treatments."

Example—"I" message: "I am concerned about how the treatments are going because I want to see you get better."

Third-Person Technique

Express a feeling in terms of a third person ("he," "she," "they"). This is less threatening than directly asking children how they feel, because it gives them an opportunity to agree or disagree without being defensive.

Example—"Sometimes when a person is sick a lot, he feels angry and sad because he cannot do what others can." Either wait silently for a response or encourage a reply with a statement such as "Did you ever feel that way?"

This approach allows children three choices: (1) to agree and possibly express how they feel; (2) to disagree; or (3) to remain silent, which means they probably have such feelings but are unable to express them at this time.

Facilitative Response

Listen carefully and reflect back to patients the feelings and content of their statements.

Responses are empathic and nonjudgemental and legitimize the person's feelings.

Formula for facilitative responses: "You feel ____________ because ____________."

Example—If the child states, "I hate coming to the hospital and getting needles," a facilitative response is "You feel unhappy because of all the things that are done to you."

Storytelling

Use the language of children to probe into areas of their thinking while bypassing conscious inhibitions or fears.

The simplest technique is asking the child to relate a story about an event, such as "being in the hospital."

Other approaches:

- Show the child a picture of a particular event, such as a child in a hospital with other people in the room, and ask the child to describe the scene.
- Cut out comic strips, remove words, and have the child add statements for scenes.

Mutual Storytelling

Reveal the child's thinking and attempt to change the child's perceptions or fears by retelling a somewhat different story (more therapeutic approach than storytelling).

Begin by asking the child to tell a story about something, then tell another story that is similar to the child's tale but with differences that help the child in problem areas.

Example—The child's story is about going to the hospital and never seeing his or her parents again. The nurse's story is also about a child (using different names but similar circumstances) in a hospital, but whose parents visit every day, in the evening after work, until the child is better and goes home with them.

Bibliotherapy

Use books in a therapeutic and supportive process.

Provide children with an opportunity to explore an event that is similar to their own but sufficiently different to allow them to distance themselves from it and remain in control.

General guidelines for using bibliotherapy are as follows:

1. Assess the child's emotional and cognitive development in terms of readiness to understand the book's message.
2. Be familiar with the book's content (intended message or purpose) and the age for which it is written.
3. Read the book to the child if he or she is unable to read.
4. Explore the meaning of the book with the child by having child do the following:
    - Retell the story
    - Read a special section with the nurse or parent
    - Draw a picture related to the story and discuss the drawing
    - Talk about the characters
    - Summarize the moral or meaning of the story

Dreams

Dreams often reveal unconscious and repressed thoughts and feelings.

Ask the child to talk about a dream or nightmare.

Explore with the child what meaning the dream could have.

"What If" Questions

Encourage the child to explore potential situations and to consider different problem-solving options.

Example—"What if you got sick and had to go the hospital?" Children's responses reveal what they know already and what they are curious about, providing an opportunity for them to learn coping skills, especially in potentially dangerous situations.

Three Wishes

Ask, "If you could have any three things in the world, what would they be?"

If the child answers, "That all my wishes come true," ask the child for specific wishes.

Rating Game

Use some type of rating scale (numbers, sad to happy faces) to have the child rate an event or feeling.

Example—Instead of asking youngsters how they feel, ask how their day has been "on a scale of 1 to 10, with 10 being the best."

Word Association Game

State key words and ask children to say the first word they think of when they hear the word.

Start with neutral words and then introduce more anxiety-producing words, such as "illness," "needles," "hospitals," and "operation."

Select key words that relate to some relevant event in the child's life.

Continued

BOX 33-3 CREATIVE COMMUNICATION TECHNIQUES WITH CHILDREN—cont'd

Sentence Completion

Present a partial statement and have the child complete it. Some sample statements are as follows:

- The thing I like best (least) about school is ________.
- The best (worst) age to be is ________.
- The most (least) fun thing I ever did was ________.
- The thing I like most (least) about my parents is ________.
- The one thing I would change about my family is ________.
- If I could be anything I wanted, I would be ________.
- The thing I like most (least) about myself is ________.

Pros and Cons

Select a topic, such as "being in the hospital," and have the child list "five good things and five bad things" about it.

This is an exceptionally valuable technique when applied to relationships, such as things family members like and dislike about each other.

Nonverbal Techniques

Writing

Writing is an alternative communication approach for older children and adults. Specific suggestions include the following:

- Keep a journal or diary.
- Write down feelings or thoughts that are difficult to express.
- Write "letters" that are never mailed (a variation is making up a pen pal to write to).
- Keep an account of the child's progress from both a physical and an emotional viewpoint.

Drawing

Drawing is one of the most valuable forms of communication—both nonverbal (from looking at the drawing) and verbal (from the child's story of the picture).

Children's drawings tell a great deal about them because they are projections of their inner selves.

Spontaneous drawing involves giving the child a variety of art supplies and providing the opportunity to draw.

Directed drawing involves a more specific direction, such as "draw a person" or the "three themes" approach (state three things about the child and ask the child to choose one and draw a picture).

Guidelines for Evaluating Drawings

Use spontaneous drawings and evaluate more than one drawing whenever possible.

Interpret drawings in light of other available information about the child and family, including the child's age and stage of development.

Interpret drawings as a whole rather than focusing on specific details of the drawing.

Consider individual elements of the drawing that may be significant:

Gender of figure drawn first—Usually relates to child's perception of his or her own gender role

Size of individual figures—Expresses importance, power, or authority

Order in which figures are drawn—Expresses priority in terms of importance

Child's position in relation to other family members—Expresses feelings of status or alliance

Exclusion of a member—May denote feeling of not belonging or desire to eliminate a family member

Accentuated parts—Usually express concern for areas of special importance (e.g., large hands may be a sign of aggression)

Absence of or rudimentary arms and hands—Suggest timidity, passivity, or intellectual immaturity; tiny, unstable feet may express insecurity, and hidden hands may mean guilt feelings

Placement of drawing on the page and type of stroke—Free use of paper and firm, continuous strokes express security, whereas drawings restricted to a small area and lightly drawn in broken or wavering lines may be a sign of insecurity

Erasures, shading, or cross-hatching—Expresses ambivalence, concern, or anxiety with a particular area

Magic

Use simple magic tricks to help establish rapport with the child, encourage cooperation with health interventions, and provide effective distraction during painful procedures.

Although the magician talks, no verbal response from the child is required.

Play

Play is the universal language and "work" of children.

It tells a great deal about children because they project their inner selves through the activity.

Spontaneous play involves giving the child a variety of play materials and providing the opportunity to play.

Directed play involves a more specific direction, such as providing medical equipment or a dollhouse for focused reasons, such as exploring the child's fear of injections or exploring family relationships.

consistency and accuracy of the information provided, which can better enable parents to participate in their child's medical care. Canadian researchers audited the appropriateness of advice given by telephone triage nurses and found that 90% of the advice was appropriate (Beaulieu & Humphries, 2008). With the use of telephone triage, unnecessary physician office visits have decreased, reducing medical costs and time spent (along with less absence from work) for families in need of health care. The most common telephone triage call placed is for a fever.

Telenurses need to have communication skills training in telephone consultation and learn how to structure a call. A well-designed telephone triage program is essential for safe, prompt, and consistent-quality health care. Typically, guidelines for telephone triage include asking screening questions; determining when to immediately refer to emergency medical services (dial 911); and determining when to refer to same-day appointments, appointments in 24 to 72 hours, appointments in 4 days or more, or home care (Box 33-4).

BOX 33-4 TELEPHONE TRIAGE GUIDELINES FOR ASSESSMENT

Date and time
Background
- Name, age, sex
- Chronic illness
- Allergies, current medications, treatments, or recent immunizations

Chief health concern
General symptoms
- Severity
- Duration
- Other symptoms
- Pain

Systems review
Steps taken
- Advised to call emergency medical services (911)
- Advised to see practitioner
- Advice given for home care
- Call back if symptoms worsen or fail to improve

Resources for Telephone Triage Protocols

Briggs, J. K. (2011). *Telephone triage protocols for nurses* (4th ed.). Philadelphia: Lippincott Williams & Wilkins.
Schmitt, B. D. (2009). *Pediatric telephone protocols: Office version* (12th ed.). Elk Grove Village, IL: American Academy of Pediatrics.

Computer Privacy and Applications in Nursing

The use of computer technology to store and retrieve health information has become widespread. Throughout the health care community, the privacy and security of this health information has become a growing concern. Any person accessing confidential health information is charged with managing safeguards for disclosure, since violations might incur civil damages.

In 2005, the Pan-Canadian Health Information Privacy and Confidentiality Framework was developed by Deputy Ministers of Health to inform and influence any private legislative process regarding health information and to provide more consistent privacy protocols among health care jurisdictions. This framework includes the development of electronic health record systems and primary health care reform (Health Canada, 2015).

Many institutions use computerized information and applications in nursing (nursing informatics), such as electronic medical records, to record care and access information. Two health care applications are record transmission, via fax or email, and telemedicine. Telemedicine can be used for two-way video conferencing, transmission of radiographs, and clinical consultation between remote sites and centralized resources.

HISTORY TAKING

Performing a Health History

The format used for history taking may be (1) *direct*, where the nurse asks for information via direct interview with the child, parent(s), or both; or (2) *indirect*, where the patient or authorized family member supplies the information by completing some type of questionnaire. The direct method is superior to the indirect approach or a combination of both. However, in view of time constraints of health assessments the direct approach is not always practical. If the direct approach cannot be used, the parents' written responses should be reviewed and the parents questioned regarding any unusual answers. The categories listed in Box 33-5 encompass children's current and past health status and information about their psychosocial environment.

Identifying Information

Much of the identifying information may already be available from other recorded sources. However, if the parent and youngster seem anxious, history taking provides an opportunity to ask about such information and to help them feel more comfortable.

One of the important elements of identifying information is the informant, the person(s) who furnish the information. The nurse should record (1) who the person is (child, parent, or other), (2) an impression of reliability and willingness to communicate, and (3) any special circumstances, such as the use of an interpreter or conflicting answers by more than one person.

Health Issue or Concern

The chief health concern is the specific reason for the child's visit to the clinic, office, or hospital. It may be viewed as the theme, with the present illness viewed as the description of the problem. The health issue is elicited by asking open-ended, neutral questions, such as "What seems to be the matter?" "How may I help you?" or "Why did you come here today?" Labelling-type questions, such as "How are you sick?" and wording such as "What is the problem?" should be avoided; it is possible that the reason for the visit is not an illness or problem.

Occasionally, it is difficult to isolate one symptom or problem as the health issue because the parent may identify many. In this situation, the nurse should be as specific as possible when asking questions. For example, asking informants to state which one problem or symptom prompted them to seek help now may help them focus on the most immediate concern.

Present Illness

The history of the present illness is a narrative of the health issue from its earliest onset through its progression to the present. The term *illness* is used in its broadest sense to denote any problem of a physical, emotional, or psychosocial nature. It is actually a history of the health issue. The four major components are (1) the details of onset, (2) a complete interval history, (3) the present status, and (4) the reason for seeking help now. The focus of the present illness is on all factors relevant to the main issue, even if they have disappeared or changed during the onset, interval, and present.

Analyzing a symptom. Because pain is often the most characteristic symptom denoting the onset of a physical problem, it is used as an example for analysis of a symptom. Assessment includes (1) type, (2) location, (3) severity, (4) duration, and (5) influencing factors (see Guidelines box; see also Pain Assessment, Chapter 34).

BOX 33-5 OUTLINE OF A PEDIATRIC HEALTH HISTORY

Identifying information
- Name
- Address
- Telephone and email address
- Birth date and place
- Race/ethnic group
- Sex
- Religion
- Date of interview
- Informant

Presenting health issue—To establish the major specific reason for the child's and parents' seeking professional health attention

History of Present illness (PI)—To obtain all details related to the chief health concern

Past history (PH)—To elicit a profile of the child's previous illnesses, injuries, or operations
- Birth history (pregnancy, labour and birth, perinatal history)
- Previous illnesses, injuries, or operations
- Allergies
- Current medications
- Immunizations
- Growth and development
- Habits

Family medical history—To identify genetic traits or diseases that have familial tendencies and to assess exposure to a communicable disease in a family member and family habits that may affect the child's health, such as smoking and chemical use

Family history—To develop an understanding of the child as an individual and as a member of a family and a community.
- Family composition
- Home and community environment
- Occupation and education of family members
- Cultural and religious traditions
- Family function and relationships

Review of systems (ROS)—To elicit information concerning any potential health problem
- General
- Integument
- Head
- Eyes
- Ears
- Nose
- Mouth
- Throat
- Neck
- Chest
- Respiratory
- Cardiovascular
- Gastrointestinal
- Genitourinary
- Gynecological
- Musculoskeletal
- Neurological
- Endocrine

Psychosocial history—To elicit information about the child's self-concept

Sexual history—To elicit information about the child's sexual concerns or activities and any pertinent data regarding adults' sexual activity that influences the child

Nutritional assessment—To elicit information on the adequacy of the child's nutritional intake and needs
- Dietary intake
- Clinical examination

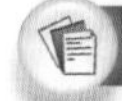

GUIDELINES

Analyzing the Symptom: Pain

Type

Be as specific as possible. With young children, asking the parents how they know the child is in pain may help describe its type, location, and severity. For example, a parent may state, "My child must have a severe earache because she pulls at her ears, rolls her head on the floor, and screams. Nothing seems to help." Help older children describe the "hurt" by asking them if it is sharp, throbbing, dull, or stabbing. Record whatever words they use in quotes.

Location

Be specific. "Stomach pains" is too general a description. Children can better localize the pain if they are asked to "point with one finger to where it hurts" or to "point to where Mommy or Daddy would put a Band-Aid." Determine if the pain radiates, by asking, "Does the pain stay there or move? Show me with your finger where the pain goes."

Severity

Severity is best determined by finding out how it affects the child's usual behaviour. Pain that prevents a child from playing, interacting with others, sleeping, and eating is most often severe. Assess pain intensity using a rating scale, such as a numeric or FACES scale (see Chapter 34).

Duration

Include the duration, onset, and frequency of the pain. Describe this in terms of activity and behaviour, such as "pain reported to last all night, child refused to sleep and cried intermittently."

Influencing Factors

Include anything that causes a change in the type, location, severity, or duration of the pain: (1) precipitating events (those that cause or increase the pain), (2) relieving events (those that lessen the pain, such as medications), (3) temporal events (times when the pain is relieved or increased), (4) positional events (standing, sitting, lying down), and (5) associated events (meals, stress, coughing).

History

The **history** contains information relating to all previous aspects of the child's health status and concentrates on several areas that are ordinarily passed over in the history of an adult. Since a great deal of information is included in this section, a combination of open-ended and fact-finding questions should be used. For example, interviewing for each section can start with an open-ended statement, such as "Tell me about your child's birth," to provide the informants with the opportunity to relate what they think is most important. Fact-finding questions related to specific details can be asked whenever necessary to focus the interview on certain topics.

Birth history. The birth history includes all data concerning (1) the mother's health during pregnancy, (2) the labour and birth, and (3) the infant's condition immediately after birth. Since prenatal influences have significant effects on a child's physical and emotional development, a thorough investigation of the birth history is essential. Because parents may question what relevance pregnancy and birth have on the child's present condition, particularly if the child is past infancy, the nurse needs to explain why such questions are included. An appropriate statement may be "I will be asking you some questions about your pregnancy and ____'s [refer to child by name] birth. Your answers will give me a more complete picture of your child's overall health."

Because emotional factors also affect the outcome of pregnancy and the subsequent parent–child relationship, it is important to investigate (1) concurrent crises during pregnancy and (2) prenatal attitudes toward the fetus. It is best to approach the topic of parental acceptance of pregnancy through indirect questioning. Asking parents if the pregnancy was planned is a leading statement because they may respond affirmatively for fear of criticism if the pregnancy was unexpected. Rather, parents should be encouraged to disclose their true reactions by referring to specific facts relating to the pregnancy, such as the spacing between offspring, an extended or short interval between marriage and conception, or the concurrent experience of pregnancy and adolescence. Parents can choose to explore such statements with further explanations or, for the moment, may not be able to reveal related feelings. If the parents or parent remains silent, this topic can be revisited later in the interview.

Previous illnesses, injuries, and operations. When inquiring about past illnesses, the nurse should begin with a general statement, such as "What other illnesses has your child had?" Since parents are most likely to recall serious health problems, they should be asked specifically about colds; earaches; and childhood diseases such as measles, rubella (German measles), chicken pox, mumps, pertussis (whooping cough), diphtheria, tuberculosis, scarlet fever, strep throat, tonsillitis, or allergic manifestations.

In addition to illnesses, the nurse needs to ask about injuries that required medical intervention, operations, and any other reason for hospitalization, including the dates of each incident. It is important to focus on injuries such as accidental falls, poisoning, choking, or burns, since these may be potential areas for parental guidance.

GUIDELINES
Taking an Allergy History

- Has your child ever taken any medications or tablets that have disagreed with him or her or caused an allergic response? If yes, can you remember the name(s) of these medications?
- Can you describe the reaction?
- Was the medication taken by mouth (as a tablet or syrup), or was it an injection?
- How soon after starting the medication did the reaction happen?
- How long ago did this happen?
- Did anyone tell you it was an allergic reaction, or did you decide for yourself?
- Has your child ever taken this medication, or a similar one, again? If yes, did your child experience the same problems?
- Have you told the doctors or nurses about your child's reaction or allergy?

Modified from Cantrill, J. A., & Cottrell, W. N. (1997). Accuracy of drug allergy documentation. *American Journal of Health-System Pharmacy, 54*, 1627–1629.

Allergies. It is important to ask about commonly known allergic disorders, such as hay fever and asthma; unusual reactions to medications, food, or latex products; and reactions to other contact agents, such as poisonous plants, animals, household products, or fabrics. If asked appropriate questions, most people can give reliable information about medication reactions (see Guidelines box).

! NURSING ALERT

Information about allergic reactions to medications or other products is essential. Failure to document a serious reaction places the child at risk if the medication is given.

Current medications. The nurse should inquire about current medication regimens, including prescription medications, over-the-counter medications, vitamins, minerals, herbal remedies, supplements, and illegal or illicit drugs (appropriate to age). All medications need to be listed, including name, dose, schedule, duration, and reason for administration. Often parents are unaware of the medication's actual name. Whenever possible, parents should bring the containers with them to the next visit, or the nurse can ask for the name of the pharmacy and call for a list of all the child's recent prescription medications. However, this list will not include over-the-counter medications or herbal remedies, which are important to know.

Immunizations. A record of all immunizations is essential. Since many parents are unaware of the exact name and date of each immunization, the most reliable source of information is a private practitioner's record or an "Immunization Record" provided to the family to keep and updated after each vaccine. All immunizations and "boosters" will be listed, stating (1) the name of the specific disease, (2) the number of injections, (3) the dosage (sometimes lesser amounts are given if a reaction is anticipated), (4) the ages when administered, and (5) the occurrence of any reaction following the immunization. See

Chapter 35 for more information on specific age-group immunizations.

NURSING ALERT

Inquire about previous administration of any horse or other foreign serum. Inquire about recent administration of immune gamma globulin or blood transfusion, which would necessitate a delay in giving live vaccines. Also ask about anaphylactic reactions to neomycin, eggs, or any other component of a vaccine.

Growth and development. The most important previous growth patterns to record are the following:

- Approximate weight at 1 week, 2 months, 4 months, 6 months, 12 to 13 months, and 18 months, then yearly (Canadian Paediatric Society [CPS], 2010)
- Approximate length at 1 week, 2 months, 4 months, 6 months, 12 to 13 months, and 18 months, then yearly (CPS, 2010)
- Dentition, including age of onset, number of teeth, and symptoms during teething
- Developmental milestones include the following:
  - Age of holding up head steadily
  - Age of sitting alone without support
  - Age of walking without assistance
  - Age of saying first words with meaning
- Present grade in school
- Scholastic grades
- If the child has a best friend
- Interactions with other children, peers, and adults

The nurse should use specific and detailed questions when inquiring about each developmental milestone. For example, "sitting up" can mean many different activities, such as sitting propped up, sitting in someone's lap, sitting with support, sitting up alone but in a hyperflexed position for assisted balance, or sitting up unsupported with the back slightly rounded. A clue to misunderstanding of the requested activity may be an unusually early age of achievement. See Developmental Assessment tools later in this chapter.

Habits. Habits are an important area to explore during the interview (Box 33-6). Parents frequently express concerns during this part of the history. The nurse needs to encourage their input, by saying, "Please tell me any concerns you have about your child's habits, activities, or development." Any concerns expressed should be investigated further.

One of the most common concerns relates to sleep. Many children develop a normal sleep pattern, and all that is required during the assessment is a general overview of nighttime sleep and nap schedules. However, a number of children also develop sleep problems (see Sleep Problems, Chapters 35 to 39). When sleep problems do occur, a more detailed sleep history is required to guide appropriate interventions.

Habits related to misuse of substances apply primarily to older children and adolescents. If a youngster admits to smoking, drinking, or drug use, he or she should be asked about the quantity and frequency. Questions such as "Have you ever had a drinking or drug problem?" or "When was the last time you had a drink or took drugs?" may yield more reliable data than questions such as "How much do you drink?" or "How often do you drink or take drugs?" The nurse needs to clarify that "drinking" includes all types of alcohol, such as beer and wine. When quantities such as a "glass" of wine or a "can" of beer are given, the size of the container needs to be determined.

If older children deny use of substances, they should be asked about past experimentation. Asking, "You mean you never tried to smoke or drink?" implies that the nurse expects some such activity, and the youngster may be more inclined to answer truthfully. It is important to be aware of the confidential nature of such questioning, the adverse effect that the parents' presence may have on the adolescent's willingness to answer, and the fact that self-reporting may not be an accurate account of substance use.

BOX 33-6 HABITS TO EXPLORE DURING A HEALTH INTERVIEW

- Behaviour patterns such as nail biting, thumb sucking, pica (habitual ingestion of nonfood substances), rituals ("security" blanket or toy), and unusual movements (head banging, rocking, overt masturbation, walking on toes)
- Activities of daily living, such as the hour of going to sleep and arising, duration of nighttime sleep and naps, type and duration of exercise, regularity of stools and urination, age of toilet training, and daytime or nighttime bed-wetting
- Unusual disposition; response to frustration
- Use of alcohol, drugs, coffee, or tobacco

Family Medical History

The family medical history is used primarily for discovering the potential existence of hereditary or familial diseases in the parents and child. In general, it is confined to first-degree relatives (parents, siblings, grandparents, and immediate aunts and uncles). Information for each family member includes age, marital status, state of health if living, cause of death if deceased, and any evidence of the following conditions: heart disease, hypertension, cancer, diabetes mellitus, obesity, congenital anomalies, allergy, asthma, seizures, tuberculosis, sickle cell disease, syphilis, rheumatic fever, cognitive impairment, mental disorders such as depression or psychosis, or emotional problems. The nurse needs to confirm the accuracy of the reported disorders by inquiring about the symptoms, course, treatment, and sequelae of each diagnosis.

Geographic location. One of the important areas to explore when assessing the family health history is geographic location, including the patient's birthplace and travel to different areas in or outside of the country, for identification of possible exposure to endemic diseases. Although the primary interest focuses on the child's temporary residence in various localities, the nurse should also inquire about close family members' travel, especially travel during tours of military service or business trips. Children are particularly susceptible to parasitic infestation in areas of poor sanitary conditions and to vector-borne diseases, such as those from mosquitoes or ticks in warm and humid or heavily wooded regions.

Family Structure

Assessment of the family, both its structure and function, is an important component of the history-taking process. Because the quality of the relationship between the child and family members is a major factor in emotional and physical health, family assessment is discussed here separately and in greater detail apart from the more traditional health history.

Family assessment is the collection of data about the family's composition and the relationships among its members. In its broadest sense, *family* refers to all those individuals who are considered by the patient to be significant to the nuclear unit, including relatives, friends, and social groups such as the school and church. Although family assessment is not family therapy, it can be therapeutic. Involving family members in the discussion of family characteristics and activities can provide insight into family dynamics and relationships.

The Calgary Family Assessment Model (CFAM) is fundamentally a "map of the family" that provides a framework as the nurse and the family explore issues in terms of the family history. This model can be used to identify any emotional, physical, or spiritual distress or disruption that is caused by a family crisis or a developmental milestone (Wright & Leahey, 2012). See Chapter 2, p. 17, for more information on this model and further family assessment models.

Because of the time involved in performing an in-depth family assessment as presented here, the nurse needs to be selective in deciding when knowledge of family function may facilitate nursing care (see Guidelines box). During brief contacts with families, a full assessment is not appropriate; screening with one or two questions from each category may reflect the health of the family system or the need for additional assessment.

The most common method of eliciting information on the family structure is to interview family members. The principal areas of concern (Box 33-7) are (1) family composition, (2) home and community environment, (3) occupation and education of family members, and (4) cultural and religious traditions.

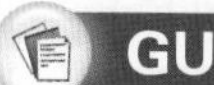

GUIDELINES

Initiating a Comprehensive Family Assessment

Perform a comprehensive assessment on the following:

- Children receiving comprehensive well-child care
- Children experiencing major stressful life events (e.g., chronic illness, disability, parental divorce, death of a family member)
- Children requiring extensive home care
- Children with developmental delays
- Children with repeated accidental injuries and those with suspected child abuse
- Children with behavioural or physical problems that could be caused by family dysfunction

NURSING ALERT

In assessing family composition, it is sometimes difficult to ascertain the status of the adult relationships. If the parent fails to mention the other parent, ask, "Where is the child's father [or mother]?" Avoid saying "husband" or "wife" because this assumes that only marital relationships exist.

Psychosocial History

The traditional medical history includes a personal and social section that concentrates on children's personal status, such as school adjustment and any unusual habits, and the family and home environment. Since several personal aspects are covered under development and habits, only those issues related to children's ability to cope and their self-concept are presented here.

Through observation, the nurse can obtain a general idea of how confident children are in dealing with others, answering questions, and coping with new situations. It is important to observe the parent–child relationship for the types of messages sent to children about their coping skills and self-worth. Do the parents treat the child with respect, focusing on strengths, or is the interaction one of constant reprimands, with emphasis on weaknesses and faults? Do the parents help the child learn new coping strategies or support the ones the child uses?

Parent–child interactions also convey messages about body image. Do the parents label the child and body parts, such as "bad boy," "skinny legs," or "ugly scar"? Do the parents handle the child gently, using soothing touch to calm an anxious child, or do they treat the child roughly, using slaps or restraint to force compliance? If the child touches certain parts of the body, such as the genitalia, do the parents make comments that suggest a negative connotation?

With older children many of the communication strategies discussed earlier in the chapter are useful in eliciting more definitive information about their coping and self-concept. Children can write down five things they like and dislike about themselves. The nurse can use sentence completion statements, such as "The thing I like best (or least) about myself is ____________," "If I could change one thing about myself, it would be ____________," or "When I am scared, I ____________."

Mental Health Screening. During the interview and history taking, the nurse may become concerned about potential psychosocial or mental health issues in the child or family being assessed. There are preliminary mental health screening tools available that can help the nurse assess potential concerns in areas such as sleep habits, social skills, family relationships, and learning difficulties. These tools are outlined later in this chapter (see also Additional Resources at the end of this chapter). More detailed information on mental health concerns in children is provided in Unit 10 and Chapter 50.

Review of Systems

The *review of systems* is a specific review of each body system, following an order similar to that of the physical examination (see Guidelines box). Often the history of the present illness provides a complete review of the system involved in the chief

BOX 33-7 FAMILY ASSESSMENT INTERVIEW

General Guidelines

Schedule the interview with the family at a time that is most convenient for all parties; include as many family members as possible; clearly state the purpose of the interview.

Begin the interview by asking each person's name and their relationship to one another.

Restate the purpose of the interview and the objective.

Keep the initial conversation general to put members at ease and to learn the "big picture" of the family.

Identify major concerns and reflect these back to the family to be certain that all parties receive the same message.

Terminate the interview with a summary of what was discussed and a plan for additional sessions, if needed.

Structural Assessment Areas

Family Composition

Immediate members of the household (names, ages, and relationships)

Significant extended family members

Previous marriages, separations, death of spouses, or divorces

Home and Community Environment

Type of dwelling, number of rooms, occupants

Sleeping arrangements

Number of floors, accessibility of stairs and elevators

Adequacy of utilities

Safety features (fire escape, smoke and carbon monoxide detectors, guardrails on windows, use of car restraint)

Environmental hazards (e.g., chipped paint, poor sanitation, pollution, heavy street traffic)

Availability and location of health care facilities, schools, play areas

Relationship with neighbours

Recent crises or changes in home

Child's reaction and adjustment to recent stresses

Occupation and Education of Family Members

Types of employment

Work schedules

Work satisfaction

Exposure to environmental or industrial hazards

Sources of income and adequacy

Effect of illness on financial status

Highest degree or grade level attained

Cultural and Religious Traditions

Religious beliefs and practices

Cultural and ethnic beliefs and practices

Language spoken in home

Assessment questions include the following:

- Does the family identify with a particular religious or ethnic group? Are both parents from that group?
- How is religious or ethnic background part of family life?
- What special religious or cultural traditions are practised in the home (e.g., food choices and preparation)?
- Where were family members born, and how long have they lived in this country?
- What language does the family speak most often?
- Do they speak and understand English?
- What do they believe causes health or illness?
- What religious or ethnic beliefs influence the family's perception of illness and its treatment?
- What methods are used to prevent or treat illness?
- How does the family know when a health problem needs medical attention?
- Whom does the family contact when a member is ill?
- Does the family rely on cultural or religious healers or remedies? If so, ask them to describe the type of healer or remedy.
- Whom does the family go to for support (clergy, medical healer, relatives)?
- Does the family experience discrimination because of their race, beliefs, or practices? Ask them to describe.

Functional Assessment Areas

Family Interactions and Roles

Interactions refer to ways in which family members relate to each other. The chief concern is the amount of intimacy and closeness among the members, especially spouses. *Roles* refer to behaviours of people as they assume a different status or position.

Observations include the following:

- Family members' responses to each other (cordial, hostile, cool, loving, patient, short tempered)
- Obvious roles of leadership versus submission
- Support and attention shown to various members

Assessment questions include the following:

- What activities does the family perform together?
- Whom do family members talk to when something is bothering them?
- What are members' household chores?
- Who usually oversees what is happening with the children, such as at school or for health care?
- How easy or difficult is it for the family to change or accept new responsibilities for household tasks?

Power, Decision Making, and Problem Solving

Power refers to individual member's control over others in the family; it is manifested through family decision making and problem solving. The chief concern is clarity of boundaries of power between parents and children. One method of assessment involves offering a hypothetical conflict or problem, such as a child failing school, and asking the family how they would handle this situation. Assessment questions include the following:

- Who usually makes the decisions in the family?
- If one parent makes a decision, can the child appeal to the other parent to change it?
- What input do children have in making decisions or discussing rules?
- Who makes and enforces the rules?
- What happens when a rule is broken?

Communication

Communication is concerned with clarity and directness of communication patterns. Further assessment includes periodically asking family members if they understood what was just said and to repeat the message.

Observations include the following:

- Who speaks to whom?
- If one person speaks for another or interrupts

BOX 33-7 FAMILY ASSESSMENT INTERVIEW—cont'd

- If members appear uninterested when certain individuals speak
- If there is agreement between verbal and nonverbal messages

Assessment questions include the following:

- How often do family members wait until others are through talking before "having their say"?
- Do parents or older siblings tend to lecture and preach?
- Do parents tend to "talk down" to the children?

Expression of Feelings and Individuality

Expressions are concerned with personal space and freedom to grow with limits and structure needed for guidance.

Observing patterns of communication offers clues to how freely feelings are expressed.

Assessment questions include the following:

- Is it OK for family members to get angry or sad?
- Who gets angry most of the time? What do they do?
- If someone is upset, how do other family members try to comfort this person?
- Who comforts specific family members?
- When someone wants to do something, such as try out for a new sport or get a job, what is the family's response (offer assistance, discouragement, or no advice)?

GUIDELINES

Review of Systems

General—Overall state of health, fatigue, recent or unexplained weight gain or loss (period of time for either), contributing factors (change of diet, illness, altered appetite), exercise tolerance, fevers (time of day), chills, night sweats (unrelated to climatic conditions), frequent infections, general ability to carry out activities of daily living

Integument—Pruritus, pigment or other colour changes, acne, eruptions, rashes (location), tendency for bruising, petechiae, excessive dryness, general texture, disorders or deformities of nails, hair growth or loss, hair colour change (for adolescents, use of hair dyes or other potentially toxic substances, such as hair straighteners)

Head—Headaches, dizziness, injury (specific details)

Eyes—Visual problems (behaviours indicative of blurred vision, such as bumping into objects, clumsiness, sitting close to television, holding a book close to the face, writing with head near the desk, squinting, rubbing the eyes, bending head in an awkward position), cross-eyes (strabismus), eye infections, edema of lids, excessive tearing, use of glasses or contact lenses, date of last optic examination

Ears—Earaches, discharge, evidence of hearing loss (ask about behaviours, such as need to repeat requests, loud speech, inattentive behaviour), results of any previous auditory testing

Nose—Nosebleeds (epistaxis), constant or frequent runny or stuffy nose, nasal obstruction (difficulty breathing), alteration or loss of sense of smell

Mouth—Mouth breathing, gum bleeding, toothaches, tooth brushing, use of fluoride, difficulty with teething (symptoms), last visit to dentist (especially if temporary dentition is complete), response to dentist

Throat—Sore throat, difficulty swallowing, choking (especially when chewing food—may be from poor chewing habits), hoarseness or other voice irregularities

Neck—Pain, limitation of movement, stiffness, difficulty holding head straight (torticollis), thyroid enlargement, enlarged nodes or other masses

Chest—Breast enlargement, discharge, masses, enlarged axillary nodes

Respiratory—Chronic cough, frequent colds (number per year), wheezing, shortness of breath at rest or on exertion, difficulty breathing, sputum production, infections (pneumonia, tuberculosis), date of last chest x-ray examination, skin reaction from tuberculin testing

Cardiovascular—Cyanosis or fatigue on exertion, history of heart murmur or rheumatic fever, anemia, date of last blood count, blood type, recent transfusion

Gastrointestinal (questions in regard to appetite, food tolerance, and elimination habits are asked elsewhere)—Nausea, vomiting (not associated with eating, may be indicative of brain tumour or increased intracranial pressure), jaundice or yellowing skin or sclera, belching, flatulence, recent change in bowel habits (blood in stools, change of colour, diarrhea, or constipation)

Genitourinary—Pain on urination, frequency, hesitancy, urgency, hematuria, nocturia, polyuria, unpleasant odour to urine, force of stream, discharge, change in size of scrotum, date of last urinalysis (for adolescents, sexually transmitted infection, type of treatment)

Gynecological—Menarche, date of last menstrual period, regularity or problems with menstruation, vaginal discharge, pruritus, if sexually active, type of contraception, sexually transmitted disease and type of treatment

Musculoskeletal—Weakness, clumsiness, lack of coordination, unusual movements, back or joint stiffness, muscle pains or cramps, abnormal gait, deformity, fractures, serious sprains, activity level

Neurological—Seizures, tremors, dizziness, loss of memory, general affect, fears, nightmares, speech problems, any unusual habits

Endocrine—Intolerance to weather changes, excessive thirst or urination, excessive sweating, salty taste to skin, signs of early puberty

health concern. Since asking questions about other body systems may appear unrelated and irrelevant to the parents or child, the questioning should be preceded by an explanation of why the data are needed (similar to the explanation concerning the relevance of the birth history) and the parents reassured that the child's main problem has not been forgotten.

The review of a specific system begins with a broad statement such as "How has your child's general health been?" or "Has your child had any problems with his eyes?" If the parent states that the child has had problems with some body function, this should be pursued with an encouraging statement, such as "Tell me more about that." If the parent denies any problems, the nurse can query for specific symptoms: "No headaches, bumping into objects, or squinting?" If the parent reconfirms the absence of such symptoms, the nurse should record positive statements in the history, such as "Mother denies headaches, bumping into objects, or squinting." In this way, anyone who reviews the health history is aware of exactly what symptoms were investigated.

Sexual History

The sexual history is an essential component of adolescents' health assessment. The history uncovers areas of concern related to sexual activity, alerts the nurse to circumstances that may indicate screening for sexually transmitted infections (STIs) or testing for pregnancy, and provides information related to the need for sexual counselling, such as safer sex practices. Guidelines for anticipatory guidance topics for parents and adolescents are found in Box 33-8.

One approach to initiating a conversation about sexual concerns is to begin with a history of peer interactions. Open-ended statements such as "Tell me about your social life" or "Who are your closest friends?" generally lead into a discussion of dating and sexual issues. To probe further, the nurse can include questions about the adolescent's attitudes on such topics as sex education, having a boy- or girlfriend, living together, and premarital sex. Such questions should be phrased to reflect concern rather than judgement or criticism of sexual practices.

In any conversation regarding sexual history, it is important be aware of the language used in either eliciting or conveying sexual information. For example, the nurse should avoid asking whether the adolescent is "sexually active," because this term is broadly defined. "Are you having sex with anyone?" is probably the most direct and best understood question. Since same-sex experimentation may occur, all sexual contacts should be referred to in nongender terms, such as "anyone" or "partners," rather than "girlfriends" or "boyfriends."

A detailed account of sexual partners is needed if the patient has a history of, displays any symptoms of, or asks for treatment of an STI. A difficult but necessary part of the interview is to determine the sites of possible infection. Since sexual diseases can be contracted in any of the body orifices, the adolescent should be informed that an STI can be acquired without visible signs of disease at nongenital sites.

BOX 33-8 ANTICIPATORY GUIDANCE—SEXUALITY

Ages 12 to 14 Years

Have the adolescent identify a supportive adult to discuss sexuality issues and concerns with.
Discuss advantages of delaying sexual activity.
Discuss making responsible decisions regarding normal sexual feelings.
Discuss roles of gender, peer pressure, and the media in sexual decision making.
Discuss contraceptive options (advantages and disadvantages).
Provide education regarding sexually transmitted infections (STIs) and human immunodeficiency virus (HIV) infection; clarify risks, and discuss the use of condoms.
Discuss abuse prevention: avoiding dangerous situations, the role of drugs and alcohol, and the use of self-defence.
Have the adolescent clarify values, needs, and the ability to be assertive.
If the adolescent is sexually active, discuss the use of condoms and contraceptive options.
Have a confidential interview with the adolescent (including a sexual history).
Discuss the evolution of sexual identity and expression.

Ages 15 to 18 Years

Clarify values; encourage responsible decision making.
Discuss alternatives to intercourse.
Discuss "When are you ready for sex?"
Discuss consequences of unprotected sex: early pregnancy; STIs, including HIV infection.
Discuss negotiating with the partner and barriers to safer sex.
If the adolescent is sexually active, discuss the use of condoms and contraceptive options.
Emphasize that sex should be safe and pleasurable for both partners.
Have a confidential interview with the adolescent.
Discuss concerns about sexual identity and expression.

Data from Fonseca, H., Greydanus, D. (2007). Sexuality in the child, teen and young adult: Concepts for the clinician. *Primary Care Clinical Office Practice, 34,* 275–292; Wright, K. (1997). Anticipatory guidance: Developing a healthy sexuality. *Pediatric Annals, 26*(2 Suppl), S142–S144, C3.

Performing a Nutritional Assessment

Dietary Intake

Food consumption patterns of children have changed over the past 30 years, and the prevalence of overweight and obesity among children and adolescents has significantly increased (CPS, 2013). Knowledge of the child's dietary intake is an essential component of a nutritional assessment. However, it is also one of the most difficult factors to assess. Individuals' recall of food consumption, especially amounts eaten, is frequently unreliable. The food intake history of children and adolescents is prone to reporting error, mostly in the form of underreporting. Also, people from different cultures may have difficulty adequately describing the types of food they eat. Despite these obstacles, a dietary evaluation is an important component of the child's assessment.

Specific questions used to conduct a nutritional assessment are included in Box 33-9. Every nutritional assessment should begin with a dietary history. The exact questions used to elicit a dietary history vary with the child's age. In general, the younger the child, the more specific and detailed the history should be. The overview elicited from the dietary history can be helpful in evaluating food frequency records. The history should also be concerned with financial and cultural factors that influence food selection and preparation (see Cultural Awareness box).

The most common and probably easiest method of assessing daily intake is the 24-hour recall. The child or parent recalls every item eaten in the past 24 hours and the approximate amounts. The 24-hour recall is most beneficial when it represents a typical day's intake. Some of the difficulties with a daily recall are the family's inability to remember exactly what was eaten and inaccurate estimation of portion size. To increase

BOX 33-9 DIETARY ASSESSMENT FOR AN INDIVIDUAL

Dietary History

What are the family's usual mealtimes?
Do family members eat together or at separate times?
Who does the family grocery shopping and meal preparation?
How much money is spent to buy food each week?
How are most foods prepared—baked, broiled, fried, other?
How often does the family or child eat out?

- What kinds of restaurants do they go to?
- What kinds of food does the child typically eat at restaurants?

Does the child eat breakfast regularly?
Where does the child eat lunch?
What are the child's favourite foods, beverages, and snacks?

- What are the average amounts eaten per day?
- What foods are artificially sweetened?
- What are the child's snacking habits?
- When are sweet foods usually eaten?
- What are the child's tooth-brushing habits?

What special cultural practices are followed? What ethnic foods are eaten?
What foods and beverages does the child dislike?
How would parents describe the child's usual appetite (hearty eater, picky eater)?
What are the child's feeding habits (breast, bottle, cup, spoon, eats by self, needs assistance, any special devices)?
Does the child take vitamins or other supplements? Do they contain iron or fluoride?
Does the child have any known or suspected food allergies? Is the child on a special diet?
Has the child lost or gained weight recently?
Are there any feeding problems (excessive fussiness, spitting up, colic, difficulty sucking or swallowing)? Are there any dental problems or appliances, such as braces, that affect eating?
What types of exercise does the child do regularly?
Is there a family history of cancer, diabetes, heart disease, high blood pressure, or obesity?

Additional Questions Regarding Infants

What was the infant's birth weight? When did it double? Triple?
Was the infant preterm?
Is the mother breastfeeding or has she breastfed her infant? For how long?
If formula is used, what is the brand?

- When was formula feeding started?
- How many millilitres does the infant drink a day?
- Is the infant receiving cow's milk (whole, low fat, skim)?
- When was it started?

Does the infant receive extra fluids (water, juice)?
If the infant takes a bottle to bed at nap time or nighttime, what is in the bottle?
At what age did the child start on cereal, meat or other protein sources, vegetables, fruit or juice, finger food, table food?
Do the parents make their own baby food or use commercial foods, such as infant cereal?
Does the infant take a vitamin or mineral supplement? If so, what type?
Has the infant had an allergic reaction to any food(s)? If so, list the foods and describe the reaction.
Does the infant spit up frequently; have unusually loose stools; or have hard, dry stools? If so, how often?
How often is the infant fed?
How would the parents describe their infant's appetite?

Modified from Murphy, S. P., & Poos, M. I. (2002). Dietary reference intakes: Summary of applications in dietary assessment. *Public Health Nutrition, 5*(6A), 843–849.

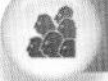

CULTURAL AWARENESS
Food Practices

Because cultural practices are prevalent in food preparation, the kinds of questions asked and the judgements made during counselling need to be considered carefully (see Food Customs, Chapter 31). For example, some First Nations, Métis, and Inuit people eat food that is different from food listed in *Eating Well With Canada's Food Guide.* Health Canada has thus adapted the *Food Guide* for First Nations, Metis, and Inuit people to include foods such as moose stew, char, and bannock. The *Food Guide* includes traditional as well as store-bought foods that are usually affordable, available, and accessible across Canada. This guide is also available in Inuktitut, Ojibwe, Plains Cree, and Woods Cree languages. For more information, visit the *Food Guide* website: http://www.hc-sc.gc.ca/fn-an/pubs/fnim-pnim/index-eng.php.

accuracy of reporting portion sizes, the use of food models and additional questioning are recommended. In general, this method is most useful in providing qualitative information about the child's diet.

To improve the reliability of the daily recall, the family can complete a food diary by recording every food and liquid consumed for a certain number of days. A 3-day record consisting of 2 weekdays and 1 weekend day is representative for most people. Providing specific charts to record intake can improve the ability to complete the chart. The family should record items immediately after eating. A food frequency questionnaire or record provides information about the number of times in a day, week, or month a child consumes items from the different food groups. In general, it provides a qualitative overview but has the advantage of avoiding recall based on a "typical" day. It can be especially useful when verifying a food history or diary.

Clinical Examination of Nutrition

A significant amount of information regarding nutritional deficiencies can be elicited from a clinical examination, especially from assessing the skin, hair, teeth, gums, lips, tongue, and eyes. The hair, skin, and mouth are vulnerable because of the rapid turnover of epithelial and mucosal tissue. Table 33-1 summarizes clinical signs of possible nutritional deficiency or excess. Few are diagnostic for a specific nutrient, and if suspicious signs are found, they must be confirmed with dietary and

TABLE 33-1 CLINICAL ASSESSMENT OF NUTRITIONAL STATUS

EVIDENCE OF ADEQUATE NUTRITION	EVIDENCE OF DEFICIENT OR EXCESS NUTRITION	DEFICIENCY OR EXCESS*
General Growth		
Between 5th and 95th percentiles for height, weight, and head circumference	Below 5th or above 95th percentile for growth	Protein, calories, fats, and other essential nutrients, especially vitamin A, pyridoxine, niacin, calcium, iodine, manganese, zinc
Steady gain with expected growth spurts during infancy and adolescence	Absence of or delayed growth spurts; poor weight gain	
Sexual development appropriate for age	Delayed sexual development	Excess vitamins A, D
Skin		
Smooth, slightly dry to touch	Hardening and scaling	Vitamin A
Elastic and firm	Seborrheic dermatitis	Excess niacin
Absence of lesions	Dry, rough, petechiae	Riboflavin
Colour appropriate to genetic background	Delayed wound healing	Vitamin C
	Scaly dermatitis on exposed surfaces	Riboflavin, vitamin C, zinc
	Wrinkled, flabby	Niacin
	Crusted lesions around orifices, especially nares	Protein, calories, zinc
	Pruritus	Excess vitamin A, riboflavin, niacin
	Poor turgor	Water, sodium
	Edema	Protein, thiamine Excess sodium
	Yellow tinge (jaundice)	Vitamin B_{12} Excess vitamin A, niacin
	Depigmentation	Protein, calories
	Pallor (anemia)	Pyridoxine; folic acid; vitamins B_{12}, C, E (in preterm infants); iron Excess vitamin C, zinc
	Paresthesia	Excess riboflavin
Hair		
Lustrous, silky, strong, elastic	Stringy, friable, dull, dry, thin	Protein, calories
	Alopecia	Protein, calories, zinc
	Depigmentation	Protein, calories, copper
	Raised areas around hair follicles	Vitamin C
Head		
Even moulding, occipital prominence, symmetrical facial features	Softening of cranial bones, prominence of frontal bones, skull flat and depressed toward middle	Vitamin D
Fused sutures after 18 mo	Delayed fusion of sutures	Vitamin D
	Hard, tender lumps in occiput	Excess vitamin A
	Headache	Excess thiamine
Neck		
Thyroid not visible, palpable in midline	Thyroid enlarged, may be grossly visible	Iodine
Eyes		
Clear, bright	Hardening and scaling of cornea and conjunctiva	Vitamin A
Good night vision	Night blindness	Vitamin A
Conjunctiva—Pink, glossy	Burning, itching, photophobia, cataracts, corneal vascularization	Riboflavin
Ears		
Tympanic membrane—Pliable	Calcified (hearing loss)	Excess vitamin D
Nose		
Smooth, intact nasal angle	Irritation and cracks at nasal angle	Riboflavin Excess vitamin A

TABLE 33-1 CLINICAL ASSESSMENT OF NUTRITIONAL STATUS—cont'd

EVIDENCE OF ADEQUATE NUTRITION	EVIDENCE OF DEFICIENT OR EXCESS NUTRITION	DEFICIENCY OR EXCESS*
Mouth		
Lips—Smooth, moist, darker colour than skin	Fissures and inflammation at corners	Riboflavin Excess vitamin A
Gums—Firm, coral pink, stippled	Spongy, friable, swollen, bluish red or black, bleed easily	Vitamin C
Mucous membranes—Bright pink, smooth, moist	Stomatitis	Niacin
Tongue—Rough texture, no lesions, taste sensation	Glossitis	Niacin, riboflavin, folic acid
	Diminished taste sensation	Zinc
Teeth—Uniform white colour, smooth, intact	Brown mottling, pits, fissures	Excess fluoride
	Defective enamel	Vitamins A, C, D; calcium; phosphorus
	Caries	Excess carbohydrates
Chest		
In infants, shape almost circular	Depressed lower portion of rib cage	Vitamin D
In children, lateral diameter increased in proportion to anteroposterior diameter	Sharp protrusion of sternum	Vitamin D
Smooth costochondral junctions	Enlarged costochondral junctions	Vitamins C, D
Breast development—Normal for age	Delayed development	See under General Growth; especially zinc
Cardiovascular System		
Pulse and blood pressure (BP) within normal limits	Palpitations	Thiamine
	Rapid pulse	Potassium Excess thiamine
	Arrhythmias	Magnesium, potassium Excess niacin, potassium
	Increased BP	Excess sodium
	Decreased BP	Thiamine Excess niacin
Abdomen		
In young children, cylindrical and prominent	Distended, flabby, poor musculature	Protein, calories
	Prominent, large	Excess calories
In older children, flat	Potbelly, constipation	Vitamin D
Normal bowel habits	Diarrhea	Niacin Excess vitamin C
	Constipation	Excess calcium, potassium
Musculoskeletal System		
Muscles—Firm, well developed, equal strength bilaterally	Flabby, weak, generalized wasting	Protein, calories
	Weakness, pain, cramps	Thiamine, sodium, chloride, potassium, phosphorus, magnesium Excess thiamine
	Muscle twitching, tremors	Magnesium
	Muscular paralysis	Excess potassium
Spine—Cervical and lumbar curves (double S curve)	Kyphosis, lordosis, scoliosis	Vitamin D
Extremities—Symmetrical; legs straight with minimum bowing	Bowing of extremities, knock-knees	Vitamin D, calcium, phosphorus
	Epiphyseal enlargement	Vitamins A, D
	Bleeding into joints and muscles, joint swelling, pain	Vitamin C
Joints—Flexible, full range of motion, no pain or stiffness	Thickening of cortex of long bones with pain and fragility, hard tender lumps in extremities	Excess vitamin A
	Osteoporosis of long bones	Calcium Excess vitamin D

Continued

TABLE 33-1 CLINICAL ASSESSMENT OF NUTRITIONAL STATUS—cont'd

EVIDENCE OF ADEQUATE NUTRITION	EVIDENCE OF DEFICIENT OR EXCESS NUTRITION	DEFICIENCY OR EXCESS*
Neurological System		
Behaviour—Alert, responsive, emotionally stable	Listless, irritable, lethargic, apathetic (sometimes apprehensive, anxious, drowsy, mentally slow, confused)	Thiamine, niacin, pyridoxine, vitamin C, potassium, magnesium, iron, protein, calories Excess vitamins A, D; thiamine; folic acid; calcium
Absence of tetany, convulsions	Masklike facial expression, blurred speech, involuntary laughing	Excess manganese
	Convulsions	Thiamine, pyridoxine, vitamin D, calcium, magnesium Excess phosphorus (in relation to calcium)
Intact peripheral nervous system	Peripheral nervous system toxicity (unsteady gait, numb feet and hands, fine motor clumsiness)	Excess pyridoxine
Intact reflexes	Diminished or absent tendon reflexes	Thiamine, vitamin E

*Nutrients listed are deficient unless specified as excess.

biochemical data. Generally, the clinical examination does not reveal children's risk for a deficiency or excess.

Anthropometry, an essential parameter of nutritional status, is the measurement of height, weight, head circumference, proportions, skin fold thickness, and arm circumference in young children. Height and head circumference reflect past nutrition, whereas weight, skin fold thickness, and arm circumference reflect present nutritional status, especially of protein and fat reserves. Skin fold thickness is a measurement of the body's fat content; approximately half the body's total fat stores are directly beneath the skin. The upper arm muscle circumference is correlated with measurements of total muscle mass. Since muscle serves as the body's major protein reserve, this measurement is considered an index of the body's protein stores. Ideally, growth measurements are recorded over time, and comparisons are made regarding the velocity of growth based on previous and present values. Numerous biochemical tests available for assessing nutritional status include analysis of plasma; blood cells; urine; and tissues from liver, bone, hair, and fingernails. Many of these tests are complicated and are not performed routinely. Common laboratory procedures for nutritional status include measurement of hemoglobin, hematocrit, transferrin, albumin, creatinine, and nitrogen. Laboratory values for these tests and more specific nutrient measurements are given in Appendix D.

Evaluation of Nutritional Assessment

After collecting the data needed for a thorough nutritional assessment, the nurse needs to evaluate the findings to plan appropriate counselling. From the data, assessment can be made as to whether the child is (1) malnourished, (2) at risk for becoming malnourished, or (3) well nourished with adequate reserves or (4) overweight or obese.

The Dietary Reference Intakes (DRIs) are a set of four nutrient-based reference values that provide quantitative estimates of nutrient intake for use in assessing and planning dietary intake (Health Canada, 2010). The specific DRIs include the following:

Estimated Average Requirement (EAR)—Nutrient intake estimated to meet the requirement of half the healthy individuals (50%) for a specific age and gender group. The EAR is used to examine the possibility of inadequacy.

Recommended Dietary Allowance (RDA)—Average daily dietary intake sufficient to meet the nutrient requirement of nearly all (97 to 98%) of healthy individuals for a specific age and gender group. Dietary intake at or above this level usually has a low probability of inadequacy.

Adequate Intake (AI)—Recommended intake level based on estimates of nutrient intake by healthy groups of individuals. Dietary intake at or above this level usually has a low probability of inadequacy.

Tolerable Upper Intake Level (UL)—Highest average daily nutrient intake level likely to pose no risk of adverse health effects. As intake increases above the UL, risk of adverse effects increases. Dietary intake above this level usually places an individual at risk of adverse effects from excessive nutrient intake.

Another resource for assessing nutrition is Health Canada's (2012) *Eating Well With Canada's Food Guide*. The *Food Guide* is based on current nutritional science and is intended to help individuals make good food choices that promote health and prevent nutrition-related illnesses (see Appendix A). The *Food Guide* provides special recommendations for children, women of child-bearing age, and adults over age 50. There are also different adaptations of the *Food Guide*, including one for First Nations, Métis, and Inuit populations. In addition to the English and French versions, the *Food Guide* has been translated into Arabic, Chinese (traditional or simplified), Farsi, Korean, Russian, Punjabi, Spanish, Tagalog, Tamil, and Urduhas. When assessing a child's food intake, it is important to analyze the daily food diary for the variety and amounts of foods suggested in *Eating Well With Canada's Food Guide*. For example, if the list includes no vegetables, the nurse can inquire about this rather than assuming that the child dislikes vegetables, since it could be that none were served that day. Also, information should be evaluated in terms of the family's ethnic practices and financial resources. Encouraging increased protein intake with additional meat may be unfeasible for families on a limited budget or in conflict with food practices in which meat is used sparingly.

DEVELOPMENTAL ASSESSMENT

One of the essential components of a complete health appraisal is the assessment of developmental function. Screening procedures are designed to quickly and reliably identify whether a child's developmental level is normal for their age and whether the child requires further investigation because of not meeting normal developmental levels. They also provide a means of recording objective measurements of present developmental function for future reference. Nurses play a vital role in providing a developmental assessment of children, particularly children with disabilities. The procedures discussed in this section can be administered in a variety of settings, such as home, school, day care centres, hospitals, health care providers' offices, or clinics. Parents and teachers sometimes complete them as well and the information is analyzed by the practitioner.

Developmental Assessment Screening Tools

There are a variety of standardized developmental screening tools that have been reviewed by the CPS (2015) and are commonly used to provide consistent and accurate data across Canada. These tools are presented in Table 33-2.

Most physicians and nurse practitioners perform a developmental assessment of some kind, during the well-child visits, but it is unknown how many use a consistent, standardized assessment. Often nurses perform the developmental assessments (Limbos, Joyce, & Roberts, 2010).

All children need to be assessed for developmental disabilities. Developmental delay affects between 4 and 16% of children and is the leading cause of disability among children younger than 4 years of age in Canada (Limbos et al., 2010). Early diagnosis and intervention are critical to improve long-term outcomes. However, only 30% of children with disabilities are identified before starting school (Limbos et al., 2010). Furthermore, it is estimated that up to one quarter of first-grade children have learning, health, and behavioural problems that will interfere with their academic and social performance (Limbos et al., 2010).

HEALTH SUPERVISION GUIDES

Rourke Baby Record

The Rourke Baby Record is a guide for health care providers in their health supervision of children in the first 5 years of life (CPS, 2014). The Rourke Baby Record consists of guides for charting well-baby/child visits, an immunization chart, and resources pages and includes growth monitoring, nutrition, physical examination, education, and advice issues. It also can be used to chart development, behaviour, parenting resources, immunization, and infectious diseases (see Additional Resources at the end of this chapter for checklists and record forms).

Greig Health Record

The Greig Health Record is an evidence-based health promotion guide for clinicians caring for children and adolescents aged 6 to 17 years (Greig, Constantin, Carsley, et al., 2010). It provides a template for periodic health visits that is easy to use and is easily adaptable for electronic medical records. On the Greig Health Record, evidence-based information is provided, and levels of evidence are indicated whenever possible. The checklist templates include sections for weight, height, and body mass index; psychosocial history and development; nutrition; education and advice; specific concerns; examination; an assessment, immunization; and medications. The College of Family Physicians of Canada and the CPS endorse the Greig Health Record and its supporting literature (see Additional Resources at the end of this chapter).

PHYSICAL ASSESSMENT

General Approaches to Examining the Child

Although the approach to and sequence of the physical examination differs according to the child's age, the traditional model for physical assessment, outlined here, can be used for all pediatric age groups and as a baseline for conducting assessments that are more age specific (see Chapter 26 for a detailed discussion of a newborn assessment).

Children need to have periodic health checkups, conducted by health care providers, in order to optimize their health. These checkups are means of trending health patterns, providing preventive care, and making early diagnoses of health issues. Such visits customarily occur at 1 and 2 weeks of age; at 1, 2, 4, 6, 9, 12, and 18 months of age; and subsequently at 1- or 2-year intervals.

Immunization Status

Along with physical examination, another vital part of preventive pediatric care is assessment of immunization status. Immunization requirements during infancy, early childhood, and adolescence are outlined in Chapter 35. (See Additional Resources for different Provinces and Territories's immunization schedules.)

Sequence of the Examination

Ordinarily, the sequence for examining patients follows a head-to-toe direction. The main function of such a systematic approach is to provide a general guideline for assessment of each body area to avoid omitting segments of the examination. The standard recording of data also facilitates exchange of information among different health care providers. This orderly sequence is frequently altered to accommodate the child's developmental needs, although the examination is recorded following the head-to-toe model. Using developmental and chronological age as the main criteria for assessing each body system accomplishes several goals:

TABLE 33-2 DEVELOPMENTAL ASSESSMENT SCREENING TOOLS

TYPE	DESCRIPTION	AGE GROUP	WHO PERFORMS THE TEST
Physical, Cognitive, and Social Development Assessment			
Nipissing District Developmental Screen	Tests 13 critical developmental stages. The Screen examines a child's skills in the following areas: • Vision • Hearing • Speech and language • Communication • Gross motor and fine motor • Cognitive • Social/emotional • Self-help	1, 2, 4, 6, 9, 12, 15, 18, 24 and 30 months, 3 to 6 years	Parent, caregiver, nurse, or physician See Appendix B for a sample form.
Ages and Stages Questionnaires (ASQ)	Assesses a child's global development: gross motor, fine motor, language functions and social-emotional development, adaptive skills. Screening tool for developmental delay and to identify specific strengths and weaknesses a child may have	4 months to 5 years	Parent, caregiver, nurse, physician, or teacher
Child Developmental Inventory (CDI)	Assesses development in 8 areas of functioning, including cognitive and language	15 months to 6 years	Parent, nurse, physician, or teacher
Children's Sleep Habits Questionnaire	Evaluates sleep on the basis of child's behaviour within 8 different subscales: bedtime resistance, sleep-onset delay, sleep duration, sleep anxiety, night wakenings, parasomnias, sleep-disordered breathing, daytime sleepiness	4 to 10 years	Parent
Conners Early Childhood	Assesses a child's social, emotional, and behavioural development	2 to 6 years	Parent, teacher, or caregiver
HEADSS for Adolescents	Identifies risky behaviours and used for health promotion, such as seat belt, helmet, protective gear use	12 to 18 years	Nurse or physician with the patient
PEDS: Parents' Evaluation of Developmental Status	Screens for developmental delays in children	Birth to 11 years	Parent or caregiver
Youth Resiliency: Assessing Development Strengths (YR:ADS)	Assesses factors associated with adolescent resilience: parental support/expectations, peer relationships, community cohesiveness, commitment to learning, school culture, cultural sensitivity, self-control, empowerment, self-concept, social sensitivity	13 to 18 years	Self-report
WHO Growth Charts for Canada	Charts to measure BMI for age and gender and used to assess weight relative to height	Growth chart for males and females, birth to 24 months, 2 to 19 years	Nurse or physician See Appendix C for growth charts
Preliminary Mental Health Assessment			
Achenbach Child Behaviour Checklists (CBCL)	Provides information on general functioning (e.g., social skills, family relationships, learning)	1½ to 5 and 6 to 18 years	Parent, teacher, or patient, depending on the version
Pediatric Symptom Checklist	A brief screening questionnaire used by pediatricians and other health care providers to improve recognition and treatment of psychosocial problems in children	4 years of age and older	Parent and self-report
Child/Adolescent Psychiatry Screen (CAPS)	Initial screening for 18 mental health issues	3 to 21 years	Parent
Weiss Symptom Record	A nonvalidated, comprehensive screening tool for various mental health conditions	5 to 19 years	Parent/teenager or teacher
Weiss Function Impairment Scales (Self-Report and Parent-Report)	A nonvalidated tool, recommended to collect systematic information from patient and parent about various disorders, including learning, developmental, and personality difficulties	14 to 19 years	Parent/teenager

BMI, body mass index.

- Minimizes stress and anxiety associated with assessment of various body parts
- Fosters a trusting nurse–child–parent relationship
- Allows for maximum preparation of the child
- Preserves the essential security of the parent–child relationship, especially with young children
- Maximizes the accuracy and reliability of assessment findings

Preparation of the Child

Although the physical examination consists of painless procedures, to a child the use of a tight arm cuff, probes in the ears and mouth, pressure on the abdomen, and a cold piece of metal to listen to the chest can be stressful. Therefore, the same considerations discussed in Chapter 44 for preparing children for procedures are followed here. In addition to that discussion, general guidelines related to the examining process are presented in the Guidelines box.

The physical examination should be as pleasant as possible as well as educational. The paper-doll technique is a useful approach to teaching children about the body part that is being examined (Fig. 33-4). At the conclusion of the visit, the child can bring home the paper doll as a memento.

Table 33-3 summarizes guidelines for positioning, preparing, and examining children at various ages. Because no child fits precisely into one age category, it may be necessary to vary the approach after a preliminary assessment of the child's developmental achievements and needs. Even with the best approach, many toddlers find the procedure difficult and are inconsolable for much of the physical examination. However, some seem intrigued by the new surroundings and unusual equipment and respond more like preschoolers than toddlers. Likewise, some early preschoolers may require more of the "security measures" employed with younger children, such as continued parent–child contact, and less of the preparatory measures used with preschoolers, such as playing

GUIDELINES

Performing a Pediatric Physical Examination

Perform the examination in an appropriate, nonthreatening area.
- Have the room well lit.
- Have room temperature comfortably warm.
- Place all strange and potentially frightening equipment out of sight.
- Have some toys, dolls, stuffed animals, and games available for the child.
- If possible, have rooms decorated and equipped for different-age children.
- Provide privacy, especially for school-age children and adolescents.

Provide time for play and becoming acquainted.

Observe behaviours that signal the child's readiness to collaborate:
- Talking to the nurse
- Making eye contact
- Accepting the offered equipment
- Allowing physical touching
- Choosing to sit on the examining table rather than the parent's lap

If signs of readiness are not observed, use the following techniques:
- Talk to the parent while essentially "ignoring" the child; gradually focus on the child or a favourite object, such as a doll.
- Make complimentary remarks about the child, such as appearance, dress, or a favourite object.
- Tell a funny story or play a simple magic trick.
- Have a nonthreatening "friend" available, such as a hand puppet to "talk" to the child for the nurse (see Fig. 33-25, A).

If the child refuses to collaborate, use the following techniques:
- Assess reason for behaviour; consider that a child who is unduly afraid may have had a traumatic experience.
- Try to involve the child and parent in the process.
- Avoid prolonged explanations about the examining procedure.
- Use a firm, direct approach regarding expected behaviour.
- Perform the examination as quickly as possible.
- Have an attendant gently restrain the child.
- Minimize any disruptions or stimulation.
- Limit the number of people in the room.
- Use an isolated room.
- Use a quiet, calm, confident voice.

Begin the examination in a nonthreatening manner for young children or children who are fearful:
- Use activities that can be presented as games, such as the test for cranial nerves (see Table 33-14) or parts of developmental screening tests.
- Use approaches such as "Simon Says" to encourage the child to make a face, squeeze a hand, stand on one foot, and so on.
- Use the paper-doll technique:
  1. Lay the child supine on an examining table or floor that is covered with a large sheet of paper.
  2. Trace around the child's body outline.
  3. Use body outline to demonstrate what will be examined, such as drawing a heart and listening with a stethoscope, before performing the activity on the child.

If several children in the family will be examined, begin with the child who is most willing to be examined to model desired behaviour.

Involve the child in the examination process:
- Provide choices, such as sitting on the table or in the parent's lap.
- Allow the child to handle or hold equipment.
- Encourage the child to use equipment on a doll, family member, or examiner.
- Explain each step of the procedure in simple language.

Examine the child in a comfortable and secure position:
- Sitting in parent's lap
- Sitting upright if in respiratory distress

Proceed to examine the body in an organized sequence (usually head to toe) with the following exceptions:
- Alter sequence to accommodate needs of different-age children (see Table 33-3).
- Examine painful areas last.
- In an emergency situation, examine vital functions (airway, breathing, and circulation) and injured area first.

Reassure the child throughout examination, especially about bodily concerns that arise during puberty.

Discuss findings with the family (if appropriate) at the end of the examination.

Praise the child for their assistance during the examination; give a reward such as a small toy or sticker.

TABLE 33-3 **AGE-SPECIFIC APPROACHES TO PHYSICAL EXAMINATION OF CHILDREN**

POSITION	SEQUENCE	PREPARATION
Infant		
Before able to sit alone—Supine or prone, preferably in parent's lap; before 4–6 mo, can place on examining table **After able to sit alone**—Sitting in parent's lap whenever possible; if on table, place with parent in full view	If quiet, auscultate heart, lungs, abdomen. Record heart and respiratory rates. Palpate and percuss same areas. Proceed in usual head-to-toe direction. Perform traumatic procedures last (eyes, ears, mouth [while crying]). Elicit reflexes as body part is examined. Elicit Moro reflex last.	Completely undress infant if room temperature permits. Leave diaper on male infant. Gain cooperation with distraction, bright objects, rattles, talking. Smile at infant; use soft, gentle voice. Use pacifier or feeding if necessary. Enlist parent's aid for restraining to examine ears, mouth. Avoid abrupt, jerky movements.
Toddler		
Sitting or standing on or by parent Prone or supine in parent's lap	Inspect body area through play: "count fingers," "tickle toes." Use minimum physical contact initially. Introduce equipment slowly. Auscultate, percuss, palpate whenever quiet. Perform traumatic procedures last (same as for infant).	Have parent remove outer clothing. Remove child's underwear as body part is examined. Allow child to inspect equipment; demonstrating use of equipment is usually ineffective. Perform procedures quickly, if child has difficulty cooperating. Use restraint when appropriate; request parent's assistance. Talk about examination; use short phrases. Praise for assisting.
Preschool Child		
Prefer standing or sitting Usually most helpful prone or supine Prefer parent's closeness	Proceed in head-to-toe direction unless child is having difficulty with examination. If having difficulty, proceed as with toddler.	Request self-undressing. Allow child to wear underpants if shy. Offer equipment for inspection; briefly demonstrate use. Make up story about procedure (e.g., "I'm seeing how strong your muscles are" [blood pressure]). Use paper-doll technique. Give choices when possible. Use positive statements (e.g., "Open your mouth").
School-Age Child		
Prefer sitting Helpful in most positions Younger child prefers parent's presence Older child may prefer privacy	Proceed in head-to-toe direction. May examine genitalia last in older child	Respect need for privacy. Request self-undressing. Allow to wear underpants. Give gown to wear. Explain purpose of equipment and significance of procedure, such as otoscope to see eardrum, which is necessary for hearing. Teach about body function and care.
Adolescent		
Same as for school-age child Offer option of parent's presence	Same as older school-age child May examine genitalia last	Allow to undress in private. Give gown. Expose only area to be examined. Respect need for privacy. Explain findings during examination: "Your muscles are firm and strong." Matter-of-factly comment about sexual development: "Your breasts are developing as they should be." Emphasize normalcy of development. Examine genitalia as any other body part; may leave to end.

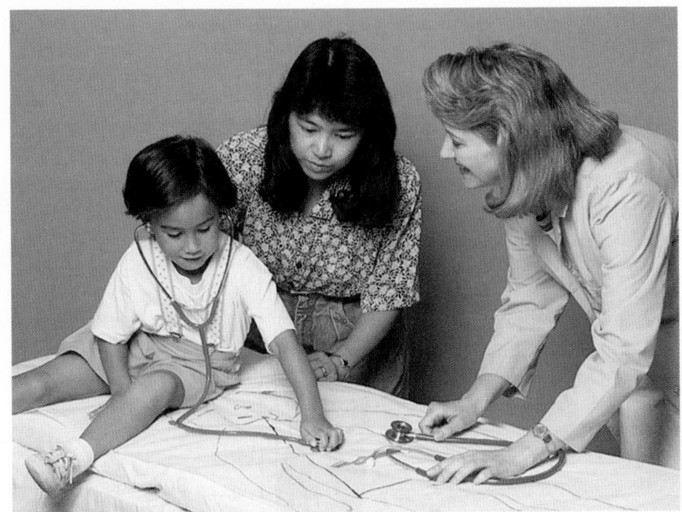

FIGURE 33-4 Using paper-doll technique to prepare child for physical examination.

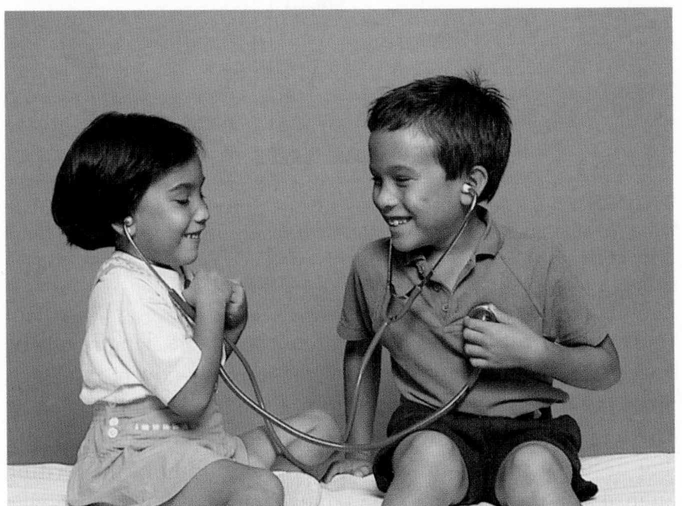

FIGURE 33-5 Preparing children for physical examination.

with the equipment before and during the actual examination (Fig. 33-5).

Although the variations in the general approaches are numerous, some common ones are elaborated on here. For example, the suggested sequence may change considerably when the child is in pain or when obvious physical defects are present. In either situation, the affected area needs to be examined last, to minimize distress early in the examination and to focus on normal, healthy, functioning body parts.

Growth Measurements

Measurement of physical growth in children is a key element in evaluating their health status. Physical growth parameters include weight, height (length), skin fold thickness, arm circumference, and head circumference. Values for these growth parameters are plotted on percentile charts, and the child's measurements in percentiles are compared with those of the general population.

Growth Charts

The growth charts used in Canada have been adapted from the 2006 and 2007 World Health Organization (WHO) Growth Standards and Growth References (see Appendix C). The charts were adapted in order to provide health care providers with consistent practices in monitoring growth and assessing patterns of linear growth and weight gain to support healthy children. These new charts reflect the 0 to 19 years of age population with optimal health conditions. It also reflects an increase in the multiethnic international population and an improvement in the tool to identify children at risk for obesity. (See Additional Resources at the end of this chapter for a parent handout on using growth charts.)

> **! NURSING ALERT**
>
> The BMI-for-age values that suggest overweight (BMI of 25 kg/m2) and obesity (BMI of 30 kg/m2) match the adult cut-offs for overweight and obesity at 19 years (Dietitians of Canada, 2014). BMI in children has been linked to future obesity and resultant negative impact on health. A BMI of 28 begins to decrease in later infancy and reaches a low at around 4 to 6 years of age. There is then an increase throughout childhood and adolescence (Dietitians of Canada, 2014).

Special groups. The WHO growth charts do not include premature infants or very low-birth-weight infants who weigh less than 1500 g. These infants do not grow in the same manner as full-term infants. Once these preterm infants are discharged from the neonatal intensive care unit, the WHO charts can then be used for them. Measurements should be plotted with the corrected postnatal age for prematurity (40 weeks—gestational age in weeks) until the child is 24 to 36 months of age. As an alternative, Fenton's growth chart (Fenton, 2003) can be used for plotting growth from 22 gestational weeks to 10 weeks post-term (Dietitians of Canada, 2014). Children with specific intellectual, developmental, genetic, or other conditions often have growth patterns that are different from those of healthy children. Their growth can also be plotted on the WHO growth charts alone or in conjunction with specific growth curves that exist for some of these disorders (Dietitians of Canada, 2014).

Children whose growth may be questionable include the following:

- Children whose height and weight percentiles are widely disparate (e.g., height in the tenth percentile and weight in the ninetieth percentile, especially with above-average skin fold thickness)
- Children who fail to show the expected growth rates in height and weight, especially during the rapid growth periods of infancy and adolescence
- Children who show a sudden increase (except during puberty) or decrease in a previously steady growth pattern

Because growth is a continuous but uneven process, the most reliable evaluation lies in comparing growth measurements over time. It is important to remember that normal growth patterns vary among children of the same age (Fig. 33-6).

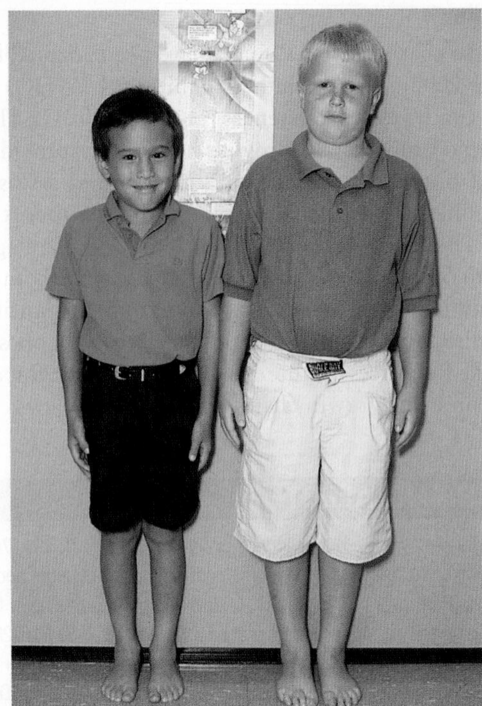

FIGURE 33-6 These children of identical age (8 years) are markedly different in size. The child on the left, of Asian descent, is at the fifth percentile for height and weight. The child on the right is above the ninety-fifth percentile for height and weight. However, both children demonstrate normal growth patterns.

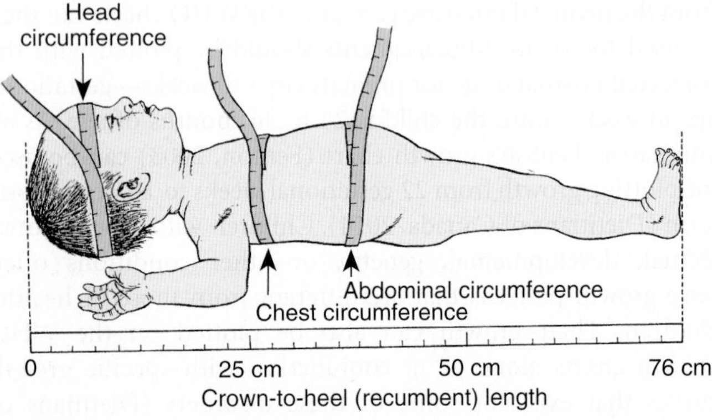

FIGURE 33-7 Measurement of head, chest, and abdominal circumference and crown-to-heel (recumbent) length.

Length

The term *length* refers to measurements taken when children are supine (also referred to as *recumbent length*). Until children are 24 months old (or 36 months if using the chart for birth to 36 months), recumbent length is measured. Because of the normally flexed position during infancy, the body should be fully extended by (1) holding the head in midline, (2) grasping the knees together gently, and (3) gently pushing down on the knees until the legs are fully extended and flat against the table. If using a measuring board, the nurse should place the head firmly at the top of the board and the heels of the feet firmly against the footboard.

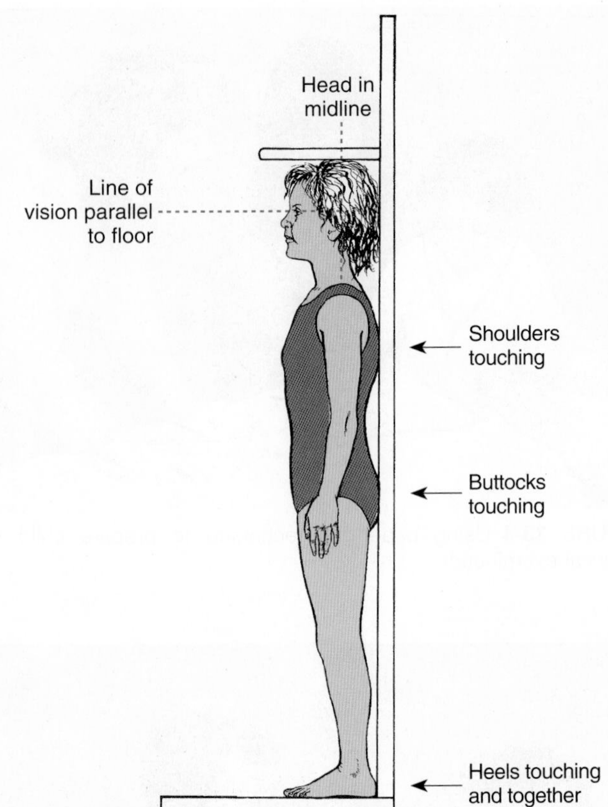

FIGURE 33-8 Measurement of height. (From Wilson, S. [2013]. *Health assessment for nursing practice* [5th ed.]. St. Louis: Mosby.)

If such a measuring device is not available, length can be measured by placing the child on a paper-covered surface, marking the end points of the top of the head and the heels of the feet, and measuring between these two points (Fig. 33-7). For accurate measurement, the nurse should hold the writing utensil at a right angle to the table when marking the cephalic point; the feet are positioned with the toes pointing directly to the ceiling when marking the heel point. Regardless of the method used, someone needs to assist the nurse in holding the child's head in midline while extending the legs and taking the measurements.

Height

The term *height* (or *stature*) refers to the measurement taken when children are standing upright. Height is measured by having the child, with shoes removed, stand as tall and straight as possible, with the head in midline and the line of vision parallel to the ceiling and floor. The child's back needs to be against the wall or other vertical flat surface, with the heels, buttocks, and back of the shoulders touching the wall and the medial malleoli touching, if possible (Fig. 33-8). The nurse should check for and correct bending of the knees, slumping of the shoulders, or raising of the heels.

For the most accurate measurement, a wall-mounted unit (stadiometer; see Fig. 33-8) can be used. The movable measuring rod of platform scales is accurate only if it maintains a parallel position to the floor and rests securely on the topmost part of the head. To improvise a flat surface for measuring length, the nurse should attach a paper or metal tape or yardstick to the wall, position the child adjacent to the tape, and place a three-dimensional object, such as a thick book or box, on top of the head. The side of the object should rest firmly against the wall to form a right angle. Length or stature should be measured to the nearest 1 mm.

Weight

Weight is measured with an appropriately sized beam balance scale, which measures weight to the nearest 10 g for infants and 100 g for children or using a digital scale. With a balance scale, before the child is weighed, the nurse needs to zero the scale prior to use. When precise measurements are needed, two nurses should take the weight independently; if there is a discrepancy, a third reading should be taken.

Measurements should be taken in a comfortably warm room. From birth to 36 months, children should be weighed nude. Older children are usually weighed while wearing their underpants or a light gown. However, the privacy of all children should always be respected. If the child must be weighed wearing some article of clothing or some type of special device, such as a prosthesis or an armboard for an intravenous device, the nurse needs to note this when recording the weight. Children who are measured for recumbent length are usually weighed on an infant platform scale and placed in a lying or sitting position. When weighing an infant, the nurse should place a hand lightly above the infant's body to prevent the child from accidentally falling off the scale (Fig. 33-9, A). When weighing a toddler, the nurse should stand close to the child, ready to prevent a fall (see Fig. 33-9, B). For maximum asepsis, the scale should be covered with a clean sheet of paper and cleaned between each child's measurement.

Skin Fold Thickness and Arm Circumference

Measures of relative weight and stature cannot distinguish between adipose (fat) tissue and muscle. One convenient measure of body fat is skin fold thickness, which is increasingly recommended as a routine measurement. Skin fold thickness is measured with special calipers, such as the Lange calipers. The most common sites for measuring skin fold thickness are the triceps (most practical for routine clinical use), subscapula, suprailiac, abdomen, and upper thigh. For greatest reliability, the nurse needs to follow the exact procedure for measurement and record the average of at least two measurements of one site.

Arm circumference is an indirect measure of muscle mass. Measurement of arm circumference follows the same procedure as that for skin fold thickness, except the midpoint is measured with a paper or steel tape. The tape is placed vertically, along the posterior aspect of the upper arm from the acromial process to the olecranon process; half the measured length is the midpoint.

Head Circumference

Head circumference in children is measured up to 36 months of age and in any child whose head size is questionable. The head is measured at its greatest circumference, usually slightly above the eyebrows and pinna of the ears and around the occipital prominence at the back of the skull (see Fig. 33-7). Because head shape can affect the location of the maximum circumference, more than one measurement at points above the eyebrows may be needed to obtain the most accurate measure. A paper or metal tape should be used, since a cloth tape can stretch and give a falsely small measurement. For greatest accuracy, devices with tenths of a centimetre are best, since the percentile charts have only 0.5-cm increments.

The nurse can plot the head size on the appropriate growth chart under head circumference. Generally, head and chest circumferences are equal at about 1 to 2 years of age. During childhood, chest circumference exceeds head size by about 5 to 7 cm. (For newborns, see Table 26-2.)

Vital Signs

Physiological measurements, key elements in evaluating physical status of vital functions, include temperature, pulse, respiration, and BP. Each physiological recording should be compared with normal values for that age group. In addition, the values taken on preceding health visits need to be compared with present recordings. For example, a falsely elevated BP reading may not indicate hypertension if previous recent readings have been

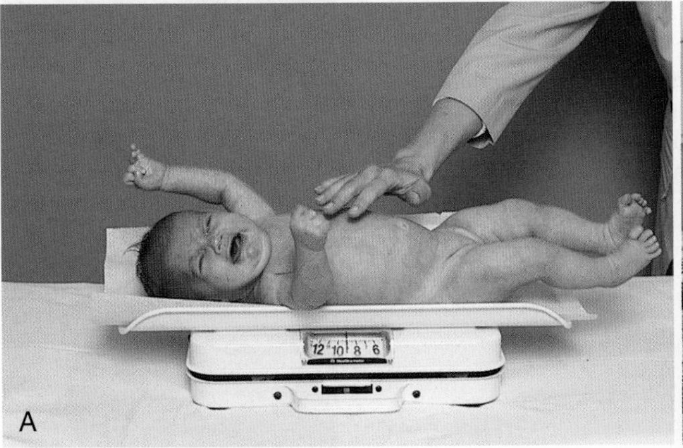

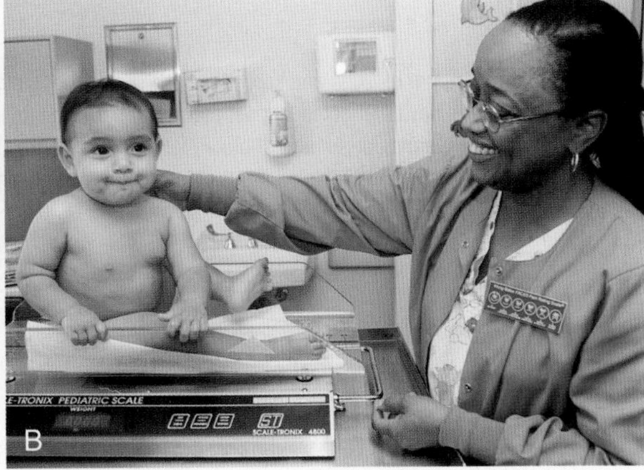

FIGURE 33-9 A: Infant on scale. **B:** Toddler on scale. Note presence of nurse to prevent falls. (**B,** Courtesy Paul Vincent Kuntz.)

ATRAUMATIC CARE

Reducing Young Children's Fears

Young children, especially preschoolers, fear intrusive procedures because of their poorly defined body boundaries. Therefore, avoid invasive procedures, such as measuring rectal temperature, whenever possible. Also, avoid using the word "take" when measuring vital signs, since young children interpret words literally and may think that their temperature or other function will be taken away. Instead, say, "I want to know how warm you are."

within normal limits. The isolated recording may indicate some stressful event in the child's life.

As in most procedures carried out with children, older children and adolescents are treated much the same as adults. However, special consideration must be given to preschool children (see Atraumatic Care box). For best results in taking vital signs of infants, the nurse should count respirations first (before the infant is disturbed), take the pulse next, and measure temperature last. If vital signs cannot be taken without disturbing the child, the nurse should record the child's behaviour, such as crying, along with the measurement.

Temperature

Temperature is the measure of heat content within an individual's body. The core temperature most closely reflects the temperature of the blood flow through the carotid arteries to the hypothalamus. Core temperature is relatively constant despite wide fluctuations in the external environment. When a child's temperature is altered, receptors in the skin, spinal cord, and brain respond in an attempt to achieve *normothermia*, a normal temperature state. In pediatrics, there is a lack of consensus on what temperature constitutes normothermia for every child. For rectal temperatures in children, 36.6°C to 38°C is an acceptable range, where heat loss and heat production are balanced (Leduc, Woods, & CPS Community Paediatrics Committee, 2000/2015). For newborns, an axillary temperature between 36.5° and 37.5°C (97.7° to 99.5°F) is a desirable range (see Chapter 26). In the newborn, temperature measurements are obtained for monitoring adequacy of thermoregulation, not fever; therefore, temperature measurements in each infant should be carefully considered in the context of the purpose and the environment. Temperature definitions of fever that are based on age are found in Table 33-4.

Temperature in healthy children can be measured at several body sites via the oral, rectal, axillary, ear canal, tympanic membrane, temporal artery, or skin route (Box 33-10). For the ill child, other sites for temperature measurement that have been used include the urinary bladder, pulmonary artery, and esophageal and nasopharyngeal sites (Box 33-11). One of the most important influences on the accuracy of temperature is improper temperature-taking technique. Detailed discussion of

TABLE 33-4 TEMPERATURE MEASUREMENT LOCATIONS FOR INFANTS AND CHILDREN

TEMPERATURE SITE

Oral

Place tip under tongue in right or left posterior sublingual pocket, not in front of tongue. Have child keep the mouth closed without biting on thermometer. Oral method is used only when a child is capable of holding onto a thermometer.

Pacifier thermometers measure intraoral or supralingual temperature and are available but lack support in the literature.

Several factors affect mouth temperature: eating and mastication, hot or cold beverages, open-mouth breathing, and ambient temperature.

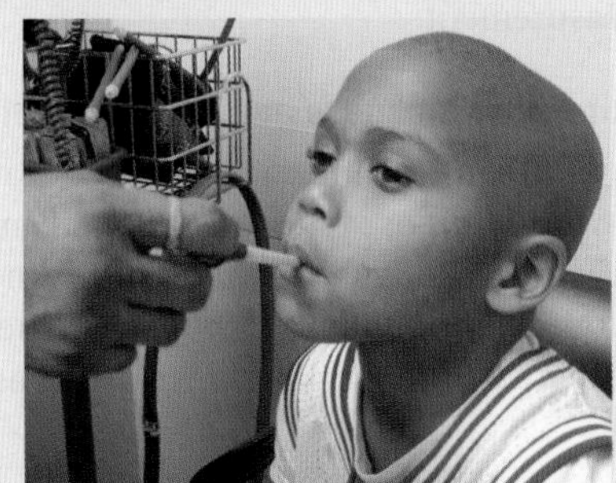

Axillary

Place tip under the arm in centre of axilla and keep close to the skin, not clothing. Hold child's arm firmly against side. Temperature may be affected by poor peripheral perfusion (results in lower value), clothing or swaddling, use of radiant warmer, or amount of brown fat in cold-stressed newborns (results in higher value).

The advantage is that use of this site avoids an intrusive procedure and eliminates the risk of rectal perforation.

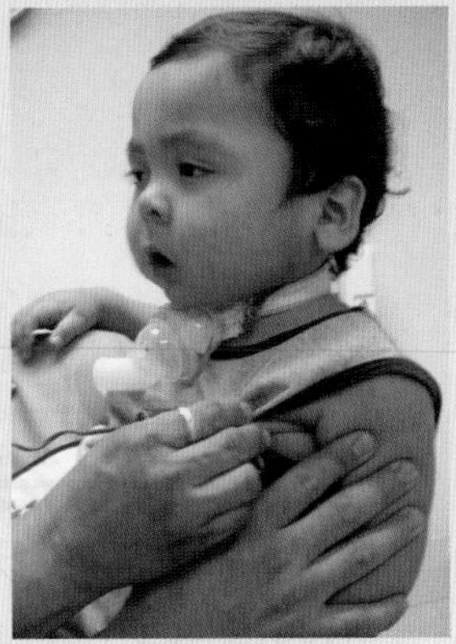

TABLE 33-4 TEMPERATURE MEASUREMENT LOCATIONS FOR INFANTS AND CHILDREN—cont'd

TEMPERATURE SITE

Ear Based (Aural)

Insert small infrared probe deeply into canal to allow sensor to obtain measurement. The size of probe (most are 8 mm) may influence accuracy of the result. In young children this may be a problem because of the small diameter of the canal. For proper placement of the ear, it is debated as to whether the pinna should be pulled in a manner similar to that used during otoscopy (see Fig. 33-23). Aural thermometers are not recommended for children under age 2 because of small diameter of ear canal, which makes the temperature more inaccurate.

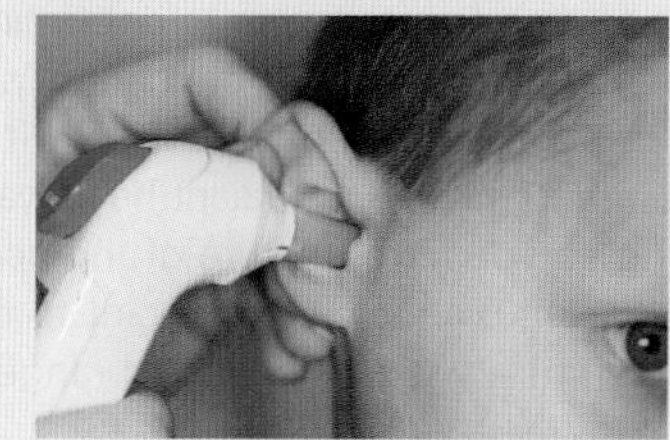

Rectal

Place well-lubricated tip at maximum 2.5 cm into rectum for children and 1.5 cm for infants; securely hold thermometer close to anus.

Child may be placed in side-lying, supine, or prone position (i.e., supine with knees flexed toward abdomen); cover the penis, since the procedure may stimulate urination. A small child may be placed prone across the parent's lap.

Rectal temperatures are slow to change in relation to changing core temperature. Rectal readings are affected by the depth of a measurement, conditions affecting local blood flow, and the presence of stool. Rectal perforation has occurred.

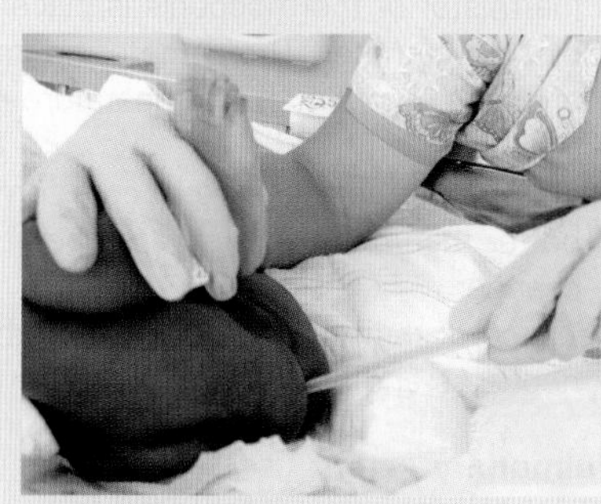

Temporal Artery

An infrared sensor probe scans across the forehead, capturing heat from arterial blood flow. The temporal artery is the only artery close enough to the skin's surface to provide access for accurate temperature measurement. A reading of 37.7°C or greater for fever in temporal measurement is equivalent to rectal temperature ≥38.3°C.

These probes have been shown to be more accurate than tympanic thermometry and are better tolerated than rectal thermometry. There is limited sensitivity in children younger than 3 years of age and as yet is not recommended for this age group.

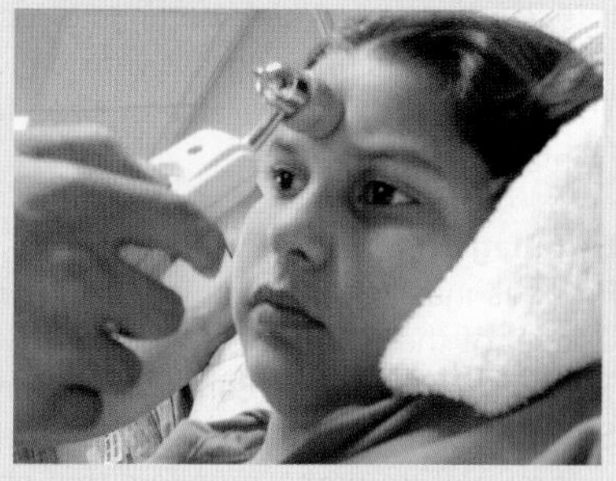

Oral, axillary, rectal, and temporal artery images courtesy Paul Vincent Kuntz.
Data from Leduc, D., Woods, S., & Canadian Paediatric Society, Community Paediatrics Committee. (2000). *Temperature measurement in paediatrics.* Reaffirmed 2015. Retrieved from http://www.cps.ca/documents/position/temperature-measurement

BOX 33-10 RECOMMENDED TEMPERATURE SCREENING ROUTES IN INFANTS AND CHILDREN

Birth to 2 Years
Axillary
Rectal—if definitive temperature reading is needed

2 to 5 Years
Oral—when a child is able to hold a thermometer under the tongue
Axillary
Tympanic or temporal artery—if in hospital for screening
Rectal—if definitive temperature reading is needed

Over 5 Years
Oral—definitive
Axillary, tympanic or temporal artery—if in hospital for screening

Adapted from Leduc, D., Woods, S., & Canadian Paediatric Society, Community Paediatrics Committee. (2000). *Temperature measurement in paediatrics.* Reaffirmed 2015. Retrieved from http://www.cps.ca/documents/position/temperature-measurement

BOX 33-11 ALTERNATIVE TEMPERATURE MEASUREMENT SITES FOR THE ILL CHILD

Skin

Probe is placed on the skin to determine heat output in response to changes in the patient's skin temperature.

Skin temperature sensors are most often used for neonates and infants placed in radiant heat warmers or isolettes (using servocontrol feature of the apparatus). In turn, the heater unit warms to a set point to maintain the infant's temperature within a specified range.

Urinary Bladder

A thermistor or thermocouple is placed within the in-dwelling bladder catheter. The catheter tip immersed in the bladder provides a continuous temperature readout on the bedside monitor.

This is not a true measure of core temperature but responds better than rectal and skin temperatures to core body changes.

Because of thermistor sizes, this method is unusable in neonates and small infants.

Pulmonary Artery

A catheter is placed into the heart to obtain a reading in the pulmonary artery.

It is used in critical care settings or operating rooms only in patients requiring aggressive monitoring.

The catheter is not available in sizes for neonates or small infants.

Esophageal Site

Probe is inserted into the lower third of the esophagus at the level of the heart.

This is used in critical care settings or operating rooms.

Several companies have esophageal stethoscopes with temperature probe monitors that show a continuous temperature reading for patients in the operating room.

Nasopharyngeal Site

Probe is inserted into the nasopharynx, posterior to the soft palate, and provides an estimate of hypothalamic temperature.

This is used in critical care settings or operating rooms.

Data from Kumar, P. R., Nisarga, R., & Gowda, B. (2004). Temperature monitoring in newborns using ThermoSpot. *Indian Journal of Pediatrics, 71*(9), 795–796; Martin, S. A., & Kline, A. M. (2004). Can there be a standard for temperature measurement in the pediatric intensive care unit? *AACN Clinical Issues, 15*(2), 254–266; Maxton, F. J., Justin, L., & Gilles, D. (2004). Estimating core temperature in infants and children after cardiac surgery: A comparison of six methods. *Journal of Advanced Nursing, 45*(2), 214–222.

temperature-taking methods and visual examples of proper techniques are shown in Table 33-4. For a critical review of the evidence on temperature-taking methods, see the Research Focus box.

Temperature depends on the time of day, age, and physical activity. In general, fever is defined as a temperature of 38°C or greater (100.4°F) rectally.

TABLE 33-5 NORMAL TEMPERATURE RANGES

MEASUREMENT METHOD	NORMAL TEMPERATURE RANGE
Rectal	36.6°C to 38°C (97.9°F to 100.4°F)
Ear	35.8°C to 38°C (96.4°F to 100.4°F)
Oral	35.5°C to 37.5°C (95.9°F to 99.5°F)
Axillary	36.5°C to 37.5°C (97.8°F to 99.5°F)

Data from Leduc, D., Woods, S., & Canadian Paediatric Society, Community Paediatrics Committee. (2000). *Temperature measurement in paediatrics.* Reaffirmed 2015. Retrieved from http://www.cps.ca/documents/position/temperature-measurement#ref38

The normal temperature ranges from the Canadian Paediatric Society are listed in Table 33-5.

The most frequently used temperature measurement devices in infant and children include the following:

Electronic intermittent thermometers—Measure the patient's temperature at oral, rectal, and axillary sites and are used as primary diagnostic indicators

Infrared thermometers—Measure the patient's temperature by collecting emitted thermal radiation from a particular site (e.g., ear canal)

Electronic continuous thermometers—Measure the patient's temperature during the administration of general anaesthesia, treatment of hypothermia or hyperthermia, and other situations that require continuous monitoring

Box 33-12 provides a detailed description of these devices.

! NURSING ALERT

The belief that core temperature can be estimated by adding 1°C to the temperature taken in the axilla is incorrect. Do not add a degree to the finding obtained by taking a temperature by the axillary route.

Pulse

A satisfactory pulse can be taken radially in children older than 2 years of age. However, in infants and young children, the apical impulse (heard through a stethoscope held to the chest at the apex of the heart) is more reliable (see Fig. 33-31 for location of apical pulse). The pulse is counted for 1 full minute in infants and young children because of possible irregularities in rhythm. However, when frequent apical rates are needed, shorter counting times (e.g., 15- or 30-second intervals) can be used. Pulses may be graded according to the criteria in Table 33-6. Radial and femoral pulses need to be compared at least once during infancy to detect the presence of circulatory impairment, such as coarctation of the aorta. (See Appendix E for normal rates for pediatric age groups.)

Respiration

The respiratory rate in children is measured in the same manner as for the adult patient. However, in newborns and infants, respirations are auscultated at the same time as observing the abdomen for movement, since respirations are primarily diaphragmatic. Because the movements are irregular, they

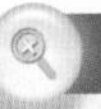

RESEARCH FOCUS

Temperature Measurement in Pediatrics

Ask the Question

In infants and children, what is the most accurate method for measuring temperature in febrile children?

Search for Evidence

Search Strategies

Clinical research strategies related to this issue were identified by searching for English-language publications for infants and children populations; comparisons to gold standard: rectal thermometry

Databases Used

PubMed, Cochrane Collaboration, MD Consult, Joanna Briggs Institute, National Guideline Clearinghouse (AHRQ), TRIP Database Plus, PedsCCM, BestBETs

Critically Analyze the Evidence

Rectal temperature—Rectal measurement remains the clinical gold standard for the precise diagnosis of fever in infants and children compared with other methods (Fortuna, Carney, Macy, et al., 2010; Greenes & Fleisher, 2004; Holzhauer, Reith, Sawin, et al., 2009; Riddell & Eppich, 2003; University of Michigan, 2003). However, this procedure is more invasive and is contraindicated for infants less than 1 month old in some agencies, children with recent rectal surgery, children with diarrhea or anorectal lesions, and children receiving chemotherapy (cancer treatment usually affects mucosa and causes neutropenia). The Canadian Paediatric Society (CPS) (Leduc, Woods, & CPS Community Paediatrics Committee, 2000/2015) recommends rectal measurement from birth to 2 years of age for high-risk screening.

Oral temperature (OT)—OT indicates rapid changes in core body temperature, but accuracy may be an issue when compared with that using the rectal site (Jensen, Jensen, Madsen, et al., 2000). OT is considered the standard for temperature measurement (Gilbert, Barton, & Counsell, 2002) but is contraindicated in children who have an altered level of consciousness, are receiving oxygen, are mouth breathing, are experiencing mucositis, had recent oral surgery or trauma, or are under 2 years of age (El-Radhi & Barry, 2006). Limitations of OT include the effect of ambient room temperature and recent oral intake (Martin & Kline, 2004).

Axillary temperature—In newborns with fever, the axillary temperature cannot be used interchangeably with rectal measurement (Muller, Van Berkel, & de Beaufort, 2008). Despite its low sensitivity and specificity in detecting fever, the axillary site is recommended by the CPS (Leduc et al., 2000/2015) as a low screening test for fever in children from birth to 2 years of age.

Ear (aural) temperature—This is not a precise measurement of body temperature. Meta-analysis of 101 studies comparing tympanic membrane temperatures with rectal temperatures in children concluded that the tympanic method demonstrated a wide range of variability, limiting its application in a pediatric setting (Craig, Lancaster, Taylor, et al., 2002). Other published reviews continue to find poor sensitivity using infrared ear thermometry (Devrim, Kara, Ceyhan, et al., 2007; Dodd, Lancaster, Craig, et al., 2006). Diagnosis of fever without a focus should not be made on the basis of tympanic thermometry, since it is not an accurate measure of core temperature (Craig et al., 2002; Devrim et al., 2007; Dodd et al., 2006).

Temporal artery temperature (TAT)—TAT was not predictable in the assessment of fever in children under 3 months of age but could be used as a screening tool for detecting fever less than 38°C in children 3 months to 4 years of age (Al-Mukhaizeem, Allen, Komar, et al., 2004; Callanan, 2003; Fortuna et al., 2010; Greenes & Fleisher, 2001; Hebbar, Fortenberry, Rogers, et al., 2005; Holzhauer et al., 2009; Schuh, Komar, Stephens, et al., 2004; Siberry, Diener-West, Schappell, et al., 2002; & Titus, Hulsey, Heckman, et al., 2009).

Apply the Evidence: Nursing Implications

No single site used for temperature assessment provides unequivocal estimates of core body temperature.

Studies show that the axillary and tympanic measures demonstrate poor agreement when these modes are compared with more accurate core temperature methods. The differences are more evident as temperature increases, regardless of age.

TAT is not predictable for fever and should be used only as a screening tool in young children over 2 years of age.

When an accurate method of obtaining a correct reflection of core temperature is needed, the rectal temperature is recommended in younger children and the oral route in older children. For infants less than 1 month of age, the CPS (Leduc et al., 2000/2015) recommends axillary temperatures for low-risk screening.

References

Al-Mukhaizeem, F., Allen, U., Komar, L., et al. (2004). Comparison of temporal artery, rectal and esophageal core temperatures in children: Results of a pilot study. *Paediatrics and Child Health, 9*(7), 461–465.

Callanan, D. (2003). Detecting fever in young infants: Reliability of perceived, pacifier, and temporal artery temperatures in infants younger than 3 months of age. *Pediatric Emergency Care, 19*(4), 240–243.

Craig, J. V., Lancaster, G. A., Taylor, S., et al. (2002). Infrared ear thermometry compared with rectal thermometry in children: A systemic review. *Lancet, 360*, 603–609.

Devrim, I., Kara, A., Ceyhan, M., et al. (2007). Measurement accuracy of fever by tympanic and axillary thermometry. *Pediatric Emergency Care, 23*(1), 16–19.

Dodd, S. R., Lancaster, G. A., Craig, J. V., et al. (2006). In a systematic review, infrared ear thermometry for fever diagnosis in children finds poor sensitivity. *Journal of Clinical Epidemiology, 59*, 354–357.

El-Radhi, A. S., & Barry, W. (2006). Thermometry in paediatric practice. *Archives of Diseases in Childhood, 91*(4), 351–356.

Fortuna, E. L., Carney, M. M., Macy, M., et al. (2010). Accuracy of non-contact infrared thermometry versus rectal thermometry in young children evaluated in the emergency department for fever. *Journal of Emergency Nursing, 36*(2), 101–104. doi:10.1016/j.jen.2009.07.017.

Gilbert, M., Barton, A. J., & Counsell, C. M. (2002). Comparison of oral and tympanic temperatures in adult surgical patients. *Applied Nursing Research, 15*(1), 42–47.

Greenes, D. S., & Fleisher, G. R. (2001). Accuracy of a noninvasive temporal artery thermometer for use in infants. *Archives of Pediatrics and Adolescent Medicine, 155*(3), 376–381.

Greenes, D. S., & Fleisher, G. R. (2004). When body temperature changes, does rectal temperature lag? *Journal of Pediatrics, 144*(6), 824–826.

Hebbar, K., Fortenberry, J. D., Rogers, K., et al. (2005). Comparison of temporal artery thermometer to standard temperature measurement in pediatric intensive care unit patients. *Pediatric Critical Care Medicine, 6*(5), 557–561.

Holzhauer, J. K., Reith, V., Sawin, K. J., & Yen, K. (2009). Evaluation of temporal artery thermometry in children 3–36 months old. *Journal for Specialists in Pediatric Nursing, 14*, 239–244. doi:10.1111/j.1744-6155.2009.00204.x.

Jensen, B. N., Jensen, F. S., Madsen, S. N., et al. (2000). Accuracy of digital tympanic, oral, axillary, and rectal thermometers compared with standard rectal mercury thermometers. *European Journal of Surgery, 166*(11), 848–851.

Leduc, D., Woods, S., & Canadian Paediatric Society, Community Paediatrics Committee (2000). *Temperature measurement in paediatrics.* Reaffirmed in 2015. Retrieved from <http://www.cps.ca/documents/position/temperature-measurement#ref38>.

Martin, S. A., & Kline, A. M. (2004). Can there be a standard for temperature measurement in the pediatric intensive care unit? *AACN Clinical Issues, 15*(2), 254–266.

Muller, P. C. E., Van Berkel, L. H., & de Beaufort, A. J. (2008). Axillary and rectal temperature measurements poorly agree in newborn infants. *Neonatology, 94*, 31–34.

Riddell, A., & Eppich, W. (2003). *Should tympanic temperature measurement be trusted? BestBETs.* Retrieved from <http://www.bestbets.org/cgi-bin/bets.pl?record=00340>.

Schuh, S., Komar, L., Stephens, D., et al. (2004). Comparison of the temporal artery and rectal thermometry in children in the emergency department. *Pediatric Emergency Care, 20*(11), 736–741.

Siberry, G. K., Diener-West, M., Schappell, E., et al. (2002). Comparison of temple temperatures with rectal temperatures in children under 2 years of age. *Clinical Pediatrics, 41*(6), 405–414.

Titus, M. O., Hulsey, T., Heckman, J., & Losek, J. D. (2009). Temporal artery thermometry utilization in pediatric emergency care. *Clinical Pediatrics (Philadelphia), 48*(2), 190–193. doi:10.1177/0009922808327056.

BOX 33-12 TYPES OF THERMOMETERS USED TO MEASURE TEMPERATURE IN INFANTS AND CHILDREN

Electronic Thermometer

Temperature is sensed with an electronic component called a thermistor, which is mounted at the tip of a plastic and stainless steel probe and is connected to an electronic recorder. A disposable plastic cover is used for infection control.

Temperature measurement appears on a digital display within 60 seconds.

Probe can be placed in the mouth, axilla, or rectum.

Infrared Thermometer

Thermal radiation is measured from the axilla, ear canal, or tympanic membrane.

Temperature measurement appears on a digital display in approximately 1 second.

Three types are available for ear-based use: tympanic, ear canal, and arterial heat balance via the ear canal (AHBE).

Often these devices are all inappropriately referred to as tympanic thermometers.

Temperatures measured in this way reflect arterial (bloodstream) temperature.

Ear-Based Temperature Sensor

Although this is frequently used in pediatric settings (especially ambulatory clinics), debate still continues on the reliability of ear-based thermometry in screening febrile children.

Most models use "offsets" for internal calculations that transform ear temperature into supposedly equivalent oral or rectal temperatures.

Ear Sensor (LighTouch LTX)

This measures the infrared heat energy radiating from the canal opening, scans the canal for the highest temperature reading, and then calculates the arterial temperature (which correlates highly with core or internal body temperature).

It is available in two sizes; the smaller size of LighTouch Pedi-Q is for infants and toddlers.

Axillary Sensor (LighTouch LTN)

This measures the infrared heat energy radiating from the axilla.

It can be used on wet skin; in incubators; or under radiant heaters, warming pads, or other heat sources.

Digital Thermometer

Probe is connected to a microprocessor chip, which translates signals into degrees and sends temperature measurement to a digital display.

It is used like an oral electronic thermometer and can be used for measuring oral, rectal, and axillary temperature.

It is more accurate and easier to read, but somewhat more expensive than a plastic strip thermometer.

Liquid Crystal Skin Contact Thermometer (Chemical Dot Thermometer)

This single-use, disposable, flexible thermometer has a specific chemical mixture in each circle that changes colour to measure temperature increments of 2/10 of a degree.

There are two types:

1. Kept in mouth (1 minute), axilla (3 minutes), or rectum (3 minutes); colour change is read 10 to 15 seconds after removing thermometer
2. Wearable, continuous-use thermometer, which is placed in the axilla; may be read within 2 to 3 minutes after placement and continuously thereafter; discard and replace every 48 hours

TABLE 33-6 GRADING OF PULSES

GRADE	DESCRIPTION
0	Not palpable
+1	Difficult to palpate, thready, weak, easily obliterated with pressure
+2	Difficult to palpate, may be obliterated with pressure
+3	Easy to palpate, not easily obliterated with pressure (normal)
+4	Strong, bounding, not obliterated with pressure

should be counted for 1 full minute for accuracy (see also Appendix E).

Blood Pressure

BP measurement by noninvasive methods is part of a routine vital sign determination. Routine yearly BP screening in the pediatric population to reduce the risk of cardiovascular disease is not supported by adequate evidence. However, the American Medical Association, American Academy of Pediatrics, and the American Heart Association recommend yearly BP screenings to detect early, treatable causes of secondary hypertension (CPS, 2010; Van Cleave, Heisler, Devries, et al., 2007). See Appendix E for parameters on what BP values require further evaluation.

Measurement devices. BP monitoring in children and adolescents is a valuable method for assessing and managing suspected hypertension. BP can also be measured using electronic devices that employ oscillometric or Doppler techniques. In oscillometry, pressure changes are transmitted through the arterial wall to the pressure cuff, and the oscillations are detected by a pressure-sensitive indicator. Oscillometers have digital readouts for systolic, diastolic, and mean arterial pressures (MAP) and for pulse. The MAP is not the same as the mean BP (arithmetic average of systolic and diastolic pressures). Rather, it is a value somewhat lower than the arithmetic mean. The oscillometric BP monitoring method is a reliable screening tool used in a variety of age groups (Midgley, Wardhaugh, Macfarlane, et al., 2009). See Appendix E for pediatric parameters of blood pressure values.

Doppler ultrasound translates changes in ultrasound frequency caused by blood movement within the artery to audible sound by means of a transducer in the cuff. This technique is useful for systolic pressure measurement but is unreliable for diastolic pressure measurement. Oscillometric and Doppler instruments are useful in measuring BP in infants and have largely replaced the flush method, which reflects only the mean BP, and the auscultatory method.

Selection of cuff. No matter what type of noninvasive technique is used, the most important factor in accurately measuring BP is the use of an appropriately sized cuff (cuff size refers only to the inner inflatable bladder, not the cloth covering). A technique to establish an appropriate cuff size is to choose a cuff having a bladder width that is approximately 40% of the arm circumference midway between the olecranon and the acromion. This will usually be a cuff bladder that covers 80 to 100% of the circumference of the arm (Fig. 33-10). Cuffs that are either too narrow or too wide affect the accuracy of BP measurements. If the cuff size is too small, the reading on the device is falsely high. If the cuff size is too large, the reading is falsely low (Table 33-7).

Using limb circumference for selecting cuff width more accurately reflects direct arterial BP than using limb length, since this method takes into account variations in arm thickness and the amount of pressure required to compress the artery. For measurement sites other than the upper arms, the limb circumference guidelines can be used, although the shape of the limb (e.g., conical shape of the thigh) may prevent appropriate placement of the cuff and inaccurately reflect intra-arterial BP.

When another site is used, BP measurements using noninvasive techniques may differ. Generally, systolic pressure in the lower extremities (thigh or calf) is greater than pressure in the upper extremities, and systolic BP in the calf is higher than that in the thigh, although diastolic pressure should be similar (Fig. 33-11). These differences are listed in Table 33-8 and apply to oscillometric measurements taken on the right extremities with the child supine and the cuff size, based on the circumference method.

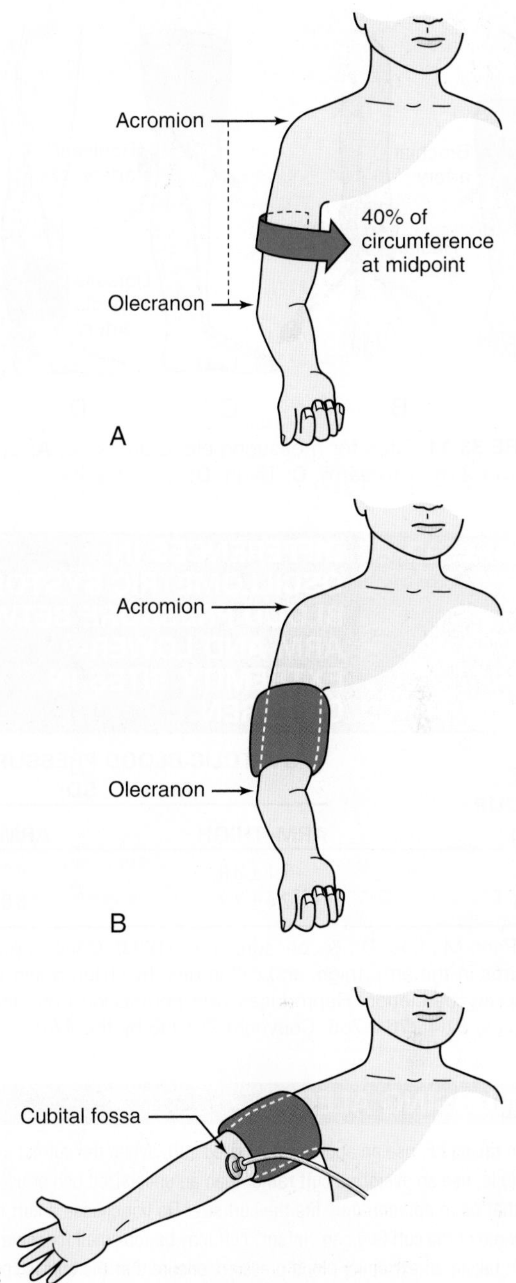

FIGURE 33-10 Determination of proper cuff size. **A:** Cuff bladder width should be approximately 40% of circumference of arm measured at a point midway between olecranon and acromion. **B:** Cuff bladder length should cover 80 to 100% of circumference of arm. **C:** Blood pressure should be measured with cubital fossa at heart level. The arm should be supported. The stethoscope bell is placed over brachial artery pulse, proximal and medial to cubital fossa and below bottom edge of cuff. (From National Institutes of Health, National Heart, Lung, and Blood Institute. [1996, September]. Update on the Task Force Report [1987] on high blood pressure in children and adolescents: A working group report from the National High Blood Pressure Education Program [NIH Pub No 96-3790]. Bethesda, MD: Author.)

TABLE 33-7 RECOMMENDED DIMENSIONS FOR BLOOD PRESSURE CUFF BLADDERS

AGE RANGE	WIDTH (CM)	LENGTH (CM)	MAXIMUM ARM CIRCUMFERENCE (CM)*
Newborn	4	8	10
Infant	6	12	15
Child	9	18	22
Small adult	10	24	26
Adult	13	30	34
Large adult	16	38	44
Thigh	20	42	52

*Calculated so that largest arm would still allow bladder to encircle arm by at least 80%.

From National High Blood Pressure Education Program Working Group on High Blood Pressure in Children and Adolescents. (2004). The fourth report on the diagnosis, evaluation, and treatment of high blood pressure in children and adolescents. Reproduced with permission from Journal *Pediatrics, 114*(2 Suppl 4th Rep), 555–576. Copyright © 2004 by the AAP.

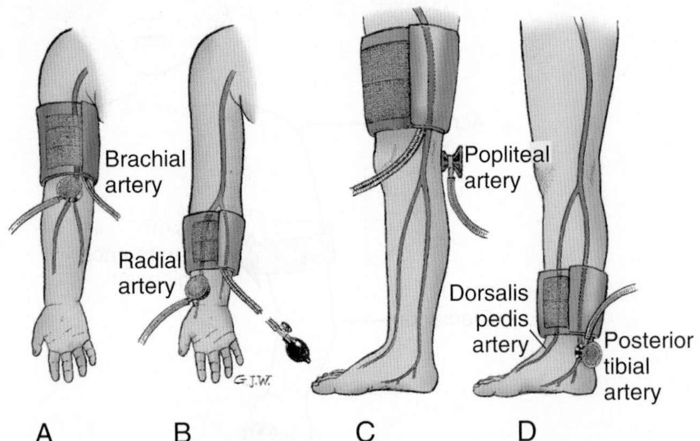

FIGURE 33-11 Sites for measuring blood pressure. **A:** Upper arm. **B:** Lower arm or forearm. **C:** Thigh. **D:** Calf or ankle.

TABLE 33-8 DIFFERENCES IN OSCILLOMETRIC SYSTOLIC BLOOD PRESSURE BETWEEN ARM AND LOWER-EXTREMITY SITES IN CHILDREN

AGE GROUP (YR)	SYSTOLIC BLOOD PRESSURE × (MEAN ± SD)	
	ARM–THIGH	ARM–CALF
4–8	−7.1 ± 6.8	−9.3 ± 7.4
9–16	−2.4 ± 7.7	−5.0 ± 26.9

From Park, M., Lee, D., & Johnson, G. A. (1993). Oscillometric blood pressures in the arm, thigh, and calf in healthy children and those with aortic coarctation. Reproduced with permission from Journal *Pediatrics, 91*(4), 761–765. Copyright © 1993 by the AAP.

! NURSING ALERT

When taking BP, use an appropriately sized cuff. When the correct size is not available, use an oversized cuff rather than an undersized one or use another site that more appropriately fits the cuff size. Do not choose a cuff based on the name of the cuff (e.g., an "infant" cuff may be too small for some infants). When taking an extremity blood pressure, ensure that the cuff is specific for taking extremity blood pressure measurements.

! NURSING ALERT

Comparing BP in the upper and lower extremities will help detect abnormalities, such as coarctation of the aorta, in which the lower extremity pressure is less than the upper extremity pressure.

Measurement and interpretation. Measuring and interpreting BP in infants and children requires additional attention to correct procedure because (1) limb sizes vary and cuff selection must accommodate the circumference; (2) excessive pressure on the antecubital fossa affects the Korotkoff sounds; (3) children easily become anxious, which can elevate BP; and (4) BP values change with age and growth. In children and adolescents, the normal range of BP is determined by body size and age. BP standards that are based on gender, age, and height provide a more precise classification of BP according to body size. This approach avoids misclassifying children who are very tall or very short. See Appendix E for BP measurements that require further investigation based on age and gender.

Orthostatic hypotension. Orthostatic hypotension (OH), also called *postural hypotension* or *orthostatic intolerance*, is often manifested as syncope (fainting), vertigo (dizziness), or lightheadedness and is caused by decreased blood flow to the brain (cerebral hypoperfusion). Normally, blood flow to the brain is maintained at a constant level by a number of compensating mechanisms that regulate systemic BP. When one assumes a sitting or standing position from a supine or recumbent position, peripheral capillary vasoconstriction occurs, and blood that was pooling in the lower vasculature is returned to the heart for redistribution to the head and remainder of the body. When this mechanism fails or is slow to respond, the person may experience vertigo or syncope. One of the most common causes of OH is hypovolemia, which may be induced by medications such as diuretics, vasodilators, and prolonged immobility or bedrest. Other causes of OH include dehydration, diarrhea, emesis, fluid loss from sweating and exertion, alcohol intake, dysrhythmias, diabetes mellitus, sepsis, and hemorrhage.

BP measurements taken with the child supine then standing (at least 2 minutes in each position) may demonstrate variability and assist in the diagnosis of OH. The child with a sustained drop in systolic pressure of more than 20 mm Hg or in diastolic pressure of more than 10 mm Hg after standing for 2 minutes without an increase in heart rate of more than 15 beats/min most likely has an autonomic deficit. Non-neurogenic causes of OH have a compensatory increase in pulse of more than 15 beats/min as well as a drop in BP, as noted previously. For the child or adolescent who is seen with vertigo, lightheadedness, nausea, syncope, diaphoresis, and pallor, it is important to monitor BP and heart rate to determine the original cause. BP is an important diagnostic measurement in children and adolescents and must be a part of the routine monitoring of vital signs.

General Appearance

The child's general appearance is a cumulative, subjective impression of the child's physical appearance, state of nutrition, behaviour, personality, interactions with parents and nurse (also siblings if present), posture, development, and speech. Although general appearance is recorded at the beginning of the physical examination, it encompasses all the observations of the child during the interview and physical assessment.

The nurse should note the facies (the child's facial expression and appearance). For example, the facies may give clues to children who are in pain; have difficulty breathing; feel frightened, discontented, or unhappy; are emotionally delayed; or are acutely ill.

The posture, position, and types of body movement should also be observed. The child with hearing or vision loss may characteristically tilt the head in an awkward position to hear or see better. The child in pain may favour a body part. The child with low self-esteem or a feeling of rejection may assume

TABLE 33-9 DIFFERENCES IN COLOUR CHANGES OF RACIAL GROUPS

DESCRIPTION	APPEARANCE IN LIGHT SKIN	APPEARANCE IN DARK SKIN
Cyanosis—Bluish tone through skin; reflects reduced (deoxygenated) hemoglobin	Bluish tinge, especially in palpebral conjunctiva (lower eyelid), nail beds, earlobes, lips, oral membranes, soles, and palms	Ashen grey lips and tongue
Pallor—Paleness; may be sign of anemia, chronic disease, edema, or shock	Loss of rosy glow in skin, especially face	Ashen grey appearance in black skin More yellowish brown colour in brown skin
Erythema—Redness; may be result of increased blood flow from climatic conditions, local inflammation, infection, skin irritation, allergy, or other dermatoses, or may be caused by increased numbers of red blood cells as compensatory response to chronic hypoxia	Redness easily seen anywhere on body	Much more difficult to assess; rely on palpation for warmth or edema
Ecchymosis—Large, diffuse areas, usually black and blue, caused by hemorrhage of blood into skin; typically result of injuries	Purplish to yellow-green areas; may be seen anywhere on skin	Very difficult to see unless in mouth or conjunctiva
Petechiae—Same as ecchymosis except for size: small, distinct, pinpoint hemorrhages ≤2 mm in size; can denote some type of blood disorder, such as leukemia	Purplish pinpoints most easily seen on buttocks, abdomen, and inner surfaces of arms or legs	Usually invisible except in oral mucosa, conjunctiva of eyelids, and conjunctiva covering eyeball
Jaundice—Yellow staining of skin usually caused by bile pigments	Yellow staining seen in sclerae of eyes, skin, fingernails, soles, palms, and oral mucosa	Most reliably assessed in sclerae, hard palate, palms, and soles

a slumped, careless, and apathetic pose. Likewise, a child with confidence, a feeling of self-worth, and a sense of security usually demonstrates a tall, straight, well-balanced posture. While observing such body language, the nurse should not interpret too freely but rather record objectively.

The child's hygiene is noted in terms of cleanliness; unusual body odour; the condition of the hair, neck, nails, teeth, and feet; and the condition of the clothing. Such observations are excellent clues to possible instances of neglect, inadequate financial resources for child care, housing difficulties (e.g., no running water), or lack of knowledge concerning children's needs.

Behaviour includes the child's personality, activity level, reaction to stress, requests, frustration, interactions with others (primarily the parent and nurse), degree of alertness, and response to stimuli. Some questions the nurse can keep in mind that serve as reminders for observing behaviour include:

- What is the child's overall personality?
- Does the child have a long attention span, or is he or she easily distracted?
- Can the child follow two or three commands in succession without the need for repetition?
- What is the youngster's response to delayed gratification or frustration?
- Does the child use eye contact during conversation?
- What is the child's reaction to the nurse and family members?
- Is the child quick or slow to grasp explanations?

Skin

Skin is assessed for colour, texture, temperature, moisture, and turgor. Examination of the skin and its accessory organs primarily involves inspection and palpation. Touch allows the nurse to assess the texture, turgor, and temperature of the skin. The normal colour in light-skinned children varies from a milky white and rose to a deeply hued pink. Dark-skinned children, such as those of Aboriginal, Latin American, or African descent, have inherited various brown, red, yellow, olive green, and bluish tones in their skin. Asian persons have skin that is normally of a yellow tone. Several variations in skin colour can occur, some of which warrant further investigation. The types of colour change and their appearance in children with light or dark skin are summarized in Table 33-9.

Normally the skin texture of young children is smooth, slightly dry, and not oily or clammy. Skin temperature is evaluated by symmetrically feeling each part of the body and comparing upper areas with lower ones. Note any difference in temperature.

Tissue turgor, or elasticity in the skin, can be determined by grasping the skin on the abdomen between the thumb and index finger, pulling it taut, and quickly releasing it. Elastic tissue immediately assumes its normal position without residual marks or creases. In children with poor skin turgor, the skin remains suspended or tented for a few seconds before slowly falling back on the abdomen. Skin turgor is one of the best estimates of adequate hydration and nutrition.

Accessory Structures

Inspection of the accessory structures of the skin may be performed while the skin is being examined or when the scalp and extremities are being assessed.

The hair is inspected for colour, texture, quality, distribution, and elasticity. Children's scalp hair is usually lustrous, silky, strong, and elastic. Genetic factors affect the appearance of hair. For example, the hair of Black children is usually curlier and coarser than that of White children. Hair that is stringy, dull, brittle, dry, friable, and depigmented may suggest poor nutrition. The nurse should record any bald or thinning spots. Loss of hair in infants may indicate lying in the same position and may be a clue for counselling parents concerning the child's stimulation needs.

The hair and scalp are inspected for general cleanliness. Persons in various ethnic groups condition their hair with oils or lubricants that, if not thoroughly washed from the scalp, can clog the sebaceous glands, causing scalp infections. The area should also be examined for lesions; scaliness; evidence of infestation, such as lice or ticks; and signs of trauma, such as ecchymosis, masses, or scars.

In children who are approaching puberty, the nurse should look for growth of secondary hair as a sign of normally progressing pubertal changes. Precocious or delayed appearance of hair growth should be noted because, although not always suggestive of hormonal dysfunction, it may be of great concern to the early- or late-maturing adolescent.

The nails are inspected for colour, shape, texture, and quality. Normally the nails are pink, convex, smooth, and hard but flexible (not brittle). The edges, which are usually white, should extend over the fingers. Dark-skinned individuals may have more deeply pigmented nail beds. Short, ragged nails are typical of habitual biting.

The palm normally shows three flexion creases (Fig. 33-12, A). In some situations, such as Down syndrome, the two distal horizontal creases are fused to form a single horizontal crease (the single palmar crease, or transpalmar crease, called a *Simian crease*) (see Fig. 33-12, B). If grossly abnormal lines or folds are observed, the nurse should sketch a picture to describe them and refer the finding to a specialist for further investigation.

Lymph Nodes

Lymph nodes are usually assessed when the part of the body in which they are located is examined. The body's lymphatic drainage system is extensive; the usual sites for palpating accessible lymph nodes are shown in Figure 33-13.

Nodes are palpated using the distal portion of the fingers and gently but firmly pressing in a circular motion along the regions where nodes are normally present. During assessment of the nodes in the head and neck, the child's head is tilted upward slightly but without tensing the sternocleidomastoid or trapezius muscles. This position facilitates palpation of the submental, submandibular, tonsillar, and cervical nodes. The nurse should palpate the axillary nodes with the child's arms relaxed at the sides but slightly abducted. The inguinal nodes are assessed with the child in the supine position. The nurse needs to note size, mobility, temperature, and tenderness, as well as reports by the parents regarding any visible change of enlarged nodes. In children, small, nontender, movable nodes are usually normal. Tender, enlarged, warm lymph nodes generally indicate infection or inflammation close to

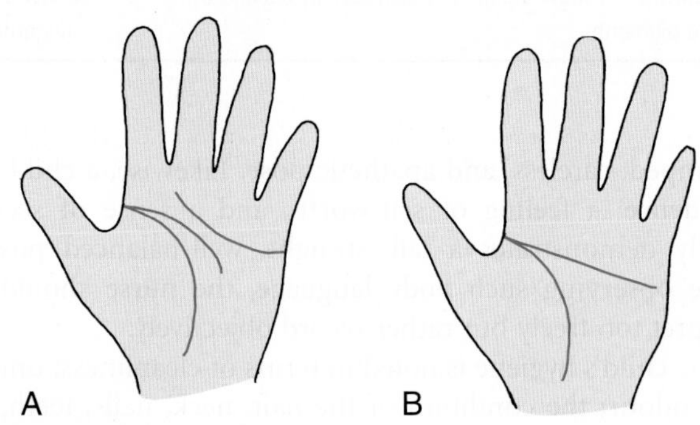

FIGURE 33-12 Examples of flexion creases on palm. **A:** Normal. **B:** Transpalmar crease.

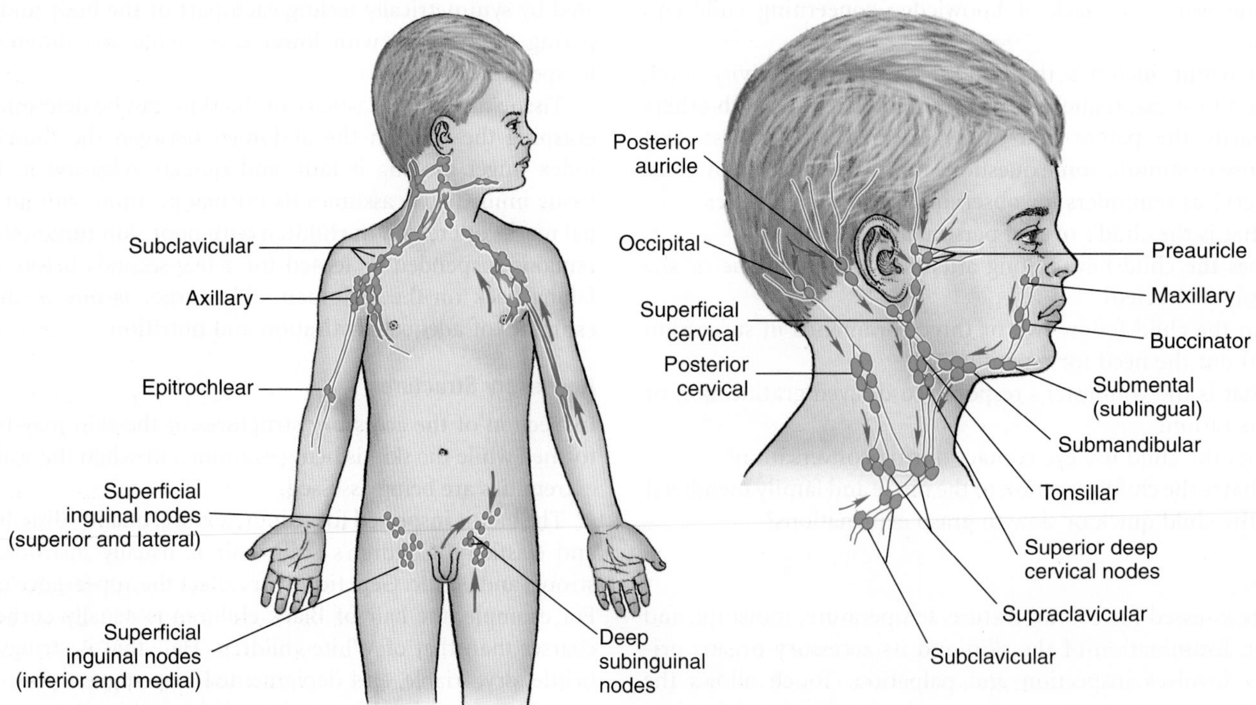

FIGURE 33-13 Location of superficial lymph nodes. *Arrows* indicate directional flow of lymph.

their location. Such findings need to be reported for further investigation.

Head and Neck

The head is observed for general shape and symmetry. A flattening of one part of the head, such as the occiput, may indicate that the child continually lies in this position. Marked asymmetry is usually abnormal and may indicate premature closure of the sutures (craniosynostosis).

NURSING ALERT

Significant head lag after 6 months of age strongly indicates cerebral injury and is referred for further evaluation.

The nurse should note head control in infants and head posture in older children. Most infants by 4 months of age should be able to hold the head erect and in midline when in a vertical position.

Range of motion is evaluated by asking the older child to look in each direction (to either side, up, and down) or by manually putting the younger child through each position. Limited range of motion may indicate wryneck, or torticollis, in which the child holds the head to one side with the chin pointing toward the opposite side as a result of injury to the sternocleidomastoid muscle.

NURSING ALERT

Hyperextension of the head (opisthotonos) with pain on flexion is a serious indication of meningeal irritation and needs to be referred for immediate medical evaluation.

The skull is palpated for patent sutures, fontanels, fractures, and swellings. Normally the posterior fontanel closes by the second month of life, and the anterior fontanel fuses between 12 and 18 months of age. When lightly palpated, the fontanels normally feel firm and very slightly curved inward to the touch. The fontanels may look like they are bulging when an infant is crying, or vomiting. However, they should return to normal when the infant is in a calm, head-up position. A tense or bulging fontanel occurs when fluid builds up in the brain or the brain swells, causing increased pressure inside the skull, and a depressed fontanel can indicate dehydration. Early or late closure should be noted, since either may be a sign of a pathological condition.

While examining the head, the nurse should observe the face for symmetry, movement, and general appearance. The nurse should ask the child to "make a face," to assess symmetrical movement and disclose any degree of paralysis. Any unusual facial proportion, such as an unusually high or low forehead; wide- or close-set eyes; or a small, receding chin needs to be noted.

In addition to assessment of the head and neck for movement, the neck is inspected for size and its associated structures palpated. The neck is normally short, with skin folds between the head and shoulders during infancy; however, it lengthens during the next 3 to 4 years.

NURSING ALERT

If any masses are detected in the neck, report them for further investigation. Large masses can block the airway.

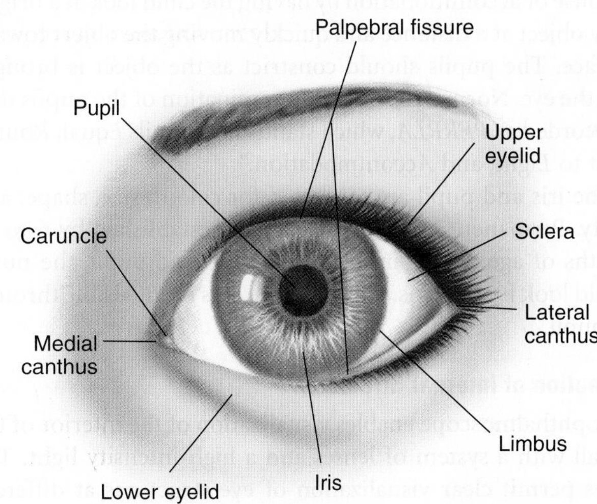

FIGURE 33-14 External structures of the eye.

Eyes

Inspection of External Structures

The lids should be inspected for proper placement on the eye. When the eye is open, the upper lid should fall near the upper iris (Fig. 33-14). When the eyes are closed, the lids should completely cover the cornea and sclera.

The general slant of the palpebral fissures or lids is determined by drawing an imaginary line through the two points of the medial canthus and across the outer orbit of the eyes and aligning each eye on the line. Usually the palpebral fissures lie horizontally. However, in Asians the slant is normally upward.

The inside lining of the lids, the *palpebral conjunctiva*, also needs to be inspected. To examine the lower conjunctival sac, the lid is pulled down while the patient looks up. To evert the upper lid, the nurse should hold the upper lashes and gently pull *down* and *forward* as the child looks down. Normally the conjunctiva appears pink and glossy. Vertical yellow striations along the edge are the *meibomian*, or *sebaceous*, glands near the hair follicle. Located in the inner or medial canthus and situated on the inner edge of the upper and lower lids is a tiny opening, the *lacrimal punctum*. Any excessive tearing, discharge, or inflammation of the lacrimal apparatus should be noted.

The *bulbar conjunctiva*, which covers the eye up to the limbus, or junction of the cornea and sclera, should be transparent. The *sclera*, or white covering of the eyeball, should be clear. Tiny black marks in the sclera of heavily pigmented individuals are normal.

The *cornea*, or covering of the iris and pupil, should be clear and transparent. The nurse needs to record opacities because they can be signs of scarring or ulceration, which can interfere with vision. The best way to test for opacities is to illuminate the eyeball by shining a light at an angle (obliquely) toward the cornea.

The pupils are compared for size, shape, and movement. They should be round, clear, and equal. Their reaction to light is tested by quickly shining a light toward the eye and removing it. As the light approaches, the pupils should constrict; as the light fades, the pupils should dilate. The pupil is tested for any response of accommodation by having the child look at a bright, shiny object at a distance and quickly moving the object toward the face. The pupils should constrict as the object is brought near the eye. Normal findings on examination of the pupils may be recorded as *PERRLA*, which stands for "*P*upils *E*qual, *R*ound, *R*eact to *L*ight, and *A*ccommodation."

The iris and pupil are inspected for colour, size, shape, and clarity. Permanent eye colour is usually established by 6 to 12 months of age. While inspecting the iris and pupil, the nurse should look for the lens. Normally the lens is not visible through the pupil.

Inspection of Internal Structures

The ophthalmoscope enables visualization of the interior of the eyeball with a system of lenses and a high-intensity light. The lenses permit clear visualization of eye structures at different distances from the nurse's eye and correct visual acuity differences in the examiner and child. Use of the ophthalmoscope requires practice to know which lens setting produces the clearest image.

The ophthalmic and otic heads are usually interchangeable on one "body" or handle, which encloses the power source, either disposable or rechargeable batteries. The nurse should practise changing the heads, which snap on and are secured with a quarter turn, and replacing the batteries and light bulbs. Nurses who are not directly involved in physical assessment are often responsible for ensuring that the equipment functions properly.

Preparing the child. The nurse can prepare the child for the ophthalmoscopic examination by showing the child the instrument, demonstrating the light source and how it shines in the eye, and explaining the reason for darkening the room. For infants and young children who do not respond to such explanations, it is best to use distraction to encourage them to keep their eyes open. Forcibly parting the lids results in a watery-eyed child who is even less likely to cooperate. Usually, with some practice, the nurse can elicit a red reflex almost instantly while approaching the child and may also gain a momentary inspection of the blood vessels, macula, or optic disc.

Funduscopic examination. Figure 33-15 shows the structures of the back of the eyeball, or the *fundus*. The fundus is immediately apparent as the red reflex. The intensity of the colour increases in darkly pigmented individuals. Figure 33-16 is an illustration of a normal left retina.

NURSING ALERT

A brilliant, uniform red reflex is an important sign because it rules out many serious defects of the cornea, aqueous chamber, lens, and vitreous chamber. Any dark shadows or opacities should be recorded because they indicate some abnormality in any of these structures.

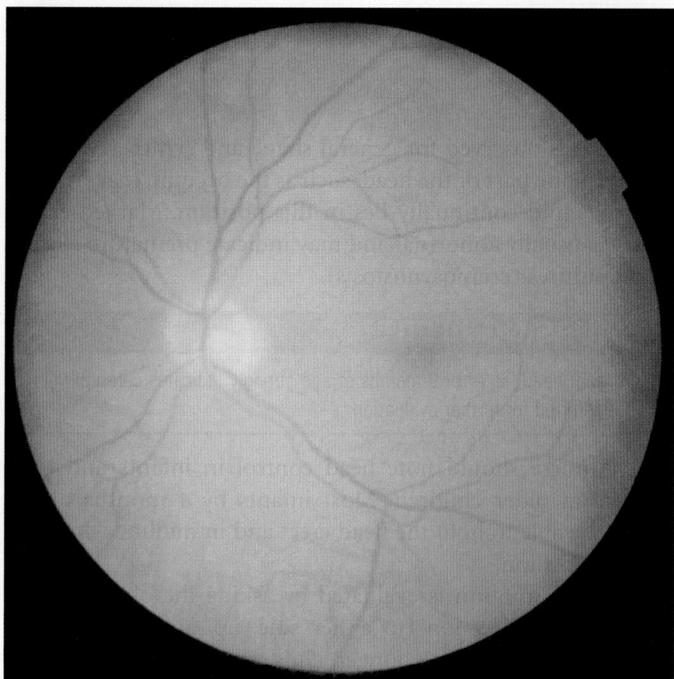

FIGURE 33-15 Normal left fundus. (From Lemmi, F. O., & Lemmi, C. A. [2009]. *Physical assessment findings* [CD-ROM]. Philadelphia: Saunders; Ball, J. W., Dains, J. E., Flynn, J. A., et al. [2015]. *Seidel's guide to physical examination* [8th ed., p. 217]. St. Louis: Mosby [Fig 11-27B].)

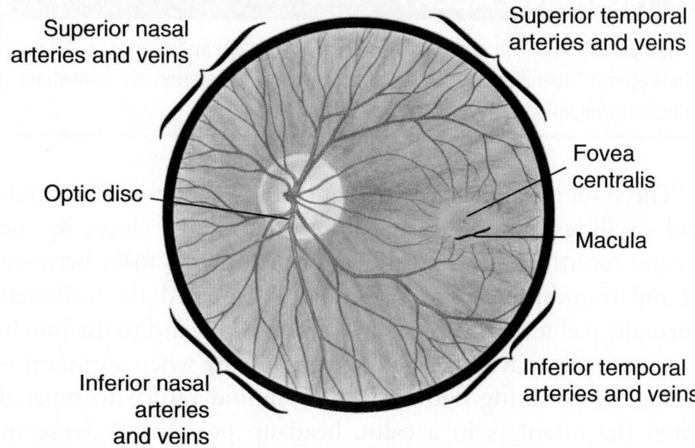

FIGURE 33-16 Structures of the fundus. (From Ball, J. W., Dains, J. E., Flynn, J. A., et al. [2015]. *Seidel's guide to physical examination*, [8th ed.]. St. Louis: Mosby.

As the ophthalmoscope is brought closer to the eye, the most conspicuous feature of the fundus is the optic disc, the area where the blood vessels and optic nerve fibres enter and exit from the eye. The colour of the disc is creamy pink; it is lighter in colour than the surrounding fundus. Normally it is round or vertically oval.

After the optic disc is located, the area is inspected for blood vessels. The central retinal artery and vein appear in the depths of the disc and emanate outward with visible branching. The veins are darker and about one fourth larger than the arteries. Normally the branches of the arteries and veins cross one another.

Other structures that may be seen are the *macula*, the area of the fundus with the greatest concentration of visual receptors; and, in the centre of the macula, a minute glistening spot of reflected light called the *fovea centralis*, which is the area of most perfect vision.

Vision Testing

Several tests are available for assessing vision. This discussion focuses on four areas: (1) ocular alignment, (2) visual acuity, (3) peripheral vision, and (4) colour vision. Vision screening should be performed at the earliest possible age and at regular intervals. A recent survey in Canada has identified that most children under the age of 4 years have yet to visit an optometrist. A common myth is that parents think that children need to be able to read in order to have their eyes examined. Guidelines recommend routine eye examinations starting at the age of 6 months (Canadian Association of Optometrists, 2014). It has been estimated that about 25% of school-age children have vision problems. Behavioural and physical signs of visual impairment are discussed in Chapter 41.

Ocular alignment. Normally, by the age of 3 to 4 months, children are able to fixate on one visual field with both eyes simultaneously (binocularity). One of the most important tests for binocularity is alignment of the eyes to detect nonbinocular vision, or strabismus. In **strabismus**, or cross-eye, one eye deviates from the point of fixation. If the misalignment is constant, the weak eye becomes "lazy," and the brain eventually suppresses the image produced by that eye. If strabismus is not detected and corrected by ages 4 to 6 years, blindness from disuse, known as **amblyopia**, may result.

Tests commonly used to detect misalignment are the corneal light reflex and the cover tests. To perform the corneal light reflex test, or Hirschberg test, the examiner shines a flashlight or the light of the ophthalmoscope directly into the patient's eyes from a distance of about 40.5 cm. If the eyes are orthophoric, or normal, the light falls symmetrically within each pupil (Fig. 33-17, A). If the light falls off centre in one eye, the eyes are misaligned. *Epicanthal folds*, excess folds of skin that extend from the roof of the nose to the inner termination of the eyebrow and that partially or completely overlap the inner canthus of the eye, may give a false impression of misalignment (pseudostrabismus) (see Fig. 33-17, B). Epicanthal folds are often found in Asian children.

In the cover test, one eye is covered, and the movement of the *uncovered* eye is observed while the child looks at a near (33 cm) or distant (6 m) object. If the uncovered eye does not move, it is aligned. If the uncovered eye moves, a misalignment is present because, when the stronger eye is temporarily covered, the misaligned eye attempts to fixate on the object.

In the cover-uncover test, occlusion shifts back and forth from one eye to the other, and movement of the eye that was covered is observed as soon as the occluder is removed while the child focuses on a point in front of him or her (Fig. 33-18). If normal alignment is present, shifting the cover from one eye to the other will not cause the eye to move. If misalignment is present, eye movement will occur when the cover is moved. This test takes more practice to perform than the other cover test because the occluder must be moved back and forth quickly and accurately to see the eye move. Because deviations can occur at different ranges, it is important to perform the cover tests at both close and far distances.

NURSING ALERT

The cover test is usually easier to perform if the examiner uses his or her own hand rather than a card-type occluder (see Fig. 33-18). Attractive occluders fashioned like an ice cream cone or happy-face lollipop cut from cardboard are also well received by young children.

Photoscreening is a technique used to screen for amblyopia, refractive disorders, and media opacities. Using a camera, the examiner obtains images of the pupillary reflexes (reflections) and red reflexes (Bruckner test). Photoscreening offers an effective way to screen infants, preverbal children, and those with developmental delays who are difficult to screen. The CPS (Amit & CPS Community Paediatrics Committee, 2009/2016) recommends photoscreening but states that is not practical for office-based primary care of children.

Visual acuity testing in children beyond infancy. The most common test for measuring visual acuity is the Snellen letter

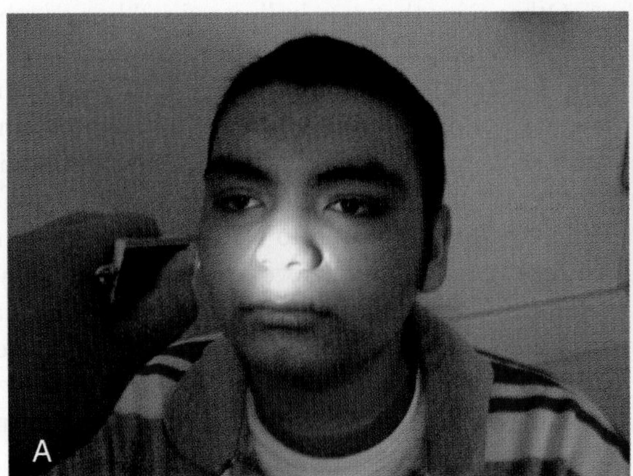

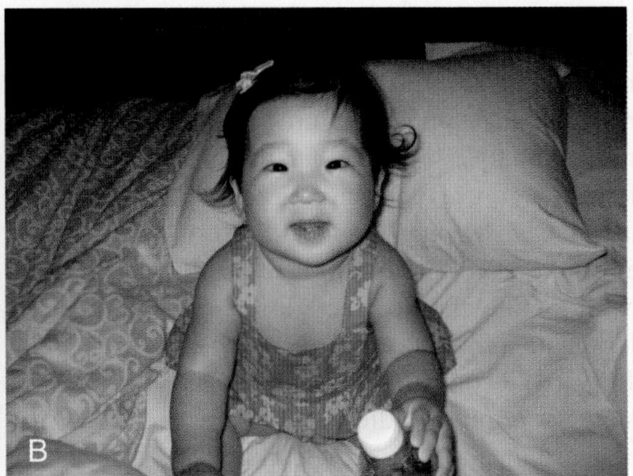

FIGURE 33-17 A: Corneal light reflex test demonstrating orthophoric eyes. **B:** Pseudostrabismus. Inner epicanthal folds cause eyes to appear misaligned; however, corneal light reflexes fall perfectly symmetrically.

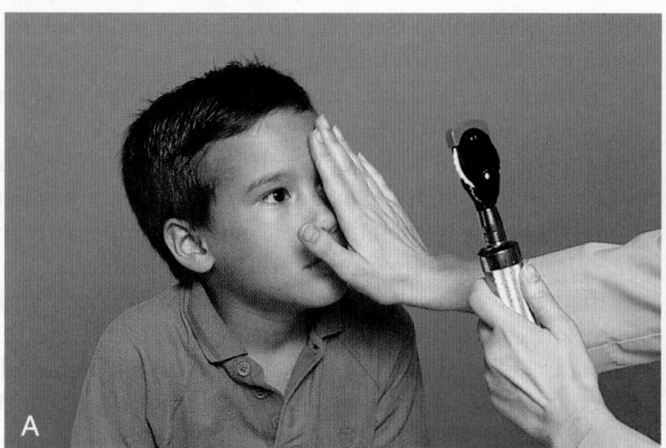

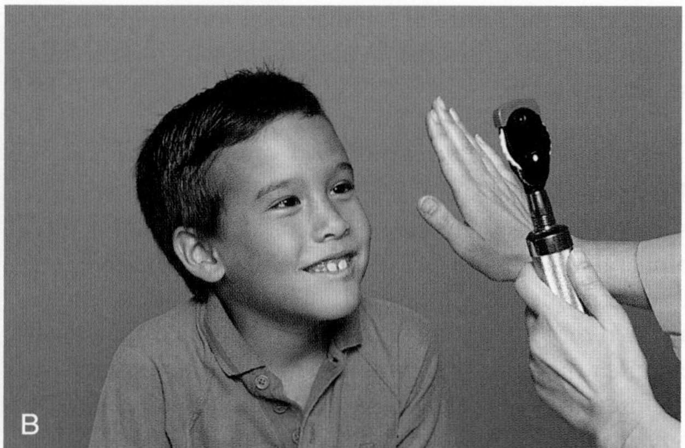

FIGURE 33-18 Alternate-cover test to detect amblyopia in patient with strabismus. **A:** Eye is occluded, and child is fixating on light source. **B:** If eye does not move when uncovered, eyes are aligned.

chart, which consists of lines of letters of decreasing size (see Additional Resources at the end of this chapter). Normally, children stand 3 metres from the chart with their heels at the 3-metre line. When screening for visual acuity in children, the right eye is tested first by covering the left eye. Children who wear glasses should be screened with them on. The child needs to keep both eyes open during the examination. The child begins moving down the chart until he or she fails to read the line. To pass each line, the child must correctly identify four of six symbols on the line. The procedure is repeated, with the child covering the right eye. Table 33-10 provides a list of visual screening tests for children and guidelines for referral. The CPS (Amit et al., 2009/2016) recommends that vision testing be done during periodic health review and when concerns are noted.

For children unable to read letters and numbers, the tumbling E or HOTV test is useful. The tumbling E test uses the capital letter E pointing in four different directions. The child is asked to point in the direction that the E is facing. The HOTV test consists of a wall chart composed of the letters H, O, T, and V. The child is given a board containing a large H, O, T, and V. The examiner points to a letter on the wall chart, and the child matches the correct letter on the board held in his or her hand. The tumbling E and HOTV tests are excellent tests for preschool-age children.

When a child is unable to perform the tumbling E or HOTV test, the LEA symbol or Allen card test may be used. The Allen card test uses common figures to test the child's vision. It is important to assess whether the child is able to identify the pictures before actual vision testing. The examiner walks backward slowly, flipping through the cards and presenting different pictures to the child. The examiner continues to move backward as the child correctly calls out the figures. When the child begins to miss the figure on the cards, the examiner moves forward to confirm that the child is able to identify the figures at that point. All Allen card figures are 20/30 in size. The farthest distance at which the child is able to accurately identify the pictures becomes the numerator, and 30 becomes the denominator. For example, if the child is able to identify the pictures accurately at 4.5 metres, the visual acuity is recorded as 15/30. This is equivalent to 20/40 or 10/20 visual acuity.

Visual acuity testing in infants and difficult-to-test children. In newborns, vision is tested mainly by checking for light perception by shining a light into the eyes and noting responses such as pupillary constriction, blinking, following the light to midline, increased alertness, or refusal to open the eyes after exposure to the light. Although the simple manoeuvre of checking light perception and eliciting the pupillary light reflex indicates that the anterior half of the visual apparatus is intact, it does not confirm that the infant can see. In other words, this test does not assess whether the brain receives the visual message and interprets the signals.

Another test of visual acuity is the infant's ability to fix on and follow a target. Although any brightly coloured or patterned object can be used, the human face is excellent. To do this the infant is held upright while the examiner moves his or her face slowly from side to side.

! NURSING ALERT

If visual fixation and following are not present by 3 to 4 months of age, further ophthalmological evaluation is needed.

Other signs that may indicate visual loss or other serious eye problems include fixed pupils, strabismus, constant nystagmus, the setting-sun sign, and slow lateral movements. Unfortunately, it is difficult to test each eye separately; the presence of such signs in one eye could indicate unilateral blindness.

Special tests are available for testing infants and other difficult-to-test children to assess acuity or confirm blindness. For example, in visually evoked potentials, the eyes are stimulated with a bright light or pattern, and electrical activity to the visual cortex is recorded through scalp electrodes. Acuity is assessed by using progressively smaller patterns.

Peripheral vision. In children who are old enough to collaborate, peripheral vision, or the visual field of each eye, can be estimated by having children fixate on a specific point directly in front of them as an object, such as a finger or a pencil, is moved from beyond the field of vision into the range of

TABLE 33-10 EYE EXAMINATION GUIDELINES*

FUNCTION	RECOMMENDED TESTS	REFERRAL CRITERIA	COMMENTS
Ages 3–5 Yr			
Distance visual acuity	Snellen letters Snellen numbers Tumbling E HOTV test Picture test • Allen figures • LEA symbols	1. Fewer than 4 of 6 correct on 6-m line with either eye tested at 3 m monocularly (i.e., <10/20 or 20/40) or 2. Two-line difference between eyes, even within passing range (i.e., 10/12.5 and 10/20 or 20/25 and 20/40)	1. Tests are listed in decreasing order of cognitive difficulty; highest test that child is capable of performing should be used; in general, tumbling E or HOTV test should be used for children 3–5 yr of age and Snellen letters or numbers for children 6 yr and older. 2. Testing distance of 3 m is recommended for all visual acuity tests. 3. Line of figures is preferred over single figures. 4. Nontested eye should be covered by occluder held by examiner or by adhesive occluder patch applied to eye; examiner must ensure that it is not possible to peek with nontested eye.
Ocular alignment	Cover-uncover test at 3 m Random dot E stereo test at 40 cm Simultaneous red reflex test (Bruckner test)	Any eye movement Fewer than 4 of 6 correct Any asymmetry of pupil colour, size, brightness	Child must be fixing on a target while cover-uncover test is performed. Use direct ophthalmoscope to view both red reflexes simultaneously in a darkened room from 60–90 cm away; detects asymmetrical refractive errors as well.
Ocular media clarity (cataracts, tumours, etc.)	Red reflex	White pupil, dark spots, absent reflex	Use direct ophthalmoscope in a darkened room. View eyes separately at 30–45 cm; white reflex indicates possible retinoblastoma.
6 Yr and Older			
Distance visual acuity	Snellen letters Snellen numbers Tumbling E HOTV test Picture test • Allen figures • LEA symbols	1. Fewer than 4 of 6 correct on 4.5-m line with either eye tested at 3 m monocularly (i.e., <10/15 or 20/30) or 2. Two-line difference between eyes, even within the passing range (i.e., 10/10 and 10/15 or 20/20 and 20/30)	1. Tests are listed in decreasing order of cognitive difficulty; highest test that child is capable of performing should be used; in general, tumbling E or HOTV test should be used for children 3–5 yr of age and Snellen letters or numbers for children 6 yr and older. 2. Testing distance of 3 m is recommended for all visual acuity tests. 3. Line of figures is preferred over single figures. Nontested eye should be covered by occluder held by examiner or by adhesive occluder patch applied to eye; examiner must ensure that it is not possible to peek with nontested eye.
Ocular alignment	(See Ages 3–5 Yr)	(See Ages 3–5 Yr)	(See Ages 3–5 Yr)
Ocular media clarity (cataracts, tumours, etc.)	(See Ages 3–5 Yr)	(See Ages 3–5 Yr)	(See Ages 3–5 Yr)

*The Canadian Paediatric Society has adapted these guidelines to be used by physicians, nurses, educational institutions, public health departments, and other health care providers who perform vision evaluation services.

From American Academy of Pediatrics, Committee on Practice and Ambulatory Medicine, Section on Ophthalmology. (2003). Eye examination in infants, children, and young adults. Reproduced with permission from Journal *Pediatrics, 111*(4), 902–907.

peripheral vision. Each eye is checked separately and for each quadrant of vision. As soon as children see the object, they should say "stop." At that point, the examiner measures the angle from the anteroposterior axis of the eye (straight line of vision) to the peripheral axis (point at which the object is first seen). Normally, children see about 50 degrees upward, 70 degrees downward, 60 degrees nasalward, and 90 degrees temporally. Limitations in peripheral vision may indicate blindness from damage to structures within the eye or to any of the visual pathways.

Colour vision. Another important test is for colour vision. It is estimated that 8 to 10% of White males and less than half that percentage of Black males inherit the X-linked disorder known as *colour vision deficit* (also known as *colour blindness*, a less acceptable term). From 0.5 to 1% of White females are affected. Although the severity of impaired perception of colour varies considerably, the two most common types are *protanomaly*, in which the child confuses grey with pink or pale blue with green, and *deuteranomaly*, in which the child confuses grey with pale purple or green. In most of these individuals the colour vision deficit causes no major problems. However, some individuals with more severe deficits may be unable to distinguish amber or red traffic lights, fail to see a red brake light on the rear of a car, have difficulty distinguishing green traffic lights from certain types of incandescent street lamps, and have a poor sense of colour coordination of clothing.

The tests available for colour vision include the Ishihara test and the Hardy-Rand-Rittler test. Each consists of a series of cards (pseudoisochromatic) on which is printed a colour field composed of spots of a certain "confusion" colour. Against the field is a number or symbol similarly printed in dots but of a colour likely to be confused with the field colour by the person with a colour vision deficit. As a result, the figure or letter is invisible to an affected individual but is clearly seen by a person with normal vision.

Ears

Inspection of External Structures

The entire external earlobe is called the *pinna*, or *auricle*; one is located on each side of the head. The height alignment of the pinna is measured by drawing an imaginary line from the outer orbit of the eye to the occiput, or most prominent protuberance of the skull. The top of the pinna should meet or cross this line. Low-set ears are commonly associated with renal anomalies or cognitive impairment. The angle of the pinna is measured by drawing a perpendicular line from the imaginary horizontal line and aligning the pinna next to this mark. Normally, the pinna lies within a 10-degree angle of the vertical line (Fig. 33-19) (see also Table 26-2). If it falls outside this area, the nurse should record the deviation and look for other anomalies.

Normally the pinnae extend slightly outward from the skull. Except in newborn infants, ears that are flat against the head or protruding away from the scalp may indicate problems. Flattened ears in an infant may suggest a frequent side-lying position and, just as with isolated areas of hair loss, may indicate a need to investigate parents' understanding of the child's stimulation needs.

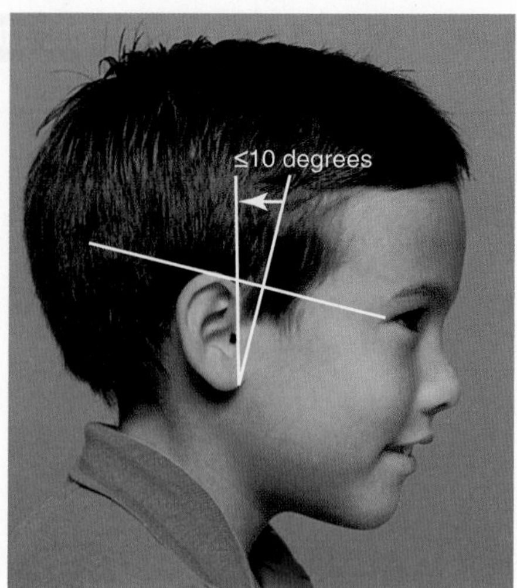

FIGURE 33-19 Ear alignment.

The skin surface around the ear should be inspected for small openings, extra tags of skin, or sinuses. If a sinus is found, the nurse should note this because it may represent a fistula that drains into some area of the neck or ear. Cutaneous tags represent no pathological process but may cause parents concern in terms of the child's appearance.

The ear should also be assessed for hygiene. An otoscope is not necessary for looking into the external canal to note the presence of cerumen, a waxy substance produced by the ceruminous glands in the outer portion of the canal. Cerumen is usually yellow-brown and soft. If an otoscope is used and any discharge is seen, its colour and odour are noted. The nurse can prevent transmission of potentially infectious material to the other ear or to another child through hand hygiene and using disposable specula or sterilizing reusable specula between each examination.

Inspection of Internal Structures

The head of the otoscope enables visualization of the tympanic membrane by use of a bright light, a magnifying glass, and a speculum. Some otoscopes have an attachment for a pneumonic device to insert air into the canal to determine membrane compliance (movement). The speculum, which is inserted into the external canal, comes in a variety of sizes to accommodate different canal widths. The largest speculum that fits comfortably into the ear is used to achieve the greatest area of visualization. The lens, or magnifying glass, is movable, allowing the examiner to insert an object, such as a curette, into the ear canal through the speculum while still viewing the structures through the lens.

Positioning the child. Before the start of the otoscopic examination, the child should be properly positioned and gently restrained (the child can sit on the parent's lap and hold parent's hand), if necessary. Older children are usually able to assist. However, the nurse should prepare them for the procedure by allowing them to play with the instrument, demonstrating how it works, and stressing the importance of remaining still. It may

ATRAUMATIC CARE

Reducing Distress From Otoscopy in Young Children

Make examining the ear a game by explaining that you are looking for a "big elephant" in the ear. This kind of make-believe is an absorbing distraction and usually elicits cooperation. After examining the ear, clarify that "looking for elephants" was only pretend and thank the child for letting you look in his or her ear. Another great distraction technique is asking the child to put a finger on the opposite ear to keep the light from getting out.

be helpful to have them observe the nurse examining the parent's ear. Restraint may be needed for younger children because the ear examination upsets them (see Atraumatic Care box).

As the speculum is inserted into the meatus, the examiner moves it around the outer rim to accustom the child to the feel of something entering the ear. If examining a painful ear, the examiner can touch a nonpainful part of the affected ear, then examine the unaffected ear, and finally return to the painful ear. By this time the child is usually less fearful of anything causing discomfort to the ear and will be more helpful.

For their protection and safety, infants and toddlers must be restrained for the otoscopic examination. There are two general positions of restraint. In one, the child is seated sideways in the parent's lap with one arm hugging the parent and the other arm at the side. The ear to be examined is toward the nurse. With one arm, the parent holds the child's head firmly against his or her chest, and with the other arm hugs the child, thereby securing the child's free arm (Fig. 33-20, A). The ear is examined using the same procedure for holding the otoscope as described in the discussion that follows.

The other position involves placing the child on the side, back, or abdomen with the arms at the side and the head turned so that the ear to be examined points toward the ceiling. The examiner leans over the child, uses the upper part of the body to restrain the arms and upper trunk movements, and uses the examining hand to stabilize the head. This position is practical for young infants or for older children who need minimum restraint, but it may not be feasible for other children who protest vigorously. For safety, the examiner can enlist the parent's or an assistant's help in immobilizing the head by firmly placing one hand above the ear and the other on the child's side, abdomen, or back (see Fig. 33-20, B).

With children who are able to help, the ear is examined with the child in a side-lying, sitting, or standing position. One disadvantage to standing is that the child may "walk away" as the otoscope enters the canal. If the child is standing or sitting, the head should be tilted slightly toward the child's opposite shoulder to achieve a better view of the drum (Fig. 33-21).

With the thumb and forefinger of the free (usually nondominant) hand, the examiner grasps the auricle. For the two positions of restraint, the otoscope is held upside down at the junction of its head and handle with the thumb and index finger. The other fingers are placed against the skull to allow the otoscope to move with the child in case of sudden movement. In examining a child who is helpful, the examiner can hold the

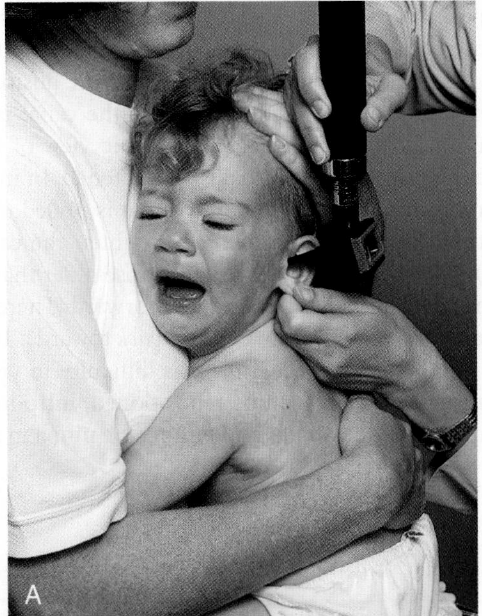

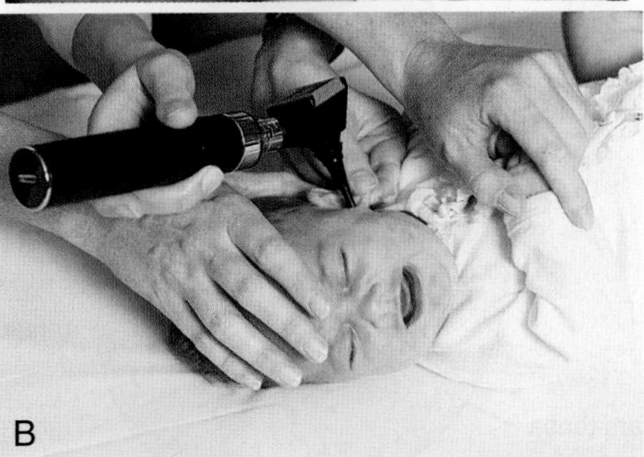

FIGURE 33-20 Position for restraining child **(A)** and infant **(B)** during otoscopic examination.

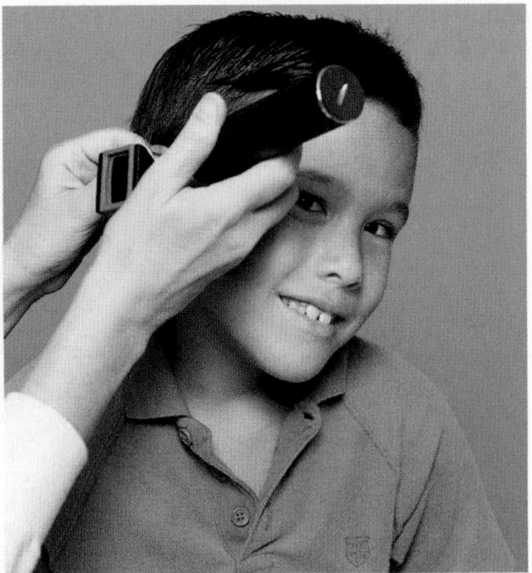

FIGURE 33-21 Positioning head by tilting it toward opposite shoulder for full view of tympanic membrane.

handle with the otic head upright or upside down. The examiner can use the dominant hand to examine both ears or reverse hands for each ear, whichever is more comfortable.

Before using the otoscope, the examiner needs to visualize the external ear and the tympanic membrane as being superimposed on a clock (Fig. 33-22). The numbers become important geographic landmarks. The speculum is introduced into the meatus between the 3 and 9 o'clock positions in a *downward* and *forward* position. Because the canal is curved, the speculum does not permit a panoramic view of the tympanic membrane unless the canal is straightened. In infants the canal curves upward. Therefore, the pinna is pulled *down* and *back* to the 6 to 9 o'clock range to straighten the canal (Fig. 33-23, A). With older children, usually those older than 3 years of age, the canal curves downward and forward. Therefore, the examiner should pull the pinna *up* and *back* toward a 10 o'clock position (see Fig. 33-23, B). If there is difficulty in visualizing the membrane, the head can be repositioned, introducing the speculum at a different angle, and pulling the pinna in a slightly different direction. The speculum should not be inserted past the cartilaginous (outermost) portion of the canal, usually a distance of 0.60 to 1.25 cm in older children. Insertion of the speculum into the posterior or bony portion of the canal causes pain.

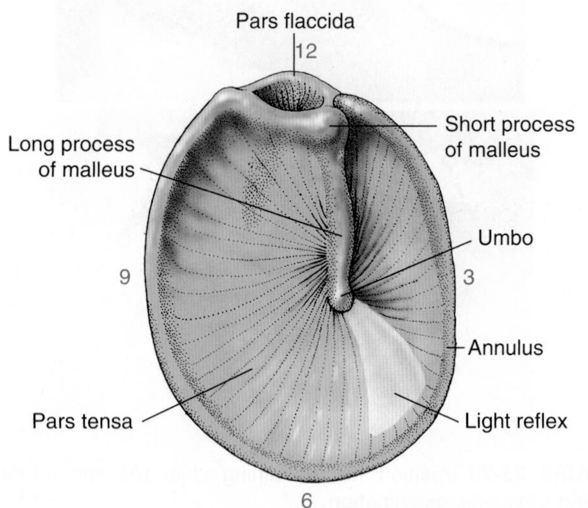

FIGURE 33-22 Landmarks of tympanic membrane with "clock" superimposed. (Adapted from Rothrock, J. C. [2015]. *Alexander's care of the patient in surgery* [15th ed.]. St. Louis: Mosby.)

In newborns and young infants, the walls of the canal are pliable and floppy because of the underdeveloped cartilaginous and bony structures. Therefore, the very small 2-mm speculum usually needs to be inserted deeper into the canal than in older children. Great care must be exercised not to damage the walls or drum. For this reason, only an experienced examiner should insert an otoscope into the ears of very young infants.

Otoscopic examination. As the speculum is introduced into the external canal, the examiner inspects the walls of the canal, the colour of the tympanic membrane, the light reflex, and the usual landmarks of the bony prominences of the middle ear. The walls of the external auditory canal are pink, although they are more pigmented in dark-skinned children. Minute hairs are evident in the outermost portion, where cerumen is produced. Signs of irritation, foreign bodies, or infection should be noted.

Foreign bodies in the ear are not uncommon in children and range from erasers to beans. Symptoms may include pain, discharge, and affected hearing. Soft objects, such as paper or insects, can be removed with forceps. Small, hard objects, such as pebbles, can be removed with a suction tip, a hook, or irrigation. However, irrigation is contraindicated if the object is vegetative matter, such as beans or pasta, which swells when in contact with fluid.

! NURSING ALERT

If there is any doubt about the type of object in the ear and the appropriate method to remove it, refer the child to the appropriate practitioner.

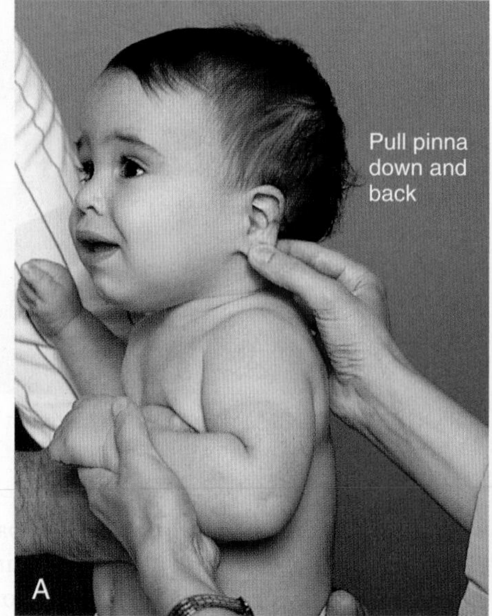

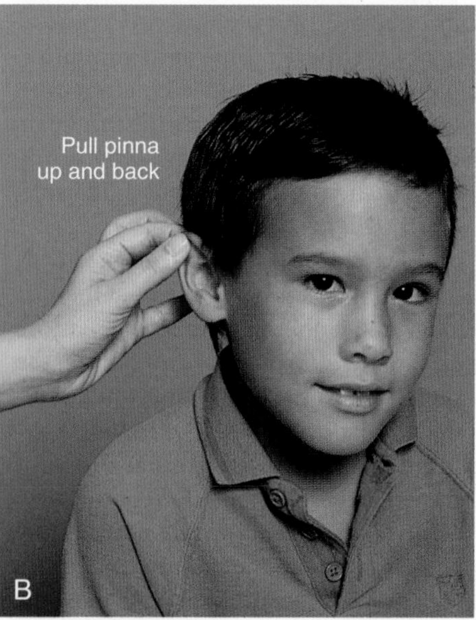

FIGURE 33-23 Positioning for visualizing eardrum in infant **(A)** and in child older than 3 years of age **(B)**.

The *tympanic membrane* is a translucent, light pearly pink or grey. Marked erythema (which may indicate suppurative otitis media), a dull nontransparent greyish colour (sometimes suggestive of serous otitis media), or ashen grey areas (signs of scarring from a previous perforation) should be noted. A black area usually suggests a perforation of the membrane that has not healed.

The characteristic tenseness and slope of the tympanic membrane cause the light of the otoscope to reflect at about the 5 or 7 o'clock position. The light reflex is a fairly well-defined, cone-shaped reflection, which normally points away from the face.

The bony landmarks of the drum are formed by the *umbo*, or tip of the malleus. It appears as a small, round, opaque, concave spot near the centre of the drum. The *manubrium* (long process or handle) of the malleus appears to be a whitish line extending from the umbo upward to the margin of the membrane. At the upper end of the long process near the 1 o'clock position (in the right ear) is a sharp, knoblike protuberance, representing the short process of the malleus. Absence of the light reflex or loss or abnormal prominence of any of these landmarks should be noted.

Auditory Testing

Several types of hearing tests are available and recommended for screening in infants and children (Patel, Feldman, & CPS Community Paediatrics Committee, 2011/2016) (Table 33-11). Many provinces and territories have mandatory hearing screening for newborns before discharge in order to detect hearing loss (see Chapter 26). The nurse must have a high index of suspicion for those children who appear to have conditions associated with hearing loss and who may have developed behaviours that indicate auditory impairment. Chapter 41 has more information on hearing loss.

Nose

Inspection of External Structures

The nose is located in the middle of the face just below the eyes and above the lips. Its placement and alignment are compared by drawing an imaginary vertical line from the centre point between the eyes down to the notch of the upper lip. The nose should be directly centred on this line, with each side exactly symmetrical. Its location, any deviation to one side, and asymmetry in overall size and in diameter of the nares (nostrils) should be noted. The bridge of the nose is sometimes flat in Asian and Black children. The nurse should observe the alae nasi for any sign of flaring, which indicates respiratory difficulty; any flaring of the alae nasi should be reported. Figure 33-24 illustrates the landmarks used in describing the external structures of the nose.

Inspection of Internal Structures

The anterior vestibule of the nose is inspected by pushing the tip upward, tilting the head backward, and illuminating the cavity with a flashlight or otoscope without the attached ear speculum. The colour of the mucosal lining should be noted, which is normally redder than the oral membranes, as well as any swelling, discharge, dryness, or bleeding. There should be no discharge from the nose.

On looking deeper into the nose, the nurse should inspect the *turbinates*, or concha, plates of bone that jut into the nasal cavity and are enveloped by mucous membrane. The turbinates greatly increase the surface area of the nasal cavity as air is inhaled. The spaces or channels between the turbinates are

TABLE 33-11 AUDIOLOGICAL TESTS FOR INFANTS AND CHILDREN

AGE	AUDITORY TEST AND AVERAGE TIME	TYPE OF MEASUREMENT	PROCEDURE
All ages	Evoked otoacoustic emissions, 10-min test	Physiological test specifically measuring cochlear (outer hair cell) response to presentation of stimulus	Small probe containing sensitive microphone is placed in ear canal for stimulus delivery and response detection
Birth–9 mo	Auditory brainstem response, 15-min test	Electrophysiological measurement of activity in auditory nerve and brainstem pathways	Placement of electrodes on child's head detects auditory stimuli presented though earphones one ear at a time
9 mo–2½ yr	Conditioned oriented responses or visual reinforced audiometry, 30-min test	Behavioural tests measuring child's responses to speech and frequency-specific stimuli presented through speakers	Both techniques condition child to associate speech or frequency-specific sound with reinforcement stimulus, such as a lighted toy
2½–4 yr	Play audiometry, 30-min test	Behavioural test measuring auditory thresholds in response to speech and frequency-specific stimuli presented through earphones and/or bone vibrator	Child is conditioned to put peg in peg board or drop block in a box when stimulus tone is heard
4 yr–adolescence	Conventional audiometry, 30-min test	Behavioural test measuring auditory thresholds in response to speech and frequency-specific stimuli presented through earphone and/or bone vibrator	Patient is instructed to raise hand when stimulus is heard

Modified with permission from Bachmann, K. R., & Arvedson, J. C. (1998). Early identification and intervention for children who are hearing impaired. Reproduced with permission from Journal *Pediatrics in Review, 19*(5), 155–165. Copyright © 1998 by the AAP.

called the *meatus* and correspond to each of the three turbinates. Normally the front end of the inferior and middle turbinate and the middle meatus are seen. They should be the same colour as the lining of the vestibule.

The septum is also inspected, which should divide the vestibules equally. Any deviation should be noted, especially if it causes an occlusion of one side of the nose. A perforation may be evident within the septum. If this is suspected, the examiner should shine the light of the otoscope into one naris and look for admittance of light to the other. Because olfaction is an important function of the nose, testing for smell may be done at this point or as part of the cranial nerve assessment (see Table 33-14).

Mouth and Throat

With a child who is helpful, almost the entire examination of the mouth and throat can be accomplished without the use of a tongue blade. The nurse can ask the child to open the mouth wide; to move the tongue in different directions for full visualization; and to say "ahh," which depresses the tongue for full view of the back of the mouth (tonsils, uvula, and oropharynx) (Fig. 33-25, B). For a closer look at the buccal mucosa, or lining of the cheeks, children can be asked to use their fingers to move the outer lip and cheek to one side (see Atraumatic Care box).

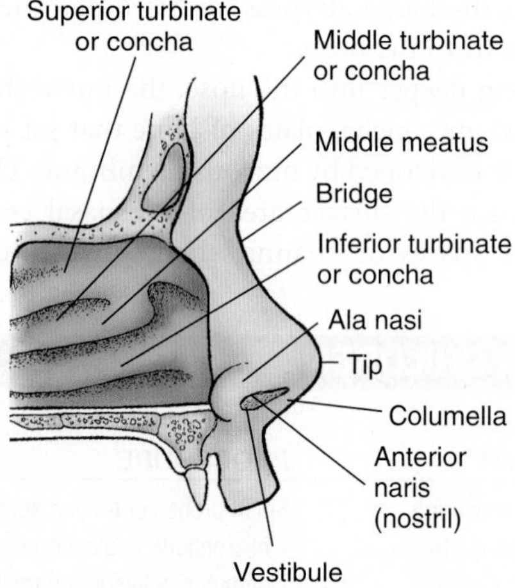

FIGURE 33-24 External landmarks and internal structures of the nose.

Infants and toddlers usually resist attempts to keep the mouth open. Because inspection of the mouth is upsetting, it should be left for the end of the physical examination (along with examination of the ears) or done during episodes of crying. However, the use of a tongue blade (preferably flavoured) to depress the tongue is necessary. The tongue blade is placed along the *side* of the tongue, not in the centre back area where the gag reflex is elicited. Figure 33-25, B illustrates proper positioning of the child for the oral examination.

The major structure of the exterior of the mouth is the lips. The lips should be moist, soft, smooth, and pink, or a deeper hue than the surrounding skin. The lips should be symmetrical when relaxed or tensed. The nurse can assess symmetry when the child talks or cries.

Inspection of Internal Structures

The major structures visible within the oral cavity and oropharynx are the mucosal lining of the lips and cheeks, gums (or gingiva), teeth, tongue, palate, uvula, tonsils, and posterior oropharynx (Fig. 33-26). The nurse needs to inspect all areas lined with mucous membranes (inside the lips and cheeks, gingiva, underside of the tongue, palate, and back of the pharynx) for colour, any areas of white patches or ulceration, bleeding, sensitivity, and moisture. The membranes should be bright pink, smooth, glistening, uniform, and moist.

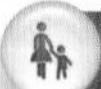

ATRAUMATIC CARE

Encouraging Opening the Mouth for Examination

- Perform the examination in front of a mirror.
- Let the child first examine someone else's mouth, such as in the parent, the nurse, or a puppet (see Fig. 33-25, A), and then examine the child's mouth.
- Instruct the child to tilt the head back slightly, breathe deeply through the mouth, and hold the breath; this action lowers the tongue to the floor of the mouth without the use of a tongue blade.
- Lightly brushing the palate with a cotton swab also may open the mouth for assessment.

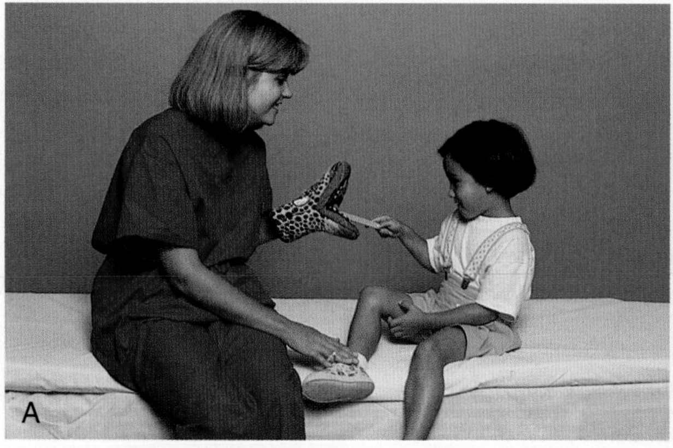

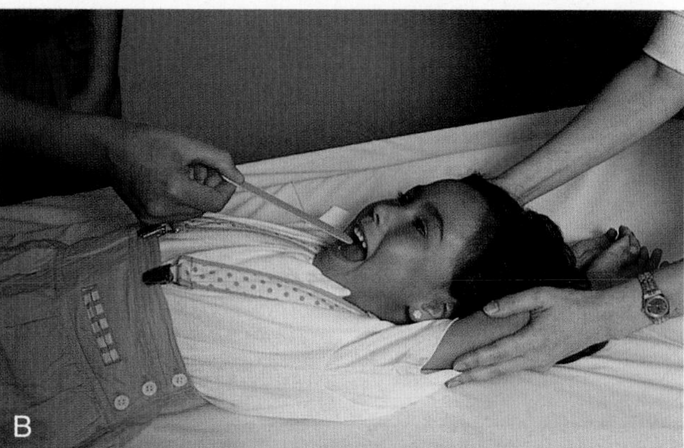

FIGURE 33-25 A: Encouraging child to assist. **B:** Positioning child for examination of the mouth.

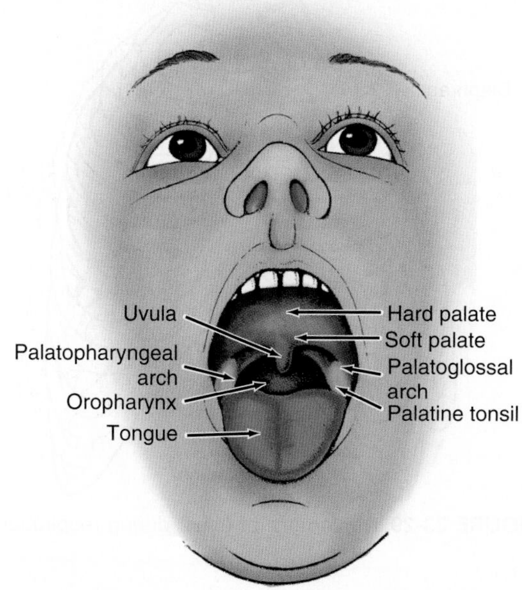

FIGURE 33-26 Interior structures of the mouth.

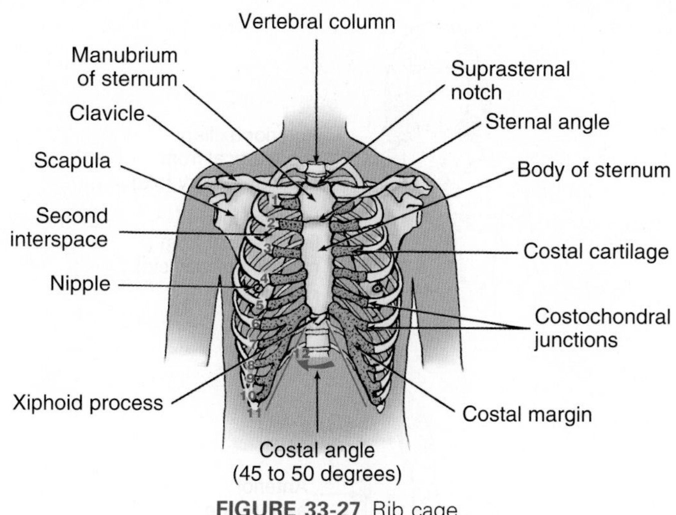

FIGURE 33-27 Rib cage.

The teeth are inspected for number in each dental arch, for hygiene, and for occlusion or bite. Discolouration of tooth enamel with obvious plaque (whitish coating on the surface of the teeth) is a sign of poor dental hygiene and indicates a need for counselling. Brown spots in the crevices of the crown of the tooth or between the teeth may be **caries** (cavities). Chalky white to yellow or brown areas on the enamel may indicate fluorosis (excessive fluoride ingestion). Teeth that appear greenish black may be stained temporarily from ingestion of supplemental iron.

The gums (gingiva) surrounding the teeth should also be examined. The colour is normally coral pink, and the surface texture is stippled, similar to the appearance of an orange peel. In dark-skinned children the gums are more deeply coloured, and a brownish area is often observed along the gum line.

The tongue is inspected for papillae, small projections that contain several taste buds and give the tongue its characteristic rough appearance. The size and mobility of the tongue should be noted. Normally the tip of the tongue should extend to the lips or beyond.

The roof of the mouth consists of the *hard palate*, which is located near the front of the oral cavity, and the *soft palate*, which is located toward the back of the pharynx and has a small midline protrusion called the *uvula*. The nurse should carefully inspect the palates to ensure that they are intact. The arch of the palate should be dome shaped. A narrow, flat roof or a high, arched palate affects the placement of the tongue and can cause feeding and speech problems. Movement of the uvula is tested by eliciting a gag reflex. The uvula should move upward to close off the nasopharynx from the oropharynx.

The nurse should examine the oropharynx and note the size and colour of the palatine tonsils. They are normally the same colour as the surrounding mucosa; glandular, rather than smooth in appearance; and barely visible over the edge of the palatoglossal arches. The size of the tonsils varies considerably during childhood. However, any swelling, redness, or white areas on the tonsils should be reported.

Chest

The chest is inspected for size, shape, symmetry, movement, breast development, and the bony landmarks formed by the ribs and sternum. The rib cage consists of 12 ribs on each side and the sternum, or breast bone, located in the midline of the trunk (Fig. 33-27). The sternum is composed of three main parts. The *manubrium*, the uppermost portion, can be felt at the base of the neck at the suprasternal notch. The largest segment of the sternum is the *body*, which forms the sternal angle (angle of Louis) as it articulates with the manubrium. At the end of the body is a small, movable process called the *xiphoid*. The angle of the costal margin as it attaches to the sternum is called the *costal angle* and is normally about 45 to 50 degrees. These bony structures are important landmarks in the location of ribs and *intercostal spaces* (ICSs), which are the spaces between the ribs. They are numbered according to the rib directly above the space. For example, the space immediately below the second rib is the second ICS.

The thoracic cavity is also divided into segments by drawing imaginary lines on the chest and back. Figure 33-28 illustrates the anterior, right lateral, and posterior divisions.

The size of the chest is measured by placing the measuring tape around the rib cage at the nipple line (see Fig. 33-7). For greatest accuracy, two measurements are needed—one during inspiration and the other during expiration—and the average recorded. The nurse should always report marked disproportions because most are caused by abnormal head growth, although some may be a result of altered chest shape, such as barrel chest (chest is round). There are two common structural findings of the rib cage. *Pigeon chest* (pectus carinatum) is a prominent sternal protrusion. The other finding is a *funnel chest* (pectus excavatum), which is an indentation of the lower sternum above the xiphoid process.

During infancy, the chest's shape is almost circular, with the anteroposterior (front-to-back) diameter equalling the transverse, or lateral (side-to-side), diameter. As the child grows, the

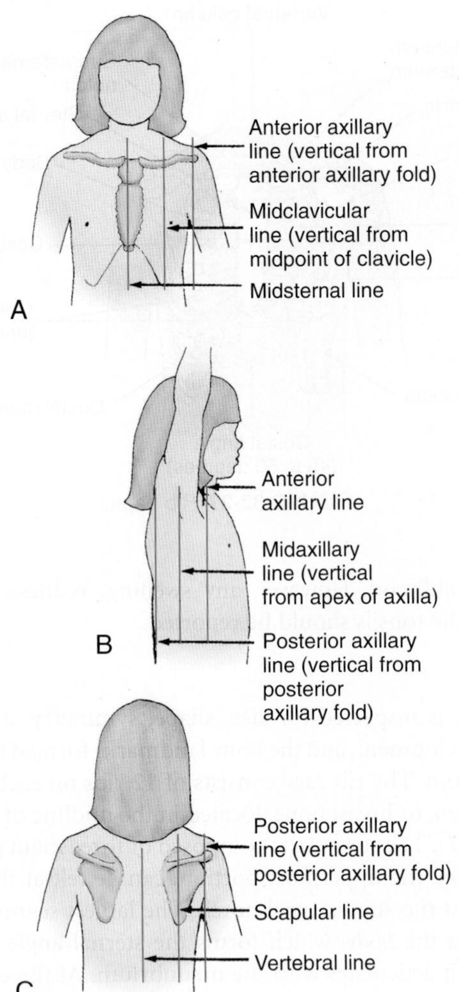

FIGURE 33-28 Imaginary landmarks of the chest. **A:** Anterior. **B:** Right lateral. **C:** Posterior.

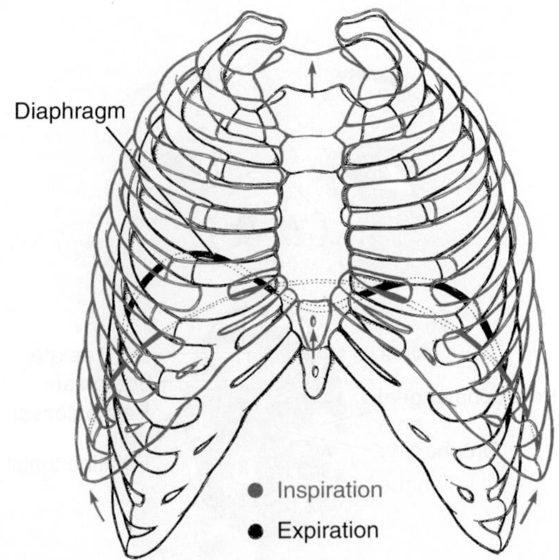

FIGURE 33-29 Movement of chest during respiration.

chest normally increases in the transverse direction, causing the anteroposterior diameter to be less than the lateral diameter. The nurse should note the angle made by the lower costal margin and the sternum and palpate the junction of the ribs with the costal cartilage (costochondral junction) and sternum, which should be fairly smooth.

Movement of the chest wall should be symmetrical bilaterally and coordinated with breathing. During inspiration, the chest rises and expands, the diaphragm descends, and the costal angle increases. During expiration, the chest falls and decreases in size, the diaphragm rises, and the costal angle narrows (Fig. 33-29). In children younger than 6 or 7 years of age, respiratory movement is principally abdominal or diaphragmatic. In older children, particularly girls, respirations are chiefly thoracic. In either type the chest and abdomen should rise and fall together. Any asymmetry of movement must be reported.

While inspecting the skin surface of the chest, the nurse should observe the position of the nipples and any evidence of breast development. Normally the nipples are located slightly lateral to the midclavicular line, between the fourth and fifth ribs. Symmetry of nipple placement should be noted as well as normal configuration of a darker pigmented areola surrounding a flat nipple in the prepubertal child.

Pubertal breast development usually begins in girls between 10 and 14 years of age. Early (precocious) or delayed breast development should be recorded, as well as evidence of any other secondary sexual characteristics. In males, breast enlargement (gynecomastia) may be caused by hormonal or systemic disorders, but more commonly it is a result of adipose tissue from obesity or a transitory body change during early puberty. In either situation, the nurse should investigate the child's feelings regarding breast enlargement.

In adolescent girls who have achieved sexual maturity, the breasts need to be palpated for evidence of any masses or hard nodules. Most palpable masses are benign, thus it is important to convey this tendency, to decrease any fear or concern that results when a mass is felt.

The stages of development of secondary sex characteristics and genital development have been defined as a guide for estimating sexual maturity and are referred to as the Tanner stages. Details on assessing Tanner stages in adolescents are found in Chapter 39.

Lungs

The lungs are situated inside the thoracic cavity, with one lung on each side of the sternum. Each lung is divided into an *apex*, which is slightly pointed and rises above the first rib; a *base*, which is wide and concave and rides on the dome-shaped diaphragm; and a *body*, which is divided into lobes. The right lung has three lobes: the upper, middle, and lower. The left lung has only two lobes, the upper and lower, because of the space occupied by the heart (Fig. 33-30).

Inspection of the lungs primarily involves observation of respiratory movements, which were discussed previously. Respirations are evaluated for rate (number per minute), rhythm (regular, irregular, or periodic), depth (deep or shallow), and quality (effortless, automatic, difficult, or laboured). The nurse should note the character of breath sounds, such as noisy, grunting, snoring, or heavy.

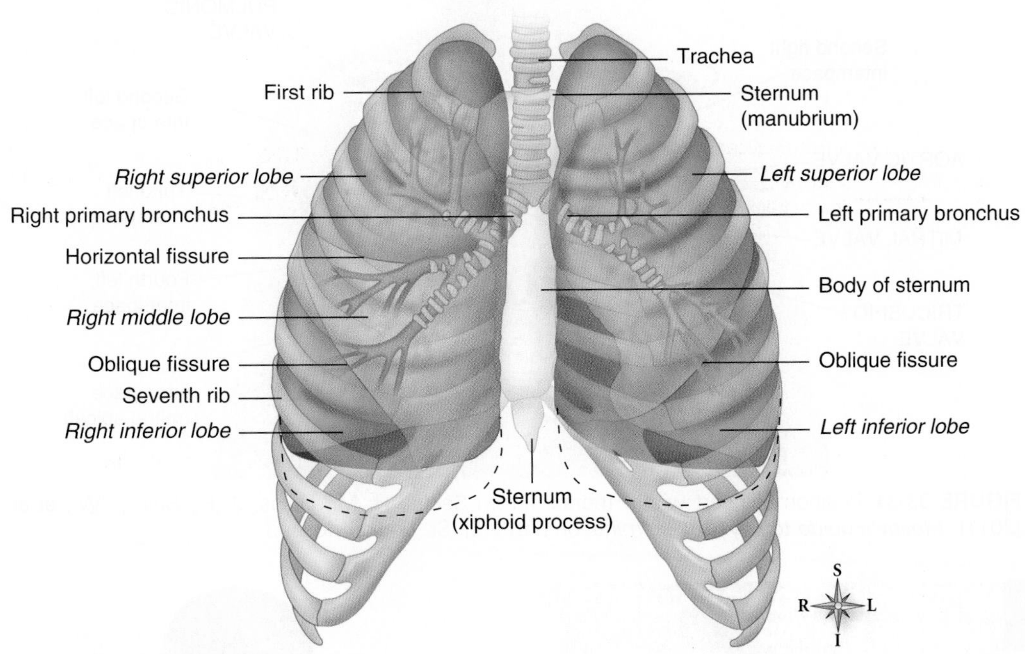

FIGURE 33-30 Location of lobes of lungs within thoracic cavity. (From Patton, K. T. [2013]. *Anatomy and physiology* [8th ed.]. St. Louis: Mosby.)

Respiratory movements are evaluated by placing each hand flat against the back or chest with the thumbs in midline along the lower costal margin of the lungs. The child should be sitting during this procedure and should take several deep breaths. During respiration, the examiner's hands will move with the chest wall. The amount and speed of respiratory excursion should be assessed and any asymmetry of movement noted.

Experienced examiners may percuss the lungs. The anterior lung is percussed from apex to base, usually with the child in the supine or sitting position. Each side of the chest is percussed in sequence to compare the sounds. When the posterior lung is percussed, the procedure and sequence are the same, although the child should be sitting. Resonance is heard over all the lobes of the lungs that are not adjacent to other organs. Any deviation from the expected sound should be recorded and reported.

Auscultation

Auscultation involves using the stethoscope to evaluate breath sounds (see Guidelines box). Breath sounds are best heard if the child inspires deeply (see Atraumatic Care box). In the lungs, breath sounds are classified as vesicular, bronchovesicular, or bronchial (Box 33-13).

Absent or diminished breath sounds are always an abnormal finding warranting investigation. Fluid, air, or solid masses in the pleural space all interfere with the conduction of breath sounds. Diminished breath sounds in certain segments of the lung can alert the nurse to pulmonary areas that may benefit from chest physiotherapy. Increased breath sounds after pulmonary therapy indicate improved passage of air through the respiratory tract. See Appendix E for normal pediatric respiratory rates.

GUIDELINES

Effective Auscultation

- Make certain the child is relaxed and not crying, talking, or laughing. Record if the child is crying.
- Check that the room is comfortable and quiet.
- Warm the stethoscope before placing it against the skin.
- Apply firm pressure on chest piece but not enough to prevent vibrations and transmission of sound.
- Avoid placing the stethoscope over hair or clothing, moving it against skin, breathing on tubing, or sliding fingers over chest piece, which may cause sounds that falsely resemble pathological findings.
- Use a symmetrical and orderly approach for comparing sounds.

ATRAUMATIC CARE

Encouraging Deep Breaths

- Ask the child to "blow out" the light on an otoscope or pocket flashlight; discreetly turn off the light on the last try so that the child feels successful.
- Place a cotton ball in the child's palm; ask the child to blow the ball into the air and have the parent catch it.
- Place a small tissue on the top of a pencil and ask the child to blow the tissue off.
- Have the child blow a pinwheel, a party horn, or bubbles.

Heart

The heart is situated in the thoracic cavity between the lungs in the mediastinum and above the diaphragm (Fig. 33-31). About two thirds of the heart lies within the left side of the rib cage, with the other third on the right side as it crosses the

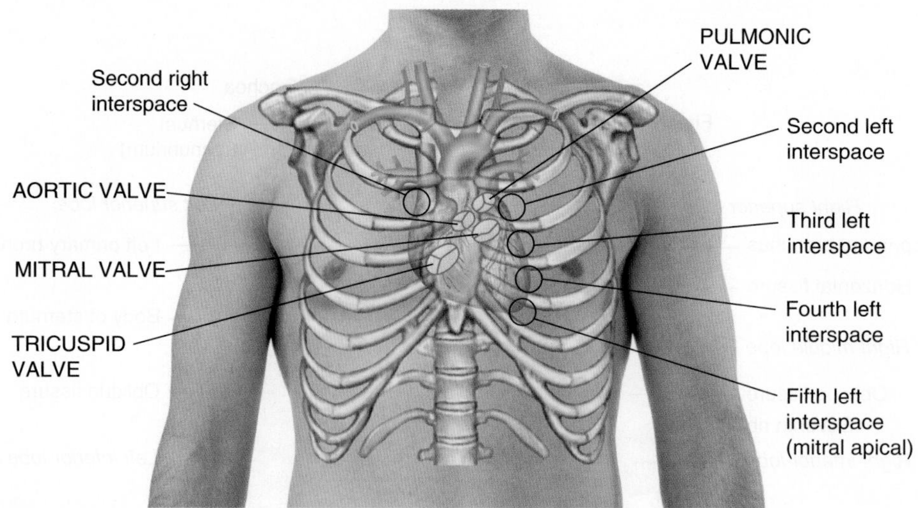

FIGURE 33-31 Position of heart within thorax. (From Seidel, H. M., Dains, J. E., Ball, J. W., et al. [2011]. *Mosby's guide to physical examination* [7th ed.]. St. Louis: Mosby.)

BOX 33-13 CLASSIFICATION OF NORMAL BREATH SOUNDS

Vesicular Breath Sounds

These sounds are heard over the entire surface of the lungs, with the exception of the upper intrascapular area and area beneath the manubrium.

Inspiration is louder, longer, and higher pitched than expiration.

Sound is a soft, swishing noise.

Bronchovesicular Breath Sounds

These sounds are heard over the manubrium and in the upper intrascapular regions where the trachea and bronchi bifurcate.

Inspiration is louder and higher pitched than in vesicular breathing.

Bronchial Breath Sounds

These sounds are heard only over the trachea near the suprasternal notch.

The inspiratory phase is short, and expiratory phase is long.

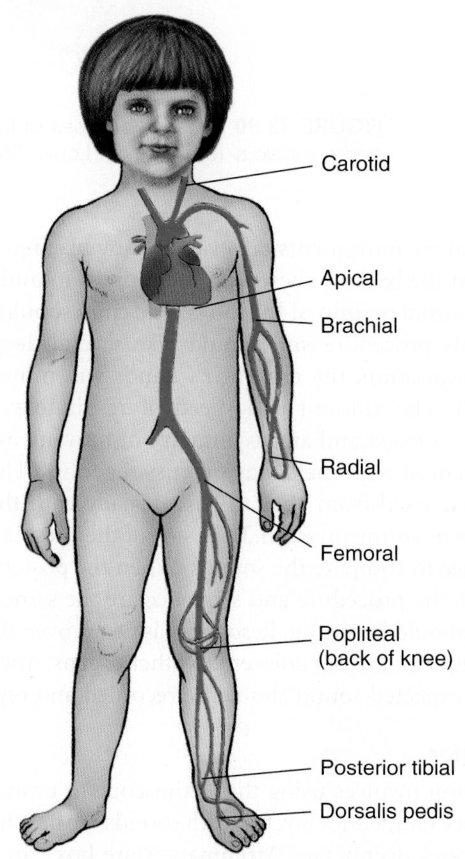

FIGURE 33-32 Location of pulses.

sternum. The heart is positioned in the thorax like a trapezoid:

- *Vertically* along the right sternal border (RSB) from the second to the fifth rib
- *Horizontally* (long side) from the lower right sternum to the fifth rib at the left midclavicular line (LMCL)
- *Diagonally* from the left sternal border (LSB) at the second rib to the LMCL at the fifth rib
- *Horizontally* (short side) from the RSB and LSB at the second ICS—base of the heart

Inspection is best done with the child sitting in a semi-Fowler position. The anterior chest wall is assessed from an angle, comparing both sides of the rib cage with each other. Normally they should be symmetrical. In children with thin chest walls, a pulsation may be visible. Because comprehensive evaluation of cardiac function is not limited to the heart, other findings such as the presence of all pulses (especially the femoral pulses) (Fig. 33-32), distended neck veins, clubbing of the fingers, peripheral cyanosis, edema, BP, and respiratory status need to be considered.

Palpation is used to determine the location of the apical impulse (AI), the most lateral cardiac impulse that may correspond to the apex. The AI is found:

- Just lateral to the LMCL and fourth ICS in children over 7 years of age.

- At the LMCL and fifth ICS in children less than 7 years of age.

Although the AI gives a general idea of the size of the heart (with enlargement, the apex is lower and more lateral), its normal location is variable, making it an unreliable indicator of heart size.

The **point of maximum impulse (PMI)**, as the name implies, is the area of most intense pulsation. Usually the PMI is located at the same site as the AI, but it can occur elsewhere. For this reason, the two terms should not be used synonymously.

Capillary refill time, an important test for peripheral circulation, is assessed by pressing the skin lightly on a central site, such as the forehead, or a peripheral site, such as the top of the hand, to produce a slight blanching. The time it takes for the blanched area to return to its original colour is the capillary refill time.

NURSING ALERT

Capillary refill should be brisk—less than 2 seconds; prolonged refill may be associated with poor systemic perfusion or a cool ambient temperature.

Auscultation

Origin of heart sounds. The heart sounds are produced by the opening and closing of the valves and the vibration of blood against the walls of the heart and vessels. Normally two sounds—S_1 and S_2—are heard, which correspond, respectively, to the familiar "lub dub" often used to describe the sounds. S_1 is caused by closure of the tricuspid and mitral valves (sometimes called the *atrioventricular valves*). S_2 is the result of closure of the pulmonic and aortic valves (sometimes called *semilunar valves*). Normally the split of the two sounds in S_2 is distinguishable and widens during inspiration. Physiological splitting is a significant normal finding.

NURSING ALERT

Fixed splitting, in which the split in S_2 does not change during inspiration, is an important diagnostic sign of atrial septal defect.

Two other heart sounds—S_3 and S_4—may be produced. S_3 is normally heard in some children; S_4 is rarely heard as a normal heart sound; it usually indicates the need for further cardiac evaluation.

Differentiating normal heart sounds. Figure 33-33 illustrates the approximate anatomical position of the valves within the heart chambers. The anatomical location of valves does not correspond to the area where the sounds are heard best. The auscultatory sites are located in the direction of the blood flow through the valves. It is important to not limit auscultation to only the four valve traditional locations. Heart sounds produced by the valves may be heard all over the precordium and many experts discourage naming the valve sites. The heart auscultation revised approach is to learn to inch the stethoscope in a rough Z pattern, from the base of the heart across and down, then over to the apex. Alternatively, the examiner can start at the apex and work upwards. Normally, S_1 is louder at the apex of the heart in the mitral and tricuspid area, and S_2 is louder near the base of the heart in the pulmonic and aortic area (Table 33-12). The nurse should listen to each sound by inching down the chest. The following areas should also be auscultated for sounds, such as murmurs, which may radiate to these sites: sternoclavicular area above the clavicles and manubrium, area along the sternal border, area along the left midaxillary line, and area below the scapulae.

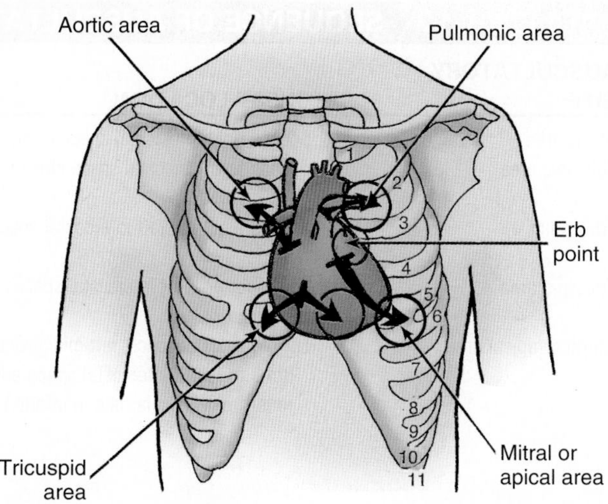

FIGURE 33-33 Direction of heart sounds for anatomical valve sites and areas (circled) for auscultation.

NURSING ALERT

To distinguish between S_1 and S_2 heart sounds, simultaneously palpate the carotid pulse with the index and middle fingers and listen to the heart sounds; S_1 is synchronous with the carotid pulse.

The nurse should auscultate the heart with the child in at least two positions: sitting and reclining. If adventitious sounds are detected, they should be further evaluated with the child standing, sitting and leaning forward, and lying on the left side. For example, atrial sounds such as S_4 are heard best with the person in a recumbent position and usually fade if the person sits or stands.

Heart sounds are evaluated for (1) quality (they should be clear and distinct, not muffled, diffuse, or distant); (2) intensity, especially in relation to the location or auscultatory site (they should not be weak or pounding); (3) rate (they should have the same rate as the radial pulse); and (4) rhythm (they should be regular and even). A particular arrhythmia that occurs normally in many children is *sinus arrhythmia*, in which the heart rate increases with inspiration and decreases with expiration. This rhythm is differentiated from a truly abnormal arrhythmia by having children hold their breath. In sinus arrhythmia, cessation of breathing causes the heart rate to remain steady.

Heart murmurs. Another important category of the heart sounds is murmurs, which are produced by vibrations within

TABLE 33-12 SEQUENCE OF AUSCULTATING HEART SOUNDS*

AUSCULTATORY SITE	CHEST LOCATION	CHARACTERISTICS OF HEART SOUNDS
Aortic area	Second right intercostal space close to sternum	S_2 heard louder than S_1; aortic closure heard loudest
Pulmonic area	Second left intercostal space close to sternum	Splitting of S_2 heard best, normally widens on inspiration; pulmonic closure heard best
Erb's point	Second and third left intercostal spaces close to sternum	Frequent site of innocent murmurs and those of aortic or pulmonic origin
Tricuspid area	Fifth right and left intercostal spaces close to sternum	S_1 heard as louder sound preceding S_2 (S_1 synchronous with carotid pulse)
Mitral or apical area	Fifth intercostal space, left midclavicular line (third to fourth intercostal space and lateral to left midclavicular line in infants)	S_1 heard loudest; splitting of S_1 may be audible because mitral closure is louder than tricuspid closure S_3 heard best at beginning of expiration with child in recumbent or left side-lying position; occurs immediately after S_2; sounds like word S_1 S_2 S_3: "Ken-tuc-ky" S_4 heard best during expiration with child in recumbent position (left side-lying position decreases sound); occurs immediately before S_1; sounds like word S_4 S_1 S_2: "Ten-nes-see"

*Use both diaphragm and bell chest pieces when auscultating heart sounds. Bell chest piece is necessary for low-pitched sounds of murmurs, S_3, and S_4. See Fig. 33-33 for sites.

the heart chambers or in the major arteries from the back-and-forth flow of blood. Murmurs are classified as follows:

Innocent—No anatomical or physiological abnormality exists.

Functional—No automatic cardiac defect exists, but a physiological abnormality such as anemia is present.

Organic—A cardiac defect with or without a physiological abnormality exists.

The description and classification of murmurs are skills that require considerable practice and training. In general, the nurse should recognize murmurs as distinct swishing sounds that occur in addition to the normal heart sounds and record the (1) location, or the area of the heart in which the murmur is heard best; (2) time of the occurrence of the murmur within the S_1–S_2 cycle; (3) intensity (evaluate in relationship to the child's position); and (4) loudness. The usual subjective method of grading the loudness or intensity of a murmur is listed in Table 33-13.

TABLE 33-13 GRADING OF THE INTENSITY OF HEART MURMURS

GRADE	DESCRIPTION
I	Very faint; often not heard if child sits up
II	Usually readily heard; slightly louder than grade I; audible in all positions
III	Loud, but not accompanied by a thrill
IV	Loud, accompanied by a thrill
V	Loud enough to be heard with a stethoscope barely touching the chest; accompanied by a thrill
VI	Loud enough to be heard with the stethoscope not touching the chest; often heard with the human ear close to the chest; accompanied by a thrill

Abdomen

Examination of the abdomen involves inspection, followed by auscultation and then palpation. Palpation should be performed last because it may distort the normal abdominal sounds, assessed during auscultation. Knowledge of the anatomical placement of the abdominal organs is essential to differentiate normal, expected findings from abnormal ones (Fig. 33-34).

Inspection

The contour of the abdomen is inspected with the child erect and supine. Normally the abdomen of infants and young children is cylindrical and, in the erect position, fairly prominent because of the physiological lordosis of the spine. In the supine position, the abdomen appears flat. A midline protrusion from the xiphoid to the umbilicus or symphysis pubis is usually diastasis recti, or failure of the rectus abdominis muscles to join in utero. In a healthy child, a midline protrusion is usually a variation of normal muscular development.

! NURSING ALERT

A tense, boardlike abdomen is a serious sign of paralytic ileus and intestinal obstruction.

The skin covering the abdomen should be uniformly taut, without wrinkles or creases. Sometimes silvery, whitish striae ("stretch marks") are seen, especially if the skin has been stretched, as in obesity. Superficial veins are usually visible in light-skinned, thin infants, but distended veins are an abnormal finding.

The nurse should observe movement of the abdomen. Normally, chest and abdominal movements are synchronous. In infants and thin children, peristaltic waves may be visible through the abdominal wall; they are best observed by standing at eye level to and across from the abdomen. This finding should always be reported.

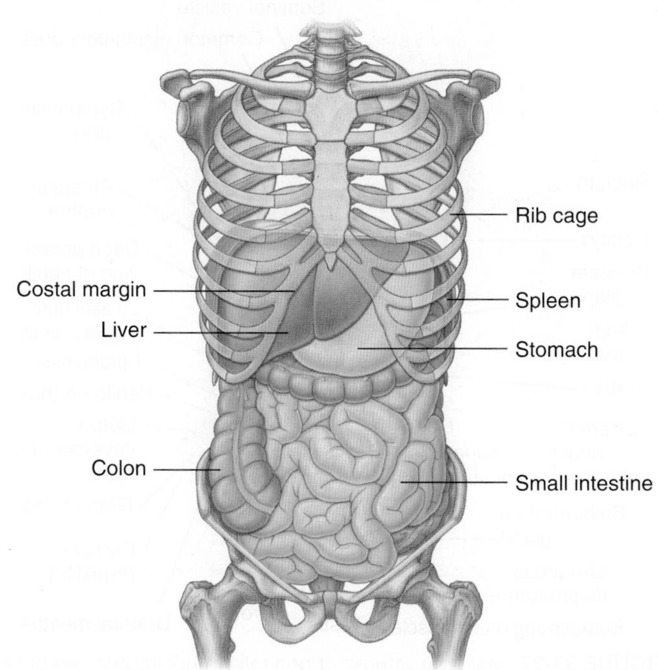

FIGURE 33-34 Location of structures in the abdomen. (From Drake, R. L., Vogl, W., & Mitchell, A. W. M. [2005]. *Gray's anatomy for students.* New York: Churchill Livingstone.)

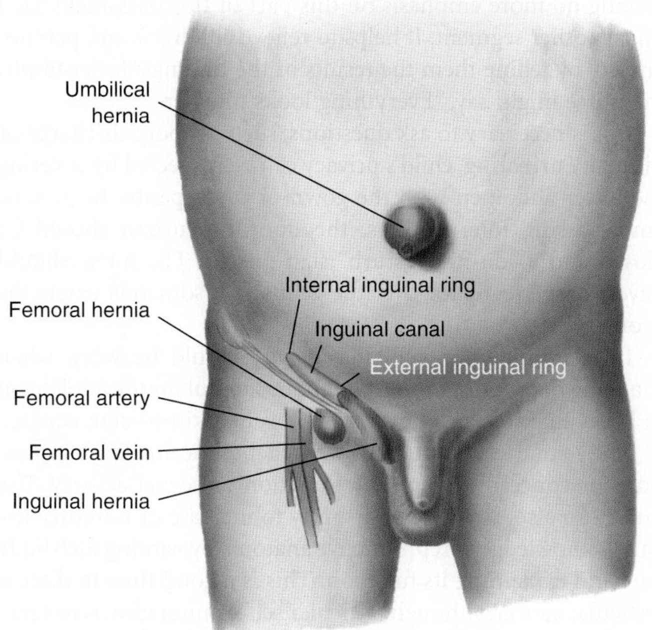

FIGURE 33-35 Location of hernias.

The umbilicus is examined for size, hygiene, and evidence of any abnormalities, such as hernias. The umbilicus should be flat or only slightly protruding. If a herniation is present, the nurse should palpate the sac for abdominal contents and estimate the approximate size of the opening. Umbilical hernias are common in infants, especially in Black children.

Hernias may exist elsewhere on the abdominal wall (Fig. 33-35). An *inguinal hernia* is a protrusion of peritoneum through the abdominal wall in the inguinal canal. It occurs mostly in males, is frequently bilateral, and may be visible as a mass in the scrotum. To locate a hernia, the examiner slides the little finger into the external inguinal ring at the base of the scrotum and asks the child to cough. If a hernia is present, it will hit the tip of the finger.

A *femoral hernia*, which occurs more frequently in girls, is felt or seen as a small mass on the anterior surface of the thigh just below the inguinal ligament in the femoral canal (a potential space medial to the femoral artery). To feel for a hernia, the examiner places the index finger of his or her right hand on the child's right femoral pulse (left hand for left pulse) and the middle finger flat against the skin toward the midline. The ring finger lies over the femoral canal, where the herniation occurs. Palpation of hernias in the pelvic region is often part of the genital examination.

Auscultation

The most important finding to listen for is *peristalsis*, or bowel sounds, which sound like short metallic clicks and gurgles. Their frequency per minute should be recorded (e.g., 5 sounds/min). Bowel sounds may be stimulated by stroking the abdominal surface with a fingernail. Absence of bowel sounds or hyperperistalsis should be reported, since either usually denotes an abdominal disorder.

Palpation

Two types of palpation are performed: superficial and deep. For superficial palpation, the examiner should lightly place the hand against the skin and feel each quadrant, noting any areas of tenderness, muscle tone, and superficial lesions such as cysts. Because superficial palpation is often perceived as tickling, several techniques can be used to minimize this sensation and relax the child (see Atraumatic Care box). Admonishing the child to stop laughing only draws attention to the sensation and may make it more difficult to complete the assessment.

Deep palpation is used for palpating organs and large blood vessels and for detecting masses and tenderness that were not discovered during superficial palpation. Palpation usually begins in the lower quadrants and proceeds upward to avoid missing the edge of an enlarged liver or spleen. Except for palpating the liver, successful identification of other organs, such as the spleen, kidney, and part of the colon, requires considerable practice with tutored supervision. Any questionable mass should be reported. The lower edge of the liver is sometimes felt in infants and young children as a superficial mass 1 to 2 cm below the right costal margin (the distance is sometimes measured in fingerbreadths). Normally, the liver descends during inspiration as the diaphragm moves downward. This downward displacement should not be mistaken as a sign of liver enlargement.

> **! NURSING ALERT**
>
> If the liver is palpable 3 cm below the right costal margin or the spleen is palpable more than 2 cm below the left costal margin, these organs are enlarged—a finding that is always reported for further medical investigation.

ATRAUMATIC CARE

Promoting Relaxation During Abdominal Palpation

- Position the child comfortably, such as in a semi-reclining position in the parent's lap, with knees flexed.
- Warm the hands before touching the skin.
- Use distraction, such as telling stories or talking to the child.
- Teach the child to use deep breathing and to concentrate on an object.
- Give infants a bottle (if being bottle-fed) or pacifier.
- Begin with light, superficial palpation and gradually progress to deeper palpation.
- Palpate any tender or painful areas last.
- Have the child hold the parent's hand and squeeze it if palpation is uncomfortable.
- Use the nonpalpating hand to comfort the child, such as placing the free hand on the child's shoulder while palpating the abdomen.
- To minimize sensation of tickling during palpation:
  - Have children "help" with palpation by placing a hand over the palpating hand.
  - Have them place a hand on the abdomen with the fingers spread wide apart, and palpate between their fingers.

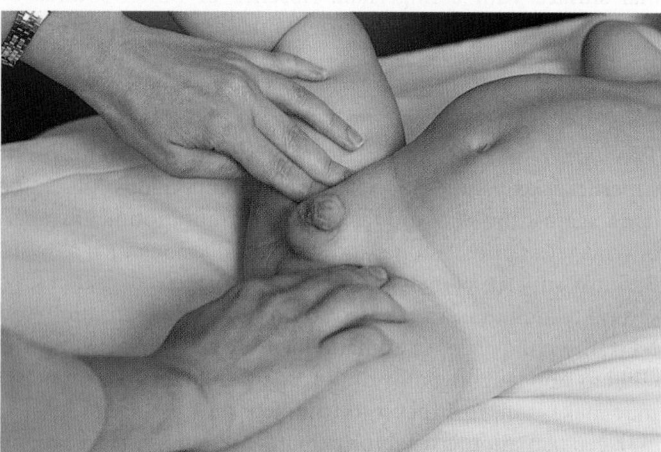

FIGURE 33-36 Palpating femoral pulses.

The femoral pulses are palpated by placing the tips of two or three fingers (index, middle, or ring) along the inguinal ligament about midway between the iliac crest and symphysis pubis. Both pulses should be felt simultaneously to make certain that they are equal and strong (Fig. 33-36).

NURSING ALERT

Absence of femoral pulses is a significant sign of coarctation of the aorta and needs to be referred for medical evaluation.

Genitalia

Examination of genitalia conveniently follows assessment of the abdomen while the child is still supine. In adolescents, inspection of the genitalia may be left to the end of the examination. The best approach is to examine the genitalia matter-of-factly,

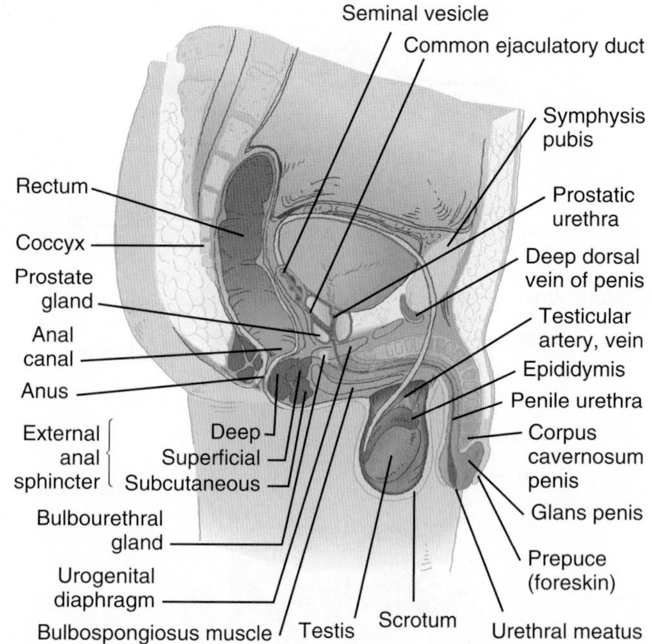

FIGURE 33-37 Major structures of genitalia in uncircumcised post-pubertal male. (From Black, J. M. [2008]. *Medical-surgical nursing: Clinical management for positive outcomes* [8th ed.]. St. Louis: Saunders.)

placing no more emphasis on this part of the assessment than on any other segment. It helps to relieve children's and parents' anxiety by telling them the results of the findings; for example, the nurse might say, "Everything looks fine here."

If it is necessary to ask questions, such as about discharge or difficulty urinating, child's privacy can be respected by covering the lower abdomen with the gown or underpants. To prevent embarrassing interruptions, the door or curtain should be closed and a "do not disturb" sign posted. The nurse should have a drape ready to cover the genitalia if someone enters the room.

In examining the genitalia, gloves should be worn when touching body substances. It might be helpful for the adolescent to know that wearing gloves also prevents skin-to-skin contact.

The genital examination is an excellent time for eliciting questions or concerns about body function or sexual activity. The nurse can also use this opportunity to increase or reinforce the child's knowledge of reproductive anatomy by naming each body part and explaining its function. This is a good time to discuss testicular cancer, although testicular self-examination is not recommended, it is important for the male to know what is normal.

Male Genitalia

In examining the male genitalia, the nurse should note the external appearance of the glans and shaft of the penis, the prepuce, the urethral meatus, and the scrotum (Fig. 33-37). The penis is generally small in infants and young boys until puberty, when it begins to increase in both length and width. In an obese child, the penis often looks abnormally small because of the folds of skin partially covering it at the base. It is important to be familiar with normal pubertal growth of the external male genitalia in order to compare the findings with the expected sequence of maturation.

The glans (head of the penis) and shaft (portion between the perineum and prepuce) are examined for signs of swelling, skin lesions, inflammation, or other irregularities. Any of these signs may indicate underlying disorders, especially STIs.

The urethral meatus is carefully inspected for location and evidence of discharge. Normally it is centred at the tip of the glans. Hair distribution should also be noted. Normally, before puberty, no pubic hair is present. Soft, downy hair at the base of the penis is an early sign of pubertal maturation. In older adolescents, hair distribution is diamond shaped from the umbilicus to the anus.

The location and size of the scrotum should be noted. The scrota hang freely from the perineum behind the penis, and the left scrotum normally hangs lower than the right. In infants, the scrota appear large in relation to the rest of the genitalia. The skin of the scrotum is loose and highly rugated (wrinkled). During early adolescence, the skin normally becomes redder and coarser. In dark-skinned children, the scrota are usually more deeply pigmented.

Palpation of the scrotum includes identification of the testes, epididymis, and, if present, inguinal hernias. The two testes are felt as small, ovoid bodies about 1.5 to 2 cm long—one in each scrotal sac. They do not enlarge until puberty, when they approximately double in size.

When palpating for the presence of the testes, the nurse should avoid stimulating the cremasteric reflex, which is stimulated by cold, touch, emotional excitement, or exercise. This reflex pulls the testes higher into the pelvic cavity. Several measures are useful in preventing the cremasteric reflex during palpation of the scrotum. First, the hands should be warmed. Second, if the child is old enough, he should be examined in a "tailor" position, which stretches the muscle, preventing its contraction (Fig. 33-38, A). Third, the examiner can block the normal pathway of ascent of the testes by placing the thumb and index finger over the upper part of the scrotal sac along the inguinal canal (see Fig. 33-38, B). If there is any question concerning the existence of two testes, the index and middle fingers can be placed in a scissors fashion to separate the right and left scrota. If, after using these techniques, the testes have not been palpated, the examiner should feel along the inguinal canal and perineum to locate masses that may be undescended testes. Although undescended testes may descend at any time during childhood and are checked at each visit, failure to palpate testes should be reported.

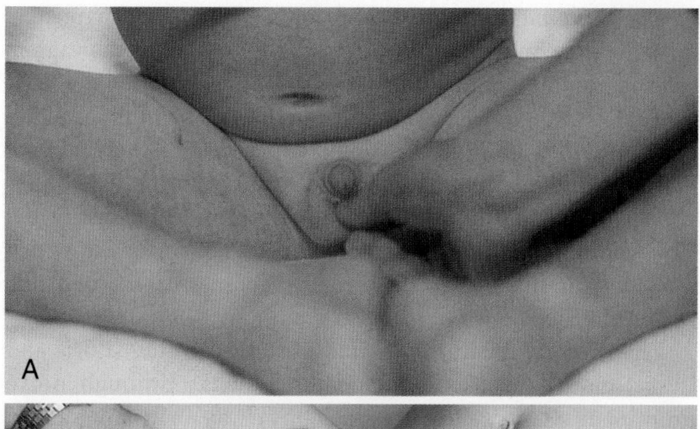

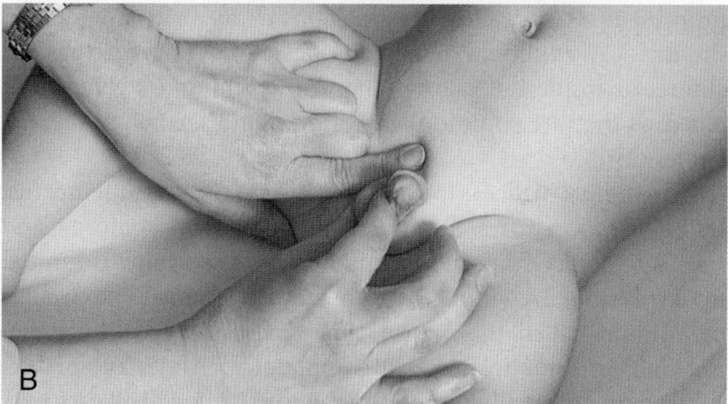

FIGURE 33-38 A: Preventing cremasteric reflex by having child sit in "tailor" position. **B:** Blocking inguinal canal during palpation of scrotum for descended testes.

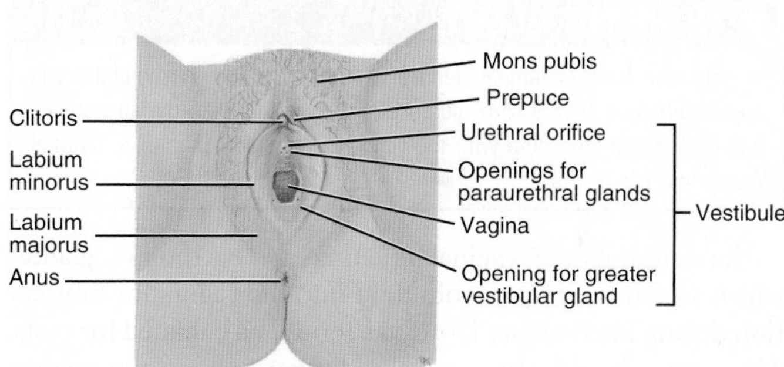

FIGURE 33-39 External structures of genitalia in postpubertal female. Labia are spread to reveal deeper structures. (From Applegate, E. [2006]. *The anatomy and physiology learning system* [3rd ed.]. St. Louis: Mosby.)

Female Genitalia

The examination of female genitalia is limited to inspection and palpation of external structures. If a vaginal examination is required, an appropriate referral is made unless the nurse is qualified to perform the procedure.

A convenient position for examination of the genitalia involves placing the young child supine on the examining table or in a semi-reclining position on the parent's lap with the feet supported on the nurse's knees as the nurse sits facing the child. The child's attention can be diverted from the examination by instructing her to try to keep the soles of her feet pressed against each other. The nurse should separate the labia majora with the thumb and index finger and retract outward to expose the labia minora, urethral meatus, and vaginal orifice.

The female genitalia are examined for size and location of the structures of the vulva, or pudendum (Fig. 33-39). The *mons pubis* is a pad of adipose tissue over the symphysis pubis. At puberty, the mons is covered with hair, which extends along the labia. The usual pattern of female hair distribution is an inverted triangle. The appearance of soft, downy hair along the labia majora is an early sign of sexual maturation. The nurse should note the size and location of the *clitoris*, a small, erectile organ located at the anterior end of the labia minora. It is covered by a small flap of skin, the *prepuce*.

The *labia majora* are two thick folds of skin running posteriorly from the mons to the posterior commissure of the vagina. Internal to the labia majora are two folds of skin called the *labia minora*. Although the labia minora are usually prominent in the newborn, they gradually atrophy, which makes them almost invisible until their enlargement during puberty. The inner surface of the labia should be pink and moist. The size of the labia should be noted as well as any evidence of fusion, which may suggest male scrota. Normally, no masses are palpable within the labia.

The urethral meatus is located posterior to the clitoris and is surrounded by Skene's glands and ducts. Although not a prominent structure, the meatus appears as a small V-shaped slit. Its location should be noted, especially if it opens from the clitoris or inside the vagina. The glands should be gently palpated, as they are common sites of cysts and sexually transmitted lesions.

The vaginal orifice is located posterior to the urethral meatus. Its appearance varies depending on individual anatomy and sexual activity. Ordinarily, examination of the vagina is limited to inspection. In virgins, a thin crescent-shaped or circular membrane, called the *hymen*, may cover part of the vaginal opening. In some instances it completely occludes the orifice. After rupture, small rounded pieces of tissue called *caruncles* remain. Although an imperforate hymen denotes lack of penile intercourse, a perforate one does not necessarily indicate sexual activity.

! NURSING ALERT

In girls who have undergone female genital mutilation the genitalia will appear different. Do not show surprise or disgust, but note the appearance and discuss the procedure with the young woman (see Chapter 5, Cultural Awareness box, p. 75).

Surrounding the vaginal opening are Bartholin's glands, which secrete a clear, mucoid fluid into the vagina for lubrication during intercourse. The ducts should be palpated for cysts. The nurse should also note the discharge from the vagina, which is usually clear or white.

Anus

After examination of the genitalia, the anal area is easily examined, although the child should be placed on the abdomen. The general firmness of the buttocks and symmetry of the gluteal folds should be noted. The tone of the anal sphincter can be assessed by eliciting the anal reflex. Gently scratching the anal area results in an obvious quick contraction of the external anal sphincter.

Back and Extremities

Spine

The general curvature of the spine is noted. Normally, the back of a newborn is rounded or C-shaped from the thoracic and pelvic curves. The development of the cervical and lumbar curves approximates development of various motor skills, such as cervical curvature with head control, and gives the older child the typical double S curve.

Marked curvatures in posture are abnormal. *Scoliosis*, lateral curvature of the spine, is an important childhood problem, especially in girls. Although scoliosis may be identified by observing and palpating the spine and noting a sideways displacement, more objective tests include:

- With the child standing erect, clothed only in underpants (and bra if older girl), observe from behind, noting asymmetry of the shoulders and hips.
- With the child bending forward so that the back is parallel to the floor, observe from the side, noting asymmetry or prominence of the rib cage.

A slight limp, a crooked hemline, or complaints of a sore back are other signs and symptoms of scoliosis.

The back should be inspected, especially along the spine, for any tufts of hair, dimples, or discolouration. Mobility of the vertebral column is easily assessed in most children because of their propensity for constant motion during the examination. However, mobility can be tested by asking the child to sit up from a prone position or to do a modified sit-up exercise.

Movement of the cervical spine is an important diagnostic sign of neurological problems, such as meningitis. Normally, movement of the head in all directions is effortless.

NURSING ALERT

Hyperextension of the neck and spine, or *opisthotonos*, which is accompanied by pain when the head is flexed, is always referred for immediate medical evaluation.

Extremities

Each extremity needs to be inspected for symmetry of length and size; any deviation should be referred for orthopaedic evaluation. The nurse should count the fingers and toes to be certain of the normal number. This is so often taken for granted that an extra digit (*polydactyly*) or fusion of digits (*syndactyly*) may go unnoticed.

The arms and legs are inspected for temperature and colour, which should be equal in each extremity, although the feet may normally be colder than the hands.

The shape of bones should also be assessed. Several variations of bone shape may be observed in children. Although many of them cause parents concern, most are benign and require no treatment. *Bowleg*, or genu varum, is lateral bowing of the tibia. It is clinically present when the child stands with the medial malleoli (rounded prominence on either side of the ankle) opposite each other and the space between the knees is greater than approximately 5 cm (Fig. 33-40). Toddlers are usually bowlegged after beginning to walk until all their lower back and leg muscles are well developed. Unilateral or asymmetrical bowlegs that are present beyond the age of 2 to 3 years, particularly in Black children, may represent pathological conditions requiring further investigation.

Knock-knee, or genu valgum, appears as the opposite of bowleg, in that the knees are close together but the feet are spread apart. It is determined clinically by using the same method as for genu varum but by measuring the distance between the malleoli, which normally should be less than

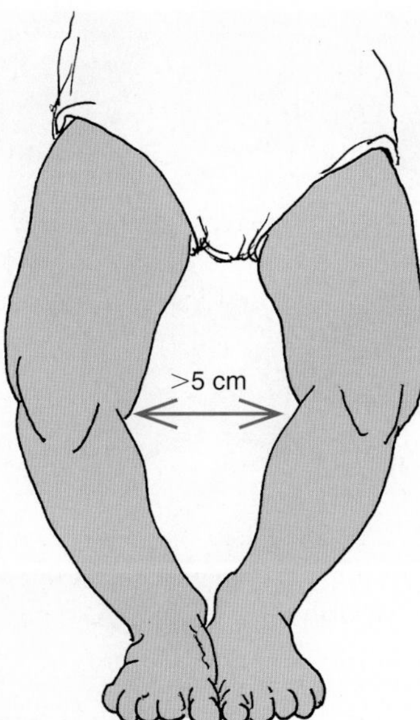

FIGURE 33-40 Bowleg.

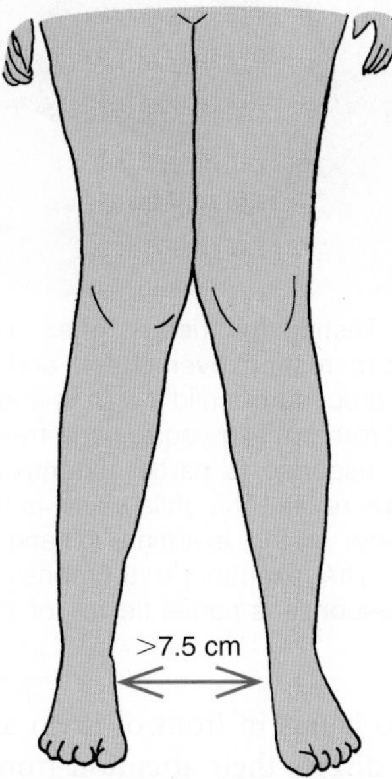

FIGURE 33-41 Knock-knee.

7.5 cm (Fig. 33-41). Knock-knee is normally present in children from about 2 to 7 years of age. Knock-knee that is excessive, asymmetrical, accompanied by short stature, or evident in a child nearing puberty requires further evaluation.

Next, the feet are inspected. Infants' and toddlers' feet appear flat because the foot is normally wide and the arch is covered by a fat pad. Development of the arch occurs naturally from the action of walking. Normally, at birth the feet are held in a valgus (outward) or varus (inward) position. To determine whether a foot deformity at birth is a result of intrauterine position or development, the examiner scratches the outer, then inner, side of the sole. (See Chapter 53 for a discussion of clubfoot and Fig. 53-12.) If the foot position is self-correctable, it will assume a right angle to the leg. As the child begins to walk, the feet turn outward less than 30 degrees and inward less than 10 degrees.

Toddlers have a "toddling" or broad-based gait, which facilitates walking by lowering the centre of gravity. As the child reaches preschool age, the legs are brought closer together. By school age the walking posture is much more graceful and balanced.

The most common gait problem in young children is *pigeon toe*, or toeing in, which usually results from torsional deformities, such as internal tibial torsion (abnormal rotation or bowing of the tibia). Tests for tibial torsion include measuring the thigh–foot angle, which requires considerable practice for accuracy.

The plantar or grasp reflex can be elicited by exerting firm but gentle pressure with the tip of the thumb against the lateral sole of the foot from the heel upward to the little toe and then across to the big toe. The normal response in children who are walking is flexion of the toes. *Babinski sign*, dorsiflexion of the big toe and fanning of the other toes, is normal during infancy but abnormal after about 1 year of age or when locomotion begins (see Fig. 35-6).

Joints

The joints are evaluated for range of motion. Normally this requires no specific testing if the nurse has observed the child's movements during the examination. However, the hips should be routinely investigated in infants for developmental dysplasia by a qualified health care provider (physician or nurse practitioner) (see Fig. 25-12 and Chapter 53). Any evidence of joint immobility or hyperflexibility needs to be reported.

The joints are palpated for heat, tenderness, and swelling. These signs, as well as redness over the joint, warrant further investigation.

Muscles

The symmetry and quality of muscle development, tone, and strength should be noted. Development is observed by looking at the shape and contour of the body in both a relaxed and a tensed state. Tone is estimated by grasping the muscle and feeling its firmness when it is relaxed and contracted. A common site for testing tone is the biceps muscle of the arm. Children are usually willing to "make a muscle" by clenching their fist.

Strength can be estimated by having the child use an extremity to push or pull against resistance, as in the following examples:

Arm strength—Child holds the arms outstretched in front of the body and tries to raise the arms while downward pressure is applied.

Hand strength—Child shakes hands with nurse and squeezes one or two fingers of the nurse's hand.

Leg strength—Child sits on a table or chair with the legs dangling and tries to raise the legs while downward pressure is applied.

Symmetry of strength in the extremities, hands, and fingers should be noted and evidence of paresis, or weakness, needs to be reported.

BOX 33-14 TESTS FOR CEREBELLAR FUNCTION

Finger-to-nose test—With the child's arm extended, ask the child to touch the nose with the index finger with eyes open and then closed.
Heel-to-shin test—Have the child stand and run the heel of one foot down the shin or anterior aspect of the tibia of the other leg, both with eyes opened and then closed.
Romberg test—Have the child stand with eyes closed and heels together; falling or leaning to one side is abnormal and is called the Romberg sign.

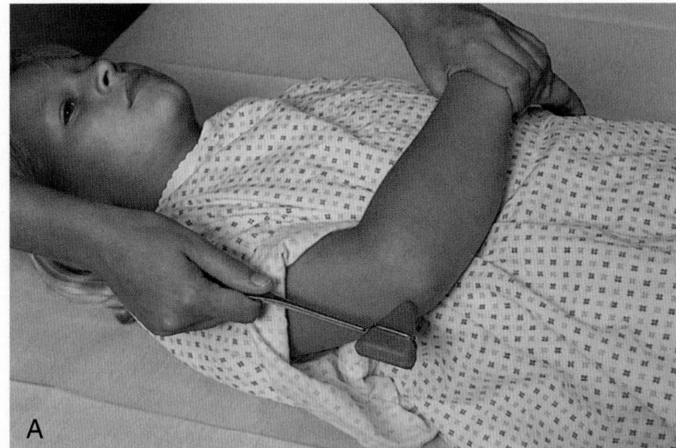

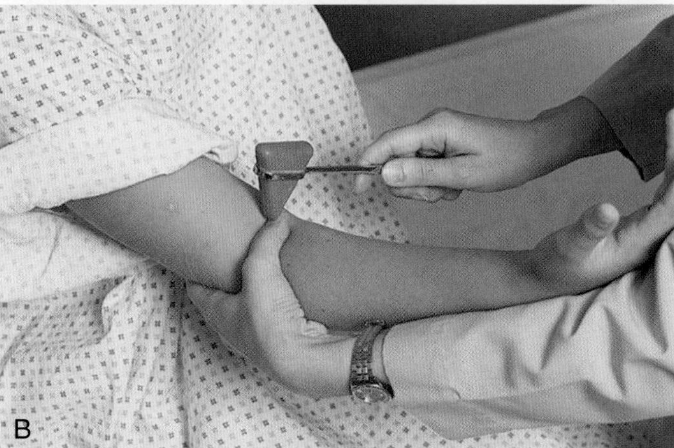

FIGURE 33-42 A: Testing for triceps reflex. The child is placed supine, with forearm resting over chest, and triceps tendon is struck. Alternative procedure: child's arm is abducted, with upper arm supported and forearm allowed to hang freely. Triceps tendon is struck. Normal response is partial extension of the forearm. **B:** Testing for biceps reflex. The child's arm is held by placing the partially flexed elbow in the examiner's hand with thumb over antecubital space. The examiner's thumbnail is struck with a hammer. Normal response is partial flexion of the forearm.

Neurological Assessment

The assessment of the nervous system is the broadest and most diverse part of the examination process, since every human function, both physical and emotional, is controlled by neurological impulses. Much of the neurological examination has already been discussed, such as assessment of behaviour, sensory testing, and motor function. The following discussion focuses on a general appraisal of cerebellar function, deep tendon reflexes, and the cranial nerves.

Cerebellar Function

The cerebellum controls balance and coordination. Much of the assessment of cerebellar function is included in observing the child's posture, body movements, gait, and development of fine and gross motor skills. Tests such as balancing on one foot and the heel-to-toe walk assess balance. Coordination is tested by asking the child to reach for a toy, button clothes, tie shoes, or draw a straight line on a piece of paper (provided the child is old enough to do these activities). Coordination can also be tested by any sequence of rapid, successive movements, such as quickly touching each finger with the thumb of the same hand.

Several tests for cerebellar function can be performed as games (Box 33-14). When a Romberg test is done, the nurse stays beside the child if there is a possibility that the child may fall. School-age children should be able to perform these tests, although in the finger-to-nose test, preschoolers normally can only bring the finger within 5 to 7.5 cm of the nose. Difficulty in performing these exercises indicates poor sense of position (especially with the eyes closed) and incoordination (especially with the eyes opened).

Reflexes

Testing reflexes is an important part of the neurological examination. Persistence of primitive reflexes, loss of reflexes, or hyperactivity of deep tendon reflexes is usually a result of a cerebral insult.

Reflexes can be elicited by using the rubber head of the reflex hammer, flat of the finger, or side of the hand. If the child is easily frightened by equipment, a hand or finger can be used. Although testing reflexes is a simple procedure, the child may inhibit the reflex by unconsciously tensing the muscle. To avoid tensing, younger children can be distracted with toys or talk to them. Older children can concentrate on the exercise of grasping their two hands in front of them and trying to pull them apart. This diverts their attention from the testing and causes involuntary relaxation of the muscles.

Deep tendon reflexes are stretch reflexes of a muscle. The most common deep tendon reflex is the knee jerk, or patellar reflex (sometimes called the quadriceps reflex). The reflexes normally elicited are described in Figures 33-42 and 33-43. Any diminished or hyperreflexive response should be reported for further evaluation.

Cranial Nerves

Assessment of the cranial nerves (Fig. 33-44) is an important area of neurological assessment (Table 33-14). With young children, the nurse can present the tests as games to foster trust and security at the beginning of the examination. Alternatively, the cranial nerve test can be included when each system is examined, such as tongue movement and strength, gag reflex, swallowing, cardinal positions of gaze (Fig. 33-45), and position of the uvula during examination of the mouth.

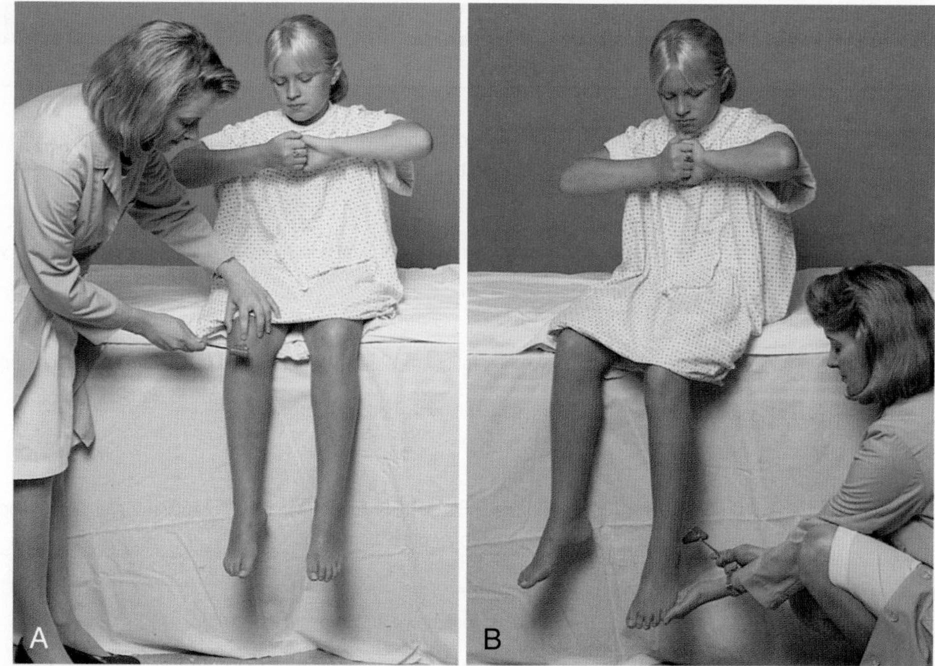

FIGURE 33-43 A: Testing for patellar, or knee jerk, reflex, using distraction. The child sits on edge of the examining table (or on parent's lap) with lower legs flexed at the knee and dangling freely. The patellar tendon is tapped just below the kneecap. Normal response is partial extension of the lower leg. **B:** Testing for Achilles reflex. The child should be in the same position as for knee jerk reflex. The foot is supported lightly in the examiner's hand, and the Achilles tendon is struck. Normal response is plantar flexion of the foot (foot pointing downward).

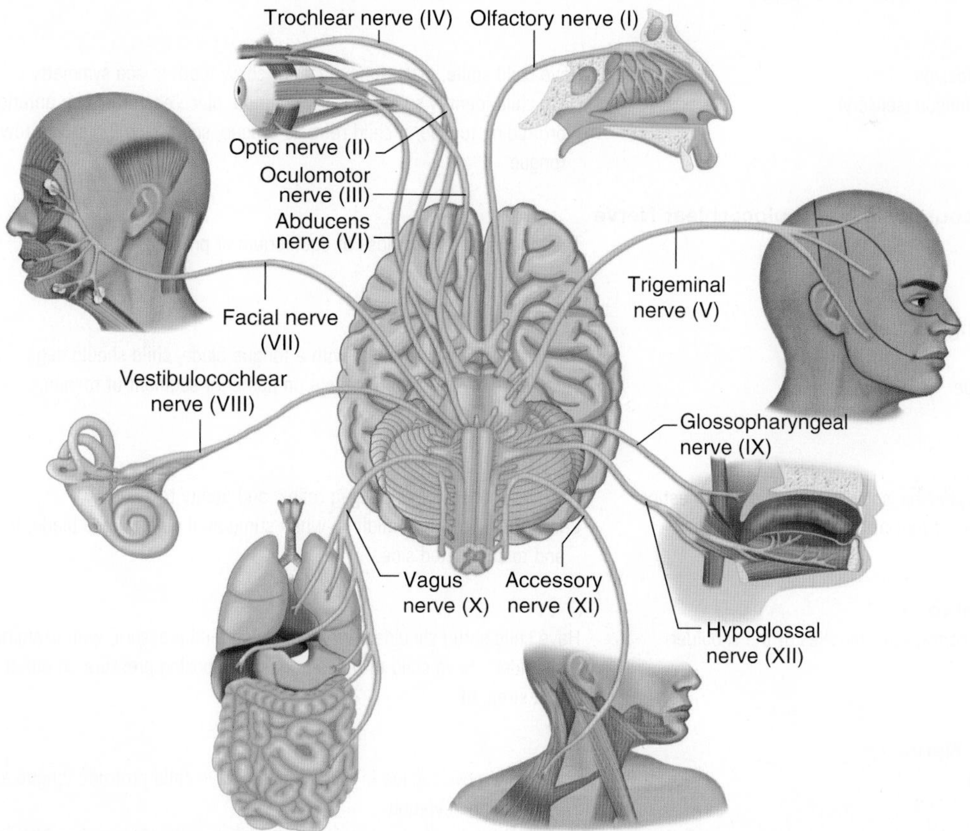

FIGURE 33-44 Cranial nerves. (From Patton, K. T., & Thibodeau, G. A. [2013]. *Anatomy & physiology* [8th ed.]. St. Louis: Mosby.)

TABLE 33-14 ASSESSMENT OF CRANIAL NERVES

DESCRIPTION AND FUNCTION	TESTS
I—Olfactory Nerve	
Olfactory mucosa of nasal cavity Smell	With eyes closed, have child identify odours such as coffee, alcohol from a swab, or other smells; test each nostril separately.
II—Optic Nerve	
Rods and cones of retina, optic nerve Vision	Check for perception of light, visual acuity, peripheral vision, colour vision, and normal optic disc.
III—Oculomotor Nerve	
Extraocular muscles of the eye: Superior rectus (SR)—moves eyeball up and in Inferior rectus (IR)—moves eyeball down and in Medial rectus (MR)—moves eyeball nasally Inferior oblique (IO)—moves eyeball up and out	Have child follow an object (toy) or light in six cardinal positions of gaze (see Fig. 33-45).
Pupil constriction and accommodation	Perform PERRLA (*P*upils *E*qual, *R*ound, *R*eact to *L*ight, and *A*ccommodation).
Eyelid closing	Check for proper placement of lid.
IV—Trochlear Nerve	
Superior oblique muscle (SO)—moves eye down and out	Have child look down and in (see Fig. 33-45).
V—Trigeminal Nerve	
Muscles of mastication	Have child bite down hard and open jaw; test symmetry and strength.
Sensory—face, scalp, nasal and buccal mucosa	With child's eyes closed, see if child can detect light touch in mandibular and maxillary regions. Test corneal and blink reflex by touching cornea lightly (approach from the side so that child does not blink before cornea is touched).
VI—Abducens Nerve	
Lateral rectus (LR) muscle—moves eye temporally	Have child look toward temporal side (see Fig. 33-45)
VII—Facial Nerve	
Muscles for facial expression	Have child smile, make funny face, or show teeth to see symmetry of expression.
Anterior two thirds of tongue (sensory)	Have child identify sweet or salty solution; place each taste on anterior section and sides of protruding tongue; if child retracts tongue, solution will dissolve toward posterior part of tongue.
VIII—Auditory, Acoustic, or Vestibulocochlear Nerve	
Internal ear Hearing and balance	Test hearing; note any loss of equilibrium or presence of vertigo.
IX—Glossopharyngeal Nerve	
Pharynx, tongue	Stimulate posterior pharynx with a tongue blade; child should gag.
Posterior third of tongue Sensory	Test sense of sour or bitter taste on posterior segment of tongue.
X—Vagus Nerve	
Muscles of the larynx, pharynx, some organs of gastrointestinal system, sensory fibres of root of tongue, heart, and lung	Note hoarseness of voice, gag reflex, and ability to swallow. Check that uvula is in midline; when stimulated with tongue blade, it should deviate upward and to stimulated side.
XI—Accessory Nerve	
Sternocleidomastoid and trapezius muscles of the shoulder	Have child shrug shoulders while applying mild pressure; with examiner's hands placed on shoulders, have child turn head against opposing pressure on either side; note symmetry and strength.
XII—Hypoglossal Nerve	
Muscles of the tongue	Have child move tongue in all directions; have child protrude tongue as far as possible; note any midline deviation. Test strength by placing tongue blade on one side of tongue and having child move it away.

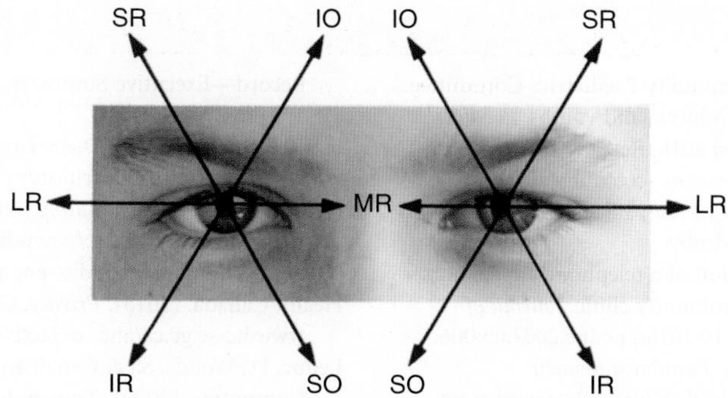

FIGURE 33-45 Testing cardinal positions of gaze. Muscles responsible for movement: *SR*, superior rectus; *IR*, inferior rectus; *MR*, medial rectus; *IO*, inferior oblique; *SO*, superior oblique; *LR*, lateral rectus.

KEY POINTS

- In order to effectively establish a setting for communication, nurses must make an appropriate introduction and ensure privacy and confidentiality.
- When communicating with parents, nurses need to encourage parental involvement, listen carefully, use silence, and be empathic.
- Communication with children needs to reflect their developmental stage.
- Nonverbal communication with children may take the form of writing, drawing, and play.
- The objectives of performing a health history are to identify pertinent information, determine the chief health concern, analyze the present illness, secure the patient's health history, review biological systems, and record a family medical history and child psychosocial and sexual history.
- Family assessment is the collection of data about family composition and relationships among its members; it also focuses on home and community environment, parents' occupation and education, and cultural and religious traditions.
- Nutritional assessment is performed by determination of dietary intake, clinical examination, and biochemical analysis.
- Developmental screening tools are valuable in identifying infants and children who are at risk of developmental delays.
- Growth measurements during the physical examination focus on length or height, weight, skin fold thickness, and arm and head circumference. Assessment of growth is measured against standard growth charts to determine a child's status in comparison with that of other children the same age.
- Measurements of temperature, pulse, respiration, and BP constitute the physiological approach to assessment.
- The child's general appearance is a cumulative, subjective impression of physical appearance, state of nutrition, behaviour, personality, interactions with parents and nurse, posture, development, and speech.
- Assessment of the skin, which primarily involves inspection and palpation, focuses on colour, texture, temperature, moisture, and turgor. The nurse needs to be aware of both physiological and ethnic factors that may affect these areas.
- In assessment of the lymph nodes, the nurse examines, by palpation, the part of the body in which the glands are located.
- The head is inspected for shape, symmetry, mobility, and muscle control.
- Examination of the eyes includes placement and alignment, inspection of external and internal structures, and vision testing.
- The ear examination encompasses placement and alignment, external and internal structures, and auditory testing.
- The lungs are examined by inspection, palpation, percussion, and auscultation.
- Auscultation is the most important procedure for examining the heart.
- Abdominal assessment follows an orderly sequence of inspection, auscultation, percussion, and, finally, palpation, since palpation may distort normal abdominal sounds assessed during auscultation.
- Examination of the genitalia may provoke anxiety in the child, and the nurse must avoid any transference of anxiety.
- Neurological assessment addresses behaviour; motor, sensory, and cerebellar function; reflexes; and cranial nerves.

evolve WEBSITE

Visit the Evolve website for additional resources related to the content in this chapter such as Case Studies, Critical Thinking Case Study Answers, Nursing Care Plans, Nursing Processes, Nursing Skills, and Review Questions for Exam Preparation at: *http://evolve.elsevier.com/Canada/Perry/maternal/*

REFERENCES

Amit, M., & Canadian Paediatric Society, Community Paediatrics Committee. (2009/2016). Vision screening in infants, children, and youths. *Paediatrics & Child Health, 14*(4), 246–248. Reaffirmed 2016. Retrieved from <http://www.cps.ca/documents/position/children-vision-screening#authors>.

Ball, J. W., Dains, J. E., Flynn, J. A., et al. (2014). *Mosby's Seidel's guide to physical examination* (8th ed.). St. Louis: Mosby.

Beaulieu, R., & Humphreys, J. (2008). Evaluation of a telephone advice nurse in a nursing faculty managed pediatric community clinic. *Journal of Pediatric Health Care, 22*(3), 175–181. doi:10.1016/j.pedhc.2007.05.006.

Canadian Association of Optometrists. (2014). *Position statement: Comprehensive vision examination of preschool children.* Retrieved from <https://opto.ca/sites/default/files/cao_position_statement_-_comprehensive_vision_examination_of_preschool_children.pdf>.

Canadian Nurses Association. (2008). *Nursing ethics. Code of ethics for registered nurses* (2008 centennial edition). Retrieved from <http://cna-aiic.ca/~/media/cna/page-content/pdf-fr/code-of-ethics-for-registered-nurses.pdf>.

Canadian Paediatric Society. (2010). The Greig health record. *Paediatrics and Child Health, 15*(3), 157–159. Retrieved from <http://www.cps.ca/tools-outils/greig-health-record>.

Canadian Paediatric Society. (2013). *Healthy kids, active kids.* Retrieved from <http://www.cps.ca/issues-questions/healthy-active-living>.

Canadian Paediatric Society. (2014). *Rourke Baby Record.* <http://www.cps.ca/tools-outils/rourke-baby-record>.

Canadian Paediatric Society. (2015). *Behavioural and general developmental screening tools.* Retrieved from <http://www.cps.ca/en/tools-outils/behavioural-and-general-developmental-screening-tools>.

Dietitians of Canada. (2014). *WHO growth charts.* Retrieved from <http://www.dietitians.ca/Dietitians-Views/Prenatal-and-Infant/WHO-Growth-Charts.aspx>.

Fenton, T. R. (2003). A new growth chart for preterm babies: Babson and Benda's chart updated with recent data and a new format. *BMC Pediatrics, 3*, 13. doi:10.1186/1471-2431-3-13. Retrieved from <http://www.biomedcentral.com/1471-2431/3/13>.

Greig, A., Constantin, E., Carsley, S., et al. (2010). Preventive health care visits for children and adolescents aged six to 17 years: The Greig Health Record—Executive Summary. *Paediatrics & Child Health, 15*(3), 157–162.

Health Canada. (2010). *Dietary reference intake tables.* Retrieved from <http://hc-sc.gc.ca/fn-an/nutrition/reference/table/index-eng.php>.

Health Canada. (2012). *Eating well with Canada's food guide.* Ottawa: Author. Retrieved from <http://www.hc-sc.gc.ca/fn-an/food-guide-aliment/order-commander/index-eng.php>.

Health Canada. (2015). *Privacy.* Ottawa: Author. Retrieved from <http://www.hc-sc.gc.ca/ahc-asc/activit/atip-aiprp/priv-prot/index-eng.php>.

Leduc, D., Woods, S., & Canadian Paediatric Society, Community Paediatrics Committee. (2000). *Temperature measurement in paediatrics.* (Reaffirmed 2015). Retrieved from <http://www.cps.ca/documents/position/temperature-measurement>.

Limbos, M. M., Joyce, D. P., & Roberts, G. J. (2010). Nipissing District Developmental Screen. Patterns of use by physicians in Ontario. *Canadian Family Physician, 56*(2), e66–e72.

Midgley, P. C., Wardhaugh, B., Macfarlane, C., et al. (2009). Blood pressure in children aged 4-8 years: Comparison of Omron HEM 711 and sphygmomanometer blood pressure measurements. *Archives of Diseases of Children, 94*(12), 955–958. doi:10.1136/adc.2008.137059.

Office of the Privacy Commissioner of Canada. (2015). *A guide for individuals: Protecting your privacy.* Ottawa: Author. Retrieved from <https://www.priv.gc.ca/information/pub/guide_ind_e.asp>.

Patel, H., Feldman, M., & Canadian Paediatric Society, Community Paediatrics Committee. (2011). Universal newborn hearing screening. *Paediatrics & Child Health, 16*(5), 301–305. Reaffirmed 2016. Retrieved from <http://www.cps.ca/documents/position/universal-hearing-screening-newborns>.

Van Cleave, J., Heisler, M., Devries, J. M., et al. (2007). Discussion of illness during well-child care visits with parents of children with and without special health care needs. *Archives of Pediatric Adolescent Medicine, 161*, 1170–1175. doi:10.1001/archpedi.161.12.1170.

Wright, L. M., & Leahey, M. (2012). *Nurses and families: A guide to family assessment and intervention* (6th ed.). Philadelphia: F. A. Davis.

ADDITIONAL RESOURCES

Canada's Food Guides: <http://healthycanadians.gc.ca/eating-nutrition/food-guide-aliment/index-eng.php?_ga=1.223021970.868197850.1432519476>.

Canadian Nursing Informatics Association: <http://www.cnia.ca/about.htm>.

Canadian Paediatric Society—Behavioural and general developmental screening tools: <http://www.cps.ca/en/tools-outils/behavioural-and-general-developmental-screening-tool>.

Canadian Paediatric Society—Mental health screening tools and rating scales: <http://www.cps.ca/en/tools-outils/mental-health-screening-tools-and-rating-sc>.

Dietitians of Canada—Is My Child Growing Well? Questions and Answers for Parents (parent handout on WHO Growth Charts for Canada): <https://www.dietitians.ca/Downloads/Factsheets/DC_ChildGrowParentsE.aspx>.

Greig Health Record: <http://www.cps.ca/tools-outils/greig-health-record>.

Public Health Agency of Canada—The Canadian Immunization Guide, and schedules for each province and territory: <http://www.phac-aspc.gc.ca/publicat/cig-gci/index-eng.php>.

Office of Privacy Commissioner of Canada (Information on the Privacy Act and PIPEDA): <http://www.priv.gc.ca/information/02_05_d_08_e.cfm>.

Rourke Baby Record: <http://www.rourkebabyrecord.ca/pdf/RBR2014Nat_Eng.pdf>.

Snellen Letter Chart: <http://www.allaboutvision.com/eye-test/>.

Telehealth Ontario: <https://www.ontario.ca/page/get-medical-advice-telehealth-ontario>.

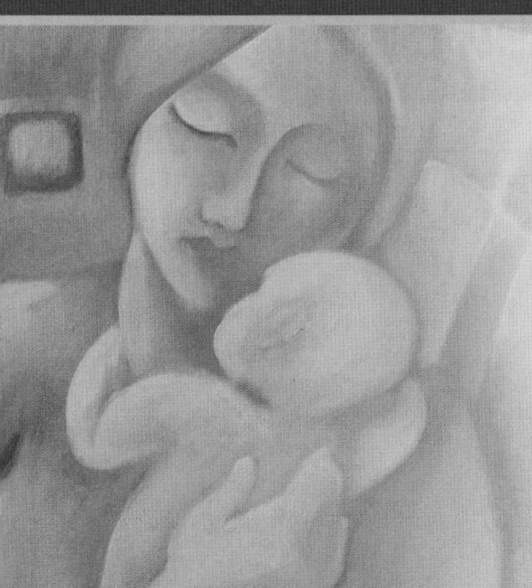

CHAPTER

34

Pain Assessment and Management

Denise Harrison, Cheryl Sams

evolve WEBSITE

Visit the Evolve website for additional resources related to the content in this chapter such as Case Studies, Critical Thinking Case Study Answers, Nursing Care Plans, Nursing Processes, Nursing Skills, and Review Questions for Exam Preparation at: http://evolve.elsevier.com/Canada/Perry/maternal/

OBJECTIVES

On completion of this chapter the reader will be able to:

- Identify measures to assess pain in infants and children.
- List various types of pain assessment tools that are used with infants and children.
- Outline essential pain management strategies of reducing pain in infants and children.
- Review common types of pain experienced.
- Discuss evidence supporting specific pain management strategies.

PAIN ASSESSMENT

Knowledge about pain assessment and availability of valid pain assessment tools for infants and children have improved dramatically in recent years. Yet pain assessment continues to be complex and challenging (Registered Nurses Association of Ontario [RNAO], 2013). Studies throughout Canada steadily report inconsistent documentation of pain assessment as well as undertreatment of pain in children in the pediatric hospital setting (Harrison, Joly, Chretien, et al., 2014; Stevens, Abbott, Yamada, et al., 2011; Stevens, Harrison, Rashotte, et al., 2012; Taylor, Boyer, & Campbell, et al., 2008). Optimal pain management begins with systematic and consistent assessment and reassessment following pain treatment and painful procedures to guide the selection of treatments and allow evaluation of the effectiveness or ineffectiveness of pain treatments (RNAO, 2013). Although there are now more than 90 different measures of pain for infants, children, and youth (Stevens et al., 2012), pain assessment remains challenging, particularly for children with complex pain that may be chronic, recurrent, or persistent. Pain assessment and management in these age groups will be discussed in this chapter; pain management for specific conditions is covered in Unit 12.

Assessment of Acute Pain

Acute pain in children may have several causes, such as medical procedures (immunization, venipuncture, for blood tests or intravenous therapy, lumbar puncture for diagnosis or treatment, bone marrow aspiration, skin debridement for severe burns); surgical (appendectomy, tonsillectomy) and orthopaedic (spinal fusion) procedures; medical treatments (chemotherapy-induced mucositis or peripheral neuropathy); injury (such as falls, burns, injury from motor vehicle accidents, other traumatic injuries); infection; and exacerbation of disease-related pain, such as arthritis, sickle cell disease, and cancer.

Pain Intensity

Traditionally, assessment measures are defined as behavioural measures, physiological measures, and measures of self-report. These measures predominantly address the domain of pain intensity. Behavioural measures of pain (for infants and children younger than 4 years; see Table 34-1) and self-reports of pain (for children 4 years and older; see Table 34-2) have been developed, validated, and widely used. Young children under 3 years of age cannot self-report pain using a pain scale, as they

TABLE 34-1 SUMMARY OF SELECTED BEHAVIOURAL PAIN MEASUREMENT SCALES FOR INFANTS AND YOUNG CHILDREN

AGES OF USE	PURPOSE/CONTEXT	ITEMS	SCORING RANGE
Children's Hospital of Eastern Ontario Pain Scale (CHEOPS) (McGrath, Johnson, Goodman, et al., 1985)			
1–7 years	Originally developed for measurement of postoperative pain Subsequently used to assess pain during brief pain episodes (e.g., vaccinations) and major procedural pain (e.g., bone marrow biopsies; severe pain (e.g., sickle cell)	Cry (1–3) Facial (0–2) Child verbal (0–2) Torso (1–2) Touch (1–2) Legs (1–2)	4 = no pain; 13 = worst pain
Modified Behavioural Pain Scale (MBPS) (Taddio, Nulman, Koren, et al., 1995)			
2–6 months	Modified from the Behavioural Pain Score (Robieux, Kumar, Radhakrishnan, et al., 1991) Developed for measurement of vaccination pain	Facial expression (0–3) Cry (0–4) Movements (0, 2, 3)	0 = no pain; 10 = worst pain
Face, Legs, Activity, Cry, and Consolability (FLACC) (Merkel, Voepel-Lewis, Shayevitz, et al., 1997)			
2 months–7 years	Originally developed for measurement of postoperative pain Subsequently used to assess pain during brief pain episodes and in critically ill patients and for infants from 15 days of age through to adults	Face (0–2) Legs (0–2) Activity (0–2) Cry (0–2) Consolability (0–2)	0 = no pain; 10 = worst pain
FLACC Scale–Revised (Malviya, Voepel-Lewis, Burke, et al., 2006)			
4–19 years	Originally developed for measurement of postoperative pain in children with cognitive impairment Subsequently used to assess pain during brief pain episodes and in critically ill patients	Same scale as for FLACC, however, further individual behaviour descriptors noted: Face 1: appears sad or worried Face 2: distressed-looking face; expression of fright or panic Legs 2: marked increase in spasticity, constant tremors, or jerking	0 = no pain; 10 = worst pain
Non-Communicating Children's Pain Checklist (NCCPC) (McGrath, Rosmus, Canfield, et al., 1998)			
5–29 years	Checklist to be used by primary caregivers to assess pain in children and young adults with cerebral palsy	31 items grouped into seven categories: Vocal; Eating/Sleeping; Social/Personality; Facial Expressions; Activity; Body and Limbs; Physiological	Checklist only; no aggregate score
Non-Communicating Children's Pain Checklist—Postoperative Version (NCCPC-PVO) (Breau, Finley, McGrath, et al., 2002)			
	Nonverbal children with intellectual disabilities	As in NCCPC, with removal of Eating/Sleeping category, therefore, 29 items grouped into six categories During a 10-minute observation, frequency of occurrence of each item scored: 0 = not at all; 1 = just a little; 2 = often; 3 = very often	0–87 Scores ≥30 considered moderate to severe pain

lack the ability to quantify pain using self-report measures. Other reasons for inability to self-report include cognitive impairment, inability to communicate, and critical illness (Crellin, Harrison, Santamaria, et al., 2015).

Behavioural measures. Distress behaviours such as crying, facial expression, and body movements occur in response to acute painful procedures and are associated with pain (see Fig. 26-19) (Box 34-1). The facial expressions of brow bulge, eye squeeze, nasolabial furrow, and stretched open lips are the most frequently occurring and specific behavioural indicators of acute procedural pain in infants regardless of gestational age or severity of illness (Harrison, Bueno, & Reszel, 2015). Behavioural indicators of pain are helpful in evaluating pain in infants and children with limited communication skills. However, discriminating between pain behaviours and reactions from other sources of distress, such as hunger, anxiety, or other types of discomfort, depends on the context of the situation and is not always easy.

Behavioural assessment is useful for measuring pain in infants and preverbal children who do not have the language skills to communicate that they are in pain or in children with limited ability to communicate meaningfully. Behaviour

TABLE 34-2 PAIN RATING SCALES FOR CHILDREN

PAIN SCALE, DESCRIPTION	INSTRUCTIONS	RECOMMENDED AGE, COMMENTS
Wong-Baker FACES® Pain Rating Scale		
Uses six cartoon faces ranging from smiling face for "no pain" to tearful face for "worst pain"	Explain to the child that each face represents a face of a person with no pain (hurt), some pain, or a lot of pain. Ask child to choose face that best describes own pain and record appropriate number.	Children as young as 3 yr The numbers are for parents and health care providers to quantify the pain. The words are included as a guide to explain how to use the faces.
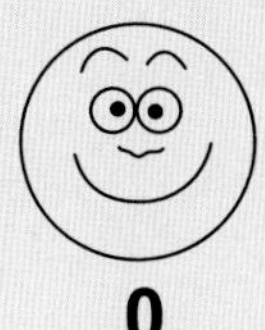 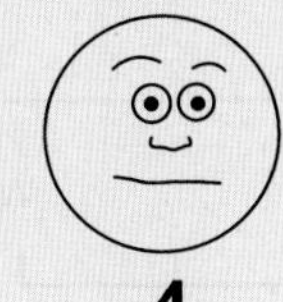 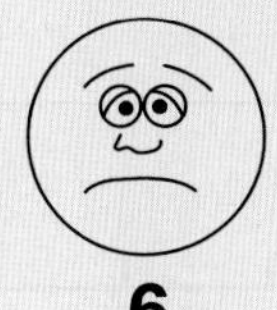 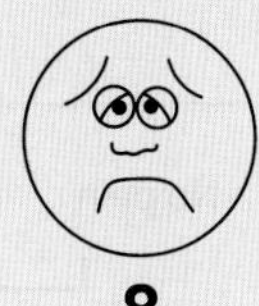 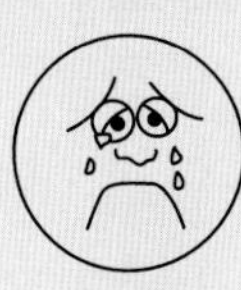 **0** No Hurt · **2** Hurts Little Bit · **4** Hurts Little More · **6** Hurts Even More · **8** Hurts Whole Lot · **10** Hurts Worst		
©1983 Wong-Baker FACES Foundation. www.WongBakerFACES.org. Used with permission. Originally published in *Whaley & Wong's Nursing Care of Infants and Children.* © Elsevier Inc.		
FACES Pain Scale-Revised (FPS-R)		
Made up of six faces depicting increasing gradation of pain severity, from 0 = "no pain" on the left face to 10 = "most pain possible" on the right face. The "no pain" 'anchor' face is a neutral face.	These faces show how much something can hurt. This face [**point to left-most face**] shows no pain. The faces show more and more pain [**point to each from left to right**] up to **this** one [**point to right-most face**]. It shows very much pain. Point to the face that shows how much you hurt [**right now**]. (International Association for the Study of Pain [IASP], 2001).	Well validated for children as young as 3 years. Do not use words like *happy* and *sad* when explaining tool to children. The scale is intended to measure how children feel, not how their face looks.
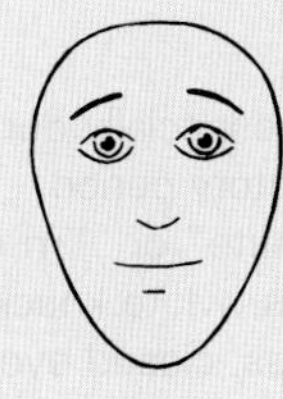 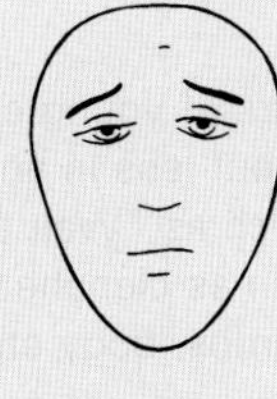 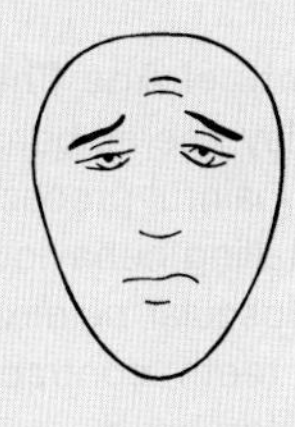 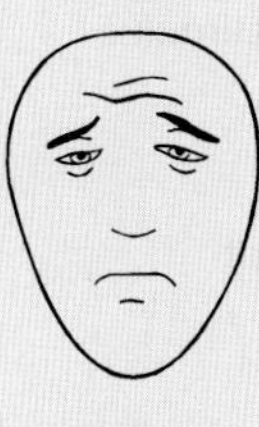 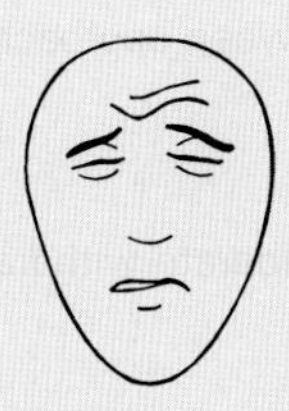 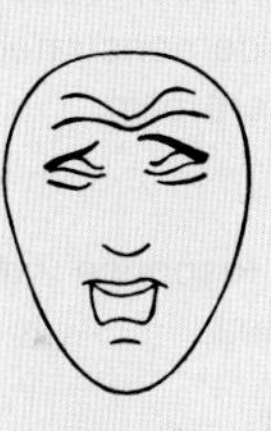 0 · 2 · 4 · 6 · 8 · 10		
Faces Pain Scale - Revised (FPS-R). www.iasp-pain.org/fpsr. Copyright © 2001, International Association for the Study of Pain®. Reproduced with permission.		
Numeric Scale		
Uses straight line with end points identified as "no pain" and "worst pain" and sometimes "medium pain" in the middle; divisions along line marked in units from 0 to 10 (high number may vary)	Explain to child that at one end of line is 0, which means that person feels no pain (hurt). At other end is usually 5 or 10, which means the person feels worst pain imaginable. The numbers 1–5 or 1–10 are for very little pain to a whole lot of pain. Ask child to choose number that best describes own pain.	Children as young as 5 yr, as long as they can count and have some concept of numbers and their values in relation to other numbers Scale may be used horizontally or vertically Number coding should be the same as in other scales used in facility.
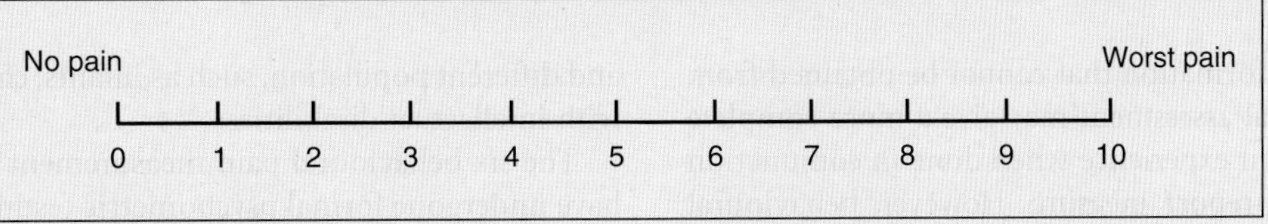		

Continued

TABLE 34-2 PAIN RATING SCALES FOR CHILDREN—cont'd

PAIN SCALE, DESCRIPTION	INSTRUCTIONS	RECOMMENDED AGE, COMMENTS
Visual Analogue Scale (VAS) (Cline, Herman, Shaw, et al., 1992)		
A vertical or horizontal line is drawn to a certain length, such as 10 cm, and anchored by items that represent extremes of the subjective phenomenon, such as pain, that is measured.	Ask child to place mark on line that best describes amount of own pain. With centimeter ruler measure from "no pain" end to the mark and record this measurement as the pain score.	Children as young as 4 to 5, up to 7 years. Vertical or horizontal scale may be used Research shows that children ages 3–18 yr prefer VAS less than other scales (Luffy & Grove, 2003; Wong & Baker, 1988).

No pain ——————— Worst pain

*Wong-Baker FACES Pain Rating Scale reference manual describing development and research of the scale is available from City of Hope Pain/Palliative Care Resource Center, 1500 East Duarte Road, Duarte, CA 91010; (626) 359-8111, ext. 3829; fax (626) 301-8941; http://www.elsevierhealth.com/WOW/. Use of FACES with children is demonstrated in *Whaley and Wong's Pediatric Nursing Video Series,* "Pain Assessment and Management," narrated by Donna Wong, PhD, RN. Available from Elsevier, 3251 Riverport Lane, Maryland Heights, MO, 63043; (800) 426-4545; fax (800) 535-9935; http://www.elsevierhealth.com.

BOX 34-1 DEVELOPMENTAL CHARACTERISTICS OF CHILDREN'S RESPONSES TO PAIN

Young Infant

- Generalized body response of rigidity or thrashing, possibly with local reflex withdrawal of stimulated area
- Crying
- Facial expression of pain (brows lowered and drawn together, eyes tightly closed, mouth stretched open and squarish)
- No association demonstrated between approaching stimulus and subsequent pain

Older Infant

- Localized body response with deliberate withdrawal of stimulated area
- Loud crying
- Facial expression of pain or anger
- Physical resistance, especially pushing the stimulus away after it is applied

Young Child

- Loud crying, screaming
- Verbal expressions such as "Ow," "Ouch," "It hurts"
- Thrashing of arms and legs
- Attempts to push stimulus away before it is applied
- Requests for termination of procedure
- Clinging to parent, nurse, or other significant person
- Requests for emotional support, such as hugs or other forms of physical comfort
- Becoming restless and irritable with continuing pain
- Behaviours occurring in anticipation of actual painful procedure

School-Age Child

- May see all behaviours of young child, especially during actual painful procedure, but less in anticipatory period
- Stalling behaviour, such as "Wait a minute" or "I'm not ready"
- Muscular rigidity, such as clenched fists, white knuckles, gritted teeth, contracted limbs, body stiffness, closed eyes, wrinkled forehead

Adolescent

- Less vocal protest
- Less motor activity
- More verbal expressions, such as "It hurts" or "You're hurting me"
- Increased muscle tension and body control

Data from Craig, K. D., et al. (1984). Developmental changes in infant pain expression during immunization injections. *Social Science and Medicine, 19*(12), 1331–1337; Katz, E. R., Kellerman, J., & Siegel, S. E. (1980). Behavioral distress in children with cancer undergoing medical procedures: Developmental considerations. *Journal of Consulting and Clinical Psychology, 48*(3), 356–365.

provides important information that cannot be obtained from self-report. Behavioural assessment may give a more complete picture of the total pain experience when done in conjunction with a subjective self-report measure. However, behavioural pain scales may be more time consuming to conduct than obtaining self-reports. These measures depend on a trained observer to watch and record children's behaviours, such as vocalization, facial expression, and body movements that suggest discomfort.

Table 34-1 lists and summarizes a selection of validated behavioural pain measurement scales used to assess pain intensity in different contexts (such as procedural, postoperative) and different population, such as infants, children, and children with intellectual disabilities.

The six behavioural pain measurement scales in Table 34-1 have undergone formal psychometric testing, and all have been used to various degrees in clinical care and research. The scales are developed for different populations of children, undergoing different procedures.

The CHEOPS was developed in collaboration with experienced recovery room nurses to measure postoperative pain in children (McGrath et al., 1985). The scale ranges from 4 (no pain) to 13 (worst pain) and includes indicators of cry, facial expressions, verbalization about pain, torso position and movements, touching (e.g., reaching, grabbing, need for restraint), and movement of legs. The MBPS, modified from the Behavioural Pain Scale (Robieux et al., 1991), was specifically developed for measurement of vaccination pain in infants (Taddio et al., 1995). The 0–10 scale includes the items of cry, facial expressions, and body movements. The FLACC has been used extensively in clinical practice and research (Crellin et al., 2015) and includes five categories of behaviour: *F*acial expression, *L*eg movement, *A*ctivity, *C*ry, and *C*onsolability (Manworren & Hynan, 2003). It measures pain by quantifying pain behaviours with scores ranging from 0 (no pain behaviours) to 10 (most possible pain behaviours). The FLACC scale-revised includes behaviours specific to individuals with cognitive impairment (Malviya et al., 2006). The Non-communicating Children's Pain Checklist (NCCPC) (McGrath et al., 1998) and the revised postoperative version (Breau et al., 2002) measure pain in nonverbal children. A 10-minute observation period by caregivers is recommended to score 31 items in seven categories on the original scale and 29 items in six categories in the revised postoperative version. Such items include moaning, whining, crying (Vocal category); irritable, withdrawn, difficult to distract (Social Category); and furrowed brow and clenching or grinding teeth (Facial Category).

In critical care settings the COMFORT scale (Ambuel, Hamlett, Marx, et al., 1992) or the revised modified COMFORT scale (Carnevale & Razack, 2002) is recommended. The modified COMFORT scale is a behavioural, unobtrusive method of measuring distress in unconscious and ventilated patients. It has six indicators: alertness, calmness/agitation, respiratory response, physical movement, muscle tone, and facial tension. Each indicator is scored between 1 and 5, based on the behaviours exhibited by the patient. Patients are observed unobtrusively for 2 minutes, and the total score is derived by adding the scores of each indicator. The total scores can range between 6 and 30, and scores of 11 generally indicate adequate sedation and pain control.

Self-report measures. Although children who are 4 or 5 years old are able to use self-report measures (Table 34-2), their ability to use them may be influenced by the cognitive characteristics of the preoperational stage (Stanford, Chambers, & Craig, 2006). The child's thinking tends to be egocentric, concrete, and perceptually dominated. Simple, concrete anchor words, such as "no hurt" to "biggest hurt," are more appropriate than "least pain sensation to worst intense pain imaginable."

The ability to discriminate degrees of pain in facial expressions appears to be reasonably established by 3 years of age (Stanford et al., 2006). For children age 3 to 4 years the most frequently used measure of pain intensity is the Faces Pain Scale. There are many different "faces" scales. Faces scales provide a series of facial expressions depicting gradations of pain. They are appealing to children and easy to use because children can simply point to the face that represents how they feel. Two Faces scales, the Bieri Faces Pain Scale–Revised (Hicks, von Baeyer, Spafford, et al., 2001) and the Wong-Baker FACES Pain Scale (Wong & Baker, 1988), are widely used. The scales range from 0 to 10. The Faces Pain Scale–Revised shows six faces depicting increasing gradation of pain severity, from 0 = "no pain" on the left face to 10 = "very much pain" on the right face. The "no pain" "anchor" face is a neutral face and does not depict the emotion of "happiness", and, similarly, none of the faces have tears, depicting the emotion of "sadness". The Wong-Baker FACES Pain Scale consists of six cartoon faces ranging from a smiling face for "no pain" to a tearful face for "worst pain." The child is asked to choose a face that describes his or her pain (see Table 34-2).

For children aged 8 years and older the numeric rating scale (NRS), specifically the 0-to-10 scale, is most widely used in clinical practice, is easy to use and document, and is well supported for use in this age group (von Baeyer, 2014). The visual analogue scale (VAS), a 10-centimetre line anchored by numbers or words "no pain" on the left and "worst pain" on the right, is another well-established measure of pain intensity in normally developing children aged 8 years and older (von Baeyer, 2014).

Global Judgement of Improvement and of Satisfaction With Treatment

Although pain intensity is the dimension that is most commonly assessed, patients or patient surrogates should also be asked to rate a global judgement of the pain and satisfaction with pain treatment. These ratings mean something different from one patient or surrogate to another. Some may focus on the relief of pain, whereas others may consider adverse effects of the treatment. The global question should be posed with indications of what should be considered in the answer, such as "Considering pain relief, adverse effects, physical recovery, and emotional recovery, how satisfied were you with the treatments your child is receiving for pain?"

Physical Recovery

Physical recovery, which includes aspects of physical functioning that are influenced by the procedure or injury, can cause acute pain. For example, swallowing 50 mL of water is important after tonsillectomy yet is painful. Sufficient preparation and instruction as well as appropriate analgesia are essential to facilitate activities that promote return to normal function. Possible assessments of the physical domain include the time taken to achieve sitting or ambulation, time to resume swallowing (post-tonsillectomy), and times to normal spirometry, oral intake, and full return to expected functioning. However, measures such as tolerance of physical therapy may be inconsistent. One child may be intolerant of physical therapy because he or she did not want to go when asked, whereas another might be considered intolerant to it if he or she cried and refused to continue with it. These measures of physical recovery should be assessed consistently and systematically to evaluate pain treatment interventions during and following procedures and injuries that have specific effects on physical functioning.

Assessment of Chronic and Recurrent Pain

The definition of *chronic pain* is prolonged pain that lasts for 3 months or more beyond the period of healing (National Institutes of Health [NIH] Medline Plus, 2011). Headache, abdominal pain, and limb pain are consistently reported to be the most common chronic pain conditions in children (Schechter, 2014). Pain that is episodic and recurs is defined as *recurrent pain*. The time frame within which episodes of pain recur is at least 3 months. Identified reasons for recurrent pain in children include headaches, migraine headaches, abdominal pain, sickle cell pain and sickle cell crisis, and "growing pains" in the long bones. van Dijk, McGrath, Pickett, et al. (2006) identified that 57% of school-age children had at least one recurrent pain episode (headaches, stomach pains, growing pains), and at least 6% had one or more chronic pain causes (disease related, back pain). Chronic and recurrent pain can have a detrimental effect on the psychosocial and physical well-being of children. Assessment of chronic or recurrent pain includes pain location and intensity; impact on physical and psychological functioning and on role functioning, such as school attendance and friendships; depression; impact on sleep; global judgement of satisfaction with treatment; and economic factors. Because the time course of chronic and recurrent pain is different from that of acute pain, measures used to assess the impact of chronic and recurrent pain must take into account timing and duration as key factors.

Pain diaries have been used to assess pain symptoms and response to treatment in children and adolescents with chronic and recurrent pain (Stinson, Stevens, Feldman, et al., 2008). Most pain diaries use an NRS or a VAS with faces or words. Children as young as 6 years have been included in pain diary studies. Conventional paper-and-pencil measures have been associated with several limitations, such as poor completion, missing data, hoarding responses, problems with recall, and back-and-forward filling (Stinson, 2009). Research has been conducted using electronic diaries with school-age children and adolescents with recurrent or chronic pain (Stinson, 2009). Such diaries facilitate real-time data collection, therefore reducing the need for recall; better capture periods of "no pain"; allow for collection of longitudinal data and investigation of within-person variability; and may facilitate rapid and responsive follow-up, support, and treatment for episodes of exacerbation of pain or difficulties managing pain. Challenges and limitations to using electronic diaries for research and clinical practice include increased costs, training, technical skills, and risk of technical malfunction (Stinson, 2009).

The physical functioning domain assessment is focused on activities of daily living, such as sitting or walking, or more vigorous exercise, such as running or sports. The Functional Disability Inventory (Walker & Greene, 1991) is recommended for assessing physical functioning in school-age children. This inventory assesses the child's ability and has established psychometrics properties with different populations (Claar & Walker, 2006; Vervoort, Goubert, Eccleston, et al., 2006). For children under 7 years of age, the PedsQL, developed by Varni, Seid, and Rode (1999), tests the physical functioning domain as it relates to pain. The PedsQL is a multidimensional scale with parent- and child-report versions. It assesses (1) physical functioning, (2) emotional functioning, (3) social functioning, and (4) school functioning.

The emotional functioning domain usually refers to depression and anxiety. Depression and anxiety are associated with chronic and recurrent pain and can occur concurrently (Palmero, 2000). However, most of these children do not have clinical levels of anxiety or depression. The Children's Depression Inventory (Kovacs, 1981) and the Revised Child Anxiety and Depression Scale (Chorpita, Yim, Moffitt, et al., 2000) have been used to assess anxiety and depression in children and adolescents with chronic or recurrent pain.

Chronic and recurrent pain can significantly interfere with the roles that children and adolescents perform, such as being a student, friend, and family member. School attendance can be used as a measure of role functioning in school-age children with chronic or recurrent pain. Other measures, such as the PedsQL and PedMIDAS (Hershey, 2001), have been validated for measurement of role functioning in these children.

Sleep disruption is also a frequent problem in chronic and recurrent pain. More than half of children with pain-related conditions (headache, juvenile idiopathic arthritis, or sickle cell disease) report difficulties sleeping (Butbul, Stremler, Benseler, et al., 2011). Sleep diaries, in which the child (or parent) records bedtimes and time to fall asleep and wake up, are useful for assessment of pain interference with sleep. In addition, the Sleep Habits Questionnaire (Owens, Spirito, & McGuinn, 2000) may be useful for assessing sleep behaviours in school-age children with chronic or recurrent pain.

Multidimensional Measures

Several cognitive skills, such as measurement, classification, and seriation (the ability to accurately place in ascending or descending order), become explicit between approximately 7 and 10 years of age. Children in this age range are therefore usually able to use a 0-to-10 numeric rating scale, currently used with adolescents and adults. However, use of this scale is only an assessment of pain intensity, which may not change in some pain states. Other dimensions such as pain quality, pain location, and spatial distribution of pain may change without a change in pain intensity.

Two multidimensional assessment tools that assess not only pain intensity but also pain location and pain quality have been well validated in children 8 years and older. Modelled after the McGill Pain Questionnaire (Melzack, 1975), the *Adolescent Pediatric Pain Tool (APPT)* is a multidimensional pain instrument for children and adolescents that is used to assess three dimensions of pain—location, intensity, and quality (Fig. 34-1)—and has been used in children of different ages, in a variety of settings, and with different health conditions (Fernandes, De Campos, Batalha, et al., 2014). The APPT is composed of three independent measures: a front and back view body outline diagram, for children to mark the location of their pain; a 10-cm word-graphic pain intensity rating scale, anchored by "no pain" and "worst possible pain"; and a pain descriptor list that includes qualitative descriptors to assess three dimensions of pain: sensory (e.g., aching, burning), affective (e.g., sickening, terrifying), evaluative (e.g., uncomfortable), as well as temporal (e.g., off and on, steady). Each of the three components of the APPT is scored separately. The total number of words on the descriptor list is counted, with scores ranging from 0 to 56. The clinician then counts the number of words selected from the categories and calculates a percentage score for each one (Savedra, Holzemer, Tesler, et al., 1993).

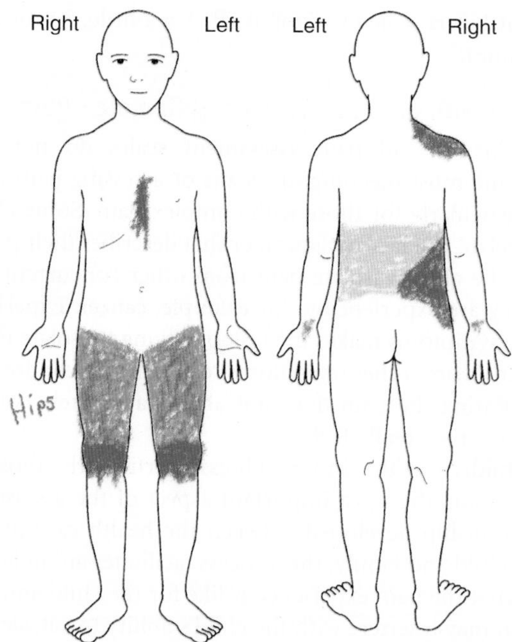

FIGURE 34-1 Adolescent Pediatric Pain Tool (APPT): Body outlines for pain assessment. Instructions: "Colour in the areas on these drawings to show where you have pain. Make the marks as big or as small as the place where the pain is." (From Savedra, M. C., Tesler, M. D., Holzemer, W. L., & Ward, J. A. School of Nursing, University of California–San Francisco; copyright 1989, 1992.)

An advantage to using the APPT is that in some pain states pain-intensity ratings do not change, but pain location and spatial distribution of pain may change over time. The total surface area may decrease, but some children may perceive the remaining sites as equal in pain intensity. In addition to pain location, assessments of pain quality may be able to distinguish the presence of the different dimensions of pain (temporal, affective, evaluative, and sensory). Words may not be quantifiable on an NRS yet represent the pain experience, such as *horrible* and *terrible* from the evaluative dimension, *screaming* and *terrifying* from the affective dimension, or *sharp* and *stabbing* from the sensory dimension. The different qualities of pain may also represent whether pain is of an ischemic and inflammatory nature in the cutaneous, subcutaneous, and musculoskeletal tissues as opposed to pain that is more neuropathic, which may be described using words such as *shooting, burning,* or *shocklike*.

The *Pediatric Pain Questionnaire (PPQ)* is a multidimensional pain instrument to assess patient and parental perceptions of the pain experience in a manner appropriate for the cognitive-developmental level of children and adolescents. The PPQ represents an attempt to assess the complexities of pediatric chronic, recurrent pain and targeted chronic musculoskeletal pain in children with juvenile rheumatoid arthritis. It consists of eight questions: (1) the pain history, (2) pain language, (3) the colours that children associate with pain, (4) the emotions they experience, (5) their worst pain experiences, (6) the ways in which they cope with pain, (7) the positive aspects of pain, and (8) the location of their current pain. The PPQ includes three components: (1) VASs; (2) colour-coded rating scales; and (3) verbal descriptors to provide information about the sensory, affective, and evaluative dimensions of chronic pain (Varni, Thompson, & Hanson, 1987). It also has information about the child's and family's pain history, symptoms, pain-relief interventions, and socioenvironmental situations that may influence pain. The child, parent, and health care provider complete the form separately.

The number of pain measures available for use in infants and young children has increased dramatically and adds a layer of complexity to the assessment of pain in children. Scales for pain measurement instruments mostly consist of 0 for no pain but a variable top score anchor (most severe pain) ranging from 4 to 160. A pain score of 5 may mean a lot of pain (if a 0-to-5 scale is used) or very little (if a 0-to-100 scale is used). This highlights the need to clearly specify which score corresponds to which scale and, at an organizational level, making it clear which pain assessment measures have been adopted for which populations. A common metric, such as a 0-to-10 score, may facilitate using pain scores to guide treatment, as a certain score may be considered the point at which an intervention is required or a point at which pain may be considered to be well controlled (von Baeyer & Hicks, 2000). A 0-to-10 system was reported to be preferred by health care providers and would make pain scores easier to read, interpret, and integrate into research and practice (von Baeyer & Hicks, 2000).

PAIN ASSESSMENT IN SPECIFIC POPULATIONS

Cultural Differences

While the experience of pain is universal, everyone has a unique experience with pain that is influenced by many dynamic factors, including family, community, and culture. Language and cultural differences between health care providers and the children they treat can make pain assessment and treatments more challenging. Several barriers to effective pain treatment that have been documented among non-English-speaking patients in general include inadequate assessment of pain, patient concern about adverse effects and tolerance of analgesics, patient and family reluctance to report pain, fear that pain means worse disease, reluctance to take pain medications, and lack of adherence to prescribed analgesics (Abbe, Simon, Angiolilo, et al., 2006; Bruera, Willey, Ewert-Flannagan, et al., 2005). One particular challenge in the assessment and management of pain in children is the cultural appropriateness of pain assessment tools that have been validated predominantly in White and English-speaking children. Observational scales and interview questionnaires for pain may not be as reliable for pain assessment as self-report scales in non-White and non-English-speaking children.

Aboriginal children tend to have pronounced vulnerabilities related to pain due to (a) the high prevalence of painful conditions among these children, (b) potential cultural differences in how they express pain, (c) the lack of culturally relevant validated pain assessments, and (d) inadequate pain care resulting in persistent pain (Latimer, Simandl, Finley, et al.,

2014). Westernized pain assessment tools may not accurately reflect the indigenous cultural differences in the pediatric Aboriginal population, resulting in inaccurate pain assessment and inadequate pain management. Further research is required to develop more accurate pain measurement tools that have a "two eyed lens approach" that blend Westernized pain management with the Canadian Aboriginal cultural understanding of pain (Latimer et al., 2014).

Children With Communication and Cognitive Impairment

The assessment of pain in children with communication and cognitive impairment can be challenging. Children who have difficulties communicating with others about their pain include those with significant neurological impairments, such as cerebral palsy, cognitive impairment, metabolic disorders, autism, or severe brain injury, and those with communication barriers, such as critically ill children who are on ventilators or heavily sedated or have neuromuscular disorders, loss of hearing, or loss of vision. These children are at greater risk than other children for undertreatment of pain because, in addition to potential communication difficulties, they have medical problems that cause pain and they may require repeated painful procedures. Pain may also occur during daily living activities, such as assisted stretching and walking; independent standing; toileting; putting on splints; and doing occupational therapy, range-of-motion exercises, or physical therapy. These children may experience spasticity, contractures, and orthopaedic surgical treatment that can be painful.

Mothers, fathers and partners, and other primary caregivers are important aids in helping health care providers understand and identify pain behaviours and provide optimal pain care for children with cognitive impairments and communication challenges (Breau, 2014). Behaviours related to pain include crying, moaning, irritability, changes in facial expression, and changes in social behaviour such as cooperation, activity, play, eating and sleeping, and engagement with family, friends, and others (Breau, 2014).

The *Non-communicating Children's Pain Checklist (NCCPC)* is a pain measurement tool specifically designed for children with cognitive impairments (Breau, McGrath, Camfield, et al., 2002). The scale discriminates between periods of pain and calm and can be used to predict behaviour during subsequent episodes of pain (Fig. 34-2). The scale consists of six subscales (vocal, social, facial, activity, body and limbs, physiological), which are scored on the basis of number of times the items are observed over a 10-minute period (0 = not at all; 1 = just a little; 2 = fairly often; 3 = very often).

Another tool, the *Pain Indicator for Communicatively Impaired Children (PICIC)*, is used to distinguish between pain and nonpain in communicatively impaired children with life-threatening illness (Stallard, Williams, Velleman, et al., 2002a, 2002b). The PICIC has six core pain cues: (1) crying with or without tears; (2) screaming, yelling, groaning, or moaning; (3) screwed-up or distressed-looking face; (4) body appearing stiff or tense; (5) difficulty in being comforted or consoled; and (6) flinching or moving away if touched. The items are rated using a 4-point Likert scale (1 = not at all, 2 = a little, 3 = often, 4 = all the time).

Children With Chronic Illness and Complex Pain

Questionnaires and pain assessment scales do not always provide the most meaningful means of assessing pain in children, particularly for those with complex pain. Some children cannot relate to a face or a number that describes their pain and may not be able to isolate pain from other concurrent symptoms they are experiencing, for example, cancer. Experiencing multiple symptoms makes the task of having to isolate the pain symptom from other symptoms difficult in children with cancer. Rating the pain does not always accurately convey to others how they really feel.

In children with chronic illness, particularly those with complex pain, the most important aspect of the assessment is the relationship developed between the health care providers and the child and family; this process facilitates an understanding of what the pain experience is like for the child and family. The pain may interfere with the child's ability to eat, sleep, and perform daily activities and routines.

Important questions to ask the family include those relating to the (1) onset of pain (i.e., was the onset sudden, unexpected, off and on, ongoing); (2) pain duration or pattern (i.e., when did the pain start; how long does it last); (3) effectiveness of the current treatment (i.e., which medications and doses help; what other strategies that have been tried have worked); (4) factors that aggravate or relieve the pain (i.e., which situations, positions, events, or activities make the pain worse, what makes the pain better); (5) other symptoms (e.g., nausea) and complications (e.g., fever, difficulty with breathing) that occur concurrently; and (6) interference with the child's sleep, mood, function, and interactions with family. Asking if the pain is better or worse at certain times during the day or night can also give clues to variations and rhythms of pain. Other factors warranting assessment that may pose barriers to effective pain management include family issues and relationships, fears and concerns about addiction (see further discussion on p. 980), the clinician's and family's lack of knowledge about pain, inappropriate use of pain medications, ineffective management of adverse effects from medications, and the use of various pain interventions.

PAIN MANAGEMENT

Unrelieved pain may lead to potential long-term physiological, psychosocial, and behavioural consequences, highlighting that management of pain should be a priority for all clinicians.

Nonpharmacological Management

Pain is often associated with fear, anxiety, and stress. A number of nonpharmacological techniques (see Guidelines box), such as distraction, relaxation, guided imagery, and cutaneous stimulation, provide coping strategies that may help reduce pain perception, make pain more tolerable, decrease anxiety, and enhance the effectiveness of pharmacological treatments

Non-communicating Children's Pain Checklist — Postoperative Version (NCCPC-PV)

NAME:________________ UNIT/FILE #: __________ DATE:______________ (dd/mm/yy)

OBSERVER:______________ START TIME:__________ AM/PM STOP TIME:____________AM/PM

How often has this child shown these behaviours in the last 10 minutes? Please circle a number for each behaviour. If an item does not apply to this child (for example, this child cannot reach with his/her hands), then indicate "not applicable" for that item.

	0 = NOT AT ALL	1 = JUST A LITTLE	2 = FAIRLY OFTEN	3 = VERY OFTEN	NA = NOT APPLICABLE
I. Vocal					
1. Moaning, whining, whimpering (fairly soft)	0	1	2	3	NA
2. Crying (moderately loud)	0	1	2	3	NA
3. Screaming/yelling (very loud)	0	1	2	3	NA
4. A specific sound or word for pain (e.g., a word, cry, or type of laugh)	0	1	2	3	NA
II. Social					
5. Not cooperating, cranky, irritable, unhappy	0	1	2	3	NA
6. Less interaction with others, withdrawn	0	1	2	3	NA
7. Seeking comfort or physical closeness	0	1	2	3	NA
8. Being difficult to distract, not able to satisfy or pacify	0	1	2	3	NA
III. Facial					
9. A furrowed brow	0	1	2	3	NA
10. A change in eyes, including squinching of eyes, eyes opened wide, eyes frowning	0	1	2	3	NA
11. Turning down of mouth, not smiling	0	1	2	3	NA
12. Lips puckering up, tight, pouting, or quivering	0	1	2	3	NA
13. Clenching or grinding teeth, chewing, or thrusting tongue out	0	1	2	3	NA
IV. Activity					
14. Not moving, less active, quiet	0	1	2	3	NA
15. Jumping around, agitated, fidgety	0	1	2	3	NA
V. Body and Limbs					
16. Floppy	0	1	2	3	NA
17. Stiff, spastic, tense, rigid	0	1	2	3	NA
18. Gesturing to or touching part of the body that hurts	0	1	2	3	NA
19. Protecting, favouring, or guarding part of the body that hurts	0	1	2	3	NA
20. Flinching or moving the body part away, being sensitive to touch	0	1	2	3	NA
21. Moving the body in a specific way to show pain (e.g., head back, arms down, curls up, etc.)	0	1	2	3	NA
VI. Physiological					
22. Shivering	0	1	2	3	NA
23. Change in colour, pallor	0	1	2	3	NA
24. Sweating, perspiring	0	1	2	3	NA
25. Tears	0	1	2	3	NA
26. Sharp intake of breath, gasping	0	1	2	3	NA
27. Breath holding	0	1	2	3	NA

SCORE SUMMARY

Category	I	II	III	IV	V	VI	TOTAL
Score							

FIGURE 34-2 Non-communicating Children's Pain Checklist (NCCPC). (Copyright 2004, Lynn Breau, Patrick McGrath, Allen Finley, & Carol Camfield. Reprinted with permission.)

Continued

USING THE NCCPC-PV

The NCCPC-PV was designed to be used for children age 3 to 18 years who are unable to speak because of cognitive (mental/intellectual) impairments or disabilities. It can be used *whether or not* a child has physical impairments or disabilities. Descriptions of the types of children used to validate the NCCPC-PV can be found in: Breau, L.M., Finley, G.A., McGrath, P.J., & Camfield, C.S. (2002). Validation of the Non-communicating Children's Pain Checklist — Postoperative Version. *Anesthesiology, 96* (3), 528-535. The NCCPC-PV was designed to be used without training by parents and caregivers (carers), or by other adults who are not familiar with a specific child (do not know them well).

The NCCPC-PV may be freely copied for clinical use or use in research funded by not-for-profit agencies. For-profit agencies should contact Lynn Breau: Pediatric Pain Research, IWK Health Centre, 5850 University Avenue, Halifax, Nova Scotia, Canada, B3J 3G9 (lbreau@ns.sympatico.ca).

The NCCPC-PV was intended for use for pain after surgery or due to other procedures conducted in hospital. If short- or long-term pain is suspected for a child at home or in a long-term residential setting, the **Non-communicating Children's Pain Checklist — Revised** may be used. It can be obtained by contacting Lynn Breau. Information regarding the NCCPC-R can be found in: Breau, L.M., McGrath, P.J., Camfield, C.S. & Finley, G.A. (2002). Psychometric Properties of the Non-communicating Children's Pain Checklist—Revised. *Pain, 99,* 349-357.

ADMINISTRATION

To complete the NCCPC-R, base your observations on the child's behaviour over **10 minutes**. ***It is not necessary to watch the child continuously for this period***. However, it is recommended that the observer be in the child's presence for the majority of this time (e.g., be in the same room with the child). Although shorter observation periods may be used, the cut-off scores described below may not apply.

At the end of the observation time, indicate how frequently (how often) each item was seen or heard. This should not be based on the child's typical behaviour or in relation to what he or she usually does. A guide for deciding the frequency of items is below:

0 = Not present at all during the observation period. (Note: If the item is not present because the child is not capable of performing that act, it should be scored as "NA").
1 = Seen or heard rarely (hardly at all), but is present.
2 = Seen or heard a number of times, but not continuous (not all the time).
3 = Seen or heard often, almost continuous (almost all the time); anyone would easily notice this if they saw the child for a few moments during the observation time.
NA = Not applicable. This child is not capable of performing this action.

SCORING

1. Add up the scores for each subscale and enter below that subscale number in the Score Summary at the bottom of the sheet. Items marked "NA" are scored as "0" (zero).
2. Add up all subscale scores for Total Score.
3. Check whether the child's score is greater than the cut-off score.

CUT-OFF SCORE

Based on the scores of 24 children age 3 to 18 (Breau, Finley, McGrath, & Camfield, 2002), a **Total Score of 11 or more** indicates a child has **moderate to severe pain**. Based on unpublished data from this same sample, a ***Total score of 6-10*** indicates a child has **mild pain**. When parents and caregivers completed the NCCPC-PV in hospital for the study group, this was accurate 88% of the time. When other observers completed the NCCPC-PV, this was accurate 75% of the time. A Total Score of 10 or less indicates less than moderate/severe pain. This was correct in the study group for parents and caregivers 81% of the time and for other observers 63% of the time.

USE OF CUT-OFF SCORES

As with all observational tools, caution should be taken in using cut-off scores, because they may not be 100% accurate. They should not be used as the only basis for deciding whether a child should be treated for pain. In some cases children may have lower scores when pain is present. For more detailed instructions for use of the NCCPC-PV in such situations, please refer to the full manual, available from Lynn Breau: Pediatric Pain Research, IWK Health Centre, 5850 University Avenue, Halifax, Nova Scotia, Canada, B3J 3G9 (lbreau@ns.sympatico.ca).

FIGURE 34-2, cont'd

(**analgesics**) or reduce the dosage required. In addition, these techniques decrease the perceived threat of pain, provide a sense of control, enhance comfort, and promote rest and sleep. Although there is limited rigorous research on the effectiveness of many of these interventions, the strategies are safe, non-invasive, inexpensive, simple, and feasible to use. Environmental and psychological factors may play a large role in children's pain perceptions and may be modified by using psychosocial strategies, education, parental support, and cognitive-behavioural interventions. For children undergoing repeated painful procedures, cognitive-behavioural interventions are effective for decreasing anxiety and distress.

GUIDELINES

Nonpharmacological Strategies for Pain Management

General Strategies

- Prepare the child before conducting potentially painful procedures but avoid "planting" the idea of pain.
- For example, instead of saying, "This is going to (or may) hurt," say, "Sometimes this feels like pushing, sticking, or pinching, and sometimes it doesn't bother people. Tell me what it feels like to you."
- Use "nonpain" descriptors when possible (e.g., "It feels like heat" rather than "It's a burning pain"). This allows for variation in sensory perception, avoids suggesting pain, and gives child control in describing reactions.
- Avoid evaluative statements or descriptions (e.g., "This is a terrible procedure" or "It really will hurt a lot").
- Stay with the child during a painful procedure.
- Support parents to stay with the child whenever possible; support and encourage parent to breastfeed or hold their baby skin-to-skin if possible, comfort child, hold child if possible and feasible, talk softly to the child, and remain near the child's head.
- Educate the child about the pain, especially when explanation may lessen anxiety (e.g., that pain may occur after surgery and does not indicate that something is wrong); reassure the child that he or she is not responsible for the pain.
- It may help to give the child a medical play doll, which represents "the patient," and allow the child to first do the procedures on the doll. Pain treatment can be emphasized through the doll by stating, "Dolly feels better after the medicine."

Specific Strategies

Distraction

- Involve the parent and child in identifying their preferred distracters.
- Involve the child in play; use a radio, CD player, MP3 player, electronic tablet, or computer game; have the child sing or use rhythmic breathing.
- Have the child take a deep breath and blow it out until told to stop.
- Have the child blow bubbles to "blow the hurt away."
- Have the child concentrate on yelling or saying "ouch," with instructions to "yell as loud or soft as you feel it hurt; that way I know what's happening."
- Have the child look through a kaleidoscope (one with glitter suspended in fluid-filled tube) and encourage him or her to concentrate, by asking, "Do you see the different designs?"
- Use humour, such as watching cartoons, telling jokes or funny stories, or acting silly with the child.
- Have the child read, play games, or visit with friends.

Relaxation

With an infant or a young child:

- Hold the child in a comfortable, well-supported position, such as vertically against the chest and shoulder.
- Rock the child in a wide, rhythmic arc in a rocking chair or sway back and forth, rather than bouncing the child.
- Repeat one or two words softly, such as "Mommy's here."

With a slightly older child:

- Ask the child to take a deep breath and "go limp as a rag doll" while exhaling slowly; then ask the child to yawn (demonstrate if needed).
- Help the child assume a comfortable position (e.g., pillow under neck and knees).
- Begin progressive relaxation: starting with the toes, systematically instruct the child to let each body part "go limp" or "feel heavy"; if the child has difficulty relaxing, instruct the child to tense or tighten each body part and then relax it.
- Allow the child to keep eyes open, since children may respond better if eyes are open rather than closed during relaxation.

Guided Imagery

- Have the child identify some highly pleasurable real or imaginary experience.
- Have the child describe details of the event, including as many senses as possible (e.g., "feel the cool breezes," "see the beautiful colours," "hear the pleasant music").
- Have the child write down or record the script.
- Encourage the child to concentrate only on the pleasurable event during the painful time; enhance the image by recalling specific details through reading the script or playing the recording.
- Combine with relaxation and rhythmic breathing.

Positive Self-Talk

- Teach the child positive statements to say when in pain (e.g., "I will be feeling better soon," "When I go home, I will feel better, and we will eat ice cream").

Thought Stopping

- Identify positive facts about the painful event (e.g., "It does not last long").
- Identify reassuring information (e.g., "If I think about something else, it does not hurt as much").
- Condense positive and reassuring facts into a set of brief statements and have the child memorize them (e.g., "short procedure, good veins, little hurt, nice nurse, go home").
- Have the child repeat the memorized statements whenever thinking about or experiencing the painful event.

Behavioural Contracting

Informal—May be used with children as young as 4 or 5 years of age:

- Use stars, tokens, or cartoon character stickers as rewards.
- Give a child who has difficulty assisting or is procrastinating during a procedure a limited time (measured by a visible timer) to complete the procedure.
- Proceed as needed if the child is unable to comply.
- Reinforce assistance with a reward if the procedure is accomplished within a specified time.

Formal—Use a written contract, which includes:

- Realistic (seems possible) goal or desired behaviour
- Measurable behaviour (e.g., agreeing not to hit anyone during procedures)
- Date and signature of all persons involved in any of the agreements
- Identified rewards or consequences that are reinforcing
- Goals that can be evaluated
- Commitment and compromise requirements for both parties (e.g., while timer is used, the nurse will not nag or prod the child to complete the procedure)

If the child cannot identify a familiar coping technique, the nurse can describe several strategies and let the child select the most appealing one. Experimentation with several strategies that are suitable to the child's age, pain intensity, and abilities is often necessary to determine the most effective approach. Parents should be involved in the selection process; they may be familiar with the child's usual coping skills and can help identify potentially successful coping strategies. Involving parents also encourages their participation in learning the relevant skill with the child and acting as coach. If the parent cannot assist the child, other appropriate persons may include a grandparent, older sibling, nurse, or child life specialist.

Children should learn to use a specific strategy before pain occurs or before it becomes severe. To reduce the child's effort, instructions for a strategy, such as distraction or relaxation, can be recorded and played during a period of comfort. However, even after they have learned an intervention, children often need help using it during a painful procedure. The intervention can also be used after the procedure. This gives the child a chance to recover, feel mastery, and cope more effectively.

For newborns, there is high-quality evidence of analgesic effects of breastfeeding, kangaroo (skin-to-skin) holding, and oral sucrose or glucose, with or without non-nutritive sucking, during painful procedures (Harrison et al., 2015) (Fig. 34-3). When it is not possible or feasible to use these strategies, facilitated tucking can help the infant return to a calm state following a painful procedure (Pillai Riddell, Racine, Gennis, et al., 2015). *Facilitated tucking*, which is holding the infant's extremities flexed and contained close to the trunk during heel lance procedures, has been demonstrated to decrease heart rate, decrease crying time, and promote stability in the sleep–wake cycles after the lance (Cignacco, Sellam, Stoffel, et al., 2012). See Chapter 26, p. 705, Pain in the Newborn, and Research Focus box, p. 707, for further information, as well as Additional Resources at the end of this chapter.

The administration of concentrated sucrose or glucose with or without non-nutritive sucking has been extensively shown to have calming and analgesic effects for painful invasive procedures in neonates. A small volume (0.1 mL up to 2 mL) of sufficiently sweet sucrose or glucose solutions (minimum 20%), given prior to and throughout the procedure, consistently reduces crying time, facial expression scores, and pain scores during a heel lance, venipuncture, or intramuscular injection (Bueno, Yamada, Harrison, et al., 2013; Stevens Yamada, Lee, et al., 2013). For more major and invasive procedures, such as circumcision, the use of multimodal therapy, such as sucrose in combination with swaddling or non-nutritive sucking, as well as pharmacological strategies, such as topical anaesthetics and a penile nerve block, are recommended for effective prevention and treatment of pain.

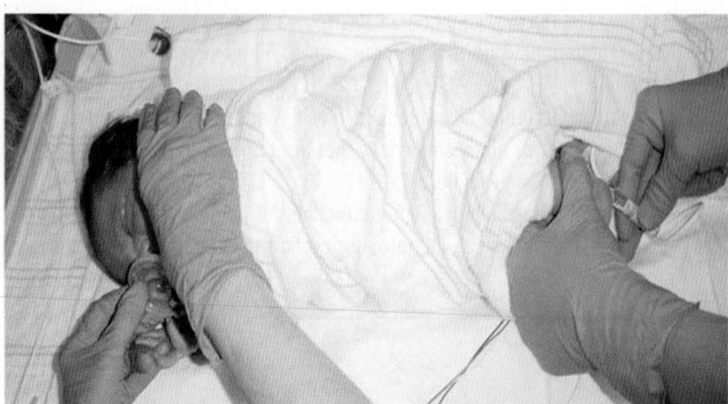

FIGURE 34-3 Oral sweet solutions (sucrose or glucose), with or without non-nutritive sucking, effectively reduces pain during a heel stick in a preterm infant.

Kangaroo care is skin-to-skin holding of infants, dressed only in diapers, against their mother's or other parent's chest (Johnston, Campbell-Yeo, Fernandes, et al., 2014) (see Chapter 26, Research Focus box). Skin-to-skin care, when commenced before a painful procedure and continued throughout and following the procedure, reduces behavioural responses to pain (crying, facial expressions, and pain scores) (Fig. 34-4) (Johnston et al., 2014).

Breastfeeding, when feasible and possible, during heel lance, venipuncture, or intramuscular injection is a simple and easy method of effective pain treatment for term newborn and young infants (Shah, Herbozo, Aliwalas, et al., 2012). Supporting and facilitating mothers to breastfeed during administration of minor painful procedures to an infant, and mothers and other family members to hold babies in kangaroo care, when feasible, during painful procedures, are strategies that not only effectively reduce pain in infants but can also help empower the mother and family in caring for their infant.

Complementary Pain Medicine

Many terms are used to describe approaches to health care that are outside the realm of conventional medicine as practised in

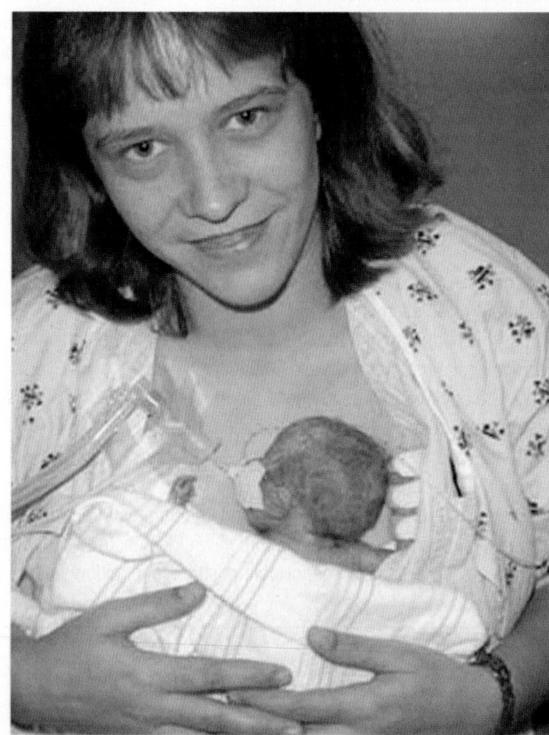

FIGURE 34-4 Mother using kangaroo hold with her newborn infant. Note placement of the infant directly on the mother's skin.

Canada. *Complementary and alternative medicine (CAM)*, as defined by the Canadian Interdisciplinary Network for Complementary and Alternative Medicine Research (INCAM), is a group of diverse medical and health care systems, practices, and products that are not currently considered part of conventional medicine. Although some scientific evidence exists regarding the efficacy of some CAM therapies, questions remain to be answered through well-designed scientific studies, such as whether these therapies are safe and whether they work for the diseases or medical conditions for which they are used.

CAM therapies may be grouped into five classes:

1. **Biologically based**—Foods, special diets, herbal or plant preparations, vitamins, other supplements
2. **Manipulative treatments**—Chiropractic, osteopathy, massage
3. **Energy based**—Reiki, bioelectric or magnetic treatments, pulsed fields, alternating and direct currents
4. **Mind–body techniques**—Mental healing, expressive treatments, spiritual healing, hypnosis, relaxation
5. **Alternative medical systems**—Homeopathy; naturopathy; ayurvedic; and traditional Chinese medicine, including acupuncture and moxibustion

Current use of pediatric CAM in Canada is estimated to be 11%. Homeopathy is one of the more popular alternative therapies used in children for dermatological; ear, nose and throat; respiratory; and emotional disorders (Spigelblatt & Canadian Paediatric Society [CPS] Community Paediatrics Committee, 2005/2016). Other therapies that are used include herbal medicine, massage, megavitamins, self-help groups, traditional remedies, and energy healing.

A Canadian study comparing the use of CAM in a western provincial pediatric and a central provincial ambulatory hospital found that CAM use is high among pediatric specialty clinic outpatients and that there was much higher use in the western province than in the central hospital (Adams, Dagenais, Clifford, et al., 2013). Most participants felt that their CAM use was helpful with few or no harm effects associated. Among parents in the study 50% were using CAM along with their medically prescribed treatments but in many cases were not informing their physicians about the usage. The most popular CAM products used were vitamins and minerals, herbal products, and homeopathic remedies. The most popular practices were massage, faith healing, chiropractic manipulation, aromatherapy, and relaxation techniques (Adams et al., 2013). To reduce risk of harmful interactions, health care providers working with children and their families need to ask about use of CAM.

Pharmacological Management

For mild pain (≤3 on 0-to-10 scale) or moderate pain (4 to 6 on 0-to-10 scale) acetaminophen (Tylenol, Tempra) and nonsteroidal anti-inflammatory drugs (NSAIDs) are suitable (Table 34-3). For moderate (5 to 6) to severe pain (7 to 10 on 0-to-10 scale) opioids are recommended (Table 34-4). The combination

TABLE 34-3 NONOPIOID AND NONSTEROIDAL ANTI-INFLAMMATORY DRUGS (NSAIDS) APPROVED FOR USE IN CHILDREN*

DRUG	DOSAGE	COMMENTS
Nonopioids		
Acetaminophen (Tylenol)	Oral: 10–15 mg/kg/dose q4–6h Rectal: 10–15 mg/kg/dose q4–6h Not to exceed 5 doses in 24 hr or 65 mg/kg/day	Available in numerous preparations Nonprescription Higher dosage range may provide increased analgesia. Physician dosage consultation is recommended for infants to 6 mo.
Nonsteroidal Anti-inflammatory Drugs (NSAIDS)		
Ibuprofen (children's Motrin, children's Advil)	Children 6 mo to 12 yr: 5–10 mg/kg/dose q6–8h; not to exceed: 40 mg/kg/day	Available in numerous preparations Available in suspension (100 mg/5 mL) and drops (100 mg/2.5 mL) Nonprescription
Naproxen (Naprosyn)	Children over 2 yr: 10 mg/kg/day PO divided into 2 doses at 12-hour intervals Naprosyn not recommended for use under 2 years of age	Available in suspension (25 mg/mL) and several different dosages for tablets (125 mg, 250 mg, 375 mg, 500 mg) Nonprescription

Acetylsalicylic acid (aspirin) is also an NSAID but is not recommended for children because of its possible association with Reye's syndrome. The NSAIDs in this table have no known association with Reye's syndrome. However, caution should be exercised in prescribing any salicylate-containing drug for children with known or suspected viral infection.

Adverse effects of ibuprofen and naproxen include nausea, vomiting, diarrhea, constipation, gastric ulceration, bleeding nephritis, and fluid retention.

Acetaminophen is well tolerated in the gastrointestinal tract and does not interfere with platelet function. NSAIDs should not be given to patients with allergic reactions to salicylates. All the NSAIDs should be used cautiously in patients with renal impairment.

PO, orally; *q,* every.

*All NSAIDs in this table have significant anti-inflammatory, antipyretic, and analgesic actions. Acetaminophen has a weak anti-inflammatory action. Patients respond differently to various NSAIDs; thus changing from one drug to another may be necessary for maximum benefit.

Data from *Drug facts and comparisons.* Philadelphia: Lippincott Williams & Wilkins, 2008. Dosages from *The Sick Kids Drug Handbook and Formulary*, Toronto: The Hospital for Sick Children, 2012; Canadian Pharmacists Association. (2016). *Compendium of Pharmaceuticals and Specialties (CPS).* Ottawa, Ontario. Retrieved from http://www.e-therapeutics.ca; Health Canada. (2015). *Drug product database online query.* Retrieved from http://webprod5.hc-sc.gc.ca/dpd-bdpp/start-debuter.do?lang=eng

TABLE 34-4 DOSAGE OF SELECTED OPIOIDS FOR CHILDREN

DRUG	APPROPRIATE EQUIANALGESIC	APPROXIMATE EQUIANALGESIC PARENTERAL DOSE	RECOMMENDED STARTING DOSAGE (CHILDREN <50 kg BODY WEIGHT)* ORAL	PARENTERAL*
Morphine	30 mg q3–4h	10 mg q3–4h	0.2–0.5 mg/kg q3–4h 0.3–0.6 mg/kg time released q12h	If no concurrent infusion running, 0.05–0.1 mg/kg/dose IV q2–4h; if a concurrent infusion is running, 0.02–0.05 mg/kg/dose IV q4h prn
Fentanyl	Not available	0.1 mg IV		0.5–1.5 mcg/kg IV bolus q30min 1–2 mcg/hr IV infusion
Hydromorphone (Dilaudid)†	7.5 mg q3–4h	1.5 mg q3–4h	0.04–0.08 mg/kg q4h	0.015–0.02 mcg/kg/dose q2–4h, max 1.0 mg bolus, infusion 4–6 mcg/kg/hr, PCA PCA: 3–5 mcg/kg/PCA dose (start at 3), 3–5 mcg/kg/hr infusion (start at 3), 6-minute lockout and 2-hr dose limit of 80% of 2-hr max
Oxycodone HCl	6–12 yr: 0.625 mg oxycodone hydrochloride	Not available	0.05–0.15 mg/kg/dose q4–6h, maximum 10 mg/dose**	Not available

Note: Published tables vary in suggested doses that are equianalgesic to morphine. Clinical response is the criterion that must be applied for each patient; titration to clinical response is necessary. Because there is not complete cross-tolerance among these drugs, it is usually necessary to use a lower than equianalgesic dose when changing drugs and to retitrate to response.

Caution: Recommended dosages do not apply to patients with renal or hepatic insufficiency or other conditions affecting drug metabolism and kinetics.

Caution: Codeine is no longer recommended as a pain relief medication for children. Codeine is converted into morphine; however, the conversion is highly variable. Therefore, some children obtain no analgesia and some rapidly metabolize codeine into morphine and are therefore at high risk of toxic levels of morphine (MacDonald & MacLeod, 2010).

IM, intramuscular; *IV,* intravenous; *PCA,* patient-controlled analgesia; *prn,* as needed; *q,* every

* *Caution:* Dosages listed for patients with body weight <50 kg cannot be used as initial starting doses in infants <6 months of age. For nonventilated infants younger than 6 months, the initial opioid dose should be about one fourth to one third of the dose recommended for older infants and children. For example, morphine could be used at a dose of 0.03 mg/kg instead of the traditional 0.1 mg/kg.

†For morphine, hydromorphone, and oxymorphone, rectal administration is an alternative route for patients unable to take oral medications, but equianalgesic doses may differ from oral and parenteral doses because of pharmacokinetic differences.

** *Caution:* Doses of aspirin and acetaminophen in combination with opioid or nonsteroidal anti-inflammatory drug preparations must also be adjusted to patient's body weight. Daily dose of acetaminophen should not exceed 75 mg/kg or 4000 mg.

Data from Acute Pain Management Guideline Panel. (1992). *Acute pain management: Operative or medical procedures and trauma: Clinical practice guideline* [AHCPR Pub No 92-0032]. Rockville, MD.

of NSAIDs and opioids provides increased analgesia without increased adverse effects, as nonopioids act at the peripheral nervous system and opioids act at the central nervous system. Oxycodone is available without a nonopioid in an immediate-release and controlled-release preparation. Morphine is considered the gold standard for the management of severe pain. When morphine is not a suitable opioid, drugs such as hydromorphone (Dilaudid) and fentanyl (Sublimaze) are effective substitutes. Although fentanyl is used as an anaesthetic in the operating room, it is classified as an analgesic. It can be safely administered by nurses by the intravenous (IV), intramuscular (IM), transmucosal, and transdermal routes.

Several drugs known as *coanalgesics* or **adjuvant** *analgesics* may be used alone or with opioids for pain management and to reduce opioid adverse effects. Medications frequently used to relieve anxiety, cause sedation, and provide amnesia are diazepam (Valium) and midazolam (Versed). However, these drugs are not analgesics and should be used to enhance the effects of analgesics, not as a substitute for analgesics. Other adjuvants include tricyclic antidepressants, such as amitriptyline and imipramine, and antiepileptics, such as gabapentin, carbamazepine, and clonazepam, for neuropathic pain; stool softeners and laxatives for constipation; antiemetics for nausea and vomiting; diphenhydramine for itching; and steroids for inflammation and bone pain.

! NURSING ALERT

The optimum dosage of an analgesic is one that controls pain without causing severe adverse effects. This usually requires *titration,* the gradual adjustment of drug dosage (usually by increasing the dose), until optimum pain relief without excessive sedation is achieved. Dosage recommendations are only safe initial dosages (see Tables 34-3 and 34-4), not optimum dosages.

Children (except infants younger than about 3 to 6 months) metabolize drugs more rapidly than adults; younger children may require higher doses of opioids to achieve the same analgesic effect. Therefore, the therapeutic effect and duration of analgesia vary. Children's dosages are usually calculated

TABLE 34-5 MANAGEMENT OF OPIOID ADVERSE EFFECTS

ADVERSE EFFECT	ADJUVANT DRUGS	NONPHARMACOLOGICAL TECHNIQUES
Constipation	**Senna and docusate sodium** *Tablet:* 2–6 yr: Start with ½ tablet once a day; maximum: 1 tablet twice a day 6–12 yr: Start with 1 tablet once a day; maximum: 2 tablets twice a day >12 yr: Start with 2 tablets once a day; maximum: 4 tablets twice a day *Liquid:* 1 mo–1 yr: 1.25–5 mL qhs 1–5 yr: 2.5–5 mL qhs 5–15 yr: 5–10 mL qhs >15 yr: 10–25 mL qhs **Bisacodyl:** PO or PR 3–12 yr: 5 mg/dose/day >12 yr: 5–10 mg/dose/day **Lactulose** 5–10 mL/day PO, double daily dose until stool produced Adult: 15–30 mL/day PO **Mineral oil:** 1–2 tsp/day PO **Magnesium citrate** <6 yr: 1–3 mL/kg PO OD 6–12 yr: 100–150 mL PO once/day >12 yr: 150–300 mL PO once/day follow with 250 mL water **Milk of Magnesia** <2 yr: 0.5 mL/kg/dose PO once/day 2–5 yr: 5–15 mL/day PO 6–12 yr: 15–30 mL PO once/day >12 yr: 30–60 mL PO once/day	Increase water intake. Prune juice, bran cereal, vegetables Increase ambulation.
Sedation (without respiratory depression)	*Consider dose reduction and monitor analgesia closely; if analgesia is inadequate at reduced dose, consider opioid switch and continue to monitor analgesia and sedation closely.* **Caffeine:** single dose of 1–1.5 mg PO **Dextroamphetamine:** 2.5–5 mg PO in AM and early afternoon **Methylphenidate:** 2.5–5 mg PO in AM and early afternoon*	Caffeinated drinks (e.g., cola drinks)
Nausea, vomiting	**Ondansetron:** 0.1–0.15 mg/kg IV or PO q4h; maximum: 8 mg/dose **Granisetron:** 10–40 mcg/kg q2–4h; maximum: 1 mg/dose **Droperidol:** 0.05–0.06 mg/kg IV q4–6h; can be very sedating	Imagery, relaxation Deep, slow breathing
Pruritus	**Diphenhydramine:** 1 mg/kg IV or PO q4–6h prn; max: 25 mg/dose **Hydroxyzine:** 0.6 mg/kg/dose PO q6h; maximum: 50 mg/dose **Naloxone:** 0.25– 2mcg/kg/hr not to exceed upper dose recommendation or else analgesia may reverse **Butorphanol:** 0.3–0.5 mg/kg IV (use cautiously in opioid-tolerant children; may cause withdrawal symptoms); maximum: 2 mg/dose because mixed agonist-antagonist	Oatmeal baths, good hygiene Exclude other causes of itching. Change opioids.
Respiratory depression: mild to moderate	Hold dose of opioid Reduce subsequent doses by 25%	Arouse gently, give oxygen, encourage to deep breathe.
Respiratory depression: severe	**Naloxone** *During disease pain management:* 0.5 mcg/kg in 2-min increments until breathing improves Reduce opioid dose if possible Consider opioid switch *During sedation for procedures:* 5–10 mcg/kg until breathing improves Reduce opioid dose if possible Consider opioid switch	Oxygen, bag and mask if indicated

Continued

TABLE 34-5 MANAGEMENT OF OPIOID ADVERSE EFFECTS—cont'd

ADVERSE EFFECT	ADJUVANT DRUGS	NONPHARMACOLOGICAL TECHNIQUES
Dysphoria, confusion, hallucinations	Evaluate medications, eliminate adjuvant medications with central nervous system effects as symptoms allow Consider opioid switch if possible **Haloperidol** (Haldol): 0.05–0.15 mg/kg/day divided in 2–3 doses; maximum: 2–4 mg/day	Rule out other physiological causes.
Urinary retention	Evaluate medications, eliminate adjuvant medications with anticholinergic effects (e.g., antihistamines, tricyclic antidepressants) Occurs more frequently with spinal analgesia than with systemic opioid use	Rule out other physiological causes. In/out or in-dwelling urinary catheter

hs, at bedtime; *IV,* intravenously; *PO,* by mouth; *PR,* by rectum; *prn,* as needed; *q,* every.
*Although pharmacological treatment options for sedation do exist as noted in this table, in the pediatric population this is not the recommended treatment approach. For patients with light sedation but adequately controlled pain, consider a dose reduction. If pain is not well controlled and the patient is sedated, consider changing to a different opioid.
Sources: Lau, E. (Ed.). (2016). *2016 SickKids Drug Handbook and Formulary*. Toronto: The Hospital for Sick Children; Canadian Pharmacists Association. (2016). *Compendium of Pharmaceuticals and Specialties (CPS)*. Ottawa: Author. Retrieved from http://www.e-therapeutics.ca

according to body weight, except in children with a weight greater than 50 kg, where the weight formula may exceed the average adult dosage. In this case, the adult dosage is used. Conversion factors for selected opioids must be used when a change is made from IV (preferred) or IM to oral. Immediate conversion from IM or IV to the suggested equianalgesic oral dose may result in a substantial error. For example, the dose may be significantly more or less than that which the child requires. Small changes ensure small errors. Several routes of analgesic administration can be used (Box 34-2); the most effective and least traumatic route should be selected.

Patient-Controlled Analgesia

A significant advance in the administration of IV, epidural, or subcutaneous analgesics is the use of patient-controlled analgesia (PCA). As the name implies, the patient controls the amount and frequency of the analgesic, which is typically delivered through a special infusion device. Children who are physically able to "push a button" (i.e., 5 to 6 years of age) and who can understand the concept of pushing a button to obtain pain relief can use PCA. Although controversial, the IV PCA system for children has been used by parents and nurses. Children can use the IV PCA system if they are old enough and capable of effectively managing their own pain. Nurses can efficiently use the infusion device on a child of any age to administer analgesics to avoid signing for and preparing opioid injections every time one is needed (Fig. 34-5). When PCA is used as "nurse- or parent-controlled" analgesia, the concept of patient control is negated, and the inherent safety of PCA needs to be monitored. Researchers have reported safe and effective analgesia in children when the PCA was controlled by the patient, parent, or nurse.

PCA infusion devices typically allow for three methods or modes of drug administration to be used alone or in combination:

1. Patient-administered boluses that can only be infused according to the preset amount and *lockout interval* (time between doses). More frequent attempts at self-administration usually mean that the patient may need the dose and time adjusted for better pain control.
2. Nurse-administered boluses that are typically used to give an initial loading dose to increase blood levels rapidly and to relieve *breakthrough pain* (pain not relieved with the usual programmed dose)
3. Continuous basal rate infusion that delivers a constant amount of analgesic and prevents pain from returning during those times, such as sleep, when the patient cannot control the infusion

As with any type of analgesic management plan, continued assessment of the child's pain relief is essential for the greatest benefit from PCA. Typical uses of PCA are for controlling pain from surgery, sickle cell crisis, trauma, and cancer. Morphine is the drug of choice for PCA and is usually prepared in a concentration of 10 mcg/mL. Other options are hydromorphone (2 mcg/mL) and fentanyl (0.1 mcg/mL). Hydromorphone is often used when patients are not able to tolerate the adverse effects, such as pruritus and nausea, from the morphine PCA.

Epidural Analgesia

Epidural analgesia may also be used to manage pain, in selected cases. Although an epidural catheter may be inserted at any vertebral level, it is usually placed into the epidural space of the spinal column at the lumbar or caudal level (Fig. 34-6). The thoracic level is usually reserved for older children or adolescents who have had an upper abdominal or thoracic procedure, such as a lung transplant. An opioid (usually fentanyl, hydromorphone, or preservative-free morphine, which is often combined with a long-acting local anaesthetic such as bupivacaine or ropivacaine) is instilled via single or intermittent bolus, continuous infusion, or patient-controlled epidural analgesia.

BOX 34-2 ROUTES AND METHODS OF ANALGESIC DRUG ADMINISTRATION

Oral

Oral route preferred because of convenience, cost, and relatively steady blood levels

Higher dosages of oral form of opioids required for equivalent parenteral analgesia

Peak drug effect after 1 to 2 hours for most analgesics

Delay in onset is a disadvantage when rapid control of severe pain or of fluctuating pain is desired

Sublingual, Buccal, or Transmucosal

Tablet or liquid placed under tongue (sublingual), between cheek and gum (buccal), or through the mucous membrane (transmucosal)

Highly desirable because more rapid onset than with oral route

- Produces less first-pass effect through liver than with oral route, which normally reduces analgesia from oral opioids (unless sublingual or buccal form is swallowed, which occurs often in children)

Few drugs are commercially available in this form

Many drugs can be compounded into sublingual troche or lozenge

- Actiq—Oral transmucosal fentanyl citrate in hard confection base on a plastic holder; indicated only for management of breakthrough cancer pain in patients with malignancies who are already receiving and are tolerant of opioid therapy, but can be used for preoperative or preprocedural sedation and analgesia

Intravenous (IV) (Bolus)

Preferred for rapid control of severe pain

Provides most rapid onset of effect, usually in about 5 minutes

Advantage for acute pain, procedural pain, and breakthrough pain

Needs to be repeated hourly for continuous pain control

Preferable for drugs with short half-life (morphine, fentanyl, hydromorphone) to avoid toxic accumulation of drug

Intravenous (Continuous)

Preferred over bolus and intramuscular injection for maintaining control of pain

Provides steady blood levels

Easy to titrate dosage

Subcutaneous (Continuous)

Used when oral and IV routes not available

Provides equivalent blood levels to continuous IV infusion

Suggested initial bolus dose to equal 2-hour IV dose; total 24-hour dose usually requires concentrated opioid solution to minimize infused volume; use smallest-gauge needle that accommodates infusion rate

Patient-Controlled Analgesia (PCA)

Generally refers to self-administration of drugs, regardless of route

Typically involves programmable infusion pump (IV, epidural, subcutaneous [SC]) that permits self-administration of boluses of medication at preset dose and time interval (*lockout interval* is time between doses)

PCA bolus administration is often combined with initial bolus and continuous (basal or background) infusion of opioid

Optimum lockout interval is not known but must be at least as long as time needed for onset of drug

- Should effectively control pain during movement or procedures
- Longer lockout requires larger dose

Family-Controlled Analgesia

One family member (usually a parent) or other caregiver is designated as child's primary pain manager with responsibility for pressing PCA button

Guidelines for selecting a primary pain manager for family-controlled analgesia:

- Spends a significant amount of time with the patient
- Is willing to assume responsibility of being primary pain manager
- Is willing to accept and respect patient's reports of pain (if able to provide) as best indicator of how much pain the patient is experiencing; knows how to use and interpret a pain rating scale
- Understands the purpose and goals of patient's pain management plan
- Understands concept of maintaining a steady analgesic blood level
- Recognizes signs of pain and adverse reactions to opioid

Nurse-Activated Analgesia

Child's primary nurse is designated as primary pain manager and is only person who presses PCA button during that nurse's shift

Guidelines for selecting primary pain manager for family-controlled analgesia are also applicable to nurse-activated analgesia

May be used in addition to a basal rate to treat breakthrough pain with bolus doses; patients assessed every 30 minutes for the need for a bolus dose

May be used without a basal rate as a means of maintaining analgesia with around-the-clock bolus doses

Intramuscular

Not recommended for pain control; not current standard of care

Painful administration (hated by children)

Tissue and nerve damage possible with some drugs

Wide fluctuation in absorption of drug from muscle

Faster absorption from deltoid than from gluteal sites

Shorter duration and more expensive than oral drugs

Time consuming for staff and unnecessary delay for child

Intranasal

Available commercially as butorphanol (Stadol NS); approved for those older than 18 years of age

Should not be used in patient receiving morphine-like drugs because butorphanol is partial antagonist that will reduce analgesia and may cause withdrawal

Intradermal

Used primarily for skin anaesthesia (e.g., before lumbar puncture, bone marrow aspiration, arterial puncture, skin biopsy)

Local anaesthetics (e.g., lidocaine) cause stinging, burning sensation

Continued

BOX 34-2 ROUTES AND METHODS OF ANALGESIC DRUG ADMINISTRATION—cont'd

Duration of stinging dependent on type of "caine" used

To avoid stinging sensation associated with lidocaine:

- Buffer the solution by adding 1 part sodium bicarbonate (1 mmol/mL) to 9 or 10 parts 1% or 2% lidocaine with or without epinephrine

Normal saline with preservative, benzyl alcohol, used to anaesthetize venipuncture site

Use same dose as for buffered lidocaine

Topical or Transdermal

EMLA (eutectic mixture of local anaesthetics [lidocaine and prilocaine]) cream and anaesthetic disk or LMX4 (4% lidocaine cream)

- Eliminates or reduces pain from most procedures involving skin puncture
- Must be placed on intact skin over puncture site and covered by occlusive dressing or applied as anaesthetic disk for 1 hour or more before procedure
- May cause skin blanching and vasoconstriction therefore may make venous access more difficult

AMETOP (4% tetracaine)

- Eliminates or reduces pain from most procedures involving skin puncture
- Must be placed on intact skin over puncture site and covered by occlusive dressing or for 40 minutes or more before procedure
- May cause vasodilation, therefore, may make venous access easier

LAT (lidocaine-adrenaline-tetracaine) or tetracaine-phenylephrine (tetraphen)

- Provides skin anaesthesia about 15 minutes after application on nonintact skin
- Gel (preferable) or liquid placed on wounds for suturing
- Adrenaline not for use on end arterioles (fingers, toes, tip of nose, penis, earlobes) because of vasoconstriction

Numby Stuff system

- Uses iontophoresis to transport lidocaine 2% and epinephrine 1:100,000 (Iontocaine) into the skin
- Current delivered by small battery-powered device that has an electrode with Iontocaine and a ground electrode
- Produces local dermal anaesthesia in about 10 minutes to a depth of approximately 10 mm at maximum setting
- May be frightening to young children when they see the device and feel the current
- Observe child during iontophoresis and remove all metal, such as jewellery, from application site to prevent burns

Transdermal fentanyl (Duragesic)

- Available as patch for continuous pain control
- Safety and efficacy not established in children younger than 12 years of age
- Not appropriate for initial relief of acute pain because of long interval to peak effect (12 to 24 hours); for rapid onset of pain relief, an immediate-release opioid is given
- Orders for "rescue doses" of an immediate-release opioid recommended for breakthrough pain (a flare of severe pain that breaks through the medication being administered at regular intervals for persistent pain)
- Has duration of up to 72 hours for prolonged pain relief
- If respiratory depression occurs, possible need for several doses of naloxone
- Patch should not be cut or modified in any way. Gloves needed to handle. Soap, alcohol, or any other solvent should not be used on the skin before application as this may affect drug absorption. Patch should be applied only to intact skin. Patch should not be exposed to external heat sources as this may increase drug release and has resulted in fatalities. Must be removed before MRI.

Vapocoolant

- Use of prescription spray coolant, such as fluorimethane (Spray and Stretch) or ethyl chloride (Pain Ease)
- Applied to the skin for 10 to 15 seconds immediately before the needle puncture; anaesthesia lasts about 15 seconds
- Cold disliked by some children; may be more comfortable for child to spray coolant on a cotton ball and then apply this to the skin
- Application of ice to the skin for 30 seconds found to be ineffective

Rectal*

Alternative to oral or parenteral routes

Variable absorption rate

Generally disliked by children

Regional Nerve Block

Use of long-acting local anaesthetic (bupivacaine or ropivacaine) injected into tissue surrounding nerves to block pain at site

Provides prolonged analgesia postoperatively, such as after inguinal herniorrhaphy

May be used to provide local anaesthesia for surgery, such as dorsal penile nerve block for circumcision or for reduction of fractures

Inhalation

Use of anaesthetics, such as nitrous oxide, to produce partial or complete analgesia for painful procedures

Adverse effects (e.g., headache) possible from occupational exposure to high levels of nitrous oxide

Epidural or Intrathecal

Involves catheter placed into epidural, caudal, or intrathecal space for continuous infusion or single or intermittent administration of opioid with or without a long-acting local anaesthetic (e.g., bupivacaine, ropivacaine)

Analgesia primarily from drug's direct effect on opioid receptors in spinal cord and from action of local anaesthetic on spinal nerves

Respiratory depression is rare but may have slow and delayed onset; can be prevented by checking level of sedation and respiratory rate and depth hourly for initial 24 hours and decreasing dose when excessive sedation is detected

Nausea, itching, and urinary retention are common dose-related adverse effects from the epidural opioid

Mild hypotension, urinary retention, and temporary motor or sensory deficits are common unwanted effects of epidural local anaesthetic

Catheter for urinary retention is inserted during surgery to decrease trauma to child; if inserted when child is awake, anaesthetize urethra with lidocaine

*Many drugs can be compounded into rectal suppositories. For further information about compounding drugs in troche or suppository form, contact Professional Compounding Centers of America (PCCA), Canada, 744 Third Street, London, ON, N5V 5J2, 800.668.9453, http://www.pccarx.ca/

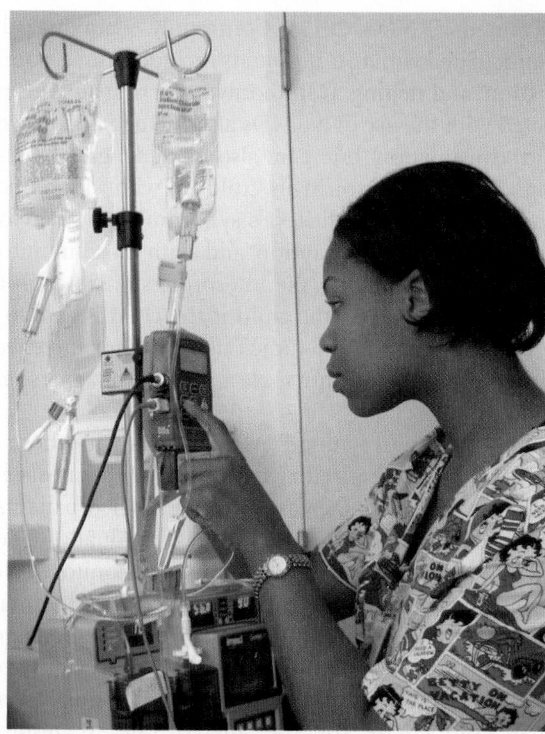

FIGURE 34-5 Nurse programming a patient-controlled analgesia pump to administer analgesic.

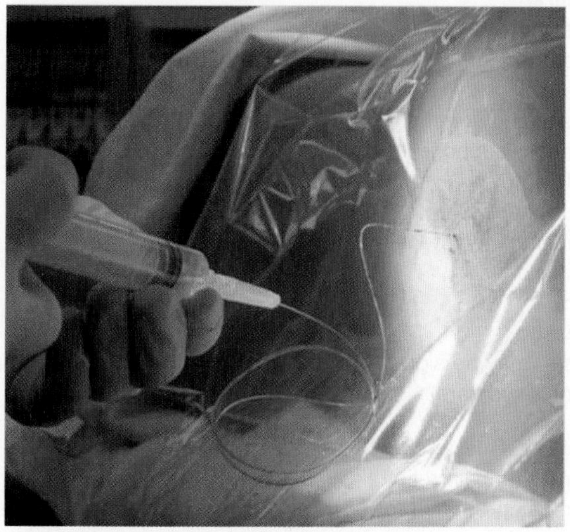

FIGURE 34-6 Epidural analgesia catheter placement.

Analgesia results from the drug's effect on opiate receptors in the dorsal horn of the spinal cord, rather than the brain. As a result, respiratory depression is rare, but if it occurs, it develops slowly, typically 6 to 8 hours after administration. Careful securing of the epidural catheter with an occlusive dressing decreases the possibility of soiling or inadvertently displacing the catheter. Careful monitoring of sedation level and respiratory status is critical to prevent opioid-induced respiratory depression. Assessment of pain and of the skin condition around the catheter site is an important aspect of related nursing care.

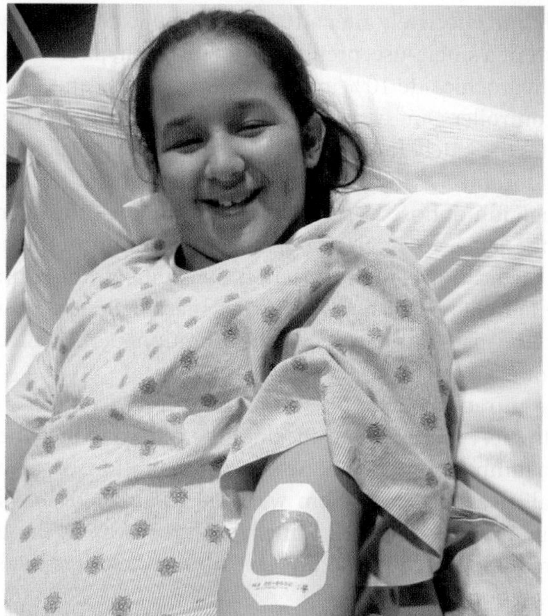

FIGURE 34-7 LMX is an effective analgesic before intravenous insertion or blood draw.

Transmucosal and Transdermal Analgesia

Oral transmucosal fentanyl (Oralet) provides nontraumatic preoperative and preprocedural analgesia and sedation. Fentanyl is also available as a transdermal patch (Duragesic). Although contraindicated for acute pain management, it may be used for older children and adolescents who have cancer pain or sickle cell pain or for patients who are opioid tolerant.

One of the most significant improvements in the ability to provide atraumatic care to children is the anaesthetic cream LMX (a 4% liposomal lidocaine cream) or EMLA (a eutectic mixture of local anaesthetics). The eutectic mixture (lidocaine 2.5% and prilocaine 2.5%), whose melting point is lower than that of the two anaesthetics alone, permits effective concentrations of the drug to penetrate intact skin (Fig. 34-7).

A needle-free system containing 0.5 mg of sterile lidocaine powder (Zingo) is available and provides a rapid onset of action to reduce pain associated with peripheral IV insertions or blood draws. Two randomized, double-blind, placebo-controlled studies conducted at 15 centres across the United States found significant reduction in procedural pain compared with placebo in children 3 to 18 years of age (Migdal, Chudzynska-Pomianowska, Vause, et al., 2006; Zempsky, Bean-Lijewski, Kauffman, et al., 2008).

In some situations, refrigerant sprays such as ethyl chloride and fluorimethane can be used. When sprayed on the skin, these sprays vaporize, rapidly cooling the area and providing superficial anaesthesia. Hospital formularies may have other products with lidocaine, prilocaine, or amethocaine topical preparations that require less time for application.

The LidoSite Topical System is another method used to help reduce needle-related pain associated with procedures such as IV cannulation, venipuncture, or laser ablation of superficial skin lesions for patients aged 5 years and older. The LidoSite system delivers numbing medication to the procedure site quickly and effectively after a 10-minute application. The system consists of a single-use, prefilled LidoSite patch, filled with lidocaine hydrochloride 10% and epinephrine 0.1%, and the LidoSite controller, an easy-to-use preprogrammed device that activates the patch. It provides pain reduction equivalent to that of a lidocaine (Xylocaine) injection, without the needlestick. Through iontophoresis, a mild current from the controller activates the patch to accelerate delivery of lidocaine—the anaesthetic medication—to the injection site. Epinephrine contained in the LidoSite patch helps focus the anaesthetic effect directly under the patch and extends the duration of the effect for one hour.

The intradermal route is sometimes used to inject a local anaesthetic, typically lidocaine, into the skin to reduce the pain from a lumbar puncture, bone marrow aspiration, or venous or arterial access. One problem with the use of lidocaine is the stinging and burning that initially occur. However, the use of buffered lidocaine with sodium bicarbonate reduces the stinging sensation

Timing of Analgesia

The right timing for administering analgesics depends on the type of pain. For continuous pain control, such as for postoperative or cancer pain, a preventive schedule of medication around the clock (ATC) is effective. The ATC schedule avoids the low concentrations of medications in plasma that permit breakthrough pain. If analgesics are administered only when pain returns (a typical use of the prn, or "as needed," order), pain relief may take several hours. The patient may then require higher doses, leading to a cycle of undermedication of pain, alternating with periods of overmedication and drug toxicity. This cycle of erratic pain control also promotes "clock watching," which may be erroneously equated with addiction. Nurses can effectively use prn (as needed) orders by giving the drug at regular intervals, since "as needed" should be interpreted as "as needed to prevent pain," not "as little as possible."

Preventive pain control is best provided through continuous IV infusion rather than intermittent boluses. If intermittent boluses are given, the intervals between doses should not exceed the drug's expected duration of effectiveness. For extended pain control with fewer administration times, drugs that provide longer duration of action (e.g., some NSAIDs, time-released morphine or oxycodone, methadone, levorphanol) can be used.

Continuous analgesia is not always appropriate, since not all pain is continuous. Frequently, temporary pain control or conscious sedation is needed to provide analgesia before a scheduled procedure. When pain can be predicted, the drug's peak effect should be timed to coincide with the painful event. For example, with opioids the peak effect is approximately a half-hour for the IV route; with nonopioids the peak effect occurs about 2 hours after oral administration. For rapid onset and peak of action, opioids that quickly penetrate the blood–brain barrier (e.g., IV fentanyl) provide excellent pain control.

Monitoring Adverse Effects of Analgesic Management

Anticipation and early management of adverse effects of pharmacological interventions is an important and vital aspect of pain treatment (RNAO, 2013). Commonly occurring adverse effects anticipated with use of opioids include nausea, vomiting, constipation, and itching. Commonly occurring adverse events anticipated with the use of NSAIDs also include nausea, vomiting, and constipation but can also include gastrointestinal bleeding. The use of aspirin in children with chickenpox or influenza is associated with Reye's syndrome and, therefore, if used, must be used with caution and with close monitoring. Nurses, in partnership with the interprofessional health team, the family/caregivers, and the child if the child is able to contribute information, need to judiciously monitor the effectiveness of the treatment and anticipate and monitor adverse effects of treatment.

The major concern with adverse effects is with those from opioids (Box 34-3). Respiratory depression is the most serious complication and poses increased risk in sedated patients and infants. The respiratory rate may decrease gradually, or respirations may cease abruptly, and thus must be monitored closely. Lower limits of normal are not established for children, but any significant change from a previous rate calls for increased vigilance. A slower respiratory rate does not necessarily reflect decreased arterial oxygenation; an increased depth of ventilation may compensate for the altered rate. If respiratory

BOX 34-3 ADVERSE EFFECTS OF OPIOIDS

General
Constipation (possibly severe)
Respiratory depression
Sedation
Nausea and vomiting
Agitation, euphoria
Confusion
Hallucinations
Orthostatic hypotension
Pruritus
Urticaria
Sweating
Miosis (may be sign of toxicity)
Anaphylaxis (rare)

Signs of Tolerance
Decreasing pain relief
Decreasing duration of pain relief

Signs of Withdrawal Syndrome in Patients With Physical Dependence
Initial Signs of Withdrawal
Lacrimation
Rhinorrhea
Yawning
Sweating

Later Signs of Withdrawal
Restlessness
Irritability
Tremors
Anorexia
Dilated pupils
Gooseflesh
Nausea, vomiting

depression or arrest occurs, the nurse must be prepared to intervene quickly (see Guidelines box).

Although respiratory depression is the most feared adverse effect, constipation is a common, and sometimes serious, adverse effect of opioids. If ongoing use of opioids is expected, prevention with stool softeners and laxatives is more effective than treatment once constipation occurs. Dietary treatment, such as increased fibre, is usually not sufficient to promote regular bowel evacuation. However, dietary measures, such as greater fluid and fruit intake, and physical activity are encouraged. Another common adverse effect is pruritus from epidural or IV infusion. Pruritus can be treated with low doses of IV naloxone, nalbuphine, or diphenhydramine. Nausea, vomiting, and sedation usually subside after 2 days of opioid administration; however, oral or rectal antiemetics may be necessary.

Both tolerance and physical dependence can occur with prolonged use of opioids (see Family-Centred Teaching box). When opioids are abruptly discontinued without weaning, withdrawal symptoms occur. Symptoms of withdrawal usually occur around 24 hours after abrupt discontinuation and reach a peak within 72 hours. Withdrawal symptoms can be anticipated and prevented by following an opioid weaning protocol for patients that were administered opioids for more than 5 to 10 days. A weaning flow sheet may be used to assess the efficacy of opioid weaning in neonates (Fig. 34-8). In infants and young children (7 months to 10 years) the Withdrawal Assessment Tool–1 may be used to assess and monitor withdrawal symptoms in pediatric critically ill children who are exposed to opioids and benzodiazepines for prolonged periods (Franck, Harris, Soetenga, et al., 2008). See Chapter 29, p. 802, for more information on care of the drug-exposed newborn.

GUIDELINES

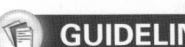

Managing Opioid-Induced Respiratory Depression

If Respirations Are Depressed

- Assess sedation level.
- Reduce infusion by 25% when possible.
- Stimulate patient (shake shoulder gently, call by name, ask to breathe).

If Patient Cannot Be Aroused or Is Apneic

Administer naloxone (Narcan).

- For children weighing less than 40 kg, dilute 0.1 mg naloxone in 10 mL sterile saline to make 10 mcg/mL solution, and give 0.5 mcg/kg.
- For children weighing more than 40 kg, dilute 0.4-mg ampule in 10 mL sterile saline, and give 0.5 mL.

Administer bolus by slow intravenous push every 2 minutes until effect is obtained.

Closely monitor patient. Naloxone's duration of antagonist action may be shorter than that of opioid, requiring repeated doses of naloxone.

Tolerance occurs when the dose of an opioid needs to be increased to achieve the same analgesic effect that was previously achieved at a lower dose (see Family-Centred Teaching box). Tolerance may develop after 10 to 21 days of morphine administration. Treatment of tolerance involves increasing the dose or decreasing the duration between doses. Treatment of physical dependence involves gradually reducing the dose over several days to prevent withdrawal symptoms. Following are guidelines for treating physical dependence from morphine (Max, Payne, Edwards, et al., 1999):

- Gradually reduce dose (similar to tapering of steroids).
- Give half of previous daily dose every 6 hours for first 2 days.
- Then reduce dose by 25% every 2 days. Continue this schedule until total daily dosage of 0.6 mg/kg/day of morphine (or equivalent) is reached. After 2 days on this dose discontinue opioid.
- May also switch to oral methadone, using one-fourth equianalgesic dose as initial weaning dose and proceeding as described previously.

Note: Respiratory depression caused by benzodiazepines (e.g., diazepam [Valium] or midazolam [Versed]) can be reversed with flumazenil (Romazicon). Pediatric dosing experience suggests 0.01 mg/kg (0.1 mL/kg); if there is no (or inadequate) response after 1 to 2 minutes, administer the same dose and repeat as needed at 60-second intervals for a maximum dose of 1 mg (10 mL).

Adapted from Yaster, M., et al. (1997). *Pediatric pain management and sedation handbook*. St. Louis: Mosby.

FAMILY-CENTRED TEACHING

Fear of Opioid Addiction

One of the reasons for the unfounded but prevalent fear of addiction from opioids used to relieve pain is a misunderstanding of the differences between physical dependence, tolerance, and addiction. Health care providers and the community members often confuse addiction with the physiological effects of opioids, when in reality physical dependence, tolerance, and addiction are unrelated. The Canadian Pain Society defines these terms as follows:

Physical dependence is a state of adaptation that often includes tolerance and is manifested by a drug class–specific withdrawal syndrome that can be produced by abrupt cessation, rapid dose reduction, decreasing blood level of the drug, or administration of an antagonist. It is not the same thing as addiction. The symptoms of withdrawal include signs of neurological excitability (irritability, tremors, seizures, increased motor tone, insomnia), gastrointestinal dysfunction (nausea, vomiting, diarrhea, abdominal cramps), and autonomic dysfunction (sweating, fever, chills, tachypnea, nasal congestion, rhinitis), hypertension, and muscle aches. These symptoms can be minimized by slowly decreasing the dose of opioids. Weaning should be planned for any patient who has been taking opioids for more than 1 week.

Tolerance is a state of adaptation in which exposure to a drug induces changes that result in a diminution of one or more of the drug's effects over time. This is also not the same as addiction.

Addiction is a primary, chronic, neurobiological disease, with genetic, psychosocial, and environmental factors influencing its development and manifestations. Addiction is characterized by behaviours that include one or more of the following (4 C's):

- Impaired Control over drug use
- Compulsive use
- Craving
- Continued use despite harm (Consequences)

Unfortunately, individuals who have severe, unrelieved pain may become intensely focused on finding relief. Sometimes behaviours such as "clock watching" make patients appear to others to be preoccupied with obtaining opioids. However, this preoccupation centres on finding relief of pain, not on using opioids for reasons other than pain control. This phenomenon has been termed *pseudoaddiction* and must not be confused with real addiction.

Nurses are in an ideal position to educate children, parents, and other health care providers about the extremely low risk of real addiction (less than 1%) from the use of opioids to treat pain. Helping families and caregivers to understand that infants, young children, and comatose or terminally ill children simply cannot become addicted is integral to the role of the nurse caring for these children.

Data from The Canadian Pain Society. (2005). *Accreditation pain standard: Making it happen!* Retrieved from http://c.ymcdn.com/sites/www.canadianpainsociety.ca/resource/resmgr/Docs/accreditation_manual.pdf

Children's Hospital Oakland Opioid Weaning Flowsheet and Guidelines for Use of the Form

Analgesia/sedation orders (drug/dose/frequency)

Date		
Drug		
Administration time		
Dose ↑ or ↓ or freq change		

	Time:		
Choose one: Crying/agitated 25%–50% of interval Crying/agitated >50% of interval	 2 3		
Choose one: Sleeps ≤25% of interval Sleeps 26%–75% of interval Sleeps >75% of interval	 3 2 1		
Choose one: Hyperactive Moro Markedly hyperactive Moro	 2 3		
Choose one: Mild tremors, disturbed Moderate/severe tremors, disturbed	 1 2		
Increased muscle tone	2		
Temperature 37.2°–38.4°C	1		
Temperature >38.4°C	2		
Respiratory rate >60 (extubated)	2		
Suction >twice/interval (intubated)	2		
Sweating	1		
Frequent yawning (>3–4/interval)	1		
Sneezing (>3–4/interval)	1		
Nasal stuffiness	1		
Emesis	2		
Projectile vomiting	3		
Loose stools	2		
Watery stools	3		
TOTAL SCORE			
ADJUSTED SCORE			
INITIALS OF PERSON SCORING			

Directions: Score every 2–4 hours per guideline
Score greater than 8–12 may indicate withdrawal

Guidelines for use of the flow sheet

Use of form

Use the flowsheet for all infants who have received continuous or around-the-clock opioid medication for 3 days or more, or more than 3 doses per day for more than 5 days. This patient population will most often include postoperative patients, agitated intubated infants, and all post-ECMO patients.

Instructions

1. Write drug, dose, and frequency of analgesics and sedatives ordered
2. Enter date, name of drug (abbreviated MS=morphine sulfate or FENT=fentanyl), and administration time of drugs given in the appropriate boxes; indicate if dose frequency given is an increase or decrease from the ordered dose
3. Scoring must be performed every 4 hours during weaning of opioids, every 2 hours if score is 8 or greater. The score for each item indicates the presence of the sign during the previous 2–4 hours (depending on the scoring interval). Every 4–hour scoring should continue until the patient is off all opioids for 48-72 hours. Place a "0" in the column after the sign if it is not seen during the scoring period.

Central nervous system

Crying behaviour: Score 2 points if patient exhibits crying or cry behaviour for a duration of ≤50% of the scoring interval. Score 3 points if cumulative crying behaviour totals >50% of the scoring interval.
NOTE: Crying behaviour is accompanied by the facial expressions associated with crying, but without audible sounds because of endotracheal intubation.
Sleeping: Score 3 points if patient sleeps for ≤25% of the scoring interval. Score 2 points if patient sleeps for 26%–75% of the scoring interval. Score 1 point if patient sleeps for >75% of the scoring interval.
Moro (startle) reflex: Score 2 points if patient has some arm and/or leg extension when touched or when disturbed by loud noises. Score 3 points if patient has marked arm and/or leg extension that is accompanied by crying behaviour, hyperalert state, or continued arm and/or leg tremors after being startled.
Tremors—disturbed: Score 1 point if patient has mild tremors when disturbed. Score 2 points if patient has moderate to severe tremors when disturbed. NOTE: Tremors are alternating movements that are rhythmic, of equal rate and amplitude, and can usually be stopped by flexion of the limb.
Increased muscle tone: Score 2 points if patient exhibits fisting or tight flexion of extremities that are difficult to extend.

Metabolic

Temperature: Score 1 point if patient's temperature is 37.2°–38.4°C. Score 2 points if patient's temperature is >38.4°C.
Respiratory rate: Score 1 point if patient's spontaneous respiratory rate is >60/minute. Score 2 points if patient's spontaneous respiratory rate is >60/minute and accompanied by retractions.
Suction: Score 2 points if patient is suctioned more than twice during a 4-hour period.
Sweating: Score 1 point if patient exhibits any type of sweating, including beads of sweat, or if skin is moist to touch.
Yawning: Score 1 point if patient yawns >3–4 times in succession or yawns 1–2 times often during a 4-hour period.
Sneezing: Score 1 point if patient sneezes >3–4 times in succession or sneezes 1–2 times during a 4-hour period.
Nasal stuffiness: Score 1 point for nasal stuffiness.

Gastrointestinal

Emesis of formula/stomach contents: Score 2 points if patient has 1 or more episodes of emesis during a 4-hour period.
Projectile vomiting: Score 3 points if patient has 1 or more episodes of projectile vomiting.
Loose stools: Score 2 points if patient has loose stools characterized by a water ring around some solid stool. The stools will often be frequent. NOTE: Do not score for "breast milk" stools: frequent, small, seedy, yellow stools.
Watery stools: Score 3 points if patient has stools that consist of only liquid. The stools will often be frequent.

Total score: Add up all the scores in the column and place the total score in this box. Clinical signs that appear continuously, such as respiratory rate >60 or regular poor feeding, should be included in the total score.
Adjusted score: The adjusted score is used when a sign is detected that is expected to occur independently of withdrawal, due to a pre-existing condition (high respiratory rate in infant with bronchopulmonary dysplasia). The decision to adjust the score should be made after discussion with the healthcare team during rounds, and the rationale should be recorded in a problem-oriented note. Circle the signs to be excluded and deduct the points from the total score to obtain the adjusted score.
Initials of person scoring: The person scoring should write his/her initials in this space.

FIGURE 34-8 Weaning flow sheet to monitor weaning in infants.

Parents and older children may fear addiction when opioids are prescribed (see Family-Centred Teaching Box). The nurse should address these concerns with assurance that any such risk is extremely low. It may be helpful to ask the question, "If you did not have this pain, would you want to take this medicine?" The answer is invariably no, which reinforces the solely therapeutic nature of the drug. It is also important to avoid making statements to the family such as "We don't want you to get used to this medicine," or "By now you shouldn't need this medicine," which may reinforce the fear of becoming addicted. Whereas both physical dependence and tolerance are physiological states, *addiction* or *psychological dependence* is a psychological state and implies a "cause–effect" mode of thinking, such as "I need the drug because it makes me feel better." Infants and children do not have the cognitive ability to make the cause–effect association and therefore cannot become addicted. The use of opioid analgesics early in life has not been demonstrated to increase the risk for addiction later in life. Nurses need to explain to parents the differences between physical dependence, tolerance, and addiction and allow parents to express concerns about the use and duration of use of opioids. Infants and children, when treated appropriately with opioids, may be at risk for physical tolerance and physical dependence, but not psychological dependence or addiction.

Evaluation of Effectiveness of Pain Regimen

The effectiveness of analgesics can be enhanced by a supportive attitude toward the child. By reinforcing the cause and effects of the medication and analgesia, the nurse in partnership with the family and interprofessional health care team can help the child understand what to expect and ways to optimize effectiveness of analgesics in conjunction with nonpharmacological measures. A pain scale or periodic ratings of pain intensity should be used for evaluation of effectiveness of pain regimens.

The response to therapy should be evaluated 15 to 30 minutes after each analgesic dose, and titration should continue to the point of highest achievable amount of relief (Turner, 2015).

Consistent use of effective pain interventions in children is suboptimal. Many children undergo painful procedures with no effective pain treatment. A nationwide study conducted in eight Canadian pediatric hospitals investigated 2987 children who had undergone at least one painful procedure in the previous 24 hours. The results showed that only 28.3% of the children received one or more pain management interventions, despite the large majority of children requiring a painful procedure (Stevens et al., 2011).

Several harmful effects occur with unrelieved pain, particularly when pain is prolonged. A number of physiological stress responses in the body are triggered during pain, which can lead to negative consequences that involve multiple systems. Unrelieved pain may prolong the stress response and adversely affect an infant or child's recovery, whether it is from trauma, surgery, procedures, or disease. In a landmark study by Anand and Hickey (1992), 30 neonates received deep intraoperative anaesthesia with high doses of the opioid sufentanil, followed postoperatively by an infusion of opioids for 24 hours, and 15 neonates received lighter anaesthesia with halothane and morphine, followed postoperatively by intermittent morphine and diazepam. The 15 neonates who received the lighter anaesthesia and intermittent postoperative opioids had more severe hyperglycemia and lactic acidemia, and four postoperative deaths occurred in the group. The 30 neonates who received deep anaesthesia had a lower incidence of complications (sepsis, metabolic acidosis, disseminated intravascular coagulation) and no deaths.

Poorly controlled acute pain can predispose patients to *chronic pain syndromes.* A guiding principle in pain management is that prevention of pain is always better than treatment. Pain that is established and severe is often more difficult to control. When pain is unrelieved, sensory input from injured tissues reaches spinal cord neurons and may enhance subsequent responses. Long-lasting changes in cells within spinal cord pain pathways may occur after a brief painful stimulus and may lead to the development of chronic pain conditions.

In a study of nursing practice related to pain assessment and management in different pediatric specialty units, Jacob and Puntillo (2000) noted that nurses were aware of patients' indications of pain but seldom documented patient-specific pain scores or notations about responses to analgesics after administration. Pain scores were not available before and after giving analgesics, and it was thus not possible to conclude whether analgesics were effective. Nurses need to evaluate and monitor pain in a timely fashion after administration of analgesics; titrate dosage to effect; or make recommendations for an alternative analgesic, addition of another analgesic, or for a combination of analgesics, adjuvants, and nonpharmacological strategies.

KEY POINTS

- Behavioural assessments are used to measure pain in infants, preverbal children, children with cognitive impairments who do not have the language skills to communicate that they are in pain, and children who for any reason have limited ability to communicate.
- Physiological measures, although less specific to pain than behavioural measures, contribute to the overall assessment of pain.
- Pain assessment and pain care are best managed as a partnership between the child, family, nurse, physician, and other clinicians.
- Knowledge about pain assessment and the number and array of pain measures available for use in infants and young children have increased dramatically; these add a layer of complexity to the assessment of pain in children.

- Important components of assessment include the onset of pain; pain duration or pattern; effectiveness, or otherwise, of the current treatment; factors that aggravate or relieve the pain; other symptoms and complications concurrently felt; and interference with the child's mood, function, and interactions with family.
- Nonopioids, including acetaminophen and NSAIDs, are suitable for mild to moderate pain; opioids are needed for moderate to severe pain.
- Several drugs—coanalgesics or adjuvant analgesics—may be used alone or with opioids to control pain symptoms and opioid adverse effects.
- A significant advance in the administration of IV, epidural, or subcutaneous analgesics is the use of PCA.
- For procedural pain in infants, breastfeeding or skin-to-skin care, if feasible and possible, or sucrose or glucose effectively reduce pain during commonly performed minor painful procedures.
- For procedural pain in children, topical anaesthetic creams, applied as directed before needle-related painful procedures, along with age- and developmentally appropriate distraction, reduce pain and distress associated with needle-related procedures.
- Anticipation and early management of commonly occurring adverse effects of pharmacological agents is crucial to effective pain management.
- Consistent use of known recommended effective, age-appropriate pain treatment is important, as untreated or poorly treated pain is harmful.

evolve WEBSITE

Visit the Evolve website for additional resources related to the content in this chapter such as Case Studies, Critical Thinking Case Study Answers, Nursing Care Plans, Nursing Processes, Nursing Skills, and Review Questions for Exam Preparation at: http://evolve.elsevier.com/Canada/Perry/maternal/

REFERENCES

Abbe, M., Simon, C., Angiolilo, A., et al. (2006). A survey of language barriers from the perspective of pediatric oncologists, interpreters, and parents. *Pediatric Blood & Cancer, 47*(6), 819–824.

Adams, D., Dagenais, D., Clifford, T., et al. (2013). Complementary and alternative medicine use by pediatric specialty outpatients. *Pediatrics, 131*(2), 225–232. doi:10.1542/peds.2012-1220.

Ambuel, B., Hamlett, K. W., Marx, C. M., et al. (1992). Assessing distress in pediatric intensive care environments: The COMFORT scale. *Journal of Pediatric Psychology, 17*(1), 95–109.

Anand, K. J., & Hickey, P. R. (1992). Halothane-morphine compared with high-dose sufentanil for anaesthesia and postoperative analgesia in neonatal cardiac surgery. *New England Journal of Medicine, 326*(1), 1–9.

Breau, L. M. (2014). Parents of non-verbal children with learning disability (LD) most commonly recognise their child's pain through vocalisations, social behaviour and facial expressions. *Evidence-Based Nursing, 17*(4), 111. doi:10.1136/eb-2013-101553.

Breau, L. M., Finley, G. A., McGrath, P. J., et al. (2002). Validation of the Non-communicating Children's Pain Checklist–Postoperative Version. *Anesthesiology, 96*(3), 528–535.

Breau, L. M., McGrath, P. J., Camfield, C. S., et al. (2002). Psychometric properties of the Non-communicating Children's Pain Checklist—Revised. *Pain, 99*, 349–357.

Bruera, E., Willey, J. S., Ewert-Flannagan, P. A., et al. (2005). Pain intensity assessment by bedside nurses and palliative care consultants: A retrospective study. *Supportive Care in Cancer, 13*(4), 228–231.

Bueno, M., Yamada, J., Harrison, D., et al. (2013). A systematic review and meta-analyses of non-sucrose sweet solutions for pain relief in neonates. *Pain Research & Management, 18*(3), 153–161.

Butbul, Y., Stremler, R., Benseler, S. M., et al. (2011). Sleep and fatigue and the relationship to pain, disease activity and quality of life in juvenile idiopathic arthritis and juvenile dermatomyositis. *Rheumatology, 50*(11), 2051–2060. doi:10.1093/rheumatology/ker256.

Carnevale, F. A., & Razack, S. (2002). An item analysis of the COMFORT scale in a pediatric intensive care unit. *Pediatric Critical Care Medicine, 3*(2), 177–180. doi:10.1097/00130478-200204000-00016.

Chorpita, B. F., Yim, L., Moffitt, C., et al. (2000). Assessment of symptoms of DSM-IV anxiety and depression in children: A revised child anxiety and depression scale. *Behaviour Research and Therapy, 38*(8), 835–855.

Cignacco, E. L., Sellam, G., Stoffel, L., et al. (2012). Oral sucrose and "facilitated tucking" for repeated pain relief in preterms: A randomized controlled trial. *Pediatrics, 129*(2), 299–308. doi:10.1542/peds.2011-1879.

Claar, R. L., & Walker, L. S. (2006). Functional assessment of pediatric pain patients: Psychometric properties of the functional disability inventory. *Pain, 121*(1–2), 77–84.

Cline, M. E., Herman, J., Shaw, E. R., et al. (1992). Standardization of the visual analogue scale. *Nursing Research, 41*(6), 378–380.

Crellin, D. J., Harrison, D., Santamaria, N., & Babl, F. E. (2015). Systematic review of the FLACC scale for assessing pain in infants and children. *Pain, 156*, 2132–2151. doi:10.1097/j.pain.0000000000000305.

Fernandes, A. M., De Campos, C., Batalha, L., et al. (2014). Pain assessment using the adolescent pediatric pain tool: A systematic review. *Pain Research & Management, 19*(4), 212–218.

Franck, L. S., Harris, S. K., Soetenga, D. J., et al. (2008). The Withdrawal Assessment Tool-1 (WAT-1): An assessment instrument for monitoring opioid and benzodiazepine withdrawal symptoms in pediatric patients. *Pediatric Critical Care Medicine, 9*(6), 573–580.

Harrison, D., Bueno, M., & Reszel, J. (2015). Prevention and management of pain and stress in the neonate. *Research and Reports in Neonatology, 5*, 9–16. doi:10.2147/RRN.S52378.

Harrison, D., Joly, C., Chretien, C., et al. (2014). Pain prevalence in a pediatric hospital: Raising awareness during Pain Awareness Week. *Pain Research & Management, 19*(1), e24–e30. doi:10.1155/2014/737692.

Hershey, A. D. (2001). PedMIDS: Development of a questionnaire to assess disability of migraines in children. *Neurology, 57*(11), 2034–2039.

Hicks, C. L., von Baeyer, C. L., Spafford, P. A., et al. (2001). The FACES pain scale—revised: Toward a common metric in pediatric pain measurement. *Pain, 93*(2), 173–183.

International Association for the Study of Pain (IASP). (2001). *Faces Pain Scale–Revised (FPS-R)*. Retrieved from http://iasp.files.cms-plus.com/Content/ContentFolders/Resources2/FPSR/facepainscale_english_eng-au-ca.pdf.

Jacob, E., & Puntillo, K. A. (2000). Variability of analgesic practices for hospitalized children on different pediatric specialty units. *Journal of Pain Symptom Management*, *20*(1), 59–67.

Johnston, C., Campbell-Yeo, M., Fernandes, A., et al. (2014). Skin-to-skin care for procedural pain in neonates. *The Cochrane Database of Systematic Reviews*, (1), CD008435 doi:10.1002/14651858.CD008435.pub2.

Kovacs, M. (1981). Rating scales to assess depression in school-aged children. *Acta Paedopsychiatric*, *46*(5–6), 305–315.

Latimer, M., Simandl, D., Finley, A. F., et al. (2014). Understanding the impact of the pain experience on Aboriginal children's wellbeing: Viewing through a two-eyed seeing lens. *First Peoples Child & Family Review*, *9*(1), 22–37.

Luffy, R., & Grove, S. K. (2003). Examining the validity, reliability, and preference of three pediatric pain measurement tools in African-American children. *Pediatric Nursing*, *29*(1), 54–60.

MacDonald, N., & MacLeod, S. M. (2010). Has the time come to phase out codeine? *Canadian Medical Association Journal*, *182*(17), 1825. doi:10.1503/cmaj.101411.

Malviya, S., Voepel-Lewis, T., Burke, C., et al. (2006). The revised FLACC observational pain tool: Improved reliability and validity for pain assessment in children with cognitive impairment. *Paediatric Anaesthesia*, *16*(3), 258–265. doi:10.1111/j.1460-9592.2005.01773.x.

Manworren, R., & Hynan, L. (2003). Clinical validation of FLACC: Preverbal patient pain scale. *Pediatric Nursing*, *29*(2), 140–146.

Max, M. B., Payne, R., Edwards, W. T., et al. (1999). *Principles of analgesic use in the treatment of acute pain and cancer pain*. Glenview, IL: American Pain Society.

McGrath, P. J., Johnson, G., Goodman, J. T., et al. (1985). CHEOPS: A behavioral scale for rating postoperative pain in children. In H. L. Fields, R. Dubner, & F. Cerveri (Eds.), *Advances in Pain Research and Therapy* (Vol. 9, pp. 395–402). New York: Raven Press.

McGrath, P. J., Rosmus, C., Canfield, C., et al. (1998). Behaviours caregivers use to determine pain in non-verbal, cognitively impaired individuals. *Developmental Medicine and Child Neurology*, *40*(5), 340–343.

Melzack, R. (1975). The McGill pain questionnaire: Major properties and scoring methods. *Pain*, *1*, 277–299.

Merkel, S. I., Voepel-Lewis, T., Shayevitz, J. R., et al. (1997). The FLACC: A behavioral scale for scoring postoperative pain in young children. *Pediatric Nursing*, *23*(3), 293–297.

Migdal, M., Chudzynska-Pomianowska, E., Vause, E., et al. (2006). Rapid, needle-free delivery of lidocaine for reducing the pain of venipuncture among pediatric subjects. *Pediatrics*, *115*(4), e393–e398. doi:10.1016/j.jpeds.2007.07.018.

National Institute of Health, Medline Plus. (2011). Chronic pain: Symptoms, diagnosis, and treatment. *Medline Plus*, *6*(1), 5–6.v. Retrieved from <http://www.nlm.nih.gov/medlineplus/magazine/issues/spring11/articles/spring11pg5-6.html>.

Owens, J. A., Spirito, A., & McGuinn, M. (2000). The children's sleep habits questionnaire (CSHQ): Psychometric properties of a survey instrument foe school-aged children. *Sleep*, *23*(8), 1043–1051.

Palmero, T. M. (2000). The impact of recurrent and chronic pain on child and family daily functioning: A critical review of the literature. *Journal of Developmental Behaviour Pediatrics*, *21*(1), 58–69.

Pillai Riddell, R., Racine, N. M., Gennis, H. G., et al. (2015). Non-pharmacological management of infant and young child procedural pain. *The Cochrane Database of Systematic Reviews*, (12), CD006275, doi:10.1002/14651858.CD006275.pub3.

Registered Nurses' Association of Ontario. (2013). *Assessment and management of pain* (3rd ed.). Toronto: Registered Nurses' Association of Ontario. Retrieved from <http://rnao.ca/sites/rnao-ca/files/AssessAndManagementOfPain_15_WEB-_FINAL_DEC_2.pdf>.

Robieux, I., Kumar, R., Radhakrishnan, S., & Koren, G. (1991). Assessing pain and analgesia with a lidocaine-prilocaine emulsion in infants and toddlers during venipuncture. *Journal of Pediatrics*, *118*(6), 971–973.

Savedra, M. C., Holzemer, W. L., Tesler, M. D., & Wilkie, D. J. (1993). Assessment of post operation pain in children and adolescents using the adolescent pediatric pain tool. *Nursing Research*, *42*(1), 5–9.

Schechter, N. L. (2014). Chronic pain syndromes in childhood: One trunk, many branches. In P. J. McGrath, B. J. Stevens, S. M. Walker, & W. T. Zempsky (Eds.), *Oxford textbook of paediatric pain* (pp. 228–236). Oxford, UK: Oxford University Press.

Shah, P. S., Herbozo, C., Aliwalas, L. I., & Shah, V. S. (2012). Breastfeeding or breast milk for procedural pain in neonates. *The Cochrane Database of Systematic Reviews*, (12), CD004950, doi:10.1002/14651858.CD004950.pub3.

Spigelblatt, L., & Canadian Paediatric Society, Community Paediatrics Committee. (2005). Homeopathy in the paediatric population. *Paediatrics & Child Health*, *10*(3), 173–177. Reaffirmed in 2016. Retrieved from <http://www.cps.ca/en/documents/position/homeopathy#authors>.

Stallard, P., Williams, L., Velleman, R., et al. (2002a). The development and evaluation of the Pain Indicator for Communicatively Impaired Children (PICIC). *Pain*, *98*(1–2), 145–149.

Stallard, P., Williams, L., Velleman, R., et al. (2002b). Intervening factors in caregivers' assessments of pain in non-communicating children. *Developmental Medicine and Child Neurology*, *44*(3), 213–214.

Stanford, E. A., Chambers, C. T., & Craig, K. D. (2006). The role of developmental factors in predicting young children's use of a self-report scale for pain. *Pain*, *120*(1–2), 16–23. doi:10.1016/j.pain.2005.10.004.

Stevens, B., Abbott, L., Yamada, J., et al. (2011). Epidemiology and management of painful procedures in children in Canadian hospitals. *Canadian Medical Association Journal*, *183*(7), E403–E410. doi:10.1503/cmaj.101341.

Stevens, B. J., Harrison, D., Rashotte, J., et al. (2012). Pain assessment and intensity in hospitalized children in Canada. *Journal of Pain*, *13*(9), 857–865. doi:10.1016/j.jpain.2012.05.010.

Stevens, B., Yamada, J., Lee, G. Y., & Ohlsson, A. (2013). Sucrose for analgesia in newborn infants undergoing painful procedures. *The Cochrane Database of Systematic Reviews*, (1), CD001069. doi:10.1002/14651858.CD001069.pub4.

Stinson, J. N. (2009). Improving the assessment of pediatric chronic pain: Harnessing the potential of electronic diaries. *Pain Research & Management*, *14*(1), 59–64.

Stinson, J. N., Stevens, B., Feldman, B. M., et al. (2008). Construct validity of a multidimensional electron pain diary for adolescent with arthritis. *Pain*, *136*(3), 281–292.

Taddio, A., Nulman, I., Koren, B. S., et al. (1995). A revised measure of acute pain in infants. *Journal of Pain Symptom Management*, *10*(6), 456–463.

Taylor, E. M., Boyer, K., & Campbell, F. A. (2008). Pain in hospitalized children: A prospective cross-sectional survey of pain prevalence, intensity, assessment and management in a Canadian pediatric teaching hospital. *Pain Research & Management*, *13*(1), 25–32. doi:10.1016/j.acpain.2008.05.042.

Turner, F. (2015). *Supporting best practice for patient care: A multiple branch implementation of the RNAO assessment and management of pain best practice guideline*. Retrieved from <http://rnao.ca/bpg/get-involved/acpf/executive-summaries/flora-turner>.

Varni, J. W., Seid, M., & Rode, C. A. (1999). The PedsQL: Measurement model for the pediatric quality of life inventory. *Medical Care*, *37*(2), 126–129.

Varni, J. W., Thompson, K. L., & Hanson, V. (1987). The Varni/Thompson Pediatric Pain Questionnaire. I. Chronic musculoskeletal pain in juvenile rheumatoid arthritis. *Pain*, *28*(1), 27–38. doi:10.1016/0304-3959(87)91056-6.

van Dijk, A., McGrath, P., Pickett, W., et al. (2006). Pain prevalence in 9- to 13-year-old schoolchildren. *Pain Research and Management*, *11*(4), 234–240.

Vervoort, T., Goubert, L., Eccleston, C., et al. (2006). Catastrophic thinking about pain is independently associated with pain severity, disability, and somatic complaints in school children and children with chronic pain. *Journal Pediatric Psychology*, *31*(7), 674–683.

von Baeyer, C. L. (2014). Self-report: The primary source in assessment after infancy. In P. J. McGrath, B. J. Stevens, S. M. Walker, & W. T. Zempsky (Eds.), *Oxford textbook of paediatric pain* (pp. 370–378). Oxford, UK: Oxford University Press.

von Baeyer, C., & Hicks, C. (2000). Support for a common metric for pediatric pain intensity scales. *Pain Research & Management, 4*(2), 157–160.

Walker, L. S., & Green, J. W. (1991). The functional disability inventory: Measuring a neglected dimension of child health status. *Journal of Pediatric Psychology, 16*(1), 39–58.

Wong-Baker FACES Foundation (2016). *Wong-Baker FACES® Pain Rating Scale.* Retrieved August 30, 2016, with permission from <http://www.WongBakerFACES.org>.

Wong, D. L., & Baker, C. M. (1988). Pain in children: Comparison of assessment scales. *Pediatric Nursing, 14*(1), 9–17.

Zempsky, W. T., Bean-Lijewski, J., Kauffman, R. E., et al. (2008). Needle-free powder lidocaine delivery system provides rapid effective analgesic for venipuncture or cannulation pain in children: Randomized, double-blind comparison of venipuncture and venous cannulation pain after fast-onset needle-free powder lidocaine or placebo treatment trial. *Pediatrics, 121*(5), 978–987.

ADDITIONAL RESOURCES

Aboutkidshealth—Pediatric health resource from The Hospital for Sick Children: <http://www.aboutkidshealth.ca/En/HealthAZ/Pages/default.aspx?name=p>.

Topics include:

- Pain After an Operation: Taking Care of Your Child's Pain at Home
- Pain at Home: Taking Care of Your Child
- Pain Diary: Pain After an Operation
- Pain Medicines
- Pain Relief: Comfort Kit
- Pain: How to Talk to Kids About Their Pain

Be Sweet to Babies (video showing parents how to help babies during blood sampling): <https://www.youtube.com/watch?v=HmJGQJ8ayL8&feature=youtu.be>.

Centre for Pediatric Pain Research: Summary of pediatric pain assessment scales: <http://pediatric-pain.ca/resources/our-measures/>.

Centre for Pediatric Research—Resources for parents and healthcare providers on how to help support children during painful procedures: <http://pediatric-pain.ca/about-us/>.

CHEO Vaccination Pain—Reducing Pain During Vaccination: <http://www.cheo.on.ca/en/reduce-vaccination-pain>.

HELP Eliminate Pain in Kids & Adults—Information about pain treatment during vaccination; resources for healthcare professionals and for families: <http://phm.utoronto.ca/helpinkids/publications.html>.

RNAO Assessment and Management of Pain (Third Edition): <http://rnao.ca/bpg/guidelines/assessment-and-management-pain>.

UNIT 10

Health Promotion and Special Health Problems

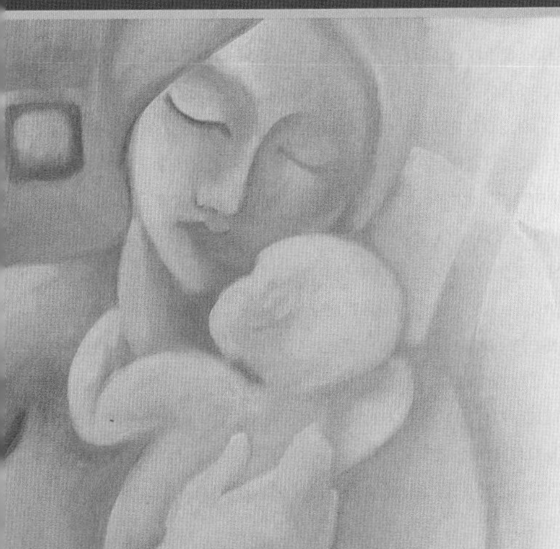

CHAPTER 35

The Infant and Family

Karen Marie Breen-Reid

evolve WEBSITE

Visit the Evolve website for additional resources related to the content in this chapter such as Case Studies, Critical Thinking Case Study Answers, Nursing Care Plans, Nursing Processes, Nursing Skills, and Review Questions for Exam Preparation at: http://evolve.elsevier.com/Canada/Perry/maternal/

OBJECTIVES

On completion of this chapter the reader will be able to:

- Identify the major biological, psychosocial, cognitive, and social developments that occur during the first year of life.
- Relate parent–child attachment, separation anxiety, and stranger fear to developmental achievements during infancy.
- Provide anticipatory guidance to parents regarding common parental concerns during infancy.
- Provide anticipatory guidance to parents regarding recommendations for feeding infants.
- Outline immunization requirements during infancy, early childhood, and adolescence.
- List general contraindications, precautions, and administration routes for immunizations.
- Provide anticipatory guidance to parents regarding injury prevention based on the infant's developmental achievements.
- Provide anticipatory guidance in the care of the family with an infant who is experiencing colic.
- Plan nursing care that can meet the physical and emotional needs of the child with growth failure as well as needs of the family.
- Provide anticipatory guidance for the prevention of sudden infant death syndrome.
- Provide nursing care that aims to meet the immediate and long-term needs of the family that has lost a child from sudden infant death syndrome.
- Identify needs of the family whose child is home monitored for apnea.

PROMOTING OPTIMUM GROWTH AND DEVELOPMENT

Biological Development

At no other time in life are physical changes and developmental achievements as dramatic as during infancy. All major body systems undergo progressive maturation, and there is concurrent development of skills that increasingly enable infants to respond to and cope with the environment. Acquisition of these fine and gross motor skills occurs in an orderly head-to-toe and centre-to-periphery (**cephalocaudal** and **proximodistal**) sequence.

Proportional Changes

Growth is very rapid during the first year, especially during the initial 6 months. Infants gain 150 to 200 grams weekly until approximately age 5 to 6 months, when the birth weight has at least doubled. An average weight for a 6-month-old child is 7.0 kg. Weight gain slows during the second 6 months. By 1 year of age the infant's birth weight has tripled, for an average weight of 9.75 kg. Height increases by 2.5 cm a month during the first 6 months and then slows during the second 6 months. Increases in length occur in sudden spurts, rather than in a slow, gradual pattern. Average height is 65 cm at 6 months and 74 cm at 12 months. By age 1 year the birth length has increased by almost

50%. This increase occurs mainly in the trunk, rather than in the legs, and contributes to the infant's characteristic physique.

It is important for individual children to have specific measurements taken so that their growth pattern can be accurately tracked. These measurements need to be done on a regular basis with a growth chart that gives a basis for comparing them with the average measurements of other children. The Dietitians of Canada, Canadian Paediatric Society (CPS), College of Family Physicians, Community Health Nurses of Canada, and Canadian Pediatric Endocrine Group have developed Canadian pediatric growth charts from the World Health Organization (WHO) 2006 Child Growth Standards and the 2007 WHO International Growth Reference charts (see Appendix C for the 2014 growth charts). There are also growth charts that have been developed for specialized conditions, such as Down syndrome, where the growth pattern is different (Myrelid, Gustafsson, Ollars, et al., 2002). However, the CPS advises caution when using these charts because of potential inaccuracies (from out-of-date data and small sample sizes) that could hide issues related to failure to grow. The CPS recommends using both the standard and specialized growth charts when tracking growth in children with such conditions.

Head growth in infants is also rapid. During the first 6 months, head circumference increases approximately 1.5 cm a month, but the rate of increase falls to only 0.5 cm monthly during the second 6 months. The average size is 43 cm at 6 months and 46 cm at 12 months. By 1 year of age, head size has increased by almost 33%. Closure of the cranial sutures occurs, with the posterior fontanel closing by 6 to 8 weeks of age and the anterior fontanel closing by 12 to 18 months of age (the average age being 14 months).

Expanding head size reflects the growth and differentiation of the nervous system. By the end of the first year, the brain has increased in weight about 2½ times. Maturation of the brain is exhibited in the dramatic developmental achievements of infancy (see Table 35-1). Primitive reflexes are replaced by voluntary, purposeful movement and new reflexes that influence motor development appear.

The chest assumes a more adult contour, with the lateral diameter becoming larger than the anteroposterior diameter. The chest circumference approximately equals the head circumference by the end of the first year. The heart grows less rapidly than the rest of the body. Its weight is usually doubled by 1 year of age; in comparison, body weight triples during the same period. The size of the heart is still large in relation to the chest cavity; its width is approximately 55% of the chest width.

The developmental process during the first 12 months is complex. Table 35-1 presents the physical, motor, sensory, and social traits as they develop throughout an infant's first year, along with average monthly age at which various skills are attained. Although all milestones are important, some represent essential integrative aspects of development that lay the foundation for achievement of more advanced skills. These essential milestones are designated by an asterisk (*) in the table. It must be remembered that although the sequence is the same, the rate will vary among children.

Maturation of Systems

Other organ systems also change and grow during infancy. The respiratory rate slows somewhat (see Appendix E) and is relatively stable. Respiratory movements continue to be abdominal. Several factors predispose the infant to more severe and acute respiratory problems. Because of the close proximity of the trachea to the bronchi and its branching structures, infectious agents can be rapidly transmitted from one anatomical location to another. The short, straight eustachian tube closely communicates with the ear, allowing infection to ascend from the pharynx to the middle ear. In addition, because the infant's immune system is unable to produce sufficient immune globulin A (IgA) in the mucosal lining, there is less protection against infection in infancy than during later childhood.

The heart rate slows (see Appendix E), and the rhythm is often sinus arrhythmia (i.e., rate increases with inspiration and decreases with expiration). Blood pressure also changes during infancy (see Appendix E). Systolic pressure rises during the first 2 months as a result of the increasing ability of the left ventricle to pump blood into the systemic circulation. Diastolic pressure decreases during the first 3 months then gradually rises to values close to those at birth. Fluctuations in blood pressure occur during varying states of activity and emotion.

Significant hematopoietic changes occur during the infant's first year (see Appendix D). Fetal hemoglobin (HgbF) is present in large quantities for the first 5 months, with adult hemoglobin steadily increasing through the first half of infancy. Fetal hemoglobin has a shorter lifespan than that of adult hemoglobin; thus there is an increased turnover of these cells and a gradual decrease in hemoglobin. This process results in a physiological anemia around 3 to 6 months of age. High levels of HgbF depress the production of erythropoietin, a hormone released by the kidney that stimulates red blood cell production. Hemoglobin levels decrease to a point at which tissue oxygenation needs stimulate erythropoietin, and erythropoiesis resumes, forming new red blood cells (Blackburn, 2013).

Maternally derived iron stores are present for the infant's first 5 to 6 months and then gradually diminish, which also accounts for lowered hemoglobin levels toward the end of the first 6 months. The occurrence of physiological anemia is not affected by an adequate supply of iron. However, when erythropoiesis is stimulated, iron supplies are necessary for the formation of hemoglobin.

The digestive processes are immature at birth. Although term newborn infants have some limitations in digestive function, human milk has properties that partially compensate for decreased digestive enzymatic activity, thus enabling breastfed infants to receive optimal nutrition during the first several months of life. Saliva is secreted in small amounts, but most of the digestive processes do not begin functioning until age 3 months, when drooling is common because of the poorly coordinated swallowing reflex. The enzyme amylase (also called ptyalin) is present in small amounts but usually has little effect on the foodstuffs because of the small amount of time the food stays in the mouth. Gastric digestion in the stomach consists

Text continued on p. 993

TABLE 35-1 GROWTH AND DEVELOPMENT DURING INFANCY

AGE (mo)	PHYSICAL	GROSS MOTOR	FINE MOTOR	SENSORY	VOCALIZATION	SOCIALIZATION/ COGNITION
Birth –6 mo	Weight gain of 140–200 g weekly for first 6 mo Height gain of 2.5 cm monthly for first 6 mo Head circumference increases by 1.5 cm monthly for first 6 mo Primitive reflexes present and strong Doll's eye reflexes and dance reflex fading Obligatory nose breathing (most infants)	Assumes flexed position with pelvis high but knees not under abdomen when prone (at birth, knees flexed under abdomen)* Can turn head from side to side when prone; lifts head momentarily from bed (see Fig. 35-3, A)* Has marked head lag, especially when pulled from lying to sitting position (see Fig. 35-2, A) Holds head momentarily parallel and in midline when suspended in prone position Assumes asymmetrical tonic neck reflex position when supine When held in standing position, body is limp at knees and hips In sitting position, back is uniformly rounded, absence of head control	Hands predominantly closed Grasp reflex strong Hand clenches on contact with rattle	Able to fixate on moving object in range of 45 degrees when held at a distance of 20–25 cm Visual acuity approaches 20/100† Follows light to midline Quiets when hears a voice	Cries to express displeasure Makes small, throaty sounds Makes comfort sounds during feeding	Is in sensorimotor phase—stage I, use of reflexes (birth–1 mo), and stage II, primary circular reactions (1–4 mo) Watches parent's face intently as parent talks to infant
2	Posterior fontanel closed Crawling reflex disappears	Assumes less flexed position when prone—hips flat, legs extended, arms flexed, head to side* Less head lag when pulled to sitting position (see Fig. 35-2, B) Can maintain head in same plane as rest of body when held in ventral suspension When prone, can lift head almost 45 degrees off table When moved to sitting position, head is held up but bends forward (see Fig. 35-5, B) Assumes asymmetrical tonic neck reflex position intermittently	Hands often open Grasp reflex fading	Binocular fixation and convergence to near objects beginning When supine, follows dangling toy from side to point beyond midline Visually searches to locate sounds Turns head to side when sound is made at level of ear	Vocalizes, distinct from crying* Crying becomes differentiated Coos Vocalizes to familiar voice	Demonstrates social smile in response to various stimuli*

Continued

TABLE 35-1 GROWTH AND DEVELOPMENT DURING INFANCY—cont'd

AGE (mo)	PHYSICAL	GROSS MOTOR	FINE MOTOR	SENSORY	VOCALIZATION	SOCIALIZATION/ COGNITION
3	Primitive reflexes fading	Able to hold head more erect when sitting, but still bobs forward Has only slight head lag when pulled to sitting position Assumes symmetrical body positioning Able to raise head and shoulders from prone position to a 45- to 90-degree angle from table; bears weight on forearms When held in standing position, able to bear slight fraction of weight on legs Looks at own hand	Actively holds rattle but will not reach for it* Grasp reflex absent Hands kept loosely open Clutches own hand; pulls at blankets and clothes	Follows object to periphery (180 degrees)* Locates sound by turning head to side and looking in same direction* Begins to have ability to coordinate stimuli from various sense organs	Squeals aloud to show pleasure* Coos, babbles, chuckles Vocalizes when smiling "Talks" a great deal when spoken to Less crying during periods of wakefulness	Displays considerable interest in surroundings Ceases crying when parent enters room Can recognize familiar faces and objects Shows awareness of strange situations
4	Drooling begins Moro, tonic neck, and rooting reflexes have disappeared*	Has almost no head lag when pulled to sitting position (see Fig. 35-2, C)* Balances head well in sitting position (see Fig. 35-5, C)* Back less rounded, curved only in lumbar area Able to sit erect if propped up Able to raise head and chest off surface to angle of 90 degrees (see Fig. 35-3, B) Assumes predominant symmetrical position Rolls from back to side*	Inspects and plays with hands; pulls clothing or blanket over face in play* Tries to reach objects with hand but overshoots Grasps object with both hands Plays with rattle placed in hand, shakes it, but cannot pick it up if dropped Can carry objects to mouth	Able to accommodate to near objects Binocular vision fairly well established Can focus on a 1.25-cm block Beginning eye–hand coordination	Makes consonant sounds *n, k, g, p, b* Laughs out loud* Vocalization changes according to mood	Is in stage III, secondary circular reactions Demands attention by fussing; becomes bored if left alone Enjoys social interaction with people Anticipates feeding when sees bottle or mother if breastfeeding Shows excitement with whole body, squeals, breathes heavily Shows interest in strange stimuli Begins to show memory
5	Beginning signs of tooth eruption Birth weight doubles	No head lag when pulled to sitting position When sitting, able to hold head erect and steady Able to sit for longer periods when back is well supported Back straight When prone, assumes symmetrical positioning with arms extended Can turn over from abdomen to back* When supine, puts feet to mouth	Able to grasp objects voluntarily* Uses palmar grasp, bidextrous approach Plays with toes Takes objects directly to mouth Holds one cube while looking at a second one	Visually pursues a dropped object Is able to sustain visual inspection of an object Can localize sounds made below ear	Squeals Makes cooing vowel sounds interspersed with consonant sounds (e.g., *ah-goo*)	Smiles at mirror image Pats breast or bottles with both hands More enthusiastically playful, but may have rapid mood swings Is able to discriminate strangers from family Vocalizes displeasure when object is taken away Discovers parts of body

TABLE 35-1 GROWTH AND DEVELOPMENT DURING INFANCY—cont'd

AGE (mo)	PHYSICAL	GROSS MOTOR	FINE MOTOR	SENSORY	VOCALIZATION	SOCIALIZATION/ COGNITION
6	Growth rate may begin to decline Weight gain of 85–140 g weekly for next 6 mo Height gain of 1.25 cm monthly for next 6 mo Teething may begin with eruption of two lower central incisors* Chewing and biting occur*	When prone, can lift chest and upper abdomen off surface, bearing weight on hands (see Fig. 35-3, C) When about to be pulled to a sitting position, lifts head Sits in high chair with back straight Rolls from back to abdomen When held in standing position, bears almost all of weight Hand regard absent	Re-secures a dropped object Drops one cube when another is given Grasps and manipulates small objects Holds bottle Grasps feet and pulls to mouth	Adjusts posture to see an object Prefers more complex visual stimuli Can localize sounds made above ear Will turn head to the side, then look up or down	Begins to imitate sounds* Babbling resembles one-syllable utterances—*ma, mu, da, di, hi** Vocalizes to toys, mirror image Takes pleasure in hearing own sounds (self-reinforcement)	Recognizes parents; begins to fear strangers Holds arms out to be picked up Has definite likes and dislikes Begins to imitate (cough, protrusion of tongue) Excites on hearing footsteps Laughs when head is hidden in a towel Briefly searches for a dropped object (object permanence beginning)* Frequent mood swings—from crying to laughing with little or no provocation
7	Eruption of upper central incisors	When supine, spontaneously lifts head off surface Sits, leaning forward on hands (see Fig. 35-5, D)* When prone, bears weight on one hand Sits erect momentarily Bears full weight on feet (see Fig. 35-6, A) When held in standing position, bounces actively	Transfers objects from one hand to the other (see Fig. 35-5, E)* Has unidextrous approach and grasp Holds two cubes more than momentarily Bangs cube on table Rakes at a small object	Can fixate on very small objects* Responds to own name Localizes sound by turning head in a curving arch Beginning awareness of depth and space Has taste preferences	Produces vowel sounds and chained syllables—*baba, dada, kaka** Vocalizes four distinct vowel sounds "Talks" when others are talking	Increasing fear of strangers; shows signs of fretfulness when parent disappears* Imitates simple acts and noises Tries to attract attention by coughing or snorting Plays peekaboo Demonstrates dislike of food by keeping lips closed Exhibits oral aggressiveness in biting and mouthing Demonstrates expectation in response to repetition of stimuli
8	Begins to show regular patterns in bladder and bowel elimination Parachute reflex appears (see Fig. 35-4)	Sits steadily unsupported (see Fig. 35-5, E)* Readily bears weight on legs when supported; may stand holding onto furniture Adjusts posture to reach an object	Has beginning pincer grasp using index, fourth, and fifth fingers against lower part of thumb Releases objects at will Rings bell purposely Retains two cubes while regarding third cube Secures an object by pulling on a string Reaches persistently for toys out of reach		Makes consonant sounds *t, d, w* Listens selectively to familiar words Utterances signal emphasis and emotion Combines syllables, such as *dada*, but does not ascribe meaning to them	Increasing anxiety over loss of parent, particularly mother, and fear of strangers Responds to word "no" Dislikes dressing, diaper change

Continued

TABLE 35-1 GROWTH AND DEVELOPMENT DURING INFANCY—cont'd

AGE (mo)	PHYSICAL	GROSS MOTOR	FINE MOTOR	SENSORY	VOCALIZATION	SOCIALIZATION/ COGNITION
9	Eruption of upper lateral incisor may begin	Creeps on hands and knees Sits steadily on floor for prolonged time (10 min) Recovers balance when leaning forward but cannot do so when leaning sideways Pulls self to standing position and stands holding onto furniture (see Fig. 35-6, B and C)*	Uses thumb and index fingers in crude pincer grasp (see Fig. 35-1)* Preference for use of dominant hand now evident Grasps third cube Compares two cubes by bringing them together	Localizes sounds by turning head diagonally and directly toward sound Depth perception increasing	Responds to simple verbal commands Comprehends "no-no"	Parent (mother) is increasingly important for own sake Shows increasing interest in pleasing parent Begins to show fears of going to bed and being left alone Puts arms in front of face to avoid having it washed
10	Labyrinth-righting reflex is strongest—when infant is in prone or supine position, is able to raise head	Can change from prone to sitting position Stands while holding onto furniture, sits by falling down Recovers balance easily while sitting While standing, lifts one foot to take a step (see Fig. 35-6, D)	Crude release of an object beginning Grasps bell by handle		Says "dada," "mama" with meaning* Comprehends "bye-bye" May say one word (e.g., "hi," "bye," "no")	Inhibits behaviour to verbal command of "no-no" or own name Imitates facial expressions; waves bye-bye Extends toy to another person but will not release it Develops object permanence* Repeats actions that attract attention and cause laughter Pulls clothes of another to attract attention Plays interactive game such as pat-a-cake Reacts to adult anger; cries when scolded Demonstrates independence in dressing, feeding, locomotive skills, and testing of parents Looks at and follows pictures in a book
11	Eruption of lower lateral incisor may begin	When sitting, pivots to reach toward back to pick up an object Cruises or walks holding onto furniture or with both hands held*	Explores objects more thoroughly (e.g., clapper inside bell) Has neat pincer grasp Drops object deliberately for it to be picked up Puts one object after another into a container (sequential play) Able to manipulate an object to remove it from tight-fitting enclosure		Imitates definite speech sounds	Experiences joy and satisfaction when a task is mastered Reacts to restrictions with frustration Rolls ball to another on request Anticipates body gestures when a familiar nursery rhyme or story is being told (e.g., holds toes and feet in response to "This little piggy went to market") Plays game up-down, "so big," or peek-a-boo Shakes head for "no"

TABLE 35-1 GROWTH AND DEVELOPMENT DURING INFANCY—cont'd

AGE (mo)	PHYSICAL	GROSS MOTOR	FINE MOTOR	SENSORY	VOCALIZATION	SOCIALIZATION/ COGNITION
12	Birth weight tripled* Birth length increased by 50%* Head and chest circumference equal (head circumference 46 cm) Has total of six to eight deciduous teeth Anterior fontanel almost closed Landau reflex fading Babinski reflex disappears Lumbar curve develops; lordosis evident during walking	Walks with one hand held* Cruises well May attempt to stand alone momentarily; may attempt first step alone* Can sit down from standing position without help	Releases cube in cup Attempts to build two-block tower but fails Tries to insert a pellet into a narrow-necked bottle but fails Can turn pages in a book, many at a time	Discriminates simple geometric forms (e.g., circle) Amblyopia may develop with lack of binocularity Can follow rapidly moving object Controls and adjusts response to sound; listens for sound to recur	Says three to five words besides "dada," "mama"* Comprehends meaning of several words (comprehension always precedes verbalization) Recognizes objects by name Imitates animal sounds Understands simple verbal commands (e.g., "Give it to me," "Show me your eyes")	Shows emotions such as jealousy, affection (may give hug or kiss on request), anger, fear Enjoys familiar surroundings and explores away from parent Is fearful in strange situation; clings to parent May develop habit of "security blanket" or favourite toy Has increasing determination to practise locomotor skills Searches for an object even if it has not been hidden, but searches only where object was last seen*

*Milestones that represent essential integrative aspects of development that lay the foundation for the achievement of more advanced skills.
†Degree of visual acuity varies according to vision measurement procedure used.

primarily of the action of hydrochloric acid and rennin, an enzyme that acts specifically on the casein in milk to cause the formation of curds (i.e., coagulated semisolid particles of milk). The curds cause the milk to be retained in the stomach long enough for digestion to occur.

Digestion also takes place in the duodenum, where pancreatic enzymes and bile begin to break down protein and fat. Secretion of the amylase, which is needed for digestion of complex carbohydrates, is deficient until about the fourth to sixth month of life. Lipase is also limited, and infants do not achieve adult levels of fat absorption until 4 to 5 months of age. Trypsin is secreted in sufficient quantities to catabolize protein into polypeptides and some amino acids.

The immaturity of the digestive processes is evident in the appearance of stools. During infancy, solid foods (e.g., peas, carrots, corn, and raisins) are passed incompletely broken down in the feces. An excess quantity of fibre easily disposes the child to loose, bulky stools. During infancy, the stomach enlarges to accommodate a greater volume of food. By the end of the first year, the infant is able to tolerate three meals a day and an evening feeding by breast or bottle and may have one or two bowel movements daily. With any type of gastric irritation, however, the infant is vulnerable to diarrhea, vomiting, and dehydration (see Chapter 46).

The liver is the most immature of all the gastrointestinal organs throughout infancy. The ability to conjugate bilirubin and secrete bile is achieved after the first couple of weeks of life. However, the capacities for gluconeogenesis, formation of plasma protein and ketones, storage of vitamins, and deamination of amino acids remain relatively immature for the first year of life.

Maturation of the suckling, sucking, and swallowing reflexes and the eruption of teeth (see Teething, p. 1005) parallel the changes in the gastrointestinal tract and prepare the infant for the introduction of solid foods.

The immunological system undergoes numerous changes during the first year. The full-term newborn receives significant amounts of maternal immunoglobulin G (IgG), which for approximately 3 months confers immunity against **antigens** to which the mother was exposed. During this time, the infant begins to synthesize IgG; approximately 40% of adult levels are reached by 1 year of age. Significant amounts of IgM are produced at birth, and adult levels are reached by 9 months of age. Secretory IgA is not present at birth but is found in saliva and tears by 2 to 5 weeks.

Prebiotic oligosaccharides found in breast milk produce probiotic bacteria such as bifidobacteria and lactobacilli, which in turn stimulate synthesis and secretion of secretory IgA (sIgA). Secretory IgA is present in large amounts in colostrum; IgA confers protection to the mucous membranes of the gastrointestinal tract (Blackburn, 2013; Lawrence & Lawrence, 2015) against many bacteria, such as *Escherichia coli,* and viruses, such as rubella, poliovirus, and the enteroviruses. The development of the mucosa-associated lymphoid tissue occurs during infancy; in part, this system is believed to prevent colonization and passage of bacteria across the infant's mucosal barrier (Lawrence & Lawrence, 2015). The function and quantity of T-lymphocytes, lymphokines, interferon-γ, interleukins, tumour necrosis factor-α, and complement are reduced in early infancy, thus preventing optimal response to certain bacteria and viruses. The production of IgA and immunoglobulins D and E (IgD and IgE) is much more gradual, and maximum levels are not attained until early childhood. Probiotics may have a significant role in helping the gastrointestinal tract establish a "good" bacterial colonization in the gut to prevent many illnesses, including antibiotic-induced diarrhea and possibly *Helicobacter pylori* gastritis (Thomas, Greer, & American Academy of Pediatrics, Committee on Nutrition and Section on Gastroenterology, Hepatology, and Nutrition, 2010).

There is evidence that vernix caseosa, a white oily substance that coats the term infant's body and is often found in abundance in the creases of the axilla and groin, has innate immunological properties that serve to protect the newborn from infection (Hoath & Narendran, 2011). Vernix also appears to have a role in maintaining the integrity of the stratum corneum and facilitating acid mantle development. The epidermis of the full-term infant undergoes maturation during the first month of life; the newborn's skin acts as a barrier to infection, assists in thermal regulation, and prevents transepidermal water loss in term infants.

During infancy, *thermoregulation* becomes more efficient; the ability of the skin to contract and of muscles to shiver in response to cold increases. The peripheral capillaries respond to changes in ambient temperature to regulate heat loss. The capillaries constrict in response to cold, conserving core body temperature and decreasing potential evaporative heat loss from the skin surface. The capillaries dilate in response to heat, decreasing internal body temperature through evaporation, conduction, and convection. Shivering (**thermogenesis**) causes the muscles and muscle fibres to contract, generating metabolic heat that is distributed throughout the body. Increased adipose tissue during the first 6 months insulates the body against heat loss.

A shift in the total body fluid also occurs. At birth, 75% of the term infant's body weight is water, and there is an excess of **extracellular fluid (ECF)**. As the percentage of body water decreases, so does the amount of ECF—from 40% at term to 20% in adulthood. The high proportion of ECF, which is composed of blood plasma, **interstitial fluid**, and lymph, predisposes the infant to a more rapid loss of total body fluid and, consequently, dehydration. The loss of 5 to 10% of the term newborn's initial birth weight in the first 5 days of life is attributed to ECF compartment contraction, enhanced renal tubular function, and rapidly increasing glomerular filtration rate.

The immaturity of the renal structures also predisposes the infant to dehydration. Complete maturity of the kidney occurs during the latter half of the second year, when the cuboidal epithelium of the glomeruli becomes flattened. Before this time the glomeruli's filtration capacity is reduced. Urine is voided frequently and has a low specific gravity (i.e., 1.000 to 1.010). At term, most infants produce and excrete approximately 15 to 60 mL/kg/24 hr; an output of less than 0.5 mL/kg/hr after 48 hours of age is considered to be oliguria (Blackburn, 2013).

Auditory acuity is at adult levels during infancy. Visual acuity begins to improve, and binocular fixation is established. Binocularity, or the fixation of two ocular images into one cerebral picture (fusion), begins to develop by 6 weeks of age and should be well established by age 4 months. Depth perception (**stereopsis**) begins to develop by age 7 to 9 months but may exist earlier as an innate safety mechanism against accidental falling (see Table 35-1).

Fine Motor Development

Fine motor behaviour includes the use of the hands and fingers in the prehension (grasp) of an object, as discussed in Table 35-1. Grasping occurs during the first 2 to 3 months as a reflex and gradually becomes voluntary. At 1 month of age the hands are predominantly closed, and by 3 months they are mostly open. If a rattle is placed in the hand, the infant will actively hold onto it. By 5 months the infant is able to voluntarily grasp an object.

Gradually the palmar grasp (using the whole hand) is replaced with a **pincer grasp** (using the thumb and index finger). The infant uses a crude pincer grasp by 8 to 9 months of age and has progressed to a neat pincer grasp by 11 months (Fig. 35-1).

By 6 months of age, infants have increased manipulative skill: they can hold a bottle, grasp their feet and pull them to their mouth, and feed themselves a cracker. By 7 months they transfer objects from one hand to the other, enjoy banging objects, and will explore the movable parts of a toy.

By 10 months of age, the pincer grasp is sufficiently established to enable infants to pick up a raisin and other finger foods. By 11 months they can put objects into a container and

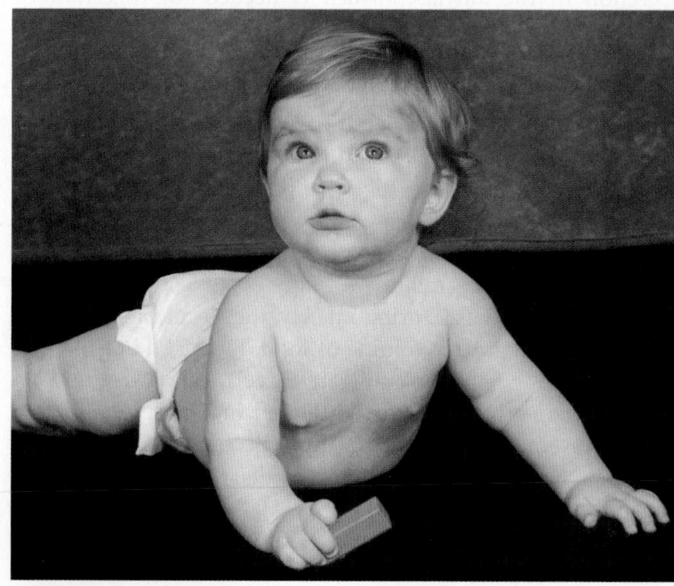

FIGURE 35-1 Crude pincer grasp at 8 to 10 months. (Photo by Paul Vincent Kuntz.)

like to remove them. By age 1 year, infants try, but may fail, to build a tower of two blocks.

Gross Motor Development

Head control. The full-term newborn can momentarily hold the head in midline and parallel when the body is suspended ventrally and can lift and turn the head from side to side when prone. This is not the case when the infant is lying prone on a pillow or soft surface; infants do not have the head control to lift their head out of the depression of the object and thus risk possible suffocation in the prone position early in infancy (see Sudden Infant Death Syndrome, p. 1032, and Chapter 26, p. 711). Marked head lag is evident when the infant is pulled from a lying to a sitting position. By 3 months of age, infants can hold their head well beyond the plane of the body. By 4 months infants can lift the head and front portion of the chest approximately 90 degrees above the table, bearing their weight on the forearms. Only slight head lag is evident when the infant is pulled from a lying to a sitting position, and by 4 to 6 months head control is well established (Figs. 35-2 and 35-3).

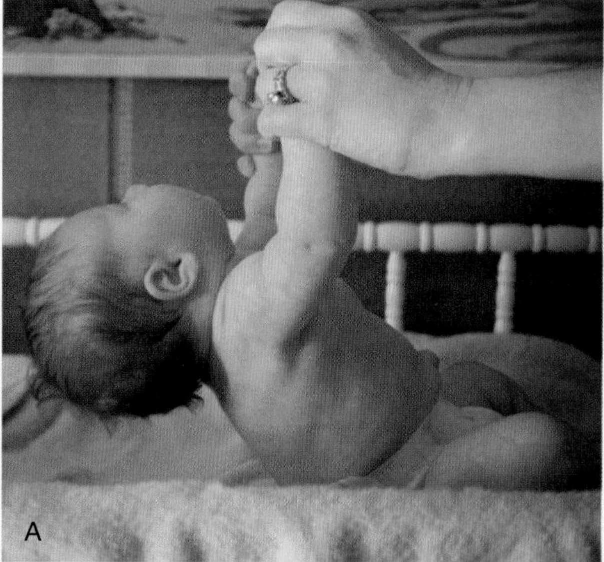

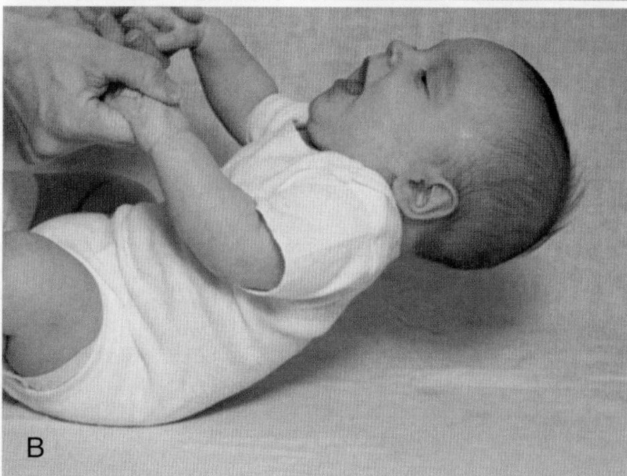

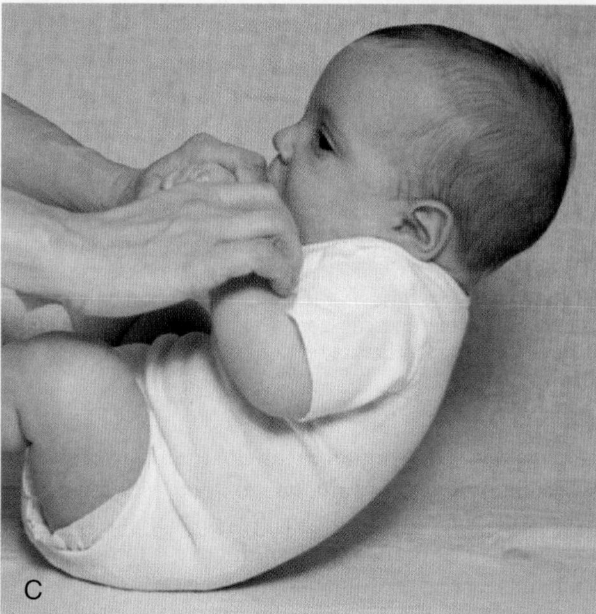

FIGURE 35-2 Head control while pulled to sitting position. **A:** Complete head lag at 1 month. **B:** Partial head lag at 2 months. **C:** Almost no head lag at 4 months.

! NURSING ALERT

An infant who displays head lag at 6 months of age should have a developmental and neurological evaluation.

Rolling over. Newborns may roll over accidentally because of their rounded back. The ability to willfully turn from the abdomen to the back generally occurs at 5 months, and the ability to turn from the back to the abdomen occurs at 6 months. Infants put to sleep on their sides may easily roll over to a prone (face-down) position, thus placing them at higher risk for sudden infant death syndrome (SIDS). It is therefore important to place infants in a supine position for sleep. While the infant is awake and being observed, a prone position is acceptable to enhance achievement of milestones such as head control, crawling, creeping, and turning over. The parachute reflex (Fig. 35-4), a protective response to falling, appears at 7 months.

 **NURSING ALERT**

In the first several months, before the infant can roll over, the head should be positioned on alternating sides to prevent positional plagiocephaly (when asleep or awake in the supine position).

Sitting. The ability to sit follows progressive head control and straightening of the back (Fig. 35-5). For the first 2 to 3 months the back is uniformly rounded. The convex cervical curve forms at approximately 3 to 4 months of age, when head control is established. The convex lumbar curve appears when the child begins to sit, at about age 4 months. As the spinal column straightens, the infant can be propped in a sitting position. By age 7 months infants can sit alone, leaning forward on their hands for support. By age 8 months they can sit well while unsupported and begin to explore their surroundings in this position rather than in a lying position. By 10 months they can manoeuvre from a prone to a sitting position.

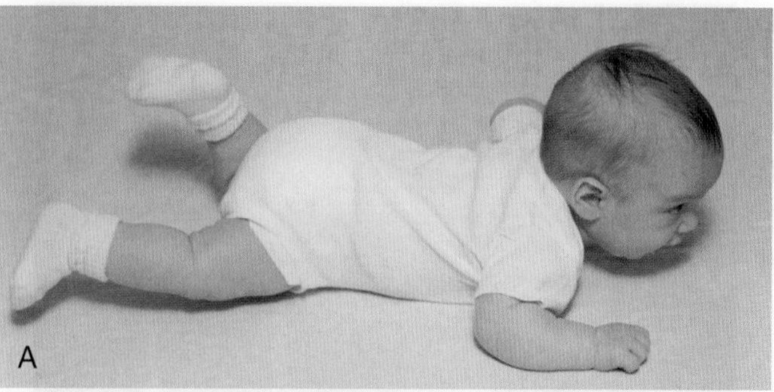

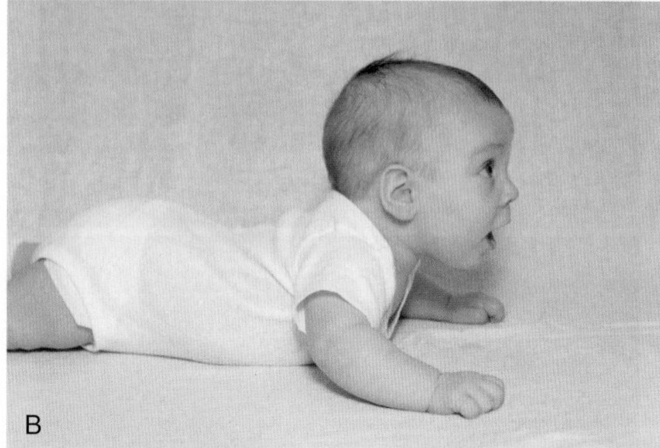

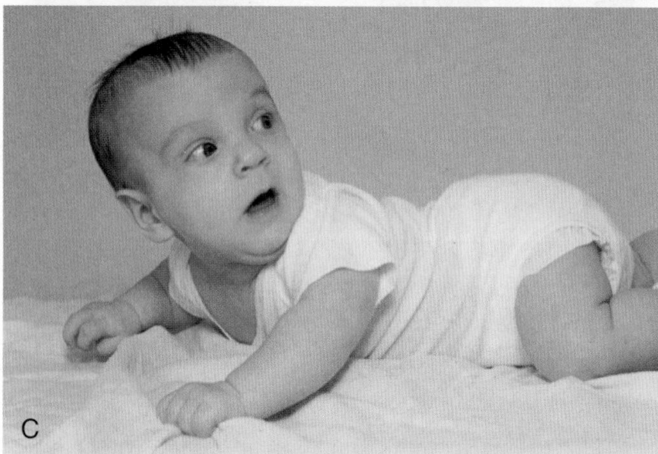

FIGURE 35-3 Head control while prone. **A:** Infant momentarily lifts head at 1 month. **B:** Infant lifts head and chest 90 degrees and bears weight on forearms at 4 months. **C:** Infant lifts head, chest, and upper abdomen and can bear weight on hands at 6 months. Note how this position facilitates turning from abdomen to back.

Locomotion. Locomotion involves acquiring the ability to bear weight, propel forward on all four extremities, stand upright with support, and, finally, walk alone (Fig. 35-6). Following a cephalocaudal pattern, infants 4 to 6 months old develop increasing coordination in their arms. Initial locomotion results in infants propelling themselves backward by pushing with the arms. By 6 to 7 months of age, they are able to bear all their weight on their legs with assistance. Crawling (propelling forward with belly on floor) progresses to creeping (on hands and knees with belly off floor) by 9 months. At this time, they stand while holding onto furniture and can pull themselves to the standing position, but they are unable to manoeuvre back down except by falling. By 11 months they can usually walk while holding onto furniture or with both hands held, and by age 1 year they may be able to walk with one hand held. A number of infants attempt their first independent steps by their first birthday. Although there is considerable variation among infants for the achievement of these milestones, they provide guidelines for early intervention.

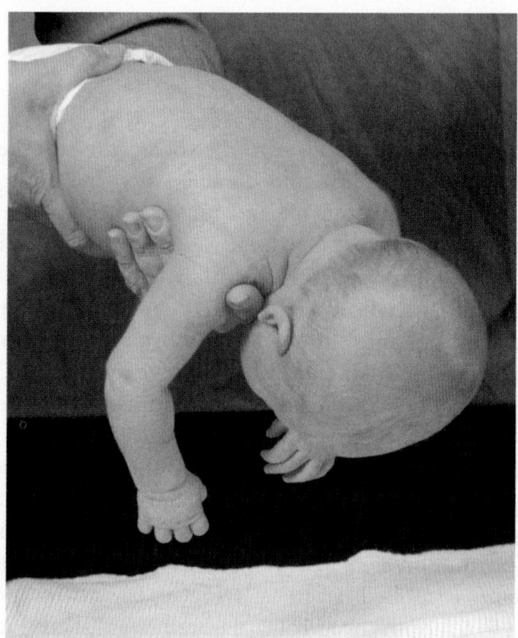

FIGURE 35-4 Parachute reflex. (Photo by Paul Vincent Kuntz.)

> **! NURSING ALERT**
>
> An infant who does not pull to a standing position by 11 to 12 months of age should be further evaluated for possible developmental **dysplasia** of the hip (see Fig. 53-10. Although there is considerable variation among infants for the achievement of these milestones, they provide guidelines for early intervention.

Psychosocial Development

Developing a Sense of Trust (Erikson)

Erikson's (1963) phase I (birth to 1 year) is concerned with *acquiring a sense of* **trust** while *overcoming a sense of* **mistrust** (termed "trust versus mistrust") (see Chapter 32). The trust that develops is a trust of self, of others, and of the world. Infants "trust" that their feeding, comfort, stimulation, and caring needs will be met. The crucial element for the achievement of this task is the quality of both the parent–child (or caregiver–child) relationship and the care that the infant receives. The provision of food, warmth, and shelter alone is inadequate for the development of a strong sense of self. The infant and parent must jointly learn to satisfactorily meet their needs in order for mutual regulation of frustration to occur. When this synchrony fails to develop, mistrust is the eventual outcome.

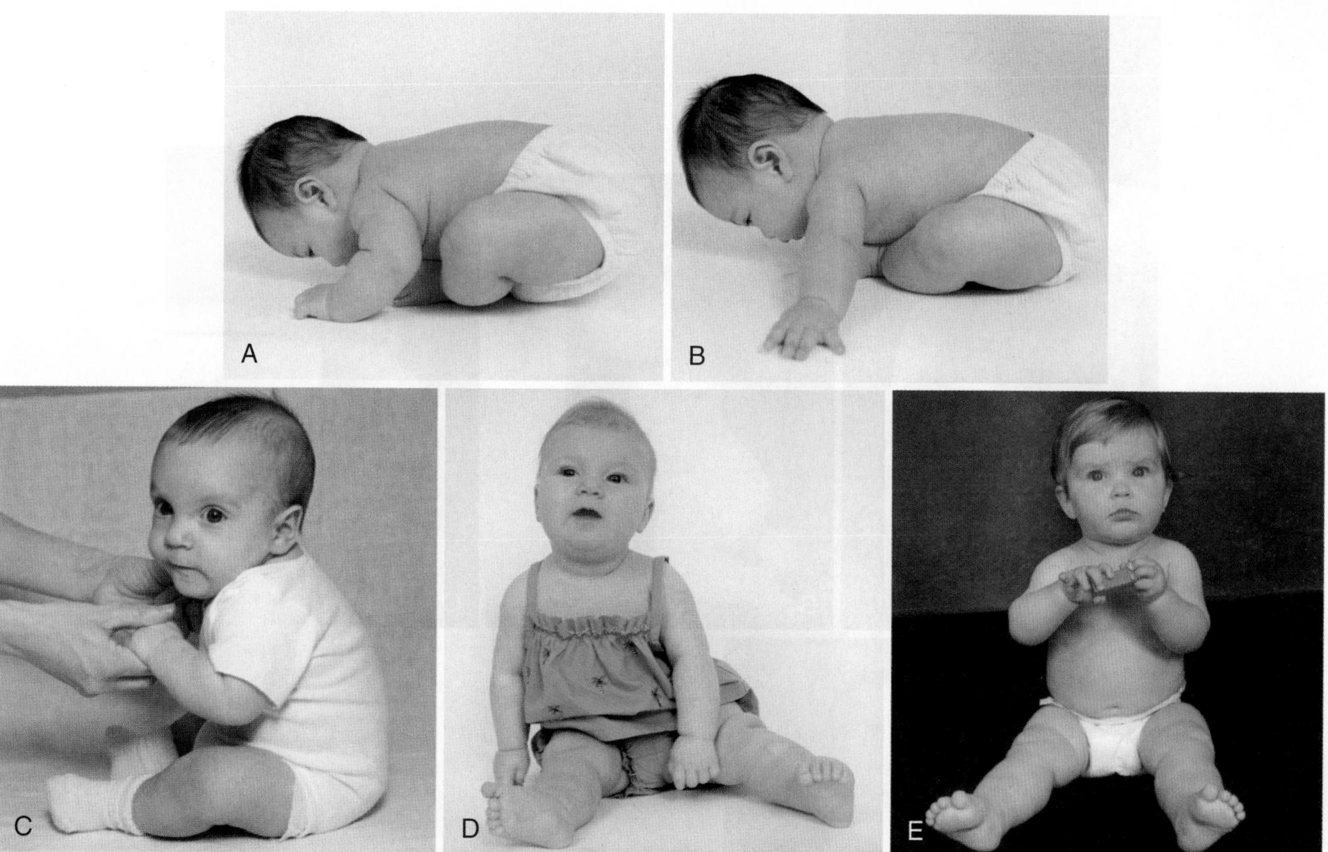

FIGURE 35-5 Development of sitting. **A:** Back is completely rounded, and infant has no ability to sit upright at 1 month. **B:** At 2 months, infant exhibits more control; back is still rounded, but infant can sit up momentarily with some head control. **C:** Back is rounded only in lumbar area, and infant is able to sit erect with good head control at 4 months. **D:** Infant can sit alone, leaning on hands for support, at 7 months. **E:** Infant sits without support at 8 months. Note the transferring of objects that occurs, beginning at 7 months. (Photos by Paul Vincent Kuntz.)

Mistrust can result either from too much or too little frustration. If parents always meet their children's needs before the children signal their readiness, infants will never learn to test their ability to control the environment. If the delay is prolonged, infants experience constant frustration and eventually mistrust others in their efforts to satisfy them. Therefore, consistency of care is essential.

The trust acquired in infancy provides the foundation for all succeeding phases. Trust gives infants a feeling of physical comfort and security, which assists them in experiencing unfamiliar situations with a minimum of fear. Erikson divided the first year of life into two oral/social stages. During the first 3 to 4 months, food intake is the most important social activity in which the infant engages. The newborn can tolerate little frustration or delay of gratification. Primary **narcissism** (total concern for oneself) is at its height. However, as bodily processes such as vision, motor movements, and vocalization become better controlled, infants use more advanced behaviours to interact with others. For example, rather than cry, infants may put their arms up to signify a desire to be held.

The next social modality involves a mode of reaching out to others through grasping. *Grasping* is initially reflexive, but even as a reflex it has a powerful social meaning for the parents. The reciprocal response to the infant's grasping is the parents' holding on and touching. Both the child and parents experience pleasurable tactile stimulation.

Tactile stimulation is extremely important in the total process of acquiring trust. The degree of mothering skill, the quantity of food, or the length of sucking does not determine the quality of the experience. Rather, it is the overall quality of the interpersonal relationship that influences the infant's formulation of trust.

During the second stage, the more active and aggressive modality of biting occurs. Infants learn that they can hold onto what is their own and can more fully control their environment. During this stage, infants may be confronted with one of their first conflicts. If they are breastfeeding, they quickly learn that biting causes the mother to become upset and withdraw the breast. Yet biting also brings internal relief from teething discomfort and a sense of power or control.

This conflict may be solved by teaching the infant not to bite and by the mother saying "no" and withdrawing the nipple from the baby's mouth. The successful resolution of this conflict strengthens the mother–child relationship because it occurs at a time when infants are recognizing the mother as the most significant person in their life.

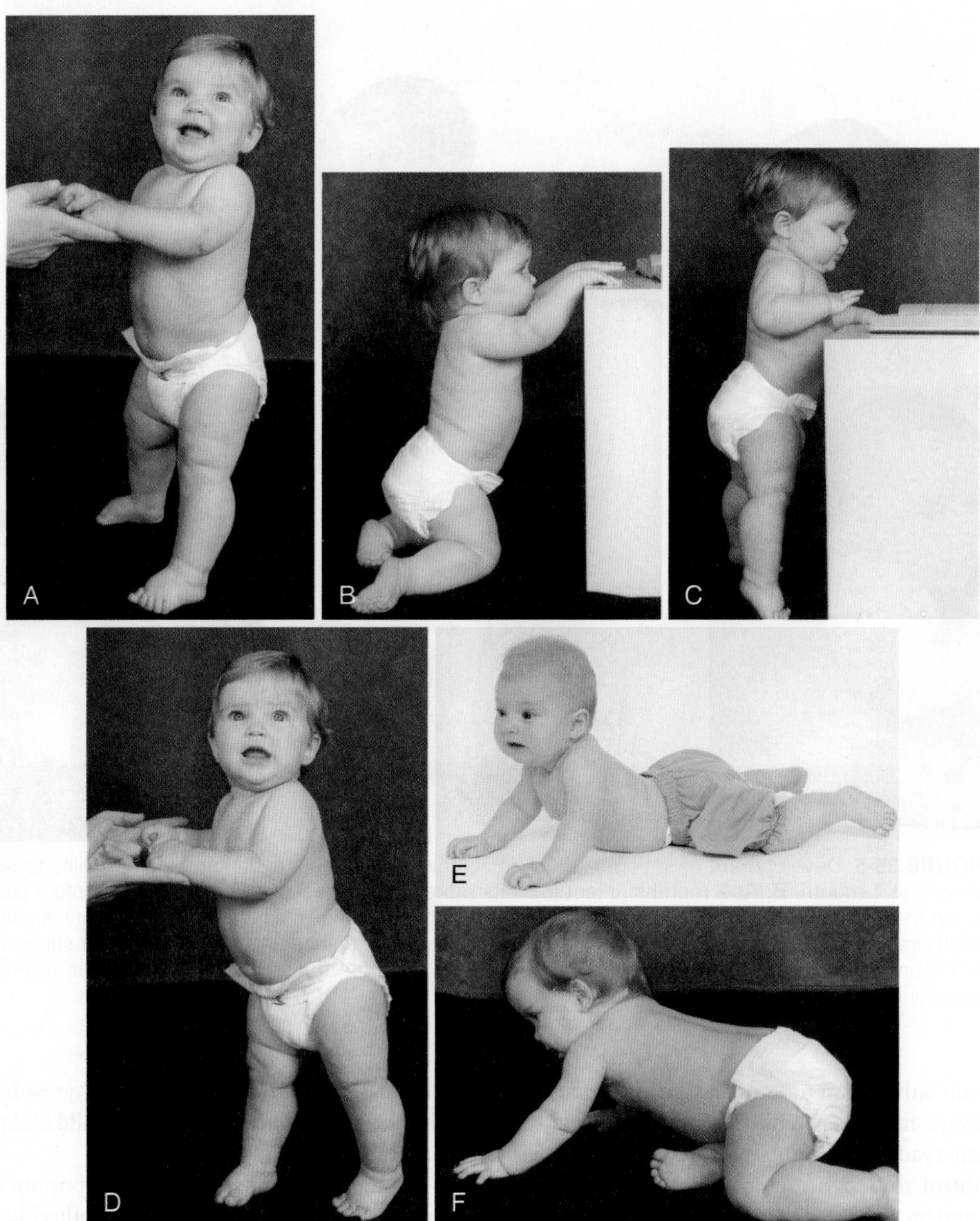

FIGURE 35-6 Development of locomotion. **A:** Infant bears full weight on feet by 7 months. **B:** Infant can manoeuvre from sitting to kneeling position. **C:** Infant can stand holding onto furniture at 9 months. **D:** While standing, infant takes deliberate step at 10 months. **E:** Infant crawls with abdomen on floor and pulls self forward, and then **(F)** creeps on hands and knees at 9 months. (Photos by Paul Vincent Kuntz.)

Cognitive Development

The theory most commonly used to explain *cognition*, or the ability to know, is that of Piaget (1952) (see Chapter 32). The period from birth to 24 months is termed the sensorimotor phase and is composed of six stages; however, because this discussion is concerned with ages birth to 12 months, only the first four stages are discussed here. The last two stages (tertiary circular reactions and invention of new means) occur during the toddler period of 12 to 24 months and are discussed in Chapter 36.

During the sensorimotor phase, infants progress from reflex behaviours to simple repetitive acts to imitative activity. Three crucial events take place during this phase. The first event involves *separation*, in which infants learn to separate themselves from other objects in the environment. They realize that others besides themselves control the environment and that certain readjustments must take place for mutual satisfaction to occur. This coincides with Erikson's concept of the formation of trust.

The second major accomplishment is achieving the concept of object permanence, or the realization that objects that leave the visual field still exist. A typical example of the development of object permanence is when infants are able to pursue objects they observe being hidden under a pillow or behind a chair

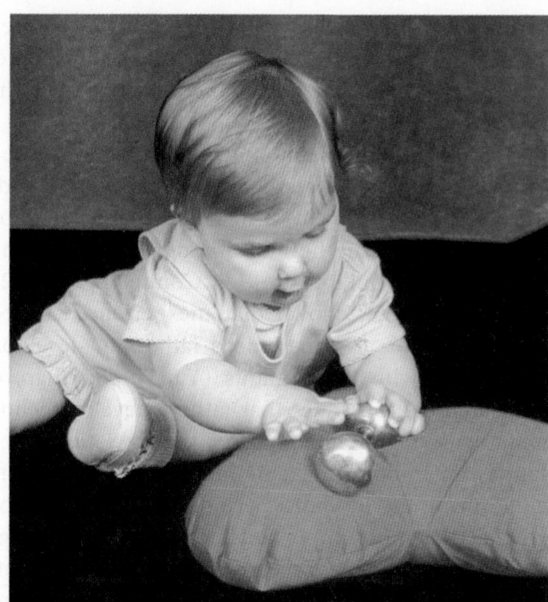

FIGURE 35-7 Nine-month-old infant actively searches for object hidden behind pillow. (Photo by Paul Vincent Kuntz.)

(Fig. 35-7). This skill develops at approximately 9 to 10 months of age, which corresponds to the time of increased locomotion skills.

The last major intellectual achievement of this period is the ability to use *symbols*, or *mental representation*. The use of symbols allows the infant to think of an object or situation without actually experiencing it. The recognition of symbols is the beginning of the understanding of time and space.

Piaget's first stage, from birth to 1 month, is identified by the infant's *use of reflexes*. At birth, the infant's individuality and temperament are expressed through the physiological reflexes of sucking, rooting, grasping, and crying. The repetitious nature of the reflexes is the beginning of associations between an act and a sequential response. When infants cry because they are hungry, a nipple is put in the mouth, and they suck, feel satisfaction, and sleep. They are assimilating this experience while perceiving auditory, tactile, and visual cues. This experience of perceiving certain patterns, or "ordering," provides a foundation for the subsequent stages.

The second stage, *primary circular reactions*, marks the beginning of the replacement of reflexive behaviour with voluntary acts. During the period from 1 to 4 months, activities such as sucking or grasping become deliberate acts that elicit certain responses. The beginning of accommodation is evident. Infants incorporate and adapt their reactions to the environment and recognize the stimulus that produced a response. Previously they would cry until the nipple was brought to the mouth. Now they associate the nipple with the sound of the parent's voice. They accommodate this new piece of information and adapt by ceasing to cry when they hear the voice—before receiving the nipple. What is taking place is a realization of causality and a recognition of an orderly sequence of events. The environment is taken in with all of the senses and with whatever motor ability is present.

The *secondary circular reactions* stage is a continuation of primary circular reactions and lasts until 8 months of age. In this stage, the primary circular reactions are repeated and prolonged for the resulting response. Grasping and holding now become shaking, banging, and pulling. Shaking is performed to hear a noise, not solely for the pleasure of shaking. The quality and quantity of an act become evident. More or less shaking produces different responses. Understanding of causality, time, deliberate intention, and separateness from the environment begins to develop.

Three new processes of human behaviour occur. *Imitation* requires the differentiation of selected acts from several events. By the second half of the first year, infants can imitate sounds and simple gestures. *Play* becomes evident as they take pleasure in performing an act after they have mastered it. Many of the infant's waking hours are absorbed in sensorimotor play. *Affect* (the outward manifestation of emotion and feeling) is seen as infants begin to develop a sense of permanency. During the first 6 months, infants believe that an object exists only for as long as they can visually perceive it—in other words, out of sight, out of mind. Affect in relation to external objects is evident when the object continues to be present or remembered even though it is beyond the range of perception. Object permanence is a critical component of parent–child attachment and is seen in the development of **separation anxiety** at 6 to 8 months of age.

During the fourth sensorimotor stage, *coordination of secondary schematas and their application to new situations*, infants use previous behavioural achievements primarily as the foundation for adding new intellectual skills to their expanding repertoire. This stage is largely transitional. Increasing motor skills allow for greater exploration of the environment. They begin to discover that hiding an object does not mean that it is gone but that removing an obstacle will reveal the object. This marks the beginning of intellectual reasoning. Furthermore, they can experience an event by observing it, and they begin to associate symbols with events (e.g., "bye-bye" with "Daddy or Mommy goes to work"), but the classification is purely their own. In this stage, they learn from the object itself; this is in contrast to the second stage, in which infants learn from the type of interaction between objects or individuals. Intentionality is further developed, in that infants now actively attempt to remove a barrier to the desired (or undesired) action (see Fig. 35-7). If something is in their way, they attempt to climb over it or push it away. Previously, an obstacle would have caused them to give up any further attempt to achieve the desired goal.

Development of Body Image

The development of body image parallels sensorimotor development. Infants' kinesthetic and tactile experiences are the first perceptions of their body, and the mouth is the principal area of pleasurable sensations. Other parts of the body are primarily objects of pleasure—the hands and fingers to suck and the feet to play with. As physical needs are met, they feel comfort and satisfaction with their body. Messages conveyed by the caregivers reinforce these feelings. For example, when infants smile, they receive emotional satisfaction from others who smile back.

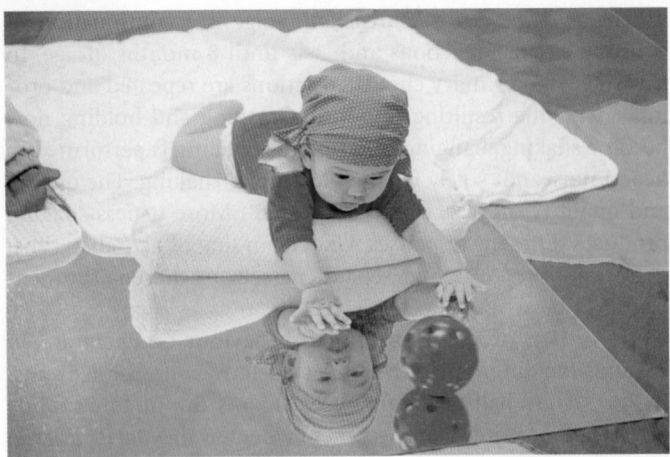

FIGURE 35-8 Nine-month-old infant enjoying own image in mirror.

Achieving the concept of object permanence is basic to the development of self-image. By the end of the first year, infants recognize that they are distinct from their parents. At the same time, they have increasing interest in their own image, especially in the mirror (Fig. 35-8). As motor skills develop, they learn that parts of the body are useful; for example, the hands bring objects to the mouth, and the legs help them move to different locations. All of these achievements transmit messages to them about themselves. Therefore, it is important to transmit positive messages to infants about their bodies.

Social Development

Infants' social development is initially influenced by their reflexive behaviour, such as the grasp, and eventually depends primarily on the interaction between them and the principal caregivers. **Attachment** to the parent is increasingly evident during the second half of the first year, and tremendous strides are made in communication and personal–social behaviour. Whereas crying and reflexive behaviour are initial ways in which newborns meet their needs, the social smile is an early step in social communication. This has a profound effect on family members and is stimulus for evoking continued responses from others. By 4 months of age, infants can laugh out loud.

Play is a major socializing agent and provides stimulation needed to learn from and interact with the environment. By age 6 months infants are personable. They can play games such as peek-a-boo when their head is hidden behind a towel, signal their desire to be picked up by extending their arms, and show displeasure when a toy is removed or their face is being washed.

Attachment

The importance to infants of human physical contact cannot be overemphasized. Parenting is not an instinctual ability but a learned, acquired process. The attachment of parent and child, which begins before birth, assumes even greater importance at birth and during the first year (see Chapter 23, Parental Attachment, Bonding, and Acquaintance). In the following discussion of attachment, the term *mother* is used in the broad context of the consistent caregiver with whom the child relates more than anyone else. However, in society's changing social climate and sex-role stereotypes, this person may very well be the father or a grandparent.

Studies on paternal–infant attachment demonstrate that stages similar to those in maternal attachment occur and that fathers are often more involved in child care when mothers are employed outside the home (although mothers continue to do the majority of infant care) (McConnell & Moss, 2011). Additional research has shown that inexperienced, first-time fathers are as capable as experienced fathers of developing a close attachment with their infants (Yu, Hung, Chan, et al., 2012). Research demonstrates that fathers develop feelings of attachment with their children, and their relationship with the infant is an important factor in the mother's emotional well-being during the newborn period. Breastfeeding mothers reported that the most important factor in establishing and maintaining breastfeeding in early infancy was the father's acceptance of breastfeeding and support for the mother (Feldman-Winter, 2013). In single-parent families, a grandmother (or other significant caregiver) may become the primary caregiver. It is important for nurses to recognize that infant–parent attachments may be present or absent in situations in which caregiver roles are less well defined by those involved.

When the infant is not provided a safe haven and consistent and loving care, an *insecure attachment* develops; such infants do not feel they can trust the world in which they live. This insecure attachment may result in psychosocial difficulties as the child grows and may persist even into adulthood. Insecure attachment may also exist in homes where there is domestic violence and maternal perinatal mood disorder.

Attachment progresses during infancy, with the child assuming an increasingly significant role. Two components of cognitive development are required for attachment: (1) the ability to discriminate the mother from other individuals, and (2) the achievement of object permanence. Both of these processes prepare the infant for an equally important aspect of attachment: separation from the parent. Separation–individuation should occur as a harmonious, parallel process with emotional attachment.

During the formation of attachment to the parent, the infant progresses through four distinct but overlapping stages. For the first few weeks, infants respond indiscriminately to anyone. Beginning at approximately 8 to 12 weeks of age, they cry, smile, and vocalize more to the mother than to anyone else but continue to respond to others, whether familiar or not. At approximately 6 months of age, infants show a distinct preference for the mother. They follow her more, cry when she leaves, enjoy playing with her more, and feel most secure in her arms. About 1 month after showing attachment to the mother, many infants begin attaching to other members of the family, most often the other parent.

Infants acquire other developmental behaviours that influence the attachment process. These include the following:

- Differential crying, smiling, and vocalization (more to the mother than to anyone else);

- Visual-motor orientation (looking more at the mother, even if she is not close);
- Crying when the mother leaves the room;
- Approaching through locomotion (crawling, creeping, or walking);
- Clinging (especially in the presence of a stranger); and
- Exploring away from the mother while using her as a secure base.

Reactive attachment disorder (RAD) is a psychological and developmental problem that stems from maladaptive or absent attachment between the infant and parent (or primary caregiver) and may persist into childhood and even adulthood (Smyke, Zeanah, Fox, et al., 2010). Infants at risk for RAD include those who have been victims of physical abuse, sexual abuse, or neglect; infants exposed to parental alcoholism, mental illness, or substance use; and infants who have experienced the absence of a consistent primary caregiver as a result of foster care, institutionalization, parental abandonment, or parental incarceration. RAD is a form of extreme insecure attachment with two separate disorders identified: disinhibited social engagement disorder of childhood and reactive attachment disorder of infancy or early childhood (Gleason, Fox, Drury, et al., 2011). It is postulated that children who experience grossly inadequate child care will develop severe attachment disorder. Signs of RAD are usually seen before the age of 5 years in infants who had insecure attachments to the mother or other primary caregiver. The child may manifest behaviours such as not being cuddly with parents, failing to make eye contact with significant others, having poor impulse control, and being destructive to self and others. Without early intervention, some of these children fail to develop a conscience and suffer from an antisocial personality disorder that may lead to criminal acts.

Separation anxiety. Between ages 4 and 8 months, the infant progresses through the first stage of separation–individuation and begins to have some awareness of self and mother as separate beings. At the same time, the sense of object permanence is developing, and the infant is aware that the parent can be absent. Thus, separation anxiety develops and is manifested through a predictable sequence of behaviours.

During the early second half of the first year, infants usually protest when placed in their crib, and a short time later they will object when the mother leaves the room. Infants may not notice the mother's absence if they are absorbed in an activity. However, when they realize her absence, they may protest. From this point on, they become very alert to her activities and whereabouts. By 11 to 12 months of age, they are able to anticipate her imminent departure by watching her behaviours, and they may begin to protest before she leaves. At this point, many parents learn to postpone alerting the child to their departure until just before leaving.

Fear of strangers. As infants demonstrate attachment to one person, they correspondingly exhibit less friendliness to others. Between 6 and 8 months of age, fear of strangers and **stranger anxiety** become prominent and are related to infants' ability to discriminate between familiar and unfamiliar people. Behaviours such as clinging to the parent, crying, and turning away from the stranger are common (Fig. 35-9).

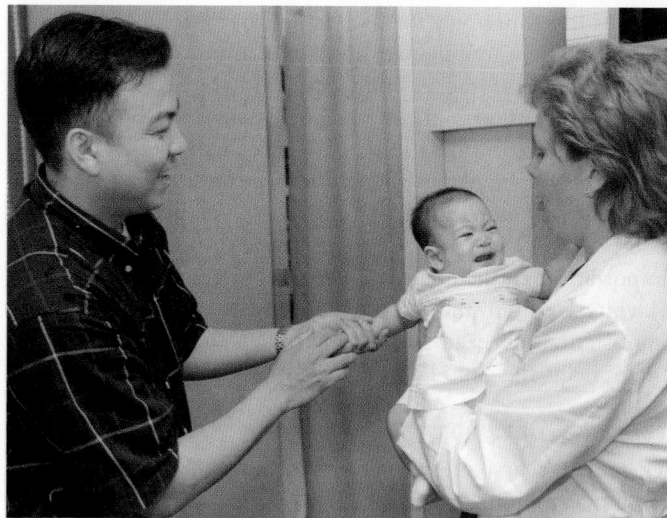

FIGURE 35-9 Behaviours related to fear of strangers include clinging to the parent and turning away from the stranger. (Photo by Paul Vincent Kuntz.)

Play

Play during infancy represents the various social modalities observed during cognitive development (see Chapter 32, Role of Play in Development). Infants' activity is primarily narcissistic and revolves around their own body. As discussed under Development of Body Image (p. 999), body parts are primarily objects of play and pleasure.

During the first year, play becomes more sophisticated and interdependent. From birth to 3 months of age, infants' responses to the environment are global and largely undifferentiated. Play is dependent; pleasure is demonstrated by a quieting attitude (1 month), a smile (2 months), or a squeal (3 months). From 3 to 6 months, infants show more discriminate interest in stimuli and begin to play alone with a rattle or a soft stuffed toy or with someone else. There is much more interaction during play. By 4 months of age, they laugh out loud, show a preference for certain toys, and become excited when food or a favourite object is brought to them. They recognize an image in a mirror, smile at it, and vocalize to it.

By age 6 months to 1 year, play involves sensorimotor skills. Actual games such as peekaboo and pat-a-cake are played. Verbal repetition and imitation of simple gestures occur in response to demonstration. Play is much more selective, not only in terms of specific toys but also in terms of "playmates." Although play is solitary or one-sided, infants choose with whom they will interact. At 6 to 8 months of age they usually refuse to play with strangers. Parents are definite favourites, and infants know how to attract their attention. At 6 months they will extend the arms to be picked up, at 7 months cough or squeal to make their presence known, at 10 months pull the parent's clothing, and at 12 months call them by name. This represents a tremendous advance from the newborn, who signalled biological needs by merely crying to express displeasure.

Stimulation is important for psychosocial growth. Knowledge of **developmental milestones** enables nurses to guide parents in proper play for infants. For instance, it is not sufficient to place a mobile over a crib and toys in a playpen for a child's optimum social, emotional, and intellectual development. Play must provide interpersonal contact and recreational and educational stimulation. Infants need to be *played with*, not merely *allowed to play*. Although the type of play infants engage in is called *solitary*, this is a figurative, not literal, term to denote one-sided play. The type of toys given to the child is much less important than the quality of personal interaction that occurs. Having a parent that is interactive with the infant is very important—for example, smiling often and directly at the infant helps the child learn to be responsive.

Language Development

The infant's first means of verbal communication is crying. Crying as a biological sign conveys a message of urgency and signals displeasure, such as hunger. However, crying is also a social event that affects the development of the parent–infant relationship—either by its absence, which usually has a positive effect on parents, or its presence, which may involve a negative response or persuade parents to minister to the child's physical or emotional needs.

In the first few weeks of life, crying has a reflexive quality and is mostly related to physiological needs. Infants cry for 1 to 1.5 hours a day up to 3 weeks of age, then build up to 2 and even 4 hours a day by 6 weeks. Crying tends to decrease by 12 weeks of age. It is thought that the increase in crying for no apparent reason during the first few months may be related to the discharge of energy and the maturational changes in the central nervous system. During the end of the first year, infants cry for attention; from fear (especially stranger fear); and from frustration, usually in response to their developing but inadequate motor skills.

NURSING ALERT

Be alert to parents' reports about maternal perinatal mood disorder and infant crying, since these concerns may indicate a stressed mother–infant relationship. Depression or anxiety is a serious issue that may have started earlier in the pregnancy. See Chapter 24 (Postpartum Complications) for further information.

Infants vocalize as early as 5 to 6 weeks of age by making small throaty sounds. See Table 35-1 for discussion of language ability. By 8 months they can imitate sounds; add the consonants *t*, *d*, and *w*; and combine syllables (e.g., "dada"), but they do not ascribe meaning to the word until 10 to 11 months of age (see Family-Centred Teaching box).

Temperament

The infant's temperament or behavioural style influences the type of interaction that occurs between the child and parents, especially the mother (see general discussion of temperament in Chapter 32). In assessments of a child's temperament, it is the parents' perception of the child and the degree of fit between their expectations and the child's actual temperament that are important. The more dissonance, or lack of harmony, between the child's temperament and the parent's ability to accept and deal with the behaviour, the more risk there is for subsequent parent–child conflicts.

FAMILY-CENTRED TEACHING

Child's Developing Language Skills

During the acquisition of new language skills the child temporarily may stop using other recently learned sounds or words. This is often distressing for parents, who have waited in anticipation for the words "dada" or "mama," because these sounds are commonly replaced by other vocalizations and may not be repeated for several weeks. Nurses can reassure parents that the child will again say these special words, and with increased meaning.

Although most behavioural researchers agree that there is a strong biological component to temperament, researchers also suggest that temperament may be modified by the environment, particularly the family (Megel, Wilson, Bravo, et al., 2011). Family interaction with the infant is perceived as a circular process in which family members affect each other and the family as a unit. With these concepts in mind, the nurse has an important role in helping the family understand the infant's temperament as it relates to family dynamics and the eventual well-being of the child and family unit (Megel et al., 2011).

Some researchers speculate that infant temperament may contribute to maternal depression. Indeed, when reciprocity is lacking between the infant and the mother or when the infant's behaviour does not meet maternal expectations, there is increased risk for discord. McGrath, Records, and Rice (2008) found that depressed mothers (compared with nondepressed mothers) rated their infant's temperament at 2 and 6 months of age as more difficult. Thus depressed mothers need to be identified and assisted in making the transition to motherhood and in developing synchronicity with their newborn infants. Researchers have also correlated fussy infant temperament with the introduction of early complementary feedings (at 3 months of age) (Wasser, Bentley, Borja, et al., 2011).

The Revised Infant Temperament Questionnaire (RITQ) (Carey & McDevitt, 1978) can be used as a screening tool with parents. The questionnaire focuses on nine temperament variables, and the 95 questions relate specifically to activities such as sleeping, feeding, playing, diapering, and dressing. The scores from the RITQ help identify the child's temperament style. Use of the RITQ is well accepted by parents and should be accompanied by an adequate explanation of the results. In discussing the results, the nurse should avoid descriptors such as *difficult* and instead describe such infants using terms such as *intense* or *less predictable*. The Early Infancy Temperament Questionnaire, a 76-item parent questionnaire, was adapted from the RITQ to specifically evaluate temperament characteristics of infants 1 to 4 months old. The RITQ is best suited for infants aged 4 months and older (Medoff-Cooper, Carey, & McDevitt, 1993).

With knowledge of the infant's temperament, nurses are better able to (1) provide parents with background information that will help them see their child in a better perspective, (2) offer a more organized picture of their child's behaviour and possibly reveal distortions in their perceptions of the behaviour, and (3) guide parents in appropriate child-rearing techniques.

Appropriate counselling based on awareness of the child's temperament can greatly enhance the quality of interactions between parents and infant. Even letting parents know that "difficult" traits are innate can relieve feelings of guilt and incompetence.

Coping With Concerns Related to Normal Growth and Development

Knowledge of the developmental sequence allows the nurse to assess normal growth and minor or abnormal deviations. It also helps parents gain realistic expectations of their child's ability and provides guidelines for suitable play and stimulation. Parents who lack knowledge of child growth and development may set inappropriate behavioural expectations for their child. Emphasizing the child's developmental rather than chronological age strengthens the parent–child relationship by fostering trust and lessening frustration. Therefore, thorough understanding and appreciation of children's growth and development are essential.

Separation and Fear of Strangers

A number of fears can appear during infancy. However, the fear that causes parents the most concern is fear related to strangers and separation. Although erroneously interpreted by some as a sign of undesirable, antisocial behaviour, fear of strangers and separation anxiety are important components of a strong, healthy, parent–child attachment. Nevertheless, this period can present difficulties for the parent and child. Parents may experience guilt at having to leave the infant because he or she violently protests having a babysitter. To accustom the infant to new people, parents can have close friends or relatives visit often. This gives the child the opportunity to become comfortable with other persons and can give parents time for themselves.

Infants also need opportunities to safely experience strangers. Usually toward the end of the first year, infants begin to venture away from the parent and demonstrate curiosity about strangers. If allowed to explore at their own rate, many infants eventually "warm up" to strangers. The best approach for the stranger (who may be the nurse) is to talk softly; meet the child at eye level (to appear smaller); maintain a safe distance from the infant; and avoid sudden, intrusive gestures, such as holding the arms out and smiling broadly.

Parents also may wonder whether they should encourage the child's clinging, dependent behaviour, especially if there is pressure from others who view this as "spoiling the baby." Parents need to be reassured that such behaviour is healthy, desirable, and necessary for the child's optimum emotional development. If parents can reassure the infant of their presence, the infant will learn to realize that they are still there even if not physically present. Talking to infants when leaving the room, allowing them to hear one's voice on the telephone, and using transitional objects (e.g., a favourite blanket or toy) reassures them of the parent's continued presence.

Alternative Child Care Arrangements

For many parents, especially working parents, locating safe and competent child care facilities for the infant is an increasingly difficult problem—one that is compounded by the number of families with both parents working outside the home.

The basic types of care are in-home care, either in the parents' or caregivers' home, and centre-based care, usually in a day care centre. *In-home care* may consist of a full-time babysitter who lives in the home, a full-time babysitter who comes to the home, cooperative arrangements such as exchange babysitting, and family day care. A licensed in-home day care typically provides care and protection for up to six children for part of a day and does not include informal arrangements such as exchange babysitting or caregivers in the child's own home. The six children rule is expected to include the day care provider's own children younger than 6 years of age living in the home. If the children are less than 1 year of age, the ratio may be smaller (i.e., 3 : 1). Unfortunately, many day care homes operate without a licence and may care for large numbers of infants without adequate staff and facilities.

Child centre–based care usually refers to a licensed day care facility that provides care for six or more children, for 6 or more hours a day. *Work-based group care* is another option that is becoming increasingly popular as employers recognize the benefit of providing high-quality and convenient child care to their employees. *Sick-child care* may also be available for times when the youngster is ill.

Nurses may fulfill a unique role in guiding parents in locating suitable facilities that have a well-qualified staff. Provincial licensing regulations exist in most provinces and territories to ensure that facilities meet minimum standards for such things as staff qualifications, the ratio of staff to children, the safety and cleanliness of the care environment, and behaviour management. These regulations help ensure that any potential risks to the child's well-being are kept to a minimum. Community agencies can assist parents in identifying day care centres that accept children of specific age groups and that are convenient to home and work. Their records should be available to the public and provide reports from the health, safety, and fire departments; periodic evaluations from the licensing agency; complaints filed against the centre; and qualifications of the centre's employees. Early-childhood programs may also belong to a voluntary accreditation system, for example, the Association of Day Care Operators of Ontario, which serves as a model for optimum care. References from other parents are helpful, provided that they have investigated the centre carefully and have remained involved with the centre's activities. Information for parents on what to consider when selecting a child care facility can be found in the Additional Resources section at the end of the chapter.

The same attention should be applied to locating competent babysitters. References from other parents are essential, and there is no substitute for observing the interaction between the individual and the child. Although very young infants need little if any preparation for the introduction of a new caregiver, older infants may benefit from a gradual placement to reduce stranger anxiety.

Some child care centres provide a service whereby the parent may log on to the Internet and view the child's activity at the centre for reassurance that the child is well. At all times, the parent should have the right to visit the child, and regular conferences should be established to review the child's progress. Important areas for parents to evaluate are the centre's daily program, teacher qualifications, nurturing qualities of caregivers, child-to-staff ratio, discipline policy, environmental safety precautions, provision of meals, sanitary conditions, adequate indoor and outdoor space per child, and fee schedule. Resources to familiarize parents with characteristics of quality child care and checklists to systematically evaluate the centre and compare it with other facilities can help parents make successful choices.

One of the areas that is increasingly important in selecting child care is the day care centre's health practices; however, parents often do not check the centre for health and safety features. The CPS (Lang & CPS, Community Paediatrics Committee, 2008/2016) has described factors characterizing high-quality child care centres and the developmental and behavioural outcomes of children in these centres. Children in day care centres, especially those under 3 years of age, tend to have more illnesses—especially diarrhea, otitis media, respiratory tract infections (especially if the caregiver smokes), hepatitis A, meningitis, and cytomegalovirus—than children cared for in their own home (Lang & CPS, Community Paediatrics Committee, 2009/2016). The strongest predictor of risk of illness is the number of unrelated children in the room. Proactive infection control measures and education of staff have been effective in reducing the incidence of upper respiratory tract infections, diarrhea, and rotavirus in day care centres. Families who have children in out-of-home child care may lose several days of work per year as a result of childhood infections. Parents should inquire about the centre's policy regarding the attendance and care of sick children. Parents with infants in day care or in-home care need to discuss safe sleep positions and environments in order to prevent SIDS (Matthews & Moore, 2013).

Limit-Setting and Discipline

As infants' motor skills advance and mobility increases, parents face the need to set safe limits to protect the child and establish a positive and supportive parent–child relationship (see Nurse's Role in Injury Prevention, p. 1010).

Parents must recognize the child's cognitive and behavioural limitations; adequate protection from hazards must be implemented because infants and toddlers do not understand a cause–effect relationship between dangerous objects and physical harm. Children will innately test limits and explore during the exploratory phase of growth; instead of discouraging exploration, parents should provide safe alternatives, put away dangerous household items, and provide consistent discipline and nurturing.

Effective teaching for injury prevention optimally begins in infancy, by helping parents understand the nature of their child's normal development. Parents need to be reminded that infants cry because a need is not being met, not to intentionally irritate an adult. The fussy or irritable infant may be a potential victim of shaken baby syndrome (or other bodily harm) since adults and caregivers may not understand the nature of the infant's crying. Parents need to reassure caregivers that it is acceptable to call them if the child is causing increased frustration in the caregiver. See Additional Resources for information on shaken baby syndrome.

Thumb-Sucking and Use of a Pacifier

Sucking is the infant's chief pleasure and may not be satisfied by breastfeeding or bottle-feeding. It is such a strong need that infants who are deprived of sucking, such as those with a cleft lip repair, will suck on their tongues. Some newborns are born with sucking blisters on their hands from in utero sucking activity.

Problems arise when parents are overly concerned about the sucking of the fingers, thumb, or pacifier and attempt to restrain this natural tendency. Before giving advice, nurses should investigate the parents' feelings and base guidance on this information.

Pacifier use, particularly in the early days after birth and in the birth hospital, has gained considerable attention in the scientific literature. Lawrence and Lawrence (2015), as well as other experts in breastfeeding, recommend that health care workers not introduce pacifiers to breastfed infants unless at the request of the parent. Pacifier use is not recommended as part of the WHO Baby-Friendly Hospital Initiative (Breastfeeding Committee for Canada, 2012). However, in a Cochrane review, the investigators concluded that pacifier use in full-term and healthy infants, started from birth or after lactation was established, did not significantly affect the prevalence or duration of exclusive or partial breastfeeding up to 4 months of age (Jaafar, Jahanfar, Angolkar, et al., 2012). (For further discussion of the relation between breastfeeding and pacifier use, see Chapter 27, Bottles and Pacifiers, p. 736).

Researchers have found that infants put to sleep with a pacifier had a reduced risk of SIDS (see Sudden Infant Death Syndrome: Etiology, p. 1033). Based on SIDS research, investigators have postulated the following reasons why pacifiers help to prevent SIDS: pacifiers lower the auditory arousal threshold; they may provide a mechanical barrier to rolling over into the prone position; sucking on a pacifier keeps the tongue forward, maintaining upper airway patency; an infant who is soothed by a pacifier may not move as often during sleep, thus limiting the chance of becoming covered by blankets; pacifiers might reduce gastroesophageal reflux and subsequent apnea; pacifier use could lead to slight carbon dioxide retention and increase the respiratory drive. The CPS (Ponti & CPS, Community Paediatrics Committee, 2003/2016) has also stated that pacifier use may decrease the risk of SIDS, but given the lack of definitive research on pacifiers the decision on their use is left to the parents. If pacifiers are used, they should not be given to the child until breastfeeding is well established and should be restricted if infants and children experience frequent or recurrent otitis media (Ponti & CPS, Community Paediatrics Committee, 2003/2016). Pacifier use should not replace actual feeding or suckling; prohibiting pacifier use will not ensure an increase in the length of breastfeeding; and there should be an emphasis on allowing the infant to control the pace, frequency, and termination of feeding rather than allowing the pacifier (or anything else) to become the focus of the interaction.

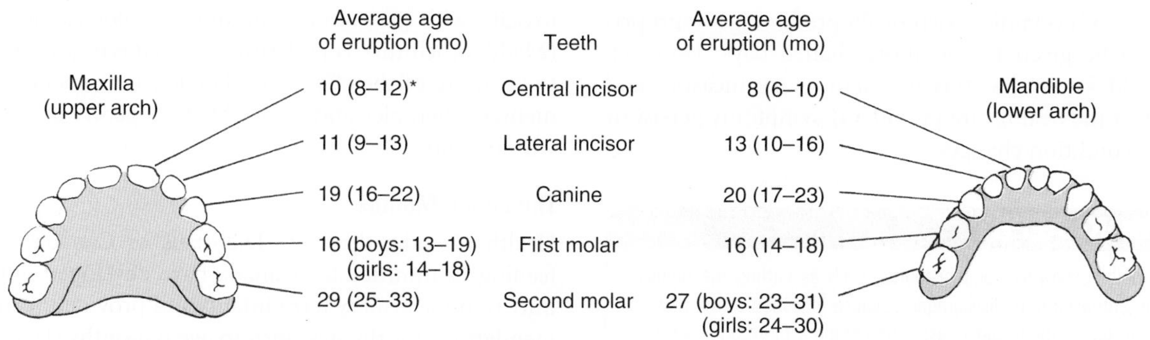

FIGURE 35-10 Sequence of eruption of primary teeth. *Range represents ±1 standard deviation, or 67% of subjects studied. (From American Dental Association. [n.d.]. *Eruption charts.* Retrieved from http://www.mouthhealthy.org/en/az-topics/e/eruption-charts.)

Pacifier use during painful procedures in newborns has been shown to produce an analgesic effect when combined with a concentrated sucrose solution (Harrison et al., 2015) (see Chapter 34).

The infant's use of a pacifier has also been suggested as a causative factor in the increase in episodes of acute otitis media, and pacifier use appears to be a risk factor in the development of otitis media when there is extended and more frequent use (Ponti & CPS, Community Paediatrics Committee, 2003/2016). Regarding other possible correlations with pacifier use, such as increased risk of infections or dental **malocclusion**, researchers have been unable to make any recommendations for or against pacifier use, given the limited number of studies (Hanzer, Zotter, Sauseng, et al., 2010; Jenik, Vain, Gorestein, et al., 2009).

To decrease dependence on non-nutritive sucking in young infants, sucking pleasure can be increased by prolonging feeding time.

Families need to receive instruction on the safe and appropriate use of pacifiers (CPS, 2012a), and safety considerations in purchasing one must be stressed (see Fig. 26-24). Parents should be cautioned against altering a pacifier, thus making it more dangerous. See Additional Resources at the end of this chapter for further information from Health Canada on the safety of baby equipment, including pacifiers.

During infancy and early childhood there is no need to restrain non-nutritive sucking of the fingers. Malocclusion may occur if thumb-sucking persists past 4 to 6 years of age, or when the permanent teeth erupt. Pacifiers may be perceived by some parents as less damaging because they are discarded by 2 to 3 years of age, whereas thumb-sucking may persist well into school-age years. Both pacifier use and thumb-sucking may also have significant cultural variations. Thumb-sucking reaches its peak at age 18 to 20 months and is most prevalent when the child is hungry, tired, or feeling insecure. Persistent thumb-sucking in a listless, apathetic child always warrants investigation. It may be a sign of an emotional problem between parent and child or of boredom, isolation, and lack of stimulation.

At the time of this writing, there is no evidence that pacifier use and non-nutritive sucking in *preterm infants* have any effect on the initiation and length of breastfeeding. Non-nutritive sucking should not be withheld from preterm infants, especially when used in conjunction with concentrated sucrose for pain management (see Atraumatic Care, p. 1022).

Teething

One of the more difficult periods in the infant's (and parents') life is the eruption of the deciduous (primary) teeth, often referred to as *teething*. The age of tooth eruption varies considerably among children, but the order of tooth appearance is fairly regular and predictable (Fig. 35-10). The first primary teeth to erupt are the lower central incisors, which appear at approximately 6 to 10 months of age (average 8 months). These are followed by the upper central incisors. The following is a quick guide to assessment of deciduous teeth during the first 2 years:

Age of the child in months − 6 = Number of teeth

For example: 8 months of age − 6 = 2 teeth

Teething is a physiological process; some discomfort is common as the crown of the tooth breaks through the periodontal membrane. Some children show minimum evidence of teething, such as drooling, gum rubbing, increased finger sucking, or biting on hard objects. Others are very irritable, have difficulty sleeping, and refuse to eat. Generally, signs of illness such as fever, vomiting, or diarrhea are not symptoms of teething but of illness and may warrant further investigation. Parents need to be cautioned not to overdiagnose teething; the ill-appearing child or child with a temperature over 38°C should be evaluated by a health care provider.

Because teething pain is a result of **inflammation**, application of cold is soothing. Giving the child a cold teething ring helps relieve the inflammation (but liquid-filled teaching rings should not be frozen). Several nonprescription topical anaesthetic ointments are available, although parents and health practitioners should be aware of the risks of using topical anaesthetic products, as absorption rates vary in infants and the active ingredient, benzocaine, can rarely cause methemoglobinemia (a condition in which an abnormal amount of methemoglobin, a type of hemoglobin, is produced) (Markman, 2009). If such products are used, parents are advised to apply them according to the product recommendations. The CPS (2013) does not recommend the use of topical anaesthetics because of the risk of the infant swallowing it. In the event of persistent irritability that affects sleeping and feeding, systemic analgesics such as acetaminophen or ibuprofen (age-appropriate dose) can be given for no more than 3 days. However, parents should know that this is a temporary measure and should contact the health care provider if symptoms persist or if the child's condition changes.

! NURSING ALERT

The use of teething powders or procedures, such as cutting the gums or rubbing them with aspirin, is discouraged because ingestion of the powder, infection or irritation of the tissue, or aspiration of the aspirin can occur. Hard candy may cause accidental choking or aspiration and should be avoided at this age.

PROMOTING OPTIMUM HEALTH DURING INFANCY

Nutrition

Ideally, discussion of optimum nutrition should begin prenatally, with a discussion regarding maternal intake of adequate nutrition in the form of a balanced diet and adequate amounts of protein, vitamins, and minerals, all of which have an impact on the growing fetus. Nurses should encourage and provide information for parents to discuss the options of breastfeeding or bottle-feeding the infant well in advance of the birth date. The choice for either is highly individual and is discussed in Chapter 27. This section is concerned primarily with infant nutrition during the months when growth needs and developmental milestones ready the child for introduction of solid food.

Among health care providers there is concern that, despite adequate availability of optimum nutrient sources, infants are not being fed appropriately. Certain chronic health conditions have been linked to feeding practices in infancy. Some poor nutrition examples are feeding solids before their digestive system is mature enough to absorb it, and providing fluids that are not enriched milk and consist of empty calories. These examples could contribute to future cardiovascular disease, obesity, iron-deficiency anemia, vitamin D deficiency, and rickets. A survey of infant feeding practices found that about 40% of the infants had eaten infant cereal, fruit, or vegetables by 4 months of age, and 50% were eating cake, fried potatoes, candy, and cookies by age 12 months (Fein, Li, Chen, et al., 2014). Nurses need to be proactive in teaching parents about what constitutes adequate and appropriate infant nutrition as well as positive nutritional habits to support healthy growth and development.

Health care providers have become more aware of the use of complementary and alternative medical therapies in children that may not be as beneficial as indicated in various media sources. One concern is children's intake of megavitamins and herbs; parents may assume that the word *natural* in reference to ingredients means the product is safe, when this may not be the case. One report cited the home administration of star anise tea to treat colic as the cause of adverse neurological reactions. Chinese star anise (*Illicium verum*) is a popular herbal remedy for infantile colic. Contamination with a related species of Japanese star anise (*Illicium anisatum*) has been related to infant toxicity with gastrointestinal and neurological adverse effects (Madden, Schmitz, & Fullerton, 2012). It is important for nurses to be aware of the effects, availability, and practice of complementary therapies and to be able to cogently discuss their use with parents.

The First 6 Months

Health Canada, the CPS, Dietitians of Canada, and Breastfeeding Committee for Canada have developed guidelines on nutrition for healthy term infants and provided related recommendations for the newborn to age 6 months (Health Canada, 2015a). This collaborative group recommends breast milk exclusively for the first 6 months and that it be given for up to 2 years or longer with appropriate complementary feeding. Human milk is the most desirable complete diet for the infant during the first 6 months, and it provides nutrition, immunological protection, growth, and development for infants and toddlers (Health Canada, 2015a). See Chapter 27 for more information on human milk and feeding. The healthy term infant receiving breast milk usually requires no vitamin and mineral supplements, with a few exceptions. Daily supplementation of vitamin D is indicated because many Canadian mothers and babies, especially those in northern communities, do not get enough vitamin D. It is recommended that all breast milk–fed infants receive a daily supplement of 400 International Units (IU) (10 mcg) of vitamin D, beginning in the first few days of life, to prevent rickets and vitamin D deficiency. Concentrated vitamin D drops are available with the entire 400 IU dose in one drop; this can be placed on the nipple (breast or bottle). Non-breast-milk–fed infants who are taking less than 1 L/day of vitamin D–fortified formula should also receive a daily vitamin D supplement of 400 IU (10 mcg) and should receive more if living in a northern community.

Indigenous groups, as well other individuals who live in the northern regions, continue to need extra vitamin D. The CPS (Godel & CPS, First Nations, Inuit and Métis Health Committee, 2007/2015) recommends increasing vitamin D to 800 IU/day from all sources between October and April for all infants up to 1 year of age living north of the fifty-fifth parallel. This 800 IU dosage is also recommended for individuals who live between the fortieth and fifty-fifth parallel with risk factors for vitamin D deficiency other than latitude alone. Vitamin D deficiency continues to be a problem among Indigenous mothers during pregnancy as well.

NURSING ALERT

There are reports of accidental overdose of liquid vitamin D in infants because of packaging errors; the syringe for liquid administration may not be labelled clearly for 400 IU. Nurses need to teach parents how to read the syringe accurately.

Up until the age of 6 months, term infants should have adequate maternal stores of iron in their bodies. Beyond 6 months of age, these stores of iron will be depleted and breast milk alone can no longer meet all of the nutritional requirements for the rapidly growing infant. To prevent iron deficiency, at 6 months, iron-rich foods should be introduced to the diet. Iron-rich cereals, meat, and fish all contain absorbable iron (Health Canada, 2015b).

Whether breastfed or bottle-fed, infants do not require additional fluids, especially water or juice, during the first 6 months of life. Excessive intake of water in infants may result in water intoxication and hyponatremia.

An alternative to breastfeeding is commercial iron-fortified formula. It supplies the nutrients needed by the infant for the first 6 months. Unmodified whole cow's milk, low-fat cow's milk, skim milk, other animal milks, and imitation milks are not acceptable as a major source of nutrition for infants because of infants' limited ability to digest these foods, the increased risk of contamination, and the lack of nutritional components in animal milk that are needed for appropriate growth. Pasteurized whole cow's milk is deficient in iron, zinc, and vitamin C and has a high renal solute load, which makes it undesirable for infants less than 12 months of age (American Academy of Pediatrics [AAP], 2009).

! NURSING ALERT

Neither infant formula nor breast milk should be warmed in a microwave oven because this may cause infant oral burns as a result of uneven heating in the container. The bottle or container may remain cool while hot spots develop in the formula. To thaw breast milk, it should be placed in a container under a lukewarm water bath (less than 40.5°C) or placed in the refrigerator overnight. Warming expressed breast milk in a microwave oven also decreases the availability of anti-infective properties and vitamin C and causes a separation of the milk layers that affect fat content (Lawrence & Lawrence, 2015).

NURSING ALERT

Dietary fat should not be restricted in infancy unless such restriction is under medical supervision. Feeding the infant skim or low-fat milk is unacceptable because the essential fatty acids are inadequate and the solute concentration of protein and electrolytes, such as sodium, is too high.

The amount of formula per feeding and the number of feedings per day vary among infants. Infants on demand feeding usually determine their own feeding schedule, but some infants may need a more planned schedule based on average feeding patterns to ensure their receiving sufficient nutrients. In general, the number of feedings per day decreases from six at 1 month of age to four or five at 6 months. Regardless of the number of feedings, the total amount of formula ingested will usually level off at about 960 mL/day. (See discussion of formula-feeding in Chapter 27, p. 748.)

Bottled water for mixing powdered or concentrated formula is a relatively safe alternative to tap water if available tap water has a high content of contaminants such as lead. Bottled water, however, should not be assumed to be sterile unless specifically stated on the container. Fluoridated bottled water is not necessary for mixing powdered formula unless the local water source is low in fluoride, in which case fluoride supplementation is recommended after age 6 months (see Dental Health, p. 1010). If powdered formula is being used, parents should be instructed in its safe preparation (see Chapter 27, Patient Teaching box, p. 752). Powdered formula has a greater risk of contamination by microorganisms than concentrated formula and is only recommended to be used for infants who are healthy and full term. For low-birth-weight and immunocompromised infants, liquid formula is recommended for the first 2 months (Health Canada, 2015a). Recommendations for preparation of powdered infant formula in the home or in a professional setting (i.e., hospitals and day care centres) are provided by Health Canada (2015a).

Health Canada, the CPS, and Dietitians of Canada advise that potential serious health risks are associated with infants' intake of homemade noncommercial formulas and thus their use is not recommended. The health risks include severe malnutrition and potentially fatal illness from receiving inadequate nutrients and from contamination by harmful bacteria. Recipes for these formulas are being promoted by some practitioners and are available on the Internet (Health Canada, 2014).

Parents should be cautioned to not feed their infant juices and non-nutritive drinks such as fruit-flavoured drinks or carbonated beverages (soft drinks). Many of these drinks do not provide sufficient caloric intake for infants less than 12 months of age. Such drinks do not replace the nutrients in milk (formula), and their use may lead to growth or health problems.

The addition of solid foods before 6 months of age is also not recommended (Health Canada, 2015a). During the first months of an infant's life, solid foods are not compatible with the ability of the gastrointestinal tract and the infant's nutritional needs. Developmentally, infants are not ready for solid food. The extrusion (protrusion) reflex is strong and causes food to be pushed out of the mouth. Early introduction of solid foods is a type of forced feeding that may lead to excessive weight gain and iron-deficiency anemia. Despite these recommendations, and lacking evidence-based information to support such practices, many parents introduce solids as early as 2 weeks of age. In such cases, rice cereal is often added to the formula to help the infant sleep better at night or to enhance weight gain; however, this practice is not substantiated by any scientific evidence (Health Canada, 2015a).

The Second 6 Months

During the second half of the infant's first year, human milk or formula continues to be the primary source of nutrition. Fluoride supplementation should begin, depending on the infant's intake of fluoridated tap water (see Dental Health, p. 1010). If breastfeeding is discontinued, a commercial iron-fortified formula should be substituted. Follow-up or transition formulas specially marketed for older infants offer no special advantages over other infant formulas (AAP, 2009).

The major change in feeding habits is the addition of solid foods to the infant's diet. Physiologically and developmentally, the infant at 6 months of age is in a transition period. By this time, the gastrointestinal tract has matured sufficiently to handle more complex nutrients. Tooth eruption is beginning and facilitates biting and chewing. The extrusion reflex has disappeared, and swallowing is more coordinated to allow the infant to accept solids easily. Head control is well developed, which permits infants to sit with support and purposely turn the head away to communicate disinterest in food. Voluntary grasping and improved eye–hand coordination gradually allow infants to pick up finger foods and feed themselves. Their increasing sense of independence is evident in their desire to hold the bottle and try to "help" during feeding.

Selection and preparation of solid foods. The choice of solid foods to introduce first is variable but should meet the criteria for feeding solids, such as supplying nutrients not found in formula or breast milk. Infants should be offered iron-fortified cereal as well as meat, poultry, and fish or meat alternatives on a daily basis at 6 months, gradually working up to two or more times each day (Health Canada, 2015b). Iron-fortified infant cereal is generally introduced first because of its high iron content (7 mg prepared dry cereal). Commercially prepared ready-to-serve dry cereals for infants include rice, barley, oatmeal, and high-protein cereals. Cereals such as cream of farina should not be used because infant commercial cereals are a better source of iron. Some of the commercial baby cereals are combined with fruit, but there is little nutritional benefit from these preparations; they are more expensive; and some may contain additional, unneeded calories and sugar. Infant cereal (iron fortified) should be mixed with formula until whole milk is given. If the infant is being breastfed, the cereal can be mixed with expressed breast milk or water. The addition of solid foods to the exclusively breastfed infant's diet does not significantly increase overall caloric intake or weight gain. After 6 months of age, small amounts of fruit juices can be mixed with the dry cereal; the vitamin C content of the juice enhances the absorption of iron in the cereal. Infants should be offered breast milk or formula first for the first 6 to 12 months before the solids are given.

The CPS (Chan, Cummings, CPS, Community Paediatrics Committee, 2013/2016) has stated that delaying the introduction of certain "trigger" foods is shown to have no protective effect on allergic sensitization or disease development. Rather, they recommend not delaying any specified solid food beyond 6 months of age. When feeding an infant food that is a potential allergen, only one new food per day should be given; 2 days should pass before introducing another allergenic food (Health Canada, 2015a, b).

Following is a recommended sequence for parents to follow for introducing foods (CPS, 2014; Health Canada, 2015a):

- **Grain products**—At 6 to 9 months, offer up to 30 to 60 mL of iron-fortified infant cereal, twice a day. Then try other grain products such as small pieces of dry toast or unsalted crackers. At 9 to 12 months, offer other plain cereals, whole-grain bread, rice, and pasta.
- **Meat and alternatives**—At 6 to 9 months, offer cooked meat, fish, chicken, tofu, mashed beans, and egg yolk. At 9 to 12 months, mince or dice these foods.
- **Vegetables**—At 6 to 9 months, offer cooked vegetables—yellow, green, or orange. At 9 to 12 months, progress to soft, mashed cooked vegetables.
- **Fruits**—At 6 to 9 months, offer cooked fruits, very ripe mashed fruits (such as bananas). At 9 to 12 months, try soft fresh fruits, peeled, seeded, and diced or canned fruit, packed in water or juice (not syrup). Avoid whole grapes, as they are a choking hazard.
- **Milk and milk products**—At 6 to 9 months, offer dairy foods like yogurt (3.25% or higher), cottage cheese, or grated hard cheese. Wait until the infant is 9 to 12 months old before introducing whole cow's milk (3.25%). After 12 months of age, the infant should not take more than 720 mL of milk products per day. Too much milk can lead to iron-deficiency anemia.

The introduction of solid foods into the infant's diet at this age is primarily for taste and chewing experience, not for growth. The majority of the infant's caloric needs are derived from the primary milk source (breast or formula); therefore, solids should not be perceived as a substitute for milk until the child is older than 12 months. Portion sizes may vary according to the infant's taste. In general, 15 to 20 mL is adequate for most infants. In most cases, larger amounts may be served, but because of the infant's focus on the texture and feel of the food, smaller amounts will be consumed. Food with a lumpy texture should be offered no later than 9 months of age and table food is encouraged from age 6 months.

Parents should be cautioned to avoid reliance on foods and supplements marketed as iron- or vitamin-fortified as primary sources of minerals. Instead, they should be encouraged to offer the child a variety of fruits, vegetables, whole grains, meats, and those known to naturally be rich in iron.

Infants and toddlers should not be given low-calorie foods unless a strict, medically prescribed diet is required. The infant's growth during this phase is crucial to future development, and curtailing dietary fat should be done with great caution.

! NURSING ALERT

Infants under 12 months should not be given honey or corn syrup as these may contain the bacterium *Clostridium botulinum*, a source of foodborne botulism. Botulism is a serious illness caused by the bacterium's toxin, which affects the nervous system. Botulism can cause paralysis. Thus a pacifier should not be coated with honey or corn syrup to encourage the infant to take it.

Introduction of solid foods. When the spoon is first introduced, infants often push it away and appear dissatisfied. Patience and skill are required to overcome this initial response. As infants become accustomed to the spoon, they more eagerly accept the food and eventually will open the mouth in anticipation (or keep it closed in dislike). Because the first introduction of food is a new experience, spoon feeding should be attempted after ingestion of some breast milk or formula to associate this activity with a pleasurable and satisfying experience. During the toddler years, eating becomes less of an adventure, and strong food preferences become evident.

Infants know when they are hungry and when they are full. Parents need to be able to pick up signs of hunger and fullness in their infant to avoid under- or overfeeding. Hungry infants may open their mouths for food and protest if the food is taken away. Infants who are full may close their mouths, turn head away, or push food away (Health Link BC, 2014).

FAMILY-CENTRED TEACHING

Introducing Solid Foods to Infants

- Introduce solid foods when the infant is hungry.
- Begin spoon feeding by pushing food to the back of the tongue because of the infant's natural tendency to thrust the tongue forward.
- Use a small spoon with a straight handle; begin with 5 or 10 mL of food; gradually increase to a couple of tablespoons per feeding.
- Feed new foods in small amounts, from 5 to 30 mL. As the amount of solid food increases, the quantity of milk is decreased to less than 1 L daily to prevent overfeeding.
- Do not introduce foods by mixing them with formula in the bottle.
- Encourage the eating of table food and promote finger food so the infant can feed self.
- Ensure foods with lumpy textures are introduced by 9 months of age.

Because feeding is a learning process, as well as a means of nutrition, new foods should be given alone, not mixed with others, to allow the child to learn new tastes and textures. Food should not be mixed in the bottle and fed through a nipple with a large hole. This can cause poor chewing of food later in life because of lack of experience. Guidelines for the introduction of new foods are given in the Family-Centred Teaching box.

The infant's first, second, and often twentieth try at self-feeding or cup feeding is a sloppy experience. Finger foods such as soft fruits or vegetables are just as good as playthings as they are food. However, all of this is part of learning, and mastery follows many accidents.

Parents need to be encouraged to interpret their infant's signals of discomfort and intervene in ways other than through feeding. Crying, fussiness, and sucking do not necessarily indicate hunger. Rocking, stroking, holding, and offering a toy or a pacifier may be more appropriate than automatically responding with food.

Weaning

Defined as the process of giving up one method of feeding for another, *weaning* usually refers to relinquishing the breast or bottle for a cup (see Chapter 27). In Western societies this is generally regarded as a major task for infants; it is psychologically significant because the infant is required to give up a major source of oral pleasure and gratification.

Upon receiving solid foods, infants have learned that good things come from a spoon. Their increasing desire for freedom of movement may lessen their desire to be held close for feedings. They eventually acquire more control over their actions and can easily manipulate a cup to their lips. Imitation becomes a powerful motivator by age 8 or 9 months, and they enjoy using a cup or glass with sips of water like others do (Lawrence & Lawrence, 2015). In an infant under 6 months, no extra oral fluids are required other than breast milk or formula, which provides enough hydration. At 6 months to 12 months, the only fluids that are recommended are sips of water so that the infant will drink adequate breast milk or formula and eat adequate solid food. After 12 months, the child can have water liberally. Fruit juice is not recommended because it can lead to other health problems such as poor nutrition, obesity, and tooth decay (AAP, 2015).

Weaning should be individualized and gradual. A child should not be allowed to take a bottle of milk to bed, as this is a major cause of caries. If breastfeeding is discontinued, weaning should be to a bottle to provide for sucking needs. If breastfeeding is discontinued later, weaning can be directly to a cup, especially by age 12 to 14 months.

Sleep and Activity

Sleep patterns vary among infants, with active infants sleeping typically less than placid children. Newborns and infants up to 6 months of age sleep approximately 16 hours per day, 3 to 4 hours at a time, with about three naps a day. Infants aged 6 months to 1 year sleep approximately 14 hours per day and gradually will require only two naps (CPS, 2012b). Breastfed infants usually sleep for less prolonged periods, with more frequent waking, especially during the night, than do formula-fed infants.

Most infants are naturally active and need no encouragement to be mobile. If devices such as playpens, strollers, and commercial swings are used excessively, they can restrict movement and prevent infants from exploring and developing gross motor skills. Health Canada (2007) has banned the sale of infant walkers because of the large number of associated injuries. Newer models of infant walkers have been designed without wheels to decrease infant injuries.

Sleeping Concerns

The discussion here focuses on minor sleep issues in infants, such as refusal to go to sleep or frequent waking during the night.

Parental concerns regarding sleep are common during infancy. It has been reported that between 15 and 35% of parents report problems with their infant's sleep during the first 6 months of life (Cook, Bayer, Le, et. al., 2012). Sometimes these concerns are as basic as parents' questioning whether the infant needs additional sleep. In this case, it is best to investigate the reason for their concern, stressing each child's individual needs. Infants who are active during wakeful periods and growing normally are sleeping a sufficient amount of time.

Sleep problems in early infancy have been positively correlated with higher maternal depression scores and poorer general and mental health in both mothers and fathers (Della Vedova, 2014). Therefore, nurses should discuss infant sleep problems with the mother and family in addition to other developmental aspects of newborn care both before and after the baby is born.

When a sleeping problem exists, a careful assessment is helpful to ascertain the perception of the problem (Stremler, Hodnett, Kenton, et al., 2013). Recording sleep habits both before and after interventions is also an important strategy. Questions regarding the frequency and duration of waking, the usual bedtime routine, the number of nighttime feedings, the perceived problem (e.g., how much disruption the behaviour generates), and the attempted interventions are useful in planning effective approaches designed for the specific sleep problem.

Several interventions to assist families have been studied and compared. A common suggestion given for any type of sleep problem—"Let the child cry until he or she falls asleep"—is difficult to implement and inappropriate for certain conditions, such as for an infant in the first 3 to 6 months when feeding routines are still being established.

One intervention considered to be an atraumatic approach to night crying, known as *graduated extinction*, is to let the child cry for progressively longer times between brief parental interventions that consist only of reassurance—not rocking, holding, or using a bottle or pacifier (Matthey & Črnčec, 2012). For example, the parents may check on the child every 5 minutes during the first night and progressively extend this interval by 5 minutes on successive nights until the infant can self-soothe.

Children who learn to fall asleep on their own at bedtime have longer sustained sleep periods than those who fall asleep with a parent present (Moore, Meltzer, & Mindell, 2008). In addition, comforting children outside their own bed at night once they awaken has been associated with poor sleep consolidation. For example, feeding 5-month-old children after awakening at night resulted in fewer consecutive sleep hours (Touchette, Petit, Tremblay, et al., 2009). The authors of this study recommend parental presence at bedtime until the child is drowsy, then placing the child in his or her own bed for a night's sleep. Infants can develop effective and healthy self-soothing techniques when provided a pacifier or a soft toy or blanket to hold and placed in their own crib (Cook et al., 2012).

Some researchers indicate that the best way to prevent sleep problems is to encourage parents to establish healthy sleep habits in their infant that fit with normal circadian rhythms (Whittingham & Douglas, 2014). They suggest providing parents with education on the biology of sleep, to expose the infant to normal circadian cues of daylight and noise in order to prevent oversleeping during the day and help consolidate sleep at nights. For example, the infant would be exposed to natural light early in the day, and both caregiver and infant would have appropriately timed exercise and relaxation. Parents can also be encouraged to identify and remove barriers to overall health functioning, such as eating and crying problems (colic), and to learn the cues for sleepiness in their infant so that they can adapt to those cues instead of developing rigid preset schedules. Finally, a safe sleep environment is recommended, where the infant is near the caregivers but not in the same bed.

There are many interventions to regulate infant sleep; however, it is not confirmed that any one intervention is more effective over another. A supportive environment and following good sleep habits may end up being the best advice a nurse can provide to the family once all physical causes for the sleep disturbances are eliminated.

Dental Health

Good dental hygiene begins with good maternal dental health and with counselling during early infancy regarding dietary intake for the promotion of optimal oral hygiene (Canadian Dental Association, 2016). Parents also need to be counselled on feeding practices that increase the risk of poor dental health, such as not propping the milk bottle or giving the milk bottle in the bed, and not giving fruit juices in a bottle, especially before 6 months of age.

Mouth cleaning can commence right after birth: parents should be taught to clean the infant's gums with a piece of gauze or cloth so that children become accustomed to cleaning of the mouth. Once the primary teeth erupt, the teeth and gums are initially cleaned by wiping with a damp cloth; tooth brushing is too harsh for the tender gingiva. The caregiver can stabilize the infant by cradling the child with one arm and using the free hand to cleanse the teeth. Oral hygiene can be made pleasant by singing or talking to the infant.

The Canadian Dental Association (2016) recommends that all children have their first visit to a dentist in their first year of life. It is generally recommended that a small, soft-bristled toothbrush be used as more teeth erupt and the infant adjusts to the routine of cleaning. Water is preferred to toothpaste, which the infant will swallow (and if the toothpaste is fluoridated, the infant will ingest excessive amounts of fluoride).

Fluoride, an essential mineral for building caries-resistant teeth, needs to be supplemented beginning at 6 months of age if the infant does not already receive water with adequate fluoride content. The Canadian Dental Association (2016) recommends that parents discuss their infant's fluoride needs with a dentist. Many communities fluoridate public drinking water. Thus if bottled water is used to reconstitute powdered or concentrated formula, it should either be fluoride free or contain low levels of fluoride (Canadian Dental Association, 2012).

Dietary considerations are also important to dental health because habits begun during infancy tend to continue into later years. Foods with added concentrated sugar should be used sparingly (if at all) in the infant's diet. Parents need to be counselled regarding the detrimental effects of frequent and prolonged bottle-feeding or breastfeeding during sleep, when the sweet milk or other fluid, such as juice, bathes the teeth, producing caries. (See Chapter 36 for a more extensive discussion of dental care, including nursing caries.)

Safety Promotion and Injury Prevention

Injuries are a major cause of death during infancy, especially for children 6 to 12 months old. The main causes of death in children under 1 year of age are threats to breathing (54%), being a passenger in a motor vehicle accident (18%), and drowning (15%). Falls are the main reason for visits to the hospital for children under age 1 year (46%) (Yanchar, Warda, & Fuselli, 2012). According to a recent Cochrane study, one third of all injuries occur in the home, yet there is insufficient evidence to demonstrate that modification of the home environment has an impact on the rate of injuries (Turner, Arthur, Lyons, et al., 2011). Constant awareness and supervision are essential as the child gains increased locomotor and manipulative skills that are coupled with an insatiable curiosity about the environment. Box 35-1 lists the major developmental achievements of each period during infancy

BOX 35-1 INJURY PREVENTION DURING INFANCY

Birth to 4 Months

Major Developmental Accomplishments

Exhibits involuntary reflexes (e.g., crawling reflex may propel infant forward or backward; startle reflex may cause the body to jerk)

May roll over

Has increasing eye–hand coordination and voluntary grasp reflex

Injury Prevention

Aspiration

Aspiration is not as great a danger to this age group as in older infants, but parents should begin practising safeguarding early (see under Age 4 to 7 Months).

Baby powder should be cornstarch-based and never shaken directly on the infant; powder should be placed in the hand and then on the infant's skin; store container closed and out of infant's reach.

Hold the infant for feeding; do not prop bottle.

Know emergency procedures for choking.

Use a pacifier with one-piece construction and loop handle.

Burns

Install smoke detectors in the home.

Do not microwave infant formula or breast milk because this can cause burns because of uneven warming.

Check bathwater temperature.

Do not pour, hold, or drink hot liquids and keep them out of reach when the infant is close by, such as when sitting on your lap.

Beware of cigarette ashes that may fall on the infant.

Do not leave infant in the sun for more than a few minutes; keep skin covered.

Wash flame-retardant clothes according to label directions.

Use cool-mist vaporizers.

Check surface heat of the car restraint before placing child in the seat.

Drowning and Suffocation

Keep all plastic bags stored out of the infant's reach; discard large plastic garment bags after tying in a knot.

Do not cover mattress with plastic.

Use firm mattress and loose light blankets, with no pillows. Minimize the number of items in the crib.

Make certain the crib design follows government regulations and the mattress fits snugly. No crib manufactured before September 1986 should be used for infants (Government of Canada, 2016a).

Position the crib away from other furniture and away from radiators.

Keep all cords and strings out of reach and do not tie pacifier on a string around infant's neck.

Remove bibs at bedtime.

Never leave an infant alone in the bath.

Do not leave an infant under age 1 year alone on an adult or youth mattress or "beanbag"-type seats.

Install carbon monoxide monitor

Motor Vehicles

Transport infant in a Transport Canada–approved, rear-facing car seat, preferably in the back seat.

Do not place infant on the seat (of car) or in your lap.

Do not place child in a carriage or stroller behind a parked car.

Do not place infant or child in the front passenger seat with an activated air bag.

Do not leave child unattended in car.

Falls

Crib rails should be fixed and firmly latched. As of 2012, only beds with fixed rails are recommended, but some older models may be in use (suggest purchasing a rail-latching mechanism for older models).

Never leave an infant alone on a raised, unguarded surface.

When in doubt as to where to place the child, use the floor.

Restrain child in an infant seat or stroller, and never leave child unattended while the seat is resting on a raised surface.

Avoid using a high chair until the child can sit well with support.

Poisoning

Poisoning is not as great a danger in this age group as in older infants, but parents should begin practising safeguards early (see under Age 4 to 7 Months).

Bodily Damage

Keep sharp or jagged objects such as knives and broken glass out of child's reach.

Keep diaper pins closed and away from the infant.

Age 4 to 7 Months

Major Developmental Accomplishments

Rolls over

Sits momentarily

Grasps and manipulates small objects

Resecures a dropped object

Has well-developed eye–hand coordination

Can focus on and locate small objects

Places objects in mouth (hand-to-mouth)

Can push up on hands and knees

Crawls backward

Injury Prevention

Aspiration

Keep buttons, beads, syringe caps, and other small objects out of infant's reach.

Keep floor free of any small objects.

Do not feed infant hard candy, nuts, food with pits or seeds, or whole or circular pieces of hot dog or grapes.

Exercise caution when giving teething biscuits, since large chunks may be broken off and aspirated.

Do not feed the infant while he or she is lying down.

Inspect toys for removable parts. Use only toys approved for the age of your child.

Use only cornstarch baby powder, if powder is needed, and keep out of reach.

Suffocation

Keep all latex balloons out of reach.

Remove all crib toys that are strung across the crib or playpen when the child begins to push up on hands or knees or is 5 months old.

Continued

BOX 35-1 INJURY PREVENTION DURING INFANCY—cont'd

Burns

Keep water faucets out of reach.

Place hot objects (cigarettes, candles, incense) on a high surface out of the child's reach.

Limit exposure to sun; apply sunscreen.

Falls

Restrain in a high chair.

Keep crib rails fixed and firmly latched.

Motor Vehicles

See under Birth to 4 Months.

Poisoning

Make certain that paint for furniture or toys does not contain lead.

Place toxic substances on a high shelf or in locked cabinet.

Keep medication vials and bottles locked in a secure place.

Hang plants or place them on a high surface rather than on the floor.

Avoid storing large quantities of cleaning fluid, paints, pesticides, and other toxic substances.

Discard used containers of poisonous substances.

Do not store toxic substances in food or drink containers.

Discard used button-size batteries; store new batteries in a safe area.

Know the telephone number of the provincial or territorial poison control centre (usually listed in front of telephone directory).

Bodily Damage

Give the child toys that are smooth and rounded, preferably made of wood or plastic.

Avoid long, pointed objects as toys.

Avoid toys that are excessively loud.

Keep sharp objects out of infant's reach.

Age 8 to 12 Months

Major Developmental Accomplishments

Crawls or creeps

Stands, holding onto furniture

Stands alone

Cruises around furniture

Walks

Climbs

Pulls on objects

Throws objects

Is able to pick up small objects; has pincer grasp

Explores by putting objects in mouth

Dislikes being restrained

Explores away from parent

Increasingly understands simple commands and phrases

Injury Prevention

Aspiration

Keep small objects off the floor, off furniture, and out of reach of children.

Take care when feeding solid table food.

Do not use beanbag toys or allow the child to play with dried beans.

See also under Age 4 to 7 Months.

Bodily Damage

See under Age 4 to 7 Months.

Avoid placing televisions or other large objects on top of furniture, which may be overturned when the infant pulls self to standing position.

Falls

Avoid walkers (illegal in Canada), especially near stairs.*

Ensure that furniture is sturdy enough for the child to pull self to standing position.

Fence stairways at the top and bottom if the child has access to either end.

Dress infant in safe shoes and clothing (soles that do not "catch" on floor, tied shoelaces, pant legs that do not touch floor).

Suffocation and Drowning

Keep doors of the oven, dishwasher, refrigerator, cooler, and front-loading clothes washer and dryer closed at all times.

If storing an unused large appliance, such as a refrigerator, lock or remove the door.

Supervise contact with inflated balloons; immediately discard popped balloons, and keep uninflated balloons out of reach.

Fence swimming pools and other bodies of standing water such as decorative fountains; lock gates to swimming pools so only adult can gain access.

Always supervise the child when near any source of water, such as cleaning buckets, drainage areas, ponds, and toilets.

Keep bathroom doors closed.

Eliminate unnecessary pools of water.

Keep one hand on the child at all times when in the tub. Never leave them unattended.

Poisoning

Administer medications as a drug, not as a candy.

Do not administer medications unless prescribed by a practitioner.

Return medications and poisons to a safe storage area immediately after use; replace caps properly if a child-protector cap is used.

Have the provincial or territorial poison control centre number on the telephone and refrigerator.

Burns

Place guards in front of or around any heating appliance, fireplace, or furnace.

Keep electrical wires hidden or out of reach.

Place plastic guards over electrical outlets; place furniture in front of outlets.

Keep hanging tablecloths out of reach (the child may pull down hot liquids or heavy or sharp objects).

*Information on many items such as cribs or walkers is available from Health Canada, at http://www.hc-sc.gc.ca/cps-spc/pubs/cons/child-enfant/safe-securite-eng.php

and the appropriate corresponding injury prevention plan that parents can implement.

Motor Vehicle Injuries

Automobile injuries are the leading cause of accidental death in children in Canada between the ages of 1 and 9 years (Yanchar et al., 2012). A significant number of nonfatal vehicle-related injuries in children between 1 and 4 years of age occur as a result of a car backing out while children are playing in a driveway (Centers for Disease Control and Prevention [CDC], 2005). In addition, a significant number of infants are injured or die from improper restraint within the vehicle, most often from riding on the lap of another occupant or from riding unrestrained in the back seat of the vehicle. All infants must be secured in a Transport Canada–approved restraint rather than being held or placed on the seat of the car (see Additional Resources at the end of this chapter). There is no safe alternative. Misuse rates range from 44 to 81% for car seats and 30 to 50% for booster seats (van Schaik & CPS, Injury Prevention Committee, 2008).

According to the CPS, when used correctly, child seats reduce the risk of fatal injury by 71% and risk of serious injury by 67%. Many unfortunate outcomes of motor vehicle–related accidents can be prevented with increased public education and clinician advocacy (van Schaik & CPS, Injury Prevention Committee, 2008). Parents and caregivers need to know that all provinces and territories have child restraint legislation as well as guidelines on how to properly install and use child restraint systems.

Infant restraints are designed either as an infant-only model or as a convertible infant-toddler model (Fig. 35-11). Either restraint is a semireclined seat that faces the rear of the car. A rear-facing car seat provides the best protection for the disproportionately heavy head and weak neck of a young child. This position minimizes the stress on the neck by spreading the forces of a frontal crash over the entire back, neck, and head; the spine is supported by the back of the car seat. If the seat were faced forward, the head would whip forward because of the force of the crash, creating enormous stress on the neck.

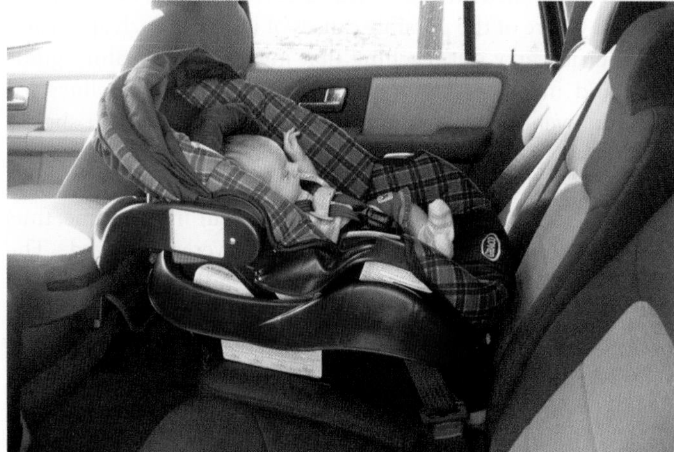

FIGURE 35-11 A rear-facing infant car restraint that is approved by Transport Canada and placed in the back seat provides the best protection. (Courtesy of Brian and Mayannyn Sallee.)

Infants and toddlers should ride in rear-facing car safety seats until they outgrow the height and weight limit of the car seat. The earliest a child should move to a forward-facing car seat is at 10 kg, but toddlers up to 24 months of age are safer riding in convertible seats in the rear-facing position (Transport Canada, 2015).

The restraint is anchored to the vehicle with the vehicle's seat belt, and the restraint has a harness system for securing the infant. Some harness systems require a clip to keep the shoulder straps correctly positioned. Newer vehicles (manufactured after 1999) have tether straps that attach to anchors in the car seat to better secure the seat and minimize forward movement of the forward-facing convertible seats in the event of an accident. The LATCH (lower anchor and tether for children) system provides car seat anchors between the front cushion and backrest so that the seat belt does not have to be used. However, Transport Canada (2015) recommends that the seat belt be used to anchor the car seat instead of the LATCH system, based on the vehicle and car seat manufacturer's recommendations. If no recommendations are given then the car seat belt should be used if the child's weight exceeds 18 kg. Some automobiles have tether straps for rear-facing infant-only seats as well. Although many infant restraints can be recliners, they are used in the car only in the position specified by the manufacturer.

! NURSING ALERT

Infants should ride in a rear-facing car seat from birth to a weight of 10 kg and until at least 1 year of age. If the child weighs 10 kg but is not 1 year old, the rear-facing position is still recommended. Infants and children must be in a car seat or booster seat until age 8 years. All children's car seats and booster seats sold in Canada must have a Transport Canada sticker on them and will have an expiration or useful life date on them. Manufacturers place expiratory or useful-life dates to inform current owners and prospective buyers of the potential risks of using car seats and booster seats that may be missing important parts, labels, or instructions or that may have an unknown history that could lead to inadequate performance when needed. People should not use children's car seats and booster seats past their expiration or useful-life date or that have previously been in a car accident (Transport Canada, 2015).

Severe injuries and deaths in children have occurred from air bags deploying on impact in the front passenger seat; thus the back seat is the safest area of the car for children. For restraints to be effective, they must be used properly. Dressing the infant in a light-weight outfit with sleeves and legs allows the harness to hold the child securely in the seat. A small blanket or towel rolled tightly can be placed on either side of the head to minimize movement and keep the infant's hips against the back of the seat. Padding between the infant's legs and crotch can be added to prevent slouching. Thick, soft padding should not be placed under the infant or behind the back, and the infant should not be wearing a snowsuit or heavy coat because during the impact, the padding will compress, leaving the harness straps loose. Only padding that came with the car seat should be used. Preterm infants being discharged home should be placed in an appropriate car seat restraint as it would be placed in the car, and the infant's heart rate and oxygen saturations should be monitored for a determined period to detect any potential problems with airway occlusion. (For further discussion of car seat restraints, see Chapter 36.) See Additional Resources for more information on motor vehicle restraints.

NURSING ALERT

Rear-facing infant safety seats must not be placed in the front seats of cars equipped with an air bag on the passenger side. If an infant safety seat is placed in the passenger seat with an air bag, the child could be seriously injured if the air bag is released, since rear-facing infant seats extend closer to the dashboard.

Another automobile-related hazard for infants is overheating (hyperthermia) and subsequent death when left in a vehicle in hot weather (over 26°C). Infants dissipate heat poorly, and an increase in body temperature may cause death in a few hours. Parents should be cautioned against leaving infants in a vehicle alone *for any reason.* A small sign or placard has been designed to hang in the rear-view mirror to remind the parent that there is a child in the back seat. Busy parents may forget that the child is in the back when preoccupied with other thoughts.

Shaken Baby Syndrome

Shaken baby syndrome (SBS), also known as "shaken impact syndrome" or "abusive head trauma") (PHAC, 2011), is a serious form of child abuse caused by violent shaking of infants and young children. This shaking can be easily recognized by others as dangerous (PHAC, 2011) and is most often a result of the caregiver's frustration with an infant's crying. Shaken babies can have serious neurological injuries with significant morbidity and mortality.

It is important to understand what happens in SBS. Infants have a large head-to-body ratio, weak neck muscles, and a large amount of water in the brain. Violent shaking causes the brain to rotate within the skull, resulting in shearing forces that tear blood vessels and neurons. The characteristic injuries that occur are intracranial bleeding (subdural and subarachnoid hematomas) and retinal hemorrhages, but they may also include fractures of the ribs and long bones. Most often there are no external signs of injury. SBS is often not an isolated event; in one study, 45% of the children with inflicted traumatic brain injury caused by shaking showed some evidence of prior injury (CPS, Child and Youth Maltreatment Section, 2001/2005).

Victims of SBS can manifest a variety of symptoms, from generalized flulike symptoms to unresponsiveness with impending death (CPS, Child and Youth Maltreatment Section, 2001/2005). Many of the presenting symptoms, such as vomiting, irritability, poor feeding, and listlessness, are often mistaken for common infant and childhood ailments. In more severe forms, presenting symptoms may include seizures, posturing, alterations in level of consciousness, apnea, bradycardia, or death. The long-term outcomes of SBS include seizure disorder; visual impairments, including blindness; developmental delays; hearing loss; cerebral palsy; and mild to profound mental, cognitive, and motor impairments (CPS, Child and Youth Maltreatment Section, 2001/2005). See Chapter 31 for information on child maltreatment.

Nurses can take an active role in preventing SBS by teaching all caregivers about infant crying and techniques to safely cope with inconsolable crying, such as checking the infant for obvious signs of upset (such as hunger, need to burp, illness, discomfort from clothes or pinching, dirty diaper); calling a friend or family member to talk if frustrated; placing the baby safely in his or her crib on the back and leaving the child, checking every 5 to 10 minutes; and talking to a help line or health care provider for support. The Period of PURPLE Crying program has been implemented in many provinces; see Chapter 26, Family-Centred Teaching box, p. 716, for information on the Period of PURPLE Crying (also see Additional Resources at the end of the chapter). This program is designed to help parents understand increased levels of crying that occur at about 2 weeks of age and continue until about 3 to 4 months of age, which is a normal developmental stage when infants cry more and turn purple. The program provides tips on how to soothe infants, such as carrying the infant over the shoulder. Health Link BC (2015) provides tips for parents dealing with children who cry from being overstimulated or overtired. One such tip involves taking the child to a quiet, dark, and safe space, closing the door, and setting a kitchen timer for 15 to 20 minutes. If the child has not settled down after 15 to 20 minutes, parents should check to see whether there is another reason for the crying (see Chapter 26).

NURSING ALERT

Nurses should emphasize to parents the danger of shaking an infant (shaking can cause SBS). Education must include coping mechanisms for caring for children with inconsolable crying.

Nurse's Role in Prevention of Injury

The task of injury prevention can be appreciated only when the potential environmental dangers to which infants are vulnerable are considered. Injury prevention and parent education should be handled on a growth and developmental basis. Nurses must be aware of the possible causes of injury in each age group in order to carry out teaching that involves anticipatory guidance and injury prevention. For example, the guidelines for injury prevention during infancy presented in Box 35-1 should be discussed before the child reaches each age group. Preventive teaching ideally occurs during pregnancy.

Two thirds of all injuries to children occur in the home, thus the importance of safety cannot be overemphasized. The Family-Centred Teaching box contains a home safety checklist that can be presented to parents to increase their awareness of danger areas in the home and assist them in implementing safety devices and practices before their absence leads to injury in infants. In addition, displays such as a safety demonstration board can be helpful in familiarizing parents with inexpensive commercial devices that can be used in the home to prevent injuries (Fig. 35-12). To help parents appreciate the dangers to young children that are present in their home, the nurse can

FAMILY-CENTRED TEACHING

Child Safety Home Checklist

Safety: Fire, Electrical, Burns

__ Guards in front of or around any heating appliance, fireplace, or furnace (including electric heaters)*
__ Electrical wires are hidden or out of reach*
__ No frayed or broken wires; no overloaded sockets
__ Plastic guards or caps over electrical outlets, furniture in front of outlets*
__ Hanging tablecloths are out of reach, away from open fires*
__ Smoke detectors tested and operating properly
__ Kitchen matches stored out of child's reach*
__ Large, deep ashtrays throughout house (if used)
__ Small stoves, heaters, and other hot objects (cigarettes, candles, coffee pots, slow-cookers) are placed where they cannot be tipped over or reached by children
__ Hot water heater is set at 49°C or lower
__ Pot handles are turned toward back of stove, centre of table
__ No loose clothing is worn near stove
__ No cooking or eating of hot foods or liquids with the child standing nearby or sitting in lap
__ All small appliances, such as irons, are turned off, disconnected, and placed out of reach when not in use
__ Cool, not hot, mist vaporizer is used
__ Fire extinguisher is available on each floor and checked periodically
__ Electrical fuse box and gas shutoff accessible
__ Family escape plan in case of a fire is practised periodically; fire escape ladder is available on upper-level floors
__ Telephone number of fire or rescue squad and address of home with nearest cross street posted near phone

Safety: Suffocation and Aspiration

__ Small objects are stored out of reach*
__ Toys inspected for small removable parts or long strings*
__ Hanging crib toys and mobiles placed out of reach
__ Plastic bags are stored away from young child's reach, large plastic garment bags discarded after tying in knots*
__ Mattress or pillow is not covered with plastic or in manner accessible to child*
__ Crib design is according to government regulations (crib slats less than 6 cm apart) with snug-fitting mattress*
__ Crib is positioned away from other furniture or windows*
__ Portable playpen gates are up at all times while in use*
__ Accordion-style gates are not used*
__ Bathroom doors are kept closed and toilet seats down*
__ Faucets are turned off firmly*
__ Pool is fenced with locked gate
__ Proper safety equipment is at poolside
__ Electric garage door openers are stored safely and garage door adjusted to rise when door strikes object
__ Doors of oven, trunks, dishwasher, refrigerator, and front-loading clothes washer and dryer are kept closed*
__ Unused appliance, such as a refrigerator, is securely locked or doors are removed*
__ Food is served in small, noncylindrical pieces*
__ Toy chests are without lids or with lids that securely lock in open position*
__ Buckets and wading pools are kept empty when not in use*
__ Clothesline is above head level
__ At least one member of household is trained in basic life support (cardiopulmonary resuscitation), including first aid for choking

Safety: Poisoning

__ Toxic substances, including batteries, are placed on a high shelf, preferably in locked cabinet
__ Toxic plants are hung or placed out of reach*
__ Excess quantities of cleaning fluids, paints, pesticides, medications, and other toxic substances are not stored in home
__ Used containers of poisonous substances discarded where child cannot obtain access
__ Telephone number of local poison control centre and address of home with nearest cross street posted near phones
__ Medicines are clearly labelled in childproof containers and stored out of reach
__ Household cleaners, disinfectants, and insecticides are kept in their original containers, separate from food, and out of reach
__ Smoking takes place in areas away from children, with no smoking in home

Safety: Falls

__ Nonskid mats, strips, or surfaces in tubs and showers
__ Exits, halls, and passageways in rooms are kept clear of toys, furniture, boxes, or other items that could be obstructive
__ Stairs and halls are well lit, with switches at both top and bottom
__ Sturdy handrails for all steps and stairways
__ Nothing stored on stairways
__ Treads, risers, and carpeting in good repair
__ Glass doors and walls are marked with decals
__ Safety glass is used in doors, windows, and walls
__ Windows and balcony doors are secure and locked
__ Gates are on top and bottom of staircases and elevated areas, such as porch, fire escape*
__ Guardrails are on upstairs windows with locks that limit height of window opening and access to areas such as fire escape*
__ Crib side rails are raised to full height; mattress lowered as child grows*
__ Restraints are used in high chairs or other baby furniture; preferably, walkers with wheels are not used*
__ Scatter rugs are secured in place or used with nonskid backing
__ Walks, patios, and driveways are in good repair

Safety: Bodily Injury

__ Knives, power tools, and unloaded firearms are stored safely or placed in locked cabinet
__ Garden tools are returned to storage racks after use
__ Pets are properly restrained and immunized for rabies
__ Swings, slides, and other outdoor play equipment are kept in safe condition
__ Yard is free of broken glass, nail-studded boards, other litter
__ Cement birdbaths and large flower pots are placed where young child cannot tip them over*

*Safety measures are specific for homes with young children. All safety measures should be implemented in homes where children reside and visit frequently, such as those of grandparents or babysitters. Information about home safety can be obtained at http://www.cdc.gov/parents/infants/safety.html, and related Government of Canada information can be found at http://www.hc-sc.gc.ca/cps-spc/pubs/cons/child-enfant/safe-securite-eng.php.

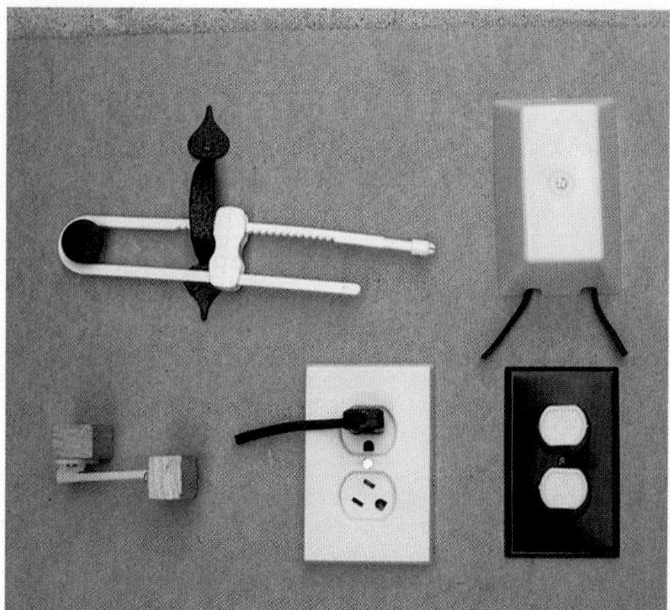

FIGURE 35-12 Safety demonstration board. Clockwise from lower left: Two types of cabinet latches, a shock guard for an electrical outlet in use, and two types of outlet covers (the one with the white cover has passive devices that automatically cover the outlet when a plug is removed).

suggest that they get down on the floor at the child's eye level to survey the environment from a child's viewpoint, looking for any signs of danger.

Injury prevention requires protection of the child and education of the caregiver. Nurses in ambulatory care settings and health maintenance centres and community health nurses are in a favourable position to provide injury education and infant care. Community health nurses are in an ideal role to give anticipatory guidance for injury prevention and infant care, provide immunizations and other services, and monitor growth and development. This is particularly true in rural areas where community health nurses provide essential health care at nursing stations. Nurses in inpatient facilities can use visiting times as an opportunity for discussing injury prevention.

One approach to teaching prevention of injury is to relate why children in various age groups are prone to specific types of injuries. Stressing prevention is just as important as emphasizing the "why" of the injury. However, injury prevention must also be practical. Asking parents for their ideas can lead to realistic suggestions to be followed. For instance, bathroom cleaning agents, cosmetics, and personal care items can be placed on a top shelf in the linen closet and towels or sheets can be stored on the lower shelves and floor.

! NURSING ALERT

Parents should know the telephone number of the local poison centre, place the number on the phone, and call this number in the event of a suspected poisoning. Ipecac, used to induce vomiting, is no longer a standard recommendation. If the child is not breathing, the parent should call 911 immediately.

If an injury has occurred, the nurse should not be too quick to admonish the parent; injuries do not always indicate neglect. It is a difficult task to watch children carefully without overprotecting or unnecessarily confining them. Allowing children to explore while maintaining consistent, age-appropriate limits is sound advice.

Parents need to remember that infants and young children cannot anticipate danger or understand when it is or is not present. Also, infants have no cognitive concept of cause and effect and therefore cannot relate meaning to experiences or potential dangers. A dead electrical wire may present no actual harm; but if the child is allowed to play with it, a poor behaviour develops and may be practised when the child encounters a live wire. Although it is always wise to explain why something is dangerous, it must be remembered that small children need to be physically removed from the situation.

It is not easy to teach safety, supervise closely, and refrain from saying "no" multiple times a day. Parents become acutely aware of this dilemma as soon as the infant learns to crawl. Preventing injuries to children is usually the first reason for limit-setting and discipline, but limits are also set to prevent danger to valuable household objects. When small children are in the home, dangerous objects must be removed or guarded and valuable articles placed out of reach.

When children are taught the meaning of "no," they should also be taught what "yes" means. Children should be praised for playing with suitable toys, their efforts at behaving or listening should be reinforced, and innovative and creative recreational toys should be provided for them. Infants love to tear paper and avidly pursue books, magazines, or newspapers left on the floor. Instead of always scolding them for destroying a valued book, child-safe books (such as those constructed of fabric) can be kept available for them to play with. If they enjoy pots and pans, a cabinet can be arranged with safe utensils for them to explore.

One additional factor must be stressed concerning injury prevention and education: Children are imitators; they copy what they see and hear. *Practising safety teaches safety*. This applies to parents and their children and to nurses and their patients. Saying one thing but doing another confuses children and can lead to difficulties as the child grows older.

Immunizations

One of the most dramatic advances in pediatrics has been the decline of infectious diseases during the twentieth century because of the widespread use of immunization for preventable diseases. In recent years, however, childhood vaccines have been widely criticized, and fear related to vaccine components has prompted some families to avoid childhood vaccination. In addition, many of the diseases for which children are vaccinated are rarely seen on a large-scale basis, leading some parents to believe that such vaccines are no longer necessary in the twenty-first century. A variety of information is available suggesting that parents avoid childhood vaccines altogether; a number of "vaccine myths" exist, which are based on erroneous information. It is the nurse's responsibility to provide parents with accurate information about childhood illnesses and available vaccines; the parents must then make an informed decision about the child's vaccinations. Nurses should address parents' concerns about childhood vaccines and avoid judgemental attitudes regarding the parents' decision to not vaccinate their children.

Although many of the immunizations can be given to individuals of any age, the recommended primary schedule begins during infancy and, with the exception of boosters, is completed during early childhood. Therefore, the discussion of childhood immunizations for diphtheria, tetanus, pertussis (DTaP); polio; measles, mumps, rubella (MMR); *Haemophilus influenzae* type b (Hib); hepatitis A virus (HAV), hepatitis B virus (HBV); pneumococcus; influenza; meningococcus; and chickenpox is included here, under health promotion during infancy. Selected vaccines generally reserved for children considered at high risk for the respective disease are also discussed here and as appropriate throughout the text. The Public Health Agency of Canada (2015a) has a nationally notifiable diseases list that are communicable diseases that have been identified by the federal government and all provinces and territories as priorities for monitoring and control efforts. The public can access the website and discover the trends in these communicable diseases since 1924. (See also Chapter 37, Communicable Diseases, for a discussion of several of the diseases for which vaccines are available.)

Schedule for Immunizations

In Canada, recommendations for immunization are from the National Advisory Committee on Immunization, under the authority of the Minister of Health and Public Health Agency of Canada (PHAC) (see Additional Resources at the end of this chapter). These recommendations are interpreted differently among the provinces and territories. Most countries have different immunization recommendations. Thus, with the increasing number of children in Canada who come from other countries, it is important that nurses obtain detailed immunization information from the family when their children are being immunized. Nurses also need to keep informed of the latest advances and changes in immunization policies and guidelines (PHAC, 2015b).

Children who began primary immunization at the recommended age but then fail to receive all of the doses do not need to begin the series again but instead should receive only the missed doses. When there is doubt that the child will return for immunization according to the optimum schedule, any of the recommended vaccines can be administered simultaneously. Parenteral vaccines are given in separate syringes in different injection sites.

Recommendations for Routine Immunizations

Because of constant changes in the pharmaceutical industry, trade names of some single and combination vaccines in this section may differ from those currently available. The reader is encouraged to access the Canadian Immunization Guide (PHAC, 2015b), which is updated periodically.

Hepatitis B virus (HBV). Hepatitis B virus (HBV) is a highly infectious disease that can be transmitted by blood and infected body fluids. This virus can be prevented by vaccination. While Canada is a region of low endemicity, certain vulnerable populations, including Indigenous peoples, men who have sex with men, street youth, and people who are or have been incarcerated, are disproportionately affected. The low prevalence is mainly attributable to Canada's universal HBV immunization programs. About 60% of individuals with chronic hepatitis B infection are not aware of their status and transmit the infection (PHAC, 2014a). See Chapter 46 for more information on hepatitis.

HBV is a significant pediatric disease because HBV infections that occur during childhood and adolescence can lead to fatal consequences from cirrhosis or liver cancer during adulthood. Up to 90% of infants infected perinatally and 25 to 50% of children infected before age 5 years become HBV carriers. In addition, the incidence of HBV infection increases rapidly during adolescence (AAP, Committee on Infectious Diseases, & Pickering, 2015). The child with hepatitis B has few or no symptoms.

It is recommended that newborns receive the hepatitis B vaccine (HepB) within 12 hours of birth if the mother is infected with hepatitis B, because of the high risk of long-term complications if infection occurs (see Chapter 26 , Medication Guide: Hepatitis B Vaccine, p. 702). Both full-term and preterm infants born to mothers whose HBsAg status is positive should also receive hepatitis B immune globulin (HBIG), 0.5 mL (see Chapter 26, Medication Guide: Hepatitis B Immune Globulin, p. 702). The HepB vaccine and HBIG should be given at two different injection sites. Parental consent must be obtained before administering the medication. If the mother's status is unknown, testing should be done at the time of delivery. If maternal HBV status is not available within 12 hours of delivery, serious consideration should be given to administering HepB vaccine and HBIG while the results are pending, taking into account the mother's risk factors and erring on the side of providing vaccine and HBIG if there is any suspicion that the mother could be infected (PHAC, 2015b). Because the immune response to HepB is not optimum in newborns weighing less than 2000 g, the first HepB dose should be given to such infants at 1 month, as long as the mother's hepatitis B surface antigen (HBsAg) status is negative (PHAC, 2015b). In the event that the preterm infant is given a dose at birth, the current recommendation is that the infant be given the full series (three additional doses) at 1, 2, and 6 months of age. The PHAC (2015b) encourages immunization of all children before or in early adolescence. Since the early 1990s, all provinces and territories have had either a universal school-based hepatitis B vaccination program aimed at children aged 9 to 13 or an infant vaccination program (PHAC, 2015b).

The vaccine is given intramuscularly in the vastus lateralis in newborns (see Fig. 26-15) or in the deltoid for older infants and children. Regardless of age, the dorsogluteal site should never be used for intramuscular injections, because it has been associated with low antibody **seroconversion** rates, indicating a reduced immune response. No data exist regarding the seroconversion when the ventrogluteal site is used. The vaccine can be safely administered simultaneously at a separate site with DTaP, MMR, and Hib vaccines.

Hepatitis A virus (HAV). HAV has been recognized as a significant child health problem, particularly in communities where widespread childhood HepA immunization has not been historically recommended. HAV is spread by the fecal–oral route and from person-to-person contact, by ingestion of contaminated food or water, and rarely by blood transfusion. The illness has an abrupt onset, with fever, malaise, anorexia, nausea, abdominal discomfort, dark urine, and jaundice being the most common clinical signs of infection. In children under 6 years of age the disease may be asymptomatic, and jaundice is rarely evident.

In Canada, universal HepA vaccination is not recommended. Individuals at risk, such as those living in communities where hepatitis A is endemic, such as specific Canadian Indigenous regions or those travelling to countries where hepatitis A is endemic, should be immunized (PHAC, 2015b). If HepA vaccine is given, it is given in a two-dose series with the second dose administered no sooner than 6 months after the first dose.

Diphtheria. Although cases of diphtheria are rarely seen in Canada, the disease can result in significant morbidity. Respiratory manifestations include respiratory nasopharyngitis or obstructive laryngotracheitis with upper airway obstruction. The cutaneous manifestations of the disease include vaginal, otic, conjunctival, or cutaneous lesions, which are primarily seen in the tropics (PHAC, 2014b). Diphtheria vaccine is commonly administered (1) in combination with tetanus and acellular pertussis vaccines (DTaP) or DTaP and Hib vaccines for children younger than 7 years of age, (2) in combination with a conjugate Hib vaccine, (3) in a combined vaccine with tetanus (DT) for children younger than 7 years of age who have some contraindication to receiving pertussis vaccine, or (4) as a single antigen when combined antigen preparations are not indicated. Although the diphtheria vaccine does not produce absolute immunity, protective antitoxin persists for 10 years or more when given according to the recommended schedule, and boosters are given every 10 years for life (see discussion below for adolescent diphtheria and acellular pertussis and tetanus toxoid recommendation). Several vaccines contain diphtheria toxoid (Hib, meningococcal, pneumococcal), but this does not confer immunity to the disease.

Tetanus. Tetanus (also known as lockjaw) is an infection spread by a bacterium. The bacterium is present in dirt, soil, and dust but can also be found in human and animal feces. The tetanus bacteria can enter the body through a cut in the skin. Tetanus affects the nerves that control muscles and they become stiff and painful and also make swallowing and breathing difficult. Additional symptoms include headache, seizures, fever, diaphoresis, high blood pressure, and tachycardia. Without proper intervention, tetanus can be fatal. Tetanus is preventable through vaccination (PHAC, 2014c).

Two forms of tetanus vaccine—tetanus toxoid and tetanus immune globulin (TIG) (human)—are available. Tetanus toxoid is used for routine primary immunization, usually in one of the combinations listed for diphtheria, and provides protective antitoxin levels for approximately 10 years.

For wound management, passive immunity is available with TIG. This is recommended for children who have immune deficiency, in addition to the vaccine. In persons with a history of two previous doses of tetanus toxoid, a booster dose of the toxoid can be given. Separate syringes and different sites are used when tetanus toxoid and TIG are given concurrently.

Pertussis. Pertussis (whooping cough) is a highly contagious infection of the respiratory tract caused by the bacterium *Bordetella pertussis*. It is preventable by vaccination. *B. pertussis* is a Gram-negative aerobic bacterium. Pertussis is a toxin-mediated disease in which toxins produced by the bacteria are responsible for the majority of its symptoms. The initial catarrhal stage is characterized by runny nose, sneezing, low-grade fever, and a mild cough, similar to a cold. After 1 to 2 weeks of gradually worsening cough, the paroxysmal stage begins with bursts of rapid coughing, ending with an inspiratory whoop and sometimes post-tussive vomiting. This stage can last from 2 to 8 weeks. The last stage is convalescent recovery; it is gradual and may take weeks to months (PHAC, 2014d).

Pertussis vaccine is recommended for all children 6 weeks through 6 years of age (up to the seventh birthday) who have no neurological contraindications to its use. Concerns over outbreaks of the disease in the past decade have prompted discussion about vaccinating infants and adults; many cases of pertussis have been seen in children less than 6 months or persons over 7 years of age, both groups falling in the category for which there was inadequate vaccine protection from pertussis infection (PHAC, 2015b).

Pertussis vaccine is only available in combined form with other agents such as diphtheria (D) and tetanus (T) toxoids with or without inactivated polio vaccine (IPV) and Hib conjugate vaccine (Hib).

The acellular pertussis vaccine contains one or more immunogens derived from the *B. pertussis* organism. Health care workers who may be susceptible to pertussis as a result of waning immunity and who have potential exposure to children or adults with pertussis should take the necessary protective precautions against droplet contamination (wear procedural or surgical masks and practise hand hygiene). The diagnosis of pertussis may be missed or delayed in unvaccinated infants, who often are seen with respiratory distress and apnea without the typical cough. Additional guidelines for prevention and treatment of pertussis among health care workers and close contacts are found in the *Canadian Immunization Guide* (PHAC, 2015b) and the *2015 Red Book: Report of the Committee on Infectious Diseases* (AAP, Committee on Infectious Diseases, & Pickering, 2015).

Polio. Poliomyelitis is a disease that may cause irreversible paralysis in less than 1% of infected individuals. It is a highly infectious disease that is spread from person to person, principally through the fecal-oral route (PHAC, 2016). Canada was certified polio-free in 1994. The last major Canadian epidemic of wild poliovirus occurred in 1959, with 1887 paralytic cases reported. Smaller clusters occurred after that time.

An all-inactivated polio virus (IPV) schedule for routine childhood polio vaccination is now recommended; oral poliovirus (OPV) is no longer used in Canada. For routine immunization beginning in infancy, four doses of IPV are recommended, in combination with other routinely administered vaccines

(DTaP and Hib) at 2 months, 4 months, 18 months, and 4 to 6 years of age (preschool booster). The fourth dose is not needed if the third dose is given on or after the fourth birthday. It is acceptable to give an additional dose of IPV at 6 months of age for convenience of administration in combination with DTaP and Hib (PHAC, 2016).

The change from the exclusive use of OPV to the exclusive use of IPV is related to the rare risk of vaccine-associated polio paralysis (VAPP) from OPV.

It is important for all health care providers to remain vigilant about polio vaccinations. One infected child puts children in all countries at risk and could result in as many as 200,000 new cases every year, and within 10 years, all over the world. Afghanistan and Pakistan remain the only two countries with individuals with active polio infections (World Health Organization, 2016).

Measles. Measles is a highly contagious, serious respiratory viral disease characterized by fever, cough, coryza, conjunctivitis, and generalized maculopapular erythematous rash. Measles infection can result in serious complications such as blindness, encephalitis, or severe respiratory infections such as pneumonia. Measles is a preventable disease by vaccination (PHAC, 2013).

For routine immunization of all children, two doses of measles vaccine should be given. Infants should receive a first dose combined with mumps and rubella vaccines (MMR) on or shortly after their first birthday; the second dose should be given after 15 months of age but before school entry. It is convenient to link this dose with other routinely scheduled immunizations. Options include giving it with the scheduled immunization at 15 or 18 months of age, with school entry immunization at 4 to 6 years, or at any intervening age that is practicable (such as entry to day care).

Two doses of vaccine given at least 4 weeks apart are recommended for children who

- Have missed MMR immunization on the routine schedule
- Are without an immunization record
- Are without reliable records of measles immunization (e.g., migrants)
- Were given live measles vaccine and immune globulin (Ig) separated by an inappropriate interval (PHAC, 2015b).

Vaccine may be recommended for children less than 12 months of age during outbreaks or before international travel to an area where measles is common. MMR may be given as early as 6 months of age. Under these circumstances, or if vaccine was inappropriately given before the child's first birthday, two doses of MMR should still be given after the first birthday.

Individuals born before 1970 are thought to be immune from exposure to natural measles virus. Because of the continuing occurrence of measles in older children and young adults, potentially susceptible adolescents and young adults should be identified and immunized if two doses of measles vaccine have not been administered previously or the person had a confirmed case of the illness (PHAC, 2015b).

In 2014, between January and May, 103 cases of measles were reported among several Canadian provinces (PHAC, 2014e). This was due to several factors: increased travel of Canadians importing the disease, an increased incidence of measles in countries with a high population exchange with Canada (France, the Netherlands, the Philippines), and suboptimal immunization coverage in small pockets across Canada (PHAC, 2014e). Parents who have infants under 1 year of age who have not been immunized need to be encouraged to be vigilant about exposure of their child to nonimmunized children and watch for the signs and symptoms of measles, if exposed.

Mumps. Mumps is an acute infectious disease caused by the mumps virus. The symptoms include the swelling of one or more of the salivary glands, typically the parotid glands. Usually the infection is mild, although it can result in complications such as viral meningitis and orchitis/oophoritis. It is preventable by vaccination.

One dose of MMR vaccine should be administered for the purpose of mumps protection, with the second dose given for full measles protection. The first dose should be given on or after the first birthday and the second dose given at least 1 month after the first dose and before school entry. The standard dose is 0.5 mL.

In Canada, since the approval of mumps vaccine in 1969, the number of reported mumps cases has decreased by more than 99%, from an average of nearly 33,000 cases reported per year from 1951 to 1955 to approximately 180 cases per year from 2011 to 2013. Large Canadian outbreaks have been rare in recent years, but from 2007 to 2010, large mumps outbreaks were reported in several Canadian provinces, including British Columbia, Alberta, Ontario, Quebec, Nova Scotia, and New Brunswick. In several of the outbreaks, the most mumps occurred in individuals aged 20 to 29 years, many of whom had received only one dose of a mumps-containing vaccine. Other outbreaks occurred in communities that were largely unimmunized for religious or philosophical reasons. These outbreaks tended to be in a younger age group and similar to outbreaks that were seen in the pre-vaccine era (PHAC, 2014f).

Rubella. Rubella is a relatively mild infection in children. The main goal of immunization is the prevention of rubella infection in pregnancy, which may give rise to congenital rubella syndrome (CRS). This syndrome can result in miscarriage, stillbirth, and fetal malformations, including congenital heart disease, cataracts, deafness, and mental disabilities. Fetal infection can occur at any stage of pregnancy, but the risk of fetal damage following maternal infection is particularly high in the earliest months after conception (85% in the first trimester). One dose of rubella-containing vaccine (MMR) is recommended routinely for all children on or as soon as practical after their first birthday. The second dose, given for measles protection, should be given after 15 months of age and before school entry. The acceptable minimum interval between the first and second dose is at least 1 month. All nonimmunized prepubertal children, susceptible adolescents, and adult women in the child-bearing age group should be vaccinated, particularly those who have emigrated from countries that do not routinely vaccinate for rubella. Because the live attenuated virus may cross the placenta and theoretically present a risk to the developing fetus, rubella vaccine is not given to any pregnant woman (PHAC, 2015b).

Varicella. Varicella (chickenpox) is a common and highly infectious disease of childhood. It is caused by varicella-zoster virus (VZV). Symptoms appear in 10 to 21 days after infection and last about 2 weeks and include an irritating blister-like rash. The majority of children have a relatively mild illness, but severe illness may occur in adults and people with depressed immunity due to existing illness or because of a treatment that they are receiving, such as chemotherapy (PHAC, 2012a). It is preventable by vaccination.

Unlike the United States, Canada does not have as a goal the elimination of varicella, and the National Advisory Committee on Immunization (NACI) continues to recommend a single-dose vaccine strategy for children (two doses for adults and adolescents at least 13 years of age). Administration of the cell-free live-attenuated varicella vaccine (Varivax) is recommended for any susceptible child (one who lacks proof of varicella vaccination or has a reliable history of varicella infection). A single dose of varicella vaccine is recommended for children ages 12 to 15 months. The NACI does not recommend booster doses (PHAC, 2015b). A single dose of 0.5 mL should be given by subcutaneous injection. Children 13 years of age or older who are susceptible should receive two doses administered at least 4 weeks apart. The vaccine should be kept frozen in the lyophilic form (stable particles that readily go into solution) and used within 30 minutes of being reconstituted to ensure viral potency.

Varicella vaccine may be administered simultaneously with MMR. However, separate syringes and injection sites should be used. If they are not administered simultaneously, the interval between administration of varicella vaccine and MMR should be at least 1 month. Varicella vaccine may also be given simultaneously with DTaP, IPV, HBV, or Hib (PHAC, 2015b).

Pneumococcal infections. Streptococcal pneumococci are responsible for a number of bacterial infections in children under 2 years of age, which may cause serious morbidity and mortality. Among these are generalized infections such as septicemia and meningitis or localized infections such as otitis media, sinusitis, and pneumonia. These illnesses are particularly problematic in children who attend day care facilities (the incidence among children in day care centres is two to three times higher than in children not attending out-of-home day care) and in those who are immunocompromised.

A pneumococcal conjugate vaccine (Prevnar) is approved for use in Canada for children from 6 weeks to 9 years of age and is composed of the purified polysaccharides of the capsular antigens of seven *Streptococcus pneumoniae* serotypes, individually conjugated to CRM197 (cross-reacting material 197), a purified nontoxic variant of diphtheria toxin (PHAC, 2015b).

The recommended optimal schedule for infants is four doses of the conjugate vaccine administered at 2, 4, 6, and 12 to 15 months of age. Infants of very low birth weight (<1500 grams) should be given their first dose according to their chronological age and not their calculated gestational age. Children 7 to 11 months old who have not been previously immunized against invasive pneumococcal disease (IPD) should receive two doses at least 4 weeks apart, followed by a third dose after 12 months of age and at least 2 months after the second dose. Children 12 to 23 months of age not previously immunized should receive two doses at least 2 months apart. For children 2 to 5 years old, one dose is sufficient for healthy children, but two doses given 2 months apart are recommended for children with chronic conditions that place them at higher risk of IPD (PHAC, 2015b). The long-term efficacy of the conjugate pneumococcal vaccines is not known, but immunological memory has been demonstrated 18 months after two to three doses in infancy and up to 20 months after one dose in children 2 to 3 years of age.

Conjugate pneumococcal vaccine is recommended for routine administration to all children 23 months of age or younger. It is also recommended for children 24 to 59 months of age at higher risk of IPD: those who attend child care centres; Indigenous children; those who have sickle cell disease and other sickle cell hemoglobinopathies or who have other types of functional or anatomical asplenia, HIV infection, immunocompromising conditions (e.g., primary immunodeficiencies; malignancies; conditions resulting from immunosuppressive therapy, solid organ transplantation, or the use of long-term systemic corticosteroids; nephrotic syndrome), or chronic medical conditions (e.g., chronic cardiac and pulmonary disease such as bronchopulmonary dysplasia, diabetes mellitus, chronic renal disease, or cerebrospinal fluid leak); and children with cochlear implants or those receiving cochlear implants (PHAC, 2015b).

The polysaccharide vaccine (PPV) is not recommended for children less than 2 years of age, as it is relatively ineffective and the conjugate vaccine is superior. Children aged 2 years to less than 5 years of age who are at increased risk of IPD should receive the conjugate vaccine with the polysaccharide vaccine being used as a booster dose in this age group to increase the serotype coverage.

The polysaccharide vaccine should be given to all individuals older than 5 years of age who have not received the vaccine previously and who are at higher risk of IPD (PHAC, 2015b).

Haemophilus influenzae *type B (Hib).* Hib conjugate vaccines protect against a number of serious infections caused by Hib, especially bacterial meningitis, epiglottitis, bacterial pneumonia, septic arthritis, and sepsis (Hib is not associated with the viruses that cause influenza, or "flu"). Hib vaccines that are currently available in Canada include PedvaxHIB, Pentacel, and ActHIB. These conjugate vaccines connect Hib to a nontoxic form of another organism, such as meningococcal protein or diphtheria protein. While there is no antibody response to these nontoxic proteins, they significantly improve the antibody response to Hib, especially in infants. The use of combination vaccines provides equivalent immunogenicity and decreases the number of injections an infant receives; however, it is important that they be given to the appropriate-age child.

All Canadian provinces and territories include Hib conjugate vaccine in their immunization program for children.

The 2009 Centers for Disease Control and Prevention (CDC) immunization guidelines indicate limited data for administering the Hib vaccine to persons 5 years and older. However, children with sickle cell disease, leukemia, or HIV infection or children who have had a splenectomy may benefit from one dose of the Hib vaccine (PHAC, 2015b).

When possible, the Hib conjugate vaccine used at the first vaccination should be used for all subsequent vaccinations in the primary series. All Hib vaccines are administered by intramuscular injection using a separate syringe and at a site separate from any concurrent vaccinations.

Influenza. Influenza vaccine may be administered to any healthy individual for whom contraindications are not present. To reduce the morbidity and mortality associated with influenza and the impact of illness in communities, immunization programs should focus on those at high risk of influenza-related complications, those capable of transmitting influenza to individuals at high risk of complications, and those who provide essential community services. However, significant morbidity and societal costs are also associated with seasonal interpandemic influenza illness and its complications occurring in healthy children and adults. For this reason, healthy children and adults should be encouraged to receive the vaccine annually, particularly children aged 6 months to 18 years (PHAC, 2015b). Children who have a reported anaphylactic hypersensitivity to eggs should not receive the vaccine.

The vaccine is administered in early fall before the flu season begins and is repeated yearly for ongoing protection. The intramuscular vaccine is administered as two separate doses 4 weeks apart in first-time recipients under the age of 9 years (PHAC, 2015b). The dose is 0.25 mL for children ages 6 to 35 months and 0.5 mL for children 3 years and above. The vaccine may be given simultaneously with other vaccines but at a separate site. The vaccine is administered yearly because different strains of influenza are used each year in the manufacture of the vaccine.

Meningococcal infections. Invasive meningococcal disease (IMD) is an acute and serious communicable disease caused by the bacterium *Neisseria meningitides.* This bacterium results in meningitis, septicemia (meningococcemia), or both. Meningococcal infections are also responsible for significant morbidities, including limb or digit amputation, skin scarring, hearing loss, and neurological disabilities. Symptoms include sudden fever, drowsiness, irritability or agitation, intense headache, nausea and vomiting, stiff neck, and photophobia. Most commonly, invasive disease leads to meningitis or septicemia, as well as a characteristic nonblanching petechial or purpuric rash (PHAC, 2015c). The NACI recommends routine immunization against meningococcal disease and the Committee to Advise on Tropical Medicine and Travel (CATMAT) recommends immunization before travel to high-risk meningococcal destinations (PHAC, 2015c).

IMD is endemic in Canada, showing periods of increased activity roughly every 10 to 15 years with no consistent pattern. The incidence rate varies considerably with different serogroups of *Neisseria meningitidis,* age groups, geographical locations, and time. Implementation of universal meningococcal C immunization programs will also affect disease epidemiology (PHAC, 2015b).

Since 1985, the overall incidence of IMD has remained at or below 2 per 100,000 per year. Overall, the incidence rate has been highest among children less than 1 year of age and then declines as age increases, except for a smaller peak in the 15- to 19-year age group. An average of 298 cases of meningococcal disease have been reported annually. Disease occurs year round, but with seasonal variation, with most cases occurring in the winter months (PHAC, 2015b).

Meningococcal C conjugate vaccines are recommended for routine immunization of infants. The recommended schedule differs depending on the vaccine used. Three doses of either Meningitec or Menjugate are recommended to be given to infants beginning no earlier than 2 months of age and separated by at least 1 month. Two doses of NeisVac-C should be administered at least 2 months apart, with the first dose not to be administered before 2 months of age. At least one dose of the primary immunization series should be given after 5 months of age. Infants 4 to 11 months of age who have not previously received the vaccine should be immunized with two doses given at least 4 weeks apart. Infants born prematurely should receive the vaccine at the same chronological age as term infants. Polysaccharide vaccine is not recommended for routine infant immunization.

There have been recent concerns regarding reports of an association between quadrivalent meningococcal conjugate vaccine (Menactra) and cases of Guillain-Barré syndrome in vaccinated persons 11 to 19 years of age; onset of symptoms occurred within 2 to 23 days of vaccination. A preliminary survey by the CDC (Strikas & CDC, 2015) indicates insufficient data to change the 2005 recommendation for adolescents, college freshmen residing in dormitories, and other high-risk populations.

Tuberculosis. Active, infectious tuberculosis (TB) disease is caused by a bacterium spread through the air from person to person. The TB infection is most infectious and is transmitted by an individual who has active TB disease of the lungs or airways via coughing, sneezing, singing, playing a wind instrument, or sometimes even just talking. Active TB is most infectious when it is found in the person's sputum. The symptoms of active, infectious TB disease of the lungs or airways include a significant cough lasting longer than 3 weeks, pain in the chest, coughing up blood or sputum, weakness or feeling very tired, weight loss, lack of appetite, chills, fever, and night sweats (PHAC, 2012b).

Bacille Calmette-Guérin (BCG) is the collective term applied to a family of live, attenuated vaccines derived from the passage of *Mycobacterium bovis.* In Canada there has been a longstanding interest in BCG vaccinations and was at one time universal. However, researchers have questioned the efficacy of the vaccine. In recent years its use has been limited to the Indigenous populations, in which it has been part of a TB elimination plan. There have been reports of disseminated BCG in children born with congenital immunodeficiencies and the vaccinations are now being phased out of this group. Vaccination of Indigenous infants has now been discontinued in the Atlantic Provinces and in Quebec and British Columbia. In Alberta, the rationale for continued use of the BCG has been challenged and systematic withdrawal has begun. On the prairies and in the territories, the benefits of BCG vaccination in preventing severe forms of TB in infants and young children may still outweigh any risks (PHAC, 2014g).

Recommendations for Selected Immunizations

Two additional vaccines are recommended for children and adolescents at high risk for particular diseases. Two rotavirus vaccines, RotaTeq and Rotarix, are available for distribution in Canada. Rotavirus is one of the leading causes of severe diarrhea in infants and young children. RotaTeq is licensed for administration to infants 6 to 12 weeks of age, with two additional doses administered at 4- to 10-week intervals but not after 32 weeks of age. The dose is 2 mL, and the product must be protected from light until administration. Rotarix (1 mL) may be administered beginning at 6 weeks of age, with a second dose at least 4 weeks after the first dose but before 24 weeks of age. Both vaccines are administered orally. At the time of publication, the rotavirus vaccine was covered by all provincial or territorial health care plans, except for New Brunswick, Nova Scotia, and Nunavut, where it must be paid for out of pocket (Government of Canada, 2016b).

Reactions

Vaccines used for routine immunizations are among the safest and most reliable medications available. However, minor adverse effects do occur after many of the immunizations, and, rarely, a serious reaction may result from the vaccine (PHAC, 2015b).

With inactivated antigens, such as DTaP, adverse effects are most likely to occur within a few hours or days of administration and are usually limited to local tenderness, **erythema**, and swelling at the injection site; low-grade fever; and behavioural changes (e.g., drowsiness, fretfulness, eating less, and prolonged or unusual cry). Local reactions tend to be less severe when the deltoid (except in small infants) rather than the vastus lateralis site is used and when a needle of sufficient length to deposit the vaccine in the muscle is used (see Atraumatic Care box). Rarely, more severe reactions may occur, especially with pertussis (Table 35-2). Reactions to DTaP tend to be more severe if they occurred with a previous immunization; fever, swelling, irritability, and pain are more common after the fourth DTaP vaccination in the series. Acetaminophen may help reduce this discomfort and should be given in an age-appropriate dose and time interval.

Hib vaccine is one of the safest vaccines available but may be associated with low-grade fever and mild local reactions at the site of injection, which resolve rapidly. Fever (temperature higher than 38.5°C) may rarely occur.

A number of inactive components are incorporated in vaccines to enhance their effectiveness and safety. Some of these components include preservatives, stabilizers, adjuvants, antibiotics, and purified culture medium proteins to enhance effectiveness. A child may react to the preservative in the vaccine rather than the vaccine component; an example of this is the HepB vaccine, which is prepared from yeast cultures. Yeast hypersensitivity would preclude one from receiving that particular vaccine. Trace amounts of neomycin are used to decrease bacterial growth within certain vaccine preparations, and

ATRAUMATIC CARE
Immunizations

Needle length and gauge size are important factors and must be considered for each individual child; fewer reactions to immunizations are observed when the vaccine is given deep into the muscle rather than into subcutaneous tissue. Deep intramuscular tissue has a better blood supply and fewer pain receptors than adipose tissue, thus providing an optimum site for immunizations with fewer adverse effects.

To minimize local reactions from vaccines:

- The recommended needle length for newborn to 2 months is 16 mm (5/8 inch).
- Select a needle of adequate length (16 mm in infants) to deposit the antigen deep in the muscle mass.
- Toddlers and older children require a needle length of 16 to 25 mm for deltoid, or 25 to 32 mm for vastus lateralis.
- Adolescents require a needle length of 25 to 38 mm in deltoid or vastus lateralis.
- Inject into the vastus lateralis or ventrogluteal muscle; the deltoid may be used in children 18 months of age or older. Do not withdraw plunger in syringe after injecting needle into the muscle.

Use one or more of the following techniques to minimize pain:

- Apply a topical anaesthetic such as EMLA (lidocaine-prilocaine) or Maxilene to the injection site and cover with an occlusive dressing for at least 1 hour.
- Apply the topical anaesthetic LMX4 (4% lidocaine) to the injection site 30 minutes before the injection; there is no evidence that an occlusive dressing is required except to prevent ingestion or accidental application to the eyes in infants.
- Apply a vapocoolant spray (e.g., ethyl chloride or FluoriMethane) directly to the skin or to a cotton ball, which is placed on the skin for 15 seconds immediately before the injection.
- There is evidence that a concentrated oral sucrose solution (24%) and non-nutritive sucking (NNS) (pacifier) decrease the pain related to minor invasive procedures in newborns and infants (Harrison, Yamada, & Stevens, 2010). Hatfield (2008) found that 2- and 4-month-old infants who received a 0.6 mL/kg dose of 24% sucrose and NNS 2 minutes before immunization administration had decreased pain behavioural responses in comparison to a control group of infants who received only sterile water and NNS 2 minutes before the injection. Liaw, Zeng, Yang, et al. (2011) found that NNS and oral sucrose provided analgesia to newborns receiving the hepatitis B vaccine. Therefore, it is recommended that a concentrated oral sucrose solution (1 to 2 mL) be administered orally 2 minutes before the injection, during the injection, and up to 3 minutes after the procedure to decrease newborn pain with immunizations.
- NOTE: Changing the needle on the syringe after drawing up the vaccine and before injecting it has not been shown to make a difference with local reactions.

persons with documented anaphylactic reactions to neomycin should avoid those vaccines. Most vaccine preparations now contain vial stoppers with a synthetic rubber to prevent latex allergy reactions; however, health care personnel administering vaccines should make sure that the package insert specifies there is no latex in the stopper. In the event that an individual has had a severe reaction to a vaccine and subsequent immunizations are required, an allergist should be consulted to determine the best course of action. The influenza vaccine contains small amounts of egg protein; thus children who have severe allergy

TABLE 35-2 CONTRAINDICATIONS AND PRECAUTIONS TO VACCINATIONS*

TRUE CONTRAINDICATIONS	PRECAUTIONS†	NOT CONTRAINDICATIONS (VACCINES MAY BE ADMINISTERED)
General for All Vaccines (DTaP, IPV, MMR, Hib, HepB, Varicella, PCV, HepA, Influenza, Meningococcal)		
Anaphylactic reaction to vaccine is contraindication to further doses of that vaccine or to use of vaccines containing that substance Moderate or severe illnesses with or without fever		Mild to moderate local reaction (soreness, redness, swelling) after a dose of injectable antigen Mild acute illness with or without low-grade fever Current antimicrobial therapy Convalescent phase of illnesses Prematurity (same dosage and indications as for normal, full-term infants) Recent exposure to infectious disease History of penicillin or other nonspecific allergies or family history of such allergies
Diphtheria, Tetanus, and Pertussis or Acellular Pertussis Vaccine (DTP or DTaP)		
Encephalopathy within 7 days of administration of previous dose of DTaP	Fever of ≥40.5°C within 48 hr after vaccination with prior dose of DTaP Collapse or shock-like state (hypotonic-hyporesponsive episode) within 48 hr of receiving prior dose of DTaP Seizures within 3 days of receiving prior dose of DTaP‡ Persistent, inconsolable crying lasting ≥3 hr within 48 hr of receiving prior dose of DTaP	Temperature of <40.5°C after previous dose of DTaP Family history of seizures‡ Family history of sudden infant death syndrome Family history of adverse event after DTaP administration
Diphtheria, Tetanus (DT, Td)		
Severe allergic reaction after a previous dose or to a vaccine component	GBS ≤6 wk after previous dose of tetanus toxoid–containing vaccine Moderate or severe acute illness with or without fever	Same as DTaP or DTP
Inactivated Poliovirus Vaccine (IPV)		
Anaphylactic reaction to neomycin or streptomycin	Pregnancy	Breastfeeding Diarrhea
Measles, Mumps, Rubella Vaccine (MMR)		
Pregnancy Known altered immunodeficiency (hematological and solid tumours, congenital immunodeficiency, long-term immunosuppressive therapy)	Recent immune globulin administration Immune globulin products and MMR should not be given simultaneously; if unavoidable, give at different sites and revaccinate or test for seroconversion in 3 mo; if immune globulin is given first, MMR should not be given for at least 3–6 mo, depending on dose; if MMR is given first, immune globulin should not be given for 2 wk. Thrombocytopenia or thrombocytopenic purpura	Tuberculosis or positive tuberculin skin test Simultaneous tuberculosis skin testing§ Breastfeeding Pregnancy of mother of recipient Immunodeficient family member or household contact Infection with HIV Nonanaphylactic reactions to eggs or neomycin Consider MMR for mildly symptomatic HIV-infected children (PHAC, 2015b)

Continued

TABLE 35-2 CONTRAINDICATIONS AND PRECAUTIONS TO VACCINATIONS—cont'd

TRUE CONTRAINDICATIONS	PRECAUTIONS†	NOT CONTRAINDICATIONS (VACCINES MAY BE ADMINISTERED)
***Haemophilus influenzae* Type b Vaccine (Hib)**		
None identified		History of Hib disease
Hepatitis B Virus Vaccine (HepB)		
Anaphylactic reaction to common baker's yeast	Preterm birth	Pregnancy‖
Pneumococcal Vaccine (PCV)		
Severe allergic reaction after a previous dose or to a vaccine component	Moderate or severe acute illness with or without fever A child who has received pneumococcal polysaccharide vaccine (PPV) previously should wait at least 2 mo before receiving PCV.	Minor illnesses with or without fever Mild upper respiratory tract infection Allergic rhinitis
Varicella Vaccine		
Severe allergic reaction after a previous dose or to a vaccine component (e.g., neomycin or gelatin) Infection with HIV Known altered immunodeficiency (hematological and solid tumours, congenital immunodeficiency, and long-term immunosuppressive therapy) Pregnancy Children receiving corticosteroids	Recent immune globulin administration (see MMR, above) (PHAC, 2015b) Family history of immunodeficiency	Breastfeeding
Rotavirus Vaccine		
Severe allergic reaction after a previous dose or to a vaccine component Infants born to HIV-positive mother Known or suspected weakened immune system caused by radiation; medications; or conditions such as leukemia, blood disorders, cancer	Altered immunocompetence Moderate to severe acute gastroenteritis Moderate to severe febrile illness Chronic gastrointestinal diseases Intussusception	Pregnancy Previous history of rotavirus infection; history of intussusception; temperature ≥38°C; close contact with immunocompromised person(s); blood transfusion or immune globulins within previous 42 days
Influenza Vaccine (Inactivated/Live-Attenuated)¶		
Severe allergic reaction after a previous dose or to a vaccine component, including eggs Egg hypersensitivity LAIV should not be administered to persons taking salicylates, with known or suspected immunodeficiency, with a history of GBS, or with a reactive airway disease or other chronic disorder considered high risk for severe influenza.	GBS within 6 wk after previous influenza immunization	Pregnancy
Meningococcal Vaccine		
MCV4—Allergy to vaccine components, including diphtheria toxoid, and possible reaction to latex stopper; history of GBS		Pregnancy
MPSV4—Allergy to vaccine components		Pregnancy

TABLE 35-2 **CONTRAINDICATIONS AND PRECAUTIONS TO VACCINATIONS—cont'd**

TRUE CONTRAINDICATIONS	PRECAUTIONS†	NOT CONTRAINDICATIONS (VACCINES MAY BE ADMINISTERED)
Tetanus (Booster Toxoid), Reduced Diphtheria Toxoid, Acellular Pertussis Adsorbed (Tdap)		
Serious reaction to any vaccine component History of encephalopathy (e.g., coma, prolonged seizures) within 7 days of administration of a pertussis vaccine that is not attributable to another identifiable cause	GBS ≤6 wk after previous dose of a tetanus toxoid vaccine Progressive neurological disorder, uncontrolled epilepsy, or progressive encephalopathy until the condition has stabilized	Temperature ≥40.5°C within 48 hr after DTP/DTaP immunization not attributable to another cause Collapse or shocklike state within 48 hr after DTP/DTaP immunization Persistent crying lasting ≥3 hr, occurring within 48 hr after DTP/DTaP immunization Seizures with or without fever, occurring within 3 days after DTaP/DTP immunization History of entire limb swelling reaction after pediatric DTaP/DTP or Td immunization that was not an Arthus hypersensitivity reaction Stable neurological disorder, including well-controlled seizures, history of seizure disorder, and CP Brachial neuritis Latex allergy other than anaphylactic allergies (e.g., history of contact to latex gloves) Immunosuppression, including persons with HIV Antibiotic use Intercurrent minor illness
Human Papillomavirus Vaccine		
Pregnancy Hypersensitivity to yeast or any vaccine component		Immunosuppressed female Minor acute illness Lactation

See also the National Advisory Committee on Immunizations (Public Health Agency of Canada) at http://www.phac-aspc.gc.ca/naci-ccni/

CP, cerebral palsy; *GBS,* Guillain-Barré syndrome; *HIV,* human immunodeficiency virus; *LAIV,* live-attenuated influenza vaccine; *PPD,* purified protein derivative.

*This information is based on the recommendations of the Advisory Committee on Immunization Practices (ACIP) and those of the Committee on Infectious Diseases (Red Book Committee) of the American Academy of Pediatrics. Sometimes these recommendations vary from those contained in manufacturer's package inserts. For more detailed information, consult published recommendations of the ACIP and American Academy of Pediatrics and manufacturer's package inserts.

†Events or conditions listed as precautions, although not contraindications, should be carefully reviewed. Benefits and risks of administering a specific vaccine to an individual under the circumstances should be considered. If risks are believed to outweigh benefits, vaccination should be withheld; if benefits are believed to outweigh risks (e.g., during an outbreak or foreign travel), vaccination should be administered. Whether and when to administer DTaP to children with proven or suspected underlying neurological disorders should be decided on an individual basis. It is prudent on theoretical grounds to avoid vaccinating pregnant women.

‡Acetaminophen given before administering DTaP and thereafter every 4 hours for 24 hours should be considered for children with a personal history of seizures or family history of seizures in siblings or parents.

§Measles vaccination may temporarily suppress tuberculin reactivity. If testing cannot be done the day of MMR vaccination, the test should be postponed for 4 to 6 wk.

ǁ Birth weight <2000 g and unknown or hepatitis B surface antigen–positive mother is not a contraindication for vaccination.

¶See James, J. M., et al. (1998). Safe administration of influenza vaccine to patients with egg allergies. *Journal of Pediatrics, 133*(5), 624–628.

Modified from American Academy of Pediatrics, Committee on Infectious Diseases & Pickering, L. (Ed.). (2009). *2009 Red book: Report of the Committee on Infectious Diseases* (28th ed.). Elk Grove Village, IL: Author.

to egg should seek the advice of an allergist regarding this vaccine. Most children with egg allergy are reported to be likely to develop a tolerance to small amounts over time (Settipane, Siri, & Bellanti, 2009).

Some vaccines contain a preservative, *thimerosal*, which contains ethylmercury. Concerns regarding possible mercury poisoning in the 1990s prompted many to put off vaccination of infants and small children for fear of childhood developmental problems such as autism. A number of manufacturers have since stopped producing vaccines containing thimerosal. No local hypersensitivity reactions to thimerosal have been recorded, and studies on thimerosal and the potential link to autism or any other pervasive developmental disorder failed to establish a causal relationship between the two (Price, Thompson, Goodson, et al., 2010; Schultz, 2010). The Institute of Medicine (2004), following an in-depth 3-year study, concluded that there was no link between autism and the MMR vaccine or vaccines containing the preservative thimerosal.

A commonly observed reaction includes localized erythema and induration, which may occur when the vaccine is not administered deeply enough into the muscle. This reaction can be prevented by ensuring that needle length is appropriate for the child's muscle size. Although many vaccine preparations are commercially available in prepackaged form, the enclosed needle may not be of adequate length to penetrate the muscle in certain children (see Atraumatic Care box above and Administration).

Unlike the inactivated antigens, live attenuated virus vaccines such as MMR multiply for days or weeks, and unfavourable reactions and vaccine-associated disorders can occur for 30 to 60 days. These reactions are usually mild, although reactions to rubella tend to be more troublesome in older children and adults than in infants.

Contraindications and Compliance

Nurses need to be aware of the reasons for withholding immunizations—both for the child's safety in terms of avoiding reactions and for the child's maximum benefit from receiving the vaccine. Unfounded fears and lack of knowledge of contraindications can needlessly prevent a child from having protection from life-threatening diseases. Issues that have surfaced regarding vaccines include the misconception that administering combination vaccines may overload the child's immune system; the combined vaccines have undergone rigorous study in relation to adverse effects and immunogenicity rates following administration. Others may express concern that vaccines are not a part of the individual's natural immunity and that administering too many vaccines may decrease the child's immunity to such diseases. Another concern of parents is the number of vaccines or "shots" given to infants at any given time and the pain and discomfort this may cause.

Parents must be given appropriate information about vaccine safety, benefits, and risks so that they can make informed decisions regarding vaccinations for their children. The advantage of widespread media via television and the Internet is that information is readily available at any given moment; the disadvantage is that some of this information may be incorrect, incomplete, or misleading and may influence parents to make decisions that may have deleterious consequences on their children's health. To help parents make informed decisions about immunizations for their children, parents may be directed to resources such as the Canadian Paediatric Society's *A Parent's Guide to Immunization Information on the Internet* (CPS, 2015a).

Strategies that may ensure parents follow immunization guidelines include giving parents vaccine information at the time of the newborn's discharge, mailing reminder cards, making immunization services readily available, removing barriers to vaccination (such as long waiting times and appointment-only systems), and taking every opportunity to immunize children when they enter a health care facility (such as emergency departments, clinics, private offices, and hospitals).

A *contraindication* is considered a condition in an individual that increases the risk for a serious adverse reaction (e.g., not administering a live virus vaccine to a severely compromised child). A *precaution* is a condition in a recipient that might increase the risk for a serious adverse reaction or that might compromise the ability of the vaccine to produce immunity. For contraindications and precautions to the usual childhood vaccines, see Table 35-2.

Administration

The principal precautions in administering immunizations include proper storage of the vaccine to protect its potency and the institution of recommended procedures for injection. The nurse must be familiar with the manufacturer's directions for storage and reconstitution of the vaccine. For example, if the vaccine is to be refrigerated, it should be stored on a centre shelf and not in the door, where frequent temperature increases from opening the refrigerator can alter the vaccine's potency. For protection against light, the vial can be wrapped in aluminum foil. Periodic checks should be scheduled to ensure that no vaccine is used after its expiration date.

The DTaP vaccines contain the adjuvant *alum* to retain the antigen at the injection site and to prolong the stimulatory effect. Because subcutaneous or intracutaneous injection of the adjuvant can cause local irritation, inflammation, or abscess formation, excellent intramuscular injection technique must be used (see Atraumatic Care box, p. 1022). Ipp, Parkin, Lear, et al. (2009) evaluated the administration order of the vaccines diphtheria-tetanus–acellular pertussis–*Haemophilus influenzae* type b (DTaP-Hib) and pneumococcal conjugate vaccine (PCV) and pain perception in 120 infants 2 to 6 months of age. The infants who were given the primary DTaP-Hib vaccine before the PCV vaccine had significantly lower pain scores as measured by the Modified Behavioural Pain Scale than those who received the PCV vaccine first. Both groups of infants were given both vaccines. Additional pain measures included crying as measured by video recording and parent perception of child pain using the Visual Analog Scale. The researchers recommend giving the primary DTaP-Hib vaccine before the PCV to reduce pain in infants receiving routine immunizations.

The total series requires several injections, and every attempt is made to rotate the sites and administer the injections as painlessly as possible. When two or more injections are given at separate sites, the order of injections is arbitrary. Because allergic reactions can occur after injection of vaccines, appropriate precautions need to be taken (see Chapter 47, Anaphylaxis).

Another important nursing responsibility is accurate documentation. Each child should have an immunization record for parents to keep, especially for families who move often. Although immunization rates have increased significantly, health care providers should use every opportunity to encourage complete immunization of all children. Blank immunization records may be downloaded from a number of websites, including Immunize Canada (see Additional Resources at the end of the chapter), which has vaccine information and records.

The following information is documented on the medical record: day, month, and year of administration; manufacturer and lot number of vaccine; expiration date of vaccine; and the name, work address, and title of the person administering the vaccine. Additional data to record are the site and route of administration and evidence that the parent or legal guardian gave informed consent before the immunization was administered.

Practitioners are required to fully inform families of the risks and benefits of the vaccines. Any adverse reactions after the administration of any vaccine should be reported to the Canadian Adverse Events Following Immunization Surveillance System (CAEFISS) (PHAC, 2015d). See the Additional Resources section at the end of this chapter for additional information on immunization.

Anticipatory Guidance—Care of Families

Child-rearing is no easy task; it presents challenges to both new and "seasoned" parents. Society's changing roles and mores, combined with a highly mobile population, leave little stability for traditional role models and time-honoured methods of raising children. As a result, parents look to health care providers for guidance. Nurses are in an advantageous position to render assistance and offer suggestions. For parents of an infant, some challenges centre on dependency, discipline, increased mobility, and safety. Major areas for parental guidance during the first year are listed in the Family-Centred Teaching box.

FAMILY-CENTRED TEACHING

Guidance During Infant's First Year

First 6 Months

- Teach car safety with use of a government-approved restraint, facing toward the rear, in the middle of the back seat—not in a front seat with an air bag.
- Understand each parent's adjustment to the newborn, especially the mother's postpartum emotional needs.
- Teach care of the infant and help parents understand the infant's individual needs and temperament and that the infant expresses wants through crying.
- Reassure parents that the infant cannot be spoiled by too much attention during the first 4 to 6 months.
- Encourage parents to establish a schedule that meets the needs of the child and themselves.
- Help parents understand the infant's need for stimulation in the environment.
- Support parents' pleasure in seeing the child's growing friendliness and social response, especially smiling.
- Plan anticipatory guidance for safety.
- Stress the need for routine childhood immunizations.
- Prepare parents for the introduction of solid foods.

Second 6 Months

- Prepare parents for the child's "stranger anxiety."
- Encourage parents to allow the child to cling to them and avoid long separation from either parent.
- Guide parents concerning discipline because of the infant's increasing mobility.
- Encourage use of negative voice and eye contact rather than physical punishment as a means of discipline.
- Encourage showing the most attention when the infant is behaving well, rather than when the infant is crying.
- Teach injury prevention, because of the child's advancing motor skills and curiosity.
- Encourage parents to leave the child with a suitable caregiver to allow them some free time.
- Discuss readiness for weaning (as desired).
- Explore parents' feelings about their infant's sleep patterns.

SPECIAL HEALTH PROBLEMS

Colic (Paroxysmal Abdominal Pain)

Colic is reported to occur in 15 to 40% of all infants (Morin, 2009). The condition is generally described as paroxysmal abdominal pain or cramping that is manifested by loud crying and drawing the legs up to the abdomen. Other definitions include variables such as duration of cry greater than 3 hours a day, occurring more than 3 days per week, and parental dissatisfaction with the child's behaviour. Some studies report an increase in symptoms (fussiness and crying) in the late afternoon or evening; however, in some infants the onset of symptoms occurs at another time. Colic is more common in infants under 3 months of age than in older infants, and infants with so-called difficult temperaments are more likely to be colicky. Despite the obvious behavioural indications of pain, the infant with colic gains weight and usually thrives. There is no evidence of a residual effect of colic on older children, except perhaps a strained parent–child relationship in some cases (Megel et al., 2011); in other words, infants who are colicky grow up to be normal children and adults. Colic is self-limiting and in most cases resolves as infants mature, generally around 12 to 16 weeks of age (O'Connor, 2009).

Among the theories that have been investigated as potential causes are too-rapid feeding, overeating, swallowing excessive air, improper feeding technique (especially in positioning and burping), disrupted sleep patterns, and emotional stress or tension between parent and child. Although all of these may occur, there is no evidence that one factor is consistently present. Infants with cow's milk allergy (CMA) symptoms have a high rate of colic (44%), and eliminating cow's milk products from the infant's diet can reduce the symptoms. However, there is considerable controversy about the role of allergy and colic because there does not appear to be an increased incidence of atopy in infants with colic.

Keefe, Lobo, Froese-Fretz, et al. (2006) proposed that colic has origins in the infant's inability to self-regulate the sleep–wake cycles based on central nervous system (CNS) immaturity rather than gastrointestinal system dysfunction. These researchers implemented a home-based intervention program aimed at promoting infant state regulation (sleep–wake cycles), promoting synchrony between parent and child, providing parental support, and decreasing infant irritability. The results of the study found that infants in the treatment group cried 1.7 hours less per day than infants in the control group. In addition, families in both the treatment and control group reported benefitting from a nurse visiting in the home and listening to parents' concerns about the infant's and the family's well-being.

Parental smoking, strained parent–infant interaction, lactase deficiency, consumption of fruit juices (carbohydrate malabsorption), difficult infant temperament, difficulty regulating emotions, CNS immaturity, and neurochemical dysregulation in the brain have all been proposed as potential causes of colic. The consensus of most experts who study colic is that it is multifactorial in nature and no single treatment for every colicky infant will be effective in alleviating the symptoms. New information suggests that what used to be called colic is actually a normal part of an infant's development (CPS, 2015b). All infants go through a time period early in life when they cry more than at any other time, and some infants generally cry more often than others. See more information on crying in the Shaken Baby Syndrome section (p. 1014).

Therapeutic Management

Management of colic should begin with an investigation of possible organic causes, such as CMA, intussusception, or other gastrointestinal problem. If a sensitivity to cow's milk is strongly suspected, a trial substitution of another formula, such as an extensively hydrolyzed (e.g., Nutramigen, Alimentum, Pregestimil), whey hydrolysate, or amino acid (e.g., Neocate, EleCare) formula, is warranted. Soy formulas are usually avoided because of the possibility of sensitivity to soy protein as well. Oral administration of *Lactobacillus reuteri* to colicky exclusively breastfed infants decreased crying symptoms to less than 3 hours per day within 21 days of initiation in a randomized, double-blind, placebo-controlled trial of 50 colicky infants (Savino, Cordisco, Tarasco, et al., 2010). When no specific inciting agent can be found, the supportive measures discussed under Nursing Care are used.

The use of medications, including sedatives, antispasmodics, antihistamines, and antiflatulents, is sometimes recommended. The most commonly used sedatives are phenobarbital, hydroxyzine hydrochloride (Atarax), and chloral hydrate. Simethicone (Mylicon) may also help allay the symptoms of colic. However, in most controlled studies, none of these medications completely eliminated the symptoms of colic. Behavioural interventions have not proved effective at reducing symptoms of colic but have helped parents deal with the crying infant in a more positive manner. The addition of lactase to infant formula has produced mixed results in the abatement of overall symptoms.

The use of complementary medicines for infantile colic, namely fennel extract, herbal tea, and sugar solutions, reportedly lack sufficient evidence to recommend their use (Perry, Hunt, & Ernst, 2011). One study found that a combination of interventions—massage, herbal tea, sucrose solution, and hydrolyzed formula—decreased crying in reported colicky infants; the administration of the hydrolyzed formula achieved best results, whereas massage was least effective at reducing crying (Arikan, Alp, Gözüm, et al., 2008).

In a position statement, Critch and the CPS Nutrition and Gastroenterology Committee (2011/2016) concluded that dietary modifications are beneficial in some cases but not all. The CPS does not recommend making nutrition interventions in the majority of infants with colic unless the infant has CMA symptoms. Breastfeeding mothers could try eliminating cow's milk from their diet as a trial for 3 to 5 days.

NURSING CARE

The initial step in managing colic is to take a thorough, detailed history of the usual daily events. Areas that should be examined include (1) the infant's diet; (2) the diet of the breastfeeding mother; (3) the time of day when crying occurs; (4) the relationship of the crying to feeding time; (5) the presence of specific family members during the crying and habits of family members, such as smoking; (6) activity of the mother or usual caregiver before, during, and after the crying; (7) characteristics of the cry (e.g., duration, intensity); (8) measures used to relieve the crying and their effectiveness; and (9) the infant's stooling, voiding, and sleeping patterns. Of special emphasis is a careful assessment of the feeding process via demonstration by the parent.

If cow's milk sensitivity is suspected, breastfeeding mothers should follow a milk-free diet for a minimum of 3 to 5 days in an attempt to reduce the infant's symptoms. Mothers need to be cautioned that some nondairy creamers may contain calcium caseinate, a cow's milk protein. If a milk-free diet is helpful, lactating mothers may need calcium supplements to meet their body's requirement. Formula-fed infants may improve with the same dietary modifications as for the child with CMA (Critch & CPS, Nutrition and Gastroenterology Committee, 2011/2016). Additional approaches for managing colic are listed in the Family-Centred Care box. Parents should be encouraged to try as many of these approaches as possible, since not all are effective for every infant.

Perhaps the most important nursing intervention (before or after an organic cause has been eliminated) is reassurance of both parents that they are not doing anything wrong and that the infant is not experiencing any physical or emotional harm. Parents, especially mothers, can become easily frustrated with the infant's crying and perceive this as a sign that there is something horribly wrong, when this may be part of an infant's normal development. In addition, colicky infants may be at increased risk for being shaken or otherwise abused by their caregivers and experiencing traumatic brain injury. A survey of fathers of colicky infants revealed that professional assistance was limited. The fathers described the experience of having a

FAMILY-CENTRED CARE

Caring for the Colicky Infant

- Place the awake infant prone over a covered hot-water bottle, heated towel, or covered heating pad set on "low."
- Massage the infant's abdomen.
- Respond immediately to the crying.
- Change the infant's position frequently; walk with the child's face down and body across the parent's arm, with the parent's hand under the infant's abdomen, applying gentle pressure (Fig. 35-13).
- Use a front carrier for transporting the infant.
- Place the infant in an electric (or wind-up) infant swing for short periods.
- Take the infant for car rides or outside for a change in environment.
- Use bottles that minimize air swallowing (curved bottle or inner collapsible bag).
- Use a commercial device in the crib that stimulates the vibration and sound of a car ride or plays soothing "noise," in utero sounds, or music.
- Provide smaller, frequent feedings; burp the infant during and after feedings using the shoulder position or sitting upright, and place the infant in an upright seat after feedings.
- Introduce a pacifier for added sucking.
- In breastfed infants, the mother could try avoiding all milk products for a trial period (3 to 5 days).
- If household members smoke they should avoid smoking near the infant; smoking must be done outside the home.
- Give an appropriate dose of acetaminophen elixir or suppository if suggested by the health care provider; this is not recommended for daily use.
- If nothing reduces the crying, place the infant in the crib and allow to cry; periodically hold and comfort the child and put down again.
- Maintain a brief diary of the time of day the crying starts; events going on in household; time, amount, and type of last feeding; length of crying; and characteristics of cry. Although this will not stop the crying, it may help the practitioner identify a possible cause.

colicky infant as similar to falling into an abyss from which they had to climb with the assistance of family and friends, thus reinforcing the importance of empathetic nurses (Ellett, Appleton, & Sloan, 2009). An empathetic, gentle, and reassuring attitude, in addition to suggestions for treatment, will help allay parents' anxieties, which are usually exacerbated by loss of sleep and preoccupation over the infant's welfare. Colic disappears spontaneously, usually by 3 to 4 months of age, although guarantees should never be given since it may continue for much longer. Other support persons and extended family members may be enlisted to help support the parents during this difficult time.

Growth Failure (Failure to Thrive)

Growth failure, or *failure to thrive* (FTT), is a sign of inadequate growth resulting from an inability to obtain or use calories required for growth. FTT has no universal definition, although one of the more common parameters is a weight (and sometimes height) that falls below the fifth percentile for the child's age. Another definition of FTT includes a weight for age (height) z-value of less than −2.0 (a z-value is a standard deviation value that represents anthropometric data normalizing for sex and age with greater precision than growth percentile curves)

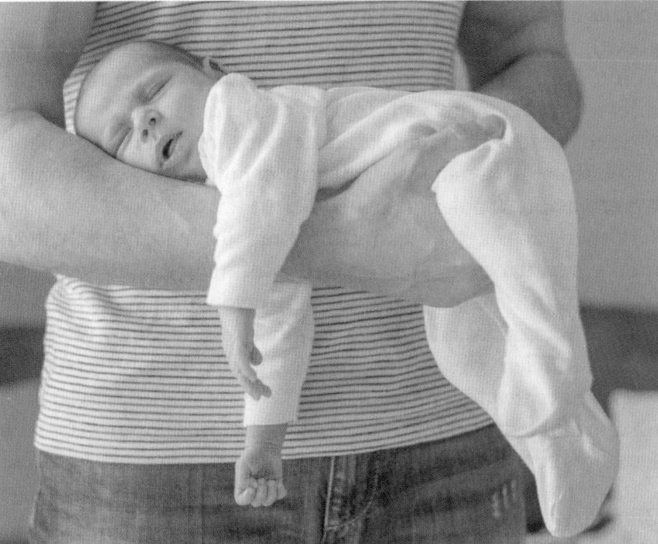

FIGURE 35-13 The "colic carry" may be comforting to an infant with colic. (OndroM/Shutterstock.com.)

(Markowitz, Watkins, & Duggan, 2008). The Canadian growth charts (see Appendix A) should be used to measure growth. Growth measurements alone, however, are not used to diagnose children with FTT. Rather, the finding of a pattern of persistent deviation from established growth parameters is cause for concern. In addition to lack of consensus on the precise definition of FTT, there are those who advocate for a change in terminology; thus terms such as *growth failure* and *pediatric undernutrition* are used in the literature for FTT. According to Cole and Lanham (2011), approximately 5 to 10% of children in primary care have FTT, with the majority presenting before the age of 18 months.

It has been suggested that FTT be classified according to pathophysiology in the following categories: (1) inadequate caloric intake—incorrect formula preparation, neglect, food fads, excessive juice consumption, poverty, behavioural problems affecting eating, or CNS problems affecting intake; (2) inadequate absorption—cystic fibrosis, celiac disease, vitamin or mineral deficiencies, biliary atresia, or hepatic disease; (3) increased metabolism—hyperthyroidism, congenital heart defects, or chronic immunodeficiency; and (4) defective utilization—genetic anomaly such as trisomy 21 or 18, congenital infection, or metabolic storage diseases (Cole & Lanham, 2011).

The cause of growth failure is often multifactorial and involves a combination of infant organic disease, dysfunctional parenting behaviours, subtle neurological or behavioural problems, and disturbed parent–child interactions (Marchand & CPS, Nutrition and Gastroenterology Committee, 2012/2015). However, the primary etiology is inadequate caloric intake, regardless of the cause.

Infants who are premature and have a very low birth weight (VLBW) or extremely low birth weight (ELBW), as well as those with intrauterine growth restriction (IUGR), are often referred for FTT within the first 2 years of life because they typically do not grow physically at the same rate as term normal weight infants even after discharge from the acute care facility. Catch-up growth has been shown to be much more difficult to achieve in ELBW and VLBW infants. Children with congenital heart disease are also more likely to develop FTT in infancy as a result of inadequate caloric intake, malabsorption, increased energy expenditure that superseded caloric intake, and pulmonary hypertension (Cook & Higgins, 2010).

Other factors that can contribute to inadequate caloric intake in infancy include inadequate financial resources for food, health or child-rearing beliefs involving fad diets, inadequate nutritional knowledge, family stress, feeding resistance, and insufficient breast milk intake. In infants younger than 8 weeks, breastfeeding problems as a result of inadequate latch or uncoordinated sucking and swallowing may occur (Cole & Lanham, 2011).

Diagnostic Evaluation

Diagnosis is initially made from evidence of growth failure. If FTT is recent, the weight, but not the height, is below accepted standards (usually the fifth percentile); if FTT is long-standing, both weight and height are low, indicating chronic malnutrition. The use of weight velocities (according to the World Health Organization growth charts) may be a better indicator of short-term growth failure while considering age-dependent changes in growth (Cole & Lanham, 2011) (see Additional Resources at the end of this chapter). Perhaps as important as anthropometric measurements are a complete health and dietary history (including perinatal history), physical examination for evidence of organic causes, developmental assessment, and family assessment. A dietary intake history, either a 24-hour food intake or a history of food consumed over a 3- to 5-day period, is also essential. In addition, the child's activity level, perceived food allergies, and dietary restrictions, as well as parental height, should be explored. An assessment of household organization and mealtime behaviours and rituals is important in the collection of pertinent data. It is also helpful to obtain the growth patterns of parents and siblings. An assessment of the home environment and child–parent interaction may be helpful as well. Other tests (lead toxicity, anemia, stool-reducing substances, occult blood, ova and parasites, alkaline phosphatase, and zinc levels) are selected only as indicated to rule out organic problems. To prevent the overuse of diagnostic procedures, FTT should be considered early in the differential diagnosis. To avoid the social stigma of FTT during the early investigative phase, many health care practitioners use the term *growth delay* (or *failure*) until the actual cause is established.

Therapeutic Management

The primary management of FTT is aimed at reversing the cause of the growth failure. If malnutrition is severe, the initial treatment is directed at reversing the malnutrition without going into a refeeding syndrome. The goal is to provide sufficient calories to support "catch-up" growth—a rate of growth greater than the expected rate for age. Any coexisting medical problems are treated. The child might require a high-calorie diet with supplementary vitamins and minerals and treatment of any other existing medical issues.

In most cases of FTT, an interdisciplinary team of physician, nurse, dietitian, child life specialist, occupational therapist, pediatric feeding specialist, and social worker or mental health care provider is needed to deal with the multiple problems in order to provide comprehensive care that addresses the biological, psychiatric, and socioeconomic aspects of the child's life. Efforts are made to relieve any additional stresses on the family by offering referrals to welfare agencies or supplemental food programs. In some cases, family therapy may be required; temporary placement in a foster home may relieve the family's stress, protect the child, and allow the child some stability if insurmountable obstacles are preventing appropriate family functioning. Behaviour modification aimed at mealtime rituals (or lack thereof) and family social time may be required. Hospitalization admission is indicated for (1) evidence (anthropometric) of severe acute malnutrition, (2) child abuse or neglect, (3) significant dehydration, (4) caretaker substance use or psychosis, (5) serious intercurrent infection, or (6) outpatient management that does not result in weight gain.

Prognosis

The prognosis for FTT is related to the cause. If the parents have simply not understood the infant's needs, teaching may remedy the child's limited caloric intake and permanently reverse the growth failure. Inadequate or infrequent feeding periods by the infant's primary caregiver, in conjunction with family disorganization, are often the cause of FTT.

Few long-term studies provide evidence on the prognosis for children with FTT. Low-birth-weight preterm infants have demonstrated long-term detrimental effects, such as poor growth, cognitive delays, and poor academic performance (Cole & Lanham, 2011). The research is unclear if normal-birth-weight infants who develop FTT and then recover have similar long-term consequences (Cole & Lanham, 2011).

Factors related to poor prognosis are severe feeding resistance, lack of awareness in and cooperation from the parent(s), low family income, low maternal educational level, adolescent mother, preterm birth, IUGR, and early age of onset of FTT. Because later cognitive and motor function is affected by malnourishment in infancy, many of these children may be below normal in intellectual development, have poorer language development and less developed reading skills, attain lower social maturity, and have a higher incidence of behavioural disturbances (Markowitz et al., 2008). Such findings indicate that a long-term plan and follow-up care are needed for the optimum development for all of these children.

NURSING CARE

Nurses play a critical role as part of the interdisciplinary team in the diagnosis of FTT through their assessment of the child, parents, and family interactions. Knowledge of the characteristics of children with FTT and their families is essential in helping identify these children and hastening the confirmation of a diagnosis (Box 35-2). Accurate assessment of initial weight and height and daily weight, as well as recording of all food intake, is essential. The nurse documents the child's feeding

BOX 35-2 CLINICAL MANIFESTATIONS OF GROWTH FAILURE (FAILURE TO THRIVE)

Growth failure (see p. 1029 for definitions)
Undernutrition
Developmental delays—social, motor, adaptive, language
Apathy
Withdrawn behaviour
Feeding or eating disorders, such as vomiting, feeding resistance, anorexia, pica, rumination
No fear of strangers (at age when stranger anxiety is normal)
Avoidance of eye contact
Wide-eyed gaze and continual scan of the environment ("radar gaze")
Stiff and unyielding or flaccid and unresponsive
Minimal smiling

behaviour and the parent–child interaction during feeding, other caregiving activities, and play.

Besides showing signs of malnutrition and delayed social development, children with FTT may exhibit altered behavioural interactions. They may display intense interest in inanimate objects, such as toys, but much less interest in social interactions. They are often watchful of people at a distance but become increasingly distressed as others come closer. They may dislike being touched or held and avoid face-to-face contact. However, when held, they protest briefly on being put down and are apathetic when left alone.

Children with FTT may have a history of difficult feeding, vomiting, sleep disturbances, and excessive irritability. Patterns such as crying during feeds, vomiting, hoarding food in the mouth, rumination after feeding, refusing to switch from liquids to solids, and displaying aversion behaviour such as turning from food or spitting food become attention-seeking ways to prolong attention received at meals. In some cases, the child may use feeding as a control mechanism in a poorly organized or chaotic family situation; parents may allow the child to dictate the norms for behaviour and feeding because of inexperience with parenting or poor parenting role models. Thus refusing to eat or eating only sweets and snacks with non-nutritive value may be the child's norm based on food availability and family tradition. In such cases, family therapy is essential to reverse the trend and assist the parents and child in understanding each other's roles.

Some parents are at increased risk for attachment problems because of (1) isolation and social crisis; (2) inadequate support systems, such as for teenage and single mothers; and (3) poor parenting role models as a child. Other factors that should be considered are lack of education; physical and mental health problems such as physical and sexual abuse, depression, or drug dependence; immaturity, especially in adolescent parents; and lack of commitment to parenting, such as giving priority to entertainment or employment. Often these parents and their families are under stress and in multiple chronic emotional, social, and financial crises.

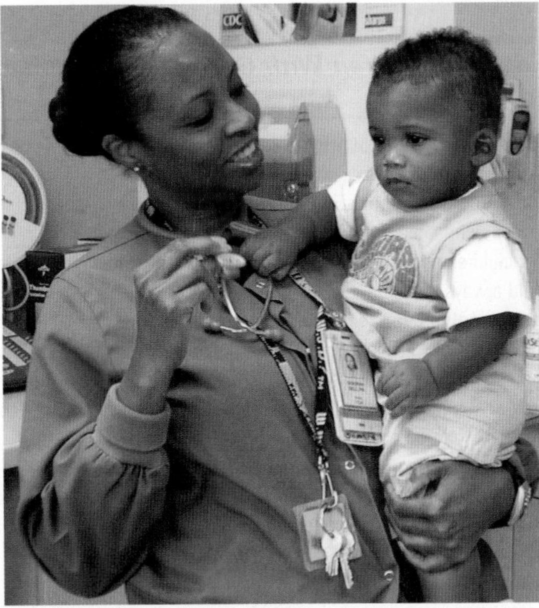

FIGURE 35-14 Consistent nursing contact is important in developing trust in infants with failure to thrive.

Because part of the difficulty between parent and child is dissatisfaction and frustration, the child should have a primary core of nurses (Fig. 35-14). The nurses caring for the child can learn to perceive the child's cues and reverse the cycle of dissatisfaction, especially in the area of feeding.

Because many of these children are responding to stimuli that have led to the negative feeding patterns, an important primary intervention is to structure the feeding environment in such a way to encourage healthful eating. Initially staff members and a feeding specialist may need to feed these children to assess thoroughly the difficulties encountered during the feeding process and to devise strategies that eliminate or minimize such problems. General guidelines for the feeding process are outlined in the Guidelines box.

Four primary goals in the nutritional management of FTT are to (1) correct nutritional deficiencies and achieve ideal weight for height, (2) provided adequate calories for catch-up growth, (3) restore optimum body composition, and (4) educate the parents or primary caregivers regarding the child's nutritional requirements and appropriate feeding methods. To increase caloric intake in formula-fed infants, supplements such as Polycose or medium-chain triglycerides may be added slowly. For infants, 24 kcal/30 mL formulas may be provided to increase caloric intake; older children (1 to 6 years) may benefit from a 30 kcal/30 mL formula (Marchand & CPS, Nutrition and Gastroenterology Committee, 2012/2015). Other carbohydrate additives include fortified rice cereal and vegetable oil. Because vitamin and mineral deficiencies may be present, multivitamin supplementation, including zinc and iron, is recommended. For toddlers, a high-calorie milk drink such as PediaSure may be used to increase caloric intake. Signs of intolerance to the formula should be carefully monitored.

Because maladaptive feeding practices often contribute to growth failure, parents need to be given specific step-by-step

GUIDELINES

Feeding Children With Growth Failure (Failure to Thrive)

Provide a primary core of staff to feed the child. The same nurses are able to learn the child's cues and respond consistently.

Provide a quiet, unstimulating atmosphere. A number of these children are very distractible, and their attention is diverted with minimal stimuli. Older children do well at a feeding table; bottle-fed infants and children should always be held.

Maintain a calm, even temperament throughout the meal. Negative outbursts may be commonplace in this child's habit formation. Limits on eating behaviour definitely need to be provided, but they should be stated in a firm, calm tone. If the nurse is hurried or anxious, the feeding process will not be optimized.

Talk to the child by giving directions about eating. "Take a bite, Lisa" is appropriate and directive. The more distractible the child, the more directive the nurse should be to refocus attention on feeding. Positive comments about feeding need to be actively given.

Be persistent. This is perhaps one of the most important guidelines. Parents often give up when the child begins negative feeding behaviour. Calm perseverance through 10 to 15 minutes of food refusal will eventually diminish negative behaviour. Although forced feeding is avoided, "strictly encouraged" feeding is essential.

Maintain a face-to-face posture with the child when possible. Encourage eye contact and remain with the child throughout the meal.

Introduce new foods slowly. Often these children have been exclusively bottle-fed. If acceptance of solids is a problem, begin with puréed food and, once accepted, advance to junior and regular solid foods.

Follow the child's rhythm of feeding. The child will set a rhythm when the previous conditions are met.

Develop a structured routine. Disruptions in their other activities of daily living have great impact on feeding responses, so bathing, sleeping, dressing, and playing, as well as feeding, should be structured. The nurse should feed the child in the same way and place as often as possible. The length of the feeding should also be established (usually 30 minutes).

directions for formula preparation, as well as a written schedule of feeding times. Juice intake in children with FTT should be restricted until adequate weight gain has been achieved with appropriate milk sources; thereafter no more than 120 mL/day of juice should be given.

Behaviour modification techniques may be used with older infants and toddlers to interrupt poor feeding patterns. Feeding times may actually involve "struggles of will" in cases of maladaptive feedings that result in FTT. These behaviours are different from the occasional toddler behaviour of food refusal, which is primarily developmental, not pathological. The association of appropriate food with good or bad behaviours and consequent rewards may be part of the complex problem. In severe cases of malnourishment, tube feedings or intravenous therapy may be required.

Besides attending to the physical needs of the child, the interdisciplinary team must plan care for appropriate developmental stimulation. After an approximate developmental age is established, a planned program of play is begun. Ideally, a child life specialist is involved to implement and supervise the stimulation program. Every effort should be made to teach the parent how to play and interact with the child.

Nursing care of these children involves a family systems approach. In other words, for the entire family to become healthy, each member must be helped to change. Care of the parents is aimed at helping them increase their feelings of self-esteem through positive, successful parenting skills. Initially this necessitates providing an environment in which they feel welcomed and accepted. Because these parents are often distrustful of authority figures, it may take some time before they trust the nurse. One approach is to empathize with the parent about the difficulties of child-rearing. For example, the nurse may state that many parents find adjusting to parenthood a trying time or that the demands of caring for an infant can become overwhelming.

The nurse provides infant care techniques to the parents through example and demonstration. As the nurse perceives the infant's cues, he or she can emphasize these to the parents. For example, during a feeding the nurse might comment that the infant is still hungry because the child sucks vigorously and looks at the nurse. When the infant is satisfied, the nurse can point out that the infant is signalling this by releasing the strong suck, closing the eyes, and breathing deeply and more slowly.

Sudden Infant Death Syndrome

Sudden infant death syndrome (SIDS) is defined as the sudden death of an infant younger than 1 year of age that remains unexplained after a complete postmortem examination, including an investigation of the death scene and a review of the case history. Since 2002, the data have included another term, *sudden unexplained death in infants* (SUDI). SIDS and SUDI combined are the third leading cause of infant deaths (birth to 12 months) and the first leading cause of postneonatal deaths (between 1 and 12 months). In 2008, SIDS claimed the lives of 107 infants and in 2012 there were 51 deaths in Canada (Statistics Canada, 2016). The PHAC has reported that the infant mortality rates due to SIDS have fallen in Canada in recent decades; this decrease is attributed to the Back to Sleep campaign, initiated in 1999. (See Additional Resources at the end of this chapter for further information on Back to Sleep teaching programs.) The SIDS rates vary greatly among the different provinces and territories. Recent data indicate that Quebec has the lowest rate, while Nunavut has the highest rate. SIDS mortality declined from 1.0 per 1000 live births in 1981 to 0.3 per 1000 live births in 2009 (a 71% reduction) (PHAC, 2014h).

During the same period, postneonatal mortality declined from 3.5 to 1.3 per 1000 newborn survivors (a 64% reduction). The decrease in the occurrence of SIDS may be due to a decrease in the risk factors. For example, maternal smoking rates during pregnancy have declined while protective behaviours such as sleep position (changing infants to sleeping on their backs) have increased, along with higher rates of breastfeeding (PHAC, 2014h).

Table 35-3 summarizes the major epidemiological characteristics of SIDS.

TABLE 35-3 EPIDEMIOLOGY OF SUDDEN INFANT DEATH SYNDROME (SIDS)

FACTORS	OCCURRENCE
Incidence	0.3 per 1000 live births in 2009 in Canada*
Peak age	2 to 3 months and 95% occur by 6 months. Premature infants die at mean age 6 weeks later than mean age of death from SIDS for term infants
Sex	Higher percentage of males affected
Time of death	During sleep
Time of year	Increased incidence in winter
Socioeconomic	Increased occurrence in lower socioeconomic class
Birth	Higher incidence in: • Preterm infants, especially infants of extremely and very low birth weight • Multiple births† • Newborns with low Apgar scores • Infants with central nervous system disturbances and respiratory disorders such as bronchopulmonary dysplasia • Increasing birth order (subsequent siblings as opposed to firstborn child) • Infants with a recent history of illness, lower incidence in immunized infants
Sleep habits	Highest risk associated with prone position; use of soft bedding; overheating (thermal stress); co-sleeping with adult, especially on sofa or noninfant bed; higher incidence of co-sleeping with an adult smoker Infants co-sleeping with adult at higher risk if they are younger than 11 weeks
Feeding habits	Lower incidence in breastfed infants
Pacifier	Lower incidence in infants put to sleep with pacifier
Siblings	May have greater incidence in siblings with SIDS
Maternal	Young age; cigarette smoking, especially during pregnancy; poor prenatal care; substance use (heroin, methadone, cocaine); a few studies have shown an increased risk in infants exposed to second-hand environmental tobacco smoke

*Data from Public Health Agency of Canada. (2014). Sudden infant death syndrome (SIDS) fact sheet. Retrieved from http://www.phac-aspc.gc.ca/rhs-ssg/factshts/mat_sids-smsn_mat-eng.php
†Although rare, twins can die simultaneously of SIDS.
Data from Canadian Paediatric Society, Community Paediatrics Committee. (2004). Recommendations for safe sleeping environments for infants and children. *Paediatrics & Child Health, 9*(9), 659–663; Statistics Canada. (2014). *Leading causes of death, infants, by sex, Canada, annual.* Retrieved from http://www5.statcan.gc.ca/cansim/pick-choisir?lang=eng&p2=33&id=1020562

Etiology

Numerous theories have been proposed regarding the etiology of SIDS; however, the cause remains unknown. One compelling hypothesis is that SIDS is related to a **brainstem** abnormality in the neurological regulation of cardiorespiratory control. This abnormal development affects the arousal and physiological responses to a life-threatening situation during sleep (PHAC, 2012c). Abnormalities include prolonged sleep apnea, increased frequency of brief inspiratory pauses, excessive **periodic breathing**, and impaired arousal responsiveness to increased carbon dioxide or decreased oxygen. However, sleep apnea is not the cause of SIDS. The vast majority of infants with apnea do not die, and only a minority of SIDS victims have documented apparent life-threatening events (ALTEs) (see Apnea and Apparent Life-Threatening Events, p. 1037). Numerous studies indicate that there is no association between SIDS and any childhood vaccine.

A genetic predisposition to SIDS has been postulated as a cause. In one study, a genetic mutation on chromosome 6q 22.1-22.31 was positively linked to a syndrome of SIDS and dysgenesis of the testis (Puffenberger, Hu-Lince, Parod, et al., 2004). Infants who are male, premature, or of low birth weight, as well as infants from socioeconomically disadvantaged and Indigenous populations, have a higher incidence of SIDS (PHAC, 2014h).

Three triple-threat hypotheses have been proposed to explain the etiology of SIDS. Proposed factors include an underlying infant vulnerability factor (e.g., brain abnormality), a critical incidence in fetal development period or in early newborn life, and an environment stressor such as prone sleeping (Matthews & Moore, 2013). However, the triple-risk theories have not been fully accepted by all experts as a cause for SIDS, and further data are needed to identify a single cause or combination of causes for SIDS deaths.

Maternal smoking during pregnancy has emerged in numerous epidemiological studies as a major factor in SIDS, and tobacco smoke in the infant's environment after birth has also been shown to have a possible relationship with the incidence of SIDS (PHAC, 2014h). It has been postulated that 12% of all SIDS deaths could be prevented with prenatal maternal smoking cessation.

Bed sharing refers to a child sharing a bed with an adult or older child on a noninfant bed. Bed sharing has been reported to have an increased association with SIDS; there is a high association between infant deaths, use of nonstandard beds (sofa, day bed), and bed sharing; a large percentage of infants were found dead on their backs when bed sharing, which suggests suffocation. Studies have correlated higher incidences of SIDS in the context of infant bed sharing when there is also maternal smoking, bed sharing with multiple family members, maternal overweight, soft bedding, or unintentional asphyxiation resulting from adult intoxication (overlaying) (PHAC, 2014i).

Room sharing refers to a situation in which an infant is sleeping in close proximity to another person in the same room but in a different bed. Room sharing with infants in the age range when most SIDS deaths occur has been shown to be preventive. The term *co-sleeping* can refer to a range of sleeping practices that include both bed sharing and room sharing (PHAC, 2014i). Co-sleeping occurs in many cultures, and the nurse needs to ask parents about this practice to provide appropriate health teaching. The latest recommendation for prevention of SIDS from the PHAC (2014i) is that the infant's crib or bassinette be placed in close proximity to the mother's bed and that the infant be placed in the adult bed only for breastfeeding, then placed to sleep in his or her own crib once the feeding session is completed.

Other studies have linked sleep position with an increased risk of SIDS. Prone sleeping may cause oropharyngeal obstruction or affect thermal balance or arousal state. Healthy full-term infants may have significantly impaired arousal from active and quiet sleep states when sleeping prone. Rebreathing of carbon dioxide by infants in the prone position is another possible cause for SIDS. Infants sleeping prone and on soft bedding may not be able to move their heads to the side, thus increasing the risk of suffocation and lethal rebreathing. Evidence from other countries and the United States shows an increased incidence of SIDS in infants placed in a side-lying position; these infants are able to turn to a prone position. Thus the side-lying position is no longer recommended for infants sleeping at home or in day care centres or hospitals (unless medically indicated); healthy infants should be placed to sleep in the supine position (on the back) (PHAC, 2014i). Most preterm infants being discharged from the hospital should be placed in a supine sleeping position unless special factors predispose them to airway obstruction.

Parents need to know that certain sleep environments (prone sleeping, tobacco smoke exposure, soft bedding, noninfant bed surface, use of certain drugs by the individual sharing the bed with the infant, and thermal stress) can increase the risk for SIDS. Soft bedding such as waterbeds, sheepskins, beanbags, pillows, or quilts should be avoided for infant sleeping surfaces. Bedding items such as stuffed animals or toys should be removed from the crib while the infant is asleep. Head covering by a blanket has also been found to be a risk factor for SIDS, thus supporting the recommendation to avoid extra bed linens or other items. Crib bumper pads have not been shown to reduce infant injury and should therefore be avoided (PHAC, 2014i).

Research has indicated that breastfeeding during the first 16 weeks of life decreased the likelihood of SIDS. Some studies have found pacifier use in infants to be a protective factor against the occurrence of SIDS; the data for pacifier use in this population of infants (first year of life) are more compelling than data linking pacifier use to the development of dental complications and the inhibition of breastfeeding (PHAC, 2014i). Therefore, the CPS (2012a) has provided a parent guide on the safe use of nonsweetened pacifiers after successful breastfeeding, should parents want to give their infant a pacifier (see Thumb-sucking and Use of a Pacifier, p. 1004).

Although the etiology of SIDS is ultimately unknown, autopsies have revealed consistent pathological findings, such as pulmonary edema and intrathoracic hemorrhages, that confirm the diagnosis of SIDS. Consequently, autopsies should be performed on all infants suspected of dying of SIDS. The findings should be shared with the parents as soon as possible after the death.

Whether subsequent siblings of an infant who has died of SIDS are at increased risk for SIDS is unclear. Even if the increased risk is correct, families have a 99% chance that their subsequent child will *not* die of SIDS. Recurrence risks for a SIDS death in a family with a previous infant SIDS death range from 2 to 6% (AAP Task Force on Sudden Infant Death Syndrome, 2011). Home apnea monitoring is not recommended for this group of children, but it is often used by practitioners and may even be requested by parents. There is no evidence that home apnea monitoring prevents SIDS (Strehle, Gray, Gopisetti, et al., 2012). Monitoring is best initiated on an individual basis.

NURSING CARE

Nurses have a vital role in preventing SIDS, by educating families about the risk of prone sleeping position in infants from birth to 6 months of age, the use of appropriate bedding surfaces, the association with maternal smoking, and the dangers of bed sharing on noninfant surfaces with adults or other children. Also, nurses have an important role in modelling behaviours for parents to foster practices that decrease the risk for SIDS, including placing infants in a supine sleeping position in the hospital. There are still a small percentage of nurses who place healthy infants in a side-lying position in the hospital. A survey of levels II and III neonatal intensive care unit (NICU) nurses found that nurses still positioned infants in a side-lying position for fear of aspiration (29%), for comfort reasons (28%), and for infant safety (20%) (Grazel, Phalen, & Palomano, 2010). Nurses must be proactive in further decreasing the incidence of SIDS; after-birth discharge planning, newborn discharges, follow-up home visits, well-baby clinic visits, and immunization visits provide excellent opportunities to educate parents in these matters. The Family-Centred Teaching box gives families ways to reduce the potential incidence of SUDI.

A concern of many health care providers is that infants placed on their back to sleep will aspirate emesis or mucus; studies have failed to show an increase in infant deaths, spitting up during sleep, aspiration, asphyxia, or respiratory failure as a result of supine sleep positioning. (AAP Task Force on Sudden Infant Death Syndrome, 2011).

Loss of a child from SIDS presents several crises for the parents. In addition to grief and mourning the death of their child, the parents must face a tragedy that was sudden, unexpected, and unexplained. The psychological intervention for the family must deal with these additional variables. The discussion here focuses primarily on the objectives of care for families experiencing SIDS, rather than on the process of grief and mourning, which is explored in Chapter 40.

Care of the Family of a SIDS Infant

The first persons to arrive may be the police and emergency medical service personnel. Ideally, they will handle the situation by asking few questions; giving no indication of wrongdoing, abuse, or neglect; making sensitive judgements concerning any resuscitation efforts for the child; and comforting the members of the family as much as possible. A compassionate, sensitive approach to the family during the first few minutes can help spare them some of the overwhelming guilt and anguish that commonly follow this type of death.

The medical examiner or coroner may go to the home or place of death and make the death pronouncement; until then, the sleep environment should remain as it was when the infant was initially found. If the infant is not pronounced dead at the scene, he or she may be transported to the emergency department to be pronounced by a physician. Usually there is no

FAMILY-CENTRED CARE

Safe Sleep for Infants—Reducing the Incidence of Sudden Unexpected Death in Infants

- Always place your baby to sleep on the back. Side and tummy positions are not safe.
- Use a crib that meets current safety standards. The mattress should be firm and fit snugly in the crib. Cover the mattress with only a tight-fitting crib sheet.
- Do not put anything soft, loose, or fluffy in your baby's sleep space. This includes pillows, blankets, comforters, soft or pillow-like bumpers, stuffed animals, and other soft items.
- Use a sleep sack or other type sleeper instead of blankets to keep your baby warm and safe. Make sure your baby doesn't get too warm during sleep.
- Place your baby's separate, safe sleep space near your bed to help you protect her or him and to make breastfeeding easier. This is called room sharing. Bed sharing is not recommended.
- Never place your baby to sleep on top of any soft surface. This includes adult beds, waterbeds, pillows, cushions, comforters, and sheepskins.
- Do not use anything to prop your baby up or keep him or her on the back.
- Offer your baby a nonsweetened pacifier every time you place her or him down to sleep. If you are breastfeeding, wait until nursing is well established before using a pacifier (usually around 1 month).
- Avoid smoking.
- Educate everyone who cares for your baby about these safe sleep rules!

Adapted from About Kids Health. (2015). *Sudden infant death syndrome.* Retrieved from http://www.aboutkidshealth.ca/En/ResourceCentres/PregnancyBabies/NewbornBabies/HealthIssuesinYourNewbornBaby/Pages/Sudden-Infant-Death-Syndrome.aspx; Canadian Paediatric Society, Canadian Foundation for the Study of Infant Deaths, Canadian Institute of Child Health, Health Canada, & Public Health Agency of Canada. (2012). *The joint statement on safe sleep: Preventing sudden infant deaths in Canada.* Retrieved from http://www.phac-aspc.gc.ca/hp-ps/dca-dea/stages-etapes/childhood-enfance_0-2/sids/jsss-ecss-eng.php

attempt at resuscitation in the emergency department. While they are in the emergency department, the parents should be asked only factual questions, such as when they found the infant, how he or she looked, and whom they called for help. The nurse should avoid any remarks that may suggest responsibility, such as "Why didn't you go in earlier?" "Didn't you hear the infant cry out?" "Was the head buried in a blanket?" or "Were the siblings jealous of this child?" It is the coroner's responsibility to document these findings at the scene rather than have parents recount the experience in the emergency department (Koehler, 2008). Parents may also express feelings of guilt about administering cardiopulmonary resuscitation (CPR) correctly or the timing of CPR in relation to finding the infant.

At this time, the physician should initiate the discussion of an autopsy, often with the nurse being present to support the family. The physician or medical examiner, depending on the circumstances, should emphasize that a diagnosis cannot be confirmed until the postmortem examination is completed. Nurses may balk at the idea of requesting an autopsy because of the parents' emotional state; however, an autopsy may clear up possible misconceptions regarding the death. Instructions about the autopsy and funeral arrangements may need to be repeated or put in writing. If the mother was breastfeeding, she needs information about abrupt discontinuation of lactation. The nurse or physician should contact the primary care practitioner for the infant and the mother to avoid any miscommunications or telephone calls at a later date inquiring about the child's health status.

A review of 60 studies indicates that parents experiencing perinatal death perceive health care workers' responses as having a significant impact on the parents' grieving process; parents perceived the behaviour of many health care workers as thoughtless or insensitive. The findings suggest that nurses and physicians would benefit from more bereavement training (Gold, 2007).

Another important aspect of compassionate care for these parents is allowing them to say good-bye to their child. These are the parents' last moments with their child, and they should be as quiet, meaningful, peaceful, and undisturbed as possible. Parents should be encouraged to hold their infant before leaving the emergency department. Because the parents leave the hospital without their infant, it is helpful to accompany them to the car or arrange for someone else to take them home. A debriefing session may help health care workers who dealt with the family and deceased infant to cope with emotions that are often engendered when a SIDS victim is brought into the acute care facility. Comprehensive guidelines have been published for health care providers involved in SIDS investigations to assist the family and at the same time determine that the infant's death was not the result of other factors, such as child maltreatment (see Additional Resources at the end of this chapter).

When the parents return home, they should be visited by a competent, qualified health care provider as soon after the death as possible. Printed material and websites that contain excellent information about SIDS (available from national organizations) should be provided. Baby's Breath is a resource listed in the Additional Resources section at the end of this chapter.

During the initial visit, the parents should be helped in gaining an intellectual understanding of the condition. The nursing objectives are to assess what the parents have been told about SIDS; what they think happened; and how they explained this to the other siblings, family members, and friends. One question that the nurse will never be able to answer and therefore should not attempt to is "Why did this happen to our baby?" or "Who is responsible for this tragedy?" These and other questions may linger in the parents' minds for months or even years.

When the unexpected death of a child occurs, it is common for one parent to blame the other for the child's death. Parents may also experience guilt over the child's death; if they had checked earlier, the child might still be alive. It is important that the nurse assist parents in working through these feelings to prevent marital disruption in addition to the loss of the loved child.

Some parents are able to discuss their feelings openly, and the nurse should be supportive of this coping skill. However, others may be reluctant to express their grief, and the nurse can encourage the expression of emotions by asking about crying and feeling sad, angry, or guilty. This is an attempt to provoke a display of emotion, not just an admission of a feeling. During this session, the parents should be helped to explore their usual coping mechanisms and, if these are ineffectual, to investigate new approaches. For example, one parent may refrain from discussing the death for fear of upsetting the other parent, but each may need to hear how the other feels.

Ideally, the number of visits and plans for subsequent intervention need to be flexible. Parents facing the question of having a subsequent child will need support. Both the birth of a subsequent child and the survival of that child, especially past the age of death of the previous child, are important transitional stages for parents.

Positional Plagiocephaly

Since the Back to Sleep campaign began in 1999 in Canada, which advocates nonprone sleeping for infants to prevent SIDS, an increase in the incidence of positional plagiocephaly has been observed. The prevalence of positional plagiocephaly at 4 months is reported to range from slightly less than 20% to as much as 48% (Robinson & Proctor, 2009). The term *plagiocephaly* connotes an oblique or asymmetrical head; *positional plagiocephaly, deformational plagiocephaly*, or *nonsynostotic plagiocephaly* implies an acquired condition that occurs as a result of cranial moulding during infancy. Because the infant's sutures are not closed, the skull is pliable and, when the infant is placed on the back to sleep, the posterior occiput flattens over time (Fig. 35-15, A); a transient typical bald spot will develop. As a result of prolonged pressure on one side of the skull, that side becomes misshapen; mild facial asymmetry may develop. The sternocleidomastoid muscle may tighten on the preferential side, and torticollis may also develop. Congenital or acquired torticollis may cause plagiocephaly; the discussion here centres only on plagiocephaly caused by the supine sleeping position.

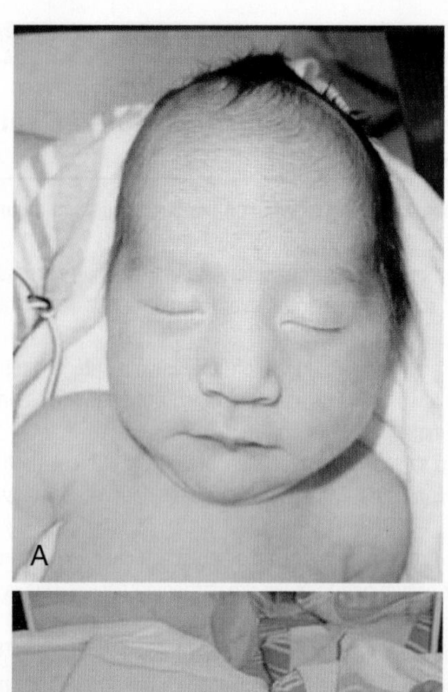

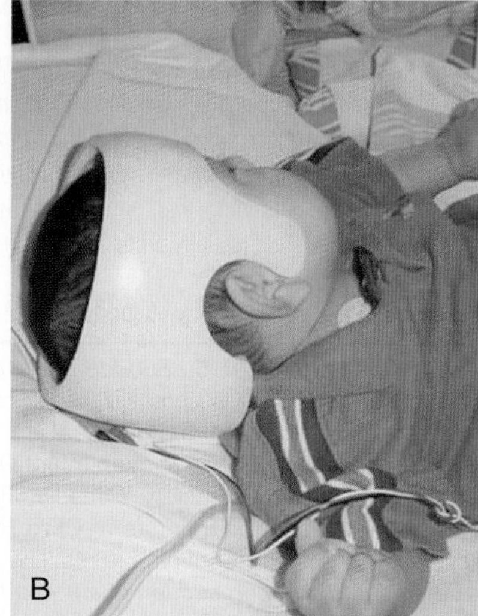

FIGURE 35-15 **A:** Plagiocephaly. **B:** Helmet used to correct plagiocephaly. (Courtesy Dr. Gerardo Cabrera-Meza, Department of Neonatology, Baylor College of Medicine.)

Diagnostic Evaluation

The diagnosis of positional plagiocephaly may be made on physical examination of the infant's head; the infant's head is viewed frontally and from above. The typical infant's head shape will resemble a parallelogram, with unilateral flattening of the occiput, frontal and parietal bossing, a prominent cheekbone, and an anterior ear displacement. An evaluation of neck movement and range of motion is also made to determine the presence of torticollis. In most cases, skull films and further radiological studies (computed tomographic scan) are used only to rule out craniosynostosis or any other cranial deformity that may affect brain growth.

Therapeutic Management

Prevention of positional plagiocephaly may begin shortly after birth by placing the infant to sleep supine and alternating the infant's head position nightly, avoiding prolonged placement in car safety seats and swings, and using prone positioning or "tummy time" for approximately 30 to 60 minutes per day when the infant is awake (Laughlin, Luerssen, Dias, et al., 2011; PHAC, 2014i).

Treatment of torticollis and plagiocephaly initially involves exercises to loosen the tight muscle and changing head position from side to side during feeding, carrying, and sleep. If the plagiocephaly is not resolved within 4 to 8 weeks of physiotherapy, a customized helmet may be worn to decrease the pressure on the affected side of the skull (Fig. 35-15, B). If no improvement occurs with physiotherapy or a moulded helmet over a period of 2 to 3 months, the infant may be referred to a pediatric neurosurgeon or craniofacial surgeon; the referral should optimally occur by 4 to 6 months of age (Laughlin et al., 2011).

The helmet is worn 23 hours a day for a prescribed period (usually 3 months). Repositioning and physical therapy are said to be more effective when used before the infant can roll over or move his or her head alone (i.e., before approximately 3 to 4 months of age) (Robinson & Proctor, 2009). Reports of developmental delay in infants with positional plagiocephaly (nonsynostotic) vary in regard to outcomes, but current studies do not conclusively prove that such infants are at higher risk for developmental delays (Robinson & Proctor, 2009).

NURSING CARE

When a nurse or parent notices plagiocephaly, a consultation with the primary health care provider is recommended to evaluate the head shape and ascertain the need for early intervention.

Nurses are in a unique position in well-child care settings to encourage parents to follow guidelines for preventing plagiocephaly, to demonstrate alternating head placement for sleeping, to demonstrate sternocleidomastoid muscle exercises (as appropriate to the condition), and to encourage supervised tummy time for infants during awake periods. Most important, nurses should continue to encourage parents to place the infant in a supine sleep position despite the development of plagiocephaly. Nurses can also assist parents in the proper use of a skull-moulding helmet and reassure them of the high rate of success with the helmet. Parents should be encouraged to express concerns and feelings related to the health status of the child as well as provision of current best practice is an important nursing function. Parents should not become so alarmed by plagiocephaly that they abandon the supine sleeping position for the infant; instead, they should consult with the practitioner for further advice.

Apnea and Apparent Life-Threatening Events

An *apparent life-threatening event* (ALTE), formerly referred to as *aborted SIDS death* or *near-miss SIDS*, generally refers to an event that is sudden and frightening to the observer, in which the infant exhibits a combination of apnea, change in colour (pallor, cyanosis, redness), change in muscle tone (usually hypotonia), choking, gagging, or coughing, and which usually involves a significant intervention and even CPR by the caregiver who witnesses the event. The definition of ALTE may include apnea, but ALTE may occur without apnea (Silvestri, 2012). It is erroneous to characterize ALTE as a near-miss SIDS incident (Adams, Good, & Defranco, 2009). Infants with ALTE are at increased risk for SIDS; the risk for SIDS may be three to five times greater in infants who experienced an ALTE (Hunt & Hauck, 2016).

Infants with a history of ALTEs may be at increased risk for SIDS, but these children constitute only approximately 7 to 12% of all SIDS victims. Most infants with ALTE are less than 6 months of age, and although there has been a significant decrease in SIDS since 1992, the incidence of ALTE has not changed (Hunt & Hauck, 2016). A diagnosis of apnea of infancy or idiopathic ALTE is often made when no cause is found.

Results from the Collaborative Home Infant Monitoring study (CHIME) found that apnea and bradycardia occurred at conventional and extreme alarm thresholds in all groups of infants studied: siblings of SIDS infants, infants with ALTEs, symptomatic (of apnea and bradycardia) and asymptomatic preterm infants weighing less than 1750 g at birth, and healthy term infants. The researchers concluded that many infants experience apnea and bradycardia in each of these groups yet do not die (Ramanathan, Corwin, Hunt, et al., 2001). Furthermore, it was reported that apnea does not appear to be an immediate precursor to SIDS and that cardiorespiratory monitoring is not an effective tool for identifying infants at greater risk for SIDS. CHIME data indicate that infants with ALTE did not have some of the typical characteristics associated with SIDS infants; these include fewer infants with low birth weight and who are small for gestational age at birth, fewer teenage pregnancies, and a younger infant age at the time of ALTE. The researchers concluded that despite some similar characteristics between ALTE and SIDS, the differences warrant a separate focus on ALTEs (Esani, Hodgman, Ehsani, et al., 2008).

Diagnostic Evaluation

An essential component of the diagnostic process includes a detailed description of the event—who witnessed the event, where the infant was during the event, and what, if any, activities were involved (such as during or after a feeding, riding in a car seat restraint, presence of siblings or any minor children, what clothing the infant was wearing). In addition, a prenatal and postnatal history must be obtained. A short period of observation in the emergency department may be appropriate to observe the infant's respiratory pattern and response to feeding. A careful evaluation of the preterm infant in a car restraint is essential; upper airway occlusion and subsequent apnea and cyanosis may occur if the infant is not positioned properly. Reported diagnoses in infants with ALTE include a neurological event such as a seizure (30% of cases seen); gastrointestinal problem, including gastroesophageal reflux (50%); respiratory conditions (20%); and metabolic, cardiac, or child abuse (each less than 5%). In some cases, multiple diagnoses may be made (Hunt & Hauck, 2016).

In the event that an underlying diagnosis is not established, home monitoring may be recommended. The most commonly used monitoring is continuous recording of cardiorespiratory patterns (cardiopneumogram, or pneumocardiogram). Four-channel pneumocardiograms (or multichannel pneumogram) monitor heart rate, respirations (chest impedance), nasal airflow, and oxygen saturation. A more sophisticated test, polysomnography (sleep study), also records brain waves, eye and body movements, esophageal manometry, and end-tidal carbon dioxide measurements. However, none of these tests can predict risk. Some children with normal results may still have subsequent apneic episodes.

Therapeutic Management

The treatment of the infant with an ALTE depends on the underlying condition (see above). Treatment of recurrent apnea (without an underlying organic problem) usually involves continuous home monitoring of cardiorespiratory rhythms and in some cases the use of methylxanthines (respiratory stimulant drugs, such as theophylline or caffeine). The decision to discontinue the monitoring is based on the infant's clinical condition. A general guideline for discontinuation is when infants with ALTEs have gone 2 or 3 months without significant numbers of episodes requiring intervention. Silvestri (2012) notes that the challenge in treating an infant with an ALTE is to determine if the infant is at further risk for a recurrent event and significant morbidity and death.

Newer home apnea monitors allow downloading of information that assists the practitioner in deciding when to discontinue home monitoring. It is imperative to remember that the home apnea monitor will not predict or prevent SIDS deaths. Furthermore, impedance-based monitors detect chest wall movement and will not detect obstructive apnea unless the episode involves significant bradycardia (see Family-Centred Teaching box). Monitors with respiratory impedance plethysmography (RIP) are capable of detecting obstruction as well as central apnea (Silvestri, 2012).

NURSING CARE

The diagnosis of an ALTE engenders great anxiety and concern in parents, and the institution of home monitoring presents additional physical and emotional burdens. Parents of infants on home apnea monitors report experiencing emotional distress, especially depression and hostility, during the first few weeks after hospital discharge. For parents of a SIDS victim who have a new infant on home apnea monitoring, the anxiety is compounded by the uncertainty of the future of the living child and grief for the lost child. Home apnea monitoring may offer some predictability and control over the current child's survival through the period of uncertainty.

If home monitoring is required, the nurse can be a major source of support to the family in terms of education about the equipment; education regarding observation of the infant's status; and instruction regarding immediate intervention during apneic episodes, including CPR. Several reports indicate that the first week to month after discharge is the most stressful period for parents, particularly when the rate of false alarms is high. To help the family cope with the numerous procedures they must learn, adequate preparation before discharge and written instructions are essential. In the first few weeks after discharge, parents may benefit by having a practitioner readily available to answer questions regarding false alarms and for other technical assistance.

Several types of home monitors are available and are set up by either a home monitor equipment company or home health staff. Nurses, especially those involved in the care at home, must become familiar with the equipment, including its advantages and disadvantages. Safety is a major concern because monitors can cause electrical burns and electrocution (see Family-Centred Teaching box). Parents also need information about travelling or running necessary errands with an infant on an apnea monitor, what to do in case of power failure, and whom to contact if the monitor alarm goes off continuously but the infant appears well.

Siblings should also be supervised when near the infant and taught that the monitor is not a toy. Other safety practices include informing local utility and rescue squads of the home monitoring in case of an emergency. Telephone numbers for these services should be posted near all telephones in the home. Instructions for infant CPR should be posted in a central location of the house. Parents should be encouraged to tell visitors and other family members about the location of such instructions. If a cellular phone is the main house phone, it should stay in a central location for all family members to access in an emergency.

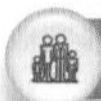

FAMILY-CENTRED TEACHING

Using Apnea Monitors or Home Oxygen Saturation Monitors

Use the monitor as instructed by the practitioner.
If the alarm goes off, look at the infant first to ensure the infant is breathing and then determine the cause of the alarm.
Do not adjust the monitor to eliminate false alarms. Adjustments could compromise the monitor's effectiveness.
Place the monitor on a firm surface away from the crib and drapes; plug the power cord directly into a wall socket with a three-pronged outlet.
Do not sleep in the same bed as a monitored infant.
Keep pets and children away from the monitor and infant.
Keep the monitor away from possible electrical interferences such as appliances (e.g., electric blankets, televisions, air conditioners, cellphones).
Check the monitor several times a day to be sure that the alarm is working and that it can be heard from room to room. Be certain the caregiver can reach the monitor quickly (in less than 30 seconds).
Periodically check the monitor's breath detection indicator and battery or charger connections.
Be aware that strong signals from nearby radio and television stations, airports, ham radios, cellular phones, or police stations could interfere with the monitor. Check for interference if the monitor is to be operated in these areas.
Read the monitor's user manual carefully; report problems promptly.
Inform community utility and rescue squads of home monitoring as appropriate.
Keep emergency rescue numbers near phones in the home.
Practise safety precautions:

- Remove leads when the infant is not attached to the monitor.
- Unplug the power cord from the electrical outlet when the cord is not plugged into the monitor.
- Use safety covers on electrical outlets to prevent children from inserting objects into a socket.

! NURSING ALERT

If the infant is apneic, gently stimulate the trunk by patting or rubbing it. Call loudly for help even if alone. If the infant is prone, turn to the back and flick the feet. If there is still no response, immediately begin CPR. After approximately 2 minutes of CPR, activate the emergency medical service—"Call 911!" and then resume CPR until emergency responders arrive or the infant starts breathing. Never vigorously shake the child. No more than 10 seconds are spent on stimulation before implementing CPR.

Caregivers need detailed information regarding proper attachment of the electrodes to the infant's chest. The electrodes are placed in the midaxillary line, at a space one or two fingerbreadths below the nipple. For home use, electrodes attached to a belt that is placed around the child's trunk are preferred (Fig. 35-16). The belt is positioned so that the electrodes contact the skin in the same area. Monitors may have memory chips that

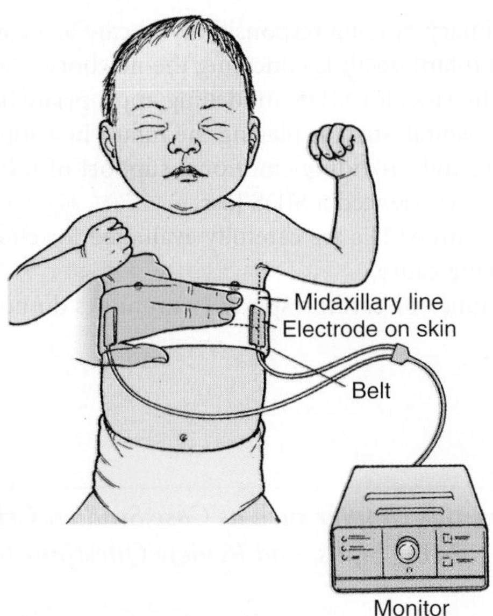

FIGURE 35-16 Electrode placement for apnea monitoring. In small infants, one fingerbreadth may be used.

allow for event recording, which can be an effective tool in evaluating the use of the monitor, events immediately before and after the event, and reported frequency of alarms.

Monitors are effective only if they are used. They do not prevent death but alert the caregiver to the ALTE in time to intervene. The need to use the monitor and to respond appropriately to alarms must be stressed. The inability to use the monitor properly can result in the infant's death.

Family support. Many of the stresses observed during the monitoring period are characteristic of those of families with chronically ill children. The child with an apnea or cardiorespiratory monitor may have additional health care needs, such as a gastrostomy, tracheostomy, ostomy, and myriad medications or treatments that exacerbate the parents' stress. Parents of these infants report increased stress, including concern for their child's survival, fear of incompetence in assuming home responsibility, inadequate respite care, lack of time for other children and the spouse, social isolation from friends and extended family, constant work, and fatigue. The monitored child is at risk for vulnerable child syndrome, which may lead to lack of parental separation and preferential treatment, causing further family disruption. To deal with these potential effects, nurses need to employ the same interventions as those discussed for children with chronic illness and to be aware of the need for referral when difficulties are suspected.

To lessen the continuous responsibility of monitoring, other family members, such as grandparents, should be taught how to manipulate the equipment, read and interpret the signals, and administer CPR. They should be encouraged to stay with the infant for regular periods to give parents respite. Support groups of other families who have successfully completed monitoring can also be of benefit. Because babysitters may be difficult to locate, support group members or nursing students may be potential sources of qualified caregivers.

KEY POINTS

- Biological development of the child encompasses proportional changes; sensory changes, including binocularity, depth perception, and visual preference; maturation of biological systems; fine motor development; and gross motor development.
- Erikson's theory of psychosocial development (birth to 1 year) is concerned with acquiring a sense of trust while overcoming a sense of mistrust.
- Piaget's theory of cognitive development, as it applies to the infant, focuses on the sensorimotor phase, which includes the use of reflexes, primary circular reactions, secondary circular reactions, and coordination of secondary schemata and their application to new situations.
- Development of body image begins in infancy; by 1 year of age, infants recognize that they are distinct from their parents.
- Social development of the infant is guided by attachment, language development, personal-social behaviour, and participation in play.
- Temperament influences the type of interaction that occurs between the child and parents and siblings.
- Parents are faced with many concerns, including selecting an appropriate day care, limit-setting and discipline, thumb-sucking and pacifier use, and teething.
- Breast milk provides optimum nutrition for the infant during the first 6 months; introduction of solid food occurs during the second 6 months. Commercial iron-fortified infant formula is an alternative to human milk. Whole milk is not recommended until after 1 year of age.
- Cleaning the teeth regularly in early childhood and appropriate dietary intake promote good dental health.
- Recommended routine immunizations include those for HBV, HAV, diphtheria, influenza, tetanus, pertussis, polio, measles, mumps, rubella, pneumococcus, meningococcus, chickenpox, and Hib.
- Recommended immunizations for selected groups of children are rotavirus and HPV vaccines.
- Because injuries are a major cause of death during infancy, parents should be alerted to the possibility of aspiration of foreign objects, suffocation, falls, poisoning, burns, motor vehicle injuries, and bodily damage, as well as preventive actions needed to make the environment safe for infants.
- Treatment of colic may involve change in feeding practices, correction of a stressful environment, behaviour modification, and support of the parent.
- Growth failure, or FTT, may occur in children who have a chronic illness, or it may occur in a family environment in which healthy infant feeding practices are poorly managed or understood. FTT is often multifactorial and not always

associated with a pattern of a disturbed maternal–infant relationship.
- SIDS is the third leading cause of infant death.
- Factors that place the infant at high risk for SIDS/SUDI include prone sleeping position, soft bedding, sleeping in a noninfant bed with an adult or older child, poor socioeconomic status, and maternal prenatal smoking.
- Positional plagiocephaly can be easily prevented by allowing the awake infant to have periods of supervised tummy time and by alternating the infant's head position during sleep.
- The primary nursing responsibility in care associated with sudden infant death is educating the newborn's family about the risks for SIDS, modelling appropriate behaviours in the hospital, such as placing the infant in a supine sleep position, and providing emotional support of the family that has experienced a SIDS loss.
- Infants with ALTEs are carefully evaluated for clues to the underlying cause.
- Home apnea or cardiorespiratory monitors do not prevent SIDS.

evolve WEBSITE

***Visit the Evolve website for additional resources related to the content in this chapter such as Case Studies, Critical Thinking Case Study Answers, Nursing Care Plans, Nursing Processes, Nursing Skills, and Review Questions for Exam Preparation at:** http://evolve.elsevier.com/Canada/Perry/maternal/*

REFERENCES

Adams, S. M., Good, M. W., & Defranco, G. M. (2009). Sudden infant death syndrome. *American Family Physician, 79*(10), 870–874.

American Academy of Pediatrics. (2009). *Pediatric nutrition handbook* (6th ed.). Elk Grove Village, IL: Author.

American Academy of Pediatrics. (2015). *How to prevent tooth decay in your baby*. Retrieved from <https://www.healthychildren.org/English/ages-stages/baby/teething-tooth-care/Pages/How-to-Prevent-Tooth-Decay-in-Your-Baby.aspx>.

American Academy of Pediatrics, Committee on Infectious Diseases, & Pickering, L. (Eds.), (2015). *2015 Red book: Report of the Committee on Infectious Diseases* (30th ed.). Elk Grove Village, IL: Author.

American Academy of Pediatrics, Task Force on Sudden Infant Death Syndrome. (2011). SIDS and other sleep-related infant deaths: Expansion of recommendations for a safe infant sleeping environment. *Pediatrics, 128*(5), e1341–e1367. doi:10.1542/peds.2011-2285.

Arikan, D., Alp, H., Gözüm, S., et al. (2008). Effectiveness of massage, sucrose solution, herbal tea or hydrolyzed formula in the treatment of infantile colic. *Journal of Clinical Nursing, 17*(13), 1754–1761. doi:10.1111/j.1365-2702.2007.02093.x.

Blackburn, S. T. (2013). *Maternal, fetal, and neonatal physiology: A clinical perspective* (4th ed.). St. Louis: Saunders.

Breastfeeding Committee of Canada. (2012). *Summary: Integrated 10 steps practice outcome indicators for hospitals and community health services*. Retrieved from <http://breastfeedingcanada.ca/documents/2012-05-14_BCC_BFI_Ten_Steps_Integrated_Indicators.pdf>.

Canadian Dental Association. (2012). *CDA position on use of fluorides in caries prevention*. Retrieved from <http://www.cda-adc.ca/_files/position_statements/fluoride.pdf>.

Canadian Dental Association. (2016). *Dental care for children*. Retrieved from <http://www.cda-adc.ca/en/oral_health/cfyt/dental_care_children/>.

Canadian Paediatric Society. (2012a). *Pacifiers (soothers): A user's guide for parents*. Retrieved from <http://www.caringforkids.cps.ca/handouts/pacifiers>.

Canadian Paediatric Society. (2012b). *Healthy bodies: Healthy sleep for your baby and child*. Retrieved from <http://www.caringforkids.cps.ca/handouts/healthy_sleep_for_your_baby_and_child>.

Canadian Paediatric Society. (2013). *Healthy teeth for children*. Retrieved by <http://www.caringforkids.cps.ca/handouts/healthy_teeth_for_children>.

Canadian Paediatric Society. (2014). *Feeding your baby in the first year*. Retrieved from <http://www.caringforkids.cps.ca/handouts/feeding_your_baby_in_the_first_year>.

Canadian Paediatric Society. (2015a). *A parent's guide to immunization information on the Internet*. Retrieved from <http://www.caringforkids.cps.ca/handouts/immunization_information_on_the_internet>.

Canadian Paediatric Society. (2015b). *Colic and crying*. Retrieved from <http://www.caringforkids.cps.ca/handouts/colic_and_crying>.

Canadian Paediatric Society, Child and Youth Maltreatment Section. (2001). Reaffirmed 2005. Joint statement on shaken baby syndrome. *Paediatrics & Child Health, 6*(9), 663–667. Reaffirmed 2005. Retrieved from <http://www.cps.ca/documents/position/shaken-baby-syndrome>.

Carey, W. B., & McDevitt, S. C. (1978). Revision of the infant temperament questionnaire. *Pediatrics, 61*(5), 735–739.

Centers for Disease Control and Prevention. (2005). Nonfatal motor-vehicle-related backover injuries among children—United States, 2001–2003. *MMWR. Morbidity and Mortality Weekly Report, 54*(6), 144–146.

Chan, E. S., Cummings, C., & Canadian Paediatric Society, Community Paediatrics Committee. (2013). Dietary exposures and allergy prevention in high-risk infants. *Paediatrics & Child Health, 18*(10), 545–549. Reaffirmed 2016. Retrieved from <http://www.cps.ca/documents/position/dietary-exposures-and-allergy-prevention-in-high-risk-infants>.

Cole, S. Z., & Lanham, J. S. (2011). Failure to thrive: An update. *American Family Physician, 83*(7), 829–834.

Cook, F., Bayer, J., Le, H. N. D., et al. (2012). Baby Business: A randomized controlled trial of a universal parenting program that aims to prevent early infant sleep and cry problems and associated parental depression. *BMC Pediatrics, 12*(13), doi:10.1186/1471-2431-12-13.

Cook, E. H., & Higgins, S. S. (2010). Congenital heart disease. In P. J. Allen, J. A. Vessey, & N. A. Schapiro (Eds.), *Primary care of the child with a chronic condition* (5th ed.). St. Louis: Mosby.

Critch, N., & Canadian Paediatric Society, Nutrition and Gastroenterology Committee. (2011). Infantile colic: Is there a role for dietary interventions? *Paediatrics & Child Health, 16*(1), 47–49. Reaffirmed 2016. Retrieved from <http://www.cps.ca/documents/position/infantile-colic-dietary-interventions>.

Della Vedova, A. M. (2014). Maternal psychological state and infant's temperament at three months. *Journal of Reproductive and Infant Psychology, 32*(5), 520–534.

Ellett, M. L., Appleton, M. M., & Sloan, R. S. (2009). Out of the abyss of colic: A view through the father's eyes. *MCN: The American Journal of Maternal Child Nursing, 34*(3), 164–171.

Erikson, E. H. (1963). *Childhood and society* (2nd ed.). New York: Norton.

Esani, N., Hodgman, J. E., Ehsani, N., et al. (2008). Apparent life-threatening events and sudden infant death syndrome: Comparison of risk factors. *Journal of Pediatrics, 152*(3), A2. doi:10.1016/j.jpeds.2007.07.054.

Fein, S. B., Li, R., Chen, J., et al. (2014). Methods for the year 6 follow-up study of children in the Infant Feeding Practices Study II. *Pediatrics, 134*(Suppl. 1), S4–S12. doi:10.1542/peds.2014-0646C.

Feldman-Winter, L. (2013). Evidence-based interventions to support breast feeding. *Pediatric Clinics of North America, 60*(1), 169–187. doi:10.1016/j.pcl.2012.09.007.

Gleason, M. M., Fox, N. A., Drury, S., et al. (2011). Validity of evidence-derived criteria for reactive attachment disorder: Indiscriminately social/disinhibited and emotionally withdrawn/inhibited types. *Journal of the American Academy of Child and Adolescent Psychiatry, 50*(3), 216–231. doi:10.1016/j.jaac.2010.12.012.

Godel, J. C., & Canadian Paediatric Society, First Nations, Inuit and Métis Health Committee. (2007). Vitamin D supplementation: Recommendations for Canadian mothers and infants. *Paediatrics & Child Health, 12*(7), 583–589. Reaffirmed 2015. Retrieved from <http://www.cps.ca/documents/position/vitamin-d>.

Gold, K. J. (2007). Navigating care after a baby dies: A systematic review of parent experiences with health providers. *Journal of Perinatology, 27*(4), 230–237. doi:10.1038/sj.jp.7211676.

Government of Canada. (2016a). *Cribs, cradles and bassinets regulations (SOR/2010-261)*. Retrieved from <http://laws-lois.justice.gc.ca/eng/regulations/SOR-2010-261/>.

Government of Canada. (2016b). *Canada's provincial and territorial routine (and catch-up) vaccination programs for infants and children*. Retrieved from <http://healthycanadians.gc.ca/healthy-living-vie-saine/immunization-immunisation/children-enfants/schedule-calendrier-table-1-eng.php?_ga=1.181545134.868197850.1432519476>.

Grazel, R., Phalen, A. G., & Palomano, R. C. (2010). Implementation of the American Academy of Pediatrics recommendations to reduce sudden infant death syndrome risk in neonatal intensive care units: An evaluation of nursing knowledge and practice. *Advances in Neonatal Care, 10*(6), 332–342.

Hanzer, M., Zotter, H., Sauseng, W., et al. (2010). Non-nutritive sucking habits in sleeping infants. *Neonatology, 97*(1), 61–66. doi:10.1159/000231518.

Harrison, D., Yamada, J., & Stevens, B. (2010). Strategies for the prevention and management of neonatal and infant pain. *Current Pain and Headache Reports, 14*(2), 113–123.

Harrison, D., Bueno, M., & Reszel, J. (2015). Prevention and management of pain and stress in the neonate. *Research and Reports in Neonatology, 5*, 9–16. doi:10.2147/RRN.S52378.

Hatfield, L. A. (2008). Sucrose decreases infant neurobehavioural pain response to immunizations: A randomized controlled trial. *Journal of Nursing Scholarship, 40*(3), 219–225. doi:10.1111/j.1547-5069.2008.00229.x.

Health Canada. (2007). *Injury data analysis leads to baby walker ban*. Retrieved from <http://www.hc-sc.gc.ca/sr-sr/activ/consprod/baby-bebe-eng.php>.

Health Canada. (2014). *Safety of homemade infant formulas in Canada*. Retrieved from <http://www.hc-sc.gc.ca/fn-an/nutrition/infant-nourisson/formula-safety_innocuite-nourrisons-eng.php>.

Health Canada. (2015a). *Nutrition for healthy term infants: Recommendations from birth to six months. A joint statement of Health Canada, Canadian Paediatric Society, Dietitians of Canada, and Breastfeeding Committee for Canada*. Retrieved from <http://www.hc-sc.gc.ca/fn-an/nutrition/infant-nourisson/recom/index-eng.php#a7>.

Health Canada. (2015b). *Nutrition for healthy term infants: Recommendations from 6 to 24 months. A joint statement of Health Canada, and Breastfeeding Committee for Canada*. Retrieved from <http://www.hc-sc.gc.ca/fn-an/nutrition/infant-nourisson/recom/recom-6-24-months-6-24-mois-eng.php>.

Health Link BC. (2014). *Feeding your baby*. Retrieved from <http://www.healthlinkbc.ca/healthyeating/feeding-baby.html#resources>.

Health Link BC. (2015). *Crying: Tired or overstimulated*. Retrieved from <http://www.healthlinkbc.ca/healthtopics/content.asp?hwid=not42047>.

Hoath, S. B., & Narendran, V. (2011). The skin. In R. J. Martin, A. A. Fanaroff, & M. C. Walsh (Eds.), *Fanaroff and Martin's neonatal-perinatal medicine* (9th ed.). St. Louis: Mosby.

Hunt, C. E., & Hauck, F. R. (2016). Sudden infant death syndrome. In R. M. Kliegman, et al. (Eds.), *Nelson textbook of pediatrics* (20th ed.). Philadelphia: Saunders.

Institute of Medicine. (2004). *Immunization safety review: Vaccines and autism*. Washington, DC: National Academies Press.

Ipp, M., Parkin, P. C., Lear, N., et al. (2009). Order of vaccine injection and infant pain response. *Archives of Pediatrics & Adolescent Medicine, 163*(5), 469–472.

Jaafar, S. H., Jahanfar, S., Angolkar, M., et al. (2012). Effect of restricted pacifier use in breastfeeding term infants for increasing duration of breastfeeding. *The Cochrane Database of Systematic Reviews*, 16(3), CD007202, doi:10.1002/14651858.CD007202.pub2.

Jenik, A., Vain, N., Gorestein, A. N., et al. (2009). Does the recommendation to use a pacifier influence the prevalence of breastfeeding? *The Journal of Pediatrics, 155*(3), 350–354. doi:10.1016/j.jpeds.2009.03.038.

Keefe, M. R., Lobo, M. L., Froese-Fretz, A., et al. (2006). Effectiveness of an intervention for colic. *Clinical Pediatrics, 45*(2), 123–133.

Koehler, S. A. (2008). Sudden infant death syndrome deaths: The role of forensic nurses. *Journal of Forensic Nursing, 4*(3), 141–142.

Lang, M., & Canadian Paediatric Society, Community Paediatrics Committee. (2008). Health implications of children in child care centres Part A: Canadian trends in child care, behaviour and developmental outcomes. *Paediatrics & Child Health, 13*(10), 863–867. Reaffirmed 2016. Retrieved from <http://www.cps.ca/documents/position/child-care-centres-trends-behaviour-development>.

Lang, M., & Canadian Paediatric Society, Community Paediatrics Committee. (2009). Health implications of children in child care centres Part B: Injuries and infections. *Paediatrics & Child Health, 14*(1), 40–43. Reaffirmed 2016. Retrieved from <http://www.cps.ca/documents/position/child-care-centres-injuries-infections#authors>.

Laughlin, J., Luerssen, T. G., Dias, M. S., & Committee on Practice and Ambulatory Medicine, Section on Neurological Surgery. (2011). Prevention and management of positional skull deformities in infants. *Pediatrics, 128*(6), 1236–1241. doi:10.1542/peds.2011-2220.

Lawrence, R. A., & Lawrence, R. M. (2015). *Breastfeeding: A guide for the medical profession* (8th ed.). St. Louis: Mosby.

Liaw, J. J., Zeng, W. P., Yang, L., et al. (2011). Nonnutritive sucking and oral sucrose relieve neonatal pain during intramuscular injection of hepatitis vaccine. *Journal of Pain and Symptom Management, 42*(6), 918–930.

Madden, G. R., Schmitz, K. H., & Fullerton, K. (2012). A case of infantile star anise toxicity. *Pediatric Emergency Care, 28*(3), 284–285. doi:10.1097/PEC.0b013e3182495ba7.

Marchand, V., & Canadian Paediatric Society, Nutrition and Gastroenterology Committee. (2012). The toddler who is falling off the growth chart. *Paediatrics & Child Health, 17*(8), 447. Reaffirmed 2015. Retrieved from <http://www.cps.ca/en/documents/position/toddler-falling-off-the-growth-chart>.

Markman, L. (2009). Teething: Facts and fiction. *Pediatric Review, 30*(8), 359–364.

Markowitz, R., Watkins, J. B., & Duggan, C. (2008). Failure to thrive: Malnutrition in the pediatric setting. In R. Markowitz, J. B. Watkins, & C. Duggan (Eds.), *Nutrition in pediatrics* (4th ed.). Hamilton, ON: Decker.

Matthews, R., & Moore, A. (2013). Babies are still dying of SIDS. *American Journal of Nursing, 113*(2), 59–64.

Matthey, S., & Črnčec, R. (2012). Comparison of two strategies to improve infant sleep problems, and associated impacts on maternal experience, mood and infant emotional health: A single case replication design study. *Early Human Development, 88*(6), 437–442. doi:10.1016/j.earlhumdev.2011.10.010.

McConnell, M., & Moss, E. (2011). Attachment across the life span: Factors that contribute to stability and change. *Australian Journal of Educational & Developmental Psychology, 11*, 60–77.

McGrath, J. M., Records, K., & Rice, M. (2008). Maternal depression and infant temperament characteristics. *Infant Behavior & Development*, *31*(1), 71–80.

Medoff-Cooper, B., Carey, W. B., & McDevitt, S. C. (1993). The Early Infancy Temperament Questionnaire. *Journal of Developmental and Behavioral Pediatrics*, *14*(4), 230–235.

Megel, M. E., Wilson, M. E., Bravo, K., et al. (2011). Baby lost and found: Mothers' experiences of infants who cry persistently. *Journal of Pediatric Health Care*, *25*(3), 144–152.

Moore, M., Meltzer, L. J., & Mindell, J. A. (2008). Bedtime problems and night wakings in children. *Primary Care*, *35*(3), 569–581, viii. doi:10.1016/j.pop.2008.06.002.

Morin, K. (2009). The challenge of colic in infants. *MCN: The American Journal of Maternal Child Nursing*, *34*(3), 192.

Myrelid, A., Gustafsson, J., Ollars, B., et al. (2002). Growth charts for Down's syndrome from birth to 18 years of age. *Archives of Disease in Childhood*, *87*(2), 97–103.

O'Connor, N. R. (2009). Infant formula. *American Family Physician*, *79*(7), 565–570.

Perry, R., Hunt, K., & Ernst, E. (2011). Nutritional supplements and other complementary medicines for infantile colic: A systematic review. *Pediatrics*, *127*(4), 720–733.

Piaget, J. (1952). *The origins of intelligence in children*. New York: International Universities Press.

Ponti, M., & Canadian Paediatric Society, Community Paediatrics Committee. (2003). Recommendations for the use of pacifiers. *Paediatrics & Child Health*, *8*(8), 515–519. Reaffirmed 2016. Retrieved from <http://www.cps.ca/en/documents/position/pacifiers#authors>.

Price, C. S., Thompson, W. W., Goodson, B., et al. (2010). Prenatal and infant exposure to thimerosal from vaccines and immunoglobulins and risk of autism. *Pediatrics*, *126*(4), 656–664.

Public Health Agency of Canada. (2011). *Shaken baby syndrome*. Retrieved from <http://www.phac-aspc.gc.ca/hp-ps/dca-dea/cht-sse/shaken-secoue/index-eng.php>.

Public Health Agency of Canada. (2012a). *Varicella (chickenpox)*. Retrieved from <http://www.phac-aspc.gc.ca/im/vpd-mev/varicella-eng.php>.

Public Health Agency of Canada. (2012b). *Tuberculosis fact sheets: Active infectious TB disease*. Retrieved from <http://www.phac-aspc.gc.ca/tbpc-latb/fa-fi/infecttb-eng.php>.

Public Health Agency of Canada. (2012c). *Joint statement on safe sleep: Preventing sudden infant deaths in Canada*. Retrieved from <http://www.phac-aspc.gc.ca/hp-ps/dca-dea/stages-etapes/childhood-enfance_0-2/sids/jsss-ecss-eng.php>.

Public Health Agency of Canada. (2013). Guidelines for the prevention and control of measles outbreaks in Canada. *Canada Communicable Disease Report*, *39*, ACS–3. Retrieved from <http://www.phac-aspc.gc.ca/publicat/ccdr-rmtc/13vol39/acs-dcc-3/assets/pdf/meas-roug-eng.pdf>.

Public Health Agency of Canada. (2014a). *Summary of the primary care management of hepatitis B—Quick reference*. Retrieved from <http://www.phac-aspc.gc.ca/publicat/ccdr-rmtc/14vol40/dr-rm40-13/dr-rm40-13-clin-1-eng.php>.

Public Health Agency of Canada. (2014b). *Diphtheria: For health professionals*. Retrieved from <http://www.phac-aspc.gc.ca/im/vpd-mev/diphtheria-diphterie/professionals-professionnels-eng.php>.

Public Health Agency of Canada. (2014c). *Tetanus*. Retrieved from <http://www.phac-aspc.gc.ca/im/vpd-mev/tetanus-tetanos-eng.php>.

Public Health Agency of Canada. (2014d). *Pertussis (whooping cough): For health professionals*. Retrieved from <http://www.phac-aspc.gc.ca/im/vpd-mev/pertussis/professionals-professionnels-eng.php>.

Public Health Agency of Canada. (2014e). *Canada communicable disease report CCDR*. Measles activity in Canada: January–June 2014. Retrieved from <http://www.phac-aspc.gc.ca/publicat/ccdr-rmtc/14vol40/dr-rm40-12/dr-rm40-12-rc-cr-eng.php>.

Public Health Agency of Canada. (2014f). *Mumps: For health professionals*. Retrieved from <http://www.phac-aspc.gc.ca/im/vpd-mev/mumps-oreillons/professionals-professionnels-eng.php>.

Public Health Agency of Canada. (2014g). *Canadian tuberculosis standards* (7th ed). Retrieved from <http://www.phac-aspc.gc.ca/tbpc-latb/pubs/tb-canada-7/tb-standards-tb-normes-ch16-eng.php#s1-2>.

Public Health Agency of Canada. (2014h). *Sudden infant death syndrome (SIDS) in Canada fact sheet*. Retrieved from <http://www.phac-aspc.gc.ca/rhs-ssg/factshts/mat_sids-smsn_mat-eng.php>.

Public Health Agency of Canada. (2014i). *Safe sleep*. Retrieved from <http://www.phac-aspc.gc.ca/hp-ps/dca-dea/stages-etapes/childhood-enfance_0-2/sids/index-eng.php>.

Public Health Agency of Canada. (2015a). *Notifiable diseases online*. Retrieved from <http://dsol-smed.phac-aspc.gc.ca/dsol-smed/ndis/charts.php?c=pl>.

Public Health Agency of Canada. (2015b). *Canadian immunization guide*. Retrieved from <http://www.phac-aspc.gc.ca/publicat/cig-gci/index-eng.php>.

Public Health Agency of Canada. (2015c). *Invasive meningococcal disease: For health professionals*. Retrieved from <http://www.phac-aspc.gc.ca/im/vpd-mev/meningococcal/professionals-professionnels-eng.php>.

Public Health Agency of Canada. (2015d). *Canadian Adverse Events Following Immunization Surveillance System (CAEFISS)*. Retrieved from <http://www.phac-aspc.gc.ca/im/vs-sv/index-eng.php>.

Public Health Agency of Canada. (2016). *Poliomyelitis*. Retrieved from <http://www.phac-aspc.gc.ca/im/vpd-mev/poliomyelitis-eng.php>.

Puffenberger, E. G., Hu-Lince, D., Parod, J. M., et al. (2004). Mapping of sudden infant death with dysgenesis of the testis syndrome (SIDDT) by a SNP genome scan and identification of TSPYL loss of function. *Proceedings of the National Academy of Sciences of the United States of America*, *101*(32), 689–691, 694.

Ramanathan, R., Corwin, M. J., Hunt, C. E., et al. (2001). Cardiorespiratory events recorded on home monitors: Comparison of healthy infants with those at increased risk for SIDS. *Journal of the American Medical Association*, *285*(17), 2199–2207.

Robinson, S., & Proctor, M. (2009). Diagnosis and management of deformational plagiocephaly: A review. *Journal of Neurosurgery: Pediatrics*, *3*(4), 284–295.

Savino, F., Cordisco, L., Tarasco, V., et al. (2010). *Lactobacillus reuteri* DSM 17938 in infantile colic: A randomized, double-blind, placebo-controlled trial. *Pediatrics*, *126*(3), e526–e533.

Schultz, S. T. (2010). Does thimerosal or other mercury exposure increase the risk for autism? *Acta Neurobiologiae Experimentalis*, *70*(2), 187–195.

Settipane, R. A., Siri, D., & Bellanti, J. A. (2009). Egg allergy and influenza vaccination. *Allergy and Asthma Proceedings*, *30*(6), 660–665.

Silvestri, J. M. (2012). Indications for home apnea monitoring (or not). *Clinics in Perinatology*, *36*(1), v87–v99. doi:10.1016/j.clp.2008.09.012.

Smyke, A. T., Zeanah, C. H., Fox, N. A., et al. (2010). Placement in foster care enhances quality of attachment among young institutionalized children. *Child Development*, *81*(1), 212–223. doi:10.1111/j.1467-8624.2009.01390.x.

Statistics Canada. (2016). *Leading causes of death, infants, by sex, Canada, annual*. Retrieved from <http://www5.statcan.gc.ca/cansim/pick-choisir?lang=eng&p2=33&id=1020562>.

Strehle, E. M., Gray, W. K., Gopisetti, S., et al. (2012). Can home monitoring reduce mortality in infants at increased risk of sudden infant death syndrome? A systematic review. *Acta Paediatrica*, *101*(1), 8–13.

Stremler, R., Hodnett, E., Kenton, L., et al. (2013). Effect of behavioural-educational intervention on sleep for primiparous women and their infants in early postpartum: Multisite randomized controlled trial. *British Medical Journal*, *346*, f1164. doi:10.1136/bmj.f1164.

Strikas, R. A., & Centers for Disease Control and Prevention (CDC), Advisory Committee on Immunization Practices (ACIP), ACIP Child/Adolescent Immunization Work Group. (2015). Advisory committee on immunization practices recommended immunization schedules for persons aged 0 through 18 years–United States, 2015. *MMWR. Morbidity and Mortality Weekly Report*, *64*(4), 93–94.

Thomas, D. W., Greer, F. R., & American Academy of Pediatrics (AAP) Committee on Nutrition and Section on Gastroenterology, Hepatology, and Nutrition. (2010). Probiotics and prebiotics in pediatrics. *Pediatrics*, *126*(6), 1217–1231.

Touchette, E., Petit, D., Tremblay, R. E., et al. (2009). Risk factors and consequences of early child dyssomnias: New perspectives. *Sleep Medicine Reviews*, *13*(5), 355–361. doi:10.1016/j.smrv.2008.12.001.

Transport Canada. (2015). *Keep kids safe*. Retrieved from <https://www.tc.gc.ca/eng/motorvehiclesafety/safedrivers-childsafety-car-time-stages-1083.htm>.

Turner, S., Arthur, G., Lyons, R. A., et al. (2011). Modification of the home environment for the reduction of injuries. *The Cochrane database of systematic reviews [electronic resource]*, (2), CD003600, doi:10.1002/14651858.CD003600.pub3.

van Schaik, C., & Canadian Paediatric Society, Injury Prevention Committee. (2008). Transportation of infants and children in motor vehicles. *Paediatrics & Child Health, 13*(4), 313–318.

Wasser, H., Bentley, M., Borja, J., et al. (2011). Infants perceived as "fussy" are more likely to receive complementary foods before 4 months. *Pediatrics, 127*(2), 229–237.

Whittingham, K., & Douglas, P. (2014). Optimizing parent–infant sleep from birth to 6 months: A new paradigm. *Infant Mental Health Journal, 35*(6), 614–623. doi:10.1002/imhj.21455.

World Health Organization. (2016). *Poliomyelitis: Fact sheet N 114*. Retrieved from <http://www.who.int/mediacentre/factsheets/fs114/en/>.

Yanchar, N. L., Warda, L. J., & Fuselli, P. (2012). Child and youth injury prevention: A public health approach. Canadian Paediatric Society Injury Prevention Committee Abridged version. *Paediatrics & Child Health, 17*(9), 511.

Yu, C. Y., Hung, C. H., Chan, T. F., et al. (2012). Prenatal predictors for father–infant attachment after childbirth. *Journal of Clinical Nursing, 21*, 1577–1583. doi:10.1111/j.1365-2702.2011.04003.x.

ADDITIONAL RESOURCES

Baby's Breath Canada: <http://www.babysbreathcanada.ca/grievingfamilies.html>.

Canadian Growth Charts for 2014 and the health professional guide on how to accurately utilize the charts: <http://www.dietitians.ca/Dietitians-Views/Prenatal-and-Infant/WHO-Growth-Charts.aspx>.

Canadian Coalition for Immunization Awareness and Promotion: <http://www.immunize.cpha.ca/en/default.aspx>.

Canadian Partnership for Children's Health and Environment—Working to Protect Children from Environmental Contaminants: <http://www.healthyenvironmentforkids.ca/>.

Caring for Kids—Back to Sleep: <http://www.caringforkids.cps.ca/handouts/safe_sleep_for_babies>.

Caring for Kids—Never Shake a Baby: <http://www.caringforkids.cps.ca/handouts/never_shake_a_baby>.

Health Canada—Baby Car Seat Carrier Safety Belts Pose Risk of Serious Injury to Infants: <http://www.hc-sc.gc.ca/ahc-asc/media/advisories-avis/_2011/2011_126-eng.php>.

Health Canada Consumer Product Safety—Is Your Child Safe: <http://www.hc-sc.gc.ca/cps-spc/pubs/cons/child-enfant/safe-securite-eng.php>.

Healthlink BC—Safe Sleeping for Babies: <http://www.healthlinkbc.ca/healthfiles/hfile107.stm>.

Immunize Canada: <http://immunize.ca/en/learn/records.aspx>.

Information for parents on what to consider when selecting a child care facility:
<http://www.healthlinkbc.ca/kb/content/special/aa43308.html>.
<http://www.senecacollege.ca/community/KOLTguidetochoosingchildcare.html>
<http://childcaretoday.ca/index.php>.

Parachute—Child passenger safety: <http://www.parachutecanada.org/policy/item/child-passenger-safety>.

Parents coping with the loss of their baby—Resources: <http://www.aboutkidshealth.ca/En/ResourceCentres/BrainTumours/TreatmentofBrainTumours/PalliativeCare/Pages/Grieving.aspx>.

Period of PURPLE Crying: <http://www.purplecrying.info/>.

Public Health Agency of Canada—Child maltreatment publications: <http://phac-aspc.gc.ca/cm-vee/index-eng.php>.

Public Health Agency of Canada—Injury prevention: <http://www.phac-aspc.gc.ca/inj-bles/index-eng.php>.

Public Health Agency of Canada—The Canadian Immunization Guide, schedules for each province and territory: <http://www.phac-aspc.gc.ca/publicat/cig-gci/index-eng.php>.

Transport Canada—Legal Requirements for Children's Motor Vehicle Restraints: <http://www.tc.gc.ca/eng/roadsafety/safedrivers-childsafety-programs-index-874.htm>.

World Health Organization—Growth velocities charts: <http://www.who.int/childgrowth/standards/en/>.

CHAPTER 36

The Toddler and Family

Cheryl Dika

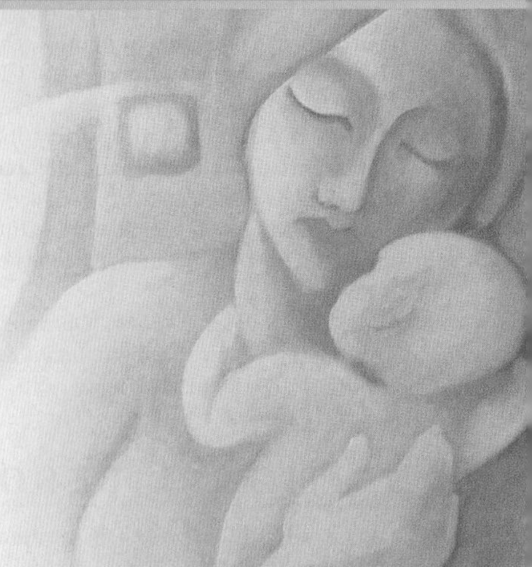

evolve WEBSITE

Visit the Evolve website for additional resources related to the content in this chapter such as Case Studies, Critical Thinking Case Study Answers, Nursing Care Plans, Nursing Processes, Nursing Skills, and Review Questions for Exam Preparation at: http://evolve.elsevier.com/Canada/Perry/maternal/

OBJECTIVES

On completion of this chapter the reader will be able to:

- Identify the major biological, psychosocial, cognitive, and social developments during the toddler years.
- Relate separation anxiety and negativism to developmental tasks.
- Recognize a child's readiness for toilet training and offer parents guidelines.
- Prepare parents of toddlers for the birth of a sibling.
- Provide parents with guidelines for handling temper tantrums.
- Provide parents with feeding recommendations for the toddler.
- Outline a preventive dental hygiene plan for toddlers.
- Provide anticipatory guidance to parents regarding injury prevention that is based on the toddler's developmental achievements.

PROMOTING OPTIMUM GROWTH AND DEVELOPMENT

For children aged 12 to 36 months, it is a time of intense exploration of the environment as they attempt to figure out how things work and learn how to control others through their behaviour, which can include temper tantrums, negativism, and obstinacy. The term *terrible twos* has often been used to describe the toddler years, the period from 12 to 36 months of age. Although the term may be used to describe the toddler's *behaviour*, it is not meant to typify or label the child. Toddlers can also be very lovable, but because of their search for autonomy, they may test parents' and caregivers' patience. This can be a challenging time for parents and child as each comes to know the other better. It is also an important period for developmental achievement and intellectual growth. Neuroscientists are building a knowledge base supporting the strong relationship between a child's earliest development and environment and the long-term effects later in life on the child's physical and mental health, school performance, and behaviour (Williams, Clinton, & Canadian Paediatric Society [CPS], Early Years Task Force, 2011). The CPS has recommended specific evidence-based clinical tools to collect standardized developmental data that are used across Canada. Currently, different tools are being used in various parts of the country. The most commonly used tools include the Nipissing District Developmental Screening (NDDS), the Ages and Stages Questionnaires (ASQ), PEDS/PEDS: DM, and the Rourke Baby Record and these can be used to assess the toddler stage of growth and development (see Additional Resources at the end of this chapter). See Chapter 33 for more information on the developmental screening tools.

Nurses have an important role in assessing the development of children. They provide the assessment, interventions, family education, and connection of the child and family to community resources. Child development centres across Canada play a key role in assessing, treating, and supporting children and their families.

Biological Development

Proportional Changes

Growth slows considerably during toddlerhood. The average weight gain is 1.8 to 2.7 kg per year. The birth weight is quadrupled by 2½ years of age. The rate of increase in height also slows. The usual increment is an addition of 7.5 cm per year and occurs mainly in elongation of the legs rather than the trunk. The average height of a 2-year-old is 86.6 cm. In general, adult height is about twice the 2-year-old child's height. Accurate measurement of height and weight during the toddler years should reveal a steady growth curve that is steplike in nature rather than linear, which is characteristic of the growth spurts during the early childhood years. It is important that individual children have specific measurements taken to accurately track their growth patterns. These measurements need to be recorded on a regular basis using a growth chart that compares them with the averages of other children. The Dietitians of Canada, CPS, College of Family Physicians, and Community Health Nurses of Canada have put forward a joint recommendation to use the WHO 2006 Child Growth Standards and the 2007 WHO Growth Reference growth charts for Canadian children (Dietitians of Canada, 2016) (see Appendix C).

The rate of increase in head circumference slows somewhat by the end of infancy; head circumference is usually equal to chest circumference by 1 to 2 years of age. The usual total increase in head circumference during the second year is 2.5 cm. The anterior fontanel closes between 12 and 18 months of age.

Chest circumference continues to increase in size and exceeds head circumference during the toddler years. After the second year the chest circumference exceeds the abdominal measurement; this, in addition to the growth of the lower extremities, gives the child a taller, leaner appearance. However, the toddler still appears relatively squat and "pot-bellied" because of the less well-developed abdominal musculature and short legs. The legs remain slightly bowed or curved during the second year from the weight of the relatively large trunk.

Sensory Changes

Visual acuity of 20/40 is considered acceptable during the toddler years. Full binocular vision is well developed, and any evidence of persistent strabismus requires professional attention as early as possible to prevent amblyopia. Depth perception continues to develop but, because of the child's lack of motor coordination, falls from heights are a persistent danger.

The senses of hearing, smell, taste, and touch become increasingly well developed, coordinated with each other and associated with other experiences. All of the senses are used to explore the environment. Toddlers will visually inspect an object by turning it over; they may taste it, smell it, and touch it several times before they are satisfied with their investigation. They will shake it to see if it makes noise and vigorously test its durability.

Another example of the integrated function of the senses is the toddler's development of specific taste preferences. The toddler is much less likely than an infant to try a new food because of its appearance, texture, or smell, not just its taste.

Maturation of Systems

Most of the physiological systems are relatively mature by the end of toddlerhood. The volume of the respiratory tract and growth of associated structures continue to increase during early childhood, lessening some of the factors that predisposed the child to frequent and serious infections during infancy. The internal structures of the ear and throat continue to be short and straight, and the lymphoid tissue of the tonsils and adenoids continues to be large. As a result, otitis media, tonsillitis, and upper respiratory tract infections are common. The respiratory and heart rates slow, and the blood pressure increases (see Appendix E). Respirations continue to be abdominal.

Under conditions of moderate variation in temperature, the toddler is able to maintain body temperature. The mature functioning of the renal system serves to conserve fluid under times of stress, decreasing the risk of dehydration.

The digestive processes are fairly complete by the beginning of toddlerhood. The acidity of the gastric contents continues to increase and has a protective function, since they are capable of destroying many types of bacteria. Stomach capacity increases to allow for the usual schedule of three meals a day.

One of the more prominent changes of the gastrointestinal system is the voluntary control of elimination. With complete myelination of the spinal cord, control of the anal and urethral sphincters is gradually achieved. The physiological ability to control the sphincters probably occurs somewhere between ages 18 and 24 months. Bladder capacity also increases considerably, and by 14 to 18 months of age the child is able to retain urine for up to 2 hours or longer.

The defence mechanisms of the skin and blood, particularly phagocytosis, are much more efficient in toddlers than in infants. The production of antibodies is well established. However, many young children demonstrate a sudden increase in colds and minor infections when they enter preschool or other group situations, such as day care, because of their exposure to pathogens and the lack of understanding of general hygiene measures such as hand washing.

Gross and Fine Motor Development

The major gross motor skill during the toddler years is the development of locomotion. By 12 to 13 months of age, toddlers try to walk alone using a wide stance for extra balance, and by 18 months they try to run but fall easily (Fig. 36-1). At age 2 years, toddlers can walk up and down stairs; by age 2½ years they can jump using both feet, stand on one foot for a second or two, and manage a few steps on tiptoe.

Mastery of gross and fine motor skills is evident in all phases of the child's activity, such as play, dressing, language comprehension, response to discipline, social interaction, and propensity for injuries. Fine motor development is demonstrated in increasingly skillful manual dexterity. Activities occur less in isolation and more in conjunction with other physical and mental abilities to produce a purposeful result. For example, the toddler will walk to reach a new location, release a toy to pick it up or to choose a new one, and scribble to look at the image produced. The possibilities of the exploration, investigation, and manipulation of the environment—and its hazards—are endless.

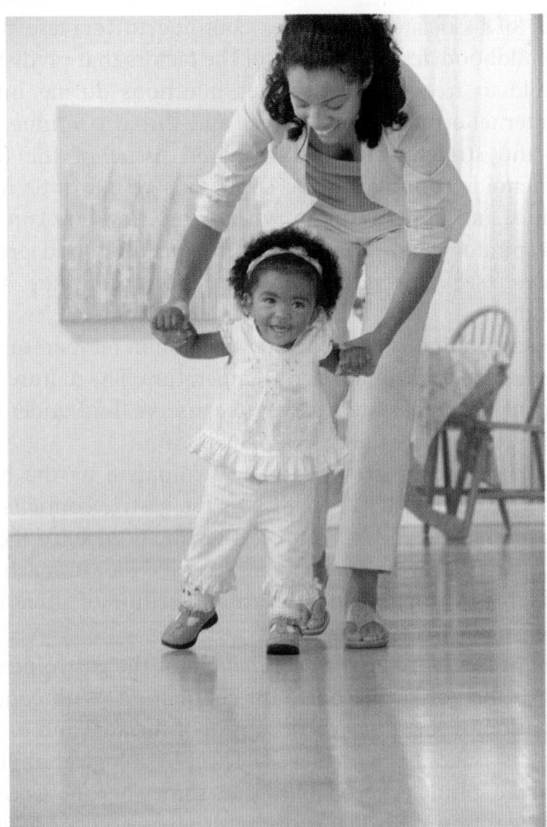

FIGURE 36-1 Typical toddling gait. (Blend Images/Shutterstock.com.)

The major features of growth and development for the age groups of 15, 18, 24, and 30 months are summarized in Table 36-1.

Psychosocial Development

Toddlers are faced with the mastery of several important tasks. If the need for basic trust has been satisfied, they are ready to give up dependence for control, independence, and autonomy. Some of the specific tasks to be dealt with include the following:

- Differentiation of self from others, particularly the mother
- Toleration of separation from the parent
- Ability to delay gratification
- Control over bodily functions
- Acquisition of socially acceptable behaviour
- Verbal means of communication
- Ability to interact with others in a less egocentric manner

Mastery of these goals is only begun during late infancy and the toddler years, and tasks such as developing interpersonal relationships with others may not be completed until adolescence. However, crucial foundations for successful completion of such developmental tasks are established during these early formative years.

Developing a Sense of Autonomy (Erikson)

According to Erikson (1963), the developmental task of toddlerhood is acquiring a sense of autonomy while overcoming a sense of doubt and shame. As infants gain trust in the predictability and reliability of their parents, environment, and interaction with others, they begin to discover that their behaviour is their own and that it has a predictable, reliable effect on others. However, although they realize their will and control over others, they are confronted with the conflict of exerting autonomy and relinquishing the much-enjoyed dependence on others. Exerting their will has definite negative consequences, whereas retaining dependent, submissive behaviour is generally rewarded with affection and approval. At the same time, continued dependency creates a sense of doubt regarding their potential capacity to control their actions. This doubt is compounded by a sense of shame for feeling this urge to revolt against others' will and a fear that they will exceed their own capacity for manipulating the environment.

Just as the infant has the social modalities of grasping and biting, the toddler has the newly gained modality of holding on and letting go. To hold on and let go is evident with the use of the hands, mouth, eyes, and, eventually, the sphincters, when toilet training is begun. These social modalities are expressed constantly in the child's play activities, such as casting or throwing objects; taking objects out of boxes, drawers, or cabinets; holding on tighter when someone says, "No, don't touch"; and spitting out food as taste preferences become strong.

Several characteristics, especially negativism and ritualism, are typical of toddlers in their quest for autonomy. As toddlers attempt to express their will, they often act with *negativism*, the persistent negative response to requests. The words "no" or "me do" can be the sole vocabulary. Emotions are strongly expressed, usually in rapid mood swings. One minute, toddlers can be engrossed in an activity, and the next minute they might be extremely frustrated because they are unable to manipulate a toy or open a door. If scolded for doing something wrong, they can have a temper tantrum and almost instantaneously pull at the parent's legs to be picked up and comforted. Understanding and coping with these swift changes in behaviour is often difficult for parents. Many parents find the negativism exasperating and, instead of dealing constructively with it, give in to it, which further threatens children in their search for learning acceptable methods of interacting with others (see Temper Tantrums and Negativism, pp. 1055–1056).

In contrast to negativism, which often disrupts the environment, *ritualism*, the need to maintain sameness and reliability, provides a sense of comfort. Toddlers can venture out with security when they know that familiar people, places, and routines still exist. One can easily understand why change, such as hospitalization, represents such a threat to these children. Without the comfortable rituals, there is little opportunity to exert autonomy. Consequently, dependency and regression occur (see Regression, p. 1056).

Erikson focused on the development of the *ego*, which may be thought of as reason or common sense, during this phase of psychosocial development. There is a struggle as the child deals with the impulses of the id and attempts to tolerate frustration and learn socially acceptable ways of interacting with the environment. The ego is evident as the child is able to tolerate delayed gratification.

There is also a rudimentary beginning of the *superego*, or conscience, which is the incorporation of the morals of society

TABLE 36-1 GROWTH AND DEVELOPMENT DURING TODDLER YEARS

AGE (mo)	PHYSICAL	GROSS MOTOR	FINE MOTOR	SENSORY	LANGUAGE	SOCIALIZATION
15	Steady growth in height and weight Head circumference 48 cm Weight 11 kg Height 78.7 cm	Walks without help (usually since age 13 mo) Creeps up stairs Kneels without support Cannot walk around corners or stop suddenly without losing balance Cannot throw ball without falling Runs clumsily; falls often	Constantly casting objects to floor Builds tower of two cubes Holds two cubes in one hand Releases a pellet into a narrow-necked bottle Scribbles spontaneously Uses cup well but rotates spoon before it reaches mouth	Able to identify geometric forms; places round object into appropriate hole Binocular vision well developed Displays an intense and prolonged interest in pictures	Uses expressive jargon Says four to six words, including names "Asks" for objects by pointing Understands simple commands May use head-shaking gesture to denote "no" Uses "no" even while agreeing to the request Uses common repetitive gestures such as putting cup to mouth when empty	Tolerates some separation from parent Less likely to fear strangers Beginning to imitate parents, such as cleaning house (sweeping, dusting), folding clothes May discard bottle Kisses and hugs parents; may kiss pictures in a book
18	Picky eater from decreased growth needs Anterior fontanel closed Physiologically able to control sphincters	Assumes standing position without support Walks up stairs with one hand held Pulls and pushes toys Jumps in place with both feet Seats self on chair Throws ball overhand without falling	Builds tower of three or four cubes Release, prehension, and reach are well developed Turns pages in a book two or three at a time In drawing, makes stroke imitatively Manages spoon without rotation		Says 10 or more words Points to a common object, such as a shoe or ball, and to two or three body parts Forms word combinations Forms gesture–word combinations Forms gesture–gesture combinations	Expresses emotions; has temper tantrums Great imitator (domestic mimicry) Takes off gloves, socks, and shoes and unzips Beginning awareness of ownership ("my toy") May develop dependence on transitional objects, such as "security blanket"
24	Head circumference 49–50 cm Chest circumference exceeds head circumference Lateral diameter of chest exceeds anteroposterior diameter Usual weight gain of 1.8–2.7 kg; birth weight quadruples by age 2½ years Usual gain in height of 10–12.5 cm; height at age 2 is approximately 50% of eventual adult height May have achieved readiness for beginning daytime control of bowel and bladder Primary dentition of 16 teeth	Goes up and down stairs alone with two feet on each step Runs fairly well, with wide stance Picks up object without falling Kicks ball forward without overbalancing	Builds tower of six or seven cubes Aligns two or more cubes like a train Turns pages of book one at a time In drawing, imitates vertical and circular strokes Turns doorknob; unscrews lid	Accommodation well developed In geometric discrimination, able to insert square block into oblong space	Has vocabulary of approximately 300 words Uses two- or three-word phrases Uses pronouns "I," "me," "you" Understands directional commands Gives first name; refers to self by name Verbalizes need for toileting, food, or drink Talks incessantly	Stage of parallel play Has sustained attention span Temper tantrums decreasing Pulls people to show them something Increased independence from parent Dresses self in simple clothing Develops visual recognition and verbal self-reference ("Me big")

Continued

TABLE 36-1 GROWTH AND DEVELOPMENT DURING TODDLER YEARS—cont'd

AGE (mo)	PHYSICAL	GROSS MOTOR	FINE MOTOR	SENSORY	LANGUAGE	SOCIALIZATION
30	Birth weight quadrupled Primary dentition (20 teeth) completed May have daytime bowel and bladder control	Jumps with both feet Jumps from chair or step Stands on one foot momentarily Takes a few steps on tiptoe	Builds tower of eight cubes Adds chimney to train of cubes Good hand–finger coordination; holds crayon with fingers rather than fist Moves fingers independently In drawing, imitates vertical and horizontal strokes; makes two or more strokes for cross		Gives first and last name Refers to self by appropriate pronoun Uses plurals Names one colour	Separates more easily from parent In play, helps put things away; can carry breakable objects; pushes with good steering Begins to notice sex differences; knows own sex May attend to toilet needs without help except for wiping Emotions expand to include pride, shame, guilt, embarrassment

and the process of acculturation. With the development of the ego, children further differentiate themselves from others and expand their sense of trust within themselves. But as they begin to develop awareness of their own will and capacity to achieve, they also become aware of their ability to fail. This ever-present awareness of potential failure creates doubt and shame. Successful mastery of the task of autonomy necessitates opportunities for self-mastery while withstanding the frustration of necessary limit setting and delayed gratification. Opportunities for self-mastery are present in appropriate play activities, toilet training, the crisis of sibling rivalry, and successful interactions with significant others.

Cognitive Development

Sensorimotor and Preoperational Phase (Piaget)

The period from 12 to 24 months of age is a continuation of the final two stages of Piaget's (1952) sensorimotor phase. During this time, the cognitive processes develop rapidly and at times seem similar to those of mature thinking. However, reasoning skills are still primitive and need to be understood in order to effectively deal with the typical behaviours of a child of this age.

Tertiary circular reactions. In the fifth stage of the sensorimotor phase (13 to 18 months of age), the child uses active experimentation to achieve previously unattainable goals. Newly acquired physical skills are increasingly important for the function they serve rather than for the acts themselves. The child incorporates the old learning of secondary circular reactions with new skills and applies the combined knowledge to new situations, with emphasis on the results of the experimentation. In this way, there is the beginning of rational judgement and intellectual reasoning. During this stage, there is further differentiation of one's self from objects. This is evident in the child's increasing ability to venture away from the parent and to tolerate longer periods of separation.

The child also starts to develop awareness of a causal relationship between two events. After flipping a light switch, toddlers are aware that a reciprocal response occurs. However, they are not able to transfer that knowledge to new situations. Therefore, every time they see what appears to be a light switch, they must reinvestigate its function. Such behaviour demonstrates the beginning of categorizing data into distinct classes and subclasses. Examples of this type of behaviour are innumerable as toddlers continuously explore the same object each time it appears in a new place.

Because classification of objects is still rudimentary, the appearance of an object denotes its function. For example, if the child's toys are stored in a paper bag or large container, that toy receptacle is no different from the garbage pail or laundry basket. If allowed to turn over the toy receptacle, the child will just as quickly do the same to other similar containers because, in the child's mind, there is no difference. Expecting the child to judge which receptacles are permissible to explore and which are not is inappropriate for this age group. Instead, the forbidden object, such as the garbage pail, should be placed out of reach. This has significance in relation to protecting the toddler from injury; the toddler is not able to differentiate between what is a safe object to play with in any given situation and what is unsafe in another. For example, if the child is allowed to throw a toy ball, he or she does not necessarily understand why a different toy that may harm someone cannot be thrown as well.

The discovery of objects as objects leads to the awareness of their spatial relationships. Children are able to recognize different shapes and their relationship to each other. For example, they can fit slightly smaller boxes into each other (nesting) and can place a round object into a hole, even if the board is turned around, turned upside down, or reversed. Children are also aware of space and the relationship of their body to dimensions such as height. They will stretch, stand on a low stair or stool, and pull a string to reach an object.

Object permanence has also advanced. Although they still cannot find an object that has been invisibly displaced or moved from under one pillow to another without their seeing the change, toddlers are increasingly aware of the existence of objects behind closed doors, in drawers, on countertops, and under tables. Parents are usually acutely aware of this developmental achievement and find high places and locked cabinets the only places inaccessible to toddlers.

Invention of new means through mental combinations. From ages 19 to 24 months, the child is in the final sensorimotor stage. During this stage, the child completes the more primitive, autistic-like thought processes of infancy and is prepared for the more complex mental operations that occur during the phase of preoperational thought. One of the most dramatic achievements of this stage is in the area of object permanence. Children will now actively search for an object in several potential hiding places. In addition, they can infer a cause when only experiencing the effect. They can infer that an object was hidden in any number of places even if they only saw the original hiding place.

Imitation displays deeper meaning and understanding. There is greater symbolization to imitation. The child is acutely aware of others' actions and attempts to copy them in gestures and in words. Domestic mimicry (imitating household activities) and gender-role behaviour become increasingly common during this stage, especially during the second year. Identification with the parent of the same gender becomes apparent by the second year and represents the child's intellectual ability to identify different models of behaviour and to imitate them appropriately (Fig. 36-2).

While the concept of time is still embryonic, children have some sense of timing in terms of anticipation, memory, and a limited ability to wait. They may listen to the command, "Just a minute," and behave appropriately. However, their sense of time is exaggerated—1 minute can seem like an hour. Toddlers' limited attention spans also indicate their sense of immediacy and concern for the present.

Preoperational phase. At approximately 2 years of age, the child enters the *preconceptual phase* of cognitive development, which lasts until about age 4 years. The preconceptual phase is a subdivision of the *preoperational phase*, which spans ages 2 to 7 years. The preconceptual phase is primarily one of transition that bridges the purely self-satisfying behaviour of infancy and the rudimentary socialized behaviour of latency. *Preoperational thought* implies that children cannot think in terms of operations—the ability to manipulate objects in relation to each other in a logical fashion. Rather, toddlers think primarily on the basis of their perception of an event. Problem solving is based on what they see or hear directly rather than on what they recall about objects and events. Several characteristics are unique to preoperational thought (Box 36-1).

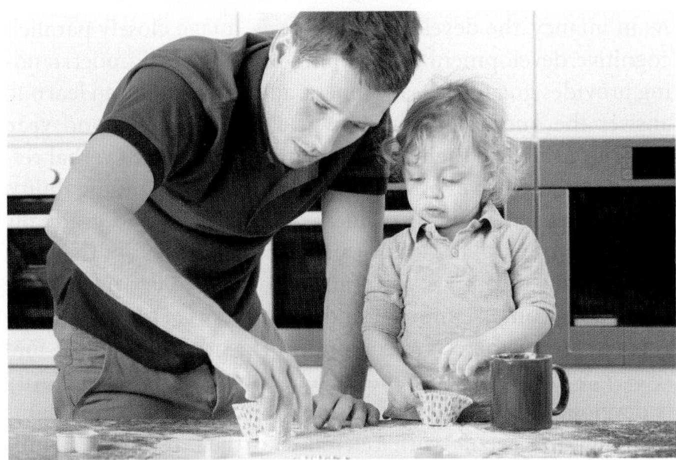

FIGURE 36-2 Domestic mimicry and gender-role behaviour are common during toddlerhood. (Photographee.eu/Shutterstock.com.)

Within the second year, the child increasingly uses language symbolically and is concerned with the "why" and "how" of things. For example, a pencil is "something to write with," and food is "something to eat." However, such mental symbolization is closely associated with prelogical reasoning. For instance, a needle is "something that hurts." Such painful experiences take on new significance because memory is associated with the specific event, and fears are likely to develop, such as resistance to people who wear a uniform or rooms that look like the practitioner's office. Because of the vulnerability of these early years, it is essential to prepare children for any new experience, whether it is a new babysitter or a visit to the health care practitioner or dentist.

Spiritual Development

Spiritual development in children is often discussed in terms of the child's developmental level because the evolution of spirituality often parallels cognitive development. The child's family and environment strongly influence the child's perception of the world around him or her, and this often includes spirituality. Furthermore, family values, beliefs, customs, and expressions of these will influence the child's perception of his or her spiritual self. Neuman (2011) proposes that Fowler's stages of faith (Fowler, 1981) be used to better understand children and spirituality; she provides an excellent overview of the stages of faith in childhood. The relationship between spirituality, illness in childhood, and nursing has been studied in the context of suffering, terminal illness such as cancer, and end-of-life care. There is more emphasis on understanding of the influence of one's spirituality on health, illness, and well-being. For instance, the Canadian Virtual Hospice website provides information on how to talk to children, including toddlers, about serious illness (see Additional Resources at the end of this chapter).

Toddlers learn about God or other spiritual powers through the words and the actions of those closest to them. They have only a vague idea of God or greater powers and religious teachings because of their immature cognitive processes; however, if God or the divine is spoken about with reverence, young children associate that with something special. During this period, the designation of powerful religious symbols and images is strongly influenced by the manner in which they are presented; therein lies the potential for the development of guilt and fear or, conversely, love and companionship with religious symbols (Roehlkepartain, King, Wagener, et al., 2006). Toddlers are said to be in the intuitive-projective phase of Fowler's faith

BOX 36-1 CHARACTERISTICS OF PREOPERATIONAL THOUGHT

Egocentrism—Inability to envision situations from perspectives other than one's own

Example—If a person is positioned between the toddler and another child, the toddler, who is facing the person, will explain that both children can see the middle person's face. The young child is unable to realize that the other person views the middle person from a different perspective, the back.

Implication—Avoid moralizing about "why" something is wrong if it requires an understanding of someone else's feelings or opinion. Telling a child to stop hitting because hitting hurts the other person is often ineffective because, to the aggressor, it feels good to hit someone else. Instead, emphasize that hitting is not allowed.

Transductive reasoning—Reasoning from the particular to the particular

Example—Child refuses to eat a food because something previously eaten did not taste good.

Implication—Accept the child's reasoning; offer refused food at a different time.

Global organization—Reasoning that changing any one part of the whole changes the entire whole

Example—Child refuses to sleep in his or her room because the location of the bed is changed.

Implication—Accept the child's reasoning; use the same bed position or introduce change slowly.

Centration—Focusing on one aspect rather than considering all possible alternatives

Example—Child refuses to eat a food because of its colour, even though its taste and smell are acceptable.

Implication—Accept the child's reasoning.

Animism—Attributing lifelike qualities to inanimate objects

Example—Child scolds stairs for making the child fall down.

Implication—Join the child in the "scolding." Keep frightening objects out of view.

Irreversibility—Inability to undo or reverse the actions initiated physically

Example—When told to stop doing something, such as talking, the child is unable to think of positive activity.

Implication—State requests or instructions positively (e.g., "Be quiet.")

Magical thinking—Believing that thoughts are all-powerful and can cause events

Examples—Child wishes someone died; then if the person dies, the child feels at fault because of the "bad" thought that made the death happen.

- Calling children "bad" because they did something wrong makes children feel as if they are bad.

Implications—Clarify that thoughts do not make things happen and that the child is not responsible.

- Use "I" messages rather than "you" messages to communicate thoughts, feelings, expectations, or beliefs, without imposing blame or criticism. Emphasize that the *act* is bad, not the child.

Inability to conserve—Inability to understand the idea that a mass can be changed in size, shape, volume, or length without losing or adding to the original mass (instead, children judge what they see by the immediate perceptual clues given to them)

Example—If two lines of equal length are presented in such a way that one appears longer than the other, the child will state that one line is longer, even if the child measures both lines with a ruler or yardstick and finds that each has the same length.

Implications—Change the most obvious perceptual clue to reorient the child's view of what is seen. For example, give medicine in a small medicine cup, rather than a large cup, since the child will imagine that the large vessel contains more liquid. If the child refuses the medicine in the small cup, pour it into a large cup, because the liquid will appear to be less in a tall, wide container.

- Give a large, flat cookie rather than a thick, small one, or do the reverse with meat or cheese; the child will usually eat a larger size of favourite food and a smaller size of less favourite food.

construct (Fowler, 1981) in which thinking is largely based on fantasy and is fluid in relation to reality and fantasy. God or the divine may be described as being around like air by the toddler because of the fluidity in dividing fantasy and reality (Neuman, 2011).

Toddlers begin to assimilate behaviours associated with the divine (e.g., folding hands in prayer). Routines such as saying prayers before meals or at bedtime can be important and comforting. Because toddlers tend to find solace in ritualistic behaviour and routines, they incorporate routines associated with religious practices into their behavioural patterns without understanding all of the implications of the rituals until later. Near the end of toddlerhood, when children use preoperational thought, there is some advancement of their understanding of God or other religious figures. Religious teachings, such as reward or fear of punishment (heaven or hell) and moral development (see Chapter 31), may influence their behaviour.

Development of Body Image

As in infancy, the development of **body image** closely parallels cognitive development. Developing psychological understanding provides greater self-awareness, and young children learn to answer the question "Who am I?" During their second year, children recognize themselves in a mirror and make verbal references to themselves ("Me big"). With increasing motor ability, toddlers recognize the usefulness of body parts and gradually learn their names. They also learn that certain parts of the body have various meanings; for example, during toilet training the genitalia become significant and cleanliness is emphasized. By 2 years of age there is recognition of gender differences and reference to self by name and then by pronoun. Gender identity is developed by age 3 years. Also by this time, the child begins to remember events with reference to their personal significance, forming an autobiographic memory that helps establish a continuous identity throughout life's events.

Once they begin preoperational thought, toddlers can use symbols to represent objects, but their thinking may lead to inaccuracies. For example, if someone who is pregnant is called "fat," they will describe all "fat" women as having babies. There is a beginning recognition of words used to describe physical appearance, such as "pretty," "handsome," or "big boy." Such expressions eventually influence how children view their own bodies.

Although little research has been done on body-image development in young children, it is evident that body integrity is poorly understood and that intrusive experiences are threatening. For example, toddlers forcefully resist procedures such as examination of the ear or mouth and taking of an axillary temperature. The procedure itself (e.g., taking vital signs) is not hurting the child, but it represents an intrusion into the child's personal space, which will elicit a strong protest. Toddlers also have unclear body boundaries and may associate nonviable parts, such as feces, with essential body parts. This can be seen in a toddler who is upset by flushing the toilet and watching the stool disappear.

Nurses can assist parents in fostering a positive body image in their child by encouraging them to avoid negative labels, such as "skinny arms" or "chubby legs," self-perceptions that can last a lifetime. Body parts, especially those related to elimination and reproduction, should be called by their correct names. Respect for the body should be practised.

Development of Gender Identity

Just as toddlers explore their environment, they also explore their bodies and find that touching certain body parts is pleasurable. Genital fondling (masturbation) can occur and involves manual stimulation of genitalia and posturing movements (especially in young girls) such as tightening the thighs or applying mechanical pressure to the pubic or suprapubic area. Other demonstrations of pleasurable activities include rocking, swinging, and hugging people and toys. Parental reactions to toddlers' sexual behaviour influence the children's own attitudes and should be accepting rather than critical. If such acts are performed in public, parents should not condone or bring attention to the behaviour but should teach the child that it is more acceptable to perform the behaviour in private.

Children in this age group are learning vocabulary associated with anatomy, elimination, and reproduction. Certain associations between words and functions become significant and can influence future sexual attitudes. For example, if parents refer to the genitalia as dirty, especially in the context of elimination, this association between "genitalia" and "dirty" may be transferred to sexual functions. Gender-role differences become obvious to children and are evident in much of their imitative play. Although current research indicates that prenatal exposure to testosterone strongly influences the individual's gender identity, researchers also indicate that there are sensitive periods (e.g., puberty) that may influence the development of gender identity (Berenbaum, & Beltz, 2011; Hines, 2011; Savic, Garcia-Falqueras, & Swaab, 2010). A sense of maleness or femaleness, *gender identity*, is usually formed by age 3 years. Early attitudes are formed about affectionate behaviours between adults from observing parental and other adult sexual or sensual activities (see also Chapter 37, Sex Education). The quality of relationships with parents is important to the child's capacity for sexual and emotional relationships later in life.

Social Development

A major task of the toddler period is differentiation of self from significant others, usually the mother. The differentiation process consists of two phases: *separation*, the child's emergence from a symbiotic fusion with the mother; and *individuation*, those achievements that mark the child's expressions of his or her individual characteristics in the environment. Although the process begins during the latter half of infancy, the major achievements occur during the toddler years (see Table 36-1).

Toddlers have an increased understanding and awareness of object permanence and have some ability to withstand delayed gratification and tolerate moderate frustration. As a result, toddlers react differently to strangers than do infants. The appearance of unfamiliar persons does not represent such a significant threat to their attachment to the mother. They have learned from experience that parents still exist when physically absent. Repetition of events such as going to bed without the parents but waking to find them there again (in the household) reinforces the reliability of such brief separations. Consequently, toddlers are able to venture away from their parents for brief periods.

According to Harpaz-Rotem and Bergman (2006), the separation–individuation phase encompasses the phenomenon of rapprochement; as the toddler separates from the mother and begins to make sense of experiences in the environment, he or she is drawn back to the mother for assistance in verbally articulating the meaning of the experiences. Developmentally the term *rapprochement* means the child moves away and returns for reassurance. If the mother's response to the toddler is inappropriate, the toddler may experience insecurity and confusion.

Transitional objects, such as a favourite blanket or toy, provide security for children, especially when they are separated from parents, dealing with a new stress, or just fatigued (Fig. 36-3). Security objects often become so important to toddlers that they refuse to have them taken away. Such behaviour is normal; there is no need to discourage this tendency. During separations such as day care, hospitalization, or even overnight stays with relatives, transitional objects should be provided to minimize any feelings of fear or loneliness.

Learning to tolerate and master brief periods of separation is an important developmental task of children in this age group. In addition, it is a necessary component of parenting, since brief periods of separation allow parents to regain their energy and patience and to minimize any tendency to direct their irritations and frustrations at the children.

Language

The most striking characteristic of language development during early childhood is the increasing level of comprehension (see Table 36-1). Although the number of words acquired—from about 4 at 1 year of age to approximately 300

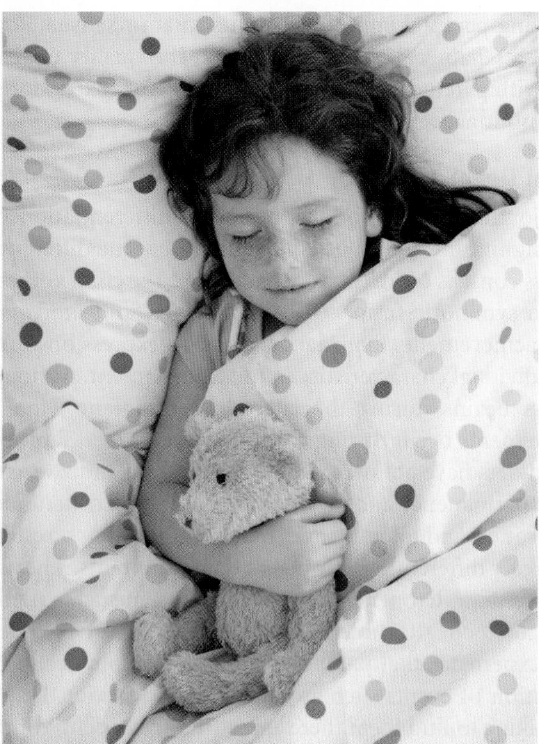

FIGURE 36-3 Transitional objects such as a fuzzy stuffed animal are sources of security to a toddler. (Copyright © 2011 Photos.com, a division of Getty Images. All rights reserved.)

at age 2 years—is notable, the ability to *comprehend and understand speech is much greater than the number of words the child can say*. Bilingual children also achieve their early linguistic milestones in each of the languages at the same time and produce a substantial number of semantically corresponding words in each of their two languages from the very first words or signs.

At age 1 year the child uses one-word sentences, or *holophrases*. The word "up" can mean "pick me up" or "look up there." For the child, the one word conveys the meaning of a sentence, but to others it may mean many things or nothing. At this age about 25% of the vocalizations are intelligible. By the age of 2 years the child uses multiword sentences by stringing together two or three words, such as the phrases "mama go bye-bye" or "all gone," and approximately 65% of the speech is understandable. By 3 years of age the child puts words together into simple sentences, begins to master grammatical rules, and acquires five or six new words daily, knows their age and gender, and can count three objects correctly. Looking at books during this period provides an ideal setting for further language development (Feigelman, 2016). Authorities have evaluated the impact of television viewing on toddler language development and found that those who started watching television at younger than 12 months of age and who watched longer than 2 hours per day had significant language delays (Chonchaiya & Pruksananonda, 2008). Adult–child conversations with infants and toddlers have been shown to positively affect language development; reading, storytelling, and interactive adult–child communication during this period provides an ideal setting for further language development (Feigelman, 2016; Zimmerman, Gilkerson, Richards, et al., 2009).

Gestures precede or accompany each of the language milestones up to 30 months of age (putting phone to ear, pointing). Once language is sufficiently mastered, gestures phase out and the pace of word learning increases (Goodrich & Hudson, 2009).

Personal-Social Behaviour

One of the most dramatic aspects of development in the toddler is personal-social interaction. Parents often wonder why their manageable, docile, lovable infant has turned into a determined, strong-willed, volatile little tyrant. In addition, the tyrant of the terrible twos can swiftly and unpredictably revert to the adorable, cuddly child. All of this is part of growing up and is evident in such areas as dressing, feeding, playing, and establishing self-control.

Toddlers are developing skills of independence, and these are evident in all areas of behaviour. By 15 months children feed themselves, drink well from a covered cup, and manage a spoon with considerable spilling. By 24 months they use a spoon well and by 36 months may be using a fork. Between ages 2 and 3 years they like to help with chores, such as setting the table or removing dishes from the dishwasher. However, they lack appropriate table etiquette at times and may find it difficult to sit through the family's entire meal.

In dressing, toddlers also demonstrate strides in independence. The 15-month-old child helps by putting the arm or foot out for dressing and pulls shoes and socks off. The 18-month-old child removes gloves, helps with pullover shirts, and may be able to unzip. By age 2 years the toddler removes most articles of clothing and puts on socks, shoes, and pants without regard to right or left and back or front. Help is still needed to fasten clothes.

Toddlers also begin to develop concern for the feelings of others and develop an understanding of how adult expectations for behaviour apply to specific situations (e.g., causing a sibling to cry while playing rough). As parents foster their understanding, they are able to develop control. Age-appropriate discipline contributes to healthy social and emotional development. Positive reinforcement, redirecting, and time-out are appropriate for most toddlers. Early screening and intervention promote more positive developmental outcomes as the young child grows and develops.

Play

Play magnifies the toddler's physical and psychosocial development. Interaction with people becomes increasingly important. The solitary play of infancy progresses to parallel play—the toddler plays alongside, not with, other children (see Fig. 32-7). Although sensorimotor play is still prominent, there is much less emphasis on the exclusive use of one sensory modality. The toddler inspects the toy, talks to the toy, tests its strength and durability, and invents several uses for it. Imitation is one of the more distinguishing characteristics of play and enriches the child's opportunity to engage in fantasy. With less emphasis on gender-stereotyped toys, play objects such as dolls, carriages,

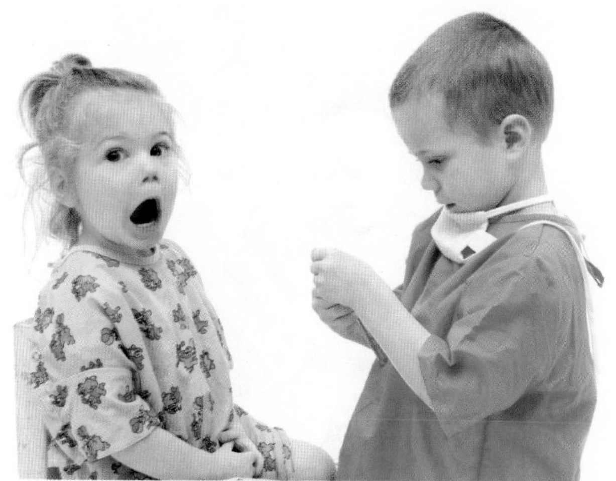

FIGURE 36-4 Young children enjoy dressing up. (© Can Stock Photo Inc./nameinfame.)

dollhouses, dishes, balls, clay, cooking utensils, child-size furniture, trucks, and dress-up clothes (Fig. 36-4) are suitable for both genders. However, some children may be more interested in activities associated with the opposite gender.

Increased locomotive skills make push-pull toys, straddle trucks or cycles, a small gym and slide, balls of various sizes, and rocking horses appropriate for the energetic toddler. Finger paints; thick crayons; chalk; a blackboard; paper; and puzzles with large, simple pieces use the child's developing fine motor skills. Interlocking blocks in various sizes and shapes provide hours of fun and, during later years, are useful objects for creative and imaginative play. The most educational toy is the one that fosters the interaction of an adult with a child in supportive, unconditional play. Toys are never substitutes for the attention of devoted caregivers, but toys can enhance these interactions (Milteer, Ginsburg, & Council on Communications and Media Committee on Psychosocial Aspects of Child and Family Health, 2012). Parents and other providers are encouraged to allow children to play with a variety of simple toys that foster creative thinking (e.g., blocks, dolls, and clay) rather than passive toys that the child observes (battery-operated or mechanical toys). Active play time should also be encouraged over the use of computer or video games, which are more passive.

Certain aspects of play are related to emerging linguistic abilities. Talking is a form of play for toddlers who enjoy musical toys, such as age-appropriate music players, "talking" dolls and animals, and toy telephones. Toddlers also enjoy "reading" stories from a picture book and imitating the sounds of animals. Children's television programs are appropriate for some children over 2 years of age who learn to associate words with visual images. However, total media or screen time should be limited to less than 1 hour of quality programming per day for children ages 2 to 4 years (Lipnowski, LeBlanc, & CPS, Healthy Active Living and Sports Medicine Committee, 2012). The CPS discourages screen-based activities (television, video games, handheld devices, etc.) for children under 2 and encourages active and interactive games (Lipnowski et al., 2012). Excessive television watching can affect children's sleep, cause behaviour problems, and leaves less time for active play. See Additional Resources at the end of the chapter for tips for parents on managing children's television watching.

Tactile play is also important for the exploring toddler. Water toys, a sandbox with pail and shovel, finger paints, soap bubbles, and clay provide excellent opportunities for creative and manipulative recreation. Adults sometimes forget the fascination of feeling slippery cream, mud, or pudding; catching airy bubbles; squeezing and reshaping clay; or smearing paints. These types of unstructured activities are as important as educational play to allow children freedom of expression.

The selection of appropriate toys must involve safety factors, especially in relation to size and sturdiness. Toddlers' oral activity puts them at risk for aspirating small objects or for ingesting toxic substances. Parents need to be especially careful to keep toys of older siblings or those played with in other children's homes away from toddlers. Toys are a potential source of serious bodily damage to toddlers, who may have the physical strength to manipulate them but not the knowledge to appreciate their danger (see Family-Centred Teaching box, p. 1071). Government agencies do not inspect and police all toys on the market. Therefore, adults who purchase play equipment, supervise purchases, or allow children to use play equipment (including toys that are gifts or are purchased by the children themselves) need to evaluate their safety. Adults should also be alert to notices of toys determined to be defective and recalled by the manufacturers. Parents and health care workers can report potentially dangerous toys and child products on Health Canada's website. Health Canada also has a consumer product recall list available for reference (see Additional Resources at the end of chapter).

Coping With Concerns Related to Normal Growth and Development

Toilet Training

One of the major tasks of toddlerhood is toilet training. Anticipatory guidance and clinical interventions for families regarding toilet training should begin during routine well-child visits before the toddler has the readiness to start the training. Preparation and education reveal and allay misconceptions, lead to the development of appropriate expectations, and provide information, guidance, and support to parents for managing this potentially frustrating process.

Voluntary control of the anal and urethral sphincters is achieved sometime after the child is walking, probably between ages 18 and 24 months. However, complex psychophysiological factors are required for readiness. The child must be able to recognize the urge to let go and hold on and be able to communicate this sensation to the parent. In addition, there may be some necessary motivation in the desire to please the parent by holding on, rather than pleasing oneself by letting go (Clifford, Gorodzinsky, & CPS, Community Paediatrics Committee, 2000/2016).

Five markers signal a child's readiness to toilet train: motor, language, social milestones, demeanour, and relationship with the parents (Clifford et al., 2000/2016). According to some experts, physiological and psychological readiness is not complete until age 28 months. By this time, the child has mastered

GUIDELINES

Assessing Toilet Training Readiness

Physical Readiness

- Voluntary control of anal and urethral sphincters, usually by 18 to 24 months of age
- Ability to stay dry for 2 hours; decreased number of wet diapers; waking dry from nap
- Regular bowel movements
- Gross motor skills of sitting, walking, and squatting
- Fine motor skills to remove clothing

Cognitive Readiness

- Recognizing urge to defecate or urinate
- Verbal or nonverbal communicative skills to indicate when wet or has urge to defecate or urinate
- Cognitive skills to imitate appropriate behaviour and follow directions

Psychological Readiness

- Expressing willingness to please parent
- Ability to sit on toilet for 5 to 10 minutes without fussing or getting off
- Curiosity about adults' or older sibling's toilet habits
- Impatience with soiled or wet diapers; desire to be changed immediately

Parental Readiness

- Recognizing child's level of readiness
- Willingness to invest time required for toilet training
- Absence of family stress or change, such as a divorce, moving, new sibling, or imminent vacation

the majority of essential gross motor skills, can communicate intelligibly, is in less conflict with parents in terms of self-assertion and **negativism**, and is aware of the ability to control the body and please the parent. The CPS recommends starting toilet training no sooner than 18 months of age and suggests that the child must be interested in the process (Kiddoo, 2012). There is no universal right age to begin toilet training or an absolute deadline to complete training. One of the nurse's most important responsibilities is to help parents identify the readiness signs in their child and how to facilitate toilet learning (see Guidelines box). On average, girls are developmentally ready to begin toilet training 2 to 2½ months before boys (Clifford et al., 2000/2016). The CPS has a helpful parent guide to toilet training (see Additional Resources at the end of this chapter).

Nighttime bladder control normally takes several months to years after daytime training. This is because the sleep cycle needs to mature to the point that the child can awaken in time to urinate. Feigelman (2016) indicates that bed-wetting is normal in girls up to age 4 years and boys up to age 5 years. Few children will have night wetting episodes after daytime dryness is achieved; however, those children who do not have nighttime dryness by the age of 6 years are likely to require intervention.

Bowel training is usually accomplished before bladder training because of its greater regularity and predictability. The sensation for defecation is stronger than that for urination and easier for children to recognize. A well-balanced diet that includes dietary fibre helps keep stools soft and supports the development and maintenance of regular bowel movements.

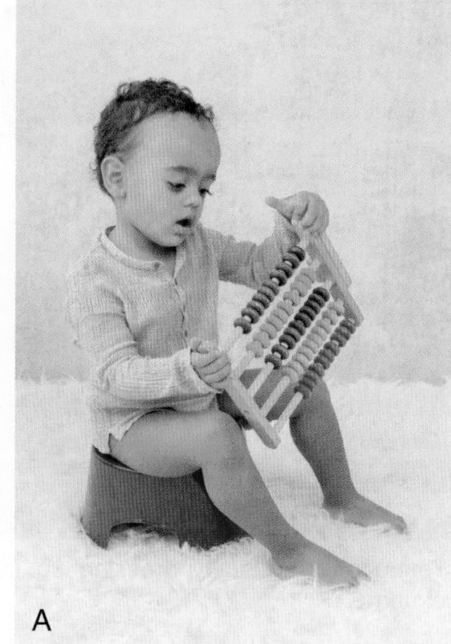

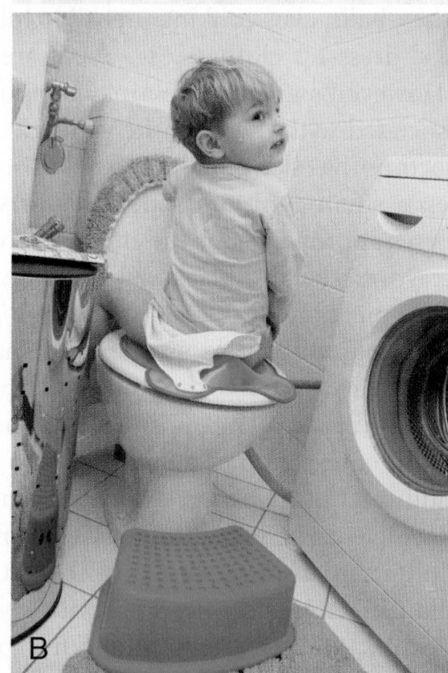

FIGURE 36-5 A: Children may begin toilet training sitting on a small potty chair. **B:** Sitting in reverse fashion on a regular toilet provides additional security to a young child. (A, Anneka/Shutterstock.com. B, aleksandr hunta/Shutterstock.com.)

A number of techniques can be helpful when initiating training, and cultural differences should be considered in this process. The following discussion of toilet training methods includes suggestions from the child-oriented approach to toilet training. Parents should begin the readiness phase of toilet training by teaching the child how the body functions in relation to voiding and having a bowel movement. Parents should talk about how adults and animals perform such functions on a routine basis. Another suggestion is to make toilet training as easy and simple as possible. Important considerations are the selection of the child's clothing and the potty chair or use of the toilet. A freestanding potty chair allows children a feeling of security (Fig. 36-5, *A*). Planting the feet firmly on the floor also facilitates defecation. Another option is a portable seat attached to the regular toilet, which may ease the transition from potty chair to regular toilet (Fig. 36-5, *B*). Placing a small bench under the feet helps stabilize the child's position. It is probably best to keep the potty chair in the bathroom and to let the child observe the excreta being flushed down the toilet to associate these activities with usual practices. If a potty chair is not available, having the child sit facing the toilet tank provides added support. Practice sessions should be limited to 5 to 8 minutes, and a parent should stay with the child, practising sanitary habits after every session. Children should be praised for their behaviour and successful evacuation. Dressing children in easily removed clothing; using training pants, "pull-on" diapers, or underwear; and encouraging imitation by watching others are other helpful suggestions. Another method emerging in the literature involves early assisted toilet training of infants around 2 to 3 weeks of age, but there are no studies assessing this method (Kiddoo, 2012).

When the child begins to experience regular daytime dryness, parents may experiment with the child wearing underwear during the day. Daytime accidents are common, particularly during periods of intense activity. Young children become so engrossed in play that, if they are not reminded, they will wait until it is too late to reach the bathroom. Therefore, frequent reminders and trips to the toilet are necessary. Parents often forget to plan ahead when the toddler is being toilet trained; before trips outside the house it is important to remind the child to at least try to urinate, to decrease the chance of needing to use the toilet while the car is stuck in traffic.

As the child develops each step of toileting (discussion, undressing, going, wiping, dressing, flushing, and hand washing), he or she gains a sense of accomplishment that parents should reinforce. If the parent–child relationship becomes strained, both may need a break from toilet training to focus on enjoyable activities together. Regression may coincide with a stressful family situation or may occur if the child is being pushed too hard and too fast. Regression is a normal part of toilet training and does not mean failure but should be viewed as a temporary setback to a more comfortable place for the child.

Day care providers also play a role in the support and education of parents regarding toilet-training practices. It is important for parents to inform all caregivers of their individual family values and the child's specific needs when planning for training away from home. Ensuring consistency in care of the toddler and healthy practices in a sanitary environment allows for safe and effective toilet practices in all settings.

Once the child has been successfully toilet trained for bladder control, sudden wetting accidents and frequent urinating urges may require further investigation for a possible urinary tract infection (UTI), especially in girls. Younger children often have a UTI without accompanying fever or painful urination.

Temper Tantrums

Toddlers may assert their independence by violently objecting to discipline. They may lie down on the floor, kick their feet, and scream as loud as possible. Some have learned the effectiveness of holding their breath until the parent relents. Although holding one's breath may cause fainting from lack of oxygen, the accumulation of carbon dioxide will stimulate the respiratory control centre, resulting in no physical harm. Tantrums can occur as a result of the child seeking attention or feeling tired, hungry, or uncomfortable. Children may feel frustrated by their inability to achieve something and are unable to express themselves. As their cognitive, physical, and language skills improve, tantrums will decrease.

The best approach toward tapering temper tantrums requires consistency and developmentally appropriate expectations and rewards. Ensuring consistency among all caregivers in expectations, prioritizing what rules are important, and developing consequences that are reasonable for the child's level of development can help manage the behaviour (Nieman, Shea, & CPS, Community Paediatrics Committee, 2004/2016). For example, a common time for a tantrum is bedtime; mealtime is also a common time for temper tantrums to occur. Active toddlers often have trouble slowing down and, when placed in bed, resist staying there. Parents can reinforce consistency and expectations by stating, "After this story it is bedtime." Starting at 18 months time-outs work well for managing temper tantrums. One key to handling the child's behaviour is to demonstrate consistency in dealing with both the behaviour and the situation that seemingly precipitated the tantrum; inconsistency reinforces the negative behaviour because the child cannot cognitively comprehend the ambiguous messages being received from the parents. Another favourite time for temper tantrums is in the store, especially at the end of the day when the child is tired. The "set-up" for a negative outcome can be avoided by recognizing the child's limitations and working around the situation for a positive outcome.

During tantrums parents should ignore the behaviour, provided the behaviour is not injurious to the child, such as violently banging the head on the floor. Parents should continue to be present to provide a feeling of control and security to the child once the tantrum has subsided. When the child starts demonstrating appropriate behaviour, he or she should be given positive feedback about that behaviour. During periods of no tantrums developmentally appropriate positive reinforcement can be practised. The Patient Teaching box outlines other behaviour strategies that parents can use to manage their toddler's tantrums.

Temper tantrums are common during the toddler years and essentially represent normal developmental behaviours.

PATIENT TEACHING

Temper Tantrums

Other suggestions for handling tantrums include the following (Kids Health, 2012):

- Make sure your child isn't acting up simply because he or she isn't getting enough attention.
- Try to give toddlers some control over little things.
- Keep off-limits objects out of sight and out of reach to make struggles less likely to develop over them.
- Distract your child.
- Set the stage for success when the child is playing or trying to master a new task.
- Consider the request carefully when your child wants something.
- Know your child's limits.

However, temper tantrums can be signs of serious problems. Nurses should be alert to situations that require further evaluation.

Negativism

One of the more difficult aspects of rearing children in this age group is their persistent "no" response to every request. The negativism is not an expression of being stubborn or insolent but a necessary assertion of self-control. Children test limits to gain understanding of the world and to learn to modify their behaviour to fit the expectations of society. Negativism begins to subside as most children prepare to enter kindergarten.

One method of dealing with the negativism is to reduce the opportunities for a "no" answer. Asking the child, "Do you want to go to sleep now?" is an almost certain example of a question that will be answered with an emphatic "no." Instead, the parent should tell the child that it is time to go to sleep and proceed accordingly. In their attempt to exert control, children like to make choices. When confronted with appropriate choices, such as "You may have a peanut-butter-and-jelly sandwich or chicken-noodle soup for lunch," they are more likely to choose one rather than automatically say "no." However, if their response is negative, parents should make the choice for the child.

Nurses working with children and parents can help parents understand this concept by role modelling. For example, when the nurse approaches the toddler to take vital signs, instead of asking, "Can I listen to your heart?" the nurse can say, "I'm going to listen to your heart." Because of normal developmental behaviour, toddlers vigorously resist first attempts at taking vital signs because it is an intrusion on their bodies. Second, they are most likely going to answer "no," not because they necessarily fear the procedure itself but because of the tendency to answer all questions with a negative response. If the nurse asks the question, and the toddler says, "No," but the nurse proceeds anyway, the toddler starts to mistrust the nurse's actions because they contradict his or her words.

Sibling Rivalry

The natural jealousy and resentment of children to a new child in the family is referred to as *sibling rivalry*. The arrival of a new infant represents a crisis for even the best-prepared toddlers. It is not the infant that toddlers resent but the changes that this additional sibling produces, especially the separation from the mother during the birth. The parents now share their love and attention with someone else, the usual routine is disrupted, and toddlers may lose their crib or room, all at a time when they thought they were in control of their world. Sibling rivalry tends to be most pronounced in the firstborn, who experiences *dethronement* (i.e., loss of sole parental attention). It also seems to be most difficult for young children, particularly in terms of mother–child interaction.

Preparation of children for the birth of a sibling is individual, but age dictates some important considerations. Time for toddlers is a vague concept. Tomorrow could be yesterday or next week, and a month from now could be never. Preparing children too soon for the birth may lessen their interest by the time the event occurs. A good time to start talking about the new baby is when the toddler becomes aware of the pregnancy and the changes taking place in the home in anticipation of the new member (see Chapter 11, Patient Teaching Box: Tips for Sibling Preparation, p. 233).

Toddlers need to have a realistic idea of what the newborn will be like. Telling them that a new playmate will come home soon sets up unrealistic expectations. Rather, parents should stress the activities that will take place when the baby arrives home, such as diapering, feeding, bathing, and dressing. At the same time, parents should emphasize which routines will stay the same, such as reading stories or going to the park. The disruption of the toddler's routine is significant but can be restored with some effort by the parents. It may be helpful for the father or partner to spend more quality time with the toddler in anticipation of the mother's time being occupied with the new baby. If toddlers have had no contact with an infant, it is a good idea to introduce them to one, if feasible.

A new sibling in the home is stressful, so any additional stresses for the toddler should be avoided or minimized. For example, moving the toddler to a regular bed or to a different room should be done well in advance of the infant's arrival.

Pregnancy is an abstraction for toddlers. They need concrete illustrations of how the baby is growing inside the mother. It is an excellent opportunity for introducing aspects of reproduction and sexuality. Seeing simple pictures of the uterus and fetus and feeling the fetus move can help the child feel involved in the experience (see Fig. 11-3). Children also benefit from classes for siblings that may be part of prenatal sessions.

When the newborn arrives, toddlers keenly feel the changed focus of attention. Visitors may initiate problems when they inadvertently shower the infant with attention and presents while neglecting the older child. Parents can minimize this by alerting visitors to the toddler's needs and by including the child in the visits as much as possible. The toddler can also help with the care of the newborn by getting diapers and doing other small tasks (Fig. 36-6).

How children exhibit jealousy is complex. Some will overtly hit the infant, push the child off the mother's lap, or pull the breast or bottle from the infant's mouth. For this reason, infants must be protected by parental supervision of the interaction between the siblings. More often the expressions of hostility and resentment are more subtle and covert. Toddlers may verbally express a wish that the infant "go back inside mommy," or they will revert to more infantile forms of behaviour, such as demanding a bottle, soiling their underpants, clinging for attention, using baby talk, or aggressively acting out toward others.

Regression

The retreat from one's present pattern of functioning to past levels of behaviour is referred to as *regression*. It usually occurs in instances of discomfort or stress when one attempts to conserve psychic energy by reverting to patterns of behaviour that were successful in earlier stages of development. Regression is common in toddlers because almost any additional stress hinders their ability to master present developmental tasks. Any threat to their autonomy, such as illness, hospitalization,

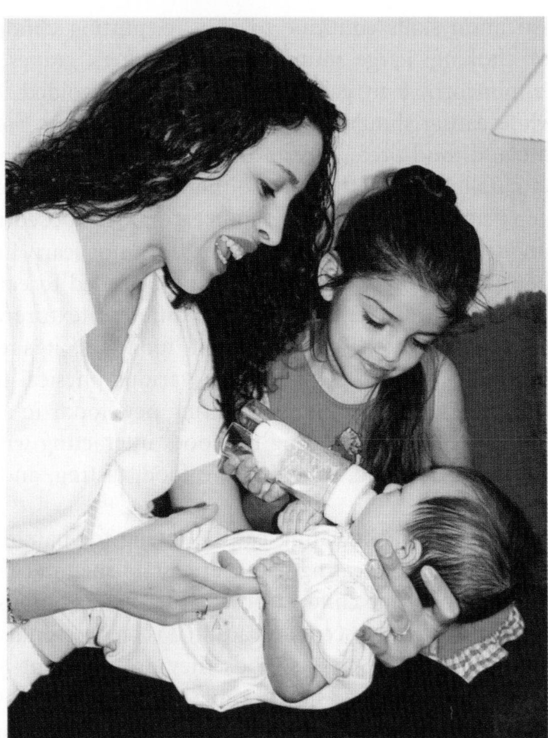

FIGURE 36-6 To minimize sibling rivalry, parents should include the toddler during caregiving activities.

separation from parents, or adjustment to a new sibling, represents a need to revert to earlier forms of behaviour, such as increased dependency; refusal to use the potty chair; temper tantrums; demand for the bottle, stroller, or crib; and loss of newly learned motor, language, social, and cognitive skills.

At first, such regression appears acceptable and comfortable for children, but the loss of newly acquired achievements is actually frightening and threatening because children are aware of their helplessness. Parents become concerned about regressive behaviour and often, in their efforts to deal with it, force the child to cope with an additional source of stress—the pressure to live up to expected standards. Brazelton (1999) suggests that these predictable times of regression, or *touchpoints*, are an opportunity to prepare parents for the next step in their child's development.

When regression does occur, the best approach is to ignore it while praising existing patterns of appropriate behaviour. Regression is a child's way of saying, "I can't cope with this present stress and perfect this skill as well, but I will if given patience and understanding." For this reason, it is advisable not to attempt new areas of learning when an additional crisis is present or expected, such as beginning toilet training shortly before a sibling is born or attempting new areas of learning during a brief period of hospitalization.

Mental Health

A child with mental health concerns can have symptoms in this age group that may need to be carefully investigated. For example, there is evidence that autism spectrum disorders (ASDs) can sometimes be seen at 18 months or younger and can be diagnosed by age 2 (Autism Canada, 2015). Early treatment is critical to all mental health disorders in order to optimize interventions successfully.

The well-baby visits and developmental screening tools are very important for picking up any unusual developmental delays or behaviours that would indicate a mental health issue. See Chapter 33 for more information on developmental assessment tools. Nurses play an important role in assessing the child and the family and helping families understand the developmental norms for the age and stage. The signs of mental illness in children vary by age and type of illness, with some psychiatric disorders appearing in preschoolers. See Chapter 37 for more information on the preschooler and mental health.

PROMOTING OPTIMUM HEALTH DURING TODDLERHOOD

Nutrition

During the period from 12 to 18 months of age, the growth rate slows, decreasing the child's need for calories, protein, and fluid. However, the protein (13 g/day) and energy requirements are still relatively high to meet the demands for muscle tissue growth and a high activity level. The need for minerals such as iron, calcium, and phosphorus may be difficult to meet, considering the characteristic food habits of children in this age group. Parents may be tempted to rely on vitamin supplementation rather than a well-balanced diet to meet these requirements. Toddlers usually require three meals and two snacks per day; however, the portions consumed are generally much smaller than those of older children. Canada's *Food Guide* gives guidance on how to provide good nutrition for children (see Appendix A).

At approximately 18 months of age, most toddlers manifest this decreased nutritional need with a decrease in appetite, a phenomenon known as *physiological anorexia*. They become picky, fussy eaters with strong taste preferences. They may eat large amounts one day and almost nothing the next. They become increasingly aware of the non-nutritive function of food (i.e., the pleasure of eating, the social aspect of mealtime, and the control of refusing food).

Toddlers are influenced by factors other than taste when choosing food. If a family member refuses to eat something, toddlers are likely to imitate that response. If the plate is overfilled, they are likely to push it away, overwhelmed by its size. If food does not appear or smell appetizing, they will probably not agree to try it. In essence, mealtime is more closely associated with psychological components than with nutritional components.

The **ritualism** of this age also dictates certain principles in feeding practices. Toddlers like to have the same dish, cup, or spoon every time they eat. They may reject a favourite food simply because it is served in a different dish. If one food touches another, they often refuse to eat it.

Mixed foods, such as stews or casseroles, are rarely favourites. Because toddlers have unpredictable table manners, it is best to use plastic dishes and cups for both economical and safety reasons. For some children a regular mealtime schedule also contributes to their desire and need for predictability and ritualism.

Developmentally, by 12 months of age most children are encouraged to be eating the same food prepared for the rest of the family. Some may have mastered using a cup, with occasional spilling; most cannot adeptly use a spoon until 18 months of age or later and generally prefer using their fingers.

Nutritional Counselling

It is now recognized that lifetime eating habits may be established in early childhood, and health care workers are increasingly emphasizing the role of food selection, exercise, stress reduction, and other lifestyle choices (such as tobacco and alcohol use) on the quality of adult life and survival. Conditions such as obesity and cardiovascular disease can be decreased by encouraging healthy eating habits in toddlers and their families.

If food is used as a reward or sign of approval, a child may overeat for non-nutritive reasons. If food is forced and mealtime is consistently unpleasant, the usual pleasure associated with eating may not develop. Mealtimes should be enjoyable rather than times for discipline or family arguments. The social aspect of mealtime may be distracting for young children; therefore an earlier feeding hour may be appropriate. Young children are unable to sit through a long meal and will become restless and disruptive. This is particularly common when children are brought to the table just after active play. Calling them in from play 15 minutes before mealtime allows them ample opportunity to get ready for eating while settling down their active minds and bodies.

The method of serving food also takes on more importance during this period. Toddlers need to have a sense of control and achievement in their abilities. Giving them large, adult-size portions can be overwhelming. In general, what is eaten is much more significant than how much is consumed. Toddlers usually restrict their food preference to four or five main foods and rarely try new foods; in some cases a toddler may insist on one food such as mashed potatoes for lunch and dinner. Small amounts of meat and vegetables supply greater food value than a large consumption of bread or potato. Serving sizes need to be appropriate for age (see Appendix A).

To determine serving size for young children, the following guidelines should be used:

- A general guide to the serving size of food is 15 mL (1 tablespoon) of solid food per year of age, or one fourth to one third of the adult portion size.
- Use the 15-mL guide for easily measured foods such as vegetables or rice.

Young children tend to like less spicy, bland food, although this is a culturally determined preference. Substitutions can be provided for foods that they do not enjoy, although this practice should not cater to all of their desires. Frequent nutritious *planned* snacks may provide adequate caloric intake at this age. *Grazing*—nibbling and snacking—is a good way to ensure proper nutrition, provided that appropriate foods are offered; giving the child something to eat merely to pacify the child is not recommended.

Mastication skills continue to mature, putting children at risk for choking. Large round foods (hot dogs, grapes, peas, carrots, popcorn, fruit gel snacks) should be avoided. Active play while eating should be discouraged, to prevent choking. Appetite and food preferences are sporadic. Often the interest in food parallels a growth spurt, so that periods of good eating are interspersed with phases of poor eating. If exposed to the same food every day, a young toddler does not learn how to manage the complex sensory information needed to eat new, more difficult foods (vegetables with a different texture versus puréed, slippery fruits). To help prevent "food jags," it is recommended that parents present food in various physical forms. The child may need to progress to eating new foods in a stepwise fashion: visually tolerating the food, interacting with the food, smelling the food, touching the food, tasting, and then eating the food.

This period of picky eating can be trying for parents and children alike. Because eating habits are established in early life and affect not only the child's future eating habits but also the child's health as an adolescent and adult, it is recommended that toddlers not be forced to eat foods they are reluctant to eat. Evidence indicates that toddlers are able to regulate their hunger and satiety needs internally and that forcing foods during this period may exacerbate or lead to future eating problems. It has also been suggested that parents plan a nutritionally balanced week instead of day because of the way toddlers will restrict food intake in their effort to exert control over their environment (Morin, 2007).

Nutrition Guidelines

Nutrition guidelines are necessary to promote adequate energy and nutrient intake to support physical, emotional, psychological, and cognitive development. A number of new nutrition guidelines have been developed to address the issue of childhood obesity, sedentary lifestyles, and increase in cardiovascular disease mortality in Canada (see Additional Resources at the end of this chapter).

Nutrition during toddlerhood involves a transition as a young toddler is weaned off milk- or formula-dependent diets. The CPS recommends breastfeeding until age 24 months or older, but if the child is weaned earlier the introduction of cow's milk should be delayed until age 9 to 12 months and 500 mL offered per day (Critch & CPS, Nutrition and Gastroenterology Committee, 2014). Milk intake for a toddler is the chief source of calcium and phosphorus and should average two or three servings (700 to 900 mL) a day. However, more than 750 mL of milk consumption daily considerably limits the intake of solid foods, resulting in a deficiency of dietary iron and other **nutrients** (Critch & CPS, Nutrition and Gastroenterology Committee, 2014). Water is an important option for quenching thirst in the toddler. After 2 years of age, children can be given a lower-fat milk to reduce daily total fat to less than 30% of calories, saturated fatty acids to less than 10% of calories, and cholesterol to less than 300 mg. Fat restriction of trans fatty acids and of saturated fats is important in the protection of toddlers' cardiovascular health. However, for the first 2 years homogenized milk provides an important part of essential nutrients required for energy and brain development. Other measures to reduce dietary fat include eating lean meats and fat-modified foods (such as low-fat cheese) and cooking with low-fat products. Because less fat in children's diet can also mean fewer calories and nutrients, caregivers must know what kinds of food to choose. *Eating Well With Canada's Food Guide* still recommends using 2% milk in the toddler age group and not restricting nutritious foods because of fat content (see Appendix A) (Health Canada, 2011).

Iron-fortified cereals and iron-rich foods are recommended for all children beyond 6 months of age a couple of times a day. Parents are encouraged to provide an iron-rich diet that includes heme and nonheme iron sources (red meats, poultry, fish, green leafy vegetables, dried fruit, beans) and limit whole-milk consumption after 2 years of age. Iron supplementation may be necessary in some cases.

Calcium and vitamin D are essential for healthy bone development. Research findings have indicated the need for a higher dietary intake of calcium and vitamin D. As well, vitamin D deficiency may play an important role in the development of systemic conditions later in life, such as cancer (Godel & CPS, First Nations, Inuit and Métis Health Committee, 2007/2015). It is well known that vitamin D deficiency is common in adults and children in Canada. At particular risk are Indigenous populations and others who live in the high Arctic regions where cold-weather clothing and a lack of light decrease the amount of vitamin D produced in the skin. At the same time, these populations have decreased dietary intake of their traditional vitamin D–rich foods. Children who have high body mass indices (BMIs) and are overweight or obese have lower levels of vitamin D as well (Godel & CPS, First Nations, Inuit and Métis Health Committee, 2007/2015).

Research carried out by the U.S. Institute of Medicine on vitamin D and calcium levels has led to new joint recommendations on increased calcium and vitamin D intakes (Health Canada, 2012). The recommendation for adequate intake of calcium for a child 1 to 3 years of age has increased to 700 mg per day; the tolerable upper intake per day is 2500 mg. Whole milk, cheese, yogurt, legumes (beans), and vegetables (broccoli, collard greens, kale) are good sources of calcium. Popular calcium-fortified foods include waffles, cereals and cereal bars, orange juice, and some white breads. Adequate vitamin D intake is essential to prevent rickets; the new vitamin D recommendation for children aged 1 to 3 years is 600 International Units (IU) (15 mcg) per day, with a tolerable upper level per day at 2500 IU (62.5 mcg). For children under the age of 2 years who live above a northern latitude of 55°, those with dark skin, and those avoiding sunlight, 800 IU (20 mcg) of vitamin D per day should be provided in the winter months (Godel & CPS, First Nations, Inuit and Métis Health Committee, 2007/2015). Supplements may be required if food intake is poor or exposure to sunlight is minimal. Sources of vitamin D include fish, fish oils, and egg yolks; additionally, the consumption of 1 litre of vitamin D–fortified milk will provide 400 IU (10 mcg) of vitamin D. Fortified cereals, dairy products, and meat are also good sources of zinc and vitamin E.

Eating Well With Canada's Food Guide (see Appendix A) recommends that children have four servings of fruit and vegetables each day. Vitamin C enhances iron absorption. Fruit and vegetables are recommended over fruit juices. Toddlers should consume a maximum of 120 to 180 mL of juice per day. A 180-mL glass of fruit juice equals one fruit serving; however, juices lack the fibre of whole fruit and should not be used as a substitute. High intake of juice can contribute to diarrhea, overnutrition or undernutrition, and the development of caries (Critch & CPS, Nutrition and Gastroenterology Committee, 2014). Beverages called "fruit cocktail," "fruit punch," or "fruit drink," or "pop" should be avoided given the high sugar content. Also, children should be offered beverages in a regular cup instead of a bottle or sippy cup (Critch & CPS, Nutrition and Gastroenterology Committee, 2014).

Vegetarian Diets

Vegetarian diets have become increasingly prevalent for many reasons: people are concerned about hypertension, cholesterol, obesity, cardiovascular disease, and cancer of the stomach, intestine, and colon; the influence of the animal rights movement; and for cultural or religious reasons (see Chapter 46). For families who eat a vegetarian diet, careful planning is needed to ensure that growing children have their nutritional requirements met. These families may also benefit from consultation with a dietitian (Health Canada, 2015).

Activity and Sleep

The toddler's activity level is high, and too little physical exercise is rarely a problem as long as inappropriate restrictions are not instituted. However, recently there has been concern that decreased time spent in actual physical play and more time involved with computers and television watching have increased the tendency toward being overweight. This is especially true in large urban centres during the winter months where there may not be adequate "safe" play and physical exercise space. With increasing numbers of young children being cared for outside the home, attention to the kinds of activity provided is important. For example, children with high activity levels may benefit from an environment in which outdoor play is encouraged.

Total sleep decreases only slightly during the second year and averages about 12 hours a day. Most toddlers take one nap a day, and by the end of the second or third year, many relinquish this habit. Children reach an adult pattern of sleep by 3 years of age.

Sleep problems are common among toddlers, especially going to bed and falling asleep, and are probably related to fears and awareness of separation. Toddlers are more prone to having bedtime resistance (refusal to go to bed) and frequent night waking; during later toddlerhood this group of children may become more resistant about going to bed and express fears about monsters. Fears can be provoked by a child's daily stressors, such as pressure to toilet train, moves, sibling birth, experiences of loss, or separation from parents. Bedtime rituals (e.g., same hour of sleep, snack, and quiet activity) are helpful, and transitional objects, such as a favourite stuffed animal or blanket, can help ease the child's insecurity at bedtime (see Fig.

36-3). Children may need a light snack before bedtime; a heavy meal immediately before bedtime may interfere with sleep. Other suggestions to help small children sleep better include keeping the television out of the child's room, making the hour before bedtime a quiet time of reading stories, and avoiding stimulating activities, such as computer games and roughhousing (Owens, 2016). Toddlers no longer sleeping in a crib may come out of their rooms after being put to bed. Prolonging of bedtime rituals can be limited by defining the length of time and set of activities (one more story, one more drink of water). Toddlers who are too immature to respond to such measures may need their doorways gated.

As with infants, a safe sleeping environment is important at the toddler stage. Many factors affect sleeping arrangements, including parental and cultural values and socioeconomic factors. All of these factors need to be taken into consideration when health care providers are offering guidance on the physical and emotional security of sleeping environments. Although rare, sudden infant death syndrome (SIDS) can occur in children over 1 year of age, as can accidental suffocation or entrapment. Therefore, families need to be educated about the CPS's (2015) recommendations on safe sleeping environments. These recommendations include using cribs that meet the Canadian government's safety regulations, not makeshift temporary beds; dressing the child in sleepers with a thin blanket without pillow-like items and toys for sleep; and preventing exposure to passive smoke (CPS, 2015). (See Chapter 35 for more information on the relation between a safe sleeping environment and the occurrence of SIDS.)

When a sleeping problem is presented, a careful assessment is essential. Charting sleep habits both before and after interventions is also an important strategy. Questions regarding the frequency and duration of waking, the usual bedtime routine, the number of nighttime feedings, the perceived problem (e.g., how much disruption the behaviour generates), and the attempted interventions are important in planning effective approaches designed for the specific sleep problem.

The best way to prevent sleep problems is to encourage parents to establish bedtime rituals that do not foster problematic patterns. One of the most constructive routines is placing infants awake in their own crib. When infants are accustomed to falling asleep somewhere else, such as in their parent's arms, and then transferred to their crib, they awaken in unfamiliar surroundings and are unable to fall asleep until the routine is repeated. In addition, the bed should be used for sleeping only—not as a play area. Playthings should not be hung over the bed or placed in it, so the child associates the bed with sleep and not with activity. It is much easier to prevent a sleep problem with appropriate counselling from the nurse and actions by parents during the early months of the infant's life.

Dental Health

Regular Dental Examinations

Oral health is an important cornerstone of health for all Canadians. The Health Canada Oral Health Report Card (Canadian Dental Association [CDA], 2010) indicates that most Canadians have access to professional dental care and have good oral health. However, a minority of the population has difficulty accessing adequate oral health care; these groups include individuals with low income; people with special needs; some children; and Indigenous peoples. Indigenous peoples generally have the poorest oral health within Canada and have a lower rate of accessing dental coverage (CDA, 2010).

The Canadian Dental Association (CDA) recommends that dental visits begin within 6 months of the eruption of the first tooth or within the first year, for prevention of dental decay. Families need to have education on how to provide a healthy diet and good oral hygiene for their child. Children at high risk for dental problems should be identified by nurses, nurse practitioners, family doctors, pediatricians, and community health agencies. The number one cause of day surgeries in Canadian children is preventable early childhood dental caries.

Initial visits to the dentist should be nontraumatizing. Because toddlers react negatively to new and potentially frightening experiences, the initial visit can centre on meeting the dentist, seeing the equipment, and sitting in the chair. If the child will cooperate, the dentist may just look at the teeth but reserve a more thorough examination for another visit. *Modelling*, in which the child observes procedures performed on the parent or a sibling, can also be effective but may not work for some toddlers.

Removal of Plaque

Oral hygiene measures should be implemented to remove *plaque*, or soft bacterial deposits that adhere to the teeth and cause dental **caries** (decay or cavities) and periodontal (gum) disease. Poor oral hygiene and poor dietary habits are associated with the development of caries in children.

The most effective methods for plaque removal are brushing and flossing. Several brushing techniques exist, although there is no universal agreement regarding the best method. One that is suitable for cleaning the primary teeth is the scrub method. The tips of the bristles are placed firmly at a 45-degree angle against the teeth and gums and moved back and forth in a vibratory motion. The ends of the bristles should be wiggling but not moving forcefully back and forth, as this can damage the gums and enamel. All the surfaces of the teeth should be cleaned in this manner except the lingual (inner) surfaces of the anterior teeth. To clean these surfaces, the toothbrush is placed vertical to the teeth and moved up and down. Only a few teeth are brushed at one time, using six to eight strokes for each section. A systematic approach should be used so that all surfaces are thoroughly cleaned (Fig. 36-7).

For young children, the most effective cleaning is done by parents (Fig. 36-8). Several positions can be used that facilitate access to the mouth and help stabilize the head for comfort:

- Standing with the child's back toward the adult. (When done in front of a bathroom mirror, both the child and adult can see what is being done in the mirror.)
- Sitting on a couch or bed with the child's head resting in the adult's lap.
- Sitting on the floor or a stool with the child's head resting between the adult's thighs.

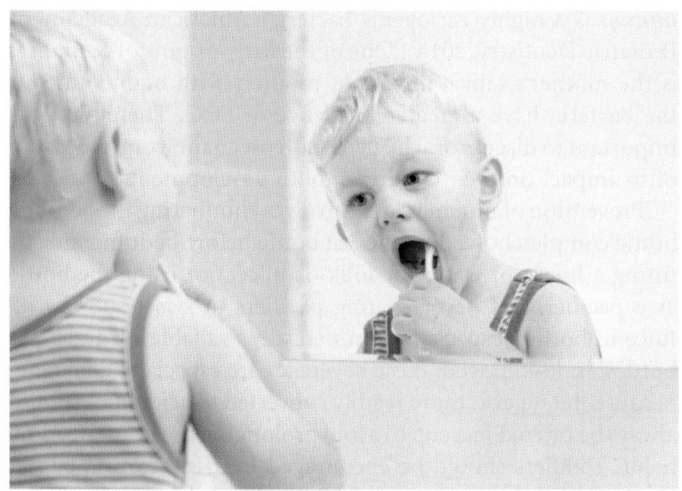

FIGURE 36-7 Young children can participate in tooth brushing, but parents need to brush all the child's teeth thoroughly. (Oksana Kuzmina/Shutterstock.com.)

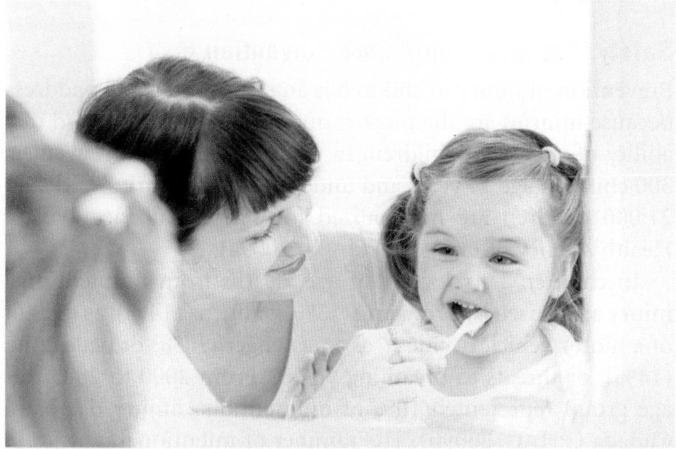

FIGURE 36-8 The most effective cleaning of the teeth is done by parents. (Oksana Kuzmina/Shutterstock.com.)

With all positions, one hand cups the chin and the other brushes the teeth. For easier access to back teeth, the mouth is held partially open.

For effective cleaning, a small toothbrush with soft, rounded, multitufted nylon bristles that are short and uniform in length is recommended. Nylon bristles dry more rapidly after use and retain their shape better than natural bristles. Toothbrushes should be replaced as soon as the bristles are frayed or bent.

If a child up to age 3 is identified by a health care provider to be at risk of developing tooth caries, then a minimal amount (the size of a grain of rice) of fluoridated toothpaste should be used (CDA, 2012). Use of fluoridated toothpaste in a small amount has been determined to achieve a balance between the benefits of fluoride and the risk of developing fluorosis. When using toothpaste, children should select the flavour they like, to encourage the brushing habit. If the child is not considered to be at risk, the teeth should be brushed by an adult using a toothbrush moistened only with water.

After the teeth have been cleaned, flossing with dental floss is done to remove plaque and debris from between the teeth and below the gum margin, where brushing is ineffective. Since young children do not have the dexterity to manipulate the floss, parents should be taught the procedure to use in children.

Ideally, the teeth should be cleaned after each meal and especially before bedtime, and the child should be given nothing to eat or drink after the night brushing, except water. When brushing is impractical, the "swish-and-swallow" method of cleaning the mouth can be taught: with a mouthful of water, the child rinses the mouth and swallows, repeating the procedure three or four times.

Fluoride

In Canada, public water systems have fluoride added to the drinking water. The Federal-Provincial-Territorial Committee on Drinking Water recommends the optimal level of fluoride that is added to public drinking water to prevent tooth decay. The Government of Canada's guideline for fluoride in drinking water indicates a maximum acceptable concentration of 1.5 milligrams per litre (Health Canada, 2016). All health care providers should know the level of fluoridation in their regional drinking water; this information is available from their local public health agency. Fluoride supplements, in the form of chewable tablets, lozenges, or drops, are not recommended for the majority of Canadians. However, health professionals may wish to prescribe fluoride supplements to high-risk patients in nonfluoridated communities where individuals are not able to obtain fluoride in any other form (CDA, 2012). The CDA (2012) recommends that for young children the total daily fluoride intake from all sources not exceed 0.05 to 0.07 mg fluoride/kg body weight, to minimize the risk of dental fluorosis.

Increased fluoride ingestion, such as when children swallow fluoridated toothpaste, leads to enamel protein retention, hypomineralization of the enamel and dentin, and disturbance of crystal formation. The effects caused by this change range from barely discernible white fibrelike lines or spots to grey-brown stains or pitted areas. Parents should be cautioned against regular use of fluoridated water or beverages such as bottled water containing fluoride if the community water supply already has an adequate amount of fluoride.

Dietary Factors

Nutrition is critical to developing good teeth because carious development depends primarily on fermentable sugars, especially sucrose and other carbohydrates. Refined table sugar, honey, molasses, corn syrup, and dried fruits such as raisins are highly cariogenic. Complex carbohydrates such as breads, potatoes, and pasta also contribute to caries because they lower the plaque pH. Beverages and snacks that are commonly consumed by children and adolescents are also highly cariogenic and may contribute to the incidence of overweight and obesity (American Academy of Pediatric Dentistry, 2014).

Ideally, highly cariogenic foods, especially those containing complex sugars, should be eliminated from the child's diet. However, since this is impractical, some suggestions can be helpful. First, *the frequency with which sugar is consumed is more important than the total amount eaten*. Therefore, when sweets are eaten, they are less damaging if consumed immediately after a meal rather than as a snack between meals. When sweets are served as the dessert, the teeth should be cleaned afterward, decreasing the amount of time the sugar is in the mouth.

Second, the form of sugar (sucrose) is important. The more cariogenic foods are those that are sticky or hard, since they remain in the mouth longer. Consequently, sucking on lollipops is more cariogenic than eating a chocolate bar. Sometimes the source of the sugar is "hidden," as in numerous prescription and nonprescription medications and in many popular cereals, including the "all-natural" variety. Reading food labels is essential in identifying and eliminating sources of sucrose.

Some snacks do not contribute to tooth decay. Aged cheeses such as cheddar may alter the pH and slow bacterial growth. Sugarless gum chewed after eating may actually protect against cavities by stimulating saliva that neutralizes acid.

A special form of tooth decay in children between 18 months and 3 years of age is early childhood caries (ECC) (historically called *nursing caries* or *baby bottle tooth decay*). This occurs when the child is routinely given a bottle of milk or juice at naptime or bedtime or uses the bottle as a pacifier while awake. Frequent nocturnal breastfeeding for prolonged periods also leads to extensive destruction of the teeth. The practice of coating pacifiers in honey or corn syrup can also contribute to the development of caries and may be a potential source of botulism poisoning in infants. As the sweet liquid pools in the mouth, the teeth are bathed for several hours in this cariogenic environment. Prolonged bottle-feeding well into toddler years in some cultures may contribute to significant ECC (Brotanek, Schroer, Valentyn, et al., 2009). The maxillary (upper) incisors and molars are affected most, since the mandibular (lower) incisors are protected by the lower lip, tongue, and saliva (Fig. 36-9). Severely decayed teeth may require the application of stainless steel bands to preserve the spacing until the permanent teeth erupt.

Early childhood caries is now considered to be an infectious disease of childhood. There is evidence that *Streptococcus mutans* is a highly cariogenic bacteria (American Academy of Pediatric Dentistry, 2014). One of the early origins of *S. mutans* is the mother's saliva; infants of mothers with high counts of the bacteria have a greater incidence of ECC. Therefore, it is important to discuss oral hygiene with pregnant women because of its impact on their children's tooth development.

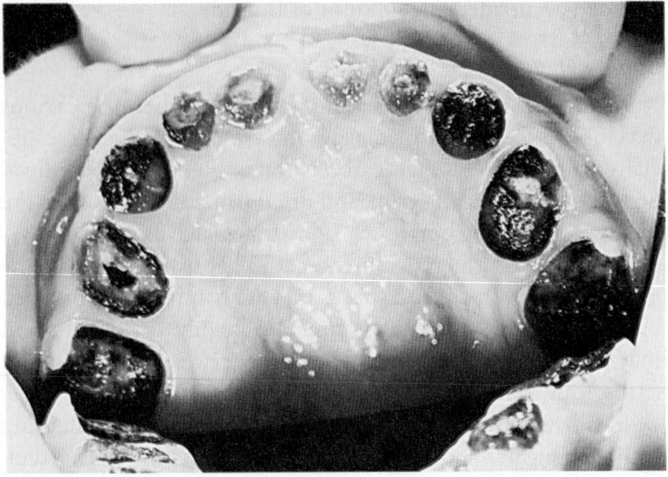

FIGURE 36-9 Nursing caries. Note extensive carious involvement of maxillary primary incisors. (Courtesy Bruce Carter, DDS, Texas Children's Hospital.)

Prevention of nursing caries involves eliminating the bedtime bottle completely, feeding the last bottle before bedtime, substituting a bottle of water for milk or juice, not using the bottle as a pacifier, and never coating pacifiers in sweet substances. Juice in bottles, especially commercially available ready-to-use bottles, is discouraged; these beverages are especially damaging because the sugar is more readily converted to acid. Juice should always be offered in a cup to avoid prolonging the bottle-feeding habit. Toddlers should be encouraged to drink from a cup at the first birthday and weaned from a bottle by 14 months of age. Nurses are in an excellent position to counsel parents regarding the dangers of poor dietary habits and other aspects of dental care.

Safety Promotion and Injury Prevention

Prevention of injury in children is an important area to address because injuries are the most common cause of death and disability of Canadian children. In Canada, annually, on average, 300 children age 14 years and under die from injuries, and over 21,000 children are hospitalized for serious injuries (Public Health Agency of Canada [PHAC], 2009a).

In children 1 to 4 years of age, deaths from unintentional injury are caused by drowning (23%) or burns (14%); as a result of a motor vehicle accident, as a passenger (14%) or pedestrian (14%); or threats to breathing (11%). From 2000 to 2005 this age group represented 10% of unintentional injury deaths in Canada (PHAC, 2009b). The number of intentional injuries in children, including from maltreatment, peaks at 1 to 2 years of age (PHAC, 2009a).

A major factor in the critical increase in the number of injuries during early childhood is the unrestricted freedom achieved through locomotion combined with an unawareness of danger within the environment. Toddlers delight in the repetitive use of gross motor skills, and with increasing age these skills are refined. This age group is also very curious about how things work, and exploration of previously unknown or unseen objects and places is common. Toddlers also have not fully developed or do not understand the cause-and-effect principles that older children have and often are unable to gauge danger; poorly developed depth perception may also contribute to falls and tumbles, as does the general bodily structure of toddlers. Specific categories of injuries and appropriate prevention are best understood by associating them with the major developmental achievements of young children (Table 36-2). The discussions of injuries in Chapters 35 and 37 are also relevant to safety concerns at this age.

Motor Vehicle Injuries

Motor vehicle injuries cause more accidental deaths in all pediatric age groups older than 1 year of age than any other type of injury or disease and are responsible for almost half of all

TABLE 36-2 INJURY PREVENTION DURING EARLY CHILDHOOD

DEVELOPMENTAL ABILITIES RELATED TO RISK OF INJURY	INJURY PREVENTION
Motor Vehicles	
Walks, runs, and climbs Able to open doors and gates Can ride tricycle and other toy vehicles Can throw ball and other objects	Use federally approved car restraint. Supervise child while playing outside. Do not allow child to play on curb or behind a parked car. Do not permit child to play in a pile of leaves, snow, or large cardboard container in trafficked area. Supervise tricycle riding. Lock fences and doors if not directly supervising children. Teach child to obey pedestrian safety rules: • Obey traffic regulations; cross only at crosswalks and only when traffic signal indicates it is safe. • Stand back a step from the curb until it is time to cross. • Look left, right, and left again and check for turning cars before crossing the street. • Use sidewalks; when there is no sidewalk, walk on the left, facing traffic. • Wear light colours at night and attach fluorescent material to clothing.
Submersion Injuries	
Able to explore if left unsupervised Has great curiosity Helpless in water; unaware of its danger—may consider "play" in any body of water the same as in the bath; depth of water has no significance	Supervise closely when near any source of water regardless of depth, including buckets. Keep bathroom doors closed and lid down on toilet (or install latch). Have fence around swimming pool and lock gate. Teach swimming and water safety (this is, however, not a substitute for safety).
Burns	
Able to reach heights by climbing, stretching, and standing on toes Pulls objects Explores any holes or opening Can open drawers and closets Unaware of potential sources of heat or fire Plays with mechanical objects	Turn pot handles toward back of stove. Place electrical appliances, such as coffee maker and popcorn machine, toward back of counter. Place guardrails in front of radiators, fireplaces, or other heating elements. Store matches and cigarette lighters in locked or inaccessible area; discard carefully. Place burning candles, incense, hot foods, and cigarettes out of reach. Do not let tablecloth hang within child's reach. Do not let electric cord from iron, curling iron, or other appliance hang within child's reach. Cover electrical outlets with protective plastic caps. Keep electrical wires hidden or out of reach. Do not allow child to play with electrical appliance, wires, or lighters. Stress danger of open flames; teach what "hot" means. Always check bathwater temperature; adjust water heater temperature to 49°C or lower; do not allow children to play with faucets. Apply a sunscreen when child is exposed to sunlight.
Accidental Poisoning	
Explores by putting objects in mouth Can open drawers, closets, boxes, and most containers Climbs Cannot read labels Does not know safe dose or amount	Place all potentially toxic agents out of reach or in a locked cabinet. Caution against eating nonedible items, such as plants. Replace medications or poisons immediately in proper storage and out of the child's reach; replace child-guard caps properly. Administer medications as a drug, not as a candy. Do not store surplus toxic agents. Promptly discard empty poison containers; never reuse to store a food item or other poison. Teach child not to play in trash containers. Never remove labels from containers of toxic substances. Do not store toxic liquids in containers not specifically intended for their storage (e.g., an empty pop bottle that the child may drink from, unaware of the difference in contents). Know the number of the nearest poison control centre (http://capcc.ca/)

Continued

TABLE 36-2 INJURY PREVENTION DURING EARLY CHILDHOOD—cont'd

DEVELOPMENTAL ABILITIES RELATED TO RISK OF INJURY	INJURY PREVENTION
Falls	
Able to open doors and some windows Goes up and down stairs Depth perception unrefined Climbs on higher surfaces	Use window guardrail; fasten securely. Place gates at top and bottom of stairs. Keep doors locked or use child-proof doorknob covers at the entry to stairs, high porch, or other elevated area, including laundry chute. Remove unsecured or scatter rugs. Apply nonskid decals in the bathtub or shower. Crib rails should be fixed and firmly latched. As of 2012, only beds with fixed rails are recommended, but some older models may be in use (suggest purchasing a rail-latching mechanism for older models). Place carpeting under the crib and in the bathroom. Keep large toys and bumper pads out of the crib or playpen (child can use these as "stairs" to climb out), then move the child to a youth bed when he or she is able to climb out of the crib. Dress in safe clothing (soles that do not "catch" on the floor, tied shoelaces, pant legs that do not touch the floor). Keep child restrained in vehicles; never leave the child unattended in a shopping cart. Supervise the child at playgrounds; select play areas with a soft ground cover and safe equipment.
Choking and Suffocation	
Puts things in mouth May swallow hard or nonedible pieces of food	Avoid large, round chunks of meat, such as whole hot dogs (slice lengthwise into short pieces). Avoid fruit with pits, fish with bones, dried beans, hard candy, chewing gum, nuts, popcorn, grapes, marshmallows. Choose large, sturdy toys without sharp edges or small removable parts. Discard old refrigerators, ovens, and other appliances after removing the door. Select safe toy boxes or chests without heavy, hinged lids. Keep blind cords out of child's reach. Use split cords. Remove drawstrings from clothing.
Bodily Damage	
Still clumsy in many skills Easily distracted from tasks Unaware of potential danger from strangers or other people	Avoid giving the child sharp or pointed objects, such as knives, scissors, or toothpicks, especially when walking or running. Do not allow lollipops or similar objects in the child's mouth when walking or running. Teach safety precautions (e.g., to carry knife or scissors with pointed end away from face). Store all dangerous tools, garden equipment, and firearms in a locked cabinet. Be alert to danger of supervised animals and household pets. Use safety glass and decals on large glassed areas, such as sliding glass doors. Teach the child his or her name, address, and phone number and to ask for help from appropriate people (cashier, security guard, police) if lost; have identification on child (sewn in clothes, inside shoe). Teach stranger safety: • Avoid personalized clothing in public places. • Never go with a stranger. • Tell parents if anyone makes the child feel uncomfortable in any way. Always listen to the child's concerns regarding others' behaviour. Teach the child to say "no" when confronted with uncomfortable situations.

accidental deaths among children ages 1 to 4 years. Many of the deaths are caused by injuries within the car when restraints have not been used or have been used improperly. Unrestrained children riding in the front seat of the vehicle are at highest risk for injury. Approved restraints properly installed and applied can prevent many fatalities and injuries. Motor vehicle back-over injuries and deaths, along with deaths or serious injury resulting from heat stroke when left in a car, account for a large number of motor vehicle–related injuries in children.

To reduce the incidence of these injuries, mandatory child car seat legislation was implemented in Canada in 1993, resulting in a decrease of 58% in childhood deaths (PHAC, 2009a). When car seats are installed correctly, the seats decrease the risk of death by 71% in this age group (van Schaik & CPS, Injury Prevention Committee, 2008). The use of correctly installed car seats has also decreased the risk of hospitalization, by 67% for children age 4 and under. Booster seats provide up to 60% more protection than seat belts (CPS, 2011). Despite this added protection, however, in Canada, 44 to 81% of car seats and 30 to 50% of booster seats are not installed correctly (CPS, 2011).

Nurses have a responsibility to educate parents about the importance of using car restraints for children under 8 years of

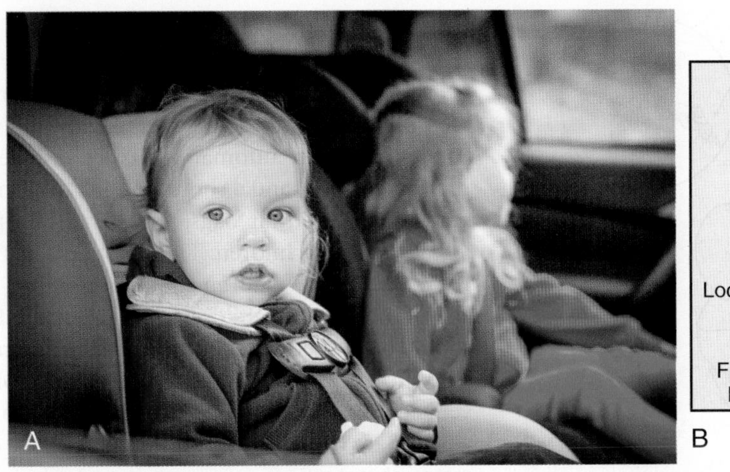

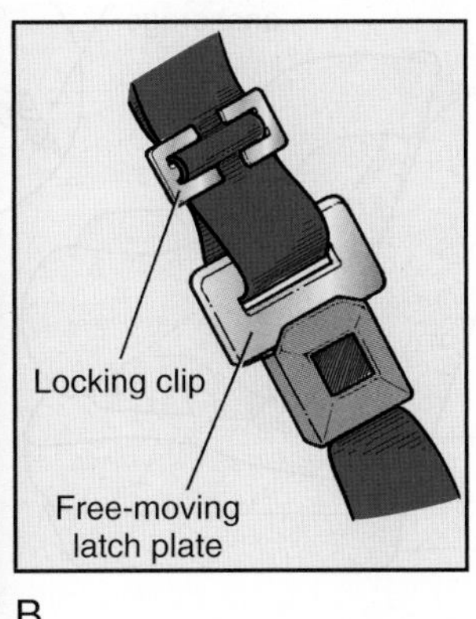

FIGURE 36-10 **A:** Convertible car safety seat in forward-facing position. **B:** Use of locking clip. (A, Sokolova Maryna/Shutterstock.com.)

age and the proper use of car restraints. Five types of restraints are available: (1) infant-only devices, (2) convertible models for both infants and toddlers, (3) boosters, (4) safety belts, and (5) devices for children with special needs (see Chapter 40). Infant-type restraints are discussed in Chapter 35 (p. 1013); convertible restraints and boosters are discussed here. The convertible restraint is suitable for infants and toddlers in the rearward-facing position and when height or weight requirements are not met in the forward-facing position. The transition point for switching to the forward-facing position is defined by the manufacturer but is generally at a body weight of at least 10 kg and a minimum of 1 year of age. Infants who weigh 10 kg before 1 year of age should continue to ride in a rear-facing seat (van Schaik & CPS, Injury Prevention Committee, 2008). It is strongly recommended that children older than 1 year continue to ride rear-facing as long the child continues to fit in the car seat. Many rear-facing car safety seats can accommodate children weighing up to a maximum of 16 kg (according to manufacturer specifications). Studies indicate that toddlers up to 24 months of age are safer riding in convertible seats in the rear-facing position (Bull & Durbin, 2008; Henary, Sherwood, Crandall, et al., 2007).

Children who have outgrown the rear-facing height or weight limit for their car safety seat should use a forward-facing car safety seat with a harness up to the maximum height or weight recommended by the manufacturer (Durbin & American Academy of Pediatrics Committee on Injury, Violence, and Poison Prevention, 2011) (Fig. 36-10). Convertible safety seats should be used until the child weighs at least 13.6 kg or more regardless of age and as long as the child fits properly into the seat (van Schaik & CPS, Injury Prevention Committee, 2008). The next stage in child restraints is the forward-facing infant/child seats. These can be used for children between 10 kg and at least 22 kg and up to 122 cm in height, which varies according to the manufacturer's instructions. Some models are a combination of forward-facing infant/child seats that will convert to a child booster seat when the child reaches the appropriate booster weight and height.

Convertible restraints have different types of harness systems: a five-point harness that consists of a strap over each shoulder, one on each side of the pelvis, and one between the legs (all five come together at a common buckle); and a padded shield that uses shoulder straps attached to a shield that is held in place by a crotch strap. With both the infant and toddler restraints, it is important not to add extra blankets, head cushions, or padding between the child and the restraint straps that did not come as original equipment because these "add-ons" create spaces of air between the child and the restraint and decrease support for the back, head, and neck.

Built-in seats are available in some cars and vans. They may be used for children who are at least 1 year of age and weigh at least 10 kg. Built-in seats eliminate installation problems. However, weight and height limits vary. Owners must verify with vehicle manufacturers the details about built-in seats to ensure that the seats will adequately protect their child.

Starting in 2003, the Universal Anchorage System (UAS) (also known as LATCH [Lower Anchors and Tethers for Children]) universal child safety seat system was implemented as a requirement for all new automobiles and child safety seats. The LATCH system provides car seat anchors between the front cushion and backrest so that the seat belt does not have to be used (Fig. 36-11). However, Transport Canada (2015) recommends that the seat belt be used to anchor the car seat instead of the LATCH system, based on the recommendations of the vehicle and car seat manufacturer's recommendations. If no recommendations are given, then the car seat belt should be used if the child's weight exceeds 18 kg.

The third stage in child car restraints is booster car seats. Booster seats are not restraint systems like the convertible devices because they depend on the vehicle belts to hold the child and booster seat in place. These should be used for children who have surpassed the weight or height limits of their forward-facing car seat and weigh at least 18 kg. Booster seats should be used until children are at least 36 kg. Some booster models accommodate children up to 45 kg. It is necessary to always check the label for the lower and upper weight and height limits because they vary depending on the manufacturer. Booster seat legislation varies among provinces and territories; some do not have booster seat requirements, although it is

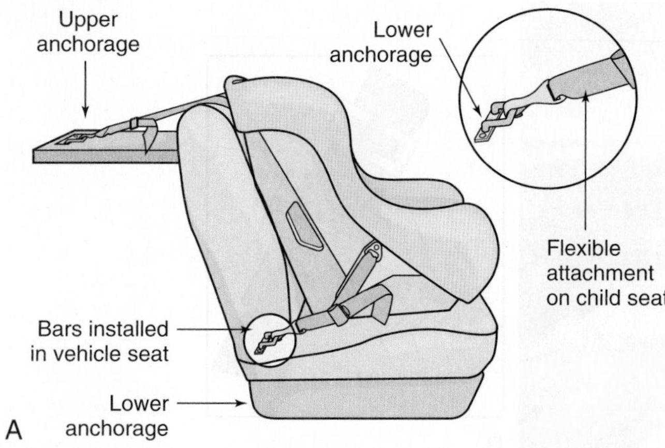

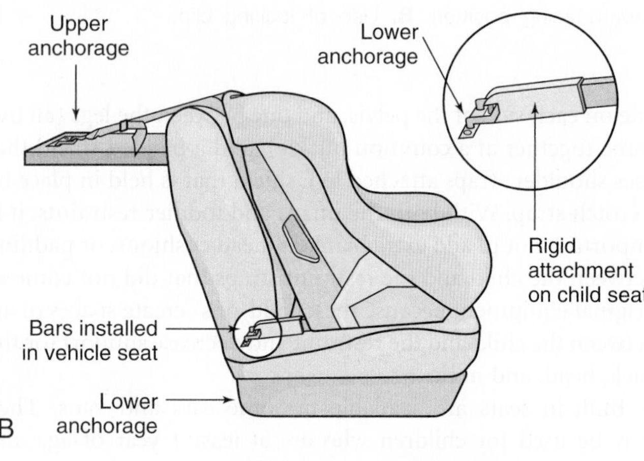

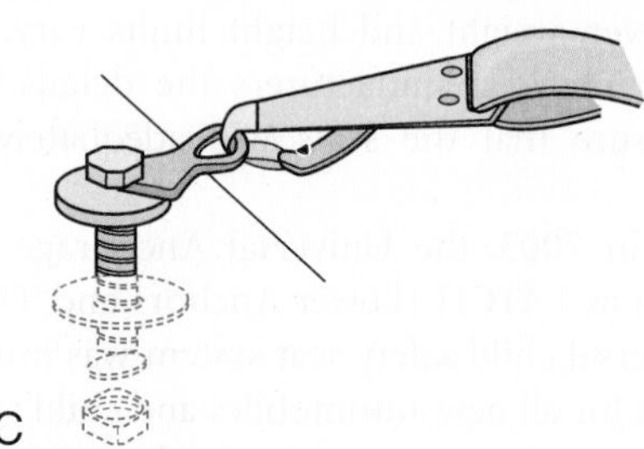

FIGURE 36-11 Universal anchorage system (UAS). **A:** Flexible two-point attachment with top tether. **B:** Rigid two-point attachment with top tether. **C:** Top tether. (Courtesy U.S. Department of Transportation, National Highway Traffic Safety Administration.)

recommended that children stay in their booster seats until they are 8 years old.

A booster seat should be used until the child is able to sit against the back of the seat with feet hanging down and legs bent at the knees (approximately 145 cm in height). The belt-positioning booster model raises a child higher in the seat, moving the shoulder part of the belt off the neck and the lap portion of the belt off the abdomen onto the pelvis. Children who outgrow the convertible restraint may still be able to ride safely in a booster seat until the midpoint of the head is higher than the vehicle seat back. Cars with free-sliding latch plates on the lap or shoulder belt require the use of a metal locking clip to keep the belt in a tight-holding position. The locking clip is threaded onto the belt above the latch plate (see Fig. 36-10, B). If parents have newer cars with automatic lap and shoulder belts, they need to have additional lap belts installed to properly secure the restraint.

Shoulder-only automatic belts are designed to protect adults. If children use manual shoulder belts they should sit in the rear seat, as deployed air bags, which face the front seats, can be lethal to young children. The safest area of the car for children is the back seat. Children should ride in the back seat until the age of 12 years. If children do ride in the front seat, the seat should be pushed as far back as possible to prevent serious harm or critical injury from the air bags. Many of the newer-model vehicles have side impact air bags for collision protection; these air bags are reported to be safe as long as the child is in a proper restraint system.

The Government of Canada has enacted safety regulations for motor vehicles and booster seat safety that require manufacturers to modify car seats and booster seats in order to improve their safety. These regulations include an expiration date for car seats; for further information on Canadian regulations regarding child booster seats see Additional Resources at the end of the chapter. It is important that every car seat and booster seat be bought in Canada, to meet Transport Canada regulations, and not be purchased from other countries such as the United States because the regulations vary between the two countries. For any restraint to be effective, it must be used consistently and properly. Examples of misuse include misrouting the vehicle seat belt through the restraint; failing to use the vehicle seat belt to secure the restraint; failing to use the restraint's harness system; and incorrectly positioning the child, especially by facing infants and toddlers forward instead of toward the rear. Nurses are in an excellent position to advise parents in using car restraints correctly (see Family-Centred Teaching box). There are child care seat clinics across Canada to help families choose approved car seats, install them, and position the child in the seat. For additional information about

FAMILY-CENTRED TEACHING

Using Car Safety Seats

- Read manufacturer's directions and follow them exactly.
- Anchor the safety seat securely to the car's seat and apply harness snugly to the child.
- Do not start the car until everyone is properly restrained.
- Always use the restraint, even for short trips.
- If the child begins to climb out or undo the harness, firmly say, "No." It may be necessary to stop the car to reinforce the expected behaviour. Use rewards, such as stars or stickers, to encourage appropriate behaviour.
- Encourage the child to help attach buckles, straps, and shields, but always double-check fastenings.
- Decrease boredom on long trips. Keep soft toys in the car for quiet play; talk to the child; point out objects and teach the child about them. Stop periodically. If the child wishes to sleep, make certain the child stays in the restraint.
- Insist that others who transport children also follow these safety rules.

child safety restraints see the Additional Resources section at the end of this chapter.

Children with special needs may require a restraint system that secures them appropriately in the event of a crash. Examples of such devices include car bed restraints for infants who cannot tolerate a semi-reclining position and specially adapted moulded-plastic chairs for children who have spica casts. The E-Z-On vest is a special safety harness for larger children with poor trunk control.

Motor vehicle–related injuries. Injuries to children may also occur during sudden stops when objects are left unrestrained. On sudden impact, a loose toy or package can become a projectile missile. Therefore, all items should be secured or stored in the trunk.

Children over 3 years of age are often involved in pedestrian traffic injuries. Because of their gross motor skills of walking, running, and climbing and their fine motor skills of opening doors and fence gates, they are likely to be in hazardous areas when unsupervised. Unaware of danger and unable to approximate the speed of cars, they are hit by moving vehicles. Running after a ball, riding a tricycle, and playing behind a parked car are common activities that may result in a vehicular tragedy.

Toddlers playing in driveways or farmyards are at risk of back-over injury from vehicles in reverse gear. A precaution when children are playing in driveways is attaching to the tricycle a pole with a bright flag that is high enough to be visible through the back window of an automobile. Another safeguard is the use of a device that beeps when the vehicle is driven in reverse to alert children to the oncoming car, van, tractor, or truck. Some models now come equipped with rearview motion cameras so the driver can see the driveway clearly while backing out.

Another dangerous situation that has become more commonplace is children crawling into an open trunk and pulling it closed. Asphyxia may occur in such cases; therefore, car trunks should not be left open when children are near and not being supervised. Some cars come equipped with a safety switch that can be activated from inside the trunk to open a closed trunk door.

Overheating (hyperthermia) of toddlers and their subsequent death can occur when they are left in a vehicle in hot weather (more than 27°C). Small children dissipate heat poorly, and an increase in body temperature can cause death in a few hours. Canadian statistics for vehicular hyperthermia are not available. In the United States in 2011, however, 33 children died of vehicular hyperthermia. From 1998 to 2011, more than 50% of the deaths were of children under 2 years of age. During this time period, 23% of the victims were 1 year of age; 20% were 2 years; and 13% were 4 years of age (Null, 2016). According to a study funded by General Motors of Canada, the air temperature in a previously air-conditioned small car can exceed 50°C within 20 minutes on a day with temperatures of 35°C and up to 65.5°C within 40 minutes (Canada Safety Council, n.d.). In a study of 171 child fatalities from overheating in a car, 50% of adults who left a child in a car either forgot or were unaware that the child was still in the car. A significant number of those children (32) were left by family members who intended to take the child to day care but forgot the child in the car at the workplace; 22 children were left in the car by a day care worker or driver (Guard & Gallagher, 2005). In addition, leaving children unsupervised in a parked vehicle, especially in a private driveway, provides an opportunity for the child to release the brake or put the car in gear. Parents should be cautioned against leaving children alone in a vehicle *for any reason*.

Prevention of vehicular injuries involves protecting and educating children and adults about the dangers of moving or parked vehicles. Children in bicycle-towed trailers or bicycle-mounted child seats can also be injured by collisions or falls and should always wear an approved, well-fitted helmet and harness (Parachute, n.d.a). Although preschool children are too young to be trusted to always obey, parents should emphasize looking for moving vehicles before crossing the street, recognizing the stop and go colours of traffic lights, and following traffic officers' signals. Physical barriers that limit children from playing near vehicles can help prevent these injuries. Most important, what is preached must be practised. Children learn through imitation, and consistency reinforces learning.

Drowning

Drowning ranks as the second most common cause of fatalities (15%) from unintentional injuries in the 1- to 4-year age group (PHAC, 2009b). With well-developed skills of locomotion, toddlers are able to reach potentially dangerous areas, such as bathtubs, toilets, buckets, swimming pools, hot tubs, and lakes. Their intense drive for exploration and investigation, combined with an unawareness of the danger of water and their helplessness in water, makes drowning always a viable threat. It is also one category of injuries that results in death within minutes, diminishing the chance for rescue and survival. Children under 5 years of age have a small lung capacity; their lungs can fill fast with water and they can drown in 2.5 cm of water. Close adult supervision of children when near any source of water is essential; teaching swimming and water safety can be helpful but cannot be regarded as sufficient protection. To ensure safety around water, toddlers need to be kept within arm's length with proper adult supervision at all times. It is important to use approved lifejackets and personal flotation devices that are properly fitted as well as choose a safe place to swim.

Burns

In Canada, burns are the third leading injury-related cause for hospital admissions of children ages 0 to 4 years (Parachute, n.d.b). Because of their thinner skin, children are more vulnerable to burns than adults. Consequently, significant burns can cause permanent scarring with contracting of underlying tissues due to rapid growth and can lead to emotional scarring and physical disabilities. Please see Chapter 52 for information on how to care for a child with a burn.

Toddlers' ability to climb, stretch, and reach objects above their heads makes any hot surface a potential source of danger.

Scald burns, the most common type of thermal injury in small children, can result from children pulling hot pots from the stove on top of themselves; of all scald injuries needing hospitalization, 83% were in children under age 5 years (Parachute, n.d.b). As a precaution, pot handles should be turned toward the back of the stove. Ideally, the knobs for controlling the range burners should be out of reach, not on the front panel where nimble fingers can turn them on and accidentally touch the hot burner. Oven doors should be closed whenever the oven is turned on or when it is cooling. The outside of doors of automatic self-cleaning ovens may become hot and, if touched, could cause a burn. It is also important to keep appliance cords out of reach, to use baby gates, and to keep toddlers seated in the kitchen.

Scald burns are also often caused by exposure to high-temperature tap water. Children come in contact with hot tap water by turning on the hot-water faucet or falling into a bathtub of hot water or through parental deliberate abuse. Youngsters must always be supervised when they are near tap water, and bathwater temperatures need to be checked. Limiting household water temperatures to 49°C is also recommended for gas or oil-fired heaters and 60°C if using electric heaters. It is not advisable to run the heaters at lower than these temperatures because of the risk of Legionnaire's disease (Parachute, n.d.c). At 49°C it takes 10 minutes of exposure to the water to cause a full-thickness burn. Conversely, water temperatures of 55°C, a common setting of most water heaters, can cause third-degree burns to children within 5 seconds. Nurses can help prevent such burns by advising parents of this common household danger and recommending that they readjust the water heater to a safe temperature. An easy-to-read hot-water gauge that changes colour to show water temperatures between 49° and 60°C is also available; it shows a "hot," "cool," or "OK" water temperature. A special device can be added to the faucet that reduces the water flow once the set temperature is reached, or guards that block access to the faucet can be used. There are also mixing valves available that can be installed in the plumbing to mix hot and cold water. Scalding can also occur when a curious child tries to sip a parent's coffee or tea and spills the boiling liquid down the chin and chest. Thus lidded travelling cups are a safe choice.

Other sources of heat, such as radiators, fireplaces, accessible furnaces, kerosene heaters, or wood-burning stoves, should have a guard placed in front of them. Portable electrical heaters must be placed in a high area, well out of reach of climbing young children. Hair curling irons and hot curlers may easily burn the hands of curious toddlers when left within easy reach.

Hot objects such as candles, incense, cigarettes, pots of tea or coffee, or irons must be placed away from children. The flame of a candle and the smoke of a cigarette invite investigation. Ashtrays with a centre well are preferred to prevent the cigarette from falling off the rim, and adults should try not to smoke, to cook, or to drink hot liquids when children are physically close. If tablecloths are used, the edges should be placed out of reach to prevent injuries from both burns and falling objects.

Flame burns represent one of the most fatal types of burns and commonly occur when children play with matches and accidentally set themselves (and the home) on fire. In Canada, approximately 40 children aged 14 years and under die from fire or other burns annually. Another 770 children are hospitalized for serious injuries related to fire exposure (Parachute, n.d.d). To prevent flame burns, matches and lighters must be stored safely away from children, and parents need to teach children the dangers of playing with such objects. In addition, all homes, apartments, and any other type of dwelling where people sleep should have smoke detectors installed to alert the occupants of a fire. A safety plan for immediate escape is also essential.

Electrical burns also represent an immediate danger to children. Young toddlers may explore outlets and wires by mouthing them, and since water is an excellent conductor, the chance for a severe circumoral electrical burn is great. Electrical outlets should have protective guards plugged into them when not in use (Fig. 36-12) or be made inaccessible by having furniture placed in front of them, when feasible.

Sunburns are a year-round concern in certain regions. Children spend a large amount of time outdoors. Their increased mobility makes it difficult to prevent sun exposure. Sunburn can be prevented by applying a sunscreen with a sun protection factor (SPF) of 15 or greater, dressing the child in protective clothing (wide-brimmed hat, protective cotton clothing with a tight weave), and avoiding sun exposure between 1000 and 1400 hours (see Chapter 52 for more information).

Accidental Poisoning

Poisoning is a significant cause of injuries in children. According to Health Canada, approximately 7 children under the age of 14 years die from poisoning every year; another 1700 children require hospitalization for poison-related injuries. Children ages 1 to 4 years constitute 64% of these poisonings (Government of Canada, 2014). Poisoning is the second highest cause of unintentional injury requiring hospitalization for ages 1 to 4 (Yanchar, Warda, Fuselli, et al., 2012).

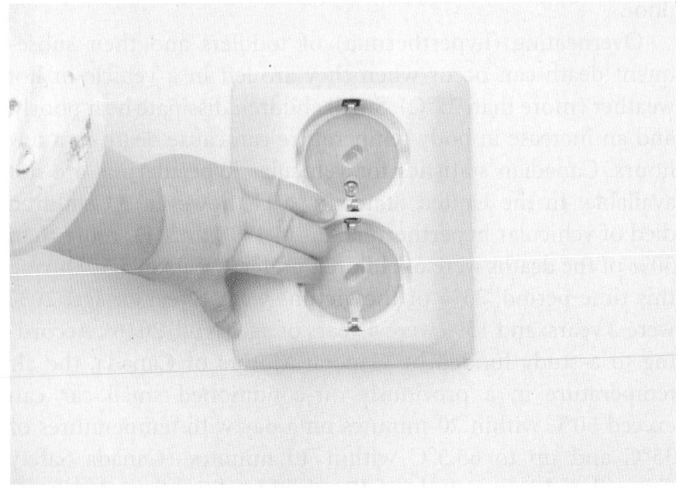

FIGURE 36-12 Special plastic caps in electrical sockets prevent young fingers from exploring dangerous areas. (Ioannis Pantzi/Shutterstock.com.)

Toddlers are at highest risk for accidental poisoning because of their innate curiosity and ability to open "childproof" containers. Mouthing activity continues to be prevalent after 1 year of age, and exploring objects by tasting them is part of children's natural investigation. Toddlers' curiosity and inability to understand logical consequences further place them at risk for ingesting harmful substances. Many household products, medications, and plants can be poisonous if swallowed, if they come in contact with the skin or eyes, or if inhaled. Although in many instances poisoning does not result in death, it may cause significant morbidity, such as esophageal stricture from lye ingestion. Toddlers are able to climb most heights, open most drawers or closets, and unscrew most lids. By trial and error, younger children also manage to undo tops of bottles, plastic containers, aerosol cans, and jars, including those with child-resistant lids. Newer forms of medications, such as transdermal patches and cough-suppressant lozenges, have created additional dangers, since they are not packaged with safety caps and the lozenges look like candy. Unintentional medication ingestion causes 64% of the poisonings in children 14 years and younger. Ingestion of iron pills is of special concern as it is the leading cause of death (Parachute, n.d.e).

The major reason for poisoning is improper storage, particularly when the substance is taken out of the original container (Fig. 36-13). The guidelines suggested in Chapter 35 apply to children in this age group as well (p. 1015). However, unlike the infant, who was confined to certain heights and unable to unlatch inventive locks, young children manage to find access to many high-level, tight-security places. For this age group, only a locked cabinet is safe.

Recent attention has focused on the use of over-the-counter (OTC) medications used for cough and colds as a common cause of accidental poisonous ingestion in toddlers. Ingestion of acetaminophen is also a common cause of morbidity because it is found in many combination OTC products; caregivers may unknowingly administer a dose of acetaminophen in addition to an OTC drug containing the product without knowing the danger.

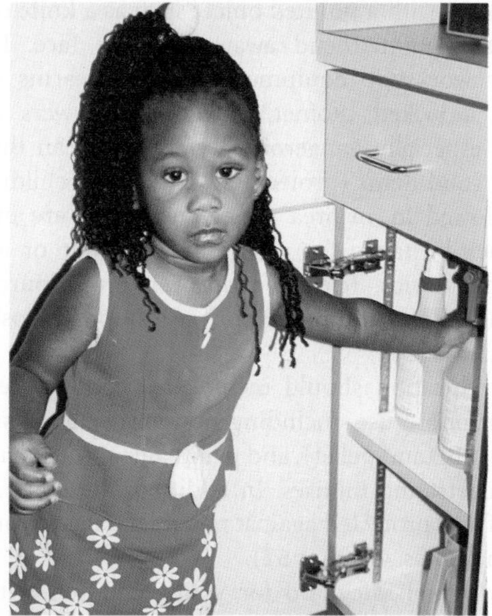

FIGURE 36-13 Children are most likely to ingest substances that are on their level, such as cleaning agents stored under sinks, rat poison, plants, or diaper pail deodorants.

Carbon monoxide is a rare cause of poisoning in children in Canada but is very serious and can cause a coma or death (Parachute, n.d.f). This toxic gas is colourless and has no odour. Defective appliances, clothes dryers, furnaces, and exhaust fumes from cars in home garages are sources of carbon monoxide poisoning. Unlike smoke detectors, carbon monoxide detectors are becoming mandatory, and they can save the lives of entire families. The detectors should be installed on every level and near sleeping areas and should be replaced every 5 to 7 years. Fuel-burning appliances should be checked once a year for carbon monoxide leakage (Parachute, n.d.f).

Emergency and preventive measures for accidental poisoning are discussed in Chapter 35.

> **! NURSING ALERT**
>
> Parents should have ready access to the telephone number on their telephone for the local poison control centre. These telephone numbers are in the telephone book under emergency numbers for each individual provincial or territorial poison control centre. They are also available on the Canadian Association of Poison Control Centres website (http://www.capcc.ca). Parents should be prepared to act on the centre's advice.

Falls

Falls are still a hazard to children in this age group, although by the later part of early childhood, gross and fine motor skills are well developed, decreasing the incidence of falls down stairs or from chairs. Nonetheless, from 1990 to 2007 in Canada, 527,456 (32.7%) children 0 to 4 years of age had injuries that required emergency care. Of these injuries, 56.5% were in boys, 6.7% required observation or admission to the hospital, 14.2% were closed-head injuries, and 12.0% were skull fractures (PHAC, 2009b). Cribs, bassinets, and play yards were associated with a large number of accidental falls (66% of all fall injuries to children) (Yeh, Rochette, McKenzie, et al., 2011).

Playground injuries are common and can be serious. More than 28,000 children are injured every year on playgrounds across Canada. The hospitalization rate has risen by 8% and the rate of hospitalizations has gone up by 8% between 2007 and 2012 (Parachute n.d.g). These injuries usually are caused by falls and can include fractured bones and brain and spinal injuries. In children under 5 years of age, head and face injuries are most common (Fuselli, Yanchar, & CPS, Injury Prevention Committee, 2012). Children need to be taught safety at play areas, such as no horseplay on high slides or jungle gyms, *sitting* on swings, and staying away from moving swings. Passive prevention of injury includes placement of grass, sand, or wood chips under play equipment, which lessens injuries. Swing seats should be made of plastic, canvas, or rubber and have smooth or rounded edges. Slides should not exceed an incline of 30 degrees and should have evenly spaced rungs for climbing and protective "tunnels." See Additional Resources at the end of the chapter for more information on playground safety.

The climbing and running of the typical toddler are complicated by the child's total lack of appreciation of danger. Thus gates must be placed at both ends of stairs. Accessible windows that are left open during warm weather must be guarded with a rail. Falling from open windows is a major cause of accidental death in children; parents should be advised that a screened window is not a safety device to prevent falls. Doors leading to stairwells or porches must be locked because preschoolers can easily open them. A convenient type of lock is a sliding bar or hook that can be attached to the door and frame at a level higher than what the child can reach; such locks also have safety clasps or devices that prevent children from opening them. Falls from balconies, porches, decks, and bleachers are all possible for active toddlers.

Cribs and vehicles are other sources of falls. To avoid injury, crib rails should be locked in raised position, the mattress should be kept at the lowest position, and toys or bumper pads that may be used as steps to climb out should be removed. Ideally the floor under the crib should be carpeted or have a throw rug. Once children reach a height of 89 cm, they should sleep in a bed rather than a crib. If a bunk bed is selected, parents should be aware of possible dangers such as falls from the top bed and the ladder, and head entrapment between the mattress and guardrail or between the supporting mattress slats. Please see Chapter 35 for a discussion on crib safety and the legislative requirements for cribs.

Children can fall from high chairs, shopping carts, carriages, car seats, and strollers if not properly restrained or if the balance changes when the object is weighted down with heavy items. Therefore, proper restraint and adequate supervision are essential. Children, especially older infants who are mobile, should not be placed in an infant seat on top of a shopping cart because the infant seat may fall off the cart; the safest place for an infant seat is inside the bed of the cart.

Aspiration and Suffocation

Threats to breathing are the fourth major cause of hospitalization and fatalities in Canadian children. These threats include strangulation, suffocation, choking, aspiration, entrapment, and traumatic asphyxia. The incidence peaks at 9 to 11 months of age with the majority of choking and suffocation deaths occurring in the first year of life. The majority of hospitalizations occur in children aged 3 years or under, with an elevated risk continuing until 6 years of age (Cyr & CPS, Injury Prevention Committee, 2012). For survivors there can be long-term consequences with brain damage due to oxygen deprivation.

Small children often put small objects, such as coins, batteries, small toys, and toy parts, into their mouths. Foreign-body aspiration is most common during the second year of life. Usually by 1 year of age children chew well, but they may have difficulty with large pieces of food, such as meat and whole hot dogs, and with hard foods, such as nuts. Young children cannot discard pits from fruit or bones from fish. It takes practice to learn how to chew gum without swallowing it. Common foods causing choking include nuts, raw carrots, and popcorn kernels. Therefore, the same precautions as discussed for infants regarding food selection must be used for toddlers (see Chapter 35).

As with infants, play objects for toddlers must be chosen with an awareness of danger from small parts. A toy should not be able to fit into a toilet paper roll, otherwise it could be a choking hazard. Large, sturdy toys without sharp edges or removable parts are safest. Coins, paper clips, pins, bells, button (round) batteries, toy magnets, pull-tabs on cans, thumbtacks, nails, screws, jewellery (especially pierced earrings), and all types of pins are common household objects that can cause significant harm if swallowed or aspirated. Small items such as coloured beads, green peas, pellets, or beans are often placed into the nose by toddlers and may present a danger if aspirated into the airway. Because of the danger of aspiration, parents should be taught emergency procedures for choking (see Airway Obstruction, Chapter 45).

Suffocation from causes seen during infancy is less frequent, but old refrigerators, ovens, and other large appliances are a threat. Toddlers can climb inside these appliances and, if they close the door behind them, can be trapped inside. Removing all doors before discarding or storing old appliances can prevent such tragic deaths. Toddlers may also suffocate when unsafe toy box lids accidentally close on their head or neck (see Table 36-2).

Bodily Damage

Toddlers are still clumsy in many of their skills and can seriously harm themselves by walking while holding a sharp or pointed object or by having food or objects such as spoons in their mouths. Preventing such occurrences is the best approach with toddlers. The child should be taught that, when walking with a pointed object such as a knife or scissors, to hold the pointed end away from the face. Dangerous garden or workshop equipment and all firearms should be stored in a locked cabinet. Power lawnmowers and weed eaters are especially dangerous because they can throw rocks and other solid items (projectiles), and young children should not be allowed in an area where such tools are in use, nor should they be taken for a ride on a mower or allowed to operate that device. Television tip-overs are a source of head trauma in toddlers and preschool age group (Rutkoski, Sippey, & Gaines, 2011).

Safety education should include respect for firearms and their appropriate use, including nonpowder guns such as air guns, rifles (BB and pellet), and paintball guns, which can cause serious penetrating injuries. In addition, the child should be warned of and protected against potential danger from animals (see Animal Bites, Chapter 52).

An additional safeguard for young children is the use of safety glass in doors, windows, and tabletops and the application of decals on glass doors and windows to reduce the likelihood of running through glass. In addition, children should not be allowed to run, jump, wrestle, or play ball near glass structures.

A discussion of bodily injury must also include alerting the parent to threats to the child's well-being from adults or other children who might take advantage of the toddler who cannot protect himself or herself. Because toddlers are often not able to verbalize their emotions and feelings or may not understand inappropriate touching behaviour by a family member or friend, it is important for parents to protect children by not leaving them in situations where there is a potential for bodily harm. The "stranger danger" concept is still important to teach, yet statistics show that personal harm more often comes from relatives or family friends who are not considered strangers. Therefore, it is important to discuss appropriate and inappropriate touching (what feels comfortable and what does not) in a manner that will not frighten or overwhelm the child.

Toys can also be a source of danger, and safety must be a prime consideration when selecting toys. While most toys have age ranges written on them to designate their safety, this information must be used with knowledge of the specific child's readiness. Please see Additional Resources at the end of this chapter for government regulations and recalls for defective toys.

Household safety should be practised and includes the usual precautions recommended for any age group.

Anticipatory Guidance—Care of Families

Understanding toddlers' development, abilities, and limits is fundamental to successful child-rearing. Nurses, particularly those in ambulatory or child health centres, are in a favourable position to assist parents in facilitating the tasks and meeting the needs of children in this age group. Prevention yields better results than treatment. Anticipatory guidance is paramount to prevent future problems and injuries (see Family-Centred Teaching box).

Advice, however, is sometimes not the sole answer. Actual assistance, such as being available for telephone consulting, should be part of the nurse's flexible repertoire of interventions. Whether parents are experiencing the child-rearing dilemmas of a first or a subsequent child, they benefit from sharing their feelings, frustrations, and satisfactions. They need adult companionship, occasional freedom from child-rearing responsibilities, and periodic separations from their children. Part of a nurse's responsibility is to provide opportunities for parents to express their feelings and support them in meeting their parental responsibilities.

FAMILY-CENTRED TEACHING

Guidance During Toddler Years

Ages 12 to 18 Months

Prepare parents for expected behavioural changes of the toddler, especially negativism and ritualism.

Assess present feeding habits and encourage gradual weaning from the bottle and increased intake of solid foods.

Stress expected feeding changes of picky eating habits, food fads and strong taste preferences, need for scheduled routine at mealtimes, inability to sit through an entire meal, and lack of table manners.

Prepare parents for potential dangers of the home, particularly those contributing to motor vehicle injuries, poisoning, and falling injuries; give appropriate suggestions for safety proofing the home.

Discuss the need for firm but gentle discipline and ways to deal with negativism and temper tantrums; stress positive benefits of appropriate discipline.

Emphasize the importance for both the child and parents of brief, periodic separations.

Discuss new toys that use developing gross and fine motor, language, cognitive, and social skills.

Emphasize the need for dental supervision, the types of basic dental hygiene at home, and food habits that predispose to caries; stress the importance of supplemental fluoride when required.

Ages 18 to 24 Months

Stress the importance of peer companionship in play.

Explore the need for preparation for an additional sibling (as appropriate); stress the importance of preparing the child for new experiences.

Assess sleep patterns at night, particularly the habit of a bedtime bottle, which is a major cause of dental caries, and behaviours that delay the hour of sleep.

Discuss present discipline methods, their effectiveness, and parents' feelings about the child's negativism; stress that negativism is an important aspect of developing self-assertion and independence and is not a sign of parental spoiling.

Discuss signs of readiness for toilet training; emphasize the importance of waiting for physical and psychological readiness.

Discuss development of fears, such as fear of darkness or loud noises, and of habits, such as security blanket or thumb-sucking; stress normalcy of these transient behaviours.

Prepare parents for signs of regression in time of stress.

Assess the child's ability to separate easily from parents for brief periods under familiar circumstances.

Allow parents the opportunity to express their feelings of weariness, frustration, and exasperation; be aware that it is often difficult to love toddlers when they are not asleep!

Point out some of the expected changes of the next year, such as longer attention span, somewhat less negativism, and increased concern for pleasing others.

Ages 24 to 36 Months

Discuss the importance of imitation and domestic mimicry and the need to include the child in activities.

Discuss approaches toward toilet training, particularly realistic expectations and the parents' attitude toward accidents.

Stress uniqueness of toddlers' thought processes, especially through their use of language, poor understanding of time, view of causal relationships in terms of proximity of events, and inability to see events from another's perspective.

Stress that discipline still must be structured and concrete and that relying solely on verbal reasoning and explanation leads to injuries, confusion, and misunderstanding.

Discuss investigation of preschool or a day care centre toward completion of the child's second year.

KEY POINTS

- The toddler stage, extending from 12 to 36 months, is a period of intense exploration of the environment.
- Biological development during the toddler years is characterized by the acquisition of fine and gross motor skills that allow children to master a wide range of activities.
- Although most of the physiological systems are mature by the end of toddlerhood, development of certain areas of the brain is still occurring, allowing for greater intellectual capacity.
- Locomotion is the major gross motor skill acquired during toddlerhood, followed by increased eye–hand coordination.
- Specific tasks in the psychosocial development of a toddler include differentiating self from others, tolerating separation from the parent, coping with delayed gratification, controlling bodily functions, acquiring socially acceptable behaviour, communicating verbally, and interacting with others in a less egocentric manner.
- According to Erikson, the major developmental task of toddlerhood is acquiring a sense of autonomy while overcoming a sense of doubt and shame.
- In Piaget's sensorimotor and preconceptual phases of development, the toddler experiments by incorporating the old learning of secondary circular reactions with new skills and applies this knowledge to new situations. There is the beginning of rational judgement, an understanding of causal relationships, and discovery of objects as objects.
- Preconceptual thought is characterized by egocentrism, centration, global organization of thought processes, animism, and irreversibility.
- Language is the major cognitive achievement in toddlerhood.
- The most striking characteristic of language development during early childhood is the increasing level of comprehension.
- Development of body image occurs with increasing motor ability, at which point toddlers recognize the importance and capacity of body parts.
- The two phases of differentiation of self from significant others are separation and individuation.
- Parental concerns during the toddler years include toilet training; coping with sibling rivalry; limit setting and discipline; and dealing with temper tantrums, negativism, and regression.
- Effective discipline techniques for toddlers include reward, ignoring, and time-out.
- Nutrition is important during the toddler stage because eating habits established in this period have lasting effects in subsequent years.
- Regular dental examinations, fluoride supplementation, removal of plaque, and provision of a low-cariogenic diet promote optimum dental health.
- Common sleep problems that develop during early childhood (and that are easily prevented) are associated with night crying and refusal to go to sleep.
- Because of increased locomotion, toddlers are at high risk for sustaining injuries. Fatal injuries are primarily a result of motor vehicle accidents, drowning, and burns.
- Motor vehicle injuries are responsible for many of all accidental deaths among toddler age.

evolve WEBSITE

Visit the Evolve website for additional resources related to the content in this chapter such as Case Studies, Critical Thinking Case Study Answers, Nursing Care Plans, Nursing Processes, Nursing Skills, and Review Questions for Exam Preparation at: http://evolve.elsevier.com/Canada/Perry/maternal/

REFERENCES

American Academy of Pediatric Dentistry (AAPD). (2014). *Guideline on infant oral health care.* Retrieved from <http://www.aapd.org/media/Policies_Guidelines/G_InfantOralHealthCare.pdf>.

Autism Canada. (2015). *Autism physician handbook*, Canadian Edition. Retrieved from <http://autismcanada.org/wp-content/uploads/2015/11/PhysicianHandbook_2015.pdf>.

Berenbaum, S. A., & Beltz, A. M. (2011). Sexual differentiation of human behavior: Effects of prenatal and pubertal organizational hormones. *Frontiers in Neuroendocrinology, 32*(2), 183–200. doi:10.1016/j.yfrne.2011.03.001.

Brazelton, T. B. (1999). How to help parents of young children: The touchpoints model. *Journal of Perinatology, 19*(6 Pt. 2), S6–S7.

Brotanek, J. M., Schroer, D., Valentyn, L., et al. (2009). Reasons for prolonged bottle-feeding and iron deficiency among Mexican-American toddlers: An ethnographic study. *Academic Pediatrics, 9*(1), 17–25.

Bull, M. J., & Durbin, D. R. (2008). Rear-facing car safety seats: Getting the message right. *Pediatrics, 121*(3), 619–620.

Canada Safety Council. (n.d.). *Hot car warning.* Retrieved from <https://canadasafetycouncil.org/child-safety/hot-car-warning>.

Canadian Dental Association. (2010). *A position paper on access to oral health care for Canadians.* Retrieved from <http://www.cda-adc.ca/en/about/position_statements/accesstocare/>.

Canadian Dental Association. (2012). *CDA position on the use of fluorides in caries prevention.* Retrieved from <http://www.cda-adc.ca/_files/position_statements/fluoride.pdf>.

Canadian Paediatric Society. (2011). *Caring for kids: Car seat safety.* Retrieved from <http://www.caringforkids.cps.ca/handouts/car_seat_safety>.

Canadian Paediatric Society. (2015). *Safe sleep for babies.* Retrieved from <http://www.caringforkids.cps.ca/handouts/safe_sleep_for_babies>.

Chonchaiya, W., & Pruksananonda, C. (2008). Television viewing associates with delayed language development. *Acta Paediatrica, 97*(7), 977–982. doi:10.1111/j.1651-2227.2008.00831.

Clifford, T., Gorodzinsky, F. P., & Canadian Paediatric Society, Community Paediatrics Committee. (2000). Toilet learning: Anticipatory guidance with a child-oriented approach. *Paediatrics & Child Health, 5*(6), 333–335. Reaffirmed 2016. Retrieved from <http://www.cps.ca/documents/position/toilet-learning>.

Critch, J. N., & Canadian Paediatric Society, Nutrition and Gastroenterology Committee. (2014). Nutrition for healthy term infants, six to 24 months: An overview. *Paediatrics & Child Health, 19*(10), 547–549.

Cyr, C., & Canadian Paediatric Society, Injury Prevention Committee. (2012). Preventing choking and suffocation in children. *Paediatrics & Child Health, 17*(2), 91–92.

Dietitians of Canada. (2016). *WHO growth charts.* Retrieved from <http://www.dietitians.ca/Dietitians-Views/Prenatal-and-Infant/WHO-Growth-Charts.aspx>.

Durbin, D. R., & American Academy of Pediatrics (AAP) Committee on Injury, Violence, and Poison Prevention. (2011). Technical report—child passenger safety. *Pediatrics, 127*(4), e1050–e1066.

Erikson, E. H. (1963). *Childhood and society* (2nd ed.). New York: Norton.

Feigelman, S. (2016). The second year. In R. M. Kliegman, B. F. Stanton, J. W. St. Geme, et al. (Eds.), *Nelson textbook of pediatrics* (20th ed.). St. Louis: Saunders.

Fowler, J. W. (1981). *Stage of faith: The psychology of human development and quest for meaning.* San Francisco: Harper and Row.

Fuselli, P., Yanchar, N. L., & Canadian Paediatric Society, Injury Prevention Committee. (2012). Preventing playground injuries. *Paediatrics & Child Health, 17*(6), 328. Retrieved from <http://www.cps.ca/documents/position/playground-injuries>.

Godel, J. C., & Canadian Paediatric Society, First Nations, Inuit and Métis Health Committee. (2007). Vitamin D supplementation: Recommendations for Canadian mothers and infants. *Paediatrics & Child Health, 12*(7), 583–589. Reaffirmed 2015. Retrieved from <http://www.cps.ca/en/documents/position/vitamin-d>.

Goodrich, W., & Hudson, C. L. (2009). Co-speech gesture as input in verb learning. *Developmental Science, 12*(1), 81–87.

Government of Canada. (2014). *Government of Canada reminds Canadians how to protect children from dangerous household chemicals—Products should be locked out of sight and out of reach.* Retrieved from <http://news.gc.ca/web/article-en.do?nid=826029&_ga=1.220557201.868197850.1432519476>.

Guard, A., & Gallagher, S. S. (2005). Heat related deaths in young children in parked cars: An analysis of 171 fatalities in the United States, 1995–2002. *Injury Prevention, 11*(1), 33–37. doi:10.1136/ip.2003.004044.

Harpaz-Rotem, I., & Bergman, A. (2006). On an evolving theory of attachment: Rapprochement—theory of a developing mind. *Psychoanalysis Study Child, 61*, 170–189.

Health Canada. (2011). *Eating well with Canada's food guide: Children.* Retrieved from <http://www.hc-sc.gc.ca/fn-an/food-guide-aliment/choose-choix/advice-conseil/child-enfant-eng.php#>.

Health Canada. (2012). *Vitamin D and calcium: Updated dietary reference intakes.* Retrieved from <http://www.hc-sc.gc.ca/fn-an/nutrition/vitamin/vita-d-eng.php>.

Health Canada. (2015). *Nutrition for healthy term infants: Recommendations from six to 24 months.* Retrieved from <http://www.hc-sc.gc.ca/fn-an/nutrition/infant-nourisson/recom/recom-6-24-months-6-24-mois-eng.php#a2>.

Health Canada. (2016). *Fluoride and human health.* Retrieved from <http://www.hc-sc.gc.ca/hl-vs/iyh-vsv/environ/fluor-eng.php>.

Henary, B., Sherwood, C. P., Crandall, J. R., et al. (2007). Car safety for children: Rear facing for best protection. *Injury Prevention, 13*(6), 398–402. doi:10.1136/ip.2006.015115.

Hines, M. (2011). Gender development and the human brain. *Annual Review of Neuroscience, 34*, 69–88. doi:10.1146/annurev-neuro-061010-113654.

Kiddoo, D. A. (2012). Toilet training children: When to start and how to train. *Canadian Medical Association Journal, 184*(5), 511–512.

Kids Health. (2012). *Temper tantrums.* Retrieved from <http://kidshealth.org/parent/emotions/behavior/tantrums.html#>.

Lipnowski, S., LeBlanc, C. M., & Canadian Paediatric Society, Healthy Active Living and Sports Medicine Committee. (2012). Healthy active living: Physical activity guidelines for children and adolescents. *Paediatrics & Child Health, 17*(4), 209–210. Retrieved from <http://www.cps.ca/documents/position/physical-activity-guidelines>.

Milteer, R. M., Ginsburg, K. R., & Council on Communications and Media Committee on Psychosocial Aspects of Child and Family Health. (2012). The importance of play in promoting healthy child development and maintaining strong parent–child bond: Focus on children in poverty. *Pediatrics, 129*(1), e204–e213. doi:10.1542/peds.2011-2953.

Morin, K. (2007). Infant nutrition: Toddlers: Start off on the right foot. *American Journal of Maternal Child Nursing, 32*(2), 122. doi:10.1097/01.NMC.0000264294.79845.2f.

Neuman, M. E. (2011). Addressing children's beliefs through Fowler's stages of faith. *Journal of Pediatric Nursing, 26*(1), 44–50. doi:10.1016/j.pedn.2009.09.002.

Nieman, P., Shea, S., & Canadian Paediatric Society, Community Paediatrics Committee. (2004). Effective discipline for children. *Paediatrics & Child Health, 9*(1), 37–41. Reaffirmed 2016. Retrieved from <http://www.cps.ca/documents/position/discipline-for-children>.

Null, J. (2016). *Heatstroke deaths of children in vehicles.* San Francisco: San Francisco State University. Retrieved from <http://www.ggweather.com/heat>.

Owens, J. A. (2016). Sleep medicine. In R. M. Kliegman, B. F. Stanton, J. W. St. Geme, et al. (Eds.), *Nelson textbook of pediatrics* (20th ed.). St. Louis: Saunders.

Parachute. (n.d.a). *Bike carriers & trailers.* Retrieved from <http://www.parachutecanada.org/injury-topics/item/bike-carriers-and-trailers>.

Parachute. (n.d.b). *Child injury prevention (ages 0–6): Burns and scalds prevention.* Retrieved from <http://www.parachutecanada.org/child-injury-prevention/item/burns-and-scalds-prevention>.

Parachute. (n.d.c). *Lowering hot water temperature.* Retrieved from <http://www.parachutecanada.org/injury-topics/item/lowering-hot-water-temperature>.

Parachute. (n.d.d). *Protect your child from flame burns.* Retrieved from <http://www.parachutecanada.org/injury-topics/item/flame-burns>.

Parachute. (n.d.e). *Child injury prevention (ages 0–6): Child poisoning prevention.* Retrieved from <http://www.parachutecanada.org/child-injury-prevention/item/child-poisoning-prevention>.

Parachute. (n.d.f). *Carbon monoxide poisoning.* Retrieved from <http://www.parachutecanada.org/policy/item/carbon-monoxide-poisoning>.

Parachute. (n.d.g). *Fall prevention.* Retrieved from <http://www.parachutecanada.org/injury-topics/topic/C20>.

Piaget, J. (1952). *The origins of intelligence in children.* New York: International Universities Press.

Public Health Agency of Canada (2009a). *Injury and child maltreatment analysis of Statistics Canada mortality data and Canadian Institute for Health Information Hospitalization data (2000–2005).* Ottawa: Author.

Public Health Agency of Canada. (2009b). *Child and youth injury in review, 2009 edition—Spotlight on consumer product safety.* Retrieved from <http://www.parachutecanada.org/downloads/research/reports/ChildYouthInjuryinReview2009.pdf>.

Roehlkepartain, E. C., King, P. E., Wagener, L., et al. (Eds.), (2006). *The handbook of spiritual development in childhood and adolescence.* Thousand Oaks, CA: SAGE. doi:10.4135/9781412976657.

Rutkoski, J. D., Sippey, M., & Gaines, B. A. (2011). Traumatic television tip-overs in the pediatric population. *Journal of Surgical Research, 166*(2), 199–204.

Savic, I., Garcia-Falqueras, A., & Swaab, D. F. (2010). Sexual differentiation of the human brain in relation to gender identity and sexual orientation. *Progress in Brain Research, 186*, 41–62.

Transport Canada. (2015). *Keep kids safe.* Retrieved from <https://www.tc.gc.ca/eng/motorvehiclesafety/safedrivers-childsafety-car-time-stages-1083.htm>.

van Schaik, C., & Canadian Paediatric Society, Injury Prevention Committee. (2008). Transportation of infants and children in motor vehicles. *Paediatrics & Child Health, 13*(4), 313–318. Retrieved from <http://www.cps.ca/en/documents/position/car-seat-safety>.

Williams, R., Clinton, J., & Canadian Paediatric Society, Early Years Task Force. (2011). Getting it right at 18 months: In support of an enhanced well-baby visit. *Paediatrics & Child Health, 16*(10), 647–650. Retrieved from <http://www.cps.ca/en/documents/position/enhanced-well-baby-visit>.

Yanchar, N. L., Warda, L. J., Fuselli, P., & Canadian Paediatric Society, Injury Prevention Committee. (2012). Child and youth injury prevention: A public health approach. Abridged version. *Paediatr Child Health, 17*(9), 511.

Yeh, E. S., Rochette, L. M., McKenzie, L. B., et al. (2011). Injuries associated with cribs, playpens, and bassinets among young children in the US—1990–2008. *Pediatrics, 127*(3), 479–486.

Zimmerman, F. J., Gilkerson, J., Richards, J. A., et al. (2009). Teaching by listening: The importance of adult–child conversations to language development. *Pediatrics, 124*(1), 342–349. doi:10.1542/peds.2008-2267.

ADDITIONAL RESOURCES

Ages and Stages Questionnaires (ASQ): <http://www.brookespublishing.com/resource-center/screening-and-assessment/asq/>.

Canadian Association of Poison Control Centres: <www.capcc.ca>.

Canadian Dental Association—Dental Care for Children: <http://www.cda-adc.ca/en/oral_health/cfyt/dental_care_children>.

Canadian Hospitals Injury Reporting and Prevention Program (CHIRPP) (national database of circumstances of injuries that require hospital emergency treatment): <http://www.phac-aspc.gc.ca/injury-bles/chirpp/index-eng.php>.

Canadian Paediatric Society—How to promote good television habits: <http://www.caringforkids.cps.ca/handouts/promote_good_television_habits>.

Canadian Paediatric Society—Parent guide to toilet training: <http://www.caringforkids.cps.ca/handouts/toilet_learning>.

Canadian Virtual Hospice—Emotional Health (talking with children and youth about serious illness): <http://www.virtualhospice.ca/en_US/Main+Site+Navigation/Home/Topics/Topics/Emotional+Health/Talking+with+Children+and+Youth.aspx>.

City of Brampton—Car Seat: Child Safe & Secure Video: <http://www.brampton.ca/EN/residents/fire-emergency-services/Fire-Safety/Pages/Child-Safe-and-Secure-Video.aspx>.

Government of Canada—Childhood Obesity: <www.healthycanadians.gc.ca/healthy-living-vie-saine/obesity-obesite/index-eng.php>.

Health Canada—Eating Well With Canada's Food Guide: <http://www.hc-sc.gc.ca/fn-an/food-guide-aliment/index-eng.php>.

Health Canada—Healthy Living—Oral Health: <http://www.hc-sc.gc.ca/hl-vs/oral-bucco/index-eng.php>.

Health Canada—Report an Incident Involving a Consumer Product: <http://www.hc-sc.gc.ca/cps-spc/advisories-avis/incident/index-eng.php>.

Healthy Canadians—Search Recalls and Safety Alerts: <http://healthycanadians.gc.ca/recall-alert-rappel-avis/index-eng.php>.

Nipissing District Developmental Screen: <http://www.ndds.ca/language.php>.

Parachute—Information on how to prevent injuries: <http://www.parachutecanada.org/>.

PEDS/PEDS DM—Tools for developmental/behavioural screening and surveillance: <http://www.pedstest.com/default.aspx>.

Peel Region Health Department—Car Seat Safety: <http://www.peelregion.ca/health/carseat/index.htm>.

Region of Peel Health Services: Toddlers and Preschoolers—Behaviour: Jealousy and Sibling Rivalry: <http://www.peelregion.ca/health/family-health/toddlers-and-preschoolers/behaviour/jealousy.htm>.

Transport Canada—Child Car Seat Clinics in Canada: <https://www.tc.gc.ca/eng/motorvehiclesafety/safedrivers-childsafety-seat-clinics-1058.htm>.

Transport Canada—Regulations for child car seats and restraints: <http://www.tc.gc.ca/media/documents/roadsafety/TP14772e.pdf>.

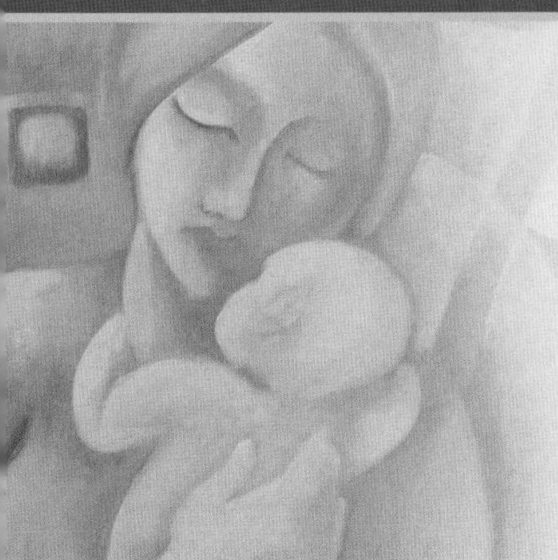

CHAPTER 37

The Preschooler and Family

Cheryl Sams

evolve WEBSITE

Visit the Evolve website for additional resources related to the content in this chapter such as Case Studies, Critical Thinking Case Study Answers, Nursing Care Plans, Nursing Processes, Nursing Skills, and Review Questions for Exam Preparation at: http://evolve.elsevier.com/Canada/Perry/maternal/

OBJECTIVES

On completion of this chapter the reader will be able to:

- Identify the major biological, psychosocial, cognitive, moral, spiritual, and social developments that occur during the preschool years.
- List the benefits of imaginary playmates.
- Discuss how to prepare preschoolers for preschool or day care experience.
- Provide parents with guidelines for their child's sex education.
- Provide parents with guidelines for dealing with a child's fears, stresses, aggression, and sleep problems.
- Recognize causes of stuttering during preschool years.
- Offer parents suggestions for preventing speech problems.
- Recognize feeding patterns of preschoolers.
- Provide anticipatory guidance to parents regarding safety promotion and injury prevention based on preschoolers' developmental achievements.
- Provide parents with information on early signs of mental health concerns.

PROMOTING OPTIMUM GROWTH AND DEVELOPMENT

The combined biological, psychosocial, cognitive, and social achievements during the preschool period (3 to 5 years of age) prepare preschoolers for their most significant change in lifestyle: entrance into school. Their control of bodily functions, experience of brief and prolonged periods of separation, ability to interact cooperatively with other children and adults, use of language for mental symbolization, and increased attention span and memory prepare them for the next major period: school years. Successful achievement of previous levels of growth and development is essential for preschoolers in order to refine many of the tasks that were mastered during the toddler years.

Biological Development

The rate of physical growth slows and stabilizes during the preschool years. See Table 37-1 for preschooler heights and weights. The World Health Organization (WHO) Child Growth Standards 2006 and WHO Growth Reference charts are used to measure and track Canadian preschooler's growth patterns and were revised in 2014 by the Dietitians of Canada, Canadian Paediatric Society (CPS), College of Family Physicians, and Community Health Nurses of Canada, and Canadian Pediatric Endocrine Group. See these growth charts in Appendix C.

The physical proportions of the preschooler no longer resemble the squat, pot-bellied toddler. The preschooler is slender but sturdy, graceful, agile, and posturally erect. There is little difference in physical characteristics according to gender.

Most organ systems can adjust to moderate stress and change. During this period, most children are toilet trained. Motor development mainly consists of increases in strength and refinement of previously learned skills. Muscle development and bone growth are still not mature. Excessive activity and overexertion can injure delicate tissues. Good posture, appropriate exercise, and adequate nutrition and rest are essential for optimum development of the musculoskeletal system.

TABLE 37-1 GROWTH AND DEVELOPMENT DURING PRESCHOOL YEARS

PHYSICAL	GROSS MOTOR	FINE MOTOR	LANGUAGE	SOCIALIZATION	COGNITION	FAMILY RELATIONSHIPS
Age 3 Yr						
Usual yearly weight gain of 1.8–2.7 kg Average weight of 14.5 kg Usual gain in height of 5 to 7.5 cm per year Birth length doubles by age 4 Average height of 95 cm May have achieved nighttime control of bowel and bladder	Rides tricycle Jumps off bottom step Stands on one foot for a few seconds Goes up stairs using alternate feet; may still come down using both feet on step Broad jumps May try to dance, but balance may not be adequate	Builds tower of 9–10 cubes Builds bridge with 3 cubes Adeptly places small pellets in narrow-necked bottle In drawing, copies a circle, imitates a cross, names what has been drawn; cannot draw stick figure but may make circle with facial features	Has vocabulary of about 900 words Uses primarily telegraphic speech Uses complete sentences of three or four words Talks incessantly regardless of whether anyone is paying attention Repeats sentence of six syllables Asks many questions	Dresses self almost completely if helped with back buttons and told which shoe is right or left Pulls on shoes Has increased attention span Feeds self completely Can prepare simple meals, such as cold cereal and milk Can help to set table; can dry dishes without breaking any May have fears, especially of dark and going to bed Knows own gender and gender of others Play is parallel and associative; begins to learn simple games, but often follows own rules; begins to share	Is in preconceptual phase Is egocentric in thought and behaviour Has beginning understanding of time; uses many time-oriented expressions, talks about past and future as much as about present, pretends to tell time Has improved concept of space, as demonstrated by understanding of prepositions and ability to follow directional command Has beginning ability to view concepts from another perspective	Attempts to please parents and conform to their expectations Is less jealous of younger sibling; may be opportune time for birth of additional sibling Is aware of family relationships and gender-role functions Boys tend to identify more with father or other male figure Has increased ability to separate easily and comfortably from parents for short periods
Age 4 Yr						
Pulse and respiration rates decrease slightly Growth rate is similar to that of previous year Average weight of 16.7 kg Average height of 103 cm Length at birth is doubled Maximum potential for development of amblyopia	Skips and hops on one foot Catches ball reliably Throws ball overhead Walks down stairs using alternate footing	Uses scissors successfully to cut out picture following outline Can lace shoes but may not be able to tie bow In drawing, copies a square, traces a cross and diamond, adds three parts to stick figure	Has vocabulary of 1500 words or more Uses sentences of four or five words Questioning is at peak Tells exaggerated stories Knows simple songs May be mildly profane if associates with older children Obeys four prepositional phrases, such as *under, on top of, beside, in back of,* or *in front of* Names one or more colours Comprehends analogies, such as, "If ice is cold, fire is _______"	Very independent Tends to be selfish and impatient Aggressive physically and verbally Takes pride in accomplishments Has mood swings Shows off dramatically, enjoys entertaining others Tells family tales to others with no restraint Still has many fears Play is associative Imaginary playmates are common Uses dramatic, imaginative, and imitative devices Sexual exploration and curiosity demonstrated through play, such as being "doctor" or "nurse"	Is in phase of intuitive thought Causality is still related to proximity of events Understands time better, especially in terms of sequence of daily events Unable to conserve matter Judges everything according to one dimension, such as height, width, or order Immediate perceptual clues dominate judgement Is beginning to develop less egocentrism and more social awareness May count correctly but has poor mathematical concept of numbers Obeys because parents have set limits, not because of understanding of right and wrong	Rebels if parents expect too much, such as impeccable table manners Takes aggression and frustration out on parents or siblings Do's and don'ts become important May have rivalry with older or younger siblings; may resent older sibling's privileges and younger sibling's invasion of privacy and possessions May "run away" from home Identifies strongly with parent of opposite sex Is able to run simple errands outside home

Age 5 Yr						
Pulse and respiration rates decrease slightly Average weight of 18.7 kg Average height of 110 cm Eruption of permanent dentition may begin Handedness is established (about 90% are right-handed)	Skips and hops on alternate feet Throws and catches ball well Jumps rope Skates with good balance Walks backward with heel to toe Jumps from height of 30 cm and lands on toes Balances on alternate feet with eyes closed	Ties shoelaces Uses scissors, simple tools, or pencil very well In drawing, copies a diamond and triangle; adds seven to nine parts to stick figure; prints a few letters, numbers, or words, such as first name	Has vocabulary of about 2100 words Uses sentences of six to eight words, with all parts of speech Names coins (e.g., nickel, dime) Names four or more colours Describes drawing or pictures with much comment and elaboration Knows days of week, months, and other time-associated words Knows composition of objects, such as "A shoe is made of _____." Can follow three commands in succession	Less rebellious and quarrelsome than at age 4 yr More settled and eager to get down to business Not as open and accessible in thoughts and behaviour as in earlier years Independent but trustworthy, not foolhardy; more responsible Has fewer fears; relies on outer authority to control world Eager to do things right and to please; tries to "live by rules" Has better manners Cares for self totally, occasionally needing supervision in dress or hygiene Not ready for concentrated close work or small print because of slight farsightedness and still unrefined eye–hand coordination Play is associative; tries to follow rules but may cheat to avoid losing	Begins to question what parents think by comparing them with age-mates and other adults May notice prejudice and bias in outside world Is more able to view other's perspective but tolerates differences rather than understanding them May begin to show understanding of conservation of numbers through counting objects regardless of arrangement Uses time-oriented words with increased understanding Cautious about accepting or believing information	Gets along well with parents May seek out parent more often than at age 4 yr for reassurance and security, especially when entering school Begins to question parents' thinking and principles Strongly identifies with parent of same sex, especially boys with their fathers Enjoys activities such as sports, cooking, and shopping with parent of same sex

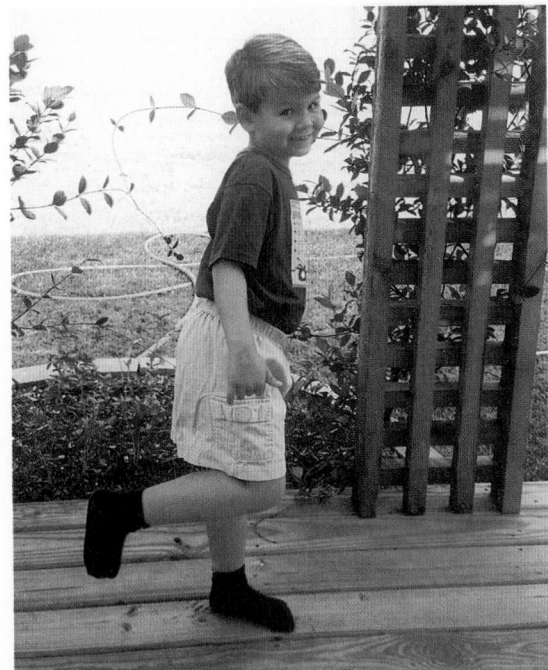

FIGURE 37-1 A 4-year-old child has sufficient balance to stand or hop on one foot.

Gross and Fine Motor Skills

Walking, running, climbing, and jumping are well established by age 36 months. Refinement in eye–hand and muscle coordination is evident in several areas (see Table 37-1 and Fig. 37-1). Fine motor development is evident in these children's increasingly skilful manipulation, such as in drawing and dressing. These skills provide readiness for learning and independence for entry into school.

Psychosocial Development

Developing a Sense of Initiative (Erikson)

After preschoolers have mastered the tasks of the toddler period, they are ready to face the developmental endeavours of the preschool period. Erikson (1963) maintained that the chief psychosocial task of this preschool period is acquiring a sense of initiative. Children are in a stage of energetic learning. They play, work, and live to the fullest and feel a real sense of accomplishment and satisfaction in their activities. Conflict arises when children overstep the limits of their ability and inquiry and experience a sense of guilt for not having behaved appropriately. Feelings of guilt, anxiety, and fear may also result from thoughts that differ from expected behaviour.

A particularly stressful thought for the preschooler is wishing one's parent dead. As a sense of rivalry or competition develops between the child and the same-sex parent, the child may think of ways to get rid of the interfering parent. In most situations this rivalry is resolved when the child strongly identifies with the same-sex parent and peers during the school years. However, if that parent dies before the identification process is completed, the preschooler may be overwhelmed with guilt for having wished and therefore "caused" the death. Clarifying for children that wishes cannot and do not make events occur is essential in helping them overcome their guilt and anxiety.

CULTURAL AWARENESS

Learning Sociocultural Mores

Developing a conscience implies learning sociocultural mores of the family's heritage. Depending on the type of attitudes conveyed, children will learn not only appropriate behaviours but also tolerance-based, biased, or prejudicial values concerning their ethnic, religious, and social background and those of other groups. Much of this influence may remain dormant until they associate with children or adults of a different heritage. Depending on the particular group, they may be accepted or ostracized for their attitudes.

Development of *superego*, or *conscience*, begins toward the end of the toddler years and is a major task for preschoolers (see Cultural Awareness box). Learning right from wrong and good from bad is the beginning of a sense of morality (see Moral Development section).

Cognitive Development

One task related to the preschool period is readiness for school and scholastic learning.

Preoperational Phase (Piaget)

Piaget's cognitive theory (1952) does not include a period specifically for children who are 3 to 5 years old. The *preoperational phase* covers the age span from 2 to 7 years and is divided into two stages: *preconceptual phase*, ages 2 to 4, and the phase of *intuitive thought*, ages 4 to 7. One main transition during these two phases is the shift from totally egocentric thought to social awareness and the ability to consider other viewpoints. However, egocentricity is still evident.

Language continues to develop during the preschool stage. Speech remains primarily a vehicle of egocentric communication. Preschoolers assume that everyone thinks as they do and that a brief explanation of their thinking makes the entire thought understood by others. Because of this self-referenced, egocentric verbal communication, it is often necessary to explore and understand a young child's thinking through other, nonverbal approaches. For children in this age group, the most enlightening and effective method is *play*, which becomes the child's way of understanding, adjusting to, and working out life's experiences.

Preschoolers increasingly use language without comprehending the meaning of words, particularly concepts of right and left, causality, and time. Children may use the concepts correctly but only in the circumstances in which they have learned them. For example, they may know how to put on shoes by remembering that the buckle is always on the outside of the foot. If different shoes have no buckles, they cannot reason which shoe fits which foot. In other words, they do not understand the concepts of *right and left*.

Superficially, *causality* resembles logical thought. Preschoolers explain a concept as they heard it described by others, but understanding is limited. An example is the concept of time. Because *time* is still incompletely understood, children interpret it according to their own frame of reference. Consequently, time is best explained in relationship to an event, such as "Your mother will visit you after you finish your lunch." Avoiding words such as *yesterday, tomorrow, next week*, or a named day of the week to express when an event is expected to occur and instead associating time with expected daily events can help children learn about temporal relationships while increasing their trust in others' predictions.

Preschoolers' thinking is often described as *magical thinking*. Because of their egocentrism and **transductive reasoning**, they believe that thoughts are all-powerful. Such thinking places them in the vulnerable position of feeling guilty and responsible for bad thoughts, which may coincide with the occurrence of a wished event. Their inability to logically reason cause and effect of an illness or injury makes it especially difficult for them to understand such events.

Preschoolers believe in the power of words and accept their meaning literally. An example of this type of thinking is when children are called "bad" because they did something wrong: In preschoolers' minds, calling them "bad" means they are a bad person; it is better to say that their actions were bad by saying, for example, "That was a bad thing to do."

NURSING ALERT

Counselling children whose parents are going through a divorce or separation should involve a discussion with the child about her or his role. Because of magical thinking the child may believe that she or he wished the other parent away. The child should be reassured that this is not the case.

Moral Development

Preconventional or Premoral Level (Kohlberg)

Young children's development of moral **judgement** is at the most basic level. They have little, if any, concern about why something is wrong. They behave because of freedom or restriction that is placed on actions. In the *punishment and obedience orientation*, children (from about 2 to 4 years) judge whether an action is good or bad depending on whether it results in reward or punishment. If children are punished for it, the action is bad. If they are not punished, the action is good, regardless of the meaning of the act. For example, if parents allow hitting, children will perceive that hitting is good because it is not associated with punishment.

From approximately 4 to 7 years of age, children are in the stage of *naive instrumental orientation*, in which actions are directed toward satisfying their needs and, less frequently, the needs of others. They have a concrete sense of justice and fairness during this period of development.

Spiritual Development

Children generally learn about faith and religion from significant others in their environment, usually from parents and their religious beliefs and practices. However, young children's understanding of spirituality is influenced by their cognitive level. Preschoolers have a concrete concept of a God or other deity with physical characteristics, often like an imaginary friend. They understand simple religious stories and memorize short prayers, but their understanding of the meaning of these rituals is limited. Preschoolers benefit from concrete representations of religious practices, such as picture books, small statues, and other related objects. They will imitate religious practices of their parents without fully understanding the significance of these acts.

Observing religious traditions and participating in a religious community can help children cope during stressful periods, such as illness, hospitalization, and other traumatic events. In many religious faiths and belief systems, cultural practices and religion are closely intertwined and are an important part of the child's and family's life.

Development of Body Image

The preschool years play a significant role in the development of **body image**. With increasing comprehension of language, preschoolers recognize that individuals have undesirable and desirable appearances. They are aware of the meaning of words such as *pretty* or *ugly*, and they reflect opinions of others regarding their own appearance. By 5 years of age, children compare their size with that of their peers and can become conscious of being large or short, especially if others refer to them as "so big" or "so little" for their age. Research indicates that girls as young as preschool age already show concern about appearance and weight (Skouteris, McCabe, Swinburn, et al., 2010). Because these are formative years for boys and girls, parents should make the efforts to instill positive attitudes about body image, give their children encouraging feedback regarding their appearance, and emphasize the importance of accepting individuals no matter how their appearances differ. Children at this age should be educated about the benefits of physical activity and nutrition on health instead of focusing on weight.

Despite advances in body image development, preschoolers have poorly defined body boundaries and little knowledge of their internal anatomy. Intrusive experiences are frightening, especially those that disrupt the integrity of the skin, such as injections and surgery. They fear that if their skin is "broken," all of their blood and "insides" can leak out. Bandages are critical to "keep everything from coming out."

Development of Sexuality

Sexual development during these years is an important phase in the formation of a person's overall sexual identity and beliefs. *Sex-typing*, or the process by which an individual develops behaviour, personality, attitudes, and beliefs appropriate for his or her culture and sex, occurs through several mechanisms during this period. Probably the most powerful mechanisms are child-rearing practices and imitation. Gender identification is a result of complex prenatal and postnatal psychological factors and biological or genetic factors. Most children are aware of their gender and the expected sets of related behaviours by 1.5 to 2.5 years.

As sexual identity develops beyond gender recognition, modesty may become a concern. Gender-role imitation and "dressing up" like Mommy or Daddy are important activities.

Attitudes and responses of others to role-playing can condition children to accept the views of others. For example, comments such as "Boys shouldn't play with dolls" can influence a boy's self-concept of masculinity.

Sexual exploration may be more pronounced now than ever before, particularly in terms of exploring and manipulating genitalia. Questions about sexual reproduction may come to the forefront in preschoolers' search for understanding (see Chapters 38 and 39).

Social Development

During the preschool period, the *separation–individuation process* is completed. Preschoolers have overcome much of the anxiety associated with strangers and the fear of separation of earlier years. They relate to unfamiliar people easily and tolerate brief separations from parents with little or no protest. However, they still need parental security, reassurance, guidance, and approval, especially when entering preschool or elementary school. Prolonged separation, such as that imposed by illness and hospitalization, is difficult, but preschoolers respond to anticipatory preparation and concrete explanation. Maintaining an established routine is still important for early preschoolers regardless of home, school, or hospital environment. They can cope with changes in daily routine much better than toddlers, although they may develop more imaginary fears. Preschoolers gain security and comfort from familiar objects, such as toys, dolls, or photographs of family members. They are able to work through many of their unresolved fears, fantasies, and anxieties through play, especially if guided with appropriate play objects (e.g., dolls, puppets) that represent family members, other adults, and other children.

Language

During preschool years, language becomes more sophisticated and complex and the major mode of communication and social interaction (Fig. 37-2). Through language, preschool children learn to express feelings of frustration or anger without acting them out. Both cognitive ability and environment, particularly consistent role models, influence vocabulary, speech, and comprehension. Vocabulary increases dramatically from 300 words at age 2 years to more than 2100 words at the end of 5 years. Sentence structure, grammatical usage, and intelligibility also advance to a more adult level. Language development during these early years predicts school readiness (Harrison & McLeod, 2010) and sets the stage for later success in school (Reilly, Wake, Ukoumunne, et al., 2010).

Children between 3 and 4 years of age form sentences of about three or four words and include only the most essential words to convey a meaning. Such speech is often termed *telegraphic* for its brevity. Three-year-old children ask many questions and use plurals, correct pronouns, and the past tense of verbs. They name familiar objects such as animals, parts of the body, relatives, and friends. They can give and follow simple commands. They talk incessantly regardless of whoever is listening or answering them. They enjoy musical or talking toys or dolls and imitate new words proficiently. Preschoolers also benefit from "reading" picture books with a parent or adult figure; this provides immediate feedback to the child and helps develop vocabulary as the child hears the pronunciation of words from adults (Feigelman, 2016). There is evidence that reading and speaking to a child in early life programs words into the child's memory bank for use at a later time.

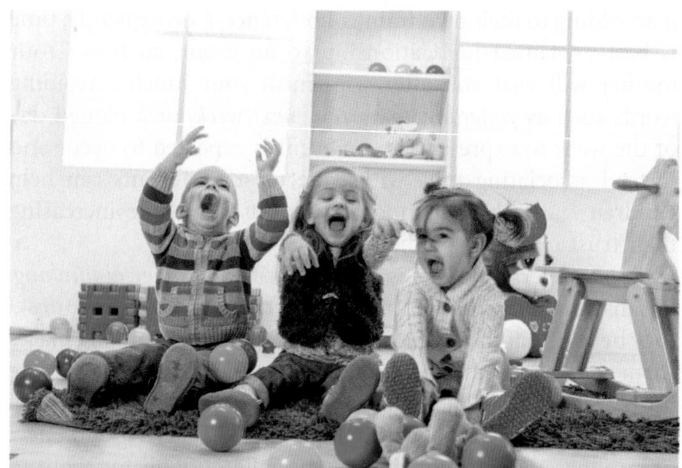

FIGURE 37-2 Preschool children enjoy friends and often use nonverbal messages to communicate. (Goran Bogicevic/Shutterstock .com.)

From ages 4 to 5 years, preschoolers use longer sentences of four or five words and more parts of speech to convey a message (e.g., prepositions, adjectives, and a variety of verbs). They can follow simple directional commands, such as "Put the ball on the chair," but can carry out only one request at a time. They answer questions such as "What do you do when you're hungry?" by describing the appropriate action. The pattern of asking questions is at its peak, and children usually repeat a question until they receive an answer. Preschoolers also are incapable of understanding figurative speech and are very literal in their understanding of the meaning of words (Feigelman, 2016). For example, saying that an intravenous (IV) cannula is to be inserted for hydration is a straw is interpreted by the preschoolers as literally a drinking straw because that is their common frame of reference for that object.

By age 6, children can use all parts of speech correctly, except for deviations from the rules. They can define simple things by describing the use, shape, or general category of classification, rather than simply describing their outward appearance. For example, they may define a ball as "round," "something you bounce," or "a toy," rather than only describing its colour. They understand the concept of opposites and they can describe an object according to its composition, such as "A spoon is made of metal."

While Canada is bilingual with two official languages, English and French, a multitude of other languages are also spoken in this multicultural country. Children can learn two languages at home, at school, or in the community. Often children will learn both languages well but may have a dominant language depending on how often the languages are practised. Learning two languages does not cause speech or language problems. If there is a concern about the child's language skills, then the child likely has a speech or language delay that is not related

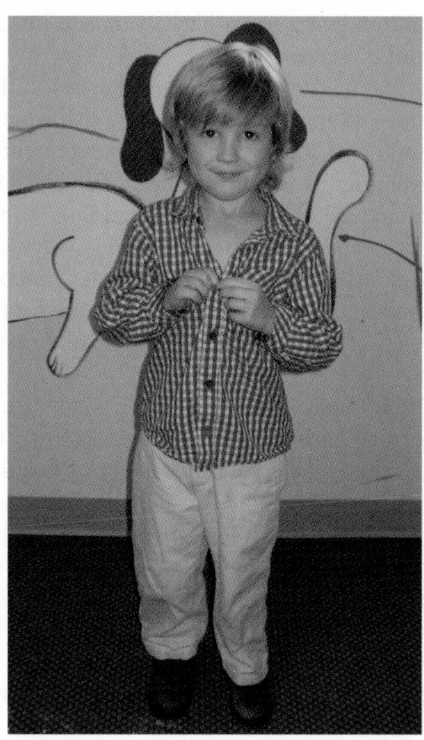

FIGURE 37-3 Most preschoolers are able to dress themselves but need help with more difficult items of clothing.

to bilingualism and needs an assessment (American Speech-Language-Hearing Association, n.d.).

Personal-Social Behaviour

The pervasive ritualism and negativism of toddlerhood gradually diminish during the preschool years. Although self-assertion is still a major theme, preschoolers demonstrate their sense of autonomy differently. They are able to verbalize their request for independence and perform independently because of their much-refined physical and cognitive development. By 4 or 5 years of age, they need little if any assistance with dressing, eating, or toileting (Fig. 37-3). They can also be trusted to obey warnings of danger, although 3- or 4-year-old children may exceed their boundaries at times.

Preschoolers are much more sociable and willing to please than toddlers. They have internalized many standards and values of family and culture. By the end of early childhood they begin to question parental values and compare them with those of their peer group and other authority figures. As a result, they may be less willing to abide by the family's code of conduct. Preschoolers become increasingly aware of their position and role within the family. Although this is a more secure age for experiencing the addition of another sibling, relinquishing the position of only or youngest is still difficult and requires special parental attention to prevent feelings of desertion and resentment (see Chapter 36, Sibling Rivalry).

Play

Various types of play are typical of this period, but preschoolers especially enjoy associative play—group play in similar or identical activities but without rigid organization or rules

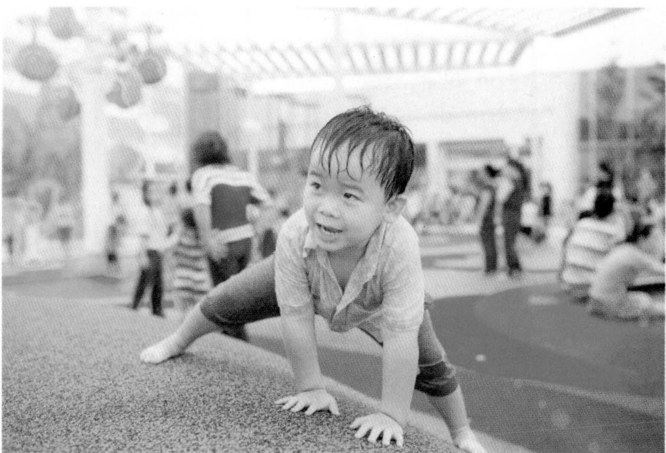

FIGURE 37-4 Preschoolers enjoy play activities that promote motor skills such as jumping and running. (Makistock/Shutterstock .com.)

(see Fig. 32-8). Play should foster physical, social, and mental development.

Play activities for physical growth and refinement of motor skills include jumping, running, and climbing. Tricycles, wagons, gym and sports equipment, sandboxes, wading pools, and activities at water parks can help develop muscles and coordination (Fig. 37-4). Activities such as swimming and skating teach safety and enhance muscle development and coordination. Children involved in the work of play do not require expensive toys and gadgets to keep them entertained but often enjoy playing with common household items such as a broom handle or even items that adults consider junk (boxes, sticks, rocks, and dirt). The imaginative mind of the preschooler enjoys playing for playing's sake.

Manipulative, constructive, creative, and educational toys provide for quiet activities, fine motor development, and self-expression. Easy construction sets, large blocks of various sizes and shapes, a counting frame, alphabet or number flash cards, paints, crayons, simple carpentry tools, musical toys, illustrated books, simple sewing or handicraft sets, large puzzles, and clay are suitable toys. Electronic games and computer programs are especially valuable in helping children learn basic skills such as letters and simple words.

Probably the most characteristic and pervasive preschool activity is *imitative, imaginative*, and dramatic play. Dress-up clothes, dolls, housekeeping toys, dollhouses, play store toys, telephones, farm animals and equipment, village sets, trains, trucks, cars, planes, hand puppets, and medical kits provide hours of self-expression (Fig. 37-5). Probably at no other time is reproduction of adult behaviour as faithful and absorbing as in 4- and 5-year-old children. Toward the end of the preschool period, children are less satisfied with make-believe or pretend objects and enjoy doing the actual activity, such as cooking and carpentry, with the aid of an adult.

Television and other media also have their place in children's play, although each should be only one part of children's total repertoire of social and recreational activities (see Chapter 32). Parents and other caregivers should supervise the selection of programs, watch and discuss programs with their children,

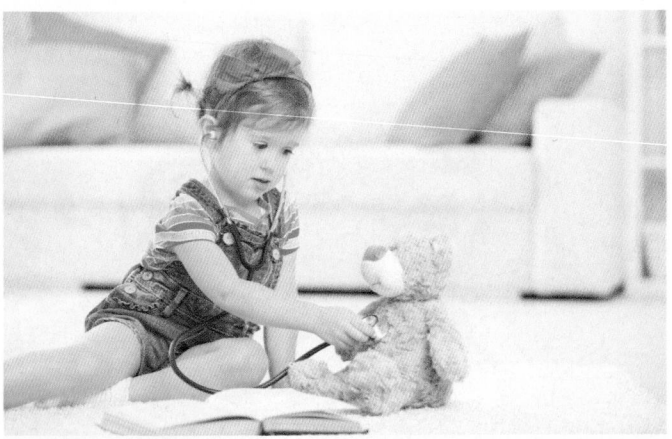

FIGURE 37-5 Imaginative and imitative play is typical of preschoolers. (Evgeny Atamanenko/Shutterstock.com.)

schedule limited time for television viewing, and set a good example of television viewing (Nieman & CPS, Psychosocial Paediatrics Committee, 2003/2011). Television viewing, however, may limit time spent in meaningful activities such as reading, story-telling, physical activity, and socialization (Lipnowski, LeBlanc, & CPS, Healthy Active Living and Sports Medicine, 2012). Prolonged television viewing among young children has been linked to an increase in psychological distress and decreased time spent in active playing, which can increase the risk for obesity among certain children (Hamer, Stamatakis, & Mishra, 2009). Watching fast-paced television cartoons has been linked to a temporary decrease in executive functioning (self-regulation and working memory) in 4-year-olds (Lillard & Peterson, 2011). Because of the significant increase in media accessibility through the various portable electronic devices and cell phones, parents need to be aware of the potential positive and negative effects of media exposure. The Canadian Society for Exercise Physiology recommends that children 2 to 4 years of age be limited to under 1 hour per screen (television, computers, and video games) per day (Tremblay, Leblanc, Carson, et al., 2012).

Although the potential negative effects of television viewing have been well documented in literature, research has also shown that prosocial behaviour and later academic achievement can result from viewing educational media during the preschool years. However, positive effects depend on the media content, the age of the viewer, the length of viewing time, and the presence of a co-viewing parent (Kirkorian, Wartella, & Anderson, 2008). When parents view media with their children, the activity can become interactive, with parents and children discussing program content.

Play is so much a part of a young child's life that reality and fantasy become blurred. Make-believe is reality during play and only becomes fantasy when toys are put away or dress-up clothes are removed. It is no wonder that imaginary playmates are so much a part of this age period. The appearance of imaginary companions usually occurs between ages 2½ and 3 years, and, for the most part, such playmates are relinquished when the child enters school. Birth order and number of siblings may influence the creation of imaginary companions, with firstborn and only children being more likely to create imaginary playmates (Trifonfi & Reese, 2009).

Imaginary companions serve many purposes: they become friends in times of loneliness, they accomplish what the child is still attempting, and they experience what the child wants to forget or remember. It is not unusual for the "friend" to have myriad vices and be blamed for wrongdoing. Sometimes the child hopes to escape punishment by saying, "My friend George broke the glass." At other times the child may fantasize that the companion misbehaved and play the role of the parent. This becomes a way of assuming control and authority in a safe situation.

Parents often worry about imaginary playmates, not realizing how normal and useful they are. Parents need to be reassured that the child's fantasy is a sign of health that helps differentiate make-believe and reality. Parents can acknowledge an imaginary companion's presence by calling him or her by name and even agreeing to simple requests, such as setting an extra place at the table, but they should not allow the child to use the "playmate" to avoid punishment or responsibility. For example, if the child blames the companion for messing up a room, parents need to state clearly that the child is the only one they see; therefore the child is responsible for cleaning up.

Children also benefit from play that occurs between them and a parent. *Mutual play* fosters development from birth through the school years and provides enriched opportunities for learning. Through mutual play, parents can provide tactile and kinesthetic experiences, maximize verbal and language abilities, and offer praise and encouragement for exploration of the world. In addition, mutual play encourages positive interactions between parent and child, strengthening their relationship.

Coping With Concerns Related to Normal Growth and Development

Preschool and Kindergarten Experience

While some children are home-schooled, many children attend some type of early childhood program, usually preschool or a day care centre. Group care has become commonplace with large numbers of parents being employed outside the home (see Chapter 35, Alternative Child Care Arrangements). Researchers have identified that at least 70% of Canadian children, aged 6 months to 6 years, are in nonparental care (Cleveland, Forer, Hyatt, et al., 2008). The effects of early education and stimulation on children have increasingly gained recognition. Because social development widens to include age-mates and other significant adults, preschool provides an excellent vehicle for expanding children's experiences with others. It is also excellent preparation for entrance into elementary school.

In preschool or day care centres, children are exposed to opportunities for learning group cooperation, adjusting to sociocultural differences, and coping with frustration, dissatisfaction, and anger. If activities are tailored to provide mastery and achievement, children increasingly have feelings of success, self-confidence, and personal competence. Whether structured learning is imposed is less important than the social climate, type of guidance, and attitude toward children that is fostered by the teacher or leader. With a teacher who is aware of preschoolers' developmental abilities and needs, children will learn from the activity that is provided. Most programs incorporate a daily schedule of quiet play, active outdoor activity, group activities such as games and projects, creative or free play, and snack and rest periods. Preschool is particularly beneficial for children who lack a peer-group experience and for children from impoverished homes.

One issue that all parents face is their child's readiness for preschool or kindergarten. While there are no absolute indicators for school readiness, the child's social maturity, especially attention span, is as important as his or her academic readiness. Use of a developmental screening tool such as the Nipissing District Developmental Screen (NDDS) that addresses cognitive (especially language), social, and physical milestones can help identify children who may benefit from diagnostic testing and early intervention programs before they start school (see Table 33-2 and see Additional Resources at the end of the chapter). The NDDS is for children up to 6 years of age and can be used by all health care providers to assess level of development. Also assisting with school readiness and child development are innovative programs such as the Human Early Learning Partnership (HELP), which researches the many factors related to child development and makes related program and policy recommendations (see Additional Resources at the end of this chapter).

Parents play an integral role in their children's school readiness by promoting a positive attitude toward learning, reading to their children, encouraging their children to participate in a variety of activities to explore their talents, and choosing appropriate child care or preschool programs. Family income and the availability of quality child care and early childhood education can be factors in such choices. Nurses and other health care providers can guide parents in selecting enriched social and educational early-intervention programs.

An Aboriginal Head Start preschool program for Indigenous families has demonstrated that locally controlled early-intervention strategies can improve the health of these children by providing supports in order for them to gain confidence toward attaining life goals. Such strategies include support for physical, personal, and social development (Health Canada, 2011).

When parents are considering an early-childhood development program, areas to evaluate include the facility's daily program, teacher qualifications, staff-to-student ratio, discipline policy, environmental safety precautions, provision of meals, sanitary conditions, whether there is adequate indoor and outdoor space per child, safety and injury prevention, and fee schedule (Fig. 37-6) (see Chapter 35, Alternative Child Care Arrangements).

Children need preparation for the preschool or kindergarten experience. For young children, it represents a change from their usual home environment and a prolonged separation from parents. Before children begin school, parents should present the idea as exciting and pleasurable. Talking to children about activities such as painting, building with blocks, or enjoying swings and outdoor equipment allows children to fantasize about the event in a positive manner. When the first day of school arrives, parents should behave confidently. Such behaviour requires parents to have resolved their own feelings regarding the experience.

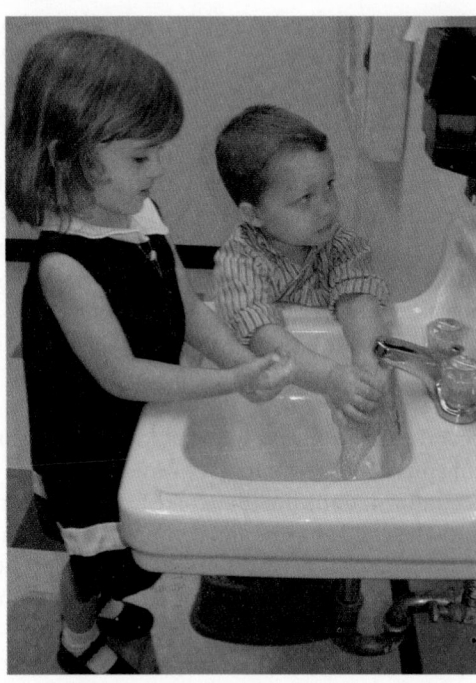

FIGURE 37-6 Thorough hand hygiene is the single most effective method of preventing infection.

Parents should introduce their child to the teacher and the facility. In some instances, it is helpful for parents to remain with the child for at least part of the first day until the child is comfortable and at ease. Other specific actions that can help reduce separation anxiety include providing the school with detailed information about the child's home environment, such as familiar routines, favourite activities, food preferences, names of siblings or pets, and personal habits. Such information helps the teacher make the child feel familiar in strange surroundings. When schools automatically request this information, the parent has a valuable clue to the quality of the program—the request represents the staff's awareness of each child's needs. Transitional objects, such as a favourite toy, may also help the child bridge the gap from home to school.

Sex Education

Preschoolers have assimilated a tremendous amount of information during their short lifetimes. Although their thinking may not be mature, they search constantly for explanations and reasons that are logical and reasonable to them. The word "why" seems to supplant the word "no," which was common in toddlerhood. It is only natural that as they learn about "me" they will also want to know "why me" and "how me." Questions such as "Where do babies come from?" are as casual as "What makes it rain?" or "Who is that?" It is the way in which questions about origins of human life are answered that conditions children, even the youngest, to separate these questions from others about their world.

Two rules govern answering sensitive questions about topics such as sex. The first is to *find out what children know and think*. By investigating the theories that children have produced as a reasonable explanation, parents can give correct information and help children understand why their explanation is inaccurate. Another reason for ascertaining what the child thinks before offering any information is that the "unasked for" answer may be given. For example, 4-year-old Kristen asked her father, "Where did I come from?" Both parents quickly took this inquiry as a clue for offering sex education. After the explanation Kristen exclaimed, "I don't know about all that! All I know is that Charlotte came from Winnipeg, and I want to know where I was born."

The second rule for giving information is to *be honest*. It is true that the preschooler will forget or misunderstand much of the correct information, but the correct information can be restated until the child absorbs and comprehends the facts. Even though correct anatomical words may be hard to pronounce or even more difficult to remember, they become the foundational content for explaining other concepts at a later time.

Honesty does not imply imparting to children every fact of life or allowing excessive permissiveness in sexual curiosity. When children ask one question, they are looking for one answer. When they are ready, they will ask about the other "unfinished" parts of the story. Sooner or later they will wonder how the "sperm meets the egg" and "how the baby gets out," but during this period it is best to wait until they ask.

Regardless of whether children are given sex education, they will engage in games of sexual curiosity and exploration. At about 3 years of age, children are aware of anatomical differences between sexes and are concerned with how the other "works." This is not really "sexual" curiosity because many children are still unaware of the reproductive function of genitalia. Their curiosity is for the eliminative function of anatomy. Little boys wonder how girls can urinate without a penis, so they watch girls go to bathroom. Because they cannot see anything but the stream of urine coming out, they want to observe further.

One question that parents often have is how to handle such sexual curiosity. A positive approach is to neither condone nor condemn it but to express that if children have questions, they should ask the parents. Parents should also encourage their child to engage in some other activity. In this way, children can be helped to understand that there are ways to satisfy their sexual curiosity other than through investigative games. This in no way condemns the act but stresses alternative methods to seek solutions and answers. Allowing children unrestricted permissiveness only intensifies their anxiety and concern, since exploring and searching usually yield little evidence to satisfy their curiosity.

There are many variable cultural influences on sex education. Some cultures encourage open discussion and other cultures are more reticent. For example, Indigenous peoples have generally an open view of sexuality, sexual practices, and sexual orientation. Sex is seen as a way to express an individual's spiritual, emotional, physical, and mental being. Many excellent books on sex education are available for preschool children at public libraries. The Action Canada for Sexual Health and Rights website contains information on how to talk about sex with various age groups (see Additional Resources at the end of the chapter). Parents should read a children's book on sex education themselves *before* giving or reading it to a child.

Another concern for some parents is *masturbation*, or self-stimulation of the genitalia. This occurs at any age for a variety of reasons and, if not excessive, is normal and healthy. It is most common at 4 years of age and during adolescence. For preschoolers, it is a part of sexual curiosity and exploration. If parents are concerned about their children masturbating, the nurse needs to investigate circumstances associated with the activity because it may be an expression of anxiety, boredom, or unresolved conflicts. Children who openly and publicly masturbate are inviting a reaction, such as discipline, punishment, or criticism. They may be overwhelmed by their sexual feelings and are asking others to help channel them into more constructive outlets. Masturbation, like other forms of sex play, is a private act, and parents should emphasize this to children when teaching them socially acceptable behaviour.

Fears

During the preschool years, a great number and variety of real and imagined fears are present, including fear of the dark, being left alone (especially at bedtime), animals (particularly large dogs), ghosts, sexual matters (castration), and objects or persons associated with pain. The exact cause of children's fears is often unknown. Parents often become perplexed about handling these fears because no amount of logical persuasion, coercion, or ridicule will send away the ghosts, boogeymen, monsters, and devils. Inappropriate television viewing by preschoolers may increase fears and anxieties because of their inability to separate reality-based experiences from fantasy portrayed on television.

The concept of *animism*, ascribing lifelike qualities to inanimate objects, helps explain why children fear objects. For example, a child may refuse to use the toilet after watching a television commercial in which the toilet bowel is portrayed as turning into a monster.

Preschoolers also experience fear of annihilation. Because of poorly defined body boundaries and improved cognitive abilities, young children develop concerns related to the loss of body parts. They fear losing body parts with certain medical procedures, such as an intravenous insertion or cast application on a limb, and may see these procedures as real threats to their existence. Preschoolers are often fearful when approaching the health care environment (office or hospital) and are especially fearful of pain. Because of their inability to sometimes discern reality from the imagined, a painful procedure such as a vaccination may be perceived as the end of existence (death) to the child; the preschooler is often unable to see beyond that experience. It is helpful to discuss the child's fears but maintain honesty and openness when working with preschoolers in the health care setting.

The best way to help children overcome their fears is by actively involving them in finding practical methods to deal with the frightening experience. This may be as simple as keeping a night light on in child's bedroom for assurance that no monsters lurk in the dark. Exposing children to the feared object in a safe situation also provides a type of conditioning, or *desensitization*. For instance, children who are afraid of dogs should never be forced to approach or touch one, but they may be gradually introduced to the experience by watching other children play with an animal. This type of modelling, with others demonstrating fearlessness, can be effective if the child is allowed to progress at his or her own rate.

Usually by 5 or 6 years of age, children relinquish many fears. Explaining the developmental sequence of fears and their gradual disappearance may help parents feel more secure in handling preschoolers' fears. Sometimes fears do not subside with simple measures or developmental maturation. When children experience severe fears that disrupt family life, professional help is required.

Stress

Although for parents preschool years generally are less troublesome than toddlerhood, this period of life presents children with many unique stresses. Some, such as fears, are innate and stem from preschoolers' unique understanding of the world. Others, such as beginning school, are imposed. Although minimal amounts of stress are beneficial during the early years to help children develop effective coping skills, excessive stress is harmful. Young children are especially vulnerable because of their limited capacity to cope. Expression of frustration, fear, or anxiety is hampered by inadequate expressive language.

To help parents deal with stress in their child's life, they must be aware of the signs of stress (see Chapter 32, Stress in Childhood) and be helped to identify the source. Any number of stressors may be present, such as the birth of a sibling, marital discord, divorce and separation, relocation, or illness.

The best approach to dealing with stress is prevention—monitoring the amount of stress in children's lives so that levels do not exceed their coping ability. In many instances, structuring children's schedules to allow rest and preparing them for change, such as entering school, are sufficient measures.

Aggression

The term *aggression* refers to behaviour with the intent to hurt a person or destroy property. Aggression differs from anger, which is a temporary emotional state, but anger may be expressed through aggression. Hyperaggressive behaviour in preschoolers is characterized by unprovoked physical attacks on other children and adults, destruction of others' property, frequent intense temper tantrums, extreme impulsivity, disrespect, and noncompliance. Aggression is influenced by a complex set of biological, sociocultural, and familial variables. Factors that tend to increase aggressive behaviour are gender, frustration, modelling of such behaviour, and reinforcement.

Evidence indicates that types of aggression differ between genders. Boys exhibit more physical aggression than girls during preschool years (Benzies, Keown, & Magill-Evans, 2009). However, preschool girls exhibit more relational aggression than preschool boys (Ostrov & Bishop, 2008). *Frustration*, or continual thwarting of self-satisfaction by disapproval, humiliation, punishment, or insults, can lead children to act out against others as a means of release. Especially if they fear their parents, these children will displace their anger onto others, particularly peers and other authority figures. This type of aggression often applies to the child who is well behaved at home but is a discipline problem at school or a bully among playmates.

Modelling, or imitating the behaviour of significant others, is a powerful influencing force in preschoolers. Children who see their parents as physically abusive are observing behaviour that they come to know as acceptable, and they may exhibit this behaviour with others (Benzies et al., 2009). Another aspect of modelling is the "double standard" for acceptable conduct. For example, in some families, aggression is synonymous with masculinity, and boys are encouraged to defend themselves. Television is also a significant source for modelling at this age. Research indicates that there is a direct correlation between media exposure, both violent and educational media, and preschoolers exhibiting physical and relational aggression (Ostrov, Gentile, & Crick, 2006). Therefore, parents should be encouraged to supervise television viewing.

Reinforcement can also shape aggressive behaviour. Sometimes reward for aggression is negative (e.g., punishment) yet reinforcing because it brings attention. For example, children who are ignored by a parent until they hit a sibling or the parent learn that this act garners attention.

When children exhibit extreme behaviours, such as aggression, parents may be concerned about the need for professional help. Generally, the difference between "normal" and "problematic" behaviour is not behaviour itself but its *quantity* (number of occurrences), *severity* (interference with social or cognitive functioning), *distribution* (different manifestations), *onset* (when behaviour started), and *duration* (at least 4 weeks).

Speech Issues

The most critical period for speech development occurs between 2 and 4 years of age. During this period, children are using their rapidly growing vocabulary faster than they can produce the words. Failure to master sensorimotor integrations results in stuttering or stammering as children try to say the word they are already thinking about. This **dysfluency** in speech pattern is a normal characteristic of language development in children ages 2 to 5 years, affects boys more frequently than girls, and usually resolves during childhood (Canadian Association of Speech-Language Pathologists and Audiologists, n.d.). When parents or other significant persons place undue emphasis on a child's dysfluency, an abnormal speech pattern may develop. The Canadian Association of Speech-Language Pathologists and Audiologists (n.d.) encourages parents and caregivers of children who stutter to speak slowly, refrain from correcting or criticizing the child's speech, resist the temptation to complete the child's sentences, provide the opportunity for the child to speak frequently, and take time to listen attentively.

The best therapy for speech problems is prevention and early detection. Common causes of speech problems include hearing loss or impairment, oropharyngeal structural anomalies, developmental disorders such as autism, brain injuries and other neuromotor impairments, lack of a verbally stimulating environment, and change in language exposure as in international adoption (Sharp & Hillenbrand, 2008). Most provinces and territories have newborn hearing screening, which enables early identification of children with hearing problems (see Chapter 26, p. 697); treatment can then begin at birth. Referral for further evaluation and treatment may be necessary to prevent a problem from interfering with learning. Anticipatory preparation of parents for expected developmental norms may allay caregiver concerns.

Children pressured into producing sounds ahead of their developmental level may develop *dyslalia* (articulation problems) or revert to using infantile speech. Prevention involves educating parents about the usual achievement of speech production during childhood. The NDDS is an excellent tool for assessing articulation skills in the child and for explaining to parents the expected progression of sounds (see Additional Resources at the end of the chapter).

Mental Health

Various mental health issues can begin in early childhood, including depression, anxiety, attention-deficit/hyperactivity disorder (ADHD), autism spectrum disorders (ASD), and disruptive behaviour problems such as aggression, opposition, and defiance. It can be difficult for parents to differentiate between normal growth and development behaviours and early mental health concerns. Developmental screenings tools that are detailed in Chapter 33 may help nurses and other health care providers pick up potential mental health issues. Early interventions may improve treatment outcomes.

The early signs of mental health issues include ongoing changes in behaviours that have an impact on how children function, such as fluctuations in mood, energy levels, sleep patterns, attitude, and appetite. For example, ASD symptoms usually appear before age 3 years. The signs vary in severity, but ASD often affects children's ability to communicate and interact with others. Mental health concerns are covered in more detail in Chapters 38 and 39, in the section Special Health Problems, and ASD is discussed in Chapter 41.

PROMOTING OPTIMUM HEALTH DURING PRESCHOOL YEARS

Nutrition

Nutritional requirements for preschoolers are fairly similar to those for toddlers. The required number of calories per unit of body weight continues to decrease slightly. The active 2- to 3-year-old boy will need 1500 calories and girls of the same age will need 1400 calories. The active male 4- to 5-year-old will need 1650 calories and the active girl of the same age will need 1500 calories (Health Canada, 2014). Fluid requirements may also decrease slightly to approximately 100 mL/kg/day but depend on the activity level, climatic conditions, and state of health. Protein requirements increase with age; the recommended intake for preschoolers is 13 to 19 g/day (Health Canada, 2007).

Eating Well With Canada's Food Guide (see Appendix A) supports reducing the amount of saturated fats in children's diets in order to decrease risks of future coronary artery disease. The *Food Guide* recommends that a variety of nutritious foods be offered to children, including some choices that contain fat, such as 2% milk, peanut butter, and avocado, to meet children's nutrient requirements (Appendix A). But children should only have an average saturated fat content of 8 to 9% total energy (Health Canada, 2007).

It is important that all diets contain adequate nutrients such as calcium. The recommendation for daily calcium intake for children 1 to 3 years of age is 700 mg, and the recommendation for children 4 to 8 years of age is 1000 mg (Health Canada, 2012). Milk and dairy products are excellent sources of calcium and vitamin D (fortified). Low-fat milk may be substituted so that the quantity of milk may remain the same while limiting fat intake overall. *Canada's Food Guide* recommends 500 mL of milk daily to meet young children's need for vitamin D (Health Canada, 2007).

Excessive consumption of fruit juices has been associated with adverse health effects such as dental caries and gastrointestinal symptoms; *Canada's Food Guide* recommends giving children ages 2 to 4 years four servings of fruit or vegetables and to offer whole fruit instead of fruit juices. Young children's intake of high sugar content or acidic carbonated beverages contributes to the development of dental caries, and consumption of large amounts of non-nutritive calories may displace or preclude intake of nutrients necessary for growth.

Some preschoolers still have food habits that are typical of toddlers, such as food fads and strong taste preferences. When children reach 4 years of age, they seem to enter another period of finicky eating, which is generally characteristic of the more rebellious behaviour of children in this age group. As with the toddler, small portions should be offered of each item being served. The practice of having the child remain at the table until the "plate is clean" should be avoided because this may contribute to overeating and the development of poor eating habits that contribute to poor health later in life. By age 5 years, children are more agreeable to trying new foods, especially if they are encouraged by an adult who allows them to help with food preparation or experiment with a new taste or different dish (Fig. 37-7). Mealtimes can become battlegrounds if parents expect perfect table manners. Usually the 5-year-old child is ready for the "social" side of eating, but the 3- or 4-year-old child still has difficulty sitting quietly through a long family meal.

The amount and variety of foods consumed by young children vary greatly from day to day. Consequently, parents sometimes worry about the quantity and quality of food that preschoolers consume. Preschoolers can self-regulate their energy intake needs. In general, quality is much more important than quantity, a fact that should be stressed during nutritional counselling. Eating habits are well established by 5 years of age, with the major contributing factor being the family, especially the parents.

The Dietitans of Canada (2014) suggest the following tips:

- Eat together at regular times often as possible without distractions such as electronics.

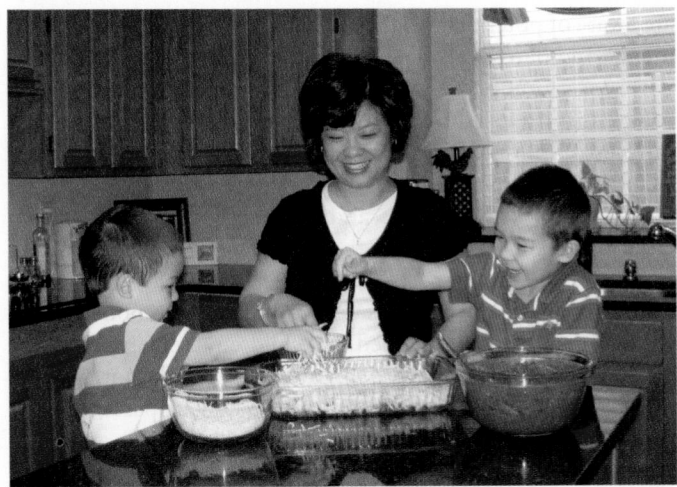

FIGURE 37-7 Preschool-age children enjoy helping adults and are more likely to try new foods if they can assist in the preparation.

- Let preschoolers eat with their fingers and do not expect good table manners.
- Offer three meals and three snacks and do not let the child graze or eat throughout the day.
- Remove food calmly if it has not been eaten within 15 minutes.
- Always serve one food the child will eat.
- Serve foods in different ways, such as adding grated carrots to a muffin or soup.

One way to lessen parental concern about their child's diet is to advise parents to keep a weekly record of everything the child eats. In particular, the parents can measure the amount of food, such as setting aside 120 mL of vegetables and serving the child from this premeasured amount, to provide a more accurate estimate of food intake at each meal. When parents look at the food chart at the end of the week, they are usually amazed by how much the child has consumed. In general, preschoolers consume only slightly more than toddlers, or about half an adult's portion.

The incidence of obesity has nearly tripled over the last 25 years, with up to 26% of young people from ages 2 to 17 years of age being overweight or obese, and 41% of the same age group of Indigenous people (Katzmarzyk, 2008). Childhood obesity has major negative health outcomes, including insulin resistance, type 2 diabetes, cardiovascular disease, dyslipidemia, hypertension, obstructive sleep apnea, nonalcoholic steatohepatitis, poor self-esteem, and a lower health-related quality of life (Katzmarzyk, 2008; Lipnowski et al., 2012). Childhood obesity is an important predictor of adult obesity, so preventing overweight and obesity in childhood is essential.

> **! NURSING ALERT**
>
> Obesity has increased over the past several decades in young children. Efforts to provide a healthy diet and to encourage physical activity should begin early to help children achieve optimum health (Lipnowski et al., 2012).

In addition to unhealthy eating habits, experts recognize that a sedentary lifestyle contributes to cardiovascular disease and obesity. Therefore, the Canadian sedentary behaviour guidelines recommend that children 1 to 4 years old should have both structured and unstructured activity (free play) for at least 180 minutes per day at any intensity (Lipnowski et al., 2012; Tremblay et al., 2012).

Sleep and Activity

While sleep patterns vary widely, the average preschooler sleeps about 12 hours a night and may still take daytime naps. The *Day Nurseries Act* mandates a sleep/rest time, and most day care centres enforce this. The child who is sleeping 1 to 2 hours at day care may not be ready to sleep at the usual bedtime. Waking during the night is common throughout early childhood and may be related to social rather than developmental or physiological factors.

Motor activity levels continue to be high and allow preschoolers to explore their environment, begin learning physical games and sports, and interact with others. Sedentary activities, such as television and video or computer games, are appealing and can become an unhealthy substitute for active play. Physical activity improves motor skills, body composition, and aspects of metabolic health and social development in children younger than 5 years of age (Lipnowski et al., 2012; Tremblay et al., 2012).

Preschoolers' increased gross motor abilities and coordination allow them to engage in many physical activities, if only at a novice level. Whether young children should begin formalized training in an activity at this early age is controversial. Training programs must consider the child's physical and psychological immaturity, and readiness to participate in organized sports should be determined individually. The decision to participate should be based on the child's, not the parent's, motivation and enjoyment. The preschooler learns best with egocentric activities and with auditory and visual cues. Activities that should be focused on include running, throwing, catching, and tumbling. Activities need to be fun, encourage exploration and experimentation, and avoid competition in a variety of environments.

Sleep Problems

Preschool years are a prime time for sleep disturbances. Such disturbances are typically related to increasing autonomy, negative sleep associations, nighttime fears, inconsistent bedtime routines, and lack of limit setting (Moore, Meltzer, & Mindell, 2008). Sleep disturbances may also be caused by nightmares and sleep terrors. Consequences of inadequate sleep include daytime tiredness, irritability, hyperactivity, difficulty concentrating, impaired learning ability, poor control of emotions and impulses, and strain on family relationships (Mindell, Kuhn, Lewin, et al., 2006). Interventions vary greatly; for example, *nightmares* (frightening dreams that are followed by full arousal) and *sleep terrors* (partial arousal from deep, nondreaming sleep) require different approaches.

For children who delay going to bed, a recommended approach involves counselling parents about the importance of a consistent bedtime ritual and emphasizing the normalcy of this type of behaviour in young children. Parents should ignore attention-seeking behaviour and not take children into the parents' bed or allow children to stay up past a reasonable hour. Other measures that may be helpful include keeping a light on in the room, providing transitional objects such as a favourite toy, or leaving a drink of water by the bed. Parental consistency is paramount to all treatment approaches.

Helping children slow down *before* bedtime also reduces the resistance to going to bed. One strategy is to establish limited rituals that signal readiness for bed, such as a bath or story. Parents can reinforce the pattern by stating, "After this story it's bedtime," and consistently carrying out the routine. If anticipated extra stimulation such as having visitors arrive at bedtime disrupts this routine, it is advisable to settle children in bed beforehand. Television viewing before bedtime may cause bedtime resistance and delay sleep.

Dental Health

By the beginning of the preschool period, the eruption of the deciduous (primary) teeth is complete. Dental care is essential to preserve these temporary teeth and to teach good dental habits (see Chapter 36, p. 1060). Although preschoolers' fine motor control is improved, they still require assistance and supervision with brushing, and parents should floss the teeth. Professional care and prophylaxis, especially fluoride supplements (if needed), should be continued. Routine dental care should be well established during preschool years and assessment by a dentist is recommended at 6- to 12-month intervals depending on the family history, the child's dental development, and the presence or absence of dental caries. For children cared for away from home, parents should be encouraged to monitor the dental care provided by others, including minimizing cariogenic foods. Trauma to teeth during this period is not uncommon, and prompt evaluation by a dentist is warranted if oral trauma occurs. Preservation of the space previously occupied by an avulsed tooth is necessary for proper eruption of the secondary tooth.

Canadian children continue to have a high rate of dental disease. In 2010, the Canadian Health Measures Survey identified that 57% of Canadian children 6 to 11 years of age have had a cavity, with an average of 2.5 teeth affected by decay (Public Health Agency of Canada [PHAC], 2010).

Dental disease is disproportionately represented by children of lower socioeconomic status whose families are less likely to have dental insurance. This is true particularly of those in Indigenous communities and new immigrants. In Canada, there has been a decrease in the proportion of public funding for dental care; publicly funded provincial/territorial dental plans for Canadian children are restricted and show substantial variability in coverage. The CPS has called for improvement in government-sponsored dental programs (Rowan-Legg & CPS, Community Paediatrics Committee, 2013).

Safety Promotion and Injury Prevention

Because of improved gross and fine motor skills, coordination, and balance, preschoolers are less prone to falls than toddlers. They tend to be less reckless; listen more to parental rules; and are aware of potential dangers, such as hot objects, sharp instruments, and dangerous heights. Putting objects in the mouth as part of exploration has all but ceased, although accidental poisoning is still a danger. The number of pedestrian motor vehicle injuries among preschoolers tends to increase because they spend a lot of time playing in the parking lot, driveway, or street and riding tricycles, bicycles, and other play vehicles. Preschoolers also run after balls in the street and may forget safety regulations when crossing streets. Children in rural areas are likely to be riding all-terrain vehicles (ATVs) and snowmobiles in the winter. It is not recommended that children under 16 years ride on ATVs. Children younger than 6 years of age do not have the strength or stamina to be transported safely as passengers on snowmobiles and no one should be towed on a tube, tire, sled, or saucer by a snowmobile (Stanwick & CPS, Injury Prevention Committee, 2004/2013).

In general, the guidelines suggested for injury prevention for toddlers apply to children in this age group as well. However, emphasis is now on *education* concerning safety and potential hazards, in addition to appropriate protection. This is an excellent time to start enforcing the use of safety items such as bicycle helmets to prevent head trauma; children are less likely to warm to the idea later in life because of peer pressure. Because preschoolers are great imitators, it is essential that parents set a good example by "practising what they preach." Children quickly observe discrepancies in what they are told to do and what they see others do. Establishing habits at this time, such as wearing protective equipment, can create long-term safety behaviours.

Anticipatory Guidance—Care of Families

The preschool years present fewer child-rearing difficulties than do earlier years. This stage of development is facilitated by appropriate anticipatory guidance in the areas discussed in previous sections (see Family-Centred Teaching box). There is a shift in child-rearing practices from protection to education. Whereas injury prevention previously focused on safeguarding the immediate environment, with less emphasis on reasoning, now the protective guardrails or electrical outlet caps may be replaced by verbal explanations of why danger exists and how to avoid it.

During this period, an emotional transition between parent and child occurs. Although children are still attached to their parents and accept all their values and beliefs, they are nearing the period of life when they will question previous teachings and prefer the companionship of peers. Entry into school marks a separation for parents and for children. Parents may need help in adjusting to this change, particularly if one parent has focused his or her daily activities primarily on home responsibilities. All family members must adjust to changes, which is part of the process of growth and development.

INFECTIOUS DISORDERS

Communicable Diseases

The incidence of childhood communicable diseases has declined significantly since the advent of immunizations. Serious complications resulting from such infections have been further

FAMILY-CENTRED TEACHING

Guidance During Preschool Years

Age 3 Years

Prepare parents for child's increasing interest in widening relationships.
Encourage enrollment in preschool.
Emphasize the importance of setting limits.
Prepare parents to expect exaggerated tension-reduction behaviours, such as the need for a "security blanket."
Encourage parents to offer the child choices.
Prepare parents to expect marked changes at 3½ years, when the child becomes insecure and exhibits emotional extremes.
Prepare parents for normal dysfluency in speech and advise them to avoid focusing on the pattern.
Prepare parents to expect extra demands on their attention as a reflection of the child's emotional insecurity and fear of loss of love.
Warn parents that the equilibrium of a 3-year-old will change to the aggressive, out-of-bounds behaviour of a 4-year-old.
Inform parents to anticipate a more stable appetite with more food selections.
Stress need for protection and education of the child to prevent injury

Age 4 Years

Prepare parents for more aggressive behaviour, including motor activity and offensive language.
Prepare parents to expect resistance to parental authority.
Explore parental feelings regarding the child's behaviour.
Suggest some type of respite for primary caregivers, such as placing the child in preschool for part of the day.
Prepare parents for the child's increasing sexual curiosity.
Emphasize the importance of realistic limit setting on behaviour and appropriate disciplinary techniques.
Prepare parents for the highly imaginative 4-year-old who indulges in "tall tales" (to be differentiated from lies) and develops imaginary playmates.
Help parents prepare children for entrance into school environment.
Prepare parents to expect nightmares or an increase in them.
Provide reassurance that a period of calmness begins at about 5 years of age.

Age 5 Years

Inform parents to expect a tranquil period at around 5 years of age.
Make certain that immunizations are up to date before the child enters school.
Suggest that unemployed parental caregivers consider their own activities when children begin school.
Suggest swimming lessons for the child.

reduced with the use of antibiotics and antitoxins. However, infectious diseases do occur, and nurses must be familiar with the particular infectious agent to recognize the disease and to institute appropriate preventive and supportive interventions (Table 37-2).

NURSING CARE

The more common communicable diseases of childhood, their therapeutic management, and specific nursing care are described in Table 37-2. The following is a general discussion of nursing care management for communicable diseases.

Identification of the infectious agent is of primary importance to prevent exposure to susceptible individuals. Nurses in ambulatory care settings, child care centres, and schools are often the first persons to see signs of a communicable disease, such as a rash or sore throat. The nurse must operate under a high index of suspicion for common childhood diseases to identify potentially infectious cases and to recognize diseases that require medical intervention. An example is the common symptom of sore throat. Although most often a symptom of a minor viral infection, it can signal diphtheria or a streptococcal infection, such as scarlet fever. Each of these bacterial conditions requires appropriate medical treatment to prevent serious sequelae.

When a communicable disease is suspected, it is important to assess the following:

- Recent exposure to a known case
- **Prodromal** symptoms (symptoms that occur between early manifestations of the disease and its overt clinical syndrome) or evidence of constitutional symptoms, such as a fever or rash (see Table 37-2)
- Immunization history
- History of having the disease

Immunizations are available for many diseases, and infection usually confers lifelong immunity; therefore, the possibility of many infectious agents can be eliminated on the basis of these two criteria.

Preventing Spread

Prevention consists of two components: prevention of the disease and control of its spread to others. Primary prevention rests almost exclusively on immunization (see Additional Resources at the end of the chapter for a complete immunization schedule). (The nurse's role in immunization of children is discussed in Chapter 35.)

Control measures to prevent the spread of disease should include techniques to reduce the risk of cross-transmission of infectious organisms between patients and to protect health care workers from organisms harboured by patients. If the child is hospitalized, the facility's policies for infection control should be followed (see Chapter 44, Infection Control). The most important procedure is hand hygiene. Persons directly caring for the child or handling contaminated articles must wash their hands and practise effective routine precautions in care of their patients.

The child should be instructed to practise good hand hygiene technique before eating and after toileting. For diseases spread by droplets, the parents should be instructed in measures to reduce airborne transmission. Children who are old enough should use a tissue and then discard it. The nurse needs to stress to the family the usual hygiene measures of not sharing eating and drinking utensils.

NURSING ALERT

If a child is admitted to the hospital with an undiagnosed exanthema, strict additional precautions (contact, airborne, and droplet) and routine precautions are instituted until a diagnosis is confirmed. Childhood communicable diseases requiring these precautions include diphtheria, chickenpox, measles, tuberculosis, adenovirus, *Haemophilus influenzae* type b, influenza, mumps, *Mycoplasma pneumoniae*, pertussis, plague, streptococcal pharyngitis, pneumonia, and scarlet fever (PHAC, 2013).

Text continued on p. 1096

TABLE 37-2 COMMUNICABLE DISEASES OF CHILDHOOD

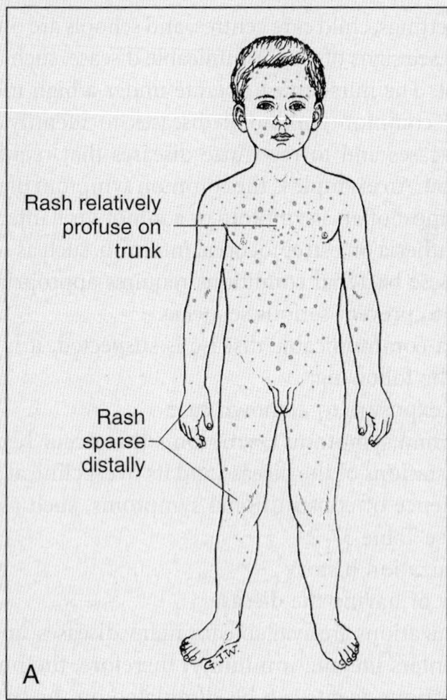

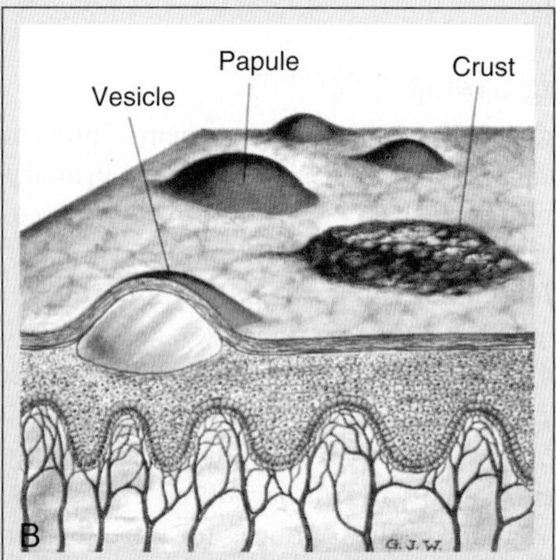

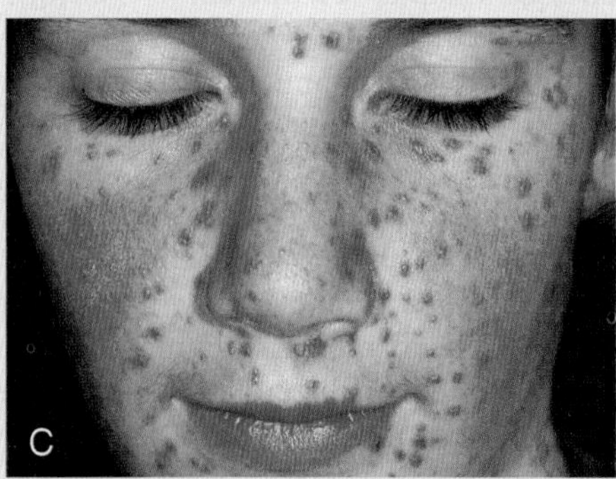

FIGURE 37-8 Chickenpox (varicella). **A:** Progression of disease. **B:** Simultaneous stages of lesions. **C:** Clinical view. (**C,** From Habif, T. P. [2010]. *Clinical dermatology: A color guide to diagnosis and therapy* [5th ed.], St. Louis: Mosby.)

DISEASE

Chickenpox (Varicella) (Fig. 37-8)

Agent—Varicella-zoster virus (VZV)

Source—Primary secretions of respiratory tract of infected persons; to a lesser degree, skin lesions (scabs not infectious)

Transmission—Direct contact, droplet (airborne) spread, and contaminated objects

Incubation period—2–3 wk, usually 14–16 days

Period of communicability—Probably 1–2 days before eruption of lesions (prodromal period) until all lesions have crusted

Diphtheria

Agent—*Corynebacterium dipthitheriae*

Source—Discharges from mucous membranes of nose and nasopharynx, skin, and other lesions of infected person

Transmission—Direct contact with infected person, a carrier, or contaminated articles

Incubation period—Usually 2–5 days, possibly longer

Period of communicability—Variable; until virulent bacilli are no longer present (identified by three negative cultures); usually 2 wk but as long as 4 wk

***Erythema Infectiosum* (Fifth Disease) (Fig. 37-9)**

Agent—Human parvovirus B19

Source—Infected persons, mainly school-age children

Transmission—Respiratory secretions, blood, blood products

Incubation period—4–14 days; may be as long as 21 days

Period of communicability—Uncertain but before onset of symptoms in children with aplastic crisis

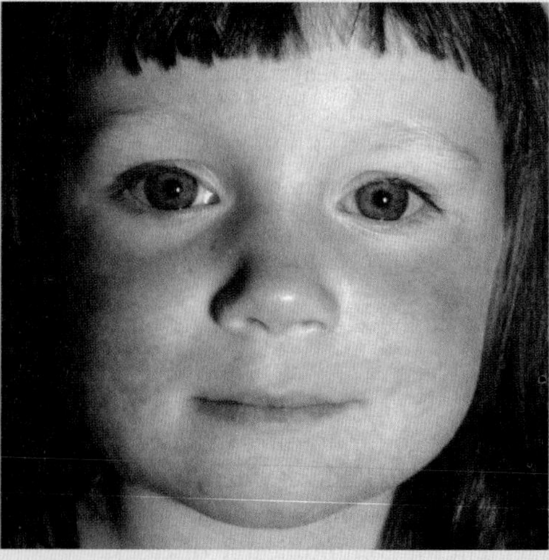

FIGURE 37-9 *Erythema infectiosum* ("Slapped face" appearance). (From Habif, T. P. [2010]. *Clinical dermatology: A color guide to diagnosis and therapy* [5th ed]. St. Louis: Mosby.)

CLINICAL MANIFESTATIONS	THERAPEUTIC MANAGEMENT AND COMPLICATIONS	NURSING CARE
Prodromal stage—Slight fever, malaise, and anorexia for first 24 hr; rash highly pruritic; begins as macule, rapidly progresses to papule and then vesicle (surrounded by erythematous base, becomes umbilicated and cloudy, breaks easily and forms crusts); all three stages (papule, vesicle, crust) present in varying degrees at one time **Distribution**—Centripetal, spreading to face and proximal extremities but sparse on distal limbs and less on areas not exposed to heat (i.e., from clothing or sun) **Constitutional signs and symptoms**—Elevated temperature from lymphadenopathy, irritability from pruritus Breakthrough varicella seen in previously vaccinated; primarily maculopapular, with 50 lesions or fewer that often appear to be insect bites; heals faster than varicella and fever lasts fewer days; one-third less contagious to other people	**Specific**—Antiviral agent acyclovir (Zovirax); varicella-zoster immune globulin (VariZIG) or immune globulin intravenous (IGIV) after exposure in high-risk children **Supportive**—Diphenhydramine hydrochloride or antihistamines to relieve itching; skin care to prevent secondary bacterial infection **Complications**—Secondary bacterial infections (abscesses, cellulitis, necrotizing fasciitis, pneumonia, sepsis) Encephalitis Varicella pneumonia (rare in normal children) Hemorrhagic varicella (tiny hemorrhages in vesicles and numerous petechiae in skin) Chronic or transient thrombocytopenia	Maintain routine, airborne, and contact precautions if hospitalized, until all lesions are crusted; for immunized child with mild breakthrough varicella, isolate until no new lesions are seen. Keep child in home away from susceptible individuals until vesicles have dried (usually 5–7 days after onset of disease), and isolate high-risk children from infected children. Administer skin care; give bath and change clothes and linens daily; administer topical calamine lotion; keep child's fingernails short and clean; apply mittens if child scratches. The goal is to prevent secondary infection and make child comfortable. Administer antipyretics and antihistamine for pruritus. Keep child cool (may decrease number of lesions). Minimize pruritus; keep child distracted; use oatmeal or baking soda baths to minimize pruritus. Remove loose crusts that rub and irritate skin. Teach child to apply pressure to pruritic area rather than scratching it. Avoid use of aspirin (possible association with Reye syndrome). Administer acetaminophen for fever.
Vary according to anatomical location of pseudomembrane **Nasal**—Resembles common cold, serosanguineous mucopurulent nasal discharge without constitutional symptoms; may be frank epistaxis **Tonsillar/pharyngeal**—Malaise; anorexia; sore throat; low-grade fever; pulse increased above that expected for temperature within 24 hr; smooth, adherent, white or grey membrane; lymphadenitis possibly pronounced ("bull's neck"); in severe cases, toxemia, septic shock, and death within 6–10 days **Laryngeal**—Fever, hoarseness, cough, with or without previous signs listed; potential airway obstruction, apprehensive, dyspneic retractions, cyanosis	Equine antitoxin (usually intravenously); preceded by skin or conjunctival test to rule out sensitivity to horse serum Antibiotics (penicillin G procaine or erythromycin) in addition to equine antitoxin Tracheostomy for airway obstruction Treatment of infected contacts and carriers **Complications**—Toxic cardiomyopathy (second to third week) Toxic neuropathy	Follow routine and droplet precautions until two cultures are negative for *C. diphtheriae*; contact precautions with cutaneous manifestations. Administer antibiotics in timely manner. Participate in sensitivity testing; have epinephrine available. Observe respiration for signs of obstruction. Administer humidified oxygen as prescribed.
Rash appearing in three stages: **I**—Erythema on face, chiefly on cheeks, "slapped face" appearance; disappears by 1–4 days (Fig. 37-9) **II**—About 1 day after rash appears on face, maculopapular red spots appear, symmetrically distributed on upper and lower extremities; rash progresses from proximal to distal surfaces and may last a week or more **III**—Rash is subsiding but reappears if skin is irritated or traumatized (sun, heat, cold, friction). In children with aplastic crisis, rash is usually absent and prodromal illness includes fever, myalgia, lethargy, nausea, vomiting, and abdominal pain. Child with sickle cell disease may have concurrent vaso-occlusive crisis.	**Symptomatic and supportive**—Antipyretics, analgesics, anti-inflammatory medications Possible blood transfusion for transient aplastic anemia **Complications**—Self-limited arthritis and arthralgia (arthritis may become chronic); more common in adult women May result in serious complications (anemia, hydrops) or fetal death if mother infected during pregnancy (primarily second trimester) Aplastic crisis in children with hemolytic disease or immunodeficiency Myocarditis (rare)	Isolation of child is not necessary, except hospitalized child (immunosuppressed or with aplastic crises) suspected of parvovirus infection is placed on routine and droplet precautions. Pregnant women need not be excluded from workplace where parvovirus infection is present; they should not care for patients with aplastic crises; explain low risk of fetal death to those in contact with affected children; assist with routine fetal ultrasound for detection of fetal hydrops. Neonate with intrauterine hydrops does not need to be isolated.

Continued

DISEASE

Exanthem Subitum (*Roseola Infantum*; Sixth Disease) (Fig. 37-10)

Agent—Human herpesvirus type 6 (HHV-6; rarely HHV-7)

Source—Possibly acquired from saliva of healthy adult; entry via nasal, buccal, or conjunctival mucosa

Transmission—Year round; no reported contact with infected individual in most cases (virtually limited to children under age 3 yr but peak age is between 6 and 15 mo)

Incubation period—Usually 5–15 days

Period of communicability—Unknown

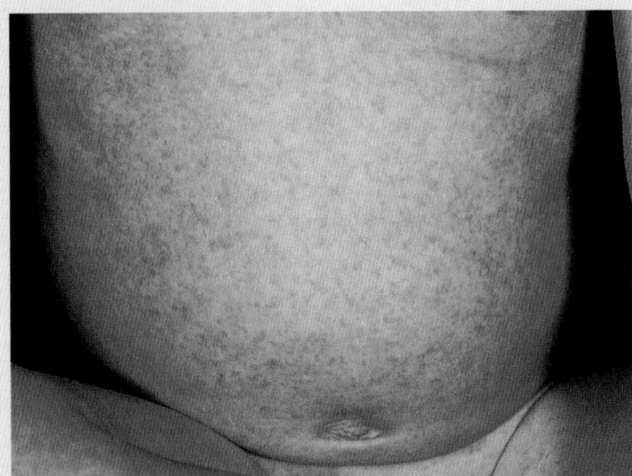

FIGURE 37-10 *Roseola infantum.* (From Habif, T. P. [2010]. *Clinical dermatology: A color guide to diagnosis and therapy* [5th ed]. St. Louis: Mosby.)

Measles (Rubeola) (Fig. 37-11)

Agent—Virus

Source—Respiratory tract secretions, blood, and urine of infected person

Transmission—Usually by direct contact with droplets of infected person; primarily in winter

Incubation period—8–12 days

Period of communicability—From 4 days before to 4 days after rash appears but mainly during prodromal (catarrhal) stage

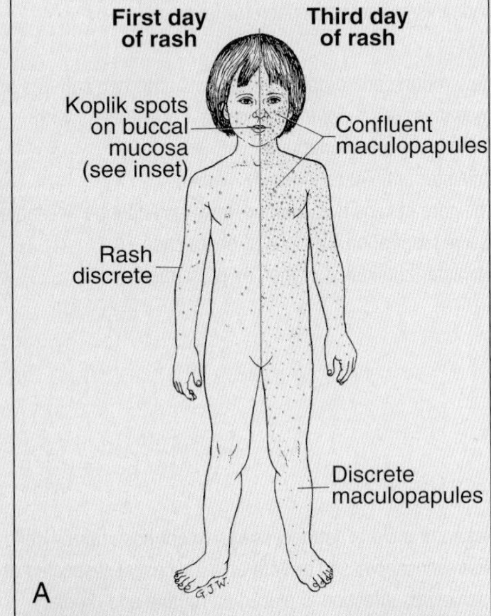

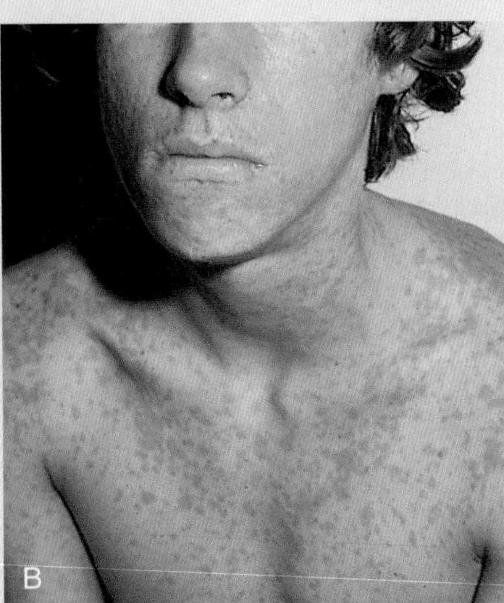

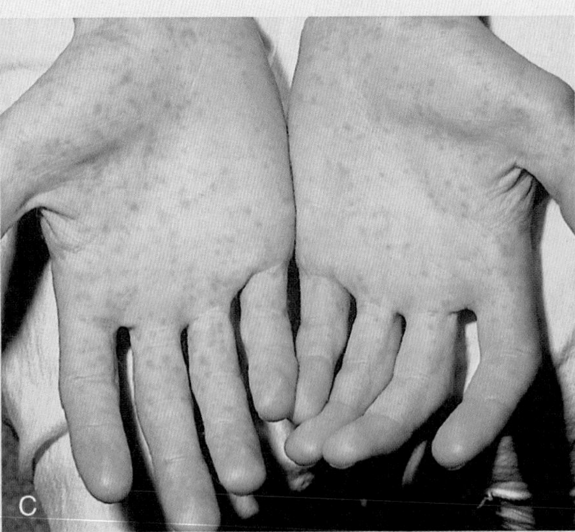

FIGURE 37-11 Measles (rubeola). **A:** Progression of disease. **B:** Exanthem first appears at hairline and spreads from head to toe over 3 days. **C:** Measles ultimately involves palms and soles. (**B** and **C,** from Zitelli, B. J., & Davis, H. W. [2012]. *Atlas of pediatric physical diagnosis* [6th ed.]. St. Louis: Mosby; courtesy Michael Sherlock, M.D., Lurville, MD.)

CLINICAL MANIFESTATIONS	THERAPEUTIC MANAGEMENT AND COMPLICATIONS	NURSING CARE
Persistent high fever for 3–4 days in child who appears well Precipitous drop in fever to normal with appearance of rash **Rash**—Discrete rose-pink macules or maculopapules appearing first on trunk, then spreading to neck, face, and extremities; nonpruritic, fades on pressure, lasts 1–2 days **Associated signs and symptoms**—Cervical/postauricular lymphadenopathy, inflamed pharynx, cough, coryza	Nonspecific Antipyretics to control fever **Complications**—Recurrent febrile seizures (possibly from latent infection of central nervous system that is reactivated by fever) Encephalitis, myocarditis, hepatitis, acute cerebellitis (all rare)	Teach parents measures for lowering temperature (antipyretic medications); ensure adequate parental understanding of specific antipyretic dosage to prevent accidental overdose. If child is prone to seizures, discuss appropriate precautions and possibility of recurrent febrile seizures. Ensure adequate oral fluid intake.
Prodromal (catarrhal) stage—Fever and malaise, followed in 24 hr by coryza, cough, conjunctivitis, Koplik's spots (small, irregular red spots with a minute, bluish white centre first seen on buccal mucosa opposite molars 2 days before rash); symptoms gradually increasing in severity until second day after rash appears, when they begin to subside (Fig. 37-11, A) **Rash**—Appears 3–4 days after onset of prodromal stage; begins as erythematous maculopapular eruption on face and gradually spreads downward; more severe in earlier sites (appears confluent) and less intense in later sites (appears discrete); after 3–4 days assumes brownish appearance, and fine desquamation occurs over area of extensive involvement **Constitutional signs and symptoms**—Anorexia, abdominal pain, malaise, generalized lymphadenopathy	Vitamin A supplementation for children with acute illness (see p. 1098) **Supportive**—Bedrest during febrile period; antipyretics Antibiotics to prevent secondary bacterial infection in high-risk children **Complications**—Otitis media Pneumonia (bacterial) Obstructive laryngitis and laryngotracheitis Encephalitis (rare but has high mortality)	Isolate until fourth day of rash; if hospitalized, institute droplet precautions. Encourage rest during prodromal stage; provide quiet activity. **Fever**—Instruct parents to administer antipyretics; avoid chilling; if child is prone to seizures, institute appropriate precautions. **Eye care**—Dim lights if photophobia present; clean eyelids with warm saline solution to remove secretions or crusts; keep child from rubbing eyes. **Coryza, cough**—Use cool-mist vaporizer; protect skin around nares with layer of petrolatum; encourage fluids and soft, bland foods. **Skin care**—Keep skin clean.

Continued

TABLE 37-2 COMMUNICABLE DISEASES OF CHILDHOOD—cont'd

DISEASE

Mumps

Agent—Paramyxovirus

Source—Saliva of infected persons

Transmission—Direct contact with other droplet spread from an infected person

Incubation period—16–18 days

Period of communicability—Most communicable immediately before and after swelling begins

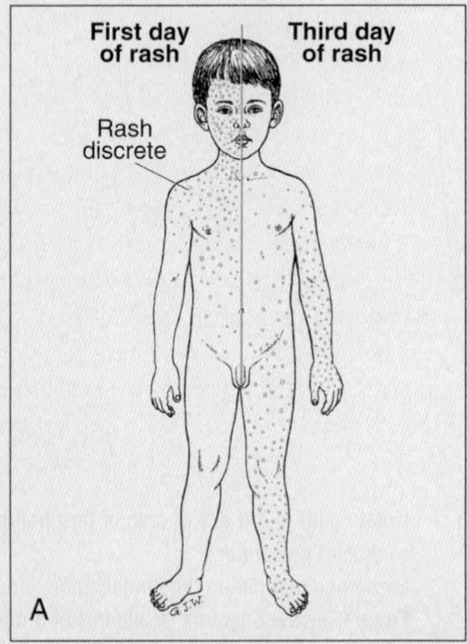

B

FIGURE 37-12 Rubella (German measles). **A:** Progression of rash. **B:** Clinical view. (**B,** from Zitelli, B. J., & Davis, H. W. [2012]. *Atlas of pediatric physical diagnosis* [6th ed.]. St. Louis: Mosby; courtesy Michael Sherlock, MD, Lurville, MD.)

Pertussis (Whooping Cough)

Agent—*Bordetella pertussis*

Source—Discharge from respiratory tract of infected person

Transmission—Direct contact or droplet spread from infected person; indirect contact with freshly contaminated articles

Incubation period—7–10 days, range 5–21 days

Period of communicability—Greatest during catarrhal stage and the first 2 weeks after cough onset

Rubella (German Measles) (Fig. 37-12)

Agent—Rubella virus

Source—Primarily nasopharyngeal secretions of person with apparent or inapparent infection; virus also present in blood, stool, and urine

Incubation period—14–21 days

Period of communicability—2–3 days before to about 7 days after appearance of rash

CLINICAL MANIFESTATIONS	THERAPEUTIC MANAGEMENT AND COMPLICATIONS	NURSING CARE
Prodromal stage—Fever, headache, malaise, and anorexia for 24 hr, followed by "earache" that is aggravated by chewing **Parotitis**—Parotid gland(s) (either unilateral or bilateral) enlarges and reaches maximum size in 1–3 days; accompanied by pain and tenderness; or exocrine glands (submandibular) may also be swollen	**Symptomatic and supportive**—Analgesics for pain and antipyretics for fever Intravenous fluid may be necessary for child refusing to drink or child vomiting because of meningoencephalitis **Complications**—Sensorineural deafness Postinfectious encephalitis Myocarditis Arthritis Hepatitis Orchitis Oophoritis Pancreatitis Sterility (extremely rare in adult males) Meningitis Thyroiditis (rare)	Isolate during period of communicability; institute droplet and contact precautions during hospitalization. Encourage rest and decreased activity during prodromal phase until swelling subsides. Give analgesics for pain; if child is unable to swallow pills or tablets medication, use elixir form. Encourage fluids and soft, bland foods; avoid foods requiring chewing. Apply hot or cold compresses to neck or groin, whichever are more comforting.
Catarrhal stage—Begins with symptoms of upper respiratory tract infection, such as coryza, sneezing, lacrimation, cough, and low-grade fever; symptoms continue for 1–2 wk, when dry, hacking cough becomes more severe **Paroxysmal stage**—Cough most often occurs at night and consists of short, rapid coughs followed by sudden inspiration associated with a high-pitched crowing sound or "whoop"; during paroxysms, cheeks become flushed or cyanotic, eyes bulge, and tongue protrudes; paroxysm may continue until thick mucous plug is dislodged; vomiting frequently follows attack; stage generally lasts 4–6 wk, followed by convalescent stage. Infants under 6 mo of age may not have characteristic whoop cough, but have difficulty maintaining adequate oxygenation with amount of secretions, frequent vomiting of mucus and formula or breast milk (see also Chapter 39, Immunizations, for discussion of pertussis in adolescents).	Antimicrobial therapy (e.g., erythromycin, clarithromycin, azithromycin) **Supportive treatment**—Hospitalization sometimes required for infants, children who are dehydrated, or those who have complications Supplemental oxygen Adequate fluid intake Intensive care and mechanical ventilation may be necessary for infant <6 mo **Complications**—Pneumonia (usual cause of death) Atelectasis Otitis media Seizures Hemorrhage (scleral, conjunctival, epistaxis; pulmonary hemorrhage in neonate) Weight loss and dehydration Hernias (umbilical and inguinal) Prolapsed rectum	Isolate during catarrhal stage; if hospitalized, institute droplet and routine precautions. Obtain nasopharyngeal culture for diagnosis. Encourage oral fluids; offer small amount of fluids frequently. Ensure adequate oxygenation during paroxysms; position infant on side to decrease chance of aspiration with vomiting. Provide high humidity (humidifier); suction as needed to prevent choking on secretions. Observe for signs of airway obstruction (infants), such as increased restlessness, apprehension, retractions, cyanosis. Encourage household contacts to complete antibiotic therapy. Encourage adolescents to obtain pertussis booster (Tdap) (see also Chapter 39, Immunizations). Health care workers should use routine precautions when exposed to children with persistent cough and high suspicion of pertussis.
Constitutional signs and symptoms—Occasionally low-grade fever, headache, malaise, and lymphadenopathy **Prodromal stage**—Absent in children, present in adults and adolescents; consists of low-grade fever, headache, malaise, anorexia, mild conjunctivitis, coryza, sore throat, cough, and lymphadenopathy; lasts 1–5 days, subsides 1 day after appearance of rash **Rash**—First appears on face and rapidly spreads downward to neck, arms, trunk, and legs; by end of first day, body is covered with discrete, pinkish red maculopapular exanthema; disappears in same order as it began and is usually gone by third day	No treatment necessary other than antipyretics for low-grade fever and analgesics for discomfort **Complications**—Rare (arthritis, encephalitis, or purpura); most benign of all childhood communicable diseases but can be serious for some children; greatest danger is teratogenic effect on fetus; miscarriage and fetal death may occur	Reassure parents of benign nature of illness in affected child. Use comfort measures as necessary. Avoid contact with pregnant women and unimmunized or immunocompromised children. Monitor rubella titre in pregnant adolescent. Routine precautions for hospitalized child; droplet precautions for 7 days after onset of rash. Contact isolation for infant with suspected or confirmed congenital rubella or until two cultures are negative for rubella.

Continued

TABLE 37-2 COMMUNICABLE DISEASES OF CHILDHOOD—cont'd

DISEASE
Scarlet Fever (Fig. 37-13) **Agent**—Group A *β-hemolytic streptococci* (GAS) **Source**—Usually from nasopharyngeal secretions of infected persons and carriers **Transmission**—Direct contact with infected person or droplet spread; indirectly by contact with contaminated articles or ingestion of contaminated milk or other food **Incubation period**—2–5 days, with range of 1–7 days **Period of communicability**—During incubation period and clinical illness, approximately 10 days; during first 2 wk of carrier phase, although may persist for months Severe cases now rare

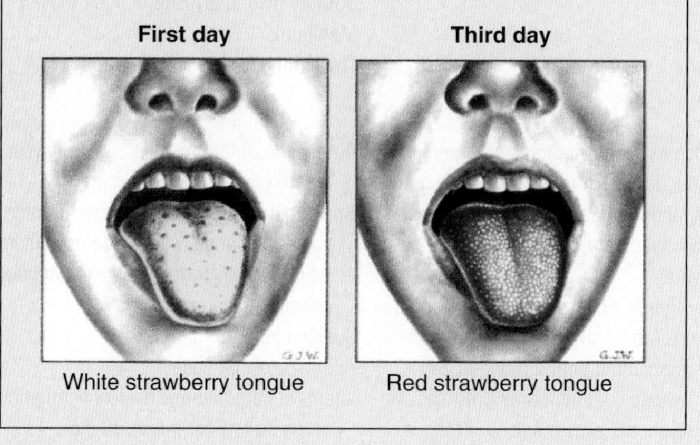

FIGURE 37-13 Scarlet fever.

Preventing Complications

Although most children recover without difficulty, certain groups are at risk for serious, even fatal, complications from communicable diseases, especially the viral diseases chickenpox and *erythema infectiosum* (fifth disease) caused by human parvovirus B19.

Children with immunodeficiency—those receiving steroid or other immunosuppressive therapy, those with a generalized malignancy such as leukemia or lymphoma, or those with an immunological disorder—are at risk for viremia from replication of the varicella-zoster virus (VZV) in the blood. VZV is so named because it causes two distinct diseases: varicella (chickenpox) and zoster (herpes zoster, or shingles). Varicella occurs primarily in children younger than 15 years of age. However, it leaves the threat of herpes zoster, an intensely painful varicella that is localized to a single dermatome (body area innervated by a particular segment of the spinal cord). In children, the dermatomes most likely affected by herpes zoster are the cervical and sacral dermatomes (Leung, Robson, & Leong, 2006). Immunocompromised patients and healthy infants younger than 1 year of age (who also have reduced immunity) are at a higher risk for reactivation of VZV causing herpes zoster, probably as a result of a deficiency in cellular immunity (American Academy of Pediatrics [AAP], Committee on Infectious Diseases, & Pickering, et al., 2015). One population-based study found that the incidence of herpes zoster infection in children was rare; rates were higher among children vaccinated after 5 years of age (versus those vaccinated at 12 to 18 months of age), children with severe asthma, or those with developmental disorders (Tseng, Smith, Marcy, et al., 2009). Complications of herpes zoster virus in children include secondary bacterial infection, depigmentation, and scarring. Postherpetic neuralgia in children is uncommon. Fetal infection after maternal varicella, especially if infection occurs before the twentieth week of gestation, may be fatal or result in congenital varicella syndrome. Varicella infection occurring in infants exposed to maternal varicella from a period 5 days before birth to 2 days after birth have an increased likelihood of becoming infected and should be treated with varicella-zoster immunoglobulin intravenous (IGIV) (AAP et al., 2012).

The use of varicella-zoster immune globulin (VariZIG) or IGIV is recommended for children who are immunocompromised, who have no previous history of varicella, and who are likely to contract the disease and have complications as a result (Salvadori & CPS, Infectious Diseases and Immunization Committee, 2005/2014). The antiviral agent acyclovir (Zovirax) may be used to treat varicella infections in susceptible immunocompromised persons; it is effective in decreasing the number of

CLINICAL MANIFESTATIONS	THERAPEUTIC MANAGEMENT AND COMPLICATIONS	NURSING CARE
Prodromal stage—Abrupt high fever, pulse increased out of proportion to fever, vomiting, headache, chills, malaise, abdominal pain, halitosis Tonsils enlarged, edematous, reddened, and covered with patches of exudates; in severe cases appearance resembles membrane seen in diphtheria; pharynx edematous and beefy red; during first 1–2 days tongue coated and papillae become red and swollen (white strawberry tongue); by fourth or fifth day white coat sloughs off, leaving prominent papillae (red strawberry tongue); palate covered with erythematous punctate lesions **Exanthema**—Rash appears within 12 hr after prodromal signs; red pinhead-sized punctate lesions rapidly become generalized but are absent on face, which becomes flushed with striking circumoral pallor; rash more intense in folds of joints; by end of first week desquamation begins (fine, sandpaper-like on torso; sheetlike sloughing on palms and soles), which may be complete by 3 wk or longer	**Treatment of choice**—Full course of penicillin (or erythromycin in penicillin-sensitive children), or oral cephalosporin **Supportive measures**—Rest during febrile phase, analgesics for sore throat; antipruritics for rash if bothersome **Complications**—Peritonsillar and retropharyngeal abscess Sinusitis Otitis media Acute glomerulonephritis Acute rheumatic fever Polyarthritis (uncommon) Toxic shock syndrome Osteomyelitis	Institute routine and droplet precautions until 24 hr after initiation of treatment. Ensure compliance with oral antibiotic therapy; intramuscular benzathine penicillin G [Bicillin] may be given if difficulty in giving oral medications as prescribed. Encourage rest during febrile phase; provide quiet activity during convalescent period. Relieve discomfort of sore throat with analgesics, gargles, lozenges, and antiseptic throat sprays. Encourage oral fluids during febrile phase; avoid irritating liquids (certain citrus juices) or rough foods (chips); when child is able to eat, begin with soft diet. Advise parents to consult practitioner if fever persists after beginning therapy. Discuss procedures for preventing spread of infection—discard toothbrush; avoid sharing drinking and eating utensils. Monitor for sequelae of GAS-acute rheumatic fever and acute glomerulonephritis.

lesions, shortening the duration of fever, and decreasing itching, lethargy, and anorexia. The CPS (Salvadori & CPS, Infectious Diseases and Immunization Committee, 2005/2014) recommends that oral acyclovir be considered for immunocompromised children who cannot receive VariZIG.

Children with hemolytic disease, such as sickle cell disease, are at risk for aplastic anemia from *erythema infectiosum*. Human parvovirus B19 (fifth disease) infects and lyses red blood cell (RBC) precursors, thus interrupting the production of RBCs. Thus the virus may precipitate a severe aplastic crisis in patients who need increased RBC production to maintain normal RBC volumes. Thrombocytopenia and neutropenia may also occur as a result of human parvovirus B19 infection. Fetuses have a relatively high rate of RBC production and immature immune systems; they may develop severe anemia and hydrops as a result of maternal human parvovirus infection. Fetal death rates as a result of human parvovirus B19 have been estimated to be between 2 and 6% (AAP et al., 2012).

The past decade has seen an increase in the incidence of pertussis, particularly in infants less than 6 months old and children 10 to 14 years of age. Early clinical manifestations of pertussis in infants may include gagging, coughing, emesis, and apnea; the typical whooping cough associated with the disease is absent (The Hospital for Sick Children, 2014). In older children, the disease may manifest as a common cold (see Table 37-2). It is now recommended that children ages 11 to 18 receive a booster pertussis vaccine (Tdap—tetanus, diphtheria, pertussis) to prevent the disease (see Chapter 39, Immunizations). Because pertussis is contagious, especially among close household members, pertussis should be identified early and treatment initiated for the child and those who have been exposed. Azithromycin (for infants under 1 month) and erythromycin are administered to infants and children with pertussis. Although the risk of contracting hypertrophic pyloric stenosis is increased in infants younger than 1 month old taking azithromycin, it remains the drug of choice for the treatment of pertussis in this age group (AAP et al., 2012).

Prevention of complications from diseases such as diphtheria, pertussis, and scarlet fever requires adherence to antibiotic therapy. With oral preparations, the need to complete the entire course of therapy needs to be stressed.

There is evidence that vitamin A supplementation reduces both morbidity and mortality in individuals with measles and that all children with severe measles should be given vitamin A supplements. A single oral dose of 200,000 International Units (6000 mcg) for children at least 1 year old (or half that dose for children 6 to 12 months of age) is recommended. The higher dose may be associated with vomiting and headache for a few hours. The dose should be repeated the next day and only repeated for a third time at 4 weeks if the child has ophthalmological evidence of vitamin A deficiency (AAP et al., 2012).

NURSING ALERT

Although the risk of vitamin A toxicity from these doses (they are 100 to 200 times the recommended dietary allowance) is relatively low, nurses should instruct parents on safe storage of the medication. Ideally, vitamin A should be dispensed in the age-appropriate unit dose, to prevent excessive administration and possible toxicity.

Providing Comfort

Many communicable diseases cause skin manifestations that are bothersome to the child. The chief discomfort from most rashes is itching, and measures such as cool baths (usually without soap) and lotions (e.g., calamine) are helpful.

NURSING ALERT

When lotions with active ingredients such as diphenhydramine in Caladryl are used, they should be applied sparingly, especially over open lesions, where excessive absorption can lead to drug toxicity. These lotions should be used with caution in children who are simultaneously receiving an oral antihistamine. Cooling the lotion in the refrigerator beforehand often makes it more soothing on the skin than using it at room temperature.

To avoid overheating, which increases itching, children should wear lightweight, loose, nonirritating clothing and keep out of the sun. If the child persists in scratching, the nails should be kept short and smooth; mittens and clothes with long sleeves or legs may be needed. For severe itching, antipruritic medication, such as diphenhydramine (Benadryl) or hydroxyzine (Atarax), may be required, especially when the child has trouble sleeping because of itching. Loratadine, cetirizine, and fexofenadine do not cause drowsiness and may be preferred for urticaria during the day.

An elevated temperature is common, and both antipyretic medicine (acetaminophen or ibuprofen) and environmental manipulation should be implemented (see Chapter 44, Controlling Elevated Temperatures). The acetaminophen is effective in lowering the fever but does not significantly reduce the symptoms of itching, anorexia, abdominal pain, fussiness, or vomiting.

A sore throat, another frequent symptom, is managed with lozenges, saline rinses (if the child is old enough to assist), and analgesics. Because most children have a decreased appetite during an illness, bland foods and increased liquids are usually preferred. During the early stages of the disease, children voluntarily curtail their activity, and although bedrest is beneficial, it should not be imposed unless specifically indicated. During periods of irritability, quiet activity (e.g., reading, music, television, video games, puzzles, colouring) helps distract children from the discomfort.

Supporting Child and Family

Most communicable diseases are benign but may produce considerable concern and anxiety for parents. Often the occurrence of a disease such as chickenpox is the first time the child is acutely uncomfortable. Parents need assistance to cope with manifestations of the illness, such as intense itching. The family and child need reassurance that recovery is generally rapid. However, visible signs of the dermatosis may be present for some time after the child is well enough to resume usual activities.

NURSING ALERT

The occurrence of a communicable disease provides the opportunity to ask parents about the child's immunization status and reinforce the benefits of vaccines for children. The Canadian Paediatric Society (MacDonald, Bortolussi, & CPS, Infectious Diseases and Immunization Committee, 2011/2014) notes the urgent need for a national harmonized immunization schedule for Canada. Although the Public Health Agency of Canada (2016) has a minimum immunization schedule, each province and territory has variable schedules, which can be confusing and put the public at risk (see Additional Resources at the end of the chapter).

KEY POINTS

- The preschool years consist of the period from 3 to 5 years of age, a time considered critical for emotional and psychological development.
- Biological development in the preschool period is characterized by mature body systems and refinement in gross and fine motor behaviour, as evidenced by activities such as running, riding a tricycle, and drawing.
- According to Erikson, acquiring a sense of initiative is the chief psychosocial task of the preschooler. Development of the superego occurs during this period, as conscience begins to emerge.
- According to Piaget, the preschool age is characterized by intuitive (or prelogical) thinking and a move toward logical thought processes through advanced, complex learning; language; and understanding of causality.
- The seeds of moral development are planted during the preschool period. According to Kohlberg, these children are in the stage of naive instrumental orientation, in which they are concerned with satisfying their own needs and, less frequently, the needs of others.
- Social development includes further separation–individuation; more sophisticated language; greater independence; and more complex, imaginative forms of play.
- Areas of special concern to parents during the preschool period are the preschool and kindergarten experience, sex education, fears, stress, and speech problems.

- In selecting an early learning program, parents should inquire about daily activities, teacher qualifications, accreditation, student–staff ratio, safety, meals, fees, and health practices.
- Two rules that govern how parents answer questions about sex and other sensitive issues are to find out what the children know and to be honest.
- Fears constitute a great part of the preschool period; fear of objects or potential annihilation and parent-induced fears are common.
- Preschool aggression may result from frustration, modelling behaviour, and reinforcement.
- Hesitancy or dysfluency in speech patterns is a normal characteristic of language development. Speech problems can occur when parents express excessive concern over this pattern.
- Preschoolers can exhibit early signs of mental health issues, which include ongoing behaviour changes that affect how children function, such as fluctuations in mood, energy levels, sleep patterns, attitude, and appetite.
- Health promotion continues to be directed toward proper nutrition, adequate sleep, proper dental care, and injury prevention.

evolve WEBSITE

Visit the Evolve website for additional resources related to the content in this chapter such as Case Studies, Critical Thinking Case Study Answers, Nursing Care Plans, Nursing Processes, Nursing Skills, and Review Questions for Exam Preparation at: http://evolve.elsevier.com/Canada/Perry/maternal/

REFERENCES

American Academy of Pediatrics (AAP), Committee on Infectious Diseases, Pickering, L., Baker, C. J., et al. (Eds.). (2015). *2015 red book: Report of the Committee on Infectious Diseases* (30th ed.). Elk Grove Village, IL: Author.

American Speech-Language-Hearing Association. (n.d.). *Learning two languages*. Retrieved from <http://www.asha.org/public/speech/development/BilingualChildren/>.

Benzies, K., Keown, L. A., & Magill-Evans, J. (2009). Immediate and sustained effects of parenting on physical aggression in Canadian children aged 6 years and younger. *Canadian Journal of Psychiatry*, *54*(1), 55–64.

Canadian Association of Speech-Language Pathologists and Audiologists. (n.d.). *Preschool stuttering*. Retrieved from <http://sac-oac.ca/sites/default/files/resources/Preschool-Stuttering.pdf>.

Cleveland, G., Forer, B., Hyatt, D., et al. (2008). New evidence about child care in Canada: Use patterns, affordability and quality. *Institute for Research on Public Policy Choices*, 14.

Dietitians of Canada. (2014). *Tips on feeding your picky toddler or preschooler*. Retrieved from <http://www.dietitians.ca/Downloads/Factsheets/Tips-Feeding-Picky-Toddler.aspx>.

Erikson, E. H. (1963). *Childhood and society* (2nd ed.). New York: Norton.

Feigelman, S. (2016). The preschool years. In R. M. Kliegman, B. F. Stanton, J. W. St. Geme, et al. (Eds.), *Nelson textbook of pediatrics* (20th ed.). Philadelphia: Saunders.

Hamer, M., Stamatakis, E., & Mishra, G. (2009). Psychological distress, television viewing, and physical activity in children aged 4 to 12 years. *Pediatrics*, *123*(5), 1263–1268. doi:10.1542/peds.2008-1523.

Harrison, L. J., & McLeod, S. (2010). Risk and protective factors associated with speech and language impairment in a nationally representative sample of 4- to 5-year-old children. *Journal of Speech, Language, and Hearing Research*, *53*(2), 508–529. doi:10.1044/1092-4388(2009/08-0086).

Health Canada. (2007). *Eating well with Canada's food guide: How much food you need every day*. Retrieved from <http://www.hc-sc.gc.ca/fn-an/food-guide-aliment/basics-base/quantit-eng.php>.

Health Canada. (2011). *Aboriginal head start on reserve*. Retrieved from <http://www.hc-sc.gc.ca/fniah-spnia/famil/develop/ahsor-papa_intro-eng.php>.

Health Canada. (2012). *Vitamin D and calcium: Updated dietary reference intakes*. Retrieved from <http://www.hc-sc.gc.ca/fn-an/nutrition/vitamin/vita-d-eng.php#t5>.

Health Canada. (2014). *Estimated energy requirements: Canada's food guide*. Retrieved from <http://hc-sc.gc.ca/fn-an/food-guide-aliment/basics-base/1_1_1-eng.php>.

The Hospital for Sick Children. (2014). *About kids' health. Pertussis (whooping cough)*. Retrieved from <http://www.aboutkidshealth.ca/En/HealthAZ/ConditionsandDiseases/InfectiousDiseases/Pages/Pertussis-Whooping-Cough.aspx>.

Katzmarzyk, P. T. (2008). Obesity and physical activity among Aboriginal Canadians. *Obesity*, *16*(1), 184–190. doi:10.1044/1092-4388(2009/08-0086).

Kirkorian, H. L., Wartella, E. A., & Anderson, D. R. (2008). Media and young children's learning. *The Future of Children*, *18*(1), 39–61.

Leung, A. K., Robson, W. L., & Leong, A. G. (2006). Herpes zoster in childhood. *Journal of Pediatric Health Care*, *20*(5), 300–303.

Lillard, A. S., & Peterson, J. (2011). The immediate impact of different types of television on young children's executive function. *Pediatrics*, *128*(4), 644–649. doi:10.1542/peds.2010-1919.

Lipnowski, S., LeBlanc, C. M., & Canadian Paediatric Society, Healthy Active Living and Sports Medicine. (2012). Healthy active living: Physical activity guidelines for children and adolescents. *Paediatrics & Child Health*, *17*(2), 209–210. Retrieved from <http://www.cps.ca/documents/position/physical-activity-guidelines>.

MacDonald, N. E., Bortolussi, R., & Canadian Paediatric Society, Infectious Diseases and Immunization Committee. (2011). A harmonized immunization schedule for Canada: A call for action. *Paediatrics & Child Health*, *16*(1), 29–31. Reaffirmed 2014. Retrieved from <http://www.cps.ca/documents/position/harmonized-immunization-schedule-Canada>.

Mindell, J. A., Kuhn, B., Lewin, D. S., et al. (2006). Behavioral treatment of bedtime problems and night wakings in infants and young children. *Sleep*, *29*(10), 1263–1276.

Moore, M., Meltzer, L. J., & Mindell, J. A. (2008). Bedtime problems and night wakings in children. *Primary Care*, *35*(3), 569–581, viii. doi:10.1016/j.pop.2008.06.002.

Nieman, P., & Canadian Paediatric Society, Psychosocial Paediatrics Committee. (2003). Impact of media use on children and youth. *Paediatrics & Child Health*, *8*(5), 301–306. Reaffirmed 2011.

Ostrov, J. M., & Bishop, C. M. (2008). Preschoolers' aggression and parent-child conflict: A multi-informant and multimethod study. *Journal of Experimental Child Psychology*, *99*(4), 309–322. doi:10.1016/j.jecp.2008.01.001.

Ostrov, J. M., Gentile, D. A., & Crick, N. R. (2006). Media exposure, aggression and prosocial behavior during early childhood: A longitudinal study. *Social Development*, *15*(4), 612–627. doi:10.1111/j.1467-9507.2006.00360.x.

Piaget, J. (1952). *Origins of intelligence in children*. New York: International Universities Press.

Public Health Agency of Canada. (2010). *Canadian Health Measures Survey results—Oral health statistics, 2007–2009.* Retrieved from <http://www.phac-aspc.gc.ca/publicat/hpcdp-pspmc/30-4/preface2-eng.php>.

Public Health Agency of Canada. (2013). *The Chief Public Health Officer's report on the state of public health in Canada, 2013. Infectious disease—The never-ending threat.* Retrieved from <http://www.phac-aspc.gc.ca/cphorsphc-respcacsp/2013/infections-eng.php#a8>.

Public Health Agency of Canada. (2016). *Canadian immunization guide.* Retrieved from <http://www.phac-aspc.gc.ca/publicat/cig-gci/p01-12-eng.php>.

Reilly, S., Wake, M., Ukoumunne, O. C., et al. (2010). Predicting language outcomes at 4 years of age: Findings from Early Language in Victoria Study. *Pediatrics, 126*(6), 1530–1537. doi:10.1542/peds.2010-0254.

Rowan-Legg, A., & Canadian Paediatric Society, Community Paediatrics Committee. (2013). Oral health care for children—a call for action. *Paediatrics & Child Health, 18*(1), 37–43.

Salvadori, M. I., & Canadian Paediatric Society, Infectious Diseases and Immunization Committee. (2005). Prevention of varicella in children and adolescents. *Paediatrics & Child Health, 10*(7), 409–412. Reaffirmed 2014. Retrieved from <http://www.cps.ca/documents/position/preventing-varicella>.

Sharp, H. M., & Hillenbrand, K. (2008). Speech and language development and disorders in children. *Pediatric Clinics of North America, 5*, 1159–1173, viii. doi:10.1016/j.pcl.2008.07.007.

Skouteris, H., McCabe, M., Swinburn, B., et al. (2010). Healthy eating and obesity prevention for preschoolers: A randomised controlled trial. *BMC Public Health, 28*(10), 220. doi:10.1186/1471-2458-10-220.

Stanwick, R., & Canadian Paediatric Society, Injury Prevention Committee. (2004). Recommendations for snowmobile safety. *Paediatrics & Child Health, 9*(9), 639–642. Reaffirmed 2013. Retrieved from <http://www.cps.ca/en/documents/position/snowmobile-safety>.

Tremblay, M. S., Leblanc, A. G., Carson, V., et al. (2012). Canadian sedentary behaviour guidelines for the early years (aged 0–4 years). *Applied Physiology, Nutrition, and Metabolism, 37*(2), 370–391. doi:10.1139/h2012-019.

Trionfi, G., & Reese, E. (2009). A good story: Children with imaginary companions create richer narratives. *Child Development, 80*(4), 1301–1313. doi:10.1111/j.1467-8624.2009.01333.x.

Tseng, H. F., Smith, N., Marcy, S. M., et al. (2009). Incidence of herpes zoster among children vaccinated with varicella vaccine in a prepaid health care plan in the United States, 2002–2008. *Pediatric Infectious Disease Journal, 28*(12), 1069–1072. doi:10.1097/INF.0b013e3181acf84f.

ADDITIONAL RESOURCES

Action Canada for Sexual Health and Rights: <http://www.sexualhealthandrights.ca/topics/#comprehensive-sexuality-education>.

Canadian Physical Activity Guidelines and Canadian Sedentary Behaviour Guidelines: <http://www.csep.ca/cmfiles/guidelines/csep_guidelines_handbook.pdf>.

Canadian Society for Exercise Physiology—Recommendations for healthy television viewing: <http://www.csep.ca/CMFiles/Guidelines/SBGuidelinesBackgrounder_EY2012_E.pdf>.

Canada's Provincial and Territorial Routine (and Catch-up) Vaccination Programs for Infants and Children: <http://healthycanadians.gc.ca/healthy-living-vie-saine/immunization-immunisation/schedule-calendrier/infants-children-vaccination-enfants-nourrissons-eng.php>.

Encyclopedia of Early Childhood Development—Information on Canadian child development and behaviour: <http://www.child-encyclopedia.com/en-ca/child-aggression/perspectives.html?RId=CA&CId=169>.

Human Early Learning Partnerships (HELP): <http://www.earlylearning.ubc.ca>.

Kids Help Phone—Phone line that children can call to reach a counsellor, 24 hours a day, across Canada: <http://www.kidshelpphone.ca/teens/home/splash.aspx>; phone 1-888-668-6868.

Nipissing District Developmental Screen: <http://www.ndds.ca/canada/>.

Public Health Agency of Canada—Provincial and Territorial Immunization Schedule: <http://healthycanadians.gc.ca/healthy-living-vie-saine/immunization-immunisation/children-enfants/alt/schedule-calendrier-table-1-eng.pdf>.

Teacher Created Resources—Quick and fun learning activities books (suggestions on mutual play): <http://www.teachercreated.com>.

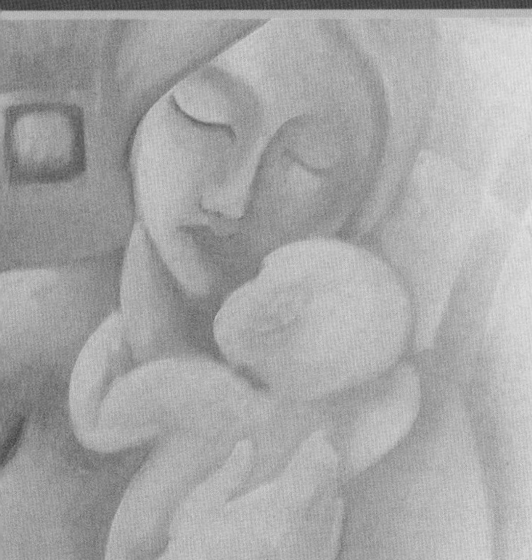

CHAPTER 38

The School-Age Child and Family

Cheryl Sams, with contributions from Marilyn J. Hockenberry

evolve WEBSITE

Visit the Evolve website for additional resources related to the content in this chapter such as Case Studies, Critical Thinking Case Study Answers, Nursing Care Plans, Nursing Processes, Nursing Skills, and Review Questions for Exam Preparation at: http://evolve.elsevier.com/Canada/Perry/maternal/

OBJECTIVES

On completion of this chapter the reader will be able to:

- Describe the physical, cognitive, and moral changes that take place during the middle childhood years.
- Describe ways to help a child develop a sense of accomplishment.
- Demonstrate an understanding of the changing interpersonal relationships of school-age children.
- Discuss the role of the peer group in the socialization of the school-age child.
- Discuss the role of schools in the development and socialization of the school-age child.
- Demonstrate an understanding of the types, causes, and prevention of sports injuries in middle childhood.
- Describe the most common causes of growth and maturation failure in later childhood.
- Discuss the manifestations and nursing management of selected emotional and behavioural problems.
- Outline an appropriate health teaching plan for the school-age child.
- Plan a sex education session for a group of school-age children.
- Identify the causes and discuss the preventive aspects of injury in middle childhood.
- Describe health concerns of particular relevance to school-age children of Indigenous background.

PROMOTING OPTIMUM GROWTH AND DEVELOPMENT

The segment of the lifespan that extends from age 6 years to approximately 12 years has a variety of labels, each of which describes an important characteristic of the period. These middle years are most often referred to as *school-age* or the *school years*. This period begins with entrance into the school environment, which has a significant impact on children's development and relationships. While the biological, social, emotional, and cognitive changes discussed throughout the chapter help us understand development during the school-age years, limiting our attention to these aspects of children's lives may divert attention from vital differences affecting health and well-being. School-age children vary in many ways according to race, gender, ethnicity, and class, and these differences have important implications. Thus, in this chapter, growth and development in the school-age years are discussed within the context of these differences. Also addressed is how nurses can support children and their families in ways that attend to diversity while acknowledging the developmental changes that are ongoing in these children's lives.

Biological Development

Physiologically the middle years begin with the shedding of the first deciduous tooth and end at puberty with the acquisition of the final permanent teeth (with the exception of the wisdom teeth). Before 5 or 6 years of age, children have progressed from helpless infants to sturdy, complicated individuals with an ability to communicate, conceptualize in a limited way, and become involved in complex social and motor behaviours. Physical growth is also rapid during the preschool-age years. In contrast, the period of middle childhood, between the rapid growth of early childhood and the prepubescent growth spurt, is a time of gradual growth and development with more even progress in both physical and emotional aspects.

During middle childhood, growth in height and weight assumes a slower but steady pace as compared with that of the earlier years. Between ages 6 and 12, children will grow an average of 5 cm per year to gain 30 to 60 cm in height and will almost double their weight, increasing 2 to 3 kg per year. The average 6-year-old child is about 116 cm tall and weighs about 21 kg; the average 12-year-old child is about 150 cm tall and weighs approximately 40 kg. During this period, girls and boys differ little in size, although boys tend to be slightly taller and heavier than girls. Toward the end of the school-age years, both boys and girls begin to increase in size, although most girls begin to surpass boys in both height and weight.

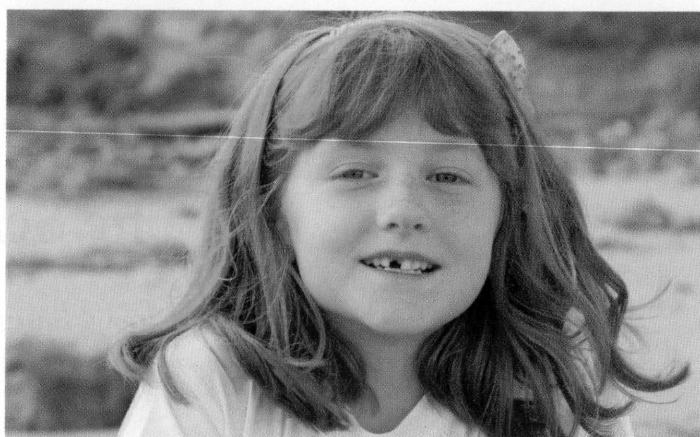

FIGURE 38-1 Middle childhood is the stage of development when deciduous teeth are shed. (S Curtis/Shutterstock.com.)

Proportional Changes

School-age children are more coordinated than they were as preschoolers and are steadier on their feet. Their body proportions take on a slimmer look, with longer legs, varying body proportion, and a lower centre of gravity. Posture improves over that of the preschool period to facilitate locomotion and efficiency in using the arms and trunk. These proportions make climbing, bicycle riding, and other activities easier. Fat gradually diminishes, and its distribution patterns change, contributing to the thinner appearance of the child during the middle years.

Accompanying the skeletal lengthening and fat diminution is an increase in the percentage of body weight represented by muscle tissue. By the end of this age period, both boys and girls double their strength and physical capabilities, and their steady and relatively consistent development of coordination increases their poise and skill. However, this increased strength can be misleading. Although strength increases, muscles are still functionally immature when compared with those of the adolescent, and they are more readily damaged by muscular injury caused by overuse.

The most pronounced changes that indicate increasing maturity in children are a decrease in head circumference in relation to standing height, a decrease in waist circumference in relation to height, and an increase in leg length in relation to height. These observations often provide a clue to a child's degree of physical maturity and have proved useful in predicting readiness for meeting the demands of school.

Specific physiological and anatomical characteristics are typical of children in middle childhood. Facial proportions change as the face grows faster in relation to the remainder of the cranium. The skull and brain grow very slowly during this period and increase little in size. Because all of the primary (deciduous) teeth are lost during this age span, middle childhood is sometimes known as the age of the loose tooth (Fig. 38-1). In the early years of middle childhood, the new secondary (permanent) teeth appear to be too large for the face.

Maturation of Systems

Maturity of the gastrointestinal system is reflected in fewer stomach upsets; better maintenance of blood glucose levels; and an increased stomach capacity, which permits retention of food for longer periods. The school-age child does not need to be fed as carefully, as promptly, or as frequently as the preschool-age child. Caloric needs are less than what they were in the preschool years.

Physical maturation is evident in other body tissues and organs. Bladder capacity, although differing widely among individual children, is generally greater in girls than in boys. The heart grows more slowly during the middle years and is smaller in relation to the rest of the body than at any other period of life. Heart and respiratory rates steadily decrease and blood pressure increases from ages 6 to 12 (see Appendix E).

The immune system becomes more competent in its ability to localize infections and to produce an antibody–antigen response. However, children may have several infections in the first 1 to 2 years of school because of increased exposure to other children with infectious diseases.

Bones continue to ossify throughout childhood but yield to pressure and muscle pulls more readily than with mature bones. Children need ample opportunity to move around and should observe caution in carrying heavy loads. For example, they should shift books or tote bags from one arm to the other or consider backpacks that distribute weight more evenly.

Wider differences between children are observed at the end of middle childhood than at the beginning. These differences become increasingly apparent and, if they are extreme or unique, may create emotional problems. The associated characteristics of height and weight relationships, rapid or slow growth, and other important features of development should be discussed with children and their families.

Prepubescence. *Preadolescence* is the period of approximately 2 years that begins at the end of middle childhood and ends with the thirteenth birthday. Because puberty signals the beginning of the development of secondary sex characteristics, prepubescence typically occurs during preadolescence.

Toward the end of middle childhood, the discrepancies in growth and maturation between boys and girls become apparent. On average, there is a difference of approximately 2 years between girls and boys in the age of onset of pubescence. This is a period of rapid growth in height and weight, especially for girls.

There is no universal age at which children assume the characteristics of prepubescence. The first physiological signs appear at about 9 years of age (particularly in girls) and are usually clearly evident in 11- to 12-year-old children. Although preadolescent children do not want to be different, variability in physical growth and physiological changes between children of the same sex and between the two sexes is often striking at this time. This variability, especially in relation to the onset of secondary sexual characteristics, is often noticed by the preadolescent. Either early or late appearance of these characteristics can be a source of discomfort to both sexes.

Preadolescence is a period of considerable overlapping of developmental characteristics of both middle childhood and early adolescence. However, several unique characteristics set this period apart from others. Generally, puberty begins at age 10 years in girls and 12 years in boys, but it can be normal for either sex after the age of 8 years. Boys experience little visible sexual maturation during preadolescence.

Table 38-1 summarizes the major developmental achievements of the school-age years.

Psychosocial Development

Freud described middle childhood as the latency period, a time of tranquility between the Oedipal phase of early childhood and the eroticism of adolescence. During this time, children experience relationships with same-sex peers following the indifference of earlier years and preceding the sexual fascination that occurs for most boys and girls in puberty.

Developing a Sense of Industry (Erikson)

Successful mastery of Erikson's first three stages of psychosocial development is important in terms of development of a healthy personality. Successful completion of these stages requires a loving environment within a stable family unit. These initial experiences prepared the child to engage in experiences and relationships beyond the intimate family group.

A sense of industry, or a stage of accomplishment, is achieved somewhere between age 6 and adolescence. School-age children are eager to develop skills and participate in meaningful and socially useful work. They acquire a sense of personal and

TABLE 38-1 GROWTH AND DEVELOPMENT DURING SCHOOL-AGE YEARS

PHYSICAL AND MOTOR	MENTAL	ADAPTIVE	PERSONAL-SOCIAL
Age 6 Yr			
Height and weight gain continues slowly Weight gain is 2 to 3 kg per year Height gain is 5 cm per year after age 7 and birth length triples by about age 13 Central mandibular incisors erupt Loss of first tooth Gradual increase in dexterity Active age; constant activity Often returns to finger feeding More aware of hand as a tool Likes to draw, print, colour Vision reaches maturity	Develops concept of numbers Easily counts 13 pennies Knows whether it is morning or afternoon Defines common objects such as fork and chair in terms of their use Obeys three commands in succession Knows right and left hands Says which is pretty and which is ugly of a series of face drawings Describes the objects in a picture rather than simply enumerating them Attends first grade	At the table, uses knife to spread butter or jam on bread At play, cuts, folds, pastes paper; sews crudely if the needle is threaded Takes a bath without supervision; performs bedtime activities alone Reads from memory; enjoys oral spelling game Likes table games, checkers, simple card games Giggles a lot Sometimes steals money or attractive items Has difficulty owning up to misdeeds Tries out own abilities	Can share and cooperate better Has great need for children of own age Will cheat to win Often engages in rough play Often jealous of younger brother or sister Does what adults are seen doing May have occasional temper tantrums Is a boaster Is more independent, probably influenced by school Has own way of doing things Increases socialization
Age 7 Yr			
Begins to grow at least 5 cm in height per year Weight 17.7–30 kg Height 112–130 cm Maxillary central incisors and lateral mandibular incisors erupt More cautious in approaches to new activities Repeats performances to master them Jaw begins to expand to accommodate permanent teeth	Notices that certain items are missing from pictures Can accurately copy a diamond Repeats three numbers backward Develops concept of time; reads ordinary clock or watch correctly to nearest quarter hour; uses clock for practical purposes Attends second grade More mechanical in reading; often does not stop at the end of a sentence; skips words such as "it," "the," and "he"	Uses table knife for cutting meat; may need help with tough or difficult pieces Brushes and combs hair acceptably without help Likes to help and have a choice Is less resistant and stubborn	Is becoming an active member of the family group Takes part in group play Most boys prefer playing with boys; most girls prefer playing with girls Spends a lot of time alone; does not require a lot of companionship

Continued

TABLE 38-1 GROWTH AND DEVELOPMENT DURING SCHOOL-AGE YEARS—cont'd

PHYSICAL AND MOTOR	MENTAL	ADAPTIVE	PERSONAL-SOCIAL
Ages 8–9 Yr			
Continues to gain 5 cm in height per year Weight 19.5–39.5 kg Height 117–142 cm Lateral incisors (maxillary) and mandibular cuspids erupt Movement is fluid; often graceful and poised Always on the go; jumps, chases, skips Increased smoothness and speed in fine motor control; uses cursive writing Dresses self completely Likely to overdo; hard to quiet down after recess More limber; bones grow faster than ligaments	Gives similarities and differences between two things from memory Counts backward from 20 to 1; understands concept of reversibility Repeats days of the week and months in order; knows the date Describes common objects in detail, not merely their use Makes change out of a quarter Attends third and fourth grades Reads more; may plan to wake up early just to read Reads classic books, but also enjoys comics More aware of time; can be relied on to get to school on time Can grasp concepts of parts and whole (fractions) Understands concepts of space, cause and effect, nesting (puzzles), conservation (permanence of mass and volume) Classifies objects by more than one quality; has collections Produces simple paintings or drawings	Makes use of common tools such as a hammer, saw, screwdriver Uses household and sewing utensils Helps with routine household tasks such as dusting and sweeping Assumes responsibility for share of household chores Looks after all of own needs at the table Buys useful articles; exercises some choice in making purchases Runs useful errands Likes pictorial magazines Likes school; wants to answer all the questions Is afraid of failing a grade; is ashamed of bad grades Is more critical of self Takes music and sport lessons	Is easy to get along with at home Likes the reward system Dramatizes Is more sociable Is better behaved Is interested in relationships with person of the same sex and/or opposite sex but will not admit it Goes about home and community freely, alone or with friends Likes to compete and play games Shows preference in friends and groups Plays mostly with groups of own sex but is beginning to mix Develops modesty Compares self with others Enjoys organizations, clubs, and group sports
Ages 10–12 Yr			
Weight 24.5–58 kg Height 127–162.5 cm Posture is more similar to an adult's; will overcome lordosis Remainder of teeth will erupt and tend toward full development (except wisdom teeth) Girls—Pubescent changes may begin to appear; body lines soften and round out Boys—Slow growth in height and rapid weight gain; may become obese in this period	Writes brief stories Attends fifth to seventh grades Writes occasional short letters to friends or relatives on own initiative Responds to magazine, television, or other advertising Reads for practical information or own enjoyment—stories of adventure, fantasy, science fiction, or romance	Makes useful tools or does easy repair work Cooks or sews in small way Raises pets Washes and dries own hair; is responsible for a thorough job of cleaning hair, but may need reminding to do so Is sometimes left alone at home for an hour or so Is successful in looking after own needs or those of other children left in his or her care	Loves friends; talks about them constantly Chooses friends more selectively; may have a "best friend" Enjoys conversation Develops beginning interest in opposite sex (if heterosexual) Is more diplomatic Likes family; family has significant meaning Likes mother and wants to please her in many ways Demonstrates affection Likes father, who is admired and may be idolized Respects parents

interpersonal competence; receive the systematic instruction prescribed by their individual cultures; and develop the skills needed to become useful, contributing members of their social communities.

Interests expand in the middle years, and with a growing sense of independence, children want to engage in tasks that can be carried through to completion (Fig. 38-2). They gain satisfaction from independent behaviour in exploring and manipulating their environment and from interaction with peers. Often the acquisition of skills provides a way to achieve success in social activities. Reinforcement in the form of grades, material rewards, additional privileges, and recognition provides encouragement and stimulation.

A sense of accomplishment also involves the ability to cooperate, to compete with others, and to cope effectively with people. Middle childhood is the time when children learn the value of doing things with others and the benefits derived from division of labour in the accomplishment of goals. Peer approval is a strong motivating power.

The danger inherent in this period of development is the occurrence of situations that might result in a sense of inferiority. Children with physical and mental limitations may be at a

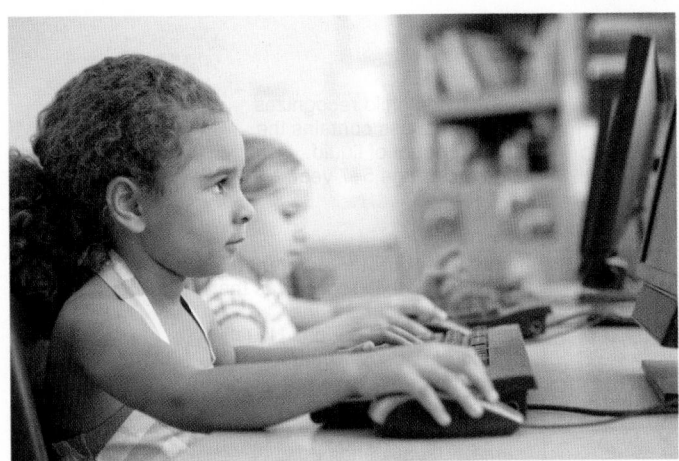

FIGURE 38-2 School-age children are motivated to complete tasks working alone. (Monkey Business Images/Shutterstock.com.)

disadvantage in the acquisition of certain skills. When the reward structure is based on evidence of mastery, children who are incapable of developing these skills risk feeling inadequate and inferior. Even children without chronic disabilities may experience feelings of inadequacy in some areas. No child is able to do everything well, and children must learn that they will not be able to master every skill they attempt. All children, even children who usually have positive attitudes toward work and their own abilities, will feel some degree of inferiority when they encounter specific skills that they cannot master.

Children need and want a sense of real achievement. Children achieve a sense of industry when they have access to tasks that need to be done and when they are able to complete the tasks well despite individual differences in their innate capacities and emotional development.

Cognitive Development

When children enter the school years, they begin to acquire the ability to relate a series of events to mental representations that can be expressed both verbally and symbolically (see Table 38-1). This is the stage Piaget (1952) describes as "concrete operations," when children are able to use thought processes to experience events and actions. The rigid, egocentric view of the preschool years is replaced by mental processes that allow children to see things from another's point of view.

During this stage, children develop an understanding of relationships between things and ideas. They progress from making judgements based on what they see (perceptual thinking) to making judgements based on what they reason (conceptual thinking). They are able to master symbols and to use their memories of past experiences to evaluate and interpret the present.

One cognitive task of school-age children is mastering the concept of conservation (Fig. 38-3). At an early age (about 5 to 7 years), children grasp the concept of reversibility of numbers as a basis for simple mathematics problems (e.g., $2 + 4 = 6$ and $6 - 4 = 2$). They learn that simply altering their arrangement in space does not change certain properties of the environment, and they are able to resist perceptual cues that suggest alterations in the physical state of an object. For example, they recognize that changing the shape of a substance such as a lump of clay does not alter its total mass. They no longer perceive a tall, thin glass of water as containing a greater volume than a short, wide glass; they can distinguish between the weights of items regardless of their size. They recognize that size is not necessarily related to weight or volume. There is a developmental sequence in children's capacity to conserve matter. Conservation of mass usually is accomplished first, weight some time later, and volume last.

School-age children also develop classification skills. They can group and sort objects according to the attributes they share, place things in a sensible and logical order, and hold a concept in mind while making decisions based on that concept. Another characteristic of middle childhood is that children derive enjoyment from classifying and ordering their environment. They become occupied with collections of objects, such as stickers, shells, dolls, cars, cards, and stuffed animals. Depending on their cultural background, they may even begin to order friends and relationships (e.g., best friend, second-best friend).

They also develop the ability to understand relational terms and concepts, such as bigger and smaller; darker and paler; heavier and lighter; to the right of and to the left of; first, last, and intermediate relationships; and more than and less than. They view family relationships in terms of reciprocal roles (e.g., to be a brother, one must have a sibling).

School-age children learn the alphabet and the world of symbols called words, which can be arranged in terms of structure and their relationship to the alphabet. They learn to tell time, to see the relationship of events in time (history) and places in space (geography), and to combine time and space relationships (geology and astronomy).

The ability to read is usually achieved during the school years and becomes the most significant and valuable tool for independent inquiry. Children's capacity to explore, imagine, and expand their knowledge is enhanced by reading.

Moral Development

As children move from egocentrism to more logical patterns of thought, they also move through stages in the development of conscience and moral standards (Kohlberg, 1968). Young children do not believe that standards of behaviour come from within themselves but that rules are established and set down by others. During the preschool years, children adopt and internalize the moral values of their parents. They learn standards for acceptable behaviour, act according to these standards, and feel guilty when they violate them. Although children 6 or 7 years of age know the rules and behaviours expected of them, they do not understand the reasons behind them. Rewards and punishments guide their judgement; a "bad act" is one that breaks a rule or causes harm. This description of moral development includes the aspect that young children believe that what other people tell them to do is right and that what they themselves think is wrong. Consequently, children 6 or 7 years old may interpret accidents or misfortunes as punishment for "bad" acts.

Older school-age children are able to judge an act by the intentions that prompted it rather than just its consequences.

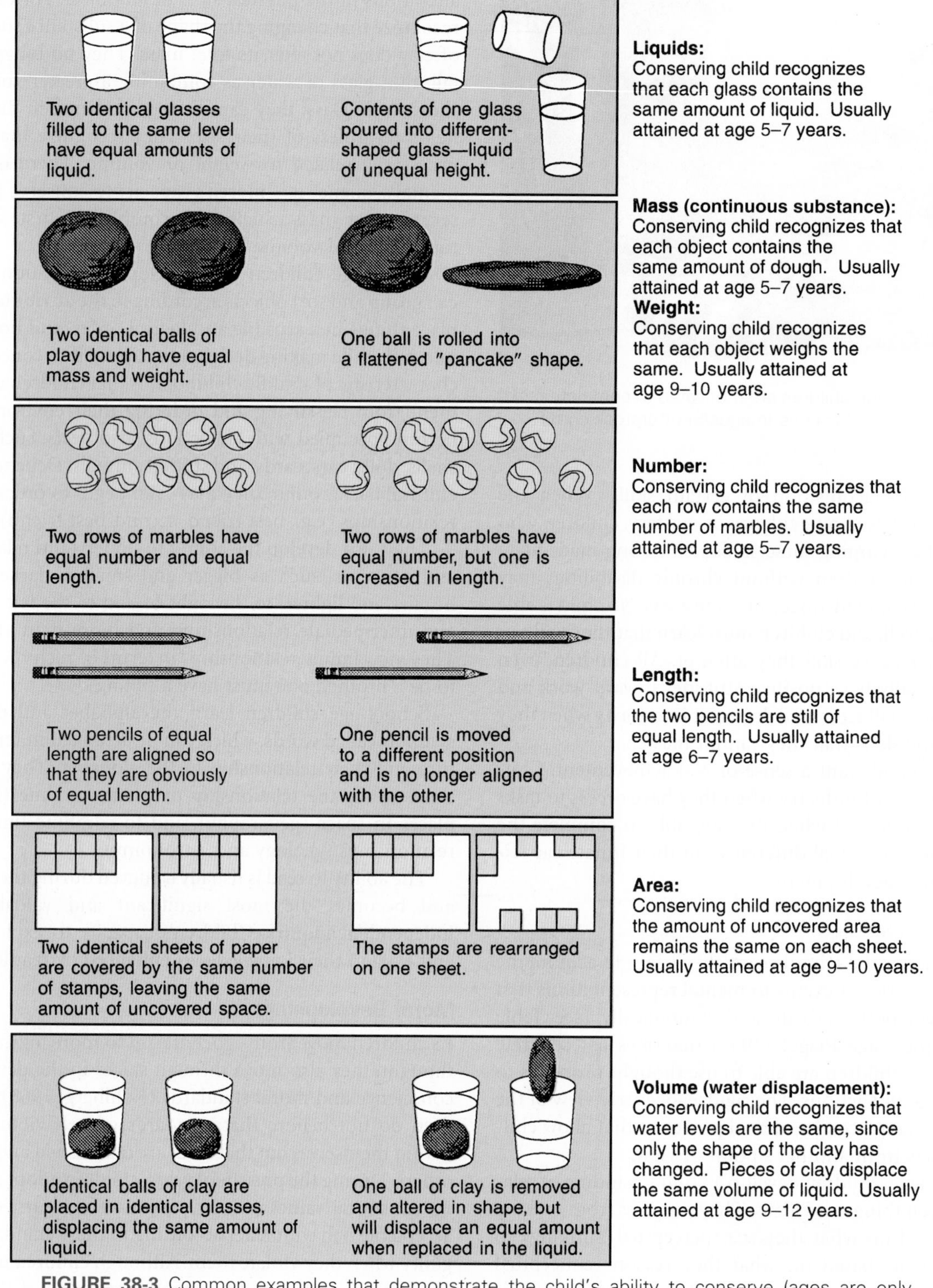

Two identical glasses filled to the same level have equal amounts of liquid.
Contents of one glass poured into different-shaped glass—liquid of unequal height.
Liquids:
Conserving child recognizes that each glass contains the same amount of liquid. Usually attained at age 5–7 years.
Two identical balls of play dough have equal mass and weight.
One ball is rolled into a flattened "pancake" shape.
Mass (continuous substance):
Conserving child recognizes that each object contains the same amount of dough. Usually attained at age 5–7 years.
Weight:
Conserving child recognizes that each object weighs the same. Usually attained at age 9–10 years.
Two rows of marbles have equal number and equal length.
Two rows of marbles have equal number, but one is increased in length.
Number:
Conserving child recognizes that each row contains the same number of marbles. Usually attained at age 5–7 years.
Two pencils of equal length are aligned so that they are obviously of equal length.
One pencil is moved to a different position and is no longer aligned with the other.
Length:
Conserving child recognizes that the two pencils are still of equal length. Usually attained at age 6–7 years.
Two identical sheets of paper are covered by the same number of stamps, leaving the same amount of uncovered space.
The stamps are rearranged on one sheet.
Area:
Conserving child recognizes that the amount of uncovered area remains the same on each sheet. Usually attained at age 9–10 years.
Identical balls of clay are placed in identical glasses, displacing the same amount of liquid.
One ball of clay is removed and altered in shape, but will displace an equal amount when replaced in the liquid.
Volume (water displacement):
Conserving child recognizes that water levels are the same, since only the shape of the clay has changed. Pieces of clay displace the same volume of liquid. Usually attained at age 9–12 years.

FIGURE 38-3 Common examples that demonstrate the child's ability to conserve (ages are only approximate).

Rules and judgements become less absolute and authoritarian and begin to be founded on the needs and desires of others. For older children, a rule violation is likely to be viewed in relation to the total context in which it appears. The situation, as well as the morality of the rule itself, influences reactions. Although younger children judge an act only according to whether it is right or wrong, older children take into account a different point of view. They are able to understand and accept the concept of treating others as they would like to be treated.

Spiritual Development

School-age children begin to learn the difference between the natural and the supernatural but have difficulty understanding symbols. Consequently, religious concepts must be presented to

CULTURAL AWARENESS

Religious Orientation

Many schools and communities in Canada have a Christian or Jewish orientation toward prayer, holidays, and values. For children of other religious backgrounds, the predominance of these practices and values may result in their feeling conflict and discomfort. It is important that schools and communities exercise sensitivity so as not to offend and confuse children from other religious backgrounds, such as Buddhism, Hinduism, and Islam, or those with no religious background. In Canada, awareness of and openness to the spiritual diversity of Indigenous groups is also important.

them in concrete terms. Prayer or other religious rituals comfort them, and if these activities are a part of their daily lives, they may help them cope with threatening situations. Their petitions to their God in prayers tend to be for tangible rewards. Although younger children expect their prayers to be answered, as they get older, they begin to recognize that this does not always occur and become less concerned when prayers are not answered. School-age children want and expect to be punished for misbehaviours and, when given the option, tend to choose a punishment that is relevant to the misdemeanour. However, they may view illness or injury as a punishment for a real or imagined misdeed. The beliefs and ideals of family and religious persons are more influential than those of their peers. They are able to discuss their feelings about their faith and how it relates to their lives (see Cultural Awareness box).

Social Development

One of the most important socializing agents in the school-age years is the peer group. In addition to parents and the schools, the peer group conveys a substantial amount of information to its members. Peer groups have a culture of their own, with secrets, traditions, and codes of ethics that may promote feelings of solidarity and detachment from adults. Through peer relationships, children often learn how to deal with dominance and hostility, how to relate to persons in positions of leadership and authority, and how to explore ideas and the physical environment.

Peer group identification is an important factor in gaining independence from parents. The aid and support of the group provide the child with enough security to risk the moderate parental rejection brought about by small victories in the development of independence.

A child's concept of the appropriate gender role is also influenced by relationships with peers. During the early school years few gender differences exist in the play experiences of children. Both girls and boys shares games and other activities. In the later school years the differences in the play of boys and girls may become more marked.

Social Relationships and Cooperation

Daily relationships with peers provide important social interactions for school-age children. Now children join group activities with unrestrained enthusiasm and steady participation. Previous interactions were limited to short periods under considerable adult supervision. With increased skills and wider opportunities, school-age children become involved with one or more peer groups in which they can gain status as respected members.

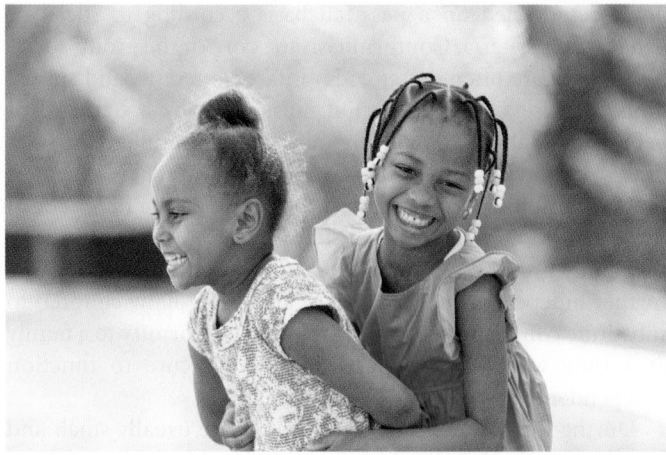

FIGURE 38-4 School-age children enjoy engaging in activities with a "best friend." (Samuel Borges Photography/Shutterstock.com.)

Valuable lessons are learned from daily interaction with age-mates. First, children learn to appreciate the numerous and varied points of view that are represented in the peer group. As children interact with peers who see the world in ways that are somewhat different from their own, they become aware of the limits of their own point of view. Because age-mates are peers and are not forced to accept each other's ideas as they are expected to accept those of adults, other children have a significant influence on decreasing the egocentric outlook of the child. Consequently, children learn to argue, persuade, bargain, cooperate, and compromise to maintain friendships.

A second lesson that children learn is increasing sensitivity to the social norms and pressures of the peer group. The peer group establishes standards for acceptance and rejection, and children are often willing to modify their behaviour to be accepted by the group. The need for peer approval becomes a powerful influence toward conformity. Children learn to dress, talk, and behave in a manner acceptable to the group. A variety of roles, such as class joker or class hero, may be assumed by individual children to gain approval from the group.

Finally, the interaction among peers leads to the formation of intimate friendships between peers—the school-age period is the time when children may have "best friends" with whom they share secrets, private jokes, and adventures; they come to one another's aid in times of trouble. In the course of these friendships children also fight, threaten each other, break up, and reunite. These relationships, in which the child experiences love and closeness for a peer, may be important as a foundation for relationships in adulthood (Fig. 38-4).

Clubs and peer groups. In contemporary Western society, one of the outstanding characteristics of middle childhood seems to be the formation of formalized groups, or clubs. A prominent feature of these groups is the rigid rules imposed on the members. There is exclusiveness in the selection of persons who have the privilege of joining. Acceptance in the group is often determined on a pass-fail basis according to social or behavioural criteria. Conformity is the core of the group structure. There are often secret codes, shared interests, and special modes of dress, and each child must abide by a standard of behaviour established by the members. Conforming to the rules provides children with feelings of security and relieves them of the responsibility of making decisions. By merging their identities with those of their peers, children are able to move from the family group to an outside group, as a step toward seeking further independence. Peer groups and clubs allow children to substitute conformity to a peer group for conformity to a family at a time when children are still too insecure to function independently.

During the early school years, groups are usually small and loosely organized, with changing membership and no formal structure. The clubs and groups usually do not display elements of cooperation and order that are seen in groups of older children. Although there may be a mixture of both sexes in the early school years, the groups of later school years are composed predominantly of children of the same sex. Common interests are the basis around which the group is structured.

Bullying. Peer-group identification and association are essential to a child's socialization. Poor relationships with peers and a lack of group identification can contribute to bullying. *Bullying* is any recurring activity that is intended to harm or bother someone where there is a perceived imbalance of power between the aggressor and the victim (Lamb, Pepler, & Craig, 2009).

Between the ages of 4 and 11, bullying often begins when children are forming their self-identities at school and through other social activities. Research has shown that a higher percentage of students engage in bullying behaviours while in middle school and high school than in elementary school, but the percentage of students victimized gradually decreases with age. Boys in elementary school report higher levels of bullying than that for girls in middle and high school. During middle school and high school, boys practise and are the victims of bullying almost twice as much as girls (Government of Canada, 2015). Among adult Canadians, 38% of males and 30% of females reported having experienced occasional or frequent bullying during their school years (Canadian Institutes of Health Research [CIHR], 2012). Although bullying can occur in any setting, it most often occurs at school during unstructured times such as recess (Arseneault, Bowes, & Shakoor, 2010).

Bullies are generally defiant toward adults, antisocial, and likely to break school rules. They have dominant personalities, may come from homes where parental involvement and nurturing are lacking, and may experience or witness violence or abuse at home (Bowes, Arseneault, Maughan, et al., 2009). Boys who bully tend to use physical force, referred to as *direct bullying*, but girls usually use indirect bullying methods such as exclusion, gossip, or rumours (Arseneault et al., 2010). Cyberbullying is a new form of bullying and involves the use of cellular telephones, digital cameras, or social networking Internet sites to cause distress in an individual (American Academy of Pediatrics [AAP] Committee on Injury, Violence, and Poison Prevention, 2009). The use of social media for mass communication has escalated the gravity of many methods of bullying.

Children who are targeted for bullying may have internalizing characteristics such as withdrawal, anxiety, depression, low self-esteem, and reduced assertiveness that may make them an easy target for bullying (Arseneault et al., 2010). Children who are bullied are vulnerable and may have characteristics that are different from the group norm, such as obesity, learning problems, a minority sexual orientation, or different family background (Lamb et al., 2009). Children with less obvious disabilities such as developmental coordination disorder, specific language impairment, or attention deficit/hyperactivity disorder may receive less protection from their peer group in contrast to a child with a visible disability, such as spina bifida (Frederickson, 2010).

Canada does not have a good record of effectively managing bullying. The World Health Organization global survey of health behaviours of school-age children ranks Canada twenty-sixth out of 35 countries for number of bullying incidents (CIHR, 2012). A Canadian federal network, called PrevNET (Promoting Relationships and Eliminating Violence), has been established to prevent bullying, by bridging the gap between research and practice (see Additional Resources at the end of this chapter). Bullying needs to be managed directly by adults who will acknowledge the problem and step in to stop it. Children also need empowerment strategies that can give them peer support and that help them in bullying situations. School personnel can play an important role in implementing antibullying interventions in elementary schools, before bullying becomes a part of the school culture (Lamb et al., 2009).

The long-term consequences of bullying are significant. Victims of bullying often experience psychological distress, such as worry, sadness, anxiety, depression, and nightmares, and can have increased self-harm behaviours, social isolation, suicidal ideation, and violent behaviours (Arseneault et al., 2010). Chronic bullies may continue their behaviours into adulthood, and such behaviours negatively influence their ability to develop and maintain relationships. Researchers have recognized that involving the whole family in antibullying programs greatly increases success (Arseneault et al., 2010).

Relationships With Families

Although the peer group is influential and necessary for normal child development, parents are usually the primary influence in shaping the child's personality, setting standards for behaviour, and establishing value systems. Family values usually take precedence over peer value systems. Although children may appear to reject parental values while testing the new values of the peer group, ultimately they retain and incorporate into their own value systems the parental values they have found to be of worth.

In the middle school years, children want to spend more time in the company of peers and they often prefer peer-group activities to family activities. This can be disturbing to parents. Children may become intolerant and critical of their parents, especially when their parents' ways deviate from those of the group. They discover that parents can be wrong, and they begin to question the knowledge and authority of their parents, who were previously often considered to be all-knowing and all-powerful.

Although increased independence is the goal of middle childhood, children are not prepared to abandon all parental control. They need and want restrictions placed on their behaviour, and they are not prepared to cope with all the problems of their expanding environment. They feel more secure knowing there is an authority figure to implement controls and restrictions. Children may complain loudly about restrictions and try to break down parental barriers, but they are uneasy if they succeed in doing so. They respect adults who prevent them from acting on every urge. Children view this behaviour as an expression of love and concern for their welfare.

Children need stable, secure guidance provided by mature adults to whom they can turn during troubled relationships with peers or stressful changes in their world (see Family-Centred Teaching box). Children also need their parents to be adults, not friends. Sometimes parents, hurt by their children's rejection, attempt to maintain their love and gratitude by assuming the role of a friend.

Play

Play takes on new dimensions that reflect a new stage of development in the school years (see Table 38-1). Play involves increased physical skill, intellectual ability, and fantasy. In addition, children develop a sense of belonging to a team or club by forming groups and cliques.

Rules and rituals. The need for conformity in middle childhood is strongly manifested in the activities and games of school-age children. In the preschool years, children's games were either invented for them or played in the company of a friend or an adult. Now children begin to see the need for rules, and their games have fixed and unvarying rules that may be bizarre and extraordinarily rigid. Part of the enjoyment of the game is knowing the rules because knowing means belonging. Conformity and ritual permeate their play and are also evident in their behaviour and language. Childhood is full of chants and taunts, such as "Eeeny, meeny, miney, mo," "Last one is a rotten egg," and "Step on a crack, break your mother's back." Children derive a sense of pleasure and power from such sayings, which have been handed down with few changes through generations.

Team play. A more complex form of play that evolves from the need for peer interaction is team games and sports. A referee, umpire, or person of authority may be required so that the rules can be followed more accurately. Team play teaches children to modify or exchange personal goals for goals of the group; it also teaches them that division of labour is an effective

FAMILY-CENTRED TEACHING

Guidance for Parents During School Years

Age 6 Years

- Prepare parents for potential strong food preferences and potential refusal of specific food items.
- Prepare parents to expect an increasingly ravenous appetite.
- Prepare parents for emotionality as the child experiences mood changes.
- Help parents anticipate the child's continued susceptibility to illness.
- Review immunization schedule with the parents—if tetanus schedule of four initial doses is completed before age 4, a fifth dose of tetanus toxoid is recommended at school entry by age 6 (Public Health Agency of Canada, 2015).
- Teach injury prevention and safety, especially bicycle safety.
- Encourage parents to respect the child's need for privacy.
- Prepare parents for the child's increasing interests outside the home.
- Help parents understand the need to support the child's interactions with peers.

Ages 7 to 10 Years

- Prepare parents to expect an improvement in their child's health with fewer illnesses, although allergies may increase or become apparent.
- Prepare parents to expect an increase in minor injuries.
- Advise parents to use caution in selecting and maintaining sports equipment, and re-emphasize focus on safety.
- Prepare parents to expect increased involvement with peers and interest in activities outside the home.
- Emphasize the need to encourage independence in the child while maintaining limit-setting and discipline.
- Prepare mothers to expect more demands from the child at age 8 years.
- Prepare fathers to expect increasing admiration from the child at age 10 years; encourage father–child activities.
- Prepare parents for prepubescent changes in girls.

Ages 11 to 12 Years

- Help parents prepare the child for body changes of pubescence.
- Prepare parents to expect a growth spurt in girls.
- Make certain the child's sex education is adequate with accurate information.
- Prepare parents to expect energetic and stormy behaviour at age 11 years, possibly becoming more even-tempered at age 12 years.
- Encourage parents to support the child's desire to "grow up" but to allow regressive behaviour when needed.
- Prepare parents to expect an increase in the child's masturbation.
- Instruct parents that the amount of rest the child needs may increase.
- Help parents educate the child regarding experimentation with potentially harmful activities.

Health Guidance

- Provide information regarding human papilloma virus (HPV) immunization. Health Canada recommends HPV immunization in girls and women between ages 9 and 26, preferably before sexual activity has commenced (see Chapter 7). Health Canada is now recommending the HPV vaccine for males between 9 and 26 years as well. At the date of this publication, the vaccine is covered by all provincial and territorial health plans for females and in Alberta, Nova Scotia, and Prince Edward Island for males and females (see Chapter 35) (Public Health Agency of Canada, 2015).Help parents understand the importance of regular health and dental care for the child.
- Encourage parents to teach and model sound health practices, including diet, rest, activity, and exercise.
- Stress the need to encourage children to engage in appropriate physical activities.
- Emphasize the importance of providing a safe physical and emotional environment.

strategy for attaining a goal. Children learn about competition and the importance of winning—an attribute highly valued in some cultures and by some individuals.

Team play can also contribute to children's social, intellectual, and skill growth. Children work hard to develop the skills needed to become team members, to improve their contribution to the group, and to anticipate the consequences of their behaviour for the group. Team play helps stimulate cognitive growth because children are called on to learn many complex rules, make judgements about those rules, plan strategies, and assess the strengths and weaknesses of members of their own team and members of the opposing team.

Quiet games and activities. Although play at this age is highly active, school-age children also enjoy quiet and solitary activities. The middle years are a time for collections, which constitute another ritual. Young school-age children's collections can be an odd assortment of unrelated objects in messy, disorganized piles. Collections of later school years are more orderly, selective, and may be organized in scrapbooks, on shelves, or in boxes.

School-age children become fascinated with complex board, card, video, or computer games that they can play alone, with a best friend, or with a group. As in all games, adherence to the rules is strict. Disagreements over rules can cause much discussion and argument, but may be easily resolved by reading the rules of the game.

The newly acquired skill of reading becomes increasingly satisfying as school-age children expand their knowledge of the world through books (Fig. 38-5). School-age children never tire of stories and, as with preschool children, love to have stories read aloud. They also enjoy sewing, cooking, carpentry, gardening, and creative activities such as painting. Many creative skills, such as music and art, as well as athletic skills, such as swimming, karate, dancing, and skating, are learned during these years and continue to be enjoyed into adolescence and adulthood (Fig. 38-6).

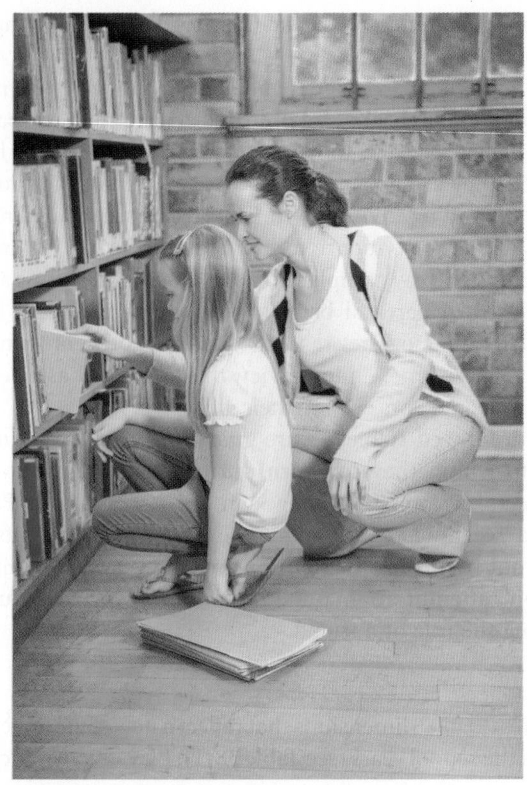

FIGURE 38-5 Selecting a book with the assistance of an adult. (wavebreakmedia/Shutterstock.com.)

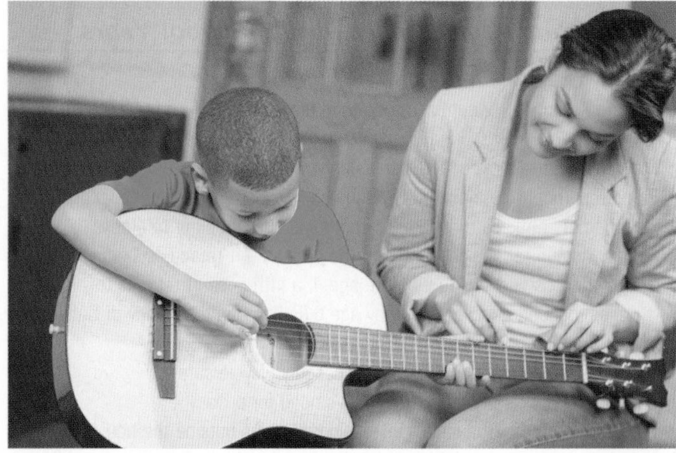

FIGURE 38-6 School-age children take pride in learning new skills. (wavebreakmedia/Shutterstock.com.)

Development of a Self-Concept

The term *self-concept* refers to a conscious awareness of self-perceptions, such as one's physical characteristics, abilities, values, self-ideals and expectations, and idea of self in relation to others. It also includes one's body image, sexuality, and self-esteem. Although primary caregivers continue to exert influence on children's self-evaluation, the opinions of peers and teachers provide valuable input during middle childhood. With the emphasis on skill building and broadened social relationships, children are continually engaged in the process of self-evaluation.

Significant adults can often manage to unobtrusively manipulate the environment so that children experience success. Each small success increases a child's self-image. The more positive children feel about themselves, the more confident they will remain in trying for success in the future. All children profit from feeling that they are in some way special to a significant adult. A positive self-concept makes children feel likable, worthwhile, and capable of significant contributions. These feelings lead to self-respect, self-confidence, and happiness.

Development of a Body Image

School-age children have a relatively accurate and positive perception of their physical selves, but in general they like their physical selves less as they grow older. The head appears to be the most important part of the school-age child's perceived image of self, with hair and eye colour being the characteristics used most frequently to describe the physical self.

Body image is influenced, but not solely determined, by significant others. The number of significant others influencing one's perception of the physical self increases with age. Children are acutely aware of their own body, the bodies of their peers, and those of adults. They are also aware of deviations from the norm. It is important that children learn about bodily functions and that adults provide correct information. Physical impairments, such as hearing or visual defects, ears that "stick out," or birthmarks, assume great importance during this age span. Increasing awareness of these differences, especially when accompanied by unkind comments and taunts from others, may cause a child to feel inferior and less desirable. This is especially true if the defect interferes with the child's ability to participate in games and activities.

Coping With Concerns Related to Normal Growth and Development

School Experience

School constitutes an important part of the experience of children 6 to 12 years of age. Schools serve as a significant agent in the transmitting of values of society to children. School is also the setting for building relationships with peers. After the family, schools are the second most important socializing agent in the lives of children.

Entrance into school causes a sharp break in the structure of the child's world. For many children, it is their first experience with conforming to a group pattern imposed by an adult who is not a parent and who has responsibility for too many children to be constantly aware of each child as an individual. Most children want to go to school and usually adapt to the new conditions with little difficulty. Successful adjustment is related to the child's physical and emotional maturity and the parent's readiness to accept the separation associated with school entrance. Unfortunately, some parents express their unconscious attempts to delay the child's maturity by clinging behaviour, particularly with their youngest child.

By the time they enter school, most children have a fairly realistic concept of what school involves. They receive information regarding the role of a student from parents, siblings, playmates, and the media. In addition, most children have had some experience with day care, preschool, or kindergarten. Middle-class children generally have fewer adjustments to make and less to learn about expected behaviour, since schools tend to reflect dominant middle-class customs and values. If the child has attended a preschool program, the focus of the preschool program also affects the child's adjustment. Some preschool programs provide custodial care only, whereas others emphasize emotional, social, and intellectual development.

Classmates have a significant impact on the socialization of children. For some children, school is their first experience of becoming members of a large group of individuals their own age. Peer relationships become increasingly important and influential as children proceed through school (see section Social Relationships and Cooperation, earlier in this chapter). The specific influence exerted by the peer group depends on the individual child's background, interests, and abilities.

Some children in Canada are home-schooled. There are many reasons why parents choose this type of education, including educational liberty to form their own curriculum; religious freedom to integrate their values and beliefs into their child's learning; formation of a closer family relationship; potential for less peer pressure and bullying; and flexible scheduling. Some disadvantages include the amount of time required for parents to teach, less income if one parent has to stay at home to teach, limited access for the child to organized sports, and criticism from others, as home-schooling remains controversial. The children must be able to meet the legal conditions and pass standardized tests in accordance with the individual province's or territory's educational requirements. It is essential for home-schooled children to have opportunities to socialize and build peer relationships in order to foster their social development. Organized sports, play dates with neighbourhood children, and group swimming lessons are examples of common ways to help children develop friendships and social skills with others.

Teachers. Children respond best to teachers who possess the characteristics of a warm, loving parent. Teachers in the early grades perform many of the activities formerly assumed by the parent, such as recognizing the child's personal needs (e.g., the need to go to the bathroom, need for help with clothing) and helping to develop their social behaviour (e.g., manners).

Teachers, like parents, are concerned about the child's psychological and emotional welfare. Although the functions of teachers and parents differ, both place constraints on behaviour, and both are in a position to enforce standards of conduct. However, unlike parents, the teacher's primary responsibility involves stimulating and guiding children's intellectual development, not providing for their physical welfare beyond the school setting.

Teachers serve as models that children often try to emulate. Children seek their teachers' approval and avoid their disapproval. The teacher is a significant person in the life of the early schoolchild, and hero worship of a teacher may extend into late childhood and preadolescence. Teachers who make supportive statements that reassure or commend children, use accepting and clarifying statements that help children refine ideas and feelings, and provide assistance that aids children with their own problem solving contribute to the development of a positive self-concept in the school-age child.

Parents. Parents share responsibility for helping children develop innate capabilities and social awareness. Parents can supplement academic education in numerous ways (see Family-Centred Care box). Cultivating responsibility is one goal of parental assistance, as being responsible for schoolwork helps children learn to keep promises, meet deadlines, and succeed at their jobs as adults. Children may occasionally ask for help (e.g., with a spelling list), but usually they prefer to think through their work by themselves. Excessive pressure or lack of encouragement from parents may inhibit development of these desirable traits.

Latchkey Children

The term *latchkey children* is used to describe children in elementary school who are left to care for themselves before or after school without the supervision of an adult. The increasing numbers of lone-parent families and families in which both parents work outside the home, together with the lack of available child care, have created a stress-provoking situation for many school-age children.

Inadequate adult supervision after school leaves children at greater risk for injury and delinquent behaviour. In some

FAMILY-CENTRED CARE

Helping Children in School

General Guidelines

- Be supportive—Provide companionship; share ideas and thoughts.
- Be positive—Every child should experience some success each day.
- Share an interest in reading—Use the library; discuss books they are reading.
- Support and encourage activity rather than passivity.
- Encourage originality—Help children make their own projects from discarded articles or other available materials.
- Foster the development of hobbies and collections.
- Encourage children to wonder and reflect during free time.
- Initiate family trips to places of interest.
- Encourage asking of questions—Help children discover sources for information or places to explore and investigate.
- Stimulate creative thinking and problem solving—Help children try out new solutions to problems without fear of making mistakes.
- Use rewards rather than punishment.

Specific Guidelines

- Meet the teacher at the beginning of school and plan to visit the school to see what is taught and expected.
- Demonstrate an interest in what the child is learning.
- Demonstrate an interest in content of school education and in the child's growth, more than in grades.
- Make it clear to the child that schoolwork is between the child and the teacher; the teacher and child should set goals for better school performance so that the child feels responsible for school successes and failures.
- Take advantage of situations that support and reinforce school learning.
- Share information with teachers that will help them understand the child better.
- Communicate with the teacher if there appears to be a problem; avoid waiting for a scheduled conference.
- Provide a quiet, well-lit area for study that is safe from interruption.
- Avoid dictating a study time, but do enforce rules, such as no television until homework is done; accept the child's word that work is complete.
- Help with homework should focus on explaining the question, not giving the answer.
- Teach the child to break large tasks (e.g., a report) down into smaller, manageable tasks spread over the allotted time rather than attempting the entire project the night before it is to be completed.
- Limit home tutoring to special circumstances, such as when the teacher requests parental assistance after a child's prolonged absence.
- Request special help for children with learning problems.
- Support the school staff by showing respect for both the school system and the teacher, especially in the child's presence.

instances, outside activities are curtailed and relationships with peers may be significantly diminished. Latchkey children may feel more lonely, isolated, and fearful than children who have someone to care for them. To cope with their fears and anxieties while alone, these children may devise strategies such as hiding, playing the television at loud volume, or using pets for comfort. In addition, some latchkey children may have a chronic illness or other health problem that remains improperly treated.

Many communities and persons concerned about the welfare of latchkey children are trying to help these children and their parents deal with this potentially serious problem. Some communities and employers have implemented after-school programs or telephone "hotlines" that provide check-in and reassurance for children. Nurses should be aware of these community services and encourage parents to teach self-help skills to their children.

Limit-Setting and Discipline

Many factors influence the amount and manner of discipline and limit-setting imposed on school-age children. Some of these factors are the parents' psychosocial maturity, the parents' childhood and child-rearing experiences, the children's temperament, the context of the children's misconduct, and the children's response to rewards and punishments. When children develop an ability to see a situation from another's point of view, they are also able to understand the effects of their reactions on others and themselves.

Discipline should take place in a positive, supportive environment with the use of strategies to instruct and guide desired behaviours and eliminate undesired behaviours (Knox, 2010). Parents can set the stage for this environment and encourage good behaviour by establishing the following: (1) a calm, organized space with age-appropriate toys; (2) an organized schedule along with the child that includes some quiet activities and some outdoor and other physical activities; (3) standard sleep routines that ensure adequate nighttime sleep; and (4) regular mealtimes and healthy snacks to avoid irritability from hunger. In addition, peer relationships affect a child's behaviour, so parents should get to know the child's friends and explain the house rules and expect respectful behaviour from everyone. Parents also need to limit screen time to high-quality shows and limit violent video games and shows that can make a child anxious or may encourage aggressive behaviour. Parents need to respect their child's feelings, thoughts, ideas, and contributions and be honest with and listen to the child (Canadian Paediatric Society [CPS], 2013).

Reasoning is an effective technique for older school-age children. With advancing cognitive skills, they are able to benefit from more complex disciplinary strategies. For example, withholding privileges, requiring compensation, imposing penalties, and contracting can be used with great success. Problem solving is the best approach to limit-setting, and children themselves can be included in the process of determining appropriate disciplinary measures.

Dishonest Behaviour

During middle childhood, children may engage in what is considered to be antisocial behaviour. Previously well-behaved children may engage in lying, stealing, and cheating. Such behaviours are disturbing and challenging to parents.

Lying can occur for a number of reasons. By the time children enter school, they still "tell stories," often exaggerating a story or situation as a means of impressing their family or friends. However, during middle childhood, children become able to distinguish between fact and fantasy. If children do not develop this characteristic, parents need to teach them what is real and what is make-believe.

Young children may lie to escape punishment or to get out of some difficulty even when their misbehaviour is evident. Older children may lie to meet expectations set by others to which they have been unable to measure up. However, most children know that lying and cheating are wrong, and they are concerned when it is observed in their friends. They can be quick to report others when they detect cheating.

Parents need to be reassured that all children lie occasionally and that sometimes children may have difficulty separating fantasy from reality. Parents should be helped to understand the importance of being truthful in their relationships with children.

Cheating is most common in children who are 5 to 6 years of age. They find it difficult to lose at a game or contest, so they may cheat to win. They have not yet realized that this behaviour is wrong, and they do it almost automatically. This behaviour usually disappears as they mature. However, because children model observed behaviours, parents need to be aware of their own behaviour. When parents set examples of honesty, children are more likely to conform to these standards.

As with other ethically related behaviour, stealing is not unexpected in the younger child. Between 5 and 8 years of age, children's sense of property rights is limited, and they tend to take something simply because they are attracted to it or to take money for what it will buy. They are equally likely to give away something valuable that belongs to them. When young children are caught and punished, they are penitent—they "didn't mean to" and "promise to never do it again"—but they are likely to repeat the performance the following day. Often they not only steal but also lie about their behaviour or attempt to justify it with excuses. It is seldom helpful to trap children into admission by asking directly if they committed the offence. Children do not take responsibility for these types of behaviours until the end of middle childhood. Stealing can be an indication that something is seriously wrong or lacking in the child's life. For example, children may steal to make up for love or another satisfaction that they feel is lacking. Or if they are not receiving adequate food, they may steal food because they are hungry. In most situations it is wise not to attempt to attach a hidden or deep meaning to the stealing. An admonition, together with an appropriate and reasonable punishment, such as having the older child pay back the money or return the stolen items, takes care of most cases. Most children can be taught to respect the property rights of others with little difficulty despite numerous temptations and opportunities. If children's personal rights are respected, they are likely to respect the rights of others. Some children simply need more time to learn the rules regarding private property.

Stress and Fear

Children today experience significant amounts of stress, which can cause long-term adjustment and health problems. Stress in childhood comes from a variety of sources, such as conflict within the family, interpersonal relationships, poverty, and chronic illness. The school environment and participation in multiple organized activities can be additional sources of stress. The demands from coaches and parents, in addition to school requirements and pressure from teachers to do well on proficiency testing, can place unrealistic expectations on the school-age child. In addition, with increasing exposure to sexuality and provocative clothing and behaviours, children of this age group may feel pressured to have a girlfriend or boyfriend, which their maturity level cannot handle and which causes additional stress (McLeod & Knight, 2010).

Increasing violence in society has also spilled over into the school setting. In the present information age, in which tragedy is broadcast daily in the media, children come to school knowing more about the latest world events than any previous generation of children. In addition, today's children are often personally aware of violence in their families or communities. Some children know other children who have been killed or children who have brought weapons to school. School-age children can be victims of teasing, bullying, and physical abuse in the school environment.

To help children cope with stress, parents, teachers, and health care providers need to frequently reassure children that they are safe, have honest and open communication with them, encourage children to express their feelings, and promote a daily routine and reliable limits. It is important that adults help children build coping strategies to foster self-confidence and overcome fears, by providing practical solutions, encouraging a sense of self-control, praising accomplishments, and avoiding criticism (CPS, 2013). Adults need to recognize signs indicating that a child is undergoing stress, identify the source of the stress promptly, and refer children who need specialized treatment.

> **! NURSING ALERT**
>
> The nurse who observes the following signs of stress in a child should explore the situation further:
> - Stomach pains or headache
> - Changes in sleep patterns or nightmares
> - Bedwetting
> - Changes in eating habits
> - Aggressive or stubborn behaviour
> - Withdrawal or reluctance to participate
> - Regression to earlier behaviours (e.g., thumb-sucking)
> - Trouble concentrating or changes in academic performance

Children 7 to 12 years of age are capable of identifying their own physiological responses to stress with terms that have meaning to them. They may describe their body's reaction to stress in terms of having tight muscles; being hot or red in the face; tingling; having chills or goose bumps; or experiencing shakiness, a heart beating fast, headache, or stomachache. Some children may experience headaches or get angry more easily. Children should be taught to recognize these signs as indicators of stress and to use techniques to manage their stress. Children can learn relaxation techniques such as deep-breathing exercises, progressive relaxation of muscle groups, and positive imagery to immediately reduce stress. "Blowing off steam" through physical activity can reduce tension and anxiety. Children can also be encouraged to observe effective coping strategies in others and adopt them for their own use. When an effective strategy has been developed for one situation, parents can show the child how to transfer the coping strategy or technique to other situations (Psychology Foundation of Canada, 2016).

In addition to stress, school-age children experience a wide variety of fears, including fear of the dark, excessive worry about past behaviour, self-consciousness, social withdrawal, and an excessive need for reassurance. These fears are considered normal for children this age. During the middle range of the school-age years, children become less fearful of body safety than they were as preschoolers, but they still fear being hurt, being kidnapped, or having to undergo surgery. They also fear death and are fascinated by all aspects of death and dying. Fears of noises, darkness, storms, and dogs lessen, while new fears related predominantly to school and family can bother children at this age.

PROMOTING OPTIMUM HEALTH DURING THE SCHOOL YEARS

Nutrition

Although caloric needs are diminished in relation to body size during middle childhood, resources are being laid down at this time for the increased growth needs of adolescence. Parents and children need to be aware of the value of a balanced diet toward promoting growth, because children usually eat what their family members eat (see Family-Centred Teaching box, p. 1109). The quality of the child's diet depends on the family's pattern of eating.

Likes and dislikes established at an early age tend to continue in middle childhood, although preferences for single foods subside and children develop a taste for a variety of foods. Unfortunately, the easy availability of fast-food restaurants, the influence of the mass media, and the temptation of "junk food" make it easy for children to fill up on empty calories. Foods that do not promote growth, such as sugars, starches, and excess fats, are common in the school-age child's diet. As discussed in Chapter 30, the easy availability of high-calorie foods, combined with the tendency toward more sedentary activities, has contributed to an epidemic of childhood obesity. This problem is discussed further in Chapter 39.

Parents are unable to monitor what their children eat when they are away from home. A parent may pack a lunch for school but is unaware of how much is eaten, traded, sold, or thrown away. Nutrition education can and should be integrated in the school curriculum throughout the school years. Important aspects of nutrition education include the relationship of nutrition to activity, fitness, and health; elements of a wholesome diet; and how food products are grown, processed, and prepared. A good resource for this is *Eating Well With Canada's Food Guide* (see Appendix A). In addition, some schools are seeking to provide healthy, nutritious meals at school, in the cafeteria. This effort includes the implementation of school policies related to vending machines, corporate sponsorships, and school and sports events. Some schools have initiated "breakfast clubs" for children who do not have access to breakfast at home. These programs are particularly important for children from impoverished families. Such programs are linked with greater student engagement in the classroom.

The community health nurse can take an active role in nutrition education by working with teachers to plan and implement units on nutrition instruction and by working with parents and children to give nutritional guidance.

Sleep and Rest

The amount of sleep and rest required during middle childhood is highly individualized. The amount of sleep depends on the child's age, activity level, and state of health. The growth rate slows in the school-age years, and less energy is expended in growth than during preceding years.

School-age children usually require approximately 10 to 12 hours of sleep from 5 to 10 years of age (CPS, 2012a). Although fewer bedtime problems occur during these years, occasional difficulties are still associated with the bedtime ritual. Usually children 6 or 7 years old exhibit few bedtime problems, and encouraging quiet activity before bedtime, such as colouring or reading, facilitates the task of going to bed. However, most children in middle childhood must be reminded frequently to go to bed; 8- to 11-year-old children can be particularly resistant. Often these children are unaware that they are tired; if they are allowed to remain up later than usual, they are fatigued the following day. Sometimes, bedtime resistance can be resolved by allowing a later bedtime as the child gets older. Twelve-year-old children usually offer no resistance at bedtime; some even retire early to read a book or listen to music.

Exercise and Activity

Because of the improved capabilities and adaptability of the school-age child, these children have greater speed and exert more effort in motor activities. Larger, stronger muscles enable longer and increasingly strenuous play without exhaustion. While school-age children acquire the coordination, timing, and concentration that are needed to participate in adult-type activities, they may lack the strength, stamina, and control of the adolescent and adult. Parents, teachers, and coaches must remember that, although children this age are large and appear strong, they may not be ready for strenuous competitive athletics.

All growing children need regular exercise and opportunities for satisfying experiences consistent with individual likes and dislikes. Positive reinforcement achieved by experiencing increasingly smooth, rhythmic, and efficient use of the body conditions the child toward regular physical activity. Exercise is essential for muscle development and tone, refinement of balance and coordination, increased strength and endurance, and stimulation of body functions and metabolic processes. Children need ample space to run, jump, skip, and climb, in addition to safe indoor and outdoor facilities and equipment. Most children have abundant energy and need little encouragement to engage in physical activity. Children from 5 to 11 years of age require an accumulation of 60 minutes per day of moderate to vigorous activity and vigorous-intensity activities three times a week (Canadian Society for Exercise Physiology, 2012). Children with disabling conditions or those who hesitate to become involved in active play (such as obese children) require special assessment so that activities appeal to them and are

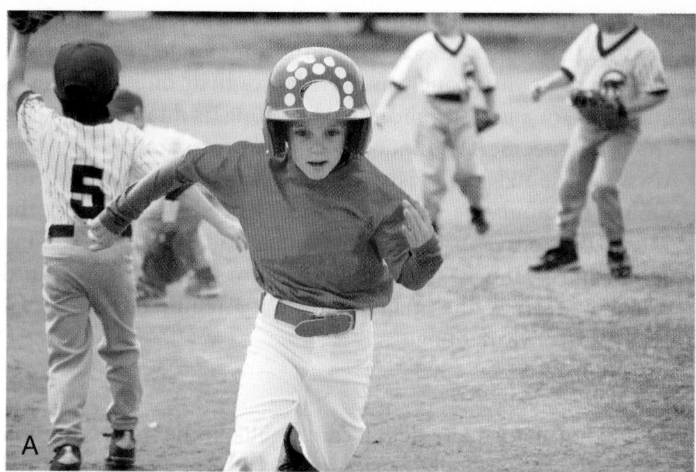

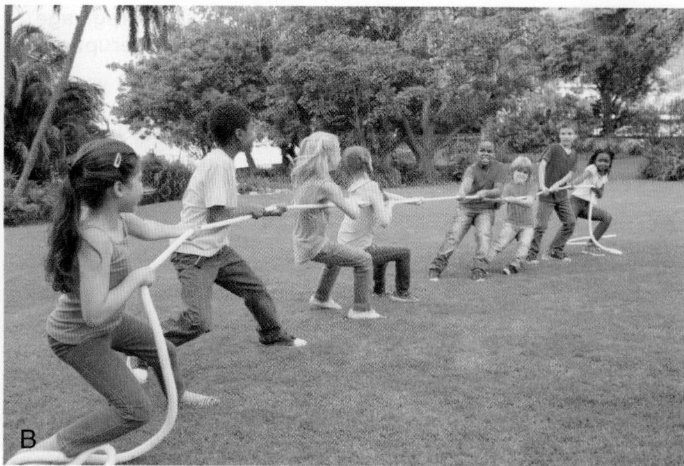

FIGURE 38-7 The activities engaged in by school-age children vary according to interest and opportunity. **A:** Little League competitors. **B:** Playing tug-of-war. (A, tammykayphoto/Shutterstock.com. B, wavebreakmedia/Shutterstock.com.)

compatible with their limitations while also meeting their developmental needs.

Sports

Considerable controversy surrounds the trend toward early participation in competitive athletics and the amount and type of competitive sports that are appropriate for children in the elementary grades. The current view is that virtually every child is suited for some sport, and authorities do not discourage participation if children are matched to the type of sport appropriate to their abilities and to their physical and emotional constitution. School-age children tend to enjoy competition (Fig. 38-7). However, teachers and coaches must understand the physical limitations of children this age and teach them the proper techniques and safety measures needed to avoid injuries. A safe and appropriate sport can be identified for even the most unskilled and uncompetitive child, including children with chronic illnesses and cognitive impairments. Common activities for school-age children include hockey, skiing, softball, soccer, gymnastics, and swimming. Equipment must be maintained in safe condition, and protective gear should be worn to prevent serious injury.

The Canadian Paediatric Society (CPS) (Warda, Yanchar, & CPS, Injury Prevention Committee 2012) recommends that children wear helmets when skiing and snowboarding and that they also wear wrist splints when snowboarding. These activities can lead to significant head and limb injuries and there is evidence that helmets and wrist splints prevent injuries (see Chapter 53, Traumatic Injury). It is important that parents provide approved helmets for winter temperatures and not use bike helmets for winter sports.

During the school-age years, girls have the same basic body structure as that of boys and have a similar response to systematic exercise training. However, at puberty, boys become larger and have more muscle mass, and at this stage it is usually recommended that girls compete only against other girls, in most sports. Before puberty there is no essential difference in strength and size between girls and boys, making these precautions unnecessary.

Preadolescence is a time to teach fundamental motor skills; develop fitness in a practical, safe, and gradual manner; and promote healthy attitudes and values. Activities should include both practice sessions and unstructured play; the actual game or event should be managed in a manner that stresses mastery of the sport, fun, and enhancement of self-image rather than winning or pleasing others. All children should have an opportunity to participate, and special ceremonies should recognize all participants, not just individuals who excel in sports or athletics.

Acquisition of Skills

School-age children demonstrate increasing fine-motor abilities and complex artistic skills. Handedness is well established by the beginning of the school years, and children make great strides in writing and drawing during this period. It is a time of energetic and vibrant creative productivity. With the tools of language and reading, children create poems, stories, and plays. With more advanced fine-motor skills, they are able to master an unlimited variety of handicrafts, such as ceramics, needlework, wood carving, and beadwork. They avidly pursue these skills in solitude; with a friend; or through organized groups, such as boys' or girls' clubs, or special interest groups that use crafts or other activities as a means to occupy, entertain, and educate children.

School-age children are capable of assuming responsibility for their own needs. School-age children can and want to assume their share of household tasks, which may be related to male and female roles defined by their culture. Parents may choose to role model open and flexible gender expectations. Many children also assume responsibility for tasks outside the home, such as babysitting, mowing lawns, or having paper routes.

Dental Health

The first permanent (secondary) teeth erupt at about 6 years of age, beginning with the 6-year molar, which erupts posterior to the deciduous molars. Other permanent teeth appear in approximately the same order as eruption of the primary teeth

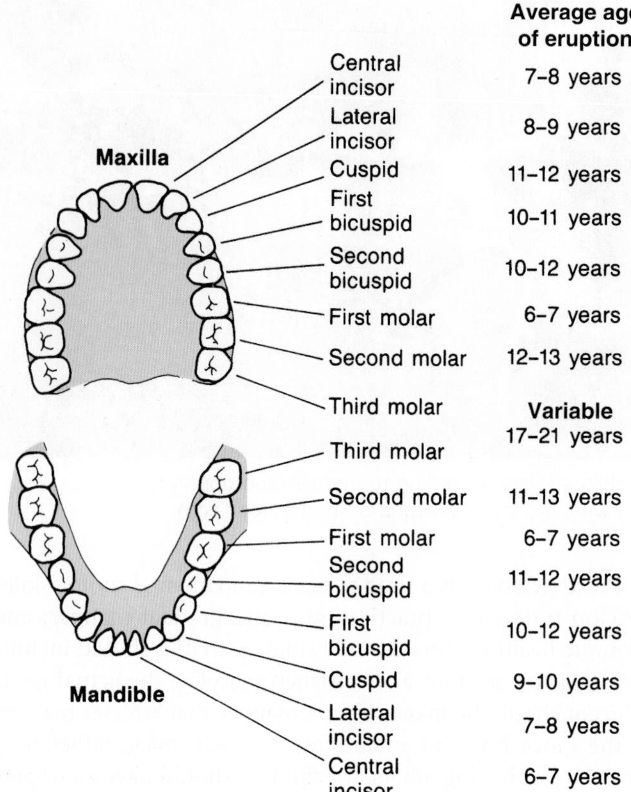

FIGURE 38-8 Sequence of eruption of secondary teeth. (Data from American Dental Association [2014]. *Eruption charts.* Retrieved from http://www.mouthhealthy.org/en/az-topics/e/eruption-charts.)

and follow shedding of the deciduous teeth (Fig. 38-8). With the appearance of the second permanent (12-year) molar, most permanent teeth are present. Permanent dentition is more advanced in girls than in boys.

Because the permanent teeth erupt during the school-age years, dental hygiene and regular attention to dental caries are important parts of health supervision during this period. Correct brushing techniques should be taught or reinforced, and the role that fermentable carbohydrates play in production of dental caries should be emphasized. It is important to be alert to possible malocclusion problems that may result from irregular eruption of permanent teeth and that may impair function. Regular dental supervision and continued fluoride supplementation are integral parts of the health maintenance program.

The most effective means of preventing dental caries is proper oral hygiene. Children should be taught to perform their own dental care, with the supervision and guidance of the parents. Parents should learn the correct brushing technique with their children, and they should monitor their child's efforts until the child can assume full responsibility.

Teeth should be brushed after meals, after snacks, and at bedtime. Children who brush their teeth frequently and become accustomed to the feel of a clean mouth at an early age usually maintain the habit throughout life. For the school-age child with mixed and permanent dentition, the best toothbrush is one with soft nylon bristles and should be comfortable for the child to hold and reach all teeth. Several methods of brushing have been described and recommended for children, but there is no conclusive evidence that one method is superior to another. Thorough cleaning is more important than the specific technique used, and professionals like dentists and dental hygienists should assess factors such as the child's manipulative skills and special needs and suggest the most appropriate brushing technique and regimen. Flossing follows brushing. Parents should perform the flossing until children acquire the manual dexterity required (usually at about 8 or 9 years of age).

Dental Problems

Limited or inadequate dental care results in the most common dental problems: dental caries, malocclusion, and periodontal disease. Trauma, especially tooth avulsion, is another important dental problem. All of these conditions benefit from early intervention to prevent tooth loss.

Dental caries (cavities) is the principal oral problem in children and adolescents. Reducing the incidence and consequences of dental caries is extremely important in childhood. If untreated, dental caries can result in the total destruction of the involved teeth. The prevalence rate of caries increases steadily across the lifespan.

Because many children are exposed to health care but not dental care, oral inspection is an integral part of the physical assessment of every child. Recent research indicates a high incidence of dental caries in baby teeth of Indigenous children; the prevalence of early-childhood caries exceeds 90% in Indigenous communities (Schroth, Harrison, & Moffatt, 2009). The CPS recommends that action be taken at the first age that caries are observed (Irvine, Holve, Krol, et al., 2011/2016). If there is any evidence of dental caries or other unhealthy dental state, the child should be referred for dental services. An alarming number of children do not receive regular dental supervision, and a significant number reach adulthood without having undergone dental examinations or treatment by a dentist.

Periodontal disease, an inflammatory and degenerative condition involving the gums and tissues supporting the teeth, often begins in childhood and accounts for a significant amount of tooth loss in adulthood. The more common periodontal problems are *gingivitis* (simple inflammation of the gums) and *periodontitis* (inflammation of the gums and loss of connective tissue and bone in the supporting structures of the teeth). Gingivitis, the most prevalent periodontal disease, is a reversible inflammatory disease that can begin in early childhood and is most often associated with the buildup of plaque on the teeth. Changes take place in the plaque bacteria, in both the type and number of organisms, causing them to release destructive exotoxins, enzymes, and other noxious agents. These substances produce an inflammatory reaction in the gingival tissues, causing the gums to become red, edematous, tender, and subject to bleeding at the slightest irritation. Management is directed toward prevention by conscientious brushing and flossing, including the use of fluoride. The child should see the dentist at any signs of inflammation or irritation.

Malocclusion occurs when teeth of the upper and lower dental arches do not approximate in the proper relationships. As a result, the physiological function of chewing is less effective and the cosmetic effect is displeasing. Teeth that are uneven, crowded, or overlapping are unable to meet their counterparts in the opposite jaw in the appropriate relationships and may be predisposed to disease in later years.

Orthodontic treatment is most successful when it is started in the late school-age or early teenage years, after the last primary teeth have been shed and before growth ceases. However, referral should be made as soon as malocclusion is evident, since some deformities can be corrected at an earlier age or require treatment in stages over the years. For families with few financial resources, such as new immigrant families, orthodontic corrects are hard to afford.

Dental injury may occur in childhood and includes fractures of varying degrees of severity, chipping, dislocation, or avulsion. All tooth injuries should be treated as a dental emergency requiring prompt treatment by a competent dentist to prevent permanent displacement or loss. Delayed examination and diagnosis of tooth damage can result in infection or pulp involvement. Because the loss can affect the remaining teeth, replacement of the lost tooth is needed to maintain normal alignment and position of the other teeth.

A tooth that is avulsed (exarticulated, or "knocked out") should be replanted by the child, parent, or nurse and stabilized as soon as possible so that the blood supply to the tooth can be re-established and the tooth kept alive (see Emergency box). A tooth that is replanted promptly has a good survival rate. Avulsed primary teeth are usually not reimplanted.

As with all injuries to the mouth, an avulsed tooth causes a large amount of bleeding, which is frightening to children and their families. Therefore, the nurse or anyone faced with dental trauma should be prepared to provide support and reassurance during the dental trauma.

EMERGENCY

Avulsed Permanent Tooth

Recover the tooth.
Hold tooth by the crown; avoid touching root area.
If the tooth is dirty, rinse it gently under running water or saline; be certain to insert a stopper in the sink or basin (to avoid losing tooth).

To Reimplant Tooth

Insert tooth into the socket; be certain that the lip side (or convex surface) is facing front.
Have child maintain tooth in place by slowly biting down on a piece of gauze.
Transport child to dentist immediately.
Avoid sudden stops or sharp turns to prevent dislodging the tooth.

If Reluctant to Reimplant Tooth

Place avulsed tooth in a suitable medium for transport:

- Cold milk
- Saliva—under the child's or parent's tongue

If child is holding tooth in the mouth, avoid sudden stops to prevent swallowing of tooth.
DO NOT FORGET TO TAKE THE TOOTH.

Sex Education

Many children experience some form of sex play during or before preadolescence, as a response to normal curiosity, not as a result of love or sexual urges. Children are experimentalists by nature, and sex play is incidental and transitory. Any adverse emotional consequences or guilt feelings depend on how the behaviour is managed by the parents; whether it is discovered; or whether children view their actions as wrong in the eyes of significant persons, particularly the parents.

The child's attitude toward sex is acquired indirectly at an early age. Initial curiosity about differences in body structure between boys and girls and between children and adults arises in the preschool years. Middle childhood is an ideal time for formal sex education, and many authorities believe that the topic is best presented from a lifespan approach. Information about sexual maturation and the process of reproduction minimizes the child's uncertainty, embarrassment, and feelings of isolation that often accompany puberty.

An important component of ongoing sex education is effective communication with parents. If parents either repress the child's sexual curiosity or avoid dealing with it, the sexual information that the child receives may be acquired almost entirely from peers. When peers are the primary source of sexual information, it is often transmitted and exchanged in secret conversation and contains a large amount of misinformation.

Nurse's Role in Sex Education

No matter where nurses practise, they can provide information on human sexuality to both parents and children. To discuss the topic adequately, nurses must have an understanding of the physiological aspects of sexuality; knowledge of the cultural and societal values; and an awareness of their own attitudes, feelings, and biases about sexuality.

When presenting sexual information to school-age children, nurses should treat sex as a normal part of growth and development. They should answer questions honestly, matter-of-factly, and to the same extent as questions about other topics. Answers should be at the child's level of understanding. There may be times when boys and girls should be taught content separately.

Children need help differentiating sex and sexuality. Exercises on clarifying values, identifying role models, engaging in problem-solving skills, and practising responsibility are important to prepare children for early adolescence and puberty. In addition, children need explanations of sexual information provided via the media or jokes. Information concerning pregnancy, contraceptives, and sexually transmitted infections (STIs), including human immunodeficiency virus (HIV) and human papillomavirus (HPV), should be presented in simple, accurate terms.

Preadolescents need precise and concrete information that will allow them to answer questions such as "What if I start my period in the middle of class?" or "How can I keep people from telling I have an erection?" It is important to tell children what they want to know and what they can expect to happen as they become mature sexually.

During interactions with parents, nurses should be open and available for questions and discussion. They can set an example by the language they use in discussing body parts and their function and by the way in which they deal with problems that have emotional overtones, such as exploratory sex play and masturbation. Parents may need help understanding normal behaviours and viewing sexual curiosity in their children as a part of the developmental process. Assessment of the parents' level of knowledge and understanding of sexuality can provide cues to their need for supplemental information that will prepare them for the increasingly complex explanations they will need to provide as their children grow older.

School Health

Child health maintenance is ultimately the responsibility of the parents; however, public schools and health departments in Canada have contributed to the improvement of child health by providing a healthful school environment, health services, and health education that emphasize sound health practices. Varying by province, territory, and school district, most of these functions constitute major components of community health services and involve public funding and health care providers, including nurses. School health programs are involved in ongoing health maintenance through assessment, screening, and referral activities. Health services provided by many schools include health appraisal by consultation, emergency care, safety education, communicable disease control, counselling, and follow-up care. Health education of school-age children is directed toward providing knowledge of health and influencing habits, attitudes, and conduct in relation to health promotion and injury prevention. School districts may allocate their money to programs aimed at improving learning by improving nutrition—for example, some inner city schools in Vancouver and Toronto have breakfast programs for all children.

Today, community health nurses may manage and coordinate care required by regular students and students with special health care needs. In many settings, school health services have enlarged into community health centres that meet the needs of not only school-age children but also their families and the community. In these settings, schools provide health care that includes assessment of physical, psychological, emotional, behavioural, and learning problems, as well as comprehensive well-child care.

The level of integration of children with chronic illness or disability into regular classrooms varies among the provinces and territories in Canada. Community health nurses are usually available for consultation on integrating the child into the classroom, although the individual parent may need to make arrangements with their local community health nursing organization if their child requires nursing care at school. Community health nurses can develop, implement, and evaluate individualized health care plans for these children. Most health jurisdictions aim to provide unregulated care providers such as special education assistants (EAs) to be with all children who require such assistance. Delegation and supervision of unregulated care providers requires skillful nursing assessment, effective communication, and professional judgement.

Injury Prevention

Because school-age children have developed more refined muscular coordination and control and can apply their cognitive capacities to their behaviour, the number of injuries in middle childhood is less than that in early childhood. Currently, data related to accidents in Canada are collected and analyzed by the Canadian Hospitals Injury Reporting and Prevention Program (CHIRPP), a program of the Public Health Agency of Canada (2009a). Much of the data relates to children seen in Canada's 10 pediatric hospitals. Nurses and other health care providers can use these data to help prevent injury in children, as the details collected relate to the pre-event context of injury. In Canada, the leading cause of death for children under 14 years of age is child pedestrian accidents. On average, annually more than 30 child pedestrians under age 14 are killed and 2400 are injured, with most accidents happening between the hours of 1500 and 1800, when children are walking home from school and drivers are going home from work (Parachute, 2009). Hand-held devices such as cell phones put children at a higher risk of pedestrian injury. This equipment along with ear plugs are distractors and lessen traffic sounds and can result in pedestrian injury.

To help reduce the number of injuries in children as passengers in motor vehicle accidents, nurses need to emphasize to parents the three automobile safety measures found to reduce the severity of injuries: effective car restraint systems, use of door-lock mechanisms, and appropriate passenger-seating locations in the motor vehicle. The CPS position statement on motor vehicle safety advises that the back seat is the safest place for children under the age of 12 years. Children should use specially designed car restraints until they are 145 cm in height or are 8 to 12 years old, and they should not sit in the front seat until they are at least 12 years of age (Government of Canada, 2016; van Schaik & CPS, Injury Prevention Committee, 2008). Shoulder-lap safety belts should be worn low on the hips, snug, and not on the abdominal area. Children should be taught to sit up straight to allow for proper fit. The shoulder belt is used only if it does not cross the child's neck or face.

The school-age child's frequent bicycle-riding activity increases the risk of injury. Other serious injuries include accidents on skateboards, roller skates, in-line skates, scooters, and other sports equipment. Most injuries occur in or near the home or school. Skateboarders need to use a specific helmet for that sport. All-terrain vehicles (ATVs), popular with children younger than 16 years of age, are unstable, difficult to handle, and responsible for an increasing number of childhood injuries. In some Canadian jurisdictions, children are not allowed to operate ATVs if they are under 16 years of age. The CPS advocates a Canada-wide ban on ATV operation by those under 16 years of age (Yanchar & CPS, Injury Prevention Committee, 2012). The IWK Health Centre in Halifax reported a 50% decrease in ATV injuries among youth under age 14 after the Nova Scotia government restricted youth younger than 14 from operating ATVs; the injury rate was unchanged in 14- to 15-year-olds, which suggests that the restriction be raised to 16 years of age (Parachute, n.d.). Snowmobiles are also a source of serious injury to a child; the CPS recommends that youth under 16 years not operate a snowmobile (Stanwick & CPS, Injury Prevention Committee, 2004/2014). See Chapter 39 for more information on ATV and snowmobile safety.

The most effective means of injury prevention is education of the child and family about the hazards of risk taking and the improper use of equipment. Safety helmets, protective eye and mouth shields, and protective padding are strongly recommended for children engaging in active sports, even though they may not be required equipment. Falls from bicycles, ATVs, and skateboards are the cause of a significant number of head injuries in school-age children. Because head injury is the major cause of bicycle-related fatalities, the most important aspect of bicycle safety is to encourage the rider to wear a protective helmet. Wearing of a properly fitting helmet can decrease the risk of serious head injury by over 85%; this means that four out of five head injuries could be prevented by the use of helmets (Parachute, 2014). British Columbia, Ontario, New Brunswick, Nova Scotia, Alberta, Prince Edward Island, and Manitoba all require cyclists under 18 years of age to wear a bike helmet. Some provinces require helmets for all age groups, as do some municipalities. It is also important that children ride bicycles that are the correct size for their bodies (Fig. 38-9). The Family Centred Teaching boxes provide guidelines for bicycle, skateboard, and in-line skate safety and guidance during the school years.

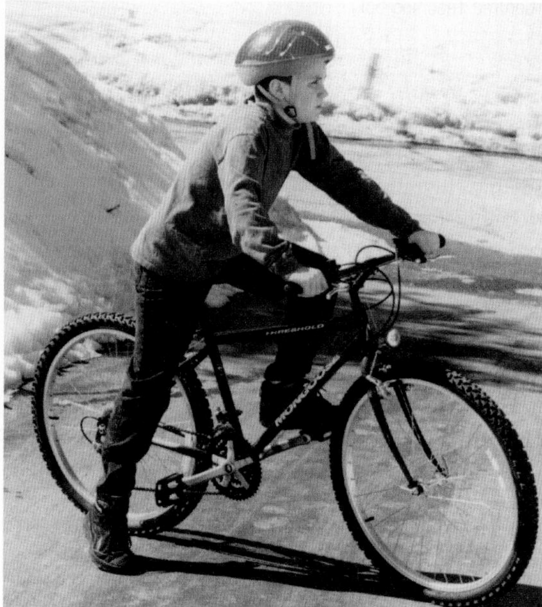

FIGURE 38-9 The right-size bike is important; the child should be able to sit on the bike and place the balls of both feet on the ground. The foot should comfortably reach and manipulate the pedal in the down position. Wearing a protective helmet should be mandatory. The helmet should be positioned so it sits low on the forehead and parallel to the ground when the head is held upright. It should not rock back and forth or shift from side to side. The strap should fasten securely under the chin.

Physically active school-age children are also highly susceptible to cuts and abrasions; the incidence of childhood fractures, strains, and sprains is high. Trampoline injuries occur most frequently in children ages 5 through 14 years and account for numerous fractures, sprains, and head injuries. Trampolines in the home environment, routine physical education classes, or outdoor playgrounds are not recommended for children of any age (Eberl, Schalamon, Singer, et al., 2009).

Table 38-2 lists characteristics of school-age children that make them prone to injury and provides suggestions for injury prevention.

Injury prevention is particularly important in Indigenous communities in Canada, as the leading cause of death for all Indigenous people aged 1 to 44 years is injuries. In this group, 26% of all deaths are caused by injuries, compared with 6% for the rest of the Canadian population. The majority of hospital admissions in this population are for falls in most age groups. School-age Indigenous children commonly fall

FAMILY-CENTRED TEACHING

Bicycle Safety

- Always wear a properly fitted bicycle helmet that is certified, e.g., by the Canadian Standards Association (CSA); look for the CSA approval sticker on the inside liner of the helmet and to find out if helmet use is legally mandated (legislation varies across provinces) (Public Health Agency of Canada, 2009b).
- Replace a helmet every 5 years or sooner if the manufacturer recommends it. **Never use a damaged or outgrown helmet**. Bike helmets can be used for in-line skating and scooter riding but skateboarding has its own specific helmet (Parachute, n.d.).
- Ride bicycles with traffic and away from parked cars.
- Ride single file.
- Walk bicycles through busy intersections only at crosswalks.
- Give hand signals well in advance of turning or stopping.
- Keep as close to the curb as practical.
- Watch for drain grates, potholes, soft shoulders, loose dirt, or gravel.
- Keep both hands on the handlebars, except with signalling.
- Never ride double on a bicycle.
- Do not carry packages that interfere with vision or control; do not drag objects behind the bike.
- Watch for and yield to pedestrians.
- Watch for cars backing up or pulling out of driveways; be especially careful at intersections.
- Look left, right, then left, before turning into traffic or road.
- Never hitch a ride on a truck or other vehicle.
- Learn rules of the road and respect traffic officers.
- Obey all local ordinances.
- Wear shoes that fit securely while riding.
- Wear light colours at night and attach fluorescent material to clothing and the bicycle.
- Equip the bicycle with proper lights and reflectors.
- Be certain the bicycle is the correct size for rider (see Fig. 38-9).
- Have the bicycle inspected to ensure good mechanical condition.
- Children riding as passengers must wear appropriate-size helmets and sit in specially designed protective seats.

Modified from American Academy of Pediatrics, Committee on Injury and Poison Prevention. (2001). Bicycle helmets. *Pediatrics, 108*(4), 1030–1032.

FAMILY-CENTRED TEACHING

Skateboard, In-Line Skate, and Scooter Safety

- Children younger than 5 years of age should not use skateboards or in-line skates because they are not developmentally prepared to protect themselves from injury. Children ages 6 to 10 years should use these only with adult supervision.
- Children younger than 8 years should ride scooters only with close adult supervision.
- Children who ride skateboards, in-line skates, or scooters should wear helmets and other protective equipment, especially on the knees, wrists, and elbows, to prevent injury.
- Skateboards, in-line skates, and scooters should never be used near traffic or in streets. Their use should be prohibited at night. Activities that bring skateboards together (e.g., "catching a ride") are especially dangerous.
- Some types of use, such as riding homemade ramps on hard surfaces, may be particularly hazardous.

Data from American Academy of Pediatrics, Committee on Injury and Poison Prevention. (2006). Skateboard injuries. *Pediatrics, 109*(3), 542–543; American Academy of Pediatrics, Committee on Injury and Poison Prevention. (2006). In-line skating injuries in children and adolescents. *Pediatrics, 117*(5), 1846–1847; Public Health Agency of Canada. (2014). Bicycle injuries and injury prevention. *Chronic Diseases and Injuries in Canada, 34*(2–3), 71–73. Retrieved from http://www.phac-aspc.gc.ca/publicat/hpcdp-pspmc/34-2-3/assets/pdf/CDIC_MCC_Vol34_2-3-eng.pdf

TABLE 38-2 INJURY PREVENTION DURING SCHOOL-AGE YEARS*

DEVELOPMENTAL ABILITIES RELATED TO RISK OF INJURY	INJURY PREVENTION
Motor Vehicle Accidents	
Is increasingly involved in activities away from home Is excited by speed and motion Is easily distracted by environment Can be reasoned with	Educate child regarding proper use of seat belts while a passenger in a vehicle. Children should ride in the back seat of a car until age 12. Maintain discipline while a passenger in a vehicle (e.g., keep arms inside, do not lean against doors, do not interfere with driver). Remind parents and children that no one should ride in the bed of a pickup truck. Emphasize safe pedestrian behaviour. Insist on child wearing safety apparel (e.g., helmet) when applicable, such as when riding a bicycle, motorcycle, moped, or all-terrain vehicle (see Family Centred Teaching box).
Drowning	
Is apt to overdo May work hard to perfect a skill Has cautious, but not fearful, gross motor actions Likes swimming	Teach child to swim. Teach basic rules of water safety. Select safe and supervised places to swim. Check sufficient water depth for diving. Swim with a companion. Use an approved flotation device. Advocate for legislation requiring fencing around pools. Learn cardiopulmonary resuscitation. Teach winter ice safety, for example, when ice skating, playing pond hockey, and snowmobiling
Burns	
Has increasing independence Is adventurous Enjoys trying new things	Make certain the home has smoke and carbon monoxide detectors. Set water heaters at 49°C to avoid scald burns. Do not lower the temperature of water heater below 49°C or a medium setting or below 60 degrees if electric heater because lower settings can lead to the growth of the bacteria that causes Legionnaires' disease. Instruct child in behaviour in areas involving contact with potential burn hazards (e.g., gasoline, matches, bonfires or barbecues, lighter fluid, firecrackers, cigarette lighters, cooking utensils, chemistry sets). Instruct child to avoid climbing or flying a kite around high-tension or electrical wires. Instruct child in proper behaviour in the event of a fire (e.g., fire drills at home and school). Teach child safe cooking (use low heat; avoid any frying; be careful of steam burns, scalds, or exploding foods, especially from microwaving).
Accidental Poisoning	
Adheres to group rules May be easily influenced by peers Has strong allegiance to friends	Educate child regarding hazards of taking nonprescription drugs and chemicals, including aspirin and alcohol. Teach child to say "no" if offered illegal or dangerous drugs or alcohol. Keep potentially dangerous products in properly labelled receptacles, preferably out of reach.

TABLE 38-2 INJURY PREVENTION DURING SCHOOL-AGE YEARS—cont'd

DEVELOPMENTAL ABILITIES RELATED TO RISK OF INJURY	INJURY PREVENTION
Bodily Damage	
Has increased physical skills Needs strenuous physical activity Is interested in acquiring new skills and perfecting attained skills Is daring and adventurous, especially with peers Frequently plays in hazardous places Confidence often exceeds physical capacity Desires group loyalty and has strong need for friends' approval Attempts hazardous feats Accompanies friends to potentially hazardous facilities Is likely to overdo Growth in height exceeds muscular growth and coordination	Help provide facilities for supervised activities. Encourage playing in safe places. Keep firearms safely locked up except under adult supervision. Teach proper care of, use of, and respect for devices with potential danger (e.g., power tools, firecrackers). Teach children not to tease or surprise dogs, invade their territory, take dogs' toys, or interfere with dogs' feeding. Stress eye, ear, or mouth protection when using potentially hazardous objects or devices or when engaging in potentially hazardous sports. Teach safety regarding use of corrective devices (glasses); if the child wears contact lenses, monitor duration of wear to prevent corneal damage. Stress careful selection, use, and maintenance of sports and recreation equipment, such as skateboards and in-line skates (see Family-Centred Teaching box). Emphasize proper conditioning, safe practices, and use of safety equipment for sports or recreational activities. Caution against engaging in hazardous sports, such as those involving trampolines. Use safety glass and decals on large glassed areas, such as sliding glass doors. Use window guards to prevent falls. Teach child that he or she should ask for help from appropriate people (e.g., cashier, security guard, police) if lost; have identification on the child (e.g., sewn in clothes, inside shoe). Teach stranger safety: • Avoid clothing displaying the child's name or family name in public places. • Caution child to never go with a stranger. • Have child tell parents if anyone makes child feel uncomfortable in any way. Always listen to child's concerns regarding others' behaviour. Teach child to say "no" when confronted by uncomfortable situations—practise this with them.

*See also Public Health Agency of Canada. (2011). *The chief public health officer's report on the state of public health in Canada 2009. Growing up well—Priorities for a healthy future.* Retrieved from http://www.phac-aspc.gc.ca/cphorsphc-respcacsp/2009/fr-rc/pdf/cphorsphc-respcacsp-eng.pdf

from playground equipment, fences, and trees (Health Canada, 2008).

Use of Social Media and the Internet

Children are very familiar with different forms of media, and this contact with the media brings benefits as well as risks. Social media sites abound, including Facebook, Twitter, Instagram, Snapchat, blogs, gaming sites, and virtual worlds such as Club Penguin, Second Life, and The Sims. Children also frequent video sites such as YouTube. The benefits of social media and Internet use to children include entertainment as well as development of communication and technical skills. However, there are also risks to children with these media sites, such as cyberbullying. Sexual predators lurk on the Internet and can make dangerous contact with children.

It is recommended that parents talk to their children about their use of the Internet and the dangers that children may face online. Parents also need to address cyberbullying, "sexting," and time management of using social media. Families can create a "family online-use plan" that emphasizes good citizenship and healthy behaviour. Children need parental monitoring with participation and discussion of their online activity (O'Keeffe, Clarke-Pearson, & Council on Communications and Media, 2011). (See Additional Resources at the end of the chapter for a guide for parents.)

SPECIAL HEALTH PROBLEMS

Health Problems Related to Sports Participation

Every sport has the potential for injury to the participant—whether the youngster engages in serious competition or participates for enjoyment. Serious injury occurs most often during rough contact sports or to persons who are not physically prepared for the activity. Injuries also occur to children or adolescents when their body is not suited to the sport, when their muscles and body systems (respiratory and cardiovascular) are not conditioned to endure physical stress, or when they lack the insight and judgement to recognize that an activity exceeds their physical abilities. More injuries occur during recreational sports participation than during organized athletic competition.

Acute overload injuries are those that occur suddenly during an activity and produce immediate symptoms. A blow or overstretching, twisting, or sudden stress to tissues can cause these injuries. For descriptions and management of traumatic injuries, see Chapter 53.

Head Injuries and Concussion

There is increasing concern about the risk of injury when children are playing sports, particularly with sports where there is a risk of head injury.

Clinical manifestations of concussion can be subtle and easily missed by athletes, coaches or trainers, parents, and even health care providers. Often, injured athletes do not recognize the signs or symptoms of a concussion or choose not to get medical treatment. Any child who sustains a concussion needs to be removed from play immediately and undergo a medical assessment as soon as possible. Cognitive and physical rest are recommended to allow symptoms to resolve. Cognitive rest may require a temporary school absence, as well as modified class work or homework. After symptoms have entirely resolved at rest, a child can return to school with a medically supervised, stepwise exertion program to return to play (Purcell & CPS, Healthy Active Living and Sports Medicine Committee, 2014). See Chapter 50 for more information on head injuries.

Overuse Syndromes

To excel in sports, the young athlete is forced to train longer, harder, and earlier in life than previously. The rewards are an increased level of fitness, better performances, faster times, and the satisfaction of attaining a personal goal. However, the risk of overuse injury is always present and is related to several factors: training errors, muscle–tendon imbalance, anatomical malalignment, incorrect footwear or playing surface, an associated disease state, and growth.

A common feature in overuse injuries is the repetitive microtrauma that occurs to a particular anatomical structure when the same movements are performed over a long period of time. The result is inflammation of the involved structure with symptoms of chronic pain, tenderness, swelling, and disability. Examples of overuse syndromes include "Little League elbow" (tendonitis and osteochondritis from repetitive throwing), "tennis elbow" (lateral epicondylitis from repetitive elbow strain), and Osgood-Schlatter disease (traction apophysitis of the tibial tubercle).

Stress fractures. Stress fractures occur as a result of repeated muscle contraction and are seen most often in repetitive weight-bearing sports such as running, gymnastics, and basketball. They occur less often in swimmers. The most common symptoms are a sharp, persistent, progressive pain or a deep, persistent, dull ache located over the bone. Sometimes there is pain on impact (heel strike), but the most important clinical sign is pain over the involved bony surface. Diagnosis is established on the basis of clinical observation, but occasionally a bone scan is performed.

Therapeutic management. Inflammation is common in all overuse syndromes, and management is directed toward rest or alteration of activities, physiotherapy, and medication. Rest is the primary therapy and is usually interpreted as reduced activity and the use of alternative exercise—not bedrest or immobilization with casting. The primary purpose is to alleviate the repetitive stress that initiated the symptoms. It is important to keep the youngster mobile, and training can be continued. Alternative exercise that maintains conditioning without aggravating the injury is selected. For example, pool running (treading water in the deep end of a pool) is an excellent alternative to running. Pool running involves the same movements as running without weight bearing. Other therapies include cryotherapy; cold whirlpools; and sometimes taping, bracing, splinting, or other orthoses. Treatment is specific to the injury. Nonsteroidal anti-inflammatory drugs (NSAIDs) are prescribed to reduce pain and inflammation. Topical medications are of questionable value.

NURSING CARE

Nurses' involvement in children's sports activities often entails preparation and evaluation for activities, prevention of injury, treatment of injuries, and rehabilitation after injury. For example, nurses work with parents and children in these roles in emergency rooms, orthopaedic clinics, and inpatient units. Community health nurses work with individuals and groups performing these roles as well. Selecting an appropriate sport for both recreation and competition is a joint effort of the youngster, parents, and health care providers. The best approach to counselling children and parents regarding sports participation is to encourage activities that are most likely to provide pleasure and physical benefits throughout childhood and into adulthood. Exposure to a variety of activities is better for young children than limiting them to one sport. Parents should be cautioned against overcommitting children to sports activities so that they have time for other activities.

When children sustain athletic injuries, nurses are often responsible for instructions in care. The instructions (e.g., schedule for appointments, application of ice, and any restrictions in activity) should be clear and accompanied by written directions. The importance of taking medications as prescribed should also be emphasized, especially if medications are needed for an extended period and if adherence is an issue. Medications given an hour before practice or competition may be advantageous to children who are continuing their activities.

Prevention of sports injuries is the most important aspect of athletic programs. Children should be suited to the activity, and the environment and equipment must be safe. Children should be prepared for the sport, especially if it requires strenuous or continuous physical exertion. Nurses, coaches, and athletic trainers must collaborate to ensure that safety measures are implemented. Stretching exercises, warm-up and cool-down activities, and appropriate training are requirements for safe participation. Protective measures such as pads, taping, and wrapping are also important to prevent injury.

Altered Growth and Maturation

The absence of physical or sexual maturation at a time when other children are experiencing positive evidence of sexual development and its associated spurt in growth and physical strength can be a concern to both the parents and their affected child. Fortunately, in most instances, the delay in development is a simple physiological or constitutional delay that represents one end of the normal genetically influenced variation of pubertal growth. These children will go through a delayed but normal puberty and finally catch up, in their late teens, with their more rapidly developing age-mates. Less benign causes of delayed development may be the result of endocrine disorders or chromosomal abnormalities. Delayed development can also be a result of chronic diseases (such as malabsorption or chronic asthma) that are serious enough to slow development or a result of environmental factors (such as stress or poor nutrition).

Rates of maturation are important during the school years, but at puberty it assumes larger proportions to both teens and their parents. Girls or boys who lag behind their peers in physical maturation are painfully aware of their difference in growth.

Tall Stature

Despite the fact that the average height of boys and girls is steadily increasing, there is a small group of children who, because of some organic disorder or a familial tendency, are excessively tall compared with their peers.

When the rate of height change before puberty suggests the probability of excessive adult height, treatment with hormones may be considered, although there is considerable controversy regarding the use of hormones for this purpose. The use of estrogens is effective in controlling height when therapy is initiated before menarche and before the end of the adolescent growth spurt that normally precedes menarche. The selection of children for hormonal therapy is made on the basis of a careful evaluation of physical, psychological, and social factors.

Short Stature

Short stature is a nonspecific finding that may be the first manifestation of a serious disorder, or it may be of no consequence medically. On a worldwide scale, the most common cause of short stature or delayed development is inadequate nutrition. The major physical disorders that produce delayed development are chronic diseases, endocrine dysfunction, and syndromes of primary gonad failure.

Chronic diseases can interfere with growth, but unless the illness is unduly prolonged, catch-up growth occurs. Diseases and disorders that cause some degree of growth delay include asthma, cystic fibrosis, gastrointestinal diseases (such as parasitic infections), celiac disease, malabsorption syndromes, cardiac anomalies, and chronic renal disturbances. The duration of the illness is more significant than the intensity in terms of the effect on growth, although the precise length of time necessary to affect growth permanently has not been determined.

Skeletal disorders that affect growth in stature are those described as dwarfism. Most disorders are caused by congenital defects and disorders, such as achondroplasia, and by inborn errors of metabolism, such as Hurler's syndrome or Hunter's syndrome.

Psychosocial or deprivation dwarfism is a stress-induced growth failure. It is defined as growth restriction in children over 2 years of age that is caused by environmental (emotional) stress and is associated with a marked delay in physical growth, delayed developmental skills, and immature behaviour. When these children are removed from the deprived environment, their growth proceeds at a normal or increased rate. (See also Growth Failure [Failure to Thrive], Chapter 35, and Child Maltreatment, Chapter 31.)

Management involves continued medical observation, attention to general health and nutrition, and psychological support. When growth delay is accompanied by poor self-esteem, many authorities recommend hormonal therapy. Testosterone in carefully regulated doses is effective in some cases. Growth hormone is capable of increasing height and is used to treat growth hormone deficiency (see Chapter 51, Hypopituitarism). Its use with children who have constitutional delay is highly controversial.

NURSING CARE

One difficulty related to size being incongruent with chronological and mental age is the manner in which others relate to the child. People often respond to children with short stature as though they are younger than their age. Consequently, these children may react with babyish or juvenile behaviour, thus establishing a circular pattern of behaviour and response. Conversely, children who are tall or physically advanced for their age are frequently treated as though they were more advanced than their years. They are often considered to be cognitively impaired or immature when they perform according to the normal behavioural expectations for their age.

Listening to distressed adolescents and conveying interest in and concern about them are important interventions. Counselling and therapy need to be individualized for each youth. Encouraging these children to focus on the positive aspects of their bodies and personalities and to adopt sound health practices and practise good grooming fosters a more positive self-image.

Sex Chromosome Abnormalities

Most sex chromosome abnormalities are caused by an alteration in sex chromosome number (Table 38-3). Most of these conditions are due to nondisjunction. An alteration in the number of sex chromosomes usually does not produce the profound defects associated with the autosomal trisomies. Intelligence may be normal or low normal or the child may have some learning disabilities. Moderate or severe cognitive impairment is less common.

Turner Syndrome

Turner syndrome is caused by absence of one of the X chromosomes. Most girls who have this disorder have one X chromosome missing from all cells (45,X). This disorder is often recognized at birth if the newborn has a webbed neck, low posterior hairline, widely spaced nipples, and edema of the hands and feet. It can also be diagnosed at puberty because of three features: short stature, sexual infantilism, and amenorrhea. Girls with Turner syndrome are generally infertile. They may also have difficulty with peer relationships and understanding social cues. They frequently exhibit behavioural problems, especially in relation to their immature, socially isolated behaviour. Diagnosis is confirmed on the basis of a negative sex chromatin test (see Chapter 9, p. 183).

Therapy is individualized for these girls and consists primarily of hormone treatment and psychological counselling for

TABLE 38-3 COMMON SEX CHROMOSOME ABNORMALITIES

SYNDROME	CHROMOSOMAL NOMENCLATURE	PHENOTYPE	INCIDENCE (LIVE BIRTHS)	CLINICAL MANIFESTATIONS
Turner	45,X or 45XO	Female	1:2500 female births*	Short stature; webbed neck; low posterior hairline; shield-shaped chest with widely spaced nipples; sterile; no development of secondary sex characteristics
Triple X, or superfemale	47,XXX (can also be 48,XXXX or 49,XXXXX)	Female	1:850–1250 female births	Normal female characteristics; usually tall; variable mental capacity and behaviour; at risk for impaired language, learning difficulties; fertile
XYY male	47,XYY (can also be 48,XYYY or mosaic)	Male	1:900 male births*	Usually normal sexual development; tendency to be tall with long head; poor coordination; may demonstrate aberrant behaviour
Klinefelter	47,XXY (48,XXYY, 48,XXXY, 49,XXXXY, and so on, mosaics)	Male	1:850 male births*	Tall with long legs; hypogenitalism; sterile; male secondary sex characteristics may be deficient; may demonstrate aberrant behaviour; learning disabled; possible gynecomastia

*Data from Nora, J. J., & Fraser, F. C. (1989). *Medical genetics: Principles and practice* (3rd ed.). Philadelphia: Lea & Febiger.

both the child and parents. Linear growth can be increased by the administration of growth hormone if therapy is begun early. Estrogen therapy is initiated during the usual time for puberty to promote the development of secondary sex characteristics. Responses to estrogen therapy vary from girl to girl, but gradual feminization is accomplished to some degree in most individuals.

Klinefelter Syndrome

Klinefelter syndrome, the most common of all sex chromosome abnormalities, is caused by the presence of one or more additional X chromosomes. Most males with this syndrome have a chromosome complement of 47, XXY. The disorder is seldom recognized before puberty, at which time varying degrees of failure of adolescent virilization occur. Some males are not diagnosed until they appear for evaluation for infertility. All have absence of sperm in the semen (azoospermia), small testes, and defective development of secondary sex characteristics. In 80% of these boys there is a chromatin-positive buccal smear, and the extra chromosome is apparent on chromosome analysis.

Cognitive impairment is a frequent clinical finding and appears to be related to the number of X chromosomes. Boys may also have gross motor skill difficulties, a developmental language delay, poor verbal skills, reduced auditory memory, shyness, passivity, behavioural problems, and school difficulties. Therapy is directed toward enhancing the masculine characteristics through administration of testosterone.

NURSING CARE

The nursing care of children with Turner syndrome or Klinefelter syndrome is primarily supportive. Nurses can assist in diagnosis, explain tests and therapies, and provide support and encouragement to the child and the family. Because the disorders render the individual unable to reproduce, psychological counselling is an important aspect of care. Marriage and sexual relationships are possible, but alternative reproductive options, such as artificial insemination and adoption, should be discussed.

School-Age Disorders With Behavioural Components

Attention-Deficit/Hyperactivity Disorder and Learning Disability

Attention-deficit/hyperactivity disorder (ADHD) refers to developmentally inappropriate degrees of inattention, impulsiveness, and hyperactivity. A **learning disability (LD)** refers to a heterogeneous group of disorders manifested by significant difficulties in the acquisition and use of listening, speaking, reading, writing, reasoning, or mathematic skills.

ADHD and LDs affect every aspect of the child's life but are most obvious in the classroom. Early identification of affected children is important because the characteristics of these disorders significantly interfere with the normal course of emotional and psychological development. Many children develop maladaptive behaviour patterns that impede psychosocial adjustment while they try to cope with cognitive dysfunction. Their behaviour evokes negative responses from others, and repeated exposure to negative feedback adversely affects their self-concept. The characteristics of ADHD can affect the child's written and adaptive skills, social status, and self-esteem (Urion, 2016).

Diagnostic evaluation. The behaviours exhibited by the child with ADHD are not unusual. The difference lies in the quality of motor activity and developmentally inappropriate inattention, impulsivity, and hyperactivity displayed by children with ADHD. The manifestations may be numerous or few, mild or severe, and will vary with the child's developmental level. Any

BOX 38-1 ATTENTION-DEFICIT/ HYPERACTIVITY DISORDER

Diagnostic Features

Inattention

Manifests behaviourally in ADHD as wandering off task, lacking persistence, having difficulty sustaining focus, and being disorganized and is not due to defiance or lack of comprehension

Hyperactivity

Excess motor activity (such as a child running about) when it is not appropriate, or excessive fidgeting, tapping, or talkativeness

Impulsivity

Hasty actions that occur in the moment without forethought and that have high potential for harm to the individual (e.g., darting into the street without looking). Impulsivity may reflect a desire for immediate awards or an inability to delay gratification.

Reprinted with permission from the *Diagnostic and statistical manual of mental disorders*, Fifth Edition, (Copyright ©2013). American Psychiatric Association.

given child will not have every symptom of the condition and the degree of severity is highly variable. Mild manifestations of symptoms may not be apparent in some educational and family environments, but severe symptoms will be recognizable in most environments. Every child with ADHD is different from all other children. The clinical manifestations of ADHD are outlined in Box 38-1.

Most behavioural manifestations of ADHD are apparent at an early age, but the LDs may not become evident until the child enters school. The disorder is unpredictable; it may remit spontaneously at any age, and the number of years that a child will require treatment is unknown.

A major clinical manifestation is distractibility. The stimuli may come from external or internal sources. Children often demonstrate immaturity relative to chronological age. Selective attention is often seen, in which the child has difficulty attending to "nonpreferred" tasks such as completing chores or finishing homework. The child may not consider the consequences of behaviour, may take excessive physical risks (often beginning early in life), and may demonstrate inappropriate social skills.

Children with ADHD demonstrate one of three subtypes (APA, 2013) (Box 38-1).

1. Combined type—six or more symptoms of inattention and six or more symptoms of hyperactivity-impulsivity that last at least 6 months. Most children and adolescents with ADHD have the combined type hyperactivity-impulsivity.
2. Predominantly inattentive type—six or more symptoms of inattention but fewer than six symptoms of hyperactivity-impulsivity that persist for at least 6 months
3. Predominantly six or more symptoms of hyperactivity-impulsivity inattention but fewer than six symptoms of inattentiveness that last at least 6 months. Inattention may often still be a significant clinical feature in such cases.

A diagnosis of ADHD is established on the basis of characteristics in the American Psychiatric Association's (2013) *Diagnostic and Statistical Manual of Mental Disorders* (*DSM-5*) and a thorough evaluation of the child (Box 38-1). It is important to emphasize the need for a complete and thorough multidisciplinary evaluation that incorporates the efforts of the pediatrician (often a developmental pediatrician or pediatric neurologist), psychologist, pediatric nurse, classroom teacher, reading and math specialist, special education teacher, possibly a speech therapist, and the child's parents. The clinicians and professionals must first determine whether the child's behaviour is age appropriate or truly problematic.

A history, both developmental and medical, and a description of the child's behaviour should be obtained from as many observers of the child as possible (especially the parents and the teachers, along with the health care providers involved). Descriptions of the child's behaviour in home and school situation should be included. In obtaining descriptive materials, the interviewer must question observers carefully because some persons, especially parents, may be so concerned with gross behaviours that they overlook less distressing but equally important symptoms. For example, parents may report a child who began to run soon after walking, a toddler who was compelled to touch everything in sight, and a child who resisted sleep until exhausted. A pregnancy and birth history may provide clues to a situation that might have produced a hypoxic episode.

A physical examination including vision and hearing screening and a detailed neurological evaluation will help rule out any severe neurological disorder. Psychological testing, especially projective tests, is valuable in identifying visual or perceptual difficulties, problems with spatial organization, and other phenomena that suggest cortical or diencephalic involvement; it also helps to identify the child's intelligence and achievement levels.

Behavioural checklists and adaptive scales are helpful in measuring social adaptive functioning in children with ADHD. Psychiatric disorders, medical problems, and traumatic experiences are ruled out, including lead poisoning, seizure, partial hearing loss, psychosis, and the witnessing of sexual activity or violence.

Therapeutic management. Management of the child with ADHD usually involves multiple approaches that include family education and counselling, medication, proper classroom placement, environmental manipulation, and sometimes behavioural therapy or psychotherapy for the child. Interventions for children with LDs are primarily educational.

Pharmacological therapy. The most frequently prescribed medications are the psychostimulants methylphenidate hydrochloride (Ritalin) and dextroamphetamine sulphate (Dexedrine). The majority of patients with ADHD are treated with the psychostimulant methylphenidate (AAP, 2011). These medications increase dopamine and norepinephrine levels, which leads to stimulation of the inhibitory system of the central nervous system (CNS). Children are given a small dosage initially and the dosage is gradually increased until the desired response is achieved. Children who receive stimulants should be monitored carefully for the development of tics during initial treatments, and stimulants should be avoided in children who have a history of ticlike behaviours, a family history of Tourette syndrome (TS), or ADHD combined with TS.

The stimulant dextroamphetamine may be used in children younger than 6 years to treat ADHD, but evidence of its safety and efficacy in young children and adolescents has been questioned. Lisdexamfetamine reportedly has less substance misuse potential than dextroamphetamine; it is metabolized to dextroamphetamine only after ingestion and thus may be more suitable for children and adolescents who may misuse dextroamphetamine (AAP, 2011). Other medications include mixed amphetamine salts (Adderall), which are available in extended-release form. In some cases a nonstimulant may be added to the medication regimen along with a stimulant to achieve optimal therapeutic effects. Many of the stimulant drugs are available in short-acting or long-acting form to better meet the child's need for therapeutic management. The CPS recommends the long-acting version of the drugs as first-line treatment, to improve adherence; decrease stigma, since the child does not need to take medication at school; and reduce school staff's need to administer and store controlled substances (Feldman, Bélanger, & CPS, Community Paediatrics Committee, 2009/2016). The long-acting drugs are expensive and are inaccessible to many families, as not all public and medical insurance companies cover the long-acting version. An additional consideration in the administration of medications is the child's ability to swallow pills; some drugs come in capsule form and can be sprinkled on applesauce (Ryan-Krause, 2011).

In addition, atomoxetine, a presynaptic norepinephrine transport inhibitor, is available for use in children with ADHD (Feldman et al., 2009/2016). The α_2-adrenergic agonists (clonidine and guanfacine) are second-line medications and are available in extended-release form but are reported to have limited evidence of efficacy and safety in preschool children with ADHD (AAP, 2011). Concerns have been raised that ADHD drugs could potentially reduce growth and cause weight loss. Generally, these drugs are not considered to have a major impact on growth and weight and the effectiveness of the treatment for school and social improvements outweighs the risk. Children on these medications need to have their growth and weight closely monitored (Damiani, Damiani, & Casella, 2010).

Except for atomoxetine, these medications are not prescribed on the basis of the child's weight but rather the resolution of symptoms. It is important to follow the child closely and evaluate for therapeutic effects and potential adverse effects. With all of these medications, regularly scheduled re-evaluation of the child is essential to determine medication effectiveness, detect and evaluate any adverse effects, monitor development and health status (especially growth and blood pressure), and assess family interaction (see Critical Thinking Case Study). Children taking stimulant drugs for ADHD should undergo an extensive physical examination and history, including family history of cardiac disease. Currently electrocardiography screening is recommended only for children

CRITICAL THINKING CASE STUDY

Attention Deficit Hyperactivity Disorder

Johnnie, age 8 years, is a third grader who was recently diagnosed with ADHD. He has been taking methylphenidate (Ritalin) for about 1 month. In the short time that Johnnie has been taking this medication, his math teacher has noticed an improvement in his performance in math class. He is receiving a grade of B instead of his previous grades of D on most math quizzes. The math teacher has also noted that Johnnie is socializing more with his classmates and now has a "best friend" in math class. Johnnie usually receives his methylphenidate from the school office staff before lunch. Yesterday Johnnie's mother told the school staff person that he has not eaten his lunch for the past week and is not hungry. The staff person spoke to the community health nurse who was following this child and his medication administration at the school about his lack of appetite.

What important issues regarding Johnnie's medication should the nurse consider in her discussions with Johnnie's mother?

QUESTIONS

1. Evidence—Is there sufficient evidence to draw conclusions about Johnnie's medication from his behaviour?
2. Assumptions—Describe some underlying assumptions about the following:
   a. Pharmacological action of methylphenidate in ADHD
   b. Adverse effects of methylphenidate
   c. Management of adverse effects
3. What implications for nursing care can be drawn at this time?
4. Does the evidence objectively support your conclusion?

ADHD, attention deficit hyperactivity disorder.

taking stimulant drugs for ADHD who have a close member with a history of cardiac arrhythmia or structural heart defect (Perrin, Friedman, Knilans, et al., 2008).

Some families prefer to use alternative therapies. The CPS (2012b) has indicated that essential fatty acids, such as fish oil or primrose oil, may be helpful in the treatment of ADHD, but more research is needed. Biofeedback is still considered to be experimental. The following alternative therapies have little to no evidence that they will help children with ADHD or LDs but are nonetheless used:

- Diet without sugar or additives—May help some children with allergies, food sensitivities, or migraines (little evidence)
- Vitamin supplements (no evidence)
- Valerian, blue-green algae, ginkgo biloba (should not be used in children with clotting conditions)—Herbs that can be calming and may aid memory and thinking but do not alleviate ADHD symptoms. Herbs are not regulated, and pharmacists need to be asked about their strength, safety, and toxicity.
- Antioxidants or anti-aging remedies help protect nerve cells but have no proven direct effect on ADHD symptoms. Pyncogenol should not be used in children with a blood disorder. Melatonin may help with sleep problems but can also cause headaches, fatigue, irritability, and sleepiness, trigger seizures, and possibly delay puberty.
- Hypnotherapy may help with some common ADHD symptoms.

- Homeopathy remedies are a blend of plant, animal, or mineral extracts. No studies have shown that this treatment works for symptoms of ADHD.

Regularly scheduled evaluations with the child and family are essential to assess the effects of medications, behaviour strategies, parent guidance, education programs, and individual and family alternative therapies. Medication therapy alone is not adequate to manage the child's symptoms, and other treatment modalities such as behavioural therapy should also be used for successful treatment.

Behavioural therapy. Behavioural therapy focuses on the prevention of undesired behaviour. The nurse should help families identify new appropriate contingencies and reward systems to meet the child's developing needs. They may also receive instruction in effective parenting skills, such as delivering positive reinforcement, rewarding small increments of desired behaviour, and providing age-appropriate consequences (e.g., time-out, response cost). The use of organizational charts for completing self-care activities and the use of a word processor instead of manually writing assignments are emphasized. Through collaborative teamwork, parents learn techniques to help the child become more successful at home and in school.

Counselling or therapy can be helpful for children who demonstrate signs of anxiety or depression. Therapy can help children develop healthier self-esteem and practise problem-solving strategies. Adolescents may benefit from group work that focuses on social skill development. Parents of children with ADHD can face a lot of stress, and therapy may be indicated for parents and other family members.

Multimodal treatments. The results of several studies suggest that multimodal treatment that involves the use of pharmacotherapy and behavioural interventions as well as close follow-up and feedback from school personnel is more effective than intensive behavioural treatment alone (Selekman, 2010).

Environmental manipulation. Families should be encouraged to learn how to modify the home environment with the aim of enabling the child to be more successful. Consistency is especially important for children with ADHD. Consistency between families and teachers in terms of reinforcing the same goals is essential. Fostering improved organizational skills requires a more highly structured environment than most children need. Children should be encouraged to make more appropriate choices and take responsibility for their actions.

Other helpful nursing interventions include teaching parents how to make organizational charts (e.g., listing all activities that must be performed before leaving for school) and to decrease distractions in the home while the child is completing homework (e.g., turning off television, having a consistent study area equipped with needed supplies). The nurse can also assist parents in modelling positive behaviours and problem solving. The focus is on using strategies that help the child succeed and cope with deficits while emphasizing strengths.

Classroom education. Children with ADHD need an orderly, predictable, and consistent classroom environment with clear and consistent rules. Homework and assignments may need to be reduced, and more time may need to be allotted for tests, to allow the child to complete the task. Verbal instructions should be accompanied by visual references, such as written instructions on the blackboard. Schedules may need to be arranged so that academic subjects are taught in the morning when the child has the morning medication dose working. Low-interest and high-interest classroom activities should be intermingled to maintain the child's attention and interest. Regular and frequent breaks in activity are helpful because sitting in one place for an extended time may be difficult. Computers are helpful for children who have difficulty with writing (**dysgraphia**) and fine motor skills; in such children, handwriting will *not* improve. They also need alternatives to physical competition that requires coordination of movement.

If the child has an LD, special training activities may be accomplished in self-contained classes limited to six to eight children, in special resource rooms with equipment and teaching teams, by mobile consultants who move from room to room to provide assistance to teachers and children, and in special first-grade programs in which high-risk children receive special attention to prevent or reduce the need for services as they progress. The purpose of programs for children with LDs is to assist them toward more successful achievement, personal adjustment, and retention in the regular classroom. Selekman (2010) lists additional behavioural, educational, and environmental strategies for children and adolescents with ADHD.

Growth and development. Children with ADHD who are taking stimulant medications need to be assessed for the achievement of appropriate growth and development milestones at least every 6 months (Selekman, 2010). The adverse effects of these drugs often include appetite suppression, nausea, and vomiting; suppression of growth acceleration and sleep disturbances have also been recorded in children taking stimulant drugs (Selekman, 2010).

Prognosis. With appropriate intervention, ADHD is relatively stable through early adolescence for most children. Some children experience decreased symptoms during late adolescence and adulthood, but a significant number of these children carry their symptoms into adulthood. The goal for children with LDs is to help them identify their areas of weakness and learn to compensate for them.

NURSING CARE

Nurses are active participants in all aspects of management of the child with ADHD or LDs. Nurses in the community work with families and school personnel on a long-term basis to help plan and implement therapeutic regimens and to evaluate the effectiveness of therapy. They coordinate services and serve as a liaison between health and education professionals directly involved in the child's therapy program. Nurses in any setting (community, school, hospital, practitioner's office) provide support and guidance to children and families during the difficult period of the child's growing up with a disabling condition.

Nursing care begins with an explanation to the parents and the child about the diagnosis, including the nature of the problem. Most parents are confused and feel some measure of guilt. To some parents, a diagnosis of ADHD is confirmation of the fear that their child has some irreversible, serious disease; to others, it is a relief. All parents need the opportunity to vent their feelings and suspicions. A common complaint of parents is that health care providers do not listen to what they have to say about their children. The health care provider should focus on building the family's self-esteem by encouraging the family to focus on developing the child's strengths (e.g., sports, hobbies, and talents) rather than just the weaknesses (Jellinek, 2008).

Parents need to be informed of the possible adverse effects of medications. The psychostimulants have similar adverse effects, including weight loss, abdominal pain, headaches, decreased appetite, sleeplessness, increased crying and irritability, nervous stimulation, and cardiovascular stimulation. The use of caffeine decreases the efficacy of these drugs, and insulin requirements may also be altered. If decreased appetite is a concern, helpful interventions include giving the psychostimulants with or after meals rather than before, encouraging consumption of nutritious snacks in the evening when the effects of the medication are decreasing, and serving frequent small meals with healthy "on-the-go" snacks. Sleeplessness is reduced by administering the medication early in the day.

Children and adolescents with ADHD are at increased risk for accidents and unintentional injuries because of their impulsivity and decreased judgement of dangerous activities. Therefore, measures should be taken to protect such children from personal injury (Selekman, 2010).

Children taking tricyclic antidepressants display a dramatic increase in the incidence of dental caries. The marked anticholinergic action of the drugs increases saliva viscosity and produces a dry mouth. Emphasis on rigorous dental hygiene, regular visits to the dentist, limited intake of refined carbohydrates, and use of artificial saliva is an important nursing function. The child should drink plenty of fluids and be well hydrated.

Parents often express concern that their children will become addicted to the psychostimulants or antidepressant drugs. Both types of drugs have the potential for misuse, and all children taking these drugs should be monitored closely for psychological dependence, tolerance, depression, and other adverse behaviour changes or idiosyncratic effects. Most children with ADHD are not interested in misusing their drugs because the effect of the drugs in these children is opposite that produced in normal individuals. However, parents should be cautioned to keep these drugs safely stored away from young children who may inadvertently ingest them and adolescents who may misuse them.

If a child has an LD, nurses must understand which type of LD a child has, in order to provide direction for the child, parents, and teachers. Children with an auditory perceptual deficit are often unable to follow directions or to comprehend large amounts of verbal teaching. These children need diagrams, pictures, demonstration, and written lists. Children with visual perceptual deficits may have difficulty reading, lining up numbers for mathematic operations, or judging distance. These children may have dyslexia (letter reversals) and do better with demonstration and a verbal approach. Children with an integrative deficit may have difficulty sequencing data or storing and retrieving sensory data. Multisensory techniques should be used, and comprehension should be checked frequently throughout instruction. They need to find an alternative to physical competition that requires coordination of movement (Learning Disabilities Association of Ontario, 2015).

Parents need information about the prognosis and an understanding of the treatment plan. The greater their understanding of the disorder and its effects, the more likely they will be to carry out the recommended program of therapy. It is important that they understand that the therapy is not necessarily a panacea and that it will extend over a long period. This has particular significance for changes they need to make in environmental management.

Enuresis

Enuresis is defined as involuntary urination. *Nocturnal enuresis* (bedwetting) is a common and troublesome disorder that is defined as the involuntary passage of urine at night by children who are beyond the age when voluntary bladder control should normally have been acquired. The inappropriate voiding of urine occurs at least twice a week for at least 3 months, and the chronological or developmental age of the child must be at least 5 years.

Enuresis can also be defined as primary (bedwetting in children who have never been dry for extended periods) or secondary (the onset of wetting after a period of established urinary continence). The passage of urine may be monosymptomatic and occur only during nighttime sleep, with the child remaining dry during the day; or it may be polysymptomatic, in which the child has daytime urinary urgency and an occasional daytime accident in conjunction with other conditions, such as sleep apnea, urinary tract infection, neurological impairment, constipation, or emotional stressors (Elder, 2016). The nocturnal, monosymptomatic type is most common. The condition may be particularly distressing to adolescents, who may refuse therapy. Although enuresis may occur during the daytime (*diurnal enuresis*), the following discussion focuses primarily on nocturnal enuresis.

Organic causes that may be related to enuresis should be ruled out before psychogenic factors are considered. Organic causes include structural disorders of the urinary tract; urinary tract infection; neurological deficits; disorders that increase the normal output of urine, such as diabetes; and disorders that impair the concentrating ability of the kidneys, such as chronic renal failure or sickle cell disease.

Therapeutic techniques used to manage nocturnal enuresis include medications, complementary and alternative medicine techniques (such as hypnotherapy), restriction or elimination of fluids after the evening meal, avoidance of caffeinated and sugar-containing beverages after the hour of 1600, purposeful interruption of sleep to void, motivational therapy, and various devices designed to establish a conditioned reflex response to waken the child at the initiation of voiding (alarms).

NURSING CARE

No matter what techniques are used, the nurse can help both children and parents to understand the problem of enuresis, the treatment plan, and the difficulties they may encounter in the process. Essential to the success of any method is the supportive care of parents and their children. Both need encouragement and patience. The problem is discussed with both the parent and child because all treatments involve and require the child's active participation. In some treatment interventions, the child is in charge of the intervention; therefore parents must learn to support the child rather than intervene themselves. For example, children can strip their wet covers, limit fluids, and use the toilet before bedtime. Parents should encourage the child to maintain a regular bowel evacuation regimen; constipation can contribute to nocturnal enuresis (Elder, 2016). A calendar with wet and dry nights may be helpful to motivate the child to stay dry and to maintain a positive perspective on the problem; positive rewards are also helpful.

Parents need to understand that punishment such as scolding, shaming, and threatening is contraindicated because of its negative emotional impact and limited success in reducing the behaviour. Positive reinforcement of the desired behaviour may be beneficial. Children need to believe they are helping themselves, and they need to sustain feelings of confidence and hope. Many parents believe enuresis is caused by an emotional disturbance and fear that they have somehow produced the situation by using improper child-rearing practices. They need reassurance that bedwetting is not a manifestation of an emotional disturbance and does not represent willful misbehaviour. Parents need to be encouraged to be patient and understanding and to communicate love and support to the child.

Communication with children is directed toward eliminating the emotional impact of the problem, relieving feelings of shame and guilt and the burden of parental disapproval, building self-confidence, and motivating children toward independent control. More important, the nurse can provide consistent support and encouragement to help children through the inconsistent and unpredictable treatment process.

Parents should also be taught to observe for adverse effects of any medications used.

Anxiety Disorders

All children have normal worries and fears. The child may fear a monster under the bed, a math test at school, or being picked for a baseball team. However, some children develop anxiety disorders that interfere with their enjoyment of life and get in the way of accomplishing the tasks they need to do. Some of the signs that a child has an anxiety disorder include expressing worry or showing anxiety on most days, for weeks at a time; difficulty sleeping at night or being unusually tired and sleepy in the daytime; trouble concentrating; and being unusually irritable or easy to upset.

Children and adolescents can have more than one type of anxiety disorder at the same time. Some types of school-age and adolescent anxiety disorders include separation anxiety, generalized anxiety, obsessive-compulsive, panic, phobia, post-traumatic stress. Approximately 6% of children and youth have an anxiety disorder that is serious enough to need treatment (Children's Mental Health Ontario, 2016). Anxiety disorders often occur in individuals with depression. Some of the anxiety disorders that begin in childhood can continue into adulthood if no treatment is given.

Anxiety disorders have complex causes, including a genetic base. Children and adolescents are particularly apt to develop anxiety disorders if they have a parent with depression or anxiety. The beliefs and behaviours that add to and help to maintain anxiety and depression can be reinforced by the parent as well (Children's Mental Health Ontario, 2016).

Post-Traumatic Stress Disorder

Post-traumatic stress disorder (PTSD) refers to the development of characteristic symptoms after exposure to an extremely traumatic experience or catastrophic event. The traumatic experience is typically life threatening to self or a significant other and may involve grotesque mutilation or death, serious injury, or physical coercion (e.g., an assault, a natural disaster, sexual abuse, or witnessing violence). It is important to note that PSTD is not limited to children who have lived in "war-torn" countries. Events such as automobile, school, or recreational accidents and bullying have been identified as causes of PTSD. The characteristic symptoms are persistent re-experiencing of the traumatic event, avoidance of stimuli associated with the event or trauma, numbing of general responsiveness, and increased arousal.

Acute PTSD is diagnosed if symptoms are present after the first month but before the third month after the initial traumatic event. Acute stress disorder may also occur with acute PTSD. Chronic PTSD is diagnosed if the symptoms persist beyond 3 months (Cohen, Bukstein, & AACAP Work Group on Quality Issues, 2010).

The response to the event takes place in three stages. The initial response involves intense arousal, which usually lasts for a few minutes to 1 or 2 hours. The stress hormones are at the maximum as the individual prepares for "fight" or "flight." A prolonged arousal phase may indicate **psychosis**.

The second phase, which lasts approximately 2 weeks, is one in which defence mechanisms are mobilized. It is a period of quiescence in which the event appears to have produced no impression. The child feels numb, and stress hormone secretion is absent. Defence mechanisms are less adaptive to specific situations and may not be what the situation demands. Denial that anything is wrong is a frequently observed defence mechanism.

The third phase is one of coping and consciously directed inquiry, which normally extends over 2 to 3 months. The victims want to know what happened and appear to be getting worse, when actually they are getting better. Numerous psychological symptoms, such as depression, phobia, anxiety, and conversion reactions, may be present. Children frequently display repetitive actions. They play out the situation over and over again in an attempt to come to terms with their fear. Flashbacks are common. This phase can be self-perpetuating, and a prolonged reaction can develop into an obsession with the traumatic event. Some traumatic effects remain indefinitely.

Trauma-focused psychotherapy is considered first-line therapy, and selective serotonin reuptake inhibitor (SSRI) drugs may be considered on an individual basis.

NURSING CARE

Children need to deal with any traumatic event. Their reactions depend heavily on their social environment and the way in which their caretaking adults react to the event. In the second phase of PTSD, the appropriateness of the defence mechanism must be assessed, and children must be assisted in application of their defence. If children do not engage in some catharsis, or if their defence phase is prolonged, they need referral for special psychological help.

Coping is a learned response, and children in the third phase can be helped to deal with their fear. Children usually are willing to accept reasoning. Those who are assisted in their catharsis and allowed expression will survive without serious lasting effects. They should be encouraged to play out the stress and to discuss their feelings about the event. If they are unable to do this, they may become obsessed with the traumatic event and require professional help. Conversion reactions are common obsessive behaviours in children suffering from PTSD (see Conversion Reactions below).

Children need professional help if any of the phases of PTSD are prolonged. Boys tend to have a prolonged defence phase more often than girls. Occasionally the event will be unrecognized, and the affected child will engage in what is considered to be unusual behaviour. Children exhibiting any sudden change in behaviour need to be assessed for having experienced a traumatic event. When the change in behaviour is traced to a traumatic event, treatment can be implemented.

Nurses in settings such as the emergency department, pediatric critical care unit, and neonatal intensive care unit should also recognize that parents of children who experience a traumatic acute trauma, life-threatening illness, or chronic illness may also experience symptoms of PTSD. PTSD may occur more often in mothers than in fathers, but some evidence indicates that fathers may have delayed symptoms (Mowery, 2011). Appropriate nursing interventions include allowing parents to discuss their feelings about the incident or threat (to themselves or their children), encouraging support from other parents in similar situations, avoiding interjecting one's own experience or feelings, and evaluating the child's reaction to the parents' symptoms (Mowery, 2011).

School Phobia

Children, other than beginning students, who resist going to school or who demonstrate extreme reluctance to attend school for a sustained period as a result of severe anxiety or fear of school-related experiences are said to have school phobia. The terms *school refusal* and *school avoidance* are also used to describe this behaviour. School phobia occurs in children of all ages but is more common in children 10 years of age and older. School-avoidance behaviours occur in both boys and girls and in children from all socioeconomic levels.

Anxiety that often verges on panic is a constant manifestation, and children can develop symptoms as a protective mechanism to keep them from facing the situation that distresses them. Physical symptoms are prominent and may affect any part of the body (e.g., anorexia, nausea, vomiting, diarrhea, dizziness, headache, leg pains, abdominal pains, or even a low-grade fever). A striking feature of school phobia is the prompt subsidence of symptoms when it is evident that the child can remain at home. Another significant observation is absence of symptoms on weekends and holidays unless they are related to other places such as Sunday school or parties. Occasional mild reluctance is not uncommon among schoolchildren, but if the fear continues for longer than a few days, it must be considered a serious problem.

The onset of school phobia is usually sudden and precipitated by a school-related incident. By taking a careful history, nurses find out whether a poor attendance record is caused by trivial reasons.

NURSING CARE

Treatment for school phobia depends on the cause. The primary goal is to return the child to school. The longer a child is permitted to stay out of school, the more difficult it is for the child to re-enter. Parents must be convinced gently but firmly that immediate return is essential and that it is their responsibility to insist on school attendance.

A school re-entry protocol may be necessary for the child with severe symptoms. In re-entry programs, the child role-plays routines involved in getting ready for school and that occur at school. Relaxation techniques are also used. The child usually goes to school initially for a half-day and then progresses to a full day. Often a school nurse may be asked to provide support to the parents and the teacher during the re-entry process. If the problem persists, professional help is recommended.

Eating Disorders

While 13 years is the average age of onset of anorexia nervosa and bulimia, these eating disorders are being identified in children as young as 8 or 9. Epidemiological evidence has shown that the incidence of anorexia nervosa in adolescents has been increasing over the past 50 years; it is now the third most chronic illness affecting adolescent females. A surveillance survey conducted for the CPS indicated that 161 children younger than 13 years from across Canada had been diagnosed with an eating disorder, with six girls to every boy. The average age was 11 years (Pinhas, Morris, Crosby, et al., 2011).

Because of the social determinants related to eating disorders, health care providers must be aware of the current risk status in their area and of the potential development of eating disorders. Please refer to Chapter 39 for detailed information on eating disorders in adolescents.

Recurrent Abdominal Pain

Recurrent abdominal pain (RAP) is a condition often attributed to a psychogenic etiology, although it can be a symptom of either psychosomatic or organic disease. *RAP* is defined as three or more separate episodes of abdominal pain during a 3-month period, similar to the "spastic" or "irritable" colon syndrome of adulthood. Children with RAP have real pain that is usually located in the periumbilical or epigastric area (or both). On palpation the pain is likely to be experienced in the epigastric area or in the lower right or left quadrant and is accompanied by vague tenderness without muscle guarding. The pain is irregular in time, duration, and intensity and associated with either loose or pellet-formed stools. Other symptoms that may accompany the pain are headache, pallor, dizziness, dysuria, flushing, vomiting, diarrhea, and fatigue.

Treatment involves providing reassurance and reducing or eliminating the symptoms. Hospitalization may be necessary, and the child frequently shows improvement in the hospital. Initial efforts are directed toward ruling out organic causes of the pain, relieving discomfort, and attempting to determine the situations that precipitate attacks. A high-fibre diet, psyllium bulk agents, lubricants such as mineral oil, and bowel training are emphasized. Other therapies include cognitive-behavioural therapy and biofeedback. There is limited evidence for the use of probiotics or antispasmodic medications. However, if there are significant symptoms for an irritable colon, then anti-spasmodic and antidiarrheal medications may be used (Sandhu & Paul, 2014).

NURSING CARE

Once the diagnosis has been established, the parents and the child need an explanation of the pain, which can be compared to a skeletal muscle cramp or "charley horse." Reassurance that the symptoms are not unique to their child and that the pain can be expected to subside is helpful in relieving parental fears and anxieties.

The simple measure of having the child rest in a peaceful, quiet environment and providing comfort will often relieve the symptoms in a short time. A heating pad may also help ease the discomfort (see Chapter 34, Nonpharmacological Management). When pain is not relieved by these simple measures, the parents need to be taught how to administer antispasmodics, if prescribed. For example, if pain is precipitated by meals, having the child take the medication 20 to 30 minutes before mealtime may prevent an episode.

The most valuable assistance that the nurse can provide is support and reassurance to the family. When open communication is established and families appreciate the relationship between stress-provoking situations and the child's symptoms, the chance for remedial action is enhanced. Follow-up care and continued support are essential, since the symptoms tend to remit and exacerbate. The availability of a supportive health care provider can be a source of comfort to the child and family.

Conversion Reaction

Conversion reaction, also known as *hysteria, hysterical conversion reaction*, and *childhood hysteria*, is a psychophysiological disorder with a sudden onset that can usually be traced to a precipitating environmental event. In childhood the disorder is observed with equal frequency in both sexes, although girls outnumber boys during adolescence. Manifestations of conversion reaction involve primarily the voluntary musculature and special senses and include abdominal pain, fainting, pseudoseizures, paralysis, headaches, and visual field restriction. Once considered rare in childhood, this disorder occurs more frequently than has generally been acknowledged. The most common symptom is seizure activity, which can be differentiated from symptoms of neurogenic origin by formal tests. A normal electroencephalogram indicates that the origin is not neurogenic.

Many children with a conversion reaction have experienced a major family crisis (such as the loss of a parent or other significant person through death, divorce, or moving) before the onset of symptoms. Children with conversion reaction characteristically come from families with communication problems or have a parent with depression or hypochondriasis.

Educating the child and family about the cause of emotional stresses or feelings and alternative approaches to coping with stress may alleviate the child's symptoms.

NURSING CARE

Nursing care is similar to that for the child with RAP. If significant personality problems are evident, psychiatric consultation is indicated.

Childhood Depression

Depression in childhood is often difficult to detect because children may be unable to express their feelings and tend to act out their problems and concerns. Some states of depression are temporary (e.g., acute depression precipitated by a traumatic event). This might be related to a period of hospitalization; loss of a parent through death or separation; or loss of a significant relationship with something (a pet), someone (a friend or family member), or a place (due to a move from a familiar home, neighbourhood, or city). Children with depression may demonstrate a variety of behaviours (Box 38-2). Most responses in children are not sustained and can be modified with social and family support.

More serious and less common are the depressive responses to chronic stress and loss; these are frequently observed in children with chronic illness or complex conditions when other family members are in denial and often depressed. There is no apparent precipitating event, but there is often a history of frequent disruptions in important relationships. Often, there is also a history of depressive illness in one or both parents. Manifestations in the child are similar to those observed in acute depression, but they occur more frequently and extend over a longer time.

Depressed children are cared for by a health team especially prepared in the care of children with mental disorders. Children who answer affirmatively to queries about a distressing life experience or a depressed or irritable mood should be offered the opportunity to talk about the situation. By engaging in active listening the health care provider can assess the severity of the symptoms and associated dangerousness, distress, and functional impairment. Treatment is highly individualized and undertaken in the least restrictive environment. Suicidal children need to be admitted to the hospital for protection if the family is unable to provide constant monitoring. Two SSRIs, fluoxetine and escitalopram, are the first-line medication used

BOX 38-2 CHARACTERISTICS OF CHILDREN WITH DEPRESSION

Behaviour

Predominantly sad facial expression with absence or diminished range of affective response
Solitary play or work; tendency to be alone; lack of interest in play
Withdrawal from previously enjoyed activities and relationships
Lowered grades in school; lack of interest in doing homework or achieving in school
Diminished motor activity; tiredness
Tearfulness or crying
Dependent and clinging or aggressive and disruptive
Irritability or anger
Anxiety is often present

Internal States

Utterance of statements reflecting lowered self-esteem, sense of hopelessness, or guilt
Suicidal ideations

Physiology

Constipation
Nonspecific complaints of not feeling well
Change in appetite resulting in weight loss or gain
Alterations in sleeping pattern; sleeplessness or hypersomnia

to treat depression in adolescents, although sertraline or citalopram may also be used (Walter, Bogdanovic, Moseley, et al., 2016). There have been reports that antidepressant medications may cause increased suicidal thinking and behaviours in pediatric patients, but DeMaso and Walter (2016) have stated that it is usually more beneficial to treat with SSRIs than not.

NURSING CARE

Nurses should be aware that depression can easily be overlooked in the child and can interrupt normal growth and development. Recognizing depression and suicidal tendencies in depressed children and making appropriate referrals are important nursing functions. Identification of the depressed child requires a careful history (health, growth and development, social, and family health); interviews with the child; and observations by the nurse, parents, and teachers. If antidepressants are prescribed, the child and family need to know that antidepressants must be at a therapeutic level for 2 to 4 weeks to achieve a beneficial effect. The child and family also need to monitor the child for adverse effects of the drug prescribed and for any interactions with other drugs.

Childhood Schizophrenia

Childhood schizophrenia is a term that refers to severe deviations in ego functioning and is generally reserved for psychotic disorders that appear in children younger than 15 years of age. Childhood schizophrenia is a rare illness among children in the general population; among children with mental illness, only about 2 in every 1000 have childhood schizophrenia.

Childhood schizophrenia is characterized by symptoms that last for at least 6 months and seriously interfere with the child's functioning in school, at home, or in other social situations. The basic disturbance is a lack of contact with reality and the subsequent development of a world of the child's own. Other areas of development that may be impaired include cognition, perception, emotion, language, and physical motor control. The most common manifestations involve language disturbances, impaired interpersonal relationships, and inappropriate affect (outward expression of emotion). Treatment involves management of the symptoms, prevention of relapse, and social and occupational rehabilitation. Antipsychotic drugs that may be used include haloperidol, clozapine, chlorpromazine, olanzapine, quetiapine fumarate, and risperidone. Family interventions and family therapy often result in improvements in psychotic symptoms, thought disorders, and social functioning among children with schizophrenia.

NURSING CARE

Nursing care of children with psychotic disorders is a highly specialized area. Nurses should be alert to the possibility that schizophrenia can occur in children and should refer children to a psychiatrist for evaluation if they consistently demonstrate abnormal behaviour. In addition, nurses need to teach family members of children taking antipsychotic medications to observe for possible adverse effects. Common adverse effects include dizziness, drowsiness, tachycardia, hypotension, and extrapyramidal effects such as abnormal movements and seizures.

KEY POINTS

- Middle childhood, also known as the school years, is the period of life that extends from 6 to 12 years of age.
- Although growth is slower than in previous years, there is a steady gain in height and weight, with maturation of body systems; primary teeth are lost and replaced by permanent teeth.
- A major task during the middle school years is developing a sense of industry or accomplishment (Erikson).
- Piaget's period of concrete operations refers to the school-age period, when children are able to use their thought processes to experience events and actions and make judgements based on reasoning.
- The child develops a conscience and is able to understand and adhere to rules and standards set by others.
- Entertaining different points of view, becoming sensitive to cultural norms, and forming peer friendships are important features of social development during the school years.
- Cooperative play, team activities, and the acquisition of skills are prime elements of play during the school years; rules and rituals assume greater importance.

- Parental concerns during middle childhood include lying, cheating, stealing, bullying, and school achievement.
- The availability of junk foods, irregular family meals, and schedules of working parents often interfere with optimum nutrition and may lead to obesity.
- Activities involving physical movement should be encouraged; sedentary activities, such as watching television or playing video games for long periods of time, contribute to health problems in this age group.
- Dental care is important during this time; potential dental problems include caries, periodontal disease, malocclusion, and dental injury.
- Increased socialization and media exposure make the school years an ideal time for sex education.
- Ideally, school health programs include health appraisal, emergency care, safety education, lifestyle support, recommended immunizations, communicable disease control, counselling, guidance, and health education with adjustment to individual student needs.
- Injury prevention is directed toward safety education, provision of safe play areas and equipment, and supervision of sports activities.
- Education related to appropriate uses of social media is important.
- Alterations in growth and maturation may be manifested as short or tall stature or as delayed sexual development.
- Behaviour problems in middle childhood can result from ADHD, enuresis, school phobia, RAP, anxiety disorder, childhood depression, conversion reaction, or childhood schizophrenia.
- Eating disorders are being seen in younger children; an index of suspicion is important to diagnosis.

evolve WEBSITE

Visit the Evolve website for additional resources related to the content in this chapter such as Case Studies, Critical Thinking Case Study Answers, Nursing Care Plans, Nursing Processes, Nursing Skills, and Review Questions for Exam Preparation at: *http://evolve.elsevier.com/Canada/Perry/maternal/*

REFERENCES

American Academy of Pediatrics (AAP). (2011). Clinical practice guideline. ADHD: Clinical practice guideline for the diagnosis, evaluation, and treatment of attention-deficit/hyperactivity disorder in children, and adolescents. *Pediatrics*, *128*(5), 1007–1022. doi:10.1542/peds.2011-2654.

American Academy of Pediatrics (AAP) Committee on Injury, Violence, and Poison Prevention. (2009). Policy statement: Role of the pediatrician in youth violence prevention. *Pediatrics*, *124*(1), 393–402.

American Psychiatric Association. (2013). *Diagnostic and statistical manual of mental disorders* (5th ed.). Washington, DC: Author. (DSM-5).

Arseneault, L., Bowes, L., & Shakoor, S. (2010). Bullying victimization in youths and mental health problems: 'much ado about nothing'? *Psychological Medicine*, *40*, 717–729.

Bowes, L., Arseneault, L., Maughan, B., et al. (2009). School, neighborhood, and family factors are associated with children's bullying involvement: A nationally representative longitudinal study. *Journal of the American Academy of Child & Adolescent Psychiatry*, *48*(5), 545–553.

Canadian Institutes of Health Research. (2012). *Canadian bullying statistics*. Retrieved from <http://www.cihr-irsc.gc.ca/e/45838.html>.

Canadian Paediatric Society. (2012a). *Healthy sleep for your baby and child*. Retrieved from <http://www.caringforkids.cps.ca/handouts/healthy_sleep_for_your_baby_and_child>.

Canadian Paediatric Society. (2012b). *Alternative treatments for attention deficit hyperactivity disorder*. Retrieved from <http://www.caringforkids.cps.ca/handouts/alternative_treatments_adhd>.

Canadian Paediatric Society. (2013). *Guiding your child with positive discipline*. Retrieved from <http://www.caringforkids.cps.ca/handouts/guiding_with_positive_discipline>.

Canadian Society for Exercise Physiology. (2012). *Canadian physical activity guidelines and Canadian sedentary behaviour guidelines*. Retrieved from <http://www.csep.ca/guidelines>.

Children's Mental Health Ontario. (2016). *Learn more about child and youth mental health*. Retrieved from <http://www.kidsmentalhealth.ca/parents/resources_parents.php>.

Cohen, J. A., Bukstein, A., & AACAP Work Group on Quality Issues. (2010). Practice parameter for the assessment and treatment of children and adolescents with posttraumatic stress disorder. *Journal of American Academy of Child & Adolescent Psychiatry*, *49*(4), 414–430.

Damiani, D., Damiani, D., & Casella, E. (2010). Attention deficit disorder and hyperactivity—Does the treatment affect the statural growth? *Arquivos Brasileiros de Endocrinologia & Metabologia*, *54*(3), 262–268. Retrieved from <http://www.scielo.br/scielo.php?script=sci_arttext&pid=S0004-27302010000300003&lng=en&nrm=iso&tlng=en>.

DeMaso, D. R., & Walter, H. J. (2016). Psychopharmacology. In R. M. Kliegman, B. F. Stanton, J. W. St. Geme, et al. (Eds.), *Nelson textbook of pediatrics* (20th ed.). Philadelphia: Saunders.

Eberl, R., Schalamon, J., Singer, G., et al. (2009). Trampoline-related injuries in childhood. *European Journal of Pediatrics*, *168*, 1171–1174.

Elder, J. (2016). Enuresis and voiding dysfunction. In R. M. Kliegman, B. F. Stanton, J. W. St. Geme, et al. (Eds.), *Nelson textbook of pediatrics* (20th ed.). Philadelphia: Saunders.

Feldman, M., Bélanger, S., & Canadian Paediatric Society, Community Paediatrics Committee. (2009). Extended-release medications for children and adolescents with attention-deficit hyperactivity disorder. *Paediatrics & Child Health*, *14*(9), 593–597. Retrieved from <http://www.cps.ca/documents/position/extended-release-medications-ADHD>. Reaffirmed 2016.

Frederickson, N. (2010). Bullying or befriending? Children's responses to classmates with special needs. *British Journal of Special Education*, *37*, 4–12.

Government of Canada. (2015). *Bullying*. Retrieved from <http://healthycanadians.gc.ca/healthy-living-vie-saine/bullying-intimidation/index-eng.php?_ga=1.185279392.868197850.1432519476>.

Government of Canada. (2016). *Car seat safety*. Retrieved from <https://www.tc.gc.ca/eng/motorvehiclesafety/safedrivers-childsafety-car-index-873.htm>.

Health Canada. (2008). *First Nations, Inuit, and Aboriginal health: Keeping safe—Injury prevention*. Retrieved from <http://www.hc-sc.gc.ca/fniah-spnia/promotion/injury-bless/index-eng.php>.

Irvine, D., Holve, S., Krol, D., et al. (2011). Early childhood caries in indigenous communities. *Paediatrics & Child Health*, *16*(6), 351–357. Retrieved from <http://www.cps.ca/documents/position/oral-health-indigenous-communities>. Reaffirmed 2016.

Jellinek, M. (2008). ADHD treatments: Going beyond the meds. *Contemporary Pediatrics*, *25*(5), 39–48.

Knox, M. (2010). On hitting children: A review of corporal punishment in the United States. *Journal of Pediatric Health Care*, *24*(2), 103–107.

Kohlberg, L. (1968). Moral development. In D. L. Sills (Ed.), *International encyclopedia of the social sciences*. New York: Macmillan.

Lamb, J., Pepler, D. J., & Craig, W. (2009). Approach to bullying and victimization. *Canadian Family Physician*, *55*(4), 356–360.

Learning Disabilities Association of Ontario. (2015). *Dysgraphia: The handwriting learning disability*. Retrieved from <http://www.ldao.ca/introduction-to-ldsadhd/articles/about-lds/dysgraphia-the-handwriting-learning-disability/>.

McLeod, J. D., & Knight, S. (2010). The association of socioemotional problems with early sexual initiation. *Perspectives on Sexual and Reproductive Health*, *42*(2), 93–101. doi:10.1363/4209310.

Mowery, B. D. (2011). Post-traumatic stress disorder (PTSD) in parents: Is this a significant problem? *Pediatric Nursing*, *37*(2), 89–92.

O'Keeffe, G. S., Clarke-Pearson, K., & Council on Communications and Media. (2011). Clinical report—The impact of social media on children, adolescents, and families. *Pediatrics*, *127*(4), 800–804. doi:10.1542/peds.2011-0054.

Parachute. (2009). *Child pedestrian injuries report 2007–2008*. Retrieved from <http://www.parachutecanada.org/downloads/injurytopics/ChildPed_Report_07:08.pdf>.

Parachute. (2014). *Bike helmet legislation chart*. Retrieved from <http://www.parachutecanada.org/downloads/policy/Bike%20Helmet%20Legislation%20Chart-2014.pdf>.

Parachute. (n.d.). *ATV safety*. Retrieved from <http://www.parachutecanada.org/policy/item/atv-safety>.

Perrin, J. M., Friedman, R. A., Knilans, T. K., et al. (2008). Cardiovascular monitoring and stimulant drugs for attention-deficit/hyperactivity disorder. *Pediatrics*, *122*(2), 451–453. doi:10.1542/peds.2008-1573.

Piaget, J. (1952). *The origins of intelligence in children*. New York: International Universities Press.

Pinhas, L., Morris, A., Crosby, R. D., et al. (2011). Incidence and age-specific presentation of restrictive eating disorders in children. A Canadian paediatric surveillance program study. *Archives of Pediatric Adolescent Medicine*, *165*(10), 895–899. doi:10.1001/archpediatrics.2011.145.

Psychology Foundation of Canada. (2016). *Kids have stress too! (KHST!)*. Retrieved from <http://psychologyfoundation.org/Public/Programs/Kids_Have_Stress_Too/Public/Programs/Kids_Have_Stress_Too/Kids_Have_Stress_Too_.aspx?hkey=281a7065-a1dd-486d-8e83-f4b0da83ac56>.

Public Health Agency of Canada. (2009a). *Child and youth injury in review: Spotlight on consumer product safety*. Ottawa: Author.

Public Health Agency of Canada. (2009b). *The Chief Public Health Officer's Report on the state of public health in Canada. Growing up well—Priorities for a healthy future 2009*. Retrieved from <http://www.phac-aspc.gc.ca/cphorsphc-respcacsp/2009/fr-rc/pdf/cphorsphc-respcacsp-eng.pdf>.

Public Health Agency of Canada. (2015). *Canadian immunization guide*. Retrieved from <http://www.phac-aspc.gc.ca/publicat/cig-gci/index-eng.php>.

Purcell, L. K., & Canadian Paediatric Society, Healthy Active Living and Sports Medicine Committee. (2014). Sport-related concussion: Evaluation and management. *Paediatrics & Child Health*, *19*(3), 153–158. Retrieved from <http://www.cps.ca/en/documents/position/sport-related-concussion-evaluation-management>.

Ryan-Krause, P. (2011). Attention deficit hyperactivity disorder: Part III. *Journal of Pediatric Health Care*, *25*(1), 50–56. doi:10.1016/j.pedhc.2010.10.00.

Sandhu, B. K., & Paul, S. P. (2014). Irritable bowel syndrome in children: Pathogenesis, diagnosis and evidence-based treatment. *World Journal of Gastroenterology*, *20*(20), 6013–6230. doi:10.3748/wjg.v20.i20.6013.

Schroth, R. J., Harrison, R. L., & Moffatt, M. (2009). Oral health of indigenous children and the influence of early childhood caries on childhood health and wellbeing. *Pediatric Clinics of North America*, *56*, 1481–1499.

Selekman, J. (2010). Attention deficit/hyperactivity disorder. In P. Jackson, J. A. Vessey, & N. A. Shaprio (Eds.), *Primary care of children with chronic conditions* (5th ed.). St. Louis: Mosby.

Stanwick, R., & Canadian Paediatric Society, Injury Prevention Committee. (2004). Recommendations for snowmobile safety. *Paediatrics & Child Health*, *9*(9), 639–642. Retrieved from <http://www.cps.ca/en/documents/position/snowmobile-safety> Reaffirmed 2014.

Urion, D. K. (2016). Attention-deficit/hyperactivity disorder. In R. M. Kliegman, B. F. Stanton, J. W. St. Geme, et al. (Eds.), *Nelson textbook of pediatrics* (20th ed.). Philadelphia: Saunders.

van Schaik, C., & Canadian Paediatric Society, Injury Prevention Committee. (2008). Transportation of infants and children in motor vehicles. *Paediatrics & Child Health*, *13*(4), 313–318. Retrieved from <http://www.cps.ca/en/documents/position/car-seat-safety>.

Walter, H. J., Bogdanovic, N., Moseley, L. R., & DeMaso, D. R. (2016). Major and other depressive disorders. In R. M. Kliegman, B. F. Stanton, J. W. St. Geme, et al. (Eds.), *Nelson textbook of pediatrics* (20th ed.). Philadelphia: Saunders.

Warda, L. J., Yanchar, N. L., & Canadian Paediatric Society, Injury Prevention Committee. (2012). *Skiing and snowboarding injury prevention*. Retrieved from <http://www.cps.ca/en/documents/position/skiing-snowboarding-injury>.

Yanchar, N. L., & Canadian Paediatric Society, Injury Prevention Committee. (2012). *Preventing injuries from all-terrain vehicles*. <http://www.cps.ca/documents/position/preventing-injury-from-atvs>.

ADDITIONAL RESOURCES

Canadian ADHD Resource Alliance: <http://caddra.ca/>.

Canadian Mental Health Association—Children, Youth, and Depression: <http://www.cmha.ca/mental_health/children-and-depression/>.

Canadian Paediatric Society—Social Media: What Parents Should Know: <http://www.caringforkids.cps.ca/handouts/social_media>.

Health Canada—Eating Well With Canada's Food Guide: <http://www.hc-sc.gc.ca/fn-an/food-guide-aliment/index-eng.php>.

Health Canada—Natural and Non-prescription Health Products: <http://www.hc-sc.gc.ca/dhp-mps/prodnatur/index-eng.php>.

Human Early Learning Partnerships (HELP): <http://www.earlylearning.ubc.ca>.

Learning Disabilities Association of Canada: <http://www.ldac-acta.ca/>.

National Eating Disorder Information Centre: <http://www.nedic.ca/>.

Parenting and Behaviour—How to Foster Your Child's Self-Esteem: <http://www.caringforkids.cps.ca/handouts/foster_self_esteem>.

PrevNET—Canada's authority on bullying: <http://www.prevnet.ca>.

Public Health Agency of Canada—Injury Prevention: <http://www.phac-aspc.gc.ca/inj-bles/index-eng.php>.

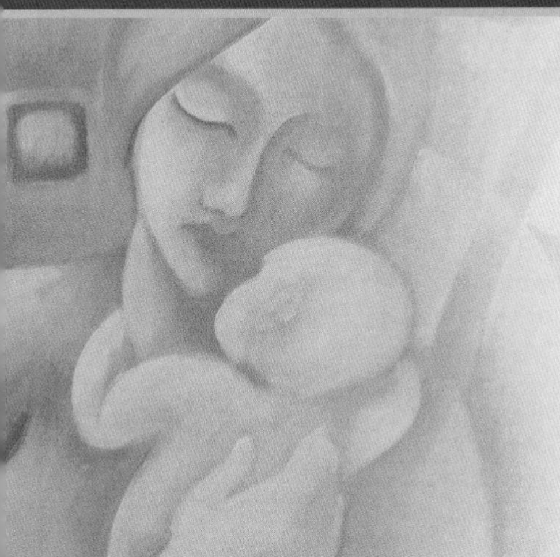

CHAPTER

39

The Adolescent and Family

Cheryl Dika, with contributions from David Wilson

evolve WEBSITE

Visit the Evolve website for additional resources related to the content in this chapter such as Case Studies, Critical Thinking Case Study Answers, Nursing Care Plans, Nursing Processes, Nursing Skills, and Review Questions for Exam Preparation at: http://evolve.elsevier.com/Canada/Perry/maternal/

OBJECTIVES

On completion of this chapter the reader will be able to:

- Describe the usual physical changes that occur throughout the adolescent years.
- Discuss the reactions of adolescents to the physical changes that take place at puberty.
- Demonstrate an understanding of the processes by which adolescents develop a sense of identity.
- Discuss the significance of changing interpersonal relationships and the role of peer groups during adolescence.
- Outline a health teaching plan for adolescents.
- Identify the causes and discuss the preventative aspects of injuries during adolescence.
- Demonstrate an understanding of common disorders of the male and female reproductive systems.
- Demonstrate an understanding of health challenges related to adolescent sexuality.
- Outline a care plan for the child or adolescent with an eating disorder.
- Discuss the manifestations and nursing management of selected emotional or behavioural problems.

PROMOTING OPTIMUM GROWTH AND DEVELOPMENT

Adolescence is a period of transition between childhood and adulthood—a time of rapid physical, cognitive, social, and emotional maturing. In Canada, social determinants of health, such as family income, education, literacy, ethnicity, and gender, have a profound impact on adolescents' health and help set the stage for adult health. Raphael (2010) has described how these social determinants can bring about health inequalities among Canadian children, having an impact into adulthood. See Chapter 1 for more information on the social determinants of health.

The precise boundaries of adolescence are difficult to define, but this period is customarily viewed as beginning with the gradual appearance of secondary sex characteristics at about 11 or 12 years of age and ending with cessation of body growth at 18 to 20 years. Several terms are used to refer to this stage of growth and development. Puberty refers to the maturational, hormonal, and growth process that occurs when the reproductive organs begin to function and the secondary sex characteristics develop. This process is sometimes divided into three stages: *prepubescence*, the period of about 2 years immediately before puberty when the child is developing preliminary physical changes that herald sexual maturity; *puberty*, the point at which sexual maturity is achieved, marked by the first menstrual flow in girls but by less obvious indications in boys; and *postpubescence*, a 1- to 2-year period following puberty during which skeletal growth is completed and reproductive functions become fairly well established. Adolescence, which literally means "to grow into maturity," is generally regarded as the psychological, social, and maturational process initiated by the pubertal changes. It involves three distinct subphases: early adolescence (ages 11 to 14), middle adolescence (ages 15 to 17), and late adolescence (ages 18 to 20). The term *teenage years* is used synonymously with *adolescence* to describe ages 13 through 19.

Biological Development

The physical changes of puberty are primarily the result of hormonal activity under the influence of the central nervous system, although all aspects of physiological functioning are mutually interacting. The obvious physical changes are noted in increased physical growth and in the appearance and development of secondary sex characteristics; less obvious are physiological alterations and neurogonadal maturity, accompanied by the ability to procreate. Physical distinction between the sexes is made on the basis of distinguishing characteristics. **Primary sex characteristics** are the external and internal organs that carry out the reproductive functions (e.g., ovaries, uterus, breasts, penis). **Secondary sex characteristics** are the changes that occur throughout the body as a result of hormonal changes (e.g., voice alterations, development of facial and pubertal hair, fat deposits) but that play no direct part in reproduction.

Hormonal Changes of Puberty

The events of puberty are caused by hormonal influences that are controlled by the anterior pituitary (adenohypophysis) in response to stimuli from the hypothalamus. Hormonal stimulation of the **gonads** has two effects: (1) production and release of gametes—production of sperm in the male and maturation and release of ova in the female; and (2) secretion of sex-appropriate **hormones**—estrogen and progesterone from the ovaries (female) and testosterone from the testes (male).

The ovaries, testes, and adrenals secrete sex hormones. These hormones are produced in varying amounts by both sexes throughout the lifespan. The adrenal cortex is responsible for the small amounts secreted before the pubescent years, but the sex hormone production that accompanies maturation of the gonads is responsible for the biological changes observed during puberty.

Estrogen, the feminizing hormone, is found in low quantities during childhood. This hormone is secreted in slowly increasing amounts until about age 11 years. In males this gradual increase continues through maturation. In females the onset of estrogen production in the ovary causes a pronounced increase that continues until about 3 years after the onset of menstruation, at which time it reaches a maximum level that continues throughout the reproductive life of the female.

Androgens, the masculinizing hormones, are also secreted in small and gradually increasing amounts up to about 7 or 9 years of age, at which time there is a more rapid increase in both sexes, especially boys, until about age 15 years. These hormones appear to be responsible for most of the rapid growth changes of early adolescence. With the onset of testicular function, the level of androgens (principally testosterone) in boys increases over that in girls and continues to increase until a maximum level is attained at maturity.

Sexual Maturation

The visible evidence of sexual maturation is achieved in an orderly sequence, and the state of maturity can be estimated on the basis of the appearance of these external manifestations. The age at which these changes are observed and the time required to progress from one stage to another vary among children. The time from the appearance of breast buds to full maturity may be up to 6 years for adolescent girls. It may take 2 to 5 years for male genitalia to reach adult size. The stages of development of secondary sex characteristics and genital development have been defined as a guide for estimating sexual maturity and are referred to as the *Tanner stages*. The usual sequence of appearance of maturational changes is presented in Box 39-1.

BOX 39-1 USUAL SEQUENCE OF MATURATIONAL CHANGES

Girls

Breast changes
Rapid increase in height and weight
Growth of pubic hair
Appearance of axillary hair
Menstruation (usually begins 2 years after first signs)
Abrupt deceleration of linear growth

Boys

Enlargement of testicles
Growth of pubic hair, axillary hair, hair on upper lip, hair on face and elsewhere on body (facial hair usually appears about 2 years after appearance of pubic hair)
Rapid increase in height
Changes in the larynx and consequently the voice (usually take place along with the growth of the penis)
Nocturnal emissions
Abrupt deceleration of linear growth

Sexual maturation in girls. In most girls the initial indication of puberty is the appearance of breast buds, an event known as *thelarche*, which occurs after 8 years of age (Fig. 39-1). This is followed in approximately 2 to 6 months by the growth of pubic hair on the mons pubis, known as *adrenarche* (Fig. 39-2). In a minority of normally developing girls, however, pubic hair may precede breast development. The average age for thelarche varies depending on many factors.

The initial appearance of menstruation, or **menarche**, occurs about 2 years after the appearance of the first pubescent changes, approximately 9 months after attainment of peak height velocity and 3 months after attainment of peak weight velocity. Menarche has been related to a critical gain in body fat content (more fat content, earlier menarche), although this association is controversial. The normal age range of menarche is usually 10½ to 15 years, with the average age of onset of menarche in Canadian girls is 12.72 years, with British Columbia having the lowest average age at less than 11.5 years (Al-Sahab, Ardern, Hamadeh, et al., 2010). Ovulation and regular menstrual periods usually occur 6 to 14 months after menarche. Girls may be considered to have pubertal delay if breast development has not occurred by age 13 or if menarche has not occurred within 4 years of the onset of breast development.

There is evidence that puberty is occurring at an earlier age, and considerable literature supports the rise of obesity rates as an important factor in this change. Other variables besides genetics and weight have been associated with earlier puberty, including certain intrauterine conditions and exposures,

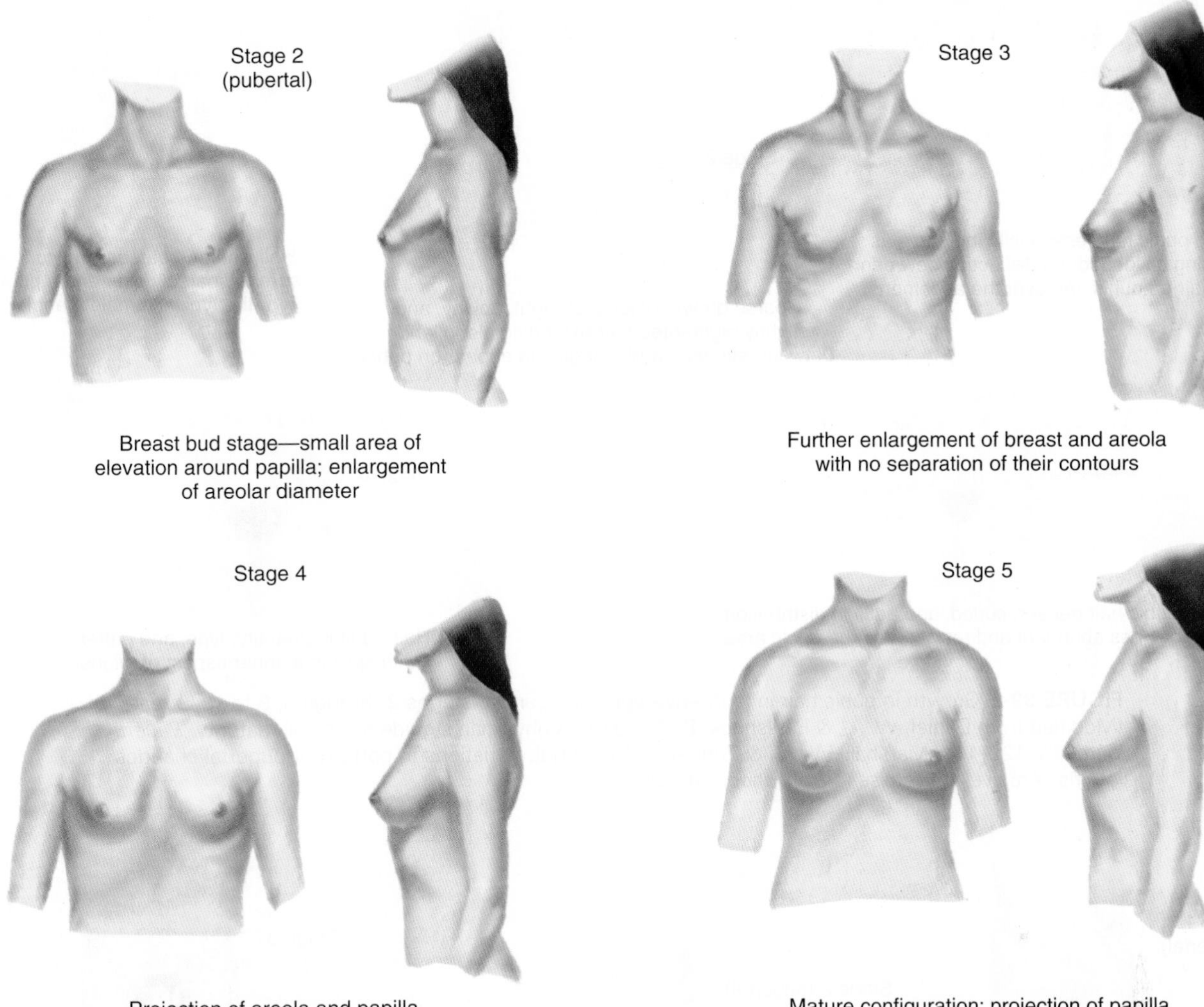
Stage 2
(pubertal)
Breast bud stage—small area of elevation around papilla; enlargement of areolar diameter
Stage 3
Further enlargement of breast and areola with no separation of their contours
Stage 4
Projection of areola and papilla to form a secondary mound (may not occur in all girls)
Stage 5
Mature configuration; projection of papilla only caused by recession of areola into general contour

FIGURE 39-1 Development of the breast in girls—average age span: 9 to 13½ years. Stage 1 (prepubertal, elevation of papilla only) is not shown. (Modified from Daniel, W. A., & Paulshock, B. Z. [1979]. A physician's guide to sexual maturity. *Patient Care, 13,* 122–124; Marshall, W. A., & Tanner, J. M. [1969]. Variations in pattern of pubertal changes in girls. *Archive of Diseases in Childhood, 44,* 291.)

preschool high-meat diet, intake of dairy products, low fibre intake, exposure to isoflavones, living in a high-stress family, the father being absent, certain endocrine disruptors, hormone-laced hair products, insulin resistance, activity level, and geographical location (Biro, Greenspan, & Galvez, 2012; Herman-Giddens, 2013; Roberts, Shields, de Groh, et al., 2012).

Sexual maturation in boys. The first pubescent changes in boys are testicular enlargement accompanied by thinning, reddening, and increased looseness of the scrotum (Fig. 39-3). These events usually occur between 9½ and 14 years of age. Early puberty is also characterized by the initial appearance of pubic hair. Penile enlargement begins, and testicular enlargement and pubic hair growth continue throughout midpuberty. During this period increasing muscularity, early voice changes, and development of early facial hair also occur. Temporary breast enlargement and tenderness, *gynecomastia*, are common during midpuberty, occurring in up to one third of boys. The spurts in height and weight occur concurrently toward the end of midpuberty. For most boys, breast enlargement disappears within 2 years. By late puberty there is a definite increase in the length and width of the penis, testicular enlargement continues, and first ejaculation occurs. Axillary hair develops, and facial hair extends to cover the anterior neck. Final voice changes occur secondary to the growth of the larynx. Concerns about pubertal delay should be considered for boys who exhibit no enlargement of the testes or scrotal changes by 13½ to 14 years of age, or if genital growth is not complete 4 years after the testicles begin to enlarge.

Physical Growth

A constant phenomenon associated with sexual maturation is a dramatic increase in growth. The final 20 to 25% of height is

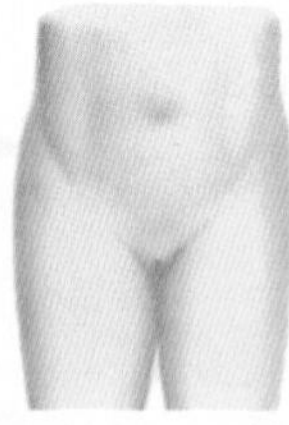

No pubic hair; essentially the same as during childhood; no distinction between hair on pubis and over the abdomen

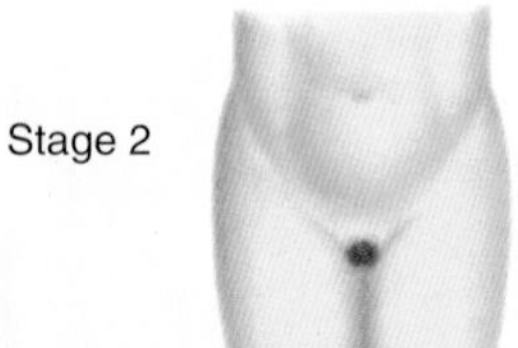

Sparse growth of long, straight, downy, and slightly pigmented hair extending along labia; between stages 2 and 3 begins to appear on pubis

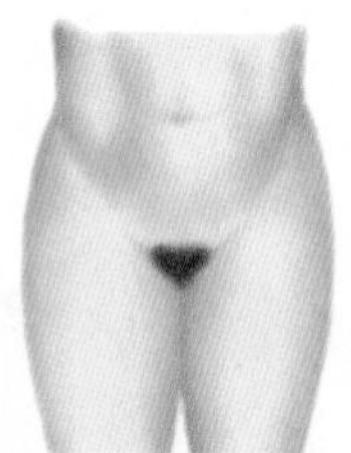

Hair darker, coarser, and curly and spread sparsely over entire pubis in the typical female triangle

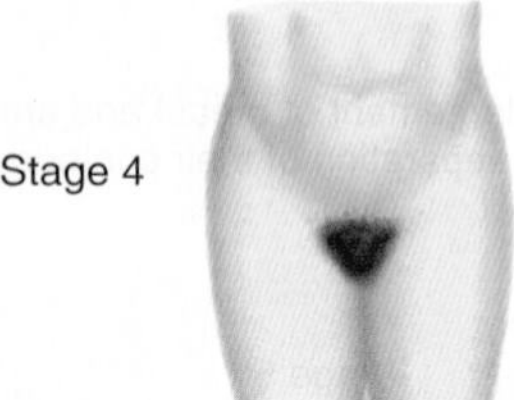

Pubic hair denser, curled, and adult in distribution but less abundant and restricted to the pubic area

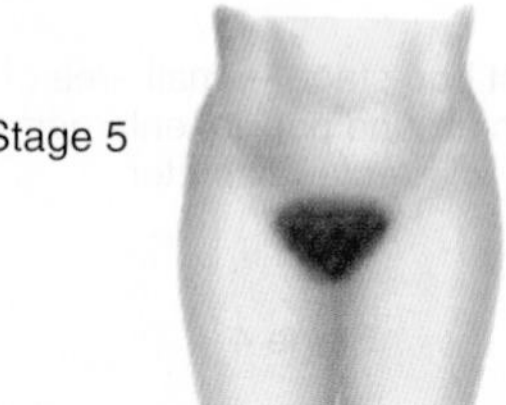

Hair adult in quantity, type, and pattern with spread to inner aspect of thighs

FIGURE 39-2 Growth in pubic hair in girls—average age span for stages 2 through 5: 9 to 13½ years. (Modified from Daniel, W. A., & Paulshock, B. Z. [1979]. A physician's guide to sexual maturity. *Patient Care, 13,* 122–124; Marshall, W. A., & Tanner, J. M. [1969]. Variations in pattern of pubertal changes in girls. *Archive of Diseases in Childhood, 44,* 291.)

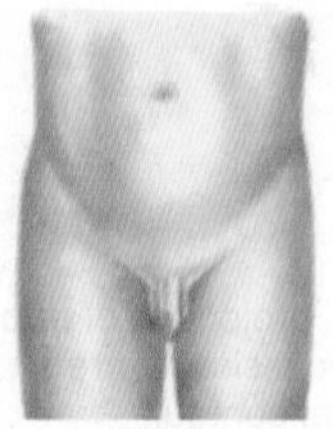

No pubic hair; essentially the same as during childhood; no distinction between hair on pubis and over the abdomen

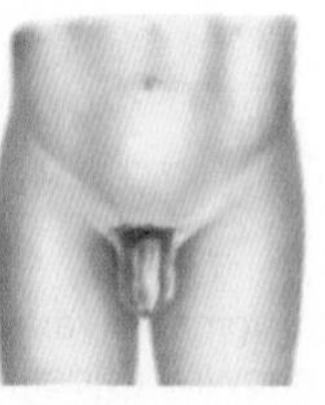

Initial enlargement of scrotum and testes; reddening and textural changes of scrotal skin; sparse growth of long, straight, downy, and slightly pigmented hair at base of penis

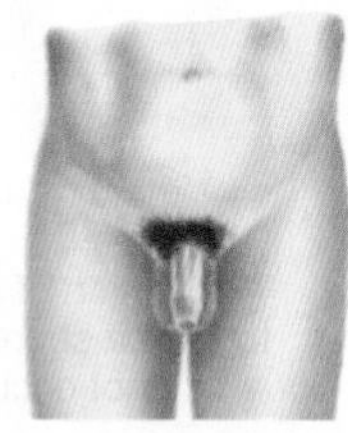

Initial enlargement of penis, mainly in length; testes and scrotum further enlarged; hair darker, coarser, and curly and spread sparsely over entire pubis

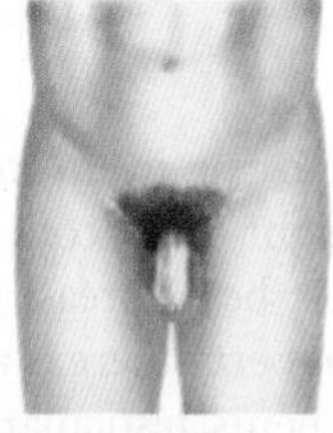

Increased size of penis with growth in diameter and development of glans; glans larger and broader; scrotum darker; pubic hair more abundant with curling but restricted to pubic area

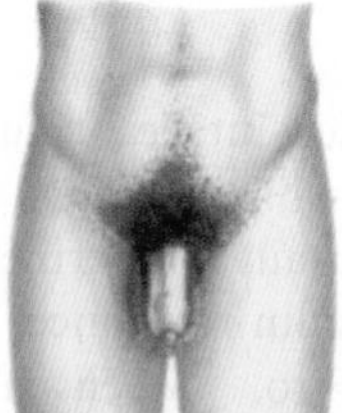

Testes, scrotum, and penis adult in size and shape; hair adult in quantity and type with spread to inner surface of thighs

FIGURE 39-3 Developmental stages of secondary sex characteristics and genital development in boys—average age span, 9½ to 14 years. (Modified from Daniel, W. A., & Paulshock, B. Z. [1979]. A physician's guide to sexual maturity. *Patient Care, 13,* 122–124; Marshall, W. A., & Tanner, J. M. [1969]. Variations in pattern of pubertal changes in girls. *Archive of Diseases in Childhood, 44,* 291.)

achieved during puberty, and most of this growth occurs during a 24- to 36-month period—the adolescent growth spurt. This accelerated growth occurs in all children but, as in other areas of development, is highly variable in age of onset, duration, and extent. The growth spurt begins earlier in girls, usually between ages 9½ and 14½ years; on average it begins between ages 10½ and 16 years in boys. During this period, the average boy gains 10 to 30 cm in height and 7 to 30 kg in weight. The average girl, in whom the growth spurt is slower and less extensive, gains 5 to 20 cm in height and 7 to 25 kg in weight. Growth in height typically ceases 2 to 2½ years after menarche in girls and at age 18 to 20 years in boys.

This increase in size is acquired in a characteristic sequence. Growth in length of the extremities and neck precedes growth in other areas, and since these parts are first to reach adult length, the hands and feet appear larger than normal during adolescence. Increases in hip and chest breadth take place in a few months, followed several months later by an increase in shoulder width. These changes are followed by increases in the length of the trunk and depth of the chest. This sequence of changes is responsible for the characteristic long-legged, gawky appearance of the early adolescent child.

Sex differences in general growth patterns. Sex differences in general growth and distribution patterns are apparent in skeletal growth, muscle mass, adipose tissue, and skin. Skeletal growth differences between boys and girls are apparently a function of hormonal effects at puberty and are evident primarily in limb length. The earlier cessation of growth in girls is caused by epiphyseal unity under the potent effect of estrogen secretion, and the hormonal effect on female bone growth is much stronger than the similar effect of testosterone in boys. In boys the prolonged growth period before puberty and the less rapid epiphyseal closure are reflected in their greater overall height and longer arms and legs. Other skeletal differences are increased shoulder width in boys and broader hip development in girls.

Hypertrophy of the laryngeal mucosa and enlargement of the larynx and vocal cords occur in both boys and girls to produce voice changes. Girls' voices become slightly deeper and considerably fuller. The effect in boys is particularly striking, occurring as boys mature, with the voice often shifting uncontrollably from deep to high tones in the middle of a sentence.

Growth of lean body mass, principally muscle, which tends to occur after the bone growth spurt, takes place steadily during adolescence. Lean body mass is both quantitatively and qualitatively greater in boys than in girls at comparable stages of pubertal development. Muscle development, under the influence of androgenic hormones, increases steadily. Muscles become remarkably well developed in boys, whereas in girls, muscle mass increase is proportionate to general tissue growth.

Growth of nonlean body mass, primarily fat, is also increased but follows a less orderly pattern. There may be a transient increase in subcutaneous fat just before the skeletal growth spurt, especially in boys. This is followed 1 to 2 years later by a modest to marked decrease, which is again more notable in boys. Later, variable amounts of fat are deposited to fill out and contour the mature physique in patterns characteristic of the adolescent's sex, particularly in the regions over the thighs, hips, and buttocks and around the breast tissue. Girls with thelarche as the first sign of puberty have earlier menarche and greater body fat and body mass index (BMI) at menarche than girls with adrenarche as the first pubertal sign. This may have long-term effects for increased risk of adult adiposity and obesity (Biro et al., 2012) although the relationship between early pubescence and obesity has yet to be fully understood (Kaplowitz, 2008).

Hormonal influences during puberty cause acceleration in growth and maturation of the skin and its structural appendages. Sebaceous glands become extremely active at this time, especially those on the genitalia and in the "flush areas" of the body (i.e., face, neck, shoulders, upper back, and chest). This increased activity and the structural nature of the glands are important in the pathogenesis of a common problem of puberty: acne (see Chapter 52). The eccrine sweat glands, present almost everywhere on the human skin, become fully functional and respond to emotional and thermal stimulation. Heavy sweating appears to be more pronounced in boys than in girls. The apocrine sweat glands, nonfunctional in childhood, reach secretory capacity during puberty. Unlike the eccrine sweat glands, the apocrine glands are limited in distribution and grow in conjunction with hair follicles in the axillae, around the areola of the breast, around the umbilicus, on the external auditory canal, and in the genital and anal regions. Apocrine glands secrete a thick substance as a result of emotional stimulation that, when acted on by surface bacteria, becomes highly odorous.

Body hair assumes very characteristic distribution patterns and changes texture during puberty. Under the influence of gonadal and adrenal androgens, hair coarsens, darkens, and lengthens at sites related to secondary sex characteristics. Pubic and axillary hair appears in both sexes, although pubic hair is more extensive in boys than in girls. Beard, moustache, and body hair on the chest, upward along the linea alba, and sometimes on other areas (e.g., back and shoulders) appears in boys and is androgen dependent. Extremity hair appears in varying amounts in both sexes but is also more prolific in boys.

Physiological Changes

A number of physiological functions are altered in response to some of the pubertal changes. The size and strength of the heart, blood volume, and systolic blood pressure increase, whereas the pulse rate and basal heat production decrease (see Appendix E). Blood volume, which increases steadily during childhood, reaches a higher value in boys than in girls, a fact that may be related to the increased muscle mass in pubertal boys. Adult values are reached for all formed elements of the blood. Respiratory rate and basal metabolic rate, which decrease steadily throughout childhood, reach the adult rate in adolescence. Respiratory volume and vital capacity are increased and to a far greater extent in males than in females. During this period, physiological responses to exercise change drastically: performance improves, especially in boys, and the body is able to make the physiological adjustments needed for normal functioning after exercise is completed. These capabilities are a result of the increased size and strength of muscles and the increased level of cardiac, respiratory, and metabolic functioning.

Norms related to the changes that occur during the early, middle, and late phases of adolescence are summarized in Table 39-1.

Psychosocial Development

Developing a Sense of Identity (Erikson)

Traditional psychosocial theory holds that the developmental crisis of adolescence leads to the formation of a sense of identity (Erikson, 1963). Adolescents come to see themselves as distinct

TABLE 39-1 GROWTH AND DEVELOPMENT DURING ADOLESCENCE

EARLY ADOLESCENCE (11–14 YR)	MIDDLE ADOLESCENCE (15–17 YR)	LATE ADOLESCENCE (18–20 YR)
Growth		
Rapidly accelerating growth Reaches peak velocity Secondary sex characteristics appear	Growth decelerating in girls Stature reaches 95% of adult height Secondary sex characteristics well advanced	Physically mature Structure and reproductive growth almost complete
Cognition		
Explores new-found ability for limited abstract thought Groping for new values and energies Comparison of "normality" with peers of same sex	Developing capacity for abstract thinking Enjoys intellectual powers, often in idealistic terms Concern with philosophical, political, and social problems	Established abstract thought Can perceive and act on long-range options Able to view problems comprehensively Intellectual and functional identity established
Identity		
Preoccupied with rapid body changes Trying out of various roles Measurement of attractiveness by acceptance or rejection of peers Conformity to group norms	Modifies body image Very self-centred; increased narcissism Tendency toward inner experience and self-discovery Has a rich fantasy life Idealistic Able to perceive future implications of current behaviour and decisions; variable application	Body image and gender-role definition nearly secured Mature sexual identity Phase of consolidation of identity Stability of self-esteem Comfortable with physical growth Social roles defined and articulated
Relationships With Parents		
Defining independence–dependence boundaries Strong desire to remain dependent on parents while trying to detach No major conflicts over parental control	Major conflicts over independence and control Low point in parent–child relationship Greatest push for emancipation; disengagement Final and irreversible emotional detachment from parents; mourning	Emotional and physical separation from parents completed Independence from family with less conflict Emancipation nearly secured
Relationships With Peers		
Seeks peer affiliations to counter instability generated by rapid change Upsurge of close, idealized friendships with members of the same sex Struggle for mastery takes place within peer group	Strong need for identity to affirm self-image Behavioural standards set by peer group Acceptance by peers extremely important—fear of rejection Exploration of ability to attract sexual partner	Peer group recedes in importance in favour of individual friendship Testing of romantic relationships against possibility of permanent alliance Relationships characterized by giving and sharing
Sexuality		
Self-exploration and evaluation Limited dating, usually group Limited intimacy	Multiple plural relationships Internal identification of heterosexual, homosexual, or bisexual attractions Exploration of "self appeal" Feeling of "being in love" Tentative establishment of relationships	Forms stable relationships and attachment to another Growing capacity for mutuality and reciprocity Dating as a romantic pair May publicly identify as gay, lesbian, or bisexual Intimacy involves commitment rather than exploration and romanticism
Psychological Health		
Wide mood swings Intense daydreaming Anger outwardly expressed with moodiness, temper outbursts, and verbal insults and name-calling	Tendency toward inner experiences; more introspective Tendency to withdraw when upset or feelings are hurt Vacillation of emotions in time and range Feelings of inadequacy common; difficulty in asking for help	More constancy of emotion Anger more apt to be concealed

individuals, somehow unique and separate from every other individual.

Adolescence begins with the onset of puberty and extends to relative physical and emotional stability at or near graduation from high school. During this time, the adolescent is faced with the crisis of group identity versus alienation. In the period that follows, the individual strives to attain autonomy from the family and develop a sense of personal identity instead of role diffusion. A sense of group identity appears to be essential to developing a sense of personal identity. Young adolescents must resolve questions concerning relationships with a peer group before they are able to resolve questions about who they are in relation to family and society.

Group identity. During the early stage of adolescence, pressure to belong to a group is intensified. Teenagers find it essential to have a group to which they can belong and that provides them with status. They dress as the group dresses and wear makeup and hairstyles according to group criteria, all of which are different from those of the parental generation. Language, music, and dancing reflect a culture that is exclusive to the adolescent. Adolescent conformity to the peer group and nonconformity to the adult group provides teenagers with a frame of reference in which they can display their own self-assertion while rejecting the identity of their parents' generation. To be different from the group, however, is to be unaccepted and alienated from the group.

Individual identity. The quest for personal identity is an ongoing process. As adolescents establish identity within a group they also attempt to incorporate multiple body changes into a concept of the self. In addition, as part of their search for identity, adolescents will take stock of their current and past relationships, as well as the directions they hope to take in the future.

The evolving of a personal identity is fraught with periods of confusion, excitement, depression, and discouragement. Determining an identity and a place in the world is a critical feature of adolescence. However, as the pieces gradually shift and settle into place, an identity eventually emerges. Role diffusion results when the individual is unable to formulate a satisfactory identity from the multiplicity of aspirations, roles, and influences.

Gender-role identity. Adolescence is the time for consolidation of a gender-role identity. During early adolescence the peer group will begin to communicate expectations regarding relationships, and as development progresses, adolescents will encounter expectations for mature gender-role behaviour from both peers and adults. Adolescents will explore their identities and gender orientation, working to identify whether they are gay, lesbian, transgender, or bisexual. Expectations vary from culture to culture, between geographic areas and socioeconomic groups.

Emotionality. Adolescents vacillate in their emotional states between considerable maturity and childlike behaviour. One minute they are exuberant and enthusiastic; the next minute they are depressed and withdrawn. Unpredictable, but essentially normal, mood swings are common during this time. As the tension is relieved, individuals can bring the emotion under control and individuals may retreat to review what has happened, to attempt to master their anger, and to increase their ability to control their emotions and gain from the new experience. Because of these mood swings, adolescents are frequently labelled unstable, inconsistent, and unpredictable. Little things can cause an emotional upheaval and, depending on the teenager's interpretation, can mean a great deal.

Teenagers are generally better able to control their emotions in later adolescence. They can approach problems more calmly and rationally, and although they are still subject to periods of sadness, their feelings are less vulnerable and they begin to demonstrate more mature emotions. Whereas early adolescents react immediately and emotionally, older adolescents can control their emotions until socially acceptable times and places for expression present themselves. They are still subject to heightened emotion, and when it is expressed, their behaviour can reflect feelings of insecurity, tension, and indecision.

Cognitive Development

Cognitive thinking culminates with the capacity for abstract thinking. This stage, the period of formal operations, is Piaget's (1952) fourth and last stage. Adolescents are no longer restricted to the real and actual, which was typical of the period of concrete thought. They now have the capacity to think beyond the present. Without having to centre attention on the immediate situation, they can imagine a sequence of events that might occur, such as college and occupational possibilities; how things might change in the future, such as relationships with parents; and the consequences of their actions, such as dropping out of school. At this time their thoughts can be influenced by logical principles rather than just their own perceptions and experiences. They become increasingly capable of scientific reasoning and formal logic.

Adolescents are capable of mentally manipulating more than two categories of variables at the same time. For example, they can consider the relationship between speed, distance, and time in planning a trip. They can detect logical consistency or inconsistency in a set of statements and evaluate a system or set of values in a more analytical manner. For instance, they question the parent who insists on honesty in the teenager but at the same time cheats on an income tax report or expense account.

In adolescence, young people begin to think about both their own thinking and the thinking of others. They wonder what opinion others have of them, and they are able to imagine the thoughts of others. With this capacity comes the ability to differentiate between others' thoughts and their own and to interpret the thoughts of others more accurately. They are able to understand that few concepts are absolute or independent of other influencing factors. As they become aware that other cultures and communities have different norms and standards from their own, it becomes easier for them to accept members of these other cultures, and the decision to behave in their own culture in an accepted manner becomes a more conscious commitment.

Moral Development

Although younger children tend to accept the decisions or point of view of adults, adolescents, in their efforts toward autonomy, must substitute their own set of morals and values. According to Kohlberg (1968), when old principles are challenged but new independent values have not yet emerged to take their place, young people search for a moral code that preserves their personal integrity and guides their behaviour, especially in the face of strong pressure to violate the old beliefs. Their decisions involving moral dilemmas must be based on an internalized set of moral principles that provides them with the resources to evaluate the demands of the situation and to plan actions that are consistent with their ideals.

Late adolescence is characterized by serious questioning of existing moral values and their relevance to society and the individual. Adolescents can easily take the role of another. They understand duty and obligation based on the reciprocal rights of others, as well as the concept of justice that is founded on making amends for misdeeds and repairing or replacing what has been spoiled by wrong-doing. However, they seriously question established moral codes, often as a result of observing that adults verbally ascribe to a code but do not adhere to it.

Spiritual Development

As adolescents move toward independence from parents and other authorities, some begin to question their families' values and ideals. Others cling to these values as a stable element in their lives as they struggle with the conflicts of this turbulent period. Adolescents need to work out these conflicts for themselves, but they also need support from authority figures and peers for their resolution.

Adolescents are capable of understanding abstract concepts and of interpreting analogies and symbols. They are able to empathize, philosophize, and think logically. Most teens search for ideals and speculate about illogical statements and conflicting ideologies. Their tendency toward introspection and emotional intensity often makes it difficult for others to know what they are thinking. They tend to keep their thoughts private, fearing that no one will understand these feelings that they perceive to be unique and special. However, they may reveal deep spiritual concerns. They need support and encouragement in their struggle for understanding as well as the freedom to question without censure.

Generally, the stated importance of participation in organized religions declines somewhat during the adolescent years. More high school students than post–secondary school young people attend religious services regularly, and, not surprisingly, the younger the adolescents, the more likely they are to view religion as being important to them. Among older adolescents, the importance of organized religion declines more among college students than among those not in college. Late adolescence appears to be a time when individuals re-examine and re-evaluate many of the beliefs and values of their childhood. Consistent with developmental changes in value autonomy, the religious beliefs of young people are likely to become more personalized and less bound to the traditional religious practices they may have been exposed to when they were younger. As adolescents mature and form an identity, they may either reject their family's traditional beliefs or they may decide to conform to those beliefs (Neuman, 2011). Religious beliefs in adolescence are also strongly influenced by interpersonal relationships with peers as well as adults in their environment.

Nurses can play an important role in providing an opportunity to discuss issues dealing with spirituality with this age group.

Social Development

Adolescents gradually reconfigure their relationship with their families and develop a sense of themselves that allows them to exist separately from their parents. However, this process is fraught with ambivalence on the part of both teenagers and their parents. Adolescents want to grow up and be free of parental restraints, but they are fearful as they try to comprehend the responsibilities that are linked with independence. Feelings of immortality and exemption from the consequences of risk-taking behaviour, while usually viewed as negative, can serve an important developmental function at this time. These feelings may give adolescents the courage to separate from their parents and become independent. Part of this emancipation involves developing social relationships outside the family that help teenagers identify their role in society and have a sense of belonging outside of their family bonds. For many, adolescence is a time of intense sociability and often a time of equally intense loneliness. Acceptance by peers, a few close friends, and the secure love of a supportive family support interpersonal maturation.

Relationships With Parents

During adolescence the parent–child relationship changes from one of protection and dependency to one of mutual affection and equality (see Table 39-1). The process of achieving independence often involves turmoil and ambiguity as both parent and adolescent learn to play new roles and work toward this end while, at the same time, resolving the often painful series of rifts essential to establishing the ultimate relationship.

Most behaviour observed is related to the struggle for independence and the external restrictions and checks that are placed on this spontaneous maturation process. They are allowed privileges previously denied, and they are provided with increasing responsibilities. On the other hand, because of their unpredictability and insecurity in evaluating situations and making sound judgements, they are required to adhere to certain regulations and restrictions set by adults. In many families, this state of affairs is exemplified by the struggle between parents and adolescents concerning curfews, the use of social media, and the use of the family car.

As teenagers assert their rights for grown-up privileges, they frequently create tensions within the home. They resist parental control, and conflicts can arise from almost any situation or any subject. Favourite topics of dispute include Internet and cell phone use, manners, dress, chores and duties, homework, disrespectful behaviour, friendships, dating and relationships, money, automobiles, alcohol and other substance use, and time schedules. Present in these areas of conflict is the overriding argument that "everyone else has one" or is allowed the desired item or privilege and the ever-present assertions that "You don't understand me or trust me" and "You always treat me like a child." Spoken or unspoken, parents' reactions consist of "Is this all the thanks I get for what I have done for you?"

Adolescents' earliest attempts to achieve emancipation from parental controls are manifested in a period of rejection of the parents. They absent themselves from home and family activities and spend increasing time with the peer group. They confide less in their parents, but parents continue to play an important role in their personal and health-related decision making.

With advancing adolescence, teenagers become more competent, and with this competence comes a need for more autonomy. Although they may be psychologically prepared for independence, they are often thwarted in their efforts by lack of money or other barriers. Conflict may arise in relation to the teenager's independent activities as well as the needs of privacy and trust. Parental supervision remains important throughout adolescence and may have a direct influence on adolescent sexual and substance use behaviour. Parents should be guided toward a style of parenting in which authority is used to guide the adolescent while allowing developmentally appropriate levels of freedom and providing clear, consistent messages about expectations. Consistency in guidance and establishing ground rules is important for adolescents, even though they may fiercely reject the parents' wishes. An authoritative style of parenting has been shown to have both immediate and long-term protective effects toward adolescent risk reduction (Newman, Harrison, Dashiff, et al., 2008). However, to gain the trust of adolescents, parents must respect their adolescent's privacy and show an honest and sincere interest in what the adolescent believes and feels (see Family-Centred Teaching box).

FAMILY-CENTRED TEACHING

Communication With Teens: The Art of Listening

Conflicts between parents and their adolescents are often a result of a natural characteristic of parenthood: the desire to protect one's children from harm or from simply doing something "stupid" or embarrassing or something they may later regret. Teenagers sometimes bounce their thoughts and ideas off adults. At times they really want some feedback; at other times they simply want to elicit a reaction.

I found it easy to listen openly, thoughtfully, and without interrupting when my teenagers' friends discussed troublesome topics. However, one day, when one of my own teenagers had a similar conversation with me, the parent part kicked in. I felt responsible and spoke my piece on the spot. This brought communication to a halt and resulted in defensiveness. It was a long time before my child tried to talk to me about anything controversial again. The next time one of my teenagers started a similar conversation, I decided to try to trick myself.

Throughout the entire conversation, I told myself over and over again to act as if this were not my teenager, but rather someone else's child. I found this actually worked quite well, and I was able to listen without interrupting. I continued to use the system, sometimes with more success than at other times.

—Mother of Four

Relationships With Peers

Although parents remain the primary influence in their lives, for most teenagers, peers assume a more significant role in adolescence than they did during childhood (see Table 39-1). For many adolescents, the peer group serves as a strong support providing them with a sense of belonging and a feeling of strength and power. The peer group forms the transitional world between dependence and independence.

Peer groups. Adolescents are usually social, gregarious, and group minded. Thus the peer group has an intense influence on adolescents' self-evaluation and behaviour. To gain acceptance by a group, younger teenagers tend to conform completely in such things as mode of dress, hairstyle, taste in music, and vocabulary. Teenagers use the peer group as a yardstick of what is normal.

The school is psychologically important to adolescents as a focus of social life. Teenagers usually distribute themselves into a relatively predictable social hierarchy. They know to which groups they and others belong. School connectedness is correlated with caring teachers and the absence of prejudice or discrimination from peers; it is less dependent on class size, attendance, academic preparation, and parental involvement (Waters, Cross, & Shaw, 2010).

Within the larger peer groups are smaller, distinct, and rather exclusive crowds or cliques of selected close friends who are emotionally attached to each other (Fig. 39-4). The selection tends to follow common tastes, interests, and background. Although cliques may become formalized, most of them remain informal and small. However, each has an identifying feature that proclaims its difference from others and its solidarity within itself, in much the same manner as the adolescent generation as a whole sets itself apart from the adult generation. Cliques are usually made up of one gender. Within the intimacy of the group, adolescents gain support in learning about themselves, consideration for the feelings of others, and increased ego development and self-reliance.

To belong is of utmost importance; thus adolescents behave in ways that will ensure their establishment in a group. Adolescents are highly susceptible to social approval, acceptance, and

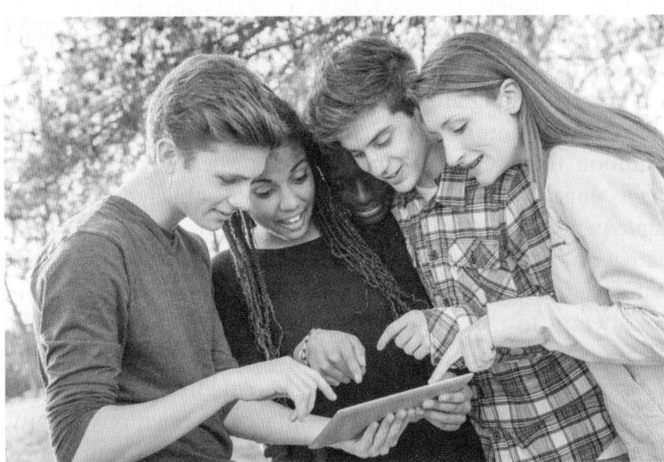

FIGURE 39-4 Teenagers often like to gather in small groups. (Riccardo Piccinini/Shutterstock.com.)

demands. Being ignored or criticized by peers can create feelings of inferiority, inadequacy, and incompetence.

Close friendships. Personal friendships between individuals usually develop between same-sex and opposite-sex adolescents. These relationships tend to be closer and more stable than those of middle childhood and are important in the quest for identity. A best friend is the best audience on whom to try out possible roles and identities that an adolescent wants to test. Best friends may try a social role together, each supporting the other. Each cares about what the other thinks and feels. Because a sense of intimacy grows within a permanent relationship, the stability of this friendship is an important link in the progress toward intimate relationships in young adulthood.

Interests and Activities

Adolescents spend a large amount of time engaging in leisure-time activities—sports, video games, parties, and nonstructured time spent with friends. As teenagers progress through the developmental stages of adolescence, these leisure-time activities move from being family centred to being peer centred. In addition to providing teenagers with fun and enjoyment, leisure-time activities assist in the development of social, physical, and cognitive skills. Leisure-time activities also allow teenagers the opportunity to learn to set priorities and structure their time.

The role of social media and advanced technology is nowhere more prominent than in the lives of today's adolescents. Most adolescents in Canada are connected to others through electronic means: cell phones, gaming consoles, personal tablets, and computers (Fig. 39-5). The large availability of social media through Facebook, Snapchat, Twitter, and Instagram have created virtual communities and ways for young people to interact with others, occasionally anonymously; Web cameras allow those interactions to include real-time video communication. Cellular telephones offer more mobile opportunities to talk on the phone, send text messages or instant messaging, send photos, or use video phone capabilities. These can create opportunities for those who have limited access to friends (because of rural location, shyness, or rare chronic conditions) to interact with other people. However, most teenagers appear to be using online social media to interact with the same peers they spend their day with at school.

Text messaging and instant messaging via cell phones have become a common activity and can be disruptive at school. In addition, these activities can be used for cyberbullying, in which teens engage in insults, harassment, and publicly humiliating statements online or on cell phones. There is also increased danger of adolescents coming in contact and sharing personal information with sexual predators who pose as adolescents in an attempt to make contact with underage victims or engage them in sexting (sending sexually explicit or suggestive pictures or messages online) (Dowdell, Burgess, & Flores, 2011). Adolescent sexting, rather than being an innocent anonymous activity, has been linked in some studies to risky sexual behaviours (Rice, Rhoades, Winetrobe, et al., 2012; Temple, Paul, van den Berg, et al., 2012).

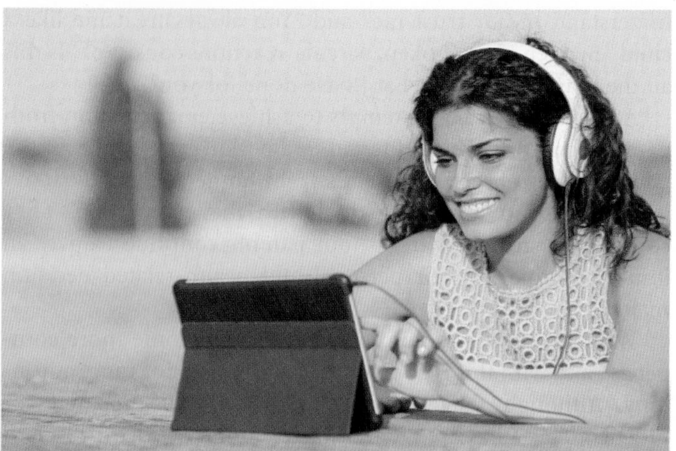

FIGURE 39-5 Cell phones and social media create ways for adolescents to communicate with peers. (Antonio Guillem/ Shutterstock.com.)

Today, many adolescents must learn to juggle their time between school, extracurricular activities, and the responsibilities of a job. Adolescent work experiences can provide the benefits of time management, teamwork skills, and increased income. It is generally recommended that adolescents limit their work to no more than 20 hours per week during the school year.

Adolescent Sexuality

Adolescence represents a critical time in the development of sexuality. Hormonal, physical, cognitive, and social changes that occur during adolescence all have an impact on sexual development. Of all the developmental changes that affect adolescent sexuality, none is more obvious than the impact of puberty. Adolescents must come to terms with hormonal influences, physiological manifestations such as menstruation and ejaculation, and physical changes such as breast and genital development. All of these changes have a profound impact on the way in which teenagers perceive their bodies (i.e., **body image**). In addition to transitions in body image, higher levels of pubertal hormones contribute to increased levels of sexual motivation among both boys and girls.

Changes in sexual motivations and feelings, happening at the same time as shifts in cognitive skills, contribute to painful conjectures ("Is what I'm feeling normal?"), self-conscious concern ("Am I good looking enough?"), and hypothetical thinking ("What if she wants to have sex?"). The emergence of formal operational thinking also increases adolescents' decision-making capabilities concerning sexual issues. As they mature, teenagers become better able to think through potential risks and benefits of sexual behaviours before they engage in any behaviour. Older adolescents may also be able to conceptualize more long-term consequences of present behaviours. One of the important goals of adolescence is to incorporate sexuality successfully into close, intimate relationships. This is made possible by the advanced cognitive abilities that emerge over the course of adolescence (see Table 39-1).

Many teenagers begin to make a shift toward intimate relationships during middle adolescence. The type and degree of seriousness of partner relationships vary by age and maturity level.

An integrated sexual identity often emerges during late adolescence as individuals incorporate sexual experiences, feelings, and knowledge. For most, this identity is consistent with their own physical and mental capacities and with societal limits and expectations. Most older adolescents identify themselves as being predominantly heterosexual or bisexual, with a smaller number self-identifying as gay or lesbian and an even smaller group still unsure of their sexual orientation, although this varies somewhat by ethnicity (Canadian Paediatric Society [CPS], 2011). Whatever their sexual orientation, many older teenagers possess the capacity to have intimate relationships that satisfy the emotional and sexual needs of both partners.

Gender identification refers to how an individual sees himself or herself as a man or a woman and affects one's feelings and behaviours (Johnson & Oliffe, 2012). During adolescence individuals commonly begin to identify their sexual orientation as part of their developing sexual identity. This identification process is generally profoundly influenced by cultural beliefs and values, by societal and family pressures, and by peers. Sexual orientation is an important aspect of sexual identity. **Sexual orientation** is defined as a pattern of sexual arousal or romantic attraction toward persons of the opposite gender (heterosexual), of the same gender (homosexual, often called *gay* or *lesbian*), or of both genders (bisexual). Sexual orientation encompasses several dimensions, including attraction, fantasy, actual sexual behaviour, and self-labelling or group affiliation. In individuals, the direction and intensity of each dimension are not necessarily consistent with any of the others. For example, individuals may be attracted most strongly to their same gender, fantasize about both genders, have sexual activity only with the opposite gender, and identify as gay or lesbian. Other individuals may engage in same-gender sexual behaviour and fantasize about both genders but identify as heterosexual. As with all aspects of sexual identity, the dimensions of sexual orientation are influenced by cultural meaning and expectation, by gender, by peer groups, and by other environmental contexts. For adolescents whose orientation encompasses any same-sex dimensions, the identity process during adolescence can be complicated, especially when community norms disapprove of orientations other than heterosexual. Adolescents who have witnessed harassment or violence directed at gay, lesbian, bisexual, and transgender people, for example, may be reluctant to self-identify as belonging to any of these groups, even when their attractions and behaviours are exclusively same-sex or bisexual. *Transgender* is defined as a person whose gender identity, outward appearance, expression, or anatomy does not fit into conventional expectations of male or female (Public Health Agency of Canada [PHAC], 2010). For example, a transgender adolescent boy may dress as a girl in order to satisfy his female sense of identity.

The development of sexual orientation as part of sexual identity includes several developmental milestones during late childhood and throughout adolescence. These milestones do not necessarily occur in the same order for everyone, nor are they completed in the same amount of time. They include (1) the realization of romantic or erotic attraction to people of one or both genders; (2) erotic daydreaming about one or both genders; (3) romantic partners or dates without sexual activity; (4) sexual activity with people of the preferred gender or genders (also, for some teens, sexual activity with a nonpreferred gender, out of curiosity or through social pressure); (5) self-identification of the orientation that best fits one's current circumstances and understanding; (6) publicly self-identifying that orientation, usually to intimate friends and family first, then the wider social group; and (7) an intimate, committed, sexual relationship with a person of the gender appropriate to one's orientation.

There is no evidence that gay, lesbian, bisexual, or transgender adults are more or less likely to create long-term, stable relationships than are heterosexual couples. It should be noted that bisexual adolescents and adults do not generally engage in sexual relationships with both genders concurrently; self-identification as bisexual usually refers to the ability to be attracted to either gender but does not imply that such a person requires partners of both genders, or that one must be equally attracted to and have sexual experience with both genders.

Although the order of these milestones varies greatly among adolescents, adolescents who identify as gay, lesbian, bisexual, or transgender tend to publicly self-identify later than heterosexual peers. Without positive gay, lesbian, bisexual, or transgender role models or a supportive peer group, sexual-minority teens can feel isolated, and they may not share their orientation with anyone for fear of rejection or violence (see Critical Thinking Case Study). The best available Canadian research statistics are from an Adolescent Health Survey of 289,767 students from public schools done in British Columbia. Out of all of the boys in the survey, 1.5% identified themselves as bisexual, mostly homosexual, or 100% homosexual. However, 3.5% of the sexually active boys stated that they had had sex with an individual of the same gender in the past year. Out of all the girls, 3% identified themselves as bisexual, mostly homosexual, or 100% homosexual. However, 6.4% of sexually active girls identified themselves as having had sex with someone of the same gender in the past year (CPS, 2011; Saewyc, Poon, Wang, et al., 2007).

A comparison of bisexual youth and heterosexual youth found that bisexual adolescents, especially girls, reported lower levels of connection to family and school than did heterosexual adolescents. Nurses should be alert to these lower levels of protective relationships for bisexual youth because it may lead to poor health outcomes (Saewyc, Homma, Skay, et al., 2009). It is also important for health care providers to be cognizant of the significant psychological, social, and medical issues that confront young people who are gay, lesbian, bisexual, or transgender. Almost all of these concerns are the result of stigmatization that these youth face, rather than from the orientation itself (CPS, 2011). It is important for nurses to have specific strategies to help these youth open up for a nonjudgemental, sensitive, and respectful discussion on gender identity and sexuality. For example, not referring to or calling the individual "he" or "she" but perhaps "they" can present a respectful approach. Asking the questions "What gender were you assigned at birth?" and "What gender do you associate with now?" is a sensitive way for

CRITICAL THINKING CASE STUDY

Discussing Sexual Orientation With Adolescents

John, a 17-year-old adolescent, comes into the school-based clinic and tells the nurse practitioner that he thinks he is gay. What is the most appropriate response for the nurse practitioner?

1. Evidence—Is there sufficient evidence to draw any conclusions about John's sexual orientation at this time?
2. Assumptions—Describe an underlying assumption about each of the following issues:
   a. Sexual orientation in adolescents
   b. Societal reactions toward self-identifying as gay
   c. Health care providers and sexuality
3. What implications and priorities for nursing care can be drawn at this time?
4. Does the evidence support your argument (conclusion)?

nurses to begin performing a health assessment of an individual considering identifying as transgender.

Development of Self-Concept and Body Image

The sudden growth that takes place in early adolescence creates feelings of confusion. The security of a familiar body is lost and the adolescent may feel uncomfortable within their altered body. Consequently, some adolescents may try to either hide their body or advertise it, or they may alternate between the two extremes. Teenagers tend to be acutely aware of their appearance as they begin to acquire images of themselves as adults, but they see discrepancies between their ideal and actual skills and abilities.

Adolescents are continually comparing themselves with their peers and making judgements about their own normality based on these observations. Most youth feel most comfortable when they are just like their friends and age-mates. Perceived defects or deviations from the group average can threaten their idealized image. Any blemish may be magnified out of proportion, and any delay of the visible evidence of maturity is cause for worry. Unfortunately, this is also the time when the hormonal effect of the sebaceous glands produces acne, and even the most insignificant pimple may be viewed as a disfigurement. The diagnosis of chronic disease or a permanent physical disability has special significance during adolescence and creates additional stresses for both adolescents with the condition and health care providers.

The body image that is established during adolescence is the one that individuals retain throughout life. Much of adolescents' search for identity takes a variety of forms. For some, much of this process unfolds in front of a mirror as they try to read from the reflected features just who they are and what they look like to other people. Adolescents may practise facial expressions and postures, try out hair arrangements, worry about a pimple, and in other ways attempt to assess the best means to achieve a maximum effect—to reveal the "true self."

The self-concept becomes more differentiated as adolescents acquire a more complex picture of themselves, one that takes situational factors into account. The self-concept gradually becomes more individualized and more distinct from the concepts of others. Although younger teenagers describe themselves in terms of similarities with peers, as adolescence advances, young people tend to describe themselves in terms of their special characteristics.

Responses to Puberty

The response to the physical changes of pubertal growth and development is manifested differently depending on the stage of development. During early adolescence, young adolescents may be preoccupied with the rapid changes in their body and are interested in the anatomy, physiology, and function of their sexual organs. Boys must also confront the sexual feelings and tensions that accompany puberty, and the appearance of nocturnal emissions may be puzzling, troublesome, or embarrassing. Unless the boy has been prepared in advance, he may find it difficult to discuss his feelings with his parents and may turn to his friends for information and guidance. Many girls also find the rapid changes in their body to be sources of concern. Some girls perceive the increase in weight and associated fat deposition as evidence of obesity and may indulge in fad diets. Although many girls look forward to menstruation and take this event in stride, others may find the first menstrual period a distressing and frightening event. All teenagers, regardless of gender, are concerned with the question, "Am I normal?" To answer this question, they compare their body with those of their peers and with images in the media. This leads to a great deal of uncertainty about their appearance and attractiveness.

If an adolescent does not enter puberty at the same time as his or her peers, considerable inner conflict may occur. Early-maturing girls and boys have higher rates of sexual risk-taking behaviours, delinquency, and substance use than their on-time peers (Costello, Sung, & Worthman, 2007; Lynne, Graber, Nicols, et al., 2007). Early puberty onset in females who are daughters of adolescent mothers may also be a significant factor in teenage pregnancies (de Genna, Larkby, & Cornelius, 2011). Nurses who work with adolescents must provide teaching and health care interventions that are appropriate for the adolescent's chronological and cognitive development rather than the stage of physical maturation.

As growth and development proceed through middle adolescence, the rapid body changes diminish. The adolescent has time to try to make the body more attractive. Adolescents strive to achieve the perfect body within their own cultural norms; the "right" clothes and hairstyle become very important. By late adolescence the heightened concern with body image generally subsides and the youth develops a more comfortable relationship with his or her body.

PROMOTING OPTIMUM HEALTH DURING ADOLESCENCE

The major causes of morbidity and mortality in adolescence are not diseases but, instead, health-damaging behaviours. Important sources of morbidity in adolescence include injury, depression, violence, and **sexually transmitted infections (STIs)**;

obesity may begin in childhood or adolescence, but the health consequences are more evident in early and middle adulthood. Health promotion for this age group often consists mainly of teaching and guidance to avoid risk-taking activities and health-damaging behaviours. Adolescence provides an opportunity for teenagers to learn and incorporate healthy lifestyle behaviours that will benefit them not only during the teenage years but also throughout the lifespan.

Effective health education for adolescents should incorporate a developmentally appropriate, multifaceted approach. Motivational interviewing has been shown to improve adherence to health care advice by using a collaborative approach (Resnicow & McMaster, 2012). In this process the adolescent is encouraged to introspectively explore feelings of ambivalence and, on the basis of his or her insights, to develop solutions for effecting change. Education alone, however, is not enough to change behaviour. Effective programs for adolescents must include opportunities to improve communication skills and enhance their social network to make more positive connections (Bröning, Kumpfer, Kruse, et al., 2012).

As young people progress through adolescence, they assume increasing responsibility for their own health, including maintaining health practices, taking prescribed medications, keeping appointments, and performing procedures, when necessary. Health care providers who work with adolescents should consider the adolescent's increasing independence and responsibility and maintain their privacy and ensure confidentiality (see Guidelines box and Critical Thinking Case Study). Parents should also respect their teenager's independence and move toward the role of consultant about health issues while also maintaining some level of parental involvement in their health care throughout their child's adolescence.

GUIDELINES
Interviewing Adolescents

- Ensure confidentiality and privacy; interview the adolescent without the parents.
- Show concern for the adolescent's perspective with statements such as "First, I'd like to talk about your main concerns" and "I'd like to know what you think is happening."
- Offer a nonthreatening explanation for the questions you ask: "I'm going to ask a number of questions to help me better understand your health."
- Maintain objectivity; avoid assumptions, judgements, and lectures.
- Ask open-ended questions when possible; move to more directive questions if necessary.
- Begin with less sensitive issues and proceed to more sensitive ones.
- Use language that both the adolescent and you understand. Clarify terms, such as "having sex" or "hooking up."
- Restate: reflect back to adolescents what they have said, along with feelings that may be associated with their descriptions.
- Ask the adolescent if he or she minds if the practitioner shares general (or specific) information gathered in the health examinations and interview with the parents. Reiterate that the teen's confidentiality will be maintained if he or she refuses to give permission (unless life-threatening information is shared).

Immunizations

Immunization updates are a significant part of adolescent preventive care and, in Canada, most vaccines are included in publicly funded immunizations programs. Immunization schedules vary slightly among the provinces and territories (PHAC, 2015a) (see Additional Resources at the end of the chapter). The following guidelines are based on the recommendations of the National Advisory Committee on Immunization (NACI).

Adolescents 11 to 16 years of age should receive a single tetanus–diphtheria–acellular pertussis (Tdap) vaccine if they have received the recommended childhood series of diphtheria–tetanus–acellular pertussis (DTaP) immunizations. This vaccine is now required because of the increased incidence of pertussis seen in adolescents and adults who were previously immunized with the DTaP series. Adolescents who have received Td but not Tdap vaccine should also receive a single dose of the Tdap vaccine, provided 5 years have elapsed between the tetanus-diptheria (Td) and Tdap vaccination (PHAC, 2015b).

A booster dose of meningococcal vaccine (Men-C or Men-C-ACYW, depending on jurisdiction) should be given to preteens at 12 years of age (PHAC, 2015a). If not previously vaccinated, they should receive one dose between 13 and 18 years of age.

A quadrivalent human papillomavirus (HPV) vaccine has been approved and is recommended for female children and adolescents to prevent HPV-related cervical cancer (see Chapter 7). The HPV vaccine is also recommended in males between 9 and 26 years of age. HPV is the most common STI: the overall prevalence of HPV infection in Canada ranges between 11 and 29%, with peak prevalence in adolescents and young adults (younger than 25 years of age). The vaccine is administered intramuscularly in three separate doses; the first dose in the series may be given at 11 to 12 years of age (minimum age 9 years), the second dose is administered 2 months after the first, and the third dose is given 6 months after the first dose (PHAC, 2015b). As of September 2015, the schedule is decreased to two doses of vaccine rather than three in 50% of the provinces and territories. The vaccine is covered by all provincial

CRITICAL THINKING CASE STUDY
Respecting Privacy

Jamie, a 17-year-old girl, arrives at the adolescent clinic with her mother, Mrs. S, for a routine history and physical examination with the nurse practitioner. As the nurse practitioner walks with Jamie to an examination room, Mrs. S whispers to the nurse practitioner, "I need to speak with you in private." What principles should guide the nurse practitioner's response to Mrs. S's request?

1. Evidence—Is there sufficient evidence to formulate a response to Jamie's mother?
2. Assumptions—Describe an underlying assumption about each of the following topics:
    a. The role of the adolescent in health care
    b. The role of parents in the health of their adolescent
    c. Adolescents and confidentiality
3. What implications for nursing care should be established at this time?
4. Does the evidence support your conclusion?

and territorial health plans for females; in Alberta, Nova Scotia, and Prince Edward Island it is covered for males and females (Government of Canada, 2016).

All adolescents who have not previously received two doses of hepatitis B vaccine should be vaccinated against hepatitis B virus. The age at which children and youth are offered the vaccine varies between provinces (see Chapter 7).

In Canada, the hepatitis A vaccine is recommended for individuals of all ages considered to be at risk of exposure.

Annual influenza vaccination with either the live attenuated influenza vaccine or trivalent influenza vaccine is now encouraged for all children and adolescents.

All adolescents should be assessed for previous history of varicella infection or vaccination. Vaccination with the varicella vaccine is recommended for those with no previous history; for those with no previous infection or history of immunization, the varicella vaccine may be given in a single dose (PHAC, 2015b).

Any adolescent who has not completed the immunization series for hepatitis A, hepatitis B, poliovirus, and influenza should receive these immunizations according to the latest catch-up schedule (see also Chapter 35, Immunizations).

Nutrition

The rapid and extensive increase in height, weight, muscle mass, and sexual maturity of adolescence is accompanied by increased nutritional requirements. Because nutritional needs are closely related to the increase in body mass, the peak requirements occur in the years of maximum growth, during which the body mass almost doubles. The caloric and protein requirements during this time are higher than at almost any other time of life. As a result of this increased anabolic need, the adolescent is highly sensitive to caloric restrictions.

Eating Well With Canada's Food Guide outlines recommended dietary intake for adolescents (see Appendix A). However, not all adolescents' diets meet these recommendations. In a survey of seventh- to tenth-grade students in Alberta, a large portion (42%) of adolescents were not receiving the minimum dietary recommendations outlined in *Canada's Food Guide* (Storey, Forbes, Fraser, et al., 2009). Compared to youth whose diets met the minimum dietary recommendations, these teenagers tended have lower intakes of protein and fibre, higher intakes of carbohydrates and fats, a lower frequency of consuming breakfast, higher numbers of meals eaten away from home, and a lower level of physical activity. Dietary intervention should promote the regular consumption of breakfast and a balanced intake of a variety of foods.

There is a substantial increase in the need for the minerals *calcium, iron,* and *zinc* during periods of rapid growth: calcium for skeletal growth, iron for expansion of muscle mass and blood volume, and zinc for the generation of both skeletal and bone tissue (see Table 12-1). Girls with heavy or frequent menses may be especially susceptible to iron deficiency resulting from blood loss. Calcium intake from food sources is essential during adolescence to assist in building bone mass; the calcium deposited during these years determines the risk for osteoporosis as an older adult.

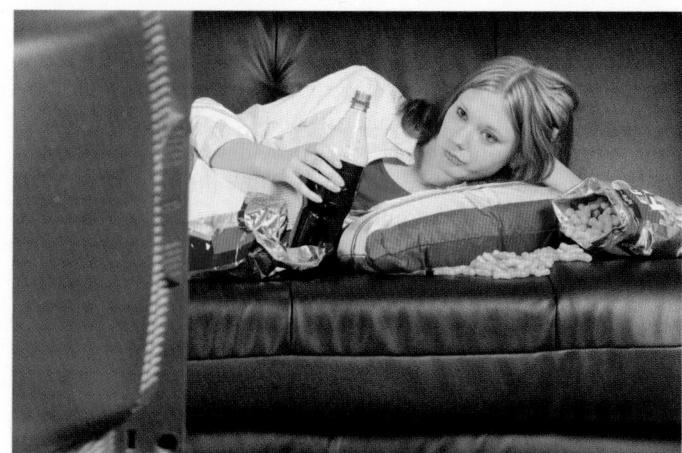

FIGURE 39-6 Snacking on empty calories is common among adolescents, especially during inactivity. (runzelkorn/Shutterstock.com.)

Eating Habits and Behaviour

Eating and attitudes toward food are primarily family centred during early and middle childhood, and food habits are largely related to cultural and individual family preferences and patterns. With adolescence and the move toward independence, family influences on the individual may diminish. Adolescents' interests, attitudes, and routines are altered as an increasing number of meals are eaten away from home. These changes are largely a result of the high value that teenagers place on peer acceptability and sociability. Their peers may easily influence the adolescent's eating habits.

Pressure for time and commitments to activities can adversely affect the teenager's eating habits. Snacks, usually selected on the basis of accessibility rather than nutritional merit, can become a greater part of the habitual eating pattern during adolescence (Fig. 39-6). Excess intake of calories, sugar, fat, cholesterol, and sodium is common among adolescents and is found in all income and racial or ethnic groups and in both genders. Inadequate intake of certain vitamins (folic acid, vitamin B_6, vitamin A) and minerals (iron, calcium, zinc) is also evident, particularly among girls and teenagers of low socioeconomic status. Milk is often passed over in favour of soft drinks.

Overeating or undereating during adolescence presents special problems. When teenage girls experience the normal increase in weight and fat deposition of a growth spurt, they often resort to dieting. The desire for a slim figure and a fear of becoming "fat" can prompt teenage girls to embark on nutritionally inadequate weight-reducing regimens that drain their energy and deprive their growing bodies of essential nutrients. They may resort to diets on their own or with peers in an effort to conform. Many adopt current fad diets and are victims of food misinformation. Boys may be less inclined to undereat; they are more concerned about gaining size and strength. However, they tend to eat foods high in calories but low in other essential nutrients.

Obesity has increased significantly among both children and adolescents in Canada. The obesity currently seen is not a result of metabolic disturbances but of poor dietary habits and sedentary lifestyles. A contributing factor to the increase in obesity is the fact that, over the past two decades, the overall portion size for foods has increased, the largest portions for most foods being at fast-food restaurants. In addition, a study of adolescents showed that the increased amount of time they spent looking at electronic screens after school resulted in more snacking and greater portion sizes along with consumption of foods with overall poor nutrition (Ciccone, Woodruff, Fryer, et al., 2013). With these high levels of obesity there are reports of increasing occurrences of hypertension and risk factors that can lead to the development of cardiovascular disease (Bassareo & Mercuro, 2014; LaRosa & Meyers, 2010).

Hypertension and Hyperlipidemia

As adolescents experience sexual maturation, along with increases in height and weight, blood pressure increases from the onset of adolescence and continues to rise until the end of pubertal growth. This trend is especially apparent among males. Approximately 1% of adolescents have sustained **hypertension**, defined as a blood pressure greater than the ninety-fifth percentile of standards. The detection of hypertension during adolescence is important because hypertension is one of the major preventable risk factors for adult cardiovascular disease. With increasing levels of obesity, smoking, and elevated serum cholesterol and triglyceride levels, there have been reports of increasing incidence of hypertension among adolescents (Hansen, Gunn, & Kaelber, 2007; LaRosa & Meyers, 2010). Children of all ages need to have their blood pressure checked and be followed during episodic practitioner office visits, using the Canadian Heart and Stroke Foundation guidelines (see Chapter 47 for more information; see Appendix E for normal values).

NURSING CARE

Adolescents should receive an annual assessment of weight, height, and BMI for age, plotted on a standard growth chart (see Appendix C). Healthy dietary habits should be discussed with all adolescents. The frequency of eating at fast-food restaurants, consumption of sweetened beverages, and consumption of excessive portion sizes should be identified. A growing concern among children and adolescents is the availability of high-fat, high-carbohydrate snack foods and drinks within the school environment, which may further contribute to obesity; such foods compete with school meals yet are often favourites of adolescents (Beaulieu & Godin, 2012). In addition to food intake, the nurse should assess the adolescent's level of physical activity and sedentary behaviours. Readiness to change; environmental supports and barriers; and family history of diabetes, heart disease, and early stroke must be considered when planning nutritional education and guidance.

In general, adolescents are body conscious and concerned about their appearance. Concrete messages about the relationship between an attractive appearance and the benefits of a healthy lifestyle are most effective. However, helping adolescents arrive at a decision for change is more difficult than providing information. They respond best when the counsellor provides straightforward information, uses instructional methods that actively involve them, talks with them and not at them, and listens to what they have to say.

Sleep and Rest

Adolescents vary in their need for sleep and rest. Rapid physical growth, the tendency toward overexertion, and the overall increased activity of this age contribute to fatigue in adolescents. During growth spurts the need for sleep is increased.

There is some evidence that there is a shift in the circadian rhythm and increase in melatonin in adolescence, which results in this group falling asleep later at night and finding it hard to wake up early in the morning (Crowley, Acebo, & Carskadon, 2007). The CPS (2013) recommends 9 to 10 hours of sleep during the adolescent years. Teenagers who lack adequate sleep are more apt to struggle in school, have trouble with memory and concentration, feel depressed, and lack motivation. In addition, sleepiness affects reaction time and can cause car accidents or other accidents. To establish healthy sleep patterns, adolescents can do the following:

- Have a relaxing bedtime routine with a light snack, in a cool, dark room.
- Go to bed and wake up at approximately the same time every night.
- Use bed for sleeping only.
- Avoid watching television, doing homework, or using a computer before going to bed.
- Open curtains and let light into the room in the morning.
- Avoid napping during the day and after dinner; this can make it difficult to fall asleep. If a nap is needed it should be less than 30 minutes.
- Exercise daily but avoid heavy exercise activities in the evening.
- Build in some time for fun activities.
- Avoid drinking caffeine after the middle of the afternoon.
- On weekends, no matter how late going to bed, try to get up within 2 to 4 hours of usual rising time.
- Write a to-do list to help decrease worries (CPS, 2013).

Exercise and Activity

Although today's youth are said to be less fit than children 20 years ago, adolescents probably spend more time and energy practising and participating in sports activities than members of any other age group. Many adolescents participate in sports within school settings (Fig. 39-7). School-based, health-oriented physical education may provide both immediate effects of the activity and sustained effects through encouragement of lifelong activity patterns. Canadian schools average 170 minutes of physical education per week (grades 11–12). However, the percentage of students taking at least one physical education class per week drops significantly in higher secondary grades (57% among grade 11–12 students) compared to other grades (99% in grades 1–8) (Active Healthy Kids Canada, 2012). The amount of time spent being sedentary also increases with age. Canadian preschoolers spend an average of 5.8 hours a day being sedentary; this increases to 7.6 hours for ages 5–11 and 9.3 hours for ages 12–17 (Active Healthy Kids Canada, 2014). To improve health outcomes, school-age children and

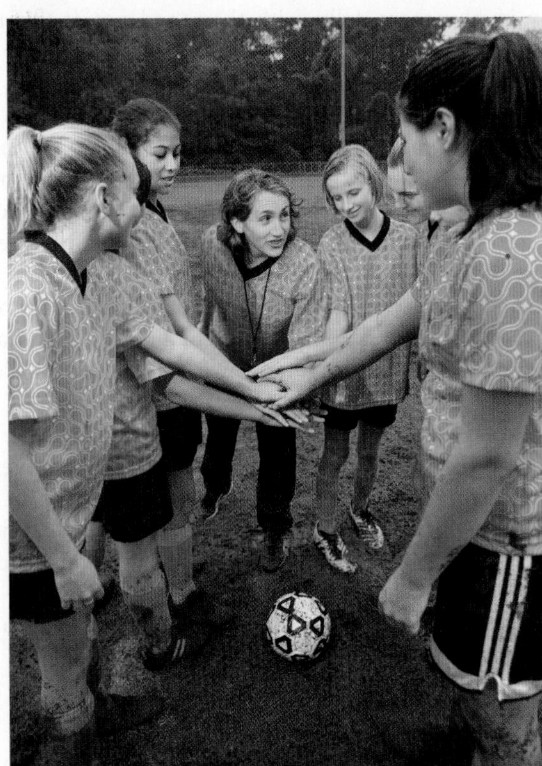

FIGURE 39-7 Adolescents should be encouraged to participate in activities that contribute to lifelong physical fitness. (Jupiterimages/Stockbyte/Thinkstock.)

adolescents should engage in 60 minutes or more of moderate to vigorous physical activity daily (Canadian Society for Exercise Physiology, 2015).

The practice of sports, games, and even dancing contributes significantly to growth and development, the education process, and better health. These activities provide exercise for growing muscles, interactions with peers, and a socially acceptable means of enjoying stimulation and conflict. In addition, competitive activities help teenagers conduct their own self-appraisal and develop self-respect and concern for others. Because physical fitness appears to be a major influence on one's lifelong health status, children and adolescents should be encouraged to participate in activities that contribute to lifelong physical fitness. Nurses can encourage participation as a way to promote health and build self-esteem. However, adolescents should not be encouraged to engage in physical activities that are beyond their physical or emotional capacity (see Health Problems Related to Sports Participation, Chapter 38).

Dental Health

Dental health should not be neglected during adolescence, even though the rate of caries formation is not as great as in childhood. The rate of caries formation may be significant due to poor nutritional habits (e.g., increased intake of cariogenic substances) and inadequate oral hygiene. Flossing and regular tooth brushing in adolescence serve to remove plaque and prevent periodontal disease. Additional factors that may influence oral health during adolescence include the use of tobacco (particularly chewing tobacco), pregnancy, eating disorders, increased risk for traumatic dental injury and periodontal disease, and increased awareness of appearance (American Academy of Pediatric Dentistry, Clinical Affairs Committee, 2015). Dental care is an aspect of preventive care that substantial proportions of children in Canada do not receive. It is recommended that an evaluation for caries take place at a minimum of every year and optimally at 6-month intervals. Pit and fissure sealants are a safe and effective technique for dental caries prevention.

Corrective orthodontic appliances (braces) are a fact of life for many teens, particularly during the early adolescent years. These may be a source of embarrassment and concern; however, in some cases these may be considered trendy, depending on the individual's and peers' attitudes toward their cosmetic effects. Reassurance regarding the temporary nature of the annoyance and anticipation of an improved appearance can help make the inconvenience tolerable. It is also important to reinforce the orthodontist's directions regarding use and care of the appliances and to emphasize careful attention to oral hygiene during this time.

Adequate fluoride remains important throughout the adolescent years. While most teens no longer require oral supplements, the Canadian Dental Association (2016) recommends that adolescents with high caries risk receive oral supplementation—this includes teens who do not brush their teeth or have not brushed with a fluoridated toothpaste twice a day, and those who are assessed as being susceptible to high caries activity due to community or family history.

Personal Care

Body-conscious teenagers are highly amenable to discussion and counselling about personal care and hygiene. Body changes associated with puberty bring special needs for cleanliness. The hyperactive sebaceous glands and newly functioning apocrine glands make frequent bathing or showering a necessity, and underarm deodorants and antiperspirants assume an important place in personal care. The adolescent discovers that hair requires more frequent shampooing, and girls often have questions about hair removal, use of cosmetics, and menstrual hygiene. Peer group discussions centre on the advantages of particular products or methods. Adolescents are continually bombarded with messages from the media regarding the best way to enhance their popularity and attractiveness. Nurses are in a position to help them evaluate the relative merits of commercial products.

Vision

Regular vision testing is an important part of health care and supervision during adolescence. During this time, visual refractive difficulties reach a high level that is not exceeded until the fifth decade of life. The increased demands of schoolwork make adequate vision essential for academic success. Consequently, teenagers are more likely to be referred for visual evaluation. The need for corrective lenses can create psychological problems for teenagers if they believe that glasses spoil their appearance or do not fit their body image. Contact lenses may be a preferred solution; a wide variety of lenses are now available at fairly reasonable prices.

Hearing

Considerable concern has focused on current teenage practices that cause hearing damage. Cochlear damage from relatively continuous exposure to loud sound levels of music has been documented. The popularity of handheld devices with ear bud earphones are of particular concern. When these units are used for extended periods, permanent hearing loss can occur. Although appeals for more judicious use are not always successful, teenagers should be informed of the risk. Efforts directed toward legislating legal limits of noise exposure that can be achieved through earphones may be another possible solution. (See Chapter 41 for a discussion of noise-related hearing loss.)

Posture

Many adolescents demonstrate altered posture. Rapid skeletal growth is often associated with slower muscular growth, and as a result, some teenagers may appear awkward or slump and fail to stand or sit upright. However, some postural defects of adolescence require early medical intervention. Scoliosis is a defect of the spine that occurs frequently in adolescence and is more common in girls than in boys (see Idiopathic Scoliosis, Chapter 53). Most cases are idiopathic, and the defect manifests as a painless curvature of the spine. Fortunately, most of these spinal curvatures will not require treatment. However, because there is no way to predict which curvatures will progress, all curvatures of the spine should be referred for further evaluation.

Body Art

Body art (piercing and tattooing) is generally associated with adolescents' alignment with particular groups and reflects their shifting sense of identity. The adolescent often seeks body art as an expression of his or her personal identity and style. Tattoos may mark significant life events such as new relationships, births, and deaths. Piercing of the ear, nose, nipple, eyebrow, navel, labia, penis, or tongue may sometimes create a health problem. It is a nursing responsibility to caution girls and boys against having piercings performed by friends, parents, or themselves. Although in most cases piercings have few, if any, serious adverse effects, there is always a danger of complications such as infection, abscess formation, cyst or keloid formation, bleeding, dermatitis, or metal allergy. Using the same unsterilized needle to pierce body parts of multiple persons presents the same risk of human immunodeficiency virus (HIV), hepatitis C, and hepatitis B virus transmission as occurs with other needle-sharing activities. A recent report highlighted the danger of contaminated tattoo ink, which occurred in association with an outbreak of nontuberculous *Mycobacterium chelonae* skin infections (Kennedy, Bedard, Younge, et al., 2012).

A qualified operator using proper sterile technique should perform the procedure. This is especially important if the adolescent has a history of diabetes, allergies, or skin disorders. Adolescents should be informed about the approximate time for healing after body piercing and the care of the pierced area during and after healing. Some body sites require extra precautions. For example, cartilage (ear, nose) has a poor blood supply and heals slowly and scars easily; nipple piercing puts the adolescent at risk for breast abscess. Penile piercing often penetrates the urethra. Finally, migration of the piercing is common with navel and other flat skin surface piercing. Piercing guns should not be used for piercing anything other than the earlobe because guns place the piercing too deeply.

The presence of body art in the form of tattoos and branding is common among adolescents and young adults. Although there are no recent statistics for body piercing and tattooing among Canadian youth, studies of distinct populations of young adults and adolescents report body art rates as high as 23% (Braverman, 2006). Professionals as well as amateur artists administer tattoos. The risk to the adolescent receiving a tattoo is low. The greatest risk is for the tattoo artist who comes in contact with the patient's blood. Adolescents who are amateur tattoo artists benefit from discussions about **routine practices** and the hepatitis B vaccination. Many provinces and territories either have no regulations or do not enforce existing regulations for piercing and tattooing facilities. Health Canada (2015a) regulates the dyes used for tattoos or permanent makeup, which are considered to be cosmetic products and must meet the requirements of the *Food and Drugs Act* and its cosmetics regulations. The definition of a cosmetic is "any substance or mixture of substances manufactured, sold, or represented for use in cleansing, improving or altering the complexion, skin, hair or teeth, and includes deodorants and perfumes." The local health department is a source of information about local regulatory requirements. Comprehensive guidelines on tattooing can be found through the Simcoe Muskoka District Health Unit (2015) (see Additional Resources section at the end of this chapter).

Health Canada (2015b) has issued a health warning to alert consumers to the potential risks of using tattoo removal products, which include gels, creams or solutions, applied topically or injected through the skin using a tattoo needle. Incident reports concerning adverse reactions related to the use of tattoo removal products have included skin irritation and scarring. Health Canada does not recommend the use of any tattoo-removing product.

Tanning

The quest for an attractive appearance leads many teenagers to excessive sunbathing and artificial means for tanning. A Canadian Cancer Society (2007) study showed that nearly 65% of Ontario students in grades 7 to 12 tan by one means or another. Seven percent of girls and 4% of boys had used an artificial tanning bed, and the use of artificial tanning among adolescents is rising. This practice has serious long-term risks, and the adolescent should be educated regarding the detrimental effects of sunlight on the skin (see Sunburn, Chapter 52). Long-term effects include premature aging of the skin; increased risk of skin cancer; and, in susceptible individuals, phototoxic reactions. Cutaneous melanoma, the most common fatal form of skin cancer, is associated with ultraviolet light exposure and affects an increasing number of Canadians (Canadian Dermatology Association, 2011).

The increasing popularity of artificial tanning has prompted concern from health care providers regarding the use of tanning machines. The long-term effects of tanning machines are similar to those of the sun; dermatologists do not recommend tanning by these means. For individuals under 35 years of age there is a 75% increased risk of developing melanoma from exposure to indoor tanning equipment. Nova Scotia, New Brunswick, Prince Edward Island, Ontario, and British Columbia have banned the use of artificial tanning devices by people under the age of 18. Those who insist on using tanning equipment should be warned that goggles must be worn in tanning booths to prevent serious corneal burning (Taddeo, Stanwick, & CPS, Adolescent Health Committee, 2012/2016). The Canadian federal government has mandated warning labels of radiation exposure on all of the tanning beds in Canada (Health Canada, 2014).

Adolescents require education on the use of sunscreens, including hypoallergenic products, with a sun protective factor (SPF) of at least 30 and a nonalcohol base without lanolin, parabens, or fragrance. Broad-spectrum sunscreens that protect against both ultraviolet A and B are most effective. Self-tanning creams safely simulate the appearance of a tan; however, teens using these products should be cautioned that sun protection is still required. The Canadian Dermatology Association (CDA) has a list of sunscreens that the association has approved and has the CDA logo on it (see Additional Resources at the end of this chapter). Targeting health education messages to adolescents and incorporating educational components relating to sun protection behaviours in school health curricula and in health care visits can help to increase adolescent knowledge and awareness.

Mental Health

During this time of transition from childhood to becoming an adult, adolescents experience many physiological and emotional changes. This age group often will have a sense of pressure to achieve success at home, school, and in social groups yet lack the experience required to help them realize that these challenges can be overcome as they gain that life experience (Canadian Mental Health Association, 2016a). With these changes and pressures, some adolescents may be more vulnerable to developing an **emotional disorder**.

In May 2006, a Senate committee chaired by Senator Michael Kirby released a comprehensive report on mental health and mental illness in Canada, titled "Out of the Shadows: Report of the Senate Committee on Social Affairs, Science and Technology." It concluded that "children and youth are at a significant disadvantage when compared to other demographic groups affected by mental illness, in that the failings of the mental health system affect them more acutely and severely" (Parliament of Canada, Standing Senate Committee on Social Affairs, Science and Technology, 2006). It is important for nurses to not only assess the mental health of adolescent patients but also support those who struggle with mental disorders (see also Serious Health Problems with a Behavioural Component, later in this chapter). Given the varied emotions of adolescents, identifying mental health concerns can be a challenge. For instance, adolescent depression is underdiagnosed and undertreated; it should be identified with symptoms of low mood, anhedonia, insomnia, or low energy lasting for 2 weeks or more. For teens symptoms such as insomnia are more marked than in children. The Guideline for Adolescent Health—Primary Care (GLAD-PC) is endorsed by the Canadian Paediatric Society to provide resources and support for diagnosis and treatment of depression and other mental health disorder in teens (American College of Preventive Medicine, 2011).

A significant number of young people and their families are affected by mental, emotional, or behavioural disorders, which can be caused by biology, environment, or a combination of the two. In Canada, it is estimated that as many as one in five children and adolescents have a mental health disorder that requires interventional treatment. These disorders include anxiety disorders, severe depression, bipolar disorder, attention-deficit hyperactivity disorder, learning disorder, conduct disorder, eating disorders, autistic spectrum disorders, and schizophrenia (Mental Health Canada, n.d.). It is thus important for nurses to incorporate mental health assessment into their practice. See Table 33-2 for mental health assessment tools that can help nurses comprehensively screen for these mental health disorders.

Stress Reduction

The multiple changes occurring in adolescence can result in much stress (Fig. 39-8 and Box 39-2). Adolescents are faced with pressures from peers that often involve flouting adult authority and taking serious health risks, including pressures for sexual experimentation and use of drugs, alcohol, and tobacco, as well as potentially dangerous physical activities.

Early-maturing girls and late-maturing children are especially sensitive to the stresses of being different from their peers. Many feel intense anxiety over their identity. Both early- and late-maturing children can feel out of place among their classmates, but slow-maturing children appear to suffer the most pronounced inner turmoil and may be hesitant to voice their

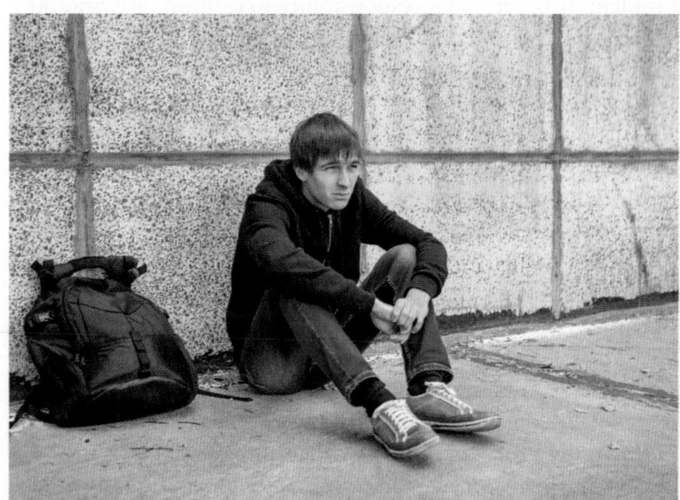

FIGURE 39-8 Adolescents may use being alone as a method of coping with stress. Health care providers need to assess whether this indicates clinical depression. (Sabphoto/Shutterstock.com.)

BOX 39-2 AREAS OF STRESS IN ADOLESCENCE

- Body image
- Sexuality conflicts
- Academic pressures
- Competitive pressures
- Relationships with parents
- Relationships with siblings
- Relationships with peers
- Dating
- Finances
- Decisions about present and future roles
- Career planning
- Ideological conflicts

concerns. Slow-maturing adolescents need support and reassurance that they are not abnormal and need only be patient until the time comes when they, too, will mature physically.

Sexual Health

Youth sexual health is a critical consideration for nurses working directly with adolescents and for those involved in creating programs and shaping policy that affects services to youth. The World Health Organization (WHO) defines sexual health as "a state of physical, mental and social well-being in relation to sexuality [requiring] a positive and respectful approach to sexuality and sexual relationships, as well as the possibility of having pleasurable and safe experiences, free of coercion, discrimination and violence" (WHO, 2015). When it comes to the sexual health of youth, STIs, pregnancy, birth control, abortion, and sexual practices need to be considered.

The province of Nova Scotia has developed a comprehensive strategy to promote the sexual health of adolescents (Nova Scotia Roundtable on Youth Sexual Health, 2011). This framework is intended to address youth sexual health on a number of levels, but is particularly directed toward individuals who make decisions affecting youth health. Among the key components of this plan are an emphasis on school-based sexual health education; the involvement of youth in discussion, initiative, and decision making; and developing and sustaining services that will ensure that adolescents have access to education, direct services, and other resources.

Sexuality Education

To put adolescents' need for sexuality education into context, the average North American teenager spends more than 7 hours every day in front of some type of medium, which often contains unrealistic sexual messages and images. In addition, some evidence indicates that teenagers express sexual experimentation online, by sending and receiving sexually explicit messages, photographs, or images via cell phones, tablets, and computers (O'Keeffe & Clarke-Pearson, 2011). All media sources can provide adolescents with information that may be inaccurate, riddled with cultural and moral judgements, and not very helpful. Adolescents may feel societal pressure to start dating, and their own inner sex drive urges them toward exploration. This is often exacerbated by peer pressure to be involved in sexual relationships and the adolescent's need to fit in.

The responsibility for providing sexuality education has been assumed by parents, schools, churches, community agencies such as the Canadian Federation for Sexual Health, and health care providers, including nurses. Many adolescents perceive nurses, especially school nurses, as individuals who possess important information and who are willing to discuss sex with them. To be able to discuss the topic adequately, nurses must have not only an understanding of the physiological aspects of sexuality and a knowledge of cultural and societal values but also an awareness of their own attitudes, feelings, and biases about sexuality.

Guidelines for sexual health education and STIs have been developed by the Public Health Agency of Canada (2016). These guidelines are based on an understanding that sexual health education should be culturally sensitive and respectful of sexual diversity, abilities, and choices. Other resources for information about sexuality, STIs, sexual health, and sexuality education are the Sex Information and Education Council of Canada (SIECCAN) and Sexualityandu.ca (sponsored by the Society of Obstetricians and Gynaecologists of Canada) (see Additional Resources section at the end of this chapter).

Nurses may counsel young people on an individual basis, in mixed groups, or in groups segregated by gender. Ideally, boys and girls should be able to discuss sexuality objectively with one another and in groups, but this is not always possible. The differences in the rate of maturation between boys and girls and between different members of the same sex often make it desirable to discuss certain aspects of sexuality in segregated groups. As a rule, the need for separate discussion groups diminishes as young people mature.

Sexuality education should consist of instruction concerning normal body functions and should be presented in a straightforward manner using correct terminology. When discussing sex and sexual activities, nurses should use simple but correct language, not street language (although it may be helpful to know), highly scientific terminology, or evasive jargon. Once the meanings of biological terms such as *uterus*, *testicles*, and *vagina* are understood, most teenagers prefer to use them in their discussions.

Many girls arrive at menarche with ambivalent attitudes, myths, and illogical beliefs. Even girls adequately prepared for menstruation do not always understand its relationship to the total process of reproduction. Many are under the incorrect impression that the "safe" time for sexual intercourse is midway between menstrual periods.

Teenagers' curiosity and their desire for information extend beyond the need for anatomical and physiological knowledge. They need to know more than the mechanics of conception, pregnancy, and birth. Adolescents, girls in particular, want answers to questions such as "What is it like?" "Does it hurt?" "What happens when ...?" and "Is it all right if you ...?" Boys are often concerned about the fallacy that a relationship exists between penis size and sexual function. They need reassurance that masturbation is a normal and common practice and that oral–genital relations can be normal substitutes for intercourse but still carry risks of transmitting STIs.

Teenagers need to discuss intercourse, alternative methods of sexual satisfaction, and how to resist peer pressure. With the increased incidence of STIs, especially HIV infection, the topic of "safer sex," especially abstinence or the use of condoms, is essential. Role-playing may help teenagers learn effective approaches to dealing with difficult situations. Sex and sexuality cannot be taught without discussions of mature decision making, sexual responsibility, and values clarification. Adolescents may receive inaccurate and ambiguous messages regarding sexual behaviour; for example, an adolescent may be told that abstinence from vaginal intercourse will prevent transmission of an STI. Accurate and unbiased information about sexual practices should be provided in a setting where the adolescent feels comfortable asking questions without being degraded or made to feel uncomfortable for seeking information.

Most importantly, adolescents need problem-solving experience and decision-making skills so that they can anticipate the positive and negative outcomes of a decision. These types of experience can help teenagers become sexually responsible young adults. Adolescents who receive comprehensive sexual education are less likely to become pregnant or get someone else pregnant; programs that focus only on abstinence have not had any effect on rates of sexual abstinence. Adolescents can receive information on contraception and abortion from community health units, community health clinics, and Planned Parenthood Centres.

Pregnancy, Abortion, and Birth Control

The rate of live births to mothers aged 15 to 17 years decreased steadily from 11.0 to 7.4 per 1000 females between 1999 and 2005, and increased to 8.2 per 1000 females in 2008. Similar trends have occurred among teenagers who are 18 and 19 years old (PHAC, 2012). Many factors shape the likelihood of whether a young woman who is sexually active will become pregnant. In research with high school students in Nova Scotia, Langille, Corbett, Wilson, et al. (2010) found that 52.3% of students reported being sexually active. Among girls, 84.7% reported using some sort of contraception (hormonal contraception or condoms). Other important findings from this study include the following:

- Many sexually active youth (7.2%) reported reluctance to buy condoms because of feeling embarrassed.
- 35.8% of sexually active youth reported unplanned or unintentional sex as a result of intoxication (drugs or alcohol) in the past year.
- Casual sex was common, with 25.3% of sexually active students reporting having intercourse with someone they did not know particularly well.
- 40.4% of sexually active youth reported having more than one sexual partner within the same time period.
- Clear links exist between alcohol or drug use and sexual risk taking.

While this survey reflects the sexual health of youth in one community in Nova Scotia, the findings alert nurses and other health care providers to the kinds of issues that are important in the development and delivery of services for youth and in the provision of nursing care to adolescents.

Safety Promotion and Injury Prevention

Physical injuries are the greatest single cause of death among Canadian youth, claiming more lives than all other causes combined. The most vulnerable ages are the years 15 to 24, when accidental injuries account for about 64% of all deaths (PHAC, 2009). In addition, for every youth that dies from trauma, many more have serious injuries.

Injury prevention during adolescence requires a multidimensional approach. To begin, education of youth about potential risks is vital (Box 39-3). Education, however, is not enough; engaging with youth about the motivations for risk-taking behaviour is useful. For such discussions to be effective, the adult must be seen as credible and the tone must be nonjudgemental. Finally, advocating for provincial, territorial, and federal legislation is another avenue through which nurses can work to reduce injuries among youth. For instance, the introduction of a comprehensive staged and graduated driver's licensing system has resulted in some reduction of motor vehicle deaths among youth. All provinces and territories have enacted distracted driving laws to ban the use of cellular phones and texting (Hands Free Info, 2016), which may further reduce rates of motor vehicle injury among youth.

Motor Vehicle-Related Injuries

The adolescent's newly acquired ability to drive and the normal developmental need for independence and freedom make the automobile an attractive but potentially dangerous part of many adolescents' lives. Motor vehicle collisions (MVC) continue to be the leading cause of injury-related deaths for this age group (Yanchar, Warda, Fuseli, et al., 2012). Many factors contribute to the higher rate of crashes among teen drivers, including lacking driving experience and maturity, following too closely, driving too fast, having other teen passengers in the car, texting or answering a cell phone while driving, and driving under the influence of alcohol (Parachute, n.d.). Studies have shown that drivers using handheld devices are considerably more distracted and spend less time looking at the road or paying attention to driving conditions (Hosking, Young, & Regan, 2009; Owens, McLaughlin, & Sudweeks, 2011).

Several provinces have enacted graduated driver licence laws with restrictions on younger adolescent driving. In most provinces, adolescents may obtain a learner's licence by successfully passing a knowledge test. Upon passing a road test, the teen may drive supervised with certain imposed conditions (only one other nonfamily member in the car, zero blood alcohol level, no electronic devices). The age at which an adolescent can first drive varies among provinces and territories.

Nurses should educate teenagers and their parents about the risk of driving while drinking alcohol or of riding in an automobile with a drunk driver. Many families arrange a no-questions-asked ride home to prevent an adolescent from riding with a drunk driver. Families should also require adolescents to log several hours of supervised practice driving before taking

BOX 39-3 INJURY PREVENTION DURING ADOLESCENCE

Developmental Abilities Related to Risk for Injury

Need for independence and freedom
Testing independence
Age permitted to drive a motor vehicle (varies)
Inclination for risk-taking behaviours
Feeling of indestructibility
Need for discharging energy, often at expense of logical thinking and other control mechanisms
Strong need for peer approval
Desire to attempt hazardous feats
Peak incidence for practice and participation in sports
Access to more complex tools, objects, and locations
Can assume responsibility for own actions

Injury Prevention

Pedestrian

Emphasize and encourage safe pedestrian behaviour.

- At night, walk with a friend.
- If someone is following you, go to the nearest place with people.
- Do not walk in secluded areas; take well-travelled walkways.

Motor or Nonmotor Vehicles

Passenger—Promote appropriate behaviour while riding in a motor vehicle.
Driver—Provide competent driver education; encourage judicious use of vehicle; discourage drag racing, "playing chicken"; discourage cell phone usage and text messaging; maintain vehicle in proper condition (brakes, tires, etc.).
Reinforce not to drink and then drive or to get into a vehicle driven by someone who has been drinking.
Teach and promote safety and maintenance of two-wheeled vehicles.
Encourage wearing of safety apparel such as helmet and long trousers.
Reinforce the dangers of drugs, including alcohol, when operating a motor vehicle.
Reinforce the pedestrian risks when using cellular phones and listening to music with ear phones when walking.

Falls

Teach and encourage general safety measures in all activities.

Drowning

Teach nonswimmers to swim.
Teach basic rules of water safety:

- Select carefully a place to swim.
- Ensure sufficient water depth for diving.
- Swim with a companion.
- Wear a life vest during water sports (e.g., boating, skiing).
- Avoid swimming, boating, or other water sports after alcohol consumption or illicit drug use.

Burns

Reinforce proper behaviour in areas involving contact with burn hazards (gasoline, electric wires, and fires).
Advise regarding excessive exposure to natural or artificial sunlight (ultraviolet burn).
Discourage smoking.
Encourage use of sunscreen.
Discourage use of tanning beds.

Poisoning

Educate in hazards of drug use, including alcohol.

Other Sources of Physical Harm

Promote proper instruction in sports and use of sports equipment.
Instruct in safe use of and respect for firearms and other devices with potential danger (e.g., power tools, fireworks).
Provide and encourage use of protective equipment when using potentially hazardous devices (e.g., motorcycles, ATVs, power tools) or when engaging in sports activities such as skate boarding.
Promote access to and provision of safe sports and recreational facilities.
Be alert for signs of depression (potential suicide).
Instruct in proper use of corrective devices (e.g., glasses, contact lenses, hearing aids).
Encourage judicious application of safety principles and prevention.

the car out alone. Educational efforts should also convey that the major risk for death in a motor vehicle accident is failure to use a safety restraint. Teenage seat belt use, especially among boys, is lower than adult seat belt usage. An exception to this pattern is research findings in British Columbia, which suggest that increasing numbers of adolescents are always wearing seatbelts (66% in 2008 versus 54% in 2003) (Smith, Stewart, Peled, et al., 2009).

Teens with attention-deficit/hyperactivity disorder (ADHD) may have difficulty with driver competency. Individuals with the disorder may have impaired driving performance, leading to a greater risk for adverse driving outcomes. Effective treatment of ADHD and the positive effects of stimulant medications on driving performance may minimize the driving safety risk (Barkley & Cox, 2007).

Other vehicle injuries. The increasing use of motorized bicycles, all-terrain vehicles, jet skis, and snowmobiles has caused an increase in injuries among teenagers below the legal age for driving automobiles.

Many adolescents ride bicycles without helmets and without lights at night, and the overwhelming majority of deaths from bicycle injuries (primarily head injuries) involve teenagers. In-line skating and skateboarding without protective gear also contribute to a significant number of traumatic brain injuries in adolescents and young people.

Firearms

Currently, most deaths involving firearms are suicides. The relatively low rates of death from injuries involving firearms can be attributed to Canada's gun laws. A valid firearms licence is required to own, borrow, or store a firearm, and many firearms are prohibited or restricted (notably automatic guns and handguns). Potential gun owners also must pass the Canadian Firearms Safety course (Royal Canadian Mounted Police, 2014).

Youth access to firearms is generally through family members and acquaintances. Gun availability in the home is strongly correlated to unintentional death and injury to children and youth (Laws, 2005/2014). In addition, the presence of a gun in the home increases the risk of adolescent suicide and homicide. When guns are in the home, adults must take preventive action to be certain that the guns are never loaded, that they are locked up in a safe place, and that ammunition is stored and locked up separately in a location where only appropriate adults have access to it.

Nonpowder firearms. Guns that do not use powder (e.g., airguns and airsoft guns), while viewed as toys by many, account for almost as many injuries as powder guns. The regulations regarding use of nonpowder guns are relaxed; they can be purchased legally by adolescents and are labelled as suitable for children as young as 8 years of age. In Canada, some provinces, such as Ontario, restrict the sale of airguns to persons under the age of 18 years. Many cities have bylaws against discharging airguns within city limits. Paintball guns have also increased in popularity, and safety equipment with their use, such as helmets and goggles, is recommended (Frappier, Austin Leonard, Sacks, et al., 2005/2016).

Nurses are in a good position to advocate for laws regulating the sale of these potentially dangerous "toys."

Sports Injuries

Because the degree of physical maturity, size, coordination, and endurance varies greatly among adolescents of the same age, sports competition can result in predictable and unnecessary injuries for those not fit for or suited to particular sports. The matching of adolescent candidates with individual sports should be done relative to physical maturity, height, weight, and physical fitness and skills, particularly in a sport involving rigorous body contact. Age is a less important consideration.

Every sport has some potential for injury, whether one participates in serious competition or for pure enjoyment. Overuse injuries are common in adolescents and result in more time missed from the activity than do fractures. The increase in strength and vigour in adolescence may tempt adolescents to overextend themselves. The range of injuries sustained in sports or recreational activities can involve any part of the body and extend from relatively minor cuts, bruises, and abrasions to totally incapacitating central nervous system injuries or death. Recently, attention has focused on traumatic brain injuries resulting from concussions incurred in contact sports (see Chapter 38).

The increase in girls' competitive sports in high schools in Canada has resulted in an increase in sports-related injuries among this population. Research shows that 48% of grade 10 Canadian girls were injured while playing or training for sports, compared with 10% being injured while running or walking, 1% while biking, 3% while skating, 5% while fighting, 3% while riding in or driving a car, and 2% while doing paid or unpaid work (PHAC, 2011a).

NURSING CARE

Safety promotion and injury prevention is an ongoing part of nursing responsibility throughout the teenage years. Anticipatory guidance with parents and children regarding the expected problems and hazards related to growth and development does not end as children approach maturity. They need education in basic safety precautions and instruction in skills required in the performance of activities such as sports, instruction in handling motor vehicles, proper protective equipment, and instruction in proper maintenance of equipment. During adolescence, however, health and safety education and guidance are more effective when the young people are involved directly. Parents and health care providers can emphasize the importance of safety during performance of activities and the proper conditioning and preparation for sports.

Prevention can occur on a variety of levels. Safety advocacy, changes in public policy, and legislation can help curtail injuries. Examples of such approaches are laws that mandate wearing seat belts, requiring the wearing of a helmet while driving moving vehicles other than automobiles, keeping the legal minimum drinking age (age 18 in Alberta, Manitoba, Québec and age 19 in the rest of the provinces and territories), and instituting curfews for teen drivers. In addition, health education for teenagers and significant adults is essential. Helping adolescents understand their need for engaging in risky behaviour, exploring possible negative outcomes of such behaviour, and weighing possible alternatives are critical components of injury prevention.

Anticipatory Guidance—Care of Families

Both adolescents and their parents are often confused and perplexed about the changes and behaviour of this stage of development. Parents need support and guidance to help them through this trying time. They need to understand the changes taking place in their teenage children and to accept the expected behaviours that accompany the process of detachment. Parents may need help in "letting go" and in promoting the changed relationship from one of dependence to one of mutuality (see Family-Centred Teaching box).

SPECIAL HEALTH PROBLEMS

Disorders of the Female Reproductive System

Disorders related to the female reproductive system, such as amenorrhea and dysmenorrhea, are discussed in Chapter 7. Sexually transmitted infections are also discussed in Chapter 7.

Disorders of the Male Reproductive System

Most of the obvious anomalies, such as hypospadias, hydrocele, phimosis, and cryptorchidism, are identified with corrective measures instituted during early childhood. The most frequent problems related to the reproductive organs in adolescence are (1) infections, such as urethritis (see Urinary Tract Infection,

FAMILY-CENTRED TEACHING

Guidance During Adolescence

Encourage Parents To:

- Accept the adolescent as a unique individual
- Respect the adolescent's ideas, likes and dislikes, and wishes
- Be involved with school functions and attend the adolescent's performances, whether it be a sporting event or a school play
- Listen and try to be open to the teenager's views, even when they disagree with parental views
- Avoid criticism about no-win topics
- Provide an opportunity for choosing options and accept natural consequences of these choices
- Allow the young person to learn by doing, even when choices and methods differ from those of adults
- Provide the adolescent with clear, reasonable limits
- Clarify house rules and consequences for breaking them
- Let society's rules and consequences teach responsibility outside the home
- Allow increasing independence within limitations of safety and well-being
- Be available but avoid pressing the teenager too far
- Respect the adolescent's privacy
- Try to share the adolescent's feelings of joy or sorrow
- Respond to feelings, as well as words
- Be available to answer questions, give information, and provide companionship
- Try to make communication clear
- Avoid comparisons with siblings
- Assist the adolescent in selecting appropriate career goals and preparing for an adult role
- Welcome the adolescent's friends into the home and treat them with respect
- Provide unconditional love
- Be willing to apologize when mistaken

Be Aware That Adolescents:

- Are subject to turbulent, unpredictable behaviour
- Are struggling for independence
- Are extremely sensitive to feelings and behaviour that affect them
- May receive a different message from what was sent
- Consider friends extremely important
- Have a strong need to belong to a peer group of friends and not necessarily to family (except in certain circumstances)

Chapter 49); (2) hematuria; (3) penile problems, such as nonretractable foreskin in uncircumcised males, carcinoma, and trauma; (4) scrotal conditions, such as varicocele (elongation, dilation, and tortuosity of the veins superior to the testicle); and (5) testicular torsion (a condition in which the testicle hangs free from its vascular structures, which can result in partial or complete venous occlusion with rotation).

Tumours of the testes are not common (Feldman, Bosl, Sheinfeld, et al., 2008), but when manifested in adolescence, they are generally malignant and demand immediate evaluation. Testicular cancer is the most common solid tumour in adolescent boys and men 15 to 34 years of age. The usual presenting symptom for testicular cancer is a heavy, hard mass (either smooth or nodular) that is palpated on the testis; approximately 40% of men present with a painful mass. If a firm swelling is noted, the adolescent should be evaluated by ultrasonography and immediately referred for direct biopsy if the mass is found to be solid. Treatment involves surgical removal of the affected testicle (orchiectomy) and adjacent lymph nodes (if affected) and possibly chemotherapy and radiation following surgery (Gray & Moore, 2009). Fertility may be regained after chemotherapy and surgery; however, sperm banking before the initiation of chemotherapy is recommended. Assisted reproduction is also an option, and successful paternity is reported to be between 50% and 85% (Feldman et al., 2008). Recurrence of testicular cancer in the contralateral testis may occur; therefore follow-up is essential.

NURSING CARE

Most adolescent boys are self-conscious about their changing bodies. Preparation is crucial before performing a genital examination. Generally, the most effective approach is to assume a matter-of-fact attitude toward the examination, explain precisely what will take place, and maintain a continuous commentary about what is being done and the findings at each phase of the examination.

The routine health assessment of every adolescent boy should include teaching about testicular cancer. The Canadian Cancer Society (2016) recommends that young men age 15 years and older be taught the signs and symptoms of testicular cancer. They should also know how their testicles normally look and feel. Testicular tumours may be detected by the individual male. There is not enough evidence to recommend regular testicular exams, but it is important for men to know what is normal for them (see Additional Resources for an effective video from the Canadian Cancer Society that can be used in teaching). This fact is particularly important if the male adolescent may be at a higher risk of developing testicular cancer (undescended testicle(s), a family member with testicular cancer, or a history of testicular cancer. Young men should be taught to examine their testes while they are in a warm shower or bath, which relaxes the scrotum and helps testes to descend (Canadian Cancer Society, 2016). Any of the following findings should be reported to a health care provider: a lump on the testicle, a painful testicle, a feeling of heaviness or dragging in the lower abdomen or scrotum, or a dull ache in the lower abdomen and groin. This rare malignancy is curable if detected early.

The normal testicle is a firm organ with a smooth, egg-shaped contour; the epididymis is palpated as a raised swelling on the superior aspect of the testicle and should not be confused with an abnormality.

Gynecomastia

The male breast, although not strictly part of the male reproductive system, responds to hormonal changes. Some degree of bilateral or unilateral breast enlargement occurs frequently in boys during puberty. It is estimated that approximately half of adolescent boys have transient gynecomastia, which subsides spontaneously in less than one year with achievement of male development. A careful assessment of the pubertal stage at the onset of gynecomastia; medication history, including anabolic steroids, calcium, channel blockers, cancer chemotherapy, histamine receptor blockers, and oral ketoconazoles; and the exclusion of renal, liver, thyroid, and endocrine disorders or dysfunction allow the examiner to reassure the adolescent that the changes are pubertal gynecomastia and no further assessment is indicated. Gynecomastia may also be drug induced; calcium channel blockers, cancer chemotherapeutic agents, histamine$_2$-receptor blockers, and oral ketoconazoles have all been shown to cause the condition.

If the condition persists or is extensive enough to cause embarrassment or to produce doubts about gender identity in the young boy, plastic surgery may be indicated for cosmetic and psychological considerations. Administration of testosterone has no effect on breast development or regression and may aggravate the condition.

NURSING CARE

Treatment usually consists of assuring the adolescent and his parents that this is a benign and temporary situation. A physical examination with palpation is necessary to differentiate gynecomastia from increased adiposity caused by being overweight. Adolescents who are distressed about physical integrity and masculinity may benefit from the knowledge that this condition occurs in more than 50% of all adolescent boys.

Obesity

Few problems in childhood and adolescence are so obvious to others, are so difficult to treat, and have such effects on current and long-term health as obesity. According to the Public Health Agency of Canada (2011b) childhood obesity rates have tripled in Canada over the last 25 years, with rates among Indigenous children and youth being two to three times higher than the Canadian average. The World Health Organization defines *overweight* as a BMI greater than 25, and *obesity* as a BMI greater than 30. BMI measurements provide the most accurate method for screening children and adolescents for obesity. The new WHO growth charts have been adapted for use in Canada and adopted by health authorities in most provinces and territories. These charts include ideal BMI standards according to age and gender (see Appendix C for BMI charts). Children and adolescents with a BMI between the eighty-fifth and ninety-seventh percentile are considered overweight, those between the ninety-fifth and 99.9th percentile are considered obese, and those above the 99.9th percentile are categorized as severely obese.

Because adult obesity is associated with increased mortality and morbidity from a variety of complications, both physical and psychological, adolescent obesity is a serious condition. Research indicates that overweight children and adolescents are at risk for continuing to be obese as adults, thereby experiencing the health and social consequences of obesity much earlier than children and adolescents of normal weight. Obesity in childhood and adolescence has been related to elevated blood cholesterol; high blood pressure; respiratory disorders; orthopaedic conditions (Fennoy, 2010); cholelithiasis; some types of adult-onset cancer; sleep issues like obstructive sleep apnea (CPS, 2013; Owens & Committee on Adolescence, 2014); non-alcoholic fatty liver disease (Na, Park, Kang, et. al., 2014); and type 2 diabetes mellitus (Canadian Diabetes Association, 2016). The incidence of metabolic syndrome is also high in overweight and obese adolescents. Common emotional consequences of obesity include poor body image, low self-esteem, social isolation, and feelings of depression and rejection (Lipnowski, LeBlanc, & CPS, Healthy Active Living and Sports Medicine Committee, 2012).

Etiology and Pathophysiology

Obesity results from a caloric intake that consistently exceeds caloric requirements and expenditure and may involve a variety of interrelated influences, including metabolic, hypothalamic, hereditary, social, cultural, and psychological factors (Fig. 39-9). Because the etiology of obesity is multifactorial, the treatment requires multilevel interventions.

Familial influence is an epidemiological consideration in regard to children's weight. Twin studies suggest that approximately 35 to 50% of the tendency toward obesity is inherited (Beaty, 2007). When both parents are obese, there is a 60 to 80% increase in the likelihood of the child becoming obese (Wardle, Carnell, Haworth, et al., 2008). The specific influences of genes and environment within developing children are not well defined. The increasing rates of obesity within genetically stable populations suggest that environmental and some perinatal factors (e.g., formula feeding) are contributors to the current increases in childhood obesity.

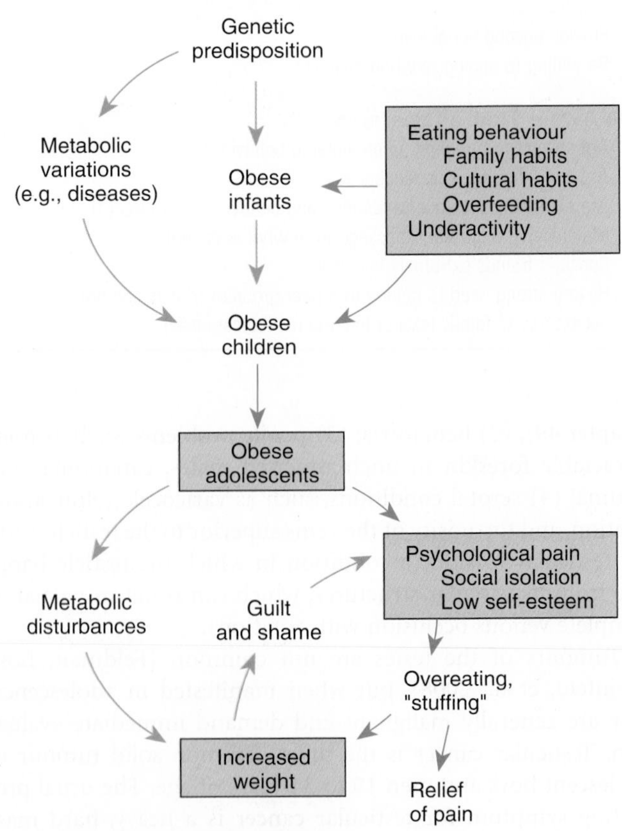

FIGURE 39-9 Complex relationships in obesity.

Birth weight does not seem to be a long-term contributing factor in detection and prediction of childhood obesity (Kain, Corvalán, Lera, et al., 2009; McCarthy, Hughes, Tilling, et al., 2007); obese children do not have higher birth weights than nonobese children. There is, however, a high correlation between childhood adiposity and parental adiposity (Bouchard, 2009). One study found that the best determinant of adult obesity was the child's weight at 5 years of age or an increased weight gain from 1 to 5 years of age (McCarthy et al., 2007).

Fewer than 5% of the cases of childhood obesity can be attributed to an underlying disease. Such diseases include hypothyroidism; adrenal hypercorticoidism; hyperinsulinism; and dysfunction of the central nervous system as a result of tumour, injury, infection, or vascular accident. Obesity is a frequent complication of muscular dystrophy, paraplegia, Down syndrome, spina bifida, and other chronic illnesses that limit mobility.

A major focus of obesity research has been on appetite regulation. The expression of appetite is chemically coded in the hypothalamus by distinctive circuitry. Orexigenic substances produce signals that promote eating behaviours, and anorexigenic substances promote the cessation of eating behaviours. Feedback loops between signals have been identified where one signal peptide is able to alter the secretion of another signal peptide. No one signal has been identified as the gatekeeper of appetite. It is apparent that an entire network of signals, including their frequency and amplitude, is responsible for triggering eating behaviours.

Others have explored and found little evidence to support a relationship between obesity and "low metabolism." No differences in basal metabolic rate, sleeping metabolic rate, respiratory quotient, heart rate, or total energy expenditure have been found in normal-weight children with or without a familial predisposition to overweight.

The tendency toward obesity is manifested whenever environmental conditions are favourable to excessive caloric intake, such as an abundance of food, limited access to low-fat foods, increased availability of high-fat foods, reduced or minimal physical activity, and snacking combined with excessive television viewing.

A report by the Government of Canada Standing Committee on Health (2007) has drawn attention to the links between childhood obesity and the key determinants of overall health. In particular, family income, education, social support, geographic location, cultural norms and values, biological and genetic factors, accessibility of services for health, and gender are important determinants of body weight among Canadian children and adolescents. Table 39-2 summarizes some of these influences.

Family and cultural eating patterns play a role in whether a child becomes obese; many families and cultures consider fat to be an indication of good health. It is not uncommon for obese children to come from families that provide large meals or admonish children for leaving food on their plates. Parents may have an exaggerated concept of the amount of food children require and expect them to eat more than they need. Lower socioeconomic groups have a greater prevalence of obesity than that of higher-income groups, especially for girls. This difference between groups is often apparent before children are 6 years of age. Food outlets that are found in lower-income

TABLE 39-2 DETERMINANTS OF HEALTH THAT INFLUENCE FOOD INTAKE AND PHYSICAL ACTIVITY IN CHILDHOOD AND ADOLESCENCE

Income	Family income determines access to quality food. In isolated and northern communities, food costs are higher and fresh fruits and vegetables are very difficult to obtain.
	Family income shapes access to physical activity facilities and organized sports.
Education	Increased education increases resources (i.e., literacy and numeracy) available for decision making related to food and activity choices.
Social environment	Strong communities can strengthen localized food systems.
	Lack of control over personal lives and communities limits opportunities to promote health (i.e., in many Indigenous communities).
Physical environment/geographic location	Children and youth living in advantaged neighbourhoods have a far lower risk of becoming obese than those in disadvantaged neighbourhoods.
	Parental perceptions of public safety influence child and youth physical activity.
	The cost of food varies widely according to community location, with prices far higher in isolated and northern communities.
	Access to low-fat, nutritious foods varies by location.
Values and norms	Values and norms vary widely and affect food and physical activity patterns among children and youth.
Biological/genetic factors	Indigenous and South Asian populations have a genetic susceptibility to type 2 diabetes.
Accessibility of services for health	Availability and accessibility of quality health promotion and health intervention services vary.
	Availability of basic health care services varies.
Culture	Availability of television, computers and tablets, and video games varies.
	Family eating patterns vary by culture.
	Peer group activities and eating patterns vary by culture.
Gender	Adolescent boys, on average, are more active than adolescent girls.

Adapted from Government of Canada, Standing Committee on Health. (2007). *Healthy weights for healthy kids.* Ottawa: Parliament of Canada.

neighbourhoods tend to be fast-food outlets and convenience stores. It may also be difficult for these families to find transportation to shop elsewhere, which could also lead to fewer food choices in their neighbourhood.

Children from families with low physical activity levels may adopt these patterns of their parents and other adults. Parental obesity and low levels of physical activity are correlated with decreased physical activity in children. The higher rates of sedentary activities such as screen viewing, which coincides with increased intake of low-nutritive value foods, during the teen years also contribute to obesity (Lipnowski et al., 2012). The CPS asserts that media time, especially advertisements of food products, has a direct correlation with the increased incidence of childhood obesity in Canada. Lack of green space, extreme climates, heavy traffic, and local crime can discourage physical activity. The type and level of adolescents' physical activity may also be influenced by sociocultural factors. A study of two Canadian provinces reported sex-based differences of youth with girls achieving less physical activity during the week (Comtes, Hobin, Majumdar, et al., 2013). The difference was not seen on the weekend or with younger children.

Psychological factors also affect eating patterns. In infancy, children experience relief from discomfort through feeding and learn to associate eating with a sense of well-being, security, and the comforting presence of a nurturing person. Eating is soon associated with the feeling of being loved. In addition, the pleasurable oral sensation of sucking provides a connection between emotions and early eating behaviour. Many parents use food as a positive reinforcer for desired behaviours. This practice may become a habit, and the child may continue to use food as a reward, a comfort, and a means of dealing with depression or hostility. Many individuals eat when they are not hungry or in response to boredom, loneliness, sadness, depression, or tiredness. Difficulty determining feelings of satiety can lead to weight problems and may compound the factor of eating in response to emotional rather than physical hunger cues.

Eating behaviours are closely related to memory. Memory and appetite are chemically encoded, with each individual having his or her own circuitry relating to eating behaviours. Like memory, the circuitry can be modified over time.

Diagnostic Evaluation

A careful history should be obtained regarding the development of obesity and a physical examination performed to differentiate simple obesity from increased fat due to organic causes. A family history of obesity, diabetes, coronary heart disease, and dyslipidemia should be obtained for all children who are overweight or at risk for being overweight. Specific information from the patient and family about the effects of obesity on daily functioning—for example, problems with nighttime breathing and sleep, daytime sleepiness, joint pain, inability to keep up with family activities and peers at school—is helpful. The physical examination should focus on identifying comorbid conditions and identifiable causes of obesity. For some, psychological assessment, by interviews and standardized personality tests, may provide insight into the personality and emotional problems that contribute to obesity and that might interfere with therapy.

It is useful to estimate the degree of obesity to determine the component of body weight that can be modified. All of the following methods have been used to assess obesity: BMI, body weight, weight–height ratios, weight–age ratios, hydrostatic (underwater) weight, skin fold measurements, bioelectrical analysis, computed tomography (CT), magnetic resonance imaging (MRI), and neutron activation. Each of these methods has advantages and disadvantages. Hydrostatic, or underwater, weighing provides the most accurate measurement of lean body weight.

BMI is currently considered the best method to assess weight in children and adolescents. The calculation is based on the individual's height and weight (see Appendix C). In adults, BMI definitions are fixed measures without regard for sex and age. The BMI in children and adolescents varies to accommodate age- and gender-specific changes in growth. The formula for BMI calculation is as follows:

$$\text{Weight in kilograms} \div [\text{Height in metres}]^2$$

BMI measures in children and adolescents are plotted on growth charts that enable heath care providers to determine the patient's BMI-for-age.

The initial assessment of obese children and adolescents should include screening to evaluate for comorbidities. The history is an important guide to determine the workup. The physical examination should focus on identifying **comorbid** conditions and identifiable causes of obesity. Some areas to focus on include (1) skin for stretch markings and discolourations (e.g., acanthosis nigricans), (2) joints for swelling and evidence of pain, and (3) airway for evidence of obstruction and enlarged tonsils. Basic laboratory studies include a fasting lipid panel; fasting insulin level; fasting glucose hepatic enzymes, including γ-glutamyltransferase; and, in some institutions, hemoglobin A_{1c}. Other studies, such as a sleep study, metabolic studies, and radiographic evaluations, may be added on the basis of the history and physical examination.

Therapeutic Management

The best approach to the management of obesity is a preventive one. Early recognition and control measures are essential before the child or adolescent reaches an obese state. Health care providers must educate families about the medical complications of obesity, and families should be encouraged to be involved in the treatment plan.

The treatment of obesity is difficult. Many approaches do not achieve long-term success. The average individual loses only about 5 to 10% of his or her weight with available therapies. Losing weight can have a significant positive effect on many comorbidities, but unfortunately, the lost weight is frequently regained in a year or two.

Diet modification is an essential part of weight-reduction programs. Nutrition counselling is directed toward improving the nutritional quality of the diet rather than dietary restriction. Educating youth about the limits and risks of fad diets is important. *Eating Well With Canada's Food Guide* recommends that for youth ages 14 to 18, daily consumption should include seven to eight servings of vegetables and fruit, six to seven servings of grain products, three to four servings of milk and milk alternatives, and two to three servings of meat and meat alternatives (see Appendix A). Many programs recommend using a food diary as a helpful tool to increase awareness of food choices and eating behaviours. The goal is to encourage the individual to make healthier choices in foods selection and discourage eating food by habit or to appease boredom. The Dietitians of Canada (2014) have published "5 steps to a healthy body weight for teens":

1. Follow the science of *Eating Well With Canada's Food Guide.*
2. Take charge of your lunch.
3. Be a healthy snacker.
4. Eating out? Eat smart.
5. Practise active living.

For adolescents who are severely obese, a strict, nutrition-based diet may need to be implemented, such as the protein-sparing modified fast, a hypocaloric, ketogenic diet designed to provide enough protein to minimize loss of lean body mass during weight loss. Such diets need to be closely monitored and should be used only with a multidisciplinary team that includes a physician, nutritionist, and behavioural therapist. Generally, the diet consists of 1.5 to 2.5 g of protein per kilogram. The intake of carbohydrates is low enough to induce ketosis. The benefits of the diet are relatively rapid weight loss and anorexia induced by ketosis. Potential complications include protein losses, hypokalemia, hypoglycemia, inadequate calcium intake, and orthostatic hypotension. Potassium and calcium supplements and adequate calorie-free beverages can minimize these complications. It is difficult to sustain such diets over a long period of time, and the long-term outcomes of using these diets have not been established.

Researchers continue searching for medications that will successfully treat obesity. Sibutramine, an appetite suppressant, has been used in adolescents 16 years old and older for the treatment of obesity. Orlistat, a lipase inhibitor, has been used for adolescents 12 to 18 years of age who have a BMI more than 2 units above the ninety-fifth percentile for age and sex; however, adverse effects of the drug include fatty or oily stools and possible malabsorption of fat-soluble vitamins (Kanekar & Sharma, 2010). There are currently no drugs approved for use in overweight or obese children younger than the age of 12 years. Other medications have been used to promote weight loss in children with certain conditions; examples include metformin in obese adolescents with insulin resistance and hyperinsulinism, octreotide for hypothalamic obesity caused by intracranial tumours, growth hormone in children with Prader-Willi syndrome, and leptin for congenital leptin deficiency.

Combining behavioural modifications with pharmacological therapy in children 12 years and older has produced mixed results in regard to total weight loss maintained over a significant period of time (U.S. Preventive Services Task Force, 2010). Reports suggest modest benefits with moderate to high behavioural interventions (measured in number of contact hours) in decreasing mean BMI of children and adolescents involved in such programs over a period of 6 to 12 months (Whitlock, O'Connor, Williams, et al., 2010). Programs including family-based behavioural modification, dietary modification, and exercise have been shown to be successful in reducing obesity in some children.

Bariatric surgery may be the only practical alternative for increasing numbers of severely overweight adolescents who have failed organized attempts to lose or maintain weight loss through conventional nonoperative approaches and who have serious life-threatening conditions. Until recently, there were few studies in adolescents that suggested surgical weight loss improved the early mortality of patients with severe obesity. In 2010, Toronto's Hospital for Sick Children began offering bariatric surgery to patients who (a) are between the ages of 12 and 17 years; (b) have a BMI greater than the ninety-fifth percentile for their age and gender; and (c) have at least one coexisting chronic condition, or for any adolescent between the ages of 12 and 17 years with a BMI above the ninety-ninth percentile. Australian researchers (Nobili, Vajro, Dezsofi, et al., 2015; O'Brien, Sawyer, Laurie, et al., 2010) have found that gastric banding surgery in adolescents can be safe and effective if combined with lifestyle changes and interdisciplinary support. Data suggest that bariatric surgery in adolescents results in sustained weight loss and a decrease in BMI and comorbidities such as type 2 diabetes (Barnett, 2011). Physicians must define clear, realistic, and restrictive guidelines to apply with younger patients when surgery is considered. Candidates for surgery should be referred to centres that offer a multidisciplinary team experienced in the management of childhood and adolescent obesity.

NURSING CARE

Nurses play a key role in the adherence and maintenance phases of weight-reduction programs for overweight adolescents and may assess, manage, and evaluate their progress. Nurses also play an important role in recognizing potential weight problems and assisting parents and adolescents in preventing obesity. Nursing care of the adolescent who is overweight is outlined in the Nursing Process box available on the Evolve site. 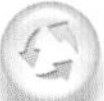

The presence of obesity may not be obvious from appearance alone. Regular assessment of height and weight and computation of the BMI facilitate early recognition. Children with a BMI greater than or equal to the ninety-fifth percentile for age and sex should receive in-depth medical assessment. Children with a BMI in the eighty-fifth to ninety-fifth percentile range should be evaluated for secondary complications, such as hypertension and hyperlipidemia, and family history. Evaluation should include a height and weight history of the adolescent and family members, eating habits, appetite and hunger patterns, and physical activities. A psychosocial history is also helpful in understanding the impact of obesity on the child's life.

Before initiating a treatment plan, it is important to establish that the family is ready for change. Lack of readiness may result in failure, frustration, and reluctance to address the problem in the future. The nurse should explore with the adolescent the reasons behind the desire to lose weight, since motivation to lose weight is the key to success. Adolescents need to take personal responsibility for their dietary habits and physical activity. Teens who are forced by their parents to seek help are seldom motivated, can become rebellious, and are usually unwilling to control their dietary intake.

Nutritional Counselling

Preventing an increase in body fat during growth is a realistic approach. This is often accomplished by adjusting four aspects of eating:

1. Reducing the quantity eaten, by purchasing, preparing, and serving smaller portions
2. Altering the quality consumed by substituting low-calorie, low-fat foods for high-calorie foods (especially for snacks)
3. Eating regular meals and snacks, particularly breakfast
4. Altering situations by severing associations between eating and other stimuli, such as eating while watching television

The most successful diets are those that use ordinary foods in controlled portions rather than diets that require the avoidance of specific foods.

The nurse can teach adolescents and parents how to incorporate favourite foods into their diet and to select satisfying substitutes. The dieting teen should eat what the rest of the family eats, but less of it. When parents buy and prepare smaller amounts, they eliminate tempting second helpings and leftovers. To maintain a healthy diet, it is necessary to encourage the consumption of high-nutrient foods, such as fruits, vegetables, whole grains, and low-fat dairy protein products. Calories and fat should be kept to a healthy level without being significantly restricted. To be successful, a dietary program should be nutritionally sound with sufficient satiety value, produce the desired weight loss, and be accompanied by nutrition education and continued support. Children and adolescents should not initiate a reduction diet without health assessment and counselling (Whitlock et al., 2010).

Behavioural Therapy

Altering eating behaviour, including reducing inappropriate eating habits, is essential to weight reduction, especially in maintaining long-term weight control. Most behavioural modification programs include the following concepts:

- A description of the behaviour to be controlled, such as eating habits
- Attempts to modify and control the stimuli that govern eating
- Development of eating techniques designed to control the speed of eating
- Positive reinforcement for these modifications through a suitable reward system

Specific strategies to modify eating habits are listed in the Patient Teaching box.

Group Involvement

Commercial groups (e.g., Weight Watchers) or diet workshops composed primarily of adults may be helpful to some teenagers; however, a group of other dieting adolescents is often more effective. Teenage groups include summer camps designed for obese young people and conducted by health care providers, school groups organized and led by a community health nurse, and groups associated with special clinics.

These groups are concerned not only with weight loss but also with the development of a positive self-image and encouragement of physical activity. Nutrition education, planning, and improvement of social skills are essential components of these groups. Improvement is determined by positive changes in all aspects of behaviour.

PATIENT TEACHING

Helpful Suggestions to Promote Healthy Eating Habits

Identify current eating patterns and behaviours by keeping a food diary and then look for areas to change. Record everything eaten, including where and when, and associated activities.

Change eating patterns.

- Choose sugar-free beverages or low-fat milk only.
- Limit fast-food consumption to no more than once a week.
- Do not skip meals.
- Eat three meals and one or two snacks per day.
- Try the plate method: one-half plate of vegetables, one-fourth plate of lean meat, and one-fourth plate of starch or starchy vegetables (potatoes, peas).
- Take second helpings of fruits and vegetables (not potatoes) only.
- Avoid low-fat food (these are usually high in sugars).
- Use whole-grain breads, cereals, and pastas.
- Pack your lunch for school.
- Buy healthy foods for snacking.

Change the act of eating.

- Eat meals at the family dinner table.
- Avoid distractions (e.g., television).
- Slow down; meals may last at least 20 to 30 minutes.

Substitute other activities for managing stress, such as hobbies, walking, listening to music, talking to friends on the phone, reading, or playing a game.

Provide alternative rewards for reinforcement or accomplishments (e.g., music or video downloads, movie, concert, new clothes, new games).

Think positively.

Enlist family involvement and support.

Family Involvement

There is a definite correlation between family environment, interaction, and obesity. The nurse needs to educate parents in the purposes of the therapeutic measures and their role in supporting such measures. The family needs nutrition education and counselling regarding the reinforcement plan, alterations in the food environment, and ways to maintain helpful attitudes. They can support their child in efforts to change eating behaviours, food intake, and physical activity.

Research indicates that family meals may also play a role in decreasing obesity and high-risk behaviours among adolescents by promoting healthy eating habits; however, more quality research is needed to clarify the protective role of such interactions in regard to adolescent obesity (Fulkerson, Neumark-Sztainer, Hannan, et al., 2008).

Physical Activity

Regular physical activity is incorporated into all weight-reduction programs. Any form of increased physical activity is beneficial, provided that the activities are age appropriate and enjoyable. In recommendations for physical activity, the current health status and developmental level of the child or adolescent need to be considered. The best choice for exercise is any form that is enjoyable and likely to be sustainable. Aerobic and endurance exercises help oxidize body fats. Light exercise such as walking may provide an opportunity for the family to increase time together and increase caloric expenditure. Walking for 30 minutes each day and decreasing caloric intake by 500 calories per day may significantly reduce the risk of chronic disease. Weight training can increase basal metabolic rate and replace fat mass with muscle mass. However, weight training is not generally recommended for prepubertal children until they have reached physical and skeletal maturity. Adolescents should get at least 60 minutes of moderate- to vigorous-intensity physical activity daily, including vigorous-intensity activities at least 3 days/week and activities that strengthen muscle and bone at least 3 days/week (Lipnowski et al., 2012).

Prevention

Weight loss programs do not enjoy the success of therapeutic interventions for other disorders. Gradual accumulation of adipose tissue during childhood establishes a pattern of eating that is difficult to reverse in adolescence. Prevention of adolescent obesity is thus best accomplished by early identification of obesity in the preschool, school-age, and preadolescent periods and by development of healthy eating habits and regular exercise patterns at an early age. Health care providers should encourage frequent health care visits for children who are overweight or obese and should incorporate a dietary history and counselling into each well-child and well-adolescent visit.

Anorexia Nervosa, Bulimia Nervosa, and Binge-Eating Disorder

Anorexia nervosa and bulimia nervosa are most common among adolescent girls, although boys tend to have a substantial incidence of binge-eating disorders. It is estimated that 0.3% of adolescent females are anorexic or bulimic, and the rates appear to increase during the transition from adolescence to young adulthood (Hoek, 2007). A Canadian research team found that 37% of ninth-grade girls and 40% of tenth-grade girls perceived themselves as too fat. For students with normal weight (based on BMI), 19% perceived that they were too fat, and 12% of these students reported trying to lose weight (Boyce, King, & Roche, 2008).

Anorexia nervosa (AN) is an eating disorder characterized by an inability to maintain a minimally normal body weight and by severe weight loss in the absence of obvious physical causes. The average age of onset is 13 years, but the disorder can occur as early as 10 years of age and as late as 25 years of age. Individuals with AN are often described as perfectionists, academically high achievers, conforming, and conscientious. Typically, they have high energy levels, even with marked emaciation. Patients with anorexia may eventually develop bulimia.

Adolescents with **bulimia nervosa (BN)** (from the Greek meaning "ox hunger") undertake binge eating and then use compensatory behaviours to prevent weight gain, such as self-induced vomiting; misuse of laxatives, diuretics, or other medications; fasting; or excessive exercise. BN is observed more commonly in older adolescent girls and young women; males with bulimia are less common. Patients with BN may be of average or slightly above average weight. The binge-eating behaviour consists of secretive, frenzied consumption of large amounts of high-calorie (or "forbidden") foods during a brief time (usually less than 2 hours). The binge is counteracted by a variety of weight-control methods (purging). These binge–purge cycles are followed by self-deprecating thoughts, a depressed mood, and an awareness that the eating pattern is abnormal.

Although persons with BN have many issues in common with those who have other eating disorders, impulse control and satiety regulation are particularly important issues in BN. Many individuals with BN begin with only occasional binges and purges, enjoying the control over their weight while eating amounts of food that would normally produce obesity. As the condition progresses, the frequency of binges increases, the amount of food consumed increases, and they gradually lose control over the binge–purge cycle. The frequency of binging can be anywhere from once per week to seven or eight times per day. Because persons with BN usually binge on high-calorie foods, especially sweets, ice cream, and pastries, insulin production is stimulated to cope with the added carbohydrates. When the food is vomited, the unused insulin stimulates hunger and the desire to eat.

A third eating disorder, identified as eating disorder not otherwise specified (EDNOS), has components of both AN and BN with varying degrees of symptomatology that are not always characteristic of the established diagnostic criteria for AN and BN (National Eating Disorder Information Centre, 2014). Binge-eating disorder (BED) is a type of EDNOS. Persons with BED may diet in an attempt to control their weight but without the extreme weight-control compensatory practices of vomiting, laxative use, diuretics, and excessive exercise (Forman, 2012; National Eating Disorder Information Centre, 2014). The American Psychiatric Association (APA) has now defined BED as a separate category of eating disorders (APA, 2013).

A fourth type of eating disorder, avoidant/restrictive food intake disorder (ARFID), has been proposed. In this disorder, there is an apparent lack of interest in eating or food with significant weight loss, nutritional deficiency, and dependence on enteral feeding; there is also significant psychosocial functioning with this disorder, and it is not associated with AN or BN (APA, 2013).

Etiology and Pathophysiology

The cause of these disorders remains unclear. There is a distinct psychological component, and the diagnosis is based primarily on psychological and behavioural criteria. Dieting appears to be common to the initiation of both AN and BN. The disorders appear to be caused by a combination of genetic, neurochemical, psychodevelopmental, and sociocultural factors. The dominant aspects of AN are a relentless pursuit of thinness and a fear of fatness, usually preceded by a period of mood disturbances and behaviour changes.

Weight loss may be triggered by a typical adolescent crisis, such as the onset of menstruation, or a traumatic interpersonal incident that precipitates serious, out-of-control dieting. Situations of severe family stress (such as parental separation or divorce) or circumstances in which the adolescent perceives a lack of personal control (such as teasing at school, changing schools, or going to college) may precipitate a desire for control and the decision not to eat. Frequently, there is an exaggerated misinterpretation of the normal fat deposition characteristic of early adolescence or anxiety because of comments that the adolescent is putting on weight.

Many experts have associated the development of an eating disorder with family characteristics such as an adolescent perception of high parental expectations for achievement and appearance, difficulty managing conflict and poor communication styles, enmeshment and occasionally estrangement between family members, devaluation of the mother or the maternal role, and marital tension. Families struggling with an eating disorder have been characterized as having difficulties responding positively to the adolescent's changing physical and emotional needs. Family stress of any kind may become a significant factor in the development of an eating disorder (Forman, 2012).

Individuals with eating disorders commonly have psychiatric problems, including affective disorder, anxiety disorder, obsessive-compulsive disorder (OCD), and personality disorder. Adult women with eating disorders have been found to have higher than average rates of obsessive-compulsive behaviour traits in their childhood. Patients with eating disorders also tend to have higher than average reported rates of substance use, with alcohol problems being more common in those with BN than in those with AN (Forman, 2012). Many of the clinical findings are directly related to the state of starvation and improve with weight gain.

Many sports and artistic endeavours that emphasize leanness (e.g., ballet and running) and sports in which the scoring is partly subjective (e.g., skating and gymnastics) have been associated with a higher incidence of eating disorders, such as AN. The term **female athlete triad**, characterized by disordered eating behaviour, amenorrhea, and osteoporosis, has been applied to young women with restrictive eating disorders and amenorrhea (Female Athlete Triad Coalition, 2011; Landry, 2016) (see Chapter 7, p. 108).

A genetic role has been postulated for eating disorders; a significant number of young females with a first-degree relative having an eating disorder had a significantly higher rate of eating disorders (Forman, 2012). However, some consider these eating disorders to not be a direct result of family inheritance but, rather, a secondary effect of the manifestations of conditions such as anxiety, depression, and OCD that may be modulated through the internal milieu of puberty (Landry, 2016).

Diagnostic Evaluation

Diagnosis of AN and BN is made on the basis of clinical manifestations and conformity to the criteria established by the APA's *Diagnostic and Statistical Manual of Mental Disorders* (2013). Table 39-3 presents the characteristics of individuals with eating disorders.

TABLE 39-3 CHARACTERISTICS OF INDIVIDUALS WITH EATING DISORDERS

FACTORS	ANOREXIA NERVOSA	BULIMIA
Food	Turns away from food to cope	Turns to food to cope
Personality	Introverted Avoids intimacy Negates feminine role	Extroverted Seeks intimacy Aspires to feminine role
Behaviour	"Model" child Obsessive-compulsive	Often acts out Impulsive
School	High achiever	Variable school performance
Control	Maintains rigid control	Loses control
Body image	Body image distortion	Less frequent body image distortion
Health	Denies illness	Recognizes illness Health fluctuates
Weight	Body weight <85% of expected norm	Within 2.3–7 kg (5–15 lb) of normal body weight or may be overweight
Sexuality	Usually not sexually active	Often sexually active

A complete history and physical examination are important for ruling out other causes of weight loss. The medical assessment of an eating disorder should focus on the complications of altered nutritional status and purging. A careful history includes weight changes, dietary patterns, and the frequency and severity of purging and excessive exercise. The patient's weight and height should be measured and evaluated for appropriateness according to standard weight for height, age, and sex charts, determined according to the percentile of his or her expected body weight or BMI (see Appendix C). Box 5-7 provides the SCOFF screening tool for nurses to use in assessing for eating disorders.

The diagnosis of eating disorder is made clinically, but additional laboratory diagnostic tests may be obtained to identify malnutrition or other associated complications. Additional diagnostic measures may include a complete blood count to evaluate for anemia and other hematological abnormalities; erythrocyte sedimentation rate or C-reactive protein to detect evidence of inflammation; electrolytes, calcium, magnesium, phosphorus, blood urea nitrogen, and creatinine; urinalysis, including specific gravity; and bone density studies for osteopenia, which is commonly observed in patients with AN. In patients with prolonged amenorrhea, human chorionic gonadotropin is assessed to check for pregnancy. Other tests for patients with amenorrhea include thyroid function tests and measurement of serum prolactin and follicle-stimulating hormone to help rule out prolactinoma (hormone-secreting pituitary tumour), hyperthyroidism, hypothyroidism, or ovarian failure. In addition, a comprehensive cardiac evaluation is often recommended in those with AN. Further diagnostic tests may be required on the basis of the history and findings from the diagnostic tests discussed above.

Therapeutic Management

The treatment and management of AN involve three major goals: (1) reinstitution of normal nutrition or reversal of the severe state of malnutrition, (2) resolution of disturbed patterns of family interaction, and (3) individual psychotherapy to correct deficits and distortions in psychological functioning. The treatment of eating disorders requires the collaborative efforts of an interdisciplinary team composed of a primary care practitioner, nurse, dietitian, and mental health care provider with pediatric and adolescent health care experience. Because of the psychogenic nature of the disorder, the treatment may be long. Recent studies suggest that family-based therapy is more effective than individual cognitive-behavioural therapy in reducing the maladaptive eating behaviours in adolescents with AN (Lock, 2010).

Most adolescents are treated on an outpatient basis, but those with problems requiring immediate medical attention, such as severe malnutrition or electrolyte or psychiatric disturbances (severe depression or suicidal ideation), require hospitalization. Persons with BN may benefit from cognitive-behavioural therapy, other psychotherapy, antidepressant medications, or a combination of antidepressant medication and psychotherapy (Forman, 2012).

Nutrition education and meal planning may help the person with BN maintain an adequate weight and accept foods that are often considered bad or forbidden.

Nutrition therapy. The most important goal is to treat any life-threatening malnutrition and to restore dietary stability and weight gain. This may require the administration of tube feedings or intravenous fluids if the malnutrition is severe. In most cases, it is best to reintroduce food and snacks slowly in a stepwise manner. A reasonable goal is to reach an eventual intake of 2000 to 3000 kcal/day and a weight gain of 0.22 to 0.45 kg per week (American Dietetic Association, 2006). When restoring nutrition, health care providers must avoid the **refeeding syndrome**, which consists of cardiovascular, neurological, and hematological complications that occur when nutritional replacement is given too rapidly. This syndrome can be avoided with slow refeeding and the addition of phosphorus when total body phosphorus is depleted. Treatment goal weights should be individualized and based on age, height, stage of puberty, premorbid weight, and previous growth charts. In girls who have reached menarche, resumption of menses is an objective measure of return to biological health.

Dietary interventions need to be combined with psychotherapy to improve the underlying psychological misconceptions about weight loss. Another aspect of treatment is to relieve the anxiety related to eating and the depression that accompanies the disorder. The administration of antianxiety or antidepressant medications can be beneficial. However, when these drugs are used, patients should be carefully monitored for cardiovascular adverse effects.

Cognitive behavioural therapy. Behavioural interventions are often necessary to encourage patients to accomplish the desired caloric intake and weight gain. Weight restoration on an outpatient basis is accomplished with behavioural contracts negotiated between the therapists and the patient. The goal is to increase the patient's feelings of personal control and his or her responsibility for achieving recovery. The contract can stipulate at what weight tube feedings will be implemented, if needed. Individual psychotherapy is aimed at helping the young person resolve the adolescent identity crisis, particularly as it relates to a distorted body image. If the disorder is related to a dysfunctional family situation, therapy is most successful when it is started soon after the onset of illness and directed toward disengagement from and redirection of malfunctioning processes in the family.

Pharmacological therapy. Pharmacotherapy in the treatment of AN has been disappointing so far. None of the randomized controlled trials have shown improvement in weight gain in adults treated with pharmacotherapy, and no studies have been conducted in children and adolescents (Golden & Attia, 2011). The few studies that have been done have primarily evaluated medications' efficacy in the treatment of comorbid disorders, such as OCD and depression. Anxiolytic medications may be helpful before meals to relieve some patients' anxiety.

Tricyclic antidepressants and fluoxetine belong to a group of medications known as selective serotonin reuptake inhibitors (SSRIs), which have been more successful in treating BN. There is also some evidence that tricyclic antidepressants such as desipramine, imipramine, and amitriptyline; monoamine oxidase inhibitors; and buspirone are more effective than a placebo in decreasing binging and vomiting in patients with BN. Some of the latter medications, however, may have adverse effects that may preclude their utility in such patients (Golden & Attia, 2011). Topiramate, an antiepileptic agent, and the selective serotonin antagonist ondansetron may have some benefit in treating BN. As with AN, pharmacotherapy should be an adjunct to behavioural therapy.

NURSING CARE

Nurses must maintain a kind and supportive, yet firm, manner in managing the care of the adolescent with an eating disorder, without creating a passive-dependent attitude. The individual requires sustained support and reassurance to cope with ambivalent feelings related to body concept and the desire to be seen as cooperative, reliable, and worthy of receiving kindness. Encouraging the adolescent with education and activities that strengthen self-esteem can facilitate the resocialization process and promote social acceptance among peers. (See the Nursing Care Plan on Evolve.)

It is important for nurses to be aware of the physical side effects of AN. Patients frequently limit their fluid intake. Urinary tract problems are common, and ketones and protein may be detected in the urine as a result of breakdown of fat and protein. Vital-sign instability can be severe and can include orthostatic hypotension; the pulse becomes irregular, and the rate decreases markedly. Electrolyte imbalances can be life threatening, and

CRITICAL THINKING CASE STUDY

Anorexia Nervosa

Jane is a 13-year-old whose grades have been excellent and whom the teachers describe as a "model student." Recently, Jane's teacher told the nurse practitioner that Jane's parents were in the middle of a "messy divorce." In addition, several of Jane's friends told the nurse practitioner that they are concerned about Jane because she runs every day at lunchtime and seldom eats lunch with them. Jane told her friends that she gained weight over the winter months and that she is running because she wants to qualify for the track team this spring. At the time of her routine health interview and sports physical, the nurse practitioner notes that Jane's oral temperature is 36°C and that she weighs 35 kg. Jane has lost 9 kg since her last sports physical. When discussing her menstrual periods with the nurse practitioner, Jane states that she has not had her period for 3 months.

1. Evidence—Is there sufficient evidence to draw any conclusions about Jane's behaviour?
2. Assumptions—Describe some underlying assumptions about the following:
   a. Personality characteristics of individuals with anorexia nervosa (AN)
   b. Factors influencing the development of AN
   c. Clinical manifestations of AN
   d. Treatment of AN
3. What implications for nursing care should be established for Jane at this time?
4. Does the evidence support your conclusion?

bradycardia and hypothermia can result in cardiac arrest (see Critical Thinking Case Study).

The health care team responsible for the management of young people with AN should arrange a carefully structured environment. First, there must be consistency. The team needs to decide on an approach and adhere to it. The plan must be structured with reality testing regarding caloric intake and body-image perception. Team members need to provide a unified front, to avoid any possibility of manipulation or inconsistency. Second, all team members need to be involved in the treatment; responsibility for the program cannot be left to one person. The role and boundaries of each member must be clearly spelled out. Third, continuity of team members is important; it is helpful to have the same team members all the time.

Finally, communication among team members is essential. Communication with the patient regarding what is expected is also important. Sometimes the limit-setting may seem unreasonable; if the adolescent does not understand the rationale for the limits, he or she may sabotage the entire program. It is also important to communicate with the family. The plan must also provide support of the adolescent, the family, and team members. The adolescent's efforts should be supported, and positive feedback should be provided for accomplishments made in normalizing eating habits. Meetings should be held to discuss the feelings and concerns of the patient, immediate caregivers, and team members.

A *behavioural contract*, an agreement that the adolescent makes with others to change a maladaptive behaviour, has proved to be effective in some cases. The written contract is constructed by the therapeutic team and is approved and signed by the adolescent. Unless the adolescent agrees to its terms, the contract can become the source of a power struggle. However, it can be an effective tool that places the responsibility for weight gain or other behavioural change on the adolescent.

Family-based therapy is often used in the treatment of adolescent eating disorders, specifically in the treatment of AN. In particular, the aim of the Maudsley approach is to help parents rediscover their own resources and take an active role in their children's recovery. Families are encouraged to explore how following the normal developmental course of their family life cycle has become problematic, by looking at how the eating disorder and the interactional patterns in the family have become entangled.

Nursing care of the adolescent with BN is similar to care of the patient with AN. Acute care involves careful monitoring of fluid and electrolyte alterations and observation for signs of cardiac complications. Nutritional consultation and follow-up care are essential. The nurse should encourage the adolescent and family members to structure the environment in such a way as to reduce the binging behaviour. Getting rid of binge foods, restricting eating to one room of the house, and not engaging in other activities while eating may be helpful interventions.

Health care providers, patients, and families can find assistance and information on the prevention, identification, and treatment of eating disorders from the National Eating Disorder Information Centre in Canada (see Additional Resources at the end of this chapter).

SERIOUS HEALTH PROBLEMS WITH A BEHAVIOURAL COMPONENT

Substance Use

Although experimentation with drugs during childhood and adolescence is widespread, most children and teens do not become high-risk users. Research by the McCreary Centre Society in British Columbia indicates that alcohol and marijuana use has declined throughout the past decade, as has the use of certain drugs, such as cocaine, amphetamines, and mushrooms. The use of other drugs, however, including certain hallucinogens, is on the rise (Smith, Stewart, Peled, et al., 2009). Health Canada (2011) reports in the Canadian Alcohol and Drug Use Monitoring Survey that 85% of Canadian teenagers have consumed alcohol and 50% have consumed illegal drugs.

Drug use, misuse, and addiction are culturally defined and are voluntary behaviours. Drug tolerance and physical dependence are involuntary physiological responses to the pharmacological characteristics of the drugs, such as opioids and alcohol. Consequently, an individual can be addicted to a narcotic with or without being physically dependent. A person can also be physically dependent on a narcotic without being addicted (e.g., patients who use opioids to control pain).

Indigenous youth tend to be at particular risk for substance use. Compared with non-Indigenous youth, they have a two to six times greater risk for all alcohol-related problems. They are also more likely to use illicit drugs and use tobacco, alcohol, and cannabis at a younger age than that of non-Indigenous youth (Canadian Centre on Substance Abuse, 2014).

Most drug use begins with experimentation. The drug may be used only once, may be used occasionally, or may become part of a drug-centred lifestyle. Children and adolescents initiate drug use out of curiosity. Adolescents who use drugs may fall into one of two broad categories—experimenters and compulsive users—or they may fall into a third category somewhere on the continuum between these extremes, as recreational users, principally of drugs such as marijuana, cocaine, alcohol, and prescription medications. For many the goal is peer acceptance; these users fit more closely with the experimenting, intermittent users. For others the goal is intoxication or the sustained intense effects from using a particular drug; these users resemble the compulsive users. They may engage in periodic heavy use, or binges. The groups of greatest concern to health care providers are those whose patterns of use involve high doses or mixed drugs with the danger of overdose, and those compulsive users vulnerable to dependence, withdrawal syndromes, and altered lifestyle.

There are two common developmental pathways that substance use disorders follow. One is characterized by high levels of impulsive risk-taking behaviours and the other is an internalizing behaviour of anxiety or depression (Canadian Centre on Substance Abuse, 2014). Co-occurring mental health problems can antagonize one's susceptibility to substance use disorders.

Any drug can be used for nonmedical purposes, and most are potentially harmful to adolescents still going through formative life experiences. Although rarely considered drugs by society, the chemically active substances frequently used are the xanthines and theobromines contained in chocolate, tea, coffee, and colas. Ethyl alcohol and nicotine are other drugs that are legal and socially sanctioned. Any of these substances can produce mild to moderate euphoric or stimulant effects and can lead to physical and psychological dependence.

Drugs with mind-altering abilities that are available on the "street" and are of medical and legal concern are the hallucinogenic, narcotic, hypnotic, and stimulant drugs. In addition, there has been a notable increase in the use of alcohol and volatile substances that are inhaled to achieve an altered sensation (such as gasoline, antifreeze, plastic model airplane cement, typewriter correction fluid, and organic solvents). Nonmedical use of prescription and synthetic medications such as oxycodone, alprazolam (Xanax), and amphetamine-dextroamphetamine (Adderall) has become a concern for professionals who work with children and adolescents. Studies show that adolescents prefer pain relievers to stimulants, sedatives, or tranquilizers; females tend to prefer pain relievers to stimulants, and misuse of these substances was also strongly correlated with other illicit substances (Young, Glover, & Havens, 2012). Others report that adolescents believe that prescription medications, although not taken under practitioner orders, are safer than illicit substances. Many of the prescription medications are available at a cheaper cost than that of the more exotic drugs of use and are often found in the medicine cabinet at home. Some websites also promote the "safe use" of some psychoactive drugs and supply information on new "designer" drugs that are not detectable on a standard urine drug screening test.

Tobacco

Cigarette smoking has continued to decline since the late 1990s, in part because of increased costs, changes in community attitudes about smoking among adults, decreased advertising of cigarettes to children, and increased antismoking advertising as a result of the government lawsuits against tobacco companies (Johnston, O'Malley, Miech, et al., 2015). In a province-wide survey in 2008, 74% of British Columbian youth reported that they had never smoked a single cigarette (Smith et al., 2009). Studies have also shown that family-based interventions affect children's and adolescents' use of cigarettes (Thomas, Baker, Thomas, et al., 2015).

Although the number of adult and adolescent smokers has declined in recent years, cigarette smoking is still considered the chief avoidable cause of death. The hazards of smoking at any age are undisputed; a preventive approach to teenage smoking is especially important. Because of its addictive nature, smoking begun in childhood and adolescence can result in a lifetime habit, with increased morbidity and early mortality. Research indicates an association between current use of tobacco and the development of depression (Chaiton, Cohen, O'Loughlin, et al. 2010) and sleep problems (Region of Waterloo, Public Health, 2015) in adolescence. Cigarettes are considered to be a gateway drug; teenagers who smoke are 11.4 times more likely to use illicit drugs.

Youth in the Indigenous populations smoke at a rate of 24.9% compared with 19.7% for non-Indigenous youth. They were less likely than non-Indigenous youth to have tried to stop smoking. It is likely that smoking among Indigenous youth is significantly underreported in the off-reserve population (Elton-Marshall, Leatherdale, & Burkhalter, 2011).

Etiology. Teenagers begin smoking for a variety of reasons, including imitation of adult behaviour; peer pressure; a desire to imitate behaviours and lifestyles portrayed in movies and advertisements; and a desire to control weight, especially among young women. Teenagers who do not smoke usually have family members and friends who do not smoke or who oppose smoking. Most teens who refrain from smoking have a desire to succeed in academics or athletics (particularly high-performance sports, such as basketball, swimming, and track) and plan to go to college (see Community Focus box). Although smoking among college students has increased in recent years, rates of smoking are highest among adolescents who do not complete high school.

Electronic cigarettes. Electronic cigarette (e-cigarette) use is on the rise among youth in Canada. These cigarettes are tobacco free and do not produce secondhand smoke but may contain nicotine and different flavourings. Various other chemicals and metals in the e-cigarettes are harmful especially to children and adolescents. Flavourings and propylene glycol (a chemical) in the e-liquid can irritate the lungs and worsen breathing problems like bronchitis and asthma; when heated, these ingredients change form and create toxins; formaldehyde (a colourless gas) can be produced at levels higher than those seen with regular cigarettes. The heating process also releases heavy metals from the materials used in the manufacturing of the e-cigarettes, at levels higher than in regular cigarettes; and

COMMUNITY FOCUS

Early Sexual Maturation, Alcohol, and Cigarettes

Cigarette smoking and alcohol use by adolescents are complex behaviours not explained by any one factor. Some theorists and investigators believe there is a relationship between biological maturation and risk-taking behaviours. For example, girls who are sexually mature at an earlier age than their peers are often attracted to older girls and boys who may engage in risk-taking behaviours. If older teens smoke, drink, and drive while under the influence of alcohol with no adverse consequences (e.g., no motor vehicle accidents), younger teens may believe that they, too, will be safe while smoking, drinking, or riding in an automobile with friends who are drinking.

Although parents and nurses cannot influence the time of biological maturation, they can identify young girls who are at risk for the initiation of risk-taking behaviours because of early puberty. Parents need to understand that an early-maturing daughter might be uncomfortable with her body, and they should take advantage of opportunities to build her self-esteem. Parental sensitivity to the importance of peer-group acceptance and parental support of a teenage daughter who feels left out or different are crucial. School nurses can provide anticipatory guidance to these girls and help them role play coping strategies for situations that involve offers to smoke and drink. In addition, school nurses can provide information about physical development during puberty and emphasize that not all teenagers mature at the same time or rate.

Teachers, coaches, and community and church leaders can provide opportunities for these girls to "fit in" with their same-age peers through activities that stress mutual goals. For example, an early-maturing girl is typically taller than her age-mates and can be an asset in sports such as basketball and track-and-field events.

the vapour can be harmful to the user and to people exposed to the secondhand e-cigarette smoke.

E-cigarettes remain controversial; there is debate over how effective they are and whether they are a gateway to tobacco smoking. The CPS (2015) warns against the growing industry of e-cigarettes and the misperceived safety of their use.

Smokeless tobacco. The term *smokeless tobacco* refers to tobacco products that are placed in the mouth but not ignited (e.g., chewing tobacco). This substitute for cigarettes continues to pose a hazard to adolescents. While smokeless tobacco use has decreased by a significant amount, there was a rebound in use from the mid-2000s through 2010. Since 2010, prevalence levels have continued to decrease modestly but have remained level since 2014.

Many children and adolescents believe that smokeless tobacco is a safe alternative to cigarette smoking and is not addictive, and they believe they can stop using it at any time. However, the number of adolescents who identify it as a health risk has increased since the mid-1990s, with nearly half now agreeing it has health risks (Johnston et al., 2015). These products have also been proved to be carcinogenic, and regular use can cause dental problems, foul-smelling breath, and tooth erosion or loss.

NURSING CARE

Prevention of regular smoking among teenagers is the most effective way to reduce the overall incidence of smoking. A variety of methods have been employed. Posters, charts, displays, statistics, and the use of examples of actual damaged lungs to communicate the hazards of smoking all have their supporters and doubters. The use of films and demonstrations may also be useful.

For the most part, smoking-prevention programs that focus on the negative, long-term effects of smoking on health have been ineffective. Youth-to-youth programs and those emphasizing the immediate consequences are more effective but primarily in improving teenagers' attitudes toward not smoking. Because smoking and smoking-related behaviours are social symbols, antismoking campaigns must address the norms of potential smokers. Anything that ridicules or threatens the social norms of the peer group can be unproductive or counterproductive. Investigators have found that teaching resistance to peer pressure to smoke is effective in early adolescence. Although the effects of these programs may decrease with time, the effects can be enhanced in older adolescents by presenting information in class instead of simply handing out written material to the students (Thomas, McLellan, & Perera, 2013).

Two areas of focus for antismoking programs are peer-led programs and the use of media in smoking prevention (e.g., television and Internet antismoking ads, and films). Peer-led programs emphasizing the social consequences of smoking have proved most successful. If a significant number of influential peers can "sell" their classmates on the idea that the habit is not popular, the followers will imitate their behaviour. Such programs emphasize short-term rather than long-term consequences (e.g., the effects of smoking on personal appearance, such as unattractive stains on teeth and hands and the unpleasant odour of breath and clothing).

Pharmacological agents used for smoking cessation include nicotine replacement therapy, bupropion, and varenicline. Varenicline taken orally for 12 weeks was shown to be safe and effective in assisting persons who wish to stop smoking (Cahill, Stead, & Lancaster, 2011), but adverse effects such as nausea and abdominal distension may make the drug less palatable for some. None of these three drugs has been specifically approved for use in children and adolescents for smoking cessation. The CPS (2015) does not recommend e-cigarette use as a smoking cessation tool as there is no evidence it is an effective smoking-cessation strategy.

The impact of school-based antismoking programs can be strengthened by expanding these programs to include parents, mass media, youth groups, and community organizations. For example, mass media efforts that involve antismoking radio campaigns have been identified as the most cost-effective mass media intervention. The more effective interventions included young spokespeople, a single message containing information that was previously shown to be effective, and clear language (Thomas et al., 2013).

Smoking bans in schools accomplish several goals: (1) they discourage students from starting to smoke, (2) they reinforce knowledge of the health hazards of cigarette smoking and exposure to environmental tobacco smoke, and (3) they promote a smoke-free environment as the norm (see Community Focus box).

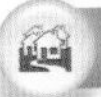

COMMUNITY FOCUS

Nonsmoking Strategies

Nurses who work in schools, hospitals, and community agencies can take advantage of all opportunities to provide education about the dangers of smoking, discourage smoking initiation by children and adolescents, encourage smoking cessation, and promote smoke-free environments. In particular, community or school nurses must be alert to the vulnerability of young preteens when they enter junior high or middle school. These nurses are in an ideal position to assess stress, personal conflict, weight concerns, peer pressures, and other factors that place preteens at risk for smoking initiation. (See Chapter 5 for RNAO Best Practice Guidelines on this topic.) Nurses should serve as counsellors to student, teacher, and parent groups and as advocates for antismoking legislative efforts. The following additional strategies are recommended*:

- Provide only brief information about long-term health consequences (e.g., cardiovascular and cancer risks).
- Discuss immediate physiological consequences (e.g., changes in heart rate, blood pressure, respiratory symptoms, and blood carbon monoxide concentrations).
- Mention alternatives to smoking that also establish a self-image that appears independent, mature, or sophisticated (e.g., weight lifting; jogging; dancing; joining a boys' or girls' club; engaging in volunteer work for a hospital, political, religious, or community group).
- Mention the negative effects in detail (e.g., earlier wrinkling of skin; yellow stains on teeth and fingers; tobacco odour on breath, hair, and clothing).
- Mention the increasing ostracism of smokers by nonsmokers, both legal and informal, in the workplace and in public places.
- Mention the increasing evidence that secondhand smoke is injurious to the health of nonsmokers who are regularly exposed, especially small children.
- Acknowledge that many adults who were enticed to start smoking as teenagers because of its social benefits now wish they could stop smoking.
- Give adolescents effective arguments to deal with peer pressure (e.g., by not smoking, a teenager demonstrates independence and nonconformity, traits normally prized by youth).
- Request posters or pamphlets from local agencies (e.g., Canadian Cancer Society, Canadian Heart and Stroke Foundation, and Canadian Lung Association) to display in prominent places at school.

*Health Canada has information on the effects of tobacco, smoking cessation, and tobacco control programs at http://www.hc-sc.gc.ca/hc-ps/tobac-tabac/index-eng.php

Alcohol

Acute or chronic use of alcohol (ethanol) is responsible for many acts of violence, suicide, accidental injury, and death. Alcohol drinking is likely to begin in the middle-school years and increases with age. By 18 years of age, 80 to 90% of adolescents have tried alcohol. Ethanol is a depressant that reduces inhibitions against aggressive and sexual acting out. Severe physical and psychological symptoms accompany abrupt withdrawal, and long-term use leads to slow tissue destruction, especially of the brain and liver cells. The most noticeable effects of alcohol occur within the central nervous system and include changes in cognitive and autonomic functions such as judgement, memory, learning ability, and other intellectual capacities.

Young alcoholics often drink alone and cannot control their use of alcohol. They often rely on the substance as a defence against depression, anxiety, fear, or anger. Not all of these characteristics are observed in the adolescent who is using alcohol, but if several signs are evident, the child or adolescent should be considered at risk. Referral to a health care provider and detoxification therapy may be necessary. Various groups provide support and counselling for families, including Al-Anon, Ala-Teen, and Alcoholics Anonymous (an organization that has listings in all local telephone directories and via the Internet).

Cocaine

Although cocaine is not pharmacologically considered a narcotic, it is legally categorized as such. Cocaine is available in two forms: water-soluble cocaine hydrochloride, which is administered by "snorting" or intravenous injection, and nonsoluble alkaloid (freebase) cocaine, which is used primarily for smoking. Crack, or "rock," is a purer, more dangerous form of the drug. It can be produced cheaply and smoked in either water pipes or mentholated cigarettes.

The use of cocaine has increased in recent years because of its availability and affordability, its association with persons in glamorous occupations, peer pressure, and its reputation as a sexually enhancing drug.

Cocaine creates a sense of euphoria, or an indefinable high. Withdrawal does not produce the dramatic symptoms observed in withdrawal from other substances. The effects are those commonly seen in depression, including lack of energy and motivation, irritability, appetite changes, decrease in psychomotor activity, and irregular sleep patterns. More serious symptoms include cardiovascular manifestations and seizures. Physical withdrawal should not be confused with the so-called crash after a cocaine high, which consists of a long period of sleep.

Narcotics

Narcotic drugs include **opiates**, such as heroin and morphine, and opioids (opiate-like drugs), such as hydromorphone (Dilaudid), hydrocodone, fentanyl, meperidine (Demerol), and codeine. These drugs produce a state of euphoria by removing painful feelings and creating a pleasurable experience and a sense of success accompanied by clouding of the consciousness and a dreamlike state. Physical signs of narcotic use include constricted pupils, respiratory depression, and, often, cyanosis. Needle marks may be visible on the arms or legs of chronic users. Physical withdrawal from opiates is extremely unpleasant unless controlled with supervised tapering doses of the opioid or substitution of methadone.

As important as the physical effects are the indirect consequences related to the illegal status of narcotic use and the problems associated with securing the drug (e.g., the time-consuming searches to obtain the drug and the often illegal methods used to meet the high cost of purchasing it). Health problems also result from self-neglect of physical needs (nutrition, cleanliness, dental care); overdose; contamination; and infection, including HIV and hepatitis B and C infection (see Additional Resources section at the end of this chapter).

Central Nervous System Depressants

Central nervous system depressants include a variety of hypnotic drugs that produce physical dependence and withdrawal symptoms on abrupt discontinuation. They create a feeling of relaxation and sleepiness but impair general functioning. Drugs in this category include barbiturates, nonbarbiturates, and alcohol. Barbiturates combined with alcohol produce a profound depressant effect. Flunitrazepam (Rohypnol), known as the "date rape drug," is a hypnotic drug used by some adolescents. Many women report being raped after unknowingly being given flunitrazepam in a drink. Flunitrazepam is 10 times more powerful than diazepam (Valium). It produces prolonged sedation, a feeling of well-being, and short-term memory loss.

Central Nervous System Stimulants

Amphetamines and cocaine do not produce strong physical dependence and can be withdrawn without much danger. However, psychological dependence is strong, and acute intoxication can lead to violent aggressive behaviour or psychotic episodes characterized by paranoia, uncontrollable agitation, and restlessness. When combined with barbiturates, the euphoric effects are particularly addictive.

Methamphetamine can be snorted, injected, swallowed, or smoked and produces a burst of energy in its users, along with intense, alternating attacks of boldness and paranoia. It provokes excitement far more intense than that caused by cocaine. The drug, with the street names speed, crank, meth, ice, and crystal, is inexpensive and has a longer period of action than that of cocaine. Instead of a short (few minutes) high, as achieved with cocaine, a user can remain "up" for hours on a similar dose of crank.

The use of various volatile substances, or inhalants such as gasoline, model airplane cement, and organic solvents, is also of concern. Adolescents breathe or place these substances into paper or plastic bags or soft drink cans from which they rebreathe the fumes to produce a feeling of euphoria and altered consciousness. These substances contain chemical solvents and are extremely hazardous. Dusters contain Freon, a substance that can cause fatal cardiac arrhythmias. Common inhalant substances are inexpensive and easily obtained, such as gasoline, paint, propane/butane, air fresheners, and formalin (Baydala & CPS, First Nations, Inuit and Métis Health Committee, 2010/2016). Unfortunately, the use of inhalants is increasing, after nearly a decade of decline (Baydala & CPS, First Nations, Inuit and Métis Health Committee, 2010/2016). Inhalants are becoming a gateway drug for young children and preteens, who often progress to other harder drugs such as heroin and cocaine. One in five Indigenous youth reported having used inhalant solvents (one out of three users were under 15 years of age) and over half had started to use solvents before age 11. In response to this danger to Indigenous youth, the National Youth Solvent Program was established by Health Canada and Indigenous communities to promote a stronger cultural identity and cultural healing.

Many young children are unaware of the dangers of "sniffing" or "huffing." In addition to rapid loss of consciousness and respiratory arrest, these substances may cause visual-scanning problems, language deficiencies, motor instability, memory deficits, and attention and concentration problems.

Mind-Altering Drugs

Hallucinogens (psychedelics, psychotomimetics, psychotropics, or illusionogenics) are drugs that produce vivid hallucinations and euphoria. These drugs do not produce physical dependence, and they can be abruptly withdrawn without ill effect. However, the acute and long-term effects are variable, and in some individuals the dissociative behaviour may be prolonged. Cannabis (marijuana, hashish) and lysergic acid diethylamide (LSD) are also included in this category of drugs. According to a report from British Columbia, by age 18 years, 15% had tried ecstasy (Stewart, Vallance, Stockwell, et al., 2009).

NURSING CARE

Nurses who have contact with children and adolescents are in an excellent position to provide information about substance use and to serve as patient advocates (see Additional Resources section at the end of this chapter). The nurse most often encounters young drug users when they are (1) experiencing overdose or withdrawal symptoms, (2) manifesting bizarre behaviour or confusion secondary to drug ingestion, (3) worried that they are or will become addicted, or (4) worried about a friend or family member who is addicted.

In particular, nurses who care for hospitalized adolescents need to know if these youths use drugs compulsively. Drug withdrawal can seriously complicate other illnesses. Nurses should be on the alert for any physical or behavioural clues that indicate the onset of withdrawal or the effects of drugs. Nurses who work in schools or in the community can play an essential role in identifying children, adolescents, and families with substance use problems. These nurses may be the first to identify a child or adolescent who has ingested a particular drug by the child's erratic behaviour in class or on the school grounds. Early identification of those at risk for substance use problems is an essential aspect of prevention. Pediatric health care providers can also prevent substance use by creating trusting relationships with children and adolescents so that they feel comfortable asking questions about drugs. Health care providers can alert them to websites and other aspects of society that may actually encourage experimentation with drugs.

Acute Care

Adolescents experiencing toxic drug effects or withdrawal symptoms are usually seen initially in the emergency department. Experienced emergency department personnel are familiar with the management of acute drug toxicity and the signs, symptoms, and behavioural characteristics associated with a variety of substances. When the drug is questionable or unknown, such expertise can help facilitate management and treatment. Often, observation or a description of the child or adolescent's behaviour is more valuable than reports by patients or their friends.

The treatment for drug toxicity or withdrawal varies according to the drug and the method used. Every effort should be made to determine the type and amount of drug taken, the time of ingestion, the mode of administration, and factors related to the onset of presenting symptoms. It is helpful to know the individual's pattern of use. For example, if two types of drugs are involved, they may require different treatments. Gastric lavage may be employed when the drug has been ingested recently and the cough reflex is intact, but it is of little value when the drug has been administered by the intravenous ("mainlined") or intranasal ("sniffed") route.

Single-dose activated charcoal has been used for acute poisoning, but there is considerable controversy regarding the benefits and effects over time (Isbister & Kumar, 2011). Some experts recommend supportive care as the mainstay of overdose treatment in pediatrics (Hanhan, 2008). The administration of a drug antidote such as naloxone and the early (within 1 to 2 hours of ingestion) administration of activated charcoal may be used for opioid overdose. Because the actual content of most street drugs is highly questionable, other pharmaceutical agents should be administered with caution, except perhaps the narcotic antagonists in cases of suspected opiate overdoses. It is also necessary to assess for possible trauma sustained while the patient was under the influence of the drug. See Chapter 46, Ingestion of Injurious Agents for more information on nursing care.

Long-Term Management

A major factor in the treatment and rehabilitation of young drug users is careful assessment during the nonacute stage to determine the function the drug plays in the adolescent's life. The motivation phase is directed toward exploring the factors that influence drug use. It also involves establishing a feeling of self-worth in the teenager as well as a commitment to self-help.

Rehabilitation begins when adolescents decide that they can and are willing to change. Rehabilitation involves fostering healthy interdependent relationships with caring and supportive adults and exploring alternative mechanisms for problem solving while simultaneously reducing or eliminating drug use. Persons working with troubled youth must be prepared for *recidivism*, or the tendency to relapse, and maintain a plan for re-entry into the treatment process.

Family Support

Most treatment programs for substance users are based on adult 12-step models such as Alcoholics Anonymous. Research is needed to determine whether these adult models are effective for adolescents. Tough Love is a program based on the premise that parents have the right and responsibility to be the policymakers in the family, to set limits on their children's behaviour, and to take control of the household from out-of-control adolescents. By allowing teenagers to experience the negative consequences of their behaviour, they may become more willing to accept help or to change their behaviour. Another group that provides support and counselling for families affected by a child's substance use is Parents Anonymous. The Government of Canada has a National Anti-Drug Strategy that also provides help for parents seeking to prevent youth substance use. Another source of information is the U.S. National Institute on Drug Abuse. For further information on all of these resources see Additional Resources at the end of this chapter.

Prevention

Nurses play an important role in education as well as in individual observation, assessment, and therapy related to substance use. In recent years, a variety of educational programs have been applied, with promising results. The most effective prevention strategies are part of a broader, more general effort to promote overall health and success. Health-compromising behaviours are often interconnected and have common antecedents. Prevention efforts that focus on changing only one behaviour (e.g., alcohol, other drug use) are less likely to be successful. Successful programs are those that have promoted parenting skills, social skills among distractible children, academic achievement, and skills to resist peer pressure.

Peer pressure is a powerful tool and can be used effectively in substance use prevention. A group that has had some success in reducing injury from drunk driving is Mothers Against Drunk Driving (MADD). Techniques used by this group include peer counselling, parental guidelines for teenage parties, and community awareness. Nurses can encourage the formation of Students Against Destructive Decision (SADD) chapters in high schools in their communities (see Additional Resources section).

Suicide

Suicide is defined as the deliberate act of self-injury with the intent that the injury results in death. Most experts distinguish between suicidal ideation, suicide attempt (or parasuicide), and suicide. *Suicidal ideation* involves a preoccupation with thoughts about committing suicide and may be a precursor to suicide. Although it is not uncommon for adolescents to experience occasional suicidal thoughts, expressions of preoccupation with suicide should be taken seriously, and an assessment should be conducted for appropriate referral. A *suicide attempt* is intended to cause injury or death. The term *parasuicide* refers to behaviours ranging from gestures to serious attempts to kill oneself. Parasuicide is a preferred term because it makes no reference to intent and because a person's motive may be too difficult or complex to determine. All parasuicidal activity should be taken seriously.

> **! NURSING ALERT**
>
> A history of a previous suicide attempt is a serious indicator for possible suicide completion in the future. Studies of adolescent suicides have found that as many as half of the adolescents had made previous attempts.

Results from the 2008 British Columbia Adolescent Health Survey indicate that the proportion of youth who seriously consider suicide may be decreasing, at least among certain groups. In 2008, 12% of youth reported seriously considering suicide, which is a drop from 16% in 1992 (Smith et al., 2009). In Canada, among 15- to 24-year-olds, suicide is the cause of death from injury in 24% of all deaths (Canadian Mental Health Association, 2016a). Suicide is currently the third leading cause of death in adolescents aged 15 to 19 years, surpassed only by death from motor vehicle crash and homicide (see Chapter 31). On average, 294 Canadian youths die yearly from suicide, and many more attempt suicide. Although the youth suicide rate as a whole is decreasing in Canada, including the rate for male adolescents, the rate for adolescent girls is slightly increasing.

Etiology

Individual, family, and social or environmental factors have all been implicated in suicide. The single most important individual factor is the presence of an active psychiatric disorder (depression, bipolar disorder, psychosis, substance use, or conduct disorder). Comorbidity of an affective disorder and substance use also increases the risk for suicide. Approximately 90% of adolescents who completed suicide met criteria for a psychiatric disorder before the suicide (Shain & AAP Committee on Adolescence, 2007). Depression is considered the highest single risk factor for adolescent suicide (Canadian Mental Health Association, 2016a). Child and adolescent suicide victims are reported to have higher rates not only of depression but also of conduct disorders; bipolar disorders; substance misuse; interpersonal problems with parents; and a family history of depression, substance misuse, and suicidal behaviour. See Chapter 38 for more information on depression.

Indigenous teens and gay, lesbian, bisexual, and transgender teens may be at a particularly high risk for suicide completion, depending on their own sense of self-esteem and the community in which they reside (Mental Health Commission of Canada, 2015) (see Community Focus box). Among Indigenous youth the suicide rate is approximately five to seven times and for the Inuit population 11 times that of the non-Indigenous population (Bhatia, 2010). Family factors contributing to suicide risk include parental loss; family disruption; a family history of suicide, depression, substance use, or emotional disturbance; child abuse or neglect; unavailable parents; poor communication and isolation within the family; family conflict; and unrealistically high parental expectations or parental indifference with low expectations. Families who respect individuality, are cohesive and caring, balance discipline with a supportive and understanding relationship, have good systems of communication, and have at least one attentive and caring parent available to the child can help protect adolescents from suicidal outcomes. Social or environmental factors include incarceration, isolation, acute loss of a boyfriend or girlfriend, lack of future options, and availability of firearms in the home. Cyberbullying and messages on some Internet sites that encourage suicide may also have an impact on suicide rates in the adolescent population (Kirmayer, 2012).

Methods

Hanging or suffocation is the most common means of suicide among male and female adolescents. Other methods include firearms, poisoning by gas, and overdose. Adolescents may play a choking game in which there is a temporary cutting off of the airway in order to cause euphoria; some suicides may actually be unintentional deaths but are impossible to differentiate from suicide (Kirmayer, 2012).

The most common method of suicide *attempt* is overdose or ingestion of a potentially toxic substance, such as drugs. The second most common method of suicide attempt is self-inflicted laceration.

COMMUNITY FOCUS

Suicide, Sexual Identity, and Sexual Orientation

A significant number of teenage suicides occur among lesbian, gay, bisexual, transgender, and queer (LGBTQ) youths. LGBTQ adolescents who live in families or communities that do not accept them are likely to suffer low self-esteem, self-loathing, depression, and hopelessness as a result. Such internalization, without treatment and support, can lead to substance use and, eventually, suicide. Youths most at risk are those who struggle with gender identity issues, such as LGBTQ identity formation at a young age, intrapersonal conflict regarding sexuality, nondisclosure of orientation to others, and identifying as transgender.

LGBTQ youth face approximately 14 times the risk of suicide and substance abuse compared to that of their heterosexual peers. Bisexual and transgender individuals are also overrepresented among low-income Canadians. For example, an Ontario-based study found that half of transgender people were living on less than $15,000 a year. LGBTQ youth can experience stigma and discrimination, and can be targets of sexual and physical assault, harassment, and hate crimes (Canadian Mental Health Association, 2016b).

Supportive parents and friends serve as protective factors against suicide. However, many LGBTQ adolescents do not feel supported, understood, or accepted by their friends, parents, and families. Nurses who interact with adolescents must be aware of the association between suicide and adolescent LGBTQ sexuality and gender nonconformity. School nurses may be the first individuals to discuss issues of sexual identity and orientation with adolescents or their families. In their professional capacity, nurses can serve as support persons for these adolescents. Nurses can also provide guidance and resources to families so that they understand how best to nurture and support their child.

Nurses must also capitalize on opportunities or experiences that promote the healthy development of self-esteem in youths who have a nontraditional sexual orientation. Educational programs to raise the level of consciousness about the risk factors for and warning signs of suicide are one example. Another possibility is programs conducted in or outside of school that are designed to foster peer relationships and competency in social skills among high-risk adolescents and young adults, such as support groups and social organizations for these young people.

NURSING ALERT

Given what is known about youth suicide, nurses should ask parents, especially those with at-risk teenagers, if firearms are available in the house and, if so, recommend their removal. Parents must ensure that their children—especially those who are depressed, have poor problem-solving skills, or use drugs or alcohol—do not have access to firearms. Parents must be educated on the warning signs of suicide (Box 39-4).

Motivation

Suicidal ideation is common in adolescents. It represents numerous fantasies, such as relief from suffering, a means of gaining comfort and sympathy, or a means of revenge against those who

BOX 39-4 WARNING SIGNS OF SUICIDE

- Preoccupation with themes of death—focuses on morbid thoughts
- Wants to give away cherished possessions
- Talks of own death, desire to die
- Loss of energy, loss of interest, listlessness
- Exhaustion without obvious cause
- Changes in sleep patterns—too much or too little
- Increased irritability, argumentativeness, or stubbornness
- Physical complaints—recurrent stomach aches, headaches
- Repeated visits to the physician, nurse practitioner, or emergency department for treatment of injuries
- Reckless behaviour
- Antisocial behaviour—engages in drinking, uses drugs, fights, commits acts of vandalism, runs away from home, becomes sexually promiscuous
- Sudden change in school performance—lowered grades, cutting classes, dropping out of activities
- Resists or refuses to go to school
- Remains distant, sad, remote—flat affect, frozen facial expression
- Describes self as worthless
- Sudden cheerfulness following deep depression
- Social withdrawal from friends, activities, interests that were previously enjoyed
- Impaired concentration
- Dramatic change in appetite

BOX 39-5 CHARACTERISTICS OF CHILDREN OR ADOLESCENTS WITH DEPRESSION

Behaviour

Predominantly sad facial expression with absence or diminished range of affective response (most of the day)
Solitary play or work; tendency to be alone; lack of interest in play with friends
Withdrawal from previously enjoyed activities and relationships
Lowered grades in school; lack of interest in doing homework or achieving in school; refuses to wake up for school
Diminished motor activity; tiredness
Tearfulness or crying
Inability to concentrate
Dependent and clinging or aggressive and disruptive
Recurrent suicidal thoughts or talk

Internal States

Utterance of statements reflecting lowered self-esteem, sense of hopelessness, or guilt
Suicidal ideations

Physiology

Constipation
Loss of energy; fatigue
Nonspecific complaints of not feeling well
Change in appetite resulting in weight loss or gain
Alterations in sleeping pattern, sleeplessness, or hypersomnia

have hurt them. Adolescents have the erroneous perception that the act of suicide will evoke remorse and pity and that they will be able to return and witness the grief. Angry children who are unable to directly punish those who have injured or insulted them may take revenge on those who love them through self-destruction ("They'll be sorry when they find me dead"; "They'll be sorry they were mean to me").

For adolescents who are severely depressed, suicide seems to be the only release from their despair. These adolescents rarely provide evidence of their intent and frequently conceal their suicidal thoughts. Some adolescents, however, tell their peers of their suicidal thoughts or plans but avoid telling adults. Social isolation is a significant factor in distinguishing adolescents who will kill themselves from those who will not. It is also more characteristic of those who complete suicide than of those who make attempts or threats.

The frequency of contagion, or copycat suicides (i.e., an increase in youth suicide that occurs after the suicide of one teenager is publicized), is disturbing and may indicate that teenagers perceive suicide as glamorous. In addition, young people may not realize the finality of suicide because they have become desensitized from constantly viewing violence and death on television, in video games, or in movies.

Diagnostic Evaluation

Depression is common among adolescents who attempt suicide. It is estimated that in those 15 to 18 years of age, approximately 7.6% had experienced depression and 13.5% had been diagnosed as having suicidal tendencies. Among Canadian female adolescents the rate of depression was 11.1%, with 18.4% exhibiting suicidality, and 8.8% of adolescent boys had depression (Cheung & Dewa, 2006). Depression is characterized by both subjective symptoms and objective signs that reflect the adolescent's sadness and despair. Adolescents describe feelings of sadness, despair, helplessness, hopelessness, boredom, loss of interest, and isolation. They may also feel self-reproach, self-deprecation, and guilt. Subjective symptoms of depression or specific changes in behaviour place an adolescent at risk for suicide (Box 39-5).

Therapeutic Management

Threats of suicide should always be taken seriously. There has been a tendency to dismiss a suicide attempt as an impulsive act resulting from a temporary crisis or depression. If a suicide attempt fails to draw attention to their problems or makes them worse, the child or adolescent may conclude that suicide is the only answer. Children and adolescents need to know that someone cares, and they must be provided with swift and efficient crisis intervention. Although ordinary practitioners can manage an acute depressive reaction without difficulty, the adolescent who has made a serious attempt or has a specific plan for suicide should receive immediate attention and competent psychiatric care.

Youths who are actively suicidal need inpatient care, monitoring, and treatment. Medications for depression and bipolar disorder often take several weeks to reach therapeutic levels. The time until medications and therapy begin to take effect can be trying for the adolescent and the family. It is important to encourage families to support their teen in adherence to the regimen prescribed. The selective serotonin reuptake inhibitors are often prescribed for depression, but teens who are taking such medications need careful, frequent monitoring.

> **! NURSING ALERT**
>
> Adolescents who express suicidal feelings and have a specific plan should be monitored at all times. They should not have access to firearms, prescription or over-the-counter medications, belts, scarves, shoestrings, sharp objects, matches, or lighters. If they are intoxicated, they must be restrained or placed in a protective environment until a psychiatrist or psychologist can assess them.

NURSING CARE

Nurses play a pivotal role in reducing adolescent suicide. Nurses have the opportunity to provide anticipatory guidance to parents and adolescents. They can teach parents to be supportive and to develop positive communication patterns that help teens feel connected with and loved by their families. To foster healthy development, parents can be encouraged to provide teens with creative outlets and to assist young people in accepting strong emotions—pain, anger, and frustration—as a normal part of the human experience.

Care of the suicidal adolescent includes early recognition, management, and prevention. The most important aspect of management is the recognition of warning signs that indicate an adolescent is troubled and might attempt suicide. Health care providers must be alert to the signs of depression, and anyone who exhibits such behaviour should be referred for thorough psychological assessment. Depression is manifested differently in children and adolescents than in adults. In teens it may be masked by impulsive, aggressive behaviours. Defiance, disobedience, behaviour problems, and psychosomatic disturbances can indicate underlying depression, suicidal ideation, and impending suicide attempts.

No threat of suicide should be ignored or challenged. Too often, suicidal threats or minor attempts are confused with bids for attention. It is also a mistake to be lulled into a false sense of security when the adolescent's depression is apparently relieved. The improvement in attitude may mean that the adolescent has made the decision and found the means to carry out the threat. Nurses have an ethical and legal obligation to report attempted or suspected attempted suicides (Canadian Nurses Association, 2008). The mechanism of reporting varies by province and territory, and each nurse must be aware of the appropriate channels for reporting (for example, in British Columbia, nurses and others report to the Ministry for Children and Family Development).

Peers or other confidants are valuable observers and excellent sources of information about **suicide potential**. They may not be able to diagnose depression, but they can sense when a friend has undergone a marked personality change. The peer who detects any changes in a friend is a potential rescuer and should not remain silent about the observations. Friendship does not imply collusion. A peer who believes that a friend may be suicidal should alert someone who can help (e.g., a parent, teacher, guidance counsellor, school nurse), and nurses should be supportive of peers who come forward with such information.

Routine health assessments of adolescents should include questions that assess the presence of suicidal ideation or intent. The following questions can be asked (American Foundation for Suicide Prevention, 2016):

- Do you consider yourself more a happy person, an unhappy person, or somewhere in the middle?
- Have you ever been so unhappy or upset that you felt like being dead?
- Have you ever thought about hurting yourself?
- Have you ever developed a plan to hurt yourself or kill yourself?
- Have you ever attempted to kill yourself?

If children or adolescents express suicidal intent to a nurse, the nurse needs to make a contract, asking them to sign an agreement that they will not attempt suicide during an agreed-on period and that they will call the 24-hour crisis line immediately if they feel that they cannot keep their contract. The amount of time that an adolescent feels comfortable contracting is usually an indication of his or her risk and stability.

Because a suicide attempt is frequently an outgrowth of family distress, it is essential to intervene with the family. It is important to assess family interactions and to recognize disturbed relationships. The most effective approach is recognition of susceptible adolescents during the early stages of family distress so that family counselling can be started. Prevention must be directed toward improving child-rearing practices through support and education of parents and changing societal conditions that generate defeat, despair, and maladaptive behaviour.

Although confidentiality is an essential part of adolescent counselling, in the case of self-destructive behaviours, confidentiality cannot be honoured. Suicidal behaviour needs to be reported to the family and other professionals and adolescents informed that this will be done. Such action conveys an important message to the youth: that the professionals understand and care.

Many schools have instituted suicide prevention programs. These programs include services such as drop-in counselling and a peer-counselling telephone line. Information can also be obtained from the Canadian Mental Health Association (see Additional Resources section at the end of this chapter).

KEY POINTS

- The pubescent growth spurt that begins around age 10 in girls and age 12 in boys signals the beginning of adolescence.
- Biological development during puberty is characterized by increased activity of the pituitary gland, which results in sexual maturity and the appearance of secondary sex characteristics.
- Development of body image is closely tied to body changes and social interactions.
- According to Erikson, the major developmental crisis of adolescence is establishing a sense of identity.
- Cognitive development in adolescence includes abstract thought, thinking beyond the present, logical reasoning, and a sense of idealism.
- According to Kohlberg's theory of moral development, adolescents begin to question existing moral values and learn to make their own choices.
- Spiritual development is characterized by the questioning of one's family's values and ideals and a move toward more philosophical thinking.
- Adolescent relationships with parents may be strained; the influence of the peer group increases and intimate relationships assume importance.
- Teenagers demonstrate a wide variety of interests, and their increased physical and cognitive skills allow them to engage in increasingly difficult and complex activities.
- Adolescents' emotions fluctuate.
- Nutritional needs may not be met by teenagers' eating habits, such as snacking and irregular mealtimes.
- Motor vehicle injuries are the primary cause of death from injury in the adolescent years.
- The rapid changes, growth, and stress accompanying the transition to adulthood may predispose adolescents to faulty problem solving.
- The most common health problems related to the female reproductive system during adolescence involve menstrual dysfunction; male reproductive health problems include testicular cancer and gynecomastia.
- Eating disorders observed in middle and late childhood are obesity, anorexia nervosa, bulimia nervosa, and eating disorder not otherwise specified.
- Tobacco smoking is a widespread problem among teenagers. Reasons for smoking include social pressure and mass media influence.
- The substances used by children and adolescents are alcohol, marijuana, narcotics, central nervous system depressants, central nervous system stimulants, hydrocarbons and fluorocarbons, and mind-altering drugs.
- Suicide, the deliberate act of self-injury with the intent to kill, may occur because of difficulties coping with stress, disturbed family environment, substance use or dependency, or mental health disorder.
- No threat of suicide by an adolescent should be ignored or challenged.
- Signs of depression in children and adolescents are often subtle and require astute observation by parents and health care professionals.

evolve WEBSITE

Visit the Evolve website for additional resources related to the content in this chapter such as Case Studies, Critical Thinking Case Study Answers, Nursing Care Plans, Nursing Processes, Nursing Skills, and Review Questions for Exam Preparation at: http://evolve.elsevier.com/Canada/Perry/maternal/

REFERENCES

Active Healthy Kids Canada. (2012). *Is active play extinct? Active Healthy Kids Canada report card on physical activity for children and youth.* Retrieved from <http://dvqdas9jty7g6.cloudfront.net/reportcards2012/AHKC%20 2012%20-%20Report%20Card%20Short%20Form%20-%20FINAL.pdf>.

Active Healthy Kids Canada. (2014). *Report card on physical activity for children and youth.* Retrieved from <http://www.participaction.com/wp-content/uploads/2015/03/AHKC_2014_ReportCard_ENG.pdf>.

Al-Sahab, B., Ardern, C., Hamadeh, M., et al. (2010). Age at menarche in Canada: Results from the national longitudinal survey of children and youth. *BMC Public Health, 10,* 736. doi:10.1186/1471-2458-10-736.

American Academy of Pediatric Dentistry, Clinical Affairs Committee. (2015). *Guideline on adolescent oral health care. Clinical practice guidelines.* Retrieved from <http://www.aapd.org/media/Policies_Guidelines/G_Adoleshealth.pdf>.

American College of Preventive Medicine. (2011). *Adolescent depression—Enhancing outcomes in primary care.* Retrieved from <https://c.ymcdn.com/sites/www.acpm.org/resource/resmgr/timetools-files/adolescentdepressionclinical.pdf>.

American Dietetic Association. (2006). Position of the American Dietetic Association: Nutrition intervention in the treatment of anorexia nervosa, bulimia nervosa, and other eating disorders. *Journal of the American Dietetic Association, 106*(12), 2073–2082. doi:10.1016/j.jada.2006.09.007.

American Foundation for Suicide Prevention. (2016). *About suicide: Risk factors and warning signs.* Retrieved from <http://www.afsp.org/preventing-suicide/suicide-warning-signs>.

American Psychiatric Association. (2013). *Diagnostic and statistical manual of mental disorders* (5th ed.) (DSM-5). Washington, DC: Author.

Barkley, R. A., & Cox, D. (2007). A review of driving risks and impairments associated with attention-deficit/hyperactivity disorder and the effects of stimulant medication on driving performance. *Journal of Safety Research, 38*(1), 113–128.

Barnett, S. J. (2011). Contemporary surgical management of the obese adolescent. *Current Opinions in Pediatrics, 23*(3), 351–355.

Bassareo, P. P., & Mercuro, G. (2014). Pediatric hypertension: An update on a burning problem. *World Journal of Cardiology, 6*(5), 253–259. doi:10.4330/wjc.v6.i5.253.

Baydala, L., & Canadian Paediatric Society, First Nations, Inuit and Métis Health Committee. (2010). Inhalant abuse. *Paediatrics & Child Health, 15*(7), 443–448. Reaffirmed 2016. Retrieved from <http://www.cps.ca/en/documents/position/inhalant-abuse>.

Beaty, T. H. (2007). Invited commentary: Two studies of genetic control of birth weight where large data sets were available. *American Journal of Epidemiology, 165*(7), 753–755.

Beaulieu, D., & Godin, G. (2012). Staying in school for lunch instead of eating in fast-food restaurants: Results of a quasi-experimental study among high-school students. *Public Health Nutrition, 15*(12), 2310–2319. doi:10.1017/S1368980012000821.

Bhatia, J. (2010). Canada: Aboriginal suicides hit crisis rate. *Global Voices*, January 18, 2010. Retrieved from <https://globalvoices.org/2010/01/18/canada-aboriginal-youth-suicides-hit-crisis-rate/>.

Biro, F. M., Greenspan, L. C., & Galvez, M. P. (2012). Puberty in girls of the 21st century. *Journal of Pediatric Adolescence Gynecology, 25*(5), 289–294. doi:10.1016/j.jpag.2012.05.009.

Bouchard, C. (2009). Childhood obesity: Are genetic differences involved? *American Journal of Clinical Nutrition, 89*(5), 1494S–1501S.

Boyce, W. F., King, M. A., & Roche, J. (2008). *Healthy living and healthy weight. In healthy settings for young people in Canada.* Ottawa: Public Health Agency of Canada. Retrieved from <http://publications.gc.ca/collections/collection_2008/phac-aspc/HP35-6-2007E.pdf>.

Braverman, P. K. (2006). Body art: Piercing, tattooing, and scarification. *Adolescent Medicine, 17*, 505–519. doi:10.1016/j.admecli.2006.06.007.

Bröning, S., Kumpfer, K., Kruse, K., et al. (2012). Selective prevention programs for children from substance-affected families: A comprehensive systematic review. *Substance Abuse Treatment and Prevention Policy, 7*, 23. doi:10.1186/1747-597X-7-23.

Cahill, R., Stead, L. F., & Lancaster, T. (2011). Nicotine receptor partial agonists for smoking cessation. *The Cochrane Database of Systematic Reviews*, (4), CD006103, doi:10.1002/14651858.CD006103.

Canadian Cancer Society. (2007). *Sun bed usage and attitudes among students in Ontario grades 7 to 12: Youthograph—Summary results.* Retrieved from <http://cancer.ca/~/media/ccs/ontario/files%20list/liste%20de%20fichiers/pdf/youthography%20survey_1856550887.ashx>.

Canadian Cancer Society. (2016). *Detecting testicular cancer.* Retrieved from <http://www.cancer.ca/en/prevention-and-screening/early-detection-and-screening/finding-cancer-early/detecting-testicular-cancer/?region=on>.

Canadian Centre on Substance Abuse. (2014). *Childhood and adolescent pathways to substance use disorders.* Retrieved from <http://www.ccsa.ca/Resource%20Library/CCSA-Child-Adolescent-Substance-Use-Disorders-Report-2014-en.pdf>.

Canadian Dental Association. (2016). *Fluoride and your child.* Retrieved from <http://www.cda-adc.ca/en/oral_health/cfyt/dental_care_children/fluoride.asp?intPrintable=1>.

Canadian Dermatology Association. (2011). *2011 Melanoma fact sheet.* Retrieved from <http://www.dermatology.ca/wp-content/uploads/2012/01/2011-Melanoma-Factsheet-EN.pdf>.

Canadian Diabetes Association. (2016). *Children and type 2 diabetes.* Retrieved from <https://www.diabetes.ca/diabetes-and-you/kids-teens-diabetes/children-type-2-diabetes>.

Canadian Mental Health Association. (2016a). *Children, youth, and depression.* Retrieved from <http://www.cmha.ca/mental_health/children-and-depression/#.VRGztuFuOT8>.

Canadian Mental Health Association. (2016b). *Lesbian, gay, bisexual, trans & queer identified people and mental health.* Retrieved from <http://ontario.cmha.ca/mental-health/lesbian-gay-bisexual-trans-people-and-mental-health/>.

Canadian Nurses Association. (2008). *Code of ethics for registered nurses.* Ottawa: Author.

Canadian Paediatric Society. (2011). *Your teen's sexual orientation.* Retrieved from <http://www.caringforkids.cps.ca/handouts/teens_sexual_orientation>.

Canadian Paediatric Society. (2013). *Teens and sleep: Why you need it and how to get enough.* Retrieved from <http://www.caringforkids.cps.ca/handouts/teens_and_sleep>.

Canadian Paediatric Society. (2015). *E-cigarettes: A danger to children and youth.* Retrieved from <http://www.caringforkids.cps.ca/handouts/e-cigarettes-a-danger-to-children-and-youth>.

Canadian Society for Exercise Physiology. (2015). *Canadian physical activity guidelines: For youth 12–17 years.* Retrieved from <http://www.csep.ca/english/view.asp?x=804>.

Chaiton, M., Cohen, J., O'Loughlin, J., et al. (2010). Use of cigarettes to improve affect and depressive symptoms in a longitudinal study of adolescents. *Addictive Behaviours, 36*(12), 1054–1064. doi:10.1016/j.addbeh.2010.07.002.

Cheung, A. H., & Dewa, C. (2006). Canadian community health survey: Major depressive disorder and suicidality in adolescents. *Healthcare Policy, 2*(2), 76–89.

Ciccone, J., Woodruff, S., Fryer, K., et al. (2013). Associations among evening snacking, screen time, weight status, and overall diet quality in young adolescents. *Applied Physiology Nutrition Metabolism, 38*(7), 789–794. doi:10.1139/apnm-2012-0374.

Comtes, M., Hobin, E., Majumdar, S., et al. (2013). Patterns of weekday and weekend physical activity in youth in 2 Canadian provinces. *Applied Physiology Nutrition Metabolism, 38*(2), 115–119.

Costello, E. J., Sung, M., & Worthman, C. (2007). Pubertal maturation and the development of alcohol use and abuse. *Drug & Alcohol Dependence, 88*(4 Suppl. 1), S50–S59. doi:10.1016/j.drugalcdep.2006.12.009.

Crowley, S. J., Acebo, C., & Carskadon, M. A. (2007). Sleep, circadian rhythms, and delayed phase in adolescence. *Sleep Medicine, 8*(6), 602–612. doi:10.1016/j.sleep.2006.12.002.

de Genna, N. M., Larkby, C., & Cornelius, M. D. (2011). Pubertal timing and early sexual intercourse in the offspring of teenage mothers. *Journal of Youth and Adolescent, 40*(10), 1315–1328. doi:10.007/s10964-010-9609-3.

Dietitians of Canada. (2014). *5 Steps to a healthy body weight.* Retrieved from <http://archive-ca.com/page/3652539/2014-02-06/http://www.dietitians.ca/Nutrition-Resources-A-Z/Factsheets/Teens/5-Steps-to-a-Healthy-Body-Weight-for-Teens.aspx>.

Dowdell, E. B., Burgess, A. W., & Flores, J. R. (2011). Original research: Online social networking patterns among adolescents, young adults, and sexual offenders. *American Journal of Nursing, 111*(7), 28–36. Quiz, 37–38. doi:10.1097/01.NAJ.0000399310.83160.73.

Elton-Marshall, T., Leatherdale, S., & Burkhalter, R. (2011). Tobacco, alcohol and illicit drug use among Aboriginal youth living off-reserve: Results from the Youth Smoking Survey. *Canadian Medical Association Journal, 183*(8), E480–E486. doi:10.1503/cmaj.101913.

Erikson, E. H. (1963). *Childhood and society* (2nd ed.). New York: W. W. Norton.

Feldman, D. R., Bosl, G. J., Sheinfeld, J., & Motzer, R. J. (2008). Medical treatment of advanced testicular cancer. *Journal of the American Medical Association, 299*(6), 672–684. doi:10.1001/jama.299.6.672.

Female Athlete Triad Coalition. (2011). *The female triad athlete.* Retrieved from <http://www.femaleathletetriad.org/wp-content/uploads/2010/03/FATC_Slideshow_2011.pdf>.

Fennoy, I. (2010). Metabolic and respiratory comorbidities of childhood obesity. *Pediatric Annals, 39*(3), 140–146. doi:10.3928/00904481-20100223-08.

Forman, S. F. (2012). *Eating disorders: Epidemiology, pathogenesis, and clinical features.* Retrieved from <http://www.uptodate.com/contents/eating-disorders-treatment-and-outcome>.

Frappier, Y., Austin Leonard, K., Sacks, D., & Canadian Paediatric Society, Adolescent Health Committee. (2005). Youth and firearms in Canada. *Paediatrics & Child Health, 10*(8), 473–477. Reaffirmed 2016. Retrieved from <http://www.cps.ca/en/documents/position/youth-and-firearms>.

Fulkerson, J. A., Neumark-Sztainer, D., Hannan, P., et al. (2008). Family meal frequency and weight status among adolescents: Cross-sectional and 5-year longitudinal associations. *Obesity, 16*(11), 2529–2534.

Golden, N. H., & Attia, E. (2011). Psychopharmacology of eating disorders in children and adolescents. *Pediatric Clinics of North America, 58*(1), 121–138.

Government of Canada. (2016). *Canada's provincial and territorial routine (and catch-up) vaccination programs for infants and children.* Retrieved from <http://healthycanadians.gc.ca/healthy-living-vie-saine/immunization-immunisation/schedule-calendrier/infants-children-vaccination-enfants-nourrissons-eng.php?_ga=1.181545134.868197850.1432519476>.

Government of Canada, Standing Committee on Health. (2007). *Healthy weights for healthy kids*. Ottawa: Parliament of Canada.

Gray, M., & Moore, K. N. (2009). *Urologic disorders: Adult and pediatric care*. St. Louis: Mosby.

Hands Free Info. (2016). *Canadian distracted driving updates*. Retrieved from <http://handsfreeinfo.com/canadian-cell-phone-law-updates/>.

Hanhan, U. A. (2008). The poisoned child in the pediatric intensive care unit. *Pediatric Clinics of North America, 55*(3), 669–686.

Hansen, M. L., Gunn, P. W., & Kaelber, D. C. (2007). Underdiagnosis of hypertension in children and adolescents. *Journal of the American Medical Association, 298*(8), 874–879.

Health Canada. (2011). *Canadian alcohol and drug use monitoring survey*. Ottawa: Author.

Health Canada. (2014). *Environmental and workplace health: Guidelines for tanning salon owners, operators and users*. Retrieved from <http://www.hc-sc.gc.ca/ewh-semt/pubs/radiation/tan-bronzage/index-eng.php#a9>.

Health Canada. (2015a). *Consumer product safety: Cosmetics*. Retrieved from <http://www.hc-sc.gc.ca/cps-spc/cosmet-person/index-eng.php>.

Health Canada. (2015b). *Consumer product update: Health Canada warns of potential risks of tattoo removal products*. Retrieved from <http://healthycanadians.gc.ca/recall-alert-rappel-avis/hc-sc/2015/43873a-eng.php?_ga=1.142748860.868197850.1432519476>.

Herman-Giddens, M. E. (2013). The enigmatic pursuit of puberty in girls. *Pediatrics, 132*(6), 1125–1126. doi:10.1542/peds.2013-3058.

Hoek, H. (2007). Incidence, prevalence and mortality of anorexia and other eating disorders. *Current Opinion in Psychiatry, 19*(4), 389–394.

Hosking, S. G., Young, K. L., & Regan, M. A. (2009). The effects of text messaging on young drivers. *Human Factors, 51*(4), 582–592.

Isbister, G. K., & Kumar, V. V. (2011). Indications for single-dose activated charcoal administration in acute overdose. *Current Opinion in Critical Care, 17*(4), 351–357.

Johnson, J. L., & Oliffe, J. L. (2012). Gender and community health. In L. L. Stamler & L. Yiu (Eds.), *Community health nursing: A Canadian perspective* (3rd ed., pp. 300–310). Toronto: Pearson.

Johnston, L. D., O'Malley, P. M., Miech, R. A., et al. (2015). *Monitoring the future national survey results on drug use: 1975–2014. Overview, key findings on adolescent drug use*. Ann Arbor: Institute for Social Research, University of Michigan. Retrieved from <http://monitoringthefuture.org/pubs/monographs/mtf-overview2014.pdf>.

Kain, J., Corvalán, C., Lera, L., et al. (2009). Accelerated growth in early life and obesity in preschool Chilean children. *Obesity, 17*(8), 1603–1608.

Kanekar, A., & Sharma, M. (2010). Pharmacological approaches for management of child and adolescent obesity. *Journal of Clinical Medicine Research, 2*(3), 105–111.

Kaplowitz, P. B. (2008). Link between body fat and the timing of puberty. *Pediatrics, 121*(Suppl. 3), S208–S217. doi:10.1542/peds.2007-1813F.

Kennedy, B. S., Bedard, B., Younge, M., et al. (2012). Outbreak of *Mycobacterium chelonae* infection associated with tattoo ink. *New England Journal of Medicine, 367*(11), 1020–1024.

Kirmayer, L. J. (2012). Changing patterns in suicide among young people. *Canadian Medical Association Journal, 184*, 1015–1016. doi:10.1503/cmaj.120509.

Kohlberg, L. (1968). Moral development. In D. L. Sills (Ed.), *International encyclopedia of the social sciences*. New York: Macmillan.

Landry, G. L. (2016). Female athletes: Menstrual problems and the risk of osteopenia. In R. M. Kliegman, B. F. Stanton, J. W. St. Geme, et al. (Eds.), *Nelson textbook of pediatrics* (20th ed.). Philadelphia: Saunders.

Langille, D. B., Corbett, E., Wilson, K., et al. (2010). *Determinants of adolescent pregnancy: Factors influencing youth sexual behaviours in a rural Nova Scotia community*. Halifax: Dalhousie University Faculty of Medicine.

LaRosa, C., & Meyers, K. (2010). Epidemiology of hypertension in children and adolescents. *Lebanese Medical Journal, 58*(3), 132–136.

Laws, C. (2005). Youth and firearms in Canada. *Paediatrics & Child Health, 10*(8), 473–477. Reaffirmed 2014.

Lipnowski, S., LeBlanc, C., & Canadian Paediatric Society, Healthy Active Living and Sports Medicine Committee. (2012). Healthy active living: Physical activity guidelines for children and adolescents. *Paediatrics & Child Health, 17*(4), 209–210. Retrieved from <http://www.cps.ca/documents/position/physical-activity-guidelines>.

Lock, J. (2010). Treatment of adolescent eating disorders: Progress and challenges. *Minerva Psychiatrica, 51*(3), 207–216.

Lynne, S. D., Graber, J., Nicols, T. R., et al. (2007). Links between pubertal timing, peer influences and externalizing behaviors among urban students followed through middle school. *Journal of Adolescent Health, 40*(2), 181.e7–181.e13. doi:10.1016/j.jadohealth.2006.09.008.

McCarthy, A., Hughes, R., Tilling, K., et al. (2007). Birth weight; postnatal, infant, and childhood growth; and obesity in young adulthood: Evidence from the Barry Caerphilly Growth Study. *American Journal of Clinical Nutrition, 86*(4), 907–913.

Mental Health Canada. (n.d.). *Children and adolescents with mental, emotional, and behavioural disorders*. Retrieved from <http://mentalhealthcanada.com/ConditionsandDisordersDetail.asp?lang=e&category=70>.

Mental Health Commission of Canada. (2015). *Informing the future: Mental health indicators for Canada*. Retrieved from <http://www.mentalhealthcommission.ca/English/informing-future-mental-health-indicators-canada>.

Na, J., Park, S., Kang, Y., et al. (2014). The clinical significance of serum ferritin in pediatric non-alcoholic fatty liver disease. *Pediatric Gastroenterology, Hepatology & Nutrition, 17*(3), 248–256.

National Eating Disorder Information Centre. (2014). *Definitions*. Retrieved from <http://nedic.ca/know-facts/definitions>.

Neuman, M. E. (2011). Addressing children's beliefs through Fowler's stages of faith. Review. *Journal of Pediatric Nursing, 26*(1), 44–50. doi:10.1016/j.pedn.2009.09.002.

Newman, K., Harrison, L., Dashiff, C., & Davies, S. (2008). Review. Relationships between parenting styles and risk behaviors in adolescent health: An integrative literature. *Revista Latino Americano de Enfermagem, 16*(1), 142–150.

Nobili, V., Vajro, P., Dezsofi, A., et al. (2015). Indications and limitation of bariatric intervention in severely obese children and adolescents with and without non-alcoholic steatohepatitis: The ESPGHAN hepatology committee position statement. *Pediatric Gastroenterology Nutrition Journal, 60*(4), 550–561. doi:10.1097/MPG.0000000000000715.

Nova Scotia Roundtable on Youth Sexual Health. (2011). *Nova Scotia health promotion and protection, guidelines for youth sexual health*. Retrieved from <http://www.pmcs.ca/nova-scotia-health-promotion-and-protection-guidelines-for-youth-sexual-health>.

O'Brien, P. E., Sawyer, S. M., Laurie, C., et al. (2010). Laparoscopic adjustable gastric banding in severely obese adolescents. *Journal of the American Medical Association, 303*(6), 519–526.

O'Keeffe, S. G., & Clarke-Pearson, K. C. (2011). Clinical report: The impact of social media on children, adolescents and families. *Pediatrics, 127*(4), 800–804.

Owens, J., & Committee on Adolescence. (2014). *Insufficient sleep in adolescents and young people: An update on causes and consequences. American Academy of Pediatrics*. Retrieved from <htpp://www.pediatrics.org/cgi/doi/10.1542/peds.2014-1696>.

Owens, J., McLaughlin, S. B., & Sudweeks, J. (2011). Driver performance while text messaging using handheld and in-vehicle systems. *Accident: Analysis and Prevention, 43*(3), 939–947.

Parachute. (n.d.). *Motor vehicle collisions—What can be done?* Retrieved from <http://www.parachutecanada.org/injury-topics/item/motor-vehicle-collisions-what-can-be-done>.

Parliament of Canada, Standing Senate Committee on Social Affairs, Science and Technology. (2006). *Out of the shadows at last. Transforming mental health, mental illness and addiction services in Canada*. Ottawa: Author. Retrieved from <http://www.parl.gc.ca/Content/SEN/Committee/391/soci/rep/rep02may06-e.htm>.

Piaget, J. (1952). *Origins of intelligence in children*. New York: International Universities Press.

Public Health Agency of Canada. (2009). *Child and youth injury in review, 2009 edition—Spotlight on consumer product safety*. Retrieved from <http://phac-aspc.gc.ca/publicat/cyi-bej/2009/index-eng.php>.

Public Health Agency of Canada. (2010). *Questions and answers: Sexual orientation in schools*. Ottawa: Author. Retrieved from <http://sieccan.org/pdf/phac_orientation_qa-eng.pdf>.

Public Health Agency of Canada. (2011a). *Investing in child and youth injury prevention recreation*. Retrieved from <http://www.phac-aspc.gc.ca/about_apropos/evaluation/reports-rapports/2013-2014/asipi-ipbas/index-eng.php>.

Public Health Agency of Canada. (2011b). *Curbing childhood obesity: A federal, provincial and territorial framework for action to promote healthy weights*. Retrieved from <http://www.phac-aspc.gc.ca/hp-ps/hl-mvs/framework-cadre/2011/hw-os-2011-eng.php>.

Public Health Agency of Canada. (2012). *Perinatal health indicators for Canada 2011* (Cat. No. HP7-1/2011). Ottawa: Author.

Public Health Agency of Canada. (2015a). *Publicly funded immunization programs in Canada—Routine schedule for infants and children including special programs and catch-up programs*. Retrieved from <http://www.phac-aspc.gc.ca/im/ptimprog-progimpt/table-1-eng.php>.

Public Health Agency of Canada. (2015b). *Canadian immunization guide*. Retrieved from <http://www.phac-aspc.gc.ca/publicat/cig-gci/index-eng.php>.

Public Agency of Canada. (2016). *Canadian guidelines on sexually transmitted infections*. Retrieved from <http://www.phac-aspc.gc.ca/std-mts/sti-its/>.

Raphael, D. (2010). The health of Canada's children. Part II: Health mechanisms and pathways. *Paediatrics & Child Health, 15*(2), 71–76.

Region of Waterloo, Public Health. (2015). *Youth and smoking*. Retrieved from <http://chd.region.waterloo.on.ca/en/healthylivinghealthprotection/youth-and-smoking.asp>.

Resnicow, K., & McMaster, F. (2012). Motivational Interviewing: Moving from why to how with autonomy support. *International Journal of Behavioral Nutrition and Physical Activity, 2*(9), 19. doi:10.1186/1479-5868-9-19.

Rice, E., Rhoades, H., Winetrobe, H., et al. (2012). Sexually explicit cell phone messaging associated with sexual risk among adolescents. *Pediatrics, 130*(4), 667–673. doi:10.1542/peds.2012-0021.

Roberts, K., Shields, M., de Groh, M., et al. (2012). Overweight and obesity in children and adolescents: Results from the 2009 to 2011 Canadian health measures survey. *Health Reports, 23*(3), 37–41.

Royal Canadian Mounted Police. (2014). *Canadian firearms program*. Retrieved from <http://www.rcmp-grc.gc.ca/cfp-pcaf/information/lic-per-eng.htm>.

Saewyc, E., Homma, Y., Skay, C. L., et al. (2009). Protective factors in the lives of bisexual adolescents in North America. *American Journal of Public Health, 99*(1), 110–117.

Saewyc, E., Poon, C., Wang, N., et al. (2007). *Not yet equal: The health of lesbian, gay, & bisexual youth in BC*. Vancouver: McCreary Centre Society. Retrieved from <http://www.mcs.bc.ca/pdf/not_yet_equal_web.pdf>.

Shain, B., & American Academy of Pediatrics Committee on Adolescence. (2007). Suicide and suicide attempts in adolescents. *Pediatrics, 120*(3), 669–676. doi:10.1542/peds.2007-1908.

Simcoe Muskoka Health Unit. (2015). *Tattooing and piercing: Make it safe*. Retrieved from <http://www.simcoemuskokahealth.org/Topics/SexualHealth/NeedlesSharps/TattooingAndPiercing.aspx>.

Smith, A., Stewart, D., Peled, M., et al. (2009). *A picture of health: Highlights from the 2008 BC Adolescent Health Survey*. Vancouver, BC: McCreary Centre Society.

Stewart, D., Vallance, K., Stockwell, T., et al. (2009). Adolescent substance use and related harms in British Columbia. *CARBC Bulletin 5*. Victoria: University of Victoria, Centre for Addictions Research of BC. Retrieved from <http://www.saravyc.ubc.ca/2009/08/11/stewart-d-vallance-k-stockwell-t-reimber-b-smith-a-reist-d-saewyc-e-2009-adolescent-substance-use-and-related-harms-in-bc-carbc-and-mccreary-centre-society-statistical-bulletin-victoria/>.

Storey, K. E., Forbes, L. E., Fraser, S. N., et al. (2009). Diet quality, nutrition and physical activity among adolescents: The Web-SPAN (Web-Survey of Physical Activity and Nutrition) project. *Public Health Nutrition, 12*(11), 2009–2017. doi:10.1017/S1368980009990292.

Taddeo, D., Stanwick, R., & Canadian Paediatric Society, Adolescent Health Committee. (2012). Banning children and youth under the age of 18 years from commercial tanning facilities. *Paediatrics & Child Health, 17*(2), 89. Reaffirmed 2016. Retrieved from <http://www.cps.ca/en/documents/position/tanning-facilities>.

Temple, J. R., Paul, J. A., van den Berg, P., et al. (2012). Teen sexting and its association with sexual behaviors. *Archives of Pediatric & Adolescent Medicine, 166*(9), 828–833.

Thomas, R., Baker, P., Thomas, B., et al. (2015). Family-based programmes for preventing smoking by children and adolescents (review). *The Cochrane Database of Systematic Reviews*, (2), doi:10.1002/14651858.CD004493.pub3.

Thomas, R., McLellan, J., & Perera, R. (2013). School-based programmes for preventing smoking (review). *The Cochrane Database of Systematic Reviews*, (4), doi:10.1002/14651858.CD001293.pub3.

U.S. Preventive Services Task Force. (2010). Screening for obesity in children and adolescents: U.S. Preventive Services Task Force recommendation statement. *Pediatrics, 125*(2), 361–367.

Wardle, J., Carnell, S., Haworth, C. M., et al. (2008). Evidence for a strong genetic influence on childhood adiposity despite the force of the obesogenic environment. *American Journal of Clinical Nutrition, 87*(2), 398–404.

Waters, S., Cross, D., & Shaw, T. (2010). Does the nature of schools matter? An exploration of selected school ecology factors on adolescent perceptions of school connectedness. *British Journal of Educational Psychology, 80*(Pt3), 381–402. doi:10.1348/000709909X484479.

Whitlock, E., O'Connor, E., Williams, S., et al. (2010). Effectiveness of weight management programs in children: A targeted systematic review for the USPSTF. *Pediatrics, 125*(2), e396–e418.

World Health Organization. (2015). *Sexual Health*. Retrieved from <http://www.who.int/topics/sexual_health/en/>.

Yanchar, N. L., Warda, L. J., Fuseli, P., & Canadian Paediatric Society, Injury Prevention Committee. (2012). Child and youth injury prevention: A public health approach. *Paediatrics & Child Health, 17*(9), 511. Retrieved from <http://www.cps.ca/documents/position/child-and-youth-injury-prevention>.

Young, A. M., Glover, N., & Havens, J. R. (2012). Nonmedical use of prescription medications among adolescents in the United States: A systematic review. *Journal of Adolescent Health, 51*(1), 6–17.

ADDITIONAL RESOURCES

Action Canada for Sexual Health and Rights: <http://www.sexualhealthandrights.ca/>.

Al-Anon Family Groups: <http://al-anon.org/>.

Canadian Cancer Society: Detecting Testicular Cancer: <http://www.cancer.ca/en/prevention-and-screening/early-detection-and-screening/finding-cancer-early/detecting-testicular-cancer/?region=on>.

Canadian Dermatology Association—Sun exposure and sunscreens: <http://www.dermatology.ca/programs-resources/>.

Canadian Mental Health Association—Mental Health: <http://www.cmha.ca/mental-health/>.

Canadian Mental Health Association—Suicide Prevention: <http://www.cmha.ca/mental_health/preventing-suicide/#.VzOE7Y-cHIU>.

Canadian Partnership Against Cancer—Canada Moving Forward With a Unique Approach to Address Childhood Obesity: <http://www.partnershipagainstcancer.ca/canada-moving-forward-with-a-unique-approach-to-address-childhood-obesity/>.

Centers for Disease Control and Prevention: NIOSH Science Blog—Body Art: <http://blogs.cdc.gov/niosh-science-blog/2008/02/body-art/>.

Centre for Addiction and Mental Health: <http://www.camh.ca/en/hospital/Pages/home.aspx>.

Kids Help Phone—24-hour bilingual hotline for children and youth for referral to resources on a variety of issues: 1-800-668-6868; <http://www.kidshelpphone.ca/Teens/Home.aspx>.

MADD Canada (Mothers Against Drunk Driving): <http://www.madd.ca/madd2/>.

National Anti-Drug Strategy: <http://www.healthycanadians.gc.ca/anti-drug-antidrogue/index-eng.php?utm_source=vanity_url&utm_medium=url_en&utm_content=redirect_justice_nationalantidrugstrategy.gc.ca&utm_campaign=pidu_14>.

National Association of Friendship Centres: <http://www.nafc.ca/>.

National Eating Disorder Information Centre: <http://www.nedic.ca/>.

National Institute on Drug Abuse: <http://www.drugabuse.gov/>.

National Youth Solvent Program: <http://www.hc-sc.gc.ca/fniah-spnia/substan/ads/nysap-pnlasj-eng.php>.

Parachute: Preventing Injuries: <http://www.parachutecanada.org/>.

Parents Anonymous: <http://ww2.parentsanon.org/>.

Public Health Agency of Canada—The Canadian Immunization Guide, and schedules for each province and territory: <http://www.phac-aspc.gc.ca/publicat/cig-gci/index-eng.php>.

Public Health Agency of Canada: The Health of Canada's Young People: A Mental Health Focus: <http://www.phac-aspc.gc.ca/hp-ps/dca-dea/publications/health-young-people-sante-jeunes-canadiens/index-eng.php>.

SADD (Students Against Destructive Decisions): <http://www.sadd.org/>.

Sex Information and Education Council of Canada (SIECCAN): <http://www.sieccan.org>.

SexualityandU.ca: <http://www.sexualityandu.ca/>.

Simcoe Muskoka District Health Unit—Tattoo and Body Art: <http://www.simcoemuskokahealth.org/Topics/InfectiousDiseases/BeautyAndBodyArt/TattooPiercingIntroduction.aspx>.

Tough Love: <http://www.toughlove.com>.

UNIT 11

Special Needs, Illness, and Hospitalization

CHAPTER

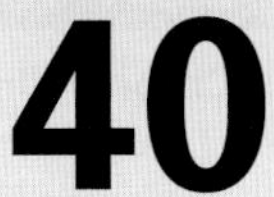

Chronic Illness, Complex Conditions, and End-of-Life Care

Karen Marie Breen-Reid, with contributions from Marilyn J. Hockenberry

evolve WEBSITE

Visit the Evolve website for additional resources related to the content in this chapter such as Case Studies, Critical Thinking Case Study Answers, Nursing Care Plans, Nursing Processes, Nursing Skills, and Review Questions for Exam Preparation at: http://evolve.elsevier.com/Canada/Perry/maternal/

OBJECTIVES

On completion of this chapter the reader will be able to:

- Identify the scope of and changing trends in the care of children with special needs.
- Identify the major reactions of and effects on the family of a child with special needs.
- Define the stages of adjustment to the diagnosis of a chronic or complex medical condition.
- Recognize the impact of the illness or condition on the developmental stages of childhood.
- Outline nursing interventions that promote the family's optimum adjustment to the child's chronic illness or complex condition.
- Outline nursing interventions that support the family at the time of the child's death.
- Define the usual symptoms of grief.

PERSPECTIVES ON THE CARE OF CHILDREN WITH SPECIAL NEEDS

Scope of the Problem

Over the years, a number of terms and defining characteristics have been used to describe chronic illness and complex conditions in children (Box 40-1). More recently researchers have sought to develop a definition that better acknowledges the number of children living with chronic conditions and the impact on health and social services (Strickland, van Dyck, Kogan, et al., 2011). Currently, *children with special health care needs* are defined as children who have or are at increased risk for a chronic physical, developmental, behavioural, or emotional condition and who also require health and related services of a type or amount beyond that generally required by children. Children with chronic illnesses and disability are described as having chronic and complex conditions (Elias, Murphy, & Council on Children with Disabilities, 2012).

Ongoing progress in medical and technological disease management has contributed to the growing number of children with special health care needs. Technological advances have substantially increased the survival of extremely-low- and very-low-birth-weight infants, and Canadian children with chronic and complex conditions have the highest survival rates of all time, with 98% now living to early adulthood. These higher survival rates have led to greater numbers of children with special needs (Carnevale, Rehm, Kirk, et al., 2008). It is estimated that 4% of Canadian children aged 5 to 14 years have a physical or cognitive disability (Statistics Canada, 2008), and approximately 30% of school-age children have a chronic illness (Martinez & Ercikan, 2009). Children with chronic and complex conditions are more likely to be in poorer health than children without disabilities (Halfon & Newacheck, 2010).

The most commonly occurring conditions causing disability are asthma, diabetes, cancer, obesity, unintentional injuries, and mental illness. In Canada, it is estimated that as many as 15% of Canadian children and youth are affected by a mental disorder at any given time. An estimated 29% of Indigenous children on reserve aged 0 to 11 years were reported by a parent or guardian as having behavioural or emotional problems (Public Health Agency of Canada, 2009).

BOX 40-1 COMMON TERMS REGARDING CHILDREN WITH SPECIAL NEEDS

Chronic illness—A long-term condition that interferes with daily functioning and that has lasted or is expected to last 6 months or more (Statistics Canada, 2003)

Congenital anomaly—Also known as birth defects, congenital disorders, or congenital malformations. Congenital anomalies can be defined as structural or functional anomalies (such as metabolic disorders) that occur during intrauterine life and can be identified prenatally, at birth, or later in life (World Health Organization [WHO], 2015).

Developmental delay (applicable to children under 5 years of age)—Child has a delay in his or her development that is either a physical, intellectual, or another type of delay in achieving milestones (Statistics Canada, 2003)

Developmental disability or disorder (applicable to children aged 5 to 14 years of age)—Cognitive limitations due to the presence of a developmental disability, such as Down syndrome, autism, or mental impairment (Statistics Canada, 2003)

Disability—A health problem that has lasted or is expected to last for 6 months or more in which daily activities are limited by long-term conditions, health problems, and task-based difficulties related to seeing, hearing, mobility, flexibility, dexterity, pain, learning, development, mental/psychological issues, or memory (Statistics Canada, 2015)

Handicap—Refers to the social and environmental consequences of an individual's impairment

Life-limiting illness—Any illness or condition developed in childhood whereby the child is likely to die before adulthood or that results in a limited expectation of life thereafter (Danvers, Freshwater, Cheater, et al., 2003). (For more information see Additional Resources section at the end of this chapter.)

Medically complex—A child from birth to 21 years of age with four characteristics: presence of one or more complex chronic conditions that are multisystem and severe; functional limitations that are significant and reliant on technology, such as feeding tubes and tracheostomies; high health care utilization both in the hospital and at home; and use of coordinated care by a specialized interdisciplinary team of health care providers (Dewan & Cohen, 2013)

References

Danvers, L., Freshwater, D., Cheater, F., et al. (2003). Providing seamless service for children with life-limiting illness: Experiences and recommendations of professional staff at the Diana Princess of Wales Children's Community Service. *Journal of Clinical Nursing, 12*(3), 351–359.

Dewan, T., & Cohen, E. (2013). Children with medical complexity in Canada. *Paediatrics & Child Health, 18*(10), 518–522.

Statistics Canada. (2003). *Profile of disability among children.* Retrieved from <http://www.statcan.gc.ca/pub/89-577-x/4065023-eng.htm>.

Statistics Canada. (2015). *Canadian survey on disability, 2012: Concepts and methods guide.* Retrieved from <http://www.statcan.gc.ca/pub/89-654-x/89-654-x2014001-eng.htm>.

World Health Organization. (2015). *Congenital anomalies.* Retrieved from <http://www.who.int/mediacentre/factsheets/fs370/en/>.

These children require specialized health care of a type or amount beyond that generally required by children with no disability. To help provide this care, nurses are moving into highly specialized community roles and families are requiring continuous support and training, as these children usually receive their care in home settings.

The impact of chronic and complex conditions in children is wide ranging. For some families, the impact is minimal but for many other families, chronic conditions in children present families with additional tasks, responsibilities, and concerns. A child's activity level and developmental opportunities can be affected. Days can be lost from school. Children with chronic illness and complex conditions may be at increased risk for behavioural or emotional problems. Parents may lose days from work, experience financial and relationship strains, and be challenged both emotionally and physically as they cope with care of the child.

Families who have children with special needs and who live in rural or remote locations in Canada have the additional stressors of trying to access services that are far away or obtain resources and assistance within their own communities (Hoogsteen & Woodgate, 2013; Skinner & Slifkim, 2007). In Canada, nearly 9 million Canadians live in rural or remote areas where the availability of community resources is often limited (Health Canada, 2008). Strategies that have been recommended to address this issue include building partnerships to optimize local resources and build capacity; mobilizing systems integration by accessing resources outside the community; and using technology to train, provide guidance, and support family caregivers and health care teams (Canadian Home Care Association, 2006). Two options available to families living in rural or remote areas are to travel to a major health care facility and attempt to coordinate all appointments in a clustered approach (which may not be an option for children with more severe disabilities and multiple services involved) or to access travelling services such as satellite clinics from specialty hospitals. A third option, which many families are forced to do, is to move closer to an urban centre, given the difficulties of getting services otherwise.

Siblings are also affected by having a "different" brother or sister and may simultaneously feel guilt and anger or jealousy toward their ill sibling. Additionally, they may suffer secondary losses such as the ability to participate in extracurricular activities or social events because of routines imposed by the affected child's chronic condition (Emerson & Giallo, 2014).

Trends in Care

Developmental Focus

In focusing on the child's developmental level rather than the **chronological age** or diagnosis, the child's abilities and strengths are emphasized, rather than disabilities. Attention is directed toward normalizing experiences, adapting the environment, and promoting **coping** skills. Nurses are often in vital positions to redirect efforts away from the pathological model, with its focus on weaknesses and problems, and toward the developmental model to meet the unique needs of the child and family.

A developmental focus also considers family development. The life cycle of the family unit reflects changing ages and needs of family members, as well as changing external demands. A family member's serious illness or disability can cause significant stress or crisis at any stage of the family life cycle. Just as with individual development, family development may be interrupted or even regress to an earlier level of functioning. Nurses can use the concept of family development to plan meaningful interventions and to evaluate care (see Chapter 2).

Family-Centred Care

Children's physical and emotional health, as well as cognitive and social functioning, is strongly influenced by how well their families function. The importance of family-centred care—a philosophy that considers the family as the constant in the child's life—is especially evident in the care of children with special needs. As parents learn about the youngster's health care needs, they often become experts in delivering care. Health care providers, including nurses, are adjuncts to the child's care and need to form partnerships with parents. Through these partnerships the parents are integral in communicating the child's "normal" responses and actions to assist the health care team. Effective communication and negotiation between parents and nurses are essential to forming trusting and effective partnerships and finding the best ways to meet the needs of the child and family (Giambra, Stiffler, & Broome, 2014). Collaborative relationships are characterized by communication, dialogue, active listening, awareness, and acceptance of differences.

The role of culture in family-centred care. Issues related to culture, ethnicity, and race can affect access to services, utilization, and follow-through with referrals and recommendations (Strickland et al., 2011). For some ethnic and minority populations, cultural understandings of illness and disability, structure of family life, social roles for individuals who are disabled, and other factors related to the perception of children may differ from those of mainstream North American culture. These factors may affect family needs and family choices regarding the care of their child with special needs.

Although culture cannot completely explain how an individual will think and act, an understanding of cultural perspectives can help the nurse anticipate and comprehend why families may make certain decisions. Cultural attributes can affect a family's response to the child's illness or disability; these include values and beliefs regarding illness or disability and its cause, social roles for the ill or disabled person, family structure, the role of children, and spirituality (Gerlach, 2008; Grossoehme, Ragsdale, Cotton, et al., 2010).

When parents not fluent in the health care provider's language are informed of their child's chronic illness, interpreters familiar with both cultures and languages should be used during clinic visits and hospitalization. Children, family members, and friends of the family should not be used as translators because their presence may prevent parents from openly discussing the issues, or they may not be able to accurately translate the medical terminology used or the meaning of what the health care provider is trying to relay. When nurses are working with people of cultural backgrounds different from their own, nurses must listen carefully and take into account their own constructs of bias and belief, with an initial goal of understanding and articulating the family's perspective (see Chapter 2). The ability to interpret mainstream medical culture to the family is also important. Furthermore, every effort should be made to incorporate a family's traditional cultural beliefs into the treatment plans. Developing a care plan in conjunction with the family that considers their preferences and priorities is an important first step in formulating a plan that best meets the family's needs (Daudji, Eby, Foo, et al., 2011).

Faith traditions, beliefs, and practices. It is important for the nurse to discuss with the family their faith and to ask whether or how they would like their religious beliefs and practices integrated into the child's care. Most religions have common rituals and traditions regarding illness and death, but every family has their own perspective on how they would like their faith practised. Table 40-1 outlines such beliefs and rituals

TABLE 40-1 FAITH TRADITIONS, BELIEFS, AND PRACTICES REGARDING ILLNESS, DYING, AND DEATH

RELIGION	ILLNESS AND DEATH RITES AND RITUALS
Buddhism*	Family presence is important. May chant mantras as infant or child becomes seriously ill The child's body should not be touched after death. Family may take the body home to prepare it for burial. The body should not be moved for 8 hours after death.
Catholicism†	Sacrament of the sick with anointing of oil, communion, and final blessing by priest
Hinduism*	It is ideal to be surrounded by family and friends who sing sacred hymns and say prayers or chant the dying person's mantra. When death is near, the family spiritual leader is asked to conduct final rites. The body should be as close to the ground as possible to help the soul absorb into the ground.
Islam*	Body is washed three times Muslim burial performed within 24 hours Cremation forbidden
Judaism†	Prayers for the sick No cremation Living person always with body after death Burial as soon after death as possible
Protestantism‡	Variable; may include prayer, anointing body with oil, communion, laying on of hands, final blessing Family presence may be important.

Modified from Wiener, L., McConnell, D. G., Latella, L., Ludi, E. (2013). Cultural and religious considerations in pediatric palliative care. *Palliative Support Care, 11*(1), 47–67. Reproduced with permission.
*Kongnetiman, L., Lai, B., & Berg, B. (2008). Cultural competency in palliative care: A literature review. Alberta: Alberta Health Services. Retrieved from http://fcrc.albertahealthservices.ca/publications/cultural/Cultural-Competency-in-Palliative-Paediatric-Care-Literature-Review.pdf
†Pulchalski, C. M., Dorff, R. E., & Hendi, I. Y. (2004). Religion, spirituality, and healing in palliative care. *Clinics in Geriatric Medicine, 20*, 689–714.
‡Johnson, C. J., & McGee, M. (1998). *How different religions view death and afterlife.* Philadelphia: The Charles Press.

of the major faith traditions. The table is meant to be a guide only as every family needs to be approached on an individual basis for their preferences.

Family–health care provider communication. Disclosure of a child's serious, acute, or chronic illness is one of the most stressful aspects of communication between families and health care providers. Often, parents have suspected for some time that something is wrong with their child and believe that their concerns were minimized or ignored by health care providers. Parents may not be satisfied with the way in which the information is given. The communication may have been flawed by unsympathetic and brief diagnostic interviews, a lack of privacy during diagnostic discussions, and lack of opportunity for the parents to ask questions. Conversely, parents report satisfaction when they perceive health care providers to be giving information in an open and honest manner with respect for the parents' need for privacy and time to express emotions and ask questions.

Providing information to families with a chronically ill child should be a process of repeated discussions, to enable the family to process the information and their reactions to that information and allow them to ask for clarification and further information. Nurses play an important role in ensuring that families' needs are met during discussions related to a child's diagnosis, condition, and treatment. The family should be assessed regarding how much information they are comfortable with, what they understand of the information already given to them, and how they are coping with the information, both cognitively and emotionally. Nurses should ensure that the appropriate health care providers address any concerns or further questions that the family may have (Young, Eden, Hill, et al., 2012).

Establishing therapeutic relationships. Another important aspect of family-centred care of chronically ill children is establishing a therapeutic relationship with the child and family, which can improve health-related outcomes. Families, most often the mother, take on enormous responsibility in providing technical care and symptom management of their child's condition outside the health care institution. To build a successful therapeutic relationship with a family, the nurse needs to recognize the parents' level of experience in understanding their child's condition and meeting his or her needs, and the parents need to recognize the nurse's expertise as a collaborative partner. Care conferences, especially interdisciplinary meetings that include family members and key health care providers as the centre of the care team, provide an opportunity for sharing ideas and information and for expressing feelings or concerns (Kratz, Uding, Trahms, et al., 2009).

Shared Decision Making

Shared decision making among the child, family, and health care team can result from open, honest, culturally sensitive communication and the establishment of a therapeutic relationship between the family and health care providers. In a shared decision-making model, the health care providers provide honest, clear information regarding the diagnosis, prognosis, treatment options, and risk–benefit assessment. The patient and family share information with the health care team about important family values, acceptable levels of discomfort or inconvenience, and their ability to adhere to treatments being recommended (Kon, 2010; Kratz et al., 2009). This process allows them to discuss all options in terms of the risks and benefits to the child and family, the prognosis or expected course of the illness, and the impact on the family's resources (Box 40-2). Together the parents and health care team can make decisions that are best for the family and child (Kon, 2010).

BOX 40-2 FACILITATING SHARED DECISION MAKING

- Continually assess the impact of the child's illness and treatment on the family.
- Provide honest, accurate information regarding the trajectory of the disease, anticipated complications, and prognostic information.
- Discuss what the family desires for the child's quality of life.
- Avoid personal opinion or judgement of the family's questions and decisions.
- Be aware of nurses' personal and cultural assumptions and the ways these assumptions impact communication, decision making, and judgement.

Normalization

Normalization refers to the efforts that family members make to create a normal family life, their perceptions of the consequences of these efforts, and the meanings they attribute to their management efforts (Knafl, Darney, Gallo, et al., 2010). For chronically ill children, such behaviours could include attending school, pursuing hobbies and recreational interests, and achieving employment and a level of independence. For their families, it may entail adapting the family routine to accommodate the ill or disabled child's health and physical needs. Children with chronic illness and complex conditions and their families face numerous challenges in achieving normalization. Families move between the "normal" of living with the experience of chronic childhood illness and the "normal" of the outside world; they often redefine "normal" on the basis of their particular experiences, needs, and circumstances. Normalization may be an important mediator of illness-related stressors (e.g., treatment demands, uncertainty) on family outcomes.

Nurses can assist families in normalizing their lives by assessing the family's everyday life, social support systems, coping strategies, family cohesiveness, and family and community resources. Interventions could include encouraging families to reduce stress through delegation of care and family tasks, identifying ways to incorporate care into current routines, structuring the home environment to foster the child's engagement in age-appropriate activities, and ensuring that families have access to appropriate community support services (Spalding & Salib, 2008).

Home care represents the return to a system and set of priorities in which a family's values are as important in the care of a child with a chronic health problem as they are in the care of other children (Spalding & Salib, 2008). To best partner with families of children with special health care needs, health care providers need to understand the family environment and challenges of managing a medical environment in the home. One way to educate health care providers about the unique needs these families have is to invite parents to serve as guest faculty in classes on family-centred care. This approach helps health care providers learn from those who know the children and their needs best (Kube, Bishop, Roth, et al., 2013). The goals for home care include the following:

- Normalize the life of a child with special needs, including those with technologically complex care, in a family and community context and setting
- Minimize the disruptive impact of the child's condition on the family
- Foster the child's maximum growth and development

Paralleling normalization and home care can be the process of *mainstreaming*, or integrating children with special needs into regular classrooms. Just as the home is the natural environment for children, the school must also be included as an essential component of children's overall physical, intellectual, and social development. Children who attend school have the advantages of learning and socializing with a wide group of peers. There is an increased focus on individualization as plans are made to meet the academic needs of these children along with those of the rest of the students.

A variety of supplemental programs have been designed in school systems to accommodate the special needs of children of school age and younger through *early intervention*. These programs consist of any sustained and systematic effort to assist children from birth to age 3 years who are disabled and developmentally vulnerable. These programs, as well as increasing opportunities for normalization for children with special needs, resulted in large part from examination of the *Charter of Rights and Freedoms*; Canada signed the United Nations *Convention on the Rights of the Child* on May 28, 1990, and ratified it on December 13, 1991 (United Nations, 1989). The *Charter* continues to be used as a basis for supporting children with disabilities. Each province and territory has different laws that govern education and health care for children. It is important for nurses to be aware of the laws within their jurisdiction and how these laws might affect their patients. Nurses can provide parents with information about the relevant laws and rights and, in some cases, may participate in the development of individualized educational programs (IEPs) or individualized family service plans for children with special needs.

Coordinated Care

It can be challenging for parents and other caregivers of children with special health care needs to coordinate the many professionals, programs, and agencies that may be involved with their child's care (Doig, McLennan, & Urichuk, 2009; Woodgate, Edwards, Ripat, et al., 2015). The assistance of a knowledgeable case manager or service coordinator can ease the stress of navigating the various systems. In Canada there are three major issues facing children and youth who need home care: (1) lack of specialized pediatric professionals; (2) lack of timely access to services, which can result in long waits for treatment; and (3) integration of these complex services (Hollander & Prince, 2008; Spalding & Salib, 2008). Nurses can play a key role in helping families access the appropriate services in a way that causes as little disruption in health care as possible—for example, clustering appointments with different services at a health care facility on the same day to avoid multiple visits for routine care.

THE FAMILY OF THE CHILD WITH A CHRONIC OR COMPLEX CONDITION

A major goal in working with the family of a child with a chronic or complex illness is to support the family's effective coping and promote their optimal functioning throughout the child's life. Long-term, comprehensive, family-centred approaches extend beyond supporting the child and family during only the critical periods of diagnosis and hospitalization. Rather, comprehensive care involves forming parent–health care provider partnerships that can support a family's adaptation to the many changes that may be necessary in day-to-day life. This includes ongoing reassessment and reviewing and adjusting expectations of and for the child while providing continued support based on the child's strengths and abilities.

The impact of a child's medical or developmental condition is often experienced over time, initially as a crisis at the time of diagnosis, which may occur at birth, after a long period of physical or psychological testing, or immediately after a tragic injury or illness. The impact may also be felt before the diagnosis is made, when parents are aware that something is wrong with their child but before receiving medical confirmation of the condition.

The diagnosis and initial discharge home can be a critical time for parents. Several factors can make it difficult, including a long duration of uncertainty in the diagnostic process, negative perceptions of chronic illness and complex conditions, insufficient information, and lack of trust between parents and their child's health care team (Nuutila & Salanterä, 2006). Parental feelings of shock, helplessness, isolation, fear, and depression are common (Nuutila & Salanterä, 2006). Throughout the first year, parents may struggle to accept the child's diagnosis and care needs and the uncertainty of the future. The provision of explicit and uncomplicated information to parents using an empathic approach yields more positive outcomes with the development of a collaborative relationship. Providing optimal support at the time of diagnosis and initial discharge home includes assessment of the family's daily routine, living conditions, background knowledge, skills and abilities, and coping behaviours, and evaluation of the family's understanding of the information. It is also necessary to reassess parental needs for information and support on a routine basis.

Impact of the Child's Chronic Illness and Complex Conditions

Each member of a family who has a child with special needs is affected by the experience. The effects on the parents and their

BOX 40-3 ANTICIPATED PARENTAL STRESS POINTS

Diagnosis of the condition—Parents require considerable education while dealing with an emotional response.

Developmental milestones—Times that children normally achieve walking, talking, and self-care are delayed or impossible for the child.

Start of schooling—Particularly stressful are situations in which appropriate schooling will not be in a regular class placement.

Reaching the ultimate attainment—Parents must deal with difficult situations, such as realizing that ambulation will be impossible or that the child will not learn to read.

Adolescence—Issues such as sexuality and independence become prominent.

Future placement—Decisions about placement must be made when the child becomes an adult or when the parents can no longer care for the child.

Death of the child—Parents coping with the death of a child can suffer enormous loss with physical and psychological effects, including higher levels of depression.

responses are so critical that they directly influence the other members' reactions and the child's own coping.

Parents

Parents may grieve for the loss of the child they expected. Many parents of children with special needs feel satisfaction and fulfillment from their role as parents. For others, parenting may be a series of unrewarding experiences that contribute to feelings of inadequacy and failure (Box 40-3). These responses may be most evident in the parents who are most responsible for the child's care. Parents may become preoccupied with their ability to carry out certain procedures, overlooking the child's personal comfort and satisfaction or failing to offer praise for anything less than perfect cooperation or performance. They may pursue a frustrating activity until they achieve "success"—long after the child has become irritable and uncooperative. Parents can become caught in a pattern of interaction that is mutually unrewarding and minimally productive. For these parents, several strategies may be helpful: education regarding what can reasonably be expected of their child, assistance in identifying the child's strengths, praise for a parental job well done, and respite care so that parents can renew their energy.

Parental roles. Parenting a child with a complex chronic condition requires much more than raising a typical child. In addition to attending to the routine aspects of parenting, parents of chronically ill children take on the added responsibility of performing complex technical care and symptom management, advocating for their child, and seeking and coordinating health and social services for their ill or disabled child. These added responsibilities must then be balanced with the needs of other family members and friends and with personal health and obligations, to minimize consequences to the overall functioning of the family (Woodgate et al., 2015). Enormous demands may be placed on parental time, energy, and financial resources.

Often one parent or partner remains at home to manage existing family responsibilities while the other remains with the ill child in the hospital or other care facility. The partner who is not included in the caregiving activities may feel neglected because all of the attention is directed toward the child. The partner may feel resentful that he or she is not sufficiently informed to be competent in the child's care. Without active participation in the child's care, this parent has little appreciation of the time and energy involved in performing these activities. When this partner does attempt to participate, the other parent may criticize the less skillful efforts. As a result, communication and support for one another can be adversely affected.

The nurse can assist parents in avoiding role conflicts by providing anticipatory guidance early on in the child's illness. Teaching should address stressors often identified as having an impact on the marriage: (1) the burden of care at home assumed by primarily one parent, (2) the financial burden, (3) the fear of the child dying, (4) pressure from relatives, (5) the hereditary nature of the disease (if applicable), (6) fear that the parents may become ill and unable to care for their child, and (7) fear of pregnancy. Other causes of tension may centre on the inconveniences associated with care, such as long waits for an appointment, lack of parking (or available handicapped parking) near care facilities, or lack of affordable overnight accommodations. Certainly, these last stressors are within health care providers' domain to try to minimize.

Mother–father differences. Mothers and fathers or partners in the same family often adjust and cope differently as parents of a child with special needs. Some mothers experience a periodic crisis pattern, whereas most fathers tend to experience a steady, gradual recovery. Some research suggests that mothers of children with certain conditions may be more susceptible to psychological distress and fatigue than fathers. Frequently, mothers are the primary caregivers and are more likely than fathers to give up their job to care for their child, which can result in their social isolation. It can be hard for mothers to get out of the house because of the difficulty in finding alternative caregivers. Also, travelling with the child may require extensive equipment, and there may be physical-access barriers. Some mothers may not have a social network of people who can help with child care, adding to their feelings of isolation.

The father of a child with special needs may struggle with issues that are distinct from those of the mother. He may think that his role of protector is challenged because he does not know how to help and cannot protect the family from the seemingly overwhelming recurring problems. With today's increased emphasis on fathers' involvement in the lives of their children, this vulnerability is felt more profoundly than in the past. Extensive stresses in the family can leave the father feeling depressed, weak, guilty, powerless, isolated, embarrassed, and angry. Fearful that he will lose control or be viewed as weak or ineffectual, the father will often hide feelings and display an outward confidence that may lead others to believe that everything is fine. Fathers may worry about what the future holds for their children, their ability to manage the increasing financial burden, and the daily disruptions of the entire family (Swallow, Macfadyen, Santacroce, et al., 2012). Some fathers escape in their work as a means of dulling the pain. Common coping strategies tend to be problem oriented and include praying, getting information, looking at options, and weighing choices, in addition to withdrawal (Gerlach, 2008).

Lone-parent families. Lone-parent families are of special concern. As the only parent of a child who may require extensive, sophisticated, and lifelong care, lone parents may feel an enormous burden. Available financial and emotional resources may already be stretched to the limit. A special effort should be made to assist lone parents in finding financial and support services that can ease the burden of care. Lone parents often have fewer opportunities to get involved in community and outside activities, contributing to diminished support networks and feelings of social isolation. This and the burden of care can lead to negative physiological effects further increasing stress responses when caring for a child with special needs (Brown, Wiener, Kupst, et al., 2008). Nurses can involve social workers and assist in seeking out support options, such as online support networks, for the lone parent. Nurses can also assist the lone parent in identifying helping roles that may be acceptable to relatives and friends.

Siblings

Results of studies on how siblings are affected by having a brother or sister with special needs are mixed (Dykens, 2015; Emerson & Giallo, 2014). Generally, the evidence indicates a negative effect on siblings of children with a chronic illness when compared with siblings of healthy children (Gold, Treadwell, Weissman, et al., 2011). More recently, this effect has appeared to decrease in significance—most likely because of changes in public attitudes toward the ill and disabled. Newer research has shown that being a sibling of a child with special needs can have a positive impact on the sibling's life, in being generally more mature and independent and accepting of individual differences. For example, a literature review indicated that siblings of children with Down syndrome were well adjusted to living with their siblings. By contrast, results on the adjustment of siblings of children with cancer and autism were mixed. Siblings of children with chronic illness or disability also report depression and anxiety more often than peers with no ill siblings, and they can experience guilt at not having their sibling's condition. A number of factors increase the risk of negative effects for siblings of ill children. Responsibility for caregiving, differential treatment by parents, and decreased family resources and recreational time are often the experience of siblings of chronically ill or disabled children (Emerson & Giallo, 2014) (Box 40-4). Thus being mindful of the potential harmful effects that some siblings can experience, health care providers need to provide interventions that support siblings' physical and emotional well-being (O'Brien, Duffy, & Nicholl, 2009).

An important factor in a sibling's adjustment to and coping with a brother's or sister's illness or complex condition is receiving adequate information about the condition. Siblings may be worried about what the disability or condition means and wonder if they can "catch it." They can also worry about how their sibling will fare in the future. While parents are usually in the best position to impart information, they are often overwhelmed with the medical crisis at hand. Nurses can encourage parents to talk with the siblings about how they perceive their sick brother or sister and to be accepting of the siblings' feelings. Nurses can also be educators and counsellors of siblings during the course of their brother's or sister's illness.

Coping With Ongoing Stress and Periodic Crises

Health care providers can help families cope with stress by providing anticipatory guidance and emotional support, assisting the family in assessing and identifying specific stressors, aiding the family in developing coping mechanisms and problem-solving strategies, and working collaboratively with parents so that they become empowered in the process (Anderson & Davis, 2011).

Concurrent Stresses Within the Family

The ability to deal with the overwhelming stress of a lifelong disability or illness is challenged further when additional stresses are present. Stressors may be situational or developmental. They may be related to marital difficulties, sibling needs, homelessness, or social isolation. Even relatively minor stressors, such as arranging care for siblings, managing the home, and travelling to distant treatment centres, can challenge a family's ability to cope successfully.

Most families, regardless of their income or insurance coverage, have financial concerns. The costs of caring for a child with special needs can be overwhelming. Nurses and social workers can help a family review options for financial assistance, including insurance and other financial resources, disease-related associations and support groups, and local philanthropic organizations.

Coping Mechanisms

Coping mechanisms are behaviours aimed at reducing the tension caused by a crisis. *Approach behaviours* are coping mechanisms that result in movement toward adjustment and resolution of the crisis. *Avoidance behaviours* result in movement away from adjustment and represent maladaptation to the crisis. Several approach and avoidance behaviours used in coping with a chronic or complex condition are listed in the Guidelines box. Each behaviour must be viewed in the context of all of the variables affecting the family. For example, the observation of several avoidance behaviours in an emotionally healthy family with a solid support system may denote significantly less risk to the successful resolution of the crisis than an equal number of avoidance behaviours in an individual who has few available supports.

Parental Empowerment

Empowerment can be seen as a process of recognizing, promoting, and enhancing competence. For parents of children with chronic conditions, empowerment may occur gradually as strength and capabilities are drawn on to master the child's care, manage family life, and plan for the future. Advocating for the

BOX 40-4 SUPPORTING SIBLINGS OF CHILDREN WITH SPECIAL NEEDS

Promote Healthy Sibling Relationships

- Value each child individually and avoid comparisons. Remind each child of his or her positive qualities and contribution to other family members.
- Help siblings see the differences and similarities between themselves and the child with special needs. Create a climate in which children can achieve successes without feeling guilty.
- Teach siblings ways to interact with the child.
- Seek to be fair in terms of discipline, attention, and resources; require the affected child to do as much for himself or herself as possible.
- Let siblings settle their own differences; intervene only to prevent siblings from hurting one another.
- Legitimize reasonable anger. Even children with special needs behave badly sometimes.
- Respect a sibling's reluctance to be with or to include the child with special needs in activities.

Help Siblings Cope

- Listen to siblings to let them know that their thoughts and suggestions are valued.
- Praise siblings when they have been patient, have sacrificed, or have been particularly helpful. Do not expect them to always act in this manner.
- Acknowledge the personal strengths that siblings have and their ability to cope with stress successfully.
- Provide age-appropriate information about the child's condition and update it when appropriate.
- Let teachers know what is happening so they can be understanding and helpful.
- Recognize special stress times for siblings and plan to minimize negative effects.
- Schedule special time with siblings; have a friend or family member substitute when the parent is unavailable.
- Encourage siblings to join or help establish a sibling support group.
- Use the services of professionals when needed. If parent thinks that such a service is necessary, it should be provided in as vigorous a manner as a service for the child with special needs.

Involve Siblings

- Seek out ways to realistically include siblings in the care and treatment of the child with special needs.
- Limit caregiving responsibilities and give recognition when siblings perform them.
- Develop a library of children's books on special needs.
- Invite siblings to attend meetings to develop plans for the child with special needs (e.g., individualized educational program, individualized family service plan).
- Discuss future plans with the siblings.
- Solicit their ideas on treatment and service needs.
- Have them visit professionals who work with the child.
- Help them develop competencies to teach the child new skills.
- Provide opportunities for siblings to advocate for the child.
- Allow siblings to set their own pace for learning and involvement.

Data from Powell, T., & Ogle, P. (1985). *Brothers and sisters—A special part of exceptional families.* Baltimore: Paul H. Brooks; Spokane Washington Deaconess Medical Center, Pediatric Oncology Unit. (1987). Tips for dealing with siblings. *Candlelighters Childhood Cancer Foundation—A Newsletter, 11*(3,4), 7; Carlson, J., Leviton, A., & Mueller, M. (1993). Services to siblings: An important component of family-centered practice, *Association for the Care of Children's Health Advocate, 1*(1), 53–56.

GUIDELINES

Assessing Coping Behaviours

Approach Behaviours

- Asks for information regarding diagnosis and child's present condition
- Seeks help and support from others
- Anticipates future problems; actively seeks guidance and answers
- Endows the illness or disability with meaning
- Shares burden of disorder with others
- Plans realistically for the future
- Acknowledges and accepts child's awareness of diagnosis and prognosis
- Expresses feelings such as sorrow, depression, and anger and realizes reason for the emotional reaction
- Realistically perceives child's condition; adjusts to changes
- Recognizes own growth through passage of time, such as earlier denial and nonacceptance of diagnosis
- Verbalizes possible loss of child

Avoidance Behaviours

- Fails to recognize seriousness of child's condition despite physical evidence
- Refuses to agree to treatment
- Intellectualizes about the illness, but in areas unrelated to child's condition
- Is angry and hostile to members of the staff, regardless of their attitude or behaviour
- Avoids staff, family members, or child
- Entertains unrealistic future plans for child, with little emphasis on the present
- Is unable to adjust to or accept a change in progression of the disease
- Continually looks for new cures with no perspective toward possible benefit
- Refuses to acknowledge child's understanding of disease and prognosis
- Uses magical thinking and fantasy; may seek "occult" help
- Places complete faith in religion to point of relinquishing own responsibility
- Withdraws from outside world; refuses help
- Punishes self because of guilt and blame
- Makes no change in lifestyle to meet needs of other family members
- Resorts to excessive use of alcohol or drugs to avoid problems
- Expresses suicidal intent
- Is unable to discuss possible loss of child or previous experiences with death

child and developing parent–professional partnerships are part of the promotion of empowerment. Families of children with special health care needs want to be active members of the health care team and to be actively engaged in decision making. Nurses can ensure that they are included in meetings related to their child's care and in all aspects of their child's care as they are able (Kratz et al., 2009; LeGrow, Hodnett, Stremler, et al., 2014).

Parents of children with complex medical conditions are very aware of their child's needs and should be included in making all decisions for their child. In addition, studies have shown that health care providers can learn much from listening and partnering with parents in the planning and provision of health care for children with disabilities (Kube et al., 2013).

Helping Family Members in Managing Their Feelings

Although previous research has postulated stages of adaptation to a chronic or complex condition, there is a great deal of variation in individuals' responses to the child's diagnosis, in the adjustments they make, and in the time frame for coming to terms with a diagnosis. It is important that health care providers recognize and respect a wide range of reactions and coping mechanisms. In fact, members of the family of a child with a complex chronic condition may experience a number of difficult emotions, including fear, guilt, anger, resentment, and anxiety. Learning to manage these emotions promotes adaptive coping (see Guidelines box). Support from health care providers, other family members, and friends can assist family members in managing their feelings. The following discussion examines some common phases of adjustment and emotional reactions.

Shock and Denial

The initial diagnosis of a chronic illness or complex condition is often met with intense emotion and is characterized by shock, disbelief, and sometimes **denial**, especially if the disorder is not obvious, as in chronic illness. Denial as a defence mechanism is necessary to prevent disintegration and is a normal response to grieving for any type of loss. Probably all family members experience various degrees of adaptive denial as they learn of the impact that the diagnosis has and will have on their lives.

Shock and denial can last from days to months, sometimes even longer. Examples of denial that may be exhibited at the time of diagnosis include the following:

- Health care provider shopping
- Attributing the symptoms of the actual illness to a minor condition
- Refusing to believe the diagnostic tests
- Delaying consent for treatment
- Acting happy and optimistic despite the revealed diagnosis
- Refusing to tell or talk to anyone about the condition
- Insisting that no one is telling the truth regardless of others' attempts to do so
- Denying the reason for admission
- Asking no questions about the diagnosis, treatment, or prognosis

Generally, these mechanisms should be respected as short-term responses that allow individuals to distance themselves from the emotional impact of the news and to collect and mobilize their energies toward goal-directed, problem-solving behaviours.

In children, the importance of denial has repeatedly been demonstrated as a factor in their positive coping with the diagnosis. Denial allows the child to maintain hope in the face of overwhelming odds and to function adaptively and productively. Like hope, denial may be an adaptive mechanism for dealing with loss that persists until a family or patient is ready for or needs other responses.

Denial is probably the least understood and most poorly dealt-with reaction. Health care providers typically label denial as maladaptive and act inappropriately by attempting to strip it away by giving repeated and sometimes blunt explanations of the prognosis. Denial becomes maladaptive only when it prevents recognition of treatment or rehabilitative goals necessary for the child's optimal survival or development.

Anger

Other common and normal reactions to a diagnosis are bitterness and anger. Anger directed inward may be evident as self-reproaching or punitive behaviour, such as neglecting one's health and verbally degrading oneself. Anger directed outward may be manifested in either open arguments or withdrawal from communication and may be evident in the person's relationship with the spouse, the child, and siblings. Passive anger toward the ill child may be evident in decreased hospital visiting, refusal to believe how sick the child is, or an inability to provide comfort. Among the more common targets for parental anger are members of the health care staff. Parents may complain about the nursing care, the insufficient time physicians spend with them, or the lack of skill of those who draw blood or start intravenous infusions.

Children are likely to respond with anger as well, and this includes the affected child and the well siblings. Children are aware of the loss engendered by their illness or disability and may react angrily to the restrictions imposed or the feelings of being different. Siblings may also feel anger and resentment toward the ill child and the parents for the loss of routine and parental attention. This anger may be directed at parents, the ill child, or at school, such as acting out in class. It is difficult for older children and almost impossible for younger children to comprehend the plight of the affected child. Their perception is of a brother or sister who has the undivided attention of their parents, is showered with cards and gifts, and is the focus of everyone's concern.

Adjustment

For most families, adjustment gradually follows shock and is usually characterized by an open admission that the condition exists. This stage may be accompanied by several responses, which are normal parts of the adaptation process. Probably the most universal of these feelings are guilt and self-accusation. Guilt is often greatest when the cause of the disorder is directly traceable to the parent, as in genetic diseases or accidental injury. It can occur even without any scientific or realistic basis for parental responsibility. Frequently the guilt stems from a false assumption that the illness is a result of personal failure or wrongdoing, such as not doing something correctly during the pregnancy or birth. Guilt may also be associated with cultural or religious beliefs. Some parents are convinced that they are being punished for some previous misdeed. Others may see the disorder as a test of their religious strength and faith. With correct information, support, and time, most parents master guilt and self-accusation. The ability to master resentful and self-accusatory feelings of having "caused" the child's disorder is a crucial factor in determining the parents' acceptance of their child.

Children, too, may interpret their serious illness as retribution for past misbehaviour. The nurse should be particularly sensitive to the child who passively accepts all painful procedures. This child may believe that such acts are inflicted as deserved punishment. It is vital that parents and health care providers reassure children that their illness is not their fault.

During the period of adjustment, four types of parental reactions to the child influence the child's eventual response to the disorder:

1. Overprotection, in which the parents fear letting the child achieve any new skill, avoid all discipline, and cater to every desire to prevent frustration (Box 40-5)
2. Rejection, in which the parents detach themselves emotionally from the child but usually provide adequate physical care or constantly nag and scold the child
3. Denial, in which parents act as if the disorder does not exist or attempt to have the child overcompensate for it
4. Gradual acceptance, in which parents place necessary and realistic restrictions on the child, encourage self-care activities, and promote reasonable physical and social abilities

Reintegration and Acknowledgement

For many families the adjustment process culminates in the development of realistic expectations for the child and reintegration of family life with the illness or disability in a manageable perspective. Because a large portion of this phase is one of grief for a loss, total resolution is not possible until the child dies or leaves home as an independent adult. Therefore, one can regard adjustment as "increased comfort" with everyday living rather than a complete resolution.

This adjustment phase also involves social reintegration in which the family broadens its activities to include relationships outside the home, with the child as an accepted and participating member of the group. This last criterion often differentiates the reaction of gradual acceptance during the adjustment period from total acceptance, or perhaps is more descriptive of the acknowledgement process.

Many parents of children with chronic illnesses experience **chronic sorrow**, feelings of sorrow and loss that recur in waves over time. As the child's condition progresses, parents may experience repeated losses that represent further declines and new caregiving demands. Consequently, families must be assessed on an ongoing basis and offered appropriate support and resources as their needs change over time (Doig et al., 2009). This represents a critical period of time, as the approach and support provided by the nursing and medical team during this period can directly impact the experience of complicated grief after the death of the child. *Complicated grief* (Meert, Shear, Newth, et al., 2011), characterized as persistent distress and chronic stress response, may last 6 months or longer after the death of a child and has a significant impact on quality of life of the family left behind.

Establishing a Support System

The diagnosis of a child with a complex chronic condition is a major **situational crisis** that affects the entire family system. Families can experience positive outcomes as they successfully deal with the many challenges that accompany a child with chronic illness.

One nursing goal is to assess which families are at greater or lesser risk for succumbing to the effects of the crisis. Several variables—available support system, perception of the event, coping mechanisms, reactions to the child, available resources, and concurrent stresses within the family—influence the resolution of a crisis. Although most families cope well, the needs of families at risk are great. If they receive emotional support and guidance early, there is an increased likelihood that they will also cope successfully.

Although it is easy to assume that families of children with the most severe illnesses or disabilities would have the poorest adjustment, the severity of the condition reflects only one part of the overall picture. The level of adjustment is significantly influenced by the *functional burden* on the individual family (Baillargeon & Bernier, 2010; Brehaut, Kohen, Garner, et al., 2009; Lach, Kohen, Garner, et al., 2009). This concept involves the issues related to caring for and living with the child in relation to the family's resources and ability to cope (Box 40-6). The family of a child with multiple disabilities demanding complex care, yet having many resources and coping skills, may adjust more successfully to the child's situation than the family of a child with a less serious condition and few resources to

BOX 40-5 CHARACTERISTICS OF PARENTAL OVERPROTECTION

- Sacrifices self and rest of family for the child
- Continually helps the child, even when the child is capable
- Is inconsistent with regard to discipline or employs no discipline; frequently applies different rules to the siblings
- Is dictatorial and arbitrary, making decisions without considering the child's wishes, such as keeping the child from attending school
- Hovers and offers suggestions; calls attention to every activity, overdoes praise
- Protects the child from every possible discomfort
- Restricts play, often out of fear that the child will be injured
- Denies the child opportunities for growing up and assuming responsibility, such as learning to give own medications or perform treatments
- Does not understand the child's capabilities and sets goals too high or too low
- Monopolizes the child's time, such as sleeping with the child, permitting few friends, or refusing participation in social or educational activities

BOX 40-6 CONCEPT OF FUNCTIONAL BURDEN

Impact of the Child With Special Needs on the Family
Child's need for medical and nursing care
Child's fixed deficits
Child's age-appropriate dependency in activities of daily living
Disruptions in the family routine caused by the care
Psychological burden of the prognosis on the family

Family Resources and Ability to Cope
Family's physical resources
Family's emotional resources
Family's educational resources
Family's social supports and available help
Competing demands for family members' time and energy

Data from Doig, J. L., McLennan, J. D., & Urichuk, L. (2009). "Jumping through hoops": Parents' experiences with seeking respite care for children with special needs. *Child: Care, Health and Development, 35*(2), 234–242; Dewan, T., & Cohen, E. (2013). Children with medical complexity in Canada. *Paediatrics & Child Health, 18*(10), 518–522.

counterbalance the situation. If a family of a child with a high level of technology dependence who demands complex care has many resources and coping skills, they may adjust more successfully to the child's situation than the family of a child with a less serious condition and fewer resources. Little is available in the literature regarding the impact of the child's intellectual or developmental disabilities on the families of these children. Considerable need and opportunity exist to conduct research in the area of family coping and resilience, for the purpose of enhancing family resources (Dykens, 2015).

Intrafamilial resources, social support from friends and relatives, parent-to-parent support, parent–professional partnerships, and community resources interweave to provide a flexible web of support for the family of a child with a chronic condition. However, nurses should be aware that rare conditions often have fewer parent-to-parent support networks or online resources, leaving parents feeling frustrated and alone.

THE CHILD WITH A CHRONIC OR COMPLEX CONDITION

The child's reaction to chronic illness depends to a great extent on his or her developmental level, temperament, and available coping mechanisms; on the reactions of family members or significant others; and, to a lesser extent, on the condition itself. A child's conceptual understanding of his or her own illness is based not only on age and developmental level but also on the duration and type of experience accumulated with the disease. Knowledge of these variables is essential in providing the kind of information and support these children need in order to cope with a sometimes overwhelming situation.

Developmental Aspects

The impact of a chronic complex illness is influenced by the age at onset. While chronic illness affects children of all ages, the developmental aspects of each age group dictate particular

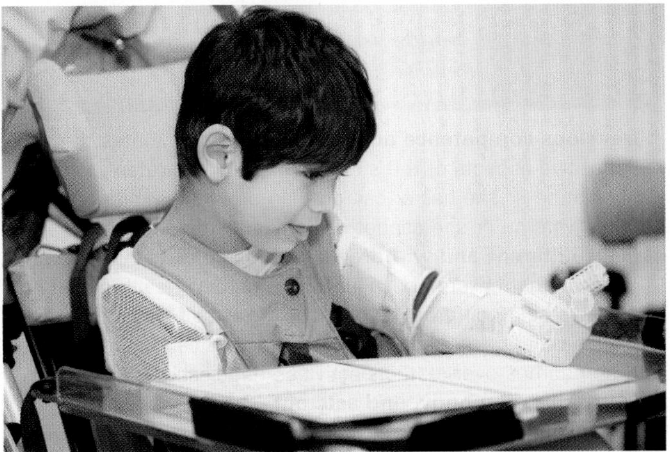

FIGURE 40-1 Children with any type of impairment should have the opportunity to develop their skills. (Jaren Jai Wicklund/Shutterstock.com.)

stresses and risks for the child. The nurse must recognize that children need to redefine their condition and its implications as they develop and grow. For example, appearance, skills, and abilities are highly valued by peers (Fig. 40-1); a teenager who is limited in any of these qualities is subject to rejection or bullying. While bullying is a large topic at any developmental age, the need to address it in the special needs population is of particular importance, yet there are few resources available on bullying and the special needs child (Lund & Vaughn-Jensen, 2012). Some children with special needs are aware of the bullying behaviour, while others may not realize it is occurring, because of their limited developmental capacity. Parents can ask their child about daily interactions with other children through inquiry such as "Tell me some of the nicknames the other children have for you at school," in order to detect potential bullying. (See Additional Resources at the end of this chapter for further information on bullying and the special needs child.)

Coping Mechanisms

Children with chronic conditions tend to use five distinct patterns of coping (Box 40-7). Children with more positive and accepting attitudes about their chronic illness use a more adaptive coping style characterized by optimism, competence, and compliance. They show fewer behavioural problems at home and at school. The two maladaptive coping patterns—"Feels different and withdraws" and "Is irritable, is moody, and acts out"—are associated with poorer adaptation; children using these strategies have poorer self-concepts, more negative attitudes about their conditions, and more behavioural problems at home and at school.

Well-adapted children gradually learn to accept their physical limitations and find achievement in a variety of compensatory motor and intellectual pursuits. They function well at home, at school, and with peers. They understand their disorder, which allows them to accept their limitations, assume responsibility for care, and assist in treatment and rehabilitation regimens. They express appropriate emotions, such as sadness, anxiety, and anger, at times of exacerbations, but confidence and guarded optimism during periods of clinical stability (Fig. 40-2). They

BOX 40-7 COPING PATTERNS USED BY CHILDREN WITH SPECIAL NEEDS

Develops competence and optimism—Accentuates the positive aspects of the situation and concentrates more on what he or she has or can do than on what is missing or on what he or she cannot do; is as independent as possible

Feels different and withdraws—Sees self as being different from other children because of the chronic health condition; views being different as negative; sees self as less worthy than others; focuses on things he or she cannot do and sometimes over-restricts activities needlessly

Is irritable, is moody, and acts out—Uses proactive and self-initiated coping behaviours, although usually counterproductive in that the behaviours are not ego enhancing or socially responsible and do not result in desired outcomes; acts out irritably, which may or may not be associated with condition's symptoms

Adheres to treatment—Takes necessary medications, treatments; adheres to activity restrictions; also uses behaviours that indicate developing independence (e.g., assumes responsibility for taking medication)

Seeks support—Talks with adults, children, physicians, and nurses; develops plans to handle problems as they occur; uses downward comparison (i.e., realizes that others have it worse)

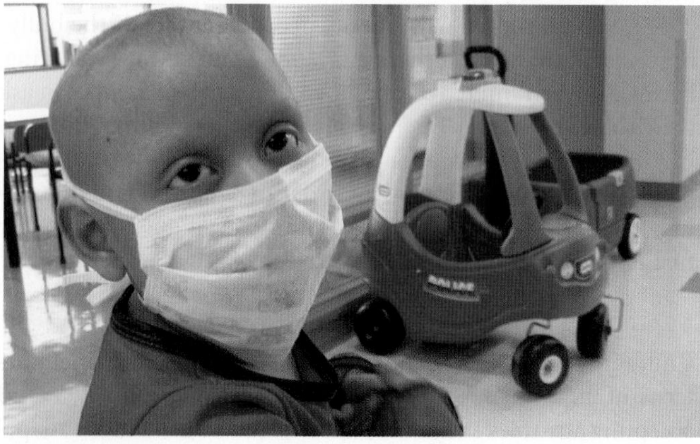

FIGURE 40-2 Periods of sadness and anger are appropriate in the child's adjustment to a chronic illness or complex condition, especially during exacerbations of the disorder.

are able to identify with other similarly affected individuals, promoting positive self-images and displaying pride and self-confidence in their ability to lead a productive, successful life despite their illnesses.

Health Education and Self-Care

Health education is an intervention that promotes better skilled coping. Children need information about their condition, the therapeutic plan, and how the disease or the therapy might affect their particular situation. Children nearing puberty also need to understand the maturation process and how their disability may alter this event. A youngster with Crohn's disease should understand that this disorder is associated with growth failure and delayed puberty; a child with diabetes needs to know that hormonal changes and increased growth needs will alter food and insulin requirements at this time; and a sexually active girl with sickle cell anemia or systemic lupus erythematosus needs to be aware of the risks of pregnancy. The information should not be given all at once but should be timed appropriately to meet the changing needs of the youth, and it should be described and repeated as often as the situation requires.

NURSING CARE OF THE FAMILY AND CHILD

Performing an Assessment

Because the nurse may meet a family during any phase of the adjustment process, several assessment areas are important. The family's ability to cope with previous stresses will influence the current situation, and answers to questions about their usual coping skills can provide insight into their ability to cope with having a child with special needs. Knowledge of concurrent stresses, such as financial, marital, and career or unemployment, will help the nurse identify families who may have fewer resources to cope with the child's needs.

Finally, awareness of family members' reactions to the child and the illness is important. Sample questions that the nurse and family can use to evaluate the support system, perception of the illness, coping mechanisms, resources, and concurrent stresses are listed in Table 40-2. Because factors affecting the family's response may change at any point during the illness, assessment must be a continual process.

Special challenges exist in assessing the child's feelings about having a chronic condition. Chapter 33 presents several approaches to encouraging a child to discuss feelings about the condition. The nurse should use a variety of communication techniques, such as drawing and play, as assessment tools rather than relying solely on parental reports. Often, children are neglected partners in their care, and their unique needs are not identified.

The needs of working parents and siblings also should be assessed, a goal that requires flexibility in scheduling appointments to include these important family members. When working parents know that their input is valuable, they will often change their work schedule to meet with a health care provider; but this may not always be possible and should be accommodated. Because siblings can be of any age, the use of appropriate communication strategies for assessment must be considered. Nonverbal techniques such as those discussed in Chapter 33 should be considered for these children.

The main objective in working with the family is to help them cope effectively with the stresses related to the child's special needs. To achieve this goal, the entire family should be considered in every aspect of the implementation process. Encouraging questions from each family member, including siblings, enables open dialogue while developing trust, a cornerstone to family engagement.

Providing Support at the Time of Diagnosis

The diagnosis is a critical time for parents and can influence how they perceive their health care providers throughout care.

TABLE 40-2 ASSESSMENT OF FACTORS AFFECTING FAMILY ADJUSTMENT

FACTORS AFFECTING ADJUSTMENT	ASSESSMENT QUESTIONS
Available Support System	
Status of marital relationship	With whom do you talk when you have something on your mind? (If answer is not the spouse, ask for the reason.)
Alternative support systems	When something is worrying you, what do you do? What helps you most when you are upset?
Ability to communicate	Does talking seem to help when you feel upset?
Perception of the Illness or Disability	
Previous knowledge of disorder	Have you ever heard the word (name of diagnosis) before? Tell me about it (if answer is yes).
Imagined cause of disorder	What are your thoughts about the causes of the disorder?
Effects of illness or disability on family	How has your child's illness or disability affected you and your family? How has your lifestyle changed?
Coping Mechanisms	
Reactions to previous crises	Tell me about a time when you've had another crisis (problem, bad time) in your family. How did you solve that problem?
Reactions to the child	Do you find yourself being a little more cautious with this child than with your other children?
Child-rearing practices	Do you feel as comfortable disciplining this child as your other children?
Influence of religion	Has your religion or faith been of help to you? Tell me how (if answer is yes).
Attitudes	How is this child different from the siblings or other children of similar age? Describe your child's personality. When you think of your child's future, what thoughts come to mind?
Available Resources	What parts of your child's care are causing the most difficulty for you or your family? What services are available to help? What services do you need that currently are not available?
Concurrent Stresses	What other problems are you facing now? (Be specific; ask about financial, marital, or sibling stresses, and concerns around extended family or friends.)

Although they may not hear or remember all that is said to them, they can sense the health care provider's attitude—whether it be acceptance, rejection, hope, or despair—and this may influence their ability to absorb the shock and begin adapting to the family's altered future.

Parents may be encouraged to be together when they are informed of their child's condition, thus avoiding the problem of one parent having to interpret or convey complex findings and deal with the initial emotional reaction of the other. The informing session should take place in a private, comfortable setting free of distractions and interruptions, in an atmosphere in which the parents feel free to express their emotions. Their emotional needs require acknowledgement through acceptance of such expressions as crying, sadness, anger, and disappointment. Emotional support can be offered by having tissues available if a family member cries and demonstrating through facial and body language that this is a difficult and painful period. Although touching is a powerful expression of empathy, it must be used wisely. For example, it can prematurely terminate free expression of feelings, especially when combined with statements such as "Everything will be all right." Nurses should also be aware of cultural issues regarding touching; some individuals of certain cultures or backgrounds may not welcome being touched, particularly if the person is of the opposite sex. Regardless, the nurse should always ask permission prior to providing touch.

Parents should receive the kind of information they desire. This can be assessed by asking questions such as "Do you prefer to hear detailed information?" Parents or other family members may have different preferences regarding the amount of information they wish to hear. Most parents want a clear, simple explanation of the diagnosis; a prediction of possible futures for the child; advice on what to do next; an opportunity to ask questions; a warm, sympathetic listener; and, most important, time. Understanding of explanations is elicited with such questions as "Can you tell me in your own words what you think I told you?" or "Can you explain to me what you have heard so far? What questions do you still have at this time?" Technical terms should be clarified with simple, written definitions.

Finally, the informing conference does not end with the presentation of devastating news. Instead, the child's strengths, appealing behaviours, and potential for development need to be stressed, as well as available rehabilitation efforts or treatment. Parents can be encouraged to view their experiences as a series of challenges that they are capable of handling, particularly with available professional feedback. Parents need to be assured that the nurse will be available to answer questions and provide further assistance. Because of the need for long-term follow-up, the initial informing interview is only one in a series of continuing discussions. In all interactions the family's input needs to be solicited and incorporated into the care plan. Some situations require consideration of special problems.

Supporting the Family's Coping Methods

For the family to meet the stresses while optimally adjusting to the child's condition, each member must be individually supported so that the family system is strong. Although the family can indefinitely support a member who is in need of assistance, its greatest strength lies in every member supporting each other. The nurse should bear in mind that the family member in greatest need is not necessarily the affected child but may be a parent or sibling who is dealing with stresses that require intervention.

Parents. The nurse can provide support by being attentive to families' responses to their children. Mothers and fathers or partners need to experience success, joy, and pride in their children in order to give the support they need. Their attempts to get to know their care providers and to communicate their needs to them must be reinforced with support.

It is important for nurses to continuously examine their attitudes to determine their ability to engage in parent–professional partnerships. An essential characteristic for this partnership is the belief that parents are equal to professionals and are experts in caring for their child (see Family-Centred Teaching box).

Communication among all family members is also encouraged. Parent group sessions can help parents express thoughts and feelings to each other but often do not take into account siblings' or the child's viewpoint. Therefore, the nurse may need to set up a family session, such as during a home or clinic visit. Although the ideal situation is to have all the members present at one time, often this is not possible. Inviting members to participate at various visits is an appropriate alternative, or arranging a teleconference or videoconference to support participation.

Parents can be encouraged to discuss their feelings toward the child, the impact of this event on their relationship with their spouse or partner, and associated stresses such as financial burdens. In addition, the family wage earner may have to sacrifice job opportunities to remain close to a medical facility or to avoid losing insurance benefits.

The nurse needs to regard both parents as able, effective parents, competent and capable of coping with the challenges they face. Every effort should be made to include the parent working outside the home in visits, such as to the nursery, clinic, special school, and stimulation programs. This parent needs to be included in the assessment process, with specific emphasis on having him or her describe the child's strengths and difficulties. It is not unusual to find two parents who have differing views of the child's abilities, especially in the area of developmental disabilities.

Numerous volunteer and community resources are available that provide assistance, rehabilitation, equipment, and funding for a variety of health problems (see Additional Resources at the end of this chapter). National and local disease-oriented organizations may provide needed assistance and support to families that qualify. Provincial and federal departments of health, mental health, social services, and labour may be able to help locate appropriate regional resources. For example, provincial or territorial programs for children with special health needs can provide financial assistance for children with many disabling conditions. Local and national sources of respite care and medical day care may also be useful to families. Nurses should become acquainted with these resources in their communities and with vocational programs for special groups so that they can effectively guide the families who wish to access these resources.

Parent-to-parent support. Just being with another parent who has shared similar experiences can be helpful. It may not need to be a parent of a child with the same diagnosis, since parents in the process of adjusting to a child with special needs—or finding respite services, educational or rehabilitative services, special equipment vendors, and financial counselling—tread a common path.

A parent self-help group can be a means of promoting parent-to-parent support. Group members usually feel less alone and have the opportunity to observe both coping and mastery from other members. Parents' groups are also rich resources for information. Even if parents are unable to attend meetings, they can still benefit from group newsletters, blogs, and other resources that often accompany membership.

The nurse can foster parent participation in support groups by serving as a referral agent, a group advisory board member, a resource person, a group member, or an assistant in founding a group. Sometimes all that is required to start a group is identifying one or two parents as leaders; sharing with them the names, telephone numbers, and e-mail addresses of other families who have expressed both an interest and a willingness to release this information; and guiding them in how to initiate a first meeting.

Advocate for empowerment. Nurses can advocate for methods that foster opportunities for parent empowerment. For example, nurses can suggest reimbursement options for travel and child care, plus stipends to enable parents' voices to

FAMILY-CENTRED TEACHING

Developing Successful Parent–Professional Partnerships

- Promote primary nursing; in nonhospital settings designate a case manager.
- Acknowledge parents' overall competence and their unique expertise with their child.
- Respect parents' time as having value equal to that of other members of child's health care team.
- Explain or define any medical, technical, or discipline-specific terms. Provide written information or diagrams to augment explanations.
- Tell families, "I am not sure" or "I don't know," when appropriate, then seek an answer if possible.
- Facilitate the family's effectiveness in team meetings (e.g., provide parents with same information as other participants).

be heard at meetings and conferences. They can encourage parent membership on relevant committees and boards. They can also keep parents informed of pending legislation on child health issues or take action when parents inform them of such initiatives.

The child. Through ongoing contacts with the child, the nurse will be able to (1) observe the child's responses to the disorder, ability to function, and adaptive behaviours within the environment and with significant others; (2) explore the child's own understanding of his or her illness or condition; and (3) provide support while the child learns to cope with his or her feelings. Children should be encouraged to express their concerns rather than allowing others to express them for them, since open discussions may reduce anxiety.

One of the most important interventions is alleviating the child's feeling of being different and normalizing his or her life as much as possible (see Guidelines box). Whenever possible, the nurse should assist the family in assessing the child's daily routine for indications of a need for normalizing practices. For example, the child who remains in a bedroom all day requires a restructured daily routine to provide activities in different parts of the house, such as eating in the kitchen or dining room with the family. Such children may also be deprived of social, recreational, and academic activities that can be better accommodated by applying normalization practices. For example, home and out-of-home health-related treatments should be planned at times that interfere as little as possible with normal daily activities.

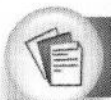

GUIDELINES

Promoting Normalization

Preparation—Prepare child in advance for changes that may occur from the illness or disability.

Example—Tell the child in advance the possible adverse effects of medication therapy.

Participation—Include child in as many decisions as possible, especially those relating to his or her care regimen.

Example—The child is responsible for taking medications or scheduling home treatments.

Sharing—Allow family members and the child's peers to be a part of the care regimen whenever possible.

Examples—Give the child his or her medication when the other siblings receive their vitamins.

The parent cooks the same menu for the whole family.

If the child is invited to another's home, the parent advises the family of the child's dietary restrictions.

Control—Identify areas where child can be in control, to decrease feelings of uncertainty, passivity, and helplessness.

Example—The child identifies activities that are appropriate to his or her energy level and chooses to rest when fatigued.

Expectation—Apply the same family rules to the child with a chronic or complex condition as those used with the well siblings or peers.

Example—The child is disciplined, is expected to fulfill household responsibilities, and attends school in accordance with abilities.

Children who are concerned that their condition detracts from their physical attractiveness need attention focused on the positive or conventional aspects of appearance and capabilities. Health care providers can help strengthen and consolidate a child's self-image and help the child fit in with his or her peer group, while allowing the child to express anger, isolation, fear of rejection, feelings of sadness, and loneliness. Children need positive reinforcement for their efforts at enhancing their self-image and for any evidence of improvement. Anything that might improve a personal sense of attractiveness and contribute to a positive self-image should be employed, such as makeup for a teenager with a scar, clothing that disguises a prosthesis, or a hairstyle, scarf, hat, or wig to cover a deformity or lost hair.

Siblings. The presence of a child with special needs may result in parents paying less attention to the other children in a family. Siblings may respond by developing negative attitudes toward the child or by expressing anger in different forms. The nurse can help by using anticipatory guidance—questioning the parents about what they believe is the best way to have siblings respond to the child and guiding them through ways to meet their other children's needs for attention. This supportive questioning should take place before serious negative effects occur.

Siblings may also experience embarrassment associated with having a brother or sister with a chronic illness or complex medical condition. Parents are then faced with the difficulty of responding to this embarrassment in an understanding and appropriate manner without punishing the siblings for how they feel. Parents should be encouraged to talk with the siblings about how they view their affected sibling. For example, siblings of a child who is cognitively impaired may express fears about their ability to bear normal children. Adolescents in particular may not be able to discuss these vital issues with their parents and may prefer to consult with the nurse. Many siblings benefit from sharing their concerns with other young people who are in a similar situation. Support groups for siblings can help decrease isolation, promote expression of feelings, and provide examples of effective coping skills.

Many parents express concern about when and how to inform the other children in the family about a sibling's illness or disability. The answer depends on each child's level of sophistication and understanding. However, it is usually best to inform the siblings before a neighbour or other nonfamily member does so. Uninformed siblings may fantasize or develop apprehensions that are out of proportion to the child's actual condition. Furthermore, if parents choose to be silent or deceptive about the issue, they are setting a negative precedent for the siblings to follow rather than encouraging them to cope with the experience in a healthy and nurturing way.

The nurse needs to be sensitive to the reactions of siblings and, whenever possible, intervene to promote more positive adjustment. For example, siblings often mention that they are expected to take on additional responsibilities to help the parents care for the child. It is not unusual for them to express a positive reaction to assuming the extra duties but a negative response to feeling unappreciated for doing so. Such feelings can often be minimized by encouraging siblings to discuss this with the parents and by suggesting to parents ways of showing gratitude, such as an increase in allowance, special privileges, and, most significantly, verbal praise.

Educating About the Disorder and General Health Care

Educating the family about the disorder is actually an extension of revealing the diagnosis. Education involves not only supplying technical information but also discussing how the condition will affect the child. Parents and other family members may be able to digest only so much information at a time. It may be helpful to provide essential information and then follow by asking, "What else would you like to know about your child's condition?" Responding to the parents' and families' questions and concerns ensures that their information needs are met.

Activities of daily living. Parents also need guidance with how the condition may interfere with or alter activities of daily living, such as eating, dressing, sleeping, and toileting. One area frequently affected is nutrition. Common problems are undernutrition and overnutrition. Undernutrition results from food being inappropriately restricted, or loss of appetite, vomiting, or motor deficits that interfere with feeding. Overnutrition may also occur, usually because of a caloric intake in excess of energy expenditure or boredom and lack of stimulation in other areas. Although the child requires the same basic nutrients as other children, daily requirements may differ. Special nutritional considerations are discussed as appropriate throughout the text.

Safe transportation. Modifications may also be needed regarding car safety. Children with conditions such as low birth weight or orthopedic, neuromuscular, or respiratory problems often cannot safely use conventional car restraints. For example, children with hip spica casts cannot sit properly in child safety seats (see Developmental Dysplasia of the Hip, Chapter 53). Families will need assistance in determining the modifications allowed in their vehicles without affecting safety and insurance coverage (see Chapter 35). Transport Canada strictly limits the amount a car seat can be modified after sale. Parachute Canada (n.d.), dedicated to injury prevention, has valuable information for families on car seat safety (see Additional Resources at the end of this chapter).

If a child requires a wheelchair, the family should consult the wheelchair manufacturer for specific instructions regarding safe transportation by car. Considerations for wheelchairs used with vehicle transportation include securing both the wheelchair and the occupant in the wheelchair. Wheelchairs should be secured facing forward with tie downs at four points. The tie-down system should be dynamically crash tested, as should the occupant securement system that secures the child in the wheelchair. For example, the use of trays would not be recommended for transportation. With children who must travel with additional medical equipment (e.g., oxygen, monitors, or ventilators), this equipment should be anchored to the floor or underneath the vehicle seat or wheelchair. Soft padding should be added around the equipment to reduce movement. A second adult should be present to monitor the condition of a medically fragile child while travelling (Transport Canada, 2008).

Primary health care. Children with special needs require all the usual health care recommended for any child. Attention to injury prevention, immunizations, dental health, and regular physical examinations is essential. Nurses can play an important role in reminding parents of these aspects that are so often neglected when the concern is focused on the child's chronic condition. Specific discussions of nutrition, sleep, and activity, dental health, and injury prevention are presented in the chapters on health promotion for specific age groups (see Chapters 35–39). Immunizations are discussed in Chapter 35.

Dental hygiene is a particularly important and often overlooked concern for the child with complex chronic illness (Thikkurissy & Lal, 2009). Dental and oral hygiene are even more important in children with chronic conditions such as cardiac failure, immunosuppressive disorders, and development issues such as cerebral palsy. Untreated dental caries can lead to painful abscesses and overwhelming infections. Parents should be referred within the child's first year of life to a qualified pediatric dental team with expertise in managing care for children with special health care needs. Some children may have developed oral aversion as a result of tube feeding or secondary to developmental conditions such as autism spectrum disorder, where they do not tolerate touch. Nurses in a hospital and community setting can help manage these challenges by ensuring oral care is part of the child's daily routine and helping parents develop ways to effectively provide oral health. When assessing the child, the nurse should perform a risk assessment related to the child's oral health, assist with desensitization of touch and the oral check experience, and examine the oral cavity at each visit to check for hygiene, risk of caries, and dental and gum abscess. The nurse can also provide anticipatory guidance in addressing the parents' concerns and assist with planning and implementing a graduated approach to oral care. Before performing oral hygiene in the child, he or she should be gently prepared for what will happen. Oral hygiene can start with a moist cloth wrapped around the finger or sponge-wrapped soft applicator to gently wipe the gums, starting with front outer teeth and gums then moving to the back and inner regions. Once this is tolerated, then the caregiver can advance to a toothbrush and small amount of toothpaste. For some children who may move or thrash their arms, providing the care from behind may be easier with another caregiver providing gentle restraint and reassurance from the front (Ferguson & Cinotti, 2009).

Parents also need to be aware of the importance of communicating the child's condition in the event of a medical emergency. Young children are unable to give information about their disorder, and although older children may be reliable sources, after an accident they may be physically unable to speak. Therefore, all children with any type of chronic illness or complex condition that may affect medical care should wear some type of identification, such as a MedicAlert bracelet (see Additional Resources at the end of the chapter), and carry a card in their wallet that lists the medical condition and a phone number as well as Internet links for accessing emergency medical records and other personal information.

Promoting Normal Development

Aside from having knowledge of the condition and its effect on the child's abilities, the parents need to foster appropriate development in their child. Although each stage may take longer to achieve, parents should be guided toward helping the child reach his or her potential. Table 40-3 outlines developmental aspects of chronic illness or complex conditions along with supportive interventions. With appropriate planning and knowledge of strategies to improve the child's functional abilities, most children can live fulfilling and productive lives.

One important aspect of promoting development is to encourage the child's self-care abilities in both activities of daily living and the medical regimen. An assessment of the child's age and physical, emotional, and mental capacities, as well as the support and structure provided by the family, should be considered in determining the appropriate level of self-care in the medical regimen. Even toddlers can be involved in their own care, for example, by holding supplies for the parent during a procedure. Over time, children should be encouraged toward greater autonomy in their own self-care.

Early childhood. During infancy the child is achieving basic trust through a satisfying, intimate, consistent relationship with his or her parents. However, affected children's early existence may be stressful, chaotic, and unsatisfying. Consequently, he or she may need more parental support and expressions of affection to achieve trust. Likewise, the parents may require assistance in finding ways to meet the infant's needs, such as how to hold a rigid or flaccid infant, how to feed a child with tongue thrust or episodes of dyspnea, and how to stimulate a child who seems incapable of achieving any skills. If hospitalizations are frequent or prolonged, every effort is made to preserve the parent–child relationship (see Chapter 43). Hospital policies should promote visitation by and involvement of families.

During early childhood the goal is to achieve separation from parents, autonomy, and initiative. The natural parental response to having a sick child is overprotection. Parents need help in realizing the importance of allowing brief separations of the child from them and from others involved in the child's care and of providing social experiences outside the home whenever possible. Respite care, which provides temporary relief for family members, can be essential in allowing caregivers time away from the daily burdens.

Young children also need the opportunity to develop independence. Frequently the child is able to learn self-help skills, such as holding the bottle, finger feeding, and removing simple articles of clothing, but the parent continues to perform the act. The nurse can guide parents to the usual milestones

TABLE 40-3 DEVELOPMENTAL EFFECTS OF CHRONIC ILLNESS OR COMPLEX CONDITIONS ON CHILDREN

DEVELOPMENTAL TASKS	POTENTIAL EFFECTS OF CHRONIC ILLNESS OR COMPLEX CONDITION	SUPPORTIVE INTERVENTIONS
Infancy		
Develop a sense of trust	Multiple caregivers and frequent separations, especially if hospitalized	Encourage consistent caregivers in hospital or other care settings.
	Deprived of consistent nurturing	Encourage parental presence, "rooming in" during hospitalization, and participation in care.
Bond, or attach, to parent	Delayed because of separation; parental grief for loss of "dream" child; parental inability to accept the condition, especially a visible defect	Emphasize healthy, perfect qualities of infant. Help parents learn special care needs of infant for them to feel competent.
Learn through sensorimotor experiences	More exposure to painful experiences than pleasurable ones	Expose infant to pleasurable experiences through all senses (touch, hearing, sight, taste, movement). Use skin-to-skin contact as appropriate.
	Limited contact with environment from restricted movement or confinement	Encourage age-appropriate developmental skills (e.g., holding bottle, finger feeding, crawling).
Begin to develop a sense of separateness from parent	Increased dependency on parent for care	Encourage all family members to participate in care to prevent overinvolvement of one member.
	Overinvolvement of parent in care	Encourage periodic respite from demands of care responsibilities.
Toddlerhood		
Develop autonomy	Increased dependency on parent	Encourage independence in as many areas as possible (e.g., toileting, dressing, feeding).
Master locomotor and language skills	Limited opportunity to test own abilities and limits	Provide gross motor skill activity and modification of toys or equipment, such as a modified swing or rocking horse.
Learn through sensorimotor experience; beginning preoperational thought	Increased exposure to painful experiences	Give choices to allow simple feeling of control (e.g., choice of what book to look at, what kind of sandwich to eat). Institute age-appropriate discipline and limit-setting. Recognize that negative and ritualistic behaviours are normal. Provide sensory experiences (e.g., water play, sandbox play, finger painting).

Continued

TABLE 40-3 DEVELOPMENTAL EFFECTS OF CHRONIC ILLNESS OR COMPLEX CONDITIONS ON CHILDREN—cont'd

DEVELOPMENTAL TASKS	POTENTIAL EFFECTS OF CHRONIC ILLNESS OR COMPLEX CONDITION	SUPPORTIVE INTERVENTIONS
Preschool		
Develop initiative and purpose Master self-care skills	Limited opportunities for success in accomplishing simple tasks or mastering self-care skills	Encourage mastery of self-care skills. Provide devices that make task easier (e.g., self-dressing).
Begin to develop peer relationships	Limited opportunities for socialization with peers; may appear "like a baby" to age-mates Protection within tolerant and secure family causing child to fear criticism and withdraw	Encourage socialization (e.g., inviting friends to play, day care experience, trips to park). Provide age-appropriate play, especially associative play opportunities. Emphasize child's abilities; dress appropriately to enhance desirable appearance.
Develop sense of body image and sexual identification	Awareness of body centring on pain, anxiety, and failure Gender-role identification focused primarily on mothering skills	Encourage relationships with peers and adults.
Learn through preoperational thought (magical thinking)	Guilt (thinking he or she caused the illness or disability or is being punished for wrongdoing)	Help child deal with criticisms; realize that too much protection prevents child from learning to cope with realities of the world. Clarify that child's illness is not his or her fault or a punishment.
School Age		
Develop a sense of accomplishment	Limited opportunities to achieve and compete (e.g., many school absences, inability to join regular athletic activities)	Encourage school attendance; schedule medical visits at times other than school; encourage child to make up missed work.
Form peer relationships	Limited opportunities for socialization	Educate teachers and classmates about child's condition, abilities, and special needs. Encourage sports activities (e.g., Special Olympics). Encourage socialization (e.g., Girl Guides, Boy Scouts, 4-H Club; having a best friend or club membership).
Learn through concrete operations	Incomplete comprehension of the imposed physical limitations or treatment of the disorder	Provide child with information about his or her condition. Encourage creative activities (e.g., VSA Arts, Ontario and Québec affiliates; see Additional Resources).
Adolescence		
Develop personal and sexual identity	Increased sense of feeling different from peers and reduced ability to compete with peers in appearance, abilities, special skills	Help child realize that many of the difficulties the teenager is experiencing are part of normal adolescence (rebelliousness, risk taking, lack of cooperation, hostility toward authority).
Achieve independence from family	Increased dependency on family; limited job or career opportunities	Provide instruction on interpersonal and coping skills. Encourage increased responsibility for care and management of the disease or condition (e.g., assuming responsibility for making and keeping appointment [ideally alone], sharing assessment and planning stages of health care delivery, contacting resources). Discuss planning for future and how condition can affect choices.
Form healthy sexual relationships	Limited opportunities for healthy sexual friendships; less opportunity to discuss sexual concerns with peers Increased concern with issues such as why did the teen get this disorder, can he or she have a relationship and have a family	Encourage socialization with peers, including peers with special needs and those without special needs. Encourage activities appropriate for age (e.g., attending mixed-gender parties, sports activities, driving a car). Be alert to cues that signal readiness for information regarding implications of condition on sexuality and reproduction. Emphasize good appearance and wearing stylish clothes, use of makeup. Understand that the adolescent has the same sexual needs and concerns as any other teenager.
Learn through abstract thinking	Decreased opportunity for earlier stages of cognition impeding achievement of level of abstract thinking	Provide instruction on decision making, assertiveness, and other skills necessary to manage personal plans.

expected for the child. When a child is unable to perform a skill independently, functional aids should be used. With innovation, many adaptations can be implemented in children's environments to increase their mobility and independence and allow them to play like other children their age. For example, with slight modifications, a child with physical limitations may be able to ride a tricycle (Fig. 40-3).

Another critical component for normal child development is discipline. Discipline and guidance serve several purposes, such as providing children with boundaries at which to test their behaviour and teaching them socially acceptable behaviour. Resentment and hostility can arise among siblings if different standards are applied to each child. The nurse's responsibility is to help parents learn successful methods of managing a child's behaviours before they become problems.

School age. For school-age children, the major tasks are entry into school and achieving a sense of industry. Although the importance of school in the life of all children is well known, school absences are significantly higher among children with chronic illness than among their healthy peers. The more school absences the child experiences, the more difficult it is to resume attendance, and school phobia may result. The child should return to school as soon as possible after diagnosis or treatments. Discussion with the child on how he or she wants to proceed should be included within the development of the return to school preparation.

Preparation for entry into or resumption of school is best accomplished through a team approach with the parents, child, teacher, community health nurse, and primary nurse in the hospital. Ideally, this planning should begin before hospital discharge, provided that the child is well enough to resume usual activities. A structured plan should be developed, with attention to those aspects of care that must be continued during school hours, such as administration of medication or other treatments.

Children also need preparation before entering or resuming school. Having a tutor in the hospital or home as soon as children are physically able helps them realize that school will continue and gives them time to consider this prospect (Fig. 40-4). They need to investigate possible answers to the many questions others will ask. One method of anticipatory preparation is to role-play, with the child as the "returned pupil" and the nurse or parent as "other schoolmates." If the child returns to school with some obvious physical change, such as hair loss, amputation, or visible scar, the nurse might also ask questions about these alterations to prompt preparatory responses from the child.

Classroom peers also need preparation, and a joint plan involving the teacher, nurse, and child is best. At a minimum, classmates should be given a description of the child's

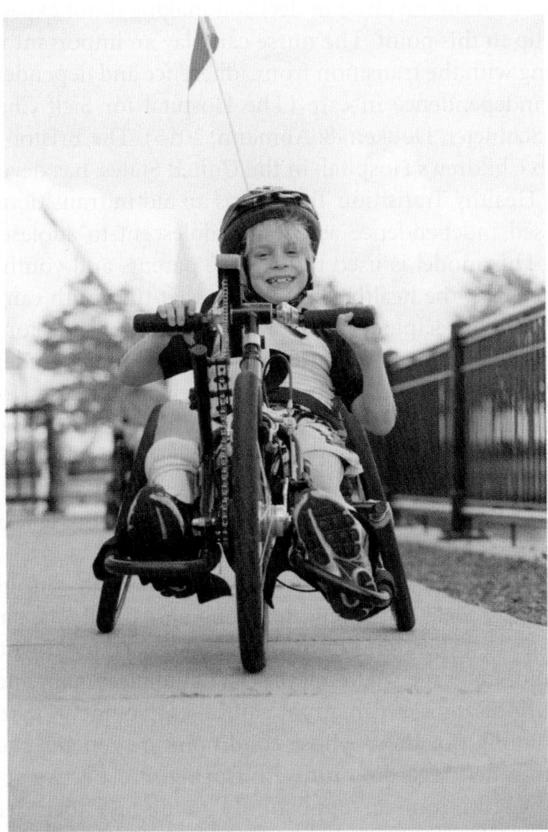

FIGURE 40-3 A modified tricycle with block pedals, self-adhesive straps for support, and modified seat and handle bars can help a child with disabilities gain mobility. (Disability Images/Science Source.)

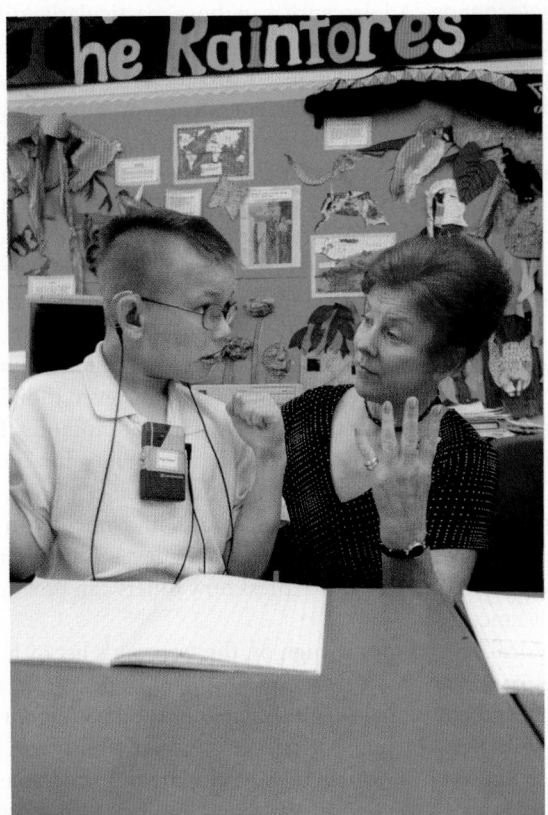

FIGURE 40-4 Children with special needs should continue their schooling as soon as their condition permits.

condition, prepared for any visible changes in the child, and allowed an opportunity to ask questions. The child should have the option of attending this session. As the child's condition changes, particularly if the illness is potentially fatal, school personnel, including the students, need periodic appraisal of the child's status and preparation for what to expect.

Children with special needs should be encouraged to maintain or re-establish relationships with peers and to participate according to their capabilities in any age-appropriate activities. Alternative activities may be substituted for those that are impossible or that place a strain on the child's condition. Programs such as the Special Olympics offer children an opportunity to compete with their peers and to achieve athletic skill. Summer camps give children with special needs the opportunity to associate with peers and develop a wide variety of skills (see Additional Resources at the end of this chapter). These children can derive enormous benefits from expressive activities, such as art, music, poetry, dance, and drama. With adaptive equipment and imagination, children can participate in a variety of activities. Organizations such as VSA Arts (with Ontario and Quebec affiliates) enable children to celebrate and share their accomplishments (see Additional Resources).

Children need the opportunity to interact with healthy peers and to engage in activities with groups or clubs composed of similarly affected age-mates. Such organizations as ostomy clubs, diabetes clubs, and cerebral palsy groups share information and provide support related to the special problems the members face.

Adolescence. Adolescence can be a particularly difficult period for the teenager with special needs and for his or her family. All of the needs discussed previously apply to this age group as well. Developing independence or autonomy is a major task for the adolescent as planning for the future becomes a prominent concern. For these children, the emphasis in the past was on achieving independence from physical assistance. However, recent developments in the fields of special education, adolescent development, and family systems suggest that autonomy be redefined in terms of individuals' capacities to take responsibility for their own behaviour, make decisions regarding their own lives, and maintain supportive social relationships. Given this understanding, even individuals with severe impairment can be viewed as autonomous if they perceive their own needs and take responsibility for meeting them, either directly or by engaging the assistance of others. As adolescents become more autonomous, the nurse can help them articulate their needs, participate in developing their own care plan, and discover and express how others can be of greatest assistance.

Physical symptoms are high on the teenager's list of health-related concerns. Because adolescence is a time of enormous physical and emotional changes, it is important for the nurse to distinguish between body changes related to disability and those that are a result of normal body development. It can be a great comfort for teenagers with disabling conditions to know that many of the changes they experience are normal developmental outcomes.

A sense of feeling different from peers can lead to loneliness, isolation, and depression. Participation in groups of teenagers with chronic conditions or disabilities can help alleviate feelings of isolation and smooth the transition to meaningful relationships in adulthood.

Establishing Realistic Future Goals

One of the most difficult adjustments for the child and for those involved in his or her continued care is setting realistic future goals. Sometimes the impact of such planning does not surface until the child finishes school or the parents approach retirement, when a crisis can arise because of disruption of all of the family roles and relationships that maintained stability.

Planning for the future should be a gradual process. All along, parents should cultivate realistic vocations for their child. For example, if children have physical disabilities, they could be directed toward undertaking intellectual, artistic, or musical pursuits. Children with developmental disabilities need to be taught manual skills. In this way, the child's development proceeds in the direction of self-support through gainful employment.

Transition to care from a pediatric- to adult-focused care environment can be stressful for the child and family. They will have developed strong relationships with the pediatric care team and must change to an environment that is more patient- than family-centric. Parents may be concerned about being left out of decisions, and the young adult may be stressed by the need to be more involved in decision making if not expected to do so up to this point. The nurse can play an important role in assisting with the transition from adherence and dependency to more independence in care (The Hospital for Sick Children, 2014; Schlucter, Dokken, & Ahmann, 2015). The Bristol-Myers Squibb Children's Hospital, in the United States, has developed a "My Healthy Transition Toolkit" as an aid in transitioning to increased independence as the preadolescent-to-adolescent is ready. This model is used to help the parents and youth work together with the health care team so that the youth can move from being a recipient of care to being responsible for some self-management and then full management of care independently. A similar model has been effectively used at the Hospital for Sick Children, Toronto to assist youths and their parents in adjusting to and managing care effectively, to the best of their abilities. This model is being used for the hospital's transition clinic (Good 2 Go; see Additional Resources at the end of this chapter).

With prolonged survival, young people with chronic illnesses must deal with new decisions and problems, such as marriage or other long-term relationships, employment, and insurance coverage. With appropriate guidance, many individuals with disabilities can attain gainful employment, marriage, and a family. For those whose conditions are genetic, counselling is needed regarding future offspring. Prospective spouses often benefit from an opportunity to discuss their feelings about marriage to an individual with continued health needs and possibly a limited lifespan. Health insurance coverage can be a critical issue if extra health care is needed, such as medications or treatments. Life insurance is another dilemma, especially when children have serious defects, such as congenital heart anomalies.

PALLIATIVE AND END-OF-LIFE CARE FOR CHILDREN

Although most childhood illnesses and many injuries and other types of trauma respond favourably to treatment, some do not. When a child and family face a prolonged and possibly terminal illness, health care providers must confront the challenge of providing the best possible care to meet the physical, psychological, spiritual, and emotional needs of the child and family during the uncertain course of the illness and at the time of death. When death is sudden and unexpected, nurses are challenged to respond to the grief and shock that families experience and to provide comfort and support in the absence of a prior relationship.

There are many factors contributing to childhood and adolescent death that nurses are likely to encounter: developmental factors, medical advances and technology, and changing social patterns.

A child who is diagnosed with a life-threatening illness or who is suffering serious, life-threatening trauma needs medical diagnosis and intervention, as well as nursing assessment and care—sometimes for a short time and sometimes over a lengthy period. Regardless of whether the child ultimately survives or dies from the condition, the principles of palliative care can and should be incorporated from the time of diagnosis, in order to provide the best possible care to both the child and family.

Principles of Palliative Care

The World Health Organization (WHO, 2016) defines palliative care as "an approach that improves the quality of life of patients and their families facing the problems associated with life-threatening illness, through the prevention and relief of suffering by means of early identification and impeccable assessment and treatment of pain and other problems—physical, psychosocial, and spiritual. Palliative care:

- provides relief from pain and other distressing symptoms;
- affirms life and regards dying as a normal process;
- intends neither to hasten or postpone death;
- integrates the psychological and spiritual aspects of patient care;
- offers a support system to help patients live as actively as possible until death;
- offers a support system to help the family cope during the patients' illness and in their own bereavement;
- uses a team approach to address the needs of patients and their families, including bereavement counselling, if indicated;
- will enhance quality of life, and may also positively influence the course of illness;
- is applicable early in the course of illness, in conjunction with other therapies that are intended to prolong life, such as chemotherapy or radiation therapy, and includes those investigations needed to better understand and manage distressing clinical complications.

Palliative care for children represents a special, albeit closely related field to adult palliative care. The WHO's definition of palliative care appropriate for children and their families is as follows:

- Palliative care for children is the active total care of the child's body, mind, and spirit and involves giving support to the family.
- It begins when illness is diagnosed and continues regardless of whether or not a child receives treatment directed at the disease.
- Health providers must evaluate and alleviate the child's physical, psychological, and social distress.
- Effective palliative care requires a broad multidisciplinary approach that includes the family and makes use of available community resources; it can be implemented successfully even if resources are limited.
- It can be provided in tertiary care facilities, in community health centres, and even in children's homes."

A distinction can be made between palliative and end-of-life care. End-of-life care is a part of palliative care, but the goals of *palliative care* extend to all aspects of a patient's quality of life and can be established early in the trajectory of a patient's disease. *End-of-life care* refers to care provided in the last weeks, days, or hours of a person's life. It is important to note that families may continue to hope and search for a miracle cure even while making decisions about where they would like the child to receive care and making plans for the child's funeral during the end-of-life period. Discussions during this time can be framed around continuing to hope and plan for the best, but also planning for the worst—just in case.

All health care providers should have a generalist level of knowledge related to the principles of palliative care so that children and families receive optimal support throughout the trajectory of a life-threatening illness. When pain or other symptoms are complex and difficult to manage, or family members are having particular challenges in coping with life-threatening illness, or staff are struggling to cope with providing care to a family, specialist pediatric palliative care providers can be contacted for assistance. Nearly all tertiary pediatric hospitals in Canada now have a specialist pediatric palliative care team. These team members have additional training and experience to assist with particularly difficult symptoms or quality-of-life issues and to provide support to children, families, and staff. These interprofessional teams generally act as consultants, providing support and advice to the primary health care team rather than taking over provision of front-line care. These teams also provide consultation over wide geographical areas, using telehealth or other technology to support children and health professionals who may not be located near a tertiary hospital. These teams may provide perinatal palliative care where they meet with families when a severe fetal anomaly has been diagnosed, in order to discuss options for care at the time of birth (Wool, 2013). The implementation of consulting services within hospitals has led to enhanced quality of life and end-of-life care for children and their families, as well as support for their care providers (Harrison, Evan,

Hughes, et al., 2014). Some pediatric palliative care teams also provide care to children in a free-standing hospice that may be associated with the tertiary hospital. Development of hospice care in Canada has followed the model of hospice care in the United Kingdom, where respite care may be provided as an additional component of palliative care (Steele, Derman, Cadell, et al., 2008). Respite care may involve scheduled time for the family to leave the ill child in the homelike setting of a hospice while they go on a holiday or spend more time with a spouse or siblings that may not be possible when caring directly for the ill child. Respite care may also be offered on an emergency basis, such as when the primary caregiver becomes ill, until other arrangements can be made for care of the ill child. Parents of children with life-threatening illness report that provision of respite care benefits the entire family and contributes to maintaining relationships and personal health so they can continue to care for the ill child in the future (Steele et al., 2008).

Decision Making at the End of Life

Discussions concerning the possibility that a child's illness or condition is not curable and that death is an inevitable outcome cause everyone involved a great deal of stress. The impending death of a child is out of the natural order of things for most people. Children represent health and hope, and their death calls into question the understanding of life. Physicians, other members of the health care team, and families must consider all information regarding the child's situation in order to make decisions that all parties can agree to, particularly those that will have a profound impact on the child and family. Nurses play a significant role as advocates, ensuring information and support are provided to the child and family while collaborating on the end-of-life care plan (Registered Nurses Association of Ontario [RNAO], 2011).

Ethical Considerations in End-of-Life Decision Making

A number of ethical concerns arise when parents and health care providers are deciding on the best course of care for the dying child. Many parents and health care providers are concerned that not offering treatment that would cause potential pain and suffering, but might extend life, would be considered euthanasia or assisted suicide. To eliminate such concerns, it is necessary to understand the various terms. *Euthanasia* involves an action carried out by a person other than the patient to end the life of the patient suffering from a terminal condition. This action is based on the belief that the act is "putting the patient out of his [or her] misery"; this action has also been called *mercy killing*. *Assisted suicide* is when someone provides the patient with the means to end his or her life and the patient uses that means to do so. The important distinction between these two actions involves who is actually acting to end the person's life.

The Canadian Nurses Association (2008) Code of Ethics for Registered Nurses does not address the active intent on the part of a nurse to end a person's life. It does indicate the nurse's role in maintaining patient dignity by providing interventions to provide comfort and relieve symptoms in the dying patient. When the prognosis for a patient is poor and death is the expected outcome, it is ethically acceptable to withhold or withdraw treatments that may cause pain and suffering and to provide interventions that promote comfort and quality of life.

Palliative care interventions do not serve to hasten death; rather, they provide pain and symptom management and address issues faced by the child and family with regard to death and dying. A primary aim of palliative care is to promote optimal functioning and quality of life during the time the child has remaining.

Physician–Health Care Team Decision Making

Decisions by physicians regarding care are often made on the basis of the progression of the disease or amount of trauma, the availability of treatment options that would provide cure from disease or restoration of health, the impact of such treatments on the child, and the child's overall prognosis. Often the main determinants prompting physicians to discuss end-of-life issues and options for children with critical illnesses include the child's age, premorbid cognitive condition and functional status, pain or discomfort, probability of survival, and quality of life. When the physician discusses this information openly with families, a shared decision-making process can occur regarding no cardiopulmonary resuscitation (CPR) (also referred to as *do-not-resuscitate [DNR]*) orders and care that is focused on the comfort of the child and family during the dying process (Tsai & Canadian Pediatric Society [CPS], Bioethics Committee, 2008/2016).

Unfortunately, many families are not given the option of terminating life-sustaining treatment and pursuing care focused on comfort and quality of life when cure is unlikely, and staff may be reluctant to raise the question of no CPR orders. The staff may believe that not being able to "save" a child is a "failure." Also, the physician and other members of the health care team may lack knowledge of and experience with the principles of palliative care (Sanderson, Hall, & Wolfe, 2016; Tsai & CPS, Bioethics Committee, 2008/2016). At times, parental decisions do not match the health care teams' recommendations. If this occurs, the team or family can request assistance from the hospital/institutional ethics committee or an ethics consultant (Canadian Bioethics Society, 2014; Harrison & CPS, Bioethics Committee, 2004/2016).

Parental Decision Making

Rarely are families prepared to cope with the numerous decisions that must be made when a child is dying. When the death is unexpected, as in the case of an accident or trauma, the confusion of emergency services and possibly a critical care setting presents challenges to parents as they are asked to make difficult choices. If the child has either experienced a life-threatening illness such as cancer or lived with a chronic illness that has now reached its terminal phase, parents are often unprepared for the reality of their child's impending death (see Family-Centred Teaching box). Numerous studies have found that families facing the impending death of a child depend on information provided to them by the health care team, particularly an honest

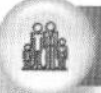

FAMILY-CENTRED TEACHING

Family of the Dying Child

No matter whether you have a PhD or many children, when your child dies, it is a new experience and nothing can prepare you for it. Like so many things in life, experience is the best teacher.

Three of our children have died, and by the time the third was dying, we handled many things differently. We learned a lot about dignity and the rights of the child and family. For example, at first, we didn't know that we had a right to have our child die at home. We also didn't understand pain medications and that if children are taking these medicines and are still in agony, they have not overdosed on the medication.

We learned a lot about case management. With our first two children, lots of different people were making decisions and disagreeing about what was best and what should be done. No one had primary authority. With our third child, one doctor took a primary role. Any questions and problems were handled by one person. I could call him 24 hours a day. It made a lot of difference, and I felt our concerns and needs were better heard and respected.

The nurses caring for our third child at home enabled me to step back and just be his mommy. When I could do this, I realized that we were fighting so hard for his life that we weren't really letting him die. His nurses had worked with him for a long time and really loved him. It was hard for them when we decided to let him die. In his last several days we wanted a lot of family time with our son, and I think the nurses felt left out. Something about their reaction to our increased time with him in the last few days made us feel guilty. If we had all been able to communicate a little more openly, I would have understood that they needed more time with him at the end, too. Everyone's needs could have been met.

–Jeni Stepanek, Mother
Upper Marlboro, MD

appraisal of the child's prognosis, to make difficult decisions regarding care options for their child (Tsai & CPS, Bioethics Committee, 2008/2016).

As the group of health care providers who are most involved with families, nurses are in an excellent position to ensure that families are presented with the relevant options available to them. The nurse's first responsibility is to explore the family's wishes related to goals of care. This discussion is best done in concert with the physician, but at times may need to be initiated by the nurse. Nurses can explore with families what they might be hoping for in relation to the child's illness as well as what they are worried or fearful about. Families who are hoping for a cure can also be guided to talk about other hopes, such as being pain free, spending more time at home, or getting to do a specific activity. Fears may include not being cured or being in pain. The discussion can move on to the specifics of where the family would like to receive care and the interventions that may or may not be used as part of the plan of care to both support hopes and address fears.

The Dying Child

Children need honest and accurate information about their (or a sibling's) illness, treatments, and prognosis; this information needs to be given in clear, simple language. In most situations this best occurs as a gradual process over time, characterized by increasingly open dialogue among parents, health care providers, and the child. Providing an atmosphere of open communication early in the course of an illness facilitates answering difficult questions as the child's condition worsens. Providing appropriate literature about the disease and the experience of illness and possible death is also helpful. Exactly how and when to involve children in decisions regarding care during their or a sibling's dying process and death is an individual matter. The children's ages or developmental level is an important consideration in the process (Table 40-4). In general, parents should be asked how they would like their child to be told of the prognosis, how siblings of the dying child should be informed, and how they all can be included in the child's care. Some parents may request that their child not be told that he or she is dying, even if the child asks. This often places health care providers in a difficult situation. Children, even at a young age, are perceptive. Even if they are not told outright that they are dying, they realize that something is seriously wrong and that it involves them. Often, when parents are helped to understand that honesty and shared decision making between them and their child are important to the child and family's emotional health, the parents may then allow discussion of dying with their child. Parents may require professional support and guidance in this process from a nurse, social worker, or child life specialist who has a good relationship with the child and family.

If given the opportunity, children will tell others how much they want to know. Asking questions such as "If the disease came back, would you want to know?" "Do you want others to tell you everything, even if the news isn't good?" or "If someone were not getting better [or more directly, "were dying"], do you think he would want to know?" helps children set the limits of how much truth they can accept and cope with. Children need time to process many feelings and much information so that they can assimilate, and ideally accept, the inevitable fact of mortality.

Care of the dying adolescent requires the nurse to become knowledgeable about any possible delays or alterations in normal growth and development. Legal and ethical issues, such as informed consent, also come to the forefront with respect to the age at which an adolescent should have autonomy in decision making about care and treatment. Effective communication between the patient, family, and health care team is an important part of optimal care for the dying adolescent.

Treatment Options for Children at the End of Life

Based on the child and family's decision regarding their wishes for end-of-life care, they have several options from which to choose. It is important to note that families may choose different locations for end-of-life care and death. For example, a family may wish to be home for as long as possible but not actually want the child to die there and want him or her to be admitted to the hospital or hospice when death appears to be imminent. Conversely, a family may prefer to be in the hospital and continue to pursue therapies aimed at curing the disease, but wish to be transferred to home or hospice when it becomes clear that the child is actively dying. Families need to be aware, however, that children can change very quickly and anticipating the time of death can be a challenge, so the timing of late transfers in settings of care can be very difficult. Families should also be aware that the child's condition or their own comfort level may change during this time, and they may want and need to change plans for the location of care and of death. For example, if the child has severe symptoms that are difficult to manage at home, they may wish to receive care in the hospital or hospice. As well, a family that initially worries about their ability to cope with having the child die at home may find that with time and the proper supports, they actually want the child to remain at home at the time of death. Research suggests that the opportunity to make plans for location of care and death may be more important to families than the actual location of the death (Dussel, Kreicbergs, Hilden, et al., 2009).

Hospital Care

Families may choose to remain in the hospital to receive care if the child's illness or condition is unstable and home care is not an option or the family is uncomfortable with providing care at home. If a family chooses to remain at the hospital for end-of-life care, the setting should be made as homelike as possible. Some hospitals have specially designated rooms that are larger, more private, or decorated differently to allow for a more home-like environment and more space for the family to be together in the child's last days or hours of life. Families should be encouraged to bring familiar items from the child's room at

TABLE 40-4 CHILDREN'S UNDERSTANDING OF AND REACTIONS TO DEATH

CONCEPTS OF DEATH	REACTIONS TO DEATH	NURSING CARE MANAGEMENT
Infants and Toddlers		
Death has least significance to children <6 mo of age. After parent–child attachment and trust are established, the loss, even if temporary, of the significant person is profound. Prolonged separation during the first several years is thought to be more significant in terms of future physical, social, and emotional growth than at any subsequent age. Toddlers are egocentric and can only think about events in terms of their own frame of reference—living. Their egocentricity and vague separation of fact and fantasy make it impossible for them to comprehend absence of life. Instead of understanding death, this age group is affected more by any change in lifestyle.	With the death of someone else, they may continue to act as though the person is alive. As children grow older, they will be increasingly able and willing to let go of the dead person. Ritualism is important; a change in lifestyle could be anxiety producing. This age group reacts more to the pain and discomfort of a serious illness than to the probable fatal prognosis. This age group also reacts to parental anxiety and sadness.	Help parents deal with their feelings, allowing them greater emotional reserves to meet the needs of their children. Encourage parents to remain as near to the child as possible, yet be sensitive to parents' needs. Maintain as normal an environment as possible to retain ritualism. If a parent has died, promote arrangements for a consistent caregiver for the child. Promote primary nursing.
Preschool Children		
Preschoolers believe their thoughts are sufficient to cause death; the consequence is the burden of guilt, shame, and punishment. Their egocentricity implies a tremendous sense of self-power and omnipotence. They usually have some understanding of the meaning of death. Death is seen as a departure, a kind of sleep. They may recognize the fact of physical death but do not separate it from living abilities. Death is seen as temporary and gradual; life and death can change places with one another. They have no understanding of the universality and inevitability of death.	If they become seriously ill, they conceive of the illness as a punishment for their thoughts or actions. They may feel guilty and responsible for the death of a sibling. Their greatest fear concerning death is separation from parents. They may engage in activities that seem strange or abnormal to adults. Because they have fewer defence mechanisms to deal with loss, young children may react to a less significant loss with more outward grief than to the loss of a very significant person. The loss is so deep, painful, and threatening that the child must deny it for a time to survive its overwhelming impact. Behaviour reactions such as giggling, joking, attracting attention, or regressing to earlier developmental skills indicate children's need to distance themselves from tremendous loss.	Help parents deal with their feelings, allowing them greater emotional reserves to meet the needs of their children. Help parents understand their children's behavioural reactions. Encourage parents to remain near the child as much as possible, to minimize the child's great fear of separation from parents. If a parent has died, promote arrangements for a consistent caregiver for the child. Promote primary nursing.

TABLE 40-4 CHILDREN'S UNDERSTANDING OF AND REACTIONS TO DEATH—cont'd

CONCEPTS OF DEATH	REACTIONS TO DEATH	NURSING CARE MANAGEMENT
School-Age Children		
The children still associate misdeeds or bad thoughts with causing death and feel intense guilt and responsibility for the event. Because of their higher cognitive abilities, they respond well to logical explanations and comprehend the figurative meaning of words. They have a deeper understanding of death in a concrete sense. They particularly fear the mutilation and punishment they associate with death. They personify death as the devil, a monster, or the bogeyman. They may have naturalistic or physiological explanations of death. By age 9–10, children have an adult concept of death, realizing that it is inevitable, universal, and irreversible.	Because of their increased ability to comprehend, they may have more fears, for example: • The reason for the illness • Communicability of the disease to themselves or others • Consequences of the disease • The process of dying and death itself Their fear of the unknown is greater than their fear of the known. The realization of impending death is a tremendous threat to their sense of security and ego strength. They are likely to exhibit fear through verbal uncooperativeness rather than physical aggression. They are interested in postdeath services. They may be inquisitive about what happens to the body.	Help parents deal with their feelings, allowing them greater emotional reserves to meet their children's needs. Encourage parents to remain near the child as much as possible, yet be sensitive to parents' needs. Because of children's fear of the unknown, anticipatory preparation is important. Because the developmental task of this age is industry, interventions of helping children maintain control over their bodies and increasing their understanding can enable them to achieve independence, self-worth, and self-esteem and avoid a sense of inferiority. Encourage children to talk about their feelings, and provide aggressive outlets. Encourage parents to honestly answer questions about dying rather than avoiding the subject or fabricating euphemisms. Encourage parents to share their moments of sorrow with their children. Provide preparation for postdeath services.
Adolescents		
Adolescents have a mature understanding of death. They are still influenced by remnants of magical thinking and are subject to guilt and shame. They are likely to see deviations from accepted behaviour as reasons for their illness.	Adolescents straddle the transition from childhood to adulthood. They have the most difficulty in coping with death. They are least likely to accept cessation of life, particularly if it is their own. Concern is for the present much more than for the past or the future. They may consider themselves alienated from their peers and unable to communicate with their parents for emotional support, feeling alone in their struggle. Adolescents' orientation to the present compels them to worry about physical changes even more than the prognosis. Because of their idealistic view of the world, they may criticize funeral rites as barbaric, money making, and unnecessary. They may have strong opinions of what postdeath rituals they want observed for them.	Help parents deal with their feelings, allowing them greater emotional reserves to meet their children's needs. Avoid alliances with either parent or child. Structure hospital admission to allow for maximum self-control and independence. Answer adolescents' questions honestly, treating them as mature individuals and respecting their needs for privacy, solitude, and personal expressions of emotions. Help parents understand their child's reactions to death and dying, especially that concern for present crises, such as loss of hair, may be much greater than for future ones, including possible death.

home. In addition, there should be a consistent and coordinated care plan for the child and family's comfort that includes interventions for any symptoms (e.g., pain, breathlessness, bleeding, seizures) that may occur during the end-of-life period given the child's underlying condition.

Home Care

Some families prefer to take their child home and receive services from a home care agency. Generally, these services entail periodic nursing visits to administer a treatment or provide medications, equipment, or supplies. Many home care agencies can provide nurses and other health care providers who are specially trained in palliative care support for patients and their families. The child's care frequently continues to be directed by the primary physician. Most specialist pediatric palliative care teams are able to continue to provide support to the child, family, and staff when the child receives care at home. As with end-of-life care provided in the hospital, there should be a plan in place to manage any expected symptoms, and the family should be aware of the symptoms associated with impending death (e.g., decreased interactions, decreased intake and output, changes in colour, and changes in breathing patterns). The family should also have contact information and directions for whom to call if the child experiences symptoms that they are not able to manage or they need additional support, as well as whom to call when the child dies (e.g., palliative care team, family physician, funeral home).

Hospice Care

There are only a few pediatric hospices currently available in Canada, but some adult hospices also provide care to children if additional supports are available for their staff. When pediatric hospices are available, 40% of families choose this option for the location of their child's death. Hospice may be an important alternative for families who are not comfortable being at home or where home care services are lacking but they do not wish to be in the hospital (Rapoport, 2008; Siden, Miller, Straatman, et al., 2008). In some cases, children can even be transferred to a hospice for withdrawal of ventilatory support. As noted above, families may receive respite care through hospice at earlier stages of an illness. A return to the hospice for end-of-life care means the family is in a familiar setting with familiar caregivers. There is space for the family to stay with the child, and they may choose to continue to provide the medical aspects of care as they did at home, or they may allow the staff to take over those aspects of care, allowing them to be "just" a parent. See Additional Resources at the end of this chapter for resources on palliative care and hospice resources.

NURSING CARE

Regardless of where the child receives end-of-life care, both the child and the family usually experience fear of (1) pain and suffering, (2) dying alone (child) or not being present when the child dies (parent), and (3) actual death. Nurses can help reduce families' fears through attention to the care needs of the child and family (see Evolve website for Nursing Care Plan).

Fear of Pain and Suffering

The presence of unrelieved pain in an ill child can have detrimental effects on the quality of life experienced by the child and family. Parents believe that having their child in pain is unendurable and results in feelings of helplessness and a sense that they must be present and vigilant to get the necessary pain medications. Persistent pain also creates more stress for the family as a whole. Nurses can alleviate the fear of pain and suffering by providing interventions aimed at treating the pain and symptoms associated with the dying process in children.

Pain and symptom management. Pain control for children in the terminal stages of illness or injury must be given the highest priority. Despite ongoing efforts to educate physicians and nurses on pain management strategies in children, studies have reported that children continue to be undermedicated for their pain. Nearly all children experience some amount of pain in the final stages of their illness. The current standard for treating children's pain follows the World Health Organization's (2012) guidelines on the pharmacological treatment of persistent pain in children with medical illnesses, which promotes tailoring the pain interventions to the child's level of reported pain. Children's pain should be assessed frequently and medications adjusted as necessary. Pain medications should be given on a regular schedule, and extra doses for breakthrough pain should be available to maintain comfort. Opioid drugs such as morphine should be given for severe pain, and the dose should be increased as necessary to maintain optimal pain relief. Techniques such as distraction, relaxation techniques, and guided imagery should be combined with drug therapy to provide the child and family strategies to control pain (see Chapter 34 for further discussion of pain-management strategies).

In addition to pain, children experience a variety of signs and symptoms during their terminal course as a result of their disease process or as an adverse effect of medicines used to manage pain or other symptoms. These symptoms include pain, fatigue, nausea and vomiting, constipation, anorexia, dyspnea, congestion, anxiety, depression, restlessness, agitation, and confusion (Heath, Clarke, Donath, et al., 2010; RNAO, 2011). Each of these symptoms should be aggressively managed with appropriate medications or treatments and with interventions such as repositioning, relaxation, massage, and other measures to maintain the child's comfort and quality of life (see Research Focus box).

Occasionally, children require very high doses of opioids to control their pain. The child on long-term opioid pain management can develop physical **tolerance** of the medication, meaning that it is necessary to give more drugs to maintain the same level of pain relief. This should not be confused with **addiction**, which is a psychological dependence on the adverse effects of opioids. Addiction is not a factor in managing terminal pain in children. Other obvious reasons for requiring increased doses of opioids include progression of disease and other physiological experiences of pain. It is important to understand that there is no maximum dose that can be given to control pain. Nurses often express concern that administering doses of opioids that exceed what they are familiar with will hasten the child's death. In cases where the child is terminally ill and in severe pain, use of large doses of opioids and sedatives to manage pain is justified when no other treatment options are available that would relieve the pain but make the risk of death less likely.

Parents' and siblings' need for education and support. Parents are the primary caregivers when the child is at home, and nurses providing care to the child and family need to teach the family about the medications being given to the child, how to administer medications, and the use of nonpharmacological techniques to control pain and other symptoms. Parents should be kept informed of all medications and treatments given to a child in the hospital or hospice and should be encouraged to participate in the child's care to the extent that they desire. This empowers parents and provides a sense of control over the child's comfort and well-being, reducing their fear that their child will be in pain or suffering as he or she is dying. Additionally, better bereavement outcomes (e.g., resilience; adaptive coping; family cohesion; less anxiety, stress, and depression) have been reported by parents who were actively involved in

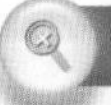

RESEARCH FOCUS

Pediatric Pain and Symptom Management at the End of Life

Ask the Question

In children, what is the pain and symptom experience at the end of life?

Search for Evidence

Search Strategies

Published studies from 2011 to 2015 using the subject terms *child, palliative care, pain,* and *symptoms*; findings dominated by retrospective descriptive studies describing infants and children's end-of-life experiences through the use of medical record reviews and provider and parental surveys

Databases Searched

CINAHL. EMBASE

Critically Analyze the Evidence

Children experienced many symptoms during their last month of life. Pain, dyspnea, and fatigue were the most frequently documented symptoms, experienced by most children at the end of life (Mahmood, Dozier, Casey, et al., 2015; Vern-Gross, Lam, Graff, et al., 2015).

A multipronged approach to help relieve physical as well as psychological and spiritual distress is necessary to provide optimum care to this very vulnerable population and their families. To achieve this aim, it is important to engage with patients and families, improve communication and relationships, and involve patients and families in the decision-making process as much as possible about needed services and treatment interventions (Epelman, 2012). Physicians reported reliance on trial and error as they learned to care for children at the end of life and the need for specialty consults with palliative care service providers (Jones, 2011). Researchers identified five of the most significant barriers that prevented nursing staff from providing optimal pain management: insufficient physician (MD) orders, insufficient MD orders before procedures, insufficient time to premedicate patients before procedures, the perception of a low priority given to pain management by medical staff, and parents' reluctance to have their child receive pain medication (Czarnecki, Simon, Thompson, et al., 2011). One study (Mahmood et al., 2015) reported that the involvement of a palliative care plan was successful in helping to manage pain, with 75% of patients achieving successful pain treatment.

Apply the Evidence: Nursing Implications

Although the philosophy of palliative care encompasses pain and symptom management for infants and children who may not outlive their disease, the provision of that care to ease suffering and provide comfort to those who will die continues to lag. Studies show that children experience significant pain and other distressing symptoms at the end of life that are not well managed. Discrepancies in perceptions of infant and child pain and suffering continue to exist between providers and parents. Barriers to the provision of pediatric palliative care exist, but involvement of palliative care approaches to assist with symptom management is increasing. Improvements are needed in the management of pain and symptoms at the end of life for infants and children.

References

Czarnecki, M. L., Simon, K., Thompson, J. J., et al. (2011). Barriers to pediatric pain management: A nursing perspective. *Pain Management Nursing, 12*(3), 154–162.

Epelman, C. L. (2012). End of life management in pediatric cancer. *Pediatrics, 129*(4), e975–e982.

Jones, B. W. (2011). The need for increased access to pediatric hospice and palliative care. *Dimensions of Critical Care Nursing, 30*(5), 231–235.

Mahmood, L., Dozier, A., Casey, D., et al. (2015). Early palliative care involvement for children with cancer. *Journal of Pain and Symptom Management, 49*(2), 439–440.

Vern-Gross, T. Z., Lam, C. G., Graff, Z., et al. (2015). Patterns of end-of-life children with advanced solid tumor malignancies enrolled on a palliative care service. *Journal of Pain and Symptom Management, 50*(3), 305–312.

their child's care and who had positive interactions and open communication with health professionals (Rosenberg, Wolfe, Bradford, et al., 2014). Assisting bereaved families is of utmost importance for the home care nurse. Providing psychological support to parents and siblings in the month prior to the child's death has been shown to facilitate the grieving process (Contro, Kreicbergs, Reichard, et al., 2011). Recognizing that parents experience bereavement and grief in varying ways will assist the nurse in providing appropriate and focused education and support (Contro et al., 2011). For example, fathers tend to speak mainly to their spouse about their feelings while mothers confide in friends, support groups, and other family members (Contro et al., 2011).

Siblings may feel isolated and displaced while their brother or sister is dying. Parents devote most of their time to the dying child's care and comfort, causing siblings to feel left out of the parent–sick child relationship. Siblings may become resentful of their sick sibling and begin to feel guilty or ashamed about such feelings. Nurses can assist the family by helping the parents identify ways to involve siblings in the caring process, perhaps by bringing some supplies or a favourite toy, game, or food item. Parents should also be encouraged to schedule time to spend with the other children where their focus is on them (Brennan, Hugh-Jones, & Aldridge, 2012). Helping parents identify a trusted friend or family member who can sit with the ill child for a short period will allow them to attend to their own needs or those of their other children.

Fear of Dying Alone or of Not Being Present When the Child Dies

The dying child may need reassurance that he or she will not be left alone as death approaches (Fig. 40-5). Often, as the child's condition declines, family members begin the "death vigil." Rarely is a child left alone for any length of time, which can be exhausting for family members. Nurses may be able to sit with the child while the family members take a shower or have a meal or nurses can assist the family by helping them arrange shifts so that friends or family members can be present with the child and allow others to rest. If the family has limited resources, community organizations such as churches often have volunteers who are willing to visit and sit with children. It is important that whoever is sitting with the child be aware of when the parent(s) would like to be notified to return to the child's bedside if death appears to be imminent.

When a child is dying in the hospital, parents should be given full access to the child at all times. If parents leave, they should be provided with a pager or other means of immediate communication and alerted if staff members note any change in the

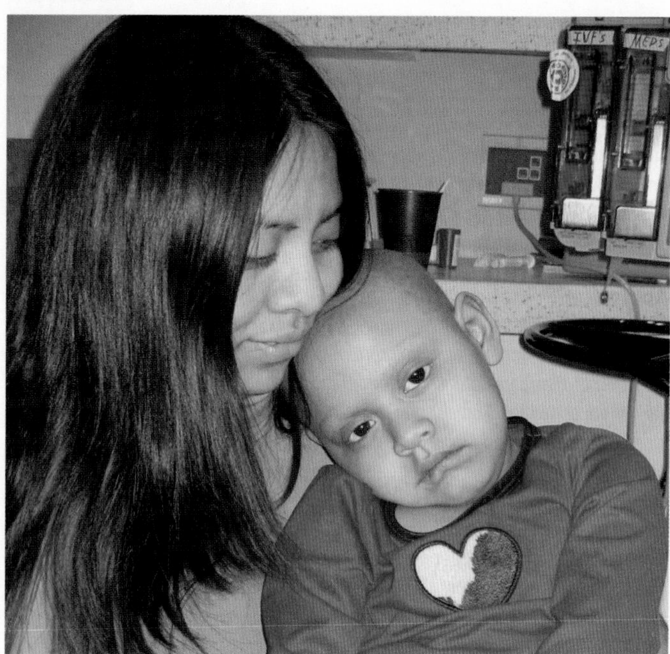

FIGURE 40-5 For the dying child there is no greater comfort than the security and closeness of a parent.

child that may indicate imminent death. Nurses must advocate for parents' presence in critical care and emergency departments and attend to parents' needs for food, drinks, comfortable chairs, blankets, and pillows.

Fear of Actual Death

The physical process of dying can be distressing to parents because often the child slowly becomes less alert in the days before the actual death. The nurse can assist the family by providing them with information about what changes will occur as the child progresses through the dying process (Box 40-8). During this time, nursing presence in the hospital or visits to the home often become more frequent and longer in duration to provide the family with additional support as the death nears. The most distressing change for parents to observe is the change in the respiratory pattern. In the final hours of life, the dying patient's respirations may become laboured, with deep breaths and long periods of apnea, referred to as *Cheyne-Stokes respirations.* Families need to be reassured that this is not distressing to the child and that it is a normal part of the dying process. Scopolamine, usually applied as a topical patch, can help reduce noisy respirations, known as the "death rattle." Noisy respirations are more likely to occur if the child is overhydrated. Symptom management should be planned with an interprofessional approach and family involvement along with specialist assessment as needed (Singh Jassal, 2011).

Death resulting from accident, trauma, or acute illness in settings such as the emergency department or critical care unit often requires the active withdrawal of some form of life-supporting intervention, such as a ventilator or bypass machine. These situations often raise difficult ethical issues, and parents are often less prepared for the actual moment of death. Nurses can assist these parents by providing detailed information about what will happen as supportive equipment is withdrawn, ensuring that appropriate pain medications are administered to prevent pain during the dying process, and allowing the parents time before the start of the withdrawal to be with and speak to their child. It is important that the nurse attempt to control the environment around the family at this time by providing privacy, asking if they would like to play music, softening lights, monitoring noises, encouraging the family to get into bed with or hold the child, and arranging for any religious or cultural rituals that the family may want performed.

After the child's death, the family should be allowed to remain with the body and hold or rock the child if they desire. After the nurse has removed all tubes and equipment from the body, parents should be given the option of assisting with the preparation of the body, such as bathing and dressing. It is important for the nurse to determine whether the family has any specific needs, since many cultures have adopted specific methods for coping with death and mourning, and impeding these practices may interfere with the grieving process. The nurse should also see if siblings or other family members not already present need to be called to see the child before the child is moved to the funeral home.

If the child is at home, arrangements for pronouncement of the death and whom to call when the child dies (e.g., a particular funeral home) should be in place before discharge home. Funeral arrangements can also be made prior to death in the hospital or hospice. If the death is sudden, following an accident or acute illness, parents may need assistance with identifying and contacting a funeral home. Parents often have concerns about the funeral, such as siblings' involvement in the death rituals. Although there are no absolute answers to the question of siblings attending the funeral or burial services, the

BOX 40-8 PHYSICAL SIGNS OF APPROACHING DEATH

Loss of sensation and movement in the lower extremities, progressing toward the upper body
Sensation of heat, although body feels cool
Loss of senses:
- Tactile sensation decreasing
- Sensitivity to light
- Hearing is the last sense to fail

Confusion, loss of consciousness, slurred speech
Muscle weakness
Loss of bowel and bladder control
Decreased appetite and thirst
Difficulty swallowing
Change in respiratory pattern:
- Cheyne-Stokes respirations (waxing and waning of depth of breathing with regular periods of apnea)
- "Death rattle" (noisy chest sounds from accumulation of pulmonary and pharyngeal secretions)

Weak, slow pulse; decreased blood pressure

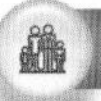

FAMILY-CENTRED TEACHING

Children Need to Say Goodbye

As a nurse and grief counsellor, I conduct grief workshops with children who have experienced the death of someone special. Children often communicate their feelings of being excluded through drawings. They may draw a picture of the dying person in a hospital bed that is raised too high for them to see the person's face clearly. Sometimes children reveal that they did not get to say goodbye because a family member told them, for example, "You don't want to see your grandma this way. She is too sick for you to visit." If the special person died at home, the children had to stay in their room when the funeral home staff took away the body.

I have learned to never underestimate the importance of allowing children to be involved with the dying person and the significance of a child's loss. Once, when I asked a 6-year-old girl to draw a picture with the theme "This is what I was doing when my ________ died," she drew a picture and completed the sentence with "when my home died." Her grandmother had been like her mother; to the child, her home was gone. We need to give children the choice of being included in the family's activities of saying goodbye.

–Barbara Bilderback, MS, MA, RN, Bereavement Supervisor, Saint Francis Hospice
Tulsa, OK

consensus is that the surviving children benefit from being involved in these events. Children need preparation for post-death services. They should be told what to expect, particularly how the deceased person will look if the coffin is open; allowed their private time to say goodbye; and permitted to stay as long as they wish. Ideally, the parents should prepare the siblings. If the parents' grief prevents this communication, a significant family member or friend should prepare the siblings (see Family-Centred Teaching box).

Organ or Tissue Donation and Autopsy

For some families, organ or tissue donation may be a meaningful act—one that benefits another human being despite the loss of their child. Unfortunately, initiating a discussion about tissue donation is often stressful for staff, and there may be confusion regarding whose responsibility this is. In centres in which transplants are performed, a transplant coordinator is usually available to inform the family about organ donation and to take care of details. If such services are not available, the staff needs to determine which members should discuss this topic with the family. Ideally, the person who knows the family best, knows when the death is expected, or has the opportunity to spend time with the family when the death is unexpected takes this role. Often nurses are in an optimal position to suggest tissue donation after consultation with the attending physician. When possible, the topic should be raised before death occurs. The request should be made in a private and quiet area of the hospital and should be simple and direct, with questions such as "Are you a donor family?" or "Have you ever considered organ donation?"

Some provinces and territories have guidelines concerning requests for organ or tissue donation when a child dies, especially if the patient is brain dead. In Canada, there is a list of provincial tissue and organ donor agencies (see Additional Resources at the end of this chapter). Written consent from the family is required before donation can proceed. When requests for organ donation are made, health care practitioners must address common misunderstandings families have about brain death and organ donation. Training health care providers on sensitive approaches to requests for organ donation has been shown to increase families' willingness to consent to organ donation. The option to donate organs should always be separate from the communication of impending or actual death.

Nurses need to be aware of common questions about organ donation to help families make an informed decision. Healthy children who die unexpectedly are excellent candidates for organ donation. Children with cancer, chronic disease, or infection or those who have suffered prolonged cardiac arrest may not be suitable candidates for organ donation but may be able to donate tissues, although this is individually determined. The nurse should ask whether organ donation was discussed with the child or whether the child ever expressed such a wish. Any number of body tissues or organs can be donated (for example, skin, corneas, bone, kidney, heart, liver, pancreas), and their removal does not mutilate or desecrate the body or cause any suffering. The family may still have an open casket, and there is no delay in the funeral. There is no cost to the donor family, but organ donation does not eliminate funeral or cremation responsibilities. Most religions permit organ donation as long as the recipient benefits from the transplant, although Orthodox Judaism forbids it (see Table 31-1).

In cases of unexplained death, violent death, or suspected suicide, autopsy is required by law. In other instances it may be optional, and parents should be informed of this choice. The procedure, as well as the forms that must be signed, should be explained. The family should know that the child can be in an open casket after an autopsy.

Grief and Mourning

Grief is a process, not an event, of experiencing physiological, psychological, behavioural, social, and spiritual reactions to a personal loss—in this case, the loss of a child. Grief is highly individualized, encompassing a broad range of manifestations from person to person. It is a natural and expected reaction to loss. It is neither orderly nor predictable. Grieving in any form is necessary for healing to occur. When death is the expected or a possible outcome of a disorder, the child and family members may experience anticipatory grief. Anticipatory grief may be manifested in varying behaviours and intensities and may include denial, anger, depression, and other psychological and physical symptoms.

Anticipatory guidance may assist grieving family members. Health care providers should emphasize that grief reactions such as hearing the dead person's voice, feeling distant from others, or seeking reassurance that they did everything possible for the lost person are normal, necessary, and expected. In no way do these reactions signify poor coping, insanity, or an approaching mental breakdown. On the contrary, such behaviours signify that the survivor is working through the acute grief. Anticipatory guidance regarding the mourning process may help families recognize the normalcy of their experiences.

It is important to recognize that some family members may experience complicated grief. *Complicated grief reactions* (more than a year after the loss) include such symptoms as intense intrusive thoughts, pangs of severe emotion, distressing yearnings, feelings of excessive loneliness and emptiness, unusual sleep disturbance, and maladaptive levels of loss of interest in personal activities (Bruce, Gumley, Isham, et al., 2011). Bereaved persons experiencing such prolonged and complicated grief should be referred to an expert in grief and bereavement counselling.

Another important aspect of grief is the individual nature of the grief experience. Each member of the family will experience the grief of the child's death in his or her own way based on the particular relationship with that child. This can create potential conflict for families, since each family member can have expectations that the other family members should feel and grieve as they do. Nurses caring for families experiencing grief should be aware of the different grieving styles and help the family learn to recognize and support the uniqueness of each other's grief.

Parental Grief

Parental grief after the death of a child can be the most intense, complex, long-lasting, and fluctuating grief experience compared with that of other bereaved individuals. Although parents experience the primary loss of their child, many secondary losses are felt, such as the loss of part of one's self, hopes and dreams for the child's future, the family unit, prior social and emotional community supports, and often spousal support. It is common for parents of the same child to experience different grief reactions.

Studies with bereaved parents have shown that grieving does not end with the severing of the bond with the deceased child, but rather involves a continuing bond between the parent and the deceased child (Foster, Gilmer, Davies, et al., 2011). Parental resolution of grief is a process of integrating the dead child into daily life, where the pain of losing a child is never completely gone, but lessens in intensity. There are occasions of brief relapse, but not to the degree experienced when the loss initially occurred. Thus parental grief work is never completed and is a timeless process of accommodating the new reality of being without a child, as it changes over time. A child's death can also challenge the relationship between partners and spouses in several ways. Maternal and paternal reactions often differ (DaSilva, Jacob, & Nascimento, 2010; Reilly, Huws, Hastings, et al., 2010). Different grieving styles between the couple may hinder communication and support for each other. Differing needs and expectations can place a strain on the relationship.

Sibling Grief

Each child grieves in his or her own way and on his or her own timeline. Children, even adolescents, grieve differently than adults. Adults and children differ more widely in their reactions to death than in their reactions to any other phenomenon. Children of all ages grieve the loss of a loved one, and their understanding and reactions to death depend on their age and developmental level. Children often revisit their grief as they grow and develop new understandings of death. They grieve in spurts and can be emotional and sad in one instance and then, just as quickly, off and playing. Children can be exquisitely attuned to their parents' grief and will try to protect them by not asking questions or by trying not to upset them. This can set the stage for a sibling to try to become the "perfect child." Children exhibit many of the grief reactions of adults, including physical sensations and illnesses, anger, guilt, sadness, loneliness, withdrawal, acting out, sleep disturbances, isolation, and search for meaning. Again, nurses should be attentive to signs that siblings are struggling with their grief and provide guidance to parents when possible.

At times family members may need assistance in their grieving (see Guidelines box). Communication with the bereaved family is essential, but often nurses do not know what to say and feel helpless in offering words of comfort. The most supportive approach is to avoid judging the family's reactions or offering advice or rationalizations and to focus on feelings. Perhaps the most valuable supportive measure the nurse can enact for families is to listen. Families understand that no words will relieve their pain; all they want is acceptance, understanding, and respect for their grief.

It is important for families to understand that mourning takes a long time. Whereas acute grief may last only weeks or months, resolving the loss is measured in years. Holidays and anniversaries can be particularly difficult, and people who previously had been supportive may now expect the family to have "adjusted." Consequently, prolonged mourning is often silent and lonely.

Many families never receive the support and guidance that could help them resolve the loss. A plan for regular follow-up with bereaved families can be beneficial. At minimum, one follow-up phone call or meeting with the family should be arranged. Families can also be referred to support groups. When such groups are not available, nurses can be instrumental in bringing families together or facilitating parent and sibling groups. Formal bereavement programs or bereavement counselling can be helpful as well.

For more information on end-of-life care, refer to Additional Resources, at the end of the chapter.

Nurses' Reactions to Caring for Dying Children

The death of a patient can be one of the most stressful aspects of nursing (see Family-Centred Teaching box). Nurses experience reactions to a fatal illness that are very similar to the responses of family members, including denial, anger, depression, guilt, and ambivalent feelings. It is acceptable and important to seek support from colleagues and other resources in the workplace. It is important to not use the family of the dying child as a source of comfort. Seeking support from the child's family is not acceptable, as it puts the therapeutic relationship at risk and crosses professional boundaries for appropriate nurse–patient relationships.

GUIDELINES

*Supporting Grieving Families**

General

- Stay with the family; sit quietly if they prefer not to talk; cry with them if that is acceptable to them.
- Accept the family's grief reactions; avoid judgemental statements (e.g., "You should be feeling better by now").
- Avoid offering rationalizations for the child's death (e.g., "Your child isn't suffering anymore").
- Avoid artificial consolation (e.g., "I know how you feel," or "You are still young enough to have another baby").
- Deal openly with feelings such as guilt, anger, and loss of self-esteem.
- Focus on feelings by using a feeling word in the statement (e.g., "You're still feeling all the pain of losing a child").
- Refer the family to an appropriate support group or for professional help, if needed.

At the Time of Death

- Reassure the family that everything possible is being done for the child, if they want lifesaving interventions.
- Do everything possible to ensure the child's comfort, especially relieving pain.
- Provide the child and family with the opportunity to review special experiences or memories in their lives.
- Express personal feelings of loss (e.g., "We will miss him so much," "We tried everything; we feel sad that we couldn't save her").
- Provide information that the family requests, and be honest.
- Respect the emotional needs of family members, such as siblings, who may need brief respites from the dying child.
- Make every effort to arrange for family members, especially parents, to be with the child at the moment of death, if they want to be present.
- Allow the family to stay with the dead child for as long as they wish and to rock, hold, or bathe the child.
- Provide practical help when possible, such as collecting the child's belongings.
- Arrange for spiritual support, based on the family's religious beliefs; pray with the family if no one else can stay with them.

After Death

- Attend the funeral or visitation if there was a special closeness with the family.
- Initiate and maintain contact (e.g., sending cards, telephoning, inviting them back to the unit, making a home visit).
- Refer to the dead child by name; discuss shared memories with the family.
- Discourage the use of drugs or alcohol as a method of escaping grief.
- Encourage all family members to communicate their feelings rather than remaining silent to avoid upsetting another member.
- Emphasize that grieving is a painful process that often takes years to resolve.

* *Family* refers to all significant persons involved in the child's life, such as the parents, siblings, grandparents, or other close relatives or friends.

FAMILY-CENTRED TEACHING

A Dying Child: A Nurse's Perspective

Claire was unresponsive with slow, gasping breathing. Her mother asked me what I thought was happening. I replied honestly, "Your baby is dying because of her brain tumour." The mother put her arms around me and cried. We arranged for Claire to be baptized.

Honesty. As painful as the loss of a child is, my job is to assist the family through this experience. Although I usually wait until a private moment, such as driving home, I found tears streaming down my face as family and friends gathered for Claire's baptism. I went into the kitchen to compose myself, only to find several of my colleagues crying as well. Saying goodbye to a dying child will always be a difficult but shared experience.

–Jeanne O'Connor Egan, RN, MSN, Pediatric Clinical Specialist, Children's Hospital
Washington, DC

Strategies that can assist the nurse in remaining able to work effectively in these settings include maintaining good general health, developing well-rounded interests, using distancing techniques such as taking time off when needed, developing and using professional and personal support systems, cultivating the capacity for empathy, focusing on the positive aspects of the caregiver role, and basing nursing interventions on sound theory and empirical observations. Attending shared-remembrance rituals can assists some nurses in resolving grief. Similarly, attending the funeral service for a patient who has died can be a supportive act for both the family and the nurse and in no way detracts from the professionalism of care.

KEY POINTS

- Trends in the treatment of children with chronic illness or complex conditions have focused on developmental age, the child's strengths and uniqueness, family-centred care, normalization, early discharge, home care, mainstreaming, and early intervention.
- Families' reactions to chronic illness or complex conditions are manifested in the following stages: shock and denial, adjustment, reintegration, and acknowledgement.
- The child's reaction to chronic illness or complex conditions depends on the child's developmental level, coping mechanisms, others' reactions, and the illness itself.
- In response to the child with chronic illness or a complex condition, parents may be affected by feelings of inadequacy and failure; excessive demands on time, energy, and financial resources; and strain on the marital relationship.

- Assessment of the family's adjustment to a child's chronic illness, complex condition, or death includes the availability of a support system, their perception of the event, their coping mechanisms, concurrent stressors, and their response to the child.
- To help parents cope with their child's chronic illness or complex condition, nurses must be attentive to parents' needs, give empathic support, solicit suggestions for care, facilitate communication, provide an opportunity to express feelings, and provide referrals to volunteer and community agencies.
- Supporting the child involves encouraging self-expression, alleviating feelings of being different, and strengthening the child's self-image.
- Palliative care focuses on improving the quality of lives of children and families who are facing a life-threatening illness and should be instituted early in the management of care of a dying child.
- Children's concept of death is determined by their cognitive ability and their experience with life-threatening illness.
- Young children see death as temporary and reversible and mainly fear separation.
- School-age children view death as irreversible but not necessarily inevitable and may fear mutilation.
- Children beyond 9 to 10 years of age realize that death is irreversible, universal, and inevitable but may resist the thought of their own death.
- Siblings have special needs, including the need for information, reassurance about their own health status, assurance that they are not responsible for the illness or death, and support for their own grieving process.
- Special needs of the family facing the unexpected death of a child include support while awaiting news of the child's status; a sensitive pronouncement of death; acknowledgement of feelings of denial, guilt, and anger; an opportunity to view the body; and referrals for support.
- Special decisions at the time of dying and death may involve location of care and death, viewing of the body, tissue donation and autopsy, and siblings' attendance at the funeral.
- Acute grief is a syndrome with intense and distressing psychological and somatic symptoms that appear at the time of death.
- Complicated grief is a prolonged, intense grief that can impede an individual's ability to function on a daily basis.
- In dealing with the stress related to a dying young patient, the nurse can cope successfully through self-awareness, knowledge and practice, an available support system, and maintenance of general good health and by focusing on the rewards of involvement with dying children and their families.

evolve WEBSITE

Visit the Evolve website for additional resources related to the content in this chapter such as Case Studies, Critical Thinking Case Study Answers, Nursing Care Plans, Nursing Processes, Nursing Skills, and Review Questions for Exam Preparation at: http://evolve.elsevier.com/Canada/Perry/maternal/

REFERENCES

Anderson, T., & Davis, C. (2011). Evidence-based practice with families of chronically ill children: A critical literature review. *Journal of Evidence-Based Social Work, 8*(4), 416–425.

Baillargeon, R. H., & Bernier, J. (2010). The burden of disability in children and youths associated with impairments of psychological functions. *Psychiatry Research, 177*, 199–205. doi:10.1016/j.psychres.2010.03.001.

Brehaut, J. C., Kohen, D. E., Garner, R. E., et al. (2009). Health among caregivers of children with health problems: Findings from a Canadian population-based study. *American Journal of Public Health, 99*(7), 1254–1259. doi:10.2105/AJPH.2007.129817.

Brennan, C., Hugh-Jones, S., & Aldridge, J. (2012). Paediatric life-limiting conditions: Coping and adjustment in siblings. *Journal of Health Psychology, 18*(6), 813–824.

Brown, R. T., Wiener, L., Kupst, M. J., et al. (2008). Single parenting and children with chronic illness: An understudied phenomenon. *Journal of Pediatric Psychology, 33*(4), 408–421.

Bruce, M., Gumley, D., Isham, L., et al. (2011). Post-traumatic stress symptoms in childhood brain tumour survivors and their parents. *Child: Care, Health and Development, 37*(2), 244–251. doi:10.1111/j.1365-2214.2010.01164.x.

Canadian Bioethics Society. (2014). *Accessing an ethics consultation.* Retrieved from <https://www.bioethics.ca/healthcare/consult.html>.

Canadian Home Care Association. (2006). *The delivery of home care services in rural and remote communities in Canada.* Retrieved from <http://www.cdnhomecare.ca/media.php?mid=2172>.

Canadian Nurses Association. (2008). *Code of ethics for registered nurses.* Retrieved from <https://www.cna-aiic.ca/~/media/cna/page-content/pdf-fr/code-of-ethics-for-registered-nurses.pdf?la=en>.

Carnevale, F. A., Rehm, R. S., Kirk, S., et al. (2008). What we know (and do not know) about raising children with complex continuing care needs. *Journal of Child Health Care, 12*(1), 4–6. doi:10.1177/1367493508088552.

Contro, N., Kreicbergs, U., Reichard, W. J., & Sourkes, B. M. (2011). Anticipatory grief and bereavement. In J. Wolfe, P. S. Hinds, & B. M. Sourkes (Eds.), *Textbook of interdisciplinary pediatric palliative care* (pp. 42–43). Philadelphia: Saunders.

Da Silva, F. M., Jacob, E., & Nascimento, C. (2010). Impact of childhood cancer on parents' relationships: An integrative review. *Journal of Nursing Scholarship, 42*(3), 250–261. doi:10.1111/j.1547-5069.2010.01360.x.

Daudji, A., Eby, S., Foo, T., et al. (2011). Perceptions of disability among south Asian immigrant mothers of children with disabilities in Canada: Implications for rehabilitation service delivery. *Disability and Rehabilitation, 33*(6), 511–521. doi:10.3109/09638288.2010.498549.

Doig, J. L., McLennan, J. D., & Urichuk, L. (2009). "Jumping through hoops": Parents' experiences with seeking respite care for children with special needs. *Child: Care, Health and Development, 35*(2), 234–242. doi:10.1111/j.1365-2214.2008.00922.x.

Dussel, V., Kreicbergs, U., Hilden, J., et al. (2009). Looking beyond where children die: Determinants and effects of planning a child's location of death. *Journal of Pain and Symptom Management, 37*(1), 33–43.

Dykens, E. M. (2015). Family adjustment and interventions in neurodevelopmental disorders. *Current Opinion in Psychiatry, 28*, 121–126.

Elias, E. R., Murphy, N. A., & Council on Children with Disabilities. (2012). Home care of children and youth with complex health care needs and technology dependencies. *Pediatrics, 129*(5), 996–1005.

Emerson, E., & Giallo, R. (2014). The wellbeing of siblings of children with disabilities. *Research in Developmental Disabilities, 35*(9), 2085–2092.

Ferguson, F., & Cinotti, D. (2009). Home oral health practice: The foundation for desensitization and dental care for special needs. *Dental Clinics of North America, 53*(2), 375–387.

Foster, T. L., Gilmer, M. J., Davies, B., et al. (2011). Comparison of continuing bonds reported by parents and siblings after a child's death from cancer. *Death Studies, 35*(5), 420–440.

Gerlach, A. (2008). "Circle of caring": A First Nations worldview of child rearing. *Canadian Journal of Occupational Therapy, 75*(1), 18–25.

Giambra, B. K., Stiffler, D., & Broome, M. E. (2014). An integrative review of communication between parents and nurses of hospitalized technology-dependent children. *Worldviews on Evidence-Based Nursing, 11*(6), 369–375. doi:10.1111/wvn.12065.

Gold, J. I., Treadwell, M., Weissman, L., et al. (2011). The mediating effects of family functioning on psychosocial outcomes in healthy siblings of children with sickle cell disease. *Pediatric Blood & Cancer, 57*(6), 1055–1061.

Grossoehme, D. H., Ragsdale, J., Cotton, S., et al. (2010). Parents' religious coping styles in the first year after their child's cystic fibrosis diagnosis. *Journal of Health Care Chaplaincy, 16*(3–4), 109–122. doi:10.1080/08854726.2010.480836.

Halfon, N., & Newacheck, P. (2010). Evolving notions of childhood chronic illness. *Journal of the American Medical Association, 2003*(7), 665–666. doi:10.1001/jama.2010.130.

Harrison, C., & Canadian Paediatric Society, Bioethics Committee. (2004). Treatment decisions regarding infants, children and adolescents. *Paediatrics & Child Health, 9*(2), 99–103. Reaffirmed 2016. Retrieved from <http://www.cps.ca/documents/position/treatment-decisions>.

Harrison, J., Evan, E., Hughes, A., et al. (2014). Understanding communication among health care professionals regarding death and dying in pediatrics. *Palliative and Supportive Care, 12*(5), 387–392. doi:10.1017/S1478951513000229.

Health Canada. (2008). *Just for you—Rural Canadians.* Retrieved from <http://www.hc-sc.gc.ca/hl-vs/jfy-spv/rural-rurale-eng.php>.

Heath, J. A., Clarke, N. E., Donath, S. M., et al. (2010). Symptoms and suffering at the end of life in children with cancer: An Australian perspective. *The Medical Journal of Australia, 192*(2), 71–75.

Hollander, M., & Prince, M. (2008). Organizing healthcare delivery systems for persons with ongoing care needs and their families. *Healthcare Quarterly, 11*(1), 44–54.

Hoogsteen, L., & Woodgate, R. L. (2013). The lived experience of parenting a child with autism in a rural area: Making the invisible, visible. *Paediatric Nursing, 39*(5), 233–237.

The Hospital for Sick Children. (2014). *Complex care transition resource guide.* Retrieved from <http://www.sickkids.ca/Good2Go/For-Youth-and-Families/Just-for-Parents-and-Caregivers/Complex-Care-Transition-Resource-Guide/Index.html>.

Knafl, K., Darney, B. G., Gallo, A. M., et al. (2010). Parental perceptions of the outcome and meaning of normalization. *Research in Nursing & Health, 33*(2), 87–98.

Kon, A. A. (2010). The shared decision-making continuum. *Journal of the American Medical Association, 304*(8), 903–904.

Kratz, L., Uding, N., Trahms, C., et al. (2009). Managing childhood chronic illness: Parent perspectives and implications for parent-provider relationships. *Families, Systems & Health, 27*(4), 303–313.

Kube, D. A., Bishop, E. A., Roth, J. M., et al. (2013). Evaluation of a parent led curriculum in developmental disabilities for pediatric and medicine/pediatric residents. *Maternal and Child Health Journal, 17*, 1304–1308. doi:10.1007/s10995-012-1133-5.

Lach, L. M., Kohen, D. E., Garner, R. E., et al. (2009). The health and psychosocial functioning of caregivers of children with neurodevelopmental disorders. *Disability and Rehabilitation, 31*(8), 607–618.

LeGrow, K., Hodnett, E., Stremler, R., et al. (2014). Evaluating the feasibility of a parent-briefing intervention in a paediatric acute care setting. *Journal for Specialists in Pediatric Nursing, 19*(2014), 219–228.

Lund, E. M., & Vaughn-Jensen, J. E. (2012). Victimisation of children with disabilities. *Lancet, 380*(9845), 867–869.

Martinez, Y. J., & Ercikan, K. (2009). Chronic illness in Canadian children: What is the effect of illness on academic achievement, and anxiety and emotional disorders? *Child: Care, Health and Development, 35*(3), 391–401.

Meert, K. L., Shear, K., Newth, C. J., et al. (2011). Eunice Kennedy Shriver National Institute of Child Health and Human Development Collaborative Pediatric Critical Care Research Network. Follow-up study of complicated grief among parents eighteen months after a child's death in the pediatric intensive care unit. *Journal of Palliative Medicine, 14*(2), 207–214.

Nuutila, L., & Salanterä, S. (2006). Children with a long-term illness: Parents' experiences of care. *Journal of Pediatric Nursing, 21*(2), 153–160. doi:10.1016/j.pedn.2005.07.005.

O'Brien, I., Duffy, A., & Nicholl, H. (2009). Impact of childhood chronic illnesses on siblings: A literature review. *British Journal of Nursing, 18*(22), 1358, 1360–1365.

Parachute Canada. (n.d.). *Information on car seats.* Retrieved from <http://www.parachutecanada.org/policy/item/child-passenger-safety>.

Public Health Agency of Canada. (2009). The health of Canadian children. *The Chief Public Health Officer's Report on the State of Public Health in Canada.* Retrieved from <http://www.phac-aspc.gc.ca/cphorsphc-respcacsp/2009/fr-rc/cphorsphc-respcacsp06-eng.php#c3-1>.

Rapoport, A. (2008). A place to die: The case for paediatric inpatient hospices. *Paediatrics & Child Health, 13*(5), 369–370.

Registered Nurses Association of Ontario. (2011). *Clinical best practice guidelines: End-of-life care during the last days and hours.* Retrieved from <http://rnao.ca/sites/rnao-ca/files/End-of-Life_Care_During_the_Last_Days_and_Hours_0.pdf>.

Reilly, D., Huws, J., Hastings, R., et al. (2010). Life and death of a child with Down syndrome and a congenital heart condition: Experiences of six couples. *Intellectual and Developmental Disabilities, 48*(6), 403–416.

Rosenberg, A. R., Wolfe, J., Bradford, M. C., et al. (2014). Resilience and psychosocial outcomes in parents of children with cancer. *Pediatric Blood & Cancer, 61*, 552–557.

Sanderson, A., Hall, A. M., & Wolfe, J. (2016). Advance care discussions: Pediatric clinician preparedness and practices. *Journal of Pain and Symptom Management, 51*(3), 520–528. doi:10.1016/j.jpainsymman.2015.10.014.

Schlucter, J. S., Dokken, D., & Ahmann, E. (2015). Transitions from pediatric to adult care: Programs and resources. *Pediatric Nursing, 41*(2), 85–88.

Siden, H., Miller, M., Straatman, L., et al. (2008). A report on location of death in paediatric palliative care between home, hospice and hospital. *Palliative Medicine, 22*, 831–834.

Singh Jassal, S. (Ed.). (2011). *Basic symptom control in paediatric palliative care.* Retrieved from <http://www.rainbows.co.uk/wp-content/uploads/2011/06/Rainbows-Hospice-Basic-Symptom-Control-In-Paediatric-Palliative-Care-8th-Ed-2011-protected.pdf>.

Skinner, A. C., & Slifkim, R. T. (2007). Rural/urban differences in barriers to and burden of care for children with special health care needs. *The Journal of Rural Health, 23*(2), 150–157.

Spalding, K., & Salib, D. (2008). *Children and youth home care in Canada.* Canadian Research. Network for Care in the Community. Retrieved from <http://www.ryerson.ca/content/dam/crncc/knowledge/infocus/factsheets/In_Focus_Children_and_Youth_Homecare_FINAL.pdf>.

Statistics Canada. (2008). *Educational services and the disabled child.* Retrieved from <http://www.statcan.gc.ca/pub/81-004-x/2006005/9588-eng.htm>.

Steele, R., Derman, S., Cadell, S., et al. (2008). Families' transition to a Canadian pediatric hospice. Part two: Results of a pilot study. *International Journal of Palliative Nursing, 14*, 287–295.

Strickland, B. B., van Dyck, P. C., Kogan, M. D., et al. (2011). Assessing and ensuring a comprehensive system of services for children with special health care needs: A public health approach. *American Journal of Public Health, 101*(2), 224–231. doi:10.2105/AJPH.2009.177915.

Swallow, V., Macfadyen, A., Santacroce, S. J., et al. (2012). Fathers' contributions to the management of their child's long-term medical condition: A narrative review of the literature. *Health Expectations, 15*(2), 157–175.

Thikkurissy, S., & Lal, S. (2009). Oral health burden in children with systemic diseases. *Dental Clinics of North America, 53*(2), 351–357.

Transport Canada. (2008). *Transporting infants and children with special needs in personal vehicles: A best practices guide for healthcare practitioners.* Retrieved from <http://www.parachutecanada.org/downloads/injurytopics/SpecialNeeds_TransportCanada.pdf>.

Tsai, E., & Canadian Paediatric Society, Bioethics Committee. (2008). Advance care planning for paediatric patients. *Paediatrics & Child Health, 13*(9), 791–796. Reaffirmed 2016.

United Nations. (1989). *Convention on the Rights of the Child.* Retrieved from <http://www.refworld.org/docid/3ae6b38f0.html>.

Woodgate, R. L., Edwards, M., Ripat, J. D., et al. (2015). Intense parenting: A qualitative study detailing the experiences of parenting children with complex care needs. *BMC Pediatrics, 15*(197), 1–15.

Wool, C. (2013). State of the science on perinatal palliative care. *Journal of Obstetric, Gynecologic, and Neonatal Nursing, 42*, 372–382. doi:10.1111/1552-6909.12034.

World Health Organization. (2012). *WHO guidelines on the pharmacological treatment of persisting pain in children with medical illnesses.* Retrieved from <http://apps.who.int/iris/bitstream/10665/44540/1/9789241548120_Guidelines.pdf>.

World Health Organization. (2016). *WHO definition of palliative care.* Retrieved from <http://www.who.int/cancer/palliative/definition/en/>.

Young, B., Eden, T., Hill, J., et al. (2012). Communicating in a way that parents find supportive: Is the guidance mistaken? *Pediatric Blood & Cancer, 59*(6), 984.

ADDITIONAL RESOURCES

Canadian Virtual Hospice—Information and support for families and health professionals on palliative and end-of-life care: <www.virtualhospice.ca>

Canadian Virtual Hospice—Programs and Services: <http://www.virtualhospice.ca/en_US/Main+Site+Navigation/Home/Support/Resources/Programs+and+Services.aspx>

Children's Wish—Canadian charity that grants favourite wish of a child diagnosed with a life-threatening illness: <http://www.childrenswish.ca>

Council of Canadians with Disabilities: <http://www.ccdonline.ca>

Easter Seals Canada: <http://easterseals.ca/english/>

Family Support Institute of BC: <http://www.familysupportbc.com/resources>

Government of Canada—Blood, Organ, and Tissue Donation: <http://healthycanadians.gc.ca/diseases-conditions-maladies-affections/donation-contribution-eng.php>

Holland Bloorview Kids Rehabilitation Hospital: Family resource centre: <http://www.hollandbloorview.ca/Home>

Introducing a Lexicon of Terms for Pediatric Palliative Care: <http://www.pulsus.com/journals/pdf_frameset.jsp?jnlKy=5&atlKy=13380&isArt=t&jnlAdvert=Paeds&adverifHCTp=&sTitle=Introducing%20a%20lexicon%20of%20terms%20for%20paediatric%20palliative%20care%2C%20Pulsus%20Group%20Inc&HCtype=&pdfType=fulltextpdf>

Medic Alert Foundation: <http://www.medicalert.org/>

My Summer Camps—Directory of private, paying camps for children with chronic illnesses or general physical disabilities: <http://www.mysummercamps.com/camps/Special_Needs_Camps/index.html>

Our Kids—Summer Camps for Kids With Special Needs: <http://www.ourkids.net/special-needs-camps.php>

Parentbooks—Books for siblings of children with special needs: <http://www.parentbooks.ca/Siblings_of_Children_with_Special_Needs.html>

Special Need Child Canada: <http://www.special-need-child-canada.com/special-need-child-blog.html>

Special Olympics Canada: <http://www.specialolympics.ca>

Staying Connected: A Guide for Families When a Sick Child Has Trouble Communicating: <http://www.aboutkidshealth.ca/En/Documents/Staying-Connected.PDF>

The Hospital for Sick Children—Good To Go Transition Program. Complex Care Transition Resource Guide: <http://www.sickkids.ca/pdfs/good2go/45804-CCRWebsiteOctober.pdf>

Together for Short Lives—Resources to assist health care providers in palliative and end-of-life care for children: <http://www.togetherforshortlives.org.uk/professionals/resources?section=143§ionTitle=Resources+and+shop>

VSA Arts—International Organization on Arts and Disability (affiliate chapters in Ontario and Québec): <http://www.kennedy-center.org/education/vsa/>

Walk a Mile in Their Shoes: Bullying and the Child With Special Needs: <http://www.abilitypath.org/areas-of-development/learning--schools/bullying/articles/walk-a-mile-in-their-shoes.pdf>

World Health Organization: Palliative Care: Symptom Management and End-of-Life Care: <http://www.who.int/hiv/pub/imai/genericpalliativecare082004.pdf>

CHAPTER

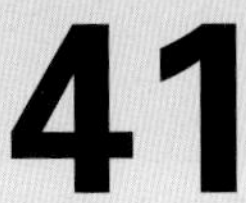

Cognitive and Sensory Impairment

Cheryl Sams

evolve WEBSITE

***Visit the Evolve website for additional resources related to the content in this chapter such as Case Studies, Critical Thinking Case Study Answers, Nursing Care Plans, Nursing Processes, Nursing Skills, and Review Questions for Exam Preparation at:** http://evolve.elsevier.com/Canada/Perry/maternal/*

OBJECTIVES

On completion of this chapter the reader will be able to:

- Define the classifications of intellectual disability.
- Outline nursing interventions for the child with cognitive impairment that promote optimum development, including during hospitalization.
- Identify the major biological and cognitive characteristics of the child with Down syndrome.
- Outline nursing interventions for the child with Down syndrome.
- Identify the major characteristics associated with fragile X syndrome.
- List the general classifications of hearing impairment and the effect on speech.
- Outline nursing interventions for the child with hearing impairment, including during hospitalization.
- List the common types of visual impairments in children.
- Outline nursing interventions for the child with visual impairment, including during hospitalization.
- Outline nursing interventions for the child with retinoblastoma.
- Outline nursing interventions for the child with autism spectrum disorder.

COGNITIVE IMPAIRMENT

General Concepts

Cognitive impairment (CI) is a general term that encompasses any type of mental difficulty or deficiency. In this chapter the term is used synonymously with intellectual disability and replaces the term *mental retardation*; this term should not be used as it is stigmatizing (Shapiro & Batshaw, 2016). This chapter discusses the characteristics and diagnosis of specific types of CI as well as the nursing care required for children with CI. Although the family's needs and concerns are also a primary focus throughout this chapter, the reader is encouraged to review Chapter 40, which details the family's adjustment to chronic illness and complex conditions in general.

The definition of CI in children consists of three components: intellectual functioning, functional strengths and weaknesses, and age younger than 18 years at time of diagnosis. Intellectual functioning is measured by the intelligence quotient (IQ) of 70 to 75 or below. The child with an intellectual disability must demonstrate functional impairment in at least 2 of 10 different adaptive skill areas: communication, self-care, home living, social skills, leisure, health and safety, self-direction, functional academics, community use, and work (American Psychiatric Association [APA], 2013) or have deficits in one or more adaptive domains (American Association on Intellectual and Developmental Disabilities [AAIDD], 2010). The classification system by the AAIDD allows for identification of the individual's specific needs in four established dimensions of care (Box 41-1). It is anticipated that the functional capabilities of children with CI will improve over time when support is provided.

Diagnosis and Classification

The diagnosis of CI is usually made after a period of suspicion, by professionals or the family, that the child's developmental progress is delayed. In some cases it is confirmed at birth

BOX 41-1 DIMENSIONS OF CARE FOR THE INTELLECTUALLY DISABLED

Dimension I—Intellectual functioning and adaptive skills
Dimension II—Psychological and emotional considerations
Dimension III—Physical, health, and etiological considerations
Dimension IV—Environmental considerations

BOX 41-2 EARLY BEHAVIOURAL SIGNS SUGGESTIVE OF COGNITIVE IMPAIRMENT

- Dysmorphic features (e.g., Down syndrome, fragile X syndrome)
- Major organ system dysfunction (e.g., feeding and breathing)
- Failure to interact with the environment
- Concerns about hearing or vision impairment
- Gross motor delay
- Decreased alertness to voice or movement
- Language difficulties or delay

Shapiro, B., & Batshaw, M. (2016). Intellectual disability. In R. M. Kliegman, B. F. Stanton, J. W. St. Geme, et al. (Eds.), *Nelson textbook of pediatrics* (20th ed.). Philadelphia: Saunders.

because of recognition of distinct syndromes, such as Down syndrome and fetal alcohol spectrum disorder. At the other extreme, the diagnosis is made when problems such as speech delays arouse concern. In all cases a high index of suspicion for developmental delay and behavioural signs (Box 41-2) is necessary for early diagnosis; routine developmental screening can assist in early identification (see Chapter 33). Delays are typically seen in gross and fine motor and speech development, although the latter is most predictive. Developmental delay can be described as any significant lag in a child's physical, cognitive, behavioural, emotional, or social development, when compared against developmental norms. CI is a permanent impairment encompassing cognitive ability and adaptive behaviour that are functioning significantly below average (see Box 41-2). In the absence of clear-cut evidence of CI, it is more appropriate to use a diagnosis of developmental delay.

The formal diagnosis of CI requires the administration of individual tests of intelligence and adaptive functioning. Results of standardized tests are used in making the diagnosis of intellectual disability based on cognitive deficits. The Bayley Scales of Infant Development (BSID-III) is the most commonly used infant intelligence scale, and for children older than 3 the most commonly used psychological tests are the Wechsler Scales (Shapiro & Batshaw, 2016). Tests for assessing adaptive behaviours include the Vineland Social Maturity Scale, which involves semistructured interviews with parents and/or caregivers and teachers that assess adaptive behaviour in four domains: communication, daily living skills, socialization, and motor skills (Shapiro & Batshaw, 2016). Informal appraisal of adaptive behaviour may be made by those fully familiarized with the child (e.g., teachers, parents, other care providers). Frequently these observations lead parents to seek evaluation of the child's development. In addition, the Nunavik Adaptive Behaviour Scale is available to assess adaptive behaviour in Inuit school-age children and in adults in whom intellectual disability is suspected (Maurice, Bouffard, Desjardins, et al., 2007).

A more useful approach for clinical application is classification based on educational potential or symptom severity. For educational purposes the term *educable CI* corresponds to the mildly impaired group, which constitutes about 85% of all people with CI. *Trainable CI* generally applies to children with moderate levels of CI and accounts for about 10% of the intellectually disabled population (APA, 2013; Katz & Lazcano-Ponce, 2008). Although nurses may be familiar with the approximate range of IQ for classifying severity, they should refrain from using numbers as the criterion for assessing or evaluating a child's abilities, since numbers are of little value in counselling parents or training these children.

Etiology

The causes of severe CI are primarily genetic, biochemical, and infectious. Although the etiology is unknown in most cases, familial, social, environmental, and organic causes may predominate. Among individuals with CI, a sizable proportion of the cases are linked to Down syndrome, fragile X syndrome, or fetal alcohol spectrum disorder. General categories of events that may lead to cognitive impairment include the following (Katz & Lazcano-Ponce, 2008):

- Infection and intoxication, such as congenital rubella, syphilis, Zika virus, maternal drug consumption (e.g., fetal alcohol spectrum disorder), chronic lead ingestion, or kernicterus
- Trauma or physical agent (i.e., injury to the brain suffered during the perinatal period)
- Inadequate nutrition and metabolic disorders, such as phenylketonuria or congenital hypothyroidism
- Gross postnatal brain disease, such as neurofibromatosis and tuberous sclerosis
- Unknown prenatal influence, including cerebral and cranial malformations, such as microcephaly and hydrocephalus
- Chromosomal abnormalities resulting from radiation, viruses, chemicals, parental age, and genetic mutations, such as Down syndrome and fragile X syndrome
- Gestational disorders, including prematurity, low birth weight, and postmaturity
- Psychiatric disorders that have their onset during the child's developmental period up to age 18 years, such as autism spectrum disorders (ASDs)
- Environmental influences, including evidence of a deprived environment associated with a history of CI among parents and siblings

NURSING CARE

Nurses play a major role in identifying children with CI. In the newborn and early infancy periods, few signs are present, with the exception of Down syndrome (p. 1221). After this age, however, delayed developmental milestones are the major clues to CI. In addition, nurses must have a high index of suspicion for early behavioural patterns that may suggest CI (see Box 41-2). Parental concerns, such as delayed development compared with that of siblings, need to be taken seriously. All children should receive regular developmental assessment, and the nurse is often the person responsible for performing such assessments (see Chapter 33). When delays are found, the nurse must use sensitivity and discretion in revealing this finding to parents.

Educating the Child and Family

To teach children with CI, it is necessary to investigate their learning abilities and deficits. This is important for the nurse who may be involved in a home care program or who may be caring for the child in a health care setting. The nurse who understands how these children learn can effectively teach them basic skills or prepare them for various health-related procedures.

Children with CI have a marked deficit in their ability to discriminate between two or more stimuli because of difficulty in recognizing the relevance of specific cues. However, these children can learn to discriminate if the cues are presented in an exaggerated, concrete form and if all extraneous stimuli are eliminated. For example, the use of colours to emphasize visual cues or the use of singing or rhymes to stress auditory cues can help them learn. Their deficit in discrimination also implies that concrete ideas are learned much more effectively than abstract ideas. Therefore, demonstration is preferable to verbal explanation, and learning should be directed toward mastering a skill rather than understanding the scientific principles underlying a procedure.

Another cognitive deficit is in short-term memory. Whereas children of average intelligence can remember several words, numbers, or directions at one time, children with CI are less able to do so. Therefore, they need simple, one-step directions. Learning through a step-by-step process requires a task analysis, in which each task is separated into its necessary components and each step is taught completely before proceeding to the next activity.

One critical area of learning that has had a tremendous impact on education for cognitively impaired individuals is motivation. Programs based on the motivational principles of behaviour modification, employing positive reinforcement for specific tasks or behaviours, have demonstrated marked improvement in children's ability to learn. Advances in technology have greatly aided in providing reinforcement, especially in children with severe disabilities and who may have physical disabilities that limit their range of capabilities. For example, with the use of specially designed switches, children can be given control of some event in the environment, such as turning on the computer or television. The screen becomes reinforcement for activating the switch. Repetitive use of these switches provides an early, simple association with a technical device that may progress to increasingly complex aids.

The care strategies for children with an intellectual disability should be multimodal, with efforts directed at all aspects of the child's life: health, education, social and recreational activities, behaviour problems, and associated impairments. Support for parents and siblings should also be provided (Shapiro & Batshaw, 2016). Early intervention programs comprise a systematic program of therapy, exercises, and activities designed to address developmental delays in children with disabilities in order to help them achieve their full potential (Canadian Down Syndrome Society, 2009; Weijerman & de Winter, 2010). Nurses working with these families need to be aware of the types of programs in their community. Under the *Education Act* (1956–1996) and the *Canadian Human Rights Act* (1977), provinces and territories are required to provide educational opportunities for all children with disabilities (see Additional Resources at the end of this chapter). Although early intervention programs are available in Canada, Canadian provinces and territories vary widely in their support, thus many expenses may fall to the parents. Services may be provided by private organizations such as the Canadian Down Syndrome Society and Easter Seals Canada (see Additional Resources). Parents should inquire about these programs by contacting the appropriate agencies. The child's education should begin as soon as possible. As children grow older, their education should be directed toward vocational training that prepares them for as independent a lifestyle as possible that is within their scope of abilities. When school age, children with CI often will have an Individual Education Plan (IEP) developed for the school setting. IEPs are created on a case-by-case basis, identifying specific learning needs and outlining any accommodations required for the student, including how the school will ensure these are met. These plans require communication and collaboration between the parents, health care team and teaching team, and the child if he or she is able to contribute (see Additional Resources for links to information related to IEP).

Teaching the Child Self-Care Skills

When a child with CI is born, parents need assistance in promoting normal developmental skills that are almost automatically learned by other children. These include self-care skills such as feeding, toileting, dressing, and grooming. In order to teach these skills, a basic knowledge of the developmental sequence in learning the skills demonstrated by children of average intelligence is required. For example, children with lower than average intelligence would not be expected to dress themselves as early as unaffected youngsters.

Teaching self-care skills also necessitates a working knowledge of the individual steps needed to master a skill. For example, before beginning a self-feeding program, the nurse needs to perform a task analysis. After a task analysis, the child is observed in a particular situation, such as eating, to determine what skills are possessed and the child's developmental readiness to learn the task. Family members are included in this process because their "readiness" is as important as the child's. Numerous self-help aids are available to facilitate independence and can help eliminate some of the difficulties of learning, such as using a plate with suction cups to prevent accidental spills (see Additional Resources at the end of this chapter).

Promoting Child's Optimum Development

Optimum development involves more than achieving independence. It requires appropriate guidance for establishing acceptable social behaviour and personal feelings of self-esteem, worth, and security. These attributes are not simply learned through a stimulation program. Rather, they must arise from the genuine love and caring of family members. However, families need guidance in providing an environment that fosters optimum development. Often the nurse can provide this help.

Another important area for promoting optimum development and self-esteem is ensuring the child's physical well-being. Any congenital defects, such as cardiac, gastrointestinal, or orthopaedic anomalies, should be repaired. Plastic surgery may be considered when the child's appearance can be substantially improved. Dental health is significant, and orthodontic and restorative procedures can often improve facial appearance immensely.

Encouraging Play and Exercise

Children who are cognitively impaired have the same needs for recreation and exercise as other children. However, because of the children's slower development, parents may be less aware of the need to provide such activities (Fig. 41-1). Therefore, the nurse needs to guide parents toward selection of suitable play and exercise activities. Because play for children in each age group has been discussed in earlier chapters (see Chapter 32, Role of Play in Development, and Chapters 35–38), only the exceptions are presented here.

The type of play is based on the child's developmental age, although the need for sensorimotor play may be prolonged for several years. Parents should use every opportunity to expose the child to as many different sounds, sights, and sensations as possible. Appropriate play includes musical mobiles, stuffed toys, water play, floating toys, a rocking chair or horse, a swing, bells, and rattles. The child should be taken on outings, such as trips to the grocery store or shopping centre; other people should be encouraged to visit in the home; and the child should be related to directly, such as by cuddling, holding, and rocking the child; talking to the child in the en face (face-to-face) position; and giving the child "rides" on the parents' shoulders.

Toys can be selected for their recreational and educational value. For example, a large inflatable beach ball is a good water toy; it encourages interactive play and can be used to learn motor skills, such as balance, rocking, kicking, and throwing. A doll with removable clothes and different types of closures can help the child learn dressing skills. Musical toys that mimic animal sounds or respond with social phrases are excellent ways of encouraging speech. Toys should be simple in design so that the child can learn to manipulate them without help. For children with severe cognitive and physical impairment, electronic switches can be used to allow them to operate toys (Fig. 41-2).

Suitable activities for physical activity should be based on the child's size, coordination, physical fitness and maturity, motivation, and health (Fig. 41-3). Some children may have physical problems that prevent participation in certain sports, such as atlantoaxial instability in children with Down syndrome. These children often have greater success in individual and dual sports than in team sports and enjoy themselves most with children of the same developmental level. The Special Olympics provides children with a unique competitive opportunity (see Additional Resources section at the end of this chapter).

Safety is a major consideration in selecting recreational and exercise activities. For example, toys that may be appropriate developmentally may present dangers to a child who is strong enough to break them or use them incorrectly.

Providing Means of Communication

Verbal skills are typically delayed more than other physical skills. Speech requires hearing and interpretation (receptive

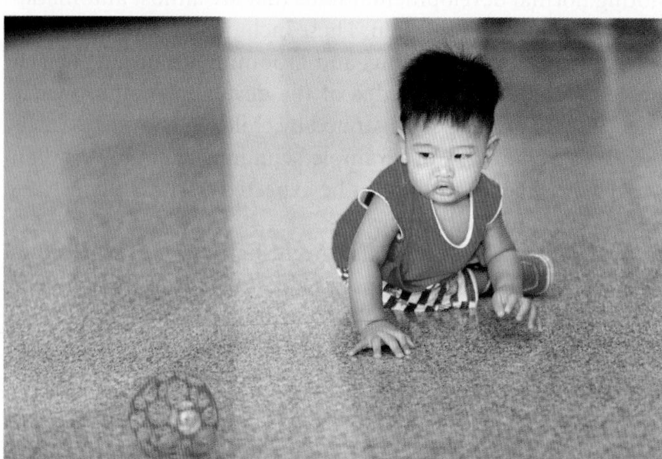

FIGURE 41-1 Placing an attractive object outside the child's reach encourages crawling movements. (Wichai Sittipan/Shutterstock .com.)

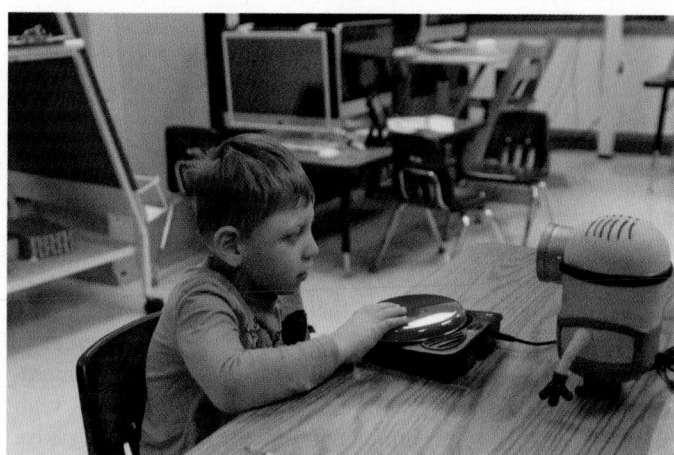

FIGURE 41-2 A manual switch allows a child with cognitive impairment to play with a battery-operated toy. (© 2015 AbleNet Inc. All Rights Reserved.)

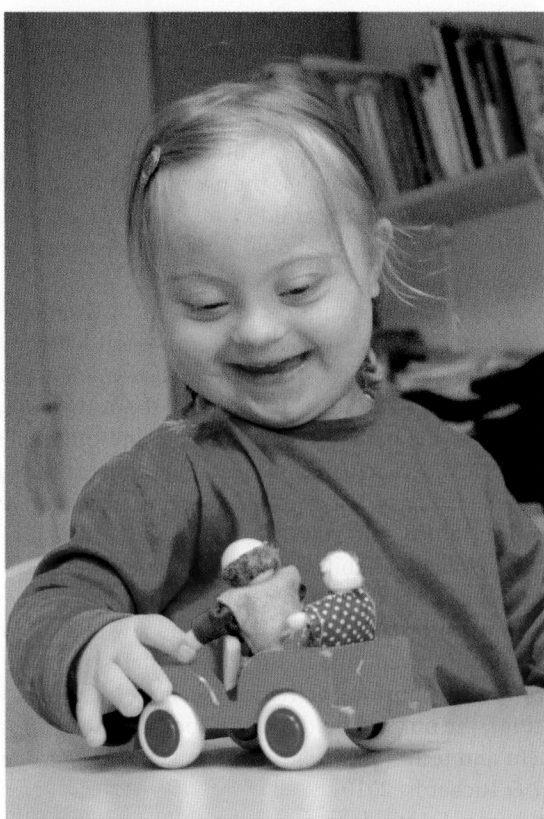

FIGURE 41-3 A favourite toy provides stimulation for a young child. (© Agencja Fotograficzna Caro/Alamy Stock Photo.)

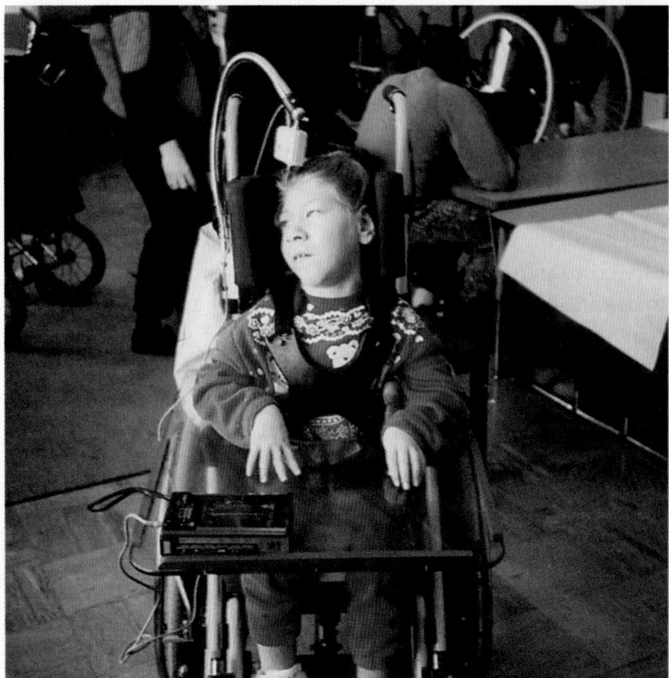

FIGURE 41-4 A child with cognitive and physical impairments can activate electronic and communication equipment by moving a device near her head.

skills) and facial muscle coordination (expressive skills). Because both types of skills may be impaired, these children need frequent audiometric testing and should be fitted with hearing aids if indicated. In addition, they may need help in learning to control their facial muscles. For example, some children may need tongue exercises to correct the tongue thrust or gentle reminders to keep the lips closed.

Nonverbal communication may be appropriate for some of these children, and various devices are available. For the child without associated physical disabilities, a talking picture board is helpful. For children with physical limitations, several adaptations or types of communication devices are available to facilitate selection of the appropriate picture or word (Fig. 41-4). Some children may be taught sign language or Blissymbols—a highly stylized system of graphic symbols that represent words, ideas, and concepts. Although the symbols require education to learn their meaning, no reading skill is needed. The symbols are usually arranged on a board, and the person points or uses some type of selector to convey a message.

Establishing Discipline

Discipline must begin early. Limit-setting measures need to be simple, consistently applied, and appropriate for the child's mental age. Control measures are based primarily on teaching a specific behaviour rather than on understanding the reasons behind it. Stressing moral lessons is of little value to a child who lacks the cognitive skills to learn from self-criticism or from a lesson based on previous wrong-doing. Behaviour modification, especially reinforcement of desired actions, and time-out are appropriate forms of behaviour control.

Encouraging Socialization

Acquiring social skills is a complex task, as is learning self-care procedures. Active rehearsal with role-playing and practice sessions and positive reinforcement for desired behaviour have been the most successful approaches. Parents should be encouraged early to teach their child socially acceptable behaviour: waving goodbye, saying "hello" and "thank you," responding to his or her name, greeting visitors, and sitting modestly. The teaching of socially acceptable sexual behaviour is especially important in order to minimize sexual exploitation. Parents also need to expose the child to strangers so that he or she can practise manners, as there is generally no automatic transfer of learning from one situation to another.

Dressing and grooming are also important aspects of socialization. A child who is dressed in age-appropriate clothing and is well groomed is much more likely to be accepted and to develop good self-esteem. Many attractive outfits can be adapted with self-adhering fasteners and elastic openings to facilitate self-dressing.

As soon as possible, parents should enroll the child in an appropriate preschool program. Not only do these programs provide education and training, but they also offer an opportunity for social experiences among children. As children grow older, they should have peer experiences similar to those of other children, including group outings, sports, and organized activities such as Scouts and Special Olympics. Nurses can assess the child's abilities and encourage others (e.g., parents, teachers) to promote developmentally appropriate peer interaction (Shapiro & Batshaw, 2016).

Providing Information on Sexuality

Adolescence may be a particularly difficult time for the family, especially in terms of the child's sexual behaviour, possibility of pregnancy, future plans to marry, and ability to be independent. Frequently, little anticipatory guidance has been offered to parents to prepare the child for physical and sexual maturation. The nurse can help in this area by providing parents with information about sexuality education that is geared toward the child's developmental level. For example, the adolescent girl needs a simple explanation of menstruation and instructions on personal hygiene during the menstrual cycle.

These adolescents also need practical sexual information regarding anatomy, physical development, and conception. Because of their easy persuasion and lack of judgement, they need a well-defined, concrete code of conduct. The subtleties of social sexual behaviour are less beneficial than specific instructions for handling certain situations. For example, an adolescent should be firmly told never to go alone anywhere with any person he or she does not know well. To protect him or her from abusive sexual activities, parents must closely observe their teenager's activities and associates. The question of contraceptive protection for these adolescents is often a parental concern.

Parents of these adolescents are often concerned about the advisability of marriage between two individuals with an intellectual disability. There is no conclusive answer; each situation must be judged individually. In some instances marriage is possible, but parenthood may not be desirable because of the complexity of child-rearing and the potential problem of perpetuating CI. The nurse should discuss this topic with parents and with the prospective couple, stressing suitable living accommodations and contraceptive methods to prevent pregnancy. If children are conceived, these parents require specialized assistance in learning to meet the needs of their offspring.

Helping Family Adjust to Future Care

Not all families are able to cope with home care of their affected child, especially one who is severely or profoundly impaired or has multiple disabilities (see Chapter 40 for strategies to support families of children with chronic illnesses). Older parents may not be able to assume care responsibilities after they reach retirement or older age. For these parents, the decision regarding residential placement is a difficult one, and the availability of such facilities varies widely. The nurse working with a family should help them investigate and evaluate various programs, in addition to assisting them in adjusting to the decision for placement.

Care for Child During Hospitalization

Caring for the child during hospitalization can be a special challenge. Frequently, nurses are unfamiliar with children who are cognitively impaired, and they may cope with their feelings of insecurity and fear by ignoring or isolating the child. Not only is this approach nonsupportive, but it may also be destructive for the child's sense of self-esteem and optimum development, and it may hamper the parents' ability to cope with the stress of the experience. One method that successfully avoids this nontherapeutic approach is the use of the mutual participation model in planning the child's care. Parents are encouraged to stay with their child but should not be made to feel as if the responsibility is theirs alone.

When the child is admitted, a detailed history should be taken (see Chapter 33), especially in terms of all self-care activity. During the interview the child's developmental age is assessed. It is best to avoid asking directly about IQ levels, since this may make the parents uncomfortable and often tells little about the child's actual abilities. Questions need to be approached positively. For example, rather than asking, "Is your child toilet trained yet?" the nurse may state, "Tell me about your child's toileting habits." The assessment should also focus on any special devices the child uses, effective measures of limit-setting, unusual or favourite routines, and any behaviours that may require intervention. If the parent states that the child engages in self-injurious activities (such as head banging or self-biting), the nurse should inquire about events that precipitate them and techniques that the parents use to manage them (Oliver & Richards, 2010).

The nurse also needs to assess the child's functional level of eating and playing; ability to express needs verbally; progress in toilet training; and relationship with objects, toys, and other children. The child should be encouraged to be as independent as possible in the hospital.

Realizing that the child may be lonely in the hospital, the nurse can make certain that toys and other activities are provided. The child should be placed in a room with other children of approximately the same developmental age, preferably a room with only two beds, to avoid overstimulation. The nurse should discuss with the other parents the child's abilities and introduce the parents and children to each other. By the nurse's example of treating the child with dignity and respect, others who may be fearful of what they do not understand are encouraged to accept the child.

Procedures should be explained to the child through methods of communication that are at the appropriate cognitive level. Generally, explanations should be simple, short, and concrete, emphasizing what the child will experience physically. Demonstration either through actual practice or with visual aids is always preferable to verbal explanation. The nurse needs to repeat instructions often and evaluate the child's understanding by asking questions such as "What will it feel like?" "Show me how you must lie," or "Where will the dressing be?" Parents should be included in preprocedural teaching for their own learning and to help the nurse learn effective methods of communicating with the child.

During hospitalization, the nurse should also focus on growth-promoting experiences for the child. For example, hospitalization may be an excellent opportunity to emphasize to parents the abilities that the child does have but has not had the opportunity to practise, such as self-dressing. It may also be an opportunity for social experiences with peers, group play, or new educational and recreational activities. For example, one child who had the habit of screaming and kicking demonstrated a definite decrease in these behaviours after he learned to pound pegs and use a punching bag. Through social services, the parents may become aware of specialized programs for the child. Hospitalization may also offer parents a respite from everyday care responsibilities and an opportunity to discuss their feelings with a concerned professional.

Assisting in Measures to Prevent Cognitive Impairment

Besides having a responsibility to families who have a child with CI, nurses also need to be involved in programs aimed at preventing CI. Many of the familial, social, and environmental factors known to cause mild impairment are preventable. Counselling and education of pregnant women and of women considering pregnancy can reduce or eliminate factors (e.g., poor nutrition, cigarette smoking, substance use) that increase the risk of prematurity and intrauterine growth restriction. Interventions should be directed toward improving maternal health by educating women about the dangers of chemicals, including prenatal alcohol exposure, which affects organogenesis, craniofacial development, and cognitive ability (Defendi, 2010). Other preventive strategies that play an important role include adequate prenatal care; optimal medical care of high-risk newborns; rubella immunization; genetic counselling and prenatal screening, especially for Down or fragile X syndrome; use of folic acid supplements to prevent neural tube defects during pregnancy and during the child-bearing years; newborn screening for treatable inborn errors of metabolism, such as congenital hypothyroidism, phenylketonuria, and galactosemia; and early appropriate therapies and rehabilitation services for children with developmental disabilities.

Down Syndrome

Down syndrome is the most common chromosomal abnormality of a generalized syndrome, occurring in 1 in every 830 live births worldwide (Bacino & Lee, 2016). In Canada, birth prevalence of Down syndrome for 1998–2007 was relatively constant, with an average of 14.1 per 10,000 total births (Public Health Agency of Canada [PHAC], 2013). There are currently 35,000 Canadians with Down syndrome (Canadian Down Syndrome Society, n.d.a). It occurs in people of all races and economic levels. Despite the national increasing rates of advanced maternal age at birth, the Down syndrome national birth prevalence rates have remained stable over the 1998–2007 time period. This stability has most likely resulted from increased access to and utilization of prenatal screening and testing and subsequent termination of pregnancies affected with Down syndrome (PHAC, 2013).

Etiology

While the cause of Down syndrome is not known, evidence from cytogenetic and epidemiological studies supports the concept of multiple causality. Approximately 95% of all cases of Down syndrome are attributable to an extra chromosome 21, thus the name nonfamilial trisomy 21 (Canadian Down Syndrome Society, 2009; PHAC, 2013). Although children with trisomy 21 are born to parents of all ages, there is a statistically greater risk in older women, particularly those older than 35 years of age (see Chapter 9, p. 182). For example, in women 35 years of age, the chance of conceiving a child with Down syndrome is about 1 in 400 live births, but in women age 40 it is about 1 in 110. However, the majority (about 80%) of infants with Down syndrome are born to women younger than age 35 because younger women have higher fertility rates. Approximately 3 to 4% of cases may be caused by translocation of chromosomes 15 and 21 or 22. This type of genetic aberration is usually hereditary and is not associated with advanced parental age. Between 1 and 2% of affected persons demonstrate *mosaicism*, which refers to the mixture of normal and abnormal cell types. The degree of cognitive and physical impairment is related to the percentage of cells with the abnormal chromosome makeup.

Diagnostic Evaluation

Down syndrome can usually be diagnosed by the clinical manifestations alone (Box 41-3 and Fig. 41-5), but a chromosome analysis should be done to confirm the genetic abnormality.

Several physical problems are associated with Down syndrome. Many of these children have congenital heart malformations, the most common being septal defects. Congenital heart defects were reported in 40.9% of Down syndrome cases, of which 98% were reported as live births in Canada (PHAC, 2013). Respiratory tract infections are prevalent and, when combined with cardiac anomalies, are the chief causes of death, particularly during the first year of life. Hypotonicity of chest and abdominal muscles and dysfunction of the immune system probably predispose the child to the development of respiratory tract infections. Other physical problems include thyroid dysfunction, especially congenital hypothyroidism, and an increased incidence of leukemia.

Therapeutic Management

Although no cure exists for Down syndrome, a number of therapies are advocated, such as surgery to correct some congenital anomalies (e.g., heart defects, strabismus). These children also benefit from an evaluative echocardiogram soon after birth and regular medical care. Evaluation of sight and hearing is essential, and treatment of otitis media is required to prevent auditory loss, which can influence cognitive function. Periodic testing of thyroid function is recommended, especially if growth is severely delayed. Some additional nursing considerations include providing ongoing assessment and monitoring of specific systems, including heart, gastrointestinal, and orthopaedic, throughout early childhood. Therefore, the nurse should be aware of specific ailments that are most closely associated with Down syndrome (Ranweiler & Merritt, 2009). Children participating in sports that may involve stress on the head and neck, such as gymnastics, diving, butterfly stroke in swimming, high jump, and soccer, should be evaluated radiologically for atlantoaxial instability. Symptoms of the disorder include neck

BOX 41-3 CLINICAL MANIFESTATIONS OF DOWN SYNDROME

Head and Eyes
Separated sagittal suture
Brachycephaly
Rounded and small skull
Flat occiput
Enlarged anterior fontanel
Oblique palpebral fissures (upward, outward slant)
Inner epicanthal folds
Speckling of iris (Brushfield's spots)

Nose and Ears
Small nose
Depressed nasal bridge (saddle nose)
Small ears and narrow canals
Short pinna (vertical ear length)
Overlapping upper helices
Conductive hearing loss

Mouth and Neck
High, arched, narrow palate
Protruding tongue
Hypoplastic mandible
Delayed tooth eruption and microdontia
Abnormal alignment of teeth common
Periodontal disease
Neck skin excess and laxity
Short and broad neck

Chest and Heart
Shortened rib cage
Twelfth rib anomalies
Pectus excavatum or carinatum
Congenital heart defects common (e.g., atrial septal defect, ventricular septal defect)

Abdomen and Genitalia
Protruding, lax, and flabby abdominal muscles
Diastasis recti abdominis
Umbilical hernia
Small penis
Cryptorchidism
Bulbous vulva

Hands and Feet
Broad, short hands and stubby fingers
Incurved little finger (clinodactyly)
Transverse palmar crease (Simian crease)
Wide space between big and second toes
Plantar crease between big and second toes
Broad, short feet and stubby toes

Musculoskeletal and Skin
Short stature
Hyperflexibility and muscle weakness
Hypotonia
Atlantoaxial instability
Dry, cracked, and frequent fissuring
Cutis marmorata (mottling)

Other
Reduced birth weight
Learning difficulty (average intelligence quotient of 50)
Hypothyroidism common
Impaired immune function
Increased risk of leukemia
Early-onset dementia (in one third)
Increased prevalence of gastrointestinal disorders/complications (i.e., Hirschsprung disease, tracheoesophageal fistula, imperforate anus, celiac disease, constipation, decreased motility)

Adapted from Bacino, C. A., & Lee, B. (2016). Cytogenetics. In R. M. Kliegman, B. F. Stanton, J. W. St. Geme, et al. (Eds.), *Nelson textbook of pediatrics* (20th ed.). Philadelphia: Saunders.

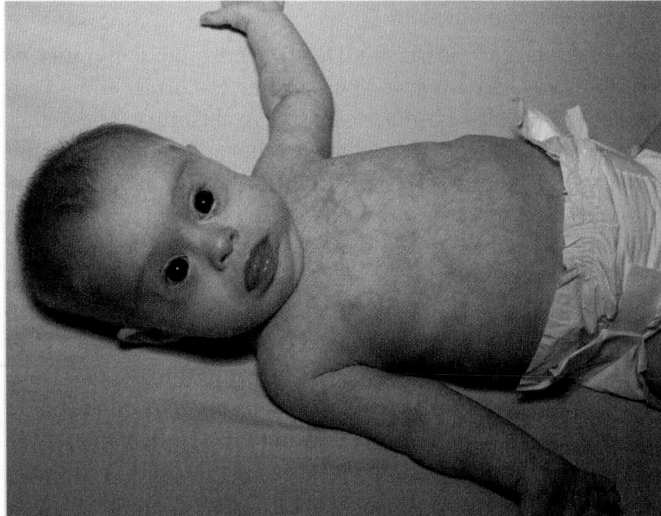

FIGURE 41-5 Down syndrome in an infant. Note small, square head with upward slant to eyes, flat nasal bridge, protruding tongue, mottled skin, and hypotonia.

pain, weakness, and torticollis. Affected children are at risk for spinal cord compression.

! NURSING ALERT

Report immediately any child with the following signs of spinal cord compression:

- Persistent neck pain
- Loss of established motor skills and bladder or bowel control
- Changes in sensation

Prognosis

Life expectancy for those with Down syndrome has improved in recent years but remains lower than for the general population. More than 80% survive to age 60 years and beyond. As the prognosis continues to improve for these individuals, it will be important to provide for their long-term health care, social, and leisure needs (National Down Syndrome Society, 2012; Weijerman & de Winter, 2010).

NURSING CARE

Supporting the Family at the Time of Diagnosis

Because of the unique physical characteristics, the infant with Down syndrome is usually diagnosed at birth if a prenatal diagnosis had not been established. Parents should be informed of the diagnosis at this time. Parents usually prefer that both of them be present during the informing interview so that they can support one another emotionally. They appreciate receiving reading material about the syndrome and being referred to parent groups or professional counselling for help or advice (see Additional Resources section at the end of this chapter). The Canadian Down Syndrome Society (CDSS) (n.d.a) recommends that "Congratulations!" be the health care providers' first words to any new parent; this can have a lifelong impact when speaking to the family of a child determined to have Down syndrome. The use of positive words and value-neutral language—not saying "I'm sorry" or "I have bad news"—can create a lasting impression with families. Nurses need to ensure that they include the positive aspects of having a child with Down syndrome, such as most children with this syndrome are healthy (see Chapter 40 for more information on how to help parents cope with chronic illness in their child).

After parents are aware of the diagnosis, they are confronted with the fact of losing their "perfect" or "dream" child and accepting the child that they have. Parents' responses to the child may greatly influence decisions regarding future care. The nurse must carefully answer questions concerning the child's developmental potential. Institutionalization is no longer an option. For families unable or unready to take the newborn home, specialized foster care or adoption are other options (see Critical Thinking Case Study).

Assisting the Family in Preventing Physical Problems

Many of the physical characteristics of infants with Down syndrome present nursing problems. The hypotonicity of muscles and hyperextensibility of joints complicate positioning. The limp, flaccid extremities resemble the posture of a rag doll; as a result, holding the infant is difficult. Sometimes parents perceive this lack of moulding to their bodies as evidence of inadequate parenting. The nurse needs to discuss with the parents their feelings concerning attachment to the child, emphasizing that the child's lack of clinging or moulding is a physical characteristic, not a sign of detachment or rejection. The child's extended body position promotes heat loss because more surface area is exposed to the environment. Parents should be encouraged to swaddle or wrap the infant tightly in a blanket before picking up the child to provide security and warmth.

Decreased muscle tone compromises respiratory expansion. In addition, the underdeveloped nasal bone causes a chronic problem of inadequate drainage of mucus. The constant stuffy nose forces the child to breathe by mouth, which dries the oropharyngeal membranes, increasing the susceptibility to upper respiratory tract infections. Measures to lessen these problems include clearing the nose with a bulb-type syringe, rinsing the mouth with water after feedings, increasing fluid intake, and using a cool-mist vaporizer to keep the mucous membranes moist and the secretions liquefied. Other helpful measures include changing the child's position frequently, performing postural drainage with percussion if necessary, practising good hand hygiene, and properly disposing of soiled articles such as tissues. If antibiotics are ordered, the nurse needs to stress to the parents the importance of completing the full course of therapy for successful eradication of the infection and the prevention of the growth of resistant organisms.

Inadequate drainage resulting in pooling of mucus in the nose also interferes with feeding. Because the child breathes by mouth, sucking for any length of time is difficult. When eating solids, the child may gag on the food because of mucus in the oropharynx. Parents are advised to clear the nose before each feeding; give small, frequent feedings; and allow opportunities for rest during mealtime.

The protruding tongue also interferes with breast feeding and with eating solid foods. Parents need to know that the tongue thrust is not an indication of refusal to feed but a physiological response. For optimum growth and immune protection, breast feeding is recommended for all infants and is particularly important for an infant with Down syndrome given their susceptibility to respiratory infections. In addition to increased nutrition, the repetitive sucking action during breastfeeding will strengthen the infant's lips, tongue, and face, which will help in the future with speech development. Infants with Down syndrome often have low muscle tone, which reduces muscle strength in their tongue and lips, thus they need good head, neck, and upper back support during feeding. A gentle, steady pressure on the base of the infant's head will help to improve sucking and decrease fatigue. Different holds, such as the cross-cradle and football holds, may provide better support. Some infants with Down syndrome have difficulties with gulping and coughing when feeding. To avoid such difficulties the mother can hold the infant so that the throat and neck are above the nipple line, or she can lean back farther, such as in a rocking chair (Canadian Down Syndrome Society, n.d.b). See Chapter 27 for more breastfeeding tips. For solid foods, parents are advised to use a small but long, straight-handled spoon to push the food toward the

CRITICAL THINKING CASE STUDY

Diagnosis of Down Syndrome

The parents of Melissa, a newborn diagnosed as having Down syndrome, ask the nurse, "What are we supposed to do with her?" They further state that they already have three other children at home.

1. Evidence—Is there sufficient evidence to draw conclusions about the parents' concerns regarding their newborn daughter?
2. Assumptions—Describe an underlying assumption about each of the following:
   a. Newborn diagnosed with Down syndrome
   b. Parental care of a newborn with Down syndrome
   c. Newborn with Down syndrome and older siblings
3. What priorities for the nursing response should be established?
4. Does the evidence support your nursing intervention?

back and side of the mouth. If food is thrust out, it should be refed.

Dietary intake also needs supervision. Decreased muscle tone affects gastric motility, predisposing the child to constipation. Dietary measures such as increased fibre and fluid promote evacuation. The child's eating habits may need careful scrutiny to prevent obesity. Height and weight measurements should be obtained on a serial basis, especially during infancy. Because these children grow more slowly than the general pediatric population, their growth should be assessed using the Canadian growth charts, which were adapted from the World Health Organization (WHO) in 2006 (see Appendix C).

During infancy the child's skin is pliable and soft. However, it gradually becomes rough and dry and is prone to cracking and infection. Skin care involves the use of minimal soap and application of lubricants. Lip balm should be applied to the lips, especially when the child is outdoors, to prevent excessive chapping.

Assisting in Prenatal Diagnosis and Genetic Counselling

The Society of Obstetricians and Gynaecologists of Canada (SOGC) recommends that all pregnant women in Canada, regardless of age, be informed and offered the choice of a prenatal screening test for the most common clinically significant fetal aneuploidies (Chitayat, Langlois, Wilson, et al., 2011) (see Chapter 13, Prenatal Screening, p. 294)

If prenatal testing indicates that the fetus is affected, the nurse should encourage the parents to express their feelings about considering elective abortion and support their decision to terminate or proceed with the pregnancy.

Fragile X Syndrome

Fragile X syndrome (FXS) is the most common inherited cause of CI and the second most common genetic cause of CI after Down syndrome. It has been described in all ethnic groups and races. The incidence of affected males is 1 in 3600; the incidence of affected females is 1 in 4000 to 6000; the incidence of carrier females is 1 in 100 to 260, and the incidence of carrier males is 1 in 250 to 800 worldwide (Hagerman, 2008). It is estimated that 50 to 100 new cases are reported every year in Canada (Canadian Paediatric Society [CPS] & PHAC, 2012).

The syndrome is caused by an abnormal gene on the lower end of the long arm of the X chromosome. Chromosome analysis may demonstrate a fragile site (a region that fails to condense during mitosis and is characterized by a nonstaining gap or narrowing) in the cells of affected males and females and in carrier females. This fragile site has been determined to be caused by a gene mutation that results in excessive repeats of nucleotide in a specific DNA segment of the X chromosome. The number of repeats in a normal individual is between 6 and 50. An individual with 50 to 200 base-pair repeats is said to have a permutation and is thus a carrier. When passed from a parent to a child, these base-pair repeats can expand to 200 or more, which is termed a *full mutation*. This expansion occurs only when a carrier mother passes the mutation to her offspring; it does not occur when a carrier father passes the mutation to his daughters.

The inheritance pattern has been termed X-linked dominant with reduced penetrance. This is in distinct contrast to the classic X-linked recessive pattern in which all carrier females are normal and all affected males have symptoms of the disorder; no males are carriers. Therefore, genetic counselling of affected families is more complex than for families with a classic X-linked disorder such as hemophilia.

Prenatal diagnosis of the fragile X gene mutation is now possible with direct DNA testing in a family with an established history, using amniocentesis or chorionic villus sampling. Both affected sexes are fertile and thus capable of transmitting the fragile X disorder. Increased newborn screening and new pharmaceutical agents in clinical trials may lead to targeted treatments being available in the next few years (CPS & PHAC, 2013). In Canada, newborn screening for FXS, similar to Down syndrome, is available and recommended (Arbour & CPS Bioethics Committee, 2003/2015), to provide early intervention treatment and genetic counselling to families for future pregnancy planning. The Canadian Paediatric Society and Public Health Agency of Canada are investigating the demographics, clinical features, geographic distribution, and management of FXS in Canada, as well as determining the potential for newborn screening (CPS & PHAC, 2012). Guidelines for genetic testing in healthy children are in Box 41-4.

Clinical Manifestations

The classic trend of physical findings in adult men with fragile X syndrome consists of a long face with a prominent jaw (prognathism); large, protruding ears; and large testes (macroorchidism). In prepubertal children, however, these features may be less obvious, and behavioural manifestations may initially suggest the diagnosis (Box 41-5). In carrier females the clinical manifestations vary greatly.

Therapeutic Management

Fragile X syndrome has no cure. Medical treatment may include the use of serotonin agents such as carbamazepine (Tegretol) or fluoxetine (Prozac) to control violent temper outbursts and the use of central nervous system stimulants or clonidine (Catapres) to improve attention span and decrease hyperactivity. Protein replacement and gene therapy are treatment options that are being investigated. The new pharmacological targeted treatments to correct underlying neural dysfunction for FXS that are currently in clinical trials may be helpful for autism as well as other cognitive disorders (Berry-Kravis, 2014).

All affected children require referral to early intervention programs (speech and language therapy, occupational therapy, and special education assistance) and multidisciplinary assessment, including cardiology (i.e., mitral valve prolapse), neurology (i.e., seizures), and orthopedic anomalies.

Prognosis

Individuals with FXS are expected to live a normal lifespan. Their CI may be improved through behavioural and educational interventions that usually begin in preschool-age children.

BOX 41-4 GUIDELINES FOR GENETIC TESTING OF HEALTHY CHILDREN

- Parents need to be informed of potential psychological and social risks when genetic testing of healthy children is being considered.
- Open discussion of familial genetic risk should be encouraged within the context of the family unit and done in an age-appropriate manner.
- The best interests of the child should be the primary consideration when contemplating testing.
- Genetic testing should be done to confirm a diagnosis in a child with symptoms, to allow for adequate medical monitoring, prophylaxis, or treatment.
- Genetic testing should be deferred if it is predicted that a genetic condition will not be present until adulthood, until the child is competent to decide if the genetic information is wanted.
- For carrier status for conditions that will be important in reproductive decision making, the testing should be discouraged until the child can fully participate in the decision to be tested.
- A request for genetic testing by a competent, well-informed adolescent for the purpose of reproductive decision making should be considered, accompanied by appropriate counselling. The decision to include his or her family in the decision making should be made by the adolescent.
- Parents rarely insist that genetic testing of healthy children be carried out where there is no medical or other benefit to the child; in this instance, the physician is not obligated to carry out testing that is not in the best interests of the child. In exceptional circumstances, not testing may create more harm than testing, and in these cases a referral for ethics or legal opinion may be appropriate.
- Infants and children being considered for adoption should not be subjected to genetic testing where there is no timely medical benefit.

Adapted from Arbour, L., & Canadian Paediatric Society Bioethics Committee. (2003). Guidelines for genetic testing of healthy children. *Paediatrics & Child Health, 8*(1), 42–45 Addendum. Reaffirmed 2015.

BOX 41-5 CLINICAL MANIFESTATIONS OF FRAGILE X SYNDROME

Physical Features

Increased head circumference
Long, wide, and protruding ears
Long, narrow face with prominent jaw
Strabismus
Mitral valve prolapse, aortic root dilation
Hypotonia
Enlarged testicles (especially postpubertally)

Behavioural Features

Mild to severe cognitive impairment
Speech delay; may have rapid speech with stuttering, word repetition
Short attention span, hyperactivity
Hypersensitivity to taste, sounds, and touch
Intolerance to change in routine
Autistic-like behaviours such as social anxiety and gaze aversion

NURSING CARE

Because CI is a fairly consistent finding in individuals with FXS, the care given to these families is the same as for any child with CI. Because the disorder is hereditary, genetic counselling is necessary to inform parents and siblings of the risks of transmission. In addition, any male or female with unexplained or nonspecific mental impairment should be referred for genetic testing and, if needed, counselling. Families with a member affected by the disorder should be referred to the Fragile X Research Foundation of Canada (see Additional Resources at the end of this chapter).

Autism Spectrum Disorders

Autism spectrum disorders (ASDs) are complex neurodevelopmental disorders of unknown etiology characterized by impairments in social interaction and communication as well as repetitive behaviours and restricted interests (APA, 2013). This new definition of ASD in the *Diagnostic and Statistical Manual of Mental Disorders* (5th ed.) (*DSM-5*) (APA, 2013) does not distinguish subtypes of ASD, such as autistic disorder and Asperger disorder, as it did in *DSM-IV-TR* but instead classifies a single category of ASD. As well, the *DSM-5* recognizes only two domains of impairment, one being persistent deficits in social communication and the other being restricted interaction, repetitive patterns of behaviour, interests, or activities. This change in definition by the APA is controversial, and there is concern that ASD prevalence estimates may be lower under the new criteria. This change could lead to inaccurate statistical gathering and delay some early diagnoses of ASD (Maenner, Rice, Arneson, et al., 2014).

ASD is typically noticed during early childhood, primarily from 24 to 48 months of age. It occurs in 1 in 166 children; is about four times more common in males than in females (although females are more severely affected); and is not related to socioeconomic level, race, or parenting style (Centers for Disease Control and Prevention, 2009).

Etiology

The cause of ASD is unknown. Researchers are investigating a number of theories, including a link between hereditary, genetics, and medical problems. Immune and environmental factors (e.g., viral infections) may interact with the genetic susceptibility to increase the incidence of ASD (DiCicco-Bloom, Lord, Zwaigenbaum, et al., 2006). Individuals with ASD may have abnormal electroencephalograms, epileptic seizures, delayed development of hand dominance, persistence of primitive reflexes, metabolic abnormalities (elevated blood serotonin), cerebellar vermal hypoplasia (part of the brain involved in regulating motion and some aspects of memory), and infantile abnormal head enlargement (Rutter, 2013).

The strong evidence for a genetic basis in twins is consistent with an autosomal recessive pattern of inheritance. Twin studies demonstrate a high concordance (60 to 96%) for monozygotic (identical) twins and less than 5% concordance for dizygotic (nonidentical) twins (Clifford, Dissanayake, Bui, et al., 2007). There is a relatively high risk of recurrence of ASD in families with one affected child (Rutter, 2013).

The scientific evidence to date supports that there is no link between ASD and the measles-mumps-rubella (MMR) and thimerosal-containing vaccines (Price, Thompson, Goodson, et al., 2010). ASD has been reported in association with a number of conditions such as fragile X syndrome, tuberous sclerosis, metabolic disorders, fetal rubella syndrome, *Haemophilus influenzae* meningitis, and structural brain anomalies (Dawson, 2007). Recent reports have retrospectively tied ASD to prenatal and perinatal events such as maternal and paternal age over 40 years (for fathers, 1 in 116 births; for mothers, 1 in 123 births), uterine bleeding during pregnancy, low Apgar score, fetal distress, and neonatal hyperbilirubinemia (Amin, Smith, & Wang, 2011; Rutter, 2013). These same researchers, however, urge caution in interpreting these findings.

Clinical Manifestations and Diagnostic Evaluation

Children with ASD demonstrate several peculiar and often seemingly bizarre characteristics, primarily in social interactions, communication, and behaviour. Parents of autistic children have noted that their infants have difficulties with eye contact, avoid body contact, and exhibit language delay at a very early age (Kirchner, Hatri, Heekeren, et al., 2011). Children with ASD also display limited functional play and may interact with toys in an unusual or odd manner. Children with ASD may have significant gastrointestinal symptoms. Constipation is a common symptom and can be associated with acquired megarectum (Buie, Fuchs, Furuta, et al., 2010).

Children with autism do not always have the same manifestations; cases vary from mild forms requiring minimal supervision to severe forms in which self-abusive behaviour is common. The majority (50 to 70%) of children with autism have some degree of CI, with scores typically in the moderate to severe range. More females than males tend to have very low intelligence scores. Despite their relatively moderate to severe disability, some children with autism (known as *savants*) excel in particular areas, such as art, music, memory, mathematics, or perceptual skills, such as puzzle building.

Speech and language delays are also common in children with ASD. Any child who does not display such language skills as babbling or gesturing by 12 months, single words by 16 months, and two-word phrases by 24 months should undergo hearing and language evaluation. A sudden deterioration in extant expressive speech is also a red-flag event for further evaluation.

Diagnosis is based on the diagnostic criteria of the American Psychiatric Association (2013). Early recognition, referral, diagnosis, and intensive early intervention tend to improve outcomes for children with ASD (Maccabee-Ryaboy & Golnik, 2010; Zwaigenbaum, 2010). Unfortunately, diagnosis is often not made until 2 to 3 years after symptoms are first recognized. At the present time there is no universal screening for autism in Canada. Increasingly, youth and adults whose ASD was not previously identified are now being diagnosed (Autism Society Canada, 2010).

Prognosis

ASD is usually a severely disabling condition. However, some children improve with acquisition of language skills and communication with others (Maccabee-Ryaboy & Golnik, 2010). Some ultimately achieve independence, but most require lifelong adult supervision. Aggravation of psychiatric symptoms occurs in about half of the children during adolescence, with girls having a tendency for continued deterioration.

Early recognition of behaviours associated with ASD is critical to implementing appropriate interventions and family involvement. See Box 41-6 for a summary of these early ASD behaviours in young children. The prognosis is most favourable for children with higher intelligence, functional speech, and less behavioural impairment (Solomon, Buaminger, & Rogers, 2011).

NURSING CARE

Therapeutic intervention for the child with ASD is a specialized area involving professionals with advanced training. Although

BOX 41-6 EARLY SIGNS OF AUTISM SPECTRUM DISORDER IN YOUNG CHILDREN

- Emotional disconnection with others such as having difficulties picking up on facial social cues and not smiling in response to others.
- Sensitivity to external stimuli, such as becoming agitated to certain noises, lights, smells, tastes, or textures.
- Ostensible lack of empathy with others with limited range of emotions.
- Unresponsiveness to the usual human interactions such as socializing and imitating others.
- Difficulties in controlling emotions and physical reactions particularly in stressful circumstances such as throwing temper tantrums or physical aggression on themselves with head banging and biting.
- Delayed language development such as lack of mimicking and babbling.
- Tendency to use nonverbal instead of verbal communication such as the use of gestures or drawings.
- Diminished ability to decipher the meaning of others' facial expression or demeanor.
- Tendency to exhibit repetitive behaviours such reorganizing the same toys, rocking themselves frequently, repeating the same hand gestures, and repeating the same words.

there is no cure for ASD, numerous therapies have been used. The most promising results have been through highly structured and intensive behaviour modification programs. In general, the objective in treatment is to promote positive reinforcement, increase social awareness of others, teach verbal communication skills, and decrease unacceptable behaviour. Providing a structured routine for the child to follow is key in the management of ASD.

When these children are hospitalized, the parents are essential to planning care and, ideally, should stay with the child as much as possible. Nurses should recognize that not all children with ASD are the same; they will require individual assessment and treatment. Decreasing stimulation by using a private room, avoiding extraneous auditory and visual distractions, and encouraging the parents to bring in possessions the child is attached to may lessen the disruptiveness of hospitalization. Because physical contact often upsets these children, minimal holding and eye contact may be necessary to avoid behavioural outbursts. Care must be taken when performing procedures on, administering medicine to, or feeding these children, since they may be either fussy eaters who willfully starve themselves or gag to prevent eating, or indiscriminate hoarders, swallowing any available edible or inedible items, such as a thermometer. Eating habits of children with ASD may be particularly problematic for families and may involve food refusal accompanied by mineral deficiencies, mouthing objects, eating nonedibles, and smelling and throwing food (Herndon, DiGuiseppi, Johnson, et al., 2009).

Children with ASD need to be introduced slowly to new situations; visits with staff caregivers should be kept short whenever possible. Because these children have difficulty organizing their behaviour and redirecting their energy, they need to be told directly what to do. Communication should be at the child's developmental level, brief, and concrete.

Family Support

As with so many other chronic conditions, ASD involves the entire family and often becomes "a family disease." Nurses can help alleviate the guilt and shame often associated with this disorder by stressing what is known from a biological standpoint and by providing family support. It is imperative to help parents understand that they are not the cause of the child's condition.

Parents need expert counselling early in the course of the disorder and should be referred to Autism Canada, which provides information about education, treatment programs and techniques, and facilities such as camps and group homes (see Additional Resources at the end of this chapter).

As much as possible, the family should be encouraged to care for the child in the home. With the help of family support programs, which are in some provinces and territories, families are often able to provide home care and assist with the educational services the child needs. As the child approaches adulthood and parents become older, the family may require assistance in locating a long-term live-in facility. Autism groups and parents of autistic children are lobbying the Canadian government through the courts to provide more financial support to help families pay for the comprehensive treatment costs.

SENSORY IMPAIRMENT

Hearing Impairment

In Canada over 23,000 children have some form of hearing impairment, and almost a third of these children have additional disabilities, such as visual or cognitive deficits (Statistics Canada, 2009). Hearing loss is a common major abnormality at birth; approximately 1 to 3 in 1000 term infants are profoundly deaf and another 3 in 1000 have serious hearing loss (CPS, 2014).

Definition and Classification

Hearing impairment is a general term indicating disability that may range in severity from mild to profound and includes the subsets of deaf and hard-of-hearing. *Slight to moderately severe hearing loss* describes a person who has residual hearing sufficiently enough to enable successful processing of linguistic information through audition, generally with use of a hearing aid. *Severe to profound hearing loss* describes a person whose hearing disability precludes successful processing of linguistic information through audition with or without a hearing aid. Hearing-impaired persons who are speech impaired tend not to have a physical speech problem other than that caused by the inability to hear.

Hearing defects may be classified according to etiology, pathology, or symptom severity. Each is important in terms of treatment, possible prevention, and rehabilitation.

Etiology

Hearing loss may be caused by a number of prenatal and postnatal conditions: a family history of childhood hearing impairment, anatomical malformations of the head or neck, low birth weight, severe perinatal asphyxia, perinatal infection (cytomegalovirus, rubella, herpes, syphilis, toxoplasmosis, bacterial meningitis), chronic ear infection, cerebral palsy, Down syndrome, prolonged neonatal oxygen supplementation, or administration of ototoxic medications (Botelho, Bouzada, Resende, et al., 2010; Weijerman & de Winter, 2010).

In addition, high-risk newborns who survive formerly fatal prenatal or perinatal conditions may be susceptible to hearing loss from the disorder or its treatment. For example, sensorineural hearing loss may be a result of continuous humming noises or high noise levels associated with isolettes, oxygen hoods, or intensive care units, especially when combined with the use of potentially ototoxic antibiotics.

Environmental noise is a special concern. Sounds loud enough to damage sensitive hair cells of the inner ear can produce irreversible hearing loss. Very loud, brief noise, such as gunfire, can cause immediate, severe, and permanent loss of hearing. Longer exposure to less intense but still hazardous sounds, such as loud persistent music via headphones, sound systems, concerts, or industrial noises, can also produce hearing loss (Henderson, Testa, & Hartnik, 2011). Loud noises combined with the toxic substances such as smoking or secondhand smoke produce a synergistic effect on hearing that causes hearing loss (Fabry, Davila, Arheart, et al., 2011).

Pathology

Disorders of hearing are divided according to the location of the defect. **Conductive** (or middle-ear) **hearing loss** results from interference of transmission of sound to the middle ear. It is the most common of all types of hearing loss and most frequently a result of recurrent serous otitis media. Conductive hearing impairment involves mainly interference with the loudness of sound.

Sensorineural hearing loss involves damage to the inner ear structures or the auditory nerve. The most common causes are congenital defects of inner ear structures or consequences of acquired conditions, such as kernicterus, infection, administration of ototoxic medications, or exposure to excessive noise. Sensorineural hearing loss results in distortion of sound and problems in discrimination. Although the child hears some of everything going on around him or her, the sounds are distorted, severely affecting discrimination and comprehension.

Mixed (conductive-sensorineural) **hearing loss** results from interference with the transmission of sound in the middle ear and along neural pathways. It frequently results from recurrent otitis media and its complications.

Central auditory imperception (**central hearing loss**) includes all hearing losses that are not linked to defects in the conductive or sensorineural structures. They are usually divided into organic or functional losses. In the organic type of central auditory imperception, the defect involves the reception of auditory stimuli along the central pathways and the expression of the message into meaningful communication. Examples are *aphasia*, the inability to express ideas in any form, either written or verbal; *agnosia*, the inability to interpret sound correctly; and *dysacusis*, difficulty in processing details or discriminating among sounds. In the functional type of hearing loss, no organic lesion exists to explain a central auditory loss. Examples of functional hearing loss are conversion hysteria (an unconscious withdrawal from hearing to block remembrance of a traumatic event), infantile autism, and childhood schizophrenia.

Symptom severity. Hearing impairment is expressed in terms of sound intensity in decibels (dB), a unit of loudness; hearing is measured at various frequencies, such as 500, 1000, and 2000 cycles/sec, the critical listening speech range. Hearing impairment can be classified according to hearing threshold level (the measurement of an individual's hearing threshold by means of an audiometer) and the degree of symptom severity as it affects speech (Table 41-1). These classifications offer only general guidelines regarding the effect of the impairment on any individual child, since children differ greatly in their ability to use residual hearing.

TABLE 41-1 CLASSIFICATION OF HEARING LOSS BASED ON SYMPTOM SEVERITY

HEARING LEVEL (dB)	EFFECT
Slight—16–25	Has difficulty hearing faint or distant speech Usually is unaware of hearing difficulty Likely to achieve in school but may have problems No speech defects
Mild to moderate—26–55	May have speech difficulties Understands face-to-face conversational speech at 0.9–1.5 m
Moderately severe—56–70 (hard of hearing)	Unable to understand conversational speech unless loud Considerable difficulty with group or classroom discussion Requires special speech training
Severe—71–90 (deaf)	May hear a loud voice if nearby May be able to identify loud environmental noises Can distinguish vowels but not most consonants Requires speech training
Profound—91 (deaf)	May hear only loud sounds Requires extensive speech training

Therapeutic Management

Conductive hearing loss. Treatment of hearing loss depends on the cause and type of hearing impairment. Many conductive hearing defects respond to medical or surgical treatment, such as antibiotic therapy for acute otitis media or insertion of tympanostomy tubes for chronic otitis media. When the conductive loss is permanent, hearing can be improved with the use of a hearing aid to amplify sound.

The nurse should be familiar with the types, basic care, and handling of hearing aids, especially when the child is hospitalized (see Additional Resources at the end of this chapter). Types of aids include those worn in or behind the ear, models incorporated into an eyeglass frame, or types worn on the body with a wire connection to the ear (Fig. 41-6). One of the most common problems with a hearing aid is acoustic feedback, an annoying whistling sound usually caused by improper fit of the ear mould. Sometimes the whistling may be at a frequency that the child cannot hear but that is annoying to others. In this case, if children are old enough, they can be told of the noise and asked to readjust the aid.

As children grow older, they may become self-conscious about the device. Every effort should be made to make the aid inconspicuous if this is a concern, such as having an appropriate hairstyle to cover behind-the-ear or in-the-ear models; wearing attractive frames for glasses; and placing the on-the-body type where it is not seen, such as under a shirt or sweater. Children should be given responsibility for the care of the device as soon as they are able, since fostering independence is a primary goal of rehabilitation.

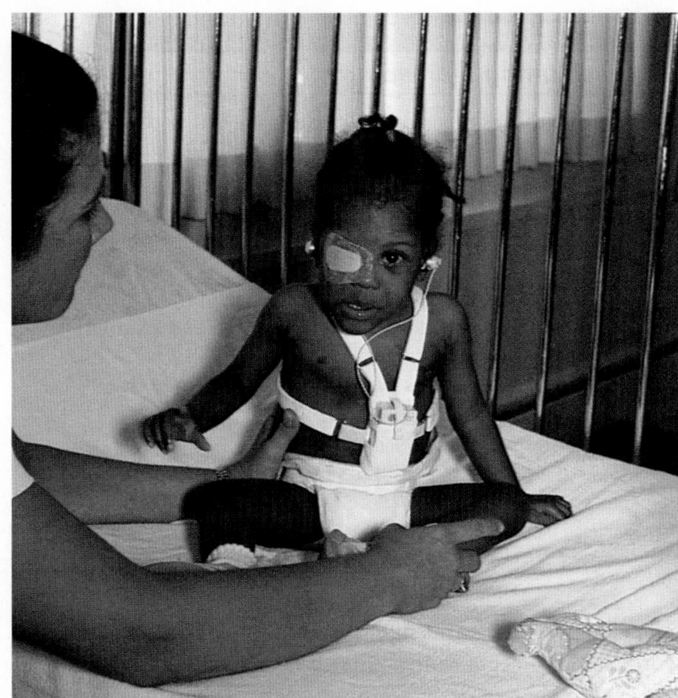

FIGURE 41-6 On-the-body hearing aids are convenient for young children, such as this child with severe bilateral hearing loss. Note eye patching for strabismus.

> **! NURSING ALERT**
>
> Stress to parents the importance of storing batteries for hearing aids in a safe location out of reach of children and of teaching children not to remove the battery from the hearing aid (or supervising young children when they do so). Battery ingestion requires immediate emergency management.

Sensorineural hearing loss. Treatment for sensorineural hearing loss is much less satisfactory. Because the defect is not one of intensity of sound, hearing aids are of less value in this type of defect. The use of cochlear implants (a surgically implanted prosthetic device) provides a sensation of hearing for individuals who have severe or profound hearing loss (Gifford, Holmes, & Bernstein, 2009) (see Additional Resources at the end of this chapter). Children with sensorineural hearing loss have lost or damaged some or all of their hair cells or auditory nerve fibres. Often these children cannot benefit from conventional hearing aids because they only amplify sound that cannot be processed by a damaged inner ear. A cochlear implant bypasses the hair cells to directly stimulate surviving auditory nerve fibres so that they can send signals to the brain. These signals can be interpreted by the brain to produce sound and sensations (Baldassari, Schmidt, Schubert, et al., 2009; Gifford et al., 2009).

Multichannelled implants are now available. This more sophisticated device stimulates the auditory nerve at a number of locations with differently processed signals. This type of stimulation allows a person to use the pitch information present in speech signals, leading to better understanding of speech. The trend is toward early use of cochlear implants, usually by 18 months of age, to give the child maximum opportunity to develop listening, language, and speaking skills.

NURSING CARE

Assessment of children for hearing impairment is a critical nursing responsibility. Early detection of hearing loss, preferably within the first 3 to 6 months of life, is essential to improve the language and educational outcomes of those with hearing impairments. Without early intervention, children with hearing impairment have irreversible deficits in communication and in psychosocial skills, cognition, and literacy (Patel, Feldman, & CPS, Community Paediatrics Committee, 2011/2016). Currently, British Columbia, Ontario, Nova Scotia, New Brunswick, and Prince Edward Island have mandatory newborn hearing screening, and the other provinces have partial programs. In the territories, there are staffing shortages and only partial programs can be implemented. Usually the screening is done before discharge from the hospital (see Chapter 26). The Canadian Paediatric Society strongly recommends that universal newborn hearing screening be done across Canada (Patel et al., 2011/2016).

The discussion here focuses on developmental and behavioural indices associated with hearing impairment. Auditory testing is presented in Chapter 33.

Infancy

At birth the nurse can observe the newborn's response to auditory stimuli, as evidenced by the startle reflex, head turning, eye blinking, and cessation of body movement. The infant may vary in the intensity of the response, depending on the state of alertness. However, a consistent absence of a reaction should lead to suspicion of hearing loss. Box 41-7 summarizes other clinical manifestations of hearing impairment.

Childhood

The child who is profoundly deaf is much more likely to be diagnosed during infancy than the less severely affected one. If the defect is not detected during early childhood, it likely will become evident during entry into school, when the child has difficulty learning. Unfortunately, some of these children are mistakenly placed in special classes for students with learning disabilities or CI. Therefore, it is essential that the nurse consider a hearing impairment in any child who demonstrates the behaviours listed in Box 41-7.

Of primary importance is the effect of hearing impairment on speech development. A child with a mild conductive hearing loss may speak fairly clearly but in a loud, monotone voice. A child with a sensorineural defect usually has difficulty with articulation. For example, inability to hear higher frequencies may result in the word *spoon* being pronounced "poon." Children with articulation problems need to have their hearing tested.

BOX 41-7 CLINICAL MANIFESTATIONS OF HEARING IMPAIRMENT

Infants

Lack of startle or blink reflex to a loud sound
Failure to be awakened by loud environmental noises
Failure to localize a source of sound by 6 months of age
Absence of babble or voice inflections by age 7 months
Lack of response to the spoken word; failure to follow verbal directions
Response to loud noises as opposed to the voice

Children

Use of gestures rather than verbalization to express desires
Failure to develop intelligible speech by age 24 months
Monotone and unintelligible speech; lessened laughter
Vocal play, head banging, or foot stamping for vibratory sensation
Yelling or screeching to express pleasure, needs, or annoyance (tantrum)
Asking to have statements repeated or answering them incorrectly
Greater response to facial expression and gestures than to verbal explanation
Avoidance of social interaction; preference for playing alone
Inquiring, sometimes confused facial expression
Suspicious alertness alternating with cooperation
Frequent stubbornness because of lack of comprehension
Irritability at not making themselves understood
Shy, timid, and withdrawn behaviour
Frequently appearing "dreamy," "in a world of their own," or exhibiting inattentiveness

NURSING ALERT

When parents express concern about their child's hearing and speech development, refer the child for a hearing evaluation. Absence of well-formed syllables (da, na, yaya) by 11 months of age should result in immediate referral.

Communication Strategies

Lipreading. Even though the child may become an expert at lipreading, only about 40% of the spoken word is understood, and less is understood if the speaker has an accent, a moustache, or a beard. Exaggerating pronunciation or speaking in an altered rhythm further reduces comprehension. Parents can help the child understand the spoken word by using the suggestions in the Guidelines box. The child learns to supplement the spoken word with sensitivity to visual cues, primarily body language and facial expression (e.g., tightening the lips, muscle tension, eye contact).

Cued speech. This method of communication is an adjunct to straight lipreading. Hand signals are used to help the child with a hearing impairment distinguish between words that look alike when formed by the lips (e.g., mat, bat). It is most often used by children with hearing impairments who are using speech, rather than those who are nonverbal.

Sign language. Sign language, such as American Sign Language (ASL) or British Sign Language (BSL), is a visual gestural language in which hand signals roughly correspond to specific words and concepts in the English language. Family members are encouraged to learn signing because using or watching hands requires much less concentration than lipreading or talking. Also, a symbol method enables some children to learn more and to learn faster. Learning a language promotes cognitive development.

GUIDELINES

Facilitating Lipreading

- Attract the child's attention before speaking; use light touch to signal speaker's presence.
- Stand close to the child.
- Face the child directly or move to a 45-degree angle.
- Stand still; do not walk back and forth or turn away to point or look elsewhere.
- Establish eye contact and show interest.
- Speak at eye level and with good lighting on the speaker's face and no light at the back of the speaker's head.
- Be certain nothing interferes with speech patterns, such as chewing food or gum.
- Speak clearly and at a slow and even rate.
- Use facial expression to assist in conveying messages.
- Keep sentences short.
- Rephrase message if the child does not understand the words.

Speech language therapy. The most formidable task in the education of a child who is profoundly hearing impaired is learning to speak. Speech is learned through a multisensory approach, using visual, tactile, kinesthetic, and auditory stimulation. Parents should be encouraged to participate fully in the learning process. One form of speech training includes the use of a speech language pathologist (SLP). An SLP can provide evaluation and treatment of the language difficulties associated with children who have some form of CI or hearing loss. The SLP can work closely with schools, the family, and the health care team to implement effective programs to help children with CI develop stronger communication skills (see Additional Resources at the end of this chapter).

Additional aids. Everyday activities present problems for older children with hearing impairment. For example, they may not be able to hear the telephone, doorbell, or alarm clock. Several commercial devices are available to help them adjust to these dilemmas. A new visual fire alarm is now available as an additional safety device. Flashing lights can be attached to a telephone or doorbell to signal its ringing, and cellular phones can be set on vibrate. Trained hearing ear dogs can provide great assistance because they alert the person to sounds, such as someone approaching, a moving car, a signal to wake up, or a child's cry. Special teletypewriters or telecommunications devices for the deaf (TDD or TTY) help people with impaired hearing communicate with each other over the telephone; the typed message is conveyed via the telephone lines and displayed on a small screen. Information on available electronic aids and new equipment is available on the Canadian Hearing Society website. Please see Additional Resources for this address. Cellular phones and smartphones also offer means of sending text and visual messages.

Any audiovisual medium presents dilemmas for these children, who can see the picture but cannot hear the message. However, with closed captioning a special decoding device is attached to the television, and the audio portion of a program is translated into subtitles that appear on the screen. There are also closed-caption applications available for smartphones and software for computers for closed captioning with video games and online streaming.

Socialization. As children learn to compensate for their lack of hearing, they become extremely perceptive to visual and vibratory changes. They often know when another person wants to talk to them because the person walks close by but does not pass. They learn to be alert to other people approaching them by seeing their shadows or feeling the vibrations of their footsteps. They are acutely aware of facial expressions and may comprehend unspoken messages more quickly than the spoken word.

Because socialization is extremely important to the child's development, the nurse should discuss with the family methods of fostering social contact. If children attend a special school for the deaf, they are able to socialize with peers in that setting. Classmates become a potential source of close friendships because they communicate more easily among themselves. Parents should be encouraged to promote these relationships whenever possible.

Children with a hearing impairment may need special help with school or social activities. For children wearing hearing aids, background noise should be kept to a minimum. Because many of these children are able to attend regular classes, the teacher may need assistance in adapting methods of teaching for the child's benefit. The nurse is often in an optimal position to emphasize methods of facilitated communication, such as lipreading (see Guidelines box above). Because group projects and audiovisual teaching aids may hinder the child's learning, these educational methods should be carefully evaluated.

In a group setting, it is helpful for the other class members to sit in a semicircle in front of the child. Because one of the difficulties in following a group discussion is that the child is unaware of who will speak next, someone should point out each speaker. Speakers can also be given numbers or their names can be written down as each person talks. If one person writes down the main topic of the discussion, the child is able to follow lipreading more closely. Such suggestions can increase the child's ability to participate in sports, organizations such as Scouts, and group projects.

Supporting the Child and Family

After the diagnosis of hearing impairment is made, parents need extensive support to adjust to the shock of learning about their child's disability and an opportunity to realize the extent of the hearing loss. If the hearing loss occurs during childhood, the child also requires sensitive, supportive care during the long and often difficult adjustment to this sensory loss. Early rehabilitation is one of the best strategies for fostering adjustment. However, progress in learning communication may not always coincide with emotional adjustment. Depression or anger is common, and such feelings are a normal part of the grieving process. (See also Chapter 43 for an extensive discussion of the emotional support of the child and family.) The Canadian Hearing Society offers a youth transition program to support career planning.

Care for the Child During Hospitalization

The needs of the hospitalized child with impaired hearing are the same as those of any other child, but the disability presents special challenges to the nurse (see Critical Thinking Case Study). For example, verbal explanations must be supplemented by tactile and visual aids, such as books or actual demonstration and practice. Children's understanding of the explanation needs to be constantly reassessed. If their verbal skills are poorly developed, they can answer questions through drawing, writing, or gesturing. For example, if the nurse is attempting to clarify where a spinal tap is done, the child is asked to point to where the procedure will be done on the body. Because these children often need more time to grasp the full meaning of an explanation, the nurse needs to be patient, allowing ample time for understanding.

When communicating with the child, the nurse should use the same principles as those outlined for facilitating lipreading. The child's hearing aid should be checked to ensure that it is working properly. If it is necessary to awaken the child at night, the nurse can gently shake the child or turn on the hearing aid before arousing the child. The nurse should always make certain that the child can see him or her before any procedures, even routine ones such as changing a diaper or regulating an infusion. It is important to remember that the child may not be aware of one's presence until alerted through visual or tactile cues.

Ideally, parents should be encouraged to room-in with the child. However, it must be conveyed to them that this is not to serve as a convenience to the nurse but as a benefit to the child. Although the parents' aid can be enlisted in familiarizing the child with the hospital and explaining procedures, the nurse also needs to talk directly to the youngster, encouraging expression of feelings about the experience. If the child's speech is difficult to understand, the nurse should make an effort to become familiar with his or her pronunciation of words. Parents often can be helpful by explaining the child's usual speech habits. Nonverbal communication devices that employ pictures or words that the child can point to are also available. Such boards can be made by drawing pictures or writing the words of common needs on cardboard, such as *parent, food, water,* or *toilet.*

The nurse has a special role as child advocate and is in a strategic position to alert other health care team members and other patients to the child's special needs regarding communication. For example, the nurse should accompany other practitioners on visits to the child's room to ensure that they speak to the child and that the child understands what is said. Caregivers sometimes forget that the child has the ability to perceive and learn despite a hearing loss; consequently they communicate only with the parents. As a result, the child's needs and feelings remain unrecognized and unmet.

CRITICAL THINKING CASE STUDY

Hearing Impairment

Four-year-old Jamel has a severe congenital hearing impairment. Jamel has been admitted to the outpatient surgery, post-anaesthetic care unit (PACU) after a herniorrhaphy and regional block. As he emerges from anaesethesia, he becomes more and more agitated.

1. Evidence—Is there sufficient evidence to draw conclusions about Jamel's increasing agitation after surgery?
2. Assumptions—Describe an underlying assumption about each of the following:
   a. Severe congenital hearing impairment in a preschool child
   b. Preschooler with severe congenital hearing impairment awakening in the PACU after surgery
   c. Preschooler with severe congenital hearing impairment awakening from his herniorrhaphy and after regional block
3. What priorities for nursing care should be established for Jamel?
4. Does the evidence support your nursing interventions?

Because children with impaired hearing may have difficulty forming social relationships with other children, the child should be introduced to roommates and encouraged to engage in play activities. The hospital setting can provide growth-promoting opportunities for social relationships. With the assistance of a child life specialist, the child can learn new recreational activities, experiment with group games, and engage in therapeutic play. The use of puppets, dollhouses, role playing with dress-up clothes, building with a hammer and nails, finger painting, and water play can help the child express feelings that previously were suppressed.

Assisting in Measures to Prevent Hearing Impairment

A primary nursing role is to prevent hearing loss. Because the most common cause of impaired hearing is chronic otitis media, it is essential that appropriate measures be instituted to treat existing infections and prevent recurrences. Children with a history of ear or respiratory tract infections or any other condition known to increase the risk of hearing impairment should receive periodic auditory testing.

To prevent the causes of hearing loss that begin prenatally and perinatally, pregnant women need counselling regarding the necessity of early prenatal care, including genetic counselling for known familial disorders; avoidance of all ototoxic medications, especially during the first trimester; tests to rule out syphilis, rubella, or blood incompatibility; medical management of maternal diabetes; strict control of alcohol intake; adequate dietary intake; and avoidance of smoke exposure. The necessity of routine immunization during childhood to eliminate the possibility of acquired sensorineural hearing loss from rubella, mumps, or measles (encephalitis) needs to be stressed.

Excessive noise pollution is a well-established cause of sensorineural hearing loss. The nurse should routinely assess the possibility of environmental noise pollution and advise children and parents of the potential danger. When individuals engage in activities associated with high-intensity noise, such as flying model airplanes, target shooting, or snowmobiling, they should wear ear protection such as earmuffs or earplugs. Even common household equipment, such as lawn mowers, vacuum cleaners, and cordless telephones and cell phones, may cause noise-induced hearing loss. Children should ensure that when using headphones to listen to music the noise should not be heard outside of the headset as this increases the risk of hearing deficits.

NURSING ALERT

Suspect hazardous noise if the listener experiences (1) difficulty in communication while hearing the sound, (2) ringing in the ears (tinnitus) after exposure to the sound, or (3) muffled hearing after leaving the sound.

Visual Impairment

Visual impairment is a common problem during childhood. Seeing disabilities are reported at a rate of 9.1% for males and 10.2% for females aged 5 to 14 years (Statistics Canada, 2009). Vision impairment such as refractive error, strabismus, and **amblyopia** occur in 5 to 10% of all preschoolers, who are usually identified through vision screening programs (Rahi, Cumberland, Perkham, et al., 2010; U.S. Preventive Services Task Force, 2011). The nurse's role is one of early assessment and detection, prevention, referral, and, in some instances, rehabilitation.

Definition and Classification

Visual impairment is a general term that encompasses both partial sight and legal blindness. Partial sight or partial visual impairment is defined as a visual acuity between 20/70 and 20/200. The child can generally use normal-sized print because near vision is almost always better than distance vision. *Legal blindness or* severe permanent visual impairment is defined as visual acuity of 20/200 or lower or a visual field of 20 degrees or less in the better eye. It is important to keep in mind that legal blindness is not a medical diagnosis but a legal definition. It allows special considerations with regard to taxes, entrance into special schools, eligibility for aid, and other benefits.

Etiology

Visual impairment can be caused by a number of genetic and prenatal or postnatal conditions. These include perinatal infections (herpes, chlamydia, gonococci, rubella, syphilis, toxoplasmosis); retinopathy of prematurity; trauma; postnatal infections (meningitis); and disorders such as sickle cell disease, juvenile rheumatoid arthritis, Tay-Sachs disease, albinism, and retinoblastoma. In many instances, such as with **refractive errors**, the cause of the defect is unknown.

Refractive errors are the most common types of visual disorders in children. The term *refraction* means bending and refers to the bending of light rays as they pass through the lens of the eye. Normally, light rays enter the lens and fall directly on the retina. However, in refractive disorders the light rays either fall in front of the retina (**myopia**) or beyond it (**hyperopia**). Other eye problems, such as **strabismus**, may or may not include refractive errors, but they are important because, if untreated, they result in severe permanent visual impairment from amblyopia. These, along with other less frequent visual disorders, are summarized in Box 41-8. In addition to these

BOX 41-8 TYPES OF VISUAL IMPAIRMENT

Refractive Errors

Myopia

Nearsightedness—Ability to see objects clearly at close range but not at a distance

Pathophysiology

Results from eyeball that is too long, causing image to fall in front of retina

Clinical Manifestations

Excessive eye rubbing
Head tilt or forward head thrusts
Difficulty in reading or in doing other close work
Headaches
Dizziness
Clumsiness; walking into objects
Blinking more than usual or irritability when doing close work
Inability to see objects clearly
Poor school performance, especially in subjects that require demonstration, such as math

Treatment

Corrected with biconcave lenses that focus rays on retina
May be corrected with laser surgery

Hyperopia

Farsightedness—Ability to see objects at a distance

Pathophysiology

Results from eyeball that is too short, causing image to focus beyond retina

Clinical Manifestations

Because of accommodative ability, usually an ability to see objects at all ranges
Most children are normally hyperopic until about 7 years of age

Treatment

When required, corrected with convex lenses that focus rays on retina
May be corrected with laser surgery

Astigmatism

Unequal curvatures in refractive apparatus

Pathophysiology

Results from unequal curvatures in cornea or lens that cause light rays to bend in different directions

Clinical Manifestations

Depend on severity of refractive error in each eye
Possible clinical manifestations of myopia

Treatment

Corrected with special lenses that compensate for refractive errors
May be corrected with laser surgery

Anisometropia

Different refractive strength in each eye

Pathophysiology

May develop amblyopia as weaker eye is used less

Clinical Manifestations

Depend on severity of refractive error in each eye
Possible clinical manifestations of myopia

Treatment

Treated with corrective lenses, preferably contact lenses, to improve vision in each eye so the eyes work as a unit
May be corrected with laser surgery

Amblyopia

Lazy eye—Reduced visual acuity in one eye

Pathophysiology

Results when one eye does not receive sufficient stimulation
Each retina receives different images, resulting in diplopia (double vision)
Brain accommodates by suppressing less intense image
Visual cortex eventually does not respond to visual stimulation in that eye, with resultant loss of vision

Clinical Manifestations

Poor vision in affected eye

Treatment

Preventable if treatment of primary visual defect, such as anisometropia or strabismus, begins before 6 years of age

Strabismus

"Squint" or cross-eye—Malalignment of eyes
Estropia—Inward deviation of eye
Exotropia—Outward deviation of eye

Pathophysiology

May result from muscle imbalance or paralysis, poor vision, or congenital defect
Because visual axes are not parallel, brain receives two images, and amblyopia can result

Clinical Manifestations

Squints eyelids together or frowns
Has difficulty focusing from one distance to another
Inaccurate judgement in picking up objects
Unable to see print or moving objects clearly
Closes one eye to see
Tilts head to one side
If combined with refractive errors, may see any of the manifestations listed for refractive errors
Diplopia
Photophobia
Dizziness
Headaches

Treatment

Depends on cause of strabismus
May involve occlusion therapy (patching stronger eye) or surgery to increase visual stimulation to weaker eye
Early diagnosis essential to prevent vision loss

Continued

BOX 41-8 TYPES OF VISUAL IMPAIRMENT—cont'd

Cataracts
Opacity of crystalline lens

Pathophysiology
Prevents light rays from entering eye and refracting on retina

Clinical Manifestations
Gradual decrease in ability to see objects clearly
Possible loss of peripheral vision
Nystagmus (with severe permanent visual impairment)
Grey opacities of lens
Strabismus
Absence of red reflex

Treatment
Requires surgery to remove cloudy lens and replace lens (with intraocular lens implant, removable contact lens, prescription glasses)
Must be treated early to prevent severe permanent visual impairment from amblyopia

Glaucoma
Increased intraocular pressure

Pathophysiology
Congenital type results from defective development of some component related to flow of aqueous humour
Increased pressure on optic nerve causes eventual atrophy and severe permanent visual impairment

Clinical Manifestations
Loss of peripheral vision—mostly seen in acquired types
Possible bumping into objects
Perception of halos around objects
Possible complaint of pain or discomfort (pain, nausea, or vomiting if sudden rise in pressure)
Eye redness
Excessive tearing (epiphora)
Photophobia
Spasmodic winking (blepharospasm)
Corneal haziness
Enlargement of eyeball (buphthalmos)

Treatment
Requires surgical treatment (goniotomy) to open outflow tracts
May require more than one procedure

disorders, other visual problems can be a result of infection or trauma.

Trauma. Trauma is a common cause of visual impairment in children. Injuries to the eyeball and adnexa (supporting or accessory structures, such as eyelids, conjunctiva, or lacrimal glands) can be classified as penetrating or nonpenetrating. Penetrating wounds are most often a result of sharp instruments, such as sticks, knives, or scissors; propulsive objects, such as firecrackers, bullets from guns, arrows, or rocks from slingshots; or a powerful contusion by a blunt object, which may occur during a fight or from a serious car accident. Nonpenetrating injuries may be a result of foreign objects in the eyes, lacerations, a blow from a blunt object such as a ball (from baseball, softball, basketball, or racquet sports) or fist, or thermal or chemical burns.

Treatment is aimed at preventing further ocular damage and is primarily the responsibility of the ophthalmologist. It involves adequate examination of the injured eye (with the child sedated or anaesthetized in severe injuries); appropriate immediate intervention, such as removal of the foreign body or suturing of the laceration; and prevention of complications, such as administration of antibiotics or steroids and complete bedrest to allow the eye to heal and blood to reabsorb (see Emergency box). The prognosis varies according to the type of injury. It is usually guarded in all cases of penetrating wounds because of the high risk of serious complications.

Infections. Infections of the adnexa and structures of the eyeball or globe may occur in children. The most common eye infection is conjunctivitis. Treatment is usually with ophthalmic antibiotics. Severe infections may require systemic antibiotic therapy. Steroids are used with caution because they exacerbate viral infections such as herpes simplex, increasing the risk of damage to the involved structures.

NURSING CARE

Assessment of children for visual impairment is a critical nursing responsibility. Discovery of a visual impairment as early as possible is essential to prevent social, physical, and psychological damage to the child. Assessment involves (1) identifying those children who by virtue of their history are at risk, (2) observing for behaviours that indicate a vision loss, and (3) screening all children for visual acuity and signs of other ocular disorders such as strabismus. The discussion here focuses on clinical manifestations of various types of visual problems (see Box 41-8). Vision testing is discussed in Chapter 33.

Infancy

At birth, the nurse should observe the newborn's response to visual stimuli, such as following a light or object and cessation of body movement. The infant may vary in the intensity of the response, depending on the state of alertness.

Of special importance in detecting visual impairment during infancy are the parents' concerns regarding visual responsiveness in their child. Their concerns, such as lack of eye contact from the infant, must be taken seriously. During infancy the child should be tested for strabismus. Lack of binocularity after 4 months of age is considered abnormal and must be treated to prevent amblyopia.

! NURSING ALERT

Suspect visual impairment in an infant that does not react to light and in a child of any age if the parents express concern.

Childhood

Because the most common visual impairment during childhood is refractive errors, testing for visual acuity is essential.

EMERGENCY

Eye Injuries

Foreign Object

Examine eye for presence of a foreign body (evert upper lid to examine upper eye).

Remove a freely movable object with the pointed corner of a gauze pad lightly moistened with water.

Do not irrigate the eye or attempt to remove a penetrating object (see following section).

Caution child against rubbing the eye.

Chemical Burns

Irrigate the eye copiously with tap water for 20 minutes.

Evert upper lid to flush thoroughly.

Hold the child's head with the eye under tap of running lukewarm water.

Take child to emergency department.

Have child rest with eyes closed.

Keep the room darkened.

Ultraviolet Burns

If skin is burned, patch both eyes (make certain lids are completely closed); secure dressing with Kling bandages wrapped around the head rather than tape.

Have child rest with eyes closed.

Refer to an ophthalmologist.

Hematoma ("Black Eye")

Use a flashlight to check for gross hyphema (hemorrhage into anterior chamber; visible fluid meniscus across iris; more easily seen in light-coloured than in brown eyes).

Apply ice for the first 24 hours to reduce swelling if no hyphema is present.

Refer to an ophthalmologist immediately if hyphema is present.

Have child rest with eyes closed.

Penetrating Injuries

Take child to emergency department.

Never remove an object that has penetrated the eye.

Follow strict aseptic technique in examining the eye.

Observe for the following:

- Aqueous or vitreous leaks (fluid leaking from point of penetration)
- Hyphema
- Shape and equality of pupils, reaction to light, prolapsed iris (not perfectly circular)

Apply a Fox shield if available (not a regular eye patch) and apply a patch over the unaffected eye to prevent bilateral movement.

Maintain bedrest with child in 30-degree Fowler's position.

Caution child against rubbing the eye.

Refer to an ophthalmologist.

The community health nurse usually assumes major responsibility for vision testing in schoolchildren, but only some provinces and territories have these vision programs in place. Preschool vision screening is important for early detection of amblyopia and to prevent long-term major eye damage, including severe permanent visual impairment from this condition. The Public Health Association of Canada recommends universal preschool screening across Canada (Mema, McIntyre, & Musto, 2012). In addition to refractive errors, the nurse should be aware of signs and symptoms that indicate other ocular problems.

The shock of learning that their child has severe permanent visual impairment precipitates a crisis for families. The family is encouraged to investigate appropriate stimulation and educational programs for their child as soon as possible. Sources of information include local schools for children with visual impairments and the Canadian National Institute for the Blind (CNIB) (see Additional Resources at the end of this chapter).

Promoting Parent–Child Attachment

A crucial time in the life of infants with visual impairment is when they and their parents are getting acquainted with each other. Pleasurable patterns of interaction between the infant and parents may be lacking if there is not enough reciprocity. For example, if the parent gazes fondly at the infant's face and seeks eye contact but the infant fails to respond because he or she cannot see the parent, a troubled cycle of responses may occur. The nurse can help parents learn to look for other cues that indicate the infant is responding to them, such as whether the eyelids blink; whether the activity level accelerates or slows; whether respiratory patterns change, such as faster or slower breathing, when the parents come near; and whether the infant makes throaty sounds when the parents speak to the infant. In time, parents learn that the infant has unique ways of relating to them. They should be encouraged to show affection using nonvisual methods, such as talking or reading, cuddling, and walking with the child.

Promoting the Child's Optimum Development

Promoting the child's optimum development requires rehabilitation in a number of important areas, including learning self-help skills and appropriate communication techniques to become independent. Although nurses may not be directly involved in such programs, they can provide direction and guidance to families regarding the availability of programs and the need to promote these activities in their child.

Development and independence. Motor development depends on sight almost as much as verbal communication depends on hearing. From earliest infancy, parents are encouraged to expose the infant to as many visual-motor experiences as possible, such as sitting supported in an infant seat or swing and being given opportunities for holding up the head, sitting unsupported, reaching for objects, and crawling.

Despite visual impairment, the child can become independent in all aspects of self-care. The same principles used for promoting independence in sighted children apply, with additional emphasis on nonvisual cues. For example, the child may need help in dressing, such as special arrangement of clothing for style coordination and braille tags to distinguish colours and prints.

The severely visually impaired child also must learn to become independent in navigational skills. The two main techniques are the tapping method (use of a cane to survey the environment for direction and to avoid obstacles) and guides, such as a sighted human guide or a dog guide, such as a seeing eye dog. Children who are partially sighted may benefit from ocular aids, such as a monocular telescope.

Play and socialization. Children with severe permanent visual impairment do not learn to play automatically. Because they cannot imitate others or actively explore the environment as sighted children do, they depend much more on others to stimulate and teach them how to play. Parents need help in selecting appropriate play materials, especially those that encourage fine and gross motor development and stimulate the senses of hearing, touch, and smell. Toys with educational value such as dolls with various clothing closures are especially useful.

Children with severe permanent visual impairments have the same needs for socialization as sighted children. Because they have little difficulty in learning verbal skills, they are able to communicate with age-mates and participate in suitable activities. The nurse should discuss with parents opportunities for socialization outside the home, especially regular preschools. The trend is to include these children with sighted children to help them adjust to the outside world for eventual independence.

To compensate for inadequate stimulation, these children may develop self-stimulatory activities, such as body rocking, finger flicking, or arm twirling. Such habits restrict the child's social acceptance and are discouraged. Behaviour modification is often successful in reducing or eliminating self-stimulatory activities.

Education. The main obstacle to the child's learning is the child's total dependence on nonvisual cues. Although the child can learn via verbal lecturing, he or she is unable to read the written word or to write without special education. Therefore, the child must rely on braille, a system that uses raised dots to represent letters and numbers. The child can then read the braille with the fingers and can write a message using a braille writer. However, unless others read braille, this system is not useful for communicating with others. A more portable system for written communication is the use of a braille slate and stylus, or an iPod or smartphone with a recording device app. A recorder is especially helpful for leaving messages for others and taking notes during classroom lectures. For mathematical calculations, portable calculators with voice synthesizers are available.

Audio books, other recordings and even CDs are significant sources of reading material other than braille books, which are large and cumbersome. The Canadian National Institute for the Blind (CNIB) has the Library for the Blind and provides audio books, E-books, and braille books online, or they will mail the materials. Many local libraries also provide audio and E-books (see Additional Resources at the end of this chapter). Various talking watches and clocks are also available. For written communication children can use a computer with a voice synthesizer, which "speaks" each letter or word that has been typed.

The child with partial sight can benefit from specialized visual aids that produce a magnified retinal image. The basic devices are accommodation (e.g., bringing the object closer), special plus lenses, handheld and stand magnifiers, telescopes, video projection systems, and large print. E-readers and computer tablets can be easily adjusted to increase the font size. Special equipment is also available to enlarge print. Information about services for the partially sighted is available from the CNIB.

Children with diminished vision often prefer to do close work without their glasses and compensate by bringing the object very near to their eyes. This practice should be allowed. The exception is the child with vision in only one eye, who should always wear glasses for protection.

Caring for the Child During Hospitalization

Because nurses are more likely to care for children who are hospitalized for procedures that involve temporary loss of vision than for children who have severe permanent visual impairment, the following discussion concentrates primarily on the needs of such children. The nursing care objectives in either situation are to (1) reassure the child and family throughout every phase of treatment, (2) orient the child to the surroundings, (3) provide a safe environment, and (4) encourage independence. Whenever possible, the same nurse should care for the child to ensure consistency in the approach.

When sighted children temporarily lose their vision, almost every aspect of the environment becomes bewildering and frightening. They are forced to rely on nonvisual senses for help in adjusting to the visual impairment without the benefit of any special training. Nurses have a major role in minimizing the effects of temporary loss of vision. They need to talk to the child about everything that is occurring, emphasizing aspects of procedures that are felt or heard. They should approach the child by always identifying themselves as soon as they enter the room. Because unfamiliar sounds are especially frightening, these should be explained. Parents should be encouraged to room with their child and participate in the care. Familiar objects, such as a teddy bear or doll, should be brought from home to help lessen the strangeness of the hospital. As soon as the child is able to be out of bed, he or she can be oriented to the immediate surroundings. If the child is able to see on admission, significant aspects of the room should be pointed out. The child needs to be encouraged to practise ambulation with the eyes closed to become accustomed to this experience.

The room should be arranged with safety in mind. For example, a stool or chair can be placed next to the bed to help the child climb in and out of bed. The furniture should always be placed in the same position to prevent collisions. Cleaning personnel need to be reminded to keep the room in the same order. If the child has difficulty navigating by feeling the walls, a rope can be attached from the bed to the point of destination, such as the bathroom. Attention to details such as well-fitting slippers or robes that do not drag on the floor is important in order to prevent tripping. Unlike children who have permanent visual impairments, children with temporary vision loss are not familiar with navigating with a cane.

The child should be encouraged to be independent in self-care activities, especially if the visual loss may be prolonged or potentially permanent. For example, during bathing the nurse can set up all the equipment and encourage the child to participate. At mealtime the nurse should explain where each food item is on the tray, open any special containers, prepare cereal or toast, and encourage the child in self-feeding. Favourite finger foods, such as sandwiches, hamburgers, hot dogs, or pizza, may be good selections. The child needs to be praised for his or her efforts at working together and being independent. Any improvements made in self-care, no matter how small, should be stressed.

Appropriate recreational activities should be provided, and if a child life specialist is available, such planning can be done jointly. Because children with temporary visual impairment have a wide variety of play experiences to draw on, they should be encouraged to select activities. For example, if they like to read, they may enjoy being read to. If they prefer manual activity, they may appreciate playing with clay or building blocks or feeling different textures and naming them. If they need an outlet for aggression, activities such as pounding or banging on a drum can be helpful. Simple board and card games can be played with a "seeing partner" or an opponent who helps with the game. They should have familiar toys from home to play with, since familiar items are more easily manipulated than new ones. If parents want to bring presents, they should be objects that stimulate hearing and touch, such as a radio, music box, or stuffed animal.

Occasionally, children who are visually impaired come to the hospital for procedures to restore their vision. Although this is an extremely happy time, it also requires intervention to help them adjust to sight. They need an opportunity to take in all that they see. They should not be bombarded with visual stimuli. They may need to concentrate on people's faces or their own to become accustomed to this experience. They often need to talk about what they see and to compare the visual images with their mental ones. These children may also go through a period of depression, which must be respected and supported. The nurse or parents should encourage the child to discuss how it feels to see, especially in terms of seeing themselves.

Newly sighted children also need time to adjust to the ability to engage in activities that were impossible before. For example, they may prefer to use braille to read, rather than learning a new "visual approach," because of familiarity with the touch system. Eventually, as they learn to recognize letters and numbers, they will integrate these new skills into reading and writing. However, parents and teachers must be careful not to push them before they are ready. This applies to social relationships and physical activities as well as learning situations.

Assisting in Measures to Prevent Visual Impairment

An essential nursing goal regarding sight in children is to prevent visual impairment. This involves many of the same interventions discussed under hearing impairments:

- Prenatal screening for pregnant women at risk, such as those with rubella or syphilis infection and family histories of genetic disorders associated with visual loss
- Adequate prenatal and perinatal care to prevent prematurity
- Periodic screening of all children, especially newborns through preschoolers, for congenital and acquired visual impairments caused by refractive errors, strabismus, and other disorders
- Rubella immunization of all children
- Safety counselling regarding the common causes of ocular trauma and safe practices when working with, playing with, or carrying objects such as scissors, knives, and balls

> **! NURSING ALERT**
>
> A helmet with a face mask should be required for children playing football, hockey, baseball, and lacrosse.

After detection of eye problems, the nurse has a responsibility to prevent further ocular damage by ensuring that corrective treatment is used. For the child with strabismus, occlusion patching of the stronger eye is often needed. Compliance with the procedure is greatest during the early preschool years. It is more difficult to encourage school-age children to wear the occlusive patch because the poor visual acuity of the uncovered weaker eye interferes with school work and the patch sets them apart from their peers. In school they benefit from being positioned favourably (closer to the board or other visual media) and allowed extra time to read or complete an assignment. If treatment of the eye disorder requires instillation of ophthalmic medication, the family should be taught the correct procedure (see Chapter 44).

The nurse can help children with refractive errors adjust to wearing glasses. Young children who often pull glasses off benefit from temporal pieces that wrap around the ears or an elastic strap attached to the frames and around the back of the head to hold the glasses on securely. After children appreciate the value of clear vision, they are more likely to wear the corrective lenses.

Glasses should not interfere with any activity. Special protective guards are available during contact sports to prevent accidental injury, and all corrective lenses should be made from safety glass, which is shatterproof. Often, corrective lenses improve visual acuity so dramatically that children are able to compete more effectively in sports. This in itself is an inducement to continue wearing glasses.

Contact lenses are a popular alternative, especially for adolescents. Several types are available, such as hard lenses, including gas-permeable ones, and soft lenses, which may be designed for daily or extended wear. Contact lenses offer several advantages over glasses, such as greater visual acuity, total corrected field of vision, convenience (especially with the extended-wear type), and optimal cosmetic benefit. Unfortunately, they are usually more expensive and require much more care than glasses, including considerable practice to learn techniques for insertion and removal. If they are prescribed, the nurse can be helpful in teaching parents or older children how to care for the lenses.

Because trauma is the leading cause of visual impairment in children, the nurse has major responsibility in preventing further eye injury until specific treatment is instituted. The major principles to follow when caring for an eye injury are outlined in the Emergency box earlier in the chapter. Because patients with a serious eye injury fear visual impairment, the nurse should stay with the child and family to provide support and reassurance.

Hearing–Visual Impairment

The most traumatic sensory impairment is loss of both vision and hearing, which may have profound effects on the child's development. They interfere with the normal sequence of physical, intellectual, and psychosocial growth. Although such children often achieve the usual motor milestones, their rate of development is slower. These children learn communication only with specialized training. Finger spelling is one desirable method often taught to these children. Some children with hearing–visual impairment, especially those with residual hearing or sight, can learn to speak. Whenever possible, speech is encouraged because it allows communication with other individuals.

The future prospects for children with hearing–visual impairment are, at best, unpredictable. Congenital hearing–visual impairment may be accompanied by other physical or neurological problems, which further diminish the child's learning potential. The most favourable prognosis is for children who have acquired hearing–visual impairment as these children tend to have few, if any, associated disabilities. Their learning capacity is greatly potentiated by their developmental progress before the sensory impairments. Although total independence, including gainful vocational training, is the goal, some children with hearing–visual impairment are unable to develop to this level. The nurse working with such families can help them deal with future goals for the child, including possible alternatives to home care during the parents' advancing years.

Retinoblastoma

Retinoblastoma, which arises from the retina, is the most common congenital malignant intraocular tumour of childhood. It occurs in approximately 1 in 20,000 babies. Retinoblastoma is caused by a mutation in a gene and may occur sporadically or be inherited (Hurwitz, Shields, & Shields, 2016). Retinoblastoma develops when the mutated gene is unable to produce the natural signals to stop the growth of retinal cells. The majority of cases are nonhereditary and unilateral, with the remainder divided between hereditary and unilateral, and hereditary and bilateral. Hereditary retinoblastomas are transmitted with few exceptions as an autosomal dominant trait with high but incomplete penetrance (Hurwitz et al., 2016).

Diagnostic Evaluation

Retinoblastoma has few grossly obvious signs (Box 41-9). Typically, the most common sign is observed by the parent as a whitish "glow" in the pupil, known as the white reflex or **leukokoria**. Leukokoria represents visualization of the tumour as the light momentarily falls on the mass (Fig. 41-7). The second most common sign of retinoblastoma is acquired strabismus (Hurwitz et al., 2016).

BOX 41-9 CLINICAL MANIFESTATIONS OF RETINOBLASTOMA

- White eye reflex (most common sign)
- Strabismus (second most common sign)
- Red, painful eye, often with glaucoma
- Severe permanent visual impairment (late sign)

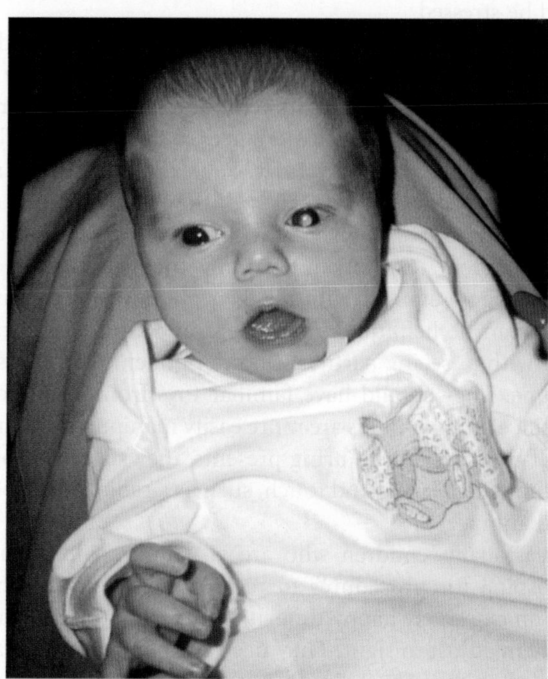

FIGURE 41-7 White reflex. Whitish appearance of lens is produced as light falls on tumour mass in left eye.

The first step in diagnosis is carefully listening to and recognizing the significance of reports from family members regarding suspected abnormalities within the eye. Eye abnormalities, including white reflex, strabismus, decreased vision, and persistent painful erythematous eyes, are referred to an ophthalmologist. Definitive diagnosis is usually based on ophthalmoscopic examination with the patient under **general anaesthesia**. Imaging studies, including ultrasonography and computed tomography of the orbit, are done to determine the extent of the disease.

Therapeutic Management

Treatment of retinoblastoma is complex. Enucleation may be used to treat advanced disease with optic nerve invasion in which there is no hope for salvage of vision. Irradiation can be used when there is vitreous seeding. Chemotherapy has been used more recently to decrease the size of the tumour, as has photocoagulation (use of a laser beam to destroy retinal blood vessels that supply nutrition to the tumour) and cryotherapy (freezing of the tumour, which destroys the microcirculation to the tumour and the cells themselves through microcrystal formation). The use of chemotherapy in advanced disease is controversial and has not shown improved survival.

Prognosis

The overall prognosis for retinoblastoma is favourable, with a survival rate of nearly 95% for both unilateral and bilateral tumours. Retinoblastoma is one of the tumours that may spontaneously regress. Of major concern in long-term survivors is the development of decreased visual acuity; facial disfiguration; and secondary tumours, especially osteogenic sarcoma, other sarcomas, and melanoma. Children with bilateral disease (hereditary form) are more likely to develop secondary cancers than are children with unilateral disease. It is thought that these individuals are predisposed to developing cancer and that radiation increases their risk.

NURSING CARE

One of the most important nursing goals is to have a high index of suspicion for this rare malignancy. If parents report noticing a strange light in the eye or expression, these concerns must be taken seriously. Families with a history of retinoblastoma require follow-up; the nurse can be instrumental in reminding parents of appointments and the importance of genetic counselling.

Because the tumour is usually diagnosed in infants or very young children, most of the preparation for diagnostic tests and treatment involves parents. After indirect ophthalmoscopy, the child may not see clearly, or the eyes may be sensitive to light because of pupillary dilation. Parents should be made aware of these normal reactions before the procedure.

The treatment plan may include focal intraocular therapy with or without chemotherapy, external beam radiation, and, if necessary, enucleation. Enucleation is the treatment of choice if there is extensive disease threatening metastasis or no chance for useful vision. The enucleation procedure and the positive benefits of a prosthesis should be explained to the parents. Showing them pictures of another child with an artificial eye may help them adjust to the thought of disfigurement (Fig. 41-8).

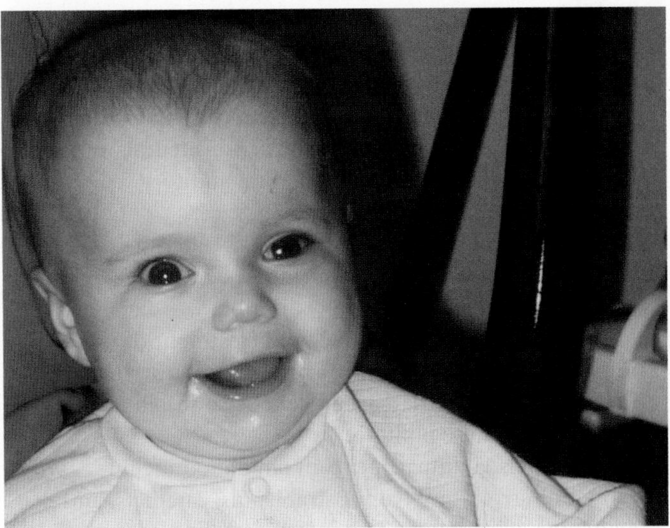

FIGURE 41-8 The same infant as in Figure 41-7, with a left prosthetic eye.

After surgery, the parents should be prepared for the child's facial appearance. An eye patch is in place, and the child's face may be edematous or ecchymotic. Parents often fear seeing the surgical site because they imagine a cavity in the skull. A surgically implanted sphere maintains the shape of the eyeball, and the implant is covered with conjunctiva. When the lids are open, the exposed area resembles the mucosal lining of the mouth. After the child is fitted for a prosthesis, usually within 3 weeks, the facial appearance returns to normal. Initial instructions for care of the prosthesis are given by the ocularist who fits and manufactures the device.

Care of the socket is minimal and easily accomplished. The wound itself is clean and has little or no drainage. If an antibiotic ointment is prescribed, it is applied in a thin line on the surface of the tissues of the socket. To cleanse the site, an irrigating solution may be ordered and is instilled daily or more frequently, before application of the antibiotic ointment. The dressing, consisting of an eye pad taped over the surgical site, needs to be changed daily. After the socket has healed completely, a dressing is no longer necessary, although it is a preventive measure against infection.

KEY POINTS

- *Intellectual disabilities* refers to the challenges that some people face in learning and in communication that are usually present from the time they are born or from an early age.
- Causes of severe CI are primarily genetic, biochemical, and infectious. Mild CI is associated primarily with familial, social, and environmental causes, whereas severe CI is more likely to be associated with specific syndromes.
- Education of children with CI emphasizes sensory and verbal discrimination, improvement of short-term memory, motivation, and technological support.
- Optimum development for the child with CI may be promoted through family guidance regarding play, communication, discipline, socialization, and sexuality.
- Prevention of CI focuses on support for the preterm newborns and other high-risk newborns, rubella immunization, genetic counselling, and maternal education regarding the risks of chemical use (e.g., alcohol ingestion) and the importance of adequate nutrition.
- Down syndrome, a chromosomal abnormality, is characterized by mild to moderate CI (most often), physical characteristics, slowed language development, congenital anomalies, sensory problems, and diminished growth and sexual development.
- Fragile X syndrome is characterized by CI and phenotypic findings in affected males. It is considered the most common hereditary cause and the second leading chromosomal cause of CI after Down syndrome.

- ASDs are a complex neurodevelopmental disorder of brain function accompanied by a broad range and severity of intellectual and behavioural deficits.
- Hearing disorders may be classified according to the location of the defect: conductive, sensorineural, mixed conductive-sensorineural, and central auditory imperception.
- Rehabilitation for hearing loss involves parent education and support, hearing aids, lipreading, sign language, speech therapy, and promotion of socialization.
- Prevention of hearing loss includes treatment of infection, universal newborn screening and child auditory testing, immunization, pregnancy and genetic counselling, and reduction of noise pollution.
- Common visual impairments in childhood include refractive errors, amblyopia, strabismus, cataracts, and glaucoma, with trauma and infections being common causes of visual impairment.
- Prevention of visual impairment focuses on prenatal screening, prenatal and perinatal care, periodic vision screening, immunization, and safety counselling.
- Nursing goals in visual rehabilitation include helping the family and child adjust to the child's visual impairment, promoting parent–child attachment, fostering optimum development and independence, providing for play and socialization, and being aware of educational facilities.
- For the child undergoing ocular surgery, nursing care is aimed at reassuring the child and family throughout treatment, orienting the child to the surroundings, providing a safe environment, and encouraging independence.
- Retinoblastoma is a rare congenital malignant tumour; its most common clinical manifestations are white pupil reflex and strabismus.

evolve WEBSITE

Visit the Evolve website for additional resources related to the content in this chapter such as Case Studies, Critical Thinking Case Study Answers, Nursing Care Plans, Nursing Processes, Nursing Skills, and Review Questions for Exam Preparation at: *http://evolve.elsevier.com/Canada/Perry/maternal/*

REFERENCES

American Association on Intellectual and Developmental Disabilities [AAIDD]. (2010). *Intellectual disability: Definition, classification, and systems of supports* (11th ed.). Washington, DC: Author.

American Psychiatric Association (APA). (2013). *Diagnostic and statistical manual of mental disorders* (5th ed.). Washington, DC: Author.

Amin, S. B., Smith, T., & Wang, H. (2011). Is neonatal jaundice associated with autism spectrum disorders: A systematic review. *Journal of Autism and Developmental Disorders, 41*(11), 1455–1463. doi:10.1007/s10803-010-1169-6.

Arbour, L., & Canadian Paediatric Society Bioethics Committee. (2003). Guidelines for genetic testing of healthy children. *Paediatrics & Child Health, 8*(1), 42–45 Addendum. Retrieved from <http://www.cps.ca/en/documents/position/guidelines-for-genetic-testing-of-healthy-children> Reaffirmed 2015.

Autism Society Canada. (2010). *Canadian charter of rights for persons with autism.* Retrieved from <http://www.autism.net/images/servicesforadults/pdp/Canadian_Charter_for_Persons_with_Autism_March_2009.pdf>.

Bacino, C. A., & Lee, B. (2016). Cytogenetics. In R. M. Kliegman, B. F. Stanton, J. W. St. Geme, et al. (Eds.), *Nelson textbook of pediatrics* (20th ed.). Philadelphia: Saunders.

Baldassari, C. M., Schmidt, C., Schubert, C. M., et al. (2009). Receptive language outcomes in children after cochlear implantation. *Otolaryngology—Head and Neck Surgery, 140,* 114–119.

Berry-Kravis, E. (2014). Mechanism-based treatments in neurodevelopmental disorders: Fragile X syndrome. *Pediatric Neurology, 50*(4), 297–302. doi:10.1016/j.pediatrneurol.2013.12.001.

Botelho, F. A., Bouzada, M. C., Resende, L. M., et al. (2010). Prevalence of hearing impairment in children at risk. *Brazilian Journal of Otorhinolaryngology, 76*(6), 739–744.

Buie, T., Fuchs, G. J., Furuta, G. T., et al. (2010). Recommendations for evaluation and treatment of common gastrointestinal problems in children with ASDs. *Pediatrics, 125*(Suppl. 1), S19–S29. doi:10.1542/peds.2009-1878DBuie.

Canadian Down Syndrome Society. (2009). *Parents helping parents: New parent visiting program.* Retrieved from <http://www.cdss.ca/services/new-parent-programs/parents-helping-parents-new-parent-visiting-program.html>.

Canadian Down Syndrome Society. (n.d.a). *Celebrate about Down syndrome.* Retrieved from <http://www.cdss.ca/images/pdf/brochures/english/celebrate_being_about_down_syndrome_english.pdf>.

Canadian Down Syndrome Society. (n.d.b). *Breastfeeding a baby with Down syndrome.* Retrieved from <http://www.cdss.ca/images/pdf/brochures/english/CDSS_breastfeeding_brochure.pdf>.

Canadian Paediatric Society. (2014). *Your baby's hearing.* Retrieved from <http://www.caringforkids.cps.ca/handouts/your_babys_hearing>.

Canadian Paediatric Society & Public Health Agency of Canada. (2012). *2012 results: Canadian Paediatric Surveillance Program.* Retrieved from <http://www.cpsp.cps.ca/uploads/publications/Results-2012.pdf>.

Canadian Paediatric Society & Public Health Agency of Canada. (2013). *2013 results: Canadian Paediatric Surveillance Program.* Retrieved from <http://www.cpsp.cps.ca/uploads/publications/Results-2013.pdf>.

Centers for Disease Control and Prevention. (2009). Prevalence of autism spectrum disorders: Autism and developmental disorders monitoring network—United States. *MMWR. Surveillance Summaries, 58*(SS10), 1–20.

Chitayat, D., Langlois, S., Wilson, D., et al. (2011). Clinical practice guideline: Screening for fetal aneuploidy in singleton pregnancies. *Journal of Obstetricians and Gynaecologists of Canada, 33*(7), 736–750.

Clifford, S., Dissanayake, C., Bui, Q. M., et al. (2007). Autism spectrum phenotype in males and females with fragile X full mutation and premutation. *Journal of Autism and Developmental Disorders, 37*(4), 738–747.

Dawson, G. (2007). Despite major challenges, autism research continues to offer hope. *Archives of Pediatrics & Adolescent Medicine, 161,* 411–412.

Defendi, G. L. (2010). Fetal alcohol spectrum syndrome: How to recognize the various manifestations. *Consultant for Pediatricians, 9*(1), 343–351.

DiCicco-Bloom, E., Lord, C., Zwaigenbaum, L., et al. (2006). The developmental neurobiology of autism spectrum disorder. *The Journal of Neuroscience*, *26*(26), 6897–6906. doi:10.1523/JNEUROSCI.1712-06.2006.

Fabry, D. A., Davila, E. P., Arheart, K. L., et al. (2011). Secondhand smoke exposure and the risk of hearing loss. *Tobacco Control*, *20*(1), 82–85. doi:10.1136/tc.2010.035832.

Gifford, K. A., Holmes, M. G., & Bernstein, H. H. (2009). Hearing loss in children. *Pediatrics in Review*, *30*(6), 207–215, quiz 216. doi:10.1542/pir.30-6-207.

Hagerman, P. J. (2008). The fragile X prevalence paradox. *Journal of Medical Genetics*, *45*(8), 498–499. doi:10.1136/jmg.2008.059055.

Henderson, E., Testa, M. A., & Hartnick, C. (2011). Prevalence of noise-induced hearing-threshold shifts and hearing loss among US youths. *Pediatrics*, *127*(1), 39–46. doi:10.1542/peds.2010-0926.

Herndon, A. C., DiGuiseppi, C., Johnson, S. L., et al. (2009). Does nutritional intake differ between children with autism spectrum disorders and children with typical development? *Journal of Autism and Developmental Disorders*, *39*(2), 212–222. doi:10.1007/s10803-008-0606-2.

Hurwitz, R. L., Shields, C. L., & Shields, J. A. (2016). Retinoblastoma. In P. A. Pizzo & D. G. Poplack (Eds.), *Principles and practice of pediatric oncology* (7th ed.). Philadelphia: Lippincott.

Katz, G., & Lazcano-Ponce, E. (2008). Intellectual disability: Definition, etiological factors, classification, diagnosis, treatment and prognosis. *Salud Publica de Mexico*, *50*(Suppl. 2), s132–s141.

Kirchner, J. C., Hatri, A., Heekeren, H. R., & Dziobek, I. (2011). Autistic symptomatology, face processing abilities, and eye fixation patterns. *Journal of Autism and Developmental Disorders*, *41*(2), 158–167. doi:10.1007/s10803-010-1032-9.

Maccabee-Ryaboy, N., & Golnik, A. (2010). Autism: Clinical pearls for primary care. *Contemporary Pediatrics*, *11*, 42–60.

Maenner, M. J., Rice, C. E., Arneson, C. L., et al. (2014). Potential impact of DSM-5 criteria on autism spectrum disorder prevalence estimates. *Journal of the American Medical Association Psychiatry*, *71*(3), 292–300. doi:10.1001/jamapsychiatry.2013.3893.

Maurice, P. R., Bouffard, C., Desjardins, S., et al. (2007). *Nunavik Adaptive Behaviour Scale (NABS): Evaluation of adaptive behaviour in Inuit population with suspected mental retardation*. Presented at the 19th IUHPE World Conference on Health Promotion and Health Education. Vancouver, BC.

Mema, S. C., McIntyre, L., & Musto, R. (2012). Childhood vision screening in Canada: Public health evidence and practice. *Canadian Journal of Public Health*, *103*(1), 40–45.

National Down Syndrome Society. (2012). *Aging matters*. Retrieved from <http://www.ndss.org/Resources/Aging-Matters/>.

Oliver, C., & Richards, C. (2010). Self-injurious behaviour in people with intellectual disability. *Current Opinion in Psychiatry*, *23*(5), 412–416. doi:10.1097/YCO.0b013e32833cfb80.

Patel, H., Feldman, M., & Canadian Paediatric Society, Community Paediatrics Committee. (2011). Universal newborn screening. *Paediatrics & Child Health*, *16*(5), 301–305. Retrieved from <http://www.cps.ca/documents/position/universal-hearing-screening-newborns> Reaffirmed 2016.

Price, C. S., Thompson, W. W., Goodson, B., et al. (2010). Prenatal and infant exposure to thimerosal from vaccines and immunoglobulins and risk of autism. *Pediatrics*, *126*(4), 656–664. doi:10.1542/peds.2010-0309.

Public Health Agency of Canada. (2013). *Congenital anomalies in Canada 2013. A perinatal health surveillance report*. Retrieved from <http://publications.gc.ca/collections/collection_2014/aspc-phac/HP35-40-2013-eng.pdf>.

Rahi, J. S., Cumberland, P. M., Peckham, C. S., et al. (2010). Improving detection of blindness in childhood: The British childhood vision impairment study. *Pediatrics*, *12*, e895–e903.

Ranweiler, R., & Merritt, L. (2009). Assessment and care of the newborn with Down syndrome. *Advances in Neonatal Care*, *9*(1), 17–24.

Rutter, M. L. (2013). Changing concepts and findings on autism. *Journal of Autism and Developmental Disorders*, *43*(8), 1749–1757. doi:10.1007/s10803-012-1713-7.

Shapiro, B. K., & Batshaw, M. L. (2016). Intellectual disability. In R. M. Kliegman, B. F. Stanton, J. W. St. Geme, et al. (Eds.), *Nelson textbook of pediatrics* (20th ed.). Philadelphia: Saunders.

Solomon, M., Buaminger, N., & Rogers, S. J. (2011). Abstract reasoning and friendship in high functioning preadolescents with autism spectrum disorders. *Journal of Autism and Developmental Disorders*, *41*(1), 32–43. doi:10.1007/s10803-010-1017-8.

Statistics Canada. (2009). *Facts on seeing limitations*. Retrieved from <http://www.statcan.gc.ca/pub/89-628-x/2009013/fs-fi/fs-fi-eng.htm>.

U.S. Preventive Services Task Force. (2011). Vision screening for children 1 to 5 years of age. *Pediatrics*, *127*, 340–346.

Weijerman, M. E., & de Winter, J. P. (2010). Clinical practice. The care of children with Down syndrome. *European Journal of Pediatrics*, *169*(12), 1445–1452. doi:10.1007/s00431-010-1253-0.

Zwaigenbaum, L. (2010). Advances in the early detection of autism. *Current Opinion in Neurology*, *23*(2), 97–102.

ADDITIONAL RESOURCES

Alexander Graham Bell Association for the Deaf and Hard of Hearing: <http://www.agbell.org>

Autism Canada: <http://www.autismcanada.org/>

Canadian Down Syndrome Society: <http://www.cdss.ca>

Canadian Down Syndrome Society—Breastfeeding Assistance: <http://www.cdss.ca/images/pdf/brochures/english/CDSS_breastfeeding_brochure.pdf>

Canadian Hearing Society—Information on hearing aids and hearing loss: <http://www.chs.ca>

Canadian National Institute for the Blind (CNIB)—Products available for people with vision problems: <http://www.cnib.ca>

Canadian Organizations for Deafblind People: <http://www.deafblind.com/canada.html>

Canadian Radio-Television and Telecommunications Commission: Toll free: *1-877 249 CRTC (2782); Toll-free TTY line: 1-877 909 CRTC (2782).* <http://www.crtc.gc.ca>

Down Syndrome Research Foundation: <http//www.dsrf.org>

Easter Seals Canada: <http://www.easterseals.ca>

Fragile X Research Foundation of Canada: <http://www.fragilexcanada.ca/index.php?home&lng=en>

Government of Canada—Canadian Human Rights Act: <http://laws-lois.justice.gc.ca/eng/acts/H-6/page-1.html>

Individualized education plans: <http://www.edu.gov.on.ca/eng/general/elemsec/speced/guide/resource/>

Learning Disabilities Association of Canada (LDAC): <http://www.ldac-acta.ca/>

Special Olympics Canada: <http://www.specialolympics.ca>

Speech-Language and Audiology Canada: <http://www.caslpa.ca>

CHAPTER 42

Family-Centred Home Care

Katherine Bertoni, with contributions from Marilyn J. Hockenberry

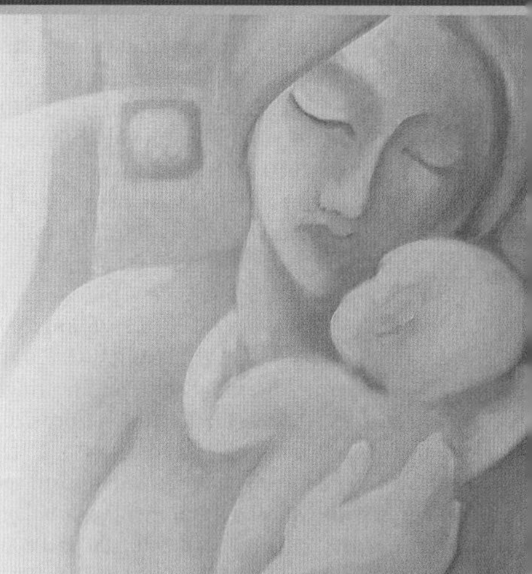

evolve WEBSITE

Visit the Evolve website for additional resources related to the content in this chapter such as Case Studies, Critical Thinking Case Study Answers, Nursing Care Plans, Nursing Processes, Nursing Skills, and Review Questions for Exam Preparation at: http://evolve.elsevier.com/Canada/Perry/maternal/

OBJECTIVES

On completion of this chapter the reader will be able to:

- List at least three factors contributing to the increasing emphasis on home care services.
- Describe case management, or care coordination, and its importance in home care.
- List general principles of a family-centred assessment and planning process.
- Identify five key characteristics of collaborative relationships.
- Describe approaches to promoting optimum development, self-care, and education in home care.
- Outline six areas in need of attention for promoting safety in home care.

GENERAL CONCEPTS OF HOME CARE

Definition

Home care has become a routine option for the child patient in today's health care environment. The Canadian Home Care Association (CHCA) (2013a) defines *home care* as "an array of services for people of all ages, provided in the home and community setting, that encompass health promotion and teaching, curative intervention, end-of-life care, rehabilitation, support and maintenance, social adaptation and integration, and support for family caregivers."

With the many advances in medical technology, along with restructuring of the Canadian health care system, there has been a rapid increase in the number of children and youth with acute and continuing home care needs across Canada. The growing demand for home care services is in part a result of increasing costs of institutionalized care. More importantly, home-based health care enables the family's valuable contribution to the child's overall health in his or her natural environment. It is not meant to replace but rather to complement self-care (CHCA, 2013b). Therefore, home care programs lead to greater parent satisfaction, improved quality of life, and a reduction in the length of hospital stays. Parab, Cooper, Woolfenden, et al. (2013) suggest that there is limited evidence that home care reduces access to hospital-based services or hospital admissions.

Home care is not a new concept in pediatrics. Over the past decades the term has referred to parents caring for mildly ill children at home; to home nursing visits after children are discharged from the hospital; and, more recently, to care at home for children with more serious chronic illness and dependence on medical technology. Providing quality home health care for children generally requires the parents' desire for it and the ability to carry out their part of the care, as well as professional assistance and community preparedness. A natural family environment optimizes growth and development when stress is minimal and support is optimal. The role of the community health or home care nurse in home care is to promote health and prevent disease; develop individual, family, and community relationships; build on the capacity of the individual and community; facilitate access and equity; and demonstrate professional responsibility and accountability (Canadian Public Health Association, 2010; Community Health Nurses Association of Canada [CHNA], 2008).

Home Care Trends and Needs

The shift toward home-based health care has been propelled by numerous factors. As stated earlier, advances in medical technology have enabled increased survival for children with congenital and acquired illnesses. Preterm infants or children who are ventilator dependent were once cared for indefinitely in a critical care unit or long-term care facility. These children are now able to live with their families in their own home.

Children with chronic conditions such as cancer, kidney disorders, cystic fibrosis, spina bifida, cardiac and respiratory disorders, gastrointestinal disorders, neurodegenerative diseases, and human immunodeficiency virus (HIV) infection may have ongoing home care needs as a result of the disease, its treatment, or adverse effects of treatment. Children with acquired injuries that result in chronic impairment, such as an acquired brain injury due to accidents and/or trauma, are also in need of ongoing health care.

Parents frequently have ongoing stressors after a child's hospitalization for diagnosis and treatment. Subsequent needs may include reinforcing teachings about the disease process, addressing the child's physical care needs, and providing emotional support during this change in parental role. In addition, home-based nutrition programs are useful, safe, and well tolerated. These programs can provide a better quality of life, decrease cost of therapy, and improve survival.

Improving the quality of life for both the child and the family is one of the driving forces in the effort to move technology-dependent children from the hospital to the home setting. Part of this process involves **normalization**, whereby, over time, families of children with chronic illness begin to perceive the child and their family life as normal (see Chapter 40). This has important implications for pediatric home care nurses in terms of assessment of family function and dynamics. The normalized family tends to be more flexible with treatments and incorporates the child with a complex illness into the usual routines of daily living.

Other factors contributing to the increase in home care are the rising cost of institutionalized health care and shifts in the financing of health care delivery. Inpatient hospital stays have become shorter, in part because of the overwhelming cost of lengthy hospitalizations and because children who have been hospitalized have an increased risk of developing health care–acquired and antibiotic-resistant infections (Chen, Wu, Chang, et al., 2008). Children may not be admitted to the hospital at all or are returned home as soon as possible after their illness. Likewise, a portion of the financial burden is shifted to the family. Third-party insurance may cover part or all of the costs at home. In some cases, the family may be forced to absorb the costs of certain medications, supplies, transportation, shelter, utilities, food, laundry, and housekeeping, as well as a portion of the nursing care. There is no home care legislation specific to children across the provinces or territories; this lack of legislation creates significant differences across jurisdictions in terms of types of home and community care services available to children that are funded (Peter, Spalding, Kenny, et al., 2007).

Home health care of children is not restricted to children with chronic and complex health care needs. Several short-term, intermittent therapies, such as dressing changes, phototherapy, chemotherapy, apnea monitoring, intravenous medication or fluid administration, and pain and symptom management, may be successfully delivered in a home setting, where the child may remain with the family, rather than in an acute-care setting. For instance, home health nurses providing asthma education to families of children frequently hospitalized for asthma exacerbations can increase the family's knowledge about asthma symptoms, triggers, and management. With this knowledge families may be able to reduce the triggers that cause acute exacerbations that often result in hospitalization (see Asthma, Chapter 45).

Currently, a major issue in providing home care is the shortage of qualified pediatric nurses in the home care field. According to a report released by the Canadian Nurses Association (2013), less than 5% of registered nurses in Canada work in community health, and less than 3% work in pediatrics. This shortage is particularly true in rural or remote areas. Agencies and families are facing much difficulty in staffing required home care services; thus more of the home care must be carried out by family members or other caregivers. The lack of pediatric training in some nursing programs, increased acuity of home care patients, and increased pay for nurses working in acute care settings have contributed to a greater than ever nursing shortage in pediatric home health care. Other health care providers that may be needed for home care, such as speech-language pathologists, respiratory therapists, audiologists, psychologists, social workers, and dietitians, are slowly growing in number within Canada (Canadian Institute for Health Information [CIHI] 2011), whereas occupational therapists and physiotherapists remain in short supply in some provincial and territorial jurisdictions (CIHI, 2011),

Given the nationwide shortage of home care nurses, there has been increased focus on the role of the family caregiver in providing home care. In 2012, it was estimated that eight million Canadians were providing care for a family member with chronic health conditions (Sinha & Statistics Canada, Social and Aboriginal Statistics Division, 2013). Caregivers have the following four responsibilities when caring for a family member who has a chronic illness:

Managing the illness—Providing daily hands-on care, monitoring the child's medical condition, and educating others to care for the child

Identifying, accessing, and coordinating resources—Locating appropriate resources in the community to meet the needs of the child and of the family as the child's caregiver

Maintaining the family unit—Continuing to nurture the family unit: siblings' needs, spousal relationships, and household maintenance

Maintaining self—Grieving the loss of the healthy child; balancing caregiver responsibilities with their own physical, emotional, mental, and personal needs; recognizing stressors and potential caregiver burnout.

Nurses need to understand the magnitude of responsibilities facing the caregiving family and assist them in finding resources to provide some respite from caring for the child in order to care for each other and maintain self and family integrity.

The Canadian Paediatric Society (CPS) (Ponti & CPS, Community Paediatrics Committee, 2008/2016) recommends that physicians advocate for *permanency planning*, through which children and youth with special health care needs obtain placement stability and personal intervention plans, should the family be unable to support the child. Options can include family-based care: adoption, nonrelative foster care, kinship foster care, or guardianship foster care. Health care providers are encouraged to collaborate with child welfare professionals, foster parents, group home staff, and the child's parents and family members, as appropriate, to provide optimum care to these children who are at increased risk for special health care needs (Ponti & CPS, Community Paediatrics Committee, 2008/2016). Each province and territory has its own home care–related legislation and policies associated with child welfare services. The exception is Indigenous children and youth, who are supported through the federal government. When compared to group residential options, family-based care is the preferred placement option for these children.

Another CPS recommendation is that health care providers be aware of community resources available to assist the caregivers of special needs children (Ponti & CPS, Community Paediatrics Committee, 2008/2016). *Respite care* provides temporary relief to parents and gives them a break from the responsibilities of caring for their child on a daily basis. Respite care can be costly, as it is not considered an insured service under the *Canada Health Act*. Respite care for caregivers of children with special care needs has been slow in its development and availability and is not always an option, due to limited financial and human resources.

Respite care for ventilator-dependent children and those with skilled technological care requirements is in short supply in some provincial and territorial jurisdictions, given the lack of skilled care providers, early discharge from the hospital, and high health needs (Canadian Healthcare Association [CHA], 2012). Nurses can play an important role in advocating for the provision of high-quality respite care, which enables families and caregivers to maintain appropriate family function, care for themselves, and continue to provide care for their child, as necessary. Family-focused respite care is considered most effective when various cultural and ethnic practices and values are taken into consideration (CHA, 2012).

Effective Home Care

In providing home-based care for children, the nurse has an opportunity to assess and interact with the family in their own environment. This assessment can provide the health care team with valuable information about safety, support systems, nutrition, parenting ability, and actual health care practices. Such information will determine future decisions for individualized care and realistic outcomes.

The pediatric home care nurse has two distinct arrangements for implementation of care. Nurses who perform *intermittent skilled nursing* visits may see different types and numbers of patients each day. These nurses typically have an assigned patient caseload and accept responsibility for implementing the care plan. Most home visits focus on helping the patient and caregiver achieve independence with care in the home, including home care by therapists, home infusion teaching by nurses, and care management, instead of providing direct physical care. Nurses who perform *private-duty nursing*, or block nursing, are usually assigned individual patients, and they remain in the home for a predetermined time, such as an 8- or 12-hour block of time, to provide patient care. The care plan is implemented over the course of the time in the home. Required nursing skills are determined by patient need, parental ability, complexity of family, and the home environment. In both types of home care, the pediatric nurse is responsible for patient and family assessment and evaluating the appropriateness of the care plan (Canadian Public Health Association, 2010) (Box 42-1).

Consideration of the caregiver's willingness and ability to provide care and of his or her limitations is of utmost importance when assessing the appropriateness of the care plan. It is

BOX 42-1 HOME CARE ASSESSMENT

Health Care Need

Child at risk—Parental substance use; child's failure to thrive; social or family situation that is potentially detrimental to child's well-being

Chronically ill, but medically stable child with multiple care needs

Education and competency validation of caregiver skills

Skilled procedures—Regularly scheduled injections or infusions, dressing changes, reinforcement of home care teaching; evaluation of caregiver's skills

Technology-dependent child (e.g., ventilator or tracheostomy, home total parenteral nutrition, or enteral feedings by pump, peritoneal dialysis)

Chronically ill child with multiple skilled nursing needs, including pain symptom management and palliative care

Intervention

Regularly scheduled visits to assess patient status, evaluate home environment, teach care provider skills, determine status of growth and development, set goals with family for positive health outcomes

As-needed home visits during exacerbation of illness to assess physical status and determine appropriate intervention in collaboration with the health care team

Assistance with transportation of child to ambulatory centre or practitioner's office for evaluation and diagnostic services

Regular visits of limited duration to perform skilled nursing intervention, assess parental ability and desire to perform procedure, teach procedure technique, supervise parental performance of procedure

Assessment of patient status; evaluation of safety of home environment; teaching, evaluation, and reinforcement of caregivers' skills; determination of status of growth and development; goal setting with family for positive health outcomes

Assessment of family status; evaluation of family coping skills and continued ability to manage care of the child at home

BOX 42-2 SERVICES THAT SUPPORT EFFECTIVE HOME CARE

- Adequate family training and preparation
- Primary care physician willing to oversee medical aspects of home care
- Professional caregivers adequately trained in relevant nursing and communication skills
- Developmental intervention such as physiotherapy and occupational and speech therapy; early intervention
- Appropriately designed and well-maintained equipment
- Supportive therapies (e.g., respiratory therapy, pharmacy, rehabilitation services, parenteral therapy, physiotherapy, durable medical and infusion supplies, nutritional support) that are accessible and that families are able to contact when needed
- Adequate social and psychological support services
- High-quality respite care
- Appropriate home renovation
- Telephone service in the home
- Internet and computer access
- Appropriate transportation
- Appropriate locally available emergency facilities
- Competent case management services
- Safe environment (electricity, refrigeration, cleanliness)

Modified from Office of Technology Assessment (OTA), Congress of the United States. (1987). *Technology dependent children: Hospital v. home care—a technical memorandum* (OTA-TM-H-38). Washington, DC: US Government Printing Office; Bakewell-Sachs, S., & Porth, S. (1995). Discharge planning and home care of the technology-dependent infant. *Journal of Obstetric, Gynecologic, & Neonatal Nursing 24*(1), 77–83.

vital to ensure that patients and families build a good support network and have access to resources such as social services (Box 42-2). An increasing concern in pediatric home health care is having a managing practitioner to oversee the home care. Shorter hospital stays have increased patients' rapid movement through the continuum of care; a patient may be seen in the emergency department or neonatal intensive care unit, then be discharged to home health without ever seeing a primary care physician. Thus, it is imperative that the provision of care for home patients involves multidisciplinary collaboration and communication among health care workers.

Discharge Planning and Selection of a Home Care Agency

Identification of appropriate local community resources is critical to a successful transfer to home care (Box 42-3). The ultimate goal of discharge planning is for the family to become familiar with the child's needs and to be competent in providing that care. A discharge plan should include emergency management and provision of social and emotional support. The CPS emphasizes that the goal for a home health care program for infants, children, or adolescents with chronic illness or complex conditions is the provision of community-based, culturally sensitive, comprehensive, and cost-effective health care within a nurturing home environment that maximizes the capabilities of the individual and minimizes the effects of the disabilities (Ponti & CPS, Community Paediatrics Committee, 2008/2016).

BOX 42-3 CHARACTERISTICS OF A HIGH-QUALITY PEDIATRIC HOME CARE AGENCY

- Fully trained pediatric staff to provide for all aspects of care (nursing, rehabilitation therapies, pharmacy, nutrition, social work, home medical equipment)
- Prompt, responsive staff with 24-hour availability
- Family-centred care
- Comprehensive continuing education programs
- Certification by local, provincial, territorial, and federal regulatory agencies
- Accreditation by Accreditation Canada Home Care Services

Much of the success of home care, particularly for the child who is dependent on medical technology or who has complex medical problems, depends on careful planning and preparation. Discharge planning must begin early; it should be based on the criteria of child and family readiness; it must be a multidisciplinary process, including representatives from acute care, home care, and community settings; and it must involve the family. Predischarge assessment (Box 42-4) and planning should include the following:

- The child's medical, nursing, educational, and other therapeutic needs
- Family members' (including siblings') education and training, coping skills, and adjustment needs
- Community readiness in areas such as accessibility of equipment, appropriate nursing and allied health personnel, educational and developmental services, respite care, and emergency plans
- Financial arrangements

Creative financial planning, including negotiating arrangements with the insurance company and community programs, may be required.

! NURSING ALERT

If home care equipment is different from hospital equipment, have the portable equipment delivered to the hospital to allow family use before discharge.

The preparation for hospital discharge and home care begins during the admission assessment. Short- and long-term goals are established to meet the child's physical and psychosocial needs. For children with complex care needs, discharge planning focuses on obtaining appropriate equipment and health care personnel for the home. It is also concerned with treatments that parents or children are expected to continue at home. In planning appropriate teaching, nurses need to assess (1) the actual and perceived complexity of the skill, (2) the parents' or child's ability to learn the skill, and (3) the parents' or child's previous or present experience with such procedures. See Family-Centred Teaching box on how to prepare the family for discharge.

BOX 42-4 EXAMPLE OF PREDISCHARGE ASSESSMENT FOR A TECHNOLOGY-DEPENDENT CHILD

The Child's Family

Identification and training of primary caregivers
Identification and training of caregivers for respite and emergency care
Parent employment status while caring for child at home
Family financial picture, especially if one parent must stop working
Sibling preparation
Availability of psychosocial support services

Technical Equipment and Supplies for the Home

Home care company's availability and experience
Home care company's coordination of services with local health care provider and others
24-hour availability and coverage for unexpected situations

Community Nursing and Support Services

Availability, training, and experience
Adequacy of number of personnel to meet needs
Additional training of staff, if needed
24-hour availability of ambulance services and emergency medical services

Physical Environment of the Home

Adequacy of space for equipment and supplies
Heavy equipment (e.g., ventilator, oxygen tanks, compressor) accessibility
Layout of home (e.g., number of floors, stairways, room accessibility, room sizes)
Location and layout of bedrooms
Adequacy of apartment building elevator and fire escape
Telephone access
Type of transportation family uses
Possibility of modifying living space to minimize invasiveness of technology without isolating child
Adequacy of heating and cooling systems
Adequacy of electrical system to accommodate equipment

Emergency Plan

Identification and training of those involved
Written implementation plan: who, what, where, when, how (include telephone numbers)
Notification of utility companies for priority repairs and maintenance
Notification of local emergency medical facility or calling 911
Emergency drill

Primary Care Provider

Identification of local primary provider or pediatrician who is able to assume direct care responsibility and coordination of other care providers
Inclusion of local provider in discharge planning
Information needs of local provider before child's discharge

FAMILY-CENTRED TEACHING

Preparation for Discharge

- For parents who choose to care for their child at home, planning for home care begins early in the recovery process.
- The family should become involved with the child's care as soon as they indicate an interest and ability to do so.
- They need education and support in learning to care for the child, regular follow-up observation and assessment of the home management, and planning for some respite care of the child.
- Parents need to understand that it is important to plan for periodic relief from the continual care of the child.

The teaching plan incorporates levels of learning such as observing, participating with assistance, and acting without help or guidance. The skill is divided into discrete steps, and each step is taught to the family member until it is learned. Return demonstration of the skill is requested before new skills are introduced. A record of teaching and performance provides an efficient checklist for evaluation. All families need to receive detailed *written* instructions about home care with telephone numbers for assistance before they leave the hospital. Communication between the nurse performing discharge planning and home health care is essential for ensuring a smooth transition for the child and family.

After the family is competent in performing the skill, they are given responsibility for the care. When possible, the family should have a transition or trial period to assume care with minimal health care supervision. This may be arranged on the unit, during a home pass, or in a facility such as a motel near the hospital. Such transitions provide a safe practice period for the family, with assistance readily available when needed, and are especially valuable when the family lives far from the hospital.

In many instances parents need only simple instructions and understanding of follow-up care. However, the often overwhelming care assumed by some families, coupled with other stressors they may be experiencing, necessitates continued professional support after discharge. A follow-up home visit or telephone call gives the nurse an opportunity to individualize care and provide information in perhaps a less stressful learning environment than the hospital. Early involvement of the home care agency in the discharge planning process promotes continuity of care and a smooth transition from hospital to home (Box 42-5). Before discharge, a general plan, sometimes called an *individualized home care plan*, should be developed with multidisciplinary input. This care plan should address the range of needs identified as part of the comprehensive predischarge assessment. Sharing the important issues surrounding the child's and family's needs is essential. Referral summaries should be concise, specific, and factual. When numerous support services are required, periodic collaboration among the professionals involved and the family is an excellent strategy to ensure efficient use and comprehensive delivery of services.

When providing education to the primary caregiver and family members, it is important to use materials that meet the

BOX 42-5 CRITICAL HOME CARE REFERRAL INFORMATION

- Scheduled medications
- Durable medical equipment
- Medical supplies
- Transportation needs
- Adaptive equipment
- Respiratory therapy
- Rehabilitation therapies (occupational, physical, and speech therapy)
- Psychological counselling
- Social work referral
- Respite plans
- Key family members
- Demographic information
- Reimbursement information

needs and the ability of the learner. An excellent method of providing home care instructions is with video recordings. Once the family masters the procedures, consider video recording their performance; if they have a smartphone the recording can be made on the phone. Visual learning is most helpful for people who cannot read or who are not fluent in English. The video recording can also serve as a secondary support or follow-up to written instructions.

A predischarge home visit allows the home care nurse to meet the family, help them assess their preparedness and the preparedness of the home environment, discuss plans for arranging the child's equipment at home (Fig. 42-1), reinforce prior discharge teaching, and implement any additional teaching that may be necessary. Additional factors that should be considered in discharge planning include parents' work schedule, whether extended family are available to assist in the care, and child care arrangements for siblings.

Care Coordination (Case Management)

Traditional definitions of case management generally focus on cost control, attainment of desired clinical outcomes, and monitoring and evaluation of care provided. However, for optimum home care of the child who is technology dependent, case management—or care coordination—should be viewed more broadly.

Often services are provided by multiple organizations and multiple vendors with different missions and a consistent lack of single systems linking home health care. In addition, eligibility criteria for funding and services are complex and vary from one province or territory to another. As a result, coordination of home care can be challenging, frustrating, and complicated for the family (Ponti & CPS, Community Paediatrics Committee, 2008/2016).

The concept of *care coordination* in home care for children is to link children with special home health care needs (and their families) to community services and resources in a coordinated effort to provide the child with optimum care. Care coordination has several purposes. Its primary goal is to ensure continuity for the child and family across hospital, home, educational, therapeutic, and other settings. Other goals involve facilitating timely access to services and enhancing child and family well-being (CHCA, 2013b). Care should be coordinated among multiple providers to reduce the complexity of care for the child, reduce fragmentation of care, prevent duplication of services, and decrease the burden of care for the family. Case managers from a number of agencies may be involved in the patient's care, which may add to the parents' confusion; the home care nurse should attempt to coordinate meetings between all case managers, the family, and a nurse care coordinator in order to minimize confusion and prevent duplication. Knowing how to access community resources is often confusing for families, given the multiple points of access and provincial or territorial ministries involved (CHCA, 2013b). Care coordination should ensure that the child's medical, nursing, and health maintenance needs, as well as the financial issues, psychosocial concerns, and educational needs of the child and family, are addressed. The coordinating case manager is often provided by the community care agency to help bring all of the resources together and help with funding information (CHCA, 2013b).

Although professionals must always see part of their role as ensuring that integrated, coordinated care is provided, care coordination should promote the family's role as primary decision maker and enhance the family's capability to meet the special needs of the child and the family unit. Many parents take on increasing responsibility for care coordination over time; they should be encouraged and supported in this role. Home care nurses and case managers should be aware that the termination of private-duty or home care nursing can be a difficult transition for which families may need preparation. A gradual reduction in services allows patients and families to adjust favourably to the changes.

Role of the Nurse, Training, and Standards of Care

The home care nurse must share a level of technical expertise with the critical care nurse while being able to adapt equipment, procedures, and the nursing process to the home setting. (See Chapter 44 for specific technical skills that may be required in home care practice.) The need for technical expertise must be matched with knowledge of child development and the ability to work creatively with the child challenged by chronic illness and technology dependence. When caring for patients in the home setting, the nurse must be comfortable making independent nursing judgements and solving problems with no immediate assistance, within the nursing scope of practice. At the same time, the nurse must have excellent interpersonal skills; an ability to work with other professionals and the family; and, most important, an ability to respect family autonomy. Being able to coordinate, facilitate, and advocate for appropriate resource allocation while considering broader determinants of health that influence the health of the child and family are vital qualities of a pediatric home care nurse. Patient outcomes are also more readily achievable with a balance of nursing skills demonstrating clinical excellence; adaptability; accountability; and the development of positive relationships with physicians, patients, and families.

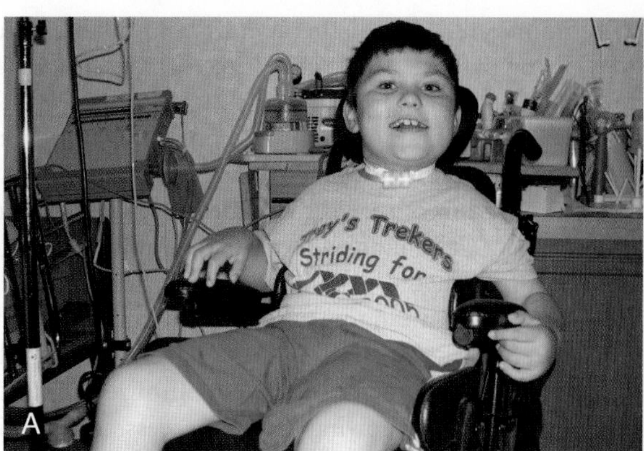

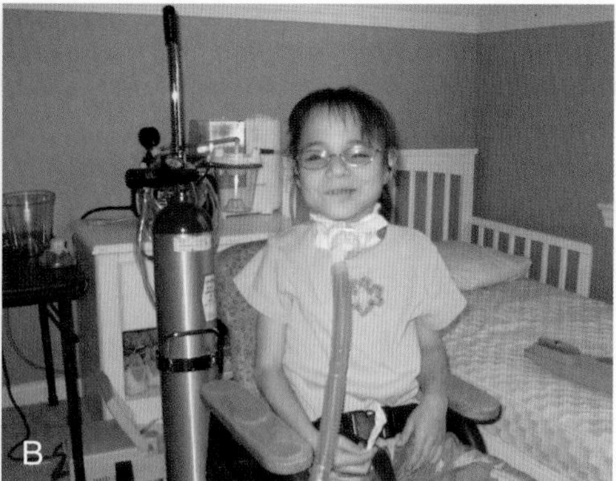

FIGURE 42-1 A: An essential aspect of preparation for home care is the arrangement of equipment and supplies. **B:** The nurse in the home care setting requires expertise to care for a child who is technology dependent.

The planning, management, and delivery of home health care services in Canada vary among provinces and territories. Currently, four provinces have legislation or an *Order in Council* regulating home care services; however, there is no national legislated framework (CHCA, 2016). Nursing standards for professional practice and conduct are governed by provincial and territorial regulatory bodies. Community health nursing standards of practice have been developed by recognized associate members of the Canadian Nurses Association (CNA) (see Chapter 3). The CNA also offers national certification in community health nursing, rehabilitation nursing, and hospice palliative care nursing, among others. Despite important differences between pediatric and adult care in the home, as of this writing no national standards specific to pediatric home care practice have been developed.

FAMILY-CENTRED HOME CARE

Technology dependence, chronic illness, and complex care requirements cross social, cultural, spiritual, and economic boundaries. Regardless of a family's background, the family's values must be respected in the provision of home care services. *The home is the family's domain*, and the child is at home because the family's central role is to nurture and raise their child. The ultimate responsibility for managing the child's health, developmental, and emotional needs lies with the family. Roush and Cox (2000) have developed a framework for helping the home health care nurse understand the significance of the home to the family. The three central concepts of the model are as follows:

Home as familiar—The environment where one is comfortable and at ease because of the familiarity with living arrangements and routines of home

Home as centre—The location of everyday experiences related to time, space, and one's social life

Home as protector—The environment that preserves privacy, safety, and identity

The philosophical basis for family-centred practice is the recognition that the family is the constant in the child's life, whereas the service systems and personnel within those systems fluctuate. The Calgary Family Assessment Model may be helpful to nurses in assessing families and assisting in their management of the complex health care needs of their children (see Chapter 2, p. 17). The model demonstrates tools such as genograms to outline a family structure and provides a visual representation of the family and their resources (Wright & Leahy, 2013). Families have the most intimate knowledge of the child's strengths and abilities, the challenges of providing care, and the abilities and needs of other family members. Honouring the belief that no one knows the child better than the family is critical to the success of any health care plan.

Respect for Diversity

Respect for varied family structures and for racial, ethnic, cultural, spiritual, and socioeconomic diversity among families is essential in home care (see also Chapter 31). Home care nurses work in close relationship with family members and in the family's own domain. The nurse shares in these relationships, participating in care throughout the course of illness (see Family-Centred Teaching box).

Health Canada has researched the First Nation and Inuit populations' home care needs and found that this population was generally younger and received fragmented care. The gaps in home and community care included mental health services, palliative and end-of-life care, rehabilitative care, and respite care. Health Canada has recommended the introduction of specialized training for service providers to help meet the needs for this population (Health Canada, 2012). Most caregivers provide a great deal of care each week, and about one in three caregivers support two or more persons needing care.

> **! NURSING ALERT**
>
> One should not assume that everyone who speaks English can read the language. Colour-coded medication bottles, written schedules, and pillboxes or oral syringes may aid family members' ability to follow through with prescription administration. Pictures or special symbols may be helpful when providing instructions for procedures and medication administration.

FAMILY-CENTRED TEACHING

Developing Relationships With Culturally Diverse Families

I work in the inner city, and my home care patients come from a variety of racial and ethnic backgrounds. I am White, from Australia. Often, when I first visit a family, there is an initial coolness or apprehension toward me. This is understandable because I am a stranger, and perhaps families think I'll judge them in one way or another. By the end of the first visit, however, there is usually a smile as I leave; by the second visit they often greet me with a smile at the door; and by the third visit, we usually have a friendship, trust, and an ease of communication.

If I'm working on a case for an extended time, I use a holistic nursing approach. This involves being aware of how the child's illness affects the entire family. As I listen over many weeks to their fears and questions, and often as I share faith perspectives, a bond begins to form. I find it a privilege to share in their joys and their pain, and I feel rewarded by the trust that they invest in me.

–Julie Edgerton, RN, Home Care Nurse

Modified from Ahmann, E. (1994). Thinking critically about family-centered home care nursing. *Pediatric Nursing, 20*(6), 588–590.

Families may also differ in their cultural views of children; health care; child-rearing practices; and illness, its causes, and its meaning. The family's health care practices and beliefs may influence the level of investment a family will make in the child's care. The family's religion or spirituality can also have a major influence on a family's response to the child's special health care needs. Some families will look for spiritual meaning in relation to the illness and purpose for the illness. Other families may choose to reject past religious ties. In some cultures, religion and beliefs about health care and illness are closely intertwined; thus it is important that home care nurses assess the relationships among culture, religion, and the family's beliefs about the child's illness.

The home care nurse, aware that personal values drive behaviour, must learn about the family's culture, ask questions without implying judgement, interpret the mainstream medical culture, and help families design interventions that meet their preferences (CNA, 2010) (see Chapter 2). When possible, culture-specific teaching materials should be used. Respect for family diversity and awareness of family developmental stages and the stages of a family's adjustment to illness in a child (see Chapter 40) will assist the home care nurse in recognizing and promoting family strengths and in respecting varied coping mechanisms. Use of labels such as "dysfunctional," "difficult," and "noncompliant" can reinforce negative expectations and shape behaviours of both parents and professionals. By contrast, emphasizing, identifying, and building on family strengths and coping mechanisms can promote a central goal in nursing care of the child and family: family empowerment.

Parent–Professional Collaboration

Family-centred nursing practice is built on a foundation of parent–professional collaboration, which represents a shift from the traditional unidirectional relationships between health care providers and families. The Collaborative Family Health Care Association has developed core competencies for health care providers collaborating with families that may also be used as a guide toward family-centred nursing practice (see Additional Resources at the end of this chapter).

Communication with the family should be clear and respectful. The nurse should explain to families the reason for questions, particularly those they may perceive as intrusive, and should tell families who will have access to the information. The nurse must also assure families that they have a right to expect confidentiality in regard to the data collected. When working in the home, the nurse must respect the privacy of family communications that may be overheard. It is essential that nurses adhere to the standards of practice related to privacy and confidentiality according to their provincial or territorial nursing regulatory body.

Communication with family members should include sharing with the family, in a supportive manner, complete and unbiased information about all aspects of the child's condition and care. Parents often feel overwhelming frustration related to obtaining accurate information about their child's illness and its management. Parents want information given slowly and repeated as necessary over time; they want explanations in terms they can understand; and they want the opportunity to ask questions, which should be answered in a straightforward manner. Stating "I don't know" or "I will find out" is better than pretending to know or giving excuses.

A plan can be made with the parents to gather relevant information when necessary. Information should be shared with families in a way that has meaning in their cultural context. Families vary in the amount and delivery of information they can tolerate about their child's status.

! NURSING ALERT

Home care nurses should restrict their communications with other health care providers to clinically relevant information about the family.

On occasion, disagreements may arise between parents and nurses over proper procedures for the child's care (see Critical Thinking Case Study). Nurses should respect parental preferences in any situation that do not pose danger or risk for the child (see Family-Centred Teaching box). It is important for the nurse to ensure that parents have adequate information in order to make an informed choice. If parents wish to alter a treatment plan that is part of medical orders, the nurse and parents should negotiate the change with the ordering practitioner and in collaboration with other members of the health care team. If disagreements cannot be resolved, a home care supervisor or case manager (care coordinator) should be contacted to assist with problem solving. Increasingly, home care agencies are developing ethics committees and policies for managing difficult situations such as treatment refusal.

The Nursing Process

In the home, the family is a partner in each step of the nursing process. Assessment should address family strengths and

CRITICAL THINKING CASE STUDY

Family-Centred Home Care and Conflicts

A family wants to begin oral feeding with a tracheostomy of their 3-year-old daughter, Sarah, who is ventilator dependent and is being tube fed through a skin-level gastrostomy feeding tube (MIC-KEY). The mother, who has assumed the role of Sarah's primary caregiver, is adamant about starting oral feedings so Sarah can be more like other children her age. One day, the mother asks you, the nurse case manager overseeing the child's home care, to feed Sarah baby food by mouth to see how she tolerates the feeding. The child is alert and sociable yet cannot communicate her wishes except through crying and whining. She has a seizure disorder and has had several episodes of aspiration pneumonia since birth. Sarah appears to have a considerable amount of tongue thrusting and copious amounts of oral mucus that must be suctioned frequently to prevent aspiration; her cough reflex is compromised and usually elicited only with tracheal suctioning.

1. Evidence—Is there sufficient evidence to draw any conclusions about the issue of feeding Sarah at this time?
2. Assumptions—Describe some underlying assumptions about the following:
   a. Sarah's readiness for oral feedings
   b. Sarah's ability to tolerate oral feedings
   c. The mother's request for Sarah to start oral feedings
3. What implications and priorities for nursing care may be drawn at this time?
4. Does the evidence objectively support your argument (conclusion)?

FAMILY-CENTRED TEACHING

Knowledgeable Parents

It is not unusual for parents, particularly those whose children have chronic illnesses or complex care regimens, to be more knowledgeable about their child's condition than a nurse who is assigned to the child's care. This can be disconcerting for both the parents and the nurse. It is important to remember and reinforce that, regardless of the condition, parents will always know more about their child than the professional caring for the child. The nurse and parents can set goals for care in an atmosphere of mutual respect. If the parents' goal is respite from prolonged caregiving, they are less likely to want to give long explanations about their child's care, and assistance from an experienced peer may be more appropriate for the nurse to seek. If the parents wish to maintain maximum participation in care delivery, the nurse and the parents can negotiate the collaboration.

When teaching parents to perform complex chronic care regimens at home, include teaching them to expect to know more about their child's care than professionals who may come to assist them, whether that be home health, hospital, or outpatient personnel. At the same time, assure them that various professionals who work with them will have a scientific knowledge base and a wealth of options for addressing and solving care problems from working with a multitude of families.

–Teresa L. Hall, MS, RN

resources. The principles of communication discussed previously need to guide data collection.

All the information gathered as part of the assessment process should be shared with the family. The nurse needs to recognize that the family's perception of their most important need will generally guide their behaviour and consume their attention and energy. Family priorities should guide the planning process.

Both short- and long-term goals should be outlined and agreed on by the child, family, and health care providers involved. The care plan should integrate various disciplines that may be involved with the child to eliminate duplication and coordinate and consolidate care requirements. Cross-training of health care providers and an interdisciplinary mode of treatment can also be useful when a child has multiple and complex care requirements. For example, certain physiotherapy or occupational therapy routines may be incorporated into the child's morning nursing procedures, or speech therapy interventions may be conducted by the parent or nurse around eating times so that the entire day is not occupied by procedures. A written schedule of daily routines should be developed and followed by all caregivers.

! NURSING ALERT

At each home visit, physically handle and look at all medications. Check them against the medical orders and read the labels. There may be discrepancies, duplications, or changes between hospitalizations. Clarify medication purpose, effect, and dosages for the family.

Goals of care and achievement of established outcomes are supported by intervention strategies that reflect normalization (see Chapter 40) and the interests and abilities of the child and family. Nurses can help the family explore a range of alternative strategies, services, and resources so that the family can choose the best match for their situation. Families can participate in evaluating a home care plan on several levels. Families and care providers should regularly review the goals of care and update the care plan as required. As part of the evaluation process, families should be acknowledged for their successes and accomplishments. Finally, families should be given an opportunity to evaluate individual home care nurses, the home care agency, and other service providers periodically. The evaluation should address the nurse's knowledge, skills, and respect for the family's choices. The agency should use the evaluations to improve the quality of care (see Family-Centred Teaching box).

In addition to maintaining a sense of control over their child's care, families need to control their home and personal lives. For this reason, nurses should inquire about "house rules" with the family and address issues such as the physical environment, private areas in the home, responsibility for maintaining the child's environment, and interactions with siblings. One of the more important aspects of the nurse's relationship with the family is maintaining professional boundaries and a therapeutic role that is supportive but not intrusive.

Technological trends that influence the nursing process in home care include the use of laptop computers (notebooks) and personal tablets to document the home visit; smart phones or small hand-held computers that store large amounts of data, including addresses, appointments, patient tracking systems, textbooks, and pharmacological databases (Government of Canada, 2013); Internet and e-mail services, which increase patient–practitioner accessibility and communication; and

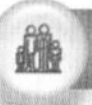

FAMILY-CENTRED TEACHING

What I Learned About Home Care

I learned many things as a result of having home care for four children over a period of 8 years. Two of the major areas I learned about were communication and families' rights. It took a long time to learn some of these things.

Initially I tried very hard to be sensitive to the professionals and often put my own feelings and needs aside. It took a while to learn that I could stand up for myself and my family and that my child could continue to receive good care. One area that was important to me was to have nurses withhold judgement on our parenting style, even if they might have parented differently.

Communication needs to be open and two-way. Families and nurses ought to tell each other what is going well. For example, "Thanks for keeping the room so neat while you're here" can help a nurse see a family's appreciation. There was so little I could do as just "Mommy" that it really meant a lot to me when nurses would say, "That's such a cute outfit you picked out for him today." Communicating about little things, even inconsequential topics such as favourite TV shows, makes it easier to communicate about more important things and about problems. Communication has to be open about problems, too.

–Jeni Stepanek, Mother

telemedicine or telehealth, which has various features, including electronic systems that can transmit physiological data directly to the practitioner via the telephone. The CNA (2007) has developed a position statement on telehealth and the role of the nurse that includes relevant guidelines and standards of practice (see Chapter 3).

Promotion of Optimum Development, Self-Care, and Education

There is little question that living at home offers most children with complex medical problems great social and emotional advantages over living in the hospital or other institutional setting. However, in infancy and throughout the developmental stages, a child's medical condition and dependence on medical technology can place constraints on and pose challenges to normal development. For example, the child may have lengthy and repeated hospitalizations; developmental regression can occur in response to stress; fatigue may result from an underlying pathological condition, the exacerbation of an illness, or medication adverse effects; and equipment requirements may impede mobility, exploration, and independence. The challenge of providing support for normal development in a child who is chronically ill and technology dependent requires the best use of opportunities for developmentally appropriate experiences within these constraints.

Home care plans are designed to promote optimum child development through assessment, planning, and referrals, and through interventions that address normalization issues and self-care. General principles for a family-centred assessment and planning process, addressed earlier in this chapter, are also applied in developmental assessment and planning.

Some parents may not pursue early developmental intervention because they do not believe their child needs the services. In this case, health care providers need to explain the child's developmental needs to parents in ways that are meaningful

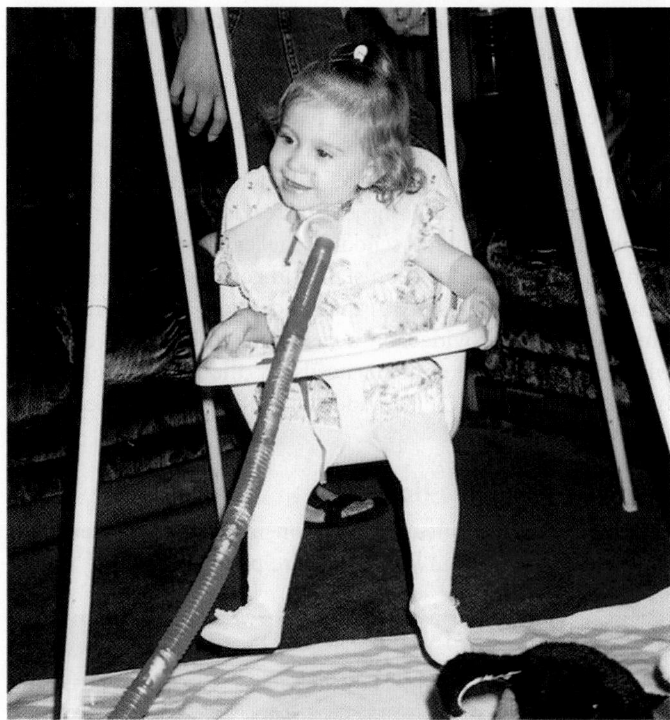

FIGURE 42-2 Use of lengthy tubing facilitates a child's freedom of movement.

from the parents' own cultural and socioeconomic perspectives. Only then can parents make truly informed decisions. Once parents have been fully informed of the child's condition, likely developmental sequelae, and the expected benefits of intervention, developmental goals outlined by the child and family should guide planning and intervention. The impact of chronic illness on development is discussed in Chapter 40.

The promotion of coping skills and capability can buffer stress and contribute to good mental health and self-esteem in a child with a chronic illness. The extent to which a child is involved in his or her own care depends on many factors, including parental comfort and support and the child's developmental age, level of interest, and physical ability. Self-care, both in activities of daily living and in regard to the medical condition, is important. The goal for self-care in activities of daily living should be the attainment of age-appropriate competence. Some modifications in the environment, the medical equipment, or the techniques for daily activities are often required to promote and support self-care (Fig. 42-2). Effective teaching for self-care is focused at the child's own level of conceptual understanding and may be augmented by the use of dolls, other models and diagrams, simple explanations, and repetition.

Educational planning is important for the child who has a chronic medical condition. Laws governing education in Canada are provincially and territorially legislated; there is no federal law governing education. Regulations, ministry guidelines, policies, and protocols, including support services and funding resources, are controlled at the local and provincial/territorial levels. Most provinces and territories have their own *Education Act* that requires school boards to provide special education programs and services for children with special needs. The home care nurse should refer the family to local educational and rehabilitation programs, as appropriate.

When a child requiring special medical care is to be placed in an educational setting, the parents, child, school health coordinator, educational evaluation team, and education and administrative staff should meet to determine safe and appropriate placement and the necessary services and personnel to enable the child to attend school in the least restrictive environment. Training of education staff and caregivers is essential to ensuring the child's safety in the educational setting. In-school nursing care is provided on a case-by-case basis for children who have advanced nursing needs by the Community Care Access Centre (CCAC) (see Additional Resources at the end of this chapter).

Safety Issues in the Home

Safety is an important consideration in child home care and should be addressed in the home care plan.

> **! NURSING ALERT**
>
> Arrangements should be made to ensure that, in an emergency, the family has adequate methods of communicating with properly trained emergency medical personnel, such as a telephone. A cellular phone may be used in place of a landline, but it is advisable to check with the local emergency facilities regarding policies for cell phone use and emergency 911 calls.

The telephone and electric companies (if the use of medical equipment requires electricity) must be notified that the family needs to be placed on a priority service list. In this way the family will learn of any anticipated interruptions in service and will receive priority in reinstatement of interrupted services. Prior contact with rescue squad and local emergency facility personnel can help ensure prompt and appropriate interventions if required. This is especially important if the family lives in a rural or remote location that may not be familiar to local emergency responders. It is recommended that local authorities be given a map marked with key landmarks and intersections for rapid access to the home.

Before hospital discharge, emergency protocols should be developed and reviewed with the parents and professional caregivers. Cardiopulmonary resuscitation guidelines, if appropriate, should be posted near the child's bedside or in another accessible location. A list of emergency telephone numbers can be placed near each home phone and entered into cellular phone contact lists and should include those of the emergency medical services and fire department, emergency department, managing physician(s), nursing agency, and equipment vendor(s) or providers. Additional issues to consider are advance directives and out-of-hospital end-of-life care orders (which may vary by province or territory), as indicated. If the patient and family desire enforcement of an advance directive, they must follow specific guidelines, which could prevent undesired life-saving measures for children with terminal illnesses.

Another aspect of safety relates to the provision of care by appropriately trained individuals. Family members should receive thorough training in the child's care requirements and have the opportunity to demonstrate knowledge and confidence before hospital discharge. One study found that although technology-dependent children cared for in the home received adequate care, the time demands of such care had negative effects on the caregiver's school, employment, and social life. Furthermore, a shortage of skilled caregivers often leads to disrupted sleep patterns and increased stress (Woodgate, Edwards, Ripat, et al., 2015). Thus professional staff caring for the child should have the appropriate background and training for the child's particular care needs. Because of the child's body size, special skill and caution are required in the performance of procedures (e.g., gastrostomy feedings, suctioning) and in monitoring the use of equipment (e.g., ventilator settings, intravenous flow rates, and total fluid volumes).

The activity level and curiosity of young children raise additional safety considerations in the provision of home care. All medications, needles, syringes, and contaminated materials must be securely stored well out of the reach of curious hands. Arrangements for the disposal of sharp items or contaminated materials can be made with the home health agency. Special attention should be given to childproofing the control panels on ventilators, pumps, monitors, and other equipment. The use of clear plastic tape, covers, or panels to cover control knobs or buttons reduces the risk of accidental changes in settings. Much of the medical equipment now in use has special lock-out capabilities that may be used to prevent accidentally altering settings. Electrical cords need to be kept short and out of reach, and safety covers should be used on any open outlets. Equipment should be unplugged when not in use and any wires (e.g., lead wires for an apnea monitor) stored out of reach.

Care at night poses other safety concerns. Parents or other caregivers need to be able to clearly hear monitor, ventilator, or pump alarms at night; an inexpensive intercom system or baby monitor can be used. Steps must be taken to prevent accidental strangulation by apnea, oximeter, or cardiac monitor wires or lengthy intravenous tubing during sleep.

See also Chapter 36, Motor Vehicle Injuries, p. 1062, for discussion of transportation of children with special needs.

> **NURSING ALERT**
>
> Coiling extra tubing and taping it at the exit site, as well as running wires or tubes out the bottoms of pyjamas or one-piece infant suits, are precautions against strangulation.

Family-to-Family Support

Family-to-family support networks can be an important source of emotional and instrumental support and empowerment for families of children with chronic health problems. Family-to-family support does not replace professional sources of support but rather is a unique resource that promotes family strengths through shared experience.

Families will most likely experience increased emotional stress as the result of living with and caring for a child with special needs. A tool that might be helpful to the pediatric home care nurse is the Caregiver Strain Index, a 13-item assessment tool designed to ascertain caregiver stress and subsequently develop appropriate strategies for individual and family coping (Onega, 2008) (see Additional Resources at the end of this chapter). Other issues that are likely to arise as a result of the child's illness and the constant attention required include labelling the child as being vulnerable, in which parents spend too much time preoccupied with the child's welfare while ignoring other family members' needs. As the child with special health care needs develops and grows, parents should impose the same disciplinary rules on the child receiving home care as on siblings, to avoid further conflict within the family.

The nurse can assist the family in their involvement in online or local community social networks. For example, a referral to a parent support group may assist a family in maintaining a sense of normalcy. Support from such a group may enhance the caregiver–child relationship and help prevent the social disruption that can occur from having a child with complex care needs in the home. The nurse should educate the parents about the group's goals so that they can determine whether they might benefit from this connection. Parents need to evaluate the quality of online support groups to ensure that they meet their needs. In addition, informal support networks can be extremely beneficial. A link to a family in the same or a similar situation allows the sharing of common experiences. This in itself may decrease the sense of isolation and provide a connection with someone who can truly identify with family struggles.

The nurse should remember that each family member's needs differ. The care plan should acknowledge the needs of each family member (mother, father, siblings, grandparents). Peer support for school-age children and adolescents with complex care needs may be beneficial. These connections can be expanded to include letter writing, e-mails, telephone calls, or specialty camp programs. Most school-age children and adolescents just want to be accepted by their peers and fit in as a part of the group. Same-age peers may at first be standoffish to children with disabilities, but this is likely out of fear and lack of understanding; helping others see that they have the same dreams, desires, goals, and interests can promote group cohesiveness and understanding.

KEY POINTS

- Effective home care depends on many factors, including the child's medical stability; the family's willingness, training, and ability to accommodate the child's care requirements; and professional, financial, and community support.
- Comprehensive, multidisciplinary discharge planning should begin early and should include the family and a home care coordinator in addition to hospital personnel.
- Thorough education and training of the family or primary caregiver can ease the transition to home.
- Care coordination ensures continuity of care, prevents duplication of services, and reduces fragmentation of services. The family may assume responsibility for varying degrees of care coordination over time.
- The home care nurse must possess a high level of technical expertise while being able to adapt equipment, procedures, and the nursing process to the home setting.
- Accreditation standards apply to agencies that provide home care; standards of practice by the Canadian Nurses Association and other professional nursing organizations can guide nurses in the home setting.
- Family-centred nursing practice is applied in the home setting; diversity in family structures, cultural backgrounds, strengths, and coping mechanisms needs to be respected.
- Collaborative relationships among parents, home care providers, and other health care providers are characterized by effective communication strategies including open discussion, active listening, awareness and acceptance of differences, and negotiation.
- The nursing process should be adapted to involve the family in each step and to preserve the family's central role in decision making.
- House rules agreed on by the nurse, child, and family enable the family to maintain a feeling of control over their own environment when health care providers are present.
- Individualized home care plans are designed to promote optimum development of the child and to focus on normalization—assessing and incorporating the impact of the child's medical condition and technological requirements on development, self-care, and educational needs.
- Safety in the provision of home care services involves emergency preparations and protocols, appropriate training of family and home care personnel, and the safe use and childproofing of medical equipment.
- Family-to-family support networks can provide emotional and instrumental support and foster family empowerment.

evolve WEBSITE

Visit the Evolve website for additional resources related to the content in this chapter such as Case Studies, Critical Thinking Case Study Answers, Nursing Care Plans, Nursing Processes, Nursing Skills, and Review Questions for Exam Preparation at: *http://evolve.elsevier.com/Canada/Perry/maternal/*

REFERENCES

Canadian Healthcare Association. (2012). *Respite care in Canada*. Ottawa: Author.

Canadian Home Care Association. (2013a). *Backgrounder—Portraits of home care in Canada 2013*. Retrieved from <http://www.cdnhomecare.ca/content.php?doc=274>.

Canadian Home Care Association. (2013b). *Portraits of home care in Canada*. Retrieved from <http://www.cdnhomecare.ca/media.php?mid=3394>.

Canadian Home Care Association. (2016). *Advocacy*. Retrieved from <http://www.cdnhomecare.ca/content.php?doc=259>.

Canadian Institute for Health Information. (2011). *Canada's health care providers, 2000–2009: A reference guide*. Ottawa: Author.

Canadian Nurses Association. (2007). *Telehealth: The role of the nurse*. Retrieved from <https://www.nurseone.ca/~/media/nurseone/page-content/pdf-en/ps89_telehealth_e.pdf?la=en>.

Canadian Nurses Association. (2010). *Position statement: Promoting culturally competent care*. Ottawa: Author.

Canadian Nurses Association. (2013). *2011 Workforce profile of registered nurses in Canada*. Ottawa: Author.

Canadian Public Health Association. (2010). *Public health—Community health nursing practice in Canada: Roles and activities*. Retrieved from <http://www.chnc.ca/documents/PublicHealth-CommunityHealthNursinginCanadaRolesandActivities2010.pdf>.

Chen, S. Y., Wu, G. H., Chang, S. C., et al. (2008). Bacteremia in previously hospitalized patients: Prolonged effect from previous hospitalization and risk factors for antimicrobial-resistant bacterial infections. *Annals of Emergency Medicine, 51*(5), 639–646.

Community Health Nurses Association of Canada. (2008). *Canadian community health nursing standards of practice*. Toronto: Author.

Government of Canada. (2013). *E-health technologies and Canada: The future is here*. Retrieved from <http://publications.gc.ca/site/eng/296468/publication.html>.

Health Canada. (2012). *Summative evaluation of the First Nations and Inuit home and community care*. Retrieved from <http://hc-sc.gc.ca/fniah-spnia/pubs/services/fnihcc-psdmcpni/index-eng.php#sum_som>.

Onega, L. L. (2008). Helping those who help others: The modified caregiver strain index. *American Journal of Nursing, 108*(9), 62–69, quiz 69–70. doi:10.1097/01.NAJ.0000334528.90459.9a.

Parab, C. S., Cooper, C., Woolfenden, S., et al. (2013). Specialist home-based nursing services for children with acute and chronic illnesses (review). *The Cochrane Database of Systematic Reviews*, (6), Art. No.: CD004383, doi:10.1002/14651858.CD004383.pub3.

Peter, E., Spalding, K., Kenny, N., et al. (2007). Neither seen nor heard: Children and homecare policy in Canada. *Social Science & Medicine, 64*(8), 1624–1635.

Ponti, M., & Canadian Paediatric Society, Community Paediatrics Committee. (2008). Position statement: Special considerations for the health supervision of children and youth in foster care. *Pediatrics & Child Health, 13*(2), 129–132. Reaffirmed 2016. Retrieved from <http://www.cps.ca/documents/position/foster-care-health-supervision>.

Roush, C. V., & Cox, J. E. (2000). The meaning of home: How it shapes the practice of home and hospice care. *Home Healthcare Nurse, 18*(6), 388–394.

Sinha, M., & Statistics Canada, Social and Aboriginal Statistics Division. (2013). *Portrait of caregivers, 2012*. Catalogue no. 89-652 X- No. 001. Ottawa: Statistics Canada.

Woodgate, R. L., Edwards, M., Ripat, J. D., et al. (2015). Intense parenting: A qualitative study detailing the experiences of parenting children with complex care needs. *BMC Pediatrics, 5*, 197. doi:10.1186/s12887-015-0514-5.

Wright, L. M., & Leahy, M. (2013). *Nurses and families: A guide to family assessment and intervention* (6th ed.). Philadelphia: FA Davis.

ADDITIONAL RESOURCES

Canadian Home Care Association: <http://www.cdnhomecare.ca>.

Caregiver Strain Index: <http://www.npcrc.org/files/news/caregiver_strain_index.pdf>.

Carers Canada: <http://www.carerscanada.ca/about-us/>.

Collaborative Family Healthcare Association: <http://www.cfha.net>.

Community Care Access Centre: School Services: <http://www.health.gov.on.ca/english/providers/pub/manuals/ccac/ccac_9.pdf>.

First Nations and Inuit Home and Community Care (FNIHCC), Quality Resource Kit (QRK): <http://hc-sc.gc.ca/fniah-spnia/pubs/services/qualit-kit-trousse/index-eng.php>.

Yaldei Developmental Center—Early Intervention: <http://www.yaldei.org/index.php/early-intervention-services/>.

CHAPTER

43

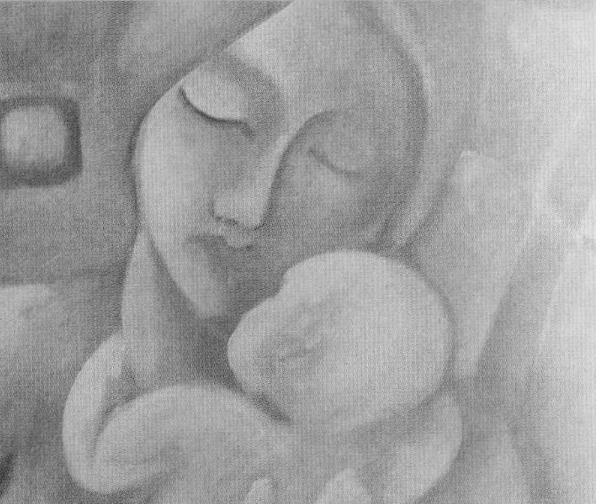

Reaction to Illness and Hospitalization

Cheryl Sams, with contributions from Marilyn J. Hockenberry

evolve WEBSITE

Visit the Evolve website for additional resources related to the content in this chapter such as Case Studies, Critical Thinking Case Study Answers, Nursing Care Plans, Nursing Processes, Nursing Skills, and Review Questions for Exam Preparation at: *http://evolve.elsevier.com/Canada/Perry/maternal/*

OBJECTIVES

On completion of this chapter the reader will be able to:

- Identify the stressors of illness and hospitalization for children during each developmental stage.
- List essential priorities of nursing care for a child on admission to the hospital.
- Review nursing interventions that prevent or minimize the stress of separation during hospitalization.
- Discuss nursing interventions that minimize the stress of loss of control during hospitalization.
- Describe nursing interventions that minimize the fear of bodily injury during hospitalization.
- Outline nursing interventions that support parents, siblings, and other family members during a child's illness and hospitalization.
- Describe nursing interventions needed when children are admitted to special units such as the emergency department.

STRESSORS OF HOSPITALIZATION AND CHILDREN'S REACTIONS

For many children, illness and hospitalization can be the first crises they face. Young children are particularly vulnerable to these crises because (1) they are experiencing stress from a change in the usual state of health and environmental routine and (2) they have a limited number of coping mechanisms to resolve *stressors* (those events that produce stress). Major stressors of hospitalization include separation, loss of control, fear of bodily injury, and pain. Children's reactions to these stressors are influenced by their developmental age; their previous experience with illness, separation, or hospitalization; their innate and acquired coping skills; the seriousness of the diagnosis; and the support system available. Children may also express fears caused by the unfamiliar environment or lack of information; child–staff relations; and the physical, social, and symbolic environment (Salmela, Aronen, & Salanterä, 2011).

Separation Anxiety

The major stress from middle infancy throughout the preschool years, especially for children ages 6 to 30 months, is separation anxiety, also called *anaclitic depression*. The principal behavioural responses to this stressor during early childhood are summarized in Box 43-1. During the stages of *protest*, children react aggressively to separation from the parent. They cry and scream for their parents, refuse the attention of anyone else, and are inconsolable in their grief (Fig. 43-1). In contrast, through the stage of *despair*, the crying stops and depression is evident. The child is much less active, is uninterested in play or food, and withdraws from others (Fig. 43-2).

The third stage is *detachment*, also called denial. Superficially it appears that the child has finally adjusted to the loss. The child becomes more interested in the surroundings, plays with others, and seems to form new relationships. However, this behaviour is the result of resignation and is not a sign of contentment. The child detaches from the parent in an effort to escape the emotional pain of desiring the parent's presence and copes by

BOX 43-1 MANIFESTATIONS OF SEPARATION ANXIETY IN YOUNG CHILDREN

Stage of Protest

Behaviours observed during later infancy include the following:

- Crying
- Screaming
- Searching for parent with eyes
- Clinging to parent
- Avoiding and rejecting contact with strangers

Additional behaviours observed during toddlerhood include the following:

- Verbally attacking strangers, such as saying "Go away"
- Physically attacking strangers, such as kicking, biting, hitting, pinching
- Attempting to escape to find parent
- Attempting to physically force parent to stay

Behaviours may last from hours to days.

Protest, such as crying, may be continuous, ceasing only with physical exhaustion.

Approach of a stranger may precipitate increased protest.

Stage of Despair

Observed behaviours include the following:

- Being inactive
- Withdrawing from others
- Being depressed, sad
- Lacking interest in environment
- Being uncommunicative
- Regressing to earlier behaviour, such as thumb sucking, bed-wetting, use of pacifier, use of bottle

Behaviours may last for a variable length of time.

The child's physical condition may deteriorate from refusal to eat, drink, or move.

Stage of Detachment (Denial)

Observed behaviours include the following:

- Showing increased interest in surroundings
- Interacting with strangers or familiar caregivers
- Forming new but superficial relationships
- Appearing happy

Detachment usually occurs after prolonged separation from the parent; it is rarely seen in hospitalized children.

Behaviours represent a superficial adjustment to loss.

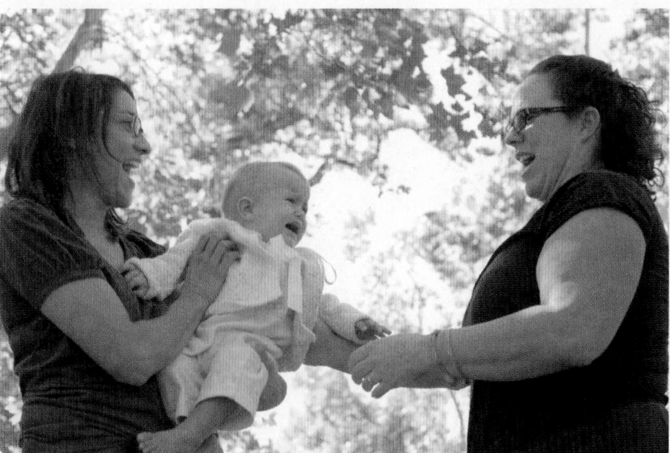

FIGURE 43-1 In the protest phase of separation anxiety, children cry loudly and are inconsolable in their grief for the parent. (© Christina Kennedy/Alamy Stock Photo.)

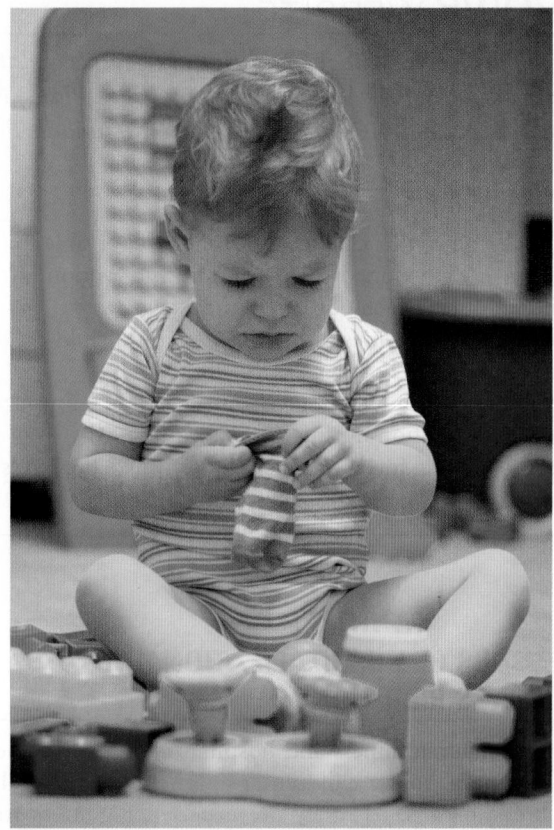

FIGURE 43-2 During the despair phase of separation anxiety, children are sad, lonely, and uninterested in food and play. (Vladimir Mucibabic/Shutterstock.com.)

forming shallow relationships with others, becoming increasingly self-centred, and attaching primary importance to material objects. This is the most serious stage in that reversal of the potential adverse effects is less likely to occur after detachment is established. However, in most situations, the temporary separations imposed by hospitalization do not cause such prolonged parental absences that the child enters into detachment. In addition, considerable evidence suggests that even with stressors such as separation, children are remarkably adaptable, and permanent ill effects are rare.

Although progression to the stage of detachment is uncommon, the initial stages are frequently observed even with brief separations from either parent. Unless health care team members understand the meaning of each stage of behaviour, they may erroneously label the behaviours as positive or negative. For example, they may see the loud crying of the protest phase as "bad" behaviour. Because the protests increase when a stranger approaches the child, they may interpret that reaction as meaning they should stay away. During the quiet, withdrawn phase of despair, health care team members may think that the child is finally "settling in" to the new surroundings, and they may see the detachment behaviours as proof of a "good

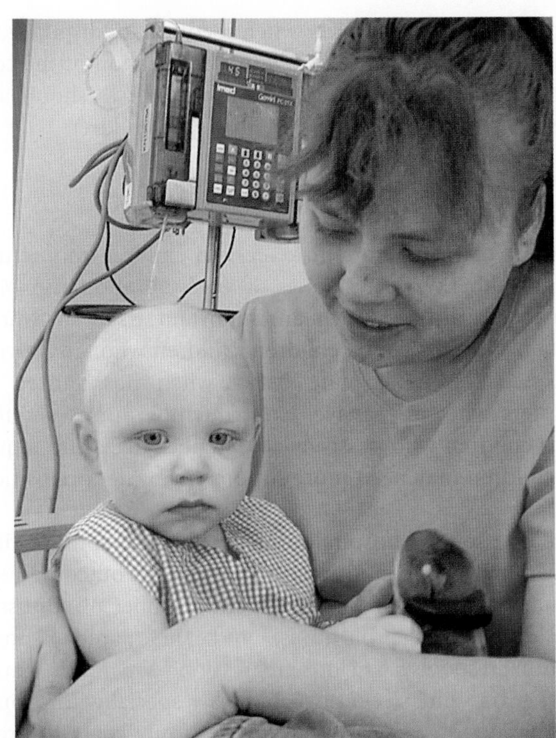

FIGURE 43-3 In the protest phase of separation anxiety, young children may appear withdrawn and sad even in the presence of a parent. (Courtesy E. Jacob, Texas Children's Hospital.)

adjustment." The faster this stage is reached, the more likely it is that the child will be regarded as the "ideal patient."

Because children seem to react "negatively" to visits by their parents, uninformed observers feel justified in restricting parental visiting privileges. For example, during the protest stage, children outwardly do not appear happy to see their parents (Fig. 43-3). In fact, they may even cry louder. If they are depressed, they may reject their parents or begin to protest again. Often they cling to their parents in an effort to ensure their continued presence. Consequently, such reactions may be regarded as "disturbing" the child's adjustment to the new surroundings. If the separation has progressed to the phase of detachment, children will respond no differently to their parents than they would to any other person.

Such reactions are distressing to parents, who are unaware of their meaning. If parents are regarded as intruders, they will see their absence as "beneficial" to the child's adjustment and recovery. They may respond to the child's behaviour by staying for only short periods, visiting less frequently, or deceiving the child when it is time to leave. The result is a destructive cycle of misunderstanding and unmet needs.

Early Childhood

Separation anxiety is the greatest stress imposed by hospitalization during early childhood. If separation is avoided, young children have a tremendous capacity to withstand any other stress. During this period, the typical reactions just described are seen. However, children in the toddler stage demonstrate more goal-directed behaviours. For example, they may plead with the parents to stay and physically try to keep the parents with them or try to find parents who have left. They may demonstrate displeasure on the parents' return or departure by having temper tantrums; refusing to follow with the usual routines of mealtime, bedtime, or toileting; or regressing to more primitive levels of development. However, temper tantrums, bed-wetting, or other behaviours may also be expressions of anger, a physiological response to stress, or symptoms of illness.

Because preschoolers are more secure interpersonally than toddlers, they can tolerate brief periods of separation from their parents and are more inclined to develop substitute trust in other significant adults. However, the stress of illness usually renders preschoolers less able to cope with separation; as a result, they manifest many of the stage behaviours of separation anxiety, although in general the protest behaviours are more subtle and passive than those seen in younger children. Preschoolers may demonstrate separation anxiety by refusing to eat, experiencing difficulty in sleeping, crying quietly for their parents, continually asking when the parents will visit, or withdrawing from others. They may express anger indirectly by breaking their toys, hitting other children, or refusing to cooperate during usual self-care activities. Nurses need to be sensitive to these less obvious signs of separation anxiety in order to intervene appropriately.

Later Childhood and Adolescence

Previous research, usually based on adult recollections, indicated that the family does not play as important a role for school-age children as it does during the toddler and preschool years. However, in a study that asked children about their fears when hospitalized, children listed their greatest fears regarding hospitalization as being separated from family and friends, being in an unfamiliar environment, receiving investigations or treatments, and losing self-determination or choices (Coyne & Kirwan, 2012). In a qualitative study of children ages 5 to 9, children described hospitalizations in stories that focused on being alone and feeling afraid, sad, or angry. These children also described the need for protection and companionship while hospitalized (Wilson, Megel, Eneback, et al., 2010).

Although school-age children are better able to cope with separation in general, the stress and often accompanying regression imposed by illness or hospitalization may increase their need for parental security and guidance. This is particularly true for young school-age children who have only recently left the safety of the home and are struggling with the crisis of school adjustment. Middle and late school-age children may react more to the separation from their usual activities and peers than to the absence of their parents. These children have a high level of physical and mental activity that frequently finds no suitable outlets in the hospital environment, and even when they dislike school, they admit to missing its routine and worry that they will not be able to compete or "fit in" with their classmates when they return. Feelings of loneliness, boredom, isolation, and depression are common. Such reactions may occur more as a result of separation than of concern over the illness, treatment, or hospital setting.

School-age children may need and desire parental guidance or support from other adult figures but may be unable or unwilling to ask for it. Because the goal of attaining independence is so important, they are reluctant to seek help directly, fearing that they will appear weak, childish, or dependent. Cultural expectations to "act like a man" or to "be brave and strong" weigh heavily on these children, especially boys, who tend to react to stress with stoicism, withdrawal, or passive acceptance. Often the need to express hostile, angry, or other negative feelings finds outlets in alternative ways, such as irritability and aggression toward parents, withdrawal from hospital personnel, inability to relate to peers, rejection of siblings, or subsequent behavioural problems in school.

For adolescents, separation from home and parents may produce varied emotions, ranging from difficulty coping to welcoming the event. However, loss of peer-group contact may pose a severe emotional threat because of loss of group status, inability to exert group control or leadership, and loss of group acceptance. Deviations within peer groups are poorly tolerated, and although group members may express concern for the adolescent's illness or need for hospitalization, they will continue their group activities, quickly filling the gap of the absent member. During the temporary separation from their usual group, ill adolescents may benefit from group associations with other hospitalized teens.

Effects of Hospitalization on the Child

Children may react to the stresses of hospitalization before admission, during hospitalization, and after discharge (Box 43-2). A child's concept of illness is even more important than age and intellectual maturity when it comes to hospitalization. This may or may not be affected by the duration of the condition or prior hospitalizations; therefore, nurses should avoid overestimating the concepts of illness in children who have prior medical experience.

Individual Risk Factors

A number of risk factors make certain children more vulnerable than others to the stresses of hospitalization (Box 43-3). Because separation is such an important issue surrounding hospitalization for young children, children who are active and strong willed tend to fare better when hospitalized than youngsters who are passive. Consequently, nurses should be alert to children who passively accept all changes and requests; these children may need more support than the "oppositional" child.

The stressors of hospitalization may cause young children to experience short- and long-term negative outcomes; stressors may be related to the length and number of admissions, multiple invasive procedures, and the parents' anxiety. Common responses include regression, separation anxiety, apathy, fears, and sleep disturbances, especially for younger children. Supportive practices, such as family-centred care and frequent family visiting, may lessen the detrimental effects. Nurses should attempt to identify those children at risk for poor coping strategies. In a study of health care providers' perceptions of children's stress level in health care settings, the data indicated that one third of the participating health care providers were unaware or did not think that their health care setting could cause stress for pediatric patients. It is essential that pediatric health care providers know how to minimize stress for children and their parents (Al-Yateem, Banni, & Rossiter, 2015). Recommended practices to minimize stress for children and parents include providing focused information for both children and health care providers, adapting the environment and systems to fit children's needs, and improving the interpersonal skills and attitudes of health care providers (Al-Yateem et al., 2015).

Children can be prepared for hospitalization through stories and colouring books and a variety of preparation materials. Many hospitals have virtual tours and online materials that parents and children can access to help decrease a child's anxiety. See the Additional Resources at the end of this chapter for

BOX 43-2 POSTHOSPITAL BEHAVIOURS IN CHILDREN

Young Children

Show initial aloofness toward parents; this may last from a few minutes (most common) to a few days. This is frequently followed by dependency behaviours:

- Tendency to cling to parents and demand attention from parents
- Vigorous opposition to any separation, such as staying at preschool or with a babysitter

Other negative behaviours include the following:

- New fears such as nightmares
- Resistance to going to bed, night waking
- Withdrawal and shyness
- Hyperactivity
- Temper tantrums
- Food peculiarities
- Attachment to a blanket or toy
- Regression in newly learned skills such as self-toileting

Older Children

Negative behaviours include the following:

- Emotional coldness, followed by intense, demanding dependence on parents
- Anger toward parents
- Jealousy toward others such as siblings

BOX 43-3 RISK FACTORS THAT INCREASE CHILDREN'S VULNERABILITY TO STRESSES OF HOSPITALIZATION

- "Difficult" temperament
- Lack of bonding between child and parent
- Age (especially between 6 months and 5 years)
- Male gender
- Developmental delays
- Multiple and continuing stresses (e.g., frequent hospitalizations)

materials developed by the Hospital for Sick Children that help prepare children for hospitalization.

Changes in the Pediatric Population

The pediatric population in hospitals has changed dramatically over the past two decades. With a growing trend toward shortened hospital stays and outpatient surgery, a greater percentage of the children hospitalized today have more serious and complex problems than those hospitalized in the past. Many of these children are fragile newborns and children with severe injuries or complex conditions who have survived because of major technological advances, yet have been left with chronic or disabling conditions that require frequent and lengthy hospital stays. The nature of their conditions increases the likelihood that they will experience more invasive and traumatic procedures while they are hospitalized. These factors make them more vulnerable to the emotional consequences of hospitalization and result in their needs being significantly different from those of the short-term patients of the past (see Chapter 40 for further discussion on children with special needs). Most of these children are infants and toddlers, the age group most vulnerable to the effects of hospitalization.

Concern has focused on the increasing length of hospitalization due to complex medical and nursing care, elusive diagnoses, and complicated psychosocial issues. Without special attention devoted to meeting the child's psychosocial and developmental needs in the hospital environment, the detrimental consequences of prolonged hospitalization may be severe.

Beneficial Effects of Hospitalization

Although hospitalization usually is stressful for children, it can also be beneficial. The most obvious benefit is the recovery from illness, but hospitalization also can present an opportunity for children to master stress and feel competent in their coping abilities. The hospital environment can provide children with new socialization experiences that can broaden their interpersonal relationships. The psychological benefits need to be considered and maximized during hospitalization. Appropriate nursing strategies to achieve this goal are presented on pp. 1261–1270.

Parents and caregivers can often experience burnout when caring for a chronically ill child in the home setting. Hospitalization of the child can be perceived as beneficial to the parent or caregiver as an opportunity for nurses and social workers to help with meals, rooming-in, and "breaks."

STRESSORS AND REACTIONS OF THE FAMILY OF THE HOSPITALIZED CHILD

Parental Reactions

The crisis of childhood illness and hospitalization affects every member of the family. Parents' reactions to illness in their child depend on a variety of factors. Although one cannot predict which factors are most likely to influence their response, a number of possible variables have been identified (Box 43-4).

BOX 43-4 FACTORS AFFECTING PARENTS' REACTIONS TO THEIR CHILD'S ILLNESS

- Seriousness of the threat to the child
- Previous experience with illness or hospitalization
- Medical procedures involved in diagnosis and treatment
- Available support systems
- Personal ego strengths
- Previous coping abilities
- Additional stresses on the family system
- Cultural and religious beliefs
- Communication patterns among family members

Common themes among parents whose children have been hospitalized include feeling an overall sense of helplessness, questioning the skills of staff, accepting the reality of hospitalization, needing to have information explained in simple language, dealing with fear and guilt, coping with uncertainty, and seeking reassurance from caregivers. This reassurance involves staff being compassionate, expressing concern for the child, and attending to detail in the child's care (Stratton, 2004). Additional important strategies that nurses can use to build relationships and encourage shared parent–nurse communication include involving parents in care decisions, expressing trust and respect for each other's expertise, having a caring attitude, being an advocate for the child, and negotiating roles (Giambra, Stiffler, & Broome, 2014).

Sibling Reactions

Siblings' reactions to a sister's or brother's illness or hospitalization are discussed in Chapter 40, and they differ little from those when a child becomes temporarily ill. Siblings experience loneliness, fear, and worry, as well as anger, resentment, jealousy, and guilt. Illness may also result in a sibling's loss of status within their family or social group. Various factors have been identified that influence the effects of the child's hospitalization on siblings. Although these factors are similar to those seen when a child has a chronic illness, Commodari (2010) has reported that siblings can feel greater effects from the hospital experience, based on the following factors:

- Being younger and experiencing many changes
- Being cared for outside the home by care providers who are not relatives
- Receiving little information about their ill sibling
- Perceiving that their parents treat them differently compared with before their sibling's hospitalization

Parents are often unaware of the number of effects that siblings experience during the sick child's hospitalization and the benefit of simple interventions to minimize such effects, such as giving explicit explanations about the illness and providing for adequate care for siblings to remain at home. Sibling visitation is usually beneficial to the patient and sibling, as the visit may allow the child to see that their fears are unfounded. Siblings should be prepared for the visit with developmentally appropriate information and be given the opportunity to ask questions.

NURSING CARE FOR THE CHILD AND FAMILY

Preparation for Hospitalization

Children and families require individualized care to minimize the potential negative effects of hospitalization. One action that can decrease negative feelings and fear in children is preparing them for hospitalization. The rationale for preparing children for the hospital experience and related procedures is based on the principle that fear of the unknown (fantasy) exceeds fear of the known. When children do not have paralyzing fear to cope with, they are better able to direct their energies toward dealing with the other, unavoidable stresses of hospitalization.

Although preparation for hospitalization is a common practice, there is no universal standard or program for all settings. The preparation process may be elaborate with tours, puppet shows, and playtime with miniature hospital equipment; it may involve the use of books, videos, or films; or it may be limited to a brief description of the major aspects of any hospital stay. No consensus exists on the timing of preparation. Some authorities recommend preparing children 4 to 7 years of age about 1 week in advance (when possible) so that they can assimilate the information and ask questions. For older children the time may be longer. However, for young children, who may begin to fantasize about what they observed, 1 or 2 days before admission is sufficient time for anticipatory preparation. The length of the session should be tailored to the children's attention span—the younger the child, the shorter the program. The optimal approach is one that is individualized for each child and family (see Additional Resources at the end of this chapter).

It is essential for families to prepare for the hospitalization as well as the child. Parents who are unsure or anxious about the hospital will transmit those emotions to the child. Nurses play an important role in helping children and families understand the reason for the hospitalization and what to expect during the admission.

Regardless of the specific type of program, all children, even those who have been hospitalized before, benefit from an introduction to the environment and routine of the unit. Sometimes it is not possible to prepare the child, as in the event of sudden, acute illness or an accident. However, care should be taken to orient the child and family to hospital routines, establish expectations, and allow for questions.

> **! NURSING ALERT**
>
> In many hospitals, child life specialists—health care providers with extensive knowledge of child growth and development and of the special psychosocial needs of children who are hospitalized and their families—help prepare children for hospitalization, surgery, and procedures. Although the structure of a program may vary, depending on the size of the pediatric facility, the patient population, and the availability of ancillary services, the two primary program objectives for child life are consistent: (1) to reduce the stress and anxiety related to the hospitalization or health care–related experiences, and (2) to promote normal growth and development in the health care setting and at home (Thompson, 2009).

A collaborative effort between the nurse, child life specialist, and other members of the child's health care team can help ensure the best possible hospital experience for the child and family.

Preparing the Child for Admission

The preparation that children require on the day of admission depends on the kind of prehospital counselling they have received. If they have been prepared in a formalized program, they will usually know what to expect in terms of initial medical procedures, inpatient facilities, and nursing staff. However, prehospital counselling does not preclude the need for support during procedures such as obtaining blood specimens, x-ray tests, or physical examinations. For example, undressing young children before they feel comfortable in their new surroundings can be upsetting to them. Causing needless anxiety and fear during admission may adversely affect the nurse's establishment of trust with these children. Nursing assistance during the admission procedure is vital, regardless of how well prepared any child is for the experience of hospitalization. In addition, spending this time with the child gives the nurse an opportunity to evaluate the child's understanding of subsequent procedures (Fig. 43-4). Ideally, a primary nurse is assigned whenever possible to allow for individualized care and provide a substitute support person for the child.

When a child is admitted, nurses need to follow admission procedures (Box 43-5). One particularly important decision is room assignment. The minimum considerations for room assignment are age, sex, and nature of the illness, including type of infectious precautions required. No absolute rules govern room selection, but, in general, placing children of the same age group and with similar types of illness in the same room is both psychologically and medically advantageous. However, there are many exceptions. For example, a child in traction may be therapeutic for another child confined to bed because of a serious illness. A child who is independent despite physical disabilities may help another child with similar or different limitations, and the parents of the child with disabilities

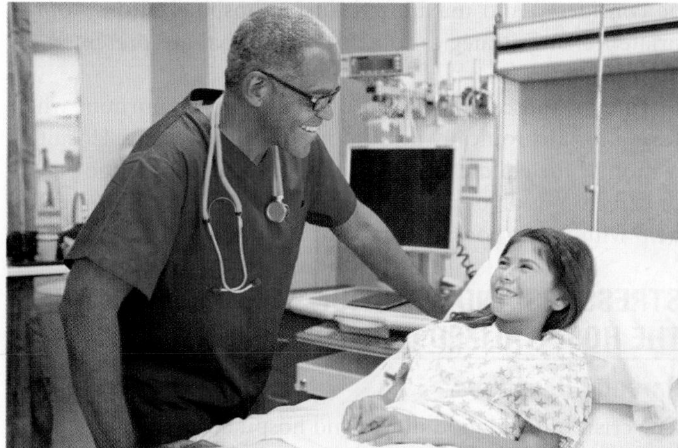

FIGURE 43-4 The initial admission procedures give the nurse an opportunity to get to know the child and to assess the child's understanding of the hospital experience. (Monkey Business Images/Shutterstock.com.)

BOX 43-5 GUIDELINES FOR ADMISSION

Preadmission

Assign a room based on developmental age, seriousness of diagnosis, communicability of illness, and projected length of stay.

Prepare roommate(s) for the arrival of a new patient; when children are too young to benefit from this consideration, prepare parents.

Prepare room for child and family, with admission forms and equipment nearby to eliminate need to leave child.

Admission

Introduce primary nurse to child and family.

Orient child and family to inpatient facilities, especially to the assigned room and unit; emphasize positive areas of pediatric unit.

Room—Explain call light, bed controls, television, bathroom, telephone, etc.

Unit—Direct to playroom, desk, dining area, or other areas.

Introduce family to roommate and his or her parents.

Apply identification band to child's wrist, ankle, or both (if not already done).

Explain hospital guidelines and schedules, such as visiting hours, mealtimes, bedtime, limitations (give written information and website if available).

Perform nursing admission history (see Box 43-6).

Take vital signs, blood pressure, height, and weight.

Obtain specimens as needed and order needed laboratory work.

Support child and assist practitioner with physical examination (for purposes of nursing assessment).

may achieve deeper insight and acceptance of their child's disorder.

Age-grouping is especially important for adolescents. Many hospitals make an effort to place teenagers on their own unit or in a separate, designated section of the pediatric or general unit whenever possible.

Admission Assessment

The nursing admission history refers to a systematic collection of data about the child and family that enables the nurse to plan individualized care. The nursing admission history is presented in Box 43-6. The questions are directed to both the child and the child's parents or other primary caregivers. One of the main purposes of the history is to assess the child's usual health habits at home in order to promote a more normal environment in the hospital. Therefore, questions related to activities of daily living in the nutrition–metabolic, elimination, sleep–rest, and activity–exercise patterns are a major part of the assessment. The questions found under the health perception–health management pattern are directed toward evaluation of the child's preparation for hospitalization and are key factors in determining whether additional preparation is needed. The questions included in the self-perception–self-concept and role–relationship patterns address the child's potential reaction to hospitalization, especially in terms of separation.

The nurse should also inquire about the use of any medications at home, including complementary medicine practices (Box 43-7), as the use of complementary and alternative medicine (CAM) has been increasing in popularity across Canada. A Health Canada (2015) survey identified that 73% of Canadians take natural health products such as vitamins and minerals, herbal products, and homeopathic medicines on a regular basis. Common CAM practices include taking natural health products, homeopathy, traditional Chinese medicine, and chiropractic treatment. It is also important that the use of any herbal or complementary therapy be noted in a preoperative assessment because of possible **anaesthesia** or surgical complications related to use of herbal products. For more information on natural health products, see the Additional Resources section at the end of this chapter.

Besides completing the nursing admission history, nurses should also perform a physical assessment (see Chapter 33) before planning care. At the very least, the nurse's physical assessment of the child should include observation of the body for any deformities or physical limitations. The nurse should also listen to the heart and lungs to assess overall physical status to provide baseline data. It is important for nurses to be on alert for any signs of maltreatment, such as bruises or signs of neglect, which must be reported to child authorities.

Nursing Interventions

Preventing or Minimizing Separation

A primary nursing goal is to prevent separation anxiety, particularly in children younger than 5 years of age by providing family-centred care. This philosophy of care recognizes the integral role of the family in a child's life and acknowledges the family as an essential part of the child's care and illness experience. The family is considered a partner in the child's care (see Chapter 30). Family-centred care also supports the family by respecting the individual needs of the child and the family and establishing priorities based on the needs and values of the family unit. Many hospitals provide facilities such as a chair or bed for at least one person per child, a unit kitchen, and other amenities that create a welcoming atmosphere for parents. Additionally, many units have a communication board outlining special activities or upcoming events for the families, as well as personal communication boards for each room. However, not all hospitals provide such amenities, and parents' own schedules may prevent rooming-in. In such instances, strategies to minimize the effects of separation must be implemented. There are out-of-hospital supports across Canada for families of seriously ill children receiving ongoing hospital care, such as Ronald McDonald House Charities Canada, which create a home-away-from-home atmosphere as well as the ability to make connections with and receive support from other families in similar situations (see Additional Resources at the end of this chapter).

Nurses need to have an appreciation of the child's separation behaviours. As discussed earlier, the phases of protest and despair are normal. The child should be allowed to cry. Even if the child rejects strangers, the nurse can provide support through physical presence. *Presence* is defined as spending time

BOX 43-6 NURSING ADMISSION HISTORY

Health Perception—Health Management

What has your child been admitted?
How has your child's general health been?
What does your child know about this hospitalization?
- Ask the child why he or she came to the hospital.
- If the answer is "For an operation or for tests," ask the child to tell you about what will happen before, during, and after the operation or tests.

Has your child ever been in the hospital before?
- How was that hospital experience?
- What things were important to you and your child during that hospitalization? How can we be most helpful now?

What medications does your child take at home?
- Why are they given?
- When are they given?
- How are they given (if a liquid, with a spoon; if a tablet, swallowed with water; or other)?
- Does your child have any trouble taking medication? If so, what helps?
- Is your child allergic to any medications?

What, if any, forms of complementary medicine practices are being used?

Nutrition

What are the family's usual mealtimes?
What are your child's favourite foods, beverages, and snacks?
- Average amounts consumed or usual size of portions
- Special cultural practices, such as family eating only ethnic food

What foods and beverages does your child dislike?
What are your child's feeding habits (bottle, cup, spoon, eating by self, needing assistance, any special devices)?
How does your child like the food served (warmed, cold, one item at a time)?
How would you describe your child's usual appetite (hearty eater, picky eater)?
- Has being sick affected your child's appetite? In what ways?

Are there any known or suspected food allergies?
Is your child on a special diet?
Are there any feeding problems (excessive fussiness, spitting up, colic); any dental or gum problems that affect feeding?
- What do you do for these problems?

Elimination

What are your child's toilet habits (diaper, toilet trained—day only or day and night, use of word to communicate urination or defecation, potty chair, regular toilet, other routines)?
What is your child's usual pattern of elimination (bowel movements)?
Do you have any concerns about elimination (bed-wetting, constipation, diarrhea)?
- What do you do for these problems?

Have you ever noticed that your child sweats a lot?

Sleep

What is your child's usual hour of sleep and awakening?
What is your child's type of bed and schedule for naps; length of naps?
Is there a special routine before sleeping (bottle, drink of water, bedtime story, nightlight, favourite blanket or toy, prayers)?
Is there a special routine during sleep time, such as waking to go to the bathroom?
In which type of bed does your child sleep?
Does your child have a separate room or share a room; if shares, with whom?
Does your child sleep with someone or alone (sibling, parent, other person)?
What is your child's favourite sleeping position?
Are there any sleeping problems (falling asleep, waking during night, nightmares, sleep walking)?
Are there any problems in awakening and getting ready in the morning?
- What do you do for these problems?

Activity and Exercise

What is your child's schedule during the day (preschool, day care centre, regular school, extracurricular activities)?
What are your child's favourite activities or toys (both active and quiet interests)?
What is your child's usual television-viewing schedule and restrictions? Favourite programs at home?
Are there any television restrictions?
Does your child have any illness or disabilities that limit activity? If so, how?
What are your child's usual habits and schedule for bathing (bath in tub or shower, sponge bath, shampoo)?
What are your child's dental habits (brushing, flossing, fluoride supplements or rinses, favourite toothpaste); schedule of daily dental care?
Does your child need help with dressing or grooming, such as hair combing?
Are there any problems with any hygiene activities (dislike of or refusal to bathe, shampoo hair, or brush teeth) and how do you manage them?
Are there special devices that your child requires help in managing (eyeglasses, contact lenses, hearing aid, orthodontic appliances, artificial elimination appliances, orthopedic devices)?

Cognition and Perception

Does your child have any hearing difficulty?
- Does your child use a hearing aid?
- Have "tubes" been placed in your child's ears?

Does your child have any vision problems?
- Does your child wear glasses or contact lenses?

Does your child have any learning difficulties?
- What is the child's grade in school?

Self-Concept

How would you describe your child (e.g., takes time to adjust, settles in easily, shy, friendly, quiet, talkative, serious, playful, stubborn, easygoing)?
What makes your child angry, annoyed, anxious, or sad? What helps when your child feels this way?
How does your child act when annoyed or upset?
What have been your child's experiences with and reactions to temporary separation from you (parent) and his or her reactions to it?

BOX 43-6 NURSING ADMISSION HISTORY—cont'd

Does your child have any fears (places, objects, animals, people, situations)?
- How do you handle them?

Do you think your child's illness has changed the way he or she thinks about self, such as being more shy, embarrassed about appearance, or less competitive with friends, or staying at home more?

Relationships

Does your child have a favourite nickname?
What are the names of other family members or others who live in the home (relatives, friends, pets)?
Who usually takes care of your child during the day and night (especially if other than parent, such as babysitter, relative)?
What are the parents' occupations and work schedules?
Are there any special family considerations (adoption, foster child, step-parent, divorce, lone parent)?
Have any major changes in the family occurred lately (death, divorce, separation, birth of a sibling, loss of a job, financial strain, parent beginning a career, other)? Describe the child's reaction.
Who are your child's play companions or social groups (peers, younger or older children, adults, prefers to be alone)?
Do things generally go well for your child in school or with friends?
Does your child have "security" objects at home (pacifier, bottle, blanket, stuffed animal, or doll)? Did you bring any of these to the hospital?
How do you handle discipline problems at home? Are these methods always effective?
Does your child have any condition that interferes with communication? If so, what are your suggestions for communicating with your child?
Will your child's hospitalization affect the family's financial support or care of other family members?
What concerns do you have about your child's illness and hospitalization?
Will anyone be staying with your child while hospitalized?
How can we contact you or another close family member outside the hospital?

Sexuality

(Answer questions that apply to your child's age group.)
Has your child begun puberty (developing physical sexual characteristics, menstruation)? Have you or your child had any concerns?
How have you approached topics of sexuality with your child?
Do you think you might need some help with some topics?
Has your child's illness affected the way he or she feels about being a boy or a girl? If so, how?
Do you have any concerns about behaviours of your child, such as masturbation, asking many questions or talking about sex, not respecting others' privacy, or wanting too much privacy?
(Questions to an adolescent: answer questions about sexual concerns that apply to you)
Who are your closest friends? (If one friend is identified, the nurse could ask more about that relationship, such as how much time they spend together, how serious they are about each other, if the relationship is going the way the teenager hoped.)
What are your views on sexuality education, living together, "hooking up," having an intimate friend or partner, or premarital sex? (The nurse should use the terms *friends* or *partners* rather than *girlfriend* or *boyfriend*.)
Which friends would you like to have visit in the hospital?

Coping and Stress

(Answer questions that apply to your child's age group.)
What does your child do when tired or upset?
- If upset, does your child want a special person or object?
- If so, explain.

If your child has temper tantrums, what causes them and how do you handle them?
To whom does your child talk when worried about something?
How does your child usually handle problems or disappointments?
Have there been any big changes or problems in your family recently? If so, how have you handled them?
Has your child ever had a problem with drugs or alcohol or tried to commit suicide?
Do you think your child is "accident prone"? If so, explain.

Values and Beliefs

Is religion important to you? If so, what is your religion?
Is religion or faith important in your child's life? If so, how?
What, if any, religious practices would you like continued in the hospital (e.g., prayers before meals or bedtime; visit by minister, priest, rabbi, or other spiritual leader; prayer group)?

BOX 43-7 COMPLEMENTARY MEDICINE PRACTICES AND EXAMPLES

Nutrition, diet, and lifestyle or behavioural health changes—Macrobiotics, megavitamins, diets, lifestyle modification, health risk reduction and health education, wellness

Mind–body control therapies—Biofeedback, relaxation, prayer therapy, guided imagery, hypnotherapy, music or sound therapy, massage, aromatherapy, education therapy, meditation, mindfulness-based meditation

Traditional and ethnomedicine therapies—Acupuncture, ayurvedic medicine, herbal medicine, homeopathic medicine, Indigenous medicine, natural products, traditional Asian medicine

Structural manipulation and energetic therapies—Acupressure, chiropractic medicine, massage, reflexology, rolfing, therapeutic touch, Qi Gong

Pharmacological and biological therapies—Antioxidants, cell treatment, chelation therapy, metabolic therapy, oxidizing agents

Bioelectromagnetic therapies—Diagnostic and therapeutic application of electromagnetic fields (e.g., transcranial electrostimulation, neuromagnetic stimulation, electroacupuncture)

being physically close to the child while using a quiet tone of voice, appropriate choice of words, eye contact, and touch in ways that establish rapport and communicate empathy. If detachment behaviours are evident, the nurse can help maintain the child's contact with the parents by talking about them frequently with the child; encouraging the child to remember them; and stressing to the parents the significance of their visits, telephone calls, or letters. The use of cellular phones and personal tablets can increase the contact between the hospitalized child and parents or other significant family members and friends. A Canadian qualitative research study evaluated the use of videophones with families with limited access to visit their hospitalized child because of being geographically separated. The videophones connected the children with their families and decreased feelings of isolation and anxiety and increased feelings of connection between family members (Nicholas, Fellner, Koller, et al., 2011).

Separation may be equally difficult for parents, especially when they do not understand the behaviours of separation anxiety. To avoid the child's immediate protest, parents may sneak out or lie to the child about leaving. As a result, instead of learning that absence is associated with a guaranteed return, the child learns that absence means loss of parents. Helping parents recognize that separation behaviours are normal and expected can decrease the parents' anxiety and may ease their fears about leaving their child. Explaining to parents how the child reacts after they leave may also be helpful. Many parents imagine that the child cries for hours after they leave, whereas in reality the child may cry for a few minutes but settle down when comforted by someone else.

Toddlers and preschoolers have a limited concept of time. Time is measured in associations, such as eating dinner "when Daddy comes home." Therefore, when helping parents with children's fears of separation, nurses need to suggest ways of explaining leaving and returning. For example, if parents must leave to go to work or to make meals for other family members, they should tell the child the reason for leaving. They also need to convey the expected time of return in terms of anticipated events. For example, if the parents will return in the morning, they can say to the child, "We'll see you after the sun comes up" or "We'll come back when [a favourite program] is on television."

The young child's ability to tolerate parental absence is limited. Thus parental visits should be frequent, such as visiting three times a day for short periods rather than once a day for an extended time. This may necessitate that each parent visit at different times in order to lessen the length of separation. When parents cannot visit, the presence of other significant people can be most comforting for the child.

Older children who know how to tell time may find it helpful to have a clock or watch. However, these children have the same need for honesty from their parents regarding visiting schedules. For adolescents, peer groups are important, thus they often appreciate planning visiting hours with their parents to ensure that they have some private time for friends.

Familiar surroundings also increase the child's adjustment to separation. If parents cannot stay with the child, they should leave favourite articles from home with the child, such as a blanket, toy, bottle, feeding utensil, or article of clothing. Because young children associate such inanimate objects with significant people, they gain comfort and reassurance from these possessions. They make the association that if the parents left this, the parents will surely return. Placing an identification band on the toy lessens the chances of its being misplaced and provides a symbol that the toy is experiencing the same needs as the child. Other reminders of home include photographs, audio or video recordings, or live video online streaming of family members reading a story, singing a song, saying prayers before bedtime, relating events at home, or taking a "talking walk" through the home. The recordings can be played at lonely times, such as on awakening or before sleeping. Some units allow pets to visit, which can have therapeutic benefits for a child. Older children also appreciate familiar articles from home, particularly photographs, a smartphone or tablet, a favourite toy or game, and their own pyjamas. Often the importance of treasured objects to school-age children is overlooked or criticized. However, many school-age children have a special object to which they formed an attachment in early childhood. Such treasured or transitional objects can help even older children feel more comfortable in a strange environment.

The strange sights, smells, and sounds in the hospital that are commonplace for the nurse can be frightening and confusing for children. It is important for the nurse to try to evaluate stimuli in the environment from the child's point of view (considering also what the child may see or hear happening to other patients) and to make every effort to protect the child from frightening and unfamiliar sights, sounds, and equipment. The nurse should offer explanations or prepare the child for those experiences that are unavoidable. Combining familiar or comforting sights with the unfamiliar can relieve much of the harshness of medical equipment.

Helping children maintain their usual contacts also minimizes the effects of separation imposed by hospitalization. This includes continuing school lessons during the illness and confinement, visiting with friends either directly or through email, text messaging, or telephone calls, and participating in stimulating projects whenever possible (Fig. 43-5). For extended hospitalizations, youngsters enjoy personalizing the hospital room to make it "home" by decorating the walls with posters and cards, rearranging the furniture (when possible), and displaying a collection or hobby.

Minimizing Loss of Control

Feelings of loss of control result from separation, physical restriction, changed routines, enforced dependency, and magical thinking. Although some of these cannot be prevented, most can be minimized through individualized planning of nursing care.

Promoting freedom of movement. Younger children react most strenuously to any type of physical restriction or immobilization. Although temporary immobilization may be necessary for some interventions, such as maintaining an intravenous line, most physical restriction can be prevented if the nurse and child work together.

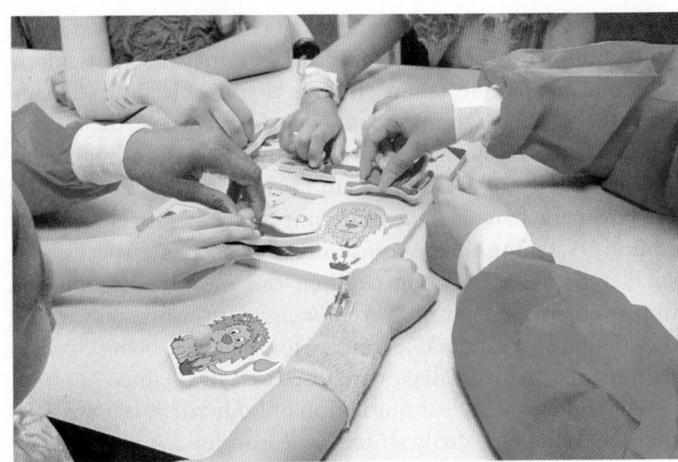

FIGURE 43-5 For extended hospitalizations children enjoy having projects with other patients to occupy time. (© Image Source/Alamy Stock Photo.)

Eric's Daily Schedule

7:30 AM	– Breakfast, morning bath	3:00 PM	– Tutor (M, W, F) – Study time (T, Th)
9:00	– Medications, dressing change	4:00	– Physical therapy
11:00	– Physical therapy	5:30	– Dinner
12:00 PM	– Lunch	9:00	– Medications, dressing change
		9:15	– Bedtime

FIGURE 43-6 Time structuring is an effective strategy for normalizing the hospital environment and increasing the child's sense of control.

For young children, particularly infants and toddlers, preserving parent–child contact is the best means of decreasing the need for or stress of restraint. For example, almost the entire physical examination can be done with the child in a parent's lap, with the parent hugging the child for procedures such as otoscopy. For painful procedures, the nurse should assess the parents' preferences for assisting, observing, or waiting outside the room.

Environmental factors may also restrict movement. Keeping children in cribs or playpens may not represent immobilization in a concrete sense, but it certainly limits sensory stimulation. Increasing mobility by transporting children in carriages, wheelchairs, carts, or wagons provides them with a sense of freedom.

In some cases, physical restraint or isolation is necessary because of the child's medical diagnosis. In these cases, the environment can be altered to increase sensory freedom such as moving the bed toward the window; opening window shades; or providing musical, visual, or tactile activities.

Maintaining the child's routine. Altered daily schedules and loss of rituals are particularly stressful for toddlers and early preschoolers and may increase the stress of separation. The nursing admission history will provide a baseline for planning care around the child's usual home activities. A frequently neglected aspect of altered routines is the change in the child's daily activities. A typical child's day, especially during the school years, is structured with specific times for eating, dressing, going to school, playing, and sleeping. However, this time structure vanishes when the child is hospitalized. Although nurses have a set schedule, the child is frequently unaware of it, and the new schedules that are imposed may be rigid. For example, some units have uniform nap times and bedtimes for all children, whereas others allow children to stay up late at night. Many children obtain significantly less sleep in the hospital than at home; the primary causes are delay in sleep onset and early termination of sleep because of hospital routines. Not only are hours of sleep disrupted, but waking hours are spent in passive activities. For example, few institutions impose any limits on the amount of time the child spends watching television or using a handheld device. This may lead to the child being less "tired" at bedtime and can delay the onset of sleep.

One technique that can minimize the disruption in the child's routine is establishing a daily schedule. This approach is most suitable for the non–critically ill school-age or adolescent child who has mastered the concept of time. It involves scheduling the child's day to include all those activities that are important to the child and nurse, such as treatment procedures, schoolwork, exercise, television, playroom, and hobbies. Together, the nurse, parent, and child can then plan a daily schedule with times and activities written down (Fig. 43-6) and left in the child's room, with a clock or watch. Whenever possible, a calendar should also be constructed with special events marked, such as favourite television programs, visits by friends or relatives, events in the playroom, and holidays or birthdays. If specific changes in treatment are expected such as, "beginning physiotherapy in 2 days," these can be added.

Encouraging independence. The dependent role of the hospitalized patient can instill tremendous feelings of loss in older children. Principal interventions should focus on respect for individuality and the opportunity for decision making. Although these sound simple to carry out, their efficacy lies with nurses who are flexible and tolerant. It is also important for the nurse to empower the patient while not feeling threatened by a sense of lessened control.

Enabling children's sense of control involves helping them maintain independence and promoting the concept of self-care. *Self-care* refers to the practice of activities that individuals personally initiate and perform on their own behalf in maintaining life, health, and well-being. Although self-care is limited by the child's age and physical condition, most children beyond infancy can perform some activities with little or no help in the hospital. Other approaches include jointly planning care, time structuring, having the child wear street clothes and make choices in food selections and bedtime, continuing school activities, and placing the child in a room with an appropriate age-mate.

Promoting understanding. A sense of loss of control can occur from feelings of having too little influence on one's destiny or from sensing overwhelming control or power over one's fate. Although preschoolers' cognitive abilities predispose

BOX 43-8 THE RIGHTS OF THE CHILD IN THE HEALTH CARE SYSTEM

The Rights of the Child in the Health Care System, which were developed by the Canadian Institute of Child Health, are based on the United Nations Convention on the Rights of the Child and are listed below:

- Right to live and to have my pain and suffering treated, regardless of my age, gender, or income
- Right to be viewed first as a child, then as a patient
- Right to be treated as a unique individual with my own abilities, culture, and language
- Right not be afraid and to cry when I feel hurt
- Right to be safe in an environment that is unfamiliar to me
- Right to ask questions and receive answers that I can understand
- Right to be cared for by people who perceive and meet my needs even though I may be unable to explain what they are
- Right to speak for myself when I am able and to have someone speak on my behalf when I am unable
- Right to have those dear to me close by when I need them
- Right to play and learn even if I am receiving care
- Need to have rights fulfilled

Adapted from the Canadian Institute of Child Health. (2002). *The rights of the child in the health care system* [pamphlet]. Retrieved from http://www.cich.ca/PDFFiles/RightHospitalizedENG.pdf

them most to magical thinking and delusions of power, all children are vulnerable to misinterpreting causes for stresses such as illness and hospitalization.

Most children feel more in control when they know what to expect, since the element of fear is reduced. Anticipatory preparation and provision of information can help to lessen stress and increase understanding (see Preparation for Diagnostic and Therapeutic Procedures, Chapter 44).

Informing children of their rights while they are hospitalized fosters greater understanding and may relieve some of the feelings of powerlessness they typically experience. Hospitals providing services to children should have a hospital-wide policy on the rights and responsibilities of these patients and of their parents or guardians. The Canadian Institute of Child Health (2002) has developed the Rights of the Child in the Health Care System (Box 43-8).

Preventing or Minimizing Fear of Bodily Injury

Beyond early infancy, all children fear bodily injury from mutilation, bodily intrusion, body-image change, disability, or death. In general, preparation of children for painful procedures decreases their fears and increases the child's ability to cooperate. Modifying procedural techniques for children in each age group also minimizes the fear of bodily injury. For example, toddlers and young preschoolers are traumatized by insertion of a rectal thermometer, thus axillary or tympanic temperatures can effectively be substituted. Whenever procedures are performed on young children, the most supportive intervention is to do the procedure as quickly as possible while maintaining parent–child contact.

Because of toddlers' and preschool children's poorly defined body boundaries, the use of bandages may be particularly helpful. For example, telling children that the bleeding will stop after the needle is removed does little to relieve their fears, whereas applying a small Band-Aid usually reassures them. The size of bandages is also significant to children in this age group; the larger the bandage, the more importance is attached to the wound. Watching their surgical dressings become successively smaller is one way young children can measure healing and improvement. Prematurely removing a dressing may cause these children considerable concern for their well-being. Specific pain management strategies are discussed in Chapter 34.

For children who fear mutilation of body parts, it is essential that the nurse repeatedly stress the reason for a procedure and evaluate their understanding. For example, explaining cast removal to preschoolers may seem simple enough, but children's comprehension of the details may vary considerably. Asking them to draw a picture of what they think will happen can present substantial evidence of how they perceive events.

Children may fear bodily injury from a great variety of sources. Imaging machines, strange equipment used for examination, unfamiliar rooms, or awkward positions can be perceived as potentially hazardous. In addition, thoughts and actions can be imagined sources of bodily damage. Therefore, it is important to investigate imagined reasons, particularly of a sexual nature, for illness. Because children may fear revealing such thoughts, using techniques such as drawing or doll play may elicit previously undisclosed misconceptions.

Older children fear bodily injury of both internal and external origins. For example, school-age children are aware of the significance of the heart and may fear the actual operation as much as the pain, the stitches, and the possible scar. Adolescents may express concern about the actual procedure but be much more anxious over the resulting scar.

Children can grasp information only if it is presented on or close to their level of cognitive development. This requires an awareness of the words used to describe events or processes. For example, young children told that they are going to have a CAT (i.e., CT, computed tomography) scan may wonder, "Will there be cats? Or something that scratches?" It is clearer to describe the procedure in simple terms and explain what the letters of the common name stand for. Therefore, to prevent or alleviate fears, nurses must be keenly aware of the medical terminology and vocabulary that they use every day.

When children are upset about their illness, their perception can be changed by (1) providing a somewhat different and less negative account of the disease or (2) offering an explanation that is characteristic of the next stage of cognitive development. An example of the first strategy is reassuring a preschooler who fears that, after a tonsillectomy, another sore throat means a second operation. Explaining that after tonsils are "fixed" they do not need fixing again can help relieve the fear. An example of the latter strategy is to explain that germs made the tonsils sick, and even though germs can cause another sore throat, they cannot cause the tonsils to ever be sick again. This higher-level explanation is based on the school-age child's concept of germs as a cause of disease.

Providing Developmentally Appropriate Activities

A primary goal of nursing care for the child who is hospitalized is to minimize threats to the child's development. Children who experience prolonged or repeated hospitalization are at greater risk for developmental delays or regression. The nurse who provides opportunities for the child to participate in developmentally appropriate activities further normalizes the child's environment and helps reduce interference with the child's development.

Interference with normal development may have long-term implications for the infant and toddler. The nurse can play a primary role in identifying children at risk and helping to plan, implement, and evaluate developmental interventions.

School is an integral part of the school-age child's and adolescent's development. A key factor in accreditation for hospitals serving children is whether the hospital provides access to appropriate educational services when a child's treatment requires a significant absence from school (Accreditation Canada, 2010). For example, BC Children's Hospital provides provincial school services to school-age children and youth (kindergarten to grade 12) while they or their siblings are staying in the hospital (BC Children's Hospital, 2016). The nurse can encourage children to resume schoolwork as their condition permits, help them schedule time for studies, and help the family coordinate hospital educational services with their children's schools. Children should have the opportunity to continue art and music classes as well as their academic subjects.

To meet the unique developmental needs of adolescents, special units may be designated that provide both privacy and increased socialization and appropriate activities. Teenagers should not share space with younger children, who are often perceived as a threat to their maturity.

In caring for the adolescent patient, it is essential to provide flexible routines and activities, such as more group activity, wearing of street clothes, and access to the items so critical to adolescents—cell phones, DVD players, laptops, personal tablets, video games, and televisions. Because adolescents' food habits are rarely limited to the three traditional meals a day, a ready supply of snacks should be available. However, the most important benefit of these units is increased socialization with peers. In addition, staff members usually enjoy working with this age group and are able to establish the trust that is so essential for communication.

! NURSING ALERT

When adolescents must share a common activity room with younger patients, referring to the area as the "activity" room rather than the "playroom" may entice them to visit the room and participate in activities.

Although regression is expected and normal for all age groups, nurses have the responsibility for fostering the child's growth and development. Hospitalization can become a significant opportunity for learning and advancing. Extended hospitalizations for long-term chronic illness or situations of failure to thrive, abuse, or neglect represent instances in which regression must be seen as an adjustment period, to be followed by plans for promoting appropriate developmental skills.

BOX 43-9 FUNCTIONS OF PLAY IN THE HOSPITAL

- Provides diversion and brings about relaxation
- Helps the child feel more secure in a strange environment
- Lessens the stress of separation and the feeling of homesickness
- Provides a means for release of tension and expression of feelings
- Encourages interaction and development of positive attitudes toward others
- Provides an expressive outlet for creative ideas and interests
- Provides a means for accomplishing therapeutic goals (see Use of Play in Procedures, Chapter 44)
- Places child in active role and provides an opportunity to make choices and be in control

Providing Opportunities for Play and Expressive Activities

Play is one of the most important aspects of a child's life and is an effective tool for managing stress. Because illness and hospitalization constitute crises in a child's life and often involve overwhelming stresses, children need to act out their fears and anxieties as a means of coping with these stresses. Play is essential to children's mental, emotional, and social well-being; it does not stop when children are ill or in the hospital. On the contrary, play in the hospital serves many functions, including to promote well-being (Box 43-9). Of all hospital facilities, no room alleviates the stressors of hospitalization more than the playroom (or activity room). In the playroom, children temporarily distance themselves from their illness, hospitalization, and the associated stressors. This room should be a safe haven for children, free from medical or nursing procedures, strange faces, and probing questions. The playroom then becomes a sanctuary in an otherwise frightening environment.

Engaging in play activities also gives children a sense of control. In the hospital environment, most decisions are made for the child; play and other expressive activities offer the child opportunities to make choices for themselves. Even if a child chooses not to participate in a particular activity, the nurse has offered the child a choice, perhaps one of only a few real choices the child has had that day.

The hospitalized child typically has lower energy levels than those of healthy children of the same age. Hospitalized children may not appear engaged and enthusiastic about an activity, even though they are enjoying the experience. Activities may need to be adjusted or limited according to the child's age, endurance, and special needs.

Diversional activities. Almost any form of play can be used for diversion and recreation, but the activity should be selected on the basis of the child's age, interests, and limitations (Fig. 43-7). Children do not necessarily need special direction for using play materials. Small children enjoy a variety of small, colourful toys that they can play with in bed or in their room,

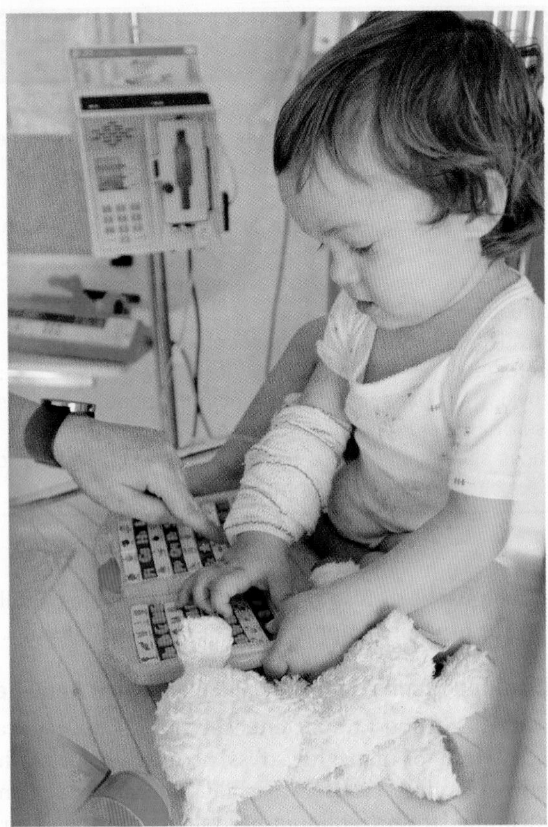

FIGURE 43-7 Play materials for children in the hospital need to be appropriate for their age, interests, and limitations. (© BSIP SA/ Alamy Stock Photo.)

or more elaborate play equipment, such as playhouses, sandboxes, rhythm instruments, or large boxes and blocks, that may be a part of the hospital playroom.

Games that can be played alone or with another child or an adult are popular with older children, as are puzzles; reading material; quiet, individual activities, such as sewing, stringing beads, and weaving; and Lego blocks and other building materials. Assembling models is an excellent pastime, but one should make certain that all pieces and necessary materials are included in the package so the child is not disappointed and frustrated.

Well-selected books are of infinite value to the child. Children never tire of stories; having someone read aloud to them gives them much pleasure and is of special value to the child who has limited energy to expend in play. A radio, MP3 player, tablet computer, electronic games, and television are useful tools for entertaining a child. Computers with access to the Internet can provide diversion, educational opportunities, and online support groups.

When supervising play for ill or convalescent children, it is best to select activities that are simpler than would normally be chosen for the child's specific developmental level. These children usually do not have the energy to cope with more challenging activities. Other limitations also influence the type of activities. Special consideration must be given to the child who is confined in terms of movement, has a restricted extremity, or is isolated. Toys for isolated children must be disposable or need to be disinfected after every use.

Toys. Parents of hospitalized children often ask nurses about the types of toys that would be best to bring for their child. Although they want to buy new toys for the hospitalized child to offer cheer and comfort, it is often better to wait to bring new things, especially in the case of younger children. Small children need the comfort and reassurance of familiar things, such as the stuffed animal the child hugs for comfort and takes to bed at night. All toys brought into the hospital should be assessed for safety.

Children who are hospitalized for an extended time benefit from changes in toys. Rather than a confusing accumulation of toys, older toys should be replaced periodically as interest wanes.

A highly successful diversion for a child who is hospitalized is having the parents bring a box with several small, inexpensive, brightly wrapped items with a different day of the week printed on the outside of each package. The child will eagerly anticipate the time for opening each one. If the parents know when their next visit will be, they can provide the number of packages that corresponds to the time between visits. In this way the child knows that the diminishing packages also represent the anticipated visit from the parent.

Expressive activities. Play and other expressive activities provide one of the best opportunities for encouraging emotional expression, including the safe release of anger and hostility. Nondirective play that allows children freedom for expression can be tremendously therapeutic. However, **therapeutic play** should not be confused with play therapy, a psychological technique reserved for use by trained and qualified therapists as an interpretative method with emotionally disturbed children. On the other hand, therapeutic play is an effective, nondirective modality for helping children deal with their concerns and fears; at the same time it often helps the nurse gain insights into children's needs and feelings.

Tension release can be facilitated through almost any activity; with younger ambulatory children, large-muscle activity through use of tricycles and wagons is beneficial. Much aggression can be safely directed into pounding and throwing games or activities. Beanbags are often thrown at a target or open receptacle with surprising vigour and hostility. A pounding board can be a favourite item for young children; clay and play dough are beneficial for use at any age.

Creative expression. Although all children derive physical, social, emotional, and cognitive benefits from engaging in art or other creative activities, children's need for such activities is intensified when they are hospitalized. Drawing and painting are excellent media for expression (Fig. 43-8). Children are more at ease expressing their thoughts and feelings through art, since humans think first in images and later learn to translate these images into words. Children can work individually or work together on a group project, such as a mural painted on a long piece of paper.

Although interpretation of children's drawing requires special training, observing changes in a series of the child's drawings over time can be helpful in assessing psychosocial adjustment and coping. The nurse can use children's drawings, stories, poetry, and other products of creative expression as a springboard for discussion of thoughts, fears, and

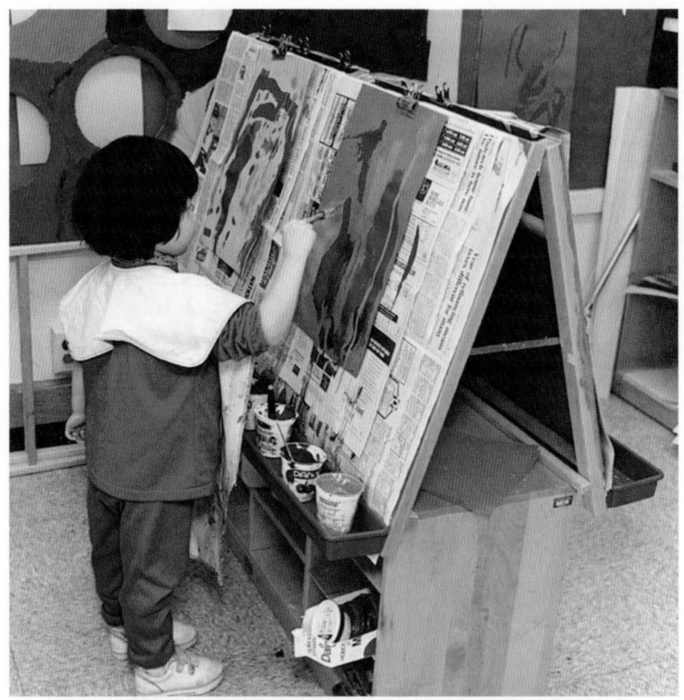

FIGURE 43-8 Drawing and painting are excellent media for expression.

CRITICAL THINKING CASE STUDY

Playroom and Hospital Procedures

Hannah, a 7-year-old with cystic fibrosis, has been hospitalized numerous times with complications from the condition. She is playing a board game with her brother, sister, and several other children in the playroom on the pediatric unit. A pediatric phlebotomist enters the playroom and says, "Hannah, I need to take some blood. I can see that you are playing a game, so I'll just do it while you play. It will just take a minute." Hannah nods her head indicating that she agrees to let the phlebotomist draw the blood at this time. The playroom is usually off-limits for invasive procedures. As Hannah's nurse, you are aware that the physician wants the results of the laboratory studies as soon as possible to make a decision about her course of therapy.

1. Evidence—Is there sufficient evidence to draw any conclusions about this situation at this time?
2. Assumptions—What are some underlying assumptions about the following?
   a. Children and painful procedures such as venipunctures
   b. The function of play for a hospitalized child
   c. The priority in performing the procedure
   d. Implications of performing the procedure in the playroom
3. What implications and priorities for nursing care can be drawn at this time (i.e., what will you do)?
4. Does the evidence objectively support your argument (conclusion)?

understanding of concepts or events (see Communication Techniques, Chapter 33). For example, a child's drawing before surgery may reveal unvoiced concerns about mutilation, body changes, and loss of self-control.

Nurses can incorporate opportunities for musical expression into routine nursing care. For example, simple musical instruments, such as bracelets with bells, can be placed on infants' legs for them to shake to accompany mealtime music or dressing changes. The nurse can suggest dance or movement to encourage a child to ambulate.

Dramatic play. Dramatic play is a well-recognized technique for emotional release, allowing children to re-enact frightening or puzzling hospital experiences. Through the use of puppets, replicas of hospital equipment, or some actual hospital equipment, children can act out the situations that are a part of their hospital experience. Dramatic play enables children to learn about procedures and events that concern them and to assume the roles of the adults in the hospital environment.

Puppets are universally effective for communicating with children. Most children see them as peers and readily communicate with them. Children will tell the puppet feelings that they hesitate to express to adults. Puppets can share children's own experiences and help them find solutions to their problems. Puppets dressed to represent figures in the child's environment—for example, a physician, nurse, child patient, therapist, and members of the child's own family—are especially useful. Small, appropriately attired dolls are equally effective in encouraging the child to play out situations, although puppets are usually best for direct conversation.

When choosing play for a child, medical needs must be considered, but at times a procedure can be postponed briefly to allow the child to complete a special activity (see Critical Thinking Case Study). In addition, any limitations imposed by the child's condition need to be taken into account. For example, small children may eat paste and other creative media; therefore a child who is allergic to wheat should not be given finger paint made from wallpaper paste or modelling dough made with flour. A child on a restricted salt intake should not play with modelling dough because salt is one of its major constituents. At home the play program can be planned around the therapy regimen. Play can be satisfactorily incorporated into the child's care if the nurse and others involved allow some flexibility and use creativity in planning for play.

Maximizing Potential Benefits of Hospitalization

Although hospitalization generally represents a stressful time for children and families, it also represents an opportunity for facilitating positive change within the child and among family members. For some families the stress of a child's illness, hospitalization, or both can lead to strengthening of family coping behaviours and the emergence of new coping strategies.

Fostering parent–child relationships. The crisis of illness or hospitalization can mobilize parents into more acute awareness of their child's needs. For example, hospitalization provides opportunities for parents to learn more about their children's growth and development. When parents are helped to understand children's usual reactions to stress, such as regression or aggression, they are not only better able to support the child through the hospital experience but also may extend their insights into child-rearing practices after discharge.

Difficulties in parent–child relationships that existed before hospitalization that are characterized by feeding problems, negative behaviour, and sleep disturbances may decrease during hospitalization. The temporary cessation of such problems sometimes alerts parents to the role they may be playing in promoting the negative behaviour. With help from health care providers, parents can restructure ways of relating to their children to foster more positive behaviour.

Hospitalization may also represent a temporary reprieve or refuge from a disturbed home. Typically, abused or neglected children's dramatic physical and social improvement during hospitalization is proof of the benefits and potential growth that can occur during such times. These children temporarily are able to seek support, reassurance, and security from new relationships, particularly with nurses and hospitalized peers.

Providing educational opportunities. Illness and hospitalization represent excellent opportunities for children and other family members to learn more about their bodies, each other, and the health professions. For example, during a hospital admission for a diabetic crisis, the child may learn about the disease; the parents may learn about the child's needs for independence, normalcy, and appropriate limits; and each of them may find a new support system in the hospital staff.

Promoting self-mastery. The experience of facing a crisis such as illness or hospitalization, coping successfully with it, and maturing as a result of it constitutes an opportunity for self-mastery. Younger children have the chance to test fantasy-versus-reality fears. They realize that they were not abandoned, mutilated, or punished. In fact, they were loved, cared for, and treated with respect for their individual concerns. It is not unusual for children who have undergone hospitalization or surgery to tell others that "it was nothing" or to display proudly their scars or bandages. For older children, hospitalization may represent an opportunity for decision making, independence, and self-reliance. They are proud of having survived the experience and may feel a genuine self-respect for their achievements. Nurses can facilitate such feelings of self-mastery by emphasizing aspects of personal competence in the child and not focusing on negative behaviour.

Providing socialization. Hospitalization may offer children a special opportunity for social acceptance. Lonely, asocial, and even delinquent children find a sympathetic environment in the hospital. Children who have a physical disability or are in some other way "different" from their age-mates may find an accepting social peer group (Fig. 43-9). Although this does not always spontaneously occur, nurses can structure the environment to foster a supportive child group. For example, selection of a compatible roommate can help children gain a new friend and learn more about themselves. Forming relationships with significant members of the health care team, such as the physician, nurse, child life specialist, or social worker, can greatly enhance children's adjustment in many areas of life.

Parents may also encounter a new social group in other parents who have similar problems. The waiting room or hallway "support" groups are inherent to every institution. Parents meet while in the hospital or clinic and discuss their children's illnesses and treatments. Nurses can capitalize on this informal gathering by encouraging parents to discuss collectively their concerns and feelings. Nurses can also refer parents to organized parent groups or can use the help and support of parents of recovered hospitalized patients. It is important that nurses emphasize to families that each child responds differently to disease, treatments, and care. Questions raised during group discussions can be clarified with a nurse or health care provider.

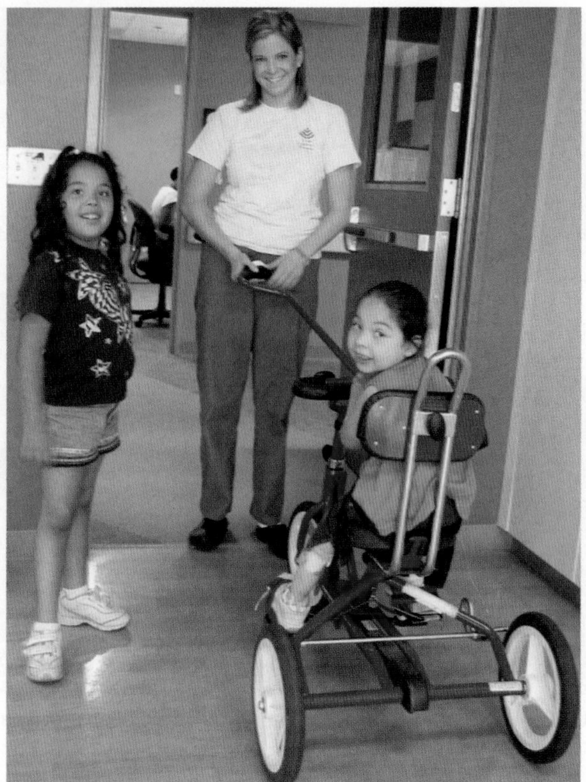

FIGURE 43-9 Placing children of the same age group with similar illnesses near each other on the unit is both psychologically and medically supportive. (Courtesy E. Jacob, Texas Children's Hospital.)

Providing Support for the Family

Although it is not possible to predict exactly which factors are most likely to have an effect on the family's reactions, important variables are (1) the seriousness of the child's illness, (2) the family's previous experience with hospitalization, and (3) the medical procedures involved in the diagnosis and treatment. Important information is also obtained in the nursing admission history (see Box 43-6).

Support for family members involves the willingness to stay and listen to parents' verbal and nonverbal messages. Sometimes the nurse does not give this support directly. For example, the nurse may offer to stay with the child to allow the parents time alone or may discuss with other family members the parents' need for extra relief. Often relatives and friends want to help but do not know how. Suggesting ways to be of assistance, such as babysitting, preparing meals, doing laundry, or transporting the siblings to school, can prompt others to help reduce responsibilities that burden parents.

Parents with religious beliefs may appreciate the counsel of a clergy member, but because of stress they may not have sufficient time and energy to initiate the contact. Nurses can be supportive by arranging for clergy to visit.

Support also involves accepting cultural, socioeconomic, and ethnic values. Health and illness are defined differently by various ethnic groups. For some, a disorder that has few outward manifestations of illness, such as diabetes, hypertension, or cardiac problems, is not a sickness. Consequently, following a prescribed treatment may be seen as unnecessary. Nurses who appreciate the influences of culture are more likely to intervene therapeutically. (See also Chapter 31, Cultural and Religious Influences on Health Care.)

Parents may need help in accepting their own feelings toward the ill child. If given the opportunity, parents often disclose their feelings of loss of control, anger, and guilt. They often resist admitting to such feelings because they expect others to disapprove of behaviour that is less than perfect. Unfortunately, health personnel, including nurses, sometimes exercise little tolerance for deviation from the expected norm. This only increases the psychological impact of a child's illness on family members. Helping parents identify the specific reason for such feelings and emphasizing that each is a normal and healthy response to stress may reduce the parents' emotional burden. Often a social worker, who may become involved early on in the hospital experience, can provide families with links to community resources and organizations that provide financial help and other supports. They can also help the child and family members talk through personal issues related to the hospitalization.

The needs of siblings should also be addressed. Support may involve preparing siblings for hospital visits, assessing their adjustment, and providing appropriate interventions or referrals when needed. The Family-Centred Teaching box suggests ways that parents can support siblings during hospitalization.

FAMILY-CENTRED TEACHING

Supporting Siblings During Hospitalization

Trade off staying at the hospital with your partner or have a surrogate who knows the siblings well stay in the home.

Offer information about the child's condition to siblings; respect the sibling who avoids information as a means of coping with the situation.

Arrange for children to visit their brother or sister in the hospital if possible.

Encourage phone visits, mail, email, and text messages between brothers and sisters; provide children with phone numbers, email addresses, writing supplies, and stamps.

Help each sibling identify an extended family member or friend to be their support person and provide extra attention during parental absence.

Make or buy inexpensive toys or trinkets for siblings, one gift for each day the child will be hospitalized.

- Wrap each gift separately and place in a basket, box, or other container at each child's bedside.
- Instruct siblings to open one gift each night at bedtime and to remember that he or she is in the parent's thoughts.

If the child's condition is stable and distance is not prohibitive, plan a special time at home with the siblings or have your partner or another relative or friend bring the children to meet you at a restaurant or other location near the hospital.

- Have extended family members or friends schedule a visit by siblings to the child in the hospital during parental absence.
- Arrange a pass for the child to leave the hospital to join the family if the child's condition permits.

Data from Craft, M., & Craft, J. (1989). Perceived changes in siblings of hospitalized children: A comparison of sibling and parent reports. *Child Health Care, 18*(1), 42–48; Rollins, J. (1992). *Brothers and sisters: A discussion guide for families.* Landover, MD: Epilepsy Foundation of America.

Providing Information

One of the most important nursing interventions is providing information about (1) the disease, its treatment, the prognosis, and home care; (2) the child's emotional and physical reactions to illness and hospitalization; and (3) the probable emotional reactions of family members to the crisis.

For many families the child's illness is the first contact they have with the hospital experience. Often parents are not prepared for the child's behavioural reactions to hospitalization, such as separation behaviours, regression, aggression, and hostility. Providing the parents with information about these normal and expected behavioural responses can lessen the parents' anxiety during the hospitalization. The family is equally unfamiliar with hospital routines and policies, which often compounds their confusion and anxiety. Thus, the family needs clear explanations about what to expect and what is expected of them.

Parents also need to be aware of the effects of illness on the family and of strategies to prevent negative changes. Specifically, parents should keep the family well informed and communicate with everyone as much as possible. They should try to treat all the children equally and in the same way as before the illness occurred. Discipline, which initially may be lessened for the ill child, should be continued to provide a measure of security and predictability. When ill children know that their parents expect certain standards of conduct from them, they feel certain that they will recover. Conversely, when all limits are removed, they fear that something catastrophic will happen.

Helping parents understand the meaning of posthospitalization behaviours of the sick child can help them tolerate and support such behaviours. In addition, parents should be forewarned of common reactions following discharge (see Box 43-2). Parents who do not expect such reactions may misinterpret them as evidence of the child's "being spoiled" and demand perfect behaviour at a time when the child is still reacting to the stress of illness and hospitalization. If the behaviours, especially the demand for attention, are dealt with in a supportive manner, most children are able to relinquish them and assume precrisis levels of functioning.

Nurses should also prepare parents for the reactions of siblings—particularly anger, jealousy, and resentment. Older siblings may deny such reactions because they provoke feelings of guilt. However, everyone needs outlets for emotions, and the repressed feelings may surface as problems in school or with agemates, as psychosomatic illnesses, or in delinquent behaviour.

Encouraging Parent Participation

Preventing or minimizing separation is a key nursing goal for the child who is hospitalized, but maintaining parent–child contact is also beneficial for the family. One of the best

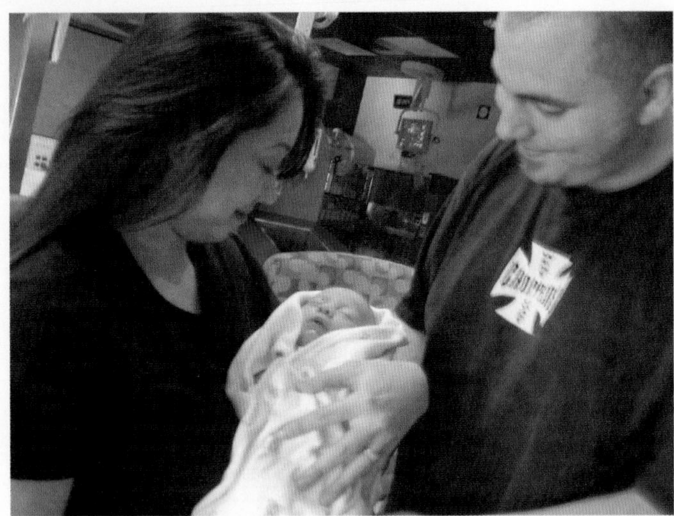

FIGURE 43-10 Parental presence during hospitalization provides emotional support for the child and increases the parent's sense of empowerment in the caregiver role. (Courtesy E. Jacob, Texas Children's Hospital.)

approaches is encouraging parents to stay with their child and to participate in the care whenever possible (Fig. 43-10). Although some health facilities provide special accommodations for parents, the concept of rooming-in can be instituted anywhere. The first requirement is the staff's positive attitude toward parents. A negative attitude toward parent participation can create barriers to collaborative working relationships.

When hospital staff members genuinely appreciate the importance of continued parent–child attachment, they foster an environment that encourages parents to stay. When parents are included in the care planning and understand that they are contributing to the child's recovery, they are more inclined to remain with their child and have more emotional reserves to support themselves and the child through the crisis. In an empowerment model of helping, the nurse focuses on parents' strengths and seeks ways to promote growth and family functioning so that the parents can gain more confidence in caring for their child. Strategies such as bedside reporting that allow parents to be involved in the discussion of the child's current status are moving health care settings closer to family-centred care (Uhl, Fisher, Docherty, et al., 2013).

Not all parents feel equally comfortable assuming responsibility for their child's care. Some may be under such great emotional stress that they need a temporary reprieve from total participation in caregiving activities. Others may feel insecure in participating in specialized areas of care, such as bathing the child after surgery. On the other hand, some parents may feel a great need to control their child's care. Individual assessment of each parent's preferred involvement is necessary to prevent the effects of separation while supporting parents in their needs.

With lifestyles and gender roles changing, fathers may assume all or some of the usual "mothering" roles in the household, and it may be the father–child relationship that requires preservation. Fathers need to be included in the care plan and respected for their parental role. For some fathers the child's hospitalization may represent an opportunity to alter their usual caregiving role and increase their involvement. In lone-parent families the caregiver may not be a parent but an extended family member, such as a grandparent or aunt.

One of the potential problems with continuous parent involvement is neglect of the parent's need for sleep, nutrition, and relaxation. Often the sleeping accommodations are limited to a chair, and sleep is disrupted by nursing procedures. Encouraging the parents to leave for brief periods, arranging for sleeping quarters on the unit but outside the child's room, and planning a schedule of alternating visits with another family member can minimize the stresses for the parent.

All too often, nurses respond to parent participation by abandoning their patient responsibilities. Nurses need to restructure their roles to complement and augment the parents' caregiving functions. Even in units structured to provide care by parents, parents frequently feel anxiety in their caregiving responsibilities. Therefore, 24-hour responsibility may be too much for some parents. Assistance and relief by nursing personnel should always be available to these families, and nurses may need to work to establish the strong bond of trust that some parents need in order to take advantage of these opportunities.

Preparing for Discharge and Home Care

Most hospitalizations necessitate some type of discharge preparation. Often this involves education of the family regarding continued care and follow-up in the home. Depending on the diagnosis, this may be relatively simple or highly complex. Preparing the family for home care demands a high degree of competence in planning and implementing discharge instructions.

Nurses are often key individuals in initiating and carrying out the discharge process. They collaborate with others in the planning and implementation phases to ensure appropriate care after hospitalization. Throughout the hospitalization the nurse should be aware of the need for discharge planning and those assessment factors that affect the family's ability to provide home care. (See Chapter 42 for more information on home care referrals and preparation.)

CARE OF THE CHILD AND FAMILY IN SPECIAL HOSPITAL SITUATIONS

In addition to a general pediatric unit, children may be admitted to special facilities such as an ambulatory or outpatient setting, an isolation room, or critical care.

Ambulatory or Outpatient Setting

The ambulatory or outpatient setting provides needed medical services for the child while eliminating the necessity of overnight admission. The benefits of ambulatory care are (1) minimized stressors of hospitalization, especially separation from the family; (2) reduced chances of infection; and (3) increased cost savings. Admission to the ambulatory or outpatient hospital setting usually is for surgical or diagnostic procedures, such as insertion of tympanostomy tubes, hernia repair, adenoidectomy, tonsillectomy, cystoscopy, or bronchoscopy.

In the ambulatory or outpatient setting, adequate preparation is particularly challenging. Ideally, the child and parents should receive preadmission preparation, including a tour of the facility and a review of the day's events. Parents need information in advance to help prepare the child and themselves for surgery and enable them to care for the child at home after the procedure. Parents also appreciate suggestions for items to bring to the hospital, such as blankets or stuffed animals. When preadmission preparation is not possible, time should be allowed on the day of the procedure for children to become acquainted with their surroundings and for nurses to assess, plan, and implement appropriate teaching.

Explicit discharge instructions are important after outpatient surgery (see Family-Centred Teaching box and Preparing for Discharge and Home Care, above). Parents need guidelines on when to call their practitioner regarding a change in the child's condition. A follow-up telephone call enables nurses to check on the child's progress within 48 to 72 hours after discharge. It also provides an opportunity for the nurse to review discharge information and answer questions.

Isolation

Admission to an isolation room increases all of the stressors typically associated with hospitalization. There is further separation from familiar persons; additional loss of control; and added environmental changes, such as sensory deprivation and the strange appearance of visitors. Orientation to time and place is affected. These stressors are compounded by children's limited understanding of isolation. Preschool children have difficulty understanding the rationale for isolation because they cannot comprehend the cause-and-effect relationship between germs and illness. They are likely to view isolation as punishment. Older children understand the causality better but still require information to decrease fantasizing or misinterpretation.

When a child is placed in isolation, preparation is essential for the child to feel in control. With young children the best approach is a simple explanation, such as "You need to be in this room to help you get better. This is a special place to make all the germs go away. The germs made you sick, and you could not help that."

All children, but especially younger ones, need preparation in terms of what they will see, hear, or feel in isolation. They should be shown the mask, gloves, and gown and be encouraged to "dress up" in them. Playing with the strange apparel lessens the fear of seeing "ghostlike" people walk into the room. Before entering the room, nurses and other health personnel should introduce themselves and let the child see their face before

FAMILY-CENTRED TEACHING

Discharge From Ambulatory Settings

Before beginning the discharge, explain that all instructions will also be presented in writing for the family to refer to later.

Provide an overview of the typical trajectory (expected pattern) of recovery.

Discuss expected progression of the child's activity level during the postdischarge period, such as "Sophia will probably sleep for the rest of the day, feel kind of tired most of tomorrow, but be back to her usual activities the next day."

Explain which activities the child is allowed to do and what is not permitted (e.g., bedrest, bathing).

Discuss dietary restrictions, being very specific and giving examples of "clear fluids" or what is meant by a "full liquid diet."

Discuss nausea and vomiting, if applicable, explaining how much is "normal" and what to do if more occurs, such as "Juan may be sick to his stomach and vomit. This is normal. However, if he vomits more than three times, please call us at this number right away."

Discuss fever and appropriate comfort measures, explaining how much fever is considered "normal," and specifically what to do if the child goes beyond the range.

Explain the amount, location, and kind of pain or discomfort the child may experience.

- Send an age-appropriate pain scale home with the family.
- Explain how much pain and discomfort is "normal" and what to do if the child surpasses that level or if pain management interventions are unsuccessful.
- Discuss pain management, including dosages for pain medications and details on how to administer them.
- Describe appropriate nonpharmacological comfort measures, such as holding, or rocking. Give any prescribed medication before leaving the facility.

Provide information about each medication that the child will be taking at home.

- Review the details, including dose and route.
- Demonstrate how to administer medications, if necessary (e.g., how to take wrapping off suppositories, how to insert).
- Discuss guidelines for requesting other medications.
- Request that all prescriptions be filled and given to the family before discharge.

Make certain the family has all of the equipment and supplies (e.g., gauze and tape for dressing changes) they will need at home.

Discuss complications that may occur and the steps to take if they do.

Ensure that appropriate measures are in place for safe transport home.

- Remind the family to use a seat belt or car seat for the child.
- Determine whether there will be one person whose sole responsibility is helping ensure the child's safety and comfort during transport.
- Discuss measures the driver may need to take if this is impossible (e.g., be certain a basin is within the child's reach should vomiting occur; take a route that permits slower traffic and has places along the roadside to stop, if necessary).
- Determine the availability of a blanket, pillow, and cup with a lid and straw for the child's use in the car.
- Provide a basin or plastic bag in case of vomiting.

Provide emergency phone numbers for the family to call with any concerns.

Explain that the family will be contacted (give an approximate time) to follow up on the child but that they should not hesitate to call if concerns arise before then.

Ask the family and child, if appropriate, if they have any questions, and problem solve with family members to meet their unique needs.

donning a mask. In this way, the child associates them with significant experiences and gains a sense of familiarity in an otherwise strange and lonely environment.

When the child's condition improves, appropriate play activities should be provided to minimize boredom, stimulate the senses, provide a real or perceived sense of movement, orient the child to time and place, provide social interaction, and reduce depersonalization. For example, the environment can be manipulated to increase sensory freedom by moving the bed toward the door or window. Opening window shades; providing musical, visual, or tactile toys; and increasing interpersonal contact can substitute mental mobility for the limitations of physical movement. Rather than dwelling on the negative aspects of isolation, the child can be encouraged to view this experience as challenging and positive. For example, the nurse can help the child look at isolation as a method of keeping others out and letting only special people in. Children often think of intriguing signs for their doors, such as "Enter at your own risk." These signs also encourage people "on the outside" to talk with the child about the ominous greeting.

Emergency Admission

One of the most traumatic hospital experiences for the child and parents is an **emergency** admission. The sudden onset of an illness or the occurrence of an injury leaves little time for preparation and explanation. Sometimes the emergency admission is compounded by admission to a critical care unit (CCU) or the need for immediate surgery. However, even in those instances requiring only outpatient treatment, the child is exposed to a strange, frightening environment and to experiences that may elicit fear or cause pain.

There is a wide discrepancy between what constitutes a medically defined emergency and a patient-defined emergency. A growing concern is the use of major emergency departments for routine primary care health visits. To offset overcrowding in emergency departments, many facilities have minor emergency units or pediatric minor emergency units for after-hours health care. Telephone triage for minor illnesses for patients is also emerging as a health care delivery mode to differentiate illnesses such as a common cold from true life-threatening conditions that require immediate practitioner attention and intervention. Other factors contributing to the overuse of emergency departments (as opposed to the primary practitioner's office) include the increasing number of households in which both parents work full time and cannot afford to take time off during the daytime to take the sick child to a practitioner.

In pediatric populations most visits to an emergency department are for respiratory infections. The most common reason parents give for bringing the child to the emergency department is concern about the illness worsening. However, practitioners may not think that the progressive symptoms necessitate immediate or emergency care. One of the nurse's primary goals is to assess the parents' perception of the event and their reasons for considering it serious or life threatening.

Lengthy preparatory admission procedures are often inappropriate for emergency situations. In such instances, nurses must focus their nursing interventions on the essential components of admission counselling (Box 43-10) and complete the process as soon as the child's condition has stabilized.

Unless an emergency is life threatening, children need to participate in their care to maintain a sense of control. Because emergency departments are frequently hectic, there is a tendency to rush through procedures to save time. However, the extra few minutes needed to allow children to participate may save many more minutes of resistance during subsequent procedures. Other supportive measures include ensuring privacy; accepting various emotional responses to fear or pain; preserving parent–child contact; explaining all events before or as they occur; and remaining calm. Pain management strategies are discussed in Chapter 34.

At times, because of the child's physical condition, little or no preparatory counselling for emergency hospitalization can be done. In such situations counselling subsequent to the event has therapeutic value. Counselling should focus on evaluating children's thoughts regarding admission and related procedures. It is similar to precounselling techniques; however, instead of supplying information, the nurse listens to the explanations offered by the child. Projective techniques such as drawing, doll play, or storytelling are especially effective. The nurse can then base additional information on what has already been understood.

Critical Care Unit

Admission to a CCU can be traumatic for both the child and parents. The nature and severity of the illness and the circumstances surrounding the admission are major factors, especially for parents. Parents experience significantly more stress when the admission is unexpected rather than expected. Stressors for the child and parent are described in Box 43-11. The most effective strategy to assist with overcoming parental stress levels may be to simply ask parents what is stressful and implement interventions that will enhance their ability to cope. Assessment should be repeated periodically to account for changes in perceptions over time. In one study, the use of daily patient goal sheets was successful in improving communication among health care providers caring for children in the CCU (Rehder, Uhl, Meliones, et al., 2012). By clearly defining daily patient care goals, health care providers believed that care was improved.

The family's emotional needs are paramount, and family-centred care is needed when a child is admitted to a critical care unit. A major stressor for parents of a child in the CCU is the child's appearance (Latour, van Goudoever, Schuurman, et al., 2011). Although the same interventions discussed earlier for the stressors of separation and loss of control apply here, additional interventions may also benefit the family and child (see Box 43-11). In a qualitative study of 19 parents of 10 children in a critical care unit, parents reported that they simply wanted nurses to nurture the child in the same way the family would (Harbaugh, Tomlinson, & Kirschbaum, 2004). Nurse behaviours that exemplified caring and affection were perceived as helpful in decreasing stress. Behaviours perceived as not helpful included separating the child from the parents and communicating poorly with parents. Another research study evaluated parental concerns when their children were admitted to a CCU.

BOX 43-10 GUIDELINES FOR SPECIAL HOSPITAL ADMISSION

Emergency Admission

Focus assessment on airway, breathing, and circulation; weigh child whenever possible for calculation of drug dosages.

Unless an emergency is life threatening, children need to participate in their care to maintain a sense of control.

Focus on essential components of admission counselling:

- Appropriate introduction to the family
- Use of child's name, not terms such as "honey" or "dear"
- Determination of child's age and some judgement about developmental age (If the child is of school age, asking about the grade level will offer some evidence of intellectual ability.)
- Information about child's general state of health, any problems that may interfere with medical treatment (e.g., allergies), and previous experience with hospital facilities
- Information about the chief concern, from both the parents and the child

Admission to Critical Care Unit

Prepare child and parents for elective critical care unit (CCU) admission, such as for postoperative care after cardiac surgery.

Prepare child and parents for unanticipated CCU admission by focusing primarily on the sensory aspects of the experience and on the usual family concerns (e.g., persons in charge of child's care, visiting guidelines, area where family can stay).

Prepare parents for child's appearance and behaviour when they first visit their child in the CCU.

Accompany family to bedside to provide emotional support and answer questions.

Prepare siblings for their visit; plan length of time for sibling visitation; monitor siblings' reactions during visit to prevent them from becoming overwhelmed.

Encourage parents to stay with their child:

- If visiting hours are limited, allow flexibility in the schedule to accommodate parental needs.
- Give family members a written schedule of visiting guidelines.
- If visiting hours are liberal, be aware of family members' needs and suggest periodic respites.
- Assure family that they can call the unit at any time.

Prepare parents for expected role changes and identify ways for parents to participate in the child's care without overwhelming them with responsibilities:

- Help with bath or feeding.
- Touch and talk to the child.
- Help with procedures.

Provide information about the child's condition in understandable language:

- Repeat information often.
- Seek clarification of understanding.
- During bedside conferences, interpret information for family members and the child or, if appropriate, conduct report outside the room.

Prepare child for procedures, even if this involves explanation while the procedure is performed.

Assess and manage pain; recognize that a child who cannot talk, such as an infant or child in a coma or on mechanical ventilation, can be in pain.

Establish a routine that maintains some similarity to daily events in the child's life whenever possible:

- Organize care during normal waking hours.
- Keep regular bedtime schedules, including quiet times when television or radio volume is lowered or turned off.
- Provide uninterrupted sleep cycles (60 minutes for infant, 90 minutes for older child).
- Close and open drapes and dim lights to establish day–night pattern.
- Place curtain around bed for privacy.
- Orient child to day and time; have clocks or calendars in easy view for older children.

Schedule a time when the child is left undisturbed (e.g., during naps, visits with family, playtime, or favourite programs).

Provide opportunities for play.

Reduce stimulation in environment:

- Refrain from loud talking or laughing.
- Keep equipment noise to a minimum:
  - Turn alarms as low as safely possible.
  - Perform treatments requiring equipment at one time.
  - Turn off bedside equipment that is not in use, such as suction and oxygen.
- Avoid loud, abrupt noises.

The parents experienced a variety of stressors, including trauma, anxiety about where the child is, post-traumatic stress symptoms, and transfer to the ward, but admission to the unit and discharge from the unit created the most anxiety (Oxley, 2015). It is important that visiting hours be liberal and flexible enough to accommodate parental needs and involvement.

Critically ill children become the focus of the parents' lives, and parents' most pressing need is for information. They want to know if their child will live and, if so, whether the child will be the same as before. They need to know why various interventions are being done for the child, that the child is being treated for pain or is comfortable, and that the child may be able to hear them even though not awake. Ideally, the nurse should answer any questions.

Despite the stresses normally associated with CCU admission, a special security develops from being carefully monitored and receiving individualized care. Therefore, planning for transition to the regular unit is essential and should include the following:

- Assignment of a primary nurse on the regular unit
- Continued visits by the CCU staff to assess the child's and parents' adjustment and to act as a temporary liaison with the nursing staff
- Explanation of the differences between the two units and the rationale for the change to less intense monitoring of the child's physical condition
- Selection of an appropriate room, such as one that is close to the nursing station, and a compatible roommate

BOX 43-11 NEONATAL OR PEDIATRIC CRITICAL CARE UNIT STRESSORS FOR THE CHILD AND FAMILY

Physical Stressors

Pain and discomfort (e.g., injections, intubation, suctioning, dressing changes, other invasive procedures)
Immobility (e.g., use of restraints, bedrest)
Sleep deprivation
Inability to eat or drink
Changes in elimination habits

Environmental Stressors

Unfamiliar surroundings (e.g., crowding)
Unfamiliar sounds
- Equipment noise (e.g., monitors, telephone, suctioning, computer printout)
- Human sounds (e.g., talking, laughing, crying, coughing, moaning, retching, walking)

Unfamiliar people (e.g., health care providers, patients, visitors)
Unfamiliar and unpleasant smells (e.g., alcohol, adhesive remover, body odours)
Constant lights (disturb day–night rhythms)
Activity related to other patients
Sense of urgency among staff
Unkind or thoughtless comments from staff

Psychological Stressors

Lack of privacy
Inability to communicate (if intubated)
Inadequate knowledge and understanding of situation
Severity of illness
Parental behaviour (expression of concern)

Social Stressors

Disrupted relationships (especially with family and friends)
Concern with missing school or work
Play deprivation

Data primarily from Shudy, M., de Almeida, M. L., Ly, S., et al. (2006). Impact of pediatric critical illness and injury on families: A systematic literature review, *Pediatrics, 118*(3), 203–218.

KEY POINTS

- Children are particularly vulnerable to the stressors of illness and hospitalization because stress represents a change from the usual state of health and routine and because they possess limited coping mechanisms for handling stress.
- The major stressors of hospitalization for children include fear of separation, loss of control, bodily injury and pain.
- The three phases of separation anxiety are protest, despair, and detachment.
- Feelings of loss of control are caused by unfamiliar environmental stimuli, physical restriction, altered routine, and dependency.
- Because of their separation from significant people, children who are hospitalized may lack the opportunity to form new attachments in the strange environment of the hospital and exhibit negative behaviours after discharge.
- Nursing care of the child in the hospital is aimed at preventing or minimizing separation, decreasing loss of control, minimizing fear of bodily injury, using play or expressive activities to lessen stress, and maximizing the potential benefits of hospitalization.
- The nurse can maximize potential benefits of hospitalization by fostering parent–child relations, providing educational opportunities, promoting self-mastery, and encouraging socialization.
- Family reactions are influenced by the seriousness of the illness, experience with illness or hospitalization and diagnostic or therapeutic procedures, available support systems, personal ego strengths, coping abilities, presence of additional stressors, cultural and religious beliefs, and family communication patterns.
- Siblings' fear of contracting illness, their younger age, a close relationship with the ill sibling, substitute child care, minimal explanation of the illness, and perceived changes in parenting all increase the deleterious effects of a brother's or sister's illness and hospitalization on siblings.
- Nursing care of the family involves listening to parents' verbal and nonverbal messages; providing clergy support; accepting cultural, socioeconomic, and ethnic values; giving information to families and siblings; and preparing them for discharge and home care.
- Admission to an outpatient setting, emergency department, isolation room, or CCU requires additional intervention strategies to meet the child's and family's needs.

evolve WEBSITE

***Visit the Evolve website for additional resources related to the content in this chapter such as Case Studies, Critical Thinking Case Study Answers, Nursing Care Plans, Nursing Processes, Nursing Skills, and Review Questions for Exam Preparation at:** http://evolve.elsevier.com/Canada/Perry/maternal/*

REFERENCES

Accreditation Canada. (2010). *Standards*. Retrieved from <https://accreditation.ca/quality-matters>.

Al-Yateem, N. S., Banni, I., & Rossiter, R. (2015). Childhood stress in healthcare settings: Awareness and suggested interventions. *Issues in Comprehensive Pediatric Nursing, 38*(2), 36–53. doi:10.3109/01460862.2015.1035465.

BC Children's Hospital. (2016). *School services*. Retrieved from <http://www.bcchildrens.ca/our-services/support-services/school-services>.

Canadian Institute of Child Health. (2002). *The rights of the child in the health care system (pamphlet)*. Retrieved from *Journal of Obstetric, Gynecologic & Neonatal Nursing*.

Commodari, E. (2010). Children staying in hospital: A research on psychological stress of caregivers. *Italian Journal of Pediatrics, 36*, 40. doi:10.1186/1824-7288-36-40.

Coyne, I., & Kirwan, L. (2012). Ascertaining children's wishes and feelings about hospital life. *Journal of Child Health Care, 16*(3), 293–304. doi:10.1177/1367493512443905.

Giambra, B. K., Stiffler, D., & Broome, M. E. (2014). An integrative review of communication between parents and nurses of hospitalized technology-dependent children. *Worldviews on Evidence-based Nursing, 11*(6), 369–375. doi:10.1111/wvn.12065.

Harbaugh, B. L., Tomlinson, P. S., & Kirschbaum, M. (2004). Parents' perceptions of nurses' caregiving behaviors in the pediatric intensive care unit. *Issues in Comprehensive Pediatric Nursing, 27*(3), 163–178.

Health Canada. (2015). *Natural and non-prescription health products*. Retrieved from <http://www.hc-sc.gc.ca/dhp-mps/prodnatur/index-eng.php/>.

Latour, J. M., van Goudoever, J. B., Schuurman, B. E., et al. (2011). A qualitative study exploring the experiences of parents of children admitted to seven Dutch pediatric intensive care units. *Intensive Care Medicine, 37*(2), 319–325. doi:10.1007/s00134-010-2074-3.

Nicholas, D. B., Fellner, K. D., Koller, D., et al. (2011). Evaluation of videophone communication for families of hospitalized children. *Social Work Health Care, 50*(3), 215–229. doi:10.1080/00981389.2010.531998.

Oxley, R. (2015). Parents' experiences of their child's admission to paediatric intensive care. *Nursing Children and Young People, 27*(4), 16–21. doi:10.7748/ncyp.27.4.16.e564.

Rehder, J. K., Uhl, T. L., Meliones, J. N., et al. (2012). Targeted interventions improved shared agreement of daily goals in the pediatric intensive care unit. *Pediatric Critical Care Medicine, 13*(1), 6–10.

Salmela, M., Aronen, E. T., & Salanterä, S. (2011). The experience of hospital-related fears of 4- to 6-year-old children. *Child: Care, Health & Development, 37*(5), 719–726. doi:10.1111/j.1365-2214.2010.01171.x.

Stratton, K. M. (2004). Parents' experiences of their child's care during hospitalization. *Journal of Cultural Diversity, 11*(1), 4–11.

Thompson, R. (2009). *The handbook of child life: A guide for pediatric psychosocial care*. Springfield, IL: Charles C. Thomas.

Uhl, T., Fisher, K., Docherty, S. L., et al. (2013). Insights into patient and family-centered care through the hospital experiences of parents. *Journal of Obstetric, Gynecologic & Neonatal Nursing, 42*(1), 121–131. doi:10.1111/1552-6909.12001.

Wilson, M. E., Megel, M. E., Eneback, L., et al. (2010). The voices of children: Stories about hospitalization. *Journal of Pediatric Health Care, 24*(2), 95–102.

ADDITIONAL RESOURCES

Health Canada: About Natural Health Products: <http://www.hc-sc.gc.ca/dhp-mps/prodnatur/about-apropos/cons-eng.php>.

Ronald McDonald House Charities Canada: <http://www.rmhccanada.ca/>.

The Hospital for Sick Children: About Kids' Health: <http://www.aboutkidshealth.ca/En/HealthAZ/Pages/default.aspx?name=A>.

CHAPTER

44

Pediatric Variations of Nursing Interventions

Cheryl Sams, with contributions from Marilyn J. Hockenberry

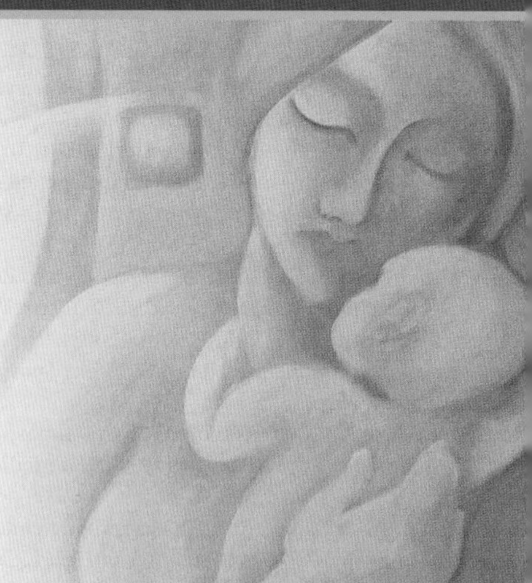

evolve WEBSITE

Visit the Evolve website for additional resources related to the content in this chapter such as Case Studies, Critical Thinking Case Study Answers, Nursing Care Plans, Nursing Processes, Nursing Skills, and Review Questions for Exam Preparation at: http://evolve.elsevier.com/Canada/Perry/maternal/

OBJECTIVES

On completion of this chapter the reader will be able to:

- Identify those instances in which informed consent is required from parents or legal guardians and when minors may be considered emancipated and can provide their own informed consent.
- Formulate general guidelines for preparing children for procedures, including surgery.
- Implement play in therapeutic procedures for children.
- List general strategies for ensuring that children and families make informed choices regarding a treatment plan and are able to follow it.
- Outline general hygiene and care procedures for hospitalized children.
- Implement feeding techniques that encourage a child's food and fluid intake.
- Describe methods of reducing the temperature of a child with fever or hyperthermia.
- Describe the body's systems that can be used for infection control.
- Describe safe methods of administering oral, parenteral, rectal, optic, otic, and nasal medications to children.
- Identify nursing responsibilities in maintaining fluid balance in pediatric patients.
- Demonstrate correct procedures for postural drainage and tracheostomy care in children.
- Describe the procedures involved in providing nutrition via gavage, gastrostomy, and parenteral routes.
- Describe the procedures involved in administering an enema and ostomy care to children.

GENERAL CONCEPTS RELATED TO PEDIATRIC PROCEDURES

Informed Consent

Before undergoing any invasive procedure, the patient, the patient's legal surrogate, or both must receive sufficient information on which to make an informed health care decision. All decisions should be based on a combination of known facts and personal values. In health care, treatment decisions relate to medical information and personal evaluation of this information. In order to make appropriate decisions, individuals and families must have pertinent information, be able to understand how it applies to themselves or their children, and then make a voluntary decision. The following guidelines of medical decision making define the three hallmarks of informed choice (Fernandez & Canadian Paediatric Society [CPS], Bioethics Committee, 2008/2016):

1. **Appropriate information:** Appropriate decisions can only be made with sufficient information.
2. **Decision-making capacity:** The person with decision-making capacity must have more than the simple ability to understand. He or she must be able to realize the purpose of the intervention, the consequences of consent or refusal, the alternatives, and the magnitude and probabilities of harm and benefit.
3. **Voluntariness:** The decision maker should not be manipulated or coerced, and the option to change one's mind should always be available.

The patient or legal guardian has the right to accept or refuse any health care. If a patient is treated without consent, the hospital or health care provider may be charged with battery. *Battery* is defined as any intentional physical contact with a person without that person's consent, which can create a situation in which the patient or legal guardian could sue the nurse. The contact can be harmful to the patient and cause an injury, or it can be considered to be offensive to the patient's personal dignity (Shapiro, 2014; Sneiderman, Irvine, & Osborne, 2003). *Assault* is conduct (such as a physical or verbal threat) that creates in another person apprehension or fear of imminent harmful or offensive contact. No actual contact is necessary in order for damages for assault to be awarded to the patient or legal guardian (Shapiro, 2014; Sneiderman et al., 2003) and held liable for damages in a lawsuit.

Requirements for Obtaining Informed Consent

Written informed consent is usually required for medical or surgical treatment, including many diagnostic procedures. One universal consent for all procedures is not sufficient. For example, when a child is admitted to a hospital, the child or parents or legal guardian needs to sign an informed general consent for noninvasive tests and procedures such as radiographs and urine testing. Separate informed permissions must be obtained for each surgical or invasive diagnostic procedure, including major or minor surgery; diagnostic tests with an element of risk, such as bronchoscopy; and medical treatments with an element of risk, such as blood transfusion and radiotherapy.

Children who have partial skills to make decisions should be recognized as having some authority over their own health care. This can be achieved through the concept of *assent*, whereby children are given both information that they can understand and some appropriate choice in their treatment. Assent should include the following elements:

- Helping the patient achieve a developmentally appropriate awareness of the nature of his or her condition
- Telling the patient what he or she can expect
- Making a clinical assessment of the patient's understanding
- Soliciting an expression of the patient's willingness to accept the proposed procedure of care

Multiple methods should be used to provide information, including age-appropriate resources such as DVDs, Internet sources, peer discussion, diagrams, and written materials.

Eligibility for Giving Informed Consent

Informed consent for minors. In most parts of Canada, there is no specific legal age for medical consent; instead, the patient's ability to understand and make decisions regarding their own condition, the treatment, and its consequences is more important than his or her chronological age. Québec is the only exception to this practice and stipulates an age of consent (14 years) (Canadian Medical Protective Association, 2006). It is important for the nurse to be aware of the procedures and laws that govern informed consent for the province or territory and institution in which they work.

Evidence of consent. In obtaining informed consent, it is the health care provider's responsibility to explain the procedure, risks, benefits, and alternatives to the parents or legal guardians and to the child, if he or she is able to understand this information. This information needs to be conveyed in a way that is fitting to their personal circumstances and ensures their understanding of the treatment and alternatives, including associated risks and benefits. A physician witnesses the patient's, parent's, or legal guardian's signature on the signed consent and the nurse may reinforce what the patient and parents have been told. A signed *consent form* is the legal document that signifies that the process of informed consent has occurred. If parents are unavailable to sign consent forms, verbal consent may be obtained via telephone by a physician and the nurse can sign as the witness. When the nurse signs a consent form as a witness, she or he is not legally assuming the responsibility of informed consent, only that the patient or guardian signature is authentic and that the patient or guardian appears to be competent to give consent (Sneiderman et al., 2003).

Informed consent of emancipated minors. *Emancipated minors* are those who are no longer dependent on their parents or legal guardians. They may be supporting themselves or living independently from their families.

Emergency treatment without consent. An emergency exists if the patient is apparently experiencing severe suffering or is at risk of suffering serious bodily harm if treatment is not administered promptly. In cases of emergency when the patient is unable to consent and a substitute decision maker (guardian) is not readily available, a health practitioner must do what is immediately necessary without consent.

Conflicts in decision making for children. In some situations, conflict may arise if the values and beliefs of the parents differ from those of the health care team or even from each other. Although most conflicts involve a remediable breakdown in communication, sometimes a genuine clash in values exists. Parental decision making should be accepted by the health care team unless it is obvious to many that the decision is not in the best interest of the child or adolescent. If the health care team feels that the parental decisions are clearly inconsistent with the child's or adolescent's best interests and collaboration with other resources, ethics committees, or consultants has not resolved the situation, involvement of local child protection authorities and the legal system may be unavoidable, although this should only be used as a last resort (Harrison & CPS, Bioethics Committee, 2004/2016).

Consent and confidentiality. The *Personal Health Information Protection Act* of 2004 (PHIPA) was passed to help protect and safeguard the security and confidentiality of a person's health information. A capable individual, regardless of age, can consent to the collection, use, or disclosure of their own personal health information. If a child is incapable of consenting, a parent or legal guardian may do so on their behalf.

Consent for health research in children. Pediatric health research involves some special challenges. The researcher must take into consideration the vulnerability of the population and needs to mitigate any potential risks (see Chapter 1, Ethical Guidelines for Nursing Research, p. 12). There must not be any conflict of interest. A fully informed consent and assent must be signed by the parent or legal guardian or the child, if capable of consent. The Tri-Council Policy Statement on Ethical Conduct for Research Involving Humans is the tool researchers in Canada are required to utilize to ensure governance of both ethical and regulatory practices (see Additional Resources at the end of this chapter). Attaining an informed consent is the responsibility of the researchers and must follow the same principles as obtaining a medical consent (Fernandez & CPS, Bioethics Committee, 2008/2016). It is also important that the researchers take into consideration the cultural and community differences in various groups and populations, such as with Indigenous participants.

Preparation for Diagnostic and Therapeutic Procedures

Technological advances and changes in health care delivery have resulted in more pediatric procedures being performed in a variety of settings. Many of these procedures are both stressful and painful experiences. For most procedures the focus of care is on psychological preparation of the child and family.

Psychological Preparation

Preparation of children for procedures has the aim of decreasing their anxiety, promoting their assistance, supporting their coping skills, and facilitating a feeling of mastery in experiencing a potentially stressful event. Many institutions have developed preadmission teaching programs designed to educate children and their families by offering hands-on experience with hospital equipment, information about the procedure to be performed, and an overview of departments they may visit. Most preparation strategies used by nurses are informal, focus on providing information about the experience, and are directed at the child undergoing stressful or painful procedures. The most effective preparation is to provide sensory-procedural information and help the child develop coping skills, such as imagery, distraction, or relaxation.

Many pediatric hospitals offer a preoperative preparation program for children and families. A child life specialist and preanaesthesia nurse may be present to help prepare the child for the operative experience. There is often a tour of the operating room area, and children are able to play with medical equipment. Hospitals recommend that, if possible, any child requiring these services come to the tour about 1 to 2 weeks before the surgery. If for travel or medical reasons the family cannot make the tour in person, virtual tours are often available online. For example, the SickKids website has a video tour of the hospital and the operative suite as well as helpful tips for families on how to verbally prepare their child. See Additional Resources at the end of this chapter for more information.

General guidelines for preparing children for procedures are described in the Guidelines box, and age-specific preparation that takes into account children's developmental needs and cognitive abilities is presented in Box 44-1. In addition to these suggestions, nurses should consider the child's temperament, existing coping strategies, and previous experiences. Children who are distractible and highly active, as well as those who need more time to adapt, may need individualized sessions that are shorter for the active child or more slowly paced for the shy child. Youngsters who tend to cope well may need more emphasis on using their present skills, whereas those who appear to cope less adequately can benefit from more time devoted to simple coping strategies, such as relaxing, breathing, counting, squeezing a hand, or singing. Children with previous health-related experiences still need preparation for repeat or new procedures; the nurse must assess what they know, correct their misconceptions, supply new information, and introduce new coping skills as indicated by their previous reactions. Especially for painful procedures, the most effective preparation includes providing sensory-procedural information and helping the child develop coping skills, such as imagery or relaxation.

Children differ in their "information-seeking dimension." Some actively ask for information about the intended procedure, while others characteristically avoid it. Parents can often guide nurses in deciding how much information is enough for their child, because they know whether he or she is typically inquisitive or satisfied with short answers. Asking older children their preferences about the amount of explanation is also important.

The exact timing of the preparation for a procedure varies with the child's age and type of procedure. While no exact guidelines govern timing, in general, the younger the child, the closer the explanation should be to the actual procedure, to prevent undue fantasizing and worrying. With complex procedures, more time may be needed for assimilation of information, especially with older children. For example, the explanation for an injection can immediately precede the procedure for all ages, whereas preparation for surgery may begin the day before for young children and a few days before for older children (although older children's preferences should be elicited).

Establish trust and provide support. The nurse who has spent time with and established a positive relationship with a child will usually find it easier to work together with the child. If the relationship is based on trust, the child will associate the nurse with caregiving activities that provide comfort and pleasure most of the time, rather than discomfort and stress. If the nurse does not know the child, it is best to be introduced by another staff person whom the child trusts. The first visit with the child should not include any painful procedure and ideally should focus on the child first, then on the explanation of the procedure.

Parental presence and support. Children need support during procedures, and for young children the greatest source of support is the parents. They represent security, safety, protection, and comfort. A British research study found that children who had their parents present during invasive procedures had lowered respirations and heart rate levels, felt less pain, and were in less distress (Matziou, Chrysostomou, Vlahioti, et al., 2013). However, the nurse should assess the parents' preferences for assisting, observing, or waiting outside the room, as well as the child's preference for parental presence. The child's and parents' choices should be respected. Parental presence is preferable as it can reduce patient and parent anxiety and decrease the need for sedation. Parents who wish to stay should be given an appropriate explanation about the procedure and coached

BOX 44-1 AGE-SPECIFIC PREPARATION OF CHILDREN FOR PROCEDURES, BASED ON DEVELOPMENTAL CHARACTERISTICS

Infant: Developing a Sense of Trust and Sensorimotor Thought

Attachment to Parent

Involve parent in procedure, if desired.*

Keep parent in infant's line of vision.

If parent is unable to be with infant, place a familiar object with infant (e.g., stuffed toy).

Stranger Anxiety

Have usual caregivers perform or assist with procedure.*

Make advances slowly and in a nonthreatening manner.

Limit number of strangers entering the room during procedure.*

Sensorimotor Phase of Learning

During procedure, use sensory soothing measures such as stroking skin, talking softly, giving pacifier.

Use analgesics, such as topical anaesthetic, intravenous opioid, to control discomfort.*

Cuddle and hug infant after stressful procedure; encourage parent to comfort infant.

Increased Muscle Control

Expect an older infant to resist.

Restrain adequately.

Keep harmful objects out of reach.

Memory for Past Experiences

Realize that older infants may associate objects, places, or persons with prior painful experiences and will cry and resist at the sight of them.

Keep frightening objects out of view.*

Perform painful procedures in a separate room, not in crib (or bed).*

Use nonintrusive procedures whenever possible, such as axillary temperatures, oral medications.*

Imitation of Gestures

Model desired behaviour, such as opening mouth.

Toddler: Developing a Sense of Autonomy and Sensorimotor to Preoperational Thought

Use the same approaches as for an infant, plus the following.

Egocentric Thought

Explain procedure in relation to what the child will see, hear, taste, smell, and feel.

Emphasize those aspects of procedure that require cooperation, such as lying still.

Tell the child it is okay to cry, yell, or use other means to express discomfort verbally.

Designate one health care provider to speak during procedures. Hearing more than one can be confusing for the child.*

Negative Behaviour

Expect treatments to be resisted; the child may try to run away.

Use a firm, direct approach.

Ignore temper tantrums.

Use distraction techniques, such as singing a song with the child.

Restrain adequately.

Animism

Keep frightening objects out of view (young children believe objects have lifelike qualities and can harm them).

Limited Language Skills

Communicate using gestures or demonstrations.

Use a few simple terms familiar to the child.

Give the child one direction at a time, such as "Lie down," then "Hold my hand."

Use small replicas of equipment; allow the child to handle equipment.

Use play; demonstrate on a doll but avoid using the child's favourite doll, since the child may think that the doll is really "feeling" the procedure.

Prepare parents separately to avoid child's misinterpreting of words.

Limited Concept of Time

Prepare the child shortly or immediately before procedure.

Keep teaching sessions short (about 5 to 10 minutes).

Have preparations completed before involving child in procedure.

Have extra equipment nearby, such as alcohol swabs, new needle, adhesive bandages, to avoid delays.

Tell the child when the procedure is completed.

Striving for Independence

Allow choices whenever possible; the child may still be resistant and negative.

Allow child to participate in care and to help whenever possible, such as drink medicine from a cup, hold a dressing.

Preschooler: Developing Initiative and Preoperational Thought

Egocentric

Explain procedure in simple terms and in relation to how it affects the child (as with toddler, stress sensory aspects).

Demonstrate use of equipment.

Allow child to play with miniature or actual equipment.

Encourage "playing out" experience on a doll both before and after procedure to clarify misconceptions.

Use neutral words to describe the procedure.

Increased Language Skills

Use verbal explanation; avoid overestimating comprehension.

Encourage child to express ideas and feelings.

Limited Concept of Time and Frustration Tolerance

Implement the same approaches as for toddlers but a longer teaching session (10 to 15 minutes) may be planned; information may be divided into more than one session.

Continued

BOX 44-1 AGE-SPECIFIC PREPARATION OF CHILDREN FOR PROCEDURES, BASED ON DEVELOPMENTAL CHARACTERISTICS—cont'd

Illness and Hospitalization Viewed as Punishment

Clarify why each procedure is performed; a child will find it difficult to understand how medicine can make him or her feel better and can taste bad at the same time.

Ask child his or her thoughts about why a procedure is performed.

State directly that procedures are never a form of punishment.

Animism

Keep equipment out of sight, except when shown to or used on the child.

Fears of Bodily Harm, Intrusion, and Castration

Point out on drawing, doll, or child where procedure is performed.

Emphasize that no other body part will be involved.

Use nonintrusive procedures whenever possible, such as axillary temperature, oral medication.

Apply an adhesive bandage over the puncture site.

Encourage parental presence.

Realize that procedures involving genitalia provoke anxiety.

Allow child to wear underpants with gown.

Explain unfamiliar situations, especially noises or lights.

Striving for Initiative

Involve child in care whenever possible, such as holding equipment, removing dressing.

Give choices whenever possible but avoid excessive delays.

Praise child for helping and attempting to cooperate; never shame a child for lack of cooperation.

School-Age Child: Developing Industry and Concrete Thought

Increased Language Skills; Interest in Acquiring Knowledge

Explain procedures, using correct scientific or medical terminology.

Explain reason for procedure, using simple diagrams and photographs.

Explain function and operation of equipment in concrete terms.

Allow child to manipulate equipment; use doll or another person as a model to practise, using equipment whenever possible (doll play may be considered childish by older school-age child).

Allow time before and after procedure for questions and discussion.

Improved Concept of Time

Plan for longer teaching sessions (about 20 minutes).

Prepare up to 1 day in advance of procedure to allow for processing information.

Increased Self-Control

Gain child's trust.

Tell child what is expected.

Suggest several ways of maintaining control from which the child may select, such as deep breathing, relaxation, counting.

Striving for Industry

Give the child responsibility for simple tasks, such as collecting specimens.

Include child in decision making, such as time of day to perform procedure, preferred site.

Encourage active participation removing dressings, handling equipment, opening packages.

Developing Relationships With Peers

Prepare two or more children for the same procedure or encourage one peer to help prepare another.

Provide privacy from peers during procedure to maintain self-esteem.

Adolescent: Developing Identity and Abstract Thought

Increasing Abstract Thought and Reasoning

Supplement explanations with reasons why the procedure is necessary or beneficial.

Explain long-term consequences of procedures; include information about body systems working together.

Realize that the adolescent may fear death, disability, or other potential risks.

Encourage questioning regarding fears, options, and alternatives.

Consciousness of Appearance

Provide privacy; describe how the body will be covered and what will be exposed.

Discuss how the procedure may affect appearance, such as scarring, and what can be done to minimize it.

Emphasize any physical benefits of procedure.

Concern More With Present Than With Future

Realize that immediate effects of the procedure are more significant than future benefits.

Striving for Independence

Involve adolescent in decision making and planning, such as time and place of procedure, individuals present during procedure, clothing.

Impose as few restrictions as possible.

Explore which coping strategies have worked in the past; adolescents may need descriptions to identify various techniques.

Accept regression to more childish methods of coping.

Realize that the adolescent may have difficulty accepting new authority figures and may resist complying with procedures.

Developing Peer Relationships and Group Identity

This is the same as for school-age children but assumes greater significance.

Allow adolescents to talk with other adolescents who have had the same procedure.

*Applies to any age.

GUIDELINES

Preparing Children for Procedures

- Determine details of exact procedure to be performed.
- Review parents' and child's current understanding.
- Base teaching on developmental age and existing knowledge.
- Incorporate parents in the teaching if they desire, especially if they plan to participate in care.
- Inform parents of their supportive role during the procedure, such as standing near the child's head or in the child's line of vision and talking softly to the child.
- Allow for ample discussion to prevent information overload and ensure adequate feedback.
- Use concrete, not abstract, terms and visual aids to describe the procedure. For example, use a simple line drawing of a boy or girl and mark the body part that will be involved in the procedure. Use nonthreatening but realistic models.
- Emphasize that no other body part will be involved.
- If the body part is associated with a specific function, stress the change in or noninvolvement of that ability, such as after tonsillectomy, the child can still speak.
- Use words appropriate to the child's level of understanding. (Rule of thumb: the number of words in a child's sentence is equal to his or her age in years plus 1.)
- Avoid words and phrases with dual meanings unless the child understands such words.
- Clarify all unfamiliar words, such as "Anaesthesia is a special sleep."
- Emphasize sensory aspects of the procedure—what the child will feel, see, hear, smell, and touch and what the child can do during the procedure, such as lie still, count out loud, squeeze a hand, hug a doll.
- Allow the child to practise procedures that require some assistance (e.g., turning, deep breathing, incentive spirometry).
- Introduce anxiety-laden information last, such as starting an intravenous line.
- Be honest with the child about unpleasant aspects of a procedure but avoid creating undue concern. When discussing that a procedure may be uncomfortable, state that it feels differently to different people.
- Emphasize the end of the procedure and any pleasurable events afterward (e.g., going home, seeing parents).
- Stress positive benefits of the procedure, such as "After your tonsils are fixed, you won't have as many sore throats."
- Provide a positive ending, praising efforts at being helpful and coping.

about what to do, and what to say in order to help the child through the procedure. Simple instructions such as clarifying where parents can stand or sit in the room and positioning them where they have eye contact with the child can provide support and lessen anxiety. Parents who do not want to be present or participate should be supported in their decision and encouraged to remain close by so that they can be available to console the child immediately after the procedure. Parents should also know that someone, such as another nurse or child life specialist, will be with their child to provide support. Ideally, this person should inform the parents after the procedure about how the child did.

Provide an explanation. Age-appropriate explanations are one of the most widely used interventions for reducing anxiety in children undergoing procedures. Teaching sessions should be planned at times most conducive to the child's learning, such as after a rest period, and for the usual span of attention. It is also important for nurses to communicate with nonthreatening language when preparing children for procedures (see Table 44-1).

TABLE 44-1 SELECTING NONTHREATENING WORDS OR PHRASES

WORDS AND PHRASES TO AVOID	SUGGESTED SUBSTITUTIONS
Shot, bee sting, stick	Medicine under the skin
Organ	Special place in body
Test	To see how (specify body part) is working
Incision, cut	Special opening
Edema	Puffiness
Stretcher, gurney	Rolling bed, bed on wheels
Stool	Child's usual term
Dye	Special medicine
Pain	Hurt, discomfort, "owie," "boo-boo," sore, achy, scratchy
Deaden	Numb, make sleepy
Fix	Make better
Take (as in "take your temperature")	See how warm you are
Take (as in "take your blood pressure")	Check your pressure; hug your arm
Put to sleep, anaesthesia	Special sleep so you won't feel anything
Catheter	Tube
Monitor	Television screen
Electrodes	Stickers, ticklers
Specimen	Sample

Special equipment is not necessary for preparing a child; but for young children who cannot yet think conceptually, using objects to supplement verbal explanation is important. Allowing children to handle actual items that will be used in their care, such as a stethoscope, sphygmomanometer, or oxygen mask, helps them develop familiarity with these items and reduces the fear often associated with their use. Miniature versions of hospital items such as stretchers and x-ray and intravenous (IV) equipment can be used to explain what the children can expect and permit them to safely experience situations that are unfamiliar and potentially frightening. Displayed photographs of children in different areas of the hospital (e.g., radiology department, operating room) can be used to give children a more realistic idea of equipment they may encounter.

Physical preparation. One area of special concern is the administration of sedation and analgesia before stressful procedures. Refer to Chapter 34 for information on sedating children.

Performance of the Procedure

Supportive care should continue during the procedure and can be a major factor in a child's ability to assist. Ideally, the same nurse who explains the procedure should perform or assist with the procedure.

Traumatic procedures should never be performed in "safe" areas, such as the playroom or the child's room, unless the child is a young infant or cannot be safely moved. If the procedure is lengthy, conversation that could be misinterpreted by the child should be avoided. As the procedure is nearing completion, the child needs to be informed that it is almost over, in language the child understands.

Expect success. Nurses who approach children with confidence and who convey the impression that they expect to be successful are less likely to encounter difficulty. It is best to approach a child with a welcoming and inclusive demeanour that encourages the child to assist with the proposed procedure. Children sense anxiety and uncertainty in an adult and may respond by striking out or actively resisting. Although it is not possible to eliminate such behaviour in every child, a firm approach with a positive attitude tends to convey a feeling of security to most children.

Involve the child. Involving children helps to gain their confidence and willingness to work together. When they are given choices they have some measure of control. However, a choice should be given only in situations in which one is available. Asking children, "Do you want to take your medicine now?" leads them to believe they have an option of not taking it and provides them with the opportunity to legitimately refuse or delay the medication. This places the nurse in an awkward, if not impossible, position. It is much better to state firmly, "It's time to drink your medicine now" and add a choice that they do indeed have, such as "Do you want to drink your medicine plain or with a little water?"

Many children respond to tactics that appeal to their maturity or courage. This also gives them a sense of participation and achievement. For example, preschool and school-age children will be proud that they can hold the dressing during the procedure or remove the tape.

Provide distraction. Distraction is a powerful coping strategy during painful procedures (Uman, Birnie, Noel, et al., 2013). It is accomplished by focusing the child's attention on something other than the procedure. Singing favourite songs, listening to music, counting out loud, or blowing bubbles to "blow the hurt away" are effective techniques. For other nonpharmacological interventions that may lessen discomfort, see Pain Management, Chapter 34.

Allow expression of feelings. The child should be allowed to express feelings of anger, anxiety, fear, frustration, or any other emotion. It is natural for children to strike out in frustration or to try to avoid stress-provoking situations. The child needs to know that it is all right to cry. Behaviour is children's primary means of communication and coping and should be permitted unless it inflicts harm on them or those caring for them.

Postprocedural Support

After the procedure, the child needs reassurance that he or she performed well and is accepted and loved. If the parents did not participate, the child should be united with them as soon as possible so that they can provide comfort.

Encourage expression of feelings. Planned activity after the procedure is helpful in encouraging constructive expression of feelings. For verbal children, reviewing the details of the procedure can clarify misconceptions and garner feedback for improving the nurse's preparatory strategies. Play is an excellent activity for all children. Infants and young children should be given the opportunity for gross motor movement. Older children are able to vent their anger and frustration in acceptable pounding or throwing activities. One of the most effective interventions is **therapeutic play**, which includes well-supervised activities, such as permitting the child to give an injection to a doll or stuffed toy to reduce the stress of injections (Fig. 44-1).

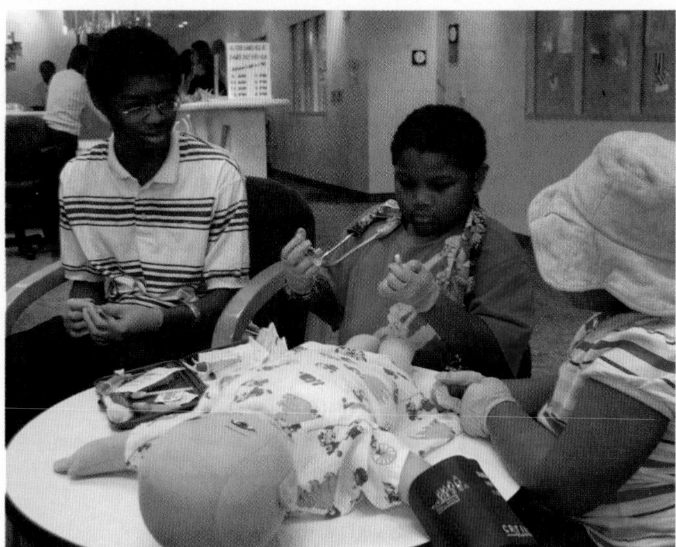

FIGURE 44-1 Playing with hospital equipment provides children with the opportunity to play out fears and concerns.

Provide positive reinforcement. Children need to hear from adults that they did the best they could in the situation, no matter how they behaved. It is important for children to know that their worth is not being judged on the basis of their behaviour in a stressful situation. Reward systems, such as earning stars, stickers, bravery beads, or a badge of courage, are appealing to children.

Returning to the child a short while after the procedure can help the nurse strengthen a supportive relationship. Relating with the child during a relaxed and nonstressful period allows the child to see the nurse not only as someone associated with stressful situations but as someone with whom to share pleasurable experiences.

Use of Play in Procedures

The use of play is an integral part of relationships with children. As such, its value in specific situations is discussed throughout this book, such as in Chapter 43, in relation to hospitalization. Many institutions have elaborate and well-organized play areas and programs under the direction of child life specialists. No matter what the institution provides for children, nurses can include play activities as part of nursing care. Play can be used to teach, express feelings, or achieve a therapeutic goal. Play sessions after procedures can be structured, as directed toward syringe play, or general, with a wide variety of equipment available for children to play with. Routine procedures such as measuring blood pressure and administering oral medication may be of concern to children. Box 44-2 offers suggestions for incorporating play into nursing procedures and activities for the hospitalized child that facilitate learning and adjustment to a new situation. Small play objects such as marbles or coins, as well as latex gloves or balloons, are unsafe for young children because of possible aspiration. Latex products also carry the risk of an allergic reaction.

Surgical Procedures

Preoperative Care

Children experiencing surgical procedures require both psychological and physical preparation. In general, psychological preparation is similar to that previously discussed for any procedure and employs many of the same techniques used in preparing a child for hospitalization, such as films, books, brochures, play, and tours. However, some important differences exist. Even though children are asleep for the actual surgical intervention, they are subjected to numerous preoperative and postoperative procedures. Stress points before and after surgery include the admission process, blood tests, IV insertions, injection of preoperative medication (if prescribed), transport to the operating room, and the stay in the postanaesthesia care unit (PACU).

Surprisingly little research has been conducted on children's perception of the surgical experience and their fears of the event. Although fear of **anaesthesia** is thought to be a major concern among children, little evidence exists to support this. School-age children report few remembered events and even fewer fears. Those events recalled most often were riding to and arriving in the operating room, receiving the preoperative or induction injection, waking up in pain, and not being allowed to eat or drink. The most feared events were the preoperative injection and the mask on the face.

Parental presence during induction of anaesthesia is allowed in some institutions (Fig. 44-2). The results on the benefit of parental presence during induction of anaesthesia are mixed; the authors of a recent Cochrane review concluded that parental presence during induction did not reduce a child's anxiety. There are other nonpharmacological interventions that hold promise for reducing anxiety, such as presence of clowns, hypnotherapy, low sensory stimulation, and playing hand-held video games (Manyande, Cyna, Yip, et al., 2015).

Appropriate education is essential to help parents understand the stages of anaesthesia, what to expect, and how to support their child. When parents choose not to or are not allowed to attend the induction, leaving a favourite possession with the child and uniting the child and parents as soon as possible after surgery (preferably in the PACU) are important actions. During surgery, the family should have a designated place to wait and should be kept informed of the child's progress. They also should know where and when they can visit the child after surgery.

Aside from possibly being separated from the parents before and after surgery, children may be cared for by a number of unfamiliar practitioners, which can instill fear and uncertainty. Although the same supportive nurse should remain with the child through as many of the procedures as possible, the child may have other nurses, especially if he or she returns to a special care unit postoperatively.

An important concern is restriction of food and fluids before surgery to avoid aspiration during anaesthesia. Infants require special attention to fluid needs. They should not be without oral fluids for an extended period preoperatively, to avoid glycogen depletion and dehydration. In a review of evidence from preoperative trials, the researchers concluded that drinking clear fluids up to a few hours before an anaesthetic did not increase the risk of regurgitation during or after surgery. These children were also less thirsty and hungry (Brady, Kinn, Ness, et al., 2009). Current preoperative fasting guidelines are found in Table 44-2. In some facilities guidelines may be different from those listed here.

Preoperative sedation. Historically, the most upsetting event for children has been the preoperative injection. Increasingly, more anaesthesiologists are using preoperative sedatives, usually midazolam (Versed), and including parental presence for children who are about to undergo surgery (Cox, Nemish, Ewen, et al., 2006). When medications are administered, they should be delivered atraumatically via oral or IV routes that have been previously initiated.

The goals for using preoperative medications include (1) anxiety reduction, (2) amnesia, (3) sedation, (4) antiemetic effect, and (5) reduction of secretions. Numerous preanaesthetic drug regimens are used with children, and no consensus exists on the optimal method (Strom, 2012). However, if children have no preoperative pain, are well prepared psychologically for surgery, and have their parents nearby, preoperative medication may be unnecessary.

Induction of anaesthesia in the pediatric patient is commonly accomplished by administering inhalation agents in combination with nitrous oxide and oxygen by mask. Children may fear induction of anaesthesia by mask. Practices that can minimize anxiety related to the inhalation of anaesthesia are (1) disguising the unpleasant odour of anaesthetic gases by applying a pleasant-smelling substance on the mask; (2) using a transparent plastic mask rather than an opaque black mask and gradually bringing it toward the face; (3) directing a stream of gas toward the child's face from the bare tube until the child becomes drowsy, then using the mask; (4) allowing the child to sit up rather than lie down for anaesthesia induction; and (5) allowing preoperative play with a mask and a doll or manikin.

Postoperative Care

Various psychological and physical interventions and observations are required to prevent or minimize possible untoward effects from anaesthesia and the surgical procedure (see Guidelines box). Although the incidence of serious postoperative complications in healthy children undergoing surgery is rare, continuous monitoring of cardiopulmonary status is essential during the immediate postoperative period. Postanaesthesia complications such as airway obstruction, postextubation croup, laryngospasm, and bronchospasm make maintaining a patent airway and maximum ventilation critical.

BOX 44-2 PLAY ACTIVITIES FOR SPECIFIC PROCEDURES*

Fluid Intake

Make ice pops using the child's favourite juice.
Cut gelatin into fun shapes.
Make a game out of taking a sip when turning the page of a book or in games such as Simon Says.
Use small medicine cups; decorate the cups.
Colour water with food colouring or powdered drink mix.
Have a tea party; pour at a small table.
Let the child fill a syringe and squirt into mouth or use it to fill small cups.
Cut straws in half and place in a small container (much easier for child to suck liquid).
Use a "crazy" straw.
Make a "progress poster"; give rewards for drinking a predetermined quantity.

Deep Breathing

Blow bubbles with a bubble blower.
Blow bubbles with a straw (no soap).
Blow on a pinwheel, feather, whistle, harmonica, balloon, horn, or party blower.
Practise band instruments.
Have a blowing contest using boats, cotton balls, feathers, ping-pong balls, or pieces of paper; blow objects on a table top over a goal line, over water, through an obstacle course, into the air, against an opponent, or up and down a string.
Suck paper or cloth from one container to another using a straw.
Use blow bottles with coloured water to transfer water from one side to the other.
Dramatize stories such as "I'll huff and puff and blow your house down" from the Three Little Pigs.
Do straw-blowing painting.
Take a deep breath and "blow out the candles" on a birthday cake.
Use a little paint brush to "paint" nails with water and blow nails dry.

Range of Motion and Use of Extremities

Throw beanbags at a fixed or movable target or throw wadded-up paper into a wastebasket.
Touch or kick Mylar balloons held or hung in different positions (if the child is in traction, hang balloon from a trapeze).
Play "tickle toes"; have child wiggle them on request.
Play Twister game or Simon Says.
Play pretend and guessing games (e.g., imitate a bird, butterfly, horse).
Have tricycle or wheelchair races in a safe area.
Play kickball or catch with a soft foam ball in a safe area.
Position bed so that the child must turn to view the television or doorway.
Climb wall like a "spider."
Pretend to teach "aerobic" dancing or exercises; encourage parents to participate.
Encourage swimming, if feasible.
Play video games or pinball (fine motor movement).
Play "hide and seek": hide a toy somewhere in the bed (or room if ambulatory) and have child find it using specified hand or foot.
Provide clay to mould with fingers.
Paint or draw on large sheets of paper placed on the floor or wall.
Encourage combing own hair; play "beauty shop" with the "customer" in different positions.

Soaks

Play with small toys or objects (cups, syringes, soap dishes) in water.
Wash dolls or toys.
Pick up marbles or coins from the bottom of a bath container.
Make designs with coins on the bottom of a container.
Pretend a boat is a submarine by keeping it immersed.
During soaks, read to the child; sing with the child; or play a game, such as cards, checkers, or other board game (if both of the child's hands are immersed, move board pieces for the child).
During a sitz bath, when soaking the perineal and rectal area, give the child something to listen to (music, stories) or look at books or tablets.
Punch holes in the bottom of a plastic cup, fill with water, and let it "rain" on the child.

Injections

Let child handle the syringe, vial, and alcohol swab and give an injection to a doll or stuffed animal.
Use syringes to decorate cookies with frosting, squirt paint, or target shoot into a container.
Draw a "magic circle" on the area before injection; draw a smiling face in the circle after injection, but avoid drawing on the puncture site.
Allow child to have a "collection" of syringes (without needles); make creative objects with syringes.
If the child has multiple injections or venipunctures, make a "progress poster"; give rewards for a predetermined number of injections.
Have the child count to 10 or 15 during injection.

Ambulation

Give the child something to push.
- Toddler—Push-pull toy
- School-age child—Wagon or a doll in a stroller or wheelchair
- Adolescent—Decorated intravenous stand

Have a parade; make hats, drums, etc.

Extending Environment (e.g., for Patients in Traction)

Make bed into a pirate ship or an airplane with decorations.
Put up mirrors so that the patient can see around the room.
Move the bed frequently to the playroom, hallway, or outside.

*Small objects such as marbles or coins, as well as latex gloves or balloons, are unsafe for young children because of possible aspiration. Latex products also carry the risk of an allergic reaction.

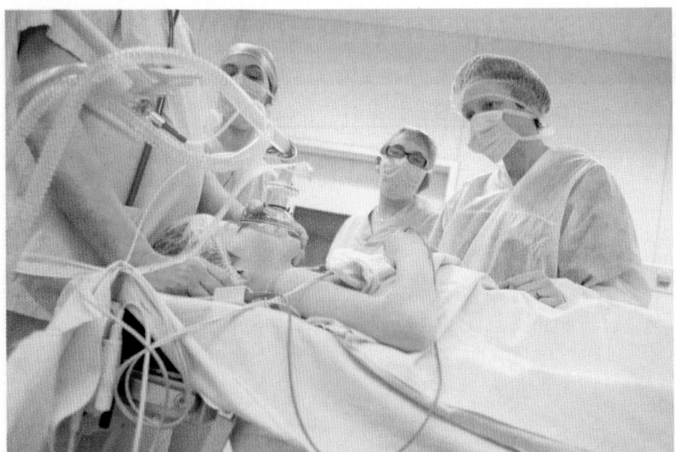

FIGURE 44-2 Parental presence during induction of anaesthesia can minimize the child's and parents' anxiety during the preoperative period. (Phanie/Alamy Stock Photo.)

TABLE 44-2 FASTING RECOMMENDATIONS TO REDUCE THE RISK OF PULMONARY ASPIRATION

TIME	WHAT CHILDREN CAN EAT AND DRINK
Midnight before receiving anaesthesia	The child must not have any solid food. Children could drink clear liquids (e.g., water with Pedialyte or apple juice) up until 3 hours before surgery.
6 hours before receiving anaesthesia	The baby must not have formula.
4 hours before receiving anaesthesia	The baby must not have breast milk.
2-3 hours before receiving anaesthesia	The child must not have clear liquids. Children must not drink anything until they wake up from the anaesthetic.
Ask your health care provider about when and how to give the medicine if the child takes prescription medicine.	

Based on About Kids Health. (2016). *General anaesthesia.* Retrieved from http://www.aboutkidshealth.ca/En/HealthAZ/TestsAndTreatments/PainReliefSedationAnaesthesia/Pages/General-Anaesthesia.aspx; and Nagelhout, John. (2003). Aspiration prophylaxis: Is it time for changes in our practice? *AANA Journal, 71*(4), 301.

Monitoring the patient's oxygen saturation and providing supplemental oxygen as needed, maintaining body temperature, and promoting fluid and electrolyte balance are important aspects of immediate postoperative care. Vital signs should be continuously monitored, and each vital sign should be evaluated in terms of adverse effects from anaesthesia, shock, or respiratory compromise (Table 44-3).

A change in vital signs that demands immediate attention in the perioperative period is caused by malignant hyperthermia (MH), a potentially fatal pharmacogenetic disorder involving a defective calcium channel in the sarcoplasmic reticulum membrane. In susceptible children, inhaled anaesthetics and the muscle relaxant succinylcholine trigger the disorder, producing hypermetabolism. Succinylcholine is rarely administered, except to provide rapid relief of laryngospasm. Intubation of the airway is enabled by a short-acting muscle relaxant, such as rocuronium (Wetzel, 2016). Symptoms of MH include hypercarbia (increased end-tidal carbon dioxide), elevated temperature, tachycardia, tachypnea, acidosis, muscle rigidity, and rhabdomyolysis (Wetzel, 2016). A family or previous history of sudden high fever associated with a surgical procedure and certain neuromuscular disorders increase the risk for MH; children who have successfully undergone prior surgery without adverse effects may still be considered susceptible.

Treatment of MH includes immediate discontinuation of the triggering agent, hyperventilation with 100% oxygen, and IV dantrolene sodium. If the child is hyperthermic, cooling measures such as ice packs to the groin, axillae, and neck and iced nasogastric (NG) lavage should be initiated. The surgery may be discontinued; or, if it is emergent, it may be continued with

GUIDELINES

Postoperative Care

Ensure that preparations are made to receive the child:
- Bed or crib is ready.
- Intravenous pumps and poles, suction apparatus, and oxygen flow meter are at bedside.

Obtain baseline information:
- Take vital signs, including blood pressure; keep blood pressure cuff in place and deflated to lessen amount of disturbance to child.
- Take and record vital signs more frequently if any value fluctuates, and as per hospital protocol.
- Inspect operative area.
- Check dressing, if present:
  - Outline any bleeding area on dressing or cast with pen.
  - Reinforce, but do not remove, loose dressing.
  - Observe areas below surgical site for blood that may have drained toward bed.
- Assess for bleeding and other symptoms in areas not covered with a dressing, such as throat after tonsillectomy.
- Assess skin colour and characteristics.
- Assess level of consciousness and activity.

Notify physician or nurse practitioner of any irregularities in the child's condition.

Assess for evidence of pain (see Pain Assessment, Chapter 34).

Review surgeon's orders after completing initial assessment, and check that any preoperative orders, such as seizure or cardiac medications, have been reordered and can be given by available routes (oral preparations may be contraindicated).

Monitor vital signs as ordered and more often if indicated.

Check dressings for bleeding or other abnormalities.

Check bowel sounds.

Observe for signs of shock, abdominal distension, and bleeding.

Assess for bladder distension.

Observe for signs of dehydration.

Detect presence of infection:
- Take vital signs, as ordered or more frequently as necessary.
- Collect or request needed specimens.
- Inspect wound for signs of infection—redness, swelling, heat, pain, and purulent drainage.

TABLE 44-3 POTENTIAL CAUSES OF POSTOPERATIVE VITAL SIGN ALTERATIONS IN CHILDREN

ALTERATION	POTENTIAL CAUSE	COMMENTS
Heart Rate		
Increase	Decreased perfusion (shock) Elevated temperature Pain Respiratory distress (early) Medications (atropine, morphine, epinephrine)	Heart rate may increase to maintain cardiac output.
Decrease	Hypoxia Vagal stimulation Increased intracranial pressure Respiratory distress (late) Medications	In the young child, bradycardia is of more concern than tachycardia.
Respiratory Rate		
Increase	Respiratory distress Fluid volume excess Hypothermia Elevated temperature Pain	Body responds to respiratory distress primarily by increasing rate.
Decrease	Anaesthetics, opioids Pain	Decreased respiratory rate from opioids may be compensated for by increase depth of respiration.
Blood Pressure		
Increase	Excess intravascular volume Increased intracranial pressure Carbon dioxide retention Pain Medication (ketamine, epinephrine)	This is serious in preterm infants because it increases risk of intraventricular hemorrhage.
Decrease	Vasodilating anaesthetic agents (halothane, isoflurane, enflurane) Opioids (morphine)	Decreased blood pressure is a late sign of shock because of elasticity and constriction of vessels to maintain cardiac output.
Temperature		
Increase	Shock (late sign) Infection Environmental causes (warm room, excess coverings) Malignant hyperthermia	Fever associated with infection usually occurs later than fever of noninfectious origin. Absence of fever does not rule out infection, especially in infants. Malignant hyperthermia requires immediate treatment.
Decrease	Vasodilating anaesthetic agents (halothane, isoflurane) Muscle relaxants Environmental causes (cool room) Infusion of cool fluids or blood	Newborns are especially susceptible to hypothermia, with serious or fatal consequences.

a different anaesthetic agent. The patient should be transferred to a critical care unit (CCU) and closely monitored for stabilization of vital signs, metabolic state, and possible recurrence of symptoms.

Managing pain is a major nursing responsibility after surgery (see Chapter 34). The nurse should assess pain frequently and administer analgesics to provide comfort and facilitate postoperative care routines, such as ambulation and deep breathing. **Opioids** are the most commonly used analgesics. Routinely scheduled IV analgesics, patient-controlled analgesia, and epidural infusions, rather than as needed (prn) orders, provide excellent analgesia in postoperative pediatric patients.

Because respiratory infections are a potential complication, every effort should be taken to aerate the lungs and remove secretions. The lungs should be auscultated regularly to identify abnormal sounds or any areas of diminished or absent breath sounds. To prevent pneumonia, respiratory movement should be encouraged with the use of incentive spirometers or other motivating activities (see Box 44-2). If these measures are presented as games, the child is more likely to work with the nurse. The child's position needs to be changed every 2 hours and deep breathing encouraged.

GENERAL HYGIENE AND BASIC CARE

Maintaining Healthy Skin

Maintaining an IV line, removing a dressing, positioning a child in bed, changing a diaper, using electrodes, and using restraints all have the potential to contribute to skin injury. Skin care must go beyond the daily bath and become a part of each nursing

GUIDELINES
Skin Care

- Cleanse skin with mild nonalkaline soap or soap-free cleaning agents for routine bathing.
- Keep skin dry and free of excess moisture such as urine, stool, excessive perspiration, and wound drainage (may apply absorbent powder such as cornstarch]) and use soft, smooth bed linen and clothes.
- Provide daily cleansing of eyes, oral, and diaper or perineal areas, and any areas of skin breakdown.
- Apply non-alcohol-based moisturizing agents after cleansing to retain moisture and rehydrate skin.
- Use minimum amount of tape and adhesives. On very sensitive skin, use a protective, pectin-based or hydrocolloid skin barrier between skin and tape or adhesives.
- Use water or adhesive remover (if skin is not fragile) when removing tape or adhesives.
- Place pectin-based or hydrocolloid skin barriers directly over excoriated skin. Leave barrier undisturbed until it begins to peel off, or for 5 to 7 days. With wet, oozing excoriations, place a small amount of stoma powder on site, remove excess powder, and apply skin barrier. Hold barrier in place for several minutes to allow barrier to soften and mould to skin surface.
- Alternate electrode and probe placement sites and thoroughly assess underlying skin, typically every 8 to 24 hours.
- Eliminate pressure secondary to medical devices such as tracheostomy, tubes, wheelchairs, braces, and gastrostomy tubes. Be certain fingers or toes are visible whenever extremity is used for an intravenous (IV) or arterial line.
- Use a slider sheet to move a child in bed or onto a stretcher; do not drag the child from under the arms.
- Position in neutral alignment; pillows, cushions, or wedges may be needed to prevent hip abduction and pressure to bony prominences such as heels, elbows, and sacral and occipital areas. When child is positioned laterally, placement of pillows or cushions between knees, under head, and under upper arm helps promote neutral body alignment. Avoid using doughnut cushions because they can cause tissue ischemia. Elevate head of bed 30 degrees or less to reduce pressure unless contraindicated.
- Do not massage reddened bony prominences because this can cause deep tissue damage; provide pressure relief to those areas instead.
- Routinely assess the child's nutritional status. A child who is NPO (nothing by mouth) for several days and is receiving only IV fluids is nutritionally at risk, which can also affect the ability of the skin to maintain its integrity. Consider parenteral nutrition.
- Identify children at risk for skin breakdown before it occurs and implement prevention interventions. The Braden Q Scale may be used to assess risk for skin breakdown as well as for assessing the severity of formed ulcers (see Additional Resources at the end of this chapter).

intervention (see Guidelines box). See Chapter 26, p. 715, for discussion of newborn skin care.

Assessment of the skin is most easily accomplished during the bath. The nurse should examine the skin for early signs of injury. Risk factors include impaired mobility, protein malnutrition, edema, incontinence, sensory loss, anemia, infection, failure to turn the patient, and intubation. Critically ill children often are at high risk of pressure ulcers and skin breakdown, since they often have several risk factors combined. Identification of risk factors helps to determine those children who need a more thorough skin assessment. Several risk assessment scales are available for use in pediatrics, such as the Braden Q Scale (Curley, Razmus, Roberts, et al., 2003) and the Glamorgan Scale (Willock, Baharestani, & Anthony, 2009). Assessment should be performed during the admission interview so that pressure ulcers and wounds that occurred before admission can be identified (Registered Nurses' Association of Ontario [RNAO], 2011). Pressure ulcers in children typically occur on the occiput, ears, sacrum, and scapula.

Pressure ulcers can develop when the pressure on the skin and underlying tissues is greater than the capillary closing pressure, causing capillary occlusion. If the pressure remains unrelieved, vessels can collapse, resulting in tissue anoxia and cellular death. Pressure ulcers most often occur over bony prominences and are usually very deep, extending into subcutaneous tissue or even deeper into muscle, tendon, or bone.

When capillary blood flow is interrupted by pressure, the blood flows back into the tissue when the pressure is relieved. As the body attempts to reoxygenate the area, a bright red flush appears. This reactive hyperemia, or flush, is the earliest sign of tissue compromise and pressure-related ischemia. If pressure is prolonged, reactive hyperemia will not be sufficient to revitalize ischemic tissue (RNAO, 2011). Pressure ulcers in hospitalized children are uncommon, with reported rates of 1 to 13% (Noonan, Quigley, & Curley, 2006). Risk factors associated with pressure ulcers in pediatric CCU patients include edema, length of stay, increasing positive end-expiratory pressure, lack of turning, and weight loss. Medical devices such as pulse oximeter probes, bilevel and continuous positive airway pressure masks, oxygen cannulas, feeding tubes, stomas, orthotics, and casts can also cause pressure ulcers.

Pressure ulcers are staged to classify the amount of tissue damage that has occurred. Necrotic tissue must be removed so that the tissue depth can be accurately assessed. Accurate documentation of redness or obvious skin breakdown is essential. Colour, size (diameter and depth), location, presence of sinus tracts, odour, exudate, and response to treatment should be observed and recorded at least daily (RNAO, 2011). A *pressure-reduction device* reduces pressure but does not prevent pressure from causing capillary closure; thus turning and repositioning the patient are always included when using these devices. A *pressure-relief device* such as a pressure-relief bed maintains pressure below that which would cause capillary closure. These devices are usually high-technology beds that are used for patients who have multiple problems and cannot be turned effectively.

Friction and shear contribute to pressure ulcers. *Friction* occurs when the skin's surface rubs against another surface, such as the bedsheets. The skin may have the appearance of an abrasion. Skin damage is usually limited to the epidermal and upper layers. It most often occurs over the elbows, heels, or occiput. Prevention of friction injury includes the use of customized splinting over infants heels; gel pillows under the head of toddlers; moisturizing agents; transparent dressings over susceptible areas; and soft, smooth bed linen and clothing. By itself, friction does not cause tissue necrosis; however, when it acts with gravity, it results in shear injury.

Shear is the result of the force of gravity pushing down on the body and friction of the body against a surface, such as the bed or chair. For example, when a patient is in the semi-Fowler position and begins to slide to the foot of the bed, the skin over the sacral area remains in the same place because of the resistance of the bed surface. The blood vessels in the area are stretched and may cause small-vessel thrombosis and tissue death (RNAO, 2011). Prevention of shear injury includes using lift sheets when repositioning a patient, elevating the bed no more than 30 degrees for short periods, and using the knee gatch to interrupt the pull of gravity on the body toward the foot of the bed.

Epidermal stripping results when the epidermis is unintentionally removed with tape removal. These lesions are usually shallow and irregularly shaped and may blister or weep. Babies are at increased risk for epidermal injury. Prevention of injury includes using no tape when possible and securing dressings with laced binders (Montgomery straps) or stretchy netting (Spandage or stockinette). Use of porous or low-tack tapes (e.g., Medipore, paper, hydrogel) and alcohol-free skin sealants (No Sting Barrier Film) or picture framing wounds with hydrocolloid or wafer barriers (e.g., DuoDERM, Coloplast, Stomahesive) and then taping on top of the barrier will also reduce epidermal stripping.

Tape should be placed so that there is no tension, traction, or wrinkles on the skin. To remove tape, it should be slowly peeled away while stabilizing the underlying skin. Adhesive remover may be used to break the adhesive bond but may be drying to the skin; adhesive removers should be avoided in preterm neonates, since absorption rates vary and toxicity may occur. The adhesive is removed with water to prevent absorption and irritation. Wetting the tape with water or alcohol-based foam hand cleansers may facilitate removal.

Chemical factors can also lead to skin damage. Fecal incontinence, especially when mixed with urine; wound drainage; or gastric drainage around gastrostomy tubes can erode epidermis. The skin can quickly progress from redness to denudement if exposure continues. Moisture barriers, gentle cleansing as soon after exposure as possible, and skin barriers can be used to prevent damage caused by chemical factors. In addition, foam dressings that wick moisture away from the skin are helpful around gastrostomy tubes and tracheostomy sites.

Bathing

Most infants and children can be bathed in a basin at the bedside, on the bed, or in a standard bathtub or shower. For infants and young children confined to bed, the towel method can be used. Two towels are immersed in a diluted soap solution and wrung damp. With the child lying supine on a dry towel, one damp towel is placed on top of the child and used to gently clean the body. This towel is discarded, and the child is dried and turned prone. The procedure is repeated using the second damp towel. Commercially available bath cloths may also be used.

Infants and small children should *never* be left unattended in a bathtub, and infants who are unable to sit alone need to be securely held with one hand during the bath. The nurse should securely support the infant's head with one hand, or grasp the farther arm firmly while the head rests comfortably on the nurse's arm. Children who are able to sit without assistance need close supervision and a pad placed in the bottom of the tub to prevent slipping and loss of balance.

School-age children and adolescents may shower or bathe. Nurses need to use judgement regarding the amount of supervision the child requires. Some can assume this responsibility unaided, whereas others will need someone in constant attendance. Children with cognitive impairments, physical limitations, or suicidal or psychotic problems (who may commit bodily harm) require close supervision.

Areas that require special attention are the ears, between skinfolds, the neck, the back, and the genital area. The genital area should be cleansed carefully and dried, with particular care given to skinfolds. In uncircumcised boys, usually those older than 3 years of age, the foreskin should be retracted gently, the exposed surfaces cleansed, and the foreskin then replaced, but only if the foreskin retracts comfortably.

Children who are ill or debilitated need more extensive assistance with bathing, but should be encouraged to perform as much as they can without overtaxing their energies. Increasing involvement can be expected with improved strength and endurance.

Oral Hygiene

Mouth care is an integral part of daily hygiene and should be continued in the hospital. Infants and debilitated children require the nurse or a family member to perform mouth care. Although young children can manage a toothbrush and should be encouraged to use it, most need assistance to perform oral hygiene satisfactorily. Older children, although capable of brushing and flossing without assistance, sometimes need to be reminded.

Hair Care

Children should have their hair brushed and combed at least once daily. The hair should not be cut without parental permission, especially if clipping hair is necessary to provide access to a scalp vein for IV insertion.

If children are hospitalized for more than a few days, the hair may need shampooing. With infants the hair may be washed during the bath. For most children, washing the hair and scalp once or twice weekly is sufficient unless there is an indication for more frequent washing, such as following a high fever and profuse sweating. Adolescents normally have increased oily sebaceous secretions that require frequent hair care and more frequent shampoos.

Most children can be transported to an accessible sink for shampooing. Those who are unable to be transported can receive a shampoo in their beds with adequate protection, specially adapted equipment or positioning, or dry shampoo caps.

Feeding the Sick Child

Loss of appetite is a symptom common to most childhood illnesses. Because an acute illness is usually short, the nutritional state is seldom compromised. Urging foods on the sick child may precipitate nausea and vomiting, and in most cases children can be permitted to determine their own need for food and to avoid future aversions.

Refusing to eat may also be one way that children can exert power and control in an otherwise helpless situation. For young children, loss of appetite may be related to the depression caused by separation from their parents. Parents' concern with eating can intensify the problem. Forcing a child to eat can be met with rebellion and reinforces the behaviour as a control mechanism. Parents should be encouraged to relax any pressure surrounding oral or nutritional intake during an acute illness. Although it is best to encourage high-quality nutritious foods, the child may desire foods and liquids that contain mostly empty or non-nutritional calories. Some well-tolerated foods include gelatin, diluted clear soups, carbonated drinks, flavoured ice pops, dry toast, and crackers. Even though these substances are not nutritious, they can provide necessary fluid and calories.

Dehydration is always a hazard when children have a fever or anorexia, especially when accompanied by vomiting or diarrhea. For diarrhea episodes the use of Pedialyte or Enfylate is most recommended and can even be made as popsicles. Fluids should not be forced, and the child is not awakened to take fluids. Forcing fluids may create the same difficulties as with urging unwanted food. Gentle persuasion with preferred beverages will usually meet with success. Using play techniques can also be effective (see Guidelines box).

Once the child is feeling better the appetite usually begins to improve. It is best to take advantage of any hungry period by serving high-quality foods and snacks. If the child still refuses to eat, nutritious fluids, such as prepared breakfast drinks, should be encouraged. Parents can help by bringing in food items from home, especially if the family's cultural eating habits differ from the hospital food. A clinical dietitian may also be consulted for alternative food choices.

When children are placed on special diets, such as clear liquids after surgery or during episodes of diarrhea, it is essential to assess their intake and readiness to advance to more complex foods. Regardless of the type of diet, charting of the amount consumed is an important nursing responsibility. Descriptions need to be detailed and accurate, such as "120 mL of orange juice, one pancake, and 240 mL of milk." Comments such as "ate well" or "ate poorly" are inadequate. Charting the percentage of the meal eaten is also inadequate unless food is measured before serving.

If parents are involved in the child's care, they should be encouraged to keep a list of everything eaten. Use of a premeasured cup for fluids ensures a more accurate estimate of intake. A comparison of the intake at each meal can isolate food deficiencies, such as insufficient intake of meat or vegetables. Behaviours associated with mealtime also may point to possible factors influencing appetite. For example, the observation that "child eats well when with other children but plays with food if left alone in room" can help the nurse plan mealtime activities that stimulate the appetite.

Hospitalization provides many opportunities for the nurse to explore parental knowledge of nutrition. If necessary, the nurse can provide nutritional information to the family that will improve the child's level of nutrition after hospitalization.

GUIDELINES

Feeding the Sick Child

Take a dietary history (see Chapter 33) and use information to make eating time as much like home as possible.

Encourage parents or other family members to feed the child or to be present at mealtimes.

Make mealtimes pleasant; avoid any procedures immediately before or after eating; make certain the child is rested and pain free.

Serve small, frequent meals rather than three large meals, or serve three meals and nutritious between-meal snacks.

Provide finger foods for young children.

Involve children in food selection and preparation whenever possible.

Serve small portions, and serve each course separately, such as soup first; followed by meat, potatoes, and vegetables; and ending with dessert.
- With young children, camouflage size of food by cutting meat thicker so that less appears on the plate or by folding a cheese slice in half.
- Offer second helpings.

Ensure a variety of foods, textures, and colours.

Provide food selections that are favourites of most children, such as peanut butter and jelly sandwiches, hot dogs, hamburgers, macaroni and cheese, pizza, spaghetti, tacos, chicken fingers, corn, and fruit yogurt.

Avoid foods that are highly seasoned, have strong odours, or are all mixed together, unless typical of cultural practices.

Provide fluid selections that are favourites of most children, such as fruit punch, cola, ginger ale, sweetened tea, flavoured ice pops, sherbet, ice cream, milk, milkshakes, eggnog, pudding, gelatin, clear broth, or creamed soups.

Offer nutritious snacks, such as frozen yogurt or pudding, oatmeal, hot cocoa, cheese slices, pieces of raw vegetable or fruit, and dried fruit or cereal.

Make food attractive and different; for example:
- Serve a "picnic lunch" in a paper bag.
- Pack food in a take-out container; decorate the container.
- Put a "face" or a "flower" on a hamburger or sandwich with pieces of vegetable.
- Use a cookie cutter to shape a sandwich.
- Serve pudding, yogurt, or juice frozen as an ice pop.
- Make slurpies or snow cones by pouring flavoured syrup on crushed ice.
- Add food colouring to water or milk.
- Serve fluids through brightly coloured or unusually shaped straws.
- Make "bowtie" sandwiches by cutting them in triangles and placing two points together.
- Slice sandwiches into "fingers."
- Grate mounds of cheese.
- Cut apples horizontally to make circles.
- Put a banana on a hot dog bun and spread with peanut butter.
- Break uncooked spaghetti into toothpick lengths and skewer cheese, cold meat, vegetables, or fruit chunks.

Praise children for what they do eat.

Do not punish children for not eating by removing their dessert or putting them to bed.

Controlling Elevated Temperatures

An elevated temperature, most frequently from fever but occasionally caused by hyperthermia, is one of the most common symptoms of illness in children. This manifestation is of great concern to parents. To facilitate an understanding of fever, the following terms are defined:

Set point—The temperature around which body temperature is regulated by a thermostat-like mechanism in the hypothalamus

Fever (hyperpyrexia)—An elevation in set point such that body temperature is regulated at a higher level; may be arbitrarily defined as temperature above 38°C (100.4°F)

Hyperthermia—Body temperature exceeding the set point, which usually results from the body or external conditions creating more heat than the body can eliminate, as in heatstroke, aspirin toxicity, seizures, or hyperthyroidism

Body temperature is regulated by a thermostat-like mechanism in the hypothalamus. This mechanism receives input from centrally and peripherally located receptors. When temperature changes occur, these receptors relay the information to the thermostat, which either increases or decreases heat production to maintain a constant set point temperature. However, during an infection, pyrogenic substances cause an increase in the body's normal set point, a process that is mediated by prostaglandins. Consequently, the hypothalamus increases heat production until the core temperature reaches the new set point.

During the fever (febrile) state shivering and vasoconstriction generate and conserve heat during the chill phase of the fever, raising central temperatures to the level of the new set point. The temperature reaches a plateau when it stabilizes in the higher range. When the temperature is greater than the set point or when the pyrogen is no longer present, a crisis, or defervescence, of the temperature occurs.

Most fevers in children are of brief duration with limited consequences and are viral in origin. When fever is caused by bacteria, endotoxins are produced that activate the inflammatory process and produce fever. Fever has physiological benefits, including increased white blood cell activity, interferon production and effectiveness, and antibody production and enhancement of some antibiotic effects (Considine & Brennan, 2007). Contrary to popular belief, neither the rise in temperature nor its response to antipyretics indicates the severity or cause of infection, which casts doubt on the value of using fever as a diagnostic or prognostic indicator.

Therapeutic Management

Therapeutic management of elevated temperature depends on whether it is due to a fever or hyperthermia. Because the set point is normal in hyperthermia but increased in fever, different approaches must be used to lower body temperature successfully.

Fever. The principal reason for treating fever is the relief of discomfort. Relief measures include pharmacological or environmental intervention. The most effective intervention is the use of antipyretics to lower the set point.

Antipyretic medications include acetaminophen, aspirin, and nonsteroidal anti-inflammatory drugs (NSAIDs). Acetaminophen is the preferred medication; aspirin should not be given to children because of its association with influenza virus or chickenpox and Reye's syndrome. One nonprescription NSAID, ibuprofen, is approved for fever reduction in children as young as 6 months of age. Ibuprofen dosage is based on the initial temperature level: 5 mg/kg of body weight for temperatures less than 39.2°C or 10 mg/kg for temperatures greater than 39.2°C. The recommended dosage for pain is 10 mg/kg every 6 to 8 hours, and the recommended maximum daily dose for pain and fever is 40 mg/kg. The duration of fever reduction is generally 6 to 8 hours and is longer with the higher dose. The recommended dose should never be exceeded. Acetaminophen should be given every 4 hours but no more than five times in 24 hours. Because body temperature normally decreases at night, three or four doses at 10 to 15 mg/kg in 24 hours will control most fevers. The nurse should retake the temperature 45 to 60 minutes after the antipyretic is given to assess its effect, but temperature should not be repeatedly measured; the child's level of discomfort is the best indication for continued treatment. Since pediatric dosages are decided on the basis of accurate and current body weights, it is recommended that weighing be repeated at a minimum of once per week or more if severe dehydration or edema exists.

Environmental measures to reduce fever may be used if tolerated by the child and if they do not induce shivering. Compensatory shivering greatly increases metabolic requirements above those already caused by the fever.

Traditional cooling measures, such as wearing minimum clothing, exposing the skin to the air, reducing room temperature, increasing air circulation, and applying cool, moist compresses to the skin (e.g., the forehead, neck and axilla, hands, femoral, and feet areas), are effective if used approximately 1 hour *after* an antipyretic is given so that the set point is lowered. Cooling procedures such as sponging or tepid baths are ineffective in treating febrile children (these measures are effective for hyperthermia) when used either alone or in combination with antipyretics, and they cause considerable discomfort (CPS, 2013a).

Seizures associated with a fever occur in 2 to 5% of all children between the ages of 6 months and 5 years (CPS, 2013b). These febrile seizures usually stop completely by age 5. The older the child is when the first seizure occurs, the lower the chance of further seizures. A family history of febrile seizures is associated with recurring episodes (CPS, 2013b). There is little evidence to support the use of antipyretic drugs or anticonvulsants to prevent a second febrile seizure; nursing interventions should focus on ways to provide care and comfort during a febrile illness. Simple febrile seizures lasting less than 10 minutes do not cause brain damage or other debilitating effects. However, there are some special febrile seizure syndromes that can have some long-term neurological abnormalities. Unless a possible serious central nervous system infection is suspected, a medical extensive workup is not required (Khair & Elmagrabi, 2015).

Hyperthermia. Unlike in fever, antipyretics are of no value in hyperthermia because the set point is already normal. Consequently, cooling measures are used. Cool applications to the skin help reduce the core temperature. Cooled blood from the skin surface is conducted to inner organs and tissues, and warm blood is circulated to the surface, where it is cooled and recirculated. The surface blood vessels dilate as the body attempts to dissipate heat to the environment and facilitate the cooling process.

Commercial cooling devices, such as cooling blankets or mattresses, are available to reduce body temperature. They should be placed on the bed and covered with a sheet or lightweight blanket. Frequent temperature monitoring is essential to prevent excessive cooling of the body.

Tepid baths are also used to decrease high temperature. For tepid tub baths it is usually best to start with warm water and gradually add cool water until the desired water temperature of 37°C is reached to accustom the child to the lower water temperature. Generally, the temperature of the water only has to be 1°C less than the child's temperature to be effective. The child should be placed directly in the tub of tepid water for approximately 20 minutes while water is gently squeezed from a washcloth over the back and chest or gently sprayed over the body from a sprayer. In the bed or crib, tepid washcloths or towels are used, exposing only one area of the body at a time. The sponging is continued for approximately 20 minutes.

After the tub or sponge bath, the child can be dried and dressed in lightweight pyjamas, a nightgown, or a diaper and placed in a dry bed. The child is dried by gently rubbing the skin surface with a towel to stimulate circulation. The temperature should be retaken 30 minutes after the tub bath or sponge bath. The tub or sponge bath should not be continued or restarted until the skin surface is warm or if the child feels chilled. Chilling causes vasoconstriction, which defeats the purpose of the cool applications. In this condition, little blood is carried to the skin surface; the blood remains primarily in the viscera to become heated.

Whether a temperature elevation in the critically ill child is caused by fever or hyperthermia, it should be treated aggressively. The metabolic rate increases 10% for every 1°C increase in temperature and three to five times during shivering, thus increasing oxygen, fluid, and caloric requirements. If the child's cardiovascular or neurological system is already compromised, these increased needs are especially hazardous. In all children with elevated temperature, attention to adequate hydration is essential. Most children's needs can be met through ingestion of additional oral fluids.

Family Teaching and Home Care

Fever is one of the most common problems for which parents seek health care. High levels of parental anxiety (fever phobia) surrounding potential complications of fever such as seizures and dehydration are prevalent and can result in overuse of antipyretics (Purssell, 2009). Parents need to know that sponging is indicated for elevated temperatures from hyperthermia, rather than fever, and that ice water and alcohol are inappropriate, potentially dangerous solutions (CPS, 2013a). Parents should know how to take the child's temperature and read the thermometer accurately and should have guidelines for seeking professional care (see Family-Centred Teaching box). Some of the newer temperature-measuring devices, such as plastic strips or digital thermometers, may be better suited for home use than hospital use (see Temperature, Chapter 33). If acetaminophen or ibuprofen is indicated, the parents need instruction in administering the medication. The nurse needs to emphasize accuracy in both the amount of medication given and the time intervals at which it is administered. The Canadian Paediatric Society (CPS) (2013a) does not recommend that parents alternate giving their child ibuprofen and acetaminophen because this practice can lead to dosage errors.

FAMILY-CENTRED TEACHING

The Child With Fever

Contact your health care provider or go to emergency if your child has any of the following symptoms:

- Your child is younger than 3 months old and has a fever of a temperature over 38.5°C.
- Your child develops a rash and does not go away when you apply pressure to it with your fingers (blanching).
- Your child cannot keep down fluids and looks dehydrated or your child's skin looks very pale or grey.
- Your child is having constant pain, is very weak, or you are unable to wake your child up easily.
- Your child has a stiff neck.
- Your child has a seizure associated with fever.
- Your child has sore, swollen, or unresponsive limbs.
- Your child has problems breathing.
- Your child is crying in a high pitch and cannot be settled.
- Your child is looking or acting very sick.

Call within 24 hours if your child has a fever over 38.5°C and:

- Your child is between 3 and 6 months old.
- Your child has an earache that doesn't improve.
- Your child has had a fever for more than 3 days.
- The fever went away for over 24 hours and then came back.
- Your child has a bacterial infection that is being treated with an antibiotic, but the fever has not gone away in 2 to 3 days.
- Your child cries when going to the bathroom or the urine smells bad.
- You have other questions or concerns.

Based on AboutKidsHealth. (2013). *Fever* (by Ellie Berger, BA, MD, FRCPC, FAAP, MHPE). Retrieved from http://www.aboutkidshealth.ca/En/HealthAZ/ConditionsandDiseases/Symptoms/Pages/Fever.aspx; and The College of Family Physicians of Canada. (2011). *Fever in infants and children.* Retrieved from http://www.cfpc.ca/ProjectAssets/Templates/Resource.aspx?id=3596.

SAFETY

While safety is an essential component of any patient's care, children have special characteristics that require an even greater concern for safety. Because small children in the hospital are separated from their usual environment and do not possess the capacity for abstract thinking and reasoning, it is the responsibility of everyone who comes in contact with them to maintain protective measures throughout their hospital stay. Nurses need to understand the age level at which each child is operating and plan for safety accordingly.

Identification bands are particularly important to use with children. Infants and unconscious patients are unable to tell or respond to their names. Toddlers may answer to any name or to a nickname only. Older children may exchange places, give an erroneous name, or choose not to respond to their own names as a form of joke, unaware of the hazards of such practices.

Environmental Factors

The hospital environment requires high vigilance by staff to avoid adverse incidents in children that may stem from the use of products and equipment used in diagnosis, prevention, and treatment. More than a decade ago, Health Canada became concerned about reports of suffocation and death in young children caused by entanglement in IV tubing and monitor leads while being treated in the hospital. In 2003, Health Canada (2003/2013) made the following recommendations for hospitals to consider when developing policies:

1. Using continuous IV administration only when necessary. For intermittent IV infusion, saline or heparin-locked IV sites should be considered.
2. Providing an appropriate level of supervision for children who have entangled themselves in tubing, including oxygen tubing or leads, or are considered to be at an increased risk of doing so. Factors to be considered might include the following:
    - The child's age and cognitive level
    - The child's mobility and state of agitation
    - The length and number of tubes and leads attached to the patient
3. Using equipment accessories that restrain or stabilize flexible lines to reduce the potential for them to become wrapped around the child's neck or limbs

All of the environmental safety measures for the protection of adults apply to children, including good illumination, floors clear of fluid or objects that might contribute to falls, and nonskid surfaces in showers and tubs. All staff members should be familiar with the area-specific fire plan. Elevators and stairways should be made safe.

All windows should be secured and blinds and curtain cord should be out of reach with split cords to prevent strangulation. Pacifiers should not be tied around the neck or attached to an infant by string.

Electrical equipment should be in good working order and only used by employees. Electrical outlets should have covers to prevent burns in small children, whose exploratory activities may extend to inserting objects into the small openings.

Staff members should practise proper care and disposal of small objects such as syringe caps, needle covers, and temperature probe covers. There should be limited use of needles for medication administration; instead, needleless syringes should be used. Vanish point needles are associated with enhanced safety and reduced needlestick injuries.

Furniture is safest when it is scaled to the child's proportions, is sturdy, and is well balanced to prevent being tipped over. A special hazard for children is the danger of entrapment under an electronically controlled bed when it is activated to descend. Infants and small children must be securely strapped into infant seats, feeding chairs, and strollers. Infants, young children, and those who are weak, paralyzed, agitated, confused, sedated, or cognitively impaired should *never* be left unattended on treatment tables, on scales, or in treatment areas. Even preterm infants are capable of surprising mobility; therefore, portholes in isolettes must be securely fastened when not in use. Beds of ambulatory patients should remain locked in place and at a height that allows easy access to the floor.

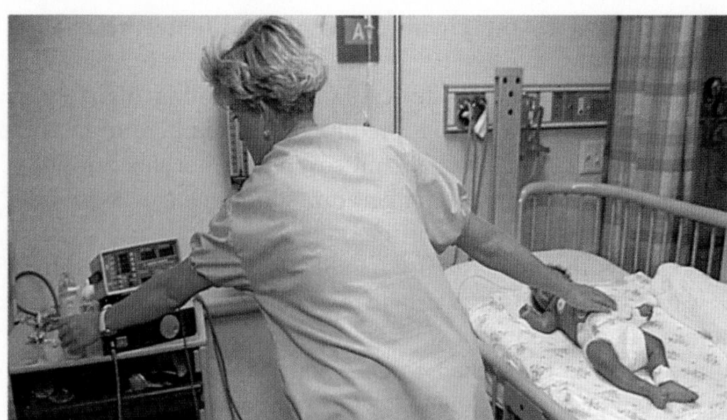

FIGURE 44-3 The nurse maintains hand contact when her back is turned.

Crib sides should be kept up and fastened securely unless an adult is at the bedside. It is safer to leave crib sides up, regardless of the child's ability to get out and when the crib is unoccupied, to remove the child's temptation to climb in. Anyone attending an infant or small child in a crib with the sides down should never turn away without maintaining hand contact with the child; that is, one hand should be kept on the child's back or abdomen to prevent the child from rolling, crawling, or jumping from the open crib (Fig. 44-3).

Toy Safety

Toys play a vital role in the everyday life of children, and they are no less important in the hospital setting. Nurses are responsible for assessing the safety of toys brought to the hospital by well-meaning parents and friends. Toys should be appropriate to the child's age, condition, and treatment. For example, if the child is receiving oxygen, electrical or friction toys are not safe, since sparks can cause oxygen to ignite. The nurse needs to inspect toys to ensure they are nonallergenic, washable, and unbreakable and have no small, removable parts that can be aspirated or swallowed or in other ways injure a child. All objects within reach of children younger than 3 years should pass the choke tube test. A toilet paper roll is a handy guide. If a toy or object fits into the cylinder (items less than 3 cm across or balls smaller than 4.5 cm), it is a potential choking danger to the child. Broken latex balloons pose a serious aspiration or choking threat to children of all ages if the child puts a piece into the mouth. Latex balloons should *never* be permitted in the hospital setting.

Preventing Falls

Prevention of falls begins with identification of children most prone to falling. Pediatric hospitals use various methods to identify a child's risk for falls, including a fall risk assessment of patients on admission and throughout hospitalization. Risk factors for hospitalized children falling include the following:

- Medication effects—Postanaesthesia or sedation; analgesics or narcotics, especially in those who have never had narcotics in the past and in whom effects are unknown
- Altered mental status—Secondary to seizures, brain tumours, or medications
- Altered or limited mobility—Reduced skill at ambulation secondary to developmental age, disease process, tubes, drains, casts, splints, or other appliances; new to ambulation with assistive devices, such as walkers or crutches
- Postoperative children—Risk of hypotension or syncope secondary to large blood loss, a heart condition, or extended bedrest
- History of falls
- Infants or toddlers in cribs with side rails down or on the daybed with family members

Once children at risk for falls have been identified, staff members need to be alerted by posting signs on the door and at the bedside, applying a special coloured armband labelled "Fall Precautions," labelling the chart with a sticker, or documenting information on the chart.

Prevention of falls requires alterations in the environment, including the following:

- The bed is in the lowest position, with brakes locked and side rails up.
- Call bell is placed within reach.
- All necessary and desired items are within reach, such as water, glasses, tissues, and snacks.
- Toileting is offered on a regular basis, especially if the patient is taking diuretics or laxatives.
- Lights are kept on at all times, including dimmed lights while patient is sleeping.
- Lock wheelchairs before transferring patients.
- Patient has an appropriate-size gown and nonskid footwear. Gowns or ties should not drag on the floor when the patient is ambulating.
- The floor is clean and free of clutter. A "Wet Floor" sign is posted if the floor is wet.
- Patient has glasses on if he or she normally wears them.

To prevent falls, patients also need relevant age-appropriate education. The child should be helped to ambulate even if he or she ambulated well before hospitalization. Patients who have been lying in bed need to get up slowly, sitting on the side of the bed before standing.

The nurse also needs to educate family members on ways to help prevent their child from falling:

- Call the nursing staff for assistance, and do not allow the child to get up independently.
- Keep the side rails of the crib or bed up whenever the child is in the crib or bed.
- Do not leave infants on the daybed; put them in the crib with the side rails up.
- When all family members need to leave the bedside, notify staff and ensure that the child is in the bed or crib with side rails up and that the call bell is within reach (if appropriate).

Infection Control

In a 2007 Canadian survey, Gravel, Matlow, Ofner-Agostini, et al. found that 91 children out of 1000 developed a health care–associated infection (HAI). And about 8% of children in Canadian hospitals have an HAI at any given time (Gravel et al., 2007; Public Health Agency of Canada [PHAC], 2013a). These infections occur when there is interaction among patients, health care personnel, equipment, and bacteria. HAIs are preventable if caregivers practise meticulous cleaning and disposal techniques.

Routine practices are used in the care of all patients to reduce the risk of transmission of microorganisms from both recognized and unrecognized sources of infection. Routine practices involve hand hygiene and the use of barrier protection, such as gloves, goggles, gowns, or masks, to prevent contamination from (1) blood; (2) all body fluids, secretions, and excretions *except sweat*, regardless of whether they contain visible blood; (3) nonintact skin; and (4) mucous membranes.

Additional precautions (*transmission-based precautions*) are designed for patients with documented or suspected infection or colonization (presence of microorganism in or on patient but without clinical signs and symptoms of infection) with highly transmissible or epidemiologically important pathogens for which additional precautions beyond routine practices are needed to interrupt transmission in hospitals. There are three types of additional precautions: airborne precautions, droplet precautions, and contact precautions. They may be combined when caring for patients with diseases that have multiple routes of transmission (Box 44-3). They are to be used in addition to routine practices.

Airborne precautions can reduce the risk of the airborne transmission of infectious agents. Airborne transmission occurs by dissemination of either airborne droplet nuclei (small-particle residue [5 microns or smaller in size] of evaporated droplets that may remain suspended in the air for long periods) or dust particles containing the infectious agent. Microorganisms carried in this manner can be dispersed widely by air currents and may become inhaled by or deposited on a susceptible host within the same room or over a longer distance from the source patient, depending on environmental factors. Special air handling and ventilation are required to prevent airborne transmission, as well as the use of respiratory masks (N95 or N100). Airborne precautions apply to patients with known or suspected infection with pathogens transmitted by the airborne route, such as measles, varicella, and tuberculosis.

Droplet precautions reduce the risk of droplet transmission of infectious agents. Droplet transmission involves contact of the conjunctivae or the mucous membranes of the nose or mouth of a susceptible person with large-particle droplets (larger than 5 microns in size) containing microorganisms generated from a person who has a clinical disease or who is a carrier of the microorganism. Droplets are generated from the source person primarily during coughing, sneezing, or talking and during procedures such as suctioning and bronchoscopy. Transmission requires close contact between source and recipient persons, since droplets do not remain suspended in the air

BOX 44-3 TYPES OF PRECAUTIONS AND PATIENTS REQUIRING THEM

Routine Practices

Routine practices are used at the level of care provided for all patients.

Airborne Precautions

In addition to routine practices, airborne precautions are used for patients known or suspected to have serious illnesses transmitted by airborne droplet nuclei. Examples of such illnesses include measles, varicella (including disseminated zoster), and pulmonary or laryngeal tuberculosis.

Health care providers must wear a respiratory mask (N95 or N100), and special air handling and ventilation are required.

Droplet Precautions

In addition to routine practices, droplet precautions are used for patients known or suspected to have serious illnesses transmitted by large-particle droplets. Practice of droplet precautions requires use of a mask when within 1 metre of an isolated patient. Droplet precautions include use of a shielded mask, and when there is a risk of the uniform becoming soiled, use of gown and gloves. Care of pediatric patients requires droplet precautions if patients are known or suspected to have any of the following:

- Invasive *Haemophilus influenzae* type b (until 24 hours of appropriate antibiotic received), including meningitis, pneumonia, epiglottitis, and sepsis
- Invasive *Neisseria meningitides* (until 24 hours of appropriate antibiotic received), including meningitis, pneumonia, and sepsis
- Other serious bacterial respiratory tract infections spread by droplet transmission, including diphtheria (pharyngeal), pertussis, streptococcal group A pharyngitis, respiratory syncytial virus, parainfluenza, and adenovirus. Droplet precautions should be practised for all definite or possible respiratory tract infections until viral infection can be ruled out in pediatric patients.
- Serious viral infections spread by droplet transmission, including adenovirus, influenza, mumps, parvovirus B19, rubella

Contact Precautions

In addition to routine precautions, contact precautions should be used for patients known or suspected to have serious illnesses easily transmitted by direct patient contact or contact with items in the patient's environment. Contact precautions require the use of gloves and gown in addition to routine precautions. Additional precautions may be indicated for certain organisms when routine practices are not sufficient to control transmission, for instance:

- If the organism has a low infective dose
- If the organism may be transmitted from the source patient's intact skin
- If there is potential for widespread environmental contamination

Pediatric patients require care with contact precautions if they are known or suspected to have any of the following:

- Diarrhea due to *Campylobacter, Rotavirus, Salmonella, Giardia, Shigella, C. difficile, Yersinia,* or pathogenic strains of *E. coli*
- Respiratory tract infections due to adenovirus, parainfluenza virus, rhinovirus, respiratory syncytial virus, or influenza (use droplet plus contact precautions)
- Hepatitis A or E, scabies, enteroviral infections, herpes simplex virus: neonatal or disseminated mucocutaneous, antimicrobial-resistant organisms
- Viral or hemorrhagic conjunctivitis
- Viral hemorrhagic infections (Ebola, Lassa, or Marburg)

From Public Health Agency of Canada. (2012). Routine practices and additional precautions for preventing the transmission of infection in healthcare settings (HP40-83/2013E-PDF), pp. 52–89. Retrieved from http://publications.gc.ca/collections/collection_2013/aspc-phac/HP40-83-2013-eng.pdf

and generally travel only short distances, usually 1 metre or less, through the air. Because droplets do not remain suspended in the air, special air handling and ventilation are not required to prevent droplet transmission although regular masks are required when within 1 metre of patient. Droplet precautions apply to any patient with known or suspected infection with pathogens that can be transmitted by infectious droplets (see Box 44-3).

Contact precautions reduce the risk of transmission of microorganisms by direct or indirect contact. Direct-contact transmission involves a skin-to-skin contact and physical transfer of microorganisms to a susceptible host from an infected or colonized person, such as occurs when turning or bathing patients. Direct-contact transmission also can occur between two patients (e.g., by hand contact). Indirect-contact transmission involves contact of a susceptible host with a contaminated intermediate object, usually inanimate, in the patient's environment. Contact precautions apply to specified patients known or suspected to be infected or colonized with microorganisms that can be transmitted by direct or indirect contact (e.g., wound infections or gastrointestinal infections). Contact precautions include the use of a gown and gloves.

NURSING ALERT

The most common piece of medical equipment, the stethoscope, can be a potent source of harmful microorganisms and health care-acquired infections. One study found that 80% of 200 stethoscopes were contaminated with at least one microbe (Maki, 2014).

Nurses caring for young children are frequently in contact with body substances, especially urine, feces, and vomitus. They should exercise judgement concerning those situations when gloves, gowns, or masks are necessary. For example, nurses should wear gloves for changing diapers and wear gowns when there is the possibility of loose or explosive stools.

Antimicrobial-resistant organisms are causing increasing numbers of HAIs. In hospitals, patients are the most significant sources of methicillin-resistant *Staphylococcus aureus* (MSRA), and the main mode of transmission is patient to patient via the hands of a health care provider. The MRSA infection rate has increased by more than 1000%, from 0.17 cases per 1000 patient admissions in 1995 to 1.96 cases in 2009 (PHAC, 2013a). Hand hygiene is the most critical infection control practice (PHAC, 2013b).

! NURSING ALERT

Hand hygiene is the most critical infection-control practice. Hand hygiene should be followed using the four moments of hand hygiene: (1) before initial contact with the patient or patient environment, (2) before a clean/aseptic procedure, (3) after body-fluid exposure risk, and (4) after contact with a patient or patient environment.

During feedings, gowns should be worn if the child is likely to vomit or spit up, which often occurs during burping. The nurse should wash hands thoroughly after removing the gloves, since gloves fail to provide complete protection. The absence of visible leakage does not indicate gloves are intact.

Another essential practice of infection control is that all needles (uncapped and unbroken) need to be disposed of in an approved sharps disposal container, often installed in patients' rooms. Since children are naturally curious, nurses need to give extra attention to disposing of sharps directly after use and preventing access to disposed needles.

Transporting Infants and Children

Infants and children need to be transported within the unit and to areas outside the pediatric unit. Infants and small children can be carried for short distances within the unit, but for more extended trips the child should be securely transported in a suitable conveyance (see hospital policy related to transport).

Small infants can be held or carried in the horizontal position (Fig. 44-4, A) or in the football hold (see Fig. 44-4, B). Both of these holds leave the nurse's other arm free for activity. The infant also can be held in the upright position in which the infant's head and shoulders are supported by the nurse's other arm in case the infant moves suddenly (see Fig. 44-4, C).

The method of transporting children is determined by their age, condition, destination, and hospital policy. Older children are safe in wheelchairs or on stretchers. Younger children can be transported in a crib, on a stretcher, in a wagon with raised sides, or in a wheelchair with a safety belt. Stretchers should be equipped with high sides and a safety belt, both of which are secured during transport. Critically ill children should always be transported on a bed or stretcher by at least two staff members with monitoring continued during transport. A blood pressure monitor or standard blood pressure cuff, pulse oximeter, and cardiac monitor/defibrillator should accompany every critically ill child. Airway equipment and emergency medication should also accompany the child.

Restraining Methods and Therapeutic Holding

A *restraint* is any method, physical or mechanical, that restricts a person's movement, physical activity, or normal access to his or her body. Before initiating use of restraint, the nurse should complete a comprehensive assessment of the patient to determine whether the need for a restraint outweighs the risk of not using one. The nurse needs to assess the child's developmental level, mental status, potential to hurt others or self, and safety. Ultimately, the nurse is responsible for selecting the means of least restraint possible.

Restraints can result in loss of dignity, violation of patient rights, psychological harm, physical harm, and even death. Thus alternative methods should first be considered and documented in the patient's record. Some examples of alternative measures include bringing a child to the nurses' station for continuous observation, providing diversional activities, such as music, encouraging the participation of the parents, or using therapeutic holding. In *therapeutic holding*, the parent or caregiver holds the child in a secure, comfortable position that provides close physical contact for 30 minutes or less (Fig. 44-5).

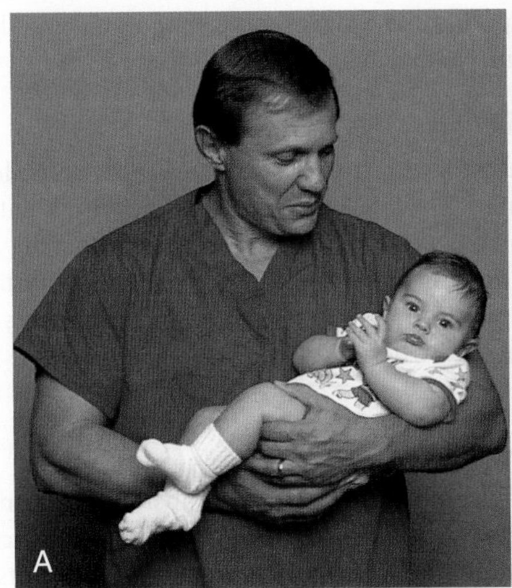

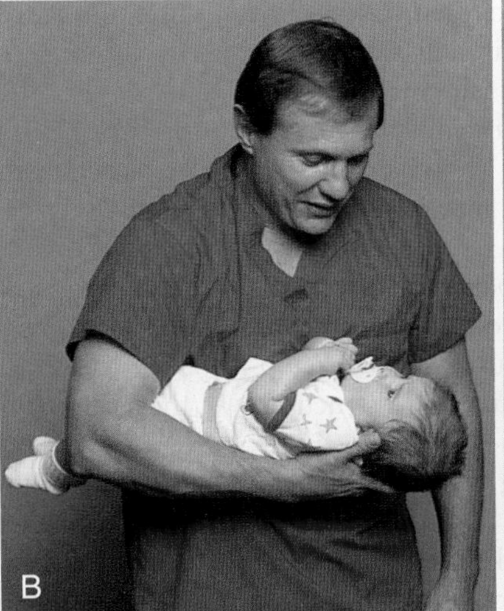

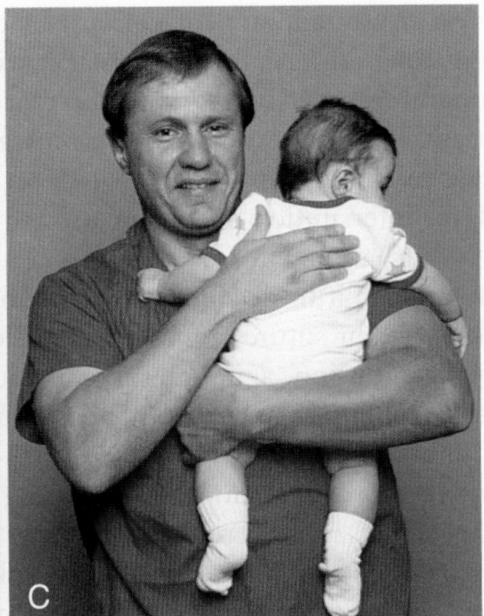

FIGURE 44-4 Transporting infants. **A:** Infant's thigh firmly grasped in nurse's hand. **B:** Football hold. **C:** Back supported.

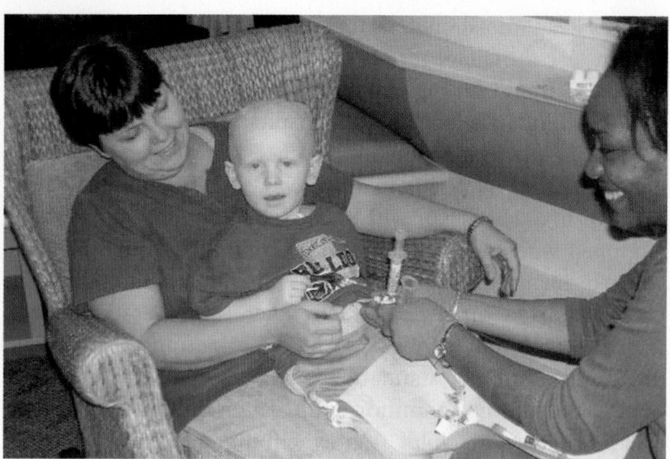

FIGURE 44-5 Therapeutic holding of child with parental assistance.

The use of restraints can often be avoided with adequate preparation of the child, parental or staff supervision of the child, or adequate protection of a vulnerable site such as an infusion device. This is often possible when the child and parents work together with the nurse.

Nurses cannot use any form of restraint without a patient's or legal guardian's informed consent except in an emergency situation in which there is a serious threat of harm to the individual or others and all other measures have been unsuccessful. It is important for nurses to know their scope of practice for their jurisdiction as well as being aware of individual agency policies in terms of restraints. The individual jurisdictions in Canada mirror the College of Nurses of Ontario (CNO) standards. In some settings, a physician's order may be required prior to the use of restraints. In other settings, it is a nursing decision (CNO, 2009). Continued use of restraints must be renewed each day. Patients need to be monitored at least every 1 hour.

The three types of restraints used with patients include physical, chemical, or environmental restraints.

Physical restraints are used for children with an artificial airway or airway adjunct for delivery of oxygen, in-dwelling catheters, tubes, drains, lines, pacemaker wires, or suture sites. The physical restraint is used to ensure that safe care is given to the patient. Physical restraints may be instituted for any of the following reasons:

- Risk for interruption of therapy used to maintain oxygenation or airway patency
- Risk of harm if in-dwelling catheter, tube, drain, line, pacemaker wire, or sutures are removed, dislodged, or ruptured
- Patient confusion, agitation, unconsciousness, or developmental inability to understand direct requests or instructions

Restraints with ties must be secured to the bed or crib frame, not the side rails. Suggestions for increasing safety and comfort while the child is in a restraint include leaving one finger breadth between skin and the device; tying knots that allow for quick release; ensuring that the restraint does not tighten as the child moves; decreasing wrinkles or bulges in the restraint; placing jacket restraints over an article of clothing; placing limb restraints below waist level, below knee level, or distal to the IV; and tucking in dangling straps. Assessment components include signs of injury associated with applying restraint, nutrition and hydration, circulation and range-of-motion of extremities, vital signs, hygiene and elimination, physical and psychological status and comfort, and readiness for discontinuation of restraint.

Chemical restraints are pharmaceutical interventions administered to keep the individual safe. Chemical restraints must be ordered by a physician and, as with all restraints, informed consent is required. Children in chemical restraints must be observed and assessed every 15 minutes. *Environmental restraint* refers to the restraining of an individual within a physical space, such as in a locked unit in a mental health facility. For example, an adolescent with a mental health issue may be admitted to an emergency department and be restricted to an examining room because of aggressive behaviour.

Mummy Restraint or Swaddle

When an infant or small child requires short-term restraint for examination or treatment, such as venipuncture, throat examination, and gavage feeding, a mummy wrap effectively controls the child's movements. A blanket or sheet is opened on the bed or crib with one corner folded to the centre. The infant is placed on the blanket with shoulders at the fold and feet toward the opposite corner. With the infant's right arm straight down against the body, the right side of the blanket is pulled firmly across the infant's right shoulder and chest and secured beneath the left side of the body. The left arm is placed straight against the infant's side, and the left side of the blanket is brought across the shoulder and chest and locked beneath the body on the right side. The lower corner is folded and brought over the body and tucked or fastened securely with safety pins. To modify the mummy restraint for chest examination, the folded edge of the blanket is brought over each arm and under the back, after which the loose edge is folded over and secured at a point below the chest to allow visualization of and access to the chest (Fig. 44-6, A). It is important that swaddling an infant in this manner is only used for short periods of time, as swaddling as a general practice is not recommended.

Jacket Restraint

A jacket restraint is sometimes used to keep the child safe in various chairs. The jacket is put on the child with the ties in back so that the child is unable to manipulate them. The jacket restraint is also useful as a means of maintaining the child in a desired horizontal position. The long tapes secured to the understructure of the crib keep the child inside the crib.

Arm and Leg Restraints

Occasionally, one or more extremities must be restrained or limited in motion. Several commercial restraining devices are available, including disposable wrist and ankle restraints (Fig. 44-6, B). The restraints must be appropriate to the child's size and padded to prevent undue pressure, constriction, or tissue

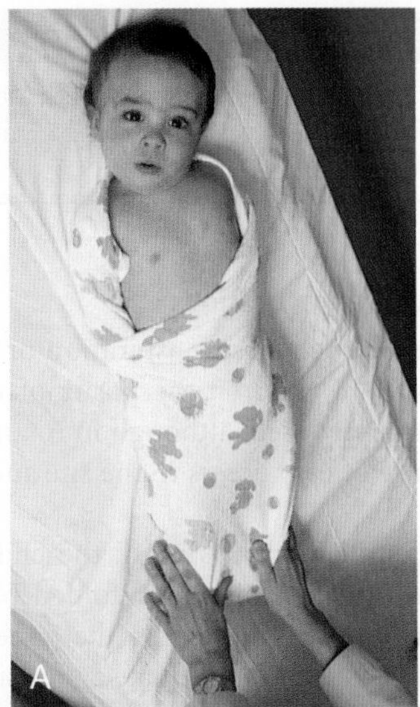

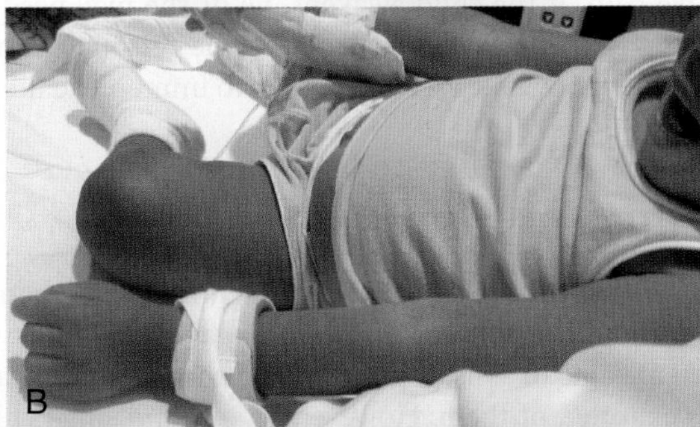

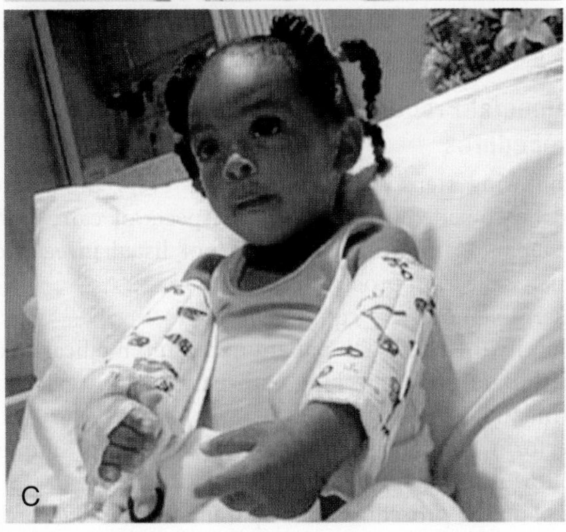

FIGURE 44-6 Restraint examples from most restrictive to least restrictive. **A:** Mummy restraint. **B:** Wrist restraints. **C:** Elbow restraints.

injury; and the extremity must be observed frequently for signs of irritation or impairment of circulation. The ends of the restraints are never tied to the side rails, since lowering the rail will disturb the extremity, frequently with a jerk that may hurt or injure the child.

Elbow Restraint

Sometimes it is important to prevent the child from reaching the head or face, such as after lip surgery, when a scalp vein

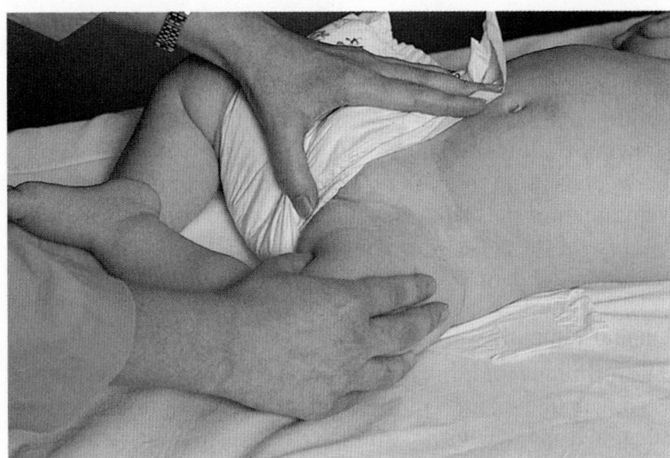

FIGURE 44-7 Restraining an infant for femoral venipuncture.

infusion is in place, or to prevent scratching in skin disorders. Elbow restraints fashioned from a variety of materials function well (Fig. 44-6, C). Commercial elbow restraints are available. An improvised form of elbow restraint consists of a piece of muslin long enough to reach comfortably from just below the axilla to the wrist with a number of vertical pockets into which tongue depressors are inserted. The restraint is wrapped around the arm and secured with tape or pins. It may be necessary to pin the top of the restraint to the undershirt sleeve to prevent the restraint from slipping.

Positioning for Procedures

Infants and small children are unable to cooperate for many procedures; therefore, the nurse is responsible for minimizing their movement and discomfort with proper positioning. A second nurse should assist with procedures required in infants or young children. Older children usually need only minimal, if any, restraint. Careful explanation and preparation beforehand and support and simple guidance during the procedure are usually sufficient. For painful procedures the child should receive adequate analgesia and sedation to minimize pain and the need for excessive restraint.

Femoral Venipuncture

The nurse places the child supine with the legs in a frog position to provide extensive exposure of the groin area. The infant's legs can be effectively held by the nurse's forearms and hands (Fig. 44-7). Only the side used for the venipuncture is uncovered, so the physician or nurse is protected should the infant urinate during the procedure. Pressure is applied to the site to prevent oozing from the site.

Extremity Venipuncture

The most common sites of venipuncture are the veins of the extremities, especially the arm and hand. If possible, it is best to use the policy of least restraint and to use some of the atraumatic techniques described in the venipuncture section of this chapter (p. 1304). If necessary, the child can be placed in the parent's (or assistant's) lap, with the child facing the parent and in the straddle position. Next, the child's arm is placed for venipuncture on a firm surface, such as a treatment table. The child's outstretched arm is partially stabilized by the technician drawing the blood. The parent should hug the child's upper body, preventing movement, and use an arm to immobilize the venipuncture site. This type of restraint also comforts the child because of the close body contact, and it allows each person to maintain eye contact.

Lumbar Puncture

The technique for lumbar puncture (LP) in infants and children is similar to that used in the adult, although modifications are suggested for newborns, who have less distress in a side-lying position with modified neck extension than in flexion or a sitting position.

Children are usually easiest to control in the side-lying position, with the head flexed and the knees drawn up toward the chest (Fig. 44-8). Even cooperative children need to be held gently to prevent possible trauma from unexpected, involuntary movement. They can be reassured that, although they are trusted, the holding will serve as a reminder to maintain the desired position. It also provides a measure of support and reassurance to them.

An alternative position used with small infants and some older children is the sitting position. The child is placed with the buttocks at the edge of the table and with the neck flexed so that the chin rests on the child's chest or the nurse's arm. The child's arms and legs are immobilized by the nurse's hands.

Specimens and spinal fluid pressure are obtained, measured, and sent for analysis in the same manner as for the adult patient. Vital signs should be taken as ordered and the child observed for any changes in level of consciousness, motor activity, or other neurological signs. Post-LP headache may occur and is related to postural changes; this is less severe when the child lies flat for a period of time. Headache is seen much less frequently in young children than in adolescents.

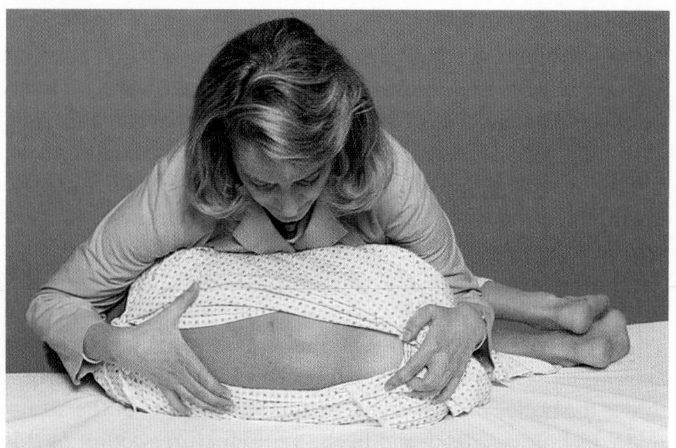

FIGURE 44-8 Child in side-lying position for lumbar puncture.

NURSING ALERT

The sitting position may interfere with chest expansion and diaphragm excursion. In infants, the soft pliable trachea may collapse, so the child must be observed for breathing difficulties.

Bone Marrow Aspiration or Biopsy

The position for a bone marrow aspiration or biopsy depends on the chosen site. In children the posterior or anterior iliac crest is most frequently used, although in infants the tibia may be selected because of easy access to the site and holding of the child.

If the posterior iliac crest is used, the child is positioned prone. Sometimes a small pillow or folded blanket is placed under the hips to facilitate obtaining the bone marrow specimen. Children should receive adequate analgesia or anaesthesia to relieve pain. If the child awakens, he or she may need to be held; this is best done with two people—one person to immobilize the upper body and a second person to immobilize the lower extremities.

COLLECTION OF SPECIMENS

Many of the specimens needed for diagnostic examination of children are collected in much the same way as for adults. Older children are able to assist if given proper instructions regarding what is expected of them. However, infants and small children are unable to follow direction or control body functions sufficiently to help in collecting some specimens.

Fundamental Procedure Steps Common to All Procedures

The following steps are important for every procedure and should be considered fundamental aspects of care. Although these steps are important, they are not listed in each of the specimen collection procedures.

1. Assemble necessary equipment.
2. Identify the child with patient name and medical record or birth date, cross-checking with parents and reviewing the armband.
3. Perform hand hygiene, maintain aseptic technique, and follow routine practices.
4. Explain the procedure to the parent and child according to the developmental level of the child; reassure the child that the procedure is not a punishment.
5. Provide atraumatic care and position the child securely.
6. Prepare the area with aseptic agent.
7. Place specimens in appropriate containers and apply a patient identification label to the specimen container in the presence of the child and family.
8. Discard puncture device in puncture-resistant container near the site of use.
9. Wash the procedural preparation agent off if povidone-iodine is used, if skin is sensitive, and for infants.
10. Remove gloves and perform hand hygiene after the procedure. Have children wash their hands if they have helped.

11. Praise the child for helping.
12. Document pertinent aspects of the procedure, such as number of attempts, site, amount of blood or urine withdrawn, and type of test performed.

Urine Specimens

Older children and adolescents can use a bedpan or urinal or can follow directions for collection in the bathroom. However, they may have special needs. School-age children are cooperative but curious. They are concerned about the reasons behind things and are likely to ask questions about the disposition of their specimen and what might be discovered from it. Self-conscious adolescents may be reluctant to carry a specimen through a hallway or waiting room and appreciate a paper bag or other means for disguising the container. The presence of menses may be an embarrassment or a concern to teenage girls; thus, it is a good idea to ask if they are menstruating and to make adjustments as necessary. The specimen can be delayed or a notation made on the laboratory slip to explain the presence of red blood cells.

Preschoolers and toddlers are usually unable to void on request. It is often best to offer them water or other liquids that they enjoy and wait about 30 minutes until they are ready to void voluntarily.

Children will better understand what is expected if the nurse uses familiar terms, such as "pee-pee," "wee-wee," or "tinkle." Some will have difficulty voiding in an unfamiliar receptacle. Potty chairs or a potty hat placed on the toilet is usually helpful. Toddlers who have recently acquired bladder control may be especially reluctant, since they undoubtedly have been admonished for "going" in places other than those approved by parents. Enlisting the parents help usually leads to success.

For infants and toddlers who are not toilet trained, special urine collection bags with self-adhering material around the opening at the point of attachment are used. To prepare the infant, the genitalia, perineum, and surrounding skin are washed and dried thoroughly because the adhesive will not stick to a moist, powdered, or oily skin surface. The collection bag is easiest to apply if attached first to the perineum, progressing to the symphysis pubis (Fig. 44-9). With girls, the perineum is stretched taut during application to the area to ensure a leak-proof fit. With boys the penis and sometimes the scrotum are placed inside the bag. The adhesive portion of the bag must be firmly applied to the skin all around the genital area to avoid leakage. For low-birth-weight infants, small bags with adhesive that is gentle to the skin are available. When a urine collection bag is used, a small slit is cut in the diaper and the bag pulled through to allow room for urine to collect and to facilitate checking on the contents. The bag is checked frequently and removed as soon as the specimen is available, since the moist bag may become loosened on an active child. When urine is collected for culture, the bag is removed immediately.

For some types of urine testing, such as specific gravity, ketones, glucose, and protein, urine can be aspirated directly from the diaper. To obtain this type of small amount of urine, the nurse can use a needleless syringe to aspirate urine directly from the diaper. If diapers with absorbent gelling material that trap urine are used, the nurse places a small gauze dressing, some cotton balls, or a urine collection device inside the diaper to collect urine, then aspirates the urine with a syringe or puts the cotton balls into the syringe and depresses the plunger to extract urine.

Clean-Catch Specimens

Clean-catch specimens traditionally refer to a urine sample obtained for culture after the urethral meatus is cleaned and the first few millilitres of urine are voided before the urine is collected (*midstream specimen*). In girls, the perineum is wiped with an antiseptic pad from front to back. In boys, the tip of the penis is cleansed.

Twenty-Four–Hour Collection

Collection bags are required to collect specimens from infants and small children for a 24-hour collection. Older children require special instruction about notifying someone when they need to void or have a bowel movement so that urine can be collected separately and not discarded. Some older school-age children and adolescents can take responsibility for collection of their own 24-hour specimens and can keep output records and transfer each voiding to the 24-hour collection container.

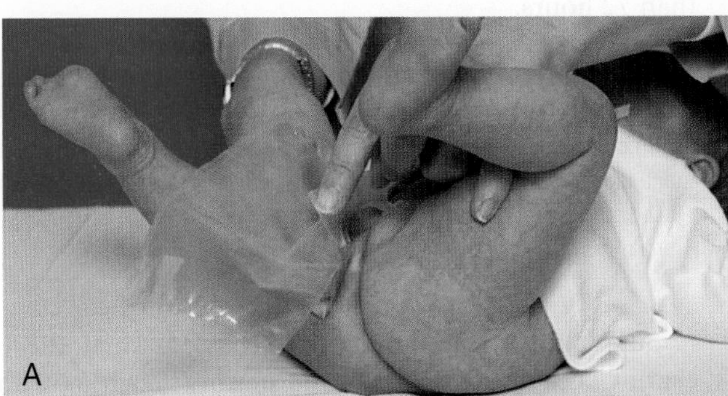

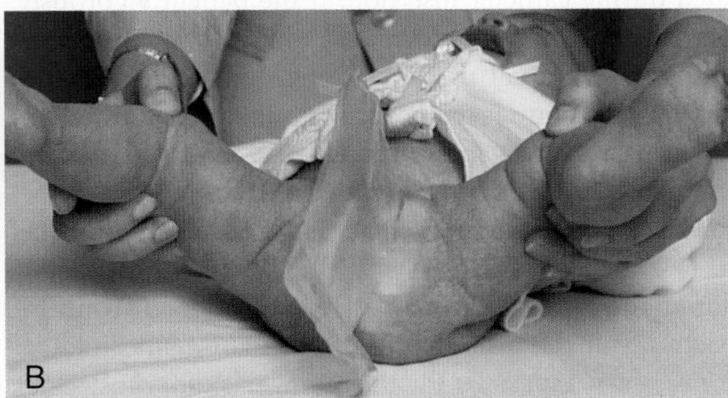

FIGURE 44-9 Application of urine collection bag. **A:** On female infants, the adhesive portion is applied to the exposed and dried perineum first. **B:** The bag adheres firmly around the perineal area to prevent urine leakage.

The collection period always starts and ends with an empty bladder. At the time the collection begins, the child is instructed to void and the specimen is discarded. All urine voided in the subsequent 24 hours is saved in a container with a preservative or is placed on ice. Twenty-four hours from the time the precollection specimen was discarded, the child is again instructed to void, the specimen is added to the container, and the entire collection is taken to the laboratory.

Infants and small children who are bagged for a 24-hour urine collection require a special collection bag. Frequent removal and replacement of adhesive collection devices can produce skin irritation. A thin coating of sealant, such as Skin-Prep, applied to the skin helps to protect it and aids adhesion, unless its use is contraindicated, such as in premature infants or children with irritated skin. Plastic collection bags with collection tubes attached are ideal when the container must be left in place for a time. These can be connected to a collecting device or emptied periodically by aspiration with a syringe. When such devices are not available, a regular bag with a feeding tube inserted through a puncture hole at the top of the bag serves as a satisfactory substitute. However, it is important to empty the bag as soon as the infant urinates to prevent leakage and loss of contents. An in-dwelling catheter may also be placed for the collection period.

Bladder Catheterization and Other Techniques

Bladder catheterization or suprapubic aspiration is employed when a specimen is urgently needed or when the child is unable to void or otherwise provide an adequate specimen. The CPS recommends that a diagnosis of urinary tract infection (UTI) made with a bag urine specimen in young infants requires confirmation with a suprapubic or urethral catheterization before treatment (Robinson, Finlay, Lang, et al., 2014).

Preparation for catheterization includes instruction on pelvic muscle relaxation, but this can be difficult to achieve in this age group. Alternatively, nurses can wait until the child relaxes with crying. If the toddler, preschooler, or younger child can follow instructions, the child is taught to blow a pinwheel and to press the hips against the bed or procedure table during catheterization to relax the pelvic and periurethral muscles. For the older child or adolescent, the location and function of the pelvic muscles are described. The patient is then taught to contract and relax the pelvic muscles, and the relaxation procedure is repeated during catheter insertion. If the patient vigorously contracts the pelvic muscles when the catheter reaches the striated sphincter (proximal urethra in boys and midurethra in girls), catheter insertion is temporarily stopped. The catheter is neither removed nor advanced; instead, the child is helped to press the hips against the bed or examining table and relax the pelvic muscles. The catheter is then gently advanced into the bladder.

Children and adolescents may experience some discomfort and anxiety during this procedure. Assistance and gentle holding may be necessary, especially for the younger child. Most children prefer to have the parents remain with them during the procedure. The parent should be encouraged to talk softly and hold the child's hand as the catheter is inserted. Using distractions such as reading a book, singing a song, or playing with small toys may decrease the child's anxiety. Older children and adolescents may wish to listen to music with headphones. Adolescents should be asked if they would like a parent to remain with them during the procedure. The decision should be made before the perineum is exposed and the sterile field is prepared.

CULTURAL AWARENESS

Bladder Catheterization

Parents may be upset when their child is catheterized. Aside from the trauma the child experiences, some parents may fear that the procedure affects the daughter's virginity. To correct this misconception, the family may benefit from a detailed explanation of the genitourinary anatomy, preferably with a model that shows the separate vaginal and urethral openings. The nurse can also indicate that catheterization has no effect on virginity.

Some parents may not understand the procedure of catheterization and may need some explanation to allay their concerns (see Cultural Awareness box).

Catheterization is a sterile procedure. If the catheter is to remain in place, a Foley catheter is used. The supplies needed for this procedure include sterile gloves, sterile lubricant anaesthetic, an appropriately sized catheter, povidone-iodine (Betadine) swabs or an alternative cleansing agent and 10×10-cm gauze squares, a sterile drape, and a syringe with sterile water if a Foley catheter is used.

NURSING ALERT

Identify patients who have allergies to povidone-iodine or alternative cleanser or latex before using these items in catheterization.

Adolescent boys and children with a history of urethral surgery may be catheterized using a coudé-tipped catheter. The child with myelodysplasia or one who has been identified as being sensitive or allergic to latex is catheterized with a catheter manufactured from an alternative material. When an in-dwelling catheter is indicated for urinary drainage, a lubricious-coated or silicone catheter is selected, because these materials produce less irritation of the urethral mucosa than does a Silastic or latex catheter when the catheter is left in place for more than 72 hours.

SAFETY ALERT

Do not advance the catheter too far into the bladder. Knotting of catheters and tubes within the bladder has been reported. Feeding tubes should not be used for urinary catheterization because they are more flexible, long, and prone to knotting than commercially designed urinary catheters.

Suprapubic aspiration is mainly used when the bladder cannot be accessed through the urethra (such as with some congenital urological birth defects, such as a fused labia) or to reduce the risk of contamination that may be present when passing a catheter. With the advent of small catheters (5 and 6

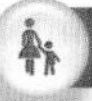

ATRAUMATIC CARE

Bladder Catheterization or Suprapubic Aspiration

- Use distraction to help the child relax (e.g., blowing bubbles, deep breathing, singing a song).
- Use lidocaine jelly to anaesthetize the area before insertion of the catheter. EMLA cream (a eutectic mix of lidocaine and prilocaine) or LMX cream (lidocaine) may lessen an infant's discomfort as the needle passes through the skin for suprapubic aspiration, but care should be taken that the site is thoroughly cleaned and prepped before the procedure.
- Children often become agitated at being restrained for either procedure. Use comfort measures through touch and voice, both during and after the procedure, to help reduce the child's distress.

French), the need for suprapubic aspiration has decreased. Access to the bladder via the urethra has a much higher success rate than suprapubic aspiration, where success depends on the practitioner's skill at assessing the location of the bladder and the amount of urine in the bladder.

Suprapubic aspiration involves aspirating bladder contents by inserting a 20- or 21-gauge needle in the midline approximately 1 cm above the symphysis pubis and directed vertically downward, performed by a physician or trained NP. The nurse prepares the skin as for any needle insertion and the bladder should contain an adequate volume of urine. This can be assumed if the infant has not voided for at least 1 hour or the bladder can be palpated above the symphysis pubis. This technique is useful for obtaining sterile specimens from young infants, since the bladder is an abdominal organ and is easily accessed. Suprapubic aspiration is painful, thus pain management during the procedure is important (Atraumatic Care). Use of distraction and comfort measure through touch and voice, during and after the procedure, help to decrease the child's distress.

Stool Specimens

Stool specimens are frequently collected from children to identify parasites and other organisms that cause diarrhea, to assess gastrointestinal function, and to check for occult (hidden) blood. Ideally, stool should be collected without contamination with urine, but in children wearing diapers this is difficult unless a urine bag is applied. Children who are toilet trained should urinate first, flush the toilet, then defecate in the toilet, a bedpan (preferably one that is placed on the toilet to avoid embarrassment), or a commercial potty hat and cover with plastic wrap to collect stool.

Stool specimens should be large enough to obtain an ample sampling, not merely a fecal fragment. Specimens should be placed in an appropriate container, which is covered and labelled. If several specimens are needed, the containers are marked with the date and time and kept in a specimen refrigerator. The specimen should be handled carefully to prevent contamination.

Blood Specimens

Whether the specimen is collected by the nurse or others, the nurse is responsible for making certain that specimens, such as serial examinations and fasting specimens, are collected on time and that the proper equipment is available. The collecting, transporting, and storing of specimens can have a major impact on laboratory results.

Venous blood samples can be obtained by venipuncture or by aspiration from a peripheral or central access device. Withdrawing blood specimens through peripheral lock devices in small peripheral veins has met with varying degrees of success and can only be performed with certain blood work. Although it avoids an additional venipuncture for the child, attempting to aspirate blood from the peripheral lock may shorten the life of the device. When using an IV infusion site for specimen collection, the type of fluid being infused needs to be considered. For example, a specimen collected for glucose level would be inaccurate if removed from a catheter through which glucose-containing solution was being administered.

The needed specimens are collected quickly, and pressure is applied to the puncture site with dry gauze until bleeding stops. The arm should be extended, not flexed, while pressure is applied for a few minutes after venipuncture in the antecubital fossa to reduce bruising. The nurse then covers the site with an adhesive bandage. In young children adhesive bandages pose an aspiration hazard; thus it is good to avoid using them or remove the adhesive bandage as soon as the bleeding stops. Applying warm compresses to ecchymotic areas increases circulation, helps remove extravasated blood, and decreases pain.

NURSING ALERT

- To obtain a blood specimen from a peripheral lock when the infusion solution may interfere with tests results, first aspirate a quantity of blood equal to the volume of fluid in the catheter and discard; then aspirate the blood sample. However, ensure that this is in accordance with hospital policy.
- For a blood culture, use the first sample of blood, since organisms are most likely to collect within the catheter itself.

NURSING ALERT

On small or anemic children, keep track of the amount drawn over time. Frequent taking of blood specimens can rapidly decrease a child's blood volume. Coordinate blood samples and ask the laboratory to save as much blood as possible to reduce the frequency.

Arterial blood samples are sometimes needed for blood gas measurement, although noninvasive techniques, such as **transcutaneous oxygen monitoring** and pulse oximetry, are used frequently. Arterial samples may be obtained by arterial puncture using the radial, brachial, or femoral arteries, or from in-dwelling arterial catheters. Adequate circulation should be assessed before arterial puncture by observing capillary refill or performing the *Allen test*, a procedure that assesses the circulation of the radial, ulnar, or brachial arteries (see Chapter 33). Because unclotted blood is required, only heparinized collection tubes are used. In addition, no air bubbles should enter the tube, since they can alter the blood gas concentration. Crying, fear, and agitation also affect blood gas values; every effort should be made to comfort the child. The nurse should pack the sample in ice to reduce blood cell metabolism and should take it to the laboratory for immediate analysis.

Capillary blood samples are taken from older children by a finger stick. A common method for taking certain peripheral blood samples from infants younger than 6 months of age is by a heel stick. Before the blood sample is taken, the heel is warmed for 3 minutes (see Fig. 26-13). The area is cleansed with alcohol, the infant's foot firmly restrained with the free hand, and the heel punctured with an automatic lancet device. An automatic device delivers a more precise puncture depth and is less painful than using a lance.

The most serious complications of infant heel puncture are necrotizing osteochondritis from lancet penetration of the underlying calcaneus bone, infection, and abscess of the heel. To avoid osteochondritis, the puncture should be no deeper than 2 mm and should be made at the outer aspect of the heel. The boundaries of the calcaneus can be marked by an imaginary line extending posteriorly from a point between the fourth and fifth toes and running parallel to the lateral aspect of the heel and another line extending posteriorly from the middle of the great toe and running parallel to the medial aspect of the heel (Fig. 44-10). Repeated trauma to the walking surface of the heel can cause fibrosis and scarring that may interfere with locomotion.

Children also dislike the discomfort associated with venous, arterial, and capillary punctures. These procedures have been identified as the ones most frequently causing pain during hospitalization and an arterial puncture as being one of the most painful of all procedures experienced. Toddlers are most distressed by venipuncture. Consequently, nurses need to institute pain reduction techniques to lessen the discomfort of these procedures (see Atraumatic Care box).

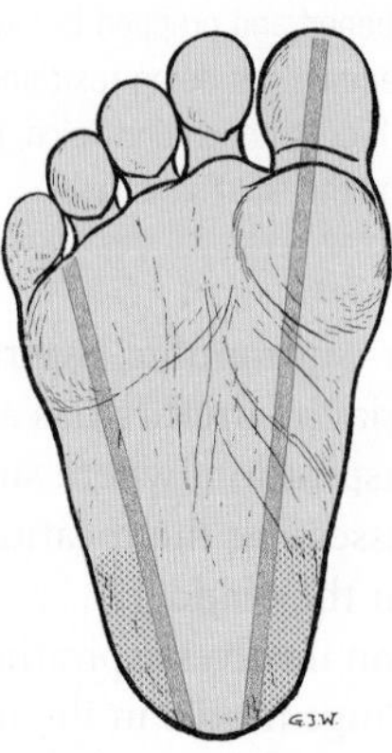

FIGURE 44-10 Puncture site (coloured stippled area) on sole of infant's foot.

ATRAUMATIC CARE

Guidelines for Skin and Vessel Punctures

For Reduction of Pain Associated With Heel, Finger, Venous, or Arterial Punctures

Apply EMLA (a eutectic mixture of lidocaine and prilocaine) topically over the site if time permits (at least 60 minutes). LMX (lidocaine) cream also may be used and requires a shorter application time (30 minutes).

To remove the transparent dressing atraumatically, grasp opposite sides of the film and pull the sides away from each other to stretch and loosen the film. After the film begins to loosen, grasp the other two sides of the film and pull.

Use iontophoresis (Numby Stuff) over the site if time permits (8 to 20 minutes), a vapocoolant spray, or buffered lidocaine (injected intradermally near the vein with a 30-gauge needle) to numb the skin.

Use nonpharmacological methods to lessen pain and anxiety, such as asking the child to take a deep breath when the needle is inserted and again when the needle is withdrawn; exhaling a large breath or blowing bubbles to "blow hurt away"; counting slowly and then faster and louder if pain is felt.

Keep all equipment out of sight until used.

Enlist parents' presence or assistance, if they wish to be present for the procedure.

Restrain child *only as needed* to perform the procedure safely; use therapeutic holding (p. 1297).

Allow the skin preparation to dry completely before penetrating the skin.

Use the smallest-gauge needle (e.g., 25 gauge) that permits free flow of blood; a 27-gauge needle can be used for obtaining 1 to 1.5 mL blood and for prominent veins (needle length is only 13 mm).

If possible, avoid putting an IV line in the dominant hand or the hand the child uses to suck the thumb.

Use an automatic lancet device for precise puncture depth of the finger or heel; press the device lightly against the skin; avoid steadying the finger against a hard surface.

Children, even some older ones, fear the loss of their blood, particularly children whose condition requires frequent blood specimens.

Have a "two-try" only policy to reduce excessive insertion attempts—two operators each have two insertion attempts; if insertion is not successful after four punctures, consider alternative venous access, such as a peripherally inserted central catheter (PICC); have a policy for identifying children with difficult access and appropriate interventions such as most experienced operator for the first attempt.

For Multiple Blood Samples

Use an intermittent infusion device (saline lock) to collect additional samples; consider PICC lines early, not as a last resort.

Coordinate care to allow several tests to be performed on one blood sample using micromethods of testing.

Anticipate tests (e.g., drug levels, chemistry, immunoglobulin levels) and ask the laboratory to save blood for additional testing.

For Heel Lancing in Newborns

Heel lancing has been shown to be more painful than venipuncture; consider venipuncture when the amount of blood from the heel would require much squeezing, such as genetic screening tests.

Place diapered newborn against the mother's bare chest in skin-to-skin contact or have mother breastfeed 10 to 15 minutes before and during heel lance.

During the procedure, allow newborn to suck a pacifier coated with a solution of 24% sucrose. Use this solution to coat the pacifier, or administer 2 mL to the tongue 2 minutes before the procedure (see Research Focus box, Chapter 26).

Respiratory Secretion Specimens

Collection of sputum or nasal discharge is sometimes required for diagnosis of respiratory infections, especially tuberculosis and respiratory syncytial virus (RSV). Older children and adolescents are able to cough and supply sputum specimens when given proper directions. It must be made clear to them that a coughed specimen, not mucus that is cleared from the throat, is needed. It is helpful to demonstrate a deep cough. Infants and small children are unable to follow directions to cough and will swallow any sputum produced; thus gastric washings (**lavage**) may be used to collect a sputum specimen. Sometimes a satisfactory specimen can be obtained using a suction device such as a mucus trap if the catheter is inserted into the trachea and the cough reflex is elicited. A catheter inserted into the back of the throat is not sufficient. For children with a tracheostomy, a specimen is easily aspirated from the trachea or major bronchi by attaching a collecting device to the suction apparatus.

Nasopharyngeal aspiration is the preferred method over nasal washings to diagnose an infection of RSV. For nasal washings, the child is placed supine, and 1 to 3 mL sterile normal saline is instilled with a sterile syringe (without needle) into one nostril. The contents are aspirated using a small, sterile bulb syringe and are placed in a sterile container. Another method involves use of a syringe with 5 cm of 18- to 20-gauge tubing. The saline is quickly instilled and then aspirated to recover the nasal specimen. To prevent additional discomfort, all of the equipment should be ready before beginning the procedure.

Other respiratory secretion collection methods include nasopharyngeal swabs to diagnose *Bordetella pertussis* and throat cultures. The nurse swabs both the tonsils and the posterior pharynx when obtaining a throat culture. The swab stick is inserted into the culture tube. Some culture kits require squeezing an ampule to release the culture medium.

ADMINISTRATION OF MEDICATION

Determination of Medication Dosage

Because the administration of medication is a nursing responsibility, nurses need to have not only knowledge of drug action and patient responses, such as adverse effects and signs of toxicity, but also resources for estimating safe dosages for children. Unlike with adult medications, there are few standardized pediatric dosage ranges.

Factors related to growth and maturation significantly alter an individual's capacity to metabolize and excrete drugs. Immaturity or defects in any of the important processes of absorption, distribution, biotransformation, or excretion can significantly alter the effects of a medication. Newborn and preterm infants with immature enzyme systems in the liver (where most drugs are broken down and detoxified), lower plasma concentrations of protein for binding with drugs, and immaturely functioning kidneys (where most drugs are excreted) are particularly vulnerable to the harmful effects of medications. Beyond the newborn period, many drugs are metabolized more rapidly by the liver, necessitating larger doses or more frequent administration. This is particularly important in pain control, since the dosage of analgesics may need to be increased or the interval between doses decreased.

Various formulas involving age, weight, and body surface area (BSA) have been devised to determine children's medication dosage. Children's dosages are most often expressed in units of measure per body weight (mg/kg). The most reliable method for determining children's dosages is to calculate the proportional amount of BSA to body weight. The ratio of BSA to weight varies inversely with length; the infant who is shorter and weighs less than an older child or adult has relatively more surface area than would be expected from the weight. The usual determination of BSA requires the use of the *West nomogram* or an electronic calculator (widely available on the Internet).

Checking Dosage

Administering the correct dosage of a medication is a shared responsibility between the practitioner who orders the medication and the nurse who carries out that order. Children react with unexpected severity to some medications, and ill children are especially sensitive to them. When a dose is ordered that is outside the usual range or when there is some question about the preparation or the route of administration, the nurse should always check with the prescribing practitioner before proceeding with the administration, since the nurse is legally liable for any medication administered.

Even when it has been determined that the dosage is correct for a particular child, many medications are potentially hazardous or lethal. Most facilities have regulations requiring specified medications to be double-checked by another nurse before they are given to the child. Among medications that require such safeguards are antiarrhythmics, anticoagulants, chemotherapeutic agents, electrolytes, and insulin. Others frequently included are epinephrine, opioids, and sedatives. Even if this precaution is not mandatory, nurses are wise to observe it. Errors in decimal point placement may occur and result in a tenfold or greater dosage error.

Identification

Before the administration of any medication, the child must be correctly identified using two identifiers (name and medical record number or birth date). With an infant, young child, or a nonverbal child, a parent can identify the child, along with the identification bracelet. After verbal verification of the child's identity (by the parent, guardian, or child), the ID band should be verified using two identifiers. Bedside computers to scan the ID bracelet for electronic record updating may also be used.

Oral Administration

The oral route is preferred for giving medications to children because of the ease of administration. Most oral medications are dissolved or suspended in liquid preparations. Although some children are able to swallow or chew solid medications at an early age, solid preparations are not recommended for young children because of the danger of aspiration.

Most pediatric medications come in palatable and colourful preparations for ease of administration. Some have a slightly unpleasant aftertaste, but most children will swallow these

ATRAUMATIC CARE

Encouraging a Child's Acceptance of Oral Medication

- Give the child a flavoured ice pop or small ice cube to suck to numb the tongue before giving the medication.
- Mix the medication with a small amount (about 5 mL) of sweet-tasting substance, such as honey (except in infants because of the risk of botulism), flavoured syrups, jam, fruit purees, sherbet, or ice cream; avoid essential food items, since the child may later refuse to eat them.
- Give a "chaser" of water, juice, soft drink, ice pop, or frozen juice bar after taking the medication.
- If nausea is a problem, give a carbonated beverage poured over finely crushed ice before or immediately after taking the medication.
- When medication has an unpleasant taste, have child pinch the nose and drink the medicine through a straw. Much of what we taste is associated with smell.
- Flavourings such as apple, banana, and bubble gum can be added at many pharmacies (e.g., FLAVORx) at nominal additional cost. An alternative is to have the pharmacist prepare the medication in a flavoured, chewable troche or lozenge.
- Infants will suck medicine from a needleless syringe or dropper in small increments (0.25 to 0.5 mL) at a time. Use a nipple or special pacifier with a reservoir for the medication.

liquids with little if any resistance. When the child dislikes the taste it can be camouflaged by various means. Most pediatric units have preparations available for this purpose (see Atraumatic Care box).

It is important to discuss with the parents how they usually give medications successfully at home. A child will often accept medications more willingly from a parent.

Preparation

The devices available to measure medicines are not always sufficiently accurate for measuring the small amounts needed in pediatric nursing practice. Moulded plastic calibrated cups offer reasonable accuracy in measuring moderate doses of liquids; paper cups are likely to have irregular shapes or crumpled bottoms and retain considerable amounts of thick medication. Measures of less than 5 mL are impossible to determine accurately with a cup.

The teaspoon is an inaccurate measuring device and is subject to error. Teaspoons vary greatly in capacity, and different persons using the same spoon will pour different amounts. Therefore, a medication ordered in teaspoons should be measured in millilitres; the established standard is 5 mL per teaspoon. A convenient hollow-handled medicine spoon is available to accurately measure and administer the medication. Household measuring spoons can also be used when other devices are not available. The volume of a drop will vary according to the *viscosity* (thickness) of the liquid measured; viscous fluids produce much larger drops than thin liquids. Many medications are supplied with caps or droppers designed for measuring each specific preparation. These are accurate when used to measure that specific medication but are not reliable for measuring other liquids. Emptying dropper contents into a medicine cup invites additional error. Because some of the liquid clings to the sides of the cup, a significant amount of the drug can be lost.

The most accurate means for measuring small amounts of medication is the plastic disposable syringe, especially the tuberculin syringe for volumes less than 1 mL. Not only does the syringe provide a reliable measure, but it also serves as a convenient means for transporting and administering the medication. The medication can be placed directly into the child's mouth from the syringe.

Young children and some older children have difficulty swallowing tablets or pills. Because a number of medications are not available in pediatric preparations, the tablet needs to be crushed before it can be given to these children. Commercial devices are available, or simple methods can be employed for crushing tablets. Not all drugs can be crushed (e.g., medication with an enteric or protective coating or formulated for slow release).

Children who must take oral medication for an extended period can be taught to swallow tablets or capsules. Training sessions include verbal instruction, demonstration, reinforcement for swallowing progressively larger candy or capsules, no attention for inappropriate behaviour, and gradual withdrawal of guidance once children can swallow their medication.

Because pediatric doses often require dividing adult preparations of medication, the nurse may be faced with the dilemma of accurate dosage. With tablets, only those that are scored can be halved or quartered accurately. If the medication is soluble, the tablet or contents of a capsule can be mixed in a small, premeasured amount of liquid and the appropriate portion given. For example, if half a dose is required, the tablet is dissolved in 5 mL water or flavoured liquid and 2.5 mL is given.

Administration

Although administering liquids to infants is relatively easy, the nurse must be careful to prevent aspiration. With the infant held in a semireclining position, the medication is placed in the mouth from a spoon, plastic cup, dropper, or syringe (without needle). The dropper or syringe is best placed along the side of the infant's tongue, and the liquid is administered slowly in small amounts, allowing the child to swallow between deposits.

Medicine cups can be used effectively for older infants who are able to drink from a cup. Because of the natural outward tongue thrust in infancy, medications may need to be retrieved from the lips or chin and refed. Techniques such as allowing the infant to suck medication that has been placed in an empty nipple or inserting the syringe or dropper into the side of the mouth, parallel to the nipple, while the infant nurses are other convenient methods for giving liquid medications to infants. Medication should not be added to the infant's formula feeding because the child may subsequently refuse the formula. Plastic covers on the ends of syringes should be disposed of, as these covers are small enough to be aspirated by young children.

The young child who refuses to take medication or resists consistently despite explanation and encouragement may require mild physical restraint. If so, it should be carried out quickly and carefully. Every effort should be made to determine

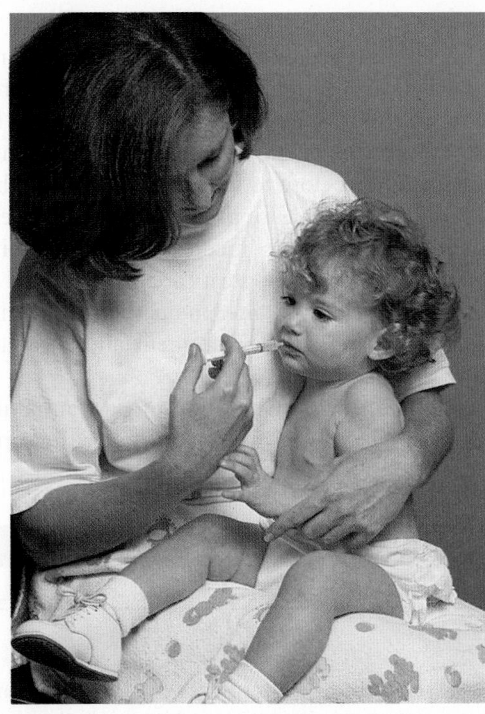

FIGURE 44-11 The nurse partially restrains child for easy and comfortable administration of oral medication.

why the child resists, and the reasons for the coercion need to be explained to the child in such a way that the child will know that it is being carried out for his or her well-being and not as a form of punishment. There is always a risk in using even mild forceful techniques. A crying child can aspirate a medication, particularly when lying on the back. If the nurse holds the child in the lap with the child's right arm behind the nurse, the left hand firmly grasped by the nurse's left hand, and the head securely restrained between the nurse's arm and body, the medication can be slowly poured into the mouth (Fig. 44-11).

Intramuscular Administration

Selecting the Syringe and Needle

The volume of medication prescribed for small children and the small amount of tissue available for injection require that a syringe be selected that can measure small amounts of solution. For volumes of less than 1 mL, the tuberculin syringe, calibrated in $\frac{1}{100}$-mL increments, is appropriate. Minute doses may require the use of a 0.5-mL, low-dose syringe. These syringes, along with specially constructed needles, minimize the possibility of inadvertently administering incorrect amounts of a drug because of dead space, which allows fluid to remain in the syringe and needle after the plunger is pushed completely forward. A minimum of 0.2 mL of the solution remains in a standard needle hub; thus when very small amounts of two drugs are combined in the syringe, such as mixtures of insulin, the ratio of the two drugs can be altered significantly. Measures that minimize the effect of dead space are as follows:

- When two drugs are combined in the syringe, always draw them up in the same order to maintain a consistent ratio between the drugs.
- Use the same brand of syringe (dead space may vary between brands).
- Use one-piece syringe units (needle permanently attached to the syringe).

Dead space is also an important factor to consider when injecting medication, since flushing the syringe with an air bubble adds an additional amount of medication to the prescribed dose. This can be hazardous when very small amounts of a medication are given. Consequently, flushing is not advisable, especially when less than 1 mL of medication is given. Syringes are calibrated to deliver a prescribed drug dose, and the amount of medication left in the hub and needle is not part of the syringe barrel calibrations. Certain drugs such as iron dextran and diphtheria and tetanus toxoid may cause irritation when tracked into the subcutaneous tissue. The Z-track method is recommended for use in infants and children rather than an air bubble. Changing the needle after withdrawing the fluid from the vial is another technique to minimize tracking.

The needle length must be sufficient to penetrate the subcutaneous tissue and deposit the medication into the body of the muscle. The needle gauge should be as small as possible to deliver fluid safely. Smaller-diameter (25- to 30-gauge) needles cause the least discomfort, but larger diameters are needed for viscous medication and prevention of accidental bending of longer needles.

Determining the Site

Factors to consider when selecting a site for an intramuscular (IM) injection on an infant or child include the following:

- The amount and character of the medication to be injected
- The amount and general condition of the muscle mass
- The frequency or number of injections to be given during the course of treatment
- The type of medication being given
- Factors that may impede access to or cause contamination of the site
- The child's ability to assume the required position safely

Older children and adolescents usually pose few problems in selecting a suitable site for IM injections, but infants, with their small and underdeveloped muscles, have fewer available sites. It is sometimes difficult to assess the amount of fluid that can be safely injected into a single site. Usually 1 mL is the maximum volume that should be administered in a single site to small children and older infants. The muscles of small infants may not tolerate more than 0.5 mL. As the child approaches adult size, volumes approaching those given to adults may be used. However, the larger the amount of solution, the larger the muscle must be into which it is injected.

Injections must be placed in muscles large enough to accommodate the medication while avoiding major nerves and blood vessels. The preferred site for infants is the vastus lateralis (the rectus femoris is not an acceptable site). However, the ventrogluteal site is also recommended as it is relatively free of major nerves and blood vessels. The ventrogluteal site is a relatively large muscle with less subcutaneous tissue than the dorsal site, is a well-defined landmarks for safe site location, is less painful than the vastus lateralis, and is easily accessible in several positions (Junqueira, Tavares, Martins, et al., 2010). Research into IM injection sites in children indicates that the ventrogluteal site has not been associated with complications and is the preferred site in children of all ages (Table 44-4). In clinical practice, this site has been safely used in children as young as newborns. The deltoid muscle, a small muscle near the axillary and radial nerves, can be used for small volumes of fluid in children as young as 18 months of age. Its advantages are less pain and fewer adverse effects from the injectate (as observed with immunizations) than with the vastus lateralis. Table 44-4 summarizes the three major injection sites and illustrates the location of the preferred IM injection sites for children.

Administration

Although injections executed with care seldom cause trauma to the child, there have been reports of serious disability related to IM injections in children. Repeated use of a single site has been associated with fibrosis of the muscle with subsequent muscle contracture. Injections close to large nerves, such as the sciatic nerve, have been responsible for permanent disability, especially when potentially neurotoxic medications are administered. When such drugs are injected, great care must be used in locating the correct site. The straighter the path of needle insertion at 90-degree angle, the less displacement and shear to tissue, and possibly less discomfort.

A potential hazard with medication in glass ampoules is the presence of glass particles in the ampoule after the container is

TABLE 44-4 INTRAMUSCULAR INJECTION SITES IN CHILDREN

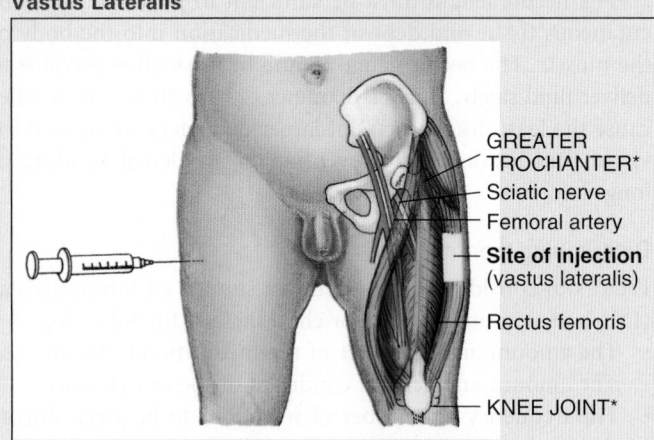

SITE	DISCUSSION
Vastus Lateralis 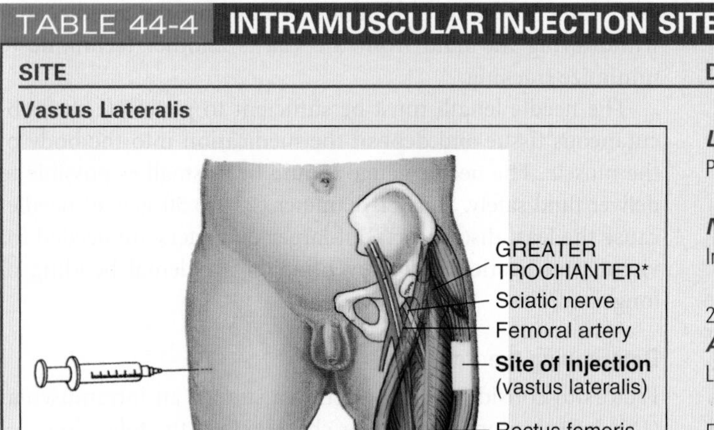 	***Location**** Palpate to find greater trochanter and knee joints; divide vertical distance between these two landmarks into thirds; inject into middle third. ***Needle Insertion and Size*** Insert needle perpendicular to knee in infants and young children or perpendicular to thigh or slightly angled toward anterior thigh. 22–25 gauge, 1.6–2.5 cm ($\frac{5}{8}$–1 inch)† ***Advantages*** Large, well-developed muscle that can tolerate larger quantities of fluid (0.5 mL [infant] to 2.0 mL [child]) Easily accessible if child is supine, side lying, or sitting ***Disadvantages*** Thrombosis of femoral artery from injection in midthigh area Sciatic nerve damage from long needle injected posteriorly and medially into small extremity More painful than deltoid or gluteal sites
Ventrogluteal 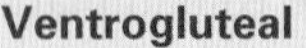 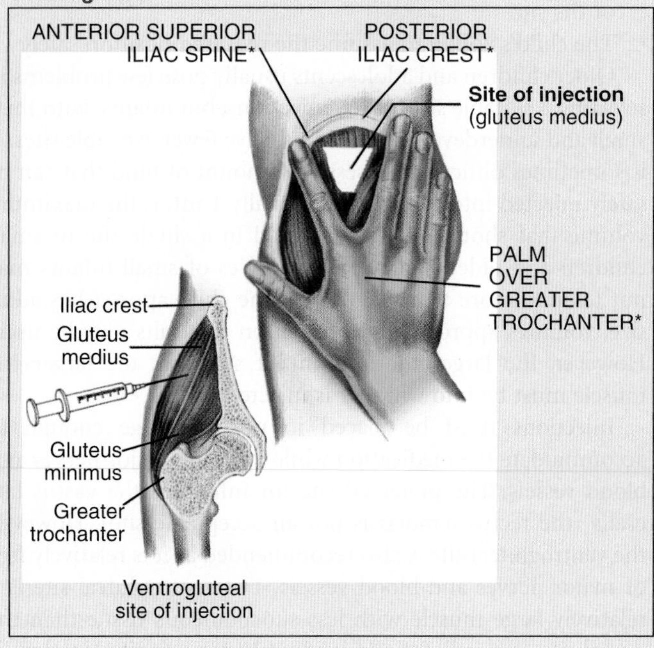 	***Location**** Palpate to locate greater trochanter, anterior superior iliac tubercle (found by flexing thigh at hip and measuring up to 1–2 cm above crease formed in groin), and posterior iliac crest; place palm of hand over greater trochanter, index finger over anterior superior iliac tubercle, and middle finger along crest of ileum posteriorly as far as possible; inject into centre of V formed by fingers. ***Needle Insertion and Size*** Insert needle perpendicular to site but angled slightly toward iliac crest. 22–25 gauge, 1.3–2.5 cm ($\frac{1}{2}$–1 inch)† ***Advantages*** Free of important nerves and vascular structures Easily identified by prominent bony landmarks Thinner layer of subcutaneous tissue than in dorsogluteal site, thus reducing chance of depositing drug subcutaneously rather than intramuscularly Can accommodate larger quantities of fluid (0.5 mL [infant] to 2.0 mL [child]) Easily accessible if child is supine, prone, or side lying Less painful than vastus lateralis ***Disadvantages*** Some health care providers' unfamiliarity with site

TABLE 44-4 INTRAMUSCULAR INJECTION SITES IN CHILDREN—cont'd

SITE	DISCUSSION
Deltoid 	***Location**** Locate acromion process; inject only into upper third of muscle that begins about 2 fingerbreadths below acromion. ***Needle Insertion and Size*** Insert needle perpendicular to site but angled slightly toward shoulder. 22–25 gauge, 1.3–2.5 cm (½ –1 inch) ***Advantages*** Faster absorption rates than gluteal sites Easily accessible with minimal removal of clothing Less pain and fewer local adverse effects from vaccines than with vastus lateralis ***Disadvantages*** Small muscle mass; can accommodate only limited amounts of medication (0.5–1.0 mL) Small margins of safety with possible damage to radial nerve and axillary nerve (not shown; lies under deltoid at head of humerus)

*Locations are indicated by asterisks on illustrations.
†A 2.5-cm (1-inch) needle is needed for adequate muscle penetration in infants 4 months old and possibly in infants as young as 2 months.

broken. When the medication is withdrawn into the syringe, the glass particles may also be withdrawn and subsequently injected into the patient. As a precaution, medication from glass ampoules should be drawn up only through a needle with a filter.

Most children are unpredictable and few can remain still when receiving an injection. Even children who appear to be relaxed and constrained can lose control under the stress of the procedure. It is advisable to have someone available to help hold the child if needed. Because children often jerk or pull away unexpectedly, the nurse should carry an extra needle to exchange for a contaminated one so that the delay is minimal. The child, even a small one, should be told that he or she is receiving an injection (preferably using a phrase such as "putting medicine under the skin"), and then the procedure carried out as quickly and skillfully as possible to avoid prolonging the stressful experience. Invasive procedures such as injections are especially anxiety provoking in young children. Because injections are painful, the nurse should employ excellent injection technique and effective pain reduction measures to reduce discomfort (see Guidelines box).

Small infants offer little resistance to injections. Although they squirm and may be difficult to hold in position, they can usually be restrained without assistance. The body of a larger infant can be securely held between the nurse's arm and body.

If the medication is given around the clock, the nurse must wake the child. Although it may seem to be easier to surprise the sleeping child and do it quickly, this can cause the child to fear going back to sleep. When awakened first, children know that nothing will be done unless they are forewarned.

A needleless injection system delivers IM or subcutaneous injections without the use of a needle and eliminates the risk of accidental needle puncture. This needle-free injection system involves a carbon dioxide cartridge that provides the power to deliver the medication through the skin. Although it is not painless, it may reduce pain and also the anxiety of seeing the needle.

Subcutaneous and Intradermal Administration

Subcutaneous and intradermal injections are frequently administered to children; the technique differs little from the method used with adults. Examples of subcutaneous injections include insulin, hormone replacement, allergy desensitization, and some vaccines. Tuberculin testing, local anaesthesia, and allergy testing are examples of frequently administered intradermal injections.

Techniques to minimize the pain associated with these injections include changing the needle if it pierced a rubber stopper on a vial, using 26- to 30-gauge needles (only to inject the solution), and injecting small volumes (up to 0.5 mL). The angle of the needle for the subcutaneous injection is typically 90 degrees.

GUIDELINES

Intramuscular Administration of Medication

Use safety precautions in administering medication (e.g., check child's identification).

Apply an eutectic mix of lidocaine and prilocaine (EMLA) topically over site if time permits or LMX cream (lidocaine) topically over site if time permits (see Pain Management, Chapter 34).

Prepare medication:

- Select needle and syringe appropriate to the following: (1) amount of fluid to be administered (syringe size), (2) viscosity of fluid to be administered (needle gauge), and (3) amount of tissue to be penetrated (needle length).
- Maximum volume to be administered in a single site is 1 mL for older infants and small children.
- Have medication at room temperature.
- If withdrawing medication from an ampule, use a needle equipped with a filter that removes glass particles; then use a new, nonfilter needle for injection.

Determine site of injection (see Table 44-4), making certain that muscle is large enough to accommodate volume and type of medication.

- Acceptable sites for infants and small or debilitated children are the vastus lateralis muscle or the ventrogluteal muscle.
- The dorsogluteal muscle is insufficiently developed to be a safe site for infants and small children.

Obtain sufficient help in restraining the child; their behaviour is usually unpredictable.

Explain briefly what is to be done and, if appropriate, what the child can do to help.

Expose injection area for unobstructed view of landmarks.

Select a site where skin is free of irritation and danger of infection; palpate for and avoid sensitive or hardened areas. With multiple injections, rotate sites.

Place child in a lying or sitting position; the child is not allowed to stand because (1) landmarks are more difficult to assess, (2) restraint is more difficult, and (3) the child may faint and fall.

- **Ventrogluteal**—Place child on side with upper leg flexed and placed in front of lower leg.
- **Vastus lateralis**—Child can be supine, lying on the side, or sitting.

Use a new, sharp needle with the smallest diameter that permits free flow of the medication.

Spread skin with thumb and index finger to displace subcutaneous tissue and grasp muscle deeply on each side. Grasp muscle firmly between the thumb and fingers to isolate and stabilize muscle for deposition of drug in its deepest part.

Allow skin preparation to dry completely before skin is penetrated.

Decrease perception of pain.

- Distract the child with conversation.
- Give the child something on which to concentrate, such as squeezing a hand or side rail, pinching own nose, humming, counting, yelling "Ouch!"
- Spray vapocoolant (e.g., ethyl chloride or fluorimethane) on site 11 to 15 seconds before injection or place a cold compress or wrapped ice cube on site about a minute before injection, or apply cold to contralateral site.
- Say to the child, "If you feel this, tell me to take it out, please."
- Have the child hold a small adhesive bandage and place it on puncture site after IM injection is given.

Insert needle quickly, using a dartlike motion at a 90-degree angle unless contraindicated.

- Use new needle, not one that has pierced the rubber stopper on vial.

Avoid tracking any medication through superficial tissues:

- Replace needle after withdrawing medication, or wipe medication from needle with sterile gauze.
- Use the Z-track or air-bubble technique as indicated.
- Avoid depressing the plunger during insertion of the needle.

Aspirate for blood, if in accordance with institutional policies and procedures.

- If blood is found, remove syringe from site, change needle, and reinsert into new location.
- If no blood is found, inject medication slowly into a relaxed muscle.

Remove needle quickly; hold gauze sponge firmly against skin near needle when removing it to avoid pulling on tissue.

Apply firm pressure to the site after injection; massage site to hasten absorption unless contraindicated, as with irritating medications.

Place a small adhesive bandage on puncture site; with young children decorate it by drawing a smiling face or other symbol of acceptance.

Hold and cuddle young child and encourage parents to comfort the child; praise an older child.

Allow expression of feelings.

Discard syringe and uncapped, uncut needle in puncture-resistant container located near site of use.

Document time of injection, medication, dose, and injection site.

In children with little subcutaneous tissue, some practitioners insert the needle at a 45-degree angle. However, the benefit of using the 45-degree angle rather than the 90-degree angle remains unsubstantiated by research. For intradermal injections the angle is 15 degrees with bevel up.

Although subcutaneous injections can be given anywhere there is subcutaneous tissue, common sites include the centre third of the lateral aspect of the upper arm, the abdomen, and the centre third of the anterior thigh. When giving an intradermal injection into the volar surface of the forearm, the nurse should avoid the medial side of the arm, where the skin is more sensitive.

Intravenous Administration

The IV route for administering medications is frequently used in pediatric therapy. It is important for nurses to follow their institution's individual nursing care protocols when delivering IV line care. For some medications it is the only effective route. This method is used for giving medications to children who:

- Have poor absorption as a result of diarrhea, dehydration, or peripheral vascular collapse
- Need a high serum concentration of a drug
- Have resistant infections that require parenteral medication over an extended time
- Need continuous pain relief

- Require emergency treatment

Insertion sites and observation of the IV infusion are discussed on pp. 1316–1317. Several factors need to be considered in relation to IV medication. When a medication is administered intravenously, the effect is almost instantaneous and further control is limited. Most drugs for IV administration require a specified minimum dilution, rate of flow, or both, and many are highly irritating or toxic to tissues outside the vascular system. In addition to the precautions and nursing observations related to IV therapy, factors to consider when preparing and administering medications to infants and children by the IV route include the following:

- Amount of drug to be administered
- Minimum dilution of drug and whether child is fluid restricted
- Type of solution in which drug can be diluted
- Length of time over which drug can be safely administered
- Rate limitations of child, vascular system, and infusion equipment
- Time that this or another drug is to be administered
- Compatibility of all drugs that child is receiving intravenously
- Compatibility with infusion fluids

Before any IV infusion, the site of insertion needs to be checked for patency. Medications are never administered with blood products. Only one antibiotic should be administered at a time. Extra fluids needed to administer IV medications can be problematic for infants and fluid-restricted children. Syringe pumps are often used to deliver IV medication because they minimize fluid requirements and more precisely deliver small volumes of medication compared with large-volume infusion pumps.

Regardless of the technique, the nurse must know the minimum dilutions for safe administration of IV medications to infants and children.

Peripheral Intermittent Infusion Device

The peripheral lock, also known as an **intermittent infusion device** or *saline lock*, is an alternative to a keep-open infusion when extended access to a vein is required without the need for continuous fluid. It is most frequently employed for intermittent infusion of medication into a peripheral venous route. A short, flexible catheter is used as the lock device, and a site is selected where there will be minimal movement, such as the forearm. The catheter is inserted and secured in the same manner as for any IV infusion device, but the hub is occluded with a stopper or injection cap.

The type of device used may vary, and the care and use of the peripheral lock are carried out according to the protocol of the institution or unit. However, the general concept is the same. The catheter remains in place and is flushed with saline after infusion of the medication.

Children may be discharged with a peripheral lock in place to continue receiving medications on a short-term basis without hospitalization. They need to be referred to a home care agency. Those with chronic illnesses who require repeated blood sampling or medications, long-term chemotherapy, or frequent hyperalimentation or antibiotic therapy are best managed with a central venous catheter.

Central Venous Access Device

Central venous access devices (CVADs) comprise different types of catheters that are inserted into and positioned within a vein in the body. Factors that can influence the type of CVAD include the reason for placement of the catheter (diagnosis), length of therapy, risk to the patient in placement of the catheter, and availability of resources to help the family maintain the catheter.

Short-term or nontunnelled catheters are used in acute care, emergency, and critical care units. These catheters are made of polyurethane and are placed in large veins such as the subclavian, femoral, or jugular vein. Insertion is by surgical incision or large percutaneous threading. A chest x-ray film should be taken to verify placement of the catheter tip before administration of fluids or medications.

Peripherally inserted central catheters (PICCs) can be used for short-term to moderate-length therapy. These catheters consist of silicone or polymer material and are placed by specially trained nurses, physicians, or interventional radiologists. The most common insertion site is above the antecubital area using the median, cephalic, or basilic vein. The catheter is threaded either with or without a guidewire into the superior vena cava. PICCs can be trimmed before insertion, and the decision can be made to insert the catheter midline, which is considered between the insertion site and the axilla. If the catheter is threaded midline, total **parenteral nutrition** (TPN) or any medication known to irritate a peripheral vein (e.g., chemotherapy drugs) should not be administered. The high concentration of glucose in TPN makes it irritating to the vessel; it should be infused through a central catheter.

The decision to insert a PICC needs to be made before several attempts at IV insertion are made. When the antecubital veins have been punctured repeatedly, they are not considered candidates for this type of catheter. Because it is the least costly and has less chance of complications than other CVADs, it is an excellent choice for many pediatric patients.

> **! NURSING ALERT**
>
> Most PICC lines are not sutured into place, so care is needed when changing the dressing. If a central venous catheter is removed accidently, apply pressure to the entry site to the vein, not the exit site on the skin.

Long-term central CVADs include tunnelled catheters and implanted infusion ports (implanted venous access devices) (Fig. 44-12). They may have single, double, or triple lumens. Several-lumens (multilumen) catheters allow more than one therapy to be administered at the same time. Reasons to use multilumen catheters include repeated blood sampling, TPN, administration of blood products or infusion of large quantities or concentrations of fluids, administration of incompatible medications or fluids at the same time (through different lumens), and central venous pressure monitoring.

With any of the central venous catheters, medication is easily instilled through the injection cap. Maintenance of the catheter

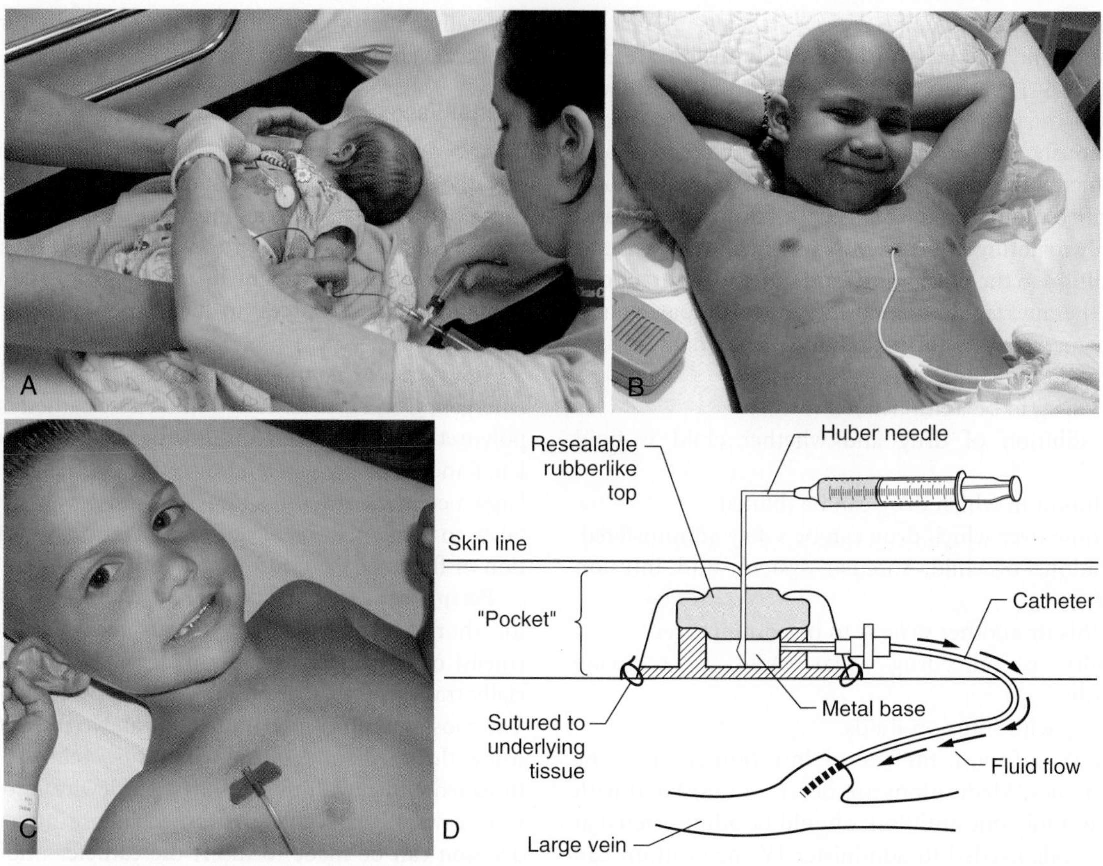

FIGURE 44-12 Venous access devices. **A:** Blood being drawn from a central venous catheter. **B:** Child with external central venous catheter. **C:** Child with implanted port with Huber needle in place. **D:** Side view of implanted port.

includes dressing changes, flushing to maintain patency, and prevention of occlusion or dislodgment.

> **! NURSING ALERT**
>
> When working with tunnelled catheters, PICCs, and peripheral intravenous lines (PIVs), avoid using scissors around the tubing or dressing. Removal is best accomplished using fingers and much patience. In the event that a tunnelled catheter is cut, use a padded clamp to clamp the catheter proximal to the exit site to avoid blood loss. Repair kits are available, which may save the catheter and avoid surgery to replace a cut catheter.

With the implanted device the port must be palpated for placement and stabilized, the overlying skin cleansed, and only special noncoring Huber needles used to pierce the port's diaphragm on the top or side, depending on the style. To avoid repeated skin punctures, a special infusion set with a Huber needle and extension tubing with a Luer connection can be used (see Fig. 44-12, C). With this attached, the injection procedure is the same as for an intermittent infusion device or a central venous catheter. To prevent infection, meticulous aseptic technique must be used any time the devices are entered, including instillation of heparin or saline to prevent clotting. There should be a protocol stating that the Huber needle needs to be changed at established intervals, usually 5 to 7 days.

The type of flushing solution that is used to maintain patency of the intravenous lines has been under review. In the past, heparin flush was used for all types of lines to maintain line patency. Normal saline (0.9%) has mostly replaced heparin in Canada (Kaasalainen, 2014). Cochrane reviewers have concluded that there is no difference between use of heparin and saline in line patency and recommend that, because heparin is more expensive, saline should be used (López-Briz, Ruiz Garcia, Cabello, et al., 2014).

The children and parents need to be taught the procedure for care of the CVAD. This teaching is provided before discharge from the hospital, including preparation and injection of the prescribed medication, the flush, and dressing changes. A protective device may be recommended for some active children, to prevent accidental dislodgment of the needle. Many children take responsibility for preparing and administering medications. Both verbal and written step-by-step instructions should be provided.

Infection and catheter occlusion are two of the most common complications of central venous catheters. They require treatment with antibiotics for infection and a fibrinolytic agent, such as alteplase, for clots (Anderson, Pesaturo, Casavant, et al., 2013). Uncapping can be prevented by taping the cap securely to the catheter and the clamped line to the dressing. Leaks can be prevented by using a smooth-edged clamp only. If the catheter leaks, the parents should be instructed to tape it above the leak and then clamp the catheter at the taped site. The child should be taken to the practitioner as soon as possible to prevent infection or clotting after a catheter leak.

Aerosol Therapy

Aerosol therapy can be effective in depositing medication directly into the airway. This route of administration can be useful in avoiding the systemic adverse effects of certain medications and in reducing the amount of drug necessary to achieve the desired effect. Bronchodilators, steroids, and antibiotics, suspended in particulate form, can be inhaled so that the medication reaches the small airways. Aerosol therapy is particularly challenging in children who are too young to be able to control the rate and depth of breathing. Administration of this therapy requires skill, patience, and creativity.

MEDICATION ALERT

Medications can be aerosolized or nebulized with air or with oxygen-enriched gas using hand-held nebulizers. The medicated mist is discharged into a small plastic mask, which the child holds over the nose and mouth. To avoid particle deposition in the nose and pharynx, the child is instructed to take slow, deep breaths through an open mouth during the treatment. For home use, an air compressor is necessary to force air through the liquid medication to form the aerosol. The **metered-dose inhaler (MDI)** is a self-contained, hand-held device that allows for intermittent delivery of a specified amount of medication and is gradually replacing nebulizer delivery via air compressors. Many bronchodilators are available in this form and are successfully used by children with asthma. Spacer devices can be used for any age group, particularly for children under the age of 5 or 6 years. This device is attached to the MDI and can help with coordination of breathing and aerosol delivery. It allows the aerosolized particles to remain in suspension longer. (See also Asthma, Chapter 45.)

Assessment of breath sounds and the work of breathing should be done before and after treatments. Young children who become upset by having a mask held close to the face may become fatigued with fighting the procedure and may actually appear worse during and immediately after the therapy. It may be necessary to spend a few minutes calming the child after the procedure and allowing the vital signs to return to baseline in order to accurately assess changes in breath sounds and the work of breathing.

Nasogastric, Orogastric, or Gastrostomy Administration

When a child has an in-dwelling feeding tube or a gastrostomy, oral medications may be given via that route. Advantages of this method include the ability to administer oral medications around the clock without disturbing the child and ensuring that the child actually takes the medication. A disadvantage of this method is the risk of occluding or clogging the tube, especially when giving viscous solutions through small-bore feeding tubes. The most important preventive measure is adequate flushing after the medication is instilled (see Guidelines box).

Rectal Administration

The rectal route for administration is less reliable but is sometimes used when the oral route is difficult or contraindicated. It is also used when oral preparations are unsuitable to control vomiting. Some of the medications available in suppository form are acetaminophen, sedatives, and antiemetics. The difficulty in using the rectal route is that, unless the rectum is empty at the time of insertion, the absorption of the drug may be delayed, diminished, or prevented by the presence of feces. Sometimes the drug is later evacuated, securely surrounded by stool.

To administer a medication rectally, the wrapper on the suppository is removed and the suppository lubricated with warm water (water-soluble jelly may affect medication absorption). Rectal suppositories are inserted with the apex (pointed end) foremost. Reverse contractions or the pressure gradient of the anal canal may help the suppository slip higher into the canal. Using a glove, the nurse inserts the suppository quickly but gently into the rectum, beyond both of the rectal sphincters. The buttocks are then held together firmly to relieve pressure on the anal sphincter until the urge to expel the suppository has passed—5 to 10 minutes. Sometimes the amount of medication ordered is less than the dosage available. The irregular shape of most suppositories makes the process of dividing them into a

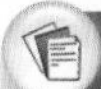

GUIDELINES

Nasogastric, Orogastric, or Gastrostomy Medication Administration in Children

Use solution, suspension, or dissolvable tablet preparations of medication whenever possible.

Dilute viscous medication or syrup with a small amount of water, if possible.

If administering tablets, crush tablet to a fine powder and dissolve drug in a small amount of warm water.

Never crush enteric-coated or sustained-release tablets or capsules.

Avoid oily medications because they tend to cling to the side of the tube.

Do not mix medication with enteral formula unless fluid is restricted. If adding a medication:

- Check with the pharmacist for compatibility.
- Shake formula well and observe for any physical reaction (e.g., separation, precipitation).
- Label formula container with name of medication, dosage, date, and time infusion started.

Check for correct placement of nasogastric or orogastric tube (see p. 1328 for placement check procedure).

Attach syringe (with adaptable tip but without plunger) to tube.

Pour medication into syringe.

Unclamp tube and allow medication to flow by gravity.

Adjust height of container to achieve desired flow rate (e.g., increase height for faster flow).

As soon as syringe is empty, pour in water to flush tubing. The amount of water depends on length and gauge of tubing.

Determine amount before administering any medication by using a syringe to fill completely an unused nasogastric or orogastric tube with water. The amount of flush solution is usually 1.5 times this volume.

With certain drug preparations (e.g., suspensions), more fluid may be needed. If administering more than one medication at the same time, flush tube between each medication with clear water.

Clamp tube after flushing unless it is left open.

desired dose difficult if not dangerous. If the suppository must be halved, it should be cut lengthwise. However, there is no guarantee that the drug is evenly dispersed throughout the petrolatum base.

If medication is administered via a retention enema, the same procedure is used. The medication should be diluted in the smallest amount of solution possible to minimize the likelihood of the child expelling it.

Optic, Otic, and Nasal Administration

There are few differences between administering eye, ear, and nose medication to children and giving them to adults. The major difficulty is in gaining children's assistance. Older children need only explanation and direction. Although the administration of optic, otic, and nasal medication is not painful, these medications can cause unpleasant sensations that can be eliminated with various techniques.

> **! NURSING ALERT**
>
> The following steps help reduce unpleasant sensations when administering medications:
>
> **Eye**—Apply finger pressure to the lacrimal punctum at the inner aspect of the lid for 1 minute to prevent drainage of medication to the nasopharynx and the unpleasant "tasting" of the medication.
>
> **Ear**—Allow medications stored in the refrigerator to warm to room temperature before instillation.
>
> **Nose**—Position the child with the head hyperextended to prevent strangling sensations caused by medication trickling into the throat, rather than up into the nasal passages.

To instill eye medication, the nurse places the child supine or sitting with the head extended, and asks the child to look up. One hand is used to pull the lower lid downward; the hand that holds the dropper rests on the head so that it may move synchronously with the child's head, thus reducing the possibility of trauma to a struggling child or of dropping medication on the child's face (Fig. 44-13). As the lower lid is pulled down, a small conjunctival sac is formed; the solution or ointment is applied to this area, never directly on the eyeball. Another effective technique is to pull the lower lid down and out to form a cup effect, into which the medication is dropped. The nurse gently closes the lids to prevent expression of the medication, and asks the child to look in all directions to enhance even distribution of the preparation. Excess medication from the inner canthus is then wiped outward to prevent contamination to the contralateral eye.

Instilling eye drops in infants can be difficult, since they often clench the lids tightly closed. One approach is to place the drops in the nasal corner where the lids meet. The medication pools in this area, and when the infant opens the lids, the medication flows onto the conjunctiva. For young children, playing a game can be helpful, such as instructing the child to keep the eyes closed until the count of three and then open them, at which time the drops are quickly instilled. Ointment can be applied by gently pulling down the lower lid and placing the ointment in the lower conjunctival sac. If both eye ointment and drops are ordered, the nurse gives the drops first, waits 3 minutes, and then applies the ointment to allow each medication to work. When possible, eye ointments should be administered before bedtime or naptime, since the child's vision will be blurred temporarily.

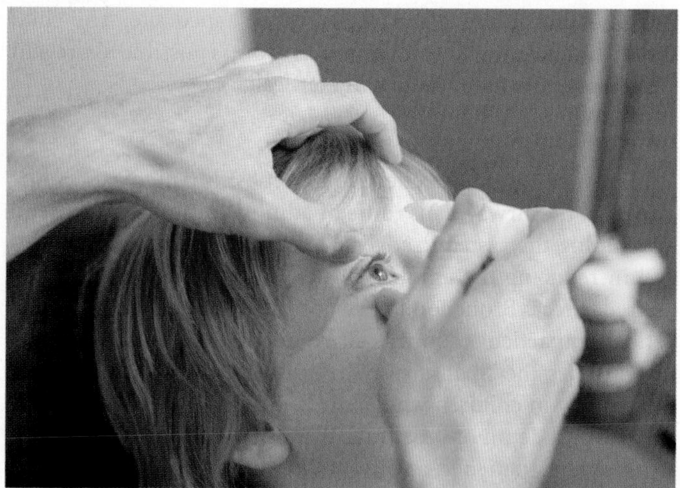

FIGURE 44-13 Administering eye drops. (Tyler Olson/Shutterstock .com.)

Ear drops are instilled with the child in the prone or supine position and the head turned to the appropriate side. For children younger than 3 years of age, the external auditory canal is straightened by gently pulling the pinna downward and straight back. The pinna is pulled upward and back in children older than 3 years of age (see Fig. 33-23, B). To place the drops deep in the ear canal without contaminating the tip of the dropper, a disposable ear speculum is placed in the canal and the drops administered through the speculum. After instillation, the child should remain lying on the unaffected side for a few minutes. Gentle massage of the area immediately anterior to the ear facilitates the entry of drops into the ear canal. The use of cotton balls prevents medication from flowing out of the external canal. However, the cotton balls should be loose enough to allow any discharge to exit from the ear. Premoistening the cotton with a few drops of medication prevents the wicking action from absorbing the medication instilled in the ear.

Nose drops are instilled in the same manner as in an adult patient. First, mucus is removed from the nose with a clean tissue or washcloth. Unpleasant sensations associated with medicated nose drops can be minimized when care is taken to position the child with the head extended well over the edge of the bed or a pillow (Fig. 44-14). Depending on the infant's size, the infant can be positioned in the football hold (see Fig. 44-4, B); in the nurse's arm with the head extended and stabilized between the nurse's body and elbow, and the arms and hands immobilized with the nurse's hands; or as shown in Figure 44-14. After instillation of the drops, the child should remain in position for 1 minute to allow the drops to come in contact with the nasal surfaces. Nasal spray dispensers are inserted into the naris vertically and then angled to avoid

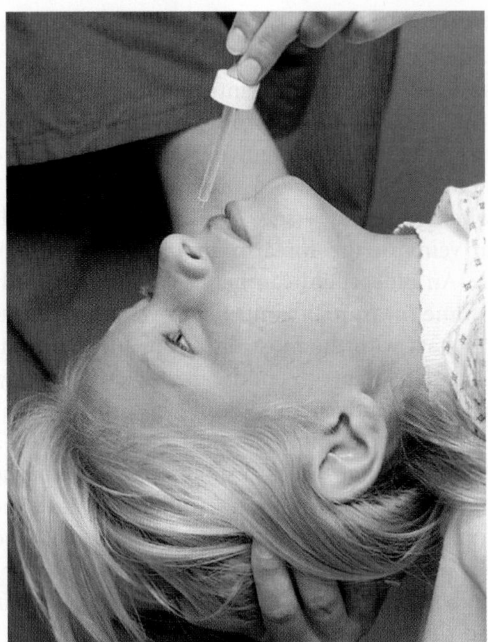

FIGURE 44-14 Proper position for instilling nose drops.

trauma to the septum and direct medication toward the inferior turbinate.

Family Teaching and Home Care

The nurse usually assumes the responsibility for preparing families to administer medications at home. The family should understand why the child is receiving the medication and the effects that might be expected, as well as the amount, frequency, and length of time the medication is to be administered. Instruction should be carried out in an unhurried, relaxed manner, preferably in an area away from a busy ward or office.

The caregiver needs to be carefully instructed in the correct dosage. Some people have difficulty understanding medical terminology; the nurse should not assume that the message is clear just because they nod or otherwise indicate an understanding. For example, it is important to ascertain their interpretation of a teaspoon and be certain they have accurate measuring devices. If the drug is packaged with a dropper, syringe, or plastic cup, the nurse should show or mark the point with tape, for example, on the device that indicates the prescribed dose and demonstrate how the dose is drawn up into a dropper or syringe, how it is measured, and how bubbles are eliminated. The parent should then give a return demonstration. This is essential when a drug such as insulin or digoxin has potentially serious consequences from incorrect dosage or when more complex administration such as parenteral injections is required. When teaching a parent to give an injection, the nurse must allot adequate time for instruction and practice.

Home modifications are often necessary because the availability of equipment or assistance can differ from the hospital setting. For example, the parent may need guidance in devising methods that allow for one person to hold the child and safely give the medication.

> **! NURSING ALERT**
>
> To administer oral, nasal, or optic medication when only one person is available to hold the child, use the following procedure:
>
> - Place child supine on flat surface (bed, couch, floor).
> - Sit facing the child so that the child's head is between the operator's thighs and the child's arms are under the operator's legs.
> - Place lower legs over the child's legs to restrain the lower body, if necessary.
> - To administer oral medication, place a small pillow under the child's head to reduce risk of aspiration.
> - To administer nasal medication, place a small pillow under the child's shoulders to aid flow of liquid through nasal passages.

The time that the medication is to be administered should be clarified with the parent. For instance, when a medication is prescribed in association with meals, the number of meals that the family is accustomed to eating influences the amount of medication the child receives. Does the child have meals twice a day or five times a day? When a medication is to be given several times during the day, together the nurse and parents can work out a schedule that accommodates the family's routine. This is particularly significant if the medication must be given at equal intervals throughout a 24-hour period. For example, telling parents that the child needs 1 teaspoon of medicine four times a day is subject to misinterpretation and a preplanned schedule based on 6-hour intervals should be set up with the number of days required for therapeutic dosage listed. Written instruction should accompany all medication prescriptions.

> **! NURSING ALERT**
>
> **Colour-Coded Instructions**
>
> If parents have difficulty reading or understanding English, use colours to convey instructions. For example, mark each medication with a colour and place the appropriate colour on a calendar chart or on a drawing of a clock to identify when the medication needs to be given. If a liquid medication and syringe are used, also mark the syringe with colour-coded tape at the place the plunger needs to be.

MAINTAINING FLUID BALANCE

Measurement of Intake and Output

Accurate measurements of fluid intake and output (I&O) are essential to the assessment of fluid balance. Measurements from all sources—intake includes gastrointestinal and parenteral and output must include that from urine, stools, vomitus, nasogastric suction, and drainage from wounds. Although the practitioner usually indicates when I&O measurements are to be recorded, it is a nursing responsibility to keep an accurate I&O record on certain children, including those:

- Receiving IV therapy
- Who have undergone major surgery
- Receiving diuretic or corticosteroid therapy
- With severe thermal burns or injuries

- With renal disease or damage
- With heart failure
- With dehydration
- With diabetes mellitus
- With oliguria
- In respiratory distress
- With chronic lung disease

Infants or small children who are unable to use a bedpan or those who have bowel movements with every voiding require the application of a collecting device. If collecting bags are not used, wet diapers or pads are carefully weighed to ascertain the amount of fluid lost, including liquid stool, vomitus, and other losses. The specific gravity as a measure of osmolality is determined with a refractometer or urine dipsticks and assists in assessing the degree of hydration.

The volume of fluid in millilitres is equivalent to the weight of the fluid measured in grams (1 g of wet diaper weight = 1 mL urine). In infants with diapers, the nurse weighs all dry diapers to be used and notes in an indelible marker the dry weight of the diaper; when there is fluid (urine or liquid stool) in the diaper, the amount of output can be approximated by subtracting the weight of the dry diaper from the weight of the wet diaper. Disadvantages of the weighed-diaper method of fluid measurement include (1) inability to differentiate one type of loss from another because of admixture, (2) loss of urine or liquid stool from leakage or evaporation (especially if the infant is under a radiant warmer), and (3) additional fluid in the diaper (superabsorbent disposable type) from absorption of atmospheric moisture (in high-humidity isolettes).

Special Needs When the Child Is NPO

Infants or children who are unable or not permitted to take fluids by mouth (NPO) have special needs. To ensure that they do not receive fluids, a sign can be placed in some obvious place, such as over their beds or on their shirts, to alert others to the NPO status. To prevent the temptation to drink, fluids should not be left at the bedside.

To keep the mouth feeling moist when the child is NPO, give ice chips (if this is permitted by the practitioner) or spray the mouth with an atomizer. To meet the need to suck, the infant can be provided with a safe commercial pacifier (if the parents agree).

Oral hygiene, a part of routine hygienic care, is especially important when fluids are restricted or withheld. For the young child who cannot brush the teeth or rinse the mouth without swallowing fluid, the mouth and teeth can be cleaned and kept moist by swabbing with saline-moistened gauze.

The child who is fluid restricted presents an equal challenge. Limiting fluids is often more difficult for the child than being NPO, especially when IV fluids are also eliminated. To make certain the child does not drink the entire amount allowed early in the day, the daily allotment is calculated to provide fluids at periodic intervals throughout the child's waking hours. Serving the fluids in small containers gives the illusion of larger servings. No extra liquid should be left at the bedside.

Parenteral Fluid Therapy

Site and Equipment

The site selected for peripheral intravenous line (PIV) infusion depends on accessibility and convenience. Although it is possible to use any accessible vein in older children, the child's developmental, cognitive, and mobility needs must be considered when selecting a site. Ideally, in older children, the superficial veins of the forearm should be used, leaving the hands free. An older child can help select the site and thereby maintain some measure of control. For veins in the extremities it is best to start with the most distal site and avoid the child's favoured hand so that the child can still do things with that hand. The child's movements should be restricted as little as possible; a site over a joint in an extremity must be avoided, such as the antecubital space. In small infants a superficial vein of the hand, wrist, forearm, foot, or ankle is usually most convenient and most easily stabilized (Fig. 44-15). Foot veins should be avoided in children learning to walk or already walking. Superficial veins of the scalp have no valves, insertion is easy, and they can be used in infants up to about 9 months of age, but they should be used only when other site attempts have failed. A transilluminator can aid in finding and evaluating veins for access (Fig. 44-16).

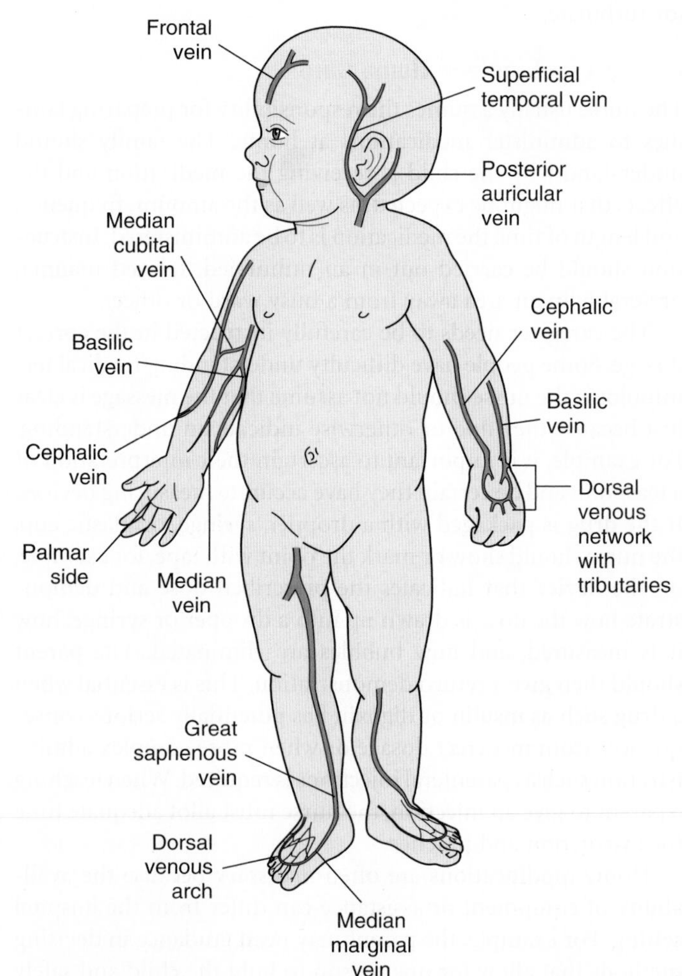

FIGURE 44-15 Preferred sites for venous access in infants.

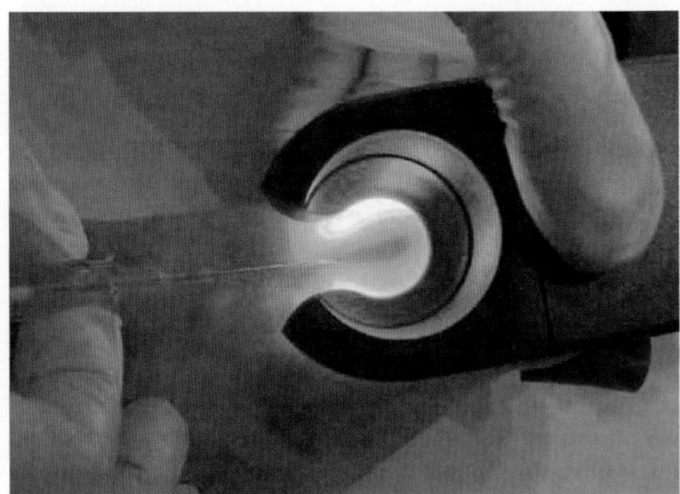

FIGURE 44-16 Transilluminator: low-heat light-emitting diode (LED) light placed on the skin to illuminate veins; an opening allows cannulation of the vein.

Selection of a scalp vein may require clipping the area around the site to better visualize the vein and provide a smoother surface on which to tape the catheter hub and tubing. Clipping a portion of the infant's hair can be upsetting to parents; therefore, they should be asked first and reassured that the hair will grow in again rapidly (the hair should be saved because parents often wish to keep it). As little hair as possible should be removed, directly over the insertion site and taping surface. A rubber band slipped onto the head from brow to occiput will usually suffice as a tourniquet, although if the vessel is visible, a tourniquet may not be necessary.

> **! NURSING ALERT**
>
> A tab of tape should be placed on the rubber band to help grasp it when removing it from the infant's head. The rubber band should be cut to avoid accidentally dislodging the catheter when moving the rubber band over the IV insertion site. The tape tab will lift the rubber band and allow it to be cut. Hold the rubber band in two places and cut between these areas to prevent the rubber band from snapping on the head.

Situations may occur in which rapid establishment of systemic access is vital, and venous access may be hampered by peripheral circulatory collapse, hypovolemic shock (secondary to vomiting or diarrhea, burns, or trauma), cardiopulmonary arrest, or other conditions. *Intraosseous infusion* provides a rapid, safe, and life-saving alternative route for administration of fluids and medications until intravascular access can be obtained, especially in children who are 6 years of age and younger. A large-bore needle, for example a bone marrow aspiration needle such as a Jamshidi or an intraosseous needle, is inserted into the medullary cavity of a long bone, most often the proximal tibia. This procedure is painful, therefore appropriate and sufficient analgesia should be administered prior to the procedure. The dependent tissue should be observed closely for swelling, since extravasation may be hidden under the leg and compartment syndrome may result.

For most IV infusions in children, a 22- to 24-gauge catheter may be used if therapy is expected to last less than 5 days. The smallest-gauge and shortest-length catheter that will accommodate the prescribed therapy should be chosen. The length of the catheter may be directly related to infection or embolus formation—the shorter the catheter, the fewer the complications. The gauge of the catheter should maintain adequate flow of the infusate into the cannulated vein while allowing adequate blood flow around the catheter walls to promote proper hemodilution of the infusate.

Determining the best catheter for the patient early in the therapy provides the best chance of avoiding catheter-related complications. As the length of therapy increases, decisions regarding the type of infusion device (short peripheral, midline, PICC, or central venous catheter) should be explored.

Safety Catheters and Needleless Systems

Over-the-needle IV inserters with hollow-bore needles carry a high risk for transmission of blood-borne pathogens from needlestick injuries. Use of safety catheters helps prevent accidental needlesticks with the use of over-the-needle IV catheters with guards.

Needleless IV systems are designed to prevent needlestick injuries during administration of IV push medications and IV piggyback medications. Some needleless devices can be used with any tubing, whereas others require the use of the entire IV delivery system for compatibility. Needleless IV systems rely on prepierced septa that are accessed by blunted plastic cannulas or systems that use valves that open and close a fluid path when activated by insertion of a syringe.

Blunt plastic cannulas and preslit injection port sites (Fig. 44-17) eliminate the need for steel needles and conventional injection port sites but remain accessible via hypodermic needles, a drawback except in emergent situations. Systems that

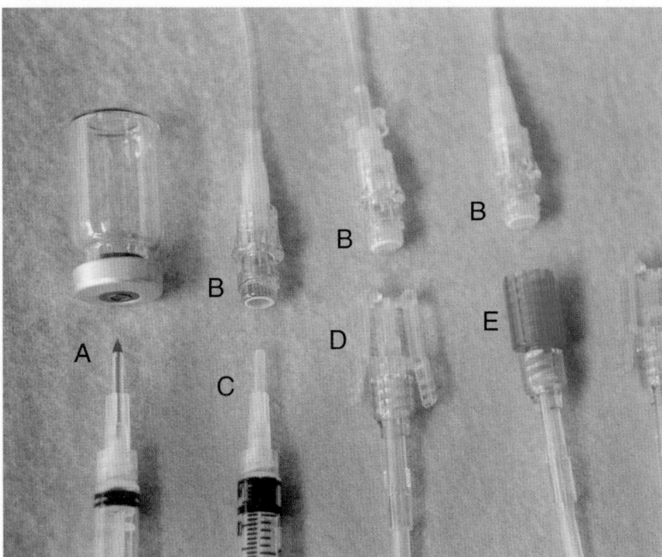

FIGURE 44-17 Interlink intravenous access systems. **A:** Blue spike syringe. **B:** Preslit injection port (needleless). **C:** Blunt plastic cannula syringe. **D:** Lever lock cannula. **E:** Threaded lock cannula.

do not permit needled access enhance safety by preventing health care workers from attempting to use needles.

> **NURSING ALERT**
>
> Misconnections of tubing have occurred, resulting in patient deaths. Many needleless IV systems allow other types of tubing, such as blood pressure and oxygen tubing, to connect and instill air directly into the IV line. Before tubing is connected or reconnected to a patient, trace it completely from the patient to the point of origin for verification.

Infusion Pumps

A variety of infusion pumps are available and used in nearly all pediatric infusions to accurately administer medication and minimize the possibility of overloading the circulation. It is important to calculate the amount to be infused in a given length of time, set the infusion rate, and monitor the apparatus frequently (at least every 1 to 2 hours) to make certain that the desired rate is maintained, the integrity of the system remains intact, the site remains intact (free of redness, edema, infiltration, or irritation), and the infusion does not stop. Continuous infusion pumps, although convenient and efficient, are not without risks. Overreliance on the accuracy of the machine can cause either too much or too little fluid to be infused; its use does not eliminate the need for careful periodic assessment by the nurse. Excess pressure can build up if the machine is set at a rate faster than the vein is able to accommodate (or continues to pump when the needle is out of the lumen).

Securement of a Peripheral Intravenous Line

To maintain the integrity of the IV line, adequate protection of the site is required. The catheter hub should be firmly secured at the puncture site with a transparent dressing and commercial securement device, for example, StatLock (Fig. 44-18), or clear, nonallergenic tape. Transparent dressings are ideal because the insertion site is easily observed. Minimal tape should be used at the puncture site and on about 2.5 to 5 cm of skin beyond the site to avoid obscuring the insertion site for early detection of infiltration.

A protective cover is applied directly over the catheter insertion site to protect the infusion site. Easy access to the IV site for frequent (1- to 2-hour) assessments must be considered. Improvised plastic cups cut in half with the ridged edges covered with tape should not be used, as they have injured patients. A commercial site protector, I.V. House, is available in different sizes (Fig. 44-19). Its ventilation holes prevent moisture from accumulating under the dome. This device is designed to protect the IV site and enables visibility of the site. It also minimizes use of padded boards, splints, or other restraints and tape and maintains skin integrity. The connector tubing or extension tubing can be looped to make it small enough to fit under the protective cover to prevent accidental snagging of the catheter. It is important to safely secure the IV tubing to prevent infants and children from becoming entangled in the tubing or from accidentally pulling the catheter or needle out. Securing the tubing in this manner also eliminates movement of the catheter hub at the insertion site (mechanical manipulation). A colourful sticker can be applied to the protecting device to add a positive note to the procedure.

Finger or toe areas should be left unoccluded by dressings or tape to allow for assessment of circulation. The thumb is never immobilized, because of the danger of contractures with limited movement later on. An extremity should never be encircled with tape. The use of roll gauze, self-adhering stretch bandages, and Ace bandages can cause the same constriction and hide signs of infiltration.

> **NURSING ALERT**
>
> Opaque covering should be avoided; however, if any type of opaque covering is used to secure the IV line, the insertion site and extremity distal to the site should be visible to detect an infiltration. If these sites are not visible, they must be checked frequently to detect problems early.

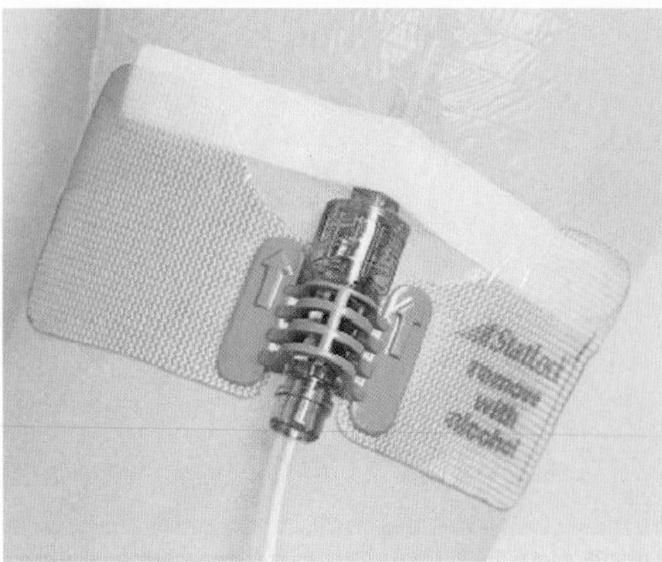

FIGURE 44-18 StatLock securement devices enhance peripheral intravenous line dwell time and decrease phlebitis.

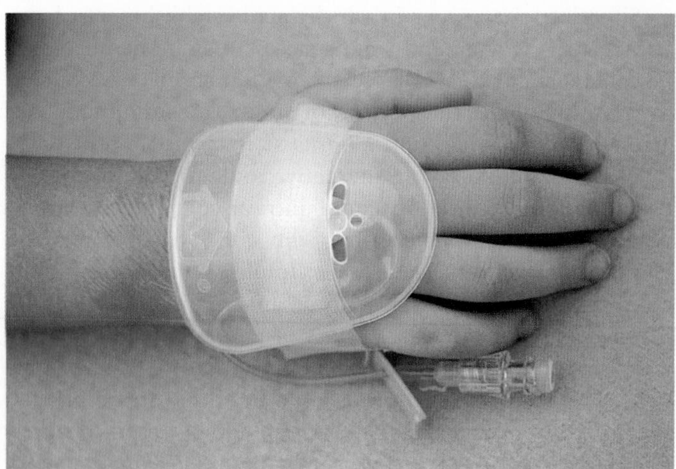

FIGURE 44-19 I.V. House used to protect intravenous site.

Traditionally padded boards and splints have been used to partially immobilize the IV site. Padded boards and splints and restraints were appropriate when metal needles were inserted into the vein to prevent the sharp end from puncturing the vessel, especially at a joint. With the more recent use of soft, pliable catheters, arm or leg boards may not be necessary and their use has several disadvantages. If they are not placed properly, they can obscure the IV site, can constrict the extremity, may excoriate the underlying tissue and promote infection, can cause a contracture of a joint, restrict useful movement of the extremity, and are uncomfortable. Unfortunately, no research has been conducted to demonstrate their proposed benefit of increasing dwell time (patency of the IV line). In most situations, the approach with the least restraint can be used, but restraint methods may be necessary to ensure patency and prevent dislodgement of IV lines. Older children who are alert and receptive can usually be trusted to protect the IV site (see Research Focus box).

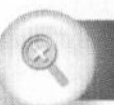

RESEARCH FOCUS

Peripheral Intravenous Care

Joy Hesselgrave; updated by Olga A. Taylor

Ask the Question

What site preparation and stabilization measures for PIV catheters are optimum for preventing complications and extending dwell time in children?

Search for Evidence

Search Strategies

Search selection criteria included English-language and research-based publications within the past 15 years that are on PIV catheter site care.

Databases Used

National Guidelines Clearinghouse (AHQR), Cochrane Collaboration, Joanna Briggs Institute, PubMed, TRIP Database Plus, MD Consult, PedsCCM, BestBETs

Critically Analyze the Evidence

Site Preparation

- The skin should be disinfected with an appropriate antiseptic before PIV catheter insertion; it should be allowed to dry before catheter insertion (Centers for Disease Control and Prevention [CDC], 2011; Infusion Nurses Society, 2011a, 2011b; Registered Nurses' Association of Ontario [RNAO], 2008).
- A 2% chlorhexidine-based preparation is preferred; but tincture of iodine, an iodophor, or 70% alcohol can be used. There is no recommendation for the use of chlorhexidine in infants younger than 2 months old (Infusion Nurses Society, 2011a).
- Cleansing the skin with a preparation that combines alcohol with either chlorhexidine gluconate or povidone-iodine before PIV catheter insertion is recommended (Infusion Nurses Society, 2011a, 2011b).
- All disinfectants have risks for neonates. Chlorhexidine gluconate with alcohol should be used with caution in premature infants or infants less than 2 months, as these products may cause chemical burns. Current CDC guidelines indicate that there is insufficient evidence to make a recommendation about a single product for all newborns (CDC, 2011). Cleansers should be removed from infants with sterile water or normal saline to prevent absorption of the disinfectant (Association of Women's Health, Obstetric and Neonatal Nurses, 2013).

Stabilization or Securement Devices

- PIV catheters must be stabilized for easy monitoring and evaluation of the access site; to promote delivery of therapy; and to prevent damage, dislodgement, or migration of the catheter (Infusion Nurses Society, 2011a; RNAO, 2008).
- To avoid catheter movement and damage, the catheter and hub should be secured firmly with Steri-Strips and clear occlusive dressing; tape should not be placed directly to the catheter (Infusion Nurses Society, 2011a; Paulson & Miller, 2008).
- The catheter site should be assessed every 7 to 8 hours to ensure that the catheter has not migrated (Infusion Nurses Society, 2011a; Paulson & Miller, 2008).
- When comparing tape, StatLock, and Hub-Guard for a 96-hour PIV protocol change, it was found that PIV catheters with StatLock produced a statistically significant improved survival rate (52%) compared with tape (8%) or HubGuard (9%) (Smith, 2006).

Dwell Time

- Evidence is insufficient regarding the effect of heparin use for extending PIV catheter use in neonates (Shah, Ng, & Sinha, 2005).
- An increase in complications and obstructions of PIV catheters was related to younger patient age, insertion into the wrist and scalp, and use of a 24-gauge catheter (Tripathi, Kaushik, & Singh, 2008).

Apply the Evidence: Nursing Implications

There is *low-quality evidence with strong recommendation* for site preparation and use of stabilization measures for PIV catheters in children. For children older than 2 months of age, chlorhexidine is the preferred skin cleanser. For younger infants the research is not conclusive regarding proper cleanser. All cleansers should be removed with sterile water or sterile normal saline to prevent absorption. The most distal vein on the extremity that allows the child optimum movement (avoid over the joint) should be selected. Veins on the scalp may be used in infants. Subsequent PIV catheters should be proximal to the previous IV site. If the child is mobile, use of a securement or protection device (e.g., StatLock, HubGuard) should be considered. The PIV catheter should be discontinued if complications occur or when it is no longer needed.

References

Association of Women's Health, Obstetric and Neonatal Nurses (AWHONN). (2013). *Neonatal skin care: Evidence-based clinical practice guideline* (3rd ed.). Washington, DC: Author.

Centers for Disease Control and Prevention. (2011). *2011 Guidelines for the prevention of intravascusular catheter-related infections.* Retrieved from <http://www.cdc.gov/hicpac/BSI/BSI-guidelines-2011.html>.

Infusion Nurses Society. (2011a). Infusion nursing standards of practice. *Journal of Infusion Nursing, 34*(1S).

Infusion Nurses Society. (2011b). *Policies and procedures for infusion nursing* (4th ed.). South Norwood, MA: Author.

Paulson, P. R., & Miller, K. M. (2008). Neonatal peripherally inserted central catheters: Recommendations for prevention of insertion and postinsertion complications. *Neonatal Network, 27,* 245–257.

Registered Nurses' Association of Ontario. (2008). *Care and maintenance to reduce vascular access complications, guideline supplement.* Toronto: Author. Retrieved from <http://rnao.ca/sites/rnao-ca/files/Care_and_Maintenance_to_Reduce_Vascular_Access_Complications.pdf>.

Shah, P. S., Ng, E., & Sinha, A. K. (2005). Heparin for prolonging peripheral intravenous catheter use in neonates. *Cochrane Database System Review,* (4), CD002774.

Smith, B. (2006). Peripheral intravenous catheter dwell times: A comparison of three securement methods for implementation of a 96-hour scheduled change protocol. *Journal of Infusion Nursing, 29*(1), 14–17.

Tripathi, S., Kaushik, V., & Singh, V. (2008). Peripheral IVs: Factors affecting complications and patency—a randomized controlled trial. *Journal of Infusion Nursing, 31,* 182–188.

IV, intravenous; *PIV,* peripheral intravenous.

Removal of a Peripheral Intravenous Line

When it comes time to discontinue an IV infusion, many children are distressed by the thought of catheter removal. They need a careful explanation of the process and suggestions for helping. Encouraging children to remove or help remove the tape from the site provides them with a measure of control and often encourages their assistance. The procedure consists of turning off any pump apparatus, occluding the IV tubing, removing the tape, pulling the catheter out of the vessel in the opposite direction of insertion, and exerting firm pressure at the site. A dry dressing (adhesive bandage strip) is placed over the puncture site. The use of adhesive-removal pads can decrease the pain of tape removal, but the skin should be washed after use to avoid irritation. To remove transparent dressings, for example, OpSite or Tegaderm, the opposing edges should be pulled parallel to the skin to loosen the bond. The nurse needs to inspect the catheter tip to ensure the catheter is intact and that no portion remains in the vein.

! NURSING ALERT

Consider the child's age, development, neurological status, and predictability (how the child responds to painful treatments) when determining the need for assistance to maintain safety. Manual removal of tape is the preferred method. Only if absolutely necessary should a small cut be made in the tape, using bandage scissors, to facilitate its removal. Before cutting the tape:

- Ensure that all digits are visible.
- Remove any barrier that hinders visibility, such as a protective covering.
- Protect the child's skin and digits by sliding your own finger(s) between the tape and the child's skin so that the scissors do not touch the patient.
- Place a cut on the tape located on the medial aspect (thumb side) of the extremity.

Complications

The same precautions regarding maintenance of asepsis, prevention of infection, and observation for infiltration need to be carried out with patients of any age. However, infiltration is more difficult to detect in infants and small children than in adults. The increased amount of subcutaneous fat and the amount of tape used to secure the catheter often obscure the early signs of infiltration. When the fluid appears to be infusing too slowly or ceases, the usual assessment for obstruction within the apparatus—kinks, screw clamps, shutoff valve, and positioning interference such as a bent elbow—often locates the difficulty. When these actions fail to detect the problem, it may be necessary to carefully remove some of the dressing to obtain a clear view of the venipuncture site. Dependent areas, such as the palm and undersides of the extremity or the occiput and behind the ears, should be examined.

Whenever possible, the IV infusion should be placed in an extremity to which the identification band (or bracelet) is not attached. Serious circulatory impairment can result from infiltrated solution distal to the band, which acts as a tourniquet, preventing adequate venous return. To check for return blood flow through the catheter, the tubing is removed from the infusion pump, and the bag is lowered below the level of the infusion site. Resistance during flushing or aspiration for blood return also indicates that the IV infusion may have infiltrated surrounding tissue. A good blood return, or lack thereof, is not always an indicator of infiltration in small infants. Flushing the catheter and observing for edema, redness, or streaking along the vein are appropriate for assessment of the IV.

IV therapy in pediatrics tends to be difficult to maintain because of mechanical factors such as vascular trauma resulting from the catheter, the insertion site, vessel size, vessel fragility, pump pressure, the patient's activity level, operator skill and insertion technique, forceful administration of boluses of fluid, and infusion of irritants or vesicants through a small vessel. These factors cause infiltration and extravasation injuries. *Infiltration* is defined as inadvertent administration of a nonvesicant solution or medication into surrounding tissue. *Extravasation* is defined as inadvertent administration of vesicant solution or medication into surrounding tissue (Infusion Nurses Society, 2016). A *vesicant* or *sclerosing agent* causes varying degrees of cellular damage when even minute amounts escape into surrounding tissue. Guidelines are available for determining the severity of tissue injury by staging characteristics, such as the amount of redness, blanching, the amount of swelling, pain, the quality of pulses below infiltration, capillary refill, and warmth or coolness of the area (Infusion Nurses Society, 2016) (see Additional Resources at the end of this chapter).

Treatment of infiltration or extravasation varies according to the type of vesicant. Guidelines are available outlining the sequence of interventions and specific treatment of infiltration or extravasation with antidotes (Infusion Nurses Society, 2016).

NURSING ALERT

When infiltration or extravasation is observed (signs include erythema, pain, edema, blanching, streaking on the skin along the vein, and darkened area at the insertion site), immediately stop the infusion, elevate the extremity, notify the practitioner, and initiate the ordered treatment as soon as possible. Remove the IV line when it is no longer needed, such as after infusing an antidote.

PROCEDURES FOR MAINTAINING RESPIRATORY FUNCTION

Inhalation Therapy

Oxygen Therapy

Oxygen is administered for hypoxemia and may be delivered by mask, nasal cannula, tent, hood, face mask, or ventilator. The mode of delivery is selected on the basis of the concentration needed and the child's ability to assist in its use. Oxygen is dry and therefore must be humidified.

Oxygen therapy is frequently administered in the hospital, although increasing numbers of children are receiving oxygen in the home.

Oxygen delivered to infants is well tolerated by using a plastic hood (Fig. 44-20). At least 4 to 5 L/min of flow is necessary to maintain oxygen concentrations and remove the exhaled carbon dioxide. The humidified oxygen should not be blown directly

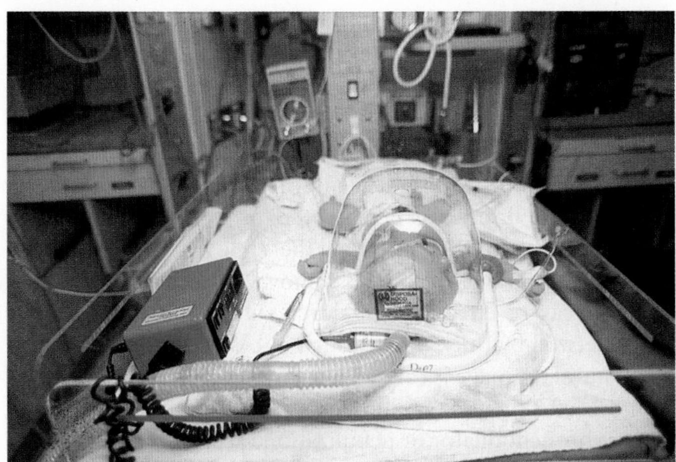

FIGURE 44-20 Oxygen administered to infant by means of a plastic hood. Note oxygen analyzer (blue machine).

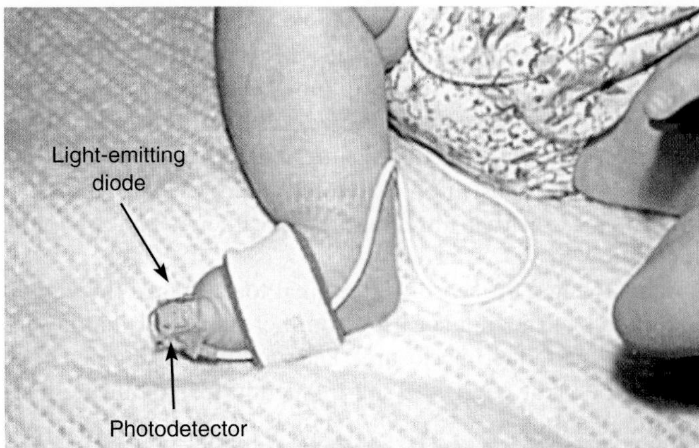

FIGURE 44-21 Pulse oximeter sensor. Note that the sensor is positioned with light-emitting diode (LED) opposite the photodetector.

into the infant's face. Older infants and children can use a nasal cannula or prongs (see Fig. 28-1), which can supply a concentration of oxygen of about 50%. A mask is not well tolerated by children.

> **MEDICATION ALERT**
>
> Prolonged exposure to high oxygen tensions can damage some body tissues and functions. The organs most vulnerable to the adverse effects of excessive oxygenation are the retina of the extremely preterm infant and the lungs of persons at any age.

Oxygen-induced carbon dioxide narcosis is a physiological hazard of oxygen therapy that may occur in persons with chronic pulmonary disease, such as cystic fibrosis. In these patients the respiratory centre has adapted to the continuously higher arterial carbon dioxide tension ($Paco_2$) levels, and hypoxia becomes the more powerful stimulus for respiration. When the arterial oxygen tension (Pao_2) level is elevated during oxygen administration, the hypoxic drive is removed, causing progressive hypoventilation and increased $Paco_2$ levels, and the child rapidly becomes unconscious. Carbon dioxide narcosis can also be induced by the administration of sedation in these patients.

Monitoring Oxygen Therapy

Pulse oximetry is a continuous, noninvasive method of determining oxygen saturation (Sao_2) to guide oxygen therapy. A sensor composed of a light-emitting diode (LED) and a photodetector is placed in opposition around a foot, hand, finger, toe, or earlobe, with the LED placed on top of the nail when digits are used (Fig. 44-21). The diode emits red and infrared lights that pass through the skin to the photodetector. The photodetector measures the amount of each type of light absorbed by functional hemoglobins. Hemoglobin saturated with oxygen (oxyhemoglobin) absorbs more infrared light than does hemoglobin not saturated with oxygen (deoxyhemoglobin). Pulsatile blood flow is the primary physiological factor that influences accuracy of the pulse oximeter. In infants, the probe should be repositioned at least every 3 to 4 hours to prevent pressure necrosis; poor perfusion and very sensitive skin may necessitate more frequent repositioning.

Another noninvasive method is *transcutaneous monitoring (TCM)*, which provides continuous monitoring of transcutaneous partial pressure of oxygen in arterial blood ($tcPao_2$) and, with some devices, of carbon dioxide in arterial blood ($tcPaco_2$). An electrode is attached to the warmed skin to facilitate arterialization of cutaneous capillaries. The site of the electrode must be changed every 3 to 4 hours to avoid burning the skin, and the machine must be calibrated with every site change. TCM is used frequently in neonatal intensive care units, but it may not reflect Pao_2 in infants with impaired local circulation or in older infants whose skin is thicker.

Oximetry is insensitive to hyperoxia because hemoglobin approaches 100% saturation for all Pao_2 readings greater than approximately 100 mm Hg, which is a dangerous situation for the preterm infant at risk for developing retinopathy of prematurity (see Chapter 28). Therefore, the preterm infant being monitored with oximetry should have upper limits identified, such as 90 to 95%, and a protocol established for decreasing oxygen when saturations are high.

Oximetry offers several advantages over TCM. It (1) does not require heating the skin, thus reducing the risk of burns; (2) eliminates a delay period for transducer equilibration; and (3) maintains an accurate measurement regardless of the patient's age or skin characteristics or the presence of lung disease.

> **NURSING ALERT**
>
> It is important to make certain that sensor connectors and oximeters are compatible. Wiring that is incompatible can generate considerable heat at the tip of the sensor, causing second- and third-degree burns under the sensors. Pressure necrosis can also occur from sensors attached too tightly. Inspect the skin under the sensor frequently.

Correct application of the sensor is essential for accurate Sao_2 measurements. Because the sensor must identify every pulse beat to calculate the Sao_2, movement can interfere with sensing. Some devices synchronize the Sao_2 reading with the heartbeat, thereby reducing the interference caused by motion. Sensors are not placed on extremities used for blood pressure monitoring or with in-dwelling arterial catheters, since pulsatile blood flow may be affected.

Infant—Secure the sensor to the great toe and tape the wire to the sole of the foot (or use a commercial holder that fastens with a self-adhering closure). Place a snugly fitting sock over the foot, but check the site frequently for colour, temperature, and pulse.

Child—Secure the sensor securely to the index finger and tape the wire to the back of the hand.

Ambient light from ceiling lights and phototherapy, as well as high-intensity heat and light from radiant warmers, can interfere with readings. Thus, the sensor should be covered to block these light sources. IV dyes; green, purple, or black nail polish; nonopaque synthetic nails; and possibly ink used for foot printing can also cause inaccurate Sao_2 measurements. The dyes should be removed or, in the case of porcelain nails, a different area used for the sensor. Skin colour, thickness, and edema do not affect the readings.

End-Tidal Carbon Dioxide

End-tidal carbon dioxide ($ETCO_2$) monitoring measures exhaled carbon dioxide noninvasively. Capnometry provides a numeric display, and continuous capnometry is available in many bedside physiological and stand-alone monitors. $ETCO_2$ differs from pulse oximetry in that it is more sensitive to the mechanics of ventilation rather than oxygenation. Hypoxic episodes can be proven through the early detection of hypoventilation, apnea, or airway obstruction.

Children who are experiencing an asthma exacerbation, receiving procedural sedation, or are mechanically ventilated may have $ETCO_2$ monitoring. Special sampling cannulas are used for nonintubated patients, and a small device is placed between the endotracheal (ET) tube and the ventilator tubing in intubated patients. Although $ETCO_2$ monitoring is not a substitute for arterial blood gases, it does provide ventilation information continuously and noninvasively. Normal $ETCO_2$ values are 30 to 43 mm Hg, which is slightly lower than normal arterial PCO_2 of 35 to 45 mm Hg. During cardiopulmonary resuscitation (CPR), $ETCO_2$ values consistently below 15 mm Hg indicate ineffective compressions or excessive ventilation. Changes in waveform and numeric display follow changes in ventilation by a very few seconds and precede changes in respiratory rate, skin colour, and pulse oximetry values.

When there is a change in $ETCO_2$ value or waveform, the nurse needs to assess the patient quickly for adequate airway, breathing, and circulation. Sedated patients may be hypoventilating and need stimulation. Intubated patients may need suctioning, have self-extubated or dislodged the tube, or have equipment failure or disconnection. Patients with asthma may have a worsening condition. Problems with the $ETCO_2$ monitoring system can include a kink in the sample line or disconnection. In general, the nurse should check the patient first and then the equipment.

Bronchial (Postural) Drainage

Bronchial drainage is indicated whenever excessive fluid or mucus in the bronchi is not being removed by normal ciliary activity and cough. Positioning the child to take maximum advantage of gravity facilitates removal of secretions. Postural drainage can be effective in children with chronic lung disease characterized by thick mucus, such as cystic fibrosis.

Postural drainage is carried out three or four times daily and is more effective when it follows other respiratory therapy, such as bronchodilator or nebulization medication (see Aerosol Therapy, p. 1313). Bronchial drainage is generally performed before meals (or 1 to 1½ hours after meals) to minimize the chance of vomiting and is repeated at bedtime. The duration of treatment depends on the child's condition and tolerance; it usually lasts 20 to 30 minutes. Several positions facilitate drainage from all major lung segments.

Chest Physical Therapy

Chest physiotherapy (CPT) usually refers to the use of postural drainage in combination with adjunctive techniques that are thought to enhance the clearance of mucus from the airway. These techniques include manual percussion, vibration, and squeezing of the chest; cough; forceful expiration; and breathing exercises. Special mechanical devices are also used to perform CPT, such as vest-type percussors. Postural drainage in combination with forced expiration has been shown to be beneficial.

Common techniques used in association with postural drainage include manual percussion of the chest wall and percussion with mechanical devices such as a high-frequency hand-held chest compression device. A "popping," hollow sound, not a slapping sound, should be the result. The procedure should be done over the rib cage only and should be painless. Percussion can be performed with a soft circular mask (adapted to maintain air trapping) or a percussion cup marketed especially for the purpose of aiding in loosening secretions. CPT is contraindicated when patients have pulmonary hemorrhage, pulmonary embolism, end-stage renal disease, increased intracranial pressure, osteogenesis imperfecta, or minimal cardiac reserves.

Intubation

Rapid-sequence intubation (RSI) is commonly performed in pediatric and some neonatal patients to induce an unconscious, neuromuscular blocked condition to avoid the use of positive-pressure ventilation and the risk of possible aspiration (Wetzel, 2016). Atropine, fentanyl, and vecuronium or rocuronium are drugs commonly used during RSI. In neonates, ET intubation is often a stressful event, and hypoxia and pain are commonly associated with it (Wetzel, 2016). RSI in neonates may prevent such adverse effects. Signs of the need for intubation include the following:

- Respiratory failure or arrest, agonal or gasping respirations, apnea

- Upper airway obstruction
- Significant increase in the work of breathing
- Potential for developing partial or complete airway obstruction—respiratory effort with no breath sounds, facial trauma, and inhalation injuries
- Potential for or actual loss of airway protection, increased risk for aspiration
- Anticipated need for mechanical ventilation related to chest trauma, shock, increased intracranial pressure
- Hypoxemia despite supplemental oxygen
- Inadequate ventilation

Mechanical Ventilation

An artificial airway is usually used in association with mechanical ventilation and in children with upper airway obstruction. ET intubation can be accomplished via the nasal (nasotracheal), oral (orotracheal), or direct tracheal (tracheostomy) routes. Although it is more difficult to place, nasotracheal intubation is preferred to orotracheal intubation because it facilitates oral hygiene and provides more stable fixation, which reduces the complication of tracheal erosion and the danger of accidental extubation. In the past, only uncuffed endotracheal tubes were used in children younger than 8 years of age, because the cuffed tubes did not fit the shape of the child's airway and created air leaks at times, and the child had to be reintubated in order to fix the leaks. Now, there are new cuffed endotracheal tubes on the market that are designed to fit the shape of the child's airway and produce less air leakage. These cuffs are recommended except for use in premature infants or infants weighing less than 3 kg (Taylor, Subaiya, & Corsino, 2011). Air or gas delivered directly to the trachea must be humidified. An artificial airway is usually used in association with mechanical ventilation and in children with upper airway obstruction.

In preparation for intubation, the child should be preoxygenated with 100% oxygen using an appropriate-size bag and mask. During intubation the cardiac rhythm, heart rate, and oxygen saturation should be monitored continuously with audible tones. ET tube placement should be verified by at least one clinical sign and at least one confirmatory technology:

- Visualization of bilateral chest expansion
- Auscultation over the epigastrium (breath sounds should not be heard) and the lung fields bilaterally in the axillary region (breath sounds should be equal and adequate)
- Water vapour in the tube (helpful, not definitive)
- Colour change on end-tidal carbon dioxide detector during exhalation after at least three to six breaths or wave form/value verification with continuous capnography
- Chest radiography

Once the ET placement has been confirmed a protective skin barrier should be applied and the ET tube secured with tape or a securement device. An NG tube typically is inserted after intubation.

Basic ongoing assessment of the mechanically ventilated patient includes observing the chest rise and fall for symmetry, bilateral breath sounds equal or unchanged from last assessment, level of consciousness, capillary refill and skin colour, and vital signs. A heart rate that is too fast or too slow is a possible indication of hypoxemia, air leak, or low cardiac output. Pulse oximetry and end-tidal carbon dioxide monitoring is also routine, along with periodic arterial blood gas analysis. If sudden deterioration of an intubated patient occurs, the nurse needs to assess for the following etiologies:

DOPE

Displacement—Tube not in the trachea or had moved into a bronchus (right mainstream is more common)

Obstruction—Secretions or kinking of the tube

Pneumothorax—Chest trauma, barotraumas, or noncompliant lung disease

Equipment failure—Check the oxygen source, AMBU bag, and ventilator

(American Heart Association, 2015).

Placement should be verified again during each transport and when patients are moved to different beds.

To maintain skin integrity in the mechanically ventilated patient, the patient needs to be repositioned at least every 2 hours as the patient's condition tolerates. The nurse can apply a hydrocolloid barrier to protect the facial cheeks. Pillows can be placed under pressure points, such as occiput, heels, elbows, and shoulder. No tubes, lines, wires, or wrinkles in bedding should be allowed under the patient. The nurse needs to provide meticulous skin care.

Analgesia and sedation are provided as needed. A system for communication can be used that includes sign boards, pointing, and opening and closing eyes. To ensure safety, soft restraints may be used, if necessary, to maintain a critical airway.

Ventilator-associated pneumonia is a complication that can be prevented through the use of aggressive hand hygiene, oral care, and elevation of the head of the bed between 30 and 45 degrees (unless contraindicated). Enteral nutrition is often provided to decrease the risk of bacterial translocation. The nurse needs to routinely assess the patient's intestine motility by auscultating bowel sound and measuring residual gastric volume or abdominal girth and adjusting the rate and volume of enteral feeding to avoid regurgitation. In high-risk patients (decreased gag reflex, delayed gastric emptying, gastroesophageal reflux, severe bronchospasm), postpyloric (duodenal, jejunal) feeding tubes are often used. To prevent the aspiration of pooled secretions, the nurse needs to suction the hypopharynx before suctioning the ET tube, before repositioning the ET tube, and before repositioning the patient. Ventilator circuits' condensate should be prevented from entering ET tube or in-line medication nebulizers.

Readiness for extubation should be assessed daily. Indications that a child is ready to be extubated include an improvement in underlying condition, hemodynamic stability, and mechanical support no longer being necessary. Level of consciousness and ability to maintain a patent airway can be assessed by having the patient mobilize pulmonary secretions through effective coughing. NPO status should be maintained 4 hours before extubation. After extubation, the child should be monitored for respiratory distress, which may develop within minutes or hours. Signs of postintubation respiratory distress

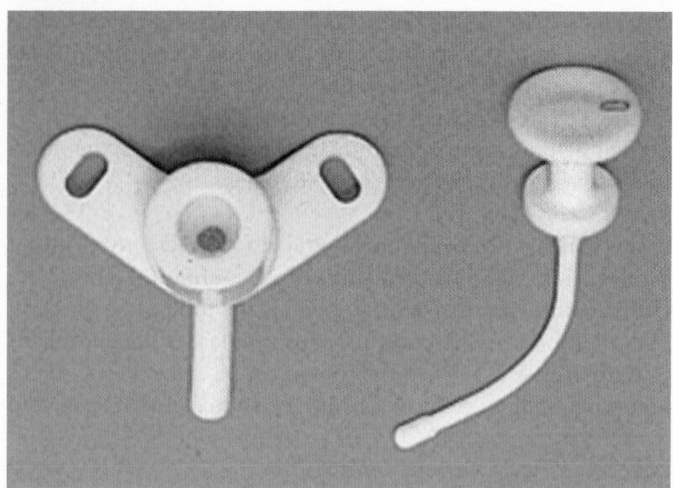

FIGURE 44-22 Silastic pediatric tracheostomy tube and obturator.

include stridor, hoarseness, increased work of breathing, unstable vital signs, and desaturations.

Tracheostomy

A *tracheostomy* is a surgical opening in the trachea; the procedure may be done on an emergency basis or may be an elective one, and it may be combined with mechanical ventilation. Pediatric tracheostomy tubes are usually made of plastic or Silastic (Fig. 44-22). The most common types are the Hollinger, Jackson, Aberdeen, and Shiley tubes. These tubes are constructed with a more acute angle than that of adult tubes, and they soften at body temperature, conforming to the contours of the trachea. Because these materials resist the formation of crusted respiratory secretions, they are made without an inner cannula.

Children who have undergone a tracheostomy must be closely monitored for complications such as hemorrhage, edema, aspiration, accidental decannulation, tube obstruction, and the entrance of free air into the pleural cavity. Nursing care focuses on maintaining a patent airway, facilitating the removal of pulmonary secretions, providing humidified air or oxygen, cleansing the stoma, monitoring the child's ability to swallow, and teaching while simultaneously preventing complications.

Because the child may be unable to signal for help, direct observation and use of respiratory and cardiac monitors are essential. Respiratory assessments include breath sounds and the work of breathing, vital signs, tightness of the tracheostomy ties, and the type and amount of secretions. Large amounts of bloody secretions are uncommon and should be considered a sign of hemorrhage. The primary practitioner should be notified immediately if this occurs.

The child is positioned with the head of the bed raised or in the position most comfortable to the child, with the call light easily available. Suction catheters, suction source, gloves, sterile saline, sterile gauze for wiping away secretions, scissors, an extra tracheostomy tube of the same size with ties already attached, another tracheostomy tube one size smaller, and the obturator are kept at the bedside. A source of humidification is provided

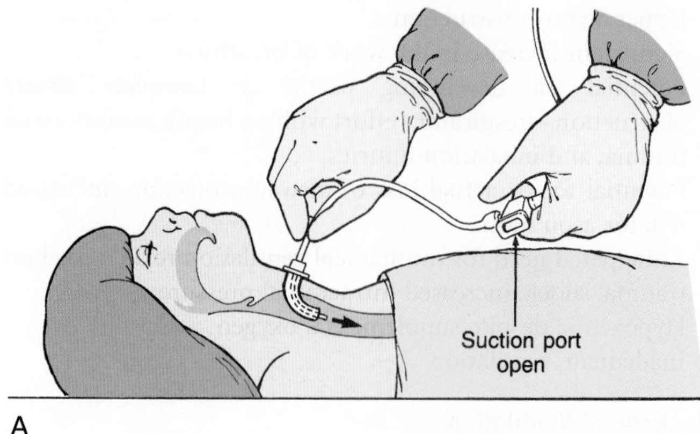

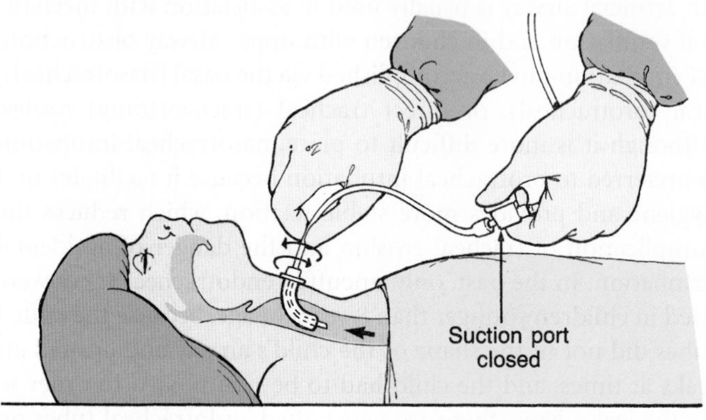

FIGURE 44-23 Tracheostomy suctioning. **A:** Insertion, port open. **B:** Withdrawal, port occluded. Note that the catheter is inserted just slightly beyond the end of the tracheostomy tube.

because the normal humidification and filtering functions of the airway have been bypassed. IV fluids ensure adequate hydration until the child is able to swallow sufficient amounts of fluids.

Suctioning

The airway must remain patent and requires frequent suctioning during the first few hours after a tracheostomy to remove mucous plugs and excessive secretions. Proper vacuum pressure and suction catheter size are important to prevent atelectasis and decrease hypoxia from the suctioning procedure. Vacuum pressure should range from 60 to 100 mm Hg for infants and children and from 40 to 60 mm Hg for preterm infants. Unless secretions are thick and tenacious, the lower range of negative pressure is recommended. Tracheal suction catheters are available in a variety of sizes. The catheter selected should have a diameter one-half the diameter of the tracheostomy tube. If the catheter is too large, it can block the airway. The catheter is constructed with a side port so that the catheter is introduced without suction and removed while simultaneous intermittent suction is applied by covering the port with the thumb (Fig. 44-23). The catheter is inserted just to the end of the tracheostomy tube. While instillation of normal saline before ET tube suctioning has been used for years as a method to loosen and dilute secretions, lubricate the suction catheter, and promote cough, there are potentially adverse effects of this procedure. The practice of instilling sterile saline in the tracheostomy tube before suctioning is not supported by research and is no longer recommended.

! NURSING ALERT

Suctioning should require no more than 5 seconds. Counting one one-thousand, two one-thousand, three one-thousand, and so on while suctioning is a simple means for monitoring the time. Without a safeguard, the airway may be obstructed for too long. Hyperventilating the child with 100% oxygen before and after suctioning (using a bag-valve-mask or increasing the fraction of inspired oxygen concentration [FiO_2] ventilator setting) may be performed to prevent hypoxia. Closed tracheal suctioning systems that allow for uninterrupted oxygen delivery may also be used.

The child should be allowed to rest for 30 to 60 seconds after each suctioning pass to allow oxygen saturation to return to normal; then the process is repeated until the trachea is clear. Suctioning should be limited to about three passes in one period. Oximetry is used to monitor suctioning and prevent hypoxia.

! NURSING ALERT

Suctioning is carried out only as often as needed to keep the tube patent. Signs of mucus partially occluding the airway include an increased heart rate, a rise in respiratory effort, a drop in SaO_2, cyanosis, and an increase in the positive inspiratory pressure on the ventilator.

In the acute care setting, aseptic technique is used during care of the tracheostomy. Secondary infection is a major concern, since the air entering the lower airway bypasses the natural defences of the upper airway. Gloves should be worn during the suctioning procedure, although a sterile glove is needed only on the hand touching the catheter. A new tube and gloves should be used each time.

Routine Care

The tracheostomy stoma requires daily care. Assessments of the stoma area include observations for signs of infection and breakdown of the skin. The skin needs to be kept clean and dry, and crusted secretions around the stoma may be gently removed with half-strength hydrogen peroxide. Hydrogen peroxide should not be used with sterling silver tracheostomy tubes because it tends to pit and stain the silver surface. The nurse should be aware of wet tracheostomy dressings, which can predispose the peristomal area to skin breakdown. Several products are available to prevent or treat excoriation.

The tracheostomy tube is held in place with tracheostomy ties made of a durable, nonfraying material. The ties can be changed daily but are normally replaced when soiled. Ties fastened with self-adhering Velcro closures are commonly used. If Velcro ties are not available, cotton ties are looped through the flanges and tied snugly in a triple knot at the side of the neck before the soiled ties are cut and removed. The ties should be tight enough to allow just a fingertip to be inserted between the ties and the neck (Fig. 44-24). It is easier to ensure a snug fit if the child's head is flexed rather than extended while the ties are being secured.

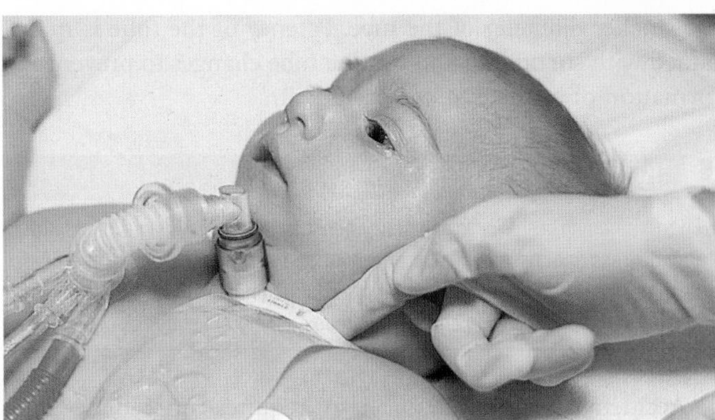

FIGURE 44-24 Tracheostomy ties are snug but allow one finger to be inserted.

Routine tracheostomy tube changes are usually carried out weekly after a tract has been formed to minimize the formation of granulation tissue. The first change is usually performed by the surgeon; subsequent changes are performed by the nurse and, if the child is discharged home with the tracheostomy, by either a parent or a visiting nurse. Ideally, two caregivers participate in the procedure to assist with positioning the child.

Changing the tracheostomy tube is accomplished using sterile technique. Tube changes should occur before meals or 2 hours after the last meal. Continuous feedings should be turned off at least an hour before a tube change. The new, sterile tube is prepared by inserting the obturator and attaching new ties. The child is suctioned before the procedure to minimize secretions, then held and positioned with the neck slightly extended. One caregiver cuts the old ties and removes the tube from the stoma. The new tube is inserted gently into the stoma (using a downward and forward motion that follows the curve of the trachea), the obturator is removed, and the ties are secured. The adequacy of ventilation must be assessed after a tube change because the tube can be inserted into the soft tissue surrounding the trachea; breath sounds and respiratory effort should be carefully monitored.

Supplemental oxygen is always delivered with a humidification system to prevent drying of the respiratory mucosa. Humidification of room air for an established tracheostomy can be intermittent if secretions remain thin enough to be coughed or suctioned from the tracheostomy. Direct humidification via a tracheostomy mask can be provided during naps and at night so that the child is able to be up and around unencumbered during much of the day. Room humidifiers are also used successfully.

The inner cannula, if used, should be removed with each suctioning, cleaned with sterile saline and pipe cleaners to remove crusted material, dried thoroughly, and reinserted.

Emergency Care: Tube Occlusion and Accidental Decannulation

Occlusion of the tracheostomy tube is life threatening, and infants and children are at greater risk than adults because of the smaller diameter of the tube. Patency of the tube is maintained with suctioning and routine tube changes to prevent the formation of crusts that can occlude it.

! NURSING ALERT

Life-threatening occlusion is apparent when the child displays signs of respiratory distress and a suction catheter cannot be passed to the end of the tube despite several attempts. This situation requires an immediate tube change, after attempting a cannula change and repositioning the child.

Accidental decannulation also requires immediate tube replacement. Some children have a fairly rigid trachea, so the airway remains partially open when the tube is removed. However, others have malformed or flexible tracheal cartilage, which causes the airway to collapse when the tube is removed or dislodged. Because many infants and children with upper airway problems have little airway reserve, if replacement of the dislodged tube is impossible, a smaller-sized tube should be inserted. If the stoma cannot be cannulated with another tracheostomy tube, oral intubation should be performed.

Chest Tube Procedures

A chest tube is placed to remove fluid or air from the pleural or pericardial space. Chest tube draining systems collect air and fluid while inhibiting a backflow into the pleura or pericardial space. Indications for chest tube placement include pneumothorax, hemothorax, chylothorax, empyema, pleural or pericardial effusion, and prevention of accumulation of fluid in the pleural and pericardial space after cardiothoracic surgery. Nursing responsibilities include assisting with chest tube placement, managing chest tubes, and assisting with chest tube removal.

Before chest tube insertion it is important to assess hematological and coagulation results for any risk of bleeding during the procedure. The health care provider should be notified of any abnormal findings. The nurse should prepare the drainage system with sterile water as described in the package insert (some systems may not require this step) and administer pain and sedation medications as ordered. Airway, breathing, circulation, and pulse oximetry need to be monitored throughout the procedure.

After the tube has been inserted and connected to the chest drainage system, the tubing should be secured so it does not become disconnected. If suction is required, connection tubing is used to join the drainage system to a wall suction adapter and suction on the drainage system adjusted as ordered (usually 10–20 cm H_2O). There should be gentle, continuous bubbling in the suction chamber. An occlusive dressing is placed over the chest tube insertion site per hospital policy. The nurse needs to note the date, time, and initials on the dressing. If gauze is used it should be presplit; gauze cut by scissors may leave loose threads in the wound. The nurse needs to ensure that the drainage system is positioned below the patient's chest and secured to the floor or bed. The drainage tubing should be kept free of dependent loops. A chest radiograph is used to confirm placement of the chest tube. Daily chest radiographs need to be scheduled to monitor placement of the chest tube and resolution of the pneumothorax or effusion.

Disposable chest drainages systems typically consist of three chambers next to one another in one drainage unit (Fig. 44-25). The fluid collection chamber collects drainage from the patient's pleural or pericardial space. The water-seal chamber is connected directly to the fluid collection chamber and acts as a

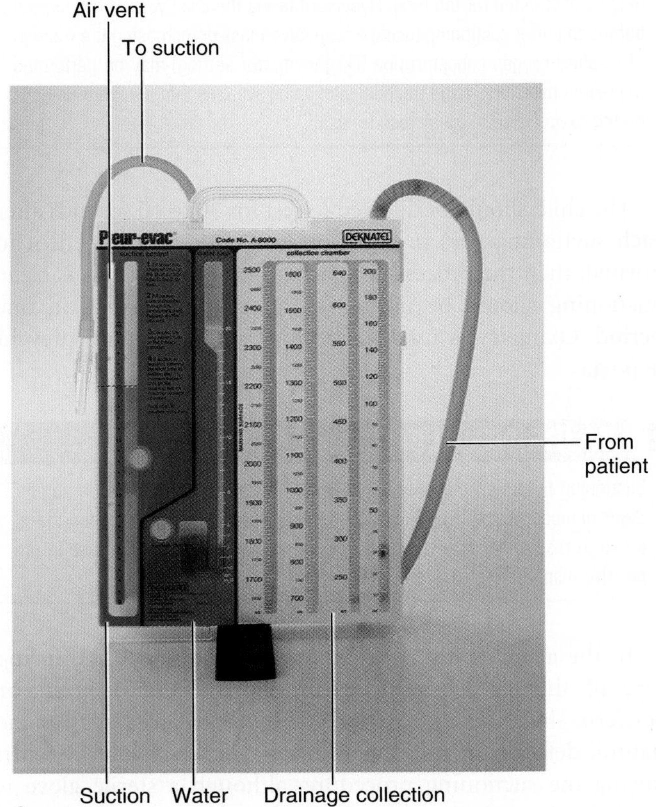

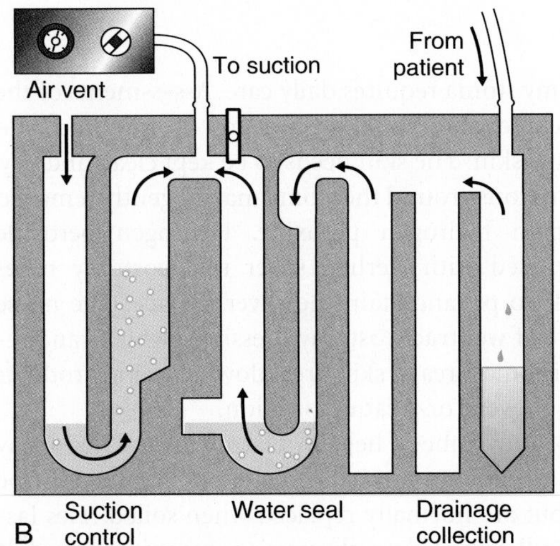

FIGURE 44-25 A: Pleur-Evac drainage system, a commercial three-bottle chest drainage device. **B:** Schematic of drainage device. (From Ignatavicius, D. D., & Workman, L. M. (2010). *Medical-surgical nursing: Patient-centered collaborative care* (6th ed.). Philadelphia: Saunders.)

one-way valve, protecting patients from air returning to the pleural or pericardial space. The suction chamber may be a dry suction or calibrated water chamber. It is connected to external vacuum suction set to the amount of suction ordered and controls the amount of suction that patients experience.

The nurse needs to assess for blood clots and fibrin strands in tubes with sanguineous or serosanguineous drainage and ensure that there are no obstructions to drainage in the tube. Chest tube clearance is maintained per hospital policy. Milking or stripping of chest tubes is not recommended for chest tube clearance because of the high negative intrathoracic pressure that is created. However, some special circumstances, such as maintaining chest tube patency while a patient is bleeding, warrant chest tube clearance with these methods. The nurse needs to notify the health care provider immediately if chest tube obstruction is suspected. Generally chest tubes should not be clamped. However, it may be necessary to clamp a chest tube when exchanging the collection chamber or determining the site of an air leak (see Guidelines box).

ALTERNATIVE FEEDING TECHNIQUES

Some children are unable to take nourishment by mouth because of anomalies of the throat, esophagus, or bowel; impaired swallowing capacity; severe debilitation; respiratory distress; or unconsciousness. These children are frequently fed by way of a tube inserted orally or nasally into the stomach (*orogastric [OG]* or *nasogastric [NG] gavage*) or duodenum-jejunum (**enteral** *gavage*), or by a tube inserted directly into the stomach (*gastrostomy*) or jejunum (*jejunostomy*). Such feedings may be intermittent or by continuous drip.

Feeding resistance is a problem that may result from any long-term feeding method that bypasses the mouth. During gavage or gastrostomy feedings, infants can be given a pacifier for non-nutritive sucking, which has several advantages, including increased weight gain and decreased crying. However, to prevent the possibility of aspiration, only pacifiers with a safe design may be used (see Fig. 26-24).

NURSING ALERT

When a child is concurrently receiving continuous-drip gastric or enteral feedings and parenteral (IV) therapy, the potential exists for inadvertent administration of the enteral formula through the circulatory system, especially when the parenteral solution is a fat emulsion, which looks milky. Safeguards to prevent this potentially serious error include the following:

- Use a separate, specifically designed enteral feeding pump mounted on a separate pole for continuous-feeding solutions.
- Label all tubing for continuous enteral feeding with brightly coloured tape or labels.
- Use specifically designed continuous-feeding bags to contain the solutions instead of parenteral equipment, such as a burette.
- Whenever access or connections are made, trace the tubing all the way from the patient to the bag to ensure that the correct tubing source is selected.

GUIDELINES

Ongoing Patient and Chest Drainage System Assessment

- Determine drainage type (sanguineous, serosanguineous, serous, chylous, empyemic), colour, amount, and consistency. If there is a marked decrease in the amount of drainage, assess for drainage around chest tube insertion site.
- Dressing clean, dry, and intact?
- Chest tube sutures intact?
- Prescribed amount of suction applied?
- Water level is at 2 cm? If water column is too high, the flow of air from the chest may be impeded.
- Bubbling in water-seal chamber is normal if chest tube was placed to evacuate a pneumothorax. Bubbling will stop when the pneumothorax has resolved.
- Fluctuations may be seen in the water column because of changes in intrathoracic pressure. Substantial fluctuations may reflect changes in a patient's respiratory status.
- Note signs and symptoms of infection or skin breakdown.
- Palpate for presence of subcutaneous air.

Interventions

- Notify health care provider of any changes in the quantity or quality of drainage.
- If 3 mL/kg/hr or greater of sanguineous drainage occurs for 2 to 3 consecutive hours after cardiothoracic surgery, it may indicate active hemorrhaging and warrants immediate attention of the physician.
- Change dressing and perform site care as per hospital policy. Typically, an occlusive dressing is applied.
- When the collection chamber is almost full, exchange existing drainage system with a new one per manufacturer instructions using sterile technique.
- To lower the water column, depress the manual vent on the back of the unit until the water level reaches 2 cm. *Do not depress the filtered manual vent when the suction is not functioning or connected.*
- If evacuation of a pneumothorax was not the indication for placement of the chest tube, bubbling in the water-seal chamber may be the result of a leak in the chest drainage system. Identify the break in the system by briefly clamping the system between the drainage unit and the system; the bubbling will stop. Tighten any loose connections. If the air leak is suspected to be at the patient's chest wall, notify the health care provider.
- Encourage patient ambulation. Secure chest tube drainage system to prevent chest tube dislodgment from patient or disconnection from drainage system.

Gavage Feeding

Infants and children can be fed simply and safely by means of a tube passed into the stomach through either the nares or the mouth. The tube can be left in place or inserted and removed with each feeding. In older children it is usually less traumatic to tape the tube securely in place between feedings. When this alternative is used, the tube should be removed and replaced with a new tube according to hospital policy, specific orders, and the type of tube used. Meticulous hand hygiene should be practised during the procedure to prevent bacterial contamination of the feeding, especially during continuous-drip feedings (see Atraumatic Care box).

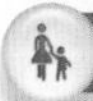

ATRAUMATIC CARE

Reducing the Distress of Nasogastric Tube Insertion

Numerous strategies can be used to decrease discomfort during nasogastric (NG) tube insertion. Most important, the nurse performing the procedure should be competent in NG tube placement. The nurse should discuss the procedure with the child in a developmentally appropriate way and give family members the details of what to expect during the procedure. A smaller-calibre, soft, flexible tube should be used. To prevent the trauma of reinsertion, make certain the NG tube is well secured after placement. Administration of sedation and analgesia should be considered before NG insertion.

Preparation

The equipment needed for gavage feeding includes the following:

- A suitable tube that is selected according to the child's size, viscosity of the solution being fed, and anticipated duration of these treatments.
- A receptacle for the fluid: for small amounts a 10- to 30-mL syringe barrel or Asepto syringe is satisfactory; for larger amounts a 60-mL syringe with a catheter tip is more convenient.
- A 10-mL syringe to aspirate stomach contents after the tube has been placed
- Water or water–soluble lubricant to lubricate the tube; sterile water is used for infants
- Paper or nonallergenic tape to mark the tube and attach the tube to the child's cheek (and nose if placed through the nares)
- pH paper to determine the correct placement in the stomach
- The solution for feeding

Not all feeding tubes are the same. Polyethylene and polyvinylchloride types lose their flexibility and need to be replaced frequently, usually every 3 or 4 days. Polyurethane and silicone tubes remain flexible; thus they can remain in place for up to 30 days. Advantages of small-bore tubes include a reduced incidence of pharyngitis, otitis media, aspiration, and discomfort. Disadvantages include difficulty during insertion (may require a stylet or metal guidewire), collapse of the tube during aspiration of gastric contents to test for correct placement, dislodgment during forceful coughing, migration out of position, knotting, occlusion, and unsuitability for thick feedings.

Procedure

It is easier to insert a feeding tube in an infant if they are first wrapped in a mummy restraint (Fig. 44-6, A). Even tiny infants with random movements can grasp and dislodge the tube. Preterm infants do not ordinarily require restraints, but if they do, a small blanket folded across the chest and secured beneath the shoulders is usually sufficient. Care should be taken so that breathing is not compromised.

Whenever possible, the infant should be held and provided with a means for non-nutritive sucking during the procedure to associate the comfort of physical contact with the feeding. When this is not possible, gavage feeding is carried out with the infant or child on the back or toward the right side and the head and chest elevated. Feeding the child in a sitting position helps to maintain placement of the tube in the lowest position, thus increasing the likelihood of correct placement in the stomach. The Guidelines box describes the procedure for gavage feeding.

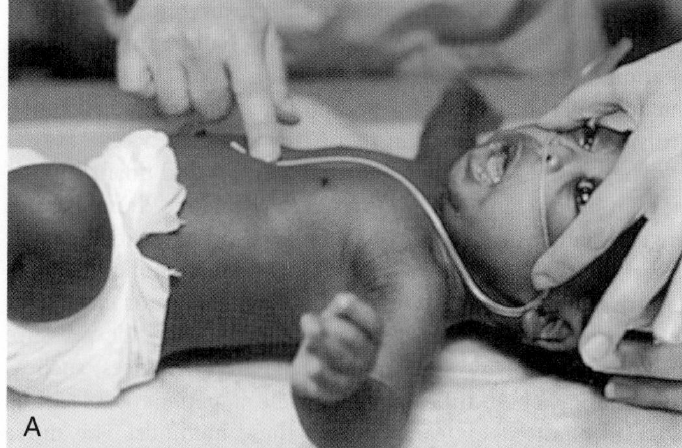

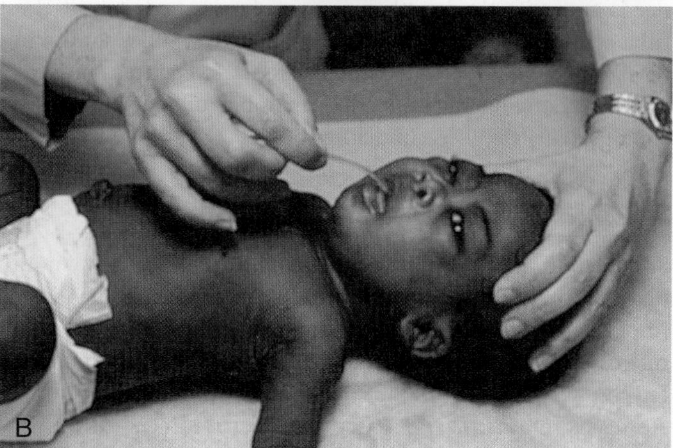

FIGURE 44-26 Gavage feeding. **A:** Measuring tube for orogastric feeding from tip of nose to earlobe and to midpoint between end of xiphoid process and umbilicus. **B:** Inserting tube.

Although the most accurate method for testing tube placement is radiography, this practice is not always possible before each feeding. In hospitalized children, there are often placement errors, particularly with children who are comatose, semiconscious, or inactive; have swallowing difficulties; or had Argyle tubes. Bedside assessment of gastrointestinal aspirate colour and pH is useful in predicting feeding tube placement. If doubt exists regarding correct placement, the practitioner should be consulted.

The morphological measure most commonly used by clinicians (i.e., nose–ear–xiphoid-distance) is often too short to reach the body of the stomach. Studies evaluating NG and OG tube length found that age-specific methods for predicting the distance based on height is the more accurate estimate of internal distance to the stomach (Beckstrand, Cirgin-Ellett, & McDaniel, 2007). However, the nose–ear–mid-ziphoid–umbilicus span is the next best measure for accuracy in lieu of the age-specific prediction equations (see Fig. 44-26, A and

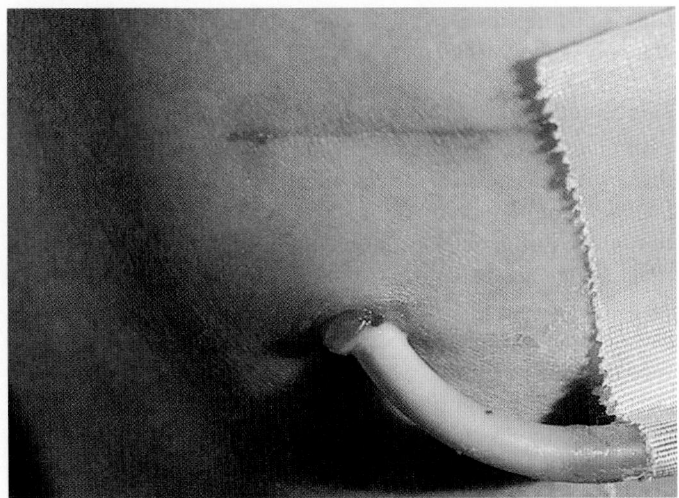

FIGURE 44-27 Appearance of healthy granulation tissue around stoma.

Guidelines box). For very low–birth-weight infants, daily weight can be used to predict insertion length.

Gastrostomy Feeding

Feeding by way of a gastrostomy, or G tube, is a variation of tube feeding that is often used for children in whom passage of a tube through the mouth, pharynx, esophagus, and cardiac sphincter of the stomach is contraindicated or impossible. It is also used to avoid the constant irritation of a gastric tube in children who require tube feeding over an extended period. Placement of a gastrostomy tube may be performed with the patient under general anaesthesia or percutaneously using an endoscope with the patient sedated and under local anaesthesia (percutaneous endoscopic gastrostomy [PEG]). The tube is inserted through the abdominal wall into the stomach about midway along the greater curvature and secured by a purse-string suture. The stomach is anchored to the peritoneum at the operative site. The tube used can be a Foley, wing-tip, or mushroom catheter. Immediately after surgery the catheter is left open and attached to gravity drainage for 24 hours or more.

Postoperative care of the wound site is directed toward prevention of infection and irritation. The area is cleansed at least daily or as often as needed to keep the area free of drainage. After healing takes place, meticulous care is needed to keep the area surrounding the tube clean and dry to prevent excoriation and infection. Daily applications of antibiotic ointment or other preparations may be prescribed to aid in healing and prevent irritation. It is important to prevent excessive pull on the catheter that might cause widening of the opening and subsequent leakage of highly irritating gastric juices. The tube is securely taped to the abdomen, leaving a small loop of tubing at the exit site to prevent tension on the site.

Granulation tissue may grow around a gastrostomy site (Fig. 44-27). This moist, beefy red tissue is not a sign of infection. However, if it continues to grow, the excess moisture can irritate the surrounding skin.

For children receiving long-term gastrostomy feeding, a skin-level device (e.g., MIC-KEY, Bard Button) offers several

GUIDELINES

Nasogastric Tube Feedings in Children

Place child supine with head slightly hyperflexed or in a sniffing position (nose pointed toward ceiling).

Measure the tube for approximate length of insertion, and mark the point with a small piece of tape.

Insert a tube that has been lubricated with sterile water or water-soluble lubricant through either the mouth or one of the nares to the predetermined mark. Because most young infants are obligatory nose breathers, insertion through the mouth causes less distress and helps to stimulate sucking. In older infants and children, the tube is passed through the nose and alternated between nostrils. An in-dwelling tube is almost always placed through the nose.

- When using the nose, slip the tube along the base of the nose and direct it straight back toward the occiput.
- When entering through the mouth, direct the tube toward the back of the throat (see Fig. 44-26, B).
- If the child is able to swallow on command, synchronize passing the tube with swallowing.
- Confirm placement by x-ray examination, if available. Document pH and colour of aspirate.

Stabilize tube by holding or taping it to the cheek, not to the forehead, because of possible damage to the nostril. To maintain correct placement, measure and record the amount of tubing extending from the nose or mouth to the distal port when the tube is first positioned. Recheck this measurement before each feeding.

Warm formula to room temperature. Do not heat it in the microwave! Document pH and colour of aspirate before each feeding to confirm tube placement. Pour formula into the barrel of the syringe attached to the feeding tube. To start the flow, give a gentle push with the plunger, but then remove the plunger and allow the fluid to flow into the stomach by gravity. The rate of flow should not exceed 5 mL every 5 to 10 minutes in preterm and very small infants and 10 mL/min in older infants and children to prevent nausea and regurgitation. The rate is determined by the diameter of the tubing and height of the reservoir containing the feeding and is regulated by adjusting the height of the syringe. A usual feeding may take 15 to 30 minutes to complete.

Flush tube with sterile water (1 or 2 mL for small tubes to 5 to 15 mL or more for large ones).

Cap or clamp in-dwelling tubes to prevent loss of feeding.

If the tube is to be removed, first pinch it firmly to prevent escape of fluid as the tube is withdrawn. Withdraw the tube quickly.

Position child with the head elevated 30 to 45 degrees or on the right side for 30 to 60 minutes in the same manner as after any infant feeding to minimize the possibility of regurgitation and aspiration. If the child's condition permits, burp the youngster after the feeding.

Record the feeding, including the type and amount of residual, the type and amount of formula, and how it was tolerated.

For most infant feedings, any amount of residual fluid aspirated from the stomach is refed to prevent electrolyte imbalance, and the amount is subtracted from the prescribed amount of feeding. For example, if the infant is to receive 30 mL and 10 mL is aspirated from the stomach before the feeding, the 10 mL of aspirated stomach contents is refed along with 20 mL of feeding. Another method can be used in children. If residual fluid is more than one fourth of the last feeding, return the aspirate and recheck in 30 to 60 minutes. When residual fluid is less than one fourth of the last feeding, give the scheduled feeding. If large amounts of aspirated fluid persist and the child is due for another feeding, notify the practitioner.

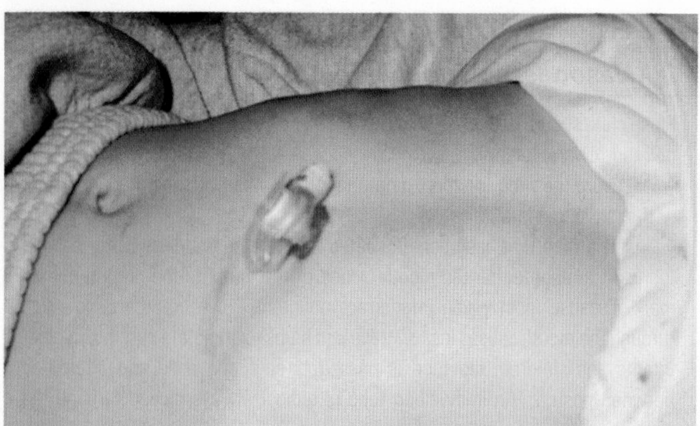

FIGURE 44-28 Child with skin-level gastrostomy device (MIC-KEY), which provides for secure attachment of extension tubing to gastrostomy opening.

advantages. The small, flexible silicone device protrudes slightly from the abdomen, is more cosmetically pleasing in appearance, affords increased comfort and mobility to the child, is easy to care for, and is fully immersible in water (Fig. 44-28). The one-way valve at the proximal end minimizes reflux and eliminates the need for clamping. However, the button requires a well-established gastrostomy site and is more expensive than the conventional tube. In addition, the valve may become clogged. When functioning, the valve prevents air from escaping; thus the child may require frequent burping. With some devices, during feedings the child must remain fairly still because the tubing easily disconnects from the opening if the child moves. With other devices, extension tubing can be securely attached to the opening. The feeding is instilled at the other end of the tubing in a manner similar to that for a regular gastrostomy. The extension tubing may also have a separate medication port. Both the feeding and the medication ports have plugs attached. Some skin-level devices require a special tube to decompress the stomach (to check residual or release air).

Feeding of water, formula, or pureed foods is carried out in the same manner and rate as in gavage feeding. A mechanical pump may be used to regulate the volume and rate of feeding. After feedings, the infant or child is positioned on the right side or in Fowler's position, and the tube may be clamped or left open and suspended between feedings, depending on the child's condition. A clamped tube allows more mobility but is appropriate only if the child can tolerate intermittent feedings without vomiting or prolonged backup of feeding into the tube. Sometimes a Y tube is used to allow for simultaneous decompression during feeding. If a Foley catheter is used as the gastrostomy tube, very slight tension is applied. The tube is securely taped to maintain the balloon at the gastrostomy opening to prevent leakage of gastric contents and to prevent the tube's progression toward the pyloric sphincter, where it may occlude the stomach outlet. As a precaution, the length of the tube should be measured postoperatively and then remeasured each shift to be certain it has not slipped. A mark can be made above the skin level to further ensure its placement. When the gastrostomy tube is no longer needed, it is removed; the skin opening usually closes spontaneously by contracture.

Nasoduodenal and Nasojejunal Tubes

Children at high risk for regurgitation or aspiration, such as those with gastroparesis, mechanical ventilation, or brain injuries, may require placement of a postpyloric feeding tube. Insertion of a nasoduodenal or nasojejunal tube is done by a trained practitioner because of the risk of misplacement and potential for perforation in tubes requiring a stylet. Accurate placement is verified by radiography. Small-bore tubes may easily clog. The tube needs to be flushed when feeding is interrupted, before and after medication administration, and routinely every 4 hours or as directed by institutional policy. Tube replacement should be considered monthly to ensure optimal tube patency. Continuous feedings are delivered by mechanical pump to regulate volume and rate. Bolus feeds are contraindicated. Tube displacement is suspected in the child showing signs of feeding intolerance, such as vomiting. Feedings should be stopped and the practitioner notified.

Total Parenteral Nutrition

TPN provides for the total nutritional needs of infants or children when feeding by the gastrointestinal tract is impossible, inadequate, or hazardous. Some common conditions associated with TPN include chronic intestinal obstruction, inadequate intestinal length, and prophylactically after surgery or during critical illness.

TPN therapy involves IV infusion of highly concentrated solutions of protein, glucose, and other nutrients. The solution is infused through conventional tubing with a special filter attached to remove particulate matter or microorganisms that may have contaminated the solution. The highly concentrated solutions require infusion into a vessel with sufficient volume and turbulence to allow for rapid dilution. The wide-diameter vessels selected are the superior vena cava and innominate or intrathoracic subclavian veins approached by way of the external or internal jugular veins. The highly irritating nature of concentrated glucose precludes the use of the small peripheral veins in most instances. However, dilute glucose-protein hydrolysates that are appropriate for infusing into peripheral veins are being used with increasing frequency. When peripheral veins are used, intralipid becomes the major calorie source. For long-term alimentation central venous catheters are usually used.

The major nursing responsibilities are the same as for any IV therapy: control of sepsis, monitoring of the infusion rate, and assessment of the patient's tolerance of the solution. The TPN solution must be prepared under sterile conditions. The infusion is maintained at a constant rate by an infusion pump to ensure the proper concentrations of glucose and amino acids. Accurate calculation of the rate is required to deliver a measured amount in a given length of time. Because alterations in flow rate are relatively common, the drip should be checked frequently to ensure an even, continuous infusion. The TPN infusion rate should not be increased or decreased without the practitioner being informed, since alterations can cause hyperglycemia or hypoglycemia.

General assessments, such as vital signs, I&O measurements, and laboratory tests, facilitate early detection of infection or fluid and electrolyte imbalance. Additional amounts of potassium and sodium chloride are often required in hyperalimentation; therefore, observation for signs of potassium or sodium deficit or excess is part of nursing care. This is rarely a problem except in children with reduced renal function or metabolic defects. Hyperglycemia may occur during the first day or two as the child adapts to the high-glucose load of the hyperalimentation solution. Although hyperglycemia occurs infrequently, insulin may be required to assist the body's adjustment. When this occurs, nursing responsibilities include blood glucose testing. To prevent hypoglycemia at the time the hyperalimentation is disconnected, the rate of the infusion and the amount of insulin are decreased gradually.

Family Teaching and Home Care

When alternative feedings are needed for an extended period, the family may need to learn how to feed the child with a nasogastric, gastrostomy, or TPN feeding regimen. Ample time must be allowed for the family to learn and perform the procedures under supervision before assuming full responsibility for the child's care at home (see Chapter 42 for further information on home care).

PROCEDURES RELATED TO ELIMINATION

Enema

The procedure for giving an enema to an infant or child does not differ essentially from that for an adult, except for the type and amount of fluid administered and the distance for inserting the tube into the rectum (see Guidelines box). Depending on the volume, a syringe with rubber tubing, an enema bottle, or an enema bag should be used.

An isotonic solution is used in children. Plain water is not used because, being hypotonic, it can cause rapid fluid shift and fluid overload. The Fleet enema (pediatric or adult sized) is not advised for children because of the harsh action of its ingredients (sodium biphosphate and sodium phosphate). Commercial enemas can be dangerous to patients with megacolon and to dehydrated or azotemic children. The osmotic effect of the Fleet enema may produce diarrhea, which can lead to metabolic acidosis. Other potential complications are extreme hyperphosphatemia, hypernatremia, and hypocalcemia, which may lead to neuromuscular irritability and coma.

Because infants and young children are unable to retain the solution after it is administered, the buttocks must be held together for a short time to retain the fluid. The enema is administered and expelled while the child is lying with the buttocks over the bedpan and with the head and back supported by pillows. Older children are usually able to hold the solution if they understand what to do and if they are not expected to hold it for too long. The nurse should have the bedpan handy or, for the ambulatory child, ensure that the bathroom is available before beginning the procedure. An enema is an intrusive procedure and thus threatening to the preschool child; a careful explanation is especially important to ease possible fear.

A preoperative bowel preparation solution given orally or through a nasogastric tube is increasingly being used instead of an enema. The polyethylene glycol–electrolyte lavage solution (GoLYTELY) mechanically flushes the bowel without significant absorption, thereby avoiding potential fluid and electrolyte imbalance. NuLYTELY, a newer form of GoLYTELY, has the same therapeutic effect but tastes better. Magnesium citrate solution is another effective cathartic.

GUIDELINES

Administration of Enemas to Children

Age	Amount (mL)	Insertion Distance
Infant	120–240	2.5 cm
2–4 yr	240–360	5 cm
4–10 yr	360–480	7.5 cm
11+ yr	480–720	10 cm

Ostomies

Children may require stomas for various health problems. The most frequent causes in infants are necrotizing enterocolitis, imperforate anus, and, less often, Hirschsprung disease. In older children the most frequent causes are inflammatory bowel disease, especially Crohn's disease (regional enteritis), and ureterostomies for distal ureter or bladder defects.

Care and management of ostomies in the older child differ little from the care of ostomies in the adult patient. The major emphases in pediatric care are preparing the child for the procedure and teaching care of the ostomy to the child and family. The basic principles of preparation are the same as for any procedure (see Guidelines on p. 1283). Simple, straightforward language is most effective, together with the use of illustrations and a replica model, such as drawing a picture of a child with a stoma on the abdomen and explaining it as "another opening where bowel movements [or any other term the child uses] will come out." At another time the nurse can draw a pouch over the opening to demonstrate how the contents are collected. Using a doll to demonstrate the process is an excellent teaching strategy, and special books are available.

Children with ileostomies are fitted immediately after surgery with an appliance to protect the skin from the proteolytic enzymes in the liquid stool. Infants may not be fitted with a pouch in the immediate postoperative period. When stomal drainage is minimal, a gauze dressing will suffice. Parents are usually given a choice of caring for the colostomy with or without an appliance. Pediatric appliances are available in a variety of sizes to ensure an adequate fit.

Ostomy equipment consists of a one- or two-piece system with a hypoallergenic skin barrier to maintain peristomal skin integrity. The pouch should be large enough to contain a moderate amount of stool and flatus but not so large as to overwhelm the infant or child. A backing helps minimize the risk of skin breakdown from moisture trapped between the skin and pouch. Small clips or rubber bands should be avoided to prevent choking in the young child.

Protection of the peristomal skin is a major aspect of stoma care. Well-fitting appliances are important to prevent leakage of contents. Before the appliance is applied, the skin is prepared with a skin sealant that is allowed to dry. Stoma paste may also be applied around the base of the stoma or the back of the wafer. The sealant and paste work together to prevent peristomal breakdown.

In infants with a colostomy left unpouched, skin care is similar to that of any diapered infant. However, the peristomal skin is protected with a wafer barrier, such as a hydrocolloid dressing (e.g., DuoDERM) or a barrier substance (e.g., zinc oxide ointment [Desitin], or a mixture of the zinc oxide ointment and stoma [Stomahesive] powder). A diaper larger than the one usually worn may be needed to extend upward over the stoma and absorb drainage. If the skin becomes inflamed, denuded, or infected, the care is similar to the interventions used for diaper dermatitis (see Chapter 52). A zinc-based product helps protect healthy skin, heal excoriated skin, and minimize pain associated with skin breakdown. The skin protectant adheres to denuded, weeping skin. The nurse can apply zinc-based products over topical antifungal and antibacterial agents if infection is present. No-sting barrier film is a skin sealant that has no alcohol base and can be used on open skin without stinging. Preventing young children from pulling off the pouch is also an important consideration. One-piece outfits keep exploring hands from reaching the pouch, and the loose waist prevents any pressure on the appliance. Keeping the child occupied with toys during the pouch change is also helpful. As children mature, their participation in ostomy care should be encouraged. Even preschoolers can assist by holding supplies, pulling paper backings from the appliance, and helping clean the stoma area. Toilet training for bladder control needs to begin at the appropriate time as for any other child.

Older children and adolescents should eventually have total responsibility for ostomy care, just as they would for usual bowel function. Adolescents may have concerns about body image and the ostomy's impact on intimacy and sexuality. The nurse should stress to teenagers that the presence of a stoma need not interfere with their activities. These youngsters can choose which ostomy equipment is best suited to their needs. Attractively designed and decorated pouch covers are well liked by teenagers.

Children with familial adenomatous polyposis may require a colectomy with ileoanal reservoir to prevent or treat carcinoma of the colon. Peristomal skin care for these children is particularly challenging because of increased liquid stools, increased digestive enzymes that may cause skin breakdown, and the stoma being at skin level rather than raised. Additional care with this condition includes close monitoring of fluid and electrolyte status and increased incidence of bowel obstruction.

An enterostomal therapy nurse specialist is an important member of the health care team and will have additional suggestions and skin care information and ostomy pouching options. Further information may be obtained by contacting the Wound, Ostomy and Continence Nurses Society (see Additional Resources at the end of this chapter).

Family Teaching and Home Care

Because these children are almost always discharged with a functioning ostomy, preparation of the family should begin as early as possible in the hospital. The family needs to be instructed in the application of the device (if used), care of the skin, and appropriate action in case skin problems develop. Early evidence of skin breakdown or stomal complications, such as ribbonlike stools, excessive diarrhea, bleeding, prolapse, or failure to pass flatus or stool, should be brought to the attention of the physician, the nurse, or the stoma specialist. The same principles are applied for discharge planning and home care (see Chapter 43).

KEY POINTS

- Before undergoing any invasive procedure, the patient (if old enough to comprehend) and the patient's legal surrogate must receive sufficient information on which to make an informed health care decision (informed consent). In Canada there is no age of consent, except for Québec, where it is 14 years.
- Informed consent is needed for major surgery, minor surgery, and diagnostic tests and medical treatments with an element of risk.
- The major principles in psychological preparation of the child for procedures are to establish trust, provide support, and give an explanation in easy-to-understand terms.
- Preparation for procedures should be based on developmental characteristics of the child and knowledge of the family, emphasizing the importance of the parents' role.
- Most parents and children want to be together during stressful procedures and should be offered this opportunity, with guidance on how the parent can comfort the child.
- The use of play activities to provide teaching about necessary nursing and medical interventions is an effective tool for use with children.
- In performing a procedure, the nurse should expect success, involve the child when possible in the procedure, provide distraction, and allow for expression of feelings.
- Proper positioning of infants and small children for procedures is essential to minimize movement and discomfort.
- In giving postprocedural support, the nurse should encourage children to express feelings and should give praise for completion of the procedure.
- Stressful times before and after surgery that produce anxiety in children are admission, blood tests, injection of preoperative medication (if used), transportation to the operating room, and return from the PACU.

- Knowledge of the ill child's eating habits and favourite foods can help in maintaining adequate nutrition.
- Skin care is essential to prevent skin breakdown.
- Control of fever may be accomplished by administration of antipyretics; hyperthermia is controlled by environmental means (minimum clothing, increased air circulation, hypothermia mattress, or cool compresses).
- Infection control is based on two systems. Routine practices provide protection when the infected person is undiagnosed. Additional precautions add extra interventions for patients diagnosed with or suspected of having an infection.
- Ensuring safety in the hospital setting is a major concern and can be achieved through environmental measures, limit setting, infection control, and safe transportation.
- Restraints should be used cautiously and require a medical order. Use of therapeutic holding can avoid the use of restraints.
- Factors that affect medication dosage determination are growth and maturation, difficulty in evaluating a medication response, and BSA.
- Family teaching regarding medication administration includes telling parents why the child is receiving the medication; its possible effects; and the amount, frequency, and length of time it is to be administered.
- The preferred sites for intramuscular injection in children are the vastus lateralis and ventrogluteal areas.
- Intermittent venous access is accomplished by means of a peripheral intermittent infusion device, a peripherally inserted central catheter, a central venous catheter, or an implanted port.
- Several safety catheters and needleless device systems are available to reduce the risk of needlestick injuries in patients and caregivers.
- Nursing assessment of fluid and electrolyte disturbances entails observation of general appearance, vital signs, and measurement of I&O.
- Oxygen can be administered by hood, mask, nasal cannula, or incubator.
- Tracheostomy suctioning involves premeasured insertion of the catheter, application of suction for 5 seconds when withdrawing the catheter, and supplemental oxygen before and after suctioning.
- Alternative forms of feeding include gavage feeding, gastrostomy feeding, and TPN.
- In the care of children with ostomies, nurses play an important role in family support and instruction in care of the stoma site.

evolve WEBSITE

Visit the Evolve website for additional resources related to the content in this chapter such as Case Studies, Critical Thinking Case Study Answers, Nursing Care Plans, Nursing Processes, Nursing Skills, and Review Questions for Exam Preparation at: http://evolve.elsevier.com/Canada/Perry/maternal/

REFERENCES

American Heart Association. (2015). CPR and ECG guidelines. *Circulation, 132*(18 Suppl. 2), S313–S314. doi:10.1161/CIR.0000000000000307. Retrieved from <https://eccguidelines.heart.org/index.php/circulation/cpr-ecc-guidelines-2/>.

Anderson, D. M., Pesaturo, K. A., Casavant, J., et al. (2013). Alteplase for the treatment of catheter occlusion in pediatric patients. *Annals of Pharmacotherapy, 47*(3), 405–409. doi:10.1345/aph.1Q483.

Beckstrand, J., Cirgin-Ellett, M. L., & McDaniel, A. (2007). Predicting internal distance to the stomach for positioning nasogastric and orogastric feeding tubes in children. *Journal of Advanced Nursing, 59*(3), 274–289.

Brady, M. C., Kinn, S., Ness, V., et al. (2009). Preoperative fasting for preventing perioperative complications in children. *Cochrane Database Systemic Review*, (4), CD005285, doi:10.1002/14651858.CD005285.pub2.

Canadian Medical Protective Association. (2006). *Consent: A guide for Canadian physicians*. Retrieved from <https://www.cmpa-acpm.ca/en/handbooks/-/asset_publisher/TayXf91AzWR2/content/consent-a-guide-for-canadian-physicians>.

Canadian Paediatric Society. (2013a). *Fever and temperature taking*. Retrieved from <http://www.caringforkids.cps.ca/handouts/fever_and_temperature_taking>.

Canadian Paediatric Society. (2013b). *Febrile seizures*. Retrieved from <http://www.caringforkids.cps.ca/handouts/febrile_seizures>.

College of Nurses of Ontario. (2009). *Practice standard: Restraints*. Retrieved from <http://www.cno.org/globalassets/docs/prac/41043_restraints.pdf>.

Considine, J., & Brennan, D. (2007). Effect of an evidence-based education programme on ED discharge advice for febrile children. *Journal of Clinical Nursing, 16*, 1687–1694.

Cox, R. G., Nemish, U., Ewen, A., et al. (2006). Evidence-based clinical update: Does premedication with oral midazolam lead to improved behavioural outcomes in children? *Canadian Journal of Anaesthesia, 53*(12), 1213–1219.

Curley, M. A., Razmus, I. S., Roberts, K. E., et al. (2003). Predicting pressure ulcer risk in pediatric patients: The Braden Q scale. *Nursing Research, 52*, 22–33.

Fernandez, C., & Canadian Paediatric Society, Bioethics Committee. (2008). Ethical issues in health research in children. *Paediatrics & Child Health, 13*(8), 707–712. Reaffirmed 2016. Retrieved from <http://www.cps.ca/documents/position/ethical-issues-in-health-research-in-children#authors>.

Gravel, D., Matlow, A., Ofner-Agostini, M., et al. (2007). A point prevalence survey of health care–associated infections in pediatric populations in major Canadian acute care hospitals. *American Journal of Infection Control, 35*, 157–162.

Harrison, C., & Canadian Paediatric Society, Bioethics Committee. (2004). Treatment decisions regarding infants, children, and adolescents. *Paediatrics & Child Health, 9*(2), 99–103. Reaffirmed 2016. Retrieved from <http://www.cps.ca/documents/position/treatment-decisions>.

Health Canada. (2003/2013). *Update: Risk of strangulation of infants by IV tubing and monitor leads–Notice to hospitals*. Retrieved from <http://

www.healthycanadians.gc.ca/recall-alert-rappel-avis/hc-sc/2003/14222a-eng.php?_ga=1.157110066.868197850.1432519476>.

Infusion Nurses Society. (2016). *Infusion therapy standards of practice* (5th ed.). Norwood, MA: Author.

Junqueira, A. L., Tavares, V. R., Martins, R. M., et al. (2010). Safety and immunogenicity of hepatitis B vaccine administered into ventrogluteal vs. anterolateral thigh sites in infants: A randomized controlled trial. *International Journal Nursing Studies, 47*(9), 1074–1079.

Kaasalainen, S. (2014). Medication administration. In P. A. Potter, A. Griffin Perry, P. A. Stockert, et al. (Eds.), *Canadian fundamentals of nursing* (5th ed.). St. Louis: Elsevier.

Khair, A. M., & Elmagrabi, D. (2015). Febrile seizures and febrile seizure syndromes: An updated overview of old and current knowledge. *Neurology Research International*, 849341. doi:10.1155/2015/849341.

López-Briz, E., Ruiz Garcia, V., Cabello, J. B., et al. (2014). Heparin versus 0.9% sodium chloride intermittent flushing for prevention of occlusion in central venous catheters in adults. *The Cochrane Database of Systematic Reviews*, (10), CD008462, doi:10.1002/14651858.CD008462.pub2.

Maki, D. (2014). Stethoscopes and health care–associated infection. *Mayo Clinic Proceeding, 89*(3), 277–280. doi:10.1016/j.mayocp.2014.01.014.

Manyande, A., Cyna, A. M., Yip, P., et al. (2015). Non-pharmacological interventions for assisting the induction of anaesthesia in children. *The Cochrane Database of Systematic Reviews*, (7), CD006447, doi:10.1002/14651858.CD006447.pub3.

Matziou, V., Chrysostomou, A., Vlahioti, E., et al. (2013). Parental presence and distraction during painful childhood procedures. *British Journal of Nursing, 22*(8), 470–475.

Noonan, C., Quigley, S., & Curley, M. A. (2006). Skin integrity in hospitalized infants and children: A prevalence survey. *Journal of Pediatric Nursing, 21*(6), 445–453.

Public Health Agency of Canada. (2013a). *Healthcare-associated infections—Due diligence*. Retrieved from <http://www.phac-aspc.gc.ca/cphorsphc-respcacsp/2013/infections-eng.php>.

Public Health Agency of Canada. (2013b). *Hand and hygiene practices in healthcare settings*. Retrieved from <http://www.ipac-canada.org/pdf/2013_PHAC_Hand%20Hygiene-EN.pdf>.

Purssell, E. (2009). Parental fever phobia and its evolutionary correlates. *Journal of Clinical Nursing, 18*, 210–218.

Registered Nurses' Association of Ontario. (2011). *Risk assessment and prevention of pressure ulcers*. Retrieved from <http://rnao.ca/bpg/guidelines/risk-assessment-and-prevention-pressure-ulcers>.

Robinson, J. L., Finlay, J. C., Lang, M. E., et al. (2014). Urinary tract infection in infants and children: Diagnosis and management. *Paediatrics & Child Health, 19*(6), 315–319.

Shapiro, C. (2014). Legal implications in nursing practice. In P. A. Potter, A. Griffin Perry, P. A. Stockert, et al. (Eds.), *Canadian fundamentals of nursing* (5th ed.). St. Louis: Elsevier.

Sneiderman, B., Irvine, J. C., & Osborne, P. H. (2003). *Canadian medical law: An introduction for physicians, nurses, and other health care professionals*. Scarborough, ON: Thomson/Carswell.

Strom, S. (2012). Preoperative evaluation, premedication, and induction of anesthesia in infants and children. *Current Opinion in Anesthesiology, 25*(3), 321–325. doi:10.1097/ACO.0b013e3283530e0d.

Taylor, C., Subaiya, L., & Corsino, D. (2011). Pediatric cuffed endotracheal tubes: An evolution of care. *The Ochsner Journal, 11*(1), 52–56.

Uman, L. S., Birnie, K. A., Noel, M., et al. (2013). Psychological interventions for needle-related procedural pain and distress in children and adolescents. *The Cochrane Database of Systematic Reviews*, (10), CD005179, doi:10.1002/14651858.CD005179.pub3.

Wetzel, R. C. (2016). Anesthesia, perioperative care, and sedation. In R. M. Kliegman, B. F. Stanton, J. St. Geme, et al. (Eds.), *Nelson textbook of pediatrics* (20th ed.). Philadelphia: Saunders.

Willock, J., Baharestani, M., & Anthony, D. (2009). The development of the Glamorgan paediatric pressure ulcer risk assessment scale. *Journal of Wound Care, 18*(1), 17–21.

ADDITIONAL RESOURCES

Body surface area calculator for medication dosages: <http://www.halls.md/body-surface-area/bsa.htm>.

Braden Q Scale—Modified Braden Q Scale (for pediatric use): <http://nursing.advanceweb.com/SharedResources/Downloads/2007/090107/NW/nng090107_p55table1.pdf>.

<http://www.marthaaqcurley.com/uploads/8/9/8/6/8986925/braden_q_scale.pdf>.

Canadian Association of Enterostomal Nurses: <https://caet.ca/>.

Canadian Paediatric Society—Preventing Choking and Suffocation in Children: <http://www.childrenssafetynetwork.org/news/preventing-choking-and-suffocation-children-canadian-paediatric-society>.

Registered Nurses' Association of Ontario—Best Practice Guideline: Risk Assessment and Prevention of Pressure Ulcers: <http://rnao.ca/bpg/guidelines/risk-assessment-and-prevention-pressure-ulcers>.

Registered Nurses' Association of Ontario—Best Practice Guideline: Assessment and Management of Stage I to IV Pressure ulcer: <http://rnao.ca/sites/rnao-ca/files/Assessment__Management_of_Stage_I_to_IV_Pressure_Ulcers.pdf>.

The Hospital for Sick Kids—Pre-Operative Preparation Program: <http://www.sickkids.ca/VisitingSickKids/Coming-for-surgery/Pre-Operative-Preparation-Program/index.html>.

Tri-Council Policy Statement—Ethical Conduct for Research Involving Humans: <http://www.pre.ethics.gc.ca/pdf/eng/tcps2/TCPS_2_FINAL_Web.pdf>.

UNIT 12

Health Problems of Children

CHAPTER

45

Respiratory Dysfunction

Cheryl Sams

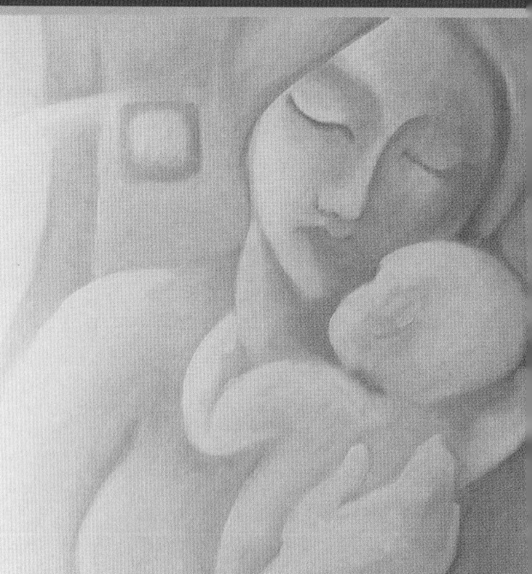

evolve WEBSITE

Visit the Evolve website for additional resources related to the content in this chapter such as Case Studies, Critical Thinking Case Study Answers, Nursing Care Plans, Nursing Processes, Nursing Skills, and Review Questions for Exam Preparation at: *http://evolve.elsevier.com/Canada/Perry/maternal/*

OBJECTIVES

On completion of this chapter the reader will be able to:

- Identify the factors leading to respiratory tract infection in the infant and young child.
- Contrast the effects of various respiratory infections observed in infants and children.
- Describe the postoperative nursing care of the child with an adenotonsillectomy.
- Outline the nursing care for a child with croup.
- Outline the nursing care for a child with acute otitis media.
- Demonstrate an understanding of the ways in which inhalation of noninfectious irritants produce pulmonary dysfunction.
- Describe the ways in which the various therapeutic measures relieve the symptoms of asthma.
- Outline a plan for teaching home care for the child with asthma.
- Describe the physiological effects of cystic fibrosis on the gastrointestinal, endocrine, reproductive, and pulmonary systems.
- Outline a plan of care for the child with cystic fibrosis.
- Describe congenital respiratory disorders and the appropriate nursing care.
- List the major signs of respiratory distress in infants and children.
- Describe the nursing care for a child with respiratory failure.

RESPIRATORY INFECTION

General Aspects of Respiratory Infections

Infections of the respiratory tract are described according to the anatomical area of involvement. The *upper respiratory tract*, or *upper airway*, consists of the oronasopharynx, pharynx, larynx, and upper part of the trachea. The *lower respiratory tract* consists of the lower trachea, mainstem bronchi, segmental bronchi, subsegmental bronchioles, terminal bronchioles, and alveoli. In this discussion, the trachea is considered with lower tract disorders, and infections of the epiglottis and larynx are categorized as croup syndromes. However, respiratory infections seldom fall into discrete anatomical areas. Infections often spread from one structure to another because of the adjoining nature of the mucous membrane lining the entire tract. Consequently, respiratory tract infections involve several areas, although the effect on one area may predominate in any given illness.

Etiology and Characteristics

Respiratory infections account for the majority of acute illnesses in children. The etiology and course of these infections are influenced by the age of the child, the season, living conditions, and pre-existing medical problems.

Infectious agents. The respiratory tract is subject to a wide variety of infective organisms. Most infections are caused by viruses, particularly respiratory syncytial virus (RSV), nonpolio enteroviruses A, B, C, and D (formerly coxsackieviruses A and B), adenoviruses, parainfluenza viruses, and human metapneumoviruses. Other agents involved in primary or secondary invasion include group A beta-hemolytic streptococci (GABHS), staphylococci, *Haemophilus influenzae*, *Chlamydia trachomatis*, *Mycoplasma* organisms, and pneumococci.

Age. Healthy full-term infants younger than 3 months of age are presumed to have a lower infection rate than that of older children, because of the protective function of maternal antibodies. However, infants may be susceptible to specific respiratory tract infections, namely pertussis, during this period. The Canadian Paediatric Society (CPS) (2016) states it is not unusual for children to get as many as 8 to 10 colds each year before they turn 2 years of age. The infection rate increases between 3 and 6 months of age, the time between the disappearance of maternal antibodies and before the infant's own antibody production matures. The viral infection rate remains high during the toddler and preschool years. By 5 years of age, viral respiratory infections are less frequent, but the incidence of *Mycoplasma pneumoniae* and GABHS infections increases. The amount of lymphoid tissue increases through middle childhood, and repeated exposures to organisms increase the level of immunity as a child grows older.

Some viral or bacterial agents produce a mild illness in older children but severe lower respiratory tract illness or croup in infants. For example, pertussis causes a relatively harmless tracheobronchitis in childhood but is a serious disease in infancy.

Size. Anatomical differences influence the response to respiratory tract infections. The diameter of the airways is smaller in young children and subject to considerable narrowing from edematous mucous membranes and increased production of secretions. The distance between structures within the respiratory tract is also shorter in the young child, and organisms may move rapidly down the respiratory tract, causing more extensive involvement. The relatively short and open eustachian tube in infants and young children allows pathogens easy access to the middle ear.

Resistance. The ability to resist invading organisms depends on several factors. Children who are breastfed have increased resistance to infections. Deficiencies of the immune system place the child at risk for infection. Other conditions that decrease resistance are malnutrition, anemia, and fatigue. Conditions that weaken defences of the respiratory tract and predispose children to infection include allergies (e.g., allergic rhinitis), preterm birth, bronchopulmonary dysplasia (BPD), asthma, history of RSV infection, cardiac anomalies that cause pulmonary congestion, and cystic fibrosis (CF). Day care attendance and exposure to secondhand smoke also increases the likelihood of infection.

Seasonal variations. The most common respiratory pathogens appear in epidemics during the winter and spring months. Mycoplasmal infections occur more often in autumn and early winter. Infection-related asthma (e.g., asthmatic bronchitis) occurs more frequently during cold weather, whereas winter and spring are typically the "RSV seasons."

Clinical Manifestations

Infants and young children, especially those between 6 months and 3 years of age, react more severely to acute respiratory tract infection than older children. Young children display a number of generalized signs and symptoms and local manifestations (Box 45-1).

NURSING CARE

Assessment of the respiratory system follows the guidelines described in Chapter 33 (for assessment of the ear, nose, mouth and throat, chest, and lungs). The assessment should include respiratory rate, depth, and rhythm; heart rate; oxygenation; hydration status; body temperature; activity level; and level of comfort. Special attention should also be given to the components and observations listed in Box 45-2. A noninvasive pulse oximeter (oxygen saturation) measurement should be performed on all children as part of the routine physical assessment. The nursing process in the case of the child with acute respiratory tract infection is outlined in the Nursing Care Plan on the Evolve site.

Ease Respiratory Efforts

Many acute respiratory infections are mild and cause few symptoms. Although children may feel uncomfortable and have a "stuffy" nose (congestion) and some mucosal swelling, respiratory distress occurs infrequently. Interventions delivered at home are usually sufficient to relieve minor discomfort and ease respiratory efforts. However, in some cases, the infant or child may require close observation by health care providers for adequate oxygenation and fluid and electrolyte status.

Warm or cool mist is a common therapeutic measure for symptomatic relief of respiratory discomfort. The moisture soothes inflamed membranes and is beneficial when there is hoarseness or laryngeal involvement. However, the use of hot steam vaporizers in the home is not recommended because of burn hazard and limited evidence to support their efficacy. As well, cool-mist vaporizers are not recommended because of the hazard of contamination from mould and bacteria unless disinfected daily.

A time-honoured method of producing warm steam is the shower. Running a shower of hot water into the empty bathtub or open shower stall with the bathroom door closed produces a quick source of steam. Keeping a child in this environment for 10 to 15 minutes humidifies inspired air and can help relieve the symptoms. A small child can be held on the parent's lap. Older children can sit in the bathroom under the supervision of an adult. Maintaining a calming environment will assist in preventing increased respiratory efforts related to emotional distress of the child.

Promote Rest

Children who have an acute febrile illness usually have limited activity. One of the cardinal signs that the child is feeling better is the increase in activity; this may, however, be temporary if a high fever returns after a few hours of increased activity. Children should be encouraged to rest or play quietly to avoid exacerbating symptoms.

Promote Comfort

Older children are usually able to manage nasal secretions with little difficulty. For very young infants, who normally breathe through their noses, an infant nasal aspirator or a bulb syringe is helpful in removing nasal secretions, especially before being

BOX 45-1 SIGNS AND SYMPTOMS ASSOCIATED WITH RESPIRATORY INFECTIONS IN INFANTS AND SMALL CHILDREN

Fever

May be absent in newborn infants
Greatest at ages 6 months to 3 years
Temperature may reach 39.5° to 40.5°C even with mild infections
Often appears as first sign of infection
Child may be listless and irritable or somewhat euphoric and more active than normal temporarily; some children talk with unaccustomed rapidity
Tendency to develop high temperatures with infection in certain families
May precipitate febrile seizures (see Chapter 50)
Febrile seizures uncommon after 3 or 4 years of age

Meningismus

Meningeal signs without infection of the meninges
Occurs with abrupt onset of fever
Accompanied by the following:

- Headache
- Pain and stiffness in the back and neck
- Presence of Kernig and Brudzinski signs

Subsides as the temperature decreases

Anorexia

Common with most childhood illnesses
Frequently the initial evidence of illness
Persists to a greater or lesser degree throughout febrile stage of illness; often extends into convalescence

Vomiting

Small children vomit readily with illness
Clue to onset of infection
May precede other signs by several hours
Usually short-lived but may persist during the illness
Frequent cause of dehydration if fluid intake is impaired

Diarrhea

Usually mild, transient diarrhea but may become severe
Often accompanies viral respiratory infections
Frequent cause of dehydration

Abdominal Pain

Common symptom
Sometimes indistinguishable from pain of appendicitis
Mesenteric lymphadenitis may be cause
Muscle spasms from vomiting may be a factor, especially in nervous, tense child

Nasal Blockage

Small nasal passages of infants easily blocked by mucosal swelling and exudation
Can interfere with respiration and feeding in infants
May contribute to the development of otitis media and sinusitis

Nasal Discharge

Frequent occurrence
May be thin and watery (rhinorrhea) or thick and purulent
Depends on the type or stage of infection
Associated with itching
May irritate upper lip and skin surrounding the nose

Cough

Common feature can be either congested in nature or a dry hacky consistency
May be evident only during acute phase
May persist several months after a disease

Respiratory Sounds

Sounds associated with respiratory disease:

- Cough
- Hoarseness
- Grunting
- Stridor
- Wheezing

Auscultation:

- Wheezing
- Crackles
- Absence of air movement

Sore Throat

Frequent symptom of older children
Young children (unable to describe symptoms) may not complain even when highly inflamed
Child will often refuse to take oral fluids or solids

put to bed to sleep and before feeding. This practice, preceded by instillation of saline nose drops as needed, may clear nasal passages and promote feeding. Saline nose drops can be prepared at home by dissolving 5 mL of salt in 1 L of warm water. Bottles of nose drops should be used for only one child and one illness because they are easily contaminated with bacteria. Medicated nose drops or sprays, oral decongestants, cough medication, or other cold products should not be administered to children under 6 years of age except after discussion with the health care provider. These medications should also not be given in the over-6 age group if individuals are on other medications or have a chronic illness without a discussion with the primary practitioner. Medicated nose drops or sprays provide only short-lived relief and should not be used for more than 2 to 3 days because they can worsen congestion with a rebound effect. None of the medicated respiratory over-the-counter (OTC) products have evidence that they are effective in children and can have detrimental effects or interact with other drugs. Natural products should not be given to children for any reason because of the lack of research supporting pediatric efficacy (CPS, 2016).

Hot or cold applications sometimes provide relief for children with painful cervical adenitis. An ice pack or heating pad applied to the neck may decrease the discomfort, but safety

BOX 45-2 COMPONENTS FOR ASSESSING RESPIRATORY FUNCTION

Respirations

The pattern of respirations is observed for rate, depth, ease, and rhythm of breathing:

Rate—Rapid (*tachypnea*), normal, or slow (bradypnea) for the particular child

Depth—Normal depth, too shallow (*hypopnea*), too deep (*hyperpnea*); usually estimated from the amplitude of thoracic and abdominal excursion

Ease—Effortless; laboured (*dyspnea*); *orthopnea* (difficult breathing except in upright position); associated with intercostal or substernal retractions (inspiratory "sinking in" of soft tissues in relation to the cartilaginous and bony thorax); nasal flaring; head bobbing (head of sleeping child with suboccipital area supported on caregiver's forearm bobs forward in synchrony with each inspiration); grunting; or wheezing

Laboured breathing—Continuous, intermittent, becoming steadily worse, sudden onset, at rest or on exertion, associated with wheezing or grunting, can be associated with pain

Rhythm—Variation in rate and depth of respirations

Other Observations

In addition to respirations, particular attention is addressed to the following:

Evidence of infection—Check for elevated temperature; enlarged cervical lymph nodes; inflamed mucous membranes; and purulent discharges from the nose, ears, or lungs (sputum).

Cough—Observe characteristics of cough (if present): under what circumstances cough is heard (e.g., night only, on arising), nature of cough (paroxysmal with or without wheeze, "barking like a seal" or "brassy"), frequency of cough, associated with swallowing or other activity, character of cough (moist or dry), and productivity.

Wheeze—Note if expiratory or inspiratory, high-pitched or musical, prolonged, slowly progressive or sudden, or associated with laboured breathing.

Cyanosis—Note distribution (peripheral, circumoral, facial, trunk, and face), degree, duration, and whether associated with activity or feeding (infant).

Abdominal pain—May be a symptom in preschooler and school-age children; it probably represents referred pain from the chest; it may be a symptom in children with pneumonia.

Chest pain—May be a symptom of older children; note location and circumstances: localized or generalized, referred to base of neck or abdomen, dull or sharp, deep or superficial, associated with rapid, shallow respirations or grunting.

Sputum—Older children may provide a sputum sample by coughing, whereas young children may need bulb suction to provide a sample; note volume, colour, viscosity, and odour.

Bad breath—May be associated with some lung infections.

Stridor—A high-pitched wheezing sound; it may be present on inspiration, exhalation or both and is a sign of upper airway edema or obstruction by mass or object.

precautions must be observed to prevent burns and frostbite. The ice bag or heating device must be covered, and the heating pad should not be set at high settings.

Reduce the Spread of Infection

Careful hand hygiene is important when caring for children with respiratory tract infections. Children and families should be taught to cough or sneeze into their arm (Public Health Agency of Canada [PHAC], 2016a), dispose of tissues properly, and wash their hands. Remembering to cover the nose or mouth is often difficult for toddlers; they should be encouraged to wash their hands frequently to prevent the spread of infection. Used tissues should be thrown into the wastebasket immediately, and tissues should not be allowed to accumulate in a pile. Children with respiratory infections should not share drinking cups, utensils, washcloths, or towels. Unaffected individuals generally should not touch their eyes or nose with unwashed hands. Parents should try to remove affected children from contact with other children. This may be a problem when living arrangements are crowded and the family has several children. An effort should be made to teach well children to stay away from ill children, to wash their hands frequently, and to avoid eating and drinking using the same utensils or cups. Parents should also keep affected children out of school and day care settings to prevent the spread of infection.

Reduce Temperature

If the child has a significantly elevated body temperature, controlling the fever is important. Parents need to know how to take a child's temperature and read the thermometer accurately. Nurses should not assume that all parents can read a thermometer and should provide education when needed.

If the health care provider prescribes acetaminophen or ibuprofen, parents may need instruction on how to administer the medication. Most parents can read the label and calculate the desired dose, but parents of infants and toddlers require detailed instruction and dosing parameters. It is important to emphasize accuracy in determining both the amount of medication to be given and the time intervals for administration. The child can be given cool liquids to reduce the temperature and minimize the chance of dehydration (see Controlling Elevated Temperatures, Chapter 44).

! NURSING ALERT

Acetaminophen is an appropriate medication for fever, pain, and aches, and it can be given every 4 hours up to five times in 24 hours. Ibuprofen can be used as well and can be given every 6 to 8 hours up to four times in a 24-hour period. Caution parents about the use of over-the-counter combination "cold" remedies, since these often include acetaminophen. Careful calculation of both the acetaminophen given separately and the acetaminophen in combination medications is necessary to avoid an overdose.

Promote Hydration

Dehydration is a potential complication when children have respiratory tract infections and are febrile or anorexic, especially when vomiting or diarrhea is present. Infants are especially prone to fluid and electrolyte deficits when they have a respiratory illness, because a rapid respiratory rate that accompanies such illnesses precludes adequate fluid intake. In addition, the presence of fever increases the total body fluid turnover in infants. If the infant has nasal secretions, this further prevents adequate respiratory effort by blocking the narrow nasal passages more so when the infant reclines to feed, which ceases the compensatory mouth breathing effort, causing the child to limit intake of fluids. Adequate fluid intake is encouraged by offering small amounts of favourite fluids (clear liquids if vomiting) at frequent intervals. Oral rehydration solutions, such as Infalyte, Pedialyte, or other pediatric rehydration brands, should be considered for infants, and water or a low-carbohydrate (<5 g per 240 cc) flavoured drink should be considered for older children. Fluids with caffeine (tea, coffee, and cola) should be avoided because these may act as a diuretic and promote fluid loss. Sports drinks and energy drinks are not recommended for oral rehydration (American Academy of Pediatrics [AAP] Committee on Nutrition and the Council on Sports Medicine and Fitness, 2011); some sports drinks may be diluted for older children. Breastfeeding infants should continue to be breastfed because human milk confers some degree of protection from infection (see Chapter 27). Fluids should not be forced, and children should not be awakened to take fluids. Forcing fluids creates the same problem as urging unwanted food. Gentle persuasion with preferred beverages or sugar-free popsicles is usually more successful. Younger children may like to drink smaller amounts from a plastic medicine cup.

To assess their child's level of hydration, parents are advised to observe the frequency of voiding and to notify a health care provider if there is insufficient voiding (see also Chapter 46). Counting the number of wet diapers in a 24-hour period is a satisfactory method to assess output in infants and toddlers. In the hospital, diapers are weighed to assess output, which should be at least 1 to 2 mL/kg per hour in children up to 30 kg in weight. Then it should be at least 30 mL per hour in older patients (The Hospital for Sick Children, 2014). The health care provider should be notified if the urine output is low.

Provide Nutrition

Loss of appetite is characteristic of children with acute infections. In most cases children can be permitted to determine their own need for food. Many children show no decrease in appetite, and others respond well to foods such as gelatin, soup, and puddings (see Feeding the Sick Child, Chapter 44). Urging foods on anorexic children may precipitate nausea and vomiting and cause an aversion to feeding that can extend into the convalescent period and beyond.

Encourage Family Support and Home Care

Young children with respiratory tract infections are irritable and difficult to comfort; the family needs support, encouragement, and practical suggestions for comfort measures and administration of medication. In addition to antipyretics and nose drops, the child may require antibiotic therapy. Parents of children receiving oral antibiotics must understand the importance of regular administration and continuing the medication for the prescribed length of time, regardless of whether the child appears ill. Parents should be cautioned against giving their child any medications that are not approved by the health care provider and to avoid giving antibiotics left over from a previous illness or prescribed for another child. Administering unprescribed antibiotics can produce serious adverse effects and lead to the development of new antibiotic-resistant organisms (see Chapter 44 for administration of medications and teaching parents).

UPPER RESPIRATORY TRACT INFECTIONS

Nasopharyngitis

Acute nasopharyngitis (the equivalent of the "common cold") is caused by rhinovirus, RSV, adenovirus, influenza virus, and parainfluenza virus. Symptoms are more severe in infants and children than in adults. Fever is common in young children, and older children have low-grade fevers, which appear early in the course of the illness. Other clinical manifestations are listed in Box 45-3. Symptoms may last up to 10 days.

Therapeutic Management

Children with nasopharyngitis are managed at home. There is no specific treatment, and effective vaccines are not available. Antipyretics are prescribed for mild fever and discomfort (see Chapter 44 for management of fever). Rest is recommended. The provision of a humidified environment and increasing oral fluids may be beneficial to some children with a cold.

Cough suppressants containing dextromethorphan should be used with caution (cough is a protective way of clearing secretions) but may be prescribed for a dry, hacking cough, especially at night. However, some preparations contain 22% alcohol and can cause adverse effects such as confusion, hyperexcitability, dizziness, nausea, and sedation. Parents should monitor the child carefully for potential adverse effects. Recent concerns regarding serious adverse effects of cough and cold preparations in young children, particularly infants, and lack of convincing evidence that such medications are effective in reducing symptoms have prompted recommendations by health care experts to carefully evaluate the benefits and risks of recommending such preparations for children younger than 6 years (Goldman & CPS, Drug Therapy and Hazardous Substances Committee, 2011/2016; Vassilev, Kabadi, & Villa, 2010; Yang & So, 2014). OTC cold preparation such as pseudoephedrine and some antihistamines are not appropriate for the treatment of the common cold in infants and toddlers; these may cause serious adverse effects in such children and have been associated with death in infants (Goldman & CPS, Drug Therapy and Hazardous Substances Committee, 2011/2016).

Antihistamines are largely ineffective in treatment of nasopharyngitis (Kinyon Munch, 2010). These drugs have a

BOX 45-3 CLINICAL MANIFESTATIONS OF NASOPHARYNGITIS AND PHARYNGITIS

Nasopharyngitis

Younger Child

Fever
Irritability, restlessness
Sneezing
Vomiting and diarrhea

Older Child

Dryness and irritation of nose and throat
Sneezing, chilling sensation
Muscular aches
Cough (productive/non-productive), sometimes

Physical Signs

Edema and vasodilation of mucosa

Pharyngitis

Younger Child

Fever
General malaise
Anorexia
Moderate sore throat
Headache

Older Child

Fever (may reach 40°C [104°F])
Headache
Anorexia
Dysphagia
Abdominal pain
Vomiting

Physical Signs

Younger Child

Mild to moderate hyperemia

Older Child

Mild to fiery red, edematous pharynx
Hyperemia of tonsils and pharynx; may extend to soft palate and uvula
Often abundant follicular exudate that spreads and coalesces to form pseudomembrane on tonsils
Cervical glands enlarged and tender

BOX 45-4 EARLY EVIDENCE OF RESPIRATORY COMPLICATIONS

Parents should be instructed to notify their regular health care provider if any of the following are noted:

- If the child is less than 3 months of age when a cold starts
- If the child has a fever for more than 5 days
- If the child has a runny nose for more than 10 days
- If the infant's nose cannot be unblocked so that the infant can drink adequate amount of fluids or the child is not eating or drinking
- If the child has a yellow discharge from the eyes
- If the child has pain in the chest
- If the child has any pain in the ear or any fluid draining from it (see p. 1346)
- If the child is having difficulty swallowing
- If the child is vomiting or choking with a cough
- If they have any concerns or need to ask questions

Parents should be instructed to go the nearest emergency department or call 911 if:

- The child is getting more ill.
- The child seems lethargic, very drowsy or irritable.
- The child is having difficulty breathing.
- The child's lips look blue (circumoral cyanosis).
- The child has a stiff or painful neck or a headache that is severe.

Modified from About Kids Health (2013). *Colds (viral upper respiratory infections)*. Retrieved from http://www.aboutkidshealth.ca/En/HealthAZ/ConditionsandDiseases/InfectiousDiseases/Pages/Colds-Viral-Upper-Respiratory-Infections.aspx

weak atropine-like effect that dries secretions, but they can cause drowsiness or, paradoxically, have a stimulatory effect on children. Second-generation antihistamines such as loratadine or cetirizine are nonsedating but also have not been shown to be effective in relieving the symptoms of the common cold in small children and are not recommended. There is no support for the usefulness of expectorants, and antibiotics are usually not indicated because most infections are viral.

The combination of supportive treatment with antipyretics, nasal saline irrigation, elevating the head of bed to promote drainage of secretions, and adequate fluid hydration is still the safest and most often recommended therapy for infants and small children with the common cold (Kinyon Munch, 2010). Parents should know the signs of respiratory complications (Box 45-4) and should notify a health care provider if complications occur.

Prevention

Nasopharyngitis is so widespread in the general population that it is impossible to prevent. Children are more susceptible because they have not yet developed resistance to many viruses. Young infants and those with decreased resistance and pulmonary illness are subject to serious complications, so attempts should be made to protect them from exposure.

Because nasopharyngitis is spread from secretions, the best means for prevention is avoiding contact with affected persons. The most frequent carriers of infection are the human hands, which deposit viruses on doorknobs, faucets, and other everyday objects. Children should be taught to wash their hands thoroughly and avoid touching their eyes, nose, and mouth.

Acute Streptococcal Pharyngitis

Children who experience GABHS infection of the upper airway (strep throat) are at risk for *rheumatic fever* (RF), an inflammatory disease of the heart, joints, and central nervous system (see Chapter 47), and *acute glomerulonephritis* (AGN), an acute kidney infection (see Chapter 49). Permanent damage can result from these sequelae, especially RF. GABHS may also cause skin manifestations, including impetigo or pyoderma.

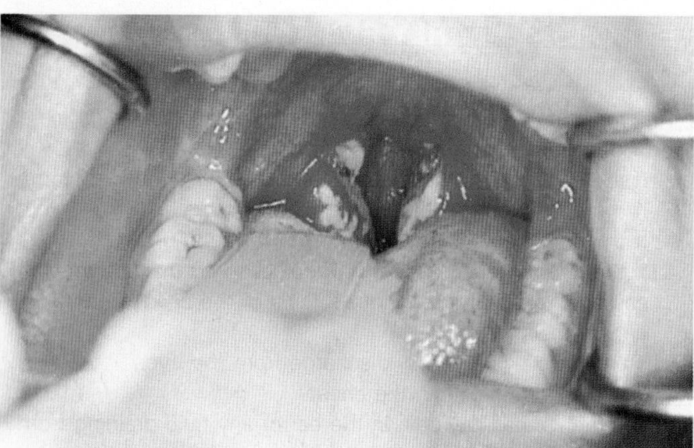

FIGURE 45-1 Tonsillitis and pharyngitis. (Courtesy Dr. Edward L. Applebaum, Head, Department of Otolaryngology, University of Illinois Medical Center.)

Clinical Manifestations

GABHS is generally a relatively brief illness that varies in severity from subclinical (no symptoms) to severe toxicity. The onset is often abrupt and characterized by pharyngitis, headache, fever, and abdominal pain (especially in small children). The tonsils and pharynx may be inflamed and covered with exudate (Fig. 45-1), which usually appears by the second day of illness. However, streptococcal infections should be suspected in children older than 2 years of age who have pharyngitis without exudate or nasal symptoms. The tongue may appear edematous and red (strawberry tongue), and the child may have a fine sandpaper rash on the trunk, axillae, elbows, and groin, seen in scarlet fever (caused by a strain of group A streptococcus). The uvula is edematous and red. Anterior cervical lymphadenopathy (in about 30 to 50% of cases) usually occurs early, and the nodes are often tender. Pain can be relatively mild to severe enough to make swallowing difficult. Clinical manifestations usually subside in 3 to 5 days unless complicated by sinusitis or parapharyngeal, peritonsillar, or retropharyngeal abscesses. Nonsuppurative complications may appear after the onset of GABHS (i.e., AGN in about 10 days and RF in an average of 18 days).

Children who are GABHS carriers may have a positive throat culture but often experience a coincidental viral illness. Although antibiotic administration is not indicated for most GABHS carriers, some conditions require antibiotic therapy; these are published in the American Academy of Pediatrics (AAP)'s *Red Book* (AAP, Committee on Infectious Diseases, Kimberlin et al., 2015).

Diagnostic Evaluation

Although 80 to 90% of all cases of acute pharyngitis are viral, a throat culture or rapid streptococcal identification test should be performed to rule out GABHS. Most streptococcal infections are short-term illnesses, and antibody responses appear later than symptoms and are useful only for retrospective diagnosis.

Rapid identification of GABHS with diagnostic test kits (rapid antigen detection test) is possible in the office or clinic setting. Because of the high specificity of these rapid tests, a positive test result generally does not require throat culture confirmation. However, the sensitivities of these kits vary considerably, and a confirmatory throat culture is recommended in patients who have a negative test result (Healthlink BC, 2015).

Therapeutic Management

If streptococcal sore throat infection is present, oral penicillin is prescribed in a dose sufficient to control the acute local manifestations and maintain an adequate level for at least 10 days to eliminate any organisms that might remain to initiate RF symptoms. Penicillin does not prevent the development of AGN in susceptible children; however, it may prevent the spread of a nephrogenic strain of GABHS to others in the family. Penicillin usually produces a prompt response within 24 hours. Patients who have a history of RF or who remain symptomatic after a full course of antibiotics may require a follow-up throat swab.

Intramuscular (IM) benzathine penicillin G is an appropriate therapy, but it is painful and is not the first choice for children. Oral erythromycin is indicated for children allergic to penicillin. Other antibiotics used to treat GABHS are azithromycin, clarithromycin, oral cephalosporins, amoxicillin, and amoxicillin with clavulanic acid (AAP, Committee on Infectious Diseases, Kimberlin et al., 2015).

NURSING CARE

The nurse will often obtain a throat swab for culture or rapid antigen testing. Parents need to be instructed about administering penicillin and analgesics as prescribed. Cold or warm compresses to the neck may provide relief. In children who can gargle, warm salt gargles offer relief of throat discomfort. Analgesics (acetaminophen or ibuprofen) can be used; these medications come in liquid or chewable form to make it easier to swallow. Pain may interfere with oral intake, but fluid intake is essential. Cool liquids or ice chips are usually more acceptable than solids.

Special emphasis should be placed on correct administration of oral medication and completing the course of antibiotic therapy (see Administration of Medication, Chapter 44). If injections are required, they must be administered deep into a large muscle mass (e.g., vastus lateralis or ventrogluteal muscle). To prevent pain, application of a topical anaesthetic cream, such as EMLA (a eutectic mixture of lidocaine and prilocaine) over the injection site 1 hour before the injection or LMX4 (4% lidocaine) over the site 30 minutes before the injection, is helpful (see Administration of Medication: Intramuscular Administration, Chapter 44). The injection site may be tender for 1 to 2 days. Local application of heat is helpful in relieving this discomfort.

Children are considered noninfectious to others after a full 24 hours of antibiotic therapy, and they should not return to school or day care until after this period has been completed. Nurses should remind the family to discard their toothbrush and replace it with a new one after they have been taking antibiotics for 24 hours. Orthodontic appliances should be washed thoroughly because they may harbour the organisms. Parents should be cautioned to prevent other household members, especially if immunocompromised, from having close contact with the sick child and to avoid sharing drinking or eating items.

If the child continues to have a high fever that does not respond to antipyretics, has an extremely sore throat, refuses liquids, and appears toxic 24 to 48 hours after starting an antibiotic, further evaluation by a health care provider is recommended.

Tonsillitis

The *tonsils* are masses of lymphoid tissue located in the pharyngeal cavity. They filter and protect the respiratory and alimentary tracts from invasion by pathogenic organisms and play a role in antibody formation. Although their size varies, children generally have much larger tonsils than those of adolescents or adults. This difference is thought to be a protective mechanism because young children are especially susceptible to upper respiratory infections.

Pathophysiology

Several pairs of tonsils are part of a mass of lymphoid tissue encircling the nasal and oral pharynx, known as the *Waldeyer tonsillar ring* (Fig. 45-2). The *palatine*, also known as *faucial, tonsils* are located on either side of the oropharynx, behind and below the pillars of the fauces (opening from the mouth). A surface of the palatine tonsils is usually visible during oral examination. The palatine tonsils are those removed during tonsillectomy. The *pharyngeal tonsils*, also known as the *adenoids*, are located above the palatine tonsils on the posterior wall of the nasopharynx. Their proximity to the nares and eustachian tubes causes difficulties in instances of inflammation. The *lingual tonsils* are located at the base of the tongue. The *tubal tonsils*, found near the posterior nasopharyngeal opening of the eustachian tubes, are not part of the Waldeyer tonsillar ring.

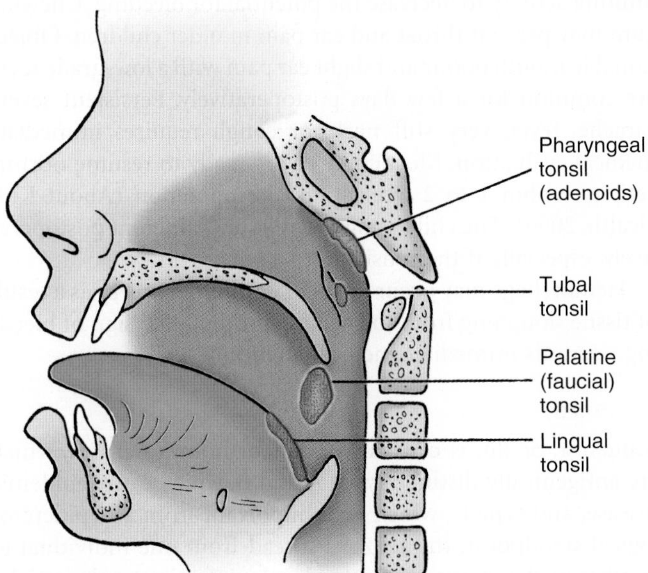

FIGURE 45-2 Location of various tonsillar masses.

Etiology

Tonsillitis often occurs with pharyngitis. The causative agent may be viral or bacterial. Because of the abundant lymphoid tissue and the frequency of upper respiratory infections, tonsillitis is a common cause of illness in young children.

Clinical Manifestations

The manifestations of tonsillitis are caused by inflammation. As the palatine tonsils enlarge from edema, they may meet in the midline (kissing tonsils), obstructing the passage of air or food. The child has difficulty swallowing and breathing. When the adenoids enlarge, the space behind the posterior nares becomes blocked, making it difficult or impossible for air to pass from the nose to the throat. As a result, the child breathes through the mouth.

Therapeutic Management

Because tonsillitis is self-limiting, treatment of viral pharyngitis is symptomatic. Throat cultures positive for GABHS infection warrant antibiotic treatment. It is important to differentiate between viral and streptococcal infection in febrile exudative tonsillitis. Because most infections are of viral origin, early rapid tests can eliminate unnecessary antibiotic administration.

Tonsillectomy is the surgical removal of the palatine tonsils. Indications for a tonsillectomy are recurrent peritonsillar abscess (six episodes per year), airway obstruction that leads to obstructive sleep apnea, and tonsils requiring tissue pathology (Canadian Society of Otolaryngology, 2013).

Adenoidectomy (the surgical removal of the adenoids) is recommended for children who have hypertrophied adenoids that obstruct nasal breathing; additional indications for adenoidectomy include recurrent adenoiditis and sinusitis, otitis media with effusion, airway obstruction and subsequent sleep-disordered breathing, and recurrent rhinorrhea. For some children the effectiveness of tonsillectomy or adenoidectomy is modest and may not justify the risk of surgery. In practice, many physicians rely on individualized decision making and do not subscribe to an absolute set of eligibility criteria for these surgical procedures. Contraindications to either tonsillectomy or adenoidectomy are (1) cleft palate, because tonsils help minimize the escape of air during speech; (2) acute infections at the time of surgery, because locally inflamed tissues increase the risk of bleeding; (3) uncontrolled systemic diseases or blood dyscrasias; and (4) poor anaesthetic risk.

NURSING CARE

Nursing care of tonsillitis involves providing comfort and minimizing activities or interventions that precipitate bleeding. A soft to liquid diet is preferred. A cool-mist vaporizer keeps the mucous membranes moist during periods of mouth breathing. Warm salt-water gargles, throat lozenges or hard candy, and analgesic-antipyretic medications such as acetaminophen or ibuprophen can be used to promote comfort. In the past, opioids were often administered after tonsillectomies to children to reduce pain so the child could drink. Health Canada (2013) no longer recommends the use of codeine in children under 12 years of age. Children and breastfeeding mothers are ultrametabolizers of codeine and convert codeine into morphine more quickly and completely than others. The use of codeine by these ultrametabolizers has the potential to cause a morphine overdose. All products in Canada that contain codeine are now labelled with the warning that they are not to be given to children under age 12. Currently, research points toward the combined use of ibuprofen and acetaminophen to provide safe and effective post-tonsillectomy pain relief in children. Post-tonsillectomy morphine should be used with caution because it may be unsafe for specific children. Research indicates that use of ibuprofen does not increase the risk of post-surgical bleeding (Kelly, Sommer, Ramakrishna, et al., 2015).

If surgery is required, the child needs the same psychological preparation and physical care as for any other surgical procedure (see Chapters 43 and 44). Most tonsillectomy and adenoidectomy (T&A) surgeries now take place in outpatient settings; however, the priorities of preoperative and postoperative care remain the same. The following discussion focuses on postoperative nursing care for T&A, although both procedures may not be performed.

Until they are fully awake, children are placed on their abdomen or side to facilitate drainage of secretions. Routine suctioning is avoided, and, when performed, it is done carefully to avoid trauma to the oropharynx. When alert, children may prefer sitting up. They should be discouraged from coughing frequently, clearing their throat, blowing their nose, or any other activity that may aggravate the operative site.

Some secretions are common, particularly dried blood from surgery. All secretions and vomitus need to be inspected for evidence of fresh bleeding (some blood-tinged mucus is expected). Dark brown (old) blood is usually present in the emesis, in the nose, and between the teeth. If parents do not expect this, they often become frightened at a time when they need to be calm and reassuring.

The throat is sore after surgery. An ice collar provides relief, but many children find it bothersome and refuse to use it. Most children experience moderate pain after a T&A and need pain medication regularly for at least the first few days. Analgesics may be given rectally or intravenously to avoid the oral route. Because pain is continuous, analgesics should be administered at regular intervals. An antiemetic such as ondansetron (Zofran) may be administered postoperatively if nausea or vomiting is present (see Pain Management, Chapter 34).

Food and fluids should be restricted until children are fully alert and there are no signs of hemorrhage. Cool water, crushed ice, flavoured ice pops, or diluted fruit juice may be given, but fluids with a red or brown colour should be avoided so that fresh or old blood in emesis can be differentiated from the ingested liquid. Raising the head of the bed helps to reduce edema. Citrus juice may cause discomfort and is usually poorly tolerated. Soft foods, particularly gelatin, cooked fruits, sherbet, soup, and mashed potatoes, are started on the first or second postoperative day or as the child tolerates feeding. The pain from surgery often inhibits fluid intake, reinforcing the need for adequate pain control. Milk, ice cream, and pudding are usually not offered, since milk products coat the mouth and throat and may cause the child to clear the throat, which can initiate bleeding.

Postoperative hemorrhage is uncommon but can occur in up to 5% of patients up to 14 days after surgery. The nurse needs to observe the throat directly for evidence of bleeding, using a good source of light and, if necessary, carefully inserting a tongue depressor. Other signs of hemorrhage are tachycardia, pallor, frequent clearing of the throat or swallowing by a younger child, and vomiting of bright red blood. Restlessness, an indication of hemorrhage, may be difficult to differentiate from general discomfort after surgery. Decreasing blood pressure is a late sign of shock.

Surgery may be required to cauterize or ligate a bleeding vessel. Airway obstruction may also occur as a result of edema or accumulated secretions and is indicated by signs of respiratory distress, such as stridor, drooling, restlessness, agitation, increasing respiratory rate, and progressive cyanosis. Suction equipment and oxygen should be available after tonsillectomy.

! NURSING ALERT

The most obvious early sign of bleeding is the child's continuous swallowing of the trickling blood. While the child is sleeping, note the frequency of swallowing. If continuous bleeding is suspected, notify the surgeon immediately.

Most children are ready to be discharged from the hospital in 6 to 8 hours after surgery (About Kids Health, 2009). Discharge instructions include (1) avoiding irritating or highly seasoned foods; (2) encouraging at least 4 cups of fluid or food with a high fluid content per day (noncitrus products for 7 to 10 days); (3) avoiding gargles or vigorous tooth brushing; (4) avoiding coughing, clearing the throat, or putting objects in the mouth such as a straw; the child should sneeze with an open mouth; (5) using analgesics or an ice collar for pain; and (6) limiting activity to decrease the potential for bleeding. Chewing gum may prevent throat and ear pain in older children. Objectionable mouth odour and slight ear pain with a low-grade fever are common for a few days postoperatively. Persistent severe earache, fever, very stiff neck, or cough requires immediate medical evaluation. Most children are ready to resume normal activity within 1 to 2 weeks after the operation (About Kids Health, 2009). The child's voice may sound different postoperatively, especially if the tonsils were large.

Hemorrhage may occur up to 14 days after surgery as a result of tissue sloughing from the healing process. Any sign of bleeding warrants immediate medical attention.

Influenza

Influenza, or flu, is caused by three orthomyxoviruses, which are antigenically distinct: types A and B, which cause epidemic disease, and type C, which is unimportant from an epidemiological standpoint. Influenza is spread from one individual to another by direct contact (large-droplet infection) or by articles recently contaminated by nasopharyngeal secretions. While there is no predilection for a specific age group, attack rates are highest in young children who have had no previous contact with a strain. Influenza is frequently most severe in infants. During epidemics, infection among school-age children is believed to be a major source of transmission in a community. The disease is more common during the winter months and has a 1- to 3-day incubation period. Affected persons are most infectious for 24 hours before and after the onset of symptoms. The virus has a peculiar affinity for epithelial cells of the respiratory tract mucosa, where it destroys ciliated epithelium with metaplastic hyperplasia of the tracheal and bronchial epithelium with associated edema. The alveoli may also become distended with a hyaline-like material. The viruses can be isolated from nasopharyngeal secretions early after the onset of infection, and serological tests identify the type by complement fixation or the subgroups by hemagglutination inhibition.

H1N1 (swine flu) is a subtype of influenza type A. In 2009, a pandemic of H1N1 caused significant morbidity and mortality, particularly in Mexico, the United States, and Canada; it was declared at an end in Canada in January 2010. A *pandemic* is defined by the World Health Organization (WHO) as the spread of a new disease to which the population has little or no immunity and that spreads rapidly from human to human. The signs and symptoms of H1N1 are the same as those mentioned below for influenza. H1N1 vaccine was combined with the seasonal influenza vaccine in the 2012 to 2013 season.

Clinical Manifestations

The manifestations of influenza may be subclinical, mild, moderate, or severe. Most patients have a dry throat and nasal mucosa, a dry cough, and a tendency toward hoarseness. A flushed face, photophobia, myalgia, hyperesthesia, and sometimes exhaustion and lack of energy accompany a sudden onset of fever and chills. Subglottal croup is common, especially in infants. The symptoms of influenza last for 4 or 5 days. Complications include severe viral pneumonia (often hemorrhagic); encephalitis; and secondary bacterial infections, such as otitis media, sinusitis, or pneumonia.

Therapeutic Management

Uncomplicated influenza in children usually requires only symptomatic treatment: acetaminophen or ibuprofen for fever and sufficient fluids to maintain hydration. Currently, zanamivir and oseltamivir (Tamiflu) are neuraminidase inhibitors and are stored in many countries to treat and prevent pandemic and seasonal influenza outbreaks before an influenza vaccine that matches the influenza strain is available. Neuraminidase inhibitors help prevent influenza A and B viruses from multiplying by interfering with the production and release of viruses from cells that line the respiratory tract. This may slow the spread of the infection within the airways and from the cells that line the respiratory tract. The WHO has declared oseltamivir to be an essential medicine. Both zanamivir and oseltamivir have been approved for the treatment of flu symptoms in children under 18 years of age. Both medications must be started within 2 days of symptom onset. Zanamivir is an inhaled medication effective for type A and B influenza. The drug is taken twice daily for 5 days and is administered by a specially designed oral inhaler (Diskhaler). Zanamivir cannot be used in children younger than 7 years of age. Oseltamivir (Tamiflu) is given orally for 5 days to children over 1 year of age and to adults to decrease the flu symptoms. It is reported to be effective for types A and B influenza (AAP, Committee on Infectious Diseases, Kimberlin et al., 2015).

Prevention

The National Advisory Committee on Immunizations (NACI) in Canada is the national surveillance program that provides information on which viral strains are put into each year's influenza vaccines. FluWatch is part of Canada's national surveillance system that provides information on the spread of influenza and influenza-like illnesses on an ongoing basis. Specific information is provided weekly on influenza viruses that are circulating across Canada (see Additional Resources at the end of this chapter). Each province or territory advises which vaccines will be made available for the publicly funded program in that jurisdiction.

The CPS recommends annual influenza vaccination for all children age 6 months or older, particularly in high-risk populations such as Indigenous peoples, those who are immunocompromised, and chronically ill populations (Moore & CPS, Infectious Diseases and Immunization Committee, 2015). In addition, the NACI has made some significant changes to their recommendations, which include the following:

- Children and adolescents with neurological or neurodevelopmental disorders were added to the list of individuals considered to be at high risk for severe influenza.
- Quadrivalent influenza vaccines are preferred over trivalent vaccines for use in children.
- An adjuvanted trivalent inactivated influenza vaccine is now available for use in children 6 to 23 months of age.

Children and adults who have been previously immunized with seasonal influenza vaccine should receive one dose of influenza vaccine each year. Children 6 months to 8 years of age receiving seasonal influenza vaccine for the first time should be given two doses, with a minimum interval of 4 weeks between doses.

Any individual who developed an anaphylactic reaction to a previous dose of influenza vaccine or to any of the vaccine components (with the exception of egg) or who developed Guillain-Barré syndrome (GBS) within 6 weeks of vaccination should not receive a further dose. The NACI recommends that individuals who are allergic to eggs may be vaccinated against influenza using trivalent inactivated influenza vaccines (TIIV) and quadrivalent inactivated influenza vaccines (QIIV) without a prior influenza vaccine skin test and with the full dose. They should receive the dose in a facility that can manage anaphylaxis, should it occur (Moore & CPS, Infectious Diseases and Immunization Committee, 2015; PHAC, 2014a).

NURSING CARE

Nursing care is the same as that for any child with an upper respiratory infection, including implementing measures to relieve symptoms. The greatest danger to affected children is development of a secondary infection. Prolonged fever or appearance of fever during early convalescence is a sign of secondary bacterial infection and should be reported to the health care provider for antibiotic therapy.

Otitis Media

Otitis media (OM) is one of the most prevalent diseases of early childhood. Its incidence is highest in the winter months. The majority of cases of bacterial OM are preceded by a viral respiratory infection. The two viruses most likely to precipitate OM are RSV and influenza. Most episodes of acute otitis media (AOM) occur in the first 24 months of life, but the incidence decreases with age, except for a small increase at age 5 or 6 years when children enter school. OM occurs infrequently in children older than 7 years of age. Preschool-age boys are affected more frequently than preschool-age girls. Children who have sibling or parents with a history of chronic OM have a higher incidence of OM. Children who live in households with many members (especially smokers) are more likely to have OM than those living with fewer persons. Passive smoking increases the risk of persistent middle ear effusion by enhancing attachment of the pathogens that cause otitis to the respiratory epithelium in the middle ear space, prolonging the inflammatory response, and impeding drainage through the eustachian tube (Le Saux, Robinson, & CPS, Infectious Diseases and Immunization Committee, 2016). Other risk factors include orofacial abnormalities, premature birth, a shorter duration of breastfeeding, prolonged bottle-feeding lying down, and **immunodeficiency** (Le Saux et al., 2016). The high rate of chronic suppurative OM among Indigenous children is likely due to the fact that Indigenous peoples have three times the smoking rates of the general Canadian population (Wong & CPS, First Nations, Inuit and Métis Committee, 2006/2016).

OM has been defined in a variety of ways. The standard terminology used to define OM is outlined in Box 45-5, and AOM treatment guidelines have been published (Lieberthal, Carroll, Chonmaitree, et al., 2013).

Etiology

Streptococcus pneumoniae, *H. influenzae*, and *Moraxella catarrhalis* are the three most common bacteria causing AOM. The etiology of noninfectious OM is unknown, although OM may occur because of blocked eustachian tubes, which results in negative ear pressure. Fluid is pulled from the mucosal lining, which accumulates and becomes colonized by infectious organisms. Predisposing factors include upper respiratory infections, allergies, Down syndrome, cleft palate, day care attendance, exposure to secondhand smoke, and bottle propping during feeding. Breastfed infants have a lower incidence of OM than formula-fed infants. Breastfeeding may protect infants against respiratory viruses and allergy because it contains secretory immune globulin A, which limits the exposure of the eustachian tube and middle ear mucosa to microbial pathogens and foreign proteins. Exclusive breastfeeding for at least 6 months shows a protective effect for prevention of OM and recurrent AOM (Lieberthal et al., 2013). Reflux of milk up the eustachian tubes is less likely in breastfed infants because of the semivertical positioning during breastfeeding compared with positioning during bottle-feeding.

BOX 45-5 STANDARD TERMINOLOGY FOR OTITIS MEDIA

Otitis media (OM)—An inflammation of the middle ear without reference to etiology or pathogenesis

Acute otitis media (AOM)—An inflammation of the middle ear with a rapid onset of the signs and symptoms of acute infection (i.e., fever and otalgia [ear pain])

Otitis media with effusion (OME)—Inflammation and fluid in the middle ear without symptoms of acute infection

Middle ear effusion (MEE)—Fluid in the middle ear without reference to etiology, pathogenesis, pathology, or duration

Pathophysiology

OM is primarily a result of malfunctioning eustachian tubes. Eustachian tubes have three functions relative to the middle ear: (1) protection of the middle ear from nasopharyngeal secretions, (2) drainage of secretions produced in the middle ear into the nasopharynx, and (3) ventilation of the middle ear to equalize air pressure within the middle ear and atmospheric pressure in the external ear canal and to replenish oxygen that has been absorbed.

Mechanical or functional obstruction of the eustachian tube causes accumulation of secretions in the middle ear. Intrinsic obstruction can be caused by infection or allergy; extrinsic obstruction is usually a result of enlarged adenoids or nasopharyngeal tumours. When the passage is not totally obstructed, contamination of the middle ear can take place by reflux, aspiration, or insufflation during crying, sneezing, nose-blowing, and swallowing when the nose is obstructed.

Diagnostic Evaluation

Careful assessment of the tympanic membrane to see if it is immobile, with a pneumatic otoscope, is essential to differentiate AOM from OM with effusion (OME). A diagnosis of AOM is made if visual inspection of the tympanic membrane reveals a purulent discoloured effusion and a bulging or full, opacified, or reddened immobile membrane, as well as an acute onset of ear pain for less than 48 hours (Le Saux et al., 2016). An immobile tympanic membrane or an orange-discoloured membrane indicates OME. Clinical symptoms of otitis are also helpful in making the diagnosis (Box 45-6). In OME, these symptoms may be absent, and other nonspecific symptoms such as rhinitis, cough, or diarrhea are often present (Le Saux et al., 2016). OME may precede AOM or predispose to its development, but OME does not represent an acute infectious process that requires antibiotic therapy (Lieberthal et al., 2013).

Therapeutic Management

Treatment for AOM is one of the most common reasons for antibiotic use in the ambulatory setting. However, concerns about drug-resistant *S. pneumoniae* and other drug resistances

BOX 45-6 CLINICAL MANIFESTATIONS OF OTITIS MEDIA

Acute Otitis Media

Follows an upper respiratory infection
Otalgia (earache)
Fever
Purulent discharge (otorrhea) may or may not be present

Infant or Very Young Child

Crying
Fussy, restless, irritable
Tendency to rub, hold, or pull affected ear
Rolls head from side to side
Difficulty comforting child
Refuses to nurse or take bottle
Loss of appetite

Older Child

Crying or expressing feelings of discomfort
Irritability
Lethargy
Loss of appetite

Chronic Otitis Media

Hearing loss
Difficulty communicating
Possible feeling of fullness, tinnitus, or vertigo

have led infectious disease authorities to recommend careful and judicious use of antibiotics for treatment of this illness. Current recommendations regarding antibiotic administration to children with AOM are as follows (Le Saux et al., 2016; Lieberthal et al., 2013):

- Prescribe antibiotics for children 6 months of age and older who have severe signs or symptoms of AOM (moderate or severe otalgia for at least 48 hours or temperature equal to or greater than 39°C).
- Prescribe antibiotics for bilateral AOM in children younger than 24 months of age who do not have severe signs or symptoms (moderate or severe otalgia for at least 48 hours or temperature equal to or greater than 39°C).
- Either prescribe antibiotics *or* offer observation with close follow-up (based on joint decision making with parent or caregiver) for unilateral AOM in children 6 months to 23 months of age who do not have severe signs or symptoms (moderate or severe otalgia for at least 48 hours or temperature equal to or greater than 39°C); if the child does not improve within 48 hours, begin antibiotic therapy.
- Either prescribe antibiotics *or* offer observation with close follow-up (based on joint decision making with parent or caregiver) for unilateral or bilateral AOM in children 24 months of age or older who do not have severe signs and symptoms (moderate or severe otalgia for at least 48 hours or temperature equal to or greater than 39°C).

It is essential that children who are on observation have medical follow-up and that parents be able to recognize a lack of improvement and treat with analgesics. The parents should be given a deferred prescription for antimicrobials if there is no improvement in the condition. Some reviews of the treatment of AOM show no clear evidence that antibiotics improve outcomes in children younger than 2 years of age with uncomplicated AOM. In addition, all cases of AOM in infants younger than 6 months of age should be treated with antibiotics because of the infant's immature immune system and the potential for infection with bacteria other than the three most common organisms found in older infants and children with AOM.

Children with AOM require comprehensive assessment and management of pain. For fever or discomfort associated with OM, analgesic-antipyretic drugs such as acetaminophen or ibuprofen may be given. The health care provider may prescribe topical pain relief drops such as benzocaine or lidocaine.

When antibiotics are warranted, oral amoxicillin in high doses (85 to 90 mg/kg/day, divided twice daily) is the treatment of choice for initial episodes of AOM in children who have not received amoxicillin within the past month. The recommendation for the duration of antibiotic therapy in severe AOM is 10 days. A 5-day course may be sufficient in children 6 years of age and older with uncomplicated mild or moderate AOM. For children with penicillin allergies, first-line antibiotics include cefuroxime-axetil 30 mg/kg/day divided twice or three times per day as tablets or suspension or ceftriaxone 50 mg/kg intramuscularly (or intravenously) daily for 3 days (Le Saux et al., 2016).

Second-line antibiotics used to treat OM include amoxicillin-clavulanate and IM or intravenous (IV) ceftriaxone if the causative organism is a highly resistant pneumococcus or if the parents have difficulty ensuring that the child receives the therapy. An important consideration with the use of single-dose IM injections is the pain involved in this therapy. One strategy to minimize pain at the injection site is to reconstitute the cephalosporin with 1% lidocaine. A topical analgesic cream such as EMLA or LMX4 can also be applied to the site beforehand to reduce pain. Alternatively, the IV route can be used. The use of steroids, decongestants, and antihistamines to treat AOM is not recommended.

Myringotomy, a surgical incision of the eardrum, may be necessary to alleviate the severe pain of AOM. A myringotomy is also performed to provide drainage of infected middle ear fluid in the presence of complications (mastoiditis, labyrinthitis, or facial paralysis) or to allow purulent middle ear fluid to drain into the ear canal for culture. A minimally invasive laser-assisted myringotomy procedure may be performed in outpatient settings.

Tympanostomy tube (t-tubes) placement and adenoidectomy are surgical procedures that may be done to treat recurrent chronic AOM (defined as three bouts in 6 months, six in 12 months, or six by 6 years of age). Tympanostomy tubes or pressure-equalizer (PE) tubes are grommets that facilitate continued drainage of fluid and allow ventilation of the middle ear. They are inserted to treat severe eustachian tube dysfunction, OM with effusion, or complications of OM (mastoiditis, facial nerve paralysis, brain abscess, labyrinthitis). Adenoidectomy is not recommended for treatment of AOM and is performed only in children with recurrent AOM or chronic OME with postnasal obstruction, adenoiditis, or chronic sinusitis.

In some children residual middle ear effusions remain after episodes of AOM. Some children have fluid that persists in the middle ear for weeks or months. Antibiotics are not required for initial treatment of OME but may be indicated for children with persistent effusion for more than 3 months (Gould & Matz, 2010). Placement of tympanostomy tubes is recommended after a total of 4 to 6 months of bilateral effusion with a bilateral hearing deficit (Gould & Matz, 2010). This therapy allows for mechanical drainage of the fluid, which promotes healing of the membrane and prevents scar formation and loss of elasticity. Myringotomy with or without insertion of PE tubes should not be performed for initial management of OME but may be recommended for children who have recurrent episodes of OME with a long cumulative duration (Gould & Matz, 2010).

OME is frequently associated with mild to moderate impairment of hearing. A hearing test should be performed if OME persists for 3 months or more or if there is evidence of language or learning delays. Follow-up examinations of children with chronic OME should be maintained on a 3- to 6-month basis until the OME is resolved, a significant hearing loss is identified, or a structural defect of the tympanic membrane or middle ear is identified (Gould & Matz, 2010). Children with hearing loss should be referred to an otolaryngologist and should receive a speech and language evaluation as necessary.

Prevention

In Canada, the pneumococcal 13-valent conjugate vaccines have been developed and approved. These vaccines have helped prevent OM from pneumococci and nontypeable *H. influenza*. There has been a significant decline in the number of AOM cases since the introduction of the pneumococcal vaccine. In Canada, AOM incidence has been reduced by 13 to 19%, because the nasopharyngeal colonization with vaccine-type *S. pneumoniae* in children has been significantly decreased, particularly among children under 2 years of age (Taylor, Marchisio, Vergison, et al., 2012). All provinces and territories have incorporated the 13-valent vaccine in their immunization programs (Kellner & CPS, Infectious Diseases and Immunization Committee, 2011/2015). The vaccine is administered as a four-dose series starting at 2 months of age.

Parents are encouraged to reduce risk factors for AOM by breastfeeding infants and avoiding propping the bottle if feeding this way, decreasing or discontinuing pacifier use after 6 months, and preventing exposure of their children to tobacco smoke (Le Saux et al., 2016).

NURSING CARE

Nursing objectives for the child with AOM include (1) relieving pain, (2) facilitating drainage when possible, (3) preventing complications or recurrence, (4) educating the family in care of the child, and (5) providing emotional support to the child and family.

Analgesic medications such as acetaminophen and ibuprofen (6 months of age and older) are used to treat mild pain. For more severe pain, a stronger analgesic may be prescribed.

If the ear is draining, the external canal may be cleaned with sterile cotton swabs or cotton balls, coupled with topical antibiotic treatment. If ear wicks or lightly rolled sterile gauze packs are placed in the ear after surgical treatment, they should be loose enough to allow accumulated drainage to flow out of the ear; otherwise, infection may be transferred to the mastoid process. The wicks need to stay dry during shampoos or baths. Occasionally, drainage is so profuse that the auricle and the skin surrounding the ear become excoriated from the exudate. This is usually prevented by frequent cleansing and application of various moisture barriers (e.g., Proshield Plus) or petrolatum jelly (e.g., Vaseline).

Tympanostomy tubes may allow water to enter the middle ear, but recommendations for earplugs are inconsistent. Research indicates that swimming without earplugs poses a slightly increased risk of infection. However, lake and river water is potentially contaminated, and the wearing of earplugs while swimming in a lake prevents total flooding of the external canal. Bathwater and shampoo water should be kept out of the ear, if possible, because soap reduces the surface tension of water and facilitates entry through the tube. Parents should be aware of the appearance of a grommet (usually a tiny, white, plastic spool-shaped tube) so that they can recognize if it falls out. They need to be reassured that this is normal and requires no immediate intervention, although they should notify the practitioner.

Prevention of recurrence requires adequate education regarding antibiotic therapy. The symptoms of pain and fever usually subside within 24 to 48 hours, but nurses need to emphasize that all of the prescribed medication must be taken. Parents should be aware that potential complications of OM, such as hearing loss, can be prevented with adequate treatment and follow-up care.

Parents also need anticipatory guidance regarding methods to reduce the risks of OM, especially in children younger than 2 years. Reducing the chances of OM is possible with simple measures, such as sitting or holding an infant upright for feedings, maintaining routine childhood immunizations, and exclusively breastfeeding until at least 6 months of age. Propping bottles is discouraged to avoid pooling of milk while the child is in the supine position and to encourage human contact during feeding. Eliminating tobacco smoke and known allergens is also recommended. Early detection of middle ear effusion is essential to prevent complications. Infants and preschool children should be screened for effusion, and all schoolchildren, especially those with learning disabilities, should be tested for hearing deficits related to a middle ear effusion.

Infectious Mononucleosis

Infectious mononucleosis is an acute, self-limiting infectious disease that is common among adolescents. The illness is characterized by an increase in the mononuclear elements of the blood and by general symptoms of an infectious process. The course is usually mild but occasionally can be severe or, rarely, accompanied by serious complications.

Etiology and Pathophysiology

The herpes-like Epstein-Barr virus (EBV) is the principal cause of infectious mononucleosis. It appears in both sporadic and epidemic forms, but the sporadic cases are more common. The mechanism of spread has not been proved, but it is believed to be transmitted in saliva by direct intimate contact, although it survives in saliva for many hours outside of the body. It is mildly contagious, but the period of communicability is unknown. The incubation period following exposure is approximately 30 to 50 days (AAP, Committee on Infectious Diseases, Kimberlin et al., 2015).

Diagnostic Tests

The onset of symptoms may be acute or insidious and may appear anywhere from 10 days to 6 weeks after exposure. The presenting symptoms vary greatly in type, severity, and duration (Box 45-7). The clinical manifestations of infectious mononucleosis are usually less severe (often subclinical or unapparent), and the convalescent phase is shorter in younger children than in older children and young adults. Heterophil antibody tests (Paul-Bunnell or Monospot) determine the extent to which the patient's serum will agglutinate sheep red blood cells; the response in these tests is primarily to immunoglobulin M, which is present in the first 2 weeks of the illness in adolescents The *spot test (Monospot)* is a slide test of venous blood that has high specificity. It is rapid, sensitive, inexpensive, and easy to perform and has an advantage over the heterophil antibody test (i.e., it can detect significant agglutinins at lower levels, thus allowing earlier diagnosis). Blood is usually obtained for the test by finger puncture or venous sampling and is placed on special paper. If the blood agglutinates, forming fragments or clumps, the test is positive for the infection.

BOX 45-7 CLINICAL MANIFESTATIONS OF INFECTIOUS MONONUCLEOSIS

Early Signs
Headache
Malaise
Fatigue
Chills
Low-grade fever
Loss of appetite
Puffy eyes

Acute Disease
Cardinal Features
Fever
Sore throat
Cervical adenopathy

Common Features
Splenomegaly (may persist for several months)
Palatine petechiae
Macular eruption (especially on trunk)
Exudative pharyngitis or tonsillitis

Therapeutic Management

No specific treatment exists for infectious mononucleosis. Simple remedies ordinarily relieve the symptoms. A mild analgesic is often sufficient to relieve the headache, fever, and malaise. Rest is encouraged for fatigue but is not imposed for any specific period. Affected persons are instructed to regulate activities according to their own tolerance unless complicating factors are present. Contact sports are discouraged in the presence of splenomegaly.

Antibiotics are contraindicated unless beta-hemolytic streptococci are present (amoxicillin or ampicillin can cause a rash in patients with EBV infection). If sore throat is severe, effective therapies include gargles; hot drinks; anaesthetic lozenges; or analgesics, including opioids. Corticosteroids have been used to treat respiratory distress from significant tonsillar inflammation, hemolytic anemia, thrombocytopenia, and neurological complications; however, routine use of steroids is not recommended (AAP, Committee on Infectious Diseases, Kimberlin et al., 2015).

Prognosis

The course of this disease is usually self-limiting and uncomplicated. Acute symptoms often disappear within 7 to 10 days, and persistent fatigue subsides within 2 to 4 weeks. Some adolescents may need to restrict vigorous activities for 2 to 3 months, but the disease rarely extends for longer periods. The adolescent is encouraged to maintain limited exercise to prevent deconditioning.

NURSING CARE

Nursing responsibilities are directed toward providing comfort measures to relieve symptoms and helping affected adolescents and their families determine appropriate activities for the stage of the disease. The child should be advised to limit exposure to persons outside the family, especially during the acute phase of illness. It may be more comfortable to limit intake to liquids during the acute phase; milk shakes are a good alternative to solid foods on a temporary basis. Throat pain may be severe enough to require a mild analgesic such as acetaminophen or ibuprofen. Careful nursing assessment of swallowing ability is essential because the edema may cause serious airway compromise.

! NURSING ALERT

Advise the family to seek medical evaluation of the child or adolescent if any of the following occur:

- Breathing becomes difficult.
- Severe abdominal pain develops.
- Sore throat pain is so severe that the child is unable to drink liquids.
- Respiratory stridor is observed.

CROUP SYNDROMES

Croup is a general term applied to a symptom complex characterized by hoarseness, a resonant cough described as "barking" or "brassy" (croupy), varying degrees of inspiratory stridor, and varying degrees of respiratory distress resulting from swelling or obstruction in the region of the larynx. Acute infections of the larynx are important to address in infants and small children because of their increased incidence in these age groups and because the small diameter of the airway in infants and children places them at risk for significant narrowing with inflammation.

Croup syndromes can affect the larynx, trachea, and bronchi. However, laryngeal involvement often dominates the clinical picture because of the severe effects on the voice and breathing. Croup syndromes are described according to the primary anatomical area affected (i.e., epiglottitis [or supraglottitis], laryngitis, laryngotracheobronchitis [LTB], and tracheitis). In general, LTB occurs in very young children, and epiglottitis is more common in older children. A comparison of croup syndromes is provided in Table 45-1.

With widespread immunization programs aimed at preventing *H. influenzae* type B, the cause of most cases of croup syndrome in Canada is now attributed to viruses (i.e., parainfluenza virus, human meta-pneumovirus, influenza types A and B, adenovirus, and measles).

Acute Epiglottitis

Acute epiglottitis, or *acute supraglottitis*, is a medical emergency It is a serious obstructive inflammatory process that occurs predominately in children ages 2 to 5 years but can occur from infancy to adulthood. The obstruction is supraglottic as opposed to the subglottic obstruction of laryngitis. The responsible organism is usually *H. influenzae*. LTB and epiglottitis do not occur together.

Clinical Manifestations

The onset of epiglottitis is abrupt, and it can rapidly progress to severe respiratory distress. The child usually goes to bed asymptomatic to awaken later with a sore throat and pain on swallowing. The child will have a fever, appear sicker than clinical findings suggest, and insist on sitting upright and leaning forward with the chin thrust out, mouth open, and tongue protruding (*tripod position*). Drooling of saliva is common because of the difficulty or pain on swallowing and excessive secretions.

! NURSING ALERT

Three clinical observations that have been found to be predictive of epiglottitis are absence of spontaneous cough, presence of drooling, and agitation.

The child tends to be irritable and extremely restless and have an anxious, apprehensive, and frightened expression. The voice is thick and muffled, with a froglike croaking sound on inspiration, but the child is not hoarse. Suprasternal and substernal retractions may be visible. The child will seldom struggle to breathe, and slow, quiet breathing provides better air exchange. The throat will appear red and inflamed, and a distinctive large, cherry-red, edematous epiglottis will be visible on careful throat inspection.

! NURSING ALERT

Throat inspection should be attempted only when immediate endotracheal intubation can be performed if needed.

TABLE 45-1 COMPARISON OF CROUP SYNDROMES

	ACUTE EPIGLOTTITIS	ACUTE LTB	ACUTE SPASMODIC LARYNGITIS	ACUTE TRACHEITIS
Age group affected	2–5 yr but varies	Infant or child under 5 yr	1–3 yr	5–7 yr
Etiological agent	Bacterial	Viral	Viral with allergic component	Viral or bacterial with allergic component
Onset	Rapidly progressive	Slowly progressive	Sudden; at night	Moderately progressive
Major symptoms	Dysphagia Stridor aggravated when supine Drooling High fever Toxic appearance Rapid pulse and respirations	URI Stridor Brassy cough Hoarseness Dyspnea Restlessness Irritability Low-grade fever Nontoxic appearance	URI Croupy cough Stridor Hoarseness Dyspnea Restlessness Symptoms awakening child but disappearing during day Tendency to recur	URI Croupy cough Purulent secretions High fever No response to LTB therapy
Treatment	Airway protection Racemic epinephrine Corticosteroids Fluids Reassurance	Racemic epinephrine Corticosteroids Fluids Reassurance	Cool mist Reassurance	Antibiotics Fluids

LTB, laryngotracheobronchitis; *URI*, upper respiratory infection.

Therapeutic Management

The course of epiglottitis may be fulminant, with respiratory obstruction appearing suddenly. Progressive obstruction leads to hypoxia, hypercapnia, and acidosis followed by decreased muscle tone; reduced level of consciousness; and, when obstruction becomes more or less complete, a sudden death.

The child who is suspected of having epiglottitis should be examined in a setting where emergency airway equipment is readily available. Examination of the throat with a tongue depressor is contraindicated until experienced personnel and equipment are available to proceed with immediate intubation or tracheostomy in the event that the examination precipitates further or complete obstruction.

Nasotracheal intubation or tracheostomy is usually considered for the child with epiglottitis with severe respiratory distress. It is recommended that the intubation or tracheostomy and any invasive procedure, such as starting an IV infusion, be performed in an area where emergency airway management can be easily and quickly accomplished. Humidified oxygen is administered as necessary either via mask in older children or blow-by in younger children, to avoid further agitation. Regardless of whether or not there is an artificial airway, the child requires intensive observation by experienced personnel. The epiglottal swelling usually decreases after 24 hours of antibiotic therapy, and the epiglottis is near normal by the third day. Intubated children are generally extubated at this time. The use of corticosteroids such as dexamethasone for 8 days to reduce edema has become a mainstay in the treatment of epiglottitis.

Children with suspected bacterial epiglottitis are given antibiotics intravenously, followed by oral administration, to complete a 7- to 10-day course. Family contacts with children younger than 4 years of age are treated with rifampin for 4 days (AAP, Committee on Infectious Diseases, Kimberlin et al., 2015).

NURSING CARE

Epiglottitis is a serious and frightening disease for the child and family. It is important to act quickly but calmly and to provide support without increasing anxiety. The child should be allowed to remain in the position that provides the most comfort and security, and parents need to be reassured that everything possible is being done to provide relief for their child.

> **! NURSING ALERT**
>
> When epiglottitis is suspected, the nurse should not attempt to visualize the epiglottis directly with a tongue depressor or take a throat culture but instead refer the child for medical evaluation immediately.

Acute care of the child is the same as that described later for the child with LTB. Continuous monitoring of respiratory status, including pulse oximetry (and blood gases if the patient is intubated), is an important part of nursing observations, and the IV infusion is maintained as described in Chapter 44.

Acute Laryngotracheobronchitis

LTB is the most common croup syndrome. It affects primarily children younger than 5 years of age, and the causative organisms are viral agents, particularly the parainfluenza virus types 2 and 3, human metapneumovirus, RSV, influenza A, and influenza B. Other causative agents include *M. pneumoniae,* pneumococcus, and staphylococcus. The disease is usually preceded by an upper respiratory infection, which gradually descends to adjacent structures. It is characterized by gradual onset of low-grade fever, and the parents often report that the child went to bed and later awoke with a barky, brassy cough. When the airway is significantly narrowed, the child inspires air past the obstruction and into the lungs, producing the characteristic inspiratory stridor and suprasternal retractions. Other classic manifestations include cough and hoarseness. Respiratory distress in infants and toddlers may be manifested by nasal flaring, intercostal retractions, tachypnea, and continuous stridor. The typical child with LTB develops the classic barking or seal-like cough and acute stridor after several days of rhinitis. When the child is unable to inhale a sufficient volume of air, symptoms of hypoxia become evident. Obstruction that is severe enough to prevent adequate ventilation and exhalation of carbon dioxide can cause respiratory acidosis and eventually respiratory failure.

Therapeutic Management

The major objective in medical management is maintaining the airway and providing adequate respiratory exchange. Children with mild croup (no stridor at rest) can be managed at home. Parents should be taught the signs of respiratory distress and instructed to summon professional help early if needed.

The application of humidity with cool mist provides relief for most children. A cool-air vaporizer can be used at home but must be disinfected daily. Riding in the car with the windows down can help relieve the respiratory symptoms. In the hospital, a nebulized mist for older infants and toddlers may be used to provide increased humidity and supplemental oxygen.

Nebulized epinephrine (racemic epinephrine) is often used in children with severe disease, stridor at rest, retractions, or difficulty breathing. The alpha-adrenergic effects cause mucosal vasoconstriction and subsequently decrease subglottic edema. The onset of action is rapid, and the peak effect is observed in 2 hours. Children may be discharged home following racemic epinephrine after a 3- to 4-hour period of observation for return of acute symptoms.

Oral steroids (dexamethasone) have proven effective in the treatment of croup (often as a single dose) and are considered standard treatment for this condition (Roosevelt, 2016). IM dexamethasone may be given to children who are unable to tolerate oral dosing. Nebulized budesonide may be administered in conjunction with IM dexamethasone.

In severe cases of LTB, the administration of heliox may be used to reduce the work of breathing and relieve airway obstruction. It reduces airway turbulence but is not recommended as a standard treatment of croup.

NURSING CARE

The most important nursing function in the care of children with LTB is continuous, vigilant observation and accurate assessment of respiratory status. Pulse oximetry is commonly used for monitoring oxygenation status. Changes in therapy are frequently based on the nurses' observations and assessments and the child's response to therapy and tolerance of procedures. The trend away from early intubation of children with LTB emphasizes the importance of nursing observations and the ability to recognize impending respiratory failure so that intubation can be implemented without delay. Intubation equipment must be readily accessible and taken with the child during transport to other areas (e.g., radiology, operating room).

NURSING ALERT

Early signs of impending airway obstruction include increased pulse and respiratory rate; substernal, suprasternal, and intercostal retractions; nasal flaring; and increased restlessness.

Infants or small children find that being treated with cool mist, are coughing, or having laryngeal spasms, and needing IV therapy are additional sources of distress. In many acute care facilities the mist tent has been abandoned, and the parent is allowed to hold the infant. If cool mist is used in the treatment, it can be administered through a tube held in front of the patient while the child is held on the parent's lap.

Children with mild croup are allowed to drink beverages they like as long as respiratory status is stable, and parents should be encouraged to try whatever comforting measures work best (e.g., holding their child, rocking, singing). If the child is unable to take oral fluids, IV fluids may be required, and steroids may need to be given intravenously.

The rapid progression of croup, the alarming sound of the cough and stridor, and the child's apprehensive behaviour and ill appearance combine to create a frightening experience for the parents. They need reassurance about their child's progress and an explanation of treatments. The family should be allowed to remain with their child as much as possible.

The nurse should provide the parents with an opportunity to express their feelings and provide them with referrals as necessary. Parents need frequent reassurance provided in a calm, quiet manner and education regarding what they can do to make their child more comfortable.

Acute Spasmodic Laryngitis

Acute spasmodic laryngitis (spasmodic croup) is distinct from laryngitis and LTB and is characterized by paroxysmal attacks of laryngeal obstruction that occur chiefly at night. Signs of inflammation are absent or mild, and it is followed by an uneventful recovery. The child usually feels well the next day. Some children appear to be predisposed to the condition; allergies or hypersensitivities may be implicated in some cases. Management is the same as for infectious croup.

Bacterial Tracheitis

Bacterial tracheitis, an infection of the mucosa of the upper trachea, is a distinct entity with features of both croup and epiglottitis. The disease occurs typically between 5 and 7 years of age and may cause severe airway obstruction (Roosevelt, 2016). It is believed to be a complication of LTB, and although *Staphylococcus aureus* is the most frequent organism responsible, *M. catarrhalis, S. pneumonia,* and *H. influenzae* have also been implicated.

Many of the manifestations of bacterial tracheitis are similar to those of LTB but are unresponsive to LTB therapy. There is a history of previous upper respiratory infection with croupy cough, stridor unaffected by position, toxicity, absence of drooling, absence of dysphagia, and high fever. A prominent manifestation is the production of thick, purulent tracheal secretions. Respiratory difficulties are secondary to these copious secretions and mucosal edema at the level of the cricoid cartilage. The child's white cell count will be elevated. Children with this condition may develop a life-threatening upper airway obstruction, respiratory failure, acute respiratory distress syndrome (ARDS), and multiple organ dysfunction (Roosevelt, 2016).

NURSING CARE

Bacterial tracheitis requires vigorous management with antipyretics and antibiotics. Many children require endotracheal intubation and mechanical ventilation. Patients are closely monitored for impending respiratory failure if not intubated. Early recognition to prevent life-threatening airway obstruction is essential.

INFECTIONS OF THE LOWER AIRWAYS

The *reactive portion* of the lower respiratory tract includes the bronchi and bronchioles in children. Cartilaginous support of the large airways is not fully developed until adolescence. Consequently, the smooth muscle in these structures represents a major factor in the constriction of the airway, particularly in the *bronchioles*, the portion that extends from the bronchi to the alveoli. Table 45-2 compares some of the major features of bronchial and bronchiolar infections.

Bronchitis

Bronchitis (sometimes referred to as *tracheobronchitis*) is inflammation of the large airways (trachea and bronchi), which is frequently associated with an upper respiratory infection. See Table 45-2 for the etiological agents and predominant characteristics.

Bronchitis is a mild, self-limiting disease that requires only symptomatic treatment, including analgesics, antipyretics, and humidity. Cough suppressants in older children and adolescents may be useful to allow rest but can interfere with clearance of secretions; parents should discuss use of these with their health care provider before administering them. Most patients recover uneventfully in 5 to 10 days. It can be associated with underlying conditions such as CF and bronchiectasis and can become chronic in nature with a cough over 3 months.

TABLE 45-2 COMPARISON OF CONDITIONS AFFECTING THE BRONCHI

	ASTHMA*	BRONCHITIS	BRONCHIOLITIS
Description	Exaggerated response of bronchi to a trigger such as URI, dander, cold air, exercise Bronchospasm, exudation, and edema of bronchi, airway obstruction Inflammatory response	Usually occurs in association with URI Seldom an isolated entity	Most common infectious disease of lower airways Maximum obstructive impact at bronchiolar level
Age group affected	Infancy to adolescence	First 4 yr of life	Usually children 2–12 mo of age; rare after age 2 yr Peak incidence approximately age 6 mo
Etiological agents	Most often viruses such as RSV in infants but may be any of a variety of URI pathogens	Usually viral Other agents (e.g., bacteria, fungi, allergic disorders, airborne irritants) can trigger symptoms	Viruses, predominantly RSVs; also adenoviruses, parainfluenza viruses, human meta-pneumovirus, and *Mycoplasma pneumonia*
Predominant characteristics	Wheezing, cough	Persistent dry, hacking cough (worse at night) becoming productive in 2–3 days	Laboured respirations, poor feeding, cough, tachypnea, retractions and flaring nares, emphysema, increased nasal mucus, wheezing, may have fever
Treatment	Inhaled corticosteroids, bronchodilators, leukotriene modifiers, allergen, control of triggers, long-term anti-inflammatory medications	Cough suppressants if needed	Provide supplemental oxygen if saturations ≤90%; bronchodilators (optional) Suction nasopharynx Ensure adequate fluid intake Maintain adequate oxygenation

RSV, respiratory syncytial virus; *URI,* upper respiratory infection.
*See Asthma, p. 1365.

Adolescents with bronchitis should be screened for tobacco or marijuana use.

Respiratory Syncytial Virus and Bronchiolitis

Bronchiolitis is an acute viral infection with maximum effect at the bronchiolar level. By age 3, most children have been infected at least once. In Canada, RSV infection is the most frequent cause of hospitalization in children less than 2 years of age with bronchiolitis. In northern Canada, Indigenous children have one of the highest rates of RSV bronchiolitis hospitalizations in the world, with a 1% mortality rate and a 3% mortality rate for children with underlying cardiac or respiratory disease, respectively. Inuit children have a bronchiolitis rate of up to 57%. The Canadian RSV season is usually from November to April (Robinson, Le Saux, & CPS, Infectious Diseases and Immunization Committee, 2015/2016). Severe RSV infections in the first year of life have been thought to represent a significant risk factor for the development of asthma up to age 13. However, a strong causal relationship between RSV and later development of asthma has not been conclusively shown (Lotz, Moore, & Peebles, 2013). RSV infection may also occur in children older than 1 year who have a chronic or serious disabling illness. Occasionally, infants with RSV may have a concurrent viral or bacterial infection (e.g., otitis media, pertussis) (Coates, Camarda, & Goodman, 2016).

Risk factors include a birth month of November, December, or January; being in day care or having siblings in day care; more than six individuals living in the home; a birth weight less than the tenth percentile for gestational age; male gender; formula-fed infants; and immediate family history with eczema (Banerj, Greenberg, White, et al., 2009; Robinson et al., 2015/2016). A Nunavut study revealed additional factors: maternal smoking during pregnancy, residing in communities outside Iqaluit, being of full Inuit lineage, and overcrowding. The risk factors for infants developing severe RSV are being less than 6 weeks old, prematurity under 6 months of age, underlying cardiac or respiratory conditions, and immunocompromise (particularly transplant patients) (Robinson et al., 2015/2016).

RSV is transmitted from exposure to contaminated secretions. RSV can live on fomites for several hours and on hands for 30 minutes (AAP, Committee on Infectious Diseases, Kimberlin et al., 2015).

Pathophysiology

RSV affects the epithelial cells of the respiratory tract. The ciliated cells swell, protrude into the lumen, and lose their cilia. RSV produces a fusion of the infected cell membrane with cell membranes of adjacent epithelial cells, thus forming a giant cell. The bronchiolar mucosa swells, and lumina are subsequently filled with mucus and exudate. The walls of the bronchi and bronchioles are infiltrated with inflammatory cells, and peribronchiolar interstitial pneumonitis is usually present. The varying degrees of obstruction produced in small air passages lead to hyperinflation, obstructive emphysema resulting from partial obstruction, and patchy areas of atelectasis. Dilation of

BOX 45-8 SIGNS AND SYMPTOMS OF RESPIRATORY SYNCYTIAL VIRUS

Initial
Rhinorrhea
Pharyngitis
Coughing/sneezing
Wheezing
Possible ear or eye drainage
Intermittent fever

With Progression of Illness
Increased coughing and wheezing
Tachypnea and retractions
Cyanosis

Severe Illness
Tachypnea greater than 70 breaths/min
Listlessness
Apneic spells
Poor air exchange; decreased breath sounds

bronchial passages on inspiration allows sufficient space for intake of air, but narrowing of the passages on expiration prevents air from leaving the lungs. Thus air is trapped distal to the obstruction and causes progressive overinflation (emphysema).

Clinical Manifestations

The illness usually begins with an upper respiratory infection after an incubation of about 5 to 8 days. Symptoms such as rhinorrhea and low-grade fever often appear first. OM and conjunctivitis may also be present. In time, a cough may develop. If the disease progresses, it becomes a lower respiratory tract infection and manifests typical symptoms (Box 45-8). Infants may have several days of upper respiratory infection symptoms or no symptoms except slight lethargy, poor feeding, or irritability.

Once the lower airway is involved, classic manifestations include signs of altered air exchange, such as wheezing, retractions, crackles, dyspnea, tachypnea, and diminished breath sounds. Apnea may be the first recognized indicator of RSV infection in very young infants (younger than 1 month).

Diagnostic Evaluation

Identification has been simplified by the development of tests done on nasal or nasopharyngeal secretions, using either rapid immunofluorescent antibody–direct fluorescent antibody (DFA) staining or enzyme-linked immunosorbent assay (ELISA) techniques for RSV antigen detection (see Respiratory Secretion Specimens, Chapter 44). Hyperinflation of the lungs is generally seen on the chest x-ray.

Therapeutic Management

Children with bronchiolitis are treated symptomatically with cool humidified oxygen, adequate fluid intake, airway maintenance, and medications. Most children with bronchiolitis can be managed at home. Hospitalization is usually recommended for children with respiratory distress or those who cannot maintain adequate hydration. Other reasons for hospitalization include complicating conditions, such as underlying lung or heart disease or associated debilitated states, or a home environment where adequate management is questionable. An infant who is tachypneic or apneic, has marked retractions, seems listless, or has a history of poor fluid intake or is dehydrated should be closely observed for respiratory failure.

Humidified oxygen is administered via mask or head hood, in concentrations sufficient to maintain adequate oxygenation (Spo_2) at or above 90% as measured by pulse oximetry. An alternative oxygen delivery system is humidified high-flow nasal cannula therapy, which may be better tolerated and potentially decrease the need for mechanical ventilation but still needs further research on efficacy. Humidified mist may be administered, but a Cochrane review has shown no evidence that either supports or negates the use of mist (Friedman, Rieder, Walton, et al., 2014). Routine chest percussion and postural drainage (formerly chest physiotherapy [CPT]) are not recommended (Roqué i Figuls, Giné-Garriga, Granados Rugeles, et al., 2012). Infants with abundant nasal secretions benefit from periodic suctioning. Fluids by mouth may be contraindicated because of tachypnea, weakness, and fatigue; thus IV fluids are preferred until the acute stage of the disease has passed. Nasogastric fluids may be required if the infant is unable to tolerate oral fluids and a peripheral IV is difficult to establish.

Clinical assessments, noninvasive oxygen monitoring, and blood gas values may guide therapy. Medical therapy for bronchiolitis is primarily supportive and aimed at decreasing airway hyperresonance and inflammation and promoting adequate fluid intake. Bronchodilators may provide short-term benefits, yet overall significant improvement in the child's condition is not always appreciable. A single dose of bronchodilator therapy is often prescribed to assess for a clinical response. If it improves symptoms, it may be prescribed on an ongoing basis. If no response is evident, no further doses are given. Racemic epinephrine has been shown to produce modest improvement in ventilation status. Nebulized hypertonic 3% saline may decrease hospital stay and improve mucociliary clearance (Wright & Piedimonte, 2011).

Corticosteroids (inhaled or systemic) and antihistamines have not been shown to be effective and are not recommended for routine use. Antibiotics are not part of the treatment of RSV unless there is a coexisting bacterial infection such as OM (Friedman et al., 2014). Additional recommendations include encouraging breastfeeding, avoiding passive tobacco smoke exposure, and promoting preventive measures, including hand hygiene.

Prevention of respiratory syncytial virus infection. The only product available in Canada for prevention of RSV is palivizumab, a monoclonal antibody, which is given monthly in an IM injection during RSV season. According to the CPS, candidates for palivizumab treatment include infants at highest risk for a severe RSV infection and children with chronic lung disease of prematurity who require ongoing medical therapy, children with hemodynamically significant congenital heart disease who are younger than 24 months of age at the start of RSV season, and infants born before 32 weeks' gestational age and who are younger than 6 months at the start of the RSV season. Prophylaxis for RSV should be initiated at the onset of the RSV season and terminated at the end of the season (November to April) (Robinson et al., 2015/2016).

At the present time, the CPS recommends palivizumab to prevent RSV in high-risk populations (Robinson et al., 2015/2016).

MEDICATION ALERT

The lyophilized powder form of palivizumab should be administered within 6 hours of being reconstituted with sterile water because it is preservative free. A new liquid form of the drug may be available for future use.

NURSING CARE

Children admitted to the hospital with suspected RSV infection may be assigned separate rooms or grouped with other RSV-infected children. Droplet, contact, and routine precautions should be used, including hand hygiene, not touching one's nasal mucosa or conjunctiva, and using gloves, mask, and gowns when entering the patient's room. Other isolation procedures of potential benefit are those aimed at diminishing the number of hospital personnel, visitors, and uninfected children in contact with the child. Another measure is to make patient assignments so that nurses assigned to children with RSV are not caring for other patients who are considered high risk.

Infants with RSV often have copious nasal secretions, making breathing and feeding difficult. The child may lose weight or stop feeding altogether. If the child is breastfeeding, the mother should be encouraged to continue feeding the infant, or if feedings are contraindicated because of the acuity of the illness, the mother should pump her milk and store it appropriately for later use (see Chapter 27). Parents should be taught how to instill normal saline drops into the nares and suction the mucus with a bulb syringe before feedings and before bedtime so that the child can eat and rest better. Unfortunately, no medications appropriate for infants can help with these symptoms. To address the issue of decreased fluid intake, parents may offer small amounts of clear fluids, 5 to 10 mL at a time, with a medication syringe every 5 to 10 minutes or so to maintain adequate hydration. Infants may cough or vomit as the secretions settle in the stomach; this may make them prone to emesis of such secretions.

Additional nursing care is aimed at monitoring oxygenation with pulse oximetry, ensuring that bronchodilator therapy is optimized by using a small mask for delivery, and providing information for the parent regarding the infant's status. For the most part, infants recover quickly from the disease and resume normal daily activities, including fluid intake. Such infants are at risk for further episodes of wheezing that may or may not involve another RSV infection; parents, however, may be concerned that the infant has another serious case of RSV infection.

Pneumonias

Pneumonia, inflammation of the pulmonary parenchyma, is common in childhood but occurs more frequently in infancy and early childhood. Clinically, pneumonia may occur either as a primary disease or as a complication of another illness. The causative agent is either inhaled into the lungs directly or comes from the bloodstream.

The most useful classification of pneumonia is based on the etiological agent (i.e., viral, bacterial, mycoplasmal, or aspiration of foreign substances) (see Aspiration Pneumonia, p. 1361). Many organisms can cause pneumonia, and these vary according to the child's age (Fleisher & Ludwig, 2010). Histomycosis, coccidioidomycosis, and other fungi also cause pneumonia. *Pneumonitis* is a localized acute inflammation of the lung without the toxemia associated with lobar pneumonia.

The clinical manifestations of pneumonia vary depending on the etiological agent, the child's age, the child's systemic reaction to the infection, the extent of the lesions, and the degree of bronchial and bronchiolar obstruction (Box 45-9). The causative agent is identified from the clinical history, the child's age, the general health history, the physical examination, radiography, and the laboratory examination.

Viral Pneumonia

Viral pneumonias, which occur more frequently than bacterial pneumonias, are seen in children of all ages and are often associated with viral upper respiratory infections. Viruses that cause pneumonia include RSV in infants and parainfluenza, influenza, human meta-pneumovirus, and adenovirus in older children. Differentiation among viruses is usually made by clinical features, such as child's age, past medical history, season of the year, and radiographic and laboratory examination.

Viral infections of the respiratory tract render the affected child more susceptible to secondary bacterial invasion, especially when there is denuded bronchial mucosa. Treatment is symptomatic and includes measures to promote oxygenation and comfort, such as oxygen administration with cool mist,

BOX 45-9 GENERAL SIGNS OF PNEUMONIA

Fever—Usually quite high (≥ 39.5°C)
Respiratory
- Cough—Nonproductive to productive with whitish sputum
- Tachypnea
- Breath sounds—Rhonchi or fine crackles
- Dullness with percussion
- Chest pain; abdominal pain with lower lobe involvement
- Retractions
- Nasal flaring
- Pallor to cyanosis (depends on severity)

Chest x-ray film—Diffuse or patchy infiltration with peribronchial distribution
Behaviour—Irritable, restless, lethargic
Gastrointestinal—Anorexia, vomiting, diarrhea, abdominal pain

antipyretics for fever management, monitoring fluid intake, and family support. Antimicrobial therapy is usually reserved for children in whom a bacterial infection is demonstrated by appropriate cultures.

Primary Atypical Pneumonia

Atypical pneumonia refers to pneumonia that is caused by pathogens other than the traditionally most common and readily cultured bacteria (e.g., *S. pneumoniae*). In the category of atypical pneumonias, *M. pneumoniae* and *Chlamydia pneumoniae* are the most common causes of community-acquired pneumonia in children age 5 years or older (Kelly & Sandora, 2016). It occurs in the fall and winter months and is more prevalent in crowded living conditions. Most affected persons recover from acute illness in 7 to 10 days with symptomatic treatment followed by a week of convalescence. The incubation period is 2 to 3 weeks, but the cough may last several weeks. Hospitalization is rarely necessary.

Chlamydial pneumonia, caused by *C. trachomatis,* can occur in infants and generally appears between 3 and 19 weeks of age. The infant contracts this from the infected genital tract of the mother at birth.

Erythromycin (for those younger than 9 years), azithromycin, and clarithromycin are the primary agents used for treating atypical pneumonia.

Bacterial Pneumonia

S. pneumoniae is the most common bacterial pathogen responsible for community-acquired pneumonia in both children and adults (Kelly & Sandora, 2016). Other bacteria that cause pneumonia in children are group A streptococcus, *S. aureus, M. catarrhalis, M. pneumoniae,* and *C. pneumoniae.*

Beyond the newborn period, bacterial pneumonias display distinct clinical patterns that facilitate their differentiation from other forms of pneumonia. The onset of illness is abrupt and generally follows a viral infection that disturbs the natural defence mechanisms of the upper respiratory tract.

The child with bacterial pneumonia usually appears ill. Symptoms include fever, malaise, rapid and shallow respirations, cough, and chest pain. The pain of pneumonia may be referred to the abdomen and confused with appendicitis. Chills and meningeal symptoms (*meningism*) are common.

Most older children with pneumonia can be treated at home if the condition is recognized and treatment is initiated early. Antibiotic therapy, bedrest, liberal oral intake of fluid, and administration of an antipyretic for fever are the principal therapeutic measures. Follow-up examination is recommended for small infants and toddlers. Hospitalization is indicated when pleural effusion or empyema accompanies the disease, when respiratory distress occurs, in situations in which compliance with therapy is difficult, in infants less than 1 month old, and when there are chronic illnesses such as heart disease or BPD (Chibuk, Cohen, Robinson, et al., 2011/2015). IV fluids may be necessary to ensure adequate hydration, and oxygen is required if the child is in respiratory distress; some children may require initial therapy with parenteral antibiotics because of the severity of illness.

Complications. At present, the classic features and clinical course of pneumonia are seen infrequently because of early and vigorous antibiotic and supportive therapy. However, some children, especially infants, with staphylococcal or GABHS pneumonia develop empyema, pyopneumothorax, or tension pneumothorax. AOM and pleural effusion are common in children with pneumococcal pneumonia.

Continuous closed-chest drainage may be instituted when purulent fluid is aspirated. If a large amount of purulent drainage is obtained, an appropriate antibiotic is instilled into the pleural space, and active chest drainage is discontinued for approximately 1 hour after the instillation. Closed drainage is continued until drainage fluid is free of pathogens, which rarely requires more than 5 to 7 days. Sometimes, repeated pleural taps are sufficient to remove fluid; however, if the purulent drainage accumulates rapidly and is highly viscous, continuous chest drainage is preferred. Thoracotomy with open debridement of the infected lung tissue may be required; if empyema and pneumothorax tend to recur, a partial thoracoscopic lobectomy may be performed. Alternatively, video-assisted thoroscopy (VATS) or insertion of a small-bore percutaneous chest tube with instillation of fibrinolytics are the best current options for and may preclude the use of open debridement and thoracotomy (Chibuk et al., 2011/2015).

Prevention. Currently, the use of the heptavalent pneumococcal conjugate vaccine (PCV-13) is recommended for infants and children (see vaccination schedule in Additional Resources at the end of this chapter). This addition has nearly eradicated invasive pneumococcal disease in children and adults. This vaccine has also decreased the rates of lobar pneumonia, pneumococcal meningitis, and OM. There has been a relatively small increase in an antibiotic-resistant strain of pneumococcal pneumonia (serotype-19) that has developed as result of the vaccine. In Quebec, in the under-5-year age group, there was a 72% drop in hospital admissions for lobar pneumonia and a 13% decline in admissions for all-cause pneumonia after the universal pneumococcal vaccine was introduced (Chibuk et al., 2011/2015; De Wals, Robin, Fortin, et al., 2008).

NURSING CARE

Nursing care of the hospitalized child with pneumonia is primarily supportive and symptomatic but necessitates thorough respiratory assessment as well as administration of supplemental oxygen (as required), fluids, and antibiotics. The child's respiratory rate and oxygenation status, as well as vital signs, pain level, and general disposition and level of activity, are frequently assessed. To prevent dehydration, fluids should be frequently administered intravenously during the acute phase.

Nursing care of the child with a chest tube requires close attention to respiratory status, as noted previously; the chest tube and drainage device used should be monitored for proper function (i.e., drainage is not impeded, vacuum setting is correct, tubing is free of kinks, dressing covering chest tube insertion site is intact, water seal is maintained [if used], and chest tube remains in place). Movement in bed and ambulation with a chest tube should be encouraged according to the child's

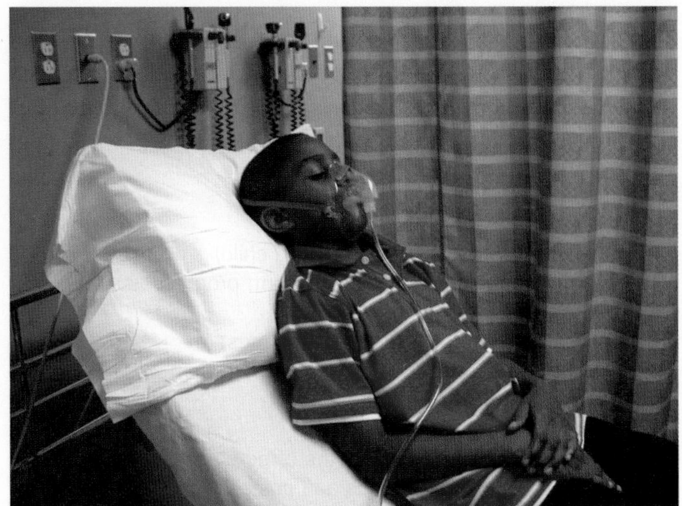

FIGURE 45-3 A child placed in a semierect position is often more comfortable, and this position enhances diaphragmatic expansion.

respiratory status; children often require a mild analgesic such as acetaminophen.

If needed, supplemental oxygen may be administered by nasal cannula, face mask, or blow-by (which is the process of wafting or blowing oxygen past a child's face). Children are usually more comfortable in a semierect position (Fig. 45-3) but should be allowed to determine the position of comfort. Lying on the affected side (if pneumonia is unilateral) splints the chest on that side and can reduce the pleural rubbing that often causes discomfort. Fever is controlled by the cool environment and administration of antipyretic medications.

Children, especially infants, with ineffectual cough or difficulty handling secretions require suctioning to maintain a patent airway. A simple bulb suction syringe is usually sufficient for clearing the nares and nasopharynx of infants, but mechanical suction should be readily available if needed. A noninvasive suction device may be used to suction the infant's nares without the danger of causing nasal trauma; the device may be connected to mechanical suction for best results. Older children can usually handle secretions without assistance. Chest percussion, incentive spirometer, postural drainage, and nebulized bronchodilator treatments may be prescribed, depending on the child's condition. Chest percussions and postural drainage currently lack research evidence for improving a patient's condition or decreasing length of stay among children with community-acquired pneumonia.

The presence of a caregiver often provides the child with a source of comfort and support. It is important to involve the entire family in the child's care, as appropriate, and to encourage questions and facilitate effective communication. Allowing the child to be involved in regular activities, such as quiet play, may help reduce the anxiety and fears of hospitalization.

For the child being cared for at home, the nurse needs to educate the parents regarding observation for worsening symptoms, antibiotic and antipyretic administration, and encouragement of oral fluid intake. Return to school or day care is usually permitted according to the type of pneumonia, severity of illness, and health care provider's recommendation. It should be emphasized that the infection may be transmitted to other children through close contact.

OTHER RESPIRATORY TRACT INFECTIONS

Pertussis (Whooping Cough)

Pertussis, or whooping cough, is an acute respiratory tract infection caused by *Bordetella pertussis* that in the past occurred primarily in children younger than 4 years of age who were not immunized. It is highly contagious and is particularly threatening in young infants, who have a higher morbidity and mortality rate. In Canada, one to four deaths each year are related to pertussis, usually in infants who are too young to be immunized or only partly immunized (PHAC, 2014b). It can result in encephalopathy, seizures, and pneumonia. Infants less than 6 months of age may not come in to the practitioner with the typical cough; in this age group, apnea is a common presenting manifestation (AAP, Committee on Infectious Diseases, Kimberlin, et al., 2015). Likewise, older children are known to manifest the disease with a persistent cough and the absence of the characteristic whoop (see Table 37-2 for clinical manifestations of pertussis and Chapter 35, p. 1018, for immunization). The incidence is highest in the spring and summer months, and a single attack confers lifetime immunity. The resurgence of pertussis in Canada, particularly in older children and adults, is due to weakening immunity from vaccines produced in the mid-1990s as well as some parents opting not to immunize their children. Two acellular pertussis booster vaccines have been approved in Canada and include one for 2 months to 7 years of age and the other for ages 11 years to 54 years (PHAC, 2015). This older population is a reservoir for pertussis, which can be passed along to the young at-risk infant. Adults should have a booster of pertussis, diphtheria, and tetanus every 10 years (PHAC, 2016b).

Most children with pertussis can be managed at home. Care is supportive and includes encouraging adequate hydration and administering antipyretics. When coughing spasms occur in small children, they can be frightening for the parents and family. Admission to the hospital occurs if respiratory symptoms are severe or if apnea occurs. Treatment with antibiotics (erythromycin, clarithromycin, or azithromycin) in the catarrhal stage may result in a milder form of the infection, but treatment also prevents spread to others (AAP, Committee on Infectious Diseases, Kimberlin et al., 2015). Family contacts may also be treated. Pertussis symptoms usually last for 6 to 10 weeks but may persist for longer.

Tuberculosis

Tuberculosis (TB) is an infectious disease that most Canadians will never develop. In Canada, there are approximately 1600 new cases of reported TB every year (Government of Canada, 2016). TB affects about 100 to 120 Canadians under the age of 15 on a yearly basis. Marginalized populations such as remote, Indigenous communities and new Canadians are particularly at risk (CPS, 2014). The risk factors for developing TB include the following populations: those with human immunodeficiency virus (HIV) or acquired immune deficiency syndrome (AIDS); those who come in close contact with individuals with known or suspected active TB, or who have a past history of TB but did not receive adequate treatment; individuals living in Indigenous communities with high rates of TB; poor, particularly urban homeless individuals; residents of long-term care and correctional facilities; individuals with transplants, diabetes mellitus, or cancer of the head and neck; those with chronic kidney disease who are on dialysis; those who have been infected by TB bacteria within the past 2 years; individuals who have undergone steroid treatments or treatment for autoimmune disorders; those who are underweight or were under age 5 when infected with TB; individuals who smoke 1 pack of cigarettes a day or more; and individuals working with any of these groups (Government of Canada, 2015).

TB is caused by *Mycobacterium tuberculosis*. Children are susceptible to the human (*M. tuberculosis*) and the bovine (*Mycobacterium bovis*) organisms. In parts of the world where TB in cattle is not controlled or milk is not pasteurized, the bovine type is a common source of infection.

Although the causative agent for TB is the tubercle bacillus, other factors influence the degree to which the organism produces an altered state in the host. These factors include heredity (resistance to the infection may be genetically transmitted), gender (higher rates among adolescent girls), age (lower resistance in infants, higher incidence during adolescence), stress (emotional or physical), nutritional state, and intercurrent infection (especially HIV, measles, and pertussis). Children with HIV infection have an increased incidence of TB, and all children with TB should be tested for HIV.

The source of TB infection in children is usually an infected member of the household or a frequent visitor to the home. The airway is the usual portal of entry for the organism. In the lungs, a proliferation of epithelial cells surrounds and encapsulates the multiplying bacilli in an attempt to wall it off, thus forming the typical tubercle. Extension of the primary lesion at the original site causes progressive tissue destruction as it spreads within the lung, discharges material from foci to other areas of the lungs (e.g., bronchi, pleura), or produces pneumonia. Erosion of blood vessels by the primary lesion can cause widespread dissemination of the tubercle bacillus to near and distant sites (miliary TB). Extrapulmonary (miliary) TB may manifest as superior lymphadenitis, meningitis, and osteoarthritis and may appear in the middle ear and mastoid and on the skin (AAP, Committee on Infectious Diseases, Kimberlin et al., 2015). With the exception of meningitis, treatment for extrapulmonary TB may be with the same medication regimen as for pulmonary TB. Infants and children younger than 3 years of age are more likely to develop miliary TB.

Diagnostic Evaluation

Diagnosis is based on information derived from physical examination, history, tuberculin skin testing, radiographic examinations, and cultures of the organism. The clinical manifestations of the disease are extremely variable (Box 45-10).

The *tuberculin skin test (TST)* is the most important indicator of whether a child has been infected with the tubercle bacillus. The standard dose of purified protein derivative (PPD) is 5 tuberculin units, which is administered using a 27-gauge needle and a 1-mL syringe intradermally into the volar aspect of the forearm. Creation of a visible wheal is crucial to accurate testing. In Canada, the current recommendations are to screen only children who are at high risk for TB infections or who are progressing from latent to active TB disease (Kakkar, Allen, Ling, et al., 2010/2015).

A *positive reaction* indicates that the individual has been infected and has developed sensitivity to the tubercle bacillus. However, it does not confirm the presence of active disease. The test is usually positive 2 to 10 weeks after initial infection with the organism. If a child received a previous bacille Calmette-Guérin (BCG) immunization he or she will always react positively. A previously negative reaction that becomes positive indicates that the person has been infected since the last test. Guidelines for interpreting the TST are listed in Box 45-11. Prompt radiographic evaluation of all children with a positive TST reaction is recommended.

The term *latent tuberculosis infection* (LTBI) is used to indicate infection in a person who has a positive TST, no physical findings of disease, and normal chest radiograph findings. The majority of children are asymptomatic when a positive skin test result is found, and most of them do not go on to develop the disease. The term *tuberculosis disease* or *clinically active TB* is used when a child has clinical symptoms or radiographic manifestations caused by the *M. tuberculosis* organism. A diagnosis of TB disease represents recent transmission of the *M. tuberculosis* organism and is an urgent event for public health. Prompt evaluation, treatment, and identification and treatment of contacts are key components to managing TB.

New blood tests have been developed to help diagnose LTBI. The two interferon-gamma-release-assay (IGRA) tests that are registered in Canada are QuantiFERON-TB Gold In-Tube assay and the T. Spot-TB test, which provide greater sensitivity and accuracy. The TST is not very sensitive for detecting LTBI and

BOX 45-10 CLINICAL MANIFESTATIONS OF TUBERCULOSIS

May be asymptomatic or produce a broad range of symptoms:
- Fever
- Malaise
- Anorexia
- Weight loss (or failure to grow in child)
- Cough (may or may not be present; progresses slowly over weeks to months)
- Aching pain and tightness in the chest
- Hemoptysis (rare)

With progression:
- Increased respiratory rate
- Poor expansion of lung on the affected side
- Diminished breath sounds and crackles
- Dullness on percussion
- Persistent fever
- Pallor, anemia, weakness, and weight loss

BOX 45-11 DEFINITION OF POSITIVE TUBERCULIN SKIN TEST (TST) RESULTS IN INFANTS, CHILDREN, AND ADOLESCENTS*

Induration 5 mm or Greater

Children in close contact with known or suspected contagious cases of tuberculosis (TB) disease

Children suspected of having TB disease:

- Findings on chest x-ray film consistent with active or previously active TB
- Clinical evidence of TB disease†

Children receiving immune suppressive therapy‡ or who have immunosuppressive conditions, including HIV infection

Induration 10 mm or Greater

Children at increased risk of disseminated disease:

- Those younger than 4 years of age
- Those with other medical risk conditions, including Hodgkin's disease, lymphoma, diabetes mellitus, chronic renal failure, or malnutrition

Children at increased risk of exposure to TB disease:

- Those born, or whose parents were born, in high-prevalence (TB) regions of the world
- Those frequently exposed to adults who are HIV infected, homeless, users of illicit drugs, residents of nursing homes, incarcerated or institutionalized, or migrant farm workers
- Those who travel to high-prevalence (TB) regions of the world

Induration 15 mm or Greater

Children 4 years of age or older without any risk factors

*These definitions apply regardless of previous Bacille Calmette-Guérin (BCG) immunization; erythema at TST site does not indicate a positive test result. TSTs should be read at 48 to 72 hours after placement.

†Evidence by physical examination or laboratory assessment that would include tuberculosis in the working differential diagnosis (e.g., meningitis).

‡Including immunosuppressive doses of corticosteroids.

From Canadian Thoracic Society. (2013). *Canadian tuberculosis standards* (7th ed.). Chapter 16, Bacille Calmette-Guérin (BCG) vaccination in Canada. Retrieved from http://www.respiratoryguidelines.ca/tb-standards-2013

can give a false-positive reading. The usefulness and ability of IGRA is limited in children under 2 years of age. The CPS recommends that the IGRA be used as a diagnostic aid in combination with the TST and other radiological and culture tests to help diagnose active TB (Kakkar et al., 2010/2015). IGRA cannot be used to diagnose TB without other positive tests. A negative IGRA test does not mean that a child does not have LTBI.

Therapeutic Management

Medical management of TB disease in children consists of adequate nutrition, pharmacotherapy, general supportive measures, prevention of unnecessary exposure to other infections that would further compromise the body's defences, prevention of reinfection, and sometimes surgical procedures. Family members and other contacts should also be assessed for symptoms by public health providers and treated accordingly.

The recommended medication regimen for LTBI in children and adolescents includes a 6- or 9-month course of isoniazid (INH) in either a daily dose or divided into two doses per week, with direct observation of therapy (DOT). DOT means that a health care worker or other responsible, mutually agreed-on individual is present when medications are administered to the patient. Rifampin (daily for 6 months; alternatively, DOT twice weekly for 6 months) may be used to treat the child or adolescent who is INH resistant (Canadian Thoracic Society & PHAC, 2013).

For the child with clinically active TB, the goal is to achieve sterilization of the tuberculous lesion. Recommended medication therapy for treating TB disease includes combinations of INH, rifampin, and pyrazinamide (PZA) and ethambutol. The Canadian Thoracic Society and Public Health Agency of Canada (2013) recommend a 6-month regimen consisting of INH, rifampin, ethambutol, and PZA given daily for the first 2 months, followed by INH and rifampin given two or three times a week by DOT for the remaining 4 months. DOT decreases the rates of relapse, treatment failures, and drug resistance and is recommended for treatment of children and adolescents with TB in Canada.

In 2010, the WHO recommended that previously treated patients should have access to drug-susceptibility testing and culture at the beginning of treatment to identify possible multidrug–TB resistance. The WHO also updated recommendations for individuals with HIV and TB; these include starting antiretroviral therapy within 8 weeks after the initiation of antituberculosis treatment and the use of a clinical algorithm to screen for TB in persons with HIV, those at high risk for HIV, or those living in congregate settings (Perez-Velez, 2012).

Surgical procedures may be required to remove the source of infection in tissues that are inaccessible to pharmacotherapy or that are destroyed by the disease. Orthopaedic procedures may be performed for correction of bone deformities, and bronchoscopy may be done for removal of a tuberculous granulomatous polyp.

Prognosis

Most children recover from primary TB infection and are often unaware of its presence. However, very young children have a higher incidence of disseminated disease. TB is a serious disease during the first 2 years of life, during adolescence, and in children who are HIV positive. Except in cases of tuberculous meningitis, death seldom occurs in treated children. Antibiotic therapy has decreased the death rate and the hematogenous spread from primary lesions.

Prevention

The only definite means of preventing TB is to avoid contact with the tubercle bacillus. Maintaining an optimal state of health with adequate nutrition and avoiding fatigue and debilitating infections promote natural resistance but do not prevent infection. Pasteurization and routine testing of milk and elimination of diseased cattle have reduced the incidence of bovine TB.

Limited immunity can be produced by the administration of BCG, a live vaccine containing bovine bacilli with reduced virulence (attenuated). In most instances, positive tuberculin reactions develop after inoculation with BCG. In more recent years, BCG use in Canada has been limited to Inuit and on-reserve Indigenous children born to mothers who tested negative for HIV prenatally. However, recommendations concerning the continued use of BCG in this and other Canadian populations have recently been revised. The vaccine is slowly being withdrawn across Canada, even from the Indigenous peoples. Currently, the National Advisory Committee on Immunization (NACI) does not recommend BCG vaccination for all Canadians. However, it allows that, in some settings, consideration of local TB epidemiology and access to diagnostic services may lead to the decision to offer BCG (Canadian Thoracic Society & PHAC, 2013).

Canada has one of the lowest TB rates in the world, although for Indigenous people living on reserve, the reported incidence of active TB was 26.6 per 100,000 in 2008, which was 29.6 times higher than the rate for the Canadian-born non-Indigenous population (Government of Canada, 2016). Rates are high among Indigenous children and young adults. Additional risk factors for this population include substance use, diabetes, HIV, overcrowding, and moving from reserve to reserve (Government of Canada, 2016).

NURSING CARE

Most hospitalized children with TB are not contagious and require only routine precautions. Children with no cough and negative sputum smears can be hospitalized in a regular patient room. However, airborne precautions and a negative-pressure room are required for children who are contagious and hospitalized with active TB disease. Infection control for hospital personnel in contagious cases should include the use of a personally fitted air-purifying N95 or N100 respirator for all patient contacts.

Asymptomatic children with TB can attend school or day care facilities if they are receiving pharmacotherapy. They can return to regular activities as soon as effective therapy has been instituted, adherence to therapy has been documented, and clinical symptoms have diminished. Children receiving pharmacotherapy for TB can receive measles and other age-appropriate live virus vaccines unless they are receiving high-dose corticosteroids, are severely ill, or have specific contraindications to immunization. Children with TB should also receive optimal nutrition and adequate rest.

Sputum specimens are either difficult or impossible to obtain from an infant or young child, because they swallow any mucus coughed from the lower respiratory tract. The best means for obtaining material for smears or culture is by gastric washing (i.e., aspiration of lavaged contents from the fasting stomach). The procedure is carried out and the specimen obtained early in the morning before the customary breakfast time. In some cases, an induced sputum specimen may be obtained by administering aerosolized normal saline for 10 to 15 minutes, followed by chest percussion and postural drainage and suctioning of the nasopharynx for sputum collection.

Because the success of therapy depends on adherence to the medication regimen, parents need to be instructed about the importance and rationale for DOT. Case finding in the community and follow-up of known contacts—individuals from whom the affected child may have acquired the disease and persons who may have been exposed to the child with the disease—are essential control measures.

PULMONARY DYSFUNCTION CAUSED BY NONINFECTIOUS IRRITANTS

Foreign Body Aspiration

Small children characteristically explore matter with their mouths and are prone to aspirate a foreign body (FB). They also place objects such as beads, paper clips, small magnets, or food items in the nose, which can easily be aspirated into the trachea. While FB aspiration can occur at any age, it is most common in children 1 to 3 years of age. Severity is determined by the location, type of object aspirated, and extent of obstruction. For example, dry vegetable matter, such as a seed, nut, or piece of carrot or popcorn, that does not dissolve and that may swell when wet creates a particularly difficult problem. The high fat content of potato chips and peanuts may cause the added risk of lipoid pneumonia. "Fun foods" are the worst offenders in terms of potential for aspiration. Offending foods in the order of frequency of aspiration are hot dog, round candy, peanut or other nut, grape, cookie or biscuit, other meat, carrot, peas, apple, and peanut butter. Objects such as small lithium or cadmium batteries may cause esophageal or tracheal corrosion.

Diagnostic Evaluation

The diagnosis of FB aspiration is suspected on the basis of the history and physical signs. Initially, a FB in the air passages produces choking, gagging, wheezing, or coughing. Laryngotracheal obstruction most commonly causes dyspnea, cough, stridor, and hoarseness because of decreased air entry. Up to half of all children with FB ingestion may be asymptomatic. Cyanosis may occur if the obstruction becomes worse. Bronchial obstruction usually produces cough (frequently paroxysmal), wheezing, asymmetrical breath sounds, decreased airway entry, and dyspnea. When an object is lodged in the larynx, the child is unable to speak or breathe. If the obstruction progresses, the child's face may become livid; if the obstruction is total, the child can become unconscious and die of asphyxiation. If obstruction is partial, hours, days, or even weeks may pass without symptoms after the initial period. Secondary symptoms are related to the anatomical area in which the object is lodged and are usually caused by a persistent respiratory tract infection distal to the obstruction. FB aspiration should also be suspected in the presence of acute or chronic pulmonary lesions.

Often, by the time secondary symptoms appear, the parents have forgotten the initial episode of coughing and gagging. Nasal FB cases are often symptomatic with unilateral purulent drainage that does not improve over time.

Radiographic examination can reveal opaque FBs but is of limited use in localizing nonradiographic matter. Bronchoscopy is required for a definitive diagnosis of objects in the larynx and trachea. Fluoroscopic examination is valuable in detecting FBs in the bronchi. The mainstay of diagnosis and management of FBs is endoscopy.

Therapeutic Management

FB aspiration may result in life-threatening airway obstruction, especially in infants because of the small diameter of their airways. Current recommendations for the emergency treatment of the choking child include the use of abdominal thrusts for children older than 1 year of age and back blows and chest thrusts for those younger than 1 year of age (see Airway Obstruction, p. 1388).

A FB is rarely coughed up spontaneously. Most frequently, it must be removed instrumentally by endoscopy. Endoscopy and bronchoscopy require sedation with an agent such as IV propofol or midazolam. The procedure is carried out as quickly as possible because the progressive local inflammatory process triggered by the foreign material hampers removal. A chemical pneumonia soon develops, and vegetable matter begins to macerate within a few days, making it even more difficult to remove. After removal of the FB, the child is usually observed for any complications, such as laryngeal edema, and discharged home within a matter of hours if vital signs are stable and recovery is satisfactory.

Prevention

Nurses are in a position to teach prevention of FB aspiration, in a variety of settings. They can educate parents singly or in groups about hazards of aspiration in relation to the developmental level of their children and encourage them to teach their children safety. Parents should be cautioned about behaviours that their children might imitate (e.g., holding foreign objects, such as pins, nails, and toothpicks, in their lips or mouth). (Prevention based on the child's age is discussed in Chapters 35, 36, and 37.)

NURSING CARE

A major role of nurses caring for a child who has aspirated an FB is to recognize the signs of FB aspiration, observe for worsening respiratory symptoms, and implement immediate measures to relieve the obstruction. Choking on food or other material should not be fatal. Back blows and chest thrusts in infants and abdominal thrusts in children are simple procedures that can be used by both health care providers and laypersons to save lives (see Fig. 45-15). To aid a child who is choking, nurses must recognize the signs of distress. A blind sweep of the child's mouth should never be performed because it may lodge the agent farther into the airway. Not every child who gags or coughs while eating is truly choking.

> **! NURSING ALERT**
>
> The child in severe distress (1) cannot speak, (2) becomes cyanotic, and (3) collapses. These three signs indicate that the child is truly choking and requires immediate action. The child can die within 4 minutes.

Aspiration Pneumonia

Aspiration pneumonia occurs when food, secretions, inert materials, volatile compounds, or liquids enter the lung and cause inflammation and a chemical pneumonitis. Aspiration of fluid or foods is a particular hazard in the child who has difficulty swallowing; is unable to swallow because of paralysis, weakness, debility, congenital anomalies, or absent cough reflex; or is force-fed, especially while crying or breathing rapidly. Clinical signs of the aspiration of oral secretions may not be distinguishable from those of other forms of acute bacterial pneumonia. For example, if vegetable matter has been aspirated, manifestations may not appear for several weeks after the event. Classic symptoms include an increasing cough or fever with foul-smelling sputum, deteriorating chest radiographs, and other signs of lower airway involvement. However, these deviations may persist for weeks while the child starts to feel better. Rarely, aspiration causes immediate death from asphyxia; more often the irritated mucous membrane becomes a site for secondary bacterial infection. In addition to fluids, food, vomitus, and nasopharyngeal secretions, other substances that may cause pneumonia are hydrocarbons, lipids, powder, and barium. The severity of the lung injury depends on the pH of the aspirated material.

NURSING CARE

Care of the child with aspiration pneumonia is the same as that described for the child with pneumonia from other causes. However, the major focus of nursing care is on the prevention of aspiration. Proper feeding techniques should be carried out for weak and debilitated children and those who cannot assist in feeding, and preventive measures should be used to prevent aspiration of any material that might enter the nasopharynx. The presence of a nasogastric feeding tube or a history of gastroesophageal reflux disease places the child at risk for aspiration. Nasogastric tubes used for feedings should be checked before the initiation of bolus feedings; continuous nasogastric tube feedings also need to be evaluated periodically for proper tube placement. Children who are at risk for swallowing difficulties as a result of illness, physical debilitation, anaesthesia, or sedation should be kept NPO (nothing by mouth) until they can properly swallow fluids effectively. The child who is at risk for vomiting and incapable of protecting the airway should be positioned in a side-lying recovery position.

Educating parents on the prevention of aspiration is important.

Pulmonary Edema

Pulmonary edema is the movement of fluid into the alveoli and interstitium of the lungs that is caused by extravasation of fluid from the pulmonary vasculature (Mazor & Green, 2016). There are two main types of pulmonary edema—cardiogenic and noncardiogenic. Cardiogenic (hydrostatic, hemodynamic) pulmonary edema is caused by an increase in pulmonary capillary pressure because of an increase in pulmonary venous pressure. It can be caused by excessive IV fluid administration, left ventricular failure, heart valve disorder (aortic regurgitation, aortic stenosis, mitral regurgitation), myocardial ischemia, myocarditis, sepsis, acute tachydysrhythmia, or coronary arteriosclerosis (Mazor &Green, 2016).

Noncardiogenic pulmonary edema is caused by various conditions that result in increased pulmonary capillary permeability. Some subtypes of noncardiogenic pulmonary edema include permeability pulmonary edema (caused by ARDS or acute lung injury [ALI]), high-altitude pulmonary edema (caused by rapid ascension to heights above 3600 metres), and neurogenic pulmonary edema (after central nervous system [CNS] insult, such as seizures, head injury, or cerebral hemorrhage). Some less common forms of PE are reperfusion pulmonary edema (after removal of thromboemboli from the lung or a lung transplant), re-expansion pulmonary edema (caused by rapid re-expansion of a collapsed lung), and pulmonary edema that results from opiate overdose (methadone or heroin), salicylate toxicity (chronic), aspiration (FB inhalation), inhalation injuries, near submersion injury, pulmonary embolism, viral infections, or pulmonary venoocclusive disease. Other causes include traumatic injury, organ dysfunction caused by sepsis, multiorgan failure, alcoholism or substance use, pregnancy (eclampsia), chronic renal impairment, malnutrition, hypertension, or a blood transfusion (transfusion-related ALI).

Pathophysiology

Fluid flows from the pulmonary vasculature into the alveolar interstitial space and then returns to the systemic circulation in a normal lung. Movement of this fluid is controlled by the net difference between hydrostatic and osmotic pressures and the permeability of the capillary membrane (Mazor & Green, 2016). Increased pulmonary hydrostatic pressure or increased permeability of the vascular membrane results in movement of fluid into the alveoli and interstitium of the lung. The pulmonary lymph system normally drains away any fluid from the alveoli, but when the amount of fluid present in the alveoli exceeds lymph drainage, pulmonary edema occurs.

Symptoms include extreme shortness of breath, cyanosis, tachypnea, diminished breath sounds, anxiety, agitation, confusion, diaphoresis, orthopnea, respiratory crackles, expiratory wheezing (in young infants), heart murmur, third heart sound (S_3) gallop, cool extremities, jugular venous distention, nocturnal dyspnea, cough, pink frothy sputum (if severe), tachycardia, hypertension, and hypotension (if caused by left ventricle dysfunction).

Therapeutic Management

Management of pulmonary edema depends on the cause but can include oxygen therapy, peak end-expiratory pressure (PEEP) via continuous positive airway pressure (CPAP), and intubation with ventilatory support if respiratory failure occurs. If ventricular failure is the cause, medications such as diuretics, digoxin, positive inotropes, and vasodilators (nitroglycerin) may be started and the child may be placed on a fluid and sodium restriction. Morphine may be prescribed to relieve dyspnea. The primary goal of management is to determine why pulmonary edema occurred and to treat the underlying condition.

NURSING CARE

Nursing care of the child with pulmonary edema is similar to that for any other acute respiratory condition. Pulse oximetry is monitored, and vital signs are observed closely for any deterioration. The nurse should note changes in oxygen saturation (Sao_2), end-tidal carbon dioxide (CO_2), and arterial blood gas (ABG) values. An ongoing assessment of the child's cardiopulmonary status is needed by checking lung sounds and observing respiratory rate, rhythm, depth, and effort. Oxygen, medications, and other respiratory treatments are administered as prescribed. Close monitoring of intake and output, electrolytes, and comfort is important. The child should be monitored for restlessness, anxiety, and air hunger. Placing the child in a high Fowler position may help with lung expansion. Because this position places pressure on bony prominences in the sacrum and hips, pressure areas must be relieved at intervals. Most of the care of pulmonary edema occurs in the critical care unit, which can be anxiety provoking for the child and family. They should be given the opportunity to express their fears and anxieties and to ask questions. (For other nursing care activities, see the following section on ARDS and ALI.)

Acute Respiratory Distress Syndrome (ARDS)/Acute Lung Injury (ALI)

ARDS and ALI are potentially life-threatening inflammatory lung conditions that may occur in both children and adults. The syndromes may be caused by direct injury to the lungs or be systemic insults that lead indirectly to lung injury, categorized by acute onset of bilateral infiltrates consistent with pulmonary edema but there is no indication of elevated left atrial pressure. They result in hypoxemia and respiratory failure. Sepsis, **trauma**, viral pneumonia, aspiration, fat emboli, drug overdose, reperfusion injury after lung transplantation, smoke inhalation, and submersion injury, among others, have been associated with ALI and ARDS. Both conditions are characterized by respiratory distress and hypoxemia that occur within 72 hours of a serious injury or surgery in a person with previously normal lungs. Acute pulmonary inflammation with alveolar capillary membrane destruction results in significant hypoxemia, and mechanical ventilation is often required. ARDS is most severe in the spectrum of illnesses in relation to the degree of hypoxemia. Mechanical ventilation is often required.

Diagnostic criteria include radiographic evidence of bilateral alveolar infiltrates, the absence of left-sided heart failure, and hypoxemia. ALI is differentiated from the more severe syndrome of ARDS by the severity of hypoxemia. In ALI, the P/F ratio is less than or equal to 300; in ARDS, the P/F ratio is less than or equal to 200. ARDS is the more severe in the spectrum of illnesses in relation to the degree of hypoxemia (Ashok, Sarnaik, Clark, et al., 2016).

Pathologically, the hallmark of ARDS is increased permeability of the alveolar-capillary membrane that results in pulmonary edema. During the acute phase of ARDS, the alveolocapillary membrane is damaged, with an increasing pulmonary capillary permeability and resulting interstitial edema. Later stages are characterized by pneumocyte and fibrin infiltration of the alveoli, with the start of either the healing process or fibrosis. When fibrosis occurs, the child may demonstrate respiratory distress and the need for mechanical ventilation. In ARDS, the lungs become stiff as a result of surfactant inactivation, gas diffusion is impaired, and eventually bronchiolar mucosal swelling and congestive atelectasis occur. The net effect is decreased functional residual capacity, pulmonary hypertension, and increased intrapulmonary right-to-left shunting of pulmonary blood flow. Surfactant secretion is reduced, and the atelectasis and fluid-filled alveoli provide an excellent medium for bacterial growth. Hypoxemia or increased work of breathing may require ventilator support.

The child with ARDS may first demonstrate only symptoms caused by an injury or infection, but as the condition deteriorates, hyperventilation, tachypnea, increasing respiratory effort, cyanosis, and decreasing oxygen saturation occur. At times, the developing hypoxemia is not responsive to oxygen administration.

Therapeutic Management

Treatment involves supportive measures such as maintenance of adequate oxygenation, administration of heliox, and pulmonary perfusion and maintenance of adequate cardiac output. After the underlying cause has been identified, specific treatment (e.g., antibiotics for infection) is initiated. Many patients require mechanical ventilatory support. This is usually achieved invasively (i.e., after endotracheal intubation), but occasionally noninvasive ventilation is used in milder cases. Patients requiring invasive mechanical ventilation usually require sedation, at least initially, to allow for ventilatory synchrony. Fluid administration to maintain adequate intravascular volume and end-organ perfusion must be balanced against the desire to decrease lung fluid to improve oxygenation. The provision of adequate nutrition, maintenance of patient comfort, and prevention of complications such as gastrointestinal ulceration are essential. Psychological support of the patient and family is also important.

Inappropriate use of mechanical ventilatory support may worsen the lung injury by causing volutrauma, barotrauma, atelectrauma, and biotrauma to the injured lungs. Protective ventilatory strategies using low tidal volumes (6 mL/kg ideal body weight) have been demonstrated to improve outcomes in adults and theoretically are also appropriate in children. PEEP is applied to decrease atelectasis and maintain an "open" lung. Permissive hypercapnia may also be used. Other strategies used in the support of patients with ARDS include maintaining them in the prone position, inhaled nitric oxide, inhaled prostaglandins, high-frequency oscillatory ventilation, and extracorporeal membrane oxygenation (ECMO), although evidence to support these therapies is scant.

Prognosis

The prognosis for patients with ARDS is improving. Nonetheless, the mortality rate remains high, and in children, ranges from 18% (after severe trauma) to 49% (Randolph, 2009). The precipitating disorder influences the outcome; the worst prognosis is associated with uncontrolled sepsis, bone marrow transplantation, cancer, and multisystem involvement with hepatic failure. Children who recover may have persistent cough and exertional dyspnea.

NURSING CARE

The child with ARDS is cared for in a critical care unit during the acute stages of illness. Nursing care involves close monitoring of oxygenation and respiratory status as well as assessment of cardiac output, perfusion, fluid and electrolyte balance, and renal function (urinary output). Acid–base status and pulse oximetry are important evaluation tools. Diuretics may be administered to reduce pulmonary fluid, and vasodilators may be administered to decrease pulmonary vascular pressure. Nutritional support is often required because of the prolonged acute phase of the illness. Nursing management also includes managing pain, monitoring the effects of the numerous parenteral fluids and medications used to stabilize the child, and monitoring for changes in the child's hemodynamic status. Most children with ARDS require invasive monitoring via a central venous line and possibly a pulmonary artery catheter to monitor oxygenation and administer medications. The nursing care of the child with ARDS involves close observance of skin condition and prevention of breakdown, passive range of motion for prevention of muscle atrophy and contractures, and nutritional support. Respiratory distress is a frightening situation for both the child and the parents, and attention to their psychological needs is a major element in the care of these children. The child is often sedated during the acute phase of the illness, and weaning from sedation requires close monitoring for anxiety reduction and comfort.

Smoke Inhalation Injury

A number of noxious substances that may be inhaled are toxic to humans. They are primarily products of incomplete combustion and cause more deaths from fires than flame injuries. The severity of the injury depends on the nature of the substances generated by the material burned, whether the victim is confined in a closed space, and the duration of contact with the smoke. Three distinct syndromes of pulmonary complications may occur in children with inhalation injury: (1) early carbon monoxide (CO) poisoning, airway obstruction, and pulmonary edema; (2) ARDS occurring at 24 to 48 hours or later in some cases; and (3) late complications of bronchopneumonia and pulmonary emboli (Antoon & Donovan, 2016).

Smoke inhalation results in three types of injury: heat, chemical, and systemic. *Heat injury* involves thermal injury to the upper airway. Air has low specific heat; thus the injury goes no farther than the upper airway. Reflex closure of the glottis prevents injury to the lower airway.

Chemical injury involves gases that may be generated during the combustion of materials such as clothing, furniture, and floor coverings. Acids, alkalis, and their precursors in smoke can produce chemical burns. These substances can be carried deep into the respiratory tract, including the lower respiratory tract, in the form of insoluble gases. Soluble gases tend to dissolve in the upper respiratory tract.

Synthetic materials are especially toxic, producing gases such as oxides of sulphur and nitrogen, acetaldehyde, formaldehyde, hydrocyanic acid, and chlorine. Heated plastics are the source of extremely toxic vapours, including (1) chlorine and hydrochloric acid from polyvinylchloride, and (2) hydrocarbons, aldehydes, ketones, and acids from polyethylene. Irritant gases such as nitrous oxide or carbon dioxide combine with water in the lungs to form corrosive acids; aldehydes cause denaturation of proteins, cellular damage, and edema of pulmonary tissues. Chemical burns to the airways are similar to burns on the skin except that they are painless because the tracheobronchial tree is relatively insensitive to pain.

Inhalation of small amounts of noxious irritants produces alveolar and bronchiolar damage that can lead to obstructive bronchiolitis. Severe exposure causes further injury, including alveolocapillary damage with hemorrhage, necrotizing bronchiolitis, inhibited secretion of surfactant, and formation of hyaline membranes—manifestations of ARDS.

Systemic injury occurs from gases that are nontoxic to the airways (e.g., CO, hydrogen cyanide). However, these gases cause injury and death by interfering with or inhibiting cellular respiration. CO is the leading cause of accidental poisonings in Canada. An estimated 414 Canadians died of carbon monoxide poisoning between 2000 and 2007 (Parachute, n.d.). CO is a colourless, odourless gas with an affinity for hemoglobin 230 times greater than that of oxygen. When it enters the bloodstream, CO combines readily with hemoglobin to form carboxyhemoglobin (COHb). Because it is released less readily, tissue hypoxia reaches dangerous levels before oxygen is available to meet tissue needs.

! NURSING ALERT

The oxygen saturation (Sao_2) obtained by pulse oximetry will be normal because the device measures only oxygenated and deoxygenated hemoglobin; it does not measure dysfunctional hemoglobin such as COHb.

Accidental CO poisoning is most often a result of exposure to fumes of heaters or smoke from structural fires, although poorly ventilated recreational vehicles with improperly operated or maintained gas lamps or stoves and cooking in underventilated areas with charcoal grills are also frequent causes. CO is produced by incomplete combustion of carbon or carbonaceous material such as wood or charcoal.

The signs and symptoms of CO poisoning are secondary to tissue hypoxia and vary with the level of COHb. Mild manifestations include headache, visual disturbances, irritability, and nausea, whereas more severe intoxication causes confusion, hallucinations, ataxia, and coma. The bright, cherry-red lips and skin often described are less often observed; pallor and cyanosis are seen more frequently.

Therapeutic Management

Treatment of children with smoke inhalation injury is largely symptomatic. The most widely accepted treatment is placing the child on humidified 100% oxygen as quickly as possible and monitoring for signs of respiratory distress and impending failure. Baseline ABGs and COHb levels need to be obtained. Pao_2 may be within normal limits unless there is marked respiratory depression. If CO poisoning is confirmed, 100% oxygen should be continued until COHb levels fall to the nontoxic range of about 10%. If CO poisoning is severe, the patient may benefit from hyperbaric oxygen therapy. This therapy may be useful in the treatment of neurological complications related to CO poisoning. See Additional Resources at the end of this chapter for more information on medical hyperbaric treatments. Pulmonary care may be facilitated by bronchodilators, inhaled corticosteroids, humidification, and chest percussion and postural drainage to enhance the removal of necrotic material, minimize bronchoconstriction, and avoid atelectasis. Bronchoscopy may be needed to clear heavy secretions.

Respiratory distress may occur early in the course of smoke inhalation as a result of hypoxia, or patients who are breathing well on admission may suddenly develop respiratory distress. Therefore, intubation equipment should be readily available. Transient edema of the airways can occur at any level in the tracheobronchial tree. Assessment and localization of the obstruction should be accomplished before severe swelling of the head, neck, or oropharynx occurs. Intubation is often necessary when (1) severe burns in the area of the nose, mouth, and face increase the likelihood of developing oropharyngeal edema and obstruction; (2) vocal cord edema causes obstruction; (3) the patient has difficulty handling secretions; and (4) progressive respiratory distress requires artificial ventilation. Controversy surrounds the use of tracheostomy in this context, but many prefer this procedure when the obstruction is proximal to the larynx and reserve nasotracheal intubation for lower tract involvement.

NURSING CARE

Nursing care of the child with inhalation injury is the same as that for any child with respiratory distress. Vital signs and other respiratory assessments (oxygenation, work of breathing, acid–base status) are performed frequently, and the pulmonary status is carefully observed and maintained. Chest physiotherapy is often part of the treatment, as well as mechanical ventilation if needed. Fluid requirements for children experiencing inhalation injury are greater than for those with surface burns alone; however, one concern is the development of pulmonary edema. Thus accurate monitoring of intake and output is essential.

In addition to observation and management of the physical aspects of inhalation injury, the nurse will also deal with the psychological needs of a frightened child and distraught parents. As with any accidental injury, the parents may feel overwhelming guilt, even when the injury occurred through no fault of their own. Parents need support, reassurance, and information regarding the child's condition, treatment, and progress.

The nurse can provide anticipatory guidance and educate families on prevention of inhalation injuries and the importance of CO detectors in the home.

Environmental Tobacco Smoke Exposure

Numerous investigations indicate that parental smoking is an important cause of morbidity in children. Children exposed to (secondhand) passive or environmental tobacco smoke have an increased number of respiratory illnesses, increased respiratory symptoms (e.g., cough, sputum, and wheezing), and reduced performance on pulmonary function tests. The incidence of AOM and OME is also increased in children who have parents who smoke (see Otitis Media, p. 1346). Maternal cigarette smoking while pregnant is associated with increased respiratory symptoms and illnesses in children; decreased fetal growth; increased births of low-birth-weight, preterm, and stillborn infants; and a greater incidence of sudden infant death syndrome (SIDS) (Government of Canada, 2015). The risk for diagnosis of early-onset asthma is associated with in utero exposure to maternal smoking. Exposure to passive smoking increases the incidence of wheezing and asthma in children and young people by at least 20%. Among children with asthma, there is an association between parental cigarette smoking and trips to the emergency department and medication use for asthma exacerbations, and impaired recovery after hospitalization for acute asthma.

Exposure to tobacco smoke during childhood may contribute to the development of chronic lung disease in the adult.

FAMILY-CENTRED TEACHING

Decreasing Childhood Exposure to Environmental Tobacco Smoke

- Maintain a smoke-free home.
- Avoid exposing an infant to environmental smoke.
- Use an air-purifying filter in the home where smoking is unavoidable.
- Encourage exclusive breastfeeding for the first 6 months.
- Do not smoke around children.
- Change clothing after smoking and before breastfeeding or holding an infant in close proximity.
- Restrict smoking to outside the home.
- Do not smoke in motor vehicles with children.

NURSING CARE

Nurses must provide information about the hazards of environmental smoke exposure in all their interactions with children and their family members. This information is especially important for children with respiratory and allergic illnesses. In families in which smokers refuse to or cannot quit, appropriate guidance should be provided for reducing exposure to smoke in the child's environment (see Family-Centred Teaching box). Nurses should set an example for children and families and become advocates for "no smoking" ordinances in public places, prohibition of advertising tobacco products in the media, and inclusion of health warnings on tobacco products packaging (see Additional Resources section at the end of this chapter). Nurses also have an important role in providing parents with affordable smoking-cessation education resources, including the appropriate use of smoking-cessation pharmacological aids.

LONG-TERM RESPIRATORY DYSFUNCTION

Asthma

Asthma is a chronic inflammatory disorder of the airways characterized by recurring symptoms, airway obstruction, and bronchial hyperresponsiveness. In susceptible children, inflammation causes recurrent episodes of wheezing, breathlessness, chest tightness, and cough, especially at night or in the early morning. The airflow limitation or obstruction is reversible either spontaneously or with treatment. Inflammation causes an increase in bronchial hyperresponsiveness to a variety of stimuli. Recognition of the key role of inflammation has made the use of anti-inflammatory agents, especially inhaled corticosteroids, a key component in the treatment of asthma.

Asthma is the most common chronic illness in childhood and is a serious disease worldwide. The WHO (2016) reported that globally there are over 235 million people with asthma, and it is estimated that over 3 million Canadians have asthma. Fortunately, in Canada, the prevalence of asthma has declined among children aged 2 to 7 and it is at its lowest level in more than a decade. In the age group 12 to 19 years, the asthma rate has declined by 0.6%. Those rates may have gone down because of reduced exposure to cigarette smoke (Thomas & Statistics Canada, 2015). Daily smoking among those aged 15 and older decreased between 2000 and 2008. During the same period the number of children regularly exposed to tobacco smoke at home decreased; the percentage of children aged 2 to 3 who live in houses where at least one parent is a daily smoker went down (Thomas & Statistics Canada, 2015). While there are more young boys than girls with asthma, in the adult population, more women than men have asthma. Asthma appears to be more prevalent in groups with poor socioeconomic status, obesity, and low levels of physical activity (Philpott, Houghton, K., Luke, et al., 2010).

In Canada, Indigenous children are affected disproportionately by respiratory infections such as viral bronchiolitis, pneumonia, and tuberculosis. However, their rates of asthma may be somewhat less than those among other Canadian children. Even so, there is a higher rate of poor asthma control in the Indigenous population (Kovesi, 2012).

Asthma is a predominant cause of hospitalization for Canadian children, with children under 5 years of age having the highest hospitalization rates. Emergency department visits for asthma peak during the third week in September; occurrence of respiratory tract infections that can trigger asthma peaks in mid-winter. Asthma continues to be a very serious condition and can be life threatening if not controlled. In Canada, approximately 500 adults and 20 children die yearly from asthma (Asthma Society of Canada, 2016). Fortunately, the number of deaths has been decreasing in all age groups since 1987.

Etiology

Studies of children with asthma indicate that allergies influence both the persistence and the severity of the disease. In fact, *atopy*, or the genetic predisposition for the development of an immune globulin E (IgE)–mediated response to common aeroallergens, is the strongest identifiable predisposing factor for developing asthma. However, 20 to 40% of children with asthma have no evidence of allergic disease. In addition to allergens, other substances and conditions can serve as triggers that may exacerbate asthma (Box 45-12). Evidence shows that viral respiratory infections, including RSV infection, may have a significant role in the development and expression of asthma (Asthma Society of Canada, 2016).

BOX 45-12 TRIGGERS TENDING TO PRECIPITATE OR AGGRAVATE ASTHMATIC EXACERBATIONS

Allergens
- Outdoor—Trees, shrubs, weeds, grasses, moulds, pollens, air pollution, spores
- Indoor—Dust or dust mites, mould, cockroach antigen

Irritants—Tobacco smoke, wood smoke, odours, sprays
Exposure to occupational chemicals
Exercise
Cold air
Changes in weather or temperature
Environmental change—Moving to new home, starting new school
Colds and infections
Animals—Cats, dogs, rodents, horses
Medications—Aspirin, nonsteroidal anti-inflammatory drugs (NSAIDs), antibiotics, beta blockers
Strong emotions—Fear, anger, laughing, crying
Conditions—Gastroesophageal reflux, tracheoesophageal fistula
Food additives—Sulphite preservatives
Foods—Nuts, milk, or dairy products
Endocrine factors—Menses, pregnancy, thyroid disease

Pathophysiology

There is general agreement that inflammation contributes to heightened airway reactivity in asthma. The mechanisms contributing to airway inflammation are multiple and involve a number of different pathways. It is unlikely that asthma is caused by either a single cell or a single inflammatory mediator; rather, it appears that asthma results from complex interactions among inflammatory cells, mediators, and the cells and tissues present in the airways. However, recognition of the importance of inflammation has made the use of anti-inflammatory agents a key component of asthma therapy.

Another important component of asthma is bronchospasm and obstruction. The mechanisms responsible for the obstructive symptoms in asthma (Fig. 45-4) include (1) inflammatory response to stimuli; (2) airway edema and accumulation and secretion of mucus; (3) spasm of the smooth muscle of the bronchi and bronchioles, which decreases the calibre of the bronchioles; and (4) airway remodelling, which causes permanent cellular changes.

Airflow is determined by the size of the airway lumen, degree of bronchial wall edema, mucus production, smooth muscle contraction, and muscle hypertrophy. Bronchial constriction is a normal reaction to foreign stimuli, but in the child with asthma it is abnormally severe, producing impaired respiratory function. Because the bronchi normally dilate and elongate during inspiration and contract and shorten on expiration, the respiratory difficulty is more pronounced during the expiratory phase of respiration.

Increased resistance in the airway causes forced expiration through the narrowed lumen. The volume of air trapped in the lungs increases as airways are functionally closed at a point between the alveoli and the lobar bronchi. This trapping of gas

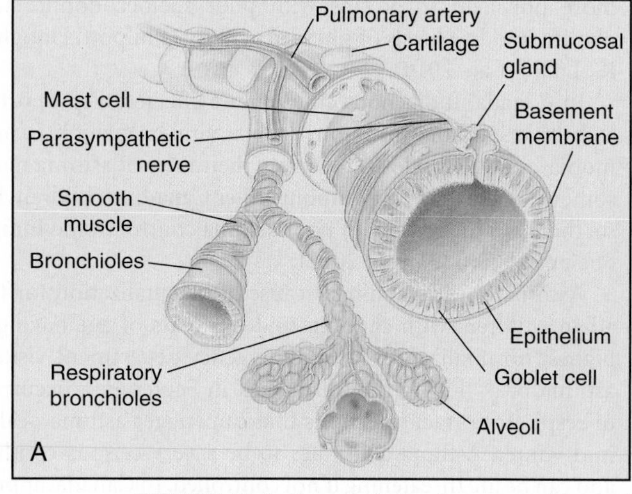

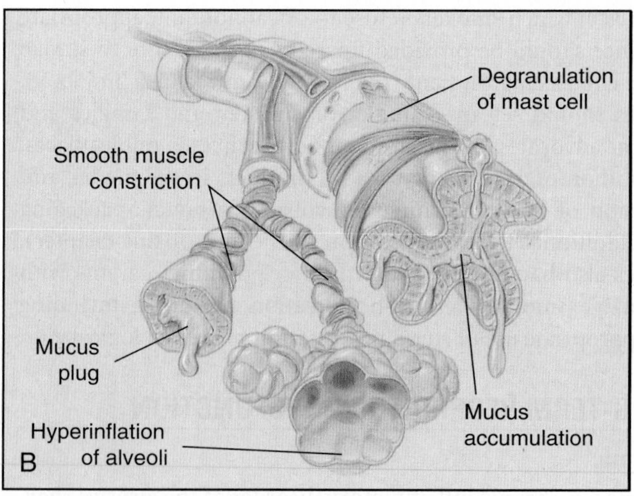

FIGURE 45-4 Airway obstruction caused by asthma. **A,** A normal lung. **B,** Bronchial asthma: thick mucus, mucosal edema, and smooth muscle spasm causing obstruction of small airways; breathing becomes laboured, and expiration is difficult. (Adapted from Des Jardins, T., & Burton, G. G. [1995]. *Clinical manifestations and assessment of respiratory disease* [3rd ed.]. St. Louis: Mosby.)

forces the individual to breathe at higher and higher lung volumes. Consequently, the person with asthma fights to inspire sufficient air. This expenditure of effort for breathing causes fatigue, decreased respiratory effectiveness, and increased oxygen consumption. The inspiration occurring at higher lung volumes hyperinflates the alveoli and reduces the effectiveness of the cough. As the severity of obstruction increases, there is reduced alveolar ventilation with carbon dioxide retention, hypoxemia, respiratory acidosis, and, eventually, respiratory failure.

Chronic inflammation may also cause permanent damage (airway remodelling) to airway structures; this remodelling cannot be prevented by and is not responsive to current treatments (Asthma Society of Canada, 2016).

Diagnostic Evaluation

The classic manifestations of asthma are dyspnea, wheezing, and coughing (Box 45-13). An attack may develop gradually or appear abruptly and may be preceded by an upper respiratory tract infection. The age of the child is often a significant factor, since the first attack frequently occurs before the age of 5 years, with some children manifesting clinical signs and symptoms in infancy. In infancy an attack usually follows a respiratory infection. Some children may experience a **prodromal** itching at the front of the neck or over the upper part of the back just before an attack, especially if the attack is related to allergies.

BOX 45-13 CLINICAL MANIFESTATIONS OF ASTHMA

Cough

Hacking, paroxysmal, irritative, and nonproductive

Becomes rattling and productive of frothy, clear, gelatinous sputum

Respiratory-Related Signs

Shortness of breath

Prolonged expiratory phase

Audible wheeze

May have a malar flush and red ears

Lips deep, dark red colour

Possible progression to cyanosis of nail beds or circumoral cyanosis

Restlessness

Apprehension

Sweating may be prominent as the attack progresses

Posture—Older children may sit upright with shoulders in a hunched-over position, hands on the bed or chair, and arms braced (tripod position)

Speech—May speak in short, panting, broken phrases

Chest

Hyperresonance on percussion

Coarse, loud breath sounds

Wheezes throughout the lung fields

Prolonged expiration

Crackles

Generalized inspiratory and expiratory wheezing; increasingly high pitched

With Repeated Episodes

Barrel chest

Elevated shoulders

Use of accessory muscles of respiration

Facial appearance: flattened malar bones, dark circles beneath the eyes, narrow nose, prominent upper teeth

! NURSING ALERT

Shortness of breath with air movement in the chest restricted to the point of absent breath sounds accompanied by a sudden rise in respiratory rate is an ominous sign indicating ventilatory failure and imminent respiratory arrest.

The diagnosis is determined primarily on the basis of clinical manifestations, history, physical examination, and, to a lesser extent, laboratory tests. Generally, chronic cough in the absence of infection or diffuse wheezing during the expiratory phase of respiration is sufficient to establish a diagnosis. The CPS classifies asthma severity as mild, moderate, or severe (Ortiz-Alvarez, Mikrogianakis, & CPS, Acute Care Committee, 2012/2015).

Pulmonary function tests (PFTs) provide an objective method of evaluating the presence and degree of lung disease, as well as the response to therapy. Spirometry can generally be performed reliably on children by the age of 5 or 6 years. The Asthma Society of Canada (2016) recommends that spirometry testing be done at the time of initial assessment of asthma, after treatment is initiated and symptoms have stabilized, and at least every 1 to 2 years to assess the maintenance of airway function.

Another measurement to consider is the *peak expiratory flow rate (PEFR)*, which measures the maximum flow of air that can be forcefully exhaled in 1 second. PEFR is measured in litres per minute using a *peak expiratory flow meter (PEFM)*. Three zones of measurement are typically used to interpret PEFR. The zone system is patterned after a traffic light to make the categories easy to understand and remember (see Guidelines box). Each child needs to establish his or her personal best value. A personal best value should be established during a 2- to 3-week period when the child's asthma is stable. During this period, the child records the PEFR at least twice a day. After the personal best value has been established, the child's current PEFR on any occasion can be compared with the personal best value. Although it can be a helpful tool in assessing a child's asthma control, it is important to note that its results depend on the child's ability to use the PEFM and willingness to participate. In some cases, a low PEFR may not truly mean that the child's asthma is poorly controlled. Each individual child's PEFR varies according to age, height, gender, and race.

Bronchoprovocation testing (i.e., direct exposure of the mucous membranes to a suspected antigen in increasing concentrations) helps to identify inhaled allergens. Exposure to methacholine, histamine, or cold or dry air may be performed to assess airway responsiveness or reactivity. Exercise challenges may be used to identify children with exercise-induced

GUIDELINES

*Interpreting Peak Expiratory Flow Rates**

- Green (80 to 100% of personal best) signals all clear. Asthma is under reasonably good control. No symptoms are present, and the routine treatment plan for maintaining control can be followed.
- Yellow (50 to 79% of personal best) signals caution. Asthma is not well controlled. An acute exacerbation may be present. Maintenance therapy may need to be increased. Call the practitioner if the child stays in this zone.
- Red (below 50% of personal best) signals a medical alert. Severe airway narrowing may be occurring. A short-acting bronchodilator should be administered. Notify the practitioner if the peak expiratory flow rate does not return immediately and stay in the yellow or green zones.

*These zones are guidelines only. Specific zones and management should be individualized for each child.

bronchospasm. Although these tests are highly specific and sensitive, they place the child at risk for an asthmatic episode and should be done under close observation in a qualified laboratory or clinic.

Skin prick testing (SPT) and serologic testing (with quantification of sIgE) for allergen-specific immunoglobulin E (sIgE) may be used to identify environmental allergens that trigger asthma (Sicherer, Wood, & AAP Section on Allergy and Immunology, 2012). It is recommended that all patients with year-round asthma symptoms be tested with skin tests or laboratory blood analysis to determine sensitization to perennial allergens (e.g., house dust mites, cats, dogs, cockroaches, moulds, and fungus) (Ortiz-Alvarez et al., 2012/2015).

In addition to these tests, other important tests include laboratory tests (complete blood count [CBC] with differential) and chest radiographs. The CBC may show a slight elevation in the white blood cell count during acute asthma episodes, but elevations of more than 12×10^9/L or an increased percentage of band cells may indicate respiratory tract infection. The presence of eosinophilia greater than 0.5×10^9/L tends to suggest an allergic or inflammatory disorder.

Frontal and lateral radiographs show infiltrates and hyperexpansion of the airways, with the anteroposterior diameter on physical examination indicating an increased diameter (suggestive of barrel chest). Additional diagnostic tests for conditions such as gastroesophageal reflux may be carried out to determine whether they may contribute to asthma symptoms. Radiography may assist in ruling out a respiratory tract infection.

Therapeutic Management

The overall goals of asthma management are to maintain normal activity levels, maintain normal pulmonary function, prevent chronic symptoms and recurrent exacerbations, provide optimal medication therapy with minimal or no adverse effects, and assist the child in living as normal and happy a life as possible. This includes facilitating the child's social adjustments in the family, school, and community and in normal participation in recreational activities and sports. To accomplish these goals, several treatment principles need to be followed (Asthma Society of Canada, 2016):

- A continuous care approach with regular visits (at least every 1 to 6 months) to the health care provider is necessary to control symptoms and prevent exacerbations.
- Prevention of exacerbations includes avoiding triggers, avoiding allergens, and using medications as needed.
- Therapy includes efforts to reduce underlying inflammation and relieve or prevent symptomatic airway narrowing.
- Therapy includes patient education, environmental control, pharmacological management, and the use of objective measures to monitor the severity of disease and guide the course of therapy.

Allergen control. Nonpharmacological therapy is aimed at the prevention and reduction of exposure to airborne allergens and irritants. House dust mites and other components of house dust are frequent agents identified in children allergic to inhalants. The cockroach, another common household inhabitant, is an important allergen in many locations. Exterminating live cockroaches, carefully cleaning kitchen floors and cabinets, putting food away after eating, and taking garbage out in the evening are essential measures to control cockroach infestation. The mouse allergen is the most recent allergen to be identified in the homes of urban children with asthma. Although some studies suggest sensitized persons should carefully evaluate having such pets in the household, the overall data are inconsistent on the effect of cat or dog exposure and subsequent asthma development (Chen, Tischer, Schnappinger, et al., 2010). Additional sources of pollutants include ozone, particulate matter produced by tobacco smoke, wood-burning stoves, pesticides, lead, mould spores, nitrogen dioxide, and sulphur dioxide; these are believed to contribute to asthma morbidity in children and should be avoided or minimized.

Living in homes close to busy roads, damp homes with mould, and exposure to tobacco smoke are significant contributing factors in the development of asthma in infants and small children (Heinrich, 2011). Recommendations for controlling allergens are found in the Family-Centred Teaching box.

Skin testing is used to identify specific allergens so steps can be taken to eliminate or avoid them. Often, simply removing the offending environmental allergens or irritants (e.g., removing carpeting from the home of a child sensitive to mould and dust particles) decreases the frequency of asthma episodes. Dehumidifiers or air conditioners may control nonspecific factors that trigger an episode, such as extremes of temperature.

Medication therapy. Pharmacological therapy is used to prevent and control asthma symptoms, reduce the frequency and severity of asthma exacerbations, and reverse airflow obstruction. A stepwise approach is recommended based on the severity of the child's asthma. Because inflammation is considered an early and persistent feature of asthma, therapy is directed toward long-term suppression of inflammation.

Asthma medications are categorized into two general classes: *long-term control medications (controllers or preventer medications)* that decrease airway swelling and prevent asthma episodes to achieve and maintain control of inflammation,

FAMILY-CENTRED TEACHING

"Allergy-Proofing" the Home and Community

- Keep humidity between 30 and 50%; use dehumidifier or air conditioner if available; keep air conditioners clean and free of mould; do not use vaporizers or humidifiers.
- Encase pillows in zippered allergen-impermeable covers or wash pillows in hot water (at least 54.4°C) every week.
- Encase mattress and box springs in zippered allergen-impermeable cover.
- Use foam rubber mattress and pillows or Dacron pillows and synthetic blankets.
- Wash bed linens every 7 to 10 days in hot water (at least 54.4°C).
- Encase polyester comforters in allergen-impermeable covers or wash in hot water (at least 54.4°C) every week; if possible, do not use comforter; use cotton blankets instead.
- Store nothing under the bed; keep clothing in a closet with the door shut.
- Use washable window shades; avoid heavy curtains; if curtains are used, launder them frequently.
- Remove all carpeting if possible; if not possible, vacuum carpet once or twice a week while the child wears a mask; have child remain out of the room while vacuuming occurs and for 30 minutes after vacuuming.
- If possible, use a central vacuum cleaner with a collecting bag outside of the home or use cleaner filters (e.g., high-efficiency particulate air [HEPA] filters).
- Have air and heating ducts cleaned annually; change or clean filters monthly; cover heating vents with filter material (e.g., cheesecloth) to prevent circulation of dust, especially when heat is turned on after summer.
- Use wipeable furniture (wood, plastic, vinyl, or leather) in place of upholstered furniture; avoid rattan or wicker furniture.
- Keep child indoors while lawn is being mowed, bushes or trees are being trimmed, or pollen count is high.
- Keep windows and doors closed during pollen season; use air conditioner if possible or go to places that are air conditioned, such as libraries and shopping malls, when the weather is hot.
- Wet-mop bare floors weekly; wet-dust and clean child's room weekly; the child should not be present during cleaning activities.
- Limit or avoid child's exposure to tobacco and wood smoke; do not allow cigarette smoking in the house or car; select day care centres, play areas, and shopping malls that are smoke free.
- Avoid cellar (basement) as a play area if it is damp; use a dehumidifier in a damp basement.
- Use pesticide sprays, roach bait traps, and boric acid powder to kill cockroaches; if living in an apartment or adjacent housing, encourage neighbours to work together to get rid of cockroaches and mice.
- Decrease child's exposure to air pollution from vehicle exhaust, outdoor grills, and environmental tobacco. Limit outside play on ozone alert days.

and *quick-relief medications (reliever medications)* to treat symptoms and exacerbations quickly (Asthma Society of Canada, 2016).

Quick-relief and long-term medications are often used in combination. Inhaled corticosteroids, cromolyn sodium and nedocromil, long-acting β_2-agonists, methylxanthines, and leukotriene modifiers are used as long-term control medications. Short-acting β_2-agonists, anticholinergics, and systemic corticosteroids are used as quick-relief or rescue medications. Bronchodilators that relax bronchial smooth muscle and dilate the airways include β_2-agonists, methylxanthines, and anticholinergics that can be used as both quick-relief and long-term medications.

Many asthma medications are given by inhalation with a nebulizer or a **metered-dose inhaler** (MDI). The MDI should always be attached to a spacer when an inhaled corticosteroid is administered, to prevent yeast infections in the mouth. Spacers are also important for children who have difficulty coordinating or learning proper inhalation technique (Canadian Thoracic Society, 2012). The spacer and holder can be equipped with a mask or a mouthpiece. An alternative propellant to the chlorofluorocarbons (CFCs) is hydrofluoroalkanes; the possible advantages include delivery of more fine particles and less oral deposition (Asthma Society of Canada, 2016). Pharmaceutical companies are currently mandated to produce inhalers that do not contain CFCs as the propellant, because CFCs have been linked to damage and depletion of the earth's ozone level. Several currently available CFC-free MDI devices use dry powder (and called *dry powder inhalers [DPIs]*); these include the Diskus inhaler and the Turbuhaler. These devices are breath activated, and the child needs to inhale as quickly and deeply as possible to use them effectively. The Diskhaler and Aerosolizer are similar, but with the Aerosolizer the medication must be loaded into the inhaler before use. Infants and very young children who have difficulty using MDIs or other inhalers can receive their asthma medications via a nebulizer, which administers the medication via compressed air or oxygen. Children are instructed to breathe normally with the mouth open to provide a direct route to the trachea. Spacers are gradually replacing nebulizers as the mechanism to deliver inhaled medications as they provide an effective way to deliver the medication. A Cochrane review concluded that nebulizer delivery produced outcomes that were not significantly better than those with spacer delivery with metered-dose inhalers for adults and children (Cates, Welsh, & Rowe, 2013).

Corticosteroids are anti-inflammatory drugs used to treat reversible airflow obstruction and control symptoms and reduce bronchial hyperresponsiveness in chronic asthma. A major change in the last two revisions of the Canadian national guidelines (Canadian Thoracic Society, 2012) is the recommendation that inhaled corticosteroids be used as first-line therapy in children over 5 years of age. Clinical studies of corticosteroids have indicated significant improvement of all asthma parameters, including decreases in symptoms, emergency visits, and medication requirements (Ortiz-Alvarez et al., 2012/2015).

Corticosteroids may be administered parenterally, orally, or by inhalation. Oral medications are metabolized slowly, with an onset of action up to 3 hours after administration and peak effectiveness occurring within 6 to 12 hours. Oral systemic steroids may be given for short periods of time (e.g., 3- or 10-day "bursts") to gain prompt control of inadequately controlled persistent asthma or to manage severe persistent asthma. These medications should be given in the lowest effective dose. They have few adverse effects (cough, dysphonia, and oral thrush), and there is strong evidence that they improve the long-term outcomes for children of all ages with mild or moderate persistent asthma. Evidence from clinical trials that monitored children for 6 years indicates that the use of inhaled corticosteroids at recommended doses does not have long-term significant effects on growth, bone mineral density, ocular toxicity, or suppression of the adrenal–pituitary axis (Ortiz-Alvarez et al., 2012/2015). However, primary care providers should frequently monitor (at least every 3 to 6 months) the growth of children and adolescents taking corticosteroids to assess the systemic effects of these medications and make appropriate reductions in dosages or changes to other types of asthma therapy when necessary. The inhaled corticosteroids include budesonide and fluticasone (Flovent).

Beta-adrenergic agonists (short acting) (primarily albuterol [Ventolin], levalbuterol [Xopenex], and terbutaline) are used for treatment of acute exacerbations and for the prevention of exercise-induced bronchospasm. These drugs bind with the beta receptors on the smooth muscle of airways, where they activate adenylate cyclase and convert adenosine monophosphate (AMP) to cyclic AMP (cAMP). It is believed that the increased cAMP enhances binding of intracellular calcium to the cell membrane, reducing the availability of calcium and thus allowing smooth muscle to relax. Other effects of these medications help stabilize mast cells to prevent the release of mediators. Most beta-adrenergics used in asthma therapy affect predominantly the β_2-receptors, which help eliminate bronchospasm and minimize effects such as increased heart rate and gastrointestinal disturbances. These medications can be given via inhalation or as oral or parenteral preparations. The inhaled medication has a more rapid onset of action than the oral form. Inhalation also reduces troublesome systemic adverse effects: irritability, tremor, nervousness, and insomnia. Inhaled beta-adrenergic agents should not be taken more than three or four times daily for acute symptoms.

Salmeterol (Serevent) is a long-acting β_2-agonist (bronchodilator) that is used twice a day (no more frequently than every 12 hours). This medication is added to anti-inflammatory therapy and used for long-term prevention of symptoms, especially nighttime symptoms, and exercise-induced bronchospasm. Salmeterol is not used in children younger than 12 years of age, and it is not used to treat acute symptoms or exacerbations. The CPS recommends the addition of a long-acting β_2-agonist to a low- or medium-dose inhaled corticosteroid to improve lung function and asthma symptoms and decrease the need for a short-acting β_2-agonist (Ortiz-Alvarez et al., 2012/2015). There is some evidence that this combination may actually allow the practitioner to lower the corticosteroid dose and manage asthma symptoms just as effectively.

Theophylline was used for decades to relieve symptoms and prevent asthma attacks; however, it is now used primarily in the emergency department when the child is not responding to maximal therapy. Therapeutic levels should be obtained with this drug because it has a narrow therapeutic window.

Cromolyn sodium is a nonsteroidal anti-inflammatory drug (NSAID) for asthma. It stabilizes mast cell membranes; inhibits activation and release of mediators from eosinophil and epithelial cells; and inhibits the acute airway narrowing after exposure to exercise, cold dry air, and sulphur dioxide. There is no way to reliably predict whether a child will respond to the drug. Cromolyn sodium has minimal adverse effects (occasional coughing on inhalation of the powder formulation) and may be given via nebulizer or MDI.

Nedocromil sodium inhibits the bronchoconstrictor response to inhaled antigens and inhibits the activity of and release of histamine, leukotrienes, and prostaglandins from inflammatory cells associated with asthma. The drug has few adverse effects and is used for maintenance therapy in asthma; it is not effective for reversal of acute exacerbations and is not used in children under 5 years of age.

Leukotrienes are mediators of inflammation that cause increases in airway hyperresponsiveness. Leukotriene modifiers (such as zafirlukast [Accolate] and montelukast sodium [Singulair]) block inflammatory and bronchospasm effects. These medications are not used to treat acute episodes but are given orally in combination with β_2-agonists and steroids to provide long-term control and prevent symptoms in mild persistent asthma. Montelukast is approved for children aged 12 months and older, whereas zafirlukast is approved for children 7 years and older.

Anticholinergics (atropine and ipratropium [Atrovent]) may also be used for relief of acute bronchospasm. However, these medications have adverse effects that include drying of respiratory secretions, blurred vision, and cardiac and CNS stimulation. The primary anticholinergic medication used is ipratropium, which does not cross the blood–brain barrier and therefore elicits no CNS effects. Ipratropium, when used in combination with albuterol, has been shown to be effective during acute severe asthma in significantly improving lung function and reducing hospitalizations in children coming to the emergency department.

Another asthma medication, omalizumab (Xolair), is a monoclonal antibody that blocks the binding of IgE to mast cells. Blocking this interaction eventually inhibits the inflammation that is associated with asthma. It is used in patients with moderate to persistent asthma who have confirmed perennial aeroallergen sensitivity and have had poor control of symptoms on inhaled steroids. Many patients with asthma are atopic and possess specific IgE antibodies to allergens responsible for airway inflammation. Xolair has been approved for use in children aged 12 years and older. The medication is administered once or twice a month by subcutaneous injection. Efficacy of omalizumab is not immediate but can be an effective therapy for patients with symptomatic moderate to severe allergic asthma that is poorly controlled with inhaled corticosteroids. There were concerns about anaphylaxis with this medication but this appears to occur infrequently. More than half of all anaphylactic reactions occurred in the first 2 hours after administration (Thomson & Chaudhuri, 2012). Some children with severe asthma and a history of severe life-threatening episodes may need a prescription for injectable EpiPen (subcutaneous epinephrine).

Exercise. *Exercise-induced bronchospasm (EIB)* is an acute, reversible, usually self-terminating airway obstruction that develops during or after vigorous activity, reaches its peak 5 to 10 minutes after stopping the activity, and usually stops in another 20 to 30 minutes. Patients with EIB have cough, shortness of breath, chest pain or tightness, wheezing, and endurance problems during exercise; an exercise challenge test in a laboratory is necessary to make the diagnosis.

The problem is rare in activities that require short bursts of energy (e.g., baseball, sprints, gymnastics, skiing) and more common in those that involve endurance exercise (e.g., soccer, basketball, distance running). Swimming is well tolerated by children with EIB because they are breathing air fully saturated with moisture and because of the type of breathing required in swimming.

Children with asthma are often excluded from exercise by parents, teachers, and practitioners, as well as by the children themselves, because they are reluctant to provoke an attack. However, this practice can seriously hamper peer interaction and physical health. Exercise is advantageous for children with asthma, and most children can participate in activities at school and in sports with minimal difficulty, provided their asthma is under control. Participation should be evaluated on an individual basis. Appropriate prophylactic treatment with beta-adrenergic agents or cromolyn sodium before exercise usually permits full participation in strenuous exertion.

Hyposensitization. The role of hyposensitization in childhood asthma has become controversial. In the past, immunotherapy was used for seasonal allergies and when single substances were identified as the offending allergen. It is not recommended for allergens that can be eliminated, such as foods, medications, and animal dander.

The Canadian Thoracic Society (2012) recommends immunotherapy for asthma patients in the following situations:

- When there is evidence of a relationship between asthma symptoms and unavoidable exposure to an allergen to which the patient is sensitive
- When symptoms occur all year or at least during a major portion of the year
- When symptom control is difficult with medication therapy because multiple medications are required, the patient is not responsive to available medications, or the patient refuses to take the medications

Injection therapy is usually limited to clinically significant allergens. The initial dose of the offending allergen(s), based on the size of the skin reaction, is injected subcutaneously. The amount is increased at weekly intervals until a maximum tolerance is reached, after which a maintenance dose is given at 4-week intervals. This may be extended to 5- or 6-week intervals during the off-season for seasonal allergens. Successful treatment is continued for a minimum of 3 years and then stopped. If no symptoms appear, acquired immunity is assumed; if symptoms recur, treatment is reinstituted. Hyposensitization injections should be administered only with emergency equipment and medications readily available in the event of an anaphylactic reaction.

Status asthmaticus. Status asthmaticus is a medical emergency that can result in respiratory failure and death if unrecognized and untreated. Children who continue to display respiratory distress despite vigorous therapeutic measures, especially the use of sympathomimetics (e.g., albuterol, epinephrine), are considered to be in status asthmaticus. The condition may develop gradually or rapidly, often coincident with complicating conditions, such as pneumonia or a respiratory virus, that can influence the duration and treatment of the exacerbation.

Therapy for status asthmaticus is aimed at improving ventilation, decreasing airway resistance and relieving bronchospasm, correcting dehydration and acidosis, allaying child and parent anxiety related to the severity of the event, and treating any concurrent infection. Humidified oxygen is recommended and should be given to maintain an oxygen saturation of greater than 90%. Inhaled aerosolized short-acting β_2-agonists are recommended for all patients. Three treatments of β_2-agonists spaced 20 to 30 minutes apart are usually given as initial therapy, and continuous administration of β_2-agonists may be initiated. A systemic corticosteroid (oral, IV, or IM) may also be given to decrease the effects of inflammation. An anticholinergic such as ipratropium bromide may be added to the aerosolized solution of the β_2-agonist. Anticholinergics have been shown to result in additional bronchodilation in patients with severe airflow obstruction. An IV infusion is often initiated to provide a means for hydration and to administer medications. Correction of dehydration, acidosis, hypoxia, and electrolyte disturbance is guided by frequent determination of arterial pH, blood gases, and serum electrolytes.

Additional therapies in acute asthma attacks include the use of IV magnesium sulphate, a potent muscle relaxant that acts to decrease inflammation and improves pulmonary function and peak flow rate among pediatric patients treated in the emergency department with moderate to severe asthma. Heliox may be administered to decrease airway resistance and thereby decrease the work of breathing; it can be delivered via a nonrebreathing face mask from premixed tanks, which may be blended in a stand-alone unit or within a ventilator. It may be used in acute exacerbations as an adjunct to β_2-agonist and IV corticosteroid therapy to improve pulmonary function until the two latter medications have time to take full effect in decreasing bronchospasm. The effects of heliox are usually seen within 20 minutes of administration, whereas other drugs may take longer to exert the desired effect. Ketamine, a dissociative anaesthetic, is believed to cause smooth muscle relaxation and decrease airway resistance caused by severe bronchospasm in acute asthma. It may be administered as an adjunct to other therapies mentioned previously. Antibiotics should not be used to treat acute asthma attacks except when a bacterial infection resulting from another condition such as pneumonia or sinusitis is present (Ortiz-Alvarez et al., 2012/2015).

A child suspected of having status asthmaticus is usually seen in the emergency department and is often admitted to a pediatric critical care unit for close observation and continuous cardiorespiratory monitoring. A key component in the prevention of morbidity is helping the child, parents, teachers, coaches, and other adults in the child's life recognize features of deteriorating respiratory status, use the correct rescue medications effectively, and immediately place the child with deteriorating respiratory status into the care of trained health care providers instead of waiting to see if the asthma gets better on its own. For the child going into early status asthmaticus, immediate medical care is required to prevent irreversible respiratory failure and possible death.

Prognosis. The outlook for children with asthma varies widely. Some children's asthma symptoms may improve at puberty, but up to two thirds of children with asthma continue to have symptoms through puberty and into adulthood. The prognosis for control or disappearance of symptoms varies in children, from those who have rare symptoms to those who are constantly wheezing or are subject to status asthmaticus. In general, when symptoms are severe and numerous, when symptoms have been present for a long time, and when there is a family history of allergy, there is a greater likelihood of a poor prognosis. Many children who outgrow their exacerbations continue to have airway hyperresponsiveness and cough as adults. Furthermore, airway hyperresponsiveness in adults appears to be associated with decreased lung function.

Risk factors for asthma deaths include early onset, frequent attacks, difficult-to-manage disease, adolescence, history of respiratory failure, psychological problems (refusal to take medications), dependency on or overuse of asthma medications, presence of physical stigmata (barrel chest, intercostal retractions), and abnormal PFTs.

NURSING CARE

Nursing care of the child with asthma begins with a review of the child's health history; the home, school, and play environment; parent and child attitudes about the child's condition; and a comprehensive physical assessment with focus on the respiratory system. (Please see the Nursing Care Plan: The Child with Asthma, available on Evolve.)

Physical assessment of asthma involves the same observations and techniques described in Chapter 33. In addition to the nursing documentation, an evaluation of physical characteristics of chronic respiratory involvement is required, including chest configuration (e.g., barrel chest), posturing (tripod), and type of breathing. A history of the current and previous episodes and precipitating factors or events provides important information.

Nurses may perform a variety of functions in asthma care, including asthma education in the primary care setting and in schools and other community settings, and care of the child with asthma in the acute care setting, ambulatory care, and critical care. Nurses also obtain information on how asthma affects the child's everyday activities and self-concept, the child's and family's adherence to the prescribed therapy, and their personal treatment goals. Every effort should be made to build a partnership between the child and family and the health care team, and effective communication is an essential part of this partnership. In particular, the child and family's satisfaction with asthma control and with the quality of care should be assessed. The nurse should also assess their perception of the severity of the disease and their level of social support.

The disease can be managed so that it does not require hospitalization or interfere with family life, physical activity, or school attendance. Children and parents need to be taught how to avoid allergens, recognize and respond to symptoms of bronchospasm, maintain health and prevent complications, and promote normal activities. The nurse should determine any cultural or ethnic beliefs or practices that influence self-management and that may necessitate modifications in educational approaches to meet the family's needs. Inconsistent home care, either on the part of the child or the parents, often leads to unnecessary emergency department visits for management (Volpe, Smith, & Sultan, 2011). Parents and older children often need education reinforced about the maintenance aspect of asthma management; children benefit from drug therapy even when asthma manifestations are not evident.

Provide Acute Asthma Care

Children who are admitted to the hospital with acute asthma are ill, anxious, and uncomfortable. The progression or resolution of status asthmaticus is variable. The importance of continual observation and assessment cannot be overemphasized.

When β_2-agonists and corticosteroids are given, the child needs to be monitored closely and continuously for relief of respiratory distress and signs of adverse effects or toxicity. Pulse oximetry is monitored along with rate and depth of breathing, auscultation of air movement, adventitious sounds, and any signs of respiratory distress (e.g., nasal flaring, tachypnea, retractions). The child on supplemental oxygen requires intermittent or continuous oxygenation monitoring depending on severity of respiratory compromise and initial oxygenation status. The child in status asthmaticus should be placed on continuous cardiorespiratory (including blood pressure) and pulse oximetry monitoring. Oral fluid intake may be limited during the acute phase; IV fluid replacement may be required to provide adequate tissue hydration.

Older children may be more comfortable standing (Fig. 45-5), sitting upright, or leaning slightly forward. When possible, the nurse should communicate in such a way that a child can reply in a few words to avoid fatigue. Shortness of breath makes talking difficult.

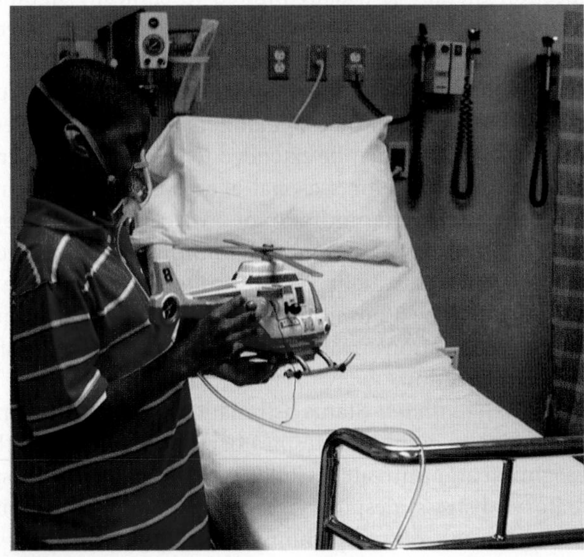

FIGURE 45-5 Child with asthma is allowed play activity as tolerated.

Children with acute asthma are generally apprehensive and anxious. The calm, efficient presence of a nurse can help reassure them that they are safe and will be cared for during this stressful period. It is important to assure children that they will not be left alone and that their parents are allowed to remain with them. Parents need reassurance and want to be informed of their child's condition and therapies. They may believe that they have in some way contributed to the child's condition or could have prevented the episode. Reassurance regarding their efforts expended on the child's behalf and their parenting capabilities can help alleviate their stress. Efforts to reduce parental apprehension also reduce the child's distress, as anxiety is easily communicated to the child from parents and members of the staff.

Avoid Allergens

One goal of asthma management is avoidance of an exacerbation. Parents need to know how to avoid allergens that precipitate asthma episodes. The nurse can assist the parents in modifying the environment to reduce contact with the offending allergen(s) (see Family-Centred Teaching box, p. 1365). Parents should be cautioned to avoid exposing a sensitive child to excessive cold, wind, or other extremes of weather; smoke; sprays; or other irritants. Foods known to provoke symptoms should be eliminated from the diet.

Approximately 2 to 6% of children with asthma are sensitive to aspirin; thus nurses should caution parents to use other analgesic–antipyretic medications for discomfort or fever and to read package labelling for ingredients. Although aspirin is rarely given to children in Canada, salicylate compounds are in other common medicines, such as Pepto-Bismol. Children with aspirin-induced asthma may also be sensitive to NSAIDs and tartrazine (yellow dye number 5, a common food colouring).

NURSING ALERT

Parents should be encouraged to avoid administering aspirin to any child unless specifically recommended by and under the supervision of a health care provider. Acetaminophen is safe for children and is the analgesic of choice.

Relieve Bronchospasm

Parents and older children should be taught to recognize early signs and symptoms of an impending attack so that it can be controlled before symptoms become distressing. Most children can recognize prodromal symptoms well before an attack (about 6 hours) and implement preventive therapy. Objective signs that parents may observe include rhinorrhea, cough, low-grade fever, irritability, itching (especially on the front of the neck and chest), apathy, anxiety, sleep disturbance, abdominal discomfort, and loss of appetite. A variety of easy-to-use, inexpensive PEFMs are available for use in the home and at school to assess changes in pulmonary function (see Patient Teaching box). Young children need to be supervised while they are learning to use their PEFM, and their technique should be checked frequently to ensure that it is correct. Children should use the same PEFM over time, and they should bring it for use at every follow-up visit. Using the same brand of meter is recommended because different brands can give significantly different values.

PATIENT TEACHING

Use of a Peak Expiratory Flow Meter

1. Before each use, make sure the sliding marker or arrow on the peak expiratory flow meter points to zero or is at the bottom of the numbered scale.
2. Stand up straight.
3. Remove gum or any food from your mouth.
4. Close your lips tightly around the mouthpiece. Be sure to keep your tongue away from the mouthpiece.
5. Blow out as hard and as quickly as you can, a "fast hard puff."
6. Note the number by the marker on the numbered scale.
7. Repeat the entire routine three times; wait 30 seconds between each routine.
8. Record the highest of the three readings, not the average.
9. Measure the peak expiratory flow rate (PEFR) close to the same time and same way each day (e.g., morning and evening; before or 15 minutes after taking medication).
10. Keep a chart of your PEFRs.

The family should obtain a PEFM and learn to use this device to monitor the child's asthma if the child is 5 years of age or older. A written *asthma action plan* that includes the three peak flow meter zones and the child's asthma medications may be obtained from the child's primary care provider (see Additional Resources at the end of this chapter for examples). A home asthma action plan may reduce the risk for asthma death by 70% (Liu, Covar, Spahn, et al., 2016). Medications used for asthma exacerbations are also included in the asthma plan. This action plan should be used to make decisions about asthma management at home and at school. The nurse may assist the child and family in understanding the written action plan, emphasizing that the child and family determine the success of the plan, not the health care providers. Parents should be taught how to read labels on prepared foods and snacks to determine the presence of allergens.

Children who use a nebulizer (Fig. 45-6), MDI, Diskus, or Turbuhaler to deliver medications need to learn how to use the device correctly. The MDI device (Fig. 45-7) delivers medication directly to the airways; thus the child needs to learn to breathe slowly and deeply for better distribution to narrowed airways (see Patient Teaching box, p. 1375).

A spacer or AeroChamber device should be used with MDI inhalers. These devices allow the parent or child to deliver the medication from the MDI and slowly inhale it. Spacers also help prevent yeast infections in the mouth when corticosteroids are inhaled via an MDI (see Fig. 45-7).

The child and parents also need to be cautioned about the adverse effects of prescribed medications and the dangers of overuse of β_2-agonists. They should know that it is important to use these medications when needed but not indiscriminately or as a substitute for avoiding the symptom-provoking allergen.

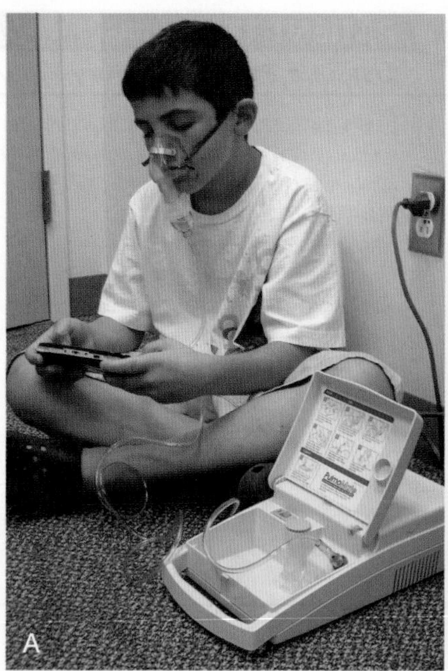

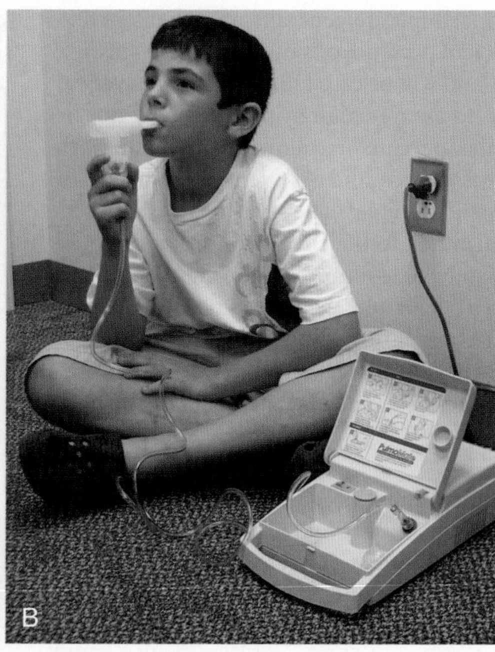

FIGURE 45-6 Children with asthma may take a nebulized aerosol treatment with a mask **(A)** or mouthpiece **(B)**. (Courtesy Texas Children's Hospital.)

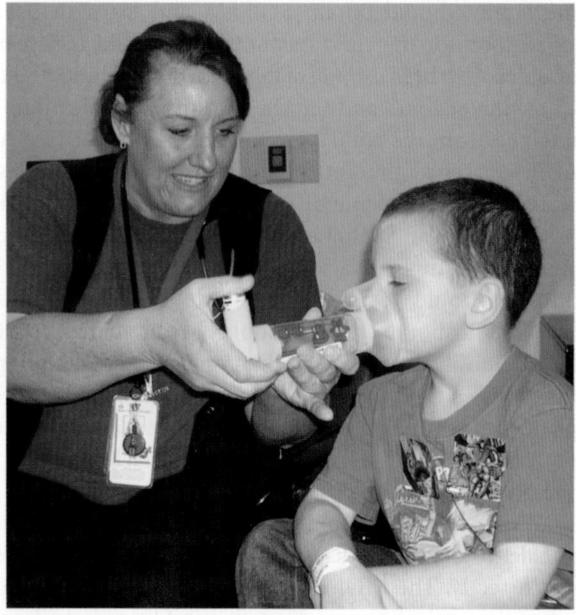

FIGURE 45-7 Child using metered-dose inhaler with spacer and face mask.

NURSING ALERT

Long-acting beta-adrenergic inhalers (salmeterol) should be used only as directed (usually every 12 hours) and not more frequently. They are not intended to relieve acute asthmatic symptoms.

The child should be protected from a respiratory tract infection, which can trigger an attack or aggravate the asthmatic state. This is especially true for young children whose airways are mechanically smaller and more reactive. Annual influenza vaccinations are recommended for children with persistent asthma (Ortiz-Alvarez et al., 2012/2015). Pneumococcal vaccines should also be maintained. Equipment used for the child, such as nebulizers, must be kept clean to decrease the chances of contamination with bacteria and fungi.

Breathing exercises and controlled breathing should be taught and encouraged for motivated children, and the nurse should provide information on activities that promote diaphragmatic breathing, side expansion, and improved mobility of the chest wall. Play techniques that can be used for younger children to extend their expiratory time and increase expiratory pressure include blowing cotton balls or a ping-pong ball on a table, blowing a pinwheel, blowing bubbles, or preventing a tissue from falling by blowing it against the wall.

Self-care and asthma self-management programs are important in helping the child and family cope with asthma. Most asthma self-management programs for children are based on the following principles:

- Asthma is a common disease that can be controlled with appropriate medication therapy, environmental control, education, and management skills.
- It is much easier to prevent than to treat an asthma episode; adherence to a therapeutic program is necessary to prevent exacerbations.
- Children with asthma can live full and active lives.

Asthma camps provide an opportunity for children with asthma to engage in physical activity while learning about their disease in a controlled environment with their peers and with health care providers. Children who attend asthma camps often demonstrate improved asthma self-management skills.

Self-contained programs, brochures, and websites for patient education are available from the Asthma Society of Canada, the Lung Association, and Canadian Allergy, Asthma, and Immunology Foundation. The Asthma Society of Canada has an

PATIENT TEACHING

*Use of a Metered-Dose Inhaler**

Steps for Checking How Much Medicine Is in the Canister

1. If the canister is new, it is full.
2. If the canister has been used repeatedly, it might be empty. (Check product label to see how many inhalations should be in each canister.)
3. The most accurate way to determine how many doses remain in a metered-dose inhaler (MDI) is to count and record each actuation as it is used.
4. Many dry-powder inhalers have a dose-counting device or dose indicator on the canister to let you know when the canister is empty.
5. Placing dry-powder inhalers or MDIs with hydrofluoroalkanes in water will destroy these inhalers.

Steps for Using the Inhaler

1. Remove the cap and hold the inhaler upright.
2. Shake the inhaler.
3. Tilt your head back slightly and breathe out slowly.
4. With the inhaler in an upright position, position the mouthpiece as follows:
   a. About 3 to 4 cm from the mouth or
   b. Into the mouth, forming an airtight seal between the lips and the mouthpiece
5. At the end of a normal expiration, depress the top of the inhaler canister firmly to release the medication (into either the AeroChamber or the mouth) and breathe in slowly (about 3 to 5 seconds). Relax the pressure on the top of the canister.
6. Hold the breath for at least 5 to 10 seconds to allow the aerosol medication to reach deeply into the lungs.
7. Remove the inhaler and breathe out slowly through the nose.
8. Wait 1 minute between puffs (if an additional one is needed).

Steps for Using the Inhaler With an AeroChamber

This approach is recommended for all age groups and for use with corticosteroids (see Fig. 45-7). A parent or caregiver helps with use of this inhaler as required according the child's age and development.

1. Remove the cap and hold inhaler upright.
2. Shake the inhaler.
3. Attach the AeroChamber.
4. With the inhaler in an upright position, insert the mouthpiece into the back of the AeroChamber.
5. Apply the AeroChamber mask to your face and make sure there is a good seal. A caregiver needs to assist younger children with this.
6. Take slow, regular breaths. Depress the top of the inhaler canister firmly to release the medication (into the AeroChamber) and breathe slowly in and out. Relax the pressure on the top of the canister.
7. Hold the AeroChamber in place over your face until six breaths have been taken. Give one puff at a time.
8. Remove the inhaler and AeroChamber.
9. Wait 1 minute between puffs (if an additional puff is needed) when using a bronchodilator.

Common Problems for Children Using Inhalers

- The child refuses or resists treatment.
- Inhalation is too rapid.
- The child is unable to coordinate the spray with inhalation.
- Breath is not held long enough after inhalation.

*Note: Some dry-powder inhalers require a different inhalation technique. To use these dry-powder inhalers, it is important to close the mouth tightly around the mouthpiece of the inhaler and inhale rapidly and deeply.

Adapted from National Asthma Education and Prevention Program. (1997). *Expert panel report II: Guidelines for the diagnosis and management of asthma* (Pub No 97-4051). Bethesda, MD: National Heart, Lung, and Blood Institute.

innovative website that teaches children about asthma. The Asthma Society participates in the Global Initiative for Asthma, which is an asthma network that works with health care providers and public health groups to decrease asthma prevalence, morbidity, and mortality. For all of these resources, see the Additional Resources section at the end of this chapter.

Support the Child or Adolescent and Family

The nurse working with children with asthma can provide support in a number of ways. Many children voice frustration because their exacerbations interfere with their daily activities and social lives. They need education about what to do to prevent an asthma episode. These children also need reassurance from the health care team that they can learn to control and cope with their asthma and live a normal life.

Children in disruptive family situations (divorce, separation, violence, custodial battles) may disregard daily asthma medication regimen or may be at higher risk for symptoms as a result of neglect by adults who are in charge of their care. Adolescents struggling with a sense of identity and body image often regard asthma as a condition that will "go away," especially if there is a time lapse between symptoms, and may abandon the therapeutic regimen. Referral for counselling and guidance is appropriate when the child or adolescent's life is potentially in harm's way and the therapeutic regimen for asthma is abandoned because of personal or family crises.

The task of living day-to-day with affected children involves the entire family. There are periodic crises and the ever-present threat of a crisis, requiring parental vigilance; sleepless nights; frequent trips to the physician, emergency department, or hospital; and often overwhelming medical expenses. Throughout these stresses, parents should be encouraged to promote as normal a life as possible for their children.

Cystic Fibrosis

Cystic fibrosis (CF) is inherited as an autosomal recessive trait; the affected child inherits the defective gene from both parents, with an overall risk of one in four if both parents carry the gene. The mutated gene responsible for CF is located on the long arm of chromosome 7. This gene codes a protein of 1480 amino acids called the *cystic fibrosis transmembrane regulator (CFTR)*. The CFTR protein is related to a family of membrane-bound glycoproteins. The glycoproteins constitute a cAMP-activated chloride channel and also regulate other chloride and sodium

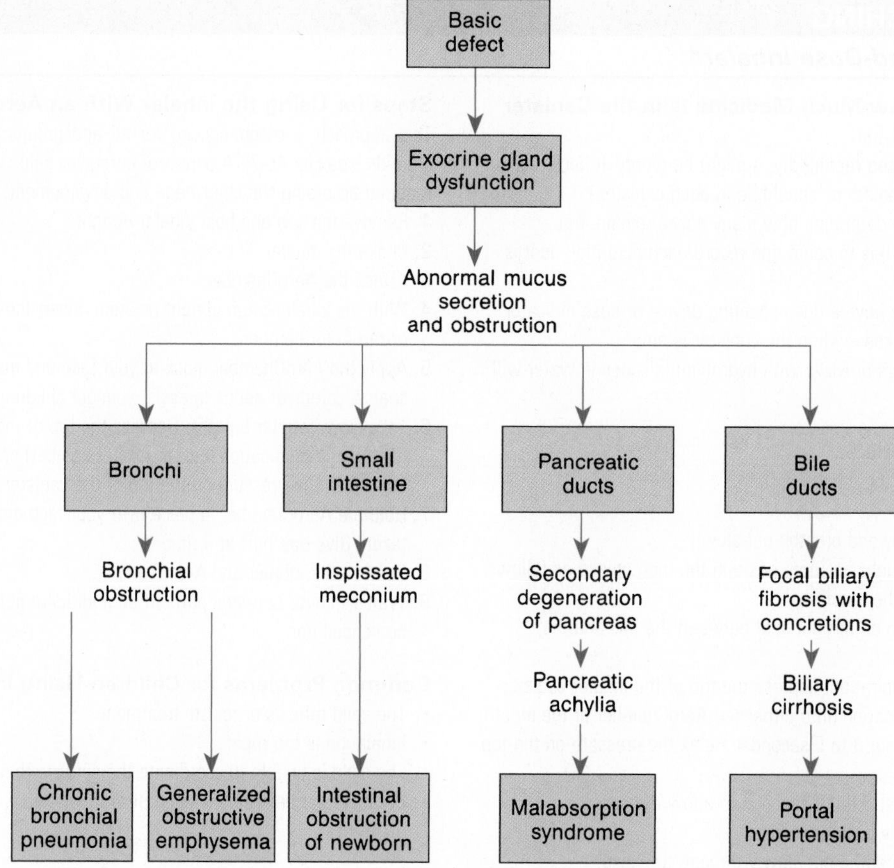

FIGURE 45-8 Various effects of exocrine gland dysfunction in cystic fibrosis.

channels at the surfaces of the epithelial cells. In Canada, 89% of individuals with CF carry at least one copy of the most common CF causing mutation, F508del (Cystic Fibrosis Canada, 2015).

It is estimated that 1 in every 3600 Canadian children is born with CF. Currently in Canada, approximately 4000 children and adults attend a CF clinic (Philpott et al., 2010). In 2013, there were 118 new diagnoses made; 68 of these were in children under 6 months of age (Cystic Fibrosis Canada, 2015).

Pathophysiology

CF is characterized by several clinical features: increased viscosity of mucous gland secretions, a striking elevation of sweat electrolytes, an increase in several organic and enzymatic constituents of saliva, and abnormalities in autonomic nervous system function. Although both sodium and chloride are affected, the defect appears to be primarily a result of abnormal chloride movement; the CFTR appears to function as a chloride channel. Children with CF demonstrate decreased pancreatic secretion of bicarbonate and chloride and an increase in sodium and chloride in both saliva and sweat. This characteristic is the basis for the sweat chloride diagnostic test. The sweat electrolyte abnormality is present from birth, continues throughout life, and is unrelated to the severity of the disease or the extent to which other organs are involved.

The primary factor, and the one that is responsible for many of the clinical manifestations of the disease, is mechanical obstruction caused by the increased viscosity of mucous gland secretions (Fig. 45-8). Instead of forming a thin, freely flowing secretion, the mucous glands produce a thick mucoprotein that accumulates and dilates them. Small passages in organs such as the pancreas and bronchioles become obstructed as secretions precipitate or coagulate to form concretions in glands and ducts. The earliest postnatal manifestation of CF is often meconium ileus in the newborn, in which the small intestine is blocked with thick, puttylike, tenacious, mucilaginous meconium.

In the pancreas the thick secretions block the ducts, eventually causing pancreatic fibrosis. This blockage prevents essential pancreatic enzymes from reaching the duodenum, which causes marked impairment in the digestion and absorption of nutrients. The disturbed function is reflected in bulky stools that are frothy from undigested fat (*steatorrhea*) and foul smelling from putrefied protein (*azotorrhea*).

The incidence of diabetes mellitus (cystic fibrosis–related diabetes [CFRD]) is greater in children with CF than in the general population; it may be caused by changes in pancreatic architecture and diminished blood supply over time. CFRD is reported to be the most common complication associated with CF. By age 30, approximately 50% of people with CF will have developed diabetes, which is associated with increased morbidity (sixfold) and mortality and poor lung function (O'Riordan, Dattani, & Hindmarsh, 2010). In 2013, 23.1% of all Canadian patients with CF had diabetes (Cystic Fibrosis Canada, 2015). The primary characteristic of CFRD is severe insulin deficiency as a result of beta-cell dysfunction; however CFRD also may demonstrate fluctuating insulin resistance, especially during acute illness. Therefore, CFRD has characteristics of both types 1 and 2 diabetes mellitus, but it is considered to be its own entity. The positive correlation between nutritional status and optimal pulmonary function in patients with CF has been described; the presence of adequate insulin appears to be a key factor in maintaining adequate nutritional status. Experts continue to recommend a high-fat, high-calorie diet for CF patients. At this time, there is no evidence to support a change in this diet for patients with CFRD (O'Riordan et al., 2010).

An uncommon gastrointestinal complication associated with CF is prolapse of the rectum, which occurs in infancy and childhood and is related to large, bulky stools; malnutrition; and increased intra-abdominal pressure secondary to paroxysmal cough. This is seen less frequently in children who receive pancreatic enzymes. Affected children of all ages are subject to intestinal obstruction from inspissated or impacted feces. Gumlike masses can obstruct the bowel and produce a partial or complete obstruction, a condition that is referred to as *distal intestinal obstruction syndrome.*

Pulmonary complications are present in almost all children with CF, but the onset and extent of involvement are variable. Symptoms are produced by stagnation of mucus in the airways, with eventual bacterial colonization leading to destruction of lung tissue. The abnormally viscous and tenacious secretions are difficult to expectorate and gradually obstruct the bronchi and bronchioles, causing scattered areas of bronchiectasis, atelectasis, and hyperinflation. The stagnant mucus offers a favourable environment for bacterial growth. The most common pathogens are *Pseudomonas aeruginosa, Burkholderia cepacia, S. aureus, H. influenzae, Escherichia coli,* and *Klebsiella pneumoniae.*

The reproductive systems of both males and females with CF are affected. Females with CF have normal fallopian tubes and ovaries, but fertility can be inhibited by highly viscous cervical secretions, which act as a plug, blocking sperm entry. Women with CF who become pregnant have an increased incidence of premature labour and birth, and low birth weight of the infant. Favourable nutritional status and pulmonary function are positively correlated with favourable pregnancy outcomes. Most adult men (95%) with CF are sterile, which may be caused by blockage of the vas deferens with abnormal secretions or by failure of normal development of the wolffian duct structures (vas deferens, epididymis, and seminal vesicles), resulting in decreased or absent sperm production.

Growth and development are often affected in children with moderate to severe forms of CF. Physical growth may be restricted as a result of decreased absorption of nutrients, including vitamins and fat; increased oxygen demands for pulmonary function; and delayed bone growth. The usual pattern is one of growth failure (failure to thrive), with increased weight loss despite an increased appetite and gradual deterioration of the respiratory system. Clinical manifestations of CF are listed in Box 45-14.

BOX 45-14 CLINICAL MANIFESTATIONS OF CYSTIC FIBROSIS

Meconium Ileus*
Abdominal distension
Vomiting
Failure to pass stools
Rapid development of dehydration

Gastrointestinal Manifestations
Large, bulky, loose, frothy, extremely foul-smelling stools
Voracious appetite (early in disease)
Loss of appetite (later in disease)
Weight loss
Marked tissue wasting
Failure to grow
Distended abdomen
Thin extremities
Sallow skin
Evidence of deficiency of fat-soluble vitamins A, D, E, and K
Anemia

Pulmonary Manifestations
Initial signs:
- Wheezing respirations
- Dry, nonproductive cough

Eventually:
- Increased dyspnea
- Paroxysmal cough
- Evidence of obstructive emphysema and patchy areas of atelectasis

Progressive involvement:
- Overinflated, barrel-shaped chest
- Cyanosis
- Clubbing of fingers and toes
- Repeated episodes of bronchitis and bronchopneumonia

*In about 10% of cases.

Diagnostic Evaluation

Traditionally, the diagnosis of CF was based on a positive sweat chloride test, absence of pancreatic enzymes, radiography, chronic obstructive pulmonary disease, and family history. Newer diagnostic methods make it possible to diagnose CF early in infancy so that therapies can be implemented to increase the child's overall survival and quality of life. In addition to the sweat chloride test and factors listed previously, diagnosis may be confirmed by any one of the following: newborn screening, DNA identification of mutant genes, and abnormal nasal potential difference measurement.

Universal newborn screening for CF has been recommended by Cystic Fibrosis Canada (2016) and all provinces except Quebec, the territories, and part of the Nunavut are doing the screening. The newborn screening test consists of an immunoreactive trypsinogen (IRT) analysis performed on a dried spot of blood, which may be followed by direct analysis of DNA for the presence of the ΔF508 mutation or other mutations on the same dried-blood spot. Benefits of early screening and detection include earlier nutritional intervention for identified infants (Southern, Mérelle, Dankert-Roelse, et al., 2009); disadvantages include the parental anxiety that false-positive results may generate. Children who are identified and treated early in infancy with aggressive nutritional support have had improved height and weight well into adolescence. An in utero diagnosis of CF is also possible, based on detection of two CF mutations in the fetus.

The consistent finding of abnormally high sodium and chloride concentrations in the sweat is a unique characteristic of CF. Parents may report that their infant tastes "salty" when they kiss the infant. The quantitative sweat chloride test (pilocarpine iontophoresis) involves stimulating the production of sweat with a special device (involves stimulation with 3-mA electric current), collecting the sweat on filter paper, and measuring the sweat electrolytes. The quantitative analysis requires a sufficient volume of sweat (more than 75 mg). Two separate samples are collected to ensure the reliability of the test for any individual. Normally, sweat chloride content is less than 40 mmol/L, with a mean of 18 mmol/L. A chloride concentration greater than 60 mmol/L is diagnostic of CF; in infants younger than 3 months a sweat chloride concentration greater than 40 mmol/L is highly suggestive of CF. In some situations DNA testing may be substituted for the sweat test. The presence of a mutation known to cause CF on each *CFTR* gene predicts with a high degree of certainty that the individual has CF; however, multiple *CFTR* mutations may also be present and detected with DNA assay.

Chest radiography reveals characteristic patchy atelectasis and obstructive emphysema. PFTs are sensitive indices of lung function, providing evidence of abnormal small airway function in CF. Other diagnostic tools that may aid in diagnosis include stool fat or enzyme analysis. Stool analysis requires a 72-hour sample with accurate recording of food intake during that time. Radiographs, including contrast dye enema, are used for diagnosis of meconium ileus.

Therapeutic Management

Improved survival among patients with CF during the past two decades can be attributed largely to antibiotic therapy and improved nutritional management. Goals of CF therapeutic management are to (1) prevent or minimize pulmonary complications, (2) ensure adequate nutrition for growth, (3) encourage appropriate physical activity, and (4) promote a reasonable quality of life for the child and the family. A multidisciplinary approach to treatment is needed to accomplish these goals.

Management of pulmonary problems. Management of pulmonary problems is directed toward prevention and treatment of pulmonary infection by improving ventilation, removing mucopurulent secretions, and administering antimicrobial agents. Many children develop respiratory symptoms by 3 years of age. The large amounts and viscosity of respiratory secretions in children with CF contribute to the likelihood of respiratory tract infections. Recurrent pulmonary infections in the child with CF result in greater damage to the airways; small airways are destroyed, causing bronchiectasis.

The most common pathogens responsible for pulmonary infections are *P. aeruginosa*, *B. cepacia*, *S. aureus*, *H. influenzae*, *E. coli*, and *K. pneumoniae*. *P. aeruginosa*, and *B. cepacia* are particularly pathogenic for children with CF, and infections with these organisms are difficult to clear. In addition, children with CF who are chronically colonized with these organisms have poorer survival rates than those of children who are not colonized. Colonization and infection with methicillin-resistant *S. aureus* (MRSA) has emerged as a critical factor in lung infection and pulmonary function in patients with CF. Patients with MRSA required longer hospitalization and multiple antibiotic regimens (Sawicki, Rasouliyan, Pasta, et al., 2008). Fungal colonization with *Candida* or *Aspergillus* organisms in the respiratory tract is also common in patients with CF.

Until recently, CPT was the cornerstone of airway clearance. However other airway clearance therapies (ACT) have replaced this modality; these treatments often require more active involvement by the patient (Newton, 2009). These ACTs include the following: percussion and postural drainage, positive expiratory pressure (PEP), active cycle-of-breathing technique, autogenic drainage, oscillatory PEP, high-frequency chest compression (HFCC), and exercise. Researchers have not found that any specific technique clears mucus better than the other. It is recommended that individualized assessments be made to determine the best ACT for each patient (Flume, Robinson, O'Sullivan, et al., 2009).

ACTs such as percussion and postural drainage are usually performed, on average, twice daily (on rising and in the evening) and more frequently if needed, especially during pulmonary infection. The Flutter mucus clearance device is a small, handheld plastic pipe with a stainless-steel ball on the inside that facilitates removal of mucus. It has the advantage of increasing sputum expectoration and being used without an assistant. Hand-held percussors may be used to loosen secretions. Another method to clear mucus is high-frequency chest compression, in which the child temporarily wears a mechanical vest device that provides high-frequency chest wall oscillation. Some children and adolescents with an implantable port may experience localized pain with the vest.

Patients with CF have been found to regress when conventional CPT is discontinued. Forced expiration, or "huffing," with the glottis partially closed helps move secretions from the small airways so that subsequent coughing can move secretions forcefully from the large airways. Several studies indicate that this manoeuvre enhances the pulmonary function of patients with CF. Autogenic drainage involves a variety of breathing techniques, which the older child can use to force mucus in lower lobes up into the airways so it can be successfully expelled. Another mucus-clearing technique involves use of a PEP mask. This technique involves breathing into a mask attached to a one-way valve, which creates resistance—as the patient exhales, the airway is kept open by the pressure, and mucus is forced into the upper airway for expulsion.

Bronchodilator medication delivered in an aerosol opens bronchi for easier expectoration and is administered before

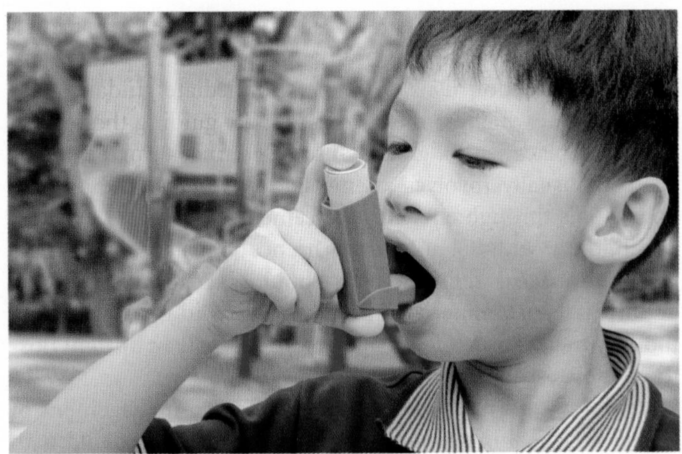

FIGURE 45-9 Bronchodilator medication delivered in an aerosol. (© Can Stock Photo Inc./parinyabinsuk.)

percussion and postural drainage when the patient exhibits evidence of reactive airway disease or wheezing (Fig. 45-9). Another aerosolized medication is recombinant human deoxyribonuclease (DNase, known generically as dornase alfa [Pulmozyme]), which decreases the viscosity of mucus. It is well tolerated and has no major adverse effects; minor reactions are voice alterations and laryngitis. This medication, given daily via nebulization, has resulted in improvements in spirometry, PFTs, dyspnea scores, and perceptions of well-being and has reduced the viscosity of sputum.

Nebulized hypertonic saline (6 to 7%) has been shown to be effective in improving airway hydration and increases mucus clearance in patients with CF; this treatment, however, causes bronchospasm and may not be recommended for patients with severe disease (Redding, 2009).

Physical exercise is an important adjunct to daily ACT. Exercise stimulates mucus excretion and provides a sense of well-being and increased self-esteem. Any aerobic exercise that the patient enjoys should be encouraged. The ultimate aim of exercise is to increase lung vital capacity, remove secretions, increase pulmonary blood flow, and maintain healthy lung tissue for effective ventilation.

Pulmonary infections need to be treated as soon as they are recognized. In patients with CF, characteristic signs of pulmonary infection—fever, tachypnea, and chest pain—may be absent; thus a careful history and physical examination are essential. The presence of anorexia, weight loss, and decreased activity should alert the practitioner to pulmonary infection and the need for an antibiotic regimen. Aerosolized antibiotics such as tobramycin, ticarcillin, and gentamicin are beneficial for patients with frequent pulmonary exacerbations.

IV antibiotics may be administered at home as an alternative to hospitalization. The use of peripherally inserted central catheters (PICCs) for the administration of antibiotics in children with CF is a viable option with limited complications and fewer needle punctures to obtain blood specimens and to maintain often lengthy treatment with parenteral antibiotics. Alternatively, an implanted port offers the advantage of access for blood draws and antibiotic infusion. When pulmonary function does not improve with outpatient management, hospitalization may be recommended for continued antibiotic therapy and vigorous postural drainage. Some health care providers hospitalize patients for IV antibiotic therapy and percussion and postural drainage periodically (a "tune-up") to keep them well; others may be treated on an outpatient basis. Oxygen administration is used for children with acute episodes but must be used cautiously because many children with CF have chronic carbon dioxide retention and the unsupervised use of oxygen can be harmful (see Oxygen Therapy, Chapter 44). With repeated infection and inflammation, bronchial cysts and emphysema may develop. These cysts may rupture, resulting in a pneumothorax.

! NURSING ALERT

Signs of a pneumothorax are usually nonspecific and include tachypnea, tachycardia, dyspnea, pallor, and cyanosis. A subtle drop in oxygen saturation (measured by pulse oximetry) may be an early sign of pneumothorax.

Children with a specific CF mutation (G551D) may benefit by taking ivacaftor (Kalydeco). This CF transmembrane conductance regulator modulator allows salt and fluid to move through the airways and prevent the buildup of thick mucus in the airways, with concomitant improvement of pulmonary function. Kalydeco is currently reimbursed in most of the provinces and the Yukon.

Blood streaking of the sputum is usually associated with increased pulmonary infection and often requires no specific treatment. Hemoptysis greater than 250 mL/24 hours for the older child (less for a younger child) indicates a potentially life-threatening event and needs to be treated immediately. Sometimes bleeding can be controlled with bedrest, IV antibiotics, replacement of acute blood loss, IV conjugated estrogens (Premarin) or vasopressin (Pitressin), and correction of any coagulation defects with vitamin K or fresh frozen plasma. If hemoptysis persists, the site of bleeding should be localized via bronchoscopy and cauterized or embolized.

Treatment of nasal polyps includes intranasal corticosteroids, oral antihistamines, and decongestants. If these measures are ineffective, surgical interventions such as cauterization may be necessary.

Treatment with corticosteroids for prolonged periods has been associated with linear growth restriction, glucose tolerance abnormalities, and cataract formation. Anti-inflammatory medications such as ibuprofen are becoming more important in the treatment of CF, but careful monitoring for adverse effects (gastrointestinal bleeding) is essential.

Management of gastrointestinal problems. Among Canadians with CF, 86% require treatment for gastrointestinal issues (Cystic Fibrosis Canada, 2015). The principal treatment for pancreatic insufficiency is replacement of pancreatic enzymes, which are administered with meals and snacks to ensure that digestive enzymes are mixed with food in the duodenum. Enteric-coated products prevent the neutralization of enzymes by gastric acids, thus allowing activation to occur in the alkaline environment of the small bowel. The amount of enzymes depends on the severity of the insufficiency, the child's response to enzyme replacement, and the practitioner's philosophy. Usually one to five capsules (or 2500 lipase units per kg) are administered with a meal, and fewer are taken with snacks. Capsules can be swallowed whole or taken apart, with the contents sprinkled on a small amount of food taken at the beginning of the meal. The amount of enzyme is adjusted to achieve normal growth and a decrease in the number of stools to one or two per day. Pancreatic enzymes should be taken within 30 minutes of eating. The enteric-coated beads should not be chewed or crushed, since destroying the enteric coating can lead to inactivation of the enzymes and excoriation of oral mucosa. The powder form should be used cautiously, because inhalation of the powder may precipitate acute bronchospasm, and if mixed with food, it predigests the food, making it unpalatable.

Children with CF require a well-balanced, high-protein, high-caloric diet (because of the impaired intestinal absorption). In the patient with minimal pulmonary disease, energy requirements up to 150% above the recommended daily allowances are necessary, depending on the severity of the disease (Cystic Fibrosis Canada, 2015). Breastfeeding with enzyme supplementation should be continued whenever possible and, when necessary, supplemented with a higher-calorie-per-mL (e.g., 24 kcal/30 mL) formula. For formula-fed infants, commercial cow's milk–based formulas may be adequate to achieve desired growth, but if growth is inadequate, a partial hydrolysate formula with medium-chain triglycerides (e.g., Progestimal, Alimentum) may be recommended. In older children with CF, three daily meals and three snacks are recommended to meet energy and growth requirements. Enzymes can be mixed into cereal or fruit such as applesauce. Because the uptake of fat-soluble vitamins is decreased, water-miscible forms of these vitamins (A, D, E, and K) are given, along with multivitamins and the pancreatic enzymes. When high-fat foods are eaten, the child should be encouraged to add extra enzymes. Growth failure despite adequate nutritional support may indicate deterioration of pulmonary status. Patients with CF may experience frequent anorexia as a result of the copious amounts of mucus produced and expectorated, persistent cough, effect of medications, fatigue, and sleep disruption. They may be placed on nighttime supplemental gastrostomy feedings or, rarely, parenteral alimentation, in an effort to build up nutritional reserves if there has been a history of inability to maintain weight. Meconium ileus and meconium ileus equivalent, or total or partial intestinal obstruction, can occur at any age. Constipation is often the result of a combination of malabsorption (either from inadequate pancreatic enzyme dosage or a failure to take the enzymes), decreased intestinal motility, and abnormally viscous intestinal secretions. These problems usually do not require surgical interventions and may be treated with GoLYTELY or Colyte (osmotic solutions given orally or by nasogastric tubes), other laxatives, stool softeners, or rectal administration of meglumine diatrizoate (Gastrografin).

Rectal prolapse occurs only in a small number of individuals; fewer are affected as result of early diagnosis and administration of pancreatic enzymes (Egan, Green, & Voynow, 2016). The first episode of rectal prolapse is frightening to both the parents and child. Its reduction usually requires immediate guidance and intervention, which is managed by simply guiding the rectum back into place with a gloved, lubricated finger. Further management usually involves attempting to decrease the bulk of daily stools through enzyme replacement.

Children with CF often experience transient or chronic gastroesophageal reflux, which should be treated with the appropriate histamine-receptor antagonist and gastrointestinal motility medication, dietary modifications, and an upright position after feedings or meals (Hazle, 2010).

Management of endocrine problems. The management of CFRD is critical in the therapeutic treatment of the child with CF. CFRD presents a combination of insulin resistance and insulin deficiency, with unstable glucose homeostasis in the presence of acute lung infection and treatment. Children with CFRD require close monitoring of blood glucose, administration of oral glucose-lowering agents or insulin injections, and diet and exercise management. Children with CF may be at increased risk for glucose management problems as a result of decreased nutrient absorption, anorexia, and severity of pulmonary illness. The prevalence of CFRD increases with age, and there is increased morbidity and mortality among children with CFRD compared to those without CFRD. Microvascular complications such as retinopathy and nephropathy may occur in children and adolescents with CFRD (O'Riordan et al., 2010). However, ketoacidosis is rare in individuals with CFRD (Egan et al., 2016). Children with CFRD should perform self-blood glucose monitoring (SBGM) three times a day and should be on an insulin regimen. Target glucose levels should be the same as for any other patient with diabetes. There is no evidence that oral glycemic agents are effective. During acute CF exacerbations, the nondiabetic child should be monitored closely for hyperglycemia. Glycosylated hemoglobin is reportedly a poor predictor of CFRD, so an oral glucose tolerance test is the preferred screening tool (Moran, Brunzell, Cohen, et al., 2010).

Bone health is of concern in children and adults with CF. The pancreatic insufficiency of CF and chronic steroid use present potential risks for less than optimum bone growth in such children. Assessment of bone health by history and bone mass density evaluation should be considered in assessing the child's (8 years old and older) health status to detect and prevent osteoporosis or osteopenia.

Prognosis

The median age of survival for Canadians with CF is currently estimated to be 50.9 years of age. Females with CF have had higher mortality rates than males with CF (Cystic Fibrosis Canada, 2016). Lung, heart, pancreas, and liver transplantation have increased survival rates among some patients with CF. Heart-lung and double-lung transplants have been successfully performed in children with advanced pulmonary vascular disease and hypoxia. The obstacles surrounding this technique are availability of donated organs; complications from surgery; pulmonary infections; and recurrence of obstructive bronchiolitis, which decreases transplanted lung function.

Despite considerable progress and a recent surge in new treatment modalities, CF remains a progressive and incurable disease. The pulmonary involvement ultimately determines the patient's outcome because pancreatic enzyme deficiency is less of a problem if adequate nutrition is ensured. With the advances in treatment technology, parents and adolescents are challenged to set future goals that may include college, careers, social relationships, and marriage. Concurrently, they are faced with increasing morbidity and higher rates of CF complications as they grow older.

NURSING CARE

Assessment of the child with CF involves both pulmonary and gastrointestinal observations. Pulmonary assessment is the same as that described for asthma, with special attention to lung sounds, observation of cough, and evidence of decreased activity or fatigue. Gastrointestinal assessment primarily involves observing the frequency and nature of the stools and abdominal distension. Evidence of growth failure (e.g., weight loss, muscle wasting, pallor, anorexia, decreased activity [from baseline norm]) also needs to be noted. Family members should be interviewed to determine the child's eating and eliminating habits and to confirm the child's history of frequent respiratory tract infections or bowel obstruction in infancy.

The nurse should assess the newborn for feeding and stooling patterns, which may indicate a potential problem such as meconium ileus. The nurse should also participate in diagnostic testing, such as the initial newborn screening, DNA analysis, or sweat chloride test. Parents are often anxious and puzzled about the diagnostic tests and the possible implications of the test results. They need careful explanations of the disease, how it might affect their family, and what they can do to provide the best possible care for their child. It is crucial to involve the parents in the follow-up for early diagnostic testing; the newborn may require several follow-up visits in the first few weeks of life if initial test results are not conclusive.

The uncertainty, fear, and initial shock associated with the diagnosis can be overwhelming to parents. They must face the impact of the chronic, life-threatening nature of the disease and the prospect of intensive treatment, for which they must assume a major part of the responsibility and are usually ill prepared. They often fear that they will be unable to provide the care that the child needs.

Hospital Care

Most patients with CF require hospitalization only for the treatment of pulmonary infection, uncontrolled diabetes, or a coexisting medical problem that cannot be treated on an outpatient basis. When patients with CF are hospitalized, routine precautions with meticulous hand hygiene should be implemented to decrease the health care–associated spread of organisms to the patient with CF and between hospitalized patients with CF (especially when MRSA is prevalent). Contact precautions may be required for specific infections.

When the child with CF is hospitalized for diagnosis or treatment of pulmonary complications, aerosol therapy, percussion, and postural drainage are instituted or continued. While respiratory therapy and physiotherapists often initiate, supervise, and provide these treatments, it is the nurse's responsibility to monitor the patient's tolerance of the procedure and evaluate its effectiveness in relation to treatment goals. The nurse may at times administer aerosol therapy, perform chest percussion and postural drainage, assist with ACTs such as the mechanical vest, and teach breathing exercises. Chest percussion and postural drainage should be done before meals and bedtime. Planning percussion and postural drainage so that it does not coincide with meals can be difficult in the hospital but is essential to the effectiveness of this treatment.

Nursing assessments, including observation of respiratory pattern, work of breathing, and lung auscultation, are vital assessments. Noninvasive pulse oximetry provides valuable data about the patient's oxygenation status. Supplemental oxygen therapy is administered to the child with mild or moderate respiratory distress, and the child requires frequent assessment of his or her tolerance of the procedure.

One of the nursing challenges in the care of the child with CF is encouraging adherence to the often daunting therapeutic medication regimen, which often includes pancreatic enzymes; vitamins A, D, E, and K; oral antifungals for *Candida* infection; antihistamines; anti-inflammatory agents; and oral antibiotics. This may be overwhelming to the child. With multiple inhaled bronchodilators, ACTs and postural and aerosol treatments, blood glucose monitoring and insulin administration, taking of various other medications, and increased mucus production during the acute phase, it is not uncommon for the child with CF to rebel and be nonadherent to this regimen. Gentle coaxing, positive reinforcement, and frank negotiation may be required to encourage the child to adhere to the required medical treatment.

The child's sleep may be disrupted frequently by hospital routines; nursing care should be flexible enough to allow him or her some quiet time without affecting vital care. In some cases a daily schedule of events, including medication administration, CPT, aerosolized therapy, and dressing changes, may need to be mutually developed with the child, nurses, and physician so that the child feels he or she has some control of the care.

The diet for the child with CF represents another challenge; careful planning with a pediatric dietitian and the child may help decrease the loss of appetite and weight loss that are often part of the condition. Children in the early stages of CF often have a good appetite. With infection and increased lung involvement, their appetite diminishes, and eventually it becomes a challenge to tempt failing appetites. When dietary intake fails to meet the child's needs for growth, enteral feedings or supplements may need to be considered. These feedings may be administered via gastrostomy tube during the night to minimize the disruption of daily activities, including school. A skin-level feeding gastrostomy affords the child few activity restrictions and minimal disruption of body image in comparison to a nasogastric tube or conventional gastrostomy tube. The child and parents should be encouraged to perceive this therapy not as a last-ditch effort but as an adjunct therapy to maintain optimum growth and prevent excessive weight loss. Some children have a nasogastric tube placed before bedtime and receive enteral feedings overnight.

The child or adolescent needs support during the many treatments and tests that are a part of the hospitalization. IV fluids, IV antibiotics and antifungals, PICC line placement or port accessing, and blood tests are almost always a part of the acute care treatment, and the child may soon associate hospitalization with these stress-provoking procedures.

Depression, anxiety, and disturbed self-image may occur in children and adolescents with CF. Young adults with severe symptoms may be especially prone to depression as a result of the realization of the poor prognosis and the reality of unmet life expectations and goals.

Providing support to both the child and the family is essential. The progressive nature of the disease makes each illness requiring hospitalization a potentially life-threatening event. Skilled nursing care and empathetic attention to the emotional needs of the child and family can help them cope with the stresses associated with repeated respiratory tract infections and hospitalizations.

The child or adolescent who is immobilized as a result of CF requires the same care and attention as the child with immobility from any other chronic or acute illness, including skin care, bowel management, passive range of motion, and positioning.

Home Care

Most children and adolescents with CF can be managed at home. The goals of care include **normalization** and daily activities, including school and peer involvement. The care plan should be flexible so that family activities are disrupted as little as possible. Parents may initially require assistance in finding and contacting durable medical equipment companies that provide home care equipment. They also need opportunities to learn how to use the equipment and to solve problems they may encounter while delivering therapy at home. The many aspects of home care for the child with CF are similar to those of home care for other children with complex conditions and are discussed in Chapter 42.

Patients and family members need education about the preferred diet of nutritious meals with tolerated fat, increased protein and carbohydrate, and the administration of pancreatic enzymes. It is important to stress to parents that the enzymes, in the amount regulated to the child's needs, should be administered at the beginning of all meals and snacks.

One of the most important aspects of educating parents for home care is teaching techniques for the removal of mucus (ACT, vest, forced expiration) and assisting with breathing exercises. The success of a therapy program depends on conscientious performance of these treatments regularly as prescribed. The number of times these therapies are performed each day is determined on an individual basis, and often parents readily learn to adjust the number and intensity of the treatments to the child's needs. For pulmonary infection, home IV antibiotics may be prescribed. Home IV care may be preferred for some families, as it reduces tension and usually brings a sense of belonging to the family members. This option depends on a number of factors, including availability of an agency with adequate staff to perform multiple daily home antibiotic infusions. With use of the venous access devices such as PICC lines and implanted ports, the parents and child can be taught the technique of direct administration into the IV line.

Families also need information about medications and possible adverse effects. Children receiving multiple antibiotics may require serum drug levels to ensure therapeutic dosing. If a child is receiving ibuprofen, observations for adverse effects such as gastrointestinal irritation are essential.

If the child has CFRD, education on SBGM, insulin therapy, diet control, and possible related complications is needed. Follow-up with a pediatric endocrinologist is recommended.

Children and adolescents with CF should receive routine primary care with special attention to diet, growth and development, and immunizations. Primary care providers should be alert to any weight loss or flattening in the growth curve associated with loss of appetite, which could indicate a pulmonary exacerbation in children with CF. In addition to all the recommended routine immunizations, patients with CF should be immunized against influenza starting at age 6 months; this should be followed by an annual booster (PHAC, 2014a). Infants with CF also meet the inclusion criteria to receive the RSV prophylaxis. Anticipatory guidance concerning issues of discipline, how to incorporate aspects of the treatment regimen into the school environment, and delayed pubertal development are also important considerations for the primary care provider.

Home palliative care for the child or adolescent with CF who is in the terminal stages may be carried out with the assistance of hospice (see Chapter 40).

The nurse can assist the family in contacting resources that provide help to families with affected children. Various special child health services, many local clinics, private agencies, service clubs, and other community groups often offer equipment and medications either free or at reduced rates. Cystic Fibrosis Canada has chapters throughout Canada to provide education and services to families and professionals (see Additional Resources at the end of this chapter).

Family Support

One of the most challenging aspects of providing care for the family of a child or adolescent with CF is meeting the emotional needs of the child and family. The diagnosis, treatment, and prognosis for CF are often associated with many problems and frustrations. The diagnosis can evoke feelings of guilt and self-recrimination in parents.

The long-range problems for an infant, child, or adolescent with CF are those encountered in any chronic illness or complex medical condition (see Chapter 40). Both the child and the family must make many adjustments, the success of which depends on their ability to cope and on the quality and quantity of support they receive from outside sources. Combined efforts of a variety of health care providers are needed to provide the most comprehensive services to families. It is often the nurse who assesses the home situation, organizes and coordinates these services, and collects the data needed to evaluate the effectiveness of the services.

The persistent need for treatment several times a day can place tremendous strain on the family. When the child is young, a family member must perform postural drainage and other ACTs. Children often struggle to accept these treatments, and the parents are placed in the position of insisting on adherence. The stress and anxiety related to this routine may produce feelings of resentment in both the child and the family members. When possible, occasional trusted respite care should be made available to allow parents to leave the situation for short periods without undue anxiety about their child's welfare.

The affected child or adolescent may become resentful about the disease, its relentless routine of therapy, and the necessary curtailment it places on activities and relationships. The child's activities are interrupted or built around treatments, medications, and diet. This imposes hardships and influences his or her quality of life. The child should be encouraged to attend school and join age-appropriate peer groups to foster a life that is as normal and productive as possible. Sports are often an important part of the child and adolescent's life; interaction with peers is a valuable life experience, especially to adolescents. The child or adolescent with CF should be encouraged to participate in sports activities as much as physical and pulmonary health allows. Exercise should be encouraged to increase pulmonary vital capacity, promote muscle development, and enhance cardiovascular function.

As the disease progresses, however, family stress should be expected, and the patient may become angry and noncompliant. It is important for the nurse to recognize the family's changing needs and the grief they may experience as the CF worsens. Families should be made aware of sources for counselling. Patients need to be guided into activities that enable them to express anger, sorrow, and fear, without guilt.

Transition to Adulthood

As life expectancy continues to rise for children and adolescents with CF, issues related to marriage, sexuality, child-bearing, and career choice have become more pressing. Males must be informed at some point that they may be unable to produce offspring. It is important that the distinction be made between sterility and impotence. Normal sexual relationships can be expected. Female patients may be able to bear children but should be informed of the possible deleterious effects on their respiratory system created by the burden of pregnancy. They also need to know that their children will be carriers of the CF gene. Adolescent females may need counselling concerning the use of oral contraceptives and other contraceptive options.

Adolescents with CF should be encouraged to take responsibility for management of the illness to maximize their life's potential. Many adolescents and young persons with the illness enroll in college or vocational and technical training school and complete degrees by either distance learning or attending a local school. Young people should be encouraged to set life goals and live normal lives to the extent their illness allows.

Anticipatory grief and other aspects related to the care of a child with a terminal illness are also part of nursing care. For example, it is important to prepare the child and family members for end-of-life decisions and care, when appropriate.

Obstructive Sleep-Disordered Breathing

Pediatric obstructive sleep-disordered breathing reportedly affects between 10 and 12% of children ages 2 to 8 years. Obstructive sleep-disordered breathing is said to form a continuum of sleep-disordered breathing, ranging from partial obstruction of the upper airway to continuous episodes of complete upper airway obstruction, with the most severe form being obstructive sleep apnea syndrome (OSAS). OSAS is defined by the Lung Association (2014) as a disorder of breathing during sleep with prolonged partial upper airway obstruction or complete obstruction that disrupts normal respiration during sleep and normal sleep patterns. Common symptoms include nightly snoring, interrupted or disturbed sleep patterns, enuresis, and daytime neurobehavioural problems (Marcus, Brooks, Draper, et al., 2012). OSAS may occur in as many as 2 to 3% of all children in Canada (The Lung Association, 2014). OSAS is to be distinguished from primary snoring, which is snoring without obstructive apnea, frequent sleep arousals, or abnormalities in gas exchange (Marcus et al., 2012). Interestingly, children with OSAS do not exhibit daytime sleepiness as do adults; the exception may be obese children. If left untreated, obstructive sleep-disordered breathing may result in complications such as failure to thrive, cardiovascular problems, hypertension, poor learning, and neurobehavioural problems such as attention-deficit hyperactivity disorder (Marcus et al., 2012).

The diagnosis of obstructive sleep-disordered breathing is made by an overnight in-laboratory sleep study (*polysomnography*), which provides evidence of sleep disturbance, respiratory pauses, and changes in oxygenation. The six-channel polysomnography can be performed in children of all ages through videotaping or audiotaping, and abbreviated (vs. full night sleep study) polysomnography, nocturnal oximetry, or daytime nap polysomnography may be useful; however, these latter methods do not predict the severity of OSAS (Marcus et al., 2012). Polysomnography can be used to distinguish between OSAS and primary snoring (Owens, 2016).

The most recent American Academy of Pediatrics (AAP) clinical practice guideline recommends adenotonsillectomy for OSAS, as long as the child has no contraindications for surgery (Marcus et al., 2012). Evidence indicates that tonsillectomy or adenoidectomy alone may not be sufficient to resolve OSAS because residual lymphoid tissue may contribute to continual obstruction (Marcus et al., 2012). Complications of these surgical interventions are discussed previously in this chapter on p. 1343. The AAP recommends that high-risk patients undergoing adenotonsillectomy be monitored as inpatients postoperatively for complications (Marcus et al., 2012). CPAP may be helpful in older children with sleep-disordered breathing whose condition persists after surgical intervention. CPAP is a long-term therapy with frequent assessments to evaluate the required amount of pressure and the overall effectiveness of the intervention. The most recent AAP guidelines also recommend the use of topical intranasal corticosteroids for children with mild OSAS (defined as an apnea hypopnea index [AHI] of less than 5 per hour) (Marcus et al., 2012).

Surgical interventions such as tracheotomy may be required for children with craniofacial syndromes such as Goldenhar, Pierre Robin, Apert, and Crouzon, in which there is partial or complete upper airway obstruction.

NURSING CARE

Nursing care of the child with sleep-disordered breathing involves early detection by observation of the infant's or child's sleep patterns and active participation in the diagnostic polysomnography. Important nursing roles are insertion of the pH probe into the esophagus, ensuring accurate placement by radiography, and monitoring the sleep study and the patient's response to diagnostic therapy. Counselling families of children with sleep-disordered breathing may involve dietary counselling for exercise programs and weight management, use of the CPAP equipment, and direct postoperative care after the surgical intervention of tonsillectomy or adenoidectomy. The nurse can be instrumental in helping the child and family cope with the chronic illness diagnosis if intervention such as CPAP is required.

CONGENITAL RESPIRATORY SYSTEM ANOMALIES

Choanal Atresia

Choanal atresia, the most common congenital anomaly of the nose, is a bony or membranous septum located between the nose and the pharynx (Fig. 45-10). The atresia may be unilateral or bilateral. Because most infants are preferential nose breathers, bilateral choanal atresia may be associated with apnea and cyanosis when the infant is at rest. When the infant cries, he or she breathes in through the mouth and pinks up. Unilateral choanal atresia may not be associated with apnea. Inability to pass a suction catheter through the nose into the pharynx or cyanosis without obvious respiratory distress usually leads to detection of choanal atresia. Nearly half of the infants with choanal atresia have other anomalies.

Congenital Diaphragmatic Hernia

Congenital diaphragmatic hernia (CDH) results from a defect in the formation of the diaphragm, allowing the abdominal organs to be displaced into the thoracic cavity. It occurs in approximately 1 in 2000 to 1 in 5000 live births (Maheshwari & Carlo, 2016). Herniation of the abdominal viscera into the thoracic cavity may cause severe respiratory distress and represent a neonatal emergency (Fig. 45-11). The defect and herniation may be minimal and easily repaired, or the defect may be so extensive that the viscera present in the thoracic cavity during embryonic life have prevented the normal development of pulmonary tissue. The defect is usually on the left because that is the side of the diaphragm that fuses last.

Most CDHs are discovered prenatally on ultrasound. Hernias may be repaired by fetal surgery, although intrauterine surgical correction of CDH has met with poor neonatal outcomes in many cases, primarily as a result of tocolysis failure and early birth. At birth, most affected infants have severe respiratory distress, and respiratory assessment reveals worsening distress as the bowel fills with air. Typically, breath sounds are diminished and bowel sounds are heard in the chest. Heart sounds may be shifted to the right side of the chest because the heart has been displaced by the abdominal contents. Physical examination reveals a flat or scaphoid abdomen and a prominent ipsilateral chest. Diagnosis can be made on the basis of the x-ray finding of loops of intestine in the thoracic cavity and the absence of intestine in the abdominal cavity.

Preoperatively, nursing interventions include assessment and stabilization of the infant's condition until surgical repair

Posterior View

FIGURE 45-10 Choanal atresia. Posterior nares are obstructed by membrane or bone, either bilaterally or unilaterally. (Used with permission of Ross Products Division, Abbott Laboratories, Inc., Columbus, OH. From Clinical Education Aid No. 6, Copyright © 1963, Ross Products Division, Abbott Laboratories, Inc.)

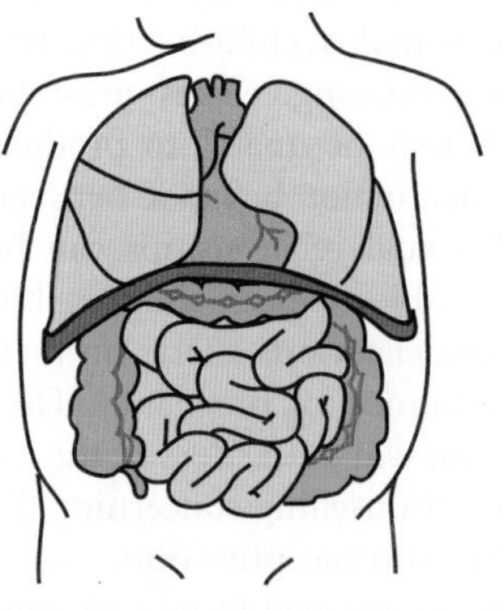

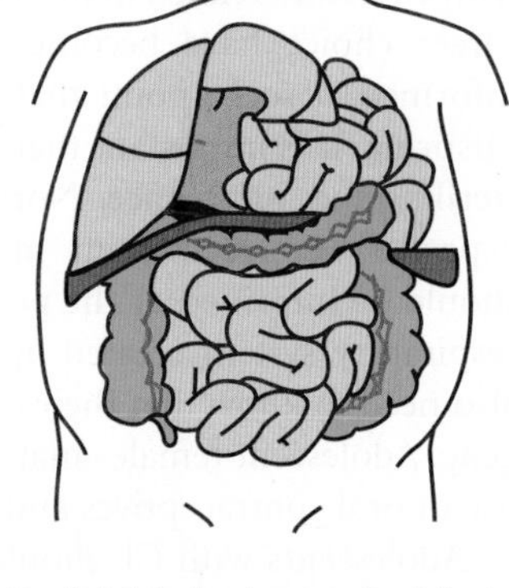

FIGURE 45-11 A: Normal diaphragm separating the abdominal and thoracic cavities. **B:** Diaphragmatic hernia with a small lung and abdominal contents in the thoracic cavity. (From Ehrlich, P. F., & Coran, A. G. [2011]. Diaphragmatic hernia. In R. M. Kliegman, B. F. Stanton, J. St. Geme, et al. [Eds.], *Nelson textbook of pediatrics* (19th ed.). Philadelphia: Saunders.

can be performed. Conventional mechanical ventilation, high-frequency oscillatory ventilation, and extracorporeal membrane oxygenation (ECMO) may be used as respiratory support. Permissive hypercapnia may be allowed as long as the pH is maintained above or equal to 7.30 (Maheshwari & Carlo, 2016). Inhaled nitric oxide to relieve pulmonary hypertension of CDH has also been used in some cases, with mixed results (see Chapter 28, page 777). Gastric contents are aspirated and suction applied to decompress the gastrointestinal tract and prevent further cardiothoracic compromise. Oxygen therapy, mechanical ventilation, and the correction of acidosis are necessary in infants with early clinical respiratory distress from CDH. ECMO may be used in infants with severe circulatory and respiratory complications. Traditional management has been early surgical repair of the defect. However, increased survival rates have been reported with surgery after a period of preoperative stabilization and resolution of pulmonary hypertension.

The prognosis depends largely on the degree of fetal pulmonary development, but the prognosis in severe cases is often poor. The overall survival rate for live-born infants is 67% (Maheshwari & Carlo, 2016). The incidence of gastroesophageal reflux disease in survivors is approximately 50%, and a significant number will have neurocognitive deficits.

RESPIRATORY EMERGENCY

Respiratory Failure

Effective pulmonary gas exchange requires clear airways, normal lungs and chest wall, and adequate pulmonary circulation. Anything that affects these functions or their relationships can compromise respiration. In general, the term *respiratory insufficiency* is applied to two situations: (1) when there is increased work of breathing but gas exchange function is near normal, and (2) when normal blood gas tensions cannot be maintained and hypoxemia and acidosis develop secondary to carbon dioxide retention.

Respiratory failure is defined as the inability of the respiratory apparatus to maintain adequate oxygenation of the blood, with or without carbon dioxide retention. This process involves pulmonary dysfunction that generally results in impaired alveolar gas exchange, which can lead to hypoxemia or hypercapnia. Respiratory failure is the most common cause of cardiopulmonary arrest in children. *Respiratory arrest* is the cessation of respiration. *Apnea* is the cessation of breathing for more than 20 seconds or for a shorter period when associated with hypoxemia or bradycardia. Apnea can be (1) central, in which respiratory efforts are absent; (2) obstructive, in which respiratory efforts are present; or (3) mixed, in which both central and obstructive components are present (see Apnea and Apparent Life-Threatening Events, Chapter 35). Respiratory dysfunction may have an abrupt or an insidious onset. Respiratory failure can occur as an emergency situation or may be preceded by gradual and progressive deterioration of respiratory function. Most clinical manifestations are nonspecific and are affected by variations among individual patients and differences in the severity and duration of inadequate gas exchange.

Diagnostic Evaluation

The diagnosis of respiratory failure is determined by the combined application of three sources of information:

1. Presence or history of a condition that might predispose the patient to respiratory failure
2. Observation of respiratory failure
3. Measurement of arterial blood gases (ABGs) and pH

Nursing observation and judgement are vital to the recognition and early management of respiratory failure. Nurses must be able to assess a situation and initiate appropriate action within moments. Signs of respiratory failure are listed in Box 45-15.

Therapeutic Management

The interventions used in the management of respiratory failure are often dramatic, requiring special skills and emergency procedures. If respiratory arrest occurs, the primary objectives are to recognize the situation and immediately initiate resuscitative measures, such as airway positioning, administration of oxygen, cardiopulmonary resuscitation (CPR), suctioning, CPAP or bilevel positive airway pressure (BIPAP), or intubation. When the situation is not an arrest, the suspicion of respiratory failure is confirmed by assessment; the severity may be defined by ABG

BOX 45-15 CLINICAL MANIFESTATIONS OF RESPIRATORY FAILURE

Cardinal Signs
Restlessness
Tachypnea
Tachycardia
Diaphoresis (except in neonates)

Early but Less Obvious Signs
Mood changes such as euphoria or depression
Headache
Altered depth and pattern of respirations
Hypertension
Exertional dyspnea
Anorexia
Increased cardiac output and renal output
Central nervous system symptoms (decreased efficiency, impaired judgement, anxiety, confusion, restlessness, irritability, depressed level of consciousness)
Flaring nares
Chest wall retractions
Expiratory grunt
Wheezing or prolonged expiration

Signs of More Severe Hypoxia
Hypotension or hypertension
Dimness of vision
Somnolence
Stupor
Coma
Dyspnea
Depressed respirations
Bradycardia
Cyanosis, peripheral or central

analysis. Interventions such as administering supplemental oxygen, positioning, stimulation, suctioning, providing positive pressure ventilation by bag and mask, and early intubation may avert an arrest. When severity is established, an attempt is made to determine the underlying cause by thorough evaluation.

The principles of management are to (1) maintain ventilation and maximize oxygen delivery, (2) correct hypoxemia and hypercapnia, (3) treat the underlying cause, (4) minimize extrapulmonary organ failure, (5) apply specific and nonspecific therapy to control oxygen demands, and (6) anticipate complications. Monitoring closely the patient's condition is critical.

NURSING CARE

For families whose child has respiratory arrest, support is aimed at keeping the family informed of the child's status and helping them cope with a near-death experience or an actual death (see Chapter 40). Knowing that their child requires CPR is a frightening and often overwhelming experience for parents. Uncertainty regarding the outcome—both mortality and morbidity—is a primary concern. Traditionally, family members were not allowed to be present during resuscitation efforts in the emergency department. However, studies indicate that family presence during emergencies alleviates the family's anger about being separated from the patient during a crisis, reduces their anxiety, eliminates doubts about what was done to help the patient, and facilitates the grieving process if the patient dies (Manqurten, Scott, Guzzetta, et al., 2006).

Regardless of whether an institution permits parental presence during CPR, nurses must consider the needs, fears, and concerns of family members during an arrest situation. Whether family presence is permitted or not permitted, nurses should arrange for someone to remain with the family during the emergency treatment. After the child's recovery or death, the family will continue to need support and thorough medical information regarding lifesaving measures, the prognosis if the child survives, and the cause of death if the child dies.

Cardiopulmonary Resuscitation

Cardiac arrest in children is less often of cardiac origin than from prolonged hypoxemia secondary to inadequate oxygenation, ventilation, and circulation (shock). Some causes of cardiac arrest include injuries, suffocation (e.g., FB aspiration), smoke inhalation, or infection. In small infants the small size of the airway may easily be compromised by improper positioning with the chin resting on the chest; this can easily be remedied by positioning the infant with the chin elevated (but not hyperextended) so the airway is open. This is common in infants who are not positioned properly in an infant seat or car restraint seat. Respiratory arrest is associated with a better survival rate than cardiac arrest. After cardiac arrest occurs, the outcome of resuscitative efforts is poor.

Complete apnea signals the need for rapid, vigorous action to prevent cardiac arrest. In such situations nurses must initiate action immediately. In the hospital, emergency equipment must be available and easily accessible in all patient care areas. The status of emergency equipment must be checked at least once daily. Regardless of the cause of the arrest, basic procedures need to be carried out and modified according to the child's size.

Resuscitation Procedure

The 2010 guidelines for **cardiopulmonary resuscitation (CPR)** and emergency cardiac care (ECC) were co-developed by the American Heart Association and the Heart and Stroke Foundation of Canada and updated in 2015 (Heart and Stroke Foundation of Canada, 2015). These organizations have implemented several changes in CPR guidelines that incorporate the use of the automatic external defibrillator (AED) as part of the treatment of cardiorespiratory arrest in children 1 year of age and older. The newer 2015 guidelines recommend using a pediatric-attenuated system first, if one is available; if it is not available the adult AED should be used. For infants less than 1 year of age, a manual defibrillator is the best one to use; if that is not available a pediatric-attenuated defibrillator should be used next, and then the AED (Heart and Stroke Foundation of Canada, 2015). The 2015 guidelines indicate that the initial shock should be 2 j/kg, then 4 j/kg strength for all of the subsequent shocks. The AED must not exceed 9 j/kg (Heart and Stroke Foundation of Canada, 2015).

In 2010, the CPR sequence was changed from airway-breathing-compression (ABC) to **compressions-airway-breathing (CAB)**. The new CAB procedure applies to all ages except newborns; this CAB routine is continued in the 2015 guide. Rescuers should continue to provide the ABC CPR sequence with a 3-to-1 ratio of compressions to breaths for the newborn age group. The ABC sequence is used because most newborns with a cardiac arrest started with a respiratory arrest (Heart and Stroke Foundation of Canada, 2015).

Open the airway. For effective CPR, the victim is placed on the back on a firm, flat surface, the rescuer using appropriate precautions. With loss of consciousness the tongue, which is attached to the lower jaw, relaxes and falls back, obstructing the airway. To open the airway, the head is positioned with a head tilt–chin lift manoeuvre by the lay rescuer. Health care providers should open the airway using either a head tilt–chin lift or jaw thrust manoeuvre.

The jaw thrust is recommended for use only by health care workers. In suspected neck injuries the jaw thrust method should be used while the cervical spine is completely immobilized (Fig. 45-12). After a patent airway has been restored by removal of foreign material and secretions (if indicated) and if the child is not breathing, maintenance of the airway is continued, and rescue breathing is initiated.

Check pulse. In children after an initial two breaths, the health care provider palpates the pulse to ascertain the presence of a heartbeat. The carotid is the most central and accessible artery in children over 1 year of age. However, the infant's short and often fat neck makes the carotid pulse difficult to palpate. In the infant it is preferable to use the brachial pulse, located on the inner side of the upper arm midway between the elbow and the shoulder (Fig. 45-13). Absence of a carotid or brachial pulse is considered sufficient indication to begin compressions.

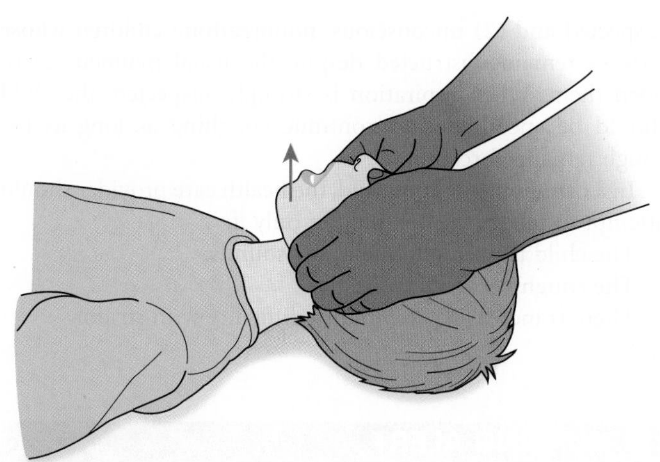

FIGURE 45-12 Open airway using jaw thrust maneouvre, and check breathing.

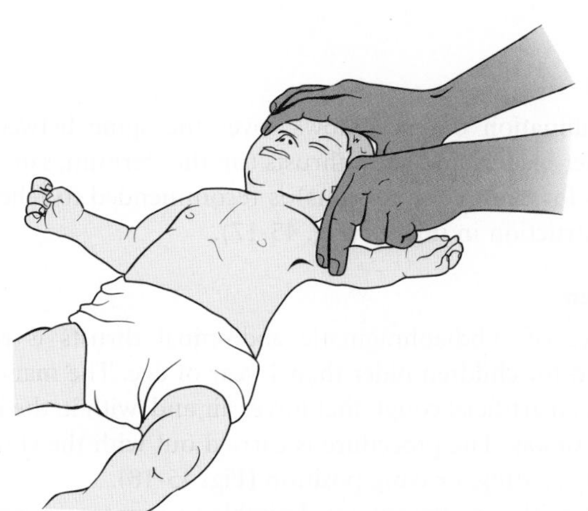

FIGURE 45-13 Locating the brachial pulse in an infant.

Perform chest compression. External chest compression consists of serial, rhythmic compressions of the chest to maintain circulation to vital organs until the child achieves spontaneous vital signs or advanced life support can be provided. *Chest compressions are always interspersed with ventilation of the lungs* (Fig. 45-14). For optimal compressions it is essential that the child's spine be supported on a firm surface during compressions of the sternum and that sternal pressure is forceful but not traumatic (Fig. 45-15). For a small infant, the hard surface can be the rescuer's hand or forearm, with the palm supporting the infant's back. The child's head is positioned for optimal airway opening using the head tilt–chin lift manoeuvre. It is essential to prevent overextension of the head of small infants because this tends to close the flexible trachea.

Give breaths. To ventilate the lungs in the infant (from birth to 1 year of age), the bag-valve mask or operator's mouth is placed in such a way that both the mouth and the nostrils are covered (Fig. 45-16). Children (over 1 year of age) are ventilated through the mouth while the nostrils are firmly pinched for airtight contact.

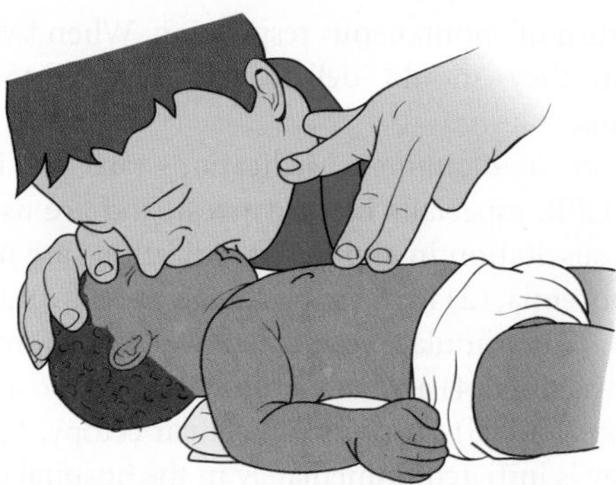

FIGURE 45-14 Combining chest compressions with breathing in an infant.

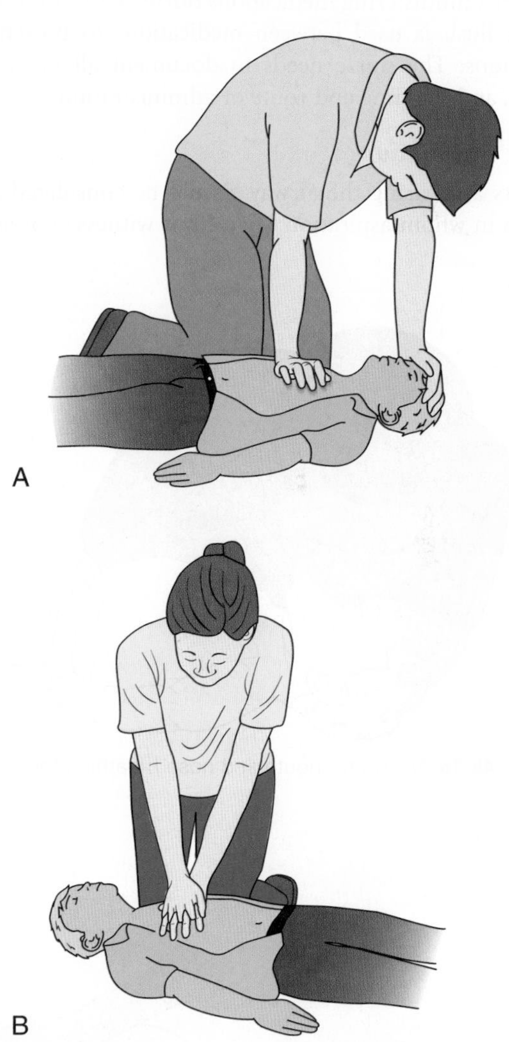

FIGURE 45-15 Chest compressions in a child: one hand for smaller child **(A)** and two hands for larger child **(B)**.

The depth of compression needs to be adapted to the child's size. The location, rate, and depth for children older than 8 years of age are the same as for adults.

Lone-rescuer CPR is continued at the ratio of two breaths to 30 compressions for all ages until signs of recovery appear. These signs include palpable peripheral pulses, return of pupils to normal size, the disappearance of mottling and cyanosis, and possibly return of spontaneous respiration. When two rescuers are present, they should deliver two breaths to each 15 compressions.

Administer medications. Medications are an important adjunct to CPR, especially cardiac arrest, and are used during and after resuscitation in children. Medications are used to (1) correct hypoxemia, (2) increase perfusion pressure during chest compression, (3) stimulate spontaneous or more forceful myocardial contraction, (4) accelerate cardiac rate, (5) correct metabolic acidosis, and (6) suppress ventricular ectopy. Appropriate fluid therapy is initiated immediately in the hospital or by EMS personnel during transport (see Parenteral Fluid Therapy, Chapter 44, and Shock, Chapter 47).

When administering medications during CPR (or a "code"), a saline flush is used between medications to prevent drug interactions. The nurse needs to document all medications, dosages, and the time and route of administration.

Airway Obstruction

Attempts at clearing the airway should be considered for (1) children in whom aspiration of an FB is witnessed or strongly suspected and (2) unconscious, nonbreathing children whose airways remain obstructed despite the usual manoeuvres to open them. When aspiration is strongly suspected, the child should be encouraged to continue coughing as long as the cough remains forceful.

In a conscious choking child, the health care provider should attempt to relieve the obstruction only if:

- The child is unable to make any sounds.
- The cough becomes ineffective.
- There is increasing respiratory difficulty with stridor.

NURSING ALERT

Blind finger sweeps should be avoided in infants and children under 8 years old.

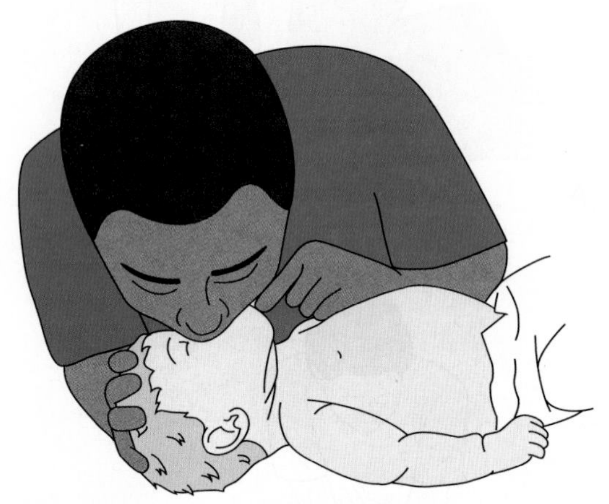

FIGURE 45-16 Mouth-to-mouth and nose breathing for an infant.

Infants

A combination of back blows (over the spine between the shoulder blades) and chest thrusts (on the sternum, same location as for chest compressions) is recommended to relieve the FB obstruction in infants (Fig. 45-17).

Children

A series of subdiaphragmatic abdominal thrusts is recommended for children older than 1 year of age. The manoeuvre creates an artificial cough that forces air and, with it, the FB out of the airway. The procedure is carried out with the child in a standing, sitting, or lying position (Fig. 45-18).

It is neither necessary nor desirable to squeeze or compress the arms during the procedure; it is not a punch or a bear hug. The child may vomit after relief of the obstruction and should be positioned to prevent aspiration (Fig. 45-19). After breathing is restored, the child should receive medical attention and be assessed for complications.

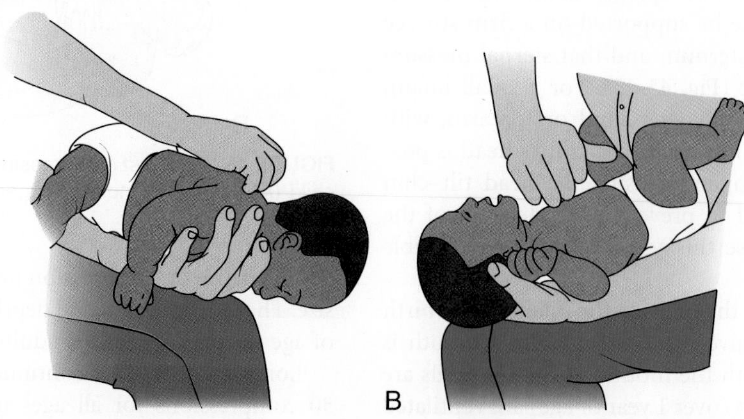

FIGURE 45-17 Relief of foreign body obstruction in an infant: back blows **(A)** and chest thrusts **(B)**.

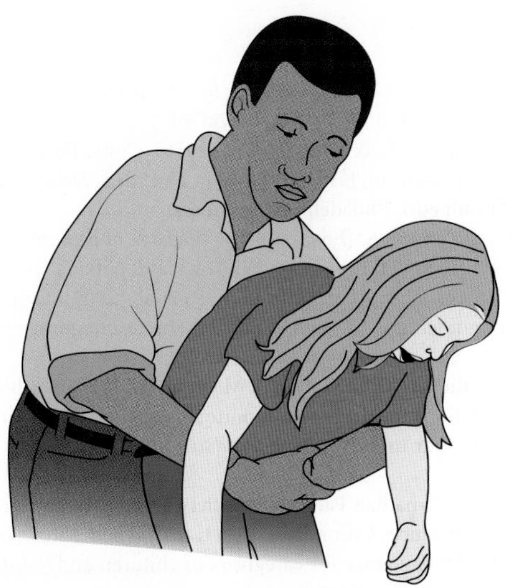

FIGURE 45-18 Abdominal thrusts in standing child for relief of foreign body obstruction.

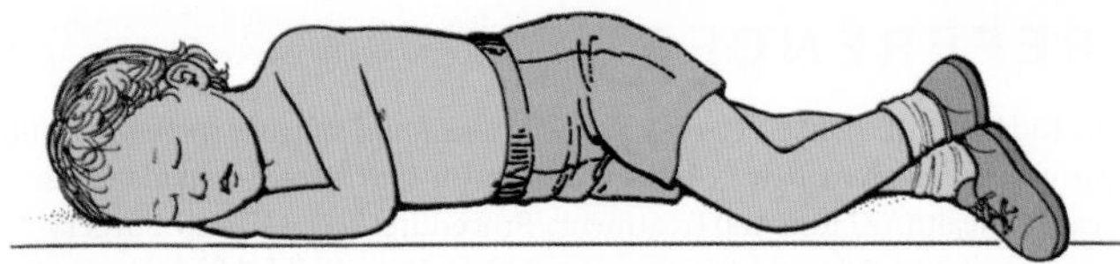

FIGURE 45-19 Recovery position for a child after respiratory emergency.

The success of the technique is primarily a result of the obstruction occurring at the end of a maximum respiration. The victim is most likely to choke on food during inspiration; thus the tidal volume plus expiratory reserve volume is present in the lungs. When pressure is exerted on the diaphragm by the thrusts, the food bolus is ejected with considerable force by this trapped air.

KEY POINTS

- Acute infection of the respiratory tract is the most common cause of illness in infancy and childhood.
- The incidence and severity of respiratory tract infections are influenced by the infectious agents involved, the child's age, and the child's natural defences.
- Common respiratory tract infections of childhood include nasopharyngitis, pharyngitis (including tonsillitis), influenza, infectious mononucleosis, and OM.
- Croup syndromes involve acute inflammation and variable degrees of obstruction of the epiglottis, larynx, or trachea.
- The primary goals in the care of children with croup are observation for signs of respiratory distress and relief of laryngeal inflammation.
- Common infections of the lower airways are bacterial tracheitis, bronchitis, and RSV-bronchiolitis.
- Pneumonias are classified according to site or by etiological agent (viral, bacterial, mycoplasmal) or are associated with aspiration of foreign material.
- In TB, susceptibility to the bacillus can be influenced by heredity, age, stress, poor nutrition, and intercurrent infection.
- Second-hand smoke exposure is a major environmental pollutant contributing to respiratory illness in children.
- Asthma is the leading cause of chronic illness in children.
- General therapeutic management of asthma includes assessment of asthma severity, allergen control, medication therapy, symptom management, and sometimes hyposensitization.
- Support for the family and the child with asthma includes education about the disease and its therapy and facilitation of self-management.
- CF is the most common inherited disease in children.
- The diagnosis of CF is based on newborn screening finding of elevated IRT, DNA analysis showing a *CFTR* mutation, and a positive sweat chloride test (increased sweat electrolyte content).
- General therapeutic management of CF is highly individualized, requiring a multidisciplinary approach and a strong support network for children and their families.
- Choanal atresia and diaphragmatic hernia are congenital respiratory conditions.
- Choking and respiratory failure are respiratory emergencies that require immediate intervention.
- Abdominal thrusts are used in children in whom FB obstruction is witnessed or strongly suspected. A combination of back blows and chest thrusts is used for infants with FB obstruction.

evolve WEBSITE

Visit the Evolve website for additional resources related to the content in this chapter such as Case Studies, Critical Thinking Case Study Answers, Nursing Care Plans, Nursing Processes, Nursing Skills, and Review Questions for Exam Preparation at: *http://evolve.elsevier.com/Canada/Perry/maternal/*

REFERENCES

About Kids Health. (2009). *Tonsil surgery or tonsil and adenoid surgery: Caring for your child after surgery*. Retrieved from <http://www.aboutkidshealth.ca/En/HealthAZ/TestsAndTreatments/Procedures/Pages/Tonsil-Surgery-or-Tonsil-and-Adenoid-Surgery-Caring-For-Your-Child-After-the-Operation.aspx>.

American Academy of Pediatrics, Committee on Infectious Diseases, Kimberlin, D. W., et al. (Eds.), (2015). *Red book: 2015 report of the Committee on Infectious Diseases* (30th ed.). Elk Grove Village, IL: Author.

American Academy of Pediatrics, Committee on Nutrition and the Council on Sports Medicine and Fitness. (2011). Clinical report: Sports drinks and energy drinks for children and adolescents: Are they appropriate? *Pediatrics*, *127*(6), 1182–1189. doi:10.1542/peds.2011-0965.

Antoon, A. Y., & Donovan, M. K. (2016). Burn injuries. In R. M. Kliegman, B. F. Stanton, J. W. Geme, et al. (Eds.), *Nelson textbook of pediatrics* (20th ed.). Philadelphia: Saunders.

Ashok, P., Sarnaik, J. A., Clark, A. A., et al. (2016). Respiratory distress and failure. In R. M. Kliegman, B. F. Stanton, J. W. Geme, et al. (Eds.), *Nelson textbook of pediatrics* (20th ed.). Philadelphia: Saunders.

Asthma Society of Canada. (2016). *About asthma*. Retrieved from <http://www.asthma.ca/adults/about>.

Banerj, A., Greenberg, D., White, L., et al. (2009). Risk factors and viruses associated with hospitalization due to lower respiratory tract infections in Canadian Inuit children: A case control study. *Pediatric Infectious Disease Journal*, *28*(8), 102, 697–701. doi:10.1097/INF.0b013e31819f1f89.

Canadian Paediatric Society. (2014). *Study examines incidence and nature of childhood tuberculosis disease*. Retrieved from <http://www.cps.ca/blog-blogue/blog-details/childhood-tuberculosis-disease>.

Canadian Paediatric Society. (2016). *Colds in children*. Retrieved from <http://www.caringforkids.cps.ca/handouts/colds_in_children>.

Canadian Society of Otolaryngology—Head and Neck Surgery. (2013). *Tonsillectomy*. Retrieved from <http://www.entcanada.org/education/general-public/public-information-sheets-2/throat/tonsillectomy/>.

Canadian Thoracic Society. (2012). *2012 CTS guideline update: Diagnosis and management of asthma in preschoolers, children and adults*. Retrieved from <http://www.respiratoryguidelines.ca/2012-cts-guideline-asthma-update>.

Canadian Thoracic Society & Public Health Agency of Canada. (2013). *Canadian tuberculosis standards*. (7th ed.). Chapter 16, Bacille Calmette-Guérin (BCG) vaccination in Canada. Retrieved from <http://www.respiratoryguidelines.ca/tb-standards-2013>.

Cates, C. J., Welsh, E. J., & Rowe, B. H. (2013). Holding chambers (spacers) versus nebulisers for beta-agonist treatment of acute asthma. *The Cochrane Database of Systematic Reviews*, (9), CD000052, doi:10.1002/14651858.CD000052.pub3.

Chen, C. M., Tischer, C., Schnappinger, M., et al. (2010). The role of cats and dogs in asthma and allergy—A systematic review. *International Journal of Hygiene and Environmental Health*, *213*(1), 1–31. doi:10.1016/j.ijheh.2009.12.003.

Chibuk, T. K., Cohen, E., Robinson, J. L., et al. (2011). Paediatric complicated pneumonia: Diagnosis and management of empyema. *Paediatrics & Child Health*, *16*(7), 425–427. Retrieved from <http://www.cps.ca/documents/position/complicated-pneumonia-empyema> Reaffirmed 2015.

Coates, B. M., Camarda, L. E., & Goodman, D. M. (2016). Wheezing in infants: Bronchiolitis. In R. M. Kliegman, B. F. Stanton, J. W. St. Geme, et al. (Eds.), *Nelson textbook of pediatrics* (20th ed.). Philadelphia: Saunders.

Cystic Fibrosis Canada. (2015). *Canadian cystic fibrosis registry. 2013 Annual report*. Retrieved from <http://www.cysticfibrosis.ca/uploads/cf%20care/Canadian-CF-Registry-2013-FINAL.pdf>.

Cystic Fibrosis Canada. (2016). *CF newborn screening*. Retrieved from <http://www.cysticfibrosis.ca/advocacy/cf-newborn-screening>.

De Wals, P., Robin, E., Fortin, E., et al. (2008). Pneumonia after implementation of the pneumococcal conjugate vaccine program in the province of Quebec, Canada. *Pediatric Infectious Disease Journal*, *27*(11), 963–968. doi:10.1097/INF.0b013e31817cf76f.

Egan, M. E., Green, D. M., & Voynow, J. A. (2016). Cystic fibrosis. In R. E. Kliegman, B. F. Stanton, J. W. St. Geme, et al. (Eds.), *Nelson textbook of pediatrics* (20th ed.). Philadelphia: Saunders.

Fleisher, G. R., & Ludwig, S. (Eds.), (2010). *Textbook of pediatric emergency medicine*. Philadelphia: Lippincott Williams and Wilkins.

Flume, P. A., Robinson, K. A., O'Sullivan, B. P., et al. (2009). Cystic fibrosis pulmonary guidelines: Airway clearance therapies. *Respiratory Care*, *54*(4), 522–537.

Friedman, J. N., Rieder, M. J., Walton, J. M., et al. (2014). Bronchiolitis: Recommendations for diagnosis, monitoring and management, in one to twenty four months of age. *Paediatrics & Child Health*, *19*(9), 485–489.

Goldman, R. D., & Canadian Paediatric Society, Drug Therapy and Hazardous Substances Committee. (2011; reaffirmed 2016). Treating cough and cold: Guidance for caregivers of children and youth. *Paediatrics & Child Health*, *16*(9), 564–566.

Gould, J. M., & Matz, P. S. (2010). Otitis media. *Pediatric Review*, *31*, 102–116. doi:10.1542/pir.31-3-102.

Government of Canada. (2015). *Dangers of second-hand smoke*. Retrieved from <http://healthycanadians.gc.ca/healthy-living-vie-saine/tobacco-tabac/avoid-second-hand-smoke-eviter-fumee-secondaire/second-hand-smoke-fumee-secondaire/dangers-eng.php>.

Government of Canada. (2016). *Tuberculosis*. Retrieved from <http://www.healthycanadians.gc.ca/diseases-conditions-maladies-affections/disease-maladie/tuberculosis-tuberculose-eng.php?_ga=1.215650078.868197850.1432519476>.

Hazle, L. A. (2010). Cystic fibrosis. In P. J. Allen, J. A. Vessey, & N. A. Schapiro (Eds.), *Primary care of the child with a chronic condition* (5th ed.). St. Louis: Mosby.

Health Canada. (2013). *Health Canada's review recommends codeine only be used in patients aged 12 and over*. Retrieved from <http://healthycanadians.gc.ca/recall-alert-rappel-avis/hc-sc/2013/33915a-eng.php>.

Healthlink, B. C. (2015). *Throat culture*. Retrieved from <http://www.healthlinkbc.ca/kb/content/medicaltest/hw204006.html>.

Heart and Stroke Foundation of Canada. (2015). *Highlights of the 2015 American Heart Association guidelines update for CPR and ECC. Heart and Stroke Foundation of Canada edition*. Retrieved from <http://www.heartandstroke.com/atf/cf/%7B99452d8b-e7f1-4bd6-a57d-b136ce6c95bf%7D/ECC%20HIGHLIGHTS%20OF%202015%20GUIDELINES%20UPDATE%20FOR%20CPR%20ECC_LR.PDF>.

Heinrich, J. (2011). Influence of indoor factors in dwellings on the development of childhood asthma. *International Journal of Hygiene and Environmental Health*, *214*(1), 1–25. doi:10.1016/j.ijheh.2010.08.009.

The Hospital for Sick Children. (2014). *Hydration assessment*. Retrieved from <http://www.sickkids.ca/Nursing/Education-and-learning/Nursing-Student-Orientation/module-two-clinical-care/hydrationassessment/index.html>.

Kakkar, F., Allen, U. D., Ling, D., et al. (2010). Tuberculosis in children: New diagnostic blood tests. *Paediatrics & Child Health*, *15*(8), 529–533. Retrieved from <http://www.cps.ca/documents/position/tuberculosis-diagnostic-blood-tests>. Reaffirmed 2015.

Kellner, J. D., & Canadian Paediatric Society, Infectious Diseases and Immunization Committee. (2011). Update on the success of the pneumococcal conjugate vaccine. *Paediatrics & Child Health*, *16*(4), 233–236. Retrieved from <http://www.cps.ca/en/documents/position/pneumococcal-conjugate-vaccine> Reaffirmed 2015.

Kelly, L. E., Sommer, D. D., Ramakrishna, J., et al. (2015). Morphine or Ibuprofen for post-tonsillectomy analgesia: A randomized trial. *Pediatrics*, *135*(2), 307–313. doi:10.1542/peds.2014-1906.

Kelly, M. S., & Sandora, T. (2016). Community-acquired pneumonia. In R. M. Kliegman, B. F. Stanton, J. St. Geme, et al. (Eds.), *Nelson textbook of pediatrics* (20th ed.). Philadelphia: Saunders.

Kinyon Munch, K. (2010). What do you tell parents when their child is sick with the common cold? *Journal for Specialists in Pediatric Nursing, 16*(1), 8–15.

Kovesi, T. (2012). Respiratory disease in Canadian First Nations and Inuit children. *Paediatrics & Child Health, 17*(7), 376–380.

Le Saux, N., Robinson, J. L., & Canadian Paediatric Society, Infectious Diseases and Immunization Committee. (2016). Management of acute otitis media in children six months of age and older. *Paediatrics & Child Health, 21*(1), 39–44. Retrieved from <http://www.cps.ca/documents/position/acute-otitis-media>.

Lieberthal, A. S., Carroll, A. E., Chonmaitree, T., et al. (2013). Clinical practice guideline: The diagnosis and management of acute otitis media. *Pediatrics, 131*(3), e964–e994.

Liu, A. H., Covar, R. A., Spahn, J. D., et al. (2016). Childhood asthma. In R. M. Kliegman, B. F. Stanton, J. W. St. Geme, et al. (Eds.), *Nelson textbook of pediatrics* (20th ed.). Philadelphia: Saunders.

Lotz, M. T., Moore, M. L., & Peebles, R. S. (2013). Respiratory syncytial virus and reactive airway disease. *Current Topics in Microbiology and Immunology, 372*, 105–118. doi:10.1007/978-3-642-38919-1_5.

The Lung Association. (2014). *Sleep apnea.* Retrieved from <https://www.lung.ca/lung-health/lung-disease/sleep-apnea>.

Maheshwari, A., & Carlo, W. A. (2016). Diaphragmatic hernia. In R. M. Kliegman, B. F. Stanton, J. St. Geme, et al. (Eds.), *Nelson textbook of pediatrics* (20th ed.). Philadelphia: Saunders.

Manqurten, J., Scott, S. H., Guzzetta, C. E., et al. (2006). Effects of family presence during resuscitation and invasive procedures in a pediatric emergency department. *Journal of Emergency Nursing, 32*(3), 225–233.

Marcus, C. L., Brooks, L. J., Draper, K. A., et al. (2012). Diagnosis and management of childhood obstructive sleep apnea syndrome. *Pediatrics, 130*(3), 576–584. doi:10.1542/peds.2012-1671.

Mazor, R., & Green, T. P. (2016). Pulmonary edema. In R. M. Kliegman, B. F. Stanton, J. W. St. Geme, et al. (Eds.), *Nelson textbook of pediatrics* (20th ed.). Philadelphia: Saunders.

Moore, D. L., & Canadian Paediatric Society, Infectious Diseases and Immunization Committee. (2015). Vaccine recommendations for children and youth for the 2015/2016 influenza season. *Paediatrics & Child Health, 20*(7), 389–391. Retrieved from <http://www.cps.ca/en/documents/position/influenza-vaccine-recommendations>.

Moran, A., Brunzell, C., Cohen, R. C., et al. (2010). Clinical care guidelines for cystic fibrosis-related diabetes: A position statement of the American Diabetes Association and a clinical practice guideline of the Cystic Fibrosis Foundation, endorsed by the Pediatric Endocrine Society. *Diabetes Care, 33*(12), 2697–2708. doi:10.2337/dc10-1768.

Newton, T. J. (2009). Respiratory care of the hospitalized patient with cystic fibrosis. *Respiratory Care, 54*(6), 769–775, discussion 775–776.

O'Riordan, S. M., Dattan, M. T., & Hindmarsh, P. C. (2010). Cystic fibrosis-related diabetes in childhood. *Hormone Research in Paediatrics, 73*(1), 15–24. doi:10.1159/000271912.

Ortiz-Alvarez, O., Mikrogianakis, A., & Canadian Paediatric Society, Acute Care Committee. (2012). Managing the paediatric patient with an acute asthma exacerbation. *Paediatrics & Child Health, 17*(5), 251–255. Retrieved from <http://www.cps.ca/documents/position/management-acute-asthma-exacerbation>. Reaffirmed 2015.

Owens, J. A. (2016). Sleep medicine. In R. M. Kliegman, B. F. Stanton, J. W. St. Geme, et al. (Eds.), *Nelson textbook of pediatrics* (20th ed.). Philadelphia: Saunders.

Parachute. (n.d.). *Carbon monoxide poisoning.* Retrieved from <http://www.parachutecanada.org/policy/item/carbon-monoxide-poisoning>.

Perez-Velez, C. M. (2012). Pediatric tuberculosis: New guidelines and recommendations. *Current Opinion in Pediatrics, 24*(3), 319–328. doi:10.1097/MOP.0b013e32835357c3.

Philpott, J., Houghton, K., Luke, A., et al. (2010). Physical activity recommendations for children with specific chronic health conditions: Juvenile idiopathic arthritis, hemophilia, asthma and cystic fibrosis. *Pediatrics & Child Health, 15*(4), 213–218. Retrieved from <http://www.cps.ca/en/documents/position/physical-activity-chronic-condition>.

Public Health Agency of Canada. (2014a). *An Advisory Committee Statement (ACS)–National Advisory Committee on Immunization (NACI) statement: Statement on seasonal influenza vaccine for 2014–2015.* Retrieved from <http://www.phac-aspc.gc.ca/naci-ccni/flu-grippe-eng.php>.

Public Health Agency of Canada. (2014b). CCDR: Volume 40-3, February 7, 2014. *Pertussis surveillance in Canada: Trends to 2012.* Retrieved from <http://www.phac-aspc.gc.ca/publicat/ccdr-rmtc/14vol40/dr-rm40-03/dr-rm40-03-per-eng.php>.

Public Health Agency of Canada. (2015). *Canadian immunization guide: Part 4 Active vaccines.* Retrieved from <http://www.phac-aspc.gc.ca/publicat/cig-gci/p04-pert-coqu-eng.php>.

Public Health Agency of Canada. (2016a). *Public health reminder: Seasonal flu 2016. Why you should take note.* Retrieved from <http://www.phac-aspc.gc.ca/phn-asp/2015/flu-grippe-1027-eng.php>.

Public Health Agency of Canada. (2016b). *Canadian immunization guide: Part 3 vaccination of specific populations.* Retrieved from <http://www.phac-aspc.gc.ca/publicat/cig-gci/p03-02-eng.php>.

Randolph, A. G. (2009). Management of acute lung injury and acute respiratory distress syndrome in children. *Critical Care Medicine, 37*(8), 2448–2454. doi:10.1097/CCM.0b013e3181aee5dd.

Redding, G. J. (2009). Bronchiectasis in children. *Pediatric Clinics of North America, 56*(1), 157–171xi. doi:10.1016/j.pcl.2008.10.014.

Robinson, J. L., Le Saux, N., & Canadian Paediatric Society, Infectious Diseases and Immunization Committee. (2015). Preventing hospitalization for respiratory syncytial virus infections. *Paediatrics & Child Health, 20*(6), 321–326. Retrieved from <http://www.cps.ca/en/documents/position/preventing-hospitalizations-for-rsv-infections>. Reaffirmed 2016.

Roosevelt, G. E. (2016). Acute inflammatory upper airway obstruction (croup, epiglottitis, laryngitis, and bacterial tracheitis). In R. M. Kliegman, B. F. Stanton, J. W. St. Geme, et al. (Eds.), *Nelson textbook of pediatrics* (20th ed.). Philadelphia: Saunders.

Roqué i Figuls, M., Giné-Garriga, M., Granados Rugeles, C., & Perrotta, C. (2012). Chest physiotherapy for acute bronchiolitis in paediatric patients between 0 and 24 months old. *Cochrane Database Systemic Review,* (2), CD004873, doi:10.1002/14651858.CD004873.pub5.

Sawicki, G. S., Rasouliyan, L., Pasta, D. J., et al. (2008). The impact of incident methicillin-resistant *Staphylococcus aureus* detection on pulmonary function in cystic fibrosis. *Pediatric Pulmonology, 43*(11), 1117–1123. doi:10.1002/ppul.20914.

Sicherer, S. H., Wood, R. A., & AAP Section on Allergy and Immunology. (2012). Allergy testing in childhood: Using allergen-specific IgE tests. *Pediatrics, 129*(1), 193–197.

Southern, K. W., Mérelle, M. M., Dankert-Roelse, J. E., et al. (2009). Newborn screening for cystic fibrosis. *The Cochrane Database of Systematic Reviews,* (1), CD001402, doi:10.1002/14651858.CD001402.pub2.

Taylor, S., Marchisio, P., Vergison, A., et al. (2012). Impact of pneumococcal conjugate vaccination on otitis media: A systematic review. *Clinical Infectious Diseases: An Official Publication of the Infectious Diseases Society of America, 12*, 1765–1773. doi:10.1093/cid/cis292.

Thomas, E. M., & Statistics Canada. (2015). *Recent trends in upper respiratory infections, ear infections, and asthma among young Canadian children.* Retrieved from <http://www.statcan.gc.ca/pub/82-003-x/2010004/article/11364-eng.htm#a1>.

Thomson, N. C., & Chaudhuri, R. (2012). Omalizumab: Clinical use for the management of asthma. *Clinical Medicine Insights. Circulatory, Respiratory and Pulmonary Medicine, 6*, 27–40. doi:10.4137/CCRPM.S7793.

Vassilev, Z. P., Kabadi, S., & Villa, R. (2010). Safety and efficacy of over-the-counter cough and cold medicines for use in children. *Expert Opinion on Drug Safety, 9*(2), 233–242.

Volpe, D. I., Smith, M. F., & Sultan, K. (2011). Managing pediatric asthma exacerbations in the ED. *American Journal of Nursing, 111*(2), 48–53.

Wong, S., & Canadian Paediatric Society, First Nations, Inuit and Métis Committee. (2006). Use and misuse of tobacco among Aboriginal peoples. *Paediatrics & Child Health, 11*(10), 681–685. Retrieved from <http://www.cps.ca/documents/position/tobacco-aboriginal-people> Reaffirmed 2016.

World Health Organization. (2016). *Chronic respiratory disease. Asthma.* Retrieved from <http://www.who.int/respiratory/asthma/en/>.

Wright, M., & Piedimonte, G. (2011). Respiratory syncytial virus prevention and therapy: Past, present, and future. *Pediatric Pulmonology*, *46*(4), 324–347.

Yang, M., & So, T. (2014). Revisiting the safety of over-the-counter cough and cold medications in the pediatric population. *Clinical Pediatrics*, *53*(4), 326–330. doi:10.1177/0009922813507998.

ADDITIONAL RESOURCES

Asthma Society of Canada—Asthma Kids.ca: <http://www.asthma.ca/global/kids.php>.

Cystic Fibrosis Canada: <http://www.cysticfibrosis.ca/>.

Cystic Fibrosis Foundation: <http://www.cff.org>.

Government of Canada—Canada's Provincial and Territorial Routine (and Catch-up) Vaccination Programs for Infants and Children: <http://healthycanadians.gc.ca/healthy-living-vie-saine/immunization-immunisation/children-enfants/schedule-calendrier-table-1-eng.php>.

Government of Canada—Second Hand Smoke: <http://healthycanadians.gc.ca/healthy-living-vie-saine/tobacco-tabac/avoid-second-hand-smoke-eviter-fumee-secondaire/second-hand-smoke-fumee-secondaire/index-eng.php>.

Hyperbaric Medical Unit: <http://www.uhn.ca/Surgery/PatientsFamilies/Clinics_Tests/Hyperbaric_Medicine_Unit>.

The Lung Association: <http://www.lung.ca>.

My Asthma Action Plan: <http://www.cheo.on.ca/uploads/asthma/files/asthma_action_plan.pdfNational> Lung Health Framework for Canada: <http://www.lunghealthframework.ca/>.

Public Health Agency of Canada—Flu Watch: <http://dsol-smed.phac-aspc.gc.ca/dsol-smed/fluwatch/fluwatch.phtml?lang=e>.

You Can Control Your Asthma—Asthma action plan examples: <https://www.ucalgary.ca/icancontrolasthma/>.

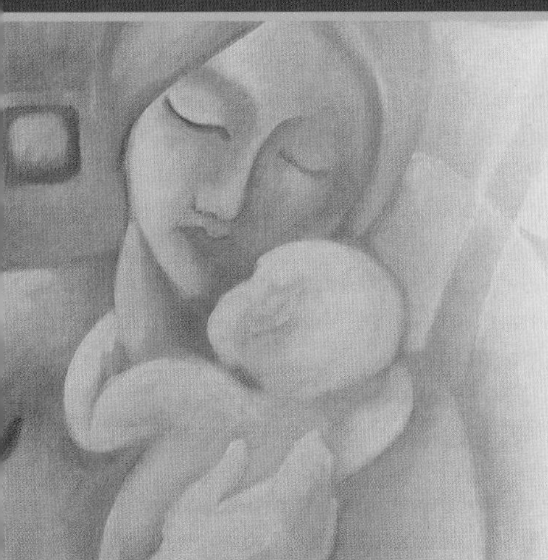

CHAPTER

46

Gastrointestinal Dysfunction

Anne Hogarth

evolve WEBSITE

Visit the Evolve website for additional resources related to the content in this chapter such as Case Studies, Critical Thinking Case Study Answers, Nursing Care Plans, Nursing Processes, Nursing Skills, and Review Questions for Exam Preparation at: *http://evolve.elsevier.com/Canada/Perry/maternal/*

OBJECTIVES

On completion of this chapter the reader will be able to:

- Identify children at increased risk of developing nutritional disorders.
- Outline a nutritional counselling plan for vitamin or mineral deficiency or excess.
- Describe the characteristics of infants that affect their ability to adapt to fluid loss or gain.
- Formulate a plan of care for the infant with acute diarrhea.
- Outline a teaching plan designed to prevent transmission of intestinal parasites.
- Describe the nursing care of the child with appendicitis.
- Compare and contrast the inflammatory bowel diseases.
- Identify the routes of transmission for hepatitis A, B, and C.
- Describe the nursing care of the child with hepatitis.
- Formulate a plan for teaching parents preoperative and postoperative care of the child with a cleft lip or cleft palate.
- Describe the nursing care for a child with a tracheoesophageal fistula or esophageal atresia.
- Formulate a plan of care for the child with an obstructive gastrointestinal disorder.
- Identify nutritional therapies for the child with a malabsorption syndrome.
- Identify the principles in the emergency treatment of accidental poisoning.
- Identify four sources of lead in the environment.
- Describe the nursing care of the child with lead poisoning.

GASTROINTESTINAL SYSTEM STRUCTURE AND FUNCTION

The gastrointestinal (GI) system has a multitude of important functions. The system includes all the structures from the mouth to the anus. The major functions are to break down and digest foods so that the nutrients may be absorbed through the digestive tract and waste products may be eliminated.

During fetal development, the GI system begins to form during the fourth week of the embryonic stage, starting with the mouth and anal tube. The GI tract becomes more mature in the last few weeks of development. Congenital anomalies of the GI tract can be present at birth or shortly after birth.

Pediatric Differences Related to the Gastrointestinal System

The mouth is highly vascular and is a common portal for infection. Infants and young children are at a higher risk of contracting infectious agents via the oral route because they may put objects in their mouths when exploring their environment.

The esophagus connects the mouth and stomach and allows for passage of food. The lower esophageal sphincter (LES) prevents regurgitation of the stomach's contents into the esophagus and mouth. LES muscle tone is not fully developed until 1 month of age, so young infants tend to regurgitate after feedings. Usually the regurgitation vanishes after 1 year of age.

A child's stomach capacity increases with age. The newborn has a capacity of 10 to 20 mL, and 2-month-olds have a 200-mL capacity, although many cannot tolerate that amount of volume per feeding. Adolescents' capacity increases to 1500 mL. By 6 months of age, the level of hydrochloric acid in gastric contents (to aid in digestion) is equal to that of adults.

A full-term newborn has approximately half the GI length of an adult. Intestinal growth spurts occur between 1 and 3 years for young children, and between 15 and 16 years of age for adolescents.

With regard to the biliary system, the liver is relatively large in the newborn. The pancreatic enzymes develop at different times postnatally and reach adult levels by 2 years of age.

NUTRITIONAL DISTURBANCES

Nurses can promote healthy eating habits early in children's lives by providing families and their children with information regarding good nutrition and healthy lifestyle. Such education covers diet and exercise that can foster good health, as well as ways to prevent morbidities associated with poor nutrient intake and a sedentary lifestyle. See Chapter 33 for conducting a nutritional assessment and Chapters 35–39 for more information regarding nutritional needs and issues specific to each stage.

Dietary Reference Intake

The **Dietary Reference Intakes (DRIs)** are quantitative estimates of nutrient requirements for planning and evaluating diets for healthy infants. The DRIs consist of four categories (see Additional Resources at the end of this chapter): Estimated Average Requirements (EARs) for age and gender categories, tolerable upper-limit (UL) nutrient intakes that are associated with a low risk of adverse effects, adequate intakes (AIs) of nutrients, and standard Recommended Daily Allowances (RDA). The guidelines present information about lifestyle factors that may affect nutrient function, such as caffeine intake and exercise, and about how the nutrient may be related to chronic disease. The first DRIs published included calcium, magnesium, phosphorus, vitamin D, and fluoride. Additional groups of nutrients include folate and other B vitamins, dietary antioxidants, micronutrients, macronutrients, trace elements, electrolytes, and food components such as dietary fibre. The comprehensive set of guidelines covers nutrient needs across the lifespan, including infancy. An important factor in the development of the DRIs that affects children, particularly infants 0 to 6 months, is that the AIs are based on the nutrient intake of term, healthy, breastfed infants (by well-nourished mothers), which now represents the gold standard for infant nutrition in this age group.

Eating Well With Canada's Food Guide (see Appendix A) was developed by Health Canada in 2007 as a guide for adult and childhood nutrition. This guide aims to simplify healthy food choices and provide guidance in both serving sizes and recommended daily servings based on age and sex. The *Food Guide* can be used to ensure that minimal recommendations for all nutrients are met for children over the age of 2 years.

Vitamin Imbalances

While most vitamin deficiencies are rare in North America, vitamin D–deficiency rickets continues to be a problem in Canada, especially among Indigenous peoples. The Canadian Paediatric Society (CPS) (Godel & CPS, First Nations, Inuit and Métis Health Committee, 2007/2015) has identified the following populations to be at risk:

- Children exclusively breastfed by mothers with an inadequate intake of vitamin D or mothers who had vitamin D deficiency during pregnancy
- Children with dark skin pigmentation
- Children with diets that are low in sources of vitamin D and calcium
- Children who live in northern communities (They have less exposure to sunlight because of fewer sunlight hours and covering the skin during sunlight hours to prevent black fly, mosquito, or other bites.)
- Children who live in polluted urban sites
- Children who cover the skin for religious purposes

Health Canada (2012a) recommends that term breastfed infants receive 400 International Units (IU)/day (10 mcg), and that this should continue until the infant receives 400 IU of vitamin D from other dietary sources or until 1 year of age. The CPS advocates an increase of vitamin intake to 800 IU/day (20 mcg) for children up to 2 years of age in northern Indigenous communities and those with dark skin during the winter months (April to October). Premature infants should receive 200 IU/kg/day to a maximum of 400 IU of vitamin D from all sources beginning shortly after birth, to prevent rickets and vitamin D deficiency (Godel & CPS, First Nations, Inuit and Métis Health Committee, 2007/2015). The CPS also recommends that children be exposed to short periods of sunlight each day (usually less than 15 minutes) to promote cutaneous production of vitamin D. For children aged 1 year through adolescence, Health Canada (2012a) recommends 200 IU of vitamin D per day, although this may be obtained through dietary sources.

Children may also be at risk for vitamin deficiencies secondary to disorders or their treatment. For example, vitamin deficiencies of the fat-soluble vitamins A and D may occur in malabsorptive disorders such as cystic fibrosis and short bowel syndrome. Preterm infants may develop rickets in the second month of life as a result of inadequate intake of vitamin D, calcium, and phosphorus. Children receiving high doses of salicylates may have impaired vitamin C storage. Environmental tobacco smoke exposure has been implicated in decreased concentrations of ascorbate in children; thus increased intake of sources of vitamin C should be encouraged even in children minimally exposed to environmental tobacco smoke (Preston, Rodriguez, & Rivera, 2006). Children with chronic illnesses resulting in **anorexia**, decreased food intake, or possible nutrient malabsorption as a result of multiple medications should be carefully evaluated for adequate vitamin and mineral intake in some form (parenteral or enteral).

Scurvy (caused by a deficiency of vitamin C) is rare in developed countries. Cases have been reported in children who were fed an organic diet deficient in vegetables and fruits (Burk & Molodow, 2007).

All women of child-bearing age are advised to take a dose of 0.4 mg of folic acid. If taken preconception and during early pregnancy, it can reduce the risk of having a child with a neural tube defect by 70%. See Chapters 12 and 54 for more information.

An excessive dose of a vitamin is generally defined as 10 or more times the RDA, although the fat-soluble vitamins, especially A and D, tend to cause toxic reactions at lower doses. With the addition of vitamins to commercially prepared foods, the potential for hypervitaminosis has increased, especially when combined with the excessive use of vitamin supplements. Hypervitaminosis of A and D presents the greatest problem, since these fat-soluble vitamins are stored in the body. High intakes of vitamin A have been linked to physeal growth arrest, which can lead to **osteoporosis**, fracture, and metaphyseal irregularity (Saltzman & King, 2007). Chronic hypervitaminosis of vitamin A can cause headaches; vomiting; dry, itching, and desquamating skin; anorexia; fissure at the corner of the mouth; weight loss; bulging fontanels; and neurological signs such as irritability and stupor. Vitamin D is the most likely of all vitamins to cause toxic reactions in relatively small overdoses. The water-soluble vitamins, primarily niacin, B_6, and C, can also cause toxicity. Poor outcomes in infants (e.g., a fatal hypermagnesemia) have been associated with megavitamin therapy with high doses of magnesium oxide, and severe anemia and **thrombocytopenia** have resulted from megadoses of vitamin A. Children with sickle cell disease with poor dietary intake can have suboptimal levels of vitamins E and D (Kawchak, Schall, Zemel, et al., 2007). Deficiencies and excesses of vitamins A, B complex, C, D, E, and K are summarized in Table 46-1. General nursing care management is discussed later in the chapter, and specific interventions are presented in Table 46-1.

Mineral Imbalances

A number of minerals are essential nutrients. The *macrominerals* refer to those with daily requirements greater than 100 mg and include calcium, phosphorus, magnesium, sodium, potassium, chloride, and sulphur. *Microminerals*, or trace elements, have daily requirements of less than 100 mg and include several essential minerals and those whose exact role in nutrition is still unclear. The greatest concern with minerals is deficiency, especially iron-deficiency anemia. However, other minerals that may be inadequate in children's diets, even with supplementation, include calcium, phosphorus, magnesium,

TABLE 46-1 VITAMINS AND THEIR NUTRITIONAL SIGNIFICANCE

PHYSIOLOGICAL FUNCTIONS AND SOURCES	RESULTS OF DEFICIENCY OR EXCESS	NURSING CARE MANAGEMENT
Vitamin A (Retinol)*		
Functions Necessary component in formation of pigment rhodopsin (visual purple) Formation and maintenance of epithelial tissue Normal bone growth and tooth development Needed for growth and spermatogenesis Involved in thyroxine formation Antioxidant ***Sources*** Natural form—Liver, kidney, fish oils, milk and nonskim milk products, egg yolk Provitamin A (carotene)—Carrots, sweet potatoes, squash, apricots, spinach, collards, broccoli, cabbage, artichokes	***Deficiency*** Night blindness Keratinization (hardening and scaling) of epithelium Xerophthalmia (hardening and scaling of cornea and conjunctiva) Phrynoderma (toad skin) Drying of respiratory, gastrointestinal, and genitourinary tracts Defective tooth enamel Delayed growth Impaired bone formation Decreased thyroxine formation Decreased resistance to infections ***Excess*** **Early signs**—Irritability, anorexia, pruritus, fissures at corners of nose and lips, dry skin **Later signs**—Hepatomegaly, jaundice, restricted growth, poor weight gain, thickening of the cortex of long bones with pain and fragility, hard tender lumps in extremities and occiput of the skull Can cause birth defects if excessive maternal intake **NOTE:** Overdose results from ingestion of large quantities of the vitamin only, not the provitamin; large amounts of carotene (carotenemia) cause yellow or orange discolouration of the skin (not the sclera, urine, or feces as in jaundice) but none of the above symptoms.	***Deficiency*** Encourage foods rich in vitamin A, such as whole cow's milk (after 12 mo). As milk consumption decreases, encourage foods rich in vitamin A. Ensure adequate intake in preterm infants. Advise parents of safe use of supplements in child with measles. It may play a role in prevention of severity of bronchopulmonary dysplasia in preterm infants (affects growth of respiratory tract epithelial cells). ***Excess*** Emphasize correct use of vitamin supplements and potential hazards of excess. Evaluate child's dietary habits to calculate approximate intake; if excessive, remove supplemental source (e.g., daily feeding of liver). Advise parents of the benign nature of carotenemia; treatment is avoidance of excess pigmented fruits or vegetables, especially carrots; skin colour returns to normal in 2 to 6 wk.

Continued

TABLE 46-1 VITAMINS AND THEIR NUTRITIONAL SIGNIFICANCE—cont'd

PHYSIOLOGICAL FUNCTIONS AND SOURCES	RESULTS OF DEFICIENCY OR EXCESS	NURSING CARE MANAGEMENT
Vitamin B_1 (Thiamine)†		
Functions Coenzyme (with phosphorus) in carbohydrate metabolism Needed for healthy nervous system Digestion and normal appetite ***Sources*** Pork, beef, liver, legumes, nuts, whole or enriched grains and cereals, green vegetables, fruits, milk, brown rice	***Deficiency*** **Gastrointestinal**—Anorexia, constipation, indigestion **Neurological**—Apathy, fatigue, emotional instability, polyneuritis, tenderness of calf muscles, partial anaesthesia, muscle weakness, paresthesia, hyperesthesia, decreased or absent tendon reflexes, convulsions, coma (in infants) **Cardiovascular**—Palpitations, cardiac failure, peripheral vasodilation, edema ***Excess*** Headache Irritability Insomnia Weakness	***Deficiency: Vitamin B Complex*** Encourage foods rich in B vitamins. Stress proper cooking and storage techniques to preserve potency, such as minimum cooking of vegetables in small amount of liquid and storage of milk in opaque container. Encourage fortified breakfast cereals and soy milk (which have B_{12}) for persons on strict vegetarian diet; dairy products and eggs contain B_{12} if these are allowed; otherwise supplementation may be required. Evaluate need for vitamin supplements when dieting, when using unfortified goat's milk exclusively for infant feeding (deficient in folic acid), or when the breastfeeding mother is a strict vegetarian (vitamin B_{12}). ***Excess*** Emphasize correct use of vitamin supplements and potential hazards of excess. Individuals with malabsorption syndrome or being treated with hemodialysis or peritoneal dialysis may have increased need for thiamine.
Vitamin B_2 (Riboflavin)†		
Functions Coenzyme (with phosphorus) in carbohydrate, protein, and fat metabolism Maintains healthy skin, especially around mouth, nose, and eyes ***Sources*** Milk and its products, eggs, organs (liver, kidney, heart), enriched cereals, some green leafy vegetables,‡ legumes	***Deficiency*** Ariboflavinosis **Lips**—Cheilosis (fissures at corners of lips), perlèche (inflammation at corners of lips) **Tongue**—Glossitis **Nose**—Irritation and cracks at nasal angle **Eyes**—Burning, itching, tearing, photophobia, blurred vision, corneal vascularization, cataracts **Skin**—Seborrheic dermatitis, delayed wound healing and tissue repair ***Excess*** Paresthesia, pruritus	Same as vitamin B complex
Niacin (Nicotinic Acid, Nicotinamide)†		
Functions Coenzyme (with riboflavin) in protein and fat metabolism Needed for healthy nervous system and skin and for normal digestion May lower cholesterol ***Sources*** Meat, poultry, fish, peanuts, beans, peas, whole or enriched grains (except corn and rice) Milk and its products are sources of tryptophan (60 mg tryptophan = 1 mg niacin)	***Deficiency*** Pellagra (rash, diarrhea, mental status changes, stomatitis) **Oral**—Stomatitis, glossitis **Cutaneous**—Scaly dermatitis on exposed areas **Gastrointestinal**—Anorexia, weight loss, diarrhea, fatigue **Neurological**—Apathy, anxiety, confusion, depression, dementia ***Excess*** Release of histamine, a vasodilator (flushing, decreased blood pressure, increased cerebral blood flow; aggravates asthma) Dermatological problems (pruritus, rash, hyperkeratosis, acanthosis nigricans) Increased gastric acidity (aggravates peptic ulcer disease) Hepatotoxicity Increased serum uric acid levels Elevated plasma glucose levels Certain cardiac arrhythmias	Same as vitamin B complex ***Excess*** If used as hypolipidemic agent, stress safe storage to prevent child's accidental ingestion.

TABLE 46-1 VITAMINS AND THEIR NUTRITIONAL SIGNIFICANCE—cont'd

PHYSIOLOGICAL FUNCTIONS AND SOURCES	RESULTS OF DEFICIENCY OR EXCESS	NURSING CARE MANAGEMENT
Vitamin B_6 (Pyridoxine)†		
Functions Coenzyme in protein and fat metabolism Needed for formation of antibodies and hemoglobin Needed for utilization of copper and iron Aids in conversion of tryptophan to niacin ***Sources*** Meats, especially liver and kidney, cereal grains (wheat, corn), yeast, soybeans, peanuts, tuna, chicken, salmon	***Deficiency*** Scaly dermatitis Weight loss Anemia Restricted growth Irritability Seizures Peripheral neuritis ***Excess*** Peripheral nervous system toxicity (unsteady gait, numb feet and hands, clumsiness of hands, sometimes perioral numbness) May cause peptic ulcer disease or seizures	Same as vitamin B complex ***Deficiency*** Stress proper cooking and storing techniques to preserve potency. Cook food covered in small amount of water. Do not soak food in water. Store in light-resistant container.
Folic Acid (Folacin; Reduced Form Called Folinic Acid or Citrovorum Factor)†		
Functions Coenzyme for single-carbon transfer (purines, thymine, hemoglobin) Necessary for formation of red blood cells May prevent neural tube defects (i.e., myelomeningocele) and facial clefts (cleft lip and palate) ***Sources*** Green leafy vegetables, beets, cabbage, asparagus, liver, kidneys, nuts, eggs, whole grain cereals, legumes, bananas	***Deficiency*** Macrocytic anemia Bone marrow depression Glossitis Intestinal malabsorption Growth failure ***Excess*** Rare because megadoses are not available over the counter May cause insomnia and irritability	Same as vitamin B complex ***Deficiency*** Stress proper cooking and storing techniques to preserve potency: Cook food covered in small amount of water. Do not soak food in water. Store in light-resistant container. Women of child-bearing age should supplement to prevent neural tube defects and orofacial clefts.
Vitamin B_{12} (Cobalamin)†		
Functions Coenzyme in protein synthesis; indirect effect on formation of red blood cells (particularly on formation of nucleic acids and folic acid metabolism) Needed for normal functioning of nervous tissue ***Sources*** Meat, liver, kidney, fish, shellfish, poultry, milk, eggs, cheese, nutritional yeast, sea vegetables	***Deficiency*** Pernicious anemia (one form of deficiency from absence of intrinsic factor in gastric secretions) General signs of severe anemia Lemon-yellow tinge to skin Spinal cord degeneration Delayed brain growth ***Excess*** Rare	Same as vitamin B complex ***Deficiency*** Consider fortified foods or supplements in persons over 50 yr of age to meet RDA because malabsorption of food-bound vitamin B_{12} is common.

Continued

TABLE 46-1 **VITAMINS AND THEIR NUTRITIONAL SIGNIFICANCE—cont'd**

PHYSIOLOGICAL FUNCTIONS AND SOURCES	RESULTS OF DEFICIENCY OR EXCESS	NURSING CARE MANAGEMENT
Vitamin C (Ascorbic Acid)†		
Functions Essential for collagen formation Increases absorption of iron for hemoglobin formation Enhances conversion of folic acid to folinic acid Affects cholesterol synthesis and conversion of proline to hydroxyproline Probably a coenzyme in metabolism of tyrosine and phenylalanine May play role in hydroxylation of adrenal steroids May have stimulating effect on phagocytic activity of leukocytes and formation of antibodies Antioxidant agent (spares other vitamins from oxidation) ***Sources*** Citrus fruits, strawberries, tomatoes, potatoes, cabbage, broccoli, cauliflower, spinach, papaya, mango, cantaloupe, watermelon, enriched fruit juice	***Deficiency*** Scurvy **Skin**—Dry, rough, petechiae; perifollicular hyperkeratotic papules (raised areas around hair follicles) **Musculoskeletal**—Bleeding muscles and joints, pseudoparalysis from pain, swelling of joints, costochondral beading (scorbutic rosary) **Gums**—Spongy, friable, swollen, bleed easily, bluish red or black, teeth loosen and fall out **General disposition**—Irritable, anorexic, apprehensive, in pain, refuses to move, assumes semi-froglike position when supine (scorbutic pose) Signs of anemia Decreased wound healing Increased susceptibility to infection ***Excess*** **Diarrhea** Increased excretion of uric acid and acidification of urine (may cause urate precipitation and formation of oxalate stones) **Hemolysis** Impaired leukocytosis activity Damage to beta cells of pancreas and decreased insulin production Reproductive failure "Rebound scurvy" from withdrawal of large amounts	***Deficiency*** Encourage foods rich in vitamin C. Evaluate child's diet for sources of vitamin, especially when cow's milk is principal source of nutrition. Tobacco smokers require an additional 35 mg/day; nonsmokers exposed to second-hand smoke should make sure they meet RDA. Stress proper cooking and storage techniques to preserve potency. Wash vegetables quickly; do not soak in water. Cook vegetables in covered pot with minimum water and for short time; avoid copper or cast iron cookware. Do not add baking soda to cooking water. Use fresh fruits and vegetables as soon as possible; store in refrigerator. Store juice in airtight, opaque container. Wrap cut fruit or eat soon after exposing to air. ***Excess*** Emphasize correct use of vitamin supplements and potential hazards of excess. Identify groups at risk for excessive vitamin C supplements (e.g., those with thalassemia or those receiving anticoagulant or aminoglycoside antibiotic therapy).
Vitamin D_2 (Ergocalciferol) and D_3 (Cholecalciferol)*		
Functions Absorption of calcium and phosphorus and decreased renal excretion of phosphorus ***Sources*** Direct sunlight Cod liver oil, herring, mackerel, salmon, tuna, sardines Enriched food sources—Milk, milk products, enriched cereals, margarine, breads, many breakfast drinks	***Deficiency*** Rickets **Head**—Craniotabes (softening of cranial bones, prominence of frontal bones [bossing]), deformed shape (skull flat and depressed toward middle), delayed closure of fontanels **Chest**—Rachitic rosary (enlargement of costochondral junction of ribs), Harrison groove (horizontal depression in lower portion of rib cage), pigeon chest (sharp protrusion of sternum) **Spine**—Kyphosis, scoliosis, lordosis **Abdomen**—Pot belly, constipation **Extremities**—Bowing of arms and legs, knock knee, sabre shins, instability of hip joints, pelvic deformity, enlargement of epiphyses at ends of long bones **Teeth**—Delayed calcification, especially of permanent teeth **Rachitic tetany**—Seizures ***Excess*** **Acute**—Vomiting, dehydration, fever, abdominal cramps, bone pain, seizures, coma **Chronic**—Lassitude, mental slowness, anorexia, failure to thrive, thirst, urinary urgency, polyuria, vomiting, diarrhea, abdominal cramps, bone pain, pathological fractures Calcification of soft tissue—Kidneys, lungs, adrenal glands, vessels (hypertension), heart, gastric lining, tympanic membrane (deafness) Osteoporosis of long bones Elevated serum levels of calcium and phosphorus	***Deficiency*** Encourage foods rich in vitamin D, especially fortified whole cow's milk (>12 mo of age). Encourage use of vitamin D supplement in all exclusively breastfed infants starting within first 2 wk of life (see text). Observe for possibility of overdose from supplements. If prescribed, supervise proper use of orthoses (splints and braces). ***Excess*** Same as vitamin A; may include low-calcium diet during initial therapy

TABLE 46-1 VITAMINS AND THEIR NUTRITIONAL SIGNIFICANCE—cont'd

PHYSIOLOGICAL FUNCTIONS AND SOURCES	RESULTS OF DEFICIENCY OR EXCESS	NURSING CARE MANAGEMENT
Vitamin E (Tocopherol)*		
Functions Production of red blood cells and protection from hemolysis Muscle and liver integrity Coenzyme factor in tissue respiration Minimizes oxidation of polyunsaturated fatty acids and vitamins A and C in intestinal tract and tissues ***Sources*** Vegetable oils, wheat germ oil, milk, egg yolk, fish, whole grains, nuts, legumes, spinach, broccoli	***Deficiency*** Hemolytic anemia from hemolysis caused by shortened life of red blood cells, especially in preterm infants; focal necrosis of tissues ***Excess*** Little is known; less toxic than other fat-soluble vitamins	***Deficiency*** Initiate early feeding in preterm infants; may need supplementation. Potential role as antioxidant in immune function, preventing or limiting the severity of retinopathy and prevention of hemolytic anemia, bronchopulmonary dysplasia, and intracranial hemorrhage
Vitamin K*		
Functions Catalyst for production of prothrombin and blood-clotting factors II, VII, IX, and X by the liver ***Sources*** Pork, liver, green leafy vegetables, cabbage, tomatoes, egg yolk, cheese	***Deficiency*** Hemorrhage ***Excess*** Hemolytic anemia in individuals who are deficient in glucose 6-phosphate dehydrogenase	***Deficiency*** Administer prophylactically to all newborns. Other indications include intestinal disease, lack of bile, prolonged antibiotic therapy; may be used in management of blood-clotting time when anticoagulants such as warfarin (Coumadin) and dicumarol (bishydroxycoumarin), which are vitamin K antagonists, are used.

Table is not intended to be all inclusive.
*Fat soluble.
†Water soluble.
‡Green leafy vegetables include spinach, broccoli, kale, turnip greens, mustard greens, collards, dandelion greens, and beet greens.
RDA, recommended dietary allowance.

and zinc. Low levels of zinc can cause nutritional growth failure (failure to thrive). Some of the macrominerals may be overlooked inadvertently when a child with intestinal failure or recent surgery is making the transition from total parenteral to enteral intake.

An imbalance in the intake of calcium and phosphorus may occur in infants who are given whole cow's milk instead of infant formula; neonatal tetany may be observed in such cases. Whole cow's milk is also a poor source of iron, and inadequate intake of iron from other food sources, such as iron-fortified cereal, may cause iron deficiency anemia.

The regulation of mineral balance in the body is complex. Dietary extremes of mineral intake can cause a number of mineral–mineral interactions that could result in unexpected deficiencies or excesses. For example, excessive amounts of one mineral such as zinc can result in a deficiency of another mineral such as copper, even if sufficient amounts of copper are ingested. Thus megadose intake of one mineral may cause deficiency of another essential mineral by blocking its absorption in the blood or intestinal wall or by competing with binding sites on protein carriers needed for metabolism.

Deficiencies can also occur when various substances in the diet interact with minerals. For example, iron, zinc, and calcium can form insoluble complexes with phytates or oxalates (substances found in plant proteins), which impair the bioavailability of the mineral. This type of interaction is important in vegetarian diets because plant foods such as soy are high in phytates. Contrary to popular opinion, spinach is not an ideal source of iron or calcium because of its high oxalate content.

Children with certain illnesses are at greater risk for growth failure, especially in relation to bone mineral deficiency as a result of the treatment of the disease, decreased nutrient intake, or decreased absorption of necessary minerals. Those at risk for such deficiencies include children who are receiving or have received radiation and chemotherapy for cancer; children with human immunodeficiency virus (HIV), sickle cell disease, cystic fibrosis, GI malabsorption, or nephrosis; and extremely low-birth-weight (ELBW) and very low–birth weight (VLBW) preterm infants.

Deficiencies and excesses of the essential macrominerals and microminerals are summarized in Table 46-2.

NURSING CARE

Identification of the adequacy of nutrient intake is the initial nursing goal and requires assessment based on a dietary history

TABLE 46-2 MINERALS AND THEIR NUTRITIONAL SIGNIFICANCE

PHYSIOLOGICAL FUNCTIONS AND SOURCES	RESULTS OF DEFICIENCY OR EXCESS	NURSING CARE MANAGEMENT
Calcium*		
Functions Bone and tooth development and maintenance (in combination with phosphorus) Muscle contractions, especially the heart Blood clotting Absorption of vitamin B_{12} Enzyme activation Nerve conduction Integrity of intracellular cement substances and various membranes ***Sources*** Dairy products, egg yolk, sardines, canned salmon with bones, green leafy vegetables† (except spinach), soybeans, dried beans, peas	***Deficiency*** Rickets Tetany Impaired growth, especially of bones and teeth Osteoporosis ***Excess*** Drowsiness, extreme lethargy Impaired absorption of other minerals (iron, zinc, manganese) Calcium deposits in tissues (renal failure)	***Deficiency*** Encourage foods rich in calcium, especially dairy products. Give vitamin D supplements in breastfed infants from birth until adequate amounts received from introduction of solid foods (see text). Caution that oxalates in leafy vegetables (spinach), oxalates in chocolates, and a high phosphorus intake (especially from carbonated beverages) can decrease calcium absorption. Discourage use of whole cow's milk or other animal milks in newborns and infants under 12 mo because the phosphorus/calcium ratio favours excretion of calcium. Advise against diets that restrict dairy products unless adequate supplementation is followed. ***Excess*** Emphasize correct use of calcium supplements, especially the possible interaction between megadoses of calcium and resulting deficiency states of other minerals.
Chloride*		
Functions Acid–base and fluid balance Enzyme activation in saliva Component of hydrochloric acid in stomach ***Sources*** Salt, meat, eggs, dairy products, many prepared and preserved foods	***Deficiency*** Acid–base disturbances (hypochloremic alkalosis, dehydration); occurs mostly in combination with sodium loss ***Excess*** Acid–base disturbance	Deficiency and excess are unusual; most diets supply adequate chloride (usually in combination with sodium). Disease states such as excessive vomiting can necessitate chloride replacement.
Copper‡		
Functions Production of hemoglobin Essential component of several enzyme systems ***Sources*** Organ meats, oysters, nuts, seeds, legumes, corn oil margarine	***Deficiency*** Anemia, leukopenia, neutropenia ***Excess*** Severe vomiting and diarrhea Hemolytic anemia	***Deficiency*** Emphasize that the correct use of any vitamin supplement with mineral because deficiency from inadequate food sources is less likely than from excess intake of other minerals, especially zinc and possibly iron. ***Excess*** Cooking acid foods in unlined copper pots can lead to chronic and toxic accumulation of copper.
Fluoride‡		
Functions Formation of caries-resistant teeth Strong bone development ***Sources*** Fluoridated water and foods or beverages prepared with fluoridated water, fish, tea	***Deficiency*** Increased susceptibility to tooth decay ***Excess*** Fluorosis (mottling or pitting of enamel) Severe bone deformities	Fluoride has the narrowest range of safe and adequate intake; therefore, stress the importance of storing supplements in a safe area. ***Deficiency*** In areas with optimally fluoridated water, encourage sufficient intake to supply recommended amount of fluoride. In areas of unfluoridated water or when ready-to-use formula, powder formula, bottled water, or breast milk is used, stress the importance of fluoride supplements (age appropriate). ***Excess*** In areas with excess fluoride in the water, consider the use of bottled water (without fluoride) in drinking and cooking to reduce the fluoride intake to safe levels.

TABLE 46-2 MINERALS AND THEIR NUTRITIONAL SIGNIFICANCE—cont'd

PHYSIOLOGICAL FUNCTIONS AND SOURCES	RESULTS OF DEFICIENCY OR EXCESS	NURSING CARE MANAGEMENT
Iodine‡		
Functions Production of thyroid hormone Normal reproduction	***Deficiency*** Goitre (enlarged thyroid from decreased thyroxine formation)	***Deficiency*** Encourage use of iodized salt for individuals living far from the sea.
Sources Seafood, kelp, iodized salt, sea salt, enriched bread, milk (from dairy processing); medications, including amiodarone, povidone-iodine, and prenatal vitamins	***Excess*** Thyrotoxicosis; goitre; hypothyroidism	***Excess*** If iodine preparations are in the home, stress the importance of safe storage.
Iron		
Functions Formation of hemoglobin and myoglobin Essential part of several enzymes and proteins ***Sources*** Liver, especially pork, followed by calf, beef, and chicken; kidney, red meat, poultry, shellfish, whole grains, iron-enriched infant formula and cereal, enriched cereals and bread, legumes, nuts, seeds, green leafy vegetables† (except spinach), dried fruits, potatoes, molasses, tofu, prune juice	***Deficiency*** Anemia (see Chapter 48) ***Excess*** Hemosiderosis (excess iron storage in various tissues of the body, especially the spleen, liver, lymph glands, heart, and pancreas) Hemochromatosis (excess iron storage with cellular damage)	***Deficiency*** Discourage excessive iron-fortified milk consumption, especially more than 1 L/day (cow's milk is a poor source of iron). If iron supplements are prescribed, teach parents factors that affect absorption. ***Excess*** Stress the importance of storing iron supplements in a safe area.
Magnesium*		
Functions Bone and tooth formation Production of proteins Nerve conduction to muscles Activation of enzymes needed for carbohydrate and protein metabolism	***Deficiency*** Tremors, spasm Irregular heartbeat Muscular weakness Lower extremity cramps Convulsions, delirium	Deficiency and excess are unusual, except in disease states such as prolonged vomiting or diarrhea or kidney dysfunction, where replacement may be needed.
Sources Whole grains, nuts, soybeans, meat, green leafy vegetables (uncooked), tea, cocoa, raisins	***Excess*** Nervous system disturbances caused by imbalance in calcium/magnesium ratio	
Phosphorus*		
Functions Bone and tooth development (in combination with calcium) Involved in numerous chemical reactions, including protein, carbohydrate, and fat metabolism Acid–base balance ***Sources*** Dairy products, eggs, meat, poultry, legumes, carbonated beverages	***Deficiency*** Weakness, anorexia, malaise, bone pain ***Excess*** Produces secondary calcium deficiency from imbalanced calcium/phosphorus ratio	***Deficiency*** Dietary deficiency is uncommon, although prolonged use of antacids can produce deficiency, in which case supplementation is recommended. To preserve calcium/phosphorus ratio in newborns and infants, discourage use of cow's milk.

Continued

TABLE 46-2 MINERALS AND THEIR NUTRITIONAL SIGNIFICANCE—cont'd

PHYSIOLOGICAL FUNCTIONS AND SOURCES	RESULTS OF DEFICIENCY OR EXCESS	NURSING CARE MANAGEMENT
Potassium*		
Functions Acid–base and fluid balance (major extracellular fluid areas) Nerve conduction Muscular contraction, especially the heart Release of energy	***Deficiency*** Cardiac arrhythmias Muscular weakness Lethargy Kidney and respiratory failure Heart failure	Dietary deficiency and excess are unlikely, although disease states such as prolonged nausea and vomiting or the use of certain diuretics can result in hypokalemia; in such instances encourage replacement with supplements of rich food sources such as bananas.
Sources Bananas, citrus fruit, dried fruits, meat, fish, bran, legumes, peanut butter, potatoes, coffee, tea, cocoa	***Excess*** Cardiac arrhythmias Respiratory failure Mental confusion Numbness of extremities	
Selenium‡		
Functions Antioxidant, especially protective of vitamin E Protects against toxicity of heavy metals Associated with fat metabolism	***Deficiency*** Keshan disease (cardiomyopathy in children; found in China)	Deficiency and excess are uncommon in North America, although selenium deficiency can occur in patients receiving prolonged total parenteral alimentation; in these instances supplementation is required.
Sources Seafood, organs, egg yolk, whole grains, chicken, meat, tomatoes, cabbage, garlic, mushrooms, milk	***Excess*** Eye, nose, and throat irritation Increased dental caries Liver and kidney degeneration	
Sodium*		
Functions Acid–base and fluid balance (major extracellular fluid cation) Cell permeability; absorption of glucose Muscle contraction	***Deficiency*** Dehydration Hypotension Convulsions Muscle cramps	***Deficiency*** Deficient intake is rare, although losses secondary to nausea, vomiting, excessive sweating, and use of diuretics can occur and require replacement.
Sources Table salt, seafood, meat, poultry, numerous prepared foods	***Excess*** Edema Hypertension Intracranial hemorrhage	***Excess*** Encourage parents to limit excessive use of salt in preparing foods and to limit commercial foods with high sodium content, such as smoked meats.
Zinc‡		
Functions Component of about 100 enzymes Synthesis of nucleic acids and protein in immune system and coagulation Release of vitamin A from liver Improved wound healing with vitamin C Normal taste sensitivity	***Deficiency*** Loss of appetite Diminished taste sensation Delayed healing Skin lesions—Erythematous, crusted lesions around body orifices (mouth, nares, anus) Alopecia Diarrhea Growth failure Delayed sexual maturity	Emphasize correct use of zinc supplements and the possible interaction with other minerals. ***Deficiency*** Encourage food sources rich in zinc, especially protein. Caution that fibre, phytates, oxalates, tannins (in tea or coffee), iron, and calcium adversely affect zinc absorption. Recognize groups at risk for zinc deficiency, such as vegetarians and those whose diets may have restricted or low meat content and high fibre and phytate content; and patients with malabsorption syndromes.
Sources Seafood (especially oysters), meat, poultry, eggs, wheat, legumes	***Excess*** Vomiting and diarrhea Malaise, dizziness Anemia, gastric bleeding Impaired absorption of calcium and copper	

Table is not intended to be all inclusive.
*Macrominerals—required intake >100 mg/day.
†Green leafy vegetables include spinach, broccoli, kale, turnip greens, mustard greens, collards, dandelion greens, and beet greens.
‡Microminerals or trace elements—required intake <100 mg/day.

and physical examination for signs of deficiency or excess. After assessment data are collected, this information is evaluated against standard intakes to identify areas of concern. DRIs are one source of standard nutrient intakes.

Standardized growth reference charts should be used in infants, children, and adolescents to compare and assess growth parameters such as height and head circumference with the percentile distribution of other children at the same ages. The World Health Organization (WHO) growth charts are a standardized growth references recommended for use with infants and toddlers up to 24 months of age and children 2 to 19 years of age (see Appendix C). These growth charts include head circumference, height/length, and weight references plus BMI calculations. The growth charts have been adopted and developed into the *WHO Growth Charts for Canada* through collaboration between the Dietitians of Canada, Canadian Pediatric Society, College of Family Physicians of Canada, and Community Health Nurses of Canada (CPS, 2014).

Infants should be exclusively breastfed for the first 6 months; breastfeeding can continue for up to 2 years. They should be introduced to some solid foods after 6 months and receive iron-fortified cereal for at least 18 months. Vitamin B_{12} supplementation is recommended if the breastfeeding mother's intake of the vitamin is inadequate or if she is not taking vitamin supplements. A variety of foods should be introduced during the early years to ensure a well-balanced intake. Infants who are identified as having particular nutritional deficits should be treated; a multidisciplinary approach should be used to determine the deficit and the etiology, and a plan needs to be established with the caregiver to promote adequate growth and development.

Protein-Energy Malnutrition

Malnutrition continues to be a major health problem in the world today, particularly in children under 5 years of age. However, lack of food is not always the primary cause for malnutrition. In many developing and underdeveloped nations, diarrhea (gastroenteritis) is a major factor. Additional factors leading to malnutrition are bottle-feeding (in poor sanitary conditions), inadequate knowledge of proper child care practices, parental illiteracy, economic and political factors, climate conditions, cultural and religious food preferences, and simply the lack of adequate food. Poverty is an important determinant of health and an underlying contributing cause of malnutrition. The most extreme forms of malnutrition, or *protein-energy malnutrition (PEM)*, are kwashiorkor and marasmus. Both of these conditions are extremely rare in Canada.

PEM may be seen in persons with chronic health problems, such as cystic fibrosis, renal dialysis, HIV, GI malabsorption; or in persons with acute illness, such as prolonged, untreated anorexia nervosa; or in children who have been fed an inappropriate diet.

Kwashiorkor is a deficiency of high-quality protein along with an adequate supply of carbohydrate calories. There is some evidence that it is caused by an interaction of nutritional deprivation, infection, oxidative stress, environment, and cultural and psychological factors that leads to radical damage. This interaction may precipitate cellular changes, leading to edema (ascites) and muscle wasting. These children are at high risk of a fatal deterioration due to diarrhea, infection, or circulatory failure.

Marasmus is caused by a general malnutrition of protein and calories. It commonly occurs in underdeveloped countries particularly where adults eat first and children have inadequate quantity and quality of food. Children with marasma exhibit a gradual wasting and atrophy of body tissues, particularly the subcutaneous fat layer. The loss of tissues creates loose and wrinkled skin. The child is irritable, apathetic, and withdrawn and prostration can occur. Intercurrent infection with debilitating disease such as tuberculosis, parasitosis, HIV, and dysentery is common. Both marasmic and kwashiorkor can occur together. Treatment includes a high-quality level of proteins, carbohydrates, vitamins, and minerals. If diarrhea is present, then rehydration using an oral rehydration solution with electrolyte replacements is required. Antibiotics are administered if infection is present. The treatment process must proceed slowly to avoid fluid overload and food intolerance and to avoid heart failure (Grover & Ee, 2009).

Vegetarian Diets

Vegetarian diets have become increasingly popular in North America, for various reasons. Many people are concerned about hypertension; cholesterol; obesity; cardiovascular disease; and cancer of the stomach, intestine, and colon. The animal rights movement has also influenced individuals to become vegetarians. The Dietitians of Canada (2014) endorses vegetarian diets for adults and children and notes that well-planned vegetarian diets are adequate for all stages of the life cycle and promote normal growth. Children and adolescents on vegetarian diets have the potential for lifelong healthy diets and have been shown to have lower intakes of cholesterol, saturated fat, and total fat and higher intakes of fruits, fibre, and vegetables than nonvegetarians (Dietitians of Canada, 2014).

The major types of vegetarianism are as follows:

Lacto-ovo vegetarians, who exclude meat from their diet but consume dairy products and rarely fish

Lactovegetarians, who exclude meat and eggs but drink milk

Pure vegetarians (vegans), who eliminate any food of animal origin, including milk, cheese, and eggs

Macrobiotics, who are even more restrictive than pure vegetarians, allowing only a few types of fruits, vegetables, and legumes

Semivegetarians, who consume a lacto-ovo vegetarian diet with some fish and poultry (This is an increasingly popular form of vegetarianism and poses little or no nutritional risk to infants unless dietary fat and cholesterol intake is severely restricted.)

Many individuals who are concerned about their health subscribe to vegetarian diets that may not be typified by these categories. During nutritional assessment it is necessary to clearly list exactly what the diet includes and excludes (see Additional Resources at the end of this chapter for further information, on the Dietitians of Canada website).

Achieving a nutritionally adequate vegetarian diet is not difficult (except with the strictest diets), but it does require careful planning and knowledge of nutrient sources. The nutritional guide *Eating Well With Canada's Food Guide* (see Appendix A) can be adapted to meet the nutrient needs of vegetarians. The introduction of solids for vegetarian infants may occur using the same guidelines as for other children (see p. 1008). Breast milk from vegetarian mothers can be deficient in vitamin B_{12}; supplementation of both mother and child is advisable. If human milk or commercial infant formula is not given, fortified soy formula is recommended only for infants who have galactosemia or who cannot consume dairy-based products for cultural or religious reasons.

To ensure sufficient protein in the diet, **incomplete protein foods** (those that do not have all the **essential amino acids**) must be eaten at the same meal with other foods that supply the missing amino acids. (**Complete protein foods** have all the essential amino acids.) The three basic combinations of foods consumed by vegetarians that generally provide the appropriate amounts of essential amino acids are as follows:

1. Grains (cereal, rice, pasta) and legumes (beans, peas, lentils, peanuts)
2. Grains and milk products (milk, cheese, yogurt)
3. Seeds (sesame, sunflower) and legumes

The major deficiencies that may occur in the stricter vegan diets are inadequate protein for growth; inadequate calories for energy and growth; poor digestibility of many of the bulky natural, unprocessed foods, especially for infants; and deficiencies of vitamin B_6, niacin, riboflavin, vitamin D, iron, calcium, and zinc. Strict vegan diets also require supplements of vitamin B_{12} and vitamin D for children aged 2 to 12 years. Vitamin D is essential if a child drinks less than 500 mL of vitamin D–fortified milk daily. Children in this category should receive 400 IU of vitamin D daily. Many of these deficiencies can be avoided in children who are not consuming 100% of the RDA of vitamins and minerals by taking a multivitamin–mineral supplement (Amit & CPS, Community Paediatrics Committee, 2010/2016).

Children on strict vegetarian and macrobiotic diets should be evaluated for iron-deficiency anemia and rickets; this may occur as a result of consuming plant foods such as unrefined cereals, which impair the absorption of iron, calcium, and zinc. Other factors that affect iron absorption are listed in Box 46-1.

BOX 46-1 FACTORS THAT AFFECT IRON ABSORPTION

Increase

Acidity (low pH)—Administer iron between meals (gastric hydrochloric acid)
Ascorbic acid (vitamin C)—Administer iron with juice, fruit, or multivitamin preparation
Vitamin A
Calcium
Tissue need
Meat, fish, poultry
Cooking in cast iron pots

Decrease

Alkalinity (high pH)—Avoid any antacid preparation
Phosphates—Milk is unfavourable vehicle for iron administration
Phytates—Found in cereals
Oxalates—Found in many fruits and vegetables (plums, currants, green beans, spinach, sweet potatoes, tomatoes)
Tannins—Found in tea, coffee
Tissue saturation
Malabsorptive disorders
Disturbances that cause diarrhea or steatorrhea
Infection

Complementary and Alternative Medicine

The misuse or overuse of vitamins as a part of complementary and alternative medicine (CAM) places some children at risk for health problems. Some parents may routinely give their children megavitamin therapy; however, more research needs to be done to determine a realistic number of children using multivitamin preparations. Many adolescent girls who have an eating disorder also use herbal supplements and other types of alternative medicines to accelerate weight loss.

There is concern among health care providers that terms often used to market supplements such as megavitamins may mislead parents regarding the actual benefits (or harm) of such therapies. It is important to ensure the safety and efficacy of supplements in children, who may experience inadvertent harm. Parents should be cautioned not to exceed the upper limits of vitamin intake according to the new DRIs (see earlier in this chapter and the Dietary Reference Intakes, available on Evolve).

The use of various herbal therapies, or intake of herbs, is also becoming more popular; many of these supplements have been a part of medicine for centuries and are beneficial in some cases.

Herbs known to have adverse effects in children include ephedra, comfrey, and pennyroyal; some herbs may not be harmful taken alone but may counteract or potentiate prescription medications when taken concurrently. Parents should be fully informed of the use of herbs to ensure that there is more benefit than potential harm in the ingredient being used. Health care providers also need to be knowledgeable about the benefits or potential harm from herbs so that they can appropriately counsel parents and address their concerns. Little research has been performed in children on many over-the-counter herbal medicines, yet some herbs are known to cause harm in children (Kemper & Gardiner, 2016).

The CPS has outlined their concerns about the use of CAMs, especially regarding homeopathic and herbal remedies. The concerns include the lack of research and safety data, particularly in relation to use in the pediatric age group, lack of standardized products, and potential drug interactions (Vohra, Clifford, & CPS, Drug Therapy and Hazardous Substances Committee, 2005/2016). For further information see Additional Resources at the end of this chapter.

Homemade Infant Formulas

The Dietitians of Canada and the CPS (2014) have warned about the risks of feeding infants homemade formula made from recipes available online. The homemade formulas may have harmful bacteria and inappropriate levels of nutrients which can cause malnutrition and illness in infants. Commercial infant formulas are the only recommended substitute for parents of infants who have made an informed decision to move from breastfeeding or breast milk. For infants 9 to 12 months of age who are no longer being breastfed, pasteurized, whole cow milk or commercial infant formula is recommended.

GASTROINTESTINAL DYSFUNCTION

The extensive surface area of the GI tract and its digestive function represent the major means of exchange between the human organism and the environment. Inflammatory and malabsorptive disorders impair the functional integrity of the GI tract. In addition, the infant's intestine is extremely vulnerable to infection. Numerous clinical observations provide clues to specific GI problems (Box 46-2). In any disorder that involves GI losses of large amounts of fluid, dehydration poses a serious threat to life and demands immediate attention.

Acute infectious diarrhea, also known as gastroenteritis, causes significant alterations in fluid and electrolyte balance in both infants and children.

Food Sensitivity

Food sensitivity is a general term that includes any type of adverse reaction to food or food additives. Food sensitivities can be divided into two broad categories:

1. **Food allergy or hypersensitivity**, which refers to reactions involving immunological mechanisms, usually immune globulin E (IgE); the reactions may be immediate or delayed and mild or severe, such as an anaphylactic reaction. *Food allergens* are defined as specific components of food or ingredients in food, such as a protein, that are recognized by allergen-specific immune cells eliciting an immune reaction that results in the characteristic symptoms (Boyce, Assa'ad, Burks, et al., 2011).
2. **Food intolerance**, which refers to reactions involving known or unknown nonimmunological mechanisms; lactose intolerance is an example of a reaction that looks like allergy but is caused by deficiency of the enzyme lactase.

However, this classification is not universally accepted; the terms *food sensitivity, hypersensitivity, allergy,* and *intolerance* are often used interchangeably. The American Academy of Allergy, Asthma, and Immunology further suggests defining food-induced reactions according to the following: adverse food reactions, food hypersensitivity (allergy), food anaphylaxis, food intolerance, food idiosyncrasy, food toxicity or poisoning,

BOX 46-2 CLINICAL MANIFESTATIONS OF GASTROINTESTINAL DYSFUNCTION IN CHILDREN

Growth failure—Weight consistently below the third percentile, body mass index below the fifth percentile, or a decrease from established growth pattern

Spitting up or regurgitation—Passive transfer of gastric contents into the esophagus or mouth

Vomiting—Forceful ejection of gastric contents; involves a complex process under central nervous system control that causes salivation, pallor, sweating, and tachycardia; usually accompanied by nausea

Projectile vomiting—Vomiting accompanied by vigorous peristaltic waves and typically associated with pyloric stenosis or pylorospasm

Nausea—Unpleasant sensation vaguely referred to the throat or abdomen with an inclination to vomit

Constipation—Delay or difficulty with the passage of stools that is present for 2 weeks or longer; associated with symptoms that may include blood-streaked stools and abdominal discomfort

Encopresis—Involuntary overflow of incontinent stool causing soiling or incontinence secondary to fecal retention or impaction

Diarrhea—Increase in the number of stools with increased water content as a result of alterations of water and electrolyte transport by the gastrointestinal (GI) tract; may be acute or chronic

Hypoactive, hyperactive, or absent bowel sounds—Evidence of intestinal motility problems that may be caused by inflammation or obstruction

Abdominal distension—Protuberant contour of the abdomen that may be caused by delayed gastric emptying, accumulation of gas or stool, inflammation, or obstruction

Abdominal pain—Pain associated with the abdomen that may be localized or diffuse, acute or chronic; often caused by inflammation, obstruction, or hemorrhage

Gastrointestinal bleeding—May be from an upper or lower GI source and may be acute or chronic

- *Hematemesis*—Vomiting of bright red or denatured blood that results from bleeding in the upper GI tract or from swallowed blood from the nose or oropharynx
- *Hematochezia*—Passage of bright red blood per rectum, usually indicating lower GI tract bleeding
- *Melena*—Passage of dark-coloured, "tarry" stools resulting from denatured blood, suggesting upper GI tract bleeding or bleeding from the right colon

Jaundice—Yellow colouration of the skin and sclerae associated with liver dysfunction in infants and in children over 4 weeks of age

Dysphagia—Difficulty swallowing caused by abnormalities in the neuromuscular function of the pharynx or upper esophageal sphincter or by disorders of the esophagus

Dysfunctional swallowing—Impaired swallowing caused by central nervous system defects or structural defects of the oral cavity, pharynx, or esophagus; can cause feeding problems or aspiration

Fever—Common manifestation of illness in children with GI disorders; usually associated with dehydration, infection, or inflammation

anaphylactoid reaction to food, pharmacological food reaction, and metabolic food reaction (Health Canada, 2012b).

In Canada, 5 to 6% of young children are estimated to have food allergies (Health Canada, 2012b). The clinical manifestations of food hypersensitivity may be divided as follows (Health Canada, 2015):

Systemic—Anaphylactic, growth failure
Gastrointestinal—Abdominal pain, vomiting, cramping, diarrhea
Respiratory—Cough, wheezing, rhinitis, infiltrates
Cutaneous—Urticaria, rash, atopic dermatitis

Food hypersensitivities usually occur either as an IgE-mediated or non–IgE-mediated immune response; some toxic reactions may occur as a result of a toxin found within the food (Health Canada, 2012b). Food allergy is caused by exposure to allergens, usually proteins (but not the smaller amino acids) that are capable of inducing IgE antibody formation (sensitization) when ingested. *Sensitization* refers to the initial exposure of an individual to an allergen, resulting in an immune response; subsequent exposure induces a much stronger response that is clinically apparent. Consequently, food hypersensitivity typically occurs after the food has been ingested one or more times. The American National Institute of Allergies and Infectious Disease states that sensitization alone is not sufficient to classify as a food allergy but it is an immune-mediated response and manifestation of specific signs and symptoms that are necessary to categorize an individual as having a food allergy (Boyce et al., 2011). The most common food allergens are listed in Box 46-3.

Cross-reactivity occurs when the proteins in one substance are similar to the proteins in another, therefore the immune system sees them as the same. With food allergies, cross-reactivity can occur between one food and another, pollen and foods, or latex and foods. There is a high degree of cross-reactivity between cow's milk and the milk from other mammals, such as goat and sheep. Cross-reactivity is rare between foods in the same animal group; for example, those individuals with a cow's milk allergy can usually eat beef. It is fairly common to be allergic to tree nuts if a child has a peanut allergy. There is a high degree of cross-reactivity among the crustacean shellfish and the risk of allergy to another crustacean shellfish. The risk may be lower for cross-reactivity between crustacean shellfish and non-crustacean shellfish (mollusks). Some people with pollen allergies (allergic rhinitis or hay fever) can develop symptoms related to the mouth and throat after eating cross-reactive raw fresh fruits, vegetables, nuts, or seeds. Allergies to latex can result in symptoms with any or several fruits cross-reactive to latex, including banana, avocado, kiwi, and chestnut. Shellfish, peanuts, and tree nuts are commonly associated with severe, potentially life-threatening reactions (Mankad, 2013).

Food allergies can occur at any time but are common during infancy because the immature intestinal tract is more permeable to proteins than the mature intestinal tract, thus increasing the likelihood of an immune response. Allergies in general demonstrate a genetic component: children who have one parent with an allergy have a 50% or greater risk of developing an allergy. Children who have two parents with an allergy have up to a 100% risk of developing an allergy. Allergies with a hereditary tendency are referred to as *atopy*. Some infants with atopy can be identified at birth from elevated levels of IgE in cord blood. Breastfeeding has been shown to decrease the risk for developing atopy.

Deaths have been reported in children who suffered an anaphylactic reaction to food, as onset of the reaction occurs shortly after ingestion (5 to 30 minutes). In most of the children the reactions did not begin with skin signs, such as hives, red rash, and flushing, but rather mimicked an acute asthma attack (wheezing, decreased air movement in airways, dyspnea). Children with food anaphylaxis should be watched closely, because a biphasic response has been recorded in a number of cases in which there is an immediate response, apparent recovery, and then acute recurrence of symptoms or symptoms may not appear for several hours after exposure (Canadian Society of Allergy and Clinical Immunology, 2014; Simmons, 2009). Parents, teachers, and day care workers should be educated about signs and symptoms of food hypersensitivity reactions. People with food sensitivity should avoid unfamiliar foods and avoid restaurants that do not disclose food ingredients. New labelling guidelines require that food additives such as spices

BOX 46-3 HYPERALLERGENIC FOODS AND FOOD SOURCES

Milk*—Ice cream, butter, margarine (if it contains dairy products), yogurt, cheese, pudding, baked goods, wieners, bologna, canned creamed soups, instant breakfast drinks, powdered milk drinks, milk chocolate
Eggs*—Mayonnaise, creamy salad dressing, baked goods, egg noodles, some cake icing, meringue, custard, pancakes, French toast, root beer
Wheat*—Almost all baked goods, wieners, bologna, pressed or chopped cold cuts, gravy, pasta, some canned soups
Legumes—Peanuts,* peanut butter or oil, beans, peas, lentils
Nuts*—Some chocolates, candy, baked goods, cherry beverages (may be flavoured with a nut extract), walnut oil
Fish or shellfish*—Cod liver oil, pizza with anchovies, Caesar salad dressing, any food fried in same oil as fish
Soy*—Soy sauce, teriyaki or Worcestershire sauce, tofu, baked goods using soy flour or oil, soy nuts, soy infant formulas or milk, soybean paste, tuna packed in vegetable oil, many margarines
Chocolate—Cola beverages, cocoa, chocolate-flavoured drinks
Buckwheat—Some cereals, pancakes
Pork, chicken—Bacon, wieners, sausage, pork fat, chicken broth
Strawberries, melon, pineapple—Gelatin, syrups
Corn—Popcorn, cereal, muffins, cornstarch, corn meal, corn bread, corn tortilla
Citrus fruits—Orange, lemon, lime, grapefruit; any of these in drinks, gelatin, juice, or medicines
Tomatoes—Juice, some vegetable soups, spaghetti, pizza sauce, ketchup
Spices—Chili, pepper, vinegar, cinnamon

*Most common allergens.

and flavouring be clearly labelled on commercially sold, store-bought foods. Hidden ingredients in prepared foods have been implicated as a potential source of food hypersensitivity. The Allergy/Asthma Information Association provides up-to-date Canadian information about food content and labelling, manufacturers' recalls because of food content or labelling errors, and "safe" substitutes for common allergenic foods (see Additional Resources at the end of this chapter).

Other symptoms of anaphylaxis to food allergens include wheezing, cough, dyspnea, **urticaria**, abdominal cramps, vomiting, diarrhea, a drop in systemic blood pressure or **shock**, and in small preverbal children, restlessness, urticaria, irritability, listlessness, and unresponsiveness. *Oral allergy syndrome* occurs when a food allergen is ingested (commonly fruits and vegetables) and there is subsequent **edema** and **pruritus** involving the lips, tongue, palate, and throat; recovery from symptoms is usually rapid. *Immediate GI hypersensitivity* is an IgE-mediated reaction to a food allergen; reactions include nausea, abdominal pain, cramping, diarrhea, vomiting, anaphylaxis, or all of these reactions. Additional food hypersensitivities seen in young children include allergic eosinophilic gastritis, allergic eosinophilic gastroenterocolitis, dietary protein enterocolitis (or milk protein intolerance), and dietary protein proctitis.

Although the reason is unknown, many children "outgrow" their food allergies, especially to milk and eggs. Approximately 50% of all infants who are intolerant to cow's milk usually develop tolerance by 3 to 5 years of age (Nowak-Wegrzyn, Sampson, & Sicherer, 2016). More than half (60%) of infants have an IgE-mediated reaction to cow's milk, and 25% retain sensitivity until the second decade of life. Children who are allergic to more than one food may develop tolerance to each food at a different time. The most common allergens, such as peanuts, are outgrown less readily than other food allergens. Because of the tendency to lose the hypersensitivity, allergenic foods should be reintroduced into the diet after a period of abstinence (usually ≥1 year) to evaluate whether the food can safely be added to the diet. However, foods that are associated with severe anaphylactic reactions continue to present a lifelong risk and must be avoided.

In a joint statement, the CPS and Canadian Society of Allergy and Clinical Immunology (CSACI) do not recommend avoiding milk, eggs, peanuts, or other foods while a mother is pregnant or breastfeeding. There is also no evidence to support the theory that avoiding certain foods during this time will prevent allergies in children (Chan, Cummings, & CPS, Community Paediatrics Committee, 2013/2016). Infants who are at high risk (defined as infants with a first-degree relative with an allergic condition) of developing a food allergy can be exposed to potential food allergens as early as 6 months of age. Delaying dietary exposure to potential allergens like peanuts, fish, or eggs will not reduce a child's risk of developing a food allergy. Once a new food is introduced, it is important to continue to offer it regularly to maintain a child's tolerance (Chan et al., 2013/2016). Parents should be advised to discuss infant feeding practices with the primary care practitioner and obtain adequate information to make an informed decision if there is a family history of atopy. The strategies listed in the Guidelines box are those recommended by most authorities for infants with a family history of atopy.

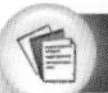

GUIDELINES

Preventing Atopy in Children

Identify Children at Risk

Family history of allergy
Increased immune globulin E (IgE) in cord blood and postnatal serum
Dry, flaky skin

Prenatal Precautions (Last Trimester)

Eat healthy; there are no known foods that should be avoided

Postnatal Precautions

Breast milk (preferred for 6 months or longer), or extensively hydrolyzed formula (Nutramigen or Alimentum) exclusively for at least 6 months
No solid food for first 6 months, and then do not delay introducing new food
One new allergy-producing food added every few days to identify possible reaction
Read commercial food product labels carefully for ingredients, preservatives

Environmental Control

Limited exposure to dust mites, moulds, furry animals, latex products, and second-hand cigarette smoke

Data from Health Link BC (2012).

EMERGENCY

Emergency Management of Anaphylaxis*

Drug—Epinephrine 0.001 mg/kg up to maximum of 0.3 mg
Dose—EpiPen Jr. (0.15 mg) intramuscularly (IM) for child weighing 10 to 25 kg; EpiPen (0.3 mg) IM for child weighing 25 kg or more
For children weighing less than 10 kg, care practitioners and families will need to judge the benefits and risks of administering epinephrine via syringes after being drawn up by a competent family member. The risks have proven to be an error in the dosage and delay in administration.
Observe for adverse reactions: tachycardia, hypertension, irritability, headaches, nausea, and tremors.

*Data from Cheng, A., & Canadian Paediatric Society, Acute Care Committee. (2011). Emergency treatment of anaphylaxis in infants and children. Reaffirmed 2016. Retrieved from http://www.cps.ca/documents/position/emergency-treatment-anaphylaxis#ref9

NURSING ALERT

The Canadian Paediatric Society (CPS) suggests that indications for the administration of intramuscular epinephrine in a child with a life-threatening anaphylactic reaction or one who is experiencing severe symptoms include any one of the following: itching sensation or tightness in throat, hoarseness, "barky" cough, difficulty swallowing, dyspnea, wheezing, cyanosis, respiratory or cardiac arrest, mild dysrhythmia or mild hypotension, severe bradycardia, hypotension, or loss of consciousness (Cheng & CPS, Acute Care Committee, 2011/2016).

Children with extremely sensitive food allergies should wear medical identification such as a Medic Alert bracelet and have an injectable epinephrine cartridge (EpiPen) readily available and know how to use it (see Emergency Box). It is also helpful

CRITICAL THINKING CASE STUDY

Food Allergy Anaphylaxis

A group of nursing students is holding a health promotion fair at a local elementary school for first, second, and third graders. The nursing students have several booths set up in the school cafeteria. Three second-grade boys are horseplaying in front of one of the booths when one of the boys, Jason, an 8-year-old child, suddenly starts coughing and clutching his throat. The students also observe that he is developing red splotches on his face, neck, and throat and that he is scratching. Jason says, "I can't breathe!" The school nurse is nearby and comes over to see what's causing the commotion. One of the boys with Jason says, "We didn't mean any harm; we were just goofing around when we put peanuts in his trail mix." One of the student nurses says, "He's in obvious distress. What should we do?"

1. Evidence—Is there sufficient evidence to draw any conclusions at this time about Jason's condition?
2. Assumptions—Describe some underlying assumptions about the following:
   a. Clinical manifestations of food allergy
   b. The emergency treatment of a food allergy "reaction," or anaphylaxis
   c. Which one of the following interventions would have highest immediate priority?
      (1) Call Jason's parents and ask them to come pick him up from school.
      (2) Call Jason's family practitioner to obtain orders for medication.
      (3) Promptly administer an intramuscular dose of epinephrine.
      (4) Call 911 and wait for the emergency response personnel to arrive.
3. What implication for nursing care exists in this situation after an intervention in the previous question has been chosen and implemented?
4. Describe the potential results of taking a "Let's observe Jason for a few minutes before we do anything" stance in this scenario.

for the child to have a copy of the individualized written treatment plan on hand for prompt diagnosis and treatment (see Critical Thinking Case Study).

Cow's Milk Allergy

Cow's milk allergy (CMA) is a multifaceted disorder representing adverse systemic and local GI reactions to cow's milk protein. The allergy may be manifested within the first 4 months of life through a variety of signs and symptoms that may appear within 45 minutes of milk ingestion or after a period of several days (Box 46-4). Approximately 2.5% of infants develop cow's milk hypersensitivity, with 60% of these being IgE mediated (Leung, Otley, & CPS, Nutrition and Gastroenterology Committee, 2009/2016). It is estimated that 50% of these children may outgrow the hypersensitivity by 3 to 4 years of age (Nowak-Wegrzyn et al., 2016). Some studies suggest that milk allergy may persist and some children may not be able to tolerate milk until they are 16 years of age (American Academy of Pediatrics [AAP], 2014). (The following discussion is centred on cow's milk protein found in commercial infant formulas; whole milk is not recommended for infants younger than the age of 12 months.)

The diagnosis may initially be made from the history, although the history alone is not diagnostic; the timing and

BOX 46-4 COMMON CLINICAL MANIFESTATIONS OF COW'S MILK SENSITIVITY

Gastrointestinal
Diarrhea
Vomiting
Colic
Abdominal pain

Respiratory
Rhinitis
Bronchitis
Asthma
Wheezing
Sneezing
Coughing
Chronic nasal discharge

Other Signs and Symptoms
Eczema
Excessive crying
Pallor (from anemia secondary to chronic blood loss in gastrointestinal tract)

diversity of clinical manifestations vary greatly. For example, CMA may be manifested as colic (see Chapter 35), diarrhea, vomiting, GI bleeding, gastroesophageal reflux (GER), chronic constipation, or sleeplessness in an otherwise healthy infant.

Diagnostic evaluation. A number of diagnostic tests may be performed, including stool analysis for blood (both frank and occult bleeding can occur from the colitis), serum IgE levels, skin-prick or scratch testing, and radioallergosorbent test (measures IgE antibodies to specific allergens in serum by radioimmunoassay). Both skin and radioallergosorbent testing help identify the offending food, but the results are not always conclusive.

The most definitive diagnostic strategy is elimination of milk in the diet, followed by challenge testing after improvement of symptoms. A clinical diagnosis is made when symptoms improve after removal of milk from the diet and two or more challenge tests produce symptoms (Kattan, Cocco, & Järvinen, 2011). If a mother is breastfeeding then she needs to eliminate cow's milk from her diet during the testing. Challenge testing involves reintroducing small quantities of milk in the diet to detect resurgence of symptoms; at times it involves the use of a placebo so that the parent is unaware of (or "blind" to) the timing of allergen ingestion. A double-blind, placebo-controlled food challenge is the gold standard for diagnosing food allergies such as CMA, yet it may not be used very often for diagnosing CMA because of the expense, time involved, and risk for further exposure and anaphylactic reaction (Kattan et al., 2011). Careful observation of the child is required during a challenge test because of the possibility of anaphylactic reaction.

Therapeutic management. Treatment of CMA is elimination of cow's milk–based formula and all other dairy products. For infants fed cow's milk formula, this primarily involves changing the formula to a casein hydrolysate milk formula or extensively hydrolyzed formula (Nutramigen or Alimentum), in which the protein has been broken down into its amino acids through enzymatic hydrolysis. Although the CPS recommends the use of hydrolyzed formulas for CMA (Leung et al., 2009/2016), many practitioners may start a soy formula instead. Approximately 50% of infants who are sensitive to cow's milk protein will also demonstrate a sensitivity to soy. Intolerance to soy is reported to be higher in infants under age 6 months with a family history of atopy and severe GI symptoms (Kattan et al., 2011).

Other choices for children who are intolerant to cow's milk–based formula are the amino acid–based formulas Neocate or EleCare, but their cost is a major consideration and they are not available in all provinces. Goat's milk is not an acceptable substitute because it cross-reacts with cow's milk protein, is deficient in folic acid, and is unsuitable as the only source of calories (Basnet, Schneider, Gazit, et al., 2010). Infants are maintained on the milk-free diet until after 1 year of age, after which time small quantities of milk can be reintroduced.

NURSING CARE

Nurses have an important role in identifying potential CMA and providing appropriate counselling of parents on the signs and symptoms of CMA and the use of substitute formulas appropriate for infants diagnosed with CMA. Parents need much reassurance regarding the needs of nonverbal infants with such an array of symptoms. Endless nights of lost sleep and a crying infant may promote feelings of parenting inadequacy and role conflict, thus aggravating the situation. Nurses can reassure parents that many of these symptoms are common and the reasons are often never found, yet the child does achieve appropriate growth and development.

The protein hydrolysate (partially hydrolyzed and extensively hydrolyzed) formulas tend to be less palatable than milk-based formulas, so the child may be reluctant to accept the new formula. This can be overcome by adding non-nutritive, hypoallergenic flavour packets or by introducing the formula gradually over a few days, using 30 mL new formula to 210 mL of old formula, then 60 mL to 180 mL, 90 mL to 150 mL, and as needed. Parents also need to be reassured that the infant will receive complete nutrition from the new formula and will suffer no ill effects from the absence of cow's milk. Protein hydrolysate formulas are also expensive; the nurse can play a role in advocating for families to government agencies to assist in paying for the formula.

Once solid foods are started, parents need guidance in avoiding milk products (see Box 46-3). The practice of carefully reading all food labels helps avoid exposure of the child to prepared foods containing milk products. Although labelled as nondairy, milk, cream, and butter substitutes may contain cow's milk protein (Kattan et al., 2011).

Lactose Intolerance

Lactose intolerance refers to at least four different entities that involve a deficiency of the enzyme *lactase*, which is needed for the hydrolysis or digestion of lactose in the small intestine; lactose is hydrolyzed into glucose and galactose. **Congenital** *lactase deficiency* occurs soon after birth, after the newborn has consumed lactose-containing milk (human milk or commercial formula). This inborn error of metabolism involves the complete absence or severely reduced presence of lactase and requires a lifelong lactose-free or extremely reduced lactose diet.

Primary lactase deficiency, sometimes referred to as *late-onset lactase deficiency*, is the most common type of lactose intolerance and occurs usually after 4 or 5 years of age, although the time of onset varies. Ethnic groups with a high incidence of lactase deficiency include Indigenous peoples, Asians, southern Europeans, Arabs, Israelis, and people of African descent; Scandinavians tend to have the lowest incidence. In Canada, researchers discovered during an Inuit health study in children under 6 years of age that 5% of Inuit children had lactose intolerance (Findlay & Janz, 2012). Lactose malabsorption manifests as lactose intolerance and is characterized by an imbalance between the ability for lactase to hydrolyze the ingested lactose and the amount of lactose ingested (Heyman & AAP Committee on Nutrition, 2006).

Secondary lactase deficiency may occur secondary to damage of the intestinal lumen, which decreases or destroys the enzyme lactase. Cystic fibrosis, sprue, celiac disease, kwashiorkor, or infections such as giardiasis, HIV, or rotavirus may cause temporary or permanent lactose intolerance.

Developmental lactase deficiency refers to the relative lactase deficiency observed in preterm infants of less than 34 weeks of gestation (Heyman & AAP Committee on Nutrition, 2006).

The primary symptoms of lactose intolerance include abdominal pain, bloating, flatulence, and diarrhea after the ingestion of lactose. The onset of symptoms occurs within 30 minutes to several hours of lactose consumption. Lactose intolerance is often perceived as an allergy; and in several studies with reports of acute GI symptoms ascribed to lactose intolerance, measurement of lactase activity is normal.

Lactose intolerance may be diagnosed on the basis of the history and improvement with a lactose-reduced diet. The breath hydrogen test is used to positively diagnose the condition. Breath samples in lactose-deficient individuals yield a higher percentage of hydrogen (20 ppm [parts per million] or more above baseline). In infants, lactose malabsorption may be diagnosed by evaluating fecal pH and reducing substances; fecal pH in infants is usually lower than in older children, but an acidic pH may indicate malabsorption (Heyman & AAP Committee on Nutrition, 2006).

Treatment of lactose intolerance is elimination of offending dairy products; however, some advocate decreasing amounts of dairy products rather than total elimination, especially in small children. In infants, lactose-free or low-lactose formula offers no special advantages over lactose-containing formula, except in the severely malnourished (Heyman & AAP Committee on Nutrition, 2006).

One concern is that dairy avoidance in children and adolescents with lactose intolerance contributes to reduced bone mineral density and osteoporosis (AAP, 2014). There is evidence that dietary lactose enhances calcium absorption and that lactose-free diets may negatively affect bone mineralization (Heyman & American Academy of Pediatrics Committee on Nutrition, 2006). It has been suggested that individuals with lactose maldigestion who do not experience lactose intolerance symptoms continue to consume small amounts of dairy products with meals to prevent reduced bone mass density and subsequent osteoporosis (AAP, 2014). There is some evidence that *probiotics* (food preparations containing microorganisms such as *Lactobacillus*, which alter the GI microflora and thus are beneficial to the host) improve lactose intolerance when live cultures are fermented in dairy products (de Vrese & Schrezenmeir, 2008). The positive attributes of probiotics for those with lactose maldigestion include delayed GI transit (slower than milk), positive effects on intestinal and colonic microflora, and a reduction of maldigestion symptoms.

Most people are able to tolerate small amounts of lactose (equal to 250 mL per day) even in the presence of deficient lactase activity and should be encouraged to continue their intake of dairy products in small amounts to obtain much-needed nutrients (Heyman & AAP Committee on Nutrition, 2006). Milk taken at meals may be better tolerated than when taken alone (see Family-Centred Teaching box). Pretreated milk (with microbial-derived lactase) is reported to be effective in improving lactose absorption. Because dairy products are a major source of calcium and vitamin D, supplementation of these nutrients is needed to prevent deficiency. Yogurt contains inactive lactase enzyme, which is activated by the temperature and pH of the duodenum; this lactase activity substitutes for the lack of endogenous lactase. Fresh, plain yogurt may be tolerated better than frozen or flavoured yogurt. Hard cheeses, lactase-treated dairy products, and lactase tablets taken with dairy products are also viable options. An important distinction between lactose intolerance and food hypersensitivity is that lactose intolerance does not manifest as an anaphylactic-type reaction.

FAMILY-CENTRED TEACHING

Controlling Symptoms of Lactose Intolerance

- In infants, substitute lactose-free or soy-based formula for cow's milk formula or human milk (only after a diagnosis of congenital lactase deficiency or secondary lactase intolerance is made).
- Limit milk consumption to one or two glasses per day.
- Drink milk with other foods rather than alone.
- Eat hard cheese, cottage cheese, or yogurt instead of drinking milk.
- Use enzyme tablets such as Lactaid or Lactrase to metabolize the lactose in milk or supplement the body's own lactose (add tablets to milk or sprinkle on dairy products such as ice cream).
- Eat small amounts of dairy foods daily to help colonic bacteria adapt to ingested lactose.
- Include a probiotic (yogurt or cultured [fermented] milk) in a meal or as a snack that has *Lactobacillus* or *Bifidobacterium* organisms.
- Take a calcium supplement if unable to consume any dairy products such as cheese.

NURSING CARE

Nursing care is similar to the interventions discussed for CMA: explaining the dietary restrictions to the family; identifying alternative sources of calcium, such as yogurt and calcium supplementation; explaining the importance of supplementation; and discussing sources of lactose, especially hidden sources, such as its use as a bulk agent in certain medications, and ways of controlling the symptoms (see Family-Centred Teaching box). Parents should be advised to check with the pharmacist regarding potential lactose bulking agents when obtaining medication.

Dehydration

Dehydration is a common body fluid disturbance in infants and children and occurs whenever the total output of fluid exceeds the total intake, regardless of the cause. Dehydration may result from a number of diseases that cause insensible losses through the skin and respiratory tract, through increased renal excretion, and through the GI tract. Although dehydration can result from lack of oral intake (especially in elevated environmental temperatures), more often it is a result of abnormal losses, such as those that occur in vomiting or diarrhea, when oral intake only partially compensates for the abnormal losses. Other significant causes of dehydration are diabetic ketoacidosis and extensive burns. Conditions in which dehydration may develop quickly include diarrhea, vomiting, sweating, fever, and disorders such as diabetes ketoacidosis, renal disease, and cardiac anomalies; administration of certain medications (such as diuretics and steroids); and trauma (major surgery, burns, and other extensive injury). In addition, any condition that causes a decrease in oral intake, such as herpangina, hand-foot-and-mouth disease, or thrush, has the potential to cause dehydration in infants and small children.

Types of Dehydration

The pathophysiology of dehydration is understood by recognizing that the distribution of water between the extracellular fluid (ECF) and intracellular fluid (ICF) spaces depends on active transport of potassium into and sodium out of cells by energy-requiring processes. Sodium is the chief solute in ECF and the primary determinant of ECF volume. It is considered a unique electrolyte in that water balance determines sodium concentration; when water is lost and sodium concentration becomes elevated, compensatory mechanisms in the kidney stop antidiuretic hormone (ADH) secretion so water is retained. The thirst mechanism (not fully functioning in infants) is also stimulated so water is replaced, thus increasing the total body water content and returning sodium to a normal level (Greenbaum, 2016). Potassium is primarily intracellular. When ECF volume is reduced in acute dehydration, the total body sodium content is almost always reduced as well, regardless of serum sodium measurements. Replacement of fluid volume should therefore be accompanied by sodium replacement as well. Sodium depletion in diarrhea occurs in two ways: out of the body in stool, and into the ICF compartment to replace potassium to maintain electrical equilibrium.

Dehydration is classified into three categories on the basis of osmolality and depends primarily on the serum sodium concentration: (1) isotonic, (2) hypotonic, and (3) hypertonic.

Isotonic (*isosmotic* or **isonatremic**) **dehydration**, the primary form of dehydration in children, occurs in conditions in which electrolyte and water deficits are present in approximately balanced proportions. Water and sodium are lost in approximately equal amounts. The observable fluid losses are not necessarily isotonic, since losses from other avenues make adjustments so that the sum of all losses, or the net loss, is isotonic. There is no osmotic force between the ICF and the ECF; thus the major loss is sustained from the ECF compartment. This significantly reduces the plasma volume and the circulating blood volume, which affects the skin, muscles, and kidneys. Shock is the greatest threat to life, and the child with isotonic dehydration displays symptoms characteristic of hypovolemic shock. Plasma sodium remains within normal limits, between 130 and 150 mmol/L.

Hypotonic (*hyposmotic* or **hyponatremic**) **dehydration** occurs when the electrolyte deficit exceeds the water deficit, leaving the serum hypotonic. Because ICF is more concentrated than ECF in hypotonic dehydration, water moves from the ECF to the ICF to establish osmotic equilibrium. This movement further increases the ECF volume loss, and shock is a frequent finding. Because there is a greater proportional loss of ECF in hypotonic dehydration, the physical signs tend to be more severe with smaller fluid losses than with isotonic or hypertonic dehydration. Serum sodium concentration is less than 130 mmol/L.

Hypertonic (*hyperosmotic* or **hypernatremic**) **dehydration** results from water loss in excess of electrolyte loss and is usually caused by a proportionately larger loss of water or a larger intake of electrolytes. This type of dehydration is the most dangerous and requires more specific fluid therapy. Hypertonic diarrhea may occur in infants who are given fluids by mouth that contain large amounts of solute or in children who receive high-protein nasogastric (NG) tube feedings that place an excessive solute load on the kidneys. In hypertonic dehydration, fluid shifts from the lesser concentration of the ICF to the ECF. Plasma sodium concentration is greater than 150 mmol/L.

Because the ECF volume is proportionately larger, hypertonic dehydration consists of a greater degree of water loss for the same intensity of physical signs. Shock is less apparent. However, neurological disturbances, including alterations in consciousness, poor ability to focus attention, lethargy, increased muscle tone with hyperreflexia, and hyperirritability to stimuli, are more likely to occur. Central nervous system (CNS) changes are serious and may result in permanent damage.

Diagnostic Evaluation of Degree of Dehydration

Diagnosis of the type and degree of dehydration is necessary to develop an effective plan of therapy. The degree of dehydration has been described as a percentage of body weight dehydrated: mild—less than 3% in older children or less than 5% in infants; moderate—5 to 10% in infants and 3 to 6% in older children; and severe—more than 10% in infants and more than 6% in older children (Greenbaum, 2016; Leung, Prince, & CPS, Nutrition and Gastroenterology Committee, 2006/2016). Water constitutes only 60 to 70% of the infant's weight. However, adipose tissue contains little water and is highly variable in individual infants and children. A more accurate means of describing dehydration is to reflect acute loss (over a period of 48 hours or less) in millilitres per kilogram of body weight. For example, a loss of 50 mL/kg is considered to be a mild fluid loss, whereas a loss of 100 mL/kg produces severe dehydration. Weight is the most important determinant of the percent of total body fluid loss in infants and younger children. However, often the preillness weight is unknown. Other predictors of fluid loss include a changing level of consciousness (irritability to lethargy), altered to response to stimuli, decreased skin elasticity and turgor, prolonged capillary refill (longer than 2 seconds), increased heart rate, and sunken eyes and fontanels. There is evidence that the clinical manifestations of abnormal capillary refill, skin turgor, and respiratory pattern are the most useful in predicting dehydration of 5% or more in children (Colletti, Brown, Sharieff, et al., 2010; Emond, 2009).

Clinical signs provide clues to the extent of dehydration (Table 46-3). Using multiple predictors increases the sensitivity of assessing the fluid deficit, and early studies have shown a reasonably high degree of agreement between experienced observers in assessment of the level of dehydration. The earliest detectable sign is tachycardia, followed by dry skin and mucous membranes, sunken fontanels, signs of circulatory failure (coolness, mottling of extremities), loss of skin elasticity, and prolonged capillary filling time. Objective signs of dehydration are present at a fluid deficit of less than 5%. Any two of the following signs—capillary refill greater than 2 seconds, abnormal skin turgor, and abnormal respiratory pattern—are predictors of a deficit of at least 5%. Generally, three or more clinical findings are present at a deficit of 5 to 9%, and four or more findings are found with a deficit of 10% or more. See Table 46-4 for clinical manifestations of dehydration. Shock, tachycardia, and very low blood pressure are common features of severe depletion of ECF volume (see Shock, Chapter 47).

Compensatory mechanisms try to maintain fluid equilibrium by adjusting to the losses. Interstitial fluid moves into the vascular compartment to maintain the blood volume in response to hemoconcentration and hypovolemia, and vasoconstriction of peripheral arterioles helps to maintain pumping pressure. When fluid losses exceed the ability of the body to sustain blood volume and blood pressure, circulation is seriously compromised and the blood pressure falls. This results in tissue hypoxia with accumulation of lactic acid, pyruvate, and other acid metabolites, which contribute to development of metabolic acidosis.

Renal compensation is impaired by decreased blood flow through the kidneys and little urine is formed. Increased serum osmolality simulates ADH to conserve fluid and initiates the renin-angiotensin mechanisms in the kidneys, leading to further vasoconstriction. Aldosterone is released to promote sodium retention and conserve water in the kidneys. If dehydration increases in severity, urine formation is greatly diminished and

TABLE 46-3 EVALUATING THE EXTENT OF DEHYDRATION

	LEVEL OF DEHYDRATION		
CLINICAL SIGNS	**MILD**	**MODERATE**	**SEVERE**
Weight loss—infants	3–5%	6–9%	≥10%
Weight loss—children	3–4%	6–8%	10%
Pulse	Normal	Slightly increased	Very increased
Respiratory rate	Normal	Slight tachypnea (rapid)	Hyperpnea (deep and rapid)
Blood pressure	Normal	Normal to orthostatic (more than 10 mm Hg change)	Orthostatic to shock
Behaviour	Normal	Irritable, more thirsty	Hyperirritable to lethargic
Thirst	Slight	Moderate	Intense
Mucous membranes*	Normal	Dry	Parched
Tears	Present	Decreased	Absent, sunken eyes
Anterior fontanel	Normal	Normal to sunken	Sunken
External jugular vein	Visible when supine	Not visible except with supraclavicular pressure	Not visible even with supraclavicular pressure
Skin*	Capillary refill less than 2 sec	Slowed capillary refill (2–4 sec [decreased turgor])	Very delayed capillary refill (more than 4 sec) and tenting; skin cool, acrocyanotic or mottled
Urine specific gravity	> 1.020	> 1.020; oliguria	Oliguria or anuria

*These signs are less prominent in patients who have hypernatremia.
Data from Jospe, N., & Forbes, G. (1996). Fluids and electrolytes—clinical aspects. *Pediatrics in Review, 17*(11), 395–403; and Steiner, M. J., DeWalt, D. A., & Byerley, J. S. (2004). Is this child dehydrated? *Journal of the American Medical Association, 291*(22), 2746–2754.

TABLE 46-4 CLINICAL MANIFESTATIONS OF DEHYDRATION

MANIFESTATION	ISOTONIC (LOSS OF WATER AND SODIUM)	HYPOTONIC (LOSS OF SODIUM IN EXCESS OF WATER)	HYPERTONIC (LOSS OF WATER IN EXCESS OF SODIUM)
Skin			
Colour	Grey	Grey	Grey
Temperature	Cold	Cold	Cold or hot
Turgor	Poor	Very Poor	Fair
Feel	Dry	Clammy	Thickened, doughy
Mucous membranes	Dry	Slightly moist	Parched
Tearing and salivation	Absent	Absent	Absent
Eyeball	Sunken	Sunken	Sunken
Fontanel	Sunken	Sunken	Sunken
Body temperature	Subnormal or elevated	Subnormal or elevated	Subnormal or elevated
Pulse	Rapid	Very rapid	Moderately rapid
Respirations	Rapid	Rapid	Rapid
Behaviour	Irritable to lethargic	Lethargic or comatose; seizures	Marked lethargy with extreme hyperirritability on stimulation

metabolites and hydrogen ions that are normally excreted by this route are retained.

Shock, caused by severe depletion of ECF volume, is preceded by tachycardia and signs of poor perfusion and tissue oxygenation (by pulse oximeter readings). Peripheral circulation is poor as a result of reduced blood volume; therefore, the skin is cool and mottled, with decreased capillary filling after blanching. Impaired kidney circulation often results in oliguria and azotemia. Low blood pressure in an infant and young child is usually a late sign of shock and could be signalling a cardiovascular collapse (see Shock, Chapter 47).

Therapeutic Management

See discussion on therapeutic management of diarrhea, p. 1418.

NURSING CARE

Whether the child is at home, in the practitioner's office or clinic, or in the hospital, nursing assessment is an essential part of the nursing care plan. The assessment of suspected or potential fluid and electrolyte disturbance begins with the observation of general appearance. Ill children usually have drawn expressions, have dry mucous membranes and lips, and "look sick." Loss of appetite is one of the first behaviours observed in most childhood illnesses, and the infant's or child's activity level is diminished from baseline or usual activities. The cry of an ill infant is less vigorous, often whining, and higher pitched than usual. The child is irritable, seeks the parent's comfort and attention, and displays purposeless movements and inappropriate responses to people and familiar objects. In some cases he or she may not protest advances by the health care worker and procedures such as taking vital signs or starting an intravenous (IV) infusion. These are signs that the child truly feels bad and that the condition is serious and immediate intervention is necessary. As the child's illness and level of dehydration become more severe, irritability progresses to lethargy and even unconsciousness.

Nursing observation and intervention are essential for detection and therapeutic management of dehydration. A variety of circumstances cause fluid losses in infants, and changes can take place quickly. An important nursing responsibility is observation for signs of dehydration. Nursing assessment should begin with observation of general appearance and proceed to more specific observations. It is important for the nurse to start isolating the symptomatic child with contact precautions to prevent the spread of infection.

Capillary filling time is assessed by pinching the abdominal skin, chest, arm, or leg and estimating the time it takes for the blood to return. Capillary filling time in mild dehydration is less than 2 seconds, increasing to more than 4 seconds in severe dehydration. The technique is effective for assessing dehydration in children of all ages. However, it can be altered in the presence of heart failure, which affects circulation time, and hypertonic dehydration, in which fluid loss is primarily intracellular. Additional clinical signs observed in children with dehydration include cool mottled extremities, sunken eyes, tachypnea, and changes in sensorium.

When caring for the ill child, the vital signs are assessed as often as every 15 to 30 minutes and fluid intake and output and body weight recorded frequently during the initial phase of therapy. Routine weights should be obtained at the same time each day. It is important to use the same scale each time the child is weighed and predetermine the weight of any equipment or devices that must remain attached during the weighing process, including elbow restraints, and any clothing the child might be wearing. Routine weights should be obtained at the same time each day using the same scales.

Accurate measurements of fluid intake and output are vital to the assessment of dehydration. This includes oral and parenteral intake and losses from urine, stools, vomiting, fistulas, NG losses, sweat, and wound drainage:

Urine—Frequency, colour, consistency, and volume (when weighing diapers, approximately 1 g wet diaper weight equals 1 mL urine)
Stools—Frequency, volume, and consistency
Vomitus—Volume, frequency, and type
Sweating—Can be only estimated from frequency of clothing and linen changes

In addition to fluid intake and output, the following observations assist in assessment of dehydration:

Vital signs—Temperature (normal, elevated, or lowered depending on degree of dehydration), pulse (tachycardia), respirations (hyperpnea), and blood pressure (hypotension)
Skin—Colour, temperature, turgor, presence or absence of edema, and capillary refill
Mucous membranes—Moisture, colour, and presence and consistency of secretions
Body weight—Decreased in relation to degree of dehydration
Fontanel (infants)—Sunken, soft, or normal
Sensory alterations—Presence of thirst

It is important to measure and record all intake, oral and parenteral, and output from all sources, including urine, stool, emesis, drainage tubes, fistulas, and wounds from which appreciable amounts of fluid are lost. Parents should be advised to observe the number of times and how much the child voids. A newborn may be expected to void at least once in the first 24 hours, two times in the second 24 hours of life, three or four times in the third and fourth days of life, and a minimum of six times by the fifth day of age. Infants younger than 1 year of age may void every 1 to 2 hours; toddlers urinate approximately every 3 hours. As children get older they void less frequently. Parents should be instructed to notify the nurse or clinician if the child appears to be voiding an insufficient amount or persistently losing fluid through vomiting or diarrhea.

DISORDERS OF MOTILITY

Diarrhea

Diarrhea is a symptom that results from disorders involving digestive, absorptive, and secretory functions. It is caused by abnormal intestinal water and electrolyte transport. Worldwide, there are an estimated 1.5 to 2.5 million deaths per year from diarrhea (Leung et al., 2006/2016). Most children living in developing countries who experience diarrhea have mild forms. However, in the United States, approximately 220,000 children younger than age 5 are hospitalized, and approximately 200 children die of diarrhea and dehydration each year, with comparable rates in Canada (Leung et al., 2006/2016). In Indigenous populations, prolonged diarrhea and malnutrition are primary causes of morbidity and mortality (Leung et al., 2006/2016).

Diarrheal disturbances involve the stomach and intestines (gastroenteritis), the small intestine (enteritis), the colon (colitis), or the colon and intestines (enterocolitis). Diarrhea is classified as acute or chronic.

Acute diarrhea, a leading cause of illness in children younger than 5 years of age, is defined as a sudden increase in frequency and a change in consistency of stools, often caused by an infectious agent in the GI tract. It may be associated with upper respiratory or urinary tract infections, antibiotic therapy, or laxative use. Acute diarrhea is usually self-limiting (less than 14 days' duration) and subsides without specific treatment if dehydration does not occur. *Acute infectious diarrhea (infectious gastroenteritis)* is caused by a variety of viral, bacterial, and parasitic pathogens (Table 46-5).

Chronic diarrhea is defined as an increase in stool frequency and increased water content for a duration of more than 14 days. It is often caused by chronic conditions such as malabsorption syndromes, inflammatory bowel disease (IBD), immunodeficiency, food allergy, lactose intolerance, or chronic nonspecific diarrhea, or it can be the result of inadequate management of acute diarrhea.

Intractable diarrhea of infancy is a syndrome that occurs in the first few months of life, persists for longer than 2 weeks with

TABLE 46-5 INFECTIOUS CAUSES OF ACUTE DIARRHEA

ORGANISM	PATHOLOGY	CHARACTERISTICS	COMMENTS
Viral Agents			
Rotavirus			
Incubation: 48 hr Diagnosis: enzyme immunoassay (EIA) and latex agglutination assay	Fecal–oral transmission Seven groups (A–G): Most group A virus replicates in mature villus epithelial cells of small intestine; leads to (1) imbalance in ratio of intestinal fluid absorption to secretion and (2) malabsorption of complex carbohydrates	Mild to moderate fever Vomiting followed by the onset of watery stools Fever and vomiting generally abate in approximately 2 days, but diarrhea persists 5–7 days Adult contacts in household may develop symptomatic infection	Most common cause of diarrhea in children <5 yr of age Infants 6–12 mo most vulnerable Peak occurrences in winter months; important cause of health care–associated infections Affects all ages; usually milder in children >3 yr of age; immune-compromised children at greater risk for complications Virus can live on toys and hard surfaces (sinks, countertops) Vaccine available for infants
Noroviruses (Formerly Norwalk-like) Caliciviruses			
Incubation: 12–48 hr Diagnosis: EIA, reverse-transcriptase polymerase chain reaction (RT-PCR)	Fecal–oral; contaminated food or water Pathology similar to rotavirus Affects villus epithelial cells of small intestine Leads to (1) imbalance in ratio of intestinal fluid absorption to secretion and (2) malabsorption of complex carbohydrates	Abdominal cramps; nausea, vomiting, malaise, low-grade fever, watery diarrhea without blood; duration brief, 2–3 days; tends to resemble food poisoning symptoms with nausea predominating	Affects all ages Multiple strains often named for the location of outbreak (e.g., Norwalk, Sapporo, Snow Mountain, Montgomery) Common in closed populations, such as day care and cruise ships
Bacterial Agents			
Escherichia coli			
Incubation: 3–4 days Variable depending on strain Diagnosis: sorbitol MacConkey agar (SMAC agar) for blood but fecal leukocytes are absent or rare	Five *E. coli* strains produce diarrhea as a result of enterotoxin production, adherence, or invasion; these strains include enterotoxigenic-producing [ETEC], enteroaggregative [EAEC], Shiga toxin–producing [STEC], enteropathogenic [EPEC], and enteroinvasive [EIEC] *E. coli*	Watery diarrhea 1–2 days; then severe abdominal cramping and bloody diarrhea STEC can progress to hemolytic uremic syndrome (HUS) and postdiarrheal thrombotic thrombocytopenia (TTP); 50% require dialysis and 3–5% die	Food-borne pathogen Traveller's diarrhea Highest incidence in summer Cause of nursery epidemics Symptomatic treatment Antibiotics may worsen course, but meta-analysis shows no harm or benefit from antibiotic therapy (AAP Committee on Infectious Diseases, Kimberlin et al., 2015) Antimotility agents and opioids should be avoided
Salmonella Groups (Nontyphoidal; Gram-Negative Rods, Nonencapsulated, Nonsporulating)			
Incubation 6–72 hr Diagnosis: Gram-stained stool culture	Invasion of mucosa in the small and large intestine; edema of the lamina propria; focal acute inflammation with disruption of the mucosa and microabscesses	Nausea, vomiting, colicky abdominal pain, bloody diarrhea, fever; symptoms variable: mild to severe May have headache, cerebral manifestations (e.g., drowsiness, confusion, meningismus, seizures) Infants may be afebrile and nontoxic May result in life-threatening septicemia and meningitis Nausea and vomiting typically of short duration; diarrhea may persist as long as 2–3 wk Typically shed virus for average of 5 wk; cases reported up to 1 yr	Incidence highest in warm months: July to November Food-borne outbreaks common Usually transmitted person to person but may be transmitted via undercooked meats or poultry Poultry and poultry products cause about half the cases In children: coming into contact with animals (e.g., snakes and turtles) that are contaminated Antibiotics not recommended in uncomplicated cases Antimotility agents also not recommended—prolong transit time and carrier state Incidence decreasing over past 10 yr

TABLE 46-5 INFECTIOUS CAUSES OF ACUTE DIARRHEA—cont'd

ORGANISM	PATHOLOGY	CHARACTERISTICS	COMMENTS
Salmonella typhi			
Produces enteric fever—systemic syndrome Incubation usually 7–14 days but could be 3–30 days, depending on size of inoculum Diagnosis: positive blood cultures; also sometimes positive stool and urine Late stage: positive bone marrow culture	Bloodstream invasion; after ingestion, organism attaches to microvilli of ileal brush borders, and bacteria invade the intestinal epithelium via Peyer's patches; organism is then transported to intestinal lymph nodes and enters bloodstream via thoracic ducts, and circulating organisms reach reticuloendothelial cells, causing bacteremia	Manifestations depend on age Abdominal pain; diarrhea; nausea, vomiting, high fever, lethargy Must be treated with antibiotics	Incidence is much lower in developed countries Ingestion of food, water, or both contaminated with human feces is most common mode of transmission Congenital and intrapartum transmission can occur Three vaccines are available
Shigella Species			
Gram-negative organisms Nonmotile Anaerobic bacilli Incubation: 1–7 days Diagnosis: stool culture Loaded with polymorphonuclear leukocytes	Enterotoxins: invade the epithelium with superficial mucosal ulcerations	Patients appear sick Symptoms begin with fever, fatigue, anorexia Crampy abdominal pain precedes watery or bloody diarrhea Symptoms usually subside in 5–10 days	Most cases in children younger than 9 yr with about one third of cases in children ages 1–4 wk Antibiotics shorten illness and lower mortality risk All patients are at risk for dehydration Acute symptoms may persist for 1 wk or more Antidiarrheal medications not recommended; may predispose to toxic megacolon
Yersinia enterocolitica			
Incubation period: dose dependent, 1–3 wk Diagnosis: stool culture serology; enzyme-linked immunosorbent assay (ELISA) Patients have leukocytosis; elevated sedimentation rate	Pathology is poorly understood; may be production of enterotoxin	Mucoid diarrhea, sometimes bloody; abdominal pain suggestive of appendicitis; fever, vomiting	Seen more frequently in winter months Transmitted by pets and food Antibiotics usually do not alter the clinical course in uncomplicated cases; they should be used in complicated infections and compromised hosts
Campylobacter jejuni and Campylobacter coli			
Microaerophilic, motile, Gram-negative bacilli Incubation period: 1–7 days Ability to cause illness appears dose related Diagnosis by stool culture, sometimes in the blood Commonly found in gastrointestinal (GI) tract of wild or domestic animals	Not fully understood; possibly (1) adherence to intestinal mucosa by toxin; (2) invasion of the mucosa in the terminal ileum and colon; (3) translocation, in which organisms penetrate the mucosa and replicate in lamina propria	Fever, abdominal pain, diarrhea, can be bloody; vomiting Watery, profuse, foul-smelling diarrhea Clinically similar to *Salmonella* or *Shigella* Fecal–oral transmission	Most infections in humans relate to consumption of contaminated foods or water; undercooked meats, particularly chicken; unpasteurized milk Also acquired from contaminated household pets (e.g., dogs, cats, hamsters) Bimodal peaks in infants <1 yr and again at ages 15–29 mo Antibiotics do not prolong the carriage of bacteria and may eliminate organism more quickly Erythromycin and azithromycin are medications of choice (5–7 days) Antimotility agents not recommended and tend to prolong symptoms
Vibrio cholerae			
Gram-negative, motile, curved bacillus living in bodies of salt water Incubation period: 1–3 days Diagnosis by stool culture	Enters via oral route in contaminated food or water; if survives acid stomach environment, travels to the small intestine, adheres to mucosa, and produces toxin	Onset abrupt; vomiting, watery diarrhea without cramping or tenesmus Dehydration can occur quickly	More prevalent in developing countries Rehydration most important treatment Antibiotics can shorten diarrhea Still no vaccine

Continued

TABLE 46-5 INFECTIOUS CAUSES OF ACUTE DIARRHEA—cont'd

ORGANISM	PATHOLOGY	CHARACTERISTICS	COMMENTS
Clostridium difficile			
Gram-positive anaerobic bacillus Diagnosis by detecting *C. difficile* toxin in stool culture	Produces two important toxins (A and B) Toxin binds to enterocyte surface receptor, resulting in alteration of permeability, protein synthesis, and direct cytotoxicity	Most cases: mild, watery diarrhea lasting few days; abdominal cramping Some cases: prolonged diarrhea and illness May cause pseudomembranous colitis Some individuals are extremely ill with high fever, leukocytosis, hypoalbuminemia	Associated with alteration of normal intestinal flora by antibiotics More common in hospitalized persons Adults tend to have more severe symptoms than children Treatment with antibiotics in symptomatic patients—metronidazole Resistant strains have developed Relapse common
Clostridium perfringens			
Incubation period: 8–24 hr; anaerobic, Gram-positive, spore-producing bacilli	Toxins produced in the intestine after ingestion of organism	Acute onset: watery diarrhea, crampy abdominal pain Fever, nausea, and vomiting rare Duration of illness usually 24 hr	Transmitted by contaminated food products, most often meats and poultry Usually self-limiting and medical intervention not needed Oral rehydration usually sufficient Antibiotics serve no purpose and should not be used
Clostridium botulinum			
Incubation period: 12–26 hr (range, 6 hr to 8 days) Gram-positive, anaerobic, spore-producing bacilli Blood and stool culture should be obtained and transmitted to special laboratory (usually provincial department) to detect toxin	Botulism caused by binding of toxin to the neuromuscular junction	Clinical presentation related to age and the strain of the botulism Abdominal pain, cramping, and diarrhea Usually infants present with constipation Other strains: respiratory compromise, central nervous system symptoms	Transmitted in contaminated food products Can be acquired via wound infection Treatment involves supportive care and neutralization of the toxin
Staphylococcus (Food Poisoning)			
Incubation period: generally short, 1–8 hr Gram-positive, nonmotile, aerobic, or facultative anaerobic bacteria Diagnosis by identifying organism in food, blood, pus, aspirate	Direct tissue invasion and production of toxin	Clinical presentation depends on site of entry In food poisoning: profuse diarrhea, nausea, and vomiting Low-grade fever and hypothermia may occur	GI illness transmitted in inadequately cooked or refrigerated foods Self-limiting in GI illness Symptomatic treatment Antibiotics not recommended

no recognized pathogens, and is refractory to treatment. The most common cause is acute infectious diarrhea that was not managed adequately.

Chronic nonspecific diarrhea (CNSD), also known as irritable colon or childhood and toddlers' diarrhea, is a common cause of chronic diarrhea in children 6 to 54 months of age. These children have loose stools, often with undigested food particles, and diarrhea greater than 2 weeks' duration. Children with CNSD grow normally and have no evidence of malnutrition, no blood in their stool, and no enteric infection. Dietary indiscretions and food sensitivities have been linked to chronic diarrhea. The excessive intake of juices and artificial sweeteners such as sorbitol, a substance found in many commercially prepared beverages and foods, may be a factor.

Etiology

Most pathogens that cause diarrhea are spread by the fecal–oral route through contaminated food or water or are spread from person to person where there is close contact (e.g., day care centres). Lack of clean water, crowding, poor hygiene, nutritional deficiency, and poor sanitation are major risk factors, especially for bacterial or parasitic pathogens. The increased frequency and severity of diarrheal disease in infants are also related to age-specific alterations in susceptibility to pathogens. For example, the immune system of infants has not been exposed to many pathogens and has not acquired protective antibodies; newborns do not have a well-developed GI mucosal barrier to many pathogens, thus increasing the predisposition to gastroenteritis. Worldwide, the most common causes of acute gastroenteritis are infectious agents, viruses, bacteria, and parasites. In developed nations, viruses, primarily rotavirus, cause 70 to 80% of infectious diarrhea.

Rotavirus is the most important cause of serious gastroenteritis among children and a significant health care–associated pathogen. Rotavirus disease is most severe in children 3 to 24 months of age. Children younger than 3 months of age have some protection from the disease because of maternally acquired antibodies. Approximately 25% of severe cases of rotavirus occur in older children.

Salmonella, Shigella, and *Campylobacter* organisms are the most frequently isolated bacterial pathogens. *Salmonella* has the highest occurrence in infants; *Giardia* and *Shigella* have the highest incidence among toddlers. *Shigella* infection is uncommon in Canada, accounting for less than 5% of diarrheal illnesses in infants and toddlers. *Campylobacter* infection has a bimodal presentation (highest in children younger than 12 months of age with a second rise in incidence at age 15 to 19 years). *Giardia* and *Cryptosporidium* organisms are parasites. *Cryptosporidium* infection is often associated with outbreaks in young children in day care centres; an increase in infections has been seen in association with outdoor swimming (pools, lakes, splash fountains) in the summer and early fall (AAP Committee on Infectious Diseases, Kimberlin, Brady, et al., 2015). *Plesiomonas* and *Yersinia* are also parasites that are frequently responsible for causing traveller's diarrhea.

Antibiotic administration is frequently associated with diarrhea because antibiotics alter the normal intestinal flora, resulting in an overgrowth of other bacteria such as *Clostridium difficile*. Antibiotic-associated diarrhea can also be caused by *Salmonella* organisms, *Clostridium porringers* type A, and *Staphylococcus aureus* pathogens. The Public Health Agency of Canada (PHAC) now identifies *C. difficile* as a reportable disease so that rates can be tracked (PHAC, 2013).

Pathophysiology

Invasion of the GI tract by pathogens results in increased intestinal secretion as a result of enterotoxins, cytotoxic mediators, or decreased intestinal absorption secondary to intestinal damage or inflammation. Enteric pathogens attach to the mucosal cells and form a cuplike pedestal on which the bacteria rest. The pathogenesis of the diarrhea depends on whether the organism remains attached to the cell surface, resulting in a secretory toxin (noninvasive, toxin-producing, noninflammatory type diarrhea), or penetrates the mucosa (systemic diarrhea). Noninflammatory diarrhea is the most common diarrheal illness, resulting from the action of enterotoxin that is released after attachment to the mucosa. The most serious and immediate physiological disturbances associated with severe diarrheal disease are (1) dehydration, (2) acid–base imbalance with acidosis, and (3) shock that occurs when dehydration progresses to the point that circulatory status is seriously impaired.

Diagnostic Evaluation

Evaluation of the child with acute gastroenteritis begins with a careful history that seeks to discover the possible cause of diarrhea, assess the severity of symptoms and the risk of complications, and elicit information about current symptoms indicating other treatable illnesses that could be causing the diarrhea. The history should include questions about recent travel, exposure to untreated drinking or washing water sources, contact with animals or birds, day care centre attendance, recent treatment with antibiotics, or recent diet changes. History questions should also explore the presence or absence of other symptoms such as fever and vomiting, frequency and character of stools (e.g., watery, bloody), urinary output, dietary habits, and recent food intake.

Extensive laboratory evaluation is not indicated in children who have uncomplicated diarrhea and no evidence of dehydration because most diarrheal illnesses are self-limiting. Laboratory tests are indicated for children who are severely dehydrated and receiving IV therapy. Watery, explosive stools suggest glucose intolerance; foul-smelling, greasy, bulky stools suggest fat malabsorption. Diarrhea that develops after the introduction of cow's milk, fruits, or cereal may be related to enzyme deficiency or protein intolerance. Neutrophils or red blood cells in the stool indicate bacterial gastroenteritis or IBD. The presence of eosinophils suggests protein intolerance or parasitic infection. Stool cultures should be performed only when blood, mucus, or polymorphonuclear leukocytes are present in the stool; symptoms are severe; there is a history of travel to a developing country; and a specific pathogen is suspected. Gross blood or occult blood may indicate pathogens such as *Shigella, Campylobacter*, or hemorrhagic *Escherichia coli* strains. An enzyme-linked immunosorbent assay (ELISA) may be used to confirm the presence of rotavirus or *Giardia* organisms. If there is a history of recent antibiotic use, the stool should be tested for *C. difficile* toxin. When bacterial and viral cultures are negative and diarrhea persists for more than a few days, stools should be examined for ova and parasites. A stool specimen with a pH of less than 6 and the presence of reducing substances may indicate carbohydrate malabsorption or secondary lactase deficiency. Stool electrolyte measurements may help identify children with secretory diarrhea.

The serum bicarbonate (HCO_3) may be useful when combined with other clinical signs. In the presence of metabolic acidosis, an anion gap may be helpful to distinguish between types of metabolic imbalance. A complete blood count (CBC), serum electrolytes, and creatinine and blood urea nitrogen (BUN) levels should be obtained for the child who has moderate-to-severe dehydration or who requires hospitalization. Urine specific gravity should be determined if dehydration is suspected. The hemoglobin, hematocrit, creatinine, and BUN levels are usually elevated in acute diarrhea and should normalize with rehydration.

Therapeutic Management

The major goals in the management of acute diarrhea include (1) assessment of fluid and electrolyte imbalance, (2) rehydration, (3) maintenance fluid therapy, and (4) reintroduction of an adequate diet. Infants and children with acute diarrhea and dehydration should be treated first with oral rehydration therapy (ORT). ORT is one of the major worldwide health care advances of the past few decades. It is more effective, safer, less painful, and less costly than IV rehydration. The World Health Organization (WHO) and the CPS recommend ORT as the treatment of choice for most cases of dehydration caused by diarrhea (Leung et al., 2006/2016). Oral rehydration solutions (ORSs) enhance and promote the reabsorption of sodium and water, and studies indicate that these solutions greatly reduce vomiting, volume loss from diarrhea, and the duration of the illness. ORSs, including reduced-osmolarity ORS, are available in Canada as commercially prepared solutions and are successful in treating the majority of infants with dehydration (Fig. 46-1). If a parent is using a commercially prepared sports drink (such as Gatorade) to rehydrate their child, the solution should be diluted 50% with water. (Commercial sports drinks are discouraged; Pedialyte is a safer alternative.)

After rehydration, children should be placed on an age-appropriate diet (Leung et al., 2006/2016). Ongoing stool losses should be replaced on a 1 : 1 basis with ORS. If the stool volume is not known, approximately 10 mL/kg of ORS should be given for each diarrheal stool.

Solutions for oral hydration are useful in most cases of dehydration, and vomiting is not a contraindication. A child who is vomiting should be given an ORS at frequent intervals and in small amounts. For young children the caregiver may give the fluid with a spoon or small syringe in 5- to 10-mL increments every 1 to 5 minutes. An ORS may also be given via NG or gastrostomy tube infusion. Infants without clinical signs of dehydration do not need ORT. However, they should receive the same fluids recommended for infants with signs of dehydration in the maintenance phase and for ongoing stool losses. The CPS suggest the use of probiotics to reduce the risk of antibiotic-associated diarrhea in children (Marchand & CPS, Nutrition and Gastroenterology Committee, 2012/2015). *Lactobacillus* GG, *Saccharomyces boulardii*, and *L. reuteri* have been shown to decrease the duration of watery diarrhea by 1 day, particularly diarrhea as a result of rotavirus (Guandalini, 2008).

! NURSING ALERT

Diarrhea is not managed by encouraging intake of clear fluids by mouth, such as fruit juices, carbonated soft drinks, and gelatin. These fluids usually have high carbohydrate content, very low electrolyte content, and high osmolality. Caffeinated soft drinks should be avoided because caffeine is a mild diuretic and may lead to increased loss of water and sodium. Chicken or beef broth is not given because it contains excessive sodium and inadequate carbohydrate. The BRAT diet (bananas, rice, applesauce, and toast or tea) is contraindicated for the child and especially for the infant with acute diarrhea because this diet has little nutritional value (low in energy and protein), is high in carbohydrates, and is low in calories (Leung et al., 2006/2016).

Early reintroduction of nutrients is desirable and is gaining more widespread acceptance. Continued feeding or early reintroduction of a normal diet has no adverse effects; it lessens the severity and duration of the illness and improves weight gain when compared with a slower reintroduction of foods (Leung et al., 2006/2016). Infants who are breastfeeding should continue to do so, and ORS should be used to replace ongoing losses in these infants. Formula-fed infants should resume their formula; formula should not be diluted or mixed with additional water. Older children who consume a regular diet, including milk, can be offered their normal foods after rehydration has been achieved. A diet of easily digestible foods such as cereals, cooked vegetables, and meats is adequate for the older child. In toddlers there is no contraindication to continuing soft or pureed foods.

In cases of severe dehydration and shock, IV fluids are initiated whenever the child is unable to ingest sufficient amounts of fluid and electrolytes to (1) meet ongoing daily physiological losses, (2) replace previous deficits, and (3) replace ongoing abnormal losses. Patients who usually require IV fluids are those with severe dehydration, those with uncontrollable vomiting, those who are unable to drink for any reason (e.g., extreme fatigue, coma), and those with severe gastric distension.

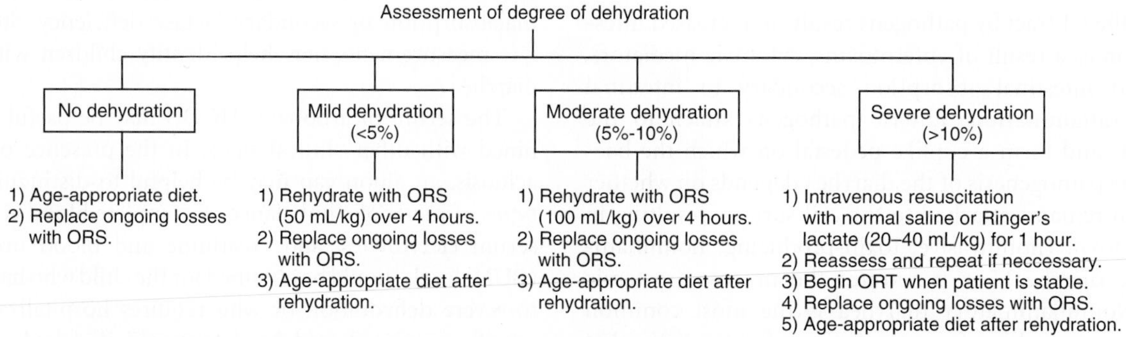

FIGURE 46-1 Algorithm for managing acute gastroenteritis in children. *ORS*, oral rehydration solution; *ORT*, oral rehydration therapy. (From Leung, A., Prince, T., & Canadian Paediatric Society, Nutrition and Gastroenterology Committee. [2006]. Oral rehydration therapy and early refeeding in the management of childhood gastroenteritis. *Journal of Paediatric and Child Health, 11*[8], 529.)

The IV solution is selected on the basis of what is known about the probable type and cause of the dehydration—normal saline solution or lactated Ringer's is used to replace volume, after which a saline solution containing 5% dextrose in normal saline with potassium chloride (20 mEq/L) may be administered as maintenance therapy. Sodium bicarbonate may be added, since acidosis is usually associated with severe dehydration. Although the initial phase of fluid replacement is rapid in both isotonic and hypotonic dehydration, rapid replacement is contraindicated in hypertonic dehydration because of the risk of water intoxication, especially in the brain cells.

After the severe effects of dehydration are under control, specific diagnostic and therapeutic measures are initiated to detect and treat the cause of the diarrhea. The use of antibiotic therapy in children with acute gastroenteritis is controversial. Antibiotics may shorten the course of some diarrheal illnesses (e.g., those caused by *Shigella* organisms). However, most bacterial diarrheas are self-limiting, and the diarrhea often resolves before the causative organism can be determined. Antibiotics may prolong the carrier period for bacteria such as *Salmonella*. However, antibiotics may be considered in patients with **immunosuppression**, severe symptoms, or persistent disease or in patients who have had transplantation. Antimotility drugs such as loperamide are not recommended in children. Because of the self-limiting nature of vomiting and its tendency to improve when dehydration is corrected, antiemetic drugs such as the phenothiazines are not recommended because of their adverse effects; however, ondansetron has few adverse effects and may be administered if vomiting persists and interferes with ORT (Bhutta, 2016).

Prevention

The best intervention for diarrhea is prevention. The fecal–oral route spreads most infections, and parents need information about preventive measures such as personal hygiene, protection of the water supply from contamination, and careful food preparation.

> **NURSING ALERT**
>
> To reduce the risk of bacteria transmitted via food, encourage parents to:
> - **Clean:** Wash hands, utensils, and work areas with hot, soapy water after contact with raw meat to keep bacteria from spreading; wash raw fruits and vegetables with clean, running water before eating.
> - **Chill:** Keep cold food cold at or below 4°C; thaw food in the refrigerator; never thaw food on the counter or let it sit out of the refrigerator for more than 2 hours.
> - **Separate:** Use one cutting board for raw meat, poultry, and seafood, and use a different cutting board for food that is ready to eat or cooked; keep raw food away from other food while shopping, and while storing, preparing, and serving foods; place raw meat, poultry, and seafood in containers on the bottom shelf of the refrigerator.
> - **Cook:** Check ground meat with a fork to make certain no pink is showing before taking a bite; cook all dishes made with ground meat until brown or grey inside or to an internal temperature of 71°C (Government of Canada, 2012).

Meticulous attention to perianal hygiene, disposal of soiled diapers, proper hand hygiene, and isolation of infected persons also minimize the transmission of infection (see Infection Control, Chapter 44).

Parents need information about preventing diarrhea in their child while travelling. They should be cautioned against giving children adult medications that are used to prevent traveller's diarrhea. Until vaccines or other prophylactic measures are proven to be safe for children, the best measure during travel to areas where water may be contaminated is to allow children to drink only bottled water and carbonated beverages (from the container through a straw supplied from home). Tap water, ice, unpasteurized dairy products, raw vegetables, unpeeled fruits, meats, and seafood should also be avoided.

To prevent contraction of rotavirus and associated diarrhea, two rotavirus vaccines are available for children. Human-bovine reassortant rotavirus vaccine (RotaTeq) and live-attenuated human rotavirus vaccine (Rotarix) may be used to prevent this infectious diarrheal disease. Infants should receive three doses of RotaTeq oral vaccine at 2, 4, and 6 months of age. Two doses of Rotarix, given at 2 and 4 months of age, will induce protective immunity (see Immunizations, Chapter 35). The CPS recommends that all babies be vaccinated (Salvadori, Le Saux, CPS, Infectious Diseases and Immunization Committee, 2010/2015). Population-based studies show a reduction of diarrhea-associated hospitalizations by as much as 87 to 96% in the years after rotavirus vaccination (Payne, Staat, Edwards, et al., 2011). Breastfeeding during the first 6 months of life has been found to have a protective effect against rotavirus infection (Plenge-Bönig, Soto-Ramírez, Karmaus, et al., 2010).

NURSING CARE

The management of most cases of acute diarrhea takes place in the home with education of the caregiver. Caregivers are taught to monitor for signs of dehydration (especially the number of wet diapers or voidings) and the amount of fluids taken by mouth and to assess the frequency and amount of stool losses. Education relating to ORT, including the administration of maintenance fluids and replacement of ongoing losses, is important (see Critical Thinking Case Study). ORS should be administered in small quantities at frequent intervals. Vomiting is not a contraindication to ORT unless it is severe. Information about the introduction of a regular diet is essential. Parents need to know that a slightly higher stool output initially occurs with continuation of a normal diet and with ongoing replacement of stool losses. The benefits of a better nutritional outcome with fewer complications and a shorter duration of illness outweigh the potential increase in stool frequency. Parents' concerns should be addressed to ensure adherence to the treatment plan.

If the child with acute diarrhea and dehydration is hospitalized, an accurate weight must be obtained, and intake and output must be carefully monitored. The child may be placed on parenteral fluid therapy with reinstitution of oral fluids and soft foods; keeping the child with gastroenteritis NPO for a long period is usually avoided to prevent changes in intestinal

CRITICAL THINKING CASE STUDY

Diarrhea

A mother brings her 8-month-old infant, Mary, to the primary care clinic. The mother reports that Mary has had a "cold" for about 2 days and this morning she began to vomit and has had diarrhea for the past 8 hours. The mother states that Mary is still breastfeeding but that she is not taking as much fluid as usual and she is having three times as many stools as usual (the stools are watery in consistency). The nurse practitioner's assessment of Mary finds that her temperature is 38.0°C, her pulse and blood pressure are in the normal range, her mucous membranes are moist, and she has tears when she cries. The nurse practitioner also notes that Mary's weight has not changed from when she was seen in the clinic 2 weeks ago for her well-child visit. What interventions should the nurse practitioner include in the initial management of Mary?

1. Evidence—Is there sufficient evidence for the nurse practitioner to draw any conclusions for the initial plan of management?
2. Assumptions—Describe some underlying assumptions about the following:
   a. Clinical manifestations of various levels of dehydration
   b. Management of acute diarrhea
   c. Breastfeeding and the management of acute diarrhea
   d. Use of antidiarrheal medications for acute diarrhea in children
3. What nursing interventions should the nurse practitioner implement at this time?
4. Does the evidence support the nurse practitioner's conclusion?

permeability as a result of infection. Monitoring the IV infusion is an important nursing function. The nurse must ensure that the correct fluid and electrolyte concentration is infused, the flow rate is adjusted to deliver the desired volume in a given time, and the IV site is maintained.

Accurate measurement of output is essential to determine whether renal blood flow is sufficient to permit the addition of potassium to the IV fluids. The nurse is responsible for examination of stools and collection of specimens for laboratory examination (see Collection of Specimens, Chapter 44). Care should be taken when obtaining and transporting stools to prevent possible spread of infection; stool specimens should be transported to the laboratory in appropriate containers and media according to hospital policy. A clean tongue depressor can be used to obtain specimens for laboratory examination or as an applicator for transfer to a culture medium.

Diarrheal stools are highly irritating to the skin, thus extra care is needed to protect the skin of the perianal and perineal region from excoriation (see Diaper Dermatitis, Chapter 52). Taking a rectal temperature should be avoided because this can stimulate the bowel, increasing passage of stool.

Support for the child and family involves the same care and consideration given all hospitalized children (see Chapter 43). Parents need to be kept informed of the child's progress and instructed in the use of frequent and proper **hand hygiene** and the disposal of soiled diapers, clothes, and bed linen. If *C. difficile* is the infecting agent, hands must be washed with soap and water and not with alcohol-based cleanser. Everyone caring for the child must be aware of "clean" areas and "dirty" areas, especially in the hospital, where the sink in the child's room is used for many purposes. Soiled diapers and linen should be discarded in receptacles close to the bedside. To remind caregivers to keep diapers and other soiled articles away from clean areas, signs can be placed identifying "clean" (e.g., bed table) and "dirty" (e.g., sink, bathroom) areas. The articles that may be stored in each area should be listed on these signs.

Constipation

Constipation is an alteration in the frequency, consistency, or ease of passing stool. Parents often define constipation as passing less than three stools per week. It is defined as infrequent, difficult, painful, or incomplete evacuation of hard stools (Rowan-Legg & CPS, Community Paediatrics Committee, 2011/2016). It may also be defined as painful bowel movements, which are often blood streaked or include the retention of stool, with or without soiling, even with a stool frequency of more than three stools per week. However, the frequency of bowel movements is not considered a diagnostic criterion because it varies widely among children. Having extremely long intervals between defecation is termed **obstipation**. Constipation with fecal soiling is referred to as **encopresis**.

Constipation may arise secondary to a variety of organic disorders or in association with a wide range of systemic disorders. Structural disorders of the intestine, such as strictures, ectopic anus, and Hirschsprung disease (HD), may be associated with constipation. Systemic disorders associated with constipation include hypothyroidism, hypercalcemia resulting from hyperparathyroidism or vitamin D excess, and chronic lead poisoning. Constipation may be associated with medications such as antacids, diuretics, antiepileptics, antihistamines, opioids, and iron supplementation. Spinal cord lesions may be associated with loss of rectal tone and sensation. Affected children are prone to chronic fecal retention and overflow incontinence.

The majority of children have **idiopathic** or *functional constipation* since no underlying cause can be identified. Chronic constipation may occur as a result of environmental or psychosocial factors or a combination of the two. Transient illness, withholding and avoidance secondary to painful or negative experiences with stooling, and dietary intake with decreased fluid and fibre all play a role in the etiology of constipation.

Infancy

Normally the newborn infant passes a first meconium stool within 24 to 36 hours of birth. Any infant who does not do so should be assessed for evidence of intestinal atresia or stenosis, HD, hypothyroidism, meconium plugs, or meconium ileus. *Meconium plugs* are caused by meconium that has reduced water content and are usually evacuated after digital examination but may require irrigation with a hypertonic solution or contrast medium.

Meconium ileus, the initial manifestation of cystic fibrosis, is the luminal obstruction of the distal small intestine by abnormal meconium. Treatment is the same as for a meconium plug; early surgical intervention may be needed to evacuate the small intestine.

CRITICAL THINKING CASE STUDY

Constipation

Jung, an 8-month-old infant, is seen by the pediatric nurse practitioner for his well-child visit. Jung's mother states that he usually has one hard stool every 4 to 5 days, which causes discomfort when the stool is passed. He has also had one episode of diarrhea and two episodes of ribbonlike stools. Abdominal distension and vomiting have not accompanied the constipation, and Jung's growth has been appropriate. Currently his diet consists of cow's milk formula only. Jung's mother reports that the infrequent passage of hard stools began approximately 6 weeks ago when she stopped breastfeeding. Which interventions should the nurse practitioner include in the initial management of Jung's problem?

1. Evidence—Is there sufficient evidence for the nurse practitioner to draw any conclusions about the management of Jung's problem?
2. Assumptions—Describe some underlying assumptions about the following:
   a. Causes of constipation in infants
   b. Factors associated with functional constipation in infants
   c. Management of functional constipation in infants
3. What interventions should the nurse practitioner implement at this time?
4. Does the evidence support these interventions?

The onset of constipation frequently occurs during infancy and may result from organic causes such as HD, hypothyroidism, and strictures. It is important to differentiate these conditions from functional constipation. Constipation in infancy is often related to dietary practices. It is less common in breastfed infants, who have softer stools than bottle-fed infants. Breastfed infants may also have fewer stools because of more complete use of breast milk with little residue. When constipation occurs with a change from human milk or modified cow's milk to whole cow's milk, simple measures, such as adding or increasing the amount of cereal, vegetables, and fruit in the infant's diet, usually corrects the problem. When a bottle-fed infant passes a hard stool that results in an anal fissure, stool-withholding behaviours may develop in response to pain on defecation (see Critical Thinking Case Study).

Childhood

Most constipation in early childhood is the result of environmental changes or normal development when a child begins to attain control over bodily functions. A child who has experienced discomfort during bowel movements may deliberately try to withhold stool. Over time, the rectum accommodates to the accumulation of stool, and the urge to defecate passes. When the bowel contents are ultimately evacuated, the accumulated feces are passed with pain, thus reinforcing the desire to withhold stool.

Constipation in school-age children may represent an ongoing problem or a first-time event. The onset of constipation at this age is often the result of environmental changes, stresses, and changes in toileting patterns. A common cause of new-onset constipation at school entry is fear of using the school bathrooms, which are noted for their lack of privacy. Early and hurried departure for school immediately after breakfast may also impede bathroom use.

The management of simple constipation consists of a plan to promote regular bowel movements. Often this is as simple as changing the diet to provide more fibre and fluids, avoiding foods known to be constipating, and establishing a bowel routine that allows for regular passage of stool. Stool-softening agents such as docusate or lactulose may also be helpful. Polyethylene glycol (PEG) 3350 without electrolytes is a chemically inert polymer that has been introduced as a laxative in recent years. It is tolerated well by children because it can be mixed in a beverage of choice (Rowan-Legg & CPS, Community Paediatrics Committee, 2011/2016). If other symptoms such as vomiting, abdominal distension, or pain and evidence of growth failure are associated with the constipation, the condition should be investigated further.

NURSING CARE

Constipation tends to be self-perpetuating. A child who has difficulty or discomfort when attempting to evacuate the bowels has a tendency to retain the bowel contents, and this may initiate a vicious cycle. Nursing assessment begins with an accurate history of bowel habits; diet; events associated with the onset of constipation; medications or other substances that the child may be taking; and the consistency, colour, frequency, and other characteristics of the stool. If there is no evidence of a pathological condition, the major tasks are to educate the parents regarding normal stool patterns and to participate in the education and treatment of the child.

Dietary modifications are essential in preventing constipation. For infants, constipation is treated on the basis of severity of the problem and how effective the treatment is. Before infants start solids, constipation can be managed fairly well with 30 mL sorbitol-containing juices (such as prune, pear, or apple) given once or twice per day (Sood, 2016). If this is unsuccessful the addition of an osmotic laxative can be useful (Sood, 2016). Glycerin suppositories should be used with caution as they can enhance anal irritation and make the problem chronic (Sood, 2016). During childhood the diet should contain increased amounts of fibre and fluid. Parents benefit from guidance in selecting foods that facilitate bowel movements (Box 46-5). They need reassurance concerning the benign nature of the condition. It is also important to discuss their attitudes and expectations regarding toilet habits.

When constipation persists despite dietary intervention, more aggressive management may be necessary. It is important to differentiate an acute episode of constipation from chronic functional constipation, which can result from chronic stool-withholding behaviour. As the rectal vault becomes distended over time, further complications such as fecal impaction and encopresis may develop (see Chapter 38).

Hirschsprung Disease

Hirschsprung disease (HD) (congenital aganglionic megacolon) is a mechanical obstruction caused by inadequate motility of part of the intestine. It accounts for about one fourth of all cases of neonatal obstruction, although it may not be diagnosed until later in infancy or childhood. The incidence is 1 in 5000 live

BOX 46-5 HIGH-FIBRE FOODS

Bread, Grains
Whole-grain bread or rolls
Whole-grain cereals
Bran
Unrefined (brown) rice

Vegetables
Raw vegetables, especially broccoli, cabbage, carrots, cauliflower, celery, lettuce, and spinach
Cooked vegetables, such as those listed previously and asparagus, beans, brussels sprouts, corn, potatoes, rhubarb, squash, string beans, and turnips

Fruits
Raw fruits, especially those with skins or seeds, other than ripe banana or avocado
Raisins, prunes, or other dried fruits

Miscellaneous
Nuts, seeds, legumes, popcorn
High-fibre snack bars

births (Fiorino & Liacouras, 2016). It is four times more common in males than in females and may follow a familial pattern in about 10% of cases. HD is usually an isolated **birth defect**, but it has been associated with other syndromes, including Down syndrome. Depending on its presentation, it may be an acute, life-threatening, or chronic condition.

Pathophysiology

The pathology of HD relates to the absence of ganglion cells in the affected areas of the intestine, resulting in a loss of the rectosphincteric reflex and an abnormal microenvironment of the cells of the affected intestine (Theocharatos & Kenny, 2008). The term *congenital aganglionic megacolon* describes the primary defect, which is the absence of ganglion cells in the myenteric plexus of Auerbach and the submucosal plexus of Meissner (Fig. 46-2).

The absence of ganglion cells in the affected bowel results in a lack of enteric nervous system stimulation, which decreases the ability of the internal sphincter to relax. Unopposed sympathetic stimulation of the intestine results in increased intestinal tone. In addition to the contraction of the abnormal bowel and the resulting lack of peristalsis, there is a loss of the rectosphincteric reflex. Normally, when a stool bolus enters the rectum, the internal sphincter relaxes and the stool is evacuated. In HD the internal sphincter does not relax. In most cases the aganglionic segment includes the rectum and some portion of the distal colon. However, the entire colon or part of the small intestine may be involved (long-segment disease). Occasionally, segments may be skipped or total intestinal aganglionosis may occur.

Diagnostic Evaluation

Most children with HD are diagnosed in the first few months of life. Clinical manifestations vary according to the age when symptoms are recognized and the presence of complications such as enterocolitis (Box 46-6). A newborn usually is seen with distended abdomen, feeding intolerance with bilious vomiting, and delay in the passage of meconium. Typically, 95% of normal-term infants pass meconium in the first 24 hours of life, whereas fewer than 10% of infants with HD do so. In older children a careful history is helpful. Radiographs, an unprepped barium enema, and anorectal manometric examinations assist in the differential diagnosis, which is confirmed by a full-thickness rectal biopsy demonstrating the absence of ganglion cells in the myenteric and submucosal plexuses.

BOX 46-6 CLINICAL MANIFESTATIONS OF HIRSCHSPRUNG DISEASE

Newborn Period
Failure to pass meconium within 24 to 48 hours after birth
Refusal to feed
Bilious vomiting
Abdominal distension

Infancy
Growth failure
Constipation
Abdominal distension
Episodes of diarrhea and vomiting
Signs of enterocolitis
Explosive, watery diarrhea
Fever
Appears significantly ill

Childhood (Symptoms Appear More Chronic)
Constipation
Ribbonlike, foul-smelling stools
Abdominal distension
Visible peristalsis
Easily palpable fecal mass
Undernourished, anemic appearance

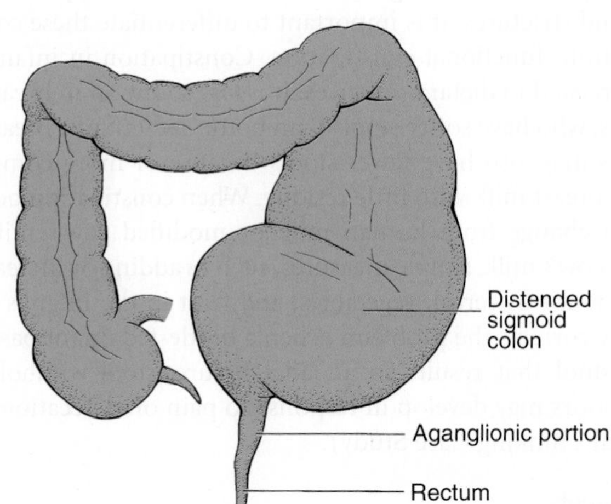

FIGURE 46-2 Hirschsprung disease.

Therapeutic Management

The majority of children with HD require surgery, rather than medical therapy with frequent enemas (Levitt, Martin,

Olesevich, et al., 2009). The child with symptoms is stabilized with fluid and electrolyte replacement prior to surgery. Surgical management consists primarily of the removal of the aganglionic portion of the bowel in order to relieve obstruction, restore normal motility, and preserve the function of the external anal sphincter. The majority of children with HD require one of the following operative procedures: a Soave transanal pull-through procedure, the Swenson procedure, or the Duhamel procedure (Gourlay, 2013). With earlier diagnosis the proximal bowel may not be extremely distended, thus allowing for a primary pull-through or one-stage procedure and eliminating the need for a temporary colostomy. Simpler operations, such as an anorectal myomectomy, may be indicated in very short–segment disease.

Prognosis

After the pull-through procedure, anal stricture and incontinence may occur and require further therapy, including dilations or bowel retraining therapy. Constipation and fecal incontinence are chronic problems in a small proportion of patients after surgical correction for HD (Fiorino & Liacouras, 2016). As these children grow older, this can significantly affect their quality of life (Mills, Konkin, Milner, et al., 2008).

NURSING CARE

The nursing concerns depend on the child's age and the type of treatment. If the disorder is diagnosed during the newborn period, the main objectives are to (1) help the parents adjust to a congenital defect in their child, (2) foster infant–parent bonding, (3) prepare them for the medical-surgical intervention, and (4) assist them in colostomy care after discharge (as applicable).

Preoperative Care

The child's preoperative care depends on the age and clinical condition. A child who is malnourished may not be able to withstand surgery until his or her physical status improves. Often this involves symptomatic treatment with enemas; a low-fibre, high-calorie, and high-protein diet; and, in severe situations, the use of total **parenteral nutrition** (TPN).

Physical preoperative preparation includes the same measures that are common to any surgery (see Surgical Procedures, Chapter 44). In the newborn, whose bowel is sterile, no additional preparation is necessary. However, in other children, preparation for the pull-through procedure involves emptying the bowel with repeated saline enemas and decreasing bacterial flora with oral or systemic antibiotics and colonic irrigations using antibiotic solution. Enterocolitis is the most serious complication of HD. Emergency preoperative care includes frequent monitoring of vital signs and blood pressure for signs of shock; monitoring fluid and electrolyte replacements and plasma or other blood derivatives; and observing for symptoms of bowel perforation, such as fever, increasing abdominal distension, vomiting, increased tenderness, irritability, dyspnea, and cyanosis.

Because progressive distension of the abdomen is a serious sign, the nurse needs to measure abdominal circumference with a paper tape measure, usually at the level of the umbilicus or at the widest part of the abdomen. The point of measurement is marked with a pen to ensure reliability of subsequent measurements. Abdominal measurement can be obtained along with the vital sign measurements and is recorded in serial order so that any change becomes obvious. To reduce stress to the acutely ill child when frequent measurements of abdominal circumference are needed, the tape measure can be left in place beneath the child rather than removed each time.

The child's age dictates the type and extent of psychological preparation. Because a colostomy is usually performed, the child who is of preschool age is told about the procedure in concrete terms with the use of visual aids (see Chapter 43). It is important to time explanations appropriately to prevent the anxiety and confusion that could result from too much information. It is also important to stress to parents and older children that the colostomy for HD is temporary, unless so much bowel is involved that a permanent ileostomy must be performed. In most instances the extent of bowel resection is known before surgery, although the nurse should be aware of cases when doubt exists concerning repair. The nurse should remember that, although a temporary colostomy is favourable in terms of future health and adjustment, it requires additional surgery, which may be stressful to parents and children.

Postoperative Care

Postoperative care is the same as that for any child or infant with abdominal surgery (see Surgical Procedures, Chapter 44). When a colostomy is part of the corrective procedure, stomal care is a major nursing task (see Ostomies, Chapter 44). To prevent contamination of an infant's abdominal wound with urine, the diaper should be pinned below the dressing. Sometimes a Foley catheter is used in the immediate postoperative period to divert the flow of urine away from the abdomen.

Discharge Care

After surgery, parents need instruction concerning colostomy care. Even a preschooler can be included in the care by handing articles to the parent, rolling up the colostomy pouch after it is emptied, or applying barrier preparations to the surrounding skin. Although the diagnosis of HD is less frequent in school-age children or adolescents, children this age can often be involved in colostomy care to the point of total responsibility.

Some institutions and communities have enterostomal therapists who provide expert assistance in planning home care. If families require financial assistance and psychological support, referral to a social worker, home health care agency, or community health nurse can provide continuity of care.

Vomiting

Vomiting is the forceful ejection of gastric contents through the mouth. It is a well-defined, complex, coordinated process that is under central nervous system control and is often accompanied by nausea and retching. Vomiting may be divided into two categories: nonbilious and bilious. Some small intestinal reflux is common in all vomiting. In *nonbilious vomiting*, the majority of bile drains into the more distal portions of the intestine. If an obstruction is present, nonbilious vomiting suggests a more proximal obstruction. *Bilious vomiting* implies a disorder of motility or distal physical blockage. Causes of nonbilious vomiting include infectious, inflammatory, metabolic or endocrinological, neurological, and psychological causes and obstructive lesions. Causes of bilious vomiting include intestinal atresia and stenosis, malrotation with or without volvulus, ileus, intussusceptions, intestinal duplication, mass lesions, incarcerated inguinal hernia, and appendicitis. Vomiting may also be associated with other processes, including acute infectious diseases, increased intracranial pressure, toxic ingestions, food intolerances and allergies, mechanical obstruction of the GI tract, metabolic disorders, and psychogenic problems. It is common in childhood, is usually self-limiting, and requires no specific treatment. However, complications may occur, including acute fluid volume loss (dehydration) and electrolyte disturbances, malnutrition, aspiration, and Mallory-Weiss syndrome (small tears in the distal esophageal mucosa).

Vomiting is a well-recognized response to psychological stress. During stress adrenaline levels rise and may stimulate the chemoreceptor trigger zone. Nausea and vomiting are likely a protective mechanism to remove toxins from the system. Vomiting may follow GI infection or toxic ingestion, or it can be a learned behavioural response.

Cyclic vomiting syndrome is a rare disorder in which bouts of vomiting occur that can last from hours to several days. There is a lack of research on this syndrome in terms of the etiology as well as evaluating the treatment protocols (Rashid, Taminiau, Benninga, et al., 2016).

Therapeutic Management

Management is directed toward detection and treatment of the cause of the vomiting and prevention of complications from the loss of fluid. Fluids are administered in the same manner as and in a similar electrolyte composition to those administered for diarrhea. Although most children respond to these measures, antiemetic medications may be needed. Antiemetics such as ondansetron (Zofran) and trimethobenzamide (Tigan) block receptors in the chemoreceptor trigger zone; others such as metoclopramide (Reglan) enhance gastroduodenal peristalsis; still others such as promethazine (Phenergan) compete for H_1-receptor sites. For children who are prone to motion sickness, it is helpful to administer an appropriate dose of dimenhydrinate (Gravol) before a trip.

NURSING CARE

The major focus of nursing care is observing and reporting vomiting behaviour and associated symptoms and implementing measures to reduce the vomiting. Accurate assessment of the type of vomiting, the appearance of the vomitus, and the child's behaviour in association with the vomiting helps to establish a diagnosis.

Nursing interventions are determined by the cause of the vomiting. When the vomiting is a manifestation of improper feeding methods, establishing proper techniques through teaching and example usually corrects the situation. If vomiting is believed to be an indication of obstruction, food is usually withheld, or special feeding techniques are implemented. In situations in which vomiting is related to concurrent infection, dietary indiscretion, or emotional factors, efforts are directed toward maintaining hydration or preventing dehydration.

The thirst mechanism is the most sensitive guide to fluid needs, and ad libitum administration of a glucose-electrolyte solution to an alert child restores water and electrolytes satisfactorily. It is important to include carbohydrate to spare body protein and avoid ketosis resulting from exhaustion of glycogen stores. Small, frequent feedings of fluids or foods are preferred. After vomiting has stopped, more liberal amounts of fluids are offered, followed by gradual resumption of the regular diet.

The vomiting infant or child should be positioned on the side or semireclining to prevent aspiration and should be observed for evidence of dehydration. Careful monitoring of fluid and electrolyte status is necessary to prevent an electrolyte disturbance.

Gastroesophageal Reflux

Gastroesophageal reflux (GER) is defined as the transfer of gastric contents into the esophagus. This phenomenon is physiological, occurring throughout the day, most frequently after meals and at night. It is important to differentiate GER from *gastroesophageal reflux disease (GERD)*, which represents symptoms or tissue damage that results from GER. Approximately 50% of infants younger than 2 months old are reported to have GER (Suwandhi, Ton, & Schwarz, 2006). This "physiological" GER usually resolves spontaneously by 1 year of age (Blanco, Davenport, & Kane, 2012). GER becomes a disease when complications such as growth failure, bleeding, or dysphagia develop. GERD is associated with respiratory symptoms, including apnea, bronchospasm, laryngospasm, and pneumonia. Heartburn is also a frequent symptom in children who are able to describe it (Box 46-7).

Certain conditions predispose children to a high prevalence of GERD, including neurological impairment, hiatal hernia, repaired esophageal atresia, and morbid obesity (Suwandhi et al., 2006). *Sandifer syndrome* is an uncommon condition, usually occurring in young children, characterized by repetitive stretching and arching of the head and neck that can be mistaken for a seizure (Blanco et al., 2012). This manoeuvre likely represents a physiological neuromuscular response attempting to prevent acid refluxate from reaching the upper portion of the esophagus.

Pathophysiology

Although the pathogenesis of GER is multifactorial, its primary causative mechanism likely involves inappropriate transient relaxation of the lower esophageal sphincter (LES) (Suwandhi et al., 2006). Factors that increase abdominal pressure, such as coughing and sneezing, scoliosis, and overeating, may contribute to GERD. Esophageal symptoms are caused by

BOX 46-7 CLINICAL MANIFESTATIONS AND COMPLICATIONS OF GASTROESOPHAGEAL REFLUX

Symptoms in Infants

May have no observable clinical signs
Spitting up, regurgitation, vomiting (may be forceful)
Excessive crying, irritability, arching of the back with neck extension, stiffening
Feeding refusal, weight loss, growth failure
Respiratory problems (cough, wheeze, stridor, gagging, choking with feedings)
Hematemesis
Apnea or apparent life-threatening event (ALTE)

Symptoms in Children

Heartburn
Dyspepsia, abdominal pain
Noncardiac chest pain
Chronic cough
Dysphagia
Nocturnal bronchospasm and asthma
Recurrent pneumonia, pneumonitis

Complications

Esophagitis
Esophageal stricture
Laryngitis
Recurrent pneumonia
Anemia
Barrett's esophagus

Adapted from Rudolph, C. D., et al. (2001). Guidelines for evaluation and treatment of gastroesophageal reflux in infants and children: Recommendations of the North American Society for Pediatric Gastroenterology and Nutrition. *Journal of Pediatric Gastroenterology & Nutrition, 32*(Suppl 2), S1–S31.

inflammation from the acid in the gastric refluxate, whereas reactive airway disease may result from stimulation of airway reflexes by the acid refluxate.

Diagnostic Evaluation

The history and physical examination are usually sufficiently reliable to establish the diagnosis of GER, but many experts recommend a combination of tests for a definitive diagnosis (Blanco et al., 2012). The upper GI series is helpful in evaluating the presence of anatomical abnormalities such as pyloric stenosis, malrotation, annular pancreas, hiatal hernia, and esophageal stricture. The 24-hour intraesophageal pH monitoring study is the gold standard in the diagnosis of GER (Blanco et al., 2012). Endoscopy with biopsy may be helpful to assess the presence and severity of esophagitis, strictures, and Barrett esophagus and to exclude other disorders such as Crohn's disease. Scintigraphy (gastroesophageal) can be used to detect radioactive substances in the esophagus after a feeding of the compound and to assess gastric emptying. It can differentiate aspiration of gastric contents from reflux and aspiration from poor oropharyngeal muscle coordination. A modified barium swallow study with video fluoroscopy may be also be a diagnostic tool for this condition.

Therapeutic Management

Therapeutic management of GER depends on its severity. No therapy is needed for the infant who is thriving and has no respiratory complications. In symptomatic bottle-fed infants, feeding manoeuvres such as thickened feedings if on a commercial formula and upright positioning can improve mild GER symptoms. Thickened feedings do not improve pH scores on 24-hour intraesophageal monitoring but may decrease the number of vomiting episodes. Feedings thickened with 5 to 15 mL of rice cereal per 30 mL of formula or a commercial thickening additive may be recommended. This may benefit infants who are underweight as a result of GERD. The American Food and Drug Administration in 2011 warned about a possible association between commercially thickened additives and necrotizing enterocolitis in preterm infants. It is not recommended that thickener be used unless approved by a health care provider (Lightdale & Gremse, 2013). NG feedings may be necessary for the infant with severe reflux and growth failure until surgery can be performed. GER occurs less frequently in breastfed infants. The infant can be breastfed as usual and may be placed in an upright position after the feeding for 2 hours. If sensitivity to cow milk protein is suspected, cow milk can be eliminated temporarily from the mother's diet while breastfeeding continues, to see if the infant improves. If the infant is on formula then extensively hydrolyzed formula may be trialled briefly to alleviate symptoms, but this trial needs to be managed by medical supervision. Small, more frequent feedings as well as frequent burping are also recommended (Lightdale & Gremse, 2013). Elevating the head of the bed 30 degrees or placing the infant in an infant seat elevated 30 degrees for 2 hours after feedings may decrease reflux-related respiratory events (Jung, Yang, Min, et al., 2012). Prone positioning of infants also decreases episodes of GER but is recommended only with extreme caution when the risk of GERD complications exceeds the risk of sudden infant death syndrome (Lightdale & Gremse, 2013). The CPS recommends supine positioning for sleep (see Chapter 35). If the prone position is used, parents need to be cautioned to avoid soft bedding.

GER is likely present in most preterm infants, with minimal clinical effects. A few preterm infants have significant symptoms of GER with aspiration and recurrent vomiting and need to be managed with standard treatments. There is evidence which suggests that GER and apnea are related, but it is controversial and not clearly proven (Jefferies & CPS, Fetus and Newborn Committee, 2014/2016).

In older children and adolescents, avoidance of certain foods that exacerbate acid reflux, such as caffeine, citrus, tomatoes, alcohol, peppermint, and spicy or fried foods; lifestyle modifications, such as weight control with a weight loss program if indicated; eating small, more frequent meals; and smoking cessation may be helpful in reducing symptoms.

Pharmacological therapy may be used to treat infants and children with GERD. Both H_2-receptor antagonists (cimetidine

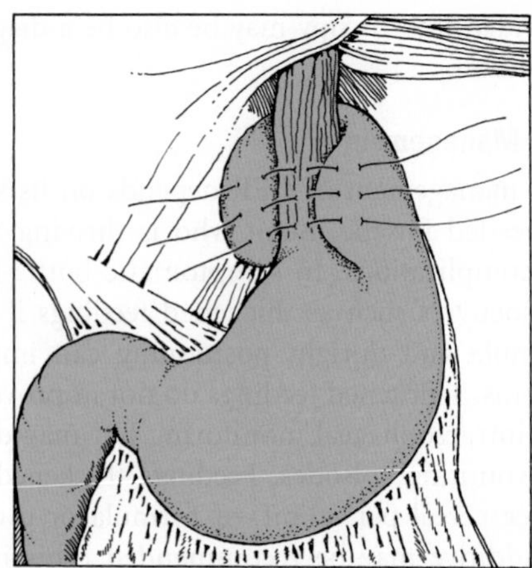

FIGURE 46-3 Nissen fundoplication sutures passing through esophageal musculature. (Redrawn from Campbell, A., & Ferrara, B. [1993]. Toupet partial fundoplication: Correcting, preventing gastroesophageal reflux. *AORN Journal, 57*(3), 671–679. Copyright 1993, with permission from Elsevier.)

[Tagamet], ranitidine [Zantac], or famotidine [Pepcid]) and proton pump inhibitors (PPIs; esomeprazole [Nexium], lansoprazole [Prevacid], omeprazole [Prilosec], pantoprazole [Protonix], and rabeprazole [Aciphex]) reduce gastric hydrochloric acid secretion and may stimulate some increase in LES tone. Use of available prokinetic medications (e.g., bethanechol [Urecholine] and metoclopramide) remains controversial. Clinical practice guidelines recommend the use of PPIs over the H_2-receptor antagonists to alleviate symptoms and to heal esophagitis (Vandenplas, Rudolph, Di Lorenzo, et al., 2009).

Surgical management of GER is reserved for children with severe complications, such as recurrent aspiration pneumonia, apnea, severe esophagitis, or growth failure, and for children who have failed to respond to medical therapy. The *Nissen fundoplication* (Fig. 46-3) is the most common surgical procedure, which is commonly performed laparoscopically with outcomes of decreased time to feedings, better cosmetic results, less pain, and fewer complications (Kane, 2009). This surgery involves passage of the gastric fundus behind the esophagus to encircle the distal esophagus. Long-term complications following fundoplication include breakdown of the wrap, small bowel obstruction, gas-bloat syndrome, infection, retching, and dumping syndrome.

NURSING CARE

Nursing care is directed at (1) identifying children with symptoms suggestive of GER, (2) educating parents in home care, including feeding, positioning, and medications, and (3) if appropriate, providing care for the child undergoing surgical repair (see Surgical Procedures, Chapter 44). Early in the treatment program, parents should be reassured that most infants and children outgrow GER and often conservative lifestyle changes are sufficient. Parents need support and reassurance to implement lifestyle changes. Although it is not known if lifestyle changes bring additional benefit to patients receiving pharmacological interventions, some changes may be helpful. To help parents cope with the inconvenience of dealing with a child who spits up frequently, simple measures such as using bibs and protective cloths during and after feedings and prone positioning when holding the infant after feeding are beneficial.

It is important to educate and reassure parents about positioning. In the past, upright positioning was encouraged during sleeping for both infants and older children. However, the supine position for sleeping continues to be recommended. Parents should not place infants on their sides as an alternative to fully supine sleeping. Infant sleep positioners have been associated with 13 infant deaths since 1997 and should not be used to position infants on their sides for GER (Lawrence, Gantt, Samuels-Reid, et al., 2012).

Rescheduling of the family's routine may be required to accommodate more frequent feeding times. If parents thicken formula with cereal, they should also enlarge the nipple opening for easier sucking. Usually breastfeeding may continue, and the mother may provide more frequent feeding times or express the milk for thickening with rice cereal. Parents should avoid feeding the child spicy foods or any foods that aggravate symptoms in general. Mothers should avoid caffeine, chocolate, tobacco smoke, and alcohol when breastfeeding. Children should also avoid vigorous play after feedings, and feeding should occur just before bedtime.

When regurgitation is severe and growth is restricted, continuous NG tube or gastrostomy feedings may be considered; these feedings decrease the amount of emesis and provide constant buffering of gastric acid. Caregivers require special preparation when this type of nutritional therapy is indicated. See Chapter 44 for more information on tube feedings.

Older children and adolescents need to know that caffeine, chocolate, and spicy foods may weaken the LES and aggravate symptoms. Exposure to tobacco and alcohol are also associated with GER. Obesity increases abdominal pressure, thus weight management may reduce GER symptoms. When medical management is necessary, parents need information about the medications and their potential adverse effects. Prokinetic medications must be given before feedings. Medications for acid control must be timed to provide coverage and given regularly and as ordered.

The nurse can support the family by providing information about all aspects of treatment. Parents often require specific information about the medications given for GER. PPIs are most effective when administered 30 minutes before breakfast so that the peak plasma concentrations occur with mealtime. If they are given twice a day, the second best time for administration is 30 minutes before the evening meal. Parents need to be reassured of their efficacy because it takes several days of administration to achieve a steady state of acid suppression. A number of new formulations available in PPIs allow for more efficient administration. Some preparations are available in dissolvable pills. Powder and granule preparations are available as well. Many pharmacies compound the medication in a liquid form for administration.

Postoperative nursing care after the fundoplication is similar to that of other laparoscopy or open abdominal surgeries.

INTESTINAL PARASITIC DISEASES

Intestinal parasitic diseases, including helminths (worms) and protozoa, constitute the most frequent infections in the world. In Canada, the incidence of intestinal parasitic disease, especially giardiasis, has increased among young children who attend day care centres. Young children are especially at risk because of typical hand–mouth activity and uncontrolled fecal activity (AboutKidsHealth, 2010).

Intestinal parasitic diseases in humans are caused by various infecting organisms. This discussion is limited to the two common parasitic infections among children in Canada: giardiasis and pinworms. Table 46-6 describes the outstanding features of selected helminths that belong to the family of nematodes.

Giardiasis

Giardiasis is caused by the protozoan *Giardia lamblia* (also called *Giardia intestinalis, Giardia duodenalis,* and *Lamblia intestinalis*) and is sometimes called "beaver fever." Giardiasis occurs worldwide. Child care centres and institutions providing care for persons with developmental disabilities are common sites for giardiasis, and the children may pass cysts for months. Children under 5 years of age and adults 25 to 39 years (usually the parents of these children) are at increased risk of infection. The greatest number of cases are reported in the warmer months of the year, such as July to October (PHAC, 2012). Giardiasis should also be considered in those with a history of recent travel to an endemic area.

The potential for transmission is great, because the *cysts*—the nonmotile stage of the protozoa—can survive in the environment for months. Chief modes of transmission are person to person; contaminated water, especially in mountain lakes and streams and swimming or wading pools frequented by diapered infants (who have the condition); food; and animals, especially puppies (PHAC, 2012). In children person-to-person transmission is the most likely cause and is commonly seen in day care centres and institutions where staff or family become infected.

TABLE 46-6 SELECTED INTESTINAL PARASITES

CLINICAL MANIFESTATIONS	COMMENTS
Ascariasis—*Ascaris lumbricoides* (Common Roundworm)	
Light infections: asymptomatic	Transferred to mouth by way of contaminated food, fingers, or toys
Heavy infections: anorexia, irritability, nervousness, enlarged abdomen, weight loss, fever, intestinal colic	Largest of the intestinal helminths
Severe infections: intestinal obstruction, appendicitis, perforation of intestine with peritonitis, obstructive jaundice, lung involvement—pneumonitis	Affects principally young children 1–4 yr of age
	Prevalent in warm climates
Hookworm Disease—*Necator americanus*	
Light infections in well-nourished individuals: no problems	Transmitted by discharging eggs on the soil, which are picked up, causing infection from direct skin contact with contaminated soil
Heavier infections: mild to severe anemia, malnutrition	Wearing shoes is recommended, although children playing in contaminated soil expose many skin surfaces
May be itching and burning followed by erythema and a papular eruption in areas to which the organism migrates	
Strongyloidiasis—*Strongyloides stercoralis* (Threadworm)	
Light infection: asymptomatic	Transmission is same as for hookworm (direct contact with human skin), except autoinfection (organism can complete its life cycle in humans) is common
Heavy infection: respiratory signs and symptoms; abdominal pain, distension; nausea and vomiting; diarrhea—large, pale stools, often with mucus	Older children and adults affected more often than young children
Threat to life in children with weakened immunological defences	Severe infections may lead to severe nutritional deficiency
Elevated eosinophils may be the only manifestation	Prevalent in warm climates
Visceral Larva Migrans—*Toxocara canis* (Dogs); Intestinal Toxocariasis—*Toxocara cati* (Cats)	
Depends on reactivity of infected individual	Transmitted by ingestion of or contact with soil containing eggs from feces of infected dog or cat
May be asymptomatic except for eosinophilia	Dogs and cats should be kept away from areas where children play; sandboxes are especially comment transmission areas
Specific diagnosis difficult	More prevalent in hot, humid environments where eggs remain in soil
	Periodic deworming of diagnosed dogs and cats
	Control of dog and cat population
	Continued education and laws to prevent indiscriminate canine and feline defecation
Trichuriasis—*Trichuris trichiura* (Whipworm)	
Light infections: asymptomatic	Transmitted from contaminated soil or from vegetables grown in soil where eggs are present
Heavy infections: abdominal pain and distension, diarrhea	Most frequent in warm, moist climates
	Occurs most often in undernourished children living in unsanitary conditions

BOX 46-8 CLINICAL MANIFESTATIONS OF GIARDIASIS

Infants and young children:
- Diarrhea
- Vomiting
- Anorexia
- Growth failure

Children older than 5 years of age:
- Abdominal cramps
- Intermittent loose stools
- Constipation
- Stools may be malodourous, watery, pale, and greasy

Most infections resolve spontaneously in 4 to 6 weeks

Rarely, chronic form occurs:
- Intermittent loose, foul-smelling stools
- Possibility of abdominal bloating, flatulence, sulphur-tasting belches, epigastric pain, vomiting, headache, and weight loss

Although some individuals infected with giardiasis may be asymptomatic, common symptoms include abdominal cramps and diarrhea (Box 46-8).

Diagnosis of giardiasis may be made by microscopic examination of stool specimens or duodenal fluid or by identification of *G. lamblia* antigens in these specimens using techniques such as enzyme immunoassay (EIA). Because the *Giardia* organisms live in the upper intestine and are excreted in a highly variable pattern, repeated microscopic examination of stool specimens may be required to identify *trophozoites* (active parasites) or cysts. Duodenal specimens are obtained by direct aspiration, biopsy, or the *string* test. In the string test, the child swallows a gelatin capsule with a nylon string attached. Several hours later, the string is withdrawn, and the contents are sent for laboratory analysis. With the availability of EIA techniques to identify *Giardia* antigens in stool specimens, other tests are being used less often.

Therapeutic Management

The medications of choice for treatment of giardiasis are metronidazole (Flagyl), tinidazole (Tindamax), paromomycin (Humatin), and nitazoxanide (Alinia). Tinidazole is said to have an 80 to 100% cure rate after a single dose and has fewer adverse effects than metronidazole. Metronidazole and tinidazole have a metallic taste and GI adverse effects, including nausea and vomiting; nitazoxanide has no bitter taste and should be taken with food to avoid GI symptoms. (AAP Committee on Infectious Diseases, Kimberlin et al., 2015).

NURSING CARE

The most important nursing consideration in prevention of giardiasis is education of parents, child care centre staff, and those who are entrusted with the daily care of small children. Nurses can play an important role in educating parents of small children and day care staff regarding appropriate sanitation practices; attention to meticulous sanitary practices during diaper changes is essential (Fig. 46-4). In addition, young children who are infected or who have diarrhea should be discouraged from swimming in community or private pools until they are infection free. Lakes and streams may contain high numbers of *Giardia* spore cysts, which can be swallowed in the water. Children should be discouraged from swimming in stagnant bodies of water and in water where children who are known to be infected are swimming. *Giardia* organisms are said to be resistant to chlorine (Eisenstein, Bodager, & Ginzl, 2008). Parents should be encouraged to take small children to the restroom frequently when swimming, to keep children in diapers out in swimming areas, and to change diapers away from the water source. After children are infected, family education regarding medication administration is essential.

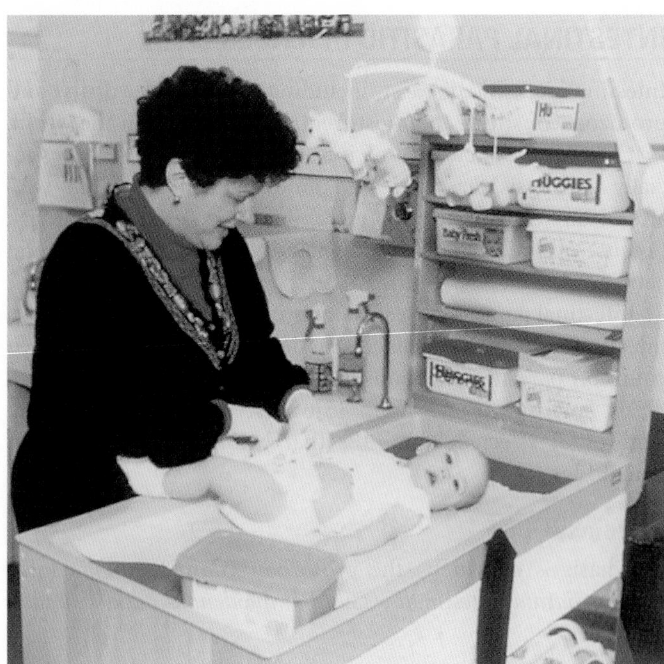

FIGURE 46-4 Prevention of giardiasis, especially in day care centres, requires sanitary practices during diaper changes, such as discarding paper diapers in a covered receptacle, changing paper covers on the diaper-changing surface, and having facilities for hand hygiene nearby. Note: Soiled cloth diapers and clothing should be stored in a plastic bag for transport home.

Enterobiasis (Pinworms)

Enterobiasis, or pinworms, caused by the nematode *Enterobius vermicularis*, is a common helminthic infection in Canada. It is universally present in temperate climatic zones and may infect more than 30% of all children at any one time. Crowded conditions such as in classrooms and day care centres favour transmission.

Infection begins when the eggs are ingested or inhaled (they float in the air). The eggs hatch in the upper intestine and then mature and migrate through the intestine. After mating, adult females migrate out the anus and lay eggs. The movement of the worms on skin and mucous membrane surfaces causes intense itching. As the child scratches, eggs are deposited on the hands and underneath the fingernails. The typical

BOX 46-9 CLINICAL MANIFESTATIONS OF PINWORMS

Intense perianal itching (principal symptom); evidence of itching in young children includes the following:
- General irritability
- Restlessness
- Poor sleep
- Bed-wetting
- Distractibility
- Short attention span

Perianal dermatitis and excoriation secondary to itching

If worms migrate, possible vaginal (vulvovaginitis) and urethral infection

hand-to-mouth activity of youngsters makes them especially prone to reinfection. Pinworm eggs persist in the indoor environment for 2 to 3 weeks, contaminating anything they contact, such as toilet seats, doorknobs, bed linen, underwear, and food. Except for the intense rectal itching associated with pinworms, the clinical manifestations are nonspecific (Box 46-9).

Diagnostic Evaluation

Diagnosis is most commonly made from the tape test (see Nursing Care). Repeated tests to collect eggs may be necessary, and if there is a possibility that other family members may be infected, a tape test should be performed on them.

Therapeutic Management

The medications available for treatment of pinworms include mebendazol (Vermox) and nonprescription pyrantel pamoate (Combatrin). The medication of choice is mebendazole, which is safe, effective, and convenient, with few adverse effects; however, it is not recommended for children younger than 2 years of age. If pyrvinium pamoate is prescribed, parents should be advised that the drug stains stool and vomitus bright red, as well as clothing or skin that comes in contact with it; it is available without prescription and should not be used in children under 2 years of age without consulting the primary practitioner. Because pinworms are easily transmitted, all household members are treated. The dose of antiparasitic medication should be repeated in 2 weeks to completely eradicate the parasite and prevent reinfection.

NURSING CARE

Nursing care is directed at identifying the parasite, eradicating the organism, and preventing reinfection. Parents need clear, detailed instructions for the tape test. A loop of transparent (not "frosted" or "magic") tape, sticky side out, is placed around the end of a tongue depressor, which is then firmly pressed against the child's perianal area. A convenient, commercially prepared tape is also available for this purpose. Pinworm specimens are collected in the morning as soon as the child awakens and *before* he or she has a bowel movement or bathes. The procedure may need to be performed on 3 or more consecutive days before eggs are collected. Parents should be instructed to place the tongue blade in a glass jar or loosely in a plastic bag so that it can be brought in for microscopic examination. For specimens collected in the hospital, practitioner's office, or clinic, the tape is placed smoothly on a glass slide, sticky side down, for examination.

Adherence to the medication regimen is usually excellent because the duration of treatment is typically only one dose. However, the family should be reminded of the need to take a second dose in 2 weeks to ensure eradication of the eggs.

To prevent reinfection, washing all clothes and bed linens in hot water and vacuuming the house may be recommended. However, there is little documentation on the effectiveness of these measures because pinworms survive on many surfaces. Helpful suggestions include hand hygiene after toileting and before eating, keeping the child's fingernails short to minimize the chance of ova collecting under the nails, dressing children in one-piece sleeping outfits, and daily showering rather than tub bathing. Families should be informed that recurrence is common. Repeated infections should be treated in the same manner as the first one.

INFLAMMATORY DISORDERS

Acute Appendicitis

Appendicitis, inflammation of the *vermiform appendix* (blind sac at the end of the cecum), is the most common cause of emergency abdominal surgery in childhood. In Canada, the pediatric appendicitis rates have been stable since 1993 at an average rate of 93.2 per 100,000 children (To & Langer, 2010). The average age of children with appendicitis is 10 years, with boys and girls equally affected before puberty and more cases occur in the spring and winter. Classically, the first symptom of appendicitis is periumbilical pain, followed by nausea, right lower quadrant pain, and later vomiting with fever. More than 50% of patients have an atypical presentation (Aiken & Oldham, 2016). Perforation of the appendix can occur within approximately 48 hours after the first sign of pain. At the time of initial presentation, about one third of all cases involve an already perforated appendix. Complications from appendiceal perforation include major abscess, phlegmon, enterocutaneous fistula, peritonitis, and partial bowel obstruction. A *phlegmon* is an acute suppurative inflammation of subcutaneous connective tissue that spreads.

Etiology

The cause of appendicitis is obstruction of the lumen of the appendix, usually by hardened fecal material (fecalith). Swollen lymphoid tissue, frequently occurring after a viral infection, can also obstruct the appendix. Another rare cause of obstruction is a parasite such as *Enterobius vermicularis*, or pinworms, which can obstruct the appendiceal lumen.

Pathophysiology

With acute obstruction, the outflow of mucus secretions is blocked, and pressure builds within the lumen, resulting in compression of blood vessels. The resulting ischemia is followed by ulceration of the epithelial lining and bacterial invasion. Subsequent necrosis causes perforation or rupture with fecal and bacterial contamination of the peritoneal cavity. The resulting inflammation spreads rapidly throughout the abdomen (*peritonitis*), especially in young children, who are unable to localize infection. Progressive peritoneal inflammation results in functional intestinal obstruction of the small bowel (*ileus*) because intense GI reflexes severely inhibit bowel motility. Because the peritoneum represents a major portion of total body surface, the loss of ECF to the peritoneal cavity leads to electrolyte imbalance and hypovolemic shock.

Diagnostic Evaluation

Diagnosis is not always straightforward. Fever, vomiting, abdominal pain, and an elevated white blood cell (WBC) count are associated with appendicitis but are also seen in IBD, pelvic inflammatory disease, gastroenteritis, urinary tract infection, right lower lobe pneumonia, mesenteric adenitis, Meckel's diverticulum, and intussusception. Prolonged symptoms and delayed diagnosis often occur in younger children, in whom the risk of perforation is greatest because of their inability to verbalize their symptoms. In addition to fever, signs of peritonitis include sudden relief from pain after perforation, subsequent increase in pain (usually diffuse and accompanied by rigid guarding of the abdomen), progressive abdominal distension, tachycardia, rapid shallow breathing, pallor, chills, and irritability.

The diagnosis is based primarily on the history and physical examination (Box 46-10). Pain, the cardinal feature, is initially generalized (usually periumbilical); however, it usually descends to the lower right quadrant. The most intense site of pain may be at *McBurney point*, located at a point midway between the anterior superior iliac crest and the umbilicus. Rebound tenderness is not a reliable sign and is extremely painful to the child. Referred pain, elicited by light percussion around the perimeter of the abdomen, indicates peritoneal irritation. Movement such as riding over bumps in an automobile or on a stretcher aggravates the pain. In addition to pain, significant clinical manifestations include fever, a change in behaviour, anorexia, and vomiting.

BOX 46-10 CLINICAL MANIFESTATIONS OF APPENDICITIS

- Right lower quadrant abdominal pain
- Fever
- Rigid abdomen
- Decreased or absent bowel sounds
- Vomiting (typically follows onset of pain)
- Constipation or diarrhea may be present
- Anorexia
- Tachycardia; rapid, shallow breathing
- Pallor
- Lethargy
- Irritability
- Stooped posture (guarding)

Laboratory studies usually include a CBC, urinalysis (to rule out a urinary tract infection), and, in adolescent females, serum human chorionic gonadotropin (to rule out an ectopic pregnancy). A WBC count greater than 10×10^6/L and an elevated C-reactive protein (CRP) are common but are not necessarily specific for appendicitis. An elevated percentage of bands (often referred to as "a shift to the left") may indicate an inflammatory process. CRP is an acute-phase reactant that rises within 12 hours of the onset of infection.

Computed tomography (CT) scan has become the imaging technique of choice, although ultrasonography may also be helpful and more often utilized in diagnosing appendicitis. Many practitioners prefer an ultrasound because of less radiation exposure than that with a CT scan (Pepper, Stanfill, & Pearl, 2012). A CT scan is considered positive in the presence of enlarged appendiceal diameter; appendiceal wall thickening; and periappendiceal inflammatory changes, including fat streaks, phlegmon, fluid collection, and extraluminal gas (Aiken & Oldham, 2016).

Therapeutic Management

Treatment of appendicitis before perforation includes rehydration, antibiotics, and surgical removal of the appendix (appendectomy). Laparoscopic surgery is now commonly used to treat nonperforated acute appendicitis and some surgeons will use laparoscopy with a perforated appendix (Aiken & Oldham, 2016). Recovery is rapid, and, if no complications occur, the hospital stay is short. A one-time dose of IV antibiotics may be administered before surgery.

Ruptured appendix. Management of the child diagnosed with peritonitis caused by a ruptured appendix often begins preoperatively with IV administration of fluid and electrolytes, systemic antibiotics, and NG compression. Postoperative management includes IV fluids, continued administration of antibiotics, and NG suction for abdominal decompression until intestinal activity returns. Sometimes surgeons close the wound after irrigation of the peritoneal cavity. Other times, they leave the wound open (delayed closure) to prevent wound infection. A Penrose drain may be used to permit transperitoneal drainage. Nonsurgical treatment for ruptured appendix is becoming more common. Treatment with antibiotics and image-guided drainage of any abdominal abscesses is now an accepted method of treatment (Whyte, Levin, & Harris, 2008).

Prognosis

Complications are uncommon after a simple appendectomy. The mortality rate for perforating appendicitis has improved from nearly certain death a century ago to less than 0.3% (Aiken & Oldham, 2016). Early recognition of the illness is essential to prevent complications.

NURSING CARE

Because abdominal pain is the most common childhood discomfort with appendicitis, it is important to assess the severity of pain (see Pain Assessment, Chapter 34). One of the most reliable estimates is the degree of change in behaviour. The younger, nonverbal child will assume a rigid, motionless, side-lying posture with the knees flexed on the abdomen, and there is decreased range of motion of the right hip. Older children may exhibit all of these behaviours along with abdominal pain. They can always indicate a point at which the pain is worse than at any other location.

> **! NURSING ALERT**
>
> In any instance when appendicitis is suspected, be aware of the danger of administering laxatives or enemas or applying heat to the area. Such measures stimulate bowel motility and increase the risk of perforation.

Postoperative Care

Postoperative care for the nonperforated appendix is the same as for most abdominal procedures. Care of the child with a ruptured appendix and peritonitis is more complex, and the course of recovery is considerably longer (usually 3 to 5 days of hospitalization). The child is maintained on IV fluids, nothing per mouth (NPO), and the NG tube is kept on low continuous gastric decompression until there is evidence of intestinal activity. Listening for bowel sounds and observing for other signs of bowel activity (e.g., passage of flatus or stool) are part of the routine assessment. Management of IV therapy is the same as for any child receiving fluids and parenteral antibiotics. A drain is often placed in the wound during surgery, and frequent dressing changes with meticulous skin care are essential to prevent excoriation of the area surrounding the surgical site. Wound care includes irrigation with antibacterial solution. If the wound is left open, a Montgomery strap or wound binder may be used to facilitate dressing changes and minimize tape removal and epidermal stripping. Early ambulation with adequate pain management assists in preventing many of the complications associated with prolonged bedrest and immobility (e.g., venous stasis, bowel hypomotility, abdominal pain from intestinal gas).

Management of pain from the incision and repeated dressing changes and irrigations are an essential part of the child's care. Psychological care of the child and parents is similar to that used in other emergency situations (see Emergency Admission, Chapter 43). Parents and older children may want to express their feelings and concerns regarding the events surrounding the illness and hospitalization. The nurse can provide education and psychosocial support to promote adequate coping and alleviate anxiety for both the child and the family. (See Nursing Care Plan: The Child with Appendicitis, available on Evolve.)

Meckel's Diverticulum

Meckel's diverticulum is a remnant of the fetal omphalomesenteric duct that connects the yolk sac with the primitive midgut during fetal life. Normally this structure is obliterated by the seventh to eighth week of gestation, when the placenta replaces the yolk sac as the source of nutrition for the fetus (Olson, Kim, & Donnelly, 2009). Failure of obliteration may result in an *omphalomesenteric fistula*, a fibrous band connecting the small intestine to the umbilicus, known as Meckel's diverticulum.

Meckel's diverticulum is a true diverticulum because it arises from the antimesenteric border of the small intestine and contains all layers of the intestinal wall with a separate blood supply from the vitelline artery. The diverticulum is usually found within 40 to 50 cm of the ileocecal valve and averages 1 to 10 cm in length.

Meckel's diverticulum is the most common congenital malformation of the GI tract and is present in 2 to 4% of the population (Pepper et al., 2012). Its occurrence in males and females is equal, but the incidence of complications is three to four times greater in males. Patients requiring surgery are generally younger than 10 years of age, and about 50% are younger than 2 years of age (Pepper et al., 2012).

Pathophysiology

Bleeding, obstruction, or inflammation causes the symptomatic complications of Meckel's diverticulum. Gastric mucosa is the most common ectopic tissue found. Bleeding, which is the most common problem in children, is caused by peptic ulceration or perforation because of the unbuffered acidic secretion. Several mechanisms can cause obstruction (Olson et al., 2009). Intussusception may be led by the diverticulum. Obstruction may also be caused by entanglement of the small intestine around a fibrous cord, trapping of a loop of intestine under the band, incarceration within a hernia sac, or volvulus of the intestinal segment containing the diverticulum. Diverticulitis occurs when peptic ulceration or obstruction leads to inflammation.

Diagnostic Evaluation

Diagnosis is usually based on the history, physical examination, and a specialized radiographic study but can be difficult to diagnose. The Meckel scan, a technetium-99m pertechnetate scan, detects the presence of gastric mucosa with an overall diagnostic accuracy of 90% but is less reliable with bleeding (Menezes, Tareen, Saeed, et al., 2008). CT scanning, wireless capsule endoscopy, and mesenteric angiography may be used to investigate complications (Thurley, Halliday, Somers, et al., 2009). Laboratory studies are usually part of the general workup to rule out any bleeding disorder and evaluate the severity of the anemia.

The most common clinical presentation in children includes painless rectal bleeding, abdominal pain, or signs of intestinal obstruction (Box 46-11). Bleeding, which may be mild or profuse, often appears as dark red or "currant jelly" stools; it may be significant enough to cause hypotension. Blood studies are performed to screen for bleeding disorders and anemia.

Therapeutic Management

The standard treatment is surgical removal of the diverticulum. When severe hemorrhage increases the surgical risk, interventions to correct hypovolemic shock, such as blood replacement, IV fluids, and oxygen, may be necessary. Antibiotics may be used preoperatively to control infection. If intestinal obstruction has occurred, appropriate preoperative measures are used to reverse electrolyte imbalances and minimize abdominal distension.

BOX 46-11 CLINICAL MANIFESTATIONS OF MECKEL'S DIVERTICULUM

Abdominal Pain
Similar to appendicitis
May be vague and recurrent

Bloody Stools*
Painless
Bright or dark red with mucus ("currant jelly" stool)
In infants, bleeding may be accompanied by pain

Sometimes
Severe anemia
Shock

*Often an initial sign.

Prognosis

If this condition is diagnosed and treated early, full recovery is likely. The mortality rate of untreated Meckel's diverticulum ranges from 2.5 to 15%. Complications of untreated Meckel's diverticulum include GI hemorrhage and bowel obstruction.

NURSING CARE

Nursing care is similar to that for any child undergoing surgery (see Chapter 43). Because the onset of this condition is often rapid, parents require psychological support. The massive intestinal bleeding that can accompany a Meckel's diverticulum is traumatic to both the child and the parents and may significantly affect their emotional reaction to hospitalization and surgery.

Specific preoperative considerations with intestinal bleeding include (1) frequent monitoring of vital signs and blood pressure for shock, (2) keeping the child on bedrest, and (3) recording the approximate amount of blood lost in stools. In the absence of frank hemorrhage, the nurse needs to test the stools for occult blood. Postoperatively, the child requires IV fluids and an NG tube for the decompression and evacuation of gastric contents. Pain management is essential.

With laparoscopic surgery use of an NG tube may be avoided. The nurse needs to monitor for signs of the return of normal bowel function.

Inflammatory Bowel Disease

Inflammatory bowel disease (IBD) is a term used for two forms of chronic intestinal inflammation: ulcerative colitis (UC) and Crohn's disease (CD). Although UC and CD have similar epidemiological, immunological, and clinical features, they are distinct disorders (Table 46-7).

TABLE 46-7 CLINICAL MANIFESTATIONS OF INFLAMMATORY BOWEL DISEASES

CHARACTERISTICS	ULCERATIVE COLITIS	CROHN'S DISEASE
Rectal bleeding	Common	Uncommon
Diarrhea	Often severe	Moderate to severe
Pain	Less frequent	Common
Anorexia	Mild or moderate	May be severe
Weight loss	Moderate	May be severe
Growth delay	Usually mild	May be severe
Anal and perianal lesions	Rare	Common
Fistulas and strictures	Rare	Common
Rashes	Mild	Mild
Joint pain	Mild to moderate	Mild to moderate

In addition to GI symptoms, both CD and UC are characterized by extraintestinal and systemic inflammatory responses. Exacerbations and remissions without complete resolution are also characteristics of IBD. Growth failure, which is particularly common in CD, is an important problem unique to the pediatric population. CD is more disabling, has more serious complications, and has less effective medical and surgical treatment than UC. Because UC is confined to the colon, theoretically it may be cured with a colectomy.

Approximately 0.5% of the Canadian population has IBD, which is one of the highest incidence and prevalence of IBD yet reported (Bernstein, Wajda, Svenson, et al., 2006). Ontario has one of the highest rates of childhood-onset IBD in the world, and there is an accelerated increase in incidence in younger children (Benchimol, Guttman, Griffiths, et al., 2009). IBD has increased in incidence in children 0 to 9 years old, but not in the 10- to 17-year age group (Benchimol, Mack, Guttmann, et al., 2015).

Etiology

Despite decades of research, the etiology of IBD is not completely understood, and there is no known cure. There is evidence to indicate a multifactorial etiology. Research has focused on theories of defective immunoregulation of the inflammatory response to bacteria or viruses in the GI tract in individuals with a genetic predisposition. In CD the chronic immune process is characterized by a T-helper-1 cytokine profile, whereas in UC the response is more humoral and mediated by T-helper-2 cells (Silbermintz & Markowitz, 2006).

There is an influence of genetics in the development of CD. Several CD susceptibility genes have been identified, including *NOD2/CARD15* on chromosome 16 associated with ileal disease, *IBD5* on chromosome 5, and *IBD6* on chromosome 6 (Sauer & Kugathasan, 2010). The influence of genetics in UC appears to be smaller than in CD; the *MDRI* gene has been associated with UC (Sauer & Kugathasan, 2010).

Environmental factors appear to play a role in the development of IBD. Breastfeeding decreases the risk of developing CD, whereas infantile diarrhea seems to increase the risk. Cigarette smoking also appears to be a risk factor for CD but appears to be protective against UC.

Pathophysiology of Ulcerative Colitis

The inflammation is limited to the colon and rectum, with the distal colon and rectum most severely affected. It affects the mucosa and submucosa and involves continuous segments along the length of the bowel with varying degrees of ulceration, bleeding, and edema. The presentation may be mild, moderate, or severe, depending on the extent of mucosal inflammation and systemic symptoms. Children with UC usually are seen with diarrhea, rectal bleeding, and abdominal pain, often associated with tenesmus and urgency. Thickening of the bowel wall and fibrosis are unusual, but long-standing disease can result in shortening of the colon and strictures. Extraintestinal manifestations are less common in UC than in CD. Toxic megacolon is the most dangerous form of severe colitis.

Pathophysiology of Crohn's Disease

The chronic inflammatory process of CD involves any part of the GI tract from the mouth to the anus but most often affects the terminal ileum. The disease involves all layers of the bowel wall (*transmural*) in a discontinuous fashion, meaning that between areas of intact mucosa there are areas of affected mucosa (*skip lesions*). The most common symptoms are abdominal pain, diarrhea, and decrease in appetite resulting in weight loss. Perianal disease, including skin tags, fistulas, and abscesses, occur in CD. Fever, growth delay, and delayed sexual development are seen commonly. Mild GI symptoms, poor growth, and extraintestinal manifestations may be present for several years before overt GI symptoms occur. The inflammation may result in ulcerations, fibrosis, adhesions, stiffening of the bowel wall, stricture formation, and fistulas to other loops of bowel, bladder, vagina, or skin. Extraintestinal manifestations include erythema nodosum, pyoderma gangrenosum, arthralgia and arthritis, uveitis and episcleritis, sclerosing cholangitis, autoimmune hepatitis, nephrolithiasis, and pneumonitis.

Diagnostic Evaluation

The diagnosis of UC and CD is derived from the history, physical examination, laboratory evaluation, and other diagnostic procedures. Laboratory tests include a CBC to evaluate anemia and an erythrocyte sedimentation rate or CRP to assess the systemic reaction to the inflammatory process. Levels of total protein, albumin, iron, zinc, magnesium, vitamin B_{12}, and fat-soluble vitamins may be low in children with CD. Stools are examined for blood, leukocytes, and infectious organisms. A serological panel is often used in combination with clinical findings to diagnose IBD and to differentiate between CD and UC. In IBD, autoantibodies called *antineutrophil cytoplasmic antibodies* (ANCAs) may be detected in the blood. The perinuclear antineutrophil cytoplasmic antibody (pANCA) is associated with UC. Approximately 60% of children with UC and 10% of those with CD are pANCA positive. Anti–*Saccharomyces cerevisiae* antibodies (ASCA) and anti–outer membrane porin of *E. coli* (anti-OmpC) have been found in up to 60% of children with CD (Anand, Russell, Tsuyuki, et al., 2008).

In patients with CD, an upper GI series with small bowel follow-through assists in assessing the existence, location, and extent of disease. Upper endoscopy and colonoscopy with biopsies are an integral part of diagnosing IBD. Endoscopy allows direct visualization of the surface of the GI tract so that the extent of inflammation and narrowing can be evaluated. CT and ultrasound also may be used to identify bowel wall inflammation, intra-abdominal abscesses, and fistulas. CD lesions may pierce the walls of the small intestine and colon, creating tracts called *fistulas* between the intestine and adjacent structures such as the bladder, anus, vagina, or skin.

Therapeutic Management

The goals of therapy are to (1) control the inflammatory process to reduce or eliminate the symptoms, (2) obtain long-term remission, (3) promote normal growth and development, and (4) allow as normal a lifestyle as possible. Treatment is individualized and managed according to the type and severity of the disease, its location, and the response to therapy. The course of IBD continues to be unpredictable with flareups that can severely impair physical and social functioning.

Medical treatment. The goal of any treatment regimen is first to induce remission of acute symptoms and then to maintain remission over time. Treatment with 5-aminosalicylates (5-ASAs) is effective in the induction and maintenance of remission in mild to moderate UC. Mesalamine, olsalazine, and balsalazide are now preferred over sulphasalazine because of reduced adverse effects (headache, nausea, vomiting, neutropenia, and oligospermia). Suppository and enema preparations of mesalamine are used to treat left-sided colitis. These medications decrease inflammation by inhibiting prostaglandin synthesis. 5-ASAs can be used to induce remission in mild CD. Corticosteroids, such as prednisone and prednisolone, are indicated in induction therapy in children with moderate to severe UC and CD. These agents inhibit the production of adhesion molecules, cytokines, and leukotrienes. Although these medications reduce the acute symptoms of IBD, they have adverse effects that relate to long-term use, including growth suppression (adrenal suppression), weight gain, and decreased bone density. High doses of IV corticosteroids may be administered in acute episodes and tapered according to clinical response. Budesonide, a synthetic corticosteroid, is designed for controlled release in the ileum and is indicated for ileal and right-sided colitis; budesonide has fewer adverse effects than prednisone and prednisolone. Rectal steroid therapy (enemas and foam-based preparations) is available for both induction and maintenance therapy in left-sided colitis.

Immunomodulators, such as azathioprine and its metabolite 6-mercaptopurine (6-MP), are used to induce and maintain remission in children with IBD who are steroid resistant or steroid dependent and in treating chronic draining fistulas. They block the synthesis of purine, thus inhibiting the ability of DNA and RNA to hinder lymphocyte function, especially that of T cells. Adverse effects include infection, pancreatitis, hepatitis, bone marrow toxicity, arthralgia, and malignancy. Methotrexate has also been shown to be useful in inducing and maintaining remission in CD patients unresponsive to standard therapies. Cyclosporine and tacrolimus have both been shown to be effective in inducing remission in severe steroid-dependent UC. 6-MP or azathioprine is then used to maintain remission. Patients on immunomodulating medications require regular monitoring of their CBC and differential to assess for changes that reflect suppression of the immune system, since many of the adverse effects can be prevented or managed by dose reduction or discontinuation of medication.

Antibiotics, such as metronidazole and ciprofloxacin, may be used as an adjunctive therapy to treat complications, such as perianal disease or small bowel bacterial overgrowth, in CD. Adverse effects of these medications are peripheral neuropathy, nausea, and a metallic taste.

Biological therapies act to regulate inflammatory and anti-inflammatory cytokines. Tumour necrosis factor-alpha (TNF-α) is believed to influence active inflammation. With the emergence of the biological agents, specifically the use of antitumour necrosis factor-alpha (TNF-α) agents such as adalimumab and infliximab, progress has been made in targeting a specific clinical response (Bradley & Oliva-Hemker, 2012; Ricart, García-Bosch, & Ordás, 2008). TNF-α is believed to influence active inflammation. Infliximab (Remicade) is a chimeric human-murine monoclonal antibody to TNF-α that is administered intravenously. Children appear to respond to infliximab similarly to adults. Infliximab is approved for the treatment of fistulas in CD and for systemic manifestations of IBD, such as ankylosing spondylitis, pyoderma gangrenosum, and chronic uveitis.

Nutritional support. Nutritional support is important in the treatment of IBD. Growth failure is a common serious complication, especially in CD. It is characterized by weight loss, alteration in body composition, restricted height, and delayed sexual maturation. Malnutrition causes the growth failure, and its etiology is multifactorial. Malnutrition occurs as a result of inadequate dietary intake, excessive GI losses, malabsorption, medication–nutrient interaction, and increased nutritional requirements. Inadequate dietary intake occurs with anorexia and episodes of increased disease activity. Excessive loss of nutrients (protein, blood, electrolytes, and minerals) occurs secondary to intestinal inflammation and diarrhea. Carbohydrate, lactose, fat, vitamin, and mineral malabsorption and vitamin B_{12} and folic acid deficiencies occur with disease episodes and with medication administration and when the terminal ileum is resected. Finally, nutritional requirements are increased with inflammation, fever, fistulas, and periods of rapid growth (e.g., adolescence).

The goals of nutritional support include (1) correction of nutrient deficits and replacement of ongoing losses, (2) provision of adequate energy and protein for healing, and (3) provision of adequate nutrients to promote normal growth. Nutritional support includes both enteral and parenteral nutrition. A well-balanced, high-protein, high-calorie diet is recommended for children whose symptoms do not prohibit an adequate oral intake. There is little evidence that avoiding specific foods influences the severity of the disease. Supplementation with multivitamins, iron, and folic acid is recommended.

Special enteral formulas, given either by mouth or continuous enteral (NG or gastrostomy) infusion (often at night), may be required. Elemental formulas are completely absorbed in the small intestine with almost no residue. Several studies have demonstrated that a diet consisting only of elemental formula not only improved nutritional status but also induced disease remission, either without steroids or with a diminished dosage of steroids required. An elemental diet is a safe and potentially effective primary therapy for patients with CD. Unfortunately, remission is not sustained when enteral feedings are discontinued unless maintenance medications are added to the treatment regimen.

TPN has also improved nutritional status in patients with IBD. Short-term remissions have been achieved after TPN, although complete bowel rest has not reduced inflammation or added to the benefits of improved nutrition by TPN. Nutritional support is less likely to induce a remission in UC than in CD. However, improvement of nutritional status is important in preventing deterioration of the patient's health status and in preparing the patient for surgery.

Surgical treatment. Surgery is indicated for UC when medical and nutritional therapies fail to prevent complications. Surgical options include a subtotal colectomy and ileostomy, leaving a rectal stump as a blind pouch. A reservoir pouch is created in the configuration of a J or S to help improve continence postoperatively. An ileoanal pull-through preserves the normal pathway for defecation. *Pouchitis*, an inflammation of the surgically created pouch, is the most common late complication of this procedure and has been reported to occur in up to 50% of cases. Metronidazole and ciprofloxacin are effective in treating pouchitis. Ciprofloxacin has fewer adverse effects. In many cases UC can be cured with a total colectomy.

Surgery may be required in children with CD when complications cannot be controlled by medical and nutritional therapy. Segmental intestinal resections are performed for small bowel obstructions, strictures, or fistulas. Partial colonic resection is not curative, and the disease often recurs.

Prognosis

IBD is a chronic disease. Relatively long periods of quiescent disease may follow exacerbations. The outcome of the disease is influenced by the regions and severity of involvement, as well as by appropriate therapeutic management. Malnutrition, growth failure, and bleeding are serious complications. The overall prognosis for UC is good.

The development of colorectal cancer (CRC) is a long-term complication of IBD. In UC the cumulative incidence of CRC is 2.5% after 20 years, increasing to 10.8% after 30 years (Rutter, Saunders, Wilkinson, et al., 2006). Surveillance colonoscopy with multiple biopsies should begin approximately 10 years after diagnosis of UC or CD and continue every 1 to 2 years. Removal of the diseased colon prevents development of CRC. However, in CD surgical removal of the affected colon does not prevent cancer from developing elsewhere in the GI tract.

NURSING CARE

The nursing considerations in the management of IBD extend beyond the immediate period of hospitalization. These interventions involve continued guidance of families in terms of (1) managing diet, (2) coping with factors that increase stress and emotional lability, (3) adjusting to a disease of remissions and exacerbations, and (4) when indicated, preparing the child and parents for the possibility of diversionary bowel surgery.

Because nutritional support is an essential part of therapy, encouraging the anorectic child to consume sufficient quantities of food is often a challenge. Successful interventions include involving the child in meal planning; encouraging small, frequent meals or snacks rather than three large meals a day; serving meals around medication schedules when diarrhea, mouth pain, and intestinal spasm are controlled; and preparing high-protein, high-calorie foods such as eggnog, milkshakes, cream soups, puddings, or custard (if lactose is tolerated) (see Feeding the Sick Child, Chapter 44). Foods that are known to aggravate the condition should be avoided. Using bran or a high-fibre diet for active IBD is questionable. Bran, even in small amounts, has been shown to worsen the patient's condition. Occasionally the occurrence of aphthous **stomatitis** (mouth ulcers) further complicates compliance with dietary management. Mouth care before eating and the selection of bland foods can help relieve the discomfort of mouth sores.

When NG feedings or TPN are indicated, nurses play an important role in explaining the purpose and expected outcomes of this therapy. The nurse should acknowledge the anxieties of the child and family members and give them adequate time to demonstrate the skills necessary to continue the therapy at home, if needed.

The importance of continued medication therapy despite remission of symptoms must be stressed to the child and family members. Failure to adhere to the pharmacological regimen can result in exacerbation of the disease. Unfortunately, exacerbation of IBD can occur even if the child and family adhere to the treatment regimen; this can be difficult for the child and family to cope with.

Family Support

The nurse needs to attend to the emotional components of the disease and assess any sources of stress. Frequently, the nurse can help children adjust to problems of growth restriction, delayed sexual maturation, dietary restrictions, feelings of being "different" or "sickly," inability to compete with peers, and necessary absence from school during exacerbations of the illness. See Chapter 40 for further information on coping with chronic illness.

If a permanent colectomy-ileostomy is required, the nurse can teach the child and family how to care for the ileostomy. The nurse can also emphasize the positive aspects of the surgery, particularly accelerated growth and sexual development, permanent recovery, eliminated risk of colon cancer in UC, and normality of life despite bowel diversion. Introducing the child and parents to other ostomy patients, especially children who are the same age, can be effective in fostering eventual acceptance. Whenever possible, continent ostomies should be offered as options to the child.

Because of the chronic and often lifelong nature of the disease, families may benefit from the educational services provided by organizations such as the Crohn's and Colitis Foundation of Canada (CCFC) (see Additional Resources at the end of this chapter). Adolescents often benefit by participating in peer-support groups, which are sponsored by the CCFC.

Peptic Ulcer Disease

Peptic ulcers may be classified as acute or chronic, and peptic ulcer disease (PUD) is a chronic condition that affects the stomach or duodenum. Ulcers are described as gastric or duodenal and as primary or secondary. A *gastric ulcer* involves the mucosa of the stomach; a *duodenal ulcer* involves the pylorus or duodenum. Most *primary ulcers* occur in the absence of a predisposing factor and tend to be chronic, occurring more frequently in the duodenum. *Stress ulcers* result from the stress of a severe underlying disease or injury (e.g., severe burns, sepsis, increased intracranial pressure, severe trauma, multisystem organ failure) and are more frequently acute and gastric. About 25% of hospitalized critically ill children have evidence of gastric bleeding (Blanchard & Czinn, 2016).

About 1.7% of children in general pediatric practices have PUD, and the disease represents about 3.4% per 10,000 of pediatric hospital admissions. Primary ulcers are more common in children older than 6 years, and stress ulcers are more common in infants younger than 6 months.

Etiology

The exact cause is unknown, although infectious, genetic, and environmental factors are important. There is an increased familial incidence, and the disease is increased in persons with blood group O.

There is a significant relationship between the bacterium *Helicobacter pylori* and ulcers. *H. pylori* is a microaerophilic, Gram-negative, slow-growing, spiral-shaped, and flagellated bacterium known to colonize the gastric mucosa in about half of the population of the world (Sung, Kuipers, & El-Serag, 2009). It has been identified in 90 to 100% of adult patients with PUD. *H. pylori* may cause ulcers by weakening the gastric mucosal barrier and allowing acid to damage the mucosa. It is believed that it is acquired via the fecal–oral route; this hypothesis is supported by finding viable *H. pylori* in feces.

In addition to ulcerogenic medications, both alcohol and smoking contribute to ulcer formation. There is no conclusive evidence to implicate particular foods such as caffeine-containing beverages or spicy foods, but polyunsaturated fats and fibre may play a role in ulcer formation. Psychological factors may play a role in the development of PUD, and stressful life events, dependency, passiveness, and hostility have all been implicated as contributing factors.

Pathophysiology

Most likely, the pathology is due to an imbalance between the destructive (cytotoxic) factors and defensive (cytoprotective) factors in the GI tract. The toxic mechanisms include acid, pepsin, medications such as aspirin and nonsteroidal anti-inflammatory drugs (NSAIDs), bile acids, and infection with *H. pylori*. The defensive factors include the mucus layer, local bicarbonate secretion, epithelial cell renewal, and mucosal blood flow. The primary mechanism that prevents the development of peptic ulcer is the secretion of mucus by the epithelial and mucous glands throughout the stomach. The thick mucus layer acts to diffuse acid from the lumen to the gastric mucosal surface, thus protecting the gastric epithelium. The stomach and duodenum produce bicarbonate, decreasing acidity on the epithelial cells and thereby minimizing the effects of the low pH. When abnormalities in the protective barrier exist, the mucosa is vulnerable to damage by acid and pepsin. Exogenous factors, such as aspirin and NSAIDs, cause gastric ulcers by inhibition of prostaglandin synthesis.

Zollinger-Ellison syndrome may occur in children who have multiple, large, or recurrent ulcers. This syndrome is characterized by hypersecretion of gastric acid, intractable ulcer disease, and intestinal malabsorption caused by a gastrin-secreting tumour of the pancreas.

Diagnostic Evaluation

Diagnosis is based on the history of symptoms, physical examination, and diagnostic testing. The focus is on symptoms such as epigastric abdominal pain, periumbilical pain, nocturnal pain, oral regurgitation, heartburn, weight loss, hematemesis, and melena (Box 46-12). History should include questions relating to the use of potentially causative substances such as NSAIDs, corticosteroids, alcohol, and tobacco. Children will often find it difficult to pinpoint the pain and move their hand in a circular motion around their stomach. The nurse can help differentiate the location by asking the child to point with one finger to the pain. Laboratory studies may include a CBC to detect anemia; stool analysis for occult blood; liver function tests (LFTs), sedimentation rate, or CRP (CRP measures the general levels of inflammation in the body) to evaluate IBD; amylase and lipase to evaluate pancreatitis; and gastric acid measurements to identify hypersecretion.

Radiographic studies such as an upper GI series may be performed to evaluate obstruction or malrotation. An upper endoscopy of the esophagus, stomach, and duodenum is the most reliable procedure to diagnose PUD. A biopsy is taken to determine the presence of *H. pylori. H. pylori* can also be diagnosed by a blood test that identifies the presence of the antigen to this organism. The C-urea breath test measures bacterial colonization in the gastric mucosa. This test is used to screen for *H. pylori* in adults and children. Polyclonal and monoclonal stool antigen tests are an accurate noninvasive method for both the initial diagnosis of *H. pylori* and the confirmation of its eradication after treatment. In children, upper endoscopy is recommended to evaluate and confirm *H. pylori* disease (Blanchard & Czinn, 2016).

BOX 46-12 CHARACTERISTICS OF PEPTIC ULCER DISEASE

Newborns

- Usually gastric and secondary to stress or critical illness
- Child commonly has a history of preterm birth, respiratory distress, sepsis, hypoglycemia, or an intraventricular hemorrhage
- Perforation may be first sign that massive bleeding may occur
- Hematemesis, feeding difficulty, crying episodes, or melena

Infants to 3-Year-Old Children

- Most likely to have a secondary ulcer located usually in the stomach or duodenum
- Primary ulcers less common and usually located in stomach
- Likely to occur in relation to illness, surgery, or trauma
- Hematemesis, melena, or perforation

3- to 6-Year-Old Children

- Primary or secondary ulcers
- Located equally in stomach and duodenum
- Perforation more likely in secondary ulcers
- Periumbilical pain, poor eating, vomiting, irritability, nighttime waking, hematemesis, melena

Children 6 Years and Older

- Usually primary and most often duodenal
- More typical of adult type
- Chance of recurrence greater
- Often associated with *Helicobacter pylori*
- Epigastric or vague abdominal pain
- Possibly nighttime waking, hematemesis, melena, and anemia

Therapeutic Management

The major goals of therapy for children with PUD are to relieve discomfort, promote healing, prevent complications, and prevent recurrence. Management is primarily medical and consists of administration of medications to treat the infection and reduce or neutralize gastric acid secretion. Antacids are beneficial medications to neutralize gastric acid. Histamine (H_2) receptor antagonists (antisecretory medications) act to suppress gastric acid production. Cimetidine (Tagamet), ranitidine (Zantac), and famotidine (Pepcid) are examples of these medications. They have few adverse effects. Cimetidine has many drug interactions so it must be used with caution.

PPIs, such as omeprazole and lansoprazole, act to inhibit the hydrogen ion pump in the parietal cells, thus blocking the production of acid. These drugs have been shown to be effective in children and adolescents but not in infants (van der Pol, Smits, Wijk, et al., 2011). They appear to be well tolerated and have infrequent adverse effects; short-term effects may include headache, diarrhea, nausea, and vomiting. Long-term implications are not yet fully known but may include decreased bone density because of decreased gastric absorption of calcium and hypergastrinemia (Hassall, Owen, Kerr, et al., 2011).

Mucosal protective agents, such as sucralfate and bismuth-containing preparations, may be prescribed for PUD. Sucralfate is an aluminum-containing agent that forms a protective barrier over ulcerated mucosa to protect against acid and pepsin. Sucralfate is available in both pill and liquid forms. Because sucralfate blocks the absorption of other medications, it should be given separately from them.

Triple medication therapy is the recommended treatment regimen for *H. pylori* (O'Connor, Gisbert, & O'Morain, 2009). Combination therapy has demonstrated 90% effectiveness in eradication of *H. pylori* when compared with antibiotic monotherapy. Examples of medication combinations used in triple therapy are (1) bismuth, clarithromycin, and metronidazole,

(2) lansoprazole, amoxicillin, and clarithromycin, and (3) metronidazole, clarithromycin, and omeprazole. Common adverse effects of medications include diarrhea, nausea, and vomiting. There is increased resistance to metronidazole and clarithromycin, which has led to failure in treatment; a 10- to 14-day treatment with bismuth-based quadruple therapy has been proposed instead (Luther, Chey, & Saad, et al., 2011). The effectiveness of probiotic treatment is still not clear, with conflicting literature on both sides (O'Connor et al., 2009).

Common adverse effects of medications include diarrhea and nausea and vomiting. In addition to medications, the child with PUD should be given a nutritious diet and advised to avoid caffeine. Adolescents should be warned about gastric irritation associated with alcohol use and smoking.

Children with an acute ulcer who have developed complications, such as significant hemorrhage, require emergency care. Surgical intervention may be required for complications such as hemorrhage, perforation, or gastric outlet obstruction.

Prognosis

The long-term prognosis for PUD is variable. Many ulcers are treated successfully with medical therapy; however, primary duodenal peptic ulcers often recur. The effect of maintenance medication therapy on long-term morbidity remains to be established with future studies.

NURSING CARE

The primary nursing goal is to promote healing of the ulcer through adherence to the medication regimen. If an analgesic–antipyretic is needed, acetaminophen, not aspirin or an NSAID, is used. Seriously ill newborns, infants, and children in critical care units should receive H_2 blockers to prevent stress ulcers. Critically ill children receiving IV H_2 blockers should have their gastric pH values checked at frequent intervals.

The role of stress in ulcer formation should be considered for nonhospitalized children with chronic illnesses. In children, many ulcers occur secondary to other conditions, and the nurse should be aware of family and environmental conditions that may aggravate or precipitate ulcers.

HEPATIC DISORDERS

Acute Hepatitis

Etiology

Hepatitis is an acute or chronic inflammation of the liver that can result from a number of different causes. These include viruses (e.g., Epstein-Barr, cytomegalovirus, HIV); metabolic, chemical, neoplastic, or anatomical issues (e.g., choledochal duct cyst and biliary atresia, medication reaction, or hemodynamic shock); heart failure and idiopathic sclerosing cholangitis and Reye syndrome; abscesses; amebiasis; autoimmune hepatitis; Wilson's disease; and α_1-antitrypsin deficiency and steatohepatitis. The following six viruses cause 90% of cases of viral hepatitis (Table 46-8):

1. Hepatitis A virus (HAV)
2. Hepatitis B virus (HBV)
3. Hepatitis C virus (HCV)
4. Hepatitis D virus (HDV)
5. Hepatitis E virus (HEV)
6. Hepatitis G virus (HGV)

Hepatitis A. Hepatitis A is the most common form of acute viral hepatitis in most parts of the world. It is a member of the picornavirus family. HAV infection is spread directly or indirectly via the fecal–oral route by ingestion of contaminated foods, direct exposure to infected fecal material, or close contact with an infected person. The virus is particularly prevalent in developing countries with poor living conditions, inadequate sanitation, crowding, and poor personal hygiene practices. The spread of HAV has been associated with improper food handling and with high-risk areas such as households with infected persons, residential centres for people with disabilities, and day care centres.

The average incubation period is about 4 weeks, with a range of 15 to 50 days. Fecal shedding of the virus can occur for 2 to 3 weeks before and for 1 week after the onset of jaundice. During this time, although the individual is asymptomatic, the virus is most likely to be transmitted. Infants with HAV infection are likely to be asymptomatic (anicteric hepatitis). Children often have diarrhea, and their symptoms are frequently attributed to gastroenteritis. Only 1 in 12 young children develops jaundice. HAV infection is self-limiting and does not result in chronic infection or chronic liver disease.

Although some cases may be prolonged, the prognosis is excellent. The HAV vaccine is highly effective. It is available in Canada and is recommended for persons at high risk of exposure or those travelling to an endemic geographical area (Cybulska, Ni, & Jimenenez-Rivera, 2011) (see Chapter 7, Hepatitis A). Usually, the hepatitis A vaccine is effective and is recommended over the immunoglobulin injection for people over 1 year of age. Immunoglobulin is the recommended postexposure immunoprophylactic agent for infants less than 1 year of age and for those in whom vaccination is contraindicated (previous adverse reactions to hepatitis A vaccine, severe latex allergy, or during a severe illness).

Hepatitis B. HBV infection can occur as an acute or chronic infection and may range from being asymptomatic and limited to causing fatal fulminant (rapid and severe) hepatitis. HBV rates vary greatly throughout the world. High-prevalence areas have been identified in Africa and Asia; Canada is considered a low-prevalence area. Transmission is usually via the parenteral route through the exchange of blood or any bodily secretions or fluids. Infections from blood transfusions have been reduced as a result of blood product–screening procedures. Transplantation of organs, intimate physical contact, transmission from mother to infant, and the splashing of contaminated fluids into the mouth or eyes are other sources of infection. Adults whose occupations are associated with exposure to blood or blood products (such as health care workers) are at increased risk for infection and should receive HBV vaccination.

Most HBV infection in children is acquired perinatally. Newborns are at risk for hepatitis if the mother is infected with HBV or was a carrier of HBV during pregnancy. Possible routes of maternal–fetal or maternal–infant transmission

TABLE 46-8 COMPARISON OF TYPES A, B, AND C HEPATITIS

CHARACTERISTICS	TYPE A	TYPE B	TYPE C
Incubation period	15–50 days, average 25–30 days	30–180 days, average 50 days	2 wk–6 mo, average 6–7 wk
Period of communicability	Believed to be later half of incubation period to first week after onset of clinical illness	Variable Virus in blood or other body fluids during late incubation period and acute stage of disease; may persist in carrier state for years to lifetime	Begins before onset of symptoms May persist in carrier state for years
Mode of transmission	Principal route—Fecal–oral Rarely—Parenteral	Principal route—Parenteral Less frequent route—Oral, sexual, any body fluid Perinatal transfer—Transplacental blood (last trimester), at birth, or during breastfeeding, especially if mother has cracked nipples	Principal route—Parenteral Nonparenteral spread possible
Clinical Features			
Onset	Usually rapid, acute	More insidious	Usually insidious
Fever	Common and early	Less frequent	Less frequent
Anorexia	Common	Mild to moderate	Mild to moderate
Nausea and vomiting	Common	Sometimes present	Mild to moderate
Rash	Rare	Common	Sometimes present
Arthralgia	Rare	Common	Rare
Pruritus	Rare	Sometimes present	Sometimes present
Jaundice	Present (many cases anicteric)	Present	Present
Other Features			
Immunity	Present after one attack; no crossover to type B or C	Present after one attack; no crossover to type A or C	Present after one attack; no crossover to type A or B
Carrier state	No	Yes	Yes
Chronic infection	No	Yes	Yes
Prophylaxis			
Immune globulin (Ig)	Passive immunity Successful, especially in early incubation period and pre-exposure prophylaxis	May provide passive immunity Inconsistent benefits; probably of no use	Not currently recommended
HAV vaccine	Two inactivated vaccines are approved for children ages 2–18 yr: Havrix and Vaqta; given in a two-dose schedule (6–12 mo between doses) Twinrix contains HAV and HBV for 18 years or older		
HBV Ig (HBIg)	No benefit	Provides passive immunity Postexposure protection possible (for 3–6 months) if given immediately after definite exposure	No benefit
HBV vaccine	No benefit	Postexposure if given immediately after definite exposure Provides active immunity Universal vaccination recommended for all children (either newborn or school age, depending on province or territory)	No benefit
Mortality Rate			
	0.1–0.2%	0.5–2.0% in uncomplicated cases; may be higher in complicated cases	1–2.0% in uncomplicated cases; may be higher in complicated case

HAV, hepatitis A virus; *HBV,* hepatitis B virus.

include (1) leakage of virus across the placenta late in pregnancy (less than 2% of cases) or during labour, and (2) ingestion of amniotic fluid or maternal blood. Infants who have HBV infection are more than 90% likely to become chronic carriers (Tran, 2009). In Canada, universal vaccination is recommended for all children (either newborn or school age, depending on province or territory). In jurisdictions where children do not receive HB vaccine in infancy, children at increased risk should be given HB-containing vaccine as soon as possible when the risk is identified (PHAC, 2016). The incubation period of HBV infection varies from 45 to 160 days (see Chapter 35, Recommendations for Routine Immunizations, p. 1017).

HBV infection occurs in children and adolescents in the following high-risk groups (see Box 7-5):

- Individuals with hemophilia and others who have received multiple transfusions
- Children and adolescents involved in IV drug use
- Institutionalized children and adolescents
- Preschool-age children in endemic areas
- Individuals engaged in sexual activity with infected partners

Hepatitis C. The highest risk factor for acquiring HCV is a history of injection drug use. HCV is transmitted through contaminated blood, especially as a result of IV drug use, and from mother to child. Approximately 5% of infected HCV mothers transmit HCV virus to their infants, but the rate varies according to the presence or absence of certain cofactors (particularly maternal coinfection with HIV) and medical conditions (Robinson & CPS, Infectious Diseases and Immunization Committee, 2008/2016) (see Chapter 7). Another common route of infection is by percutaneous exposure, which occurs through transfusion of blood or blood products, transplantation of organs or tissues, or sharing of used needles. Transfusion-associated HCV infection is low.

The clinical course of HCV infection varies. Incubation averages 6 to 7 weeks, with a range of 2 weeks to 6 months. Both acute and chronic HCV infection often produce only mild nonspecific symptoms or no symptoms at all. The length of time that maternal antibody is present in infants born to HCV-infected women must be considered, and screening should be done after the infant is 12 to 18 months old. This screening can be done after 2 months of age if there is significant parental concern or if there is a risk that the child may be lost to follow-up. However, a routine screening program, such as that for HBV, is not recommended. Current recommendations are to evaluate HCV-infected children at regular intervals to monitor for chronic hepatitis. Most children will be asymptomatic with evidence of chronic hepatitis on liver biopsy. Liver enzyme levels may fluctuate between periods of normal and elevated values (Robinson & CPS, Infectious Diseases and Immunization Committee, 2008/2016).

Hepatitis D. HDV is an important cause of acute and chronic liver disease. HDV is a defective RNA virus that requires the helper function of HBV. HDV infection occurs primarily in hemophiliac patients, people immigrating from endemic regions, and IV drug users. The incubation period is 2 to 8 weeks. Both acute and chronic forms are more severe than HBV infection and can lead to cirrhosis. Testing for HDV infection is recommended in children with chronic HBV infection or severe liver disease and in children with acute exacerbation of a previously stable liver disease.

Hepatitis E. HEV infection is enterally transmitted. Transmission may occur through the fecal–oral route or from contaminated water. The incubation period is 2 to 9 weeks. This illness is uncommon in children, does not cause chronic liver disease, is not a chronic condition, and has no carrier state. The mortality rate resulting from submassive hepatic necrosis is low except in pregnant women in their third trimester, in whom mortality reaches 10% (AAP, Committee on Infectious Diseases, Kimberlin et al., 2015).

Hepatitis G. HGV is a blood-borne virus that may also be transmitted by organ transplantation. High-risk groups include transfusion recipients, IV drug users, and individuals infected with HCV. Individuals with the virus are often asymptomatic, and most infections are chronic. The incubation period is unknown.

Pathophysiology

Pathological changes occur primarily in the parenchymal cells of the liver and result in varying degrees of swelling, infiltration of liver cells by mononuclear cells, and subsequent degeneration, necrosis, and fibrosis. Structural changes within the hepatocyte account for altered liver functions such as impaired bile excretion, elevated transaminase levels, and decreased albumin synthesis. Hepatitis can be self-limited, and complete regeneration of liver cells without scarring may occur. However, some forms of hepatitis do not result in complete return of liver function. These include *fulminant hepatitis,* which is characterized by a severe, acute course and massive destruction of the liver, resulting in liver failure and death in 1 to 2 weeks. *Subacute* or *chronic active hepatitis* is characterized by progressive liver destruction, uncertain regeneration, scarring, and potential cirrhosis.

The progression of liver disease is characterized according to histopathology by Ludwig's classification of four stages: (1) stage 1 is characterized by mononuclear inflammatory cells surrounding small bile ducts; (2) in stage 2 there is proliferation of small bile ductules; (3) stage 3 is characterized by fibrosis or scarring; and (4) stage 4 is cirrhosis (Angulo & Lindor, 2010).

The initial *anicteric* (absence of jaundice) *phase* usually lasts 5 to 7 days and is often mistaken for influenza. Symptoms include nausea, vomiting, extreme anorexia, malaise, easy fatigability, arthralgia, skin rashes, slight to moderate fever, and epigastric or upper right–quadrant abdominal pain. Dark urine is a symptom of the *icteric* (jaundice) *phase.* Pruritus may accompany jaundice and can be bothersome, but many children with acute viral hepatitis do not develop jaundice.

Diagnostic Evaluation

Diagnosis is based on the history (especially regarding possible exposure to a hepatitis virus); physical examination; and serological markers (antibodies or antigens) indicating the presence of active infection with hepatitis A, B, or C or previous infection. No LFT is specific for hepatitis, but serum aspartate

(AST) and serum aminotransferase (ALT) levels are markedly elevated. Serum bilirubin levels peak 5 to 10 days after clinical jaundice appears. When hepatitis is severe, albumin levels are depressed, and prothrombin times are increased. Histological evidence from liver biopsy may be required to establish the diagnosis and assess the severity of the liver disease. Serological markers indicate the antibodies or antigens formed in response to the specific virus and confirm the diagnosis. Serum immunological tests are not available to detect HAV antigen, but there are two HAV antibody tests: anti-HAV immunoglobulin G (IgG) and immunoglobulin M (IgM). Anti-HAV antibodies are present at the onset of the disease and persist for life. A positive anti-HAV antibody test result indicates acute infection, immunity from past infection, passive antibody acquisition (e.g., from transfusion, serum immunoglobulin infusion), or immunization. To diagnose an acute or recent HAV infection, a positive anti-HAV IgM test result that is present with the onset of the disease and that persists for only 2 or 3 days is required.

Diagnosis of hepatitis B is confirmed by the detection of various hepatitis virus antigens and the antibodies that are produced in response to the infection. These antibodies and antigens and their significance include the following:

- *HBsAg*—Hepatitis B surface antigen (found on the surface of the virus), indicating ongoing infection or carrier state
- *Anti-HBs*—Antibody to surface antigen HbsAg, indicating resolving or past infection
- *HBcAg*—Hepatitis B core antigen (found on the inner core of the virus), detected only in the liver
- *Anti-HBc*—Antibody to core antigen HbcAg, indicating ongoing or past infection
- *HBeAg*—Hepatitis Be antigen (another component of the HBV core), indicating active infection
- *Anti-HBe*—Antibody to HBeAg, indicating resolving or past infection
- *IgM anti-HBc*—IgM antibody to core antigen

Tests are available for detection of all the HBV antigens and antibodies except HBcAg. HBsAg is detectable during acute infection. The presence of HBsAg indicates that the individual has been infected with the hepatitis virus. If the infection is self-limiting, HBsAg disappears in most patients before serum anti-HBs can be detected (termed the *window phase of infection*). IgM anti-HBc is highly specific in establishing the diagnosis of acute infection and during the window phase in older children and adults. However, IgM anti-HBc usually is not present in perinatal HBV infection (AAP, Committee on Infectious Diseases, Kimberlin et al., 2015). Neonatal infection is most likely to occur in infants born to mothers who are HBeAg positive. In contrast, hepatitis B is much less likely to occur in infants whose mothers are HbsAg positive but HBeAg negative and who have antibodies to HBeAg.

Clinical improvement is usually associated with a decrease in or disappearance of these antigens followed by the appearance of their antibodies. For example, anti-HBc of the IgM class often occurs early in the disease followed by a rise in anti-HBc of the IgG class. Because the antibodies persist indefinitely, they are used to identify the carrier state (individuals with HBV who have no clinical disease but are able to transmit the organism). People with chronic HBV infection have circulating HBsAg and anti-HBc, and on rare occasions anti-HBsAg is present. Both anti-HBs and anti-HBc are detected in people with resolved infection, but anti-HBs alone is present in individuals who have been immunized with the HBV vaccine.

Hepatitis C virus RNA is the earliest serological marker for HCV. HCV-RNA can be detected during the incubation period before symptoms of HCV disease are expressed. A positive HCV-RNA result indicates active infection, and persistence of HCV-RNA indicates chronic infection. A negative test result correlates with resolution of the disease. HCV-RNA is also used to determine patient response to antiviral therapy for HCV.

An abdominal ultrasound scan provides measurement of liver size, detection of cystic lesions and stones, and imaging of the gallbladder. Cholescintigraphy radionuclide imaging detects abnormalities in liver uptake, concentration, and excretory function. Finally, a liver biopsy aids in assessing the severity of the disease.

The history of all patients should include questions to seek evidence of (1) contact with a person known to have hepatitis, especially a family member; (2) unsafe sanitation practices, such as contaminated drinking water; (3) ingestion of certain foods, such as clams or oysters (especially from polluted water); (4) multiple blood transfusions; (5) ingestion of hepatotoxic drugs, such as salicylates, sulphonamides, antineoplastic agents, acetaminophen, and anticonvulsants; and (6) parenteral administration of illicit drugs or sexual contact with a person who uses these drugs.

Therapeutic Management

Treatment options for viral hepatitis are limited. The goals of management include early detection, recognition of chronic liver disease, support and monitoring, and prevention of spread of the disease. HAV infection is an acute disease that resolves with support and management of symptoms. Treatment of HBV and HCV is directed at managing the viral load to prevent further destruction of the liver. Therapy depends on the cause and degree of inflammation. Currently, in children and adults, HBV and HCV are treated with interferons, naturally occurring proteins that exert antiviral, antiproliferative, and immunomodulatory effects. An interferon formulation, pegylated interferon, can be administered once a week and has been found to sustain plasma levels and enhance viral suppression. Interferon α-$_2$b has immunomodulatory and antiviral effects but needs a subcutaneous administration and has adverse effects of retinal changes, marrow suppression, and autoimmune disorders (Jensen & Balistreri, 2016). Lamivudine and adefovir are two other interferon analogs that suppress the replication of HBV and reduce the rate of antiviral resistance compared with lamivudine monotherapy. Telbivudine is more potent than lamivudine but has a high association with antiviral resistance compared with entocavir or tenofovir. A combination of α-pegylated interferon andribavirin may improve sustained virological response rates in children with HCV (Mack, Gonzalez-Peralta, Gupta, et al., 2012). Several specifically targeted antiviral therapies with protease and polymerase inhibitors are promising but are used with a combination of peylated and ribavirin, although further research is necessary before they can be used in children.

Another important aspect of the therapeutic management of hepatitis involves hospitalization, which is necessary if coagulopathy or fulminant hepatitis is present.

Prevention

Prophylactic use of standard immune globulin is effective in preventing HAV infection in situations of pre-exposure, such as anticipated travel to areas where HAV is prevalent, or in situations of postexposure within 2 weeks during the early part of the incubation period.

Hepatitis B immune globulin (HBIg) is effective in preventing HBV infection after one-time exposure, such as with a needlestick injury or coming in contact with mucous membrane materials, and for newborns whose mother is HBsAg positive and within 72 hours after birth. Immune globulin and HBIg must be administered less than 2 weeks after exposure.

Active immunizations are not available against HCV. It is possible to prevent HDV infection by preventing HBV infection.

Prognosis

The prognosis for children with hepatitis varies and depends on the type of virus and child's age and immune status. HAV and HEV usually cause a mild and brief illness with no carrier state. HBV causes a wide spectrum of acute and chronic illness. Approximately 5% of individuals with HBV develop chronic hepatitis B each year, and about half of these develop fulminant liver failure, leading to death in the absence of liver transplantation (PHAC, 2014). Hepatocellular carcinoma is a potentially fatal complication of HBV infection. HCV causes acute hepatitis that progresses to chronic hepatitis, but a small number of children go into spontaneous remission and others may develop cirrhosis. Of children with chronic hepatitis C, 25% develop cirrhosis, liver failure, and possible hepatocellular cancer. The highest mortality rate occurs with hepatitits D. Viral hepatitis causes approximately 50% of cases of fulminant hepatic failure and survival varies.

NURSING CARE

Nursing care depends on the severity of the hepatitis, the medical management, and factors influencing the control and transmission of the disease. Children with benign viral hepatitis are frequently cared for at home, and the nurse must explain the medical therapy and infection control measures to the family. If further assistance is needed for parents to follow through with the therapy, a home health nursing referral may be necessary.

A well-balanced diet and a realistic schedule of rest and activity adjusted to the child's condition should be encouraged. HAV is not infectious within a week after the onset of jaundice, and children may feel well enough to resume school. Parents need to be cautioned about administering any medication to the child, since normal dosages of many medications may become dangerous because of the liver's inability to detoxify and excrete them. Hand hygiene is the single most critical measure in reducing the risk of transmission. The nurse should explain to parents and children the ways in which HAV (oral–fecal route) and HBV (parenteral route) are spread. Routine precautions are carried out in the hospital, and children are not in a single room unless they have fecal incontinence. Toy sharing and sharing of personal items are discouraged.

Nurses caring for young people with HBV infection and a known or suspected history of IV drug use should help these teens realize the dangers of substance use. Nurses need to stress the parenteral mode of transmission of hepatitis and encourage patients to seek counselling through a substance use program.

HBV and HCV are chronic diseases that require frequent monitoring and management. Many communities have multidisciplinary clinics dedicated to the management of these diseases. The nurse should also address universal vaccination against HBV with the family.

Cirrhosis

Cirrhosis occurs at the end stage of many chronic liver diseases, including biliary atresia and chronic hepatitis. Cirrhosis can also result from infectious, autoimmune, or toxic factors and from chronic diseases such as hemophilia and cystic fibrosis. A cirrhotic liver is irreversibly damaged.

Clinical manifestations in children are similar to those seen with all chronic liver disorders. Children exhibit jaundice, poor growth, anorexia, muscle weakness, and lethargy. Ascites, edema, GI bleeding, anemia, and abdominal pain may be present with impaired intrahepatic blood flow. Pulmonary function may be impaired because of pressure against the diaphragm from hepatosplenomegaly and ascites. Dyspnea and cyanosis may occur, especially on exertion. Intrapulmonary arteriovenous shunts may develop and cause hypoxemia. Spider angiomas and prominent blood vessels are often present on the upper torso.

Therapeutic Management

There is no successful treatment to arrest the progression of cirrhosis. The goals of management include monitoring liver function and managing specific complications such as esophageal varices and malnutrition. Assessment of the child's degree of liver dysfunction is important so that the child can be evaluated for transplantation at the appropriate time. Liver transplantation has improved the prognosis substantially for many children with cirrhosis.

Nutritional support is important for children with cirrhosis and malnutrition. Supplements of fat-soluble vitamins and minerals are often required. Aggressive nutritional support with continuous tube feedings or parenteral nutrition may be needed.

Portal hypertension can cause esophageal and gastric varicies that are life-threatening. Acute hemorrhaging is managed with IV fluids, blood products, vasopressin, and gastric lavage. Balloon tamponade with a Senstaken-Blakemore tube may be needed. Endoscopic sclerotherapy and endoscopic banding ligation are effective in managing esophageal and gastric varices.

Ascites is treated by sodium restriction and diuretics. Severe ascites with respiratory compromise is treated by administration of albumin or by paracentesis.

Although the full mechanism of hepatic encephalopathy is unknown, failure of the damaged liver to remove endogenous toxins such as ammonia plays a role. Treatment is directed at limiting the ammonia formation and absorption that occur in the bowel, especially with the drugs neomycin and lactulose. Because ammonia is formed in the bowel by the action of bacteria on ingested protein, neomycin reduces the number of intestinal bacteria so less ammonia is produced. The fermentation of lactulose by colonic bacteria produces short-chain fatty acids, which lower the colonic pH, thereby inhibiting bacterial metabolism. This decreases the formation of ammonia from bacterial metabolism of protein.

Prognosis

Liver transplantation has revolutionized the approach to liver cirrhosis. Liver failure and cirrhosis are indications for transplantation. Careful monitoring of the child's condition and quality of life is necessary to evaluate the need for and timing of transplantation (see Family-Centred Teaching box).

Currently, liver transplant survival rates are 83 to 91% for 1-year survival and 82 to 83% for 5-year survival (Kamath & Olthoff, 2010). Increasing numbers of recipients are reaching their second decade after transplant. The increasing lifespan after transplantation is related to advances in immunosuppressants and surgical techniques as well as improved preoperative, intraoperative, and postoperative care. There still are many more children that need a liver transplant than there are available donors. One of the major issues in pediatric liver transplantation is the availability of suitable sized livers. The use of reduced-sized grafts, or split-liver donation, from liver donors has decreased the wait time for this population.

Postoperative care for liver transplantation is similar to that for other surgical procedures. There is special emphasis on prevention of infection, as patients are on multiple drugs, which cause immunosuppression.

NURSING CARE

Nursing care of the child with cirrhosis is determined by the cause of the cirrhosis, the severity of complications, and the prognosis. The prognosis for life is poor unless successful liver transplantation occurs. Nursing care of this child is similar to that for any child with a life-threatening illness (see Chapter 40). Hospitalization is required when complications such as hemorrhage, severe malnutrition, or hepatic failure occur. Nursing assessments are directed at monitoring the child's condition, and interventions are aimed at treatment of specific complications. If liver transplantation is an option, the family may need support and assistance to cope.

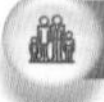

FAMILY-CENTRED TEACHING

End-Stage Liver Disease

In many cases the child and family must cope with an uncertain progression of the disease. The only hope for long-term survival may be liver transplantation. Transplantation can be successful, but the waiting period may be long, and there are many more children in need of organs than there are donors. The procedure is performed only at designated medical centres that are often far from the family's home. The nurse should recognize the unique stresses of coping with end-stage liver disease and waiting for transplantation and assist the family in coping with these stressors. The assistance of social workers and support from other parents can be beneficial.

Biliary Atresia

Biliary atresia (BA) or extrahepatic biliary atresia (EHBA) is a progressive inflammatory process that results in both intrahepatic and extrahepatic bile duct fibrosis that leads to eventual ductal obstruction. BA has been detected in 1 in 10,000 to 15,000 live births (Abdel-Kader & Balistreri, 2016). Associated malformations include polysplenia, intestinal atresia, and malrotation of the intestine. Untreated, BA usually leads to cirrhosis, liver failure, and death within the first 2 years of life.

Etiology and Pathophysiology

The exact cause of BA is unknown; it has been suggested that immune mechanisms or viral injury could cause the progressive inflammation that leads to complete obliteration of the bile ducts. Eighty-five percent of those with BA have complete obliteration of the extrahepatic biliary tree at or above the porta hepatis (Abdel-Kader & Balistreri, 2016).

Jaundice, manifesting with yellow discolouration of the skin or sclerae, is the most common early symptom of BA. Jaundice, indicating cholestasis (the accumulation of compounds that cannot be excreted because of occlusion or obstruction of the biliary tree), can be visible at a total serum bilirubin concentration as low as 85 mcmol/L. Direct hyperbilirubinemia first appears after the resolution of physiological (neonatal) jaundice. Jaundice is often associated with pale stool and dark urine. Histological study demonstrates bile duct remnants and a progressive inflammatory process.

In the fetal embryonic form of BA, which represents 10 to 35% of cases, there is a congenital absence of biliary ductal patency and an absence of bile duct remnants. Many infants have associated congenital anomalies. Varying degrees of cholestasis occur, resulting in retention of irritants and toxins. Injury to the liver occurs as the result of the inflammation caused by the cholestasis.

Diagnostic Evaluation

Early diagnosis is the key to survival of the child with BA. Infants who undergo surgery in the first 60 days of life have an 80% chance of establishing bile flow. Between 60 and 90 days of life, the chance of re-establishing flow drops to 50%, and after 90 days to 10% (Chen, Chang, Du, et al., 2006). The typical infant is thriving, appears well, and has only very mild jaundice during the first 6 to 8 weeks, but will soon begin failing to grow and thrive.

Several clinical signs may indicate the presence of BA (Box 46-13). Blood tests should include a CBC, electrolytes, bilirubin, and liver enzymes. Additional laboratory analyses,

BOX 46-13 CLINICAL MANIFESTATIONS OF EXTRAHEPATIC BILIARY ATRESIA

Jaundice
- Earliest manifestation and most striking feature of disorder
- First observed in sclera
- May be present at birth, but usually not apparent until age 2 to 3 weeks

Urine dark and stains diaper
Stools lighter than expected or white or tan
Hepatomegaly and abdominal distension common
Splenomegaly occurs later
Poor fat metabolism results in:
- Poor weight gain
- General growth failure

Pruritus
Irritability; difficulty comforting infant

including α_1-antitrypsin level, TORCH titres (see discussion of maternal infections in Chapter 29, p. 795), hepatitis serology, alpha-fetoprotein, urine cytomegalovirus, and a sweat chloride test, are indicated to rule out other conditions that cause persistent cholestasis and jaundice. Abdominal ultrasonography allows inspection of the liver and biliary system. Hepatobiliary scintigraphy demonstrates biliary patency but does not provide diagnostic certainty. Endoscopic retrograde cholangiopancreatography (ERCP) is performed in very young infants. This procedure, which is done using general anaesthesia, has an 80% reported diagnostic accuracy. Percutaneous liver biopsy is highly reliable when the biopsy contains specimens from a number of portal areas. Definitive diagnosis of BA is obtained during surgical laparotomy and an intraoperative cholangiogram.

Therapeutic Management

The primary treatment of BA is *hepatic portoenterostomy (Kasai procedure)*, in which a segment of intestine is anastomosed to the resected porta hepatis to attempt bile drainage. A Roux-en-Y jejunal limb is then anastomosed to the porta hepatis (a Y-shaped anastomosis) to provide bile drainage without reflux. This surgery has several variations, and successful bile drainage is achieved in approximately 80 to 90% of infants who undergo surgery when younger than 8 weeks of age (Abdel-Kader & Balistreri, 2016). However, progressive cirrhosis still occurs in many children, necessitating eventual liver transplantation. Prophylactic antibiotics are given after the Kasai procedure to minimize the risk of ascending cholangitis.

Medical management is primarily supportive. It includes nutritional support with breast milk or infant formulas that contain medium-chain triglycerides and essential fatty acids. Supplementation is usually required with fat-soluble vitamins (A, D, E, K), a multivitamin, and minerals, including iron, zinc, and selenium. Aggressive nutritional support with continuous gastrostomy feedings or TPN is indicated for moderate-to-severe growth failure. The enteral solution should be low in sodium. Phenobarbital may be prescribed after hepatic portoenterostomy to stimulate bile flow. Ursodeoxycholic acid is used to decrease cholestasis and treat intense pruritus and hypercholesterolemia. If the child has advanced liver damage, the management is the same as that for cirrhosis.

Prognosis

Untreated BA results in progressive cirrhosis and death in most children by 2 years of age. The Kasai procedure improves the prognosis but is not a cure. Biliary drainage can often be achieved if the surgery is done before the intrahepatic bile ducts are destroyed. Long-term survival has been reported in children who receive the Kasai procedure; however, even with successful bile drainage, many children ultimately develop liver failure.

Advances in surgical techniques and the use of immunosuppressive and antifungal medications have improved the success of transplantation. The major obstacle continues to be a shortage of donor livers. Reduced-size, split-liver transplantation, retransplantation, and increased public awareness may improve donor organ availability in the future.

NURSING CARE

Nursing interventions for the child with BA include support of the family before, during, and after surgical procedures and education regarding the treatment plan. In the postoperative period of a portoenterostomy, nursing care is similar to that after major abdominal surgery. Family members need education from the nurse regarding proper administration of medications and nutritional therapy, including special formulas, vitamin and mineral supplements, tube feedings, or parenteral nutrition in the home. In these infants, growth failure is common, and increased metabolic needs, combined with ascites, puritis, and nutritional anorexia, are major challenges for care. Pruritus can often be relieved by medication therapy or comfort measures such as colloidal oatmeal baths; trimming fingernails may help decrease the chance of secondary infection as a result of skin breakdown. The risks of BA, such as cholangitis, portal hypertension, GI bleeding, and ascites, need to be explained to the family.

Children and their families also need psychosocial support. The uncertain prognosis, discomfort, and waiting for transplantation produce stress, and hospitalizations, pharmacological therapy, and nutritional therapy impose financial burdens on the family. Families can receive help from the Canadian Liver Foundation, which provides educational materials, programs, and support systems (see Additional Resources at the end of this chapter).

STRUCTURAL DEFECTS

Cleft Lip or Cleft Palate

Clefts lip (CL) and cleft palate (CP) are facial malformations that occur during embryonic development and are the most common congenital deformities of the head and neck. They may appear separately or, more often, together. CL results from failure of the maxillary and median nasal processes to fuse; CP

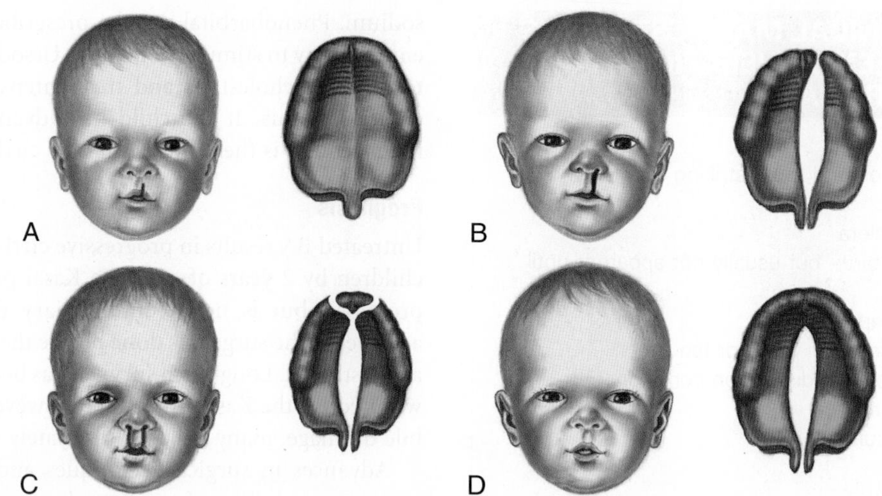

FIGURE 46-5 Variations in clefts of lip and palate at birth. **A:** Notch in vermilion border. **B:** Unilateral cleft lip and cleft palate. **C:** Bilateral cleft lip and cleft palate. **D:** Cleft palate.

is a midline fissure of the palate that results from failure of the two sides to fuse.

CL may vary from a small notch to a complete cleft extending into the base of the nose (Fig. 46-5). Clefts can be unilateral or bilateral. Deformed dental structures are associated with CL. CP alone occurs in the midline and may involve the soft and hard palates. The palate can be divided into primary and secondary palates. The primary one consists of the medial portion of the upper lip and the portion of the alveolar ridge that contains the central and lateral incisors. The secondary consists of the remaining portion of the hard palate and all of the soft palate. When associated with CL, the defect may involve the midline and extend into the soft palate on one or both sides (CL/P).

These malformations are two of the most common birth defects in Canada; the rate of CL/P is 9.4 per 10,000 and CP is 7.0 per 10,000; combined they affect 600 newborns every year. There is a higher incidence in certain ethnic groups, including the Indigenous populations (Government of Canada, 2013). Approximately 60 to 80% of children born with CL/P are male. Females have a higher frequency of isolated clefts of the secondary palate. Unilateral clefts are nine times more common than bilateral clefts and occur twice as frequently on the left side. Isolated bilateral CLs are uncommon; approximately 86% of those with bilateral CL also have palatal clefts (CL/P). Although the majority of clefts are nonsyndromic (have no associated identifiable syndrome), associated syndromes occur in varying frequencies according to the specific defect (Government of Canada, 2013). See Fig. 46-5 to see the variations in clefts of lip and palate at birth.

Etiology

Cleft deformities may be an isolated anomaly, or they may occur with a recognized syndrome. CL with or without CP is distinct from isolated CP. Clefts of the secondary palate alone are more likely to be associated with syndromes than is isolated CL or CL/P.

CL/P may be caused by exposure to teratogens such as alcohol, anticonvulsants, steroids, and retinoids and folic acid deficiency. Use of phenytoin during pregnancy is associated with a 10-fold increase in the incidence of CL. Multiple genetic and, to a lesser extent, environmental factors (e.g., maternal infection; tobacco exposure; radiation exposure; alcohol ingestion; and medications such as corticosteroids, some tranquilizers, and antiepileptics) appear to be involved in their development. Alcohol consumption (especially binge drinking) in the first trimester is associated with a higher incidence of oral clefts (DeRoo, Wilcox, Drevon, et al., 2008). The Canadian statistics suggest maternal obesity and smoking as possible risk factors for CL/P in infants (Government of Canada, 2013).

Pathophysiology

Cleft deformities represent a genetic defect in cell migration that results in a failure of the maxillary and premaxillary processes to come together between the third and twelfth week of embryonic development. Although often appearing together, CL and CP are distinct malformations embryologically, occurring at different times during the developmental process. Merging of the upper lip at the midline is completed between the seventh and eleventh weeks of gestation. Fusion of the secondary palate (hard and soft palate) takes place later, between the seventh and twelfth weeks of gestation. In the process of migrating to a horizontal position, the palates are separated by the tongue for a short time. If there is delay in this movement or if the tongue fails to descend soon enough, the remainder of development proceeds, but the palate never fuses.

Diagnostic Evaluation

CL with or without CP is apparent at birth. The defect elicits significant emotional reactions in parents. CP is less obvious than CL and may not be detected without a thorough assessment of the mouth. CP is identified when the examiner places a gloved finger directly on the palate. Clefts of the hard palate form a continuous opening between the mouth and the nasal cavity. The severity of the CP has an impact on feeding; the infant is unable to generate negative pressure and create suction in the oral cavity. This impairs feeding, even though in most cases the infant's ability to swallow is normal.

Prenatal diagnosis with fetal ultrasonography is not reliable until the soft tissues of the fetal face can be visualized at 13 to 14 weeks. The sensitivity of fetal ultrasound for facial clefting is almost 100% when CL/P is associated with other structural anomalies. In isolated CP, sensitivity may be 50%; an intact lip is the most difficult to diagnose prenatally (Robbins, Damiano, Druschel, et al., 2010).

Therapeutic Management

Treatment of the child with isolated CL is surgical and involves no long-term interventions other than possible scar revision. The management of CP involves the collaborative efforts of a multidisciplinary health care team, including pediatrics, plastic surgery, orthodontics, otolaryngology, speech/language pathology, audiology, nursing, and social work. Management is directed toward closure of the cleft(s), prevention of complications, and facilitation of normal growth and development in the child.

Surgical correction of cleft lip. The two most common procedures for repair of CL are the Tennison-Randall triangular flap (Z-plasty) and the Millard rotational advancement technique; Z-plasty is used less frequently. The difference between these two is that the Tennison-Randall procedure crosses the philtral line and the Millard procedure advances a triangle of tissue in the upper third of the lip and does not cross the midline. Surgeons often use a combination of these two techniques to address individual differences. Improved surgical techniques have minimized scar retraction, and in the absence of infection or trauma, healing occurs with little scar formation. Nasoalveolar moulding may also bring the cleft segments closer together before definitive CL repair and can reduce revisions. Optimal cosmetic results are difficult to obtain in severe defects. Surgical correction is usually performed at 10 weeks of age (or when infant weighs 4.5 kg). Additional revisions of the lip may be necessary at a later age.

Surgical correction of cleft palate. Previously, CP repair was postponed until a later age than the repair of the CL to take advantage of palatal changes that take place with normal growth. With advanced surgical and anaesthesia techniques, some surgeons are performing palatal repairs in the newborn period; however, the timing of repair remains controversial and may occur at 6 to 12 months to maximize speech production and growth of the midface (Chapman, Hardin-Jones, Goldstein, et al., 2008). Most surgeons prefer to close the cleft before the child develops faulty speech habits. Persistent velopharyngeal insufficiency, manifested by nasal regurgitation and hypernasal speech, may require a posterior pharyngeal flap procedure. Palatal bone grafting may be performed at a later time to build up bone in the alveolus.

Prognosis

Children with CL may require multiple surgeries to achieve optimal aesthetic outcomes but are still at risk for increased speech problems. Although some children with CP and CL/P do not require speech therapy, many have some degree of speech impairment that requires speech therapy at some point during childhood. Articulation errors result from a history of velopharyngeal dysfunction, incorrect articulatory placement, improper tooth alignment, and varying degrees of hearing loss. Improper drainage of the middle ear as a result of inefficient function of the eustachian tube contributes to recurrent otitis media and otitis media with effusion, which can cause scarring of the tympanic membrane, leading to hearing impairment in many children with CP. Myringotomy tubes are often used to drain the middle ear and help to prevent hearing loss (see Chapter 45). Upper respiratory tract infections require immediate and meticulous attention, and extensive orthodontics and prosthodontics may be needed to correct malposition of teeth and maxillary arches.

Long-term problems are related to the child's social adjustment. The better the physical care, the better is the chance for emotional and social adjustment, although the type of the defect and the degree of residual disability are not always directly related to a satisfactory adjustment. Physical defects can be a threat to self-image, and abnormal speech quality can be an impediment to social expression. Academic achievement, social adjustment, and behaviour should be monitored, particularly in children with syndromic cleft conditions.

NURSING CARE

The immediate nursing problems for an infant with CL or CP deformities are related to feeding. Parents of newborns with clefts place high priority on learning how to feed their infants and identify when they are sick, but they also express interest in learning about the infant's "normal" features. Whenever possible, they should be referred to a comprehensive CP team.

The nurse should encourage expression of any parental grief and fears; such expression may promote attachment in the preoperative period. It is especially important to emphasize the positive aspects of the infant's physical appearance and to express optimism regarding surgical correction while acknowledging the parents' concern. The manner of handling the infant should convey to the parents that the infant is indeed a precious human being.

Feeding

Feeding the newborn with CL, CP or CL/P can be difficult, and teaching the parent to successfully feed the child is perhaps one of the most significant and challenging nursing roles. Growth failure in infants with CL, CP, or both has been attributed to preoperative feeding difficulties. After surgical repair, most infants with isolated CL or CP and no associated syndrome gain weight successfully or achieve adequate weight and height for age.

CL may interfere with an infant's ability to achieve an adequate anterior lip seal. An infant with an isolated CL typically has no difficulty breastfeeding because the breast tissue is able to conform to the cleft. Cheek support (squeezing the cheeks together to decrease the width of the cleft) may be useful in improving lip seal during feeding.

Infants with CP and CL/P are often unable to feed using conventional methods before surgical management. CP reduces the infant's ability to suck, which interferes with breastfeeding and traditional bottle-feeding. Modifications to positioning, bottle selection, and feeder supportive techniques can help infants with CP feed efficiently. The infant with CP is placed in an upright position with the head supported by the caregiver's hand or cradled in the arm; this position allows gravity to assist with the flow of the liquid so it is swallowed instead of resulting in a loss of liquid through the nose.

Breastfeeding the infant with CL/P is a viable option and in some cases more successful than bottle-feeding. The nipple is positioned and stabilized well back in the oral cavity so that tongue action facilitates milk expression. However, the suction required to stimulate milk let-down may be absent initially; thus a breast pump may be useful before nursing to stimulate the let-down reflex. The advantages of breastfeeding include those described in Chapter 27; in addition, there is evidence that breastfeeding infants with CL/P is protective for otitis media (Lawrence & Lawrence, 2015).

Suction is almost certainly impaired in infants with CL/P because the velum is unable to elevate and separate the oral nasal cavities while generating adequate negative intraoral pressure. A number of special feeding devices are available for feeding the infant with CL/P, and some are more successful than others, depending on a number of factors (Fig. 46-6). One device is the Cleft Lip/Cleft Palate Nurser, which consists of a squeezable plastic bottle and a cross-cut nipple. The Special Needs Feeder may also be used successfully in infants with a poor or disorganized suck. The Special Needs Feeder has a specially designed valve and nipple to adjust the flow of milk to the infant and prevent choking or gagging. A Gravity Flow nipple attached to a squeezable plastic bottle allows formula to be deposited into the mouth of the infant with CL/P. The Pigeon bottle has a nipple with a Y-cut, and the nipple is slightly larger and more bulbous to fit naturally into the oral cavity. A one-way backflow valve prevents milk from flowing retrograde into the bottle to minimize the amount of air the infant swallows.

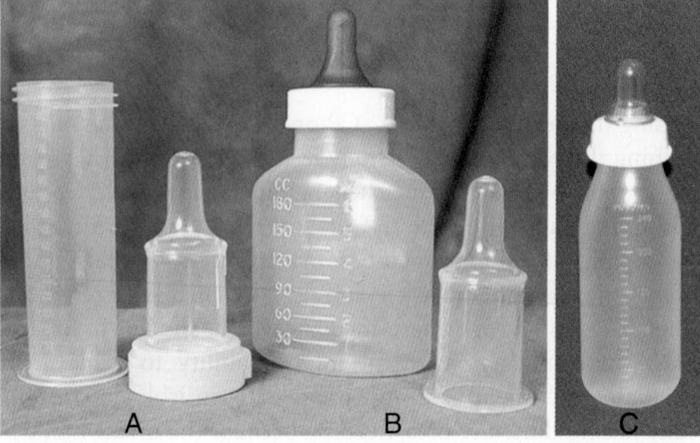

FIGURE 46-6 A: Haberman feeder. **B:** Mead-Johnson bottle used to feed infant with cleft lip and palate. **C:** Pigeon bottle. (**A** and **B**, Courtesy Texas Children's Hospital. **C**, Courtesy Paul Vincent Kuntz.)

Infants with clefts tend to swallow excessive air during feedings; thus it is important to pause during feedings and burp the infant. Some CP specialists advocate for the use of feeding obturators to help with feeding; these devices may increase compression surfaces within the oral cavity but do not improve feeding efficiency or growth within the first year of life (Masarei, Wade, Mars, et al., 2007).

Regardless of the feeding method used, the mother should begin to feed the infant as soon as possible. When maternal feeding is initiated early, the mother can help to determine the method best suited to her and the infant and can become adept in the technique before discharge from the hospital.

Preoperative Care

In preparation for surgical repair, parents are frequently taught to accustom the infant to the needs of the early postoperative period, especially if surgery is delayed for several months. The parents can use the postoperative feeding techniques a few days ahead of surgery. The infant must be positioned on the back or side postoperatively. Most infants tolerate these positions well because they are accustomed to being supine for sleeping. It is also helpful before admission to feed the infant with a rubber-tipped Asepto syringe or other device (e.g., soft Sipee cup) that will be used postoperatively.

Postoperative Care

The major efforts in the postoperative period are directed toward protecting the operative site.

For children with CL who have undergone surgery, parents may be advised to apply petroleum jelly to the operative site for several days after surgery. For infants with CL, CP, or CL/P, elbow immobilizers may be used to prevent the infant from rubbing or disturbing the suture line; they are applied immediately after surgery and may be used for 7 to 10 days. Some centres advocate using a syringe for feeding for 7 to 10 days after CL or CP repair. Adequate analgesia is required to relieve postoperative pain and prevent restlessness. Feeding is resumed when tolerated. An upright or infant seat position is helpful in the immediate postoperative period (especially for infants who have difficulty handling secretions).

The older infant or child may be discharged on a blenderized or soft diet, and parents are instructed to continue the diet until the surgeon directs them otherwise. Parents should be cautioned against allowing the child to eat hard items (e.g., toast, hard cookies, and potato chips) that can damage the repaired palate.

> **! NURSING ALERT**
>
> Avoid the use of suction or other objects in the mouth, such as tongue depressors, thermometers, pacifiers, spoons, or straws, following a palatoplasty to maintain the integrity of the surgically repaired palate.

Oral packing may be secured to the palate after palatoplasty; this packing is usually removed after 2 to 3 days. Sometimes the infant will have difficulty breathing after surgery because it is often necessary to alter an established pattern of breathing and adjust to breathing through the nose. This is frustrating but seldom requires more than positioning and support.

The expected outcomes are described in the Nursing Process: The Child With a Cleft Lip or Palate available on Evolve.

Long-Term Care

Children with any cleft often require a variety of services during recovery. Family members need support and encouragement from health care providers and guidance in activities that facilitate a normal outcome for their child. With the combined efforts of the family and the health team, most children achieve a satisfactory outcome. Many children with CL or CL/P have surgical correction that creates a near normal–appearing lip and permits good function. Parents need to understand the function of therapy, the purpose and care of all appliances, and the importance of establishing good mouth care and proper brushing habits.

Throughout the child's development, an important goal is the development of a healthy personality and self-esteem. Many communities have CP parents' groups that offer help and support to families (see Additional Resources at the end of this chapter).

Esophageal Atresia and Tracheoesophageal Fistula

Congenital atresia of the esophagus (EA) and tracheoesophageal fistula (TEF) are rare malformations that result from failed separation of the esophagus and trachea by the fourth week of gestation and failure of the trachea and esophagus to separate into distinct structures. These defects may occur as separate entities or in combination, and without early diagnosis and treatment they pose a serious threat to the infant's well-being.

Etiology

EA with or without an associated TEF is the most common esophageal malformation, occurring in approximately 1.7 per 10,000 live births (Khan & Orenstein, 2016). There appears to be an equal sex incidence, but the birth weight of most affected infants is significantly lower than average, and incidence of preterm birth is high. A history of maternal polyhydramnios is present in approximately 50% of infants with the defects.

EA/TEF is often present with the VATER or VACTERL syndromes, acronyms for syndromes involving a combination of *V*ertebral, *A*norectal, *C*ardiovascular, *T*racheo*E*sophageal, *R*enal, and *L*imb abnormalities. The cardiac and renal anomalies occur most frequently with EA/TEF. Other associated conditions include DiGeorge syndrome, Down syndrome, Pierre-Robin sequence, Fanconi syndrome, and CHARGE syndrome (*C*oloboma, *H*eart defects, choanal *A*tresia, developmental *R*estriction, *G*enital hypoplasia, and *E*ar deformities) (Guidry & McGahren, 2012).

Pathophysiology

The cause of EA/TEF is unknown. In the most frequently encountered form of EA and TEF (80 to 95% of cases), the proximal esophageal segment terminates in a blind pouch, and the distal segment is connected to the trachea or primary bronchus by a short fistula at or near the bifurcation (Fig. 46-7, C). The second most common variety (5 to 8%) consists of a blind pouch at each end, widely separated and with no communication to the trachea (see Fig. 46-7, A). Less frequently, in H-type EA (4 to 5%), an otherwise normal trachea and esophagus are connected by a common fistula (see Fig. 46-7, E). Extremely rare anomalies involve a fistula from the trachea to the upper esophageal segment (0.8%) (see Fig. 46-7, B) or to both the upper and lower segments (0.7 to 6%) (see Fig. 46-7, D).

Diagnostic Evaluation

TEF is suspected on the basis of clinical manifestations (Box 46-14). EA should also be suspected in cases of maternal polyhydramnios. Although the diagnosis is established on the basis of clinical signs and symptoms, the exact type of anomaly is determined by radiographic studies. A radiopaque catheter is inserted into the hypopharynx and advanced until it encounters an obstruction. Chest films are taken to ascertain esophageal

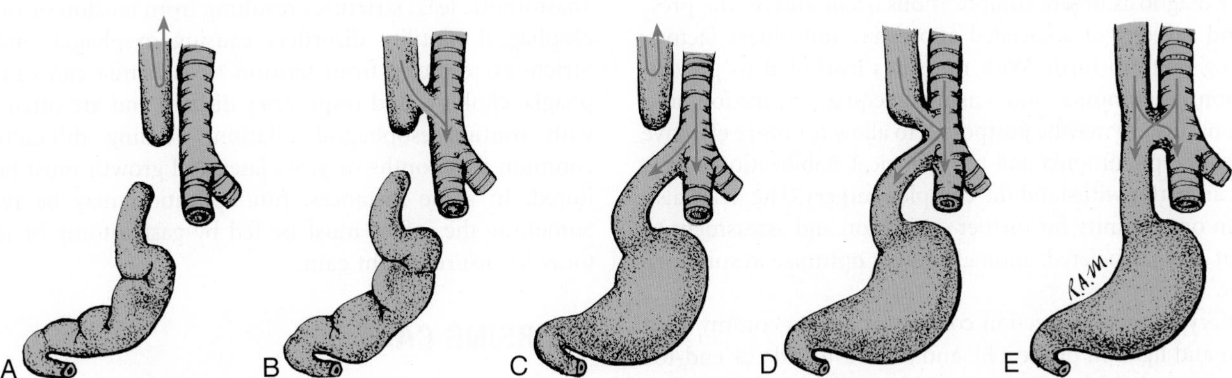

FIGURE 46-7 The five most common types of esophageal atresia and tracheosesophageal fistula. **A**: Esophageal atresia (blind pouch at each end). **B**: Fistula from upper esophageal segment to trachea. **C**: Esophageal pouch and distal segment is connected to the trachea. **D**: Fistula to upper and lower segment of esophagus from trachea. **E**: Normal esophagus and trachea connected by a fistula.

BOX 46-14 CLINICAL MANIFESTATIONS OF TRACHEOESOPHAGEAL FISTULA

Excessive salivation and drooling
Three C's of tracheoesophageal fistula:
- Coughing
- Choking
- Cyanosis

Apnea
Increased respiratory distress during and after feeding
Abdominal distension

patency or the presence and level of a blind pouch. Sometimes fistulas are not patent, which makes them more difficult to diagnose. The presence of gas in the stomach or small bowel is indicative of a coexisting TEF. Prenatal diagnosis is possible with ultrasonography or MRI, and planned delivery at a tertiary care centre is desirable (Guidry & McGahren, 2012).

Therapeutic Management

The treatment of infants with EA and TEF includes maintenance of a patent airway, prevention of pneumonia, gastric or blind pouch decompression, supportive therapy, and surgical repair of anomaly. EA is a surgical emergency. When EA/TEF is suspected, the infant is immediately taken off oral intake, started on IV fluids, and placed in the position least likely to cause aspiration of either mouth or stomach secretions (usual elevation of the head 30 to 45 degrees, as the infant's condition allows or prone). Removal of secretions from the mouth and upper pouch requires frequent or continuous suction. A double-lumen catheter should be positioned into the upper esophageal pouch and attached to intermittent or continuous low suction. The infant's head is kept upright to facilitate removal of fluid collected in the pouch and prevent aspiration of gastric contents. Aspiration pneumonia is almost inevitable in this instance and appears early; broad-spectrum antibiotic therapy is often instituted.

Most malformations can be corrected surgically in one operation or in two or more staged procedures. The success depends on early diagnosis before complications occur and on the presence and severity of associated anomalies and illness factors, including preterm birth. With measures instituted to prevent aspiration pneumonia and ensure adequate hydration and nutrition, surgery may be postponed to allow for more effective treatment of pneumonia and physiological stabilization so the infant can better withstand the complex surgery. The delay also offers an opportunity for further evaluation and assessment to rule out any associated anomalies and optimize respiratory support.

Primary surgical correction consists of a thoracotomy with division and ligation of the TEF and an end-to-side or end-to-end anastomosis of the esophagus. A chest tube may be inserted to drain intraplural fluid and air. This may consist of one operation or be staged with two or more procedures. For infants who are preterm, have multiple anomalies, or are in poor condition, a staged procedure is preferred that involves palliative measures, including gastrostomy, ligation of the TEF, and provision of constant drainage of the esophageal pouch. A delayed esophageal anastomosis is usually attempted after several weeks to months when the upper pouch elongates. Further surgical techniques may be performed later to facilitate esophageal lengthening. In some centres, thoracoscopic repair of EA/TEF has been successful, negating the need for a thoracotomy and thus minimizing associated operative complications and morbidities (Guidry & McGahren, 2012).

If an esophageal anastomosis cannot be accomplished, a gastrostomy is recommended. A cervical esophagostomy (to allow drainage of saliva through a stoma in the neck) used to be performed in cases of a long-gap atresia, but this is no longer recommended because it makes subsequent surgical repair more difficult (Kunisaki & Foker, 2012).

A primary anastomosis may be impossible because of insufficient length of the two segments of the esophagus. If the gap is 3 to 4 cm, it is called a long-gap EA, and in these cases an esophageal replacement procedure using a part of the colon or gastric tube interposition may be necessary to bridge the missing esophageal segment. An esophageal growth induction procedure may also be used (Kunisaki & Foker, 2012).

Up to 75% of infants with EA have *tracheomalacia*, but only 10 to 20% have significant *tracheomalacia*, which is a weakness in the tracheal wall that occurs when a dilated proximal pouch compresses the trachea in early fetal life or when the trachea does not develop normally because of a loss of intratracheal pressure. Signs of tracheomalacia include barking cough, stridor, wheezing, recurrent respiratory tract infections, cyanosis, and possibly apnea. If severe, surgical intervention may be required (Achildi & Grewal, 2007).

Prognosis

The prognosis is related to the birth weight, associated congenital anomalies, and time of diagnosis. The survival rate is nearly 100% in full-term infants without severe respiratory distress or other anomalies. Most deaths are the result of extreme prematurity or other lethal anomalies. In preterm low-birth-weight infants with associated anomalies, the incidence of complications is high. Complications of a primary repair include an anastomotic leak, strictures resulting from tension or ischemia, esophageal motility disorders causing dysphagia, and GER. Strictures resulting from tension or ischemia can cause dysphagia, choking, and respiratory distress and are often treated with routine esophageal dilation. Feeding difficulties are common for months or years later and growth must be monitored. In some instances, fundoplication may be required. Sometime the infant must be fed by gastrostomy or jejunostomy to ensure weight gain.

NURSING CARE

Nursing responsibility for detection of this malformation begins *immediately* after birth. Ideally, the diagnosis should be made before the initial feeding, but often it is not. If fed, the infant swallows normally but will suddenly cough and struggle, and the fluid is aspirated or returns through the nose and mouth. Early breastfeeding should not be prevented unless there is a strong suspicion of EA. If EA signs are present, the infant must have a patent airway established to prevent further respiratory compromise.

! NURSING ALERT

Any infant who has an excessive amount of frothy saliva in the mouth or difficulty with secretions and unexplained episodes of cyanosis should be suspected of having an EA/TEF and referred immediately for medical evaluation.

Cyanosis is usually the result of laryngospasm caused by overflow of saliva into the larynx from the proximal esophageal pouch. It normally clears after removal of the secretions from the oropharynx by suctioning. Any suspicion of TEF should be reported immediately. The infant is placed in an isolette or a radiant warmer, and oxygen is administered to help relieve respiratory distress. Intubation and assisted mechanical ventilation may be necessary if the infant is in respiratory distress. When a newborn is suspected of having a TEF, the most desirable position is supine with the head elevated at least 30 degrees. This position minimizes the reflux of gastric secretions up the distal esophagus into the trachea and bronchi.

It is imperative that the source of aspiration be removed at once. Oral fluids need to be withheld and the infant's fluid needs met parenterally. Until surgery, the blind pouch is kept empty by intermittent or continuous suction through an in-dwelling double-lumen nasal catheter that extends to the end of the pouch. The catheter needs attention because it has a tendency to become clogged with mucus. It is usually replaced daily. In the event that a staged repair is performed, a gastrostomy tube is inserted and left open so that air entering the stomach through the fistula can escape, thus minimizing the danger that gastric contents will be regurgitated into the trachea. The tube empties by gravity drainage. Feedings through the gastrostomy tube and irrigations with fluid are contraindicated before surgery in the infant with a distal TEF. Nursing interventions include respiratory assessment, airway management, thermoregulation, fluid and electrolyte management, and often nutritional (PN) support.

Postoperative Care

Postoperative care is essentially the same as that for any high-risk newborn. The infant is returned to the radiant warmer, and the gastrostomy tube is connected to gravity drainage until the infant can tolerate feedings. At this time, the tube is elevated and secured at a point above the level of the stomach. This allows gastric secretions to pass to the duodenum, and swallowed air can escape through the open tube. Tracheal suction should be done only using a premeasured catheter and with extreme caution to avoid injury to the suture line. If tolerated, gastrostomy feedings may be started and continued until the esophageal anastomosis is healed. Before oral feedings are initiated and the chest tube is removed, a contrast study or esophagram is performed to verify the integrity of the esophageal anastomosis. If a thoracotomy was done and a chest tube is inserted, the closed drainage system must be monitored closely. Pain control is important, particularly for the first 24 to 36 hours.

The nurse must observe the initial attempt at oral feeding carefully to make certain the infant is able to swallow without choking. Until the infant is able to take a sufficient amount by mouth, oral intake may need to be supplemented by bolus or continuous gastrostomy feedings. Ordinarily infants are not discharged until they can take oral fluids well. The gastrostomy tube may be removed before discharge or maintained for supplemental feedings at home.

Special Problems

Upper respiratory tract complications are a threat to life in both the preoperative and postoperative periods. In addition to pneumonia, there is a constant danger of respiratory distress resulting from atelectasis, pneumothorax, and laryngeal edema. Any persistent respiratory difficulty after removal of secretions is reported to the surgeon immediately. The infant is monitored for anastomotic leaks, as evidenced by purulent chest tube drainage, increased WBC count, and temperature instability.

Periodic esophageal dilations are often necessary in infants and children to manage strictures; the infant may show signs of choking or inability to swallow, thus indicating necessity for dilation. A significant number of infants develop GER after surgery and are placed on antireflux medications. Additional complications following EA repair include tracheomalacia and recurring TEFs (Achildi & Grewal, 2007).

In some infants awaiting esophageal replacement surgery, the catheter is removed, and the upper esophageal segment is drained through a cervical esophagostomy. An esophagostomy is difficult to care for because the skin becomes irritated by moisture from the continuous discharge of saliva. Frequent removal of drainage and application of a layer of protective ointment may remedy the problem. A dressing or ostomy appliance may be applied to collect the drainage, and an enterostomal therapist can provide additional guidance to prevent or treat skin breakdown.

For the infant who requires esophageal replacement, nonnutritive sucking is provided by a pacifier. Sometimes small amounts of water or formula are given orally; although the liquid drains from the esophagostomy, this process allows the infant to develop mature sucking patterns. Infants who remain NPO for an extended period or who have not received oral stimulation have difficulty eating by mouth after corrective surgery and may develop oral hypersensitivity and food aversion so oral stimulation is important. They require patient, firm guidance to learn how to take food into the mouth and swallow after repair. A referral to a multidisciplinary feeding behaviour program is often necessary.

As with any congenital anomaly, parents need support in adjusting to the child's condition. One difficulty is the immediate transfer of the sick newborn to the critical care unit and the length of hospitalization. Encouraging parents to visit the infant, participate in care when appropriate, and express their feelings regarding the infant's condition facilitates the attachment process. The nurse in the critical care unit should assume responsibility for ensuring that the parents are kept fully informed of the infant's progress.

Preparing parents for discharge involves teaching them skills they will need at home. They should be taught to observe for behaviours that indicate the need for suctioning and for signs of respiratory distress and constriction of the esophagus (e.g., poor feeding, dysphagia, drooling, regurgitation of undigested food). Discharge planning also includes obtaining the necessary equipment and home nursing services to provide home care.

Hernias

A *hernia* is a protrusion of a portion of an organ or organs through an abnormal opening. The danger from herniation arises when the organ protruding through the opening is constricted to the extent that circulation is impaired or when the protruding organs encroach on and impair the function of other structures. A hernia that cannot be reduced easily is called an *incarcerated hernia*. A *strangulated hernia* is one in which the blood supply to the herniated organ is impaired. The herniations of concern are those that protrude through the diaphragm, the abdominal wall, or the inguinal canal. The other hernias of significance to pediatric age groups are outlined in Table 46-9.

Omphalocele and Gastroschisis

Omphalocele and gastroschisis are two congenital defects that occur in the abdominal wall. They are rare, however, with omphalocele occurring in approximately 1 in 3000 to 10,000 live births, whereas the incidence of gastroschisis is 1 in 6000 live births (Blackburn, 2013). In Canada, the prevalence rate of gastroschisis between 2002 and 2009 was 3.7 per 10,000 total births. Interestingly, during this period a gradual increase in the prevalence was noted (Government of Canada, 2013).

Pathophysiology

An *omphalocele* is a covered defect of the umbilical ring into which varying amounts of the abdominal organs may herniate (Fig. 46-8). Although it is covered with a thin, often translucent peritoneal sac, the sac may rupture during or after birth. Many infants born with an omphalocele are preterm, and more than half have other defects involving the gastrointestinal, cardiac, genitourinary, musculoskeletal, and nervous systems.

Gastroschisis is the herniation of the bowel through a defect in the abdominal wall to the right of the umbilical cord. Unlike an omphalocele, there is no membrane covering the organs. In contrast to infants with omphalocele, there is less than 10 to 15% likelihood of associated anomalies, including intestinal atresia and cardiac anomalies.

Therapeutic Management and Nursing Care

The preoperative nursing care is similar for infants with either defect. Exposure of the viscera causes problems with thermoregulation and fluid and electrolyte balance. Before closure is performed, the exposed viscera are covered with moistened saline gauze and plastic wrap. Antibiotics, fluid and electrolyte replacement, gastric decompression, and thermoregulation are needed for physiological support. If complete closure is impossible because of the small size of the abdominal cavity and the large amount of viscera to be replaced, a Silastic silo pouch is created and sewn to the fascia of the abdominal defect. The defect is closed surgically after the reduction of contents is complete, which usually takes 7 to 10 days. With surgical treatment, nutritional support, and medical management, the prognosis has improved for infants born with an abdominal wall defect. It is estimated that more than 80% of infants born with omphalocele survive, as do more than 90% of those born with gastroschisis, although residual feeding difficulties such as GER are not uncommon.

OBSTRUCTIVE DISORDERS

Obstruction in the GI tract occurs when the passage of nutrients and secretions is impeded by a constricted or occluded lumen or when there is impaired motility (*paralytic ileus*). Obstructions may be congenital or acquired. Many congenital obstructions such as atresia, imperforate anus, meconium plug, and meconium ileus usually appear in the neonatal period. Other obstructions of congenital etiology such as malrotation, HD, volvulus, incarcerated hernia, and Meckel's diverticulum appear after the first few weeks of life. Intestinal obstruction from acquired causes such as intussusception, pyloric stenosis, and tumours may occur in infancy or childhood. Intestinal obstructions from any cause are characterized by similar signs and symptoms (Box 46-15).

Hypertrophic Pyloric Stenosis

Hypertrophic pyloric stenosis (HPS) occurs when the circumferential muscle of the pyloric sphincter becomes thickened, resulting in elongation and narrowing of the pyloric channel. This produces an outlet obstruction and compensatory dilation, hypertrophy, and hyperperistalsis of the stomach. This condition usually develops in the first 2 to 5 weeks of life, causing projectile nonbilious vomiting, dehydration, metabolic alkalosis, and eventually, growth failure. The precise etiology is unknown. The reported incidence is 1 per 1000 live births in Canada with a male/female ratio of 6:1 (Godwin, Sibbald, Bedard, et al., 2008). There is a genetic predisposition, and siblings and offspring of affected persons are at increased risk of developing HPS. It is more common in full-term than in preterm infants and is seen less frequently in Black and Asian infants than in White infants.

Pathophysiology

The circular muscle of the pylorus thickens as a result of hypertrophy (increased size) and hyperplasia (increased mass). This produces severe narrowing of the pyloric canal between the stomach and the duodenum, causing partial obstruction of the lumen (Fig. 46-9, A). Over time, inflammation and edema further reduce the size of the opening, resulting in complete

TABLE 46-9 SUMMARY OUTLINE OF HERNIAS

TYPE	MANIFESTATIONS/DIAGNOSTIC EVALUATION	MANAGEMENT
Diaphragmatic (Congenital)		
Protrusion of abdominal organs through opening in diaphragm, commonly on left side, causing severe respiratory compromise and inability to adequately expand affected lung, which may be hypoplastic (see Chapter 45)	**Symptoms:** Commonly severe respiratory distress at birth or within a few hours; tachypnea, cyanosis, dyspnea, absent breath sounds in affected area; impaired cardiac output; possible symptoms of shock, severe acidosis Milder cases may be seen after birth without severe respiratory distress. **Diagnosis:** Suspected on basis of symptoms—confirmed by radiographic study; often diagnosed prenatally as early as 25th week of gestation	**Therapeutic:** Provide prompt recognition, resuscitation, and stabilization. Avoid bag and mask ventilation in diagnosed or suspected CDH because this fills stomach with air and further compromises respiratory function. Provide supportive treatment of respiratory distress and correction of acidosis; possible use of endotracheal intubation, GI decompression. Additional treatments to reverse pulmonary hypertension may involve administration of inhaled nitric oxide, use of high-frequency oscillation, sildenafil, or ECMO. Administer prophylactic antibiotics. Perform surgical reduction of hernia and repair of defect after period of cardiorespiratory stabilization. **Nursing:** *Preoperative:* Monitor respiratory status; provide supplemental oxygen; assist with and monitor mechanical ventilation. Monitor cardiovascular status; support with inotropes may be necessary. Reduce stimulation—environmental and nursing care activities (cluster care to prevent constant interruptions). Maintain NG suction, oxygen, and IV fluids. Administer medications: sedation, muscular paralysis, inotropes, sildenafil (to reverse pulmonary hypertension). *Postoperative:* Carry out routine postoperative care and observation for acutely ill infant. Relieve pain and provide comfort. Support family because this is a critical illness.
Hiatal		
Sliding: Protrusion of an abdominal structure (usually stomach) through esophageal hiatus	**Symptoms:** Dysphagia, growth failure, vomiting, neck contortions, frequent unexplained respiratory problems, bleeding; usually associated with GER; may cause gastric volvulus and obstruction **Diagnosis:** Made by fluoroscopy	**Therapeutic:** Management of GER symptoms; positioning; pharmacological treatment; and dietary management Surgical treatment when complications are related to GER despite medical management **Nursing:** Be alert to significant signs and carry out routine postoperative care.
Abdominal		
Umbilical: Weakness in abdominal wall around umbilicus; incomplete closure of abdominal wall, allowing intestinal contents to protrude through opening	**Symptoms:** Noted by inspection and palpation of the abdomen High incidence in preterm and Black infants Usually closes spontaneously by 1–2 yr of age	**Therapeutic:** No treatment of small defects Operative repair if persists to age 4–6 yr or if defect is >1.5–2.0 cm by age 2 yr **Nursing:** Discourage use of home remedies (e.g., belly bands, coins) Reassure parents

Continued

TABLE 46-9 SUMMARY OUTLINE OF HERNIAS—cont'd

TYPE	MANIFESTATIONS/DIAGNOSTIC EVALUATION	MANAGEMENT
Omphalocele: Protrusion of intra-abdominal viscera into base of umbilical cord; sac is covered with peritoneum without skin	**Symptoms:** Usually obvious on inspection; however, small omphalocele may appear to be a hematoma in umbilical cord Observe for other malformations such as bladder exstrophy and hypospadias	**Therapeutic:** Surgical repair of defect *Preoperative:* Protect defect from trauma or drying. Keep sac or viscera moist with saline-soaked dressings. Maintain thermoregulation. Carry out routine care of IV fluids and line. Administer prophylactic antibiotics as prescribed. Provide nasogastric suction for gastric decompression. Keep patient NPO. Assess for associated birth defects such as CL or CP. *Postoperative:* Monitor vital signs and BP. Assess for and manage pain. Bowel decompression–NG tube IV fluid intake Monitor return of bowel function.
Gastroschisis: Protrusion of intra-abdominal contents through defect in abdominal wall lateral to umbilical ring; there is never a peritoneal sac covering the intestinal contents	Defect obvious at birth if not detected prenatally by ultrasonography	**Therapeutic:** Surgical repair of defect For large lesions provide gradual reduction of abdominal contents via Siloh pouch before surgical closure. **Nursing:** *Preoperative:* Keep sac covered with a bowel bag to prevent trauma, drying of viscera. NG decompression Maintain thermoregulation. Administer IV fluids. Administer antibiotics. Observe exposed bowel for signs of necrosis or constriction at exit site. *Postoperative:* Monitor vital signs and BP. Bowel decompression with NG tube Administer IV fluids. Assess for and manage pain. Monitor surgical closure site for infection. Monitor lower extremities for pulses and circulation (in case of vena cava compression by large bowel in small abdominal cavity). Monitor for return of bowel function and peristalsis. In event of Siloh pouch, nursing care should also include monitoring vital signs, keeping pouch clean, and aseptic technique with dressing changes (if not done by surgeon). Monitor lower extremities for circulation (as noted previously). Provide emotional support for parents. Long-term problems are associated with feeding and weight gain for gastroschisis and large omphalocele.

BP, blood pressure; *CDH,* congenital diaphragmatic hernia; *CL,* cleft lip; *CP,* cleft palate; *ECMO,* extracorporeal membrane oxygenation; *GER,* gastroesophageal reflux; *GI,* gastrointestinal; *IV,* intravenous; *NG,* nasogastric; *NPO,* nothing by mouth.

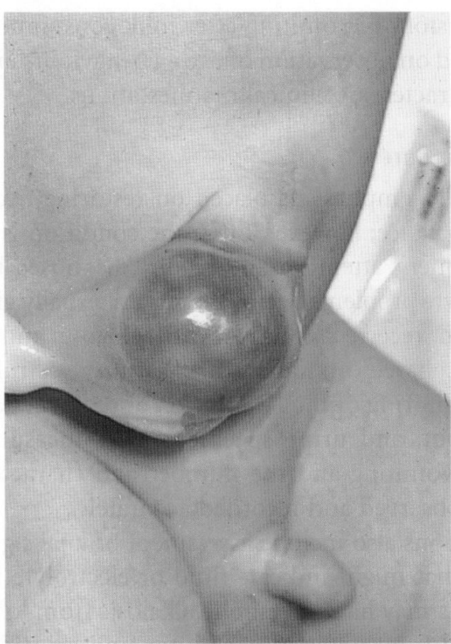

FIGURE 46-8 Omphalocele. (From O'Doherty, N. [1986]. *Neonatology: Micro atlas of the newborn*. Nutley, NJ: Hoffmann–La Roche. Used with permission of F. Hoffmann-La Roche Ltd.)

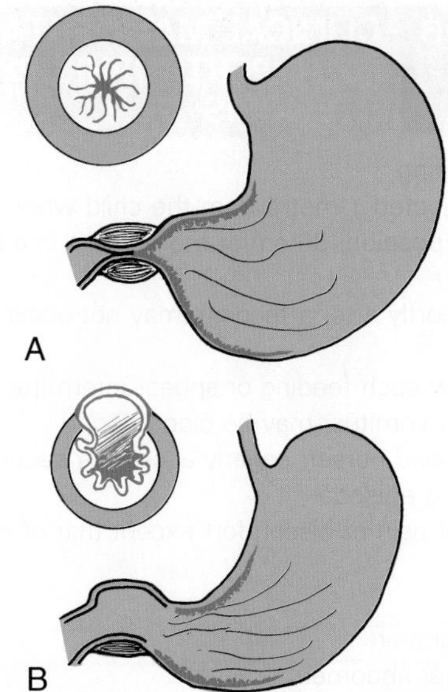

FIGURE 46-9 Hypertrophic pyloric stenosis. **A:** Enlarged muscular area nearly obliterates pyloric channel. **B:** Longitudinal surgical division of muscle down to submucosa establishes adequate passageway.

BOX 46-15 CLINICAL MANIFESTATIONS OF MECHANICAL OR PARALYTIC INTESTINAL OBSTRUCTION

Colicky abdominal pain—From peristalsis attempting to overcome the obstruction

Abdominal distension—As a result of accumulation of gas and fluid above the level of the obstruction

Vomiting—Often the earliest sign of a high obstruction; a later sign of lower obstruction (may be bilious or feculent)

Constipation and obstipation—Early signs of low obstructions; later signs of higher obstructions

Dehydration—From losses of large quantities of fluid and electrolytes into the intestine

Rigid and boardlike abdomen—From increased distension

Bowel sounds—Initially increased when peristalsis is trying to clear the obstruction. Gradually diminish and cease

Respiratory distress—Occurs as the diaphragm is pushed up into the pleural cavity

Shock—Plasma volume diminishes as fluids and electrolytes are lost from the bloodstream into the intestinal lumen (third spacing)

Sepsis—Caused by bacterial proliferation with invasion into the circulation

obstruction. The hypertrophied pylorus may be palpable as an olivelike mass in the upper abdomen. There is now substantial evidence to support decreased expression of neuronal nitric oxide synthase in the nerve fibres of the pyloric circular muscle in infants with HPS (Hunter & Liacouras, 2016). In most cases HPS is an isolated lesion; however, it may be associated with intestinal malrotation, esophageal and duodenal atresia, and anorectal anomalies. HPS has also been linked to the administration of erythromycin in the first few weeks of life as well as eosinophilic gastroenteritis, Apert syndrome, Cornelia de Lange syndrome, Zellweger syndrome, trisomy 18, and Smith-Lemli-Opitz syndrome (Hunter & Liacouras, 2016).

Diagnostic Evaluation

The diagnosis of HPS is often made after the history and physical examination. The olivelike mass is easily palpated when the stomach is empty, the infant is quiet, and the abdominal muscles are relaxed. Vomiting usually occurs 30 to 60 minutes after feeding and becomes projectile as the obstruction progresses. Emesis is nonbilious, usually consisting of stale milk. Often these infants become dehydrated and lethargic and eventually may appear significantly malnourished.

If the diagnosis is inconclusive from the history and physical signs (Box 46-16), ultrasonography will demonstrate an elongated, sausage-shaped mass with an elongated pyloric channel. The widespread availability of diagnostic ultrasonography has made the diagnosis and treatment more expedient. If ultrasound scanning fails to demonstrate a hypertrophied pylorus, upper GI radiography should be done to rule out other causes of vomiting. Laboratory findings reflect the metabolic alterations created by severe depletion of both fluid and electrolytes in the event that vomiting is prolonged and the condition remains undiagnosed. There are decreased serum levels of both sodium and potassium, although these may be masked by the hemoconcentration from ECF depletion. Of greater diagnostic value is a decrease in serum chloride levels and increases in pH and bicarbonate (carbon dioxide content) characteristic of metabolic alkalosis. The BUN level is elevated as evidence of dehydration. Hyperbilirubinemia (unconjugated) may also be present and often

BOX 46-16 CLINICAL MANIFESTATIONS OF HYPERTROPHIC PYLORIC STENOSIS

Projectile vomiting
- May be ejected 1 metre from the child when in a side-lying position, 30 cm or more when in a back-lying position
- Occurs shortly after a feeding (may not occur for several hours)
- May follow each feeding or appear intermittently
- Nonbilious vomitus; may be blood tinged

Infant hungry, avid nurser; eagerly accepts a second feeding after vomiting episode

No evidence of pain or discomfort except that of chronic hunger

Weight loss

Signs of dehydration

Distended upper abdomen

Readily palpable olive-shaped tumour in the epigastrium just to the right of the umbilicus

Visible gastric peristaltic waves that move from left to right across the epigastrium

resolves after surgical correction of the obstruction (Hunter & Liacouras, 2016).

Therapeutic Management

Surgical relief of the pyloric obstruction by **pyloromyotomy** (*Fredet-Ramstedt procedure*) is the standard treatment for this disorder. Before surgery, the infant must be rehydrated and the metabolic alkalosis must be corrected. Replacement fluid therapy may necessitate delay of surgery for 24 to 48 hours. The stomach may be decompressed by an NG tube. The procedure is performed through a right upper quadrant laparoscopic incision and consists of a longitudinal incision through the circular muscle fibres of the pylorus down to, but not including, the submucosa (see Fig. 46-9, B). The use of a small incision for the laparoscope results in shorter surgical time, more rapid postoperative feeding, and quicker discharge. The procedure has a high success rate when infants receive careful preoperative preparation to correct fluid and electrolyte imbalances.

Feedings are usually begun 3 to 6 hours postoperatively, beginning with small, frequent feedings of clear liquids followed by formula or breast milk as tolerated.

Prognosis

Most infants recover completely and rapidly after pyloromyotomy. Postoperative complications include persistent pyloric obstruction and wound dehiscence. Some infants also have GER.

NURSING CARE

The diagnosis of HPS is considered in the infant less than 6 to 8 weeks of age who appears alert but often fails to gain weight and has a history of vomiting after milk consumption. Assessment is based on observation of eating behaviours and evidence of other characteristic clinical manifestations.

Preoperative Care

Preoperatively, emphasis is placed on restoring hydration and electrolyte balance; however, often the condition is brought to the practitioner's attention and readily diagnosed before fluid and electrolyte problems occur. Infants are usually given no oral feedings and receive IV fluids with glucose and electrolyte replacement based on laboratory serum electrolyte values. Careful monitoring of the IV infusion and diligent attention to intake, output, and urine specific gravity measurements are important. Vomiting and the number and character of stools need to be observed and recorded accurately.

Observations also include assessment of vital signs, particularly those that might indicate fluid or electrolyte imbalances. These infants may have metabolic alkalosis from loss of hydrogen ions and from potassium, sodium, and chloride depletion if vomiting is prolonged. The skin, mucous membranes, and daily weight are assessed for alterations in hydration status and water gain or loss.

If stomach decompression and gastric lavage are used preoperatively, the nurse is responsible for ensuring that the tube is patent and functioning properly and for measuring and recording the type and amount of drainage. Infants who are receiving IV fluids or have an NG tube for continuous drainage must be observed to prevent the infusion device or tube from becoming dislodged.

General hygienic care, with attention to the skin and mouth in dehydrated infants, is essential. Protection from bacteria and viruses is also important because infants with impaired nutritional status tend to be more susceptible to infections. Parental involvement should be encouraged and promoted.

Postoperative Care

Postoperative vomiting may occur, and most infants, even with successful surgery, exhibit some vomiting during the first 24 to 48 hours because of edema resulting from the surgery. IV fluids are administered until the infant can retain adequate amounts by mouth. Observation of physical signs, monitoring of IV fluids, and careful recording of intake and output are maintained. The infant is also observed for evidence of pain, and appropriate analgesics are given.

Feedings are usually instituted soon after surgery, beginning with clear liquids and advancing to formula or breast milk as tolerated. They are offered slowly, in small amounts, and at frequent intervals as ordered by the practitioner. Observation and recording of feedings and the infant's responses to them are a vital part of postoperative care. Care of the operative site consists of observation for any drainage or signs of inflammation and care of the incision as directed by the surgeon.

Parents should be encouraged to remain with their child and become involved in the child's care as much as possible. Vomiting of a projectile nature is frightening to parents, and they often believe that they may have done something wrong or that surgery was not successful. Most parents need support and reassurance that the condition is caused by a structural problem and is in no way a reflection on their parenting skills and capacities.

Intussusception

Intussusception is the most common cause of intestinal obstruction in children between the ages of 3 months and 3 years (Pepper et al., 2012; Waseem & Rosenberg, 2008). Intussusception is more common in boys than in girls. Although specific intestinal lesions occur in a small percentage of the children, generally the cause is not known. More than 90% of intussusceptions do not have a pathological lead point such as a polyp, lymphoma, or Meckel's diverticulum. The idiopathic cases may be caused by hypertrophy of intestinal lymphoid tissue secondary to viral infection.

Pathophysiology

Intussusception occurs when one portion of bowel invaginates into a more distant portion of the bowel, pulling the mesentery with it. The mesentery is compressed and angled, resulting in lymphatic and venous obstruction. As the edema from the obstruction increases, pressure within the area of intussusception increases. When the pressure equals the arterial pressure, arterial blood flow stops, resulting in ischemia and the pouring of mucus into the intestine. Venous engorgement also leads to leaking of blood and mucus into the intestinal lumen, forming the classic currant jelly stools. The most common site is the ileocecal valve (ileocolic), where the ileum invaginates into the cecum and colon (Fig. 46-10). Other forms include ileoileal (one part of the ileum invaginates into another section of the ileum) and colocolic (one part of the colon invaginates into another area of the colon, usually in the area of the hepatic or splenic flexure or at some point along the transverse colon).

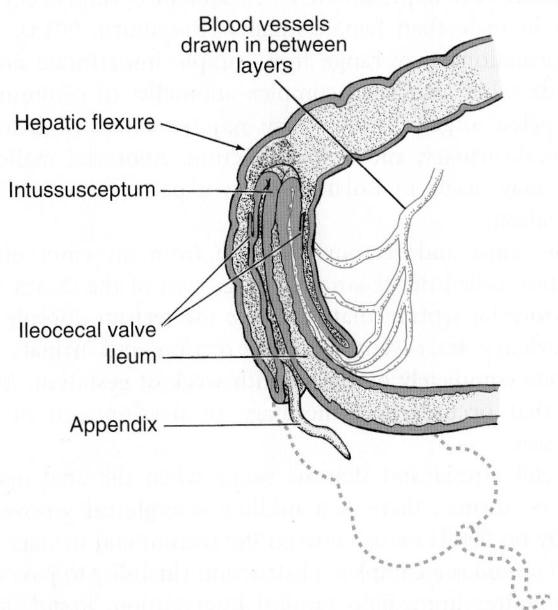

FIGURE 46-10 Ileocecal (ileocolic) intussusception.

> **! NURSING ALERT**
>
> The classic triad of intussusception symptoms (abdominal pain, abdominal mass, bloody stools) is present in 29 to 33% of children (Chu & Liacouras, 2016). Initially children might also be seen with screaming, irritability, lethargy, vomiting, diarrhea or constipation, fever, dehydration, and shock. Intussusception is potentially life-threatening; the nurse should be aware of alternative presentations; observe these children closely, and refer them for further evaluation.

Diagnostic Evaluation

Frequently subjective findings lead to the diagnosis (Box 46-17), which can be confirmed by ultrasound. Spontaneous reduction occurs in up to 10% of patients.

Therapeutic Management

Conservative treatment consists of radiologist-guided pneumoenema (air enema) with or without water-soluble contrast or ultrasound-guided hydrostatic (saline) enema to reduce the defect; the advantage of the latter is that no ionizing radiation is needed (Pepper et al., 2012). Recurrence of intussusception after conservative treatment occurs in about 1 in 10 patients; no predictable risk factors for recurrence have been identified. Herwig, Brenkert, and Losek (2009) found that hospitalized children needed minimal interventions after undergoing enema-reduced intussusception.

IV fluids, NG decompression, and antibiotic therapy may be used before hydrostatic reduction is attempted. If these procedures are not successful, the child may require surgical intervention. Surgery involves manually reducing the invagination and, when indicated, resecting any nonviable intestine.

Prognosis

Nonoperative reduction is successful in approximately 80% of cases (Huppertz, Soriano-Gabarró, Grimprel, et al., 2006). Surgery is required for patients in whom the contrast enema is unsuccessful. With early diagnosis and treatment, serious complications and death are uncommon.

> **BOX 46-17 CLINICAL MANIFESTATIONS OF INTUSSUSCEPTION**
>
> - Sudden acute abdominal pain
> - Child screaming and drawing the knees toward the chest
> - Child appearing normal and comfortable during intervals between episodes of pain
> - Vomiting
> - Lethargy
> - Passage of red, currant jelly–like stools (stool mixed with blood and mucus)
> - Tender, distended abdomen
> - Palpable sausage-shaped mass in upper right quadrant
> - Empty lower right quadrant (Dance sign)
> - Eventual fever, prostration, and other signs of peritonitis

NURSING CARE

The nurse can help establish a diagnosis by listening to the parent's description of the child's physical and behavioural symptoms. It is not unusual for parents to state that they thought something was seriously wrong before others shared their concerns. The description of the child's severe colicky abdominal pain combined with vomiting is a significant sign of intussusception.

As soon as a possible diagnosis of intussusception is made, the nurse should prepare the parents for the immediate need for hospitalization, the nonsurgical technique of hydrostatic reduction, and the possibility of surgery. It is important to explain the basic defect of intussusception. A model of the defect is easily demonstrated by pushing the end of a finger on a rubber glove back into itself or using the example of a telescoping rod. The principle of reduction by hydrostatic pressure can be simulated by filling the glove with water, which pushes the "finger" into a fully extended position.

Physical care of the child does not differ from that for any child undergoing abdominal surgery. Even though nonsurgical intervention may be successful, the usual preoperative procedures, such as maintenance of NPO status, routine laboratory testing (CBC and urinalysis), signed parental consent, and preanaesthetic sedation, are performed. For the child with signs of electrolyte imbalance, hemorrhage, or peritonitis, additional preparation, such as replacement fluids, whole blood or plasma, and NG suctioning, may be needed. Before surgery the nurse should monitor all stools.

> **! NURSING ALERT**
>
> Passage of a normal brown stool usually indicates that the intussusception has reduced itself. This should be immediately reported to the primary practitioner, who may choose to alter the diagnostic and therapeutic care plan.

Postprocedural care includes observations of vital signs, blood pressure, intact sutures and dressing, and the return of bowel sounds. After spontaneous or hydrostatic reduction, the nurse should observe for passage of water-soluble contrast material (if used) and the stool patterns, since the intussusception may recur. Children may be admitted to the hospital or monitored on an outpatient basis. A recurrence is treated with the conservative reduction techniques described previously, but a laparotomy is considered for multiple recurrences.

Malrotation and Volvulus

Pathophysiology

Malrotation of the intestine is caused by the abnormal rotation of the intestine around the superior mesenteric artery during embryological development. Malrotation may manifest in utero or may be asymptomatic throughout life. Infants with malrotation may have intermittent bilious vomiting, recurrent abdominal pain, distension, or lower GI bleeding. Malrotation is the most serious type of intestinal obstruction because, if the intestine undergoes complete volvulus (the intestine twisting around itself), compromise of the blood supply will result in intestinal necrosis, peritonitis, perforation, and death.

Diagnostic Evaluation

It is imperative that malrotation and volvulus be diagnosed promptly and surgical treatment instituted quickly. An upper GI series is the definitive procedure to diagnose this condition.

Therapeutic Management

Surgery is indicated to remove the affected area. Because of the extensive nature of some lesions, short-gut syndrome is a postoperative complication.

NURSING CARE

Preoperatively, the nursing care is the same as that provided to an infant or child with intestinal obstruction. Postoperatively, the nursing care is similar to that provided to the infant or child who has undergone abdominal surgery.

Nursing care is aimed at supporting the infant until surgical intervention can be carried out to eliminate the obstruction. Oral feedings are held, an NG tube is inserted for decompression, and IV therapy is initiated to provide needed fluids and electrolytes. In infants with an intestinal obstruction, surgery consists of resecting the obstructed area of bowel and anastomosing the unaffected bowel. In recent years, the survival rate for these infants has risen to 90 to 95% as a result of better treatments, improved neonatal intensive care, and an increased understanding of the problem.

Anorectal Malformations

Anorectal malformations are among the more common congenital malformations caused by abnormal development, with an incidence of approximately 1 in 5000 births and occur more often in male than female infants (Blackburn, 2013). These malformations may range from simple imperforate anus to include other associated complex anomalies of genitourinary and pelvic organs, which may require extensive treatment for fecal, urinary, and sexual function. Anorectal malformations may occur in isolation or as a part of the VACTERL association.

The anus and rectum originate from an embryological structure called the *cloaca*. Lateral growth of the cloaca forms the urorectal septum that separates the rectum dorsally from the urinary tract ventrally. The rectum and urinary tract separate completely by the seventh week of gestation. Anomalies that occur reflect the stage of development of these processes.

Rectal atresia and stenosis occur when the anal opening appears normal, there is a midline intergluteal groove, and usually no fistula exists between the rectum and urinary tract. *Rectal atresia* is a complete obstruction (inability to pass stool) and requires immediate surgical intervention. *Rectal stenosis* may not become apparent until later in infancy when the infant

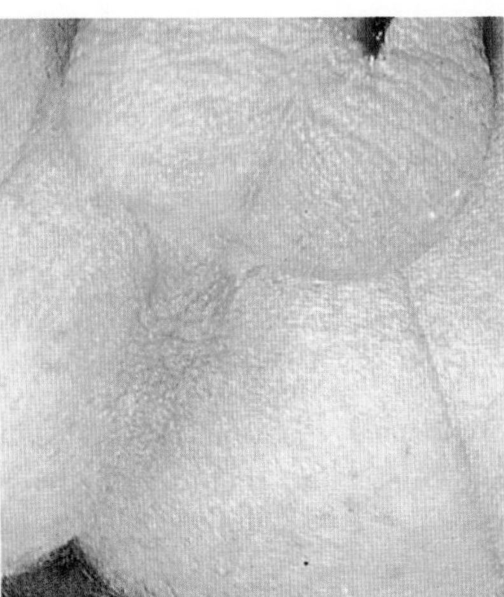

FIGURE 46-11 Anorectal malformation (imperforate anus). (From Chessell, G., Jamieson, M. J., & Morton, M. [1984]. *Diagnostic picture tests in clinical medicine: Vol. 2.* St. Louis: Mosby-Wolfe.)

has a history of difficult stooling, abdominal distension, and ribbonlike stools.

A *persistent cloaca* is a complex anorectal malformation in which the rectum, vagina, and urethra drain into a common channel that opens onto the perineum via the usual urethral site. *Cloacal exstrophy* is a rare, severe defect in which there is externalization of the bladder and bowel through the abdominal wall. Often the genitalia are indefinite, and chromosome studies are necessary to determine the child's gender, which is almost always female. The exstrophic bladder is separated into two halves by the cecum; other features may include an omphalocele, imperforate anus, and, at times, a neural tube defect.

Imperforate anus includes several forms of malformation without an obvious anal opening (Fig. 46-11). Frequently a *fistula* (an abnormal communication) leads from the distal rectum to the perineum or genitourinary system. The fistula may be evidenced when meconium is evacuated through the vaginal opening, the perineum below the vagina, the male urethra, or the perineum under the scrotum. A fistula may not be apparent at birth, but as peristalsis increases, meconium is forced through the fistula into the urethra or onto the newborn's perineum.

Anorectal anomalies are classified according to gender and abnormal anatomical features, including genitourinary and associated pelvic anomalies (Box 46-18). The level of rectal descent is determined by the relationship of the termination of the bowel to the puborectalis sling of the levator ani musculature. About 50% of children with anorectal anomalies have a urological problem.

BOX 46-18 CLASSIFICATION OF ANORECTAL MALFORMATIONS

Male Defects

Perineal fistula
Rectourethral bulbar fistula
Rectourethral prostatic fistula
Rectovesicular (bladder neck) fistula
Imperforate anus without fistula
Rectal atresia and stenosis

Female Defects

Perineal fistula
Vestibular fistula
Imperforate anus without fistula
Rectal atresia and stenosis
Cloaca

From Peña, A., & Hong, A. (2000). Advances in the management of anorectal malformations. *American Journal of Surgery, 180*(5), 370–376.

Diagnostic Evaluation

Checking for patency of the anus and rectum is a routine part of the newborn assessment and should include observations regarding the passage of meconium. Inspection of the perineal area reveals absence of the normal anal opening; however, the appearance of the perineum alone does not accurately predict the level of the lesion. Genitourinary and pelvic anomalies associated with anorectal malformations should be considered.

In the newborn, the presence of meconium on the perineum does not always indicate anal patency (particularly in girls) because a fistula may be present and allow evacuation of meconium through the vagina. Rectourinary fistulas should be suspected if there is meconium in the urine. Anal stenosis may not be identified until the child is older and comes to the physician with a history of difficult defecation, abdominal distension, and ribbonlike stools.

Abdominal ultrasonography is performed to determine the existence of other malformations. An IV pyelogram and voiding cystourethrogram are recommended for an infant with a high malformation to identify anomalies of the urinary tract. Further examination is also indicated when there is evidence of urinary tract infection or other symptoms. If a syndrome is suspected, cardiac evaluation and spinal films should be obtained.

Therapeutic Management

Successful treatment for anal stenosis is generally accomplished by manual dilations. The procedure is initiated by a physician and repeated on a regular basis by the nurses in the hospital. Parents should be taught to continue the dilations at home. Perineal fistulas are treated by anoplasty during the newborn period. The opening is moved to the centre of the external sphincter, and dilations are begun. More extensive defects are usually managed with a colostomy, and corrective surgical repair is performed later in the first year.

The type of defect, the sacral anatomy, and the quality of muscles influence the long-term prognosis. In general, if the newborn has a deep midline groove, two well-formed buttocks, and an anal dimple, the prognosis for bowel control is better than if the infant has a flat or "rocker" bottom and no midline groove because of associated neurological problems. A functioning interior anal sphincter is important to achieve continence. In its absence, the child may need a bowel program to achieve socially acceptable bowel continence. Other potential complications after surgical treatment include strictures, recurrent rectourinary fistula, mucosal prolapse, and constipation.

The surgical treatment of anorectal malformations varies according to the defect but usually involves one or a combination of several of the following procedures: anoplasty, colostomy, posterior sagittal anorectoplasty (PSARP), or other pull-through with colostomy and colostomy (take-down) closure. The PSARP is a common surgical procedure for the repair of anorectal malformations in infants approximately 1 to 2 months after the initial colostomy. In the PSARP procedure the repair is made via a posterior midline sacral approach to dissect the different muscle groups involved without damaging strategic innervation of pelvic structures so optimum postoperative bowel continence is achieved. A laparotomy may be required if the rectum is unidentifiable by the posterior approach. Laparoscopic-assisted PSARP has been described for recto–bladder neck fistula and high prostatic fistula (Bischoff, Peña, & Levitt, 2013). Additional management after successful repair involves a program of anal dilations, colostomy closure, and a bowel management program.

A primary laparoscopic repair (without colostomy) of anorectal malformation is being performed successfully in some centres. This minimizes surgical risks, associated mortality, and postoperative pain management.

NURSING CARE

The first nursing responsibility is identification of undetected anorectal malformations. A newborn who does not pass a stool within 24 to 48 hours of birth requires further assessment. In addition, meconium that appears at an inappropriate orifice should be reported. Preoperative care includes diagnostic evaluation, GI decompression, and IV fluids.

For the newborn with a perineal fistula an *anoplasty* is performed, which involves moving the fistula opening to the centre of the sphincter and enlarging the rectal opening. Postoperative nursing care after anoplasty is primarily directed toward healing the surgical site without other complications. A program of anal dilations is usually initiated when the child returns for the 2-week checkup. Feedings are started soon after surgical repair, and breastfeeding is encouraged because it causes less constipation.

In newborns with anomalies such as cloaca (girls), rectourethral prostatic fistula (boys), and vestibular fistula (girls), a descending colostomy may be performed to allow fecal elimination and avoid fecal contamination of the distal imperforate section and subsequent urinary tract infection in infants with urorectal fistulas. With a colostomy, postoperative nursing care is directed toward maintaining appropriate skin care at the stoma sites (both distal and proximal), managing postoperative pain, and administering IV fluids and antibiotics. Postoperative NG decompression may be required with laparotomy, and nursing care focuses on maintenance of appropriate drainage. (See Chapter 44 for colostomy care.)

Parents are instructed in perineal and wound care or care of the colostomy as needed. Anal dilations may be necessary for some infants. Parents should observe stooling patterns and for signs of anal stricture or complications. Information about dietary modifications and administration of medications is included in counselling. Nurses have a vital role in helping families of a child with anorectal malformations provide optimum care so that bowel management is successful and quality of life enhanced for the child and family.

Family Support, Discharge Planning, and Home Care

Long-term follow-up is important for children with complex malformations. After the definitive pull-through procedure, toilet training is delayed, and complete continence is seldom achieved at the usual age of 2 to 3 years. Prevention of constipation is important, and breastfeeding is encouraged postoperatively. If a cow's milk–based formula is used, a mild laxative may be prescribed. Bowel habit training, diet modification, and administration of stool softeners or fibre are important aspects of bowel management. Optimum bowel function may not be achieved until late childhood or adolescence. Support and reassurance are important during the slow progression to normal function. Some children never achieve bowel continence and must rely on daily bowel irrigations.

MALABSORPTION SYNDROMES

Chronic diarrhea and malabsorption of nutrients characterize malabsorption syndromes. An important complication of malabsorption syndromes in children is growth failure (failure to thrive). Most cases are classified according to the location of the supposed anatomical or biochemical defect. The term *celiac disease* is often used to describe a symptom complex with four characteristics: (1) steatorrhea (fatty, foul, frothy, bulky stools), (2) general malnutrition, (3) abdominal distension, and (4) secondary vitamin deficiencies.

Digestive defects are conditions in which the enzymes necessary for digestion are diminished or absent, such as (1) cystic fibrosis, in which pancreatic enzymes are absent, (2) biliary or liver disease, in which bile flow is affected, or (3) lactase deficiency, in which there is congenital or secondary lactose intolerance.

Absorptive defects are conditions in which the intestinal mucosal transport system is impaired. This may occur because of a primary defect (e.g., celiac disease) or as secondary to IBD, resulting in impaired absorption because bowel motility is accelerated (e.g., ulcerative colitis). Obstructive disorders (e.g., HD) also cause secondary malabsorption from enterocolitis.

Anatomical defects, such as extensive resection of the bowel or short-bowel syndrome (SBS), affect digestion by decreasing the transit time of substances and affect absorption by severely compromising the absorptive surface.

Celiac Disease (Gluten-Sensitive Enteropathy)

Celiac disease, also known as *gluten-induced enteropathy, gluten-sensitive enteropathy,* and *celiac sprue*, is a permanent intestinal intolerance to dietary wheat gliadin and related proteins that produces mucosal lesions in genetically susceptible individuals. It is second only to cystic fibrosis as a cause of malabsorption in children.

Celiac sprue used to be considered a disease of childhood, but adult presentation is becoming more common. The incidence varies and has been reported in 1 in 3000 to 1 in 4000 people. More recently the incidence has been shown to be closer to 1 in 266, as a result of improved screening tests (McCabe, Toughill, Parkhill, et al., 2012). It is seen more frequently in Europe than in North America and is rarely reported in Asians or Blacks. It is more prevalent in women than men. Although the exact cause is unknown, it is now generally accepted that celiac disease is a T-cell–mediated autoimmune and genetic small intestine enteropathy (McCabe et al., 2012). The mucosal lesions contain features that suggest both humoral and cell-mediated immunological overstimulation.

Infant feeding practices, including breastfeeding for at least 4 months and gradual introduction of gluten in the infant's diet, may play a role in the prevention of celiac disease. Infectious diseases in infancy, specifically rotavirus, have been noted to increase the incidence of this condition (Branski, Troncone, & Fasano, 2016; Ivarsson, Myléus, Norström, et al., 2013). The exact cause of celiac disease is unknown, but there appears to be an inherited predisposition with an influence by environmental factors.

Pathophysiology

Celiac disease is characterized by villous atrophy in the small bowel in response to the protein, gluten. Gluten is found in wheat, barley, rye, and oat grains. When individuals are unable to digest the gliadin component of gluten, an accumulation of a toxic substance that is damaging to the mucosal cells of the small bowel occurs. This damage leads to villous atrophy, hyperplasia of the crypts, and infiltration of the epithelial cells with lymphocytes. The atrophy leads to malabsorption caused by the reduced absorptive surface.

Membrane receptors involved in preferential antigen presentation to CD4+ T cells play a crucial role in the immune response characteristic of celiac disease. Genes located on the HLA region of chromosome 6 (i.e., HLA-DQ2 or HLA-DQ8) are found in almost 90% of those affected with celiac disease (Branski et al., 2016). Once the inflammatory reaction is activated by gluten, CD4+ T cells produce cytokines, which are likely to contribute to the intestinal damage. The damage consists of infiltration of the lamina propria, crypt hyperplasia, and villous atrophy and flattening. When there is sufficient villous atrophy, malabsorption occurs.

Classic symptoms of celiac disease are GI manifestations usually noted several months after the introduction of gluten-containing grains into the diet, usually between the ages of 6 months and 2 years (Box 46-19). Typically, children are seen with impaired growth, chronic diarrhea, abdominal distension, muscle wasting with hypotonia, poor appetite, and lack of energy. The clinical manifestations are usually insidious and chronic. The first evidence may be growth failure and diarrhea. Less typical presentation has been observed in children ages 5 to 7 years who have abdominal pain, nausea, vomiting, bloating, and constipation, or extraintestinal manifestations, including short stature, pubertal delay, iron deficiency, dental enamel defects, and abnormal LFTs. Older children have been found to have osteoporosis. Untreated celiac disease can evolve into celiac crisis, characterized by abdominal distension, explosive watery diarrhea, and dehydration with electrolyte imbalance, leading to hypotensive shock and lethargy.

BOX 46-19 CLINICAL MANIFESTATIONS OF CELIAC DISEASE

Classic Celiac Disease

- Diarrhea
- Abdominal distension
- Failure to thrive, or weight loss
- Positive serology, HLA, and villous atrophy

Atypical Celiac Disease

- Iron deficiency anemia
- Osteoporosis
- Short stature
- Arthritis
- Infertility
- Peripheral neuropathy
- Abnormal LFTs, positive serology, HLA, and varying degrees of villous atrophy

Silent Celiac Disease

- Asymptomatic but with positive serology, HLA, and villous atrophy

Latent Celiac Disease

- Variation in expression between atypical and asymptomatic
- Positive or negative serology, HLA, and no villous atrophy

HLA, Human leukocyte antigen; *LFT,* liver function test.
Modified from Scanlon, S. A., & Murray, J. A. (2011). Update on celiac disease—etiology, differential diagnosis, drug tests, and management advances. *Clinical & Experimental Gastroenterology, 4,* 297–311.

Diagnostic Evaluation

The diagnosis of celiac disease is based on a biopsy of the small intestine demonstrating the characteristic changes of mucosal inflammation, crypt hyperplasia, and villous atrophy with hyperplasia of the crypts and abnormal surface epithelium while the individual is eating adequate amounts of gluten and a full clinical remission after gluten is withdrawn (Branski et al., 2016). Within a day or two of instituting the gluten-free diet, most children with celiac disease demonstrate a favourable response, including weight gain and improved appetite. Within a few weeks diarrhea and steatorrhea resolve.

Genetic testing for the HLA genes associated with celiac disease may help in ruling out the disease in individuals at high risk for the condition. A negative test indicates the individual does not have the condition; a positive test indicates there is an increased likelihood of having the condition, and antibody screening should be considered (University of Chicago Celiac Disease Center, 2016).

Commercially available serological tests for celiac disease include antigliadin antibodies of both the immune globulin A and G classes (IgA and IgG); antiendomysium IgA; and antitissue transglutaminase IgA and IgG antibodies for screening first-degree relatives of known celiac disease patients and those with known celiac disease–associated disorders such as type 1 diabetes, thyroiditis, arthritis, primary biliary cirrhosis, Down syndrome, Turner syndrome, Williams syndrome, and osteopenia or osteoporosis. False-positive results are likely when only one serological test is used, because patients with these disorders can also test positive for these antibodies. Use of more than one test increases diagnostic accuracy (Gelfond & Fasano, 2006). Ruling out total IgA deficiency is necessary to minimize false-negative results.

Therapeutic Management

Treatment of chronic celiac disease is primarily dietary. Although the diet is called *gluten free*, it is actually low in gluten, since it is impossible to remove every source of this protein. Because gluten is found primarily in wheat and rye, but also in smaller quantities in barley and oats, these four foods are eliminated. Corn and rice become substitute grain foods.

Children with untreated celiac disease may have associated lactose intolerance related to intestinal mucosal lesions, which usually improves with gluten withdrawal and intestinal healing. Specific nutritional deficiencies such as iron, folic acid, and fat-soluble vitamin deficiencies are treated with appropriate supplements. Some patients may not respond to the gluten-free diet and exhibit refractory celiac disease; such individuals continue to have diarrhea and malabsorption and may need to rely on PN and immunosuppressants (McCabe et al., 2012).

Prognosis

Celiac disease is regarded as a chronic disease. The most severe symptoms usually occur in early childhood and again in adult life. Strict dietary avoidance of gluten prevents symptoms and may minimize the risk of developing lymphoma, the most serious complication of the disease.

NURSING CARE

The main nursing consideration is helping the child adhere to the dietary regimen of eating no wheat, barley, or rye. Oats may be safe for most patients, but contamination with other gluten products may occur in harvesting; therefore caution should be exercised with including oats. Children who have silent celiac disease without clinical manifestations should also adhere to a strict gluten-free diet (Branski et al., 2016). Considerable time is involved in explaining the disease process to the child and parents, the specific role of gluten in aggravating the disorder, and the foods that must be restricted. It is especially difficult to maintain a diet indefinitely when the child has no symptoms and temporary transgressions result in no difficulties. However, evidence indicates that most individuals who relax their diet experience a relapse of their disease and possibly exhibit growth delay, anemia, or osteomalacia. There is also the risk of developing malignant lymphoma of the small intestine or other GI malignancies.

Although the chief source of gluten is cereal and baked goods, grains are frequently added to processed foods as thickeners or fillers. To compound the difficulty, gluten is added to many foods as hydrolyzed vegetable protein, which is derived from cereal grains. The nurse must advise parents to read carefully all ingredients on labels in order to avoid hidden sources of gluten.

Many of children's favourite foods contain gluten, including bread, cake, cookies, crackers, doughnuts, pies, spaghetti, pizza, prepared soups, some processed ice cream, many types of chocolate candy, hot dogs, luncheon meats, meat gravy, and some prepared hamburgers. Many of these products can be eliminated from an infant's or young child's diet fairly easily, but monitoring the diet of a school-age child or adolescent is more difficult. Luncheon preparation away from home is particularly difficult because bread, luncheon meats, and instant soups are not allowed in the child's diet. For families on restricted food budgets, the diet adds an additional financial burden because many inexpensive and convenient foods, which often contain gluten, cannot be used.

In addition to restricting gluten, other dietary alterations may be necessary. For example, in some children who have more severe mucosal damage, the digestion of disaccharides is impaired, especially in relation to lactose. Therefore, these children often need a temporarily lactose-free diet, which necessitates eliminating all milk products. In general, dietary management includes a diet high in calories and proteins with simple carbohydrates such as fruits and vegetables but low in fats. Because the bowel is inflamed as a result of the pathological processes in absorption, the child must avoid high-fibre foods such as nuts, raisins, raw vegetables, and raw fruits with skin until inflammation has subsided.

It is important to stress long-range complications and remind parents of the child's physical status before dietary treatment and the dramatic improvement after treatment. The nurse can be instrumental in allowing the child to express concerns and frustration while focusing on ways in which he or she can still feel normal. A clinical dietitian can be consulted to provide children and their families with detailed dietary instructions and education.

Several organizations and resources are available to help families cope with this condition. The Canadian Celiac Association provides support, guidance, and educational materials to families concerning a gluten-free diet, food sources, recipes, and travel information. Several published cookbooks contain gluten-free recipes. See Additional Resources at the end of this chapter.

Short-Bowel Syndrome

Short-bowel syndrome (SBS) is a malabsorptive disorder that occurs when there is decreased mucosal surface area, usually as a result of extensive resection of the small intestine. Malabsorption may be exacerbated by other factors such as bacterial overgrowth and dysmotility. The most common causes of SBS in children are necrotizing enterocolitis (see Chapter 28, p. 778), volvulus, jejunal atresias, and gastroschisis. Other causes include midgut volvulus and diffuse small-bowel CD in older children. Less frequent causes include trauma to the GI tract and HD with extension into the small bowel.

The definition of SBS includes two important findings: (1) decreased intestinal surface area for absorption of fluid, electrolytes, and nutrients; and (2) a need for PN (Goday, 2009). The prognosis for infants with SBS has improved dramatically in the past 20 to 30 years as a result of advances in PN and enteral feeding.

Therapeutic Management

The goals of treatment are to (1) preserve as much length of bowel as possible during surgery, (2) maintain the child's optimal nutritional status, growth, and development while intestinal adaptation occurs, (3) stimulate intestinal adaptation with enteral feeding, and (4) minimize complications related to the disease process and therapy (Goday, 2009).

Nutritional support is the long-term focus of care. The initial phase of therapy includes PN as the primary source of nutrition. The second phase is the introduction of enteral feeding, which usually begins as soon as possible after surgery. Elemental formulas containing glucose, sucrose and glucose polymers, hydrolyzed proteins, and medium-chain triglycerides facilitate absorption. Usually these formulas are given by continuous infusion through an NG or gastrostomy tube. As the enteral feedings are advanced, the PN solution is decreased in terms of calories, amount of fluid, and total hours of infusion per day.

The final phase of nutritional support occurs when growth and development are sustained exclusively by enteral feedings. When PN is discontinued, there is a risk of nutritional deficiency secondary to malabsorption of fat-soluble vitamins (A, D, E, K) and trace minerals (iron, selenium, zinc). Serum vitamin and mineral levels should be obtained, and enteral supplementation of vitamins and minerals may be required. Pharmacological agents have been used to reduce secretory losses. H_2 blockers, PPIs, and octreotide inhibit gastric or pancreatic secretion. Cholestyramine is often prescribed to improve diarrhea that is associated with bile salt malabsorption. Growth factors have also been used to hasten adaptation and enhance mucosal growth, but these uses are still experimental.

Numerous complications are associated with SBS and long-term PN (see Chapter 44). Infectious, metabolic, and technical complications can occur. Catheter sepsis can occur after improper care of the catheter. The GI tract can also be a source of microbial seeding of the catheter. Bowel atrophy may foster increased intestinal permeability of bacteria. A lack of adequate sites for central lines may become a significant problem for the child in need of long-term PN. Hepatic dysfunction, hepatomegaly with abnormal LFTs, and cholestasis may also occur (Diamond, Sterescu, Pencharz, et al., 2009).

Bacterial overgrowth is likely to occur when the ileocecal valve is absent or when stasis exists as a result of a partial obstruction or a dilated segment of bowel with poor motility. Alternating cycles of broad-spectrum antibiotics are used to reduce bacterial overgrowth. This treatment may also decrease the risk of bacterial translocation and subsequent central venous catheter infections. Other complications of bacterial overgrowth and malabsorption include metabolic acidosis and gastric hypersecretion.

Many surgical interventions, such as constructing intestinal valves, tapering enteroplasty or stricturoplasty, intestinal lengthening, and interposed segments, have been used to slow intestinal transit, reduce bacterial overgrowth, or increase mucosal surface area. Intestinal transplantation has been performed successfully in children. Only children with a permanent dependence on PN or severe complications of long-term parenteral nutrition are candidates for transplantation.

Prognosis

The prognosis for infants with SBS has improved with advances in PN and with the understanding of the importance of intraluminal nutrition. Improved surgical techniques for the management of therapy-related problems and the development of more specific immunosuppressive medications for transplantation have all contributed to improved management. The prognosis depends in part on the length of the residual small intestine. An intact ileocecal valve also improves the prognosis. Mortality in infants and children with SBS is usually associated with PN-related problems, such as fulminant sepsis or severe PN cholestasis.

NURSING CARE

The most important components of nursing care are administration and monitoring of nutritional therapy. During PN therapy, care must be taken to minimize the risk of complications related to the **central venous access device** (CVAD) (i.e., catheter infections, occlusions, dislodgment, or accidental removal). Care of the enteral feeding tubes and monitoring of enteral feeding tolerance are also important nursing responsibilities.

When long-term PN is required, preparing the family for home care is a major nursing responsibility that should be initiated early to help prevent a lengthy hospitalization with subsequent delays. Many infants and children can be successfully cared for at home with enteral and parenteral nutrition when the family is prepared and provided with adequate support services. Follow-up by a multidisciplinary nutritional support service is essential. The nurse plays an active and important role in the success of a home nutrition program. Home infusion companies provide portable equipment, which enables the child and family to maintain a more normal lifestyle.

Many infants with SBS have an intestinal ostomy when the bowel was resected. Routine ostomy care is another important nursing responsibility. Maintaining skin integrity and preventing skin breakdown is accomplished by cleansing frequently and applying skin barrier creams to protect skin from the chronic diarrhea that the SBS child experiences.

When hospitalization is prolonged, the child's developmental and emotional needs must be met. This often requires special planning to promote normal family adjustment and adaptation of the hospital routines. Care of the hospitalized child is discussed in Chapter 43.

INGESTION OF INJURIOUS AGENTS

In Canada there is no national poison centre that monitors and tracks the occurrence of ingestion of injurious agents in the population. Each province and territory has its own regional centre that is responsible for both education and emergency management of these exposures. There are a total of 160,000 phone calls to the Canadian regional poison centres on a yearly basis. Unintentional poisoning is the fifth leading cause of injury deaths, hospitalization, and emergency visits for all Canadian age groups. Researchers estimate that 50% of all poison exposures occur among children less than 6 years old. In Canada, an average of seven deaths per year and 1700 serious injuries requiring hospitalization occur from unintentional poisoning in children aged 14 years and under (Government of Canada, 2014). Among Canadian children under 5 years of age the leading injurious agents causing unintentional injury and death from their ingestion are medications and household chemicals, such as bleaches, liquid detergent packs, paint thinners, ammonia, and abrasive cleansers.

Commonly ingested poisons include the following (Bronstein, Spiker, Cantilena, et al., 2012) (the most common substances in each category are in parentheses; substances ingested are not necessarily the most toxic but often are readily available):

- Cosmetics and personal care products (perfume, cologne, aftershave)
- Cleaning products (hypochlorite ["household"] bleach, pine oil disinfectants)
- Plants (nontoxic GI irritants, oxalates) (Box 46-20)
- Foreign bodies, toys, and miscellaneous substances (desiccants, thermometers, bubble-blowing solutions)

Single-use laundry detergent capsules (LCDs) have become the most common household cleaning product ingested by children (Bramuzzo, Amaddeo, Facchina, et al., 2013). The bright colours make them appealing to children and are easy to mistake for candy or toys. Ingestion of these products produces more symptoms than powdered laundry detergent, although the exact reason for this is unclear (Bonnery, Mazor, & Goldman, 2013).

Many poisonings reflect the accessibility of the product in the home, where more than 90% of poisonings occur, although a significant number of incidents take place elsewhere, such as in a grandparent's or friend's home, a school, or a health care facility.

The following five commonly used and easily available medications (the first four are over-the-counter products) can cause serious or fatal consequences if as little as 1.5 mL or a tablet is ingested: methyl salicylate, camphor, topical imidazolines (sympathomimetics such as those contained in Visine and Clear Eyes), benzocaine, and diphenoxylate-atropine (e.g., Lomotil). Parents must know the importance of keeping such medications away from children. If these agents are ingested, parents need to seek medical treatment immediately. Emesis should not be induced at home.

BOX 46-20 POISONOUS PLANTS

Poisonous Plants—Toxic Parts

Apple—Leaves, seeds
Apricot—Leaves, stem, seed pits
Azalea—All parts
Buttercup—All parts
Cherry (wild or cultivated)—Twigs, seeds, foliage
Daffodil—Bulbs
Dumb cane, Dieffenbachia—All parts
Elephant ear—All parts
English ivy—All parts
Foxglove—Leaves, seeds, flowers
Holly—Berries and leaves
Hyacinth—Bulbs
Ivy—Leaves
Mistletoe*—Berries, leaves
Oak tree—Acorn, foliage
Philodendron—All parts
Plum—Pit
Poinsettia†—Leaves, stems, sap
Poison ivy, poison oak—Leaves, fruit, stems, smoke from burning plants
Pothos—All parts
Rhubarb—Leaves
Tulip—Bulbs
Water hemlock—All parts
Wisteria—Seeds, pods
Yew—All parts

*Eating one or two berries or leaves is probably nontoxic.
†Mildly toxic if ingested in massive quantities.

The developmental characteristics of young children predispose them to poisoning by ingestion; infants and toddlers explore their environment through oral experimentation. Because the sense of taste is not discriminating at this age, many unpalatable substances are ingested. In addition, toddlers and preschoolers are developing autonomy and initiative, which increase their curiosity and misbehaving. Imitation is also a powerful motivator, especially when combined with lack of awareness of danger.

This section is primarily concerned with the immediate emergency treatment of the ingestion of injurious agents. Specific management of corrosive, hydrocarbon, acetaminophen, salicylate, iron, and plant poisoning is summarized in Box 46-21. Because of the importance of lead poisoning among young children, the ingestion of lead is discussed separately. Appropriate suggestions for poisoning prevention are discussed on p. 1466.

Principles of Emergency Treatment

A poisoning may or may not require emergency intervention, but in every instance medical evaluation is necessary to initiate appropriate action. The first action for a caregiver of a child who may have ingested a toxic substance is to consult the local

BOX 46-21 SELECTED POISONINGS IN CHILDREN

Corrosives (Strong Acids or Alkali)
Drain, toilet, or oven cleaners
Electric dishwasher detergent (liquid, because of higher pH, is more hazardous than granular)
Mildew remover
Batteries
Clinitest tablets
Denture cleaners
Bleach

Clinical Manifestations
Severe burning pain in mouth, throat, and stomach
White, swollen mucous membranes; edema of lips, tongue, and pharynx (respiratory obstruction)
Violent vomiting (hemoptysis)
Drooling and inability to clear secretions
Signs of shock
Anxiety and agitation

Comments
Household bleach is a frequently ingested corrosive but rarely causes serious damage.
Liquid corrosives cause more damage than granular preparations.

Treatment
Assess child's breathing and level of consciousness.
Contact regional poison control centre for advice.
Inducing emesis is contraindicated (vomiting redamages the mucosa).
Dilute corrosive with water or milk (usually no more than 120 mL).
Do not neutralize. Neutralization can cause an exothermic reaction (which produces heat and causes increased symptoms or produces a thermal burn in addition to a chemical burn).
Maintain patent airway if needed.
Administer analgesics.
Do not allow oral intake.
Esophageal stricture may require repeated dilations or surgery.

Hydrocarbons
Gasoline
Kerosene
Lamp oil
Mineral seal oil (found in furniture polish)
Lighter fluid
Turpentine
Paint thinner and remover (some types)

Clinical Manifestations
Gagging, choking, and coughing
Nausea
Vomiting
Alterations in sensorium, such as lethargy
Weakness
Respiratory symptoms of pulmonary involvement
- Tachypnea
- Cyanosis
- Retractions
- Grunting

Comments
Immediate danger is aspiration (even small amounts can cause bronchitis and chemical pneumonia).
Gasoline, kerosene, lighter fluid, mineral seal oil, and turpentine cause severe pneumonia.

Treatment
Contact regional poison control centre.
Inducing emesis is generally contraindicated.
Gastric decontamination and emptying are questionable, even when the hydrocarbon contains a heavy metal or pesticide; if gastric lavage must be performed, a cuffed endotracheal tube should be in place before lavage because of a high risk of aspiration.
Symptomatic treatment of chemical pneumonia includes high humidity, oxygen, hydration, and antibiotics for secondary infection.

Acetaminophen
Clinical Manifestations
Occurs in four stages:
1. Initial period (2 to 4 hours after ingestion)
   - Nausea
   - Vomiting
   - Sweating
   - Pallor
2. Latent period (24 to 36 hours)
   - Patient improves
3. Hepatic involvement (may last up to 7 days and be permanent)
   - Pain in right upper quadrant
   - Jaundice
   - Confusion
   - Stupor
   - Coagulation abnormalities
4. Patients who do not die in hepatic stage gradually recover.

Comments
It is the most common medication poisoning in children.
It occurs from acute ingestion.
Toxic dose is 150 mg/kg or greater in children.
Because of multiple formulations and concentrations, chronic acetaminophen toxicity is a significant problem.
Parents should be counselled to read product packaging carefully and to consult a health care provider to avoid inappropriate dosing.

Treatment
Antidote N-acetylcysteine (Mucomyst) can usually be given orally but is first diluted in fruit juice or a soft drink because of the antidote's offensive odour.
It is given as 1 loading dose and usually 17 maintenance doses in different dosages.
It may be given intravenously, but use is investigational.

Continued

BOX 46-21 SELECTED POISONINGS IN CHILDREN—cont'd

Aspirin (Acetylsalicylic Acid [ASA])

Clinical Manifestations

Acute poisoning

- Nausea
- Disorientation
- Vomiting
- Dehydration
- Diaphoresis
- Hyperpnea
- Hyperpyrexia
- Oliguria
- Tinnitus
- Coma
- Convulsions

Chronic poisoning

- Same as for acute poisoning but subtle onset (often mistaken for viral illness)
- Dehydration, coma, and seizures may be more severe.
- Bleeding tendencies

Comments

It may be caused by acute ingestion (severe toxicity occurs with 300 to 500 mg/kg).

It may be caused by chronic ingestion (i.e., more than 100 mg/kg/day for 2 or more days) and can be more serious than acute ingestion.

Time to peak serum salicylate level can vary with enteric aspirin or the presence of concretions (bezoars).

Treatment

Hospitalization is required for severe toxicity.

Emesis, lavage, activated charcoal, or cathartic measures may be used.

Lavage will not remove concretions of ASA.

Activated charcoal is important early in ASA toxicity.

Sodium bicarbonate (intravenous) to correct metabolic acidosis and urinary alkalinization may be effective in enhancing elimination; urinary alkalinization is very difficult to achieve.

Be aware of the risk for fluid overload and pulmonary edema.

Prescribe:

- External cooling for hyperpyrexia
- Anticonvulsants
- Oxygen and ventilation for respiratory depression
- Vitamin K for bleeding

In severe cases, hemodialysis (not peritoneal dialysis) may be used.

Iron

Mineral supplement or vitamin containing iron

Clinical Manifestations

Occurs in five stages:

1. Initial period (0.5 to 6 hours after ingestion) (if child does not develop gastrointestinal symptoms in 6 hours, toxicity is unlikely)
   - Vomiting
   - Hematemesis
   - Diarrhea
   - Hematochezia (bloody stools)
   - Gastric pain
2. Latency (2 to 12 hours)
   - Patient improves
3. Systemic toxicity (4 to 24 hours after ingestion)
   - Metabolic acidosis
   - Fever
   - Hyperglycemia
   - Bleeding
   - Shock
   - Death (may occur)
4. Hepatic injury (48 to 96 hours)
   - Seizures
   - Coma
5. Rarely, pyloric stenosis develops at 2 to 5 weeks.

Comments

Factors related to frequency of iron poisoning:

- Widespread availability
- Packaging of large quantities in individual containers
- Lack of parental awareness of iron toxicity
- Resemblance of iron tablets to candy (e.g., M&M's)

Toxic dose is based on the amount of elemental iron in various salts (sulphate, gluconate, fumarate), which ranges from 20 to 33%; ingestions of 60 mg/kg are considered dangerous.

Treatment

Emesis or lavage may be used.

For toxic doses lavage may be necessary for all chewable tablets or liquids if spontaneous vomiting has not occurred.

Chelation therapy with deferoxamine is used in severe intoxication (may turn urine a red to orange colour).

If intravenous deferoxamine is given too rapidly, hypotension, facial flushing, rash, urticaria, tachycardia, and shock may occur; stop the infusion, maintain the intravenous line with normal saline, and notify the practitioner immediately.

Plants

See Box 46-20.

Clinical Manifestations

Depends on type of plant ingested

May cause local irritation of oropharynx and entire gastrointestinal tract

May cause respiratory, renal, and central nervous system symptoms

Topical contact with plants can cause dermatitis

Comments

Plants are some of the most frequently ingested substances.

Plant ingestions rarely cause serious problems, although some can be fatal.

Plants can also cause choking and allergic reactions.

Treatment

Induce emesis.

Wash from skin or eyes.

Supportive care as needed.

Poison Control Centre (PCC). If the PCC cannot be reached, the child should be taken to the nearest emergency department. Parents are advised to call the PCC before initiating any intervention. The local PCC telephone number should be posted near each phone in the house and be included in the parent's cell phone contacts (see Critical Thinking Case Study and Emergency box).

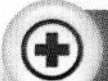

CRITICAL THINKING CASE STUDY

Poisoning

Mrs. B calls her neighbour, Mark, a community health nurse. She is very upset because her 2-year-old son has eaten several chewable multivitamins with iron. She asks the nurse if she should give her son syrup of ipecac. What should Mark advise her to do?

1. Evidence—Is there sufficient evidence to formulate an answer for Mrs. B?
2. Assumptions—Answer the following questions and describe some underlying assumptions on which your answers are based:
   a. What is the best initial response when a child ingests a potentially poisonous substance?
   b. What is syrup of ipecac?
   c. What are the dangers involved in the use of syrup of ipecac?
3. What is the priority for nursing care at this time?
4. Does the evidence support your conclusion?

EMERGENCY

Poisoning

1. Assess the victim:
   - Take vital signs; re-evaluate routinely.
   - Initiate cardiorespiratory support if needed.
   - Treat other symptoms, such as seizures.
2. Terminate exposure:
   - Empty mouth of pills, plant parts, or other material.
   - Flush eyes continuously with normal saline (or room-temperature tap water at home) for 15 to 20 minutes.
   - Flush skin and wash with soap and a soft cloth; remove contaminated clothes, especially if a pesticide, acid, alkali, or hydrocarbon is involved.
   - Bring victim of an inhalation poisoning into fresh air.
   - Give one sip of water to dilute ingested poison.
3. Identify the poison:
   - Question the victim and witnesses.
   - Look for environmental cues (empty container, nearby spill, odour on breath) and save all evidence of poison (container, vomitus, urine).
   - Be alert to signs and symptoms of potential poisoning in absence of other evidence, including symptoms of ocular or dermal exposure.
   - Call regional poison control centre or other competent emergency facility for immediate advice regarding treatment.
4. Remove poison and prevent absorption:
   - Place child in side-lying, sitting, or kneeling position with head below chest to prevent aspiration.
   - Administer activated charcoal if ordered (unless used repeatedly, usual dose is 1 g/kg unless amount of toxin is known).

! NURSING ALERT

Each province and territory has its own regional poison control centre, thus it is important to have the emergency number posted near the telephone and added to cell phone contacts.

Based on the initial telephone assessment, the PCC will counsel the parents to begin treatment at home or to take the child to an emergency facility. When a call is taken, the name and telephone number of the caller are recorded to re-establish contact if the connection is interrupted. Because most poisonings are managed in the home, expert advice is essential in minimizing adverse effects. When the exact quantity or type of ingested toxin is not known, admission to a health care facility with pediatric emergency treatment services for laboratory evaluation and surveillance is critical after ingestion.

Assessment

The first and most important principle in dealing with a poisoning is to *treat the child first, not the poison*. This requires an immediate concern for life support. Vital signs are taken, and respiratory or circulatory support is instituted as needed. The child's condition is routinely re-evaluated. Because shock is a complication of several types of household poisons, particularly corrosives, measures to reduce the effects of shock, beginning with the CAB (circulation, airway, and breathing) of resuscitation, are important (see Chapter 45). Establishing and maintaining vascular access for rapid intravascular volume expansion is vital in the treatment of pediatric shock.

The emergency department nurse's responsibility is to be prepared for immediate intervention with all of the necessary equipment. Because time and speed are critical factors in recovery from serious poisonings, anticipation of potential problems and complications may mean the difference between life and death.

Gastric Decontamination

Pediatric poisonings are common, yet they rarely result in significant morbidity and mortality (Bronstein et al., 2012; Greene, Harris, & Singer, 2008). The treatment for ingestion of poison will depend on the type of poison ingested. Gastrointestinal decontamination (GID) is used if necessary, depending on the potential toxicity of the poison and the risks versus benefits. GID is needed to remove the ingested poison, by adsorbing the toxin with activated charcoal, performing gastric lavage, or increasing bowel motility (catharsis). Because of continuing controversy regarding the use of these methods, each toxic ingestion should be treated individually (Albertson, Owen, Sutter, et al., 2011; Madden, 2008). Specific antidotes may be administered for certain poisonings.

Syrup of ipecac, an emetic that exerts its action through irritation of the gastric mucosa and by stimulation of the vomiting centre, is no longer recommended for immediate treatment of poison ingestion (Greene et al., 2008). No emetic or other substance should be given at home without consultation with a PCC or physician.

Medications such as calcium channel blockers and benzodiazepines either produce a rapid onset of adverse symptoms (e.g., sedation, seizures, coma) or exaggerate the vagal response induced by gagging, which can lead to significant bradycardia. Under either circumstance, uncontrolled vomiting becomes an undesirable and unsafe event.

A more commonly used method of GI decontamination is the use of *activated charcoal (AC)*, an odourless, tasteless, fine black powder that adsorbs many compounds, creating a stable complex. AC is mixed with water or a saline cathartic to form a slurry. Slurries are neither gritty nor distasteful but resemble black mud. To increase the child's acceptance of activated charcoal, the nurse should mix it with a diet soft drink and serve it through a straw in an opaque container with a cover (such as a disposable coffee cup and lid) or an ordinary cup covered with aluminum foil or placed inside a small paper bag. In one small study, healthy adolescents preferred the taste of activated charcoal mixed with Coca-Cola over that with water (Greene et al., 2008). Research has indicated that except in children with severe poisonings, AC has not significantly improved outcomes (Albertson et al., 2011). AC has the best results when administered 30 to 60 minutes after ingesting the poison. For small children, an NG tube may be required to administer activated charcoal. Because the charcoal solution is thick, a 12-French (or larger) NG tube should be used.

Potential complications from the use of AC include aspiration (usually in patients with impaired gag reflexes), constipation, and intestinal obstruction (in multiple doses) (Sheffield & Serwint, 2008). Superactivated charcoal products for gastric decontamination are reported to be more palatable and just as effective (Criddle, 2007). There is no clear recommendation for use of AC in the home because of the risk potential.

If the child is admitted to an emergency facility, gastric lavage may be performed to empty the stomach of the toxic agent; however, this procedure is associated with serious complications (GI perforation, hypoxia, aspiration), and it is no longer recommended in all cases of ingestion. There is no conclusive evidence that gastric lavage decreases morbidity (Criddle, 2007; Greene et al., 2008). In addition, gastric lavage may be of little use if used beyond 1 hour of ingestion (Greene et al., 2008; Sheffield & Serwint, 2008). Conditions that may be appropriate for performing gastric lavage include presentation within 1 hour of ingestion of a toxin, ingestion in a patient who has decreased GI motility, the ingestion of a toxic amount of a **sustained-release medication**, and a massive or life-threatening amount of poison (Criddle, 2007; Madden, 2008). When gastric lavage is used, the patient requires a protected airway, possible sedation, and the largest-diameter tube that can be inserted to facilitate passage of gastric contents.

Specific antidotes are available to counteract a minority of poisonings. They are highly effective and should be available in all emergency facilities. The supply of antidotes should be checked routinely and replaced as used or according to expiration dates. Antidotes available to treat toxin ingestion include N-acetylcysteine for acetaminophen poisoning, oxygen for carbon monoxide inhalation, naloxone for opioid overdose, flumazenil for benzodiazepines (diazepam) overdose, digoxin immune Fab (Digibind) for digoxin toxicity, amyl nitrate for cyanide, and antivenom for certain poisonous bites.

Prevention of Recurrence

The ultimate objective is to prevent poisonings from occurring or recurring. Education regarding home safety can be an effective method to prevent poisonings (Kendrick, Smith, Sutton, et al., 2008). One effective counselling method is first to discuss the difficulties of constantly watching and safeguarding young children (see Family-Centred Teaching box). In this way, the challenging task of raising children can lead to a discussion of injury prevention as part of the parental role. A visit to the home, especially after repeat poisonings, is recommended as part of the follow-up care to assess hazards, including family factors, and to evaluate appropriate injury-proofing measures. One method of identifying risk areas is to ask specific questions or to have the parent complete a questionnaire designed to isolate factors that predispose children to poisoning. Another approach is to encourage parents to bend down to the child's eye level and survey the home environment for potential hazards then try to open cabinets and reach shelves to access poisons.

Passive measures (those that do not require active participation) have been the most successful in preventing poisoning and include using child-resistant closures and limiting the number of tablets in one container. However, these measures alone are not sufficient to prevent poisoning, because most toxic agents in the home do not have safety closures. Therefore *active measures* (those that require participation) are essential. Guidelines for preventing the occurrence or recurrence of a poisoning are listed in the Guidelines box.

Heavy Metal Poisoning

Heavy metal poisoning can occur from the ingestion of a variety of substances, the most common being lead. Other sources that are important in terms of children are iron and mercury. *Mercury toxicity*, a rare form of heavy metal poisoning, has occurred in children from a variety of sources, such as broken thermometers or thermostats, broken fluorescent light bulbs, disk batteries, topical medications, gas regulators, cathartics,

FAMILY-CENTRED TEACHING

Poisoning

An accidental poisoning is more than a physical emergency for the child—it usually represents an emotional crisis for the parents, particularly in terms of guilt, self-reproach, and insecurity in the parenting role. The emergency department is no place to admonish the family for negligence, lack of appropriate supervision, or failure to injury-proof the home. Rather, it is a time to calm and support the child and parents while exploring the circumstances of the injury in a nonjudgemental way. If the nurse prematurely attempts to discuss ways of preventing such an incident from recurring, the parents' anxiety will block out any suggestions or offered guidance. Therefore, it is preferable for the nurse to delay the discussion until the child's condition is stabilized or, if the child is discharged immediately after emergency treatment, to make a community health referral or send a packet of information.

GUIDELINES
Poisoning Prevention

- Assess possible contributing factors in occurrence of injury, such as discipline, parent–child relationship, developmental ability, environmental factors, and behaviour problems.
- Institute anticipatory guidance for possible future injuries based on child's age and maturational level.
- Refer to community health nurse to evaluate home environment and need for injury-proofing measures.
- Provide assistance with environmental manipulation, such as lead removal, when necessary.
- Educate parents regarding safe storage of toxic substances.
- Advise parents to take medications out of sight of children.
- Teach children the hazards of ingesting nonfood items.
- Advise parents against using plants for teas or medicine.
- Discuss problems of discipline and offer strategies for effective discipline.
- Instruct parents regarding correct administration of medications for therapeutic purposes and discontinuation of medication if there is evidence of mild toxicity.
- Advise parents to contact the poison control centre or practitioner immediately when a poisoning occurs.
- Post the phone number of the regional poison control centre with emergency phone list by the telephone and add to cell phone contacts.
- Include by the telephone the home address with nearest cross street in case an ambulance is needed. (In an emergency, family members may not remember the house address, and babysitters may not be aware of the information.)

BOX 46-22 SOURCES OF LEAD*

Lead-based paint in deteriorating condition
Lead solder
Lead crystal
Battery casings
Lead fishing sinkers
Lead curtain weights
Lead bullets
The following may contain lead:
- Ceramic ware
- Water
- Pottery
- Pewter
- Dyes
- Industrial factories
- Vinyl miniblinds
- Playground equipment
- Collectible toys
- Artists' paints
- Pool cue chalk
- Some imported toys or children's metal jewellery

Occupations and hobbies involving lead:
- Battery and aircraft manufacturing
- Lead smelting
- Brass foundry work
- Radiator repair
- Construction work
- Bridge repair work
- Painting contracting
- Mining
- Ceramics work
- Stained-glass making
- Jewellery making

*Health Canada issues alerts and recalls for products that contain lead and that may unexpectedly pose a hazard to young children.

and interior latex house paint (Bose-O'Reilly, McCarthy, Steckling, et al., 2010). Elemental mercury (also called *metallic mercury* or *quicksilver*) is nontoxic if ingested and if the GI tract is healthy (e.g., has no fistulas). However, mercury is volatile at room temperature and enters the bloodstream after it is inhaled, causing toxicity (tremors, memory loss, insomnia, gingivitis, diarrhea, anorexia, weight loss). The classic form of mercury poisoning is called *acrodynia* (or "painful extremities").

NURSING ALERT

Mercury thermometers are no longer recommended because the inhaled vapours can cause toxicity if the thermometer is broken. To prevent inhalation, spilled mercury must be cleaned up quickly, using disposable towels and rubber gloves and washing the hands well after removing the spill.

Heavy metals have an affinity for certain essential tissue chemicals, which must remain free for adequate cell functioning. When metals are bound to these substances, cellular enzyme systems are inactivated. Treatment involves **chelation**, use of a chemical compound that combines with the metal for rapid and safe excretion.

Lead Poisoning

In North America, lead poisoning emerged as a problem in the early 1900s, when white lead was added to paints and tetraethyl lead was added to gasoline as an antiknock compound. Lead content in paint was decreased in 1975 in Canada; the use of lead in paint and leaded gasoline has since been banned in Canada. Blood lead levels in Canadians aged 6 to 79 years have declined over 70% since the 1970s (Government of Canada, 2011). However, children continue to be exposed to lead.

Causes of Lead Poisoning

Although there are numerous sources of lead (Box 46-22), in most instances of acute childhood lead poisoning, the source is food, drinking water, nonintact lead-based paint in an older home, or lead-contaminated bare soil in the yard. Other factors, such as whether a home has lead, copper, or plastic service lines, can affect lead exposure level. For infants and toddlers, the ingestion of soil and dust containing lead, along with food and drinking water, are the greatest sources of exposure to lead in the environment (Government of Canada, 2011). Microparticles of lead gain entrance into a child's body through ingestion or inhalation and, in the case of an exposed pregnant woman, by placental transfer. When measured, a mother's lead level is nearly the same as that of her unborn child. A level of lead not harmful to an adult woman can be harmful to the fetus.

Inhalation exposure usually occurs during renovation and remodelling activities in the home, whereas ingestion happens during normal day-to-day play and mouthing activities. Sometimes a child will actually swallow loose chips of lead-based paint because it has a sweet taste.

Because of family, cultural, or ethnic traditions, a source of lead may be a routine part of life for a child. Nurses must educate themselves about the practices of their patients and identify when such products may be a source of lead. The use of pottery or dishes containing lead may be an issue, as may the use of folk remedies for stomachaches or the use of some cosmetics. Other risk factors for having an elevated blood lead level (BLL) include poverty, age younger than 6 years, dwelling in urban areas, and living in older rental homes where lead decontamination may not be a priority. Children of immigrants and internationally adopted children may have been exposed to sources of lead in their country of origin and should also be carefully evaluated for lead exposure (Woolf, Goldman, & Bellinger, 2007). However, any child is at risk for lead poisoning if hazardous conditions for lead are present in the environment.

Pathophysiology and Clinical Manifestations

Lead can affect any part of the body, including the renal, hematological, and neurological systems (Fig. 46-12). Of most concern for young children is the developing brain and nervous system, which are more vulnerable than those of an older child or adult. Lead in the body moves via an equilibration process among the blood, the soft tissues and organs, and the bones and teeth. Lead ultimately settles in the bones and teeth, where it remains inert and in storage. This makes up the largest portion of the body burden, approximately 75 to 90%. At the cellular level it competes with molecules of calcium, interfering with the regulating action of calcium. The neurological system is of most concern when young children are exposed to lead. The developing brain is especially vulnerable. Lead disrupts the biochemical processes and may directly affect the release of neurotransmitters, may cause alterations in the blood–brain barrier, and may interfere with the regulation of synaptic activity.

The lead levels identified in children have declined since the initiation of screening for children at risk for lead poisoning. Since the late 1960s, children have rarely died of lead poisoning, and seizures and cognitive impairment have become less likely. However, even mild and moderate lead poisoning can cause a number of cognitive and behavioural problems in young children, including aggression, hyperactivity, impulsivity, delinquency, disinterest, and withdrawal. Long-term neurocognitive signs of lead poisoning include developmental delays, lowered intelligence quotient (IQ), reading skill deficits, visual–spatial problems, visual–motor problems, learning disabilities, and lower academic success. Physical growth and reproductive efficiency may also be adversely affected by chronic lead toxicity (Woolf et al., 2007).

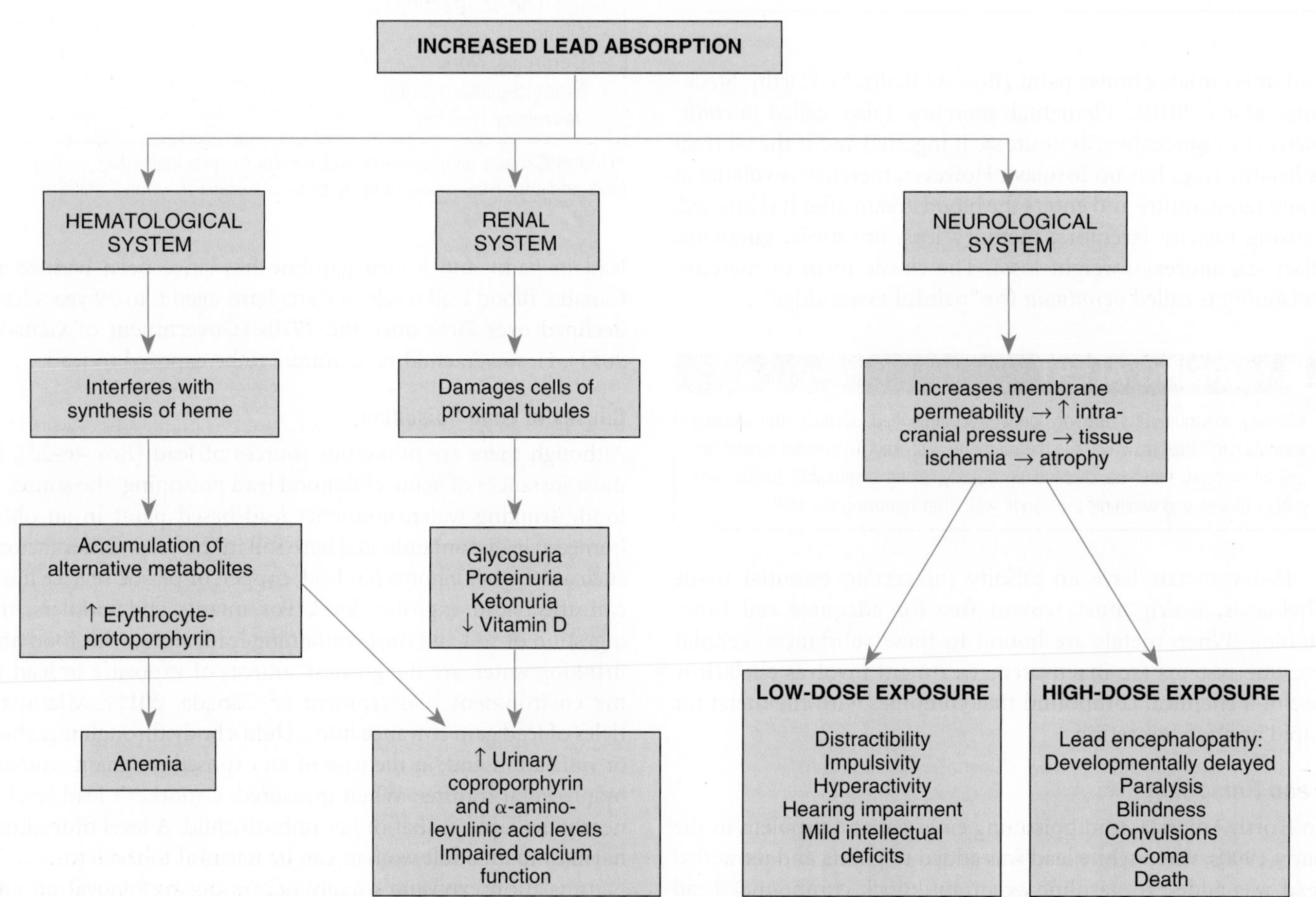

FIGURE 46-12 Main effects of lead on body systems.

There is a relationship between anemia and lead poisoning. Children who are iron deficient absorb lead more readily than those with sufficient iron stores. Lead can interfere with the binding of iron onto the heme molecule. This sometimes creates a picture of anemia, even though the child is not iron deficient. Lead toxicity to the erythrocytes leads to the release of the enzyme erythrocyte protoporphyrin (EP). Because EP is not sensitive to BLLs of lower lead levels, it is no longer used as a screening test. The BLL test is currently used for screening and diagnosis. However, elevation of the EP level is a good indicator of toxicity from lead and reflects the length of exposure and body burden of lead in the individual child.

Although adults have been shown to suffer adverse renal effects from occupational lead exposure, few studies document renal effects in children at other than extremely high lead levels. One can hypothesize that lead can affect the renal integrity of both children and adults. Thus the renal system of a child is still considered a potential target for its harmful effects.

NURSING ALERT

Acute signs of lead poisoning include nausea, vomiting, constipation, anorexia, and abdominal pain. Additional clinical manifestations are hypophosphatemia, glycosuria, and aminoaciduria (Erickson & Thompson, 2005).

Diagnostic Evaluation

Children with lead poisoning rarely have symptoms, even at levels requiring chelation therapy. A diagnosis of lead poisoning is based only on the lead testing of a venous blood specimen from a venipuncture. The collection process is important. Blood must be collected carefully to avoid contamination by lead on the skin. There is scientific evidence that health effects are occurring below the current Canadian blood lead intervention level of 10 mcg/dL. Health effects have been associated with BLLs as low as 1 to 2 mcg/dL, although there is uncertainty associated with effects observed at these levels. Although Canada has one of the lowest lead blood levels in the world, it is still important to further reduce lead exposure since there is currently no safe level of blood lead at which children may not experience adverse health effects (Health Canada, 2013).

Screening for Lead Poisoning

When primary prevention fails, the secondary prevention effort of screening for elevated BLLs can identify children much earlier than in the past. Health Canada (2013) recommends that screening may be necessary in areas where there are unusual sources of lead exposure, such as a historic or ongoing problem of soil contamination from a smelter or if higher blood lead levels have been observed.

Therapeutic Management

The degree of concern, urgency, and need for medical intervention changes as the lead level increases. Education is one of the most important elements of the treatment process. Several areas that the nurse should discuss with the family of every child who has an elevated BLL (5 mcg/dL or higher) include the following (Health Canada, 2013; Heavey, 2008):

- The child's BLL and what it means
- Potential adverse health effects of an elevated BLL
- Sources of lead exposure and suggestions on how to reduce exposure, such as importance of wet cleaning to remove lead dust on floors, window sills, and other surfaces
- Importance of good nutrition in reducing the absorption and effects of lead; for persons with poor nutritional patterns, adequate intake of calcium and iron and importance of regular meals
- Need for follow-up testing to monitor the child's BLL
- Results of an environmental investigation if applicable
- Hazards of improper removal of lead paint (dry sanding, scraping, or open-flame burning)

Treatment actions vary depending on the child's BLL. Based on a diagnosis from a venous BLL test, the Centers for Disease Control and Prevention (CDC), Advisory Committee on Childhood Lead Poison Prevention (2012) recommends that children in the 1- to 5-year age group should be checked for BLL. If the level is ≥5 mcg/dL or higher then the child needs to be checked for iron deficiency and receive an iron supplement if needed and to be checked for general nutrition (levels of vitamin C). In addition, the family should receive lead education and an environmental scan be done where they live. The CDC (2012) also recommends that a BLL of 45 mcg/dL should be considered for chelation therapy.

Chelation therapy. *Chelation* is the term used for removing lead from circulating blood and, theoretically, some lead from organs and tissues. It is unclear whether chelation affects lead stores in bones. Although not an antidote in the truest sense, it does serve a similar purpose in that the toxic substance or poison is removed from the body. However, chelation does not counteract any effects of the lead.

Historically, a chelating agent that has used consistently is calcium disodium edetate ($CaNa_2EDTA$ or calcium EDTA). British anti-Lewisite (BAL, dimercaprol, dimercaptopropanol) is used in conjunction with EDTA. All the agents have potential toxic adverse effects and contraindications. Renal, hepatic, and hematological parameters must be monitored.

Because of the equilibration process among blood, soft tissues, and other sites in the body, there is often a rebound of the BLL after chelation. After the body burden of lead is reduced enough to stabilize the BLL, rebound ceases. Multiple chelation treatments may be necessary. Adequate hydration is essential during therapy because the chelates are excreted via the kidneys.

BAL must not be used in the presence of a glucose 6-phosphate dehydrogenase (G6PD) deficiency or peanut allergy, nor should it be given in conjunction with iron. It is never used as a single-agent therapy, only in conjunction with EDTA. It must be given only at a deep intramuscular site. EDTA should be given intravenously over several hours or, when necessary to restrict fluids, intramuscularly.

An oral chelating agent, d-penicillamine, is sometimes used to treat lead poisoning, but low doses should be used in children, and monitoring of renal function and blood counts during administration is essential (Woolf et al., 2007).

COMMUNITY FOCUS

Reducing Blood Lead Levels

- Make sure the child does not have access to peeling paint or chewable surfaces painted with lead-based paint, especially window sills and wells.
- If a house was built before 1960 (possibly before 1980) and has hard-surface floors, wet mop them at least once per week. Wipe other hard surfaces (e.g., window sills, baseboards). If there are loose paint chips in an area, such as a window well, use a wet disposable cloth to pick up and discard them. Do not vacuum hard-surfaced floors or window sills or wells, because this spreads dust. Use vacuum cleaners with agitators to remove dust from rugs rather than vacuum cleaners with suction only. If a rug is known to contain lead dust and cannot be washed, it should be discarded.
- Wash and dry child's hands and face frequently, especially before eating.
- Wash toys and pacifiers frequently.
- If soil around the home is or is likely to be contaminated with lead (e.g., if the home was built before 1960 or is near a major highway), plant grass or other ground cover; plant bushes around the outside of the house so that the child cannot play there.
- During remodelling of older homes, be sure to follow correct procedures. Be certain children and pregnant women are not in the home, day or night, until the process is completed. After deleading, thoroughly clean house using cleaning solution to damp mop and dust before inhabitants return.
- In areas where lead content of water exceeds the drinking water standard and a particular faucet has not been used for 6 hours or more, "flush" the cold-water pipes by running the water until it becomes as cold as it will get (30 seconds to more than 2 minutes). The more time water has been sitting in pipes, the more lead it may contain.*
- Use only cold water for consumption (drinking, cooking, and especially for making infant formula).
- Hot water dissolves lead more quickly than cold water and thus contains higher levels of lead. First-flush water may be used for nonconsumption uses.
- Have water tested by a competent laboratory. This action is especially important for apartment dwellers; flushing may not be effective in high-rise buildings or in other buildings with lead-soldered central piping.
- Do not store food in open cans, particularly if cans are imported.
- Do not use pottery or ceramic ware that was inadequately fired or is meant for decorative use for food storage or service. Do not store drinks or food in lead crystal.
- Avoid traditional remedies or cosmetics that contain lead.
- Make sure that home exposure is not occurring from parental occupations or hobbies. Household members employed in occupations such as lead smelting should shower and change into clean clothing before leaving work. Construction and lead abatement workers may also bring home lead contaminants.
- Make sure the child eats regular meals, because more lead is absorbed on an empty stomach.
- Make sure the child's diet contains sufficient iron and calcium and does not include excessive fat.

*More information on quality of drinking water is available on Health Canada's website: http://www.hc-sc.gc.ca/ewh-semt/water-eau/drink-potab/index-eng.php

For general information on lead go to Health Canada's lead information page: http://www.hc-sc.gc.ca/ewh-semt/contaminants/lead-plomb/asked_questions-questions_posees-eng.php

Modified from Centers for Disease Control and Prevention. (2005). *Preventing lead poisoning in young children.* Atlanta, GA: Author.

Prognosis

Although most of the pathophysiological effects of lead are reversible, the most serious consequences of both high and low lead exposure are the effects on the central nervous system. In children with lead encephalopathy, permanent brain damage can result in cognitive impairment, behaviour changes, possible paralysis, and seizures. However, moderate- to low-dose exposure may also cause permanent neurological deficits. Increased distractibility, short attention span, impulsivity, reading disabilities, and school failure have been associated with lead exposure. There is some evidence that treatment of moderate levels of lead poisoning can result in cognitive improvement (CDC Advisory Committee on Childhood Lead Poison Prevention, 2012).

NURSING CARE

The primary nursing goal in lead poisoning is to prevent the child's initial or further exposure to lead. For children with low-level exposure, this requires identifying the sources of lead in the environment. Careful history-taking is the most useful and valuable tool and should concentrate on the personal risk questions. Suggestions for reducing lead in the child's environment are listed in the Community Focus box.

For children undergoing chelation therapy, the nurse prepares the child for the injections and makes all efforts to reduce injection pain. Chelating agents are administered deeply into a large muscle mass. To lessen the pain from EDTA, the local anaesthetic procaine is injected with the drug. Rotation of sites is essential to prevent the formation of painful areas of fibrotic tissue. Because EDTA and lead are toxic to the kidneys, the nurse needs to keep records of fluid intake and output and assess the results of urinalysis to monitor renal functioning.

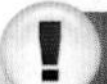

NURSING ALERT

Calcium EDTA is only administered when there is adequate urinary output. Children receiving the medication intramuscularly must be able to maintain adequate oral intake of fluids.

Discharge planning for children with lead poisoning must include thorough education of families regarding safety from lead hazards, clear instructions regarding medication administration and follow-up, and confirmation that the child will be discharged to a home without lead hazards. Although caution must be used to avoid alarming parents unnecessarily, it is important that they know the risk implications for their child's behaviour and cognitive functions. Nurses should observe the development and behaviour of children who are hospitalized. Any concerns that are identified should be thoroughly evaluated. Referral to a child development or speech and language specialist may be indicated.

As in any situational crisis, parents need support and understanding if their child is treated for lead poisoning. Many families at the highest risk for lead poisoning have the fewest resources to adhere to measures such as relocation or removing lead from the environment where the child experiences exposure.

KEY POINTS

- Common nutritional disorders of infancy and early childhood may result from vitamin and mineral deficiency or excess, some types of vegetarian diets, protein-energy malnutrition, and food intolerance.
- Food consumption varies among vegetarians; thus a detailed dietary intake is essential for planning adequate intakes, particularly in children.
- Protein-energy malnutrition may occur as a complication of underlying disease, lack of parental education about infant nutrition, inappropriate management of food allergy, or incorrect preparation of formula.
- Food intolerance encompasses food allergies and food sensitivities, which can have a number of systemic and local clinical manifestations. CMA and lactose intolerance may occur in some children.
- Infants are subject to fluid depletion because of their greater surface area relative to body mass, high rate of metabolism, and immature kidney function.
- Dehydration can be classified as isotonic, hypotonic, and hypertonic.
- Vomiting and diarrhea account for significant fluid depletion, especially in infants and small children.
- The amount, frequency, and characteristics of stool and vomitus are important nursing observations.
- Diarrhea can be caused by an inflammatory process of infectious origin, a toxic reaction to ingestion of poisonous substances, dietary indiscretions, or infections outside the alimentary tract. The primary treatment of diarrhea is the use of an oral rehydrating solution.
- HD requires surgical removal of aganglionic segments of bowel.
- Postoperative care of the child with abdominal surgery involves assessing the abdomen and providing hydration and nutrition, intravenous fluids, proper positioning, wound care, and psychological support.
- Nursing care of GER is aimed at identifying children with suggestive symptoms, helping parents with home care feeding and positioning, and caring for the child undergoing surgical intervention.
- Intestinal parasitic diseases constitute the most common infections in the world; giardiasis and enterobiasis are the most widespread parasitic infections among children in Canada.
- Although the cause of appendicitis is poorly understood, it is typically a result of obstruction of the lumen, usually by a fecalith. Common signs and symptoms are right lower quadrant abdominal pain, tenderness, and fever.
- Meckel's diverticulum is a congenital malformation of the GI tract characterized by bloody stools.
- IBD refers to UC and CD.
- Peptic ulcers are poorly understood, but contributing factors include interference with the normal protective mechanisms of the mucosal lining and the presence of *Helicobacter pylori.*
- Viral hepatitis is caused by six types of virus: HAV, HBV, HCV, HDV, HEV, and HGV.
- HAV is spread by the fecal–oral route, whereas HBV and HCV are transmitted primarily by the parenteral route. The most effective measure in prevention and control of hepatitis in any setting is hand hygiene.
- Structural disorders of the GI tract include CL, CP, EA with TEF, anorectal malformations, and BA.
- BA is a serious disorder, often causing progressive liver failure, which is an indication for liver transplantation.
- CL, CP, and CL/P are the most common facial malformations; they may involve nutritional, dental, and speech problems.
- Hernias related to the GI tract can be minor (umbilical) or life threatening (diaphragmatic, gastroschisis, omphalocele).
- General signs of obstruction include colicky abdominal pain, nausea and vomiting, abdominal distension, and decreased stool output.
- HPS is recognized by characteristic projectile vomiting, malnutrition, dehydration, and a palpable mass in the epigastrium and is relieved by pyloromyotomy.
- Intussusception is one of the most common causes of intestinal obstruction during infancy and is characterized by abdominal pain and blood in stools. Treatment is either nonsurgical hydrostatic reduction or surgical reduction.
- Malabsorption syndromes are disorders associated with some degree of impaired digestion or absorption. They include digestive, absorptive, and anatomical defects.
- Celiac disease is characterized by intolerance to gluten. It is thought to be either an inborn error of metabolism or an immunological response.
- SBS is characterized by a loss of intestine resulting in a diminished ability to absorb a regular diet normally. Specialized enteral and parenteral nutrition is a major element of care for these children.
- Although the incidence of poisoning has decreased in the past 30 years as a result of more stringent packaging regulations, childhood poisoning remains a serious health concern.

- The major principles of treatment for poisoning include assessment and the CABs of resuscitation (cardiovascular supportive measures, airway, and breathing), minimization of poison absorption, prevention of complications, family support, and prevention of recurrence.
- Communication with the area poison control centre is essential in the treatment of any poisoning.
- Acetaminophen poisoning is the most common accidental medication poisoning among children and occurs primarily from acute overdose.
- The most important factor contributing to lead poisoning is its availability in the child's environment. Lead-based paint is the most toxic source of lead.
- Because of increasing awareness of the detrimental effects of low levels of lead on the developing nervous system, acceptable BLLs have been decreasing; but children with cognitive and health effects are still seen. The latest guidelines recommend using a BLL reference value of 5 mcg/dL to guide treatment.

evolve WEBSITE

***Visit the Evolve website for additional resources related to the content in this chapter such as Case Studies, Critical Thinking Case Study Answers, Nursing Care Plans, Nursing Processes, Nursing Skills, and Review Questions for Exam Preparation at:** http://evolve.elsevier.com/Canada/Perry/maternal/*

REFERENCES

Abdel-Kader, H. H., & Balistreri, W. F. (2016). Neonatal cholestasis. In R. M. Kliegman, B. F. Stanton, J. W. St. Geme, et al. (Eds.), *Nelson textbook of pediatrics* (20th ed.). Philadelphia: Saunders.

AboutKidsHealth. (2010). *Intestinal parasites.* Retrieved from <http://www.aboutkidshealth.ca/En/HealthAZ/ConditionsandDiseases/DigestiveSystemDisorders/Pages/Intestinal-Parasites.aspx>.

Achildi, A., & Grewal, H. (2007). Congenital anomalies of the esophagus. *Otolaryngologic Clinics of North America, 40*(1), 219–244.

Aiken, J. J., & Oldham, K. T. (2016). Acute appendicitis. In R. M. Kliegman, B. F. Stanton, J. W. St. Geme, et al. (Eds.), *Nelson textbook of pediatrics* (20th ed.). Philadelphia: Saunders.

Albertson, T. E., Owen, K. P., Sutter, M. E., & Chan, A. L. (2011). Gastrointestinal decontamination in the acutely poisoned patient. *International Journal of Emergency Medicine, 4*(65), doi:10.1186/1865-1380-4-65.

American Academy of Pediatrics (AAP). (2014). *Pediatric nutrition handbook* (7th ed.). Elk Grove Village, IL: Author.

American Academy of Pediatrics, Committee on Infectious Diseases, Kimerberlin, D. W., Brady, M. T., et al. (Eds.). (2015). *Red book: 2015 report of the Committee on Infectious Diseases* (30th ed.). Elk Grove Village, IL: Author.

Amit, C., & Canadian Paediatric Society, Community Paediatrics Committee. (2010). Vegetarian diets in children and adolescents. *Paediatrics & Child Health, 15*(5), 303–314. Retrieved from <http://www.cps.ca/documents/position/vegetarian-diets>. Reaffirmed 2016.

Anand, V., Russell, A. S., Tsuyuki, R., et al. (2008). Perinuclear antineutrophil cytoplasmic autoantibodies and anti-*Saccharomyces cerevisiae* antibodies as serological markers are not specific in the identification of Crohn's disease and ulcerative colitis. *Canadian Journal of Gastroenterology, 22*(1), 33–36.

Angulo, P., & Lindor, K. D. (2010). Primary biliary cirrhosis. In M. Feldman, L. S. Friedman, & L. J. Brandt (Eds.), *Sleisenger and Fordtran's gastrointestinal and liver disease* (9th ed.). Philadelphia: Saunders.

Basnet, S., Schneider, M., Gazit, A., et al. (2010). Fresh goat's milk for infants: Myths and realities—A review. *Pediatrics, 125*(4), e973–e977.

Benchimol, E. I., Guttman, A., Griffiths, A. M., et al. (2009). Increasing incidence of paediatric inflammatory bowel disease in Ontario, Canada: Evidence from health administrative data. *Gut, 58*, 1490–1497. doi:10.1136/gut.2009.188383.

Benchimol, E. I., Mack, D. R., Guttmann, A., et al. (2015). Inflammatory bowel disease in immigrants to Canada and their children: A population-based cohort study. *American Journal of Gastroenterology, 110*(4), 553–563. doi:10.1038/ajg.2015.52.

Bernstein, C. N., Wajda, A., Svenson, L. W., et al. (2006). The epidemiology of inflammatory bowel disease in Canada: A population-based study. *American Journal of Gastroenterology, 101*(7), 1559–1568.

Bhutta, Z. A. (2016). Acute gastroenteritis in children. In R. M. Kliegman, B. F. Stanton, J. W. St. Geme, et al. (Eds.), *Nelson textbook of pediatrics* (20th ed.). Philadelphia: Saunders.

Bischoff, A., Peña, A., & Levitt, M. A. (2013). Laparoscopic-assisted PSARP—The advantages of combining both techniques for the treatment of anorectal malformations with recto-bladderneck or high prostatic fistulas. *Journal of Pediatric Surgery, 48*(2), 367–371. doi:10.1016/j.jpedsurg.2012.11.019.

Blackburn, S. (2013). *Maternal, fetal, and neonatal physiology: A clinical perspective* (4th ed.). St. Louis: Saunders.

Blanchard, S. S., & Czinn, S. J. (2016). Peptic ulcer disease in children. In R. M. Kliegman, B. F. Stanton, J. W. St. Geme, et al. (Eds.), *Nelson textbook of pediatrics* (20th ed.). Philadelphia: Saunders.

Blanco, F. C., Davenport, K. P., & Kane, T. D. (2012). Pediatric gastroesophageal reflux disease. *Surgical Clinics of North America, 92*(3), 541–558. doi:10.1016/j.suc.2012.03.009.

Bonnery, A. G., Mazor, S., & Goldman, R. D. (2013). Laundry detergent capsules and pediatric poisoning. *Canadian Family Physician, 59*(12), 1295–1296.

Bose-O'Reilly, S., McCarthy, K. M., Steckling, N., et al. (2010). Mercury exposure and children's health. *Current Problems in Pediatric and Adolescent Health Care, 40*(8), 186–215. doi:10.1016/jcppeds.2010.07.002.

Boyce, J. A., Assa'ad, A., Burks, A. W., et al. (2011). Guidelines for the diagnosis and management of food allergy in the United States: Summary of the NIAID-sponsored expert panel report. *Nutrition Research, 31*(1), 61–75.

Bradley, G. M., & Oliva-Hemker, M. (2012). Infliximab for the treatment of pediatric ulcerative colitis. *Expert Review of Gastroenterology & Hepatology, 6*(6), 659–665.

Bramuzzo, M., Amaddero, A., Facchina, G., et al. (2013). Liquid detergent capsule ingestion: A new pediatric epidemic? *Pediatric Emergency Care, 29*(3), 410–411.

Branski, D., Troncone, R., & Fasano, A. (2016). Celiac disease (gluten-sensitive enteropathy). In R. M. Kliegman, B. F. Stanton, J. W. St. Geme, et al. (Eds.), *Nelson textbook of pediatrics* (20th ed.). Philadelphia: Saunders.

Bronstein, A. C., Spiker, D. A., Cantilena, L. R., et al. (2012). 2011 Annual report of the American Association of Poison Control Centers National Poison Data System (NPDS): 29th annual report. *Clinical Toxicology, 50*(10), 911–1161. doi:10.3/09/15563650.2012.74642.

Burk, C. J., & Molodow, R. (2007). Infantile scurvy: An old diagnosis revisited with a modern dietary twist. *American Journal of Clinical Dermatology, 8*(2), 103–106.

Canadian Pediatric Society. (2014). *WHO growth charts: Promoting optimal monitoring of child growth in Canada using the WHO growth charts.* Retreived from <http://www.cps.ca/tools-outils/who-growth-charts>.

Canadian Society of Allergy and Clinical Immunology. (2014). *Anaphylaxis in schools and other child care settings* (3rd ed.). Retrieved from <http://csaci.ca/patient-school-resources/>.

Centers for Disease Control and Prevention, Advisory Committee on Childhood Lead Poison Prevention. (2012). *Low level lead exposure harms children: A renewed call for primary prevention.* Retrieved from <http://www.cdc.gov/nceh/lead/ACCLPP/Final_Document_030712.pdf>.

Chapman, K. L., Hardin-Jones, M. A., Goldstein, J. A., et al. (2008). Timing of palatal surgery and speech outcome. *Cleft Palate Craniofacial Journal, 45*(3), 297–308.

Chan, E. S., Cummings, C., & Canadian Paediatric Society, Community Paediatrics Committee, Allergy Section. (2013). Dietary exposures and allergy prevention in high-risk infants. *Paediatrics & Child Health, 18*(10), 545–549. Retrieved from <http://www.cps.ca/en/documents/position/dietary-exposures-and-allergy-prevention-in-high-risk-infants>. Reaffirmed 2016.

Chen, S. M., Chang, M. H., Du, J. C., et al. (2006). Screening for biliary atresia by infant stool color card in Taiwan. *Pediatrics, 117*(4), 1147–1154.

Cheng, A., & Canadian Paediatric Society, Acute Care Committee. (2011). Emergency treatment of anaphylaxis in infants and children. *Paediatrics & Child Health, 16*(1), 35–40. Retrieved from <http://www.cps.ca/documents/position/emergency-treatment-anaphylaxis>. Reaffirmed 2016.

Chu, C. A., & Liacouras, C. A. (2016). Ileus, adhesions, intussusceptions, and closed-loop obstructions. In R. M. Kliegman, B. F. Stanton, J. W. St. Geme, et al. (Eds.), *Nelson textbook of pediatrics* (20th ed.). Philadelphia: Saunders.

Colletti, J. F., Brown, K. M., Sharieff, G. Q., et al. (2010). The management of children with gastroenteritis and dehydration in the emergency department. *Journal of Emergency Medicine, 38*(5), 686–698. doi:10.1016/j.jemermed.2008.06.015.

Criddle, L. M. (2007). An overview of pediatric poisonings. *AACN Advanced Critical Care, 18*(2), 109–118.

Cybulska, P., Ni, A., & Jimenez-Rivera, C. (2011). Viral hepatitis: Retrospective review in a Canadian pediatric hospital. *IRSN Pediatrics, 2011*, 182964. Retrieved from <http://www.hindawi.com/isrn/pediatrics/2011/182964/>.

DeRoo, L. A., Wilcox, A. J., Drevon, C. A., et al. (2008). First-trimester alcohol consumption and the risk of infant oral clefts in Norway: A population-based case-control study. *American Journal of Epidemiology, 168*(6), 638–646.

de Vrese, M., & Schrezenmeir, J. (2008). Probiotics, prebiotics, and synbiotics. *Advances in Biochemical Engineering/Biotechnolology, 111*, 1–66.

Diamond, I. R., Sterescu, A., Pencharz, P. B., et al. (2009). Changing the paradigm: Omegaven for the treatment of liver failure in pediatric short bowel syndrome. *Journal of Pediatric Gastroenterology and Nutrition, 48*(2), 209–215. doi:10.1097/MPG.0b013e318182c8f6.

Dietitians of Canada. (2014). *Healthy eating guidelines for lacto-ovo vegetarians.* Retrieved from <http://www.dietitians.ca/Your-Health/Nutrition-A-Z/Vegetarian-Diets/Eating-Guidelines-for-Lacto-Ovo-Vegetarians.aspx>.

Dietitians of Canada & Canadian Paediatric Society. (2014). *Beware of homemade infant formulas.* Retrieved from <http://www.dietitians.ca/Media/News-Releases/2014/HomemadeFormula.aspx>.

Eisenstein, L., Bodager, D., & Ginzl, D. (2008). Outbreak of giardiasis and cryptosporidiosis associated with a neighborhood interactive water fountain—Florida, 2006. *Journal of Environmental Health, 71*(3), 18–22.

Emond, S. (2009). Dehydration in infants and young children. *Annals of Emergency Medicine, 53*(3), 395–397.

Erickson, L., & Thompson, T. (2005). A review of a preventable poison: Pediatric lead poisoning. *Journal for Specialists in Pediatric Nursing, 10*(4), 171–182.

Findlay, L. C., & Janz, T. A. (2012). The health of Inuit children under age 6 in Canada. *International Journal of Circumpolar Health, 71*, doi:10.3402/ijch.v71i0.18580.

Fiorino, K., & Liacouras, C. A. (2016). Congenital aganglionic megacolon (Hirschprung disease). In R. M. Kliegman, B. F. Stanton, J. W. St. Geme, et al. (Eds.), *Nelson textbook of pediatrics* (20th ed.). Philadelphia: Saunders.

Gelfond, D., & Fasano, A. (2006). Celiac disease in the pediatric population. *Pediatric Annals, 35*(4), 275–279.

Goday, P. S. (2009). Short bowel syndrome: How short is too short? *Clinics of Perinatology, 36*(1), 101–110. doi:10.1016/jclp.2008.09.006.

Godel, J. C., & Canadian Paediatric Society, First Nations, Inuit and Métis Health Committee. (2007). Vitamin D supplementation: Recommendations for Canadian mothers and infants. *Paediatrics & Child Health, 12*(7), 583–589. Retrieved from <http://www.cps.ca/documents/position/vitamin-d>. Reaffirmed 2015.

Godwin, K. A., Sibbald, B., Bedard, T., et al. (2008). Changes in frequencies of select congenital anomalies since the onset of folic acid fortification in a Canadian birth defect registry. *Canadian Journal of Public Health, 99*(4), 271–275.

Gourlay, D. M. (2013). Colorectal considerations in pediatric patients. *Surgical Clinics of North America, 93*(2), 251–272.

Government of Canada. (2011). *Metals of concern fact sheet series: Lead.* Retrieved from <https://www.aadnc-aandc.gc.ca/eng/1316104149117/1316104393366>.

Government of Canada. (2012). *Food safety tips—Interactive guide.* Retrieved from <http://healthycanadians.gc.ca/eating-nutrition/healthy-eating-saine-alimentation/safety-salubrite/tips-conseils/safety-interactive-salubrite-eng.php>.

Government of Canada. (2013). *Congenital anomalies in Canada 2013—A perinatal health report.* Retrieved from <http://publications.gc.ca/site/eng/443924/publication.html>.

Government of Canada. (2014). *News release: Government of Canada reminds Canadians how to protect children from dangerous household chemicals—Products should be locked up, out of sight, out of reach.* Retrieved from <http://news.gc.ca/web/article-en.do?nid=826029&_ga=1.220557201.868197850.1432519476>.

Greenbaum, L. A. (2016). Electrolyte and acid–base disorders. In R. M. Kliegman, B. F. Stanton, J. W. St. Geme, et al. (Eds.), *Nelson textbook of pediatrics* (20th ed.). Philadelphia: Saunders.

Greene, S., Harris, C., & Singer, J. (2008). Gastrointestinal decontamination of the poisoned patient. *Pediatric Emergency Care, 24*(3), 176–186.

Grover, Z., & Ee, L. C. (2009). Protein energy malnutrition. *Pediatric Clinics of North America, 56*(5), 1055–1068. doi:10.1016/j.pcl.2009.07.001.

Guandalini, S. (2008). Probiotics for children with diarrhea: An update. *Journal of Clinical Gastroenterology, 42*(Suppl. 2), S53–S57.

Guidry, C., & McGahren, E. D. (2012). Pediatric chest I: Developmental and physiologic conditions for the surgeons. *Surgical Clinics of North America, 92*(3), 615–643. doi:10.1016/j.suc.2012.03.013.

Hassall, E., Owen, D., Kerr, W., et al. (2011). Gastric histology in children treated with proton pump inhibitors long term, with emphasis on enterochromaffin cell-like hyperplasia. *Alimentary Pharmacology & Therapeutics, 33*(7), 829–836. doi:10.1111/j.1365-2036.2011.04592.x.

Health Canada. (2012a). *Vitamin D and calcium: Updated dietary reference intakes.* Retrieved from <http://www.hc-sc.gc.ca/fn-an/nutrition/vitamin/vita-d-eng.php#a15>.

Health Canada. (2012b). *Food allergies and intolerances.* Retrieved from <http://www.hc-sc.gc.ca/fn-an/securit/allerg/index-eng.php>.

Health Canada. (2013). *Lead. What is lead?* Retrieved from <http://www.hc-sc.gc.ca/ewh-semt/contaminants/lead-plomb/index-eng.php>.

Health Canada. (2015). *Food allergies: It's your health.* Retrieved from <http://www.hc-sc.gc.ca/hl-vs/iyh-vsv/food-aliment/allerg-eng.php>.

Heavey, E. (2008). Lead poisoning in children; still a threat. *Nursing, 38*(12), 17–18.

Herwig, K., Brenkert, T., & Losek, J. D. (2009). Enema-reduced intussusception management: Is hospitalization necessary? *Pediatric Emergency Care, 25*(2), 74–77.

Heyman, M. B., & American Academy of Pediatrics Committee on Nutrition. (2006). Lactose intolerance in infants, children, and adolescents. *Pediatrics, 118*(3), 1279–1286.

Hunter, A. K., & Liacouras, C. A. (2016). Pyloric stenosis and other congenital anomalies of the stomach. In R. M. Kliegman, B. F. Stanton, J. W. St. Geme, et al. (Eds.), *Nelson textbook of pediatrics* (20th ed.). Philadelphia: Saunders.

Huppertz, H. I., Soriano-Gabarró, M., Grimprel, E., et al. (2006). Intussusception among young children in Europe. *Pediatric Infectious Diseases Journal, 25*(1), S22–S29.

Ivarsson, A., Myléus, A., Norström, F., et al. (2013). Prevalence of childhood celiac disease and changes in infant feeding. *Pediatrics, 131*(3), e687–e694.

Jefferies, A. L., & Canadian Paediatric Society, Fetus and Newborn Committee. (2014). Going home: Facilitating discharge of the preterm infant. *Paediatrics & Child Health, 19*(1), 31–36. Retrieved from <http://www.cps.ca/en/documents/position/facilitating-discharge-of-the-preterm-infant>. Reaffirmed 2016.

Jensen, M. K., & Balistreri, W. G. (2016). Viral hepatitis. In R. M. Kliegman, B. F. Stanton, J. W. St. Geme, et al. (Eds.), *Nelson textbook of pediatrics* (20th ed.). Philadelphia: Saunders.

Jung, W. J., Yang, H. J., Min, T. K., et al. (2012). The efficacy of the upright position on gastro-esophageal reflux and reflux-related respiratory symptoms in infants with chronic respiratory symptoms. *Allergy Asthma Immunology Research, 4*(1), 17–23.

Kamath, B. M., & Olthoff, K. M. (2010). Liver transplantation in children: Update 2010. *Pediatric Clinics of North America, 57*(2), 401–414.

Kane, T. D. (2009). Laparoscopic Nissen fundoplication. *Minerva Chirurgica, 64*(2), 147–157.

Kattan, J. D., Cocco, R. R., & Järvinen, K. M. (2011). Milk and soy allergy. *Pediatric Clinics of North America, 58*(2), 407–426. doi:10.1016/j.pcl.2011.02.005.

Kawchak, D. A., Schall, J. I., Zemel, B. S., et al. (2007). Adequacy of dietary intake declines with age in children with sickle cell disease. *Journal of American Dietary Association, 107*(5), 843–848.

Kemper, K. J., & Gardiner, P. (2016). Complementary therapies and integrative medicine. In R. M. Kliegman, B. F. Stanton, J. St. Geme, et al. (Eds.), *Nelson textbook of pediatrics* (20th ed.). Philadelphia: Saunders.

Kendrick, D., Smith, S., Sutton, A., et al. (2008). Effect of education and safety equipment on poisoning-prevention practices and poisoning: Systematic review, meta-analysis and meta-regression. *Archives of Diseases in Childhood, 93*(7), 599–608.

Khan, S., & Orenstein, S. R. (2016). Esophageal atresia and tracheoesophageal fistula. In R. M. Kliegman, B. F. Stanton, J. W. St. Geme, et al. (Eds.), *Nelson textbook of pediatrics* (20th ed.). Philadelphia: Saunders.

Kunisaki, S. M., & Foker, J. E. (2012). Surgical advances in the fetus and neonate: Esophageal atresia. *Clinics in Perinatology, 39*(2), 349–361. doi:10.1016/j.clp.2012.04.007.

Lawrence, B., Gantt, G., Samuels-Reid, J., et al. (2012). Suffocation deaths associated with use of infant sleep positioners—United States, 1997–2011. *MMWR Morbidity & Mortality Weekly Report, 61*(46), 933–937.

Lawrence, R. A., & Lawrence, R. M. (2015). *Breastfeeding: A guide for the medical professional* (8th ed.). St. Louis: Elsevier.

Leung, A., Otley, A., & Canadian Paediatric Society, Nutrition and Gastroenterology Committee. (2009). Concerns for the use of soy-based formulas in infant nutrition. *Paediatrics & Child Health, 14*(3), 109–113. Retrieved from <http://www.cps.ca/documents/position/use-soy-based-formulas>. Reaffirmed 2016.

Leung, A., Prince, T., & Canadian Paediatric Society, Nutrition and Gastroenterology Committee. (2006). Oral rehydration therapy and early refeeding in the management of childhood gastroenteritis. *Paediatrics & Child Health, 11*(8), 527–531. Retrieved from <http://www.cps.ca/en/documents/position/oral-rehydration-therapy>. Reaffirmed 2016.

Levitt, M. A., Martin, C. A., Olesevich, M., et al. (2009). Hirschsprung disease and fecal incontinence: Diagnostic and management strategies. *Journal of Pediatric Surgery, 44*(1), 271–277.

Lightdale, J. R., & Gremse, D. A. (2013). Gastroesophageal reflux: Management guidance for the pediatrician. *Pediatrics, 131*(5), e1684–e1695. doi:10.1542/peds.2013-0421.

Luther, J., Chey, W. D., & Saad, R. J. (2011). A clinician's guide to salvage therapy for persistent *Helicobacter pylori* infection. *Hospital Practice, 39*(1), 133–140. doi:10.3810/hp.2011.02.383.

Mack, C. L., Gonzalez-Peralta, R. P., Gupta, N., et al. (2012). NASPGHAN practice guidelines: Diagnosis and management of hepatitis C infection in infants, children and adolescents. *Journal of Pediatric Gastroenterology and Nutrition, 54*(6), 838–855. doi:10.1097/MPG.0b013e318258328d.

Madden, M. A. (2008). Responding to pediatric poisoning. *Nursing, 38*(8), 52–55. doi:10.1097/01.NURSE.0000327496.01064.a9.

Mankad, V. (2013). *Food allergies and cross-reactivity.* Retrieved from <http://community.kidswithfoodallergies.org/blog/food-allergy-cross-reactivity>.

Marchand, V., & Canadian Paediatric Society, Nutrition and Gastroenterology Committee. (2012). Using probiotics in the paediatric population. *Paediatrics & Child Health, 17*(10), 575. Retrieved from <http://www.cps.ca/en/documents/position/probiotics-in-the-paediatric-population>. Reaffirmed 2015.

Masarei, A. G., Wade, A., Mars, M., et al. (2007). A randomized control trial investigating the effect of presurgical orthopedics on feeding in infants with cleft lip and/or cleft palate. *Cleft Palate & Craniofacial Journal, 44*(2), 182–193.

McCabe, M. A., Toughill, E. H., Parkhill, A. M., et al. (2012). Celiac disease: A medical puzzle. *American Journal of Nursing, 112*(19), 34–44.

Menezes, M., Tareen, F., Saeed, S., et al. (2008). Symptomatic Meckel's diverticululm in children: A 16-year review. *Pediatric Surgery International, 24*(5), 575–577.

Mills, J. L., Konkin, D. E., Milner, R., et al. (2008). Long-term bowel function and quality of life in children with Hirschsprung's disease. *Journal of Pediatric Surgery, 43*(5), 899–905.

Nowak-Wegrzyn, A., Sampson, H. A., & Sicherer, S. A. (2016). Food allergy and adverse reactions to foods. In R. M. Kliegman, B. F. Stanton, J. W. St. Geme, et al. (Eds.), *Nelson textbook of pediatrics* (20th ed.). Philadelphia: Saunders.

O'Connor, A., Gisbert, J., & O'Morain, C. (2009). Treatment of *Helicobacter pylori* infection. *Helicobacter, 14*(Suppl. 1), 46–51.

Olson, D. E., Kim, Y. W., & Donnelly, L. F. (2009). CT findings in children with Meckel's diverticulum. *Pediatric Radiology, 39*(7), 659–663. doi:10.1007/s13244-010-0017-8.

Payne, D. C., Staat, M. A., Edwards, K. M., et al. (2011). Direct and indirect effects of rotavirus vaccination upon childhood hospitalizations in 3 US counties, 2006–2009. *Clinical Infectious Diseases: An Official Publication of the Infectious Diseases Society of America, 53*(3), 245–253. doi:10.1093/cid/cir307.

Pepper, V. K., Stanfill, A. B., & Pearl, R. H. (2012). Diagnosis and management of pediatric appendicitis, intussusception, and Meckel's diverticulum. *Surgical Clinics of North America, 92*(3), 505–526. doi:10.1016/j.suc.2012.03.011.

Plenge-Bönig, A., Soto-Ramírez, N., Karmaus, W., et al. (2010). Breastfeeding protects against acute gastroenteritis due to rotavirus in infants. *European Journal of Pediatrics, 169*(12), 1471–1476. doi:10.1007/s00431-010-1245-0.

Preston, A. M., Rodriguez, C., & Rivera, C. E. (2006). Plasma ascorbate in a population of children: Influence of age, gender, vitamin C intake, and smoke exposure. *Puerto Rico Health Sciences Journal, 25*(2), 137–142.

Public Health Agency of Canada. (2012). *Giardia lambia.* Retrieved from <http://www.phac-aspc.gc.ca/lab-bio/res/psds-ftss/giardia-lamblia-eng.php>.

Public Health Agency of Canada. (2013). *Healthcare-associated infections—Due diligence.* Retreived from <http://www.phac-aspc.gc.ca/cphorsphc-respcacsp/2013/infections-eng.php>.

Public Health Agency of Canada. (2014). *Hepatitis B—Get the facts.* Retrieved from <http://www.phac-aspc.gc.ca/hcai-iamss/bbp-pts/hepatitis/hep_b-eng.php>.

Public Health Agency of Canada. (2016). *Canadian immunization. Part 4: Active vaccines. Hepatitis B vaccine.* Retrieved from <http://www.phac-aspc.gc.ca/publicat/cig-gci/p04-hepb-eng.php>.

Rashid, A. N., Taminiau, J. A., Benninga, M. A., et al. (2016). Definitions and outcome measures in pediatric functional upper gastrointestinal tract disorders: A systematic review. *Journal of Pediatric Gastroenterology and Nutrition, 62*(4), 581–587.

Ricart, E., García-Bosch, O., & Ordás, I. (2008). Are we giving biologics too late? The case for early versus late use. *World Journal of Gastroenterology, 14*(36), 5523–5527. doi:10.3748/wjg.14.5523.

Robbins, J. M., Damiano, P., Druschel, C. M., et al. (2010). Prenatal diagnosis of orofacial clefts: Association with maternal satisfaction, team care, and treatment outcomes. *Cleft Palate Craniofacial Journal, 47*(5), 476–481. doi:10.1597/08-177.

Robinson, J. L., & Canadian Paediatric Society, Infectious Diseases and Immunization Committee. (2008). Vertical transmission of the hepatitis C virus: Current knowledge and issues. *Paediatrics & Child Health, 13*(6), 529–534. Retrieved from <http://www.cps.ca/en/documents/position/vertical-transmission-of-hepatitis-C>. Reaffirmed 2016.

Rowan-Legg, A., & Canadian Paediatric Society, Community Paediatrics Committee. (2011). Managing functional constipation in children. *Paediatrics & Child Health, 6*(10), 661–665. Retrieved from <http://www.cps.ca/en/documents/position/functional-constipation>. Reaffirmed in 2016.

Rutter, M. D., Saunders, B. P., Wilkinson, K. H., et al. (2006). Thirty-year analysis of colonoscopic surveillance program for neoplasia in ulcerative colitis. *Gastroenterology, 130*(4), 1030–1038.

Saltzman, M. D., & King, E. C. (2007). Central physeal arrests as a manifestation of hypervitaminosis A. *Journal of Pediatric Orthopedics, 27*(3), 351–353.

Salvadori, M., Le Saux, N., & Canadian Paediatric Society, Infectious Diseases and Immunization Committee. (2010). Recommendations for the use of rotavirus vaccines in infants. *Paediatrics & Child Health, 15*(8), 519–523. Retrieved from <http://www.cps.ca/en/documents/position/rotavirus-vaccines>. Reaffirmed 2015.

Sauer, C. G., & Kugathasan, S. (2010). Pediatric inflammatory bowel disease: Highlighting pediatric differences in IBD. *Medical Clinics of North America, 94*(1), 35–52.

Sheffield, P., & Serwint, J. R. (2008). Emetics, cathartics, and gastric lavage. *Pediatrics in Review, 29*(6), 214–215.

Silbermintz, A., & Markowitz, J. (2006). Inflammatory bowel diseases. *Pediatric Annals, 35*(4), 268–274.

Simmons, F. E. (2009). Anaphylaxis: Recent advances in assessment and treatment. *Journal of Allergy and Clinical Immunology, 124*(4), 625–636.

Sood, M. R. (2016). Chronic functional constipation and fecal incontinence in infants and children: Treatment. *UpToDate.* Retrieved from <http://www.uptodate.com/contents/chronic-functional-constipation-and-fecal-incontinence-in-infants-and-children-treatment>.

Sung, J. J., Kuipers, E. J., & El-Serag, H. B. (2009). Systematic review: The global incidence and prevalence of peptic ulcer disease. *Aliment Pharmacology Therapies, 29*(9), 938–946. doi:10.1111/j.1365-2036.2009.03960.x.

Suwandhi, E., Ton, M. N., & Schwarz, S. M. (2006). Gastroesophageal reflux in infancy and childhood. *Pediatric Annals, 35*(4), 259–266.

Theocharatos, S., & Kenny, S. E. (2008). Hirschsprung's disease: Current management and prospects for transplantation of enteric nervous system progenitor cells. *Early Human Development, 84*(12), 801–804.

Thurley, P. D., Halliday, K. E., Somers, J. M., et al. (2009). Radiological features of Meckel's diverticulum and its complications. *Clinical Radiology, 64*(2), 109–118. doi:10.1016/j.crad.2008.07.012.

To, T., & Langer, J. C. (2010). Does access to care affect outcomes of appendicitis in children? A population-based cohort study. *BMC Health Services Research, 10*, 250.

Tran, T. T. (2009). Management of hepatitis B in pregnancy: Weighing the options. *Cleveland Clinics Journal of Medicine, 76*(Suppl. 3), S25–S29.

University of Chicago Celiac Disease Center. (2016). *Fact sheet: Genetic screening for celiac disease.* University of Chicago. Retrieved from <http://www.cureceliacdisease.org/?s=genetic+screening+for+celiac+disease+fact+sheet>.

Vandenplas, Y., Rudolph, C. D., & Di Lorenzo, C. (2009). Pediatric gastroesophageal reflux clinical practice guidelines: Joint recommendations of the North American Society for Pediatric Gastroenterology, Hepatology, and Nutrition and the European Society for Pediatric Gastroenterology, Hepatology, and Nutrition. *Journal of Pediatric Gastroenterology and Nutrition, 49*(4), 498–547. doi:10.1097/MPG.0b013e3181b7f563.

van der Pol, R. J., Smits, M. J., Wijk, M. P., et al. (2011). Efficacy of proton pump inhibitors in children with gastroesophageal reflux disease: A systematic review. *Pedatrics, 127*(5), 925–935. doi:10.1542/peds.2010-2719.

Vohra, S., Clifford, T., & Canadian Paediatric Society, Drug Therapy and Hazardous Substances Committee. (2005). Children and natural health products: What a clinician should know. *Paediatrics & Child Health, 10*(4), 227–232. Retrieved from <http://www.cps.ca/en/documents/position/natural-health-products>. Reaffirmed 2016.

Waseem, M., & Rosenberg, H. K. (2008). Intussusception. *Pediatric Emergency Care, 24*(11), 793–800.

Whyte, C., Levin, T., & Harris, B. H. (2008). Early decisions in perforated appendix in children: Lessons from a study of nonoperative management. *Journal of Pediatric Surgery, 43*(8), 1459–1463. doi:10.1016/j.jpedsurg.2007.11.032.

Woolf, A. D., Goldman, R., & Bellinger, D. C. (2007). Update on clinical management of childhood lead poisoning. *Pediatric Clinics of North America, 54*(2), 271–294. doi:10.1016/j.pcl.2007.01.008.

ADDITIONAL RESOURCES

About Face—Support for persons with cleft lip and palate and other facial differences: <http://www.aboutface.ca>.

Allergy/Asthma Information Association: <http://www.aaia.ca/en/index.htm>.

Canadian Celiac Association: <http://www.celiac.ca>.

Canadian Liver Foundation: <http://www.liver.ca>.

Crohn's and Colitis Canada: <http://www.crohnsandcolitis.ca/site/c.dtJRL9NUJmL4H/b.9012407/k.BE24/Home.htm>.

Dietitians of Canada—Information on vegetarian diets: <http://www.dietitians.ca/Your-Health/Nutrition-A-Z/Vegetarian-Diets.aspx>.

Food Allergy Canada—Information on food allergies: <http://foodallergycanada.ca/>.

Health Canada—Dietary Reference Intake Report List: <http://www.hc-sc.gc.ca/fn-an/nutrition/reference/dri_rep-rap_anref-list/index-eng.php>.

National Center for Complementary and Alternative Medicine: <http://www.nccam.nih.gov>.

Ostomy Canada Society: <http://www.ostomycanada.ca>.

Parachute—Poison prevention: <http://www.parachutecanada.org/policy/item/poison-prevention>.

CHAPTER

47

Cardiovascular Dysfunction

Anne Hogarth, with contributions from Marilyn J. Hockenberry

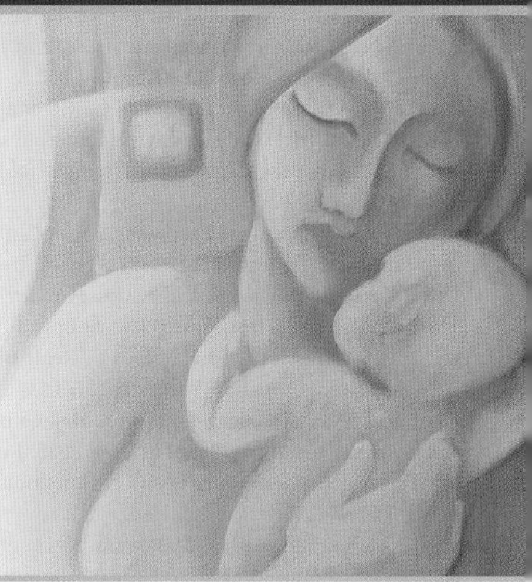

evolve WEBSITE

Visit the Evolve website for additional resources related to the content in this chapter such as Case Studies, Critical Thinking Case Study Answers, Nursing Care Plans, Nursing Processes, Nursing Skills, and Review Questions for Exam Preparation at: http://evolve.elsevier.com/Canada/Perry/maternal/

OBJECTIVES

On completion of this chapter the reader will be able to:

- Design a plan for assisting a child during a cardiac diagnostic procedure.
- Demonstrate an understanding of the hemodynamics, distinctive manifestations, and therapeutic management of congenital heart disease.
- Outline a care plan for an infant or child with heart failure.
- Describe the care for a child who has hypoxia.
- Describe the care for an infant or a child with a congenital heart defect and its surgical repair.
- Discuss the nurse's role in helping the child and family cope with congenital heart disease.
- Differentiate between rheumatic fever and rheumatic heart disease.
- List the criteria for selected cholesterol screening of children.
- Discuss the assessment and management of hypertension in children and adolescents.
- Outline a care plan for a child with Kawasaki disease.
- Describe the emergency treatment for shock, including anaphylaxis.

CARDIOVASCULAR DYSFUNCTION

Cardiovascular disorders in children are divided into two major groups: congenital heart disease and acquired heart disorders. *Congenital heart disease (CHD)* includes primarily anatomical abnormalities present at birth that result in abnormal cardiac function. The clinical consequences of congenital heart defects fall into two broad categories: heart failure (HF) and hypoxemia. *Acquired cardiac disorders* are disease processes or abnormalities that occur after birth and can be seen in the normal heart or in the presence of congenital heart defects. They result from various factors, including infection, autoimmune responses, environmental factors, and familial tendencies.

History and Physical Examination

Taking an accurate health history is an important first step in assessing an infant or child for possible heart disease. Parents may have specific concerns, such as an infant with poor feeding or fast breathing, or a 7-year-old who can no longer keep up with friends on the soccer field. Others may not realize that their child has a medical problem; their baby has always been pale and fussy.

Asking details about the mother's health history, pregnancy, and birth history are important in assessing infants. Mothers with chronic health conditions, such as diabetes or lupus, are more likely to have infants with heart disease. Some medications, such as phenytoin (Dilantin), are teratogenic to the fetus. Maternal alcohol use or illicit drug use increases the risk of congenital heart defects. Exposures to infections, such as rubella, early in pregnancy may result in congenital anomalies. Infants with low birth weight resulting from intrauterine growth restriction are more likely to have congenital anomalies. High-birth-weight infants have an increased incidence of heart disease.

A detailed family history is also important. There is an increased incidence of congenital cardiac defects if either parent or a sibling has a heart defect. Some diseases, such as Marfan syndrome, and some cardiomyopathies are hereditary. A family history of frequent fetal loss, sudden infant death, and sudden death in adults may indicate heart disease. Congenital heart defects are seen in many syndromes such as Down and Turner syndromes.

The physical assessment of suspected cardiac disease begins with observation of general appearance and proceeds with more specific observations. The following elements are supplementary to the general assessment techniques described for physical examination of the chest and heart in Chapter 33.

Inspection

Nutritional state—Failure to thrive or poor weight gain is associated with heart disease.

Colour—Cyanosis is a common feature of CHD; pallor is associated with poor perfusion.

Chest deformities—An enlarged heart sometimes distorts the chest configuration.

Unusual pulsations—Visible pulsations of the neck veins are seen in some patients.

Respiratory excursion—This refers to the ease or difficulty of respiration (e.g., tachypnea, dyspnea, expiratory grunt).

Clubbing of fingers—This is associated with cyanosis.

Palpation and Percussion

Chest—These manoeuvres help discern heart size and other characteristics (e.g., thrills) associated with heart disease.

Abdomen—Hepatomegaly or splenomegaly may be evident.

Peripheral pulses—Rate, regularity, and amplitude (strength) may reveal discrepancies.

Auscultation

Heart rate and rhythm—Listen for fast heart rates (*tachycardia*), slow heart rates (*bradycardia*), or irregular rhythms.

Character of heart sounds—Listen for distinct or muffled sounds, murmurs, and additional heart sounds.

Diagnostic Evaluation

A variety of invasive and noninvasive tests may be used in the diagnosis of heart disease. Some of the more common diagnostic tools that require nursing assessment and intervention are described in Table 47-1.

Electrocardiogram

Bedside cardiac monitoring with the electrocardiogram (ECG) is commonly used in pediatrics, especially in the care of children with heart disease. The bedside monitor provides valuable information about heart rate and rhythm through a graphic display of the ECG tracing and a digital display. An alarm can be set with parameters for individual patient requirements and will sound if the heart rate is above or below the set parameters. Gelfoam electrodes are commonly used and placed on the right side of the chest (above the level of the heart) and the left side of the chest, and a ground electrode is placed on the abdomen. Electrodes should be changed every 1 or 2 days because they irritate the skin. Bedside monitors are an adjunct to patient care and should never be substituted for direct assessment and

TABLE 47-1 PROCEDURES FOR CARDIAC DIAGNOSIS

PROCEDURE	DESCRIPTION
Chest radiograph (x-ray)	Provides information on heart size and pulmonary blood flow patterns
Electrocardiography	Graphic measure of electrical activity of heart
Holter monitor	24-hr continuous electrocardiogram (ECG) recording used to assess dysrhythmias
Echocardiography	Use of high-frequency sound waves obtained by a transducer to produce an image of cardiac structures
Transthoracic	Done with transducer on chest
M-mode	One-dimensional graphic view used to estimate ventricular size and function
Two-dimensional	Real-time, cross-sectional views of heart used to identify cardiac structures and cardiac anatomy
Doppler	Identifies blood flow patterns and pressure gradients across structures
Fetal	Imaging fetal heart in utero
Transesophageal (TEE)	Transducer placed in esophagus behind heart to obtain images of posterior heart structures or in patients with poor images from chest approach
Cardiac catheterization	Imaging study using radiopaque catheters placed in a peripheral blood vessel and advanced into heart to measure pressures and oxygen levels in heart chambers and visualize heart structures and blood flow patterns
Hemodynamics	Measures pressures and oxygen saturations in heart chambers
Angiography	Use of contrast material to illuminate heart structures and blood flow patterns
Biopsy	Use of special catheter to remove tiny samples of heart muscle for microscopic evaluation; used in assessing infection, inflammation, or muscle dysfunction disorders and to evaluate for rejection after heart transplant
Electrophysiology (EPS)	Special catheters with electrodes used to record electrical activity from within heart; used to diagnose rhythm disturbances
Exercise stress test	Monitoring of heart rate, blood pressure, ECG, and oxygen consumption at rest and during progressive exercise on a treadmill or bicycle
Cardiac magnetic resonance imaging (MRI)	Noninvasive imaging technique; used in evaluation of vascular anatomy outside of heart (e.g., coarctation of the aorta, vascular rings), estimates of ventricular mass and volume; uses for MRI are expanding

auscultation of heart sounds. The nurse should assess the patient, not the monitor.

NURSING ALERT

Electrodes for cardiac monitoring are often colour coded: white for right, green (or red) for ground, and black for left. Always check to ensure that these colours are placed correctly.

Echocardiography

Echocardiography is one of the most frequently used tests for detecting cardiac dysfunction in children. Recent improvements in echocardiographic techniques have made it increasingly possible to confirm the diagnosis without resorting to cardiac catheterization. In increasing numbers of cases a prenatal diagnosis of CHD can be made by fetal echocardiography.

Echocardiography involves the use of ultrahigh-frequency sound waves to produce an image of the heart's structure. A transducer placed directly on the chest wall delivers repetitive pulses of ultrasound and processes the returned signals (echoes).

Although the test is noninvasive, painless, and associated with no known side effects, it can be stressful for children. The child must lie quietly in the standard echocardiographic positions; crying, nursing, or sitting up often leads to diagnostic errors or omissions. Infants and young children may need a mild sedative; older children benefit from psychological preparation for the test. The distraction of a DVD or movie is often helpful.

Cardiac Catheterization

Cardiac catheterization is an invasive diagnostic procedure in which a radiopaque catheter is inserted through a peripheral blood vessel into the heart. The catheter is usually introduced through percutaneous technique, in which the catheter is threaded through a large-bore needle that is inserted into the vein. The catheter is guided through the heart with the aid of fluoroscopy. After the tip of the catheter is within a heart chamber, contrast material is injected, and films are taken of the dilution and circulation of the material (angiography). Types of cardiac catheterizations include the following:

Diagnostic catheterizations—These studies are used to diagnose congenital cardiac defects, particularly in symptomatic infants and before surgical repair. They are divided into (1) right-sided catheterizations, in which the catheter is introduced through a vein (usually the femoral vein) and threaded to the right atrium (most common), and (2) left-sided catheterizations, in which the catheter is threaded through an artery into the aorta and then into the heart.

Interventional catheterizations (therapeutic catheterizations)—A balloon catheter or other device is used to alter the cardiac anatomy. Examples include dilating stenotic valves or vessels or closing abnormal connections.

Electrophysiology studies—Catheters with tiny electrodes that record the impulses of the heart directly from the conduction system are used to evaluate dysrhythmias and sometimes destroy accessory pathways that cause some tachydysrhythmias.

NURSING CARE

Cardiac catheterization has become a routine diagnostic procedure and may be done on an outpatient basis. However, it is not without risks, especially in newborns and seriously ill infants and children. Possible complications include acute hemorrhage from the entry site (more likely with interventional procedures because larger catheters are used), low-grade fever, nausea, vomiting, loss of pulse in the catheterized extremity (usually transient, resulting from a clot, hematoma, or intimal tear), and transient dysrhythmias (generally catheter induced) (Uzark, 2001). Rare risks include stroke, seizures, tamponade, and death. Researchers from Toronto's Hospital for Sick Kids found a complication rate of 7.3% (Mehta, Lee, Chaturvedi, et al., 2008).

Preprocedural care. A complete nursing assessment is necessary to ensure a safe procedure with minimum complications. This assessment should include accurate height (essential for correct catheter selection) and weight. Obtaining a history of allergic reactions is important because some of the contrast agents are iodine based. Specific attention to signs and symptoms of infection is crucial. Severe diaper rash may be a reason to cancel the procedure if femoral access is required. Because assessment of pedal pulses is important after catheterization, the nurse should assess and mark pulses (dorsalis pedis, posterior tibial) before the child goes to the catheterization room. The presence and quality of pulses in both feet should be clearly documented. Baseline oxygen saturation using pulse oximetry in children with cyanosis is also recorded.

Preparing the child and family for the procedure is the joint responsibility of the patient care team. School-age children and adolescents benefit from a description of the catheterization laboratory and a chronological explanation of the procedure, emphasizing what they will see, feel, and hear. Older children and adolescents may bring earphones and favourite music so they can listen during the catheterization procedure. Preparation materials such as picture books, DVDs, or tours of the catheterization laboratory may be helpful. Preparation should be geared to the child's developmental level. The child's caregivers often benefit from the same explanations. Additional information, such as the expected length of the catheterization, description of the child's appearance after catheterization, and usual postprocedure care, should be outlined. (See also Prepare the Child and Family for Invasive Procedures, p. 1501.)

Methods of sedation vary among institutions and may include oral or intravenous (IV) medications (see Chapter 44). The child's age, heart defect, clinical status, and type of catheterization procedure planned are considered when sedation is determined. General anaesthesia may be needed for some interventional procedures. Children are allowed nothing by mouth (NPO) for 4 to 6 hours or more before the procedure, according to institutional guidelines. Infants and patients with polycythemia may need IV fluids to prevent dehydration and hypoglycemia.

Postprocedural care. Patients may recover from the procedure in a recovery unit, their hospital room, or, occasionally, a critical care unit. They are placed on a cardiac monitor and a pulse oximeter for the first few hours of recovery. The most important nursing responsibility is observation of the following for signs of complications:

- Pulses, especially below the catheterization site, for equality and symmetry. (Pulse distal to the site may be weaker for the first few hours after catheterization but should gradually increase in strength.)
- Temperature and colour of the affected extremity, since coolness or blanching may indicate arterial obstruction
- Vital signs, which are taken as frequently as every 15 minutes, with special emphasis on heart rate, which is counted for 1 full minute for evidence of dysrhythmias or bradycardia
- Blood pressure (BP), especially for hypotension, which may indicate hemorrhage from cardiac perforation or bleeding at the site of initial catheterization
- Dressing, for evidence of bleeding or hematoma formation in the femoral or antecubital area
- Fluid intake, both IV and oral, to ensure adequate hydration. (Blood loss in the catheterization laboratory, the child's NPO status, and diuretic actions of dyes used during the procedure put children at risk for hypovolemia and dehydration.)
- Blood glucose levels for hypoglycemia, especially in infants, who should receive dextrose-containing IV fluids

NURSING ALERT

If bleeding occurs, direct continuous pressure is applied 2.5 cm above the percutaneous skin site to localize pressure over the vessel puncture.

Depending on hospital policy, the child may be kept in bed with the affected extremity maintained straight for 4 to 6 hours after venous catheterization and 6 to 8 hours after arterial catheterization to facilitate healing of the cannulated vessel. If younger children have difficulty complying, they can be held in the parent's lap with the leg maintained in the correct position. The child's usual diet can be resumed as soon as tolerated, beginning with sips of clear liquids and advancing as the condition allows. The child should be encouraged to void to clear the contrast material from the blood. Generally, there is only slight discomfort at the percutaneous site. To prevent infection, the catheterization area is protected from possible contamination. If the child wears diapers, the dressing can be kept dry by covering it with a piece of plastic film and sealing the edges of the film to the skin with tape. However, the nurse must be careful to continue observing the site for any evidence of bleeding (see Family-Centred Teaching box).

CONGENITAL HEART DISEASE

The incidence of CHD in children is approximately 5 to 8 per 1000 live births (Park, 2015). CHD is the major cause of death (other than prematurity) in the first year of life. Although there are more than 35 well-recognized cardiac defects, the most common heart anomaly is ventricular septal defect (VSD).

FAMILY-CENTRED TEACHING

Care After Cardiac Catheterization

- Remove pressure dressing the day after catheterization. Cover site with an adhesive bandage strip for several days. Put a new bandage on every day for the next 2 days.
- Keep site clean and dry. Avoid tub baths for the first 3 days; older children may shower the first day after catheterization.
- Observe site for redness, swelling, drainage, and bleeding. Monitor for fever. Observe the catheter leg for coolness. Notify health care provider if these occur.
- Avoid strenuous exercise for several days; the child may attend school.
- Resume regular diet without restrictions.
- Use acetaminophen or ibuprofen for pain.
- Keep follow-up appointments per health care provider's instruction.

Modified from Children's Hospital (Boston) Cardiovascular Program, 2009.

The exact etiology of most congenital cardiac defects is unknown. Most are thought to be a result of multifactorial inheritance: a complex interaction of genetic and environmental factors. Some risk factors are known to increase the incidence of congenital heart defects. Maternal factors include chronic illnesses such as diabetes or poorly controlled phenylketonuria, alcohol consumption, and exposure to environmental toxins and infections. Family history of a cardiac defect in a parent or sibling increases the likelihood of a cardiac anomaly. The risk of CHD increases if a first-degree relative (parent or sibling) is affected. The familial risk is higher with left-sided obstructive lesions.

Congenital heart anomalies are often associated with chromosome abnormalities, syndromes, or congenital defects in other body systems. Trisomy 21 (Down syndrome), 13, and 18 are highly correlated with congenital heart defects. Syndromes associated with heart defects include DiGeorge syndrome, a syndrome characterized by deletion of part of chromosome 22q11 (interrupted aortic arch, truncus arteriosus, tetralogy of Fallot, and posterior malaligned VSDs); Noonan syndrome (pulmonic valve anomalies and cardiomyopathy); Williams syndrome (aortic and pulmonic stenosis); and Holt-Oram syndrome (upper limb anomalies and atrial septal defect [ASD]). Extracardiac defects such as tracheoesophageal fistula, renal abnormalities, and diaphragmatic hernia are seen in association with heart anomalies.

Circulatory Changes at Birth

During fetal life, blood carrying oxygen and nutritive materials from the placenta enters the fetal system through the umbilicus via the large umbilical vein. Oxygenated blood enters the heart by way of the inferior vena cava. Because of the higher pressure of blood entering the right atrium, it is directed posteriorly in a straight pathway across the right atrium and through the *foramen ovale* to the left atrium. In this way, the better-oxygenated blood enters the left atrium and ventricle to be pumped through the aorta to the head and upper extremities. Blood from the head and upper extremities entering the right

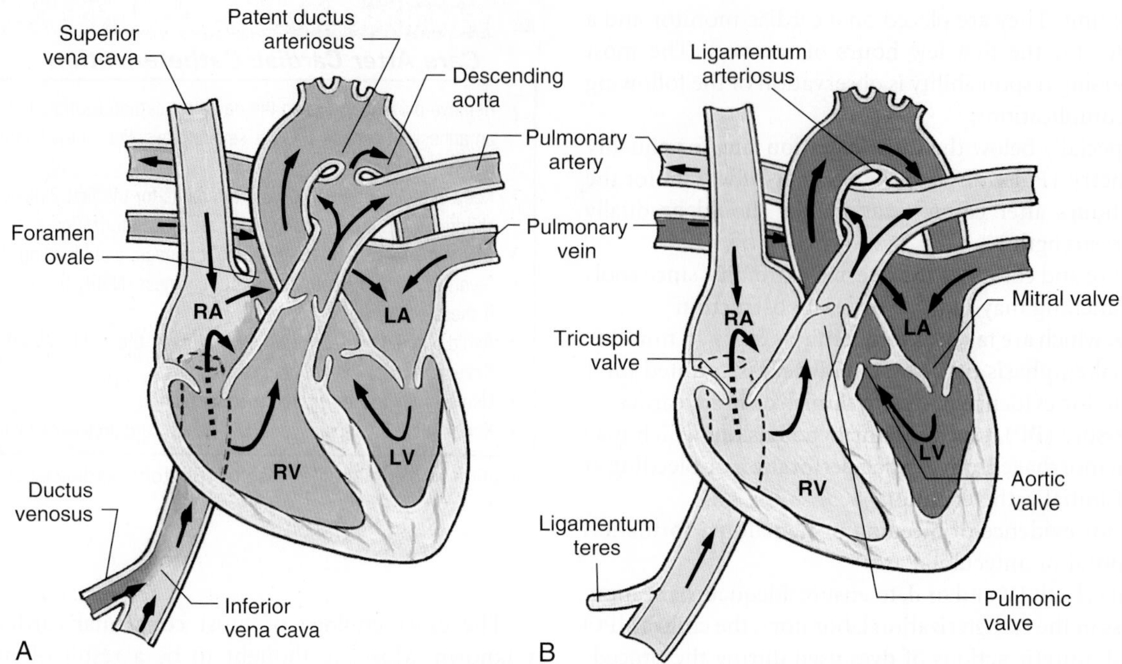

FIGURE 47-1 Changes in circulation at birth. **A:** Prenatal circulation. **B:** Postnatal circulation. *Arrows* indicate direction of blood flow. Although four pulmonary veins enter the LA, for simplicity this diagram shows only two. *LA,* left atrium; *LV,* left ventricle; *RA,* right atrium; *RV,* right ventricle.

atrium from the superior vena cava is directed downward through the tricuspid valve into the right ventricle. From here it is pumped through the pulmonary artery, where the major portion is shunted to the descending aorta via the *ductus arteriosus.* Only a small amount flows to and from the nonfunctioning fetal lungs (Fig. 47-1, A).

Before birth the high pulmonary vascular resistance created by the collapsed fetal lung causes greater pressures in the right side of the heart and the pulmonary arteries. At the same time, the free-flowing placental circulation and the ductus arteriosus produce a low vascular resistance in the remainder of the fetal vascular system. With the cessation of placental blood flow from clamping of the umbilical cord and the expansion of the lungs at birth, the hemodynamics of the fetal vascular system undergo pronounced and abrupt changes (see Fig. 47-1, B).

With the first breath, the lungs are expanded, and increased oxygen causes pulmonary vasodilation. With the removal of the placenta, pulmonary pressures start to fall as systemic pressures start to rise. Normally, the foramen ovale closes as the pressure in the left atrium exceeds the pressure in the right atrium. The ductus arteriosus starts to close in the presence of increased oxygen concentration in the blood and other factors.

Altered Hemodynamics

To appreciate the physiology of heart defects, it is necessary to understand the role of pressure gradients, flow, and resistance within the circulation. As blood is pumped through the heart, it (1) flows from an area of high pressure to one of lower pressure and (2) takes the path of least resistance. In general, the higher the pressure gradient, the greater the rate of flow; the higher the resistance, the lower the rate of flow.

Normally, the pressure on the right side of the heart is lower than that on the left side, and the resistance in the pulmonary circulation is less than that in the systemic circulation. Vessels entering or exiting these chambers have corresponding pressures. Therefore, if an abnormal connection exists between the heart chambers (such as a septal defect), blood will necessarily flow from an area of higher pressure (left side) to one of lower pressure (right side). Such a flow of blood is termed a *left-to-right shunt.* Anomalies resulting in cyanosis may result from a change in pressure so that the blood is shunted from the right to the left side of the heart (*right-to-left shunt*) because of either increased pulmonary vascular resistance or obstruction to blood flow through the pulmonic valve and artery. Cyanosis may also result from a defect that allows mixing of oxygenated and deoxygenated blood within the heart chambers or great arteries, such as occurs in truncus arteriosus.

Classification of Defects

There are typically two classification systems used to categorize congenital heart defects. Traditionally, cyanosis, a physical characteristic, has been used as the distinguishing feature, dividing the anomalies into acyanotic defects and cyanotic defects. In clinical practice, this system is problematic because children with acyanotic defects may develop cyanosis. Also, more often, those children with cyanotic defects may appear pink and have more clinical signs of HF.

A more useful classification system is based on hemodynamic characteristics (blood flow patterns within the heart). These blood flow patterns are (1) increased pulmonary blood flow;

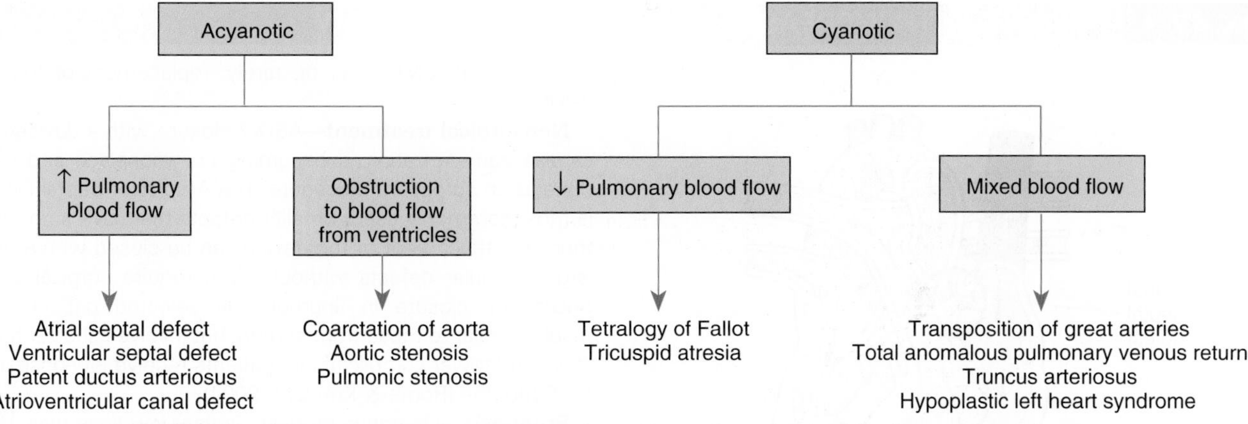

FIGURE 47-2 Comparison of acyanotic–cyanotic and hemodynamic classification systems of congenital heart disease.

(2) decreased pulmonary blood flow; (3) obstruction to blood flow out of the heart; and (4) mixed blood flow, in which saturated and desaturated blood mix within the heart or great arteries. As a comparison, both classification systems are outlined in Fig. 47-2.

With the hemodynamic classification system, the clinical manifestations of each group are more uniform and predictable. Defects that allow blood flow from the higher-pressure left side of the heart to the lower-pressure right side (left-to-right shunt) result in increased pulmonary blood flow and cause HF. Obstructive defects impede blood flow out of the ventricles; obstruction on the left side of the heart results in HF, whereas severe obstruction on the right side causes cyanosis. Defects that cause decreased pulmonary blood flow result in cyanosis. Mixed lesions present a variable clinical picture based on the degree of mixing and amount of pulmonary blood flow; hypoxemia (with or without cyanosis) and HF usually occur together. Using this classification system, the clinical presentation and management of the most common defects are outlined in the following sections.

The outcomes of surgical treatment for patients with moderate to severe disease vary. Patient risk factors for increased morbidity and mortality include prematurity or low birth weight, a genetic syndrome, multiple cardiac defects, a noncardiac congenital anomaly, and age at time of surgery (newborns are a higher risk group). For example, aortic stenosis or coarctation manifesting in the first week of life is more severe and carries a higher mortality than if it becomes apparent at 1 year of age. Outcomes for surgical repair of similar congenital heart defects also vary among treatment centres. In general, the outcomes of surgical procedures have steadily improved in the past decade, with mortality rates for many severe defects below 10%, and the incidence of complications and length of hospital stay have declined (Heart and Stroke Foundation, 2016a).

Defects With Increased Pulmonary Blood Flow

In this group of cardiac defects, intracardiac communications along the septum or an abnormal connection between the great arteries allows blood to flow from the higher-pressure left side of the heart to the lower-pressure right side of the heart (Fig. 47-3). Increased blood volume on the right side of the heart increases pulmonary blood flow at the expense of systemic blood flow. Clinically, patients demonstrate signs and symptoms of HF. Atrial septal defect (ASD), VSD, and patent ductus arteriosus (PDA) are typical anomalies in this group (Box 47-1).

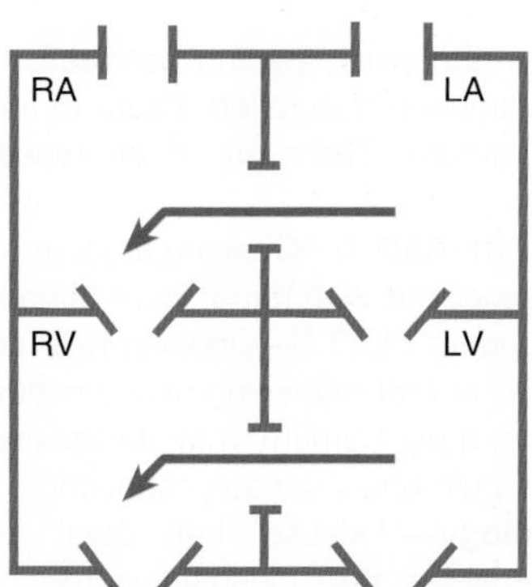

FIGURE 47-3 Hemodynamics in defects with increased pulmonary blood flow. *LA*, left atrium; *LV*, left ventricle; *RA*, right atrium; *RV*, right ventricle.

Obstructive Defects

Obstructive defects are those in which blood exiting the heart meets an area of anatomical narrowing (*stenosis*), causing obstruction to blood flow. The pressure in the ventricle and great artery before the obstruction is increased, and the pressure in the area beyond the obstruction is decreased. The location of the narrowing is usually near the valve (Fig. 47-4), as follows:

Valvular—At the site of the valve itself
Subvalvular—Narrowing in the ventricle below the valve (also referred to as the *ventricular outflow tract*)
Supravalvular—Narrowing in the great artery above the valve

Coarctation of the aorta (narrowing of the aortic arch), aortic stenosis, and pulmonic stenosis are typical defects in this

BOX 47-1 DEFECTS WITH INCREASED PULMONARY BLOOD FLOW

Atrial Septal Defect

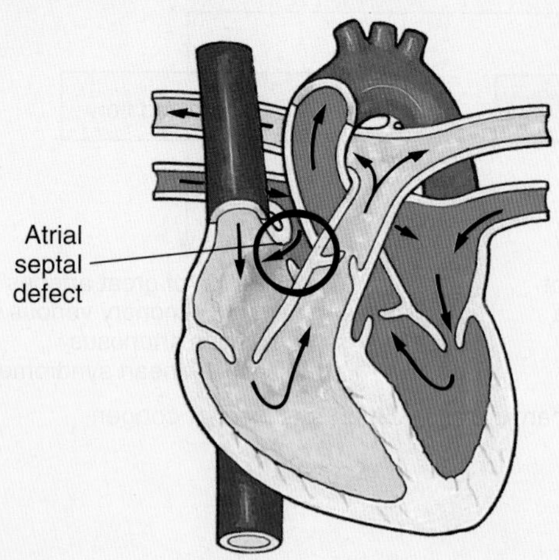

Description—Abnormal opening between the atria, allowing blood from the higher-pressure left atrium to flow into the lower-pressure right atrium. There are three types of atrial septal defects (ASDs):

Ostium primum (ASD 1)—Opening at lower end of septum; may be associated with mitral valve abnormalities

Ostium secundum (ASD 2)—Opening near centre of septum

Sinus venosus defect—Opening near junction of superior vena cava and right atrium; may be associated with partial anomalous pulmonary venous connection

Pathophysiology—Because left atrial pressure slightly exceeds right atrial pressure, blood flows from the left to the right atrium, causing an increased flow of oxygenated blood into the right side of the heart. Despite the low pressure difference, a high rate of flow can still occur because of low pulmonary vascular resistance and the greater distensibility of the right atrium, which further reduces flow resistance. This volume is well tolerated by the right ventricle because it is delivered under much lower pressure than with a ventricular septal defect (VSD). Although there is right atrial and ventricular enlargement, cardiac failure is unusual in an uncomplicated ASD. Pulmonary vascular changes usually occur only after several decades if the defect is left unrepaired.

Clinical manifestations—Patients may be asymptomatic. They may develop heart failure (HF). There is a characteristic systolic murmur with a fixed split second heart sound. There may also be a diastolic murmur. Patients are at risk for atrial dysrhythmias (probably caused by atrial enlargement and stretching of conduction fibres) and pulmonary vascular obstructive disease and emboli formation later in life from chronically increased pulmonary blood flow.

Surgical treatment—Surgical patch closure (pericardial patch or Dacron patch) is done for moderate to large defects. Open repair with cardiopulmonary bypass is usually performed before school age. In addition, the sinus venosus defect requires patch placement, so the anomalous right pulmonary venous return is directed to the left atrium with a baffle. The ASD 1 type may require mitral valve repair or, rarely, replacement of the mitral valve.

Nonsurgical treatment—ASD 2 closure with a device during cardiac catheterization is becoming commonplace and can be done as an outpatient procedure. The Amplatzer Septal Occluder is most commonly used. Smaller defects that have a rim around them for attachment of the device can be closed with a device; large, irregular defects without a rim require surgical closure. Successful closure in appropriately selected patients yields results similar to those from surgery but involves shorter hospital stays and fewer complications. Patients receive low-dose aspirin for 6 months (Rome & Kreutzer, 2004).

Prognosis—Operative mortality is very low (less than 1%).

Ventricular Septal Defect

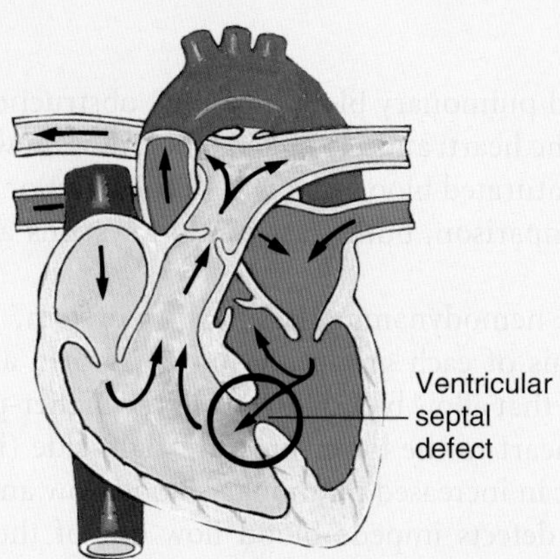

Description—Abnormal opening between the right and left ventricles. VSD may be classified according to location: membranous (accounting for 80%) or muscular. May vary in size from a small pinhole to absence of the septum, which results in a common ventricle. VSDs are frequently associated with other defects, such as pulmonary stenosis, transposition of the great vessels, patent ductus arteriosus (PDA), atrial defects, and coarctation of the aorta. Many VSDs (20 to 60%) close spontaneously. Spontaneous closure is most likely to occur during the first year of life in children having small or moderate defects. A left-to-right shunt is caused by the flow of blood from the higher-pressure left ventricle to the lower-pressure right ventricle.

Pathophysiology—Because of the higher pressure within the left ventricle and because the systemic arterial circulation offers more resistance than the pulmonary circulation, blood flows through the defect into the pulmonary artery. The increased blood volume is pumped into the lungs, which may eventually result in increased pulmonary vascular resistance. Increased pressure in the right ventricle as a result of left-to-right shunting and pulmonary resistance causes the muscle to hypertrophy. If the right ventricle is unable to accommodate the increased workload, the right atrium may also enlarge as it attempts to overcome the resistance offered by incomplete right ventricular emptying.

BOX 47-1 DEFECTS WITH INCREASED PULMONARY BLOOD FLOW—cont'd

Clinical manifestations—HF is common. A characteristic loud holosystolic murmur is heard best at the left sternal border. Patients are at risk for bacterial endocarditis and pulmonary vascular obstructive disease.

Surgical treatment

Palliative—Pulmonary artery banding (placement of a band around the main pulmonary artery to decrease pulmonary blood flow) may be done in infants with multiple muscular VSDs or complex anatomy. Improvements in surgical techniques and postoperative care make complete repair in infancy the preferred approach.

Complete repair (procedure of choice)—Small defects are repaired with sutures. Large defects usually require that a knitted Dacron patch be sewn over the opening. Cardiopulmonary bypass is used for both procedures. The approach for the repair is generally through the right atrium and the tricuspid valve. Postoperative complications include residual VSD and conduction disturbances.

Nonsurgical treatment—Device closure during cardiac catheterization is another treatment option, with being performed in some centres under investigational protocols. One device has been approved for closure of muscular defects. Early results are encouraging, with successful defect closure and few complications (Rome & Kreutzer, 2004).

Prognosis—Risks depend on the location of the defect, the number of defects, and the presence of other associated cardiac defects. Single membranous defects are associated with low mortality (less than 2%); multiple muscular defects can carry a higher risk (Jacobs, Mavroudis, Jacobs, et al., 2004).

Atrioventricular Canal Defect

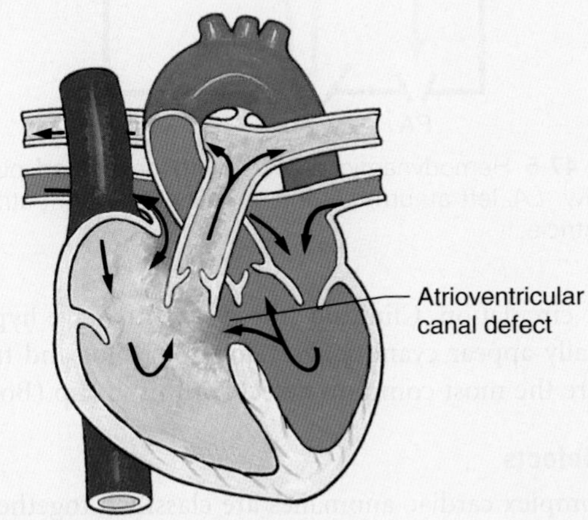

Description—Incomplete fusion of the endocardial cushions. This defect consists of a low ASD that is continuous with a high VSD and clefts of the mitral and tricuspid valves, which create a large central atrioventricular (AV) valve that allows blood to flow between all four chambers of the heart. The directions and pathways of flow are determined by pulmonary and systemic resistance, left and right ventricular pressures, and the compliance of each chamber, although flow is generally from left to right. It is the most common cardiac defect in children with Down syndrome.

Pathophysiology—The alterations in hemodynamics depend on the severity of the defect and the child's pulmonary vascular resistance. Immediately after birth, while the newborn's pulmonary vascular resistance is high, there is minimum shunting of blood through the defect. Once this resistance falls, left-to-right shunting occurs, and pulmonary blood flow increases. The resultant pulmonary vascular engorgement predisposes the child to development of HF.

Clinical manifestations—Patients usually have moderate to severe HF. There is a loud systolic murmur. There may be mild cyanosis that increases with crying. Patients are at high risk for developing pulmonary vascular obstructive disease.

Surgical treatment

Palliative—Pulmonary artery banding is occasionally done in small infants with severe symptoms. Complete repair in infancy is most common.

Complete repair—Surgical repair consists of patch closure of the septal defects and reconstruction of the AV valve tissue (either repair of the mitral valve cleft or fashioning of two AV valves). Postoperative complications include heart block, HF, mitral regurgitation, dysrhythmias, and pulmonary hypertension.

Prognosis—Operative mortality is less than 5% (Jacobs et al., 2004). A potential later problem is mitral regurgitation, which may require valve replacement.

Patent Ductus Arteriosus

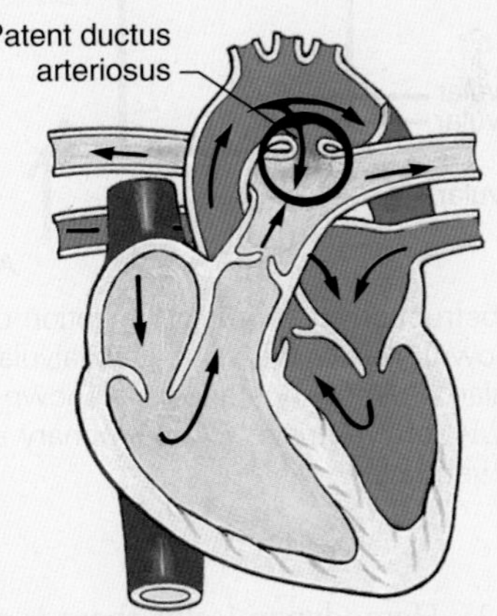

Description—Failure of the fetal ductus arteriosus (artery connecting the aorta and pulmonary artery) to close within the first weeks of life. The continued patency of this vessel allows blood to flow from the higher-pressure aorta to the lower-pressure pulmonary artery, which causes a left-to-right shunt.

Pathophysiology—The hemodynamic consequences of PDA depend on the size of the ductus and the pulmonary vascular resistance. At birth the resistance in the pulmonary and systemic

Continued

BOX 47-1 DEFECTS WITH INCREASED PULMONARY BLOOD FLOW—cont'd

circulations is almost identical so that the resistance in the aorta and pulmonary artery is equalized. As the systemic pressure comes to exceed the pulmonary pressure, blood begins to shunt from the aorta across the duct to the pulmonary artery (left-to-right shunt). The additional blood is recirculated through the lungs and returned to the left atrium and left ventricle. The effect of this altered circulation is increased workload on the left side of the heart, increased pulmonary vascular congestion and possibly resistance, and potentially increased right ventricular pressure and hypertrophy.

Clinical manifestations—Patients may be asymptomatic or show signs of HF. There is a characteristic machinery-like murmur. A widened pulse pressure and bounding pulses result from runoff of blood from the aorta to the pulmonary artery. Patients are at risk for bacterial endocarditis and pulmonary vascular obstructive disease in later life from chronic excessive pulmonary blood flow.

Medical management—Intravenous administration of indomethacin (prostaglandin inhibitor) has proved successful in closing a PDA in preterm infants and some newborns. It should be noted that this infusion should not be given via umbilical lines as this can cause a dramatic shift in the cerebral blood flow.

Surgical treatment—Surgical division or ligation of the patent vessel is performed via a left thoracotomy. In another technique, video-assisted thoracoscopic surgery, a thoracoscope and instruments are inserted through three small incisions on the left side of the chest to place a clip on the ductus. The technique is used in some centres and eliminates the need for a thoracotomy, thereby speeding postoperative recovery.

Nonsurgical treatment—In many centres, coils to occlude the PDA are placed in patients in the catheterization laboratory. Preterm or small infants (with small-diameter femoral arteries) and patients with large or unusual PDAs may require surgery.

Prognosis—Both surgical and nonsurgical procedures can be done at low risk with less than 1% mortality. PDA closure in very preterm infants has a higher mortality rate because of the additional significant medical problems. Many infants with small PDAs are asymptomatic and can be discharged home with a referral to a pediatric cardiologist, if necessary, for follow-up to ensure closure.

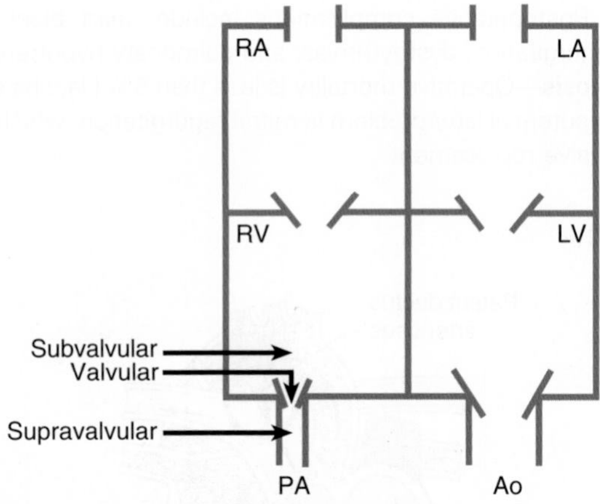

FIGURE 47-4 Obstruction to ventricular ejection can occur at the valvular level (shown), below the valve (subvalvular), or above the valve (supravalvular). Pulmonary stenosis is shown here. *Ao*, aorta; *LA*, left atrium; *LV*, left ventricle; *PA*, pulmonary artery; *RA*, right atrium; *RV*, right ventricle.

group (Box 47-2). Hemodynamically, there is a pressure load on the ventricle and decreased cardiac output. Clinically, infants and children exhibit signs of HF. Children with mild obstruction may be asymptomatic. Rarely, as in severe pulmonic stenosis, hypoxemia may be seen.

Defects With Decreased Pulmonary Blood Flow

In this group of defects, there is obstruction of pulmonary blood flow and an anatomical defect (ASD or VSD) between the right and left sides of the heart (Fig. 47-5). Because blood has difficulty exiting the right side of the heart via the pulmonary artery, pressure on the right side increases, exceeding left-sided pressure. This allows desaturated blood to shunt right to left, causing desaturation in the left side of the heart and in the systemic circulation. Clinically, these patients have hypoxemia and usually appear cyanotic. Tetralogy of Fallot and tricuspid atresia are the most common defects in this group (Box 47-3).

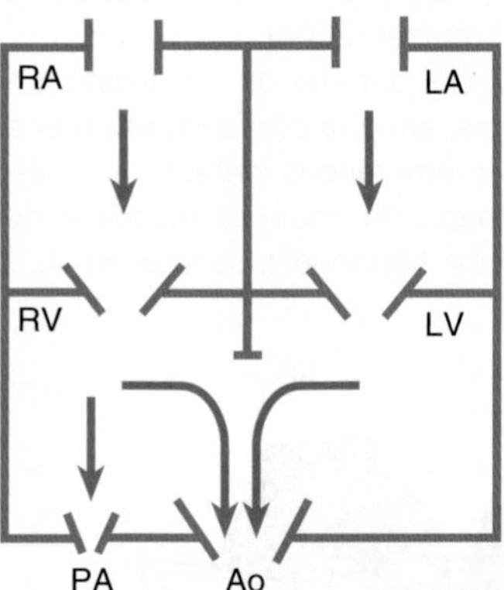

FIGURE 47-5 Hemodynamic defects with decreased pulmonary blood flow. *LA*, left atrium; *LV*, left ventricle; *RA*, right atrium; *RV*, right ventricle.

Mixed Defects

Many complex cardiac anomalies are classified together in the mixed category (Box 47-4) because survival in the postnatal period depends on the mixing of blood from the pulmonary and systemic circulations within the heart chambers. Hemodynamically, fully saturated systemic blood flow mixes with the desaturated pulmonary blood flow, causing a relative desaturation of the systemic blood flow. Pulmonary congestion occurs because the differences in pulmonary artery pressure and aortic pressure favour pulmonary blood flow. Cardiac output decreases because of a volume load on the ventricle. Clinically, these patients have a variable picture that combines some degree of desaturation (although cyanosis is not always visible) and signs of HF. Some defects, such as transposition of the great arteries

BOX 47-2 OBSTRUCTIVE DEFECTS

Coarctation of the Aorta

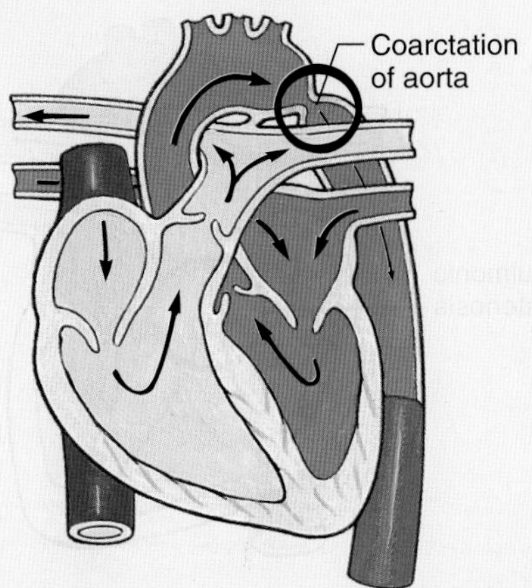

Description—There is localized narrowing near the insertion of the ductus arteriosus, which results in increased pressure proximal to the defect (head and upper extremities) and decreased pressure distal to the obstruction (body and lower extremities).

Pathophysiology—The effect of a narrowing within the aorta is increased pressure proximal to the defect and decreased pressure distal to it.

Clinical manifestations—The patient may have high blood pressure and bounding pulses in the arms, weak or absent femoral pulses, and cool lower extremities with lower blood pressure. There are signs of heart failure (HF) in infants. In infants with critical coarctation, the hemodynamic condition may deteriorate rapidly with severe acidosis and hypotension. Mechanical ventilation and inotropic support are often necessary before surgery. Older children may experience dizziness, headaches, fainting, and epistaxis resulting from hypertension. Patients are at risk for hypertension, ruptured aorta, aortic aneurysm, and stroke.

Surgical treatment—Surgical repair is the treatment of choice for infants younger than 6 months of age and for patients with long-segment stenosis or complex anatomy; it may be performed for all patients with coarctation. Repair is by resection of the coarctated portion with an end-to-end anastomosis of the aorta or enlargement of the constricted section using a graft of prosthetic material or a portion of the left subclavian artery. Because this defect is outside the heart and pericardium, cardiopulmonary bypass is not required, and a thoracotomy incision is used. Postoperative hypertension is treated with intravenous sodium nitroprusside, esmolol, or milrinone followed by oral medications, such as angiotensin-converting enzyme inhibitors or beta blockers. Residual permanent hypertension after repair of coarctation of the aorta (COA) seems to be related to age and time of repair. To prevent both hypertension at rest and exercise-provoked systemic hypertension after repair, elective surgery for COA is advised within the first 2 years of life. There is a 15 to 30% risk of recurrence in patients who underwent surgical repair as infants (Beekman, 2013). Percutaneous balloon angioplasty techniques have proved to be effective in relieving residual postoperative coarctation gradients.

Nonsurgical treatment—Balloon angioplasty is being performed as a primary intervention for COA in older infants and children. In adolescents, stents may be placed in the aorta to maintain patency. Studies have demonstrated that balloon angioplasty is effective in children and aneurysm formation is rare. The high restenosis rate in young infants limits its application in this group (Rome & Kreutzer, 2004).

Prognosis—Mortality is less than 5% in patients with isolated coarctation; risk is increased in infants with other complex cardiac defects (Jacobs et al., 2004).

Aortic Stenosis

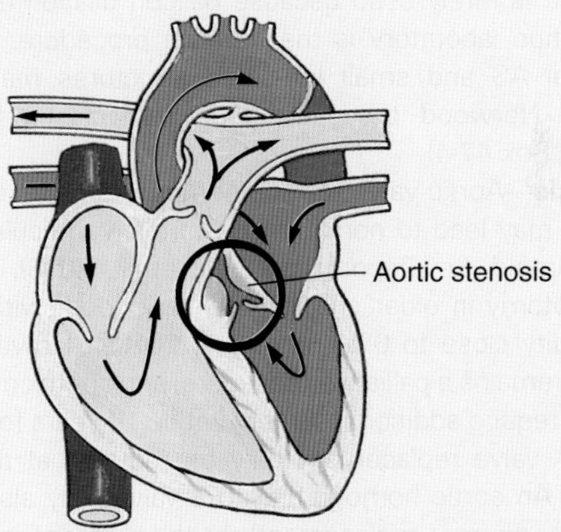

Description—Narrowing or stricture of the aortic valve, causing resistance to blood flow in the left ventricle, decreased cardiac output, left ventricular hypertrophy, and pulmonary vascular congestion. The prominent anatomical consequence of aortic stenosis (AS) is the hypertrophy of the left ventricular wall, which eventually leads to increased end-diastolic pressure resulting in pulmonary venous and pulmonary arterial hypertension. Left ventricular hypertrophy also interferes with coronary artery perfusion and may result in myocardial infarction or scarring of the papillary muscles of the left ventricle, which causes mitral insufficiency. Valvular stenosis, the most common type, is usually caused by malformed cusps that result in a bicuspid rather than tricuspid valve or fusion of the cusps. Subvalvular stenosis is a stricture caused by a fibrous ring below a normal valve; supravalvular stenosis occurs infrequently. Valvular AS is a serious defect for the following reasons: (1) the obstruction tends to be progressive; (2) sudden episodes of myocardial ischemia, or low cardiac output, can result in sudden death; and (3) surgical repair rarely results in a normal valve. This is one of the rare instances in which strenuous physical activity may be curtailed because of the cardiac condition.

Continued

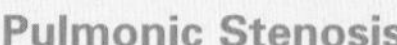

BOX 47-2 OBSTRUCTIVE DEFECTS—cont'd

Pathophysiology—A stricture in the aortic outflow tract causes resistance to ejection of blood from the left ventricle. The extra workload on the left ventricle causes hypertrophy. If left ventricular failure develops, left atrial pressure increases; this causes increased pressure in the pulmonary veins, which results in pulmonary vascular congestion (pulmonary edema).

Clinical manifestations—Newborns with critical AS demonstrate signs of decreased cardiac output with faint pulses, hypotension, tachycardia, and poor feeding. Children show signs of exercise intolerance, chest pain, and dizziness when standing for a long period. A systolic ejection murmur may or may not be present. Patients are at risk for bacterial endocarditis, coronary insufficiency, and ventricular dysfunction.

Valvular Aortic Stenosis

Surgical treatment—Aortic valvotomy is performed under inflow occlusion. It is rarely used because balloon dilation done in the catheterization laboratory is the first-line procedure. Newborns with critical AS and small left-sided structures may undergo a stage 1 Norwood procedure (see Hypoplastic Left Heart Syndrome, Box 47-4).

Prognosis—Aortic valve replacement offers a good treatment option and may lead to normalization of left ventricular size and function (Arnold, Ley-Zaporozhan, Ley, et al., 2008). Results of aortic valvotomy in older children are very good, with mortality and morbidity close to 0% (Bernstein, 2016a). However, aortic valvotomy remains a palliative procedure, and approximately 25% of patients require additional surgery within 10 years for recurrent stenosis. A valve replacement may be required at the second procedure. An aortic homograft with a valve may also be used (extended aortic root replacement), or the pulmonary valve may be moved to the aortic position and replaced with a homograft valve (Ross procedure).

Nonsurgical treatment—The narrowed valve is dilated using balloon angioplasty in the catheterization laboratory. This procedure is usually the first intervention.

Prognosis—Complications include aortic insufficiency or valvular regurgitation, tearing of the valve leaflets, and loss of pulse in the catheterized limb.

Subvalvular Aortic Stenosis

Surgical treatment—The procedure may involve incising a membrane if one exists or cutting the fibromuscular ring. If the obstruction results from narrowing of the left ventricular outflow tract and a small aortic valve annulus, a patch may be required to enlarge the entire left ventricular outflow tract and annulus and replace the aortic valve; this is known as the *Konno procedure.*

Prognosis—Mortality from surgical repairs of subvalvular AS is less than 5%; however, about 20% of these patients develop recurrent subaortic stenosis and require additional surgery (Schneider & Moore, 2013).

Pulmonic Stenosis

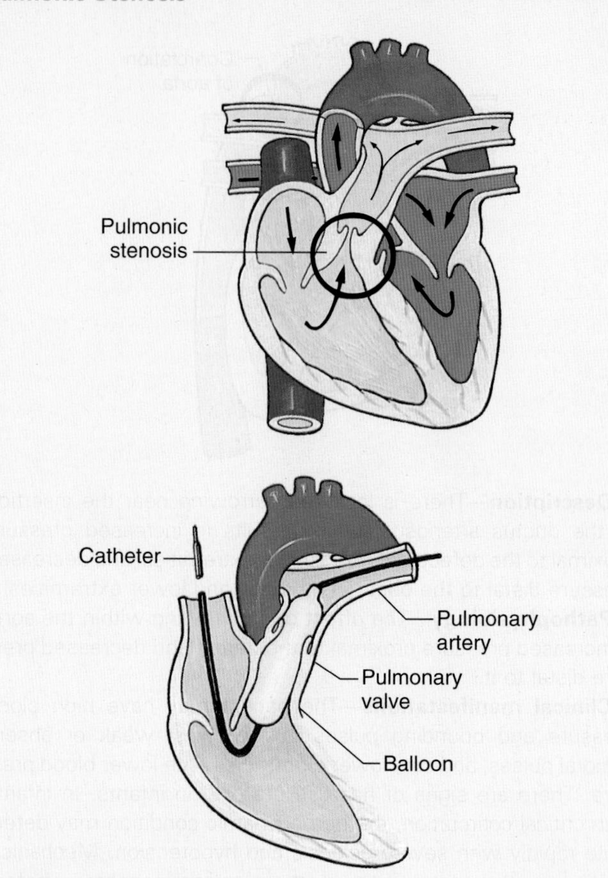

Description—Narrowing at the entrance to the pulmonary artery. Resistance to blood flow causes right ventricular hypertrophy and decreased pulmonary blood flow. Pulmonary atresia is the extreme form of pulmonic stenosis (PS) in that there is total fusion of the commissures and no blood flows to the lungs. The right ventricle may be hypoplastic.

Pathophysiology—When PS is present, resistance to blood flow causes right ventricular hypertrophy. If right ventricular failure develops, right atrial pressure increases; this may result in reopening of the foramen ovale, shunting of unoxygenated blood into the left atrium, and systemic cyanosis. If PS is severe, HF occurs, and systemic venous engorgement is noted. An associated defect such as a patent ductus arteriosus partially compensates for the obstruction by shunting blood from the aorta to the pulmonary artery and into the lungs.

Clinical manifestations—Patients may be asymptomatic; some have mild cyanosis or HF. Progressive narrowing causes increased symptoms. Newborns with severe narrowing will be cyanotic. A loud systolic ejection murmur at the upper left sternal

BOX 47-2 OBSTRUCTIVE DEFECTS—cont'd

border may be present. However, in severely ill patients the murmur may be much softer because of decreased cardiac output and shunting of blood. Cardiomegaly is evident on chest radiographic films. Patients are at risk for bacterial endocarditis.

Surgical treatment—In infants, transventricular (closed) valvotomy (Brock procedure) is used; in children, pulmonary valvotomy with cardiopulmonary bypass. The need for surgical treatment is rare with widespread use of balloon angioplasty techniques.

Nonsurgical treatment—Balloon angioplasty is done in the cardiac catheterization laboratory to dilate the valve. A catheter is inserted across the stenotic pulmonic valve into the pulmonary artery, and a balloon at the end of the catheter is inflated and rapidly passed through the narrowed opening (see figure above). The procedure is associated with few complications and has proved to be highly effective. It is the treatment of choice for discrete PS in most centres and can be done safely in newborns.

Prognosis—Risk is low for both surgical and nonsurgical procedures; mortality is lower than 1%, slightly higher in newborns. Both balloon dilation and surgical valvotomy leave the pulmonic valve incompetent because they involve opening the fused valve leaflets; however, these patients are clinically asymptomatic. Long-term problems with restenosis or valve incompetence may occur.

BOX 47-3 DEFECTS WITH DECREASED PULMONARY BLOOD FLOW

Tetralogy of Fallot

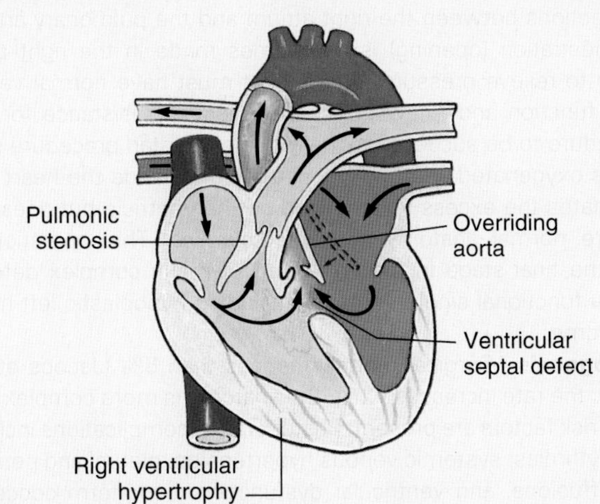

Description—The classic form includes four defects: (1) ventricular septal defect (VSD), (2) pulmonic stenosis (PS), (3) overriding aorta, and (4) right ventricular hypertrophy.

Pathophysiology—The alteration in hemodynamics varies widely, depending primarily on the degree of PS and also on the size of the VSD and the pulmonary and systemic resistance to flow. Because the VSD is usually large, pressures may be equal in the right and left ventricles. Therefore, the shunt direction depends on the difference between pulmonary and systemic vascular resistance. If pulmonary vascular resistance is higher than systemic resistance, the shunt is from right to left. If systemic resistance is higher than pulmonary resistance, the shunt is from left to right. PS decreases blood flow to the lungs and, consequently, the amount of oxygenated blood that returns to the left side of the heart. Depending on the position of the aorta, blood from both ventricles may be distributed systemically.

Clinical manifestations—Some infants may be acutely cyanotic at birth; others have mild cyanosis that progresses over the first year of life as the PS worsens. There is a characteristic systolic murmur that is often moderate in intensity. There may be acute episodes of cyanosis and hypoxia, called *blue spells* or *tet spells* (see p. 1497). Anoxic spells occur when the infant's oxygen requirements exceed the blood supply, usually during crying or after feeding. Patients are at risk for emboli, seizures, and loss of consciousness or sudden death following an anoxic spell.

Surgical treatment

Palliative shunt—In infants who cannot undergo primary repair, a palliative procedure to increase pulmonary blood flow and increase oxygen saturation may be performed. The preferred procedure is a modified Blalock-Taussig shunt operation, which provides blood flow to the pulmonary arteries from the left or right subclavian artery via a tube graft (see Table 47-3). However, in general, shunts are avoided because they may result in pulmonary artery distortion.

Complete repair—Elective repair is usually performed in the first year of life. Indications for repair include increasing cyanosis and the development of hypercyanotic spells. Complete repair involves closure of the VSD and resection of the infundibular stenosis, with placement of a pericardial patch to enlarge the right ventricular outflow tract. In some repairs the patch may extend across the pulmonary valve annulus (transannular patch), making the pulmonary valve incompetent. The procedure requires a median sternotomy and the use of cardiopulmonary bypass.

Prognosis—The operative mortality for total correction of tetralogy of Fallot is less than 3% (Jacobs et al., 2004). With improved surgical techniques there is a lower incidence of dysrhythmias and sudden death; surgical heart block is rare. Heart failure may occur postoperatively.

Continued

BOX 47-3 DEFECTS WITH DECREASED PULMONARY BLOOD FLOW—cont'd

Tricuspid Atresia

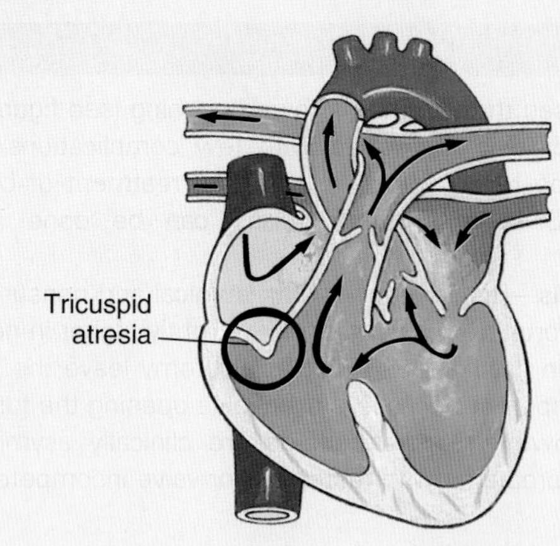

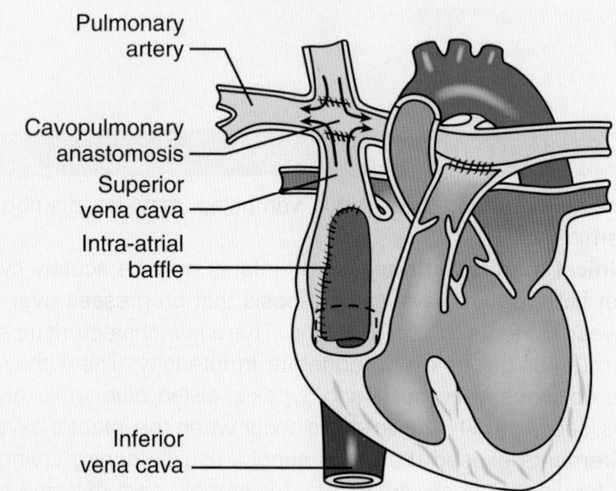

Description—The tricuspid valve fails to develop; consequently, there is no communication from the right atrium to the right ventricle. Blood flows through an atrial septal defect (ASD) or a patent foramen ovale to the left side of the heart and through a VSD to the right ventricle and out to the lungs. The condition is often associated with PS and transposition of the great arteries. There is complete mixing of unoxygenated and oxygenated blood in the left side of the heart, which results in systemic desaturation, and varying amounts of pulmonary obstruction, which causes decreased pulmonary blood flow.

Pathophysiology—At birth the presence of a patent foramen ovale (or other atrial septal opening) is required to permit blood flow across the septum into the left atrium; the patent ductus arteriosus allows blood flow to the pulmonary artery into the lungs for oxygenation. A VSD allows a modest amount of blood to enter the right ventricle and pulmonary artery for oxygenation. Pulmonary blood flow usually is diminished.

Clinical manifestations—Cyanosis is usually seen in the newborn period. There may be tachycardia and dyspnea. Older children have signs of chronic hypoxemia with clubbing.

Therapeutic management—For the newborn whose pulmonary blood flow depends on the patency of the ductus arteriosus, a continuous infusion of prostaglandin E_1 is started at 0.1 mg/kg/min until surgical intervention can be arranged.

Surgical treatment—Palliative treatment is the placement of a shunt (pulmonary–to–systemic artery anastomosis) to increase blood flow to the lungs. If the ASD is small, an atrial septostomy is performed during cardiac catheterization. Some children have increased pulmonary blood flow and require pulmonary artery banding to lessen the volume of blood to the lungs. A bidirectional Glenn shunt (cavopulmonary anastomosis) may be performed at 4 to 9 months as a second stage.

Modified Fontan procedure—Systemic venous return is directed to the lungs without a ventricular pump through surgical connections between the right atrium and the pulmonary artery. A fenestration (opening) is sometimes made in the right atrial baffle to relieve pressure. The patient must have normal ventricular function and a low pulmonary vascular resistance for the procedure to be successful. The modified Fontan procedure separates oxygenated and unoxygenated blood inside the heart and eliminates the excess volume load on the ventricle but does not restore normal anatomy or hemodynamics. This operation is also the final stage in the correction of many complex defects with a functional single ventricle, including hypoplastic left heart syndrome.

Prognosis—Surgical mortality is less than 5% (Jacobs et al., 2004); the rate increases when the anatomy is more complex and other risk factors are present. Postoperative complications include dysrhythmias, systemic venous hypertension, pleural and pericardial effusions, and ventricular dysfunction. Long-term concerns are the development of protein-losing enteropathy, atrial dysrhythmias, late ventricular dysfunction, and developmental delays.

BOX 47-4 MIXED DEFECTS

Transposition of the Great Arteries, or Transposition of the Great Vessels

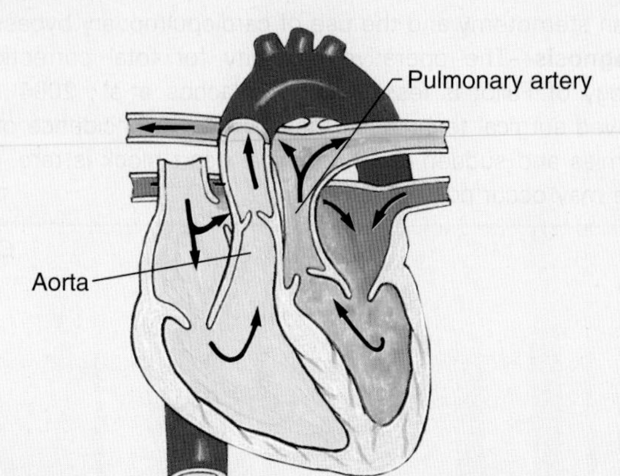

Description—The pulmonary artery leaves the left ventricle, and the aorta exits from the right ventricle, with no communication between the systemic and pulmonary circulations.

Pathophysiology—Associated defects such as septal defects or patent ductus arteriosus (PDA) must be present to permit blood to enter the systemic circulation or the pulmonary circulation for mixing of saturated and desaturated blood. The most common defect associated with transposition of the great arteries (TGA) is a patent foramen ovale. At birth there is also a PDA, although in most instances this closes after the neonatal period. Another associated defect may be a ventricular septal defect (VSD). The presence of a VSD increases the risk of heart failure (HF) because it permits blood to flow from the right to the left ventricle, into the pulmonary artery, and finally to the lungs. However, it also produces high pulmonary blood flow under high pressure, which can result in high pulmonary vascular resistance.

BOX 47-4 MIXED DEFECTS—cont'd

Clinical manifestations—These depend on the type and size of the associated defects. Newborns with minimum communication are severely cyanotic and have depressed function at birth. Those with large septal defects or a PDA may be less cyanotic but have symptoms of HF. Heart sounds vary according to the type of defect present. Cardiomegaly is usually evident a few weeks after birth.

Therapeutic management (to provide intracardiac mixing)—The administration of intravenous prostaglandin E_1 may be initiated to keep the ductus arteriosus open to temporarily increase blood mixing and provide an oxygen saturation of 75% or to maintain cardiac output. During cardiac catheterization or under echocardiographic guidance, a balloon atrial septostomy (Rashkind procedure) may also be performed to increase mixing by opening the atrial septum.

Surgical treatment—An arterial switch procedure is the procedure of choice performed in the first weeks of life. It involves transecting the great arteries, anastomosing the main pulmonary artery to the proximal aorta (just above the aortic valve), and anastomosing the ascending aorta to the proximal pulmonary artery. The coronary arteries are switched from the proximal aorta to the proximal pulmonary artery to create a new aorta. Reimplantation of the coronary arteries is critical to the infant's survival, and they must be reattached without torsion or kinking to provide the heart with its supply of oxygen. The advantage of the arterial switch procedure is the re-establishment of normal circulation, with the left ventricle acting as the systemic pump. Potential complications of the arterial switch include narrowing at the great artery anastomoses and coronary artery insufficiency.

Rastelli procedure—This procedure is the operative choice in infants with TGA, VSD, and severe pulmonic stenosis (PS). It involves closure of the VSD with a baffle, so left ventricular blood is directed through the VSD into the aorta. The pulmonic valve is then closed, and a conduit is placed from the right ventricle to the pulmonary artery to create a physiologically normal circulation. Unfortunately, this procedure requires multiple conduit replacements as the child grows.

Prognosis—Operative mortality is less than 2% (Jacobs et al., 2004). Potential long-term problems include suprapulmonic stenosis and neoaorta dilation and regurgitation.

Total Anomalous Pulmonary Venous Connection

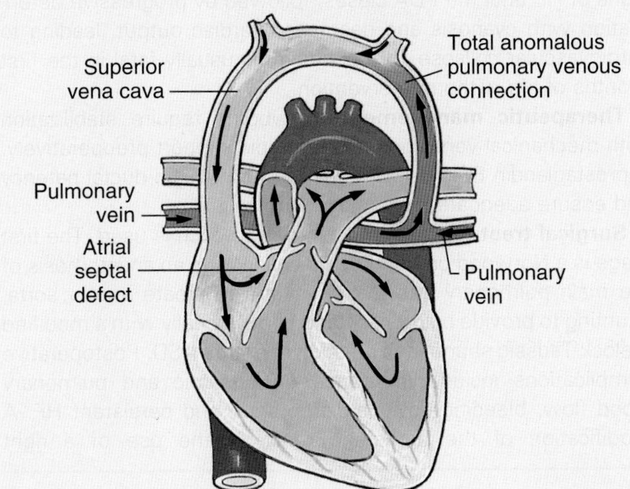

Description—Rare defect characterized by failure of the pulmonary veins to join the left atrium. Instead, the pulmonary veins are abnormally connected to the systemic venous circuit via the right atrium or various veins draining toward the right atrium, such as the superior vena cava (SVC). The abnormal attachment results in mixed blood being returned to the right atrium and shunted from the right to the left through an atrial septal defect (ASD). Total anomalous pulmonary venous connection (TAPVC; also called *total anomalous pulmonary venous return* or *total anomalous pulmonary venous drainage*) is classified according to the pulmonary venous point of attachment as follows:

Supracardiac—Attachment above the diaphragm, such as to the SVC (most common form) (see Fig. 47-9)

Cardiac—Direct attachment to the heart, such as to the right atrium or coronary sinus

Infradiaphragmatic—Attachment below the diaphragm, such as to the inferior vena cava (most severe form)

Pathophysiology—The right atrium receives all the blood that normally would flow into the left atrium. As a result, the right side of the heart hypertrophies, whereas the left side, especially the left atrium, may remain small. An associated ASD or patent foramen ovale allows systemic venous blood to shunt from the higher-pressure right atrium to the left atrium and into the left side of the heart. As a result, the oxygen saturation of the blood in both sides of the heart (and ultimately in the systemic arterial circulation) is the same. If the pulmonary blood flow is large, pulmonary venous return is also large, and the amount of saturated blood is relatively high. However, if there is obstruction to pulmonary venous drainage, pulmonary venous return is impeded, pulmonary venous pressure rises, and pulmonary interstitial edema develops and eventually contributes to HF. Infradiaphragmatic TAPVC is often associated with obstruction to pulmonary venous drainage and is a surgical emergency.

Clinical manifestations—Most infants develop cyanosis early in life. The degree of cyanosis is inversely related to the amount of pulmonary blood flow—the more pulmonary blood, the less cyanosis. Children with unobstructed TAPVC may be asymptomatic until pulmonary vascular resistance decreases during infancy, increasing pulmonary blood flow, with resulting signs of HF. Cyanosis becomes worse with pulmonary vein obstruction; once obstruction occurs, the infant's condition usually deteriorates rapidly. Without intervention, cardiac failure will progress to death.

Surgical treatment—Corrective repair is performed in early infancy. The surgical approach varies with the anatomical defect. However, in general, the common pulmonary vein is anastomosed to the back of the left atrium, the ASD is closed, and the anomalous pulmonary venous connection is ligated. The cardiac type is most easily repaired; the infradiaphragmatic type carries the highest morbidity and mortality because of the higher incidence of pulmonary vein obstruction. Potential postoperative complications include reobstruction; bleeding; dysrhythmias, particularly heart block; pulmonary artery hypertension; and persistent HF.

Prognosis—Mortality for all types is less than 10% (Jacobs et al., 2004) and is lowest for the cardiac type; morbidity increases with the presence of pulmonary vein obstruction.

Continued

BOX 47-4 MIXED DEFECTS—cont'd

Truncus Arteriosus

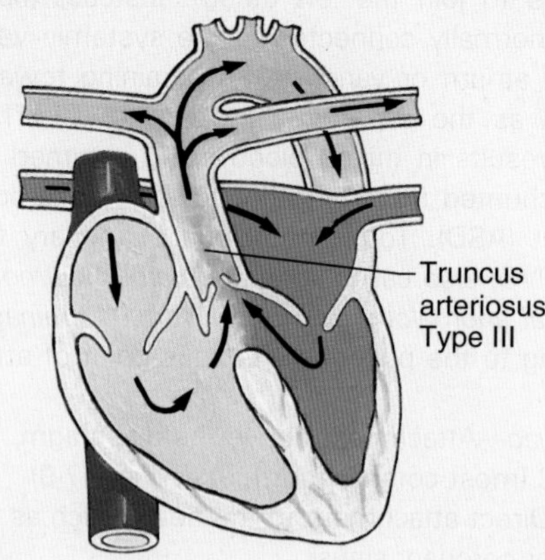

Description—Failure of normal septation and division of the embryonic bulbar trunk into the pulmonary artery and the aorta, which results in development of a single vessel that overrides both ventricles. Blood from both ventricles mixes in the common great artery, which leads to desaturation and hypoxemia. Blood ejected from the heart flows preferentially to the lower-pressure pulmonary arteries, so pulmonary blood flow is increased and systemic blood flow is reduced. There are three types:

Type I—A single pulmonary trunk arises near the base of the truncus and divides into the left and right pulmonary arteries.

Type II—The left and right pulmonary arteries arise separately but in close proximity and at the same level from the back of the truncus.

Type III—The pulmonary arteries arise independently from the sides of the truncus.

Pathophysiology—Blood ejected from the left and right ventricles enters the common trunk so that pulmonary and systemic circulations are mixed. Blood flow is distributed to the pulmonary and systemic circulations according to the relative resistances of each system. The amount of pulmonary blood flow depends on the size of the pulmonary arteries and the pulmonary vascular resistance. Generally, resistance to pulmonary blood flow is less than systemic vascular resistance, which results in preferential blood flow to the lungs. Pulmonary vascular disease develops at an early age in patients with truncus arteriosus.

Clinical manifestations—Most infants are symptomatic with moderate to severe HF and variable cyanosis, poor growth, and activity intolerance. There is a holosystolic murmur at the left sternal border with a diastolic murmur present if truncal regurgitation is present. Thirty-five percent of patients have 22q11 deletions (Goldmuntz, Crenshaw, & Lin, 2008).

Surgical treatment—Early repair is performed in the first month of life. It involves closing the VSD so that the truncus arteriosus receives the outflow from the left ventricle, excising the pulmonary arteries from the aorta and attaching them to the right ventricle by means of a homograft. Currently, homografts (segments of cadaver aorta and pulmonary artery that are treated with antibiotics and cryopreserved) are preferred over synthetic conduits to establish continuity between the right ventricle and pulmonary artery. Homografts are more flexible and easier to use during the procedure and appear less prone to obstruction. Postoperative complications include persistent heart failure, bleeding, pulmonary artery hypertension, dysrhythmias, and residual VSD. Because conduits are not living tissue, they will not grow along with the child and may also become narrowed with calcifications. One or more conduit replacements will be needed in childhood.

Prognosis—Mortality is greater than 10%; future operations are required to replace the conduits.

Hypoplastic Left Heart Syndrome

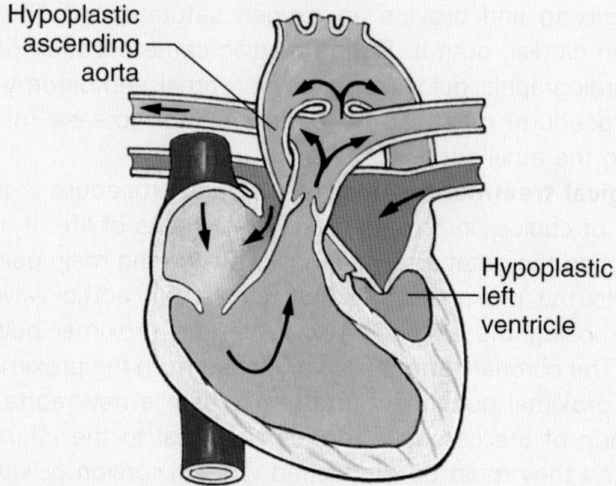

Description—Underdevelopment of the left side of the heart, resulting in a hypoplastic left ventricle and aortic atresia. Most blood from the left atrium flows across the patent foramen ovale to the right atrium, to the right ventricle, and out the pulmonary artery. The descending aorta receives blood from the PDA supplying systemic blood flow.

Pathophysiology—An ASD or patent foramen ovale allows saturated blood from the left atrium to mix with desaturated blood from the right atrium and to flow through the right ventricle and out into the pulmonary artery. From the pulmonary artery, the blood flows both to the lungs and through the ductus arteriosus into the aorta and out to the body. The amount of blood flow to the pulmonary and systemic circulations depends on the relationship between the pulmonary and systemic vascular resistances. The coronary and cerebral vessels receive blood by retrograde flow through the hypoplastic ascending aorta.

Clinical manifestations—The patient has mild cyanosis and signs of HF until the PDA closes, followed by progressive deterioration with cyanosis and decreased cardiac output, leading to cardiovascular collapse. The condition is usually fatal in the first months of life without intervention.

Therapeutic management—Newborns require stabilization with mechanical ventilation and inotropic support preoperatively. A prostaglandin E_1 infusion is needed to maintain ductal patency and ensure adequate systemic blood flow.

Surgical treatment—A multistage approach is used. The first stage is a Norwood procedure, which involves an anastomosis of the main pulmonary artery to the aorta to create a new aorta, shunting to provide pulmonary blood flow (usually with a modified Blalock-Taussig shunt), and creation of a large ASD. Postoperative complications include imbalance of systemic and pulmonary blood flow, bleeding, low cardiac output, and persistent HF. A modification of the first-stage repair is the use of a right

BOX 47-4 MIXED DEFECTS—cont'd

ventricle–to–pulmonary artery homograft conduit instead of a shunt to supply pulmonary blood flow (Sano procedure). The second stage is often a bidirectional Glenn shunt procedure (see Fig. 47-9) or a hemi-Fontan operation. Both involve anastomosing the SVC to the right pulmonary artery so that SVC flow bypasses the right atrium and flows directly to the lungs. The procedure is usually done at 3 to 6 months of age to relieve cyanosis and reduce the volume load on the right ventricle. The final repair is a modified Fontan procedure (see Tricuspid Atresia, Box 47-3).

Transplantation—Heart transplantation in the newborn period is another option for these infants. Problems include the shortage of newborn organ donors, risk of rejection, long-term problems with chronic immunosuppression, and infection (see Heart Transplantation, p. 1511).

Prognosis—For the first-stage repair, survival rates vary from 5 to 30% (Tweddell, Hoffman, Ghanayaren, et al., 2008). Improved outcomes have been associated with early diagnosis and repair and increased monitoring in the hospital and at home (Tweddell et al., 2008). Long-term problems with repair include worsening ventricular function, tricuspid regurgitation, recurrent aortic arch narrowing, dysrhythmias, and developmental delays. There is a risk of mortality between surgical procedures.

(TGA), cause severe cyanosis in the first days of life and later cause HF. Others, such as truncus arteriosus, cause severe HF in the first weeks of life and mild desaturation.

CLINICAL CONSEQUENCES OF CONGENITAL HEART DISEASE

Heart Failure

Heart failure (HF) is the inability of the heart to pump an adequate amount of blood to the systemic circulation at normal filling pressures to meet the body's metabolic demands. In children, HF most frequently occurs secondary to structural abnormalities (e.g., septal defects) that result in increased blood volume and pressure within the heart. It can also result from myocardial failure in which the contractility of the ventricle is impaired. This can occur with cardiomyopathy, dysrhythmias, or severe electrolyte disturbances. HF can also occur because of excessive demands on a normal heart muscle, such as sepsis or severe anemia.

Pathophysiology

Heart failure is often separated into two categories: right-sided and left-sided failure. In *right-sided failure*, the right ventricle is unable to pump blood effectively into the pulmonary artery, resulting in increased pressure in the right atrium and systemic venous circulation. Systemic venous hypertension causes hepatosplenomegaly and occasionally edema. In *left-sided failure*, the left ventricle is unable to pump blood into the systemic circulation, resulting in increased pressure in the left atrium and pulmonary veins. The lungs become congested with blood, causing elevated pulmonary pressures and pulmonary edema.

Although each type of HF produces different signs and symptoms, clinically it is unusual to observe solely right- or left-sided failure in children. Because each side of the heart depends on adequate function of the other side, failure of one chamber causes a reciprocal change in the opposite chamber.

If the abnormalities precipitating HF are not corrected, the heart muscle becomes damaged. Despite compensatory mechanisms, the heart is unable to maintain an adequate cardiac output. Decreased blood flow to the kidneys continues to stimulate sodium and water reabsorption, leading to fluid overload, increased workload on the heart, and congestion in the pulmonary and systemic circulations (Fig. 47-6).

The signs and symptoms of HF can be divided into three groups: (1) impaired myocardial function, (2) pulmonary congestion, and (3) systemic venous congestion (Box 47-5). Because these hemodynamic changes occur from different causes and at differing times, the clinical presentation may vary among children.

Diagnostic Evaluation

Diagnosis is made on the basis of clinical symptoms such as tachypnea and tachycardia at rest, dyspnea, retractions, activity intolerance (especially during feeding in infants), weight gain caused by fluid retention, and hepatomegaly. A chest x-ray film demonstrates cardiomegaly and increased pulmonary blood flow. Ventricular hypertrophy appears on the ECG. An echocardiogram is done to determine the cause of HF, such as a congenital heart defect or poor ventricular function.

Therapeutic Management

The goals of treatment are to (1) improve cardiac function (increase contractility and decrease afterload), (2) remove accumulated fluid and sodium (decrease preload), (3) decrease cardiac demands, and (4) improve tissue oxygenation and decrease oxygen consumption. For most infants diagnosed with HF, the cause is CHD. Infants are stabilized on medical therapy and then referred for surgical repair. Currently, many children are surgically repaired in the neonatal and early infancy stages before the onset of HF symptoms. For children newly diagnosed with HF, the cause may be worsening ventricular function after a previous cardiac repair, cardiomyopathy, dysrhythmia, or other causes. In addition to management of HF, the underlying cause is treated if possible.

Improve cardiac function. Myocardial efficiency is improved through the administration of digitalis glycosides. The beneficial effects are increased cardiac output, decreased heart size, decreased venous pressure, and relief of edema. In pediatrics, digoxin (Lanoxin) is used almost exclusively because of its more rapid onset. It is available as an elixir (0.05 mg/mL) for oral administration. For infants the dose is calculated in micrograms (1000 mcg = 1 mg).

Treatment consists of (1) a digitalizing dosage, given orally or intravenously in divided doses over 24 hours to produce

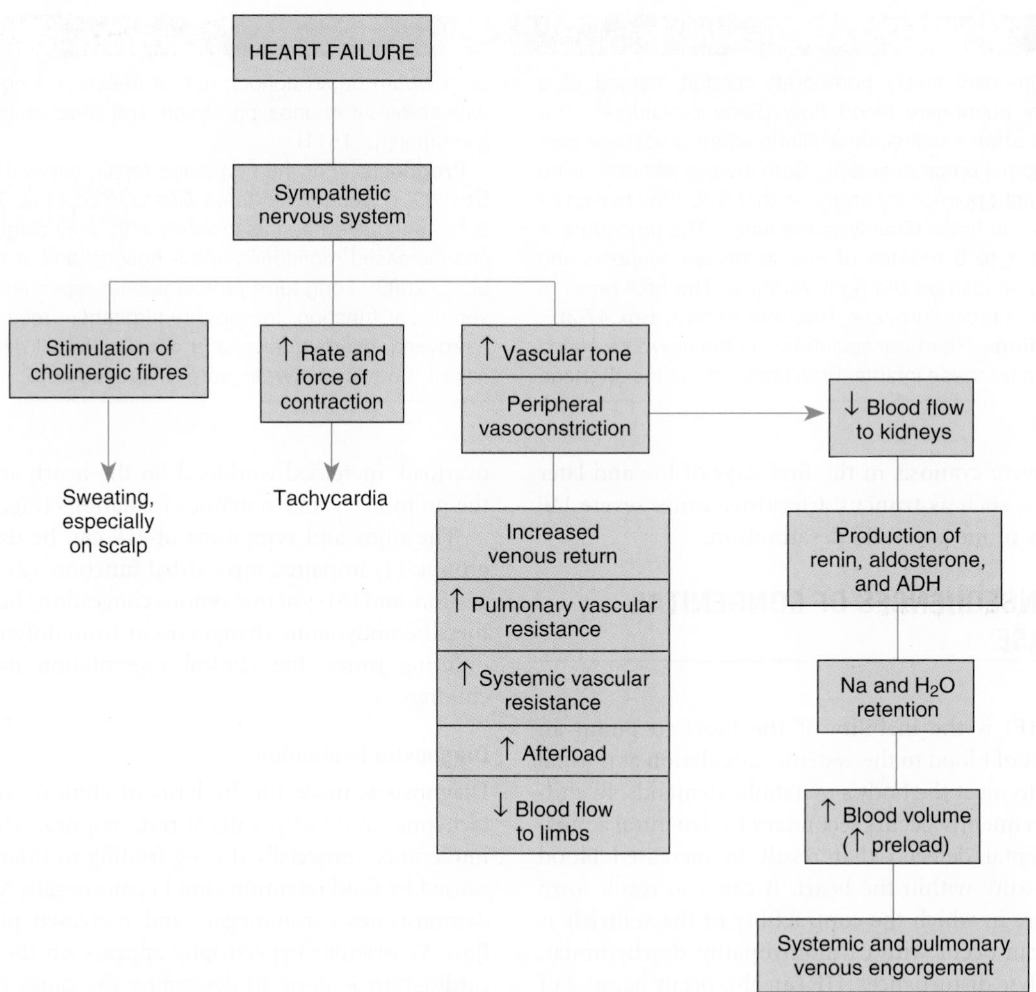

FIGURE 47-6 Pathophysiology of heart failure. *ADH*, antidiuretic hormone; Na, sodium.

optimal cardiac effects, and (2) a maintenance dosage, given orally twice a day to maintain blood levels. During digitalization the child is monitored by means of an ECG to observe for the desired effects (prolonged PR interval and reduced ventricular rate) and to detect adverse effects, especially dysrhythmias. The Canadian Cardiovascular Society Guidelines (Kantor, Loughheed, Dancea, et al., 2013) state that the addition of digoxin alone is not reported to result in improved contractility or clinical symptoms and that adjunct therapy including, but not limited to, vasodilator agents, diuretics agents, beta blockers, and angiotensin-converting enzyme (ACE) inhibitors is recommended for infants and children with HF.

ACE inhibitors are also used in the treatment of HF; these drugs inhibit the normal function of the renin-angiotensin system in the kidney. The ACE inhibitors block the conversion of angiotensin I to angiotensin II so that, instead of vasoconstriction, vasodilation occurs. Vasodilation results in decreased pulmonary and systemic vascular resistance, decreased BP, and a reduction in afterload. It also reduces the secretion of aldosterone, which reduces preload by preventing volume expansion from fluid retention and lowers the risk for hypokalemia. Common medications used in pediatrics are captopril (Capoten), enalapril (Vasotec), and lisinopril. The principal adverse effects of ACE inhibitors are hypotension, cough, and renal dysfunction.

Beta blockers, specifically metoprolol and carvedilol, are also used in the treatment of some children with chronic HF. The alpha- and beta-adrenergic receptors are blocked, causing decreased heart rate, decreased BP, and vasodilation. Beta blockers, used routinely for adults with HF, are used selectively in children, as the cause of HF in children and infants is much different from that in adults. Adverse effects include dizziness, headache, and hypotension.

Cardiac resynchronization therapy (CRT) using biventricular pacing is an effective treatment in adult patients with HF and is beginning to be applied to the pediatric population. With the pharmacological therapies discussed above, CRT has the potential to improve cardiac function in this group of patients, including those with a single ventricle (Bernstein, 2016b).

! NURSING ALERT

Because ACE inhibitors also block the action of aldosterone, the addition of potassium supplements or spironolactone (Aldactone) to the medication regimen of patients taking diuretics is usually not needed and may cause hyperkalemia.

BOX 47-5 CLINICAL MANIFESTATIONS OF HEART FAILURE

Impaired Myocardial Function
Tachycardia
Sweating (inappropriate)
Decreased urinary output
Fatigue
Weakness
Restlessness
Anorexia
Pale, cool extremities
Weak peripheral pulses
Decreased blood pressure
Gallop rhythm
Cardiomegaly

Pulmonary Congestion
Tachypnea
Dyspnea
Retractions (infants)
Flaring nares
Exercise intolerance
Orthopnea
Cough, hoarseness
Cyanosis
Wheezing
Grunting

Systemic Venous Congestion
Weight gain
Hepatomegaly
Peripheral edema, especially periorbital
Ascites
Neck vein distension (children)

Remove accumulated fluid and sodium. Treatment consists of diuretics, possible fluid restriction, and possible sodium restriction. Diuretics are the mainstay of therapy to eliminate excess water and salt in order to prevent reaccumulation. The most frequently used medications are listed in Table 47-2. Furosemide and the thiazides are potassium-losing diuretics, so potassium supplements may be prescribed, and rich sources of the electrolyte are encouraged in the diet.

! NURSING ALERT

A fall in the serum potassium level enhances the effects of digitalis, increasing the risk of digoxin toxicity. Increased serum potassium levels diminish digoxin's effect. Therefore, serum potassium levels (normal range 3.5 to 5.5 mmol/L) must be monitored carefully.

Fluid restriction may be required in the acute stages of HF and must be calculated carefully to avoid dehydrating the child, especially if cyanotic CHD and significant polycythemia are present. Infants rarely need fluid restrictions because HF makes feeding so difficult that they struggle to take maintenance fluids.

Sodium-restricted diets are used less often in children than in adults to control HF because of their potential negative effects on appetite. If salt intake is restricted, additional table salt and highly salted foods are avoided.

Decrease cardiac demands. To lessen the workload on the heart, metabolic needs are minimized by (1) providing a neutral thermal environment to prevent cold stress in infants, (2) treating any existing infections, (3) reducing the effort of breathing (by placement in semi-Fowler position), (4) using medication to sedate an irritable child, and (5) providing for rest and decreasing environmental stimuli.

TABLE 47-2 DIURETICS USED IN HEART FAILURE

ACTIONS	COMMENTS	NURSING CARE MANAGEMENT
Furosemide (Lasix)—Blocks reabsorption of sodium and water in proximal renal tubule and interferes with reabsorption of sodium	Drug of choice in severe heart failure Causes excretion of chloride and potassium (hypokalemia may precipitate digitalis toxicity)	Begin to record output as soon as drug is given. Observe for dehydration caused by profound diuresis. Observe for adverse effects (nausea and vomiting, diarrhea, ototoxicity, hypokalemia, dermatitis, postural hypotension). Encourage foods high in potassium or give potassium supplements. Monitor chloride and acid–base balance with long-term therapy. Observe for signs of digoxin toxicity.
Chlorothiazide—Acts directly on distal tubules to decrease sodium, water, potassium, chloride, and bicarbonate absorption	Less frequently used drug Causes hypokalemia, acidosis from large doses	Observe for adverse effects (nausea, weakness, dizziness, paresthesia, muscle cramps, skin eruptions, hypokalemia, acidosis). Encourage foods high in potassium or give potassium supplements, or both.
Spironolactone (Aldactone)—Blocks action of aldosterone, which promotes retention of sodium and excretion of potassium	Weak diuretic Has potassium-sparing effect; frequently used with thiazides, furosemide Poorly absorbed from gastrointestinal tract Takes several days to achieve maximum actions	Observe for adverse effects (skin rash, drowsiness, ataxia, hyperkalemia). Do not administer potassium supplements.

Improve tissue oxygenation. All of the preceding measures serve to increase tissue oxygenation, by either improving myocardial function or lessening tissue oxygen demands. In addition, supplemental cool, humidified oxygen may be administered to increase the amount of available oxygen during inspiration. Oxygen administration is especially helpful in patients with pulmonary edema, intercurrent respiratory tract infections, and increased pulmonary vascular resistance (oxygen is a vasodilator that decreases pulmonary vascular resistance).

! NURSING ALERT

Oxygen is a drug and is administered only with an appropriate order. In some uncommon circumstances in patients with complex hemodynamics, oxygen can be detrimental.

An oxygen hood, nasal cannula, or face tent is used to deliver oxygen. Nasal cannulas are ideal for long-term oxygen administration because the child can be ambulatory and can easily eat and drink. Cool humidification is necessary to counteract the drying effect of oxygen. The amount of cool humidity needs to be carefully regulated to prevent chilling.

NURSING CARE

The infant or child with HF may be acutely ill, and some children may require critical care until the symptoms improve. Expert nursing care is essential to reduce the cardiac demands that strain the failing heart muscle. During this time, the child and family require emotional support. Although the objectives of nursing care are the same, interventions differ, depending on the child's age (see Nursing Care Plan: The Child With Heart  Failure [HF] available on Evolve).

Assist in Measures to Improve Cardiac Function

The nurse's responsibility in administering digoxin includes calculating and administering the correct dosage, observing for signs of toxicity, and instituting parental teaching on medication administration at home. The child's **apical pulse rate** should always be checked before administering digoxin. As a general rule, the drug is not given if the pulse is below 90 to 110 beats per minute (bpm) in infants and young children or below 70 bpm in older children (the cutoff point for adults is 60 bpm). However, because the pulse rate varies in children in different age groups, the written medication order should specify at what heart rate the medication is withheld. The nurse should also use judgement in evaluating the pulse rate. If it is significantly lower than the previous recording, the dose should be withheld until the health care provider most responsible for the patient is notified.

The apical rate is taken because a pulse deficit (radial pulse rate lower than apical) may be present with decreased cardiac output. It is **auscultated** for a full minute to evaluate alterations in rhythm. If the child is monitored by means of an ECG, a rhythm strip is obtained and attached to the chart for rate and rhythm analysis, such as abnormal lengthening of the PR interval (more than 50% increase over predigitalization interval) and dysrhythmias.

BOX 47-6 COMMON SIGNS OF DIGOXIN TOXICITY IN CHILDREN

Gastrointestinal
Nausea
Vomiting
Anorexia

Cardiac
Bradycardia
Dysrhythmias

Digoxin is a potentially dangerous drug because of its narrow margin of safety of therapeutic, toxic, and lethal doses. Many toxic responses are extensions of its therapeutic effects. The nurse must maintain a high index of suspicion for signs of toxicity when administering digoxin (Box 47-6).

Because digoxin toxicity can occur from accidental overdose, great care must be taken in properly calculating and measuring the dosage. When converting milligrams to micrograms to millilitres, the nurse needs to carefully check the placement of the decimal point, since an error causes a significant change in dosage. For example, 0.1 mg is 10 times the dosage of 0.01 mg.

NURSING ALERT

Infants rarely receive more than 1 mL (50 mcg, or 0.05 mg) in one dose; a higher dose is an immediate warning of a dosage error. To ensure safety, always compare and check the calculation with another staff member before giving the medication.

These same principles are taught to parents in preparation for discharge, although the correct dose in millilitres is usually specified on the container, thus reducing potential errors in calculation. The nurse needs to watch the parent measure the elixir in the dropper and stress the level mark as the meniscus of the fluid that is observed at eye level. Other instructions for administering digoxin are listed in the Family-Centred Teaching box and Critical Thinking Case Study.

Parents also need to be advised of the signs of toxicity. According to the health care provider's preference, they may be taught to take the pulse before giving the medication. A return demonstration of the procedure from the parents or another principal caregiver should be included as part of the teaching plan. Their level of anxiety in counting the pulse should be assessed, since overconcern about the heart rate may result in excessive withholding of the medication.

Monitor Afterload Reduction

For patients receiving ACE inhibitors for afterload reduction, the nurse should carefully monitor BP before and after dose administration, observe for symptoms of hypotension, and notify the health care provider if BP is low. Numerous medications affecting the kidney can potentiate renal dysfunction; thus children taking multiple diuretics and an ACE inhibitor require careful assessment of serum electrolytes and renal function.

FAMILY-CENTRED TEACHING
Administering Digoxin

- Give digoxin at regular intervals, usually every 12 hours.
- Administer the drug carefully by slowly directing it to the side and back of the mouth.
- Do not mix the drug with foods or other fluids, since refusal to consume these results in inaccurate intake of the drug.
- If the child has teeth, give water after administering the drug; whenever possible, brush the teeth to prevent tooth decay from the sweetened liquid.
- If a dose is missed, do not give an extra dose or increase the dose. Stay on the same medication schedule.
- If the child vomits, do not give a second dose.
- If more than two consecutive doses have been missed, notify the physician or other designated health care provider.
- Frequent vomiting, poor feeding, or slow heart rate can be signs of toxicity; if they occur, contact the physician.
- If the child becomes ill, notify the physician or other designated health care provider immediately.
- Keep digoxin in a safe place, preferably in a locked cabinet.
- In case of accidental overdose of digoxin, call the nearest poison control centre immediately.

CRITICAL THINKING CASE STUDY
Digoxin Toxicity

A home care nurse is visiting a 3-month-old infant at home who began receiving digoxin and furosemide (Lasix) 5 days ago for management of heart failure (HF). A brief assessment indicates that the infant appears well but is not very active, has a weak suck reflex, and does not exhibit much spontaneous movement during interaction with the mother. The mother mentions that the infant is a good baby and does not cry much except when he is very hungry. She also mentions that he vomited several times yesterday and twice this morning; this was not perceived as unusual because her 3-year-old did the same thing and was diagnosed with gastroesophageal reflux. Further assessment of the infant reveals an irregular heartbeat of 86 to 104 beats/min at rest; the heart rhythm is also noted to be irregular. No murmur or other significant sounds are auscultated.

1. Evidence—Is there sufficient evidence to draw conclusions about this infant?
2. Assumptions—Describe an underlying assumption about each of the following:
   a. Adverse effects of furosemide
   b. Adverse effects of digoxin
   c. Infants with HF
3. What priorities for nursing care should be established for this infant?
4. Does the evidence support your nursing interventions?

Decrease Cardiac Demands

The infant requires rest and conservation of energy for feeding. Every effort should be made to organize nursing activities to allow for uninterrupted periods of sleep. Whenever possible, parents need to be encouraged to stay with their infant to provide the holding, rocking, and cuddling that help children sleep more soundly. To minimize disturbing the infant, changing bed linen and complete bathing should be done only when necessary. Feeding should be planned to accommodate the infant's sleep and wake patterns. The child is fed at the first sign of hunger, such as when sucking on fists, rather than waiting until he or she cries, because the stress of crying exhausts the limited energy supply. Because infants with HF tire easily and may sleep through feedings, smaller feedings every 3 hours or breastfeeding on demand may be helpful. Gavage feedings may be instituted to provide adequate nutrition and allow the infant to rest.

Every effort should be made to minimize unnecessary stress. Older children need an explanation of what is happening to them to decrease anxiety about their illness and necessary treatments such as cardiac monitoring, oxygen administration, and medications. Outlining a plan for the day, preparing the child for tests and procedures, providing quiet activities, and providing adequate rest periods are all helpful interventions with older children. Some infants and children require sedation during the acute phase of illness to allow them to rest.

Temperature needs to be monitored carefully because hyperthermia or hypothermia increases the need for oxygen. Febrile states should be reported to the primary health care provider, since infection must be treated promptly. Maintaining body temperature is of special importance in children who are receiving cool, humidified oxygen and in infants, who tend to be diaphoretic and lose heat by way of evaporation.

Skin breakdown from edema is prevented with a change of position every 2 hours (from side to side while in semi-Fowler position) and use of a pressure-relieving mattress or bed. The skin, especially over the sacrum, should be checked for evidence of redness from pressure.

Reduce Respiratory Distress

Careful assessment, positioning, and oxygen administration can reduce respiratory distress. Respirations are counted for 1 full minute during a resting state. Any evidence of increased respiratory distress should be reported, since this may indicate worsening HF.

Infants should be positioned to encourage maximum chest expansion, with the head of the bed elevated; they should sit up in an infant seat or be held at a 45-degree angle. Children prefer to sleep on several pillows and remain in a semi-Fowler or high-Fowler position during waking hours. Safety restraints, such as those used with infant seats, should be applied low on the abdomen and loosely enough to provide both safety and maximum expansion.

The infant or child is often given humidified supplemental oxygen via oxygen hood or tent, nasal cannula, or mask. The child's response to oxygen therapy needs to be carefully evaluated by noting respiratory rate, ease of respiration, colour, and especially oxygen saturation as measured by oximetry.

Respiratory tract infections can exacerbate HF and should be treated appropriately and prevented if possible. The child should be protected from persons with respiratory tract infections and have a noninfectious roommate. Good hand hygiene should be practised before and after caring for any hospitalized child. Antibiotics may be given to combat respiratory tract infection. The nurse needs to ensure that the medication is given at equally divided times over a 24-hour schedule to maintain high blood levels of the antibiotic.

Maintain Nutritional Status

Meeting the nutritional needs of infants with HF or serious cardiac defects is a nursing challenge. The metabolic rate of these infants is greater because of poor cardiac function and increased heart and respiratory rates. Their caloric needs are greater than those of the average infant because of their increased metabolic rate, yet their ability to take in adequate calories is hampered by their fatigue. Feeding for a fragile infant with serious CHD is similar to exercising for an adult, and these infants often do not have the energy or cardiac reserve to do extra work. The nurse needs to seek measures to enable the infant to feed easily without excess fatigue and to increase the caloric density of the formula.

The infant should be well rested before feeding and fed soon after awakening so as not to expend energy on crying. A 3-hour feeding schedule works well for many infants. (Feeding every 2 hours does not provide enough rest between feedings, and a 4-hour schedule requires an increased volume of feeding, which many infants are unable to take.) The feeding schedule should be individualized to the infant's needs. A feeding goal of 150 mL/kg/day and at least 120 kcal/kg/day is common for newborns with significant heart disease. Newborns can be breastfed or bottle fed. A soft preemie nipple or a slit in a regular nipple to enlarge the opening decreases the infant's energy expenditure while sucking from a bottle. Infants should be well supported and fed in a semi-upright position. The infant may need to rest frequently and may need to have the jaw and cheeks stroked to encourage sucking. Generally, giving an infant about a half-hour to complete a feeding is reasonable. Prolonging the feeding time can exhaust the infant and decrease the rest period between feedings.

Infants with feeding difficulties are often gavage fed using a nasogastric tube to supplement their oral intake and ensure adequate calories. If they are very stressed and fatigued, in respiratory distress, or tachypneic to 80 to 100 breaths/min, oral feedings may be withheld and all nutrition given by gavage feedings. Gavage feedings are usually a temporary measure until the infant's medical status improves and nutritional needs can be met through oral feedings. Some infants with severe HF, neurological deficits, or significant gastroesophageal reflux may need placement of a gastrostomy tube to allow adequate nutrition.

The caloric density of formulas is frequently increased by concentration and then adding Polycose, medium-chain triglyceride oil, or corn oil. Infant formulas provide 20 kcal/30 mL, and the use of additives can increase the calories to 30 kcal/30 mL or more. This allows the infant to obtain more calories despite a smaller volume intake of formula. The caloric density of the formula needs to be increased slowly (by 2 kcal/30 mL/day) to prevent diarrhea or formula intolerance. Breastfeeding mothers should be encouraged to provide the infant with high-calorie feedings and may feed expressed breast milk that has been fortified to increase caloric intake, which can be given using a supplemental nurser while the child nurses at the breast (see Fig. 27-10). A diet plan specific to the individual infant's needs should be calculated and prescribed by the nutritionist in collaboration with the other health personnel. The nurse needs to reinforce this information with the parents as necessary.

Assist in Measures to Promote Fluid Loss

When diuretics are given, the nurse needs to record fluid intake and output and monitor body weight at the same time each day to evaluate the benefit from the medication. Because profound diuresis may cause dehydration and electrolyte imbalance (loss of sodium, potassium, chloride, bicarbonate), the nurse should observe for signs indicating either complication, as well as signs and symptoms suggesting reactions to the medications. Diuretics should be given early in the day to children who are toilet trained, to avoid the need to urinate at night. If potassium-losing diuretics are given, the nurse can encourage foods high in potassium, such as bananas, oranges, whole grains, legumes, and leafy vegetables, and administer prescribed supplements. Serum potassium levels should be checked frequently.

Fluid restriction is rarely necessary in infants because of their difficulty in feeding. However, if fluids are restricted, the nurse can plan fluid intake schedules for a 24-hour period, allowing for most fluids during waking hours. Toddlers and preschoolers should be given small amounts of liquid in small cups so that the containers appear full. Older children can be placed in charge of recording fluid intake.

If salt is limited, the nurse needs to discuss food sources of sodium with the family and discourage their bringing salt-containing treats to the child. At mealtime, the child's tray should be checked to make sure the appropriate diet is being given.

Support the Child and Family

HF is a serious complication of heart disease. Parents and older children are usually acutely aware of the critical nature of the condition. Because stress places additional demands on cardiac function, the nurse should focus on reducing anxiety through anticipatory preparation, frequent communication with the parent regarding the child's progress, and constant reassurance that everything possible is being done.

The nurse teaches the family about the medications that need to be administered and alerts them to the signs of worsening HF that require medical attention, such as increased sweating, decreased urinary output (noted in fewer wet diapers or infrequent use of the toilet), or poor feeding. Every effort should be made to improve the family's adherence to the medication schedule by adapting the schedule to their usual home routines, avoiding medications during the night, making it as simple as possible, and using charts or visual aids to remember when to give medications (see Chapter 44). Written instructions regarding correct administration of digoxin are essential (see Family-Centred Teaching box, on previous page), including an explanation of the signs of toxicity.

If HF is the end stage of a severe heart defect, the nurse should care for this child as for any child who is terminally ill, using the principles discussed in Chapter 40.

Hypoxemia

Hypoxemia refers to an arterial oxygen tension (or pressure, Pao_2) that is less than normal and can be identified by a decreased arterial saturation or a decreased Pao_2. Hypoxia is a reduction in tissue oxygenation that is caused by low oxygen saturations and Pao_2 and results in impaired cellular processes. *Cyanosis* is a blue discolouration in the mucous membranes, skin, and nail beds of the child with reduced oxygen saturation. It results from the presence of deoxygenated hemoglobin (hemoglobin not bound to oxygen) in a concentration of blood. Cyanosis is usually apparent when arterial oxygen saturations are 80 to 85%. Determination of cyanosis is subjective. It can vary depending on skin pigment, quality of light, colour of the room, or clothing worn by the child. The presence of cyanosis may not accurately reflect arterial hypoxemia because both oxygen saturation and the amount of circulating hemoglobin are involved. Children with severe anemia may not be cyanotic despite severe hypoxemia because the hemoglobin level may be too low to produce the characteristic blue colour. Conversely, patients with polycythemia may appear cyanotic despite a near-normal Pao_2. Heart defects that cause hypoxemia and cyanosis result from desaturated venous blood (blue blood) entering the systemic circulation without passing through the lungs.

Clinical Manifestations

Over time, two physiological changes occur in the body in response to chronic hypoxemia: polycythemia and clubbing. *Polycythemia*, an increased number of red blood cells, increases the oxygen-carrying capacity of the blood. However, anemia may result if iron is not readily available for the formation of hemoglobin. Polycythemia increases the viscosity of the blood and crowds out clotting factors. *Clubbing*, a thickening and flattening of the tips of the fingers and toes, is thought to occur because of chronic tissue hypoxemia and polycythemia (Fig. 47-7). Infants with mild hypoxemia may be asymptomatic except for cyanosis and exhibit near-normal growth and development. Those with more severe hypoxemia may exhibit fatigue with feeding, poor weight gain, tachypnea, and dyspnea. Severe hypoxemia resulting in tissue hypoxia is manifested by clinical deterioration and signs of poor perfusion.

Hypercyanotic spells, also referred to as *blue spells* or *tet spells* because they are often seen in infants with tetralogy of Fallot, may occur in any child whose heart defect includes obstruction to pulmonary blood flow and communication between the ventricles. The infant becomes acutely cyanotic and hyperpneic because a sudden infundibular spasm decreases pulmonary blood flow and increases right-to-left shunting (the proposed mechanism in tetralogy of Fallot). Spells, rarely seen before 2 months of age, occur most frequently in the first year of life. They occur more often in the morning and may be preceded by feeding, crying, defecation, or stressful procedures (see Critical Thinking Case Study). Because profound hypoxemia causes cerebral hypoxia, hypercyanotic spells require prompt assessment and treatment to prevent brain damage or possibly death.

Persistent cyanosis as a result of cyanotic heart defects places the child at risk for significant neurological complications. Cerebrovascular accident (CVA, stroke), brain abscess, and developmental delays (especially in motor and cognitive development) may result from chronic hypoxia.

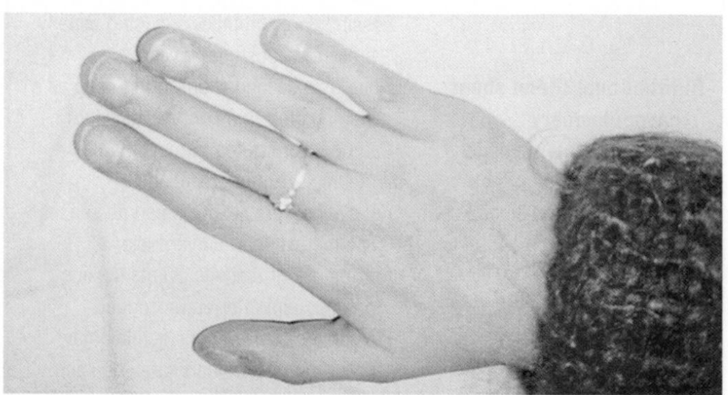

FIGURE 47-7 Clubbing of the fingers.

Diagnostic Management

Cyanosis in a newborn can be the result of cardiac, pulmonary, metabolic, or hematologic disease, although cardiac and pulmonary causes occur most often. To distinguish between the two, a hyperoxia test is helpful. The infant is placed in a 100% oxygen environment, and blood parameters are monitored. A Pao_2 of 100 mm Hg or higher suggests lung disease, and a Pao_2 lower than 100 mm Hg suggests cardiac disease (Park, 2015). An accurate history, a chest radiograph, and especially an echocardiogram contribute to the diagnosis of cyanotic heart disease.

Therapeutic Management

Newborns generally exhibit cyanosis within the first few days of life as the ductus arteriosus, which provided pulmonary blood flow, begins to close. Prostaglandin E_1, which causes vasodilation and smooth muscle relaxation, thus increasing dilation and patency of the ductus arteriosus, is administered intravenously to re-establish pulmonary blood flow. The use of prostaglandins has been life-saving for infants with ductus-dependent cardiac defects. The increase in oxygenation allows the infant to be stabilized and have a complete diagnostic evaluation performed before further treatment is needed.

CRITICAL THINKING CASE STUDY

Hypercyanotic Spell

A 4-month-old infant known to have tetralogy of Fallot is seen in the emergency department because of a 2-day history of diarrhea, low-grade fever, and poor oral intake. When blood is drawn, he becomes acutely cyanotic with rapid shallow respirations.

1. Evidence—Is there sufficient evidence to draw conclusions about this infant's condition?
2. Assumptions—Describe an underlying assumption about each of the following:
   a. Symptoms associated with tetralogy of Fallot
   b. Diarrhea, low-grade fever, and poor oral intake in a 4-month-old infant
   c. Acute cyanotic episodes in a 4-month-old infant
3. What priorities for nursing care should be established for this infant?
4. Does the evidence support your nursing interventions?

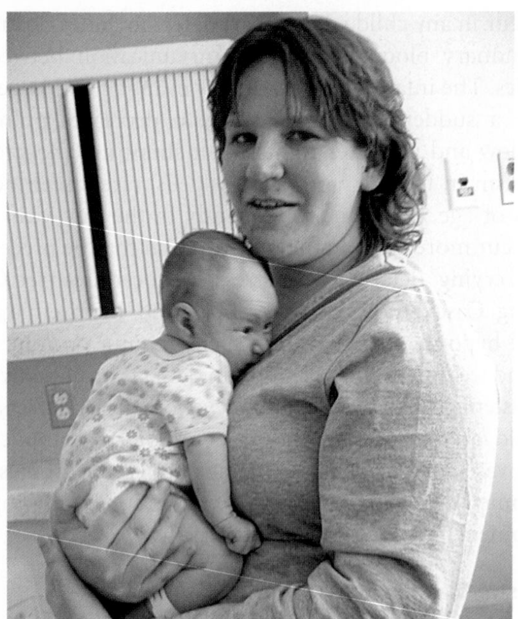

FIGURE 47-8 Infant held in knee–chest position.

GUIDELINES

Treating Hypercyanotic Spells

- Place infant in knee–chest position (see Fig. 47-8).
- Use a calm, comforting approach.
- Administer 100% oxygen by blow-by.
- Give morphine subcutaneously or through existing intravenous (IV) line.
- Begin IV fluid replacement and volume expansion if needed.
- Repeat morphine administration.

Hypercyanotic spells occur suddenly, and prompt recognition and treatment are essential. In the hospital setting, spells are often seen during blood drawing or IV insertion, when the child is highly agitated, or after cardiac catheterization. Treatment of a hypercyanotic spell is outlined in the Guidelines box. Placing the infant in the knee–chest position reduces the venous return from the legs (which is desaturated) and increases systemic vascular resistance, which diverts more blood into the pulmonary artery (Fig. 47-9). Morphine, administered subcutaneously or through an existing IV line, helps reduce infundibular spasm. A spell indicates the need for prompt surgical treatment, if possible. In infants with defects not amenable to surgical repair, a shunt may be created surgically to increase blood flow to the lungs. Several commonly used shunt procedures are described in Table 47-3 and Fig. 47-9.

The cyanotic infant and child should be well hydrated to keep the hematocrit and blood viscosity within acceptable limits to reduce the risk of CVAs. Fevers need to be carefully evaluated because bacteremia can result in bacterial endocarditis. The infant should be monitored closely for anemia because of the risk of CVAs and the reduced arterial oxygen-carrying capacity that occurs. Iron supplementation and possibly blood transfusion are used as needed.

Respiratory tract infections or reduced pulmonary function from any cause can worsen hypoxemia in the cyanotic child.

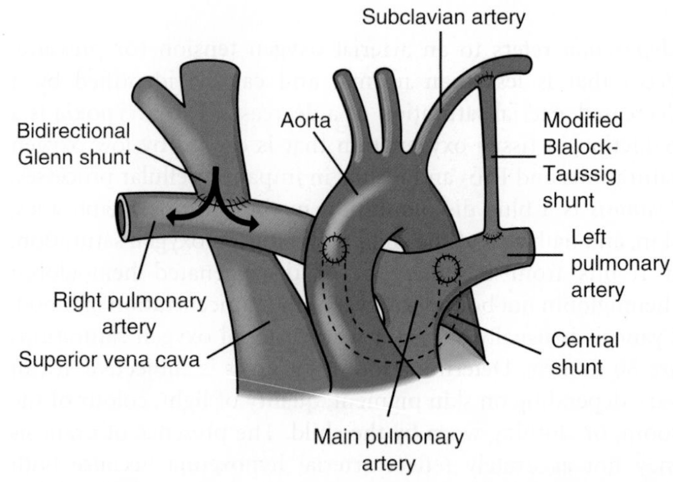

FIGURE 47-9 Schematic diagram of cardiac shunts.

TABLE 47-3 SELECTED SHUNT PROCEDURES FOR CHILDREN WITH CARDIAC DEFECTS

SHUNT TYPE	COMMENTS
Modified Blalock-Taussig shunt—Subclavian artery to pulmonary artery using Gore-Tex or Impra tube graft	Shunt flow sometimes excessive, requiring use of diuretics Possibility of thrombosis; aspirin usually prescribed postoperatively Easy to ligate at time of definitive correction Shunt size fixed and may become too small as child grows
Sano modification—Right ventricular to pulmonary artery conduit using Gore-Tex	Prevents diastolic runoff of systemic blood into the pulmonary arteries Provides a higher diastolic blood pressure and seemingly better coronary perfusion Used in place of the modified Blalock-Taussig shunt in the Norwood procedure
Central shunt—Ascending aorta to main pulmonary artery using Gore-Tex graft	Length of shunt acts to restrict blood flow; possibility of symptoms of heart failure; diuretic therapy sometimes required Uncommon; used when modified Blalock-Taussig shunt cannot be used Easy to insert and remove at time of repair Possibility of thrombosis; aspirin usually prescribed postoperatively
Bidirectional Glenn shunt (cavopulmonary anastomosis)—Superior vena cava to side of right pulmonary artery; blood flow to both lungs	Done as a second shunt; often used as a staging step to a Fontan procedure Can be incorporated into eventual modified Fontan procedure Relieves severe cyanosis and decreases volume overload on ventricle Carries risk of embolic events (mixing defect); aspirin often prescribed Pulmonary arteriovenous fistulas may occur months or years later, causing desaturation (uncommon finding)

Aggressive pulmonary hygiene, chest physical therapy, administration of antibiotics, and use of oxygen to improve arterial saturations are important interventions.

NURSING CARE

The general appearance of infants and children with significant cyanosis poses unique concerns. Blue lips and fingernails are obvious signs of their hidden cardiac defect. Clubbing and small, thin stature in older children further indicate severe heart disease. Adolescents are especially concerned about their body image; children with cyanosis are often teased about their appearance and singled out as different. When asked what surgery will do, many children reply, "Make me pink." Their joy and excitement after surgery are evident when they see their pink fingers. Parents are often fearful of their child's bluish colour because cyanosis is usually associated with lack of oxygen and severe illness. They also must deal with comments from relatives, friends, and strangers about their child's abnormal colour. They need a simple explanation of hypoxemia and cyanosis and reassurance that cyanosis does not imply a lack of oxygen to the brain. Their questions and fears need to be addressed in a calm, supportive manner, and positive aspects of their child's growth and development should be emphasized. They need to be taught the treatment for hypercyanotic spells (see Guidelines box, previous page).

Dehydration must be prevented in hypoxemic children because it potentiates the risk of CVAs. Fluid status should be monitored carefully, with accurate intake and output and daily weight measurements. Maintenance fluid therapy is the minimum requirement, supplemental fluids should be readily available, and gavage feeding or IV hydration is given to children unable to take adequate oral fluids. Fever, vomiting, and diarrhea can cause dehydration and require prompt treatment. Parents need to be instructed in the importance of adequate fluid intake and measures to prevent dehydration. An oral electrolyte solution should be available at home in the event that the infant is unable to tolerate breast milk or formula. The primary care provider should be notified of fever, vomiting, diarrhea, or other problems.

Preventive measures and accurate assessment of respiratory infection are important nursing considerations. Any compromise in pulmonary function will increase the infant's hypoxemia. Good hand hygiene and protection from individuals with an obvious respiratory tract infection are important. Aggressive pulmonary hygiene, treatment with antibiotics or antiviral agents as indicated, and supplemental oxygen to decrease hypoxemia are necessary measures. Infants may need to be gavage fed or given parenteral hydration if respiratory distress prevents oral feeding.

> **! NURSING ALERT**
>
> Intracardiac shunting of blood from the right side (desaturated) to the left side of the heart allows air in the venous system to go directly to the brain, resulting in an air embolism. Therefore, all IV lines should have filters in place to prevent air from entering the system, the entire tubing should be checked for air, all connections should be taped securely, and any air should be removed.

THE FAMILY AND CHILD WITH CONGENITAL HEART DISEASE

As the child's principal caregivers, the parents need to develop a positive, supportive working relationship with the health care team. Because most children spend the majority of their time at home, with episodic trips to the hospital, parents manage their child's illness on a daily basis. They monitor for signs of illness, give medications and treatments, bring their child to appointments, work with a variety of caregivers, and alert the team about problems. Successful relationships are partnerships between parents and caregivers that are built on mutual trust and respect. Good communication among the family, the cardiology specialists, and the primary care provider is essential. As children reach adolescence, they begin to take a larger role in managing their illness and making decisions about their care.

NURSING CARE

When a child is born with a severe cardiac anomaly, the parents are faced with the immense psychological and physical tasks of adjusting to the birth of a child with special needs. Family issues and nursing interventions to support the family are similar to those discussed in Chapter 40. The following discussion is primarily directed (1) toward the family of an infant who has a serious heart defect and requires home care before definitive repair and (2) toward preparation and care of the child and family when invasive procedures (catheterization and surgery) are performed. For nursing care related to the child with hypoxemia and HF, see earlier discussions of these topics.

Nursing care of the child with a congenital heart defect begins as soon as the diagnosis is suspected. Increasingly, this diagnosis is being made prenatally, thus nurses are having to counsel and support families as they prepare for the birth of these infants.

Help the Family Adjust to the Disorder

When parents first learn of the heart defect, they are initially in shock, then experience anxiety and fear that their child will die. The family generally needs time to grieve before they can assimilate the meaning of the defect. Unfortunately, the demands for medical treatment may not allow this process to the extent the family might like, necessitating instead that the parents immediately give **informed consent** for diagnostic-therapeutic procedures. The nurse can be instrumental in supporting parents in their loss, assessing their level of understanding, supplying information as needed, and helping other members of the health care team understand the parents' reactions (see Family-Centred Teaching box).

Severely ill newborns usually remain in the hospital. Parent–infant attachment is supported by encouraging parents to hold, touch, and look at their child and providing time for the parents to spend with their newborn in private.

The effect of a child with a serious heart defect on the family is complex. No family member, regardless of the degree of positive adjustment, is unaffected. Mothers frequently feel inadequate in their mothering ability because of the more complex

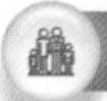

FAMILY-CENTRED TEACHING

Diagnosis of Heart Disease

Remember that we don't have your experience. We don't see children every day who have heart disease. We would have been upset finding out our child had to have his tonsils out. How could we ever be prepared for this? Please remember, we only know people who have trivial heart murmurs. How could we ever expect this to happen? And to us, this is the worst problem we've ever heard of.

We still fear most what we don't know and understand. Be honest with us. If you don't know either, tell us. But at least don't leave us wondering about what you know and we don't. Not knowing anything really can be worse than knowing something bad. Be honest, but don't strip us of hope ...

Please, remember we are trying to learn complex information in a moment of time. And trying to learn it in a context of great pain and emotional investment. This is our lives you're talking about. Please be thorough, but keep it simple. Tell us again, maybe even again and again, when we can hear better.

From Schrey, C., & Schrey, M. (1994). A parent's perspective: Our needs and our message. *Critical Care Nursing Clinics of North America, 6*(1), 113–119.

care that infants with congenital heart defects require. They often feel exhausted from the pressures of caring for these children and the other family members. Fathers or partners and siblings may feel neglected and resentful, a reaction similar to the feelings toward family members with other chronic conditions (see Chapter 40). Often, parents do not feel confident leaving the child in another's care. Although the fears are justified, they can be minimized by gradually teaching someone (a reliable relative or neighbour) how to care for the child.

The need to maintain discipline and set consistent limits can be difficult for parents. Using behaviour modification techniques in the form of either concrete awards (e.g., a favourite activity) or social reinforcement (e.g., approval) can be effective. However, these techniques are most beneficial if used *before* the child learns to control the family. It is necessary to begin discussions with parents while the child is in infancy regarding the need for discipline, to prevent later problems as the child gets older.

Another issue that may develop within family relationships is the child's overdependency. This is often the result of parental fear that the child may die. The nurse can help parents recognize the eventual hazards of continuing dependency and protectiveness as the child grows older and learn ways to foster optimum development. Unless parents are shown what activities the child can do, they may focus on physical limitations and encourage dependency.

The child also needs opportunities for normal social interaction with peers. These children do not need to be prevented from playing with other children because of concern regarding overexertion. Children usually limit their activities if allowed to set their own pace.

A child with CHD may constitute a long-term family crisis. Frequently, the continuing unremitting stresses of care—physical exhaustion, financial costs, emotional upset, fear of death, and concern for the child's future—are not fully appreciated by those caring for the family. Even when the child's condition is stabilized or corrected, the family may need to make adjustments in their lifestyle. Introducing them to other families with similarly affected children can help them adjust to the daily stresses.

Educate the Family About the Disorder

After absorbing the initial news of the CHD diagnosis, when parents are ready to hear more about the heart condition, they require a clear explanation based on their level of understanding. A review of the basic structure and function of the heart is helpful before describing the defect. A simple diagram, pictures, or a model of the heart can help parents visualize the heart and the congenital defect. Parents appreciate receiving written information about the specific condition, and a glossary of frequently used terms is helpful. Parents also require information about prognosis and treatment options.

Increasingly, families are using the Internet as a source of information about heart disease in children (see Additional Resources at the end of this chapter). They are also finding support through contacts with other parents and parent groups. It is important for parents to realize that not all websites offer medically accurate information and that information from other parents might not be applicable to their own situation. Some children with rare, complex heart defects require individualized treatment plans, and general information on the Internet or in books may not apply to their child. Parents should discuss with their health care team, in particular their cardiologist, information they have received from other sources.

Information given to the child must be tailored to his or her developmental age. As the child matures, the level of information should be revised to meet his or her cognitive level. Preschoolers need basic information about what they will experience more than what is actually occurring physiologically. School-age children benefit from a concrete explanation of the defect. Preadolescents and adolescents often appreciate a more detailed description of how the defect affects their heart. Children of all ages need to express their feelings concerning the diagnosis.

Help the Family Manage the Illness at Home

Parents should be aware of the symptoms of their child's cardiac condition and signs of worsening clinical status. They should have an information sheet, on paper and in digital form, with their child's diagnosis, significant treatments such as surgical procedures, allergies, other health care problems, current medications, and health care providers' contact numbers available in case of emergencies and to share with other caregivers such as teachers, babysitters, or day care providers.

The family also needs to be knowledgeable about the therapeutic management of the disorder and the roles that surgery, other procedures, medications, and healthy lifestyle play in maintaining good health. Medications play a critical role in managing some cardiac conditions such as dysrhythmias and severe HF; anticoagulation is used for artificial valves, and antirejection medications are needed after heart transplantation. Some patients must take multiple medications daily for their lifetime. Many medications can be dangerous if taken incorrectly and require close monitoring. Parents need to be taught the correct procedure for giving medications and cautioned to keep them in a safe area to prevent accidental ingestion.

Another area of parental concern is the child's level of physical activity. Most children do not need to restrict activity, and the best approach is to treat the child normally and allow self-limited activity. Exceptions to self-determined activity primarily involve strenuous recreational and competitive sports among children with specific cardiac problems. Activities and exercise restrictions should be discussed with the child's cardiologist.

Infants and children with CHD require good nutrition. Breastfeeding should be possible for many infants with CHD; Tandberg, Ystrom, Vollrath, et al. (2010) found that breastfeeding could be successful with adequate support and education of the mother. Nonetheless, providing adequate nutrition to infants with HF or complex congenital defects is difficult because of their high caloric requirements and inability to suck effectively because of fatigue and tachypnea. Instructing parents in feeding methods that decrease the infant's work and giving high-calorie formula are important interventions (see p. 1496 for a discussion on feeding the infant with HF). Children with severe cardiac defects are often anorexic, and encouraging them to eat can be a challenge. Consultation with a dietitian regarding this issue is often helpful. Also, the child should be given a choice of available high-nutrient foods.

Infants with heart disease should be immunized according to the current guidelines (Public Health Agency of Canada, 2016). Immunization schedules may need to be modified around times of acute illness or surgical procedures. Infants and children less than 2 years of age with unrepaired heart defects, cyanotic lesions, pulmonary hypertension, or history of prematurity should receive the vaccine for respiratory syncytial virus (RSV) monthly during RSV season (November to April in North America) (Robinson, Le Saux, & Canadian Paediatric Society [CPS], Infectious Diseases and Immunization Committee, 2015/2016).

Infants and children who have serious heart disease are at risk for developmental delays. Multiple factors can influence neurodevelopmental outcomes, including genetics (chromosome abnormalities and microdeletions), socioeconomic status, preoperative factors (including prematurity, cyanosis, shock), intraoperative factors (use of cardiopulmonary bypass, deep hypothermic circulatory arrest), and postoperative factors (hemodynamic instability, hypoxia, acidosis, cardiac arrest, stroke, ischemic events). Researchers at the Hospital for Sick Children found that the risk for arterial ischemic stroke/cerebral sinovenous thrombosis was 5.4 strokes per 1000 children undergoing a cardiac surgery (Domi, Edgell, McCrindle, et al., 2008). Efforts to limit the time of deep hypothermic circulatory arrest and provide better neuroprotection during infant surgery may improve outcomes in the future.

Prepare the Child and Family for Invasive Procedures

Chapter 44 provides an extensive discussion of the principles for preparing children for invasive procedures. The American Heart Association (2015) has published information on how to prepare a child for cardiac surgery and addresses issues specific to the child with heart disease. The following discussion highlights some important aspects of preparation for cardiac catheterization and cardiac surgery.

The expected outcomes for preprocedure preparation include reducing anxiety, improving patient collaboration with procedures, enhancing recovery, developing trust with caregivers, and improving long-term emotional and behavioural adjustments after procedures. Important factors to consider in planning preparation strategies are the child's cognitive development, previous hospital experiences, the child's temperament and coping style, timing of preparation, and involvement of the parents. The most beneficial preparation strategies usually combine information giving and coping skills training, such as conscious breathing exercises, distraction techniques, guided imagery, or other behavioural interventions.

Outpatient preoperative and precatheterization workups are common for most elective procedures. Children are then admitted on the morning of the procedure. Preprocedure teaching is often done in the clinic setting or at home and may include a tour of the critical care unit (CCU) and inpatient facilities. Children of different ages and developmental levels require different amounts of information and different approaches. Young children should be prepared close in time to the event, whereas older children and adolescents may benefit from teaching several weeks in advance. Parents should be included in the preparation session to support their child and learn about upcoming events.

Topics to include in preoperative or precatheterization preparation include information on the environment, equipment, and procedures that the child will encounter during and after the procedure. Information about what the child will see, hear, and feel should be included, especially for older children and adolescents. Some of the sensory experiences of being in a CCU or catheterization laboratory include sights (monitors, many people, much equipment), sounds (beeping noises, alarms, voices), and sensations (lines and dressings, tape, discomfort, thirst). Familiar aspects of the environment, such as BP cuffs, stethoscopes, or oximeter probes, are reviewed, and new equipment, such as monitors, IV lines, and oxygen masks, is described. Comforting aspects of the environment, such as play areas, chairs for parents, and televisions, are emphasized. Many patients who will be sedated during catheterization or receiving narcotic pain relievers after surgery will have minimal recall of that period and will not need detailed information about the equipment or procedures used. Information should be specific to the planned procedure for each patient.

A discussion of ways in which the child can cope with the experience should be included. Bringing a familiar stuffed animal or comfort object will help a young child relieve anxiety, whereas older child can be advised to bring headphones and favourite music to the catheterization laboratory as the music will help distract him or her during the procedure. Recovery topics after catheterization include lying still to prevent bleeding at the catheter site, advancing diet, controlling pain, and monitoring. After surgery, the nurse should review the importance of ambulation, coughing, deep breathing, drinking, and eating and describe pain management and monitoring routines. Simple coping strategies for use during painful procedures should be reviewed; these include distraction techniques such as counting, blowing, singing, or telling stories.

Children and their families should have a choice about taking a CCU tour. Exposure to the CCU environment can actually increase anxiety in some children, particularly young children, those with previous hospital experiences, and those who are highly anxious (LeRoy, Elixson, O'Brien, et al., 2003). The day before the procedure is usually ample time to allow the child to ask questions and to prevent undue fantasizing about the experience. The child should be protected from the frightening sights in the unit; equipment not in view after surgery, such as equipment located behind or below the bed, needs less attention. The child and parents should be encouraged to ask questions or to explore further any equipment in the room, but they should not be pushed to assimilate more information than they are able.

Provide Postoperative Care

Immediate postoperative care is usually provided by specially trained nurses in critical care units. Many of the procedures, such as arterial pressure and central venous pressure (CVP) monitoring, and the observations related to vital functions require advanced educational training (the reader should refer to critical care texts for further information). However, nurses caring for the child before surgery and during the convalescent period need to be familiar with the major principles of care. Selected complications that may occur postoperatively are described in Box 47-7.

Observe Vital Signs

Vital signs and BP are recorded frequently until the patient is stable. Heart rate and respirations are counted for 1 full minute, compared with the ECG monitor, and recorded with activity. The heart rate is normally increased after surgery. Arterial and venous pressures may be monitored. The nurse needs to observe cardiac rhythm and notify the primary health care provider of any changes in regularity. Dysrhythmias may occur postoperatively secondary to anaesthetics, acid–base and electrolyte imbalance, hypoxia, surgical intervention, or trauma to conduction pathways.

At least hourly, the lungs should be auscultated for breath sounds. Diminished or absent sounds may indicate an area of atelectasis or a pleural effusion or pneumothorax, which necessitates further medical assessment. Temperature changes are typical during the early postoperative period. Hypothermia is expected immediately after surgery from hypothermia procedures, effects of anaesthesia, and loss of body heat to the cool environment. During this period, the child needs to be kept warm to prevent additional heat loss. Infants may be placed under radiant heat warmers. During the next 24 to 48 hours the body temperature may rise to 37.7°C or slightly higher as part of the inflammatory response to tissue trauma. After this period an elevated temperature is most likely a sign of infection and warrants immediate investigation for probable cause.

BOX 47-7 SELECTED COMPLICATIONS AFTER CARDIAC SURGERY AND TREATMENT APPROACHES

Cardiac

Heart failure—Digoxin, diuretics (p. 1491)

Low cardiac output—Intravenous inotropes (Shock, p. 1515)

Dysrhythmias—Identification, drug treatment, possible pacing, cardioversion (p. 1508)

Tamponade (blood or fluid in the pericardial space constricting the heart)—Prompt removal of fluid by pericardiocentesis

Respiratory

Atelectasis—Chest physical therapy, coughing, deep breathing, ambulation

Pulmonary edema—Diuretics

Pleural effusions—Diuretics, possible chest tube drainage

Pneumothorax—Possible chest tube drainage

Neurological

Seizures—Assessment, antiepileptic drugs

Cerebrovascular accident (stroke), cerebral edema, neurological deficits—Assessment and treatment

Infectious Disease

Infections (especially wound, pneumonia, otitis media, and sepsis)—Antibiotics

Hematological

Anemia—Iron supplementation, possible transfusion

Postoperative bleeding—Initially, clotting factors, blood products; may need repeat surgery to locate and ligate source of bleeding

Other

Postpericardiotomy syndrome (syndrome of fever, leukocytosis, friction rub, pericardial and pleural effusions, and lethargy seen about 7 to 21 days after cardiac surgery; possible viral or autoimmune etiologies)—Antipyretics, diuretics, anti-inflammatory medications

Intra-arterial monitoring of BP is commonly done after open-heart surgery. A catheter is passed into the radial artery or other artery, and the other end is attached to an electronic monitoring system, which provides a continuous recording of the BP. The intra-arterial line is maintained with a low-rate, constant infusion of heparinized saline to prevent clotting.

Several IV lines are inserted preoperatively: a peripheral IV to give fluids and medications, and a CVP, which is usually inserted in a large vessel in the neck. Additional intracardiac monitoring lines are sometimes placed intraoperatively in the right atrium, left atrium, or pulmonary artery. Intracardiac lines allow assessment of pressures inside the cardiac chambers, providing vital information about volume status, cardiac output, and ventricular function. All lines must be cared for using strict aseptic technique, and patients must be carefully assessed for bleeding at the time of line removal.

Maintain Respiratory Status

Infants usually require mechanical ventilation in the immediate postoperative period, although early extubation in the operating room or early postoperative period is becoming more common. Children, especially those who did not require cardiopulmonary bypass, may be extubated in the operating room or in the first few postoperative hours. Suctioning is performed only as needed and is performed carefully to avoid vagal stimulation (which can trigger cardiac dysrhythmias) and laryngospasm, especially in infants. Suctioning is intermittent and maintained for no more than 5 seconds at a time to avoid depleting the oxygen supply. Supplemental oxygen is administered with a manual resuscitation bag before and after the procedure to prevent hypoxia. The heart rate is monitored after suctioning to detect changes in rhythm or rate, especially bradycardia. The child should always be positioned facing the nurse to permit assessment of the child's colour and tolerance of the procedure.

! NURSING ALERT

During suctioning, observe for signs and symptoms of respiratory distress, such as tachypnea, use of accessory muscles for breathing, and restlessness.

When weaning and extubation are completed, humidified oxygen is delivered by mask, hood, or nasal cannula to prevent drying of mucosa. The child should be encouraged to turn and deep breathe at least hourly. Measures such as splinting the operative site and providing analgesics can be used to enhance ventilation and decrease pain. Chest tubes are inserted into the pleural or mediastinal space during surgery or in the immediate postoperative period to remove secretions and air to allow re-expansion of the lung. Drainage should be checked hourly for colour and quantity. Immediately after surgery the drainage may be bright red, but afterward it should be serous. The largest volume of drainage occurs in the first 12 to 24 hours and is greater in extensive heart surgery.

NURSING ALERT

Chest tube drainage greater than 3 mL/kg/hr for more than 3 consecutive hours or 5 to 10 mL/kg in any 1 hour is excessive and may indicate postoperative hemorrhage. The surgeon should be notified immediately because cardiac tamponade can develop rapidly and is life threatening.

Chest tubes are usually removed on the first to third postoperative day. Removal of chest tubes is a painful, frightening experience. Analgesics such as morphine sulphate, often combined with midazolam (Versed), should be given before the procedure. Older children should be forewarned that they will feel a sharp, momentary pain. After the suture is cut, the tubes are quickly pulled out at the end of a full inspiration to prevent the intake of air into the pleural cavity. A purse-string suture (placed when the tubes were inserted) is pulled tight to close the opening. A petrolatum-covered gauze dressing is immediately applied over the wound and securely taped on all four sides to the skin so that an airtight seal is formed. It is left on for 1 or 2 days. Breath sounds need to be checked to assess for a pneumothorax, a possible complication of chest tube removal. A chest radiograph is usually obtained after removal to evaluate for possible pneumothorax or pleural effusion.

Monitor Fluids

Intake and output of all fluids must be accurately calculated. Intake is primarily IV fluids; however, a record of fluid used to flush the arterial and CVP lines or to dilute medications is also kept. Output includes hourly recordings of urine (usually a Foley catheter is inserted and attached to a closed collecting device), drainage from chest and nasogastric tubes, and blood drawn for analysis. Urine should be analyzed for specific gravity to assess the concentrating ability of the kidneys and the body's approximate degree of hydration. Renal failure is a potential risk from a transient period of low cardiac output.

NURSING ALERT

The signs of renal failure are decreased urinary output (less than 1 mL/kg/hr) and elevated levels of blood urea nitrogen and serum creatinine.

Fluids are restricted during the immediate postoperative period to prevent hypervolemia, which places additional demands on the myocardium, predisposing the patient to cardiac failure. To monitor fluid retention, the child is weighed daily, and the same scale is used at approximately the same time each day to avoid errors in measurement. The child is usually given nothing by mouth for the first 24 hours. If an endotracheal (ET) tube is inserted, oral fluids are usually withheld until the child is extubated. Fluid restriction may be imposed even when oral fluids are given. The nurse needs to calculate the distribution over a 24-hour period based on the child's preoperative weight and drinking habits. The distribution should allow for most fluid to be given during the child's most wakeful and active periods.

Provide Rest and Progressive Activity

After heart surgery, rest should be provided to decrease the workload of the heart and promote healing. The simplest way to ensure individualized, efficient, high-quality care is to plan at the beginning of the shift the nursing procedures to be done, with periods of rest identified. The schedule should be shared with parents and they should be encouraged to visit at the most advantageous times, such as after a rest period when no special treatments are anticipated.

A progressive schedule of ambulation and activity is planned, based on the child's preoperative activity patterns and postoperative cardiovascular and pulmonary function. Ambulation is initiated early, usually by the second postoperative day, when chest tubes, arterial lines, and assisted ventilatory equipment may be removed. Activity progresses from sitting on the edge of the bed and dangling the legs to standing up and sitting in a chair. Heart rate and respirations need to be carefully monitored to assess the degree of cardiac demand imposed by each activity. Tachycardia, dyspnea, cyanosis, desaturation, progressive fatigue, or dysrhythmias indicate the need to limit further energy expenditure.

Provide Comfort and Emotional Support

Heart surgery is both painful and frightening for children, and comfort is a primary nursing concern. Several incisions may be used for heart surgery. A median sternotomy is most common, following the sternum down the centre of the chest. A mini-sternotomy opens the lower sternum. It allows access to the side of the chest through an incision from under the arm around the back to the scapula.

Most patients need IV analgesics for pain control during the immediate postoperative period. Patient-controlled analgesia may be used with children old enough to understand the concept. Nonsteroidal anti-inflammatory drugs (NSAIDs) such as ketorolac (Toradol) may be used intravenously. Paralyzing agents may also be used with the analgesics for children who are agitated or hemodynamically unstable.

After extubation and the removal of lines and tubes, pain can be controlled satisfactorily with oral medications such as ibuprofen, acetaminophen, or opioids. Acetaminophen alone provides adequate pain relief for most children at discharge. Sternotomy incisions are usually well tolerated, with some discomfort when walking and coughing. Thoracotomy incisions are usually more painful because the incision is through muscle; a more aggressive pain management plan with around-the-clock medications for several days is often necessary to allow for adequate rest, ambulation, and pulmonary hygiene.

In addition to pharmacological pain control, every effort should be made to minimize the discomfort of procedures, such as using a firm pillow or favourite stuffed animal placed against the chest incision during movement and when performing treatments *after* pain medication is given, preferably at a time that coincides with the drug's peak effect. Nonpharmacological measures can be used to lessen the perception of pain, and parents should be encouraged to comfort their child as much as possible. (See also Pain Assessment; Pain Management, Chapter 34.)

Children may become depressed after surgery. This is thought to be caused by preoperative anxiety, postoperative psychological and physiological stress, and sensory overstimulation. Typically, the child's disposition improves on leaving the CCU.

Children may also be angry and unwilling to assist in any way after surgery as a response to the physical pain and the loss of control imposed by the surgery and treatments. They need an opportunity to express their feelings, either verbally or through activity. Children often regress in their behaviour during the stress of surgery and hospitalization. They also may express feelings of anger or rejection toward their parents. The nurse can support the parents by being available for information and explaining all of the procedures to them. The first few postoperative days are particularly difficult because parents see their child in pain and realize the potential risks from surgery. They often are overwhelmed by the physical environment of the CCU and feel useless because they can do so little for their child. The nurse can minimize such feelings by including parents in caregiving activities and in comfort and play activities, providing information about the child's condition, and being sensitive to the parents' emotional and physical needs. The importance of their presence in making the child feel more secure should be stressed even if they do not provide physical care.

Plan for Discharge and Home Care

Ideally, discharge planning begins on admission for cardiac surgery and includes an assessment of the parents' adjustment to the child's altered state of health. Newborns may need additional screening tests (such as newborn metabolic screen and hearing tests) and may need immunizations before discharge. The family needs both verbal and written instructions on medication, nutrition, activity restrictions, subacute bacterial endocarditis, return to school, wound care, and signs and symptoms of infection or complications (see Patient Teaching box). Referrals to community agencies may be warranted to assist parents in the transition from hospital to home and to reinforce the teaching.

The parents also need clear instructions on when to seek medical care for complications and how to contact the health care provider. Follow-up with the cardiologist and primary care provider should be arranged before discharge. Parents should have a summary, including their child's medical condition, medications, and health care providers, available for emergencies. Appropriate identification, such as a MedicAlert device, is indicated for children with a pacemaker or heart transplant and for those receiving anticoagulation therapy or antidysrhythmic medication.

Although surgical correction of heart defects has improved dramatically, it is still not possible to completely repair many of the complex anomalies. For many children, repeat procedures are required to replace conduits or grafts or to manage complications such as restenosis. Consequently, the long-term prognosis is uncertain, and full recovery is not always possible. For these families, medical follow-up and continued emotional support are essential. The nurse can often serve as an important

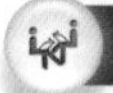

PATIENT TEACHING

Topics to Include in Discharge Teaching After Cardiac Surgery

- Medication teaching (for digoxin, see Family-Centred Teaching box, p. 1495)
- Activity restrictions
- Diet and nutrition
- Wound care (including dressings, if any; suture removal; bathing)
- Infective endocarditis prophylaxis (see Box 47-9)
- Follow-up appointments (cardiologist, primary care provider)
- Community agencies as needed (visiting nurse service, early developmental intervention)
- When to call the primary care provider; signs and symptoms of postoperative problems
- Review of cardiac defect and surgical repair
- Cardiopulmonary resuscitation (CPR) for caregivers (see Additional Resources at the end of this chapter)

primary health care provider and as a resource for referrals when needed.

ACQUIRED CARDIOVASCULAR DISORDERS

Bacterial (Infective) Endocarditis

Bacterial endocarditis (BE), or subacute bacterial endocarditis (SBE), now commonly referred to as *infective endocarditis* (IE), is an infection of the inner lining of the heart (*endocardium*), generally involving the valves. Although it can occur without underlying heart disease, it is most often a sequela of bacteremia in the child with acquired or congenital anomalies of the heart or great vessels. It especially affects children with valvular abnormalities, prosthetic valves, shunts, recent cardiac surgery with invasive lines, and rheumatic heart disease with valve involvement. The most common causative agent is *Streptococcus viridans*; other causative agents are *Staphylococcus aureus*, Gram-negative bacteria, and fungi such as *Candida albicans*.

Pathophysiology

Organisms may enter the bloodstream from any site of localized infection. In the past, endocarditis was believed to be highly associated with invasive procedures; however, it most likely occurs from routine exposure to bacteremia associated with usual daily activities, although it can also occur after procedures such as dental work (*S. viridans*); invasive procedures involving the respiratory tract; after invasive procedures involving the gastrointestinal–genitourinary tract; after cardiac surgery, especially if synthetic material is used (valves, patches, conduits); or from long-term in-dwelling catheters. The microorganisms grow on the endocardium, forming vegetations (verrucae), deposits of fibrin, and platelet thrombi. The lesion may invade adjacent tissues, such as aortic and mitral valves, and may break off and embolize elsewhere, especially in the spleen, kidney, and central nervous system.

Diagnostic Evaluation

The diagnosis of IE is suspected on the basis of clinical manifestations (Box 47-8). Several laboratory findings may suggest IE (e.g., ECG changes [prolonged PR interval], radiographic evidence of cardiomegaly, anemia, elevated erythrocyte sedimentation rate, leukocytosis, microscopic hematuria). Vegetations on the valve and abnormal valve function can often be visualized by echocardiography. Definitive diagnosis rests on growth and identification of the causative agent in the blood.

Therapeutic Management

Treatment should be instituted immediately and consists of administration of high doses of appropriate antibiotics intravenously for 2 to 8 weeks. Blood cultures are taken periodically to evaluate response to antibiotic therapy.

Prevention involves administration of prophylactic antibiotic therapy 1 hour before procedures known to increase the risk of entry of organisms in very high–risk patients. Recent guidelines recommend prophylaxis only in patients with the highest risk for poor outcome if they develop endocarditis (Box 47-9). Medications of choice for prophylaxis include amoxicillin, ampicillin, clindamycin, cephalexin, cefadroxil, azithromycin, and clarithromycin.

BOX 47-8 CLINICAL MANIFESTATIONS OF INFECTIVE ENDOCARDITIS

Onset usually insidious
Unexplained fever (low grade and intermittent)
Anorexia
Malaise
Weight loss
Characteristic findings caused by extracardiac emboli formation:
- Splinter hemorrhages (thin black lines) under the nails
- Osler nodes (red, painful intradermal nodes found on pads of phalanges)
- Janeway lesions (painless hemorrhagic areas on palms and soles)
- Petechiae on oral mucous membranes

May be present:
- Heart failure
- Cardiac dysrhythmias
- New murmur or change in previously existing one

BOX 47-9 PATIENTS AT HIGH RISK FOR ENDOCARDITIS

- Previous episode of infective endocarditis
- Prosthetic cardiac valves

Congenital heart disease (CHD), including only
- Unrepaired cyanotic CHD, including palliative shunts and conduits
- Completely repaired congenital heart defect with prosthetic material or device, during the first 6 months after the procedure

Repaired CHD with residual defects at the site of or adjacent to the site of a prosthetic patch or prosthetic device (which inhibit endothelialization)

Cardiac transplantation recipients who develop cardiac valvulopathy

Adapted from Allen, U. D., & Canadian Paediatric Society. (2010). Infective endocarditis: Updated guidelines. *Paediatrics & Child Health, 15*(4), 205–208. Reaffirmed 2016. Retrieved from http://www.cps.ca/documents/position/infective-endorcarditis-guidelines; Wilson, W., et al. (2007). Prevention of infective endocarditis: Guidelines from the American Heart Association. *Circulation, 116*(15), 1736–1754.

NURSING CARE

Ideally, the objective of nursing care is to counsel parents of high-risk children concerning the signs and symptoms of endocarditis and, in certain cases, the need for prophylactic antibiotic therapy before procedures such as dental work take place. The family's regular dentist should be advised of the child's cardiac diagnosis as an added precaution to ensure preventive treatment. As stated earlier, IE prophylaxis is now reserved for very high–risk patients; many patients who met criteria established in the past may not require prophylaxis under the new guidelines (Allen & CPS, Infectious Diseases and Immunization Committee, 2010/2016; Wilson, Taubert, Gewitz, et al., 2007) (see Box 47-9). It is important that all children with congenital or acquired heart disease maintain the highest level of oral health to reduce the chance of bacteremia from oral infections.

Parents should also have a high index of suspicion regarding potential infections. Without unduly alarming them, the nurse can stress that any unexplained fever, weight loss, or change in behaviour (lethargy, malaise, anorexia) must be brought to the primary care provider's attention. Such symptoms should not be self-diagnosed as a cold or flu. Early diagnosis and treatment are important in preventing further cardiac damage, embolic complications, and growth of resistant organisms.

Treatment of endocarditis requires long-term parenteral medication therapy. In many cases, IV antibiotics may be administered at home with nursing supervision for part of the treatment course. Nursing goals during this period are (1) preparation of the child for IV infusion, usually with an intermittent-infusion device, and several venipunctures for blood cultures; (2) observation for adverse effects of antibiotics, especially inflammation along venipuncture sites; (3) observation for complications, including embolism and HF; and (4) education regarding the importance of follow-up visits for cardiac evaluation, echocardiographic monitoring, and blood cultures.

Rheumatic Fever

Rheumatic fever (RF) is a poorly understood inflammatory disease that occurs after infection with group A beta-hemolytic streptococcal (GABHS) pharyngitis. It occurs most often in late school-age children or adolescents and is rare in adults. It is a self-limited illness that involves the joints, skin, brain, serous surfaces, and heart. Cardiac valve damage (referred to as *rheumatic heart disease*) is the most significant complication of RF. The mitral valve is most often affected.

In developed countries, such as Canada, RF and rheumatic heart disease have become uncommon and incidence rates are low. RF remains a devastating problem in developing countries.

Etiology

Strong evidence supports a relationship between upper respiratory tract infection with GABHS and subsequent development of RF (usually within 2 to 6 weeks). In almost all cases of RF a previous infection with GABHS can be documented by laboratory evidence of rising antibody titres.

Diagnostic Evaluation

Diagnosis is based on a set of guidelines recommended by the Canadian Paediatric Society (Templeton, Cooper, Human, et al., 2007). These guidelines, known as *modifications of the Jones criteria*, state that the presence of two major manifestations or one major and two minor manifestations, such as fever and arthralgia, with supportive evidence of recent streptococcal infection, indicates a high probability of RF.

Children suspected of having RF are tested for streptococcal antibodies. The most reliable and best standardized test is an elevated or rising antistreptolysin O (ASO or ASLO) titre, which occurs in 80% of children with RF.

Therapeutic Management

The goals of medical management are (1) eradication of hemolytic streptococci, (2) prevention of permanent cardiac damage, (3) palliation of the other symptoms, and (4) prevention of recurrences of RF. Penicillin is the medication of choice, either orally or intramuscularly, with erythromycin as a substitute in penicillin-sensitive children. Salicylates, naproxen, or prednisone are used to control the inflammatory process, especially in the joints, and reduce the fever and discomfort (Templeton et al., 2007). Bedrest is recommended during the acute febrile phase but need not be strictly imposed.

Children who have had acute RF are susceptible to recurrent RF for the rest of their lives and should be followed medically for at least 5 years. Repeated infections are likely to result in rheumatic heart disease.

NURSING CARE

The objectives of nursing care for the child with RF are to (1) encourage adherence to medication regimens, (2) facilitate recovery from the illness, (3) provide emotional support, and (4) prevent the disease. Because adherence is a major concern in long-term medication therapy, every effort is made to encourage the patient's adherence to the therapeutic plan. When adherence is poor, monthly injections may be substituted for daily oral administration of antibiotics and children need preparation for this often-dreaded procedure.

Interventions during home care are primarily concerned with providing rest and adequate nutrition. Usually, after the febrile stage is over, children can resume moderate activity, and their appetite improves. If carditis is present, the family must be aware of any activity restrictions and may need help in choosing less strenuous activities for the child.

One of the most disturbing and frustrating manifestations of the disease is chorea. The onset is gradual and may occur weeks to months after the illness. It may be mistaken for nervousness, clumsiness, behavioural changes, inattentiveness, and learning disability. It is usually a source of great frustration to the child because the movements, incoordination, and weakness severely limit physical ability. Of utmost importance is stressing to parents and schoolteachers that the sudden movements are involuntary, that the chorea is transitory, and that all manifestations eventually disappear.

Nurses also have a role in prevention, primarily in screening school-age children for sore throats caused by GABHS. This may involve actively participating in throat culture screening programs or referring children with a possible streptococcal infection for testing.

Hyperlipidemia/Hypercholesterolemia

Hyperlipidemia is a general term for excessive lipids (fat and fatlike substances); *hypercholesterolemia* refers to excessive cholesterol in the blood. *Dyslipidemia* is a term used to describe all abnormalities in lipid metabolism, including low levels of high-density lipoprotein (HDL), or "good" cholesterol. High lipid or cholesterol levels play an important role in producing *atherosclerosis* (fatty plaque on the arteries), which eventually can lead to coronary artery disease, a primary cause of morbidity and mortality in the adult population. A presymptomatic phase of atherosclerosis can begin in childhood. Preventive cardiology focuses on the screening and management of lipid levels in childhood; the goal is to identify children at high risk and to intervene early.

Cholesterol is part of the lipoprotein complex in plasma that is essential for cellular metabolism. Triglycerides, natural fats synthesized from carbohydrates, are used for energy. Both are major lipids transported on *lipoproteins*, a combination of lipids and proteins, which include the following:

Low-density lipoproteins (LDLs)—These contain low concentrations of triglycerides, high levels of cholesterol, and moderate levels of protein. LDL is the major carrier of cholesterol to the cells. Cells use cholesterol for synthesis of membranes and steroid production. Elevated circulating LDL is a strong risk factor in cardiovascular disease.

High-density lipoproteins (HDLs)—These contain very low concentrations of triglycerides, relatively little cholesterol, and high levels of protein. They transport free cholesterol to the liver for excretion in the bile. High levels of HDL are thought to protect against cardiovascular disease.

Diagnostic Evaluation

Hyperlipidemia is diagnosed on the basis of analysis of blood for a full lipid profile, drawn after a 12-hour fast. Hyperlipidemia can have a genetic basis or a lifestyle component or can be caused by secondary problems, such as hypothyroidism. In children with elevated cholesterol levels, a screening thyroid-stimulating hormone (TSH) is useful to rule out hypothyroidism as a cause of secondary hypercholesterolemia. In overweight children, a fasting glucose may be obtained to assess for the potential of metabolic syndrome, which is a combination of multiple symptoms that are associated with increased cardiovascular risk in adults. Blood samples should be collected after having the child sit for 5 minutes, and the tourniquet should be applied immediately before the needle puncture, since posture and vascular stasis may affect results. Diagnostic values for acceptable, borderline, and high total cholesterol and LDL cholesterol levels are listed in Table 47-4.

Screening children for hypercholesterolemia is a controversial issue; some authorities advocate universal screening, and others propose selective screening. The U.S. National Heart, Lung, and Blood Institute (NHLBI) (NHLBI, 2011) issued a recommendation for universal lipid (nonfasting or fasting) screening of all children and adolescents between the ages of 9 and 11 years and again between the ages of 17 and 21 years. LDL cholesterol–lowering drug therapy is recommended for children and adolescents 10 years of age and older whose LDL remains elevated after 6 months to 1 year on a restricted fat diet, lifestyle modification (exercise), and weight management (NHLBI, 2011).

TABLE 47-4 CLASSIFICATION OF CHOLESTEROL LEVELS IN CHILDREN FROM FAMILIES WITH A HISTORY OF HEART DISEASE

CATEGORY	TOTAL CHOLESTEROL mmol/L (g/dL)	LDL CHOLESTEROL mmol/L (g/dL)
Acceptable	<4.39 (170)	<2.8 (110)
Borderline	4.40–5.16 (170–199)	2.8–3.4 (110–129)
High	≥5.17 (200)	≥3.4 (130)

LDL, low-density lipoprotein.
From the National Cholesterol Education Program. (1992). Report of the Expert Panel on Blood Cholesterol Levels in Children and Adolescents. *Pediatrics, 89*(3 Pt 2), 527.

Therapeutic Management

The first step in the treatment of high cholesterol is oriented toward lifestyle modification. The Heart and Stroke Foundation (2016b) guidelines advocate a heart-healthy diet for all children. Children with known elevated cholesterol should have individual nutritional counselling by a nutritionist with expertise in pediatric lipids.

Research continues to support the benefit of diets low in saturated fats and trans fats and higher in monounsaturated fats (found in olive and canola oil). Current thinking favours a "Mediterranean"-type diet; whole grains, fruits, and vegetables form the foundation of this diet. In addition, this diet allows the use of monounsaturated fats, such as olive oil and canola oil, which have beneficial effects on HDL cholesterol values. The use of these fats also makes the diet more realistic. Daily aerobic exercise of at least 60 minutes a day is also recommended for children with high cholesterol. In addition, patients and parents should be counselled regarding the negative effects of smoking (both first-hand and second-hand).

For children with severe hypercholesterolemia who fail to respond to dietary modifications (after a 6- to 12-month trial) medication therapy may be necessary. Pharmacological therapy is recommended for children with LDL cholesterol over 4.9 mmol/L with a positive history of early heart disease; over 4.1 L mmol/L in patients with a positive family history and two risk factors; and over 3.4 mmol/L in patients with diabetes. In most situations, medication is reserved for those over 8 years of age (Daniels, Greer, & Committee on Nutrition, 2008).

In the past, bile acid–binding resins were the only class of drugs recommended for treatment of younger children. This class of drug acts by binding bile acids in the intestinal lumen. Because they are not absorbed by the intestine, resin binders do not produce systemic toxicity and are safe for children. Both cholestyramine and colestipol are powders that are mixed with water or juice just before ingestion. Unfortunately, bile acid–binding resins do not adequately reduce LDL cholesterol in the vast majority of patients. Many patients cannot tolerate the medication because of the taste, gritty texture, and adverse effects, the most significant being constipation, abdominal pain, gastrointestinal bloating, flatulence, and nausea. The most recent findings on lipid abnormalities in children recommend treatment with statins if pharmacological therapy is indicated, using the previously outlined guidelines for treatment (McCrindle, Urbina, Dennison, et al., 2007). Statins are much more effective at lowering LDL cholesterol and triglycerides and raising HDL cholesterol. They work by inhibiting the enzyme necessary for cholesterol synthesis, are most effective when taken in the evening, and are started at the lowest possible dose in young people. Blood work should be followed closely and should include a fasting lipid profile, liver function tests, and creatinine kinase repeated at 4- and 8-week intervals initially and with dosage changes.

A relatively new drug, ezetimibe, works by inhibiting cholesterol absorption. It lowers LDL by preventing intestinal uptake of dietary and biliary cholesterol. Recommended use is in combination therapy with a statin, further lowering LDL values. This medication is currently approved for children older than 10 years of age with extremely severe hyperlipidemia. Several large clinical trials are currently in process regarding this medication to determine the effectiveness (Leiter, Bays, Conard, et al., 2010).

Patients beginning therapy with a statin should be counselled on rare but potentially serious adverse effects such as rhabdomyolysis, elevated transaminases, and elevated creatinine kinase. They should discontinue their medication and contact their health care provider if they develop dark urine or new muscle aches. Finally, statin medications are not safe during pregnancy; thus sexually active adolescents need to take adequate birth control measures. Very long–term studies are unlikely to be available over decades; however, in the shorter-term studies that have been completed thus far, statins seem to have a safety profile for children similar to the one for adults (McCrindle et al., 2007).

NURSING CARE

Nurses play an important role in the screening, education, and support of children with hyperlipidemia and their families. When a child is referred to a lipid clinic, it is essential that the family be adequately prepared for the first visit. Generally, the parents are asked to keep a dietary history of the child before this visit. Sometimes they need to complete a questionnaire regarding the child's normal dietary habits during the preceding year. Families should be instructed to keep their child fasting for at least 12 hours before screening. Parents should also be aware that lipids should not be drawn within 3 weeks of a febrile illness because doing so can affect cholesterol values. It is important to schedule the blood test early in the morning and arrange for nourishment immediately thereafter. At the visit a full family history should be taken, including the health of both parents and all first-degree relatives. Specific questions should be asked regarding early heart disease, hypertension, strokes (CVAs), sudden death, hyperlipidemia, diabetes, and endocrine abnormalities.

Stringent dietary guidelines may become an issue of control and a source of great stress for many families. A child with a lipid disorder should not be viewed as having a disease. Rather, the positive aspects of healthy eating, exercising regularly, and avoiding smoking should be emphasized. Basic dietary changes should be encouraged for the whole family so that the affected child is not singled out. Cultural differences need to be considered, and recommendations individualized. Substitution rather than elimination should be emphasized. Visual aids (e.g., test tubes depicting the amount of fat in a hot dog) are often helpful, especially for children. Diets should be flexible and individually tailored by a nutritionist experienced in combining recommendations that meet both the nutritional demands of the growing child and the lipid modifications. Parents should be encouraged to participate in dietary and educational sessions, ask questions, and share ideas and experiences.

Parents often feel guilty about the hereditary component of hyperlipidemia. Many also believe they have failed if the diet alone is not making a significant difference in their child's lipid profile. They need to be reassured that a dietary approach alone is often not sufficient, especially for children with significantly elevated values.

Parents of children who require pharmacological therapy need to understand the purpose, dosage, and possible adverse effects of the various medications. Medication schedules should remain flexible and should not interfere with the child's daily activities. Follow-up phone calls by the nurse between visits allow parents to discuss their concerns and ask any questions that have arisen.

Cardiac Dysrhythmias

Dysrhythmias, or abnormal heart rhythms, can occur in children with structurally normal hearts, as features of some congenital heart defects, and in patients after surgical repair of congenital heart defects. They are also seen in patients with cardiomyopathy and cardiac tumours and can occur secondary to metabolic and electrolyte imbalances. They can be classified in several ways, including by heart rate characteristics (bradycardia and tachycardia) and by the origin of the dysrhythmia in the atria or ventricles. Some dysrhythmias are well tolerated and self-limited. Others may cause decreased cardiac output with associated symptoms, and some can cause sudden death. Treatment depends on the cause of the dysrhythmia and its severity.

Many advances have been made in the diagnosis and treatment of pediatric dysrhythmias. Improvements in technology have allowed better diagnosis, the development of ablation techniques, and the expansion of pacemaker capabilities. New antidysrhythmic medications have proved safe and effective in children. Radiofrequency ablation has offered a cure for some dysrhythmias. Pediatric electrophysiology has become a highly specialized field; the reader should consult more detailed sources for an in-depth discussion. The next sections address diagnostic studies and provide a general discussion of the most common tachycardia (supraventricular tachycardia [SVT]) and the most common bradycardia (complete heart block) that require treatment in the pediatric population.

Diagnostic Evaluation

Nurses must be familiar with the standards of normal heart rate for the particular age group (see Appendix E). An initial nursing responsibility is recognition of a heartbeat that is abnormal in either rate or rhythm. When a dysrhythmia is suspected, the apical rate is counted for a full minute and compared with the radial rate, which may be lower because not all of the apical beats are felt. Consistently high or low heart rates should be regarded as suspicious. The patient should be placed on a cardiac monitor with recording capabilities. A 12-lead ECG yields more information than the monitor recording and should be done as soon as possible.

The basic diagnostic procedure is the ECG, including 24-hour Holter monitoring. Electrophysiological cardiac catheterization allows for identification of the conduction disturbance and immediate investigation of medications that may control the dysrhythmia. Another procedure that may be used is transesophageal recording. An electrode catheter is passed to the lower esophagus and, when in position at a point proximal to the heart, is used to stimulate and record dysrhythmias.

Dysrhythmias can be classified according to various criteria, such as effect on heart rate and rhythm, as follows:

Bradydysrhythmias—Abnormally slow rate
Tachydysrhythmias—Abnormally rapid rate
Conduction disturbances—Irregular heart rate

Bradydysrhythmias. *Sinus bradycardia* (slower than normal rate) in children can be caused by the influence of the autonomic nervous system, as with hypervagal tone, or in response to hypoxia and hypotension. Sinus bradycardias are also known to develop after some complex cardiac surgical repairs involving extensive atrial suture lines such as the Fontan procedure.

Complete atrioventricular block (AV block) is also referred to as *complete heart block*. This can be either congenital (occurring in children with structurally normal hearts) or acquired after surgery to repair cardiac defects. AV blocks are most often related to edema around the conduction system and resolve without treatment. Temporary epicardial wires are placed in most patients at surgery; if a rhythm disturbance occurs, temporary pacing can be used. Several days after surgery, the health care provider removes the wires by pulling slowly and deliberately down on them from the site of insertion.

Some children may need a permanent pacemaker. The pacemaker takes over or assists in the heart's conduction function. The implantation of a pacemaker, in the operating room or possibly the catheterization laboratory, is usually a low-risk procedure. The pacemaker is made up of two basic parts: the pulse generator and the lead. The pulse generator is composed of the battery and the electronic circuitry. The lead is an insulated, flexible wire that conducts the electrical impulse from the pulse generator to the heart. Two types of leads are available: transvenous and epicardial. After the lead has been attached to the heart, a small incision is made, and a pocket is formed under the muscle to house and protect the generator. Continuous ECG monitoring is necessary during the recovery phase to assess pacemaker function. The nurse should be aware of the programmed rate and expected individual generator variations. The pacemaker insertion site should be monitored for signs of infection. Analgesics can be given for pain.

Pacemaker functions have become more sophisticated, and some models can adjust heart rate to activity demands or be programmed for overdrive pacing or cardioversion.

Discharge teaching includes information about the signs and symptoms of infection, general wound care, and activity restrictions. Parents and patients, if they are old enough, should be taught to take a pulse and know the settings of the pacemaker. If the patient's low rate is set at 80 bpm and the heart rate is only 68 bpm, there is a possible problem with the pacemaker that needs to be investigated. Instructions for telephone transmission of ECG readings are also given. Telephone transmission can be used to transmit ECG strips and also to monitor battery life and pacemaker function. The pacemaker generator will have to be replaced periodically because of battery depletion. Children with pacemakers should wear a medical alert device, and their parents should have a paper identification card with specific pacer data in case of an emergency. Cardiopulmonary resuscitation instruction is suggested for parents.

Tachydysrhythmias. *Sinus tachycardia* (abnormally fast heart rate) secondary to fever, anxiety, pain, anemia, dehydration, hypovolemia, hypoxia, shock, pulmonary edema, medication or any other etiological factor requiring increased cardiac output should be ruled out before diagnosing an increased heart rate as pathological. SVT is the most common tachydysrhythmia found in children and refers to a rapid regular heart rate of 200 to 300 bpm. The onset of SVT is often sudden, the duration is variable, and the rhythm may end abruptly and convert back to a normal sinus rhythm. Clinical signs in infants and young children are poor feeding, extreme irritability, and pallor. Children may experience palpitations, dizziness, chest pain, and diaphoresis. If SVT is sustained, signs of HF may be seen.

The treatment of SVT depends on the degree of compromise imposed by the dysrhythmia. In some cases vagal manoeuvres, such as applying ice to the face, massaging the carotid artery (on one side of the neck only), or having an older child perform a Valsalva manoeuvre (e.g., exhaling against a closed glottis, blowing on a thumb as if it were a trumpet for 30 to 60 seconds), have terminated SVT. If vagal manoeuvres fail or the child is hemodynamically unstable, adenosine (a drug that impairs AV conduction) may be used. Adenosine is given by rapid IV push with a saline bolus immediately after the drug because of its very short half-life. If this is unsuccessful or cardiac output is compromised, esophageal overdrive pacing or synchronized cardioversion (delivering an electrical shock to the heart) can be used in the critical care setting. Sedation is needed for both procedures. Cardioversion should never be done in a conscious patient. More long-term pharmacological treatment includes digoxin or possibly propranolol (Inderal) or amiodarone for severe or recurrent SVT.

A primary focus of nursing care is education of the family regarding the symptoms of SVT and its treatment. SVT may occur again despite therapy. Parents should be taught to take a radial pulse for a full minute. If medication is prescribed, instructions regarding accurate dosage and the importance of administering the correct dose at specified intervals should be stressed.

Radiofrequency ablation has become first-line therapy for some types of SVT. The procedure is done in the cardiac catheterization laboratory and begins with mapping of the conduction system to identify the dysrhythmia focus. A catheter delivering radiofrequency current is directed at the site, and the area is heated to destroy the tissue in the area. These are lengthy procedures, often 6 to 8 hours, and sedation or general anaesthesia is required. Preparation is similar to that for cardiac catheterization. Another procedure, cryoablation, is also used in treatment of SVT. Liquid nitrous oxide is used to cool a catheter to subfreezing temperatures, which then destroys the target tissue by freezing. This procedure is performed in the cardiac electrophysiology catheterization laboratory (Van Hare, 2016).

Pulmonary Hypertension

Pulmonary artery hypertension (PAH) describes a group of rare disorders that result in an elevation of pulmonary artery pressure above 25 mm Hg at rest after the neonatal period (Bernstein, 2016c). PAH affects the small pulmonary arteries and is characterized by vascular narrowing leading to an increase in pulmonary vascular resistance. Generally, these abnormalities result in remodelling of the pulmonary circulation, characterized by occlusion of the lumen in medium and small pulmonary arteries because of cellular proliferation (Michelakis, Wilkins, & Rabinovitch, 2008). PAH can be difficult to diagnose in the early stages. Often when patients become symptomatic and a diagnosis is made, their disease is rapidly progressing, treatment is unsuccessful, and death occurs within several years. These disorders are poorly understood, and until recently there was no treatment beyond supportive care. Significant new information about the disease process, genetic links, diagnosis, and treatment has been learned that may improve treatments and outcomes for these patients.

Why some children develop the disease and others do not is unclear. There are many possible causes of PAH. Cardiac causes occur primarily in patients with a large left-to-right shunt producing increased pulmonary blood flow. If these defects are not repaired early, the high pulmonary flow will cause changes in the pulmonary artery vessels, and the vessels will lose their elasticity. Other causes of PAH include hypoxic lung diseases, thromboembolic diseases causing pulmonary vascular obstruction, collagen vascular diseases, and exposure to toxic substances. Many patients with PAH have no identifiable cause for it and have primary or idiopathic PAH.

Clinical Manifestations

The clinical manifestations include dyspnea with exercise, chest pain, and syncope. Dyspnea is the most common symptom and is caused by impaired oxygen delivery. Chest pain is the result of coronary ischemia in the right ventricle from severe hypertrophy. Syncope reflects a limited cardiac output leading to decreased cerebral blood flow. Right-sided heart dysfunction is steadily progressive; when symptoms of venous congestion and edema are present, the prognosis is poor.

Therapeutic Management

Although no cure is known, several therapies have shown promise in slowing the progression of the disease and improving quality of life. In general, situations that may exacerbate the disease and cause hypoxia, such as exercise and high altitudes, are to be avoided. Supplemental oxygen, especially at night while sleeping, is commonly used to relieve hypoxia. Patients are at risk for thromboembolic events leading to pulmonary emboli; thus anticoagulation with warfarin (Coumadin) is often prescribed.

Vasodilator therapy (which relaxes vascular smooth muscle and reduces pulmonary artery pressure) has prolonged the survival of patients with PAH. Use of oral calcium channel blockers has been successful in some children. Continuous IV prostacyclin has been used with some success in children who did not respond to oral therapy. Although promising, both of these therapies have been used in only small numbers of patients and are expensive. Lung transplantation may be another treatment option.

Cardiomyopathy

Cardiomyopathy refers to abnormalities of the myocardium in which the cardiac muscles' ability to contract is impaired. Cardiomyopathies are relatively rare in children. Possible etiological factors include familial or genetic causes, infection, deficiency states, metabolic abnormalities, and collagen vascular diseases. Most cardiomyopathies in children are considered primary or idiopathic, in which the cause is unknown and the cardiac dysfunction is not associated with systemic disease. Some of the known causes of secondary cardiomyopathy are anthracycline toxicity (the antineoplastic agents doxorubicin [Adriamycin] and daunomycin), hemochromatosis (from excessive iron storage), Duchenne muscular dystrophy, Kawasaki disease (KD), collagen diseases, and thyroid dysfunction.

Cardiomyopathies can be divided into three broad clinical categories according to the type of abnormal structure and dysfunction present: dilated cardiomyopathy, hypertrophic cardiomyopathy, and restrictive cardiomyopathy.

Dilated cardiomyopathy is characterized by ventricular dilation and greatly decreased contractility, resulting in symptoms of HF. This is the most common type of cardiomyopathy in children. Its cause is often unknown. The clinical findings are of HF with tachycardia, dyspnea, hepatosplenomegaly, fatigue, and poor growth. Dysrhythmias may be present and may be more difficult to control with worsening HF.

Hypertrophic cardiomyopathy is characterized by an increase in heart muscle mass without an increase in cavity size, usually occurring in the left ventricle and associated with abnormal diastolic filling. It is a familial autosomal dominant genetic abnormality in most cases and is probably the most common genetically transmitted cardiovascular disease. The expression of clinical disease varies greatly among patients. Clinical symptoms usually appear in the school-age period or adolescence and may include anginal chest pain, dysrhythmias, and syncope. Sudden death is possible. In one study, unexplained syncope in children under 18 years of age with known hypertrophic cardiomyopathy had a 60% cumulative risk of sudden death within 5 years of the syncopal event (Spirito, Autore, Rapezzi, et al., 2009). Presentation in infancy includes signs of HF and has a poor prognosis. The ECG demonstrates left ventricular hypertrophy, often with ST-T changes. The echocardiogram is most helpful and demonstrates asymmetrical septal hypertrophy and an increase in left ventricular wall thickness with a small left ventricle cavity.

Restrictive cardiomyopathy, rare in children, describes a restriction to ventricular filling caused by endocardial or myocardial disease or both. It is characterized by diastolic dysfunction and absence of ventricular dilation or hypertrophy. Symptoms are similar to those of HF (see Box 47-5).

Therapeutic Management

Treatment is directed toward correcting the underlying cause whenever feasible. However, in most affected children this is not possible, and treatment is aimed at managing HF and dysrhythmias. Digoxin, diuretics, and aggressive use of afterload reduction agents have been found to be helpful in managing symptoms in those with dilated cardiomyopathy. Practice guidelines for the management of HF in children have been outlined and provide an in-depth review of available therapies (Kantor et al., 2013). Digoxin and inotropic agents are usually not helpful in the other forms of cardiomyopathy, because increasing the force of contraction may exacerbate the muscular obstruction and actually impair ventricular ejection. Beta blockers such as propranolol or calcium channel blockers such as verapamil have been used to reduce left ventricular outflow obstruction and improve diastolic filling in those with hypertrophic cardiomyopathy.

Careful monitoring and treatment of dysrhythmias are essential. The placement of an implantable defibrillator (AICD) should be considered for patients at high risk of sudden death from ventricular dysrhythmias. Anticoagulants may be given to reduce the risk of thromboemboli, a complication of the sluggish circulation through the heart. For worsening HF and signs of poor perfusion, IV inotropic or vasodilating medications may be needed. Severely ill children may require mechanical ventilation, oxygen administration, and IV medications. Heart transplantation may be a treatment option for patients who have worsening symptoms despite maximum medical therapy.

NURSING CARE

Because of the poor prognosis in many children with cardiomyopathy, nursing care is consistent with that for any child with a life-threatening disorder (see Chapter 40). One of the most difficult adjustments for the child (especially the normally active youngster with hypertrophic cardiomyopathy) may be the realization of failing health and the need for restricted activity. The child should be included in decisions regarding activity and allowed to discuss his or her feelings, particularly if the disease follows a progressively fatal course. After symptoms of HF or dysrhythmias develop, the same nursing interventions are implemented. If heart transplantation is considered, the needs of the child and family are great in terms of psychological preparation and postoperative care. The nurse plays an important role in assessing the family's understanding of the procedure and long-term consequences. Children of school age and older should be fully informed in order for them to give their assent to the procedure (see Informed Consent, Chapter 44).

HEART TRANSPLANTATION

Heart transplantation has become a treatment option for infants and children with worsening HF and a limited life expectancy despite maximum medical and surgical management. Indications for heart transplantation in children are cardiomyopathy and end-stage CHD. It is also an option for patients with some forms of complex congenital cardiac defects, such as hypoplastic left heart syndrome, for whom conventional surgical approaches have a high mortality rate.

Before transplantation, potential recipients undergo a careful cardiac evaluation to determine whether any other medical or surgical options are available to improve the patient's cardiac status. Other organ systems are assessed to identify problems that might increase the risk of or preclude transplantation. A psychosocial evaluation of the patient and family is done to assess family function, support systems, and ability to comply with the complex medical regimen after the transplant. Support services to help the family successfully care for their child are provided when possible. Parents and older adolescents need extensive education about the risks and benefits of transplantation so they can make an informed decision.

The number of heart transplants in pediatric patients has been constant for the past decade, at about 450 transplants per year internationally (Kim & Marks, 2014). This likely reflects a limit in the number of available donors. Infants are the largest group of pediatric transplant recipients and account for about one fourth of all procedures. The International Society for Heart and Lung Transplantation registry data for all pediatric heart transplant recipients from 1982 to 2005 indicated a 1-year actuarial survival rate of 85%. Early rejection within the first year post-transplant is associated with increased late mortality. There is an ongoing risk of death with time from transplant. Infants with transplants have a higher early mortality rate, and adolescents have a higher late mortality rate. Overall survival is approximately 40% for patients up to 20 years after transplantation (Kim & Marks, 2014). Surviving pediatric patients have excellent functional recovery, with less than 10% reporting activity limitations (Aurora, Edwards, Kucheryavaya, et al., 2010).

The post-transplant course is complex. Although heart function is greatly improved or normal after transplantation, the risk of rejection is serious. The leading cause of death in the first 3 years after heart transplantation is rejection, with the greatest risk being in the first 6 months (Aurora et al., 2010). Rejection of the heart is diagnosed primarily by endomyocardial biopsy in older children. Serial echocardiograms are often used in infants and young children to reduce the need for invasive biopsies. Immunosuppressants must be taken for life and have many systemic adverse effects. Triple medication therapy for immunosuppression with a calcineurin inhibitor (cyclosporine or tacrolimus), steroids, and azathioprine is most commonly used in pediatric patients, although mycophenolate mofetil is being used more frequently and replacing azathioprine. Steroids are weaned in the first year and may be discontinued in some patients.

Infection is always a risk. Potential long-term problems that may limit survival include chronic rejection, causing coronary artery disease; renal dysfunction and hypertension resulting from cyclosporine administration; lymphoma; and infection. In the short term, after successful transplantation, children are able to return to full participation in age-appropriate activities and appear to adapt well to their new lifestyle. Transplantation is not a cure because patients must live with the lifetime consequences of chronic immunosuppression.

NURSING CARE

Successfully caring for a child after a heart transplant requires the expertise and dedication of many members of the health care team. Nurses play vital roles in assessment, coordination of care, psychosocial support, and patient and family education. The heart transplant recipient must be carefully monitored for signs of rejection, infection, and the adverse effects of the immunosuppressant medications. The patient's and family's psychosocial well-being also needs to be assessed to identify issues such as increased family stress, depression, substance use, and school problems, as these patients are at risk for behavioural and psychological consequences (Conway & Dipchand, 2010). Nonadherence to an intense medication regimen, especially during adolescence, can lead to serious medical problems and can be fatal. Care of the immunosuppressed child is reviewed in Chapter 48. Psychosocial concerns and appropriate interventions for the child with a life-threatening disorder are presented in Chapter 43.

The first 6 months to 1 year after the transplant are most intense because the risk of complications is greatest and the patient and family are adjusting to a new lifestyle. Patients need to be monitored closely by the health care team, with frequent visits and laboratory tests. Care is usually shared between local health care providers and the transplant centre. Many patients are able to return to school and other age-appropriate activities within 2 to 3 months after the transplant.

VASCULAR DYSFUNCTION

Systemic Hypertension

Hypertension is defined as the consistent elevation of BP beyond values considered to be the upper limits of normal. The two major categories are *essential hypertension* (no identifiable cause) and *secondary hypertension* (subsequent to an identifiable cause). Hypertension in children and adolescents is defined as having a systolic or diastolic BP that consistently falls at or over the ninety-fifth percentile. This group is further delineated as follows:

- *Stage 1 hypertension* includes patients with BP readings between the ninety-fifth and ninety-ninth percentiles.
- *Stage 2 hypertension* describes patients with BP readings over the ninety-ninth percentile plus 5 mm Hg.

An additional group includes children and adolescents who have prehypertension (or high-normal BP). This prehypertensive group includes those with BP readings that fall consistently between the ninetieth and ninety-fifth percentiles.

Etiology

Most instances of hypertension observed in young children occur secondary to a structural abnormality or an underlying pathological process, although this association is being challenged by screening programs of relatively healthy children. The most common cause of secondary hypertension is renal disease, followed by cardiovascular, endocrine, and some neurological disorders. As a rule, the younger the child and the more severe the hypertension, the more likely it is to be secondary.

The causes of essential hypertension are undetermined, but evidence indicates that both genetic and environmental factors play a role. The incidence of hypertension has been shown to be higher in children whose parents are hypertensive. Environmental factors that contribute to the risk of developing hypertension include obesity, salt ingestion, smoking, and stress.

Diagnostic Evaluation

From the increasing numbers of hypertensive or potentially hypertensive children and adolescents being identified, a BP determination should be a routine part of annual assessment in healthy children over 3 years old. BP readings should be done in children less than 3 years old who have high-risk family histories or those with individual risk factors, including CHD, kidney disease, malignancy, transplant, certain neurological problems, or systemic illnesses known to cause hypertension. Although clinical manifestations associated with hypertension depend largely on the underlying cause, some observations can provide clues to the examiner that an elevated BP may be a factor (Box 47-10). In infants and very young children who cannot communicate symptoms, observation of behaviour provides clues, although gross behavioural changes may not be apparent until complications are present.

Appendix E provides BP values that require further investigation. These values represent the lower limits for abnormal BP ranges, according to age and gender. Any BP readings equal to or greater than these values should be further evaluated (Kaelber & Pickett, 2009). Before a diagnosis is made, BP should be measured on at least three separate occasions. Routine BP screening is not recommended in children less than 3 years of age.

BOX 47-10 CLINICAL MANIFESTATIONS OF HYPERTENSION

Adolescents and Older Children
Frequent headaches
Dizziness
Changes in vision

Infants or Young Children
Irritability
Head banging or head rubbing
Waking up screaming in the night

A careful medical and family history should be obtained to screen for other relatives with hypertension or other cardiovascular risk factors. In children with suspected hypertension, initial laboratory data include a urinalysis, renal function studies such as creatinine and blood urea nitrogen, a lipid profile, complete blood count, and electrolytes. Depending on the severity of hypertension, additional testing may be indicated. Testing may include a retinal examination, renal ultrasonography to measure kidney size and Doppler flow to detect the possibility of a renal cause, and an ECG and an echocardiogram to evaluate the presence of end-organ involvement such as left ventricular hypertrophy. Further testing for a secondary cause may be indicated on the basis of individual circumstances, especially in children with significant hypertension and normal initial screening test findings.

Therapeutic Management

Therapy for secondary hypertension involves diagnosis and treatment of the underlying cause. In cases amenable to surgical repair, the nature of the condition, the type of surgery, and the child's age are all important considerations. Children or adolescents with consistently elevated BP readings from no known cause or those with secondary hypertension not amenable to surgical correction may be treated with a combination of nonpharmacological and pharmacological interventions. Dietary practices and lifestyle changes are important in the control of hypertension for both children and adults. Nonpharmacological measures, such as weight control in overweight patients, increased exercise, limited salt intake, and avoidance of stress and smoking, carry no risk and should be instituted first, except in severe cases in which pharmacological therapy may be indicated as well.

Medication therapy needs to be instituted with caution in children with significant elevations of BP resistant to nonpharmacological intervention. The treatment should begin with one medication; other medications should be added only if control is not obtained. The oral antihypertensive medications used in children include beta blockers, ACE inhibitors, calcium channel blockers, angiotensin-receptor blockers, and diuretics. The goal is to achieve a normotensive state throughout the day without accompanying medication adverse effects.

NURSING CARE

BP measurement should always be a part of the routine assessment of children over 3 years old. To obtain an accurate reading, it is important to quiet the child or relax the adolescent while the measurement is recorded, to avoid false readings caused by excitement. BP should be measured in the sitting position with the arm at the level of the heart. Initial evaluation should also include four extremity pressures (in the supine position) to rule out coarctation of the aorta. The chief cause of falsely elevated BP readings is the use of improperly fitting, narrow cuffs. Thus attention to correct measurement technique is essential (see Blood Pressure, Chapter 33).

Home BP measurements can facilitate surveillance in youngsters with chronic hypertension and can document effectiveness of therapy. A family member can be instructed in how to take and record accurate BP measurements, thus decreasing the number of trips to a health care facility. This individual needs to understand when to contact the primary practitioner regarding elevated values. The community nurse can often be a valuable resource in monitoring BP. The nurse plays an important role in assessing individual families and providing targeted information about nonpharmacological modes of intervention, such as diet, weight loss, smoking cessation, and exercise programs. If extensive dietary counselling is required, the child should be referred to a dietician with expertise in working with children and adolescents. Exercise regimens should be individualized. Schoolchildren and young adolescents generally prefer team sports rather than individual training, which they may view as a burden rather than an enjoyable activity. If peers and family members can be encouraged to participate in any of the management strategies, the child's adherence to treatment is likely to be greater.

Hypertensive adolescents should avoid using oral contraceptives because of their pressor effects. Other options need to be presented before this form of birth control is discontinued (see Contraception, Chapter 8).

If medication therapy is prescribed, the nurse needs to provide information to the family regarding the reasons for it, how the drug works, and possible adverse effects. General instructions for antihypertensive medications include the following:

- Rise slowly from a horizontal position and avoid sudden position changes.
- Take medication as prescribed.
- Maintain adequate hydration.
- Notify the health care provider if adverse effects occur, but do not discontinue medication.
- Avoid alcohol and stay on the prescribed diet.

The need for follow-up should be stressed, especially because antihypertensive therapy can sometimes be safely discontinued if BP remains under control over time.

Kawasaki Disease (Mucocutaneous Lymph Node Syndrome)

Kawasaki disease (KD) is an acute systemic vasculitis of unknown cause. It is seen in every racial group, and about 75% of the cases occur in children younger than the age of 5 years, with peak incidence in the toddler age group. The acute disease is self-limited. Infants younger than 1 year of age are most seriously affected by KD and are at the greatest risk for heart involvement.

Although it is not spread by person-to-person contact, several factors support infectious etiological factors. It is often seen in geographic and seasonal outbreaks, with most cases reported in the late winter and early spring (Burns, Herzog, Fabri, et al., 2013).

Pathophysiology

The principal area of concern in KD is the cardiovascular system. During the initial stage of the illness, extensive inflammation of the arterioles, venules, and capillaries occurs. In

BOX 47-11 DIAGNOSTIC CRITERIA FOR KAWASAKI DISEASE

The child must have had fever for more than 5 days along with four of five clinical criteria (diagnosis may be made on day 4 by an experienced clinician if child has all the clinical criteria):

1. Changes in the extremities: in the acute phase, edema and erythema of the palms and soles, and in the subacute phase, periungual desquamation (peeling) of the hands and feet
2. Bilateral conjunctival injection (inflammation) without exudation
3. Changes in the oral mucous membranes, such as erythema of the lips, oropharyngeal reddening, or "strawberry tongue" (large papillae are exposed)
4. Polymorphous rash
5. Cervical lymphadenopathy (one lymph node larger than 1.5 cm)

Note: Kawasaki disease can be diagnosed with fewer clinical criteria when coronary artery changes are noted.

addition, segmental damage to the medium-size muscular arteries, mainly the coronary arteries, can occur, causing the formation of coronary artery aneurysms in some children. When death occurs (in less than 1% of cases), it is usually the result of myocardial ischemia from coronary thrombosis or, over time, severe scar formation and stenosis in coronary aneurysms (Son & Newburger, 2016).

Clinical Manifestations

Because no specific diagnostic test exists for KD, the diagnosis is established on the basis of clinical findings and associated laboratory results (Box 47-11). These criteria should be used as guidelines. Many children with KD do not fulfill standard diagnostic criteria and infants often have an incomplete presentation. Thus it is important to consider KD as a possible diagnosis in any infant or child with prolonged elevated temperature that is unresponsive to antibiotics and not attributable to another cause.

KD manifests in three phases: acute, subacute, and convalescent. The *acute phase* begins with the abrupt onset of high fever that is unresponsive to antibiotics and antipyretics. The child then develops the remaining diagnostic symptoms. During this stage he or she is typically very irritable. The *subacute phase* begins with resolution of the fever and lasts until all clinical signs of KD have disappeared. During this phase the child is at greatest risk for the development of coronary artery aneurysms. Echocardiograms are used to monitor myocardial and coronary artery status. A baseline echocardiogram should be obtained at the time of diagnosis for comparison with future studies. Irritability persists during this phase. In the *convalescent phase*, all the clinical signs of KD have resolved, but the laboratory values have not returned to normal. This phase is complete when all blood values are normal (6 to 8 weeks after onset). At the end of this stage the child has regained his or her usual temperament, energy, and appetite.

Cardiac involvement. Long-term complications of KD include the development of coronary artery aneurysms, disrupting blood flow. In children with aneurysms, there is the potential for myocardial infarction, which can result from thrombotic occlusion of a coronary aneurysm. Over time, as the damaged vessel tries to heal, stenosis of the aneurysm may develop and may lead to myocardial ischemia. Most of the morbidity and mortality occurs in children affected with the largest aneurysms (giant aneurysms larger than 8 mm). Symptoms of acute myocardial infarction in children may include abdominal pain, vomiting, restlessness, inconsolable crying, pallor, and shock.

Therapeutic Management

The current treatment of KD includes high-dose IV gamma-globulin along with salicylate therapy. Gamma-globulin has been demonstrated to be effective at reducing the incidence of coronary artery abnormalities when given within the first 10 days of the illness. A single large infusion of 2 g/kg over 10 to 12 hours is recommended. Retreatment with IV gamma-globulin is indicated in patients who continue with fever after treatment.

Aspirin is given initially in an anti-inflammatory dose (80 to 100 mg/kg/day in divided doses every 6 hours) to control fever and symptoms of inflammation. After fever has subsided, it is continued at an antiplatelet dose (3 to 5 mg/kg/day). Low-dose aspirin is continued in patients without echocardiographic evidence of coronary abnormalities until the platelet count has returned to normal (6 to 8 weeks). If the child develops coronary abnormalities, salicylate therapy is continued indefinitely. Additional anticoagulation (e.g., clopidogrel [Plavix], enoxaparin [Lovenox], or warfarin) may be indicated in children who have medium-size or giant coronary artery aneurysms.

Prognosis

Most children with KD recover fully after treatment. However, when cardiovascular complications occur, serious morbidity may result. Death occurs rarely but almost always results from coronary thrombosis.

NURSING CARE

In the initial phase the nurse must monitor the child's cardiac status carefully. Intake and output and daily weight measurements are recorded. Although the child may be reluctant to eat and therefore may be partially dehydrated, fluids need to be administered with care because of the usual finding of myocarditis. The child should be assessed frequently for signs of HF, including decreased urinary output, gallop rhythm (an additional heart sound), tachycardia, and respiratory distress.

Administration of gamma globulin should follow the same guidelines as for any blood product, with frequent monitoring of vital signs. Patients must be watched for allergic reactions. Cardiac status must be monitored because of the large volume being administered to patients with myocarditis and diminished left ventricular function.

Most nursing care focuses on symptomatic relief. To minimize skin discomfort, cool cloths; unscented lotions; and soft, loose clothing are helpful. During the acute phase, mouth care, including lubricating ointment to the lips, is important for mucosal inflammation. Clear liquids and soft foods can be offered.

Patient irritability is perhaps the most challenging problem. These children need a quiet environment that promotes adequate rest. Their parents need to be supported in their efforts to comfort an often inconsolable child. They may need time away from their child, and nurses can often provide respite care for the family. Parents need to understand that irritability is a hallmark of KD and that they need not feel guilty or embarrassed about their child's behaviour.

Discharge Teaching

Parents need accurate information about the progression of KD, including the importance of follow-up monitoring and when they should contact their health care provider. Irritability is likely to persist for up to 2 months after the onset of symptoms. Peeling of the hands and feet is painless and occurs primarily in the second and third weeks. Arthritis, especially of the larger weight-bearing joints, may persist for several weeks. Children are typically most stiff in the mornings, during cold weather, and after naps. Passive range-of-motion exercises in the bathtub are often helpful in increasing flexibility. Any live immunizations (e.g., measles-mumps-rubella, varicella) should be deferred for 11 months after the administration of gamma globulin because the body might not produce the appropriate amount of antibodies (American Academy of Pediatrics, Committee on Infectious Diseases, Kimberlin, Brady, et al., 2015). The decision to give the varicella (chicken pox) vaccine while the child is receiving aspirin therapy is made individually by the health care provider. Temperature should be recorded after discharge until the child has been afebrile for several days.

Parents of children with large aneurysms should be educated as to the unlikely but real possibility of myocardial infarction, as well as the signs and symptoms of cardiac ischemia in a child. At discharge, the ultimate cardiac sequelae are generally not fully known because vessels do not reach their maximum diameter until 4 to 6 weeks after the onset of KD. **Cardiopulmonary resuscitation (CPR)** should be taught to parents of children with known severe coronary artery sequelae.

Long-Term Follow-Up

The frequency and type of follow-up are based on the presence or absence of coronary damage. The long-term outlook for children without aneurysms is promising. After more than 30 years of follow-up, an increased incidence of early heart disease is not being seen in this population. However, the literature regarding subtle effects of inflammation on the vessels is conflicting, and it is recommended that these children be screened and treated for the presence of coronary risk factors as they grow older. They should have a cholesterol screen performed, BP monitored, and education recommending a heart-healthy lifestyle, including exercise, a heart-healthy diet, and avoidance of smoking. This group of patients is seen at infrequent intervals—approximately every 5 years. In patients with aneurysms, follow-up focuses on the prevention and early detection of coronary ischemia. Noninvasive modalities of coronary imaging, such as cardiac computed tomography angiography, magnetic resonance imaging, echocardiography, and stress testing, are used as much as possible. Patients with coronary aneurysms may require long-term antiplatelet or anticoagulation and possibly beta-blocker therapy or other therapies, depending on the severity of coronary involvement.

Shock

Shock, or circulatory failure, is a complex clinical syndrome characterized by inadequate tissue perfusion to meet the metabolic demands of the body, resulting in cellular dysfunction and eventual organ failure. Although the causes are different, the physiological consequences are the same: hypotension, tissue hypoxia, and metabolic acidosis. Circulatory failure in children is a result of hypovolemia, altered peripheral vascular resistance, or pump failure. Types of shock are listed in Table 47-5.

TABLE 47-5 TYPES OF SHOCK

CHARACTERISTICS	MOST FREQUENT CAUSES
Hypovolemic	
Reduction in size of vascular compartment Falling blood pressure Poor capillary filling Low central venous pressure	Blood loss (hemorrhagic shock)—Trauma, gastrointestinal bleeding, intracranial hemorrhage Plasma loss—Increased capillary permeability associated with sepsis and acidosis, hypoproteinemia, burns, peritonitis Extracellular fluid loss—Vomiting, diarrhea, glycosuric diuresis, sunstroke
Distributive	
Reduction in peripheral vascular resistance Profound inadequacies in tissue perfusion Increased venous capacity and pooling Acute reduction in return blood flow to the heart Diminished cardiac output	Anaphylaxis (anaphylactic shock)—Extreme allergy or hypersensitivity to a foreign substance Sepsis (septic shock, bacteremic shock, endotoxic shock)—Overwhelming sepsis and circulating bacterial toxins Loss of neuronal control (neurogenic shock)—Interruption of neuronal transmission (spinal cord injury) Myocardial depression and peripheral dilation—Exposure to anaesthesia or ingestion of barbiturates, tranquilizers, opioids, antihypertensive agents, or ganglionic blocking agents
Cardiogenic	
Decreased cardiac output	After surgery for congenital heart disease Primary pump failure—Myocarditis, myocardial trauma, biochemical derangements, heart failure Dysrhythmias—Supraventricular tachycardia, atrioventricular block, and ventricular dysrhythmias; secondary to myocarditis or biochemical abnormalities (occasionally)

Pathophysiology

A healthy child's circulatory system is able to transport oxygen and metabolic substrates to body tissues, which require a constant source for these essential needs. The cardiac output and distribution to the various body tissues can change rapidly in response to intrinsic (myocardial and intravascular) or extrinsic (neuronal) control mechanisms. In shock states these mechanisms are altered or challenged.

Reduced blood flow, as in hypovolemic shock, causes diminished venous return to the heart, low CVP, low cardiac output, and hypotension. Vasomotor centres in the medulla are signalled, causing a compensatory increase in the force and rate of cardiac contraction and constriction of arterioles and veins, thereby increasing peripheral vascular resistance. Simultaneously, the lowered blood volume leads to the release of large amounts of catecholamines, antidiuretic hormone, adrenocorticosteroids, and aldosterone in an effort to conserve body fluids. This causes reduced blood flow to the skin, kidneys, muscles, and viscera to shunt the available blood to the brain and heart. Consequently, the skin feels cold and clammy, there is poor capillary filling, and the glomerular filtration rate and urinary output are significantly reduced.

As a result of impaired perfusion, oxygen is depleted in the tissue cells, causing them to revert to anaerobic metabolism, producing lactic acidosis. The acidosis places an extra burden on the lungs as they attempt to compensate for the metabolic acidosis by increasing respiratory rate to remove excess carbon dioxide. Prolonged vasoconstriction results in fatigue and atony of the peripheral arterioles, which leads to vessel dilation. Venules, less sensitive to vasodilator substances, remain constricted for a time, causing massive pooling in the capillary and venular beds, which further depletes blood volume.

Complications of shock create further hazards. Central nervous system hypoperfusion may eventually lead to cerebral edema, cortical infarction, or intraventricular hemorrhage. Renal hypoperfusion causes renal ischemia with possible tubular or glomerular necrosis and renal vein thrombosis. Reduced blood flow to the lungs can interfere with surfactant secretion and result in acute respiratory distress syndrome (ARDS), characterized by sudden pulmonary congestion and atelectasis with formation of a hyaline membrane. Gastrointestinal tract bleeding and perforation are always a possibility after splanchnic ischemia and necrosis of intestinal mucosa. Metabolic complications of shock may include hypoglycemia, hypocalcemia, and other electrolyte disturbances.

Diagnostic Evaluation

The etiology of shock can be discerned from the history and physical examination. The severity of the shock is determined by measurements of vital signs, including CVP and capillary filling (Box 47-12). Shock can be regarded as a form of compensation for circulatory failure. Because of its progressive nature, it can be divided into the following three stages or phases:

1. **Compensated shock**—Vital organ function is maintained by intrinsic compensatory mechanisms; blood flow is usually normal or increased but generally uneven or maldistributed in the microcirculation.
2. **Decompensated shock**—Efficiency of the cardiovascular system gradually diminishes until perfusion in the microcirculation becomes marginal despite compensatory adjustments. The outcomes of circulatory failure that progress beyond the limits of compensation are tissue hypoxia, metabolic acidosis, and eventual dysfunction of all organ systems.
3. **Irreversible, or terminal, shock**—Damage to vital organs, such as the heart or brain, is of such magnitude that the entire organism will be disrupted regardless of therapeutic intervention. Death occurs even if cardiovascular measurements return to normal levels with therapy.

At all stages the principal differentiating signs are observed in the (1) degree of tachycardia and perfusion to extremities, (2) level of consciousness, and (3) BP. Additional signs or modifications of these more universal signs may be present, depending on the type and cause of the shock. Initially the child's ability to compensate is effective; thus early signs are subtle. As the shock state advances, signs are more obvious and indicate early decompensation.

Additional signs may be present, depending on the type and cause of the shock. In early septic shock there are chills, fever, and vasodilation, with increased cardiac output that results in warm, flushed skin (hyperdynamic, or "hot," shock). A later and ominous development is disseminated intravascular coagulation (see Chapter 48), the major hematological complication of septic shock. Anaphylactic shock is frequently accompanied by urticaria and angioneurotic edema, which is life

BOX 47-12 CLINICAL MANIFESTATIONS OF SHOCK

Compensated

Apprehensiveness
Irritability
Unexplained tachycardia
Normal blood pressure
Narrowing pulse pressure
Thirst
Pallor
Diminished urinary output
Reduced perfusion of extremities

Decompensated

Confusion and somnolence
Tachypnea
Moderate metabolic acidosis
Oliguria
Cool, pale extremities
Decreased skin turgor
Poor capillary filling

Irreversible

Thready, weak pulse
Hypotension
Periodic breathing or apnea
Anuria
Stupor or coma

threatening when it involves the respiratory passages (see Anaphylaxis, below).

Laboratory tests that assist in assessment are blood gas measurements, pH, and sometimes liver function tests. Coagulation tests are evaluated when there is evidence of bleeding, such as oozing from a venipuncture site, bleeding from any orifice, or petechiae. Cultures of blood and other sites are indicated when there is a high suspicion of sepsis. Renal function tests are performed when impaired renal function is evident.

Therapeutic Management

Treatment of shock consists of three major interventions: (1) ventilation, (2) fluid administration, and (3) improvement of the pumping action of the heart (vasopressor support). The first priority is to establish an airway and administer oxygen. After the airway is ensured, circulatory stabilization is the major concern. Establishment of adequate IV access, ideally with multilumen central lines, is essential to deliver fluids and medications.

Ventilatory support. The lung is the organ most sensitive to shock. Decreased distribution or redistribution of blood flow to respiratory muscles plus the increased work of breathing can rapidly lead to respiratory failure. Critically ill patients are unable to maintain an adequate airway. To place the lung at rest and improve ventilation, tracheal intubation is initiated early with positive-pressure ventilation. Supplemental oxygen is always given as soon as possible. Blood gases and pH are monitored frequently.

Increased extravascular lung water caused by edema contributes to the development of respiratory complications. Therapy is directed toward maintaining normal arterial blood gas measurements, normal acid–base balance, and circulation. Efforts are made to remove fluid and prevent its accumulation with the use of diuretics.

Cardiovascular support. In most cases rapid restoration of blood volume is all that is needed for resuscitation of the child in shock. An isotonic crystalloid solution (normal saline or Ringer's lactate) is the fluid of choice; colloids such as albumin are also used. Successful resuscitation is reflected by an increase in BP and a reduction in heart rate; increased cardiac output results in improved capillary circulation and skin colour. CVP measurements of right atrial pressure help guide fluid therapy, and urinary output measurement is an important indicator of adequacy of circulation. Correction of acidosis, hypoxemia, hypoglycemia, hypothermia, and any metabolic derangements is mandatory.

Temporary pharmacological support may be required to enhance myocardial contractility, reverse metabolic or respiratory acidosis, maintain arterial pressure, or do all of these. The principal agents used to improve cardiac output and circulation are catecholamines, such as dopamine or epinephrine (Adrenalin). Vasodilators that are sometimes used include nitroprusside or milrinone.

NURSING CARE

The child who is in shock requires intensive observation and care. The *initial action is to ensure adequate tissue oxygenation.* The nurse should be prepared to administer oxygen by the appropriate route and assist with any intubation and ventilatory procedures indicated. Other procedures and activities that require immediate attention are establishing an IV line, weighing the child, obtaining baseline vital signs, placing an in-dwelling catheter, obtaining blood gases and other measurements, and administering medications as indicated. The child is best positioned flat with the legs elevated.

> **! NURSING ALERT**
>
> Early clinical signs of shock include apprehension, irritability, normal BP, narrowing pulse pressure (difference between diastolic and systolic BP), thirst, pallor, diminished urinary output, unexplained mild tachycardia, and decreased perfusion of the hands and feet.

The nurse's responsibilities are to monitor the IV infusion, intake and output, vital signs (including CVP), and general systems assessments on a routine basis. IV medications are titrated according to patient responses, and vital signs are taken every 15 minutes during the critical periods and thereafter as needed. Urinary output is measured hourly; blood gases, hematocrit, pH, and electrolytes are monitored frequently to assess the child's status and the efficacy of therapy. An apnea and cardiac monitor is attached and monitored continuously. In the initial stages of acute shock, more than one nurse is often needed to manage all the necessary activities that must be carried out simultaneously (see Emergency box).

Anaphylaxis

Anaphylaxis is the acute clinical syndrome resulting from the interaction of an allergen and a patient who is hypersensitive to

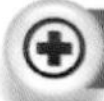

EMERGENCY

Shock

Ventilation

Establish airway; be prepared for intubation.
Administer oxygen, usually 100% by mask.

Fluid Administration

Obtain vascular access (preferably intravenous [IV]; intraosseous in emergency).
Restore fluid volume as ordered.

Cardiovascular Support

Administer vasopressors, especially IV epinephrine (dose: 0.01 mg/kg = 0.1 mL/kg of 1 : 10,000 solution).
This may be repeated every 3 to 5 minutes for patients in cardiac arrest.

General Support

Provide continuous electrocardiographic monitoring.
Monitor pulse oximetry.
Keep child flat with legs raised above level of heart.
Keep child warm and calm.

In Addition

Septic shock—Administer broad-spectrum antibiotics intravenously.
Anaphylaxis—Remove allergen if possible; provide intramuscular epinephrine and corticosteroids as ordered.

that allergen. When the antigen enters the circulatory system, a generalized reaction rapidly takes place. Vasoactive amines (principally histamine or a histamine-like substance) are released and cause vasodilation, bronchoconstriction, and increased capillary permeability.

Severe reactions are immediate in onset; are often life threatening; and frequently involve multiple systems, primarily the cardiovascular, respiratory, gastrointestinal, and integumentary systems. Exposure to the antigen can be by ingestion, inhalation, skin contact, or injection. Examples of common allergens associated with anaphylaxis include drugs (e.g., antibiotics, chemotherapeutic agents, radiological contrast media), latex, foods, venom from bees or snakes, and biological agents (antisera, enzymes, hormones, blood products).

NURSING ALERT

Penicillin allergy is associated with immediate (within an hour of administration) or accelerated (1 to 72 hours after administration) onset of skin eruption, especially a urticarial rash, or more serious symptoms such as laryngeal edema or anaphylactic shock.

Clinical Manifestations

The onset of clinical symptoms usually occurs within seconds or minutes of exposure to the antigen, and the rapidity of the reaction is directly related to its intensity: the earlier the onset, the more severe the reaction. The reaction may be preceded by symptoms of uneasiness, restlessness, irritability, severe anxiety, headache, dizziness, paresthesia, and disorientation. The patient may lose consciousness. Cutaneous signs of flushing and urticaria are common early signs, followed by angioedema, most notable in the eyelids, lips, tongue, hands, feet, and genitalia.

Bronchiolar constriction may follow, causing narrowing of the airway; pulmonary edema and hemorrhage also may occur. Laryngeal edema with severe acute upper airway obstruction may be life threatening and requires rapid intervention. Shock occurs as a result of mediator-induced vasodilation, which causes capillary permeability and loss of intravascular fluid into the interstitial space. Sudden hypotension and impaired cardiac output with poor perfusion are seen.

Therapeutic Management

A successful outcome of anaphylactic reactions depends on rapid recognition and institution of treatment. The goals of treatment are to provide ventilation, restore adequate circulation, and prevent further exposure by identifying and removing the cause when possible.

A mild reaction with no evidence of respiratory distress or cardiovascular compromise can be managed with subcutaneous administration of antihistamines, such as diphenhydramine (Benadryl) and epinephrine.

Moderate or severe distress presents a potentially life-threatening emergency. Establishing an airway is the first concern, as with all shock states. Epinephrine is given subcutaneously or intravenously as an antihistamine and to support the cardiovascular system and increase BP. Other routes for giving epinephrine are intramuscular and via the airway, either nebulized or injected through an ET tube. In severe anaphylaxis, epinephrine by any route is better than none. Fluids are given to restore blood volume. Additional vasopressors may be given to improve cardiac output.

Prevention of a reaction is preferable. Preventing exposure is more easily accomplished in children known to be at risk, including those with (1) a history of previous allergic reaction to a specific antigen; (2) a history of atopy; (3) a history of severe reactions in immediate family members; and (4) a reaction to a skin test, although skin tests are not available for all allergens. Desensitization may be recommended in certain cases.

NURSING CARE

When an anaphylactic reaction is suspected, both immediate intervention and preparation for medical therapy are nursing responsibilities. Ventilation is ensured by placing the child in a head-elevated position, unless contraindicated by hypotension, to facilitate breathing and administer oxygen. If the child is not breathing, CPR is initiated and emergency medical services are summoned.

If the cause can be determined, measures need to be implemented to slow the spread of the offending substance. An IV infusion should be established immediately. Emergency medications should be given intravenously whenever possible; however, epinephrine may be given subcutaneously (see Emergency box). Vital signs and urinary output should be monitored frequently. Medications need to be administered as prescribed, with regular assessment to monitor effectiveness and detect signs of adverse effects of medication and fluid overload.

To prevent an anaphylactic reaction, parents should always be asked about possible allergic responses to foods, latex, medications, and environmental conditions. These need to be displayed prominently on the patient's chart. The specific allergen should be noted, as well as the type and severity of the reaction. Parents are excellent historians, especially when the child has displayed a pronounced reaction to a substance. Medications, including related medications (e.g., penicillin, nafcillin), and other items such as latex that have produced a reaction previously should never be used. If the child is allergic to insect venom, the family should be instructed to purchase an emergency kit to be kept with him or her at all times. If the child is old enough, both the family and the child need to be taught how to use the equipment. The patient should carry medical identification at all times.

Septic Shock

Sepsis and septic shock are caused by an infectious organism. Normally an infection triggers an inflammatory response in a local area, which results in vasodilation, increased capillary permeability, and eventually elimination of the infectious agent. The widespread activation and systemic release of inflammatory mediators is called the *systemic inflammatory response syndrome (SIRS)*. Box 47-13 provides the exact definitions for SIRS, infection, sepsis, and severe sepsis. SIRS can occur in response to both infectious and noninfectious (e.g., trauma, burns)

BOX 47-13 DEFINITIONS OF SYSTEMIC INFLAMMATORY RESPONSE SYNDROME, INFECTION, SEPSIS, AND SEVERE SEPSIS

Systemic inflammatory response syndrome (SIRS)—The presence of at least two of the following four criteria, one of which must be abnormal temperature or leukocyte count:

1. Core temperature of more than 38.5°C (101.3°F) or less than 36°C (96.8°F)
2. Tachycardia, defined as a mean heart rate more than 2 SD above normal for age in the absence of external stimulus, chronic drugs, or painful stimuli; or otherwise unexplained persistent elevation over a 0.5- to 4-hour period; or, for children less than 1 year old: bradycardia, defined as a mean heart rate less than the tenth percentile for age in the absence of external vagal stimulus, beta-blocker drugs, or congenital heart disease; or otherwise unexplained persistent depression over a 30-minute period
3. Mean respiratory rate more than 2 SD above normal for age or mechanical ventilation for an acute process not related to underlying neuromuscular disease or the receipt of general anaesthesia
4. Leukocyte count elevated or depressed for age (not secondary to chemotherapy-induced leukopenia) or more than 10% immature neutrophils

Infection—A suspected or proven (by positive culture, tissue stain, or polymerase chain reaction test) infection caused by any pathogen; or a clinical syndrome associated with a high probability of infection. Evidence of infection includes positive findings on clinical examination, imaging, or laboratory tests (e.g., white blood cells in a normally sterile body fluid, perforated viscus, chest radiograph consistent with pneumonia, petechial or purpuric rash, or purpura fulminans)

Sepsis—SIRS in the presence or as a result of suspected or proven infection

Severe sepsis—Sepsis plus cardiovascular organ dysfunction or acute respiratory distress syndrome; or two or more other organ dysfunctions

Septic shock—Sepsis and cardiovascular organ dysfunction

From Goldstein, B., et al. (2005). International Pediatric Sepsis Consensus Conference: Definitions for sepsis and organ dysfunction in pediatrics. *Pediatric Critical Care Medicine, 6*(1), 2–8; used with permission. Copyright © 2005, The Society of Critical Care Medicine and the World Federation of Pediatric Intensive and Critical Care Societies.

TABLE 47-6 AGE-SPECIFIC VITAL SIGNS AND LABORATORY VARIABLES IN SEPTIC SHOCK*

AGE GROUP	HEART RATE (beats/min)		RESPIRATORY RATE (breaths/min)	LEUKOCYTE COUNT (leukocytes × 10^9/L)	SYSTOLIC BLOOD PRESSURE (mm Hg)
	TACHYCARDIA	BRADYCARDIA			
0 days–1 wk	>180	<100	>60	>34	<65
1 wk–1 mo	>180	<100	>40	>19.5 or <5	<75
1 mo–1 yr	>180	<90	>34	>17.5 or <5	<100
2–5 yr	>140	N/A	>22	>15.5 or <6	<94
6–12 yr	>130	N/A	>8	>13.50 or <4.5	<105
13–<18 yr	>110	N/A	>4	>11 or <4.5	<117

N/A, not applicable.
*Lower values for heart rate, leukocyte count, and systolic blood pressure are for fifth percentile, and upper values for heart rate, respiratory rate, or leukocyte count are for ninety-fifth percentile.
From Goldstein, B., et al. (2005). International Pediatric Sepsis Consensus Conference: Definitions for sepsis and organ dysfunction in pediatrics. *Pediatric Critical Care Medicine, 6*(1), 2–8; used with permission. Copyright © 2005, The Society of Critical Care Medicine and the World Federation of Pediatric Intensive and Critical Care Societies.

causes. When caused by infection, it is called *sepsis. Septic shock* is defined as sepsis with organ dysfunction and hypotension.

Most of the physiological effects of shock occur because the exaggerated immune response triggers more than 30 different mediators that result in diffuse vasodilation, increased capillary permeability, and maldistribution of blood flow. This impairs oxygen and nutrient delivery to the cells, resulting in cellular dysfunction. If the process continues, multiple organ dysfunction occurs and may result in death. Table 47-6 includes the age-specific vital signs and laboratory values reflective of septic shock in children.

The incidence of septic shock is increasing in adults and children (Hartman, Linde-Zwirble, Angus, et al., 2013), possibly as a result of greater numbers of immunosuppressed patients, more widespread use of invasive devices in the seriously ill, increased awareness of the diagnosis, and a growing number of resistant microorganisms.

Three stages have been identified in septic shock. In early septic shock the patient has chills; fever; and vasodilation with increased cardiac output, which results in warm, flushed skin that reflects vascular tone abnormalities and hyperdynamic, warm, or hyperdynamic-compensated responses. BP and urinary output are normal. The patient has the best chance for survival in this stage. The second stage—the normodynamic, cool, or hyperdynamic-decompensated stage—lasts only a few hours. The skin is cool, but pulses and BP are still normal. Urinary output diminishes, and the mental state becomes depressed. With advancing disease, certain signs of circulatory decompensation that deteriorate to signs of circulatory collapse are indistinguishable from late shock of any cause. In the hypodynamic, or cold, stage of shock, cardiovascular function progressively deteriorates, even with aggressive therapy. The patient has hypothermia, cold extremities, weak pulses, hypotension, and oliguria or anuria. Patients are severely lethargic or comatose.

Multiorgan failure is common. This is the most dangerous stage of shock.

Management of septic shock involves measures to provide hemodynamic stability and adequate oxygenation to the tissues and the use of antimicrobials to treat the infectious organism. As with other forms of shock, hemodynamic stability is achieved with fluid volume resuscitation and inotropic agents as needed. Providing adequate oxygenation often requires intubation and mechanical ventilation, supplemental oxygen, sedation, and paralysis to decrease the work of breathing. Septic shock involves activation of **complement** proteins that promote clumping of the granulocytes in the lung. The granulocytes can release chemicals that can cause direct lung injury to the pulmonary capillary endothelium. This causes a fluid leak into the alveoli, which causes stiff, noncompliant lungs. Disseminated intravascular coagulation and multiorgan dysfunction may also occur and require prompt assessment and management.

Newer therapies are being developed to modify the host immune response by attempting to block various mediators, thereby interrupting the inflammatory cascade.

Early identification of the symptoms of septic shock is critical to patient survival. A high index of suspicion is required in all critically ill patients who are at greater risk for sepsis because of multiple invasive lines and devices, poor nutrition, and impaired immune function. Subtle alterations in tissue perfusion and unexplained tachypnea and tachycardia often are early warning signs. Identification of the infectious agent and prompt treatment are also critical to patient survival. Broad-spectrum antibiotics should be given, and the site of infection should be removed if possible (e.g., drain abscesses, remove in-dwelling lines). Patients should be managed in a critical care unit, in which continuous monitoring and sophisticated cardiac and respiratory support are available. Multidisciplinary collaboration is essential in managing these critically ill patients.

KEY POINTS

- CHD is the most common form of cardiac disease in children.
- Major categories to investigate in the cardiac history are poor weight gain, poor feeding habits, and fatigue during feeding; frequent respiratory tract infections and difficulties; and evidence of exercise intolerance.
- The most common tests used in assessing cardiac function are radiography, ECG, echocardiography, and cardiac catheterization.
- Cardiac catheterization procedures can be divided into three groups: (1) diagnostic procedures, including angiography, that measure pressures and saturations to establish cardiac diagnosis; (2) interventional procedures, in which catheters or balloon devices are used to correct cardiac defects; and (3) electrophysiology studies, in which catheters with electrodes are used to evaluate dysrhythmias.
- Diagnostic cardiac catheterization provides important information about oxygen saturation of blood within the chambers and great vessels, pressure changes, changes in cardiac output or stroke volume, and anatomical abnormalities.
- Several prenatal factors may predispose children to CHD: maternal rubella during pregnancy, maternal alcoholism, maternal age older than 40 years, and maternal type 1 diabetes.
- Congenital heart defects can be divided into four main groups, as determined by hemodynamic patterns: (1) defects that result in increased pulmonary blood flow, (2) obstructive defects, (3) defects that result in decreased pulmonary blood flow, and (4) mixed defects.
- Clinical consequences of congenital heart defects include HF and hypoxemia. A child can have both hypoxemia and HF, although usually they occur independently.
- Clinical manifestations of HF are impaired myocardial function (tachycardia, cardiomegaly), pulmonary congestion (dyspnea, tachypnea, orthopnea, cyanosis), and systemic congestion (hepatosplenomegaly, edema, distended veins).
- Nursing measures in the care of a child with HF are to assist in improving cardiac function, decrease cardiac demands, reduce respiratory distress, maintain nutritional status, promote fluid loss, and provide family support.
- Clinical manifestations of hypoxemia are cyanosis, polycythemia, clubbing, and delayed growth and development. The child is at increased risk for hypercyanotic spells, CVAs, brain abscess, and infective endocarditis.
- Caring for the child with CHD and the family requires helping them to adjust to the disorder and cope with the effects of the defect, as well as fostering growth and promoting family relationships.
- Preoperative care of the child with a congenital heart defect involves introducing the child and family to the hospital and preparing them for preoperative and postoperative procedures.
- Providing postoperative care includes observing vital signs and arterial and venous pressures, maintaining respiratory status, allowing maximum rest, providing comfort, monitoring fluids, planning for progressive activities, giving emotional support, observing for complications of surgery, and planning for discharge and home care.
- Acquired cardiovascular disorders include infective endocarditis, RF, hyperlipidemia (hypercholesterolemia), and cardiac dysrhythmias.
- Prevention of infectious endocarditis in certain children with CHD involves administration of prophylactic antibiotics when specific procedures are performed.
- Acute RF is a systemic inflammatory disease that can damage the cardiac valves and is associated with previous GABHS infection.
- Cholesterol screening in children is controversial; currently, children with known risk factors for hyperlipidemia are

screened and treated as needed. The influence of childhood cholesterol levels on later development of coronary artery disease is under investigation.
- Common dysrhythmias in children include slow (bradycardias, heart block) and fast (sinus tachycardia, SVT) rhythms.
- Heart transplantation has been extended to infants and children with cardiomyopathy and complex congenital heart defects involving ventricular dysfunction, such as hypoplastic left heart syndrome.
- Education of the child with hypertension and the family focuses on drug therapy, diet control, and appropriate exercise.
- KD is an extensive inflammation of small vessels and capillaries that may progress to involve the coronary arteries, causing aneurysm formation. The administration of gamma globulin is an important aspect of treatment.
- Emergency treatment for shock includes ensuring ventilation; administering vasopressors, fluids, blood, and antibiotics as needed; and providing supportive measures, such as correct positioning, warmth, and psychological reassurance to the child and family.
- Persons at risk for anaphylaxis may be identified by a history of previous allergic reaction, history of atopy, history of severe reactions in family, and positive skin test to the allergen.

Evolve WEBSITE

Visit the Evolve website for additional resources related to the content in this chapter such as Case Studies, Critical Thinking Case Study Answers, Nursing Care Plans, Nursing Processes, Nursing Skills, and Review Questions for Exam Preparation at: http://evolve.elsevier.com/Canada/Perry/maternal/

REFERENCES

Allen, U. D., & Canadian Paediatric Society, Infectious Diseases and Immunization Committee. (2010). Infective endocarditis: Updated guidelines. *Paediatrics & Child Health, 15*(4), 205–208. Reaffirmed 2016. Retrieved from <http://www.cps.ca/documents/position/infective-endorcarditis-guidelines>.

American Academy of Pediatrics, Committee on Infectious Diseases, Kimberlin, D. W., Brady, M. T., et al. (Eds.). (2015). *Red book: 2015 report of the Committee on Infectious Diseases* (30th ed.). Elk Grove Village, IL: Author.

American Heart Association. (2015). *Preparing children for heart surgery.* Retrieved from <http://www.heart.org/HEARTORG/Conditions/CongenitalDefectsChildren&Adults/Preparing-Children-for-Surgery_UCM_307732_Article.jsp#.Vt3D1ubNx2k>.

Arnold, R., Ley-Zaporozhan, J., Ley, S., et al. (2008). Outcome after mechanical aortic valve replacement in children and young adults. *Annals of Thoracic Surgery, 85*(2), 604–610. doi:10.1016/j.athoracsur.2007.10.035.

Aurora, P., Edwards, L. B., Kucheryavaya, A. Y., et al. (2010). The registry of the International Society for Heart and Lung Transplantation: Thirteenth official pediatric lung and heart-lung transplantation report—2010. *Journal of Heart and Lung Transplantation, 29*(10), 1129–1141. doi:10.1016/j.healun.2010.08.008.

Beekman, R. H. (2013). Coarctation of the aorta. In H. D. Allen, D. J. Driscoll, R. E. Shaddy, & T. F. Feltes (Eds.), *Moss and Adams' heart disease in infants, children and adolescents* (8th ed.). Philadelphia: Lippincott Williams & Wilkins.

Bernstein, D. (2016a). Acynanotic and cyanotic congenital heart disease. In R. M. Kliegman, B. F. Stanton, J. St. Geme, et al. (Eds.), *Nelson textbook of pediatrics* (20th ed.). Philadelphia: Saunders.

Bernstein, D. (2016b). Heart failure. In R. M. Kliegman, B. F. Stanton, J. St. Geme, et al. (Eds.), *Nelson textbook of pediatrics* (20th ed.). Philadelphia: Saunders.

Bernstein, D. (2016c). Primary pulmonary hypertension. In R. M. Kliegman, B. F. Stanton, J. St. Geme, et al. (Eds.), *Nelson textbook of pediatrics* (20th ed.). Philadelphia: Saunders.

Burns, J. C., Herzog, L., Fabri, O., et al. (2013). Seasonality of Kawasaki disease: A global perspective. *PLoS ONE, 8*, doi:10.1371/journal.pone.0074529. Retrieved from <http://journals.plos.org/plosone/article?id=10.1371/journal.pone.0074529>.

Conway, J., & Dipchand, A. (2010). Heart transplantation in children. *Pediatric Clinics of North America, 57*, 353–373. doi:10.1016/j.pci.2010.01.009.

Daniels, S. R., Greer, F. R., & Committee on Nutrition. (2008). Lipid screening and cardiovascular health in childhood. *Pediatrics, 122*, 198–208.

Domi, T., Edgell, D. S., McCrindle, B. W., et al. (2008). Frequency, predictors, and neurologic outcomes of vaso-occlusive strokes associated with cardiac surgery in children. *Pediatrics, 122*(6), 1292–1298. doi:10.1542/peds.2007-1459.

Goldmuntz, E., Crenshaw, M. L., & Lin, A. (2008). Genetics of congenital heart defects. In A. D. Allen, D. J. Driscoll, R. E. Shaddy, et al. (Eds.), *Moss and Adams' heart disease in infants, children and adolescents* (7th ed.). Philadelphia: Lippincott Williams & Wilkins.

Hartman, M. E., Linde-Zwirble, W. T., Angus, D. C., et al. (2013). Trends in the epidemiology of pediatric severe sepsis. *Pediatric Critical Care Medicine, 14*(7), 686–693. doi:10.1097/PCC.0b013e3182917fad.

Heart and Stroke Foundation. (2016a). *Congenital heart disease.* Retrieved from <http://www.heartandstroke.com/site/c.ikIQLcMWJtE/b.3484063/k.E84C/Heart_disease__Congenital_heart_disease.htm>.

Heart and Stroke Foundation. (2016b). *Healthy kids.* Retrieved from <http://www.heartandstroke.com/site/c.ikIQLcMWJtE/b.3479025/k.802B/Healthy_Kids.htm>.

Jacobs, J. P., Mavroudis, C., Jacobs, M. L., et al. (2004). Lessons learned from the data analysis of the second harvest (1998–2001) of the Society of Thoracic Surgeons (STS) Congenital Heart Surgery Database. *Journal of the American College of Cardiology, 26*(1), 18–37.

Kaelber, D. C., & Pickett, F. (2009). Simple table to identify children and adolescents needing further evaluation of blood pressure. *Pediatrics, 123*(6), e972–e974.

Kantor, P. F., Loughheed, J., Dancea, A., et al. (2013). Presentation, diagnosis and medical management of heart failure in children: Canadian Cardiovascular Society Guidelines. *Journal of Cardiology, 29*(12), 1535–1552.

Kim, J. J., & Marks, S. D. (2014). Long-term outcomes of children after solid organ transplantation. *Clinics (Sao Paulo), 69*(Suppl. 1), 28–38. doi:10.6061/clinics/2014(Sup01)06.

Leiter, L. A., Bays, H., Conard, S., et al. (2010). Attainment of Canadian and European guidelines' lipid targets with atorvastatin plus ezetimibe vs. doubling the dose of atorvastatin. *International Journal of Clinical Practice, 64*(13), 1765–1772. doi:10.1111/j.1742-1241.2010.02530.x.

LeRoy, S., Elixson, E. M., O'Brien, P., et al. (2003). Recommendations for preparing children and adolescents for invasive cardiac procedures: AHA scientific statement. *Circulation, 108*, 2550–2564.

McCrindle, B. W., Urbina, E. M., Dennison, B. A., et al. (2007). Drug therapy of high-risk lipid abnormalities in children and adolescents: A scientific statement from the American Heart Association Atherosclerosis, Hypertension, and Obesity in Youth Committee, Council of Cardiovascular Disease in the Young, with the Council on Cardiovascular Nursing. *Circulation, 115*, 1948–1967. doi:10.1161/CIRCULATIONAHA.107.181946.

Mehta, R., Lee, K. J., Chaturvedi, R., & Benson, L. (2008). Complications of pediatric cardiac catheterization: A review in the current era. *Catheterization and Cardiovascular Interventions, 72*(2), 278–285.

Michelakis, E. D., Wilkins, M. R., & Rabinovitch, M. (2008). Emerging concepts and translational priorities in pulmonary arterial hypertension. *Circulation, 118*(14), 1486–1495.

National Heart, Lung, and Blood Institute (NHLBI). (2011). *Expert panel on integrated guidelines for cardiovascular health and risk reduction in children and adolescents: Summary report.* Bethesda, MD: U.S. Department of Health and Human Services, NHLBI. Retrieved from <http://www.nhlbi.nih.gov/guidelines/cvd_ped/summary.htm#chap5>.

Park, M. K. (2015). *Pediatric cardiology handbook* (5th ed.). St. Louis: Mosby.

Public Health Agency of Canada. (2016). *Canada's provincial and territorial (and catch-up) vaccination programs for infants and children.* Retrieved from <http://healthycanadians.gc.ca/healthy-living-vie-saine/immunization-immunisation/schedule-calendrier/alt/infants-children-vaccination-enfants-nourrissons-eng.pdf>.

Robinson, J. L., Le Saux, N., & Canadian Paediatric Society, Infectious Diseases and Immunization Committee. (2015). Preventing respiratory syncytial virus infections. *Paediatrics & Child Health, 16*(8), 488–490. Reaffirmed 2016. Retrieved from <http://www.cps.ca/en/documents/position/preventing-hospitalizations-for-rsv-infections>.

Rome, J. J., & Kreutzer, J. (2004). Pediatric interventional catheterization: Reasonable expectations and outcomes. *Pediatric Clinics of North America, 51*, 1589–1610.

Schneider, D. J., & Moore, J. W. (2013). Aortic stenosis. In H. D. Allen, D. J. Driscoll, R. E. Shaddy, & T. F. Feltes (Eds.), *Moss and Adams' heart disease in infants, children and adolescents* (7th ed.). Philadelphia: Lippincott Williams & Wilkins.

Son, M. B., & Newburger, J. W. (2016). Kawasaki disease. In R. M. Kliegman, B. F. Stanton, J. St. Geme, et al. (Eds.), *Nelson textbook of pediatrics* (20th ed.). Philadelphia: Saunders.

Spirito, P., Autore, C., Rapezzi, C., et al. (2009). Syncope and risk of sudden death in hypertrophic cardiomyopathy. *Circulation, 1109*, 1703–1710.

Tandberg, B. S., Ystrom, E., Vollrath, M. E., et al. (2010). Feeding infants with CHD with breast milk: Norwegian Mother and Child Cohort Study. *Acta Paediatrica, 99*(3), 373–378. doi:10.1111/j.1651-2227.2009.01605.x.

Templeton, C. G., Cooper, A. R., Human, D. G., & Canadian Paediatric Society. (2007). *Canadian Paediatric Surveillance Program: Acute rheumatic fever.* Retrieved from <http://www.cpsp.cps.ca/uploads/publications/Results-2006.pdf>.

Tweddell, J. S., Hoffman, G. M., Ghanayaren, N. S., et al. (2008). Hypoplastic left heart syndrome. In A. D. Allen, D. J. Driscoll, R. E. Shaddy, et al. (Eds.), *Moss and Adams' heart disease in infants, children and adolescents* (7th ed.). Philadelphia: Lippincott Williams & Wilkins.

Uzark, K. (2001). Therapeutic cardiac catheterization for congenital heart disease: A new era in pediatric care. *Journal of Pediatric Nursing, 16*(5), 300–307.

Van Hare, G. F. (2016). Supraventricular tachycardia. In R. M. Kliegman, B. F. Stanton, J. St. Geme, et al. (Eds.), *Nelson textbook of pediatrics* (20th ed.). Philadelphia: Saunders.

Wilson, W., Taubert, K., Gewitz, M., et al. (2007). Prevention of infective endocarditis: Guidelines from the American Heart Association. *Circulation, 116*(15), 1736–1754. doi:10.1161/CIRCULATIONAHA.106.183095.

ADDITIONAL RESOURCES

Canadian Pediatric Society. Position statement on cardiac risk assessment before the use of stimulant medications in children and youth: <http://www.ccs.ca/images/Guidelines/Guidelines_POS_Library/Peds_PS_2009.pdf>

Heart & Stroke Foundation. Canadian Resuscitation and First Aid Guidelines: <http://www.heartandstroke.com/site/c.ikIQLcMWJtE/b.9298365/k.7519/2015_Canadian_Resuscitation_and_First_Aid_Guidelines.htm>

Heart and Stroke Foundation. Heart and Soul: Your Guide to Living With Congenital Heart Disease: <http://www.heartandstroke.com/atf/cf/%7B99452D8B-E7F1-4BD6-A57D-B136CE6C95BF%7D/HeartandSoul_English.pdf>

The Hospital for Sick Kids. Congenital Heart Conditions Resource Centre: <http://www.aboutkidshealth.ca/En/ResourceCentres/CongenitalHeartConditions/Pages/default.aspx>

Western Canadian Children's Heart Network. Family Support & Resources: <http://www.westernchildrensheartnetwork.ca/family-support-resources/>

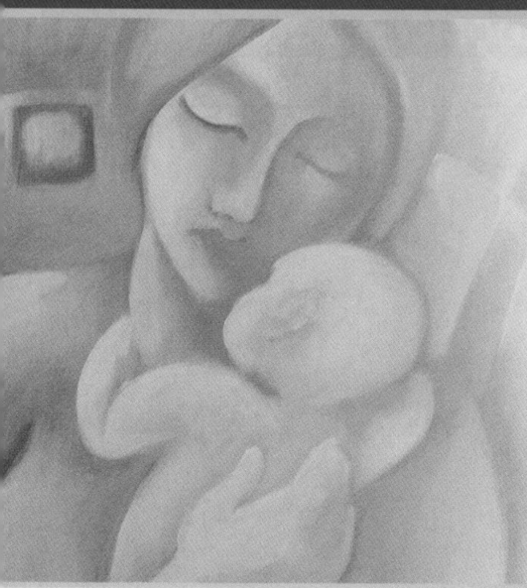

CHAPTER 48

Hematological or Immunological Dysfunction

Katherine Bertoni

evolve WEBSITE

Visit the Evolve website for additional resources related to the content in this chapter such as Case Studies, Critical Thinking Case Study Answers, Nursing Care Plans, Nursing Processes, Nursing Skills, and Review Questions for Exam Preparation at: *http://evolve.elsevier.com/Canada/Perry/maternal/*

OBJECTIVES

On completion of this chapter the reader will be able to:

- Distinguish between the various categories of anemia.
- Describe the prevention of iron-deficiency anemia and the care of the child with iron-deficiency anemia.
- Compare sickle cell anemia and beta thalassemia major in relation to pathophysiology and nursing care.
- Describe the mechanisms of inheritance and nursing care of the child with hemophilia.
- Distinguish between the pathophysiology and nursing care of idiopathic thrombocytopenic purpura (ITP) and disseminated intravascular coagulation (DIC).
- Relate the pathophysiology and clinical manifestations of aplastic anemia and leukemia.
- Demonstrate an understanding of the rationale of therapies for neoplastic disease.
- Outline a plan of care for the child with neoplastic disease and the family.
- Contrast the pathophysiology and management of the immunodeficiency disorders.
- List nursing precautions and responsibilities during blood transfusion.
- Describe the types of hematopoietic stem cell transplants.

HEMATOLOGICAL AND IMMUNOLOGICAL DYSFUNCTION

Several tests can be performed to assess hematological function, including additional procedures to identify the cause of the dysfunction. The following discussion is limited to a description of the complete blood cell count (CBC). The CBC is the most common and one of the most valuable tests used. Other procedures, such as those related to iron, coagulation, and immune status, are discussed throughout the chapter as appropriate. The nurse should be familiar with the significance of the findings from the CBC (Table 48-1) and be aware of normal values for all ages, which are listed in Appendix D.

As with any disorder, the health history and physical examination are essential to identify hematological dysfunction, and the nurse is often the first person to suspect a problem based on information from these sources. Comments by the parent(s) regarding the child's lack of energy, food diary of poor sources of iron, frequent infections, and bleeding that is difficult to control offer clues to the more common disorders affecting the blood. A careful physical appraisal, especially of the skin, can reveal findings (e.g., pallor, petechiae, bruising) that may indicate minor or serious hematological conditions. Nurses need to be aware of the clinical manifestations of blood diseases in order to assist in recognizing symptoms and establishing a diagnosis.

RED BLOOD CELL DISORDERS

Anemia

The term *anemia* describes a condition in which the number of red blood cells (RBCs) or the hemoglobin (Hgb or Hb) concentration is reduced below normal values for gender and age. This diminishes the oxygen-carrying capacity of the blood, causing a reduction in the oxygen available to the tissues. Anemia is the most common hematological disorder of infancy

TABLE 48-1 TESTS PERFORMED AS PART OF THE COMPLETE BLOOD CELL COUNT

TEST*	DESCRIPTION AND COMMENTS
Red blood cell (RBC) count	Number of RBCs per 10^{12} cells/L of blood RBCs carry oxygen from the lungs to the rest of the body Indirectly estimates Hgb content of blood Reflects function of bone marrow
Hemoglobin (Hgb) determination	Amount of Hgb g/L of whole blood Total blood Hgb primarily dependent on number of circulating RBCs but also on amount of Hgb in each cell
Hematocrit (Hct)	Percent volume of packed RBCs in whole blood Indirectly measures Hgb content
RBC indices	
Mean corpuscular volume (MCV)	Average or mean volume (size) of a single RBC MCV values are expressed as femtolitres (fL)
Mean corpuscular hemoglobin (MCH)	Average or mean quantity (weight) of Hgb in a single RBC MCH values are expressed as picograms (pg) MCV and MCH depend on accurate counts of RBCs, whereas MCHC does not; thus MCHC is often more reliable All indexes depend on average cell measurements and do not show individual RBC variations (anisocytosis)
Mean corpuscular hemoglobin concentration (MCHC)	Average concentration of Hgb in a single RBC MCHC values are expressed as g/dL
RBC volume distribution width (RDW)	Average size of RBCs Differentiates some types of anemia
Reticulocyte count	Percent reticulocytes in RBCs Index of production of mature RBCs by bone marrow • Decreased count indicates depressed bone marrow function • Increased count indicates erythrogenesis in response to some stimulus When reticulocyte count is extremely high, other forms of immature RBCs (normoblasts, even erythroblasts) may be present Indirectly estimates hypochromic anemia Usually elevated in patients with chronic hemolytic anemia
White blood cell (WBC) count	Number of WBCs × 10^9/L of blood • Increased with infection or inflammation, trauma, tissue necrosis, hemorrhage or leukemia • Decreased with viral infection, hypersplenism, bone marrow, depression Total number of WBCs less important than differential count
Differential WBC count	Inspection and quantification of WBC types present in peripheral blood Values are expressed as percentages; to obtain absolute number of any type of WBC, multiply its respective percentage by total number of WBCs
Neutrophils (polys)	Primary defence in bacterial infection; capable of phagocytizing and killing bacteria
Bands	Immature neutrophil Increased numbers in bacterial infection Also capable of phagocytosis and killing
Eosinophils	Named for their staining characteristics with eosin dye Increased in allergic disorders, parasitic diseases, certain neoplasms, and other diseases
Basophils	Named for their characteristic basophilic stippling Contain histamine, heparin, and serotonin; believed to cause increased blood flow to injured tissues while preventing excessive clotting. Can increase in cases of leukemia, during inflammatory processes, or viral infections
Lymphocytes	Involved in development of antibody and delayed hypersensitivity
Monocytes	Large phagocytic cells that are involved in early stage of inflammatory reaction
Absolute neutrophil count (ANC)	Percent neutrophils/bands × WBC count Indicates capability of body to handle bacterial infections
Platelet count	Number of platelets × 10^9/L of blood Cellular fragments that are necessary for clotting to occur
Stained peripheral blood smear	Visual estimation of amount of Hgb in RBCs and overall size, shape, and structure of RBCs Various staining properties of RBC structures may be evidence of immature forms of erythrocytes Shows variation in size and shape of RBCs: microcytic, macrocytic, poikilocytic (variable shapes)

*See Appendix D for normal values according to ages. Values may vary between Canadian laboratories.

and childhood and is not a disease itself but an indication or manifestation of an underlying pathological process.

Classification

Anemias are classified in relation to (1) *etiology* or *physiology*, manifested by erythrocyte or Hgb depletion, and (2) *morphology*, the characteristic changes in RBC size, shape, or colour (Box 48-1). Although the morphological classification is more useful in terms of laboratory evaluation of anemia, the etiological approach provides direction for planning nursing care. For example, anemia with reduced Hgb concentration may be caused by a dietary depletion of iron, and the principal intervention is replenishing iron stores. The classification of anemias is found in Fig. 48-1.

BOX 48-1 RED BLOOD CELL MORPHOLOGY

Size (Cell Size)
Variation in red blood cell (RBC) sizes (anisocytosis)
- Normocytes (normal cell size)
- Microcytes (smaller than normal cell size)
- Macrocytes (larger than normal cell size)

Shape (Cell Shape)
Variation in RBC shapes (poikilocytosis)
- Spherocytes (globular cells)
- Drepanocytes (sickle-shaped cells)
- Numerous other irregularly shaped cells

Colour (Cell Staining Characteristics)
Variation in hemoglobin concentration in the RBCs
- Normochromic (sufficient or normal amount of hemoglobin per RBC)
- Hypochromic (reduced amount of hemoglobin per RBC)
- Hyperchromic (increased amount of hemoglobin per RBC)

Consequences of Anemia

The basic physiological defect caused by anemia is a decrease in the oxygen-carrying capacity of blood and consequently a reduction in the amount of oxygen available to the cells. When the anemia has developed slowly, the child usually adapts to the declining Hgb level.

The effects of anemia on the circulatory system can be profound. Because the viscosity of blood depends almost entirely on the concentration of RBCs, the resulting hemodilution of severe anemia decreases peripheral resistance, causing greater quantities of blood to return to the heart. The increased circulation and turbulence within the heart may produce a murmur. Because the cardiac workload is greatly increased, especially during exercise, infection, or emotional stress, cardiac failure may ensue.

Children seem to have a remarkable ability to function well despite low levels of Hgb. Cyanosis (the result of the quantity of deoxygenated Hgb in arterial blood) is typically not evident. Growth restriction, resulting from decreased cellular metabolism and coexisting anorexia, is a common finding in chronic severe anemia and is frequently accompanied by delayed sexual maturation in the older child.

Diagnostic Evaluation

In general, anemia may be suspected on the basis of findings in the health history and physical examination, such as lack of energy, easy fatigability, and pallor; however, unless the anemia is severe, the first clue to the disorder may be alterations in the CBC, such as decreased RBCs, and decreased Hgb and hematocrit (Hct) levels (see Fig. 48-1). Although anemia is sometimes

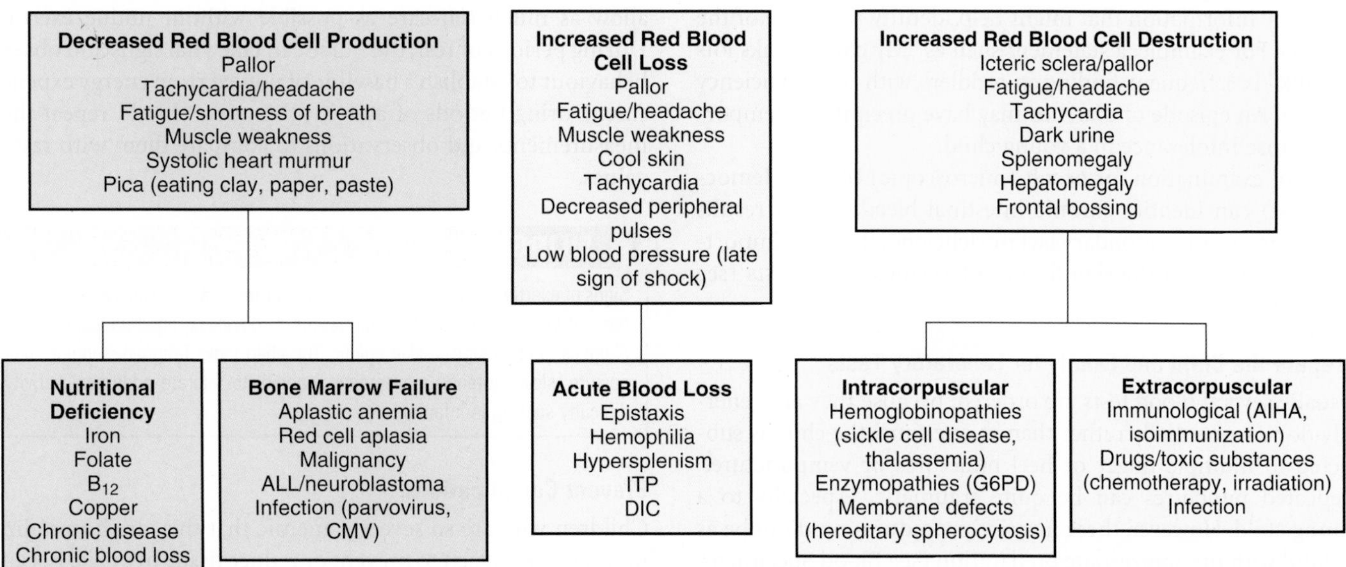

FIGURE 48-1 Classifications of anemias. *AIHA*, autoimmune hemolytic anemia; *ALL*, acute lymphoid leukemia; *CMV*, cytomegalovirus; *DIC*, disseminated intravascular coagulation; *G6PD*, glucose-6-phosphate dehydrogenase; *ITP*, idiopathic thrombocytopenic purpura.

defined as a Hgb level below 100 or 110 g/L, this arbitrary cutoff is inappropriate for all children, because Hgb levels normally vary with age and comorbid conditions (see Appendix D).

Other tests specific to a particular type of anemia are used to determine the underlying cause of anemia. These are discussed in relation to the particular disorder.

Therapeutic Management

The objectives of medical management are to reverse the anemia by treating the underlying cause and to make up for any deficiency of blood, blood component, or substance the blood needs for normal functioning. For example, blood or blood cells are replaced after hemorrhage; in nutritional anemias the specific deficiency is replaced.

In patients with severe anemia, supportive medical care may include oxygen therapy, bedrest, and replacement of intravascular volume with intravenous (IV) fluids. The prognosis for anemia depends on the correction of the cause.

NURSING CARE

The assessment of anemia includes the basic techniques that are applicable to any condition. The age of the infant or child provides some clues regarding the possible etiology of the anemia. For example, iron-deficiency anemia occurs more frequently in infants and children between 6 and 36 months of age and during the growth spurt of adolescence.

Racial or ethnic background is also significant. For example, the anemias related to abnormal Hgb levels are found in Southeast Asians and persons of African or Mediterranean ancestry. These same groups may be genetically predisposed to be deficient in the enzyme lactase after the period of infancy. Affected individuals are unable to tolerate lactose in the diet, with consequent intestinal irritation and chronic blood loss.

Special emphasis should be placed on a careful history to elicit any information that might help identify the cause of the anemia. For example, a statement such as "My child drinks lots of milk" is a frequent finding in toddlers with iron-deficiency anemia. An episode of diarrhea may have precipitated temporary lactose intolerance in a young child.

Stool examination for occult (microscopic) blood (Hemoccult test) can identify chronic intestinal bleeding that results from a primary or secondary lactase deficiency. It is also important to understand the significance of various blood tests (see Table 48-1).

Prepare the Child and Family for Laboratory Tests

Usually several blood tests are ordered; because they are generally done sequentially rather than at one time, the child is subjected to multiple finger or heel punctures or venipunctures. Repeated punctures can be quite traumatic, especially to a young child. However, these invasive procedures need not be as painful with the appropriate preparation (see Blood Specimens, Chapter 44). For example, the topical application of a eutectic mix of lidocaine and prilocaine (EMLA) before needle punctures can significantly reduce pain (see Pain Management, Chapter 34). The nurse is responsible for preparing the child and family for the tests by doing the following:

- Explaining the significance of each test, particularly why the tests are not all done at one time
- Encouraging parents or another supportive person to be with the child during the procedure
- Allowing the child to play with the equipment on a doll or participate in the actual procedure (e.g., by cleansing the finger with an alcohol swab)

Older children may appreciate the opportunity to observe the blood cells under a microscope or in photographs. This experience is especially important if a serious blood disorder, such as leukemia, is suspected, because it serves as a foundation for explaining the pathophysiology of the disorder.

Bone marrow aspiration is not a routine hematological test but is essential for definitive diagnosis of the leukemias, lymphomas, and certain anemias.

! NURSING ALERT

The following are suggested explanations for teaching children about blood components:

Red blood cells (RBCs)—Carry the oxygen you breathe from your lungs to all parts of your body

White blood cells (WBCs)—Help keep germs from causing infection

Platelets—Small parts of cells that help make bleeding stop by forming a clot (scab) over the hurt area

Plasma—The liquid portion of blood, which has clotting factors that help make bleeding stop

Decrease Tissue Oxygen Needs

Because the basic pathological process in anemia is a decrease in oxygen-carrying capacity, an important nursing responsibility is to assess the child's energy level and minimize excess demands. The child's level of tolerance for activities of daily living and play needs to be assessed and adjustments made to allow as much self-care as possible without undue exertion. During periods of rest, the nurse can take vital signs and observe behaviour to establish a baseline of nonexertion energy expenditure. During periods of activity, the nurse should repeat these measurements and observations to compare them with resting values.

NURSING ALERT

Signs of exertion include tachycardia, palpitations, tachypnea, dyspnea, shortness of breath, hyperpnea, breathlessness, dizziness, lightheadedness, diaphoresis, and change in skin colour. The child looks fatigued (sagging, limp posture; slow, strained movements; inability to tolerate additional activity; difficulty sucking in infants).

Prevent Complications

Children who are so severely anemic that they are hospitalized may require oxygen to prevent or reduce tissue hypoxia. Because these children are susceptible to infection, every effort should be made to prevent exposure to infectious agents. All the usual precautions need to be taken to prevent infection, such as practising thorough hand hygiene, selecting an appropriate room in a noninfectious area, restricting visitors or hospital personnel with active infection, and maintaining adequate nutrition. The nurse also needs to observe for signs of infection, particularly temperature elevation and leukocytosis.

Iron-Deficiency Anemia

While the rate of iron-deficiency anemia in Canada is low (3.5 to 10%), there are certain Indigenous populations in which the rate is high (Abdullah, Zlotkin, Parkin, et al., 2011). Canadian Indigenous infants and children have a prevalence of iron-deficiency anemia of up to 36% compared to 3.5 to 10% for non-Indigenous children (Christofides, Schauer, & Zlotkin, 2005; Pacey, 2009). Factors associated with an increased prevalence of iron-deficiency anemia in these children include high consumption of evaporated milk and cow's milk after 6 months of age, prolonged exclusive breastfeeding (with limited access to other food sources), and *Helicobacter pylori* infection. Other high-risk groups include children from families of low socioeconomic status, children of Asian background, low-birth-weight infants, and children who drink whole cow's milk before 12 months of age (Abdullah et al., 2011). Preterm infants are especially at risk because of their reduced fetal iron supply. Elemental iron supplementation (2 mg/kg/day to 3 mg/kg/day once the infant is on full feeds) is recommended to prevent later iron-deficiency anemia. Noninvasive monitoring for tests such as carbon dioxide and bilirubin and clustering blood samples will minimize the amount of blood being taken (Lemyre, Sample, Lacaze-Masmonteil, et al., 2015). In addition, adolescents are also at risk because of their rapid growth rate combined with possible poor eating habits.

Pathophysiology

Iron-deficiency anemia can be caused by any number of factors that decrease the supply of iron, impair its absorption, increase the body's need for iron, or affect the synthesis of Hgb. Although the clinical manifestations and diagnostic evaluations are similar regardless of the cause, the therapeutic and nursing care management depends on the specific reason for the iron deficiency. The following discussion is limited to iron-deficiency anemia resulting from inadequate iron in the diet.

During the last trimester of pregnancy, iron is transferred from mother to fetus. Most of the iron is stored in the circulating erythrocytes of the fetus, with the remainder stored in the fetal liver, spleen, and bone marrow. These iron stores are usually adequate for the first 5 to 6 months in a full-term infant but for only 2 to 3 months in preterm infants or multiple births. If dietary iron is not supplied to meet the infant's growth demands after the fetal iron stores are depleted, iron-deficiency anemia results. Physiological anemia should not be confused with iron-deficiency anemia resulting from nutritional causes.

Although most toddlers with iron-deficiency anemia are underweight, many infants are overweight because of excessive milk ingestion (known as *milk babies*). These children become anemic because milk is a poor source of iron and is given almost to the exclusion of solid foods; also, 50% of iron-deficient infants that are fed cow's milk have an increased fecal loss of blood.

Therapeutic Management

After the diagnosis of iron-deficiency anemia is made, therapeutic management focuses on increasing the amount of supplemental iron the child receives. This is usually done through dietary counselling and the administration of oral iron supplements.

In formula-fed infants, the most convenient and best sources of supplemental iron are iron-fortified commercial formula and iron-fortified infant cereal. Iron-fortified formula provides a relatively constant and predictable amount of iron and is not associated with an increased incidence of gastrointestinal (GI) symptoms, such as colic, diarrhea, or constipation. Infants younger than 9 to 12 months of age should not be given fresh cow's milk because it may increase the risk of GI blood loss occurring from allergy to the milk protein or from GI mucosal damage resulting from a lack of cytochrome iron (heme protein) (Abdullah et al., 2011). If GI bleeding is suspected, the child's stool should be guaiac tested on at least four or five occasions to identify any intermittent blood loss.

Dietary addition of iron-rich foods is usually inadequate as the sole treatment of iron-deficiency anemia, since the iron is poorly absorbed and thus provides insufficient supplemental quantities. If dietary sources of iron cannot replace body stores, oral iron supplements are prescribed for approximately 3 months. Ferrous iron, more readily absorbed than ferric iron, results in higher Hgb levels. Ascorbic acid (vitamin C) appears to facilitate the absorption of iron and may be given as vitamin C–enriched foods and juices with the iron preparation.

If the Hgb level fails to rise after 1 month of oral therapy, it is important to assess for persistent bleeding, iron malabsorption, noncompliance, improper iron administration, or other causes for the anemia. Parenteral (IV or intramuscular [IM]) iron administration is safe and effective but painful, expensive, and occasionally associated with regional lymphadenopathy or allergic reaction (Fleming, 2014). Thus parenteral iron is reserved for children who have iron malabsorption or chronic hemoglobinuria. Transfusions are indicated for the most severe anemia and in cases of serious infection, cardiac dysfunction, or surgical emergency when anaesthesia is required. Packed RBCs (2 to 3 mL/kg), not whole blood, are used to minimize the chance of circulatory overload. Supplemental oxygen is administered when tissue hypoxia is severe.

Prognosis

The prognosis for a child with this condition is very good. However, there is some evidence that, if the iron-deficiency anemia is severe and long-standing, cognitive, behavioural, and motor impairment may result. It is not clear whether these results are irreversible with treatment of iron (Abdullah et al., 2011).

NURSING CARE

An essential nursing responsibility is instructing parents in the administration of iron. Oral iron should be given as prescribed in two divided doses between meals, when the presence of free hydrochloric acid is greatest, since more iron is absorbed in the acidic environment of the upper GI tract. Citrus fruit or juice taken with the medication aids in absorption.

> **! NURSING ALERT**
>
> Cow's milk contains substances that bind the iron and interfere with absorption. Iron supplements should not be administered with milk or milk products.

An adequate dosage of oral iron turns the stools a tarry green colour. The nurse needs to advise parents of this normally expected change and inquire about its occurrence on follow-up visits. Absence of the greenish black stool may be a clue to poor administration of iron, in either schedule or dosage. Vomiting or diarrhea can occur with iron therapy. If the parents report these symptoms, the iron can be given with meals and the dosage reduced and then gradually increased until tolerated.

Liquid preparations of iron may temporarily stain the teeth. If possible, the medication should be taken through a straw or given through a syringe or medicine dropper placed toward the back of the mouth. Brushing the teeth after administration of the medication lessens the discolouration.

Diet

A primary nursing objective is to prevent nutritional anemia through education of the family about diet. Exclusively breastfed infants as well as formula-fed infants should be fed solid foods that are iron-rich, in the form of meat, fish, eggs, or iron-fortified cereals as first foods at 6 months of age (Critch & Canadian Paediatric Society [CPS], Nutrition and Gastroenterology Committee, 2013; Health Canada, 2015). Preterm infants fed human milk should begin iron supplements by 1 month of age (Abdullah et al., 2011).

It may be difficult at first to teach the infant to accept foods other than milk. Solid food should be fed before the milk (see Nutrition, Chapter 35).

A difficulty encountered in discouraging the parents from feeding milk to the exclusion of other foods is dispelling the popular myth that milk is a "perfect food." Many parents believe that milk is best for the infant and equate the weight gain with a "healthy child" and "good mothering." The nurse can also stress that overweight is not synonymous with good health.

Sickle Cell Anemia

Sickle cell anemia (SCA) is one of a group of diseases collectively termed *hemoglobinopathies*, in which normal adult Hgb (Hgb A [HbA]) is partly or completely replaced by abnormal sickle HgbS (HbS). Sickle cell disease (SCD) includes all the hereditary disorders with clinical, hematological, and pathological features that are related to the presence of HgbS. Even though the term *SCD* is sometimes used to refer to SCA, this use is incorrect. Other correct terms for SCA are *HgbSS disease* and *homozygous sickle cell disease*.

The following are the most common forms of SCD:

SCA—the homozygous form of the disease (HgbSS or SS)

Sickle cell–C disease—a heterozygous variant of SCD (HgbSC), including both HgbS and HgbC (SC), in which lysine is substituted for glutamic acid at the sixth position of the beta chain

Sickle thalassemia disease—a combination of sickle cell trait and beta thalassemia trait (Sβ-thal); β+ refers to the ability to still produce some normal HbA; β^0 indicates that there is no ability to produce HbA

Of the SCDs, SCA is the most common form in Blacks, followed by sickle cell–C disease and sickle thalassemia. Numerous other sickle syndromes exist when the HbS is paired with other mutant globins.

SCA is found in 1 in 396 births of Blacks and 1 in 36,000 births of Latin Americans, with lower incidences in other ethnic groups (DeBaun, Frei-Jones, & Vichinsky, 2016). The incidence of the disease varies in different geographic locations. In Canada, up to 1 in every 2500 births will result in sickle cell disease (Sickle Cell Disease Association of Canada, 2013). Among Blacks, the incidence of the sickle cell trait is about 9%. In West Africa, the incidence is reported to be as high as 40% among native Africans. The high incidence of the sickle cell trait in West Africans is believed to be the result of selective protection afforded trait carriers against one type of malaria.

The gene that determines the production of HgbS is situated on an autosome and, when present, is always detectable and therefore dominant. Heterozygous persons who have both normal HgbA and abnormal HgbS are said to have the *sickle cell trait*. Persons who are homozygous have predominantly HgbS and have SCA. The inheritance pattern is essentially that of an autosomal recessive disorder. Therefore, when both parents have the sickle cell trait, there is a 25% chance with each pregnancy of producing an offspring with SCA.

Although the defect is inherited, the sickling phenomenon is usually not apparent until later in infancy because of the presence of fetal Hgb (HgbF). As long as the child has predominantly HgbF, sickling does not occur because there is less HgbS. The newborn with SCA is generally asymptomatic because of the protective effect of HgbF (60 to 80% HgbF), but this rapidly decreases during the first year; thus the child is at risk for sickle cell–related complications (Heeney & Dover, 2014).

Pathophysiology

The clinical features of SCA are primarily the result of (1) obstruction caused by the sickled RBCs, (2) vascular inflammation, and (3) increased RBC destruction (Fig. 48-2). The abnormal adhesion, entanglement, and enmeshing of rigid sickle-shaped cells accompanied by the inflammatory process intermittently block the microcirculation, causing vaso-occlusion. The resultant absence of blood flow to adjacent tissues causes local hypoxia, leading to tissue ischemia and infarction (cellular death). Most of the complications seen in SCA can be traced to this process and its impact on various organs of the body. The effect of sickling and infarction on organ structures occurs in the following sequence (Box 48-2):

1. Stasis with enlargement
2. Infarction with ischemia and repeated destruction
3. Replacement with fibrous tissue (scarring)

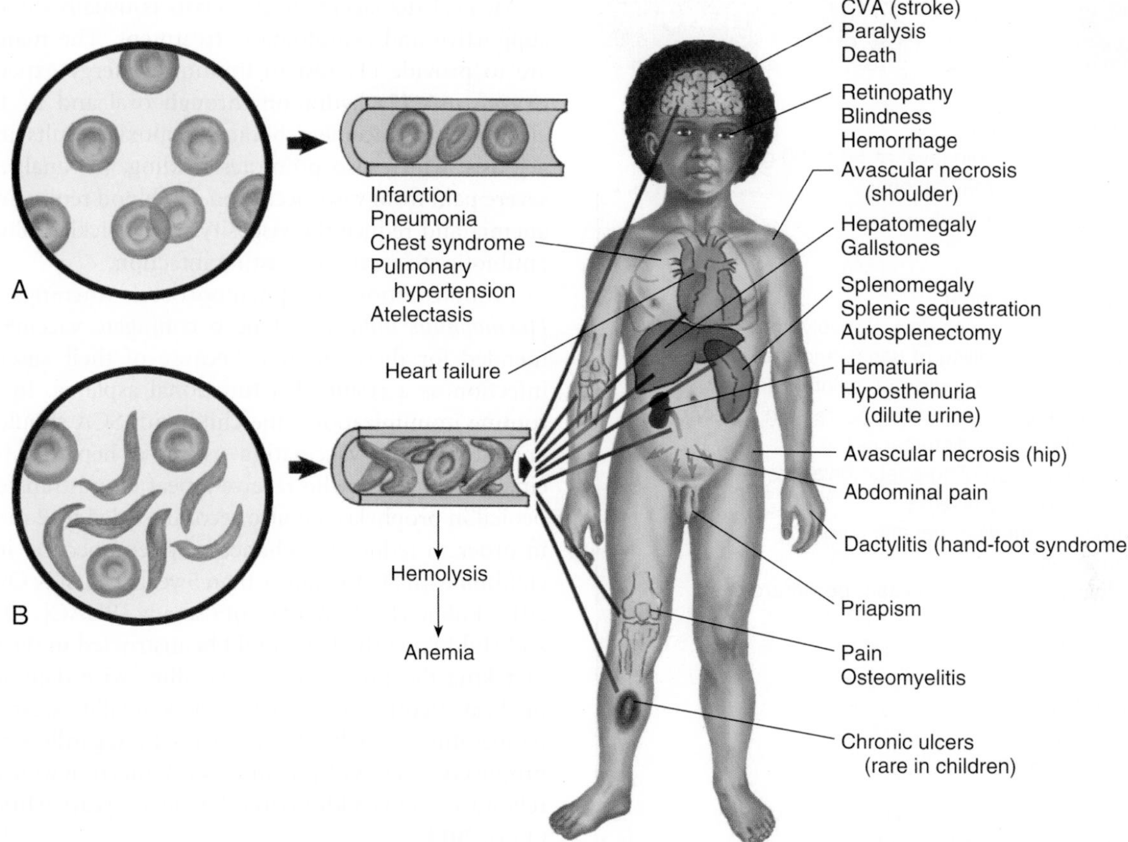

FIGURE 48-2 Differences between effects on circulation of normal **(A)** and sickled **(B)** red blood cells with related complications. *CVA*, cerebrovascular accident.

Clinical Manifestations

The clinical manifestations of SCA vary greatly in severity and frequency. The most acute symptoms of the disease occur during periods of exacerbation called *crises*. There are several types of episodic crises: vaso-occlusive, acute splenic sequestration, aplastic, hyperhemolytic, cerebrovascular accident (CVA) (stroke), chest syndrome, and infection. The crises may occur individually or concomitantly with one or more other crises. The *vaso-occlusive crisis* (VOC), preferably called a "painful episode," is characterized by ischemia causing mild to severe pain that may last from minutes to days. *Sequestration crisis* is a pooling of a large amount of blood—usually in the spleen and infrequently in the liver—that causes a decreased blood volume and ultimately shock. *Aplastic crisis* is diminished RBC production usually caused by viral infection that may result in profound anemia. *Hyperhemolytic crisis* is an accelerated rate of RBC destruction characterized by anemia, jaundice, and reticulocytosis.

Another serious complication is acute chest syndrome (ACS), which is clinically similar to pneumonia. It is the presence of a new pulmonary infiltrate and is associated with chest pain, fever, cough, tachypnea, wheezing, and hypoxia.

A CVA (stroke) is a sudden and severe complication, often with no related illnesses. Sickled cells block the major blood vessels in the brain, resulting in cerebral infarction, which causes variable degrees of neurological impairment. The current treatment for SCA children who have experienced a stroke is chronic transfusion therapy. Repeat CVAs causing progressively greater brain damage occur in approximately 70% of untreated children who have experienced one stroke and do not receive monthly transfusions (Heeney & Dover, 2014).

Diagnostic Evaluation

Currently, British Columbia, Ontario, and most of Quebec offer routine newborn screening for SCA. At birth the infant has up to 80% of HgbF, which does not carry the defect. Because levels of HgbS are low at birth, Hgb electrophoresis or other tests that measure Hgb concentrations are indicated. Nurses can use antenatal documents to identify populations at risk. Early diagnosis (before 3 months of age) enables initiation of appropriate interventions to minimize complications. The family should be taught to administer prophylactic antibiotics, to identify early signs of infection, and to seek medical therapy as soon as possible.

If SCA is not diagnosed in early infancy, it is likely to manifest symptoms during the toddler and preschool years. SCA is occasionally first diagnosed during a crisis that follows an acute respiratory tract or GI infection. Routine hematological tests are done to evaluate the anemia. Several specific tests can be used to detect the presence of the abnormal Hgb in the heterozygote or the homozygote. For screening purposes the sickle-turbidity test (Sickledex) is frequently used, because it can be

BOX 48-2 CLINICAL MANIFESTATIONS OF SICKLE CELL ANEMIA

General
Possible growth restriction
Chronic anemia (hemoglobin level of 60 to 90 g/L)
Possible delayed sexual maturation
Marked susceptibility to sepsis

Vaso-Occlusive Crisis
Pain in area(s) of involvement
Manifestations related to ischemia of involved areas
Extremities—Painful swelling of hands and feet (sickle cell dactylitis, or hand–foot syndrome), painful joints
Abdomen—Severe pain resembling acute surgical condition
Cerebrum—Stroke, visual disturbances
Chest—Symptoms resembling pneumonia, protracted episodes of pulmonary disease
Liver—Obstructive jaundice, hepatic coma
Kidney—Hematuria
Genitalia—Priapism (painful, constant penile erection)

Sequestration Crisis
Pooling of large amounts of blood
- Hepatomegaly
- Splenomegaly
- Circulatory collapse

Effects of Chronic Vaso-Occlusive Phenomena
Heart—Cardiomegaly, systolic murmurs
Lungs—Altered pulmonary function, susceptibility to infections, pulmonary insufficiency
Kidneys—Inability to concentrate urine, enuresis, progressive renal failure
Liver—Hepatomegaly, cirrhosis, intrahepatic cholestasis
Spleen—Splenomegaly, susceptibility to infection, functional reduction in splenic activity progressing to autosplenectomy
Eyes—Intraocular abnormalities with visual disturbances; sometimes progressive retinal detachment and blindness
Extremities—Avascular necrosis of hip or shoulder; skeletal deformities, especially lordosis and kyphosis; chronic leg ulcers; susceptibility to osteomyelitis
Central nervous system—Hemiparesis, seizures

performed on blood from a finger stick and yields accurate results in 3 minutes. However, if the test is positive, Hgb electrophoresis is necessary to distinguish between children with the trait and those with the disease. Hgb electrophoresis ("fingerprinting" of the protein) is an accurate, rapid, and specific test for detecting the homozygous and heterozygous forms of the disease and the percentages of the various types of Hgb.

Therapeutic Management

The aims of therapy are to (1) prevent the sickling phenomena, which are responsible for the pathological sequelae, and (2) effectively treat the medical emergencies of sickle cell crisis. The successful achievement of the aims depends on prompt nursing interventions, medical therapies, patient and family preventive measures, and use of innovative treatments.

Medical management of a crisis is usually directed toward supportive and symptomatic treatment. The main objectives are to provide (1) rest to minimize energy expenditure and oxygen use, (2) hydration through oral and IV therapy, (3) electrolyte replacement because hypoxia results in metabolic acidosis, which also promotes sickling, (4) analgesics for the severe pain from vaso-occlusion, (5) blood replacement to treat anemia and reduce the viscosity of the sickled blood, and (6) antibiotics to treat any existing infection.

Administration of pneumococcal, meningococcal, and *Haemophilus influenzae* type b conjugate vaccines is recommended for these children because of their susceptibility to infection as a result of a functional asplenia. In addition to routine immunizations, the child with SCA should receive an annual influenza vaccination, as well as hepatitis A and B vaccination for those who receive repeat blood transfusions. Oral penicillin prophylaxis is also recommended by 2 months of age in order to reduce the chance of pneumococcal infections in children with SCA younger than 5 years (Hirst & Owusu-Ofori, 2014; Public Health Agency of Canada [PHAC], 2016). Parents and children with SCA should be instructed in the importance of taking the prophylactic penicillin twice daily and seeking medical attention immediately for acute illness, especially if the temperature exceeds 38.5° C (101.3° F), regardless of the use of prophylaxis. Rates of pneumococcal infection were found to be relatively low in children over the age of 5 years (Hirst & Owusu-Ofori, 2014).

Oxygen therapy may be administered during episodes of crisis to prevent additional cell sickling, to provide comfort, and to decrease the incidence of respiratory complications (Ball, Bindler, & Cowen, 2012; Bauman, McClure, & Venner, 2013). Patients admitted for a febrile or vaso-occlusive episode should be carefully assessed and have continuous oxygen saturation monitoring. High-flow oxygen is to be administered to maintain an oxygen saturation of equal to or over 95% for early detection of clinical symptoms and/or changes in oxygenation (Canadian Haemoglobinopathy Association [CHA], 2015).

Exchange transfusion, which reduces the number of circulating sickle cells and slows down the vicious circle of hypoxia, thrombosis, tissue ischemia, and injury, has been successfully used. However, multiple transfusions carry the risk of transmission of viral infection, hyperviscosity, transfusion reactions, alloimmunization, and hemosiderosis (Driscoll, 2007; Heeney & Dover, 2014). Packed RBC transfusions may be used for treatment of splenic sequestration and stroke and preoperatively for surgical procedures in the child with SCA. Unless the child has heart failure, dyspnea, hypotension, or marked fatigue, a blood transfusion is avoided unless the hemoglobin has decreased to <50 to 60 g/L (CHA, 2015). The child with SCA should be transfused with phenotypically matched red cells to reduce the risk of alloimmunization and hemolytic transfusion reactions (CHA, 2015). To reduce iron overload from chronic transfusion therapy, chelation therapy may be started (see Chapter 46, p. 1469).

In children with recurrent life-threatening splenic sequestration, splenectomy may be a lifesaving measure. However, the spleen usually atrophies on its own through progressive fibrotic changes (functional asplenia) by 6 years of age in children with SCA. Prophylactic penicillin postsplenectomy and pneumococcal vaccines have decreased the incidence of pneumococcal sepsis.

The most common and debilitating symptom experienced by patients with SCA is vaso-occlusive pain. The chronic nature of this pain can greatly affect the child's development. A multidisciplinary approach is best for vaso-occlusive pain management, which includes pharmacological treatment, hydration, physiotherapy, and complementary treatment (e.g., prayer, spiritual healing, massage, heat, herbs, relaxation, acupuncture, and biofeedback) (Brandow, Weisman, & Panepinto, 2011). See Chapter 34 for more information on pain control.

For mild to moderate pain, nonsteroidal anti-inflammatory medication (e.g., ibuprofen, ketorolac) or acetaminophen (Tylenol) is used initially. If these medications are not effective alone, opioids can be added. The dosages of both medications are titrated (adjusted) to a therapeutic level. Opioids such as immediate- and sustained-release morphine, oxycodone, hydromorphone (Dilaudid), and methadone are administered intravenously or orally for severe pain and given around the clock. Patient-controlled analgesia (PCA) has been used successfully for sickle cell–related pain. PCA reinforces the patient's role and responsibility in managing the pain and provides flexibility in dealing with pain, which may vary in severity over time (see Pain Management, Chapter 34).

Hydroxyurea is a medication that increases the production of hemoglobin F—fetal hemoglobin that decreases endothelial adhesion of sickle cells, improves the sickle cell hydration, increases nitric oxide production (a vasodilator), and reduces leukocyte and reticulocyte counts (McGann & Ware, 2011). Hydroxyurea is a *Health Canada Food and Drug Act*–approved medication. Long-term follow-up of patients taking hydroxyurea alone revealed a 40% reduction in mortality and decreased frequency of vaso-occlusive crises (VOC), acute chest syndrome (ACS), hospital admissions, and need for transfusions, thus making SCA crises milder (CHA, 2015; McGann & Ware, 2011). Pediatric studies have shown that hydroxyurea can be safely used in children (McGann & Ware, 2011; Wang, Ware, Miller, et al., 2011).

Prognosis

The prognosis varies, but most patients with SCA live into the fifth decade. Most of the time, children are without symptoms and participate in normal activities without restrictions, but they may become fatigued more quickly than their counterparts. The greatest risk is usually in children younger than 5 years of age, and the majority of deaths in these children are caused by overwhelming infection. Consequently, SCA is a chronic illness with a potentially terminal outcome. Physical and sexual maturation are delayed in adolescents with SCA. Although adults achieve normal height, weight, and sexual function, the delay may present problems for the adolescent (Heeney & Dover, 2014). HLA-typing and storage of umbilical cord blood may be considered for siblings of children with SCA. HLA typing may be coordinated with prenatal diagnostic techniques (such as chorionic villus sampling, amniocentesis, or preimplantation genetic diagnosis) to determine if the fetus is affected with SCA (CHA, 2015).

Hematopoietic stem cell transplantation (HSCT) offers the only cure for some children, although the mortality rate is approximately 8% and graft failures after transplantation range from 9 to 14% (DeBaun, et al., 2016; Driscoll, 2007) (see p. 1542).

NURSING CARE

Educate the Family and Child

Family education begins with an explanation of the disease and its consequences. After this explanation, the most important issues to teach the family are to (1) seek early intervention for problems such as fever of 38.5°C (101.3°F) or greater, (2) give penicillin as ordered, (3) recognize signs and symptoms of splenic sequestration and respiratory problems that can lead to hypoxia, and (4) provide the same childhood experiences offered to any other child who is without illness or disease. The nurse needs to convey to the family that the child is a person like any other child but can get sick in ways that other children cannot.

The nurse should emphasize the importance of adequate hydration to prevent sickling and to delay the adhesion–stasis–thrombosis–ischemia cycle in a crisis. It is not sufficient to advise parents to "force fluids" or "encourage drinking." They need specific instructions on how many daily glasses or bottles of fluid are required. Many foods are also a source of fluid, particularly soups, flavoured ice pops, ice cream, sherbet, gelatin, and puddings.

Increased fluids combined with impaired kidney function result in the problem of enuresis. Parents who are unaware of this fact frequently use the usual measures to discourage bedwetting, such as limiting fluids at night, and may resort to punishment and shame to force bladder control. Enuresis is treated as a complication of the disease, such as joint pain or some other symptom, to alleviate parental pressure on the child.

Promote Supportive Therapies During Crises

Management of pain is especially difficult for these children. Unfortunately, these children tend to be undermedicated, resulting in "clock watching" and demands for additional doses sooner than might be expected. Often this incorrectly raises suspicions of drug addiction, when in fact the problem is one of improper dosage (see Family-Centred Teaching box). In choosing and scheduling analgesics, the goal should be *prevention* of pain.

! NURSING ALERT

Advise parents to be particularly alert to situations such as hot weather in which dehydration may be a possibility and to recognize early signs of reduced intake, such as decreased urinary output (e.g., fewer wet diapers) and increased thirst.

FAMILY-CENTRED TEACHING

Fear of Addiction

Although the pain during a sickle cell crisis is usually severe and opioids are needed, many families fear that their child will become addicted to the narcotic. Unfortunately, misinformed health care providers may foster this unfounded fear, which results in a child's needless suffering. Very few children who receive opioids for severe pain become behaviourally addicted to the drug (Lynch & Fischer, 2011). Families and older children, especially adolescents, need to be reassured that opioids are medically indicated, high doses may be needed, and children rarely become addicted.

Any pain program should be combined with psychological support to help the child deal with the depression, anxiety, and fear that may accompany the disease. This includes regular visits with the child to discuss any concerns during the hospitalization and positive reinforcement of coping skills, such as successful methods of dealing with the pain and adherence to treatment prescriptions. To reduce the negative connotation associated with the term sickle cell *crisis*, it is best to say *pain episode*.

Frequently, heat to the affected area is soothing. Cold compresses should not be applied because this enhances sickling and **vasoconstriction**. Bedrest is usually well tolerated during a crisis, although actual rest depends greatly on pain alleviation and organized schedules of nursing care. Some activity, particularly passive range-of-motion exercises, is beneficial to promote circulation. Usually the best course of action is to let children dictate their tolerance of activity.

If blood transfusions or exchange transfusions are given, the nurse has the responsibility of observing for signs of transfusion reaction (see Table 48-4). Because hypervolemia from too-rapid transfusion can increase the workload of the heart, the nurse also needs to be alert to signs of cardiac failure.

In splenic sequestration the size of the spleen is gently measured by abdominal palpation (see Abdomen, Chapter 33). The nurse should be aware of spleen size because increasing splenomegaly is an ominous sign. A decreasing spleen size denotes response to therapy. Vital signs and blood pressure are also closely monitored for impending shock. Anemia is typically not a presenting complication in vaso-occlusive crises, but it is a critical problem in other types of crises. The nurse needs to monitor for evidence of increasing anemia and institute appropriate nursing interventions (see p. 1526). Oxygen saturation level needs to be monitored carefully, and high-flow oxygen is to given if the oxygen saturation level drops below 95% (CHA, 2015).

Intake, especially of IV fluids, and output need to be recorded. The child's weight should be taken on admission to serve as a baseline for evaluating hydration. Because diuresis can result in electrolyte loss, the nurse also should observe for signs of hypokalemia and be familiar with normal serum electrolyte values to report changes.

Recognize Other Complications

Nurses also need to be aware of the signs of ACS and stroke, both potentially fatal complications. It is essential to educate parents about these symptoms.

! NURSING ALERT

Report signs of the following immediately:

Acute Chest Syndrome (ACS)

- Severe chest, back, or abdominal pain
- Fever of 38.5°C (101.3°F) or higher
- Cough
- Dyspnea, tachypnea
- Retractions
- Declining oxygen saturation (oximetry)

CVA

- Severe, unrelieved headaches
- Severe vomiting
- Jerking or twitching of the face, legs, or arms
- Seizures
- Strange, abnormal behaviour
- Inability to move an arm or leg
- Stagger or an unsteady walk
- Stutter or slurred speech
- Weakness in the hands, feet, or legs
- Changes in vision

Support the Family

Families need the opportunity to discuss their feelings about genetically transmitting a potentially fatal, chronic illness to their child. Because of the widely publicized prognosis for children with SCA, many parents express their prevalent fear of the child's death. Three manifestations of SCA that may appear in the first 2 years of life—dactylitis or painful episode, severe anemia (70 g/L), and elevated WBC count—can be predictors of disease severity (DeBaun et al., 2016; Lerner, 2016). However, nursing care for the family should be the same as for any family with a child with a life-threatening illness. The siblings' reactions, the stress on the parent's relationship, and the child-rearing attitudes displayed toward the child should be given particular emphasis (see Chapter 31). Several resources are available to the family with a sickling disorder (see Additional Resources at the end of this chapter).

The nurse needs to advise parents to inform all treating personnel of the child's condition. The use of medical identification, such as a bracelet, is another way of ensuring awareness of the disease.

If family members have the SCD trait or SCA, genetic counselling is necessary. A primary consideration in genetic counselling is informing parents of the 25% chance with each pregnancy of having a child with the disease when both parents carry the trait.

Beta Thalassemia (Cooley Anemia)

Worldwide, thalassemia is a common genetic disorder with an estimate of approximately 60,000 symptomatic individuals born annually (Galanello & Origa, 2010). The term *thalassemia*, derived from the Greek word *thalassa*, meaning "sea," is applied to a variety of inherited blood disorders characterized by deficiencies in the rate of production of specific globin chains in Hgb. The name appropriately refers to descendants of or people living near the Mediterranean Sea, who have the highest incidence of the disease (i.e., Italians, Greeks, and Syrians). Evidence suggests that the high incidence of the disorders among these groups is a result of the selective advantage the trait confers in relation to malaria, as is postulated in SCA. However, the disorder has a wide geographic distribution, probably as a result of genetic migration through intermarriage or possibly as a result of spontaneous mutation.

Beta thalassemia is the most common of the thalassemias and occurs in four forms:

- Two heterozygous forms: *thalassemia minor*, an asymptomatic silent carrier; and *thalassemia trait*, which produces a mild microcytic anemia
- *Thalassemia intermedia*, which is manifested as splenomegaly and moderate to severe anemia
- A homozygous form, *thalassemia major* (also known as *Cooley's anemia*), which results in a severe anemia that would lead to cardiac failure and death in early childhood without transfusion support

Pathophysiology

Normal postnatal Hgb is composed of two alpha- and two beta-polypeptide chains. In beta thalassemia there is a partial or complete deficiency in the synthesis of the beta chain of the Hgb molecule. Consequently, there is a compensatory increase in the synthesis of alpha chains, and gamma-chain production remains activated, resulting in defective Hgb formation. This unbalanced polypeptide unit is very unstable; when it disintegrates, it damages RBCs, causing severe anemia.

To compensate for the hemolytic process, an overabundance of erythrocytes is formed unless the bone marrow is suppressed by transfusion therapy. Excess iron from **hemolysis** of supplemental RBCs in transfusions and from the rapid destruction of defective cells is stored in various organs (*hemosiderosis*).

Diagnostic Evaluation

The onset of thalassemia major may be insidious and not recognized until the latter half of infancy. The clinical effects of thalassemia major are primarily attributable to (1) defective synthesis of HgbA, (2) structurally impaired RBCs, and (3) the shortened lifespan of erythrocytes (Box 48-3).

Hematological studies reveal the characteristic changes in RBCs (i.e., microcytosis, hypochromia, anisocytosis, poikilocytosis, target cells, and basophilic stippling of various stages). Low Hgb and Hct levels are seen in severe anemia, although they are typically lower than the reduction in RBC count because of the proliferation of immature erythrocytes. Hgb electrophoresis confirms the diagnosis, and radiographs of involved bones reveal characteristic findings.

Therapeutic Management

The objective of supportive therapy is to maintain sufficient Hgb levels to prevent bone marrow expansion and the resulting bony deformities and to provide sufficient RBCs to support normal growth and normal physical activity. Transfusions are the foundation of medical management with the goal of maintaining the Hgb level at 90–100 g/L, an aim that may require transfusions as often as every 3 to 5 weeks (Sayani, Warner, Wu, et al., 2013). The advantages of this therapy include (1) improved physical and psychological well-being because of the ability to participate in normal activities, (2) decreased cardiomegaly and **hepatosplenomegaly**, (3) fewer bone changes, (4) normal or near-normal growth and development until puberty, and (5) fewer infections.

One of the potential complications of frequent blood transfusions is iron overload (*hemosiderosis*). Because the body has no effective means of eliminating the excess iron, the mineral is deposited in body tissues. To minimize the development of hemosiderosis, the oral iron chelator deferasirox (*Exjade*) has been shown to be equivalent to *deferoxamine (Desferal)*, a parenteral iron-chelating agent, and more tolerable by patients and families (Thalassemia Foundation of Canada, 2016). Deferoxamine is given intravenously or subcutaneously at home via a portable infusion pump over a period of 8 to 10 hours (usually during sleep) for 5 to 7 days a week. Significant liver fibrosis, cardiac dysfunction, and growth impairment may be prevented if chelation therapy is adequate during childhood (Kane & Swartz, 2013).

In some children with severe splenomegaly who required repeated transfusions, a splenectomy may be necessary to decrease the disabling effects of abdominal pressure and to increase the lifespan of supplemental RBCs. Over time, the spleen may accelerate the rate of RBC destruction and thus

BOX 48-3 CLINICAL MANIFESTATIONS OF BETA THALASSEMIA

Anemia (Before Diagnosis)
Pallor
Unexplained fever
Poor feeding
Enlarged spleen or liver

Progressive Anemia
Signs of chronic hypoxia
- Headache
- Precordial and bone pain
- Decreased exercise tolerance
- Listlessness
- Anorexia

Other Features
Small stature
Delayed sexual maturation
Bronzed, freckled complexion (if not receiving chelation therapy)

Bone Changes (Older Children if Untreated)
Enlarged head
Prominent frontal and parietal bosses
Prominent malar eminences
Flat or depressed bridge of the nose
Enlarged maxilla
Protrusion of the lip and upper central incisors and eventual malocclusion
Generalized osteoporosis

increase transfusion requirements. After a splenectomy, children generally require fewer transfusions, although the basic defect in Hgb synthesis remains unaffected. A major postsplenectomy complication is severe and overwhelming infection. Therefore, these children continue to receive prophylactic antibiotics with close medical supervision for many years and should receive the pneumococcal and meningococcal vaccines in addition to the regularly scheduled immunizations. Hepatitis A and B vaccinations are also recommended for those who receive repeat blood transfusions.

! NURSING ALERT

Ensure that the family and patient understand the need to notify the health care provider of all fevers of 38.5°C (101.3°F) or greater because of the risk of sepsis in a child with asplenia.

Prognosis

Most children treated with blood transfusion and early chelation therapy survive well into adulthood. The most common cause of death is iron-induced heart disease, multiple-organ failure, postsplenectomy sepsis, liver disease, and malignancy. A curative treatment for some children is HSCT. Children with the least symptoms who are younger than 16 years of age have the best results when undergoing HSCT, with an 80% rate of complication-free survival (Gaziev & Lucarelli, 2011).

NURSING CARE

The objectives of nursing care are to (1) promote adherence to transfusion and chelation therapy, (2) assist the child in coping with the anxiety-provoking treatments and the effects of the illness, (3) foster the child's and family's adjustment to living with a chronic illness, and (4) observe for complications of multiple blood transfusions. Basic to each of these goals is explaining to parents and older children the defect responsible for the disorder, its effect on RBCs, and the potential effects of untreated iron overload (such as diabetes and heart disease). Because the prevalence of this condition is high among families of Mediterranean descent, the nurse also needs to inquire about the family's previous knowledge about thalassemia. All families with a child with thalassemia should be tested for the trait and referred for genetic counselling.

As with any chronic illness, the family's needs must be met for optimal adjustment to the stresses imposed by the disorder (see Chapter 40). Sources of information for the family include the Cooley's Anemia Foundation and the Thalassemia Foundation of Canada (see Additional Resources at the end of this chapter). Genetic counselling for the parents and fertile offspring is important, and both prenatal diagnosis using amniocentesis after 14 weeks of gestation or fetal blood sampling at 10 weeks and screening for the thalassemia trait are available.

Aplastic Anemia

Aplastic anemia (AA) refers to a bone marrow failure condition in which the formed elements of the blood are simultaneously depressed. The peripheral blood smear demonstrates **pancytopenia** or the triad of profound anemia, leukopenia, and thrombocytopenia. *Hypoplastic anemia* is characterized by a profound depression of RBCs but normal or slightly decreased WBCs and platelets.

Etiology

AA can be primary (congenital, or present at birth) or secondary (acquired). The best-known congenital disorder of which AA is an outstanding feature is *Fanconi anemia*, a rare hereditary disorder characterized by pancytopenia, hypoplasia of the bone marrow, and patchy brown discolouration of the skin resulting from the deposit of melanin and associated with multiple congenital anomalies of the musculoskeletal and genitourinary systems. Fanconi anemia is not to be used synonymously with *Fanconi syndrome*, which is a rare and serious disorder that affects the kidneys. Fanconi anemia appears to be inherited as an autosomal recessive trait with varying penetrance; thus affected siblings may demonstrate several different combinations of defects.

Several etiological factors contribute to the development of acquired hypoplastic anemia. Most of the cases are considered idiopathic (Box 48-4); however, increasing evidence suggests there is an autoimmune component (Hartung, Olson, & Bessler, 2013). Acquired AA is classified as either severe acquired AA or moderate acquired AA. The following discussion focuses on severe acquired AA, which carries a poorer prognosis and follows a more rapidly fatal course than the primary types.

Diagnostic Evaluation

The onset of clinical manifestations, which include anemia, leukopenia, and decreased platelet count, is usually insidious. Definitive diagnosis is determined from bone marrow aspiration, which demonstrates the conversion of red bone marrow to yellow, fatty bone marrow. *Severe AA* is defined as less than 25% bone marrow cellularity with at least two of the following findings: absolute **granulocyte** count less than 0.5×10^9/L, platelet count less than 20×10^9/L, and absolute **reticulocyte** count less than 25×10^9/L (McKee, 2015). *Moderate AA* is

BOX 48-4 COMMON CAUSES OF ACQUIRED APLASTIC ANEMIA

- Human parvovirus infection, hepatitis, Epstein-Barr virus, HIV, cytomegalovirus, or overwhelming infection
- Irradiation
- Immune disorders such as eosinophilic fasciitis and hypoimmunoglobulinemia
- Medications such as certain chemotherapeutic agents, anticonvulsants, and antibiotics
- Industrial and household chemicals, including benzene and its derivatives, which are found in petroleum products, dyes, paint remover, shellac, and lacquers
- Infiltration and replacement of myeloid elements, such as in leukemia or the lymphomas
- Idiopathic (In most cases no identifiable precipitating cause can be found.)

defined as more than 25% bone marrow cellularity with the presence of mild or moderate cytopenia (McKee, 2015).

Therapeutic Management

The objectives of treatment are based on the recognition that the underlying disease process is failure of the bone marrow to carry out its hematopoietic functions. Therapy is directed at restoring function to the marrow and involves two main approaches: (1) immunosuppressive therapy to remove the presumed immunological functions that prolong aplasia or (2) replacement of the bone marrow through transplantation. Bone marrow transplantation is the treatment of choice for severe AA, when a suitable donor exists (see p. 1551).

Antilymphocyte globulin (ALG) or antithymocyte globulin (ATG) and cyclosporin are the principal medication treatments used for AA. The rationale for using ATG is based on the theory that AA may be a result of autoimmunity. ATG and cyclosporine suppress T cell–dependent autoimmune responses but do not cause bone marrow suppression. Cyclosporine is administered orally for several weeks to months. ATG usually is administrated intravenously over 12 to 16 hours for 4 days, after a test dose to check for hypersensitivity. A course may be repeated, depending on the reduction in circulating lymphocytes and the patient's response. Because of the hypersensitivity response associated with ATG (i.e., fever, chills, myalgias), methylprednisolone is given intravenously to prevent these adverse effects. Colony-stimulating factor (CSF) and granulocyte-macrophage colony–stimulating factor (GM-CSF) given parenterally may be used to enhance bone marrow production. Androgens may be used with ATG to stimulate erythropoiesis if the AA is unresponsive to initial therapies.

HSCT should be considered early in the course of the disease if a compatible donor can be found. Transplantation is more successful when performed before multiple transfusions have sensitized the child to leukocyte and human leukocyte antigens (HLAs). HSCT is associated with an 85% survival rate in untransfused patients compared with a 70% survival rate in transfused patients (Velardi & Locatelli, 2016).

NURSING CARE

The care of the child with AA is similar to that of the child with leukemia (see p. 1542)—preparing the child and family for the diagnostic and therapeutic procedures, preventing complications from the severe pancytopenia, and providing emotional support in the face of a potentially fatal outcome. Information and support are available from the Aplastic Anemia and Myelodysplasia Association of Canada (see Additional Resources at the end of this chapter).

Because the aspects of nursing care are discussed in the section on leukemia, only the exceptions are presented here. The drug ATG is usually administered by way of a central vein. If not, vigilant care must be directed to the IV infusion to prevent extravasation. Meticulous care of the venous access is essential because of the child's susceptibility to infection. CSFs are usually given by subcutaneous injection over several days. Chemotherapeutic agents have been reported in the treatment of the relapsed patient with AA after ATG and CSF therapy. Many of the adverse effects associated with chemotherapy, such as nausea and vomiting, alopecia, and mucositis, are experienced by children receiving treatment for AA. Specialized care is required for children who have HSCT (see p. 1551).

DEFECTS IN HEMOSTASIS

Hemostasis is the process that stops bleeding when a blood vessel is injured. Vascular and plasma clotting factors, as well as platelets, are required. A complex system of clotting, anticlotting, and clot breakdown (*fibrinolysis*) mechanisms exists in equilibrium to ensure clot formation only in the presence of blood vessel injury and to limit the clotting process to the site of vessel wall injury. Dysfunction in these systems leads to bleeding or abnormal clotting. Although the coagulation process is complex, clotting depends on three factors: (1) vascular influence, (2) platelet role, and (3) clotting factors.

Hemophilia

The term *hemophilia* refers to a group of bleeding disorders in which there is a deficiency of one of the factors necessary for coagulation of the blood. Although the symptomatology is similar regardless of which clotting factor is deficient, the identification of specific factor deficiencies allows definitive treatment with replacement agents.

In about 80% of all cases of hemophilia, the inheritance pattern is X-linked recessive. The two most common forms of the disorder are factor VIII deficiency (hemophilia A, or classic hemophilia) and factor IX deficiency (hemophilia B, or Christmas disease). Hemophilia A affects less than 1 in 10,000 individuals, whereas hemophilia B affects approximately 1 in 50,000 individuals in Canada (Canadian Hemophilia Society, 2008). Von Willebrand disease (vWD) is another hereditary bleeding disorder characterized by a deficiency, abnormality, or absence of the protein called *von Willebrand factor* (vWF) and a deficiency of factor VIII (see Chapter 24, p. 609). Unlike hemophilia, which affects many more males than females, vWD affects both males and females equally. Approximately 1 in 100 individuals could be affected by vWD (Canadian Hemophilia Society, 2016). The following discussion is primarily concerned with factor VIII deficiency, which accounts for 80 to 85% of all hemophilia cases.

Pathophysiology

The basic defect of hemophilia A is a deficiency of factor VIII (antihemophilic factor [AHF]). AHF is produced by the liver and is necessary for the formation of thromboplastin in phase I of blood coagulation (Fig. 48-3). The less AHF found in the blood, the more severe the disease. Individuals with hemophilia have two of the three factors required for coagulation: vascular influence and platelets. Therefore, they may bleed for longer periods but not at a faster rate.

Bleeding into subcutaneous and IM tissue is common. *Hemarthrosis*, which is bleeding into a joint space (knees, elbows, ankles, shoulders, hips, wrists), is the most frequent type of internal bleeding. Bony changes and crippling

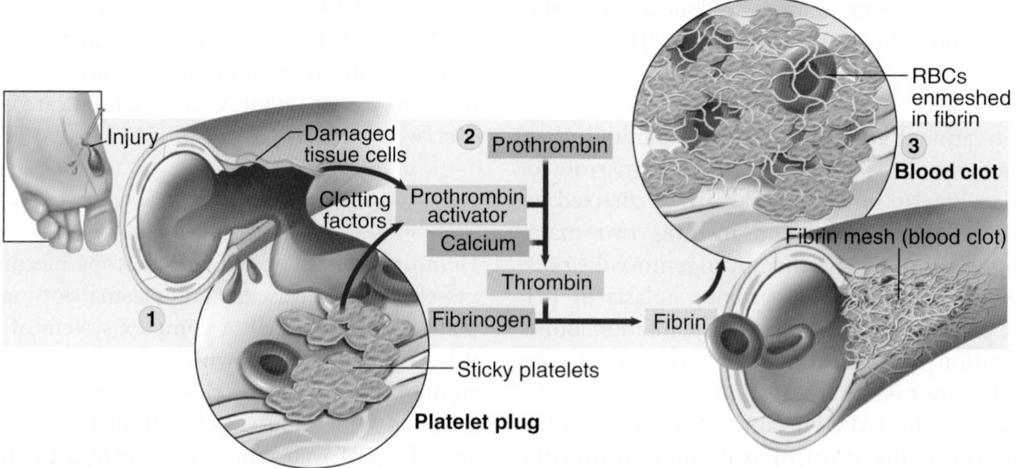

FIGURE 48-3 Blood clotting. The extremely complex clotting mechanism can be distilled into three basic steps: (1) release of clotting factors from both injured tissue cells and sticky platelets at the injury site (which form a temporary platelet plug); (2) a series of chemical reactions that eventually result in the formation of thrombin; and (3) formation of fibrin and trapping of red blood cells (RBCs) to form a clot. (From Thibodeau, G. A. [2010]. *The human body in health and disease* [5th ed.]. St. Louis: Mosby.)

BOX 48-5 CLINICAL MANIFESTATIONS OF HEMOPHILIA

- Prolonged bleeding anywhere from or in the body
- Hemorrhage from any trauma—Loss of deciduous teeth, circumcision, cuts, epistaxis, injections
- Excessive bruising, even from a slight injury, such as a fall
- Subcutaneous and intramuscular hemorrhages
- Hemarthrosis (bleeding into the joint cavities), especially the knees, ankles, and elbows
- Hematomas—Pain, swelling, and limited motion
- Spontaneous hematuria

deformities occur after repeated bleeding episodes over several years. Signs of hemarthrosis are swelling, warmth, redness, pain, and loss of movement. Bleeding in the neck, mouth, or thorax is serious because the airway can become obstructed. Intracranial hemorrhage can have fatal consequences and is one of the major causes of death. Hemorrhage anywhere along the GI tract can lead to anemia, and bleeding into the retroperitoneal cavity is especially hazardous because of the large space for blood to accumulate. Hematomas in the spinal cord can cause paralysis.

Diagnostic Evaluation

Overt, prolonged hemorrhage is readily apparent; bleeding into tissues is less apparent (Box 48-5). The diagnosis is usually made from a history of bleeding episodes, evidence of X-linked inheritance (only one third of the cases are new mutations), and laboratory findings. The tests specific for hemophilia plasma depend on specific factors for a reaction to occur, such as the partial thromboplastin time (PTT). Specific determination of factor deficiencies requires assay procedures normally performed in specialized laboratories. Carrier detection is possible in classic hemophilia using DNA testing and is an important consideration in families in which female offspring may have inherited the trait.

Therapeutic Management

The primary therapy for hemophilia is replacement of the missing clotting factor. The products available are factor VIII concentrate from pooled plasma or a genetically engineered recombinant, to be reconstituted with sterile water immediately before use. A synthetic form of vasopressin, 1-deamino-8-D-arginine vasopressin (DDAVP), increases plasma factor VIII activity and is the treatment of choice in mild hemophilia and certain types of vWD if the child shows an appropriate response. DDAVP is not effective in the treatment of severe hemophilia A, severe vWD, or any form of hemophilia B. Vigorous therapy is instituted to prevent chronic crippling effects from joint bleeding.

Other medications may be included in the therapy plan, depending on the source of the hemorrhage. Tranexamic acid is effective in both hemophilia A and B, by helping to hold a clot in place once it has formed. Corticosteroids are given for hematuria, acute hemarthrosis, and chronic synovitis. Nonsteroidal anti-inflammatory drugs (NSAIDs), such as ibuprofen, are effective in relieving pain caused by synovitis; however, they must be used with caution because they may inhibit platelet function (Health Canada, 2009; World Federation of Hemophilia, 2012). Oral administration or local application of ε-aminocaproic acid (Amicar) prevents clot destruction; however, its use is limited to mouth or trauma surgery, and a dose of factor concentrate must be given first.

A regular program of exercise and physiotherapy is an important aspect of management. Physical activity within reasonable limits strengthens muscles around joints and may decrease the number of spontaneous bleeding episodes.

Treatment without delay results in more rapid recovery and a decreased likelihood of complications; therefore, most children are treated at home. The family needs to be taught the technique of venipuncture and how to administer the AHF to children older than 2 to 3 years of age. The child can learn the procedure for self-administration at 8 to 12 years of age. Home treatment is highly successful; the rewards, in addition to the immediacy, are less disruption of family life, fewer school or work days missed, and enhancement of the child's self-esteem and independence.

Primary prophylaxis in patients with hemophilia has proved to be effective in preventing bleeding complications by administrating periodic factor replacement. Primary prophylaxis involves the infusion of factor VIII concentrate on a regular basis before the onset of joint damage. Secondary prophylaxis involves the infusion of factor VIII concentrate on a regular basis after the child experiences his or her first joint bleed. The infusions are given three times per week. Aggressive or on-demand factor replacement may be a cost-effective alternative to primary prophylaxis. This involves the infusion of a high dose of factor VIII concentrate when a joint bleed occurs, followed by 2 days of more standard doses of factor VIII concentrate, with consideration of additional treatment every other day for 1 week (Scott, 2016).

Prognosis

Although there is no cure for hemophilia, its symptoms can be controlled and its potentially crippling deformities greatly reduced or even avoided. Today, many children with hemophilia function with minimal or no joint damage. They are normal children with an average life expectancy in every respect but one: they have a tendency to bleed, which is a significant inconvenience but not necessarily a life-threatening event.

Gene therapy may prove to be a treatment option in the future. This therapy involves introducing a working copy of the factor VIII gene into a patient who has a flawed copy of the gene. Problems exist with appropriate selection of the **vector**, identification of the cell for gene expression, and control of adverse effects (Scott, 2016).

NURSING CARE

The earlier a bleeding episode is recognized, the more effectively it can be treated. Signs that indicate internal bleeding are especially important to recognize. Children are aware of internal bleeding and are reliable in telling the examiner where an internal bleed is. In addition to the manifestations described (see Box 48-5), the nurse needs to maintain a high level of suspicion when a child with hemophilia demonstrates signs such as headache, slurred speech, loss of consciousness (from cerebral bleeding), and black tarry stools (from GI bleeding).

Prevent Bleeding

The goal of the prevention of bleeding episodes is directed toward decreasing the risk of injury. Prevention of bleeding episodes is geared mostly toward appropriate exercises to strengthen muscles and joints and to allow age-appropriate activity. During infancy and toddlerhood, the normal acquisition of motor skills creates innumerable opportunities for falls, bruises, and minor wounds. Restraining the child from mastering motor development can foster more serious long-term problems than allowing the behaviour. However, the environment should be made as safe as possible, with close supervision during playtime to minimize incidental injuries.

The family usually needs assistance in preparing older children for school. A nurse who knows the family can be instrumental in discussing the situation with the teacher and jointly planning an appropriate activity schedule. The physical limitations in regard to active sports may be a difficult adjustment, and activity restrictions must be tempered with sensitivity to the child's emotional and physical needs. Use of protective equipment, such as padding and helmets, is particularly important; noncontact sports, especially recreational swimming, walking, jogging, cross-country skiing, golf, and dancing, should be encouraged (Zourikian, Jarock, & Mulder, 2010).

To prevent oral bleeding, some readjustment in dental hygiene may be needed to minimize trauma to the gums, such as use of a water irrigating device, softening the toothbrush in warm water before brushing, or using a sponge-tipped disposable toothbrush. A regular toothbrush should be small and have soft bristles.

Because any trauma can lead to a bleeding episode, all persons caring for these children must be aware of their disorder. The children should wear medical identification, and older children should be encouraged to recognize situations in which disclosing their condition is important, such as during dental extraction or injections. Health care providers need to take special precautions to prevent the use of procedures that may cause bleeding, such as IM injections. The subcutaneous route is substituted for IM injections whenever possible. Venipunctures for blood samples are usually preferred for these children. There is usually less bleeding after the venipuncture than after finger or heel punctures. Neither aspirin nor any aspirin-containing compound should be used. Acetaminophen is a suitable aspirin substitute, especially for controlling pain at home.

Recognize and Control Bleeding

As noted, the earlier a bleeding episode is recognized, the more effectively it can be treated. Factor replacement therapy should be instituted according to established medical protocol, and supportive measures—such as *RICE*, which stands for *R*est, *I*ce, *C*ompression, and *E*levation—may be implemented. When parents and older children are taught such measures beforehand, they can be prepared to initiate immediate treatment. Plastic bags of ice or cold packs should be kept in the freezer for such emergencies. However, such measures do not take the place of factor replacement.

Prevent Crippling Effects of Bleeding

As a result of repeated episodes of hemarthrosis, incompletely absorbed blood in the joints, and limitation of motion, bone and muscle changes occur that result in flexion contractures and joint fixation. During bleeding episodes the joint is elevated and immobilized. Active range-of-motion exercises are usually instituted after the acute episode. This allows the child to control the degree of exercise and discomfort. If an exercise program is instituted in the home, a physiotherapist or community health nurse may need to supervise the regimen. Rarely, orthopaedic intervention, such as casting, the application of traction, or the aspiration of blood, may be necessary to preserve joint function. Diet is also an important consideration because excessive body weight can increase the strain on affected joints, especially the knees, and predispose the child to hemarthrosis. Consequently, calories need to be supplied in accordance with energy requirements.

Support the Family and Prepare for Home Care

Genetic counselling is essential as soon as possible after diagnosis. Unlike many other disorders in which both parents carry the trait, the feeling of responsibility for this condition usually rests with the mother, and it is important that she has the opportunity to discuss her feelings. Technology is now available to identify carriers in approximately 90 to 99% of cases and may reduce the anxiety regarding child-bearing in women who may be at risk of carrying the defective gene, such as sisters or maternal aunts of an affected male. Factor concentrates have greatly changed the outlook for these children by minimizing bleeding and allowing the child to live an unrestricted life. Children are taught to take responsibility for their disease at an early age. They learn their limitations, other preventive measures, and self-administration of the prophylactic AHF.

The needs of families who have children with hemophilia are best met through a comprehensive team approach of physicians (pediatrician, hematologist, orthopedist, dentist), nurse practitioner, nurse, social worker, and physiotherapist. Parent-group discussions are beneficial in meeting the needs often best met by similarly affected families. For example, with the improved prognosis for these children, parents and adolescents with hemophilia face vocational and financial problems, in addition to concern over future child-bearing. Financial support is particularly important, as a person with severe hemophilia may require factor replacement therapy and other medical treatments that cost in excess of $70,000 to $90,000 a year. The Canadian Hemophilia Society provides numerous services and publications for both health providers and families (see Additional Resources at the end of this chapter).

Idiopathic (Autoimmune) Thrombocytopenic Purpura

Idiopathic thrombocytopenic purpura (ITP) is an acquired hemorrhagic disorder characterized by (1) *thrombocytopenia*, excessive destruction of platelets; (2) **purpura**, a discolouration caused by petechiae beneath the skin; and (3) normal bone marrow with a normal or increased number of immature platelets (megakaryocytes) and eosinophils. Although all causes of ITP are not known, it is understood that ITP involves the evolution of antibodies against multiple platelet antigens, leading to reduced platelet survival and impaired platelet production (Consolini, 2011; McCrae, 2011). It is the most frequently occurring thrombocytopenia of childhood. The greatest frequency of occurrence is between 1 and 4 years of age (Scott, 2016).

The disease occurs in one of two forms: an acute, self-limited course or a chronic condition (greater than 6 months' duration). The acute form is most often seen after upper respiratory tract infections; after immunization with the measles, mumps, rubella (MMR) vaccine; after the childhood diseases measles, rubella, mumps, and chicken pox; or after infection with parvovirus B19.

BOX 48-6 CLINICAL MANIFESTATIONS OF IDIOPATHIC THROMBOCYTOPENIC PURPURA

Easy bruising
- Petechiae
- Ecchymoses
- Hematomas over lower extremities
- Most often over bony prominences

Bleeding from mucous membranes
- Epistaxis
- Bleeding gums

Internal hemorrhage evidenced by
- Hematuria
- Hematemesis
- Melena
- Hemarthrosis
- Menorrhagia

Diagnostic Evaluation

The diagnosis is suspected on the basis of clinical manifestations (Box 48-6). In ITP the platelet count is reduced to below 20×10^9/L; thus tests that depend on platelet function, such as the tourniquet test, bleeding time, and clot retraction, are abnormal. Although there is no definitive test on which to establish a diagnosis of ITP, several are usually performed to rule out other disorders in which thrombocytopenia is a manifestation, such as systemic lupus erythematosus, lymphoma, or leukemia.

Therapeutic Management

Management of ITP is primarily supportive because the course of the disease is self-limited in most cases. Activity is restricted at the onset while the platelet count is low and while active bleeding or progression of lesions is occurring. Treatment for acute presentation is symptomatic and has included corticosteroids, IV immune globulin (IVIG), and anti-D antibody (WinRho). These are not curative therapies. Anti-D antibody is a relatively new therapy for ITP. Its infusion causes a transient hemolytic anemia in the patient. Along with the clearance of antibody-coated RBCs, there is prolonged survival of platelets resulting from the blockade of the Fc receptors of the reticuloendothelial cells. The platelet count does not increase until 48 hours after an infusion of anti-D antibody; therefore, it is not appropriate therapy for patients who are actively bleeding. The benefits of choosing anti-D antibody therapy over prednisone or IVIG are that anti-D antibody can be given in one dose over 5 to 10 minutes and is significantly less expensive than IVIG. Historically, patients who are treated with prednisone must first undergo a bone marrow examination to rule out leukemia. The

BOX 48-7 CRITERIA FOR ANTI-D ANTIBODY THERAPY

- Age between 1 and 19 years; Rh(D)-positive blood type
- Normal white blood count and hemoglobin level for age; platelet count of 20×10^9/L
- No active mucosal bleeding
- No history of reaction to plasma products
- No known immune globulin A deficiency
- No concurrent infection
- Absence of Evans syndrome (characterized by the combination of idiopathic thrombocytopenic purpura and autoimmune hemolytic anemia)
- No suspicion of lupus erythematosus or other collagen-vascular disorder
- No splenectomy

use of anti-D antibody alleviates the need for a bone marrow examination. Patients must meet certain criteria before it is administered (Box 48-7). Premedication with acetaminophen 5 to 10 minutes before infusion is recommended.

! NURSING ALERT

After administration of anti-D antibody, observe the child for a minimum of 8 hours and maintain a patent IV line. Obtain baseline vital signs before the infusion and again 5, 20, and 60 minutes after beginning the infusion. Fever, chills, hematuria, and headache may occur during or shortly after the infusion. If these symptoms occur, diphenhydramine (Benadryl) and hydrocortisone (Solu-Cortef) should be given, and the patient observed for an additional hour.

Splenectomy is reserved for patients in whom ITP has persisted for 1 year or longer. It is the only treatment associated with long-term remission for 60 to 90% of children. Splenectomy removes the risk of hemorrhage but increases the risk of septicemia (Scott, 2016; Wilson, 2014). Before considering splenectomy, it is generally recommended to wait until the child is older than 5 years of age because of the increased risk of bacterial infection. Pneumococcal and meningococcal vaccines are recommended before splenectomy. The child also receives penicillin prophylaxis after splenectomy. The length of prophylactic therapy is unsubstantiated, but in general, a minimum of 3 years is recommended.

Prognosis

Most children have a self-limited course without major complications. Approximately 20% of patients who present with acute ITP have persistent thrombocytopenia for greater than 12 months and are said to have chronic ITP and will require ongoing therapy (Scott, 2016). A splenectomy may modify the disease process, and the child will be asymptomatic.

NURSING CARE

Nursing care is largely supportive and should include teaching regarding possible adverse effects of therapy and limitation in activities while the child's platelet count is 50 to 100×10^9/L. Children with ITP should not participate in any contact sports, bike riding, skateboarding, in-line skating, gymnastics, climbing, or running. Parents should be encouraged to engage their children in quiet activities and prevent any injuries to the child's head. The harmful effects of using aspirin and NSAIDs to control pain are critical for these children; therefore, salicylate substitutes (such as acetaminophen) are always used. As in any condition with an uncertain outcome, the family needs emotional support.

Disseminated Intravascular Coagulation

Disseminated intravascular coagulation (DIC), also known as *consumption coagulopathy*, is characterized by diffuse fibrin deposition in the microvasculature, consumption of coagulation factors, and endogenous generation of thrombin and plasmin. DIC is a secondary disorder of coagulation that occurs as a complication of a number of pathological processes, such as hypoxia, acidosis, shock, and endothelial damage. It can result from surgery and trauma, cancer, many severe systemic diseases, such as congenital heart disease, necrotizing enterocolitis, Gram-negative bacterial sepsis, rickettsial infections, and some severe viral infections.

Pathophysiology

DIC occurs when the first stage of the coagulation process is abnormally stimulated. Although no well-defined sequence of events occurs, two distinct phases can be identified. First, when the clotting mechanism is triggered in the circulation, thrombin is generated in greater amounts than can be neutralized by the body. Consequently, there is rapid conversion of fibrinogen to fibrin, with aggregation and destruction of platelets. If local and widespread fibrin deposition in blood vessels takes place, obstruction and eventual necrosis of tissues occur. Second, the fibrinolytic mechanism is activated, causing extensive destruction of clotting factors. With a deficiency of clotting factors, the child is vulnerable to uncontrollable hemorrhage into vital organs. An additional complication is damage and hemolysis of RBCs (Fig. 48-4).

Diagnostic Evaluation

DIC is suspected when the patient has an increased tendency to bleed (Box 48-8). Hematological findings include prolonged prothrombin time (PT), partial thromboplastin time (PTT), serum fibrinogen, and D-dimer. Findings include a profoundly depressed platelet count, fragmented RBCs, and depleted fibrinogen.

Therapeutic Management

Treatment of DIC is directed toward control of the underlying or initiating cause, which in most instances stops the coagulation problem spontaneously. Platelets and fresh frozen plasma may be needed to replace lost plasma components, especially in the child whose underlying disease remains uncontrolled. The extremely ill newborn infant may require exchange transfusion with fresh blood. The IV administration of heparin to inhibit thrombin formation is most often restricted to patients who have not responded to treatment of

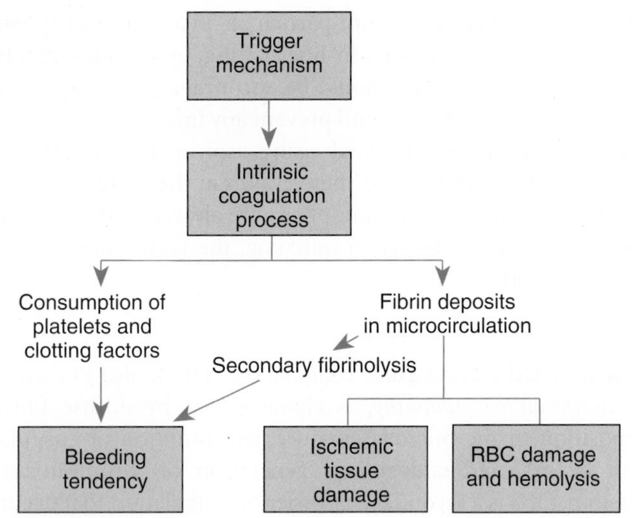

FIGURE 48-4 Effects of disseminated intravascular coagulation. *RBC*, red blood cell.

BOX 48-8 CLINICAL MANIFESTATIONS OF DISSEMINATED INTRAVASCULAR COAGULATION

Petechiae
Purpura
Bleeding from openings in the skin
- Venipuncture site
- Surgical incision

Bleeding from umbilicus, trachea (newborn)
Evidence of gastrointestinal bleeding
Hypotension
Thrombosis
Organ dysfunction from infarction and ischemia

the underlying disease or replacement of coagulation factors and platelets.

NURSING CARE

The goals of nursing care are to be aware of the possibility of DIC in the severely ill child and to recognize signs that might indicate its presence. The skills needed to monitor IV infusion and blood transfusions and to administer heparin are the same as for any child receiving these therapies. (See Chapter 40 for care of the child with a life-threatening illness.)

Epistaxis (Nosebleeding)

Isolated and transient episodes of epistaxis, or nosebleeding, are common in childhood. The nose, especially the septum, is a highly vascular structure, and bleeding usually results from direct trauma, including blows to the nose, foreign bodies, and nose picking, or from mucosal inflammation associated with allergic rhinitis and upper respiratory tract infections. The bleeding ordinarily stops spontaneously or with minimal pressure and requires no medical evaluation or therapy.

EMERGENCY

Epistaxis

- Have child sit up and lean forward (not lie down).
- Apply continuous pressure to nose with thumb and forefinger for at least 10 minutes.
- Insert cotton or wadded tissue into each nostril, and apply ice or cold cloth to bridge of nose if bleeding persists.
- Keep child calm and quiet.

Recurrent epistaxis and severe bleeding may indicate an underlying disease, particularly vascular abnormalities, leukemia, thrombocytopenia, and clotting factor–deficiency diseases (e.g., hemophilia, vWD). Nosebleeds are sometimes associated with administration of aspirin, even in normal amounts. Persistent episodes of epistaxis require medical evaluation.

NURSING CARE

In the event of a nosebleed, an essential intervention is to remain calm. Otherwise, the child will become more agitated, the blood pressure will increase, and he or she may resist treatment. Although in most instances a nosebleed is not serious, it can be upsetting to family members as well. They need reassurance that the loss of blood is not serious and that the bleeding usually stops within 10 to 15 minutes with nasal pressure.

To control the bleeding, the child is instructed to sit up and lean forward (not lie down) to avoid aspiration of blood. Most nose bleeding originates in the anterior part of the nasal septum and can be controlled by applying pressure to the soft lower portion of the nose with the thumb and forefinger (see Emergency box). During this time, the child breathes through the mouth.

In the event that hemorrhage continues, the child should be evaluated by a health care practitioner, who may pack the nose with epinephrine-soaked gauze. After a nosebleed, petroleum or water-soluble jelly can be inserted into each nostril to prevent crusting of old blood and to lessen the likelihood of the child's picking at the nose and restarting the hemorrhage. If a child has numerous nosebleeds, factors believed to increase the likelihood of bleeds should be eliminated, such as discouraging nose picking or altering the household humidity by placing a cool-mist humidifier in the child's room. Repeated bleeding episodes lasting longer than 30 minutes may be an indication to refer the child for evaluation for the possibility of a bleeding disorder.

NEOPLASTIC DISORDERS

Neoplastic disorders are the leading cause of death from disease in children past infancy, and almost half of all childhood cancers involve the blood or blood-forming organs. Leukemias and lymphomas are discussed here. Malignant solid tumours of childhood are discussed elsewhere in relation to the tissues or organs involved.

Leukemias

Leukemia, a cancer of the blood-forming tissues, is the most common form of childhood cancer. The annual incidence is 3 to 4 cases per 100,000 Caucasian children younger than 15 years of age. It is more common in males and White children, with the peak onset between 2 and 5 years of age (Rabin, Gramategs, Margolin, et al., 2016). It is one of the forms of cancer that has demonstrated dramatic improvements in survival rates. Five-year observed survival proportions for children with acute lymphoid leukemia approaches 90% (whereas acute nonlymphoid leukemia has a nearly 67% survival rate (Canadian Cancer Society, 2015). See also Prognosis, p. 1542.

Classification

Leukemia is a broad term given to a group of malignant diseases of the bone marrow and lymphatic system. Research has revealed it to be a complex disease of varying heterogeneity. Consequently, classification has become increasingly complex, sophisticated, and essential, since identification of the subtype of leukemia has therapeutic and prognostic implications. The following is a brief overview of the major classification systems currently being used.

Morphology. Two forms are generally recognized in children: acute lymphoid leukemia (ALL) and acute nonlymphoid (myelogenous) leukemia (ANLL or AML). Synonyms for ALL include lymphatic, lymphoid, lymphocytic, lymphoblastic, promyelocytic, erythroid, megakaryoblastic, and lymphoblastoid leukemia. Synonyms for the AML type include granulocytic, myelocytic, monocytic, myelogenous, monoblastic, and monomyeloblastic.

Cytochemical markers—Several chemical stains (e.g., terminal deoxynucleotidyl transferase [TdT]) aid in differentiation between ALL and AML.

Chromosome studies—Chromosome analysis has become an important tool in the diagnosis of ALL. For example, children with trisomy 21 have 20 times the risk of other children for developing ALL. Children with more than 50 chromosomes on the leukemic cells (hyperdiploid) have the best prognosis (Rabin et al., 2016). Translocations of chromosomes also found on the leukemic cells can denote a good prognosis, as in the trisomies 4 and 10, or a poor prognosis, as in the (9:22) or Philadelphia chromosome.

Cell-surface immunological markers—Cell-surface antigens have enabled differentiation of ALL into three broad classes: non-T, non-B ALL; B-cell ALL; and T-cell ALL. Children with non-T, non-B ALL have the best prognosis, especially if they have the common ALL antigen, known as CALLA positive (or CD10+), on their cell surfaces (Rabin et al., 2016).

Pathophysiology

Leukemia is an unrestricted proliferation of immature WBCs in the blood-forming tissues of the body. Although not a "tumour" as such, the leukemic cells demonstrate the same neoplastic properties as solid cancers. The resulting pathological condition and clinical manifestations are caused by infiltration and replacement of any tissue of the body with nonfunctional leukemic cells. Highly vascular organs, such as the spleen and liver, are the most severely affected.

To understand the pathophysiology of the leukemic process, it is important to clarify two common misconceptions. First, although leukemia is an overproduction of WBCs, most often in the acute form the leukocyte count is low (thus the term *leukemia*). Second, these immature cells do not deliberately attack and destroy the normal blood cells or vascular tissues. Cellular destruction takes place by infiltration and subsequent competition for metabolic elements (Table 48-2).

TABLE 48-2 PATHOLOGY AND RELATED CLINICAL MANIFESTATIONS OF LEUKEMIA

ORGAN OR TISSUE	CONSEQUENCES	MANIFESTATIONS
Bone marrow dysfunction	Decreased red blood cells—Anemia	Pallor, fatigue
	Neutropenia—Infection	Fever
	Decreased platelets—Bleeding tendencies	Hemorrhage (petechiae)
	Invasion of bone marrow—Bone weakness; invasion of periosteum	Tendency toward fractures Pain
Liver	Infiltration, enlargement, eventual fibrosis	Hepatomegaly
Spleen		Splenomegaly
Lymph glands		Lymphadenopathy
Central nervous system—Meninges	Increased intracranial pressure, ventricular enlargement	Severe headache Vomiting Irritability, lethargy Papilledema
	Meningeal irritation	Eventual coma Pain Stiff neck and back
Hypermetabolism	Cell deprivation of nutrients by invading cells	Muscle wasting Weight loss Anorexia Fatigue

In all types of leukemia the proliferating cells depress the production of formed elements of the blood in bone marrow by competing for and depriving the normal cells of the essential nutrients for metabolism. The most frequent presenting signs and symptoms of leukemia are a result of infiltration of the bone marrow. The three main consequences are (1) anemia from decreased RBCs, (2) infection from neutropenia, and (3) bleeding from decreased platelet production. The invasion of the bone marrow with leukemic cells gradually causes a weakening of the bone and a tendency toward fractures. As leukemic cells invade the periosteum, increasing pressure causes severe pain.

Leukemic cells may also invade the testes, kidneys, prostate, ovaries, GI tract, and lungs. With long-term survivors becoming more common, such sites of leukemia invasion, especially the testes, are becoming more important clinically.

Diagnostic Evaluation

Leukemia is usually suspected on the basis of the history and physical presentation, which often includes fever, signs and symptoms of low blood counts, lymph node enlargement, and an enlarged liver and spleen. Peripheral blood smear may reveal immature forms of leukocytes, frequently combined with low blood counts. Definitive diagnosis is based on bone marrow aspiration or biopsy. Flow cytometry identifies the specific type of blast cell. Typically, the bone marrow is hypercellular, with primarily **blast cells**. After the diagnosis is confirmed, a lumbar puncture is performed to determine whether there is any central nervous system (CNS) involvement. A few children have CNS involvement at diagnosis, although most are asymptomatic.

Therapeutic Management

Treatment of leukemia involves the use of chemotherapeutic agents, with or without cranial irradiation, in four phases: (1) *induction therapy*, which achieves a complete remission or less than 5% leukemic cells in the bone marrow; (2) *CNS prophylactic therapy*, which prevents leukemic cells from invading the CNS; (3) *intensification therapy* (consolidation), which eradicates residual leukemia cells, followed by delayed intensification, which prevents emergence of resistant leukemic clones; and (4) *maintenance therapy*, which serves to maintain the remission phase.

Hematopoietic stem cell transplantation. HSCT has been used successfully for treating children who have ALL and AML. It is not recommended for children with ALL during the first remission because of the excellent results possible with chemotherapy. Because of the poorer prognosis in children with AML, HSCT may be considered during the first remission when a suitable donor is available (Gottschalk, Naik, Hegde, et al., 2016).

HSCT may be not only from antigen-matched related donors but also from matched unrelated or mismatched donors. Peripheral blood stem cell transplants are capable of differentiating into specialized cells of the hematological system and can be obtained from related or unrelated donors or from umbilical cord blood. Regardless of the type of transplant, it is accompanied by significant morbidity and mortality, including graft-versus-host disease (GVHD), overwhelming infection, or severe organ damage.

Prognosis

The most important prognostic factors for determining long-term survival for children with ALL (in addition to treatment) are (1) the initial WBC count, (2) the child's age at the time of diagnosis, (3) the type of cell involved, (4) the sex of the child, and (5) karyotype analysis. Children with a normal or low WBC count and who have non-T, non-B ALL and are CALLA positive have a much better prognosis than those with a high count or other cell types. Children diagnosed between 2 and 9 years of age have consistently demonstrated a better outlook than those diagnosed before 2 or after 10 years of age, and girls appear to have a more favourable prognosis than boys. Children with a DNA index greater than 1.16 (hyperdiploid) and translocation of chromosomes 4 and 10 have a better prognosis (Rabin et al., 2016).

Late Effects of Treatment

Although vigorous treatment of childhood cancers has resulted in dramatically improved survival rates, increasing concern surrounds late effects—adverse changes related to treatment modalities—and recurrence of the disease process. Almost no organ is exempt, and almost every antineoplastic agent, especially irradiation, is responsible for some adverse effect.

The most devastating late effect is development of a second malignancy. Children who received cranial irradiation at age 5 years or younger are most susceptible to developing brain tumours (Landier, Armenian, & Bhatia, 2015). Treatment with an anthracycline is associated with cardiomyopathy; cranial irradiation and intrathecal chemotherapy are associated with endocrine, cognitive, and neuropsychological deficits; alkylating agents are associated with bone mineral density deficits, which are just a few of the long-term sequelae (Landier et al., 2015). Consequently, close monitoring for late effects is essential, especially with the advent of additional clinical trials.

NURSING CARE

Nursing care of the child with leukemia is directly related to the therapeutic regimen. The Nursing Care Plan for the child with cancer is available on Evolve.

Prepare the Child and Family for Diagnostic and Therapeutic Procedures

From the time before diagnosis to cessation of therapy, children must undergo several tests; the most traumatic tests are bone marrow aspiration, bone marrow biopsy, and lumbar punctures. Multiple finger sticks and venipunctures for blood analysis and drug infusion are common occurrences. The child needs an explanation of each procedure and what can be expected. In addition, effective pharmacological measures, including conscious and unconscious sedation, and nonpharmacological strategies can be used to reduce discomfort associated with these painful procedures (see Preparation for Diagnostic and Therapeutic Procedures, Chapter 44).

Relieve Pain

The effective use of analgesia is especially important when the malignant process is uncontrolled and causes acute pain. Dosages of opioids are adjusted, or *titrated*, to the child's needs and administered *around the clock* for optimal pain control. Nonpharmacological strategies should be implemented as needed but are not substitutes for pharmacological management. For a review of the principles of pain assessment and management, see Chapter 34.

Prevent Complications of Myelosuppression

The leukemic process and most of the chemotherapeutic agents cause myelosuppression. The reduced numbers of blood cells result in secondary problems of infection, bleeding tendencies, and anemia. Supportive care involves both medical and nursing management. Because these are so closely linked, they are discussed together.

Infection. A frequent complication of treatment for childhood cancer is overwhelming infection secondary to neutropenia. The child is most susceptible to overwhelming infection during three phases of the disease: (1) at the time of diagnosis and relapse when the leukemic process has replaced normal leukocytes; (2) during immunosuppressive therapy; and (3) after prolonged antibiotic therapy, which predisposes the child to the growth of resistant organisms. However, the use of granulocyte colony–stimulating factor (GCSF) has reduced the incidence and duration of infection in children receiving treatment for cancer.

The first defence against infection is prevention. When the child is hospitalized, the nurse needs to use all measures to control transfer of infection. These typically include the use of a private room, restriction of all visitors and health personnel with active infection, and strict hand hygiene technique with an antiseptic solution. Other measures used to help protect the child against infection include having no live plants in the child's room, cleaning and sterilizing toys, and providing education to the parents and family about healthy and safe foods for the child to eat. In some centres special germ-free environments, called *reverse isolation*, are available during complete myelosuppression from intensive chemotherapy or for bone marrow transplant.

! NURSING ALERT

Live or attenuated viral vaccines are contraindicated in immunosuppressed children and should be deferred until the child's **immune system** function has returned to normal. The administration of an attenuated vaccine (MMR, oral polio) during immunosuppression may result in overwhelming infection. There is no special risk with the administration of inactivated vaccines (pneumococcal conjugate [PCV-13], TDaP); however, the child's immune system will likely not respond adequately. Siblings and other family members can receive all routine age-appropriate vaccines except oral polio. Prophylactic measures need only be taken if the vaccinated child develops wild-type varicella infection. Revaccination is recommended 3 to 6 months after completion of chemotherapy treatment (Patel, Chisholm, & Heath, 2008).

The child should be evaluated for potential sites of infection (e.g., mucosal ulcerations, skin abrasions, or skin tears, such as a hangnail) and observed for any elevation in temperature. To identify the source of infection, chest radiographs, blood, stool, urine, and nasopharyngeal cultures are taken. IV antibiotics need to be administered; if this therapy is prolonged, a venous access device, such as a peripherally or centrally inserted catheter or intermittent infusion device (saline lock or PRN adaptor), is used to maintain IV access.

Prevention of infection continues to be a priority after discharge from the hospital. Ordinarily, the child is allowed to return to school when the WBC count is at a satisfactory level, usually when the absolute neutrophil count (ANC) is $>1.0 \times 10^9$/L. Family members need to be encouraged to practise good hand hygiene at all times to keep from introducing pathogens into the home. The child may need to be isolated from school contacts in the event of an outbreak of a childhood disease, especially chicken pox.

Nutrition is another important component of infection prevention. An adequate protein-caloric intake provides the child with better host defences against infection and increased tolerance to chemotherapy and irradiation. However, providing optimal nutrition during periods of anorexia and vomiting from chemotherapy is a tremendous challenge (see Feeding the Sick Child, Chapter 44).

Hemorrhage. Before the use of transfused platelets, hemorrhage was a leading cause of death in patients with leukemia. Now most bleeding episodes can be prevented or controlled with the administration of platelet concentrates or platelet-rich plasma.

Skin punctures should be avoided whenever possible because bleeding sites can become easily infected. When finger sticks, venipunctures, IM injections, and bone marrow aspirations are performed, aseptic technique must be used, along with continued observation for bleeding. Meticulous mouth care is essential, since gingival bleeding with resultant mucositis is a frequent problem. Because the rectal area is prone to ulceration from various medications, feces and urine are to be removed immediately and the perianal area washed. Use of rectal thermometers should be avoided to prevent trauma. Children should be advised to avoid activities that might cause injury or bleeding, such as riding bicycles or skateboards, climbing trees or playground equipment, and playing contact sports.

Platelet transfusions are generally reserved for active bleeding episodes that do not respond to local treatment and that may occur during induction or relapse therapy. Epistaxis and gingival bleeding are most common. The nurse needs to teach parents and older children measures to control nosebleeding (see p. 1540). Pressure at the site without disturbing clot formation is the general rule.

Anemia. Initially, anemia may be profound from complete replacement of the bone marrow by leukemic cells. During induction therapy, blood transfusions may be necessary. The usual precautions in caring for the child with anemia are instituted (see p. 1526).

Use Precautions in Administering and Handling Chemotherapeutic Agents

In addition to the nurse's many responsibilities in regard to the child and family, nurses must also use safeguards to protect themselves. Handling chemotherapeutic agents may present risks to handlers and their offspring, although the exact degree of risk is not known. Many chemotherapeutic agents are vesicants (sclerosing agents) that can cause severe cellular damage if even a minute amount of the drug infiltrates surrounding tissue. Only nurses who are both certified and experienced with chemotherapeutic agents should administer vesicants. Guidelines are available and must be followed exactly to prevent tissue damage to patients (see Additional Resources at the end of this chapter). Interventions for extravasation vary, but each nurse should be aware of the institution's policies and procedures and implement them at once.

In addition to extravasation, a potentially fatal complication is anaphylaxis, especially from L-asparaginase, teniposide (VM-26), etoposide (VP-16), bleomycin, and cisplatin. Nursing responsibilities include prevention of, recognition of, and preparation for serious reactions. Prevention begins with a careful history for known allergies.

Most children with cancer have a venous access device, which facilitates administration of IV medications. During treatment and remission, many medications are taken orally at home. Compliance with the medication schedule is essential; nurses play an important role in educating the family about the medications and encouraging adherence to the plan.

> **! NURSING ALERT**
>
> Chemotherapeutic drugs must be given through a free-flowing IV line. The infusion is stopped immediately if any sign of infiltration (pain, stinging, swelling, or redness at the cannulation site) occurs. When chemotherapeutic and immunological agents are given, the child must be observed for 30 minutes after the infusion for signs of anaphylaxis (cyanosis, hypotension, wheezing, severe urticaria). Emergency equipment (especially a blood pressure monitor and bag-valve-mask) and emergency medications (especially oxygen, epinephrine, antihistamine, aminophylline, corticosteroids, and vasopressors) must be available. If a reaction is suspected, the drug is discontinued, the IV line is flushed with saline, and the child's vital signs and subsequent responses are closely monitored.

Manage Problems of Drug Toxicity

Chemotherapy presents several nursing challenges. The complexity of the treatment protocols is often overwhelming to families. In addition, each therapy is associated with a number of predictable adverse effects. Nurses must be aware of these effects and use judgement in recognizing reactions and toxicities.

Nausea and vomiting. The nausea and vomiting that occur shortly after administration of several of the drugs and from cranial or abdominal radiation can be profound. The serotonin-receptor antagonists (e.g., ondansetron, granisetron) are effective in the control of nausea and vomiting occurring after emetogenic chemotherapy and radiotherapy. When combined with dexamethasone, these medications are the treatment of choice in the prevention of delayed emesis (Krane, Casillas, & Zeltzer, 2016).

The most beneficial regimen for antiemetic control has been the administration of the antiemetic before the chemotherapy begins. The goal is to prevent the child from ever experiencing nausea or vomiting, thus preventing development of anticipatory symptoms (the conditioned response of developing nausea and vomiting *before* receiving the medication). These symptoms can be prevented in nearly 70 to 80% of patients with the correct use of antiemetics (Jordan, Gralla, & Jahn, 2013).

Anorexia. Loss of appetite is a direct consequence of the chemotherapy or irradiation. It is a major problem for parents because it is the one area they feel responsible for, particularly when so many other facets of care are outside their control. There are no universally successful techniques for encouraging a sick child to eat. However, the guidelines in Chapter 44 can be helpful during the anorexic period and can prevent additional problems during the remission.

Some children still do not eat despite these approaches. When loss of appetite and weight persist, the nurse should investigate the family situation to determine whether any factors (e.g., conditioned aversion to food, environmental stress related to eating, controlling behaviour, anger) might be contributing to the problem. Nasogastric tube feedings or total parenteral nutrition may be implemented for children with significant nutritional problems.

Mucosal ulceration. One of the most distressing adverse effects of several medications is GI mucosal cell damage, which can produce ulcers anywhere along the alimentary tract. Oral ulcers greatly compound anorexia because eating is extremely uncomfortable, but the following interventions may be helpful:

- Provide a bland, moist, soft diet appropriate for the child's age and preferences.
- Use a soft sponge toothbrush (Toothettes) or cotton-tipped applicator.
- Provide frequent mouthwashes with normal saline (using a solution of 5 mL of table salt and 500 mL of water) or sodium bicarbonate mouth rinses (using a solution of 5 mL of baking soda in 1000 mL of water).
- Use local anaesthetics (e.g., Chloraseptic lozenges) or nonprescription preparations without alcohol (e.g., hydrocortisone dental paste [Orabase], antiseptic mouth rinse [UlcerEase], diphenhydramine [Benadryl], and aluminum and magnesium hydroxide [Maalox] solution).

Although local anaesthetics are effective in temporarily relieving the pain, many children dislike the taste and numb feeling they produce.

> **! NURSING ALERT**
>
> Viscous lidocaine is not recommended for young children; if applied to the pharynx, it may depress the gag reflex, increasing the risk of aspiration. Rarely, seizures have been associated with the use of oral viscous lidocaine (Krane et al., 2016).

Other preparations that may be used to prevent or treat mucositis include chlorhexidine gluconate (Peridex), because of its dual effectiveness against candidal and bacterial infections; antifungal troches (lozenges) or mouthwash; and lip balm (e.g., Aquaphor), to keep the lips moist. Agents that should not be used include lemon glycerin swabs (which irritate eroded tissue and can decay teeth), hydrogen peroxide (which delays healing by breaking down protein), and milk of magnesia (which dries mucosa).

Stomatitis may cause such difficulty with eating that the child may require hospitalization for hydration, parenteral nutrition, and pain control (often with IV morphine). The child will usually choose the foods that are best tolerated, and the nurse should encourage parents to relax any eating pressures. Because the stomatitis is a temporary condition, the child can resume good food habits after the ulcers heal. Dental hygiene can become a serious problem for children with orthodontic appliances. Sometimes it may be necessary to remove the braces to allow chemotherapy to continue.

Rectal ulcers are managed by meticulous toilet hygiene, warm sitz baths after each bowel movement, and the use of an occlusive ointment or dressing applied to the ulcerated area to promote epithelialization. Stool softeners are necessary to prevent further discomfort. Parents should record bowel movements because the child may voluntarily avoid defecation to prevent discomfort. Rectal thermometers and suppositories are contraindicated because insertion may further traumatize the area.

Neuropathy. Vincristine and, to a lesser extent, vinblastine can cause various neurotoxic effects. Nursing interventions for management of these effects include the following:

- Administering stool softeners or laxatives for severe constipation caused by decreased bowel innervation
- Maintaining good body alignment and, if the patient is on bedrest, using a footboard or high-top shoes to minimize or prevent footdrop
- Carrying out safety measures during ambulation because of weakness and numbing of the extremities, which may cause difficulty in walking or fine hand movement
- Providing a soft or liquid diet for severe jaw pain

Hemorrhagic cystitis. Sterile hemorrhagic cystitis, a side effect of chemical irritation to the bladder from cyclophosphamide, can be decreased and often prevented by (1) promoting a liberal fluid intake (at least one and a half times the recommended daily fluid requirement); (2) frequent voiding immediately after feeling the urge, before bed, and after arising; (3) administering the drug early in the day to allow for sufficient oral intake and voiding; and (4) administering mesna (an agent that provides protection to the bladder) as ordered. If oral home administration is prescribed, the family needs specific instructions regarding exactly how much fluid the child must have.

Alopecia. Hair loss is a common adverse effect of several chemotherapeutic drugs and cranial irradiation, although not all children lose their hair during drug therapy. It is better to warn children and parents of this effect than to allow them to think that it is only a remote possibility. A soft cotton cap is the most comfortable head wear for children. Polyester increases perspiration and causes itching. Other options include scarves, hats, or a wig.

The nurse should also inform the family that hair regrows in 3 to 6 months and may be of a different colour and texture. Frequently the hair is darker, thicker, and curlier than before. If the child chooses not to wear a wig, attention to some type of head covering, especially in cold climates and during exposure to sun, and scalp hygiene are important. The scalp should be washed like any other body part.

Steroid effects. Short-term steroid therapy produces no acute toxicities and two beneficial reactions: increased appetite and a sense of well-being. However, it does produce alterations in appearance, which, although not clinically significant, can be distressing to older children. One of these is "moon face," in which the child's face becomes rounded and puffy. It is helpful to reassure the child that, after cessation of the drug, the facial shape will return to normal. Unlike hair loss, little can be done to camouflage this obvious change. If the child resumes activity early in the course of treatment, the change may be less noticeable to peers than after a long absence.

Mood changes. Shortly after beginning steroid therapy, children experience a number of mood changes that range from feelings of well-being and euphoria to depression and irritability. If parents are unaware of these drug-induced changes, they may become unduly concerned. The nurse should warn them of the reactions and encourage them to discuss the behavioural changes with each other and the child.

Provide Emotional Support

An important aspect of continued emotional support involves the prognosis. Although leukemia is no longer invariably fatal, it must be remembered that survival statistics are only average estimates and apply to children treated with the latest protocols since diagnosis. For the low-risk child the chances may be better, but for the high-risk child they may be significantly poorer. Of those who do survive after discontinuing therapy, some relapse. Only the passage of time is positive confirmation of the child being ultimately "cured" of the disease. Remission, even in excess of 5 years, cannot be equated with a cure. With increasing concern regarding late effects of treatment, continued surveillance of the child's health status is needed. The nurse working with family members must individualize information regarding the "numbers" and the potential risks. An understanding of each member's emotional needs, as well as competent care of physical ones, is essential to the positive, growth-promoting support of the family. Comprehensive emotional support for the family of the child with a potentially fatal illness is discussed in Chapter 40.

LYMPHOMAS

Pediatric lymphomas are the third most common group of malignancies in children and adolescents. The lymphomas, a group of neoplastic diseases that arise from the lymphoid and hematopoietic systems, are divided into Hodgkin's disease and non-Hodgkin's lymphoma (NHL). These diseases are further subdivided according to tissue type and the extent of disease. NHL is more prevalent in children younger than 14 years of age, whereas Hodgkin's disease is prevalent in adolescence and the young-adult period, with a striking increase in incidence between ages 15 and 19 years.

Hodgkin's Disease

Hodgkin's disease is a neoplastic disease that originates in the lymphoid system and primarily involves the lymph nodes. It predictably metastasizes to non-nodal or extralymphatic sites, especially the spleen, liver, bone marrow, and lungs, although no tissue is exempt from involvement (Fig. 48-5). It is classified according to four histological types: (1) lymphocytic predominance, (2) nodular sclerosis, (3) mixed cellularity, and (4) lymphocytic depletion. Accurate staging of the extent of disease is the basis for treatment protocols and expected prognoses.

The Ann Arbor staging system assigns a stage based on the number of sites of lymph node involvement, presence of

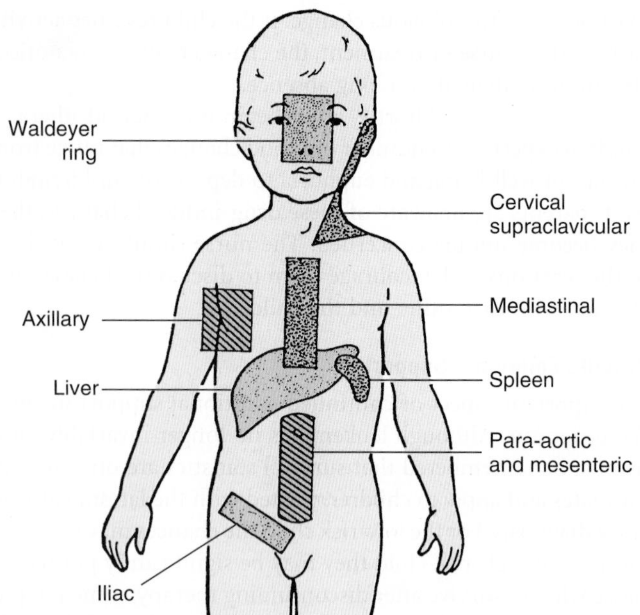

FIGURE 48-5 Main areas of lymphadenopathy and organ involvement in Hodgkin's disease.

extranodal disease, and history of any symptoms. Patients are classified as A if asymptomatic and as B if they have the following symptoms: fever, drenching night sweats, or unexplained loss of body weight (10% or more) over the preceding 6 months. Nonspecific systemic symptoms include fatigue, anorexia, mild to severe pruritus, and slight weight loss (Metzger, Krasin, Choi, et al., 2016; Woodgate, 2013).

Asymptomatic enlarged cervical or supraclavicular lymphadenopathy is the most common presentation of Hodgkin's disease. Other systemic symptoms may be manifested, including fever, weight loss, night sweats, cough, abdominal discomfort, anorexia, nausea, and pruritus. Because multiple organs may be involved, diagnosis is based on several tests and the extent of metastatic disease. Tests include a CBC, erythrocyte sedimentation rate (ESR), serum copper, ferritin level, fibrinogen, immune globulins, uric acid level, liver function tests, T-cell function studies, and urinalysis. Radiographic tests include computed tomography (CT) scans of the neck, chest, abdomen, and pelvis; a positron emission tomography (PET) scan (identifies metastatic or recurrent disease); a chest x-ray film; and, if clinically indicated, a bone scan to identify metastatic disease.

A lymph node biopsy is essential to establish histological diagnosis and staging. The presence of Reed-Sternberg cells is characteristic of Hodgkin's disease. These large cells, which are multilobed and nucleated with abundant cytoplasm and a typically halolike clear zone around the nucleolus, are often described as having an "owl's eyes" appearance (Metzger et al., 2016). A bone marrow aspiration or biopsy is usually performed. With the advent of CT and PET scans to identify metastatic disease and multi-agent therapy to eradicate metastatic disease, surgical staging involving a laparotomy with splenectomy is no longer performed.

Therapeutic Management

The primary modalities of therapy are radiation and chemotherapy. Each may be used alone or in combination, based on the clinical staging. Radiation may involve only the involved field (IF), an extended field (EF) (involved areas plus adjacent nodes), or total nodal irradiation (TNI), depending on the extent of involvement.

An effective combination of chemotherapy widely used is ABVD (doxorubicin [Adriamycin], bleomycin, vinblastine, dacarbazine) or CVPPABO (cyclophosphamide, vinblastine, procarbazine, prednisone; doxorubicin [Adriamycin], vincristine [Oncovin], bleomycin) (BC Cancer Agency, n.d.). However, the former therapy combination has caused severe late effects, especially secondary malignancies. Other drug combinations, such as COPP (cyclophosphamide, vincristine, prednisone, procarbazine), are used as a substitute and have minimized late effects.

Follow-up care of children no longer receiving therapy is essential to identify relapse and secondary cancers. In children with splenectomy resulting from laparotomy or splenic irradiation, prophylactic antibiotics are administered for an indefinite period. Also, immunizations against pneumococci and meningococci are recommended.

Prognosis

Long-term survival for all stages of Hodgkin's disease is excellent. Early-stage disease can have survival rates greater than 90%, with advanced stages having rates between 65 and 75%.

NURSING CARE

Nursing care involves the same objectives as for patients with other types of cancer, specifically (1) preparation for diagnostic and operative procedures, (2) explanation of treatment adverse effects, and (3) child and family support (see Chapter 40). Because this is most often a disease of adolescents and young adults, the nurse must have an appreciation of their psychological needs and reactions during the diagnostic and treatment phases (see Nursing Care Plan available on Evolve).

The most common adverse effect of irradiation is fatigue. This is particularly difficult for active, outgoing school-age children and adolescents because it prevents them from keeping up with their peers. Sometimes adolescents push themselves to the point of physical exhaustion rather than admit and succumb to the decreased activity tolerance. The nurse needs to caution parents to observe for behaviours such as extreme fatigue at the end of the day, falling asleep at the dinner table, inability to concentrate on homework, or an increased susceptibility to infection. A regular bedtime and scheduled rest periods are important for these children, especially during chemotherapy, when myelosuppression increases the risk of infection and debilitation. Before discharge the nurse should discuss a feasible school schedule with the parents and child.

An area of concern for adolescents is the high risk of sterility from irradiation and chemotherapy. Both drugs, particularly procarbazine and alkylating agents, and irradiation to the gonads can lead to infertility. Adolescents should be informed of these adverse effects early in the course of the diagnosis and treatment. Sperm banking is now offered through various referral programs before the initiation of treatment in adolescent boys. Sexual function is not altered, although the appearance of secondary sexual characteristics and menstruation may be delayed in the pubescent child. Delayed sexual maturation may be a sensitive and stressful issue for children and teenagers.

Non-Hodgkin's Lymphoma

NHL occurs more frequently in children than Hodgkin's disease. In Canadian children and adolescents under the age of 15, NHL made up approximately 4% of cancers in 2010, with Burkitt's lymphoma being the most common type (Leukemia & Lymphoma Society of Canada, 2013). Histological classification of childhood NHL is strikingly different from that of Hodgkin's disease:

- The disease is usually diffuse rather than nodular.
- The cell type is either undifferentiated or poorly differentiated.
- Dissemination occurs early, more often, and rapidly.
- Mediastinal involvement and invasion of meninges are common.

NHL exhibits a variety of morphological, cytochemical, and immunological features, not unlike the diversity seen in leukemia. Classification is based on the histological pattern: (1) lymphoblastic, (2) Burkitt or non-Burkitt, or (3) large cell. Immunologically these cells are also classified as T cells; B cells; or non-T, non-B cells (lacking immunological properties). The clinical staging system used in Hodgkin's disease is of little value in NHL, although it has been modified and other systems have been developed.

Diagnostic Evaluation

Because the clinical presentation of most children with NHL is widespread disseminated disease, thorough pathological staging is unnecessary. Clinical manifestations depend on the anatomical site and extent of involvement. These manifestations include many of those seen in Hodgkin's disease and leukemia, as well as organ symptoms related to pressure from enlargement of adjacent lymph nodes, such as intestinal or airway obstruction, cranial nerve palsies, and spinal paralysis.

Recommendations for staging include a surgical biopsy of an enlarged node, histopathological confirmation of disease with cytochemical and immunological evaluation, bone marrow examination, radiographic studies (especially tomograms of the lungs and GI organs), and lumbar puncture.

Therapeutic Management

The treatment protocols for NHL include aggressive use of irradiation and chemotherapy. Similar to leukemic therapy, the protocols include induction, consolidation, and maintenance phases, some with intrathecal chemotherapy. Antineoplastic agents used in the treatment of NHL include vincristine, prednisone, L-asparaginase, methotrexate, 6-mercaptopurine, cytarabine, cyclophosphamide, anthracyclines, and teniposide or etoposide (Allen, Kamdar, Bollard, et al., 2016).

Prognosis

The prognosis is excellent for children with localized disease, with an almost 100% cure rate; 75 to 90% of children with extensive disease are cured (Allen et al., 2016). Because relapse after 2 years is rare, survival after 24 months is considered a cure.

NURSING CARE

Nursing care of the child with NHL is similar to that required for children with leukemia. Many of the same medications are used, although the schedules differ. Because of the intense chemotherapy, nursing care is primarily directed toward managing the adverse effects of these agents and providing supportive care to the child and family (see Nursing Care Plan available on Evolve).

IMMUNOLOGICAL DEFICIENCY DISORDERS

A number of disorders can cause profound, often life-threatening alterations within the body's immune system. The most serious are conditions that completely depress immunity, such as severe combined immunodeficiency disease (SCID). However, the one disorder that generates the most anxiety, within both the family and the community at large, is HIV infection/AIDS.

Several classifications of immune dysfunction exist. AIDS, SCID, and Wiskott-Aldrich syndrome (WAS) are syndromes in which the body is unable to mount an immune response. The immune response can also be misdirected. In **autoimmune disorders**, antibodies, macrophages, and lymphocytes attack healthy cells.

HIV Infection and Acquired Immunodeficiency Syndrome

Since the first cases of AIDS were identified in the early 1980s, HIV infection has generated intense medical investigation. Research has led to early diagnosis of and improved medical treatments for HIV infection, changing this disease from a rapidly fatal one to a chronic, but terminal, disease.

Epidemiology

The principal modes of HIV transmission to the pediatric population are mother-to-child transmission and adolescent risky behaviours such as sexual activity and IV drug use.

According to the Canadian Perinatal HIV Surveillance Program, in 2009, 180 children were born to women who were HIV positive, with a rate of transmission of 1% (PHAC, 2014). The rate of mother-to-child transmission is decreasing even though the HIV maternal rate is increasing (PHAC, 2014). This trend may be attributed to a result of implementation of recommended HIV counselling and voluntary testing practices, optimal prenatal, antenatal and postpartum care, and the use of ART to prevent perinatal transmission (see Human Immunodeficiency Virus, Chapter 7, p. 129, and Chapter 15, p. 392).

Unsafe sexual activity and IV drug use are major sources of HIV infection in adolescents and young adults. Youth between the ages of 15 and 19 years comprise 26.5% of all reports of HIV-positive status (PHAC, 2014).

The Indigenous populations are of special concern regarding HIV infection. In 2008, this group represented 66% of all new HIV infections, primarily due to street drug injections, compared with a rate of 17% for all other Canadians. From 1998 to 2008, women represented 48.8% of all positive HIV test reports among Indigenous peoples compared with 20.6% for all other Canadians (PHAC, 2014).

Etiology

HIV is a retrovirus that is transmitted by lymphocytes and monocytes. It is found in the blood, semen, vaginal secretions, and breast milk. It has an incubation or latency period of months to years (Grace, 2014). There are different strains of HIV. HIV-2 is prevalent in Africa, whereas HIV-1 subtype B is the dominant strain in Canada. *Horizontal transmission* of HIV occurs through intimate sexual contact or parenteral exposure to blood or body fluids containing visible blood. *Perinatal (vertical) transmission* occurs when an HIV-infected pregnant woman passes the infection to her infant.

Pathophysiology

HIV primarily infects a specific subset of T lymphocytes, the CD4 T cells. The virus takes over the machinery of the CD4 lymphocyte, using it to replicate itself, rendering the CD4 cell dysfunctional. The CD4 lymphocyte count gradually decreases over time, leading to progressive immunodeficiency. The count eventually reaches a critical level below which there is substantial risk of opportunistic illnesses, followed by death.

Clinical Manifestations

Common clinical manifestations of HIV infection in children are varied (Box 48-9). The diagnosis of AIDS is associated with certain illnesses or conditions. The most common AIDS-defining conditions observed among Canadian children are listed in Box 48-10. Other problems in these children may include short stature, malnutrition, and cardiomyopathy. CNS abnormalities resulting from HIV infection may include neuropsychological deficits; developmental disabilities; and deficits in motor skills, communication, and behavioural functioning.

Diagnostic Evaluation

For children 18 months of age and older, the HIV enzyme-linked immunosorbent assay (ELISA) and Western blot immunoassay are performed to determine HIV infection. In infants born to HIV-infected mothers, these assays will be positive because of the presence of maternal antibodies derived transplacentally. Maternal antibodies may persist in infants up to 18 months of age. Thus other diagnostic tests are used, most commonly the HIV polymerase chain reaction (PCR) for detection of proviral DNA. With this technique, more than 95% of infected infants can be diagnosed by 1 to 3 months of age (Grace, 2014).

The Centers for Disease Control and Prevention (1994) developed a classification system that is still used to describe the spectrum of HIV disease in children (Table 48-3). The system indicates the severity of clinical signs and symptoms and the degree of immunosuppression. Mild signs and symptoms include lymphadenopathy, parotitis, hepatosplenomegaly, and recurrent or persistent sinusitis or otitis media. Moderate signs and symptoms include lymphoid interstitial pneumonitis (LIP) and a variety of organ-specific dysfunctions or infections. Severe signs and symptoms include AIDS-defining illnesses with the exception of LIP. Children with LIP have a better prognosis than those with other AIDS-defining illnesses. In children whose HIV infection is not yet confirmed, the letter *E* (vertically exposed) is placed in front of the classification. The immune categories are based on CD4 lymphocyte counts and percentages.

Therapeutic Management

The goals of therapy for HIV infection include slowing the growth of the virus, preventing and treating **opportunistic infections**, and providing nutritional support and symptomatic treatment. Antiretroviral medications work at various stages of the HIV life cycle to prevent reproduction of functional new virus particles. Although not a cure, these medications can suppress viral replication, preventing further deterioration of the

BOX 48-9 COMMON CLINICAL MANIFESTATIONS OF HIV INFECTION IN CHILDREN

- Lymphadenopathy
- Hepatosplenomegaly
- Oral candidiasis
- Chronic or recurrent diarrhea
- Failure to thrive
- Developmental delay
- Behavioural abnormalities
- Parotitis

BOX 48-10 COMMON DEFINING CONDITIONS FOR AIDS IN CHILDREN

- *Pneumocystis carinii* pneumonia
- Lymphoid interstitial pneumonia, pulmonary lymphoid hyperplasia, or both
- Recurrent bacterial infections
- Wasting syndrome
- Candidal esophagitis
- Human immunodeficiency virus encephalopathy
- Cytomegalovirus disease
- *Mycobacterium avium-intracellulare* complex infection
- Pulmonary candidiasis
- Herpes simplex disease
- Cryptosporidiosis

TABLE 48-3 PEDIATRIC HIV INFECTION CLASSIFICATION*

IMMUNOLOGICAL CATEGORY	N: NO SIGNS/ SYMPTOMS	A: MILD SIGNS/ SYMPTOMS	B: MODERATE SIGNS/ SYMPTOMS	C: SEVERE SIGNS/ SYMPTOMS
No evidence of suppression	N1	A1	B1	C1
Evidence of moderate suppression	N2	A2	B2	C2
Severe suppression	N3	A3	B3	C3

*Children whose HIV infection status is not confirmed are classified by using the above table with the letter *E* (for perinatally exposed) placed before the appropriate classification code (e.g., EN2).

From Centers for Disease Control and Prevention. (1994). 1994 Revised classification system for human immunodeficiency virus infection in children less than 13 years of age. *MMWR: Recommendations & Reports, 43*(RR-12), 1–10.

immune system, thus delaying disease progression. Classes of antiretroviral agents include nucleoside reverse transcriptase inhibitors (e.g., zidovudine, didanosine, stavudine, lamivudine, abacavir), non-nucleoside reverse transcriptase inhibitors (e.g., nevirapine, delavirdine, efavirenz, etravirine, rilpivirine), nucleotide reverse transcriptase inhibitors (e.g., adefovir), integrase inhibitors (dolutegravir, raltegravir), protease inhibitors (e.g., indinavir, atazanavir, saquinavir, ritonavir, nelfinavir, darunavir), and adjunctive antiretrovirals (e.g., hydroxyurea). Combinations of antiretroviral medications are used to forestall the emergence of drug resistance. ART regimens and guidelines are continually evolving. Therapy is lifelong, making adherence difficult. Laboratory markers (CD4 lymphocyte count, viral load) assist in monitoring both disease progression and response to therapy. The Canadian Paediatric Society (CPS) (Robinson & CPS, Infectious Diseases and Immunization Committee, 2010/2016) recommends following the U.S. National Institutes of Health (2015) clinical guidelines for the management of HIV.

Pneumocystis carinii pneumonia (PCP) is the most common opportunistic infection of children infected with HIV. It occurs most frequently between 3 and 6 months of age. All infants born to HIV-infected women should receive prophylaxis during the first year of life (National Institutes of Health, 2015). Trimethoprim-sulfamethoxazole (TMP-SMZ) is the agent of choice. If adverse effects are experienced with TMP-SMZ, dapsone or pentamidine can be used.

Prophylaxis is often used for other opportunistic infections, such as disseminated *Mycobacterium avium-intracellulare* complex (MAC), candidiasis, or herpes simplex. IVIG has been helpful in preventing recurrent or serious bacterial infections in some HIV-infected children.

Immunization against common childhood illnesses is recommended for all children exposed to and infected with HIV (PHAC, 2016). Varicella (chicken pox) vaccine, MMR vaccine, and herpes zoster vaccine can be administered if there is no evidence of severe immunocompromise. Because antibody production to vaccines may be poor or decrease over time, immediate prophylaxis after exposure to several vaccine-preventable diseases (e.g., measles, varicella) is warranted. Children receiving IV gamma-globulin (IVGG) prophylaxis may not respond to the MMR vaccine if given in close proximity to the IVGG dose (Centers for Disease Control and Prevention, 2003).

HIV infection often leads to marked failure to thrive and multiple nutritional deficiencies. Nutritional management may be difficult because of recurrent illness, diarrhea, and other physical problems. Intensive nutritional interventions should be instituted when the child's growth begins to slow or weight begins to decrease.

Prognosis

Early recognition and improved medical care have changed HIV disease from being a rapidly fatal illness to a chronic disease. After the introduction of combination ART, the numbers of new AIDS cases and deaths declined substantially. For example, between 1984 and 2003, there were 560 deaths among the 1987 HIV-positive individuals in Southern Alberta. Of these, 436 deaths (78%) occurred during the pre-ART era and 124 (22%) during the current ART era (Krentz, Kliewer, & Gill, 2005). Since 1998, the annual number of AIDS cases among children younger than 13 years of age has remained stable (Klause & Johnson, 2007).

NURSING CARE

Education concerning transmission and control of infectious diseases, including HIV infection, is essential for children with HIV infection and anyone involved in their care. The basic tenets of routine practices should be presented in an age-appropriate manner, with careful consideration of the educational levels of the individuals (see Infection Control, Chapter 44). Safety issues, including appropriate storage of special medications and equipment (e.g., needles and syringes), need to be emphasized.

Unfortunately, relatives, friends, and the general public may be fearful of contracting HIV infection, and the child and family may be criticized and ostracized. In an effort to protect the child, the family may limit his or her activities outside the home. Although certain precautions are justified in limiting exposure to sources of infections, they must be tempered with concern for the child's normal developmental needs. Both the family and the community need ongoing education about HIV to dispel many of the myths that have been perpetuated by uninformed persons (see Additional Resources at the end of this chapter).

Prevention is a key component of HIV education. Educating adolescents about HIV is essential in preventing HIV infection in this age group. It should include the routes of transmission, the hazards of IV and other recreational drug use, and safer sex practices. Such education should be a part of anticipatory guidance provided to all adolescent patients. Nurses can also encourage adolescents at risk to undergo HIV counselling and testing. In addition to identifying infected teenagers and getting them into care, such counselling affords adolescents an opportunity to learn about, and possibly change, their risk-related behaviours.

The multiple complications associated with HIV disease are potentially painful (Grace, 2014). Aggressive pain management is essential for these children to have an acceptable quality of life. Their pain may be caused by infections (e.g., otitis media, dental abscess), encephalopathy (e.g., spasticity), adverse effects of medications (e.g., peripheral neuropathy), or an unknown source (e.g., deep musculoskeletal pain). Sources of pain are related not only to disease processes but also to various treatments these children often undergo, including venipunctures, lumbar punctures, biopsies, and endoscopies. Ongoing assessment of pain is crucial and is most easily accomplished in older children who are able to communicate. Nonverbal and developmentally delayed children are more difficult to assess. The nurse should be alert for signs of pain such as emotional detachment, lack of interactive play, irritability, and depression. Effective pain management depends on the appropriate use of pharmacological agents, including EMLA cream, acetaminophen, NSAIDs, muscle relaxants, and opioids. Tolerance to opioids may indicate increased dosing; monitored use ensures safety. Nonpharmacological interventions (e.g., guided imagery, hypnosis, relaxation, and distraction techniques) are useful adjuncts.

Common psychosocial concerns include disclosing the diagnosis to the child, making custody plans when the parent is infected, and anticipating the loss of a family member. Other stressors may include financial difficulties, HIV-associated stigma, efforts to keep the diagnosis secret, other infected family members, and the multiple losses associated with HIV (see Family-Centred Teaching box). Family members are often involved in the care of the child, particularly if the parent has symptomatic illness. Nursing is an integral part of the multidisciplinary team necessary for the successful management of the complex medical and social problems of these families.

Children with HIV infection attend day care centres and schools. It is well established that the risk of HIV transmission in these settings is minimal. These institutions are required to follow Canada's National Workplace Health and Safety (CanOSH) guidelines for infection-control measures. Routine practices describing proper management of blood and body fluids should also be followed. It is recommended that school personnel receive current HIV information and include it in the health education curriculum for kindergarten through grade twelve. Confidentiality is a major issue in day care or school attendance. Parents and legal guardians have the right to decide whether to inform these agencies of their child's HIV diagnosis. Unfortunately, myths about HIV infection continue to exist, and the family often wishes to avoid any potential criticism or ostracism of the child.

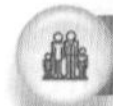

FAMILY-CENTRED TEACHING

Caregivers and the Infant With HIV Infection

Unlike other fatal pediatric diseases, human immunodeficiency virus (HIV) infection is associated with special family alterations. The infant infected in utero faces multiple physical and parental problems. Because the mother is infected, she may be coping with a chronic illness and therefore unable to care for the child. Grandparents or other relatives may assume care. Foster care is often difficult to arrange because of the nature of the disease, especially in relation to the social stigma of HIV and the child's multiple medical needs. When these children are hospitalized, the importance of consistent caregivers, especially primary nurses who attend to the youngsters' physical, developmental, and emotional needs, cannot be overemphasized. However, primary nurses may face the risk of overinvolvement and must be aware of the boundaries of a therapeutic relationship.

Severe Combined Immunodeficiency Disease

SCID is a defect characterized by the absence of both humoral and cell-mediated immunity. The terms *Swiss-type lymphopenic agammaglobulinemia* (an autosomal recessive form of the disease) and *X-linked lymphopenic agammaglobulinemia* have been used to describe this disorder, which, as the names imply, can follow either mode of inheritance.

Susceptibility to infection occurs early, most often in the first month of life. The child suffers from chronic infection, fails to completely recover from an infection, is frequently reinfected, and is infected with unusual agents. Failure to thrive is a consequence of the persistent illnesses.

Diagnosis is usually based on a history of recurrent, severe infections from early infancy; a familial history of the disorder; and specific laboratory findings, which include lymphopenia, lack of lymphocyte response to antigens, and absence of plasma cells in the bone marrow. Documentation of immune globulin deficiency is difficult during infancy because of the normally delayed response of infants in producing their own immune globulins and material transfer of immune globulin G (IgG).

Therapeutic Management

The definitive treatment for SCID is HSCT from a histocompatible donor, a haploidentical donor (usually a parent), or a matched unrelated donor. IVIG infusions and PCP prophylaxis are used to augment the humoral immunity until the transplant is performed. Several investigators are attempting gene therapy with some success, but there is a potential complication of insertional mutagenesis (Buckley, 2016).

NURSING CARE

Nursing care focuses on preventing infection and supporting the child and family. The care is consistent with that needed for HSCT for any condition. Because the prognosis for SCID is very poor if a compatible bone marrow donor is not available, nursing care is directed at supporting the family in caring for a child with a life-threatening illness (see Chapter 40). Genetic counselling is essential because of the modes of transmission in either form of the disorder.

Wiskott-Aldrich Syndrome (WAS)

WAS is an X-linked recessive disorder characterized by a triad of abnormalities: (1) thrombocytopenia, (2) eczema, and (3) immunodeficiency of selective functions of B and T lymphocytes. A defective gene has been identified and designated the WAS protein (Bonilla & Notarangelo, 2014). At birth the presenting symptom may be bloody diarrhea as a result of thrombocytopenia. As the child grows older, recurrent infection and eczema become more severe, and the bleeding becomes less frequent.

Eczema is typical of the allergic type and easily becomes superinfected. Chronic infection with herpes simplex is a frequent problem and may lead to chronic keratitis of the eye with loss of vision. Chronic pulmonary disease, sinusitis, and otitis media result from repeated infections. In children who survive the bleeding episodes and overwhelming infections, malignancy presents an additional risk to survival. Medical treatment involves the following:

- Counteracting the bleeding tendencies with platelet transfusions
- Using IV gamma-globulin to provide passive immunity
- Administering prophylactic antibiotics to prevent and control infection
- Providing aggressive local therapy for the eczema

The only curative therapy is HSCT from a matched donor (Albert, Notarangelo, & Ochs, 2011; Buckley, 2016).

NURSING CARE

Because of the poor prognosis for these children, the main nursing consideration is supporting the family in the care of a fatally ill child (see Chapter 40). Physical care is directed at controlling the problems imposed by the disorder. The measures used to control bleeding are similar to those for hemophilia and vWD (see previous discussions). Another major goal is prevention or control of infection. Because eczema is a troublesome problem, nursing measures specific to this condition are especially important (see Chapter 52). The genetic implications of this X-linked recessive disorder differ little from those of any other X-linked disorder.

TECHNOLOGICAL MANAGEMENT OF HEMATOLOGICAL AND IMMUNOLOGICAL DISORDERS

Blood Transfusion Therapy

Technological advances in blood banking and transfusion medicine enable the administration of only the blood component needed by the child, such as packed RBCs in anemia or platelets for bleeding disorders. However, regardless of the blood component infused, all transfusions have some risks. Nurses need to be aware of the possible complications and the appropriate interventions. Table 48-4 summarizes the major hazards of transfusions, the signs and symptoms typically associated with each, and nursing responsibilities. General guidelines that apply to all transfusions include the following:

- Take vital signs, including blood pressure, *before* administering blood, to establish baseline data for intratransfusion and post-transfusion comparison, and then every 15 minutes for 1 hour while blood is infusing and on completion of transfusion.
- Check the identification of the recipient with the donor's blood group and type, regardless of the blood product being used.
- Administer the first 50 mL of blood or 20% of the volume (whichever is smaller) *slowly* (and in some facilities at half rate) and stay with the child.
- Administer with normal saline on a piggyback setup or have normal saline available.
- Administer blood through an appropriate filter to eliminate particles in the blood and prevent the precipitation of formed elements; gently shake the container frequently.
- Use blood within 30 minutes of its arrival from the blood bank; if it is not used, return to the blood bank—do not store in the regular unit refrigerator.
- Infuse a unit of blood (or the specified amount) within 4 hours. If the infusion will exceed this time, the blood should be divided into appropriately sized quantities by the blood bank, and the unused portion should be refrigerated under controlled conditions.
- If a reaction of any type is suspected, take vital signs, stop the transfusion, maintain a patent IV line with normal saline and new tubing, notify the practitioner, and do not restart the transfusion until the child's condition has been medically evaluated.

Although hemolytic reactions are rare, ABO incompatibility remains the most common cause of death from blood transfusion, and human error is usually responsible (administration of the wrong type to the patient or mislabelling of the blood product) (Tondon, Paney, Mickey, et al., 2010). Hemolysis can also cause the release of large quantities of phospholipids, which are capable of stimulating DIC (see p. 1539). Acute kidney shutdown and eventual renal failure are the results of renal vasoconstriction from antigen–antibody complexes derived from the RBC surface.

Blood is usually administered to children by infusion pump; thus the usual precautions and management related to pumps apply. When the blood is started with a standard transfusion set, the filter chamber is filled to allow the total filter to be used. The drip chamber is partially filled with blood to permit counting of the drops. In adjusting the flow rate, it is important to remember that blood administration sets do not use microdrops (60 drops/mL) but regular drops (usually 10 or 15 drops/mL). The nurse must consider this when calculating the flow rate.

Hematopoietic Stem Cell (Bone Marrow) Transplantation

HSCT is used to establish healthy hemopoiesis in both malignant and nonmalignant disease. Candidates for transplantation are children who have disorders that are unlikely to be cured by other means. Most HSCT patients undergo intensive ablative therapy using high-dose combination chemotherapy with or without total body irradiation (Gottschalk et al., 2016). After the immune system is suppressed to prevent rejection of the transplanted marrow, the stem cells harvested from the bone marrow, peripheral blood, or umbilical vein of the placenta are given to the patient by IV transfusion. The newly transfused stem cells will begin to repopulate the ablative bone marrow. In essence, a new blood-forming organ will be accepted by the recipient.

TABLE 48-4 **NURSING CARE OF THE CHILD RECEIVING BLOOD TRANSFUSIONS***

COMPLICATIONS	SIGNS AND SYMPTOMS	PRECAUTIONS AND NURSING RESPONSIBILITIES
Immediate Reactions		
Hemolytic Reactions		
Most severe type, but rare Incompatible blood Incompatibility in multiple transfusions	Sudden severe headache Chills Shaking Fever Pain at needle site and along venous tract Nausea and vomiting Sensation of tightness in chest Red or black urine Flank pain Progressive signs of shock or renal failure	Identify donor blood type before transfusion is begun; verify with another nurse or practitioner. Transfuse blood slowly for first 15–20 min. Stop transfusion immediately if signs or symptoms occur, maintain patent intravenous line, and notify practitioner. Save donor blood to re-cross-match with patient's blood. Monitor for evidence of shock. Insert urinary catheter and monitor hourly outputs. Send sample of patient's blood and urine to laboratory for presence of hemoglobin (indicates intravascular hemolysis). Observe for signs of hemorrhage resulting from disseminated intravascular coagulation. Support medical therapies to reverse shock.
Febrile Reactions		
Leukocyte or platelet antibodies Plasma protein antibodies	Fever Chills Shaking Nausea Vomiting Headache	Acetaminophen may be given for prophylaxis. Leukocyte-poor red blood cells (RBCs) are less likely to cause reaction. Stop transfusion immediately; report to practitioner for evaluation.
Allergic Reactions		
Recipient reaction to allergens in donor's blood	Urticaria Pruritus Flushing Nausea/vomiting Anxiety Asthmatic wheezing Laryngeal edema	Give antihistamines for prophylaxis to children with tendency to allergic reactions. Stop transfusion immediately. Administer epinephrine for wheezing or anaphylactic reaction.
Circulatory Overload		
Too rapid transfusion (even a small quantity) Transfusion of excessive quantity of blood (even slowly)	Precordial pain Dyspnea Rales Cyanosis Dry cough Distended neck veins Hypertension	Transfuse blood slowly. Prevent overload by using packed RBCs or administering divided amounts of blood. Use infusion pump to regulate and maintain flow rate. Stop transfusion immediately if there are signs of overload. Place child upright with feet in dependent position to increase venous resistance.
Air Emboli		
May occur when blood is transfused under pressure	Sudden difficulty in breathing Sharp pain in chest Apprehension	Normalize pressure before container is empty when infusing blood under pressure. Clear tubing of air by aspirating it with syringe at nearest Y connector if it is observed in tubing; disconnect tubing and allow blood to flow until air has escaped only if a Y connector is not available.
Hypothermia		
	Chills Low temperature Irregular heart rate Possible cardiac arrest	Allow blood to warm at room temperature (<1 hr). Use approved mechanical blood warmer or electric warming coil to warm blood rapidly; never use microwave oven. Take temperature if patient has symptoms of chills; if subnormal, stop transfusion.
Electrolyte Disturbances		
Hyperkalemia (in massive transfusions or in patients with renal problems)	Nausea, diarrhea Muscle weakness Flaccid paralysis Paresthesia of extremities Bradycardia Apprehension Cardiac arrest	Use washed RBCs or fresh blood if patient is at risk.

TABLE 48-4 NURSING CARE OF THE CHILD RECEIVING BLOOD TRANSFUSIONS—cont'd

COMPLICATIONS	SIGNS AND SYMPTOMS	PRECAUTIONS AND NURSING RESPONSIBILITIES
Delayed Reactions		
Alloimmunization		
Antibody formation Occurs in patients receiving multiple transfusions	Increased risk of hemolytic, febrile, and allergic reactions	Use limited number of donors. Observe carefully for signs of reactions.
Delayed Hemolytic Reaction		
	Destruction of RBCs and fever 5–10 days after transfusion	Observe for post-transfusion anemia and decreasing benefit from successive transfusions.

*Some institutions may have more rigorous guidelines for checking blood and more frequent taking of vital signs during the initial portion of the administration. Therefore, nurses should familiarize themselves with their specific facility's policies and procedures surrounding blood transfusion administration.

From University of British Columbia. (n.d.). *Blood transfusion reactions.* Retrieved from http://learn.pediatrics.ubc.ca/body-systems/hematology-oncology/blood-transfusion-reactions/

The selection process for a suitable donor and the potential complications in transplantation are related to the *HLA system complex*. Some of the major HLAs are A, B, C, D, and DR. There is a wide diversity for each of these HLA loci. There are more than 20 different HLA-As that can be inherited and more than 40 different HLA-Bs.

The genes are inherited as a single unit or *haplotype*. A child inherits one unit from each parent; thus a child and each parent have one identical and one nonidentical haplotype. Because the possible haplotype combinations among siblings follow the laws of Mendelian genetics, there is a one-in-four chance that two siblings have two identical haplotypes and are perfectly matched at the HLA loci.

The importance of HLA matching is to prevent the serious complication known as graft-versus-host disease, or GVHD. Because the child's immune system is essentially rendered nonfunctional, there is little difficulty with bone marrow rejection by the recipient. However, the donor's marrow may contain antigens not matched to the recipient's antigens, which begin attacking body cells. The more closely the HLA systems match, the less likely GVHD will develop. However, it can occur even with a perfect HLA match because there are as yet unidentified and thus unmatched histocompatibility antigens (Gottschalk et al., 2016).

Different types of HSCT are now performed in children with cancer. Allogeneic HSCT involves matching a histocompatible donor with the recipient. However, allogeneic HSCT is limited by the presence of a suitable marrow donor.

Because of the limited numbers of patients having HLA-identical siblings, other types of allogeneic transplants have evolved. Umbilical cord blood stem cell transplantation is an established, rich source of hematopoietic stem cells for use in children with cancer. Because stem cells can be found with high frequency in the circulation of newborns, cord blood transplantation has become an alternative for some children. The benefit of using umbilical cord blood is the blood's relative immunodeficiency at birth, allowing for partially matched unrelated cord blood transplants to be successful, with a lower risk of GVHD-related problems (Frey, Guess, Allison, et al., 2009; Gottschalk et al., 2016).

Autologous HSCTs use the patient's own marrow that was collected from disease-free tissue, frozen, and sometimes treated to remove malignant cells. Children with solid tumours such as neuroblastoma, Hodgkin's disease, NHL, rhabdomyosarcoma, Ewing sarcoma, and Wilms tumour have been treated with autologous HSCTs.

Peripheral stem cell transplants (PSCTs) are also used in children with cancer. PSCT, a type of autologous transplant, differs in the way stem cells are collected from the patient. CSF is first given to stimulate the production of many stem cells. After the WBC count is high enough, the stem cells are collected by an apheresis machine. This machine filters out peripheral stem cells from whole blood, returning the remainder of the blood cells and plasma to the child. Stem cells have been collected in very small children without problems. The peripheral stem cells are then frozen until the patient is ready for the PSCT.

NURSING CARE

The care of children undergoing HSCT is similar to that of any child receiving chemotherapy and radiotherapy. The hospitalization is typically 3 to 6 weeks in an isolated environment, during which time the child is subjected to numerous procedures and adverse effects of therapy.

Throughout this long ordeal the family is concerned with successful engraftment and fear of fatal complications (see Family-Centred Teaching box). Consequently, nurses involved with the child and family need to provide sensitive care and maintain a supportive attitude during the many crises that may arise. If the procedure is not successful, the families need care consistent with that required by the family of any child with a life-threatening disorder (see Chapter 40).

Apheresis

Apheresis is the removal of blood from an individual, separation of the blood into its components, retention of one or more of

FAMILY-CENTRED TEACHING

The Decision for a Hematopoietic Stem Cell Transplant

A family's decision for a child to undergo hematopoietic stem cell transplantation (HSCT) may be fraught with challenges. Often the child is facing certain death from the malignancy. The preparation of the child for the transplant also places the patient at great medical risk.

Once the preparatory regimen is begun and the child's immune system is destroyed, there is no turning back. Unlike kidney transplantation, HSCT does not have a "rescue" procedure, such as dialysis, for supportive therapy. If the donor is a sibling, the issue of his or her marrow "saving" the brother or sister can be a concern, especially if the transplant fails. Parents often must leave the home to stay at the transplant centre and encounter additional stressors such as arranging child care, taking a leave from work, and managing finances. The patient faces the greatest stress—fear of HSCT failure or life-threatening complications.

these components, and reinfusion of the remainder of the blood into the individual. It is most often used to remove large quantities of platelets from healthy adult donors. These transfusion products have greatly prolonged the survival of patients with hematological and oncological diseases.

This technique is used to remove peripheral blood stem cells (PBSCs) from children before they receive HSCT or high-dose chemotherapy or radiotherapy, which is severely toxic to the bone marrow. These PBSCs can then be used to restore the child's bone marrow. Apheresis is also used as a therapeutic modality. The blood component that is diseased or toxic is separated from the blood, and the remainder is returned to the individual. Therapeutic apheresis is considered part of standard therapy for many diseases. Plasma is selectively removed from individuals with hyperviscosity, life-threatening complications of myasthenia gravis, Guillain-Barré syndrome, thrombotic thrombocytopenic purpura, and certain drug overdoses. WBCs are removed from individuals with high–WBC count leukemia.

NURSING CARE

Difficult venous access and small blood volume can limit the ability to use this therapy in the infant and young child. Education of the family and child includes the purposes of the therapy and the technology.

Specially trained individuals perform the apheresis procedure. Attention focuses on the rate of removal, blood component separation, and reinfusion of blood into the child. Vital signs need to be monitored and the child continuously observed for any adverse reactions secondary to the circulatory volume changes and the anticoagulant used.

When apheresis components are infused, nursing measures differ depending on whether the product is autologous (blood component from the child) or allogeneic (blood component from another individual). Autologous components are the child's own blood; thus a major precaution is proper identification to ensure the correct component. The rate of infusion should be adjusted to the child's tolerance. If the product is allogeneic, all precautions for blood transfusions apply.

KEY POINTS

- *Anemia* is defined as the reduction of RBCs or Hgb concentration to levels below normal for gender and age; disorders are classified either by etiology and physiology or by morphology.
- The nurse's role in treatment of anemia is to gather information necessary to assist in establishing a diagnosis, prepare the child for laboratory tests, administer prescribed medications, decrease tissue oxygen needs, implement safety precautions, and observe for complications.
- The main nursing goal in prevention of nutritional anemia is parent education regarding correct feeding practices.
- SCA is a hereditary hemoglobinopathy caused by normal adult Hgb (HgbA) being partly or completely replaced by sickle Hgb (HgbS).
- Nursing care of the child with SCA focuses on teaching the family how to prevent and recognize sickle cell problems; managing pain during crises; and helping the child and parents adjust to a lifelong chronic disease.
- Nursing care of the child with beta thalassemia includes observing for complications of multiple blood transfusions, assisting the child in coping with the effects of illness, and fostering parent–child adjustment to long-term illness.
- Causes of acquired AA include irradiation, medications, industrial and household chemicals, infections, and infiltration and replacement of myeloid elements; however, most cases are idiopathic.
- Clotting depends on three processes: vascular spasm, platelet aggregation, and coagulation and clot formation.
- Nursing care of the child with hemophilia involves preventing bleeding by decreasing the risk of injury, recognizing and managing bleeding with factor replacement, preventing the crippling effects of joint degeneration, and preparing and supporting the child and family for home care.
- Goals in the care of the child with leukemia are to prepare the family for diagnostic and therapeutic procedures, prevent complications of myelosuppression, manage problems of irradiation and drug toxicity, and provide continued emotional support.
- The lymphomas include Hodgkin's lymphoma and NHL and are disorders involving the lymphoid system.
- Immunodeficiency disorders render the affected individual unable to fight infectious organisms.
- HIV infection in infants is primarily acquired during pregnancy or birth from an infected mother,

and in adolescents from engaging in high-risk behaviours.
- Blood transfusions supply needed blood components.
- HSCT replaces the diseased or malfunctioning bone marrow with viable blood stem cells.
- Apheresis is the selective removal of a blood component. It can be used to supply cellular elements needed for therapy (i.e., platelets or stem cells) or to remove diseased components.

evolve WEBSITE

Visit the Evolve website for additional resources related to the content in this chapter such as Case Studies, Critical Thinking Case Study Answers, Nursing Care Plans, Nursing Processes, Nursing Skills, and Review Questions for Exam Preparation at: *http://evolve.elsevier.com/Canada/Perry/maternal/*

REFERENCES

Abdullah, K., Zlotkin, S., Parkin, P., & Grenier, D. (2011). *Iron-deficiency anemia in children.* Canadian Paediatric Surveillance Program. Retrieved from <http://www.cpsp.cps.ca/uploads/publications/RA-iron-deficiency-anemia.pdf>.

Albert, M. H., Notarangelo, L. D., & Ochs, H. D. (2011). Clinical spectrum, pathophysiology and treatment of Wiskott-Aldrich syndrome. *Current Opinion in Hematology, 18*(1), 42–48.

Allen, C. E., Kamdar, K. Y., Bollard, C. M., et al. (2016). Malignant non-Hodgkin lymphomas of childhood. In P. A. Pizzo & D. G. Poplack (Eds.), *Principles and practice of pediatric oncology* (7th ed.). Philadelphia: Lippincott.

Ball, J., Bindler, R., & Cowen, K. (2012). *Principles of pediatric nursing.* Boston: Pearson Education Inc.

Bauman, M. E., McClure, W., & Venner, M. A. (2013). Nursing care for the child with a hematologic disorder. In J. Chow, C. A. Ateah, S. D. Scott, et al. (Eds.), *Canadian maternity and pediatric nursing.* Philadelphia: Wolters Kluwer/Lippincott Williams & Wilkins.

BC Cancer Agency. (n.d.). *Chemotherapy protocols.* Retrieved from <http://www.bccancer.bc.ca/health-professionals/professional-resources/chemotherapy-protocols>.

Bonilla, F. A., & Notarangelo, L. D. (2014). Primary immunodeficiency diseases. In S. H. Oskin, D. E. Fisher, D. Ginsburg, et al. (Eds.), *Nathan and Oski's hematology of infancy and childhood* (8th ed.). Philadelphia: Saunders.

Brandow, A. M., Weisman, S. J., & Panepinto, J. A. (2011). The impact of a multidisciplinary pain management model on sickle cell disease pain hospitalizations. *Pediatric Blood & Cancer, 56*(5), 789–793.

Buckley, R. H. (2016). Evaluation of suspected immunodeficiency. In R. M. Kliegman, B. F. Stanton, J. St. Geme, et al. (Eds.), *Nelson textbook of pediatrics* (20th ed.). Philadelphia: Saunders.

Canadian Cancer Society. (2015). *Canadian cancer statistics 2015.* Toronto: Author. Retrieved from <http://www.cancer.ca/en/cancer-information/cancer-101/canadian-cancer-statistics-publication/?region=on>.

Canadian Haemoglobinopathy Association. (2015). *Consensus statement on the care of patients with sickle cell disease in Canada.* Version 2.0. Ottawa: Author. Retrieved from <http://www.sicklecelldisease.ca/wp-content/uploads/2013/04/CANHAEM-Consensus-Statement-for-SCD-Guide2015_v10.pdf>.

Canadian Hemophilia Society. (2008). *Hemophilia A and B.* Retrieved from <http://www.hemophilia.ca/en/bleeding-disorders/hemophilia-a-and-b/>.

Canadian Hemophilia Society. (2016). *An introduction to von Willebrand disease.* Retrieved from <http://www.hemophilia.ca/en/bleeding-disorders/von-willebrand-disease/an-introduction-to-von-willebrand-disease/>.

Centers for Disease Control and Prevention. (1994). 1994 revised classification system for human immunodeficiency virus infection in children less than 13 years of age. *MMWR. Morbidity & Mortality Weekly Report, 43*(RR–12), 1–10.

Centers for Disease Control and Prevention. (2003). Advancing HIV prevention: New strategies for a changing epidemic—United States. *MMWR. Morbidity & Mortality Weekly Report, 52*(15), 329–332.

Christofides, A., Schauer, C., & Zlotkin, S. H. (2005). Iron deficiency anemia among children: Addressing a global public health problem within a Canadian context. *Paediatrics & Child Health, 10*(10), 597–601.

Consolini, D. M. (2011). Thrombocytopenia in infants and children. *Pediatrics in Review, 32*(4), 135–151.

Critch, J., & Canadian Paediatric Society, Nutrition and Gastroenterology Committee. (2013). Nutrition for healthy term infants, birth to six months: An overview. *Paediatrics & Child Health, 18*(4), 206–207. Reaffirmed 2016. Retrieved from <http://www.cps.ca/en/documents/position/nutrition-healthy-term-infants-overview>.

DeBaun, M. R., Frei-Jones, M. J., & Vichinsky, E. P. (2016). Hemoglobinopathies. In R. M. Kliegman, B. F. Stanton, J. St. Geme, et al. (Eds.), *Nelson textbook of pediatrics* (20th ed.). Philadelphia: Saunders.

Driscoll, M. C. (2007). Sickle cell disease. *Pediatrics in Review, 28*(7), 259–267. doi:10.1542/pir.28-7-259.

Fleming, M. D. (2014). Disorders of iron and copper metabolism, sideroblastic anemias and lead toxicity. In S. H. Orkin, D. E. Fisher, D. Ginsburg, et al. (Eds.), *Nathan and Oski's hematology of infancy and childhood* (8th ed.). Philadelphia: Saunders.

Frey, M. A., Guess, C., Allison, J., et al. (2009). Umbilical cord stem cell transplantation. *Seminars in Oncology Nursing, 25*(2), 115–119.

Galanello, R., & Origa, R. (2010). Beta-thalassemia. *Orphanet Journal of Rare Diseases, 5*(11), doi:10.1186/1750-1172-5-11.

Gaziev, J., & Lucarelli, G. (2011). Hematopoietic stem cell transplantation for thalassemia. *Current Stem Cell Research & Therapy, 6*(2), 162–169. doi:10.2174/157488811795495413.

Gottschalk, S., Naik, S., Hegde, C. M., et al. (2016). Hematopoietic stem cell transplantation in pediatric oncology. In P. A. Pizzo & D. G. Poplack (Eds.), *Principles and practice of pediatric oncology* (7th ed.). Philadelphia: Lippincott.

Grace, R. F. (2014). Hematologic manifestations of systemic diseases. In S. H. Orkin, D. E. Fisher, D. Ginsburg, et al. (Eds.), *Nathan and Oski's hematology of infancy and childhood* (8th ed.). Philadelphia: Saunders.

Hartung, H. D., Olson, T. S., & Bessler, M. (2013). Acquired aplastic anemia in children. *Pediatric Clinics of North America, 60*(6), 1311–1336. doi:10.1016/j.pcl.2013.08.011.

Health Canada. (2009). *Basic product monograph information for nonsteroidal anti-inflammatory drugs (NSAIDS).* Retrieved from <http://hc-sc.gc.ca/dhp-mps/prodpharma/applic-demande/guide-ld/nsaid-ains/nsaids_ains-eng.php>.

Health Canada. (2015). *Nutrition for healthy term infants: Recommendations from birth to six months.* Retrieved from <http://www.hc-sc.gc.ca/fn-an/nutrition/infant-nourisson/recom/index-eng.php#a3>.

Heeney, M., & Dover, G. J. (2014). Sickle cell disease. In S. H. Orkin, D. E. Fisher, D. Ginsburg, et al. (Eds.), *Nathan and Oski's hematology of infancy and childhood* (8th ed.). Philadelphia: Saunders.

Hirst, C., & Owusu-Ofori, S. (2014). Prophylactic antibiotics for preventing pneumococcal infection in children with sickle cell disease. *The Cochrane Database of Systematic Reviews,* (11), CD003427, doi:10.1002/14651858.CD003427.pub3.

Jordan, K., Gralla, R., & Jahn, F. (2013). International antiemetic guidelines on chemotherapy induced nausea and vomiting (CINV): Content and implementation in daily routine practice. *European Journal of Pharmacology, 722*, 197–202. doi:10.1016/j.ejphar.2013.09.073.

Kane, V., & Swartz, M. K. (2013). Hematologic disorders. In C. Burns, A. M. Dunn, M. A. Brady, et al. (Eds.), *Pediatric primary care* (5th ed., p. 574). St. Louis: Saunders.

Klause, B. D., & Johnson, M. (2007). Paradigm shift: New testing guidelines for HIV. *Advance for Nurse Practitioners, 15*(3), 59–93.

Krane, J. K., Casillas, J., & Zeltzer, L. K. (2016). Pain and symptom management. In P. A. Pizzo & D. G. Poplack (Eds.), *Principles and practice of pediatric oncology* (7th ed.). Philadelphia: Lippincott.

Krentz, H. B., Kliewer, G., & Gill, M. J. (2005). Changing mortality rates and causes of death for HIV-infected individuals living in Southern Alberta, Canada from 1984 to 2003. *HIV Medicine, 6*(2), 99–106. doi:10.1111/j.1468-1293.2005.00271.x.

Landier, W., Armenian, S., & Bhatia, S. (2015). Late effects of childhood cancer and its treatment. *Pediatric Clinics of North America, 62*(1), 275–300.

Lemyre, B., Sample, M., Lacaze-Masmonteil, T., & Canadian Paediatric Society, Fetus and Newborn Committee. (2015). Minimizing blood loss and the need for transfusions in very premature infants. *Paediatrics & Child Health, 20*(8), 451–456.

Lerner, N. B. (2016). Congenital dyserythropoietic anemias. In R. M. Kliegman, B. F. Stanton, J. St. Geme, et al. (Eds.), *Nelson textbook of pediatrics* (20th ed.). Philadelphia: Saunders.

Leukemia & Lymphoma Society of Canada. (2013). *Childhood NHL*. Retrieved from <http://www.llscanada.org/#/diseaseinformation/informationforchildren/childhoodnhl/>.

Lynch, M. E., & Fischer, B. (2011). Prescription opioid abuse. What is the real problem and how do we fix it? *Canadian Family Physician, 57*(11), 1241–1242.

McCrae, K. (2011). Immune thrombocytopenia: No longer "idiopathic." *Cleveland Clinic Journal of Medicine, 78*(6), 358–373.

McGann, P. T., & Ware, R. E. (2011). Hydroxyurea for sickle cell anemia: What have we learned and what questions remain? *Current Opinion in Hematology, 18*(3), 158–165.

McKee, N. (2015). Diagnosing and treating severe aplastic anemia. *Journal of the American Academy of Physician Assistants, 28*(9), 36–38.

Metzger, M. I., Krasin, M. J., Choi, J. K., et al. (2016). Hodgkin lymphoma. In P. A. Pizzo & D. G. Poplack (Eds.), *Principles and practice of pediatric oncology* (7th ed.). Philadelphia: Lippincott.

National Institutes of Health, Panel on Antiretroviral Therapy and Medical Management of HIV-Infected Children. (2015). *Clinical guidelines portal.* Retrieved from http://www.aidsinfo.nih.gov/Guidelines/.

Pacey, A. (2009). *Iron deficiency and iron deficiency anemia among preschool aged Inuit children living in Nunavut.* Thesis for the School of Dietetics and Human Nutrition, McGill University. Retrieved from <http://www.collectionscanada.gc.ca/obj/thesescanada/vol1/QMM/TC-QMM-66931.pdf>.

Patel, S. R., Chisholm, J. C., & Heath, P. T. (2008). Vaccinations in children treated with Standard-dose cancer therapy or hematopoietic stem cell transplantation. *Pediatric Oncology, 55*(1), 169–186.

Public Health Agency of Canada. (2014). *HIV and AIDS in Canada: Surveillance report to December 31st, 2013*. Retrieved from <http://www.phac-aspc.gc.ca/aids-sida/publication/survreport/2013/dec/index-eng.php0073_CH0048_Perry_2Ce_edited.docx>.

Public Health Agency of Canada. (2016). *Canadian immunization guide. Part 3: Vaccination of specific populations*. Retrieved from <http://www.phac-aspc.gc.ca/publicat/cig-gci/p03-chroni-eng.php#a1>.

Rabin, K. R., Gramategs, M. M., Margolin, J. F., et al. (2016). Acute lymphoblastic leukemia. In P. A. Pizzo & D. G. Poplack (Eds.), *Principles and practice of pediatric oncology* (7th ed.). Philadelphia: Lippincott.

Robinson, J. L., & Canadian Paediatric Society, Infectious Diseases and Immunization Committee. (2010). Management of HIV-exposed and HIV-infected children. *Paediatrics & Child Health, 15*(6), 379. Reaffirmed 2016. Retrieved from <http://www.cps.ca/documents/position/HIV-exposed-and-HIV-infected-children>.

Sayani, F., Warner, M., Wu, J., et al. (2013). *Guidelines for the clinical care of patients with thalassemia in Canada*. Retrieved from <http://www.thalassemia.ca/wp-content/uploads/Thalassemia-Guidelines_LR.pdf>.

Scott, J. P. (2016). Platelet and blood vessel disorders. In R. M. Kliegman, B. F. Stanton, J. St. Geme, et al. (Eds.), *Nelson textbook of pediatrics* (20th ed.). Philadelphia: Saunders.

Sickle Cell Disease Association of Canada. (2013). *General knowledge*. Retrieved from <http://www.sicklecelldisease.ca/education/general-knowledge>.

Thalassemia Foundation of Canada. (2016). *Living with thalassemia*. Retrieved from <http://www.thalassemia.ca/advocacy-support/living-with-thalassemia/>.

Tondon, R., Pandey, P., Mickey, K. B., et al. (2010). Errors reported in cross match laboratory: A prospective data analysis. *Transfusion and Apheresis Science, 43*(3), 309–314.

Velardi, A., & Locatelli, F. (2016). Principles and clinical indications of hematopoietic stem cell transplantation. In R. M. Kliegman, B. F. Stanton, J. St. Geme, et al. (Eds.), *Nelson textbook of pediatrics* (20th ed.). Philadelphia: Saunders.

Wang, W. C., Ware, R. E., Miller, S. T., et al. (2011). Hydroxycarbamide in very young children with sickle-cell anaemia: A multicentre, randomized, controlled trial (BABY HUG). *Lancet, 377*(9778), 1663–1672.

Wilson, D. B. (2014). Acquired platelet defects. In S. H. Orkin, D. E. Fisher, D. Ginsburg, et al. (Eds.), *Nathan and Oski's hematology of infancy and childhood* (8th ed.). Philadelphia: Saunders.

Woodgate, R. L. (2013). Nursing care of the child with a neoplastic disorder. In J. Chow, C. A. Ateah, S. D. Scott, et al. (Eds.), *Canadian maternity and pediatric nursing*. Philadelphia: Wolters Kluwer/Lippincott Williams & Wilkins.

World Federation of Hemophilia. (2012). *Guidelines for the management of hemophilia* (2nd ed.). Montreal: Author. Retrieved from <https://www1.wfh.org/publication/files/pdf-1472.pdf>.

Zourikian, N., Jarock, C., & Mulder, K. (2010). Physical activity, exercise and sports. In C. Amesse et al. (Eds.), *Canadian Hemophilia Society's all about hemophilia: A guide for families* (2nd ed.). Retrieved from <http://www.hemophilia.ca/files/Chapter%2012.pdf>.

ADDITIONAL RESOURCES

Aplastic Anemia & Myelodysplasia Association of Canada: <http://www.aamac.ca>.

BC Cancer Agency—Cancer chemotherapy protocols: <http://www.bccancer.bc.ca/health-professionals/professional-resources/chemotherapy-protocols>.

Canadian Hemophilia Society: <http://www.hemophilia.ca>.

Canadian AIDS Society: <http://www.cdnaids.ca/>.

Canadian Paediatric Society—Rourke Baby Record: <http://www.rourkebabyrecord.ca/downloads.asp>.

Cooley's Anemia Foundation: <http://www.cooleysanemia.org>.

Oncology Nursing Society—Guideline for cancer chemotherapy administration: <https://www.ons.org/practice-resources/clinical-practice/ascoons-chemotherapy-administration-safety-standards>.

Sickle Cell Association of Ontario: <http://www.sicklecellontario.org/>.

Sickle Cell Disease Association of Canada: <http://www.sicklecelldisease.ca/>.

Thalassemia Foundation of Canada: <http://www.thalassemia.ca>.

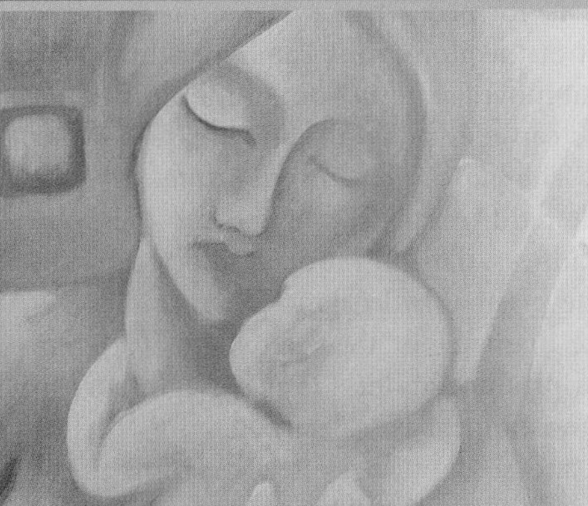

CHAPTER

49

Genitourinary Dysfunction

Cheryl Sams, with contributions from Marilyn J. Hockenberry

evolve WEBSITE

Visit the Evolve website for additional resources related to the content in this chapter such as Case Studies, Critical Thinking Case Study Answers, Nursing Care Plans, Nursing Processes, Nursing Skills, and Review Questions for Exam Preparation at: http://evolve.elsevier.com/Canada/Perry/maternal/

OBJECTIVES

On completion of this chapter the reader will be able to:

- Describe the various factors that contribute to urinary tract infections in infants and children.
- Discuss the preoperative preparation of the child and parents when the child has a structural defect of the genitourinary tract.
- Demonstrate an understanding of the causes and mechanisms of edema formation in nephrotic syndrome.
- Outline a nursing care plan for a child with nephrotic syndrome.
- Compare the child with minimal-change nephrotic syndrome and the child with acute glomerulonephritis in terms of clinical manifestations and nursing care.
- Contrast the causes, complications, and management of acute and chronic renal failure.
- List the types of renal dialysis.
- Recognize signs of kidney transplant rejection.

URINARY SYSTEM STRUCTURE AND FUNCTION

The urinary system is an excretory system that consists of the kidneys, which produce urine; the ureters, which transport urine to the bladder; and the urethra, which discharges urine from the bladder.

Kidney Structure and Function

The major purpose of the kidneys is to balance the body fluids, which include water and electrolytes. The kidneys must adapt to external and internal factors in order to maintain this equilibrium. These factors include diet, hydration variables, and extrarenal losses of water and solutes. Glomular formation produces urine, and tubular reabsorption creates equilibrium. **Reabsorption** occurs when substances are moved from the tubular lumen to the blood. **Secretion** is the movement of substances back from the blood to the lumen. Kidneys remove metabolic wastes from the blood and excrete the wastes in urine.

In addition, the kidneys help to regulate the production of red blood cells by converting plasma globulin into erythropoietin and stimulating erythropoiesis production in the bone marrow. A lack of erythropoietin decreases the number of red blood cells and can lead to anemia when significant kidney disease is present. The kidneys also aid in calcium absorption and in maintaining blood volume, composition, and pH. The enzyme *renin* is secreted by the kidneys in response to a lowered blood volume, lowered blood pressure, or an increase in the secretion of catecholamines. Renin stimulates the production of angiotensin, which creates constriction of the arterioles. This in turn leads to an increase in blood pressure and stimulates the production of aldosterone by the adrenal cortex.

The functional unit of the kidney is the **nephron**. The nephron contains a renal corpuscle and a renal tubule. Kidney and nephron structures are illustrated in Fig. 49-1. The corpuscle consists of the glomerulus and a Bowman's capsule. The glomular capillary receives blood from the afferent arteriole and passes it to the efferent arteriole. The efferent arteriole gives rise to the peritubular capillary system and loops of Henle and then into collecting ducts. Nephrons function to remove wastes, such as urea from the blood, and to regulate water and electrolyte

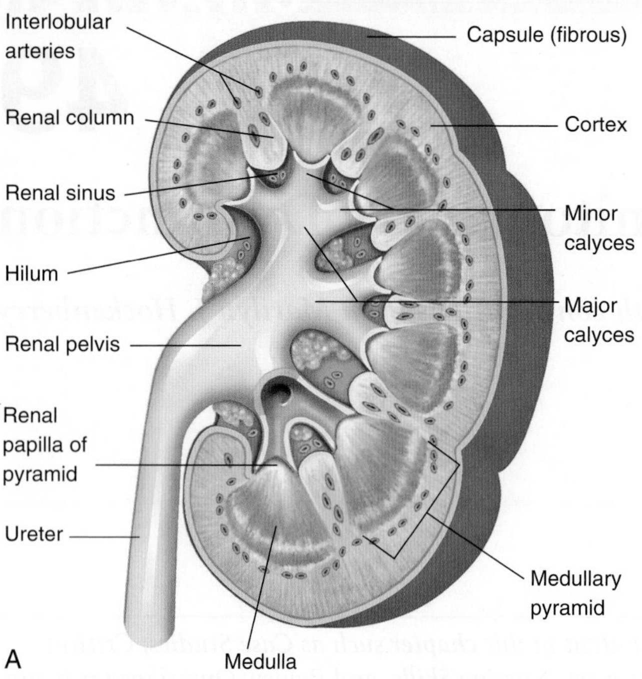

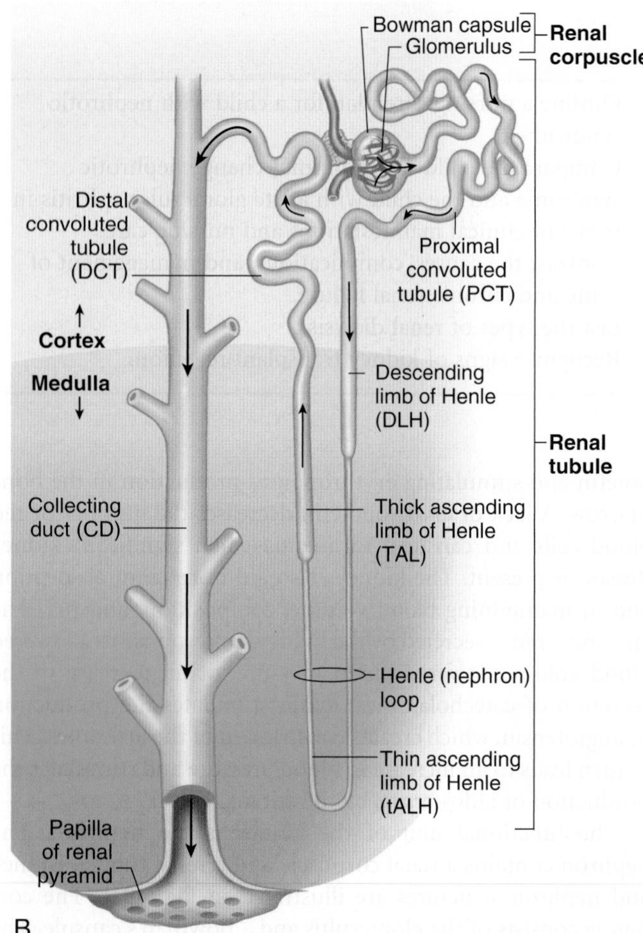

FIGURE 49-1 **A:** Kidney structure. **B:** Components of the nephron. (From Patton, K. T., & Thibodeau, G. A. [2010]. *Anatomy and physiology* [7th ed.]. St. Louis: Mosby.)

concentrations. Urine is formed when water and dissolved material are forced out of the glomerular capillaries. Filtration pressure is the force that moves materials out of the glomerulus and into the Bowman's capsule via hydrostatic pressure inside glomerular capillaries. The *glomerular filtration rate (GFR)* is the amount of fluid filtered from the capillaries into the Bowman's capsule of the kidneys. This filtration is affected by the osmotic pressure of the plasma, hydrostatic pressure in Bowman's capsule, and the diameter of the efferent and afferent arterioles. The kidneys produce about 125 mL of glomerular fluid per minute, and most of this is reabsorbed.

Glomular filtration and absorption are relatively low in the infant and do not reach adult levels until the ages of 1 or 2 years. This may be related to the glomerular epithelia cells being more shaped like a cube, a high afferent arteriole resistance, and incomplete formation of the tubules and smaller glomeruli. As a result, the newborn is at risk of being unable to excrete excess water and solutes quickly or efficiently. Substances are selectively reabsorbed by the tubules; glucose and amino acids are reabsorbed by active transport, water is reabsorbed by osmosis, and proteins are reabsorbed by pinocytosis and returned to the blood. Excess of these substances may be excreted in the urine. Sodium is mostly reabsorbed before urine is excreted and is concentrated in the renal medulla. Antidiuretic hormone (ADH), also known as *vasopressin*, from the posterior pituitary gland causes the permeability of the distal tubule and collecting ducts to increase and promotes the reabsorption of water.

Electrolytes are moved by active transport and diffusion. There is a limit to the concentration gradient against which sodium can be transported out; if there is a larger than normal amount remaining in the tubules, water stays with the sodium.

GENITOURINARY DYSFUNCTION

Clinical Manifestations

As in most disorders of childhood, the incidence and type of kidney or urinary tract dysfunction change with the child's age and maturation. In addition, the presenting health concerns and the significance of these concerns vary with maturation. For example, urinary tract infections have a greater significance in infancy than at an older age. In the newborn, urinary tract disorders are associated with a number of malformations of other body systems, including the frequent association between malformed or low-set ears and urinary tract anomalies.

While many of the clinical manifestations of renal disease are common to a variety of childhood disorders, their presence is an indication to obtain further information from the child's history, family history, and laboratory studies as part of a complete physical examination. Suspected renal disease can be further evaluated by means of radiographic studies and renal biopsy (Table 49-1).

Laboratory Tests

Both urine and blood studies contribute vital information for the detection of renal problems. The single most important test is probably routine urinalysis. Specific urine and blood tests provide additional information. Because nurses are usually the

TABLE 49-1 RADIOLOGICAL AND OTHER TESTS OF URINARY SYSTEM FUNCTION

TEST	PROCEDURE	PURPOSE	COMMENTS AND NURSING RESPONSIBILITIES
Urine culture and sensitivity	Collection of sterile specimen	Determines presence of pathogens and the medications to which they are sensitive	Does not require specific parental permission Send specimen to laboratory immediately after collection. Use catheterization, clean-catch, or suprapubic specimen.
Renal and bladder ultrasound	Transmission of ultrasonic waves through renal parenchyma, along ureteral course, and over bladder	Allows visualization of renal parenchyma and renal pelvis without exposure to external beam radiation or radioactive isotopes Visualization of dilated ureters and bladder wall also possible	Noninvasive procedure
Testicular (scrotal) ultrasound	Transmission of ultrasonic waves through scrotal contents and testis	Allows visualization of scrotal contents, including testis Testicular ultrasound is used to identify masses, and Doppler-enhanced ultrasound is used to differentiate hyperemia of epididymo-orchitis from ischemia or torsion	Noninvasive procedure
Scout film	Flat plate roentgenogram of abdomen and pelvis for kidney, ureters, bladder (KUB)	Detects and establishes renal outlines, presence of calculi, or opaque foreign bodies in bladder	Prepare as for routine x-ray film.
Voiding cystourethrography	Contrast medium injected into bladder through urethral catheter until bladder is full; films taken before, during, and after voiding	Visualizes bladder outline and urethra, reveals reflux of urine into ureters, and shows complications of bladder emptying	Prepare child for catheterization.
Radionuclide (nuclear) cystogram	Radionuclide-containing fluid injected through urethral catheter until bladder is full; images generated before, during, and after voiding	Alternative to voiding cystourethrography in children with allergy to intravesical contrast material Allows evaluation of reflux, although visualization of anatomical details is relatively poor	Prepare child for catheterization. Reassure patient and parents that allergic response to contrast materials is avoided by use of radionuclide.
Radioisotope imaging studies	Contrast medium injected intravenously; computer analysis to measure uptake or washout (excretion) for analysis of organ function	DTPA radioisotope used to measure glomerular filtration rate; estimate of differential renal function and renal washout to determine presence and location of upper urinary tract obstruction DMSA radioisotope used to visualize renal scars and differential renal function; does not visualize ureters and bladder MAG3 radioisotope combines features of DTPA (evaluation of upper urinary tract obstruction) with features of DMSA radioisotope (differential renal function)	Insert or assist with insertion of intravenous infusion. Monitor intravenous infusion. Urethral catheterization may accompany DTPA radioisotope scan; prepare child for catheterization when indicated.
Intravenous pyelography (IVP) (intravenous urogram; excretory urogram)	Intravenous injection of a contrast medium Medium secreted and concentrated by tubules X-ray films made 5, 10, and 15 min after injection; delayed films (30, 60 min, etc.) are obtained if obstruction suspected	Defines urinary tract Provides information about integrity of kidneys, ureters, and bladder Retroperitoneal masses visualized when they shift position of ureters	Preparation for test: **Infants <2 yr of age**—Give no solid food, omit one breastfeeding/bottle on morning of examination; perform studies early to avoid withholding of fluids. **Children 2–14 yr of age**—Give cathartic evening before examination, nothing orally after midnight, enema (soapsuds) morning of examination.

Continued

TABLE 49-1 RADIOLOGICAL AND OTHER TESTS OF URINARY SYSTEM FUNCTION—cont'd

TEST	PROCEDURE	PURPOSE	COMMENTS AND NURSING RESPONSIBILITIES
Computed tomography (CT)	Narrow-beam x-rays and computer analysis providing precise reconstruction of area	Visualizes vertical or horizontal cross section of kidney Especially valuable to distinguish tumours and cysts	Noncontrast scan is noninvasive. Contrast-enhanced CT scan preparation is similar to that for IVP.
Cystoscopy	Direct visualization of bladder and lower urinary tract through small scope inserted via urethra	Investigation of bladder and lower tract lesions; visualizes ureteral openings, bladder wall, trigone, and urethra	Give nothing orally after midnight. Carry out preoperative preparations. Prepare the child for cystoscopy.
Retrograde pyelography	Contrast medium injected through ureteral catheter	Visualizes pelvic calyces, ureters, and bladder	Give cathartic if ordered. Give preoperative medication if ordered. Observe for reaction to contrast medium. Monitor vital signs after procedure.
Renal angiography	Contrast medium injected directly into renal artery via catheter placed in femoral artery (or umbilical artery in newborn) and advanced to renal artery	Visualizes renal vascular system, especially for renal arterial stenosis	Prepare child for insertion of a spinal needle or perfusion catheter in renal pelvis (anaesthetic often required).
Whitaker perfusion test	Injection of contrast material through renal pelvis and ureters Measures pressures in renal pelvis and urinary bladder	Determine presence of obstruction causing upper urinary tract dilation	Give nothing orally 4–6 hr before test. Premedicate as ordered. Prepare setup for procedure. Assist with procedure. Take vital signs. Apply pressure to area with pressure dressing and, if feasible, a sandbag. Place on bedrest for 24 hr. Observe for abdominal pain, tenderness. Monitor input and output; surgical incision may be required in infants.
Renal biopsy	Removal of kidney tissue by open or percutaneous technique for study by light, electron, or immunofluorescent microscopy	Yields histological and microscopic information about glomeruli and tubules; helps distinguish between types of nephritic syndromes Distinguishes other renal disorders	Prepare child for catheterization. Insertion of a rectal tube produces feelings of rectal fullness or pressure. Insertion of needles may be required for sphincter electromyography.
Urodynamics	Set of tests designed to measure bladder filling, storage, and evacuation functions **Uroflowmetry**—Test to determine efficiency of urination **Cystometrogram**—Graphic comparison of bladder pressure as a function of volume **Voiding pressure study**—Comparison of detrusor contraction pressure, sphincter electromyelogram, and urinary flow	Determine characteristic of voiding dysfunction Used to identify type (cause) of incontinence or urinary retention Especially valuable for voiding dysfunction complicated by urinary tract infection, urinary retention, or neurogenic bladder dysfunction	Prepare child for urinary catheterization. The bladder will be filled with saline solution and filling pressures will be recorded; the child may experience fullness, coolness from the saline fluid, and urine leakage during the study. To measure sphincter EMG, it may be necessary to insert needles.

DMSA, dimercaptosuccinic acid; *DTPA*, diethylenetriamine pentaacetic acid; *EMG*, electromyography; *MAG3*, mercaptoacetyltriglycine.

persons who collect the specimens for examination and who often perform many of the screening tests, they should be familiar with the tests, their functions, and the factors that can alter or distort the results of the tests. The major urine and blood tests are outlined in Tables 49-2 and 49-3.

NURSING CARE

Nursing responsibilities in assessment of genitourinary disorders or diseases begin with observation of the child for any manifestations that might indicate dysfunction. Many conditions have specific characteristics that distinguish them from other disorders. These are discussed throughout the chapter.

The nurse is generally responsible for preparing infants, children, and parents for tests and for collecting urine and (sometimes) blood specimens for observation and laboratory analysis (see Preparation for Diagnostic and Therapeutic Procedures, and Collection of Specimens, Chapter 44). An important nursing responsibility is to maintain careful intake and output and blood pressure measurements in children with

TABLE 49-2 URINE TESTS OF RENAL FUNCTION

TEST	NORMAL RANGE	DEVIATIONS	SIGNIFICANCE OF DEVIATIONS
Physical Tests			
Volume	Age-related Infants—<1 mL/kg/hr Children—0.5 mL/kg/hr	Polyuria Oliguria	Osmotic factors (urinary glucose level in diabetes mellitus) Retention caused by obstructive disease Inadequate bladder emptying caused by neurogenic bladder or obstructive disorder
		Anuria	Obstruction of urinary tract; acute renal failure
Specific gravity	With normal fluid intake—1.016–1.022 Newborn—1.001–1.020	High	Dehydration Presence of protein or glucose Presence of radiopaque contrast medium after radiological examinations
	Others— 1.001–1.030	Low	Excessive fluid intake Distal tubular dysfunction Insufficient antidiuretic hormone Diuresis Chronic glomerular disease
Osmolality	Newborn— 274–305 mmol/kg H_2O Thereafter—282–300 mmol/kg H_2O	High or low	Same as for specific gravity More sensitive index than specific gravity
Appearance	Clear pale yellow to deep gold	Cloudy	Contains sediment
		Cloudy reddish pink to reddish brown	Blood from trauma or disease Myoglobin after severe muscle destruction
		Light	Dilute
		Dark	Concentrated
		Red	Trauma
Chemical Tests			
pH	Newborn—5–7 Thereafter— 4.8–7.8 Average—6	Weak acid or neutral	If associated with metabolic acidosis, suggests tubular acidosis If associated with metabolic alkalosis, suggests potassium deficiency Urinary infection
		Alkaline	Metabolic alkalosis
Protein level	Absent	Present	Abnormal glomerular permeability (e.g., glomerular disease, changes in blood pressure) Most kidney disease
Glucose level	Absent	Present	Diabetes mellitus Infusion of concentrated glucose-containing fluids Glomerulonephritis Impaired tubular reabsorption
Ketone levels	Absent	Present	Conditions of acute metabolic demand (stress) Diabetic ketoacidosis
Leukocyte esterase	Absent	Present	Can identify both lysed and intact white blood cells via enzyme detection
Nitrites	Absent	Present	Most species of bacteria convert nitrates to nitrites in the urine
Microscopic Tests			
White blood cell count	<1 or 2	>5 polymorphonuclear leukocytes/field	Urinary tract inflammatory process
		Lymphocytes	Allograft rejection Malignancy
Red blood cell count	<1 or 2	4–6/field in centrifuged specimen	Trauma Stones Glomerular injury Infection Neoplasms

Continued

TABLE 49-2 URINE TESTS OF RENAL FUNCTION—cont'd

TEST	NORMAL RANGE	DEVIATIONS	SIGNIFICANCE OF DEVIATIONS
Presence of bacteria	Absent to a few	>100,000 organisms/mL in centrifuged specimen	Urinary tract infection
Presence of casts	Occasional	Granular casts	Tubular or glomerular disorders Degenerative process in advanced renal disease
		Cellular casts	Pyelonephritis
		White blood cell	Glomerulonephritis
		Red blood cell	Proteinuria; usually transient
		Hyaline casts	

TABLE 49-3 BLOOD TESTS OF RENAL FUNCTION

TEST	NORMAL RANGE	DEVIATIONS	SIGNIFICANCE OF DEVIATIONS
Urea	Newborn—2.9–10.0 mmol/L Infant, child—2.0–7.1 mmol/L	Elevated	Renal disease—acute or chronic (the higher the urea, the more severe the disease) Increased protein catabolism Dehydration Hemorrhage High protein intake Corticosteroid therapy
Uric acid	Child—120–360 mcmol/L	Increased	Severe renal disease
Creatinine	Infant—10–56 mcmol/L Child—<53 mcmol/L Adolescent—<98 mcmol/L	Increased	Severe renal impairment

genitourinary dysfunction and those who might be at risk for developing renal complications (e.g., children in shock, post-operative patients). For example, any significant degree of renal disease can diminish the GFR, a measure of the amount of plasma from which a given substance is totally cleared in 1 minute. A number of substances can be used, but the most useful clinical estimation of glomerular filtration is the clearance of creatinine, an end product of protein metabolism in muscle and a substance that is freely filtered by the glomerulus and secreted by renal tubular cells. The nurse's responsibility in this test is the collection of urine, usually a 12- or 24-hour specimen.

GENITOURINARY TRACT DISORDERS AND DEFECTS

Urinary Tract Infection

Urinary tract infections (UTIs) occur in 1% of boys and 1 to 3% of girls. During the first year of life, UTIs are more common in males, particularly in uncircumcised boys (Sorokan, Finlay, Jefferies, et al. & CPS, Fetus and Newborn Committee, Infectious Diseases and Immunization Committee, 2015). Circumcision status should be assessed in male infants with unexplained fever.

UTI may involve the urethra and bladder (lower urinary tract) or the ureters, renal pelvis, calyces, and renal parenchyma (upper urinary tract). The Canadian Paediatric Society (CPS) recommends suprapubic aspiration or urethral catheterization to diagnose UTIs in young infants (see Chapter 44). Urine bagging is frequently inaccurate due to contamination (Robinson, Finlay, Lang, et al. & CPS, Community Paediatrics Committee, Infectious Diseases and Immunization Committee, 2014). Because it is often impossible to localize the infection, the broad designation *UTI* is applied to the presence of significant numbers of microorganisms anywhere within the urinary tract, except the distal third of the urethra, which is usually colonized with bacteria.

Classification

Infection of the urinary tract may be present with or without clinical symptoms. As a result, the site of infection is often difficult to pinpoint with any degree of accuracy. Various terms used to describe urinary tract disorders include the following:

Bacteriuria—Presence of bacteria in the urine

Asymptomatic bacteriuria—Significant bacteriuria (usually defined as more than 100,000 colony-forming units) with no evidence of clinical infection

Symptomatic bacteriuria—Bacteriuria accompanied by physical signs of UTI (dysuria, suprapubic discomfort, hematuria, fever)

Recurrent UTI—Repeated episode of bacteriuria or symptomatic UTI

Persistent UTI—Persistence of bacteriuria despite antibiotic treatment

Febrile UTI—Bacteriuria accompanied by fever and other physical signs of UTI; presence of a fever typically implies a pyelonephritis

Cystitis—Inflammation of the bladder

Urethritis—Inflammation of the urethra

Pyelonephritis—Inflammation of the upper urinary tract and kidneys

Urosepsis—Febrile UTI coexisting with systemic signs of bacterial illness; blood culture reveals presence of urinary pathogen

Etiology

A variety of organisms can be responsible for UTI. *Escherichia coli* (80% of cases) and other gram-negative enteric organisms are most frequently implicated; these organisms are usually found in the anal and perineal region. Other organisms associated with UTI include *Proteus, Pseudomonas, Klebsiella, Staphylococcus aureus, Haemophilus,* and coagulase-negative *Staphylococcus* organisms. Several factors contribute to the development of UTI in childhood including anatomical, physical, and chemical conditions or properties of the child's urinary tract.

Anatomical and physical factors. The structure of the lower urinary tract is believed to account for the increased incidence of bacteriuria in females. The short urethra, which measures about 2 cm in young girls and 4 cm in mature women, provides a ready pathway for invasion of organisms. In addition, the closure of the urethra at the end of micturition may return contaminated bacteria to the bladder. The longer male urethra (as long as 20 cm in an adult) and the antibacterial properties of prostatic secretions inhibit the entry and growth of pathogens.

The single most important host factor influencing the occurrence of UTI is urinary stasis. Ordinarily, urine is sterile, but at 37°C it provides an excellent culture medium. Under normal conditions the act of completely and repeatedly emptying the bladder flushes away any organisms before they have an opportunity to multiply and invade surrounding tissue. However, urine that remains in the bladder allows bacteria from the urethra to rapidly become established in the rich medium. Incomplete bladder emptying (stasis) may result from reflux (see Vesicoureteral Reflux, on next page), anatomical abnormalities (especially those involving the ureters), dysfunction of the voiding mechanism, or extrinsic ureteral or bladder compression that may be caused by constipation. The key to preventing UTI is to maintain adequate blood supply to the bladder wall through avoidance of overdistension and high bladder pressure.

Altered urine and bladder chemistry. Several mechanical and chemical characteristics of the urine and bladder mucosa help maintain urinary sterility. An increased fluid intake promotes flushing of the normal bladder and lowers the concentration of organisms in the infected bladder. Diuresis also seems to enhance the antibacterial properties of the renal medulla.

Most pathogens favour an alkaline medium. Normally, urine is slightly acidic, with a median pH of 6.0. A urine pH of about 5 hampers but does not eliminate bacterial multiplication. Much has been reported about the use of cranberry products to increase urine acidity in an effort to prevent UTI. Studies done in adults offer limited evidence for the value of cranberry products in promoting urinary tract health. A Cochrane Review concluded that the benefit of cranberry juice was too small to recommend its use for prevention of UTIs (Jepson, Williams, & Craig, 2012).

BOX 49-1 CLINICAL MANIFESTATIONS OF URINARY TRACT DISORDERS

Birth to 1 Month

Poor feeding
Vomiting
Failure to gain weight
Rapid respiration (acidosis)
Respiratory distress
Spontaneous pneumothorax or pneumomediastinum
Frequent urination
Screaming on urination
Poor urine stream
Jaundice
Seizures
Dehydration
Other anomalies or stigmata
Enlarged kidneys or bladder

1 to 24 Months

Poor feeding
Vomiting
Failure to gain weight
Excessive thirst
Frequent urination
Straining or screaming on urination
Foul-smelling urine
Pallor
Fever
Persistent diaper rash
Seizures (with or without fever)
Dehydration
Enlarged kidneys or bladder

2 to 14 Years

Poor appetite
Vomiting
Growth failure
Excessive thirst
Enuresis, incontinence, frequent urination
Painful urination
Swelling of face
Seizures
Pallor
Fatigue
Blood in urine
Abdominal or back pain
Edema
Hypertension
Tetany

Diagnostic Evaluation

The clinical manifestations of UTI depend on the child's age (Box 49-1). Diagnosis of UTI is confirmed by detection of bacteriuria in urine culture. But urine collection is often difficult, especially in infants and very small children. Unless the specimen is a first morning sample, a recent high fluid intake may indicate a falsely low organism count. Thus, children should not be encouraged to drink large volumes of water in an attempt to obtain a specimen quickly.

NURSING ALERT

A child who exhibits the following should be evaluated for UTI:
Incontinence in a toilet-trained child
Strong-smelling urine
Frequency or urgency

More accurate estimates of bacterial content are obtained from suprapubic aspiration (in children younger than 2 years of age) and properly performed bladder catheterization (as long as the first few millilitres are excluded from collection). The specimen should be taken directly to the laboratory for immediate culture.

Tests to detect bacteriuria are being used with increased frequency in screening for UTI. The dipstick tests for leukocyte esterase or nitrite are quick and inexpensive methods for detecting infection before obtaining final culture results.

Localization of the infection site may involve more specific tests, including percutaneous kidney taps and bladder wash-out procedures. Other tests such as ultrasonography, voiding cystourethrogram (VCUG), intravenous (IV) pyelogram, and dimercaptosuccinic acid (DMSA) scan may be performed after the infection subsides, to identify anatomical abnormalities contributing to the development of infection and existing kidney changes from recurrent infection.

Therapeutic Management

The objectives of treatment of children with UTI are to (1) eliminate current infection, (2) identify contributing factors to reduce the risk of recurrence, (3) prevent systemic spread of the infection, and (4) preserve renal function. Antibiotic therapy should be initiated on the basis of identification of the pathogen, the child's history of antibiotic use, and the location of the infection. Several antimicrobial medications are available for treating UTI, but all of them can occasionally be ineffective because of resistance of organisms. Common anti-infective agents used for UTI include the penicillins, sulphonamide (including trimethoprim and sulphisoxazole in combination), the cephalosporins, and nitrofurantoin.

The CPS has recommended significant changes in managing UTIs, given new research findings in children over 2 months of age with an acute UTI and no underlying urinary tract problems or risks for a neurogenic bladder (Robinson et al., 2014). The recommendations include antibiotic treatment for 7 to 10 days for a febrile UTI. Oral antibiotics may be prescribed initially if the child is not seriously ill. Children who are over 2 years of age should have a renal/bladder ultrasound with first febrile UTI to rule out any significant renal abnormalities. A voiding cystourethrogram is not required for children with a first UTI unless the renal/bladder ultrasound reveals findings suggestive of vesicoureteral reflux (VUR), renal anomalies, or obstructive uropathy.

If anatomical defects such as primary reflux or bladder neck obstruction are present, surgical correction of these abnormalities may be necessary to prevent recurrent infection. Follow-up study is an important component of medical management, since the relapse rate is high and infection tends to recur 1 to 2 months after termination of treatment. The aim of therapy and careful follow-up is to reduce the chance of renal scarring. However, recurrent infection of the urinary bladder predisposes the individual to transient episodes of VUR.

Vesicoureteral reflux. *VUR* refers to the abnormal retrograde flow of bladder urine into the ureters. During voiding, urine is swept up the ureters and then flows back into the empty bladder, where it acts as a reservoir for bacterial growth until the next void. *Primary reflux* results from congenitally abnormal insertion of ureters into the bladder; *secondary reflux* occurs as a result of an acquired condition.

It is not clear that reflux necessarily causes infections. What is clear is that reflux is more likely to be associated with recurring kidney infections than with simple bladder infections (cystitis). In the presence of reflux, infected urine (bacteria) from the bladder has access to the kidney, resulting in kidney infections (pyelonephritis). These children are usually very symptomatic with high fevers, vomiting, and chills. Reflux, when associated with UTI, is the most common cause of renal scarring in children. Renal scarring may occur with the first episode of febrile UTI. Reflux in the presence of sterile urine does not cause renal damage. Therefore, the most important concept in managing VUR is preventing bacteria from reaching the kidneys. VUR is managed conservatively with daily low-dose antibiotic therapy. A urine culture should be done every 2 to 3 months and any time the child has a fever. Many children will outgrow the reflux over a period of years. An annual VCUG is done to assess the status of the reflux.

For children with mild to moderate reflux, a minimally invasive endoscopic option, subtrigonal injection (STING), is an alternative to daily antibiotics or open surgical intervention. A bulking agent—dextranomer–hyaluronic acid polymer (Deflux)—is injected into the mucous membrane of the ureter, making retrograde flow of urine more difficult. Overall cure rates relate to the degree of reflux and range from 72 to 96% (Chen, Yeh, & Chou, 2010).

Indications for open surgical intervention include significant anatomical abnormality at the ureterovesical junction, recurrent UTIs, severe forms of VUR, difficulty adhering to medical therapy, intolerance to antibiotics, and VUR after puberty in females.

Prognosis

With prompt and adequate treatment at the time of diagnosis, the long-term prognosis for UTI is usually excellent. However, the hazard of progressive renal injury is greatest when infection occurs in young children (especially those younger than 2 years of age) and is associated with congenital renal malformations and reflux. Therefore, early diagnosis of children at risk is particularly important.

NURSING CARE

Nurses should instruct parents to observe regularly for clues suggesting UTI. Unfortunately, the signs of UTI are not as evident as those of upper respiratory tract infection. Many cases go undetected because no one thought to investigate this very common problem.

Infants and young children often are unable to express their feelings and sensations verbally, which makes it difficult to detect discomfort they may be experiencing from dysuria. A careful history regarding voiding habits, stooling patterns, and episodes of unexplained irritability may assist in detecting less obvious cases of UTI. Parents should be cautioned to observe for specific clues of UTI in suspected cases.

When infection is suspected, collecting an appropriate specimen is essential. It is the nurse's responsibility to take every precaution to obtain acceptable clean-voided specimens so that the use of other, more invasive collecting procedures can be avoided except when absolutely indicated. Given the unreliability of a specimen obtained via a urine collection bag, suprapubic aspiration of urine or sterile catheterization should be done in the infant or young child who has fever.

Frequently, additional tests are performed to detect anatomical defects. Children need to be prepared for these tests as appropriate for their age. This includes an explanation of the procedure, its purpose, and what the child will experience (see Preparation for Diagnostic and Therapeutic Procedures, Chapter 44). Sometimes a simple description of the urinary system is helpful. Especially for preschool children, the nurse needs to clarify that the urinary tract is separate from any sexual function and that the test is for a problem that they did not cause. Children may associate blame for perceived wrongdoing (e.g., masturbation) or unacceptable thoughts with the reason for the illness or the tests. For children younger than 3 to 4 years of age, the procedure can be explained on a doll. For those who are older, a simple drawing of the bladder, urethra, ureters, and kidneys makes the procedure more understandable.

Handling actual equipment, when feasible, can be helpful in allaying anxiety in children of all ages. Anticipatory instruction on distraction techniques such as deep breathing, storytelling, and imagery may help the child relax during the actual procedures. If surgery is indicated, the child's understanding of the procedure will help decrease his or her fear and anxiety concerning more extensive medical-surgical intervention.

Because antibacterial medications are indicated in UTI, the nurse needs to advise parents of proper dosage and administration. When antiseptics such as nitrofurantoin are used for prolonged therapy to maintain urine sterility, parents need an explanation of the medication's continued necessity when no signs of infection are present. For all children an adequate or increased fluid intake should be encouraged.

One adverse effect that can occur with antibiotic treatment is antibiotic-associated diarrhea (AAD). The CPS defines AAD as 3 or more loose stools/day for 2 or more days occurring for up to 2 weeks after the initiation of antibiotics; it occurs in about 30% of patients. Parents should be made aware that probiotics (specifically *Lactobacillus rhamnosus* GG and *Saccharomyces boulardii*) may decrease the incidence of AAD (Marchand & CPS, Nutrition and Gastroenterology Committee, 2012/2015).

Prevention

Prevention is the most important goal in both primary and recurrent infection, and most preventive measures are simple hygienic habits that should be a routine part of daily care (see Guidelines box). For example, parents should be taught to cleanse their infant's genital areas from front to back to avoid contaminating the urethral area with fecal organisms. Girls should be taught to wipe from front to back after voiding or defecating. Children should void as soon as they feel the urge (see Critical Thinking Case Study).

Sexually active adolescent girls should be advised to urinate as soon as possible after they have intercourse, to flush out bacteria introduced during the activity. Children who have recurrent UTIs or neurogenic bladder are frequently maintained on daily low-dose antibiotics. Giving the dose at bedtime allows the drug to remain in the bladder overnight.

GUIDELINES

Prevention of Urinary Tract Infection

Factors Predisposing to Development

- Short female urethra close to vagina and anus
- Incomplete emptying (reflux) and overdistension of bladder
- Concentrated urine
- Constipation

Measures of Prevention

- Practise good perineal hygiene: wipe from front to back.
- Avoid tight clothing or diapers; wear cotton panties rather than nylon.
- Check for vaginitis or pinworms, especially if child scratches between legs.
- Avoid "holding" urine; encourage child to void frequently, especially before long trips or other circumstances in which toilet facilities are not available.
- Empty bladder completely with each void. Have the child "double void" (void, wait a few minutes, and void again). Severe cases may require clean, intermittent catheterization or biofeedback instruction.
- Avoid straining during defecation and avoid constipation.
- Encourage generous fluid intake.

CRITICAL THINKING CASE STUDY

Urinary Tract Infection and Constipation

During the nurse's assessment of Lisa, a 5-year-old admitted to the hospital for a severe urinary tract infection (UTI), her mother tells the nurse that Lisa has bowel movements every third or fourth day. They are usually large, hard-formed stools, and Lisa sometimes has trouble evacuating the stool.

1. Evidence—Is there sufficient evidence to draw conclusions about Lisa's UTI and constipation?
2. Assumptions—Describe an underlying assumption about each of the following:
   a. UTIs and females
   b. Normal bowel patterns for 5-year-old children
   c. Association between UTIs and constipation
3. What priorities for nursing care should be established for Lisa?
4. Does the evidence support your nursing intervention?

Obstructive Uropathy

Structural or functional abnormalities of the urinary system that obstruct the normal flow of urine can produce renal disorders. When there is interference with urine flow, the backup

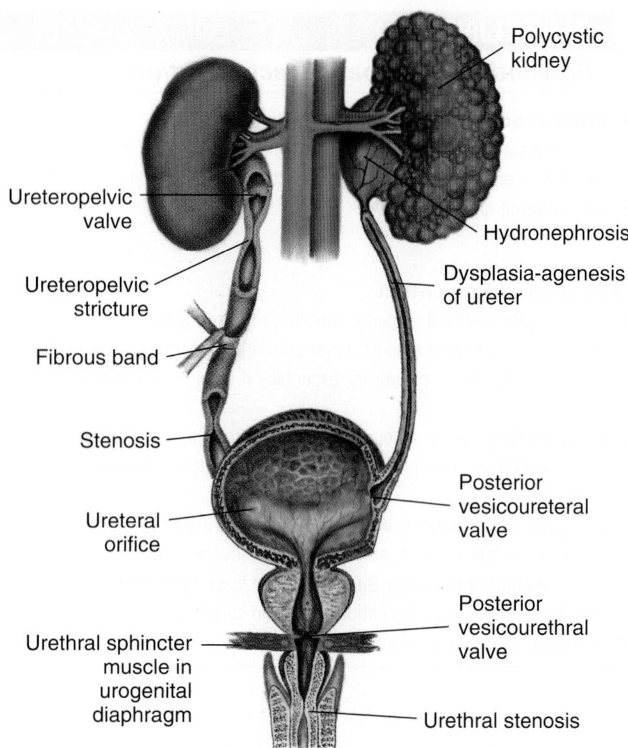

FIGURE 49-2 Major sites of urinary tract obstruction.

of urine above the obstruction causes *hydronephrosis* (dilation of the renal pelvis from distension) with eventual pressure destruction of renal parenchyma, although the dilating ureters form a reservoir that reduces the effect on the kidneys for a long time.

Obstruction may be congenital or acquired, unilateral or bilateral, complete or incomplete, with acute or chronic manifestations. The obstruction can occur at any level of the upper or lower urinary tract (Fig. 49-2). Partial obstruction may not be symptomatic unless there is a water or solute diuresis. Boys are affected more frequently than girls, and malformations should be suspected when patients have some other congenital defects (e.g., prune belly syndrome, chromosomal anomalies, anorectal malformations, defects of the pinna of the ear).

Damage to distal nephrons in chronic uropathy alters the ability to concentrate urine, contributing to increased urine flow and metabolic acidosis occurring from the decreased excretion of acid secondary to the impaired ability of the distal nephron to secrete hydrogen ions. Partial obstruction results in progressive loss of renal function as a result of irreversible damage to the nephrons. Pooled urine serves as a medium for bacterial growth; therefore, UTIs further increase the extent of renal damage.

Early diagnosis and surgical correction or procedures that divert the flow of urine to bypass the obstruction, such as placement of a temporary percutaneous nephrostomy tube or cutaneous ureterostomy, are essential to prevent progressive renal damage. Medical complications of acute or chronic renal failure (chronic kidney disease [CKD]) or infection are managed as described later for those disorders.

NURSING CARE

Nursing goals in urinary tract obstruction include helping to identify cases, assisting with diagnostic procedures, and caring for children with complications. Preparing parents and children for procedures is a major nursing responsibility. Preparation for urinary diversion procedures is of special importance (see Preparation for Diagnostic and Therapeutic Procedures, Chapter 44).

Parents and children need emotional support and counselling during the lengthy management of these disorders. Many children are discharged with ureteral drainage systems in place that must be protected from damage, and the danger of infection is a constant concern. Parents should be taught to care for the equipment and recognize the signs of possible obstruction or infection within the system. Maintaining adequate urine flow is imperative. Fluids should be encouraged. The tube should be observed frequently for indications of obstruction resulting from sediment, small blood clots, or kinking. The primary health care provider should inspect any drainage from around the tube.

Children with external diversional systems need psychological support and guidance, especially as they reach adolescence and as body image concerns assume more prominence. Peer and family support groups can be helpful. Those with progressive renal deterioration may face the prospect of dialysis or transplantation as well as the emotions that accompany these procedures.

External Defects

Defects of the external genitourinary tract are serious conditions primarily because of the psychological impact on the child. Satisfactory surgical repair is successful for the more common disorders and is carried out or initiated as early as possible. The major anomalies of the lower genitourinary tract, their description, and their management are summarized in Table 49-4.

Congenital Genitourinary System Anomalies

Hypospadias and epispadias. Hypospadias constitutes a range of penile anomalies associated with an abnormally located urinary meatus. The meatus can open below the glans penis or anywhere along the ventral surface of the penis, the scrotum, or the perineum. It is the most common anomaly of the penis, occurring in approximately 1 in 250 live births (Elder, 2016a). It is classified according to the location of the meatus and the presence or absence of chordee, which is a ventral curvature of the penis.

Mild cases of hypospadias (Fig. 49-3) are often repaired for cosmetic reasons and involve a single surgical procedure. The goals are to improve the appearance of the genitalia, make it possible for the child to urinate in a standing position, and have a sexually adequate organ. Historically these infants were not circumcised because the foreskin was used during surgical repair; the urologist should be consulted before circumcision. Repair is done early, often during or soon after the first year of life.

TABLE 49-4 **DEFECTS OF THE GENITOURINARY TRACT**

DEFECT	THERAPEUTIC MANAGEMENT
Inguinal hernia—Protrusion of abdominal contents through inguinal canal into scrotum	Detected as painless inguinal swelling of variable size Surgical closure of inguinal defect
Hydrocele—Fluid in scrotum	Surgical repair indicated if spontaneous resolution not accomplished in 1 yr
Phimosis—Narrowing or stenosis of preputial opening of foreskin	Mild cases—manual retraction of foreskin and proper cleansing of area Severe cases—circumcision or vertical division and transverse suturing of foreskin
Hypospadias—Urethral opening located behind glans penis or anywhere along ventral surface of penile shaft	Objectives of surgical correction: Enable child to void in standing position and direct stream voluntarily in usual manner Improve physical appearance of genitalia Produce a sexually adequate organ
Chordee—Ventral curvature of penis, often associated with hypospadias	Surgical release of fibrous band causing the deformity
Epispadias—Meatal opening located on dorsal surface of penis	Surgical correction, usually including penile and urethral lengthening and bladder neck reconstruction (if necessary)
Cryptorchidism—Failure of one or both testes to descend normally through inguinal canal	Detected by inability to palpate testes within scrotum Medical—Administration of human chorionic gonadotropin (older child) Surgical—Orchiopexy Objectives of therapy: Prevent damage to undescended testicle Decrease incidence of malignant tumour formation Avoid trauma and torsion Close inguinal canal Prevent cosmetic and psychological disability from empty scrotum
Exstrophy of bladder—Eversion of posterior bladder through anterior bladder wall and lower abdominal wall; associated with open pubic arch (a severe defect)	Potential objectives of surgical correction: Preserve renal function Attain urinary control Perform adequate reconstructive repair Improve sexual function (especially in males)
Disorders of Sexual Differentiation	
Masculinized female (female pseudohermaphrodite)	Assign gender as female; assign gender while avoiding irreversible surgery, realizing some children may change gender later in life; family participation essential
Incompletely masculinized male (male pseudohermaphrodite)	Assign gender while avoiding irreversible surgery, realizing some children may change gender later in life; family participation essential
True hermaphrodite (both ovaries and testes)	Assign gender while avoiding irreversible surgery, realizing some children may change gender later in life; gender assignment depends on predominant characteristics; family participation essential
Mixed gonadal dysgenesis	Assign gender while avoiding irreversible surgery, realizing some children may change gender later in life; gender assignment depends on predominant characteristics; family participation essential

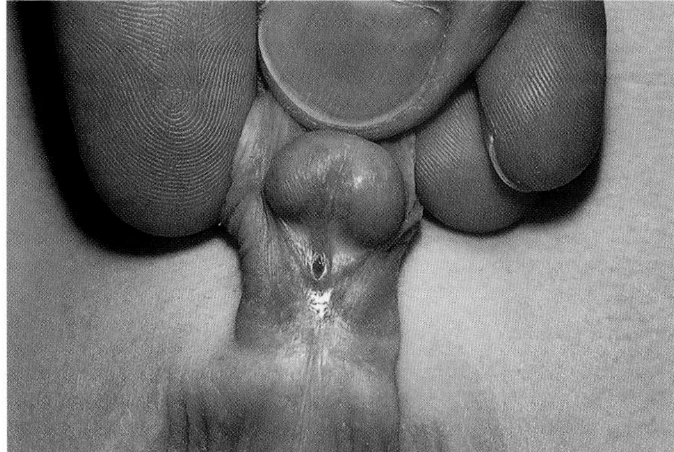

FIGURE 49-3 Hypospadias. (Courtesy H. Gil Rushton, MD, Children's National Medical Center.)

Epispadias results from failure of urethral canalization. About 55% of the affected infants are boys who have a widened pubic symphysis and a broad, spadelike penis with the urethra opening on its dorsal surface. Girls have a wide urethra and a bifid clitoris. Severity ranges from mild anomaly to a severe form associated with exstrophy of the bladder. Surgical correction is necessary, and affected male infants should not be circumcised.

Exstrophy of the bladder. The most common bladder anomaly is exstrophy (Fig. 49-4), which often occurs in conjunction with epispadias. It is rare, occurring only in about 1 in 35,000 to 40,000 live births (Elder, 2016b). It results from abnormal development of the bladder, abdominal wall, and symphysis pubis that causes the bladder, urethra, and ureteral orifices to all be exposed. The bladder is visible in the suprapubic area as a red mass with numerous folds, with urine draining from it onto the infant's skin.

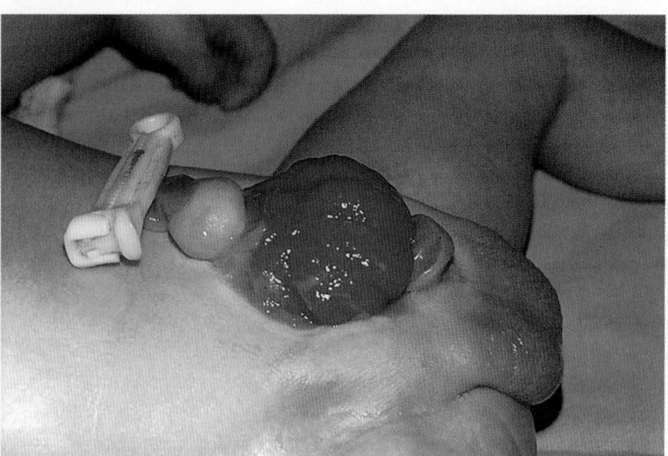

FIGURE 49-4 Exstrophy of bladder. (Courtesy H. Gil Rushton, MD, Children's National Medical Center.)

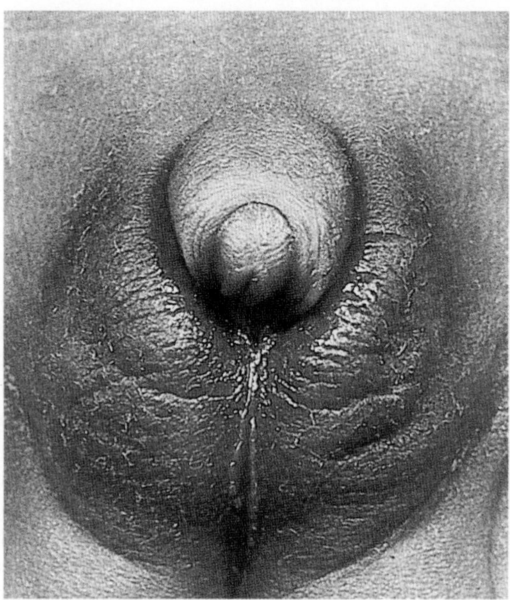

FIGURE 49-5 Ambiguous external genitalia (i.e., structure may be enlarged clitoral hood and clitoris or micropenis and bifid scrotum). (Courtesy Edward S. Tank, MD, Division of Urology, Oregon Health Sciences University.)

Immediately after birth, the exposed bladder is covered with a sterile, nonadherent dressing to protect it until closure can be performed. It is recommended that reconstructive surgery be started in the neonatal period, preferably with the bladder being closed during the first or second day of life.

Disorders of Sex Development

A disorder of sex development (DSD) in the newborn (Fig. 49-5) often is discovered by the nurse during a physical assessment. Erroneous or abnormal sexual differentiation may be a genetic defect, such as congenital adrenal hypoplasia, which can be life threatening because it involves deficiency of all adrenocortical hormones. Other possible causes of DSD include chromosomal abnormalities, defective sex hormone synthesis in males, and the placental transfer of masculinizing agents to female fetuses. Gender assignment should be based on data gathered from the following sources: maternal and family history, including the ingestion of steroids during pregnancy and relatives who had DSD or who died during the newborn period; physical examination; chromosomal analysis (results are available in 2 or 3 days); endoscopy, ultrasonography and radiographic contrast studies; biochemical tests, such as analysis of urinary steroid excretion, which helps detect several of the adrenocortical syndromes; and, in some instances, laparotomy or gonad biopsy.

Therapeutic intervention, including any counselling and surgery, should be started as soon as possible. Any child born with DSD should not receive gender assignment until a proper assessment has been done. Gender assignment should be based on age at presentation, potential for mature sexual function, potential fertility, and the long-term psychological and emotional impact on the child and family. Parents need much support as they learn to deal with this challenging situation.

Psychological Problems Related to Genital Surgery

Surgery involving sexual organs can be particularly disruptive to children, especially preschoolers fearing punishment, retaliation, body mutilation, or castration. Some of the problems of hospitalization, separation, and anxiety can be eased by hospital practices that are sensitive to the child's needs (see Chapter 43).

A child's body image is largely derived as a result of feedback from the primary caregivers, and parental anxiety regarding an acceptable physical appearance and adequate future sexual competency is readily communicated to an affected child. Children with birth defects are at risk for developing a distorted body image that reflects the caregiver's subtly communicated evaluation of their bodies. The trend toward repair of visible genital defects is based in large part on these psychological variables. The earlier a repair can be achieved, the more likely it is that the child will develop a healthy body image.

During the years from 3 to 6, the phallic-oedipal period, children show a strong interest in and concern about the genital area, sex differences, and genital normality or its lack. It is also a time when children are frightened of what they perceive to be threats to their body and bodily function. They can view any untoward happening as a punishment for real or imagined wrongdoing or unacceptable sexual feelings, such as masturbation, sex play, or erotic feelings. After extensive review of the emotional, cognitive, and body image issues that may occur in children undergoing surgical reconstruction of a genital abnormality, it is recommended that surgery be accomplished between the ages of 6 and 15 months, to minimize the psychological effects of surgery and anaesthesia.

NURSING CARE

Preparing children and their families for diagnostic and surgical procedures (see Preparation for Diagnostic and Therapeutic Procedures, Chapter 44) and for home care is a major nursing function. Most postoperative care involves care of the surgical site. Tub baths are discouraged for 1 week after simple surgeries. The surgical site needs to be kept clean and otherwise protected from infection and to be inspected for signs of infection.

Dressings, if any, should be inspected regularly. More complex surgeries require additional care and observation (e.g., catheter care for urethral reconstruction and care of urinary diversion stomas and collection devices).

Some older children's activities, such as pushing, lifting, playing with straddle toys or in sandboxes, swimming, and engaging in rough activities, may be restricted after some types of surgical repairs. Precise restrictions depend on the specific type of surgery. Activities of infants and toddlers are not limited.

In most cases the results of surgery are satisfactory. However, in some of the more severe defects, such as exstrophy and those that require stomas, additional emotional interventions may be needed. A major concern of parents and children is related to surgery affecting the genitalia directly. Concerns about penis size, appearance of the genitalia, potential ability to procreate, and rejection by peers are potential fears that require psychological adjustment, particularly during adolescence.

GLOMERULAR DISEASE

Nephrotic Syndrome

Nephrotic syndrome is a clinical state that includes massive **proteinuria**, **hypoalbuminemia**, **hyperlipidemia**, and **edema**. The disorder can occur as (1) a primary disease known as *idiopathic nephrosis, childhood nephrosis*, or *minimal-change nephrotic syndrome (MCNS)*, (2) a secondary disorder that occurs as a clinical manifestation after or in association with glomerular damage that has a known or presumed cause, or (3) a congenital form inherited as an autosomal recessive disorder. The disorder is characterized by increased glomerular permeability to plasma protein, which results in massive urinary protein loss. The glomerulus is responsible for the initial step in the formation of urine, and the filtration rate depends on an intact glomerular membrane. This discussion is devoted to MCNS because it constitutes 80% of nephrotic syndrome cases.

Pathophysiology

The onset of MCNS can occur at any age but predominantly occurs in children between 2 and 7 years of age. It is rare in children younger than 6 months of age, uncommon in infants younger than 1 year of age, and unusual after the age of 8. Patients with MCNS are twice as likely to be male.

The pathogenesis of MCNS is not understood. There may be a metabolic, biochemical, physiochemical, or immune-mediated disturbance that causes the basement membrane of the glomeruli to become increasingly permeable to protein, but the cause and mechanisms are only speculative.

The glomerular membrane, normally impermeable to albumin and other proteins, becomes permeable to proteins, especially albumin, which leak through the membrane and are lost in urine (*hyperalbuminuria*). This permeability reduces the serum albumin level (*hypoalbuminemia*), decreasing the colloidal osmotic pressure in the capillaries. As a result, the vascular hydrostatic pressure exceeds the pull of the colloidal osmotic pressure, causing fluid to accumulate in the interstitial spaces (*edema*) and body cavities, particularly in the abdominal cavity (*ascites*). The shift of fluid from the plasma to the interstitial spaces reduces the vascular fluid volume (*hypovolemia*), which in turn stimulates the renin-angiotensin system and the secretion of ADH and aldosterone. Tubular reabsorption of sodium and water is increased in an attempt to increase intravascular volume. The elevation of serum lipids is not fully understood. The sequence of events in nephrotic syndrome is diagrammed in Fig. 49-6.

Diagnostic Evaluation

The disease is suspected on the basis of clinical manifestations (Box 49-2) in children between the ages of 2 and 8 years, especially when weight gain in a previously well child increases slowly over days or weeks. The generalized edema may develop rapidly or gradually but eventually prompts the family to seek medical attention. Parents usually give a history of the child being well but steadily gaining weight; appearing edematous; and then becoming anorexic, irritable, and less active.

The hallmark of MCNS is massive proteinuria (higher than 2+ on urine dipstick). Hyaline casts, oval fat bodies, and a few red blood cells can be found in the urine of some affected children, although there is seldom gross hematuria. The GFR is usually normal or high. Total serum protein concentration is low, with the serum albumin significantly reduced and plasma lipids elevated. Hemoglobin and hematocrit are usually normal or elevated as a result of hemoconcentration. The platelet count may be elevated. Serum sodium concentration may be low.

If the patient does not respond to a 4- to 8-week course of steroids, a renal biopsy may be needed to distinguish between other types of nephrotic syndrome. The biopsy results of children with MCNS are remarkable for effacement of the foot processes of the epithelial cells lining the basement membrane, but otherwise the kidney tissue is normal.

Therapeutic Management

Objectives of therapeutic management include (1) reducing the excretion of urinary protein, (2) reducing fluid retention in the tissues, (3) preventing infection, and (4) minimizing complications related to therapies. Dietary restrictions include a low-salt diet and, in more severe cases, fluid restriction. If complications of edema develop, diuretic therapy may be initiated to provide temporary relief from edema. Sometimes infusions of 25% albumin are used. Acute infections are treated with appropriate antibiotics.

Corticosteroids are the first line of therapy for MCNS. The starting dosage for prednisone is usually 2 mg/kg body weight/day, in one or more divided doses for 6 weeks. The dose is then decreased to 1.5 mg/kg body weight per alternate days for 6 weeks (Gipson, Massengill, Yao, et al., 2009; Pais & Avner, 2016). Most children respond within 7 to 21 days. The medication is then tapered over a period of several months and eventually stopped if the child remains asymptomatic.

About two thirds of children with MCNS have a relapse, heralded first by increased urine protein. Relapses can be diagnosed early if parents are taught routine home monitoring of urine protein by dipstick. Relapses are treated with a repeated course of high-dose steroid therapy. Adverse effects of the steroids include weight gain, rounding of the face (moon face),

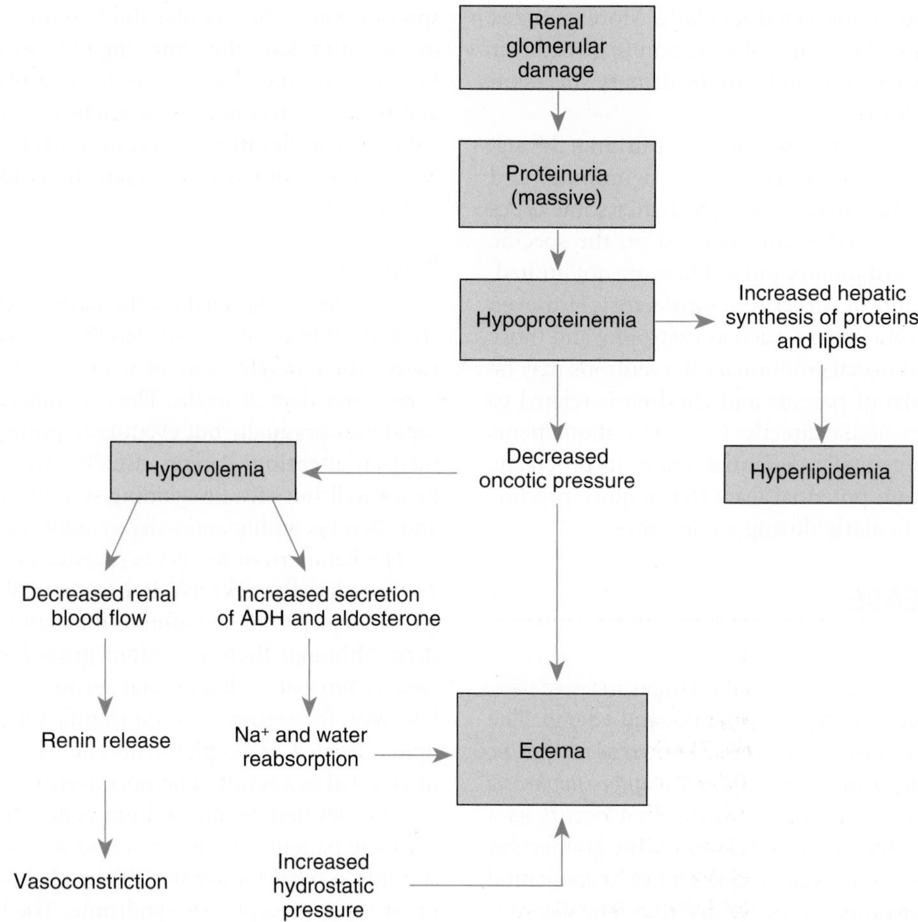

FIGURE 49-6 Sequence of events in nephrotic syndrome. *ADH,* antidiuretic hormone.

BOX 49-2 CLINICAL MANIFESTATIONS OF NEPHROTIC SYNDROME

Weight gain
Puffiness of face (facial edema):
- Especially around the eyes
- Apparent on arising in the morning
- Subsides during the day

Abdominal swelling (ascites)
Pleural effusion
Labial or scrotal swelling
Edema of intestinal mucosa, possibly causing:
- Diarrhea
- Anorexia
- Poor intestinal absorption

Ankle or leg swelling
Irritability
Tendency to fatigue easily
Lethargy
Blood pressure normal or slightly decreased
Susceptibility to infection
Urine alterations:
- Decreased volume
- Frothy

behaviour changes, and increased appetite. Long-term therapy may result in hirsutism, growth restriction, cataracts, hypertension, gastrointestinal bleeding, bone demineralization, infection, and hyperglycemia. Children who do not respond to steroid therapy, those who have frequent relapses, and those in whom the adverse effects threaten their growth and general health may be considered for a course of therapy using other immunosuppressant medications (cyclophosphamide, chlorambucil, or cyclosporine).

MCNS episodes, both the first episode and the relapse, often happen in conjunction with a viral or bacterial infection. Relapses can also be triggered by allergies and immunizations. Relapses in children with MCNS may continue over many years.

Complications of nephrotic syndrome include infection, circulatory insufficiency secondary to hypovolemia, and thromboembolism. Infections that may be seen in children with nephrotic syndrome include peritonitis, cellulitis, and pneumonia and require prompt recognition and vigorous treatment with appropriate antibiotic therapy.

Prognosis

The prognosis for ultimate recovery in most cases is good. It is a self-limiting disease, and in children who respond to steroid therapy the tendency to relapse decreases with time. With early detection and prompt implementation of therapy to eradicate proteinuria, progressive basement membrane damage is minimized, so that when the tendency to relapse is past, renal function is usually normal or near normal. It is estimated that approximately 80% of affected children have this favourable prognosis.

NURSING CARE

Continuous monitoring of fluid intake and output is an important nursing function. Strict intake and output records are essential but may be difficult to obtain from very young children. Application of collection bags is irritating to edematous skin that is readily subject to breakdown. Applying diapers or weighing wet pads may be necessary.

Other methods of monitoring progress include urine examination for albumin, daily weight, and measurement of abdominal girth. Assessment of edema (e.g., increased or decreased swelling around the eyes and dependent areas), the degree of pitting, and the colour and texture of skin are part of nursing care. Assessing for signs of skin breakdown due to severe edema is necessary. In the case of severe scrotal swelling, the use of a scrotal sling may be indicated to decrease pressure and discomfort. Vital signs need to be monitored to detect any early signs of complications such as shock or an infective process. Infection is a constant source of danger to edematous children and those receiving corticosteroid therapy. These children are particularly vulnerable to upper respiratory tract infection; they must be kept warm and dry, active, and protected from contact with infected individuals (e.g., roommates, visitors, and personnel).

Loss of appetite accompanying active nephrosis can create a perplexing problem for nurses. The combined efforts of nurse, dietitian, parents, and child are needed to formulate a nutritionally adequate and attractive diet. Salt is usually restricted (but not eliminated) during the edema phase and while the child is on steroid therapy. Fluid restriction (if prescribed) is limited to short-term use during massive edema. Every effort should be made to serve attractive meals with preferred foods and a minimum of fuss, but it usually requires considerable ingenuity to entice the child to eat (see Feeding the Sick Child, Chapter 44).

Children usually adjust activities according to their tolerance level. However, they may require guidance in selecting play activities. Suitable recreational and diversional activities are an important part of their care. Irritability and mood swings that accompany steroid therapy are not unusual in these children and may create an additional challenge for the nurse and family.

Family Support and Home Care

Continuous support of the child and family is one of the major nursing considerations. Many children are treated at home during relapses. Parents need to be taught to detect signs of relapse and to call for changes in treatment at the earliest indications. Unless the edema and proteinuria are severe or the parents are unable to care for the ill child, home care is preferred. Parents should be instructed in testing urine for albumin, administering medications, and providing general care. Parents also need to encourage the child to avoid contact with infected playmates, but the child should attend school. Psychological support may be indicated because of body image changes associated with prolonged and frequent steroid use.

The prolonged course of the relapsing form of nephrotic syndrome is taxing to both the child and the family. The up-and-down course of remissions and exacerbations with periodic disruption of family life by hospitalization places a strain on the child and the family. Success is more likely when relapses are detected and therapy is instituted early, and remissions are prolonged when care instructions are carried out.

Acute Glomerulonephritis

Acute glomerulonephritis (AGN) may be a primary event or a manifestation of a systemic disorder that can range from minimal to severe. Common features include oliguria, edema, hypertension and circulatory congestion, hematuria, and proteinuria. Most cases are postinfectious and have been associated with pneumococcal, streptococcal, and viral infections. *Acute poststreptococcal glomerulonephritis* (APSGN) is the most common of the postinfectious renal diseases in childhood and the one for which a cause can be established in most cases. APSGN can occur at any age but affects primarily early school-age children, with a peak age of onset of 6 to 7 years. It is uncommon in children younger than 2 years of age, and males outnumber females 2:1.

Etiology

APSGN is an immune-complex disease that occurs after an antecedent streptococcal infection with certain strains of the group A beta-hemolytic streptococcus. Most streptococcal infections *do not* cause APSGN. A latent period of 10 to 21 days occurs between the streptococcal infection and the onset of clinical manifestations. Disease secondary to streptococcal pharyngitis is more common in the winter or spring, but when APSGN is associated with pyoderma (principally impetigo), it may be more prevalent in later summer or early fall, especially in warmer climates. Second episodes of AGN are rare. APSGN is typically self-limiting and recovery occurs spontaneously (Reuter-Rice & Bolick, 2012).

Pathophysiology

The pathophysiology of APSGN is still uncertain. Immune complexes are deposited in the glomerular basement membrane. The glomeruli become edematous and infiltrated with polymorphonuclear leukocytes, which occlude the capillary lumen. The resulting decrease in plasma filtration results in an excessive accumulation of water and retention of sodium that expands plasma and interstitial fluid volumes, leading to circulatory congestion and edema. The cause of the hypertension associated with AGN cannot be completely explained by fluid retention. Excess renin may also be produced.

Diagnostic Evaluation

Typically, affected children are in good health until they experience the streptococcal infection. In some instances they have a history of only a mild cold or no previous infection at all. The onset of nephritis appears after an average latency period of

BOX 49-3 CLINICAL MANIFESTATIONS OF ACUTE POSTSTREPTOCOCCAL GLOMERULONEPHRITIS

Edema:
- Especially periorbital
- Facial edema more prominent in the morning
- Spreads during the day to involve extremities and abdomen

Anorexia
Urine:
- Cloudy, smoky brown (resembles tea or cola)
- Severely reduced volume

Pallor
Irritability
Lethargy
Child appearing ill
Child seldom expressing specific health concerns
Older children:
- Headaches
- Abdominal discomfort
- Dysuria

Vomiting possible
Mild to moderately elevated blood pressure

about 10 days (Box 49-3). Because the child appears to be well during the latency period, parents do not recognize the association. The edema is relatively moderate and may not be appreciated by someone unfamiliar with the child's normal appearance.

Urinalysis during the acute phase characteristically shows hematuria and proteinuria. Proteinuria generally parallels the hematuria and may be 3+ or 4+ in the presence of gross hematuria. Gross discolouration of the urine reflects red blood cell and hemoglobin content. Microscopic examination of the sediment shows many red blood cells, leukocytes, epithelial cells, and granular and red blood cell casts. Bacteria are not seen.

Azotemia that results from impaired glomerular filtration is reflected in elevated urea and creatinine levels in at least 50% of cases. Occasionally proteinuria is excessive and the patient may have nephrotic syndrome (i.e., hypoproteinemia and hyperlipidemia).

Cultures of the pharynx are rarely positive for streptococci, since the renal disease occurs weeks after the infection.

Some serological tests are necessary to make the diagnosis of APSGN. Circulating serum antibodies to streptococci indicate the presence of a previous infection. The antistreptolysin O (ASO) titre is the most familiar and readily available test for streptococcal infection. Other antibodies that may aid in diagnosis are elevated antihyaluronidase (AHase), antideoxyribonuclease B (ADNase-B), and streptozyme.

All patients with APSGN have reduced serum complement (C3) activity in the early stages of the disease. Rising C3 levels are used as a guide to indicate improvement of the disease and should be normal in almost all patients 8 weeks after disease onset.

Studies that may be useful include chest x-ray examination, which generally shows cardiac enlargement, pulmonary congestion, or pleural effusion during the edematous phase of acute disease. Renal biopsy for diagnostic purposes is seldom required but may be useful in the diagnosis of atypical cases.

Therapeutic Management

Management consists of general supportive measures and early recognition and treatment of complications. Children who have normal blood pressure and a satisfactory urine output can generally be treated at home. Those with substantial edema, hypertension, gross hematuria, or significant oliguria should be hospitalized because of the unpredictability of complications.

Dietary restrictions depend on the stage and severity of the disease, especially the extent of edema. Moderate sodium restriction and even fluid restriction may be instituted for children with hypertension and edema. Foods with substantial amounts of potassium are generally restricted during the period of oliguria.

Regular measurement of vital signs, body weight, and intake and output is essential to monitor the progress of the disease and to detect complications that may appear at any time during the course of the disease. A record of daily weight is the most useful means for assessing fluid balance. Rarely, children with APSGN will develop acute renal failure (acute kidney injury [AKI]) with oliguria that significantly alters the fluid and electrolyte balance (resulting in **hyperkalemia**, acidosis, hypocalcemia, or hyperphosphatemia). These children require careful management. Peritoneal dialysis or hemodialysis is seldom needed.

Acute hypertension must be anticipated and identified early. Blood pressure measurements should be taken every 4 to 6 hours. A variety of antihypertensive medications and diuretics can be used to control hypertension. Antibiotic therapy is indicated only for those children with evidence of persistent streptococcal infections. It is used to prevent transmission of nephritogenic streptococci to other family members.

Prognosis

Almost all children correctly diagnosed as having APSGN recover completely, and specific immunity is conferred, so that subsequent recurrences are uncommon. Some of these children have been reported to develop chronic disease, but most of these cases are now believed to be different glomerular diseases misdiagnosed as poststreptococcal disease.

NURSING CARE

Nursing care of the child with glomerulonephritis involves careful assessment of the disease status, with regular monitoring of vital signs (including frequent measurement of blood pressure), fluid balance, and behaviour.

Vital signs provide clues to the severity of the disease and early signs of complications. They need to be carefully measured, and any deviations reported and recorded. The volume and character of urine should be noted and the child weighed daily. Children with restricted fluid intake, especially those who are not severely edematous or those who have lost weight, should be observed for signs of dehydration.

Assessment of the child's appearance for signs of cerebral complications is an important nursing function, since the severity of the acute phase is variable and unpredictable. The child with edema, hypertension, and gross hematuria may be subject to complications, and anticipatory preparations such as seizure precautions and IV equipment should be included in the nursing care plan.

For most children a regular diet is allowed, but it should contain no added salt. Foods high in sodium and salted treats need to be eliminated, and parents and friends should be advised not to bring snacks such as potato chips or pretzels. The total amount of salt ingested is usually less because of poor appetite. Fluid restriction, if prescribed, is more difficult, and the amount permitted should be evenly divided throughout the waking hours. Meal preparation and service require special attention, since the child is indifferent to meals during the acute phase. Again, collaboration between parents and the dietitian and special consideration for food preferences can facilitate meal planning.

During the acute phase, children are generally content to lie in bed. As they begin to feel better and their symptoms subside, they will want to be up. Activities should be planned to allow for frequent rest periods and to avoid fatigue. Children who have mild edema and no hypertension, as well as convalescent children who are being treated at home, need follow-up care. Parents need to be instructed regarding general measures, including diet and prevention of infection.

Health supervision is continued, with weekly, followed by monthly, visits for evaluation and urinalysis. Parent education and support is needed to get the child's discharge organized and home care set up. The family needs to learn how to care for the child at home and to have the follow-up care and health supervision arranged.

MISCELLANEOUS RENAL DISORDERS

Hemolytic Uremic Syndrome

Hemolytic uremic syndrome (HUS) is an uncommon, acute renal disease that occurs primarily in infants and small children between the ages of 6 months and 5 years. HUS is one of the most frequent causes of acquired AKI in children (Duzova, Bakkaloglu, Kalyoncu, et al., 2010). The clinical features of the disease include acquired hemolytic anemia, thrombocytopenia, renal injury, and central nervous system symptoms. The etiology of HUS is thought to be associated with bacterial toxins, chemicals, and viruses. The appearance of the disease has been associated with *Rickettsia* organisms, viruses (especially coxsackievirus, echovirus, and adenovirus), *E. coli*, pneumococci, shigellae, and salmonellae and may represent an unusual response to these infections. Multiple cases of HUS caused by enteric infection of the *E. coli* O157:H7 serotype have been traced to undercooked meat, especially ground beef. Other sources are unpasteurized milk or fruit juice, especially apple; alfalfa sprouts; lettuce; and salami. Drinking or swimming in sewage-contaminated water can also cause infection. The clinical presentation is usually a history of a prodromal illness (most often gastroenteritis or an upper respiratory tract infection) followed by the sudden onset of hemolysis and renal failure.

Pathophysiology

The primary site of injury appears to be the endothelial lining of the small glomerular arterioles, which become swollen and occluded with deposits of platelets and fibrin clots (intravascular coagulation). Red blood cells are damaged as they attempt to move through the partially occluded blood vessels and are removed by the spleen, causing acute hemolytic anemia. The platelet aggregation within the damaged blood vessels or the damage and removal of platelets produce the characteristic thrombocytopenia.

Diagnostic Evaluation

The triad of anemia, thrombocytopenia, and renal failure is sufficient for diagnosis (Box 49-4). Renal involvement is evidenced by proteinuria, hematuria, and urinary casts; blood urea nitrogen (BUN) and serum creatinine levels are elevated. A low hemoglobin and hematocrit and a high reticulocyte count confirm the hemolytic nature of the anemia.

Therapeutic Management

The goals of therapy are early diagnosis and aggressive, supportive care of the AKI and hemolytic anemia. The most consistently effective treatment of HUS is hemodialysis or peritoneal dialysis, which is instituted in any child who has been anuric for 24 hours or who demonstrates oliguria with uremia or hypertension and seizures. Other treatments include use of pharmacological agents, fresh frozen plasma, and plasmapheresis. Blood transfusions with fresh, washed packed cells are administered for severe anemia but are used with caution to prevent circulatory overload from added volume.

Prognosis

With prompt treatment the recovery rate is about 95%, but residual renal impairment ranges from 10 to 50%. Long-term

BOX 49-4 CLINICAL MANIFESTATIONS OF HEMOLYTIC UREMIC SYNDROME

Vomiting
Irritability
Lethargy
Marked pallor
Hemorrhagic manifestations:
- Bruising
- Petechiae
- Jaundice
- Bloody diarrhea

Oliguria or anuria
Central nervous system involvement:
- Seizures
- Stupor or coma

Signs of acute heart failure (sometimes)

complications include CKD, hypertension, and central nervous system disorders. Death is usually caused by residual renal impairment or central nervous system injury.

NURSING CARE

Because of the sudden and life-threatening nature of the disorder in a previously well child, parents are often ill prepared for the impact of hospitalization and treatment and require support and understanding.

Wilms Tumour

Wilms tumour, or nephroblastoma, is the most common malignant renal and intra-abdominal tumour of childhood. Its frequency is estimated to be 8 cases per million in White children younger than 15 years (Daw, Huff, & Anderson, 2016). Approximately 75% of the cases occur in children younger than 5 years, with a peak incidence at 2 to 3 years of age; 2% of cases have a familial origin (Daw et al., 2016). Unfortunately, there is no method of identifying gene carriers at this time. In Canada, the Canadian Cancer Society reported that between 2006 and 2010, there were 225 cases of Wilms tumours diagnosed in children 0 to 14 years of age. In addition, there were 17 deaths from Wilms tumours in children 0 to 14 years of age from 2007 to 2011 (Canadian Cancer Society, 2016).

Etiology

Wilms tumour probably arises from a malignant, undifferentiated cluster of primordial cells capable of initiating the regeneration of an abnormal structure. Its occurrence slightly favours the left kidney, which is advantageous because surgically this kidney is easier to manipulate and remove. In about 10% of cases both kidneys are involved. Studies have shown that development of Wilms tumour is frequently associated with aniridia, hemihypertrophy, Beckwith-Wiedemann syndrome, or genitourinary anomalies (Daw et al., 2016).

Diagnostic Evaluation

In a child suspected of having Wilms tumour, special emphasis is placed on the history and physical examination for the presence of congenital anomalies, a family history of cancer, and signs of malignancy (e.g., weight loss, size of liver and spleen, indications of anemia, lymphadenopathy). Most children with Wilms tumour are brought to the health care provider because of abdominal swelling or an abdominal mass (Box 49-5). Specific tests include radiographic studies, including abdominal ultrasound and abdominal and chest computed tomography scan; hematological studies; biochemical studies; and urinalysis. Studies to demonstrate the relationship of the tumour to the ipsilateral kidney and the presence of a normal functioning kidney on the contralateral side are essential. If a large tumour is present, an inferior venacavagram is necessary to demonstrate possible tumour involvement adjacent to the vena cava. A bone marrow aspiration may be performed to rule out metastasis, which is rare in children with Wilms tumour.

BOX 49-5 CLINICAL MANIFESTATIONS OF WILMS TUMOUR

Abdominal swelling or mass:
- Firm
- Nontender
- Confined to one side

Hematuria (less than one fourth of cases)
Fatigue and malaise
Hypertension (occasionally)
Weight loss
Fever
Manifestations resulting from compression of tumour mass
Secondary metabolic alterations from tumour or metastasis
If metastasis, symptoms of lung involvement:
- Dyspnea
- Cough
- Shortness of breath
- Chest pain (sometimes)

! NURSING ALERT

To reinforce the need for caution, it may be necessary to post a sign on the bed that reads "DO NOT PALPATE ABDOMEN." Careful bathing and handling are also important in preventing trauma to the tumour site.

Therapeutic Management

Combined treatment with surgery and chemotherapy with or without radiation is based on the histological pattern and clinical stage. Surgery is scheduled as soon as possible after confirmation, usually within 24 to 48 hours of admission. A large transabdominal incision is performed for optimal visualization of the abdominal cavity. The tumour, affected kidney, and adjacent adrenal gland are removed. Great care is taken to keep the encapsulated tumour intact, since rupture can seed cancer cells throughout the abdomen, lymph channel, and bloodstream. The contralateral kidney is carefully inspected for evidence of disease or dysfunction. Regional lymph nodes are inspected, and a biopsy is performed when indicated. Any involved structures, such as part of the colon, diaphragm, or vena cava, are removed. Metal clips are placed around the tumour site for exact marking during radiotherapy.

If both kidneys are involved, the child may be treated with radiotherapy or chemotherapy before surgery to decrease the size of the tumour, allowing more conservative surgery. It may be possible to perform a partial nephrectomy on the less affected kidney, with a total nephrectomy on the opposite side. When a transplant is feasible, such as from a twin, sibling, or parent, bilateral nephrectomy is considered as a last resort.

Postoperative radiotherapy is indicated for children with large tumours, metastasis, residual postoperative disease, unfavourable histological characteristics, or recurrence. Chemotherapy is indicated for all stages. The most effective agents for treating Wilms tumour are actinomycin D (dactinomycin), vincristine, and adriamycin, with the addition of cyclophosphamide for unfavourable histological characteristics or advanced disease

(Ozan, 2015). The duration of therapy ranges from 6 to 15 months.

Prognosis

Survival rates for Wilms tumour are the highest among all childhood cancers. Children with localized tumour (stages I and II) have a 90% chance of cure with multimodal therapy. Factors that favourably affect the success of further therapy include initial treatment with only vincristine and dactinomycin, relapse to the lungs only, relapse in the abdomen of a patient who received no prior abdominal irradiation, and relapse more than 12 months after diagnosis. Wilms tumour may recur, especially in the lungs. Both chemotherapy and radiotherapy can induce second malignancies, usually in areas that have been irradiated (Ozan, 2015).

NURSING CARE

Nursing care of the child with Wilms tumour is similar to that of children with other cancers treated with surgery, irradiation, and chemotherapy. However, there are some significant differences; these are discussed for each phase of nursing care.

Preoperative Care

The preoperative period is one of swift diagnosis. The nurse faces the challenge of preparing the child and parents for all laboratory and operative procedures within 24 to 48 hours of admission. Explanations should be simple, repeated as needed, and focused on the child's actual experiences. In addition to the usual preoperative observations, blood pressure is monitored, since hypertension from excess renin production is a possibility.

There are several special preoperative concerns, the most important of which is that the *tumour is not palpated unless absolutely necessary*, because manipulation of the mass may cause dissemination of cancer cells to adjacent and distant sites.

Because radiotherapy and chemotherapy are usually begun immediately after surgery, parents need an explanation of what to expect, such as major benefits and adverse effects (see Chapter 48). The timing of the information should be considered, to avoid overwhelming the family. Ideally, the nurse should be present during physician–parent conferences to answer questions as they arise. It is usually better to postpone telling the child about these adverse effects until after surgery. Alopecia, usually of most concern to older children, does not occur until approximately 2 weeks after the initial treatment regimen. Therefore, the child can be prepared for the hair loss postoperatively.

Postoperative Care

Despite the extensive surgical intervention necessary in many children with Wilms tumour, the recovery is usually rapid. The major nursing responsibilities are the same as those after any abdominal surgery (see Surgical Procedures, Chapter 44). Because these children are at risk for intestinal obstruction from vincristine-induced ileus, radiation-induced edema, and postsurgical adhesion formation, the nurse needs to carefully monitor gastrointestinal activity, such as bowel movements, bowel sounds, distension, vomiting, and pain. The nurse should also monitor blood pressure, urine output, and signs of infection, as well as instituting pulmonary hygiene to prevent postoperative pulmonary complications.

Family Support

The postoperative period is frequently difficult for parents. The shock of seeing their child immediately after surgery may be the first realization of the seriousness of the diagnosis. It also marks the confirmation of the stage of the tumour. During this period, the nurse should be with the parents to assure them of the child's recovery after surgery and to assess their understanding of the total experience. Older children need an opportunity to deal with their feelings concerning the many procedures to which they have been subjected in rapid succession. Play therapy with dolls or puppets or through drawing can be beneficial in helping them adjust. It is not unusual for children to feel angry or stressed because of the extent of the surgery, the need for additional therapy, or the seriousness of the disorder.

> **! NURSING ALERT**
>
> After surgery the child is left with one kidney, thus certain precautions, such as wearing protective equipment for contact sports, are recommended by the Canadian Cancer Society (2012). Prompt detection and treatment of any genitourinary signs or symptoms are mandatory.

RENAL FAILURE

Renal failure is the inability of the kidneys to excrete waste material, concentrate urine, and conserve electrolytes. It can occur suddenly as acute kidney injury (AKI) in response to inadequate perfusion, kidney disease, or urinary tract obstruction, or it can develop slowly as a result of long-standing CKD or an anomaly.

Azotemia and *uremia* are terms often used in relation to renal failure. *Azotemia* is the accumulation of nitrogenous waste within the blood. *Uremia* is a more advanced condition in which retention of nitrogenous products produces toxic symptoms. Azotemia is not life threatening, whereas uremia is a serious condition that often involves other body systems.

Acute Kidney Injury

AKI is said to exist when the kidneys suddenly are unable to regulate the volume and composition of urine appropriately in response to food and fluid intake and the needs of the organism. The principal feature of AKI is *oligoanuria*, or reduced urine volume, associated with azotemia, metabolic acidosis, and diverse electrolyte disturbances. AKI is not common in childhood, but the outcome depends on the cause, associated findings, and prompt recognition and treatment.

The pathological conditions that produce AKI caused by glomerulonephritis and HUS are discussed earlier in the chapter in relation to those disorders. AKI can also develop as a result of a large number of related or unrelated clinical conditions:

poor renal perfusion; urinary tract obstruction; acute renal injury; or the final expression of chronic, irreversible renal disease. The most common cause in children is transient renal failure resulting from severe dehydration or other causes of poor perfusion that may respond to restoration of fluid volume.

Pathophysiology

AKI is usually reversible, but the deviations of physiological function can be extreme, and mortality in the pediatric age group remains high. There is severe reduction in the GFR, an elevated urea level, and a significant reduction in renal blood flow.

The clinical course is variable and depends on the cause. In reversible AKI there is a period of severe oliguria, or a low-output phase, followed by an abrupt onset of diuresis, or a high-output phase, and then a gradual return to (or toward) normal urine volumes.

Diagnostic Evaluation

In many instances of AKI the infant or child is already critically ill with the precipitating disorder, and the explanation for development of oliguria may or may not be readily apparent (Box 49-6). When a previously well child develops AKI without obvious cause, a careful history is taken to reveal symptoms that may be related to glomerulonephritis, obstructive uropathy, or exposure to nephrotoxic chemicals (e.g., ingestion of heavy metals, inhalation of carbon tetrachloride or other organic solvents, or medications such as nonsteroidal anti-inflammatory drugs [NSAIDs] [Patzer, 2008] known to be toxic to the kidneys). Significant laboratory measurements during renal shutdown that serve as a guide for therapy are urea, serum creatinine, pH, sodium, potassium, and calcium.

! NURSING ALERT

Diminished urine output and lethargy in a child who is dehydrated, is in shock, or has recently undergone surgery should be evaluated for possible AKI.

BOX 49-6 CLINICAL MANIFESTATIONS OF ACUTE RENAL FAILURE

Specific
- Oliguria
- Anuria uncommon (except in obstructive disorders)

Nonspecific (May Develop)
- Nausea
- Vomiting
- Drowsiness
- Edema
- Hypertension

Other
- Manifestations of underlying disorder or pathological condition

Therapeutic Management

Treatment of AKI is directed toward (1) treatment of the underlying cause, (2) management of the complications of renal failure, and (3) provision of supportive therapy within the constraints imposed by the renal failure.

Treatment of poor perfusion resulting from dehydration consists of volume restoration, as described in Chapter 46 in the treatment of dehydration. If oliguria persists after restoration of fluid volume or if the renal failure is caused by intrinsic renal damage, the physiological and biochemical abnormalities that have resulted from kidney dysfunction must be corrected or controlled. Initially, a Foley catheter is inserted to rule out urine retention, to collect available urine for analysis, and to monitor the results of diuretic administration. The catheter may or may not be removed during the oliguric phase.

The amount of exogenous water provided should not exceed the amount needed to maintain zero water balance. It is calculated on the basis of estimated endogenous water formation and losses from sensible (primarily gastrointestinal) and insensible sources. No allotment is calculated for urine as long as oliguria persists.

When the output begins to increase, either spontaneously or in response to diuretic therapy, the intake of fluid, potassium, and sodium must be monitored and adequate replacement provided to prevent depletion and its consequences. Some patients pass enormous amounts of electrolyte-rich urine.

Complications. The child with AKI has a tendency to develop water intoxication and hyponatremia, which makes it difficult to provide calories in sufficient amounts to meet the child's needs and reduce tissue catabolism, metabolic acidosis, hyperkalemia, and uremia. If the child is able to tolerate oral foods, food sources high in concentrated carbohydrate and fat but low in protein, potassium, and sodium may be provided. However, many children have functional disturbances of the gastrointestinal tract, such as nausea and vomiting; thus the IV route is generally preferred and usually consists of essential amino acids or a combination of essential and nonessential amino acids administered by the central venous route.

Control of water balance in these patients requires careful monitoring of accurate intake and output, body weight, and electrolyte measurements. In general, during the oliguric phase, no sodium, chloride, or potassium is given unless there are other large, ongoing losses. Regular measurement of plasma electrolyte, pH, urea, and creatinine levels is required to assess the adequacy of fluid therapy and to anticipate complications that require specific treatment.

Hyperkalemia is the most immediate threat to the life of the child with AKI. Hyperkalemia can be minimized and sometimes avoided by eliminating potassium from all food and fluid, by reducing tissue catabolism, and by correcting acidosis. Measures to reduce serum potassium levels are oral or rectal administration of an ion-exchange resin such as sodium polystyrene sulphonate (Kayexalate) and peritoneal dialysis or hemodialysis (p. 1580). The resin produces its effect by exchange of its sodium for the potassium, thus binding potassium for removal from the body. This increased sodium concentration may contribute to fluid overload, hypertension, and cardiac failure. Dialysis removes potassium and other waste products from the serum by diffusion through a semipermeable membrane.

NURSING ALERT

Any of the following signs of hyperkalemia constitute an emergency and need to be reported immediately:
- Serum potassium concentrations in excess of 7 mmol/L
- Electrocardiographic abnormalities, such as prolonged QRS complex, depressed ST segment, high peaked T waves, bradycardia, or heart block

Hypertension is a frequent and serious complication of AKI, and to detect it early, blood pressure measurements are taken every 4 to 6 hours. The most common cause of hypertension in AKI is overexpansion of extracellular fluid and plasma volume together with activation of the renin-angiotensin system. Hypertension is controlled with antihypertensive drugs. Other measures that may be used include limiting fluids and salt.

Anemia is frequently associated with AKI, but transfusion is not recommended unless the hemoglobin drops below 60 g/L. Transfusions, if used, consist of fresh washed, packed red blood cells given slowly to reduce the likelihood of increasing blood volume, hypertension, and hyperkalemia.

Seizures occur often when renal failure progresses to uremia and are also related to hypertension, hyponatremia, and hypocalcemia. Treatment is directed to the specific cause when known. More obscure causes are managed with antiepileptic drugs.

Cardiac failure with pulmonary edema is almost always associated with hypervolemia. Treatment is directed toward reduction of fluid volume, with water and sodium restriction and administration of diuretics.

Prognosis

The prognosis of AKI depends largely on the nature and severity of the causative factor or precipitating event and the promptness and competence of management. The outcome is least favourable in children with rapidly progressive nephritis and cortical necrosis. Children in whom AKI is a result of HUS or AGN recover completely, but residual renal impairment or hypertension is more often the rule. Complete recovery is usually expected in children whose renal failure is a result of dehydration, nephrotoxins, or ischemia. AKI after cardiac surgery is less favourable. It is often impossible to assess the extent of recovery for several months.

NURSING CARE

Meticulous attention to fluid intake and output is mandatory and includes all of the physical measurements discussed previously in relation to problems of fluid balance. Monitoring fluid balance and vital signs is a continuous process, and nurses need to be constantly on the alert for signs of complications so that appropriate interventions can be implemented. Because these children require intensive observation and often specialized treatment, such as dialysis, they are usually admitted to a critical care unit in which needed equipment and trained personnel are available (see Nursing Care Plan available on Evolve).

Limiting fluid intake requires ingenuity on the part of caregivers to cope with the child who is thirsty. Rationing the daily intake in small amounts of fluid served in containers that give the impression of larger volumes is one strategy. Older children who understand the rationale of fluid limits can help determine how their daily ration should be distributed.

Meeting nutritional needs is sometimes a problem; the child may be nauseated, and encouraging concentrated foods without fluids may be difficult. When nourishment is provided via the IV route, careful monitoring is essential to prevent fluid overload.

The nurse must be continually alert for changes in symptoms that indicate the onset of complications. Infection from reduced resistance, anemia, and general morbidity is a constant threat. Fluid overload and electrolyte disturbances can precipitate cardiovascular complications such as hypertension and cardiac failure. Fluid and electrolyte imbalances, acidosis, and accumulation of nitrogenous waste products can produce neurological involvement manifested by coma, seizures, or alterations in sensorium.

Although children with AKI are usually quite ill and voluntarily diminish their activity, infants may become restless and irritable, and children are often anxious and frightened. Frequent, painful, and stress-producing treatments and tests must be performed. A supportive, empathetic nurse can provide comfort and stability in a threatening and unnatural environment.

Support the Family

Providing support and reassurance to parents is among the major nursing responsibilities. The seriousness of AKI and its emergency nature are stressful to parents, and most feel some degree of guilt regarding the child's condition, especially when the illness is a result of ingestion of a toxic substance, dehydration, or a genetic disease. They also need to be kept informed of the child's progress and provided with explanations regarding the therapeutic regimen. The equipment and the child's behaviour are sometimes frightening and anxiety provoking. Nurses can do much to help parents comprehend and deal with the stresses of the situation.

Chronic Kidney Disease

The kidneys are able to maintain the chemical composition of fluids within normal limits until more than 50% of functional renal capacity is destroyed by disease or injury. Chronic kidney disease insufficiency or failure (CKD) begins when the diseased kidneys can no longer maintain the normal chemical structure of body fluids under normal conditions. Progressive deterioration over months or years produces a variety of clinical and biochemical disturbances that culminate in the clinical syndrome known as uremia.

A variety of diseases and disorders can result in CKD. The most frequent causes are congenital renal and urinary tract malformations, VUR associated with recurrent UTI, chronic pyelonephritis, hereditary disorders, chronic glomerulonephritis, and glomerulonephropathy associated with systemic diseases such as anaphylactoid purpura and lupus erythematosus. In Canada, there is an increasing concern about the higher incidence of co-diagnosis of kidney disease with children with poorly controlled diabetes. Indigenous children are particularly affected. See Chapter 51 for more information.

Pathophysiology

Early in the course of progressive nephrotic destruction, the child remains asymptomatic with only minimal biochemical abnormalities. Unless the presence of CKD is detected in the process of routine assessment, signs and symptoms that indicate advanced renal damage frequently emerge only late in the course of the disease. Midway in the disease process, as increasing numbers of nephrons are totally destroyed and most others are damaged to varying degrees, the few that remain intact are hypertrophied but functional. These few normal nephrons are able to make sufficient adjustments to stresses to maintain reasonable degrees of fluid and electrolyte balance. Definitive biochemical examination at this time will reveal limited tolerance to excesses or restrictions. As the disease progresses to the end stage, because of a severe reduction in the number of functioning nephrons, the kidneys are no longer able to maintain fluid and electrolyte balance, and the features of uremic syndrome appear.

The accumulation of various biochemical substances in the blood, those that result from diminished renal function, produces complications such as the following:

Retention of waste products, especially urea and creatinine

Water and sodium retention, which contributes to edema and vascular congestion

Hyperkalemia of dangerous levels

Metabolic acidosis of a sustained nature because of continual hydrogen ion retention and bicarbonate loss

Calcium and phosphorus disturbances, resulting in altered bone metabolism, which in turn causes growth arrest or restriction, bone pain, and deformities known as *renal osteodystrophy*

Anemia caused by hematological dysfunction, including the shortened lifespan of red blood cells, impaired red blood cell production related to decreased production of erythropoietin, prolonged bleeding time, and nutritional anemia

Growth disturbance, probably caused by such factors as renal osteodystrophy, poor nutrition associated with dietary restrictions and loss of appetite, and biochemical abnormalities

Children with CKD seem to be more susceptible to infection, especially pneumonia, UTI, and septicemia, although the reason for this is unclear. These children become extraordinarily sensitive to changes in vascular volume that may cause pulmonary overload, central nervous system symptoms, hypertension, and cardiac failure.

Diagnostic Evaluation

The diagnosis of CKD is usually suspected on the basis of any number of clinical manifestations, a history of prior renal disease, or biochemical findings. The onset is usually gradual, and the initial signs and symptoms are vague and nonspecific (Box 49-7).

BOX 49-7 CLINICAL MANIFESTATIONS OF CHRONIC KIDNEY DISEASE

Early Signs
- Loss of normal energy
- Increased fatigue on exertion
- Pallor, subtle (may not be noticed)
- Elevated blood pressure (sometimes)

As the Disease Progresses
- Decreased appetite (especially at breakfast)
- Less interest in normal activities
- Increased or decreased urine output with compensatory intake of fluid
- Pallor more evident
- Sallow, muddy appearance of skin

Child May Develop
- Headache
- Muscle cramps
- Nausea

Other Signs and Symptoms
- Weight loss
- Facial edema
- Malaise
- Bone or joint pain
- Growth restriction
- Dryness or itching of the skin
- Bruised skin
- Sensory or motor loss (sometimes)
- Amenorrhea (common in adolescent girls)

Uremic Syndrome (Untreated)
- Gastrointestinal symptoms: anorexia, nausea, and vomiting
- Bleeding tendencies: bruises, bloody diarrheal stools, stomatitis, bleeding from lips and mouth
- Intractable itching
- Uremic frost (deposits of urea crystals on skin)
- Unpleasant "uremic" breath odour
- Deep respirations
- Hypertension
- Heart failure
- Pulmonary edema
- Neurological involvement: progressive confusion, dulled sensorium, coma (ultimately), tremors, muscular twitching, seizures

Laboratory and other diagnostic tools and tests are of value in assessing the extent of renal damage, biochemical disturbances, and related physical dysfunction (see Tables 49-1 to 49-3). Often they can help establish the nature of the underlying disease and differentiate between other disease processes and the pathological consequences of renal dysfunction.

Therapeutic Management

In irreversible renal failure the goals of medical management are to (1) promote maximum renal function, (2) maintain body fluid and electrolyte balance within safe biochemical limits, (3) treat systemic complications, and (4) promote as active and normal a life as possible for the child for as long as possible. The child is allowed unrestricted activity and is allowed to set his or her own limits. School attendance is encouraged as long as the child is able, or home tutoring is arranged.

Diet regulation is the most effective means, short of dialysis, for reducing the quantity of materials that require renal excretion. The goal of diet management in renal failure is to provide sufficient calories and protein for growth while limiting the excretory demands made on the kidney, to minimize metabolic bone disease (*osteodystrophy*), and to minimize fluid and electrolyte disturbances. Dietary protein intake is limited only to the reference daily intake for the child's age. Restriction of protein intake below the Recommended Daily Allowance (RDA) is believed to negatively affect growth and neurodevelopment. Malnutrition may develop in patients with CKD even before they need dialysis.

Sodium and water are not usually limited unless there is evidence of edema or hypertension, and potassium is not usually restricted. However, restrictions of any or all three may be imposed in later stages or at any time that abnormal serum concentrations are evident.

Dietary phosphorus is controlled through reduction of protein, milk, and soft-drink intake to prevent or correct the calcium/phosphorus imbalance. Phosphorus levels can be further reduced by oral administration of calcium carbonate preparations or other phosphate-binding agents that combine with the phosphorus to decrease gastrointestinal absorption and thus the serum levels of phosphate. Treatment with 25-OH vitamin D is begun to increase calcium absorption and suppress elevated parathyroid hormone levels.

Metabolic acidosis is alleviated through the administration of alkalizing agents such as sodium bicarbonate or a combination of sodium and potassium citrate.

Growth failure is one major consequence of CKD, especially in the preadolescent. These children grow poorly both before and after the initiation of hemodialysis. The use of recombinant human growth hormone to accelerate growth in children with growth restriction secondary to CKD has been successful, with 1 year of growth hormone resulting in a 3.88-cm increase in height velocity above that of untreated patients (Hodson, Willis, & Craig, 2012). Studies were too short to determine if continuing treatment resulted in an increase in final adult height. Osseous deformities that result from renal osteodystrophy, especially those related to ambulation, are troublesome and require correction if they occur.

Dental defects are common in children with CKD, and the earlier the onset of the disease, the more severe are the dental manifestations (including hypoplasia, hypomineralization, tooth discolouration, alteration in size and shape of teeth, malocclusion, and ulcerative stomatitis). Regular dental care is especially important in these children.

Anemia in children with CKD is related to decreased production of erythropoietin. Recombinant human erythropoietin is offered to these children as thrice-weekly or weekly subcutaneous injections and replaces the need for frequent blood transfusions. The medication corrects the anemia and in turn increases appetite, activity, and general well-being. In addition, a variety of iron preparations are often administered.

Hypertension of advanced renal disease may be managed initially by cautious use of a low-sodium diet, fluid restriction, and perhaps diuretics such as hydrochlorothiazide or furosemide. Severe hypertension requires the use of antihypertensive agents, singly or in combination.

Intercurrent infections are treated with appropriate antimicrobials at the first sign of infection; however, any drug eliminated through the kidneys should be administered with caution. Other complications are treated symptomatically (e.g., central-acting antiemetics for nausea, antiepileptics for seizures, and diphenhydramine [Benadryl] for pruritus).

Once evidence of end-stage renal disease (ESRD) appears in a child, the disease runs its relentless course and results in death in a few weeks, unless waste products and toxins are removed from body fluids by dialysis or kidney transplantation. These techniques have been adapted for infants and small children and are implemented in most cases of renal failure after conservative management is no longer effective (see Technological Management of Chronic Kidney Disease, on the next page).

Prognosis

Dialysis and transplantation are the only treatments currently available for children with ESRD. Although children may survive on dialysis, it is not an ideal long-term modality. Complications include infection of access sites, growth failure, and disruption of normal socialization. Many pediatric centres encourage families of children with ESRD to consider kidney transplantation. The North American Renal Transplantation in Children Report of the North American Pediatric Renal Trials and Collaborative Studies (2010) stated a graft survival rate of 96% at 1 year and 84% at 5 years for living donor kidneys, and 95% at 1 year and 78% at 5 years for cadaver kidneys.

Post-transplantation complications include infection, hypertension, steroid toxicity, hyperlipidemia, aseptic necrosis, malignancy, and growth restriction (Dharnidharka & Araya, 2016). Long-term graft survival is not guaranteed, and many children require a second or third transplant. Successful kidney transplantation does improve rehabilitation of children with ESRD, both educationally and psychologically. Increasing use of primary or pre-emptive kidney transplants is becoming the optimal form of renal replacement therapy, leading to substantial improvement in quality of life (Sarwal, 2016).

NURSING CARE

The multiple complications of ESRD are managed according to evidence-informed clinical practice guidelines, such as the *Clinical Practice Guidelines for the Evaluation and Management of Chronic Kidney Disease* (Kidney Disease: Improving Global Outcomes, 2012). However, progressive disease places a number of stresses on the child and family, including those of a potentially fatal illness (see Chapter 40). There is a continuing need for repeated examinations that often entail painful procedures, adverse effects, and frequent hospitalizations. Diet therapy becomes progressively more restricted and intense, and the child is required to take a variety of medications. Ever present in all aspects of the treatment regimen is the agonizing realization that without treatment, death is inevitable.

Some specific stresses related to ESRD and its treatment are predictable. When it first becomes apparent that ESRD is inevitable, both the parents and child can experience depression and anxiety. Acceptance is particularly difficult if renal failure progresses rapidly after diagnosis. Denial and disbelief are usually pronounced, especially for the parents. The initiation of dialysis is usually perceived as a positive experience, and after experiencing initial concerns regarding the treatment, the child begins to feel better and parental anxiety is relieved for a time.

Initiating a dialysis regimen is a traumatic and anxiety-provoking experience for most children because it involves surgery for implantation of a vascular access (central venous line, graft, or fistula) for hemodialysis, or a peritoneal catheter for peritoneal dialysis. The initial experience with this procedure is frightening to most children. They need reassurance about the nature of the preparations for dialysis and the conduct of the treatment.

For hemodialysis, the fistula or graft requires needle insertions at each treatment. The goal is to perform pain-free venipuncture. Using buffered lidocaine with a small-gauge needle (30 gauge) to anaesthetize the area before venipuncture of the graft or fistula is one method. Using an anaesthetizing topical preparation such as EMLA (eutectic mixture of local anaesthetics [lidocaine and prilocaine]) 1 hour before venipuncture is another approach (see Pain Management, Chapter 34). Central venous lines eliminate the need for needles but are more prone to infection and other central line complications.

Adolescents, with their increased need for independence and their urge for rebellion, usually adapt less well than younger children. They may resent the control and enforced dependence imposed by the rigorous and unrelenting therapy program. They may resent being dependent on hemodialysis technology, their parents, and the professional staff. Depression or hostility is common in adolescents undergoing hemodialysis.

The availability of home peritoneal dialysis has offered a greater degree of freedom for persons undergoing long-term dialysis. Independently managing dialysis treatments at home is less disruptive to school and social activities. Patients and their families need to receive an in-depth teaching program to prepare them for assessing, implementing, and monitoring dialysis treatments.

Body changes related to the disease process, including skin discolouration, growth restriction, and lack of sexual maturation, are stress provoking. Dietary and fluid restrictions are particularly burdensome for both children and parents. Children may feel deprived when they are unable to eat foods previously enjoyed and that are unrestricted to other family members. Consequently, they may fail to adhere to their food plan. Patient, supportive, and encouraging nursing care is essential. Children, especially adolescents, should be allowed maximum participation in and responsibility for their own treatment program.

After months or years of dialysis, the parents and child may feel anxiety associated with the prognosis and continued pressures of the treatment. The time spent in transportation to and from the hemodialysis unit and the time spent undergoing dialysis treatments can interfere with the acquisition of developmental and social milestones. Vascular-access and peritoneal dialysis exit site infections may develop and present a common source of aggravation. The possibility of kidney transplantation often provides hope for relief from the rigours of hemodialysis and peritoneal dialysis.

The Kidney Foundation of Canada and other agencies provide a number of services and information for families of children with renal disease (see Additional Resources at the end of this chapter).

TECHNOLOGICAL MANAGEMENT OF CHRONIC KIDNEY DISEASE

Dialysis

Dialysis is the process of separating colloids and crystalline substances in solution by the difference in their rate of diffusion through a semipermeable membrane. Methods of dialysis currently available for clinical management of renal failure are *peritoneal dialysis*, in which the abdominal cavity acts as a semipermeable membrane through which water and solutes of small molecular size move by osmosis and diffusion according to their respective concentrations on either side of the membrane, and *hemodialysis*, in which blood is circulated outside the body through artificial membranes that permit a similar passage of water and solutes. A third type of dialysis is *hemofiltration*, in which blood filtrate is circulated outside the body by hydrostatic pressure exerted across a semipermeable membrane with simultaneous infusion of a replacement solution. Types of hemofiltration include continuous venovenous hemofiltration, continuous venovenous hemodialysis, and continuous venovenous hemodiafiltration. Hemofiltration is generally reserved for use in AKI, severe fluid overload, inborn errors of metabolism, or after bone marrow transplant.

Peritoneal dialysis is the preferred form of dialysis for infants, children, and parents who wish to remain independent, for families who live a long distance from the medical centre, and for children who prefer fewer dietary restrictions and a gentler form of dialysis. Chronic peritoneal dialysis is most often performed at home. The two types of peritoneal dialysis are continuous ambulatory peritoneal dialysis and continuous cycling peritoneal dialysis. In both methods, commercially available sterile dialysis solution is instilled into the peritoneal cavity through a surgically implanted in-dwelling catheter that is tunnelled subcutaneously and sutured into place. The warmed solution is allowed to enter the peritoneal cavity by gravity and remains a variable length of time according to the rate of solute removal and glucose absorption in individual patients. The fluid and accumulated toxic wastes are then drained from the peritoneal cavity and a new cycle of fresh dialysis solution is reinstilled. The frequency and timing of the cycles depend on the child's age, fluid balancing needs, and solute removal requirements. Performing this form of dialysis in the home can be empowering for families, especially adolescents. However, the nurse needs to carefully assess for signs of patient and caregiver burnout and arrange for respite care as necessary.

NURSING ALERT

Observe for changes in the colour of the dialysate draining from the child. The spent solution should be clear. If the colour is cloudy, notify the practitioner immediately.

Hemodialysis requires the surgical creation of a vascular access and the use of special dialysis equipment—the hemodialyzer, or so-called artificial kidney. Vascular access may be one of three types: fistulas, grafts, or external vascular access devices. An *arteriovenous fistula* is an access in which a vein and artery are connected surgically. The preferred site is the radial artery and a forearm vein that produces dilation and thickening of the superficial vessels of the forearm to provide easy access for repeated venipuncture. An alternative is the creation of a subcutaneous (internal) arteriovenous graft by anastomosing artery and vein, with a synthetic prosthetic graft for circulatory access. The most commonly used material is expanded polytetrafluoroethylene (ePTFE). Both the graft and the fistula require needle insertions with each dialysis treatment.

For external vascular access devices, percutaneous catheters are inserted in the femoral, subclavian, or internal jugular veins, even in very small children. A more permanent form of external access is available via a central catheter inserted surgically into the internal jugular vein. Catheters eliminate the need for skin punctures but require dressing changes and are prone to infection. Home care may need to be arranged to assist families with caring for their catheter at home, in between hemodialysis treatments.

Hemodialysis is best suited to children who do not have someone in the family who is able to perform peritoneal dialysis and to those who live close to a dialysis centre. The procedure is usually performed three times per week for 4 to 6 hours, depending on the child's size. Hemodialysis achieves rapid correction of fluid and electrolyte abnormalities but can cause adverse effects in association with this rapid change, such as muscle cramping, headaches, nausea and vomiting, and hypotension. Disadvantages include school absence during hemodialysis treatments and strict fluid and dietary restrictions. Boredom for the child and family is often experienced during the mobility-limiting treatments, so planned activities should be introduced (Fig. 49-7).

Most children show rapid clinical improvement with the implementation of dialysis, although it is directly related to the duration of uremia before dialysis and good nutrition. Growth rate and skeletal maturation improve, but recovery of normal growth is infrequent. In many cases, sexual development, although delayed, progresses to completion.

Transplantation

Kidney transplantation is now an acceptable and effective means of therapy in the pediatric age group. Although peritoneal dialysis and hemodialysis are life preserving, both require major alterations in lifestyle. Transplantation offers the opportunity for a relatively normal life and is the preferred form of treatment for children with ESRD. Primary or pre-emptive transplants maintain the greatest amount of normalcy in the family's life.

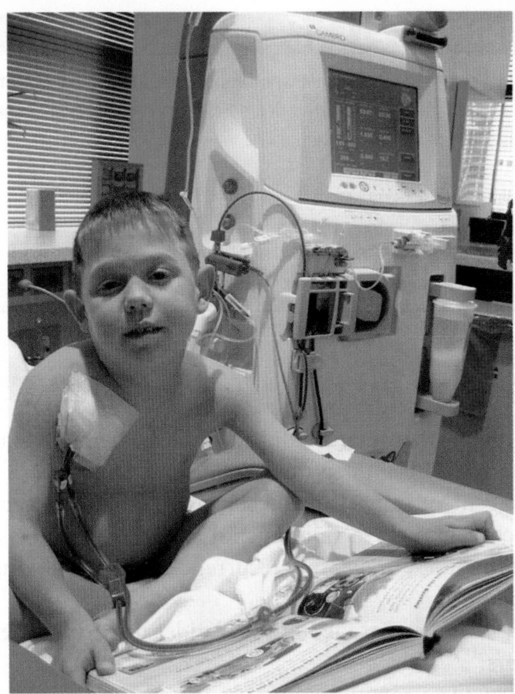

FIGURE 49-7 Diversional activities help lessen the boredom children can experience during hemodialysis.

In terms of wait time for an available kidney for transplantation, discrepancies exist between various populations. Researchers from the Pediatric Renal Outcomes Canada Group found that the time from start of dialysis to the first kidney transplant was longer for Indigenous children than for non-Indigenous children. Further research is needed to investigate individual and system barriers that contribute to the difference in the wait times (Samuel, Foster, Tonelli, et al., 2011).

Kidneys for transplant are available from two sources: a *living related donor*, usually a parent or a sibling, or a *cadaver donor*, a dead or brain-dead patient whose family consents to the donation of a healthy kidney. Retransplantation occurs frequently. The primary goal in transplantation is the long-term survival of grafted tissue by securing tissue that is antigenically similar to that of the recipient and by suppressing the recipient's immune mechanism. The immunosuppressant therapy of choice has been corticosteroids (prednisone) in conjunction with cyclosporine or tacrolimus and mycophenolate mofetil. Other therapies include antilymphoblast globulin or monoclonal antibodies. New immunosuppressant medications are rapidly coming into clinical trials and into use in large transplant centres. It is important for the nurse to learn about the medications used in the antirejection protocol(s) and about their adverse effects. Because the immunosuppressant medications are taken indefinitely, transplant patients experience many adverse effects of the medications, including hypertension, growth restriction, cataracts, risk of infection, obesity, characteristics of Cushing's syndrome, and hirsutism (McDonald, 2016).

NURSING ALERT

The child with a kidney transplant who exhibits any of the following symptoms should be evaluated immediately for possible rejection, as this the most common cause of transplant failure:

- Fever
- Swelling and tenderness over graft area
- Diminished urine output
- Elevated blood pressure
- Elevated serum creatinine

Rejection is treated aggressively with immunosuppressant medications and can often be reversed. Some patients do not respond or develop chronic rejection and must eventually return to dialysis or undergo another kidney transplant.

KEY POINTS

- Common inflammatory disorders of the genitourinary tract include UTI, nephrotic syndrome, and AGN.
- Management of UTIs is directed at eliminating infection, detecting and correcting functional or anatomical abnormalities, preventing recurrences, and preserving renal function.
- VUR is the retrograde flow of bladder urine into the ureters.
- Obstructive uropathy is a result of structural or functional abnormalities of the urinary system that obstruct the normal flow of urine.
- The more common defects of the genitourinary tract include phimosis, cryptorchidism, inguinal hernia, hydrocele, and hypospadias.
- Body image concerns and castration anxiety are particularly intense in children with defects in the genital area.
- Nephrotic syndrome is characterized by increased glomerular permeability to protein, with massive urinary loss of protein resulting in hypoproteinemia and edema.
- Management of nephrotic syndrome is aimed at reducing excretion of protein, reducing or preventing fluid retention by tissues, and preventing infection and other complications.
- Common features of AGN are oliguria, edema, hypertension, circulatory congestion, hematuria, and proteinuria.
- Therapeutic management of AGN involves maintenance of fluid balance, treatment of hypertension, and antibiotic therapy.
- Management of HUS is aimed at control of complications and hematological manifestations of renal failure.
- Wilms tumour is the most common malignant neoplasm of the kidney in infants and children.
- In AKI, management is directed at determining treatment of the underlying cause, managing complications of renal failure, and providing supportive therapy.
- Abnormalities in CKD are waste product retention, water and sodium retention, hyperkalemia, acidosis, calcium and phosphorus disturbance, anemia, and growth disturbances.
- The types of dialysis used in ESRD are peritoneal dialysis and hemodialysis.
- When the child will need home dialysis, the nurse needs to educate the family about the disease, its implications, the therapeutic plan, possible psychological effects of the disease, and the treatment and technical aspects of the procedure.
- The major concerns in kidney transplantation are tissue matching and prevention of rejection; psychological concerns involve self-image as related to possible body changes as a result of the effects of corticosteroid therapy.

evolve WEBSITE

Visit the Evolve website for additional resources related to the content in this chapter such as Case Studies, Critical Thinking Case Study Answers, Nursing Care Plans, Nursing Processes, Nursing Skills, and Review Questions for Exam Preparation at: *http://evolve.elsevier.com/Canada/Perry/maternal/*

REFERENCES

Canadian Cancer Society. (2012). Supportive care for Wilms' tumour: Fact sheet #25. Retrieved from <http://www.centreinfo.leucan.qc.ca/pdf/fiches-information-survivants/25c-wilms-tumour.pdf>.

Canadian Cancer Society. (2016). *Wilm's tumour statistics*. Retrieved from <http://www.cancer.ca/en/cancer-information/cancer-type/wilms-tumour/statistics/?region=on#ixzz3a0Fi74UJ>.

Chen, H. C., Yeh, C. M., & Chou, C. M. (2010). Endoscopic treatment of vesicoureteral reflux in children with dextranomer/hyaluronic acid—a single surgeon's 6 year experience. *Diagnostic & Therapeutic Endoscopy, pii*, 278012. doi: 10.1155/2010/278012.

Daw, N. C., Huff, V., & Anderson, P. M. (2016). Wilms tumor. In R. M. Kliegman, B. F. Stanton, J. W. St. Geme, et al. (Eds.), *Nelson textbook of pediatrics* (20th ed.). Philadelphia: Saunders.

Dharnidharka, V. R., & Araya, C. E. (2016). Complications of renal transplants. In E. D. Avner, W. E. Harmon, & P. Niaudet (Eds.), *Pediatric nephrology* (7th ed.). Heidelberg: Springer-Verlag.

Duzova, A., Bakkaloglu, A., Kalyoncu, M., et al. (2010). Etiology and outcome of acute kidney injury in children. *Pediatric Nephrology, 25*, 1453–1462. doi: 10.1007/s00467-010-1541-y.

Elder, J. S. (2016a). Anomalies of the penis and urethra. In R. M. Kliegman, B. F. Stanton, J. W. St. Geme, et al. (Eds.), *Nelson textbook of pediatrics* (20th ed.). Philadelphia: Saunders.

Elder, J. S. (2016b). Anomalies of the bladder. In R. M. Kliegman, B. F. Stanton, J. W. St. Geme, et al. (Eds.), *Nelson textbook of pediatrics* (20th ed.). Philadelphia: Saunders.

Gipson, D. S., Massengill, S. F., Yao, L., et al. (2009). Management of childhood onset nephrotic syndrome. *Pediatrics, 124*(2), 747–751. doi: 10.1542/peds.2008-1559.

Hodson, E. M., Willis, N. S., & Craig, J. C. (2012). Growth hormone for children with chronic kidney disease. *The Cochrane Database of Systematic Reviews*, (2), CD003264, doi: 10.1002/14651858.CD003264.pub3.

Jepson, R. G., Williams, G., & Craig, J. C. (2012). Cranberries for preventing urinary tract infections. *The Cochrane Database of Systematic Reviews*, (10), CD001321, doi: 10.1002/14651858.CD001321.pub5.

Kidney Disease: Improving Global Outcomes (KDIGO). (2012). *KDIGO 2012 clinical practice guideline for the evaluation and management of chronic kidney disease.* Retrieved from <http://www.kdigo.org/clinical_practice_guidelines/pdf/CKD/KDIGO_2012_CKD_GL.pdf>.

Marchand, V., & Canadian Paediatric Society, Nutrition and Gastroenterology Committee. (2012). Using probiotics in the paediatric population. *Paediatrics & Child Health, 17*(10), 575. Reaffirmed 2015. Retrieved from <http://www.cps.ca/documents/position/probiotics-in-the-paediatric-population>.

McDonald, R. A. (2016). Immunosuppression in renal transplantation in children. *UpToDate.* Retrieved from <http://www.uptodate.com/contents/immunosuppression-in-renal-transplantation-in-children>.

North American Pediatric Renal Trials and Collaborative Studies. (2010). *2010 annual report.* Retrieved from <https://web.emmes.com/study/ped/annlrept/2010_Report.pdf>.

Ozan, T. (2015). Surgery for Wilms tumor. *Medscape.* Retrieved from <http://emedicine.medscape.com/article/453076-overview>.

Pais, P., & Avner, E. D. (2016). Nephrotic syndrome. In R. M. Kliegman, B. F. Stanton, J. W. St. Geme, et al. (Eds.), *Nelson textbook of pediatrics* (20th ed.). Philadelphia: Saunders.

Patzer, L. (2008). Nephrotoxicity as a cause of acute kidney injury in children. *Pediatric Nephrology, 23*(12), 2159–2173.

Reuter-Rice, K., & Bolick, B. (2012). *Pediatric acute care: A Guide for interprofessional practice.* Mississauga, ON: Jones & Bartlett Learning.

Robinson, J. L., Finlay, J. C., Lang, M. E., et al. & Canadian Paediatric Society, Community Paediatrics Committee, Infectious Diseases and Immunization Committee. (2014). Urinary tract infection: Diagnosis and management. *Paediatrics & Child Health, 19*(6), 315–319. Retrieved from <http://www.cps.ca/documents/position/urinary-tract-infections-in-children>.

Samuel, S. M., Foster, B. J., Tonelli, M. A., et al. (2011). Dialysis and transplantation among Aboriginal children with kidney failure. *Canadian Medical Association Journal, 188*(10), E665–E672. doi: 10.1503/cmaj.101840.

Sarwal, M. M. (2016). Renal transplantation. In R. M. Kliegman, B. F. Stanton, J. W. St. Geme, et al. (Eds.), *Nelson textbook of pediatrics* (20th ed.). Philadelphia: Saunders.

Sorokan, S. T., Finlay, J. C., Jefferies, A. L., et al. & Canadian Paediatric Society, Fetus and Newborn Committee, Infectious Diseases and Immunization Committee. (2015). Newborn male circumcision. *Paediatrics & Child Health, 20*(6), 311–315. Retrieved from <http://www.cps.ca/en/documents/position/circumcision>.

ADDITIONAL RESOURCES

Kidney Foundation of Canada: <http://www.kidney.ca>.

PKD Foundation of Canada for Research in Polycystic Kidney Disease (kidney failure): <http://endpkd.ca/learn/learn-about-adpkd/just-diagnosed/>.

CHAPTER

50

Cerebral Dysfunction

Cheryl Sams, with contributions from Marilyn J. Hockenberry

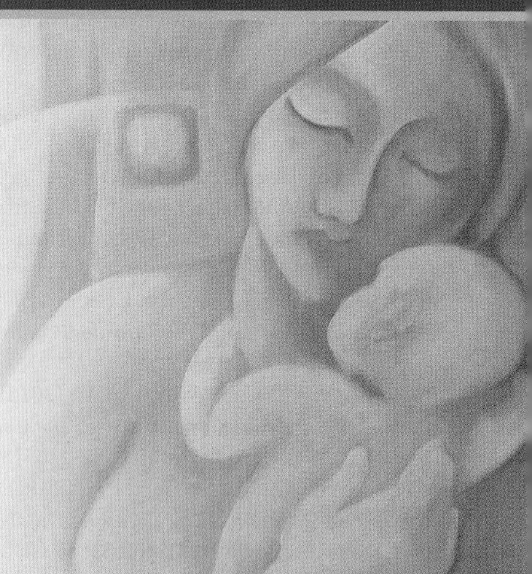

evolve WEBSITE

Visit the Evolve website for additional resources related to the content in this chapter such as Case Studies, Critical Thinking Case Study Answers, Nursing Care Plans, Nursing Processes, Nursing Skills, and Review Questions for Exam Preparation at: http://evolve.elsevier.com/Canada/Perry/maternal/

OBJECTIVES

On completion of this chapter the reader will be able to:

- Describe the various modalities for assessment of cerebral function.
- Differentiate between the stages of consciousness.
- Formulate a care plan for the unconscious child.
- Distinguish between the types of head injuries and the serious complications.
- Describe the nursing care of a child with a tumour of the central nervous system.
- Outline a care plan for the child with bacterial meningitis.
- Differentiate between the various types of seizure disorders.
- Demonstrate an understanding of the manifestations of a seizure disorder and the management of a child with such a disorder.
- Describe the preoperative and postoperative care of a child with hydrocephalus.

ASSESSMENT OF CEREBRAL FUNCTION

Most of the information about the status of the brain is obtained by indirect measurements. Some of these measurements are discussed elsewhere in relation to numerous aspects of child care (e.g., as part of the health assessment [Chapter 33], newborn status [Chapter 26], cognitive impairment [Chapter 41], cerebral palsy [Chapter 54], and attainment of developmental milestones at each stage of development). Since increased intracranial pressure (ICP) and altered states of consciousness have such prominent places in neurological dysfunction, they are described here, followed by techniques for neurological assessment and diagnostic tests.

General Aspects

Children younger than 2 years of age require special evaluation for neurological assessment, as they are unable to respond to directions designed to elicit specific responses. Early neurological responses in infants are primarily reflexive. These responses are gradually replaced by meaningful movement in the characteristic cephalocaudal direction of development. This evidence of progressive maturation reflects more extensive myelinization and changes in neurochemical and electrophysiological properties.

Most information about infants and small children is gained by observing their spontaneous and elicited reflex responses as they develop increasingly complex locomotor and fine motor skills. In addition, valuable information is also gained by eliciting progressively sophisticated communicative and adaptive behaviours. Delay or deviation from expected critical milestones helps identify children at high risk for a neurological issue. Persistence or reappearance of reflexes that normally disappear may indicate a pathological condition. In evaluating the infant or young child, it is also important to obtain the pregnancy and birth history to determine the possible impact of intrauterine environmental influences known to affect the maturation of the central nervous system (CNS). These influences include maternal infections, cigarette or alcohol consumption, drug use, toxin exposure, trauma, and metabolic insults.

General aspects of assessment that provide clues to the etiology of a neurological condition include the following:

Family history—Sometimes offers clues regarding possible genetic disorders with neurological manifestations

Health history—May provide valuable clues regarding the cause of dysfunction. Information should include Apgar scores, age of developmental milestones, trauma or injuries, acute and chronic illnesses, encounters with animals or insects, and ingestion or inhalation of neurotoxic substances.

Physical evaluation of infants—Includes assessment of the following:

- Level of alertness
- Size and shape of the head, including presence of fontanels
- Sensory responses
- Motor function, including posture, tone, and muscle strength
- Motility, including symmetry of movements and involuntary movements
- Respirations, including signs of prolonged apnea, ataxic breathing, paradoxical chest movement, or hyperventilation
- Dysmorphic facial features
- Behavioural cues, including consolability and habituation
- Primitive and deep tendon reflexes
- Cranial nerves, testing for function

Increased Intracranial Pressure

The brain, tightly enclosed in the solid bony cranium, is well protected but highly vulnerable to pressure that may accumulate within the enclosure (Fig. 50-1). The cranium's total volume—brain (80%), cerebrospinal fluid (CSF) (10%), and blood (10%)—must remain approximately the same at all times. A change in the proportional volume of one of these components (e.g., an increase or decrease in intracranial blood) must be accompanied by a compensatory change in another. In this way, the volume and pressure normally remain constant. Examples of compensatory changes are reduction in blood volume, decrease in CSF production, increase in CSF absorption, or shrinkage of brain mass by displacement of **intracellular fluid** and **extracellular fluid**. Children with open fontanels compensate by skull expansion and widened sutures. However, at any age the capacity for spatial compensation is limited. An increase in ICP may be caused by tumours or other space-occupying lesions, accumulation of fluid within the ventricular system, bleeding, or **edema** of cerebral tissues. Once compensation is exhausted, any further increase in volume will result in a rapid rise in ICP.

Early signs and symptoms of increased ICP are often subtle and assume many patterns (Box 50-1). As pressure increases, signs and symptoms become more pronounced and the level of consciousness (LOC) deteriorates.

Altered States of Consciousness

Consciousness implies awareness—the ability to respond to sensory stimuli and have subjective experiences. Consciousness has two components: *alertness*, an arousal-waking state, including the ability to respond to stimuli, and *cognitive power*, which includes the ability to process stimuli and produce verbal and motor responses.

An *altered state of consciousness* usually refers to varying states of unconsciousness that may be momentary or may extend for hours, for days, or indefinitely. *Unconsciousness* is

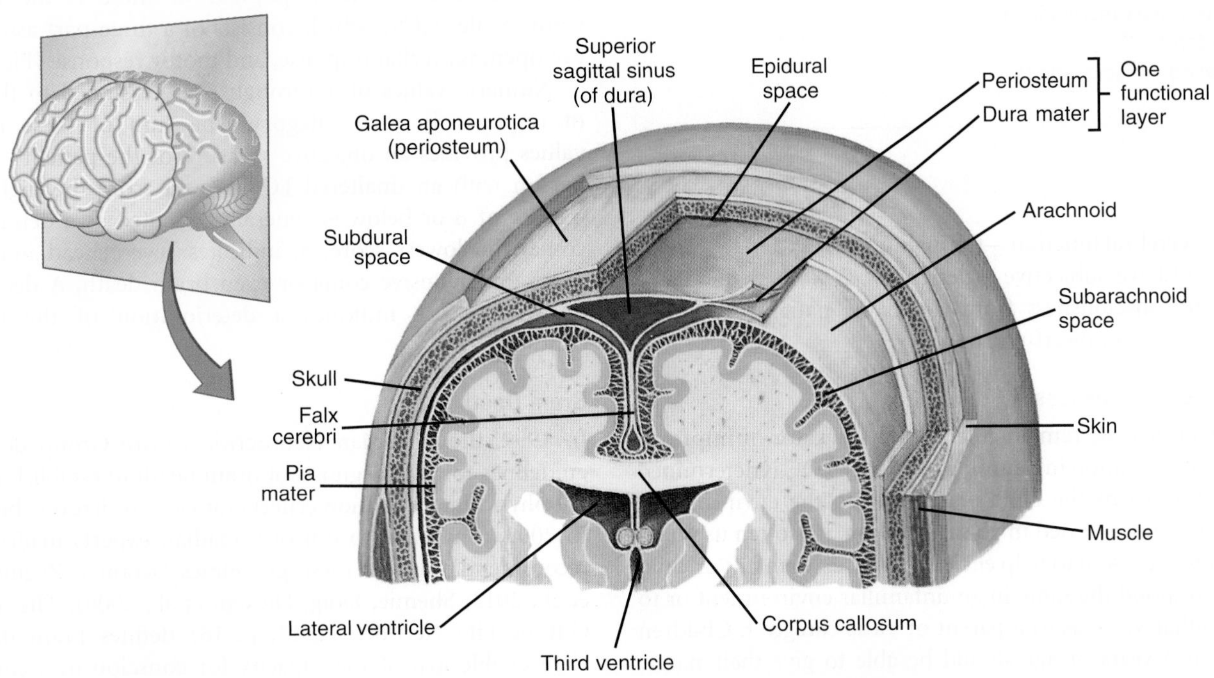

FIGURE 50-1 Coronal section of the top of the head showing meningeal layers. (From Patton, K. T., & Thibodeau, G. A. [2010]. *Anatomy and physiology* [7th ed.]. St. Louis: Mosby.)

BOX 50-1 CLINICAL MANIFESTATIONS OF INCREASED INTRACRANIAL PRESSURE IN INFANTS AND CHILDREN

Infants
Tense, bulging fontanel
Separated cranial sutures
Macewen sign (cracked-pot sound on percussion)
Irritability and restlessness
Drowsiness, increased sleeping
High-pitched cry
Increased fronto-occipital circumference
Distended scalp veins
Poor feeding
Crying when disturbed
Setting-sun sign

Children
Headache
Nausea
Forceful vomiting
Diplopia, blurred vision
Seizures
Indifference, drowsiness
Decline in school performance
Diminished physical activity and motor performance
Increased sleeping
Inability to follow simple commands
Lethargy

Late Signs in Infants and Children
Bradycardia
Decreased motor response to commands
Decreased sensory response to painful stimuli
Alterations in pupil size and reactivity
Flexion or extension posturing
Cheyne-Stokes respirations
Papilledema
Decreased consciousness
Coma

depressed cerebral function—the inability to respond to sensory stimuli and have subjective experiences. *Coma* is defined as a state of unconsciousness from which the patient cannot be roused even with powerful stimuli.

Levels of Consciousness

Assessment of LOC remains the earliest indicator of improvement or deterioration in neurological status. LOC is determined by observations of the child's responses to the environment. When it is being assessed in young children, it is often useful to have a parent present to help elicit a response. An infant or child may not respond the same in an unfamiliar environment or to an unfamiliar voice as to a parent or close caregiver. Children older than 3 years of age should be able to give their name, although they may not be cognizant of place or time. Other diagnostic tests, such as motor activity, reflexes, and vital signs,

BOX 50-2 LEVELS OF CONSCIOUSNESS

Full consciousness—Awake and alert; oriented to person, place, and time; behaviour appropriate for age
Confusion—Impaired decision making
Disorientation—Disorientation to time and place, decreased level of consciousness
Lethargy—Limited spontaneous movement, sluggish speech, drowsy, falling asleep quickly
Obtundation—A severe reduction in LOC, the child arouses with very strong stimulus but is close to a comatose state
Stupor—Remaining in a deep sleep, responsive only to vigorous and repeated stimulation or moaning responses to stimuli
Coma—No motor or verbal response or extension posturing to noxious (painful) stimuli
Persistent vegetative state (PVS)—Permanently lost function of the cerebral cortex; eyes following objects only by reflex or when attracted to the direction of loud sounds, all four limbs spastic but can withdraw from painful stimuli, hands showing reflexive grasping and groping, face grimacing, some food may be swallowed, groaning or crying but without uttering any words

Modified from Seidel, H. M., et al. (Eds.). (2011). *Mosby's guide to physical examination* (7th ed.). St. Louis: Mosby.

are more variable and do not necessarily directly parallel the depth of the comatose state. The most consistently used terms are described in Box 50-2.

Coma Assessment

Several scales have been devised in an attempt to standardize the description and interpretation of the degree of depressed consciousness. The most popular of these is the Glasgow Coma Scale (GCS), which consists of a three-part assessment: eye opening, verbal response, and motor response (Fig. 50-2).

Numeric values of 1 through 5 are assigned to the levels of response in each category. The sum of these numeric values provides an objective measure of the patient's LOC. A person with an unaltered LOC would score the highest, 15; a score of 8 or below is generally accepted as a definition of coma; the lowest score, 3, indicates severe head injury and deep, unresponsive coma or even brain death. A decrease in the GCS score indicates a deterioration of the patient's condition.

Brain Death

In 1999, the Canadian Neurocritical Care Group developed guidelines for the diagnosis of brain death to establish consistent physical examination criteria for cases of irreversible coma. In 2003, a national forum of Canadian experts made further recommendations to these guidelines (Kramer, Zygun, Doig, et al., 2013; Shemie, Doig, Dicken, et al., 2006). The Trillium Gift of Life Network (2012, p. 16) defines brain death as "irreversible loss of the capacity for consciousness combined with the irreversible loss of all brain stem functions, including the capacity to breathe." See the Guidelines box.

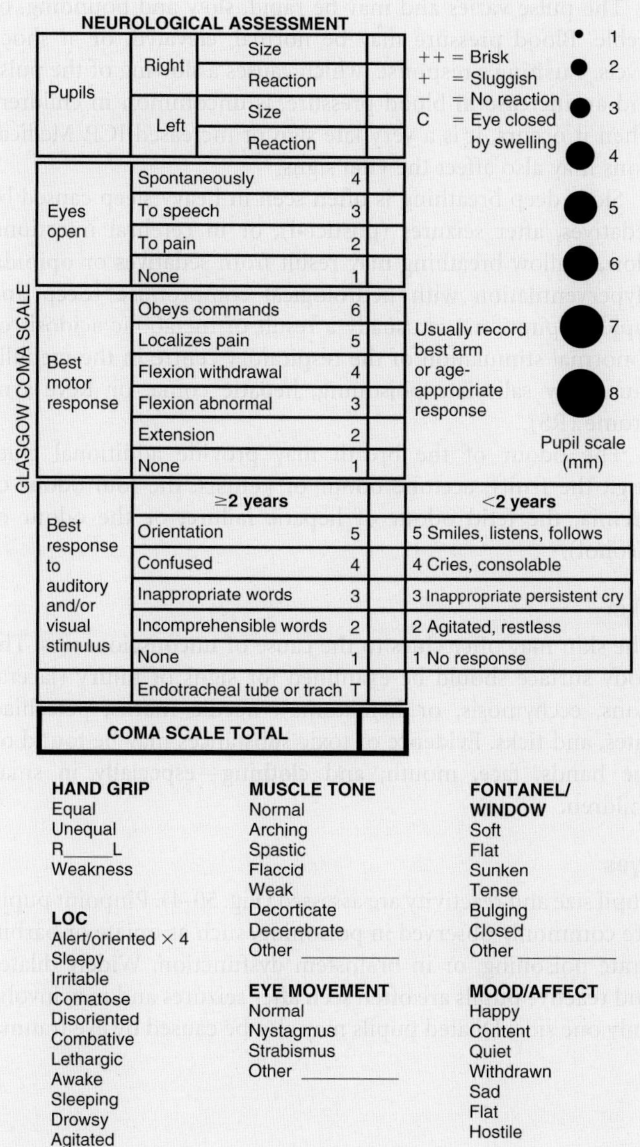

FIGURE 50-2 Pediatric coma scale. *LOC*, level of consciousness.

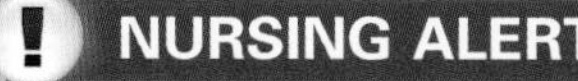

NURSING ALERT

Lack of response to painful stimuli is abnormal and should be reported immediately.

Neurological Examination

The purpose of the neurological examination is to establish an accurate, objective baseline of neurological information. It is essential that the neurological examination be documented in a fashion that is able to be reproduced by others. This allows for a comparison of the findings so the observer can detect subtle changes in the neurological status that might not otherwise be evident. Descriptions of behaviours should be simple, objective, and easily interpreted—for example: "Drowsy but awake and oriented to person, place, and time"; "Sleepy but arousable with vigorous physical stimuli. Pressure to nail base

GUIDELINES

Establishing Brain Death in Canada

Clinical criteria have primacy in the neurological determination of death (NDD) and are defined as follows:

1. Established etiology capable of causing neurological death in the absence of reversible conditions capable of mimicking neurological death
2. Deep unresponsive coma
3. Absent brainstem reflexes as defined by absent gag and cough reflexes and the bilateral absence of
   - Motor responses, excluding spinal reflexes
   - Corneal responses
   - Pupillary responses to light with pupils at midsize or greater and vestibulo-ocular responses
4. Absent respiratory effort based on the apnea test
5. Absent confounding factors
6. For the purposes of organ donation, the NDD has the following requirements:
   - Two physicians perform the examination.
   - There is no prescribed interval between determinations (except where age-adjusted criteria apply).
7. The first and second physician determinations may be performed concurrently.
8. If the determinations are performed at different points in time, a full clinical examination, including apnea testing, must be performed at each determination.
9. An ancillary test should be performed when the full clinical criteria cannot be completed. At minimum, the following two criteria must be met prior to performing an ancillary test:
   - Established etiology in the absence of reversible conditions
   - Deep unresponsive coma

Pediatric Considerations

NDD recommendations for newborns, infants, and children are similar to those for adults, and ancillary testing is not routinely recommended. NDD is a clinical evaluation. If the clinical criteria cannot be completed or if there are confounding factors, ancillary tests demonstrating absent brain blood flow are recommended for newborns, infants, and children. The recommended ancillary tests (in order of preference) are radionuclide angiography or computed tomographic (CT) angiography, traditional four-vessel angiography, magnetic resonance (MR) angiography, or Xenon CT. The Trillium Gift of Life Network provides information regarding the clinical criteria for declaration of death by neurological criteria for newborns, infants, and young children in their *Paediatric Donation Resource Manual* to support health care providers in decisions regarding NDD (Fig. 50-3).

Modified from Shemie, S. D., Doig, C., Dicken, B., et al., on behalf of the Pediatric Reference Group and the Neonatal Reference Group. (2006). Severe brain injury to neurological determination of death: Canadian forum recommendations. *Canadian Medical Association Journal, 174*(6), S1–S12. doi:10.1503/cmaj

of right hand results in upper extremity flexion/lower extremity extension."

Vital Signs

Pulse, respiration, and blood pressure provide information regarding the adequacy of circulation and the possible underlying cause of altered consciousness. Altered autonomic activity occurs most significantly in cases of deep coma or brainstem lesions.

Body temperature is often elevated, and sometimes the elevation may be extreme. High temperature is most frequently a sign of an acute infectious process or heat stroke but may be caused by ingestion of some medications (especially salicylates, alcohol, and barbiturates) or by intracranial bleeding, especially subarachnoid hemorrhage. Hypothalamic involvement may cause elevated or decreased temperature. Coma of a toxic origin may produce hypothermia.

Assessment	Neonates (>36 weeks' gestation & <30 days) requires specialist in neonatology	Infants (≥30 days & <1 year)	Children older than 1 year and adults
Deep pain stimuli	√	√	√
Pupillary response	√	√	√
Corneal reflex	√	√	√
Gag reflex	√	√	√
Cough reflex	√	√	√
Oculovestibular reflex (Cold calorics)	√	√	√
Oculocephalic reflex (Doll's eyes)	√	√	
Suck	√		
Apnea test	√	√	√*
Ancillary test	If unable to complete any of the above	If unable to complete any of the above	If unable to complete any of the above
Time of first test	48 hours post-birth	No fixed time	No fixed time
Interval between two exams	24 hours	Not specified, but at separate times	Can be done concurrently

FIGURE 50-3 Pediatric considerations for neurological determination of death (NDD). *A single apnea test may be performed in children over 1 year of age and in adults if both physicians are present at the time of the test. (Source: Trillium Gift of Life Network. [2012]. *Paediatric donation resource manual: A tool to assist hospitals with the process of organ and tissue donation*, p. 17. Retrieved from http://www.giftoflife.on.ca/resources/pdf/6752_TGLN_PedDonor_Manual_03F_Web(Sep2914).pdf. © Queen's Printer for Ontario, 2012. Reproduced with permission.)

The pulse varies and may be rapid, slow and bounding, or feeble. Blood pressure may be normal, elevated, or at shock levels. Cushing's response, which causes a slowing of the pulse and an increase in blood pressure, is uncommon in children; when it occurs, it is a very late sign of increased ICP. Medications may also affect the vital signs.

Slow, deep breathing is often seen in heavy sleep caused by sedatives, after seizures (postictal), or in cerebral infections. Slow, shallow breathing may result from sedatives or opioids. Hyperventilation with neurological compromise (deep and rapid respirations) is usually a result of metabolic acidosis or abnormal stimulation of the respiratory centre in the medulla caused by salicylate poisoning, hepatic coma, or Reye syndrome (RS).

The odour of the breath may provide additional clues (e.g., the fruity, acetone odour of ketosis; the foul odour of uremia; the fetid odour of hepatic failure; or the odour of alcohol).

Skin

The skin may offer clues to the cause of unconsciousness. The body surface should be examined for signs of injury (lacerations, ecchymosis, or hematoma), needle marks, petechiae, bites, and ticks. Evidence of toxic substances may be found on the hands, face, mouth, and clothing—especially in small children.

Eyes

Pupil size and reactivity are assessed (Fig. 50-4). Pinpoint pupils are commonly observed in poisoning, such as opiate or barbiturate poisoning, or in brainstem dysfunction. Widely dilated and reactive pupils are often seen after seizures and may involve only one side. Dilated pupils may also be caused by eye trauma.

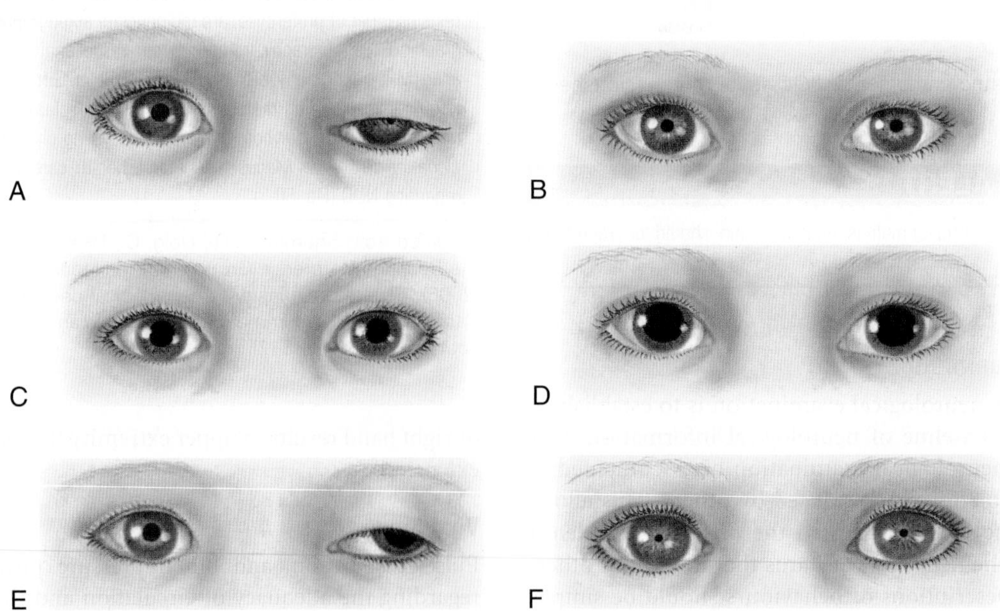

FIGURE 50-4 Variations in pupil size with altered states of consciousness. **A:** Ipsilateral pupillary constriction with slight ptosis. **B:** Bilateral small pupils. **C:** Midposition, light fixed to all stimuli. **D:** Bilateral dilated and fixed pupils. **E:** Dilated pupils, left eye abducted with ptosis. **F:** Pinpoint pupils.

Widely dilated and fixed pupils suggest paralysis of cranial nerve III secondary to pressure from herniation of the brain through the tentorium. A unilateral fixed pupil usually suggests a lesion on the same side. If pupils are fixed bilaterally for more than 5 minutes, it is usually assumed that there is brainstem damage. Dilated and nonreactive pupils are also seen in hypothermia, anoxia, ischemia, poisoning with atropine-like substances, or prior instillation of mydriatic medications.

! NURSING ALERT

The sudden appearance of a fixed and dilated pupil(s) is a neurosurgical emergency.

The description of eye movements should indicate whether one or both eyes are involved and how the reaction was elicited. The parents should be asked about pre-existing strabismus, which will cause the eyes to appear normal under compromise. Post-traumatic strabismus indicates cranial nerve VI damage.

Special tests include the following:

Doll's head manoeuvre—Elicited by rotating the child's head quickly to one side and then to the other. Conjugate (paired, or working together) movement of the eyes in the direction opposite to the head rotation is normal. Absence of this response suggests dysfunction of the brainstem or oculomotor nerve (cranial nerve III).

! NURSING ALERT

Any tests that require head movement should not be attempted until after cervical spine injury has been ruled out.

Funduscopic examination—Reveals additional clues. Papilledema is not evident early in the course of unconsciousness because it takes 24 to 48 hours to develop, if it develops at all. Papilledema is characterized by optic disc swelling, indistinct optic disc margins, hemorrhage, tortuosity of vessels, and absence of venous pulsations. The presence of preretinal (subhyaloid) hemorrhages in children is almost invariably a result of acute trauma with intracranial bleeding, usually subarachnoid or subdural hemorrhage.

Motor Function

Observing spontaneous activity, posture, and response to painful stimuli provides clues to the location and extent of cerebral dysfunction. Even subtle movements (e.g., the outward rotation of a hip) should be noted and the child observed for other signs. Asymmetrical movements of the limbs or absence of movement suggests paralysis. In hemiplegia the affected limb lies in external rotation and will fall uncontrollably when lifted and allowed to drop. In patients with cerebellum abnormalities, heel-to-toe walking is difficult. Patients with cerebellar ataxia have an unsteady, broad-based gait. These observations should be described rather than labelled.

In the deeper comatose states there is little or no spontaneous movement, and the musculature tends to be flaccid. There is considerable variability in the motor behaviour in lesser degrees of coma. For example, the child may be relatively immobile or restless and hyperkinetic; muscle tone may be increased or decreased. Tremors, twitching, and spasms of muscles are common observations. The child may display purposeless movements. Combative behaviour is common. Hyperactivity is more common in acute febrile and toxic states than in cases of increased ICP. Seizures are common in children and may be present from any cause. Any repetitive or seizure movements should be described precisely.

Posturing

Primitive postural reflexes emerge as cortical control over motor function is lost in brain dysfunction. These reflexes are evident in posturing and motor movements directly related to the area of the brain involved. Posturing reflects a balance between the lower exciting and the higher inhibiting influences, and strong muscles overcoming weaker ones. Decorticate or flexion posturing (Fig. 50-5, A) is seen with severe dysfunction of the cerebral cortex or with lesions to corticospinal tracts above the brainstem. Typical flexion posturing includes rigid flexion, with arms held tightly to the body; flexed elbows, wrists, and fingers; plantar flexed feet; legs extended and internally rotated; and possibly fine tremors or intense stiffness. Decerebrate posture or extension posturing (see Fig. 50-5, B) is a sign of dysfunction at the level of the midbrain or lesions to the brainstem. It is characterized by rigid extension and pronation of the arms and legs, flexed wrists and fingers, clenched jaw, extended neck, and possibly an arched back. Unilateral extension posturing is often caused by tentorial herniation.

Posturing may not be evident when the child is relaxed but can usually be elicited by applying painful stimuli, such as a blunt object pressed on the base of the nail. Nurses should avoid applying thumb pressure to the supraorbital region of the frontal bone (risk of orbital damage). Noxious stimuli (e.g., suctioning) can elicit a response, as may turning or touching.

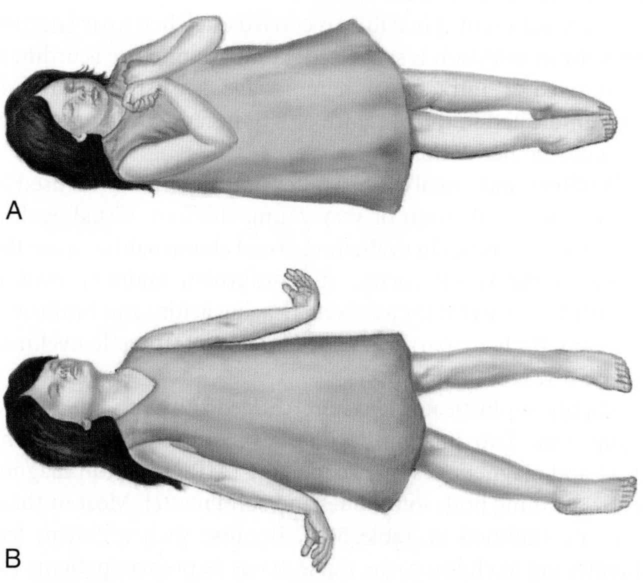

FIGURE 50-5 **A:** Flexion posturing. **B:** Extension posturing.

When the nurse is describing posturing, the stimulus needed to provoke the response is as important as the reaction.

Reflexes

Testing of some reflexes may be of limited value. In general, the corneal, pupillary, muscle-stretch, superficial, and plantar reflexes tend to be absent in deep coma. The state of reflexes is variable in lighter grades of unconsciousness and depends on the underlying pathological process and the location of the lesion. Absence of corneal reflexes and presence of a tonic neck reflex are associated with severe brain damage. The Babinski reflex (see Extremities, Chapter 33) may be of value if it is found to be present consistently in children older than 18 months. A positive Babinski reflex is significant in assessment of pyramidal tract lesions when it is unilateral and associated with other pyramidal signs.

NURSING ALERT

Three key reflexes that demonstrate healthy neurological status in young infants are the Moro, tonic neck, and withdrawal (to painful stimuli) reflexes.

Special Diagnostic Procedures

Numerous diagnostic procedures are used for assessment of cerebral function. Laboratory tests that may help delineate the cause of unconsciousness include blood glucose, urea nitrogen, electrolyte (pH, sodium, potassium, chloride, calcium, and bicarbonate) tests; clotting studies, hematocrit, a complete blood count; liver function tests; blood cultures if there is fever; urine toxicology screen; and blood lead levels if clinically indicated.

An electroencephalogram (EEG) may provide important information. For example, generalized random, slow activity suggests suppressed cortical function, and localized slow activity suggests a space-occupying lesion such as a hematoma, tumour, or infectious process. A flat tracing is one of the criteria used as evidence of brain death.

Examination of spinal fluid is carried out when toxic encephalopathy or infection is suspected. Lumbar puncture is ordinarily delayed if intracranial hemorrhage is suspected and is contraindicated in the presence of ICP because of the potential for tentorial herniation.

Auditory and visual evoked potentials are sometimes used in neurological evaluation of very young children. Visual evoked potentials are useful in evaluating visual abnormalities from the retina to the visual cortex, and brainstem auditory evoked potentials are useful for assessing hearing acuity and brainstem function. Both are particularly useful for detecting demyelinating disease and neoplasms.

Highly sophisticated tests are carried out with specialized equipment. Two imaging techniques, computed tomography (CT) and magnetic resonance imaging (MRI), assist in diagnosis by scanning both soft tissues and solid matter. Most of these tests are outlined in Table 50-1. Because such tests can feel threatening to children, the nurse needs to prepare patients for the tests and provide support and reassurance during the tests (see Preparation for Diagnostic and Therapeutic Procedures, Chapter 44). Children unfamiliar with the machines can be shown a picture beforehand. Although radiographic examinations are not painful, the machinery is often so frightening in appearance that the child protests because of anxiety. It is important to stress to the child the importance of lying still for tests. This is especially true of CT and MRI, both of which require that the child's head be placed within a special immobilizing device. Chin and cheek pads are sometimes used to prevent the slightest head movement, and straps are applied to the body to prevent a slight change in body position. The nurse can explain these events to a frightened child by comparing them to an astronaut's preparation for a space flight. It is important to emphasize to the child that at no time is the procedure painful.

Physical preparation for the diagnostic test may involve administration of a sedative. Many different agents are used for sedation of children undergoing neurological diagnostic procedures. Chloral hydrate or benzodiazepines have been used for decades as short-term sedative agents and remain safe methods in pediatric outpatient sedation (Mason, 2008). In recent years additional sedative agents have been used safely, alone and in combination. These include intravenous (IV) sodium pentobarbital (Nembutal), IV fentanyl (Sublimaze), IV midazolam (Versed), and intranasal midazolam (Bhatt, Roback, Joubert, et al., 2015). IV propofol has been added to the sedation procedural medications. Increasingly, physicians other than anaesthetists are performing procedural sedation. Concern has been raised regarding the safety of this sedation and the lack of surveillance on outcomes. Pediatric Emergency Research Canada has set up a sedation safety surveillance group to study and track effectiveness of procedural sedations in general and record frequency of adverse outcomes (Bhatt et al., 2015). Some of the adverse outcomes that have been reported include bradycardia, asystole, pulmonary aspiration, permanent neurological injury, and death. The incidence rates of these adverse outcomes are unknown because of the infrequency of their occurrence and the lack of surveillance of sedation safety.

Children scheduled to undergo sedation should be helped through the preparation and administration and be assured that someone will remain with them (if possible). Children need continual support and reinforcement during procedures in which they remain conscious. Vital signs and physiological responses to the procedure should be monitored throughout. Many diagnostic procedures performed on an outpatient basis require sedation, and children need recovery time and observation. The nurse should review written instructions with the parents before discharge. Children who have undergone a procedure with a general anaesthetic require postanaesthesia care, including positioning to prevent aspiration of secretions and frequent assessment of vital signs and LOC. In addition, other neurological functions such as pupillary responses, motor strength, and movement are tested at regular intervals. Any surgical wound resulting from the test should be checked for bleeding, CSF leakage, and other complications. Children who undergo repeated subdural taps should have their hematocrit

TABLE 50-1 NEUROLOGICAL DIAGNOSTIC PROCEDURES

TEST	DESCRIPTION	PURPOSE	COMMENTS
Lumbar puncture (LP)	Spinal needle is inserted between L3–L4 or L4–L5 vertebral spaces into subarachnoid space; CSF pressure is measured, and a sample is collected for examination.	*Diagnostic*—Measures spinal fluid pressure, obtains CSF for laboratory analysis *Therapeutic*—Injection of medication	Contraindicated in patients with ICP or infected skin over puncture site
Subdural tap	Needle is inserted into anterior fontanel or coronal suture (midline to pupil).	Helps rule out subdural effusions Removes CSF to relieve pressure	Place infant in semi-erect position after subdural tap to minimize leakage from site; prevent child from crying if possible. Check site frequently for evidence of leakage.
Ventricular puncture	Needle is inserted into lateral ventricle via coronal suture (midline to pupil).	Removes CSF to relieve pressure	Risk of intracerebral or ventricular hemorrhage
Electroencephalography (EEG)	EEG records changes in electrical potential of brain. Electrodes are placed at various points to assess electrical function in a particular area. Impulses are recorded by electromagnetic pen or digitally.	Detects spikes, or bursts of electrical activity that indicate the potential for seizures Used to determine brain death	Patient should remain quiet during procedure; may require sedation Minimize external stimuli during procedure.
Nuclear brain scan	Radioisotope is injected intravenously, then counted and recorded after fixed time intervals. Radioisotope accumulates in areas where blood-brain barrier is defective.	Identifies focal brain lesions (e.g., tumours, abscesses) Positive uptake of material with encephalitis and subdural hematoma Visualizes CSF pathways	Requires intravenous (IV) access; patient may require sedation In healthy children or children with noncommunicating hydrocephalus, no retrograde filling of ventricles occurs. Areas of concentrated uptake of material are termed *hot spots*.
Endocephalography	Pulses of ultrasonic waves are beamed through head; echoes from reflecting surfaces are recorded graphically.	Identifies shifts in midline structures from their normal positions as a result of intracranial lesions May show ventricular dilation	Simple, safe, rapid procedure Fontanel must be patent.
Real-time ultrasonography (RTUS)	RTUS is similar to CT but uses ultrasound instead of ionizing radiation.	Allows high-resolution anatomical visualization in variety of imaging planes	Produces images similar to CT scan Especially useful in neonatal central nervous system problems Anterior fontanel must be patent.
Radiography	Skull films are taken from different views—lateral, posterolateral, axial (submentoventricular), half-axial.	Shows fractures, dislocations, spreading suture lines, craniosynostosis Shows degenerative changes, bone erosion, calcifications	Simple, noninvasive procedure
Computed tomography (CT) scan	Pinpoint x-ray beam is directed on horizontal or vertical plane to provide series of images that are fed into a computer and assembled in an image displayed on a video screen. CT uses ionizing radiation.	Visualizes horizontal and vertical cross section of brain in three planes (axial, coronal, sagittal) Distinguishes density of various intracranial tissues and structures—congenital abnormalities, hemorrhage, tumours, demyelinating and inflammatory processes, calcification	Requires IV access if contrast agent is used Patient may require sedation Rapid
Magnetic resonance imaging (MRI)	MRI produces radiofrequency emissions from elements (e.g., hydrogen, phosphorus), which are converted to visual images by computer.	Permits visualization of morphological feature of target structures Permits tissue discrimination unavailable with many techniques	MRI is a noninvasive procedure except when IV contrast agent is used. No exposure to radiation occurs. Patient may require sedation. Parent or attendant can remain in room with child. MRI does not visualize bone detail or calcifications. No metal can be present in scanner.

Continued

TABLE 50-1 NEUROLOGICAL DIAGNOSTIC PROCEDURES—cont'd

TEST	DESCRIPTION	PURPOSE	COMMENTS
Positron emission tomography (PET)	PET involves IV injection of positron-emitting radionucleotide; local concentrations are detected and transformed into visual display by computer.	Detects and measures blood volume and flow in brain, metabolic activity, biochemical changes within tissue	Requires lengthy period of immobility Minimum exposure to radiation occurs. Patient may require sedation.
Digital subtraction angiography (DSA)	Contrast dye is injected intravenously; computer "subtracts" all tissues without contrast medium, leaving clear image of contrast medium in vessels studied.	Visualizes vasculature of target tissue Visualizes finite vascular abnormalities	Safe alternative to angiography Patient must remain still during procedure; may require sedation.
Single-photon emission computed tomography (SPECT)	SPECT involves IV injection of photon-emitting radionuclide; radionuclides are absorbed by healthy tissue at different rate than by diseased or necrotic tissue; data are transferred to a computer, which converts the image to film.	Provides information regarding blood flow to tissues; analyzing blood flow to organ may help determine how well it is functioning	Requires lengthy period of immobility Minimum exposure to radiation occurs. Patient may require sedation.

level monitored to detect excessive blood loss from the procedure.

THE UNCONSCIOUS CHILD

NURSING CARE

The unconscious child requires nursing observation, recording, and evaluation of changes in objective signs. These observations provide valuable information regarding the patient's progress and often serve as a guide to diagnosis and treatment. The outcome and recovery of the unconscious child may depend on the level of nursing care and observational skills. The outcome of unconsciousness may be early and complete recovery, death within a few hours or days, persistent and permanent unconsciousness, or recovery with varying degrees of residual mental or physical disability.

Emergency measures are directed toward ensuring a patent airway, breathing, and circulation; stabilizing the spine when indicated; treating shock; and reducing increased ICP. Delayed treatment often leads to increased damage. As soon as emergency measures have been implemented—and in many cases concurrently—therapies for specific causes are begun. Because nursing care is closely related to medical management, both are considered here.

Continual observation of LOC, pupillary reaction, and vital signs is essential in the care of CNS disorders. The assessment frequency depends on the cause of unconsciousness and the progression of cerebral involvement. Intervals may be as short as every 15 minutes or as long as every 2 hours. Significant alterations should be reported immediately.

Hypothalamic and brainstem disorders may affect the patient's thermoregulation. The temperature is taken every 2 to 4 hours, depending on the patient's condition. *Hypothermia* is defined as a core body temperature less than 35°C. EEG slowing is noted at 30°C and loss of pupillary light reflex is lost at 28°C. *Hyperthermia* is defined as a core temperature greater than 38.5°C and temperatures greater than 42°C can cause EEG slowing, seizures, and encephalopathy (Young, 2009).

An elevated temperature may occur in children with CNS dysfunction; thus a light covering is sufficient. Vigorous efforts, such as tepid sponge baths or application of a hypothermia blanket, are needed to prevent brain damage if temperature exceeds 40°C rectally. It is important to remember that if the child is shivering with the tepid bath that it will increase the metabolic needs, which then can further increase the temperature.

Pupils are observed for their size, symmetry, and reaction to light. Signs of meningeal irritation such as nuchal rigidity are also assessed. The presence of the oculovestibular response, corneal (blink) response, and cough and gag reflexes are evaluated. Aspects of LOC assessment include response to vocal commands, resistance to care, and response to painful stimuli. Spontaneous movement, changes in muscle tone or strength, and body position are noted. Seizure activity is described according to the duration and body areas involved. An antiepileptic medication such as phenytoin (Dilantin) or phenobarbital can be ordered to control seizure activity.

Pain management for the comatose child requires astute nursing observation and management. Signs of pain include changes in behaviour (e.g., increased agitation and rigidity, alterations in physiological parameters); increased heart rate, respiratory rate, blood pressure; and decreased oxygen saturation. Since these findings are not specific for pain, the nurse should observe for their appearance during times of induced or suspected pain and their disappearance after the end of the inciting procedure or the administration of analgesia. A pain assessment record should be used to document indications of pain and the effectiveness of interventions (see Pain Assessment, Chapter 34).

The use of opioids, such as morphine, to relieve pain is controversial because they may mask signs of altered consciousness or depress respirations. If there are concerns about assessing the LOC or respiratory depression, naloxone (Narcan) can be used to reverse the opioid effects. However, unrelieved pain activates the stress response, which can elevate ICP. To block the stress response, some authorities advocate the use of analgesics, sedatives, and, in some cases such as head injury, paralyzing agents via continuous IV infusion. A frequently used combination is fentanyl, midazolam, and vecuronium (Norcuron). Acetaminophen (Tylenol) may also be an effective analgesic for mild to moderate pain. Regardless of which medications are used, adequate dosage and regular administration are essential to provide optimal pain relief (see Pain Management, Chapter 34).

Other measures to relieve discomfort include providing a quiet, dimly lit environment; limiting visitors; and preventing any sudden, jarring movements, such as banging into the bed. Proper positioning is an effective way to prevent increased ICP during this time.

NURSING ALERT

When opioids are used, bowel elimination must be closely monitored because of the potential constipating effect. Stool softeners should be given with laxatives as needed to prevent constipation (see Chapter 34).

Respiratory Management

Respiratory effectiveness is the primary concern in the care of the unconscious child, and establishing an adequate airway is always the first priority. Carbon dioxide has a potent vasodilating effect and will increase cerebral blood flow (CBF) and ICP. Cerebral hypoxia that lasts longer than 4 minutes nearly always causes irreversible brain damage.

NURSING ALERT

Respiratory obstruction and subsequent compromise lead to cardiac arrest. Maintaining an adequate, patent airway is of critical importance.

Children in lighter states of coma may be able to cough and swallow, but those in deeper states are unable to handle secretions, which tend to pool in the throat and pharynx. Dysfunction of cranial nerves IX and X places the child at risk for aspiration and cardiac arrest; the child needs to be positioned to prevent aspiration of secretions and the stomach emptied to reduce the likelihood of vomiting. In infants, blockage of air passages from secretions can happen in seconds. In addition, upper airway obstruction from laryngospasm is a frequent complication in comatose children.

An oral airway can be used for the child who is suffering a temporary loss of consciousness, such as after a contusion, seizure, or anaesthesia. For children who remain unconscious for a longer time, a nasotracheal or orotracheal tube is inserted to maintain the open airway and facilitate removal of secretions. Insertion of an endotracheal tube (ET) should be considered when a child has a GCS of less than 8, evidence of herniation, apnea, or inability to maintain an airway (Sharma, Kochar, Sankhyan, et al., 2010). A tracheostomy is performed in cases in which laryngoscopy for introduction of an ET would be difficult or for a child who needs long-term ventilator support. Suctioning is used only as needed to clear the airway, exerting care to prevent increasing ICP.

When the respiratory centre is involved, mechanical ventilation is usually indicated (see Chapter 45). Blood gas analysis is performed regularly, and oxygen is administered when indicated. Moderately severe hypoxia and respiratory acidosis are often present but are not always evident from clinical manifestations. Hyperventilation frequently accompanies unconsciousness and may lead to respiratory alkalosis, or it may represent the body's attempt to compensate for metabolic acidosis. Thus blood gas and pH determinations are essential guides for therapy. Chest physiotherapy is carried out on a regular basis, and the child's position is changed at least every 2 hours to prevent pulmonary complications.

Intracranial Pressure Monitoring

An acute rise in ICP can cause secondary brain injury (Singhi & Tiwari, 2009); the management of the child with increased ICP is a complex and important task. ICP monitoring is used to guide therapy and provides information on intracranial compliance, cerebrovascular status, and cerebral infusion (Sankhyan, Vykunta Raju, Sharma, et al., 2010). Nonetheless, ICP monitoring is an invasive procedure that has associated risks, including infections, hemorrhage, malfunction, and obstruction (Singhi & Tiwari, 2009). A Cochrane review on traumatic encephalopathy concluded that a secondary complication of hypoxic-ischemic damage from brain swelling accompanied by raised ICP resulted in inadequate cerebral perfusion and increased brain injury. More research is needed to provide further evidence of the efficacy of early detection of raised ICP and to develop treatment interventions that would improve cerebral perfusion and reduce brain injury (Forsyth, Wolny, Rodrigues, et al., 2010). When a CSF obstruction causes increased ICP, a ventricular tap to drain excess CSF will provide relief quickly and effectively decrease the ICP (Sankhyan et al., 2010). Evacuation of a hematoma reduces pressure from this source.

Indications for inserting an ICP monitor are as follows:

- GCS evaluation of less than 8
- Traumatic brain injury with an abnormal head CT scan
- Deterioration of condition
- Subjective judgement regarding clinical appearance and response (Bhalla, Dewhirst, Sawardekar, et al., 2012)

Four major types of ICP monitors are as follows:

1. Intraventricular catheter with fibroscopic sensors attached to a monitoring system
2. Subarachnoid bolt (Richmond screw)
3. Epidural sensor
4. Anterior fontanel pressure monitor

Direct ventricular pressure measurement with an intraventricular catheter remains the gold standard of ICP monitoring. Placement of the intraventricular catheter and subarachnoid bolt occurs through a burr hole in the skull. The intraventricular method involves introduction of a catheter into the lateral ventricle on the nondominant side, if known. The subarachnoid bolt involves placement of a bolt in the subarachnoid space, and the epidural sensor involves placement of a sensor between the dura and the skull. The intraventricular catheter has the advantage of providing a means for recalibration when measurement drift occurs, but both the catheter and the bolt can be used for therapeutic CSF drainage to reduce pressure. A drainage bag attached to the system is kept at the level of the ventricles and can be lowered to decrease ICP.

NURSING ALERT

The bolt is stabilized with dressings, but these are not changed or disturbed, even to check the site. However, they can be reinforced.

The placement of the bolt is not adjusted by anyone except the neurosurgeon who placed the device. The neurosurgeon should be notified if a satisfactory waveform is not observed.

An epidural sensor provides a readout of the ICP with a stopcock assembly and transducer. In infants, a fontanel transducer can be used to detect impulses from a pressure sensor and convert them to electrical energy. The electrical energy is then converted to visible waves or numeric readings on an oscilloscope. ICP measurement from the anterior fontanel is noninvasive but may prove to be inaccurate if the equipment is poorly placed or inconsistently recalibrated.

For sustained ICP elevations greater than 20 to 25 mm Hg, several medical measures are available. Osmotic diuretics may provide rapid relief in emergency situations. Although their effect is transient, lasting only about 6 hours, they can be lifesaving in emergencies. These substances are rapidly excreted by the kidneys and carry with them large quantities of sodium and water. Mannitol (or sometimes urea) administered intravenously is the medication most frequently used for rapid reduction and can lower ICP in 1 to 5 minutes. The infusion is generally given slowly but may be pushed rapidly in cases of herniation or impending cerebral herniation. Because of the profound diuretic effect of the drug, an in-dwelling catheter is inserted to ensure bladder emptying. Hypertonic saline in concentrations of 3 to 23% has been shown to reduce ICP by its osmotic force and can be beneficial for hypovolemic and hypotensive patients by increasing intravascular volume and blood pressure (Singhi & Tiwari, 2009). Adrenocorticosteroids are not recommended for cerebral edema secondary to head trauma. $Paco_2$ should be maintained at 25 to 30 mm Hg to produce vasoconstriction, which reduces CSF, thereby decreasing ICP.

Managing Intracranial Pressure

In cases of high levels of increased ICP, nursing procedures tend to trigger reactive pressure waves in many patients. For example, increased intrathoracic or abdominal pressure will be transmitted to the cranium. Particular care should be taken in positioning these patients to avoid neck vein compression, which may further increase ICP by interfering with venous return.

The child can be propped to one side or the other, and the use of an alternating-pressure mattress reduces the chance of prolonged pressure to vulnerable areas. Frequent clinical assessment of the child cannot be replaced by an ICP monitoring device.

Nurses who are caring for patients with intracranial monitoring devices must be knowledgeable about the system, assist with insertion as per hospital policy, interpret the monitor readings, and be able to distinguish between danger signals and mechanical dysfunction.

NURSING ALERT

The head of the bed is elevated to 15 to 30 degrees, and the child is positioned so that the head is maintained in midline to facilitate venous drainage and avoid jugular compression (Bhalla et al., 2012).

It is important to avoid activities that may increase ICP by causing pain or emotional stress. Gentle range-of-motion exercises can be carried out but should not be performed vigorously. Any disturbing procedures to be performed should be scheduled to take advantage of therapies that reduce ICP, such as osmotherapy and sedation. Environmental noise should be minimized or eliminated to the degree possible (Sankhyan et al., 2010).

Suctioning and percussion are poorly tolerated and are contraindicated unless concurrent respiratory problems exist. Hypoxia and the Valsalva manoeuvre associated with cough both acutely elevate ICP. Vibration, which does not increase ICP, accomplishes excellent results and should be tried first if treatment is needed. If suctioning is necessary, it should be brief and preceded by hyperventilation with 100% oxygen, which can be monitored during suctioning with pulse oximetry to determine oxygen saturation.

Nutrition and Hydration

In the unconscious child, fluids and calories are supplied initially via the IV route (see Chapter 44). An IV infusion is started early, and the type of fluid administered is determined by the patient's general condition. Fluid therapy requires careful monitoring and adjustment based on neurological signs and electrolyte determinations. The goal of fluid therapy is *euvolemia* (normal blood volume). Often, comatose children are unable to cope with the same amounts of fluid they could tolerate at other times, and overhydration must be avoided to prevent fatal cerebral edema. When cerebral edema is a threat, fluids may need to be restricted to reduce the chance of fluid overload. Skin and mucous membranes need to be examined for signs of dehydration. Observation for signs of altered fluid balance related to abnormal pituitary secretions is also a part of nursing care.

Long-term nutrition is provided with a balanced formula via a nasogastric or gastrostomy tube. Most children have continuous feedings, but occasionally bolus feedings are used.

Altered Pituitary Secretion

An altered ability to handle fluid loads is attributed in part to the syndrome of inappropriate antidiuretic hormone secretion (SIADH) and diabetes insipidus (DI) resulting from hypothalamic dysfunction (see Chapter 51). SIADH frequently accompanies CNS diseases such as head injury, meningitis, encephalitis, brain abscess, brain tumour, and subarachnoid hemorrhage. In the patient with SIADH, scant quantities of urine are excreted, electrolyte analysis reveals hyponatremia and hyposmolality, and manifestations of overhydration are evident. It is important to evaluate all parameters, since the reduced urine output might be erroneously interpreted as a sign of dehydration. The treatment of SIADH consists of restriction of fluids until serum electrolytes and osmolality return to normal levels.

DI may occur after intracranial trauma. In DI there are large amounts of diluted urine and the accompanying danger of dehydration. Adequate replacement of fluids is essential, and observation of electrolyte balance is necessary to detect signs of hypernatremia and hyperosmolality. Exogenous vasopressin may be administered.

Medications

The cause of unconsciousness determines specific medication therapies. Children with infectious processes are given antibiotics appropriate to the disease and the infecting organism, and corticosteroids are prescribed for inflammatory conditions and edema. Cerebral edema is an indication for osmotherapy with osmotic diuretics. Sedatives or antiepileptics are prescribed for seizure activity (see p. 1620).

MEDICATION ALERT

Sedation in the combative child provides amnesic and anxiolytic properties in conjunction with a paralytic agent. The combination decreases ICP and allows treatment of cerebral edema. Usual medications include morphine, midazolam, and pancuronium (Pavulon). Midazolam is attractive because of its short half-life.

The management of ICP using a barbiturate-induced deep coma is debated among practitioners. Barbiturates are currently reserved for the reduction of increased ICP when all else has failed. Barbiturates decrease the cerebral metabolic rate for oxygen and protect the brain during times of reduced cerebral perfusion pressure. Barbiturate deep comas require extensive monitoring, cardiovascular and respiratory support, and ICP monitoring to assess response to therapy. Paralyzing agents such as pancuronium also may be needed to aid in performing diagnostic tests, improving effectiveness of therapies, and reducing risks of secondary complications.

Thermoregulation

Hyperthermia often accompanies cerebral dysfunction; if it is present, measures should be implemented to reduce the temperature to prevent brain damage and to reduce metabolic demands generated by the increased body temperature. Medically induced hypothermia assists in controlling ICP and may result in an improved outcome. Antipyretic agents are usually ineffective with hyperthermia as a result of traumatic brain injury; therefore, external cooling should be used (Badjatia, 2009). External cooling can consist of 20 to 40 cc/kg iced normal saline IV over 10 to 20 minutes and application of a cooling blanket below and occasionally on top of the patient. Additional adjunct therapies to assist in the cooling process include ice packs, a fan, lukewarm baths, and reduction of room temperature and/or ventilator humidification (Fink, Kochanek, Clark, et al., 2010). Laboratory tests and other methods can be used in an attempt to determine the cause, if any, of the hyperthermia.

Elimination

A urinary catheter is usually inserted during the acute phase, although diapers may be used and weighed to record urine output. The child who formerly had bowel and bladder control is generally incontinent. If the child remains comatose for a long period, the in-dwelling catheter may be removed and periodic bladder emptying accomplished by intermittent catheterization. Stool softeners are usually sufficient to maintain bowel function, but suppositories or enemas may be needed occasionally for adequate elimination and to prevent impaction.

Hygienic Care

Routine measures for cleansing to maintain skin integrity are an integral part of nursing of the unconscious child (see Maintaining Healthy Skin, Chapter 44). The child who is unable to move is prone to developing tissue breakdown. To help prevent this, the child can be placed on an alternating-pressure or water-filled mattress, which alleviates pressure on vulnerable areas. Assessment of pressure ulcer risk can be calculated using the modified pediatric Braden Q Scale (see Additional Resources at the end of this chapter).

Mouth care should be performed at least twice daily, because the mouth tends to become dry or coated with mucus. The teeth should be carefully brushed with a soft toothbrush or cleaned with gauze saturated with saline. Commercially prepared cleansing devices, such as Toothettes, are convenient for cleansing the mouth and teeth. Lips can be coated with ointment or other preparations to protect them from drying, cracking, or blistering. Glycerin swabs should not be used, as they break down tooth enamel.

The deeply comatose child is also prone to eye irritation. The corneal reflexes are absent; thus the eyes are easily irritated or damaged by linen, dust, or other substances that may come in contact with them. There is excessive dryness as a result of incomplete closure of the eyes or decreased secretions especially if the child is undergoing osmotherapy to reduce or prevent brain edema.

NURSING ALERT

The eyes should be examined regularly and carefully for early signs of irritation or **inflammation**. Artificial tears (methylcellulose) are placed in the eyes every 1 to 2 hours. Eye dressings may sometimes be needed to protect the eyes from possible damage.

Positioning and Exercise

The unconscious child needs to be positioned to prevent aspiration of saliva, nasogastric secretions, and vomitus and to minimize ICP. The head of the bed is elevated, and the child is placed in a side-lying or semiprone position. A small, firm pillow is placed under the head, and the uppermost limbs are flexed and supported with pillows. In the semiprone position, the child lies with the dependent arm at the side behind the body, the opposite side supported on pillows, and the uppermost arm and leg flexed and resting on the pillows. This position prevents undue pressure on the dependent extremities. The dependent position of the face encourages drainage of secretions and prevents the flaccid tongue from obstructing the airway.

Normal range-of-motion exercises help maintain function and prevent contractures of joints. Exercises should be done gently and with full range of motion. A small rolled pad can be placed in the palms to help maintain proper position of the fingers; footboards or boots can be used to help prevent footdrop; and splinting may be needed to prevent severe contractures of the wrist, knee, or ankle in decerebrate children. Extremity splints and the child's position should be changed every 1 to 2 hours.

Stimulation

Sensory stimulation is important in the care of the unconscious child, just as it is in the care of the alert child. For the temporarily unconscious or semiconscious child, sensory stimulation helps arouse the child to the conscious state and orient the child in terms of time and place. Auditory and tactile stimulation are especially valuable. Tactile stimulation is not appropriate for the child in whom it may elicit an undesirable response. However, for other children, tactile contact often has a relaxing and calming effect. When the child's condition permits, holding or rocking has a soothing effect and provides body contact needed by young children. Involving family members with the sensory stimulation can create a positive effect on the child and allows the family to participate in the care (Abbasi, Mohammadi, & Sheaykh Rezayi, 2009).

The auditory sense is often present in a state of coma. Hearing is the last sense to be lost and the first one to be regained, thus the child should be spoken to as any other child. Conversation around the child should not include thoughtless or derogatory remarks. Soft music is used frequently to provide auditory stimulation. Singing the child's favourite songs or reading a favourite story can help the child maintain contact with a familiar world. Playing songs or stories recorded in the parents' voices can provide a continuous source of familiar stimulation.

Regaining Consciousness

Awakening from a coma is a gradual process; however, sometimes children regain consciousness within a short time. Regaining orientation involves knowing person, place, and time, in that order.

Certain behaviours have been observed when children awaken from the unconscious state. The stress and anxiety they appear to feel in a strange and unfamiliar environment are consistently expressed in silent and withdrawn behaviour. Children respond to basic questioning but usually do not display their prehospitalization personality and social behaviour until they are transferred from the critical care area.

Family Support

Helping the parents of an unconscious child cope with the situation can be especially difficult. They may demonstrate all the guilt, fear, hostility, and anxiety of any parent of a seriously ill child (see Chapter 43). In addition, these parents are faced with the uncertain outcome of the cerebral dysfunction. The fear of death, intellectual disability, or other permanent disability is present. Nursing intervention with parents depends on the nature of the pathological condition, the parents' personality, and the parent–child relationship before the injury or illness.

Parents need the most intensive nursing support during periods of crisis and uncertainty. During the recovery phase they are given information clarification, and they should be encouraged to become involved in the child's care. Often the child's hospitalization is brief; however, some children require extended hospitalization for intensive therapy and rehabilitation.

The most difficult situations involve children who never regain consciousness. Family members often attempt to construct a representation of the child. They may bring items that belong to the child, such as favourite toys, music, and other objects cherished by the child. This action is an attempt to provide stimulation for the child in the hope of eliciting a response, to let the hospital staff know the child as the unique individual he or she was before losing consciousness, and to reconstitute an image of the child "lost" to them and for whom they mourn. Unlike losing a child through death, these situations lack finality, which often leaves family members in a state of prolonged grief and searching for signs of hope. An awareness of these behaviours and coping mechanisms can help nurses support the parents as they grieve.

Superimposed on the process of grieving for the "lost" child, parents may be faced with difficult decisions. When the child's brain is so severely damaged that vital functions must be maintained by artificial means, the parents, along with guidance from the health care team, must make the final decision of whether to remove life support systems. During this time nurses continue to provide specialty care that maintains the child's physiological status while addressing informational and psychological needs of the family. While the decision to remove life support is difficult for parents, having an open and honest discussion about the child's medical condition and prognosis can help parents make a decision based on their child's care and status (Young, 2009). Parent's cultural, religious, and language needs coupled with their intellectual level, decision-making preferences, and emotional state should be considered during this discussion (Truog, Campbell, Curtis, et al., 2008). Sometimes parents may choose to refuse or not initiate treatment if they believe that is best for the child and the family (informed dissent). At other times parents request that "everything possible" be done for the child.

When the child has survived the cerebral insult and is not comatose, but physical or mental capacity is limited, either minimally or severely, families must cope with the long rehabilitation process and the uncertain outcome. The drain on financial, emotional, and social resources can be enormous.

For parents who choose to care for their child at home, planning for home care begins early in the recovery process (see Chapter 42). The family should become involved with the child's care as soon as they indicate an interest and ability to do so. They need education and support in learning to care for the child, regular follow-up observation and assessment of home management, and planning for respite care. Parents need to understand that it is important to plan for periodic relief from the continual care of the child (see Family-Centred Teaching Box: Preparation for Discharge, in Chapter 42).

CEREBRAL TRAUMA

Head Injury

Head injury is a pathological process involving the scalp, skull, meninges, or brain as a result of mechanical force. According to Parachute (2015), injuries are the number one health risk for children and the leading cause of death in children in Canada who are older than 1 year of age. Tragically, almost 8000 children die every year as a result of injuries (Public Health Agency of Canada [PHAC], 2016). It has been estimated that 300 in 100,000 children per year have a traumatic brain injury. Studies indicate that as many as three fourths of the childhood deaths caused by mechanical trauma are the direct result of a brain injury. A longitudinal study done in a Montreal emergency department provided evidence that a previous head injury increases a child's risk of having a subsequent head injury within 6 to 12 months of the previous injury (Swaine, Tremblay, Platt, et al., 2007).

Etiology

The three major causes of brain damage in childhood, in order of importance, are falls, motor vehicle injuries, and bicycle injuries. Neurological injury accounts for the highest mortality rate, with boys affected twice as often as girls. In motor vehicle accidents, children younger than 2 years of age are almost exclusively injured as passengers, whereas older children may also be injured as pedestrians or cyclists. Approximately 75% of bicyclists who die each year die of brain injuries (Saskatchewan Brain Injury Association, 2010). The majority of deaths from brain trauma caused by bicycle injuries occur in children between the ages of 5 and 19 years. Bicycle helmet laws have been effective in reducing the risk of head injury by 85% and traumatic brain injury by 88% (Rivara & Grossman, 2016). However, provincial legislation on the use of bicycle helmets varies from province to province. To date, legislation mandating helmet use for all cyclists, or for cyclists under a given age (for example, 18 years), has been implemented in 6 of 10 Canadian provinces and in none of the territories. See Additional Resources for further information on mandatory bicycle helmet laws.

The exposed nature of the head renders it particularly vulnerable to external violence, and many of the physical characteristics of children predispose them to craniocerebral trauma. For example, infants may be left unattended on beds, in high chairs, and in other places from which they can fall. Because the head of an infant or toddler is proportionately larger and heavier in relation to other body parts, it is the most likely to be injured. Incomplete motor development contributes to falls at young ages, and children's natural curiosity and exuberance can also increase their risk of injury (see Chapters 36 and 37).

Pathophysiology

Primary head injuries are those that occur at the time of trauma and include skull fracture, contusions, intracranial hematoma, and diffuse injury. Subsequent complications include hypoxic brain damage, increased ICP, infection, and cerebral edema. The predominant feature of a child's brain injury is the amount of diffuse swelling that occurs. Hypoxia and hypercapnia threaten the energy requirements of the brain and increase CBF. The added volume across the blood–brain barrier, along with the loss of autoregulation, exacerbates cerebral edema. Pressure inside the skull that is greater than arterial pressure results in inadequate perfusion.

The pathology of brain injury is directly related to the force of impact. Intracranial contents (brain, blood, CSF) are damaged because the force is too great to be absorbed by the skull and musculoligamentous support of the head. The elastic, pliable skull of the infant and young child absorbs much of the direct energy of physical impact to the head and affords some protection to intracranial structures. Although nervous tissue is delicate, it usually requires a severe blow to cause significant damage.

Physical forces act on the head through acceleration, deceleration, or deformation. Acceleration or deceleration is more descriptive of the circumstances responsible for most head injuries. When the stationary head receives a blow, the sudden acceleration causes deformation of the skull and mass movement of the brain. Continued movement of the intracranial contents allows the brain to strike parts of the skull (e.g., the sharp edges of the sphenoid or the irregular surface of the anterior fossa) or the edges of the tentorium. The very young child's larger head size and insufficient musculoskeletal support render these children particularly vulnerable to acceleration–deceleration injuries.

Although the brain volume remains unchanged, significant distortion takes place as the brain changes shape in response to the force of impact to the skull. This movement can cause bruising at the point of impact (coup) or at a distance as the brain collides with the unyielding surfaces far removed from the point of impact (contrecoup) (Fig. 50-6). Thus a blow to the occipital region can cause severe injury to the frontal and temporal areas of the brain. Sudden deceleration, such as takes place during a fall, causes the greatest cerebral injury at the point of impact. Children with an acceleration–deceleration injury demonstrate diffuse generalized cerebral swelling produced by increased blood volume or a redistribution of cerebral blood volume (cerebral hyperemia) rather than by increased water content (edema), as seen in adults.

Another effect of brain movement is shearing stresses, which may tear small arteries and cause subdural hemorrhages (Fig. 50-7). Damage can also occur when severe compression of the skull forces the brain through the tentorial opening. This can produce irreparable damage to the brainstem.

The clinical manifestations of acute head injury are listed in Box 50-3.

Mild traumatic brain injury. The most common head injury is *mild traumatic brain injury (concussion)*, an alteration in neurological or cognitive function with or without loss of

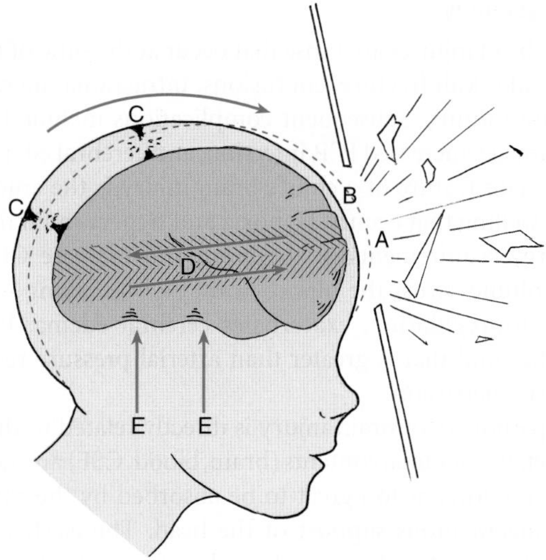

FIGURE 50-6 Mechanical distortion of cranium during closed-head injury. **A:** Preinjury contour of skull. **B:** Immediate postinjury contour of skull. **C:** Torn subdural vessels. **D:** Shearing forces. **E:** Trauma from contact with floor of cranium. (Redrawn from Grubb, R. L., & Coxe, W. S. [1974]. Central nervous system trauma: Cranial. In S. G. Eliasson, A. L. Presky, & W. B. Hardin, Jr. [Eds.], *Neurological pathophysiology*. New York: Oxford University Press.)

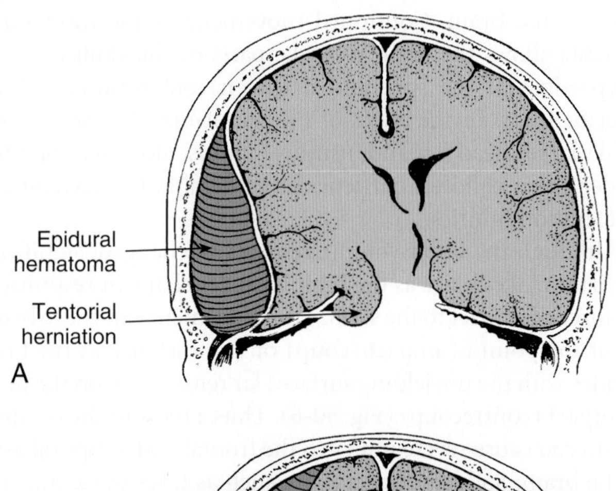

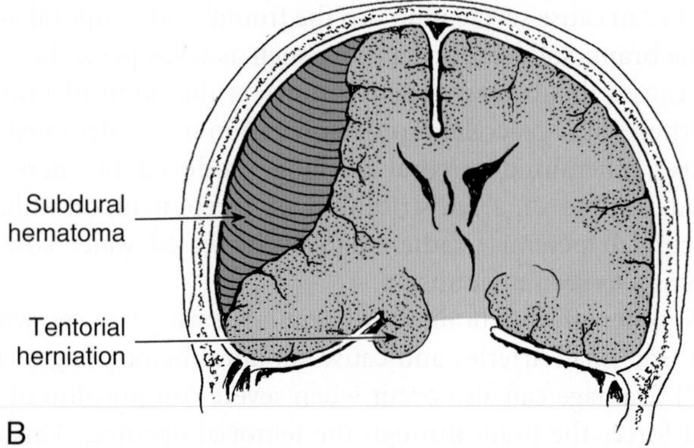

FIGURE 50-7 **A:** Epidural (extradural) hematoma and compression of temporal lobe through tentorial hiatus. **B:** Subdural hematoma.

BOX 50-3 CLINICAL MANIFESTATIONS OF ACUTE HEAD INJURY

Minor Injury

May or may not lose consciousness
Transient period of confusion
Somnolence
Listlessness
Irritability
Pallor
Vomiting (one or more episodes)

Signs of Progression

Altered mental status (e.g., difficulty rousing child)
Mounting agitation
Development of focal lateral neurological signs
Marked changes in vital signs

Severe Injury

Signs of increased intracranial pressure (see Box 50-1)
Bulging or full fontanel (infant)
Retinal hemorrhage
Extraocular palsies (especially cranial nerve VI)
Hemiparesis
Quadriplegia
Elevated temperature
Unsteady gait (older child)
Papilledema (older child)

Associated Signs

Scalp trauma
Other injuries (e.g., to extremities)

consciousness, which occurs immediately after a head injury (Landry, 2016). Confusion, dizziness, and disorientation following head injury are the most common symptoms associated with concussions. Loss of consciousness is not an accurate indicator of the presence of a concussion. Concussions usually resolve in 7 to 10 days without complications; however, some individuals may require several months to recover. There is increasing evidence that concussions in some children will persist longer with a postconcussion syndrome. A recent study reported that 11.8% of children presenting to the emergency room with a concussion remained symptomatic at 3 months postinjury. In addition, although most children reported a reduction in symptoms over time, 10% of children developed symptoms even though they initially had a good outcome (Barlow, Crawford, Brooks, et al., 2015).

The pathogenesis of concussion is still unclear but may be a result of shearing forces that cause stretching, compression, and tearing of nerve fibres, particularly in the area of the central brainstem, the seat of the reticular activating system. It has also been suggested that the anatomical alterations of nerve fibres cause the release of large quantities of acetylcholine into the CSF and a reduction in oxygen consumption with increased lactate production.

Initial concussion management begins with recognition of the injury, and the hallmark treatment of rest until the patient is asymptomatic. Once asymptomatic, a gradual step-wise

TABLE 50-2 SIGNS AND SYMPTOMS OF CONCUSSION

PHYSICAL SIGNS	CHANGE IN BEHAVIOUR	COGNITIVE IMPAIRMENT (PROBLEMS THINKING)	TROUBLE WITH SLEEP
Headache	Irritability	Slowed reaction times	Drowsiness
Nausea/vomiting	Sadness	Confusion	Trouble falling asleep
Changes in sight	Anxiety	Difficulty concentrating	Sleeping more than usual
Loss of consciousness (passing out)	Inappropriate emotions	Difficulty remembering	Sleeping less than usual
Irritation from light			
Irritation from loud sounds			
Loss of balance/poor coordination			
Amnesia			
Decreased playing ability			

Canadian Paediatric Society. (2014, March). *Sport-related concussion: Information for parents, coaches and trainers.* Retrieved from http://www.caringforkids.cps.ca/handouts/sport_related_concussion

return to activity should be followed (McCrory, Meeuwisse, Johnston, et al., 2009). According to the Canadian Paediatric Society (CPS), a child should be monitored by a responsible parent or guardian for 24 to 48 hours after the injury and observed specifically for the signs and symptoms outlined in Table 50-2 (Purcell & CPS, Healthy Active Living and Sports Medicine Committee, 2014). Knowing the signs and symptoms associated with concussions is especially pertinent when determining the status of a young child or infant, who lacks the ability to express their current state.

Contusion and laceration. The terms *contusion* and *laceration* are used to describe visible bruising and tearing of cerebral tissue. Contusions represent petechial hemorrhages along the superficial aspects of the brain at the site of impact or a lesion remote from the site of direct trauma. In serious accidents there may be multiple sites of injury.

The major areas of the brain susceptible to contusion or laceration are the occipital, frontal, and temporal lobes. Also, the irregular surfaces of the anterior and middle fossae at the base of the skull are capable of producing bruises or lacerations on forceful impact. Contusions may cause focal disturbances in strength, sensation, or visual awareness. The degree of brain damage in the contused areas varies according to the extent of vascular injury. Signs will vary from mild, transient weakness of a limb to prolonged unconsciousness and paralysis. However, the signs and symptoms may be clinically indistinguishable from those of concussion.

The lower incidence of cerebral contusion in infancy has been attributed to the infant's pliable skull with less convolutional markings of the inner space between brain tissue and bone. In addition, the infant's brain tissue has a softer consistency, which also reduces surface injury. However, infants who are roughly shaken (shaken baby syndrome) can sustain profound neurological impairment, seizures, retinal hemorrhages, and intracranial subarachnoid or subdural hemorrhages. In addition to these classic injuries, high cervical spinal cord hemorrhages and contusions can occur (Mian, Shah, Dalpiaz, et al., 2015). Cerebral lacerations are generally associated with penetrating or depressed skull fractures. However, they may occur without fracture in small children. When brain tissue is torn, with bleeding into and around the tear, more severe and prolonged unconsciousness and paralysis occur, leaving permanent scarring and some degree of disability.

Fractures. Because of its flexibility, the immature skull is able to sustain a greater degree of deformation than the adult skull before it incurs a fracture. A great deal of force is required to produce a fracture in an infant's skull. However, the undersurface of the skull contains grooves in which the meningeal arteries lie. A fracture that runs through one of these grooves may tear the artery and produce severe and damaging hemorrhage. Hypovolemic hypotension can occur in infants with skull fractures. Special attention must be paid to skull fractures in childhood when occurring near CSF large spaces, especially if a ventricle is enlarged, which could mean that hydrocephalus is present. Surgeons should evaluate for hydrocephalus before treating such fractures in order to improve the surgical result and postoperative clinical outcomes.

The types of skull fractures that occur are as follows:

Linear fractures comprise a single fracture line that starts at the point of maximal impact but does not cross suture lines. These are uncommon before 2 to 3 years of age but make up the majority of childhood skull fractures. Most linear skull fractures are associated with an overlying hematoma or soft-tissue swelling (Erlichman, Blumfield, Rajpathak, et al., 2010).

Depressed fractures are those in which the bone is locally broken, usually into several irregular fragments that are pushed inward, causing pressure on the brain. The inner portion of the bone is more extensively fragmented than the outer portion, which almost invariably produces tears in the dura or damage in the parenchyma. These are uncommon before 2 to 3 years of age. In infants and very young children, the soft, malleable bone may become dented in with a peculiar rounded or "ping-pong ball" depression, without laceration of either skin or dura. As a rule, the faster the blow, the greater the likelihood of a depressed fracture; a low-velocity impact tends to produce a linear fracture. Surgery may be needed to elevate the depressed bone fragment if there is an associated intracranial hematoma or pressure.

Comminuted fractures consist of multiple associated linear fractures. They usually result from intense impact. These types of fractures often result from repeated blows against an object and may suggest child abuse.

Basilar fractures involve the basilar portion of the frontal, ethmoid, sphenoid, temporal, or occipital bones. Because of the proximity of the fracture line to structures surrounding the brainstem, this is a serious head injury. Approximately 80% of the cases may include clinical features such as subcutaneous bleeding in the posterior neck area and over the mastoid process (battle sign). Bleeding around the eyes (raccoon eyes) or bleeding behind the tympanic membrane (hemotympanum) may occur.

Open fractures cause communication between the skull and the scalp or the surfaces of the upper respiratory tract. Open fractures increase the risk of CNS infection when the fracture creates an opening in the paranasal sinuses or middle ear that causes CSF leakage. They may have a skin laceration overlying the bone fracture called a *compound fracture*. Open fractures can also create an opening in the paranasal sinuses or middle ear that can lead to CSF rhinorrhea or otorrhea. Antibiotics are recommended to prevent osteomyelitis. Facial paralysis, vertigo, tinnitus, or hearing loss may develop.

Growing fractures are skull fractures with an underlying dural tear that fails to heal properly. The enlargement may be caused by a leptomeningeal cyst, dilated ventricles, or a herniated brain. Neurological symptoms include headache, seizures, and asymmetrical cranial growth. The majority of growing skull fractures (90%) occur before 3 years of age (Le Fournier, Hénaux, Haegelen, et al., 2015). Physical examination can reveal the development of a pulsatile mass or enlarged and sunken skull defect. Clinical neurological symptoms may be delayed for months to years after the initial skull fracture.

Complications

The major complications of trauma to the head are hemorrhage, infection, edema, and herniation through the tentorium. Infection is always a hazard in open injuries, and edema is related to tissue trauma. Vascular rupture may occur even in minor head injuries, causing hemorrhage between the skull and cerebral surfaces. Compression of the underlying brain produces effects that can be rapidly fatal or insidiously progressive.

NURSING ALERT

Post-traumatic meningitis should be suspected in children with increasing drowsiness and fever who also have basilar skull fractures.

Epidural hemorrhage. An *epidural hemorrhage* is bleeding between the dura and the skull to form a hematoma. This bleeding causes the dura to be stripped from the bone, forcing the underlying brain contents downward and inward as the brain expands (see Fig. 50-7, A). Since bleeding is generally arterial, brain compression occurs rapidly. Most often the expanding hematoma is located in the parietotemporal region, forcing the medial portion of the temporal lobe under the edge of the tentorium, where it causes pressure on nerves and blood vessels. It can also occur in the frontal or occipital posterior fossa. The lower incidence of epidural hematoma in childhood has been attributed to the fact that the middle meningeal artery is not embedded in the bone surface of the skull until approximately 2 years of age. Thus a fracture of the temporal bone is less likely to lacerate the artery. Also, the dura closely adheres to the inner table of the skull, especially at the level of the sutures, making separation from bleeding less likely. However, a child's skull can be indented with sufficient force to tear the middle meningeal artery and rebound intact without causing a fracture. Hemorrhage can also derive from dural veins or the dural sinuses, especially in infants and small children, in whom fracture is less likely to occur. In 20 to 40% of children a skull fracture is not detectable. The classic clinical picture of epidural hemorrhage (momentary unconsciousness followed by a normal period, then lethargy or coma) is seldom evident in children (see Box 50-3 for clinical manifestations). Frequently, the period of impaired consciousness is lacking, and the symptom-free period is atypical because of nonspecific symptoms such as irritability, headache, and vomiting. Physical findings can include pallor with anemia and cephalohematoma, with infants exhibiting additional findings of hypotonia and a bulging fontanel. If the severity of the child's signs and symptoms are not recognized, herniation and death will occur.

Subdural hemorrhage. A *subdural hemorrhage* is bleeding between the dura and the arachnoid membrane, usually as a result of the rupture of cortical veins that bridge the subdural space (see Fig. 50-7, B). Subdural hematomas are more common than epidural hematomas, occurring most often in infancy.

Unlike epidural hemorrhage, which develops inwardly against the less resistant brain tissue, subdural hemorrhage tends to develop more slowly and spreads thinly and widely until it is limited by the dural barriers—the falx and tentorium. Subdural hematoma is fairly common in infants, frequently as a result of birth trauma, falls, assaults, or violent shaking. Presenting signs can include irritability, vomiting, increased head circumference, bulging fontanels in infants, lethargy, or seizures. The small subdural space and dura firmly attached to the skull in this area are highly vulnerable to increased ICP. Hemiparesis, hemiplegia, and unequal pupils are signs of brainstem compression and increased ICP.

NURSING ALERT

Children with a subdural hematoma and retinal hemorrhages should be evaluated for the possibility of child abuse, especially shaken baby syndrome.

Subdural taps often provide relief in the infant, as revealed by follow-up CT scans, improved neurological status, and a flat anterior fontanel. The need for surgical evacuation of the hematoma depends on the physical examination, size of the hematoma, and CT scan abnormalities.

Cerebral edema. Some degree of brain edema is expected, especially 24 to 72 hours after craniocerebral trauma. Cerebral edema associated with traumatic brain injury may be caused by direct cellular injury leading to intracellular swelling or vascular injury leading to increased intracellular fluid. Either mechanism can result in increased ICP as a result of the increased intracranial volume and changes in cerebral blood flow.

NURSING ALERT

If a child loses consciousness or vomits more than three times following a head injury, medical attention should be sought.

Diagnostic Evaluation

A detailed health history, both past and present, is essential in evaluating the child with a craniocerebral trauma. Certain disorders, such as drug allergies, hemophilia, diabetes mellitus, or epilepsy, may produce similar symptoms. Even minor traumatic injury can aggravate a pre-existing disease process, thereby producing neurological symptoms out of proportion to the injury. Events surrounding the injury often supply significant data. It must be determined whether the infant or child exhibited alterations in consciousness; any other abnormal signs and behaviours exhibited by the child must be noted. Because head injuries are frequently accompanied by injuries in other areas, the examination needs to be performed with care to avoid further damage.

NURSING ALERT

Stabilize a child's spine after head injury until a spinal cord injury is ruled out.

Initial assessment. Priorities in the initial stabilization phase of a child with a head injury include assessment of circulation, airway, and breathing; evaluation for shock; and assessment for spinal cord injuries and a neurological examination, focusing on mental status, pupillary responses (symmetry and response to light), and motor responses. The assessment is carried out quickly in relation to vital signs (see Emergency box). Some children may have a rapid pulse, hyperventilate, appear pale, act excited or irritable, and feel clammy shortly after an injury.

NURSING ALERT

Signs of brainstem involvement include deep, rapid, periodic, or intermittent and gasping respirations; wide fluctuations or noticeable slowing of the pulse; and widening pulse pressure or extreme fluctuations in blood pressure. Note that marked hypotension may represent internal injuries.

Ocular signs such as fixed and dilated unequal pupils, fixed and constricted pupils, and pupils that are poorly reactive or nonreactive to light and accommodation indicate increased ICP or brainstem involvement. It is important to remain with the child who demonstrates fixed and dilated pupils, since these are ominous signs, with the high probability of respiratory arrest. Dilated, nonpulsating blood vessels indicate increased ICP before the appearance of papilledema. Retinal hemorrhages are seen in acute head injuries, including shaken baby syndrome.

Less urgent but important additional assessments include examination of the scalp for lacerations and palpation for other

EMERGENCY

Head Injury

For head injuries requiring resuscitation:

C—Circulation
A—Airway (with cervical-spine immobilization)
B—Bleeding

Stabilize neck and spine immediately. Use jaw thrust, not chin lift, to open airway if required.

Keep NPO (nothing by mouth) until instructed otherwise.

Assess for the following:

- Loss of consciousness
- Amnesia
- Discomfort (crying) more than 10 minutes after injury
- Headache that is severe, worsening, interferes with sleep
- Fluid leaking from ears or nose
- Blackened eyes
- Vomiting three or more times, beginning after injury, or continuing 4 to 6 hours after injury
- Swelling in front of or above earlobe or increased swelling
- Confusion or abnormal behaviour

Symptoms in a child difficult to arouse from sleep:

- Difficulty speaking
- Blurred vision or diplopia
- Unsteady gait
- Difficulty using extremities, weakness, or incoordination
- Neck pain or stiffness
- Pupils dilated, unequal, or fixed
- Infant with full or bulging fontanel
- Seizures

Do not give analgesics or sedatives.

Check pupil reaction every 4 hours (including twice during night) for 48 hours.

Interventions and treatment:

- Clean any abrasions with soap and water.
- Apply clean dressing.
- If bleeding, apply ice to relieve pain and swelling and to decrease blood flow.

Awaken twice during the night to check level of consciousness.

abnormalities. A significant amount of blood loss can occur from scalp lacerations. An underlying skull fracture should be ruled out by CT scan.

NURSING ALERT

Bleeding from the nose or ears needs further evaluation, and a watery discharge from the nose (rhinorrhea) that is positive for glucose (as tested with Dextrostix) suggests leaking of CSF from a skull fracture.

An accurate assessment of clinical signs provides **baseline data**. Serial evaluations, preferably by a single observer, help to detect changes in the neurological status. Alterations in mental status, evidenced by increased difficulty in rousing the child, mounting agitation, development of focal lateral neurological signs, or marked changes in vital signs, usually indicate extension or progression of the basic pathological process.

Special tests. After a thorough clinical examination, a variety of diagnostic tests are helpful in providing a more definitive diagnosis of the type and extent of the trauma. The severity of a head injury may not be apparent on clinical examination of a child, but it will be detectable on a CT scan. Whenever the child has a history consistent with a serious head injury (e.g., occupant in a severe motor vehicle accident or a fall from a significant height), it is important that a scan be performed even if the child initially appears alert and oriented. All children with head injuries who have any alteration of consciousness, headache, vomiting, skull fracture, seizure, or a predisposing medical condition should also undergo CT scanning.

After a head injury, an MRI may be useful in detecting and evaluating cerebral edema or structural brain abnormalities. A neurobehavioural assessment can assist in identifying any cognitive impairments. Skull x-rays are of little benefit in diagnosing skull fractures. EEG is not helpful for diagnosis of head injury but is useful for defining seizure activity. Lumbar puncture is rarely used in craniocerebral trauma and is contraindicated in the presence of increased ICP because of the possibility of herniation. See Table 50-1 for a description of tests.

Post-traumatic syndromes. Post-traumatic syndromes include post-concussion syndrome, post-traumatic seizures, and structural complications after a head injury.

Post-concussion syndrome is a common sequela to brain injury with or without loss of consciousness. Symptoms can develop within hours to days after a mild head injury but can also occur after moderate to severe head injury. The manifestations vary with the child's age and include nausea, dizziness, headache, diplopia, disorientation, fatigue, irritability, anxiety, insomnia, loss of concentration, disorientation, and memory impairment (Yeates, Taylor, Rusin, et al., 2009). Structural complications (e.g., hydrocephalus) may occur after a head injury. Clinical sequelae include cognitive deterioration, motor deficits, optic atrophy, cranial nerve palsies, and aphasia. The type of residual effect depends on the location and nature of the disorder.

The duration of manifestations can vary from several days to several months. Death from concussion is preventable unless overwhelming secondary brain injury has occurred (Blinman, Houseknecht, Snyder, et al., 2009).

Post-traumatic seizures occur in a number of children who survive a head injury and are more common in children than in adults (O'Neill, Handler, Tong, et al., 2015). Seizures are more likely to occur within the first few days after a severe head injury.

Therapeutic Management

Most children with mild to moderate concussion who have not lost consciousness can be cared for and observed at home after careful examination reveals no serious intracranial injury. Nurses should provide parents with clear explanations and instructions and should encourage them to ask questions both before and after leaving the medical facility if clarification is needed (see Family-Centred Teaching box).

The parents should be instructed to check the child every 2 hours to determine any changes in responsiveness. The sleeping child should be wakened to see if he or she can be roused normally. It is important to interpret results carefully, as young children can often display signs of confusion when awoken from a deep sleep, rather than as a result of the head injury. For children with a concussion, it is important for parents to ensure that the child rest until all symptoms are gone and not play sports, exercise, or participate in any recreational activities. As well, parents should be advised to limit their child's activities such as reading, texting, watching television, doing computer work, and playing electronic games (Purcell & CPS, Healthy Active Living and Sports Medicine Committee, 2014). Parents need to maintain contact with the health care provider, who will usually wish to examine the child again in 1 or 2 days. The manifestations of epidural hematoma in children do not generally appear until 24 hours or more after injury.

Children with severe injuries, those who have lost consciousness for more than a few minutes, and those with prolonged and continued seizures or other focal or diffuse neurological signs must be hospitalized until their condition is stable and their neurological signs have diminished. The child is maintained on nothing by mouth (NPO) or restricted to clear liquids, if able to take fluids by mouth, until it is determined that vomiting will not occur. IV fluids are indicated in the child who is comatose or displays dulled sensorium and in the child with persistent vomiting. Fluid balance is closely monitored by daily weights; accurate intake and output measurements; and serum osmolality to detect early signs of water retention, excessive dehydration, and states of hypertonicity or hypotonicity.

The volume of IV fluid needs to be carefully monitored to avoid aggravating any cerebral edema and to minimize the possibility of overhydration in case of SIADH. However, damage to the hypothalamus or pituitary gland may produce DI with its accompanying hypertonicity and dehydration.

FAMILY-CENTRED TEACHING

Maintaining Contact

Maintaining contact with parents for continued observation and re-evaluation of the child, when indicated, facilitates early diagnosis and treatment of possible complications from head injury, such as hematoma, hydrocephalus, cysts, and post-traumatic seizures. Children are generally hospitalized for 24 to 48 hours' observation if their family lives far from medical facilities or lacks transportation or a telephone that would provide access to immediate help. Other circumstances such as language or other communication barriers, or even emotional trauma, may hinder learning and make it difficult for families to feel confident in caring for their child at home.

MEDICATION ALERT

Sedating drugs are commonly withheld in the acute phase of head injuries. Headaches are usually controlled with acetaminophen, although opioids may be needed. Antiepileptics are used for seizure control and frequently in cases of suspected contusion or laceration. Antibiotics may be administered if lacerations, CSF leakage, or excessive cerebral tissue damage is present. Prophylactic tetanus toxoid is given as appropriate. Cerebral edema is managed as described for the unconscious child. Hyperthermia is controlled with tepid sponges or a hypothermia blanket.

Surgical therapy. Scalp lacerations are sutured after the underlying bone is carefully examined. Depressed fractures require surgical reduction and removal of bone fragments. Torn dura is sutured. Ping-pong ball skull fractures in very young infants ordinarily correct themselves within a few weeks; however, some may require further surgical intervention.

Prognosis

The outcome of craniocerebral trauma depends on the extent of injury and complications. More than 90% of children with concussions or simple linear fractures recover without symptoms after the initial period. The incidence of fatalities and neurological sequelae is lower in children than in adults, even in those with severe head injuries. The prognosis for recovery is primarily related to the duration of coma and the degree of injury. The combination of impaired consciousness and skull fracture carries the highest risk of complication.

The concern regarding outcome is increasingly focused on cognitive, emotional, and mental issues. Children experience a higher frequency of psychological disturbances after head injury, whereas adults are more prone to physical complaints. Children may be more vulnerable than adults to long-term cognitive and behavioural dysfunction after diffuse brain injury. Even with recovery, the effects of brain injury on a child's potential can never be known (Yeates et al., 2009).

True coma (not obeying commands, eyes closed, and not speaking) usually does not last more than 2 weeks. A child's eventual outcome can range from brain death to a persistent vegetative state to complete recovery. However, even the best recovery may be associated with personality changes, including mood lability and loss of confidence; impaired short-term memory; headaches; and subtle cognitive impairments. Many children are left with significant disabilities after a head injury that appear months later as learning difficulties, behavioural changes, or emotional disturbances (Barlow et al., 2015). Generally, within 6 months to 1 year after the injury, 90% of the long-term neurological outcome has been achieved.

NURSING CARE

The hospitalized child requires careful neurological assessment and evaluation (including vital signs) repeated at frequent intervals to provide information needed to establish a correct diagnosis, reveal signs and symptoms of increased ICP, determine clinical management, prevent complications, and provide support to the child and family during the recovery phases. Frequent examinations of vital signs, neurological signs, and LOC are extremely important nursing observations. When possible, they should be performed by a single observer to better detect subtle changes that may indicate worsening neurological status. Pupils are checked for size, equality, reaction to light, and accommodation. After the initial elevations usually seen following injury, the vital signs generally return to normal unless there is brainstem involvement. An axillary measurement of temperature is the safest method, since seizures are not uncommon and vomiting is a frequent response in children, especially when the child is disturbed.

The child is placed on bedrest, usually with the head of the bed slightly elevated and the child's head in a midline position. Appropriate safety measures, such as keeping side rails raised and maintaining seizure precautions, need to be implemented. For the extremely restless child, hard surfaces may have to be padded and restraints used to prevent the possibility of further injury. A quiet environment helps reduce restlessness and irritability and when left undisturbed, many children will fall asleep. Shining bright lights directly into the child's face is irritating and often aggravates the child, making assessment of ocular responses difficult. Care should be individualized according to the child's specific needs.

The most important nursing observation is assessment of the child's LOC. Alterations in consciousness appear earlier in the progression of an injury than alterations of vital signs or focal neurological signs. Some expected responses may be misinterpreted as deviations from normal. Frequent examinations of alertness are fatiguing to the child; thus the child will often want to fall asleep, which may be confused with depressed consciousness. It is not uncommon to observe ocular divergence through the partially closed eyelids.

A key nursing role is to provide sedation and analgesia for the child. The conflict between the need to promote comfort and relieve anxiety in the child versus the need to assess for neurological changes presents a dilemma for the nurse. However, both goals can be achieved with close observation of the child's LOC and response to analgesics, use of a pain assessment record, and effective communication with the physician. Decreasing restlessness after administration of an analgesic most likely reflects pain control rather than a declining LOC.

Observations of position and movement provide additional information. Any abnormal posturing should be noted, as well as whether it occurs continuously or intermittently. Questions nurses might consider include the following:

- Are the child's handgrips strong and equal in strength?
- Are there any signs of flexion or extension posturing?
- What is the child's response to stimulation?
- Is movement purposeful, random, or absent?
- Are movement and sensation equal on both sides or restricted to one side only?

The child may communicate having a headache or other discomfort. The child who is too young to describe a headache will be fussy and resist being handled. The child who suffers from vertigo will often assume a position of comfort and vigorously resist efforts to be moved. Forcible movement causes the child to vomit and display spontaneous nystagmus. Seizures, relatively common in children with craniocerebral trauma, may be of any type but are more often generalized, regardless of the type of injury. Any seizure activity should be carefully observed, described in detail, and recorded. Children in postictal (postseizure) states are lethargic, with sluggish pupils.

Drainage from any orifice should be noted. Bleeding from the ear suggests the possibility of a basal skull fracture. Clear nasal discharge suggests an anterior basal skull fracture. The amount and characteristics of drainage should be observed, recorded, and reported.

NURSING ALERT

Suctioning through the nares is contraindicated because of the risk of the catheter entering the brain parenchyma through a fracture in the skull.

Head trauma is frequently accompanied by other undetected injuries; thus any bruises, lacerations, or evidence of internal injuries or fractures of the extremities need to be noted and reported. Associated injuries should be evaluated and treated appropriately.

The child with normal LOC is usually allowed clear liquids unless fluid is restricted. If the child has an IV infusion, it should be maintained as prescribed. The diet is advanced to that appropriate for the child's age as soon as the condition permits. Intake and output need to be measured and recorded. Any incontinence of bowel or bladder needs to be noted in the child who has been toilet trained.

The child should be observed for any unusual behaviour, but it should be interpreted in relation to the child's normal behaviour. For example, urinary incontinence during sleep would be of no consequence for a child who routinely wets the bed but would be highly significant for one who is always dry. Parents are valuable resources in evaluating objective behaviour of their child (e.g., the ease with which the child is roused normally, the usual sleeping position and patterns, motor activities [rolling over, sitting up, climbing], hearing and visual acuity, appetite, and manner of eating [spoon, bottle, cup]).

Family Support

The emotional and educational support of the family of children who have suffered head injury presents a formidable, challenging aspect to nursing care. The nurse can encourage the family to be involved in the child's care, to bring in familiar belongings, or to make a tape recording of familiar voices and sounds. Parents may need a demonstration on how to touch or cuddle their child while being connected to monitoring equipment in a critical care unit and may want to talk about their grief. The nurse can listen attentively, reinforce what is being done to assist the child, and direct parents toward signs and symptoms of recovery. A common phenomenon is for families to seek information from all health care providers, asking, "What will she be like? What do you know?" as they search for some clue that the child is recovering. Honesty and kindness, along with competent care, can help families through this difficult time.

When the child is discharged, the parents should be advised of probable post-traumatic symptoms that may be expected, such as behavioural changes, sleep disturbances, phobias, and seizures. They should understand observations they need to make and how to contact the health care provider with follow-up questions or concerns. The importance of follow-up evaluation should be emphasized.

Rehabilitation

The rehabilitation and management of the child with permanent brain injury are essential aspects of care. Rehabilitation of brain-injured children is begun as soon as feasible and usually involves the family and a rehabilitation team. Careful assessment of the child's capabilities, limitations, and potential needs should be made as early as possible and appropriate interventions implemented to maximize the residual capacities. The Rancho Los Amigos Scale provides a **systematic assessment** of the possible progress a child may achieve after a severe head injury (see Additional Resources).

The child with a disability resulting from head trauma requires assessment on a physical, cognitive, emotional, and social level. The child has likely experienced separation, pain, sensory deprivation and overload, changes in circadian cycle, and fear of unfamiliar procedures and environment. Recovery and transition require new coping strategies at the same time that regressive and acting-out behaviour may start. A rehabilitation facility or home rehabilitation is advocated when the child has progressed beyond what can be provided in the hospital setting. The Brain Injury Association of Canada provides information and listings of rehabilitation services and support groups throughout the country (see Additional Resources at the end of this chapter).

Prevention

Tremendous strides have been made in the prevention of cerebral damage after head injury in children. The greatest benefit lies in preventing head injuries from occurring in the first place. Nurses can play a key role in promoting injury prevention. The reason many head injuries continue to occur is that unnecessary risks go unchecked; inadequate supervision combined with a child's natural sense of indestructibility and exploration can lead to lethal results. Nurses are in the unique position to educate caregivers about growth and development expectations and risk management. Public education, coupled with legislative support, can help prevent childhood injuries. (For extensive discussions of childhood injuries and prevention for specific age groups, see Chapters 35 to 39.)

Submersion Injuries

The term **submersion injury** has replaced the term *near-drowning* and should be used to describe injury occurring up until the time of drowning-related death. This term includes any person who experiences distress from near-drowning submersion or immersion in liquid that results in death (*drowning*) or survival at least 24 hours after submersion (*near-drowning*). Submersion injury is a major cause of accidental death in children over 1 year of age. Drowning is the second leading cause of injury-related death for children in Canada. Every year, approximately 60 children drown, and another 140 children must stay in the hospital because they have a submersion injury that can result in long-term health effects (Parachute, n.d.). Toddlers aged 1 to 4 years of age are at greatest risk because they are attracted to water but cannot understand the danger, can walk but cannot swim, have lungs that are smaller than adults' and fill quickly with water, and can drown in as little as 2.5 cm (1 inch) of water (Parachute, n.d.). (See Chapters 36 through 38 for more information on water safety.)

Most cases of submersion injury are accidental and usually involve the following individuals:

- Children who are helpless in water, such as inadequately attended children in or near swimming pools or infants in bathtubs or containers of fluid
- Small children who fall into ponds, streams, and flooded excavations, usually near home
- Occupants of pleasure boats who fail to wear life preservers
- Children who have diving accidents
- Children who are able to swim but overestimate their endurance

Accidental drowning occurs five times more often among boys than among girls, almost 40% of children are younger than age 5, and 90% of cases of drowning in pools occur in private swimming pools (Lifesaving Society Canada, 2015). New immigrants or visitors to Canada, especially those who have been in Canada for less than 5 years, may be more likely to be unable to swim than those born in Canada (Lifesaving Society Canada, 2015). Children younger than 1 year old who drown are most likely to have drowned in a bathtub. Buckets filled with fluid cause a risk of drowning to top-heavy toddlers, who can fall head first into the bucket (Hon & Leung, 2010). Preschoolers are at risk for drowning in swimming pools, and drowning among school-age children and adolescents most commonly occurs in natural bodies of water, such as lakes, ponds, and rivers (Caglar & Quan, 2016). The suction created at the outlet of pools, hot tubs, or whirlpool spas is strong enough to trap any child, even larger children, underwater. Drowning as a form of fatal child abuse has also been recognized as a problem.

Pathophysiology

Hypoxia is the primary cause of injury when submersion occurs and can cause damage to the brain, lungs, heart, kidneys, liver, and gastrointestinal system. Cerebral hypoxia is the major component of morbidity and mortality with submersion events. Within minutes of a submersion, a lack of oxygen leads to coma and untimely cardiac arrest (Caglar & Quan, 2016).

Pathophysiological features in submersion injuries are hypoxia, aspiration, and hypothermia. Hypoxia is related to the duration of anoxia and asphyxia. Different cells tolerate variable lengths of anoxia, causing variations of cell damage. Neurons, especially cerebral cells, sustain irreversible damage after 4 to 6 minutes of submersion. The heart and lungs can survive up to 30 minutes. Regardless of the amount of water aspirated, there is arterial hypoxemia (resulting from atelectasis with shunting of blood through the nonventilated alveoli) and a combined respiratory acidosis (resulting from retained carbon dioxide) and metabolic acidosis (caused by buildup of acid metabolites from anaerobic metabolism). Aspiration of fluid occurs in most drownings and is quickly absorbed in the pulmonary circulation, resulting in pulmonary edema, atelectasis, airway spasm, and pneumonitis. Approximately 10% of drowning victims die without aspirating fluid but succumb due to acute asphyxia as a result of prolonged reflex laryngospasm.

No clinical or physiological difference, therapy, or outcome has been noted among human survivors in the submersion of salt water versus fresh water (Caglar & Quan, 2016).

Children are at an increased risk of hypothermia because of their large surface area relative to body mass, decreased subcutaneous fat, and limited thermoregulation and partly as a result of the cold water itself (Caglar & Quan, 2016). Cold water decreases metabolic demands and activates the diving reflex, which causes blood to be shunted away from the periphery and concentrated to the brain and heart. However, prolonged submersion in cold liquids can impair cognition, coordination, and muscle strength, ultimately resulting in a loss of consciousness, decreased cardiac output, and cardiac arrest. Profound hypothermia is usually evidence of lengthy submersion (Caglar & Quan, 2016).

Therapeutic Management

The outcome of children after a submersion event depends on the circumstances and duration of the submersion and the speed and effectiveness of resuscitation efforts (Caglar & Quan, 2016). Resuscitative measures should begin at the scene, and the victim should be transported to the hospital with maximal ventilatory and circulatory support. In the hospital intensive care is implemented and continued according to the patient's needs.

In general, the management of the submersion injury victim is based on the degree of cerebral insult (Box 50-4). The first priority is to restore oxygen delivery to the cells and prevent further hypoxic damage. A spontaneously breathing child does well in an oxygen-enriched atmosphere; the more severely affected child will require endotracheal intubation

BOX 50-4 CLINICAL MANIFESTATIONS OF SUBMERSION INJURIES

Category A

Awake, minimal injury

Fully conscious; may have mild hypothermia, mild chest radiographic changes, mild arterial blood gas abnormalities

Category B

Blunted sensorium, moderate injury

Obtund, stuporous, purposeful response to painful stimuli, mild to moderate hypothermia, frequent respiratory distress, abnormal chest radiographs, arterial blood gas abnormalities

Category C

Comatose, severe anoxia

Unarousable, abnormal response to pain, abnormal respiratory pattern, seizures, shock, marked arterial blood gas abnormalities, abnormal chest radiographs, arrhythmias, metabolic acidosis, hyperkalemia, hyperglycemia, disseminated intravascular coagulation

C1—Decorticate posturing, Cheyne-Stokes respirations

C2—Decerebrate posturing, central hyperventilation

C3—Flaccid, apneic, or cluster breathing

C4—Flaccid, apneic, no detectable circulation

and mechanical ventilation. Blood gases and pH are monitored frequently as a guide to oxygen, fluid, and electrolyte therapies.

NURSING ALERT

All children who have had a submersion injury should be admitted to the hospital for observation. Almost half of asymptomatic or minimally symptomatic alert children experience complications (e.g., respiratory compromise, cerebral edema) during the first 24 hours after the incident (Caglar & Quan, 2016).

Aspiration pneumonia is a frequent complication that occurs about 48 to 72 hours after the episode. Bronchospasm, alveolocapillary membrane damage, atelectasis, abscess formation, and acute respiratory distress syndrome are other complications that occur after aspiration of fluid.

Prognosis

Studies report that the best predictors of a good outcome are length of submersion for less than 5 minutes and the presence of sinus rhythm, reactive pupils, and neurological responsiveness at the scene. The worst prognoses—for death or severe neurological impairment—are for children submerged for more than 10 minutes and not responding to advanced life support within 25 minutes. All children without spontaneous, purposeful movement and normal brainstem function 24 hours after a submersion injury sustain severe neurological deficits or die (Caglar & Quan, 2016).

NURSING CARE

Nursing care depends on the child's condition. A child who survives may need intensive respiratory nursing care with attention to vital signs, mechanical ventilation or tracheostomy or both, blood gas determination, and IV infusion. Frequently the child is comatose for an indefinite period and requires the same care as an unconscious child. A difficult aspect in the care of the child victim of submersion injury is helping the parents cope with severe guilt reactions. The magnitude of the event is so great that efforts to provide comfort and support may provide little solace. Parents need to hear that everything possible is being done to treat the child, and this message needs to be repeated often.

The parents of the child who is saved from death are also faced with the anxiety of not knowing what the outcome will be. It is important for these families to know that they are not alone. They need to be reminded frequently that there are caring people to assist them both during the crisis and later. Additional sources of support can include psychiatric and social work consultants, community services, and religious support. Support groups may be beneficial if these are available in the community.

Nurses often have difficulty relating to the parents if obvious neglect has precipitated the accident and subsequent problems. It is important for those who care for these children and their families to assess their own feelings about the situation, as well as the family's coping abilities and resources.

Prevention

Most drownings, particularly of infants or small children, can be prevented with adequate supervision. Water safety and survival training should be required for all school-age children, and nurses can be active advocates for such training in their communities. Nurses are also in a position to emphasize the importance of adequate adult supervision when children are in the water. Aquatic programs for infants and toddlers do not decrease the risk of drowning; young children should *never* be left unattended when in or near the water (Parachute, n.d.). Parents with pools should know **cardiopulmonary resuscitation (CPR)** techniques. Pool fencing, pool covers, and water entry alarms are additional ways to protect children (see also Injury Prevention, Chapters 35 to 39).

NERVOUS SYSTEM TUMOURS

Brain tumour and neuroblastoma are two major forms of childhood cancer derived from neural tissue. CNS tumours account for approximately 20% of all childhood cancers and occur most often in children under 15 years of age (Canadian Cancer Society, Advisory Committee on Cancer Statistics, 2015). Both of these tumours are difficult to treat and have not demonstrated the dramatic improvements in survival seen in other forms of childhood cancer.

Brain Tumours

Brain tumours are the most common solid tumours in children and are the second most common childhood cancer. The Canadian Cancer Society (2016a) reported that from 2006 to 2010, there were 860 Canadian children aged 0 to 14 years diagnosed with childhood brain and spinal cord cancer; 100 children were diagnosed with ependymoma; 370 children were diagnosed with astrocytoma; and 190 children were diagnosed with intracranial and intraspinal embryonal tumours. From 2007 to 2011 among Canadian children aged 0 to 14 years, 216 children died from childhood brain and spinal cord cancers (Canadian Cancer Society, 2016a).

CNS tumours can arise from any cell within the brain or spinal cord. The cell origin provides a histological classification. For instance, astrocytes (cells that form the supportive tissue for neurons) may form a common glial tumour called an *astrocytoma*. A specific type of tumour called *ependymoma* typically arises within or adjacent to the ependymoma lining of the ventricular system. CNS tumours in children are typically glial or neuronal in origin, located in the infratentorium, and generally sensitive to radiation and adjuvant chemotherapy (Merchant, Pollack, & Loeffler, 2010). *Infratentorial* brain tumours occur in the area of the brain below the tentorium cerebelli involving the cerebellum or brainstem and account for about 60% of tumours. Types of infratentorial tumours include medulloblastoma, ependymoma, cerebellar astrocytoma, and brainstem glioma. Tumours above the tentorium are referred to as *supratentorial* and may include astrocytoma, primitive neuroectodermal tumour, craniopharyngioma, and optic pathway glioma. The suprasellar and pineal regions of the brain often are at the location of germ cell tumours.

Diagnostic Evaluation

The signs and symptoms of brain tumours are directly related to their anatomical location and size and, to some extent, the child's age. In infants and very young children whose cranial sutures are still open, initial signs and symptoms of increased ICP (headache, vomiting, and lethargy) may not be evident and symptoms may include irritability, failure to thrive, and loss of developmental milestones.

Diagnosis of a brain tumour is based subjectively on presenting clinical signs, objectively on neurological tests, and histological diagnosis via surgery. Because the signs and symptoms are vague and easily overlooked, early diagnosis relies on a high index of suspicion during history taking. A number of tests may be used in the neurological evaluation, but the most common diagnostic procedure is MRI. Other tests include CT, angiography, electroencephalography, and lumbar puncture (see Table 50-1). The definitive diagnosis is based on brain tissue specimens obtained during surgery.

Therapeutic Management

Treatment may involve the use of surgery, radiotherapy, and chemotherapy or a combination of these treatment modalities. The optimal treatment is total removal of the tumour without residual neurological damage. Patients with the most complete tumour removal have the greatest chance of survival. Radiation therapy is an integral part of treatment for many brain tumours but can cause significant neurocognitive side effects and endocrinopathies. Because rapid brain development occurs during the first few years of life, radiation therapy, particularly craniospinal radiation, is avoided in children younger than 3 years of age. Chemotherapy may be used as primary treatment or in an effort to delay radiation therapy until patients are older and may experience fewer neurocognitive adverse effects. One of the challenges in using chemotherapy for CNS tumours is the blood–brain barrier, which is a natural barrier that significantly influences the penetration of substances into the CNS. Commonly used chemotherapy agents to treat brain tumours in children include cisplatin, carboplatin, vincristine, cyclophosphamide, lomustine, etoposide, and temozolomide (Parsons, Pollack, Haas-Kogan, et al., 2016). Chemotherapy is also used as adjunct therapy for residual tumour, nonresectable tumour, or recurrent tumour.

Prognosis

The prognosis for a child with a brain tumour varies greatly and depends on the type of brain tumour, the size of the tumour, the extent of the disease, the child's age, and surgical resectability. Recent advances in surgical instrumentation allowing aggressive surgical intervention (e.g., stereotactic surgery, radiosurgery), modifications in radiation (e.g., hyperfractionation, brain mapping), and use of chemotherapy (e.g., intrathecal, intratumoural) have increased the long-term survival rates for many children with brain tumours (Parsons et al., 2016). Currently, the overall survival rate for CNS tumours in children younger than 15 years of age is approximately 73% (Canadian Cancer Society, Advisory Committee on Cancer Statistics, 2015). Despite an improvement in overall survival, children with brain tumours, particularly those who are very young at diagnosis, may have significant physical, cognitive, and endocrinological sequelae because of their tumour and associated treatment (Shaw, 2009).

NURSING CARE

If a brain tumour is suspected in a child admitted to the hospital for cerebral dysfunction, establishing baseline data with which to compare preoperative and postoperative changes is an essential step. It also allows the nurse to assess the degree of physical incapacity and the family's reaction to the diagnosis.

Vital signs, including pulse pressure (the difference between systolic and diastolic pressures), need to be taken routinely and more often when any change is noted. Any sudden variations should be reported immediately. Observation for symptoms of Cushing triad (i.e., hallmark sign of increased ICP, which includes bradycardia, hypertension, and irregular respirations) is a crucial role of the nurse. It is especially important to note a change in vital signs during or after diagnostic procedures. A routine neurological assessment is performed at the same time as taking vital signs, and head circumference is measured on infants and very young children. The child should be observed for evidence of headache, vomiting, and any seizure activity. The location, severity, and duration of the headache need to be noted, as well as its relationship to activity and time of day and any associated factors noted. Behaviours such as lying flat and facing away from light or refusing to engage in play are clues to discomfort in the nonverbal child. The child's gait should be observed at least once daily. Head tilt while talking or performing an activity and other changes in posturing are always noted.

Prevention of Postoperative Complications

Usually the surgeon will prescribe specific orders for vital signs, neurological checks, positioning, fluid regulation, and medication. These vary somewhat, depending on the location of the craniotomy. The following discussion addresses general principles of care for infratentorial or supratentorial surgery. Additional aspects of care that are discussed elsewhere may include care of the child with seizures and neurological assessment of the unconscious child.

Vital signs should be taken as frequently as every 15 to 30 minutes until the child is stable. Temperature measurement is particularly important because of hyperthermia resulting from surgical intervention in the hypothalamus or brainstem and from some types of general anaesthesia. To prepare for this reaction, a cooling blanket should be placed on the bed before the child returns to the unit so that it is ready for use if required. The temperature needs to be monitored carefully when any cooling measures are taken because hypothermia can occur suddenly. Recognizing signs of other complications such as increased ICP, meningitis, and respiratory tract infection is imperative.

Neurological checks are an essential aspect of care and include pupillary reaction to light, LOC, sleep patterns, and response to stimuli. Although children may be less responsive for a few days after surgery, when they regain full consciousness there should be a steady increase in alertness. Regression to a lethargic, irritable state indicates increasing pressure, possibly caused by hemorrhage, meningitis or cerebral edema.

! NURSING ALERT

Sluggish, dilated, or unequal pupils need to be reported immediately because they may indicate increased ICP and potential brainstem herniation, a medical emergency.

Observations for function are not instituted until the child regains consciousness. However, as soon as possible the nurse should begin testing reflexes, handgrip, and functioning of the cranial nerves. Muscle strength is usually diminished as a result of general weakness after surgery but should improve daily. Ataxia may be significantly worse with cerebellar intervention, but it will slowly improve. Edema near the cranial nerves may depress important functions such as the gag, blink, or swallowing reflex.

Dressings need to be observed for evidence of drainage. If soiled, the dressing is not removed but is reinforced with dry sterile gauze. The approximate amount of drainage should be estimated and recorded. A drain may be placed in the operative site.

! NURSING ALERT

To keep an accurate account of drainage, the soiled area is circled with a pen approximately every hour. In this way, continuous bleeding is easily recognized. The presence of colourless drainage should be reported immediately, since it most likely is CSF from the incisional area. A foul odour from the dressing may indicate an infection. Such a finding should be reported, and the nurse should anticipate that a culture will be taken from the site.

Correct positioning after surgery is critical to prevent pressure against the operative site, reduce ICP, and avoid the danger of aspiration. If a large tumour was removed, the child should not be placed on the operative side, since the brain may suddenly shift to that cavity, causing trauma to the blood vessels, linings, and the brain itself. The nurse should confer with the surgeon to be certain of the correct position, including degree of neck flexion. The first 24 to 48 hours after brain surgery are critical. If the child's position is restricted, notice of this should be posted above the head of the bed. When the child is turned, every precaution should be taken to prevent jarring or malalignment and to prevent undue strain on the sutures. Two nurses are needed for repositioning the child—one supporting the head and the other supporting the body. The use of a turning sheet may facilitate turning a heavy child.

The child with an infratentorial procedure is usually positioned on either side with the bed flat. When a supratentorial craniotomy is performed, the head of the bed is elevated 20 to 30 degrees with the child on either side or on the back. In a supratentorial craniotomy the head elevation facilitates CSF drainage and decreases excessive blood flow to the brain to prevent hemorrhage. Pillows should be placed against the child's back, not head, to maintain the desired position. Ordinarily the head and neck are kept in midline with the body, and the neck should not be flexed to support venous drainage (Christie, 2008).

! NURSING ALERT

The Trendelenburg position is contraindicated in both infratentorial and supratentorial surgeries because it increases ICP and the risk of hemorrhage. If shock is impending, a primary physician knowledgeable of the child's condition should be notified immediately, before the head is lowered.

With an infratentorial craniotomy, the child is allowed nothing by mouth for at least 24 hours, or longer if the gag and swallowing reflexes are depressed or the child is comatose. With a supratentorial operation cranial neuropathy is less likely, and clear fluids may be resumed soon after the child is alert, sometimes within 24 hours. If the child vomits, oral liquids are stopped. Vomiting not only predisposes the child to aspiration, but also increases ICP and the potential for incisional rupture.

The child should be fed to conserve energy and minimize movement. If there are any cranial nerve deficits, the child should be fed slowly to prevent choking or aspiration. Thickening agents can be used if the patient experiences dysphagia with thin liquids. Sometimes enteral feeding is necessary when body functions are too depressed to permit safe oral feedings or when the child refuses to eat or drink. IV fluids should be continued until oral fluids are well tolerated or enteral feeding is established. Because of the postoperative cerebral edema and danger of increased ICP, fluid status needs to be carefully monitored.

Headache may be severe and is largely a result of cerebral edema. Measures to relieve some of the discomfort include providing a quiet, dimly lit environment; restricting visitors; preventing any sudden jarring movements, such as banging into the bed; and preventing an increase in ICP. Avoiding increased ICP is most effectively achieved by proper positioning and prevention of straining, such as during coughing, vomiting, or defecating. As stated earlier, the use of opioids, such as morphine, to relieve pain is controversial because they may mask signs of altered consciousness or depress respirations. However, they can be given safely, since naloxone can be used to reverse opioid effects, such as sedation or respiratory depression. Acetaminophen is also an effective analgesic for mild to moderate pain. The nurse must be aware that acetaminophen can mask a fever, which could indicate postoperative infection. Regardless of the medications used, adequate dosage and regular administration are essential to providing optimal pain relief (see also Pain Assessment; Pain Management, Chapter 34). Placing an ice bag on the forehead may also provide some headache relief, especially if facial edema is severe. Constipation is a common postoperative issue because of anaesthesia and immobility, and the use of narcotics for pain control may further contribute to constipation. Patients should be given a bowel regimen during the postoperative period until normal bowel function returns.

Support of the Child and Family

The family's emotional needs are immense when the diagnosis is a brain tumour; feelings can be influenced by the extent of surgery, any neurological deficits, the expected prognosis, and additional therapy (see Additional Resources at the end of this chapter). Since few definitive answers can be given before surgery, the surgeon's report is a significant finding that can vary from a completely benign, resected neoplasm to a highly malignant, invasive, and only partially removed tumour. Although parents often try to prepare themselves for the worst possible scenario, being given the news that their child has a potentially fatal tumour or may have significant neurological impairment from the necessary treatment is always devastating.

Parents should be encouraged to express their feelings about the diagnosis. Often they will express tremendous guilt for viewing the insidious onset of symptoms, such as ataxia, visual difficulty, and headache or school performance issues, as "minor complaints" by the child. The nurse needs to exercise particular care not to make any comments that insinuate that the parents should have sought medical advice sooner, because this only compounds any feelings of guilt that already exist. During this period, the nurse should also discuss with parents what they plan to tell the child. If the child was prepared honestly, the diagnosis can be expressed in an age-appropriate manner. During recovery the child will need additional explanation about the treatment and the reason for any residual neurological effects, such as ataxia or blindness. The increasing availability of child life specialists has served as a useful resource in explaining diagnoses such as brain tumours to children and helping them cope with hospitalization and necessary treatment and to understand physical sequelae they may experience (Reynolds & Boyd, 2010).

Neuroblastoma

Neuroblastomas are the most common malignant extracranial solid tumours in children and account for 8 to 10% of all childhood cancers (Mullassery, Dominici, Jesudason, et al., 2009). In Canada, from 2006 to 2010, there were 355 children and youths ages 0 to 19 years who were newly diagnosed with neuroblastoma (Canadian Cancer Society, 2016b). Approximately 95% of children with neuroblastoma manifest the disease before 10 years of age, with a median age of occurrence at 23 months (Park, Eggert, & Caron, 2010). The death rate for neuroblastoma is low; in Canada between 2007 and 2011 five deaths occurred in children and youth 0 to 19 years of age (Canadian Cancer Society, 2016b).

These tumours originate from embryonic neural crest cells that normally give rise to the adrenal medulla and the sympathetic ganglia. Consequently, the majority of tumours develop in the abdomen along the adrenal gland or the retroperitoneal sympathetic chain. Other sites may be in the head, neck, chest, or pelvis.

The signs and symptoms of neuroblastoma depend on the location and stage of the disease. Neuroblastoma is commonly referred to as a "silent" tumour because approximately half of the patients present with localized disease and display few symptoms. However, children with advanced disease are ill appearing, with symptoms of periorbital ecchymoses, proptosis, bone pain, and irritability caused by extensive tumour metastasis usually in the lymph nodes, bone marrow, skeletal system, skin, or liver (Park et al., 2010).

Diagnostic Evaluation

The objective of diagnosis is to locate the primary site and areas of metastasis. Most presenting signs are caused by compression of adjacent structures. Skeletal survey; skull, neck, chest, abdominal, and bone CT scans; and bilateral bone marrow aspirations and biopsies are used to locate a tumour mass and metastasis. A metaiodobenzylguanidine (MIBG) scan is used to determine involvement of bone, bone marrow, and soft tissue.

Urinary excretion of catecholamines is detected in approximately 95% of children with adrenal or sympathetic tumours. Analyzing the breakdown products excreted in the urine, namely vanillylmandelic acid, homovanillic acid, dopamine, and norepinephrine, enables detection of suspected tumour before and after medical-surgical intervention (Mullassery et al., 2009). Amplification of proto-oncogene, known as the *N-myc* gene, and chromosomal abnormalities correlates strongly with advanced-stage disease, rapid tumour progression, and a poor prognosis (Brodeur, Hogarty, Bagatell, et al., 2016).

Therapeutic Management

Accurate clinical staging is important for establishing initial treatment. Therefore, surgery is used both to remove as much of the tumour as possible and to obtain biopsies. In early stages, complete surgical removal of the tumour is the treatment of choice. If the tumour is large, partial resection is attempted, with a course of irradiation postoperatively to shrink the tumour in the hope of complete removal at a later date. Surgery is usually limited to biopsy in stages III and IV because of the extensive metastasis, although the use of additional surgery to assess tumour regression or remove a regressed tumour is not unlikely.

Because radiotherapy can cause vertebral damage and growth arrest, it is contraindicated with intraspinal tumours; however, it can be used for emergency management of a massive neuroblastoma that is causing spinal cord compression (Mullassery et al., 2009). Radiotherapy also offers palliation for metastatic lesions in the bones, lung, liver, or brain.

Chemotherapy is the mainstay of therapy for extensive local or disseminated disease. Agents used in various combinations include cyclophosphamide, doxorubicin, cisplatin, etoposide, vincristine, ifosfamide, carboplatin, topotecan, and teniposide. In children with high-risk disease or recurrent disease, retinoic acid, radiotherapy, and myeloablative chemotherapy with peripheral stem cell rescue may be used to obtain a longer remission, even though the overall survival rate is poor in these particular children (Brodeur et al., 2016).

Prognosis

Generally, the younger the child at diagnosis (especially younger than 1 year of age), the better the survival rate. Neuroblastoma is one of the few tumours that demonstrate spontaneous regression (especially stage IV-S), possibly as a result of maturity of the embryonic cell or the development of an active immune system.

NURSING CARE

Nursing considerations are similar to those discussed for leukemia and brain tumours, including psychological and physical preparation for diagnostic and operative procedures; prevention of postoperative complications for abdominal, thoracic, or cranial surgery; and explanation of chemotherapy, radiotherapy, and their side effects (see Chapter 48).

Because of the sometimes high degree of metastasis at the time of diagnosis, many parents suffer substantial guilt for not having recognized signs earlier. Parents need much support in dealing with these feelings and expressing them to the appropriate people.

INTRACRANIAL INFECTIONS

The nervous system is subject to infection by the same organisms that affect other organs of the body. However, the nervous system is limited in the ways in which it responds to injury. Laboratory studies are needed to identify the causative agent. The inflammatory process can affect the meninges (meningitis) or brain (encephalitis).

While meningitis can be caused by a variety of organisms, the three main types are (1) bacterial, or pyogenic, caused by pus-forming bacteria, especially meningococci, pneumococci, and *Haemophilus* organisms; (2) viral, or aseptic, caused by a wide variety of viral agents; and (3) tuberculous, caused by the *tuberculin bacillus*. Most children with acute febrile intracranial infections have either bacterial meningitis or viral meningitis as the underlying cause. Bacterial meningitis is considered much more serious than viral meningitis. Compared with viral meningitis, which typically is short lived, self-limiting, and followed by complete recovery, complications from bacterial meningitis can be quite severe and include shock, coma, seizures, intellectual deficits, hearing loss, vision loss, and death (Somand & Meurer, 2009).

Bacterial Meningitis

Bacterial meningitis is an acute inflammation of the meninges and CSF. It remains a significant cause of illness in the pediatric age groups because of the residual damage caused by undiagnosed and untreated or inadequately treated cases. Overall, the incidence rate is highest among children less than 1 year of age and then declines as age increases, except for a smaller peak in the 15- to 19-year age group, with an increased mortality risk in the adolescent and young adult. Invasive meningococcal disease is found worldwide. An average of almost 200 cases per year occur in Canada (PHAC, 2014). Suspected bacterial meningitis is a medical emergency, and immediate action must be taken to identify the causative organism and initiate prompt treatment.

The advent of antimicrobial therapy has had a significant effect on the overall clinical course and prognosis of children with bacterial meningitis. However, the introduction of vaccines has made the most significant impact on the incidence of this disease. After the introduction of the *Haemophilus influenza* type b (Hib) vaccine in 1990 and the pneumococcal conjugate vaccines in 2000, the incidence of bacterial meningitis declined in all age groups except children younger than 2 months of age. The incidence of bacterial meningitis can be caused by a variety of bacterial agents. Currently, *Haemophilus influenzae* type b, *Streptococcus pneumoniae, Neisseria meningitidis* (meningococcus), group B streptococcus (GBS), and *Listeria monocyogenes* are responsible for bacterial meningitis in 95% of children older than 2 months.

Despite the dramatic decline in incidence of bacterial meningitis, this disease can still result in death, with a fatality rate of approximately 6.9% in children. The incidence is highest among patients younger than 2 months of age, with GBS being the most common causative organism. In Canada, meningococcal outbreaks are almost exclusively due to serogroup C *Neisseria meningitidis*. Other causative organisms include beta-hemolytic streptococci, *Staphylococcus aureus*, and *Escherichia coli*.

Meningococcal meningitis occurs in epidemic form and is the only type readily transmitted by droplet infection from nasopharyngeal secretions. Although this condition may develop at any age, the risk of meningococcal infection increases with the number of contacts; therefore, it occurs predominantly in school-age children and adolescents. Post secondary students, especially those living in dormitory residences, are at moderately increased risk for meningococcal disease compared with other people their age.

There appear to be some seasonal variations in etiology. Meningitis caused by *H. influenzae* occurs primarily in autumn or early winter. Pneumococcal and meningococcal infections can occur at any time but are more common in later winter or early spring.

Pathophysiology

The most common route of infection is vascular dissemination from a focus of infection elsewhere. For example, organisms from the nasopharynx invade the underlying blood vessels and enter the cerebral blood supply or form local thromboemboli that release septic emboli into the bloodstream. Invasion by direct extension from infections in the paranasal and mastoid sinuses is less common. Organisms also gain entry by direct implantation after penetrating wounds, skull fractures that provide an opening into the skin or sinuses, lumbar puncture or surgical procedures, anatomical abnormalities such as spina bifida, or foreign bodies such as an internal ventricular shunt or an external ventricular device. After implanting, the organisms spread into the CSF, by which the infection spreads throughout the subarachnoid space.

The infective process is like that seen in any bacterial infection: inflammation, exudation, white blood cell accumulation, and varying degrees of tissue damage. The brain becomes hyperemic and edematous, and the entire surface of the brain is covered by a layer of purulent exudate that varies with the type of organism. For example, meningococcal exudate is most marked over the parietal, occipital, and cerebellar regions; the thick, fibrinous exudate of pneumococcal infection is confined chiefly to the surface of the brain, particularly the anterior lobes; and the exudate of streptococcal infections is similar to that of pneumococcal infections, but thinner. As infection extends to the ventricles, thick pus, fibrin, or adhesions may occlude the narrow passages and obstruct the flow of CSF.

Clinical Manifestations

Patients with bacterial meningitis may present with fever and signs of meningeal irritation, including nausea, vomiting, irritability, anorexia, headache, photophobia, confusion, back pain, and nuchal rigidity (Box 50-5). A history of an upper respiratory infection often precedes these symptoms. Nuchal rigidity is manifested by inability to flex the neck and to place the chin on the chest as well as by the presence of Kernig and Brudzinski signs. The Kernig sign is present if the patient, in the supine position with the hip and knee flexed at 90 degrees, cannot extend the knee more than 135 degrees and pain is felt in the hamstrings. Flexion of the opposite knee may also occur. The Brudzinski sign is present if the patient, while in the supine position, flexes the lower extremities if passive flexion of the neck is attempted (Ball, Dains, Flynn, et al., 2015).

NURSING ALERT

Any child who is ill and develops a purpuric or petechial rash may have (overwhelming) meningococcemia and must receive medical attention immediately.

Diagnostic Evaluation

A lumbar puncture is the definitive diagnostic test for meningitis. The fluid pressure is measured, and samples are obtained for culture, Gram stain, blood cell count, and determination of glucose and protein content. The findings are usually diagnostic. Culture and sensitivity testing are needed to identify the causative organism. Spinal fluid pressure is usually elevated, but interpretation is often difficult when the child is crying. Sedation with fentanyl and midazolam can alleviate the child's pain and fear associated with this procedure. If there is evidence or suspicion of increased ICP (papilledema, focal neurological deficits, bulging fontanel), a CT scan of the head may be warranted before the procedure. Lumbar puncture is contraindicated in any patient with imaging to suggest that the procedure is not safe (e.g., midline shift, mass effect, transependymal migration of CSF). However, a "normal" CT does

BOX 50-5 CLINICAL MANIFESTATIONS OF BACTERIAL MENINGITIS

Children and Adolescents

Usually abrupt onset
Fever
Chills
Headache
Vomiting
Alterations in sensorium
Seizures (often the initial sign)
Irritability
Agitation
May develop:

- Photophobia
- Delirium
- Hallucinations
- Aggressive behaviour
- Drowsiness
- Stupor
- Coma

Nuchal rigidity: May progress to opisthotonos
Positive Kernig and Brudzinski signs
Hyperactive but variable reflex responses
Signs and symptoms peculiar to individual organisms:

- Petechial or purpuric rashes (meningococcal infection), especially when associated with a shocklike state
- Joint involvement (meningococcal and *Haemophilus influenzae* infection)
- Chronically draining ear (pneumococcal meningitis)

Infants and Young Children

Classic picture (above) is rarely seen in children between 3 months and 2 years of age
Fever
Poor feeding
Vomiting
Marked irritability
Frequent seizures (often accompanied by a high-pitched cry)
Bulging fontanel
Nuchal rigidity (may or may not be present)
Brudzinski and Kernig signs not helpful in diagnosis (difficult to elicit and evaluate in this age group)
Subdural empyema (*H. influenzae* infection)

Newborns: Specific Signs

Extremely difficult to diagnose
Manifestations vague and nonspecific
Well at birth but within a few days begins to look and behave poorly
Refusal of feedings
Poor sucking ability
Vomiting or diarrhea
Poor tone
Lack of movement
Weak cry
Full, tense, and bulging fontanel sometimes appearing late in course of illness
Neck usually supple

Newborns: Nonspecific Signs That May Be Present

Hypothermia or fever (depending on the infant's maturity)
Jaundice
Irritability
Drowsiness
Seizures
Respiratory irregularities or apnea
Cyanosis
Weight loss

not always mean that a lumbar puncture is safe with bacterial meningitis. It is important to take the clinical status into careful consideration. Clinical signs including recent seizures, deteriorating LOC, or brainstem signs (posturing, pupillary changes, respiratory pattern change) are clinical predictors of when a lumbar puncture should be delayed (Joffe, 2007).

The patient with meningitis generally has an elevated white blood cell count, often predominantly polymorphonuclear leukocytes. Typically in bacterial meningitis the CSF glucose level is reduced, generally in proportion to the duration and severity of the infection. It is a common misconception that the CSF glucose is low because of bacterial consumption of glucose. However, CNS infections may alter glucose transport across the blood–CSF barrier, resulting in a low CSF glucose value. The CSF glucose value in viral meningitis is usually normal (Logan & MacMahon, 2008). Protein concentration is usually increased.

A blood culture is advisable for all children suspected of having meningitis and occasionally will be positive when CSF culture is negative. Nose and throat cultures may provide helpful information in some cases.

Therapeutic Management

Acute bacterial meningitis is a medical emergency that requires early recognition and immediate institution of therapy to prevent death or residual disabilities. The initial therapeutic management includes the following:

- Isolation precautions
- Initiation of antimicrobial therapy
- Restrict hydration
- Maintenance of ventilation
- Reduction of increased ICP
- Management of systemic shock
- Control of seizures
- Control of temperature
- Treatment of complications

The child should be placed in respiratory isolation and is usually in a critical care unit for close observation. An IV infusion is started to facilitate the administration of antimicrobial agents, fluids, antiepileptic medications, and blood, if needed (Le Saux & CPS, Infectious Diseases and Immunization Committee, 2014).

Medications. Until the causative organism is identified, the choice of antibiotic is based on the known sensitivity of the organism most likely to be the infective agent. After identification of the organism, antimicrobial agents are adjusted accordingly.

Dexamethasone can be used as an adjunctive treatment for children older than 6 weeks of age with suspected bacterial meningitis. It should be given before or within 1 hour of antibiotic administration (Le Saux & CPS, Infectious Diseases and Immunization Committee, 2014). It should not be used if aseptic or nonbacterial meningitis is suspected. The role of steroids in the management of acute bacterial meningitis in children continues to be debated, except in the case of Hib meningitis, for which there is evidence that steroids decrease hearing loss in children if they are administered just before or with the initial antimicrobial therapy (Le Saux & CPS, Infectious Diseases and Immunization Committee, 2014). Signs of gastrointestinal hemorrhage or secondary infection may complicate steroid administration. Antibiotic treatment with cephalosporins demonstrates superiority for promptly sterilizing the CSF and reducing the incidence of severe hearing impairment.

Nonspecific measures. Maintaining hydration is a primary concern; IV fluids and the type and amount of fluid are determined by the patient's condition. Children with bacterial meningitis must be monitored for electrolyte and fluid abnormalities. The optimum hydration involves correction of any fluid deficits followed by fluid restriction until normal serum sodium levels and no signs of increased ICP are present. If needed, measures to decrease ICP are implemented (see p. 1594). Long-term fluid restriction is not the standard of care because a lack of adequate fluid volume can reduce blood pressure and cerebral perfusion pressure, causing CNS ischemia (Prober, Srinivas, & Mathew, 2016).

Complications need to be treated appropriately, such as aspiration of subdural effusion in infants and disseminated intravascular coagulation syndrome. Shock is managed by restoration of circulating blood volume and maintenance of electrolyte balance. Seizures can occur during the first few days of treatment. These are controlled with the appropriate antiepileptic medication. Hearing loss is common. The patient should undergo auditory evaluation 6 months after the illness has resolved.

Lumbar puncture is carried out as needed to determine the effectiveness of therapy. The patient should be evaluated neurologically during the convalescent period.

Prognosis

Approximately 10% of cases of bacterial meningitis are fatal (PHAC, 2014). The child's age, the duration of illness before antibiotic therapy, rapidity of diagnosis after onset, type of organism, and adequacy of therapy are important in the prognosis for bacterial meningitis. Survivors can experience significant physical and neurological sequelae. The most common sequelae in children include hearing loss, intellectual disability, spasticity or paresis, and seizure disorder. Approximately half of the survivors of pediatric bacterial meningitis will have at least one sequela at a 5-year follow-up time point (Chandran, Herbert, Misurski, et al., 2011).

The sequelae of bacterial meningitis are seen most often when the disease occurs in the first 2 months of life and least often in children with meningococcal meningitis. The residual deficits in infants are primarily a result of communicating hydrocephalus and the greater effects of cerebritis on the immature brain. In older children, the residual effects are related to the inflammatory process itself or result from vasculitis associated with the disease.

Prevention

In Canada, meningococcal C conjugate vaccines are recommended for routine immunization of infants, children aged 1 to 4 years, and adolescent and young adults, to prevent the increased risk of serogroup C meningococcal disease in these age groups. The recommended schedule differs depending on the vaccine used. For children at least 5 years of age who have not reached adolescence, immunization with a single dose of MenC-conjugate vaccine may also be considered. A single dose is required for any person at least 1 year of age. Routine vaccinations for Hib and pneumococcal conjugate vaccine are recommended for all children beginning at 2 months of age (Le Saux & CPS, Infectious Diseases and Immunization Committee, 2014; PHAC, 2015) (see Immunizations, Chapter 35).

NURSING CARE

The room should be kept as quiet as possible and environmental stimuli kept to a minimum, because most children with meningitis are sensitive to noise, bright lights, and other external stimuli. Most children are more comfortable without a pillow and with the head of the bed slightly elevated. A side-lying position is more often assumed because of nuchal rigidity. The nurse should avoid actions that cause pain or increase discomfort, such as lifting the child's head. Evaluating the child for pain and implementing appropriate relief measures are important during the initial 24 to 72 hours. Acetaminophen or ibuprofen are often used. The nurse should determine if a patient is febrile before giving acetaminophen or ibuprofen because either of these medications may mask a fever, which is an important clinical indication of infection. Measures to ensure the child's safety should be observed, because the child is often restless and subject to seizures.

The nursing care of the child with meningitis is determined by the child's symptoms and treatment. Observation of vital signs, neurological signs, LOC, urine output, and other pertinent data needs to be carried out at frequent intervals. The child who is unconscious is managed as described previously (see p. 1592), and all children are observed for signs of the complications described in Box 50-5, especially increased ICP, shock, or respiratory distress. Frequent assessment of the open fontanels is needed in the infant because subdural effusions and obstructive hydrocephalus can develop as a complication of meningitis.

> **! NURSING ALERT**
>
> A major priority of nursing care of a child suspected of having meningitis is to administer antibiotics as soon as they are ordered. The child is placed on respiratory isolation for at least 24 hours after initiation of antimicrobial therapy.

Fluids and nourishment are determined by the child's status. The child with dulled sensorium is usually given nothing by mouth. Other children are allowed clear liquids initially and, if these are tolerated, progress to a diet suitable for their age. Careful monitoring and recording of intake and output are needed to determine deviations that might indicate impending shock or increasing fluid accumulation, such as cerebral edema or subdural effusion.

One of the most difficult problems in the nursing care of children with meningitis is maintaining IV infusion for the length of time needed to provide adequate antimicrobial therapy (usually 10 days). Because continuous IV fluids are usually not necessary, an **intermittent infusion device** is used. In some cases, children who are recovering uneventfully are sent home with the device, and the parents are taught IV medication administration.

Family Support

The sudden nature of the illness makes emotional support of the child and parents extremely important. Parents are upset and concerned about their child's condition and often feel guilty for not having suspected the seriousness of the illness sooner. They need much reassurance that the natural onset of meningitis is sudden and that they acted responsibly in seeking medical assistance when they did. The nurse should encourage the parents to openly discuss their feelings to minimize blame and guilt. They also need to be kept informed of the child's progress and of all procedures, results, and treatments. In the event that the child's condition worsens, they need the same psychological care as parents who face the possible death of their child (see Chapter 40).

Nonbacterial (Aseptic) Meningitis

Aseptic meningitis is caused by many different viruses, including arbovirus, herpes simplex virus (HSV), cytomegalovirus, adenovirus, and HIV. Enteroviruses are the most common cause of viral meningitis (Prober et al., 2016). The term *aseptic meningitis* refers to the onset of meningeal symptoms, fever, and pleocytosis without bacterial growth from CSF cultures. Viral meningitis can occur at any age but is most common in the very young child. It has many of the same presenting signs and symptoms as bacterial meningitis, including headache, fever, photophobia, and nuchal rigidity. It can also be accompanied by cutaneous and mucosal manifestations of enterovirus, including hand, foot, and mouth syndrome, herpangina, and maculopapular rash. The onset may be abrupt or gradual. Signs of meningeal irritation develop 1 or 2 days after the onset of illness. Onset is more insidious in infants and toddlers. Signs and symptoms are vague and are often thought to be associated with a minor illness. The clinical course of viral meningitis is much shorter and typically without any significant complications (Logan & MacMahon, 2008).

Diagnosis is based on clinical features and CSF findings. Variations in CSF values in bacterial and viral meningitis are listed in Table 50-3. It is important to differentiate this self-limited disorder from the more serious forms of meningitis.

Treatment is primarily symptomatic, such as acetaminophen for headache and muscle pain, maintenance of hydration, and positioning for comfort. Until a definitive diagnosis is made, antimicrobial agents may be administered and isolation enforced as a precaution against the possibility that the disease might be of bacterial origin. Nursing care is similar to the care of the child with bacterial meningitis.

Encephalitis

Encephalitis is an inflammatory process of the CNS that is caused by a variety of organisms, including bacteria,

TABLE 50-3 VARIATION OF CEREBROSPINAL FLUID ANALYSIS IN BACTERIAL AND VIRAL MENINGITIS

MANIFESTATIONS	BACTERIAL*	VIRAL
White blood cell count	Elevated; increased polymorphonuclears	Slightly elevated; increased lymphocytes
Protein content	Elevated	Normal or slightly increased
Glucose content	Decreased	Normal
Gram stain; bacteria culture	Positive	Negative
Colour	Cloudy	Clear

*Results may vary in the newborn.

spirochetes, fungi, protozoa, helminths, and viruses. Most infections are associated with viruses; this discussion is limited to those agents.

Etiology

Encephalitis can occur as a result of (1) direct invasion of the CNS by a virus or (2) postinfectious involvement of the CNS after a viral disease. Often the specific type of encephalitis may not be identified. The cause of more than half the cases reported in Canada is unknown. The majority of cases of known etiology are associated with the childhood diseases of measles, mumps, varicella, and rubella and, less often, with the enteroviruses, herpesviruses, and West Nile virus.

While herpes simplex encephalitis is an uncommon disease, 30% of cases involve children. The initial clinical findings are nonspecific (fever, altered mental status), but most cases evolve to demonstrate focal neurological signs and symptoms. Children may experience focal seizures. The CSF is abnormal in most cases. Because of a rise in the number of children with herpes simplex encephalitis, suspected cases require prompt attention, especially because the diagnosis can be difficult. CSF polymerase chain reaction testing can confirm the clinical diagnosis. The early use of IV acyclovir reduces mortality and morbidity. Empiric therapy with acyclovir is given before precise virological diagnosis has been established. CSF should be sent for viral titres. Approximately two thirds of children with HSV encephalitis have residual neurological deficits (James, Kimberlin, & Whitley, 2009). The variety of causes of viral encephalitis makes diagnosis difficult. Most are those involved with arthropod vectors (togaviruses and bunyaviruses) and those associated with hemorrhagic fevers (arenaviruses, filoviruses, and Hantaviruses). The vector reservoir for most agents pathogenic for humans is the mosquito (St. Louis or West Nile encephalitis); therefore, most cases of encephalitis appear during the hot summer months and subside during the autumn.

In Canada, the risk of acquiring West Nile virus is very low, particularly in children; for more information see Additional Resources at the end of this chapter.

The clinical features of encephalitis are similar regardless of the agent involved. Manifestations can range from a mild benign form that resembles aseptic meningitis, lasts a few days, and is followed by rapid and complete recovery to a fulminating encephalitis with severe CNS involvement. The onset may be sudden or may be gradual with malaise, fever, headache, dizziness, apathy, nuchal rigidity, nausea and vomiting, ataxia, tremors, hyperactivity, and speech difficulties (Box 50-6). In severe cases the patient has high fever, stupor, seizures, disorientation, spasticity, and coma that may proceed to death. Ocular palsies and paralysis also may occur.

BOX 50-6 CLINICAL MANIFESTATIONS OF ENCEPHALITIS

Onset: Sudden or Gradual
Malaise
Fever
Headache
Dizziness
Apathy
Lethargy
Nucal rigidity

Severe Cases
High fever
Stupor
Seizures
Disorientation
Nausea and vomiting
Ataxia
Tremors
Hyperactivity
Speech difficulties—mutism
Altered mental status
Spasticity
Coma (may proceed to death)
Ocular palsies
Paralysis

Diagnostic Evaluation

The diagnosis is made on the basis of clinical findings and, where possible, identification of the specific virus. Early in the course of encephalitis, CT scan results may be normal. Later, hemorrhagic areas in the frontotemporal region may be seen. Togaviruses (some of which were formerly labelled arboviruses) are rarely detected in the blood or spinal fluid, but viruses of herpes, mumps, measles, and enteroviruses may be found in the CSF. Serological testing may be required. The first blood sample should be drawn as soon as possible after onset, with the second sample drawn 2 or 3 weeks later. There are a number of characteristic EEG findings in encephalitis, particularly in HSV encephalitis, and an EEG is often part of diagnostic evaluation (Somand & Meurer, 2009).

Therapeutic Management

Patients suspected of having encephalitis are hospitalized promptly for observation. Only HSV encephalitis has specific treatment available. In other cases treatment is primarily supportive and includes conscientious nursing care, control of cerebral manifestations, and adequate nutrition and hydration, with observation and management as for other cerebral disorders. Viral encephalitis can cause devastating neurological injury. Cerebral edema, seizures, abnormal fluid and electrolyte balances, aspiration, and cardiac or respiratory arrest occurs in severe viral encephalitis, and close monitoring is needed (Prober et al., 2016).

The prognosis for the child with encephalitis depends on the child's age, the type of organism causing the disease, and residual neurological damage. Long-term outcomes of HSV encephalitis in children can be serious; deficits include visual, auditory, motor, and psychiatric (Prober et al., 2016). Very young children (younger than 2 years of age) may exhibit increased neurological disabilities, including learning difficulties and seizure disorders. Follow-up care with periodic re-evaluation is important because symptoms are often subtle, and rehabilitation is essential for patients who develop residual effects of the disease.

NURSING CARE

Nursing care of the child with encephalitis is the same as for any unconscious child and for the child with meningitis. Additional nursing interventions include observation for deterioration in consciousness. Isolation of the child is not necessary; however, good hand hygiene must be followed. A main focus of nursing management is the control of rapidly rising ICP. Neurological monitoring, administration of medications, and support of the child and parents are the major aspects of care.

Reye Syndrome

Reye syndrome (RS) is a disorder defined as acute encephalopathy associated with other characteristic organ involvement. It is characterized by fever, profoundly impaired consciousness, and disordered hepatic function.

The etiology of RS is not well understood, but most cases follow a common viral illness, most commonly influenza or varicella. RS is a condition characterized pathologically by cerebral edema and fatty changes of the liver. The onset of RS is notable for profuse vomiting and varying degrees of neurological impairment, including personality changes, seizures, and coma, that lead to increased ICP, herniation, and death (Balistreri & Ibrahim, 2016). The cause of RS is a mitochondrial insult induced by different viruses, medications, exogenous toxins, and genetic factors. Elevated serum ammonia levels tend to correlate with the clinical manifestations and prognosis.

Definitive diagnosis is established by liver biopsy. The staging criteria for RS are based on liver dysfunction and on neurological signs that range from lethargy to coma (Box 50-7). As a result of improved diagnostic techniques, children who in the past would have been diagnosed with RS are now diagnosed with other illnesses such as viral or metabolic diseases. Cases of unrecognized, drug-induced encephalopathy caused by antiemetics given to children during viral illnesses have symptoms similar to those of RS.

The potential association between acetylsalicyclic acid (ASA) therapy for the treatment of fever in children with varicella or influenza and the development of RS precludes its use in these patients. Manufacturers must label all over-the-counter products that have ASA with a warning about the dangers of giving ASA to a child under 12 years or to a teenager under 18 years if the teenager has varicella, a cold, or influenza symptoms (Health Canada, 2013). Since the labelling of aspirin with this warning, the number of Reye syndrome diagnoses has decreased, due to increased public awareness of aspirin risk.

BOX 50-7 STAGING CRITERIA FOR REYE SYNDROME

Stage I—Vomiting, lethargy, and drowsiness; liver dysfunction; type I electroencephalogram (EEG); patient follows commands; pupillary reaction is brisk

Stage II—Disorientation, combativeness, delirium, hyperventilation, hyperactive reflexes, appropriate responses to painful stimuli; evidence of liver dysfunction; type I EEG; pupillary reaction is sluggish

Stage III—Obtunded, coma, hyperventilation, decorticate rigidity, preservation of pupillary light reaction and oculovestibular reflexes (although sluggish); type II EEG

Stage IV—Deepening coma, decerebrate rigidity, loss of oculocephalic reflexes, large and fixed pupils, loss of doll's eye reflex, loss of corneal reflexes; minimal liver dysfunction; type III or IV EEG; evidence of brainstem dysfunction

Stage V—Seizures, loss of deep tendon reflexes, respiratory arrest, flaccidity; type IV EEG; usually no evidence of liver dysfunction

Prognosis

Although the incidence of RS has markedly decreased, health care providers must remind parents and caregivers to avoid using both aspirin and non-aspirin–containing salicylates during febrile illnesses in children. Recovery from RS is rapid and usually without sequelae if the diagnosis is determined early and therapy is initiated promptly. Patients who survive have full liver function recovery; however, approximately one third may have subtle neuropsychological deficits (Balistreri & Ibrahim, 2016).

NURSING CARE

The most important aspect of successful management of the child with RS is early diagnosis and aggressive therapy. Cerebral edema with increased ICP represents the most immediate threat to life. Recovery from RS is rapid and usually without sequelae given early diagnosis and implementation of therapy.

Care and observations are implemented as for any child with an altered state of consciousness (see p. 1585) and increasing ICP. Accurate and frequent monitoring of intake and output is essential for adjusting fluid volumes to prevent both dehydration and cerebral edema. Because of related liver dysfunction, laboratory studies to determine impaired coagulation, such as prolonged bleeding time, should be monitored.

Parents of children with RS need to be kept informed of the child's progress, have diagnostic procedures and therapeutic management explained, and be given concerned and empathetic support (see Additional Resources at the end of this chapter). Families need to be aware that salicylate, the alleged offending ingredient in aspirin, is contained in other products (e.g., Pepto-Bismol). They should refrain from administering any product for influenza-like symptoms without first checking the label for "hidden" salicylates.

SEIZURE DISORDERS

Seizures are the most common pediatric neurological disorder. Seizures are caused by excessive and disorderly neuronal discharges in the brain. The manifestation of seizures depends on the region of the brain in which they originate and may include unconsciousness or altered consciousness; involuntary movements; and changes in perception, behaviours, sensations, and posture. Seizures are the most common treatable neurological disorder in children and can occur with a wide variety of conditions involving the CNS. The most common cause of seizures in children is a febrile seizure.

Seizures are a symptom of an underlying disease process. Causes of seizures may be infectious, neurological, metabolic, traumatic, or related to ingestion of toxins. *Epilepsy* is a condition characterized by two or more unprovoked seizures and can be caused by a variety of pathological processes in the brain. A single seizure event should not be classified as epilepsy and is generally not treated with long-term antiepileptic medications. Some seizures may result from an acute medical or neurological illness and cease once the illness is treated. In other cases, children may have a single seizure without the cause ever being known.

Approximately 0.6% of the Canadian population has epilepsy. This includes those who take anticonvulsant drugs or who had a seizure within the past 5 years. Each year an average of 15,500 people learn they have epilepsy; 44% are diagnosed before the age of 5 years, 55% before the age of 10 years, 75 to 85% before age 18 years, and 1% of children will have recurrent seizures before age 14 (Epilepsy Canada, 2009). In approximately 50% of cases of childhood epilepsy, seizures disappear completely. In 50 to 60% of cases, the cause of epilepsy is unknown (Epilepsy Canada, 2009).

After it is determined that the child has had a seizure, it is important to classify the seizure, according to the Classification of Epileptic Seizures, and assign it to the appropriate epilepsy syndrome, according to the Classification of Epilepsies and Epileptic Syndromes (see Additional Resources at the end of this chapter). Optimum treatment and prognosis require an accurate diagnosis and a determination of the cause whenever possible.

Etiology

Seizures in children have many different causes. Seizures are classified according to not only type but also etiology. Acute symptomatic seizures are associated with an acute insult, such as head trauma or meningitis. Remote symptomatic seizures are those without an immediate cause but with an identifiable prior brain injury such as major head trauma, meningitis or encephalitis, hypoxia, stroke, or a static encephalopathy such as intellectual disability or cerebral palsy. Cryptogenic seizures are those occurring with no clear cause. **Idiopathic** seizures are genetic in origin. A partial list of causative factors is presented in Box 50-8.

Pathophysiology

Regardless of the etiological factor or type of seizure, the basic mechanism is the same. Abnormal electrical discharges (1) may

BOX 50-8 ETIOLOGY OF SEIZURES IN CHILDREN

Nonrecurrent (Acute)

Febrile episodes
Intracranial infection
Intracranial hemorrhage
Space-occupying lesions (cyst, tumour)
Acute cerebral edema
Anoxia
Toxins
Medications
Tetanus
Lead encephalopathy
Shigella, Salmonella organisms
Metabolic alterations:
- Hypocalcemia
- Hypoglycemia
- Hyponatremia or hypernatremia
- Hypomagnesemia
- Alkalosis
- Disorders of amino acid metabolism
- Deficiency states
- Hyperbilirubinemia

Recurrent (Chronic)

Idiopathic epilepsy
Epilepsy secondary to:
- Trauma
- Hemorrhage
- Anoxia
- Infections
- Toxins
- Degenerative phenomena
- Congenital defects
- Parasitic brain disease
- Hypoglycemia injury

Epilepsy—sensory stimulus
Epilepsy-stimulating states:
- Narcolepsy and catalepsy
- Psychogenic
- Tetany from hypocalcemia, alkalosis

Hypoglycemic states:
- Hyperinsulinism
- Hypopituitarism
- Adrenocortical insufficiency
- Hepatic disorders

Uremia
Allergy
Cardiovascular dysfunction or syncopal episodes
Migraine

arise from central areas in the brain that affect consciousness, (2) may be restricted to one area of the cerebral cortex, producing manifestations characteristic of that particular anatomical focus, or (3) may begin in a localized area of the cortex and spread to other portions of the brain and, if sufficiently extensive, produce generalized seizure activity.

Seizure activity begins with a group of neurons in the CNS that, because of excessive excitation and loss of inhibition, amplify their discharge simultaneously. In response to physiological stimuli, such as cellular dehydration, severe hypoglycemia, electrolyte imbalance, sleep deprivation, emotional stress, and endocrine changes, these hyperexcitable cells activate normal cells in surrounding areas and distant, synaptically related cells. A generalized seizure develops when the neuronal excitation from the epileptogenic focus spreads to the brainstem, particularly the midbrain and reticular formation. These centres within the brainstem, known as the *centrencephalic system*, are responsible for the spread of the epileptic potentials. The discharges can originate spontaneously in the centrencephalic system or be triggered by a focal area in the cortex. On the basis of these characteristic neuronal discharges (as recorded by the EEG), seizures are designated as *partial*, *generalized*, and *unclassified* epileptic seizures (Berg, Berkovic, Brodie, et al., 2010). In a large proportion of children, focal seizures spread to other areas, ultimately becoming generalized with loss of consciousness.

Hallmark early systemic changes during a generalized seizure include tachycardia, hypertension, hyperglycemia, and hypoxemia. Brief seizures rarely produce significant durable side effects. In contrast, prolonged seizures can lead to lactic acidosis rhabdomyolysis, hyperkalemia, hyperthermia, and hypoglycemia. All of these changes can cause long-term neurological damage (Mikati & Hani, 2016).

Seizure Classification and Clinical Manifestations

There are many different types of seizures, and each has unique clinical manifestations. Seizures are classified into three major categories:

1. *Partial seizures*, which have a local onset and involve a relatively small location in the brain
2. *Generalized seizures*, which involve both hemispheres of the brain and are without local onset
3. *Unclassified epileptic seizures*

Descriptions of the different types of seizures are found in Box 50-9 and Table 50-4.

Diagnostic Evaluation

Establishing a diagnosis is critical for establishing a prognosis and planning the proper treatment. The process of diagnosis in a child suspected of having epilepsy includes (1) determining whether epilepsy or seizures exist and not an alternative diagnosis and (2) defining the underlying cause, if possible. The assessment and diagnosis rely heavily on a thorough history, skilled observation, and several diagnostic tests.

It is especially important to differentiate epilepsy from other brief alterations in consciousness or behaviour. Clinical entities that mimic seizures include migraine headaches, toxic effects of medications, syncope (fainting), breath-holding spells in infants and young children, movement disorders (tics, tremor, chorea), prolonged QT syndrome, sleep disturbances (sleepwalking, night terrors), psychogenic seizures, rage attacks, and transient ischemic attacks (rare in children) (Mikati & Hani, 2016). Cocaine intoxication should be considered in the differential diagnosis of new-onset seizure activity in newborn infants.

The history of the seizure should be equally detailed, including the type of seizure or description of the child's behaviour during the event, the age at onset, and the time at which the seizure occurs (e.g., early morning, before meals, while awake, or during sleep). Any factors that may have precipitated the seizure are important, including fever, infection, head trauma, anxiety, fatigue, sleep deprivation, menstrual cycle, alcohol, and activity (e.g., hyperventilation or exposure to strong stimuli such as bright flashing light or loud noises). If the child can describe any sensory phenomena, these should be recorded. The duration and progression of the seizure (if any) and the postictal feelings and behaviour (e.g., confusion, inability to speak, amnesia, headache, and sleep) should also be recorded. It is important to determine whether more than one seizure type exists. It is often more informative to ask parents to mime the seizure rather than relying on their oral description. Miming often reveals features, such as head turning, that would otherwise go unrecognized. Some seizures are overlooked by parents. For example, some parents may not identify brief head nods or brief single jerks as seizures unless specifically asked whether their child has these symptoms. The family history should include whether other family members have had a seizure, intellectual ability, cerebral palsy, or other neurological disorders. A family history can offer clues to paroxysmal disorders, such as migraine headaches, breath-holding spells, febrile seizures, or neurological diseases.

A complete physical and neurological examination, including developmental assessment of language, learning, behaviour, and motor abilities, may provide clues to the cause of the seizures. A number of laboratory and neuroimaging tests may be ordered depending on the child's age, whether this is a new-onset seizure, characteristics of the seizure, and the history. Laboratory studies that may prove to be of value include a venous lead level if the history warrants or white blood cell count (for signs of infection). Blood glucose may give evidence of hypoglycemic episodes, and serum electrolytes, blood urea nitrogen, calcium, serum amino acids, lactate, ammonia, and urine organic acids may indicate metabolic disturbances. Blood for chromosomal analysis may also be tested if a genetic etiology is suspected. A toxic screen may be done if alcohol or drug use or withdrawal is suspected. Lumbar puncture can confirm a suspected diagnosis of meningitis. CT may be done to detect a cerebral hemorrhage, infarctions, and gross malformations. MRI provides greater anatomical detail and is used to detect developmental malformations, tumours, and cortical dysplasias.

The EEG is obtained for all children with seizures and is the most useful tool for evaluating a seizure disorder. The EEG confirms the presence of abnormal electrical discharges and provides information on the seizure type and the focus. The

BOX 50-9 CLASSIFICATION AND CLINICAL MANIFESTATIONS OF SEIZURES

Partial Seizures

Simple Partial Seizures With Motor Signs

Characterized by:
- Localized motor symptoms
- Somatosensory, psychic, autonomic symptoms
- Combination of these
- Abnormal discharges remaining unilateral

Manifestations:
- Aversive seizure (most common motor seizure in children)—Eye or eyes and head turn away from the side of the focus; awareness of movement or loss of consciousness
- Rolandic (Sylvan) seizure—Tonic-clonic movements involving the face, salivation, arrested speech; most common during sleep
- Jacksonian march (rare in children)—Orderly, sequential progression of clonic movements beginning in a foot, hand, or face and moving, or "marching," to adjacent body parts

Simple Partial Seizures With Sensory Signs

Uncommon in children younger than 8 years of age

Characterized by various sensations, including the following:
- Numbness, tingling, prickling, paresthesia, or pain originating in one area (e.g., face or extremities) and spreading to other parts of the body
- Visual sensations or formed images
- Motor phenomena such as posturing or hypertonia

Complex Partial Seizures (Psychomotor Seizures)

Observed more often in children from 3 years through adolescence

Characterized by:
- Period of altered behaviour
- Amnesia for event (no recollection of behaviour)
- Inability to respond to environment
- Impaired consciousness during event
- Drowsiness or sleep usually following seizure
- Confusion and amnesia possibly prolonged
- Complex sensory phenomena (aura)—Most frequent sensation is a strange feeling in the pit of the stomach that rises toward the throat; often accompanied by odd or unpleasant odours or tastes; complex auditory or visual hallucinations; ill-defined feelings of elation or strangeness (e.g., déjà vu, a feeling of familiarity in a strange environment); strong feelings of fear and anxiety; distorted sense of time and self; and in small children, emission of a cry or attempt to run for help

Patterns of motor behaviour:
- Stereotypical
- Similar with each subsequent seizure
- May suddenly cease activity, appear dazed, stare into space, become confused and apathetic, and become limp or stiff or display some form of posturing
- May be confused
- May perform purposeless, complicated activities in a repetitive manner (automatisms), such as walking, running, kicking, laughing, or speaking incoherently, most often followed by postictal confusion or sleep; may exhibit oropharyngeal activities, such as smacking, chewing, drooling, swallowing, and nausea or abdominal pain followed by stiffness, a fall, and postictal sleep; rarely manifests actions such as rage or temper tantrums; aggressive acts uncommon during seizure

Generalized Seizures

Tonic-Clonic Seizures (Formerly Known as Grand Mal)

Most common and most dramatic of all seizure manifestations

Occur without warning

Tonic phase: lasts approximately 10 to 20 seconds

Manifestations:
- Eyes roll upward
- Immediate loss of consciousness
- If standing, falls to floor or ground
- Stiffens in generalized, symmetrical tonic contraction of entire body musculature
- Arms usually flexed
- Legs, head, and neck extended
- May utter a peculiar piercing cry
- Apneic; may become cyanotic
- Increased salivation and loss of swallowing reflex

Clonic phase: lasts about 30 seconds but can vary from only a few seconds to a half-hour or longer

Manifestations:
- Violent jerking movements as the trunk and extremities undergo rhythmic contraction and relaxation
- May foam at the mouth
- May be incontinent of urine and feces

As event ends, movements are less intense, occurring at longer intervals, then ceasing entirely

Status epilepticus: series of seizures at intervals too brief to allow the child to regain consciousness between the time one event ends and the next begins
- Requires emergency intervention
- Can lead to exhaustion, respiratory failure, and death

Postictal state:
- Appears to relax
- May remain semiconscious and difficult to arouse
- May awaken in a few minutes
- Remains confused for several hours
- Poor coordination
- Mild impairment of fine motor movements
- May have visual and speech difficulties
- May vomit or complain of severe headache
- When left alone, usually sleeps for several hours
- On awakening is fully conscious
- Usually feels tired and has symptoms of sore muscles and headache
- No recollection of entire event

Absence Seizures (Formerly Called Petit Mal or Lapses)

Characterized by:
- Onset usually between 4 and 12 years of age
- More common in girls than in boys
- Usually cease at puberty
- Brief loss of consciousness

BOX 50-9 CLASSIFICATION AND CLINICAL MANIFESTATIONS OF SEIZURES—cont'd

- Minimum or no alteration in muscle tone
- May go unrecognized because of little change in child's behaviour
- Abrupt onset; suddenly develops 20 or more attacks daily
- Event often mistaken for inattentiveness or daydreaming
- Events possibly precipitated by hyperventilation, hypoglycemia, stresses (emotional and physiological), fatigue, or sleeplessness

Manifestations:

- Brief loss of consciousness
- Appear without warning or aura
- Usually last about 5 to 10 seconds
- Slight loss of muscle tone may cause child to drop objects
- Ability to maintain postural control; seldom falls
- Minor movements such as lip smacking, twitching of eyelids or face, or slight hand movements
- Not accompanied by incontinence
- Amnesia for episode
- May need to reorient self to previous activity

Atonic and Akinetic Seizures (Also Known as Drop Attacks)

Characterized by:

- Onset usually between 2 and 5 years of age
- Sudden, momentary loss of muscle tone and postural control
- Events recurring frequently during the day, particularly in the morning hours and shortly after awakening

Manifestations:

- Loss of tone causing child to fall to the floor violently; unable to break fall by putting out hand; may incur a serious injury to the face, head, or shoulder
- Loss of consciousness only momentary

Myoclonic Seizures

A variety of seizure episodes

May be isolated as benign essential myoclonus

May occur in association with other seizure forms

Characterized by:

- Sudden, brief contractures of a muscle or group of muscles
- Occur singly or repetitively
- No postictal state
- May or may not be symmetrical
- May or may not include loss of consciousness

Infantile Spasms

Also called infantile myoclonus, massive spasms, hypsarrhythmia, salaam episodes, or infantile myoclonic spasms

Most commonly occur during the first 6 to 8 months of life

Twice as common in boys as in girls

Numerous seizures during the day without postictal drowsiness or sleep

Poor outlook for normal intelligence

Manifestations:

- Possible series of sudden, brief, symmetrical, muscular contractions
- Head flexed, arms extended, and legs drawn up
- Eyes sometimes rolling upward or inward
- May be preceded or followed by a cry or giggling
- May or may not include loss of consciousness
- Sometimes flushing, pallor, or cyanosis
- Infants who are able to sit but not stand:
  - Sudden dropping forward of the head and neck with trunk flexed forward and knees drawn up—the salaam or jackknife seizure
- Less often: alternative clinical forms:
  - Extensor spasms rather than flexion of arms, legs, and trunk, and head nodding
  - Lightning events involving a single, momentary, shocklike contraction of the entire body

TABLE 50-4 COMPARISON OF SIMPLE PARTIAL, COMPLEX PARTIAL, AND ABSENCE SEIZURES

CLINICAL MANIFESTATIONS	SIMPLE PARTIAL	COMPLEX PARTIAL	ABSENCE
Age of onset	Any age	Uncommon before age 3 yr	Uncommon before age 3 yr
Frequency (per day)	Variable	Rarely >1–2 times	Multiple
Duration	Usually <30 sec	Usually >60 sec, rarely <10 sec	Usually <10 sec, rarely >30 sec
Aura	May be sole manifestation of seizure	Frequent	Never
Impaired consciousness	Never	Always	Always; brief loss of consciousness
Automatisms	Never	Frequent	Frequent
Clonic movements	Frequent	Occasional	Occasional
Postictal impairment	Rare	Frequent	Never
Mental disorientation	Rare	Common	Unusual

EEG is carried out under varying conditions—with the child asleep, awake, awake with provocative stimulation (flashing lights, noise), and hyperventilating. Stimulation may elicit abnormal electrical activity, which is recorded on the EEG. Various seizure types produce characteristic EEG patterns: high-voltage spike discharges are seen in tonic-clonic seizures, with abnormal patterns in the intervals between seizures; a three-per-second spike and wave pattern is observed in an absence seizure; and absence of electrical activity in an area suggests a large lesion, such as an abscess or subdural collection of fluid.

A normal EEG does not rule out seizures because the EEG is only a surface recording that represents approximately 1 hour of time; therefore it may show normal interictal activity. If there is concern about whether a child has seizures or the seizure type cannot be determined, then a long-term video EEG may be done to record the child during wakefulness and sleep. The full body image is recorded on video, with selected EEG channels displayed on the same screen for simultaneous recording and viewing. EEG monitoring is also available in digital EEG and digital video imaging, which allows for greater selection of EEG channels and is available in both routine and long-term EEGs. Although the EEG is very valuable, it should not be used alone to determine the type of seizure. Rather, the EEG interpretation, along with a thorough clinical description of the patient's behaviour during the seizure episode, can be a guide to the correct classification of the seizure and the appropriate treatment choice.

Therapeutic Management

The goal of treatment of seizure disorders is to control the seizures or to reduce their frequency and severity, discover and correct the cause when possible, and help the child live as normal a life as possible. If the seizure activity is a manifestation of an infectious, traumatic, or metabolic process, the seizure therapy is instituted as part of the general therapeutic regimen. Management of epilepsy has four treatment options: medication therapy, the ketogenic diet, vagus nerve stimulation, and epilepsy surgery.

Medication therapy. Persons predisposed to epilepsy have seizures when their basal level of neuronal excitability exceeds a critical point; no event occurs if the excitability is maintained below this threshold. The administration of antiepileptic medications serves to raise this threshold and prevent seizures. Consequently, the primary therapy for seizure disorders is administration of the appropriate antiepileptic medication or combination of medications in a dosage that provides the desired effect without causing undesirable adverse effects or toxic reactions. Antiepileptic medications are believed to exert their effect primarily by reducing the responsiveness of normal neurons to the sudden, high-frequency nerve impulses that arise in the epileptogenic focus. Thus the seizure is effectively suppressed; however, the abnormal brain waves may or may not be altered. Complete control can be achieved through medication in 70 to 80% of children with epilepsy (Curatolo, Moavero, Lo Castro, et al., 2009; Lozsadi, Von Oertzen, & Cock, 2010).

The initiation of anticonvulsant therapy is based on several factors, including the child's age, type of seizure, risk of recurrence, and other comorbid or predisposing medical issues. For children who develop recurrent seizures or epilepsy, treatment is begun with a single drug known to be effective and have the lowest toxicity (i.e., the safest adverse-effect profile for the child's particular type of seizure). The dosage is gradually increased until the seizures are controlled or the child develops adverse effects. If the medication is effective but does not sufficiently control the seizures, a second medication is added in gradually increasing doses. Once seizures are controlled, the first medication may be tapered to reduce the potential adverse effects of polytherapy. However, this decision is individualized for each child. Monotherapy remains the treatment method of choice for epilepsy, but a combination of medications may be a viable alternative for children who cannot attain seizure control with only one agent (Mikati & Hani, 2016).

Measurement of blood levels of the drug is important if the seizures continue once the child is on a therapeutic dose of medication, to adjust the dosage, and to assist in determining which medication may be causing the adverse effects if the child is on multiple antiepileptic medications. Some possible causes of low serum blood concentrations are not taking the medication, poor absorption, and drug interactions. The dosage needs to be increased as the child grows. Blood cell counts, urinalysis, and liver function tests are obtained at frequent intervals for children receiving particular antiepileptic medications that can affect organ function.

If complete seizure control is maintained on an anticonvulsant medication for 2 years, it is safe to discontinue the medication for patients with no risk factors. Risk factors include age of onset being over 12 years, history of neonatal seizures, numerous seizures before control is achieved, and the presence of a neurological dysfunction (e.g., motor or cognitive impairment). Up to 40% of children whose medications are discontinued will experience seizure recurrence. Recurrence occurs most frequently within 6 months of discontinuation (Sillanpää & Schmidt, 2006).

When seizure medications are discontinued, the dosage is decreased gradually over several weeks. Sudden withdrawal of a medication is not recommended because it can cause an increase in the number and severity of seizures.

STOP MEDICATION ALERT

Fosphenytoin is often used to treat seizures instead of IV phenytoin because of possible complications and drug interactions associated with IV phenytoin. If IV phenytoin is used, it should be administered via slow IV push at a rate that does not exceed 50 mg/min. Because phenytoin precipitates when mixed with glucose, only normal saline is used to flush the tubing or catheter. Fosphenytoin may be given in saline or glucose solutions at a rate of up to 150 mg PE (phenytoin equivalent)/min, and it may be given intramuscularly if necessary.

Ketogenic diet. The ketogenic diet is a high-fat, low-carbohydrate, and adequate-protein diet (Kossoff, Zupec-Kania, & Rho, 2009). Consumption of such a diet forces the body to shift from using glucose as the primary energy source to using fat, and the individual develops a state of ketosis. The diet is rigorous. All foods and liquids the child consumes must be carefully weighed and measured. The diet is deficient in vitamins and minerals; thus, vitamin supplements are necessary. Early adverse effects of the diet are diarrhea, hypoglycemia, dehydration, acidosis, and lethargy. Long-term effects of the diet are dyslipidemia, kidney stones, and poor growth (Kossoff et al., 2009).

The ketogenic diet has been shown to be an efficacious and tolerable treatment for medically refractory seizures (Kossoff et al., 2009). Studies have shown that as many as 56% of children on the diet had greater than a 50% reduction in seizure episodes (Hartman & Vining, 2007).

Vagus nerve stimulation. Vagus nerve stimulation (VNS) uses an implantable device that reduces seizures in individuals who have not had effective control with medication therapy. It is currently indicated as adjunct therapy in patients 12 years and older with partial-onset seizures (with or without secondary generalization) who are refractory to antiepileptic drugs (Elliott, Rodgers, Bassani, et al., 2011). A programmable signal generator is implanted subcutaneously in the chest. Electrodes tunnelled underneath the skin deliver electrical impulses to the left vagus nerve (cranial nerve X). The device is programmed noninvasively to deliver a precise pattern of stimulation. The patient or caregiver can activate the device using a magnet at the onset of a seizure. No long-term adverse effects have been reported with VNS, but dysphonia, throat or neck pain, and cough can occur during stimulation. To minimize laryngeal complications in implantation surgery for VNS devices, it has been recommended that the surgical technique be significantly modified, and lower neck incision could be implemented together with a submuscular pocket for the battery (Lotan & Vaiman, 2015). Studies show a medium reduction in seizures of 35 to 45% after 1 year of therapy (Elliott et al., 2011; Orosz, McCormick, Zamponi, et al., 2014).

Surgical therapy. When seizures are determined to be caused by a hematoma, tumour, or other cerebral lesion, surgical removal is the treatment. In children with epilepsy, surgery is reserved for those who suffer from incapacitating, refractory seizures. *Refractory seizures* are usually defined as the persistence of seizures despite adequate trials of three antiepileptic medications, alone or in combination (Mikati & Hani, 2016). An extensive medical (e.g., invasive EEG monitoring), psychosocial, and psychoneurological evaluation is required before surgery. There are several types of surgical interventions. Focal resection entails removal of the epileptogenic zone, and hemispherectomy involves removing all or most of one hemisphere in patients with catastrophic hemispheric epilepsy (Mikati & Hani, 2016). Corpus callosotomy consists of the separation of the connections between the two hemispheres in the brain to prevent seizure activity by blocking epileptic discharges. Patients undergoing surgical resection can experience a decrease in the frequency and severity of seizures, a decrease in antiepileptic medication requirements, and an improvement in their quality of life (Spencer & Huh, 2008).

Treatment for status epilepticus. *Status epilepticus* is a continuous seizure that lasts more than 30 minutes or a series of seizures from which the child does not regain a premorbid LOC (Huff & Fountain, 2011). It has been suggested that the term *impending status epilepticus* be used for a continuous seizure or series of seizures lasting between 5 and 30 minutes (Mikati & Hani, 2016). The initial treatment is directed toward support and maintenance of vital functions such as airway and breathing, administering oxygen, and gaining IV access, immediately followed by IV administration of antiepileptic agents.

MEDICATION ALERT

Lorazepam (buccal or rectally), or midazolam (buccal or intranasally), and diazepam (rectally) are quick, effective, and safe treatments for the prehospital treatment of status epilepticus (Friedman & CPS, Acute Care Committee, 2011/2016). Cessation of seizure occurs in 8 minutes with buccal midazolam and 15 minutes with rectal diazepam (Shorvon, 2011). Respiratory depression is a potential adverse effect of these medications, and patients should be monitored closely after administration (Mikati & Hani, 2016).

For in-hospital management of status epilepticus, IV lorazepam (Ativan) or midazolam, or diazepam are the first-line medications of choice (Friedman & CPS, Acute Care Committee, 2011/2016). Lorazepam is the preferred choice because of rapid onset (2 to 5 minutes) and long half-life (12 to 24 hours). It has a longer duration of action and causes less respiratory depression in children over 2 years of age. IV loading with fosphenytoin, phenytoin, or phenobarbital is usually necessary if benzodiazepines (diazepam, lorazepam, or midazolam) are not effective for sustained control of seizures. The child must be closely monitored during administration to detect early alterations in vital signs that may indicate impending respiratory depression. This combination of therapy places the child at high risk for apnea, and respiratory support is generally necessary (Friedman & CPS, Acute Care Committee, 2011/2016).

Children who continue to have seizures despite the above medication treatment may be given anaesthetizing doses of midazolam, propofol, or pentobarbital (Shorvon, 2011). In this situation, continuous EEG monitoring is typically done to monitor for and treat electrographic seizures.

NURSING ALERT

Nursing care of a child with status epilepticus includes, in addition to the CAB of life support, monitoring blood pressure and body temperature. During the first 30 to 45 minutes of the seizure the blood pressure may be elevated. Thereafter the blood pressure typically returns to normal but may be decreased, depending on the medications being administered for seizure control. Hyperthermia requiring treatment may occur as a result of increased motor activity.

Diazepam is incompatible with many medications. To give intravenously, inject slowly and directly into the vein or through tubing as close as possible to the vein insertion site.

Prognosis

Most children who experience a second seizure will experience additional seizures; as many as 72% of children have additional seizures within 5 years after the second seizure (Berg, 2008). Therefore, a history of two seizures is sufficient to diagnose epilepsy. In one study, children who had epilepsy and severe neurological disorders were 22 times more likely to die than children with epilepsy and normal neurological status (Nei & Bagla, 2007). Mortality is also associated with the severity and frequency of the child's seizures. It can be as high as 46% in patients with status epilepticus (Nei & Bagla, 2007).

NURSING CARE

An important nursing responsibility is to observe the seizure episode and accurately document the events. Any alterations in behaviour preceding the seizure and the characteristics of the episode, such as sensory-hallucinatory phenomena (e.g., an aura), motor effects (e.g., eye movements, muscular contractions), alterations in consciousness, and postictal state, should be noted and recorded (Box 50-10). The nurse should describe only what is observed, rather than trying to label a seizure type. The time that the seizure began and the duration of the seizure should be noted.

The child must be protected from injury during the seizure. Nursing observations made during the event provide valuable information for diagnosis and management of the disorder (see Emergency box). For nursing care of the child with a seizure disorder see the Nursing Care Plan available on Evolve.

It is impossible to halt a seizure once it has begun, and no attempt should be made to do so. The nurse must remain calm, stay with the child, and prevent the child from sustaining any harm during the seizure. If possible, the child should be isolated from the view of others by closing a door or pulling screens. A seizure can be upsetting to the child, other visitors, and his or her family. If other persons are present, they should be assured that everything is being done for the child. After the seizure, they can be given a simple explanation about the event as needed.

If the nurse is able to reach the child in time, a child who is standing or seated in a chair (including a wheelchair) should be eased to the floor immediately. During (and sometimes after) the tonic-clonic seizure, the swallowing reflex is lost, salivation increases, and the tongue is hypotonic. Thus, the child is at risk for aspiration and airway occlusion. Placing the child on the side facilitates drainage and helps maintain a patent airway. Suctioning the oral cavity and posterior oropharynx may be necessary. Vital signs should be taken. The child should be allowed to rest if at school or away from home. When feasible,

BOX 50-10 GENERAL OBSERVATIONS: THE CHILD DURING A SEIZURE

Observations During a Seisure

Describe

Order of events (before, during, and after)

Duration of seizure

- Tonic-clonic—from first signs of event until jerking stops
- Absence—from loss of consciousness until consciousness is regained
- Complex partial—from first sign of unresponsiveness, motor activity, automatisms until there are signs of responsiveness to environment

Onset

Time of onset

Significant precipitating events—missed medication dosage, illness, stress, sleep deprivation, menses

Behaviour

Change in facial expression

Cry or other sound

Stereotypical and automatic movements

Random activity (wandering)

Position of eyes, head, body, extremities

Unilateral or bilateral posturing of one or more extremities

Movement

Change of position, if any

Site of commencement—hand, thumb, mouth, generalized

Tonic phase—length, parts of body involved

Clonic phase—twitching or jerking movements, parts of body involved, sequence of parts involved, generalized, change in character of movements

Lack of movement or muscle tone of body part or entire body

Face

Colour change—pallor, cyanosis, flushing

Perspiration

Mouth—position, deviation to one side, teeth clenched, tongue bitten, frothing at mouth, flecks of blood or bleeding

Lack of expression

Asymmetrical expression

Eyes

Position—straight ahead, deviation upward or outward, conjugate or divergent gaze

Pupils—change in size, equality, reaction to light

Respiratory Effort

Presence and length of apnea

Other

Incontinence

Postictal Observations

Duration of postictal period

State of consciousness

Orientation

Arousability

Motor ability:

- Any change in motor function
- Ability to move all extremities
- Paresis or weakness

Speech

Sensations:

- Symptoms of discomfort or pain
- Any sensory impairment

Recollection of preseizure sensations (aura)

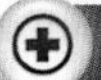

EMERGENCY

Seizures

Tonic-Clonic Seizure

During the Seizure

Remain calm.
Time seizure episode.
If child is standing or seated, ease child down to the floor.
Place pillow or folded blanket under child's head.
Loosen restrictive clothing.
Remove eyeglasses.
Clear area of any hazards or hard objects.
Allow seizure to end without interference.
If vomiting occurs, turn child to one side.
Do not:

- Attempt to restrain child or use force
- Put anything in child's mouth
- Give any food or liquids

After the Seizure

Time postictal period.
Check for breathing. Check position of head and tongue.
Reposition if head is hyperextended. If child is not breathing, give rescue breathing and call emergency medical services (EMS).
Keep child on side.
Remain with child.
Do not give food or liquids until child is fully alert and swallowing reflex has returned.
Call EMS when necessary.
Look for medical identification, and determine what factors occurred before onset of seizure that may have been triggering factors.
Check head and body for possible injuries.
Check inside of mouth to see if tongue or lips have been bitten.

Complex Partial Seizure

During the Seizure

Do not restrain child.
Remove harmful objects from area.
Redirect to safe area.
Do not agitate; instead, talk in calm, reassuring manner.
Do not expect child to follow instructions.
Watch to see if seizure generalizes.

After the Seizure

Stay with child and reassure until fully conscious.

Call Emergency Medical Services If

The child stops breathing.
There is evidence of injury or the child is diabetic or pregnant.
The seizure lasts for more than 5 minutes (unless duration of seizure is typically longer than 5 minutes).
Status epilepticus occurs.
Pupils are not equal after seizure.
The child vomits continuously 30 minutes after seizure has ended (sign of possible acute problem).
The child cannot be awakened and is unresponsive to pain after seizure has ended.
The seizure occurs in water.
This is the child's first seizure.

Modified from Epilepsy Foundation. (2001). *Seizure recognition and first aid.* Retrieved from http://www.epilepsyfoundation.org

BOX 50-11 SEIZURE PRECAUTIONS

The extent of precautions depends on type, severity, and frequency of seizures. They may include the following:

- Side rails raised when child is sleeping or resting
- Side rails and other hard objects padded
- Waterproof mattress or pad on bed or crib

Appropriate precautions during potentially hazardous activities may include the following:

- Swimming with a companion
- Taking showers; bathing only with close supervision
- Using protective helmet and padding during bicycle riding, skateboarding, in-line skating
- Supervising child during use of hazardous machinery or equipment

Have child carry or wear medical identification.
Alert other caregivers to need for any special precautions.
The child may not drive or operate hazardous machinery or equipment unless seizure free for designated period (varies by province).

the child should be integrated into the environment as soon as possible. Sending a child with a chronic seizure disorder home from school is not necessary unless requested by the parents.

Seizure precautions are required for children who are known to have seizures or who are under observation for seizures. The extent of these measures depends on the type and frequency of the seizure (Box 50-11).

NURSING ALERT

Do not move or forcefully restrain the child during a tonic-clonic seizure, and do not place a solid object between the teeth.

Long-term care. Care of the child with a recurrent seizure disorder involves physical care and instruction regarding the importance of the medication therapy and, probably more significant, the problems related to the emotional aspects of the disorder. Few diseases generate as much anxiety among relatives as epilepsy. Fears and misconceptions about the disease and its treatment are common. For many, it represents the archetype of severe hereditary affliction. Nursing care is directed toward educating the child and family about epilepsy and helping them develop strategies to cope with the psychological and sociological problems related to epilepsy.

Children with epilepsy are prescribed antiepileptic medications. These medications need to be administered at regular intervals to maintain adequate levels in the blood. The nurse can help the parents plan the administration of the medication at convenient times to avoid disruptions of family routines as much as possible. It is important to impress on the family the necessity of giving the antiepileptic medication regularly and for as long as required. In general, antiepileptic medications are continued until the child has been seizure free for 2 years (Mikati & Hani, 2016). The medication is then slowly tapered over a period of weeks to avoid the possibility of precipitating a seizure. It is sometimes easy to skip doses or omit them for a variety of reasons, especially when the child is free of seizures most of the time. This is particularly so when the child is older and assumes responsibility for his or her medication. The seizure threshold may be lowered during any illness, but particularly with fever. Parents should be aware that if their child has an illness, he or she is at increased risk for seizures. Parents should contact their health care provider if their child misses medications during an illness because of vomiting.

Rectal preparations of some antiepileptic medications are highly effective when a child is unable to take oral medications because of repeated vomiting, gastrointestinal surgery, or status epilepticus. Parents can learn to administer rectal antiepileptic medication for home treatment. Buccal midazolam or rectal diazepam is a useful adjunctive home treatment for children at risk for prolonged seizures or clusters of seizures and can minimize the need for hospitalization while enhancing parental confidence.

MEDICATION ALERT

Children taking phenobarbital or phenytoin should receive adequate vitamin D and folic acid, since deficiencies of both have been associated with these medications. Phenytoin should not be taken with milk.

Nurses should educate the child and parents about the possible adverse reactions to the medications used to treat seizures. Parents need to understand the common adverse effects and be encouraged to report their observations to their health care provider. Parents should understand that the child needs periodic physical assessment and laboratory studies. Possible adverse effects on the hematopoietic system, liver, and kidneys may be reflected in symptoms such as fever, sore throat, enlarged lymph nodes, jaundice, and bleeding (e.g., easy bruising, petechiae, ecchymoses, epistaxis). A common factor in status epilepticus is inadequate blood levels of antiepileptic medications.

Although children with epilepsy are at increased risk for injury, few limitations should be placed on activities. The degree to which activities are restricted is individualized for each child and depends on the type, frequency, and severity of the seizures; the child's response to therapy; and the length of time the seizures have been controlled. To prevent head injuries children should always wear appropriate safety devices such as helmets and avoid activities involving heights. Although bike riding is safe for most children, children with frequent seizures and impairment of consciousness should avoid it. Skating, in-line skating, and skateboarding should be restricted only in children with frequent seizures. Helmets must be worn while participating in these activities.

Children with epilepsy are at higher risk for submersion injury than children without epilepsy. Young children should never be left alone in the bathtub, even for a few seconds. Older children and adolescents should be encouraged to use a shower and reminded not to lock the bathroom door when showering. They should never swim unsupervised.

Because the child is encouraged to attend school, camp, and other normal activities, teachers should be made aware of his or her condition and therapy. They can help ensure regularity of medication administration and provision of any special care the child might need. Teachers, child care providers, camp counsellors, youth organization leaders, coaches, and other adults who assume responsibility for children should be instructed regarding care of the child during a seizure so they can act calmly for the child's welfare and influence the attitude of her or his peers.

Triggering factors. Careful and detailed documentation of seizures over time may indicate a pattern. In the general population, as many as 90% of individuals can identify at least one trigger for their seizure (Haut & Lipton, 2009). When this occurs, the nurse or responsible adult may intervene to identify the triggering factors and make changes in the environment that may prevent seizures or decrease their frequency. Often the necessary changes are simple but can make an enormous difference in the lives of the child and family.

The most common factors that may trigger seizures in children include emotional stress, sleep deprivation, fatigue, fever, and illness (Epilepsy Foundation, 2014). Other precipitating factors include flickering lights, menstrual cycle, alcohol, heat, hyperventilation, and fasting. Some individuals have pattern- or photo-sensitive epilepsy, that is, seizures precipitated by changes in dark–light patterns, such as those that occur with a flash on a camera, automobile headlights, reflections of light on snow or water, or rotating blades on a fan. Most of these individuals have absence, myoclonic, or generalized tonic-clonic seizures. Some children have seizures while playing video games. Although the actual incidence of video game–induced epilepsy is unknown, it most commonly affects children between the ages of 9 and 15 years (Shoja, Tubbs, Malekian, et al., 2007). These children are sensitive to intermittent photic stimulation (more than 3 flashes per second) that can trigger an epileptic episode (Shoja et al., 2007). The prognosis for pattern- or photo-epilepsy is good. Prevention techniques such as maintaining a 2-metre distance from the television or computer screen, using a smaller screen, and taking frequent breaks can reduce seizure incidence (Shoja et al., 2007).

Febrile Seizures

Febrile seizures are one of the most common neurological conditions of childhood, affecting approximately 2 to 5% of children between the ages of 6 and 60 months, with the peak incidence occurring at 18 months of age (Mikati & Hani, 2016; Østergaard, 2009). They are classified as simple or complex. Simple febrile seizures occur in children between the ages of 6 months and 5 years with no pre-existing neurological abnormality and consist of a general tonic-clonic seizure that occurs with a fever (>38.0°C) and resolves within 15 minutes with a return to alert mental status after the seizure and with no further seizure occurring within a 24-hour period (Mikati & Hani, 2016). Complex febrile seizures by contrast can occur in children of any age, usually with a previous neurological impairment, and consist of a prolonged seizure lasting more than 15 minutes that can recur within 24 hours and result in neurological deficits after the seizure (Fetveit, 2008).

The cause of febrile seizures is still uncertain. Risk factors for simple febrile seizures include viral infections and a family history of febrile seizures (Fetveit, 2008). Associations with chromosome mutations, premature birth, and developmental delay have been evaluated but have not demonstrated any conclusive evidence (Fetveit, 2008). Most febrile seizures have stopped by the time the child is taken to a medical facility and require no treatment. However, if the seizure continues, treatment consists of controlling the seizure with IV or rectal lorazepam or diazepam and reducing the temperature with acetaminophen or ibuprofen (Hampers & Spina, 2011). Antiepileptic prophylaxis usually is not indicated. Antipyretic therapy may lower the child's temperature and provide symptomatic relief but will not prevent a seizure, probably because the seizure often occurs as the temperature is rising or falling (Mikati & Hani, 2016). Tepid sponge baths are not recommended, for several reasons: they are ineffective in significantly lowering the temperature, the shivering effect further increases metabolic output, and cooling causes discomfort to the child (see Chapter 44, Therapeutic Management of fever, p. 1292). Parental education and emotional support are important interventions, and information may need to be repeated, depending on the parents' anxiety and education level. Parents need reassurance regarding the benign nature of simple febrile seizures. Several large studies show no difference in neurological deficits, cognitive functioning, or memory impairments in children with simple or complex febrile seizures compared with population control participants (Fetveit, 2008).

Long-term antiepileptic therapy is usually not required for children with simple febrile seizures. These children have only a 1% risk of developing epilepsy, but children with a complex febrile seizure along with a pre-existing neurological abnormality and a family history of afebrile seizure have a 10% risk of developing epilepsy (Hampers & Spina, 2011).

NURSING ALERT

If a febrile seizure lasts more than 5 minutes, parents should seek medical attention right away. Instruct them to call for emergency assistance (911) and not to place the child who is actively having a seizure in the car.

CEREBRAL MALFORMATIONS

Cranial Deformities

In the healthy newborn the cranial sutures are separated by membranous seams several millimetres wide. Up to 2 days after birth, the cranial bones are highly mobile, which allows them to mould and slide over one another. The principal sutures in the infant's skull are the sagittal, coronal, and lambdoidal sutures, and the major soft areas at the juncture of these sutures are the anterior and posterior fontanels (see Fig. 16-1, p. 402).

After birth, growth of the skull bones occurs in a direction perpendicular to the line of the suture, and normal closure occurs in a regular and predictable order. Although there are wide variations in the age at which closure takes place in individual children, normally all sutures and fontanels are ossified by the following ages:

Eight weeks—Posterior fontanel closed
Six months—Fibrous union of suture lines and interlocking of serrated edges
Eighteen months—Anterior fontanel closed
After 12 years—Sutures unable to be separated by increased ICP

A solid union of all sutures is not completed until late childhood. **Craniosynostosis** (closure of a suture before the expected time) inhibits the perpendicular growth. Since the normal increase in brain volume requires expansion, the skull is forced to grow in a direction parallel to the fused suture. This alteration in skull growth always produces a distortion of the head shape when the underlying brain growth is normal. A small head with closed and normal shape is a result of deficient brain growth; the suture closure is secondary to this brain growth failure.

Various types of cranial deformities are encountered in early infancy. These include an enlarged head with frontal protrusion (bossing; characteristic of hydrocephalus), parietal bossing that is seen in chronic subdural hematoma, a small head (microcephaly), and a variety of skull deformities. Some occur during prenatal development; in others, head circumference is usually within normal limits at birth, and the deviation from normal development becomes apparent with advancing age. The majority of infants with craniosynostosis have normal brain development. The exceptions are those with genetic disorders that involve brain pathological conditions.

Microcephaly

Microcephaly is a congenital condition that refers to a head circumference that measures more than 3 standard deviations below the mean for age and sex. Brain growth is usually restricted and thus cognitive impairment is common. Microcephaly can be the result of an autosomal-dominant disorder; a chromosomal abnormality; fetal exposure to teratogens such as radiation; maternal substance use; and congenital infections such as rubella, toxoplasmosis, cytomegalovirus, or Zika virus. Infants with microcephaly require supportive nursing care and medical observation to determine the extent of the psychomotor delay that almost always accompanies this abnormality. There is no treatment. Parents need support to learn to care for a child with cognitive impairment.

Positional Plagiocephaly

Positional plagiocephaly (PP) is a cranial asymmetry. An increase in the frequency of PP has been noted since the recommendation that infants be placed in the supine position for sleeping to reduce the incidence of sudden infant death syndrome (SIDS). There is unilateral flattening of the occiput, with ipsilateral anterior shifting of the ear. The incidence of PP is striking at 6 weeks of age but the vast majority of plagiocephaly cases resolve by 2 years of age (Cummings & CPS, Community Paediatrics Committee, 2011/2016).

The Canadian Paediatric Society (Cummings & CPS, Community Paediatrics Committee, 2011/2016) recommends the following:

- Prevention of plagiocephaly begins with positioning of the head to encourage lying on each side in the supine position.

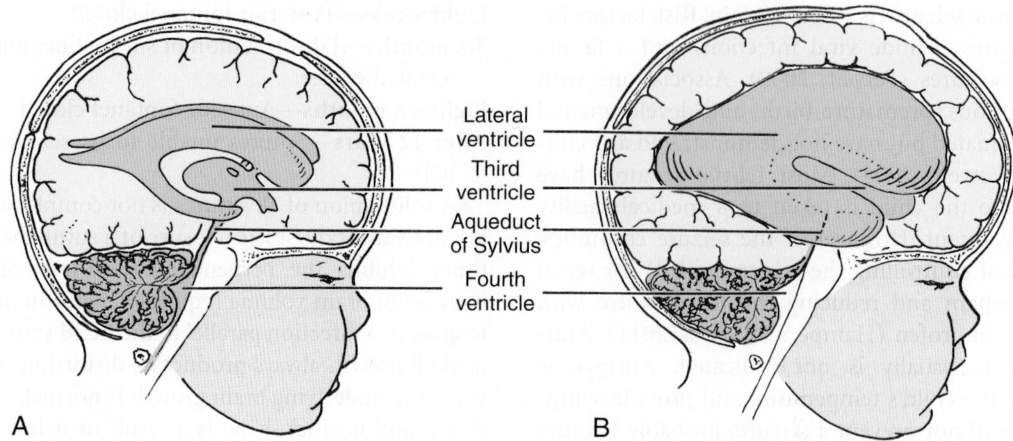

FIGURE 50-8 Hydrocephalus: a block in flow of cerebrospinal fluid. **A:** Patent cerebrospinal fluid circulation. **B:** Enlarged lateral and third ventricles caused by obstruction of circulation—stenosis of aqueduct of Sylvius.

- The child should be in a prone position during awake time (tummy time) for 10 to 15 minutes at least three times per day
- Evaluation for craniosynostosis, congenital torticollis, and cervical spine abnormalities should be part of the examination of a child with plagiocephaly.
- Repositioning therapy plus physiotherapy as needed are the interventions for children with mild or moderate PP.
- Moulding therapy (helmet therapy) may be considered for children with severe asymmetry (see Fig. 35-15).

NURSING CARE

Nursing care of families in which there is a child with a cranial defect involves identifying children with deformities and referring them for evaluation. Since no therapy is available for children with microcephaly, nursing care is directed toward helping parents adjust to rearing a child with brain damage (see Chapter 41).

Caring for infants who benefit from surgery requires special emphasis on observation for signs of anemia because of the large blood loss during surgery. Nursing care includes observation for signs of hemorrhage, infection, pain, and swelling, as well as parental education for suture care and safety. Surgical sutures should remain dry and intact. Parents need to observe for any signs of redness, drainage, or swelling and report any temperature greater than 38.4°C (101°F).

Early surgical management of craniosynostosis allows proper expansion of the brain and the creation of an acceptable appearance. Parents require special support and education during this time, especially from the health care team.

Hydrocephalus

Hydrocephalus is a condition caused by an imbalance in the production and absorption of CSF in the ventricular system. When production is greater than absorption, CSF accumulates within the ventricular system, usually under increased pressure, producing passive dilation of the ventricles.

Pathophysiology

The causes of hydrocephalus are varied, but the result is either (1) impaired absorption of CSF fluid within the subarachnoid space, obliteration of the subarachnoid cisterns, or malfunction of the arachnoid villi (communicating hydrocephalus), or (2) obstruction to the flow of CSF through the ventricular system (noncommunicating hydrocephalus) (Kinsman & Johnston, 2016). Any imbalance of secretion and absorption causes an increased accumulation of CSF in the ventricles, which become dilated (ventriculomegaly) and compress the brain substance against the surrounding rigid bony cranium. When this occurs before fusion of the cranial sutures, it causes enlargement of the skull and dilation of the ventricles (Fig. 50-8). In children younger than 10 to 12 years of age, partially closed suture lines, especially the sagittal suture, may become diastatic or opened. After 12 years of age the sutures are fused and will not open.

Most cases of noncommunicating hydrocephalus are a result of developmental malformations. Although the defect is usually apparent in early infancy, it may become evident at any time from the prenatal period to late childhood or early adulthood. Other causes include neoplasms, infections, and trauma. An obstruction to the normal flow can occur at any point in the CSF pathway to produce increased pressure and dilation of the pathways proximal to the site of obstruction.

About one third of all cases of congenital hydrocephalus result from stenosis of the aqueduct of Sylvius in the brain. Other developmental defects (e.g., Arnold-Chiari malformations, aqueduct gliosis, and atresia of the foramina of Luschka and Magendie [Dandy-Walker syndrome]) account for most other cases of hydrocephalus from birth to 2 years of age. Hydrocephalus is also often associated with myelomeningocele (see Chapter 54 for further discussion). All infants with this condition should be observed for its development. In the remainder of cases there is a history of intrauterine infection, perinatal hemorrhage, and neonatal meningoencephalitis. In older children, hydrocephalus is most often a result of intracranial masses, intracranial infections, hemorrhage, pre-existing developmental defects, such as aqueduct stenosis or the Arnold-Chiari malformation (a congenital anomaly in which the cerebellum and medulla oblongata extend down through the foramen magnum), or trauma.

Clinical Manifestations

The factors that influence the clinical picture in hydrocephalus are the time and acuity of onset, and associated structural malformations. In infancy, before closure of the cranial sutures, head enlargement is the predominant sign, whereas in older infants and children the lesions responsible for hydrocephalus produce other neurological signs through pressure on adjacent structures before causing CSF obstruction (Box 50-12).

The signs and symptoms in early to late childhood are caused by increased ICP, and specific manifestations are related to the focal lesion. Most commonly resulting from posterior fossa neoplasms and aqueduct stenosis, the clinical manifestations are primarily those associated with space-occupying lesions (i.e., headaches on awakening with improvement after emesis or being in an upright position, strabismus, and ataxia).

Diagnostic Evaluation

Hydrocephalus in infants is based on head circumference that crosses at least one percentile line on the head measurement chart within 2 to 4 weeks. In evaluation of a preterm infant specially adapted head circumference charts are consulted to distinguish abnormal head growth from normal rapid head growth. Fetal ultrasound is helpful in the detection of hydrocephalus. The primary diagnostic tools to detect hydrocephalus in older infants and children are CT and MRI. Diagnostic evaluation of children who have symptoms of hydrocephalus after infancy is similar to that used in those with suspected intracranial tumour. In newborns echoencephalography is useful in comparing the ratio of lateral ventricle to cortex.

Therapeutic Management

The treatment of hydrocephalus is directed toward relief of the hydrocephalus, treatment of complications, and management of problems related to the effect of the disorder on psychomotor development. The treatment is, with few exceptions, surgical. This is accomplished by direct removal of an obstruction (such as a tumour) or placement of a shunt that provides primary drainage of the CSF from the ventricles to an extracranial compartment, usually the peritoneum (ventriculoperitoneal [VP] shunt) (Fig. 50-9).

Most shunt systems consist of a ventricular catheter, a flush pump, a unidirectional flow valve, and a distal catheter. In all models the valves are designed to open at a predetermined intraventricular pressure and close when the pressure falls below that level, thus preventing backflow of secretions.

The initial shunt is placed to relieve CSF obstruction, and revisions are needed when signs of malfunction appear. In all mechanisms the initial success rate is relatively high; however, shunts are associated with complications that interfere with continued shunt function or threaten the child's life.

The major complications of VP shunts are infection and malfunction. All shunts are subject to mechanical difficulties, such as kinking, plugging, or separation or migration of the tubing. Malfunction is most often caused by mechanical obstruction either within the ventricles from particulate matter (tissue or exudate) or at the distal end from thrombosis or displacement as a result of growth. Revisions are needed when signs of malfunction appear. The child with a shunt obstruction is often first seen in an emergency department with clinical manifestations of increased ICP, frequently accompanied by worsening neurological status.

BOX 50-12 CLINICAL MANIFESTATIONS OF HYDROCEPHALUS

Infancy (Early)

Abnormally rapid head growth
Bulging fontanels (especially anterior) sometimes without head enlargement:
- Tense
- Nonpulsatile

Dilated scalp veins
Separated sutures
Macewen sign (cracked-pot sound on percussion)
Thinning of skull bones

Infancy (Later)

Frontal enlargement, or bossing
Depressed eyes
Setting-sun sign (sclera visible above the iris)
Pupils sluggish, with unequal response to light

Infancy (General)

Irritability
Lethargy
Infant crying when picked up or rocked and quieting when allowed to lie still
Early infantile reflex acts may persist
Normally expected responses failing to appear
May display:
- Change in level of consciousness
- Opisthotonos (often extreme)
- Lower extremity spasticity
- Vomiting

Advanced cases:
- Difficulty in sucking and feeding
- Shrill, brief, high-pitched cry
- Cardiopulmonary embarrassment

Childhood

Headache on awakening; improvement following emesis or upright posture
Papilledema
Strabismus
Extrapyramidal tract signs (e.g., ataxia)
- Irritability
- Lethargy
- Apathy
- Confusion
- Incoherence
- Vomiting

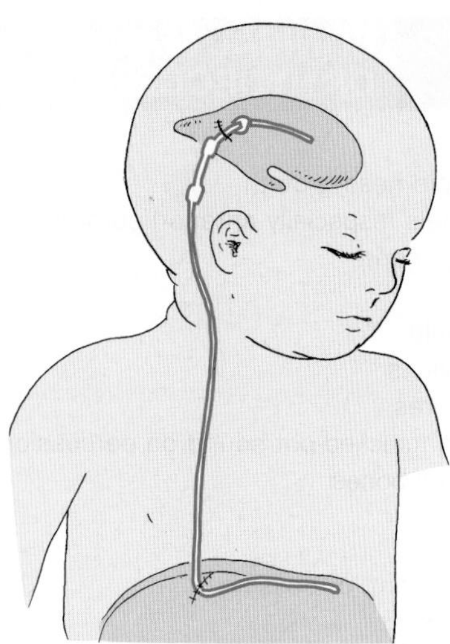

FIGURE 50-9 Ventriculoperitoneal shunt. Catheter is threaded beneath the skin.

The most serious complication, shunt infection, can occur at any time, but the period of greatest risk is 1 to 2 months after placement. The infection is generally a result of intercurrent infections at the time of shunt placement. Infections include septicemia, bacterial endocarditis, wound infection, shunt nephritis, meningitis, and ventriculitis. Meningitis and ventriculitis are of greatest concern, since any complicating CNS infection is a significant predictor of poor intellectual outcome. Infection is treated with antibiotics administered intravenously or intrathecally for a minimum of 7 to 10 days. A persistent infection requires removal of the shunt until the infection is controlled. External ventricular drainage (EVD) is used until CSF is sterile. The EVD allows for removal of CSF through a tube that is placed in the child's ventricle and flows by gravity into a collection device. The EVD drainage point is set at the prescribed level ordered by the neurosurgeon.

An alternative to shunt placement is the endoscopic third ventriculostomy in children with noncommunicating hydrocephalus. In this procedure, an endoscope is used to make a small opening in the floor of the third ventricle that allows the CSF to flow freely through the previously blocked ventricle. Endoscopic septal fenestration has an overall patency rate of 81%, which may eliminate the need for a CSF shunt. Complications include CSF leak, intraventricular hemorrhage, meningitis, cranial nerve injury, obstruction, and hypothalamic injury (Hader, Walker, Myles, et al., 2008).

Prognosis

The prognosis for children with treated hydrocephalus depends largely on the rate at which hydrocephalus develops, the duration of increased ICP, the frequency of complications, and the cause of the hydrocephalus. For example, malignant tumours may have a high mortality rate regardless of other complicating factors.

Surgically treated hydrocephalus with continued neurosurgical and medical management has a survival rate of about 80%, with the highest incidence of mortality occurring within the first year of treatment (Paulsen, Luundar, & Lindegaard, 2010). Of the surviving children, approximately one third are both intellectually and neurologically normal, and one half have neurological disabilities. Although most children with a history of hydrocephalus are good-natured and friendly, some can have aggressive or delinquent behaviour and may be depressed (Kinsman & Johnston, 2016).

NURSING CARE

Preoperatively the infant with diagnosed or suspected hydrocephalus is observed carefully for signs of increasing ICP. In infants the head is measured daily at the largest point, the occipitofrontal circumference (see Head Circumference, Chapter 33, for technique). If the infant's head is large, a special pressure-sensitive mattress and frequent position changes are necessary to prevent skin breakdown. Fontanels and suture lines are gently palpated for size, signs of bulging, tenseness, and separation. An infant with normal ICP will display bulging under certain circumstances such as straining or crying; therefore, such accompanying behaviour should be noted. Irritability, lethargy, or seizure activity, as well as altered vital signs and feeding behaviour, may indicate an advancing pathological condition.

General nursing care of the infant with hydrocephalus may present special problems. Maintaining adequate nutrition often requires flexible feeding schedules to accommodate diagnostic procedures, since feeding before or after handling can precipitate an episode of vomiting. Small feedings at more frequent intervals are often better tolerated than larger ones spaced further apart. These infants are often difficult to feed and require extra time and innovation.

In older children the most valuable indicator of increasing ICP is an alteration in the child's LOC and changes in the way the child interacts with the environment. Changes are identified by observation and by comparison of present behaviour with customary behaviour, sleep patterns, developmental capabilities, and habits, all obtained through a detailed history and a baseline assessment. This baseline information serves as a guide for postoperative assessment and evaluation of shunt function.

The nurse is responsible for preparing the child for diagnostic tests such as MRI or CT scan and assisting the practitioner with procedures such as a ventricular tap, which is often performed to relieve excessive pressure during the preoperative period and for CSF examination. Sedation is required, since the child must remain absolutely still during diagnostic testing (see Preparation for Diagnostic and Therapeutic Procedures, Chapter 44).

Postoperative Care

In addition to routine postoperative care and observation, the infant or child is positioned carefully on the unoperated side to prevent pressure on the shunt valve. The child is kept flat to avoid complications resulting from too-rapid reduction of intracranial fluid. When the ventricular size is reduced too rapidly, the cerebral cortex may pull away from the dura and tear the small interlacing veins, producing a subdural hematoma. The surgeon will indicate the position to be maintained and the extent of activity allowed. Pain management can be achieved with acetaminophen for mild to moderate pain and opioids for severe pain (see Pain Management, Chapter 34).

Observation is continued for signs of increased ICP, which indicates obstruction of the shunt. Neurological assessment includes evaluation of pupillary dilation (pressure causes compression or stretching of the oculomotor nerve, producing dilation on the same side as the pressure) and blood pressure (hypoxia to the brainstem causes variability in these vital signs). If there is increased ICP, the surgeon will prescribe elevation of the head of the bed and allow the child to sit up to enhance gravity flow through the shunt.

> **! NURSING ALERT**
>
> Arbitrary pumping of the shunt may cause obstruction or other problems and should not be performed unless indicated by the neurosurgeon.

Because infection is the greatest hazard of the postoperative period, nurses need to be on the alert for the usual manifestations of CSF infection, such as elevated temperature, poor feeding, vomiting, decreased responsiveness, and seizure activity. There may be signs of local inflammation at the operative sites and along the shunt tract. The child is also observed for abdominal distension, since CSF may cause peritonitis or a postoperative ileus as a complication of distal catheter placement. Antibiotics are administered by the IV route as ordered, and the nurse may also need to assist with intraventricular instillation. The incision site is inspected for leakage, and any suspected drainage is tested for glucose, an indication of CSF. In addition, intake and output need to be carefully monitored. Children may be placed on fluid restriction with nothing by mouth for 24 hours. The IV infusion should be closely monitored to prevent fluid overload. Routine feeding is resumed after the prescribed NPO period, but the presence of bowel sounds should be determined before feeding a child with a VP shunt.

Meticulous skin care is continued postoperatively, with extra care to prevent tissue damage from pressure. A pressure-reducing mattress or overlay pad underneath the child helps prevent pressure on prominent areas. Skin should be inspected regularly for any signs of pressure, irritation, or infection.

Family Support

Specific needs and concerns of parents during periods of hospitalization are related to the reason for the child's hospitalization (shunt revision, infection, diagnosis) and the diagnostic and surgical procedures to which the child is subjected. Parents may have little understanding of anatomy; therefore, they need further exploration and reinforcement of information that was given to them by the neurosurgeon, as well as information about what they can expect. They may be especially frightened of any procedure that involves the brain, and the fear of intellectual disability or brain damage is real and pervasive. Nurses can do much to allay their anxiety by explaining the rationale underlying the various nursing and medical activities, such as positioning or testing, and by simply being available and willing to listen to their concerns.

To prepare for the child's discharge and home care, the parents need to be instructed on how to recognize signs that indicate shunt malfunction or infection. Active children may have injuries, such as a fall, that can damage the shunt, and the tubing may pull out of the distal insertion site or become disconnected during normal growth. Contact sports should be avoided, and a helmet should be worn when outside play is vigorous.

The management of hydrocephalus in a child is a demanding task for both family and health care providers, and helping a family cope with the child is an important nursing responsibility. Children with hydrocephalus have lifelong special health care needs and require evaluation on a regular basis. The overall aim is to establish realistic goals and an appropriate educational program that will help the child to achieve his or her optimal potential.

Families can be referred to community agencies for support and guidance. The Spina Bifida and Hydrocephalus Association of Canada provides information on the condition for families and assists interested groups in establishing local organizations. Helpful booklets are available from this source (see Additional Resources at the end of this chapter).

KEY POINTS

- LOC is the most important indicator of neurological health; altered levels include full consciousness, confusion, disorientation, lethargy, obtundation, stupor, coma, and persistent vegetative state.
- Complete neurological examination includes LOC; posture; motor, sensory, cranial nerve, and reflex testing; and vital signs.
- Nursing care of the unconscious child focuses on ensuring respiratory management; performing neurological assessment; monitoring ICP; supplying adequate nutrition and hydration; providing medication therapy; promoting elimination, hygienic care, proper positioning, exercise, and stimulation; and providing family support.
- Primary head injury involves features that occur at the time of trauma, including fractured skull, contusions, intracranial hematoma, and diffuse injury. Secondary complications include hypoxic brain damage, increased ICP, infection, cerebral edema, and post-traumatic syndromes.
- Fractures resulting from head injuries may be classified as linear, depressed, comminuted, basilar, open and growing.
- The young child's response to head injury is different from that of adults because of the following features: larger head

size, expandable skull, larger blood volume to the brain, and small subdural spaces.

- Problems resulting from submersion injuries include hypoxia and asphyxiation, aspiration, and hypothermia.
- Nursing care of the child with a brain tumour includes observing for signs and symptoms related to the tumour, preparing the child and family for diagnostic tests and operative procedures, preventing postoperative complications, planning for discharge, and promoting a return to optimal health.
- Nursing care of the child with meningitis includes administering antibiotics, taking isolation precautions, removing environmental stimuli, ensuring correct positioning, monitoring vital signs, administering IV therapy, promoting adequate fluid and nutritional status, and providing supportive care to the family.
- Routine immunization of infants with *H. influenzae* type b and pneumococcal conjugate vaccines has reduced the incidence of bacterial meningitis.
- Encephalitis may result from direct invasion of the CNS by a virus or from involvement of the CNS after viral disease.
- A seizure is a symptom of an underlying pathological condition and may be manifested by sensory-hallucinatory phenomena, motor effects, sensorimotor effects, or loss of consciousness.
- Partial seizures are categorized as simple (without associated impairment of consciousness) or complex (with impaired consciousness); both types may become generalized.
- Generalized seizures are categorized as tonic, clonic, tonic-clonic, absence, atonic, and myoclonic.
- Long-term care of the child with recurrent seizure disorders includes physical care and education regarding the importance of medication therapy and concerns related to emotional aspects of the disorder.
- Febrile seizures are the most common type of childhood seizure.
- Some cranial deformities are amenable to surgical correction.
- Hydrocephalus is a symptom of an underlying brain pathological condition demonstrated by impaired absorption of CSF or obstruction to the flow of CSF within the ventricles.
- Therapy for hydrocephalus involves relief of the hydrocephalus, treatment of the underlying brain disorder if possible, prevention or treatment of complications, and management of problems related to psychomotor development.

evolve WEBSITE

Visit the Evolve website for additional resources related to the content in this chapter such as Case Studies, Critical Thinking Case Study Answers, Nursing Care Plans, Nursing Processes, Nursing Skills, and Review Questions for Exam Preparation at: http://evolve.elsevier.com/Canada/Perry/maternal/

REFERENCES

Abbasi, M., Mohammadi, E., & Sheaykh Rezayi, A. (2009). Effect of a regular family visiting program as an affective, auditory, and tactile stimulation on the consciousness level of comatose patients with a head injury. *Japan Journal of Nursing Science*, *6*(1), 21–26. doi:10.1111/j.1742-7924.2009.00117.x.

Badjatia, N. (2009). Hyperthermia and fever control in brain injury. *Critical Care Medicine*, *37*(Suppl. 7), S250–S257. doi:10.1097/CCM.0b013e3181aa5e8d.

Balistreri, W. F., & Ibrahim, S. H. (2016). Mitochondrial hepatopathies. In R. M. Kliegman, B. F. Stanton, J. W. St. Geme, et al. (Eds.), *Nelson textbook of pediatrics* (20th ed.). Philadelphia: Saunders.

Ball, J. W., Dains, J. E., Flynn, J. A., et al. (2015). *Seidel's guide to physical examination* (8th ed.). St. Louis: Mosby.

Barlow, K. M., Crawford, S., Brooks, B. L., et al. (2015). The incidence of post-concussion syndrome remains stable following mild traumatic brain injury in children. *Pediatric Neurology*, *5*(6), 491–497. doi:10.1016/j.pediatrneurol.2015.04.011.

Berg, A. T. (2008). Risk of recurrence after a first unprovoked seizure. *Epilepsia*, *49*(Suppl. 1), 13–18. doi:10.1111/j.1528-1167.2008.01444.x.

Berg, A. T., Berkovic, S., Brodie, M. J., et al. (2010). Revised terminology and concepts for organization of seizures and epilepsies: Report of the ILAE Commission on Classification and Terminology, 2005–2009. *Epilepsia*, *51*(4), 676–685. doi:10.1111/j.1528-1167.2010.02522.x.

Bhalla, T., Dewhirst, E., Sawardekar, A., et al. (2012). Perioperative management of the pediatric patient with traumatic brain injury. *Paediatric Anaesthesia*, *22*(8), 627–640. doi:10.1111/j.1460-9592.2012.03842.x.

Bhatt, M., Roback, M. G., Joubert, G., et al. (2015). The design of a multicentre Canadian surveillance study of sedation safety in the paediatric emergency department. *BMJ Open*, *5*(5), e008223. doi:10.1136/bmjopen-2015-008223.

Blinman, T. A., Houseknecht, E., Snyder, C., et al. (2009). Postconcussive symptoms in hospitalized pediatric patients after mild traumatic brain injury. *Journal of Pediatric Surgery*, *44*, 1223–1228.

Brodeur, G. M., Hogarty, M. D., Bagatell, R., et al. (2016). Neuroblastoma. In P. A. Pizzo & D. G. Pollack (Eds.), *Principles and practice of pediatric oncology* (7th ed.). Philadelphia: Lippincott Williams & Wilkins-Raven.

Caglar, D., Quan, L., et al. (2016). Drowning and submersion injury. In R. M. Kliegman, B. F. Stanton, & J. W. St. Geme (Eds.), *Nelson textbook of pediatrics* (20th ed.). Philadelphia: Saunders.

Canadian Cancer Society. (2016a). *Childhood brain and spinal tumours*. Retrieved from <http://www.cancer.ca/en/cancer-information/cancer-type/brain-spinal-childhood/statistics/?region=on>.

Canadian Cancer Society. (2016b). *Neuroblastoma*. Retrieved from <http://www.cancer.ca/en/cancer-information/cancer-type/neuroblastoma/statistics/?region=on>.

Canadian Cancer Society, Advisory Committee on Cancer Statistics. (2015). *Canadian cancer statistics 2015*. Toronto: Canadian Cancer Society. Retrieved from <https://www.cancer.ca/~/media/cancer.ca/CW/cancer%20information/cancer%20101/Canadian%20cancer%20statistics/Canadian-Cancer-Statistics-2015-EN.pdf>.

Chandran, A., Herbert, H., Misurski, D., et al. (2011). Long-term sequelae of childhood bacterial meningitis: An underappreciated problem. *The Pediatric Infectious Disease Journal*, *30*(1), 3–6.

Christie, R. J. (2008). Therapeutic positioning of the multiply-injured trauma patient in ICU. *The British Journal of Nursing*, *17*(10), 638–642.

Cummings, C., & Canadian Paediatric Society, Community Paediatrics Committee. (2011). Positional plagiocephaly. *Paediatrics & Child Health*, *16*(8), 493–494. Reaffirmed 2016. Retrieved from <http://www.cps.ca/documents/position/positional-plagiocephaly>.

Curatolo, P., Moavero, R., Lo Castro, A., et al. (2009). Pharmacotherapy of idiopathic generalized epilepsies. *Expert Opinion on Pharmacotherapy*, *10*(1), 730–734.

Elliott, R. E., Rodgers, S. D., Bassani, L., et al. (2011). Vagus nerve stimulation for children with treatment-resistant epilepsy: A consecutive series of 141 cases. *Journal of Neurosurgery. Pediatrics*, *7*(5), 491–500. doi:10.3171/2011.2.PEDS10505.

Epilepsy Canada. (2009). *Children and epilepsy*. Retrieved from <http://www.epilepsy.ca/uploads/7/0/8/6/70868839/children-new.pdf>.

Epilepsy Foundation. (2014). *Seizure triggers in children*. Retrieved from <http://www.epilepsy.com/learn/seizures-youth/about-kids/seizure-triggers-children>.

Erlichman, D. B., Blumfield, E., Rajpathak, S., et al. (2010). Association between linear skull fractures and intracranial hemorrhage in children with minor head trauma. *Pediatric Radiology*, *40*(8), 1375–1379. doi:10.1007/s00247-010-1555-4.

Fetveit, A. (2008). Assessment of febrile seizures in children. *European Journal of Pediatrics*, *167*(1), 17–27.

Fink, E. L., Kochanek, P. M., Clark, R. S., et al. (2010). How I cool children in neurocritical care. *Neurocritical Care*, *12*(3), 414–420. doi:10.1007/s12028-010-9334-5.

Forsyth, R., Wolny, S., Rodrigues, B., et al. (2010). Routine intracranial pressure monitoring in acute coma. *The Cochrane Database of Systematic Reviews*, (2), CD002043, doi:10.1002/14651858.CD002043.pub2.

Friedman, J. N., & Canadian Paediatric Society, Acute Care Committee. (2011). Emergency management of the paediatric patient with generalized convulsive status epilepticus. *Paediatrics & Child Health*, *16*(2), 91–97. Reaffirmed 2016. Retrieved from <http://www.cps.ca/documents/position/convulsive-status-epilepticus>.

Hader, W. J., Walker, R. L., Myles, S. T., et al. (2008). Complications of endoscopic third ventriculostomy in previously shunted patients. *Neurosurgery*, *63*(1 Suppl. 1), ONS168–ONS174, discussion, ONS174–175. doi:10.1227/01.neu.0000335032.31144.17.

Hampers, L. C., & Spina, L. A. (2011). Evaluation and management of pediatric febrile seizures in the emergency department. *Emergency Medicine Clinics of North America*, *29*(1), 83–93. doi:10.1016/j.emc.2010.08.008.

Hartman, A. L., & Vining, E. P. (2007). Clinical aspects of the ketogenic diet. *Epilepsia*, *48*(1), 31–42.

Haut, S. R., & Lipton, R. B. (2009). Predicting seizures: A behavioral approach. *Neurologic Clinics*, *27*(4), 925–940. doi:10.1016/j.ncl.2009.06.002.

Health Canada. (2013). *Updated labelling information for acetylsalicylic acid (ASA) products*. Retrieved from <http://www.healthycanadians.gc.ca/recall-alert-rappel-avis/hc-sc/2013/36303a-eng.php?_ga=1.144466108.868197850.1432519476>.

Hon, K. E., & Leung, A. K. (2010). Childhood accidents: Injuries and poisoning. *Advances in Pediatrics*, *57*, 33–62.

Huff, J. S., & Fountain, N. B. (2011). Pathophysiology and definitions of seizures and status epilepticus. *Emergency Medicine Clinics of North America*, *29*(1), 1–13. doi:10.1016/j.emc.2010.08.001.

James, S. H., Kimberlin, D. W., & Whitley, R. J. (2009). Antiviral therapy for herpesvirus central nervous system infections: Neonatal herpes simplex virus infection, herpes simplex encephalitis, and congenital cytomegalovirus infection. *Antiviral Research*, *83*(3), 207–213. doi:10.1016/j.antiviral.2009.04.010.

Joffe, A. R. (2007). Lumbar puncture and brain herniation in acute bacterial meningitis: A review. *Journal of Intensive Care Medicine*, *22*(4), 194–207.

Kinsman, S. L., & Johnston, M. V. (2016). Congenital anomalies of the central nervous system. In R. M. Kliegman, B. F. Stanton, J. W. St. Geme, et al. (Eds.), *Nelson textbook of pediatrics* (20th ed.). Philadelphia: Saunders.

Kossoff, E. H., Zupec-Kania, B. A., & Rho, H. M. (2009). Ketogenic diets: An update for child neurologists. *Journal of Child Neurology*, *24*(8), 979–988.

Kramer, A. H., Zygun, D. A., Doig, C. J., et al. (2013). Incidence of neurologic death among patients with brain injury: A cohort study in a Canadian health region. *Canadian Medical Association Journal*, *185*, E838–E845. doi:10.1503/cmaj.130271.

Landry, G. L. (2016). Epidemiology and prevention of injuries. In R. M. Kliegman, B. F. Stanton, J. W. St. Geme, et al. (Eds.), *Nelson textbook of pediatrics* (20th ed.). Philadelphia: Saunders.

Le Fournier, L., Hénaux, P. L., Haegelen, C., et al. (2015). Intradiploic growing skull fracture: Review of mechanisms and literature. *Child's Nervous System*, *31*(11), 2199–2205.

Le Saux, N., & Canadian Paediatric Society, Infectious Diseases and Immunization Committee. (2014). Guidelines for the management of suspected and confirmed bacterial meningitis in Canadian children older than one month of age. *Paediatrics & Child Health*, *19*(3), 141–146. Retrieved from <http://www.cps.ca/documents/position/management-of-bacterial-meningitis>.

Lifesaving Society Canada. (2015). *Canadian drowning report. 2015 edition*. Retrieved from <http://www.lifesaving.ca/wp-content/uploads/2015/07/CLS-Drowning-0615E_WEB.pdf>.

Logan, S. A., & MacMahon, E. (2008). Viral meningitis. *British Medical Journal*, *336*(7634), 36–40. doi:10.1136/bmj.39409.673657.AE.

Lotan, G., & Vaiman, M. (2015). Treatment of epilepsy by stimulation of the vagus nerve from head-and-neck surgical point of view. *The Laryngoscope*, *125*(6), 1352–1355. doi:10.1002/lary.25064.

Lozsadi, D. A., Von Oertzen, J., & Cock, H. R. (2010). Epilepsy: Recent advances. *Journal of Neurology*, *257*(11), 1946–1951. doi:10.1007/s00415-010-5740-z.

Mason, K. P. (2008). The pediatric sedation service: Who is appropriate to sedate, which medications should I use, who should prescribe the drugs, how do I bill? *Pediatric Radiology*, *38*(Suppl. 2), S218–S224. doi:10.1007/s00247-008-0769-1. Arch Dis.

McCrory, P., Meeuwisse, W., Johnston, K., et al. (2009). Consensus statement on concussion in sport, 3rd International Conference on Concussion in Sport. *Clinical Journal of Sport Medicine*, *19*(3), 185–200.

Merchant, T. E., Pollack, I. F., & Loeffler, J. S. (2010). Brain tumors across the age spectrum: Biology, therapy, and late effects. *Seminars in Radiation Oncology*, *20*(1), 58–66. doi:10.1016/j.semradonc.2009.09.005.

Mian, M., Shah, J., Dalpiaz, A., et al. (2015). Shaken baby syndrome: A review. *Fetal and Pediatric Pathology*, *34*(3), 169–175. doi:10.3109/15513815.2014.999394.

Mikati, M. A., & Hani, A. J. (2016). Seizures in childhood. In R. M. Kliegman, B. F. Stanton, J. W. St. Geme, et al. (Eds.), *Nelson textbook of pediatrics* (20th ed.). Philadelphia: Saunders.

Mullassery, D., Dominici, C., Jesudason, E. C., et al. (2009). Neuroblastoma: Contemporary management. *Archives of Disease in Childhood. Education and Practice Edition*, *94*(6), 177–185. doi:10.1136/adc.2008.143909.

Nei, M., & Bagla, R. (2007). Seizure-related injury and death. *Current Neurology and Neuroscience Reports*, *7*(4), 335–341.

O'Neill, B. R., Handler, M. H., Tong, S., et al. (2015). Incidence of seizures on continuous EEG monitoring following traumatic brain injury in children. *Journal of Neurosurgery. Pediatrics*, *16*(2), 167–176. doi:10.3171/2014.12.PEDS14263.

Orosz, I., McCormick, D., Zamponi, N., et al. (2014). Vagus nerve stimulation for drug-resistant epilepsy: A European long-term study up to 24 months in 347 children. *Epilepsia*, *55*(10), 1576–1584. doi:10.1111/epi.12762.

Østergaard, J. R. (2009). Febrile seizures. *Acta Paediatrica*, *98*(5), 771–773. doi:10.1111/j.1651-2227.2009.01200.x.

Parachute. (n.d.). *Drowning prevention*. Retrieved from <http://www.parachutecanada.org/injury-topics/topic/C3>.

Parachute. (2015). *About injuries. Why pay attention to injuries?* Retrieved from <http://www.parachutecanada.org/injury-topics>.

Park, J. R., Eggert, A., & Caron, H. (2010). Neuroblastoma: Biology, prognosis, and treatment. *Hematology/Oncology Clinics of North America*, *24*(1), 65–86. doi:10.1016/j.hoc.2009.11.011.

Parsons, D. W., Pollack, I. F., Hass-Kogan, T. Y., et al. (2016). Gliomas, ependymomas, and other nonembryonal tumours of the central nervous system. In P. A. Pizzo & D. G. Pollack (Eds.), *Principles and practice of pediatric oncology* (7th ed.). Philadelphia: Lippincott Williams & Wilkins.

Paulsen, A. H., Lundar, T., & Lindegaard, K. F. (2010). Twenty-year outcome in young adults with childhood hydrocephalus: Assessment of surgical outcome, work participation, and health-related quality of life. *Journal of Neurosurgery. Pediatrics, 6*, 527–535.

Prober, C. G., Srinivas, N. S., Mathew, R., et al. (2016). Central nervous system infections. In R. M. Kliegman, B. F. Stanton, & J. W. St. Geme, et al. (Eds.), *Nelson textbook of pediatrics* (20th ed.). Philadelphia: Saunders.

Public Health Agency of Canada. (2014). *Invasive meningococcal disease.* Retrieved from <http://www.phac-aspc.gc.ca/im/vpd-mev/meningococcal-eng.php>.

Public Health Agency of Canada. (2015). *Canadian immunization guide.* Retrieved from <http://www.phac-aspc.gc.ca/publicat/cig-gci/index-eng.php>.

Public Health Agency of Canada. (2016). *Leading causes of death, Canada, 2008, males and females combined, counts (age-specific death rate per 100,000).* Ottawa: Author.

Purcell, L. K., & Canadian Paediatric Society, Healthy Active Living and Sports Medicine Committee. (2014). Sport-related concussion: Evaluation and management. *Paediatrics & Child Health, 19*(3), 153–158. Retrieved from <http://www.cps.ca/documents/position/sport-related-concussion-evaluation-management>.

Reynolds, D., & Boyd, M. (2010). Child life specialists and nurses working together. *Imprint, 57*(1), 22–25.

Rivara, F. P., & Grossman, D. (2016). Injury control. In R. M. Kliegman, B. F. Stanton, J. W. St. Geme, et al. (Eds.), *Nelson textbook of pediatrics* (20th ed.). Philadelphia: Saunders.

Sankhyan, N., Vykunta Raju, K. N., Sharma, S., et al. (2010). Management of raised intracranial pressure. *Indian Journal of Pediatrics, 77*(12), 1409–1416. doi:10.1007/s12098-010-0190-2.

Saskatchewan Brain Injury Association. (2010). *Putting the pieces together: Brain injury*. Retrieved from <http://www.sbia.ca/pdf/pieces.pdf>.

Sharma, S., Kochar, G. S., Sankhyan, N., et al. (2010). Approach to the child with coma. *Indian Journal of Pediatrics, 77*, 1279–1287.

Shaw, S. (2009). Endocrine late effects in survivors of pediatric brain tumors. *Journal of Pediatric Oncology Nursing, 26*(5), 295–302. doi:10.1177/1043454209343180.

Shemie, S. D., Doig, C., Dicken, B., on behalf of the Pediatric Reference Group and the Neonatal Reference Group. (2006). Severe brain injury to neurological determination of death: Canadian forum recommendations. *Canadian Medical Association Journal, 174*(6), S1–S12. doi:10.1503/cmaj.045142.

Shoja, M. M., Tubbs, R. S., Malekian, A., et al. (2007). Video game epilepsy in the twentieth century: A review. *Child's Nervous System, 23*(3), 265–267.

Shorvon, S. (2011). The treatment of status epilepticus. *Current Opinion in Neurology, 24*(2), 165–170. doi:10.1097/WCO.0b013e3283446f31.

Sillanpää, M., & Schmidt, D. (2006). Prognosis of seizure recurrence after stopping antiepileptic drugs in seizure-free patients: A long term population-based study of childhood-onset epilepsy. *Epilepsy & Behavior, 8*(4), 713.

Singhi, S. C., & Tiwari, L. S. (2009). Management of intracranial hypertension. *Indian Journal of Pediatrics, 6*(5), 519–529. doi:10.1007/s12098-009-0137-7.

Somand, D., & Meurer, W. (2009). Central nervous system infections. *Emergency Medicine Clinics of North America, 27*(1), 89–100, ix. doi:10.1016/j.emc.2008.07.004.

Spencer, S., & Huh, L. (2008). Outcomes of epilepsy surgery in adults and children. *The Lancet. Neurology, 7*(6), 525–537. doi:10.1016/S1474-4422(08)70109-1.

Swaine, B. R., Tremblay, C., Platt, R. W., et al. (2007). Previous head injury is a risk factor for subsequent head injury in children: A longitudinal cohort study. *Pediatrics, 119*(4), 750–758. doi:10.1542/peds.2006-1186.

Trillium Gift of Life Network (TGLN). (2012). *Paediatric donation resource manual: A tool to assist hospitals with the process of organ and tissue donation.* Retrieved from <http://www.giftoflife.on.ca/resources/pdf/6752_TGLN_PedDonor_Manual_03F_Web(Sep2914).pdf>.

Truog, R. D., Campbell, M. L., Curtis, J. R., et al. (2008). Recommendations for end-of-life care in the intensive care unit: A consensus statement by the American College of Critical Care Medicine. *Critical Care Medicine, 36*(3), 953–963. doi:10.1097/CCM.0B013E3181659096.

Yeates, L. O., Taylor, H. G., Rusin, J., et al. (2009). Longitudinal trajectories of postconcussive symptoms in children with mild traumatic brain injuries and their relationship to acute clinical status. *Pediatrics, 123*, 735–743.

Young, G. B. (2009). Coma. *Annals of the New York Academy of Sciences, 1157*, 32–47. doi:10.1111/j.1749-6632.2009.04471.x.

ADDITIONAL RESOURCES

About Kids Health—All About Kids and Swimming: <http://www.aboutkidshealth.ca/En/JustForKids/Life/OnePagers/Pages/OnePagerSwimmingSafety.aspx>.

Brain Injury Canada: <http://braininjurycanada.ca/>.

Brain Tumour Foundation of Canada: <http://www.braintumour.ca>.

Canadian Cancer Society: <http://www.cancer.ca>.

Classification of Epilepsies and Epileptic Syndromes: <http://www.epilepsy.com/information/professionals/about-epilepsy-seizures/classifying-seizures>.

Epilepsy Canada: <http://www.epilepsy.ca/>.

Health Canada—Surveillance of West Nile Virus: <http://healthycanadians.gc.ca/diseases-conditions-maladies-affections/disease-maladie/west-nile-nil-occidental/surveillance-eng.php>.

Modified Braden Q Scale (for Pediatric Use): <http://www.therapybc.ca/eLibrary/docs/Resources/Braden%20Q%20scale%20for%20paeds.pdf>.

Neurologic Rehabilitation Institute of Ontario: <http://www.nrio.com/faq.html>.

Parachute—Injury Prevention: <http://parachutecanada.org/>.

Rancho Los Amigos Levels of Cognitive Functioning: <http://www.neuroadvance.com/rancho.htm>.

Spina Bifida and Hydrocephalus Association of Canada: <http://www.sbhac.ca>.

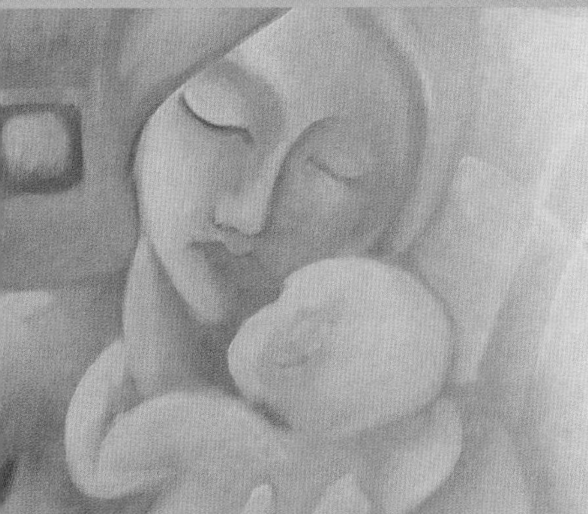

CHAPTER 51

Endocrine Dysfunction

Nancy Caprara, with contributions from Marilyn J. Hockenberry

evolve WEBSITE

***Visit the Evolve website for additional resources related to the content in this chapter such as Case Studies, Critical Thinking Case Study Answers, Nursing Care Plans, Nursing Processes, Nursing Skills, and Review Questions for Exam Preparation at:** http://evolve.elsevier.com/Canada/Perry/maternal/*

OBJECTIVES

On completion of this chapter the reader will be able to:

- Differentiate between the disorders caused by hypopituitary and hyperpituitary dysfunction.
- Describe the manifestations of thyroid hypofunction and hyperfunction and the care of children with the disorders.
- Distinguish between the manifestations of adrenal hypofunction and hyperfunction.
- Differentiate among the various categories of diabetes mellitus.
- Discuss care of the child with diabetes mellitus in the acute care setting.
- Distinguish between a hypoglycemic and a hyperglycemic reaction.
- Design a teaching plan for a child with diabetes mellitus.
- Formulate a teaching plan for the parents of a child with diabetes mellitus.

THE ENDOCRINE SYSTEM

The endocrine system consists of three components: (1) the cells, which send chemical messages by means of hormones; (2) the target cells, or end organs, which receive the chemical messages; and (3) the environment through which the chemicals are transported (blood, lymph, extracellular fluids) from the sites of synthesis to the sites of cellular action. The endocrine system controls or regulates metabolic processes governing energy production, growth, fluid and electrolyte balance, response to stress, and sexual reproduction. The pathophysiology review in Fig. 51-1 provides a summary of the principal pituitary hormones and their target organs.

Hormones

A *hormone* is a complex chemical substance produced and secreted into body fluids by a cell or group of cells that exerts a physiological controlling effect on other cells. These effects may be local or distant and may affect either most cells of the body or specific "target" tissues. Hormones are released by the endocrine glands into the bloodstream, and production is regulated by a feedback mechanism. The master gland of the endocrine system is the anterior pituitary, which is in turn controlled by the hypothalamus. Some hormones, such as insulin, are regulated by other mechanisms.

DISORDERS OF PITUITARY FUNCTION

The pituitary gland is separated into the anterior and posterior lobes and each lobe secretes different hormones. Disorders of the anterior pituitary hormones may be due to organic defects or have an idiopathic etiology and may occur as a single hormonal problem or in combination with other hormonal deficiencies. The clinical manifestations depend on the hormones involved and the age of onset. *Panhypopituitarism* is often defined clinically as the loss of all anterior pituitary hormones, leaving only posterior function intact (Toogood & Stewart, 2008).

> **! NURSING ALERT**
>
> Children with panhypopituitarism should wear a medical alert bracelet.

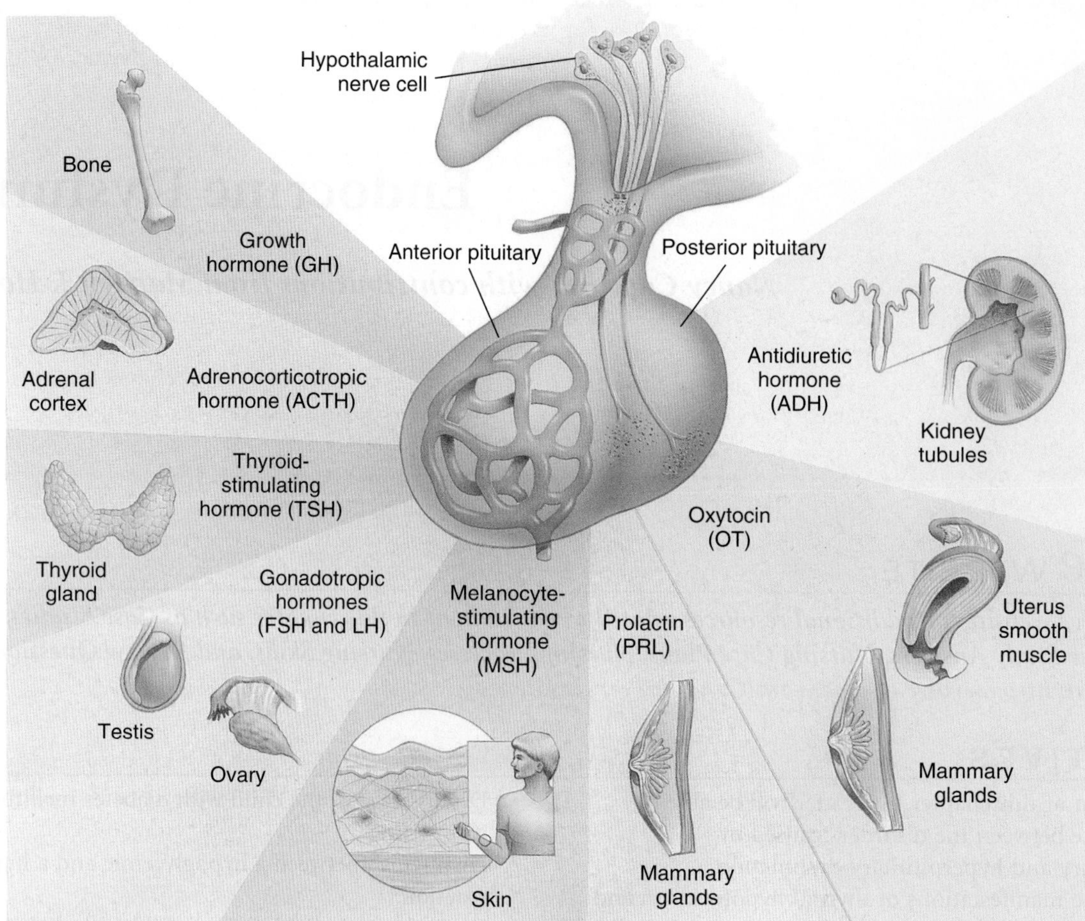

FIGURE 51-1 Principal anterior and posterior pituitary hormones and their target organs. *FSH,* follicle-stimulating hormone; *LH,* luteinizing hormone. (From Patton, K. T., & Thibodeau, G. A. [2013]. *Anatomy and physiology* [8th ed.]. St. Louis: Mosby.)

Hypopituitarism

Hypopituitarism is diminished or deficient secretion of pituitary hormones. The consequences of the condition depend on the degree of dysfunction and lead to gonadotropin deficiency with absence or regression of secondary sex characteristics. Hormones associated with this condition and the respective clinical manifestations are listed in Box 51-1. The most common organic cause of pituitary undersecretion is tumours in the pituitary or hypothalamic region, especially the craniopharyngiomas. Congenital hypopituitarism can be seen in newborn infants, often as a result of birth trauma. Symptoms of apnea, cyanosis, severe hypoglycemia, and seizure activity often manifest within the first 24 hours after birth (Parks & Felner, 2016; Toogood & Stewart, 2008).

Idiopathic hypopituitarism, or idiopathic pituitary growth failure, is usually related to growth hormone (GH) deficiency, which inhibits somatic growth in all cells of the body (Parks & Felner, 2016). *Growth failure* is defined as an absolute height of less than −2 standard deviation (SD) for age or a linear growth velocity consistently less than −1 SD for age. When this occurs without the presence of hypothyroidism, systemic disease, or malnutrition, an abnormality of the GH–insulin-like growth factor (IGF-I) axis should be considered (Richmond & Rogol, 2008). Not all children with short stature have GH deficiency. In most instances, the cause is either familial short stature or constitutional growth delay. *Familial short stature* refers to otherwise healthy children who have ancestors with adult height in the lower percentiles. *Constitutional growth delay* refers to individuals (usually boys) with delayed linear growth, generally beginning as a toddler, and skeletal and sexual maturation that is behind that of age-mates (Parks & Felner, 2016). Typically, these children will reach normal adult height. Often there is a history of a similar pattern of growth in one of the child's parents or other family members. The untreated child will proceed through normal changes as expected on the basis of bone age. Although treatment with GH is not usually indicated, its use has become controversial, especially in relation to parental and child requests for treatment to accelerate growth.

Clinical Manifestations

Children with hypopituitarism generally grow normally during the first year and then follow a slowed growth curve that is below the third percentile. Skeletal proportions and

BOX 51-1 CLINICAL MANIFESTATIONS OF PANHYPOPITUITARISM

Growth Hormone
- Short stature but proportional height and weight
- Delayed epiphyseal closure
- Delayed bone age proportional to height
- Premature aging common in later life
- Increased insulin sensitivity

Thyroid-Stimulating Hormone
- Short stature with infantile proportions
- Dry, coarse skin; yellow discolouration, pallor
- Cold intolerance
- Constipation
- Somnolence
- Bradycardia
- Dyspnea on exertion
- Delayed dentition, loss of teeth

Gonadotropins
- Absence of sexual maturation or loss of secondary sexual characteristics
- Atrophy of genitalia, prostate gland, breasts
- Amenorrhea without menopausal symptoms
- Decreased spermatogenesis

Adrenocorticotropic Hormone
- Severe anorexia, weight loss
- Hypoglycemia
- Hypotension
- Hyponatremia, hyperkalemia
- Adrenal apoplexy, especially in response to stress
- Circulatory collapse

Antidiuretic Hormone
- Polyuria
- Polydipsia
- Dehydration

Melanocyte-Stimulating Hormone
- Decreased pigmentation

weight are normal for the age, but these children may appear younger than their chronological age. Dentition is delayed, and teeth may be overcrowded and malpositioned because of the undeveloped jaw. Sexual development is usually delayed but is otherwise normal unless the gonadotropin hormones are deficient. Growth may extend into the third or fourth decade of life, but permanent height is usually diminished if the disorder is left untreated. Symptoms such as headache and vision changes may indicate the presence of a tumour. Clinical manifestations of panhypopituitarism are listed in Box 50-1.

Diagnostic Evaluation

Only a small number of children with delayed growth or short stature have hypopituitary dwarfism. In most instances the cause is constitutional delay. Diagnostic evaluation is aimed at isolating organic causes, which, in addition to GH deficiency, may include hypothyroidism, oversecretion of cortisol, gonadal aplasia, chronic illness, nutritional inadequacy, Russell-Silver dwarfism, or hypochondroplasia.

BOX 51-2 EVALUATING THE GROWTH CURVE

Ensure reliability of measurements—Accurately obtain and plot height and weight measurements.

Determine absolute height—The child's absolute height bears some relationship to the likelihood of a pathological condition. However, most children who have a height below the lowest percentile (either third or fifth percentile on the height curve) do not have a pathological growth problem.

Assess height velocity—The most important aspect of a growth evaluation is observation of a child's height over time, or height velocity. Accurate determination of height velocity requires at least 4 and preferably 6 months of observation. A substantial deceleration in height velocity (crossing several percentiles) between 3 and 12 or 13 years of age indicates a pathological condition until proven otherwise.

Determine weight-to-height relationship—Determination of the weight-to-height ratio has some diagnostic value in ascertaining the cause of growth restriction in a short child.

Project target height—The height of a child can be judged inappropriately short only in the context of his or her genetic potential. The target height of the child can be determined with the formula:

[Father's height (cm) + Mother's height (cm) + 13] /2 for boys

or

[Father's height (cm) + Mother's height (cm) − 13] /2 for girls

Most children achieve an adult stature within approximately 10 cm of the target height.

Modified from Vogiatzi, M. G., & Copeland, K. C. (1998). The short child. *Pediatrics in Review, 19*(3), 92–99.

A complete diagnostic evaluation should include a family history, a history of the child's growth patterns and previous health status, physical examination, psychosocial evaluation, radiographic surveys, and endocrine studies. Accurate measurement of height (using a calibrated stadiometer) and weight and comparison with standard growth charts are essential. Multiple height measures reflect a more accurate assessment of abnormal growth patterns (Box 51-2).

A skeletal survey in children less than 3 years of age and radiographic examination of the hand-wrist for centres of ossification (bone age) in older children are important in evaluating growth (Box 51-3).

Definitive diagnosis is based on absent or subnormal reserves of pituitary GH. Because GH levels are variable in children, GH stimulation testing is usually required for diagnosis. Initial assessment of the serum IGF-I and IGF binding protein 3 (IGFBP3) indicates a need for further evaluation of GH dysfunction if levels are less than −1 SD below the mean for age. It

BOX 51-3 BONE AGE FOR EVALUATING GROWTH DISORDERS

Bone age refers to a method of assessing skeletal maturity by comparing the appearance of representative epiphyseal centres obtained on x-ray examination with age-appropriate published standards.

Most conditions that cause poor linear growth also cause a delay in skeletal maturation and a restricted bone age. Observation of even a profoundly delayed bone age is never diagnostic or even indicative of a specific diagnosis. A delayed bone age merely indicates that the associated short stature is to some extent "partially reversible," since linear growth will continue until epiphyseal fusion is complete. In comparison, a bone age that is not delayed in a short child is of much greater concern and may, in fact, be of some diagnostic value under certain circumstances.

Modified from Vogiatzi, M. G., & Copeland, K. C. (1998). The short child. *Pediatrics in Review, 19*(3), 92–99.

is recommended that GH stimulation tests be reserved for children with low serum IGF-I and IGFBP3 levels and poor growth who do not have other causes for short stature (Richmond & Rogol, 2008). Children with poor linear growth, delayed bone age, and abnormal GH stimulation tests are considered GH deficient.

Therapeutic Management

Treatment of GH deficiency caused by organic lesions is directed toward correction of the underlying disease process (e.g., surgical removal or irradiation of a tumour). The definitive treatment of GH deficiency is replacement of GH, which is successful in 80% of affected children. Biosynthetic GH is administered subcutaneously on a daily basis. Growth velocity increases in the first year and then declines in subsequent years. Final height is likely to remain less than normal (Bryant, Baxter, Cave, et al., 2007), and early diagnosis and intervention are essential.

The decision to stop GH therapy is made jointly by the child, family, and health care team. Growth rates of less than 2.5 cm/year, a decision by the patient that he or she is tall enough, and a bone age of more than 14 years in girls and more than 16 years in boys are often used as criteria to stop GH therapy (Parks & Felner, 2016). Children with other hormone deficiencies require replacement therapy to correct the specific disorders. This may involve administration of thyroid extract, cortisone, testosterone, or estrogens and progesterone. Treatment with the sex hormones is usually begun during adolescence to promote normal sexual maturation.

NURSING CARE

The principal nursing consideration is identifying children with growth problems. Despite the fact that most growth problems are not a result of organic causes, any delay in normal growth and sexual development poses special emotional adjustments for these children.

The nurse may be a key person in helping establish a diagnosis. For example, if serial height and weight records are not available, the nurse can question parents about the child's growth compared with that of siblings, peers, or relatives.

Preparation of the child and family is especially important if a number of tests are being performed, and the child requires particular attention during provocative testing. Blood samples are usually taken every 30 minutes over a 3-hour period. Children also have difficulty overcoming **hypoglycemia** generated by tests, surgeries, and procedures, so they must be observed carefully for signs of hypoglycemia.

Child and Family Support

Children undergoing hormone replacement require additional support. The nurse should provide education for patient self-management during the school-age years. Nursing functions include family education concerning medication preparation and storage, injection sites, injection technique, and syringe disposal (see Chapter 44). Administration of GH is facilitated by family routines that include a specific time of day for the injection. Younger children may enjoy using a calendar and colourful stickers to designate received injections.

Even when hormone replacement is successful, these children attain their eventual adult height at a slower rate than that of their peers; therefore, they need assistance in setting realistic expectations regarding improvement. Because these children appear younger than their chronological age, others frequently relate to them in infantile or childish ways. Parents and teachers benefit from guidance directed toward setting realistic expectations for the child based on age and abilities. For example, in the home, such children should have the same age-appropriate responsibilities as their siblings. As they approach adolescence, they should be encouraged to participate in group activities with peers. If abilities and strengths are emphasized rather than physical size, such children are more likely to develop a positive self-image.

Pituitary Hyperfunction

Excess GH before closure of the epiphyseal shafts results in proportional overgrowth of the long bones until the individual reaches a height of 2.4 m or more. Vertical growth is accompanied by rapid and increased development of muscles and viscera. Weight is increased but is usually in proportion to height. Proportional enlargement of head circumference also occurs and may result in delayed closure of the fontanels in young children. Children with a pituitary-secreting tumour may also demonstrate signs of increasing intracranial pressure, especially headache.

If oversecretion of GH occurs after epiphyseal closure, growth is in the transverse direction, producing a condition known as *acromegaly.* Typical facial features include overgrowth of the head, lips, nose, tongue, jaw, and paranasal and mastoid sinuses; separation and **malocclusion** of the teeth in the enlarged jaw; disproportion of the face to the cerebral division of the skull; increased facial hair; thickened, deeply creased skin; and increased tendency toward **hyperglycemia** and diabetes mellitus (DM). Acromegaly develops slowly, so this may delay being diagnosed and treatment.

Diagnostic Evaluation

Diagnosis is based on a history of excessive growth during childhood and evidence of increased levels of GH. Radiographic studies may reveal a tumour in an enlarged sella turcica, normal bone age, enlargement of bones (such as the paranasal sinuses), and evidence of joint changes. Endocrine studies to confirm an excess of other hormones, specifically thyroid, cortisol, and sex hormones, should also be included in the differential diagnosis.

Therapeutic Management

If a lesion is present, surgical treatment by cryosurgery or hypophysectomy is performed to remove the tumour when feasible. Other therapies aimed at destroying pituitary tissue include external irradiation and radioactive implants. Depending on the extent of surgical extirpation and degree of pituitary insufficiency, hormone replacement with thyroid extract, cortisone, and sex hormones may be necessary.

NURSING CARE

The primary nursing consideration is early identification of children with excessive growth rates. Although medical management is unable to reduce growth already attained, further growth can be restricted. The earlier the treatment, the more control there is in predetermining a normal adult height. Nurses in ambulatory settings who are frequently involved in growth screening should refer children who demonstrate excessive linear growth for a medical evaluation. They should also observe for signs of a tumour, especially headache, and evidence of concurrent hormonal excesses, particularly the gonadotropins, which cause sexual precocity. Children with excessive growth rates require as much emotional support as those with short stature. Children and their parents need an opportunity to express their thoughts. A compassionate nurse can be supportive to these children, especially before adolescence when they are larger than their peers.

Precocious Puberty

Manifestations of sexual development before age 9 years in boys or age 8 years in girls have traditionally been considered precocious development, and these children were recommended for further evaluation (Garibaldi & Chemaitilly, 2016). Mean onset of puberty is occurring earlier and is presently 10.2 and 9.6 years in White and Black girls, respectively (Ramnitz, & Lodish, 2013). Based on this pattern, it is recommended that precocious puberty evaluation for a pathological cause be performed for White girls younger than 7 years of age and for Black girls younger than 6 years of age. There is a concern that early menarche will increase the risk of future breast cancer (Steingraber, 2007).

Normally, the hypothalamic-releasing factors stimulate secretion of the **gonadotropic hormones** from the anterior pituitary at the time of puberty. In boys, interstitial cell–stimulating hormone stimulates Leydig's cells of the testes to secrete testosterone; in girls, follicle-stimulating hormone (FSH) and luteinizing hormone (LH) stimulate the ovarian follicles to secrete estrogens. This sequence of events is known as the *hypothalamic–pituitary–gonadal axis*. If for some reason the cycle undergoes premature activation, the child will display evidence of advanced or precocious puberty. Causes of precocious puberty are found in Box 51-4.

BOX 51-4 CAUSES OF PRECOCIOUS PUBERTY

Central Precocious Puberty

Idiopathic, with or without hypothalamic hamartoma

Secondary

- Congenital anomalies
- Postinflammatory—Encephalitis, meningitis, abscess, granulomatous disease
- Radiotherapy
- Trauma
- Neoplasms

After effective treatment of long-standing pseudosexual precocity

Peripheral Precocious Puberty

Familial male-limited precocious puberty

Albright syndrome

Gonadal or extragonadal tumours

Adrenal

- Congenital adrenal hyperplasia
- Adenoma, carcinoma
- Glucocorticoid resistance

Exogenous sex hormones

Primary hypothyroidism

Incomplete Precocious Puberty

Premature thelarche

Premature menarche

Premature pubarche or adrenarche

Modified from Garibaldi, L.R. & Chemaitilly, W. (2016). Disorders of pubertal development. In R. M. Kliegman, B. Stanton, J. W. St. Geme, et al. (Eds.), *Nelson textbook of pediatrics* (20th ed.). Philadelphia: Saunders.

Isosexual precocious puberty is more common among girls than boys. Approximately 80% of children with precocious puberty have *central precocious puberty (CPP)*, in which pubertal development is activated by the hypothalamic gonadotropin-releasing hormone (GnRH) (Garibaldi & Chemaitilly, 2016). This produces early maturation and development of the gonads with secretion of sex hormones, development of secondary sex characteristics, and sometimes production of mature sperm and ova. CPP may be the result of congenital anomalies; infectious, neoplastic, or traumatic insults to the central nervous system (CNS); or treatment of long-standing sex hormone exposure. CPP occurs more frequently in girls and is usually idiopathic, with 90% demonstrating no causative factor (Garibaldi & Chemaitilly, 2016). A CNS insult or structural abnormality is found in more than 75% of boys with CPP (Garibaldi & Chemaitilly, 2016).

Peripheral precocious puberty (PPP) includes early puberty resulting from hormone stimulation other than the hypothalamic GnRH–stimulated pituitary gonadotropin release. Isolated manifestations that are usually associated with puberty may be seen as variations in normal sexual development (Garibaldi & Chemaitilly, 2016). They appear without other signs of pubescence and are probably caused by unusual end-organ sensitivity to prepubertal levels of estrogen or androgen. Included are premature thelarche (development of breasts in prepubertal girls), premature pubarche (premature adrenarche, early development of sexual hair), and premature menarche (isolated menses without other evidence of sexual development).

Therapeutic Management

Treatment of precocious puberty is directed toward the specific cause, when known. In 50% of cases, precocious pubertal development regresses or stops advancing without any treatment (Carel & Leger, 2008). If needed, precocious puberty of central (hypothalamic–pituitary) origin is managed with monthly injections of a synthetic analogue of luteinizing hormone–releasing hormone, which regulates pituitary secretions (Garibaldi & Chemaitilly, 2016). The available preparation, leuprolide acetate (Lupron Depot), is given in a dosage of 0.25 to 0.3 mg/kg intramuscularly once every 4 weeks. Longer-lasting formulations have recently been developed as well. GnRH analogue (GnRHa) histrelin has been formulated to implant in the subdermal tissue and may be useful for patients who want to avoid injections (Garibaldi & Chemaitilly, 2016; Kaplowitz, 2009).

Once treatment is initiated, breast development regresses or does not advance, and growth returns to normal rates, enhancing predicted height. Studies suggest that not all patients attain adult targeted heights and the addition of GH therapy may be warranted (Carel & Leger, 2008; Kaplowitz, 2009). Treatment is discontinued at a chronologically appropriate time, allowing pubertal changes to resume. Psychological management of the patient and family is an important aspect of care. Both parents and the affected child should be taught the injection procedure.

NURSING CARE

Psychological support and guidance of the child and family are the most important aspects of nursing care. Parents need anticipatory guidance, support and information resources, and reassurance of the benign nature of the condition. Dress and activities for the physically precocious child should be appropriate to the chronological age. Sexual interest is not usually advanced beyond the child's chronological age, and parents need to understand that the child's mental age is congruent with the chronological age.

Diabetes Insipidus

The principal disorder of posterior pituitary hypofunction is diabetes insipidus (DI), also known as neurogenic DI, resulting from undersecretion of antidiuretic hormone (ADH), also known as vasopressin, and producing a state of uncontrolled diuresis (Qureshi, Galiveeti, Bichet, et al., 2014). This disorder is not to be confused with nephrogenic DI, a rare hereditary disorder affecting primarily males and caused by unresponsiveness of the renal tubules to the hormone.

Neurogenic DI may result from a number of different causes. Primary causes are familial or idiopathic; of the total cases, approximately 45 to 50% are idiopathic. Secondary causes include trauma (accidental or surgical), tumours, granulomatous disease, infections (meningitis or encephalitis), and vascular anomalies (aneurysm). Certain drugs, such as alcohol or phenytoin (diphenylhydantoin), can cause a transient polyuria.

The cardinal signs of DI are polyuria and polydipsia. In the older child, signs such as excessive urination accompanied by a compensatory insatiable thirst may be so intense that the child does little more than go to the toilet and drink fluids. Frequently the first sign is enuresis. In the infant the initial symptom is irritability that is relieved with feedings of water but not milk. The infant is also prone to dehydration, electrolyte imbalance, hyperthermia, azotemia, and potential circulatory collapse.

Dehydration is usually not a serious problem in older children, who are able to drink larger quantities of water. However, any period of unconsciousness, such as after trauma or anaesthesia, may be life threatening because the voluntary demand for fluid is absent. During such instances careful monitoring of urine volumes, blood concentration, and IV fluid replacement is essential to prevent dehydration.

! NURSING ALERT

The child with DI complicated by congenital absence of the thirst centre must be encouraged to drink sufficient quantities of liquid to prevent electrolyte imbalance.

Diagnostic Evaluation

The simplest test used to diagnose this condition is restriction of oral fluids and observation of consequent changes in urine volume and concentration. Normally, reducing fluids results in concentrated urine and diminished volume. In DI, fluid restriction has little or no effect on urine formation but causes weight loss from dehydration. Accurate results from this procedure require strict monitoring of fluid intake and urine output, measurement of urine concentration (specific gravity or osmolality), and frequent weight checks. A weight loss between 3 and 5% indicates significant dehydration and requires termination of the fluid restriction.

NURSING ALERT

Small children require close observation during fluid deprivation to prevent them from drinking from toilet bowls, flower vases, or other unlikely sources of fluid.

If this test is positive, the child should be given a test dose of injected aqueous vasopressin, which should alleviate the polyuria and polydipsia. Unresponsiveness to exogenous vasopressin usually indicates nephrogenic DI. An important diagnostic consideration is to differentiate DI from other causes of polyuria and polydipsia, especially DM. DI may be the early sign of an evolving cerebral process (De Buyst, Massa, Christophe, et al., 2007).

Therapeutic Management

The usual treatment is hormone replacement, either with an intramuscular or subcutaneous injection of vasopressin tannate or with a nasal spray of aqueous lysine vasopressin (Breault & Majzoub, 2016). The injectable form has the advantage of lasting 48 to 72 hours, which affords the child a full night's sleep. However, it has the disadvantage of requiring frequent injections and proper preparation of the drug.

NURSING CARE

The initial objective is identification of the disorder. Because an early sign may be sudden enuresis in a child who is toilet trained, excessive thirst with bed-wetting is an indication for further investigation. Another clue is persistent irritability and crying in an infant that is relieved only by bottle-feedings of water. After head trauma or certain neurosurgical procedures, the development of DI can be anticipated; these patients must be closely monitored.

Assessment includes measurement of body weight, serum electrolytes, blood urea nitrogen (BUN), hematocrit, and urine specific gravity taken before surgery and every other day after the procedure. Fluid intake and output should be carefully measured and recorded. Alert patients are able to adjust intake to urine losses, but unconscious or very young patients require closer fluid observation. In children who are not toilet trained, collection of urine specimens may require application of a urine-collecting device.

After confirmation of the diagnosis, parents need a thorough explanation regarding the condition with specific clarification that DI is a different condition from DM. They must realize that treatment is lifelong. If children are to receive the injectable vasopressin, ideally two caregivers should be taught the correct procedure for preparation and administration of the medication. Once children are old enough, they should be encouraged to assume full responsibility for their care.

For emergency purposes, these children should wear a medical alert bracelet. Older children should carry the nasal spray with them for temporary relief of symptoms. School personnel need to be aware of the problem so they can grant children unrestricted use of the lavatory. Failure to permit this may result in embarrassing accidents that often lead to a child's unwillingness to attend school.

Syndrome of Inappropriate Antidiuretic Hormone

The disorder that results from hypersecretion of ADH from the posterior pituitary hormone is known as *syndrome of inappropriate antidiuretic hormone (SIADH)*. It is observed with increased frequency in a variety of conditions, especially those involving infections, tumours, or other CNS disease or trauma, and is a common cause of hyponatremia in the pediatric population (Rivkees, 2008).

The manifestations are directly related to fluid retention and hypotonicity. Excess ADH causes most of the filtered water to be reabsorbed from the kidneys back into central circulation. Serum osmolality is low, and urine osmolality is inappropriately elevated. When serum sodium levels are diminished to 120 mmol/L, affected children display anorexia, nausea (and sometimes vomiting), stomach cramps, irritability, and personality changes. With progressive reduction in sodium, other neurological signs, stupor, and convulsions may be evident (Rivkees, 2008). The symptoms usually disappear when the underlying disorder is corrected.

The immediate management consists of restricting fluids. Subsequent management depends on the cause and severity. Fluids continue to be restricted to one-fourth to one-half maintenance. When there are no fluid abnormalities but SIADH can be anticipated, fluids are often restricted expectantly at two-thirds to three-fourths maintenance.

NURSING CARE

The first goal of nursing management is recognizing the presence of SIADH from symptoms described in patients at risk, especially those in the pediatric critical care unit.

> **! NURSING ALERT**
>
> Nausea, vomiting, and malaise may precede the onset of more severe stages, such as disorientation, confusion, coma, and seizures.

Accurately measuring intake and output, noting daily weight, and observing for signs of fluid overload are primary nursing functions, especially in the child receiving IV fluids. Seizure precautions should be implemented, and the child and family need education regarding the rationale for fluid restrictions. The rare child with chronic SIADH will be placed on long-term ADH-antagonizing medication, and the child and family will require instructions for its administration.

DISORDERS OF THYROID FUNCTION

The thyroid gland secretes two types of hormones: thyroid hormone (TH), which consists of the hormones thyroxine (T_4) and triiodothyronine (T_3), and calcitonin. The secretion of thyroid hormones is controlled by TSH from the anterior pituitary, which in turn is regulated by thyrotropin-releasing factor (TRF) from the hypothalamus as a negative feedback response. Consequently, hypothyroidism or hyperthyroidism may result from a defect in the target gland or from a disturbance in the secretion of TSH or TRF. Because the functions of T_3 and T_4 are qualitatively the same, the term *TH* is used throughout this discussion.

The synthesis of TH depends on available sources of dietary iodine and tyrosine. The thyroid is the only endocrine gland capable of storing excess amounts of hormones for release as needed. During circulation in the bloodstream, T_4 and T_3 are bound to carrier proteins (thyroxine-binding globulin). They must be unbound before they are able to exert their metabolic effect.

The main physiological action of TH is to regulate the basal metabolic rate and thereby control the processes of growth and tissue differentiation. Unlike GH, TH is involved in many more diverse activities that influence the growth and development of body tissues. Therefore, a deficiency of TH exerts a more profound effect on growth than that seen in hypopituitarism.

Calcitonin helps maintain blood calcium levels by decreasing the calcium concentration. Its effect is the opposite of parathyroid hormone (PTH) in that it inhibits skeletal demineralization and promotes calcium deposition in the bone.

Juvenile Hypothyroidism

Hypothyroidism is one of the most common endocrine problems of childhood. It may be either **congenital** or acquired and represents a deficiency in secretion of TH.

Beyond infancy, primary hypothyroidism may be caused by a number of defects. For example, a congenital hypoplastic thyroid gland may provide sufficient amounts of TH during the first year or two but be inadequate when rapid body growth increases demands on the gland. A partial or complete thyroidectomy for cancer or thyrotoxicosis can leave insufficient thyroid tissue to furnish hormones for body requirements. Radiotherapy for Hodgkin disease or other malignancies may lead to hypothyroidism (Metzger, Krasin, Choi, et al., 2015). Infectious processes may cause hypothyroidism. It can also occur when dietary iodine is deficient, which is rare in Canada, due to iodized salt availability.

Clinical manifestations depend on the extent of dysfunction and the child's age at onset. Primary congenital hypothyroidism is characterized by low levels of circulating thyroid hormones and raised levels of TSH at birth. In Canada, all newborns are screened for hypothyroidism at birth, and this has led to earlier detection and prevention of complications. The GnRH test and baseline measurement of gonadotropin and sex hormone serum concentrations at 3 months of age are promising options for the assessment of hypothalamic–pituitary–gonadal function in infants with congenital hypothyroidism (van Tijn, Schroor, Delemarre-van de Waal, et al., 2007). Researchers associated with the Hospital for Sick Children in Toronto used an automated neuroimaging technique to determine if children with congenital hypothyroidism differ in cortical thickness. The research indicated that the children with congenital hypothyroidism had thinner and thicker areas of the cortex; these findings could potentially predict long-term deficits with neuropsychological functioning (Clairman, Skocic, Lischinsky, et al., 2015). The presenting symptoms are decelerated growth from chronic deprivation of TH or thyromegaly. Impaired growth and development are less severe when hypothyroidism is acquired at a later age, and, because brain growth is nearly complete by 2 to 3 years of age, intellectual disability and neurological sequelae are not associated with juvenile hypothyroidism. Other manifestations are myxedematous skin changes (dry skin, puffiness around the eyes, sparse hair), constipation, sleepiness, and mental decline.

Therapy is TH replacement, the same as for hypothyroidism in the infant, although the prompt treatment needed in the infant is not required in the child. In children with severe symptoms, the restoration of euthyroidism is achieved more gradually with administration of increasing amounts of L-thyroxine over a period of 4 to 8 weeks to avoid symptoms of hyperthyroidism, which can occur with treatment of chronic hypothyroidism. Children who are treated early continue to have mild delays in skills in reading, comprehension, and math but catch up by grade 6. However, adolescents may demonstrate problems with memory, attention, and visuospatial processing.

NURSING CARE

Growth cessation or restriction in a child whose growth has previously been normal should alert the nurse to the possibility of hypothyroidism. After diagnosis and implementation of thyroxine therapy, the importance of adhering to the treatment and periodic monitoring of response to therapy should be stressed to parents. Children should learn to take responsibility for their own health as soon as they are old enough, at about 9 or 10 years of age.

Goitre

A *goitre* is an enlargement or hypertrophy of the thyroid gland. It may occur with deficient (*hypothyroid*), excessive (*hyperthyroid*), or normal (**euthyroid**) TH secretion. It can be congenital or acquired. Congenital disease usually occurs as a result of maternal administration of antithyroid medications or iodides during pregnancy. Acquired disease can result from increased secretion of pituitary TSH in response to decreased circulating levels of TH or from infiltrative neoplastic or inflammatory processes. In most children, goitre is caused by chronic autoimmune thyroiditis (de Vries, Bulvik, Phillip, et al., 2009). In areas where dietary iodine (essential for TH production) is deficient, goitre can be endemic.

Enlargement of the thyroid gland may be mild and noticeable only when there is an increased demand for TH (e.g., during periods of rapid growth). Enlargement of the thyroid at birth can be sufficient to cause severe respiratory distress. Colloid goitres are diffuse and benign and occur more frequently in adolescent girls. Thyroid function is normal, and the gland will gradually decrease over several years without treatment. TH replacement is necessary to treat the hypothyroidism and reverse the TSH effect on the gland.

NURSING CARE

Large goitres are identified by their obvious appearance. In older children, each lobe of the thyroid should be approximately the same as the terminal phalanx of the child's thumb (de Vries et al., 2009). Smaller nodules may be evident only on palpation. Benign enlargement of the thyroid gland may occur during adolescence and should not be confused with pathological states. Nodules rarely are caused by a cancerous tumour but always require evaluation. Questions regarding exposure to radiation should be included in the assessment.

! NURSING ALERT

If an infant is born with a goitre, immediate precautions need to be instituted for emergency ventilation, such as giving supplemental oxygen and having a tracheostomy set nearby. Hyperextension of the neck often facilitates breathing. Immediate surgery to remove part of the gland may be lifesaving in infants born with a goitre.

Lymphocytic Thyroiditis

Lymphocytic thyroiditis (Hashimoto disease, juvenile autoimmune thyroiditis) is the most common cause of thyroid disease in children and adolescents and is associated with the largest percentage of juvenile hypothyroidism. It accounts for many of the enlarged thyroid glands formerly designated *thyroid hyperplasia of adolescence* or *adolescent goitre*. Although it can develop during the first 3 years of life, it occurs more frequently after age 6. It reaches a peak incidence during adolescence, and there is evidence that the disease is self-limiting. The presence of a goitre and elevated thyroglobulin antibody with progressive increase in both thyroid peroxidase antibody and TSH may be predictive factors for future development of hypothyroidism (Radetti, Gottardi, Bona, et al., 2006).

The presence of an enlarged thyroid gland is usually detected by the health care provider during a routine examination, although it may be noted by parents when the youngster swallows. In most children the entire gland is enlarged symmetrically (though it may be asymmetrical) and is firm, freely movable, and nontender. There may be manifestations of moderate tracheal compression (sense of fullness, hoarseness, and dysphagia), but it is extremely rare for a nontoxic diffuse goitre to enlarge to the extent that it causes mechanical obstruction. Most children are euthyroid, but some display symptoms of hypothyroidism, including delayed growth and puberty and declining school performance. Other signs suggestive of lymphocytic thyroiditis are found in Box 51-5.

Diagnostic Evaluation

Thyroid function tests are usually normal, although TSH levels may be slightly or moderately elevated. With progressive disease the T_4 decreases, followed by a decrease in T_3 levels and an increase in TSH. Most affected children have antithyroid antibody titres. However, levels in children are lower than in adults; repeated measurements may be needed in doubtful cases, since titres may increase later in the disease.

Therapeutic Management

In many cases the goitre is transient and asymptomatic and regresses spontaneously within a year or two. Therapy of a nontoxic diffuse goitre is usually simple, uncomplicated, and effective. Oral administration of TH decreases the size of the gland significantly and provides the feedback needed to suppress TSH stimulation, and the hyperplastic thyroid gland gradually regresses in size. TSH levels should be monitored with the goal of restoring normal growth and development. Surgery is contraindicated in this disorder. Untreated patients should be evaluated periodically.

BOX 51-5 CLINICAL MANIFESTATIONS OF LYMPHOCYTIC THYROIDITIS

Enlarged thyroid gland
- Usually symmetrical
- Firm
- Freely movable
- Nontender

Tracheal compression
- Sense of fullness
- Hoarseness
- Dysphagia

Hyperthyroidism (possible)
- Nervousness
- Irritability
- Increased sweating
- Hyperactivity

NURSING CARE

Nursing care consists of identifying the youngster with thyroid enlargement, reassuring the child and parents that the condition is probably only temporary, and reinforcing instructions for thyroid therapy.

Hyperthyroidism

The largest percentage of hyperthyroidism in childhood is caused by Graves' disease, which is usually associated with an enlarged thyroid gland and exophthalmos (Huang & LaFranchi, 2016). Most cases of Graves' disease in children occur between ages 6 and 15, with a peak incidence at 12 to 14 years of age, but the disease may be present at birth in children of thyrotoxic mothers. The incidence is five times higher in girls than in boys.

The hyperthyroidism of Graves' disease is apparently caused by an autoimmune response to TSH receptors, but no specific etiology has been identified. There is definitive evidence for familial association, with a high concordance incidence in twins. There may be an association with other autoimmune diseases such as rheumatoid arthritis and lupus.

The development of manifestations is highly variable. Signs and symptoms develop gradually, with an interval between onset and diagnosis of approximately 6 to 12 months. The principal clinical features are excessive motion—irritability, hyperactivity, short attention span, tremors, insomnia, and emotional lability. Clinical manifestations are presented in Box 51-6.

Exophthalmos (protruding eyeballs), observed in many children, is accompanied by a wide-eyed staring expression, increased blinking, eyelid lag, lack of convergence, and absence of wrinkling of the forehead when looking upward. As protrusion of the eyeball increases, the child may not be able to completely cover the cornea with the lid. Visual disturbances may include blurred vision and loss of visual acuity. Ophthalmopathy can develop long before or after the onset of hyperthyroidism. A consistent pathogenic link between them has not been identified. It is now thought that Graves' ophthalmopathy

BOX 51-6 CLINICAL MANIFESTATIONS OF HYPERTHYROIDISM (GRAVES' DISEASE)

Cardinal Signs
Emotional lability
Physical restlessness, characteristically at rest
Decelerated school performance
Voracious appetite with weight loss in 50% of cases
Fatigue

Physical Signs
Tachycardia
Widened pulse pressure
Dyspnea on exertion
Exophthalmos (protruding eyeballs)
Wide-eyed, staring expression with lid lag
Tremor
Goitre (hypertrophy and hyperplasia)
Warm, moist skin
Accelerated linear growth
Heat intolerance (may be severe)
Hair fine and unable to hold a curl
Systolic murmurs

Thyroid Storm
Acute onset:
- Severe irritability and restlessness
- Vomiting
- Diarrhea
- Hyperthermia
- Hypertension
- Severe tachycardia
- Prostration

May progress rapidly to:
- Delirium
- Coma
- Death

is a disorder of autoimmune origin caused by a complex interplay of endogenous and environmental factors.

Diagnostic Evaluation

The presence of a thyroid mass in a child requires a thorough history, including inquiry into prior irradiation to the head and neck and exposure to a goitrogen. The diagnosis is established on the basis of increased levels of T_4 and T_3. TSH is suppressed to unmeasurable levels. Graves' disease is confirmed by measurement of the thyroid-stimulating immunoglobulins.

Therapeutic Management

Therapy for hyperthyroidism has not been firmly established, but all methods are directed toward slowing the rate of hormone secretion. The three acceptable modes available are the antithyroid medications, including propylthiouracil (PTU) and methimazole (MTZ, Tapazole), which interfere with the biosynthesis of TH; subtotal thyroidectomy when other treatments are not effective; and ablation with radioiodine (^{131}I iodide) (Huang & LaFranchi, 2016). Each treatment is effective, but each has its own advantages and disadvantages. Pharmacological therapy may induce a remission, and treatment may be discontinued. However, relapse may occur. Radioactive iodine ablation is usually effective but response may be slower, and there have been concerns about a possible link to thyroid cancer in younger children. Surgery is often used when other treatments are not effective. These children require lifelong monitoring.

When affected children exhibit signs and symptoms of hyperthyroidism (e.g., increased weight loss, pulse, pulse pressure, and blood pressure), their activity should be limited to quiet and low-impact play and to classwork. Vigorous exercise is restricted until thyroid levels are decreased to normal or near-normal values.

Thyrotoxicosis (thyroid *crisis* or thyroid *storm*) may occur from the sudden release of the hormone. Although thyrotoxicosis is unusual in children, a crisis can be life threatening. These "storms" are evidenced by the acute onset of severe irritability and restlessness, vomiting, diarrhea, hyperthermia, hypertension, severe tachycardia, and prostration (see Box 51-6). There may be rapid progression to delirium, coma, and even death. A crisis may be precipitated by acute infection, surgical emergencies, or discontinuation of antithyroid therapy. Treatment, in addition to antithyroid medications, is administration of beta-adrenergic blocking agents (propranolol), which provide relief from the adrenergic hyperresponsiveness that produces the disturbing adverse effects of the reaction. Therapy is usually required for 2 to 3 weeks.

The Thyroid Foundation of Canada has extensive information related to the prevention, treatment, and cure of thyroid disease (see Additional Resources at the end of this chapter).

NURSING CARE

The initial nursing objective is identification of children with hyperthyroidism. Because the clinical manifestations often appear gradually, the goitre and ophthalmic changes may not be noticed, and the excessive activity may be attributed to behavioural problems. Nurses in ambulatory settings need to be alert to signs that suggest this disorder, especially weight loss despite an excellent appetite, academic difficulties resulting from a short attention span and inability to sit still, unexplained fatigue and sleeplessness, and difficulty with fine motor skills such as writing. Exophthalmos may develop long before the onset of signs and symptoms of hyperthyroidism and may be the only presenting sign. Exophthalmos is less common in adults than children.

Much of the care of these children is related to treating physical symptoms before a response to medication therapy is achieved. A regular routine is beneficial in providing frequent rest periods, minimizing the stress of coping with unexpected demands, and meeting the children's needs promptly. Physical activity is restricted. Mood swings and irritability can disrupt interpersonal relationships, creating difficulties within and outside the home. The child and parents should be encouraged to express their feelings about the behaviour and its effect on others. Heat intolerance may be minimized by the use of light cotton or moisture-wicking clothing, good ventilation, air conditioning or fans, frequent baths, and adequate hydration. Dietary requirements should be adjusted to meet the child's increased metabolic rate. Rather than three large meals, the child's appetite may be better satisfied by five or six moderate meals throughout the day.

NURSING ALERT

Children being treated with propylthiouracil or methimazole must be carefully monitored for adverse effects of the medication. Because sore throat and fever accompany the grave complication of leukopenia, these children should be seen by a health care provider if such symptoms occur. Parents and children should be taught to recognize and report symptoms immediately.

DISORDERS OF PARATHYROID FUNCTION

The parathyroid glands secrete parathyroid hormone (PTH), the main function of which, along with vitamin D and calcitonin, is homeostasis of serum calcium concentration. The effect of PTH on calcium is opposite that of calcitonin. The net result of the integrated action of PTH and vitamin D is maintenance of serum calcium levels within a narrow normal range and the mineralization of bone. Secretion of PTH is controlled by a negative feedback system involving the serum calcium ion concentration. Low ionized calcium levels stimulate PTH secretion, causing absorption of calcium by the target tissues; high ionized calcium concentrations suppress PTH.

Hypoparathyroidism

Hypoparathyroidism is a spectrum of disorders that result in deficient PTH. Congenital hypoparathyroidism may be caused by a specific defect in the synthesis or cellular processing of PTH or by aplasia or hypoplasia of the gland (Doyle, 2016).

Hypoparathyroidism can also occur secondary to other causes, including infection and autoimmune syndromes. Postoperative hypoparathyroidism may follow thyroidectomy with acute or gradual onset and be transient or permanent. Two forms of transient hypoparathyroidism may be present in the newborn, both of which are the result of a relative PTH deficiency. One type is caused by maternal hyperparathyroidism or maternal DM. A more common, later form appears almost exclusively in infants fed a milk formula with a high phosphate-to-calcium ratio.

Pseudohypoparathyroidism occurs when there is a genetic defect in the cellular receptors to PTH. The result is normal parathyroid gland and elevated PTH levels. Abnormal calcium and phosphorus levels are not affected by administration of PTH. These children typically have a short, stocky build; a round face; and abnormally shaped hands and fingers. Other endocrine dysfunction may be found concurrently (Doyle, 2016).

Clinical signs of hypoparathyroidism are found in Box 51-7. Muscle cramps are an early symptom, progressing to numbness, stiffness, and tingling in the hands and feet. A positive Chvostek or Trousseau sign or laryngeal spasms may be present. Convulsions with loss of consciousness may occur. These episodes may be preceded by abdominal discomfort, tonic rigidity, head retraction, and cyanosis. Headaches and vomiting with increased intracranial pressure and papilledema may occur and may suggest a brain tumour (Doyle, 2016).

BOX 51-7 CLINICAL MANIFESTATIONS OF HYPOPARATHYROIDISM

Pseudohypoparathyroidism

Short stature
Round face
Short, thick neck
Short, stubby fingers and toes
Dimpling of skin over knuckles
Subcutaneous soft tissue calcifications
Intellectual disability a prominent feature

Idiopathic Hypoparathyroidism

None of the above physical characteristics observed
May include papilledema
May have intellectual disability

Both Types

Dry, scaly, coarse skin with eruptions
Hair often brittle
Nails thin and brittle with characteristic transverse grooves
Dental and enamel hypoplasia
Muscle contractions:
- Tetany
- Carpopedal spasm
- Laryngospasm (laryngeal stridor)
- Muscle cramps and twitching
- Positive Chvostek sign or Trousseau's sign (see Nursing Alert on p. 1644)

Neurological:
- Headache
- Seizures (generalized, absence, or focal)
- Swings of emotion
- Loss of memory
- Depression
- Confusion possible
- Paresthesias, tingling

Gastrointestinal:
- Muscle cramps
- Diarrhea
- Vomiting

Delayed skeletal growth

Diagnostic Evaluation

The diagnosis of hypoparathyroidism is made on the basis of clinical manifestations associated with decreased serum calcium and increased serum phosphorus. Levels of plasma PTH are low in idiopathic hypoparathyroidism but high in pseudohypoparathyroidism. End-organ responsiveness is tested by the administration of PTH with measurement of urinary cyclic adenosine monophosphate (cAMP). Kidney function tests are included in the differential diagnosis to rule out renal insufficiency. Although bone radiographs are usually normal, they may demonstrate increased bone density and suppressed growth.

NURSING ALERT

The earliest indication of hypoparathyroidism may be anxiety and mental depression, followed by paresthesia and evidence of heightened neuromuscular excitability:

Chvostek sign—Facial muscle spasm elicited by tapping the facial nerve in the region of the parotid gland

Trousseau sign—Carpal spasm elicited by pressure applied to nerves of the upper arm

Tetany—Carpopedal spasm (sharp flexion of wrist and ankle joints), muscle twitching, cramps, seizures, and stridor

Therapeutic Management

The objective of treatment is to maintain normal serum calcium and phosphate levels with minimum complications. Acute or severe tetany is corrected immediately by IV and oral administration of calcium gluconate and follow-up daily doses to achieve normal levels. Twice-daily serum calcium measurements are taken to monitor the efficacy of therapy and prevent hypercalcemia. When diagnosis is confirmed, vitamin D therapy is begun. Vitamin D therapy is somewhat difficult to regulate because the drug has a prolonged onset and a long half-life. Some health care providers advocate beginning with a lower dose with stepwise increase and careful monitoring of serum calcium until stable levels are achieved. Others prefer fast induction with higher doses and rapid reduction to lower maintenance levels (Cooper & Gittoes, 2008; Doyle, 2016).

Long-term management usually consists of vitamin D and oral calcium supplementation. Serum calcium and phosphorus are monitored frequently until the levels have stabilized, then routinely thereafter. Renal function, blood pressure, and serum vitamin D levels are measured every 6 months. Serum magnesium levels are measured to detect hypomagnesemia, which may raise the requirement for vitamin D.

NURSING CARE

The initial objective is recognition of hypocalcemia. Unexplained convulsions, irritability (especially to external stimuli), gastrointestinal symptoms (diarrhea, vomiting, cramping), and positive signs of tetany should lead the nurse to suspect this disorder. Much of the initial nursing care is related to the physical manifestations and includes institution of seizure and safety precautions; reduction of aggravating environmental stimuli, such as avoiding sudden or loud noise, bright lights, and stimulating activities; and observation for signs of laryngospasm, such as stridor, hoarseness, and a feeling of tightness in the throat. A tracheostomy set and injectable calcium gluconate should be located near the bedside for emergency use. The administration of calcium gluconate requires precautions against extravasation of the drug and tissue destruction.

After initiating treatment, the nurse should discuss with the parents the need for continuous daily administration of calcium salts and vitamin D. Because vitamin D toxicity can be a serious consequence of therapy, parents are advised to watch for its signs, which include weakness, fatigue, lassitude, headache, nausea, vomiting, and diarrhea. Early renal impairment is manifested by polyuria, polydipsia, and nocturia.

BOX 51-8 CLINICAL MANIFESTATIONS OF HYPERPARATHYROIDISM

Gastrointestinal
Nausea
Vomiting
Abdominal discomfort
Constipation

Central Nervous System
Delusions
Confusion
Hallucinations
Impaired memory
Lack of interest and initiative
Depression
Varying levels of consciousness

Neuromuscular
Weakness
Easy fatigability
Muscle atrophy (especially proximal muscles of lower limbs)
Tongue twitching
Paresthesias in extremities

Skeletal
Vague bone pain
Subperiosteal resorption of phalanges
Spontaneous fractures
Absence of lamina dura around teeth

Renal
Polyuria
Polydipsia
Renal colic
Hypertension

Hyperparathyroidism

Hyperparathyroidism is rare in childhood but can be primary or secondary. The most common cause of primary hyperparathyroidism is adenoma of the gland (Doyle, 2016). The most common causes of secondary hyperparathyroidism are chronic renal disease, renal osteodystrophy, and congenital anomalies of the urinary tract. The common factor is hypercalcemia. The clinical signs of hyperparathyroidism are listed in Box 51-8.

Diagnostic Evaluation

Blood studies to identify elevated calcium and decreased phosphorus levels are routinely performed. Measurement of PTH, as well as several tests to isolate the cause of the hypercalcemia, such as renal function studies, should be included. Other procedures used to substantiate the physiological consequences of the disorder include electrocardiography and radiographic bone surveys.

Therapeutic Management

Treatment depends on the cause of hyperparathyroidism. The treatment of primary hyperparathyroidism is surgical removal of the tumour or hyperplastic tissue. Treatment of secondary hyperparathyroidism is directed at the underlying contributing cause, which subsequently restores the serum calcium balance. However, in some instances, such as in chronic renal failure, the underlying disorder is irreversible. In this case, treatment is aimed at raising serum calcium levels to inhibit the stimulatory effect of low levels on the parathyroids. This includes oral administration of calcium salts, high doses of vitamin D to enhance calcium absorption, a low-phosphorus diet, and administration of a phosphorus-mobilizing aluminum hydroxide to reduce phosphate absorption.

NURSING CARE

The initial nursing objective is recognition of the disorder. Because secondary hyperparathyroidism is a consequence of chronic renal failure, the nurse needs to be alert to signs that suggest this complication, especially bone pain and fractures. Because urinary symptoms are the earliest indication, assessment of other body systems for evidence of high calcium levels is indicated when polyuria and polydipsia coexist. Clues to the possibility of hyperparathyroidism include a change in behaviour, especially inactivity; unexplained gastrointestinal symptoms; and cardiac irregularities.

DISORDERS OF ADRENAL FUNCTION

The adrenal cortex secretes three main groups of hormones collectively called *steroids* and classified according to their biological activity: (1) glucocorticoids (cortisol, corticosterone), (2) mineralocorticoids (aldosterone), and (3) sex steroids (androgens, estrogens, and **progestins**). Alterations in the levels of these hormones produce significant dysfunction in a variety of body tissues and organs. Because the adrenocortical cells are capable of producing any of the steroids, pathological conditions may result in a deficiency or an excess of more than one type of hormone. However, most of these conditions are rare in children.

The adrenal medulla secretes the catecholamines epinephrine and norepinephrine. Both hormones have essentially the same effects on various organs as those caused by direct sympathetic stimulation, except that the hormonal effects last several times longer. Catecholamine-secreting tumours are the primary cause of adrenal medullary hyperfunction.

Acute Adrenocortical Insufficiency

The acute form of adrenocortical insufficiency (*adrenal crisis*) may have a number of causes during childhood. Although a rare disorder, some of the more common etiological factors include hemorrhage into the gland from trauma, which may be caused by a prolonged, difficult labour; fulminating infections, such as meningococcemia, which result in hemorrhage and necrosis (Waterhouse-Friderichsen syndrome); abrupt withdrawal of exogenous sources of cortisone or failure to increase exogenous supplies during stress; or congenital adrenogenital hyperplasia of the salt-losing type.

BOX 51-9 CLINICAL MANIFESTATIONS OF ACUTE ADRENOCORTICAL INSUFFICIENCY

Early Symptoms

Increased irritability
Headache
Diffuse abdominal pain
Weakness
Nausea and vomiting
Diarrhea

Generalized Hemorrhagic Manifestations (Waterhouse-Friderichsen Syndrome)

Fever (increases as condition worsens)
Central nervous system signs:
- Nuchal rigidity
- Seizures
- Stupor
- Coma

Shocklike State

Weak, rapid pulse
Decreased blood pressure
Shallow respirations
Cold, clammy skin
Cyanosis
Circulatory collapse (terminal event)

Newborn

Hyperpyrexia
Tachypnea
Cyanosis
Seizures
Gland evident as palpable retroperitoneal mass (hemorrhagic)

Early symptoms of adrenocortical insufficiency include increased irritability, headache, diffuse abdominal pain, weakness, nausea and vomiting, and diarrhea. Other clinical signs are found in Box 51-9. In the newborn, adrenal crisis is accompanied by extreme hyperpyrexia (high temperature), tachypnea, cyanosis, and seizures. Usually there is no evidence of infection or purpura. However, hemorrhage into the adrenal gland may be evident as a palpable retroperitoneal mass.

Diagnostic Evaluation

There is no rapid, definitive test for confirmation of acute adrenocortical insufficiency. Routine procedures such as measurement of plasma cortisol levels are too time consuming to be practical. Thus diagnosis is usually made on the basis of clinical presentation, especially when a fulminating sepsis is accompanied by hemorrhagic manifestations and signs of circulatory collapse despite adequate antibiotic therapy. Because there is no real danger in administering a cortisol preparation for a short period, treatment should be instituted immediately. Improvement with cortisol therapy confirms the diagnosis.

Therapeutic Management

Treatment involves replacement of cortisol, replacement of body fluids to combat dehydration and hypovolemia, administration of glucose solutions to correct hypoglycemia, and specific antibiotic therapy in the presence of infection. Initially, IV hydrocortisone (Solu-Cortef) is administered. Normal saline containing 5% glucose is given parenterally to replace lost fluid, electrolytes, and glucose. If hemorrhage has been severe, whole blood may be replaced. In the event that these measures do not reverse the circulatory collapse, vasopressors are used for immediate vasoconstriction and elevation of blood pressure.

Once the child's condition is stabilized, oral doses of cortisone, fluids, and salt are given, similar to the regimen used for chronic adrenal insufficiency. To maintain sodium retention, aldosterone is replaced by synthetic salt-retaining steroids.

NURSING CARE

Because of the abrupt onset and potentially fatal outcome of this condition, prompt recognition is essential. Vital signs and blood pressure are taken every 15 minutes to monitor the hyperpyrexia and shock-like state. Seizure precautions need to be instituted, since convulsions from the elevated temperature are not uncommon. As soon as therapy is instituted, the nurse should monitor the child's response to fluid and cortisol replacement. Too-rapid administration of fluids can precipitate cardiac failure, whereas overdosage with cortisol produces hypotension and a sudden fall in temperature.

Once the acute phase is over and the hypovolemia is corrected, the child is given oral fluids, such as small quantities of ginger ale, fruit juice, or salted broth. Too-rapid ingestion of oral fluids may induce vomiting, which increases dehydration. Therefore, the nurse should plan a gradual schedule for reintroducing liquids.

! NURSING ALERT

Monitor serum electrolyte levels and observe for signs of hypokalemia or hyperkalemia, such as weakness, poor muscle control, paralysis, cardiac dysrhythmias, and apnea. The condition is rapidly corrected with IV or oral potassium replacement.

! NURSING ALERT

When an oral potassium preparation is given, it should be mixed with a small amount of strongly flavoured fruit juice to disguise its bitter taste.

The sudden, severe nature of this disorder necessitates a great deal of emotional support for the child and family. The child may be placed in a critical care unit where the surroundings are strange and frightening. Despite the need for emergency intervention, the nurse must be sensitive to the family's psychological needs and prepare them for each procedure, even if with a brief statement such as "The intravenous infusion is necessary to replace fluid that the child is losing." Because recovery within 24 hours is often dramatic, the nurse should keep the parents apprised of the child's condition, emphasizing signs of improvement, such as a lowered temperature and elevated blood pressure.

Chronic Adrenocortical Insufficiency (Addison Disease)

Chronic adrenocortical insufficiency is rare in children. Causes include infections, destructive lesions of the adrenal gland or neoplasms, autoimmune processes, or idiopathic.

Evidence of this disorder is usually gradual in onset, since 90% of adrenal tissue must be nonfunctional before signs of insufficiency are manifested. However, during periods of stress, when demands for additional cortisol are increased, symptoms of acute insufficiency may appear in a previously well child (Box 51-10).

Definitive diagnosis is based on measurements of functional cortisol reserve. The fasting serum cortisol and urinary 17-hydroxycorticosteroid levels are low and fail to rise, and

BOX 51-10 CLINICAL MANIFESTATIONS OF CHRONIC ADRENOCORTICAL INSUFFICIENCY

Neurological Symptoms
- Muscular weakness
- Mental fatigue
- Irritability, apathy, and negativism
- Increased sleeping, listlessness

Pigmentary Changes
- Previous scars
- Palmar creases
- Hyperpigmentation over pressure points (elbows, knees, or waist)
- Less frequently, vitiligo (loss of pigmentation)

Gastrointestinal Symptoms
- Dehydration
- Anorexia
- Weight loss

Circulatory Symptoms
- Hypotension
- Small heart size
- Dizziness
- Syncopa (fainting) attacks

Hypoglycemia
- Headache
- Hunger
- Weakness
- Trembling
- Sweating

Other Signs (Seen in Some Children)
- Recurrent, unexplained seizures
- Intense craving for salt
- Acute abdominal pain
- Electrolyte imbalances

plasma adrenocorticotropic hormone (ACTH, or corticotropin) levels are elevated with ACTH stimulation, the definitive test for the disease.

Therapeutic Management

Treatment involves replacement of glucocorticoids (cortisol) and mineralocorticoids (aldosterone). Some children are able to be maintained solely on oral supplements of cortisol (cortisone or hydrocortisone preparations) with a liberal intake of salt. During stressful situations, such as fever, infection, emotional upset, or surgery, the dosage must be tripled to accommodate the body's increased need for glucocorticoids. Failure to meet this requirement will precipitate an acute crisis. Overdosage produces the appearance of cushingoid signs.

Children with more severe states of chronic adrenal insufficiency require mineralocorticoid replacement to maintain fluid and electrolyte balance. Other forms of therapy include monthly injections of desoxycorticosterone acetate or implantation of desoxycorticosterone acetate pellets subcutaneously every 9 to 12 months.

NURSING CARE

Once the disorder is diagnosed, parents need guidance with medication therapy. They must be aware of the continuous need for cortisol replacement. Sudden termination of the medication because of inadequate supplies or inability to ingest the oral form because of vomiting places the child in danger of an acute adrenal crisis. The parents should always have a spare supply of the medication in the home. Ideally, they will have a prefilled syringe of hydrocortisone and be instructed in proper technique for intramuscular administration of the medication in case of a crisis. Unnecessary administration of cortisone will not harm the child, but if it is needed, it may be lifesaving. Any evidence of acute insufficiency should be reported to the primary practitioner immediately.

Parents also need to be aware of adverse effects of the medications. Undesirable effects of cortisone include gastric irritation, which is minimized by ingestion of certain foods or the use of an antacid; increased excitability and sleeplessness; weight gain, which may require dietary management to prevent obesity; and, rarely, behavioural changes, including depression or euphoria. Parents should be aware of signs of overdose and report these to the health care provider. In addition, the medication has a bitter taste, which creates a challenge for nurses and parents in its administration.

Because the body cannot supply endogenous sources of cortical hormones during times of stress, the home environment should be stable and relatively unstressful. Parents need to be aware that during periods of emotional or physical crisis the child requires additional hormone replacement. The child should wear a medical alert bracelet, to permit medical personnel to adjust requirements during emergency care.

Cushing Syndrome

Cushing syndrome is a characteristic group of manifestations caused by excessive circulating free cortisol. It can result from a variety of causes, which generally fall under one of five categories (Box 51-11). Cushing syndrome in young children may be due to an adrenal tumour.

Cushing syndrome is uncommon in children. When seen, it is often caused by excessive or prolonged steroid therapy that produces a cushingoid appearance (Fig. 51-2). This condition

BOX 51-11 ETIOLOGY OF CUSHING SYNDROME

Pituitary—Cushing syndrome with adrenal hyperplasia, usually attributed to an excess of adrenocorticotropic hormone (ACTH)

Adrenal—Cushing syndrome with hypersecretion of glucocorticoids, generally a result of adrenocortical neoplasms

Ectopic—Cushing syndrome with autonomous secretion of ACTH, most often caused by extra pituitary neoplasms

Iatrogenic—Cushing syndrome, frequently a result of administration of large amounts of exogenous corticosteroids

Food dependent—Inappropriate sensitivity of adrenal glands to normal postprandial increases in secretion of gastric inhibitory polypeptide

Adapted from Magiakou, M. A., et al. (1994). Cushing's syndrome in children and adolescents: Presentation, diagnosis, and therapy. *New England Journal of Medicine, 331*(10), 629–636.

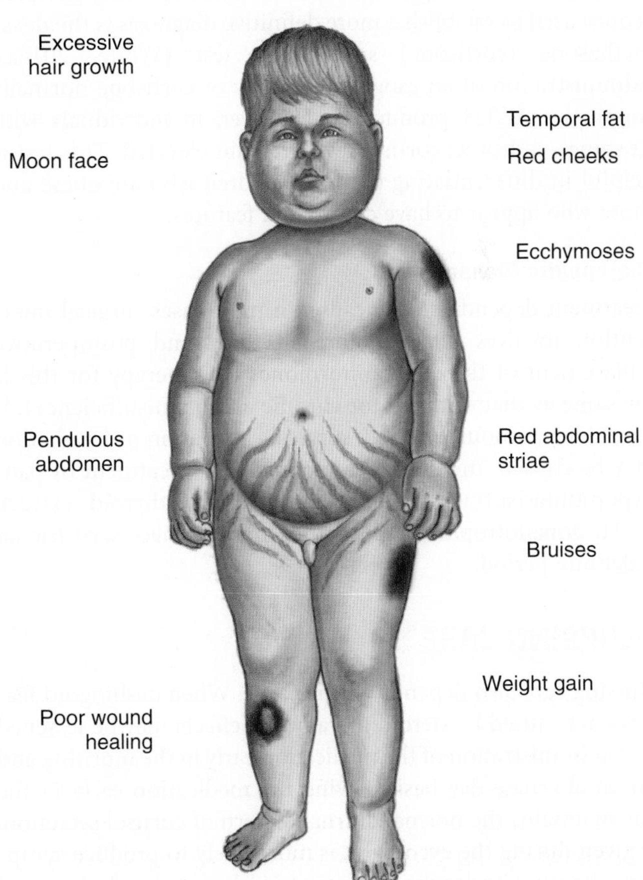

FIGURE 51-2 Characteristics of Cushing syndrome.

is reversible once the steroids are gradually discontinued. Abrupt withdrawal will precipitate acute adrenal insufficiency. Gradual withdrawal of exogenous supplies is necessary to allow the anterior pituitary an opportunity to secrete increasing amounts of ACTH to stimulate the adrenals to produce cortisol.

Clinical Manifestations

Because the actions of cortisol are widespread, clinical manifestations are equally profound and diverse. Those symptoms that produce changes in physical appearance occur early in the disorder and are of considerable concern to school-age and older children. The physiological disturbances, such as hyperglycemia, susceptibility to infection, hypertension, and hypokalemia, may have life-threatening consequences unless recognized early and treated successfully. Children with short stature may be responding to increased cortisol levels, resulting in Cushing syndrome. Cortisol inhibits the action of GH.

Diagnostic Evaluation

Several tests are helpful in confirming Cushing syndrome. Serum cortisol levels should be measured at midnight and in the morning along with corticotropin hormone, urinary free cortisol, fasting blood glucose levels for hyperglycemia, serum electrolyte levels for hypokalemia and alkalosis, 24-hour urinary levels of elevated 17-hydroxycorticoids and 17-ketosteroids, and radiographic studies of bone for evidence of osteoporosis and of the skull for enlargement of the sella turcica. Another procedure used to establish a more definitive diagnosis is the dexamethasone (cortisone) suppression test (White, 2016a). Administration of an exogenous supply of cortisone normally suppresses ACTH production. However, in individuals with Cushing syndrome, cortisol levels remain elevated. This test is helpful in differentiating between children who are obese and those who appear to have cushingoid features.

Therapeutic Management

Treatment depends on the cause. In most cases surgical intervention involves bilateral adrenalectomy and postoperative replacement of the cortical hormones (the therapy for this is the same as that outlined for chronic adrenal insufficiency). If a pituitary tumour is found, surgical extirpation or irradiation may be chosen. In either of these instances, treatment of panhypopituitarism with replacement of GH, thyroid extract, ADH, gonadotropins, and steroids may be necessary for an indefinite period.

NURSING CARE

Nursing care also depends on the cause. When cushingoid features are caused by steroid therapy, the effects may be lessened with administration of the medication early in the morning and on an alternate-day basis. Giving the medication early in the day maintains the normal diurnal pattern of cortisol secretion. If given during the evening, it is more likely to produce symptoms because endogenous cortisol levels are already low and the additional supply exerts more pronounced effects. An alternate-day schedule allows the anterior pituitary an opportunity to maintain more normal hypothalamic–pituitary–adrenal control mechanisms.

If an organic cause is found, nursing care is related to the treatment regimen. Although a bilateral adrenalectomy permanently solves one condition, it reciprocally produces another syndrome. Before surgery, parents need to be adequately informed of the operative benefits and disadvantages. Postoperative teaching regarding medication replacement is the same as that discussed in the previous section.

> **! NURSING ALERT**
>
> Postoperative complications of adrenalectomy are related to the sudden withdrawal of cortisol. Observe for shocklike symptoms (e.g., hypotension, hyperpyrexia).

Anorexia, nausea, and vomiting are common and may be improved with the use of nasogastric decompression. Muscle and joint pain may be severe, requiring use of analgesics. The psychological depression can be profound and may not improve for months. Parents should be aware of the physiological reasons behind these symptoms in order to be supportive of the child.

Congenital Adrenal Hyperplasia

Congenital adrenal hyperplasia (CAH) is a family of disorders caused by decreased enzyme activity required for cortisol production in the adrenal cortex. The adrenal glands produce excessive amounts of cortisol precursors and androgens to compensate. The most common defect is 21-hydroxylase deficiency, which leads to more than 90% of all cases of CAH (White, 2016b). This deficiency occurs in approximately 1 in 15,000 to 20,000 births. In its most severe form it can be life threatening (White, 2016b).

Excessive androgens cause masculinization of the urogenital system at approximately the tenth week of fetal development. The most pronounced abnormalities occur in the girl, who is born with varying degrees of **ambiguous** genitalia. Masculinization of external genitalia causes the clitoris to enlarge so that it appears as a small phallus. Fusion of the labia produces a saclike structure resembling the scrotum without testes. However, no abnormal changes occur in the internal sexual organs, although the vaginal orifice is usually closed by the fused labia. The label *ambiguous genitalia* should be applied to any infant with hypospadias or micropenis and no palpable gonads, and a diagnostic evaluation for CAH should be contemplated. Boys do not display genital abnormalities at birth, so it may go undetected.

Increased pigmentation of skin creases and genitalia caused by increased ACTH may be a subtle sign of adrenal insufficiency. A salt-wasting crisis frequently occurs, usually within the first few weeks of life (White, 2016b). Infants fail to gain weight, and hyponatremia and hyperkalemia may be significant. Cardiac arrest can occur.

Untreated CAH results in early sexual maturation with enlargement of the external sexual organs; development of axillary, pubic, and facial hair; deepening of the voice; acne; and a marked increase in musculature with changes toward an adult male physique. However, in contrast to precocious puberty, breasts do not develop in girls and they remain amenorrheic and infertile. In boys, the testes remain small and spermatogenesis does not occur. In both sexes, linear growth is accelerated and epiphyseal closure is premature, resulting in short stature at the end of puberty.

Diagnostic Evaluation

Clinical diagnosis is initially based on congenital abnormalities that lead to difficulty in assigning sex to the newborn and on signs and symptoms of adrenal insufficiency. Many provinces perform newborn screening of measurement of the cortisol precursor *17-hydroxyprogesterone*. Definitive diagnosis is confirmed by evidence of increased 17-ketosteroid levels in most types of CAH (Menon & Lawson, 2007). In complete 21-hydroxylase deficiency, blood electrolytes demonstrate loss of sodium and chloride and elevation of potassium. In older children bone age is advanced, and linear growth is increased. DNA analysis typing for positive sex determination and to rule out any other genetic abnormality, such as Turner syndrome, is always done in any case of ambiguous genitalia.

Another test that can be used to visualize the presence of pelvic structures is **ultrasonography**, a noninvasive, painless imaging technique that does not require anaesthesia or sedation. It is especially useful in CAH because it readily identifies the absence or presence of female reproductive organs in a newborn or child with ambiguous genitalia. Because ultrasonography yields immediate results, it has the advantage of determining the child's gender long before the more complex laboratory results for chromosome analysis or steroid levels are available.

Therapeutic Management

After diagnosis is confirmed, medical management includes administration of glucocorticoids to suppress the abnormally high secretions of ACTH and adrenal androgens (White, 2016b). If cortisone is begun early enough, it is very effective. Cortisone depresses the secretion of ACTH by the adenohypophysis, which in turn inhibits the secretion of adrenocorticosteroids, which stems the progressive virilization. The signs and symptoms of masculinization in the female gradually disappear, and excessive early linear growth is slowed. Puberty occurs normally at the appropriate age.

The recommended oral dosage is divided to simulate the normal diurnal pattern of ACTH secretion. Because these children are unable to produce cortisol in response to stress, it is necessary to increase the dosage during episodes of infection, fever, surgery, or other stresses. Acute emergencies require immediate IV or intramuscular administration. Children with the salt-losing type of CAH require aldosterone replacement, as outlined under chronic adrenal insufficiency, and supplementary dietary salt. Frequent laboratory tests are conducted to assess the effects on electrolytes, hormonal profiles, and renin levels. The frequency of testing needs to be individualized to the child.

Gender assignment and surgical intervention in the newborn with ambiguous genitalia are complex and controversial. This issue is a significant stress for families, who need support from a multidisciplinary team. Factors that influence gender assignment include genetic diagnosis, genitalia appearance, surgical options, fertility, and family and cultural preferences. Generally, genetically female (46,XX) infants should be raised as girls. Early reconstructive surgery should be considered only in the case of severe virilization. Emphasis is on functional rather than cosmetic outcomes, and surgery can often be delayed. Reports concerning sexual satisfaction after partial clitoridectomy indicate that the capacity for orgasm and sexual gratification is not necessarily impaired.

Unfortunately, not all children with CAH are diagnosed at birth and are raised in accordance with their **genetic sex**. Particularly in the case of affected girls, masculinization of the external genitalia may have led to sex assignment as a male. In boys, diagnosis is usually delayed until early childhood, when signs of virilism appear. In these situations it is advisable to continue rearing the child as a male in accordance with assigned sex and phenotype. Hormone replacement may be required to permit linear growth and to initiate male pubertal changes. Surgery is usually indicated to remove the female organs and reconstruct the phallus for satisfactory sexual relations. These individuals are not fertile.

NURSING CARE

Of major importance is recognition of ambiguous genitalia and diagnostic confirmation in newborns. Parents need assistance in understanding and accepting the condition and time to adjust to the gender ambiguity in their newborn child. As soon as the gender is determined, parents should be informed of the findings and encouraged to choose an appropriate name, and the child should be identified as a male or female, with no reference to ambiguous gender.

In general, rearing the genetically female child as a girl is preferred because of the success of surgical intervention and the satisfactory results with hormones in reversing virilism and providing a prospect of normal puberty and the ability to conceive. This is in contrast to the choice of rearing the child as a boy, in which case the child is sterile, and which can lead to the child struggling with gender identity and potentially with sexual relationships. If the parents persist in their decision to assign a male sex to a genetically female child, a psychological consultation should be requested to explore their motivations and ensure their understanding of the future consequences for the child.

Nursing care management regarding cortisol and aldosterone replacement is the same as that discussed for chronic adrenocortical insufficiency. Because infants are especially prone to dehydration and salt-losing crises, parents need to be aware of signs of dehydration and the urgency of immediate medical intervention to stabilize the child's condition. Parents should have injectable hydrocortisone available and know how to prepare and administer the intramuscular injection (see Chapter 44).

In the unfortunate situation in which the sex is erroneously assigned and the correct sex determined later, parents need a great deal of help in understanding the reason for the incorrect sex identification and the options for sex reassignment or medical-surgical intervention.

Parents should be referred for genetic counselling before they conceive again, as CAH is an autosomal recessive disorder. Prenatal diagnosis and treatments are available.

> **! NURSING ALERT**
>
> The parents should be advised that there is no physical harm in treating for suspected adrenal insufficiency that is not present; the consequence of not treating acute adrenal insufficiency can be fatal.

Pheochromocytoma

Pheochromocytoma is a rare tumour characterized by the secretion of catecholamines. The tumour most commonly arises from the chromaffin cells of the adrenal medulla but may occur wherever these cells are found, such as along the para-ganglia of the aorta or thoracolumbar sympathetic chain (White, 2016c). Approximately 10% of these tumours are located in extra-adrenal sites. In children they are frequently bilateral or multiple and are generally benign. Often there is a familial transmission of the condition as an autosomal dominant trait (White, 2016c).

The clinical manifestations of pheochromocytoma are caused by an increased production of catecholamines, producing hypertension, tachycardia, headache, decreased gastrointestinal activity with resultant constipation, increased metabolism with anorexia, weight loss, hyperglycemia, polyuria, polydipsia, hyperventilation, nervousness, heat intolerance, and diaphoresis. In severe cases, signs of heart failure are evident.

Diagnostic Evaluation

The clinical manifestations mimic those of other disorders, such as hyperthyroidism or DM. Usually the tumour is identified by computed tomography (CT) scan or magnetic resonance imaging (MRI). Definitive tests include 24-hour urinary collection for catecholamines and metanephrines.

Therapeutic Management

Definitive treatment consists of surgical removal of the tumour. In children the tumours may be bilateral, requiring a bilateral adrenalectomy and lifelong glucocorticoid and mineralocorticoid therapy. The major complications during surgery include severe hypertension, tachydysrhythmias, and hypotension. The first two are caused by excessive release of catecholamines during manipulation of the tumour, and the latter results from catecholamine withdrawal and hypovolemic shock.

Preoperative treatment to inhibit the effects of the catecholamines is done 1 to 3 weeks before surgery to prevent these complications. The medications used are alpha-adrenergic blocking agents with or without beta-adrenergic blocking agents. The most commonly used beta-adrenergic blocker is phenoxybenzamine (Dibenzyline), a long-acting medication given orally every 12 hours. The shorter-acting phentolamine (Regitine) is equally effective but less satisfactory for long-term use, although it is useful for acute hypertension. The importance of meticulous preoperative conditioning with alpha-blockers cannot be overemphasized. This intervention is largely responsible for the improvement in outcomes. In select cases, beta blockers (medications that slow the heart rate) may be added after adequate alpha-blockade has been established.

Success of therapy is judged by lowering of blood pressure to normal, absence of hypertensive attacks (flushing or blanching, fainting, headache, palpitations, tachycardia, nausea and vomiting, profuse sweating), heat tolerance, a decrease in perspiration, and disappearance of hyperglycemia. A disadvantage of these drugs is their inability to block the effects of catecholamines on beta receptors.

NURSING CARE

An initial nursing objective is identification of children with this disorder. Outstanding clues are hypertension and hypertensive attacks. Because of behavioural changes (nervousness, excitability, overactivity, and even psychosis), increased cardiac and respiratory activity may appear to be related to an acute anxiety attack. Thus a careful history of the onset of symptoms and association with stressful events is helpful in distinguishing between an organic and a psychological cause for the symptoms.

Preoperative nursing care involves frequent monitoring of vital signs and observation for evidence of hypertensive attacks and heart failure. Therapeutic effects are evidenced by normal vital signs and absence of glycosuria. Daily blood glucose levels, urine acetone, and any signs of hyperglycemia need to be noted and reported immediately.

> **NURSING ALERT**
>
> Do not palpate the mass. Preoperative palpation of the mass releases catecholamines, which can stimulate severe hypertension and tachydysrhythmias.

The environment should be made conducive to rest and free of emotional stress. This requires adequate preparation during hospital admission and before surgery. Play activities need to be tailored to the child's energy level without being overly strenuous or challenging because these can increase the metabolic rate and promote frustration and anxiety.

After surgery, the child needs to be observed for signs of shock from the removal of excess catecholamines. If a bilateral adrenalectomy was performed, the nursing interventions are those discussed for chronic adrenocortical insufficiency.

DISORDERS OF PANCREATIC HORMONE SECRETION

Diabetes mellitus (DM) is a chronic disorder of metabolism characterized by a partial or complete deficiency of the

TABLE 51-1 CHARACTERISTICS OF TYPES 1 AND 2 DIABETES MELLITUS

CHARACTERISTIC	TYPE 1	TYPE 2
Age at onset	<20 yr	Usually adult but increasingly occurring in younger children
Type of onset	Abrupt	Gradual
Sex ratio	Affects males slightly more than females	Females outnumber males
Percentage of diabetic population	5%–8%	85%–90%
Heredity:		
Family history	Sometimes	Frequently
Human leukocyte antigen	Association	No association
Twin concordance	25%–50%	90%–100%
Ethnic distribution	Primarily Whites	Increased incidence in Indigenous peoples and in people of Arab, Asian, Latin American, or African origins
Presenting symptoms	Three P's are common: polyuria, polydipsia, polyphagia	Fatigue, blurred vision, weight gain or loss, polydipsia, and polyuria
Nutritional status	Underweight	Overweight, high levels of fat or cholesterol in the blood
Insulin (natural):		
Pancreatic content	Usually none	>50% normal
Serum insulin	Low to absent	High or low
Primary resistance	Minimum	Marked
Islet cell antibodies	80%–85%	<5%
Therapy:		
Insulin	Always	20%–30% of patients
Oral agents	Ineffective	Often effective
Diet only	Ineffective	Often effective
Chronic complications	>80%	Variable
Ketoacidosis	Common	Infrequent

Panagiotopoulos, C., Riddell, M.C., & Sellers, E.A. (2013). Canadian Diabetes Association 2013 clinical practice guidelines for the prevention and management of diabetes in Canada type 2 diabetes in children and adolescents. *Canadian Journal of Diabetes, 37*(Suppl 1), S163–S167. Retrieved from http://guidelines.diabetes.ca/app_themes/cdacpg/resources/cpg_2013_full_en.pdf

hormone insulin. It is the most common metabolic disease, resulting in metabolic adjustment or physiological change in almost all areas of the body. It is also one of the most common endocrine diseases and chronic conditions in the pediatric population. Overall there are more than 3 million Canadians with diabetes (Canadian Diabetes Association [CDA], Clinical Practice Guidelines Expert Committee, 2013). Currently, no national surveillance data for children living with diabetes are available, and statistics that are available vary widely between provinces and territories (Public Health Agency of Canada [PHAC], 2012).

The different types of DM include type 1 and type 2 diabetes. The characteristics of type 1 DM and type 2 DM are outlined in Table 51-1.

Diabetes Mellitus Type 1

Over 300,000 Canadians have type 1 diabetes. In Canada, there is an annual increase of 3 to 5%, with the highest increase in children 5 to 9 years of age. Canada has the sixth highest incidence of type 1 diabetes in the world for children 14 years of age or younger (PHAC, 2011). DM in children can occur at any age but has a peak incidence between ages 10 and 15 years, with 75% of cases diagnosed before 18 years of age. In Canada there are still not enough data to determine the incidence of type 1 diabetes in relation to specific ethnic origins.

Type 1 diabetes is characterized by destruction of the pancreatic beta cells, which produce insulin; this usually leads to absolute insulin deficiency. Type 1 diabetes has two forms. *Immune-mediated DM* results from an autoimmune destruction of the beta cells; it typically starts in children or young adults who are slim, but it can arise in adults of any age. *Idiopathic type 1* refers to rare forms of the disease that have no known cause.

The symptomatology of diabetes is more readily recognizable in children than in adults, so it is surprising that the diagnosis may sometimes be missed or delayed. Diabetes is a great imitator; influenza, gastroenteritis, and appendicitis are the conditions most often diagnosed when it turns out that the disease is really diabetes (Box 51-12).

Pathophysiology

Insulin is needed to support the metabolism of carbohydrates, fats, and proteins, primarily by facilitating the entry of these substances into the cells. Insulin is needed for the entry of glucose into the muscle and fat cells, prevention of mobilization of fats from fat cells, and storage of glucose as glycogen in the cells of liver and muscle. Insulin is not needed for the entry of glucose into nerve cells or vascular tissue. The chemical composition and molecular structure of insulin are such that it fits into receptor sites on the cell membrane. Here it initiates a sequence of poorly defined chemical reactions that alter the cell membrane to facilitate the entry of glucose into the cell and stimulate enzymatic systems outside the cell that metabolize the glucose for energy production.

BOX 51-12 CLINICAL MANIFESTATIONS OF TYPE 1 DIABETES MELLITUS

Polyphagia
Polyuria
Polydipsia
Weight loss
Enuresis or nocturia
Irritability; the person is "not himself or herself"
Shortened attention span
Lowered frustration tolerance
Dry skin
Blurred vision
Poor wound healing
Fatigue
Flushed skin
Headache
Frequent infections
Hyperglycemia
- Elevated blood glucose levels
- Glucosuria

Diabetic ketosis
- Ketones and glucose in urine
- Dehydration in some cases

Diabetic ketoacidosis
- Dehydration
- Electrolyte imbalance
- Acidosis
- Deep, rapid breathing (Kussmaul)

With a deficiency of insulin, glucose is unable to enter the cell, and its concentration in the bloodstream increases (*hyperglycemia*). The increased concentration of glucose produces an osmotic gradient that causes the movement of body fluid from the intracellular space to the interstitial space and then to the extracellular space and into the glomerular filtrate to "dilute" the hyperosmolar filtrate. Normally, the renal tubular capacity to transport glucose is adequate to reabsorb all the glucose in the glomerular filtrate. When the serum glucose level exceeds the renal threshold ±10 mmol/L, glucose "spills" into the urine (*glycosuria*), along with an osmotic diversion of water (*polyuria*), a cardinal sign of diabetes. The urinary fluid losses cause the excessive thirst (*polydipsia*) observed in diabetes. This water "washout" results in a depletion of other essential chemicals, especially potassium.

Protein is also wasted during insulin deficiency. Because glucose is unable to enter the cells, protein is broken down and converted to glucose by the liver (*glucogenesis*); this glucose then contributes to the hyperglycemia. These mechanisms are similar to those seen in starvation when substrate (glucose) is absent. The body is actually in a state of starvation during insulin deficiency. Without the use of carbohydrates for energy, fat and protein stores are depleted as the body attempts to meet its energy needs. The hunger mechanism is triggered, but the increased food intake (*polyphagia*) enhances the problem by further elevating the blood glucose.

Ketoacidosis. When insulin is absent or insulin sensitivity is altered, glucose is unavailable for cellular metabolism, and the body chooses alternative sources of energy, principally fat. Consequently, fats break down into fatty acids, and glycerol in the fat cells is converted by the liver to ketone bodies (beta-hydroxybutyric acid, acetoacetic acid, acetone). Any excess is eliminated in the urine (*ketonuria*) or the lungs (*acetone breath*). The ketone bodies in the blood (*ketonemia*) are strong acids that lower serum pH, producing ketoacidosis.

Ketones are organic acids that readily produce excessive quantities of free hydrogen ions, causing a fall in plasma pH. Then chemical buffers in the plasma, principally bicarbonate, combine with the hydrogen ions to form carbonic acid, which readily dissociates into water and carbon dioxide. The respiratory system attempts to eliminate the excess carbon dioxide by increasing the depth and rate of respirations—**Kussmaul respirations**, or the hyperventilation characteristic of metabolic acidosis. The ketones are buffered by sodium and potassium in the plasma. The kidney attempts to compensate for the increased pH by increasing tubular secretion of hydrogen and ammonium ions in exchange for fixed base, thus depleting the base buffer concentration.

With cellular death, potassium is released from the cell (intracellular fluid) into the bloodstream (extracellular fluid) and excreted by the kidney, where the loss is accelerated by **osmotic diuresis**. The total body potassium is then decreased, even though the serum potassium level may be elevated as a result of the decreased fluid volume in which it circulates. Alteration in serum and tissue potassium can lead to cardiac arrest.

If these conditions are not reversed by insulin therapy in combination with correction of the fluid deficiency and electrolyte imbalance, progressive deterioration occurs, with dehydration, electrolyte imbalance, acidosis, coma, and death. **Diabetic ketoacidosis (DKA)** should be diagnosed promptly in a seriously ill patient and therapy instituted in a critical care unit.

Long-term complications. Long-term complications of diabetes involve both the microvasculature and the macrovasculature. The principal microvascular complications are nephropathy, retinopathy, and neuropathy. Microvascular disease develops during the first 30 years of diabetes, beginning in the first 10 to 15 years after puberty, with renal involvement evidenced by proteinuria and clinically apparent retinopathy.

With poor diabetic control, vascular changes can appear as early as 2½ to 3 years after diagnosis; however, with good to excellent control, changes can be postponed for 20 or more years. Glycemic control decreases the likelihood of long-term complications in patients with DM (CDA, Clinical Practice Guidelines Expert Committee, 2013). Intensive insulin therapy appears to delay the onset and slow the progression of clinically important retinopathy, nephropathy, and neuropathy. Hypertension and atherosclerotic cardiovascular disease are also major causes of morbidity and mortality in patients with DM. The postpubertal duration, not the total duration, of type 1 DM is implicated as a risk factor for the development of microvascular disease (CDA, Clinical Practice Guidelines Expert Committee, 2013).

Macrovascular disease develops after 25 years of diabetes and creates the predominant problems in patients with type 2 DM. The process appears to be one of glycosylation, in which proteins from the blood become deposited in the walls of small vessels (e.g., glomeruli), where they become trapped by "sticky" glucose compounds (glycosyl radicals). The buildup of these substances over time causes narrowing of the vessels, with subsequent interference with microcirculation to the affected areas.

Other complications have been observed in children with type 1 DM. Hyperglycemia appears to influence thyroid function, and altered function is frequently observed at the time of diagnosis and in poorly controlled diabetes. Limited mobility of small joints of the hand occurs in 30% of 7- to 18-year-old children with type 1 DM and appears to be related to changes in the skin and soft tissues surrounding the joint as a result of glycosylation.

Diagnostic Evaluation

Three groups of children who should be considered as possibly having diabetes are (1) children who have glycosuria, polyuria, and a history of weight loss or failure to gain weight despite a voracious appetite, (2) those with transient or persistent glycosuria, and (3) those who display manifestations of metabolic acidosis, with or without stupor or coma. In every case diabetes must be considered if there is glycosuria, with or without ketonuria, and unexplained hyperglycemia.

Glycosuria by itself is not diagnostic of diabetes. Other sugars, such as galactose, can produce a positive result with certain urine test strips, and a mild degree of glycosuria can be caused by other conditions, such as infection, trauma, emotional or physical stress, hyperalimentation, and some renal or endocrine diseases.

An 8-hour fasting blood glucose level of ≥7.0 mmol/L or more, a random blood glucose value of >11.1 mmol/L or more accompanied by classic signs of diabetes, or an oral glucose tolerance test (OGTT) finding of ≥11.1 mmol/L in the 2-hour sample is almost certain to indicate diabetes (CDA, Clinical Practice Guidelines Expert Committee, 2013). Postprandial blood glucose determinations and the traditional OGTTs have yielded low detection rates in children and are not usually necessary for establishing a diagnosis. Serum insulin levels may be normal or moderately elevated at the onset of diabetes; delayed insulin response to glucose indicates impaired glucose tolerance.

Ketoacidosis must be differentiated from other causes of acidosis or coma, including hypoglycemia, uremia, gastroenteritis with metabolic acidosis, salicylate intoxication encephalitis, and other intracranial lesions. There are no definitive criteria for the diagnosis of DKA but it typically includes a state of relative insulin insufficiency and may include ketonemia (strongly positive), acidosis (pH≤7.30 and bicarbonate ≤15 mmol/L, anion gap ≥12 mmol/L), glycosuria, and ketonuria. The plasma glucose is usually ≥14.0 mmol/L but can be lower and is more difficult to diagnose (CDA, Clinical Practice Guidelines Expert Committee, 2013). Tests used to determine glycosuria and ketonuria are the glucose oxidase tapes (Keto-Diastix).

Therapeutic Management

The management of the child with type 1 DM consists of a multidisciplinary approach involving the family, the child (when appropriate), and professionals, including a pediatric endocrinologist, diabetes nurse educator, nutritionist, and exercise physiologist. Often psychological support from a mental health professional may be needed. Communication among the team members is essential and extends to other individuals in the child's life, such as teachers, the school guidance counsellor, and coaches.

The definitive treatment is replacement of insulin that the child is unable to produce. However, insulin needs are also affected by emotions, nutritional intake, activity, and other life events such as illnesses and puberty. The complexity of the disease and its management requires that the child and family incorporate diabetes needs into their lifestyle. Medical and nutritional guidance are primary, but management also includes continuing diabetes education, family guidance, and emotional support.

Insulin therapy. Insulin replacement is the cornerstone of management of type 1 DM. Insulin dosage is tailored to each child through home blood glucose monitoring. The goal of insulin therapy is to maintain near-normal blood glucose values while avoiding too frequent episodes of hypoglycemia. The recommended glucose levels are listed in Table 51-2. Insulin is administered as two or more injections per day or as a continuous subcutaneous infusion using a portable insulin pump.

Healthy pancreatic cells secrete insulin at a low but steady basal rate with superimposed bursts of increased secretion that coincide with the intake of nutrients. Consequently, insulin levels in the blood increase and decrease coincidentally with rises and falls in blood glucose levels. In addition, insulin is secreted directly into the portal circulation; thus the liver, which is the major site of glucose disposal, receives the largest concentration of insulin. No matter which method of insulin replacement is used, this normal pattern cannot be duplicated. Subcutaneous injection results in absorption of the drug into the general circulation, thus reducing the concentrations of insulin to which the liver is exposed.

Insulin preparations. Insulin is available in highly purified pork preparations and in human insulin biosynthesized by and extracted from bacterial or yeast cultures. Most clinicians suggest human insulin as the treatment of choice. Insulin is available in rapid-, intermediate-, and long-acting preparations, and all are packaged in the strength of 100 units/mL. Some insulins are available as premixed insulins, such as 70/30 and 50/50 ratios, the first number indicating the percentage of intermediate-acting and the second number the percentage of rapid-acting insulin. The type of insulin prescribed depends on different factors that include the patient's age, duration of diabetes, socioeconomic factors, family lifestyle, and family, patient, and prescriber preferences. The different types of insulin are listed in Box 51-13 (see also Table 15-3).

TABLE 51-2 **RECOMMENDED GLYCEMIC GOALS FOR CHILDREN AND ADOLESCENTS WITH TYPE 1 DIABETES**

AGE IN YEARS	HEMOGLOBIN A_{1C} (%) GLYCOSYLATED HEMAGLOBIN	FASTING/PREPRANDIAL (MMOL/L) PLASMA GLUCOSE	2-HOUR POSTPRANDIAL (MMOL/L) PLASMA GLUCOSE	COMMENTS
<6	<8.0	6.0–10.0		It is important to minimize hypoglycemia because of the potential association between severe hypoglycemia and later cognitive impairment. Target of Hgb A_{1C} <8.5% should be considered if excessive hypoglycemia occurs
6–12	<7.5	4.0–10.0		Targets should be graduated to the child's age. Target of Hgb A_{1C} <8.0% should be considered if excessive hypoglycemia occurs
13–18	≤7.0	4.0–7.0	5.0–10.0	Appropriate for most adolescents

Adapted from the Canadian Diabetes Association, Clinical Practice Guidelines Expert Committee. (2013). Canadian Diabetes Association 2013 clinical practice guidelines for the prevention and management of diabetes in Canada. *Canadian Journal of Diabetes, 37*(Suppl 1), S1–S212. Retrieved http://guidelines.diabetes.ca/App_Themes/CDACPG/resources/cpg_2013_full_en.pdf

BOX 51-13 **TYPES OF INSULIN**

There are four types of insulin, based on the following criteria:

- How soon the insulin starts working (onset)
- When the insulin works the hardest (peak time)
- How long the insulin lasts in the body (duration)

However, each person responds to insulin in his or her own way. That is why onset, peak time, and duration are given as ranges.

INSULIN TYPE (TRADE NAME)	ONSET	PEAK	DURATION
Prandial (Bolus) Insulin			
Rapid-acting insulin analogues (clear)			
Insulin aspart (NovoRapid)	10–15 min	1–1.5 hr	3–5 hr
Insulin lispro (Humalog)	10–15 min	1–2 hr	3–4.75 hr
Short-acting insulin (clear)			
Humulin-R Novolin ge Toronto	30 min	2–3 hr	6.5 hr
Inhaled insulin (approved but not yet available in Canada)	10–20 min	2 hr	6 hr
Basal Insulin			
Intermediate-acting (cloudy)			
Humulin-N Novolin ge NPH	1–3 hr	5–8 hr	Up to 18 hr
Long-acting basal insulin analogues (clear)			
Insulin determir (Levemir) Insulin glargine (Lantus)	90 min	Not applicable	Up to 24 hr (glargine 24 hr, determir 16–24 hr)
Premixed Insulin			
Premixed regular insulin—NPH (cloudy)			
Humulin 30/70			
Novolin ge 30/70, 40/60/, 50/50			
Premixed analogues (cloudy)			
Biphasic insulin aspart (NovoMix 30) Insulin lispro/lispro protamine (Humalog Mix25 and Mix50)	A single vial or cartridge contains a fixed ratio of insulin (% of rapid-acting or short-acting insulin to % of intermediate-acting insulin)		

Adapted from the Canadian Diabetes Association, Clinical Practice Guidelines Expert Committee. (2013). Canadian Diabetes Association 2013 clinical practice guidelines for the prevention and management of diabetes in Canada. *Canadian Journal of Diabetes, 37*(Suppl 1), S1–S212. Retrieved from http://guidelines.diabetes.ca/App_Themes/CDACPG/resources/cpg_2013_full_en.pdf

! NURSING ALERT

The human insulins from various manufacturers may be interchangeable, but human insulin and pork insulin or pure pork insulin should never be substituted for one another.

Dosage. Conventional management has consisted of a twice-daily insulin regimen of a combination of rapid-acting and intermediate-acting insulin drawn up into the same syringe and injected before breakfast and before the evening meal. The amount of morning regular insulin is determined by patterns in the late-morning and lunchtime blood glucose values. The morning intermediate-acting dose is determined by patterns in the late-afternoon and supper blood glucose values. Fasting blood glucose patterns at breakfast help determine the evening dose of intermediate insulin, and the blood glucose patterns at bedtime help determine the evening dose of rapid-acting (regular) insulin. For some children, better morning glucose control is achieved by a later (bedtime) injection of intermediate-acting insulin.

Regular insulin is best administered at least 30 minutes before meals. This allows sufficient time for absorption and results in a significantly greater reduction in the postprandial rise in blood glucose than if the meal were eaten immediately after the insulin injection. Intensive therapy consists of multiple injections throughout the day with a once- or twice-daily dose of long-acting (Ultralente) insulin to simulate the basal insulin secretion, and injections of rapid-acting insulin before each meal. A multiple daily injection program reduces microvascular complications of diabetes in young, healthy patients who have type 1 DM.

The precise dosage of insulin needed cannot be predicted. Thus the total dosage and percentage of regular- to intermediate-acting insulin should be determined empirically for each child. Usually 60 to 75% of the total daily dose is given before breakfast and the remainder before the evening meal. Furthermore, insulin requirements do not remain constant but change continuously during growth and development; the need varies according to the child's activity level and pubertal status. For example, less insulin is required during spring and summer months, when the child is more active. Illness also alters insulin requirements. And some children require more frequent insulin administration, such as children with difficult-to-control diabetes and those going through the adolescent growth spurt.

The *insulin pump* is an electromechanical device designed to deliver fixed amounts of regular or lispro insulin continuously (basal rate), thereby more closely imitating the release of the hormone by the islet cells (see Fig. 15-2). Although the pump delivers a programmed amount of basal insulin, the child or parent must program a dose for the pump to deliver before each meal.

The system consists of a syringe to hold the insulin, a plunger, and a computerized mechanism to drive the plunger. The insulin flows from the syringe through a catheter to a needle inserted into subcutaneous tissue (the abdomen or thigh), and the lightweight device is worn on a belt or a shoulder holster. The needle and catheter are changed every 48 to 72 hours by the child or parent, using aseptic technique, and then taped in place.

Although the pump provides more consistent insulin delivery, it has certain disadvantages. Pump therapy is expensive and requires commitment from the parent and child. A certain level of math skills is required to calculate infusion rates. It should also not be removed for more than 1 hour at a time, which may limit some activities. Skin infections are common, and, as with any other mechanical device, it is subject to malfunction. However, the pumps are equipped with alarms that signal problems, such as a depleted battery, an occluded needle or tubing, or a microprocessor malfunction.

Monitoring. Daily monitoring of blood glucose levels is an essential aspect of appropriate DM management. Plasma blood glucose and hemoglobin A_{1c} goal ranges are found in Table 51-2.

Blood glucose. Self-monitoring of blood glucose (SMBG) has improved diabetes management and is used successfully by children from the onset of their diabetes. By testing their own blood, children are able to change their insulin regimen to maintain their glucose level in the euglycemic (normal) range of 4.4 mmol/L to 6.6 mmol/L. Diabetes management depends to a great extent on SMBG. In general, children tolerate the testing well.

Glycosylated hemoglobin. The measurement of hemoglobin A_{1c} levels is a satisfactory method for assessing control of the diabetes. As red blood cells circulate in the bloodstream, glucose molecules gradually attach to the hemoglobin A molecules and remain there for the lifetime of the red blood cell, approximately 120 days. The attachment is not reversible; this glycosylated hemoglobin reflects the average blood glucose levels over the previous 2 to 3 months. The test is a satisfactory method for assessing control, detecting incorrect testing, monitoring effectiveness of changes in treatment, defining patients' goals, and detecting nonadherence to the treatment regimen. Nondiabetic hemoglobin A_{1c} values are generally between 4 and 6% but can vary by laboratory. Diabetes control for children depends on age, with hemoglobin A_{1c} levels of 7 to 8% indicating a slightly elevated but acceptable range (CDA, Clinical Practice Guidelines Expert Committee, 2013). Hemoglobin A_{1c} levels of less than 7% are a well-established goal at most care centres.

Urine. Urine testing for glucose is no longer used for diabetes management; there is poor correlation between simultaneous glycosuria and blood glucose concentrations. However, urine testing can be carried out to detect evidence of ketonuria.

NURSING ALERT

It is recommended that urine be tested for ketones every 3 hours during an illness or whenever the blood glucose level is over 13.3 mmol/L or when symptoms of diabetic ketoacidosis are present.

Nutrition. Essentially the nutritional needs of children with diabetes are no different from those of healthy children. Children with diabetes need no special foods or supplements. They need sufficient calories to balance daily expenditure for energy and to satisfy the requirement for growth and development. Unlike the child without diabetes, whose insulin is secreted in response to food intake, insulin injected subcutaneously has a relatively predictable time of onset, peak effect, duration of action, and absorption rate depending on the type of insulin used. Consequently, the timing of food consumption must be regulated to correspond to the timing and action of the insulin prescribed.

Meals and snacks should be eaten according to peak insulin action, and the total number of calories and proportions of basic nutrients should be consistent from day to day. The constant release of insulin into the circulation makes the child prone to hypoglycemia between the three daily meals unless a snack is provided between meals and at bedtime. The distribution of calories should be calculated to fit each child's activity pattern. For example, a child who is more active in the afternoon will need a larger snack at that time. This larger snack might also be split to allow some food at school and some food after school. Food intake should be altered to balance food, insulin, and exercise. Extra food is needed for increased activity.

Concentrated sweets are discouraged, and because of the increased risk for atherosclerosis in persons with DM, fat is reduced to 30% or less of the total caloric requirement. Dietary fibre has become increasingly important in dietary planning because of its influence on digestion, absorption, and metabolism of many nutrients. It has been found to diminish the rise in blood glucose after meals.

Eating Well With Canada's Food Guide provides a flexible, balanced, and easy-to-follow plan that has a specific adaption for Indigenous peoples (see Appendix A). The plan has been translated into many different languages. Correctly used, the diet allows for flexibility and the incorporation of preferred foods in most instances. For the growing child, food restriction should never be used for diabetes control, although caloric restrictions may be imposed for weight control if the child is overweight. In general, the child's appetite should be the guide for the amount of calories needed, with the total caloric intake adjusted to appetite and activity.

Exercise. Exercise should be encouraged and never restricted unless indicated by other health conditions. Exercise lowers blood glucose levels, depending on the intensity and duration of the activity. An exercise plan should be included as part of diabetes management, and the type and amount of exercise should be planned around the child's interests and capabilities. However, in most instances children's activities are unplanned, and the resulting decrease in blood glucose can be compensated for by providing extra snacks before (and, if the exercise is prolonged, during) the activity. In addition to a feeling of well-being, regular exercise aids in the utilization of food and often results in a reduction of insulin requirements.

Hypoglycemia. Occasional episodes of hypoglycemia are an integral part of insulin therapy, thus an objective of diabetes management is to achieve the best possible glycemic control while minimizing the frequency and severity of hypoglycemia. Even with good control, a child may frequently experience mild symptoms of hypoglycemia. If the signs and symptoms are recognized early and promptly relieved by appropriate therapy, the child's activity should be interrupted for no more than a few minutes. Home management with mini-doses of glucagon can prevent or treat hypoglycemia. Severe hypoglycemia must be treated with IV dextrose and managed in the hospital. There is a concern that significant hypoglycemia events can lead to cognitive impairment in children (CDA, Clinical Practice Guidelines Expert Committee, 2013). Decreased cognitive functioning is more apt to occur in children with early-onset type 1 diabetes and severe hypoglycemia.

! NURSING ALERT

Hypoglycemic episodes most commonly occur before meals, or when the insulin effect is peaking.

The signs and symptoms of hypoglycemia are caused by both increased adrenergic activity and impaired brain function. The increased adrenergic nervous system activity plus increased secretion of catecholamines produces nervousness, pallor, tremulousness, palpitations, sweating, and hunger. Weakness, dizziness, headache, drowsiness, irritability, loss of coordination, seizures, and coma are more severe responses and reflect CNS glucose deprivation and the body's attempts to elevate the serum glucose levels.

It is often difficult to distinguish between hyperglycemia and a hypoglycemic reaction (Table 51-3). Because the symptoms are similar and usually begin with changes in behaviour, the simplest way to differentiate between the two is to test the blood glucose level. The blood glucose level is low in hypoglycemia, whereas in hyperglycemia the glucose level is significantly elevated. In doubtful situations it is safer to give the child some simple carbohydrate. This will help alleviate the symptoms in the case of hypoglycemia but will do little harm if the child is hyperglycemic.

Children are usually able to detect the onset of hypoglycemia, but some are too young to implement treatment. Parents should become adept at recognizing the onset of symptoms—for example, a change in a child's behaviour, such as tearfulness or euphoria. In most cases, 10 to 15 g of simple carbohydrate, such as 15 g of granulated table sugar (approximately 15 mL or 1 Tbsp), will elevate the blood glucose level and alleviate the symptoms. The simpler the carbohydrate, the more rapidly it will be absorbed (237 mL of milk equals 15 g of carbohydrate). The rapid-releasing sugar can be followed by a complex carbohydrate, such as a slice of bread or a cracker, and by a protein, such as peanut butter or milk.

For a mild reaction, milk or fruit juice is a good food to use in children. Milk supplies them with lactose or milk sugar, as well as a more prolonged action from the protein and fat (aids in decreased absorption). Other glucose sources include flavoured liquid glucose, carbonated drinks (not sugarless), sherbet, gelatin, or cake icing. All children with diabetes should carry with them glucose tabs, sugar cubes, or sugar-containing candy. A difficulty with candies or icing is that the child may learn to fake a reaction to get the sweets; thus commercial glucose treatment products may be preferred.

TABLE 51-3 COMPARISON OF MANIFESTATIONS OF HYPOGLYCEMIA AND HYPERGLYCEMIA

VARIABLE	HYPOGLYCEMIA	HYPERGLYCEMIA
Onset	Rapid (minutes)	Gradual (days)
Mood	Labile, irritable, nervous, weepy	Lethargic
Mental status	Difficulty concentrating, speaking, focusing, coordinating	Dulled sensorium
	Nightmares	Confusion
Inward feeling	Shaky feeling	Thirst
	Hunger	Weakness
	Headache	Nausea and vomiting
	Dizziness	Abdominal pain
Skin	Pallor	Flushed
	Sweating	Signs of dehydration
Mucous membranes	Normal	Dry, crusty
Respirations	Shallow, normal	Deep, rapid (Kussmaul)
Pulse	Tachycardia, palpitations	Less rapid, weak
Breath odour	Normal	Fruity, acetone
Neurological	Tremors	Diminished reflexes
		Paresthesia
Ominous signs	Late—Hyperreflexia, dilated pupils, seizure	Acidosis, coma
	Shock, coma	
Blood:		
Glucose	Low: <3.3 mmol/L	High: ≥13.8 mmol/L
Ketones	Negative	High, large
Osmolarity	Normal	High
pH	Normal	Low (≤7.25)
Hematocrit	Normal	High
Bicarbonate	Normal	<20 mmol/L
Urine:		
Output	Normal	Polyuria (early) to oliguria (late)
Glucose	Negative	Enuresis, nocturia
Ketones	Negative or trace	High
Vision	Diplopia	Blurred vision

Small doses of glucagon have been shown to be useful for treating and preventing hypoglycemia at home if there is an inability or refusal to take oral carbohydrate. Glucagon functions by releasing stored glycogen from the liver and requires about 15 to 20 minutes to elevate the blood glucose level. It is available as an emergency kit that must be mixed at the time of use and is administered intramuscularly or subcutaneously with a dose of 10 mcg per year of age, which ranges from a minimum of 20 mcg to a maximum of 150 mcg. The glucagon dose may be doubled if blood glucose does not increase within 20 minutes (CDA, Clinical Practice Guidelines Expert Committee, 2013). At home, if a severe hypoglycemia reaction occurs in an unconscious child older than 5 years, the child should be treated with 1 mg glucagon subcutaneously or intramuscularly. In children under 6 years of age, a dose of 0.5 mg of glucagon should be given. The episode should be discussed with the diabetes health care team as soon as possible (CDA, Clinical Practice Guidelines Expert Committee, 2013). In the hospital, hypoglycemia should be treated with dextrose 0.5 to 1 g/kg given over 1 to 3 minutes when IV access is available.

! NURSING ALERT

Vomiting may occur after administration of glucagon; thus precautions against aspiration must be taken (e.g., placing the child on the side), since the child often becomes unconscious.

Once the child is responsive, the lost glycogen stores are replaced by small amounts of sugar-containing fluid administered frequently until the child feels comfortable trying solid foods.

Morning hyperglycemia. The management of elevated morning blood glucose levels depends on whether the increase is a true dawn phenomenon, insulin waning, or a rebound hyperglycemia (the Somogyi effect). *Insulin waning* is a progressive rise in blood glucose levels from bedtime to morning. It is treated by increasing the nocturnal insulin dose. The *true dawn phenomenon* shows a relatively normal blood glucose level until about 0300, when the level begins to rise. The *Somogyi effect* may occur at any time but often entails an elevated blood glucose level at bedtime and a drop at 0200 with a rebound rise following. The treatment for this phenomenon is decreasing the nocturnal insulin dose to prevent the 0200 hypoglycemia. The rebound rise in the blood glucose level is a result of counterregulatory hormones (epinephrine, GH, and corticosteroids), which are stimulated by hypoglycemia. More frequent blood monitoring (especially at times of anticipated peak insulin action) will usually identify these conditions.

Illness management. Illness alters diabetes management, and maintaining control is usually related to the seriousness of the illness. In a child whose diabetes is well controlled, an illness will run its course as it does in the unaffected child. The goals during an illness are to restore euglycemia, treat urinary ketones, and maintain hydration. Blood glucose levels and urinary ketones should be monitored every 3 hours. Some hyperglycemia and ketonuria are expected in most illnesses, even with diminished food intake, and are an indication for increased insulin. Insulin should never be omitted during an illness, although dosage requirements may increase, decrease, or remain unchanged, depending on the severity of the illness and the child's appetite. Often the child will need supplemental insulin between usual dose times. If the child vomits more than once, if blood glucose levels remain above 13.3 mmol/L, or if urinary ketones remain high, the health care provider should be notified. Although insulin and diet are important tools in sick-day care, fluids are the most important intervention. Fluids must be encouraged to prevent dehydration and to flush out ketones.

Therapeutic Management of Diabetic Ketoacidosis

DKA, the most complete state of insulin deficiency, is a life-threatening situation. Management consists of rapid assessment, adequate insulin to reduce the elevated blood glucose level, fluids to overcome dehydration, and electrolyte replacement (especially potassium). The risk factors for cerebral edema include the following: being less than 5 years old; new onset of diabetes; high initial serum urea; low initial partial pressure of arterial carbon dioxide (Pco_2); rapid administration of hypotonic fluids 0.45% sodium chloride (0.45% NS commonly called half normal saline); IV bolus of insulin; early IV insulin infusion (within first hour of administration of fluids; Novolin Toronto insulin commonly used); failure of serum sodium to rise during treatment; and use of sodium bicarbonate (CDA, Clinical Practice Guidelines Expert Committee, 2013).

Because DKA constitutes an emergency situation, the child should be admitted to a critical care facility for management. The priority is to obtain venous access for administration of fluids, electrolytes, and insulin. The child should be weighed, measured, and placed on a cardiac monitor. Blood glucose and ketone levels are determined at the bedside, and samples are obtained for laboratory measurement of glucose, electrolytes, BUN, arterial pH, Po_2, Pco_2, hemoglobin, hematocrit, white blood cell count and differential, calcium, and phosphorus.

Oxygen may be administered to patients who are cyanotic and in whom arterial oxygen is less than 80%. Gastric suction is applied to unconscious children to avoid the possibility of pulmonary aspiration. Antibiotics may be administered to febrile children after appropriate specimens are obtained for culture. A Foley catheter may or may not be inserted for urine samples and measurement. Unless the child is unconscious, a collection bag is usually sufficient for accurate assessments.

Fluid and electrolyte therapy. All patients with DKA suffer from dehydration (10% of total body weight in severe ketoacidosis) because of the osmotic diuresis, accompanied by depletion of electrolytes, sodium, potassium, chloride, phosphate, and magnesium. Serum pH and bicarbonate reflect the degree of acidosis. Prompt and adequate fluid therapy restores tissue perfusion and suppresses the elevated levels of stress hormones.

The initial hydrating solution is 0.45% saline solution. Current trends suggest more cautious fluid management to reduce the risk of cerebral edema. The fluid deficit is replaced evenly over a period of 36 to 48 hours (Cooke & Plotnik, 2008).

Serum potassium levels may be normal on admission, but after fluid and insulin administration the rapid return of potassium to the cells can seriously deplete serum levels, with the attendant risk of cardiac dysrhythmias. As soon as the child has established renal function (is voiding at least 25 mL/hr) and insulin has been given, vigorous potassium replacement is implemented. The cardiac monitor is used as a guide to therapy, and configuration of T waves should be observed every 30 to 60 minutes to determine changes that might indicate alterations in potassium concentration (widening of the QT interval and the appearance of a U wave following a flattened T wave indicate hypokalemia; an elevated and spreading T wave and shortening of the QT interval indicate **hyperkalemia**).

! NURSING ALERT

Potassium must never be given until the serum potassium level is known to be normal or low and urinary voiding is observed. When required, all maintenance IV fluids should include 20 to 40 mEq/L of potassium. Potassium should never be given as a rapid IV bolus, or cardiac arrest may result.

Insulin should not be given until urinary ketones and a blood glucose level have been obtained. Continuous IV regular insulin is given at a dosage of 0.1 units/kg/hr. Insulin therapy should be started after the initial rehydration bolus, since serum glucose levels fall rapidly after volume expansion. Blood glucose levels should decrease by 2.8 mmol/L to 5 mmol/L per hour. When blood glucose levels fall to 14 mmol/L to 17 mmol/L, dextrose is added to the IV solution. The goal is to maintain blood glucose levels between 6.7 and 13.3 mmol/L by adding 5 to 10% dextrose (CDA, Clinical Practice Guidelines Expert Committee, 2013). Sodium bicarbonate is used with extreme caution because it may cause cerebral edema and should be only considered if the child is experiencing cardiac instability. Children receiving this substance must be carefully monitored for changes in their level of consciousness (CDA, Clinical Practice Guidelines Expert Committee, 2013).

When the critical period is over, the task of regulating insulin dosage in relation to diet and activity is started. Children should be actively involved in their own care and given responsibility according to their ability and the guidance of the nurse.

NURSING ALERT

Because insulin can chemically bind to plastic tubing and in-line filters, thereby reducing the amount of medication reaching the systemic circulation, an insulin mixture is run through the tubing to saturate the insulin-binding sites before the infusion is started.

NURSING CARE

Children with DM may be admitted to the hospital at the time of their initial diagnosis; during illness or surgery; or for episodes of ketoacidosis, which may be precipitated by any of a variety of factors. Many children are able to keep the disease under control with periodic assessment and adjustment of insulin, diet, and activity as needed under the supervision of a health care provider. Under most circumstances these children can be managed well at home and require hospitalization only for a serious illness or upset.

However, a small number of children with diabetes exhibit a degree of metabolic lability and have repeated episodes of DKA that require hospitalization, which interferes with their education and social development. These children appear to display a characteristic personality structure. They tend to be unusually passive and nonassertive and to come from families that are inclined to smooth over conflicts without resolution.

Hospital Management

The child with DKA requires intensive nursing care. Vital signs should be observed and recorded frequently. Hypotension caused by the contracted blood volume of the dehydrated state may cause decreased peripheral blood flow, which can be particularly hazardous to the heart, lungs, and kidneys. An elevated temperature may indicate infection and should be reported immediately, and necessary testing and treatment may be implemented.

Careful and accurate records should be maintained, including vital signs (pulse, respiration, temperature, blood pressure), weight, IV fluids, electrolytes, insulin, blood glucose level, and intake and output. A urine collection device or retention catheter is used to obtain the urine measurements, which include volume, specific gravity, and glucose and ketone values. The volume relative to the glucose content is important because 5% glucose in a 300-mL sample is a significantly greater amount than a similar reading from a 75-mL sample. The level of consciousness needs to be assessed and recorded at frequent intervals. The comatose child generally regains consciousness fairly soon after initiation of therapy but is managed like any unconscious child until then.

When the critical period is over, the task of regulating insulin dosage to diet and activity is begun. The same meticulous records of intake and output, urine glucose and acetone levels, and insulin administration should be maintained. Capable children should be actively involved in their own care and be given responsibility for keeping the intake and output record, testing the blood and urine, and, when appropriate, administering their own insulin—all under the nurse's supervision and guidance (see Family-Centred Teaching box and Nursing Care Plan on Evolve).

Medical Identification

One of the first things the nurse should call to the parents' attention is the need for the child to wear some means of medical identification. Usually recommended is the medical alert bracelet, which is an identification bracelet that is visible and immediately recognizable. It contains a telephone number that medical personnel can call around the clock for medical records and personal information.

Meal Planning

Normal nutrition is a major aspect of the family education program. Diet instruction is usually conducted by the dietitian, with reinforcement and guidance from the nurse. The emphasis is on adequate intake for age, consistent menus, inclusion of complex carbohydrates in the child's diet, and consistent eating times. The family is taught how the meal plan relates to the requirements of growth and development, the disease process, and the insulin regimen. Meals and snacks should be modified on the basis of the child's preferences and current menu, preserving cultural patterns and preferences as much as possible.

Learning about foods within specific food groups can help in making choices regarding the child's diet. Weights and measures of foods can be used as eye-training devices for defining serving sizes and their use should be practised for about 3 months, with gradual progression to estimation of food portions. Even when the child and family become competent in estimating portion sizes, reassessment should take place weekly or monthly and when there is any change of brands.

Family members should also be guided in reading labels for the nutritional value of foods and food content. They need to become familiar with the carbohydrate content of food groups, as substituting foods of equal carbohydrate content is a useful skill for successful carbohydrate counting. Substitution might be necessary, for instance, if a food is not available in sufficient quantity or if the child wishes to eat fast food with peers.

Lists of items served at major fast-food chains can be obtained from the restaurants or online to help guide food selections (the major chains' menus are remarkably uniform). It is important that the child know the nutritional value of these items, but the child should be cautioned to avoid high-fat and high-sugar/high-carbohydrate items; for example, the child could choose a plain hamburger instead of a double cheeseburger.

Children should use sugar substitutes in moderation in items such as soft drinks. Artificial sweeteners have been shown to be safe, but if there is any question about amounts, the physician, dietitian, or nurse specialist can provide guidelines based on body weight. Sugar-free chewing gum and candies made with sorbitol may be used in moderation by children with DM. Although sorbitol is less cariogenic than other varieties of sugar substitutes, it is an alcohol sugar that is metabolized to fructose and then to glucose. Furthermore, large amounts can cause osmotic diarrhea. Most dietetic foods contain sorbitol. They are more expensive than regular foods. Also, while a product may be sugar free, it is not necessarily carbohydrate free.

Travelling

Travelling requires planning, especially when a trip involves crossing time zones. Before travelling it is important to consider what will be needed from the primary practitioner before leaving, what and how much to take along, needs in transit, what to consider at the destination, and planning for when the child returns home. Planning is needed no matter what type of travel is considered—automobile, plane, bus, or train.

Insulin

Families need to understand the treatment method and the insulin prescribed, including the effective duration, onset, and

FAMILY-CENTRED TEACHING

Teaching About Diabetes

The better the parents understand the pathophysiology of diabetes and the function and action of insulin and glucagon in relation to caloric intake and exercise, the better they will understand the disease and its effects on the child. Parents need answers to a number of questions (voiced or unvoiced) to increase their confidence in coping with the disease. For example, they may want to know about the various procedures performed on their child and treatment rationale, such as what is being put in the intravenous bag and the expected effect.

peak action. They also need to know the characteristics of the various types of insulins, the proper mixing and dilution of insulins, and how to substitute another type when their usual brand is not available (insulin is a nonprescription medication). Insulin need not be refrigerated but should be maintained at a temperature between 15° and 29.5°C. Freezing renders insulin inactive.

Insulin bottles that have been "opened" (i.e., the stopper has been punctured) should be stored at room temperature or refrigerated for up to 28 to 30 days. After 1 month these vials should be discarded. Unopened vials should be refrigerated and are good until the expiration date on the label.

Injection Procedure

Learning to give insulin injections can be a source of anxiety for both parents and children. It is helpful for the learner to know that this important aspect of care will become as routine as brushing the teeth. First, the basic injection technique is taught, using an orange or similar item and sterile normal saline for practice. To gain children's confidence, the nurse can demonstrate the technique by giving a skillful injection to the parent and then having the parent return the demonstration by giving the nurse an injection. With practice and confidence, the parents will soon be able to give the insulin injection to their children and their children will trust them. Another effective strategy is to instruct the children and then have them teach the technique to the parents while the nurse observes. Both parents should participate, and as little time as possible should elapse between instruction and the actual injection, especially with parents and teenage learners.

Insulin can be injected into any area in which there is adipose (fat) tissue over muscle; the drug is injected at a 90-degree angle. Newly diagnosed children may have lost adipose tissue, and care should be exerted not to inject intramuscularly. The pinch technique is the most effective method for tenting the skin to allow easy entrance of the needle to subcutaneous tissues in children. The site selected will sometimes depend on whether children or parents administer the insulin. The arms, thighs, hips, and abdomen are usual injection sites for insulin. The children can reach the thighs, abdomen, and part of the hip and arm easily but may require help to inject other sites. For example, a parent can pinch a loose fold of skin of the arm while the child injects the insulin.

The parents and child should be helped to work out a rotation pattern to various areas of the body to enhance absorption, because insulin absorption is slowed by fat pads that develop in overused injection areas. The most efficient rotation plan involves giving about four to six injections in one area (each injection about 2.5 cm apart, or the diameter of the insulin vial from the previous injection) and then moving to another area.

It is important to remember that the absorption rate varies in different parts of the body (Table 51-4). The methodical use of one anatomical area and then movement to another minimizes variations in absorption rates. However, absorption is also altered by vigorous exercise, which enhances absorption from exercised muscles; it is recommended that a site be chosen other than the exercising extremity (e.g., avoiding legs and arms when playing in a tennis tournament).

TABLE 51-4 INSULIN'S ONSET AND DURATION OF ACTION RELATED TO INJECTION SITE

	SITE OF INJECTION			
	ABDOMEN	ARM	LEG	BUTTOCK
Rate	Very fast	Fast	Slow	Very slow
Duration	Very short	Short	Long	Very long

From Albisser, A. M., & Sperlich, M. (1992). Adjusting insulins. *Diabetes Education, 18*(3), 211–218.

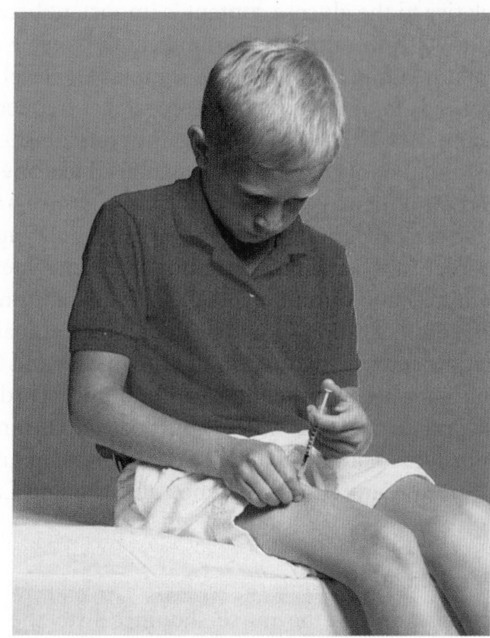

FIGURE 51-3 School-age children are able to administer their own insulin.

Injection sites for an entire month can be determined in advance on a simple chart. For example, a "paper doll" (body outline) can be constructed and insulin sites marked by the child. After injection, the child places the date on the appropriate site. To keep in practice, it is a good idea for the parent to give two or three injections a week in areas that are difficult for the child to reach.

The same basic methodology is used when teaching children to give their own insulin injections (Fig. 51-3). They should practise first on an orange or a doll, building confidence gradually. Other devices are available for insulin injection and may offer advantages to some children. Children who do not wish to give themselves injections can be taught to use a syringe-loaded injector (Inject-Ease). With the device, puncture is always automatic. Adolescents respond well to a self-contained and compact device resembling a fountain pen (NovoPen), which eliminates conventional vials and syringes. Preloaded pens may also cause less pain, since the needle is not blunted by piercing the rubber top of the insulin vial.

Continuous subcutaneous insulin infusion. Some children are considered candidates for use of a portable insulin pump, and even some young children with unsatisfactory metabolic control can benefit from its use. The child and the parents need to be taught to operate the device, including the mechanics of the pump, battery changes, and alarm systems. A number of devices are on the market that vary in the basal rates they are able to deliver and in the cost of the equipment. Families can investigate the various devices and select the model that best suits their needs.

Parents and children also need to learn the technical aspects of self-monitoring of blood glucose. Numerous blood glucose measurements (at least four times per day) are an essential part of infusion pump use. Intensive education and supervision are critical to obtaining maximum efficiency and control. This is particularly important if the family has been accustomed to a conventional insulin regimen. They must realize that simply wearing the pump will not normalize blood glucose. The pump is merely an insulin delivery device; frequent, routine blood glucose determinations are necessary to adjust the insulin delivery rate.

The major problem with use of the insulin pump is inflammation from irritation or infection at the insertion site. The site should be cleaned thoroughly before the needle is inserted and then covered with a transparent dressing. The site should be changed and rotated every 48 to 72 hours (this may vary) or at the first sign of inflammation. Nurses working where pumps are part of the therapeutic regimen should become familiar with the operation of the specific device being used and the protocol of disease management.

Monitoring

Nurses should also be prepared to teach and supervise blood glucose monitoring. SMBG is associated with few complications, and although it does not necessarily lead to improved metabolic control, it provides a more accurate assessment of blood glucose levels than can be obtained with the historical urine testing. Blood glucose monitoring has the added advantage that it can be performed anywhere (see Atraumatic Care box).

ATRAUMATIC CARE
Minimizing Pain of Blood Glucose Monitoring

- To enhance blood flow to the finger, hold it under warm water for a few seconds before the puncture.
- When obtaining blood samples, use the ring finger or thumb (blood flows more easily to these areas), and puncture the finger just to the side of the finger pad (where there are more blood vessels and fewer nerve endings).
- To prevent a deep puncture, press the platform of the lancet device lightly against the skin and avoid steadying the finger against a hard surface.
- Use lancet devices with adjustable-depth tips. Begin with the shallowest setting.
- Use glucose monitors that require small blood samples to avoid repeated punctures.

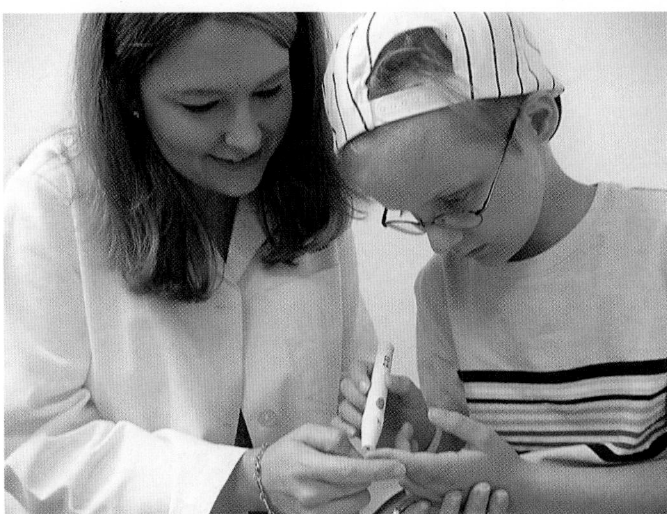

FIGURE 51-4 Child using finger-stick device to obtain blood sample.

Blood for testing can be obtained by using a mechanical bloodletting device. A mechanical device is recommended for children, although the child and family should learn to use both methods in the event of mechanical failure. Several lancet devices are available, and each provides a means for obtaining a large drop of blood for testing (Fig. 51-4).

NURSING ALERT

Caution children not to allow anyone else to use their lancet because of the risk of contracting blood-borne infections such as hepatitis B virus or human immunodeficiency virus infection.

The blood sample may be obtained from fingertips or alternative sites such as the forearm. Alternative-site testing requires a meter that can test a small volume of blood. Not all meters are capable of this.

Signs of redness and soreness at the site of finger puncture should be examined by the nurse. It may be evidence of poor technique, poor hygiene, or poor skin healing relative to poor control. Many types of blood-testing meters are available for home use (Fig. 51-5). Newer technology has brought about improvements in meter size and ease of use. The family should be shown features of several meters, including advantages and disadvantages, and allowed to choose equipment that best meets their needs.

Signs of Hyperglycemia

Severe hyperglycemia is most often caused by illness, growth, emotional upset, or missed insulin doses. Emotional stress from school examinations or a physical response to immunizations are examples that may contribute to causes of hyperglycemia. With careful glucose monitoring, any elevation can be managed by adjustment of insulin or food intake. Children and parents should understand how to adjust food, activity, and insulin at the time of illness or when the child is treated for an illness with a medication known to raise the blood glucose level (e.g.,

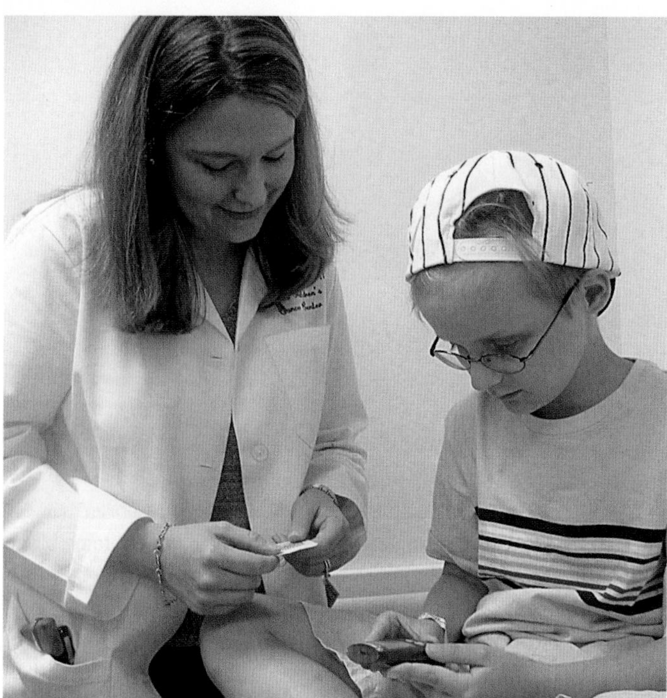

FIGURE 51-5 Child using blood glucose monitor and reagent strips to test blood for glucose.

EMERGENCY
Hypoglycemia

Mild Reaction—Adrenergic Symptoms
Give child 10 to 15 g of a simple, high-carbohydrate substance (preferably liquid, e.g., 90 mL to 180 mL of orange juice).
Follow with starch-protein snack.

Moderate Reaction—Neuroglycopenic Symptoms
Give child 10 to 15 g of a simple carbohydrate as above.
Repeat in 10 to 15 minutes if symptoms persist.
Follow with larger snack.
Watch child closely.

Severe Reaction—Unresponsive, Unconscious, or Seizures
Administer glucagon as prescribed.
Follow with planned meal or snack when child is able to eat, or add a snack of 10% of daily calories.

Nocturnal Reaction
Give child 10 to 15 g of a simple carbohydrate.
Follow with snack of 10% of daily calories.

steroids). The hyperglycemia is managed by increasing insulin soon after the increased glucose level is noted. The health care team should be aware that adolescent girls often become hyperglycemic around the time of their menses and should be advised to increase insulin dosages if necessary.

Signs of Hypoglycemia

Hypoglycemia is caused by imbalances of food intake, insulin, and activity. Ideally, hypoglycemia should be prevented, and parents need to be prepared to prevent, recognize, and treat the problem. They should be familiar with the signs of hypoglycemia and instructed in treatment, including care of the child with seizures. Early signs are adrenergic, including sweating and trembling (see Table 51-3), which help raise the blood glucose level, much like the reaction when an individual is startled or anxious. The second set of symptoms that follow an untreated adrenergic reaction is neuroglycopenic (also called *brain hypoglycemia*). These symptoms typically include difficulty with balance, memory, attention, or concentration; dizziness or lightheadedness; and slurred speech. Severe and prolonged hypoglycemia leads to seizures, coma, and possible death. Hypoglycemia can be managed effectively, as outlined in the Emergency box.

Parents need to plan for anticipated stress or exercise that could trigger a hypoglycemic event. In addition, gastroenteritis may decrease insulin needs slightly as a result of poor appetite, vomiting, or diarrhea. If the blood glucose level is low, the family should be aware of the increased need for simple carbohydrates and liquids.

Hygiene

All aspects of personal hygiene should be emphasized for the child with diabetes. The child should be cautioned against wearing shoes without socks, wearing sandals, or walking barefoot. Correct nail and extremity care tailored to the individual child (with the guidance of a podiatrist) can help the child begin using health practices that last a lifetime. Eyes should be checked once a year unless the child wears glasses, and then as directed by the ophthalmologist. Regular dental care is emphasized, and cuts and scratches should be treated with plain soap and water unless otherwise indicated. Diaper rash in infants and candidal infections in teens may indicate poor diabetes control.

Exercise

Exercise is an important component of the treatment plan. If the child is more active at one time of the day than at another time, food or insulin can be altered to meet that activity pattern. The child who is active in team sports will need a snack about a half-hour before the anticipated activity. Races or other competition may call for a slightly higher food intake than at practice times.

Food intake will usually need to be repeated for prolonged activity periods, often as frequently as every 45 minutes to 1 hour. Families should be informed that if increased food is not tolerated, decreased insulin is the next course of action. If the timing of the exercise is changed so that the supper meal is delayed, the insulin in the second or third dose of the day may be moved back to precede the mealtime. Sugar may sometimes be needed during exercise periods for quick response. Elevated blood glucose levels after extreme activity may represent the body's adrenergic response to exercise. If the blood glucose level is elevated (13 mmol/L or higher) before planned exercise, urinary ketones should be checked and the activity may need to be postponed until the blood glucose is controlled.

Record Keeping

Home records are an invaluable aid to diabetes self-management. The nurse and family can devise a method to chart insulin administered, blood glucose values, and other factors and events that affect diabetes control. The child and family should be encouraged to observe for patterns of blood glucose responses to events such as exercise. If lapses in management occur (such as eating a candy bar), the child should be encouraged to note this and not be criticized for the transgression.

Self-Management

Self-management is the key to close control. Being able to make changes when they are needed rather than waiting until the next contact with health care providers is important for self-management and gives the individual and family the feeling they have control over the disease. Psychologically this helps family members feel that they are useful and participating members of the team. Allowing the child to learn to look at records objectively promotes independence in self-management. As children grow and assume more responsibility for self-management, they develop confidence in their ability to manage their disease and confidence in themselves as persons. They learn to respond to the disease and to make more accurate interpretations and changes in treatment when they become adults.

Puberty is associated with decreased sensitivity to insulin that normally would be compensated for by an increased insulin secretion. Health care providers should anticipate that pubertal patients will have more difficulty maintaining glycemic control. Insulin doses commonly need to be increased, often dramatically. If there is chronic poor metabolic control with a hemoglobin A_{1C} over 10.0%, then the cause needs to be identified. Possible factors could include depression and eating disorders (CDA, Clinical Practice Guidelines Expert Committee, 2013). Patients should be taught to give themselves additional doses of rapid-acting insulin (5 to 10% of their daily dose) when their blood glucose levels are increased. The use of supplemental rapid-acting insulin is preferred to withholding food.

Child or Adolescent and Family Support

Just as the physiological responses affect the child, the parents and other family members of the child with newly diagnosed DM experience various emotional responses to the crisis. Care in the acute setting is short but may create fear and frustration. The prospect of a chronic illness in their child can engender all the feelings and concerns faced by parents of children with other chronic illnesses (see Chapter 40). The threat of complications and death is always present, as well as the continuing drain on emotional and financial resources.

Certain fears may develop as a result of past experiences with the disease. A severe insulin reaction with seizures can contribute to fear of repetition. If parents observe a seizure or the adolescent has one in a public place, the desire to maintain better control is reinforced. They must understand how to prevent problems and how to handle problems calmly and coolly if they occur, and they must understand the complexities of the body, the disease, and its complications. Young children usually adjust well to problems related to the disease. With toddlers and preschoolers, insulin injections and glucose testing may be difficult at first. However, they usually accept the procedures when the parents use a matter-of-fact approach, without calling attention to a "hurt," and treat the procedures like any other routine part of the child's life. After receiving an injection, giving the child some positive attention, such as reading to the child or engaging in some other pleasant activity, is one way to help children who initially refuse injections to accept them.

In the years before adolescence, children probably accept their condition most easily. They are able to understand the basic concepts related to their disease and its treatment. They are able to test blood glucose and urine, recognize food groups, give injections, keep records, and distinguish fear or excitement from hypoglycemia. They understand how to recognize, prevent, and treat hypoglycemia. However, they still need considerable parental involvement.

Adolescents appear to have the most difficulty adjusting. Adolescence is a time of stress in trying to be accepted by one's peers, and having diabetes can be viewed as being different and as an obstacle to such acceptance. Some adolescents are more upset about not being able to have a chocolate bar than about injections, diet, and other aspects of management. If children can accept the difference as a part of life—in other words, that each person is different in some way—then, with adequate parental support, they should be able to adjust well.

Diabetes Mellitus Type 2

Type 2 diabetes arises because of insulin resistance, in which the body fails to use insulin properly, combined with relative (rather than absolute) insulin deficiency leading to predominant insulin resistance. People with type 2 DM can range from predominantly insulin resistant with relative insulin deficiency to predominantly deficient in insulin secretion with some insulin resistance. In North America, the incidence of type 2 diabetes has been increasing over the past 20 years in both the adult and pediatric populations (CDA, Clinical Practice Guidelines Expert Committee, 2013).

Factors that put nonpubertal and pubertal children at greater risk of developing type 2 diabetes include obesity (BMI >95% percentile for age and gender); being a member of a high-risk ethnic group, such as Indigenous peoples and those of Asian or African descent; having a family history of type 2 diabetes or gestational diabetes; signs or symptoms of insulin resistance that include acanthosis nigricans, hypertension, and dyslipidemia; and impaired fasting and glucose tolerance test results (Amed, Dean, & Panagiotopoulos, 2010; CDA, Clinical Practice Guidelines Expert Committee, 2013; Saylor & CPS, First Nations, Inuit and Métis Health Committee, 2005/2016).

Screening and Diagnostic Evaluation

The physical signs of insulin resistance and metabolic syndrome are acanthosis nigricans (AN) (hyperpigmentation and thickening of the skin in the neck and axillary regions), polycystic ovarian syndrome (PCOS), hypertension, dyslipidemia, and steatohepatitis. While these signs do not cause type 2 diabetes, they are associated with glucose intolerance and early-onset type 2 diabetes. Although research has not proven that AN is a definitive marker, neck observation for AN is a useful community screening tool that is acceptable to most children. The at-risk AN group also has impaired glucose tolerance. Type 2 diabetes may be connected to the use of atypical neuropsychiatric medications, which are more commonly used in the pediatric populations (Amed et al., 2010; CDA, Clinical Practice Guidelines Expert Committee, 2013).

Screening of fasting plasma glucose is recommended as routine in assessment for type 2 diabetes, but an OGTT is more likely to have a higher detection rate. An OGTT test is done when fasting blood glucose is 6.1 to 6.9 mmol/L; it may be done if the level is 5.6 to 6.0 mmol/L and the type 2 diabetes risk is high (CDA, Clinical Practice Guidelines Expert Committee, 2013).

PCOS is rarely seen in Indigenous adolescent girls in Canada (Saylor & CPS, First Nations, Inuit and Métis Health Committee, 2005/2016). By contrast, AN was found in 21% of an Ontario Indigenous group of children aged 5 to 14 years. Because of their higher risk for type 2 diabetes, Indigenous children should be screened for type 2 diabetes after age 10. It is also recommended that if additional risk factors are present, physical activity should be increased and greater attention paid to sugar intake (Canadian Agency for Drugs and Technologies in Health, 2010).

Management

The management of type 2 diabetes is similar to that for type 1 diabetes. The pediatric multidisciplinary team needs to consult with the family about lifestyle, with a focus on healthy eating and physical activity. Psychological issues such as depression and smoking need to be sorted out, with interventions offered. Research has shown that when Indigenous children receive lifestyle interventions their glycemic control drops to within normal in 2 weeks (Saylor & CPS, First Nations, Inuit and Métis Health Committee, 2005/2016). Children with severe metabolic decompensation (DKA, hemoglobin A_{1C} >9.0%) and hyperglycemia who need insulin can be successfully weaned once the glycemic goals are reached, especially if their lifestyle has improved.

Short-term complications of type 2 diabetes in children include DKA and a hyperosmolar state. Children who have both at onset have high morbidity and mortality rates. There is evidence that early-onset type 2 diabetes in adolescents is associated with severe and early-onset microvascularization, which includes retinopathy, neuropathy, and nephropathy; thus these individuals need to be monitored for it. Hypertension is present in 36% of individuals with type 2 diabetes; this also needs monitoring and potential intervention. Other potential complications that require monitoring include dyslipidemia, steatohepatitis, and PCOS (CDA, Clinical Practice Guidelines Expert Committee, 2013).

Risk Reduction for Type 2 Diabetes

The CPS (Saylor & CPS, First Nations, Inuit and Métis Health Committee, 2005/2016) has recommended the following risk-reduction program for decreasing the incidence of type 2 diabetes in the Indigenous population; the more general recommendations pertain as well to all Canadian children:

- Culturally based and community-run diabetes prevention programs should be set up in Indigenous communities.
- Indigenous health care providers should provide type 2 diabetes opportunistic screening.
- In Indigenous communities, traditional values, diets (using Canada's *Food Guide*), activities, and lifestyles should be promoted; group activities with the elders may work most effectively.
- Daily physical activity for at least 60 to 90 minutes, as laid out in *Canada's Physical Activity Guide*, is recommended. Physical activity guidelines are available from the Canadian Society for Exercise Physiology (2012).
- A healthy lifestyle needs to be taught as part of the curriculum at schools, day care, and Head Start programs.
- Community leaders can act as role models and provide appropriate safe environments for physical and other recreational activities.
- Passive activities, such as watching television, working on computers, and playing video games, should be limited to 1.5 to 2 hours per day.

Camping and other special group activities are also useful to children with diabetes. At diabetes camp, children learn that they are not alone. As a result, they become more independent and resourceful in other settings. Useful information about such camps and organizations, as well as resources for children with diabetes, their families, and health care providers, can be obtained from the Canadian Diabetes Association (see Additional Resources at the end of this chapter).

Several organizations assist with education about diabetes and support for individuals with diabetes. These include the Juvenile Diabetes Research Foundation Canada and the Canadian Diabetes Educator Certification Board (see Additional Resources).

KEY POINTS

- The endocrine system has three components: the cells, which send chemical messages via hormones; target cells, which receive the messages; and the environment through which the chemicals are transported from the sites of synthesis to the sites of cellular action.
- Pituitary dysfunction is manifested primarily by growth disturbance.
- The main physiological action of TH is to regulate the basal metabolic rate and control the processes of growth and tissue differentiation.

- Disorders of thyroid function include hypothyroidism, autoimmune thyroiditis, goitre, and hyperthyroidism.
- Therapy for hyperthyroidism is directed at slowing the rate of hormone secretion and may include medication therapy, thyroidectomy, or radioiodine therapy.
- Classic forms of hypoparathyroidism in childhood are idiopathic (deficient production of PTH) and pseudohypoparathyroidism (increased PTH production with end-organ unresponsiveness to PTH).
- The adrenal cortex secretes three important groups of hormones: glucocorticoids, mineralocorticoids, and sex steroids.
- Disorders of adrenal function include acute adrenocortical insufficiency, chronic adrenocortical insufficiency, Cushing syndrome, and CAH.
- Five categories of Cushing syndrome are pituitary, adrenal, ectopic, iatrogenic, and food dependent.
- Management of CAH includes assignment of a sex according to genotype, administration of cortisone, and, possibly, reconstructive surgery.
- DM is categorized as type 1 diabetes and type 2 diabetes.
- The focus of treatment for type 1 DM is insulin replacement, diet, and exercise.
- Education of families includes explanation of diabetes, meal planning, administering insulin injections, monitoring general hygienic practices, promoting exercise, record keeping, and observing for complications.
- The focus of treatment for type 2 DM is weight reduction, diet, exercise, and possible medication administration.

evolve WEBSITE

Visit the Evolve website for additional resources related to the content in this chapter such as Case Studies, Critical Thinking Case Study Answers, Nursing Care Plans, Nursing Processes, Nursing Skills, and Review Questions for Exam Preparation at: http://evolve.elsevier.com/Canada/Perry/maternal/

REFERENCES

Amed, S., Dean, H. J., & Panagiotopoulos, C. (2010). Type 2 diabetes, medication-induced diabetes, and monogenic diabetes in Canadian children: A prospective national surveillance study. *Diabetes Care, 33*, 786–791.

Breault, D. T., & Majzoub, J. A. (2016). Diabetes insipidus. In R. M. Kliegman, B. Stanton, J. W. St. Geme, et al. (Eds.), *Nelson textbook of pediatrics* (20th ed.). Philadelphia: Saunders.

Bryant, J., Baxter, L., Cave, C. B., et al. (2007). Recombinant growth hormone for idiopathic short stature in children and adolescents. *The Cochrane Database of Systematic Reviews, 18*(3), CD004440, doi:10.1002/14651858.CD004440.

Canadian Agency for Drugs and Technologies in Health. (2010). *Diabetes in Aboriginal populations: Review of guidelines for screening and treatment.* Retrieved from <http://www.cadth.ca/media/pdf/l0205_diabetes_ifirst_nations_population_htis-2.pdf>.

Canadian Diabetes Association, Clinical Practice Guidelines Expert Committee. (2013). Canadian Diabetes Association 2013 clinical practice guidelines for the prevention and management of diabetes in Canada. *Canadian Journal of Diabetes, 37*(Suppl. 1), S1–S212. Retrieved from <http://guidelines.diabetes.ca/App_Themes/CDACPG/resources/cpg_2013_full_en.pdf>.

Canadian Society for Exercise Physiology. (2012). *Canadian physical activity guidelines. Canadian sedentary behaviour guidelines.* Retrieved from <http://www.csep.ca/CMFiles/Guidelines/CSEP_Guidelines_Handbook.pdf>.

Carel, J. C., & Leger, J. (2008). Precocious puberty. *The New England Journal of Medicine, 358*, 2366–2377.

Clairman, H., Skocic, J., Lischinsky, J., et al. (2015). Do children with congenital hypothyroidism exhibit abnormal cortical morphology? *Pediatric Research, 78*, 286–297. doi:10.1038/pr.2015.93.

Cooke, D. W., & Plotnik, L. (2008). Type I diabetes mellitus in pediatrics. *Pediatrics in Review / American Academy of Pediatrics, 29*(11), 374–384.

Cooper, M. S., & Gittoes, N. J. (2008). Diagnosis and management of hypocalcaemia. *British Medical Journal, 336*(7656), 1298–1302. doi:10.1136/bmj.a334.

De Buyst, J., Massa, G., Christophe, C., et al. (2007). Clinical, hormonal and imaging findings in 27 children with central diabetes insipidus. *European Journal of Pediatrics, 166*(1), 43–49. doi:10.1007/s00431-006-0206-0.

de Vries, L., Bulvik, S., & Phillip, M. (2009). Chronic autoimmune thryroiditis in children and adolescents: At presentation and during long term follow up. *Archives of Disease in Childhood, 94*(1), 33–37. doi:10.1136/adc.2007.134841.

Doyle, D. A. (2016). Hyperparathyroidism. In R. M. Kliegman, B. Stanton, J. W. St. Geme, et al. (Eds.), *Nelson textbook of pediatrics* (20th ed.). Philadelphia: Saunders.

Garibaldi, L. R., & Chemaitilly, W. (2016). Disorders of pubertal development. In R. M. Kliegman, B. Stanton, J. St. Geme, et al. (Eds.), *Nelson textbook of pediatrics* (20th ed.). Philadelphia: Saunders.

Huang, S. A., & LaFranchi, S. H. (2016). Hyperthyroidism. In R. M. Kliegman, B. Stanton, J. W. St. Geme, et al. (Eds.), *Nelson textbook of pediatrics* (20th ed.). Philadelphia: Saunders.

Kaplowitz, P. B. (2009). Treatment of central precocious puberty. *Current Opinion in Endocrinology, Diabetes, and Obesity, 16*(1), 31–36.

Menon, K., & Lawson, M. (2007). Identification of adrenal insufficiency in pediatric critical illness. *Paediatrics & Child Health, 15*(7), 411–412.

Metzger, M. L., Krasin, M. J., Choi, J. K., et al. (2015). Hodgkin lymphoma. In P. A. Pizzo & D. G. Poplack (Eds.), *Principles and theories of pediatric oncology* (7th ed.). Philadelphia: Lippincott, Williams & Wilkins.

Parks, J. S., & Felner, E. I. (2016). Hypopituitarism. In R. M. Kliegman, B. Stanton, J. W. St. Geme, et al. (Eds.), *Nelson textbook of pediatrics* (20th ed.). Philadelphia: Saunders.

Public Health Agency of Canada. (2011). *Chapter 5–Diabetes in children and youth.* Retrieved from <http://www.phac-aspc.gc.ca/cd-mc/publications/diabetes-diabete/facts-figures-faits-chiffres-2011/chap5-eng.php>.

Public Health Agency of Canada. (2012). *Diabetes in Canada: Facts and figures from a public health perspective.* Retrieved from <http://www.phac-aspc.gc.ca/cd-mc/publications/diabetes-diabete/facts-figures-faits-chiffres-2011/index-eng.php>.

Qureshi, S., Galiveeti, S., Bichet, D. G., et al. (2014). Diabetes insipidus: Celebrating a century of vasopressin therapy. *Endocrinology, 155*(12), 4605–46021. doi:10.1210./en2014-1385.

Radetti, G., Gottardi, E., Bona, G., et al. (2006). The natural history of euthyroid Hashimoto's thyroiditis in children. *The Journal of Pediatrics, 149*(6), 827–832.

Ramnitz, M. S., & Lodish, M. B. (2013). Racial disparities in pubertal development. *Seminars in Reproductive Medicine, 31*(5), 333–339. doi:10.1055/s-0033-1348891.

Richmond, E. J., & Rogol, A. D. (2008). Growth hormone deficiency in children. *Pituitary, 11*, 115–120.

Rivkees, S. A. (2008). Differentiating appropriate antidiuretic hormone secretion, inappropriate antidiuretic hormone secretion and cerebral salt wasting: The common, uncommon, and misnamed. *Current Opinion in Pediatrics, 20*(4), 448–452.

Saylor, K., & Canadian Paediatric Society, First Nations, Inuit and Métis Health Committee. (2005). Risk reduction for type 2 diabetes in Aboriginal children in Canada. *Paediatrics & Child Health, 10*(1), 49–52. Reaffirmed 2016. Retrieved from <http://www.cps.ca/documents/position/risk-reduction-type-two-diabetes-aboriginal-children>.

Steingraber, S. (2007). *The falling age of puberty in US girls: What we know, what we need to know.* Breast Cancer Fund. Retrieved from <http://www.breastcancerfund.org/assets/pdfs/publications/falling-age-of-puberty.pdf>.

Toogood, M., & Stewart, P. M. (2008). Hypopituitarism: Clinical features, diagnosis, and management. *Endocrinology and Metabolism Clinics of North America, 37*(1), 235–261.

van Tijn, D. A., Schroor, E. J., Delemarre-van de Waal, H. A., et al. (2007). Early assessment of hypothalamic-pituitary-gonadal function in patients with congenital hypothyroidism of central origin. *The Journal of Clinical Endocrinology and Metabolism, 92*(1), 104–109. doi:10.1210/jc.2006-0689.

White, P. C. (2016a). Cushing syndrome. In R. M. Kliegman, B. Stanton, J. W. St. Geme, et al. (Eds.), *Nelson textbook of pediatrics* (20th ed.). Philadelphia: Saunders.

White, P. C. (2016b). Congenital adrenal hyperplasia and related disorders. In R. M. Kliegman, B. Stanton, J. St. Geme, et al. (Eds.), *Nelson textbook of pediatrics* (20th ed.). Philadelphia: Saunders.

White, P. C. (2016c). Pheochromocytoma. In R. M. Kliegman, B. Stanton, J. W. St. Geme, et al. (Eds.), *Nelson textbook of pediatrics* (20th ed.). Philadelphia: Saunders.

ADDITIONAL RESOURCES

Canadian Diabetes Association: <http://www.diabetes.ca/>.

Canadian Diabetes Educator Certification Board: <http://cdecb.ca/>.

Diabetes Resource Centre: About Kids Health (updated 2014): <www.aboutkidshealth.ca/en/resourcecentres/diabetes/pages/default.aspx>.

Juvenile Diabetes Research Foundation Canada: <http://www.jdrf.ca/>.

Thyroid Foundation of Canada: <http://www.thyroid.ca/>.

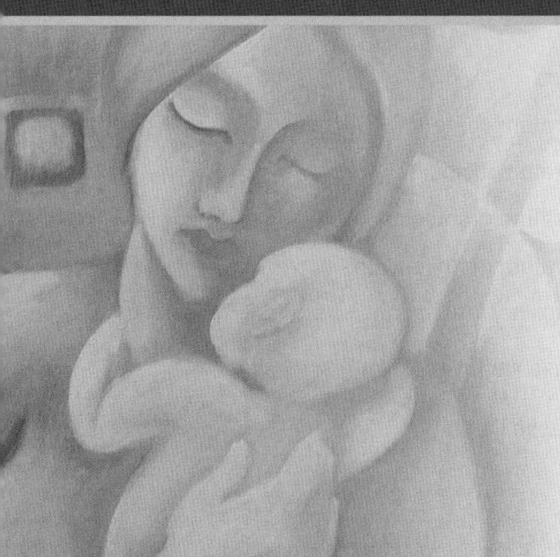

CHAPTER 52

Integumentary Dysfunction

Cheryl Sams

evolve WEBSITE

Visit the Evolve website for additional resources related to the content in this chapter such as Case Studies, Critical Thinking Case Study Answers, Nursing Care Plans, Nursing Processes, Nursing Skills, and Review Questions for Exam Preparation at: http://evolve.elsevier.com/Canada/Perry/maternal/

OBJECTIVES

On completion of this chapter the reader will be able to:

- Describe the distribution and configuration of the various skin lesions.
- List the benefits of a moist environment for wound healing.
- Discuss the nursing care related to therapies for skin disorders.
- Contrast the manifestations of and therapies for bacterial, viral, and fungal infections of the skin.
- Compare the skin manifestations related to age in children.
- Outline a care plan to prevent and treat diaper dermatitis.
- Outline a care plan for a child with atopic dermatitis.
- Formulate a teaching plan for an adolescent with acne.
- Describe the methods for assessing a burn wound.
- Discuss the physical and emotional care of a child with a severe burn wound.

INTEGUMENTARY ANATOMY AND PHYSIOLOGY

The skin is the largest organ in the body and provides a protective covering. The skin is composed of stratified epithelial cells, which are thickest on the palms and soles. The outer epidermal layer starts with the following stratum: corneum lucidum, granulosum, spinsum, and germinativum (Fig. 52-1). The skin is pigmented by melanocytes in the germinativum layer, which darken the skin (in response to sunlight) to varying degrees. Blood vessels are located in the dermis, which tint the skin pink. The dermis, which lies directly beneath the epidermis, consists of connective tissue containing white collagenous and yellow elastic fibres, blood vessels, nerves, lymph vessels, hair follicles, and sweat glands.

The skin has four functions:

- To provide sensory input—the sensations of pain, temperature, touch, and pressure—and to discriminate between the sensations through a nervous system pattern to the cerebral cortex
- For protection—the skin forms an elastic, resistant covering for protection against the external environment, inhibits excessive water loss and that of essential electrolytes, provides an acid mantle to protect skin from irritants and bacterial invasions.
- Thermoregulation and the prevention of heat loss by processes of conduction, convection, radiation, and evaporation (which occurs as either insensible water loss or visual water loss as perspiration)
- To act as a warning system for danger by sending information to the brain about the external environment

The appendages of the skin are protective and include hair, nails, and glands. Hair is composed of individual units of follicles that contain cuticle, cortex, and medulla with attached arrector pili muscles that are smooth fibre bundles. Nails are composed of hard keratin; modified layers of horny epidermal cells arise from proximal nail folds and adhere to nail beds. Skin glands include sebaceous glands, which produce sebum for skin surface lubrication and minimizes fluid loss; secretion

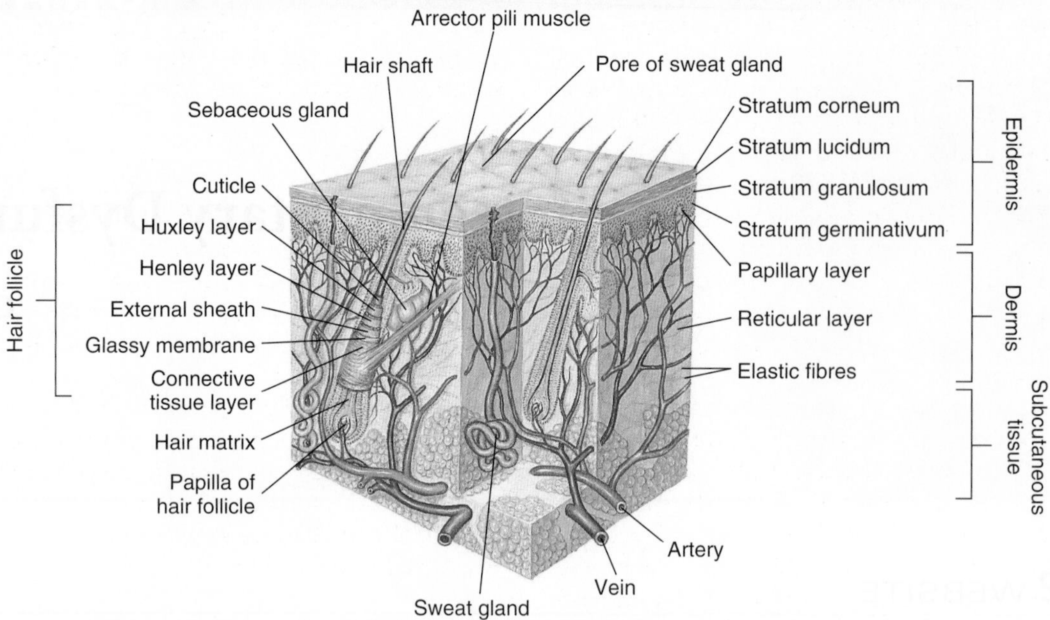

FIGURE 52-1 Anatomical structures of the skin. (From Ball, J. W., Dains, J. E., Flynn, J. A., et al. [2015]. *Seidel's guide to physical examination* [8th ed., p. 115]. St. Louis: Mosby [Fig. 8-1]).

increases at puberty and late in pregnancy and decreases in advancing age.

Young children are unable to effectively prevent fluid loss or regulate body temperature, which puts them at high risk for fluid and electrolyte imbalance; this is due to having immature sweat glands, a large body surface area, and an immature renal system. The infant has thin, delicate, and light-appearing skin from incomplete melanization. See Chapter 33 for more information on skin assessment.

Skin of Younger Children

The major skin layers arise from different embryological origins. Early in the embryonic period, a single layer of epithelium forms from the ectoderm, while simultaneously the corium develops from the mesenchyme. In the infant and small child the epidermis is loosely bound to the dermis. This poor adherence causes the layers to separate easily during an inflammatory process to form blisters. This is especially true in preterm infants, who have a propensity to blister formation and separation of the skin with minor trauma, such as with the removal of adhesive tape. In contrast, the skin of the older child is thinner, and the cells of all the strata are more compressed.

INTEGUMENTARY DYSFUNCTION

Skin Lesions

Lesions of the skin result from a variety of etiological factors. Skin lesions originate from (1) contact with injurious agents (infective organisms, toxic chemicals, and physical trauma), (2) hereditary factors, (3) external factors such as allergens, or (4) systemic diseases, such as measles, lupus erythematosus, and nutritional deficiency diseases. Responses to these agents or factors are highly individualized. An agent that is harmless to one individual may be damaging to another, and a single agent may produce varying degrees of response.

An important factor in the etiology of skin manifestations is the child's age. Infants are subject to "birthmark" malformations and atopic dermatitis (AD) that appear early in life; the school-age child is susceptible to ringworm of the scalp; and acne is a characteristic skin disorder of puberty.

Contact dermatitis, such as poison ivy, is seen only when the noxious agent is found in the environment. Tension and anxiety may produce, modify, or prolong skin conditions.

Pathophysiology of Dermatitis

More than half of the dermatological problems in children are forms of dermatitis. This implies a sequence of inflammatory changes in the skin that are grossly and microscopically similar but diverse in course and causation. Acute responses produce intercellular and intracellular edema, the formation of intradermal vesicles, and an initial infiltration of inflammatory cells into the epidermis. In the dermis there is edema, vascular dilation, and early perivascular cellular infiltration. The location and manner of these reactions produce the lesions characteristic of each disorder. The changes are usually reversible, and the skin ordinarily recovers without blemish unless complicating factors such as ulceration from the primary irritant, scratching, and infection are introduced or underlying vascular disease develops. In chronic conditions, permanent effects are seen that vary according to the disorder, the general condition of the affected individual, and the available therapy.

Diagnostic Evaluation

Although the history and subjective symptoms of skin lesions are explored first, the obvious objective characteristics of the lesions are often noted simultaneously. Many skin lesions are easily diagnosed after careful inspection.

History and subjective symptoms. Many cutaneous lesions are associated with local symptoms. The most common local symptom is itching (*pruritus*), which varies in intensity. Pain or tenderness often accompanies some skin lesions. Other skin sensations such as burning, prickling, stinging, or crawling are also described. Alterations in local feeling include absence of sensation (*anaesthesia*); excessive sensitiveness (*hyperesthesia*); diminished sensation (*hypesthesia* or *hypoesthesia*); or abnormal sensation, such as burning or prickling (*paresthesia*). These symptoms may remain localized or migrate, may be constant or intermittent, and may be aggravated by a specific activity, such as exposure to sunlight.

It is important to determine whether the child has an allergic condition such as asthma or hay fever or history of a previous skin disease. AD, often associated with allergies, frequently begins in infancy. Important questions for the parent include when the lesion or symptom first appeared; whether it occurred with ingestion of a food or other substance, including any medication; and whether the condition was related to activity such as contact with plants, insects, or chemicals.

Objective findings. The distribution, size, morphological characteristics, and arrangement of skin lesions provide significant information. Extrinsic causes usually result from physical, chemical, or allergic irritants or from an infectious agent such as bacteria, fungi, viruses, or animal parasites. Skin manifestations are also produced by intrinsic causes such as an infection (measles or chicken pox), drug sensitization, or other allergic phenomena.

Types of lesions. Skin lesions assume distinct characteristics that are related to the pathological process. Nurses should become familiar with the common terms that are used to describe skin lesions because these terms are used in the processes of record keeping and communication. These terms include the following:

Erythema—A reddened area caused by increased amounts of oxygenated blood in the dermal vasculature

Ecchymoses (bruises)—Localized red or purple discolourations caused by extravasation of blood into dermis and subcutaneous tissues

Petechiae—Pinpoint, tiny, and sharp circumscribed spots in the superficial layers of the epidermis

Primary lesions—Skin changes produced by a causative factor; primary lesions in pediatric skin disorders include macules, papules, vesicles, patches, bullae, plaque, wheals, nodules, pustules, and cysts (Fig. 52-2)

Secondary lesions—Changes that result from alteration in the primary lesions, such as those caused by rubbing, scratching, medication, or involution and healing (Fig. 52-3)

Distribution pattern—The pattern in which lesions are distributed over the body, whether local or generalized, and the specific areas associated with the lesions

Configuration and arrangement—The size, shape, and arrangement of a lesion or groups of lesions (e.g., *discrete, clustered, diffuse,* or *confluent*)

Laboratory studies. If a skin problem is related to a systemic disease such as collagen or immunodeficiency disease, laboratory studies are performed to identify the condition. Diagnostic techniques include microscopic examination, cultures, skin scrapings or biopsy, cytodiagnosis, patch testing, Wood light examination, allergic skin testing, and other laboratory tests, such as blood count and sedimentation rate.

Wounds

Wounds are structural or physiological disruptions of the skin that activate normal or abnormal tissue repair responses. Wounds are classified as acute or chronic. *Acute wounds* are those that heal uneventfully within 2 to 3 weeks. *Chronic wounds* are those that do not heal in the expected time frame or are associated with complications. Cofactors that disrupt or delay wound healing include compromised perfusion, malnutrition, and infection. In children, most wounds are acute and can be prevented from becoming chronic wounds through appropriate nursing care. Wounds are also classified as surgical and nonsurgical and then further classified in the same manner as burns: superficial, partial thickness, or full thickness (complex wounds that include muscle or bone).

Epidermal Injuries

Abrasions are the most common epidermal wounds in children, usually in the form of a skinned knee or elbow. In most injuries the margins of the abraded area are superficial, involving only the outer layers of epidermis, although the central portion may extend into the dermis. Epithelial tissue is composed of labile cells, which are constantly destroyed and replaced throughout the lifespan. Thus epidermal injuries usually result in rapid, uneventful healing and recovery.

Injury to Deeper Tissues

Tissues composed of permanent cells such as muscle and nerve cells are unable to regenerate. These tissues repair themselves by substituting fibrous connective tissue for the injured tissue. This fibrous tissue, or *scar*, serves as a patch to preserve or restore the continuity of the tissue. Wounds involving permanent cells include surgical incisions, lacerations, ulcers, evulsions, and full-thickness burns.

Factors That Influence Wound Healing

Wound care management has shifted from interventions aimed at maintaining a dry environment to those that promote a moist, crust-free environment that enhances the migration of epithelial cells across the wound and facilitates remodelling. Whereas an acute full-thickness wound kept in a moist environment usually re-epithelializes in 12 to 15 days, the same wound when kept open to the air heals in about 25 to 30 days.

Numerous factors can delay healing (Table 52-1). For example, traditional practices, such as the use of antiseptics (hydrogen peroxide and povidone-iodine [Betadine] solutions), which were once thought to prevent infection, are now known to have a cytotoxic effect on healthy cells and minimal effect on controlling infections. Povidone-iodine may also be absorbed through the skin in newborns and young children.

General Therapeutic Management

Some wounds demand aggressive therapy, but by and large the major aim of treatment is to prevent further damage,

Macule—flat; nonpalpable; circumscribed; less than 1 cm in diameter; brown, red, purple, white, or tan in colour
Examples: Freckles; flat moles; rubella; rubeola

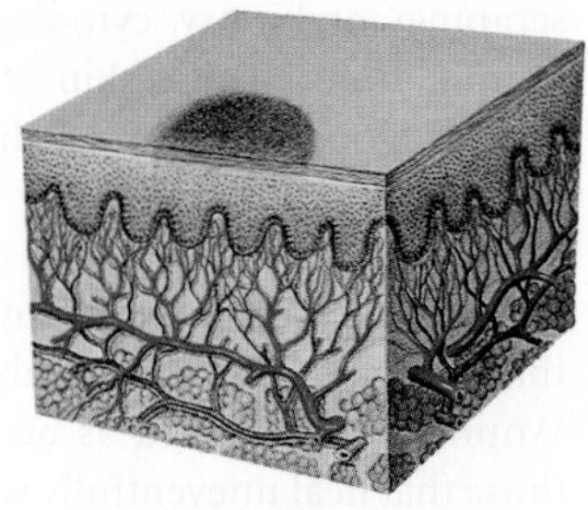

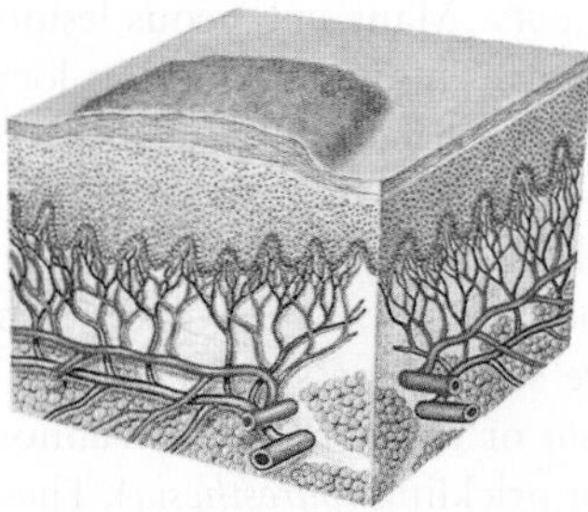

Plaque—elevated; flat topped; firm; rough; superficial papule greater than 1 cm in diameter; may be coalesced papules
Examples: Psoriasis; seborrheic and actinic keratoses

Patch—flat; nonpalpable; irregular in shape; macule that is greater than 1 cm in diameter
Examples: Vitiligo; port-wine marks

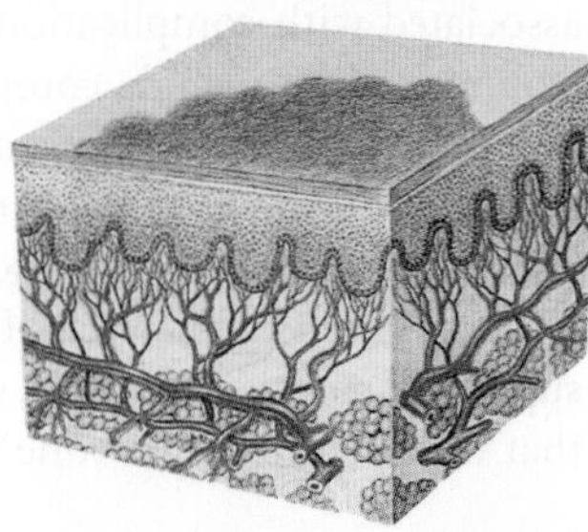

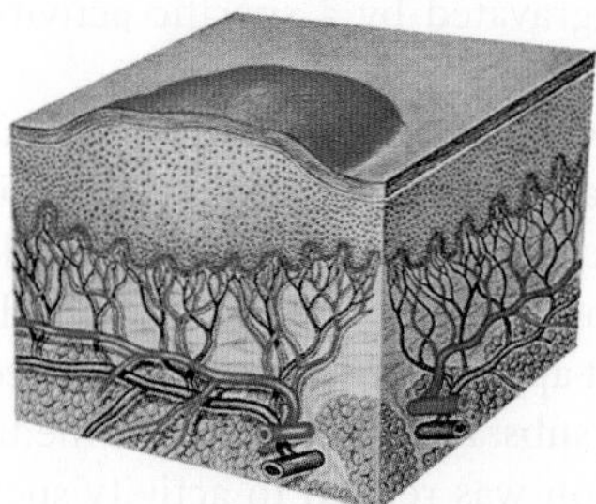

Wheal—elevated, irregularly shaped area of cutaneous edema; solid, transient, changing, variable diameter; pale pink with lighter centre
Examples: Urticaria; insect bites

Papule—elevated; palpable; firm; circumscribed; less than 1 cm in diameter; brown, red, pink, tan, or bluish red in colour
Examples: Warts; drug-related eruptions; pigmented nevi

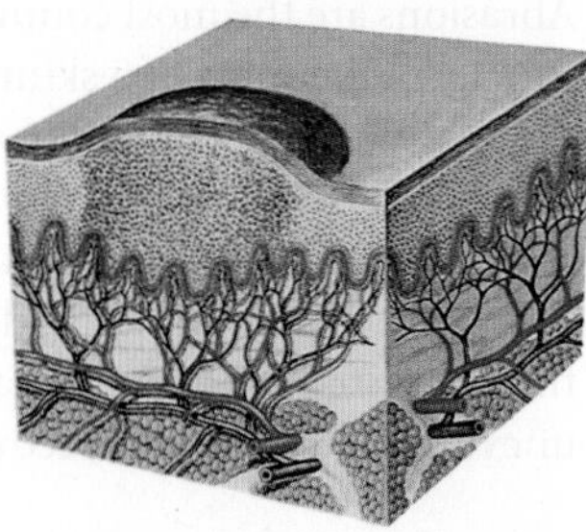

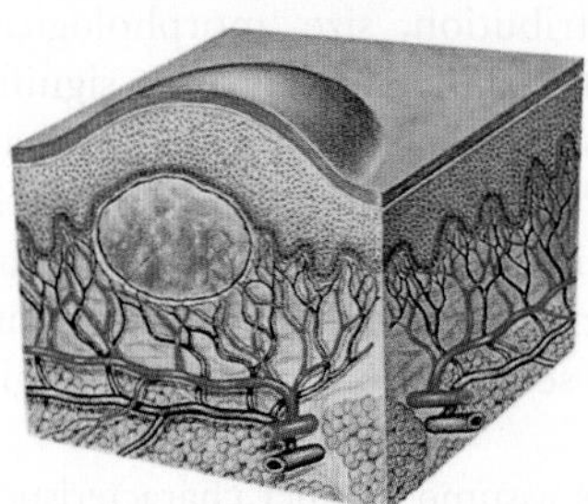

Nodule—elevated; firm; circumscribed; palpable; deeper in dermis than papule; 1 to 2 cm in diameter
Examples: Erythema nodosum; lipomas

Vesicle—elevated; circumscribed; superficial; filled with serous fluid; less than 1 cm in diameter
Examples: Blister; varicella

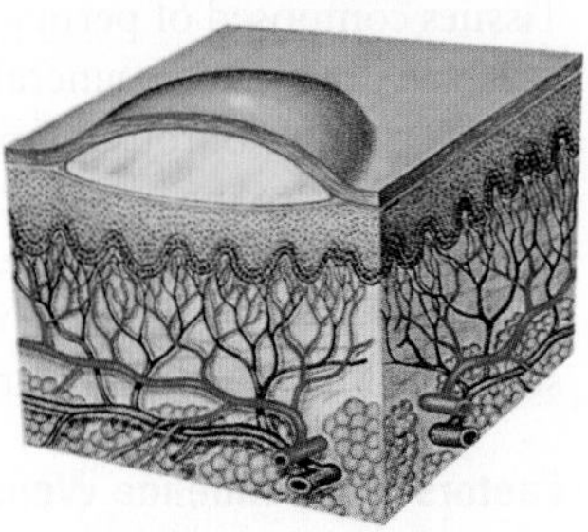

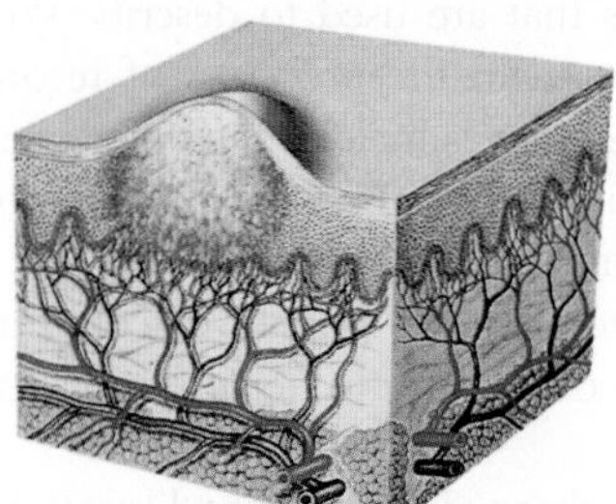

Pustule—elevated; superficial; similar to vesicle but filled with purulent fluid
Examples: Impetigo; acne; variola

Bulla—vesicle greater than 1 cm in diameter
Examples: Blister; pemphigus vulgaris

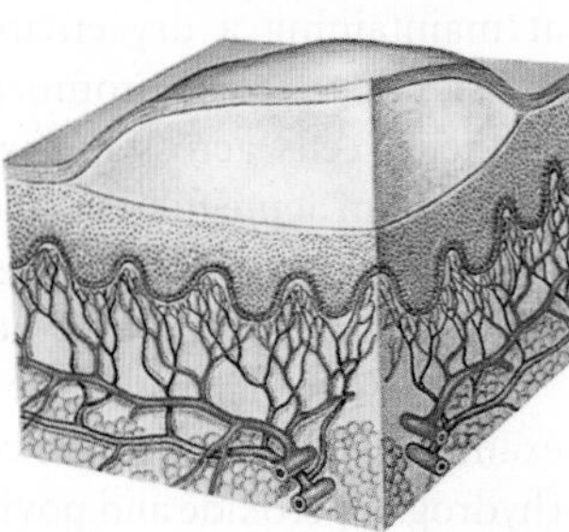

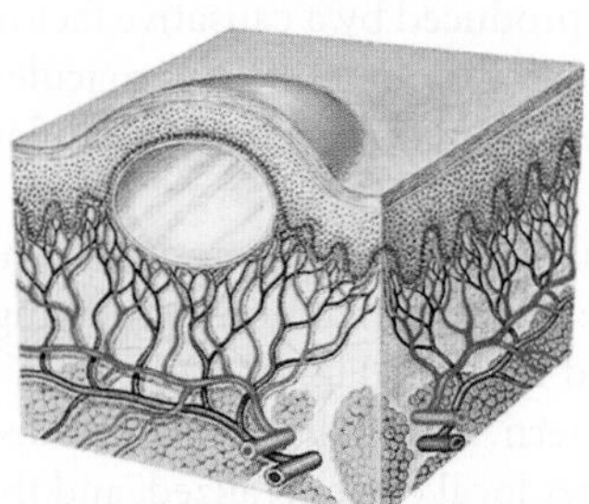

Cyst—elevated; circumscribed; palpable; encapsulated; filled with liquid or semisolid material
Example: Sebaceous cyst

FIGURE 52-2 Primary skin lesions. (From Seidel, H. M., et al. [Eds.]. [2006]. *Mosby's guide to physical examination* [6th ed., pp. 183–185]. St. Louis: Mosby [Table 8-4].)

Scale—heaped-up keratinized cells; flaky exfoliation; irregular; thick or thin; dry or oily; varied size; silver, white, or tan in colour
Examples: Psoriasis; exfoliative dermatitis

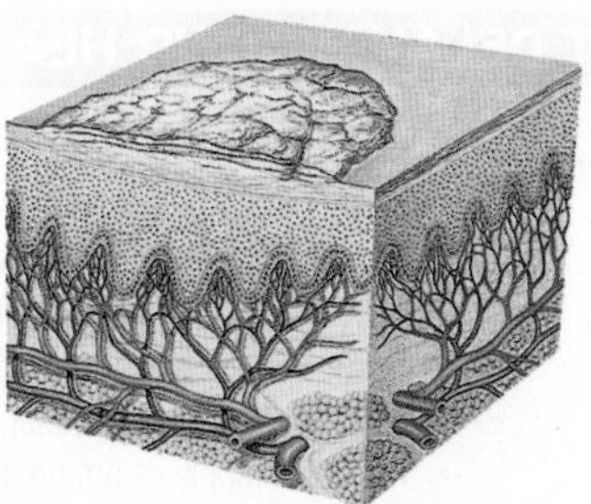

Crust—dried serum, blood, or purulent exudate; slightly elevated; size varies; brown, red, black, tan, or straw in colour
Examples: Scab on abrasion; eczema

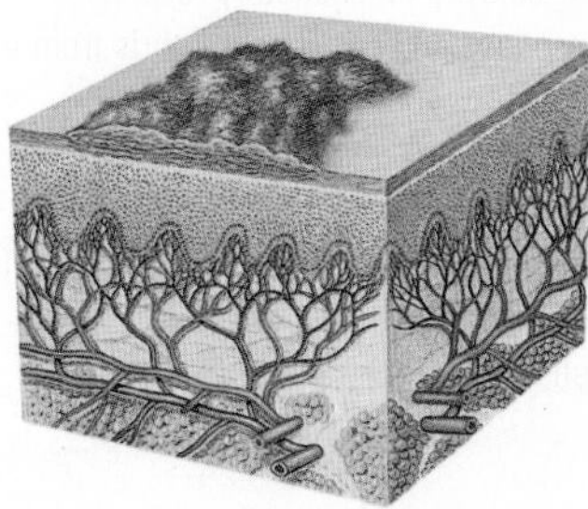

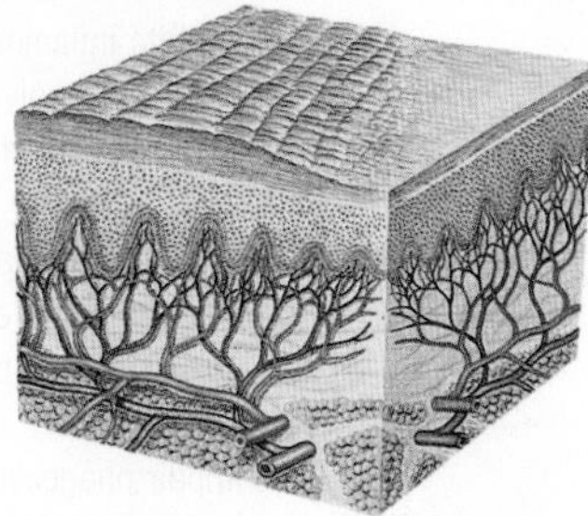

Lichenification—rough, thickened epidermis; accentuated skin markings caused by rubbing or irritation; often involves flexor aspect of extremity
Example: Chronic dermatitis

Scar—thin to thick fibrous tissue replacing injured dermis; irregular; pink, red, or white in colour; may be atrophic or hypertrophic
Example: Healed wound or surgical incision

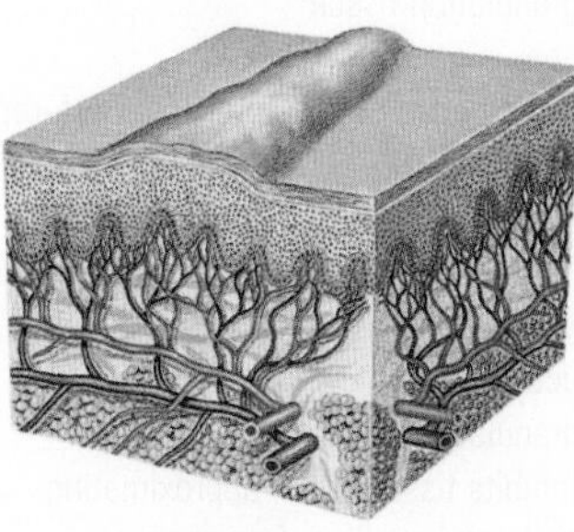

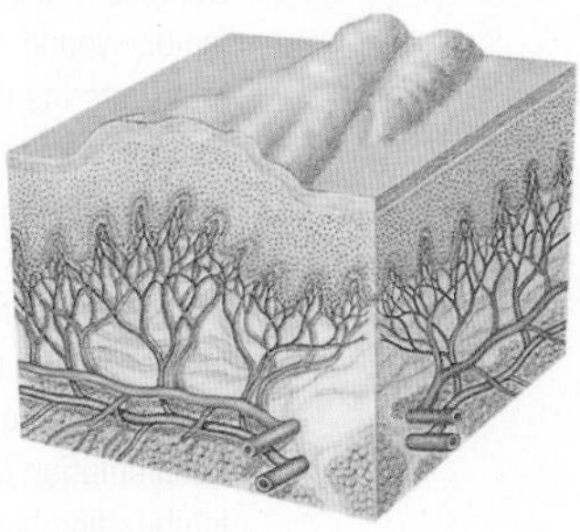

Keloid— irregularly shaped, elevated, progressively enlarging scar; grows beyond boundaries of wound; caused by excessive collagen formation during healing
Example: Keloid from ear piercing or burn scar

Excoriation—loss of epidermis; linear or hollowed-out crusted area; dermis exposed
Examples: Abrasion; scratch

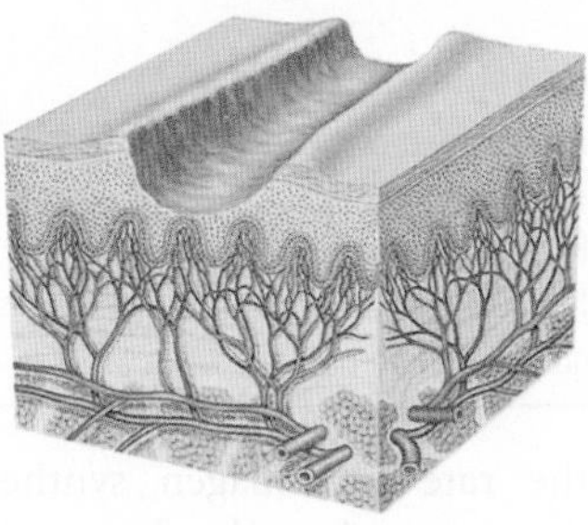

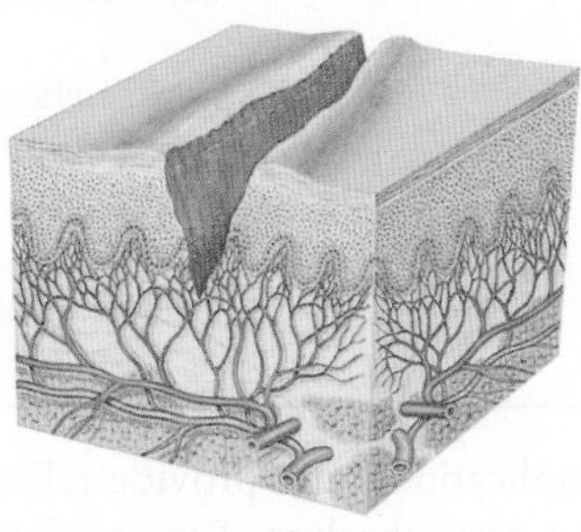

Fissure—linear crack or break from epidermis to dermis; small; deep; red
Examples: Athlete's foot; cheilosis

Erosion—loss of all or part of epidermis; depressed; moist; glistening; follows rupture of vesicle or bulla; larger than fissure
Examples: Varicella; variola following rupture

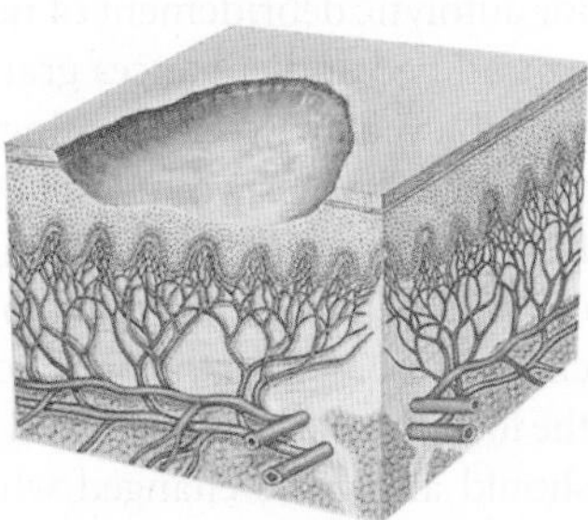

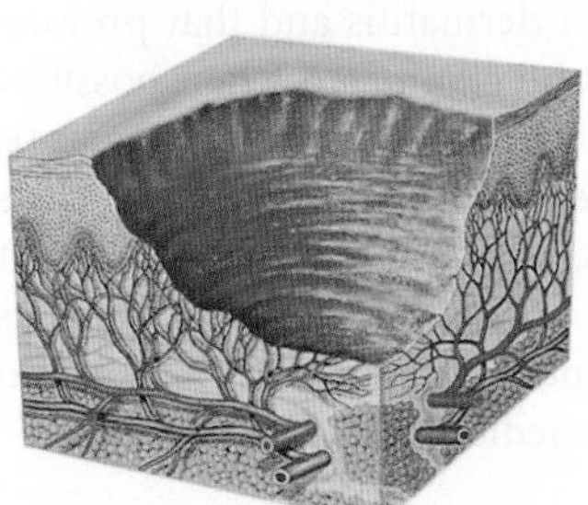

Ulcer—loss of epidermis and dermis; concave; varies in size; exudative; red or reddish blue
Examples: Decubiti; stasis ulcers

FIGURE 52-3 Secondary skin lesions. (From Seidel, H. M., et al. [Eds.]. [2006]. *Mosby's guide to physical examination* [6th ed., pp. 186–188]. St. Louis: Mosby [Table 8-5].)

TABLE 52-1 FACTORS THAT DELAY WOUND HEALING

FACTOR	EFFECT ON HEALING
Dry wound environment	Allows epithelial cells to dry out and die; impairs migration of epithelial cells across wound surface
Nutritional deficiencies	
Vitamin A	Results in inadequate inflammatory response
Vitamin B_1	Results in decreased collagen formation
Vitamin C	Inhibits formation of collagen fibres and capillary development
Protein	Reduces supply of amino acids for tissue repair
Zinc	Impairs epithelialization
Immunocompromise	Results in inadequate or delayed inflammatory response
Impaired circulation	Inhibits inflammatory response and removal of debris from wound area Reduces supply of nutrients to wound area
Stress (pain, poor sleep)	Releases catecholamines that cause vasoconstriction
Antiseptics	
Hydrogen peroxide	Toxic to fibroblasts; can cause subcutaneous gas formation (mimics gas-forming infection)
Povidone-iodine	Toxic to white and red blood cells and fibroblasts
Chlorhexidine	Toxic to white blood cells
Medications	
Corticosteroids	Impair phagocytosis Inhibit fibroblast proliferation Depress formation of granulation tissue Inhibit wound contraction
Chemotherapy	Interrupts the cell cycle; damages DNA or prevents DNA repair
Anti-inflammatory drugs	Decrease the inflammatory phase
Foreign bodies	Increase inflammatory response Inhibit wound closure
Infection	Increases inflammatory response Increases tissue destruction
Mechanical friction	Damages or destroys granulation tissue
Fluid accumulation	Accumulation in area inhibits tissues from approximating
Radiation	Inhibits fibroblastic activity and capillary formation May cause tissue necrosis
Diseases	
Diabetes mellitus	Inhibits collagen synthesis Impairs circulation and capillary growth Hyperglycemia impairs phagocytosis
Anemia	Reduces oxygen supply to tissues
Peripheral vascular disease	Reduces oxygen supply to wounds
Uremia	Decreases collagen and granulation tissue

eliminate the cause, prevent complications, and provide relief from discomfort while tissues undergo healing. Factors that contribute to the development of dermatitis and that prolong the course of the disease should be eliminated when possible. For example, the most common causative agents of dermatitis in infants, children, and adolescents are environmental factors (soaps, bubble baths, shampoos, rough or tight clothing, wet diapers, blankets, and toys) and the natural elements (such as dirt, sand, heat, cold, moisture, and wind). Dermatitis may also result from home remedies and medications.

Dressings

No one dressing meets the needs of all wounds. The traditional dry gauze dressing should not be used on open wounds because it allows the wound surface to dry, does little to prevent bacterial invasion, and adheres to the dried scab so that removal disturbs the newly regenerating epithelial cells. In most instances, traditional gauze dressings have been replaced by dressings that promote moist wound healing. Moist wound healing increases the rate of collagen synthesis and re-epithelialization and decreases pain and inflammation. It also creates an environment for autolytic debridement of necrotic tissue, which creates a clean wound bed and enhances granulation. However, a balance must be achieved between creating a moist wound bed and maintaining a dry periwound area that protects the skin and wound from maceration. The dressing type and frequency of dressing changes help to achieve this balance. The frequency of dressing changes is based on the presence of infection, the type of dressing, the location of the wound, and the amount of drainage. Dressings should always be changed when they are loose or soiled. They should be changed more frequently in areas where contamination is likely, such as the sacral area, the buttocks, the tracheal area, or when wound infection is suspected or present.

Topical Therapy

Several agents and methods are available for treatment of lesions and wounds. In selecting a therapeutic regimen, the practitioner considers (1) the choice of active ingredient, (2) the proper vehicle or base, (3) the cosmetic effect, (4) the cost, and (5) instructions for use. Several basic concepts must also be considered. Overtreatment should be avoided. For example, when dermatitis is acute, topical applications should be mild and bland to avoid further irritation. Broken or inflamed skin, especially in children, is more absorbent than intact skin, and chemicals that are nonirritating to intact skin may be quite irritating to inflamed skin.

Topical applications may be applied to treat a disorder, reduce itching, decrease external stimuli, or apply external heat or cold. The emollient action of soaks, baths, and lotions provides a soothing film over the skin surface that reduces external stimuli. Ordinarily, lukewarm or cool applications offer the greatest relief.

> **! NURSING ALERT**
>
> Application of heat tends to aggravate most conditions, and its use is usually reserved for reducing specific inflammatory processes, such as folliculitis and cellulitis.

Ointments in a petrolatum base provide protection from moisture. Therefore, this type of ointment is indicated around gastrostomy tubes, in skin folds, and in the diaper area. Creams are absorbed by the skin and are used for areas where a nongreasy "feel" is desired, such as the face and hands.

Topical corticosteroid therapy. Glucocorticoids are the therapeutic medications used most frequently for skin disorders. Their local anti-inflammatory effects are merely palliative, so the medication must be applied until the condition undergoes remission or the causative agent is eliminated. Corticosteroids are applied directly to the affected area, are essentially nonsensitizing, and have only minor adverse effects. As with the use of any steroids, their use in large amounts may mask signs of infection, and symptoms may be exacerbated after termination of the medication. Families should be cautioned that the medication cannot be used for all skin disorders. The concentrations available without prescription are not adequate for stubborn skin conditions such as psoriasis and may further aggravate inflammation caused by fungus or bacteria. Most parents and children should be counselled that it is both effective and economical to apply only a thin film and to massage it into the skin. Parents and children should also be advised to use the application for no more than 5 to 7 days, because these agents may cause depigmentation and other changes in the skin.

Other topical therapies. Other topical treatments include chemical cautery (especially useful for warts), cryosurgery, electrodesiccation (chiefly used for warts, granulomas, and nevi), ultraviolet (UV) therapy (primarily used in psoriasis and acne), laser therapy (especially for birthmarks), and acne therapies such as dermabrasion and chemical peels. New medications called *topical immunomodulators* are effective in reducing the itching of AD (eczema) and preventing "flares."

Systemic Therapy

Systemic medications may be used as an adjunct to topical therapy in some dermatological disorders. The medications most frequently used are corticosteroids, antibiotics, and antifungal medications. Corticosteroids are valuable because of their capacity to inhibit inflammatory and allergic reactions. Dosage is carefully adjusted and gradually tapered to the minimum dosage that is effective and tolerated, as prolonged use may temporarily suppress growth.

Antibiotics are used in severe or widespread skin infections. However, because these medications tend to produce hypersensitivity in some patients, they are used with caution. Antifungal medications are the only means for treating systemic fungal infections.

NURSING CARE

The child's subjective symptoms and the parent's history provide valuable information to help establish a diagnosis when caring for child with a lesion. Older children often describe the condition as painful, itching, or tingling or in other descriptive terms. However, much can be determined by also observing the younger child's behaviour. Does the child scratch? Is the child restless or irritable? Does the child favour or avoid using a body part? A careful history provides important clues. Has the child had access to chemicals or been in the woods or around a woodpile? Has the child eaten a new food? Is the child taking medication? Has the child any known allergy? Do siblings or playmates have similar lesions? What soap or bubble bath is used for bathing?

It is important for nurses to not only describe but also assess skin lesions and the associated wounds. The colour, shape, and distribution of lesions and wounds are important. Individual lesions are described according to standard terminology. Sometimes two descriptors are used for a particular characteristic, such as maculopapular rash. To confirm or amplify the findings made by inspection, the nurse may gently palpate the skin to detect characteristics such as temperature, moisture, texture, elasticity, and edema. Wounds need to be assessed for depth of tissue damage, evidence of healing, and signs of infection.

> **! NURSING ALERT**
>
> Signs of wound infection are as follows:
> - Increased erythema, especially beyond the wound margin
> - Edema
> - Purulent exudate
> - Pain
> - Increased temperature

The frequency of wound assessment depends on the severity and complexity of the wound. For example, simple or chronic wounds are assessed weekly; infected or complex wounds are assessed daily. Wounds are measured at least weekly (height, width, and depth). The wound bed is assessed for colour, drainage, odour, necrosis, granulation tissue, fibrin slough, undermining and condition of the wound edges, and the colour and condition of the surrounding skin.

Therapeutic programs are designed to include general measures such as rest, protection, and relief of discomfort, and specific treatments such as medication and physical techniques. Only a few skin diseases are contagious; thus it is usually not necessary to isolate the affected child, except from persons in danger of acquiring a secondary infection, such as a child receiving large doses of corticosteroids or other immunosuppressant medications or a child with an immunological deficiency disorder. However, if the skin manifestation is caused by a viral **exanthema**, such as measles or chicken pox, the child should be prevented from exposing other susceptible children.

Wound Care

Parents can generally manage small skin lesions or wounds at home. The parents should be instructed to wash their hands and then wash the wound gently with mild soap and water or normal saline. They should be cautioned to avoid povidone-iodine, alcohol, and hydrogen peroxide because these products are toxic to wounds.

NURSING ALERT

Do not put anything in a wound that you would not put in the eye. The safest solution is normal saline.

Open wounds are covered with a dressing, such as a commercial adhesive bandage, although larger wounds may benefit from the use of occlusive dressings. If occlusive dressings are applied, parents need to learn how to apply and remove the dressings correctly. For example, hydrocolloid dressings adhere best if a wide margin is left around the wound and the dressing is pressed against intact skin until it adheres. If a dressing needs to be secured, a nonalcohol skin barrier can be applied to protect the skin, or the wound can be "picture framed" with hydrocolloid dressing and dressing tape can be secured to the hydrocolloid. This method of securing the dressing protects the skin when the tape is removed. Montgomery straps or stretch netting can also be used to secure dressings and to avoid the use of tape.

NURSING ALERT

Advise parents that the yellow gel forming under hydrocolloid dressings may look like pus and has a distinct odour (somewhat fruity) but is normal leakage.

Dressings need to be removed carefully to protect intact skin and the epithelial surface of the wound. When removing transparent or hydrocolloid dressings, the nurse or parent should raise one edge of the dressing and pull parallel to the skin to loosen the adhesive. The longer the dressings are left on, the easier they are to remove. Less frequent dressing changes decrease wound contamination.

Lacerations present a special challenge. The injured child and family are usually distressed by the bleeding. In particular, scalp lacerations tend to bleed profusely. Parental guilt and shock usually accompany the injury. The initial nursing intervention is to apply pressure to the area and to attempt to calm the child before further examination. Unless there is bleeding from a severed artery, the wound is cleansed with a forced jet of sterile tepid water or saline (via syringe) and examined for extent, depth, and presence of foreign material such as dirt, glass, or fabric fragments.

The location of the wound facilitates assessment. Wounds over bony areas may contain bone chips, and clear fluid seeping from severe head wounds may indicate cerebrospinal fluid. A pressure dressing is applied for transfer to medical care. After the child is in a medical facility, the child is prepared for treatment.

Puncture wounds that do not require a tetanus booster are soaked in warm water and soap for several minutes. Causing the wound to rebleed may be helpful. An adhesive bandage can be applied if desired. Puncture wounds of the head, chest, or abdomen or those that could still contain a portion of the puncturing object must be evaluated carefully.

Parents should be cautioned against opening blisters or kissing a wound "to make it better." The wound can easily become contaminated from germs in the human mouth. If scabs form, they need to be allowed to slough off without assistance; picking or early removal may cause scarring and secondary infection. Parents should be advised to seek medical help if there is evidence of infection.

Relief of Symptoms

Most therapeutic regimens for skin lesions are directed toward relief of pruritus, the most common subjective complaint. Cooling the affected area and increasing the skin pH with cool baths or compresses and alkaline applications such as baking soda baths are helpful in reducing the itching. Clothing and bed linen should be soft and lightweight to decrease irritation from friction and stimulation.

During treatment, both the affected and unaffected skin should be protected from damage and secondary infection. Preventing scratching is important. Older children can refrain from scratching or rubbing, although they may need to be reminded to do so. Small children may require the use of devices such as mittens (especially during sleep) or special coverings. Keeping fingernails clean, short, and trimmed reduces the risk of secondary infection.

Antipruritic medications, such as diphenhydramine (Benadryl) or hydroxyzine (Atarax), may be prescribed for severe itching, especially if it disturbs the child's rest. Pain and discomfort are usually managed with nonpharmacological measures and mild analgesia. Severe pain requires more potent medication. Occlusive dressings over wounds reduce pain. For suturing wounds a topical anaesthetic or intradermal buffered lidocaine should be used (see Pain Management, Chapter 34).

Treatment of Skin Disorders

The specific type of topical therapy and the mode of application depend on the nature and location of the lesion. It is especially important to perform proper hand hygiene before and after application of any topical therapy. The skin should be assessed before the application and reassessed after treatment. Any observed changes need to be noted and described.

Wet compresses or dressings cool the skin by evaporation, relieve itching and inflammation, and cleanse the area by loosening and removing crusts and debris. A variety of ingredients, such as plain water or Burow solution, can be applied on Kerlix gauze, plain gauze, or freshly laundered soft cloths.

Dressings immersed in the desired solution are wrung out slightly and applied to the affected area wet but not dripping. They are applied flat and smooth in such a way that motion is not totally restricted—fingers are wrapped separately, and arms and legs are wrapped so that elbows and knees can bend. Dressings are held in place by Kerlix or other cotton wrap, tubular stockinette, mittens, and socks (two pairs—one to hold the dressings in place, the other to protect from movement). When evaporation begins to dry them, the dressings are removed, rewet in the solution, and reapplied using aseptic technique. The solution is *not* poured or applied with a syringe directly over the dressings. As fluid evaporates, the solution becomes more concentrated, and this could damage sensitive lesions.

Fresh solution at room temperature is applied at 2-, 3-, or 4-hour intervals and allowed to remain on the lesion from 20 to 90 minutes. Wet dressings are seldom continued after about 48 hours. The child needs to be protected against chilling during treatment, and no more than 20% of the body is covered with a dressing at one time, to avoid the risk of hypothermia. After treatment, the skin is dried thoroughly by patting with a towel. Lotion or other medication (if prescribed) is applied at this time.

When the use of wet dressings is not possible, soaks are often used for removal of crusts and for their mild astringent action. The same solutions are used as for wet compresses. Gaining young children's assistance with hand or foot soaks can be difficult unless the procedure is accompanied by play. Older infants and toddlers delight in playing with brightly coloured objects or poker chips scattered over the bottom of the receptacle, and preschoolers can be challenged to hold a floating item beneath the water's surface. However, these activities require supervision; infants and small children place items in their mouths, and children easily lose control with water play. Washing dishes, cars, dolls, or doll clothes will also occupy time during soaks.

Older children also need something to do during the procedure, such as listening to music or a story or watching television. Placing the solution and the extremity in a plastic sealable bag is an effective method to soak a hand or foot.

Baths are useful in the treatment of widespread dermatitis by evenly distributing the soothing antipruritic and anti-inflammatory effects of the solution, usually oatmeal or mineral oil preparations. The solution is added to a tub of lukewarm water. The temperature of the bath should be tepid, and the treatment usually lasts 15 to 30 minutes. Therapeutic baths are more interesting when toy boats, ducks, or other items for water play accompany the procedure.

Topical applications are applied to skin lesions to ease discomfort, prevent further injury, and facilitate healing. A thin application of the ointment or cream may be covered with a plastic film and anchored with adhesive, covered with a commercial transparent dressing, or wrapped in Kerlix gauze and held in place by a stretchy net dressing. Topical preparations are applied systematically with the contour of the body surface (not simply up and down). Children love to be "painted," and lotion applications can be fun when an ordinary paintbrush is used. Regardless of the type of preparation used, parents need detailed information on how to apply it and how long the preparation should remain on the skin.

! NURSING ALERT

Provide written instructions and demonstrate to parents the correct amount of topical medication to apply (e.g., size of a pea; thin film to cover). If more than one preparation is applied, mark the containers with numbers so the parents remember the correct order of application. Stress that more is not necessarily better with some medications, such as steroids.

Home Care and Family Support

Dermatological conditions always involve the family, but few situations require hospitalization and most care is delivered at home. Because the family members must carry out the treatment plan, their assistance is essential. Regimens that are simple to accomplish in the clinic, hospital, or primary care provider's office may be frustrating and baffling at home. The family may also need assistance in adapting equipment available for home therapy.

It is important that the child and family be given explanations that are as detailed as possible about both the expected and unexpected results of treatment, including any ill effects that might occur. If unexplained reactions develop, the family should be directed to discontinue treatment and report the reactions to the appropriate person. The use of over-the-counter medicines is discouraged unless the preparations have been discussed and approved by the health care provider.

Because the skin is the most visible portion of the body, defects in its surface alter its appearance and can cause distress for the child. Skin problems may also result in rejection by others. Parents of other children may fear that their children will "catch" the disorder. Occasionally the affected child's own family members reduce their interaction or physical contact with the child. This is seldom a problem with dermatitis of short duration, but chronic conditions can frequently create problems and affect the child's self-esteem.

INFECTIONS OF THE SKIN

Bacterial Infections

Normally, the skin harbours a variety of bacterial flora, including the major pathogenic varieties of staphylococci and streptococci. The degree of pathogenicity of the organism depends on its invasiveness and toxicity, the integrity of the skin, and the immune and cellular defences of the host. Children with congenital or acquired immunodeficiency disorders (such as acquired immunodeficiency syndrome [AIDS]), those in a debilitated condition, those receiving immunosuppressant therapy, and those with a generalized malignancy such as leukemia or lymphoma are at risk for developing bacterial infections. Common bacterial skin disorders are outlined in Table 52-2.

Because of the characteristic "walling-off" process of the inflammatory reaction (abscess formation), staphylococci are more difficult to treat, and the local infected area is associated

TABLE 52-2 BACTERIAL INFECTIONS

DISORDER AND ORGANISM	MANIFESTATIONS	MANAGEMENT	COMMENTS
Impetigo contagiosa—*Staphylococcus* (Fig. 52-4)	Begins as a reddish macule Becomes vesicular Ruptures easily, leaving superficial, moist erosion Tends to spread peripherally in sharply marginated irregular outlines Exudate dries to form heavy, honey-coloured crusts Pruritus common Systemic effects—Minimal or asymptomatic	Careful removal of undermined skin, crusts, and debris by softening with 1:20 Burow solution compresses Topical application of bactericidal ointment Systemic administration of oral or parenteral antibiotics (penicillin) in severe or extensive lesions	Tends to heal without scarring unless secondary infection Autoinoculable and contagious Common in toddlers and preschoolers May be superimposed on eczema
Pyoderma—*Staphylococcus, streptococcus*	Deeper extension of infection into dermis Tissue reaction more severe Systemic effects—Fever, lymphangitis	Soap and water cleansing Wet compresses Bathing with antibacterial soap as prescribed Washcloths or towels should not be shared Mupirocin to nares and lesions as prescribed Systemic antibiotics	Autoinoculable and contagious May heal with or without scarring
Folliculitis (pimple), furuncle (boil), carbuncle (multiple boils)—*Staphylococcus aureus*	Folliculitis—Infection of hair follicle Furuncle—Larger lesion with more redness and swelling at a single follicle Carbuncle—More extensive lesion with widespread inflammation and "pointing" at several follicular orifices Systemic effects—Malaise, if severe	Skin cleanliness Local warm, moist compresses Topical application of antibiotic medications Systemic antibiotics in severe cases Incision and drainage of severe lesions, followed by wound irrigation with antibiotics or suitable drain implantation	Autoinoculable and contagious Furuncle and carbuncle tend to heal with scar formation Never squeeze a lesion
Cellulitis—*Streptococcus, staphylococcus, Haemophilus influenzae* (Fig. 52-5)	Inflammation of skin and subcutaneous tissues with intense redness, swelling, and firm infiltration Lymphangitis "streaking" frequently seen Involvement of regional lymph nodes common May progress to abscess formation Systemic effects—Fever, malaise	Oral or parenteral antibiotics Rest and immobilization of both affected area and child Hot, moist compresses to area Marking the edges of the erythema to determine and track spreading of the infection	Hospitalization may be necessary for child with systemic symptoms Otitis media may be associated with facial cellulitis
Staphylococcal scalded skin syndrome—*S. aureus*	Macular erythema with "sandpaper" texture of involved skin Epidermis becoming wrinkled (in 2 days or less), and large bullae appearing	Systemic administration of antibiotics Gentle cleansing with saline, Burow solution, or 0.25% silver nitrate compresses	Infants subject to fluid loss; impaired body temperature regulation; and secondary infection, such as pneumonia, cellulitis, and septicemia Heals without scarring

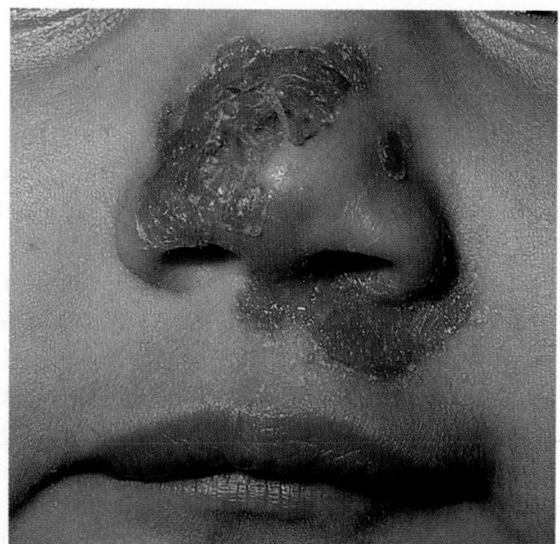

FIGURE 52-4 Impetigo contagiosa. (From Weston, W. L., Lane, A. T., & Morelli, J. G. [2002]. *Color textbook of pediatric dermatology* [3rd ed.]. St. Louis: Mosby.)

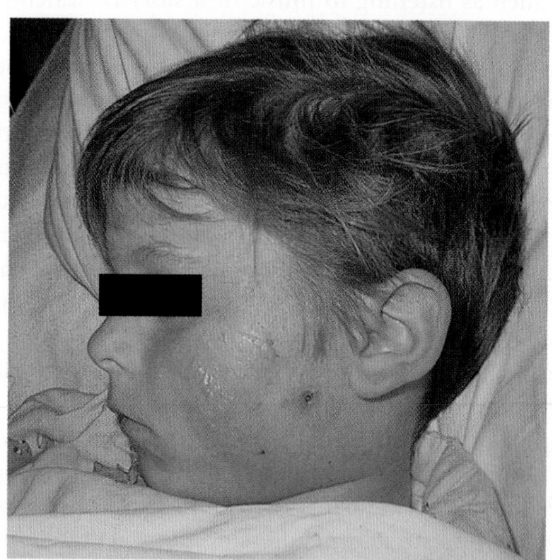

FIGURE 52-5 Cellulitis of cheek from puncture wound. (From Weston, W. L., Lane, A. T., & Morelli, J. G. [2002]. *Color textbook of pediatric dermatology* [3rd ed.]. St. Louis: Mosby.)

with an increase in bacteria all over the skin surface that serves as a source of continuing infection. In recent years, the number of community-acquired methicillin-resistant *Staphylococcus aureus* (MRSA) infections has risen. Recent outbreaks of MRSA in Canada have been seen among athletes, prisoners, military recruits, children who attend day care centres, injection drug users, and other groups of people who live in crowded settings or routinely share contaminated items. Indigenous peoples have high rates of community-acquired MRSA infections that are mostly skin and soft-tissue infections and are more virulent, resulting in significant morbidity and mortality. This increased prevalence is in part due to household overcrowding and a lack of indoor piped water, which directly affects this community's ability to maintain adequate personal and environmental hygiene (Irvine & Canadian Paediatric Society [CPS], First Nations, Inuit and Métis Health Committee, 2012/2015). There is also increasing concern about evolving resistant forms of MRSA due to overuse of antibacterials.

Thus when caring for infected children and their lesions or wounds, the importance of careful hand hygiene and cleanliness needs to be stressed, as this practice can help prevent the spread of infection and is an essential prophylactic measure in general when caring for infants and small children.

NURSING CARE

The major nursing interventions related to bacterial skin infections are to prevent the spread of infection and to prevent complications. Impetigo contagiosa and MRSA infections can easily spread by self-inoculation; thus the child must be cautioned against touching the involved area. Hand hygiene is mandatory before and after contact with an affected child. Good hand hygiene practice should also be emphasized to both the child and family. Many children with AD are colonized with MRSA in the nares and under the fingernails. Thus for many bacterial infections, and for MRSA infection in particular, the child should be provided with washcloths and towels separate from those of other family members. The child's pyjamas, underwear, and other clothes should be changed daily and washed in hot water. Razors used for shaving should be discarded after each use and not shared. To prevent recurrence, some infectious disease specialists recommend bathing in a chlorine bath once or twice weekly with approximately 120 mL of bleach that is diluted in one-quarter tub of water (Fisher, Chain, Hair, et al., 2008; Kaplan, 2008). In addition, mupirocin (Bactroban) can be applied to the nares of patients and families twice daily for 2 to 4 weeks to prevent reinfection (Huang, Abrams, Tlougan, et al., 2009).

Children and parents are often tempted to squeeze follicular lesions. They must be warned that squeezing will not hasten the resolution of the infection and that there is a risk for making the lesion worse or spreading the infection. No attempt should be made to puncture the surface of the pustule with a needle or sharp instrument. For example, a child with a sty (an abscess on the inner or outer part of the eyelid caused by a bacterial infection) may waken with the eyelids of the affected eye sealed shut with exudate. The child or the parents should be instructed to gently wipe the lid from the inner to the outer edge with warm water and a clean washcloth until the exudate is removed.

The child with limited cellulitis of an extremity is usually managed at home on a regimen of oral antibiotics and warm compresses. Children with more extensive cellulitis, especially around a joint with lymphadenitis or on the face, are usually admitted to the hospital for parenteral antibiotics, followed by continued treatment at home. Nurses are responsible for teaching the family to administer the medication and apply compresses.

Viral Infections

Viruses are intracellular parasites that produce their effect by using the intracellular substances of the host cells. Composed of only a deoxyribonucleic acid (DNA) or ribonucleic acid (RNA) core enclosed in an antigenic protein shell, viruses are unable to provide for their own metabolic needs or to reproduce themselves. After a virus penetrates a cell of the host organism, it sheds the outer shell and disappears within the cell, where the nucleic acid core stimulates the host cell to form more virus material from its intracellular substance. In a viral infection the epidermal cells react with inflammation and vesiculation (as in herpes simplex) or by proliferating to form growths (warts).

Many of the communicable viral diseases of childhood are associated with rashes, and each rash is characteristic. The type of lesion and the configuration of rubeola, rubella, and chicken pox are described in Table 37-2. Other common viral disorders of the skin are outlined in Table 52-3.

Dermatophytoses (Fungal Infections)

The dermatophytoses (ringworm) are infections caused by a group of closely related filamentous fungi that invade primarily the stratum corneum, hair, and nails. These are superficial infections that live on, not in, the skin. They are confined to the dead keratin layers and are unable to survive in the deeper layers. Because the keratin is **desquamated** constantly, the fungus must multiply at a rate that equals the rate of keratin production to maintain itself; otherwise the infection would be shed with the discarded skin cells. Common dermatophytoses are outlined in Table 52-4.

Dermatophytoses are designated by the Latin word *tinea*, with further designation related to the area of the body where they are found (e.g., tinea capitis [ringworm of the scalp]). Dermatophyte infections are most often transmitted from one person to another or from infected animals to humans. Diagnosis is made from microscopic examination of scrapings taken from the advancing periphery of the lesion, which almost always produces a scale.

NURSING CARE

When teaching families how to care for ringworm, the nurse should emphasize good health and hygiene. Because of the infectious nature of the disease, affected children should not exchange with other children grooming items, headgear, scarves,

TABLE 52-3 **VIRAL INFECTIONS**

INFECTION	MANIFESTATIONS	MANAGEMENT	COMMENTS
Verruca (warts) Cause—Human papillomavirus (various types)	Usually well-circumscribed, grey or brown, elevated, firm papules with a roughened, finely papillomatous texture Occur anywhere, but usually appear on exposed areas such as fingers, hands, face, and soles May be single or multiple Asymptomatic	Not uniformly successful Local destructive therapy, individualized according to location, type, and number—surgical removal, electrocautery, curettage, cryotherapy (liquid nitrogen), caustic solutions (lactic acid and salicylic acid in flexible collodion, retinoic acid, salicylic acid plasters), x-ray treatment, laser	Common in children Tend to disappear spontaneously Course unpredictable Most destructive techniques tend to leave scars Autoinoculable Repeated irritation will cause to enlarge Apply topical anaesthetic EMLA
Verruca plantaris (plantar wart)	Located on plantar surface of feet and, because of pressure, is practically flat; may be surrounded by a collar of hyperkeratosis	Apply caustic solution to wart and wear foam insole with hole cut to relieve pressure on wart; Soak 20 minutes after 2–3 days; repeat until wart comes out	Destructive techniques tend to leave scars, which may cause problems with walking Apply topical anaesthetic EMLA
Herpes simplex virus Type I (cold sore, fever blister) Type II (genital)	Grouped, burning, and itching vesicles on inflammatory base, usually on or near mucocutaneous junctions (lips, nose, genitalia, buttocks) Vesicles dry, forming a crust, followed by exfoliation and spontaneous healing in 8–10 days May be accompanied by regional lymphadenopathy	Avoidance of secondary infection Burow solution compresses during weeping stages Topical therapy (penciclovir) to shorten duration of cold sores Oral antiviral (acyclovir) for initial infection or to reduce severity in recurrence Valacyclovir, an oral antiviral, used for episodic treatment of recurrent genital herpes; reduces pain, stops viral shedding, and has a more convenient administration schedule than acyclovir	Heal without scarring unless secondary infection Type I cold sores prevented by using sunscreens protecting against UVA and UVB light to prevent lip blisters Aggravated by corticosteroids Positive psychological effect from treatment May be fatal in children with depressed immunity
Varicella-zoster virus (herpes zoster; shingles)	Caused by same virus that causes varicella (chicken pox) Virus has affinity for posterior root ganglia, posterior horn of spinal cord, and skin; crops of vesicles usually confined to dermatome following along course of affected nerve Usually preceded by neuralgic pain, hyperesthesias, or itching May be accompanied by constitutional symptoms	Symptomatic Analgesics for pain Mild sedation sometimes helpful Local moist compresses Drying lotions sometimes helpful Ophthalmic variety: use systemic corticotropin (adrenocorticotropic hormone) or corticosteroids Acyclovir Lidocaine (Lidoderm) topical anaesthetic	Pain in children usually minimal Postherpetic pain does not occur in children Chicken pox may follow exposure; isolate affected child from other children in a hospital or school May occur in children with depressed immunity; can be fatal
Molluscum contagiosum Cause—Pox virus Small, benign tumours	Flesh-coloured papules with a central caseous plug (umbilicated) Usually asymptomatic	Cases in well children resolve spontaneously in about 18 mo Treatment reserved for troublesome cases Apply topical anaesthetic EMLA and remove with curette Use tretinoin gel 0.01% or cantharidin (Cantharone) liquid Curettage or cryotherapy	Common in school-age children Spread by skin-to-skin contact, including autoinoculation and fomite-to-skin contact

EMLA, eutectic mix of lidocaine and prilocaine; *UVA*, ultraviolet A; *UVB*, ultraviolet B.

or other articles of apparel that have been in proximity to the infected area. Affected children should have their own towels and wear a protective cap at night to avoid transmitting the fungus to bedding, especially if they sleep with another person. Because the infection can be acquired by animal-to-human transmission, all household pets should be examined for the disorder. Other sources of infection are seats with headrests (such as theatre seats), seats in public transportation vehicles, helmets, and gymnasium mats.

Both 2% ketoconazole and 1% selenium sulphide shampoos may reduce colony counts of dermatophytes. These shampoos can be used in combination with oral therapy to reduce the transmission of disease to others. The shampoo should be applied to the scalp for 5 to 10 minutes at least three times per week. The child may return to school once the therapy is initiated.

Alternatively, if the child is treated with the drug griseofulvin, the therapy frequently continues for weeks or months, and

TABLE 52-4 DERMATOPHYTOSES (FUNGAL INFECTIONS)

DISEASE AND ORGANISM	MANIFESTATIONS	MANAGEMENT	COMMENTS
Tinea capitis—*Trichophyton tonsurans, Microsporum audouinii, Microsporum canis* (Fig. 52-6, A)	Lesions in scalp but may extend to hairline or neck Characteristic configuration of scaly, circumscribed patches or patchy, scaling areas of alopecia Generally asymptomatic, but severe, deep inflammatory reaction may occur that manifests as boggy, encrusted lesions (kerions) Pruritic Microscopic examination of scales is diagnostic	Oral griseofulvin Oral ketoconazole for difficult cases Selenium sulphide shampoos Topical antifungal medications (e.g., clotrimazole, haloprogin, miconazole)	Person-to-person transmission Animal-to-person transmission Rarely, permanent loss of hair *M. audouinii* transmitted from one human being to another directly or from personal items; *M. canis* usually contracted from household pets, especially cats Atopic individuals more susceptible
Tinea corporis—*Trichophyton rubrum, Trichophyton mentagrophytes, M. canis, Epidermophyton* organisms (see Fig. 52-6, B)	Generally round or oval, erythematous scaling patch that spreads peripherally and clears centrally; may involve nails (tinea unguium) Diagnosis—Direct microscopic examination of scales Usually unilateral	Oral griseofulvin Local application of antifungal preparation such as tolnaftate, haloprogin, miconazole, clotrimazole; apply 1 cm beyond periphery of lesion; continual application 1–2 wk after no sign of lesion	Usually of animal origin from infected pets Majority of infections in children caused by *M. canis* and *M. audouinii*
Tinea cruris ("jock itch")—*Epidermophyton floccosum, T. rubrum, T. mentagrophytes*	Skin response similar to that in tinea corporis Localized to medial proximal aspect of thigh and crural fold; may involve scrotum in males Pruritic Diagnosis—Same as for tinea corporis	Local application of tolnaftate liquid Wet compresses or sitz baths may be soothing	Rare in preadolescent children Health education regarding personal hygiene
Tinea pedis ("athlete's foot")—*T. rubrum, Trichophyton interdigitale, E. floccosum*	On intertriginous areas between toes or on plantar surface of feet Lesions vary: Maceration and fissuring between toes Patches with pinhead-sized vesicles on plantar surface Pruritic Diagnosis—Direct microscopic examination of scrapings	Oral griseofulvin Local applications of tolnaftate liquid and antifungal powder containing tolnaftate Acute infections—Compresses or soaks followed by application of glucocorticoid cream Elimination of conditions of heat and perspiration by clean, light socks and well-ventilated shoes; avoidance of occlusive shoes	Most frequent in adolescents and adults; rare in children, but occurrence increases with wearing of plastic shoes Transmission to other individuals rare Ointments not successful
Candidiasis (moniliasis)—*Candida albicans*	Grows in moist areas Inflamed areas with white exudate, peeling, and easy bleeding Pruritic Diagnosis—Characteristic appearance	Amphotericin B, nystatin ointment, or other antifungal preparations to affected areas	Common form of diaper dermatitis (see Fig. 52-12) Oral form common in infants Vaginal form in older females May be disseminated in immunosuppressed children

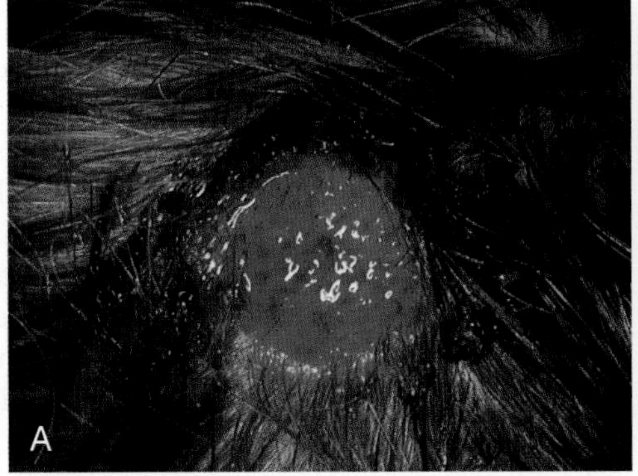

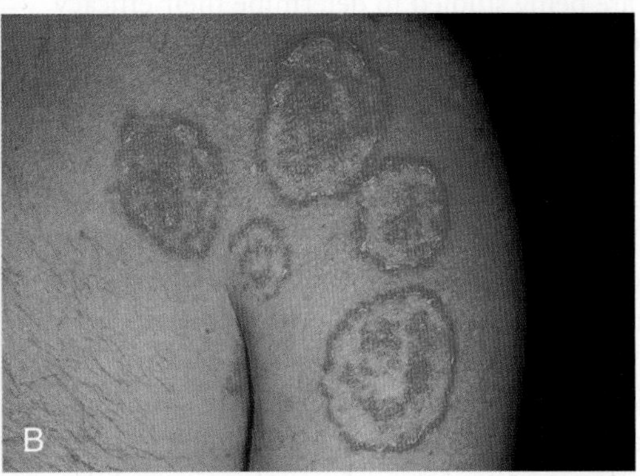

FIGURE 52-6 A: Tinea capitis. **B:** Tinea corporis. Both infections are caused by *Microsporum canis*, the "kitten" or "puppy" fungus. (From Habif, T. P. [2004]. *Clinical dermatology: A color guide to diagnosis and therapy* [4th ed.]. St. Louis: Mosby.)

TABLE 52-5 SYSTEMIC MYCOSES

DISORDER AND ORGANISM	SKIN MANIFESTATIONS	SYSTEMIC MANIFESTATIONS	MANAGEMENT	COMMENTS
North American blastomycosis—*Blastomyces dermatitidis*	Chronic granulomatous lesions and microabscesses in any part of body Initial lesion a papule; undergoes ulceration and peripheral spread	Pulmonary symptoms, such as cough, chest pain, weakness, and weight loss May have skeletal involvement, with bone destruction and formation of cutaneous abscesses	Intravenous (IV) administration of amphotericin B	Usual portal of entry is lungs Source of infection unknown Noninfectious Pulmonary infections may be mild and self-limited and require no treatment Progressive disease often fatal
Cryptococcosis—*Cryptococcus neoformans (Torula histolytica)*	Usually on face; acneiform, firm, nodular, painless eruption	Central nervous system (CNS) manifestations—Headache, dizziness, stiff neck, and signs of increased intracranial pressure Low-grade fever, mild cough, lung infiltration	IV amphotericin B; may be administered intrathecally for CNS involvement 5-Fluorocytosine for meningitis Excision and drainage of local lesions	Acquired by inhalation of dust but may enter through skin Prognosis serious Noninfectious Increased incidence in persons receiving corticosteroids with lymphoreticular malignancies, or type 2 diabetes
Histoplasmosis—*Histoplasma capsulatum*	Not distinctive or uniform, but most appear as punched-out or granulomatous ulcers	General systemic symptoms may include pallor, diarrhea, vomiting, irregular spiking temperature, hepatosplenomegaly, and pulmonary symptoms Any tissue of body may be involved with related symptoms	IV amphotericin B for severe cases Oral ketoconazole	Organism cultured from soil, especially where contaminated with fowl droppings Fungus enters through skin or mucous membranes of mouth and respiratory tract Endemic in St. Lawrence Valley region where 20 to 30% of the population test positive on a yearly basis Disseminated diseases most common in infants and children

because subjective symptoms subside, children or parents may be tempted to decrease or discontinue the medication. The nurse should emphasize to family members the importance of maintaining the prescribed dosage schedule and of taking the medication with high-fat foods for best absorption. They should also be informed of possible medication adverse effects, such as headache, gastrointestinal upset, fatigue, insomnia, and photosensitivity. For children who take the medication over many months, periodic testing is required to monitor leukopenia and assess liver and renal function. Newer antifungal medications such as terbinafine, itraconazole, and fluconazole may be used when there are adverse reactions to griseofulvin. Currently, these medications are being studied to determine their efficacy and safety in treating tinea capitis in children.

Systemic Mycotic (Fungal) Infections

Mycotic (systemic or deep fungal) infections have the capacity to invade the viscera as well as the skin. The most common infections are the lung diseases, which are usually acquired by inhalation of fungal spores. These fungi produce a variable spectrum of disease, and some are common in certain geographic areas. They are not transmitted from person to person but appear to reside in the soil, from which their spores are airborne. The cutaneous lesions caused by deep fungal infections are granulomatous and appear as ulcers, plaques, nodules, fungating masses, and abscesses. The course of deep fungal diseases is chronic with slow progression that favours sensitization (Table 52-5).

SKIN DISORDERS RELATED TO CHEMICAL OR PHYSICAL CONTACTS

Contact Dermatitis

Contact dermatitis is an inflammatory reaction of the skin to chemical substances, natural or synthetic, that evoke a hypersensitivity response or direct irritation. The initial reaction occurs in an exposed region, most commonly the face and neck, backs of the hands, forearms, male genitalia, and lower legs. Early in the reaction, there is usually a sharp delineation between inflamed and normal skin that ranges from a faint, transient erythema to massive bullae on an erythematous swollen base. Itching is a constant symptom.

The cause may be a primary irritant or a sensitizing agent. A *primary irritant* is one that irritates any skin. A *sensitizing agent* produces an irritation on those individuals who have met the irritant or something chemically related to it, have undergone an immunological change, and have become sensitized. Prior exposure is not necessarily a factor in the reaction. A sensitizer irritates in relatively low concentrations only persons who are allergic to it.

In infants, contact dermatitis occurs on the convex surfaces of the diaper area (see Diaper Dermatitis, p. 1690). Other agents that produce contact dermatitis include plants (poison ivy, oak, or sumac), animal irritants (wool, feathers, and furs), metal (nickel found in jewellery and the snaps on sleepers and denim), vegetable irritants (oleoresins, oils, and turpentine), synthetic fabrics (e.g., shoe components), dyes, cosmetics, perfumes, and soaps (including bubble baths).

The major goal in treatment is to prevent further exposure of the skin to the offending substance. Provided there is no further irritation, the skin's normal recuperative powers will often produce healing without treatment. Otherwise, treatment of contact dermatitis is based on severity. Mild cases are treated with topical steroids. Mild to moderately severe cases may require a 2-week course of strong topical corticosteroids. Very severe cases require systemic corticosteroids.

NURSING CARE

Nurses frequently detect evidence of contact dermatitis during routine physical assessments. Skin manifestations in specific areas suggest limited contact, such as around the eyes (mascara), areas of the body covered by clothing but not protected by undergarments (wool), or areas of the body not covered by clothing (UV injury). Generalized involvement is more likely to be caused by bubble bath or soap. Often nurses can determine the offending agent and counsel families regarding management. However, if the lesions persist, are extensive, or show evidence of infection, medical evaluation is indicated.

Poison Ivy, Oak, and Sumac

Contact with the dry or succulent portions of any of three poisonous plants (ivy, oak, and sumac) produces localized, streaked or spotty, oozing and painful impetiginous lesions. The offending substance in these plants is an oil, *urushiol*, that is extremely potent. Sensitivity to urushiol is not inborn but is developed after one or two exposures and may change over a lifetime. All parts of the plants contain the oil, including dried leaves and stems. Even smoke from burning brush piles can produce a reaction. Some people may react to the skin of mango, which contains uroshiol.

Animals do not seem to be affected by the oil; however, dogs or other animals that have run or played in the plants may carry the sap on their fur, and animals that eat the plants can transfer the oil in their saliva. Shoes, tools, and toys can transfer the oil. Golf balls that have been in the rough are another source of contact.

Urushiol takes effect as soon as it touches the skin. It penetrates through the epidermis and bonds with the dermal layer, where it initiates an immune response. The full-blown reaction is evident after about 2 days, with redness, swelling, and itching at the site of contact. Several days later, streaked or spotty blisters oozing serum from damaged cells produce the characteristic impetiginous lesions (Fig. 52-7). The lesions dry and heal spontaneously, and itching stops by 10 to 14 days.

Therapeutic Management

As soon as an exposure is realized, there is no time to waste. The earlier the skin is cleansed, the greater the chance of removing the urushiol before it attaches to the skin. The exposed skin can be cleansed with isopropyl alcohol or vinegar followed by water. A shower with soap and warm water should follow. Clothes, tools, shoes, and any other objects that had contact with the plants should be cleaned with alcohol and then water.

Treatment of the lesions includes calamine lotion, soothing Burow solution compresses, or Aveeno baths to relieve discomfort. Topical corticosteroid gel is effective for prevention or relief of inflammation, especially when applied before blisters form. Oral corticosteroids may be needed for severe reactions, and a sedative such as diphenhydramine may be ordered.

NURSING CARE

When it is known that the child has made contact with the plant, the area should be immediately flushed (preferably within 15 minutes) with *cold* running water to neutralize the urushiol not yet bonded to the skin. If there is a stream nearby, an effective method is to have the child enter the water (clothes and all) and allow the water to rinse the oil from both skin and clothing. Harsh soap is contraindicated because it removes protective skin oils and dilutes the urushiol, allowing it to spread; hard scrubbing irritates the skin. All clothing that has come in contact with the plant should be removed with care and thoroughly laundered in hot water and detergent. Every effort needs to be made to prevent the child from scratching the lesions. Although the lesions do not spread by contact with the blister serum or from scratching, they can become secondarily infected.

Prevention

Prevention is best accomplished by avoiding contact and removing the plant from the environment. All children, especially those known to be sensitive, should be taught to recognize the plant. The Government of Canada (2013) has information on how to eliminate the plants safely. It is important not to burn the plants because the smoke fumes can cause a severe lung reaction in sensitive individuals. The oil on dead plants can cause a reaction for up to 5 years. If poisonous plants are growing in public or community areas, the local authorities should be contacted to remove the plants.

Medication Reactions

Adverse reactions to medications are seen more often in the skin than in any other organ, although any organ of the body can be affected. The reaction may be a result of toxicity related to drug concentration, individual intolerance to the average dosage of the medication, or an allergic or idiosyncratic response. The manifestations may be associated with adverse effects or secondary effects of a medication, either of which are unrelated to its primary pharmacological actions.

Although any medication is capable of producing a reaction in the susceptible individual, some medications have a tendency to produce a particular reaction consistently, and others are more likely to produce an untoward effect. Many are allergenic responses that occur after a previous administration of the medication, even a topical application. Other factors influence a drug response in a particular individual. For example, the

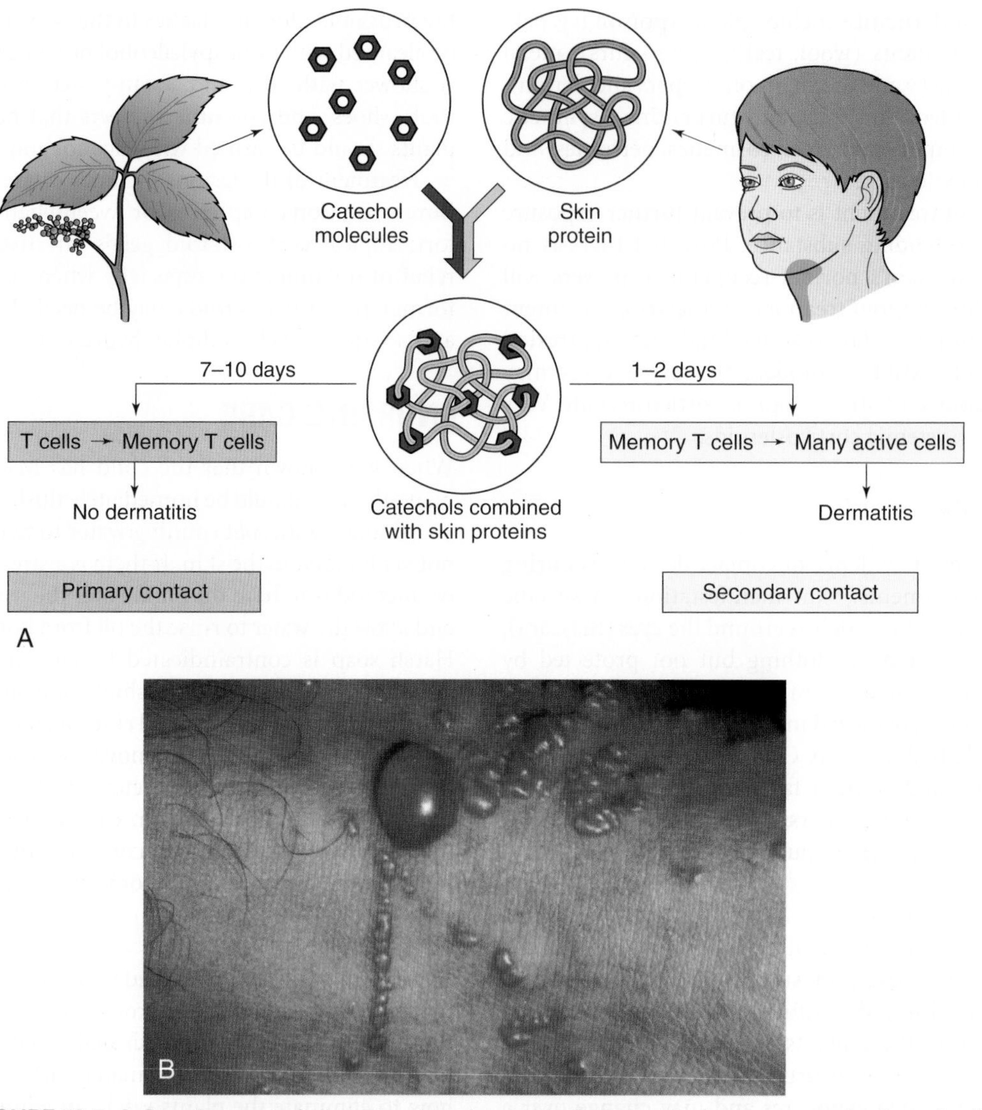

FIGURE 52-7 A: Development of allergic contact dermatitis. **B:** Poison ivy lesions; note the "streaked" blisters surrounding one large blister. (A, from McCance, K., & Huether, S. [2010]. *Pathophysiology: The biological basis for disease in adults and children* [6th ed.]. St. Louis: Mosby. B, from Habif, T. P. [2010]. *Clinical dermatology: A color guide to diagnosis and therapy* [5th ed.]. St. Louis: Mosby.)

incidence increases with the amount and number of medications given.

NURSING ALERT

Intravenous (IV) medications are more likely to cause a reaction than oral medications. Stop the medication, but maintain the infusion with normal saline.

Manifestations of medication reactions may be delayed or immediate. A period of 7 days is usually required for a child to develop sensitivity to a medication that has never been administered previously. With prior sensitivity the manifestations appear almost immediately. Rashes are the most common manifestation of adverse medication reactions in children. However, individual medication reactions may vary from a single lesion to extensive, generalized epidermal necrosis such as that seen in Stevens-Johnson syndrome. Cutaneous manifestations can resemble almost any skin disease and can appear in almost any degree of severity. With few exceptions, the distribution of a medication eruption is widespread because it results from a circulating agent, appears as an inflammatory response with itching, is sudden in onset, and may be associated with constitutional symptoms such as fever, malaise, gastrointestinal upsets, anemia, or liver and kidney damage.

In most cases treatment for simple cutaneous reactions consists of discontinuing the medication. Sometimes a decision is made to continue the medication, such as an antibiotic in an infant or small child, until the cause of the rash is clearly indicated. In urticarial-type eruptions antihistamines may be ordered, and for widespread and severe lesions corticosteroids are beneficial. Severe anaphylactic reactions are a medical emergency (see Anaphylaxis, Chapter 47).

NURSING CARE

The most effective means of management is prevention. Parents always remember a severe reaction in their child; a careful history will elicit evidence of a previous medication reaction. The history should include the medication's name, the nature of the reaction, dosage, and how soon after administration the reaction occurred (see Chapter 33).

Nurses who suspect that a rash is caused by a medication should withhold any further dose and report the eruption to the primary care provider. Frequent offenders in medication reactions are penicillin and sulphonamides, and nurses must be alert to this possibility. However, even commonplace medications, including aspirin, barbiturates, chemical agents in some foods, flavouring agents, and preservatives, are capable of producing an undesired response. Persons who have severe reactions should wear a medical identification bracelet in case of emergency or inadvertent administration of the offending medication.

Foreign Bodies

Parents can remove small wooden splinters or slivers with a needle and tweezers that have been sterilized with alcohol or a flame. The area around the sliver is washed with soap and water before removal is attempted. The sliver is exposed with the needle and then grasped firmly by tweezers and pulled out. Some foreign bodies, such as a fishhook, pieces of glass, difficult-to-see object, or a deeply embedded object such as a needle in a foot or near a joint, require medical evaluation.

SKIN DISORDERS RELATED TO ANIMAL CONTACTS

Arthropod Bites and Stings

Bites and stings account for a significant amount of mild to moderate discomfort in children. Most bites and stings are managed by simple symptomatic measures, such as compresses, calamine lotion, and prevention of secondary infection. *Arthropods* include insects and arachnids, such as mites, ticks, and spiders. Most arthropods in Canada, including tarantulas, are relatively harmless. Although all spiders produce venom that is injected via fangs, some are unable to pierce the skin and others produce venom that is insufficiently toxic to be harmful. Only two spiders—the brown recluse and the black widow—inject venom deadly enough to require immediate attention. Children bitten by these arachnids must receive medical attention as soon as possible. The black widow bite causes local, regional, or generalized pain associated with nonspecific symptoms and autonomic effects such as sweating, muscle cramps, and vomiting. Antivenoms are an important treatment for black widow spider bites. Muscle relaxants, analgesics or sedatives, and steroids are also used to treat the manifestations. The brown recluse spider bite causes pain and erythema that can become a necrotic ulcer. Systemic reactions include fever, nausea and vomiting, and joint pain. These bites are treated with antibiotics, corticosteroids, and analgesics. Wounds may require skin grafts.

When a hymenopteran (bees in particular) stings, its barbed stinger penetrates the skin. As long as the stinger remains in the skin, the muscles push the stinger deeper and the venom is pumped into the wound. The best approach is to remove the stinger as quickly as possible and to get away from the vicinity of other insects to prevent further injury. Children who have become sensitized to hymenopteran bites may demonstrate a severe systemic response that can be life threatening. One sting can produce generalized urticaria, respiratory difficulty (from laryngeal edema), hypotension, and death. Intramuscular administration of epinephrine provides immediate relief and must be available for emergency use.

Hypersensitive children should wear a medical identification bracelet. They should also have a kit that contains epinephrine and a hypodermic syringe. Families should be reminded to check the expiration date on the kit and to replace an outdated one. They should determine whether someone at the school should be designated to inject the epinephrine in case of an emergency.

Skin lesions caused by other arthropods are outlined in Table 52-6, along with manifestations and management.

Scabies

Scabies is an endemic infestation caused by the scabies mite, *Sarcoptes scabiei*. Lesions are created as the impregnated female burrows into the stratum corneum of the epidermis (never into living tissue) to deposit her eggs and feces. The inflammatory response and intense itching occur after the host becomes sensitized to the mite, approximately 30 to 60 days after initial contact. If the person has been previously sensitized to the mite, the response occurs within 48 hours after exposure. After this time, the areas over which the mite has travelled will begin to itch and develop the characteristic eruption (Box 52-1). Consequently, mites will not necessarily be located at all sites of eruption.

There is great variability in the type of lesions. Infants often develop an eczematous eruption; therefore the observer must look for discrete papules, burrows, or vesicles.

NURSING CARE

The treatment of scabies is the application of a scabicide. Currently, permethrin 5% cream (Elimite) is the medication of

BOX 52-1 CLINICAL MANIFESTATIONS OF SCABIES

Lesion

Children—Minute greyish brown, threadlike (mite burrows), pruritic

- Black dot at end of burrow (mite)

Infants—Eczematous eruption, pruritic

Distribution

Generally in intertriginous areas—Interdigital, axillary-cubital, popliteal, inguinal

Children older than 2 years of age—Primarily hands and wrists

Children younger than 2 years—Primarily feet and ankles

TABLE 52-6 SKIN LESIONS CAUSED BY ARTHROPODS

MECHANISM AND CHARACTERISTIC	MANIFESTATIONS	MANAGEMENT
Insect Bites—Flies, Gnats, Mosquitoes, Fleas		
Mechanism: Foreign protein in insects' saliva introduced when skin is penetrated for a blood-sucking meal *Distribution:* Almost everywhere—Fleas, mosquitoes, ants Suburbs and rural areas—Bees Urban areas—Hornets, wasps, yellow jackets	Hypersensitivity reaction Papular urticaria Firm papules; may be capped by vesicles or excoriated Little or no reaction in nonsensitized person	*Treatment:* Use antipruritic medications and baths. Administer antihistamines. Prevent secondary infection. *Prevention:* Avoid contact. Remove focus, such as treating furniture, mattresses, carpets, and pets, where insects may live. Apply insect repellent when exposure is anticipated.
Hymenopterans—Bees, Wasps, Hornets, Yellow Jackets, Fire Ants		
Mechanism: Injection of venom through stinging apparatus Venom contains histamine, allergenic proteins, and often a spreading factor, hyaluronidase Severe reactions caused by hypersensitivity or multiple stings	Local reaction—Small red area, wheal, itching, and heat Systemic reactions—May be mild to severe, including generalized edema, pain, nausea and vomiting, confusion, respiratory embarrassment, and shock	*Treatment:* Carefully scrape off stinger or pull out stinger as quickly as possible. Cleanse with soap and water. Apply cool compresses. Apply common household product (e.g., lemon juice, paste made with aspirin or baking soda). Administer antihistamines. Severe reactions—Administer epinephrine, corticosteroids; treat for shock. *Prevention:* Teach child to wear shoes; to avoid wearing bright clothing, flowery prints, shiny jewellery, or perfumed grooming products (cologne, scented hairspray), which might attract the insect; and to avoid places where the insect may be contacted. Hypersensitive children should wear medical identification bracelet to indicate allergy and therapy needed; family should keep emergency medication and be taught its administration.
Ticks		
Mechanism: In process of sucking blood, head and mouth parts are buried in skin *Characteristics:* Feed on blood of mammals Significant in humans because of pathological organism carried May be vectors of various infectious diseases, such as Rocky Mountain spotted fever, Q fever, tularemia, relapsing fever, Lyme disease, tick paralysis Must attach and feed for 1–2 hr to transmit disease Usual habitat is wooded area	Tick usually attached to skin, head embedded Produce firm, discrete, intensely pruritic nodules at site of attachment May cause urticaria or persistent localized edema	*Treatment:* Grasp tick with tweezers (forceps) as close as possible to point of attachment. Pull straight up with steady, even pressure; if bare hands, use a tissue to touch tick during removal; wash hands thoroughly with soap and water. Remove any remaining part (e.g., head) with sterile needle. Cleanse wounds with soap and disinfectant. Veterinarian offices sell tick removers to make removal more effective. *Prevention:* Teach children to avoid areas where prevalent. Inspect skin (especially scalp) after being in wooded areas. See discussion on p. 1687.

choice. Alternative medications are benzyl benzoate (10 to 12.5% for children), which has high efficacy and is less expensive and is widely used outside of North America; and 1% lindane cream or lotion. Lindane can be neurotoxic and should be reserved for patients who fail to respond to other therapy (Banerji & CPS, First Nations, Inuit and Métis Health Committee, 2015).

Ivermectin is an oral medication and can be used to treat scabies in patients with secondary excoriation for whom topical scabicides are irritating and not well tolerated or whose infestation is refractory and it is only available under special Health Canada permission. Safety and efficacy of ivermectin for children under 5 years or weighing less than 15 kg have not been established.

BOX 52-2 CLINICAL MANIFESTATIONS OF PEDICULOSIS

- Pruritus (caused by crawling insects and insect saliva on skin)
- Nits observable on hair shaft (see Fig. 52-8)

Distribution

- Occipital area
- Behind ears
- Nape of neck
- Eyebrows and eyelashes (occasionally) (caused by pubic lice)

Nurses instructing families in the use of scabicides should emphasize the importance of following directions carefully. Permethrin is applied to all skin surfaces from the neck down to the toes (not just areas with rash, but also areas between the fingers and toes, the umbilicus, and the cleft of the buttocks). Infants should have the cream applied to their faces as well. The cream should remain on the skin for 8 to 9 hours for children under 6 years and 8 to 14 hours for older children and is then removed by bathing.

Because of the length of time between infestation and physical symptoms (30–60 days), all persons who were in close contact with the affected child need treatment. This may include boyfriends or girlfriends, babysitters, grandparents, and immediate family members. The objective is to treat as thoroughly as possible the first time. Enough medication for the entire family should be prescribed, with 60 mL allowed for each adult and 30 mL for each child.

All clothes, bedding, and towels used by the infested person before treatment should be washed in hot water and dried in a hot dryer. Families need to know that although this treatment will kill the mite that causes scabies, it will not eliminate the rash and the itch until the stratum corneum is replaced in approximately 2 to 3 weeks. For itching, oral antihistamines can be taken and soothing ointments or lotions can be applied. Antibiotics may be given for secondary infection (Banerji & CPS, First Nations, Inuit and Métis Health Committee, 2015).

Pediculosis Capitis

Pediculosis capitis (head lice) is an infestation of the scalp by *Pediculus humanus capitis*, a common parasite in school-age children. The adult louse lives only about 48 hours when away from a human host, and the lifespan of the average female is 1 month. The female lays her eggs at night at the junction of a hair shaft and close to the skin because the eggs need a warm environment. The *nits*, or eggs, hatch in approximately 7 to 10 days. Itching is usually the only symptom. Common areas involved are the occipital area, behind the ears, and the nape of the neck (Box 52-2).

Diagnostic Evaluation

Diagnosis is made by observation of the white eggs (nits) firmly attached to the hair shafts (Fig. 52-8). Because of their brief lifespan and mobility, adult lice are more difficult to locate. Nits must be differentiated from dandruff, lint, hair spray, and other items of similar size and shape. Scratch marks or inflammatory papules, caused by secondary infection, may also be found on the scalp in the vulnerable areas.

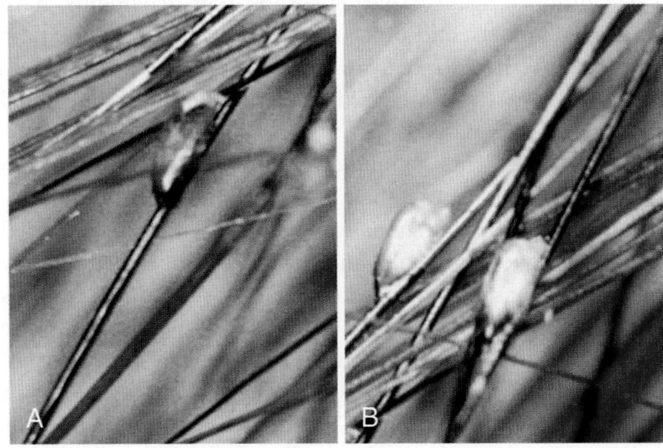

FIGURE 52-8 **A:** Empty nit case. **B:** Viable nits. (From *The contemporary approach to the control of head lice in schools and communities, Pittsburgh* [1991]. SmithKline Beecham.)

Therapeutic Management

Treatment consists of the application of **pediculicides** and manual removal of nit cases. The medication of choice for infants and children is permethrin 1% cream rinse (Nix), which kills adult lice and nits. This product and preparations of pyrethrin with piperonyl butoxide (RID or A-200 Pyrinate) can be obtained without a prescription and are more effective and safer than lindane. Most experts advise a second treatment at 7 to 10 days to ensure a cure (Finlay, MacDonald, & CPS, Infectious Diseases and Immunization Committee, 2008/2016). However, pyrethrin products are contraindicated for individuals with contact allergy to ragweed or turpentine. A new noninsecticidal product has been approved by Health Canada for treatment of head lice which contains isopropyl myristate 50% and ST-cyclomethicone 50% for age 4 years and older (Finlay et al., 2008/2016).

Because of concerns that head lice may be developing resistance to chemical shampoos and that repeated exposure of children to strong chemicals on the scalp may be unwise, effective nonchemical control measures are essential. Daily removal of nits from the child's hair with a metal nit comb at least every 2 or 3 days is a control measure to use after treatment with a pediculicide.

NURSING CARE

An important nursing role is educating the parents about pediculosis. Nurses should emphasize that *anyone* can get pediculosis; it has no respect for age, socioeconomic level, or cleanliness. Lice do not jump or fly, but they can be transmitted from one person to another on personal items and are more likely to infect people with straight hair and girls. Children need to be cautioned against sharing combs, hair ornaments, hats, caps, scarves, coats, and other items used on or near the hair. Children who share lockers are more likely to become infested, and slumber parties place children at risk. Lice are not carried or transmitted by pets.

Nurses or parents should carefully inspect children who scratch their head more than usual for bite marks, redness, and nits. The hair is systematically spread with two flat-sided sticks or tongue depressors, and the scalp is observed for any movement that indicates a louse. Nurses should wear gloves when examining the hair. Lice are small and greyish tan, have no wings, and are visible to the naked eye. The nits, or eggs, appear as tiny whitish oval specks adhering to the hair shaft about 6 mm from the scalp. The adherent nature of the nits distinguishes them from dandruff, which falls off readily. Empty nit cases, indicating hatched lice, are translucent rather than white and are located more than 6 mm from the scalp (see Fig. 52-8).

If evidence of infestation is found, it is important to treat the child according to the directions on the label of the pediculicide. Parents should read the directions carefully before beginning treatment. The child should be made as comfortable as possible during the application process because the pediculicide must remain on the scalp and hair for several minutes. Playing "beauty parlour" or "barber shop" during the shampoo is a useful strategy. The child lies supine, with the head over a sink or basin, and covers the eyes with a dry towel or washcloth. This prevents medication, which can cause chemical conjunctivitis, from splashing into the eyes. If eye irritation occurs, the eyes must be flushed well with tepid water. It is not necessary to remove the nits after treatment because only live lice cause infestation. However, because none of the pediculicides is 100% effective in killing all the eggs, the makers of some pediculicides recommend manual removal of the nits after treatment. An extra-fine-tooth comb that is included in many commercial pediculicides or is available at pharmacies facilitates manual removal. If the comb is ineffective in removing the nit cases, the examiner should remove them by scraping them off the strands of hair with his or her fingernails.

Live lice only survive for up to 48 hours away from the host, but nits are shed into the environment and are capable of hatching in 7 to 10 days; retreatment may be required (see Community Focus box). Spraying with insecticide is not recommended because of the danger to children and animals. Families should also be advised that the pediculicide is relatively expensive, especially when several members of the household require treatment. Families may be inclined to try home remedies such as vinegar or petroleum jelly to treat the lice, but most are ineffective.

Prevention

The increasing incidence of pediculosis in schoolchildren is a serious concern for school nurses, parents, and community health agencies. However, school head lice screening programs have not proven to have a significant effect on the incidence of head lice in the school setting; parent education programs may be more helpful in the management of head lice. Children with head lice should be allowed to return to school after proper treatment.

COMMUNITY FOCUS

Pediculosis Treatment

- Under a good light, check the scalp at the bottom of the neck and behind the ears for lice.
- Use pyrethrin, permethrin, or lindane insecticide to treat lice. Do not leave the insecticide on any longer than recommended on the label. Do not use lindane on children under 2 years of age. Rinse scalp well with cool water over a sink.
- Alternatively, use isopropyl myristate/cyclomethicone noninsecticide for children 4 years of age or older.
- Machine wash all objects that were in intimate contact with the head (e.g., hats, pillowcases, brushes and combs) in hot water and dry in a hot dryer for at least 15 minutes. Dry clean other nonwashable items or store items in airtight plastic bags for 14 days if unable to dry clean.
- Excessive cleaning is not required.
- In day care centres, store children's clothing items in separate cubicles and discourage sharing of clothing items.
- Provide educational programs for prevention, transmission, detection, and treatment of pediculosis.

Modified from Finlay, J., MacDonald, N. E., & Canadian Paediatric Society, Infectious Diseases and Immunization Committee. (2008). Head lice infestations: A clinical update. *Paediatric Child Health, 13*(8), 692–696. Reaffirmed 2016. Retrieved from http://www.cps.ca/documents/position/head-lice

Bed Bugs

Bed bugs, or cimicidae, are small, biting insects that feed off the blood of warm-blooded animals and birds, preferring human blood. Bed bug infestations are becoming increasingly common in Canada because of the increase in travelling (Government of Canada, 2015). Cimicidae invade homes by travelling on objects such as clothing, televisions, and mattresses, where they hide in along the folds and on box springs.

Clinical Manifestations

Cimicidae reproduce quickly and travel easily. The insects are 6 mm in length, with wingless, oval bodies that redden with blood intake (Fig. 52-9). The tiny eggs are whitish ovals and are clustered in crevices. They feed at night and bite all over the human body, particularly in the face, neck, and upper body. Cimicidae can survive up to 6 months without feeding. When the insect injects saliva into the skin, it creates localized red, itchy, flat or raised lesions, often linear in a group of three. Some individuals are more sensitive or allergic and react more with welts. Cimicidae do not transmit infection but an infection can develop from scratching the lesions. The bites do not require treatment and disappear quickly. It is important to not scratch and keep the skin clean in order to avoid infection. Antihistamines or creams can help relieve the itchiness and antibiotics can be prescribed if there is secondary infection present (Toronto Public Health Department, 2008).

Cimicidae are very difficult to get rid of (see Family-Centred Teaching box). Various chemicals or nonchemicals are usually

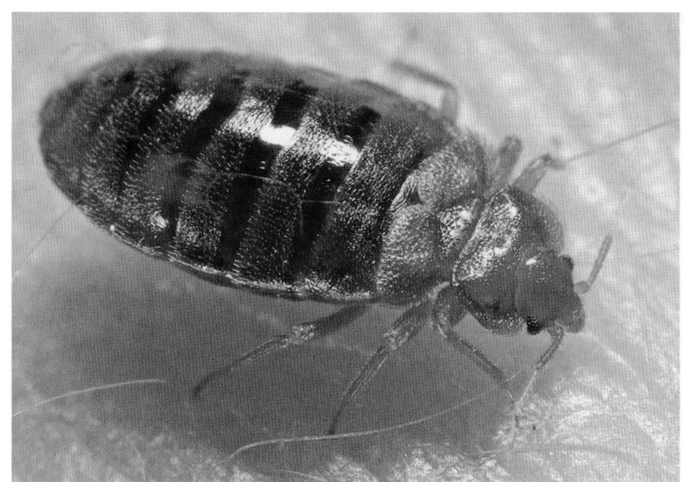

FIGURE 52-9 A bed bug biting a human.

FAMILY-CENTRED TEACHING

How to Eliminate Cimicidae in the Home

- Check with the local health department or a pesticide control company to confirm Cimicidae presence.
- Inspect mattress, frame, and underside of beds.
- Vacuum with nozzle daily in your house along any crevices such as baseboards and other crevices and immediately dispose of vacuum contents.
- Wash linens in the hottest water possible and cover pillows and mattresses with plastic.
- Remove all unnecessary clutter.
- Seal cracks and crevices.
- Monitor daily, using double-sided carpet sticky tape to catch Cimicidae.
- Inspect any objects coming into the house.
- When travelling, keep luggage off the floor and wrap in plastic. Pull the bed away from the wall, tuck in linen, and keep blankets off the floor.
- Consult professional pesticide services and choose the least risky option to humans and the environment.

Modified from Toronto Public Health. (2008). *Bed bug information for tenants.* Retrieved from http://www.toronto.ca/legdocs/mmis/2008/hl/bgrd/backgroundfile-11158.pdf

needed to eliminate these insects. Available products will usually contain the active ingredients pyrethrin or other pyrethroids or diatomaceous earth. Caution must be used that outdoor products are not used indoors (Government of Canada, 2015).

Rickettsial Diseases

Rickettsiae, the organisms responsible for a number of disorders (Table 52-7), are transmitted to human beings via arthropods. Mammals become infected only through the bites of infected lice, fleas, ticks, and mites, all of which serve as both infectors and reservoirs. Rickettsiae are intracellular parasites, similar in size to bacteria that inhabit the alimentary tract of a wide range of natural hosts. Rickettsial diseases are more common in temperate and tropical climates where humans live in association with arthropods. Infection in humans is incidental (except epidemic typhus) and not necessary for the survival of the rickettsial species. However, after the organism invades a human, it causes a disease that varies in intensity from a benign, self-limited illness to a disease that is fulminating and fatal.

Lyme Disease

Lyme disease is a tick-borne disease in Canada that is increasing in incidence although still relatively rare (Onyett & CPS, Infectious Diseases and Immunization Committee, 2014a). In 2009, Lyme disease became a nationally reportable disease in Canada. The number of reported cases has increased from 128 in 2009 to an estimated more than 500 in 2013 (Government of Canada, 2016a). It is caused by the spirochete *Borrelia burgdorferi*, which enters the skin and bloodstream through the saliva and feces of ticks, especially the deer tick. Most cases of Lyme disease are reported in parts of southern and southeastern Québec, southern and eastern Ontario, southeastern Manitoba, New Brunswick, and Nova Scotia, as well as most of southern British Columbia (Public Health Agency of Canada [PHAC], 2016).

The disease may initially appear in any of three stages:

- *Stage 1* consists of the tick bite at the time of inoculation, followed in 3 to 31 days by the development of erythema migrans at the site of the bite (Fig. 52-10).
- *Stage 2*, the most serious stage of the disease, is characterized by systemic involvement of neurological, cardiac, and musculoskeletal systems that appears several weeks after the cutaneous phase is completed.
- *Stage 3*, or the late stage, includes musculoskeletal pain that involves the tendons, bursae, muscles, and synovia. Arthritis may occur, and late neurological problems include deafness and chronic encephalopathy.

Diagnostic Evaluation

Diagnosis is best made clinically during the early stages by recognizing the characteristic rash, erythema migrans. Serological testing may be used to establish the diagnosis in later stages of the disease.

Therapeutic Management

Early and appropriate treatment is essential to prevent complications. Children are treated with oral doxycycline; amoxicillin is recommended for children younger than 8 years of age. The CPS (Onyett & CPS, Infectious Diseases and Immunization Committee, 2014a) recommends following the Infectious Diseases Society of America's treatment for Lyme disease (American Academy of Pediatrics, 2015). Most experts treat individuals with early Lyme disease for 14 to 21 days. Persons who have removed ticks from themselves should be monitored closely for signs and symptoms of tick-borne diseases for 30 days; in particular they should be monitored for erythema migrans, a red expanding skin lesion at the site of the tick bite that may suggest Lyme disease. People who develop a skin lesion or viral infection–like illness within 1 month of an attached tick should seek prompt medical attention. Treatment of erythema migrans most often prevents development of later stages of Lyme disease.

TABLE 52-7 ERUPTIONS CAUSED BY RICKETTSIAE

DISORDER, ORGANISM, AND HOST	MANIFESTATIONS	MANAGEMENT	COMMENTS
Rocky Mountain spotted fever—*Rickettsia rickettsii* *Arthropod*—Tick *Transmission*—Tick *Mammal source*—Wild rodents, dogs	*Gradual onset*—Fever, malaise, anorexia, myalgia *Abrupt onset*—Rapid temperature elevation, chills, vomiting, myalgia, severe headache Maculopapular or petechial rash primarily on extremities (ankles and wrists) but may spread to other areas, characteristically on palms and soles	*Control*—Protection from tick bite by wearing proper apparel, tick repellent Tetracycline or chloramphenicol Vigorous supportive therapy	Usually self-limited in children Onset in children may resemble that of any infectious disease. Severe disease is rare in children. Disease has been reported in Canada, particularly in the south, but the overall incidence is unknown. Inspect children and dogs regularly if they play in wooded areas. See Table 52-6 for management of ticks.
Epidemic typhus—*Rickettsia prowazekii* *Arthropod*—Body louse *Transmission*—Infected feces into broken skin *Mammal source*—Humans	Abrupt onset of chills, fever, diffuse myalgia, headache, malaise Maculopapular rash becoming petechial 4–7 days later, spreading from trunk outward	*Control*—Immediate destruction of vectors Tetracycline or chloramphenicol Supportive treatment	Patient should be isolated until deloused See discussion on p. 1685 for management of pediculosis. Excreta from infected lice also in dust; disinfect patient's clothing, bedding, and possessions and wash in hot water
Endemic typhus—*Rickettsia typhi* *Arthropod*—Rat fleas or lice *Transmission*—Flea bite; inhaling or ingesting flea excreta *Mammal source*—Rats	Headache, arthralgia, backache followed by fever; may last 9–14 days Maculopapular rash after 1–8 days of fever; begins in trunk and spreads to periphery; rarely involves face, palms, soles	*Control*—Eliminate rat reservoir, insect vectors, or both Tetracycline or chloramphenicol Supportive treatment	Rare in Canada and found mainly in warm climates Shorter duration than epidemic typhus Mild, seldom fatal illness Difficult to distinguish from epidemic typhus
Rickettsial pox—*Rickettsia akari* West Nile fever *Arthropod*—Mosquitoes *Transmission*—Mosquito bite *Mammal source*—Birds	Maculopapular rash following primary lesion; eschar at site of bite; most children do not have symptoms or get sick If illness is present, symptoms appear in 2 to 15 days; fever, headache, and body aches, mild rash, or swollen lymph nodes If illness is present in person with lower immunity, risk of meningitis and encephalitis	*Control*—Eradication of rodent reservoir and mosquitoes Tetracycline or chloramphenicol Supportive treatment	Self-limited nonfatal disease Found In British Columbia, Alberta, Saskatchewan, Manitoba, Ontario, and Quebec In 2010, only three cases in Canada (Government of Canada, 2016b)

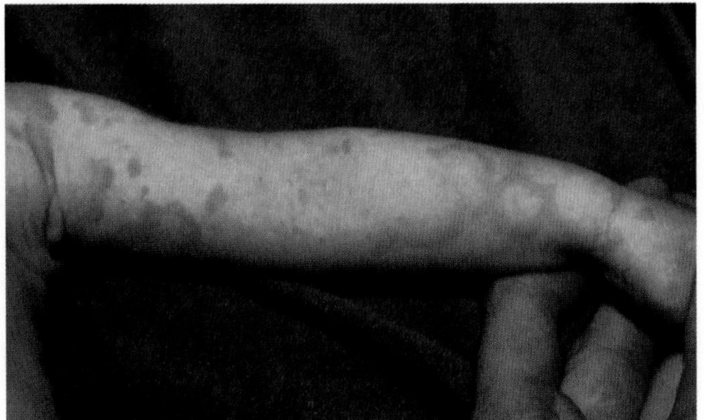

FIGURE 52-10 Lyme disease. Note annular red rings in erythema chronicum migrans. (From Weston, W. L., & Lane, A. T. [2007]. *Color textbook of pediatric dermatology* [4th ed.]. St. Louis: Mosby.)

NURSING CARE

The major thrust of nursing care should be educating parents to protect their children from exposure to ticks. Children should avoid tick-infested areas or wear light-coloured clothing so that ticks can be spotted easily, tuck pant legs into socks, and wear a long-sleeved shirt tucked into pants when in wooded areas. Parents and children need to perform regular tick checks when they are in infested areas (with special attention to the scalp, neck, armpits, and groin areas). Parents should also be alert for signs of the skin lesion, especially if their children have been in tick-infested areas. Insect repellents containing diethyltoluamide (DEET) and picardin can protect against ticks, but parents should use these chemicals cautiously (Onyett & CPS, Infectious Diseases and Immunization Committee, 2014b). DEET must not be used in children under 6 months. As well, products with citronella or lavender oil should not be used on infants (Onyett & CPS, Infectious Diseases and Immunization Committee, 2014b). All insecticides should be approved in Canada. Although there have been reports of serious neurological complications in children resulting from frequent and excessive application of DEET repellants, the risk is low when they are used properly. Products with DEET should be applied sparingly according to label instructions and not applied to a child's face or hands or to any areas of irritated skin.

After the child returns indoors, treated skin should be washed with soap and water. If a tick is found, it should be removed carefully with tweezers by gripping the head and mouth parts as closely to the skin as possible and pulling straight out or with a veterinarian tick remover. The tick should be kept in case the child develops Lyme symptoms so the tick can be identified. The area should be washed with soap and disinfected with alcohol or other disinfectant (Government of Canada, 2016a).

Pet and Wild Animal Bites

Animal bites are common in childhood. However, children are bitten more often by animals belonging to the family or to neighbours than by stray animals. Most victims of dog bites are young children (Sabhaney & Goldman, 2012). In Canada, between 1990 and 2007, 24 of 28 fatal dog bites occurred in children younger than 12 years of age (Raghavan, 2008). Most dog or cat injuries are to the upper extremities. Small children are likely to be bitten or scratched on the head, face, and neck because they tend to put their heads near the animal's head and flail their arms rather than protecting their heads (Kaye, Bela, Kirschner, et al., 2009). Animal bites are potentially serious because of the likelihood of significant infection. Injuries vary in intensity from small puncture wounds to complete evulsion of tissue that is associated with significant crush injury.

Therapeutic Management

General wound care consists of rinsing the wound with copious amounts of saline or Ringer's lactate under pressure via a large syringe and of washing the surrounding skin with mild soap. A clean pressure dressing is applied, and the extremity is elevated if the wound is bleeding. Medical evaluation is advised because of the danger of tetanus and rabies, although dogs in most urban areas must be immunized against rabies. Bites from wild animals, such as squirrels, bats, raccoons, foxes, and skunks, are also dangerous.

Prophylactic antibiotics are indicated for puncture wounds and wounds in areas that may prove to be cosmetically or functionally impaired if infected. Extensive lacerations are debrided and loosely sutured to allow drainage in the event of infection. Tetanus toxoid is administered according to standard guidelines (see Immunizations, Chapter 35), and rabies protocol is followed. Injuries to poorly vascularized areas, such as the hands, are more likely to become infected than those in more vascularized areas, such as the face; puncture wounds are more likely to become infected than lacerations.

NURSING CARE

The most important aspect related to animal bites is prevention. Children should understand animal behaviour and develop respect for animals (see Family-Centred Teaching box). Parents should monitor their children's behaviour with dogs and instruct them not to tease or surprise dogs, invade their territory, interfere with their feeding or sleeping, take their toys, or interact with sick or injured dogs or dogs with pups. Parents who are considering getting a pet, especially a dog, for themselves or their children should select a dog that has a high level of sociability with and is unlikely to be a danger to children.

FAMILY-CENTRED TEACHING

Animal Safety

The Humane Society of Canada (2007) offers the following top ten tips to help children avoid dog bites.

- Encourage children to be alert around dogs in their neighbourhood. It is important that children never pet a strange or unfamiliar animal.
- Teach children to never approach a dog that is tied up or confined to a small space; this may lead to fear in the dog and cause the dog to protect its space.
- Never allow children to tease a dog with food or toys; they may become aggravated and attack.
- Approach a dog by offering a closed hand and allowing the dog to smell it first before petting the dog.
- Never allow children to rub a dog along his side or grab his tail, which can cause fear and may lead them to attack.
- Spaying or neutering a dog can lessen any aggressive tendencies and make the dog happier and healthier.
- Never, under any circumstance, leave a family dog alone unsupervised with infants or small children. Children have been maimed and killed this way.
- Dog owners should be responsible and socialize their dogs, which will make them familiar with people and other pets in the neighbourhood.
- If ever confronted by a dog, try to stay calm and do not scream or run away. Try to place an object between you and the dog or throw food or a stick as a distraction to divert the dog's attention.
- It is important to remember that most dogs never bite anyone, but it is always better to be prepared.

Modified from Humane Society of Canada. (2007). *National dog bite awareness campaign*. Retrieved from https://www.humanesociety.com/pets/pet-info/799-national-dog-bite-awareness-campaign.html

Human Bites

Children often acquire lacerations from the teeth of other humans in rough play, during fights, or as victims of child abuse. Many preschool children bite others out of frustration or anger. Because human dental plaque and gingiva harbour pathogenic organisms, all human bites should receive attention. Delayed treatment increases the risk of infection.

If the laceration is less than 6 mm in length, the wound can be treated at home. The wound is washed vigorously with soap and water, and a pressure dressing is applied to stop bleeding. Ice applications minimize discomfort and swelling. Increased pain or redness at the wound site is an indication that the child should receive medical attention for antibiotic therapy. Tetanus toxoid is needed if the child is insufficiently immunized. Wounds larger than 6 mm should receive medical attention.

Cat-Scratch Disease

Cat-scratch disease (*Bartonella henselae*) is the most common cause of regional lymphadenitis in children and adolescents. It usually follows the scratch or bite of an animal (a cat in 99% of cases). The disease is usually a benign, self-limited illness that resolves spontaneously in about 2 to 4 months. Diagnosis is made on the basis of (1) history of contact with a cat, (2) the presence of regional lymphadenopathy for several days, and (3) serological identification of the causative organism by indirect fluorescent antibody assay or polymerase chain reaction test. The disease may persist for several months before gradual resolution. In some children, especially those who are immunocompromised, the adenitis may progress to suppuration and serious complications. Treatment is primarily supportive, but antibiotic therapy may hasten the resolution of adenopathy in the disease (PHAC, 2011).

MISCELLANEOUS SKIN DISORDERS

A number of miscellaneous skin lesions occur in children. Some occur as a result of congenital disorders and are inherited as an autosomal dominant trait (Table 52-8). *Ichthyoses* are a heterogeneous group of disorders characterized by scaling that create challenging problems in treatment. These disorders are not discussed in detail here because of their wide variability.

SKIN DISORDERS ASSOCIATED WITH SPECIFIC AGE GROUPS

Several common dermatological conditions are confined to children in specific age groups. These conditions include diaper, atopic, and seborrheic dermatitis, which occurs predominantly in infants, and acne, which is most common in adolescence.

Diaper Dermatitis

Diaper dermatitis is common in infants and is one of several acute inflammatory skin disorders caused either directly or indirectly by wearing diapers. The peak age of occurrence is 9 to 12 months of age, and the incidence is greater in formula-fed infants than in breastfed infants.

Pathophysiology and Clinical Manifestations

Diaper dermatitis is caused by prolonged and repetitive contact with an irritant (e.g., urine, feces, soaps, detergents, ointments, friction). Although the irritant in the majority of cases is urine and feces, a combination of factors contributes to irritation.

Prolonged contact of the skin with diaper wetness produces higher friction, greater abrasion damage, increased transepidermal permeability, and increased microbial counts. Healthy skin is less resistant to potential irritants.

Although ammonia was once thought to cause diaper rash because of its association with the strong odour on diapers and dermatitis, ammonia alone is not sufficient. The irritant quality of urine is related to an increase in pH from the breakdown of urea in the presence of fecal urease. The increased pH promotes the activity of fecal enzymes, principally the proteases and lipases, which act as irritants. Fecal enzymes also increase the permeability of skin to bile salts, another potential irritant in feces.

The eruption of diaper dermatitis is manifested primarily on convex surfaces or in folds. The lesions represent a variety of types and configurations. Eruptions involving the skin in most intimate contact with the diaper, such as the convex surfaces of buttocks, inner thighs, mons pubis, and scrotum but sparing the folds, are likely to be caused by chemical irritants, especially from urine and feces (Fig. 52-11). Other causes are detergents or soaps from inadequately rinsed cloth diapers or the chemicals in disposable wipes. Perianal involvement is usually the result of chemical irritation from feces, especially diarrheal stools. *Candida albicans* infection produces perianal inflammation and a maculopapular rash with satellite lesions that may cross the inguinal fold (Fig. 52-12). It is seen in up to 90% of infants with chronic diaper dermatitis and should be considered in diaper rashes that are recalcitrant to treatment.

NURSING CARE

Nursing interventions are aimed at altering the three factors that produce dermatitis: wetness (hydration), pH, and fecal irritants. The most significant factor amenable to intervention is the moist environment created in the diaper area. Changing the diaper as soon as it becomes wet eliminates a large part of the problem, and removing the diaper to expose healthy skin to air facilitates drying. The use of a hair dryer or heat lamp is not recommended because these devices can cause burns.

Contemporary diaper construction has had a significant impact on the incidence and severity of diaper dermatitis. Superabsorbent disposable diapers reduce diaper dermatitis. They contain an absorbent gelling material that binds water tightly to decrease skin wetness, maintains pH control by providing a buffering capacity, and decreases skin irritation by preventing mixing of urine and feces in the diaper.

Guidelines for controlling diaper rash are presented in the Family-Centred Teaching box. A common misconception about using cornstarch on skin is that it promotes the growth of *C. albicans*. Neither cornstarch nor talc promotes the growth of fungi under conditions normally found in the diaper area. Cornstarch is more effective in reducing friction and tends to cake less than talc when the skin is wet. On the basis of these properties and its safety in terms of inhalation injury, cornstarch is the preferred product. Talc should not be used.

Atopic Dermatitis (Eczema)

Eczema or *eczematous inflammation of the skin* refers to a descriptive category of dermatological diseases and not to a specific etiology. AD is a type of pruritic eczema that usually begins during infancy and is associated with allergy with a hereditary tendency (*atopy*). AD manifests in three forms based on the child's age and the distribution of lesions:

1. *Infantile (infantile eczema)*—Usually begins at 2 to 6 months of age; generally undergoes spontaneous remission by 3 years of age
2. *Childhood*—May follow the infantile form; occurs at 2 to 3 years of age; 90% of children have manifestations by age 5 years
3. *Preadolescent and adolescent*—Begins at about 12 years of age; may continue into the early adult years or indefinitely

TABLE 52-8 MISCELLANEOUS SKIN DISORDERS

DISEASE AND CAUSATIVE AGENT	LOCAL MANIFESTATIONS	MANAGEMENT	COMMENTS
Urticaria—Usually allergic response to medications or infection	Development of wheals Vary in size and configuration and tend to appear quickly, spread irregularly, and fade within a few hours May be constant or intermittent, sparse or profuse, small or large, discrete or confluent May be acute, chronic, or recurrent in acute attacks	Local soothing and antipruritic applications Antihistamines Epinephrine or ephedrine Cortisone in severe cases Severe upper respiratory tract involvement may require tracheostomy	Known etiological agents should be avoided May be accompanied by malaise, fever, lymphadenopathy Severe cases may involve mucous membranes, internal organs, and joints Obstruction to air passages constitutes medical emergency (see Chapter 45)
Intertrigo—Mechanical trauma and aggravating factors of excessive heat, moisture, and sweat retention	Red, inflamed, moist, partially denuded, marginated areas, the shape of which is determined by location Appears where opposing skin surfaces rub together, such as intergluteal folds, groin, neck, and axilla Excessive moisture and obesity are often factors	Affected areas kept clean and dry Skin folds kept separated with a generous supply of nonmedicated powder Expose to air and light Remove excess clothing	A form of diaper irritation Prevent recurrence by keeping susceptible areas clean and dry Frequently associated with overheating from too much clothing; common in tracheostomy patients with short necks and copious secretions
Psoriasis—Unknown; hereditary predisposition; may be triggered by stress	Round, thick, dry, reddish patches covered with coarse, silvery scales over trunk and extremities; first lesions commonly appear in scalp; facial lesions more common in children than in adults Affected cells proliferate at a much more rapid rate than normal cells	Tar preparations in combination with UVB light or natural sunlight Topical corticosteroids Topical vitamin D analog *calcipotriene* Phenol and saline solutions followed by a tar shampoo to remove scales Keratolytic agents (salicylic acid) Acitretin Emollients may provide relief	Uncommon in children younger than 6 years Patients are otherwise healthy Coal tar acts synergistically with UVB light Keratolytic agents enhance absorption of corticosteroids Humidifiers may help in winter
Alopecia*			
Alopecia areata	Sudden onset of asymptomatic, noninflammatory, round, bald patches in hairy parts of body	Psychological support Inducement of allergic contact dermatitis to stimulate growth of hair Minoxidil (peripheral vasodilator)	Family history in 10 to 26% of cases Some concern regarding medication therapy safety Refer to support groups*
Traumatic alopecia	Traction alopecia around scalp margins from tight hair styles (e.g., braids, pony tails, corn rows)	Counselling regarding hair styling, use of hair cosmetics, hot combs, rollers	More prevalent in Black children and adolescents Prolonged traction can produce fibrosis of hair root and permanent loss
Trichotillomania	Compulsive hair pulling	Determine and treat cause	Chronic hair pulling may require psychological therapy
Tinea capitis	See Table 52-4	See Table 52-4	See Table 52-4
Erythema multiforme (Stevens-Johnson syndrome)—Unknown; associated with ingestion of some medications; often follows upper respiratory tract infection	Erythematous papular rash Lesions enlarge by peripheral expansion, develop central vesicle Involves most skin surfaces except scalp May extend to mucous membranes, especially oral, ocular, and urethral	Symptomatic and supportive Maintain adequate intake of fluids (oral or intravenous), calories, and protein Moist wound care, hydrogels such as Vaseline, or Aquaphor Appropriate treatment of complications Diligent monitoring of urine volume and specific gravity, hemoglobin and hematocrit, serum electrolyte levels, total body weight	Rash often preceded by fever and malaise Complications include renal failure and severe eye disease Respiratory involvement in a number of cases Self-limiting, but recovery may extend for weeks; skin lesions may subside without scarring; mucous membrane lesions may persist for months Recurrence rate, 20%; mortality rate as high as 10% High mutation rate
Neurofibromatosis—Inherited disorder; autosomal dominant inheritance pattern	Café-au-lait spots, pigmented nevi, axillary freckling Slow-growing cutaneous and subcutaneous neurofibromas	Symptomatic treatment of associated manifestations (e.g., speech defects, seizures, skeletal defects [scoliosis, kyphosis], learning disabilities) Surgical removal of troublesome tumours	Refer to support groups† Family needs to know about genetic implications

UVB, Ultraviolet B.

*Canadian Alopecia Areata Foundation: http://www.canaaf.org/

†Children's Tumor Foundation, 95 Pine St., 16th Floor, New York, NY 10005; 800-323-7938 or 212-344-6633; fax: 212-747-0004; e-mail: info@ctf.org; www.ctf.org.

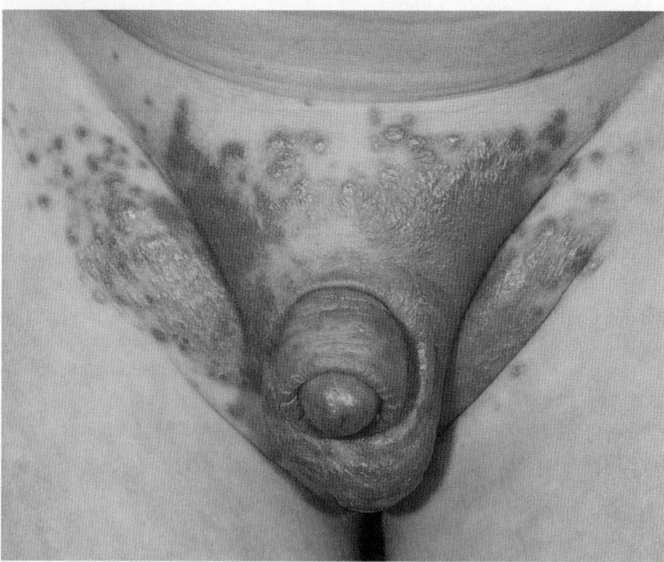

FIGURE 52-11 Irritant diaper dermatitis. Note sharply demarcated edges. (From Habif, T. P. [1996]. *Clinical dermatology: A color guide to diagnosis and therapy* [3rd ed.]. St. Louis: Mosby.)

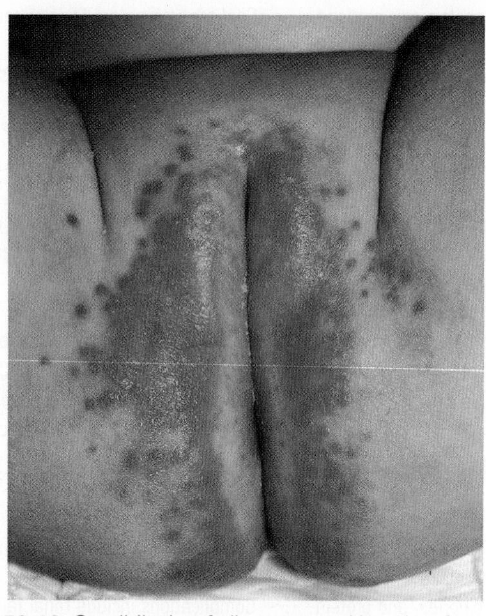

FIGURE 52-12 Candidiasis of diaper area. Note beefy red central erythema with satellite pustules. (From Paller, A. S., & Mancini, A. J. [2011]. *Hurwitz clinical pediatric dermatology* [4th ed.]. St. Louis: Saunders.)

The diagnosis of AD is based on a combination of history and morphological findings (Box 52-3). Children with AD have a lower threshold for cutaneous itching than do other children, and many authorities believe the dermatological manifestations appear subsequent to scratching from the intense pruritus (Alanne, Nermes, Söderlund, et al., 2011). For example, infants rub their faces against bed linen, and their crawling (a form of scratching) results in irritation of knees and elbows. Lesions disappear if the scratching is stopped (Fig. 52-13).

The majority of children with infantile AD have a family history of eczema, asthma, food allergies, or allergic rhinitis, which strongly supports a genetic predisposition. The cause is unknown but appears to be related to abnormal function of the skin, including alterations in perspiration, peripheral vascular function, and heat tolerance. Manifestations of the chronic disease improve in humid climates and get worse in the fall and winter, when homes are heated and environmental humidity is lower. The disease can be controlled but not cured. Research has shown that itching and scratching in infants with this disorder create sleep disturbances and can lessen the quality of life (Alanne et al., 2011).

FAMILY-CENTRED TEACHING

Controlling Diaper Rash

Keep skin dry.*

- Use superabsorbent disposable diapers to reduce skin wetness.
- If using cloth diapers, use only overwraps that allow air to circulate; avoid rubber pants.
- Change diapers as soon as soiled—especially with stool—whenever possible, preferably once during the night.
- Expose healthy or only slightly irritated skin to air, not heat, to dry completely.

Apply ointment, such as zinc oxide or petrolatum, to protect skin, if skin is very red or has moist, open areas.

- Avoid removing skin barrier cream with each diaper change; remove waste material and reapply skin barrier cream.
- To completely remove ointment, especially zinc oxide, use mineral oil; do not wash vigorously.

Avoid overwashing the skin, especially with perfumed soaps or commercial wipes, which may be irritating.

- A moisturizer or nonsoap cleanser may be used, such as cold cream or Cetaphil, to wipe urine from skin.
- Gently wipe stool from skin using water and mild soap.
- When travelling, take along an old baby wipe container filled with soft paper towels and warm water.

*Powder helps to keep the skin dry, but talc is dangerous if breathed into the lungs. Plain cornstarch or cornstarch-based powder are safer. When using any powder product, first shake it in to your hand, and then apply to the diaper area. Store the container away from the infant's reach; keep the container closed when not in use.

Therapeutic Management

The major goals of management are to (1) hydrate the skin, (2) relieve pruritus, (3) reduce flare-ups or inflammation by avoiding triggers, and (4) prevent and control secondary infection. The general measures for managing AD focus on reducing pruritus and other aspects of the disease. Management strategies include avoiding exposure to skin irritants or allergens; avoiding overheating; avoiding skin moisture loss and improving skin hydration; and administrating medications such as antihistamines, topical immunomodulators, topical steroids, and (sometimes) mild sedatives as indicated. Products with coal tar are available and are an effective topical treatment (Canadian Dermatology Association, 2016a).

Enhancing skin hydration and preventing dry, flaky skin are accomplished in a number of ways, depending on the child's skin characteristics and individual needs. A tepid bath with a mild soap, no soap, or an emulsifying oil, followed immediately

BOX 52-3 CLINICAL MANIFESTATIONS OF ATOPIC DERMATITIS

Distribution of Lesions

Infantile form—Generalized, especially cheeks, scalp, trunk, and extensor surfaces of extremities (see Fig. 52-13)

Childhood form—Flexural areas (antecubital and popliteal fossae, neck), wrists, ankles, and feet

Preadolescent and adolescent form—Face, sides of neck, hands, feet, face, and antecubital and popliteal fossae (to a lesser extent)

Appearance of Lesions

Infantile Form

Erythema
Vesicles
Papules
Weeping
Oozing
Crusting
Scaling
Often symmetrical

Childhood Form

Symmetrical involvement
Clusters of small erythematous or flesh-coloured papules or minimally scaling patches
Dry and may be hyperpigmented
Lichenification (thickened skin with accentuation of creases)
Keratosis pilaris (follicular hyperkeratosis) common

Adolescent or Adult Form

Same as childhood manifestations
Dry, thick lesions (lichenified plaques) common
Confluent papules

Other Physical Manifestations

Intense itching
Unaffected skin dry and rough
Children of African descent are likely to exhibit more papular or follicular lesions than are White children
May exhibit one or more of the following:

- Lymphadenopathy, especially near affected sites
- Increased palmar creases (many cases)
- Atopic pleats (extra line or groove of lower eyelid)
- Prone to cold hands
- Pityriasis alba (small, poorly defined areas of hypopigmentation)
- Facial pallor (especially around nose, mouth, and ears)
- Bluish discolouration beneath eyes ("allergic shiners")
- Increased susceptibility to unusual cutaneous infections (especially viral)

by application of an emollient (within 3 minutes), assists in trapping moisture and preventing its loss. Bubble baths and harsh soaps should be avoided. The bath may need to be repeated once or twice daily, depending on the child's status; excessive bathing without emollient application only dries out the skin. Some lotions are not effective, and emollients should be chosen carefully to prevent excessive skin drying. Aquaphor, Cetaphil, and Eucerin are acceptable lotions for skin hydration. A nighttime bath, followed by emollient application and dressing in soft cotton pyjamas, may help alleviate most nighttime pruritus. Sometimes colloid baths, such as the addition of 2 cups of cornstarch to a tub of warm water, provide temporary relief of itching and may help the child sleep if given before bedtime.

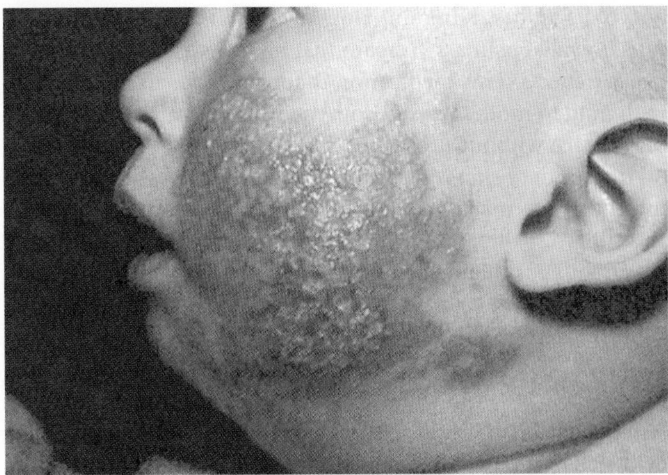

FIGURE 52-13 Infantile atopic dermatitis with oozing and crusting of lesions. (From Weston, W. L., Lane, A. T., & Morelli, J. G. [2002]. *Color textbook of pediatric dermatology* [4th ed.]. St. Louis: Mosby.)

Cool wet compresses are soothing to the skin and provide antiseptic protection. A soft cloth with several layers is soaked in water or Burow solution. The compress is left on the skin for 20 to 30 minutes. If the cloth starts to dry, more fluid is added to keep it very wet. After the removal of the cloth, the skin is patted dry and the medicated treatment or emollient applied. Phototherapy can also be an effective management tool (Canadian Dermatology Association, 2016a).

Oral antihistamine medications such as hydroxyzine or diphenhydramine usually relieve moderate or severe pruritus. Nonsedating antihistamines such as loratadine (Claritin) or fexofenadine (Allegra) may be preferred for daytime pruritus relief. Because pruritus increases at night, a mildly sedating antihistamine may be needed.

Occasional flare-ups require the use of topical steroids to diminish inflammation. Low-, moderate-, or high-potency topical corticosteroids are prescribed, depending on the degree of involvement, the area of the body to be treated, the child's age, the potential for local adverse effects (striae, skin atrophy, and pigment changes), and the type of vehicle to be used (e.g., cream, lotion, ointment). Patients receiving topical corticosteroid therapy for chronic conditions should be evaluated for risk factors for suboptimal linear growth and reduced bone density. Topical immunomodulators, a new nonsteroidal treatment for AD, are best used at the beginning of a flare-up just as the skin becomes red and itches. Two newer immunomodulator medications used in children with AD are tacrolimus and pimecrolimus (Walling & Swick, 2010). Tacrolimus is available in two ointment strengths (0.03% and 0.1%); the 0.03% concentration has been approved for use in children 2 years of age and older (Doss, Kamoun, Dubertret, et al., 2010). Pimecrolimus is available in a 1% cream that has no systemic accumulation or effects. This medication is approved for use in children with mild to moderate AD. Both medications can be used freely on the face without producing steroid adverse effects.

If secondary skin infections occur in children with AD, these infections are managed with appropriate systemic antibiotics. In a subgroup of patient with moderate to severe AD, the disease may require systemic treatment (Ricci, Dondi, Patrizi, et al., 2009).

NURSING CARE

Assessment of the child with AD includes a family history for evidence of atopy, a history of previous involvement, and any environmental or dietary factors associated with the present and previous exacerbations. The skin lesions are examined for type, distribution, and evidence of secondary infection. Parents should be interviewed regarding the child's behaviour, especially in relation to scratching, irritability, and sleeping patterns. Exploration of the family's feelings and methods of coping is also important.

The nursing care of the child with AD can be challenging. Controlling the intense pruritus is imperative if the disorder is to be successfully managed, since scratching leads to new lesions and may cause secondary infection. In addition to the medical regimen, other measures can be taken to prevent or minimize the scratching. Fingernails and toenails need to be cut short, kept clean, and filed frequently to prevent sharp edges. Gloves or cotton stockings can be placed over the hands and pinned to shirtsleeves. One-piece outfits with long sleeves and long pants also decrease direct contact with the skin. If gloves or socks are used, the child needs time to be free from such restrictions. An excellent time to remove gloves, socks, or other protective devices is during the bath or after the child receives sedative or antipruritic medication.

Conditions that increase itching should be eliminated when possible. Woollen clothes or blankets, rough fabrics, and furry stuffed animals should be removed from the child's environment. Because heat and humidity cause perspiration (which intensifies itching), proper dress for climatic conditions is essential. Pruritus is often precipitated by exposure to the irritant effects of certain components of common products such as soaps, detergents, fabric softeners, perfumes, and powders. Most children experience less itching when soft cotton fabrics are worn next to the skin. During cold months, synthetic fabrics (not wool) should be used for overcoats, hats, gloves, and snowsuits. Exposure to latex products, such as gloves and balloons, should also be avoided.

Clothes and sheets should be laundered in a mild detergent and rinsed thoroughly in clear water (without fabric softeners or antistatic chemicals). Putting the clothes through a second complete wash cycle without using detergent reduces the amount of residue remaining in the fabric.

Preventing infection is usually accomplished by preventing scratching. Baths are given as prescribed, the water kept tepid, and soaps (except as indicated) and bubble baths avoided, along with oils or powders. Skin folds and diaper areas need frequent cleansing with plain water. A room humidifier or vaporizer may benefit children with extremely dry skin. The skin lesions should be examined for signs of infection—usually honey-coloured crusts or pustules with surrounding erythema. Any signs of infection need to be reported to the health care practitioner.

Wet soaks and compresses can be applied and medications for pruritus or infection are administered as directed. The family should be given explicit instructions on the preparation and use of soaks, special baths, and topical medications, including the order of application if more than one is prescribed. It is important to emphasize that one thick application of topical medication is *not* equivalent to several thin applications, and that excessive use of a medication (particularly steroids) can be hazardous. If children have difficulty remaining still for a 10- or 15-minute soak, bath, or dressing application, these can be carried out at naptime or when the child is engrossed in watching television, listening to a story, or playing with tub toys.

Diet modification is another source of frustration to parents. When a hypoallergenic diet is prescribed, parents need help to understand the reason for the diet and the guidelines for avoiding hyperallergenic foods (see Chapter 45). Because hypoallergenic diets take time before effects are apparent, parents need reassurance that results may not be seen immediately. If airborne allergens make eczema worse, the family should be counselled about "allergy proofing" the home (see Asthma, Chapter 45).

Family Support

Parents need to be assured that the lesions will not produce scarring (unless secondarily infected) and that the disease is not contagious. However, the child may have repeated exacerbations and remissions. Spontaneous and permanent remission takes place at approximately 2 to 3 years of age in most children with the infantile disorder.

During acute phases, emotional stress can become intense for the family. They need time to discuss negative feelings and to be reassured that these feelings are normal. Stress tends to aggravate the severity of the condition. Thus efforts to relieve anxiety in both the parents and the child have a beneficial emotional and physical effect.

Seborrheic Dermatitis

Seborrheic dermatitis is a chronic, recurrent, inflammatory reaction of the skin. It occurs most commonly on the scalp (cradle cap) but may involve the eyelids (blepharitis), external ear canal (otitis externa), nasolabial folds, and inguinal region. The cause is unknown, although it is more common in early infancy, when sebum production is increased. The lesions are characteristically thick, adherent, yellowish, scaly, oily patches that may or may not be mildly pruritic. Unlike AD, seborrheic dermatitis is not associated with a positive family history for allergy and is common in infants shortly after birth and in adolescents after puberty. Diagnosis is made primarily on the basis of the appearance and the location of the crusts or scales.

NURSING CARE

Cradle cap may be prevented with adequate scalp hygiene. Frequently, parents omit shampooing the infant's hair for fear of damaging the "soft spots," or fontanels. The nurse should discuss how to shampoo the infant's hair and emphasize that the fontanel is like skin anywhere else on the body—it does not puncture or tear with mild pressure.

When seborrheic lesions are present, the treatment is directed at removing the crusts. Parents should be taught the appropriate procedure to clean the scalp. Education may need to include a demonstration. Shampooing should be done daily with a mild soap or commercial baby shampoo; medicated shampoos are not necessary, but an antiseborrheic shampoo containing sulphur and salicylic acid may be used. Shampoo is applied to the scalp and allowed to remain on the scalp until the crusts soften. Then the scalp is thoroughly rinsed. A fine-tooth comb or a soft facial brush helps remove the loosened crusts from the strands of hair after shampooing.

Acne

Acne vulgaris is the most common skin problem treated by physicians during patients' adolescence. Acne is not caused by dirt but by testosterone, a hormone present in males and females that increases during puberty. It stimulates the sebaceous glands of the skin to enlarge and increase in number or produce oil and plug the pores. Whiteheads, blackheads, and pimples are present in teenage acne.

Half of the adolescent population experiences acne by the end of the teenage years. Although the disorder can appear before the age of 10 years, the peak incidence occurs in middle to late adolescence (at age 16 to 17 years in girls and 17 to 18 years in boys). It is more common in boys than in girls. The degree to which an individual is affected may range from nothing more than a few isolated comedones to a severe inflammatory reaction. Some research studies have indicated that the earlier the acne is present the worse the acne will be (Canadian Dermatology Association, 2016b). Although the disease is self-limited and not life threatening, it has great significance to the adolescent. Health care providers should not underestimate the impact that acne has on teens.

Numerous factors affect the development and course of acne. Its distribution in families and a high degree of concordance in identical twins suggest hereditary factors. Premenstrual flares of acne occur in nearly 70% of adolescent girls, suggesting a hormonal cause. Studies do not indicate a clear association between stress and acne, but adolescents commonly cite stress as a cause for acne outbreaks. Cosmetics containing lanolin, petrolatum, vegetable oils, lauryl alcohol, butyl stearate, and oleic acid can increase comedone production. Exposure to oils in cooking grease can be a precursor in adolescents who work over fast-food restaurant hot oils. There is no known link between dietary intake and the development or worsening of acne.

Pathophysiology

Contributors to acne development include sebum secretion, abnormal desquamation of follicles, bacterial growth, and inflammation (Kim & Armstrong, 2011). *Comedogenesis* (formation of comedones) results in a noninflammatory lesion that may be either an *open comedone* ("blackhead") or a *closed comedone* ("whitehead"). Inflammation occurs with the proliferation of *Propionibacterium acnes*, which draws in neutrophils, causing inflammatory papules, pustules, nodules, and cysts.

Therapeutic Management

Successful management of acne depends on a collaborative effort between the health care provider, the adolescent, and the parents. Unlike many other dermatological conditions, acne lesions resolve slowly, and improvement may not be apparent for at least 6 weeks. Individual comedones can take several weeks to months to resolve, and papules and pustules usually resolve in about 1 week. The multifactorial causes of acne necessitate a combined approach for successful treatment. Treatment consists of general measures of care and specific treatments determined by the type of lesions involved.

General measures. Improvement of the adolescent's overall health status is part of the general management. Adequate rest, moderate exercise, a well-balanced diet, reduction of emotional stress, and elimination of any foci of infection are all part of general health promotion.

Cleansing. Dirt or oil on the surface of the skin does not cause acne. Gentle cleansing with a mild cleanser once or twice daily is usually sufficient. Antibacterial soaps are ineffective and may be too drying when used in combination with topical acne medications. For some adolescents hygiene of the hair and scalp appears to be related to the clinical activity of the acne. Acne on the forehead may improve with brushing the hair away from the forehead and more frequent shampooing.

Medications. Treatment success depends on commitment from the adolescent. Before prescribing treatment, the health care provider should determine the adolescent's level of comfort and readiness to begin treatment.

Tretinoin (Retin-A) is the only medication that effectively interrupts the abnormal follicular keratinization that produces microcomedones, the invisible precursors of the visible comedones. Tretinoin alone is usually sufficient for management of comedonal acne (Kim & Armstrong, 2011). Tretinoin is available as a cream, gel, or liquid. This medication can be extremely irritating to the skin and requires careful patient education for optimal usage. The patient should be instructed to begin with a pea-sized dot of medication, which is divided into the three main areas of the face and then gently rubbed into each area. The medication should not be applied for at least 20 to 30 minutes after washing, to decrease the burning sensation. The avoidance of sun and the daily use of sunscreen must be emphasized, since sun exposure can result in severe sunburn. Adolescents should be advised to apply the medication at night and to use a sunscreen with a sun protection factor (SPF) of at least 15 in the daytime. Topical *benzoyl peroxide* is an antibacterial medication that inhibits the growth of *P. acnes* organisms. It is effective against both inflammatory and noninflammatory acne and is an effective first-line agent. This medication is available as a cream, lotion, gel, or wash. The patient should be informed that the medication may have a bleaching effect on sheets, bedclothes, and towels. The adolescent can be reassured that skin bleaching will not occur. Accommodation to the medication can be gained with a gradual increase in the strength and frequency of application.

When inflammatory lesions accompany the comedones, a *topical antibacterial medication* may be prescribed. These agents are used to prevent new lesions and to treat pre-existing acne. Clindamycin, erythromycin, metronidazole, and azelaic acid and the combination of either benzoyl peroxide and erythromycin or benzoyl peroxide and glycolic acid are all choices for topical antibacterial therapy. The combination of 5% benzoyl peroxide and 3% erythromycin are especially beneficial, although the exact mechanism of the action is not known (Kim & Armstrong, 2011). *Systemic antibiotic therapy* is used when moderate to severe acne does not respond to topical treatments. Oral antibiotics such as tetracycline, erythromycin, minocycline, and doxycycline are considered safe to use (Leyden & Del Rosso, 2011). A gel combining 0.25% tretinoin and 1.2% clindamycin phosphate is more effective in treating acne than tretinoin or clindamycin alone (Hanna & Barankin, 2015).

Young women with mild to moderate acne may respond well to topical treatment and the addition of an *oral contraceptive pill (OCP)*. OCPs reduce the endogenous androgen production and decrease the bioavailability of the woman's circulating androgens. Both of these actions result in decreased acne.

Isotretinoin,13-cis-retinoic acid (Accutane), is a potent and effective oral medication that is reserved for severe cystic acne that has not responded to other treatments. Isotretinoin is the only agent available that affects factors involved in the development of acne. However, treatment with isotretinoin should be managed only by a dermatologist. Adolescents with multiple, active, deep dermal or subcutaneous cystic and nodular acne lesions are treated for 20 weeks. Multiple adverse effects can occur, including dry skin and mucous membranes, nasal irritation, dry eyes, decreased night vision, photosensitivity, arthralgia, headaches, mood changes, aggressive or violent behaviours, depression, and suicidal ideation. Adolescents taking this medication should be monitored for depression, depressive symptoms, and suicidal ideation (Misery, 2011). The medication should be given only at the recommended doses for no longer than the recommended duration. The most significant adverse effects of this medication are the teratogenic effects. Isotretinoin is absolutely contraindicated in pregnant women. Sexually active young women must be using an effective contraceptive method during treatment and for 1 month after treatment. Patients receiving isotretinoin should also be monitored for elevated cholesterol and triglyceride levels. Significant elevation may require discontinuation of the medication.

NURSING CARE

Because acne is a common skin condition and its appearance may seem mild, the health care provider may underestimate the relative importance of the disease to the adolescent. The nurse should assess the individual adolescent's level of distress, current management, and perceived success of any regimen before initiating a referral. If adolescents do not perceive the acne to be a problem, they may lack motivation to follow the treatment plan.

The nurse can provide ongoing support for the adolescent when a treatment plan is initiated. The family is also encouraged to support the adolescent in his or her efforts. Use of medications and basic skin care information should be discussed in detail with the adolescent. Written instructions should accompany the verbal discussion. Information to dispel myths regarding the use of abrasive cleansing products can prevent unnecessary costs and trauma to the skin.

Teenagers need education about the factors that aggravate and damage the skin, such as too vigorous scrubbing. In addition, picking, squeezing, and manual expression with fingernails break down the ductal walls of lesions and cause the acne to worsen. Mechanical irritation, such as vinyl helmet straps that rub areas predisposed to acne, can also cause the development of lesions.

THERMAL INJURY

Burns

Burn injuries are usually attributed to extreme heat sources but may also result from exposure to cold, chemicals, electricity, or radiation. Most burns are relatively minor and do not require definitive medical treatment. However, burns involving a large body surface area, critical body parts, or the older adult or pediatric population often benefit from treatment in specialized burn centres.

In Canada, researchers discovered over a 10-year period (1994 to 2003) that 10,229 children were admitted to Canadian hospitals for burn injuries. Out of that number, 494 children died from their injuries. Children who were aged 1 to 5 years had the highest risk of death. Scalds caused the most thermal injuries and represented 50% of all burn admissions. Boys and children under 5 years of age had the highest risk of burn injuries. Fortunately, there was a downward trend over that time period, with a significant reduction in burn injuries. The decrease is likely due to burn safety programs and improved burn treatments and hospital admission protocols (Spinks, Wasiak, Clelan, et al., 2008).

When burns are characterized by patients' age and type of injury, the following patterns become apparent: (1) hot-water scalds are most frequent in toddlers, (2) flame-related burns are more common in older children, (3) 10 to 20% of documented cases of child abuse include burn injuries (Herndon, 2012), and (4) children playing with matches or lighters account for 1 in 10 house fires.

The extent of tissue destruction in burns is determined by the intensity of the heat source, the duration of contact or exposure, the conductivity of the tissue involved, and the rate at which the heat energy is dissipated by the skin. A brief exposure to high-intensity heat from a flame can produce burn injuries similar to those induced by long exposure to less intense heat in hot water.

Characteristics of Burn Injury

The physiological responses, therapy, prognosis, and disposition of the injured child are all directly related to the *amount of tissue destroyed.* Thus the severity of the burn injury is assessed on the basis of the percentage of *total body surface area (TBSA)* burned and the *depth* of the burn. Among children in the school-age group or younger age groups, a burn that is 10% of TBSA can be life threatening if not treated correctly. Other important factors in determining the seriousness of the injury are the location of the wounds, the child's age and general health, the causative agent, the presence of respiratory involvement, and any associated injury or condition.

Type of injury. Most burns result from contact with thermal agents such as a flame, hot surfaces, or hot liquids. Electrical injuries caused by household current have the greatest incidence in young children, who insert conductive objects into electrical outlets and bite or suck on connected electrical cords. Burns occur most commonly during the spring and summer months and are also associated with risk-taking behaviours in boys. Direct contact with high- or low-voltage current, as well as lightning strikes, is the most frequent mechanism of injury. The resistance of the tissue and the path of the electric current are responsible for the damage incurred. Electric current travels through the body following the path of least resistance, which involves the tissues, fluid, blood vessels, and nerves. A more localized burn is produced if skin resistance is high at the area of contact, and a more systemic pattern of injury is produced if skin resistance is low. Often compared with a crush injury, serious electrical trauma results from current passing through vital organs, muscle compartments, and nerve or vascular pathways. Loss of limbs, cardiac fibrillation, respiratory collapse, and burns are common occurrences after exposure to electrical energy. Criteria for admission, as derived from evidence-informed practice for electrical burn injuries, include a history of loss of consciousness, electrocardiographic (ECG) changes, 10% TBSA affected, or the need for monitoring an affected extremity. Cardiac monitoring is thus included in standard burn care when ECG changes are identified on admission.

Chemical burns are seen in the pediatric population and can cause extensive injury. The severity of injury is related to the chemical agent (acid, alkali, or organic compound) involved and the duration of contact. The mechanism of injury differs from that in other burns in that there is a chemical disruption and alteration of the physical properties of the exposed body area. Noxious agents exist in many cleaning products commonly found in the home. In addition to concern for localized damage, the potential for systemic toxicity must be addressed. Of particular concern is the exposure of the eyes to chemical agents, the ingestion of caustic substances, and inhalation of toxic gases produced from chemicals.

Extent of injury. The extent of a burn is expressed as a percentage of the TBSA. This is most accurately estimated by using specially designed age-related charts (Fig. 52-14). It is more efficient to use a chart designed to assign body proportions to children of different ages.

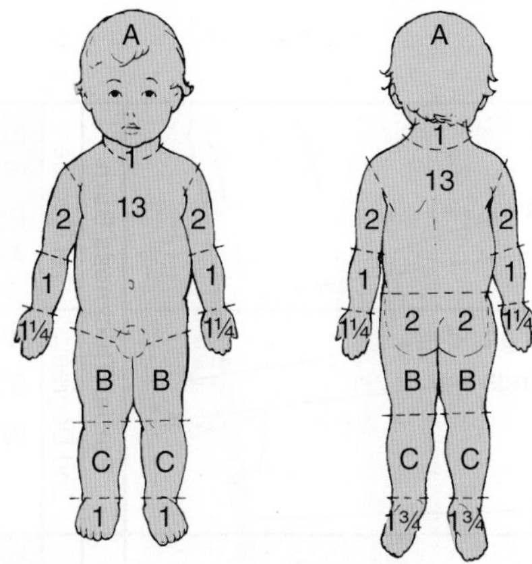

RELATIVE PERCENTAGES OF AREAS AFFECTED BY GROWTH

AREA	BIRTH	AGE 1 YR	AGE 5 YR
A = ½ of head	9½	8½	6½
B = ½ of one thigh	2¾	3¼	4
C = ½ of one leg	2½	2½	2¾

A

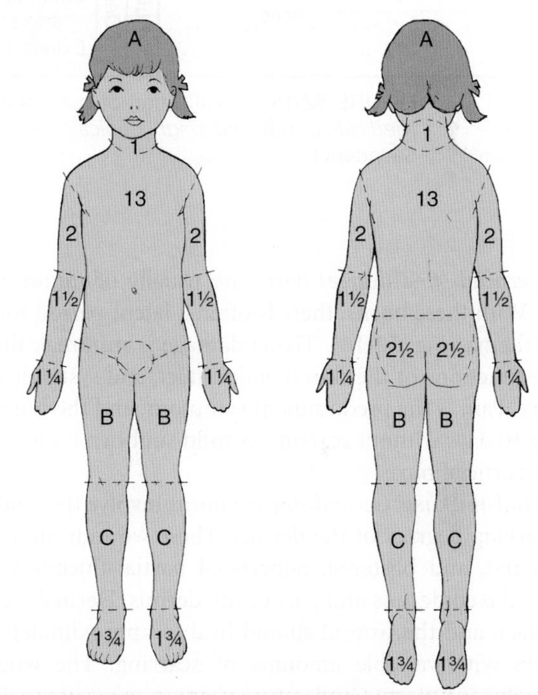

RELATIVE PERCENTAGES OF AREAS AFFECTED BY GROWTH

AREA	AGE 10 YR	AGE 15 YR	ADULT
A = ½ of head	5½	4½	3½
B = ½ of one thigh	4½	4½	4¾
C = ½ of one leg	3	3¼	3½

B

FIGURE 52-14 Estimation of distribution of burns in children. **A:** Children from birth to age 5 years. **B:** Older children.

Depth of injury. A thermal injury is a three-dimensional wound that is also assessed in relation to depth of injury. Traditionally the terms *first-*, *second-*, and *third-degree* have been used to describe the depth of tissue injury. However, with the current emphasis on wound healing, these have been replaced by more descriptive terms based on the extent of destruction to the epithelializing elements of the skin (Fig. 52-15).

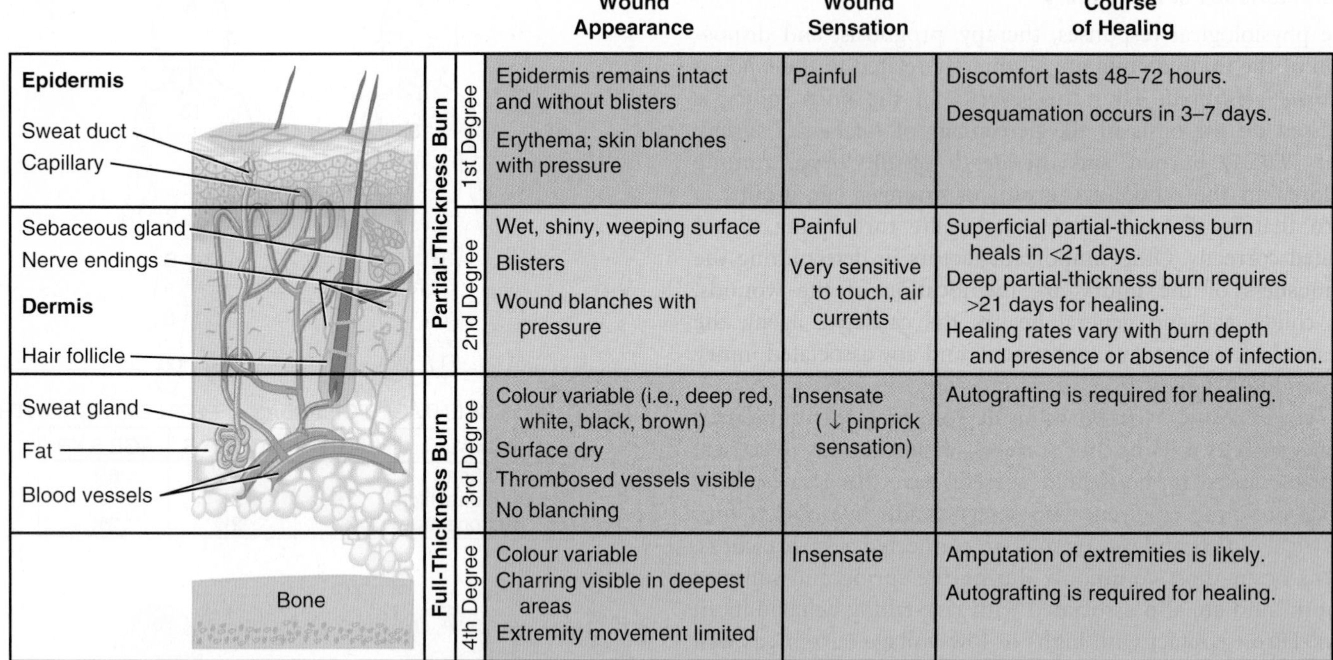

Depth	Degree	Wound Appearance	Wound Sensation	Course of Healing
Partial-Thickness Burn	1st Degree	Epidermis remains intact and without blisters Erythema; skin blanches with pressure	Painful	Discomfort lasts 48–72 hours. Desquamation occurs in 3–7 days.
Partial-Thickness Burn	2nd Degree	Wet, shiny, weeping surface Blisters Wound blanches with pressure	Painful Very sensitive to touch, air currents	Superficial partial-thickness burn heals in <21 days. Deep partial-thickness burn requires >21 days for healing. Healing rates vary with burn depth and presence or absence of infection.
Full-Thickness Burn	3rd Degree	Colour variable (i.e., deep red, white, black, brown) Surface dry Thrombosed vessels visible No blanching	Insensate (↓ pinprick sensation)	Autografting is required for healing.
Full-Thickness Burn	4th Degree	Colour variable Charring visible in deepest areas Extremity movement limited	Insensate	Amputation of extremities is likely. Autografting is required for healing.

FIGURE 52-15 Classification of burn depth according to depth of injury. (From Black, J. M. [2008]. *Medical-surgical nursing: Clinical management for positive outcomes* [8th ed.]. Philadelphia: Saunders.)

Superficial (first-degree) burns are usually of minor significance. With these burns, there is often a latent period followed by erythema (Fig. 52-16). Tissue damage is minimal, the protective functions of the skin remain intact, and systemic effects are rare. Pain is the predominant symptom, and the burn heals in 5 to 10 days without scarring. A mild sunburn is an example of a superficial burn.

Partial-thickness (second-degree) burns involve the epidermis and varying degrees of the dermis. These wounds are painful, moist, red, and blistered. Superficial partial-thickness burns involve the epidermis and part of the dermis. Dermal elements are intact, and the wound should heal in approximately 14 to 21 days with variable amounts of scarring. The wound is extremely sensitive to temperature changes, exposure to air, and light touch. Although classified as partial-thickness (or second-degree) burns, deep dermal burns resemble full-thickness injuries in many respects except that sweat glands and hair follicles remain intact. The burn may appear mottled, with pink, red, or waxy white areas exhibiting blisters and edema formation. Systemic effects are similar to those encountered with full-thickness burns. Although many of these wounds heal spontaneously, healing time may extend beyond 21 days. These burn wounds often heal with extensive scarring.

Full-thickness (third-degree) burns are serious injuries that involve the entire epidermis and dermis and extend into subcutaneous tissue (see Fig. 52-15). Nerve endings, sweat glands, and hair follicles are destroyed. The burn varies in colour from red to tan, waxy white, brown, or black and is distinguished by a dry, leathery appearance (Fig. 52-17). Normally, full-thickness burns lack sensation in the area of

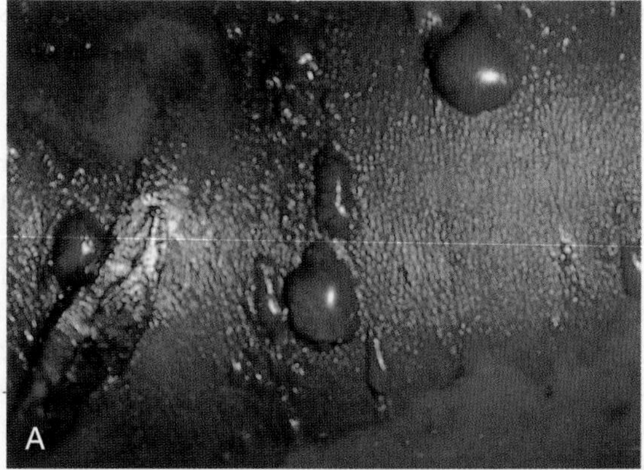

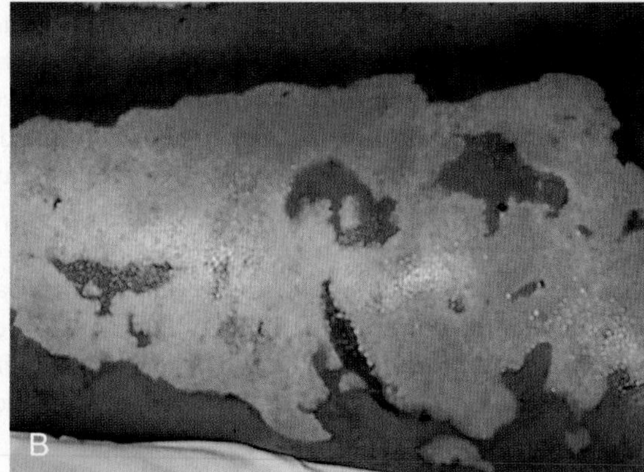

FIGURE 52-16 Superficial burns on a Black child. **A:** Blisters intact. **B:** Blisters removed. (Courtesy Hillcrest Medical Center, Tulsa, OK.)

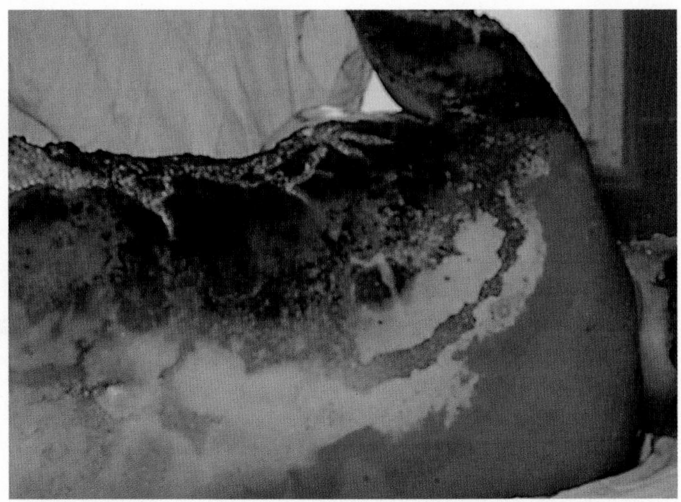

FIGURE 52-17 Bottom to top: Deep partial-thickness burn (red area); full-thickness burn (white area); full-thickness burn with eschar (brown area). (Courtesy Hillcrest Medical Center, Tulsa, OK.)

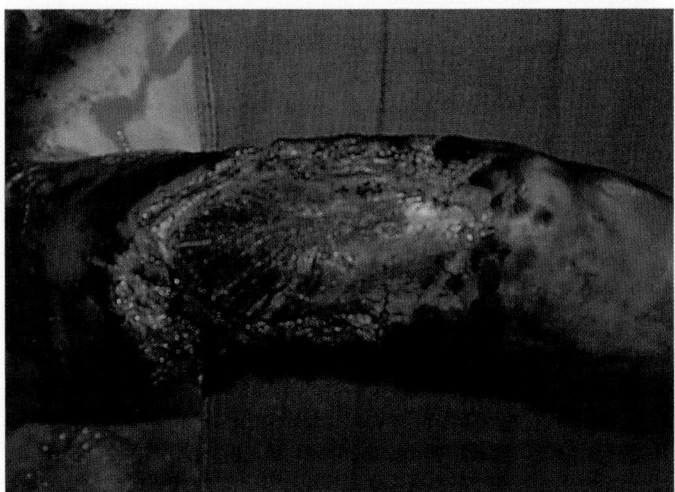

FIGURE 52-18 Full-thickness burn with muscle and fascia involved. (Courtesy Hillcrest Medical Center, Tulsa, OK.)

injury because of the destruction of nerve endings. However, most full-thickness burns have superficial and partial-thickness burned areas at the periphery of the burn, where nerve endings are intact and exposed. Excised eschar and donor sites also cause exposed nerve fibres. As the peripheral fibres regenerate, painful sensations return. Consequently, children often experience severe pain related to the size and depth of the burn. Full-thickness wounds are not capable of re-epithelialization and require surgical excision and grafting to close the wound.

Fourth-degree burns are full-thickness injuries that involve underlying structures such as muscle, fascia, and bone. The wound appears dull and dry, and ligaments, tendons, and bone may be exposed (Fig. 52-18).

Severity of injury. Burns are classified as minor, moderate, or major, which is useful in determining the disposition of the patient for treatment. Burn patients are categorized as (1) those with a *major burn injury*, who require the services and facilities of a specialized burn centre; (2) those with a *moderate burn*, who may be treated in a hospital with expertise in burn care; and (3) those with *minor injuries*, who may be treated on an outpatient basis. The extent and depth of the burn, the causative agent, the body area involved, the patient's age, and concomitant injuries and illnesses determine the severity of the injury.

As the skin of infants is so thin, it is likely to sustain deeper injuries than those of older children. Children younger than 2 years of age, especially 6 months or younger, have a significantly higher mortality rate than that of older children with burns of similar magnitude. Acute or chronic illnesses or superimposed injuries also complicate burn care and response to treatment.

Inhalation injury. Trauma to the tracheobronchial tree often follows inhalation of the heated gases and toxic chemicals produced during combustion. Although direct thermal injury to the upper airway may occur, heat damage below the vocal cords is rare. Inspired heated air is cooled in the upper airway before reaching the trachea. Reflex closure of the cords and laryngospasm also prevent full inhalation. However, evidence of direct thermal injury to the upper airway includes burns of the face and lips, singed nasal hairs, and laryngeal edema. Clinical manifestations may be delayed as long as 24 to 48 hours. Wheezing, increasing secretions, hoarseness, wet crackles, and carbonaceous secretions are signs of respiratory tract involvement. Upper airway obstruction is often associated with burn shock and fluid resuscitation. In such situations, endotracheal intubation may also be necessary to preserve a patent airway.

Inhalation of carbon monoxide is suspected when the injury has occurred in an enclosed space. Mucosal erythema and edema followed by sloughing of the mucosa are manifestations of respiratory tract injury. A mucopurulent membrane replaces the mucosal lining and seriously compromises respiration and ventilation. A significant increase in mortality has been observed when inhalation injury and pneumonia are both present. Deep burns, especially those encircling the thorax, may cause restriction of chest excursion as a result of edema and inelastic eschar formation. Young children are particularly at risk because of the pliability of the skeletal structure.

Pathophysiology

Thermal injuries produce both local and systemic effects that are related to the extent of tissue destruction. In superficial burns the tissue damage is minimal. In partial-thickness burns there is considerable edema and more severe capillary damage. With a major burn greater than 30% TBSA, there is a systemic response involving an increase in capillary permeability, allowing plasma proteins, fluids, and electrolytes to be lost. Maximum edema formation in a small wound occurs about 8 to 12 hours after injury. After a larger injury, hypovolemia, associated with this phenomenon, will slow the rate of edema formation, with maximum effect at 18 to 24 hours.

Another systemic response is anemia, caused by direct heat destruction of red blood cells (RBCs), hemolysis of injured RBCs, and trapping of RBCs in the microvascular thrombi of damaged cells. A long-term decrease in the number of RBCs may occur as a result of increased RBC fragility. Initially there is an increased blood flow to the heart, brain, and kidneys, with decreased blood flow to the gastrointestinal tract. There is an increase in metabolism to maintain body heat, providing for the body's increased energy needs.

Complications. Thermally injured children are subject to a number of serious complications, both from the wound and from systemic alterations resulting from the injury. The immediate threat to life is related to airway compromise and profound shock. During healing, infection—both local and systemic sepsis—is the primary complication. Mortality associated with thermal trauma in children increases with the severity of injury and decreases as age advances. In children older than 3 years, the mortality rate is similar to that of adults. Below this age, the survival rate with burns and their associated complications lessens considerably.

A less apparent respiratory tract injury is inhalation of carbon monoxide. Carbon monoxide has a greater affinity for hemoglobin than does oxygen, thereby depriving peripheral tissues and oxygen-dependent organs (such as the heart and brain) of the oxygen needed for survival. Treatment for either of these two problems is 100% oxygen, which reverses the situation rapidly.

Pulmonary problems are a major cause of fatality in children with either thermal burns or complications in the respiratory tract. In the early stages after a burn, most respiratory infections result from nosocomial exposure, immobility, and abdominal distension. The hematogenous type occurs later and is related to the septic burn wound or other focus, such as phlebitis at the site of an invasive IV line. Respiratory problems include inhalation injuries, aspiration in unconscious patients, bacterial pneumonia, pulmonary edema, pulmonary embolus, post-traumatic pulmonary insufficiency, and atelectasis. The most common cause of respiratory failure in the pediatric age group is bacterial pneumonia, which requires prolonged intubation and sometimes a tracheostomy. Tracheostomies increase the incidence of serious complications and are performed only in extreme cases.

A less common complication is pulmonary edema resulting from fluid overload or acute respiratory distress syndrome (ARDS) in association with Gram-negative sepsis. ARDS results from pulmonary capillary damage and leakage of fluid into the interstitial spaces of the lung. A loss of adherence to and interference with oxygenation are the consequences of pulmonary insufficiency in conjunction with systemic sepsis.

Sepsis is a critical problem in the treatment of burns and an ever-present threat following the shock phase. Decreased level of consciousness and lethargy are early signs of sepsis. Initially, burn wounds are relatively pathogen free unless they are contaminated with potentially infectious material, such as dirt or polluted water. However, dead tissue and exudate provide a fertile field for bacterial growth. On approximately the third postburn day, early colonization of the wound surface by a preponderance of Gram-positive organisms (primarily staphylococci) changes to predominantly Gram-negative opportunistic organisms, particularly *Pseudomonas aeruginosa*. By the fifth postburn day, bacterial invasion is well under way beneath the surface of the burn wound. Early surgical excision of eschar together with placement of autografts reduces the incidence of sepsis.

EMERGENCY

Burns

Minor Burns

Stop the burning process:

- Apply cool water to the burn or hold the burned area under cool running water.
- Do not use ice.

Do not disturb any blisters that form, unless the injury is from a chemical substance.

Do not apply anything to the wound.

Cover with a clean cloth if risk of damage or contamination.

Remove burned clothing and jewellery.

Major Burns

Stop the burning process:

- Flame burns—smother the fire.
- Place victim in the horizontal position.
- Roll victim in a blanket or similar object; avoid covering the head.

Assess for an adequate airway and breathing.

If child is not breathing, begin mouth-to-mouth resuscitation.

Remove burned clothing and jewellery.

Cover wound with a clean cloth.

Keep victim warm.

Transport to medical aid.

Begin intravenous and oxygen therapy as prescribed.

Therapeutic Management

Emergency care. The initial management of the burn patient begins at the scene of injury. The first priority is to stop the burning process (see Emergency box). The child should then be transported immediately to the nearest medical facility for treatment and evaluation. The child and the family are usually extremely frightened and anxious; sensitivity to their emotional state and reassurance should be provided during the transport process.

Stop the burning process. The chief aim of rescue in flame burns is to smother the fire, not fan it. Children tend to panic and run, which spreads the flames and makes assistance more difficult. The injured child should be placed in a horizontal position and rolled in a blanket, rug, or similar article, with care taken not to cover the head and face because of the danger of inhalation of toxic fumes. If nothing is available, the victim should lie down and roll over slowly to extinguish the flames. Remaining in the vertical position may cause the hair to ignite or the inhalation of flames, heat, or smoke.

Major burns with large amounts of denuded skin should not be cooled. Heat is rapidly lost from burned areas, and additional cooling leads to a drop in core body temperature and potential circulatory collapse. Wet dressings also promote vasoconstriction because of cooling, resulting in impaired circulation to the burned area and increased tissue damage. Chemical burns require continuous flushing with large amounts of water before transport to a medical facility. The use of neutralizing agents on the skin is contraindicated, since a chemical reaction is initiated and further injury may result. If the chemical is in powder form, the addition of water may spread the caustic agent. The powder should be brushed off if possible before flushing the area.

Burned clothing is removed to prevent further damage from smouldering fabric and hot beads of melted synthetic materials. Jewellery is removed to eliminate the transfer of heat from the metal and constriction resulting from edema formation. This also provides access to the wound and prevents painful removal later.

Assess the victim's condition. As soon as the flames are extinguished, the child is assessed. Circulation, airway, and breathing (CAB) are the primary concerns. Cardiopulmonary complications may result from exposure to electric current, inhalation of toxic fumes and smoke, hypovolemia, and shock. Emergency measures are instituted as appropriate.

Cover the burn. The burn wound should be covered with a clean cloth to prevent contamination, decrease pain by eliminating air contact, and prevent hypothermia. No attempt should be made to treat the burn. Application of topical ointments, oils, or other home remedies is contraindicated.

Transport the child to medical aid. The child with an extensive burn is not given anything by mouth, to avoid aspiration in the presence of paralytic ileus and upper airway edema and to prevent water intoxication. The child is transported to the nearest medical facility. If this cannot be accomplished within a relatively short period, IV access should be established, if possible, with a large-bore catheter. Oxygen is administered, if available, at 100%. A report of the initial assessment and any interventions implemented is given to the medical facility assuming care of the child.

Provide reassurance. Providing reassurance and psychological support to both the family and the child helps immeasurably during the period of postinjury crisis. Reducing anxiety conserves energy the family and child will need to cope with the physiological and emotional stress of injury.

Minor burns. Treatment of burns classified as minor can usually be managed adequately on an outpatient basis when it is determined that the parent can be relied on to carry out instructions for care and observation. Patients with less than optimum circumstances may require close follow-up to ensure they are able to manage the treatment.

The wound is cleansed with a mild soap and tepid water. Debridement of the wound includes removal of any embedded debris, chemicals, and devitalized tissue. Removal of intact blisters remains controversial. Some authorities argue that blisters provide a barrier against infection; others maintain that blister fluid is an effective medium for the growth of microorganisms. However, blisters should be broken if the injury is due to a chemical agent to control absorption. Most practitioners favour covering the wound with an antimicrobial ointment to reduce the risk of infection and to provide some form of pain relief. The dressing consists of nonadherent fine-mesh gauze placed over the ointment and a light wrap of gauze dressing that avoids interference with movement. This helps keep the wound clean and protect it from trauma. The caregiver is instructed to wash the wound, reapply the dressing, and return the child to the office or clinic as directed for wound observation. The frequency of dressing changes may vary from every other day to once a day.

Some practitioners prefer an occlusive dressing, such as a hydrocolloid, which is placed over the wound after cleansing. Hydrogel dressings, which are soothing and nonadherent, may also be used. The dressing is changed when leakage occurs—at regular intervals or at least weekly. This method eliminates the discomfort associated with frequent dressing changes but impairs visualization of the wound surface.

If there is a high probability of infection or other complications or if there is doubt about the ability to carry out instructions, the caregiver may be directed to bring the patient in daily for dressing changes and inspection. Another option is to have a nurse make a home visit to inspect the wound and perform the dressing change. Frequent removal of the dressing is an effective mode of debridement. Soaking the dressing in tepid water or normal saline before removal helps loosen the dressing and debris and reduce discomfort. Burns of the face are usually treated by an open method. The wound is washed and debrided in the same manner, and a thin film of antimicrobial ointment is applied.

A tetanus history is obtained on admission. If there is no history of immunization, or if more than 5 years have passed since the last immunization, tetanus prophylaxis is administered. A mild analgesic such as acetaminophen is usually sufficient to relieve discomfort; the antipyretic effect of the medication also alleviates the sensation of heat.

Most minor burns heal without difficulty, but if the wound margin becomes erythematous, gross purulence is noted, or the child develops evidence of systemic reaction, such as fever or tachycardia, hospitalization is indicated. The child should also be evaluated for functional impairment, and the caregiver should be instructed in the exercise and ambulation program. After wound healing, an evaluation of scar maturation and range of motion will indicate any need for further therapy.

Major burns. The first priority is airway maintenance. Respiratory burns or the inhalation of noxious agents are suggested when there is a history of injury in an enclosed space; edema of the oral and nasal membranes; thermal injury to the face, nares, and upper torso; hyperemia; and blisters or evidence of trauma to the upper respiratory passages. When respiratory involvement is suspected or evident, 100% oxygen is administered and blood gas values, including carbon monoxide levels, are determined.

If the child exhibits changes in sensorium, air hunger, or other signs of respiratory distress, an endotracheal tube is inserted to maintain the airway. When severe edema of the face and neck is anticipated, intubation is performed before swelling makes intubation difficult or impossible. Controlled intubation is preferred to an emergency procedure. Intubation allows for the delivery of humidified oxygen, the removal of secretions from respiratory passages, and the provision of ventilatory support. When full-thickness burns encircle the chest, constricting eschar may limit chest wall excursion, and ventilation of the child becomes more difficult. Escharotomy of the chest relieves this constriction and improves ventilation.

Fluid replacement therapy. The objectives of fluid therapy are to (1) compensate for water and sodium lost to traumatized areas and interstitial spaces, (2) re-establish sodium balance, (3) restore circulating volume, (4) provide adequate perfusion, (5) correct acidosis, and (6) improve renal function.

Fluid replacement is required during the first 24 hours because of fluid shifts that occur after the injury. Various formulas are used to calculate fluid needs, and the one adopted depends on practitioner preference. Crystalloid solutions are used during this initial phase of therapy. Parameters such as vital signs (especially heart rate), urine output, adequacy of capillary filling, and state of sensorium determine adequacy of fluid resuscitation.

After the initial 24-hour period, theoretically there is a capillary seal, and capillary permeability is restored. Colloid solutions such as albumin, Plasma-Lyte, or fresh frozen plasma are useful in maintaining plasma volume. However, children with burn injuries usually require fluids in excess of their calculated maintenance and replacement volume. Reasons for this may include underestimation of burn size (particularly in pediatric patients), pulmonary injury that sequesters resuscitation fluid in the lung, electrical injury with greater tissue destruction than what is visible, and a delay in the initiation of fluid resuscitation. Irreversible burn shock that persists despite aggressive fluid resuscitation remains a significant cause of death in the immediate postburn period. Fluid balance may continue to be a problem throughout the course of treatment, especially when there is considerable evaporative loss from the wound.

Nutrition. The enhanced metabolic requirements and catabolism in severe burns make nutritional needs of paramount importance and often difficult to satisfy. To avoid protein breakdown, the diet must provide sufficient calories to meet the increased metabolic needs and enough protein. Hypoglycemia can result from the stress of the burn injury because the liver glycogen stores are rapidly depleted.

A high-protein, high-calorie diet is encouraged. Many children have poor appetites and are unable to meet energy requirements solely by oral feeding. Oral feedings are encouraged unless the child is intubated or has a paralytic ileus. Most children with burns in excess of 25% TBSA require supplementation with tube feeding. Early and continued nutritional support is an important part of therapy for seriously burned patients. Enteral feeding provides direct nourishment to the gastrointestinal tract and helps reverse the defective gut barrier that accompanies burn shock (Antoon & Donovan, 2016). Children who require enteral supplementation must be monitored for feeding intolerance and tube malposition. The nurse should also monitor and report any abdominal distension, diarrhea, or electrolyte, and metabolic deviations. If nutritional requirements cannot be met entirely by the enteral route, parenteral hyperalimentation is used to supplement intake. However, enteral feeding increases blood flow in the intestinal tract, preserves gastrointestinal function, and minimizes bacterial translocation by decreasing mucosal atrophy of the intestines. These factors make enteral feeding the preferred route of nutritional support (Herndon, 2012).

To facilitate growth and proliferation of epithelial cells, the administration of vitamins A and C is begun early in the postburn period. Zinc is also supplemented because of its important role in wound healing and epithelialization.

Medication. Antibiotics are usually not administered prophylactically. The administration of systemic antibiotics to control wound colonization is not indicated, since decreased circulation to the injured area prevents delivery of the medication to areas of deepest injury. Surveillance cultures and monitoring of the clinical course provide the most reliable indicators of developing infection. Appropriate antibiotics are instituted to treat the specific identified organism. Otitis media should not be overlooked as a source of fever in the pediatric population.

Some form of sedation and analgesia is required in the care of burned children. Morphine sulphate is the medication of choice for severe burn injuries. Morphine has extensive distribution but is metabolized rapidly; continuous infusion or frequent administration is needed for pain management in burns. Morphine is administered intravenously and titrated to individual need. The unstable circulatory status and edema formation preclude intramuscular or subcutaneous administration. When combined, midazolam (Versed) and fentanyl (Sublimaze) also provide excellent IV sedation and analgesia to control procedural pain in children with burns (Herndon, 2012). The oral form of fentanyl, Oralet, provides effective analgesia in a convenient form that children can suck. Dosage monitoring is important because tolerance to opioids may develop. IV analgesics are most effective when they are administered just before the onset of procedural pain.

The use of short-acting anaesthetic agents, such as propofol (Diprivan) and nitrous oxide, has proved beneficial in eliminating procedural pain. Pharyngeal reflexes remain intact, thus ensuring a patent airway. Propofol is an IV sedative hypnotic that produces sedation in less than 1 minute and lasts only a few minutes. Nitrous oxide is a useful short-term analgesic when given in a mixture of gases on a fixed ratio of 50% nitrous oxide and 50% oxygen. Initiation of action is approximately 1 minute, with peak effect reached in 3 to 5 minutes. Nitrous oxide is useful to alleviate anxiety and raise the threshold of pain during procedures. The child may self-administer the nitrous oxide mixture with assistance. For any conscious or unconscious sedation, the child must be monitored continuously during the procedure (see Preoperative Care, Chapter 44; and Pain Assessment and Pain Management, Chapter 34).

Management of the burn wound. After the initial period of shock and the restoration of fluid balance, the primary concern is the burn wound. The objectives of wound management include prevention of infection, removal of devitalized tissue, and closure of the wound. The application of dressings and topical antimicrobial therapy reduce pain by minimizing the exposure to air.

Primary excision. In children with large, full-thickness burn wounds, excision is performed as soon as the patient is hemodynamically stable after initial resuscitation. Because the burn wound precipitates an exaggerated physiological response, many complications do not resolve until the eschar is excised and the wound is closed. Early excision of deep partial- and full-thickness burns reduces the incidence of infection and the threat of sepsis.

Debridement. Partial-thickness wounds require debridement of devitalized tissue to promote healing. Debridement is painful and requires analgesia and a sedative before the procedure. Medications given for pain need to be readily available during this procedure and may need to be titrated upward during the procedure. Hydroxyzine and diphenhydramine are often needed for itching that occurs after whirlpool and debridement. The itching becomes particularly bothersome as the burns heal.

Hydrotherapy is employed to cleanse the wound and involves soaking in a tub or showering at least once a day for no more than 20 minutes. The water loosens and removes sloughing tissue, exudate, and topical medications. Hydrotherapy helps to cleanse not only the wound but also the entire body and aids in maintenance of range of motion. Mesh gauze entraps the exudative slough and is readily removed during hydrotherapy. Any loose tissue is carefully trimmed away before the wound is redressed.

Topical antimicrobial medications. Methods used for managing the burn wound include the following:

Exposure—Wounds are left open to air; crust forms on partial-thickness wounds, and eschar forms on full-thickness burns.

Open—Topical antimicrobial medication is applied directly to the wound surface and the wound is left uncovered.

Modified—Antimicrobial medication is applied directly or impregnated into thin gauze and applied to the wound; gauze or net secures the area.

Occlusive—Antimicrobial medication is impregnated in gauze or applied directly to the wound; multiple layers of bulky gauze are placed over the primary layer and secured with gauze or net.

All of these methods provide wound coverage and employ some type of topical agent. Topical medications do not eliminate organisms from the wound but can effectively inhibit bacterial growth. To be effective, a topical application must be nontoxic, capable of diffusing through eschar, harmless to viable tissue, inexpensive, and easy to apply. A topical ointment should not encourage the development of resistant strains of bacteria and should produce minimal electrolyte derangement. A variety of specific agents are available; examples include Bacitracin, silver sulfadiazine (Thermazene), collagenase (Santyl), and mafenide acetate (Sulfamylon). Some topical agents are packaged and prepared on a fine-meshed gauze that allows ease of application. The gauze provides necessary protection for the wound, maximizes patient comfort, increases rate of healing, decreases the necessity for frequent dressing changes, and is cost effective. Examples include a nanocrystalline film of pure silver (Acticoat), a hydrofibre with ionic silver (Aquacel Ag), a flexible nylon mesh matrix with oat-beta glucan and silver (Glucan Silver Matrix), and a silicone foam dressing with silver (Mepilex Ag).

Biological skin coverings. Permanent coverage of extensive burns is a prolonged process that requires repeated operative procedures using general anaesthesia for atraumatic care in debridement and grafting. Early closure shortens the period of metabolic stress and decreases the likelihood of burn wound sepsis. In the acute phase, biological dressings cover and protect the wound from contamination, reduce fluid and protein loss, increase the rate of epithelialization, reduce pain, and facilitate movement of joints to retain range of motion.

Allograft (homograft) skin is obtained from human cadavers that are screened for communicable diseases. Allograft is particularly useful in the coverage of surgically excised deep partial- and full-thickness wounds in extensive burns when available donor sites are limited. Severe immunosuppression occurs in massively burned children, and the allograft becomes adherent. The allograft can remain in place until suitable donor sites become available. Typically, rejection is seen approximately 3 to 4 weeks after application (Antoon & Donovan, 2016). The insufficient availability of tissue banks and suitable donors limits the use of allografts.

Xenograft from a variety of species, most notably pigs, is commercially available. In large burns, the porcine xenograft is commonly applied when extensive early debridement is indicated to cover a partial-thickness burn; this provides a temporary covering for the wound until an available autograft can be applied to the full-thickness areas (Antoon & Donovan, 2016). Pigskin dressings are replaced every 1 to 3 days. They are particularly effective in children with partial-thickness scald burns of the hands and face because they allow relatively pain-free movement, which reduces contracture formation and has the added benefit of improving appetite and morale.

When applied early to a superficial partial-thickness injury, biological dressings stimulate epithelial growth and faster wound healing. However, biological dressings must be applied to clean wounds. If the dressing covers areas of heavy microbial contamination, infection occurs beneath the dressing. In the case of partial-thickness burns, such infection may convert the wound to a full-thickness injury.

Synthetic skin coverings are available for the management of partial-thickness burn wounds. Ideally, the dressing should provide the properties of human skin: adherence, elasticity, durability, and hemostasis. Synthetic skin substitutes are readily available, have an indefinite shelf life, and are relatively inexpensive. Synthetic dressings are composed of a variety of materials and can be used successfully in the management of superficial partial-thickness burns and donor sites. Examples include adherent elastic films; hydroactive materials; or colloidal suspensions that are usually permeable to air, vapour, and fluids.

Biobrane is a flexible silicone-nylon membrane bonded to collagenous peptides of porcine skin. Calcium alginate is another treatment for donor sites. As with biological dressings,

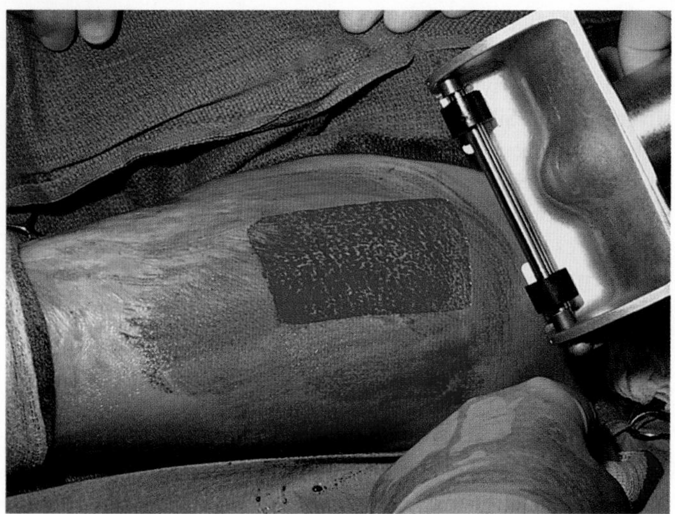

FIGURE 52-19 Removal of split-thickness skin graft with a dermatome.

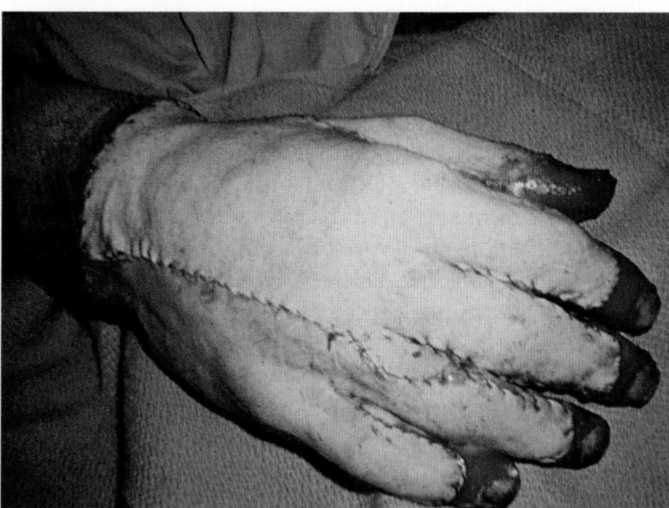

FIGURE 52-20 Sheet graft.

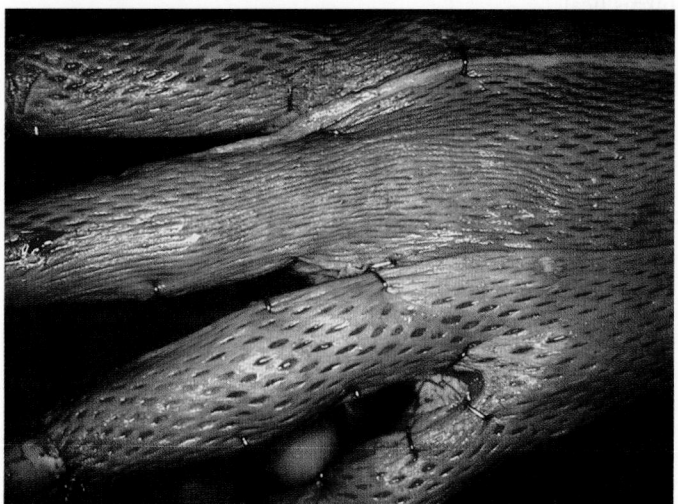

FIGURE 52-21 Mesh graft.

it is important that the wound be free of debris before the dressing is applied. Body temperature elevation or evidence of purulence, erythema, or cellulitis around the wound edges may indicate that the wound has become infected beneath the dressing. If this occurs, prompt discontinuance of the synthetic dressing is indicated. All synthetic dressings are reputed to hasten wound healing and reduce discomfort.

Permanent skin coverings. Permanent coverage of deep partial- and full-thickness burns is usually accomplished with a split-thickness skin graft. This graft consists of the epidermis and a portion of the dermis removed from an intact area of skin by a special instrument, the *dermatome* (Fig. 52-19). With extensive burns it is often difficult to find enough viable skin to cover the wounds; therefore, available donor sites and special techniques are used. Split-thickness skin grafts may be sheet graft or mesh graft.

Sheet graft. A sheet of skin, removed from the donor site, is placed intact over the recipient site and sutured in place; this is used in areas where cosmetic results are most visible (Fig. 52-20).

Mesh graft. A sheet of skin is removed from the donor site and passed through a mesher, which produces tiny slits in the skin that allow the skin to cover 1.5 to 9 times the area of the sheet graft; this results in a less desirable cosmetic and functional outcome (Fig. 52-21).

The donor site is dressed with synthetic wound coverings or fine-mesh gauze until the dressing separates at 10 to 14 days, when the wound is healed. Dressings are not changed on donor sites to avoid damage to newly healed, delicate epithelium. Healed donor sites are available for reharvesting in patients with extensive burns and limited undamaged skin, but the quality of skin is decreased when multiple grafts are taken.

Artificial skin. The development of Integra, a product that allows the dermis to regenerate, has produced significant improvement in burn wound healing and decreased scar formation. It is applied to partial- and full-thickness burns. The two-layer membrane is made of collagen (a fibrous protein from animal tendons and cartilage) and silicone rubber (i.e., Silastic). The Silastic layer is peeled off after the dermis is formed. The application of artificial skin does not replace the grafting procedure, but it prepares the burn wound to accept an ultrathin autograft. Advantages include faster healing of the burn wound when integrity of the dermis is restored, faster healing of donor sites with the use of ultrathin grafts, and restoration of sweat glands and hair follicles. A disadvantage is its high cost.

Cultured epithelium. When burns are extensive and donor sites for split-thickness skin grafting are limited, it is possible to culture cells from a full-thickness skin biopsy and produce coherent sheets that can be applied to clean, excised full-thickness wounds. Epithelial cell culture grafts offer the possibility of an unlimited source of autograph in patients with extensive burns. Cultured epithelial auto grafts are effective in early wound closure. The child's own skin is fractionated and cultured in a porcine media to form a thin epithelial layer that is applied to the burn wound. This technique offers an improved rate of survival in patients with extensive burns and limited donor sites.

Prognosis

Children differ from adults in their responses to thermal injury, and the mortality rates in young children are significantly higher than those in older children and adults. Mortality is greatest for children younger than 48 months of age. Many children who do survive have long-term functional and cosmetic impairments.

NURSING CARE

Because the care of burned children encompasses a broad range of skills, nursing care has been divided into segments that correspond with the major phases of burn treatment. The *acute phase*, also referred to as the *emergent* or *resuscitative phase*, involves the first 24 to 48 hours. The *management phase* extends from the completion of adequate resuscitation through wound coverage. The *rehabilitative phase* begins once the majority of the wounds have healed and rehabilitation has become the predominant focus of the care plan. This phase continues until all reconstructive procedures and corrective measures are accomplished (often a period of months or years).

Acute Phase

The primary emphasis during the emergent phase is the treatment of burn shock and the management of pulmonary status. Monitoring vital signs, output, fluid infusion, and respiratory parameters are ongoing activities in the hours immediately after injury. IV infusion is begun immediately and is regulated to maintain a urine output of at least 1 to 2 mL/kg in children weighing less than 30 kg; an output of 30 to 50 mL/hr is expected in children weighing more than 30 kg. Urine output and specific gravity, vital signs, laboratory data, and objective signs of adequate hydration guide the rate of fluid administration.

Children who are hospitalized with burns require constant observation and assessment for complications. Alterations in electrolyte balance produce clinical symptoms of confusion, weakness, cardiac irregularities, and seizures. Changes in respiratory function and gas exchange are reflected clinically by restlessness, irritability, increased work of breathing, and alterations in blood gas values. The loss of protective function of the skin exposes burned children to increased risk of hypothermia. Edema formation and circulatory impairment result in the loss of sensation and deep throbbing pain.

! NURSING ALERT

Evaluate the burned extremity and check the pulse every hour. If unable to palpate, use Doppler to ascertain loss of circulation and pulse. If the pulse is lost, escharotomy may be necessary to relieve the edema causing pressure on blood vessels, to restore adequate circulation.

Burn units maintain a pictorial record of the wound to record progress and for legal purposes (if child abuse is suspected). The burn wound is treated according to the protocol of the specific burn facility.

Throughout the acute phase of care, the psychosocial needs of the children and their families should not be overlooked. The child is frightened, uncomfortable, and often confused. Children may be isolated from familiar persons and surroundings; the overwhelming physical needs at this time are the primary focus of the staff and parents. In addition to feeling concern for their child, the family may experience guilt, which may be related to the fact that the parents did not or could not protect their child from injury. Consistency in the information presented and in the staff's attitude can create a sense of familiarity and stability during the acute phase of care. Consistent caregivers can also help decrease the patient's and family's anxiety and provide coordination of care. For example, when many teams of consultants and specialists are involved in the child's care, appointing one "spokesperson" decreases the confusion and enhances communication regarding the child's care.

Management and Rehabilitative Phases

After the patient's condition is stabilized, the management phase begins. The multidisciplinary team concentrates on preventing wound infections, closing the wound as quickly as possible, and managing the numerous complications. Although the rehabilitative phase begins when permanent wound closure has been achieved, rehabilitation issues are identified on admission and are included in the care plan throughout the hospital course.

Comfort Management

The severe pain of the wound and resultant therapies, the anxiety generated by these experiences, sleep deprivation, itching related to wound healing, and the conscious and unconscious interpretations of traumatic events contribute to the psychological behaviours commonly observed in children with burns. It is always difficult to deal with a child in pain, and inflicting pain on a helpless child is contrary to the empathic nature of nursing. Interventions to promote comfort may include medications (including IV morphine, fentanyl, or midazolam and short-term anaesthetics such as propofol), relaxation techniques, distraction therapy, behavioural techniques, operant conditioning such as tokens, star chart, and family participation.

Children need age-appropriate explanations before all procedures. As stated earlier, consistency in caregivers is important. If this is not possible, a carefully developed, multidisciplinary care plan is necessary to provide consistency.

Care of the Burn Wound

The nurse has a major responsibility for cleansing, debriding, and applying topical medications and dressings to the burn wound. Pain medication should be administered so that the peak effect of the drug coincides with the procedure. Children who have an understanding of the procedure to be performed

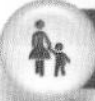

ATRAUMATIC CARE

Reducing the Stress of Burn Care Procedures

- Have all materials ready before beginning.
- Administer appropriate analgesics and sedatives.
- Remind the child of the impending procedure to allow sufficient time to prepare.
- Allow the child to test and approve the temperature of the water.
- Allow the child to select the area of the body on which to begin.
- Allow the child to request a short rest period during the procedure.
- Allow the child to remove the dressings if desired.
- Provide something constructive for the child to do during the procedure (e.g., holding a package of dressings or a roll of gauze).
- Inform the child when the procedure is near completion.
- Praise the child for their assistance.

and some perceived control demonstrate less anxious behaviour. Children also respond well to participating in decisions (see Atraumatic Care box).

Outer dressings are removed. Any dressings that have adhered to the wound can be more easily removed by applying tepid water or normal saline. Loose or easily detached tissue is debrided during the cleansing process. In dressing the wound, it is important that all areas be clean, that medication be amply applied, and that no two burned surfaces touch each other, such as fingers or toes, or ears touching the side of the head. If they are touching, the burned surfaces will heal together, causing deformity or dysfunction.

Topical medications may be applied directly to the wound with a tongue blade or gloved hand or impregnated into fine-mesh gauze before application. Dressings are then applied to assist in exudate absorption, wound debridement, and increased patient comfort. All dressings applied circumferentially should be wrapped in a distal-to-proximal manner. The dressing is applied with sufficient tension to remain in place but not so tightly as to impair circulation or limit motion. Elastic net or bandages are applied over dressings to prevent epithelial breakdown, decrease edema, stimulate circulation, and improve mobility. A stable dressing is especially important when the child is ambulatory.

Routine precautions, including the use of protective garments and barrier techniques, should be followed when caring for patients with thermal injuries. Frequent hand hygiene, including of the forearm, are the single most important elements of the infection control program. Strict policies for cleaning the environment and patient care equipment should be implemented to minimize the risk of cross-contamination. All visitors and members of other departments should be oriented to the infection control policies, including the importance of hand hygiene and forearm washing and use of protective garb. Visitors should be screened for infection and contagious diseases before patient contact.

Prevention of Complications

Acute care. The maintenance of body temperature is important to the child with burns. Core body temperature is supported when energy is conserved with an environmental temperature of 28° to 33°C. Large areas of the body should not be exposed simultaneously during dressing changes. Warmed solutions, linens, occlusive dressings, heat shields, a radiant warmer, and warming blankets assist in preventing hypothermia.

The chief danger during acute care is infection—wound infection, generalized sepsis, or bacterial pneumonia. Accurate and ongoing assessments of all parameters that provide clues to the early diagnosis and treatment of infection are essential. Symptoms of sepsis include a decreasing level of consciousness, a rising or falling white blood cell count, hyperthermia progressing to hypothermia, increasing fluid requirements, hypoactive or absent bowel sounds, a rising or falling blood glucose level, tachycardia, tachypnea, and thrombocytopenia. Infection delays the loss of the progression of wound healing.

Children are reluctant to move if movement causes pain, and they are likely to assume a position of comfort. Unfortunately, the most comfortable position often encourages the formation of contractures and loss of function. Ongoing efforts to prevent contractures include maintaining proper body alignment, positioning and splinting involved extremities in extension, providing active and passive physical therapy, and encouraging spontaneous movement when feasible. Frequent position changes are important to promote adequate bronchopulmonary hygiene and capillary perfusion to common pressure areas. Low–air loss beds are beneficial for the morbidly obese or children with posterior grafts. Special attention should be given to areas at risk for increased pressure, such as the posterior scalp, heels, sacrum, and areas exposed to mechanical irritation from splints and dressings.

Long-term care. The rehabilitative phase of care begins once wound coverage is achieved. Scar formation becomes a major problem as burn wounds heal (Fig. 52-22). Contractile properties of the scar tissue can result in disabling contractures, deformity, and disfigurement.

Uniform pressure applied to the scar decreases the blood supply. When pressure is removed, blood supply to the scar is immediately increased; therefore, periods without pressure should be brief to avoid nourishment of the hypertrophic tissue. Continuous pressure to areas of scarring can be achieved by use of elastic bandages or commercially available pressure garments. Because these custom-made garments are often worn for months, revisions may be required as the child grows. It is much easier to prevent scarring and contracture of the wound than to resolve an existing problem. Splints and appliances may also be needed until wound maturation is achieved (Fig. 52-23).

Scar tissue has certain significant properties, particularly for growing children. Intense itching occurs in healing burn wounds and scar tissue until the scar is no longer active. Itching is usually treated with $H_1$and H_2 antagonists such as cetirizine and cimetidine (Tagamet); an H_1 antagonist alone; and frequent applications of a moisturizer, such as Vaseline Intensive Care Rescue, Aveeno Baby, Alpha Keri, or Eucerin. Massage therapy during the application of moisturizers is also beneficial to stretch scar tissue and aid in contracture prevention. Scar tissue has no sweat glands, and children with extensive scarring may

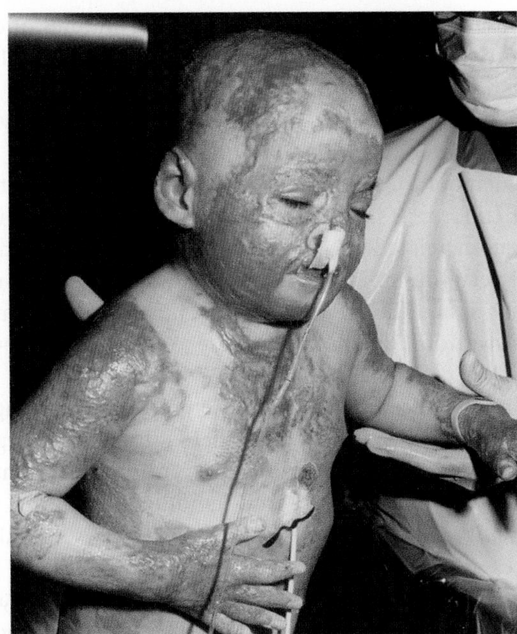

FIGURE 52-22 Extensive scars from flame burn. (Courtesy The Paul and Carol David Foundation Burn Institute, Akron, Ohio.)

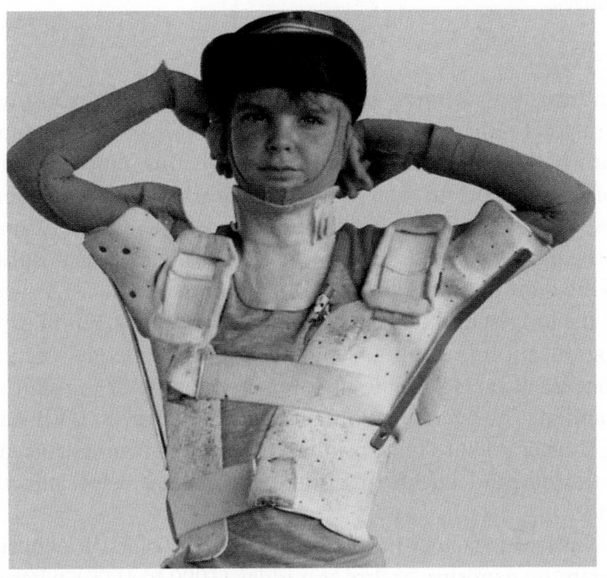

FIGURE 52-23 Child in elasticized (Jobst) garment and "airplane" splints.

experience difficulty during hot weather. Caregivers should be alerted to this possibility and be prepared to institute alternative methods of cooling when necessary.

Scar tissue does not grow and expand as normal tissue does, which may create difficulties, especially in functional areas such as on the hands and over joints. Additional surgery is sometimes required to allow independent functioning in daily activities, to improve cosmetic appearance, or to restore anatomical integrity.

The nursing activities in the rehabilitative phase of treatment focus on the child's and family's adaptation to the burn injury and their ability to transition back into home and family life. The psychological pain and sequelae of severe burn injury are as intense as the physical trauma. The impact of severe burns taxes the coping mechanisms at all ages. Very young children, who suffer acutely from separation anxiety, and adolescents, who are developing an identity, are probably most affected psychologically. Toddlers cannot understand why the parents they love and who have protected them can leave them in such a frightening and unfamiliar place. Adolescents, in the process of achieving independence from the family, find themselves in a dependent role with a damaged body. Being different from others at a time when conformity with peers is so important is difficult to accept.

Anticipation of the return to school can be overwhelming and frightening. It is essential that health care providers recognize the importance of preparing teachers and classmates for the child's return. Teachers need to be provided with information to assist the child and family and to promote the child's optimal adjustment. Hospital-sponsored school re-entry programs use a variety of methods to provide education and information about the implications of the injury, the garments and appliances, and the need for support and acceptance. Telephone calls, emails, videos, information packets, and visits by members of the health care team offer opportunities to help with reintegration into the school environment—a focal point of the child's life.

Psychosocial Support of the Child

Children should begin early to do as much for themselves as possible and to be active participants in their care. Loss of control and perceived helplessness may result in acting-out behaviours. During illness, children regress to a previous developmental level that allows them to deal with stress. As children begin to participate in their care, they gain confidence and self-esteem. Fears and anxieties diminish with accomplishment and self-confidence. If the child demonstrates nonadherence in the rehabilitative phase, a behaviour modification program can be initiated to promote or reward the child's accomplishment in care.

Children need to know that their injury and the treatments are not punishment for real or imagined transgressions and that the nurse understands their fear, anger, and discomfort. They also need body contact. This is often difficult to arrange for the child with massive burns. Stroking areas of unburned skin is comforting. Even older children enjoy sitting on the parent's lap and being cuddled and hugged. This can be a reward or a comfort in times of stress, but most of all it should be kept in mind that it is a natural part of childhood.

Psychosocial Support of the Family

Recognizing and respecting each family's strengths, differences, and methods of coping allows the nurse to respond to their unique needs by implementing a family-centred approach to care. In the acute phase, all attention is focused on the child, and the parents feel powerless and ineffectual. Most parents feel overwhelming guilt, whether or not the guilt is justified. They feel responsible for the injury. These feelings may impede the child's rehabilitation. Parents may indulge the child and allow noncompliant behaviours that affect physical and emotional recovery. Parents need to be informed of the child's progress and helped to cope with their feelings while supporting their child. The nurse can help them understand that it is not selfish to look after themselves and their own needs to meet their child's needs. It is important to recognize the parents' need to grieve the change in their child's normal appearance. Professional psychological help may be needed for parents whose response to the injury is severe or whose response to stress is manifested in destructive behaviour.

The parents are members of the multidisciplinary team and participate in the development of the care plan. It is important to facilitate their input; to consider all aspects of the physical, emotional, social, and cultural factors affecting the child and family; and to establish a realistic home therapy program. The family's willingness to assume responsibility for care and their ability to implement the therapeutic regimen needs to be assessed. Home, school, and other environmental factors should be explored; financial concerns and available community resources discussed; and a specific care plan for the child, with an anticipated follow-up program, developed.

Prevention of Burn Injuries

The best intervention is to prevent burns from occurring. Hot liquids in the kitchen and bathroom most commonly injure infants and toddlers. Hot liquids should be kept out of reach; tablecloths and dangling appliance cords are often pulled by toddlers, who spill hot grease and liquids on themselves. Electrical cords and outlets represent a potential risk to small children, who may chew on accessible cords and insert objects into outlets.

Parachute Canada (2015) recommends a reduction of water heater thermostats to a medium setting. The "dial-down" recommendation has been suggested by utility companies, burn treatment centres, medical personnel, and others interested in public safety. However, many water heaters continue to remain set at levels well above the safe level. It is important to not lower the temperature of the water heater below 49°C or a medium setting if it is a gas heater and not below 60°C if it is an electric heater. A lower setting can lead to the growth of the bacteria that causes Legionnaires' disease.

Small children are especially at risk for scald injuries from hot tap water because of their decreased reaction time and agility, their curiosity, and the thermal sensitivity of their skin. Caregivers should never leave a child unattended in a bath and without adult supervision. Water should always be tested before a child is placed in the tub or shower.

The increased use of microwave ovens has resulted in burn injuries from the extremely hot internal temperatures generated in heated items. Baby formula, jelly-filled pastries, and hot liquids and dishes may result in cutaneous scalds or the ingestion of overheated liquids. Parents should use caution when removing items from the microwave oven and should always test the food before giving it to children.

Barriers should be placed around the glass doors on gas fireplaces, and wood and pellet stoves. Fireplace doors can reach dangerous temperatures of 245°C in about 6 minutes, and it can take approximately 45 minutes before cooling down after the fireplace has been shut off.

As children mature, risk-taking behaviours increase. Matches and lighters are dangerous in the hands of the young. Adults must remember to keep potentially hazardous items out of the reach of children; a lighter, like a match, is a tool for adult use.

Education related to fire safety and survival should begin with the very young. They can practise "stop, drop, and roll" to extinguish a fire. The fire escape route, including a safe meeting place away from the home in case of fire, also should be practised.

Community activities are also helpful in supporting burn survivors and preventing burns. There are different organizations that provide important burn prevention educational programs as well as financial and emotional support to the children with burn injuries and their families (see Additional Resources at the end of this chapter). An example is TOMA Foundation for Burned Children, which is a Canadian and American organization of firefighters who fundraise and work with interdisciplinary health care providers to provide support to burn victims and their families. There are also burn camps in most of the provinces for children who have sustained burn injuries.

Sunburn

Sunburn is a common skin injury caused by overexposure to ultraviolet radiation (UVR). The sun emits a continuous spectrum of visible and nonvisible light rays that range in length from very short to very long. The shorter, higher-frequency waves are more damaging than longer wavelengths, but much of the light is filtered out as it travels through the atmosphere. Of the light that does filter through, *ultraviolet A (UVA)* waves are the longest and cause only minimum burning, but they play a significant role in photosensitive and photoallergic reactions. They are also responsible for premature aging of the skin and potentiate the effects of *ultraviolet B (UVB)* waves. UVB waves are shorter and are responsible for tanning, burning, and most of the harmful effects attributed to sunlight, especially skin cancer.

Numerous factors influence the amount of UVR exposure. Maximum exposure occurs at midday (1000 to 1600), when the distance from the sun to a given spot on the earth is shortest. There is more exposure at higher altitudes and near the equator, and less when the sky is hazy (although the amount of UVR that does penetrate is easily underestimated). Window glass effectively screens out UVB but not UVA rays. Fresh snow, water, and sand reflect UVR, especially when the sun is directly overhead.

Sunburn is usually an epidermal burn, although severe sunburn can be a partial-thickness burn with blister formation. Treatment of sunburn involves stopping the burning process, decreasing the inflammatory response, and rehydrating the skin. Local application of cool tap water soaks, or immersion in a tepid-water bath (temperature slightly below 36.7°C for 20 minutes or until the skin is cool), limits tissue destruction and relieves the discomfort. After the cool applications, a bland oil-in-water moisturizing lotion can be applied. Partial-thickness sunburns are treated the same as those from any heat source (see earlier discussion on burns).

NURSING CARE

Protection from sunburn is the major goal of management, and the harmful effects of the sun on the delicate skin of infants and children are currently receiving increased attention. To protect skin exposed to the sun for extended periods, skin should be covered with clothing and a broad-spectrum sunscreen should be applied. Children with fair skin, who usually burn and do not easily tan when out in the sun, or children with blond or red hair, freckles, or many moles, are at greatest risk of sun damage (Canadian Dermatology Association, 2016c).

The Canadian Dermatology Association (2016c) recommends that babies under 1 year of age be kept out of direct sunlight and in the shade or under cover; all children should wear wide-brimmed hats and loose-fitting clothing. Children should be taught how to find and go to shady locations, and all children should wear sunglasses with 100% UV protection and wraparound style. Canadian Dermatology Association–approved sun protection agents should be applied.

Two types of products are available for sun protection: *topical sunscreens*, which partially absorb UVR, and *sun blockers*, which block out UVR by reflecting sunlight. The most frequently recommended sun blockers are zinc oxide and titanium dioxide ointments. Sunscreens are products containing an SPF based on an evaluation of its effectiveness against UVR. The SPF is a number, such as 15, which indicates that if individuals normally burn in 10 minutes without a sunscreen, use of a sunscreen with SPF 15 allows them to remain in the sun 15 times 10, or 150 minutes (2½ hours) before acquiring the same degree of burns. The most effective sunscreens against UVB are p-aminobenzoic acid (PABA) and PABA-esters. However, many individuals are allergic to PABA, and sunscreens without PABA are encouraged to prevent these reactions in children. The Canadian Dermatology Association provides an approved list of sunscreens on their website (see Additional Resources at the end of this chapter); approved products have the Canadian Dermatology Association logo on them. The Canadian Dermatology Association (2016c) also recommends use of a sunscreen that protects against UVA and UVB, with SPF 30 or higher, but if a child develops a burn with SPF 30, the parent should try a higher SPF. Sunscreen should not be applied around a child's eyes, as it may sting and burn. Swimmers should use water-resistant sunscreens, and children can wear sun-protective bathing suits to protect their skin while swimming. Sunscreens should be applied liberally to a child's skin; lip balm with SPF 30 should be applied to a child's lips. As well, parents can work together with the day care centre for sun protection.

Sunscreens should be applied evenly to all exposed areas, with special attention to skin folds and areas that might become exposed as clothing shifts. Parents need to read labels of sunscreen products carefully for the SPF and follow the manufacturer's directions for application.

> **! NURSING ALERT**
>
> Infants should be kept out of the sun or physically shaded from it. Infants should be covered as much as possible with tightly woven fabric, such as cotton, when in the sun. Small amounts of sunscreen can be applied to sun-exposed skin, such as on the back of the hands and face, in small amounts (Canadian Dermatology Association, 2016c).

Individuals who work in the community, such as teachers, day care workers, coaches, and youth-group leaders, as well as relatives should all be made aware of sun safety for children. Sunscreens must be applied *liberally and frequently*.

The increased incidence of indoor tanning beds is of particular concern for nurses and health teaching and promotion. Teenagers are frequent visitors to tanning parlours; the majority of the users are females. The incidence of cutaneous malignant melanoma (CMM) has increased more than threefold in the last 35 years (Taddeo, Stanwick, & CPS, Adolescent Health Committee, 2012/2016). Skin damage is cumulative, and the full impact and scope of damage caused by year-round indoor tanning may take years to develop into certain skin cancers. Ontario and other provinces have banned the use of commercial tanning facilities by children and youth under the age of 18 (Taddeo et al., 2012/2016).

Cold Injury

In cold injuries the nature of the body's heat-regulating mechanisms is such that the inner portion of the body, or *core*, produces heat, and the periphery, or outer area, conserves or dissipates heat. When the body attempts to conserve heat, the outer tissues are subjected to low temperatures, and local trauma may result.

Chilblain, redness and swelling of the skin, occurs when extremities, usually the hands, are exposed to cold temperatures and moisture. The response may vary but is characterized by intense vasodilation that increases the temperature of involved tissues above that of unaffected tissue and produces edematous, reddish blue patches that itch and burn. As warming takes place, the sensations become more intense, but ordinarily they subside in a few days.

Frostbite is the term used to describe tissue damage caused when excessive heat loss to local tissues allows ice crystals to form in tissues. The frostbitten part appears white or blanched, feels solid, and is without sensation. Rapid rewarming is associated with less tissue necrosis than slow thawing. It restores blood flow and shortens the period of cellular damage. Rewarming produces a flush (sometimes deep purple) and a return of sensation, which is extremely painful. Large blisters may appear in 24 to 48 hours after rewarming and begin to reabsorb within 5 to 10 days, followed by the formation of a hard black eschar. Superficial injury often heals without incident. Rewarming is accomplished by immersing the part in well-agitated water at 37.8° to 42.2°C. Discomfort is managed with analgesics and sedatives. Care of blistered skin is similar to that described for burns. It is seldom possible to estimate the extent of tissue loss until new skin layers are revealed after the eschar layer separates.

KEY POINTS

- A variety of factors can produce lesions of the skin.
- It is important for nurses to be able to describe skin lesions accurately.
- A moist environment promotes wound healing.
- Bacterial, viral, and fungal infections are common in childhood.
- Some skin diseases are transmitted by arthropod vectors, especially ticks.
- The most common skin infestations of childhood—scabies and pediculosis capitis— affect children of any age and from any social class.
- Contact dermatitis may involve a primary irritant or a sensitizing agent.
- Adverse reactions to medications are manifested more often in the skin than in any other body organ.
- The most common skin disorders of infancy are diaper dermatitis, seborrheic dermatitis, and AD.
- Acne, a disorder affecting many adolescents, is related to hormonal fluctuation, stimulation of the sebaceous glands, excessive sebum production, the formation of comedones, and the overgrowth of the *P. acnes* organism.
- Medication and gentle facial cleansing are the treatments of choice for acne.
- Burns are caused by thermal, chemical, electric, or radioactive agents.
- Burns are assessed on the extent, depth, and severity of the wound.
- Essentials of emergency care of burn injury include stopping the burning process, covering the burn, transporting the injured child to medical aid, and providing reassurance to the child and family.
- Management of minor burns consists of facilitating wound healing, relieving discomfort, and preventing complications.
- Management of major burns consists of facilitating wound healing, relieving discomfort, replacing destroyed skin, preventing or treating complications, and providing rehabilitation.
- Sunscreen is recommended for use when the skin is exposed to the damaging effects of the sun's rays.
- Thermal injuries to the skin can result from exposure to extreme cold.

evolve WEBSITE

Visit the Evolve website for additional resources related to the content in this chapter such as Case Studies, Critical Thinking Case Study Answers, Nursing Care Plans, Nursing Processes, Nursing Skills, and Review Questions for Exam Preparation at: *http://evolve.elsevier.com/Canada/Perry/maternal/*

REFERENCES

Alanne, S., Nermes, M., Söderlund, R., et al. (2011). Quality of life in infants with atopic dermatitis and healthy infants: A follow-up from birth to 24 months. *Acta Pediatrics, 100*(8), e65–e70.

American Academy of Pediatrics (AAP). (2015). Lyme disease (*Lyme borreliosis, Borrelia burgdorferi* infection). In D. W. Kimberlin, M. T. Brady, M. A. Jackson, et al. (Eds.), *Red Book: 2015 report of the Committee on Infectious Diseases* (30th ed.). Elk Grove Village, IL: Author.

Antoon, A. Y., & Donovan, M. K. (2016). Burn injuries. In R. M. Kliegman, B. M. Stanton, J. S. Geme, et al. (Eds.), *Nelson textbook of pediatrics* (20th ed.). Philadelphia: Saunders.

Banerji, A., & Canadian Paediatric Society, First Nations, Inuit and Métis Health Committee. (2015). Scabies. *Paediatrics & Child Health, 20*(7), 395–398. Retrieved from <http://www.cps.ca/en/documents/position/scabies>.

Canadian Dermatology Association. (2016a). *Childhood eczema.* Retrieved from <http://www.dermatology.ca/skin-hair-nails/skin/eczema/#!/skin-hair-nails/skin/eczema/childhood-eczema/>.

Canadian Dermatology Association. (2016b). *Acne.* Retrieved from <http://www.dermatology.ca/skin-hair-nails/skin/acne/>.

Canadian Dermatology Association. (2016c). *Protecting your family.* Retrieved from <http://www.dermatology.ca/programs-resources/resources/sun-safety/protecting-your-family/>.

Doss, N., Kamoun, M. R., Dubertret, L., et al. (2010). Efficacy of tacrolimus 0.03% as second-line treatment for children with moderate-to-severe atopic dermatitis: Evidence from a randomized, double-blind non-inferiority trial vs. fluticasone 0.005% ointment. *Pediatric Allergy and Immunology, 21*(2 Pt. 1), 321–329.

Finlay, J., MacDonald, F. E., & Canadian Paediatric Society, Infectious Diseases and Immunization Committee. (2008). Head lice infestations: A clinical update. *Paediatrics & Child Health, 13*(8), 692–696. Retrieved from <http://www.cps.ca/documents/position/head-lice> Reaffirmed 2016.

Fisher, R. G., Chain, R. L., Hair, P. S., et al. (2008). Hypochlorite killing of community-acquired methicillin-resistant *Staphylococcus aureus* infections in children. *Pediatric Infectious Disease Journal, 27*(10), 934–935. doi:10.1097/INF.0b013e318175d871.

Government of Canada. (2013). *Poison ivy.* Retrieved from <http://healthycanadians.gc.ca/healthy-living-vie-saine/environment-environnement/home-maison/poisonivy-herbepuce-eng.php?_ga=1.253060992.868197850.1432519476>.

Government of Canada. (2015). *Bedbugs—What are they?* Retrieved from <http://www.healthycanadians.gc.ca/product-safety-securite-produits/pest-control-products-produits-antiparasitaires/pesticides/tips-conseils/bedbugs-punaises-lits-eng.php>.

Government of Canada. (2016a). *Lyme disease.* Retrieved from <http://healthycanadians.gc.ca/diseases-conditions-maladies-affections/disease-maladie/lyme/index-eng.php>.

Government of Canada. (2016b). *West Nile virus.* Retrieved from <http://www.phac-aspc.gc.ca/id-mi/westnile-virusnil-eng.php>.

Hanna, M., & Barankin, B. (2015). *What's new in acne treatment in Canada?* Retrieved from <http://www.skintherapyletter.com/fp/2012/8.1/2.html>.

Herndon, D. N. (Ed.). (2012). *Total burn care* (4th ed.). London: Saunders.

Huang, J., Abrams, M., Tlougan, B., et al. (2009). Treatment of *Staphylococcus aureus* colonization in atopic dermatitis decreases disease severity. *Pediatrics, 123*(5), e808–e814. doi:10.1542/peds.2008-2217.

Irvine, J., & Canadian Paediatric Society, First Nations, Inuit and Métis Health Committee. (2012). Community-associated methicillin-resistant *Staphylococcus aureus* in Indigenous communities in Canada. *Paediatrics & Child Health, 17*(7), 385–386. Retrieved from <http://www.cps.ca/documents/position/community-associated-MRSA-in-Indigenous-communities> Reaffirmed 2015.

Kaplan, S. L. (2008). Commentary: Prevention of recurrent staphylococcal infections. *Pediatric Infectious Diseases Journal, 27*(10), 935–937. doi:10.1097/INF.0b013e31818632b3.

Kaye, A. E., Bela, J. M., & Kirschner, R. E. (2009). Pediatric dog bite injuries: A 4 year review of experience at Children's Hospital of Philadelphia. *Plastic Reconstructive Surgery, 124*(2), 551–558.

Kim, R. H., & Armstrong, A. W. (2011). Current state of acne treatment: Highlighting lasers, photodynamic therapy, and chemical peels. *Dermatology Online Journal, 17*(3), 1–13.

Leyden, J. J., & Del Rosso, J. Q. (2011). Oral antibiotic therapy for acne vulgaris: Pharmacokinetic and pharmacodynamic perspectives. *Journal of Clinical and Aesthetic Dermatology, 4*(2), 40–47.

Misery, L. (2011). Consequences of psychological distress in adolescents with acne. *Journal of Investigative Dermatology, 131*(2), 290–292.

Onyett, H., & Canadian Paediatric Society, Infectious Diseases and Immunization Committee. (2014a). Preventing mosquito and tick bites: A Canadian update. *Paediatrics & Child Health, 19*(6), 326–328. Retrieved from <http://www.cps.ca/documents/position/preventing-mosquito-and-tick-bites>.

Onyett, H., & Canadian Paediatric Society, Infectious Diseases and Immunization Committee. (2014b). Lyme disease in Canada: Focus on children. *Paediatrics & Child Health, 19*(7), 379–383. Retrieved from <http://www.cps.ca/en/documents/position/lyme-disease-children>.

Parachute Canada. (2015). *Lowering hot water temperature.* Retrieved from <http://www.parachutecanada.org/injury-topics/item/lowering-hot-water-temperature>.

Public Health Agency of Canada. (2011). *Bartonella henselae. Pathogen safety sheet—infectious substances.* Retrieved from <http://www.phac-aspc.gc.ca/lab-bio/res/psds-ftss/bartonella-henselae-eng.php>.

Public Health Agency of Canada. (2016). *Public health reminder: Lyme disease. Why you should take note.* Retrieved from <http://www.phac-aspc.gc.ca/phn-asp/2013/lyme-0730-eng.php>.

Raghavan, M. (2008). Fatal dog attacks in Canada, 1990–2007. *Canadian Veterinary Journal, 49*(6), 577–581.

Ricci, G., Dondi, A., Patrizi, A., et al. (2009). Systemic therapy of atopic dermatitis in children. *Drugs, 69*(3), 297–306.

Sabhaney, V., & Goldman, R. D. (2012). Management of dog bites in children. *Canadian Family Physician, 58*(10), 1094–1096.

Spinks, A., Wasiak, J., Clelan, H., et al. (2008). Ten-year epidemiological study of pediatric burns in Canada. *Journal of Burn Care Research, 29*(3), 482–488.

Taddeo, D., Stanwick, R., & Canadian Paediatric Society, Adolescent Health Committee. (2012). Banning children and youth under the age of 18 years from commercial tanning facilities. *Paediatric Child Health, 17*(2), 89. Retrieved from <http://www.cps.ca/documents/position/tanning-facilities>. Reaffirmed 2016.

Toronto Public Health Department. (2008). *Fact sheet: Bed bugs.* Retrieved from <http://www1.toronto.ca/city_of_toronto/toronto_public_health/healthy_environment/bed_bugs/files/pdf/bedbugs_factsheet.pdf>.

Walling, H. W., & Swick, B. L. (2010). Update on the management of chronic eczema: New approaches and emerging treatment options. *Clinical Cosmetic Investigation Dermatology, 3*, 99–117.

ADDITIONAL RESOURCES

Canadian Dermatology Association: <http://www.dermatology.ca/>.

CanLyme Canadian Lyme Disease Foundation: <http://www.canlyme.com/>.

Parachute Canada—Prevention of burns and scalds: <http://www.parachutecanada.org/injury-topics/item/scalds-and-burns>.

Registered Nurses Association of Ontario—Best Practice Guideline. Risk Assessment and Prevention of Pressure Ulcers: <http://rnao.ca/bpg/guidelines/risk-assessment-and-prevention-pressure-ulcers>.

TOMA Foundation for Burned Children: <http://www.fondtomafound.org>.

CHAPTER

53

Musculoskeletal or Articular Dysfunction

Cheryl Sams, with contributions from David Wilson

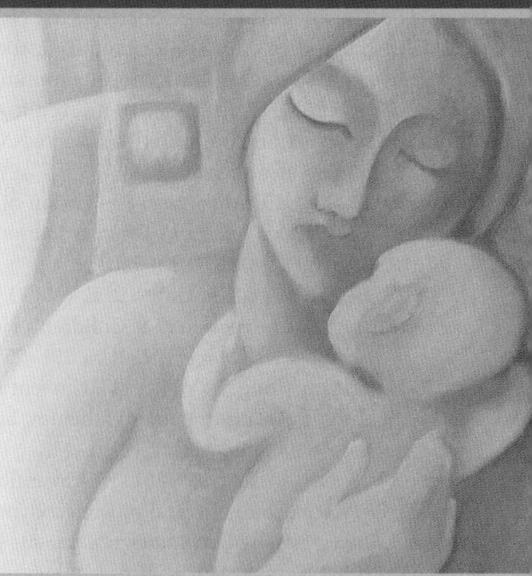

evolve WEBSITE

***Visit the Evolve website for additional resources related to the content in this chapter such as Case Studies, Critical Thinking Case Study Answers, Nursing Care Plans, Nursing Processes, Nursing Skills, and Review Questions for Exam Preparation at:** http://evolve.elsevier.com/Canada/Perry/maternal/*

OBJECTIVES

On completion of this chapter the reader will be able to:

- Outline a care plan for a child immobilized with an injury or a physically limiting condition.
- Formulate a teaching plan for the parents of a child in a cast.
- Explain the functions of the various types of traction.
- Differentiate among the various congenital skeletal defects.
- Design a teaching plan for the parents of a child with a congenital skeletal deformity.
- Describe the therapies and nursing care of a child with scoliosis.
- Outline a care plan for a child with osteomyelitis.
- Differentiate between osteosarcoma and Ewing sarcoma.
- Describe the nursing care of a child with juvenile arthritis.
- Demonstrate an understanding of the management of systemic lupus erythematosus.

THE IMMOBILIZED CHILD

One of the most difficult aspects of illness in children is the immobility it imposes. Children by nature are usually active, and immobility, however temporary, may have lasting effects on the child's developmental progress. The most frequent reasons for immobility are congenital defects (e.g., spina bifida), degenerative disorders (e.g., muscular dystrophy), and infections or injuries that impair the integumentary system (e.g., severe burns), the musculoskeletal system (e.g., multiple fractures, osteomyelitis), or the neurological system (e.g., spinal cord injury, Guillain-Barré syndrome, traumatic brain injury and coma). At times therapies such as traction and spinal fusion are responsible for prolonged immobilization, although the increasing trends in health care are early mobilization and discharge and outpatient treatment.

Physiological Effects of Immobilization

Many clinical studies have documented predictable consequences that occur after immobilization. Functional and metabolic responses to restricted movement can be noted in most of the body's systems. Each has a direct influence on the child's growth and development because homeostatic mechanisms thrive on normal use and need feedback to maintain dynamic equilibrium. Inactivity leads to a decrease in the functional capabilities of the whole body as dramatically as the lack of physical exercise leads to muscle weakness.

Disuse from illness, injury, or a sedentary lifestyle can limit function and potentially delay age-appropriate milestones. Most of the pathological changes that occur during immobilization arise from decreased muscle strength and mass, decreased metabolism, and bone demineralization, which are closely interrelated, with one change leading to or affecting the other. Some results of immobilization are primary and produce a direct effect; other pathophysiological consequences occur frequently but seem to be more indirect and are thus secondary effects. Many pathophysiological changes affect more than one body system, with the primary or secondary effect being demonstrated in both systems.

The major effects of immobilization are outlined briefly in Table 53-1 and are related directly or indirectly to decreased muscle activity, which produces numerous primary changes in the musculoskeletal system with secondary alterations in the cardiovascular, respiratory, metabolic, and renal systems. The musculoskeletal changes that occur during disuse are a result of alterations in gravity and stress on the muscles, joints, and bones. Muscle disuse leads to tissue breakdown and loss of muscle mass (**atrophy**). Muscle atrophy causes decreased strength and endurance, which may take weeks or months to restore.

During immobilization, a joint contracture begins when the arrangement of collagen, the main structural protein of connective tissues, is altered, resulting in a denser tissue that does not glide as easily. Eventually, muscles, tendons, and ligaments can shorten and reduce joint movement, ultimately producing contractures that restrict function. The daily stresses on bone created by motion and weight bearing maintain the balance between bone formation (osteoblastic activity) and bone resorption (osteoclastic activity). During immobilization, more calcium leaves the bone, causing **osteopenia** (demineralization of the bones), which may predispose bone to pathological fractures. The major musculoskeletal consequences of immobilization are as follows:

- Significant decrease in muscle size, strength, and endurance
- Bone demineralization leading to osteoporosis
- Contractures and decreased joint mobility

TABLE 53-1 SUMMARY OF PHYSICAL EFFECTS OF IMMOBILIZATION*

PRIMARY EFFECTS	SECONDARY EFFECTS	NURSING CONSIDERATIONS
Muscular System		
Decreased muscle strength, tone, and endurance	Decreased venous return and decreased cardiac output	Use antiembolism stockings or intermittent compression devices to promote venous return (monitor circulatory and neurovascular status of extremities when such devices are used).
	Decreased metabolism and need for oxygen	Plan play activities to use uninvolved extremities.
	Decreased exercise tolerance	Place in upright position as often as possible.
	Bone demineralization	Perform passive range-of-motion exercises.
Disuse atrophy and loss of muscle mass	Catabolism Loss of strength	Have patient perform active and passive range-of-motion, stretching exercises.
Loss of joint mobility	Contractures, ankylosis of joints	Maintain correct body alignment. Use joint splints as indicated to prevent further deformity. Maintain range of motion.
Weak back muscles	Secondary spinal deformities	Maintain body alignment.
Weak abdominal muscles	Impaired respiration	See nursing considerations for respiratory system.
Skeletal System		
Bone demineralization—Osteoporosis, hypercalcemia	Negative calcium balance Pathological fractures Calcium deposits	With paralysis, use upright posture on tilt table. Handle extremities carefully when turning and positioning. Administer calcium-mobilizing drugs (diphosphonates) and normal saline infusions as directed.
	Extraosseous bone formation, especially at hip, knee, elbow, and shoulder	
	Renal calculi	Ensure adequate fluid intake; monitor output. Acidify urine. Promptly treat urinary infections.
Negative calcium balance	Life-threatening electrolyte imbalance	Monitor serum calcium levels. Provide electrolyte replacement as indicated.
Metabolism		
Decreased metabolic rate	Slowing of all systems Decreased food intake	Mobilize as soon as possible. Have patient perform active and passive resistance and deep breathing exercises. Ensure adequate food intake. Provide a high-protein diet.
Negative nitrogen balance	Decline in nutritional state Impaired healing	Encourage small frequent feedings with protein and preferred foods. Monitor for and prevent pressure sores.
Hypercalcemia	Electrolyte imbalance	See nursing considerations for skeletal system.
Decreased production of stress hormones	Decreased physical and emotional coping capacity	Identify causes of stress. Implement appropriate interventions to lower physical and psychosocial stresses.

Continued

TABLE 53-1 SUMMARY OF PHYSICAL EFFECTS OF IMMOBILIZATION—cont'd

PRIMARY EFFECTS	SECONDARY EFFECTS	NURSING CONSIDERATIONS
Cardiovascular System		
Decreased efficiency of orthostatic neurovascular reflexes	Inability to adapt readily to upright position **(orthostatic intolerance)** Pooling of blood in extremities in upright posture	Monitor peripheral pulses and skin temperature changes. Use antiembolism stockings or intermittent compression devices to decrease pooling when upright.
Diminished vasopressor mechanism	Orthostatic hypotension (intolerance) with syncope—Hypotension, decreased cerebral blood flow, tachycardia	Provide abdominal support. In severe cases, use antigravitational pants. Position horizontally.
Altered distribution of blood volume	Increased cardiac workload Decreased exercise tolerance	Monitor hydration, blood pressure, and urinary output.
Venous stasis	Systemic embolus or thrombus development, pulmonary emboli	Encourage and assist with frequent position changes. Elevate extremities without knee flexion. Ensure adequate fluid intake. Have patient perform active or passive exercise or movement as needed. Prescribe routine wearing of antiembolism stockings or intermittent compression devices. Monitor for signs of *pulmonary embolism*—sudden dyspnea, chest pain, respiratory arrest. Promptly intervene to maintain adequate oxygenation if signs and symptoms of pulmonary emboli are noted. Measure circumference of extremities periodically. Give anticoagulant drugs as prescribed.
Dependent edema	Tissue breakdown and susceptibility to infection	Administer skin care. Turn every 2 hours Monitor skin colour, temperature, and integrity. Use pressure-reduction surface as necessary to prevent skin breakdown (see Chapter 52).
Respiratory System		
Decreased need for oxygen	Altered oxygen–carbon dioxide exchange and metabolism	Promote exercise as tolerated. Encourage deep breathing exercises.
Decreased chest expansion and diminished vital capacity	Diminished oxygen intake Dyspnea and inadequate arterial oxygen saturation; acidosis	Position for optimum chest expansion. Semi-Fowler's position may assist in lung expansion if the patient can tolerate it. Use prone positioning without pressure on abdomen to allow gravity to aid in diaphragmatic excursion. Ensure that patient maintains proper alignment when sitting to prevent pressure on respiratory mechanisms.
Poor abdominal tone and distension	Interference with diaphragmatic excursion	Avoid restriction of chest and abdominal musculature. Supply torso support to promote chest expansion.
Mechanical or biochemical secretion retention	Hypostatic pneumonia Bacterial and viral pneumonia Atelectasis	Change position frequently. Carry out percussion, vibration, and drainage (or suctioning) as necessary. Use incentive spirometer. Monitor breath sounds.
Loss of respiratory muscle strength	Poor cough	Encourage deep breathing and coughing. Support chest wall by splinting with pillow when patient coughs. Use incentive spirometer. Observe for signs of respiratory distress with pulse oximetry or blood gas measurement as necessary.
	Upper respiratory tract infection	Prevent contact with an infected person. Provide adequate hydration. Administer immunizations as necessary (pneumococcal, meningococcal).

TABLE 53-1 SUMMARY OF PHYSICAL EFFECTS OF IMMOBILIZATION—cont'd

PRIMARY EFFECTS	SECONDARY EFFECTS	NURSING CONSIDERATIONS
Gastrointestinal System		
Distension caused by poor abdominal muscle tone	Interference with respiratory movements	Monitor bowel sounds. Encourage having small, frequent meals.
No specific primary effect	Difficulty in feeding in prone position	Have patient sit upright in bedside chair, if possible
	Possible constipation caused by gravitational effect on feces through ascending colon and smooth muscle tone	Carry out bowel training program with hydration, stool softeners, increased fibre intake, and mild laxatives if necessary.
	Anorexia	Stimulate appetite with favoured foods.
Urinary System		
Alteration of gravitational force	Difficulty in voiding in prone or supine position	Position as upright as possible to void.
Impaired ureteral peristalsis	Urinary retention in calyces and bladder Infection Renal calculi	Hydrate to ensure adequate urinary output for age. Stimulate bladder emptying with warm running water as necessary. Catheterize only for severe urinary retention. Administer antibiotics as indicated.
Integumentary System		
No specific primary effect	Decreased circulation and pressure leading to tissue injury and decreased healing capacity	Turn and reposition at least every 2 hours. Frequently inspect total skin surface. Eliminate mechanical factors causing pressure, friction, moisture, or irritation. Place on pressure-relief mattress.
	Difficulty with personal hygiene	Assess ability to perform self-care and assist with bathing, grooming, and toileting as needed. Encourage self-care to potential ability. Ensure adequate intake of protein, vitamins, and minerals.

*Not all problems will apply in every situation.

Circulatory stasis combined with hypercoagulability of the blood, which results from factors such as damage to the endothelium of blood vessels (Virchow triad), can lead to thrombus and embolus formation. *Deep vein thrombosis (DVT)* involves the formation of a thrombus in a deep vein such as the iliac and femoral veins and can cause significant morbidity if it remains undetected and untreated. The thrombus and emboli may obstruct vessels in organs such as the lungs, kidneys, or brain. Pulmonary embolus is a life-threatening complication of immobilization. The larger the portion of the body immobilized and the longer the immobilization, the greater the hazards of immobility.

Psychological Effects of Immobilization

Throughout childhood, physical activity is an integral part of daily life and is essential for physical growth and development. The activity helps children deal with a variety of feelings and impulses and provides a mechanism by which they can exert control over inner tensions. Children respond to anxiety with increased activity. Removal of or a reduction in this power deprives them of necessary input and a natural outlet for their feelings and fantasies.

When children are immobilized by disease or as part of a treatment regimen, they experience diminished environmental stimuli with a loss of tactile input and an altered perception of themselves and their environment. Sudden or gradual immobilization narrows the amount and variety of environmental stimuli children receive by means of all of their senses: touch; sight; hearing; taste; smell; and *proprioception*, or the feeling of where they are in their environment. This sensory deprivation commonly leads to feelings of isolation and boredom and of being forgotten, especially by peers.

Physical interference with the activity of young children gives them a feeling of frustration and helplessness. Even speech and language skills require sensorimotor activity and experience. For the toddler, exploration and imitative behaviours are essential to developing a sense of autonomy; the preschooler's expression of initiative is evidenced by the need for vigorous physical activity; the school-age child's development is strongly influenced by physical achievement and competition; and the adolescent relies on mobility to achieve independence. The quest for mastery at every stage of development is related to mobility.

The monotony of immobilization can lead to sluggish intellectual and psychomotor responses, decreased communication skills, and increased fantasizing. Children are likely to become depressed over their loss of ability to function or any marked changes in body image. They may seek the attention of others by reverting to earlier developmental behaviours, such as wanting to be fed, or bed-wetting and baby talk.

Limbs in casts or traction transmit less than normal sensory data. Children who have limited ability to feel others touching them not only experience less tactile stimuli in a physical sense but are also deprived of warm, loving feelings that arise from being touched. The loss of feeling derived from touch can further add to their sense of being isolated and unwanted.

Children may react to immobility by active protest, anger, and aggressive behaviour; or they may become quiet, passive, and submissive. They may believe the immobilization is a justified punishment for misbehaviour. Children should be allowed to express their feelings, but it should be within the limits of safety to their self-esteem and not damaging to the integrity of others. For example, providing an inanimate object to attack rather than a person or a valued possession is safe and therapeutic. When children are unable to express anger and frustration, aggression is often displayed inappropriately through regressive behaviour and outbursts of crying or temper tantrums.

Effect on Families

Even brief periods of immobilization may disrupt family function, and sudden catastrophic illness or chronic disability may severely tax their resources and coping abilities.

The family's needs often must be met by the services of a multidisciplinary team, and nurses play a key role in anticipating the services they will need and in coordinating conferences to plan care. In preparation for discharge, home visits are advisable, and home management is commonly planned weeks in advance of the actual discharge (see Chapter 42).

NURSING CARE

Physical assessment of the child who is immobilized as a result of an injury or illness focuses not only on the injured part (e.g., fracture or damaged joint) but also on the functioning of other systems that may be affected secondarily (e.g., the circulatory, renal, respiratory, muscular, and gastrointestinal systems). With long-term immobilization, there may also be neurological impairment and changes in electrolytes (especially calcium), nitrogen balance, and the general metabolic rate. The psychological impact of immobilization should also be assessed.

Children who require prolonged total immobility and are unable to move themselves in bed should be placed on a special surface to prevent skin breakdown. Frequent position changes also help prevent dependent edema and stimulate circulation, respiratory function, gastrointestinal motility, and neurological sensation. Children at greater risk for skin breakdown include those with prolonged immobilization; orthotic and prosthetic devices, including wheelchairs; and casts. Additional risk factors include poor nutrition, friction (from bed linen with traction), and moist skin (from urine or perspiration). In critically ill children, factors associated with increased skin breakdown include requirement for mechanical ventilation, age less than 2 years, length of stay of 4 days or more, and a respiratory diagnosis on admission (Schindler, Mikhailov, Kuhn, et al., 2011). In newborns and infants, skin breakdown is more likely to occur on the occiput and on the nasal septum when nasal continuous positive airway pressure devices are used (Murray, Noonan, Quigley, et al., 2013). The Braden Q Scale is a reliable, objective tool that may be used in the assessment for pressure ulcer development in children who are acutely ill or at risk for skin breakdown from neurological conditions and immobilization (Noonan, Quigley, & Curley, 2011) (see Additional Resources at the end of the chapter).

The use of antiembolic stockings and intermittent compression devices prevents circulatory stasis and dependent edema in the lower extremities and the development of DVT. Anticoagulant therapy may also be implemented with low-molecular-weight heparin, vitamin K antagonists, or unfractionated heparin. The child should be allowed as much activity as possible within the limitations of the illness or treatment. Any functional mobility, however minimal, is preferred to total immobility.

High-protein, high-calorie foods are encouraged to prevent negative nitrogen balance, which may be difficult to correct by diet, especially if there is anorexia as a result of immobility and decreased gastrointestinal function (decreased motility and possibly constipation). Stimulating the appetite with small servings of attractively arranged, preferred foods may be sufficient. Sometimes supplementary nasogastric or gastrostomy feedings or intravenous (IV) fluids may be needed, but these are reserved for serious disability in which oral intake is impossible.

Adequate hydration and, when possible, an upright position and remobilization promote bowel and kidney function and help prevent complications in these systems. The child should be encouraged to do as much activity as possible within the limitations of the illness or treatment. Most children have an innate ingenuity and natural inclination toward maximizing mobility. They need the opportunity, the materials, or objects to stimulate activity and the encouragement and participation of others. Those children who are unable to move need passive exercise and movement, often in consultation with a physiotherapist.

Whenever possible, transporting the child outside the confines of the room increases environmental stimuli and allows social contact with others. Specially designed wheelchairs for increased mobility and independence are available. Children also benefit from frequent visitors, accessibility of clocks and calendars, and a program of diversional therapy to help them function more normally. A child life specialist should be consulted for recreational planning. An activity centre or slanting tray can be helpful for the child with limited mobility to use for drawing, colouring, writing, and playing with small toys. In addition to being able to do things they like to do, children can express their frustration, displeasure, and anger through play activities (see Chapter 44), which is helpful in the child's recovery. Hospitalized children should be allowed to wear their own clothes (street clothes, especially for preadolescent and adolescent girls) and resume school and preinjury activities. A parent or siblings should be allowed to stay overnight and room in with the hospitalized child to prevent the effects of family disruption caused by hospitalization; all efforts should be made to minimize this disruption. Although most of the suggestions discussed relate to hospital care, the same consultations (physiotherapist, occupational therapist, child life specialist, speech therapist) and environment may also be considered in the home to help the child and family achieve independence and normalization.

Using dolls, stuffed animals, or puppets to illustrate and explain the immobilization is a valuable tool for small children. Placing a cast, tubing, or other restraining equipment on the doll offers the child a nonthreatening opportunity to express, through the doll, feelings concerning the restrictions and feelings toward the nurse and other health care providers.

One of the most useful interventions to help children cope with immobility is participation in their own self-care; children usually welcome doing this to the extent possible. They can help plan their daily routine; select their diet (when possible); and choose clothes, including innovative adornments such as baseball caps, brightly decorated sunglasses, or brightly coloured stockings, to express their autonomy and individuality. They should be encouraged to do as much as they are able to for themselves to keep muscles active and their interest alive. Visits from significant people such as family members and friends offer occasions for emotional support and also provide opportunities for learning how to care for the child. Privacy is necessary, especially for adolescents, and most long-term health care facilities recognize that private or semiprivate rooms shared by one or two children are the best environment for rehabilitation.

For a child with greatly restricted movement (e.g., child with a large bilateral hip spica cast), nursing care is often a challenge. These situations require long-term care either in the hospital or at home; but, wherever the care occurs, consistent planning and coordination of activities with other health care workers and significant others are vital nursing functions.

With the increased trend toward early mobilization, early discharge, and home health care, many children are discharged home within a few hours or days of hospitalization. Follow-up treatment may take place in the home setting or an outpatient ambulatory facility.

Family Support and Home Care

The needs of a child with complex or chronic conditions that cause immobility can be complex, and although the optimal situation is for family members to have time to assimilate the teachings and demonstrations needed to understand the child's situation and care, this is often shortened considerably by moving the child to a rehabilitation facility or even to the home within a matter of days. Even the child who is confined on a short-term basis can be a challenge for the family, which is usually unprepared for the problems imposed by the child's special needs. Home modification is usually needed for facilitating care, especially when it involves traction, large casts, or extended confinement (see Chapter 42). Suitable child care may be needed for times when all family members work.

Just as in the hospital, the child at home should be encouraged to be as independent as possible and to follow a schedule that approximates his or her normal lifestyle as nearly as possible, such as continuing school lessons, regular bedtime, and suitable recreational activities.

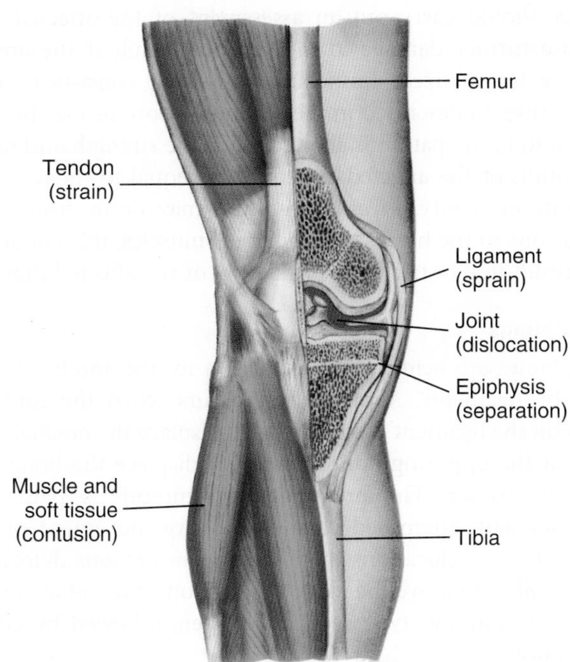

FIGURE 53-1 Sites of injuries to bones, joints, and soft tissues.

TRAUMATIC INJURY

Soft-Tissue Injury

Injuries to the muscles, ligaments, and tendons are common in children, and areas of injuries are shown in Fig. 53-1. In young children, soft-tissue injury usually results from mishaps during play. In older children and adolescents, participation in sports is the more common cause.

Contusions

A *contusion* is damage to the soft tissue, subcutaneous structures, and muscle. The tearing of these tissues and small blood vessels and the inflammatory response lead to hemorrhage, edema, and associated pain when the child attempts to move the injured part. The escape of blood into the tissues is observed as *ecchymosis*, a black-and-blue discolouration.

Contusions are crush injuries that can occur in children when they slam their fingers (in doors, folding chairs, or equipment) or hit their fingers (as when hammering a nail). A severe crush injury involves the bone, with swelling and bleeding beneath the nail (subungual) and sometimes laceration of the pulp of the distal phalanx. The subungual hematoma can be released by creating a hole at the proximal end of the nail with a battery-operated microcautery device or a heated sterile 18-gauge needle.

Large contusions that are often sustained while the child is participating in sports cause gross swelling, pain, and disability, and usually receive immediate attention from health personnel. Smaller injuries may go unnoticed, allowing continued participation; however, they can become disabling after rest because of pain and muscle spasm. The young athlete is commonly instructed to "walk it off" or disregard the pain. Instead of this approach, first a qualified health care worker or certified athletic trainer should carry out an assessment of the affected area because further damage to the site may result if the area is severely traumatized. Immediate treatment consists of cold application, as described in the section on sprains (see below). Return to participation is allowed when the strength and range of motion of the affected extremity are equal to those of the opposite extremity. *Myositis ossificans* may occur from deep contusions to the biceps or quadriceps muscles; this condition may result in a restriction of flexibility of the affected limb.

Dislocations

Long bones are held in approximation to one another at the joint by ligaments. A dislocation occurs when the force of stress on the ligament is so great as to displace the normal position of the opposing bone ends or to displace the bone end from its socket. The predominant symptom is pain that increases with attempted passive or active movement of the extremity. In dislocations there may be an obvious deformity and inability to move the joint. Dislocation of the phalanges is the most common type seen in children, followed by elbow dislocation.

One of the most common injuries in young children is subluxation of the annular ligament, also called *pulled elbow* or *nursemaid elbow*. With this injury the annular ligament slips proximally off the radial head into the joint between the radial head and ulna, causing immediate pain and limited supination (Carrigan, 2016). In most cases, the injury occurs in a child between the ages of 1 and 3 who receives a sudden longitudinal pull or traction at the wrist while the arm is fully extended and the forearm pronated. It usually occurs when an adult or older sibling who is holding the child by the hand or wrist gives a sudden pull or jerk to prevent a fall or attempts to lift the child by pulling the wrist, or when the child pulls away by dropping to the floor or ground. The child often cries, appears anxious, and refuses to use the affected limb. To treat this, the health care provider manipulates the arm by applying firm finger pressure to the head of the radius, then supinates and flexes the forearm to return the ligament to its place. A click or clunk may be heard or felt, and functional use of the arm returns within minutes. However, the longer the subluxation is present, the longer it takes for the child to recover mobility after treatment. Usually no anaesthetic is required, but a mild pain reliever such as acetaminophen may be given. In an older child, severe elbow injury or dislocation should be carefully evaluated by a health care provider immediately; likewise, a traumatic elbow injury in the younger child that is not a subluxation should be carefully evaluated.

In children younger than 5 years of age, the hip can be dislocated by a fall. The greatest risk after this injury is the potential loss of blood supply to the head of the femur. Relocation of the hip within 60 minutes after the injury provides the best chance for prevention of damage to the femoral head.

Shoulder dislocations occur most often in older adolescents and are often sports related. In a shoulder dislocation, temporary restriction of the joint, with a sling or bandage that secures the arm to the chest, can provide sufficient comfort and immobilization until medical attention is received.

Simple dislocations should be reduced as soon as possible with the child under mild (procedural) sedation and often local anaesthesia. Anaesthetics such as IV ketamine (Ketalar), midazolam (Versed), IV propofol (Diprivan), or fentanyl (Sublimaze) can be used to produce partial or complete analgesia. Nitrous oxide in concentrations of 50 to 70% has been shown to be safe for relatively short periods (15 to 20 minutes) in children ages 1 year and older (Babl, Oakley, Seaman, et al., 2008; Zier & Liu, 2011). An unreduced dislocation will be complicated by increased swelling, making reduction difficult and increasing the risk of neurovascular problems. Treatment depends on the severity of the injury.

Sprains

A *sprain* occurs when trauma to a joint is so severe that a ligament is partially or completely torn or stretched by the force created as a joint is twisted or wrenched, often accompanied by damage to associated blood vessels, muscles, tendons, and nerves. Sprains can be graded as follows: *grade 1 sprain* has minimal pain with damage to the ligaments; *grade 2 sprain* has more ligament damage and mild joint looseness; and *grade 3* has a complete tearing of the ligament with a very loose or unstable joint (About Kids Health, 2009).

The presence of joint laxity is the most valid indicator of the severity of a sprain. In a severe injury the child may describe the joint as "feeling loose" or as if "something is coming apart" and may describe hearing a "snap," "pop," or "tearing." Pain is seldom the principal subjective symptom. There is a rapid onset with swelling (often diffuse), accompanied by immediate disability and appreciable reluctance to use the injured joint.

Strains

A *strain* is a microscopic tear to the musculotendinous unit and has features in common with sprains. The area is painful to touch and swollen. Most strains are incurred over time rather than suddenly, and the rapidity of the appearance provides clues regarding severity. In general, the more rapidly the strain occurs, the more severe the injury. When the strain involves the muscular portion, there is more bleeding, often palpable soon after injury and before edema obscures the hematoma.

Therapeutic Management

The first minutes to 12 hours are the most critical period for virtually all soft-tissue injuries. Basic principles of managing sprains and other soft-tissue injuries are summarized in the acronyms *RICE* and *ICES*:

RICE	ICES
R—Rest	**I**—Ice
I—Ice	**C**—Compression
C—Compression	**E**—Elevation
E—Elevation	**S**—Support

Soft-tissue injuries should be iced immediately. This is best accomplished with crushed ice wrapped in a towel or encased in a screw-top ice bag or resealable storage bag. A plastic bag of frozen vegetables, such as peas, serves as a convenient ice pack for soft-tissue injuries. It is clean, watertight, and easily moulded to the injured part. When available, snow placed in a plastic bag may serve as an ice bag. A wet elastic wrap, which transfers cold better than dry wrap, is applied to provide compression and to keep the ice pack in place. Chemical-activated ice packs are also effective for immediate treatment but are not reusable and must be closely monitored for leakage. A cloth barrier should be used between the ice container and the skin to prevent trauma to the tissues. Ice has a rapid cooling effect on tissues and reduces the pain threshold. Ice therapy should be intermittent and should never be applied for more than 30 minutes at a time because of the body's homeostatic response to cold, which may trigger a decrease in vascularization at the injury site. Parents should be instructed to ice for 30 minutes every 4 hours for 3 days for sprains and strains.

Elevating the extremity uses gravity to facilitate venous return and to reduce edema formation in the damaged area. The point of injury should be kept several inches above the level of the heart for therapy to be effective. Several pillows can be used for elevation. Allowing the extremity to be dependent causes excessive fluid accumulation in the area of injury, delaying healing and causing painful swelling.

Bandages or an aircast can decrease swelling to an ankle injury. The child may require crutches. Ibuprofen can be used to manage pain and decrease the edema. For minor ankle sprains, the child can start strengthening ankle exercises as early as 48 hours after the injury by range-of-movement motions. Light weight bearing and easy walking can improve balance. The child can return to normal physical activities and sports when there is full range of movement and full strength to the joint. Torn ligaments, especially those in the knee, are usually treated by immobilization with a knee immobilizer or range-of-motion brace until the child is able to walk without a limp. Crutches are used for mobility to rest the affected extremity. Passive leg exercises, gradually increased to active ones, are begun as soon as sufficient healing has taken place. Parents and children should be cautioned against using any form of liniment or other heat-producing preparation before the injured area is examined. If the injury requires casting or splinting, the heat generated in the enclosed space can cause extreme discomfort and may even cause tissue damage. In some cases torn knee ligaments are managed with arthroscopy and ligament repair or reconstruction as necessary, depending on the extent of the tear, the ligaments involved, and the child's age. Surgical reconstruction of the anterior cruciate ligament (ACL) may be performed in young athletes who wish to continue in active sports (Sarwark, 2010).

Fractures

Bone fractures occur when the resistance of bone against the stress being exerted yields to the stress force. Fractures are a common injury at any age but are more likely to occur in children and older adults. Because childhood is a time of rapid bone growth, the pattern of fractures, problems of diagnosis, and methods of treatment in children differ from those in the adult. In children fractures heal much faster than in adults. Consequently, children may not require as long a period of immobilization of the affected extremity as that in an adult with a fracture.

Fracture injuries in children are most often a result of traumatic incidents at home, at school, in a motor vehicle, or in association with recreational activities. Children's everyday activities include vigorous play that predisposes them to injury—climbing, falling down, running into immovable objects, skateboarding, and receiving blows to any part of their bodies.

Aside from automobile accidents or falls from heights, true injuries that cause fractures rarely occur in infancy; thus bone injury in children of that age group warrants further investigation. In any small child, especially under the age of 12 months, radiographic evidence of fractures at various stages of healing is, with few exceptions, a result of nonaccidental trauma (child abuse). Any investigation of fractures in infants, particularly multiple fractures, should include consideration of osteogenesis imperfecta.

Fractures in school-age children are often a result of bicycle, automobile, or skateboard injuries. Adolescents are vulnerable to multiple and severe trauma because they are active in sports and mobile on bicycles, all-terrain vehicles, skateboards, skis, snowboards, bicycles, and motorcycles.

A distal forearm (radius, ulna, or both) is the most common fracture. The clavicle is also a bone that is commonly broken in childhood, with approximately half of clavicle fractures occurring in children under 10 years of age. Common mechanisms of injury include a fall with an outstretched hand or direct trauma to the bone. In newborns a fractured clavicle may occur with a large newborn and a small maternal pelvis. This may be noted in the first few days after birth by a unilateral Moro reflex or at an early well-child check, when a fracture callus is palpated on the infant's healing clavicle.

Types of Fractures

A fractured bone consists of fragments—the fragment closer to the midline, or the *proximal* fragment; and the fragment farther from the midline, or the *distal* fragment. When fracture fragments are separated, the fracture is *complete*; when fragments remain attached, the fracture is *incomplete*. The fracture line can be any of the following:

Transverse—Crosswise, at right angles to the long axis of the bone

Oblique—Slanting but straight, between a horizontal and a perpendicular direction

Spiral—Slanting and circular, twisting around the bone shaft

The twisting of an extremity while the bone is breaking results in a spiral break. If the fracture does not produce a break in the skin, it is a *simple*, or *closed*, *fracture*. *Open*, or *compound*, *fractures* are those with an open wound through which the bone is or has protruded. If the bone fragments cause damage to other organs or tissues (such as the lung or bladder), the injury is said to be a *complicated fracture*. When small fragments of bone are broken from the fractured shaft and lie in the surrounding tissue, the injury is a *comminuted fracture*. This type of fracture is rare in children. The types of fractures seen most often in children are described in Box 53-1 and in Fig. 53-2.

Immediately after a fracture occurs, the muscles contract and physiologically splint the injured area. This phenomenon

BOX 53-1 TYPES OF FRACTURES IN CHILDREN

Plastic deformation—Occurs when the bone is bent but not broken. A child's flexible bone can be bent 45 degrees or more before breaking. However, if bent, the bone will straighten slowly, but not completely, to produce some deformity but without the angulation seen when the bone breaks. Bends occur most commonly in the ulna and fibula, often in association with fractures of the radius and tibia.

Buckle, or torus, fracture—Produced by compression of the porous bone; appears as a raised or bulging projection at the fracture site. These fractures occur in the most porous portion of the bone near the metaphysis (the portion of the bone shaft adjacent to the epiphysis) and are more common in young children.

Greenstick fracture—Occurs when a bone is angulated beyond the limits of bending. The compressed side bends, and the tension side fails, causing an incomplete fracture similar to the break observed when a green stick is broken.

Complete fracture—Divides the bone fragments. These fragments often remain attached by a periosteal hinge, which can aid or hinder reduction.

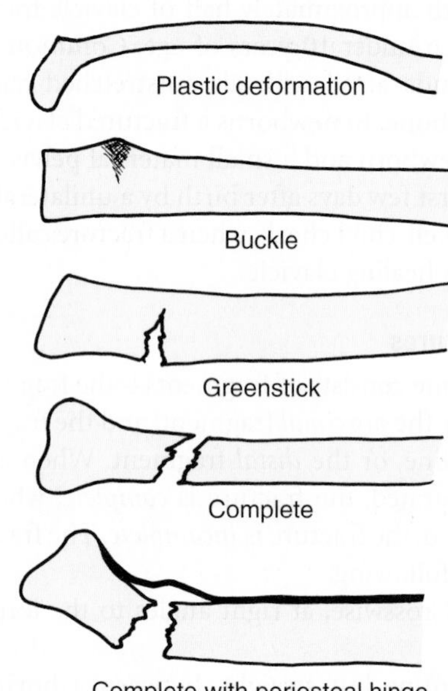

FIGURE 53-2 Types of fractures in children.

accounts for the muscle tightness observed over a fracture site and the deformity that is produced as the muscles pull the bone ends out of alignment. This muscle response must be overcome by traction or complete muscle relaxation (e.g., with anaesthesia) in order to realign the distal bone fragment to the proximal bone fragment.

Growth Plate (Physeal) Injuries

The weakest point of long bones is the cartilage growth plate, or epiphyseal plate. Consequently, this is a common site of damage during trauma. Growth plate fractures are classified with the Salter-Harris classification system (Fig. 53-3).

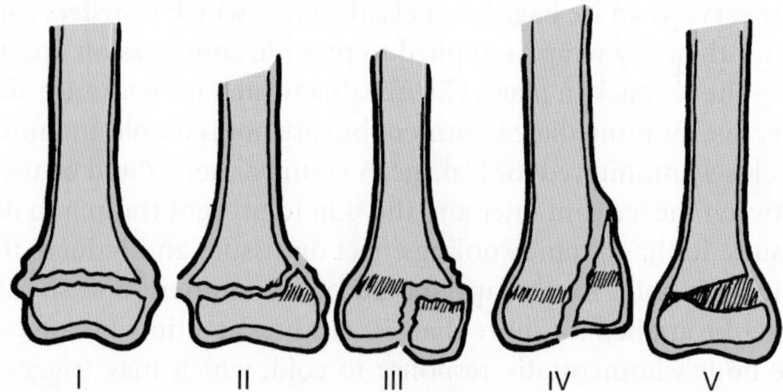

FIGURE 53-3 Salter Harris fracture classification. Types of epiphyseal injury in order of increasing risk. The injuries are classified as follows: type I, separation or slip of growth plate without fracture of the bone; type II, separation of growth plate and breaking off of section of metaphysis; type III, fracture of epiphysis extending through joint surface; type IV, fracture of growth plate, epiphysis, and metaphysis; and type V, crushing injury of epiphysis (can be diagnosed only in retrospect). This classification of epiphyseal injuries was developed by orthopedists R. B. Salter and W. R. Harris. (Salter, R. B. & Harris, W. R. [1963]. Injuries involving the physeal plate, *Journal of Bone & Joint Surgery, 45*[3], 587–622. Used with permission. Copyright © 1963 by The Journal of Bone and Joint Surgery, Incorporated.)

Detection of epiphyseal injuries is sometimes difficult, but it is critical. Close monitoring and early treatment, if indicated, are essential to prevent longitudinal or angular growth deformities (or both). Treatment of these fractures may include open reduction and internal fixation to prevent or reduce growth disturbances.

Bone Healing and Remodelling

Bone healing is characteristically rapid in children because of the thickened periosteum and generous blood supply. When there is a break in the continuity of bone, the osteoblasts are stimulated to maximum activity. New bone cells are formed in immense numbers almost immediately after the injury and, in time, are evidenced by a bulging growth of new bone tissue between the fractured bone fragments. This is followed by deposition of calcium salts to form a callus. Remodelling is a process that occurs in the healing of long bone fractures in growing children. The irregularities produced by the fracture become indistinct as the angles and bone overgrowth are smoothed out, giving the bone a straighter appearance. A general rule of thumb is that an angulated fracture in a growing child remodels by one degree per month (Mencio & Swiontkowski, 2015).

Fractures heal in less time in children than in adults. The approximate healing times for a femoral shaft are as follows:

Newborn period—2 to 3 weeks
Early childhood—4 weeks
Later childhood—6 to 8 weeks
Adolescence—8 to 12 weeks

Diagnostic Evaluation

A history may be lacking in some childhood injuries. Infants and toddlers are unable to communicate, and older children may not volunteer information (even under direct questioning)

BOX 53-2 CLINICAL MANIFESTATIONS OF A FRACTURE

Signs of injury:
- Generalized swelling
- Pain or tenderness
- Diminished functional use of affected part

May be:
- Bruising
- Severe muscular rigidity
- **Crepitus** (grating sensation at fracture site)

when the injury occurred during suspicious or forbidden activities. Whenever possible, it is helpful to obtain information from someone who witnessed the injury. In cases of nonaccidental trauma providers may give false information to protect themselves or family members.

The child may exhibit the same manifestations seen in adults (Box 53-2). However, often a fracture is remarkably stable because of an intact periosteum. The child may even be able to use an affected arm or walk on a fractured leg. Because bones have increased vascularity, a soft pliable hematoma may be felt around the fracture site.

Radiographic examination is the most useful diagnostic tool for assessing skeletal trauma. The calcium deposits in bone make the entire structure radiopaque. Radiographic films are taken after fracture reduction and, in some cases, may be taken during the healing process to determine satisfactory progress.

! NURSING ALERT

A fracture should be strongly suspected in a small child who refuses to walk or crawl.

Therapeutic Management

The goals of fracture management are as follows:
- To regain alignment and length of the bony fragments (reduction)
- To retain alignment and length (immobilization)
- To restore function to the injured parts
- To prevent further injury and deformity

The majority of children's fractures heal well, and nonunion is rare. Most fractures are splinted and casted to immobilize and protect the injured extremity. Children with displaced fractures may have immediate surgical reduction and fixation (internal or external) rather than being immobilized by traction until healing takes place. This practice is more common and holds true for all types of fractures, including femur fractures, although there is variation based on provider preference and institutional practice. Some conditions, including open fractures, compartment syndrome, fractures associated with vascular or nerve injury, and joint dislocations that are unresponsive to reduction manoeuvres, require immediate medical attention.

! NURSING ALERT

Compartment syndrome is a serious complication that results from compression of nerves, blood vessels, and muscle inside a closed space. This injury may be devastating, resulting in tissue death, and thus requires emergency treatment (fasciotomy). The five P's of ischemia from a vascular, soft tissue, nerve, or bone injury should be included in an assessment of any injury (see Emergency box, p. 1722).

In children the bone fragments are usually realigned and immobilized by traction or by closed manipulation and casting until an adequate callus is formed. The position of the bone fragments in relation to one another influences the rapidity of healing and residual deformity. Weight bearing on lower extremity fractures and active movement for the purpose of regaining function can begin after the fracture site is determined to be stable by the health care provider. The child's natural tendency to be active is usually sufficient to restore normal mobility, and physiotherapy is rarely needed. In most cases children's fractures can be managed by closed reduction and cast immobilization, which is most often provided on an outpatient basis with re-evaluation in 7 to 10 days.

Children are most frequently hospitalized for fractures of the femur and the supracondylar area of the distal humerus, which may require internal fixation and pinning. If simple reduction cannot be achieved or a neurovascular problem is detected after the injury, observation in a hospital setting may be indicated. The trend is to avoid hospitalization. The major methods for immobilizing a fracture (i.e., casting and traction) are described later in the chapter.

Wrist buckle fractures are common in children who fall and extend their arm forward to break the fall. Radius or ulna buckle fractures in children can be treated with a cast or a removable splint for 3 to 4 weeks.

NURSING CARE

Nurses are frequently the persons who make the initial assessment of a child with a suspected fracture (see Emergency box). The child and parents may be frightened and upset, and the child is often in pain. Therefore, if the child is alert and there is no evidence of hemorrhage, the initial nursing interventions are directed toward calming and reassuring the child and parents so that a more extensive assessment can be more easily accomplished. While remaining calm and speaking in a quiet voice, the nurse can ask the parents and an older child to describe how the injury occurred.

The child may arrive with the limb supported in some manner; if not, careful support or immobilization may be provided to the affected site. In the event that the limb is already supported or immobilized, it may be best not to touch the child but to ask him or her to point to the painful area and to wiggle the fingers or toes. By this time the child may feel relatively safe and will allow someone to gently touch the area just enough to feel the pulse and test for sensation. A child's anxiety is greatly influenced by previous experiences with

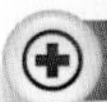

EMERGENCY

Fracture

Assess the extent of injury and the five P's of ischemia assessment:

1. **P**ain and point of tenderness
2. **P**ulselessness
3. **P**allor
4. **P**aresthesia—Sensation distal to the fracture site
5. **P**aralysis—Movement distal to the fracture site

Determine the mechanism of injury.

Move the injured part as little as possible.

Cover open wounds with a sterile or clean dressing.

Immobilize the limb, including joints above and below the fracture site; do not attempt to reduce the fracture or push protruding bone under the skin.

- Soft splint (pillow or folded towel)
- Rigid splint (rolled newspaper or magazine)
- Uninjured leg can serve as a splint for a leg fracture if no splint is available

Reassess neurovascular status.

Apply traction if circulatory compromise is present.

Elevate the injured limb if possible.

Apply cold to the injured area.

Call emergency medical services or transport patient to medical facility.

injury and with health personnel; he or she needs to be told what will happen and what to do to help. The affected limb need not be palpated, and it should not be moved unless properly splinted. Parental anxiety may be heightened by the child's pain reaction and fear, and possibly other events surrounding the accident; thus it is important to communicate to the parents that the child will receive the necessary care, including pain management.

The Child Requiring a Cast

The completeness of the fracture, the type of bone involved, and the amount of weight bearing influence how much of the extremity must be included in the cast to immobilize the fracture site completely. In most cases the joints above and below the fracture are immobilized to eliminate the possibility of movement that might cause displacement at the fracture site. Four major categories of casts are used for fractures: *upper extremity* to immobilize the wrist or elbow, *lower extremity* to immobilize the ankle or knee, *spinal* and *cervical* for immobilization of the spine, and *spica* casts to immobilize the hip and knee.

Casts are constructed from gauze strips and bandages impregnated with plaster of paris or, more commonly, from synthetic lighter weight and water-resistant materials (e.g., waterproof liners, fibreglass, and polyurethane resin). Both types of casting produce heat from the chemical reaction activated by water immediately after application. Plaster casts mould closely to the body part, take 10 to 72 hours to dry, have a smooth exterior, and are inexpensive. The newer synthetic casting material is lighter, dries in 5 to 20 minutes, permits earlier weight bearing, and is water resistant. The disadvantage of synthetic casting is its inability to mould closely to body parts; its rough exterior, which may scratch surfaces; and increased cost.

Synthetic casts have special advantages for children. They come in different colours and with designs (e.g., cartoons, stripes), and they are lightweight, durable, easy to clean, and relatively water resistant, depending on the type of inner lining used; only those with a Gore-Tex inner lining may be immersed in water without affecting the cast integrity. Bathing with a synthetic cast may be accomplished by covering the cast with a plastic bag; if the synthetic cast gets wet, it should be dried thoroughly. One drawback to immersion is the time necessary to completely dry the cast. The synthetic casts are difficult to write on.

Cast Application

The child's developmental age should be considered before the cast is applied. For preschoolers who fear bodily harm and fantasize about the loss of an extremity, it may be helpful to use a plastic doll or stuffed animal to explain the procedure beforehand. Toddlers and preschoolers do not have easily defined body boundaries; if an extremity is wrapped in a bandage, cast, or splint, to the young child the extremity often ceases to exist. It is also helpful to explain that some synthetic cast material will become warm but will not burn. During the application of the cast various distraction methods can be used, such as blowing bubbles. In this age group explanations such as "This will help your arm get better" are futile because the child has no concept of causality.

Before the cast is applied, the extremities are checked for any abrasions, cuts, or other alterations in the skin surface, and rings or other items that might cause constriction from swelling are removed. The skin may be protected by a cloth stockinette or cotton batting, which is applied liberally to the area to be casted. Particular attention is given to bony prominences, which are padded with extra cotton batting. Some practitioners use a Gore-Tex liner under a hip spica cast to prevent continuous exposure to moisture and possible skin breakdown. The stockinette is pulled over the ends of the cast to protect the skin from rough edges.

NURSING CARE

The complete evaporation of the water from a hip spica cast can take 24 to 72 hours when older types of plaster materials are used. Fibreglass cast material dries within minutes. The cast must remain uncovered to allow it to dry from the inside out. Turning the child in a plaster cast at least every 2 hours will help dry a body cast evenly and prevent complications related to immobility. A regular fan or cool-air hair dryer to circulate air may be helpful when the humidity is high.

NURSING ALERT

Heated fans or dryers are not used because they cause the cast to dry on the outside and remain wet beneath or cause burns from heat conduction by way of the cast to the underlying tissue.

A wet plaster cast should be supported by a pillow that is covered with plastic and should be handled by the palms of the hands to avoid indenting the cast, which can create pressure areas. A dry plaster-of-paris cast produces a hollow sound when it is tapped with the finger. After it has dried, "hot spots" felt on the cast surface or a foul-smelling odour may indicate an infection. This should be reported for further evaluation; if concern continues, an opening, or a "window," could be exposed over the area of concern to evaluate the site.

During the first few hours after a cast is applied, the chief concern is that the extremity may continue to swell to the extent that the cast becomes a tourniquet, shutting off circulation and producing neurovascular complications (compartment syndrome). To prevent swelling, elevation of the body part increases venous return. If edema is excessive, casts are bivalved (i.e., cut to make anterior and posterior halves that are held together with an elastic bandage). The cast and the involved extremity need to be observed frequently for neurovascular integrity and any signs of compromise. Permanent muscle and tissue damage can occur within 6 to 8 hours.

NURSING ALERT

Observations such as pain (unrelieved by pain medication 1 hour after administration), swelling, discolouration (pallor or cyanosis) of the exposed skin, decreased pulses, decreased temperature, or the inability to move the distal exposed part(s) should be reported immediately.

When an extremity that has sustained an open fracture is casted, a window is often left over the wound area to allow for observation and for dressing of the wound or a splint is used temporarily to allow for observation before casting. For the first few hours after surgery, there may be substantial bleeding that will soak through the cast. Periodically, the circumscribed blood-stained area should be outlined with a ball-point pen or pencil and the time indicated to provide a guide for assessing the amount of bleeding.

Appropriate cast care guidelines for the child's caregiver are necessary before discharge. Parents need instructions on drying and caring for the cast and on checking for signs and symptoms that indicate the cast is too tight or is too loose (see Patient Teaching box).

Nurses can help families adapt the child's home environment to meet the temporary encumbrance of a large cast or one that restricts the child's mobility (e.g., a long-leg or spica cast). Commonplace situations can become problematic (e.g., transporting a child safely and comfortably in a car). Standard seat belts and car seats may not be readily adapted for use by children in some casts and may require special seating. The adaptations must meet specific Canadian safety regulations (see Additional Resources at the end of this chapter). Alterations to standard car seats to accommodate the cast are not recommended because the structure may be adversely altered and fail to properly restrain the child.

Parents need to be taught the proper care of the cast (or immobilization device) and helped to devise means for maintaining cleanliness. With a hip spica cast, a superabsorbent

PATIENT TEACHING

Cast Care

Keep the casted extremity elevated on pillows or similar support for the first day, or as directed by the health care provider.

Avoid denting the plaster cast with fingertips (use palms of hand to handle) while it is still wet to avoid creating pressure points.

Observe the extremities (fingers or toes) for any evidence of swelling or discolouration (darker or lighter than a comparable extremity), and contact the health care provider if noted.

Check movement and sensation of the visible extremities frequently.

Follow the health care provider's orders regarding any restriction of activities.

Restrict strenuous activities for the first few days.
- Engage in quiet activities but encourage use of muscles.
- Move the joints above and below the cast on the affected extremity.

Encourage frequent rest for a few days, keeping the injured extremity elevated while resting.

Avoid allowing the affected limb to hang in a dependent position for any length of time.
- Keep an injured upper extremity elevated (e.g., in a sling) while upright.
- Elevate a lower limb when sitting and avoid standing for too long.

Do not allow the child to put anything inside the cast. Keep small items that might be placed inside the cast away from small children.

Keep a clear path for ambulation. Remove toys, hazardous floor rugs, pets, or other items the child might stumble over.

Use crutches appropriately if lower limb fracture requires non–weight bearing on affected extremity.

The crutches should fit properly, have a soft rubber tip to prevent slipping, and be well padded at the axilla.

With crutch walking, the child's body weight is supported on the hand grips, not the axilla.

disposable diaper may be tucked beneath the entire perineal opening of the cast. A larger diaper can be applied and fastened over the small diaper and cast to hold the smaller diaper in place.

For tightly fitting casts, transparent film dressings can be cut into strips with one edge applied to the cast edge and the other directly to the perineum; this forms a continuous waterproof bridge between the perineum and the cast to prevent leakage. An additional advantage to the use of this transparent dressing is that it keeps both the skin and the cast dry while allowing for observation of skin beneath the dressing.

Older infants and small children may stuff bits of food, small toys, or other items under the cast; parents should be alerted to this possibility so that suitable preventive measures can be initiated.

Feeding the infant in a hip spica cast offers problems in positioning. Very young infants can be fed in the supine position with the head elevated. With the infant's hips and legs supported on a pillow at the side, the parent can cuddle the infant in his or her arms during feeding. A somewhat similar position can be used for breastfeeding (i.e., with the infant supported on pillows or held in a "football" hold facing the mother with the legs behind her). An alternative position is to hold the infant upright on the caregiver's lap with the legs of the infant astride the adult's leg.

Children in spica casts may find the prone position easier for self-feeding from a small table placed next to the dining table; alternatively they may manage a semisitting position in a bed or wheelchair. The use of a conventional toilet is almost impossible. A bedside toilet can be adapted for use. Small bedpans or other containers offer alternatives to a toilet for elimination. The nurse may suggest waterproofing methods, using plastic wraps that can help with elimination and showers. Baths are possible only if the plaster cast is kept out of the water and covered to prevent it from becoming wet.

Cast Removal

Cutting the cast to remove it or to relieve tightness is frequently a frightening experience for children. They fear the sound of the cast cutter and are terrified that their flesh, as well as the cast, will be cut. The oscillating blade vibrates rapidly back and forth and will not cut when placed *lightly* on the skin. Children have described it as producing a "tickly" sensation. The vibration also generates heat that may be felt by the child. Both of these feelings should be explained.

Preparation for the procedure will help reduce anxiety, especially if a trusting relationship has been established between the child and the nurse. Many young children come to regard the cast as part of themselves, which intensifies their fear of removal (Fig. 53-4). Using the analogy of having fingernails trimmed or a haircut sometimes helps reduce their anxiety. They need continual reassurance that all is going well and that they are helping things go well. After the cast is removed, the parents and child should be given the option of keeping it. If the cast has been in place for a lengthy period, decreased muscle mass will be noted. The child should be reassured that resuming exercise and routine activities will return function and appearance (provided there was no significant trauma beforehand).

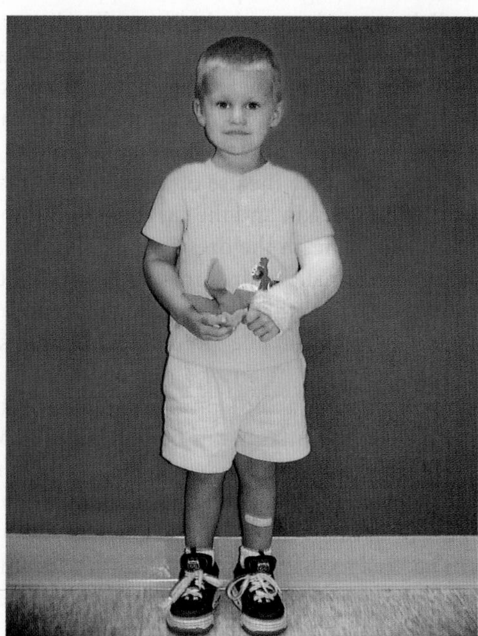

FIGURE 53-4 Young children usually adapt well to a cast but often fear the removal.

After the cast is removed, the skin surface will be caked with desquamated skin and sebaceous secretions. Simple soaking in a bathtub is usually sufficient for their removal, but several days may be required to eliminate the accumulation completely. Application of oil or skin lotion may provide comfort. The parents and child should be instructed not to pull or forcibly remove this material with vigorous scrubbing because it may cause excoriation and bleeding.

The Child in Traction

Most balanced skeletal traction is applied in children after a severe or complex injury to allow physiological stabilization, align bone fragments, and permit closer evaluation of the injured site. Newer technology has produced orthopedic fixation devices that allow partial or full mobility, thus preventing long-term immobilization and its consequences. In many situations, surgical intervention may be carried out within a matter of days; thus skeletal traction devices described here may be used infrequently in pediatrics.

Purposes of Traction

The three essential components of traction management are traction, countertraction, and friction (Fig. 53-5). To reduce or realign a fracture site, *traction* (forward force) is produced by attaching weight to the distal bone fragment. Body weight provides *countertraction* (backward force), and the patient's contact with the bed constitutes the *frictional* force. These forces are used to align the distal and proximal bone fragments by adjusting the line of pull upward or downward and adducting or abducting the extremity.

To attain equilibrium, the amount of forward force is adjusted by adding weight to or subtracting weight from the traction, and countertraction can be increased by elevating the foot of the bed to create a greater gravitational pull to the backward force.

The *all-or-none law*, characteristic of muscle contractibility, influences the complete relaxation. When muscle is stretched, muscle spasm ceases and permits the realignment of the bone ends. The continuous maintenance of traction is important during this phase because releasing the traction allows the normal contracting ability of the muscle to again cause a malpositioning of the bone ends.

The traction pull to some degree immobilizes the fracture site; however, adjunctive immobilizing devices such as splints or casts are sometimes used with skeletal traction. In injuries in which there is severe soft-tissue swelling or vascular and nerve damage, traction may be used until these complications have been resolved and it is safe to apply a cast or to perform surgical fixation.

Types of Traction (General)

The pull needed for traction can be applied to the distal bone fragment in several ways (Box 53-3). The type of traction applied is determined primarily by the child's age, the condition of the soft tissues, and the type and degree of displacement of the fracture. Fractures most commonly treated by the application of traction are those involving the femur and vertebrae.

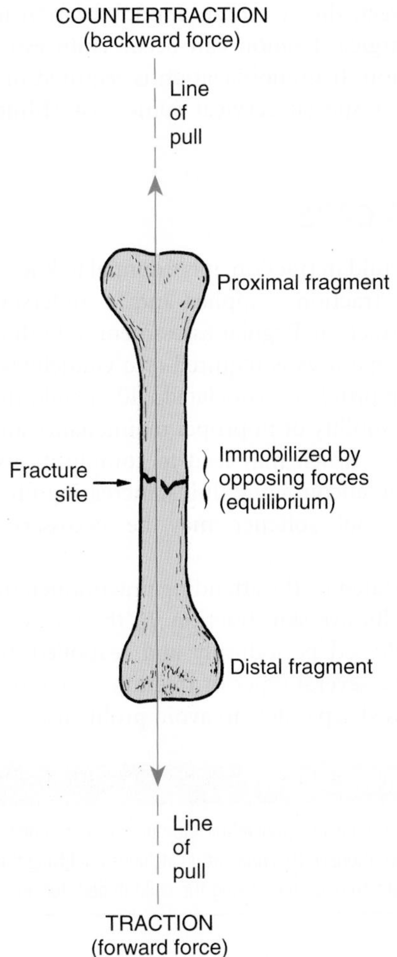

FIGURE 53-5 Application of traction for maintaining equilibrium.

BOX 53-3 TYPES OF TRACTION

Manual traction—Applied to the body part by the hands placed distal to the fracture site. Manual traction may be provided during application of a cast but more commonly when a closed reduction is performed.

Skin traction—Applied directly to the skin surface and indirectly to the skeletal structures. The pulling mechanism is attached to the skin with adhesive material or an elastic bandage. Both types are applied over soft, foam-backed traction straps to distribute the traction pull.

Skeletal traction—Applied directly to the skeletal structure by a pin, wire, or tongs inserted into or through the diameter of the bone distal to the fracture.

The major types of traction for specific fractures are discussed in the following sections.

Fractures of the femur can often be reduced with immediate application of a hip spica cast in young children. When traction is required, several types may be used, based on the initial assessment.

Bryant traction is a type of running traction in which the pull is in only one direction. Skin traction is applied to the legs, which are flexed at a 90-degree angle at the hips. The child's trunk (with the buttocks raised slightly off the bed) provides countertraction. Bryant traction may be used to treat a femoral shaft fracture in young children.

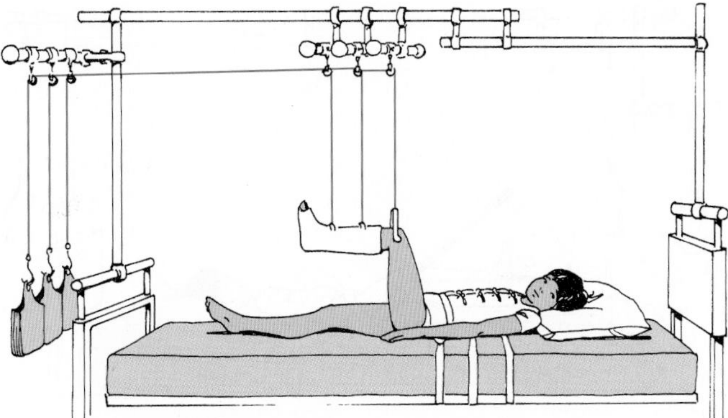

FIGURE 53-6 "Ninety-ninety" traction.

Buck extension traction is a type of skin traction with the legs in an extended position. Except for fracture cases, turning from side to side with care is permitted to maintain the involved leg alignment. Buck extension is used primarily for short-term immobilization, preoperatively with dislocated hips, for correcting contractures, or for bone deformities such as Legg-Calvé-Perthes disease. Buck traction may be accomplished with either skin straps or a special foam boot designed for traction.

Russell traction uses skin traction on the lower leg and a padded sling under the knee. Two lines of pull, one along the longitudinal line of the lower leg and one perpendicular to the leg, are produced. This combination of pulls allows realignment of the lower extremity and immobilizes the hip and knee in a flexed position. The hip flexion must be kept at the prescribed angle to prevent fracture malalignment, since there is no direct support under the fracture and the skin traction may slip.

A common type of skeletal traction is *90-degree–90-degree traction* (90-90 traction) (Fig. 53-6). The lower leg is supported by a boot cast or a calf sling, and a skeletal Steinmann pin or Kirschner's wire is placed in the distal fragment of the femur, resulting in a 90-degree angle at both the hip and the knee. From a nursing standpoint, this traction facilitates position changes, toileting, and prevention of complications related to traction.

Balanced suspension traction (Fig. 53-7) may be used with or without skin or skeletal traction. Unless used with another traction, the balanced suspension merely suspends the leg in a desired flexed position to relax the hip and hamstring muscles and does not exert any traction directly on a body part. A *Thomas splint* extends from the groin to midair above the foot, and a *Pearson attachment* supports the lower leg. When the child is lifted off the bed, the traction lifts with the child without loss of alignment. This traction requires very careful checking of splints and ropes to make certain that no slippage or fraying has occurred. The traction is of great value in an older and heavier child when it is essential to lift the patient for care.

The cervical area is a vulnerable site for flexion or extension injuries to muscle, vertebrae, or the spinal cord. Cervical muscle trauma without other complications is treated with a

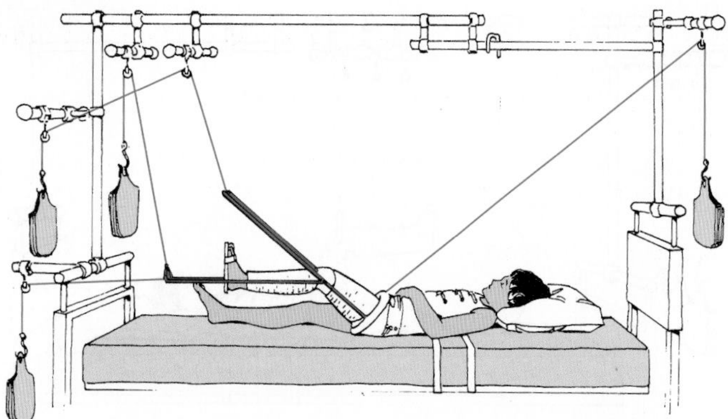

FIGURE 53-7 Balance suspension with Thomas splint and Pearson attachment.

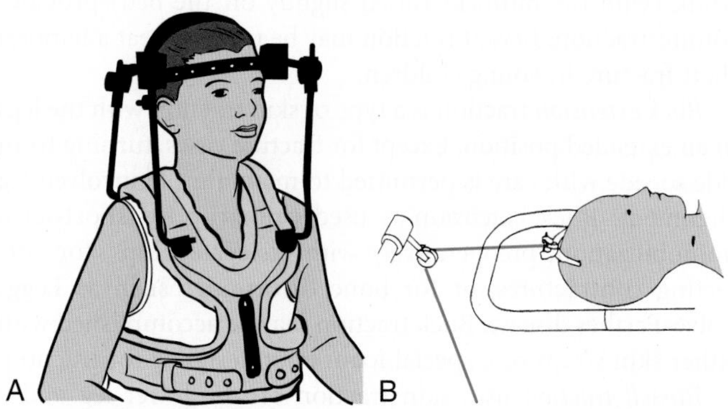

FIGURE 53-8 **A:** Halo vest. **B:** Gardner-Wells tongs.

cervical hard collar to relieve the weight of the head from the fracture site. When a child displaces or fractures a cervical vertebra, it may be necessary to reduce and immobilize the site with cervical skeletal traction. The spinal cord runs through the intravertebral canal, and dislocation or fracture of the vertebrae can also cause spinal cord injury. Nursing assessment of neurological function is essential to prevent further injury during the application and use of cervical skeletal traction. Most cervical traction is accomplished with the use of a *halo brace* or *halo vest* (Fig. 53-8, A). This device consists of a steel halo attached to the head by four screws inserted into the outer skull; several rigid bars connect the halo to a vest that is worn around the chest, thus providing greater mobility of the rest of the body while avoiding cervical spinal motion altogether. If the injury has been limited to a vertebral fracture without neurological deficit, a halo brace can be applied to permit earlier ambulation.

Gardner-Wells tongs (Fig. 53-8, B) may be used with the halo vest (Bailey, 2015). Gardner-Wells tongs are spring loaded, thus making burr holes and shaving hair are not required; a local anaesthetic may be used during application. In-line cervical traction may also be accomplished by attaching Gardner-Wells tongs to the child's head, with a 1.5- to 2-kg weight (depending on the child's weight) exerting traction on the cervical vertebrae.

As the neck muscles fatigue with constant traction pull, the vertebral bodies gradually separate so that the cord is no longer pinched between the vertebrae. Immobilization until fracture healing or surgical fixation can occur is an essential goal of cervical traction. If immobilization is required in an infant or young child, a special cervical spine cast (Minerva cast) is applied.

NURSING CARE

To assess the child in traction, it is essential to know the purpose for which the traction is applied and to understand the basic principles of traction. Regular assessment of both the child and the traction apparatus is required (see Guidelines box). Many of the nursing problems associated with a child in traction are related to immobility or improper maintenance and care of the traction device, which may lead to complications. Modifying the child's diet, encouraging fluids, increasing fibre, and offering a mild stool softener may be necessary to prevent constipation.

When indicated by the attending practitioner, the nurse may remove nonadhesive skin traction. In these cases intermittent traction is released periodically and reapplied as ordered. A child may have several types of traction at one time; each one must be assessed separately to avoid problems.

> **! NURSING ALERT**
>
> Skeletal traction is never released by the nurse (except under direct supervision by the practitioner). This precaution includes not lifting the weights that are applying traction (e.g., for moving the child in bed, for repositioning).

In addition to routine skin observation and care, the child in skeletal traction will need special skin care at the pin site according to hospital policy or practitioner preference. Pin sites should be frequently assessed and cleaned to prevent infection. Pin site infection is a common and significant complication after external fixation insertion. Health care organizations have their own pin care protocol with cleaning using an antiseptic cleaner or just normal saline. As well, some protocols have the nurse removing adherent pin scabs and others not. The frequency of cleaning varies.

When the child is first placed in traction, an increase in discomfort is common as a result of the traction pull fatiguing the muscle. Orthopedic conditions are associated with a higher-than-average number of painful events and a higher percentage of bodily symptoms than other common conditions. IV opioids, including analgesics and muscle relaxants, help during this phase of care and should be administered liberally.

> **! NURSING ALERT**
>
> For skeletal traction to be effective, ensure that the weights are hanging freely at all times. The specific nursing responsibilities for the patient in traction are outlined in the Guidelines box, on the following page.

Distraction

Unlike *traction*, which helps bones realign and fuse properly, *distraction* is the process of separating opposing bone

GUIDELINES

Traction Care

Understand Therapy

Understand the purposes of traction.

Understand the function of traction in each specific situation.

Maintain Traction

Check desired line of pull and relationship of distal fragment to proximal fragment. Check whether the fragment is being directed upward, adducted, or abducted.

Check function of each component.

- Position of bandages, frames, splints, specialized boot
- Ropes—In centre track of pulley, taut, no fraying, knots tied securely
- Pulleys—In original position on attachment bar; have not been displaced from original site
- Wheels freely moveable
- Weights—Correct amount of weight, hanging freely, in safe location

Check bed position; the head or foot should be elevated as directed for desired amount of pull and countertraction.

Do not remove skeletal traction or adhesive traction straps on skin traction.

Maintain Alignment

Observe for correct body alignment with emphasis on alignment of shoulder, hip, and leg.

Check after the child has moved.

Maintain correct angles at joints.

Skin Traction

Replace nonadhesive straps or elastic bandage on skin traction *when permitted* or absolutely necessary, but make certain that traction on limb is maintained by someone during procedure.

Assess straps or bandages to ascertain whether they are correctly applied (diagonal or spiral), not too loose or too tight, which could cause slippage and malalignment of traction.

Assess the traction boot to ensure it has not slipped and is not causing compression of the foot, thus impairing the circulation.

Skeletal Traction

Check pin sites frequently for signs of bleeding, inflammation, or infection.

Cleanse and dress pin sites per institution protocol or as ordered.

Apply topical antiseptic or antibiotic to pin sites daily as ordered.

Cover ends of pins with protective rubber or padding to prevent the child's being scratched by the pin.

Note pull of traction on the pin; pull should be even.

Check pin screws to be certain that screws are tight in metal clamp that attaches the traction apparatus to the pin.

Prevent Skin Breakdown

Provide foam overlay or alternating-pressure mattress underneath the hips and back.

Make total-body skin checks for redness or breakdown, especially over areas that receive the greatest pressure.

Wash and dry skin at least daily.

Inspect pressure points daily or more often if risk of breakdown is observed.

Use a skin breakdown assessment scale such as the Modified Braden Q.

Stimulate circulation with gentle massage over pressure areas.

Change position at least every 2 hours to relieve pressure.

Encourage increased intake of oral fluids.

Provide and encourage the patient to eat a balanced diet, including vegetables and fruits.

Prevent Complications

Check pulses in the affected area and compare with pulses in the contralateral site.

Assess circular dressings for excessive tightness.

Assess restrictive bandages or devices used to maintain traction on the affected limb.

- Make certain that they are not too loose or too tight.
- Remove periodically and check for pressure areas.

Encourage deep breathing frequently with maximum inspiratory chest expansion. Note any neurovascular changes, such as:

- Changes in colour in skin and nail beds
- Alterations in sensation, increased pain
- Alterations in motor ability

Take immediate action to correct problem or report to primary practitioner if neurovascular changes are found.

Record findings of neurovascular changes.

Carry out passive, active, or active-with-resistance exercises of uninvolved joints.

Note if any tightness, weakness, edema, or contractures are developing in uninvolved joints and muscles.

Take measures to correct or prevent further development of weakness, such as applying footboard or foot orthoses to prevent footdrop.

to encourage regeneration of new bone in the created space. Distraction can also be used when limbs are of unequal lengths and new bone is needed to elongate the shorter limb.

External Fixation

Monolateral, Taylor Spatial Frame, and Ilizarov external fixator (IEF) are common external fixation devices. The IEF uses a system of wires, rings, and telescoping rods that permits limb lengthening to occur by manual distraction (Fig. 53-9). In addition to lengthening bones, the device can be used to correct angular or rotational defects or to immobilize fractures. The device is attached surgically by securing a series of external full or half rings to the bone with wires. External telescoping rods connect the rings to each other. Manual distraction is accomplished by manipulating the rods to increase the distance between the rings. A percutaneous **osteotomy** is performed when the device is applied to create a "false" growth plate. A special osteotomy or corticotomy involves cutting only the cortex of the bone while preserving its blood supply, bone marrow, endosteum, and periosteum. Capillary blood flow to the transected area is essential for proper bone growth. Cut bone ends typically grow at a rate of 1 cm/month. The IEF can result in up to a 15-cm gain in length.

NURSING CARE

Success of external fixation devices depends on the child's and family's ability to collaborate with the health care team. Before

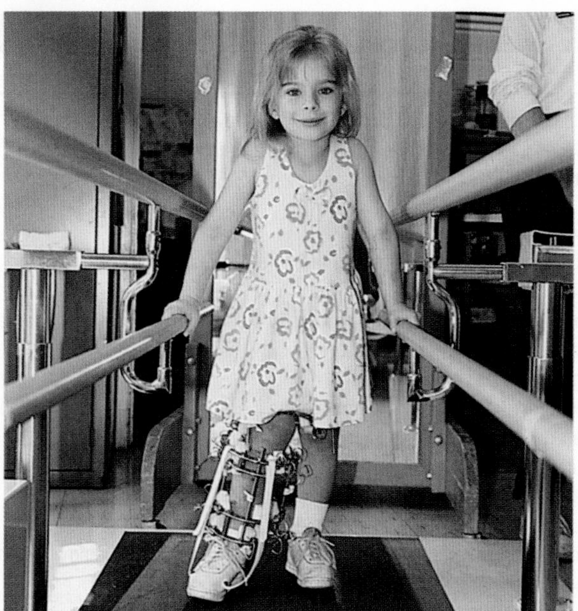

FIGURE 53-9 Child with Ilizarov external fixator (right leg) during physiotherapy on parallel bars.

surgery they must be fully informed of the appearance of the device, how it accomplishes bone growth and limits mobility, and of home and follow-up care. Children need to be involved in learning to adjust the device to accomplish distraction. Children, as well as parents, should be instructed in pin care, including observation for infection and loosening of the pins. Cleaning routines for the pin sites vary among practitioners but should not traumatize the skin. For example, the pins in IEF are thin and the child can go directly into a shower to clean the device and pins.

Children who participate actively in their care report less discomfort. Because the device is external, the child and family need to be prepared for the reactions of others and helped to camouflage it with appropriate apparel, such as wide-legged pants that close with self-adhering fasteners around it. A loose sock or stockinette may also be used over the device to help camouflage it. Partial weight bearing is allowed (see Fig. 53-9), and the child learns to walk with crutches. Alterations in activity include modifications at school and in physical education. Full weight bearing is not allowed until the distraction is completed and bone consolidation has occurred. Follow-up care is essential to maintaining appropriate distraction until the desired leg length is achieved. The device is removed surgically after the bone has consolidated, and the child may need to use crutches or have a cast for 4 to 6 weeks after removal to reduce the risk of fracture.

Amputation

A child may be born with the congenital absence of a body part, have a traumatic loss of an extremity, or need a surgical amputation for a pathological condition such as osteosarcoma (see p. 1744). With today's surgical technology and the quick thinking of bystanders who save a traumatically amputated body part, children have had fingers and arms reattached with variable degrees of functional use regained.

> **! NURSING ALERT**
>
> For an amputated limb or body part that may be reattached, do the following:
> 1. Rinse limb gently with normal saline.
> 2. Loosely wrap limb in sterile gauze.
> 3. Place wrapped limb in a watertight bag.
> 4. Cool (without freezing) bag in ice water (do not pack in ice because this may harm tissue).
> 5. Label with child's name, date, and time, and transport with the child to the hospital.

Surgical amputation or the surgical repair of a permanently severed limb focuses on constructing an adequately nourished residual limb. A smooth, healthy, padded stump, free of nerve endings, is important in prosthesis fitting and subsequent ambulation. In some situations in which there is no vascular or neurological deficit, a cast is applied to the stump immediately after the procedure, and a pylon, metal extension, and artificial foot are attached so that the patient can walk on the temporary prosthesis within a few hours.

NURSING CARE

Stump shaping is performed postoperatively with special elastic bandaging using a figure-8 bandage, which applies pressure in a cone-shaped fashion. This technique decreases stump edema, controls hemorrhage, and aids in developing the desired contours so that the child will bear weight on the posterior aspect of the skin flap rather than on the end of the stump. Stump elevation may be used during the first 24 hours, but after this time the extremity should not be left in this position because contractures will develop in the proximal joint and seriously hamper ambulation. Monitoring proper body alignment will further decrease the risk of flexion contractures.

For older children and adolescents, arm exercises (as well as parallel bars, which are used in prosthesis-training programs) help build up the arm muscles necessary for walking with crutches. Full range-of-motion exercises of joints above the amputation must be performed several times daily using active and isotonic exercises. Younger children are often spontaneously active and require little encouragement.

Depending on the child's age, children or their parents will need to learn stump hygiene, including careful soap-and-water washing every day and checking for skin irritation, breakdown, or infection. A tube of stockinette or powder is used to slide the prosthesis on more easily. Skin must be checked carefully every time the prosthesis is removed, and prosthesis tolerance time must be adjusted to prevent skin breakdown.

For children who have had an amputation, *phantom limb sensation* is an expected experience because the nerve–brain connections are still present. Gradually these sensations fade, although in many amputees they persist for years. Preoperative discussion of this phenomenon will aid a child in understanding these "unusual feelings" and in not hiding the experiences from others. Limb pain, especially pain that increases with ambulation, should be evaluated for the possibility of a neuroma at the free nerve endings in the stump, or other problems such as a poorly fitting prosthesis or joint instability.

CONGENITAL DEFECTS

Some skeletal defects may be diagnosed at birth or within days, weeks, or months after birth. In other cases the deviation may be difficult to detect without careful inspection. It is imperative that nurses become acquainted with signs of these defects and understand the principles of therapy in order to direct others in the care and management of these children.

Arthrogryposis

Arthrogryposis is a term used to describe a number of rare, congenital conditions that are characterized by stiff joints and abnormally developed muscles. It is also called *arthrogryposis multiplex congenital*, or *amyloplasia*. Research indicates that the incidence is likely 1 in every 5000 to 10,000 live births (Horstmann, Conroy, & Davidson, 2016). Arthrogryposis is not considered to be an inherited condition. While the exact etiology is unknown, there are several proposed theories: obstruction to uterine movement during pregnancy, an early viral infection during fetal development, and the result of the central nervous system or muscular system not developing appropriately.

Children experience clinical manifestations differently. The common symptoms are limited or fixed range of movement in joints, internal rotation of the shoulders, abnormal extension of the elbows, and more flexibility than usual in the wrists and fingers. These children may also have developmental congenital hip dysplasia and a club foot (Horstmann et al., 2016).

Diagnostic Evaluation

To diagnose the condition, the health care provider takes a comprehensive medical history and performs a careful physical examination. Radiography and other diagnostic imaging, blood work, and muscle biopsy may also be used.

Therapeutic Management

Treatment consists of physiotherapy and occupational therapy to increase flexibility and strengthen joints. Orthopedic surgery might be needed to increase joint function, and the child will likely have some persistent muscle and joint limitations caused by the underlying condition that may improve substantially with treatment. This condition is not progressive and will not get worse as the child gets older (Azbell & Dannemiller, 2015).

Achondroplasia

Achondroplasia is a bone disorder that is genetic; it is the most common type of dwarfism. The incidence is 1 in 20,000 infants. The arms and legs are short in proportion to the body length, and the head is often large and the trunk of normal size. The genetic mutation causes abnormal cartilage formation (Ireland, Pacey, Zankl, et al., 2014).

The average height of adult males with achondroplasia is 132 cm (52 inches [4 feet, 4 inches]), and the average height of adult females with achondroplasia is 124 cm (49 inches [4 feet, 1 inch]).

The most common clinical manifestations are as follows:

- Shortened arms and legs, with the upper arms and thighs more shortened than the forearms and lower legs
- Large head size with prominent forehead and a flattened nasal bridge; crowded or misaligned teeth
- Curved lower spine (lordosis), which may lead to *kyphosis*, or the development of a small hump near the shoulders, that usually goes away after the child begins walking; small vertebral canals bones, which may lead to spinal cord compression in adolescence. Occasionally children with achondroplasia die suddenly in infancy or early childhood in their sleep because of compression of the upper end of the spinal cord, which interferes with breathing.
- Bowed lower legs
- Flat feet that are short and broad
- Extra space between the middle and ring fingers (also called a *trident hand*)
- Poor muscle tone and loose joints
- Frequent middle ear infections, which may lead to hearing loss
- Normal intelligence
- Delayed developmental milestones, such as walking (which may occur between 18 and 24 months instead of around 1 year of age) (Ireland et al., 2014)

In some cases, the child inherits the achondroplasia from a parent with the condition, but most cases (about 80%) are caused by a new genetic mutation. This means the parents are of average height and do not have the abnormal gene. However, people with achondroplasia have a 50% chance of passing the gene to their child, resulting in the condition. Achondroplasia can be diagnosed before birth by fetal ultrasound or after birth by complete medical history and physical examination. DNA testing is available before birth to confirm fetal ultrasound findings for parents who are at increased risk for having a child with achondroplasia (Ireland et al., 2014).

Therapeutic Management

Some children may be treated with a growth hormone, although this has little effect on the height of the child. In some very specific cases, surgeries to lengthen legs may be considered (see Distraction, p. 1726). It is important to check for bone abnormalities, especially in the back region, as these can cause respiratory difficulties and leg pain. Kyphosis may need to be corrected through surgery if it does not correct itself when the child starts to walk. Surgery may also be done to help prevent bowing of the legs.

Developmental Dysplasia of the Hip

The broad term *developmental dysplasia of the hip (DDH)* describes a spectrum of disorders related to abnormal development of the hip that may develop at any time during fetal life, infancy, or childhood, in which there is a shallow acetabulum, subluxation, or dislocation. The incidence of hip instability of some kind is approximately 10 per 1000 live births. The incidence of frank dislocation or a dislocatable hip is 1 to 1.5 per 1000 live births (Sankar, Horn, Wells, et al., 2016). Girls are more commonly affected (80%) and there is a positive family history in approximately 12 to 33% of affected children (Sankar et al., 2016).

Pathophysiology

Predisposing factors associated with DDH may be divided into three broad categories:

1. Physiological factors, which include maternal hormone secretion and intrauterine positioning
2. Mechanical factors, which involve breech presentation, multiple fetuses, oligohydramnios, and large infant size (other mechanical factors may include continued maintenance of the hips in adduction and extension, which will in time cause a dislocation)
3. Genetic factors, which entail a higher incidence of DDH in siblings of affected infants, and an even greater incidence of recurrence if a sibling and one parent were affected

Some experts categorize DDH into two major groups: (1) *idiopathic*, in which the infant is neurologically intact; and (2) *teratological*, which involves a neuromuscular defect such as arthrogryposis or myelodysplasia. The teratological forms usually occur in utero and are much less common.

Three degrees of DDH are illustrated in Fig. 53-10.

1. **Acetabular dysplasia**—The mildest form of DDH, in which there is neither subluxation nor dislocation. There is a delay in acetabular development evidenced by osseous hypoplasia of the acetabular roof that is oblique and shallow, although cartilaginous roof is comparatively intact. The femoral heal remains in the acetabulum.
2. **Subluxation**—The largest percentage of DDH, subluxation, implies incomplete dislocation of the hip and is sometimes regarded as an intermediate state in the development from primary dysplasia to complete dislocation. The femoral head remains in contact with the acetabulum, but a stretched capsule and ligamentum teres cause the head of the femur to be partially displaced. Pressure on the cartilaginous roof inhibits ossification and produces a flattening of the socket.
3. **Dislocation**—The femoral head loses contact with acetabulum and is displaced posteriorly and superiorly over the fibrocartilaginous rim. The ligamentum teres is elongated and taunt.

Diagnostic Evaluation

DDH is often not detected at the initial examination after birth; thus all infants should be carefully monitored for hip dysplasia at follow-up visits throughout the first year of life. In the newborn period dysplasia usually appears as hip joint laxity rather than as outright dislocation. The clinical manifestations of DDH are outlined in Box 53-4.

The Ortolani and Barlow tests are the most reliable tests for infants from birth to 4 weeks of age (see Fig. 25-12 on p. 661). With the Barlow test the thighs are adducted; the Ortolani test involves abducting the thigh to test for hip subluxation or dislocation (Ball, Dains, Flynn, et al., 2015). Other signs of DDH are shortening of the leg on the affected side, asymmetrical thigh and gluteal folds, and broadening of the perineum (in bilateral dislocation) (see Box 53-4).

Radiographic examination in early infancy is not reliable, since ossification of the femoral head does not normally take place until the fourth to sixth month of life. However, the cartilaginous head can be visualized directly by **ultrasonography**, and it is recommended as an adjunct to other diagnostic procedures (Sankar et al., 2016). In children older than age 4 months, radiographic examination is useful in confirming the diagnosis. An upward slope in the roof of the acetabulum (the acetabular angle) greater than 40 degrees with upward and outward displacement of the femoral head is a frequent finding in older children. A computed tomography (CT) scan may be useful to assess the position of the femoral head relative to the acetabulum after closed reduction and casting.

Therapeutic Management

Treatment is begun as soon as the condition is recognized, because early intervention is more favourable to the restoration of normal bony architecture and function. The longer treatment is delayed and the more severe the deformity, the more difficult the treatment and the less favourable the prognosis.

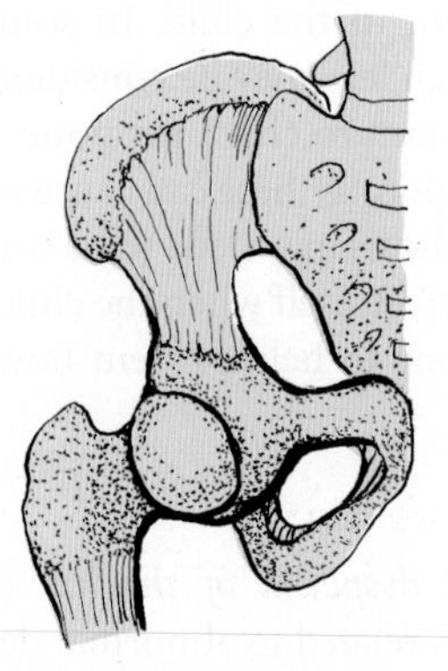

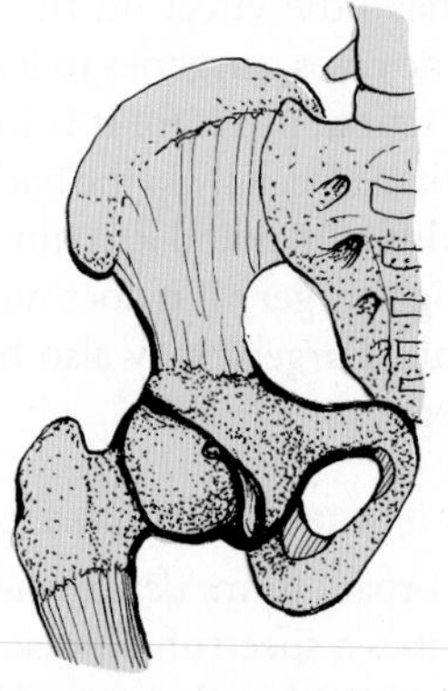

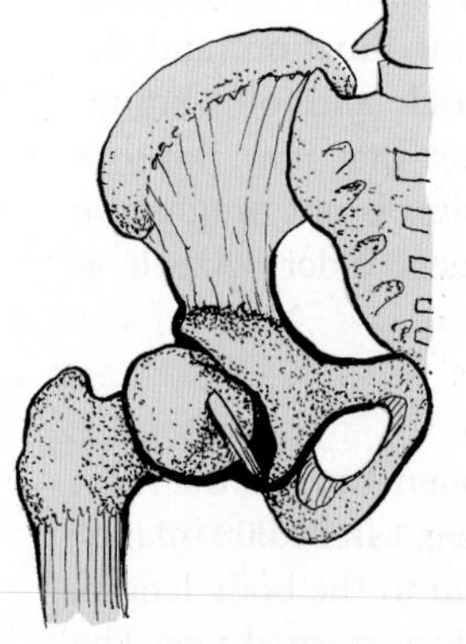

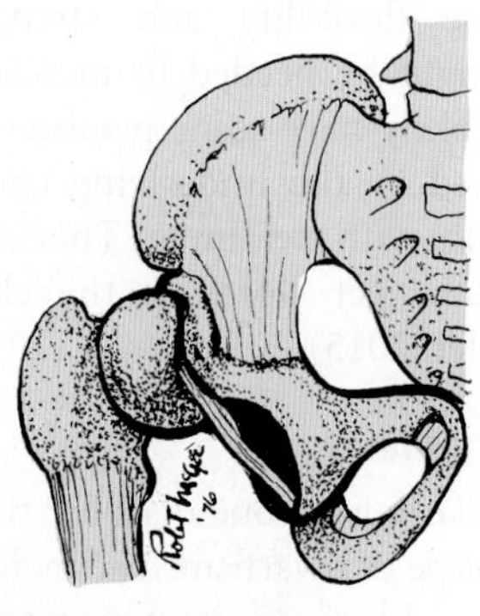

FIGURE 53-10 Configuration and relationship of structures in developmental dysplasia of the hip.

BOX 53-4 CLINICAL MANIFESTATIONS OF DEVELOPMENTAL DYSPLASIA OF THE HIP

Infant

Shortening of limb on affected side (Galeazzi sign)
Restricted abduction of hip on affected side
Unequal gluteal folds (best visualized with infant prone)
Positive Ortolani test (hip reduced by abduction)
Positive Barlow test (hip dislocated by adduction)

Older Infant and Child

Affected leg shorter than the other
Telescoping or piston mobility of joint—Head of femur felt to move up and down in buttock when extended thigh is pushed first toward child's head and then pulled distally
Trendelenburg sign—When child stands first on one foot and then on the other (holding onto a chair, rail, or someone's hands) bearing weight on the affected hip, the pelvis tilts downward on the normal side instead of upward, as it would with normal stability
Greater trochanter prominent and appearing above a line from anterosuperior iliac spine to tuberosity of ischium
Marked lordosis and waddling gait (bilateral dislocations)

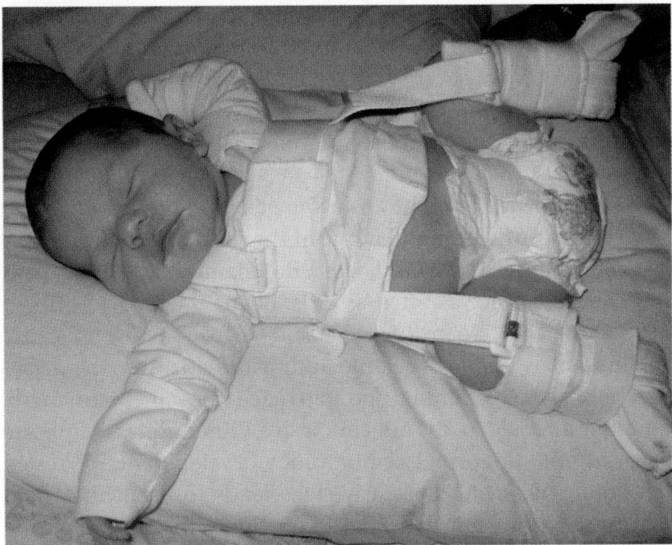

FIGURE 53-11 Child in Pavlik harness. (Courtesy Amanda Politte.)

The treatment varies with the child's age and the extent of the dysplasia. The goal of treatment is to obtain and maintain a safe, congruent position of the hip joint to promote normal hip joint development.

Newborn to age 6 months. The hip joint is maintained by splinting with the proximal femur centred in the acetabulum in an attitude of flexion. Of the numerous devices available, the *Pavlik harness* is the most widely used, and with time, motion, and gravity, the hip works into a more abducted, reduced position (Fig. 53-11). The harness is worn continuously until the hip is proved stable clinically and on ultrasound examination, usually in about 6 to 12 weeks. After the age of 6 months the Pavlik harness tends to lose its effectiveness because of the child's increasing mobility and strength (Sankar et al., 2016).

When adduction contracture is present, other devices, such as Bryant traction (see p. 1725), are used to slowly and gently stretch the hip to full abduction. After this is achieved, wide abduction is maintained until stability is attained. Maintaining stable reduction is difficult; therefore, a hip spica cast is applied and changed periodically to accommodate the child's growth. After 3 to 6 months, sufficient stability is acquired to allow transfer to a removable protective abduction brace. The duration of treatment depends on development of the acetabulum but is usually accomplished within the first year.

Ages 6 to 18 months. In this age group the dislocation may not be recognized until the child begins to stand and walk, when attendant shortening of the limb and contractures of the hip adductor and flexor muscles become apparent. A surgical closed reduction is performed, and the child is placed in a spica cast for approximately 12 weeks. An abduction orthosis may be used instead of a hip spica cast. In the event that the hip remains unstable, an open reduction is performed (Sankar et al., 2016).

Older child. Correction of the hip deformity in older children is inherently more difficult than in the preceding age groups, because secondary adaptive changes and other etiological factors (such as juvenile idiopathic arthritis or nonambulatory cerebral palsy) complicate the condition. Operative reduction, which may involve preoperative traction, tenotomy of contracted muscles, and any one of several innominate osteotomy procedures designed to construct an acetabular roof, often combined with proximal femoral osteotomy, is usually required. After cast removal and before weight bearing is permitted, range-of-motion exercises help restore movement. Successful reduction and reconstruction become increasingly difficult after the age of 4 years and are usually impossible or inadvisable in children older than 6 years of age because of severe shortening and contracture of muscles and deformity of the femoral and acetabular structures.

NURSING CARE

Nurses are in a unique position to detect DDH in early infancy. During the infant assessment process and routine nurturing activities, the hips and extremities are inspected for any deviations from normal. These observations should be reported to the attending practitioner, and the ambulatory child who displays a limp or an unusual gait should be referred for evaluation. This may indicate an orthopedic or neurological problem. Nonambulatory children with cerebral palsy should also be assessed for evidence of hip problems.

! NURSING ALERT

The Ortolani and Barlow tests must be performed by an experienced clinician (physician or nurse practitioner) to prevent further damage to the hip. If these tests are performed too vigorously in the first 2 days of life, when the hip subluxates freely, persistent dislocation may occur. An unskilled examiner can cause injury to the newborn.

The major nursing problems in the care of an infant or child in a cast or other device are related to maintenance of the device and adaptation of nurturing activities to meet his or her needs. Generally, treatment and follow-up care of these children are carried out in an outpatient setting. Hospitalization may be necessary for cast application or brace fitting but seldom exceeds 24 to 48 hours. Longer hospitalization is required for open reduction.

! NURSING ALERT

The former practice of double- or triple-diapering for DDH is not recommended because it promotes hip extension, thus impeding proper hip development. There is no evidence to support its efficacy.

The primary nursing goal is teaching parents to apply and maintain the reduction device. The Pavlik harness allows for easy handling of the infant and usually produces less apprehension in the parent than do heavy braces and casts. Because of the infant's rapid growth, the straps should be checked in the beginning of therapy every week for possible adjustments. It is important that parents understand the correct use of the appliance, which may or may not allow for its removal during bathing. Removing the harness is determined individually on the basis of the provider's recommendation, the family's level of understanding, and the degree of hip deformity. Parents should be instructed not to adjust the harness. The child should be examined by the practitioner before any adjustment is attempted to make certain the hips are in correct placement.

Skin care is an important aspect of the care of an infant in a harness. The following instructions for preventing skin breakdown are stressed:

- Always put an undershirt (or a shirt with extensions that close at the crotch) under the chest straps
- Put knee socks under the foot and leg pieces to prevent the straps from rubbing the skin.

The child's skin should be checked frequently (at least two or three times a day) for red areas under the straps and the clothing. The caregiver should gently massage healthy skin under the straps once a day to stimulate circulation. In general, use of lotions and powders is avoided because they can cake and irritate the skin. The diaper should always be placed under the straps.

Parents should be encouraged to hold the infant with a harness and continue care and nurturing activities. The nurse can assist by being available for parents' questions about the necessary adaptations to daily care to decrease their anxiety and possible feelings about the child being hurt by routine caring.

Casts and orthotics devices (harness) offer more challenging nursing problems because they cannot be removed for routine care, although sometimes a brace may be removed for bathing. Care of an infant or small child with a cast requires nursing innovation to reduce skin pressure or friction and to maintain cleanliness of both the child and the cast, particularly in the diaper area.

It is important for nurses, parents, and other caregivers to understand that children in corrective devices need to be involved in all the activities of any child in the same age group. Confinement in a cast or appliance should not exclude children from family (or unit) activities. They can be held astride the lap for comfort and transported to areas of activity. The child may be allowed to walk in a cast or orthotic device. An adapted wheelchair, stroller, or scooter can offer mobility to an older infant or child.

Clubfoot

Clubfoot is a complex deformity of the ankle and foot that includes forefoot adduction, midfoot supination, hindfoot varus, and ankle equinus. Deformities of the foot and ankle are described according to the position of the ankle and foot. The more common positions involve the following variations:

Talipes varus—An inversion or a bending inward

Talipes valgus—An eversion or bending outward

Talipes equinus—Plantar flexion, in which the toes are lower than the heel

Talipes calcaneus—Dorsiflexion, in which the toes are higher than the heel

Talipes equinovarus—Toes lower than the heel and facing inward

Most cases of clubfoot are a combination of these positions, and the most commonly occurring type of clubfoot (approximately 95%) is the composite deformity *talipes equinovarus (TEV)*, in which the foot is pointed downward and inward in varying degrees of severity (Fig. 53-12). Clubfoot may occur as an isolated deformity or in association with other disorders or syndromes, such as chromosome abnormalities, arthrogryposis, cerebral palsy, or spina bifida.

The incidence of clubfoot in the general population is 1 in 1000 births worldwide and is one of the most common congenital deformities (Mang'oli, Theuri, Kollmann, et al., 2014), with boys affected twice as often as girls. Bilateral clubfeet occur in 50% of the cases (Winell & Davidson, 2016). The precise cause of clubfoot is unknown. Some authorities attribute the defect to abnormal positioning and restricted movement in utero, although the evidence is not conclusive. Other experts implicate arrested or abnormal embryonic development. Arrested development during this early stage tends to result in a rigid deformity; however, mechanical pressures from intrauterine positioning are likely causes of more flexible deformities (Shyy, Wang, Sheffield, et al., 2010).

Classification

Clubfoot may be further divided into three categories: (1) *positional clubfoot* (also called *transitional, mild,* or *postural clubfoot*), which is believed to occur primarily from intrauterine crowding, (2) *syndromic* (or *teratological*) *clubfoot*, which is associated with other congenital anomalies such as myelomeningocele or arthrogryposis and is a more severe form of clubfoot that is often resistant to treatment, and (3) *congenital clubfoot*, also referred to as *idiopathic*, which may occur in an otherwise normal child and has a wide range of rigidity and prognosis.

The mild, or postural, clubfoot may correct spontaneously or may require passive exercise or serial casting. There is no bony abnormality, but there may be tightness and shortening

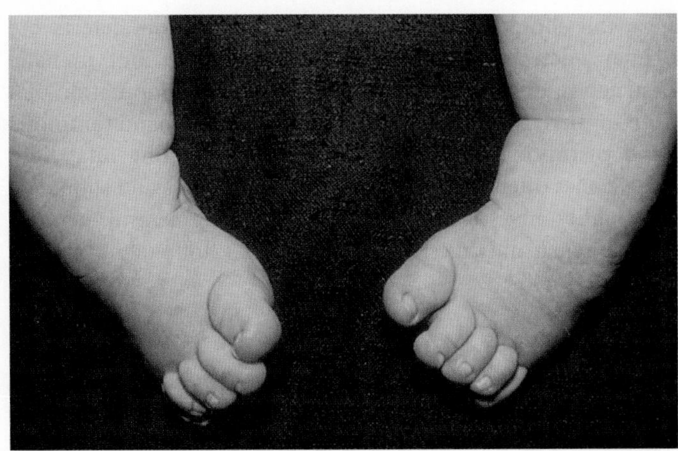

FIGURE 53-12 Bilateral congenital talipes equinovarus (congenital clubfoot) in a 2-month-old infant. (From Zitelli, B. J., & Davis, H. W. [2007]. *Atlas of pediatric physical diagnosis* [5th ed., p. 8]. St. Louis: Mosby [Fig. 1-12F].)

of the soft tissues medially and posteriorly. The teratological clubfoot usually requires surgical correction and has a high incidence of recurrence. The congenital idiopathic clubfoot, or "true clubfoot," almost always requires surgical intervention because there is bony abnormality.

Diagnostic Evaluation

The deformity is often readily apparent and easily detected prenatally through ultrasonography or at birth. However, it must be differentiated from some positional deformities that can be passively corrected or overcorrected. Paralytic changes in the lower extremity of children with neuromuscular involvement often produce equinovarus deformity. An increased risk of hip dysplasia is associated with clubfoot deformities.

Therapeutic Management

The goal of treatment for clubfoot is to achieve a painless, plantigrade, and stable foot. Treatment of clubfoot involves three stages: (1) correction of the deformity, (2) maintenance of the correction until normal muscle balance is regained, and (3) follow-up observation to avert possible recurrence of the deformity. Some feet respond to treatment readily while some respond only to prolonged, vigorous, and sustained efforts, and the improvement in others remains disappointing despite all the efforts.

A common approach to clubfoot management is the Ponseti method (Ponseti, 1996). Serial casting is begun shortly after birth. Weekly gentle manipulation and serial long-leg casts allow for gradual repositioning of the foot (Fig. 53-13). The extremity or extremities are casted until maximum correction is achieved, usually within 6 to 10 weeks. Most of the time a percutaneous heel cord tenotomy is performed at the end of the serial casting to correct the equinus. After the tenotomy, a long-leg cast is applied and left in place for 3 weeks. A Denis Browne bar with Ponseti sandals or straight-laced shoes placed in abduction is then fitted to prevent recurrence. Inability to achieve normal foot alignment after casting and tenotomy indicates the need for surgical intervention. For the Ponseti manipulation to be successful, it is important for the health care provider to support the parents and instruct them in how best to set up and apply the brace. Follow-up is also important, to identify early signs of reoccurrence and prevent full relapse by enforcing abduction bracing, recasting, or tilialis anterior tendon. Recent midterm outcome studies have shown that by following the Ponseti treatment regime in all aspects, it is possible to prevent open joint surgery in almost all cases (Radler, 2013).

Surgical intervention for clubfoot involves pin fixation and the release of tight joints and tendons. Casting of the affected foot and leg is performed, and after 2 or 3 months, a varus-prevention brace is used to maintain correction. With severe deformities, repeated surgical tendon or joint releases may be necessary.

Children with clubfoot need to be followed by a health care provider. Sometimes the original problem will reoccur, particularly at 2 to 3 years of age. There can also be long-term residual symptoms. When an adolescent is having a growth spurt, the pain may reoccur. Orthotics that are customized will be needed to support the foot.

NURSING CARE

Nursing care of the child with clubfoot is the same as for any child who has a cast (see p. 1722). Because the child will spend considerable time in a corrective device, nursing care plans include both long- and short-term goals. Conscientious observation of the skin and circulation is particularly important in young infants because of their rapid growth rate. Because treatment and follow-up care are handled in the orthopedist's office, clinic, or outpatient department, parent education and support are important in nursing care of these children.

It is important for parents to understand the overall treatment program, the importance of regular cast changes, and the role they play in the long-term effectiveness of the therapy. Reinforcing and clarifying the orthopedist's explanations and instructions, teaching parents about care of the cast or appliance (including vigilant observation for potential problems), and encouraging parents to facilitate normal development within the limitations imposed by the deformity or therapy are all part of nursing responsibilities.

Metatarsus Adductus (Varus)

Metatarsus adductus, or metatarsus varus, is probably the most common congenital foot deformity. In most instances it is a result of abnormal intrauterine positioning, particularly in the firstborn child, and is usually detected at birth. The deformity is characterized by medial adduction of the toes and forefoot, frequently in association with inversion, and by convexity of the lateral border of the foot. Metatarsus adductus may be divided into three categories: *type I*, in which the forefoot is flexible and corrects easily with manipulation; *type II*, in which there is only partial flexibility in the forefoot, and it corrects passively past neutral position but only to neutral position with active manipulation; and *type III*, in which the forefoot is rigid and will not stretch to neutral position with manipulation. Unlike

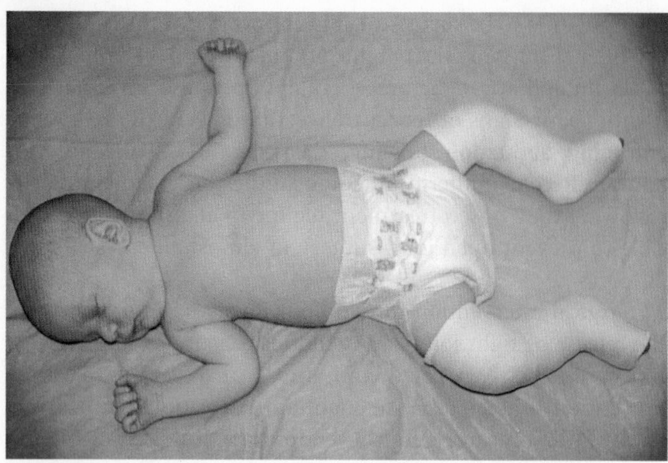

FIGURE 53-13 Feet casted for correction of bilateral congenital talipes equinovarus.

TEV, with which it is often confused, the angulation occurs at the tarsometatarsal joint, whereas the heel and ankle remain in a neutral position. Ankle range of motion is normal. This deformity often causes a pigeon-toed gait in the child.

Therapeutic management depends on the rigidity and type of the deformity. Correction with types I and II can usually be accomplished by gentle manipulation and passive stretching of the foot, which the parent is taught to perform. Repeated and consistent stretching is continued for the first 6 weeks, after which the treatment is based on the flexibility of the foot. With type III, the child will usually require serial manipulation and casting to correct the defect. Casting is performed every 1 to 2 weeks for 6 to 8 weeks, after which a corrective shoe or orthosis may be used. Surgical correction is rarely required for the condition unless there is residual deformity at 4 to 6 years of age or the child has considerable pain on ambulation or is unable to wear certain kinds of shoes as a result of the defect (Winell & Davidson, 2016).

NURSING CARE

The nursing role primarily involves identifying the defect so that early therapy and instruction of the parents can be initiated. The nurse needs to teach the parents how to hold the heel firmly and to stretch only the forefoot; otherwise, undue force on the heel may produce a valgus deformity. If casting or orthosis is required, the nurse should instruct the parents in cast care and observation of the corrective device (see p. 1722).

Skeletal Limb Deficiency

Congenital limb deficiencies, or reduction malformations (disruption defects), are manifested by varying degrees of loss of functional capacity. They are characterized by underdevelopment of skeletal elements of the extremities. The range of malformation can extend from minor defects of the digits to serious abnormalities such as *amelia*, absence of an entire extremity, or *meromelia*, partial absence of an extremity that includes *phocomelia* (seal limbs), interposed deficiency of long bones with relatively good development of hands and feet attached at or near the shoulder or the hips. Most reduction defects are primary defects of development of the limb, but prenatal destruction of the limb can occur, such as the amputation of a limb in utero from constriction of an amniotic band (amniotic band disruption sequence). Newborns with congenital limb deficiencies often have associated malformations and should be thoroughly investigated for cardiovascular, central nervous system, renal, and digestive abnormalities (Stoll, Alembik, Dott, et al., 2010).

Pathophysiology

Limb deficiencies can be attributed to both heredity and environment and can originate at any stage of limb development. Formation of limbs may be suppressed at the time of limb bud formation, or there may be interference in later stages of differentiation and growth. Heredity appears to play a prominent role, and prenatal environmental insults have been implicated in a number of cases. The latter includes the well-publicized thalidomide tragedy of the 1950s and early 1960s, which demonstrated a clear relationship between the time of exposure of the pregnant woman to the antiemetic medication and the presence and type of limb deformity in the newborn. There still are many drugs that may have similar teratogenic effects in the first trimester of pregnancy; therefore, medication administration during this period should be evaluated carefully by the health care provider.

Therapeutic Management

Children with congenital limb deficiencies should be fitted with prosthetic devices whenever possible, and the devices should be applied at the earliest possible stage of development in an attempt to match the infant's motor readiness. This favours natural progression of prosthetic use. For example, a young infant with an upper extremity deficiency is fitted with a simple passive device, such as a mitten prosthesis, to encourage limb exploration, sitting (with the extremities needed for support), and bilateral hand activities.

Lower limb prostheses are applied when the infant begins sitting up and can maintain balance. In preparation for prosthetic devices, surgical modification may be necessary to ensure the most favourable use of the device, since severe deformity can interfere with its effective use. Phocomelic digits are preserved for controlling switches of externally powered appliances in upper extremities. Digits (in both upper and lower extremities) provide the child with surfaces for tactile exploration and stimulation. Prostheses are replaced to accommodate the child's growth and increasing capabilities.

NURSING CARE

Prosthetic application training and habilitation are most successfully carried out in a centre that specializes in meeting the special needs of these children, especially very young children and those with amputations or missing limbs. Therapeutic management involves a prosthetist, who specializes in the development, fitting, and maintenance of prosthetic limbs, and other health care workers such as physiotherapists and occupational therapists.

Parents need special attention and support and should be encouraged to assist the child in making age-commensurate adjustments to the environment. Although these children need assistance, overprotection may produce overdependence, with later maladjustment to school and other situations.

Osteogenesis Imperfecta

Osteogenesis imperfecta (OI) is the most common osteoporosis syndrome in childhood. However, it is very rare. OI is a heterogeneous, autosomal dominant disorder characterized by fractures and bone deformity. There are at least eight described types of OI, which accounts for significant disease variability. Clinical features may include varying degrees of bone fragility, deformity, and fracture; blue sclerae; hearing loss; and *dentinogenesis imperfecta* (hypoplastic discoloured teeth). Although inheritance follows an autosomal dominant pattern in most cases, rare autosomal recessive exists primarily in populations with consanguineous marriages (Marini, 2016).

Classifications for OI are based on clinical features and patterns of inheritance (see Box 53-5). Clinically, type I is the most common, with wide variability of bone fragility; some affected family members have significant deformity and disability, whereas others lead agile, active lives. Type II variants are the most severe and are considered lethal in infancy. Type III OI is characterized by multiple fractures, bone deformity, and severe disability; affected individuals rarely live to 30 years of age. Type VII follows the autosomal recessive inheritance that has been described in a consanguinous Indigenous community from Northern Québec.

Therapeutic Management

The treatment for OI is primarily supportive, although patients and families are optimistic about new research advances. The use of bisphosphonate therapy with IV pamidronate to promote increased bone density and prevent fractures has become standard therapy for many children with OI; however, long bones are weakened by prolonged treatment. One of the advantages of bisphosphonate therapy is the decrease in vertebral compression and scoliosis (Marini, 2016).

The goals of a rehabilitative approach to management are directed toward preventing (1) positional contractures and deformities, (2) muscle weakness and osteoporosis, and (3) malalignment of lower extremity joints prohibiting weight bearing. Lightweight braces and splints help support limbs, prevent fractures, and aid in ambulation. Physiotherapy helps prevent disuse osteoporosis and strengthens muscles, which in turn improves bone density.

Surgery is sometimes used to help treat the manifestations of the disease. Surgical techniques are used to correct deformities that interfere with bracing, standing, or walking. For the child with recurrent fractures, inserting an intramedullary rod provides stability to bones.

NURSING CARE

Infants and children with this disorder require careful handling to prevent fractures. They must be supported when they are being turned, positioned, moved, and held. Even changing a diaper may cause a fracture in severely affected infants. These children should never be held by the ankles when being diapered but should be gently lifted by the buttocks or supported with pillows.

BOX 53-5 CLASSIFICATION OF OSTEOGENESIS IMPERFECTA

Type I*

A—Mild bone fragility, blue sclerae, normal teeth, hearing loss (occurs between ages 20 and 30 years), autosomal dominant inheritance

B—Same as A except dentinogenesis imperfecta instead of normal teeth

C—Same as B but no bone fragility

Type II

Lethal; stillborn or die in early infancy; severe bone fragility, multiple fractures at birth; 10% of cases of osteogenesis imperfecta (OI); autosomal recessive inheritance

Type III

Severe bone fragility leading to severe progressive deformities, normal sclerae, marked growth failure, most autosomal recessive inheritance, with a few autosomal dominant inheritance

Type IV

A—Mild to moderate bone fragility; normal sclerae; normal teeth; short stature; variable deformity; autosomal dominant inheritance

B—Same as A except dentinogenesis imperfecta instead of normal teeth; approximately 6% of cases of OI

Type V

Clinically similar to type IV; hyperplastic callus; collagen mutation is negative

Type VI

Sclerae and dentition normal; moderate to severe bone fragility; diagnosis by bone biopsy because of similarities to other types (Land, Rauch, Travers, et al., 2007)

Type VII and VIII (Recessive Form)

Clinically overlap types II and III but affected individuals have white sclerae, rhizomelia (shortening of proximal limb segments), and small-to-normal head circumference; severe osteochondroplasia and short stature in survivors (Marini, 2016).

*Two thirds of cases are type I.

! NURSING ALERT

Children with current fractures or healing fractures should be screened for osteogenesis imperfecta—the assumption that abuse or neglect is the cause of fractures in children must be carefully evaluated by a multidisciplinary team.

Both parents and the affected child need education regarding the child's limitations and guidelines in planning suitable activities that promote optimum development and protect the child from harm. Realistic occupational planning is part of the long-term goals of care. Because there is a 50% risk of an affected individual passing the gene to an offspring, genetic counselling is recommended.

OI is a differential diagnosis that must be ruled out in the event of multiple fractures that may be attributed to nonaccidental injury. A detailed history, no evidence of associated soft-tissue injury, and the presence of other symptoms related to OI help determine the diagnosis.

ACQUIRED DEFECTS

Legg-Calvé-Perthes Disease

Legg-Calvé-Perthes disease, sometimes called *coxa plana* or *osteochondritis deformans juvenilis*, is a self-limited disorder in which there is aseptic necrosis of the femoral head. The disease affects children ages 2 to 12 years, but most cases occur in boys (male/female ratio is 4:1 or 5:1) between 4 and 8 years of age as an isolated event. In approximately 10% of cases the involvement is bilateral; most of the affected children have a skeletal age significantly below their chronological age (Sankar et al., 2016). White children are affected 10 times more frequently than children with African origins.

Pathophysiology

The cause of the disease is unknown, but there is a disturbance of circulation to the femoral capital epiphysis that produces an ischemic aseptic necrosis of the femoral head. During middle childhood, circulation to the femoral epiphysis is more tenuous than at other ages and can become obstructed by trauma, inflammation, coagulation defects, and a variety of other causes. The pathological events seem to take place in four stages (Box 53-6). The entire process may encompass as little as 18 months or continue for several years. The reformed femoral head may be severely altered or appear entirely normal.

Clinical Manifestations and Diagnostic Evaluation

The onset of Legg-Calvé-Perthes disease is usually insidious, and the history may reveal only the intermittent appearance of a limp on the affected side or symptoms including hip soreness, ache, or stiffness (constant or intermittent). The parents may report seeing the child limping, and the limp becomes more pronounced with increased activity. The pain may be experienced in the hip, along the entire thigh, or in the vicinity of the knee joint. The pain and limp are usually most evident on arising and at the end of a long day of activities. The pain is usually accompanied by joint dysfunction and limited range of motion. There may be a vague history of trauma. The diagnosis is established by history, examination, radiographs, and rarely magnetic resonance imaging (MRI).

Therapeutic Management

Because deformity occurs early in the disease process, the aims of treatment are to eliminate hip irritability; restore and maintain adequate range of hip motion; prevent capital femoral epiphyseal collapse, extrusion, or subluxation; and ensure a well-rounded femoral head at the time of healing. Treatment varies according to the child's age at the time of diagnosis, the appearance of the femoral head vasculature and position within the acetabulum. Nonsurgical containment of the femoral head may be accomplished with abduction casts, immobilization, and nonsteroidal anti-inflammatory drugs (NSAIDs), and a pelvic or proximal femoral osteotomy may be used to contain the femoral head. Later, active motion is encouraged. In some cases traction is applied to stretch tight adductor muscles.

Containment can be accomplished in several ways. One is the use of non–weight-bearing devices, such as an abduction brace (e.g., Atlanta Scottish Rite orthosis), leg casts, or a leather harness sling, which prevent weight bearing on the affected limb. Another includes the use of various weight-bearing appliances, such as abduction-ambulation braces or casts after a period of bedrest and traction. A third option consists of surgical reconstruction and containment procedures. Conservative therapy must be continued for 2 to 4 years, although braces constructed from lightweight materials allow the child to maintain a nearly normal activity level. Surgical correction, which exposes the child to additional risks (e.g., from anaesthesia, infection, blood transfusion), returns the child to normal activities in 3 to 4 months. The use of home traction has also been explored.

Prognosis

The disease is self-limited, but the ultimate outcome of therapy depends on early and efficient treatment and the child's age at the onset of the disorder. Children 5 years and younger, whose epiphyses are more cartilaginous, have the best prognosis for complete recovery. Children 10 years and older have a significant risk for degenerative arthritis, especially with femoral head deformity at the time of diagnosis. The later the diagnosis is made, the more femoral damage will have occurred before

BOX 53-6 RADIOGRAPHIC STAGES OF LEGG-CALVÉ-PERTHES DISEASE

Stage I: initial or avascular stage—Aseptic necrosis or infarction of the capital femoral epiphysis with degenerative changes producing flattening of the upper surface of the femoral head

Stage II: fragmentation or revascularization stage—Capital bone resorption and revascularization with fragmentation (vascular resorption of the epiphysis) that gives a mottled appearance on radiographs

Stage III: reossification or reparative stage—New bone formation, which is represented on radiographs as calcification and ossification or increased density in the areas of radiolucency. This filling-in process appears to take place from the periphery of the head centrally.

Stage IV: residual or regenerative stage—Gradual reformation of the head of the femur without radiolucency and, it is hoped, to a spherical form treatment is implemented. In many cases, with adherence to the prescribed regimen, the prognosis is excellent.

NURSING CARE

Nurses may be the first health care providers to identify affected children and to refer them for medical evaluation. They are also persons on whom the child and the family can rely to help them understand and adjust to the therapeutic measures. Most of the child's care is conducted on an outpatient basis, hence the major emphasis of nursing care is teaching the family the care and management of the corrective appliance selected for therapy. The family needs to learn the purpose, function, application, and care of the corrective device and the importance of using it consistently and as instructed, to achieve the desired outcome.

One of the most difficult aspects associated with the disorder is coping with a normally active child who feels well but must remain relatively inactive. Suitable activities must be devised to meet the needs of the child in the process of developing a sense of initiative or industry.

Slipped Capital Femoral Epiphysis

Slipped capital femoral epiphysis (SCFE) refers to the spontaneous displacement of the proximal femoral epiphysis in a posterior and inferior direction. It develops most frequently before or during accelerated growth and the onset of puberty (children between the ages of 9 and 16 years; median age, 13 for boys, 12 for girls) and is most frequently observed in boys and in children who are obese. The incidence is 11 cases per 100,000 children. Bilateral involvement occurs in up to 40 to 60% of cases (Sankar et al., 2016).

Pathophysiology

Most cases of SCFE are idiopathic, although it can be associated with endocrine disorders, renal osteodystrophy, and radiotherapy. The cause of idiopathic SCFE is multifactorial and includes obesity, physeal architecture and orientation, and pubertal hormone changes that affect physeal strength. Although obesity stresses the physeal plate, SCFE can also occur in children who are not obese. Radiographs show medial displacement of the epiphysis and an uncovered upper portion of the femoral neck adjacent to the physis. There is a widened growth plate and irregular metaphysis. The capital femoral epiphysis remains in the acetabulum, but the femoral neck slips, deforming the femoral head and stretching blood vessels to the epiphysis.

Diagnostic Evaluation

The disorder is suspected when an adolescent or preadolescent displays clinical signs or complains of thigh pain. Hip pain may be referred to the knee as a result of the distribution of sensory nerves (Box 53-7). The diagnosis is confirmed by radiographic examination that reflects a change in position of the proximal femoral epiphysis.

Therapeutic Management

The treatment goals of SCFE are to (1) prevent further slipping until physeal closure, (2) avoid further complications such as avascular necrosis, and (3) maintain adequate hip function (Sankar, et al., 2016). After the diagnosis has been established, the child should be non-weight bearing to prevent further slippage. Some surgeons prefer to take the child to surgery within 24 hours of the onset of acute symptoms and avoid further risk for avascular necrosis. Surgical treatment varies with the degree of displacement. Surgical pinning in situ involves the placement of a single pin or multiple pins and screws through the femoral neck into the proximal femoral epiphysis to prevent further slippage. An osteotomy for deformity is seldom needed in the acute setting. Hip arthroscopy performed before in situ pinning has been shown to be effective in decreasing hip pain and allowing early hip movement in some children with SCFE (Jayakumar, Ramachandran, Youm, et al., 2012). Total hip arthroplasty may also be used in adolescents and young adults (Shrader, 2012). Postsurgical care includes non-weight bearing with crutch ambulation until acceptable and painless range of motion is achieved. SCFE is an emergency and requires early diagnosis and treatment to increase the likelihood of an acceptable outcome.

BOX 53-7 CLINICAL MANIFESTATIONS OF SLIPPED CAPITAL FEMORAL EPIPHYSIS

Limp on affected side
Pain in hip
Continuous or intermittent
Frequently referred to groin, anteromedial aspect of thigh, or knee
Restricted internal rotation on adduction with external rotation deformity
Loss of abduction and internal rotation as severity increases
Shortening of lower extremity

NURSING CARE

Nursing care is the same as that for a child in a cast or a child in traction, as discussed earlier in this chapter. Postoperative care involves hemodynamic stabilization and assessment for complications. The adolescent needs to be taught the proper use of crutches and the importance of avoiding any weight bearing on the affected hip (if unilateral). The adolescent may be involved in building upper body strength during the convalescent period to increase mobility from bed to wheelchair, as appropriate. Self-care and performance of activities of daily living to the person's capability are encouraged to promote confidence and decrease a sense of helplessness.

! NURSING ALERT

Children with hip issues such as Legg-Calvé-Perthes or SCFE often present with groin, thigh, or knee pain. This is often because of referred pain and is anatomically related to the obturator nerve. Any time a child presents with groin, thigh, or knee pain, a complete hip examination is paramount to rule out underlying hip pathology.

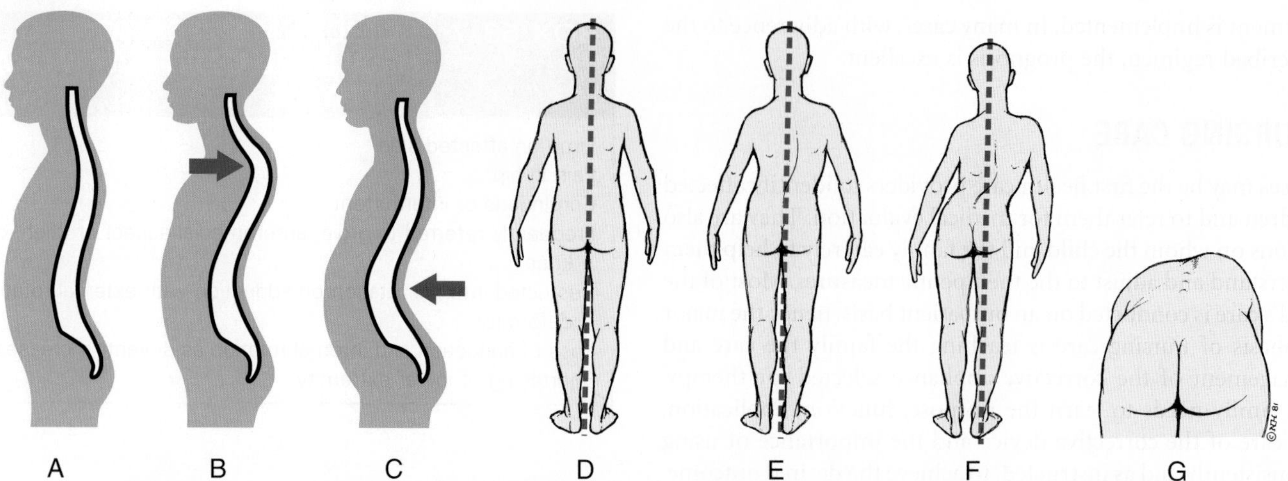

FIGURE 53-14 Spinal column curvatures. **A:** Normal spine. **B:** Kyphosis. **C:** Lordosis. **D:** Normal spine in balance. **E:** Mild scoliosis in balance. **F:** Severe scoliosis not in balance. **G:** Rib hump and flank asymmetry seen in flexion caused by rotary component. (Redrawn from Hilt, N. E., & Schmitt, E. W. [1975]. *Pediatric orthopedic nursing*. St. Louis: Mosby.)

Kyphosis and Lordosis

The spine, consisting of numerous segments, can acquire deformity curves of three types: **kyphosis, lordosis,** and **scoliosis** (Fig. 53-14).

Kyphosis is an abnormally increased convex angulation in the curvature of the thoracic spine (see Fig. 53-14, B). It can occur secondary to disease processes such as tuberculosis, chronic arthritis, osteodystrophy, or compression fractures of the thoracic spine. The most common form of kyphosis is "postural." Children are prone to exaggeration of a normal kyphosis, especially when skeletal growth outpaces growth of muscle. They assume abnormal sitting and standing positions. This is particularly common in self-conscious adolescent girls who assume a round-shouldered slouching posture in an attempt to hide their developing breasts. *Scheuermann's kyphosis* is a thoracic curve greater than 45 degrees with wedging greater than 5 degrees of at least three adjacent vertebral bodies and vertebral irregularity.

Postural (flexible) kyphosis is almost always accompanied by a compensatory postural lordosis, an abnormally exaggerated concave lumbar curvature. Treatment of kyphosis consists of exercises to strengthen shoulder and abdominal muscles and bracing for more marked deformity. With adolescents who are significantly self-conscious about their appearance, the best approach is to emphasize the cosmetic value of corrective therapy and to place the responsibility on the adolescent for carrying out an exercise program at home, with regular visits to and assessments by a therapist. Treatment with a brace may be indicated until skeletal maturity; surgical spinal fusion may be considered for severe, painful, or progressive deforming thoracic curves such as Scheuermann's kyphosis.

Lordosis is an accentuation of the cervical or lumbar curvature beyond physiological limits (see Fig. 53-14, C). It may be a secondary complication of a disease process, a result of trauma, or idiopathic. It is often seen in association with flexion contractures of the hip, scoliosis, obesity, developmental dysplasia of the hip, and slipped capital femoral epiphysis. During the pubertal growth spurt, lordosis of varying degrees is observed in teenagers, especially girls. In obese children the weight of the abdominal fat alters the centre of gravity, causing a compensatory lordosis. Unlike kyphosis, severe lordosis is usually accompanied by pain.

Treatment involves management of the predisposing cause when possible, such as weight loss and correction of deformities. Postural exercises or support garments are helpful in relieving symptoms in some cases; however, these do not usually result in a permanent cure.

Idiopathic Scoliosis

Idiopathic *scoliosis* is a complex spinal deformity in three planes, usually involving lateral curvature, spinal rotation causing rib asymmetry, and thoracic hypokyphosis. It is the most common spinal deformity and can be further classified according to age of onset: *congenital*, during fetal development; *infantile*, at birth or up to 3 years of age; *childhood (juvenile)*, in children 4 to 10 years of age; or, most commonly, *adolescent* (diagnosed at age 10 years or later), which develops during the growth spurt of early adolescence.

Scoliosis can be caused by a number of conditions and may occur alone or in association with other diseases, particularly neuromuscular conditions (neuromuscular scoliosis). In most cases, however, there is no apparent cause, thus the name *idiopathic scoliosis*. There appears to be a genetic component to the etiology of idiopathic scoliosis; however, the exact relationship has yet to be established. The following discussion involves the adolescent type, which is often called *adolescent idiopathic scoliosis*.

Idiopathic scoliosis is most noticeable during the preadolescent growth spurt. School screening is somewhat controversial, since there are no controlled studies to demonstrate improved outcomes and a reported number of false positives lead to referrals. Screenings may cause potential harm in terms of unnecessary medical evaluations and an adverse psychological impact. As a result, the Canadian Paediatric Society does not recommend routine screening (Greig, Constantin, LeBlanc, et al., 2016).

Diagnostic Evaluation

Observation is performed behind an undressed (in undergarments) standing child, noting any asymmetry of shoulder height, scapular or flank shape, or hip height and alignment. When the child bends forward at the waist (the Adams forward bend test) with hanging arms, asymmetry of the ribs and flanks may be noted. A scoliometer is also used in the initial screening to measure truncal rotation. Often a primary and a compensatory curve will place the head in alignment with the gluteal cleft. However, in the uncompensated curve the head and hips are not aligned (see Fig. 53-14, E and F). (See Spine, Chapter 33, for additional information.) Definitive diagnosis is made by radiographs of the child in the standing position and use of the Cobb technique that establishes the degree of curvature. The Risser scale is used to evaluate skeletal maturity on the radiographs; the scale assists in making a determination of the likely progression of the spinal angulature based on growth potential. Radiographic curves need to measure at least 10 degrees for diagnosis. Curves of less than 25 degrees are mild and require observation during growth.

> **! NURSING ALERT**
>
> Intraspinal conditions or other disease processes that can cause scoliosis must be ruled out. The presence of pain, sacral dimpling or hairy patches, cutaneous vascular changes, absent or abnormal reflexes, bowel or bladder incontinence, or left thoracic curve may indicate an intraspinal abnormality such as syringomyelia, diastematomyelia, or tethered cord syndrome. An MRI scan should be obtained for evaluation.

Therapeutic Management

Current management options include observation with regular clinical and radiographic evaluation, orthotic intervention (bracing), and surgical spinal fusion. Treatment decisions are based on the magnitude, location, and type of curve; the age and skeletal maturity of the child or adolescent; and any underlying or contributing disease process. Individuals with mild clinical scoliosis may not benefit from interventions such as braces and exercises (Greig et al., 2016).

Bracing and exercise. For many curves in the growing child and adolescent, bracing may be the treatment of choice. It is important to realize that *bracing is not curative*, but that it may slow the progression of the curvature to allow skeletal growth and maturity. The two most common types of bracing are (1) the *Boston* and *Wilmington braces*, which are underarm orthoses customized from prefabricated plastic shells, with corrective forces for each patient using lateral pads and decreasing lumbar lordosis, and (2) a *TLSO (thoracolumbosacral orthotic)*, which is an underarm orthosis made of plastic that is custom moulded to the body and then shaped to correct or hold the deformity (Fig. 53-15). The *Milwaukee brace*, which is an individually adapted brace that includes a neck ring, is rarely used in scoliosis but is sometimes used in the treatment of kyphosis. The *Charleston nighttime bending brace* is worn only when the child is in bed because it prevents walking because of the severity of the trunk bend. Bracing, although used as the gold standard treatment for mild to moderate curvatures, has not proved to be entirely effective in the treatment of scoliosis. Adherence to wearing the brace can be difficult because of the adolescent's age and preoccupation with body image and appearance. Bracing is also ineffective in managing curves greater than 45 degrees. However, brace treatment in some children with significant scoliosis may help avoid surgical intervention by slowing curve progression (Richards & Vitale, 2008).

Exercises, transcutaneous electrical stimulation, and chiropractic treatment are rarely of value for managing scoliosis. Exercises are of benefit when used in conjunction with bracing to maintain and increase the strength of spinal and abdominal muscles during treatment.

Surgical management. Surgical intervention may be required for correction of severe curves, which are typically greater than 45 degrees. It is required for progressive curves that do not respond to bracing and for progressive congenital and neuromuscular curves. The degree of curvature and the cause guide the decision to have surgery.

The surgical technique of spinal fusion consists of realignment with internal fixation and instrumentation combined with bony fusion (*arthrodesis*) of the realigned spine. Donor bone can be used to fuse the spine. The goals of surgical intervention are to correct the curvatures on the sagittal and coronal planes and to have a solid, pain-free fusion in a well-balanced torso, with maximum mobility of the remaining spinal segments. Surgical approaches may be posterior, anterior, or both.

Many instrumentation systems, including Harrington, Dwyer, Zielke, Luque, Cotrel-Dubousset, Isola, TSRH (Texas Scottish Rite Hospital), and Moss Miami, are available. Selection of the system is individualized according to the patient's needs and surgeon's preference.

The Luque-rod segmental spinal instrumentation provides segmental stability by the use of wires and L-shaped rods. By way of a posterior approach, the wires are threaded beneath the lamina of each vertebra and tightened around the rods resting along the transverse processes to stabilize the spine. Bone from the iliac crest or donor bone is used to fuse the spine. The advantage of this method is that the patient can be mobile within a few days and requires no postoperative immobilization. The disadvantage is the risk of nerve damage.

The Cotrel-Dubousset instrumentation is a newer generation of spinal instrumentation and implements bilateral rods and hooks at many sites. Anterior approaches using the Dwyer or Zielke instrumentation involve screws into the vertebral bodies connected by a cable or rod. These systems require postoperative immobilization with a custom-fitted plastic jacket.

NURSING CARE

Treatment for scoliosis extends over a significant portion of the affected child's period of growth. In adolescents this period is

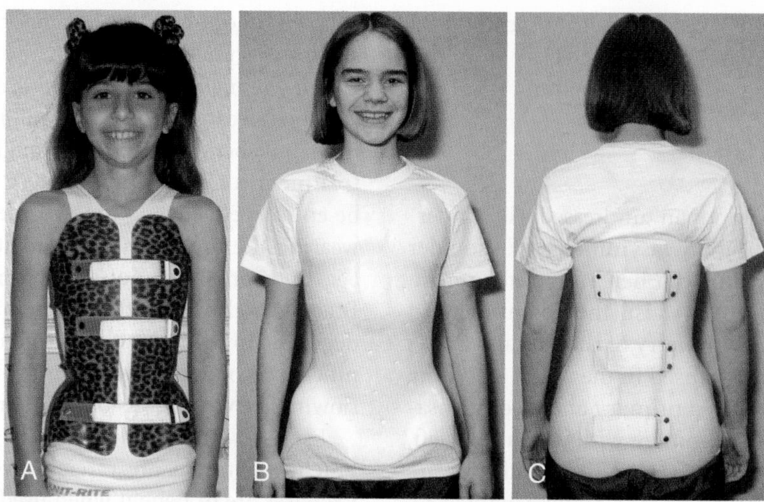

FIGURE 53-15 **A:** Standard thoracolumbosacral (TLSO) brace for idiopathic scoliosis. Note the colour and design incorporated into the brace to make it more acceptable to children and adolescents. **B:** Variation of a standard TLSO that fastens in the back **(C)** to provide needed support for the spine curvature.

the one in which their identity, physical and psychological, is formed. The identification of scoliosis as a "deformity," in combination with unattractive appliances and a significant surgical procedure, can have a negative effect on the already vulnerable adolescent body image. The adolescent and family require nursing care that meets both physical and psychological needs associated with the diagnosis, surgery, postoperative recovery, and eventual rehabilitation. Although adolescents with scoliosis are encouraged to participate in most peer activities, necessary therapeutic modifications are likely to make them feel different. Nursing care of the adolescent who is facing scoliosis surgery should address potential social isolation, pain, uncertainty, and emotions related to body image issues. See Additional Resources at the end of this chapter for a patient and family teaching tool for scoliosis.

When a child or adolescent first faces the prospect of a prolonged period in a brace, jacket, or other device, the therapy program and the nature of the device must be explained thoroughly to both the child and the parents so that they will understand the anticipated results, how the appliance corrects the defect, the freedoms and constraints imposed by the device, and what they can do to help achieve the desired goal. The management involves the skills and services of a team of specialists, including an orthopedist, physiotherapist, orthotist (a specialist in fitting orthopedic braces), nurse, social worker, and sometimes a thoracic or pulmonary specialist.

It is difficult for a child to be restricted at any phase of development, but for adolescents in particular continual positive reinforcement and encouragement are needed, along with as much independence as can be safely assumed during restriction. Guidance and assistance regarding anticipated problems, such as selection of clothing and participation in social activities, are appreciated by adolescents. Socialization with peers is strongly encouraged, and every effort should be made to help the adolescent feel attractive and of value.

Preoperative Care

The preoperative workup usually involves a radiographic series, including bending and traction films, pulmonary function studies, and a number of routine laboratory studies (including prothrombin, partial thromboplastin, and bleeding times; blood count; electrolyte levels; urinalysis and urine culture; and blood levels of any medications). Spinal surgery usually involves considerable blood loss, thus several options are considered preoperatively to maintain or replace blood volume. These options include autologous blood donations obtained from the patient before the surgery, intraoperative blood salvage, intraoperative hemodilution, erythropoietin administration, and controlled induced hypotension, which must be carefully monitored at all times to prevent physiological instability.

Surgery for spinal fusion is complex, and often adolescents who require the procedure because of idiopathic scoliosis are not familiar with medical terms, procedures, or experiences. Preoperative teaching is critical for the adolescent to be able to participate in his or her treatment and recovery. The corrective surgery is extensive so the patient must be taught how to manage his or her own patient-controlled analgesia (PCA) pump, how to log-roll, and use other equipment, such as a chest tube (for anterior repair) and Foley catheter. It is recommended that the child or adolescent bring personal items such as a favourite stuffed animal, laptop computer or personal tablet (with internet access), cell phone or iPod, or movie player for postoperative use. Meeting with a peer who has undergone a similar surgery is also valuable.

Postoperative Care

After surgery, patients are monitored in an acute care setting and log rolled when changing position to prevent damage to the fusion and instrumentation. In some cases an immobilization brace or cast is used postoperatively depending on the type of surgical intervention. Skin care is important, and pressure-relieving mattresses or beds may be needed to prevent pressure wounds (see Maintaining Healthy Skin, Chapter 44).

In addition to the usual postoperative assessments of wound, circulation, and vital signs, the neurological status of the patient's extremities requires special attention. Common post-operative problems after spinal fusion include neurological injury or spinal cord injury, hypotension from acute blood loss, wound infection, syndrome of inappropriate secretion of anti-diuretic hormone, atelectasis, pneumothorax, ileus, delayed neurological injury, and implanted hardware complications (Warner, Sawyer, & Kelly, 2012). *Superior mesenteric artery (SMA) syndrome* may occur several days after spinal surgery; this involves duodenal compression by the aorta and SMA and may result in acute partial or complete duodenal obstruction. Clinical manifestations include epigastric pain, nausea, copious vomiting, and eructation; symptoms are aggravated in the supine position and often relieved with the patient in a left lateral decubitus or prone position.

The child usually has considerable pain for the first few days after surgery and requires frequent administration of pain medication, preferably IV opioids administered on a regular schedule. For children able to understand the concept, PCA is recommended (see Pain Assessment; Pain Management, Chapter 34). In most cases the patient begins ambulation as soon as possible; depending on the instrumentation used and the surgical approach, most patients are walking by the second or third postoperative day and are discharged by 1 week after surgery. Discharge planning should include a timetable for follow-up with the orthopedic care provider and resumption of regular activities.

The patient may start physiotherapy as soon as he or she is able, beginning with range-of-motion exercises on the first postoperative day, and many of the activities of daily living in the following days. Self-care, such as washing and eating, is always encouraged. Throughout the hospitalization, age-appropriate activities and contact with family and friends are important parts of nursing care and planning (see The Immobilized Child, p. 1716).

The family should be encouraged to become involved in the patient's care in order to facilitate the transition from hospital to home management. The American Academy of Orthopaedic Surgeons and Scoliosis Research Society, an organization of physicians and scientists, have published an excellent book, *Scoliosis*, and the Scoliosis Research Society has educational information available on their website. A Canadian scoliosis support association operates from the province of British Columbia (see Additional Resources at the end of this chapter).

INFECTIONS OF BONES AND JOINTS

Osteomyelitis

Osteomyelitis, an infectious process in the bone, can occur at any age but most frequently is seen in children 10 years of age or younger. Boys are more commonly affected than girls, and the median age of diagnosis is 5 to 6 years of age. The limbs most commonly affected include the foot, femur, tibia, and pelvis. It is estimated that 1 in 5000 children younger than the age of 13 years is diagnosed each year with this condition (Zaoutis, Localio, Leckerman, et al., 2009). *Staphylococcus aureus* is the most common causative organism. Newborns are also likely to have osteomyelitis caused by group B streptococci. Children with sickle cell disease may develop osteomyelitis from *Salmonella* organisms and *S. aureus*. *Neisseria gonorrhoeae* is a potential causative organism in sexually active adolescents. *Kingella kingae* has been reported as one of the most causative organisms in children younger than age 5 years (Kaplan, 2016a).

Acute hematogenous osteomyelitis results when a blood-borne bacterium causes an infection in the bone. Common foci include infected lesions, upper respiratory tract infections, otitis media, tonsillitis, abscessed teeth, pyelonephritis, and infected burns. Exogenous osteomyelitis is acquired from direct inoculation of the bone from a puncture wound, open fracture, surgical contamination, or adjacent tissue infection. Subacute osteomyelitis has a longer course and may be caused by less virulent microbes with a walled-off abscess or Brodie's abscess, typically in the proximal or distal tibia. Chronic osteomyelitis is a progression of acute osteomyelitis and is characterized by dead bone, bone loss, drainage, and sinus tracts.

Generally, healthy bone is not likely to become infected. Factors that contribute to infection include inoculation with a large number of organisms, presence of a foreign body, bone injury, high virulence of an organism, immunosuppression, and malnutrition; certain types and locations of bone are also more vulnerable to infection.

Typically, children with acute hematogenous osteomyelitis are seen with a 2- to 7-day history of pain, warmth, tenderness, and decreased range of motion in the affected limb, along with systemic symptoms of fever, irritability, and lethargy (Box 53-8). Infants may have an adjacent joint effusion as well. Symptoms often resemble those observed in other diseases involving bones, such as arthritis, leukemia, or sarcoma.

BOX 53-8 CLINICAL MANIFESTATIONS OF ACUTE OSTEOMYELITIS

General Manifestations

History of trauma to affected bone (frequent)
Child appears very ill
Irritability
Elevated temperature
Restlessness
Rapid pulse
Dehydration

Local Manifestations

Tenderness
Increased warmth
Diffuse swelling over involved bone
Involved extremity painful, especially on movement
Involved extremity held in semiflexion
Surrounding muscles tense and resistant to passive movement

Pathophysiology

In acute osteomyelitis bacteria adhere to bone, causing a suppurative infection with inflammatory cells, edema, vascular congestion, and small-vessel thrombosis; the result is bone destruction, abscess formation, and dead bone (sequestra). Infection within the bone can rupture through the cortex into the subperiosteal space, stripping loose periosteum and forming an abscess. As dead bone is resorbed, new bone is formed along the live bone and infection borders. This surrounding sheath of live bone is called an *involucrum*. Sinus tracts from perforations in the involucrum may drain pus through soft tissue to the skin.

The pathology of osteomyelitis is different in infants, children older than 1 year of age, and adults. In infants blood vessels cross the growth plate into the epiphysis and joint space, which allows infection to spread into the joint. In children the infection is contained by the growth plate, and joint infection is less likely (unless the infection is intracapsular). In older adolescents (with a closed growth plate) the infection is poorly contained, and the joint is compromised. Adult periosteum is attached to bone; consequently, rupture through the periosteum and sinus drainage are more common in adults.

Diagnostic Evaluation

Organism identification and antibiotic susceptibility testing are essential for effective therapy. Cultures of aspirated subperiosteal pus along with cultures of blood, joint fluid, and infected skin samples should be obtained. Bone biopsy is indicated if blood culture results and radiographic findings are not consistent with osteomyelitis. Supporting evidence for osteomyelitis includes leukocytosis and an elevated erythrocyte sedimentation rate (ESR). Radiographic signs, except for soft-tissue swelling, are evident only after 2 to 3 weeks. A three-phase technetium bone scan can show areas of increased blood flow, such as occurs in early stages in infected bone, and is useful in locating multiple sites; however, it is not a diagnostic test. CT can be used to detect bone destruction, and MRI provides anatomical details useful in delineating the area of involvement, especially if surgical intervention is planned. Sometimes the osteomyelitis may be unrecognized if it occurs as a complication of a severe toxic and debilitating disease. Newborns may not present with clinical manifestations other than limited mobility of the affected extremity; fever may or may not be present, and the newborn may not appear to be sick (Kaplan, 2016a).

Therapeutic Management

After culture specimens are obtained, empiric therapy is started with IV antibiotics covering the mostly likely organisms. For *S. aureus*, nafcillin or clindamycin is generally used. Consideration should be given to the increased rates of community-acquired methicillin-resistant *S. aureus* (MRSA) in the selection of first-line antibiotic therapy, which may require vancomycin. When the infective agent is identified, administration of the appropriate antibiotic is initiated and continued for at least 3 to 4 weeks, but the length of therapy is determined by the duration of the symptoms, the response to treatment, and the organism's sensitivity; 6 weeks to 4 months may be required in some cases (Kaplan, 2016a). In selected cases oral antibiotic therapy may follow a shorter IV course. Given the prolonged duration of high-dose antibiotic therapy, it is important to monitor for hematological, renal, hepatic, ototoxic, and other potential adverse effects. To prevent antibiotic-associated diarrhea in some children, administration of a probiotic may be considered.

Surgery may be indicated if there is no response to specific antibiotic therapy, persistent soft-tissue abscess is seen, or the infection spreads to the joint. Opinions differ regarding surgical intervention, but many advocate sequestrectomy and surgical drainage to decompress the metaphyseal space before pus erupts and spreads to the subperiosteal space, forming abscesses that strip the periosteum from bone or form draining sinuses. When these complications occur, a chronic infection usually persists, which may require antibiotic therapy for several months.

NURSING CARE

During the acute phase of illness any movement of the affected limb will cause discomfort, thus the child needs to be positioned comfortably with the affected limb supported. A temporary splint or cast may be applied. Weight bearing is avoided in the acute phase, and moving and turning are carried out carefully to minimize pain. The child may require long-term pain medication to deal with the bone pain. After surgery, pain medication should be considered as with any other surgical procedure. Vital signs should be taken and recorded frequently and measures implemented to reduce a significant temperature elevation.

Antibiotic therapy requires careful observation and monitoring of the IV equipment and site. Because more than one antibiotic is usually administered, the compatibility of the medications needs to be determined and care taken to avoid mixing incompatible medications. A peripherally inserted central catheter (PICC) may be inserted for long-term antibiotic therapy. Antibiotic therapy is often continued at home.

Routine precautions are implemented for all children with osteomyelitis. If there is an open wound, it is managed according to standard wound care precautions. If a PICC line or central venous catheter (CVC) is inserted, meticulous care should be taken to prevent catheter-related infection. Administration of an antibiotic solution directly into the wound is most efficiently accomplished using a regular infusion setup that is prepared and regulated in the same manner as for any IV infusion. Intake and output should be measured and recorded, and the character of both the wound and drainage noted. The amount and character of drainage on the wound dressing also should be noted.

The child usually has a poor appetite and may be prone to vomiting. The appetite returns as the acute symptoms recede. During convalescence, adequate nutrition must be maintained to aid healing and formation of new bone.

When the acute stage subsides, children begin to feel better, appetite improves, and they become interested in their surroundings and relationships. Weight bearing on the affected limb is not permitted until healing is well under way, to avoid pathological fractures. Provision of diversional and constructive activities becomes an important nursing intervention. At this stage, the continuous IV infusion may be replaced by a heparin lock system to allow greater freedom.

As the infection subsides, physiotherapy is instituted to ensure restoration of optimum function. The child is usually discharged on a regimen of oral antibiotics, and progress is followed closely for some time.

Septic Arthritis

Septic arthritis is a bacterial infection in the joint. It usually results from hematogenous spread or from direct extension of an adjacent cellulitis or osteomyelitis. Direct inoculation from trauma accounts for 15 to 20% of septic arthritis cases. The most common causative organism is *S. aureus*. Community-acquired MRSA is commonly a cause of septic arthritis (Kaplan, 2016b). In addition to *S. aureus*, pathogens seen in newborns include group B streptococci, *Escherichia coli*, and *Candida albicans*. In children 2 months to 5 years of age, *S. aureus*, *Streptococcus pyogenes*, *Streptococcus pneumoniae*, and *Kingella kingae* are the primary organisms causing infection, whereas children older than 5 years are more likely to be infected by *S. aureus* and *S. pyogenes*; sexually active adolescents may be infected by *Neisseria gonorrhoeae* (Kaplan, 2016b).

The knees, hips, ankles, and elbows are the most common joints affected. Clinical manifestations include severe joint pain, swelling, warmth of overlying tissue, and occasionally erythema. However, an infection involving the hip is considered a surgical emergency to prevent compromised blood supply to the head of the femur (Kaplan, 2016b).

The child is resistant to any joint movement. Features of systemic illness, such as fever, malaise, headache, nausea, vomiting, and irritability, may also be present.

Therapeutic Management and Nursing Care

The affected joint is aspirated and the specimen evaluated by Gram stain, culturing (including separate cultures for *Haemophilus influenzae* and *N. gonorrhoeae*), and determination of leukocyte count. In addition, blood culture should be performed, and complete blood count with differential and ESR or C-reactive protein level should be obtained. Early radiographic findings are limited to soft-tissue swelling but may reveal a foreign body, and such films always provide a baseline for comparison. Technetium scans reveal areas of increased blood flow but will not differentiate between sites. MRI and CT scans provide more detailed images of cartilage loss, joint narrowing, erosions, and ankylosis of progressive disease. Ultrasonography is helpful in the detection of joint effusions and fluid in the soft tissue and subperiosteum (Kaplan, 2016b).

Treatment is IV antibiotic therapy based on Gram stain results and the clinical presentation. The benefits of serial aspirations to demonstrate sterility of synovial fluid and reduce pressure or pain are disputed. Pain management is an important aspect of nursing care, particularly with involvement of a large joint such as the hip. Surgical intervention may also be required if there was a penetrating wound or a possible involvement of a foreign object. Physiotherapy may be initiated for the child who is immobilized in a cast or traction to prevent flexion contractures.

Additional nursing care is the same as for osteomyelitis.

Skeletal Tuberculosis

In children, tubercular infection of the bones and joints is acquired by lymphohematogenous spread at the time of primary infection. Occasionally it is from chronic pulmonary tuberculosis (TB). Skeletal tubercular infection is not common in North America but should be considered in communities with high TB case rates. The condition is a late manifestation of TB and is most likely to involve the vertebrae, causing tubercular spondylitis. If the infection is progressive, it causes Pott disease with destruction of the vertebral bodies and results in kyphosis. Symptoms are insidious. The child may report persistent or intermittent pain. Other findings include joint swelling and stiffness; fever and weight loss are not common. Tubercular arthritis can also affect single joints such as a knee or hip and tends to cause severe destruction of adjacent bone. Infection in the fingers causes spina ventosa, a tuberculous dactylitis.

As with pulmonary TB, the index case should be located. A family and environmental history needs to be obtained and tuberculin skin tests (TSTs) performed. Results of TSTs are positive for the majority of children with tuberculous arthritis; however, the results are not diagnostic, and the clinical and laboratory features do not differentiate tubercular arthritis from a nontubercular septic arthritis. Diagnosis requires isolation of *Mycobacterium tuberculosis* from the site. Patients with the susceptible organism start treatment with combined antituberculosis chemotherapy (isoniazid, rifampin, and pyrazinamide); directly observed therapy is preferred (see also Chapter 45).

NURSING CARE

Nursing care depends on the site and extent of infection. Tuberculous spondylitis and hip infection may require immobilization, casting, and fusion. Nursing care is the same as for osteomyelitis and septic arthritis.

BONE AND SOFT-TISSUE TUMOUR

Malignant bone tumour represent less than 5% of all malignant neoplasms. Approximately 90% of all primary malignant bone tumours in children are either osteogenic sarcoma or Ewing sarcoma; osteosarcoma, the most common type, occurs in 56% of all cases. The peak age for pediatric bone tumours is 15 years, and they occur more often in boys.

Most malignant bone tumours produce localized pain in the affected site, which may be severe or dull and may be attributed to trauma or the vague complaint of "growing pains." The pain is often relieved by a flexed position, which relaxes the muscles overlying the stretched periosteum. Frequently it draws attention when the child limps, curtails physical activity, or is unable to hold heavy objects (Box 53-9). A palpable mass is also a common manifestation of bone tumours, but systemic

BOX 53-9 CLINICAL MANIFESTATIONS OF BONE TUMOUR

Pain localized at affected site
- May be severe or dull
- Often relieved by position of flexion

Frequently brought to attention when the child
- Limps
- Curtails own physical activity
- Is unable to hold heavy objects

symptoms, such as fever, and other clinical symptoms, such as spinal cord compression and respiratory distress, are more frequent in patients with Ewing sarcoma.

Diagnostic Evaluation

Diagnosis begins with a thorough history and physical examination. A primary objective is to rule out causes such as trauma or infection. Careful questioning regarding pain is essential in determining the duration and rate of tumour growth. Physical assessment focuses on functional status of the affected area, signs of inflammation, size of the mass, involvement of regional lymph nodes, and any systemic indication of generalized malignancy, such as anemia, weight loss, and frequent infection.

Definitive diagnosis is based on radiological studies, such as plain films and CT and MRI of the primary site, CT of the chest, and radioisotope bone scans to evaluate metastasis. Bone marrow examination is done in patients with suspected Ewing sarcoma. A needle or surgical biopsy is necessary to establish the diagnosis. Ewing sarcoma most commonly involves the pelvis, long bones of the lower extremities, and chest wall, and radiographically involves the diaphysis with detachment of the periosteum from the bone (Codman triangle). In osteosarcoma lesions are most commonly located in the metaphyseal region of the bone, often involving the long bones. Radial ossification in the soft tissue gives the tumour a "sunburst" appearance on plain radiograph.

Osteosarcoma

Osteosarcoma (osteogenic sarcoma) is the most common bone cancer in children and most commonly affects patients in the second decade of life, during their growth spurt (Gorlick, Janeway, & Marina, 2015). It presumably arises from bone-forming mesenchyme, which gives rise to malignant osteoid tissue. Most primary tumour sites are in the metaphysis (wider part of the shaft, adjacent to the epiphyseal growth plate) of long bones, especially in the lower extremities. More than half of cases occur in the femur, particularly the distal portion, with the rest involving the humerus, tibia, pelvis, jaw, and phalanges.

Therapeutic Management

Optimum treatment of osteosarcoma includes surgery and chemotherapy. The surgical approach consists of surgical biopsy followed by either limb salvage or amputation. To ensure local control, all gross and microscopic tumours must be resected. Depending on the tumour site, surgery includes amputation of the affected extremity at least 7.5 cm (3 inches) above the proximal tumour margin or above the joint proximal to the involved bone. With tumour of the distal femur, preservation of the hip joint may be possible. Other procedures include an above-the-knee amputation for tumour of the tibia or fibula, a hemipelvectomy for tumour of the innominate (hip) bone, and a forequarter amputation (removal of arm, scapula, and portion of the clavicle on the affected side) for tumour of the upper humerus.

A *limb salvage procedure* involves en bloc resection of the primary tumour with prosthetic replacement of the involved bone. For example, with osteosarcoma of the distal femur, a total femur and joint replacement is performed. Frequently children undergoing a limb salvage procedure will receive preoperative chemotherapy in an attempt to decrease the tumour size and make surgery more manageable (Gorlick et al., 2015).

Chemotherapy plays a vital role in the treatment of osteosarcoma. Antineoplastic medications, such as high-dose methotrexate with citrovorum factor rescue, doxorubicin, cisplatin, ifosfamide, and etoposide, may be administered singly or in combination and may be used either before or after surgical resection of the tumour. The use of chemotherapy after amputation has comparable results to those in trials using preoperative chemotherapy followed by limb salvage surgery. Preoperative chemotherapy allows for examination of the surgical specimen at the time of definitive surgery, which predicts clinical outcome. When pulmonary metastases are found, thoracotomy and chemotherapy have resulted in prolonged survival and potential cure. These combined-modality approaches have significantly improved the prognosis in osteosarcoma to approximately 78% for nonmetastatic patients (Lanzkowsky, 2015). Ongoing trials are evaluating the use of muramyl tripeptide phosphatidylethanolamine (Mifamurtide) to eradicate micrometastases by stimulating macrophages to kill tumour cells not eliminated by chemotherapy (Lanzkowsky, 2015). This drug has been used successfully in patients with nonmetastatic osteosarcoma (Anderson, Tomaras, & McConnell, 2010).

NURSING CARE

Nursing care depends on the type of surgical approach. Obviously, the family may have more difficulty adjusting to an amputation than a limb salvage procedure. In either instance, preparation of the child and family is critical. Straightforward honesty is essential in gaining the child's collaboration and trust. The diagnosis of cancer should not be disguised with falsehoods such as "infection." To accept the need for radical surgery, the child must be aware of the lack of alternatives for treatment. Although the responsibility of telling the child is generally left to the physician, the nurse should be present at the discussion or be aware of exactly what is said. The child should be told a few days before surgery to allow him or her time to think about the diagnosis and consequent treatment and to ask questions.

Sometimes children have many questions about the prosthesis, limitations on physical ability, and prognosis in terms of cure. At other times they react with silence or with a calm manner that belies their concern and fear. Either response must be accepted, since it is part of the shock and grieving process of a loss. For those who desire information, it may be helpful to introduce them to another amputee before surgery or to show them pictures of the prosthesis. However, the nurse must be careful not to overwhelm children with information. A sound approach is to answer questions without offering additional information. For those who do not pursue additional information, the nurse can express a willingness to talk.

The child should also be informed of the need for chemotherapy and its adverse effects, but without offering too much information at one time.

If an amputation is performed, the child is usually fitted with a temporary prosthesis immediately after surgery, which permits early functioning and fosters psychological adjustment. If this is not done, the child requires stump care, which is the same as for any amputee. A permanent prosthesis is usually fitted within 6 to 8 weeks. During hospitalization the child begins physiotherapy to become proficient in the use and care of the device. There is a unique "Champ Program" in Canada, developed by War Amps, which matches mothers of children who have undergone amputation and junior counsellors who provide support to such children and their families. This organization provides information, support, financial assistance, and public education programs on child safety (see Additional Resources at the end of this chapter).

Phantom limb pain may develop after amputation. This symptom is characterized by sensations such as tingling, itching, and, more frequently, pain felt in the amputated limb. The child and family need to know that the sensations are real, not imagined. Adolescent amputees identify the primary triggers of phantom sensation or pain with exercise, objects approaching the stump, cold weather, and "feeling nervous." Amitriptyline (Elavil) has been used successfully in children to decrease the pain. In addition, an epidural is often used before surgery as a nerve block in an effort to decrease or eliminate the occurrence of phantom limb pain.

Discharge planning must begin early in the postoperative period. Once the child has begun physiotherapy, the nurse should consult with the therapist and practitioner to evaluate the child's physical and emotional readiness to re-enter school. It is an opportune time to involve a community nurse in the child's home care. Every effort should be made to promote normalcy and gradual resumption of realistic preamputation activities. Role-playing is beneficial in preparing the child for questions and reactions from others. Environmental barriers, such as stairs, need to be assessed in terms of accessibility in the school and home; the child may need to use crutches or a wheelchair before complete healing and prosthetic competency are achieved.

The family and child need much support in adjusting not only to a life-threatening diagnosis but also to alteration in the child's body form and function. Loss of a limb entails a grieving process; therefore, those caring for the child need to recognize that the reactions of anger and depression are normal and necessary. Often parents view the anger as a direct affront to them for allowing the amputation to occur, or they see the depression as rejection. These are not personal attacks but the child's attempts to cope with a loss.

Ewing Sarcoma (Primitive Neuroectodermal Tumour)

Ewing sarcoma, or the Ewing sarcoma family of tumours, which include primitive neuroectodermal tumour, are the second most common malignant bone tumour in childhood (Lanzkowsky, 2015). Ewing sarcoma arises in the marrow spaces of the bone rather than from osseous tissue. The tumour originates in the shaft of long and trunk bones, most often affecting the femur, tibia, fibula, humerus, ulna, vertebrae, scapula, ribs, pelvic bones, and skull. It occurs almost exclusively in individuals under age 30 and affects White people much more often than those of other races.

Therapeutic Management

Limb salvage procedures might be feasible in extremity lesions, and amputation may be considered if the results of radiotherapy render the extremity useless or deformed (e.g., from restricted growth in young children). The treatment of choice is intensive irradiation of the involved bone, combined with chemotherapy. A widely used drug regimen includes vincristine, doxorubicin, and cyclophosphamide alternating with ifosfamide and etoposide. The addition of ifosfamide and etoposide has increased the 3-year survival to 78% for patients with localized disease (Lanzkowsky, 2015).

NURSING CARE

The psychological adjustment to Ewing sarcoma is typically less traumatic than it is to osteosarcoma because of the preservation of the affected limb. Many families accept the diagnosis with relief in knowing that this type of bone cancer does not necessitate amputation, and initially they may not be aware of the damaging effects on the irradiated site. They need preparation for the various diagnostic tests, including bone marrow aspiration and surgical biopsy, and adequate explanation of the treatment regimen. High-dose radiotherapy often causes a skin reaction of dry or moist **desquamation** followed by hyperpigmentation. The child should wear loose-fitting clothes over the irradiated area to minimize additional skin irritation. Given the increased sensitivity, the area should be protected from sunlight and sudden changes in temperature, such as from heating pads or ice packs. The child should be encouraged to use the extremity as tolerated. Occasionally the physiotherapist may plan an active exercise program to preserve maximum function.

The child needs the same considerations for adjusting to the effects of chemotherapy as any other patient with cancer. The drug regimen usually results in hair loss, severe nausea and vomiting, peripheral neuropathy, and possibly cardiotoxicity. Every effort should be made to outline a treatment plan that allows the child maximum resumption of a normal lifestyle and

activities (see also Nursing Care Plan: The Child With Cancer, from Chapter 48 available on Evolve).

Rhabdomyosarcoma

Rhabdomyosarcoma (*rhabdo*, striated) is the most common soft-tissue sarcoma in children. Striated (skeletal) muscle is found almost anywhere in the body, so these tumours occur in many sites, the most common of which are the head and neck, especially the orbit (eye). In Canada there were 145 new cases of rhabdomyosarcoma from 2006 to 2010 in children aged 0 to 14 years (Canadian Cancer Society, 2016).

Rhabdomyosarcoma arises from embryonic mesenchyme. Three subtypes are recognized: embryonal, alveolar, and pleomorphic. Soft-tissue sarcomas are the fourth most common type of solid tumour in children. These malignant neoplasms originate from undifferentiated mesenchymal cells in muscles, tendons, bursae, and fascia, or in fibrous, connective, lymphatic, or vascular tissue. They derive their name from the specific tissue(s) of origin, such as myosarcoma (*myo*, muscle).

The initial signs and symptoms are related to the site of the tumour and compression of adjacent organs (Box 53-10). Some tumour locations, particularly the orbit, produce symptoms early in the course of the illness and contribute to rapid diagnosis and an improved prognosis. Other tumours, such as those of the retroperitoneal area, produce no symptoms until they are large, invasive, and widely metastasized. Unfortunately, many of the signs and symptoms attributable to rhabdomyosarcoma are vague and frequently suggest a common childhood illness, such as "earache" or "runny nose." In some instances a primary tumour site is never identified.

BOX 53-10 CLINICAL MANIFESTATIONS OF RHABDOMYOSARCOMA ACCORDING TO TUMOUR SITE

Orbit
- Rapidly developing unilateral proptosis
- Ecchymosis of conjunctiva
- Loss of extraocular movements (strabismus)

Nasopharynx
- Stuffy nose (earliest sign)
- Nasal obstruction-dysphagia, nasal voice (obstruction of posterior nasal conchae)
- Pain (sore throat and ear)
- Epistaxis
- Palpable neck nodes
- Visible mass in oropharynx (late sign)

Paranasal Sinuses
- Nasal obstruction
- Local pain, swelling
- Discharge (may be unilateral)
- Sinusitis
- Swelling

Middle Ear
- Signs of chronic serous otitis media with effusion (OME)
- Pain
- Sanguinopurulent drainage
- Facial nerve palsy

Retroperitoneal Area
- Usually a "silent" tumour
- Abdominal mass
- Pain
- Signs of intestinal or genitourinary obstruction

Perineum
- Visible superficial mass (scrotum, vaginal, or cervical areas)
- Bowel or bladder dysfunction (from tumour compression)

Diagnostic Evaluation

Diagnosis begins with a careful history and physical examination. Radiographic studies to delineate the primary tumour should include CT or MRI. Metastatic evaluation should include a CT of the chest, bone scan, and bilateral bone marrow aspirates and biopsies. For patients with tumours in the parameningeal area, a lumbar puncture should be done to examine the spinal fluid. When possible, an excisional biopsy or surgical resection of the tumour is done to confirm the diagnosis.

Careful staging is extremely important for planning treatment and determining the prognosis. The Intergroup Rhabdomyosarcoma Study Group has developed a surgicopathological staging system, shown in Box 53-11 (Lanzkowsky, 2015; Wexler, Skapek, Meyer, et al., 2015).

With the use of contemporary multimodal therapy, more than 80% of patients with nonmetastatic disease are expected to survive (Lanzkowsky, 2015; Wexler et al., 2015). If relapse occurs, the prognosis for long-term survival is poor.

BOX 53-11 STAGING OF RHABDOMYOSARCOMA

Group I—Localized disease; tumour completely resected, and regional nodes not involved

Group II—Localized disease with microscopic residual, or regional disease with no residual or with microscopic residual

Group III—Incomplete resection or biopsy with gross residual disease

Group IV—Metastatic disease present at diagnosis

Therapeutic Management

All rhabdomyosarcomas are high-grade tumours with the potential for metastases. Therefore, multimodal therapy is recommended for all patients. Complete removal of the primary tumour is advocated whenever possible. However, because the tumour is chemosensitive, radical procedures with high morbidity should be avoided. In most cases a biopsy is followed by chemotherapy, irradiation, or both. Patients with embryonal tumours and group I disease can be treated with chemotherapy alone, but all others require chemotherapy and radiotherapy. Drugs that are used most often for the treatment of rhabdomyosarcoma include vincristine, actinomycin D, cyclophosphamide (VAC); ifosfamide; topotecan; irinotecan; and doxorubicin, which are administered for about 1 year (Lanzkowsky, 2015).

NURSING CARE

The nursing responsibilities are similar to those for other types of cancer, especially the solid tumour when surgery is used. Specific objectives include (1) careful assessment for signs of the tumour, especially during well-child examinations, (2) preparation of the child and family for the multiple diagnostic tests, and (3) supportive care during each stage of multimodal therapy.

DISORDERS OF JOINTS

Juvenile Idiopathic Arthritis (Juvenile Rheumatoid Arthritis)

Juvenile idiopathic arthritis (JIA) is a new name replacing *juvenile rheumatoid arthritis (JRA)* in the research literature and now in clinical practice. The JRA nomenclature revision to JIA was partly attributable to the minimally applicable reference to "rheumatoid" in JRA. Only a small percentage of children have a positive rheumatoid factor; furthermore, the JRA classification system focuses more on disease at onset than on disease progression, which is more important.

JIA is a chronic autoimmune inflammatory disease causing inflammation of joints and other tissue with an unknown cause. JIA starts before age 16 years with peak onset between 1 and 3 years of age. Twice as many girls as boys are affected. The worldwide incidence of JIA ranges from approximately 1 to 22 per 100,000 children per year, with an overall prevalence of approximately 7 to 401 per 100,000 children (Wu, Bryan, & Rabinovitch, 2016). The cause is unknown, but two factors are hypothesized: immunogenic susceptibility and an environmental or external trigger such as a virus (e.g., rubella, Epstein-Barr virus, parvovirus B19) (Cassidy, 2015). There are a few known genetic risk factors, including HLA class I and class II genes, the *PTPN22* gene, and the *IL2RA/CD 25* gene; however, the genetic contribution is complicated and still not well understood.

Pathophysiology

The disease process is characterized by chronic inflammation of the synovium with joint effusion and eventual erosion, destruction, and fibrosis of the articular cartilage. Adhesions between joint surfaces and ankylosis of joints occur if the inflammatory process persists.

Clinical Manifestations

The outcome of JIA is variable and unpredictable. The disease, even in severe forms, is rarely life threatening but can cause significant disability. The arthritis tends to wax and wane; however, patterns of clinical remission indicate that approximately 25% will obtain clinical remission off medication for a follow-up duration of at least 4 years. Children with arthritis in four or fewer joints had the greatest likelihood for a sustained remission. Children with extensive arthritis and a positive rheumatoid factor were less likely to have a sustained remission. Their arthritis can cause significant joint deformity and functional disability, requiring medication, physiotherapy, and perhaps future joint replacement. Chronic and acute *uveitis*, inflammation in the anterior chamber of the eye, can cause permanent vision loss if undiagnosed and not aggressively treated.

Classification of Juvenile Idiopathic Arthritis

JIA is not a single disease, but a heterogeneous group of diseases. The universal Durban classification of JIA, revised and published in 1998, lists several disease categories, each with its own set of criteria and exclusions, which continue to be revised (Firestein, Budd, Harris, et al., 2009):

Systemic arthritis is arthritis in one or more joints associated with at least 2 weeks of fever, rash, lymphadenopathy, hepatosplenomegaly, and serositis.

Oligoarthritis (or pauciarticular arthritis) is arthritis in one to four joints for the first 6 months of disease. It is subdivided to *persistent oligoarthritis* if it remains in four joints or less, and becomes *extended oligoarthritis* if it involves more than four joints after 6 months.

Polyarthritis rheumatoid factor negative affects five or more joints in the first 6 months with a negative rheumatoid factor.

Polyarthritis rheumatoid factor positive also affects five or more joints in first 6 months, but these children have a positive rheumatoid factor.

Psoriatic arthritis is arthritis with psoriasis or an associated dactylitis, nail pitting, or onycholysis or psoriasis in a first-degree relative.

Enthesitis-related arthritis is arthritis, enthesitis (inflammation at the tendon insertion site), or both associated with at least two of the following: sacroiliac or lumbosacral pain, HLA-B27 antigen, arthritis in boys older than 6 years, acute anterior uveitis, inflammatory bowel disease, Reiter's syndrome, or acute anterior uveitis in a first-degree relative.

Undifferentiated arthritis fits none of the previous categories or fits more than one category.

Diagnostic Evaluation

JIA is a diagnosis of exclusion; there are no definitive tests. Classifications are based on the clinical criteria of age of onset before 16 years, arthritis in one or more joints for 6 weeks or longer, and exclusion of other causes. Laboratory tests may provide supporting evidence of disease. The ESR may or may not be elevated. Leukocytosis is frequently present during exacerbations of systemic JIA. Antinuclear antibodies are common in JIA but are not specific for arthritis; however, they help identify children who are at greater risk for uveitis. Plain radiographs are the best initial imaging studies and may show soft-tissue swelling and joint space widening from increased synovial fluid in the joint. Later films can reveal osteoporosis, narrow joint space, erosions, subluxation, and ankylosis. A slit-lamp eye examination is necessary to diagnose sight-threatening uveitis, which is most common in antinuclear antibody–positive young girls with oligoarthritis. Routine examinations are necessary for early diagnosis and treatment to avoid sight-threatening disease (Qian & Acharya, 2010). The Canadian Paediatric Society (2008) has indicated that some children with JIA are not diagnosed early enough and can thus develop long-term complications. The late diagnosis can result in joint contractures, muscle wasting, growth disturbances, impaired functioning, undetected uveitis, and possible sight loss.

Therapeutic Management

There is no cure for JIA. The major goals of therapy are to control pain, preserve joint range of motion and function, minimize effects of inflammation, such as joint deformity, and promote normal growth and development. Outpatient care is the mainstay of therapy; lengthy hospitalizations are infrequent. The treatment plan can be exhaustive and intrusive for the child and family, including medication administration, physiotherapy and occupational therapy, ophthalmological slit-lamp examinations, splints, comfort measures, dietary management, school modifications, and psychosocial support.

Medications. Many arthritis medications are available, and most are effective in suppressing the inflammatory process and relieving pain. These medications may be given alone or in combination and are prescribed in a stepwise manner dependent on arthritis severity.

NSAIDs are the first medications used. Naproxen, ibuprofen, tolmetin, indomethacin, celecoxib, meloxicam, and aspirin are approved for use in children. They are effective with few common adverse effects other than gastrointestinal irritation and bruising; with naproxen, skin fragility is a possible adverse effect. NSAIDs must be taken with food. Aspirin, once the medication of choice, has been replaced by NSAIDs because they have fewer adverse effects and easier administration schedules.

Methotrexate is the second-line medication used in children whose symptoms are not relieved with NSAIDS alone. It is started in combination with an NSAID. It is effective, with acceptable toxicity, which requires monitoring of complete blood cell counts and liver function tests. Patient education about possible adverse effects, including discussions with teens about birth defects in offspring and avoiding alcohol, is essential.

Corticosteroids are potent immunosuppressives used for life-threatening complications, incapacitating arthritis, and uveitis. They are administered at the lowest effective dose for the briefest period and discontinued on a tapering schedule. They may be administered orally, as intra-articular joint injections, as IV pushes, or in eye drop form for uveitis. A single intra-articular injection may provide effective relief for children with pauciarticular disease unresponsive to NSAIDs. Prolonged use of systemic steroids is associated with significant adverse effects, including Cushing's syndrome, osteoporosis, increased infection risk, glucose intolerance, cataracts, and growth suppression.

Biological agents that work by several mechanisms to interrupt and minimize the inflammatory process are used in children with severe or progressive arthritis. Etanercept is a tumour necrosis factor (TNF) (inhibitor) alpha-receptor blocker and an effective medication for children with JIA whose symptoms are nonresponsive to methotrexate. It is given once or twice per week via subcutaneous injections. The long-term safety and efficacy of etanercept have been confirmed (Giannini, Howite, Lovell, et al., 2009; Kerensky, Gottlieb, Yaniv, et al., 2012). Adalimumab is a monoclonal antibody that also inhibits TNF, thereby reducing inflammation; it is a subcutaneous injection given every 2 weeks (Lovell, Ruperto, Goodman, et al., 2008). Abatacept reduces inflammation by inhibiting T cells and is given intravenously every 4 weeks. Possible adverse effects of biologicals include an increased infection risk, rare reports of demyelinating disease and pancytopenia, and allergic reactions. Because of the infection risk, children should be evaluated for TB exposure before starting these medications, and live vaccines should be avoided while taking them. There is a reported potential increased risk of malignancy with anti-TNF agents (etanercept, adalimumab, and infliximab) at high doses (U.S. Food and Drug Administration, 2011).

Physiotherapy and occupational therapy. Programs of physical management are individualized for each child and designed to reach the ultimate goal: preserving function or preventing deformity. Physiotherapy is directed toward specific joints, focusing on strengthening muscles, mobilizing restricted joint motion, and preventing or correcting deformities. Occupational therapy assumes responsibility for generalized mobility and performance of activities of daily living.

General treatment or maintenance programs vary; physiotherapists may be involved several times weekly to monthly in the management of a home program, or their visits may be limited to infrequent reviews of the home program for compliance, effectiveness, and need. Normal activities of daily living and the child's natural tendency to be active are usually sufficient to maintain muscle strength and joint mobility.

Exercising in a pool is excellent therapy, since it allows freedom of movement with support and minimal gravitational pull. If there is pain on motion, a hot pack or warm bath before therapy may help.

Health care providers may recommend nighttime splinting to help minimize pain and reduce flexion deformity. Joints most frequently splinted are the knees, wrists, and hands. Loss of extension in the knee, hip, and wrist causes special problems and requires vigilance to detect the earliest signs of involvement and vigorous attention to prevent deformity with specialized passive stretching, positioning, and resting splints.

NURSING CARE

Nursing the child with JIA involves assessment of the child's general health, the status of involved joints, and the child's emotional response to all ramifications of the disease—discomfort, physical restrictions, therapies, and self-concept.

The effects of JIA are manifest in every aspect of the child's life, including physical activities, social experiences, and personality development. Nursing interventions to support the parents may foster successful adaptation for the entire family. Parental concerns about the disease prognosis, financial and insurance issues, spouse and sibling relationships, and job and schedule conflicts must all be addressed. Referral to social workers, counsellors, or support groups may be needed.

Relieve Pain

The pain of JIA is related to several aspects of the disease: disease severity, functional status, individual pain threshold, family variables, and psychological adjustment. The aim is to provide as much relief as possible with medication and other therapies to help children tolerate the pain and cope as effectively as possible. Nonpharmacological modalities such as behavioural therapy and relaxation techniques have proved effective in modifying pain perception (see Pain Management, Chapter 34) and activities that aggravate pain. Opioid analgesics are typically avoided in juvenile arthritis; however, for children immobilized with refractory pain, short-term opioid analgesics can be part of a comprehensive plan that uses multiple pain relief techniques.

Promote General Health

The child's general health must be considered. A well-balanced diet with sufficient calories to maintain growth is essential. If the child is relatively inactive, caloric intake should match energy needs to avoid excessive weight gain, which places additional stress on affected joints. Sleep and rest are essential for children with JIA. Some children require rest during the day; however, daytime napping that interferes with nighttime sleepiness should be avoided. A bedtime routine that involves comfort measures can help induce sleep. A firm mattress, heated water bed, electric blanket, or sleeping bag helps provide warmth, comfort, and rest. Nighttime splints needed to maintain range of motion might initially be a source of bedtime conflict. The family needs to be instructed on how to use the splint appropriately; the splint should not be painful or impede sleep. Behaviour modification programs that reward splint and exercise use may be helpful in reducing barriers to use.

Well-child care to assess growth, development, and immunization requirements needs to be coordinated between the primary care provider and the rheumatologist. Common childhood illnesses, such as upper respiratory tract infections, may cause arthritis to worsen; consequently, medical attention must be sought quickly for relatively minor illness to prevent arthritis flares. Effective communication between the family, the primary care provider, and the rheumatology team is essential for care coordination.

Children should be encouraged to attend school, even on days when there may be some pain or discomfort. Split days or half days may help a child remain involved in school. Permitting the child to come to school late allows time to gain joint movement and reduces the time at school to avoid exhaustion. It is important that the child attend school to learn skills and engage in social interaction, especially if the JIA continues to limit physical skills. Arranging for two sets of textbooks eliminates the need to carry books to and from school, thus reducing discomfort and difficulty walking.

Facilitate Adherence

The child and family need to be involved in the therapeutic plan. They need to know the purpose and correct use of any splints and appliances and the medication regimen. The family should be instructed in the administration of medications and the value of a regular schedule of administration to maintain a satisfactory drug level in the body. They should be advised that NSAIDs are not be given on an empty stomach and to be alert for signs of medication toxicity. If evidence of drug toxicity is noted, the family should notify their health care provider and follow that person's instructions.

Encourage Heat and Exercise

Heat has been shown to be beneficial to children with arthritis. Moist heat is best for relieving pain and stiffness, and the most efficient and practical method is in the bathtub with warm water. In some cases a daily whirlpool bath, paraffin bath, or hot packs may be used as needed for temporary relief of acute swelling and pain. Hot packs are easily applied using a bath towel wrung out after being immersed in hot water or heated in a microwave oven, applied to the area, and covered with plastic for 20 minutes. Commercial pads that warm in only a few minutes in the microwave are also available. Painful hands or feet can be immersed in a pan of warm water for 10 minutes two or three times daily in addition to immersion in tub baths. Pool therapy is the easiest method for exercising a large number of joints. Swimming activities strengthen muscles and maintain mobility in larger joints. Very small children who are frightened of the water can carry out their exercises in the bathtub; small children love to splash, kick, and throw things in the water. Adult supervision is necessary for all water activities.

Activities of daily living provide satisfactory exercise for older children to maintain maximal mobility with minimal pain. These children should be encouraged in their efforts to be independent and allowed to dress and groom themselves, to assume daily tasks, and to care for their belongings. It is often difficult for children to manipulate buttons, comb or brush hair, and turn faucets, but unless there is an acute flare, parents and other caregivers should not offer assistance. In addition, children should learn and understand why others do not help them. Many helpful devices, such as self-adhering fasteners, tongs for manipulating difficult items, and grab bars installed in bathrooms for safety, can be used to facilitate tasks. A raised (higher) toilet seat often makes the difference between dependent and independent toileting, since weak quadriceps muscles and sore knees inhibit the ability to raise the body from a low sitting position.

A child's natural affinity for play offers many opportunities for incorporating therapeutic exercises. Throwing or kicking a ball and riding a tricycle (with the seat raised to achieve maximum leg extension) are excellent moving and stretching exercises for a very young child whose daily living activities are physically limited.

An effective approach to beginning the day's activities is to awaken children early to give them their medication and then to allow them to sleep for an hour. On arising, children can take a hot bath (or shower) and perform a simple ritual of limbering-up exercises, after which they can start the day's activities, such as going to school. Exercise, heat, and rest are spaced throughout the remainder of the day according to the child's individual needs and schedule. Parents should be instructed in exercises that meet the child's needs.

Support the Child and Family

JIA affects every aspect of life for the child and family. Physical limitations may interfere with self-care, school participation, and recreational activities. The intensive treatment plan, including multiple medications, physiotherapy, comfort measures, and medical appointments, is intrusive and disruptive to the parents' work schedule and the family routine. To prevent isolation and foster independence, the family should be encouraged to pursue their normal activities. At the same time, the adaptations necessary require resourcefulness and commitment from all family members. At diagnosis and throughout the span of JIA, it is essential to recognize signs of stress and counterproductive coping and provide the necessary support to maximize adaptation. The problems and needs of these families are discussed in Chapter 40, along with guidance in planning care. (See also Nursing Care Plan, The Child With Arthritis on  Evolve.)

In Canada, the Arthritis Society provides many services for children with arthritis and their families, including education and support groups (see Additional Resources at the end of this chapter).

Systemic Lupus Erythematosus

Systemic lupus erythematosus (SLE) is a chronic, multisystem, **autoimmune disease** of the connective tissues and blood vessels that is characterized by inflammation in potentially any body tissue. Its course and symptoms are variable and unpredictable, with mild to life-threatening complications. In addition to SLE, there are other forms of lupus, such as neonatal lupus, which occurs when maternal autoantibodies cross the placenta and cause transient lupus-like symptoms in the newborn, with the potential serious complication of heart block. The following discussion focuses on SLE.

Reports suggest that survival rates in children with SLE have significantly improved; 5-year survival rates are said to be almost 100%, and 10-year survival rates are close to 98.2% (Hashkes, Wright, Lauer, et al., 2010). SLE is more common in girls, with an approximate 2–5 : 1 female-to-male ratio before puberty, and a 9 : 1 ratio during reproductive years. SLE typically occurs between the ages of 10 and 19 years and rarely before the age of 5; however, some cases may be diagnosed in infancy (Sadun, Ardoin, & Schanberg, 2016). There is a familial tendency, although many newly diagnosed patients are unaware of other affected family members. Researchers studying the ethnicity and socioeconomic factors of SLE in Canada discovered that Asian Canadians and those with Afro-Caribbean origins had a higher frequency of renal involvement and more exposure to immunosuppressives. Indigenous people had higher frequencies of antiphospholipid antibodies and **comorbidity**. Canadians of Asian descent had the youngest onset. The results indicated that there are different lupus phenotypes in ethnic groups, but low income was the significant independent predictor for long-term physical damage (Peschken, Katz, Silverman, et al., 2009).

The cause of SLE is not known. It appears to result from a complex interaction of genetics with an unidentified trigger that activates the disease. Suspected triggers include exposure to ultraviolet (UV) light, estrogen, pregnancy, infections, and medications. Patients with JIA have been known to develop SLE symptoms as a result of the use of TNF medications such as etanercept. Genetic predisposition to SLE is evidenced in an increased concordance rate in twins (2 to 5% among dizygotic twins and 25 to 60% among monozygotic twins), although multiple genes are probably involved, and epigenetic and nongenetic factors are also important in disease expression (Sadun et al., 2016)

Clinical Manifestations and Diagnostic Evaluation

The child with SLE may have any number of clinical manifestations with mild to life-threatening severity (Box 53-12). The diagnosis is established when 4 of the 11 diagnostic criteria in Box 53-13 are met; however, children with fewer than 4 criteria who are suspected of having lupus should receive appropriate medical treatment (Sadun et al., 2016). Kidney involvement heralds progressive disease and the need for rigorous therapeutic management.

Therapeutic Management

The goal of treatment is to ensure the child's health by balancing the medications necessary to avoid exacerbation and complications while preventing or minimizing treatment-associated morbidity. Therapy involves the use of specific medications and

BOX 53-12 CLINICAL MANIFESTATIONS OF SYSTEMIC LUPUS ERYTHEMATOSUS RELATED TO TISSUES INVOLVED

Constitutional—Fever, fatigue, weight loss, anorexia
Cutaneous—Erythematous butterfly rash over bridge of nose and across cheeks, discoid rash, photosensitivity, mucocutaneous ulceration, alopecia, periungual telangiectasias
Musculoskeletal—Arthritis, arthralgia, myositis, myalgia, tenosynovitis
Neurological—Headache, seizure, forgetfulness, behaviour change, change in school performance, psychosis, chorea, stroke, cranial and peripheral neuropathy, pseudotumour cerebri
Pulmonary and cardiac—Pleuritis, basilar pneumonitis, atelectasis, pericarditis, myocarditis, endocarditis
Renal—Glomerulonephritis, nephrotic syndrome, hypertension
Gastrointestinal—Abdominal pain, nausea, vomiting, blood in stool, abdominal crisis, esophageal dysfunction, colitis
Hepatic, splenic, and nodal—Hepatomegaly, splenomegaly, lymphadenopathy
Hematological—Anemia, cytopenia
Ophthalmological—Cotton-wool spots, papilledema, retinopathy
Vascular—Raynaud's phenomenon, thrombophlebitis, livedo reticularis

BOX 53-13 CLASSIFICATION CRITERIA FOR SYSTEMIC LUPUS ERYTHEMATOSUS

Four of the following 11 criteria must be met for diagnosis:

1. **Malar rash**—Fixed malar erythema
2. **Discoid rash**—Patchy erythematous lesions
3. **Photosensitivity**—Rash with sun exposure
4. **Oral ulcers**—Painless ulcers in mouth, nose
5. **Arthritis**—Swelling, tenderness, or effusion in two or more peripheral joints (nonerosive)
6. **Serositis**—Pleuritis, pericarditis
7. **Renal disorder**—Proteinuria, casts
8. **Neurological disorder**—Psychosis, seizures
9. **Hematological disorder**—Hemolytic anemia, thrombocytopenia, leukopenia, lymphopenia
10. **Immunological disorder**—Anti-dsDNA, anti-SM, antiphospholipid antibodies, lupus anticoagulant, false-positive syphilis test (RPR)
11. **Antinuclear antibody**

general supportive care. The drugs used to control inflammation are corticosteroids administered in doses sufficient to control inflammation and then tapered to the lowest suppressive dose. Other drugs include antimalarial preparations, which are useful for rash and arthritis; NSAIDs, which relieve muscle and joint inflammation; and immunosuppressive agents such as cyclophosphamide for renal and central nervous system disease. Mycophenolate, azathioprine, and methotrexate are effective immunosuppressive drugs that may be used to control SLE and allow reduction in steroid use. Antihypertensives, aspirin, and antibiotics are just a few of the additional drugs that may be necessary to treat or avoid complications.

General supportive care includes sufficient nutrition, sleep and rest, and exercise. Exposure to the sun and ultraviolet B (UVB) light should be limited because of its association with SLE exacerbation.

NURSING CARE

The principal nursing goal is to help the child and family adjust to the disease and therapy. The child and family must learn to recognize subtle signs of disease exacerbation and potential complications of medication therapy. Patient and family education is an ongoing process initiated at diagnosis and individualized. Referral to a social worker, psychologist, or support group may help the child and family make a successful adjustment. Support groups are available through Lupus Canada and the Arthritis Society (see Additional Resources at the end of this chapter).

Key issues include therapy adherence; body-image problems associated with rash, hair loss, and steroid therapy; school attendance; vocational activities; social relationships; sexual activity; and pregnancy. (See Chapter 40 for a discussion on adjusting to a chronic illness.) Specific instructions for avoiding exposure to the sun and UVB light, such as using sunscreens, wearing sun-resistant clothing, and altering outdoor activities, must be provided with sensitivity to ensure adherence while minimizing the associated feeling of being different from peers (see Sunburn, Chapter 52). Patients need to be instructed to maintain regular medical supervision and seek attention quickly during illness or before elective surgical procedures, such as dental extraction, because of potential needs for increased steroids or prophylactic antibiotics. People with SLE should wear a medical alert bracelet for their disease and steroid dependence.

KEY POINTS

- Immobility has a profound effect on all aspects of growth and development.
- The major physical consequences of immobilization are loss of muscle strength, endurance, and muscle mass; bone demineralization; loss of joint mobility; and contractures.
- Features of children's fractures not observed in the adult include presence of growth plate, thicker and stronger periosteum, bone porosity, more rapid healing, and less joint stiffness.
- The goals of fracture management are to regain alignment and length of bony fragments, retain alignment and length, and restore function to injured parts.
- The method of fracture reduction is determined by the child's age, degree of displacement, amount of overriding, amount of edema, condition of the skin and soft tissues, sensation, and circulation distal to the fracture.
- The primary purposes of traction are to fatigue involved muscles and reduce muscle spasm, position bone ends in desired realignment, and immobilize the fracture site until realignment has been achieved to permit casting or splinting.
- The etiology of DDH appears to be related to intrauterine, genetic, and cultural factors.
- Treatment of clubfoot consists of manipulation and casting to correct the deformity, maintenance of the correction, and prevention of possible recurrence of the deformity.
- Acquired hip deformities are managed with non–weight-bearing devices (Legg-Calvé-Perthes disease) or surgical stabilization (SCFE).
- Observation for idiopathic scoliosis is an important part of an adolescent's routine physical assessment.
- Idiopathic scoliosis is managed by observation, bracing, and exercise or surgical correction.
- Bone infections are managed with vigorous antibiotic therapy, immobilization of the affected part, and (sometimes) surgical drainage.

- Osteosarcoma is a neoplasm of bone-forming tissues; Ewing sarcoma is a neoplasm that arises from bone marrow spaces.
- Rhabdomyosarcoma may occur almost anywhere in the body, but the most common sites are the head and neck.
- Nursing care of the child with juvenile arthritis consists of promoting general health, relieving discomfort, preventing deformity, and preserving function.
- SLE is a chronic autoimmune disorder that affects the collagen tissues of the body.

Evolve WEBSITE

Visit the Evolve website for additional resources related to the content in this chapter such as Case Studies, Critical Thinking Case Study Answers, Nursing Care Plans, Nursing Processes, Nursing Skills, and Review Questions for Exam Preparation at: http://evolve.elsevier.com/Canada/Perry/maternal/

REFERENCES

About Kids Health. (2009). *Ankle sprains.* Retrieved from <http://www.aboutkidshealth.ca/En/HealthAZ/ConditionsandDiseases/Injuries/Pages/AnkleSprains.aspx>.

Anderson, P. M., Tomaras, M., & McConnell, K. (2010). Mifamurtide in osteosarcoma—A practical review. *Drugs of Today (1998), 46*(5), 327–337.

Azbell, K., & Dannemiller, L. (2015). A case report of an infant with arthrogryposis. *Pediatric Physical Therapy, 27*(3), 293–301. doi:10.1097/PEP.0000000000000148.

Babl, F. E., Oakley, E., Seaman, C., et al. (2008). High-concentration nitrous oxide for procedural sedation in children: Adverse events and depth of sedation. *Pediatrics, 121*(3), e528–e532. doi:10.1542/peds.2007-1044.

Bailey, C. S. (2015). Principles of orthotic management. In B. D. Browner, J. B. Jupiter, C. Krettek, et al. (Eds.), *Skeletal trauma: Basic science, management, and reconstruction* (5th ed.). Philadelphia: Saunders.

Ball, J. W., Dains, J. E., Flynn, J. A., et al. (2015). *Seidel's guide to physical examination* (8th ed.). St. Louis: Mosby.

Canadian Cancer Society. (2016). *What is soft tissue sarcoma?* Retrieved from <http://www.cancer.ca/en/cancer-information/cancer-type/soft-tissue-sarcoma/soft-tissue-sarcoma/?region=on>.

Canadian Paediatric Society. (2008). Challenge for timely diagnosis of juvenile idiopathic arthritis in children. *Paediatrics & Child Health, 13*(3), 192.

Carrigan, R. B. (2016). The upper limb. In R. M. Kliegman, B. F. Stanton, J. W. St. Geme, et al. (Eds.), *Nelson textbook of pediatrics* (20th ed.). Philadelphia: Saunders.

Cassidy, J. T. (2015). Chronic arthritis in childhood. In R. E. Petty, R. M. Laxer, C. B. Lindsley, et al. (Eds.), *Textbook of pediatric rheumatology* (7th ed.). Philadelphia: Saunders.

Firestein, G. S., Budd, R. C., Harris, E. D., Jr., et al. (Eds.). (2009). *Kelley's textbook of rheumatology* (8th ed.). Philadelphia: Saunders.

Giannini, E. H., Ilowite, N. T., Lovell, D. J., et al. (2009). Long-term safety and effectiveness of etanercept in children with selected categories of juvenile idiopathic arthritis. *Arthritis & Rheumatology, 60*(9), 2794–2804.

Gorlick, R., Janeway, K., & Marina, N. (2015). Osteosarcoma. In P. A. Pizzo & D. G. Poplack (Eds.), *Principles and practices of pediatric oncology* (7th ed.). Philadelphia: Lippincott.

Greig, A. A., Constantin, E., LeBlanc, C., et al. (2016). An update to the Greig Health Record: Preventative health care visits for children and adolescents aged 6 to 17 years—Technical report. *Paediatrics & Child Health, 21*(5), 265–268. Retrieved from <http://www.cps.ca/en/documents/position/greig-health-record-technical-report>.

Hashkes, P. J., Wright, B. M., Lauer, M. S., et al. (2010). Mortality outcomes in pediatric rheumatology in the US. *Arthritis and Rheumatism, 62*(2), 599–608. doi:10.1002/art.27218.

Horstmann, H. M., Conroy, C. M., & Davidson, R. S. (2016). Arthrogryposis. In R. M. Kliegman, B. F. Stanton, J. W. St. Geme, et al. (Eds.), *Nelson textbook of pediatrics* (20th ed.). Philadelphia: Saunders.

Ireland, P. J., Pacey, V., Zankl, A., et al. (2014). Optimal management of complications associated with achondroplasia. *The Application of Clinical Genetics, 7*, 117–125. doi:10.2147/TACG.S51485.

Jayakumar, P., Ramachandran, M., Youm, T., et al. (2012). Arthroscopy of the hip for paediatric and adolescent disorders. *The Journal of Bone & Joint Surgery, 94*(3), 290–296.

Kaplan, S. I. (2016a). Osteomyelitis. In R. M. Kliegman, B. F. Stanton, J. W. St. Geme, et al. (Eds.), *Nelson textbook of pediatrics* (20th ed.). Philadelphia: Saunders.

Kaplan, S. I. (2016b). Septic arthritis. In R. M. Kliegman, B. F. Stanton, J. W. St. Geme, et al. (Eds.), *Nelson textbook of pediatrics* (20th ed.). Philadelphia: Saunders.

Kerensky, T. A., Gottlieb, A. B., Yaniv, S., et al. (2012). Etanercept: Efficacy and safety for approved indication. *Expert Opinion on Drug Safety, 11*(1), 121–139.

Land, C., Rauch, F., Travers, R., et al. (2007). Osteogenesis imperfecta type VI in childhood and adolescence: Effects of cyclical intravenous pamidronate treatment. *Bone, 40*(3), 638–644. doi:10.1016/j.bone.2006.10.010.

Lanzkowsky, P. (2015). *Manual of pediatric hematology and oncology* (5th ed.). San Diego: Academic Press.

Lovell, D. J., Ruperto, N., Goodman, S., et al. (2008). Adalimumab with or without methotrexate in juvenile rheumatoid arthritis. *The New England Journal of Medicine, 359*(8), 810–820.

Mang'oli, P., Theuri, J., Kollmann, T., et al. (2014). Ponseti clubfoot management: Experience with the Steenbeek foot abduction brace. *Paediatrics & Child Health, 19*(10), 513–514.

Marini, J. C. (2016). Osteogenesis imperfecta. In R. M. Kliegman, B. F. Stanton, J. W. St. Geme, et al. (Eds.), *Nelson textbook of pediatrics* (20th ed.). Philadelphia: Saunders.

Mencio, G. A., & Swiontkowski, M. F. (2015). *Green's skeletal trauma in children* (5th ed.). Philadelphia: Saunders.

Murray, J. S., Noonan, C., Quigley, S., et al. (2013). Medical device-related hospital-acquired pressure ulcers in children: An integrative review. *Journal of Pediatric Nursing, 28*(6), 585–595. doi:10.1016/j.pedn.2013.05.004.

Noonan, C., Quigley, S., & Curley, M. A. (2011). Using the Braden Q scale to predict pressure ulcer risk in pediatric patients. *Journal of Pediatric Nursing, 26*(6), 566–575. doi:10.1016/j.pedn.2010.07.006.

Peschken, C., Katz, S. J., Silverman, E., et al. (2009). The 1000 Canadian faces of lupus: Determinants of disease outcome in a large multiethnic cohort. *The Journal of Rheumatology, 36*(6), 1200–1208. doi:10.3899/jrheum.080912.

Ponseti, I. V. (1996). *Congenital clubfoot: Fundamentals of treatment.* Oxford, UK: Oxford University Press.

Qian, Y., & Acharya, N. R. (2010). Juvenile idiopathic arthritis-associated uveitis. *Current Opinion in Ophthalmology, 21*(6), 468–472.

Radler, C. (2013). The Ponseti method for the treatment of congenital club foot: Review of the current literature and treatment recommendations. *International Orthopaedics, 37*(9), 1747–1753. doi:10.1007/s00264-013-2031-1.

Richards, B. S., & Vitale, M. G. (2008). Screening for idiopathic scoliosis in adolescents: An information statement. *The Journal of Bone & Joint Surgery, 90*(1), 195–198. doi:10.2106/JBJS.G.01276.

Sadun, R. E., Ardoin, S. P., & Schanberg, L. E. (2016). Systemic lupus erythematosus. In R. M. Kliegman, B. F. Stanton, J. W. St. Geme, et al. (Eds.), *Nelson textbook of pediatrics* (20th ed.). Philadelphia: Saunders.

Sankar, W. N., Horn, B. D., Wells, L., et al. (2016). The hip. In R. M. Kliegman, B. F. Stanton, J. W. St. Geme, et al. (Eds.), *Nelson textbook of pediatrics* (20th ed.). Philadelphia: Saunders.

Sarwark, J. F. (2010). *Essentials of musculoskeletal care* (4th ed.). Rosemont, IL: American Academy of Orthopaedic Surgeons.

Schindler, C. A., Mikhailov, T. A., Kuhn, E. M., et al. (2011). Protecting fragile skin: Nursing interventions to decrease development of pressure ulcers in pediatric intensive care. *American Journal of Critical Care, 20*(1), 26–34, quiz 35. doi:10.4037/ajcc2011754.

Shrader, M. W. (2012). Total hip arthroplasty and hip resurfacing arthroplasty in the very young patient. *The Orthopedic Clinics of North America, 43*(3), 359–367.

Shyy, W., Wang, K., Sheffield, V. C., et al. (2010). Evaluation of embryonic and perinatal myosin gene mutations and the etiology of congenital idiopathic clubfoot. *Journal of Pediatric Orthopedics, 30*(3), 231–234.

Stoll, C., Alembik, Y., Dott, B., et al. (2010). Associated malformations in patients with limb reduction deficiencies. *European Journal of Medical Genetics, 53*(5), 286–290. doi:10.1016/j.ejmg.2010.07.012.

U. S. Food and Drug Administration. (2011). *Drug safety communication: Update on tumour necrosis factor (TNF) blockers and risk for pediatric malignancies.* Retrieved from <http://www.fda.gov/drugs/drugsafety/ucm278267.htm>.

Warner, W. C., Sawyer, J. R., & Kelly, D. M. (2012). Scoliosis and kyphosis. In S. T. Canale & J. H. Beaty (Eds.), *Campbell's operative orthopaedics* (12th ed.). Philadelphia: Mosby.

Wexler, L. H., Skapek, S. X., & Helman, L. J. (2015). Rhabdomyosarcoma. In P. A. Pizzo & D. G. Poplack (Eds.), *Principles and practices of pediatric oncology* (7th ed.). Philadelphia: Lippincott.

Winell, J. J., & Davidson, R. S. (2016). The foot and toes. In R. M. Kliegman, B. F. Stanton, J. W. St. Geme, et al. (Eds.), *Nelson textbook of pediatrics* (20th ed.). Philadelphia: Saunders.

Wu, E. Y., Bryan, A. R., & Rabinovitch, C. E. (2016). Juvenile idiopathic arthritis. In. In R. M. Kliegman, B. F. Stanton, J. W. St. Geme, et al. (Eds.), *Nelson textbook of pediatrics* (20th ed.). Philadelphia: Saunders.

Zaoutis, T., Localio, A. R., Leckerman, K., et al. (2009). Prolonged intravenous therapy versus early transition to oral antimicrobial therapy for acute osteomyelitis in children. *Pediatrics, 123*(2), 636–642.

Zier, J. L., & Liu, M. (2011). Safety of high-concentration nitrous oxide by nasal mask for pediatric procedural sedation: Experience with 7802 cases. *Pediatric Emergency Care, 27*(12), 1107–1112. doi:10.1097/PEC.0b013e31823aff6d.

ADDITIONAL RESOURCES

About Kids Health—Information on scoliosis: <http://www.aboutkidshealth.ca/En/HealthAZ/TestsAndTreatments/MedicalDevices/Pages/Scoliosis-Treatment-with-a-Spinal-Orthosis-Spinal-Brace.aspx>.

American Academy of Orthopaedic Surgeons and Scoliosis Research Society: <http://orthoinfo.aaos.org/main.cfm>.

Arthritis Society: <http://arthritis.ca/home>.

Canadian Spine Society: <http://spinecanada.ca/>.

Childhood Cancer Canada—Information about special programs for children with amputations: <http://www.childhoodcancer.ca>.

Health Canada—Child Car Seat Safety: <https://www.canada.ca/en/services/transport/road/child-car-seat-safety.html>.

Lupus Canada: <http://www.lupuscanada.org>.

Modified Braden Q Scale (for Pediatric Use): <http://www.therapybc.ca/eLibrary/docs/Resources/Braden%20Q%20scale%20for%20paeds.pdf>.

Scoliosis—Life, Support and Friends: <http://scoliosisnutty.blogspot.com/2009/02/scoliosis-association-of-british.html>.

Scoliosis Canada: <www.scoliosiscanada.org>.

War Amps (Child Amputee [CHAMP] Program)—Support group for children undergoing amputation: <http://www.waramps.ca/champ/home.html>.

CHAPTER

54

Neuromuscular or Muscular Dysfunction

Cheryl Sams

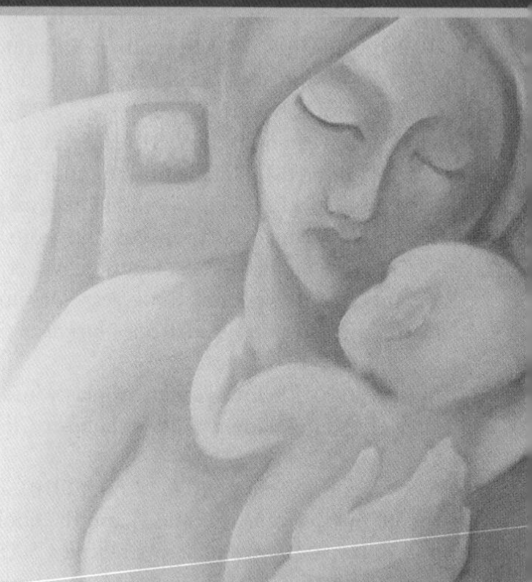

evolve WEBSITE

Visit the Evolve website for additional resources related to the content in this chapter such as Case Studies, Critical Thinking Case Study Answers, Nursing Care Plans, Nursing Processes, Nursing Skills, and Review Questions for Exam Preparation at: http://evolve.elsevier.com/Canada/Perry/maternal/

OBJECTIVES

On completion of this chapter the reader will be able to:

- Discuss the nursing role in helping parents care for a child with cerebral palsy.
- Formulate a nursing care plan for the preoperative and postoperative care of a child with myelomeningocele.
- Outline a plan of care for a child with Duchenne muscular dystrophy.
- Discuss the prevention and treatment of tetanus.
- Identify the causes of botulism in infants and children.
- List three causes of spinal cord injury in children.
- Discuss the emergent nursing care of the child or adolescent with a spinal cord injury.

CONGENITAL NEUROMUSCULAR OR MUSCULAR DISORDERS

Cerebral Palsy

Cerebral palsy (CP) is a diagnostic term used to describe a group of permanent disorders of movement and posture causing activity limitation that are attributed to nonprogressive disturbances in the developing fetal or infant brain (Johnston, 2016). In addition to motor disorders, the condition often involves disturbances of sensation, perception, communication, cognition, and behaviour; secondary musculoskeletal problems; and epilepsy. The etiology, clinical features, and course are variable and are characterized by abnormal muscle tone and coordination as the primary disturbances. A significant percentage (15 to 60%) of children with CP also have epilepsy. CP is the most common permanent motor disability of childhood (Johnston, 2016). In Canada, there are 42,679 individuals living with CP (Statistics Canada, 2012). Prevalence of CP among extremely low-birth-weight infants (less than 28 weeks' gestation) is said to be nearly 100 times the rate in term infants; however, these rates have declined in recent years (Hack & Costello, 2008).

CP is currently believed to result from existing prenatal brain abnormalities; the exact cause of these abnormalities remains elusive but may include genetic factors, including clotting disorders as well as brain malformations. It has been estimated that as many as 80% of CP cases are attributable to unidentified prenatal factors (Johnston, 2016). Intrauterine exposure to maternal chorioamnionitis is associated with an increased risk of CP in infants of normal birth weight and in preterm infants (Volpe, 2008); however, not all term infants exposed to chorioamnionitis develop CP. Perinatal ischemic stroke is also associated with a later diagnosis of CP (Golomb, 2009). One study found a higher risk for CP occurring among infants born at 42 weeks' gestation or later than among those born at 37 or 38 weeks' gestation (Moster, Wilcox, Vollset, et al., 2010). Additional factors that may contribute to the development of CP postnatally include bacterial meningitis, multiple births, viral encephalitis, being in a motor vehicle accident (MVA), and child abuse (shaken baby syndrome [traumatic brain injury]). In summary, as many as 80% of the total cases of CP may be linked to a perinatal or neonatal brain lesion or brain maldevelopment, regardless of the cause (Krägeloh-Mann & Cans, 2009).

Pathophysiology

It is difficult to establish a precise location of neurological lesions based on etiology or clinical signs because no characteristic pathological pattern exists. Some patients have gross malformations of the brain; others may have evidence of vascular occlusion, atrophy, loss of neurons, and degeneration that produce narrower gyri, wider sulci, and low brain weight. Anoxia appears to play the most significant role in the pathological state of brain damage, which is often secondary to other causative mechanisms.

There are a few exceptions. In some cases, the manifestations or etiology is related to anatomical areas. For example, CP associated with preterm birth is usually spastic diplegia caused by hypoxic infarction or hemorrhage with periventricular leukomalacia in the area adjacent to the lateral ventricles. The athetoid (extrapyramidal) type of CP is most likely to be associated with birth asphyxia but can also be caused by kernicterus and metabolic genetic disorders such as mitochondrial disorders and glutaric aciduria (Johnston, 2016). Hemiplegic (hemiparetic) CP is often associated with a focal cerebral infarction (stroke) secondary to an intrauterine or perinatal thromboembolism, usually a result of maternal thrombosis or hereditary clotting disorder (Johnston, 2016). Cerebral hypoplasia and sometimes severe neonatal hypoglycemia are related to ataxic CP. Generalized cortical and cerebral atrophy often cause severe neonatal quadriparesis with cognitive impairments and microcephaly.

Clinical Classifications

A revision of the Winter classification was proposed in 2005 to reflect the child's actual clinical problems and their severity, an assessment of the child's physical and quality-of-life status across time, and long-term support needs (Nehring, 2009). The proposed new definition has four major dimensions of classification (Nehring, 2009):

1. Motor abnormalities—Nature and typology of the motor disorder; functional motor abilities
2. Associated impairments—Seizures; hearing or vision impairment; attentional, behavioural, communicative, or cognitive deficits; oral motor and speed functions
3. Anatomical and radiological findings—Anatomy distribution of parts of the body affected by motor impairments or limitations; radiological findings sometimes including white matter lesions or brain anomaly noted on computed tomography (CT) or magnetic resonance imaging (MRI).
4. Causation and timing—Identification of a clearly identified cause, such as postnatal event (e.g., meningitis, traumatic brain injury).

CP has four primary types of movement disorder: spastic, dyskinetic, ataxis, and mixed (Johnston, 2016). The most common clinical type is spastic CP, which represents an upper motor neuron muscle weakness (Box 54-1). The reflex arc is intact, and the characteristic physical signs are increased stretch reflexes, increased muscle tone, and (often) weakness. Early neurological manifestations are usually generalized hypotonia or decreased tone that lasts for a few weeks or may extend for months or even as long as 1 year.

BOX 54-1 CLINICAL CLASSIFICATION OF CEREBRAL PALSY

Spastic (Pyramidal)

Characterized by persistent primitive reflexes, positive Babinski, ankle clonus, exaggerated stretch reflexes, eventual development of contractures

85% of all cases of cerebral palsy (CP)

- **Diplegia**—All extremities affected; lower more than upper (35% of spastic CP)
- **Tetraplegia**—All four extremities involved: legs and trunk, mouth, pharynx, and tongue (20% of spastic CP)
- **Triplegia**—Three limbs involved
- **Monoplegia**—Only one limb involved
- **Hemiplegia**—Motor dysfunction on one side of the body; upper extremity more affected than lower (25% of spastic CP)

Other features:

- **Hypertonicity** with poor control of posture, balance, and coordinated motion
- **Impairment** of fine and gross motor skills

Dyskinetic (Nonspastic, Extrapyramidal)

Athetoid—Chorea (involuntary, irregular, jerking movements); characterized by slow, wormlike, writhing movements that usually involve the extremities, trunk, neck, facial muscles, and tongue

Dystonic—Slow, twisting movements of the trunk or extremities; abnormal posture

Involvement of the pharyngeal, laryngeal, and oral muscles, causing drooling and dysarthria (imperfect speech articulation)

Ataxic (Nonspastic, Extrapyramidal)

Wide-based gait

Rapid, repetitive movements performed poorly

Disintegration of movements of the upper extremities when the child reaches for objects

Mixed Type

Combination of spastic CP and dyskinetic CP

May be labelled *mixed* when no specific motor pattern is dominant; however, this term is losing favour to more precise descriptions of motor function and affected area of brain involved (Rosenbaum, Paneth, Leviton, et al., 2007)

Data from Jones, M. W., et al. (2007). Cerebral palsy: Introduction and diagnosis, part 1. *Journal of Pediatric Health Care, 21*(3), 146–152; National Institute of Neurological Disorders and Stroke. (2016). *Cerebral palsy: Hope through research.* Retrieved from http://www.ninds.nih.gov/disorders/cerebral_palsy/detail_cerebral_palsy.htm; Nehring, W. (2009). Cerebral palsy. In P. J. Allen, J. A. Vessey, & N. A. Schapiro (Eds.), *Primary care of the child with a chronic condition* (5th ed.). St. Louis: Mosby.

Diagnostic Evaluation

Infants at risk according to known etiological factors associated with CP warrant careful assessment during early infancy to identify the signs of neuromotor dysfunction as early as possible. The neurological examination and history are the primary modalities for diagnosis. Neuroimaging of the child with suspected brain abnormality and CP is now recommended for diagnostic assessment, with MRI preferred to CT scan. Metabolic and genetic testing is recommended if no structural abnormality is identified by neuroimaging; laboratory tests are no longer recommended in the diagnostic process for CP.

Early recognition is made more difficult by the lack of reliable neonatal neurological signs. However, nurses should monitor infants with known etiological risk factors and evaluate closely in the first 2 years of life. As cortical control of movement does not occur until later in infancy, motor impairment associated with voluntary control is usually not apparent until after 2 to 4 months of age at the earliest. More often the diagnosis cannot be confirmed until the age of 2 years because motor tone abnormalities may be indicative of another neuromuscular illness. In addition, some children who show signs consistent with CP before 2 years of age do not demonstrate such signs after 2 years (Nehring, 2009). However, there is no consensus regarding an age cut-off for the onset of symptoms. Clinical manifestations of CP at the time of diagnosis are listed in Box 54-2, and early warning signs are listed in Box 54-3, but these are not considered diagnostic.

Establishing a diagnosis may be easier with the persistence of primitive reflexes: (1) either the asymmetrical tonic neck reflex or persistent Moro reflex (beyond 4 months of age), and (2) the crossed extensor reflex. The tonic neck reflex normally disappears between 4 and 6 months of age. An "obligatory" response is considered abnormal. This reflex is elicited by turning the infant's head to one side and holding it there for 20 seconds. When a crying infant is unable to move from the asymmetrical posturing of the tonic neck reflex when crying, it is considered obligatory and an abnormal response. The crossed extensor reflex, which normally disappears by 4 months, is elicited by applying a noxious stimulus to the sole of one foot with the knee extended. Normally the contralateral foot responds with extensor, abduction, and then adduction movements. The possibility of CP is suggested if these reflexes occur after 4 months.

A number of assessment instruments are now available to evaluate muscle spasticity, including functional independence in self-care, mobility, and cognition; self-initiated movements over time; and capability and performance of functional activities in self-care, mobility, and social function.

Therapeutic Management

The goals of therapy for children with CP are early recognition and optimizing development to enable affected children to attain developmental and activity levels within the limits of their existing health problems. The disorder is permanent, and therapy is primarily preventive and symptomatic.

Therapy has five broad aims:

1. To establish locomotion, communication, and self-help skills
2. To gain optimal appearance and integration of motor functions
3. To correct associated defects as effectively as possible
4. To provide educational opportunities adapted to the child's needs and capabilities
5. To promote socialization experiences with other children

Each child is evaluated and managed on an individual basis. The scope of the child's needs requires multidisciplinary planning and care coordination among professionals and the child's family.

Ankle-foot orthoses (AFOs, braces) are worn by many of these children and are used to help prevent or reduce deformity, increase the energy efficiency of gait, and control alignment.

BOX 54-2 CLINICAL MANIFESTATIONS OF CEREBRAL PALSY (AT TIME OF DIAGNOSIS)

Delayed Gross Motor Development

- A universal manifestation
- Delay in all motor accomplishments
- Increases as growth advances
- Becomes more obvious as growth advances

Abnormal Motor Performance

- Very early preferential unilateral hand preference
- Abnormal and asymmetrical crawl
- Standing or walking on toes
- Uncoordinated or involuntary movements
- Poor sucking
- Feeding difficulties
- Persistent tongue thrust

Alterations of Muscle Tone

- Increased or decreased resistance to passive movements
- Opisthotonic posturing (arching of back)
- Feels stiff on handling or dressing
- Difficulty in diapering
- Rigid and unbending at the hip and knee joints when pulled to sitting position (early sign)

Abnormal Postures

- Maintains hips higher than trunk in prone position with legs and arms flexed or drawn under the body
- Scissoring and extension of legs with feet plantar flexed in supine position
- Persistent infantile resting and sleeping position
- Arms abducted at shoulders
- Elbows flexed
- Hands fisted

Reflex Abnormalities

- Persistence of primitive infantile reflexes
- Obligatory tonic neck reflex at any age
- Persistence or hyperactivity of the Moro, plantar, and palmar grasp reflexes
- Hyperreflexia, ankle clonus, and stretch reflexes elicited in many muscle groups on fast, passive movements

Associated Disabilities

- Altered learning and reasoning
- Seizures
- Impaired behavioural and interpersonal relationships
- Sensory impairment (vision, hearing)

From Nehring, W. M. (2009). Cerebral palsy. In P. J. Allen, J. A. Vessey, N. A. Schapiro, (Eds.), *Primary care of the child with a chronic condition* (5th ed.). St. Louis: Mosby. Adapted from Jones, M. W., Morgan, E., & Shelton, J. E. (2007). Primary care of the child with cerebral palsy: A review of systems (part II). *Journal of Pediatric Health Care, 21*(4), 226–237.

BOX 54-3 EARLY WARNING SIGNS OF CEREBRAL PALSY

- Failure to meet any developmental milestones, such as rolling over, raising head, sitting up, crawling
- Persistent primitive reflexes, such as Moro, asymmetrical tonic neck reflex
- Poor head control (head lag) and clenched fists after 3 months of age
- Stiff or rigid arms or legs; scissoring legs
- Pushing away or arching back; stiff posture
- Floppy or limp body posture, especially while sleeping
- Inability to sit up without support by 8 months
- Using only one side of the body or only the arms to crawl
- Feeding difficulties
- Persistent gagging or choking when fed
- After 6 months of age, tongue pushing soft food out of the mouth
- Extreme irritability or crying
- Failure to smile by 3 months
- Lack of interest in surroundings

Data from Nehring, W. (2009). Cerebral palsy. In P. J. Allen & J. A. Vessey (Eds.), *Primary care of the child with a chronic condition* (5th ed.). St. Louis: Mosby; Jones, M. W., Morgan, E., Shelton, J. E., et al. (2007). Cerebral palsy: Introduction and diagnosis (part 1). *Journal of Pediatrics & Health Care, 21*(3), 146–152.

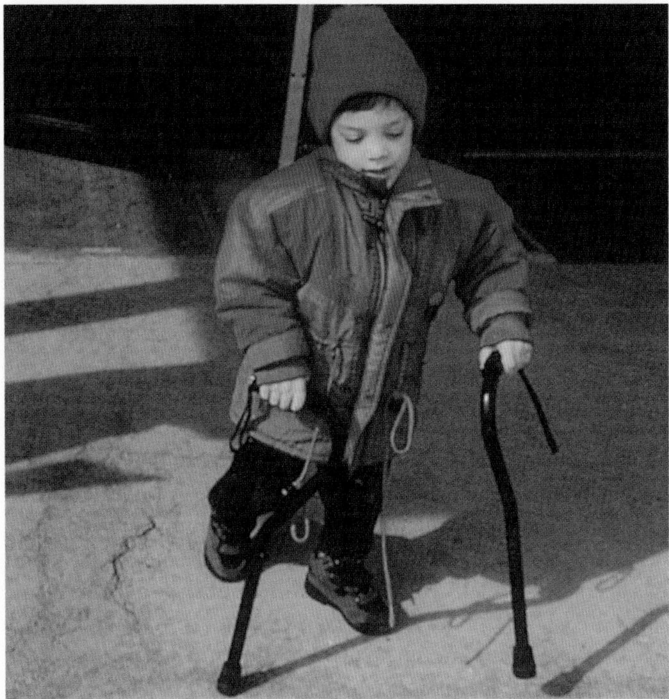

FIGURE 54-1 Mobilization device for child.

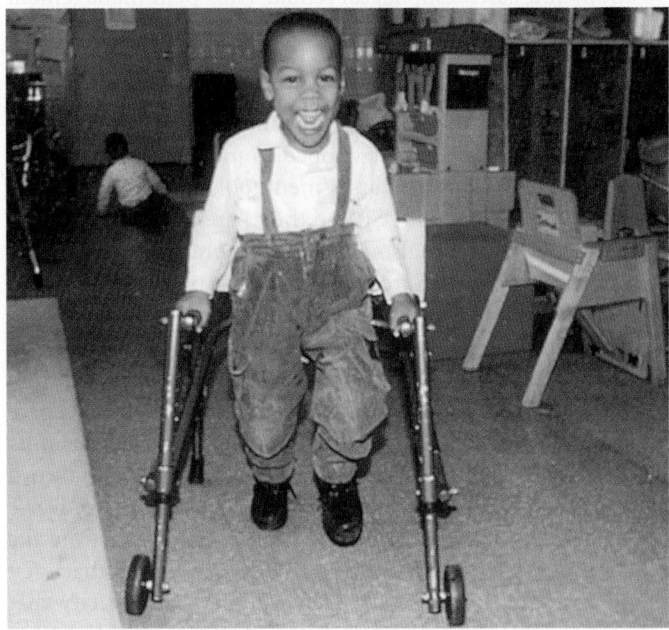

FIGURE 54-2 Child ambulating with use of assistive device.

Wheeled go-carts that provide sitting balance may serve as early "wheelchair" experience for young children. Manual or powered wheelchairs allow for more independent mobility (Figs. 54-1 and 54-2). Strollers can be equipped with custom seats for dependent mobilization.

Orthopedic surgery may be required between the ages of 5 and 7 years to correct contracture or spastic deformities, to provide stability for an uncontrollable joint, and to provide balanced muscle power. This surgery includes tendon-lengthening procedures (especially heel-cord lengthening), release of spastic wrist flexor muscles, and correction of hip and adductor muscle spasticity or contracture to improve locomotion. Hip dislocation often occurs in children with CP. Spinal fusion may be done for scoliosis. Computerized motion analysis, radiographs, and clinical findings are used to make decisions about the orthopedic surgery. Selective dorsal rhizotomy has provided marked improvement in some children with CP. The procedure involves selectively cutting dorsal column sensory rootlets that have an abnormal response to electrical stimulation. For children to achieve the most benefit from the surgery they must undergo intensive physiotherapy and the family must be committed to it. The procedure results in flaccid muscles, so the child must be retaught to sit, stand, and walk.

Surgical intervention is usually reserved for the child who does not respond to the more conservative measures such as bracing, but it is also indicated for the child whose spasticity causes progressive deformities. Surgery is primarily used to improve function and enable proper sitting, standing, and walking rather than for cosmetic purposes.

Intense pain may occur with muscle spasms in patients with CP. Pharmacological agents given orally (dantrolene sodium, baclofen, and diazepam [Valium]) have had little effectiveness in improving muscle coordination in children with CP; however, they are effective in decreasing overall spasticity. The most common adverse effects of these medications include hepatotoxicity (dantrolene), drowsiness, fatigue, and muscle weakness; less commonly, diaphoresis and constipation may be seen with baclofen. Botulinum toxin A (Botox) is also used to reduce spasticity in targeted muscles. Botulinum toxin A is injected into a selected muscle (commonly the quadriceps, gastrocnemius, or medial hamstrings) after a topical anaesthetic or sedation is used. The drug acts to inhibit the release of acetylcholine into a specific muscle group, thereby preventing muscle movement. When it is administered early in the course of the illness, affected muscle contractures may be prevented, particularly in lower extremities, thus the patient may avoid needing surgical procedures with possible adverse effects. The goal is to allow stretching of the muscle as it relaxes and enable ambulation with an AFO. The major reported adverse effect of botulinum toxin A injection is pain at the injection site and temporary weakness (Lukban, Rosales, & Dressler, 2009). Prime candidates for botulinum toxin A injections are children with spasticity confined to the lower extremities; the drug weakens spasticity so the muscles can be stretched and the child may ambulate with or without orthoses. The onset of action occurs within 24 to 72 hours, with a peak effect observed at 2 weeks and a duration of action of 3 to 6 months. Botulinum toxin injected into salivary glands may also help reduce the severity of drooling, which is seen in 10 to 30% of patients with CP and has been traditionally treated with anticholinergic agents (Johnston, 2016). Diazepam has proven to be effective on a short-term basis in reducing spasticity in children with CP (Delgado, Hirtz, Aisen, et al., 2010; Johnston, 2016).

Children with CP may also experience pain as a result of surgical procedures intended to reduce contracture deformities, position, and gastroesophageal reflux. Thus pain management is an important care priority in these children. Pain assessment can be very difficult to assess in children, particularly in children with cognitive impairment and who have communication struggles from CP. A pediatric questionnaire on pain caused by spasticity (QPS) has been developed to more accurately assess this type of pain. This pain assessment tool was developed with the input of children with CP and their parents. This enhanced pain assessment could also be used to more accurately assess the effectiveness of pain treatments, such as botulinum toxin A (Geister, Quintanar-Solares, Martin, et al., 2014).

The neurosurgical and pharmacological approach to relieving the spasticity associated with CP involves the implantation of a pump to infuse baclofen directly into the intrathecal space surrounding the spinal cord, where it reduces neurotransmission of afferent nerve fibres. Direct delivery to the spinal cord overcomes the problem of central nervous system adverse effects caused by the large oral doses needed to penetrate the blood–brain barrier (Johnston, 2016). Intrathecal baclofen therapy is best suited for children with severe spasticity that interferes with activities of daily living (ADLs) and ambulation. Relief of spasticity occurs for several hours after the infusion. If a positive effect is noted, the patient is considered a candidate for pump placement.

The implantation procedure is done in the operating room by a neurosurgeon. The pump, which is approximately the size of a hockey puck, is placed in the subcutaneous space of the midabdomen. An intrathecal catheter is tunnelled from the lumbar area to the abdomen and connected to the pump. Benefits of intrathecal baclofen include fewer systemic adverse effects than from oral medication, dosage titration for maximizing effects, and reversibility of therapy with removal of the pump if so desired. The patient may remain hospitalized for 3 to 7 days to adjust the dosage and ensure proper healing. Outpatient visits to refill the pump and make dosage adjustments should occur about every 3 to 6 months, depending on the patient's response to the treatment. This procedure is most suited for a multidisciplinary setting where rehabilitation specialists are readily available and consistently involved in the patient's ongoing care. Abrupt withdrawal of intrathecal baclofen, especially at high doses, may result in adverse effects such as rebound spasticity, pruritus, hyperthermia, rhabdomyolysis, disseminated intravascular coagulation, multiorgan failure, and death. In some cases, intrathecal baclofen withdrawal may mimic sepsis.

Oral baclofen has also been widely used in children with CP to treat spasticity. However, adverse effects are common and include systemic toxicity, drowsiness, and sedation (Delgado et al., 2010).

Antiepileptic drugs (AEDs), such as carbamazepine (Tegretol) and divalproex (valproate sodium and valproic acid; Depakote), are prescribed routinely for children who have seizures. The use of oral tizanidine in children has been limited and only a few small studies have been conducted in children with CP specifically evaluating the reduction of spasticity (Delgado et al., 2010). All medications should be monitored for maintenance of therapeutic levels and avoidance of subtherapeutic or toxic levels. Other medications used include levodopa to treat dystonia, artane for treating dystonia and for increasing the use of upper extremities and vocalizations, and reserpine for hyperkinetic movement disorders such as chorea or athetosis (Johnston, 2016).

Dental hygiene is especially important for children with CP. Regular visits to the dentist along with prophylaxis, including brushing, fluoride, and flossing, should be instituted as soon as the teeth erupt. Dental care is important for children being given phenytoin, as they often develop gum hyperplasia. Additional problems common among children with CP include constipation caused by neurological deficits and lack of exercise, poor bladder control and urinary retention, chronic respiratory tract infections, and aspiration pneumonia. These issues occur as a result of gastroesophageal reflux, abnormal muscle tone, immobility, and altered positioning; skin problems result from altered positioning, poor nutrition, and immobility. Given these issues, children with CP often toilet train later than other children.

A wide variety of technical aids are available to improve the functioning of children with CP. These include electromechanical toys that employ the concept of biofeedback and operate from a head unit. The toy is manipulated only when the head and trunk are in correct alignment. Eye–hand coordination can also be enhanced by use of computerized toys and games. Microcomputers combined with voice synthesizers help children with speech difficulties to "speak." These and other devices print messages onto screen monitors and paper.

Many other electronic devices enable independent functioning. Sensors can be activated and deactivated by using a head-stick or tongue or other voluntary muscle movement over which the child has control. Voice-activated computer technology may also allow increased mobility and ambulation with specially designed devices such as wheelchairs. The application of this technology makes it possible for persons with CP to function eventually in their own residences and can be extended into the workplace.

There is some evidence that neuromuscular electrical stimulation (NMES) in addition to dynamic splinting may result in increased muscle strength, range of motion, and function of upper limbs in children with CP. Further studies are needed in children with CP to support the use of botulinum toxin A in conjunction with NMES to decrease muscle spasticity and improve function (Wright, Durham, Ewins, et al., 2012).

Behaviour problems may occur and often interfere with the child's development. Attention deficit hyperactivity disorder and other learning problems require professional attention. In addition, children with CP may have vision difficulties such as strabismus, nystagmus, and optic atrophy (Johnston, 2016). Speech-language therapy involves the services of a speech-language pathologist who may also assist with feeding problems.

Physiotherapy is one of the most frequently used conservative treatment modalities. It requires the specialized skills of a qualified therapist with an extensive repertoire of exercise methods who can design a program to stimulate each child to achieve his or her functional goals. An active therapy program involves the family, the physiotherapist, and often other members of the health team, including the nurse. The most common approach employs traditional types of therapeutic exercises that consist of stretching, passive, active, and resistive movements applied to specific muscle groups or joints to maintain or increase range of motion, strength, and endurance.

Prognosis

The prognosis for the child with CP depends largely on the type and severity of the condition. Children with mild to moderate involvement (85%) have the capability of achieving ambulation between the ages of 2 and 7 years (Berker & Yalçin, 2008). If the child does not achieve independent ambulation by this time, chances are poor for ambulation and independence. Approximately 30 to 50% of individuals with CP have cognitive impairment, and an even higher percentage have mild cognitive and learning deficits; however, many children with severe spastic tetraplegic CP have normal intelligence. Growth is affected in children with spastic tetraplegia, and many children remain below the fifth percentile for age and gender.

Vocational rehabilitation and higher education are possible for adults with CP. Children with severe CP mobility impairment and feeding problems often succumb to respiratory tract infection in childhood (Liptak, Murphy, & Council on Children with Disabilities, 2011). The few survival rate studies on children and adults with CP show that survival is influenced by existing comorbidities (Nehring, 2009). In Canada, approximately 4300 individuals with CP live in institutions (Statistics Canada, 2013).

Neurorehabilitation involves rehabilitating and stimulating nerves (that control muscle movement) that have been damaged, to improve brain development. Brain plasticity is being examined as a possible route for reorganizing traditionally damaged neural pathways to function optimally for children with CP. Children with CP or spinal cord injuries (SCI) may benefit from therapies such as constraint-induced movement, in which a stronger extremity is constrained to force the weaker extremity to function; some children with CP who have undergone these treatments have shown improvement in their symptoms (Aisen, Kerkovich, Mast, et al., 2011).

Some progress has been made in the prevention of CP in children. Studies indicate that early neuroprotection in term infants with the use of therapeutic hypothermia (head cooling or whole-body cooling) within 6 hours of birth has improved survival without CP by approximately 40% (Johnston, Fatemi, & Wilson, 2011). Other studies have found lower death rates and less severe disability with the use of therapeutic hypothermia, but overall IQ scores at 6 or 7 years of age were not significantly changed in those receiving hypothermia (as compared with those receiving conventional treatment) (Shankarn, Pappas, McDonald, et al., 2012). Preliminary results from controlled trials of magnesium sulphate given intravenously to mothers in premature labour with birth imminent before 32 weeks' gestation have also shown a significant reduction in the risk of CP in children 2 years of age (Johnston, 2016) (see Chapter 20, Management of Inevitable Preterm Birth, p. 519).

NURSING CARE

Because CP in children is now being identified and treated at an earlier age of the child, parents are participating earlier in treatment programs for their children with such complex conditions. They are taught the proper handling and home care of young children with CP. Close work with other multidisciplinary team members is essential. Nurses can reinforce the therapeutic plan and assist the family in devising or modifying equipment at home. The nursing care of the child with CP is outlined in the Nursing Care Plan available on Evolve.

Children with CP expend much energy in their efforts to accomplish ADLs, thus more frequent rest periods should be arranged to avoid fatigue. The diet should be tailored to the child's activity and metabolic needs. Gastrostomy feedings may be necessary to supplement regular feedings and ensure adequate weight gain, particularly in the child who is at risk for growth failure or chronic malnutrition and in those with severe CP who have subsequent oral feeding difficulties. Oral feedings may be continued in order to maintain oral motor skills. Weight gain is an important measure of adequate oral feeding efficiency.

A skin-level gastrostomy is particularly suited for the child with CP (see Chapter 44). Parents may need assistance and advice regarding tube care, tube feedings, and medication administration through a gastrostomy tube to prevent clotting of the device. Jaw control is often compromised in the child with CP; more normal control can be achieved if the feeder provides stability of the oral mechanism from the side or front of the face. When directed from the front, the middle finger of the nonfeeding hand is placed posterior to the body portion of the chin, the thumb is placed below the bottom lip, and the index finger is placed parallel to the child's mandible (Fig. 54-3).

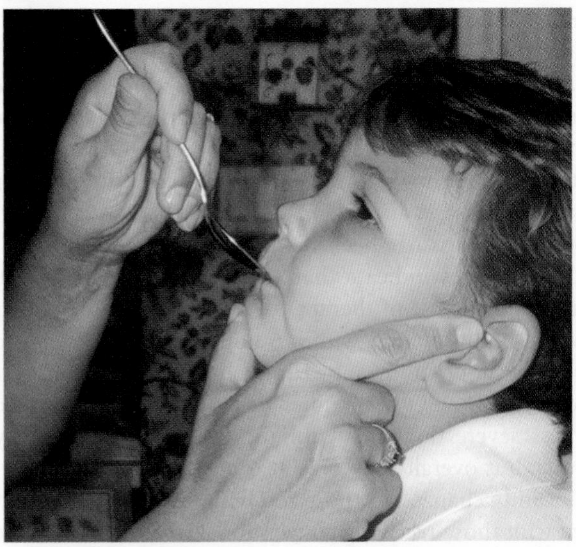

FIGURE 54-3 Manual jaw control provided anteriorly.

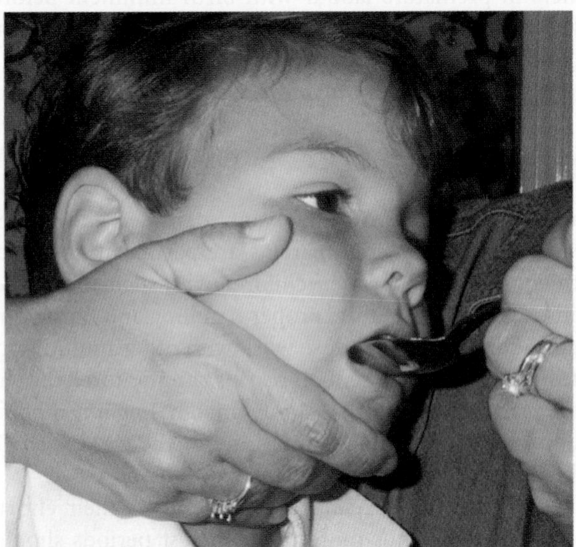

FIGURE 54-4 Manual jaw control provided from the side.

Manual jaw control from the side assists with head control, correction of neck and trunk hyperextension, and jaw stabilization. The middle finger of the nonfeeding hand is placed posterior to the bony portion of the chin, the index finger is placed on the chin below the lower lip, and the thumb is placed obliquely across the cheek to provide lateral jaw stability (Fig. 54-4).

Safety precautions need to be implemented, such as having children wear protective helmets if they are subject to falls or capable of injuring their head on hard objects. Because the child with CP is at risk for altered proprioception and subsequent falls, the home and play environment should be adapted to the child's needs to prevent bodily harm. Transportation of the child with motor problems and restricted mobility may be especially challenging for the family and child. Attention must be given to the child's safety when riding in a motor vehicle; a federally approved safety restraint should be used at all times. It is recommended that children with CP ride in a rear-facing seat as long as possible because of their poor head, neck, and trunk control (Lovette, 2008). In addition, appropriate immunizations should be administered to prevent childhood illnesses and protect against respiratory tract infections such as influenza.

The involvement of physiotherapy, speech therapy, and occupational therapy is particularly important in the establishment and maintenance of muscle function, development of adequate speech and phonation, and identification of modifications necessary for the child's environment so that ADLs can be performed to the child's satisfaction.

As in all aspects of care, educational requirements are determined by the child's needs and potential. Children with mild to moderate involvement are generally able to participate, for varying amounts of time, in regular classes. Resource rooms are available in most schools to provide more individualized attention. Integration of children with CP into regular classrooms should be the initial goal. For those who are unable to benefit from formal education, a vocational training program may be appropriate. At adolescence, prevocational and vocational counselling and guidance can be arranged. At any phase or in any setting, education is geared toward the child's abilities.

Recreation and after-school activities should be considered for the child who is unable to participate in the regular athletic programs and other peer activities. Some children can compete in athletic and artistic endeavours, and many games and pastimes are suited to their capabilities. Competitive sports are also becoming increasingly available to children with disabilities and offer an added dimension to physical activities. The Canadian Cerebral Palsy Sports Association is a national organization that provides sports opportunities for individuals with CP (see Additional Resources at the end of this chapter). Canada is ranked among the top countries for athletes with CP. The Association supports sports for these individuals at the regional, national, and international levels.

Recreational activities serve to stimulate children's interest and curiosity, help them adjust to their disability, improve their functional abilities, and build self-esteem. Any accomplishment that helps children approach a "normal" way of life can enhance their self-concept.

Support the Family

The nursing interventions that tend to be most valuable to the family are support and help in coping with the emotional aspects of the disorder, many of which are discussed in this book in relation to the child with a disability (see Chapter 40). Initially, the parents need supportive counselling directed toward understanding the implications of the diagnosis and all of the feelings that it engenders. Later they need clarification on what they can expect from the child and from health care providers. Educating families in the principles of family-centred care and parent–professional collaboration is essential. The family may require assistance in modifying the home environment for care of the child (see also Chapter 42), including modifications to facilitate the use of a wheelchair. The child or adolescent should be encouraged to be as independent as possible. Transportation in a car often requires special considerations.

Care coordination for the child and family with CP is an important nursing role. In many cases the family assumes complete care of the child and becomes adept at meeting his or her individual needs. The home health nurse or care manager has an important role in support and encouragement for families who assume the primary care of a child with CP. Having a child with CP implies numerous problems of daily management and changes in family life that require support from the nurse to help with coordinating family activities and care.

The nurse needs to support the parents in their frustration, problem solving, concerns, and approaches to helping the child; all of these aspects must be explored and discussed. Siblings of a child with a disability are also affected and may respond to the child's presence with overt or less evident behavioural issues. The family needs a relationship with nurses who can provide continued contact, support, and encouragement through the long process of habilitation.

Parents may also find help and comfort from parent groups with whom they can share problems and concerns and from whom they can derive comfort and practical information. Parent support groups are most helpful through sharing of experiences and accomplishments.

The organization Cerebral Palsy Support Canada provides support, funding, and aids in locating assistive devices for children and families. This organization also has a resource library for children with CP, their families, and health care providers. See Additional Resources at the end of this chapter for more information.

Support the Hospitalized Child

CP is not a disorder that requires hospitalization; thus when children with CP are hospitalized, they are usually admitted for another reason or for corrective surgery. Nursing care for the child with CP is the same as for any other child with a disability. Children with CP should be approached in the same manner as for any child in the hospital. Speech impairment is common in children with CP, but this may not correlate with their ability to understand. To facilitate the care and management of these children, the therapy program should be continued, insofar as their condition allows, during the time they are hospitalized. Encouraging the parent to room in and actively participate in the child's care facilitates a continuation of the home therapy program and helps the child adjust to an unfamiliar environment. However, it is equally important to remember that hospitalization may be the first time a parent can defer care to a nurse and not be the primary caregiver. This respite may be crucial to the parent's well-being. The Family-Centred Teaching box presents a story about a mother with a child with CP and the reality of accepting the diagnosis of CP.

FAMILY-CENTRED CARE

The Reality of Acceptance of Cerebral Palsy

Acceptance is rarely achieved in the length of time implied in the literature.

In the first place, what is it? To me, it is the end of comparing my son with every other child I see. I focus on his gains, not society's expectations.

It is also being able to laugh periodically at his "clumsiness." It is "gallows humour" as he achieves adulthood; jokes about CP can be funny now.

The bitterness is gone; I am now happy for people who have children without CP.

I am no longer sorry for my son, but rather for the people who cannot see him for the great person he is; the CP does not come first.

He is now a young man of 25 years and I am leaning to accept his independence.

It is a "never-ending story."

—Elaine A. Dunham, RN, Shriner's Hospitals for Children
Springfield, MA

BOX 54-4 NEURAL TUBE DEFECTS

Cranioschisis—A skull defect through which various tissues protrude

Exencephaly—Brain totally exposed or extruded through an associated skull defect; fetus usually aborted

Anencephaly—If fetus with exencephaly survives, there is degeneration of the brain to a spongiform mass with no bony covering; incompatible with life usually beyond a few days

Encephalocele—Herniation of brain and meninges through a defect in the skull producing a fluid-filled sac

Rachischisis or spina bifida—Fissure in the spinal column that leaves the meninges and spinal cord exposed

Meningocele—Hernial protrusion of a saclike cyst of meninges filled with spinal fluid (see Fig. 54-5, C)

Myelomeningocele (meningomyelocele)—Hernial protrusion of a saclike cyst containing meninges, spinal fluid, and a portion of the spinal cord with its nerves (see Fig. 54-5, D)

Neural Tube Defects

Abnormalities that derive from the embryonic neural tube (**neural tube defects** [NTDs]) constitute the largest group of congenital anomalies (Box 54-4). Normally, the spinal cord and cauda equina are encased in a protective sheath of bone and meninges (Fig. 54-5, A). Failure of neural tube closure produces defects of varying degrees (see Box 54-4). They may involve the entire length of the neural tube or may be restricted to a small area.

In Canada, the rate of NTDs decreased from 7.6 per 10,000 total births in 1997 to 4.1 per 10,000 total births in 2007 (Public Health Agency of Canada [PHAC], 2014a). Prenatal supplementation of folic acid and the increased use of prenatal diagnostic techniques and termination of pregnancies have affected the overall incidence of NTDs (see also Prevention, p. 1765).

Encephalocele and anencephaly are abnormalities resulting from failure of the anterior end of the neural tube to close. An *encephalocele* is a herniation of the brain and meninges through a skull defect, usually at the base of the neck. The defect may be associated with hydrocephalus (see Chapter 50); the resulting sequelae depend on the amount of neural tissue within the protruding sac and associated neurological defects. Treatment consists of surgical repair and shunting to relieve hydrocephalus, unless a major brain malformation is present. *Anencephaly*,

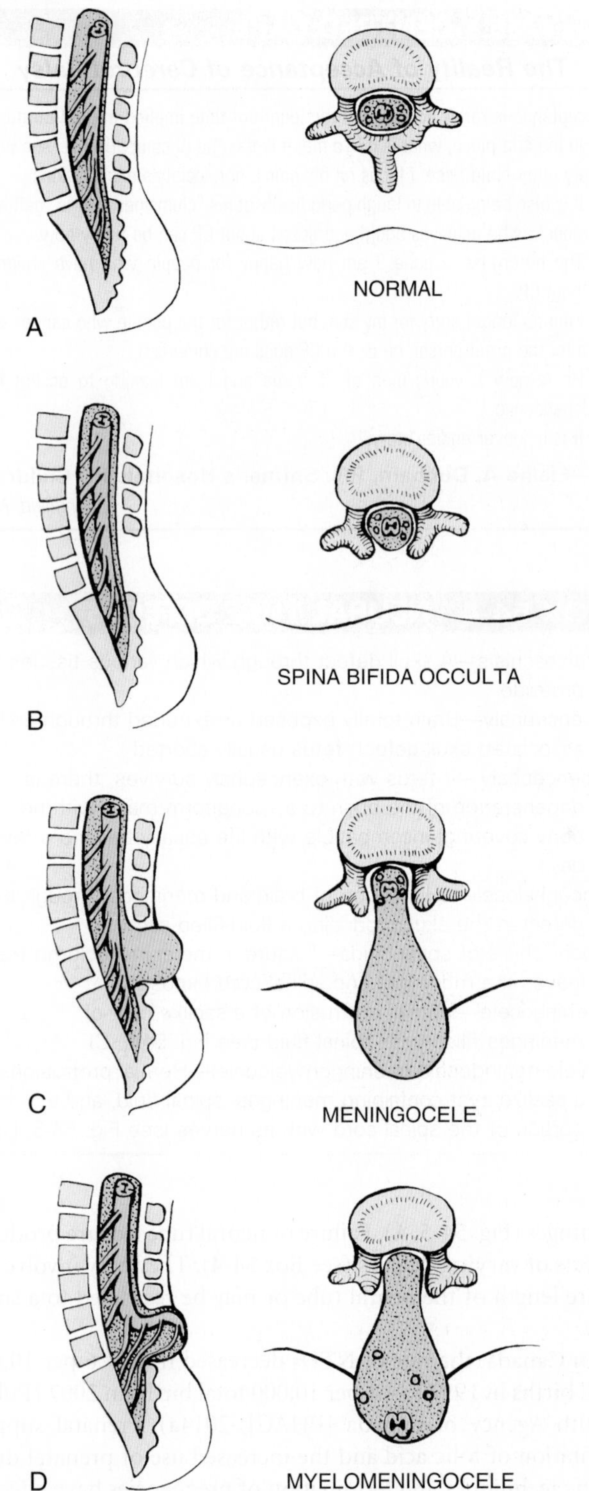

FIGURE 54-5 A through **D:** Midline defects of osseous spine with varying degrees of neural herniations.

the most serious NTD, is a congenital malformation in which both cerebral hemispheres are absent. The condition is incompatible with life, and many affected infants are stillborn. For those who survive, no specific treatment is available. The infants have a portion of the brainstem and are able to maintain vital functions (e.g., temperature regulation and cardiac and respiratory function) for a few hours to several weeks. Comfort measures are provided until the infant eventually dies of temperature instability and respiratory failure.

Myelodysplasia refers broadly to any malformation of the spinal canal and cord. Midline defects involving failure of the osseous (bony) spine to close are called *spina bifida (SB)*, the most common defect of the central nervous system. SB is categorized into two types: spina bifida occulta and spina bifida cystica.

Spina bifida occulta refers to a defect that is not visible externally. It occurs most frequently in the lumbosacral area (L5 and S1) (see Fig. 54-5, B). SB occulta may not be apparent unless there are associated cutaneous manifestations or neuromuscular disturbances.

Spina bifida cystica refers to a visible defect with an external saclike protrusion. The two major forms of SB cystica are *meningocele*, which encases meninges and spinal fluid but no neural elements (see Fig. 54-5, C), and *myelomeningocele* (or *meningomyelocele*), which contains meninges, spinal fluid, and nerves (see Fig. 54-5, D). Meningocele is not associated with neurological deficit, which occurs in varying, often serious, degrees in myelomeningocele.

Pathophysiology

The pathophysiology of NTD is best understood when related to the normal formative stages of the nervous system. At approximately 20 days of gestation, a dedicated depression, the neural groove, appears in the dorsal ectoderm of the embryo. During the fourth week of gestation, the groove deepens rapidly, and its elevated margins develop laterally and fuse dorsally to form the neural tube. Neural tube formation begins in the cervical region near the centre of the embryo and advances in both directions—caudally and cephalically—until by the end of the fourth week of gestation, the ends of the neural tube, the anterior and posterior neuropores, close.

Most experts believe that the primary defect in NTDs is a failure of neural tube closure. However, some evidence indicates that the defects are a result of splitting of the already closed neural tube as a result of an abnormal increase in cerebrospinal fluid (CSF) pressure during the first trimester.

There is evidence of multifactorial etiology, including medications, radiation, maternal malnutrition, chemicals, and possibly a genetic mutation in folate pathways in some cases, which may result in abnormal development. There is also evidence of a genetic component in the development of SB; myelomeningocele may occur in association with syndromes such as trisomy 18, PHAVER syndrome (limb pterygia, congenital heart anomalies, vertebral defects, ear anomalies, and radial defects), and Meckel-Gruber syndrome (Kinsman & Johnston, 2016). Additional factors predisposing children to an increased risk of NTDs include prepregnancy maternal obesity, maternal diabetes mellitus, previous NTD pregnancy, low maternal vitamin B_{12} status, maternal hyperthermia, and the use of AEDs (e.g., valproic acid) in pregnancy. The genetic predisposition is supported by evidence of the risk for recurrence after one affected child (3–4%) and a 10% risk for recurrence with two previously affected children (Kinsman & Johnston, 2016).

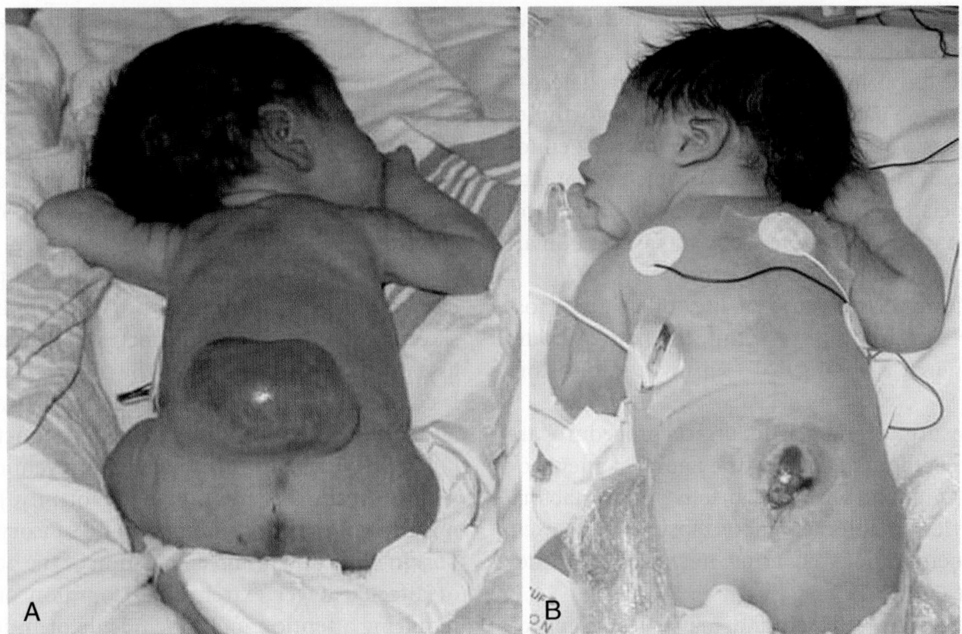

FIGURE 54-6 A: Myelomeningocele with intact sac. **B:** Myelomeningocele with ruptured sac. (Courtesy Dr. Robert C. Dauser, Neurosurgery, Baylor College of Medicine.)

The majority of myelomeningoceles (75%) involve the lumbar or lumbosacral area (Fig. 54-6). Hydrocephalus is a frequently associated anomaly in 80 to 90% of the children. About 80% of patients with myelomeningocele develop a type II Chiari malformation (Kinsman & Johnston, 2016). There is some evidence that prolonged exposure of the myelomeningocele sac to amniotic fluid predisposes an infant to the development of hindbrain herniation and Chiari II malformation (Adzick, 2013).

Diagnostic Evaluation

The diagnosis of SB is made on the basis of clinical manifestations (Box 54-5) and examination of the meningeal sac (see Fig. 54-6, A). Diagnostic measures used to evaluate the brain and spinal cord include MRI, ultrasound, and CT. A neurological evaluation will determine the extent of involvement of bowel and bladder function as well as lower extremity neuromuscular involvement. Flaccid paralysis of the lower extremities is a common finding with absent deep tendon reflexes.

Prenatal detection. It is possible to determine the presence of some major open NTDs prenatally. A second-trimester anatomical ultrasound with detailed fetal intracranial and spinal imaging and assessment is the primary screening tool for open and closed NTDs. Elevated maternal concentrations of alpha-fetoprotein (AFP, or MS-AFP), a fetal-specific γ_1-globulin, in amniotic fluid may indicate anencephaly or myelomeningocele but is only recommended for women with a body mass index >35 or women who do not have geographic or clinical access to good-quality ultrasound screening at 18 to 22 weeks (Wilson, Audibert, Brock, et al., 2014). The optimum time for performing these diagnostic tests is between 16 and 18 weeks of gestation, before AFP concentrations normally diminish and in sufficient time to permit a therapeutic abortion.

BOX 54-5 CLINICAL MANIFESTATIONS OF SPINA BIFIDA

Spina Bifida Cystica

Sensory disturbances usually parallel to motor dysfunction

- Below second lumbar vertebra—Flaccid, partial paralysis of lower extremities, varying degrees of sensory deficit, overflow incontinence with constant dribbling of urine, lack of bowel control, rectal prolapse (sometimes)
- Below third sacral vertebra—No motor impairment, may have saddle anaesthesia with bladder and anal sphincter paralysis

Associated deformities (sometimes produced in utero):

- Talipes valgus or varus contractures
- Kyphosis
- Lumbosacral scoliosis
- Hip dislocation or subluxation

Spina Bifida Occulta

Frequently no observable manifestations

May be associated with one or more cutaneous manifestations:

- Skin depression or dimple
- Port-wine angiomatous nevi
- Dark tufts of hair
- Soft, subcutaneous lipomas

May have neuromuscular disturbances:

- Progressive disturbance of gait with foot weakness
- Bowel and bladder sphincter disturbances

Therapeutic Management

Management of the child who has a myelomeningocele requires a multidisciplinary approach involving the specialties of neurology, neurosurgery, pediatrics, urology, orthopedics, rehabilitation, physiotherapy, and social services, along with intensive nursing care in a variety of specialty areas. The collaborative efforts of these specialists are focused on (1) the myelomeningocele and the problems associated with the defect—hydrocephalus, lower limb paralysis and orthopedic deformities (developmental dysplasia of the hip and club foot), and genitourinary abnormalities; (2) possible acquired problems that may or may not be associated, such as meningitis, hypoxia, and hemorrhage; and (3) other conditions, such as cardiac (Chiari II malformation) or gastrointestinal malformations.

Early closure, within several days of life, offers the most favourable outcome. Surgical closure within the first 24 hours is recommended if the sac is leaking CSF (Kinsman & Johnston, 2016).

A variety of neurosurgical and plastic surgical procedures are used for skin closure without disturbing the neural elements or removing any portion of the sac. The objective is satisfactory skin coverage of the lesion and meticulous closure. Wide excision of the large membranous covering may damage functioning neural tissue.

Associated problems are assessed and managed by appropriate surgical and supportive measures. Shunt procedures provide relief from imminent or progressive hydrocephalus (see Chapter 50). When diagnosed, ventriculitis, meningitis, urinary tract infection, and pneumonia are treated with vigorous antibiotic therapy and supportive measures. Surgical intervention for Chiari II malformation is indicated only when the child is symptomatic (i.e., high-pitched crowing cry, stridor, respiratory difficulties, oral-motor difficulties, upper extremity spasticity).

Early surgical closure of the myelomeningocele sac through fetal surgery has been evaluated in relation to prevention of injury to the exposed spinal cord tissue and improvement of neurological and urological outcomes in the affected child. Research has demonstrated that prenatal surgery has better outcomes (reduced number of shunt placements and less lower limb impairment) than those for children who had postnatal surgery. However, the surgery is not without risks to the fetus and mother, and premature birth is common. Maternal complications included oligohydramnios, chorioamniotic separation, placental abruption, and spontaneous membrane herniation (Adzick, Thom, Spong, et al., 2011; Grivell, Andersen, & Dodd, 2014).

Postnatal care. Initial care of the newborn involves prevention of infection; performing a neurological assessment, including observing for associated anomalies; and dealing with the impact of the anomaly on the family. Although meningoceles are repaired early, especially if there is danger of rupture of the sac, the opinion regarding skin closure of myelomeningocele varies. Most authorities believe that early closure, within the first 24 to 72 hours, offers the most favourable outcome. Early closure, preferably in the first 12 to 18 hours, not only prevents local infection and trauma to the exposed tissues but also avoids stretching of other nerve roots (which may occur as the meningeal sac expands during the first hours after birth), thus preventing further motor impairment. Broad-spectrum antibiotics are initiated, and neurotoxic substances such as povidone-iodine are avoided at the malformation.

Associated problems are assessed and managed by appropriate surgical and supportive measures. Improved surgical techniques do not alter the major physical disability and deformity or the chronic urinary tract and pulmonary infections that affect the quality of life for these children. Superimposed on the physical problems are the effects that the disorder has on family life and finances, including the need for long-term health care services.

Orthopedic management. Most orthopedists recommend early evaluation and treatment (where indicated) of musculoskeletal problems that will affect later locomotion. Neurological assessment will determine the neurosegmental level of the lesion and enable recognition of spasticity and progressive paralysis, potential for deformity, and functional expectations. Orthopedic management includes prevention of joint contractures, correction of the existing deformity, prevention or minimization of the effects of motor and sensory deficits, prevention of skin breakdown, and acquisition of the best possible function of affected lower extremities. Common orthopedic problems requiring attention in SB include deformities of the knees, hips (subluxation), feet (clubfeet), and spine; fractures and insensate skin further complicate orthopedic care. See Chapter 53 for more information on orthopedic management. Other problems that may occur later include kyphosis and scoliosis (Lazzaretti & Pearson, 2010). Because children with this condition often have decreased sensitivity in their lower extremities, preventive skin care is important. The status of the neurological deficit remains the most important factor in determining the child's ultimate functional abilities.

With technological advances, a variety of lightweight orthoses, including braces, special "walking" devices, and custom-built wheelchairs, are available to provide mobility to children with spinal cord lesions (see also Chapter 41). Early in infancy, intervention with passive range-of-motion exercises, positioning, and stretching exercises may help decrease the incidence of muscle contractures. Corrective surgical procedures, when indicated, are best initiated at an early age so that the child will not lag significantly behind age-mates in developmental progress. Where there is little hope for lower extremity functioning, surgery is seldom recommended unless it will improve sitting position in a wheelchair and function for ADLs and mobility.

Management of genitourinary function. Myelomeningocele is one of the most common causes of neuropathic (neurogenic) bladder dysfunction in children. In infants the goal of treatment is to preserve renal function. In older children the goal is to preserve renal function and achieve optimal urinary continence. Urinary incontinence is a chronic, often debilitating problem for the child. In addition, the neuropathic bladder may produce urinary system distress, characterized by symptomatic urinary tract infections, ureterohydronephrosis, and vesicoureteral reflux or renal insufficiency. The characteristics of bladder dysfunction in children vary according to the level of the neurological lesion and the influence of bony growth and development on the spine. Thus ongoing urological monitoring is essential. Evidence is growing that early intervention, based on evaluation during the neonatal period and before complications occur, serves to improve bladder function, reduces the risk of subsequent urinary system distress, and decreases the need for reconstructive surgery of the lower urinary tract (Snodgrass & Gargolla, 2010).

Treatment of renal problems includes (1) regular urological care with prompt and vigorous treatment of urinary tract infections; (2) a method of regular emptying of the bladder, such as clean intermittent catheterization (CIC), taught to and performed by parents, and self-catheterization taught to children; (3) medications to improve bladder storage and continence, such as oxybutynin chloride (Ditropan) and tolterodine (Detrol); and (4) surgical procedures, such as *vesicostomy* (bladder surgically brought out to the abdominal wall, allowing continuous urinary drainage) and *augmentation enterocystoplasty* (using a segment of bowel or stomach to increase bladder capacity, thereby reducing high bladder pressures).

However, despite the combined efforts of CIC, medication, and surgical intervention, some children with myelodysplasia may continue to experience debilitating urinary incontinence. Many of these children are able to attain social continence with a continent urinary diversion commonly referred to as *Mitrofanoff procedure.* In this procedure, a catheterizable channel is surgically created from the appendix, ureter, or tapered bowel. The proximal end of the channel is connected to the bladder with the distal end brought out as a small stoma on the abdominal wall, usually near the umbilicus. The bladder neck may be sutured to prevent urinary leakage from the urethra. CIC through the easily accessible abdominal route fosters greater independence in children, especially in those unable to transfer from a wheelchair to a toilet to perform CIC.

Bowel control. Some degree of fecal continence can be achieved in most children with myelomeningocele with diet modification, regular toilet habits, and prevention of constipation and impaction. It is frequently a lengthy process. Dietary fibre supplements (recommended dosage is age of child in years + 5 = g /day), laxatives, stool softeners, suppositories, or enemas aid in producing regular evacuation. Older children and adolescents seeking more independence may attain bowel continence and higher quality of life after undergoing an antegrade continence enema (ACE) procedure (Masadeh, Krein, Peterson, et al., 2013). In a procedure similar to Mitrofanoff, the appendix or ileum is used to create a catheterizable channel with attachment of the proximal end to the colon. The distal end of the channel exits through a small abdominal stoma. Every 1 or 2 days, a catheter is passed through the stoma, allowing enema solution to be instilled directly into the colon. After administration of the enema solution, the child sits on the toilet for 30 to 60 minutes as stool is flushed out through the rectum. Frequency of enemas and volume of solution used to completely evacuate the bowel vary among individuals.

Prognosis

The early prognosis for the child with myelomeningocele depends on the neurological deficit present at birth, including motor ability, bladder innervation, and associated neurological anomalies. Early surgical repair of the spinal defect, antibiotic therapy to reduce the incidence of meningitis and ventriculitis, prevention of urinary system dysfunction, and early detection and correction of hydrocephalus have significantly increased the survival rate and quality of life in such children. Children with SB have normal intelligence. Many children with SB achieve partial independent living and gainful employment. Reports of survival rates vary; many include adults who were born before medical advances and surgical techniques seen in the past 25 years.

In children and adolescents with SB, the achievement of urinary continence is associated with improved self-concept and esteem, especially among girls. This chronic condition has an array of associated complications, including hydrocephalus and shunt malfunctions, Chiari II development, scoliosis, bowel and bladder management issues, latex allergy, and epilepsy. However, based on current medical knowledge and ethical considerations, aggressive, early management for the child with myelomeningocele improves the prognosis.

Prevention

The Centers for Disease Control and Prevention (CDC) (2009) has affirmed that 50 to 70% of NTDs can be prevented by daily consumption of 0.4 mg of folic acid by women of child-bearing age. In Canada, the rate of children born with an NTD declined between 1997 and 2007, to approximately 4 per 10,000 births, mainly due to folic acid fortification of food (PHAC, 2014a). The greatest reduction was for SB at 54%, anencephaly at 38%, and encephalocele at 31% (De Wals, Tairou, Van Allen, et al., 2008). In 2008, a total of 1286 SB cases were identified: 51% livebirths, 3% stillbirths, and 46% terminations. Prevalence decreased from 0.86/1000 in the prefortification period to 4.0 per 10,000 in the full fortification period, while the proportion of upper defects decreased from 32 to 13%. Nurses and other health care workers have an important task in disseminating information that may decrease the incidence of birth defects in children by promoting maternal consumption of folic acid (see Chapter 12, p. 269). (See Additional Resources at the end of this chapter.)

Adolescent girls and women of child-bearing age need to be educated about the necessity of consuming folic acid in order to prevent NTDs. They can take a daily multivitamin supplement containing 0.4 mg folic acid; eat folic acid–fortified breakfast cereal, bread, rice, or pasta; or eat foods naturally rich in folate (green leafy vegetables and citrus fruits) (see Table 12-1). For women who have had a previous pregnancy affected by NTDs, folic acid intake is increased to 4 mg/day, under supervision of a health care provider, beginning 1 month before a planned pregnancy and continuing during the first trimester. Supplementation of 4 mg of folate should not be given in multivitamin preparations because of the risk of overdose of other vitamins. Medications that affect folic acid metabolism and increase the risk for myelomeningocele should be avoided before pregnancy (if plans are to become pregnant in the near future) and during pregnancy; these include trimethoprim and the AEDs carbamazepine, phenytoin, phenobarbital, valproic acid, and primidone (Kinsman & Johnston, 2016).

NURSING CARE

At birth an examination needs to be performed to assess the intactness of the membranous cyst. If a defect is assessed, every effort should be made to prevent trauma to this protective covering during transport to the nursery. In addition to the routine assessment of the newborn (see Chapter 26), the infant should be assessed for the level of neurological involvement. Movement of extremities or skin response, especially an anal reflex, that might provide clues to the degree of motor or sensory impairment should be noted. It is important to observe the infant's behaviour in conjunction with the stimulus, since limb movements can be induced in response to spinal cord reflex activity that has no connection with the higher centres. Observation of urine output, especially if a diaper remains dry, may indicate urinary retention. Abdominal assessment revealing bladder distension, even with a wet diaper, may indicate urinary overflow in a retentive bladder. The head circumference should be measured daily and the fontanels examined for signs of tension or bulging.

Care of the Myelomeningocele Sac

The infant is usually placed in an isolette or warmer so that temperature can be maintained without clothing or covers that might irritate the spinal defect. Before surgical closure, the myelomeningocele is prevented from drying by the application of a sterile, moist, nonadherent dressing over the defect. The moistening solution is usually sterile normal saline. When an overhead warmer is used, the dressings over the defect require more frequent moistening because of the dehydrating effect of the radiant heat.

Dressings are changed frequently (every 2 to 4 hours), and the sac is closely inspected for leaks, abrasions, irritation, or any signs of infection. The sac must be carefully cleansed if it becomes soiled or contaminated. Sometimes the sac ruptures during delivery or transport, and any opening in the sac greatly increases the risk of infection to the central nervous system (see Fig. 54-6, B).

NURSING ALERT

Avoid measuring rectal temperatures in infants with SB. Because bowel sphincter function is frequently affected, the thermometer can cause irritation and rectal prolapse.

One of the most important and challenging aspects in the early care of the infant with myelomeningocele is positioning. Before surgery the infant is kept in the prone position to minimize tension on the sac and the risk of trauma. The prone position allows for optimal positioning of the legs, especially in cases of associated hip subluxation. The infant is placed prone with the hips slightly flexed and supported to reduce tension on the defect. The legs are maintained in abduction with a pad between the knees to counteract hip subluxation, and a small roll is placed under the ankles to maintain a neutral foot position. A variety of aids, including diaper rolls, pads, small foam pads, or specially designed frames and appliances, can be used to maintain the desired position.

Prevent Complications

The prone position affects other aspects of the infant's care. For example, in this position the infant is more difficult to keep clean, pressure areas are a constant threat, and feeding becomes a problem. The infant's head is turned to one side for feeding. Fortunately, most defects are repaired early, and the infant can be held for feeding soon after surgery. Special care must be taken to avoid pressure on the operative site.

Diapering the infant may be contraindicated until the defect has been repaired and healing is well advanced or epithelialization has taken place. The padding beneath the diaper area should be changed as needed to keep the skin dry and free of irritation. When urinary retention is detected, CIC is employed. Because the bowel sphincter is frequently affected, there is continual passage of stool, often misinterpreted as diarrhea, which is a constant irritant to the skin and a source of infection to the spinal lesion.

Areas of sensory and motor impairment are subject to skin breakdown and require meticulous care. Placing the infant on a special mattress or mattress overlay reduces pressure on the knees and ankles. Periodic cleansing and gentle massage aid circulation.

Gentle range-of-motion exercises should be carried out to prevent contractures, and stretching of contractures is performed when indicated. However, these exercises may be restricted to the foot, ankle, and knee joint. When the hip joints are unstable, stretching against tight hip flexors or adductor muscles, which act much like bowstrings, may aggravate a tendency toward subluxation. Consultation with a physiotherapist is an important aspect of the short- and long-term management of infants with myelomeningocele.

Infants with unrepaired myelomeningocele may be unable to be held in the arms and cuddled as unaffected infants are; their need for tactile stimulation is met by caressing, stroking, and other comfort measures. One method to protect the sac while the parent is holding the infant is to place a pillow on the parent's lap and lay the infant on the side on the pillow.

NURSING ALERT

It is important for nurses to observe for early signs of infection, such as temperature instability (axillary), irritability, and lethargy, and for signs of increased intracranial pressure, which might indicate developing hydrocephalus.

Provide Postoperative Care

Postoperative care of the infant with myelomeningocele involves the same basic care as that of any postsurgical infant: monitoring vital signs, monitoring intake and output, providing nourishment, observing for signs of infection, and managing pain as needed. Care of the operative site is carried out under the direction of the surgeon and includes close observation for signs of leakage of CSF. To prevent stool contamination into the incision, nurses can employ a flap of surgical drape, cut to size, adhered to the lower back below the incision. General care is continued as preoperatively.

The prone position is maintained after surgical closure, although many neurosurgeons allow a side-lying or partial side-lying position unless it aggravates a coexisting hip subluxation or permits undesirable hip flexion. This offers an opportunity for position changes, which reduces the risk of pressure ulcers and facilitates feeding. If permitted, the infant can be held upright against the body, with care taken to avoid pressure on the operative site. After the effects of anaesthesia have subsided and the infant is alert, feedings may be resumed unless there are other anomalies or associated complications.

Support the Family and Educate Them About Home Care

As soon as the parents are able to assist with the infant's care, they should be encouraged to become involved. They need to learn how to continue at home the care that has been initiated in the hospital—positioning, feeding, skin care, and range-of-motion exercises when appropriate. They need to be taught CIC technique when it is prescribed. Parents also need to know the signs of complications (urinary, neurological, orthopedic) and how to obtain assistance when needed.

The mother who wishes to breastfeed the infant should be encouraged to do so. Shortly after birth, the mother is started on a program of pumping to initiate and maintain milk supply until the infant is stable enough to begin breastfeeding. This process may require considerable support from nurses, lactation consultants, physicians, and family members because of separation from the infant for surgical care and recovery.

The long-range planning and support of the parents and newborn begin in the hospital and continue throughout childhood and even into young adulthood. The life expectancy of children with SB extends well into adulthood; thus planning should involve long-term goals and plans for optimum function as an adult. Discussion about aspects of adulthood, such as receiving educational or vocational training, living independently, having a mate, having sexual relationships, and bearing and rearing children, is important and should not be overlooked. The unique service needs of adolescents with SB as they attempt to gain independence from family and establish lives of their own have not been adequately addressed in the literature (Sawyer & Macnee, 2010). Betz, Linroth, Butler, et al. (2010) interviewed young people with SB making the transition to adulthood. Some common themes that emerged among these young people were (1) challenges in preparation for self-management, (2) limited social relationships, (3) awareness of their cognitive challenges, and (4) the cost of independence.

Nurses assume an important role as a central member of the health care team. As a care manager and coordinator, the nurse reviews information with the family, takes responsibility for family teaching, and acts as a liaison between inpatient and outpatient services. The child may need numerous hospitalizations over the years, and each one will be a source of stress to which the younger child is especially vulnerable (see Chapter 40 for a discussion of care of the child with a complex condition).

Habilitation involves solving not only problems of self-help and locomotion but also the problem of urinary or bowel incontinence, which threatens the child's social acceptability. Assistance in preparing the child and the school for the child's special needs helps provide a better initial adjustment to this broader social experience.

A Life Course model has been developed for patients, families, caregivers, teachers, and clinicians to facilitate, through a developmental approach, the care of the child and young person with SB; this program has been made into a Web-based tool that can be used to assist in the transition to adulthood (Dicianno, Fairman, Juengst, et al., 2010). The Spina Bifida and Hydrocephalus Association Canada is a national centre that provides support and various services for families of children with spinal lesions (see Additional Resources at the end of this chapter).

Latex Allergy

Latex allergy or **latex hypersensitivity** was identified as a serious health hazard when a report linked intraoperative anaphylaxis with latex in children with SB. *Latex*, a natural product derived from the rubber tree, is used in combination with other chemicals to give elasticity, strength, and durability to many products. Children with SB are at high risk for developing latex allergy because of repeated exposure to latex products during surgery and procedures. Therefore, such children should not be exposed to latex products from birth onward, to minimize the occurrence of latex hypersensitivity. Allergic reactions range from urticaria, wheezing, watery eyes, and rashes to anaphylactic shock. More severe reactions tend to occur when latex comes in contact with mucous membranes, wet skin, the bloodstream, or an airway. There also can be cross-reactions to a number of foods (e.g., banana, avocado, kiwi, chestnut).

Allergic reactions to latex protein can also occur when the substance is transferred to food by food handlers wearing latex gloves. See Box 54-6 for medical conditions associated with a risk of latex allergy.

BOX 54-6 MEDICAL CONDITIONS ASSOCIATED WITH RISK OF LATEX ALLERGY

- Spina bifida
- Urogenital anomalies
- Imperforate anus
- Esophageal atresia/tracheoesophageal fistula
- VATER association (vertebral defects, imperforate anus, tracheoesophageal fistula, and radial and renal dysplasia)
- Preterm infants
- Ventriculoperitoneal shunt
- Neurocognitive impairment
- Cerebral palsy
- Tetraplegia
- Multiple surgeries
- Atopy

GUIDELINES

Identifying Latex Allergy

- Does your child have any symptoms, such as sneezing, coughing, rashes, or wheezing, when handling rubber products (e.g., balloons, tennis or Koosh balls, adhesive bandage strips) or when in contact with rubber hospital products (e.g., gloves, catheters)?
- Has your child ever had an allergic reaction during surgery?
- Does your child have a history of rashes, asthma, or allergic reactions to medication or foods, especially milk, kiwi, bananas, or chestnuts?
- How would you identify or recognize an allergic reaction in your child?
- What would you do if an allergic reaction occurred?
- Has anyone ever discussed latex or rubber allergy or sensitivity with you?
- Has your child had any allergy testing?
- When did your child last come in contact with any type of rubber product? Were you present?

The most important goals regarding latex allergy are its prevention and the identification of children with a known hypersensitivity (see Guidelines box). High-risk and latex-allergic individuals must be managed in a *latex-free* environment. Care must be taken so that they do not come in direct or secondary contact with products or equipment containing latex *at any time* during medical treatment. Allergy testing has been used to identify latex allergy with varying success. Skin prick testing and provocation testing carry the risk of allergic reaction or anaphylaxis. Several commercially available assays can be useful in confirming latex sensitivity. To date, none of these tests demonstrates complete diagnostic reliability, and they should not be the sole determinant of the presence or absence of an allergic response to latex.

Nonlatex products lists are available to parents and health care workers; these products may be substituted for those containing latex. In the health care arena, it is important to use products with the lowest potential risk for sensitizing patients and staff members. Many health care facilities are establishing latex-safe environments.

NURSING ALERT

Ask all patients, not only those at risk, about allergic reactions to latex during the health interview with the parent or child. Be certain that this is a routine part of all preoperative and preprocedural histories. Stress the importance of the allergy history to all personnel (e.g., phlebotomists).

The identification of those sensitive to latex is best accomplished through careful screening of *all* patients (see Guidelines box for questions related to latex allergy). Children with latex allergy should carry or wear some form of medical alert bracelet; those who have had serious reactions should also carry an injectable epinephrine pen and a pair of latex-free gloves for emergencies. In addition to educating caregivers about the child's exposure to medical products that contain latex, nurses need to inform them of common nonmedical latex objects, such as water toys, pacifiers, and plastic storage bags. Parents should also be given literature explaining signs and symptoms of latex hypersensitivity and appropriate emergency treatment (see Anaphylaxis, Chapter 47).

Spinal Muscular Atrophy

Spinal muscular atrophy (SMA) type 1 (Werdnig-Hoffmann disease) is a disorder characterized by progressive weakness and wasting of skeletal muscles caused by degeneration of anterior horn cells. It is inherited as an autosomal recessive trait and is the most common paralytic form of the *floppy infant syndrome* (congenital hypotonia). The sites of the pathological condition are the anterior horn cells of the spinal cord and the motor nuclei of the brainstem, but the primary effect is atrophy of skeletal muscles. The age of onset is variable, but the earlier the onset, the more disseminated and severe the motor weakness. The disorder may be manifested early—often at birth—and almost always before 2 years of age; death may occur as a result of respiratory failure by age 2 years (Lunn & Wang, 2008; Sarnat, 2016a). The manifestations (Box 54-7) and prognosis are categorized according to the age of onset, severity of weakness, and clinical course; some children may fluctuate between exhibiting symptoms of types 1 and 2 or types 2 and 3 in regard to clinical function (Sarnat, 2016a). Some experts also categorize SMA according to the highest level of motor function; type 1 includes "nonsitters," type 2 includes "sitters," and type 3, "walkers" (Kolb & Kissel, 2014). A severe rare fetal form of SMA, classified as type 0, is reported to be quite lethal in the perinatal period; motor neuron degeneration may be noted as early as midgestation in type 0 (Sarnat, 2016a). Type 4 may present between 20 and 30 years of age and may be referred to as proximal adult-type SMA (Prior, 2010).

Spinal muscular atrophy type 3 (Kugelberg-Welander disease) is a result of anterior horn cell and motor nerve degeneration. The disease is characterized by a pattern of muscular weakness similar to that of infantile SMA (see Box 54-7). Several modes of inheritance have been reported for the disease: autosomal recessive, autosomal dominant, and X-linked recessive.

The onset occurs from younger than 1 year of age into adulthood, with symptoms resembling type 2 SMA. Proximal muscle weakness (especially of the lower limbs) and muscular atrophy are the predominant features. The disease runs a slowly progressive course. Some children lose the ability to walk 8 to 9 years after the onset of symptoms, but many can still walk after age 30 years or older. One source notes that approximately half of all children with SMA type 3 lose ambulation by age 14 years and may require a wheelchair for times when falls are more frequent (Mercuri et al., 2012). Many affected persons have a normal life expectancy (Lunn & Wang, 2008).

Diagnostic Evaluation and Therapeutic Management

The diagnosis is based on the molecular genetic marker for the *SMN* (survival motor neuron) gene, which is located on chromosome 5q13. Prenatal diagnosis may be made by genetic analysis of circulating fetal cells in maternal blood or circulating fetal cells in amniotic fluid. The risk of subsequent affected offspring in carriers of the mutant gene or in families with

BOX 54-7 CLINICAL MANIFESTATIONS OF SPINAL MUSCULAR ATROPHY*

Type 1 (Werdnig-Hoffmann Disease)
Disease acquired in utero or during first 2 months of life
Hypotonia and inactivity most prominent features
Infant lying in the frog position with legs externally rotated, abducted, and flexed at knees
Weakness
Absent deep tendon reflexes
Limited movements of shoulder and arm muscles
Active movement usually limited to fingers and toes
Diaphragmatic breathing with intercostal retractions (diaphragmatic paralysis may occur)
Abnormal tongue movements
Weak cry and cough (may be absent)
Secretions tending to pool in oropharynx
Alert facies
Normal sensation and intellect
Tiring quickly during feedings (if breastfed, may lose weight before noticeable)
Affected infants failing to progress to sitting alone, rolling over, or walking
Early death (usually by 2 years of age) from respiratory failure or infection

Type 2 (Intermediate Spinal Muscular Atrophy)
Symptoms manifest between 2 and 12 months of age:
- **Early**—Weakness confined to arms and legs
- **Later**—Becomes generalized

Legs usually involved to greater extent than arms
Prominent pectus excavatum
Movements absent during complete relaxation or sleep
Some infants able to sit if placed in position, but few can ambulate
Lifespan varies from 7 months to 7 years, although may have normal life expectancy

Type 3 (Kugelberg-Welander Disease)
Onset of symptoms in late childhood or adolescence (may be initially misdiagnosed as muscular dystrophy [limb-girdle])
Normal head control and ability to sit unassisted by 6 to 8 months of age
Thigh and hip muscles weak
In those who manage to walk:
- Waddling gait
- Genu recurvatum
- Protuberant abdomen

Ambulation becomes increasingly difficult
- Age of onset influences ambulatory difficulty—the later (after 2 years) the onset, the better the prognosis
- Confined to a wheelchair by second decade (may vary)

Deep tendon reflexes may be present early but disappear
Scoliosis common

*Note: These classifications are general, and experts suggest there may be variations in lifespan and other characteristics.

known cases of SMA may also be evaluated genetically. Further diagnostic studies include muscle electromyography (EMG), which demonstrates a denervation pattern, and muscle biopsy; however, genetic analysis has become the gold standard for diagnosis of the condition.

There is no cure for the disease, and treatment is symptomatic and preventive, primarily preventing joint contractures and treating orthopedic issues, the most serious of which is scoliosis. Hip subluxation and dislocation may also occur. Many children benefit from powered chairs, lifts, special pressure-adjustable mattresses, and accessible environmental controls. Muscle and joint contractures require careful attention and care to prevent further complications. Nutritional growth failure (failure to thrive) may occur in infants and toddlers as a result of poor feeding; supplemental gastrostomy feedings may be required to maintain adequate nutritional status and maintain weight gain. The use of lower extremity orthoses may assist with ambulation, but eventually the child may be confined to a wheelchair as muscle atrophy progresses. Restrictive lung disease is the most serious complication of SMA (Kolb & Kissel, 2014). Upper respiratory tract infections often occur and are treated with antibiotic therapy; they are the cause of death in many children. Rapid eye movement (REM)–related sleep-disordered breathing is common in children with SMA type 1; this progresses to sleep-disordered breathing during REM and non-REM sleep followed by respiratory failure, which often requires nocturnal noninvasive mechanical ventilation (Schroth, 2009). Noninvasive ventilation methods such as bilevel positive airway pressure (BiPAP) have decreased the morbidity and increased the survival rate of children with SMA types 1 and 2. Children with SMA type 1 who undergo tracheotomy and invasive ventilation often remain ventilator dependent for the rest of their lives; some families choose to withdraw support when invasive ventilation becomes necessary (Mercuri, Bertini, & Iannaccone, 2012). *Palliative care* is an important aspect of care for families of children with SMA type 1. A decreased ability to cough and clear secretions may be managed with airway clearance therapies such as the cough-assist machine and manual cough assistance. Guidelines for the standardization of respiratory care for patients with SMA have been published elsewhere (Schroth, 2009).

Prognosis

Prognosis varies according to the age of onset or type as described in Box 54-7. Individuals with SMA type 1 may succumb to respiratory tract infections or failure between 1 and 24 months of age (Sarnat, 2016a); however, some may live longer with enteral feeding and noninvasive mechanical ventilation techniques. A significant number of infants with SMA require a tracheotomy, and associated medical conditions in survivors include gastroesophageal reflux, scoliosis, early-onset puberty, hip dysplasia, and recurrent oral candidiasis (Bach, 2007). Drug therapy with riluzole, valproic acid, gabapentin, and oral phenylbutyrate has been shown to slow the progression of the condition, but none has demonstrated significant overall benefits (Sarnat, 2016a; Wadman, Bosboom, van der Pol, et al., 2012).

NURSING CARE

The infant or small child with progressive muscle weakness requires nursing care similar to that of the immobilized patient (see Chapter 53). However, the underlying goal of treatment should be to assist the child and family in dealing with the illness while progressing toward a life of normalization within the child's capabilities. Special attention should be directed to preventing muscle and joint contractures, promoting independence in performance of ADLs, and incorporating the child into the mainstream of school when possible. Because children with neuromuscular disease have abnormal breathing patterns that often contribute to early death, it is important to assess adequate oxygenation, especially during the sleep phase when shallow breathing occurs and hypoxemia may develop. Home pulse oximetry may be used to assess the child during sleep, which alerts the parents to provide noninvasive ventilation as necessary (Young, Lowe, Fitzgerald, et al., 2007) (see Duchenne [Pseudohypertrophic] Muscular Dystrophy, p. 1772, for respiratory management). Supportive care also includes management of orthoses and other orthopedic equipment as required. Because children with SMA are intellectually normal, verbal, tactile, and auditory stimulation are important aspects of developmental care. Supporting children so they can see the activities around them and transporting them in appropriate equipment (e.g., wheelchair, wagon) for a change of environment are ways to provide stimulation and enhance their development.

Children who are able to sit require proper support and attention to alignment to prevent deformities and the complications. Children who survive beyond infancy need attention to educational needs and opportunities for social interaction with other children. The parents of a child who is chronically ill require much support and encouragement (see Chapter 42). Parents who have not sought genetic counselling should be encouraged to do so in order to evaluate further risk potential.

Therapeutic Management and Nursing Care

The management is primarily symptomatic and supportive and is related to maintaining mobility as long as possible, preventing complications such as skin breakdown, optimizing and maintaining respiratory function, and providing support to the child and family. The discussion of family support in the section for Duchenne muscular dystrophy is also applicable to families of children with SMA.

Muscular Dystrophies

Muscular dystrophies (MDs) constitute the largest and most important single group of muscle diseases of childhood. The MDs have a genetic origin in which there is gradual degeneration of muscle fibres, and they are characterized by progressive weakness and wasting of symmetrical groups of skeletal muscles, with increasing disability and deformity. In all forms of MD there is insidious loss of strength, but each type differs in regard to muscle groups affected (Fig. 54-7), age of onset, rate of progression, and inheritance pattern. The most common form, *Duchenne muscular dystrophy (DMD)*, is considered separately in the next section.

Facioscapulohumeral (Landouzy-Dejerine) MD is inherited as an autosomal dominant disorder with onset in early adolescence. It is characterized by difficulty in raising the arms over the head, lack of facial mobility, and a forward slope of the shoulders. The progression is slow, and the lifespan is usually unaffected.

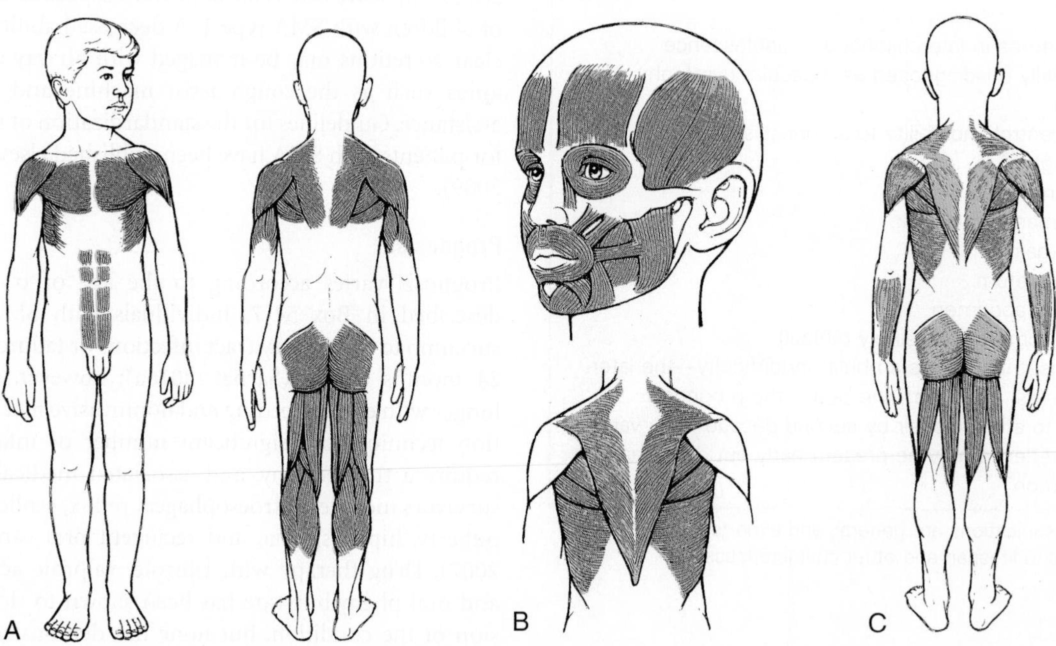

FIGURE 54-7 Initial muscle groups involved in muscular dystrophies. **A:** Pseudohypertrophic. **B:** Facioscapulohumeral. **C:** Limb-girdle.

Limb-girdle muscular dystrophy (LGMD) is a heterogeneous group of disorders with autosomal dominant and recessive inheritance whose clinical manifestations often appear in later childhood, adolescence, or early adulthood with variable but usually slow progression (Quan, 2011). All types of LGMD are characterized by weakness of proximal muscles of the pelvic and shoulder girdles.

Other forms of MD include myotonic dystrophy, scapulohumeral MD (Emery-Dreifuss MD), fascioscapulohumeral MD (Landouzy-Dejerine disease), and congenital MD.

Treatment of the MDs consists mainly of supportive measures, including physiotherapy, orthopedic procedures to minimize deformity, ventilation support, and assistance for the affected child in meeting the demands of daily living.

Duchenne (Pseudohypertrophic) and Becker Muscular Dystrophy

DMD is the most severe and the most common MD of childhood. It is inherited as an X-linked recessive trait, and the single-gene defect is located on the short arm of the X chromosome. DMD has a reportedly high mutation rate, with a positive family history in 65% of all cases; therefore, genetic counselling is an important aspect of the care of the family. In about 30% of cases, it is a new mutation and the mother is not the carrier (Sarnat, 2016b).

As in all X-linked disorders, males are affected almost exclusively. The female carrier may have an elevated creatinine kinase, but muscle weakness is usually not a problem; however, about 10% of female carriers develop cardiomyopathy (Manzur, Kinali, & Muntoni, 2008). In rare instances, a female may be identified with DMD, yet with muscular weakness that is milder than in boys (Sarnat, 2016b). At the genetic level, both DMD and Becker MD (a milder variant) result from mutations of the gene that encodes dystrophin, a protein product in skeletal muscle. Dystrophin is absent from the muscle of children with DMD and is reduced or abnormal in children with Becker MD. Children with Becker MD have a later onset of symptoms, which are usually not as severe as those seen in DMD. The incidence is approximately 1 in 3600 male births for the Duchenne form and approximately 1 in 30,000 live births for the Becker type (Sarnat, 2016b). Box 54-8 describes the characteristics of DMD.

BOX 54-8 CHARACTERISTICS OF DUCHENNE MUSCULAR DYSTROPHY

- Early onset, usually between 3 and 5 years of age
- Progressive muscular weakness, wasting, and contractures
- Calf muscle hypertrophy in most patients
- Loss of independent ambulation by 9 to 11 years of age
- Slowly progressive, generalized weakness during teenage years
- Relentless progression until death from respiratory or cardiac failure

Most children with DMD reach the appropriate developmental milestones early in life, although they may have mild, subtle delays. Evidence of muscle weakness usually appears during the third to seventh year, although there may have been a history of delay in motor development, particularly walking. Difficulties in running, riding a bicycle, and climbing stairs are usually the first symptoms noted. Typically, affected boys have a waddling gait and lordosis, fall frequently, and develop a characteristic manner of rising from a squatting or sitting position on the floor (Gower sign). Lordosis occurs as a result of weakened pelvic muscles, and the waddling gait is a result of weakness in the gluteus medius and maximus muscles (Battista, 2010). In the early years, rapid developmental gains may mask the progression of the disease.

Muscles, especially in the calves, thighs, and upper arms, become enlarged from fatty infiltration and feel unusually firm or woody on palpation (Box 54-9). The term *pseudohypertrophy* is derived from this muscular enlargement. Profound muscular atrophy occurs in the later stages; contractures and deformities involving large and small joints are common complications as the disease progresses. Ambulation usually becomes impossible by 12 years of age. The loss of mobilization further increases the spectrum of complications, which may include osteoporosis, fractures, constipation, skin breakdown, and psychosocial and behavioural problems. Atrophy of facial, oropharyngeal, and respiratory muscles does not occur until the advanced stage of the disease. Ultimately, the disease process involves the diaphragm and auxiliary muscles of respiration, and cardiomyopathy is seen in approximately 50 to 80% of patients with DMD (Sarnat, 2016b).

Obesity is a common complication that contributes to premature loss of ambulation. Children who have restricted opportunities for physical activity could potentially consume calories in excess of their needs. This may be compounded by

BOX 54-9 CLINICAL MANIFESTATIONS OF DUCHENNE MUSCULAR DYSTROPHY

Waddling gait
Lordosis
Frequent falls
Gower sign (child turning onto side or abdomen, flexing knees to assume a kneeling position, then with knees extended gradually pushing torso to an upright position by "walking" the hands up the legs)
Enlarged muscles (especially thighs and upper arms); feel unusually firm or woody on palpation
Later stages: profound muscular atrophy
Cognitive impairment
- Mild (about 20 IQ points below normal)
- IQ <70 present in 25 to 30% of patients

Complications:
- Contracture deformities of hips, knees, and ankles
- Disuse atrophy
- Obesity

overfeeding by well-meaning family and friends. Proper dietary intake and a diversified recreational program help reduce the likelihood of obesity and enable children to maintain ambulation and functional independence for a longer time.

Mild to moderate cognitive impairment is commonly associated with MD. A deficiency of dystrophin isoforms in brain tissue causes cognitive and intellectual impairment (Manzur et al., 2008). The majority of affected children have learning disabilities that still allow them to function in a regular classroom, particularly with remedial help, although more severe cognitive deficit is present in 20 to 30% of these children with an IQ of less than 70 (Sarnat, 2016b). Verbal IQ is markedly low in boys with DMD, and emotional disturbance is more common than in other children with disabilities. Patients with Becker MD present later in life than those with DMD, but they often do not survive past the middle of the second decade, with few patients living into their 40s (Sarnat, 2016b).

Diagnostic Evaluation

The diagnosis of DMD is primarily established by blood polymerase chain reaction (PCR) for the dystrophin gene mutation (Sarnat, 2016b). Prenatal diagnosis is also possible as early as 12 weeks of gestation. Serum enzyme measurement, muscle biopsy, and EMG may also be used in establishing the diagnosis. Serum creatine kinase levels are extremely high in the first 2 years of life, before the onset of clinical weakness. If the child demonstrates the usual characteristics, has a positive family history for DMD, and the PCR is positive, the muscle biopsy may be deferred.

Therapeutic Management

No effective treatment exists for childhood MD. The use of the corticosteroids prednisone and deflazacort has been evaluated as a treatment for DMD. Several clinical trials demonstrated increased muscle strength and improved performance and pulmonary function, with significant decrease in the progression of weakness, when prednisone was administered for 6 months to 2 years (Manzur, Kuntzur, Pike, et al., 2008). The American Academy of Neurology has published a practice parameter for the administration of corticosteroids in the treatment of DMD which is supported by the Canadian Paediatric Society (Manzur et al., 2008). Major adverse effects include weight gain and a cushingoid facial appearance.

Maintaining optimum function in all muscles for as long as possible is the primary goal; secondary is the prevention of contractures. Children with DMD who remain as active as possible are able to avoid wheelchair confinement for a longer time. Maintenance of function often involves stretching exercises, strength and muscle training, breathing exercises to increase and maintain vital lung capacity, range-of-motion exercises, surgery to release contracture deformities, bracing, and performance of ADLs.

Parents should be supported in making decisions about the child's care; teaching regarding home safety and prevention of falls is important as well. Parents should also be encouraged to have the child keep follow-up appointments for medical care and physical and occupational therapy. Because respiratory tract infections are most troublesome in these children, influenza and pneumococcal vaccines are encouraged and contact with persons with respiratory tract infections should be avoided. Action plans for prompt treatment of respiratory illness are important.

Eventually, respiratory and cardiac problems become the central focus of the debilitating illness. Children with neuromuscular disease have abnormal breathing patterns, particularly during REM sleep, and hypoxia may occur as a result of inadequate oxygenation. The child and parents should be involved in a discussion of long-term ventilation options. Cardiac and respiratory assessment during wake–sleep cycles is imperative. Respiratory care for children with neuromuscular conditions such as SMA and DMD may involve the use of noninvasive ventilation with BiPAP on a temporary or full-time basis, mechanically assisted coughing (MAC), or tracheotomy and relief of airway obstruction with coughing and suctioning devices; the tracheotomy, however, is associated with more complications. Home pulse oximetry may be used to monitor oxygenation during sleep or to aid in decision making regarding the use of MAC to clear the airways.

Several devices are available for children with neuromuscular disease to assist in clearing the airway when the cough reflex is ineffective or diminished. The mechanical cough in-exsufflator (MIE) has been evaluated and found to be safe and effective in the daily management of respiratory function (Kravitz, 2009). The MIE delivers positive inspiratory pressures at a set rate, followed by negative pressure exsufflation coordinated with the patient's own breathing rhythm; the exsufflation is designed to mimic a cough reflex so mucus can be effectively cleared. Airway suctioning after exsufflation is accomplished as necessary to clear the airways. In children the MIE may be connected directly to a tracheostomy or used with a mouthpiece or face mask.

Manual cough-assisting techniques breathing include glossopharyngeal breathing or air stacking (frog breathing); the abdominal thrust, which is similar to the Heimlich manoeuvre (Kravitz, 2009); and manual hyperinflation with a self-inflating resuscitation bag (without oxygen) and a mouthpiece. Hyperinflation may be used in conjunction with abdominal thrusts to improve peak cough flows (Boitano, 2009).

The use of routine chest physiotherapy (postural drainage) for DMD has not been adequately evaluated for its effectiveness in clearing the airway of mucus except when there is focal atelectasis and mucus plugging the airways (Kravitz, 2009).

Survival in individuals with DMD may be prolonged several years with the use of noninvasive ventilation and MAC as alternatives to tracheotomy and airway suctioning. The Canadian Thoracic Society has published extensive guidelines for respiratory monitoring and care of children and adults with DMD (McKim, Road, Avendano, et al., 2011).

Muscular Dystrophy Canada (2012) recommends an extensive cardiac evaluation of the child diagnosed with either DMD or Becker MD. Patients with neuromuscular conditions may not have the typical signs and symptoms of cardiac dysfunction. Thus symptoms such as weight loss, nausea and vomiting, cough, increased fatigue on performance of ADLs, and orthopnea should be carefully evaluated to detect early signs of cardiomyopathy.

Long-term care, end-of-life directives, and palliative care options are issues that must be discussed with the child and family affected by MD. Professional counselling may be required to allow frank discussion of these issues in some cases, and referrals should be made as appropriate (Bushby, Finkel, Birnkrant, et al., 2010).

NURSING CARE

The care and management of a child with MD involve the combined efforts of a multidisciplinary health care team. Nurses can help clarify the roles of these health care providers to family and others. The major emphasis of nursing care is to help the child and family cope with a chronic, progressive, incapacitating disease; to help design a program that will afford maximal independence and reduce the predictable and preventable disabilities associated with the disorder; and to help the child and family deal constructively with the limitations the disease imposes on their daily lives. Because of advances in technology, children with MD may live into early adulthood; thus the goals of care should also involve decisions regarding quality of life, achievement of independence, and transition to adulthood.

Working closely with other team members, nurses assist the family in developing the child's self-help skills to give the child the satisfaction of being as independent as possible for as long as possible. This requires continual evaluation of the child's capabilities, which are often difficult to assess. Fortunately, most children with MD instinctively recognize the need to become as independent as possible and strive to do so.

Practical difficulties faced by families are physical limitations of housing and mobility. Some families live in houses or apartments that are unsuited to wheelchairs. Transportation may also be a barrier for families of children with MD. Assisting with these challenges requires team problem solving. Diet, nutritional needs, and nutrition modification should be discussed according to the needs of the individual child and family.

Children with MD tend to become socially isolated as their physical condition deteriorates to the point that they can no longer keep up with their friends and classmates. Their physical capabilities diminish, and their dependency increases at the age at which most children are expanding their range of interests and relationships.

The parents' social activities are also restricted, and the family's activities must be continually modified to accommodate the needs of the affected child. When the child becomes increasingly incapacitated, the family may consider home-based care, an assisted living facility, or respite care. Unless the child is severely incapacitated, he or she should also be involved in the decisions regarding such care. Nurses can assist with decision making by exploring all available options and resources and supporting the child and family in their decisions. Older boys with MD may also need psychiatric or psychological counselling to deal with issues such as depression, anger, and quality of life. Parents also need to be encouraged to become involved in support groups because adequate social support from family, community, and other parents is crucial to appropriate coping in families with children with chronic illness.

Regardless of how successful the program is or how well the family adapts to the disorder, superimposed on the physical and emotional problems associated with a child with a long-term disability is the constant knowledge of the ultimate outcome of the disease. All the manifestations seen in a child with a chronic fatal illness are usually encountered in these families (see Chapter 40).

Nurses are especially valuable health care providers as they come to know the family and the family's problems. Nurses can be alert to the family's problems and needs and make necessary referrals when supplementary services are indicated. Muscular Dystrophy Canada has branches in most communities to assist families in which there is a member with MD (see Additional Resources at the end of this chapter).

ACQUIRED NEUROMUSCULAR DISORDERS

Guillain-Barré Syndrome (Infectious Polyneuritis)

Guillain-Barré syndrome (GBS), also known as *infectious polyneuritis,* is an uncommon acute demyelinating polyneuropathy with a progressive, usually ascending flaccid paralysis. The hallmark of GBS is acute peripheral motor weakness. Children are affected less often than adults; among children, those between ages 4 and 10 years have higher susceptibility. Two peak time periods have been identified with an increased incidence of GBS: late adolescence and young adulthood.

Congenital GBS is rare yet may be seen in the neonatal period and consists of hypotonia, weakness, and decreased or absent reflexes; maternal neuromuscular disease may or may not be present. Diagnosis is established by the same criteria as in older children, but the symptoms gradually subside over the first few months of life and disappear by 12 months (Sarnat, 2016c).

Chronic inflammatory demyelinating plyradiculoneuropathies (CIDPs) are chronic types of GBS that recur intermittently or do not improve over a period of months to years (Sarnat, 2016c). The following discussion focuses on GBS.

Pathophysiology

GBS is an immune-mediated disease often associated with a number of viral or bacterial infections or the administration of certain vaccines. It has been associated with infectious mononucleosis, measles, mumps, *Campylobacter jejuni* (gastroenteritis), cytomegalovirus, *Borrelia burgdorferi* (Lyme disease), Epstein-Barr virus, *Helicobacter pylori,* and *Mycoplasma* and *Pneumocystis* infections. Onset of GBS symptoms usually occurs within 10 days of the primary infection. Pathological changes in spinal and cranial nerves consist of inflammation and edema with rapid, segmented demyelination and compression of nerve roots within the dural sheath. Nerve conduction is impaired, producing ascending partial or complete paralysis of muscles innervated by the involved nerves. GBS has three phases:

1. *Acute*—Phase starts when symptoms begin and continues until new symptoms stop appearing or deterioration ceases; it may last as long as 4 weeks.

BOX 54-10 CLINICAL MANIFESTATIONS OF GUILLAIN-BARRÉ SYNDROME

Initial Symptoms
Muscle tenderness
Paresthesia and cramps (sometimes)
Proximal symmetrical muscle weakness

Paralysis
Ascending bilateral paralysis from lower extremities
Frequent involvement of muscles of trunk and upper extremities and those supplied by cranial nerves (especially facial)
Flaccid paralysis with loss of reflexes
May involve facial, extraocular, labial, lingual, pharyngeal, and laryngeal muscles
Intercostal and phrenic nerves:
- Breathlessness in vocalizations
- Shallow, irregular respirations

Other Manifestations
Tendon reflexes depressed or absent
Variable degrees of sensory impairment
Muscle tenderness or sensitivity to slight pressure
Urinary incontinence or retention and constipation

2. *Plateau*—Symptoms remain constant without further deterioration; it may last from days to weeks.
3. *Recovery*—Patient begins to improve and progress to optimum recovery; it usually lasts a few weeks to months depending on the deficits incurred by the illness.

Diagnostic Evaluation

The diagnosis of GBS is based on clinical manifestations (Box 54-10), CSF analysis, and EMG findings. CSF analysis reveals an abnormally elevated protein concentration, normal glucose, and fewer than 10 white blood cells (WBCs)/mm^3 (Sarnat, 2016c). EMG shows evidence of acute muscle denervation; other laboratory studies are usually noncontributory. The symmetrical nature of the paralysis helps differentiate this disorder from spinal paralytic poliomyelitis, which usually affects sporadic muscles.

Therapeutic Management

Treatment of GBS is primarily supportive. In the acute phase, patients are hospitalized because respiratory and pharyngeal involvement may require assisted ventilation, sometimes with a temporary tracheotomy. Treatment modalities include aggressive ventilatory support, intravenous administration of immunoglobulin (IVIG), and steroids; plasmapheresis and immunosuppressive medications may also be used. Plasmapheresis has been shown to decrease the length of recovery in patients with severe GBS; adverse effects include hypotension, fever, bleeding disorders, chills, urticaria, and bradycardia. There is evidence, however, of significant improvement in children with high-dose IVIG therapy (versus supportive treatment alone) (Hughes, Swan, & van Doorn, 2014). IVIG is now recommended as the primary treatment of GBS when administered within 2 weeks of disease onset (Hughes, 2008). Corticosteroids alone do not decrease the symptoms or shorten the duration of the disease.

Medications that may be administered during the acute phase include a low-molecular-weight heparin to prevent deep vein thrombosis, a mild laxative or stool softener to prevent constipation, pain medication such as acetaminophen, and a histamine-antagonist to prevent stress ulcer formation. Chronic neuropathic pain following GBS may be treated with gabapentin, which is reported to be more effective than carbamazepine (Sarnat, 2016c).

Rehabilitation after the acute phase may involve physiotherapy, occupational therapy, and speech therapy. Additional consideration should be given to issues of general weakness and retraining for toileting and feeding (Lyons, 2008).

Course and Prognosis

Better outcomes are associated with younger age, no requirement for mechanical respiratory assistance, slower progression of disease, normal peripheral nerve function on EMG, and treatment with either IVIG or plasmapheresis. Recovery usually begins within 2 to 3 weeks, and most patients regain full muscle strength. The recovery of muscle strength progresses in the reverse order of onset of paralysis, with lower extremity strength being the last to recover. Poor prognosis with subsequent residual effects in children is reportedly associated with cranial nerve involvement, extensive disability at time of presentation, and intubation.

Most deaths associated with GBS are caused by respiratory failure, thus early diagnosis and access to respiratory support are especially important. The rate of recovery is usually related to the degree of involvement and may extend from a few weeks to months. The greater the degree of paralysis, the longer the recovery phase.

NURSING CARE

Nursing care is primarily supportive and is the same as that required for the child with immobilization and respiratory compromise. The emphasis of care is on close observation to assess the extent of paralysis and on prevention of complications, including aspiration, ventilator-associated pneumonia (VAP), atelectasis, DVT, pressure ulcer, fear and anxiety, autonomic dysfunction, and pain.

The child's respiratory function should be closely monitored, and oxygen source, appropriate-sized resuscitation bag and mask, endotracheal intubation and suctioning equipment, tracheotomy tray, and vasoconstrictor medications need to be kept available. Vital signs, including neurological signs and level of consciousness, should be monitored frequently.

Respiratory care, should intubation be required, requires close monitoring of oxygenation status, usually by pulse oximetry and arterial blood gases; maintenance of an open airway with suctioning; and postural changes to prevent pneumonia. Consideration should be given to preventing opportunistic infections such as VAP; meticulous oral care and hypopharynx suctioning, elevation of the head of bed 30 degrees, and strict asepsis with suctioning equipment (including catheters, a Yankauer device, or both) should be implemented to prevent VAP. Children with oral and pharyngeal involvement may be fed via a nasogastric tube to ensure adequate feeding. It is also important to consider the possibility of stress ulcers in such patients and to administer a proton pump inhibitor. Immobilization, which occurs with GBS, decreases gastrointestinal function; thus problems such as decreased gastric emptying and constipation require nursing assessment and appropriate collaborative interventions. Temporary urinary catheterization may be required; urinary retention is common, and appropriate assessment of urinary output is vital. Sensory impairment and paralysis in the lower extremities make the child susceptible to skin breakdown; therefore attention should be given to meticulous skin care. Prevention of deep vein thrombosis is accomplished with pneumatic compression (antiembolism) devices, administration of a low-molecular-weight heparin, and early mobilization and ambulation. Autonomic dysfunction may be life threatening; thus close monitoring of vital signs in the acute phase is essential.

A key to recovery in the child with GBS is the prevention of muscle and joint contractures, so passive range-of-motion exercises must be carried out routinely to maintain vital function. As the disease stabilizes and recovery begins, an active physiotherapy program is implemented to prevent contracture deformities and facilitate muscle recovery. This program may include active exercise, gait training, and bracing.

Although the child may have a generalized paralysis, cognitive function remains intact; thus it is important for nursing care to involve communication with the child regarding procedures and treatments that may be frightening, especially if mechanical ventilation is required. Parents should be encouraged to talk to the child and make eye and physical contact as much as possible to reassure the child during the illness.

Pain management is essential in the care of children with GBS. Although neuromuscular impairment may make pain perception more difficult to accurately evaluate, objective pain scales should be used. Carbamazepine and gabapentin may be used to manage neuropathic pain in patients with GBS.

Throughout the course of the illness, support of the child and parents is paramount. The usual rapidity of the paralysis and the long period of recovery greatly tax the emotional reserves of all family members. The parents and child benefit from repeated reassurance that recovery is occurring and from realistic information regarding the possibility of permanent disability. In the event of a residual disability, the family needs assistance in accepting and adjusting to the child's loss of function (see Chapter 40). The GBS/CIDP Foundation of Canada is a nonprofit organization devoted to support, education, and research. It provides support to families from recovered persons, publishes informational literature and a newsletter, and maintains a list of practitioners experienced with the disease (see Additional Resources at the end of this chapter).

Tetanus

Tetanus, or *lockjaw*, is an acute, preventable, but often fatal disease caused by an exotoxin produced by the anaerobic spore-forming, Gram-positive bacillus *Clostridium tetani*. It is characterized by painful muscular rigidity primarily involving the masseter and neck muscles. There are four requirements for the development of tetanus: (1) presence of tetanus spores or vegetative forms of the bacillus, (2) injury to the tissues, (3) wound conditions that encourage multiplication of the organism, and (4) a susceptible host.

Tetanus spores are found in soil, dust, and the intestinal tracts of humans and animals, especially herbivorous animals. The organisms are more prevalent in rural areas but are readily carried to urban areas by the wind. The organisms are not invasive but enter the body by way of wounds, particularly a puncture wound, burn, or an unnoticed break in the skin (such as a thorn or needle prick, bee sting, or scratch). In the newborn, infection may occur through the umbilical cord, usually in situations in which birth occurs in severely contaminated surroundings or the mother is not adequately immunized.

Tetanus is a rare disease in Canada because of tetanus immunizations. However, serosurveys suggest that a significant number of Canadians have nonprotective levels of tetanus antitoxin. The low levels are due to increasing age, birth outside Canada, and absence of immunization records (PHAC, 2014b).

Pathophysiology

When prevention efforts are not effective and conditions are favourable, the organisms proliferate and form potent exotoxins, one of which is *tetanospasmin*. Tetanospasmin affects the central nervous system to produce the clinical manifestations of the disease. The ideal conditions for the organisms' growth are devitalized tissues without access to air, such as wounds that have not been washed or kept clean and those that have crusted over, trapping pus beneath. The exotoxin appears to reach the central nervous system by way of either the neuron axons or the vascular system. The toxin becomes fixed on nerve cells of the anterior horn of the spinal cord and the brainstem. The toxin acts at the myoneural junction to produce muscular stiffness and lower the threshold for reflex excitability.

The incubation period for tetanus varies from 2 days to months and averages 8 days; most cases occur within 14 days. In newborns it is usually 5 to 14 days. Shorter incubation periods have been associated with more heavily contaminated wounds, more severe disease, and a worse prognosis (American Academy of Pediatrics [AAP] Committee of Infectious Diseases, Kimberlin, & Long, 2015).

The manner of onset varies, but the initial symptoms are usually a progressive stiffness and tenderness of the muscles in the neck and jaw. Eventually, all voluntary muscles are affected (Box 54-11).

Therapeutic Management

Primary prevention is key and occurs through immunization and boosters (see Immunizations, Chapter 35, for age-specific recommendations). An unprotected or inadequately immunized child who sustains a "tetanus-prone" wound (including wounds contaminated with dirt, feces, soil, and saliva; puncture wounds; avulsions; and wounds resulting from missiles, crushing, burns, and frostbite) should receive tetanus

BOX 54-11 CLINICAL MANIFESTATIONS OF TETANUS

Initial Symptoms

Progressive stiffness and tenderness of muscles in neck and jaw

Characteristic difficulty in opening the mouth (trismus)

Risus sardonicus (sardonic smile) caused by facial muscle spasm

Progressive Involvement

Opisthotonic positioning (severe back arching)

Boardlike rigidity of abdominal and limb muscles

Difficulty swallowing

High sensitivity to external stimuli (slight noise, gentle touch, or bright light):

- Trigger paroxysmal muscular contractions that last seconds to minutes
- Contractions recur with increased frequency until almost continuous (sustained tetanic)

Laryngospasm and tetany of respiratory muscles:

- Accumulated secretions
- Respiratory arrest
- Atelectasis
- Pneumonia

Other Aspects

Mentation unaffected; patient alert

Pain and distress are reflected in:

- Rapid pulse
- Sweating
- Anxious expression

Fever usually absent or only mild

immunoglobulin (TIG). Concurrent administration of both TIG and tetanus toxoid at separate sites is recommended both to provide protection and to initiate the active immune process.

After the individual has received primary tetanus immunization, antitoxin (human) is believed to provide protection for at least 10 years and for a longer period after booster immunization (PHAC, 2014b). Antibiotic treatment with oral or intravenous metronidazole (Flagyl) (alternatively parenteral penicillin G) is important in the management of tetanus as an adjunct against vegetative forms of Clostridia (AAP Committee of Infectious Diseases et al., 2015).

MEDICATION ALERT

TIG and tetanus toxoid are always administered via the intramuscular route in separate syringes and at separate sites; they are never administered by intravenous route.

General supportive care is indicated, including maintaining an adequate airway and fluid and electrolyte balance, managing pain, and ensuring adequate caloric intake. In-dwelling oral or nasogastric feedings may be required to maintain adequate fluid and caloric intake; continued laryngospasm may necessitate total parenteral nutrition or gastrostomy feeding. Severe or recurrent laryngospasm or excessive secretions may require advanced airway management such as endotracheal intubation or tracheotomy.

Diazepam is the medication of choice for seizure control and muscle relaxation (Arnon, 2016a), but lorazepam (Ativan) may be used in some cases. Intrathecal baclofen, magnesium sulphate, dantrolene sodium, and midazolam may also be used in the management of tetanus. Patients with severe tetanus and those who do not respond to other muscle relaxants may require the administration of a neuromuscular blocking agent, such as rocuronium or vecuronium. Because of their paralytic effect on respiratory muscles, use of these medications requires mechanical ventilation with endotracheal intubation or tracheotomy and constant cardiopulmonary monitoring. Despite the absence of pain manifestation with these medications, it is important to administer adequate analgesia. The administration of corticosteroids has met with success in some cases.

NURSING CARE

The care of the child with tetanus requires supportive management with particular attention to airway and breathing. Respiratory status needs to be carefully evaluated for any signs of distress, and appropriate emergency equipment should be kept available at all times, as medications prescribed to treat tetanus can also cause respiratory depression. Attention to hydration and nutrition involves monitoring an intravenous infusion, monitoring nasogastric or gastrostomy feedings, and suctioning oropharyngeal secretions when indicated.

In caring for the child with tetanus during the acute phase, the nurse should make every effort to control or eliminate stimulation from sound, light, and touch. Although a darkened room is ideal, sufficient light is essential so that the child can be carefully observed; light appears to be less irritating than vibratory or auditory stimuli. The infant or child should be handled as little as possible and any sudden or loud noise eliminated to prevent seizures.

Botulism

Botulism is an acute flaccid paralysis caused by the preformed toxin produced by the anaerobic bacillus *Clostridium botulinum*. The most common source of the toxin is improperly sterilized home-canned foods. The disease has a wide variation in severity, from constipation to progressive sequential loss of neurological function and respiratory failure. Central nervous system symptoms appear abruptly approximately 12 to 36 hours after ingestion of contaminated food and may or may not be preceded by acute digestive disturbance (Box 54-12).

Human botulism is caused by neurotoxins A, B, E, and, rarely, F. In addition to foodborne botulism, other forms include wound botulism; infant botulism; and human-made botulism, usually a result of bioterrorism (Arnon, 2016b).

Treatment consists of intravenous administration of botulism antitoxin and general supportive measures, primarily respiratory and nutritional. Toxins vary in protein-binding capacity. Some have a relatively short half-life and do not bind to tissues firmly; thus therapy is continued until paralysis abates.

BOX 54-12 CLINICAL MANIFESTATIONS OF BOTULISM

General Signs
Weakness
Dizziness
Headache
Difficulty talking and speaking
Diplopia
Vomiting
Progressive, life-threatening respiratory paralysis

Infant Botulism*
Constipation (a common symptom)
Generalized weakness
Decrease in spontaneous movements
Diminished or absent deep tendon reflexes
Loss of head control
Difficulty feeding
Weak cry
Reduced gag reflex
Progressive respiratory paralysis

*Most commonly diagnosed as a "rule out sepsis" in the acute phase because of clinical presentation.

Other toxins appear to bind irreversibly to nerve endings and are not amenable to neutralization.

Infant Botulism

Infant botulism, unlike the disease in older persons, is caused by ingestion of spores or vegetative cells of *C. botulinum* and the subsequent release of the toxin from organisms colonizing the gastrointestinal tract. *C. botulinum* types A and B are the most common causative strains of infant botulism. This form of botulism has become more prevalent than any other form. Many cases of infant botulism occur in breastfed infants who are being introduced to nonhuman milk substances (AAP Committee of Infectious Diseases et al., 2015). There appears to be no common food or medication source of the organisms; however, the *C. botulinum* organisms have been found in honey. Botulism may occur in infants as young as 1 week of age up to 12 months of age, with peak incidence between 2 and 4 months of age.

The severity of the disease varies widely, from mild constipation to progressive sequential loss of neurological function and respiratory failure (see Box 54-12). The affected infant is usually well before the onset of symptoms. Constipation is a common presenting symptom, and almost all infants exhibit generalized weakness and a decrease in spontaneous movements. Deep tendon reflexes are usually diminished or absent. Cranial nerve deficits are common, as evidenced by loss of head control, difficulty in feeding, weak cry, and reduced gag reflex. SMA type 1 and metabolic disorders are often mistaken for infant botulism in the initial diagnostic phase because of the similarities in clinical manifestations of hypotonia, lethargy, and poor feeding (Arnon, 2016b). Presenting clinical signs also often mimic those of sepsis in young infants. Botulism toxin exerts its effect by inhibiting the release of acetylcholine at the myoneural junction, thereby impairing motor activity of muscles innervated by affected nerves.

Diagnosis is made on the basis of the clinical history, physical examination, and laboratory detection of the organism in the patient's stool and, less commonly, blood. However, isolation of the organism may take several days; suspicion of botulism by clinical presentation should require emergent treatment (Arnon, 2016b). EMG may be helpful in establishing the diagnosis; however, results may be normal early in the course of the illness.

Treatment consists of immediate administration of botulism immune globulin intravenously without waiting for laboratory diagnosis. In Canada, the botulism antitoxin and immune globulin are not approved for sale and are only available via Health Canada's Special Access Programme (SAP). There are four products available: (1) botulism antitoxin type AB and type E, accessed from the Butantan Institute in Brazil, (2) Novartis trivalent types ABE, (3) botulism immune globulin intravenous (human) (BIG-IV) (BabyBIG) for pediatric patients under the age of 1 year, and (4) NP-018 (heptavalent) types A to G from Cangene Corporation (PHAC, 2013). Early administration of BIG-IV neutralizes the toxin and stops the progression of the disease. The human-derived botulism antitoxin (BIG-IV) has been evaluated and is now available nationwide for use only in infant botulism. Infants treated with BIG-IV usually have a shortened hospital stay from approximately 6 weeks to 2 weeks, reportedly as a result of decreased requirements for mechanical ventilation and critical care (Arnon et al., 2016b). Approximately 50% of affected infants will require intubation and mechanical ventilation; thus respiratory support is crucial, as is nutritional support, since the infant is unable to feed. Antibiotic therapy is not part of the management because the botulinum toxin is an intracellular molecule and antibiotics would not be effective; aminoglycosides in particular should not be administered because they may potentiate the blocking effects of the neurotoxin (Arnon, 2016b).

The prognosis is generally good if the patient is adequately treated, although recovery may be slow, requiring a few weeks after severe illness. Untreated patients may require a longer hospitalization.

! NURSING ALERT

Although the precise source of *C. botulinum* spores has not been identified as originating from honey in many cases of infant botulism, it is still recommended that honey or corn syrup not be given to infants less than 12 months of age because the spores have been found in honey (CDC, 2016).

NURSING CARE

Nursing responsibilities include observing for and reporting signs of neuromuscular weakness or impairment and providing intensive nursing care when the infant is hospitalized. Parental support and reassurance are important. Most infants recover when the disorder is recognized and BIG-IV therapy is implemented. Nursing care of the infant on mechanical ventilation requires observation of oxygenation status and vigilance for any complications. Parents should be aware that, during recovery, patients tire easily when muscular action is sustained. This has important implications for timing the resumption of feedings because of the risk of aspiration. Parents should also be advised that normal bowel activity may not return for several weeks, therefore a stool softener can be beneficial.

Spinal Cord Injuries

Spinal cord injuries with major neurological involvement traditionally have not been a common cause of physical disability in children. However, a sufficient number of children with these injuries are admitted to major medical centres, and because of the increased survival rate as a result of improved management, nurses are often involved in the care and rehabilitation of children with SCI.

In 2010, there were an estimated 85,556 people in Canada living with SCI. Of that group, 43,974 people had SCI due to trauma, with 19,232 individuals living with paraplegia and 24,742 with tetraplegia (Noonan, Fingas, Farry, et al., 2012). There are very few statistics for the rates of children in Canada with SCI.

Mechanisms of Injury

Children with traumatic SCI have different mechanisms of injury and have a better neurological outcome potential than that of adults (Parent, Mac-Thiong, Roy-Beaudry, et al., 2011). The most common cause of serious spinal cord damage in children is trauma involving MVAs (including automobile–bicycle, all-terrain vehicles, and snowmobiles), sports injuries (especially from diving, trampolines, gymnastics, skiing, and snowboarding), birth trauma, or nonaccidental trauma. MVAs lead to many of the SCIs in children, often related to their being improperly restrained in the car. The increased use of recreational activities involving motorized vehicles such as jet water skis, all-terrain vehicles, and motorcycles has also increased the incidence of SCIs in children.

In MVAs, most SCIs in children are a result of indirect trauma caused by sudden hyperflexion or hyperextension of the neck, often combined with a rotational force. Trauma to the spinal cord without evidence of vertebral fracture or dislocation (SCIWORA) is particularly likely to occur in an MVA when proper safety restraints are not used. An unrestrained child becomes a projectile during sudden deceleration and is subject to injury from contact with a variety of objects inside and outside the vehicle. Individuals who use only a lap seat belt restraint are at greater risk of SCI than those who use a combination lap and shoulder restraint. High cervical spine injuries have been reported in children younger than 2 years of age who are improperly restrained in forward-facing car seats. Infants who are improperly restrained in an infant car seat may experience cervical trauma in a car crash. Small children may also be severely injured by deployment of front-seat air bags.

Another source of SCI, falling from heights, occurs less often among children than adults. Vertebral compression from blows to the head or buttocks can occur in water sports (diving and surfing), falls from horses, or other athletic activities.

There has also been concern about the level of injury-inducing contact in sports in organized leagues across Canada that results in concussions and SCI in children and teenagers. Parachute Canada (2015), through monitoring of hockey injuries, has increased awareness of the risks involved in this sport (see more on concussion in Chapter 50). The Canadian Paediatric Society recommends that in all levels of organized recreational and nonelite competitive ice hockey bodychecking be eliminated and that it be delayed (in elite competitive leagues) until players are 13 to 14 years of age (bantam level) or older (Houghton, Emery, & CPS, Healthy Active Living and Sports Medicine Committee, 2012).

Birth injuries may occur in breech deliveries from traction force on the spinal cord during delivery of the head and shoulders. Infants, when shaken, commonly sustain cervical cord damage as well as subdural hematoma and retinal hemorrhage; cognitive impairment and death may occur subsequent to the traumatic event. Infants have weak neck muscles, and during vigorous shaking their large and heavy heads rapidly wobble back and forth.

SCI before the age of 15 years is an uncommon occurrence, but it can have significant psychological and physiological consequences. Although the exact rate is unknown, SCI likely represents less than 4% of the overall incidence of SCI annually in these children. The mechanism of injury, the male–female ratio, and the level of injury are different from that in the adult population. The incidence of SCI increases rapidly with age, with greater than 30% of injuries occurring between the ages of 17 and 23, and 53% occurring between the ages of 16 and 30 (Parent et al., 2011).

Fracture or subluxation (partial dislocations) is the most common immediate cause of SCI, particularly in the lower cervical region. Although unusual in adults, SCI without fracture is common in children, whose spines are suppler, weaker, and more mobile than those of adults. Therefore, the force is more easily dissipated over a larger number of segments. Infants and small children under the age of 5 years suffer upper cervical spine fractures and spinal compressions more often, whereas youth tend to have lower cervical and thorcolumbar fracture dislocations (Rekate, 2016).

The severity of the force, the mechanism of injury, and the degree of the individual's muscular relaxation at the time of the injury greatly influence the extent of the trauma. SCIs are classified as either complete or incomplete. In a *complete injury*, there is no more motor or sensory function more than three segments below the neurological level of the injury. *Incomplete lesions* have several typical characteristics (Mathison, Kadom, & Krug, 2008):

- Central cord syndrome—Central grey matter destruction and preservation of peripheral tracts: tetraplegia with sacral sparing common; some motor recovery gained
- Anterior cord syndrome—Complete motor and sensory loss with trunk and lower extremity proprioception and sensation of pressure
- Posterior cord syndrome—Loss of sensation, pain, and proprioception with normal cord function, including motor function; able to move extremities but the person has difficulty controlling such movements

- Brown-Séquard syndrome—Unilateral cord lesion with a motor deficit on the opposite side of the body from the primary insult; absence of pain and temperature sensation on the opposite side from the injury
- Spinal cord concussion—Transient loss of neural function below the level of the acute spinal cord lesion, resulting in flaccid paralysis and loss of tendon, autonomic, and cutaneous reflex activity; may last hours to weeks

The injury sustained can affect any of the spinal nerves, and the higher the injury, the more extensive the damage. The child can be left with complete or partial paralysis of the lower extremities (*paraplegia*) or with damage at a higher level and without functional use of any of the four extremities (*tetraplegia*). A high cervical cord injury that affects the phrenic nerve paralyzes the diaphragm and leaves the child dependent on mechanical ventilation.

Clinical Manifestations

It is often difficult to determine the extent and severity of the damage at first. Immediate loss of function is caused by both anatomical and impaired physiology, and improved function may not be evident for weeks or even months. Manifestations of the initial response to acute SCI is flaccid paralysis below the level of the damage. This state is often referred to as **spinal shock syndrome** and is caused by the sudden disruption of central and autonomic pathways. Local effects of cord edema and ischemia produce a physiological transection with or without an anatomic severance. Most children with an SCI experience some spinal shock. Manifestations include the absence of reflexes at or below the cord lesion, with flaccidity or limpness of the involved muscles, loss of sensation, and motor function and autonomic dysfunction (symptoms of hypotension, low or high body temperature, loss of bladder and bowel control, and autonomic dysreflexia).

Autonomic paralysis also affects thermoregulatory functions. Afferent impulses from temperature receptors in the skin are not integrated; therefore, the child is subject to temperature increases or decreases in response to alterations in environmental temperature. Hyperthermia can result from excessive ambient temperature, such as too many covers.

Except in the situations previously mentioned, flaccid paralysis is replaced by spinal reflex activity and increasing spasticity or, in incomplete lesions, greater or lesser degree of neurological recovery.

The paralytic nature of autonomic function is replaced by autonomic dysreflexia, especially when the lesions are above the midthoracic level. This autonomic phenomenon is caused by visceral distension or irritation, particularly of the bowel or bladder. Sensory impulses are triggered and travel to the cord lesion, where they are blocked, which causes activation of sympathetic reflex action with disturbed central inhibitory control. Excessive sympathetic activity is manifested by a flushing face, sweating forehead, pupillary constriction, marked hypertension, headache, and bradycardia. The precipitating stimulus may be merely a full bladder or rectum or other internal or external sensory input. It can be a catastrophic event unless the irritation is relieved.

Additional clinical findings of SCI may include numbness, tingling, or burning; priapism; weakness; and loss of bowel and bladder control.

Neurogenic shock occurs as a result of a disruption in the descending sympathetic pathways with loss of vasomotor tone and sympathetic innervations to the cardiovascular system. Hypotension, bradycardia, and peripheral vasodilation occur as a result of neurogenic shock.

Children with suspected SCI may have suffered multiple injuries (e.g., head injury); therefore clinical manifestations may occur that mask those of an SCI.

Therapeutic Management

Initial care begins at the scene of the accident with proper immobilization of the cervical, thoracic, and lumbar spine. Because of the complexity of these injuries, it is usually recommended that those with injuries be transported to a spinal injury centre for care by specially trained health care personnel as soon as possible after the injury for appropriate diagnostic evaluation and intervention.

The initial assessment of the child with a suspected SCI should begin with an assessment of CAB: **c**irculation, **a**irway, and **b**reathing. The airway should be opened using the jaw-thrust technique to minimize damage to the cervical spine. The child is monitored for cardiovascular instability, and measures are taken to support systemic blood pressure and maintain optimal cardiac output. Because MVAs and other trauma in children may involve internal organ damage and potential bleeding, abdominal distension and other signs are acted on immediately to prevent further systemic shock. After the child is stabilized and transported to a regional trauma centre, a thorough evaluation of neurological status and any other associated trauma is carried out by the multidisciplinary team. In the emergency department, spinal immobilization should be maintained until a thorough neurological assessment has been completed and spinal cord injury is ruled out; in children, this typically involves a CT scan and possibly an MRI. Additional interventions are discussed in the Nursing Care section.

Intravenous methylprednisone may be started within the first 12 hours after the injury to decrease inflammation and minimize further injury; however, its use is controversial in small children.

A number of progressive rehabilitation modalities have been developed that have the potential for increasing the quality of life for children with SCI. One such treatment is functional electrical stimulation (FES), also referred to as *functional neuromuscular stimulation,* or *neuromuscular electrical stimulation.* With this treatment, an electrical stimulator is surgically implanted under the skin in the abdomen and electrode leads are tunnelled to paralyzed leg muscles, enabling the child to sit, stand, and walk with the aid of crutches, a walker, or other orthoses. The stimulator can also be used to elicit a voluntary grasp and release with the hand. Before the latter can be accomplished, a number of surgical tendon transfers may be required for elbow extension, wrist extension, and finger and thumb flexion. In addition, FES has therapeutic benefits, which include increased muscle strength, improved gait function, and increased cardiovascular fitness (Thrasher & Popovic, 2008). Tendon transfers have been shown to be successful in enhancing hand and arm function, increasing pinch force, and facilitating independence in ADLs (Hosalkar, Pandya, Hsu, et al., 2009). Restoration of hand and arm function enables children with SCI to perform self-catheterization and achieve greater independence in personal hygiene.

Exercise is considered an integral part of SCI rehabilitation; exercise may enhance neuroplasticity and decrease further muscle atrophy. Examples of exercise modalities in SCI patients include upper body strength training and hand cycling (Hosalkar et al., 2009).

Administration of pharmacological agents such as clonidine hydrochloride may improve ambulation in patients with partial SCIs, and exercise therapy through interactive locomotor training has helped some individuals with SCI regain ambulatory function.

A number of orthoses or ambulation aids such as braces may still be necessary to achieve upright mobility, yet as robotic technology advances, so do the chances for improved mobilization in children with SCI. Mechanical or robotic orthoses may be used in conjunction with FES to enable ambulation in persons with SCI. Gait training may be achieved with a number of different modalities, including a stationary cycle; however, no specific method has proved superior to the others. FES has also been effective in reducing complications from bladder and bowel incontinence and in assisting males in achieving penile erection. Knee-ankle-foot orthosis and reciprocating gait orthosis may also be used to assist with early rehabilitation and ambulation (Vogel, Betz, & Mulcahey, 2012).

Surgical interventions for SCI include early cord decompression (decompression laminectomy) and cervical or thoracic fusion. Crutchfield, Vinke, or Gardner-Wells tongs and skeletal traction may be used for early cervical vertebral stabilization. A halo vest may be suited for ambulation after the acute phase (see also Cervical Traction, Chapter 53). After cervical spinal fusion, a hard cervical collar or sterno-occipital-mandibular immobilizer brace may be worn until the fusion is solidified. When SCI occurs in young children and preteens, scoliosis develops over time and often requires surgical consideration (Parent et al., 2011).

SCI management guidelines and standards of care have been developed on the basis of research evidence and can be found through the Spinal Cord Injury Rehabilitation Evidence Project (2010). The Rick Hansen Foundation and Accreditation Canada are developing Canadian standards for SCI services. This foundation provides research and resources as well as information on SCI. The Canadian Paraplegic Association also offers various useful services, such as assistive devices and assistive living (see Additional Resources at the end of this chapter).

NURSING CARE

The nursing care of the paraplegic or quadriplegic child is complex and challenging. A multidisciplinary SCI team is equipped to manage the acute phase of the injury, and some members, including the nurse, may follow the patient to eventual recovery. Nursing care is concerned with ensuring adequate initial stabilization of the entire spinal column with a rigid cervical collar with supportive blocks on a rigid backboard. The traumatic event causing the injury may or may not be recalled if the child lost consciousness; such events are frightening to the child. The young child may also be frightened by the immobilization process and the inability to move the extremities; therefore, it is important to reassure and comfort the child during this process.

During the acute phase of the injury it is imperative that airway patency be maintained and respiratory function monitored. It is important to evaluate the extent of the neurological damage early to establish a baseline for neurological functioning; continual assessment of function should occur to prevent further deterioration of neurological status as a result of spinal cord edema. The American Spinal Injury Association (ASIA) Impairment Scale may be used to assess neurological function on a routine basis during the patient's recovery (see Additional Resources at the end of this chapter). Once the patient is admitted, further evaluation of the patient's abilities to perform ADLs and need for assistance is ongoing.

Nursing care during the acute phase should also focus on frequent monitoring of neurological signs to determine any changes in neurological function that require further intervention (e.g., level of consciousness using the Glasgow Coma Scale, see Chapter 50). In addition to airway maintenance, the nurse should monitor for changes in hemodynamic status that may require immediate medical attention. Neurogenic shock consists of hypotension, bradycardia, and vasodilation. Inotropic medications may be required to maintain adequate perfusion. Renal function is closely monitored by measuring urinary output and fluids administered.

The child with a head injury may experience elevated intracranial pressure; therefore, changes in neurological status are reported to the health care provider. Fluid restriction may be required if intracranial pressure is elevated, so fluid intake should be closely monitored.

The nursing care of the child with an SCI is, in most respects, the same as that of any immobilized child (see The Immobilized Child, Chapter 53). Additional aspects of care that should be addressed on an individual basis include hypercalcemia in adolescent males, deep venous thrombosis, latex sensitization, pain, spasticity, autonomic dysreflexia, and sleep-disordered breathing (Vogel et al., 2012).

Respiratory care often focuses on maintaining an adequate airway and effective ventilation. The child with a high-level cervical injury (C3 and above) requires continuous ventilatory assistance. In most instances a tracheostomy is the method of choice for greater ease in clearing secretions and for less trauma to tissues during long-term ventilatory dependence. In some children breathing pacemaker devices (phrenic nerve stimulators) are implanted to stimulate the phrenic nerve and produce diaphragmatic contractions and lung expansion without assisted ventilation. In the child who does not require mechanical ventilation, special attention to clearance of secretions is vital because of decreased pulmonary function. In addition to chest physiotherapy, the child may require a cough-assist device to clear secretions effectively (see Duchenne [Pseudohypertrophic] Muscular Dystrophy: Therapeutic Management).

Temperature is often poorly regulated in children with SCI; thus, body temperature must be monitored closely for fluctuations. Response to environmental temperature changes may be slow or absent, and the ability to dissipate heat through the process of shivering may be compromised.

Children with SCI have unique needs in relation to skin care. Because of decreased sensation and impaired mobility, they depend on others to assess and assist in the management of intact skin. Skin care practices are the same as those for any child who is immobilized. A skin score scale such as the Braden Q Scale should be used to objectively evaluate risks for skin breakdown and skin conditions (Noonan, Quigley, & Curley, 2011). (See Additional Resources at the end of the chapter.) An alternating-pressure mattress or other pressure relief or reduction device should be kept underneath the child, and the skin needs to be thoroughly inspected at least once a day (or more often if there is increased risk) for signs of pressure and breakdown, especially over bony prominences. Children and adolescents confined to a wheelchair also require meticulous skin care to prevent skin breakdown on insensate areas; frequent position changes and air or gel cushions are helpful but do not eliminate the need for close observation of skin status (McCaskey, Kirk, & Gerdes, 2011).

Bowel and bladder function is often affected in the child with SCI. CIC may be required to regularly empty the neurogenic bladder and prevent urinary tract infections. A regular bowel management program should be tailored to the child's needs.

Pain management is vital in children and adolescents with SCI. In children with upper motor neuron involvement, the spasticity that develops may require administration of an antispasmodic medication such as diazepam. Baclofen is considered the drug of choice for reducing muscle spasticity. Gabapentin may be used to treat neuropathic pain. Botulinum toxin type A and α_2-adrenergic agonists may be used in older children with SCI to decrease muscle spasticity.

The child with some lower extremity function progresses to parallel bars and then to a walker; the child with tetraplegia learns to use a wheelchair—among the most valuable aids available to the child with an SCI (Fig. 54-8). The wheelchair should be selected carefully in relation to where it will be used, the architectural barriers, and the child's functional capacity. For children with severe upper extremity paralysis, a variety of motorized wheelchairs are used; however, the more complex they are, the greater their cost, weight, and tendency to break down. Wheelchair tolerance can be gained over time and is accompanied by measures to prevent orthostatic hypotension and pressure ulcers.

A variety of orthoses and other appliances can be adapted for use by many children. The primary purpose of lower extremity bracing in the child with an SCI is for ambulation.

Children with high-level lesions are susceptible to the development of autonomic dysreflexia, which requires prompt action to prevent encephalopathy and shock. Clinical manifestations of autonomic dysreflexia include a drastic increase in systemic blood pressure, headache, bradycardia, profuse diaphoresis, cardiac dysrhythmias, flushing, piloerection, blurred vision, nasal congestion, anxiety, spots on the visual field, or absent or minimum symptoms. Small children who are unable to verbalize may only become irritable. Early recognition of autonomic dysreflexia by caregivers is essential, especially in small children who are unable to verbalize their feelings. Medications such as nitropaste, nifedipine, prazosin, or terazosin may be administered to counteract the effects of the condition depending on the child's response to interventions (Vogel et al., 2012).

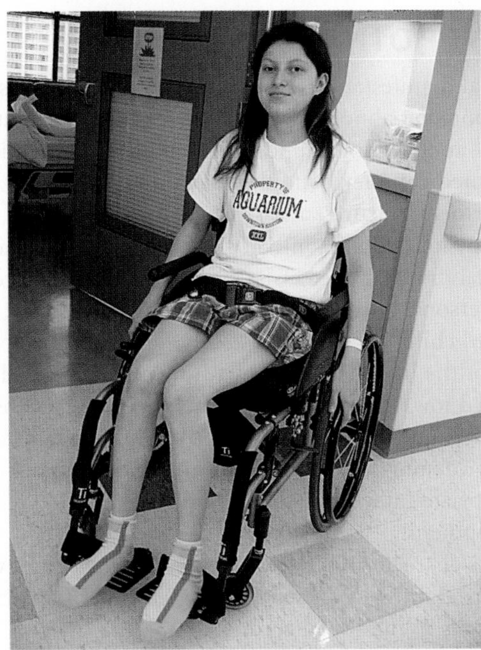

FIGURE 54-8 A wheelchair allows an adolescent mobility and independence. (Courtesy Texas Children's Hospital.)

The child and family with SCI need to be prepared for the eventual discharge from the acute care facility to a rehabilitation centre. The major aims of physical rehabilitation are to prepare the child and family to achieve normalization and resume life at home and in the community. Additional goals of rehabilitation in children with SCI are to promote independence in mobility and self-care skills, academic achievement, independent living, and employment.

The nurse is a crucial member of the health care team in helping the family cope with the magnitude of the injury and disability, understand the extent of the disability, verbalize expected outcomes, and move toward eventual rehabilitation and normalization within the child's capabilities. The goals of rehabilitation include preparing the child and family to live at home and function as independently as possible.

KEY POINTS

- Clinical manifestations of CP include delayed gross motor development; abnormal motor performance; alterations of muscle tone; abnormal postures; reflex abnormalities; and associated complex conditions such as cognitive impairment, seizures, and sensory impairment.
- Therapy for CP takes into account the nature of the physical disability, defects associated with the disorder, and interpersonal and social influences encountered by the affected child.
- Care of the infant and child with myelomeningocele is directed toward protecting the meningeal sac, preventing infection and skin breakdown, observing for signs of urological and bowel complications, and planning appropriate interventions to optimize the child's development.
- SMA is characterized by progressive weakness and wasting of skeletal muscles caused by degeneration of anterior horn cells of the spinal cord.
- MDs are the greatest and most important cause of muscular dysfunction of childhood.
- Major complications of DMD include joint contractures, disuse atrophy, obesity, and respiratory and cardiac problems.
- Nursing care of the child with GBS consists of monitoring vital signs, providing respiratory support and physiotherapy, providing reassurance, and providing support to the child and family.
- Tetanus occurs when tetanus spores or vegetative bacilli enter a wound and multiply in a susceptible host.
- Infant botulism results from the release of toxins from *C. botulinum* colonizing the gastrointestinal tract.
- Therapeutic management of SCI is directed toward immobilizing the entire spinal column at the scene of the traumatic event, safely transporting the patient by health care personnel trained to transport possible spinal trauma victims, evaluating neurological damage, preventing further neurological damage, and implementing an aggressive rehabilitation program designed to help achieve independence and movement.

evolve EVOLVE WEBSITE

Visit the Evolve website for additional resources related to the content in this chapter such as Case Studies, Critical Thinking Case Study Answers, Nursing Care Plans, Nursing Processes, Nursing Skills, and Review Questions for Exam Preparation at: *http://evolve.elsevier.com/Canada/Perry/maternal/*

REFERENCES

Adzick, N. S. (2013). Fetal surgery for spina bifida: Past, present, future. *Seminars in Pediatric Surgery*, *22*(1), 10–17. doi: 10.1053/j.sempedsurg.2012.10.003.

Adzick, N. S., Thom, E. A., Spong, C. Y., et al. (2011). A randomized trial of prenatal versus postnatal repair of myelomeningocele. *The New England Journal of Medicine*, *364*(11), 993–1004. doi: 10.1056/NEJMoa1014379.

Aisen, M. L., Kerkovich, D., Mast, J., et al. (2011). Cerebral palsy: Clinical care and neurological rehabilitation. *The Lancet. Neurology*, *10*(9), 844–852.

American Academy of Pediatrics, Committee of Infectious Diseases, Kimberlin, D. W., & Long, S. S. (Eds.). (2015). *Red book: Report of the committee on infectious diseases* (30th ed.). Elk Grove Village, IL: Author.

Arnon, S. S. (2016a). Tetanus (*Clostridium tetani*). In R. M. Kliegman, B. F. Stanton, J. W. St. Geme, et al. (Eds.), *Nelson textbook of pediatrics* (20th ed.). Philadelphia: Saunders.

Arnon, S. S. (2016b). Anaerobic bacterial infections: Botulism (*Clostridium botulinum*). In R. M. Kliegman, B. F. Stanton, J. W. St. Geme, et al. (Eds.), *Nelson textbook of pediatrics* (20th ed.). Philadelphia: Saunders.

Bach, J. R. (2007). Medical considerations of long-term survival of Werdnig-Hoffmann disease. *American Journal of Physical Medicine & Rehabilitation*, *86*(5), 349–355. doi: 10.1097/PHM.0b013e31804b1d66.

Battista, V. (2010). Muscular dystrophy: Duchenne. In P. J. Allen, J. A. Vessey, & N. A. Schapiro (Eds.), *Primary care of the child with a chronic condition* (5th ed.). St. Louis: Mosby.

Berker, A. N., & Yalçin, M. S. (2008). Cerebral palsy: Orthopedic aspects and rehabilitation. *Pediatric Clinics of North America*, *55*(5), 1209–1225. doi: 10.1016/j.pcl.2008.07.011.

Betz, C. L., Linroth, R., Butler, C., et al. (2010). Spina bifida: What we learned from consumers. *Pediatric Clinics of North America*, *57*(4), 935–944. doi: 10.1016/j.pcl.2010.07.013.

Boitano, L. J. (2009). Equipment options for cough augmentation, ventilation, and noninvasive interfaces in neuromuscular respiratory management. *Pediatrics*, *123*(Suppl. 4), S226–S230. doi: 10.1542/peds.2008-2952F.

Bushby, K., Finkel, R., Birnkrant, D. J., et al. (2010). Diagnosis and management of Duchenne muscular dystrophy, part 2: Implementation of multidisciplinary care. *The Lancet. Neurology*, *9*, 177–189.

Centers for Disease Control and Prevention (CDC). (2009). Racial/ethnic differences in the birth prevalence of spina bifida—United States, 1995–2005. *MMWR. Morbidity and Mortality Weekly Report*, *57*(53), 1409–1413.

Centers for Disease Control and Prevention (CDC). (2016). *Botulism*. Retrieved from <http://www.cdc.gov/botulism/>.

Delgado, M. R., Hirtz, D., Aisen, M., et al. (2010). Practice parameter: Pharmacological treatment of spasticity in children and adolescents with cerebral palsy (an evidence-based review). *Neurology*, *74*(1), 336–343. doi: 10.1212/WNL.0b013e3181cbcd2f.

De Wals, P., Tairou, F., Van Allen, M. I., et al. (2008). Spina bifida before and after folic acid fortification in Canada. *Birth Defects Research. Part A, Clinical and Molecular Teratology*, *82*(9), 622–626. doi: 10.1002/bdra.2048.

Dicianno, B. E., Fairman, A. D., Juengst, S. B., et al. (2010). Using the spina bifida life course model in clinical practice: An interdisciplinary approach. *Pediatric Clinics of North America*, *57*(4), 945–957. doi: 10.1016/j.pcl.2010.07.014.

Geister, T. L., Quintanar-Solares, M., Martin, M., et al. (2014). Qualitative development of the 'Questionnaire on Pain caused by Spasticity (QPS),' a pediatric patient-reported outcome for spasticity-related pain in cerebral palsy. *Quality of Life Research*, *23*, 887–896. doi: 10.1007/s11136-013-0526-2.

Golomb, M. R. (2009). Outcomes of perinatal arterial ischemic stroke and cerebral sinovenous thrombosis. *Seminars in Fetal & Neonatal Medicine, 4*(5), 318–322. doi: 10.1016/j.siny.2009.07.003.

Grivell, R. M., Andersen, C., & Dodd, J. M. (2014). Prenatal versus postnatal repair procedures for spina bifida for improving infant and maternal outcomes. *The Cochrane Database of Systematic Reviews*, (10), CD008825, doi: 10.1002/14651858.CD008825.pub2.

Hack, M., & Costello, D. W. (2008). Trends in the rates of cerebral palsy associated with neonatal intensive care of preterm children. *Clinical Obstetrics & Gynecology, 51*(4), 763–774.

Hosalkar, H., Pandya, N. K., Hsu, J., et al. (2009). Specialty update: What's new in orthopaedic rehabilitation? *Journal of Bone and Joint Surgery, 91*(9), 2296–2310. doi: 10.2106/JBJS.I.0031.

Houghton, K. M., Emery, C. A., & Canadian Paediatric Society, Healthy Active Living and Sports Medicine Committee. (2012). Bodychecking in youth ice hockey. *Paediatrics & Child Health, 17*(9), 509. Retrieved from <http://www.cps.ca/documents/position/bodychecking-ice-hockey>.

Hughes, R. (2008). The role of IVIG in autoimmune neuropathies: The latest evidence. *Journal of Neurology, 255*(Suppl. 3), 7–11.

Hughes, R. A., Swan, A. V., & van Doorn, P. A. (2014). Intravenous immunoglobulin for Guillain-Barré syndrome. *The Cochrane Database of Systematic Reviews*, (9), CD002063, doi: 10.1002/14651858.CD002063.pub6.

Johnston, M. V. (2016). Encephalopathies. In R. M. Kliegman, B. F. Stanton, J. W. St. Geme, et al. (Eds.), *Nelson textbook of pediatrics* (20th ed.). Philadelphia: Saunders.

Johnston, M. V., Fatemi, A., & Wilson, M. A. (2011). Treatment advances in neonatal neuroprotection and neurointensive care. *The Lancet. Neurology, 10*(4), 372–382.

Kinsman, S. L., & Johnston, M. V. (2016). Congenital anomalies of the central nervous system. In R. M. Kliegman, B. F. Stanton, J. W. St. Geme, et al. (Eds.), *Nelson textbook of pediatrics* (20th ed.). Philadephia: Saunders.

Kolb, S. J., & Kissel, J. T. (2014). Spinal muscular atrophy. *Neurologic Clinics, 33*(4), 831–846. doi: 10.1016/j.ncl.2015.07.004.

Krägeloh-Mann, I., & Cans, C. (2009). Cerebral palsy update. *Brain & Development, 31*(7), 537–544.

Kravitz, R. M. (2009). Airway clearance in Duchenne muscular dystrophy. *Pediatrics, 123*(Suppl. 4), S231–S235.

Lazzaretti, C. C., & Pearson, C. (2010). Myelodysplasia. In P. J. Allen, J. A. Vessey, & N. A. Schapiro (Eds.), *Primary care of the child with a chronic condition* (5th ed.). St. Louis: Mosby.

Liptak, G. S., Murphy, N. A., & Council on Children with Disabilities. (2011). Providing a primary care medical home for children and youth with cerebral palsy. *Pediatrics, 128*(5), e1321–e1329.

Lovette, B. (2008). Safe transportation for children with special needs. *Journal of Pediatric Health Care, 22*(5), 323–328. doi: 10.1016/j.pedhc.2008.05.002.

Lukban, M. B., Rosales, R. L., & Dressler, D. (2009). Effectiveness of botulinum toxin A for upper and lower limb spasticity in children with cerebral palsy: A summary of evidence. *Journal of Neural Transmission, 116*(3), 319–331.

Lunn, M. R., & Wang, C. H. (2008). Spinal muscular atrophy. *Lancet, 371*(9630), 2120–2133.

Lyons, R. (2008). Elusive belly pain and Guillain-Barré syndrome. *Journal of Pediatric Health Care, 22*(5), 310–314. doi: 10.1016/j.pedhc.2008.03.004.

Manzur, A. Y., Kinali, M., & Muntoni, F. (2008). Update on the management of Duchenne muscular dystrophy. *Archives of Disease in Childhood, 93*(11), 986–999. doi: 10.1136/adc.2007.118141.

Manzur, A. Y., Kuntzer, T., Pike, M., et al. (2008). Glucocorticoid corticosteroids for Duchenne muscular dystrophy. *The Cochrane Database of Systematic Reviews*, (1), CD003725, doi: 10.1002/14651858.CD003725.pub3.

Masadeh, M., Krein, M., Peterson, J., et al. (2013). Outcome of antegrade continent enema (ACE) procedures in children and young adults. *Journal of Pediatric Surgery, 48*(10), 2128–3213. doi: 10.1016/j.jpedsurg.2013.04.009.

Mathison, D. J., Kadom, N., & Krug, S. E. (2008). Spinal cord injury in the pediatric patient. *Clinical Pediatric Emergency Medicine, 9*(2), 106–123.

McCaskey, M. S., Kirk, L., & Gerdes, C. (2011). Preventing skin breakdown in the immobile child in the home care setting. *Home Healthcare Nurse, 29*(4), 248–255.

McKim, D. A., Road, J., Avendano, M., et al., for the Canadian Thoracic Society Home Mechanical Ventilation Committee. (2011). Home mechanical ventilation: A Canadian Thoracic Society clinical practice guideline. *Canadian Respiratory Journal, 18*(4), 197–215.

Mercuri, E., Bertini, E., & Iannaccone, S. T. (2012). Childhood spinal muscular atrophy: Controversies and challenges. *The Lancet. Neurology, 11*(5), 443–452. doi: 10.1016/S1474-4422(12)70061-3.

Moster, D., Wilcox, A. J., Vollset, S. E., et al. (2010). Cerebral palsy among term and postterm births. *Journal of the American Medical Association, 304*(9), 976–982.

Muscular Dystrophy Canada. (2012). *The diagnosis of Duchenne muscular dystrophy: A guide for families.* Retrieved from <http://www.muscle.ca/moveit/moveit-may2012/DMDstandardsofcare-E_final_lowres.pdf>.

Nehring, W. M. (2009). Cerebral palsy. In P. L. Jackson, J. A. Vessey, & N. A. Schapiro (Eds.), *Primary care of the child with a chronic illness* (5th ed.). St. Louis: Mosby.

Noonan, C., Quigley, S., & Curley, M. A. (2011). Using the Braden Q Scale to predict pressure ulcer risk in pediatric patients. *Journal of Pediatric Nursing, 26*(6), 566–575.

Noonan, V. K., Fingas, M., Farry, A., et al. (2012). Incidence and prevalence of spinal cord injury in Canada: A national perspective. *Neuroepidemiology, 38*(4), 219–226. doi:10.1159/000336014.

Parachute Canada. (2015). *About injuries. Why pay attention to injuries?* Retrieved from <http://www.parachutecanada.org/injury-topics>.

Parent, S., Mac-Thiong, J. M., Roy-Beaudry, M., et al. (2011). Spinal cord injury in the pediatric population: A systematic review of the literature. *Journal of Neurotrauma, 28*(8), 1515–1524.

Prior, T. W. (2010). Spinal muscular atrophy: Newborn and carrier screening. *Obstetrics and Gynecology Clinics of North America, 37*(1), 23–26.

Public Health Agency of Canada. (2013). *Canada's foodborne illness outbreak response protocol (FIORP) 2010: To guide a multijurisdictional approach.* Retrieved from <http://www.phac-aspc.gc.ca/zoono/fiorp-pritioa/ann1-9-eng.php>.

Public Health Agency of Canada. (2014a). *Congenital anomalies in Canada 2013: A perinatal health surveillance report.* Retrieved from <http://www.phac-aspc.gc.ca/ccasn-rcsac/cac-acc-2013-eng.php>.

Public Health Agency of Canada. (2014b). *Canadian immunization guide.* Retrieved from <http://www.phac-aspc.gc.ca/publicat/cig-gci/p04-tet-eng.php>.

Quan, D. (2011). Muscular dystrophies and neurologic diseases that present as myopathy. *Rheumatic Diseases Clinics of North America, 37*(2), 233–244. doi: 10.1016/j.rdc.2011.01.006.

Rekate, H. L. (2016). Spinal cord injuries in children. In R. M. Kliegman, B. F. Stanton, J. W. St. Geme, et al. (Eds.), *Nelson textbook of pediatrics* (20th ed.). Philadelphia: Elsevier.

Rosenbaum, P., Paneth, N., Leviton, A., et al. (2007). A report: The definition and classification of cerebral palsy, April 2006. *Developmental Medicine & Child Neurology, 49*(S109), 1–44.

Sarnat, H. B. (2016a). Spinal muscular atrophies. In R. M. Kliegman, B. F. Stanton, J. W. St. Geme, et al. (Eds.), *Nelson textbook of pediatrics* (20th ed.). Philadelphia: Saunders.

Sarnat, H. B. (2016b). Muscular dystrophies. In R. M. Kliegman, B. F. Stanton, J. W. St. Geme, et al. (Eds.), *Nelson textbook of pediatrics* (20th ed.). Philadelphia: Saunders.

Sarnat, H. B. (2016c). Guillain-Barré syndrome. In R. M. Kliegman, B. F. Stanton, J. W. St. Geme, et al. (Eds.), *Nelson textbook of pediatrics* (20th ed.). Philadelphia: Saunders.

Sawyer, S. M., & Macnee, S. (2010). Transition to adult health care for adolescents with spina bifida: Research issues. *Developmental Disabilities Research Reviews, 16*(1), 60–65.

Schroth, M. K. (2009). Special considerations in the respiratory management of spinal muscular atrophy. *Pediatrics, 123*(Suppl. 4), S245–S249. doi: 10.1542/peds.2008-2952K.

Shankarn, S., Pappas, A., McDonald, W. A., et al. (2012). Childhood outcomes after hypothermia for neonatal encephalopathy. *The New England Journal of Medicine, 366*(22), 2085–2092.

Snodgrass, W. T., & Gargollo, P. C. (2010). Urologic care of the neurogenic bladder in children. *The Urologic Clinics of North America, 37*(2), 207–214. doi: 10.1016/j.ucl.2010.03.00.

Spinal Cord Injury Rehabilitation Evidence Project. (2010). *Rehabilitation evidence.* Retrieved from <http://www.scireproject.com/rehabilitation-evidence>.

Statistics Canada. (2012). *Table 105-1300: Neurological conditions, by age group and sex, household population aged 0 and over, 2010/2011.* Retrieved from <http://www5.statcan.gc.ca/cansim/pick-choisir?lang=eng&p2=33&id=1051300>.

Statistics Canada. (2013). *Table 105-1305. Neurological conditions in institutions, by age, sex, and number of residents, Canada, provinces and territories, 2011/2012.* Retrieved from <http://www5.statcan.gc.ca/cansim/pick-choisir?lang=eng&p2=33&id=1051305>.

Thrasher, T. A., & Popovic, M. R. (2008). Functional electrical stimulation of walking: Function, exercise and rehabilitation. *Annales de Readaptation et de Medecine Physique, 51*(6), 452–460.

Vogel, L. C., Betz, R. R., & Mulcahey, M. J. (2012). Spinal cord injuries in children and adolescents. In J. Verhaagen & J. W. McDonald (Eds.), *Handbook of clinical neurology, 109* (pp. 131–148). Philadelphia: Elsevier.

Volpe, J. J. (2008). *Neurology of the newborn* (5th ed.). Philadelphia: Saunders.

Wadman, R. I., Bosboom, W. M., van der Pol, W. L., et al. (2012). Drug treatment for spinal muscular atrophy types II and III. *The Cochrane Database of Systematic Reviews,* (4), CD006282, doi: 10.1002/14651858.CD006282.pub4.

Wilson, R. D., Audibert, F., Brock, J. A., et al., Society of Obstetricians and Gynaecologists of Canada. (2014). Prenatal screening, diagnosis, and pregnancy. Management of fetal neural tube defects. *Journal of Obstetrics and Gynaecology Canada, 36*(10), 927–939.

Wright, P. A., Durham, S., Ewins, D. J., et al. (2012). Neuromuscular electrical stimulation for children with cerebral palsy: A review. *Archives of Diseases in Children, 97*(4), 364–371.

Young, H. K., Lowe, A., Fitzgerald, D. A., et al. (2007). Outcome of noninvasive ventilation in children with neuromuscular disease. *Neurology, 68*(3), 198–201. doi: 10.1212/01.wnl.0000251299.54608.13.

ADDITIONAL RESOURCES

American Spinal Injury Association (ASIA) Impairment Scale: <https://www.scireproject.com/outcome-measures-new/american-spinal-injury-association-impairment-scale-ais-international-standards>.

Association for the Neurologically Disabled of Canada: <http://www.cwhn.ca/en/node/16670>.

Canadian Cerebral Palsy Sports Association: <http://ccpsa.ca/en/>.

Cerebral Palsy Support Canada: <http://www.cpsc.ca/>.

Families of SMA Canada: <http://curesma.ca/>.

GBS/CIDP Foundation of Canada: <http://www.gbs-cidp.org/canada/>.

Modified Braden Q Scale (for Pediatric Use): <http://www.therapybc.ca/eLibrary/docs/Resources/Braden%20Q%20scale%20for%20paeds.pdf>.

Motherisk: <http://www.motherisk.org>.

Muscular Dystrophy Canada: <http://www.muscle.ca>.

Rick Hansen Foundation: <http://www.rickhansen.com/>.

Spina Bifida and Hydrocephalus Association Canada: <http://www.sbhac.ca/beta/>.

Spina Bifida and Hydrocephalus Association Canada—List of latex products and alternative products: <http://www.sbhac.ca/pdf/Latex_Allergies.pdf>.

APPENDIX A

Eating Well With Canada's Food Guide

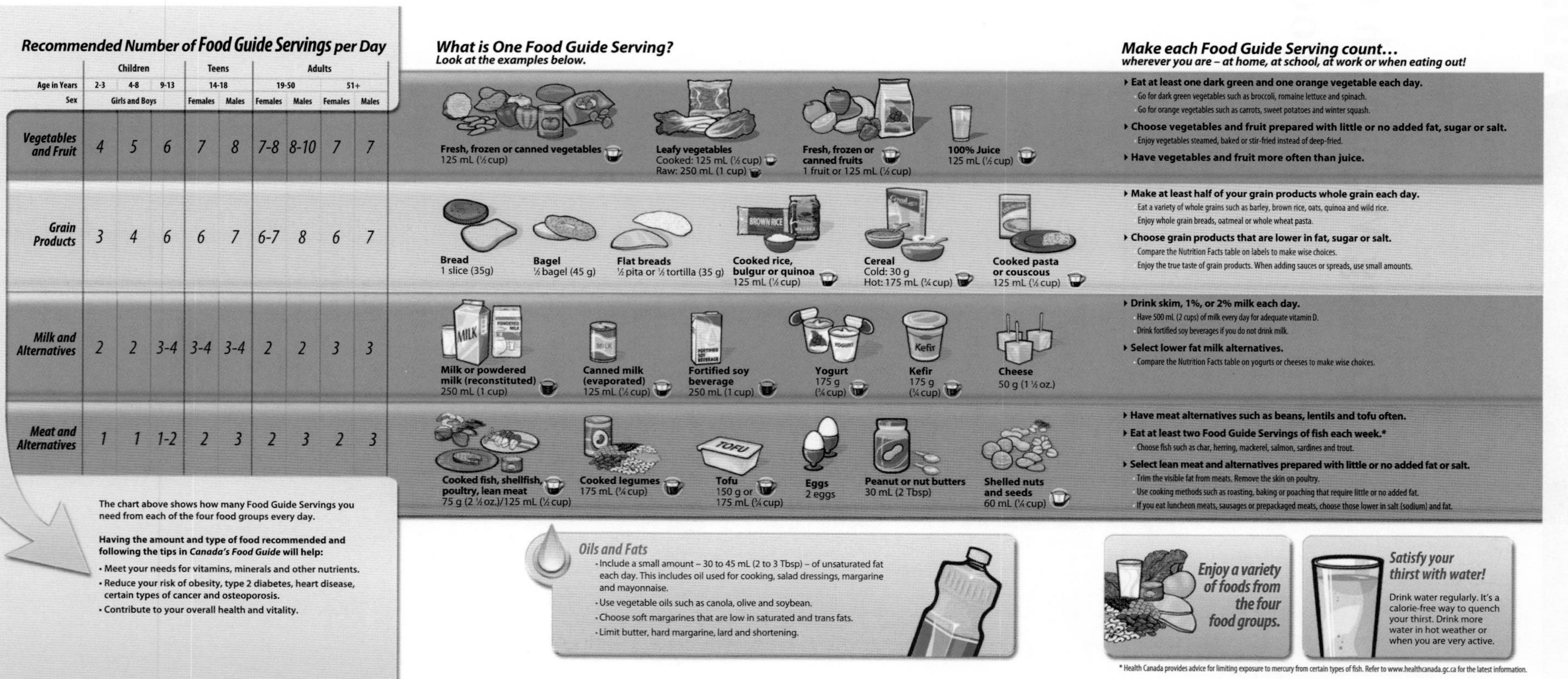

Recommended Number of Food Guide Servings per Day

Age in Years	2-3	4-8	9-13	14-18	14-18	19-50	19-50	51+	51+
	Children			Teens		Adults			
Sex	Girls and Boys			Females	Males	Females	Males	Females	Males
Vegetables and Fruit	4	5	6	7	8	7-8	8-10	7	7
Grain Products	3	4	6	6	7	6-7	8	6	7
Milk and Alternatives	2	2	3-4	3-4	3-4	2	2	3	3
Meat and Alternatives	1	1	1-2	2	3	2	3	2	3

FIGURE A-1 *Eating Well with Canada's Food Guide* recommends daily food intake for people of all ages as well as serving sizes. Using this guide will help improve overall health. Please note that there is also an *Eating Well With Canada's Food Guide—First Nations, Inuit, and Métis* (http://www.hc-sc.gc.ca/fn-an/food-guide-aliment/fnim-pnim/index-eng.php). (© All rights reserved. *Eating Well with Canada's Food Guide*. Health Canada, 2011. Adapted and reproduced with permission from the Minister of Health, 2016.)

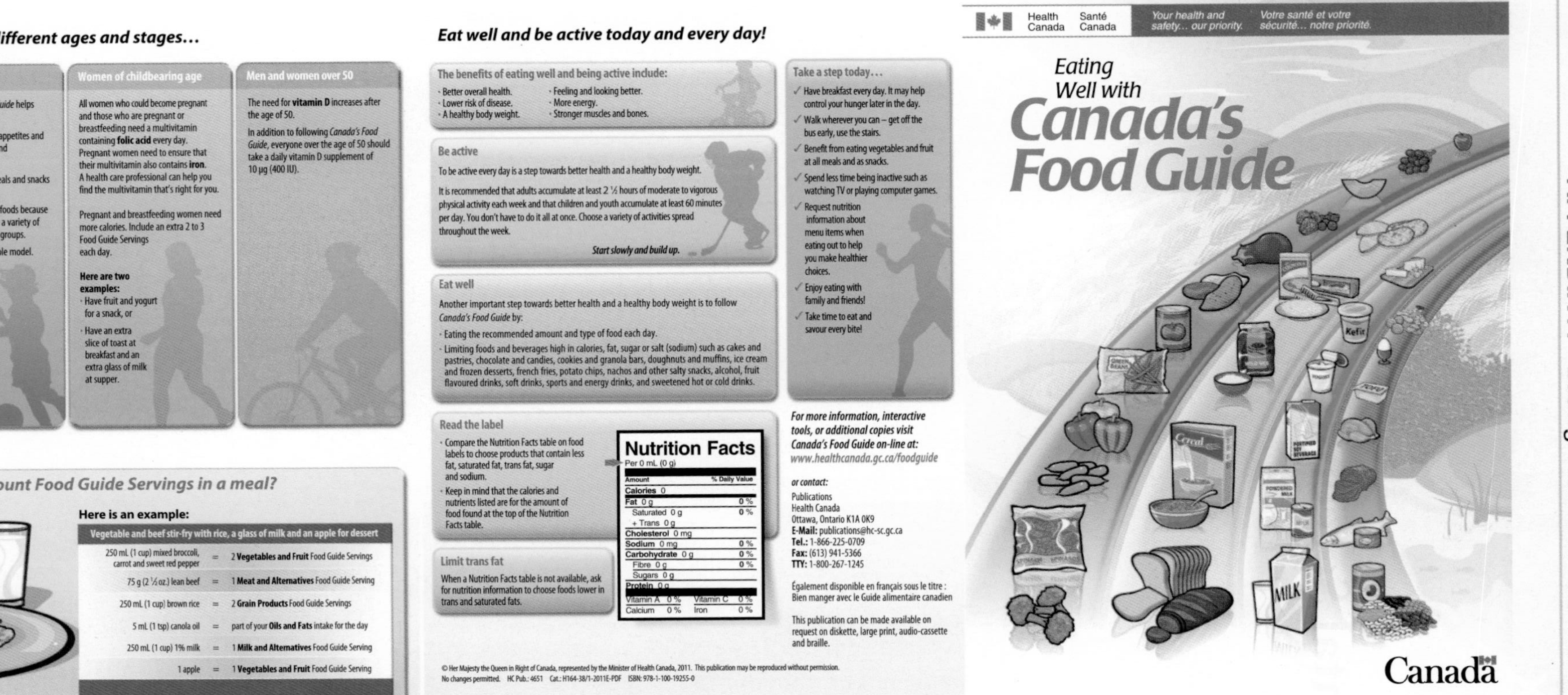

Advice for different ages and stages…

Children

Following *Canada's Food Guide* helps children grow and thrive.

Young children have small appetites and need calories for growth and development.

- Serve small nutritious meals and snacks each day.
- Do not restrict nutritious foods because of their fat content. Offer a variety of foods from the four food groups.
- Most of all... be a good role model.

Women of childbearing age

All women who could become pregnant and those who are pregnant or breastfeeding need a multivitamin containing **folic acid** every day. Pregnant women need to ensure that their multivitamin also contains **iron**. A health care professional can help you find the multivitamin that's right for you.

Pregnant and breastfeeding women need more calories. Include an extra 2 to 3 Food Guide Servings each day.

Here are two examples:

- Have fruit and yogurt for a snack, or
- Have an extra slice of toast at breakfast and an extra glass of milk at supper.

Men and women over 50

The need for **vitamin D** increases after the age of 50.

In addition to following *Canada's Food Guide*, everyone over the age of 50 should take a daily vitamin D supplement of 10 μg (400 IU).

How do I count Food Guide Servings in a meal?

Here is an example:

Vegetable and beef stir-fry with rice, a glass of milk and an apple for dessert		
250 mL (1 cup) mixed broccoli, carrot and sweet red pepper	=	2 **Vegetables and Fruit** Food Guide Servings
75 g (2 ½ oz.) lean beef	=	1 **Meat and Alternatives** Food Guide Serving
250 mL (1 cup) brown rice	=	2 **Grain Products** Food Guide Servings
5 mL (1 tsp) canola oil	=	part of your **Oils and Fats** intake for the day
250 mL (1 cup) 1% milk	=	1 **Milk and Alternatives** Food Guide Serving
1 apple	=	1 **Vegetables and Fruit** Food Guide Serving

Eat well and be active today and every day!

The benefits of eating well and being active include:

- Better overall health.
- Lower risk of disease.
- A healthy body weight.
- Feeling and looking better.
- More energy.
- Stronger muscles and bones.

Be active

To be active every day is a step towards better health and a healthy body weight.

It is recommended that adults accumulate at least 2 ½ hours of moderate to vigorous physical activity each week and that children and youth accumulate at least 60 minutes per day. You don't have to do it all at once. Choose a variety of activities spread throughout the week.

Start slowly and build up.

Eat well

Another important step towards better health and a healthy body weight is to follow *Canada's Food Guide* by:

- Eating the recommended amount and type of food each day.
- Limiting foods and beverages high in calories, fat, sugar or salt (sodium) such as cakes and pastries, chocolate and candies, cookies and granola bars, doughnuts and muffins, ice cream and frozen desserts, french fries, potato chips, nachos and other salty snacks, alcohol, fruit flavoured drinks, soft drinks, sports and energy drinks, and sweetened hot or cold drinks.

Read the label

- Compare the Nutrition Facts table on food labels to choose products that contain less fat, saturated fat, trans fat, sugar and sodium.
- Keep in mind that the calories and nutrients listed are for the amount of food found at the top of the Nutrition Facts table.

Nutrition Facts

Per 0 mL (0 g)

Amount	% Daily Value
Calories 0	
Fat 0 g	0 %
Saturated 0 g + Trans 0 g	0 %
Cholesterol 0 mg	
Sodium 0 mg	0 %
Carbohydrate 0 g	0 %
Fibre 0 g	0 %
Sugars 0 g	
Protein 0 g	
Vitamin A 0 %	Vitamin C 0 %
Calcium 0 %	Iron 0 %

Limit trans fat

When a Nutrition Facts table is not available, ask for nutrition information to choose foods lower in trans and saturated fats.

Take a step today…

- ✓ Have breakfast every day. It may help control your hunger later in the day.
- ✓ Walk wherever you can – get off the bus early, use the stairs.
- ✓ Benefit from eating vegetables and fruit at all meals and as snacks.
- ✓ Spend less time being inactive such as watching TV or playing computer games.
- ✓ Request nutrition information about menu items when eating out to help you make healthier choices.
- ✓ Enjoy eating with family and friends!
- ✓ Take time to eat and savour every bite!

For more information, interactive tools, or additional copies visit Canada's Food Guide on-line at:
www.healthcanada.gc.ca/foodguide

or contact:
Publications
Health Canada
Ottawa, Ontario K1A 0K9
E-Mail: publications@hc-sc.gc.ca
Tel.: 1-866-225-0709
Fax: (613) 941-5366
TTY: 1-800-267-1245

Également disponible en français sous le titre : Bien manger avec le Guide alimentaire canadien

This publication can be made available on request on diskette, large print, audio-cassette and braille.

 HC Pub.: 4651 Cat.: H164-38/1-2011E-PDF ISBN: 978-1-100-19255-0

FIGURE A-1, cont'd

APPENDIX B

Developmental Screening

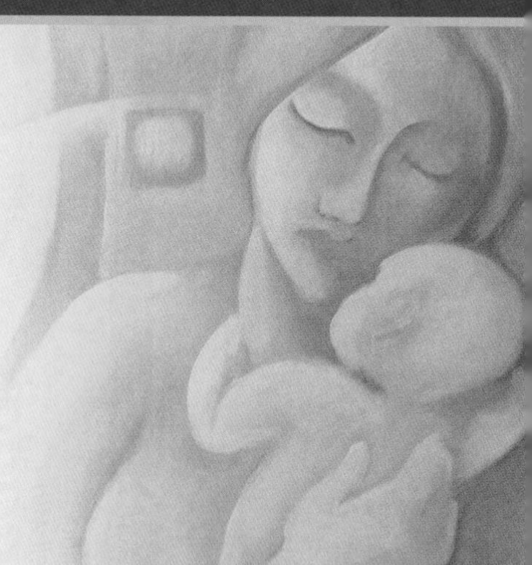

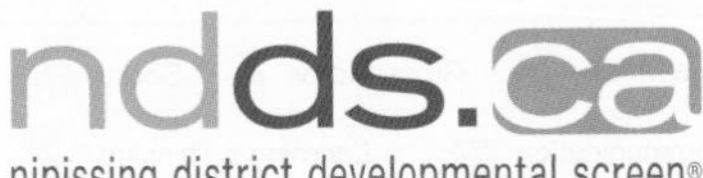

Child's Name: ______________________

Birthdate: ______________ Today's Date: ______________

The ndds checklist is designed to help monitor your child's development.

Y	N		BY **EIGHTEEN MONTHS** OF AGE, DOES YOUR CHILD:
O	O	1	Identify pictures in a book? *("show me the baby")**
O	O	2	Use a variety of familiar gestures? *(waving, pushing, giving, reaching up)**
O	O	3	Follow directions using "on" and "under"? *("put the cup on the table")**
O	O	4	Make at least four different consonant sounds? *(b, n, d, h, g, w)**
O	O	5	Point to at least three different body parts when asked? *("where is your nose?")**
O	O	6	Say 20 or more words? *(words do not have to be clear)*
O	O	7	Hold a cup to drink?**
O	O	8	Pick up and eat finger food?
O	O	9	Help with dressing by putting out arms and legs?**
O	O	10	Walk up a few stairs holding your hand?
O	O	11	Walk alone?
O	O	12	Squat to pick up a toy and stand back up without falling?
O	O	13	Push and pull toys or other objects while walking forward? *A*
O	O	14	Stack three or more blocks?
O	O	15	Show affection towards people, pets, or toys?
O	O	16	Point to show you something?
O	O	17	Look at you when you are talking or playing together?

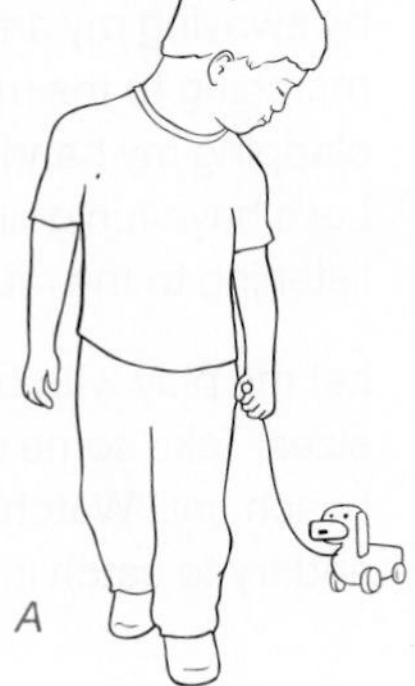

18
MONTHS
English

* Examples provided are only suggestions. You may use similar examples from your family experience.

** Item may not be common to all cultures.

Always talk to your healthcare or childcare professional if you have any questions about your child's development or well being. See reverse for instructions, limitation of liability, and product license. Source: ndds

FIGURE B-1 A: The Nipissing District Developmental Screen Checklist for the 18-month age group.

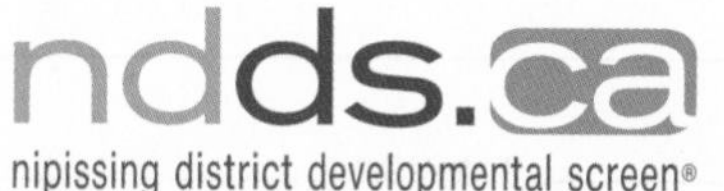

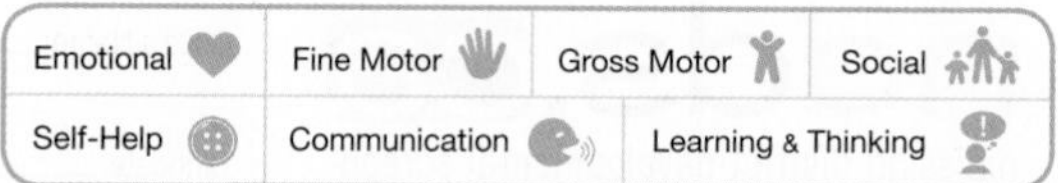

The following **activities for your child** will help you play your part in your child's development.

I feel safe and secure when I know what is expected of me. You can help me with this by following routines and setting limits. Praise my good behaviour.

I like toys that I can pull apart and put back together—large building blocks, containers with lids, or plastic links. Talk to me about what I am doing using words like "push" and "pull".

I'm not too little to play with large crayons. Let's scribble and talk about our art work.

Don't be afraid to let me see what I can do with my body. I need to practise climbing, swinging, jumping, running, going up and down stairs, and going down slides. Stay close to me so I don't get hurt.

Play some of my favourite music. Encourage me to move to the music by swaying my arms, moving slowly, marching to the music, hopping, clapping my hands, tapping my legs. Let's have fun doing actions while listening to the music.

Let me play with balls of different sizes. Take some of the air out of a beach ball. Watch me kick, throw, and try to catch it.

I want to do things just like you. Let me have toys so I can pretend to have tea parties, dress up, and play mommy or daddy.

I like new toys, so find the local toy lending library or play groups in our community.

I am learning new words every day. Put pictures of people or objects in a bag and say "1, 2, 3, what do we see?" and pull a picture from the bag.

Pretend to talk to me on the phone or encourage me to call someone.

Help me to notice familiar sounds such as birds chirping, car or truck motors, airplanes, dogs barking, sirens, or splashing water. Imitate the noise you hear and see if I will imitate you. Encourage me by smiling and clapping.

I like simple puzzles with two to four pieces and shape-sorters with simple shapes. Encourage me to match the pieces by taking turns with me.

I enjoy exploring the world, but I need to know that you are close by. I may cry when you leave me with others, so give me a hug and tell me you will be back.

I may get ear infections. Talk to my doctor about signs and symptoms.

Always talk to your healthcare or childcare professional if you have any questions about your child's development or well being. See reverse for instructions, limitation of liability, and product license.

FIGURE B-1, cont'd B: Activities that parents and caregivers can use to help play a part in an 18-month-old's development. (Source: ndds © 2011 ndds Intellectual Property Association. All rights reserved.)

APPENDIX

C

Growth Charts and Body Mass Index (BMI) Calculation

WHO GROWTH CHARTS FOR CANADA

BOYS

BIRTH TO 24 MONTHS: BOYS

Length-for-age and Weight-for-age percentiles

NAME: ______________________

DOB: ____________ **RECORD #** ________

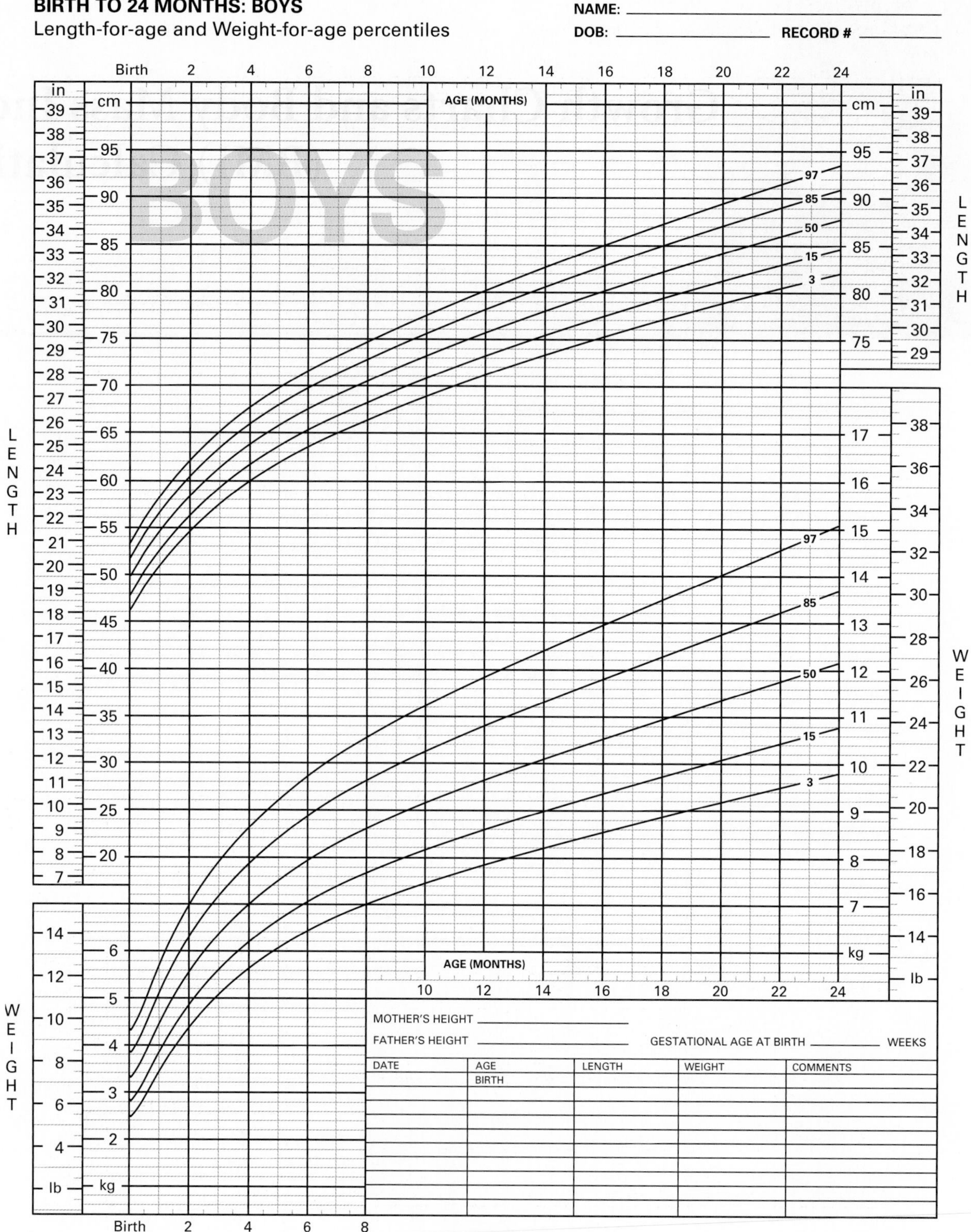

SOURCE: Based on World Health Organization (WHO) Child Growth Standards (2006) and WHO Reference (2007) and adapted for Canada by Canadian Paediatric Society, Canadian Pediatric Endocrine Group, College of Family Physicians of Canada, Community Health Nurses of Canada and Dietitians of Canada.

WHO GROWTH CHARTS FOR CANADA

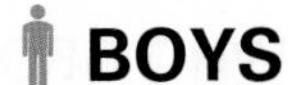

2 TO 19 YEARS: BOYS
Height-for-age and Weight-for-age percentiles

NAME: ______
DOB: ______ RECORD # ______

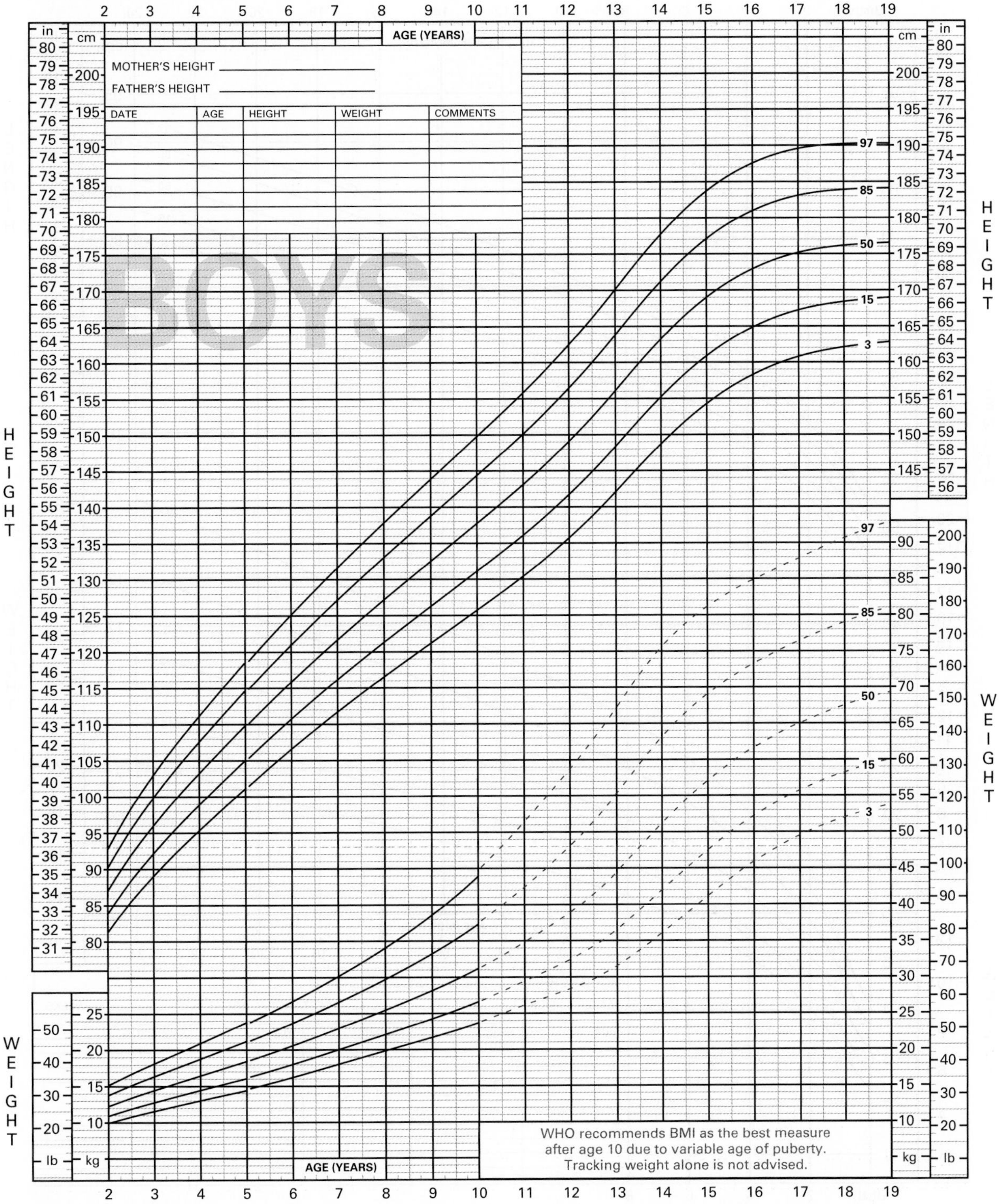

MOTHER'S HEIGHT ______
FATHER'S HEIGHT ______

DATE	AGE	HEIGHT	WEIGHT	COMMENTS

AGE (YEARS): 2 3 4 5 6 7 8 9 10 11 12 13 14 15 16 17 18 19

HEIGHT (cm): 80–200; (in): 31–80

Percentiles: 97, 85, 50, 15, 3

WEIGHT (kg): 10–90; (lb): 20–200

WHO recommends BMI as the best measure after age 10 due to variable age of puberty. Tracking weight alone is not advised.

SOURCE: The main chart is based on World Health Organization (WHO) Child Growth Standards (2006) and WHO Reference (2007) adapted for Canada by Canadian Paediatric Society, Canadian Pediatric Endocrine Group (CPEG), College of Family Physicians of Canada, Community Health Nurses of Canada and Dietitians of Canada. The weight-for-age 10 to 19 years section was developed by CPEG based on data from the US National Center for Health Statistics using the same procedures as the WHO growth charts.

WHO GROWTH CHARTS FOR CANADA

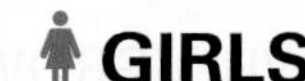

BIRTH TO 24 MONTHS: GIRLS
Length-for-age and Weight-for-age percentiles

NAME: ______
DOB: ______ RECORD # ______

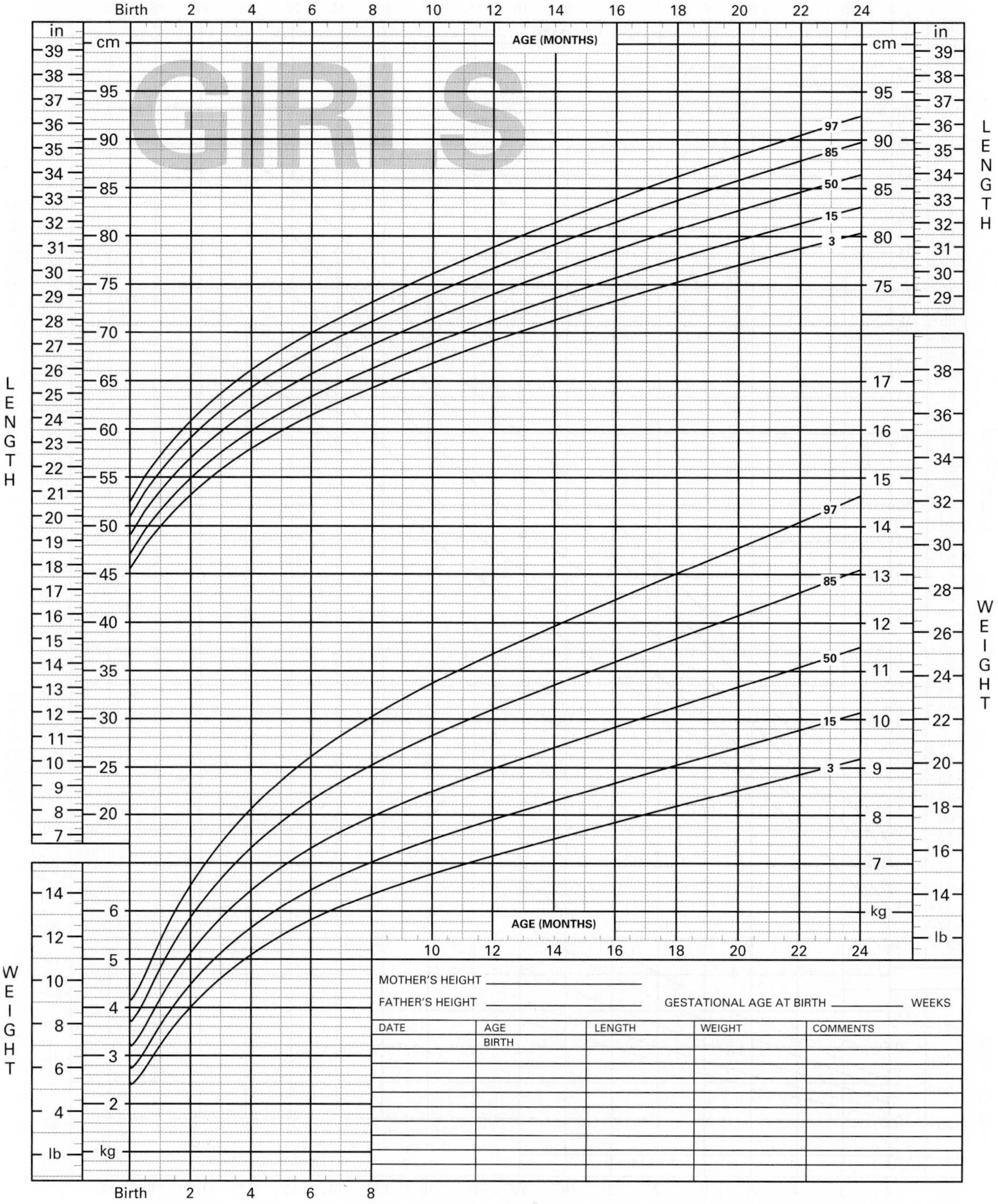

MOTHER'S HEIGHT ______
FATHER'S HEIGHT ______ GESTATIONAL AGE AT BIRTH ______ WEEKS

DATE	AGE	LENGTH	WEIGHT	COMMENTS
	BIRTH			

SOURCE: Based on World Health Organization (WHO) Child Growth Standards (2006) and WHO Reference (2007) and adapted for Canada by Canadian Paediatric Society, Canadian Pediatric Endocrine Group, College of Family Physicians of Canada, Community Health Nurses of Canada and Dietitians of Canada.

WHO GROWTH CHARTS FOR CANADA

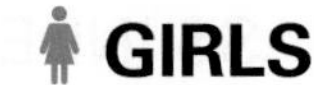
GIRLS

2 TO 19 YEARS: GIRLS

Height-for-age and Weight-for-age percentiles

NAME: ____________________

DOB: ____________ RECORD # ____________

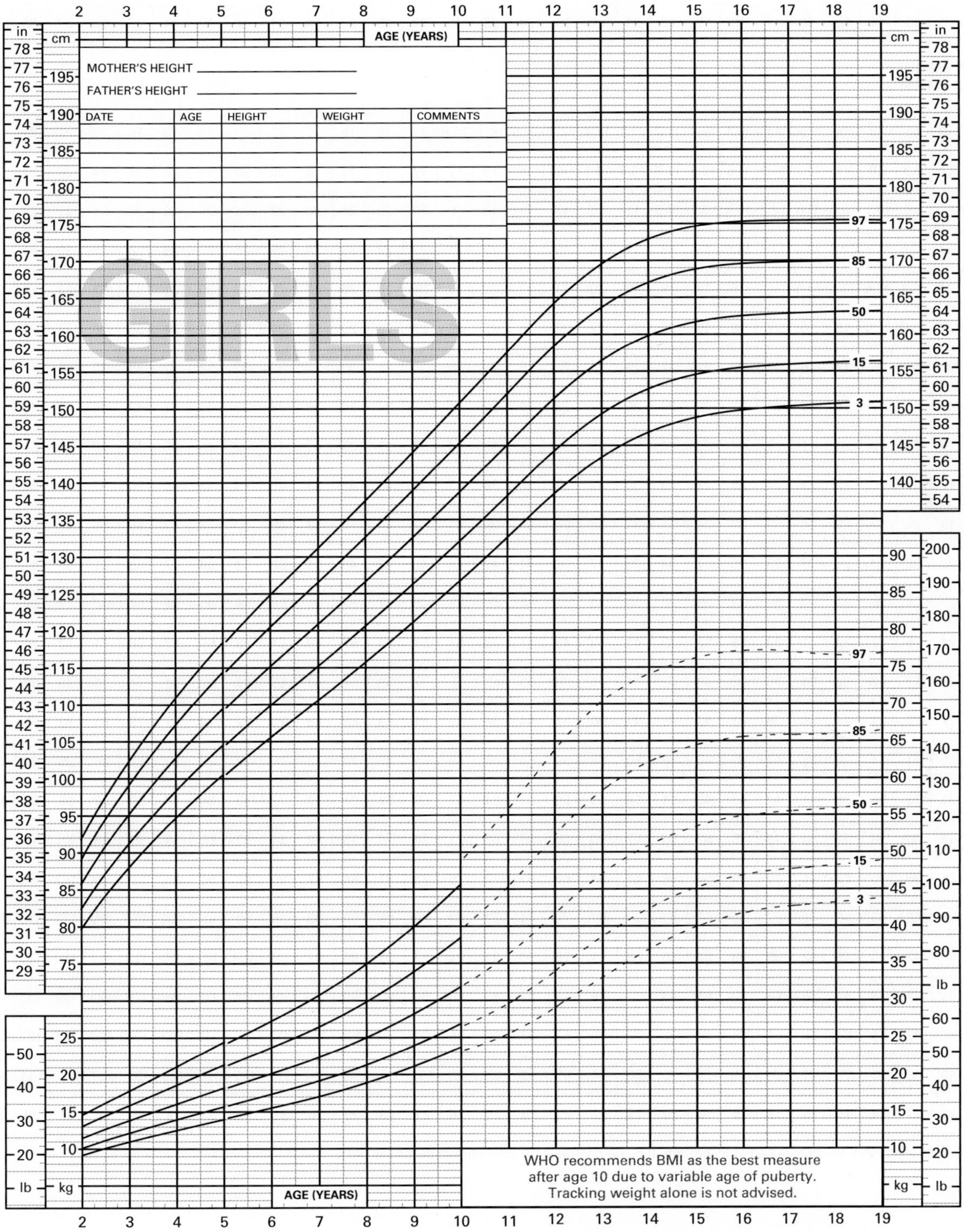

AGE (YEARS)

MOTHER'S HEIGHT ____________

FATHER'S HEIGHT ____________

DATE	AGE	HEIGHT	WEIGHT	COMMENTS

GIRLS

HEIGHT (cm, in) — percentiles 97, 85, 50, 15, 3

WEIGHT (kg, lb) — percentiles 97, 85, 50, 15, 3

WHO recommends BMI as the best measure after age 10 due to variable age of puberty. Tracking weight alone is not advised.

AGE (YEARS)

SOURCE: The main chart is based on World Health Organization (WHO) Child Growth Standards (2006) and WHO Reference (2007) adapted for Canada by Canadian Paediatric Society, Canadian Pediatric Endocrine Group (CPEG), College of Family Physicians of Canada, Community Health Nurses of Canada and Dietitians of Canada. The weight-for-age 10 to 19 years section was developed by CPEG based on data from the US National Center for Health Statistics using the same procedures as the WHO growth charts.

BODY MASS INDEX TABLE – TO CALCULATE FROM CENTIMETRES AND KILOGRAMS

USE TO CALCULATE BMI FOR THOSE AGED 2 YEARS OF AGE OR MORE

For greater precision or to calculate BMI values greater than 39, use the following equation: Weight (kg) ÷ Height (cm) ÷ Height (cm) x 10,000

BMI:	11	12	13	14	15	16	17	18	19	20	21	22	23	24	25	26	27	28	29	30	31	32	33	34	35	36	37	38	39	
HEIGHT (CM)	BODY WEIGHT (KILOGRAMS)																													HEIGHT (CM)
75	6.2	6.8	7.3	7.9	8.4	9.0	9.6	10.1	10.7	11.3	11.8	12.4	12.9	13.5	14.1	14.6	15	16	16	17	17	18	19	19	20	20	21	21	22	75
80	7.0	7.7	8.3	9.0	9.6	10.2	10.9	11.5	12.2	12.8	13.4	14.1	14.7	15	16	17	17	18	19	19	20	20	21	22	22	23	24	24	25	80
85	7.9	8.7	9.4	10.1	10.8	11.6	12.3	13.0	13.7	14.5	15	16	17	17	18	19	20	20	21	22	22	23	24	25	25	26	27	27	28	85
90	8.9	9.7	10.5	11.3	12.2	13.0	13.8	14.6	15	16	17	18	19	19	20	21	22	23	23	24	25	26	27	28	28	29	30	31	32	90
95	9.9	10.8	11.7	12.6	13.5	14.4	15	16	17	18	19	20	21	22	23	23	24	25	26	27	28	29	30	31	32	32	33	34	35	95
100	11.0	12.0	13.0	14.0	15	16	17	18	19	20	21	22	23	24	25	26	27	28	29	30	31	32	33	34	35	36	37	38	39	100
105	12.1	13.2	14.3	15	17	18	19	20	21	22	23	24	25	26	28	29	30	31	32	33	34	35	36	37	39	40	41	42	43	105
110	13.3	14.5	16	17	18	19	21	22	23	24	25	27	28	29	30	31	33	34	35	36	38	39	40	41	42	44	45	46	47	110
115	14.5	16	17	19	20	21	22	24	25	26	28	29	30	32	33	34	36	37	38	40	41	42	44	45	46	48	49	50	52	115
120	16	17	19	20	22	23	24	26	27	29	30	32	33	35	36	37	39	40	42	43	45	46	48	49	50	52	53	55	56	120
125	17	19	20	22	23	25	27	28	30	31	33	34	36	38	39	41	42	44	45	47	48	50	52	53	55	56	58	59	61	125
130	19	20	22	24	25	27	29	30	32	34	35	37	39	41	42	44	46	47	49	51	52	54	56	57	59	61	63	64	66	130
135	20	22	24	26	27	29	31	33	35	36	38	40	42	44	46	47	49	51	53	55	56	58	60	62	64	66	67	69	71	135
140	22	24	25	27	29	31	33	35	37	39	41	43	45	47	49	51	53	55	57	59	61	63	65	67	69	71	73	74	76	140
145	23	25	27	29	32	34	36	38	40	42	44	46	48	50	53	55	57	59	61	63	65	67	69	71	74	76	78	80	82	145
150	25	27	29	32	34	36	38	41	43	45	47	50	52	54	56	59	61	63	65	68	70	72	74	77	79	81	83	86	88	150
155	26	29	31	34	36	38	41	43	46	48	50	53	55	58	60	62	65	67	70	72	74	77	79	82	84	86	89	91	94	155
160	28	31	33	36	38	41	44	46	49	51	54	56	59	61	64	67	69	72	74	77	79	82	84	87	90	92	95	97	100	160
165	30	33	35	38	41	44	46	49	52	54	57	60	63	65	68	71	74	76	79	82	84	87	90	93	95	98	101	103	106	165
170	32	35	38	40	43	46	49	52	55	58	61	64	66	69	72	75	78	81	84	87	90	92	95	98	101	104	107	110	113	170
175	34	37	40	43	46	49	52	55	58	61	64	67	70	74	77	80	83	86	89	92	95	98	101	104	107	110	113	116	119	175
180	36	39	42	45	49	52	55	58	62	65	68	71	75	78	81	84	87	91	94	97	100	104	107	110	113	117	120	123	126	180
185	38	41	44	48	51	55	58	62	65	68	72	75	79	82	86	89	92	96	99	103	106	110	113	116	120	123	127	130	133	185
190	40	43	47	51	54	58	61	65	69	72	76	79	83	87	90	94	97	101	105	108	112	116	119	123	126	130	134	137	141	190
195	42	46	49	53	57	61	65	68	72	76	80	84	87	91	95	99	103	106	110	114	118	122	125	129	133	137	141	144	148	195
BMI:	11	12	13	14	15	16	17	18	19	20	21	22	23	24	25	26	27	28	29	30	31	32	33	34	35	36	37	38	39	

APPENDIX D

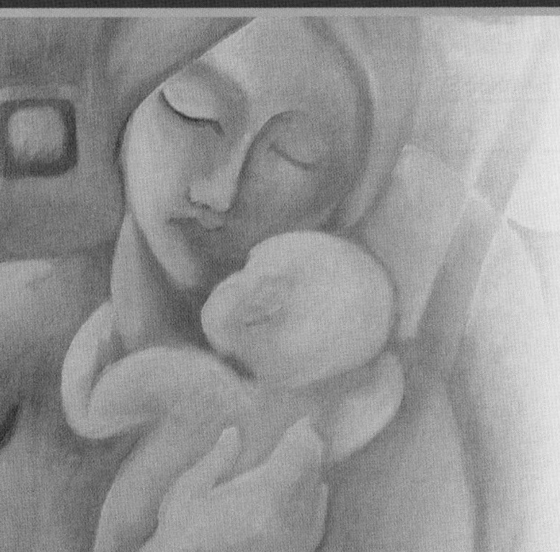

Common Laboratory Tests and Normal Ranges

TABLE D-1 CHEMISTRY: BLOOD, URINE, CEREBROSPINAL FLUID*

TEST/SPECIMEN	AGE/GENDER/ REFERENCE	NORMAL RANGES			
		INTERNATIONAL UNITS (SI)		CONVENTIONAL UNITS	
Acetaminophen					
Serum or plasma	Therap. conc.	66–200 mcmol/L		10–30 mcg/mL	
	Toxic conc.	>1300 mcmol/L		>200 mcg/mL	
Ammonia nitrogen					
Plasma or serum	Newborn	52–88 mcmol/L		90–150 mcg/dL	
	Adult/child	6–47 mcmol/L		10–80 mcg/dL	
Arterial blood gases (ABG)					
pH	Newborn	7.32–7.49		7.32–7.49	
	2 mo–2 yr	7.34–7.46		7.34–7.46	
	Adult/child	7.35–7.45		7.35–7.45	
Partial pressure of carbon dioxide (P_{CO_2})	<2 yr	26–41 mm Hg		26–41 mm Hg	
	Adult/child	35–45 mm Hg		35–45 mm Hg	
	P_{CO_2} (venous)	40–50 mm Hg		40–50 mm Hg	
Bicarbonate ion (HCO_3)	Newborn/infant	16–24 mmol/L		16–24 mEq/L	
	Adult/child	21–28 mmol/L		21–28 mEq/L	
	Venous	22–29 mmol/L		22–29 mEq/L	
Partial pressure of oxygen (P_{O_2})	Newborn	60–70 mm Hg		60–70 mm Hg	
	Adult/child	80–100 mm Hg		80–100 mm Hg	
	P_{O_2} (venous)	40–50 mm Hg		40–50 Hg	
Oxygen saturation	Newborn	85%–90%		85%–90%	
	Adult/child	95%–99%		95%–99%	
Oxygen content	Arterial	15–22 volume percent			
	Venous	11–16 volume percent			
Base excess					
Whole blood	Newborn	(–10)–(–2) mmol/L		(–10)–(–2) mEq/L	
	Infant	(–7)–(–1) mmol/L		(–7)–(–1) mEq/L	
	Child	(–4)–(+2) mmol/L		(–4)–(+2) mEq/L	
	Thereafter	(–3)–(+3) mmol/L		(–3)–(+3) mEq/L	
Bilirubin, total		**Premature** (mcmol/L)	**Full term** (mcmol/L)	**Premature** (mg/dL)	**Full term** (mg/dL)
Serum	Cord	<34	<34	<2.0	<2.0
	0–1 day	<137	<103	<8.0	<6.0
	1–2 days	<205	<137	<12.0	<8.0
	2–5 days	< 274	<205	<16.0	<12.0
	Thereafter	<340	<171	<20.0	<10.0

Continued

TABLE D-1 CHEMISTRY: BLOOD, URINE, CEREBROSPINAL FLUID—cont'd

		NORMAL RANGES			
TEST/SPECIMEN	AGE/GENDER/ REFERENCE	INTERNATIONAL UNITS (SI)		CONVENTIONAL UNITS	
Bilirubin, direct (conjugated)					
Serum		0–3.4 mcmol/L		0.0–0.2 mg/dL	
Calcium, ionized					
Serum, plasma, or whole blood	Cord	1.25–1.50 mmol/L		5.0–6.0 mg/dL	
	Newborn, 3–24 hr	1.05–1.37 mmol/L		4.20–5.58 mg/dL	
	24–48 hr	1.00–1.17 mmol/L		4.0–4.7 mg/dL	
	Thereafter	1.20–1.38 mmol/L		4.80–5.52 mg/dL	
Calcium, total					
Serum	Cord	2.25–2.88 mmol/L		9.0–11.5 mg/dL	
	Newborn, 3–24 hr	2.3–2.65 mmol/L		9.0–10.6 mg/dL	
	24–48 hr	1.75–3.0 mmol/L		7.0–12.0 mg/dL	
	4–7 days	2.25–2.73 mmol/L		9.0–10.9 mg/dL	
	Child	2.2–2.7 mmol/L		8.8–10.8 mg/dL	
	Thereafter	2.1–2.55 mmol/L		8.4–10.2 mg/dL	
Cerebrospinal fluid (CSF)					
Pressure		70–180 mm H_2O		70–180 mm H_2O	
Volume	Child	0.06–0.10 L		60–100 mL	
	Adult	0.10–0.16 L		100–160 mL	
Chloride					
Serum or plasma	Cord	96–104 mmol/L		96–104 mEq/L	
	Newborn	96–106 mmol/L		96–106 mEq/L	
	Thereafter	90–110 mmol/L		90–110 mEq/L	
Sweat	Normal (homozygote)	<40 mmol/L		<40 mEq/L	
	Marginal (e.g., asthma, Addison disease, malnutrition)	45–60 mmol/L		45–60 mEq/L	
	Cystic fibrosis	>60 mmol/L		>60 mEq/L	
Cholesterol, total		**Male** (mmol/L)	**Female** (mmol/L)	**Male** (mg/dL)	**Female** (mg/dL)
Serum or plasma	Newborn	0.98–4.50	1.45–5.04	38–174	56–195
	Infant (7–12 mo)	2.15–5.30	1.76–5.59	83–205	68–216
	10–11 yr	3.10–5.90	3.16–6.26	120–228	122–242
Creatine kinase (CK, CPK)					
Serum	Cord	70–380 U/L		70–380 U/L	
	Newborn	65–580 U/L		65–580 U/L	
	Male	55–170 U/L		55–170 U/L	
	Female	30–135 U/L		30–135 U/L	
Creatinine					
Serum	Newborn	53–97 mcmol/L		0.6–1.1 mg/dL	
	Infant	18–35 mcmol/L		0.2–0.4 mg/dL	
	Child/adolescent	18–62 mcmol/L		0.2–0.7 mg/dL	
	Adult male	53–106 mcmol/L		0.6–1.2 mg/dL	
	Adult female	44–97 mcmol/L		0.5–1.1 mg/dL	
Urine, 24 hr	Premature	72–133 mcmol/kg/24 hr		8.1–15.0 mg/kg/24 hr	
	Full term	92–174 mcmol/kg/24 hr		10.4–19.7 mg/kg/24 hr	
	1.5–7 yr	88–133 mcmol/kg/24 hr		10–15 mg/kg/24 hr	
	7–15 yr	46–362 mcmol/kg/24 hr		5.2–41 mg/kg/24 hr	
Creatinine clearance (endogenous)					
Serum or plasma and urine	Newborn	1.2 mL/sec		72 mL/min	
	Male	1.78–2.32 mL/sec		107–139 mL/min	
	Female	1.45–1.78 mL/sec		87–107 mL/min	

TABLE D-1 **CHEMISTRY: BLOOD, URINE, CEREBROSPINAL FLUID—cont'd**

TEST/SPECIMEN	AGE/GENDER/ REFERENCE	NORMAL RANGES INTERNATIONAL UNITS (SI)		CONVENTIONAL UNITS	
Digoxin					
Serum, plasma; collect at least 12 hr after dose	Therap. conc.				
	HF	1.0–1.9 nmol/L		0.8–1.5 ng/mL	
	Arrhythmias	1.9–2.6 nmol/L		1.5–2.0 ng/mL	
	Toxic conc.				
	Child	>3.2 nmol/L		>2.5 ng/mL	
	Adult	>3.8 nmol/L		>3.0 ng/mL	
Galactose					
Serum	Newborn	0–1.11 mmol/L		0–20 mg/dL	
	Thereafter	<0.28 mmol/L		<5 mg/dL	
Urine	Newborn	≤3.33 mmol/L		≤60 mg/dL	
	Thereafter	<0.08 mmol/day		<14 mg/24 hr	
Glucose					
Serum	Cord	2.5–5.3 mmol/L		45–96 mg/dL	
	Premature infant	1.1–3.3 mmol/L		20–60 mg/dL	
	Neonate (0–28 days)	1.7–3.3 mmol/L		30–60 mg/dL	
	Infant	2.2–5.0 mmol/L		40–90 mg/dL	
	Child <2 yr	3.3–5.5 mmol/L		60–100 mg/dL	
	>2 yr to Adult:	<6.1 mmol/L		<110 mg/dL	
	Fasting (no calories × 8 hours)				
	Random (any time of day)	<11.1 mmol/L		<200 mg/dL	
CSF	Adult	2.2–3.9 mmol/L		40–70 mg/dL	
Urine (quantitative)		<2.8 mmol/day		<0.5 g/day	
Urine (qualitative)		Negative		Negative	
Glucose tolerance test (GTT), oral					
Serum					
Dosages		**Normal**	**Diabetic**	**Normal**	**Diabetic**
Adult: 75 g	Fasting	4.0–6.0 mmol/L	≥7.0 mmol/L	70–110 mg/dL	≥126 mg/dL
Child: 1.75 g/kg of ideal weight up to maximum of 75 g	30 min	<11.1 mmol/L	≥11 mmol/L	<200 mg/dL	≥200 mg/dL
	60 min	<11.1 mmol/L	≥11 mmol/L	<200 mg/dL	≥200 mg/dL
	120 min	<7.8 mmol/L	≥11 mmol/L	<140 mg/dL	≥200 mg/dL
Growth hormone (GH, somatotropin)					
Plasma	0 to <7 yr	< 1–13.6 mcg/L		<1–13.6 ng/mL	
	7 to <11 yr	<1–16.4 mcg/L		<1–16.4 ng/mL	
	11 to <15 yr	<1–14.4 mcg/L		<1–14.4 ng/mL	
	15 to <19 yr	<1–13.4 mcg/L		<1–13.4 ng/mL	
	Adult male	<5 mcg/L		< 5 ng/mL	
	Adult female	<10 mcg/L		<10 ng/mL	
Iron	Age	Male mcmol/L	Female mcmol/L	Male mcg/dL	Female mcg/dL
Serum	Newborn	12.9–36.3	13.4–42.1	72–203	75–235
	Child (4–10 yr)	2.7–22.9	5.0–21.8	15–128	28–122
	Thereafter	14–32	11–29	80–180	60–160
	Intoxicated child	50.12–456.5 mcmol/L		280–2550 mcg/dL	
	Fatally poisoned child	>322.2 mcmol/L		>1800 mcg/dL	
Iron-binding capacity, total (TIBC)					
Serum	Infant	16.8–41.50 mcmol/L		94–232 mcg/dL	
	Thereafter	45–82 mcmol/L		250–460 mcg/dL	

Continued

TABLE D-1 **CHEMISTRY: BLOOD, URINE, CEREBROSPINAL FLUID—cont'd**

TEST/SPECIMEN	AGE/GENDER/ REFERENCE	NORMAL RANGES: INTERNATIONAL UNITS (SI)	NORMAL RANGES: CONVENTIONAL UNITS
Lead			
Whole blood	Child	<0.48 mcmol/L	<10 mcg/dL
Urine, 24 hr		<0.39 mcmol/L	<80 mcg/dL
Osmolality			
Serum	Child	275–290 mmol/kg	275–290 mOsm/kg
	Adult	280–300 mmol/kg	280–300 mOsm/kg
Urine, random		50–1400 mmol/kg, depending on fluid intake; after 12-hr fluid restriction: >850 mmol/kg	50–1400 mOsm/kg, depending on fluid intake; after 12-hr fluid restriction: >850 mOsm/kg
Urine, 24 hr		≅300–900 mmol/kg	≅300–900 mOsm/kg
pH			
Urine, random	Newborn	5–7	5–7
	Thereafter	4.5–8 (average ~6)	4.5–8 (average ~6)
Stool		7.0–7.5	7.0–7.5
Phenylalanine			
Serum	Premature	120–450 mcmol/L	2.0–7.5 mg/dL
	Newborn	70–210 mcmol/L	1.2–3.4 mg/dL
	Thereafter	50–110 mcmol/L	0.8–1.8 mg/dL
Urine, 24 hr	10 days–2 wk	6–12 mcmol/day	1–2 mg/day
	3–12 yr	24–110 mcmol/day	4–18 mg/day
	Thereafter	Trace–103 mcmol/day	Trace–17 mg/day
Potassium			
Serum	Newborn	3.9–5.9 mmol/L	3.9–5.9 mEq/L
	Infant	4.1–5.3 mmol/L	4.1–5.3 mEq/L
	Child	3.4–4.7 mmol/L	3.4–4.7 mEq/L
	Adult	3.5–5.0 mmol/L	3.5–5.0 mEq/L
Urine, 24 hr		2.5–125 mmol/day (varies with diet)	2.5–125 mEq/day
Protein			
Serum, total	Premature	42–76 g/L	4.2–7.6 g/dL
	Newborn	46–74 g/L	4.6–7.4 g/dL
	Infant	60–67 g/L	6.0–6.7 g/dL
	Child	62–80 g/L	6.2–8.0 g/dL
	Adult	64–83 g/L	6.4–8.3 g/dL
Total			
Urine, 24 hr		10–140 mg/L	1–14 mg/dL
		50–80 mg/day	50–80 mg/day
		<250 mg/day (after intense exercise)	<250 mg/day (after intense exercise)
CSF		Lumbar: 80–320 mg/L	8–32 mg/dL
Salicylates			
Serum, plasma	Therap. conc.	1.1–2.2 mmol/L	15–30 mg/dL
	Toxic conc.	>18.5 mmol/L	>30 mg/dL
Sodium			
Serum or plasma	Newborn	134–144 mmol/L	134–144 mEq/L
	Infant	134–150 mmol/L	134–150 mEq/L
	Child	136–145 mmol/L	136–145 mEq/L
	Thereafter	136–145 mmol/L	136–145 mEq/L
Urine, 24 hr		40–220 mmol/day (diet dependent)	40–220 mEq/L
Specific gravity			
Urine, random	Adult	1.002–1.030	1.002–1.030
	After 12-hr fluid restriction	>1.025	>1.025
Urine, 24 hr		1.015–1.025	1.015–1.025

TABLE D-1 CHEMISTRY: BLOOD, URINE, CEREBROSPINAL FLUID—cont'd

TEST/SPECIMEN	AGE/GENDER/ REFERENCE	NORMAL RANGES: INTERNATIONAL UNITS (SI)		NORMAL RANGES: CONVENTIONAL UNITS	
Theophylline					
Serum, plasma	Therap. conc.				
	Bronchodilator	56–110 mcmol/L		10–20 mcg/mL	
	Premature apnea	28–56 mcmol/L		5–10 mcg/mL	
	Toxic conc.	>110 mcmol/L		>20 mcg/mL	
Thyroxine, total (T4)					
	Age	**Male** nmol/L	**Female** nmol/L	**Male** mcg/dL	**Female** mcg/dL
Serum	1–30 days	76–276	81–276	5.9–21.5	6.3–21.5
	31 days to 1 yr	82–179	63–176	6.4–13.9	4.9–13.7
	1–3 yr	90–169	91–180	7.0–13.1	7.1–14.1
	4–6 yr	79–162	93–180	6.1–12.6	7.2–14.0
	7–12 yr	86–172	79–156	6.7–13.4	6.1–12.1
	13–15 yr	62–148	75–144	4.8–11.5	5.8–11.2
	16–18 yr	76–148	67–170	5.9–11.5	5.2–13.2
	Newborn screen (filter paper)	>90 nmol/L		>7 mcg/dL	
Triglycerides (TG)	Age (years)	**Male** (mmol/L)	**Female** (mmol/L)	**Male** (mg/dL)	**Female** (mg/dL)
Serum, after ≥2-hr fast	0–3	0.31–1.41	0.31–1.41	27–125	27–125
	4–6	0.36–1.31	0.36–1.31	32–116	32–116
	7–9	0.32–1.46	0.32–1.46	28–129	28–129
	10–11	0.27–1.55	0.44–1.58	24–137	39–140
	12–13	0.27–1.64	0.42–1.47	24–145	37–130
	14–15	0.38–1.86	0.43–1.52	34–165	38–135
	16–19	0.38–1.58	0.42–1.58	34–140	37–140
Triiodothyronine (T_3), free					
	Age	**Male** pmol/L	**Female** pmol/L	**Male** ng/dL	**Female** ng/dL
Serum	1–3 day	2.2–7.4	2.2–8.3	0.14–.048	0.14–0.54
	4–30 days	2.2–8.4	2.3–7.7	0.14–0.55	0.15–0.50
	1–12 mo	3.1–10.6	3.8–10.0	0.20–0.69	0.25–0.65
	1–5 yr	3.7–10.3	4.6–9.2	0.24–0.67	0.30–0.60
	6–10 yr	4.4–9.2	4.1–9.5	0.29–0.60	0.27–0.62
	11–15 yr	4.8–9.1	4.0–8.8	0.31–0.59	0.26–0.57
	16–18 yr	5.4–8.8	4.3–8.0	0.35–0.57	0.28–0.52
Triiodothyronine, total (T_3-RIA)					
Serum	Cord	0.46–1.08 nmol/L		30–70 ng/dL	
	Newborn	1.16–4 nmol/L		72–260 ng/dL	
	1–5 yr	1.54–4 nmol/L		100–260 ng/dL	
	5–10 yr	1.39–3.70 nmol/L		90–240 ng/dL	
	10–15 yr	1.23–3.23 nmol/L		80–210 ng/dL	
	Thereafter	1.77–2.93 nmol/L		115–190 ng/dL	
Urea nitrogen					
Serum or plasma	Cord	7.5–14.3 mmol/L		21–40 mg/dL	
	Newborn	0.7–4.6 mmol/L		2–13 mg/dL	
	Infant	1.8–6.0 mmol/L		5–17 mg/dL	
	Child	1.8–6.4 mmol/L		5–18 mg/dL	
	Adult	3.6–7.1 mmol/L		10–20 mg/dL	
Urine volume					
Urine, 24 hr	Newborn	0.05–0.3 L/day		50–300 mL/day	
	Infant	0.35–0.5 L/day		350–550 mL/day	
	Child	0.5–1 L/day		500–1000 mL/day	
	Adolescent	0.7–1.4 L/day		700–1400 mL/day	
	Thereafter: Male	0.8–1.8 L/day		800–1800 mL/day	
	Thereafter: Female	0.6–1.6 L/day (varies with intake and other factors)		600–1600 mL/day	

*For a description of abbreviations, see p. 1805.

TABLE D-2 HEMATOLOGY*

TEST/SPECIMEN	AGE/GENDER/ REFERENCE	NORMAL VALUES: INTERNATIONAL UNITS (SI)		NORMAL VALUES: CONVENTIONAL UNITS	
Bleeding time					
Blood from skin puncture					
Ivy	Normal	2–7 min		2–7 min	
	Borderline	7–11 min		7–11 min	
Simplate (G-D)		2.75–8 min		2.75–8 min	
Blood volume					
Whole blood	Male	0.052–0.083 L/kg		52–83 mL/kg	
	Female	0.050–0.075 L/kg		50–75 mL/kg	
Clotting time (Lee–White)					
Whole blood		5–8 min (glass tubes)		5–8 min	
		5–15 min (room temp)		5–15 min	
		30 min (silicone tube)		30 min	
Erythrocyte (RBC) count					
Whole blood	Newborn	$4.8–7.1 \times 10^{12}$/L		$4.8–7.1 \times 10^{6}$ mcg/L	
	2–8 wk	$4.0–6.0 \times 10^{12}$/L		$4.0–6.0 \times 10^{6}$ mcg/L	
	2–6 mo	$3.5–5.5 \times 10^{12}$/L		$3.5–5.5 \times 10^{6}$ mcg/L	
	6 mo–1 yr	$3.5–5.2 \times 10^{12}$/L		$3.5–5.2 \times 10^{6}$ mcg/L	
	1–6 yr	$4.0–5.5 \times 10^{12}$/L		$4.0–5.5 \times 10^{6}$ mcg/L	
	6–18 yr	$4.0–5.5 \times 10^{12}$/L		$4.0–5.5 \times 10^{6}$ mcg/L	
Erythrocyte sedimentation rate (ESR)					
Whole blood					
	Newborn	0–2 mm/hr		0–2 mm/hr	
Westergren (modified)	Child	0–10 mm/hr		0–10 mm/hr	
	<50 yr: Male	0–15 mm/hr		0–15 mm/hr	
	<50 yr: Female	0–20 mm/hr		0–20 mm/hr	
Fibrinogen					
Plasma	Newborn	3.68–8.82 mcmol/L		125–300 mg/dL	
	Thereafter	5.8–11.8 mmol/L		200–400 mg/dL	
Hematocrit (HCT, Hct)					
	Age	**Male** Volume fraction	**Female** Volume fraction	**Male** (%)	**Female** (%)
Whole blood	Newborn	0.37–0.47	0.38–0.48	37–47	38–48
	15–30 days	0.41–0.43	0.34–0.42	41–43	34–42
	61–180 days	0.31–0.38	0.31–0.39	31–38	31–39
	6 mo to 2 yr	0.31–0.36	0.31–0.39	31–36	31–36
	6–12 yr	0.31–0.38	0.32–0.39	31–38	32–39
	12–18 yr	0.31–0.41	0.32–0.39	31–41	32–39
Hemoglobin (Hgb)					
Whole blood	Neonate: 0–28 days	140–240 g/L		14.0–24.0 g/dL	
	Newborn (1–2 mo)	120–200 g/L		12.0–20.0 g/dL	
	2–6 mo	100–170 g/L		10.0–17.0 g/dL	
	6 mo to 1 yr	95–140 g/L		9.5–14.0 g/dL	
	1 to 6 yr	95–140 g/L		9.5–14.0 g/dL	
	6–18 yr	100–150 g/L		10.0–15.0 g/dL	
Hemoglobin A					
Whole blood		95%–98% of total Hgb		95%–98%	
Hemoglobin F					
Whole blood	Newborn	50%–80% of total Hgb		50%–80%	
	<6 mo	<8% of total Hgb		<8%	
	>6 mo	1%–2% of total Hgb		1%–2%	
	Adult	0.8%–2% of total Hgb		0.8%–2%	

TABLE D-2 **HEMATOLOGY—cont'd**

TEST/SPECIMEN	AGE/GENDER/ REFERENCE	NORMAL VALUES: INTERNATIONAL UNITS (SI)	NORMAL VALUES: CONVENTIONAL UNITS
Leukocyte count (WBC count)		$\times 10^9$/L	cells/mm^3
Whole blood	Newborn (0–6 wk)	9.0–30.0	9000–30,000
	Child ≤2 yr	6.2–17.0	6200–17,000
	Adult/child >2 yr	5.0–10.0	5000–10,000
CSF (cell count)		$\times 10^6$ cells/L	$\times$ 1000 cells/mm^3
	Premature	0–25 mononuclear	0–25
		0–10 polymorphonuclear	0–10
		0–1000 RBC	0–1000
	Neonate	0–20 mononuclear	0–20
		0–10 polymorphonuclear	0–10
		0–800 RBC	0–800
	Newborn	0–5 mononuclear	0–5
		0–10 polymorphonuclear	0–10
		0–50 RBC	0–50
	Thereafter	0–5 mononuclear	0–5
Leukocyte differential count			
Whole blood	Percentage (%)	$\times 10^9$/L	Absolute (per mm^3)
Myelocytes	0	0	0
Neutrophils	55–70	2.5–8.0	2500–8000
Lymphocytes	20–40	1.0–4.0	1000–4000
Monocytes	2–8	0.1–0.7	100–700
Eosinophils	1–4	0.0–0.5	50–500
Basophils	0.5–1.0	0.02–0.05	15–50
Mean corpuscular hemoglobin (MCH)			
Whole blood	Newborn	32–34 pg	32–34 pg
	Adult/older child/ child	27–31 pg	27–31 pg
Mean corpuscular hemoglobin concentration (MCHC)			
Whole blood	Newborn	32–33 g/dL	32%–33%
	Adult/child	32–36 g/dL	32%–36%
Mean corpuscular volume (MCV)			
Whole blood	Newborn	96–108 fL	96–108 mm^3
	Adult/Child	80–95 fL	80–95 mm^3
Partial thromboplastin time (PTT)			
Whole blood (Na citrate)			
Nonactivated		60–70 sec (Platelin)	60–70 sec
Activated (aPTT)		30–40 sec (differs with method)	30–40 sec
Plasma volume			
Plasma	Male	0.025–0.043 L/kg	25–43 mL/kg
	Female	0.028–0.045 L/kg	28–45 mL/kg
Platelet count (thrombocyte count)			
Whole blood (EDTA)	Newborn	150–300 $\times 10^9$/L	150,000–300,000/ mm^3
	Premature infant	100–300 $\times 10^9$/L	100,000–300,000/ mm^3
	Infant	200–475 $\times 10^9$/L	200,000–475,000/ mm^3
	Child/Adult	150–400 $\times 10^9$/L	150,000–400,000/ mm^3
Prothrombin time (PT)			
Whole blood		11–12.5 sec	11–12.5 sec
Red blood cell volume			
Whole blood	Male	0.020–0.036 L/kg	20–36 mL/kg
	Female	0.019–0.031 L/kg	19–31 mL/kg

Continued

TABLE D-2 HEMATOLOGY—cont'd

TEST/SPECIMEN	AGE/GENDER/ REFERENCE	NORMAL VALUES	
		INTERNATIONAL UNITS (SI)	CONVENTIONAL UNITS
Reticulocyte count			
Whole blood	Newborn	2.5%–6.5% of total number of RBCs	
	Infant	0.5%–3.1% of total number of RBCs	
	Adult/child	0.5–2% of total number of RBCs	
Thrombin time			
Whole blood (Na citrate)		Control time ±2 sec when control is 9–13 sec	Control time ±2 sec when control is 9–13 sec
WBC: see Leukocyte count (WBC count)			

*For a description of abbreviations, see p. 1805.

TABLE D-3 SEROLOGY–IMMUNOLOGY*

TEST/SPECIMEN	AGE/GENDER/ REFERENCE	NORMAL RANGES	
		INTERNATIONAL UNITS (SI)	CONVENTIONAL UNITS
Antistreptolysin O titre (ASO)			
Serum	Newborn (0–6 mo)	Similar to mother's value	Similar to mother's value
	6 mo–2 yr	≤50 Todd units/mL	≤50 Todd units/mL
	2–4 yr	≤160 Todd unit/mL	≤160 Todd unit/mL
	5–12 yr	170–330 Todd units/mL	170–330 Todd units/mL
	Adult	≤160 Todd units/mL	≤160 Todd units/mL
C-reactive protein (CRP)			
Serum		<10 mg/L	<1.0 mg/dL
Immunoglobulin A (IgA)			
Serum	1 mo	0.01–0.04 g/L	1–4 mg/dL
	2–5 mo	0.04–0.8 g/L	4–80 mg/dL
	6–9 mo	0.08–0.8 g/L	8–80 mg/dL
	1 yr	0.15–1.10 g/L	15–110 mg/dL
	2–3 yr	0.18–1.50 g/L	18–150 mg/dL
	4–12 yr	0.25–3.5 g/L	25–350 mg/dL
	Adult	0.85–3.85 g/L	85–385 mg/dL
Immunoglobulin D (IgD)			
Serum	Newborn	None detected	None detected
	Thereafter	0–80 mg/L	0–8 mg/dL
Immunoglobulin E (IgE)			
Serum		>0.35 kIU/L	>0.35 kIU/L
Immunoglobulin G (IgG)			
Serum	1 mo	2.5–9.0 g/L	250–900 mg/dL
	2–5 mo	2.0–7.0 g/L	200–700 mg/dL
	6–9 mo	2.2–9.0 g/L	220–900 mg/dL
	1 yr	3.4–12.0 g/L	340–1200 mg/dL
	2–3 yr	4.2–12.0 g/L	420–1200 mg/dL
	4–12 yr	4.6–12.0 g/L	460–1200 mg/dL
	Adult	5.65–17.65 g/L	565–1765 mg/dL
Immunoglobulin M (IgM)			
Serum	1 mo	0.20–0.80 g/L	20–80 mg/dL
	2–5 mo	0.25–1.0 g/L	25–100 mg/dL
	6–9 mo	0.35–1.25 g/L	35–125 mg/dL
	1–8 yr	0.45–2.0 g/L	45–200 mg/dL
	9–12 yr	0.50–2.5 g/L	50–250 mg/dL
	Adult	0.55–3.75 g/L	55–375 mg/dL

*For a description of abbreviations, see p. 1805.

Modified from Kliegman, R. M., et al. (Eds.). (2016). *Nelson textbook of pediatrics* (20th ed.). Philadelphia: Saunders; Crocetti, M., & Barone, M. A. (Eds.). (2006). *Oski's essential pediatrics* (4th ed.). Philadelphia: Lippincott Williams & Wilkins; Pagana, K. D., Pagana, T. J., & Pike-MacDonald, S. A. (2013). *Mosby's Canadian manual of diagnostic and laboratory tests* (1st Canadian ed.). Toronto: Elsevier.

ABBREVIATIONS USED IN LABORATORY TESTS

ABBREVIATION	TERM
cap	capillary
HF	heart failure
conc.	concentration
CSF	cerebrospinal fluid
EDTA	ethylenediaminetetraacetate
g	gram
Hgb	hemoglobin
HgbF	fetal hemoglobin
hr	hour
IU	International unit
L	litre
m	metre
mEq	milliequivalent
min	minute
mm	millimetre
mm Hg	millimetres of mercury
mm H_2O	millimetres of water
mm^3	cubic millimetre
mo	month
mol	mole
Na	sodium
Pa	Pascal
RBC	red blood cells
sec	second
temp	temperature
therap	therapeutic
U	international unit of enzyme activity
vol	volume
WBC	white blood cells
wk	week
yr	year
>	greater than
≥	greater than or equal to
<	less than
≤	less than or equal to
±	plus/minus
≅	approximately equal to

PREFIXES DENOTING DECIMAL FACTORS

PREFIX	SYMBOL	AMOUNT
Deci	d	one tenth (10^{-1})
Centi	c	one hundredth (10^{-2})
Milli	m	one thousandth (10^{-3})
Micro	mc	one millionth (10^{-6})
Nano	n	one billionth (10^{-9})
Pico	p	one trillionth (10^{-12})
Femto	f	one quadrillionth (10^{-15})

APPENDIX E

Pediatric Vital Signs and Parameters

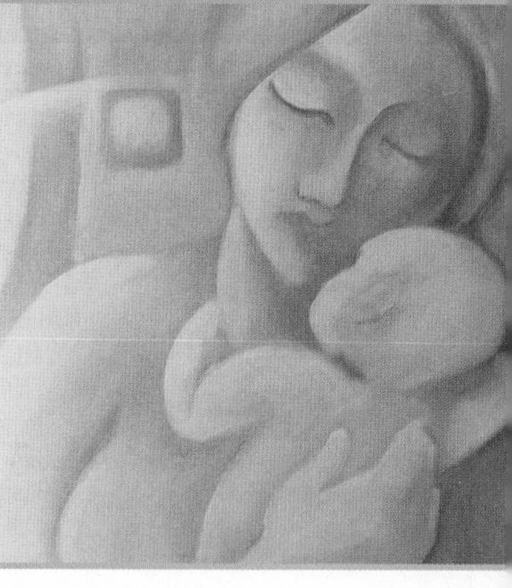

CENTIGRADE TO FAHRENHEIT TEMPERATURE CONVERSIONS

°C	°F	°C	°F	°C	°F
35.0	95.0	37.0	98.6	39.0	102.2
35.2	95.4	37.2	99.0	39.2	102.6
35.4	95.7	37.4	99.3	39.4	102.9
35.6	96.1	37.6	99.7	39.6	103.3
35.8	96.4	37.8	100.0	39.8	103.6
36.0	96.8	38.0	100.4	40.0	104.0
36.2	97.2	38.2	100.8	40.2	104.4
36.4	97.5	38.4	101.1	40.4	104.7
36.6	97.9	38.6	101.5	40.6	105.1
36.8	98.2	38.8	101.8	40.8	105.4
				41.0	105.8

Conversion Formulas

°F = (°C × 9/5) + 32 or (°C × 1.8) + 32

°C = (°F − 32) + 5/9 or (°F − 32) + 0.55

NORMAL VITAL SIGNS ACCORDING TO AGE

AGE	HEART RATE (beats/min)	BLOOD PRESSURE (mm Hg)	RESPIRATORY RATE (breaths/min)
Premature	120–170*	55–75/35–45†	40–70‡
0–3 mo	100–150*	65–85/45–55	35–55
3–6 mo	90–120	70–90/50–65	30–45
6–12 mo	80–120	80–100/55–65	25–40
1–3 yr	70–110	90–105/55–70	20–30
3–6 yr	65–110	95–110/60–75	20–25
6–12 yr	60–95	100–120/60–75	14–22
12+ yr	55–85	110–135/65–85	12–18

*In sleep, infant heart rates may drop significantly lower, but if perfusion is maintained, no intervention is required.

†A blood pressure cuff should cover approximately two thirds of the arm; too small a cuff yields spuriously high pressure readings, and too large a cuff yields spuriously low pressure readings.

‡Many premature infants require mechanical ventilatory support, making their spontaneous respiratory rate less relevant.

Source: Kliegman, R. M., Stanton, B., Geme, J., & Schor, N. (2016). *Nelson textbook of pediatrics* (20th ed.). St. Louis: Elsevier.

BLOOD PRESSURE (BP) VALUES REQUIRING FURTHER EVALUATION, ACCORDING TO AGE AND GENDER

	BLOOD PRESURE (mm Hg)			
	MALE		FEMALE	
AGE (years)	SYSTOLIC	DIASTOLIC	SYSTOLIC	DIASTOLIC
3	100	59	100	61
4	102	62	101	64
5	104	65	103	66
6	105	68	104	68
7	106	70	106	69
8	107	71	108	71
9	109	72	110	72
10	111	73	112	73
11	113	74	114	74
12	115	74	116	75
13	117	75	117	76
14	120	75	119	77
15	120	76	120	78
16	120	78	120	78
17	120	80	120	78
≥18	120	80	120	80

These values represent the lower limits for abnormal blood pressure ranges, according to age and gender. Any blood pressure readings equal to or greater than these values represent blood pressures in the prehypertensive, stage 1 hypertension, or stage 2 hypertensive stage and should be further evaluated. Routine blood pressure screening is not recommended in children less than 3 years of age.

From Kaelber, D. C., & Pickett, F. (2009). Simple table to identify children and adolescents needing further evaluation of blood pressure. Reproduced with permission from *Pediatrics, 123*(6), e972–e974.

INDEX

Page numbers followed by "*f*" indicate figures, "*t*" indicate tables, and "*b*" indicate boxes.

O

S

U

SPECIAL FEATURES

ATRAUMATIC CARE

COMMUNITY FOCUS

CRITICAL THINKING CASE STUDY

CULTURAL AWARENESS

EMERGENCY

FAMILY-CENTRED TEACHING